Body Mass Index

Height (inches)	Normal						Overweight					Obese										Extreme Obesity														
BMI	19	20	21	22	23	24	25	26	27	28	29	30	31	32	33	34	35	36	37	38	39	40	41	42	43	44	45	46	47	48	49	50	51	52	53	54
	Body Weight (pounds)																																			
58	91	96	100	105	110	115	119	124	129	134	138	143	148	153	158	162	167	172	177	181	186	191	196	201	205	210	215	220	224	229	234	239	244	248	253	258
59	94	99	104	109	114	119	124	128	133	138	143	148	153	158	163	168	173	178	183	188	193	198	203	208	212	217	222	227	232	237	242	247	252	257	262	267
60	97	102	107	112	118	123	128	133	138	143	148	153	158	163	168	174	179	184	189	194	199	204	209	215	220	225	230	235	240	245	250	255	261	266	271	276
61	100	106	111	116	122	127	132	137	143	148	153	158	164	169	174	180	185	190	195	201	206	211	217	222	227	232	238	243	248	254	259	264	269	275	280	285
62	104	109	115	120	126	131	136	142	147	153	158	164	169	175	180	186	191	196	202	207	213	218	224	229	235	240	246	251	256	262	267	273	278	284	289	295
63	107	113	118	124	130	135	141	146	152	158	163	169	175	180	186	191	197	203	208	214	220	225	231	237	242	248	254	259	265	270	278	282	287	293	299	304
64	110	116	122	128	134	140	145	151	157	163	169	174	180	186	192	197	204	209	215	221	227	232	238	244	250	256	262	267	273	279	285	291	296	302	308	314
65	114	120	126	132	138	144	150	156	162	168	174	180	186	192	198	204	210	216	222	228	234	240	246	252	258	264	270	276	282	288	294	300	306	312	318	324
66	118	124	130	136	142	148	155	161	167	173	179	186	192	198	204	210	216	223	229	235	241	247	253	260	266	272	278	284	291	297	303	309	315	322	328	334
67	121	127	134	140	146	153	159	166	172	178	185	191	198	204	211	217	223	230	236	242	249	255	261	268	274	280	287	293	299	306	312	319	325	331	338	344
68	125	131	138	144	151	158	164	171	177	184	190	197	203	210	216	223	230	236	243	249	256	262	269	276	282	289	295	302	308	315	322	328	335	341	348	354
69	128	135	142	149	155	162	169	176	182	189	196	203	209	216	223	230	236	243	250	257	263	270	277	284	291	297	304	311	318	324	331	338	345	351	358	365
70	132	139	146	153	160	167	174	181	188	195	202	209	216	222	229	236	243	250	257	264	271	278	285	292	299	306	313	320	327	334	341	348	355	362	369	376
71	136	143	150	157	165	172	179	186	193	200	208	215	222	229	236	243	250	257	265	272	279	286	293	301	308	315	322	329	338	343	351	358	365	372	379	386
72	140	147	154	162	169	177	184	191	199	206	213	221	228	235	242	250	258	265	272	279	287	294	302	309	316	324	331	338	346	353	361	368	375	383	390	397
73	144	151	159	166	174	182	189	197	204	212	219	227	235	242	250	257	265	272	280	288	295	302	310	318	325	333	340	348	355	363	371	378	386	393	401	408
74	148	155	163	171	179	186	194	202	210	218	225	233	241	249	256	264	272	280	287	295	303	311	319	326	334	342	350	358	365	373	381	389	396	404	412	420
75	152	160	168	176	184	192	200	208	216	224	232	240	248	256	264	272	279	287	295	303	311	319	327	335	343	351	359	367	375	383	391	399	407	415	423	431
76	156	164	172	180	189	197	205	213	221	230	238	246	254	263	271	279	287	295	304	312	320	328	336	344	353	361	369	377	385	394	402	410	418	426	435	443

Source: Adapted from National Heart, Lung, and Blood Institute: Clinical Guidelines on the Identification, Evaluation, and Treatment of Overweight and Obesity in Adults: the Evidence Report.
See http://www.nhlbhi.nih.gov/guidelines/obesity/bmi_tbl.pdf

CONN'S

CURRENT THERAPY

2020

CONN'S CURRENT THERAPY 2020

RICK D. KELLERMAN, MD
Professor and Chair
Department of Family and Community Medicine
University of Kansas School of Medicine–Wichita
Wichita, Kansas

DAVID P. RAKEL, MD
Professor and Chair
Department of Family and Community Medicine
University of New Mexico School of Medicine
Albuquerque, New Mexico

ELSEVIER

Elsevier
1600 John F. Kennedy Blvd.
Ste 1600
Philadelphia, PA 19103-2899

CONN'S CURRENT THERAPY 2020   ISBN: 978-0-323-71184-5
Copyright © 2020 by Elsevier, Inc. All rights reserved.

Notice

Previous editions copyrighted 2019, 2018, 2017, 2016, 2015, 2014, 2013, 2012, 2011, 2010, 2009.

978-0-323-71184-5

Senior Content Strategist: Charlotta Khryl
Senior Content Development Manager: Laura Schmidt
Publishing Services Manager: Catherine Jackson
Senior Project Manager: Kate Mannix
Design Direction: Renee Duenow

Printed in the United States

Last digit is the print number: 9 8 7 6 5 4 3 2 1

Working together
to grow libraries in
developing countries

www.elsevier.com • www.bookaid.org

Contributors

Kashif Abad, MD
Department of Internal Medicine, University of New Mexico School of Medicine, Albuquerque, New Mexico
Chronic Kidney Disease

Mustafa Abdul-Hussein, MD, MSCR
Medical University of South Carolina, Charleston, South Carolina
Gastroesophageal Reflux Disease (GERD)

Rodney D. Adam, MD
Professor of Pathology and Medicine, Aga Khan University, Nairobi, Kenya; Professor Emeritus, University of Arizona Health Sciences Center, Tucson, Arizona
Giardiasis

Paul C. Adams, MD
Professor of Medicine, University of Western Ontario; Gastroenterologist, University Hospital, London, Ontario, Canada
Hemochromatosis

Faisal I. Ahmad, MD
Head and Neck Surgical Oncologist, Baptist Health, Houston, Texas
Thyroid Cancer

Lee Akst, MD
Director, Johns Hopkins Voice Center, Assistant Professor of Otolaryngology–Head and Neck Surgery, The Johns Hopkins Medical Institute, Baltimore, Maryland
Hoarseness and Laryngitis

Kelley P. Anderson, MD
Adjunct Clinical Professor of Medicine, University of Wisconsin School of Medicine and Public Health, Madison, Wisconsin; Department of Cardiology, Marshfield Clinic, Marshfield, Wisconsin
Heart Block

Paul Andre, MD
School of Medicine, Department of Internal Medicine, University of New Mexico, Albuquerque, New Mexico
Tachycardias

Gregory M. Anstead, MD, PhD
Staff Physician, Audie L. Murphy Memorial Veterans Affairs Hospital; Professor, Department of Medicine, University of Texas Health, San Antonio, Texas
Coccidioidomycosis

Ann M. Aring, MD
Associate Program Director, Family Medicine Residency, OhioHealth Riverside Methodist Hospital, Columbus, Ohio
Drug Hypersensitivity Reactions; Rhinosinusitis

Arash Arshi, MD
Interventional Cardiology, Cardiovascular Disease, OhioHealth, Columbus, Ohio
Valvular Heart Disease

Danny Avalos, MD
Gastroenterologist, Digestive Medicine Associates, Miami, Florida
Inflammatory Bowel Disease

Cecilio M. Azar, MD
Associate in Medicine, Division of Gastroenterology, Department of Internal Medicine, American University of Beirut Medical Center, Beirut, Lebanon
Bleeding Esophageal Varices

Amir Azarbal, MD
Cardiology Fellow, Fletcher Allen Health Care, Burlington, Vermont
Pericarditis

Zachary J. Baeseman, MD, MPH
Associate Medical Director, Family Medicine with Operative Obstetrics, ThedaCare Physicians, Wild Rose and Waupaca, Wisconsin; Mosaic Family Medicine Residency Adjunct Faculty and Rural Continuity Clinic Director, Medical College of Wisconsin, Milwaukee, Wisconsin; Adjunct Faculty of Family Medicine, University of Wisconsin School of Medicine and Public Health, Madison, Wisconsin
Vaginal Bleeding in Pregnancy

Justin Bailey, MD
Clinical Faculty, Family Medicine Residency of Idaho, Boise, Idaho
Gaseousness, Indigestion, Nausea, and Vomiting; Palpitations

Mandeep Bajaj, MD
Professor of Medicine, Baylor College of Medicine, Houston, Texas
Hyperlipidemia

Vladimer Bakhutashvili, MD
West Virginia University School of Medicine, Morgantown, West Virginia
Nonalcoholic Fatty Liver Disease

Federico Balagué, MD
Médecin agree, Rheumatology, HFR Fribourg-hôpital cantonal, Fribourg, Switzerland
Spine Pain

Bradley E. Barth, MD
Associate Professor, Department of Emergency Medicine, University of Kansas Hospital, Kansas City, Kansas
Burns

Gina M. Basello, DO
Vice Chair, Department of Family Medicine, Director, Family Medicine Residency Program, Associate Director, Palliative Medicine, Jamaica Hospital Medical Center, New York, New York
Fever

Renee M. Bassaly, DO
Division Director and Fellowship Director, Associate Professor, Female Pelvic Medicine and Reconstructive Surgery, Department of Obstetrics and Gynecology, University of South Florida, Tampa, Florida
Urinary Incontinence

Adel Bassily-Marcus, MD
Associate Professor, Surgical Critical Care, The Mount Sinai Hospital, New York, New York
Targeted Temperature Management (Therapeutic Hypothermia)

Julie M. Baughn, MD
Consultant, Sleep Medicine, Mayo Clinic, Rochester, Minnesota
Pediatric Sleep Disorders

Sheryl Beard, MD
Family Medicine Physician, Ascension Medical Group Via Christi, P.A., Wichita, Kansas
Rhinitis

Aleksandr Belakovskiy, MD
Assistant Professor, Family Medicine, University of Michigan, Ann Arbor, Michigan
Erectile Dysfunction

Ronen Ben-Ami, MD
Infectious Disease Unit, Tel Aviv Sourasky Medical Center, Tel Aviv, Israel
Cat Scratch Disease

Hassan Bencheqroun, MD
Interventional Pulmonary and Critical Care Physician, Pacific Pulmonary Medical Group, Riverside, California
Pruritus

David I. Bernstein, MD
Professor Emeritus of Medicine, Division of Immunology, Allergy, and Rheumatology, University of Cincinnati College of Medicine, Cincinnati, Ohio
Hypersensitivity Pneumonitis

Jonathan A. Bernstein, MD
Department of Internal Medicine, Division of Immunology, Rheumatology and Allergy, University of Cincinnati College of Medicine, Cincinnati, Ohio
Anaphylaxis

Kristin Schmid Biggerstaff, MD
Glaucoma Staff, Michael E. DeBakey Veteran's Affairs Medical Center, Houston, Texas
Glaucoma

Clara Bloomfield, MD
Distinguished University Professor, William G. Pace III Professor of Cancer Research, Cancer Scholar and Senior Advisor, The Ohio State University Comprehensive Cancer Center –, Arthur G. James Cancer Hospital and Richard J. Solove Research Institute, The Ohio State University, Columbus, Ohio
Acute Leukemia in Adults

William Blum, MD
Professor of Hematology and Oncology, Director, Acute Leukemia Program, Winship Cancer Institute of Emory University, Atlanta, Georgia
Acute Leukemia in Adults

Diana Bolotin, MD, PhD
Associate Professor, Director of Dermatologic Surgery, Section of Dermatology, University of Chicago, Chicago, Illinois
Nonmelanoma Cancer of the Skin

Rachel A. Bonnema, MD, MS
Associate Professor of Medicine, University of Nebraska Medical Center, Omaha, Nebraska
Contraception

David Borenstein, MD
Clinical Professor of Medicine, The George Washington University Medical Center, Washington, DC
Spine Pain

Christopher Bossart, MD
Assistant Professor, Department of Emergency Medicine, University of New Mexico, Albuquerque, New Mexico
Osteoarthritis

Dee Ann Bragg, MD
Clinical Assistant Professor, Department of Family and Community Medicine, The University of Kansas School of Medicine–Wichita; Faculty, Via Christi Family Medicine Residency Program, Wichita, Kansas
Rubella and Congenital Rubella

Scott Bragg, PharmD
Associate Professor, Medical University of South Carolina (MUSC) College of Pharmacy, MUSC Department of Family Medicine, Charleston, South Carolina
Osteoporosis

Prasheda Bremjit, MD
Department of Cardiology, University of New Mexico, Albuquerque, New Mexico
Congestive Heart Failure

Takae Brewer, MD
Cancer Genomic Medicine Fellow, Genomic Medicine Institute, Cleveland Clinic, Cleveland, Ohio
Breast Cancer

Sylvia L. Brice, MD
Clinical Professor of Dermatology, University of Colorado, Denver, Colorado
Viral Diseases of the Skin

John Brill, MD, MPH
Vice-President, Population Health, Milwaukee, Wisconsin
Gonorrhea

Patricia D. Brown, MD
Professor of Medicine, Department of Internal Medicine, Division of Infectious Diseases, Wayne State University School of Medicine; Associate Chief of Staff for Medicine, John D. Dingell VA Medical Center, Detroit, Michigan
Pyelonephritis

Patrick Brown, MD
Associate Professor of Oncology and Pediatrics, The Johns Hopkins University School of Medicine; Director, Pediatric, Leukemia Program, Sidney Kimmel Comprehensive Cancer Center at Johns Hopkins Medicine, Baltimore, Maryland
Acute Leukemia in Children

Rachel Brown, MBBS
Professor and Chair, Psychiatry and Behavioral Sciences, University of Kansas School of Medicine-Wichita, Wichita, Kansas
Autism

Richard B. Brown, MD
Senior Clinician, Infectious Disease Division, Baystate Medical Center, Springfield, Massachusetts
Toxic Shock Syndrome

Peter F. Buckley, MD
Dean, School of Medicine, Virginia Commonwealth University; Executive Vice President for Medical Affairs, VCU Health, Richmond, Virginia
Schizophrenia

Sarah Burns, DO, MS
Assistant Professor, Division of Hospital Medicine, Department of Internal Medicine, University of New Mexico School of Medicine, Albuquerque, New Mexico
Acute Kidney Injury

Kenneth Byrd, DO
Assistant Professor, Department of Internal Medicine–Hematologic Malignancies and Cellular Therapeutics, University of Kansas Medical Center, Kansas City, Kansas
Disseminated Intravascular Coagulation

Diego Cadavid, MD
Senior Vice President of Clinical Development, Fulcrum Therapeutics; Affiliate Instructor in Neurology, University of Massachusetts Medical School, Worchester, Massachusetts
Relapsing Fever

Thomas R. Caraccio, PharmD
Assistant Professor of Pharmacology and Toxicology, New York College of Osteopathic Medicine, Old Westbury, New York; Associate Professor of Emergency Medicine, Stony Brook University Medical Center School of Medicine, Stony Brook, New York
Medical Toxicology

Peter J. Carek, MD, MS
Professor and Chair, Community Health and Family Medicine, University of Florida, Gainesville, Florida
Osteoporosis

Andres F. Carrion, MD
Assistant Professor of Medicine, University of Miami, Miami, Florida
Cirrhosis

Donald O. Castell, MD
Professor of Medicine, Division of Gastroenterology and Hepatology, Medical University of South Carolina, Charleston, South Carolina
Gastroesophageal Reflux Disease (GERD)

William E. Cayley Jr., MD, MDiv
Clinical Professor, University of Wisconsin School of Medicine and Public Health, Prevea Family Medicine Residency, Augusta and Eau Claire, Wisconsin
Chest Pain

Sonia Cerquozzi, MD
Clinical Assistant Professor, Division of Hematology and Hematologic Malignancies, University of Calgary, Calgary, Alberta, Canada
Polycythemia Vera

Alvaro Cervera, MD, PhD
Royal Darwin Hospital, Northern Territory, Australia
Ischemic Cerebrovascular Disease

Rachel Chamberlain, MD
Associate Program Director, Primary Care Sports Medicine Fellowship, Assistant Professor, Department of Family and Community Medicine, University of New Mexico, Albuquerque, New Mexico
Osteoarthritis

Lawrence Chan, MD
Professor, Departments of Medicine, Molecular and Cellular Biology, Biochemistry and Molecular Biology, and Molecular and Human Genetics, Baylor College of Medicine, Houston, Texas
Hyperaldosteronism; Hyperlipidemia; Hyperprolactinemia

Miriam Chan, PharmD
Director of Pharmacy Education, Family Medicine Residency Program, Riverside Methodist Hospital, Columbus, Ohio
Drug Hypersensitivity Reactions; Popular Herbs and Nutritional Supplements

Lin Yee Chen, MD, MS
Associate Professor, Cardiovascular Division, Department of Medicine, University of Minnesota Medical School, Minneapolis, Minnesota
Atrial Fibrillation

Shingo Chihara, MD
Section of Infectious Diseases, Virginia Mason Medical Center, Seattle, Washington
Anthrax

Meera Chitlur, MD
Barnhart-Lusher Hemostasis Research Endowed Chair, Director, Hemophilia Treatment Center and Hemostasis Program & Special Coagulation Laboratory, Professor of Pediatrics, Wayne State University; Division of Hematology/Oncology, Children's Hospital of Michigan, Detroit, Michigan
Hemophilia and Related Conditions

Saima Chohan, MD
Clinical Assistant Professor, Division of Clinical Education, Arizona College of Osteopathic Medicine, Glendale, Arizona
Gout and Hyperuricemia

Jacob Christensen, DO
Family Medicine, University of Mexico, Albuquerque, New Mexico
Osteoarthritis

Kuang-Yuh Chyu, MD, PhD
Staff Physician, Department of Cardiology, Heart Institute, Cedars-Sinai Medical Center; Health Sciences Clinical Professor of Medicine, University of California, Los Angeles, California
Acute Myocardial Infarction: Focus on ST-Elevation Myocardial Infarction

Joaquin E. Cigarroa, MD
Professor of Medicine, Clinical Chief, Knight Cardiovascular Institute; Division Head, Cardiology, Oregon and Health Sciences University, Portland, Oregon
Congenital Heart Disease

Peter E. Clark, MD
Associate Professor, Urologic Surgery, Vanderbilt University
Medical Center, Nashville, Tennessee
Malignant Tumors of the Urogenital Tract

Paul Cleland, MD
Clinical Assistant Professor, Department of Family and
Community Medicine, University of Kansas School of
Medicine–Wichita; Associate Director, University of Kansas
School of Medicine–Wichita Sports Medicine Fellowship,
Wichita, Kansas
Heat-Related Illness

Matthew K. Cline, MD
MUSC Affiliate Professor (Anderson/Family Medicine), Medical
University of South Carolina, Charleston, South Carolina
Antepartum Care

Kari R. Clouse, MD
Flint Hills Medical Clinic; Clinical Assistant Professor,
Department of Family and Community Medicine, University
of Kansas School of Medicine–Wichita, Wichita, Kansas
Delirium

Laura C. Coates, MBChB, PhD
NIHR Scientist, Nuffield Department of Orthopaedics,
Rheumatology and Musculoskeletal Sciences, University of
Oxford, Oxford, Great Britain
Psoriatic Arthritis

August Colenbrander, MD
Affiliate Senior Scientist, Smith-Kettlewell Eye Research
Institute, San Francisco, California
Vision Rehabilitation

Tracie C. Collins, MD, MPH, MHCDS
Dean and Professor, College of Population Health, University of
New Mexico, Albuquerque, New Mexico
Peripheral Arterial Disease

Ryan M. Commins, MD
Internal Medicine, Georgetown University Medical Center,
Washington, DC
High Altitude Illness

Christine Conageski, MD
Associate Professor, Obstetrics and Gynecology, University of
Colorado, Aurora, Colorado
Vulvar Neoplasia

John M. Conly, MD
Professor of Medicine and Microbiology, Immunology &
Infectious Diseases, University of Calgary, Calgary, Alberta,
Canada
Methicillin-Resistant Staphylococcus aureus

Carlo Contini, MD
Full Professor of Infectious Diseases, Director of Infectious
Diseases Unit, Department of Medical Sciences, University of
Ferrara, Ferrara, Italy
Toxoplasmosis

Ashley Cooper, MD
Department of Pediatrics, Division of Pediatric Rheumatology,
Children's Mercy Kansas City/University of Missouri, Kansas
City, Missouri
Juvenile Idiopathic Arthritis

Allison K. Cormier, MD
Departments of Medicine and Population Health Sciences,
University of Wisconsin–Madison, Madison, Wisconsin
Treatment and Prevention of HIV Infection

Michael L. Corriveau, MD
Assistant Clinical Professor of Internal Medicine, The Ohio State
University School of Medicine; Pulmonologist, Chalmers P.
Wylie VA Ambulatory Care Center, Columbus, Ohio
Chronic Obstructive Pulmonary Disease

Bart L. Cox, MD
Associate Professor of Medicine, Department of Cardiology,
University of New Mexico, Albuquerque, New Mexico
Congestive Heart Failure

Dustin A. Creech, MD
Assistant Professor, Belleville Family Medicine Residency, St.
Louis University/Scott Air Force Base, Belleville, Illinois
Malaria

Ana L. Creo, MD
Faculty, Pediatric Endocrinology Fellowship, Mayo Clinic,
Rochester, Minnesota
Obesity

Burke A. Cunha, MD
Professor, State University of New York School of Medicine,
Stony Brook, New York; Chief, Infectious Disease Division,
Winthrop–University Hospital, Mineola, New York
Babesiosis; Viral and Mycoplasmal Pneumonias

Cheston B. Cunha, MD
Infectious Disease Division, Alpert School of Medicine, Brown
University, Providence, Rhode Island
Babesiosis; Viral and Mycoplasmal Pneumonias

Amy E. Curry, MD
Clinical Associate Professor, Department of Family and
Community Medicine, University of Kansas School of
Medicine–Wichita; Associate Director, Via Christi Family
Medicine Residency, Wichita, Kansas
Pelvic Inflammatory Disease

Julia Dai, MD
Associate Professor, Director of Dermatologic Surgery, Section
of Dermatology, University of Chicago, Chicago, Illinois
Nonmelanoma Cancer of the Skin

Cori L. Daines, MD
Division Chief, Professor, Project Director, Pediatric Pulmonary
Center, University of Arizona, Tucson, Arizona
Cystic Fibrosis

Oriana M. Damas, MD
Assistant Professor, Director of Translational Studies for the
Crohn's and Colitis Center, Division of Gastroenterology,
Department of Medicine, University of Miami Miller School
of Medicine, Miami, Florida
Inflammatory Bowel Disease

Beth A. Damitz, MD
Associate Professor, Family and Community Medicine, Medical
College of Wisconsin, Milwaukee, Wisconsin
Immunization Practices

Natalie C. Dattilo, PhD
Assistant Professor of Psychiatry, Indiana University School of Medicine, Indianapolis, Indiana
Generalized Anxiety Disorder; Posttraumatic Stress Disorder

Raul Davaro, MD
Associate Professor of Clinical Medicine, University of Massachusetts, Worcester, Massachusetts
Smallpox

David de Berker, MRCP
Consultant Dermatologist, Bristol Dermatology, Bristol Royal Infirmary, Bristol, United Kingdom
Diseases of the Nails

André de Leon, MD
Faculty, Family Medicine, Eisenhower Family Medicine Residency, Rancho Mirage, California
Chronic Diarrhea

Tate de Leon, MD
Faculty, Family Medicine, Eisenhower Family Medicine Residency, Rancho Mirage, California
Acute Diarrhea

Alexei DeCastro, MD
Assistant Professor, Department of Family Medicine, Medical University of South Carolina, Charleston, South Carolina
Osteoporosis

Katharine C. DeGeorge, MD, MS
Associate Professor, Assistant Residency Program Director, Associate Director, Faculty Development Fellowship, Department of Family Medicine, University of Virginia, Charlottesville, Virginia
Bacterial Pneumonia; Asthma in Children

Thomas G. DeLoughery, MD
Professor of Medicine, Pathology, and Pediatrics, Oregon Health Sciences University, Portland, Oregon
Hemolytic Anemias

Atul Deodhar, MD
Professor of Medicine, Division of Arthritis & Rheumatic Diseases, Oregon Health & Science University, Portland, Oregon
Axial Spondyloarthritis

Clio Dessinioti, MD, MSc, PhD
Dermatologist, Andreas Sygros Hospital, Athens, Greece
Parasitic Diseases of the Skin

Michael P. Diamond, MD
Professor of Obstetrics and Gynecology, Leon Henri Charbonnier Endowed Chair, Associate Dean for Research, Medical College of Georgia; Senior Vice President for Research, Augusta University, Augusta, Georgia
Infertility

Geoffrey A. Donnan, MD
Department of Neurology, University of Melbourne Faculty of Medicine, Dentistry, and Health Sciences; Florey Neuroscience Institutes, Carlton South, Victoria, Australia
Ischemic Cerebrovascular Disease

John N. Dorsch, MD
Professor Emeritus, Department of Family and Community Medicine, University of Kansas School of Medicine–Wichita, Wichita, Kansas
Dry Eye Disease; Red Eye

Chad Douglas, MD, PharmD
Assistant Professor of Family and Preventive Medicine, Medical & Didactic Education Director, University of Oklahoma Health Sciences Center; Department of Family and Preventive Medicine, Medical Director-OU Physicians Health and Wellness Clinic, Oklahoma City, Oklahoma
Erythema Multiforme

Douglas A. Drevets, MD
Professor and Chief, Section of Infectious Diseases, University of Oklahoma Health Sciences Center; Staff Physician, Veterans Affairs Medical Center, Oklahoma City, Oklahoma
Plague

Samuel C. Dudley Jr., MD, PhD
Fred C. and Katherine B. Andersen Chair–Adult Cardiology, Professor and Chief, Division of Cardiology, Director of the Lillehei Heart Institute, Minneapolis, Minnesota
Atrial Fibrillation

Peter R. Duggan, MD
Associate Clinical Professor of Medicine, University of Calgary, Calgary, Alberta, Canada
Polycythemia Vera

Kim Eagle, MD
Albion Walter Hewlett Professor of Internal Medicine and Director, Cardiovascular Center, University of Michigan Health System, Ann Arbor, Michigan
Angina Pectoris

Leigh M. Eck, MD
Associate Professor of Medicine, Program Director–Internal Medicine Residency Program, Vice Chair of GME–Department of Internal Medicine, The University of Kansas Health System, Kansas City, Kansas
Thyroiditis

Genevieve L. Egnatios, MD
Affiliated Dermatology, Scottsdale, Arizona
Contact Dermatitis

Dirk M. Elston, MD
Professor and Chairman, Department of Dermatology and Dermatologic Surgery, Medical University of South Carolina, Charleston, South Carolina
Diseases of the Hair

John M. Embil, MD
Professor, Departments of Internal Medicine (Section of Infectious Diseases) and Medical Microbiology, Consultant, Infectious Diseases, Director, BSc(Med) Program, University of Manitoba; Medical Director, Infection Prevention and Control Unit, Health Sciences Centre and Winnipeg Regional Health Authority, Winnipeg, Manitoba, Canada
Blastomycosis

Scott K. Epstein, MD
Dean for Educational Affairs and Professor of Medicine, Tufts University School of Medicine, Boston, Massachusetts
Acute Respiratory Failure

Susan Evans, MD
Assistant Professor, Department of Family Medicine, University
  of Nebraska Medical Center
Iron Deficiency Anemia

Andrew M. Evens, DO, MSc
Professor of Medicine, Chief, Division of Hematology/Oncology,
  Tufts Medical Center; Director, Tufts Cancer Center, Boston,
  Massachusetts
Non-Hodgkin Lymphoma

J. Barry Fagan, MD
Service Chief, Specialty Medicine, Central Ohio VA Healthcare
  System, Columbus, Ohio
Chronic Obstructive Pulmonary Disease

Anthony J. Faugno III, MD
Instructor in Medicine, Department of Medicine, Division of
  Pulmonary, Critical Care and Sleep, Tufts Medical Center,
  Boston, Massachusetts
Acute Respiratory Failure

Kinder Fayssoux, MD
Center for Family Medicine, Eisenhower Medical Associates,
  La Quinta, California
Bacterial Infections of the Urinary Tract in Women

Dorianne Feldman, MD, MSPT
Medical Director, Inpatient Rehabilitation, Department of
  Physical Medicine and Rehabilitation, Johns Hopkins
  University School of Medicine, Baltimore, Maryland
Rehabilitation of the Stroke Patient

Terry D. Fife, MD
Director, Otoneurology and Balance Disorders, Barrow
  Neurological Institute, Phoenix, Arizona
Ménière's Disease

David J. Finley, MD
Co-Director, Complex Airway Program, Surgeon, Thoracic
  Service, Memorial Sloan Kettering Cancer Center, New York,
  New York
Pleural Effusions and Empyema Thoracis

William E. Fisher, MD
Professor, Clinical Vice-Chair and Chief, Division of General
  Surgery, George L. Jordan, MD Chair of General Surgery,
  Vice Chair, Clinical Affairs, Director, Elkins Pancreas Center,
  Michael E. DeBakey Department of Surgery, Chief, Surgery
  Service Line, Baylor St. Luke's Medical Center, Houston,
  Texas
Acute and Chronic Pancreatitis

Maria Fleseriu, MD
Professor of Medicine and Neurological Surgery, Director of
  Pituitary Center, Oregon Health and Science University,
  Portland, Oregon
Adrenocortical Insufficiency

Donald C. Fletcher, MD
Adjunct Associate Professor, Department of Ophthalmology,
  University of Kansas School of Medicine, Kansas City, Kansas
Vision Rehabilitation

Raja Flores, MD
Ames Professor of Cardiothoracic Surgery, Chief of Division
  of Thoracic Surgery, Mount Sinai School of Medicine, New
  York, New York
Pleural Effusions and Empyema Thoracis

Sarah Forsberg, PsyD
Associate Clinical Professor, Department of Psychiatry, Eating
  Disorders Program, University of California, San Francisco,
  San Francisco, California
Eating Disorders

Jeffrey Michael Foster, DO
Anesthesiology and Interventional Pain Medicine, Saint Luke's
  Hospital of Kansas City, Clinical Assistant Professor of
  Anesthesiology, University of Missouri at Kansas City, Kansas
  City, Missouri
Fibromyalgia

Daniel P. Fox, MD
Texas ENT Specialists, Katy, Texas
Obstructive Sleep Apnea

Jennifer Frank, MD
Theda Care Physicians, Neenah, Wisconsin
Syphilis; Vaginal Bleeding Late in Pregnancy

Robert S. Freelove, MD
Senior Vice President/Chief Medical Officer, Salina Regional
  Health Center, Salina, Kansas; Clinical; Associate Professor,
  Department of Family and Community Medicine, University
  of Kansas School of Medicine–Wichita, Wichita, Kansas
Pancreatic Cancer; Nongonococcal Urethritis

Ellen W. Freeman, PhD
Research Professor, Obstetrics/Gynecology, Perelman School
  of Medicine, University of Pennsylvania, Philadelphia,
  Pennsylvania
Premenstrual Syndrome

Theodore M. Freeman, MD
San Antonio Asthma and Allergy Clinic, San Antonio, Texas
Allergic Reactions to Insect Stings

Aaron Friedman, MD
Ruben Bentson Professor and Chair, Pediatrics, University of
  Minnesota, Minneapolis, Minnesota
Parenteral Fluid Therapy for Infants and Children

Ruchi Gaba, MD
Endocrinology, Diabetes and Metabolism, Baylor College of
  Medicine, Houston, Texas
Hyperaldosteronism

Melissa Gaines, MD
Cox Senior Health, Geriatrics Division, Springfield, Missouri
Constipation

R. Michael Gallagher, DO
Headache Consultant, Headache Center of Central Florida,
  Melbourne, Florida
Headache

Marc G. Ghany, MD, MHSc
Clinical Research Section, Liver Diseases Branch, National
  Institute of Diabetes and Digestive and Kidney Diseases,
  National Institutes of Health, Bethesda, Maryland
Hepatitis A, B, D, and E

Muhammad Ahmad Ghazi, MD
Family Physician, Jacksonville, Florida
Pruritus Ani and Vulvae

Lawrence M. Gibbs, MD, MSEd
Assistant Professor, Belleville Family Medicine Residency, St. Louis University/Scott Air Force Base, Belleville, Illinois
Malaria

Donald L. Gilbert, MD, MS
Professor of Pediatrics and Neurology, Cincinnati Children's Hospital Medical Center, Cincinnati, Ohio
Gilles De La Tourette Syndrome

Erin A. Gillaspie, MD, MPH
Assistant Professor, Thoracic Surgery, Vanderbilt University Medical Center, Nashville, Tennessee
Lung Cancer

Tarvinder Gilotra, MD
Department of Infectious Disease, SUNY Upstate Medical University, Syracuse, New York
Intestinal Parasites

Mark T. Gladwin, MD
Jack D. Myers Distinguished Professor and Chair, Chairman of the Department of Medicine, Director, Pittsburgh Heart, Lung, Blood and Vascular Medicine Institute, UPMC and the University of Pittsburgh School of Medicine, Pittsburgh, Pennsylvania
Sickle Cell Disease

Stephen J. Gluckman, MD
Perelman School of Medicine at the University of Pennsylvania, Philadelphia, Pennsylvania
Myalgic Encephalomyelitis/Chronic Fatigue Syndrome

Andrew W. Goddard, MD
Professor of Psychiatry, University of California, San Francisco Fresno Medical Education & Research Program, San Francisco, California
Generalized Anxiety Disorder

Danae D. Goerl, MD
Pediatric Associates, Manhattan, Kansas
Bronchiolitis

Kyle Goerl, MD
Team Physician, Sports and Family Medicine, Lafene Health Center, Kansas State University, Manhattan, Kansas; Clinical Assistant Professor, Department of Family and Community Medicine, University of Kansas School of Medicine–Wichita, Wichita, Kansas
Bursitis and Tendinopathy

Mark S. Gold, MD
Adjunct Professor, Department of Psychiatry, Washington University School of Medicine, St. Louis, Missouri
Drug Abuse

Joshua N. Goldstein, MD, PhD
Professor of Emergency Medicine, Harvard Medical School; MGH Endowed Professor of Emergency Research, Massachusetts General Hospital, Boston, Massachusetts
Intracerebral Hemorrhage

Melissa K. Gonzales, BS
Postbaccalaureate IRTA Fellow, Eunice Kennedy Shriver National Institute of Child Health and Human Development, National Institutes of Health, Bethesda, Maryland
Pheochromocytoma

Marlis González-Fernández, MD, PhD
Assistant Professor, Departments of Physical Medicine and Rehabilitation and Orthopaedic Surgery, Vice Chair, Clinical Affairs, Department of Physical Medicine and Rehabilitation, The Johns Hopkins University School of Medicine, Baltimore, Maryland
Rehabilitation of the Stroke Patient

Gregory Goodwin, MD
Assistant Professor of Pediatrics, Harvard Medical School; Senior Associate Physician in Medicine, Boston Childrens Hospital, Boston, Massachusetts
Diabetes Mellitus in Children

Aidar R. Gosmanov, MD, PhD, DMSc
Chief, Endocrinology Section, Stratton Veterans Affairs Medical Center; Associate Professor of Medicine, Division of Endocrinology, Albany Medical College, Albany, New York
Diabetic Ketoacidosis

Niyaz Gosmanov, MD
Associate Professor, Section of Endocrinology and Diabetes, The University of Oklahoma Health Sciences Center, Oklahoma City, Oklahoma
Diabetes Mellitus in Adults

Albina Gosmanova, MD
Clinical Associate Professor, Section of Endocrinology and Diabetes, The University of Oklahoma Health Sciences Center; VA Medical Center, Oklahoma City, Oklahoma
Diabetes Mellitus in Adults

Luigi Gradoni, PhD
Research Director, Unit of Vector-Borne Diseases, Department of Infectious Diseases, Istituto Superiore di Sanità, Rome, Italy
Leishmaniasis

Timothy P. Graham, MD
Program Director, Mount Carmel Family Medicine Residency; Chair, Department of Family Medicine, Mount Carmel St. Ann's Hospital, Westerville, Ohio
Hypertension

Jane M. Grant-Kels, MD
Professor of Dermatology, Pathology and Pediatrics, Founding Chair Emeritus and Vice Chair, Department of Dermatology, Director, the Cutaneous Oncology Center and Melanoma Program, University of Connecticut Health Center, Farmington, Connecticut
Nevi

Leslie A. Greenberg, MD
Associate Professor of Family and Community Medicine, University of Nevada Reno School of Medicine; Assistant Program Director, University of Nevada Reno Family Medicine Residency Program, Reno, Nevada
Keloids

William M. Greene, MD
Associate Professor, Addiction Medicine Division, Department of Psychiatry, University of Florida College of Medicine, Gainesville, Florida
Drug Abuse

Joseph Greensher, MD
Medical Director and Associate Chair, Department of Pediatrics, Long Island Regional Poison and Drug Information Center, Winthrop-University Hospital, Mineola, New York, Professor of Pediatrics, Stony Brook University Medical Center School of Medicine, Stony Brook, New York
Medical Toxicology

David S. Gregory, MD
Faculty Physician, Virginia Tech-Carilion Clinic Family Medicine Residency, Roanoke, Virginia, Assistant Clinical Professor of Family Medicine, Virginia Commonwealth University School of Medicine, Richmond, Virginia; Associate Clinical Professor of Family Medicine, University of Virginia School of Medicine, Charlottesville, Virginia
Resuscitation of the Newborn

Justin Greiwe, MD
Clinical Assistant Professor of Medicine in the Division of Immunology, Allergy, and Rheumatology, University of Cincinnati, Cincinnati, Ohio
Anaphylaxis

Tawanda Gumbo, MD
Associate Professor of Medicine, University of Texas Southwestern Medical School; Attending Physician, Parkland Memorial Hospital and University Hospital–St. Paul, Dallas, Texas
Tuberculosis and Other Mycobacterial Diseases

Melissa Hague, MD
Associate Clinical Professor, Obstetrics and Gynecology, University of Kansas School of Medicine–Wichita, Wichita, Kansas
Female Sexual Dysfunction

Rebat M. Halder, MD
Professor Emeritus and Chair Emeritus, Department of Dermatology, Howard University College of Medicine, Washington, DC
Pigmentary Disorders

Ronald Hall II, PharmD, MSCS
Associate Professor, Pharmacy Practice, Texas Tech University Health Sciences Center, Dallas, Texas
Tuberculosis and Other Mycobacterial Diseases

Lynn E. Harman, MD
Clinical Associate Professor, Department of Ophthalmology, University of South Florida, Morsani College of Medicine, Tampa, Florida
Uveitis

George D. Harris, MD, MS
Professor and Chair, Family Medicine, West Virginia University Eastern Campus, UHP Medical Director–Primary Care, Martinsburg, West Virginia
Osteomyelitis

Kari R. Harris, MD
Associate Professor of Pediatrics, Section Director, Adolescent Health, Division of Ambulatory Pediatrics, Department of Pediatrics, University of Kansas School of Medicine–Wichita, Wichita, Kansas
Adolescent Health

Taylor B. Harrison, MD
Associate Professor, Neuromuscular Division, Program Director, Clinical Neurophysiology Fellowship, Department of Neurology, Emory University, Atlanta, Georgia
Myasthenia Gravis

Adam L. Hartman, MD
Program Director, Division of Clinical Research, National Institute of Neurological Disorders and Stroke, National Institutes of Health, Bethesda, Maryland
Epilepsy in Infants and Children

James W. Haynes, MD
Professor and Chair, Department of Family Medicine, The University of Tennessee Health Sciences Center, College of Medicine; Family Medicine, Erlanger Health System, Chattanooga, Tennessee
Uterine Leiomyoma

Joel J. Heidelbaugh, MD
Clinical Professor, Departments of Family Medicine and Urology, Medical Education and Clerkship Director, Department of Family Medicine, Director, Patients and Populations Branch, University of Michigan Medical School, Ann Arbor, Michigan
Erectile Dysfunction

Nelson Iván Agudelo Higuita, MD
Associate Professor, Department of Medicine/Infectious Diseases, University of Oklahoma Health Sciences Center, Oklahoma City, Oklahoma
Plague

Stacey A. Hinderliter, MD
Associate Director, Riverside Brentwood Family Medicine Residency, Newport News, Virginia; Assistant Professor, Pediatrics, Edward Via College of Osteopathic Medicine, Blacksburg, Virginia, Clinical Assistant Professor, Family Medicine, Virginia Commonwealth University-Medical College of Virginia, Richmond, Virginia
Resuscitation of the Newborn

Molly A. Hinshaw, MD
Associate Professor of Dermatology, Section Chief of Dermatopathology, Director of Dermatology Nail Clinic, University of Wisconsin School of Medicine and Public Health, Dermatopathology Laboratory, Madison, Wisconsin
Connective Tissue Disorders; Cutaneous Vasculitis

Vanessa Ho, MD
Faculty, Eisenhower Family Medicine Residency Program, Eisenhower Medical Center, La Quinta, California
Hypopituitarism

Brandon Hockenberry, MD
University of New Mexico Health Sciences Center, Department of Family and Community Medicine, Albuquerque, New Mexico
Sports-Related Head Injuries

Raymond J. Hohl, MD, PhD
Director, Penn State Cancer Institute, Hershey, Pennsylvania
Thalassemia

Therese Holguin, MD
Assistant Professor of Dermatology, University of New Mexico, Albuquerque, New Mexico
Fungal Infections of the Skin

Sarah A. Holstein, MD, PhD
Associate Professor, Division of Oncology and Hematology, Department of Internal Medicine, University of Nebraska Medical Center, Omaha, Nebraska
Thalassemia

Marisa Holubar, MD
Clinical Assistant Professor, Division of Infectious Diseases, Stanford University School of Medicine, Stanford, California
Severe Sepsis

Gretchen Homan, MD
Associate Professor, Department of Pediatrics, University of Kansas School of Medicine–Wichita, Wichita, Kansas
Pediatric Failure to Thrive

Leora Horn, MD, MSc
Ingram Associate Professor of Cancer Research, Medicine–Hematology, Oncology, Vanderbilt Ingram Cancer Center, Nashville, Tennessee
Lung Cancer

Ahmad Reza Hossani-Madani, MD, MS
Dermatologist, Kaiser Permanente, Upper Marlboro, Maryland
Pigmentary Disorders

Steven A. House, MD
Professor, Department of Family and Geriatric Medicine, Program Director, University of Louisville/Glasgow Family Medicine Residency, Glasgow, Kentucky
Pain; Palliative and End-of-Life Care

Sarah Houssayni, MD
Clinical Associate Professor, Department of Family and Community Medicine, University of Kansas School of Medicine–Wichita, Associate Director, Pediatrics, Via Christi Family Medicine Residency, Wichita, Kansas
Encopresis

William J. Hueston, MD
Senior Associate Dean for Academic Affairs, Medical College of Wisconsin, Milwaukee, Wisconsin
Hyperthyroidism; Hypothyroidism

Alison N. Huffstetler, MD
Department of Family Medicine, University of Virginia, Charlottesville, Virginia
Bacterial Pneumonia

Scott A. Hundahl, MD
Professor of Surgery, University of California–Davis School of Medicine, Sacramento, California
Tumors of the Stomach

Stephen P. Hunger, MD
Professor of Pediatrics, University of Pennsylvania Perelman School of Medicine, Chief, Division of Pediatric Oncology, Director, Center for Childhood Cancer Research, Jeffrey E. Perelman Distinguished Chair in the Department of Pediatrics, Children's Hospital of Philadelphia, Philadelphia, Pennsylvania
Acute Leukemia in Children

Wendy S. Hupp, DMD
Associate Professor of Oral Medicine (retired), Department of General Dentistry and Oral Medicine, University of Louisville School of Dentistry, Louisville, Kentucky
Diseases of the Mouth

Gretchen M. Irwin, MD, MBA
Associate Dean for Graduate Medical Education, Associate Professor, Department of Family and Community Medicine, University of Kansas School of Medicine–Wichita, Wichita, Kansas
Otitis Media

Gerald A. Isenberg, MD
Professor of Surgery, Director, Surgical UME, Sidney Kimmel Medical College; President Medical Staff, Program Director, CRS Residency, Thomas Jefferson University Hospitals; Editor in Chief, ACS Case Reviews in Surgery, Philadelphia, Pennsylvania
Tumors of the Colon and Rectum

Alan C. Jackson, MD
Professor, Section of Neurology, Internal Medicine, University of Manitoba, Winnipeg, Manitoba, Canada
Rabies

Kurt M. Jacobson, MD
Assistant Professor of Medicine, Cardiovascular Medicine Division, University of Wisconsin School of Medicine and Public Health, Madison, Wisconsin
Mitral Valve Prolapse

Vasudha Jain, MD
Infectious Disease, Kernersville, North Carolina
Vulvovaginitis

Jose A. Jaller, MD
Department of Medicine, Division of Dermatology, Albert Einstein College of Medicine, Bronx, New York
Venous Ulcers

James J. James, MD, DrPH
Executive Director, Society for Disaster Medicine and Public Health, Bethesda, Maryland
Biologic Agents Reference Chart; Toxic Chemical Agents Reference Chart: Symptoms and Treatment

Katarzyna Jamieson, MD
Associate Professor of Medicine, Division of Hematology and Oncology, Chapel Hill
Chronic Leukemias

Xiaoming Jia, MD
Instructor, Medicine, Baylor College of Medicine, Houston, Texas
Hyperlipidemia

Lisa M. Johnson, MD
Associate Professor, Department of Family Medicine, University of Cincinnati College of Medicine, Cincinnati, Ohio
Acne Vulgaris; Rosacea

Joshua S. Jolissaint, MD
Department of Surgery, Brigham and Women's Hospital, Boston, Massachusetts
Atelectasis

R. Gregory Juckett, MD, MPH
Professor Emeritus, West Virginia University School of
Medicine, Morgantown, West Virginia
Campylobacter

Marc A. Judson, MD
Chief, Division of Pulmonary and Critical Care Medicine,
Albany Medical College, Albany, New York
Sarcoidosis

Tamilarasu Kadhiravan, MD
Additional Professor of Medicine, Jawaharlal Institute of
Postgraduate Medical Education and Research, Puducherry,
India
Typhoid Fever

Rachna Kalia, MD
Clinical Assistant Professor, Department of Psychiatry and
Behavioral Sciences, University of Kansas School of
Medicine–Wichita, Wichita, Kansas
Obsessive-Compulsive Disorder

Jessica Kanter, MD
Department of Obstetrics and Gynecology, Augusta University,
Augusta, Georgia
Infertility

Dilip R. Karnad, MD
Consultant in Critical Care, Jupiter Hospital, Thane, India
Tetanus

Andreas Katsambas, MD, PhD
Professor of Dermatology, University of Athens School of
Medicine, Athens, Greece
Parasitic Diseases of the Skin

Ben Z. Katz, MD
Professor of Pediatrics, Northwestern University Feinberg School
of Medicine, Chicago, Illinois
Infectious Mononucleosis

Rebecca Katzman, MD
Family Physician, Clearwater Valley Hospital and Clinics,
Orofino, Idaho
Palpitations

Daniel I. Kaufer, MD
Chief, Cognitive & Behavioral Neurology, Director, UNC
Memory Disorders Program, Departments of Neurology and
Psychiatry, University of North Carolina, Chapel Hill, North
Carolina
Alzheimer's Disease

Andrew M. Kaunitz, MD
University of Florida Term Professor and Associate Chairman,
Department of Obstetrics and Gynecology, University of
Florida College of Medicine–Jacksonville, Medical Director
and Director of Menopause and Gynecologic Ultrasound
Services, UF Women's Health Specialists–Emerson,
Jacksonville, Florida
Menopause

B. Mark Keegan, MD
Division Chair, Multiple Sclerosis and Autoimmune Neurology,
Professor of Neurology, Mayo Clinic College of Medicine,
Rochester, Minnesota
Multiple Sclerosis

Rick D. Kellerman, MD
Professor and Chair, Department of Family and Community
Medicine, University of Kansas School of Medicine–Wichita,
Wichita, Kansas
Chikungunya; Zika Virus Disease

Scott Kellermann, MD, MPH
Faculty, University of San Francisco, San Francisco, California;
Founder, Bwindi Community Hospital, Buhoma, Uganda
Chikungunya; Zika Virus Disease

Christina M. Kelly, MD
Department of Family Medicine, Womack Army Medical Center
Family Medicine Residency, Fort Bragg, North Carolina
Ectopic Pregnancy

Arthur Y. Kim, MD
Associate Professor of Medicine, Harvard Medical School;
Division of Infectious Diseases, Massachusetts General
Hospital, Boston, Massachusetts
Hepatitis C

Haejin Kim, MD
Senior Staff Allergist, Division of Allergy and Clinical
Immunology, Department of Internal Medicine, Henry Ford
Health System, Detroit, Michigan
Hypersensitivity Pneumonitis

Jongoh Kim, MD
Instructor in Medicine, Division of Diabetes, Endocrinology
and Metabolism, Department of Medicine, Baylor College of
Medicine, Houston, Texas
Hyperaldosteronism; Hyperlipidemia

Robert S. Kirsner, MD, PHD
Chair & Harvey Blank Professor, Dr. Phillip Frost Department
of Dermatology & Cutaneous Surgery, University of Miami
Miller School of Medicine, Miami, Florida
Venous Ulcers

Sonam Kiwalkar, MBBS
Clinical Instructor, Division of Arthritis and Rheumatology,
Oregon Health and Science University, Portland, Oregon
Axial Spondyloarthritis

Amanda Kolb, MD
Instructor, Department of Family Medicine, University of
Virginia, Charlottesville, Virginia
Asthma in Children

Bhanu Prakash Kolla, MD, MRCPsych
Senior Associate Consultant, Center for Sleep Medicine,
Department of Psychiatry and Psychology, Mayo Clinic and
Foundation; Assistant Professor of Psychiatry and Psychology,
Mayo Clinic College of Medicine, Rochester, Minnesota
Sleep Disorders

Frederick K. Korley, MD
Robert E. Meyerhoff Assistant Professor of Emergency
Medicine, The Johns Hopkins University School of Medicine;
Staff, The Johns Hopkins Medical Institutions, Baltimore,
Maryland
Disturbances due to Cold

Adrienne N. Kovalsky, DO, MPH
Hospitalist, Amita Saints Mary and Elizabeth Medical Center, Chicago, Illinois
High Altitude Illness

Megan Krause, MD
Assistant Professor, Division of Allergy, Clinical Immunology, and Rheumatology, University of Kansas School of Medicine, Kansas City, Kansas
Rheumatoid Arthritis

Eric H. Kraut, MD
Professor of Medicine, Director, Benign Hematology, Division of Hematology, The Ohio State University, Columbus, Ohio
Platelet-Mediated Bleeding Disorders

Lakshmanan Krishnamurti, MD
Professor of Pediatrics, Division of Hematology/Oncology, Children's Hospital of Pittsburgh, University of Pittsburgh Medical Center, Pittsburgh, Pennsylvania
Sickle Cell Disease

Kumar Krishnan, MD
Assistant Professor of Medicine, Harvard Medical School; Division of Gastroenterology, Massachusetts General Hospital, Boston, Massachusetts
Dysphagia and Esophageal Obstruction

Zachary Kuhlmann, DO
Residency Program Director, Clinical Associate Professor, Department of Obstetrics and Gynecology, University of Kansas School of Medicine–Wichita, Wichita, Kansas
Endometriosis

Roshni Kulkarni, MD
Professor Emerita, Michigan State University Center for Bleeding and Clotting Disorders, Department of Pediatrics and Human Development, College of Human Medicine, Michigan State University, East Lansing, Michigan
Hemophilia and Related Conditions

Seema Kumar, MD
Professor of Pediatrics, Pediatric and Adolescent Medicine, Mayo Clinic, Rochester, Minnesota
Obesity

Mary R. Kwaan, MD, MPH
Health Sciences Associate Clinical Professor of Surgery, David Geffen School of Medicine at University of California, Los Angeles, Los Angeles, California
Hemorrhoids, Anal Fissure, and Anorectal Abscess and Fistula

Robert A. Kyle, MD
Professor of Medicine, Laboratory Medicine, and Pathology, Mayo Clinic College of Medicine, Rochester, Minnesota
Multiple Myeloma

Lucius M. Lampton, MD
Private Practice, Magnolia Clinic, Magnolia, Mississippi; Clinical Professor of Family Medicine, William Carey University College of Osteopathic Medicine, Hattiesburg, Mississippi; Clinical Associate Professor of Family and Community Medicine, Tulane University School of Medicine, New Orleans, Louisiana
Yellow Fever

Richard A. Lange, MD, MBA
President, Texas Tech University Health Sciences Center El Paso; Dean, Paul L. Foster School of Medicine, El Paso, Texas
Congenital Heart Disease

Fabienne Langlois, MD
Assistant Professor, Division of Endocrinology, Department of Medicine, Universite de Sherbrooke, Sherbrooke, Quebec, Canada
Adrenocortical Insufficiency

Julius Larioza, MD
Assistant Professor of Medicine, Attending Physician, Bay State Medical Center, Springfield, Massachusetts
Toxic Shock Syndrome

Jerome Larkin, MD
Assistant Professor of Medicine, Infectious Diseases, Alpert Medical School, Brown University, Providence, Rhode Island
Severe Sepsis

Christine L. Lau, MD
Associate Professor of Surgery, University of Virginia Health System, Charlottesville, Virginia
Atelectasis

Susan Lawrence-Hylland, MD
Clinical Assistant Professor, Rheumatology Section, University of Wisconsin Hospital and Clinics, Madison, Wisconsin
Connective Tissue Disorders; Cutaneous Vasculitis

Lydia U. Lee, MD
MetroHealth, Case Western Reserve University, Cleveland, Ohio
Postpartum Depression

Jerrold B. Leikin, MD
Director of Medical Toxicology, NorthShore University HealthSystem–OMEGA, Glenbrook Hospital, Glenview, Illinois; Clinical Professor of Medicine, Pritzker School of Medicine, University of Chicago, Chicago, Illinois
Disturbances due to Cold

Scott Leikin, DO
Critical Care Medicine Fellow, Icahn School of Medicine at Mount Sinai, New York, New York
Targeted Temperature Management (Therapeutic Hypothermia); Disturbances due to Cold

Alexander K.C. Leung, MBBS
Clinical Professor of Pediatrics, University of Calgary, Calgary, Alberta, Canada
Nocturnal Enuresis

Martin M. LeWinter, MD
Professor of Medicine and Molecular Physiology and Biophysics, University of Vermont Larner College of Medicine; Attending Cardiologist, University of Vermont Medical Center, Burlington, Vermont
Pericarditis

Jennifer Lewis, MD, MPH
Instructor in Medicine, Vanderbilt University Medical Center, Nashville, Tennessee
Lung Cancer

Ming Li, MD, PhD
Section of Endocrinology, Phoenix VA Health Care System; Department of Internal Medicine, University of Arizona College of Medicine at Phoenix, Phoenix, Arizona
Hyperprolactinemia

Tyler K. Liebenstein, PharmD
Department of Pharmacy, University of Wisconsin Health, Madison, Wisconsin
Treatment and Prevention of HIV Infection

Albert P. Lin, MD
Assistant Professor, Ophthalmology, Baylor College of Medicine; Staff Physician, Eye Care Line, Michael E. DeBakey Veterans Affairs Medical Center, Houston, Texas
Glaucoma

Janet C. Lindemann, MD, MBA
Dean of Medical Student Education, Professor of Family Medicine, University of South Dakota Sanford School of Medicine, Sioux Falls, South Dakota
Fatigue

Jeffrey A. Linder, MD, MPH
Chief, Division of General Internal Medicine and Geriatrics, Michael A. Gertz Professor of Medicine, Northwestern University Feinberg School of Medicine, Chicago, Illinois
Influenza

James Lock, MD, PhD
Professor of Psychiatry, Stanford University, Stanford, California
Eating Disorders

M. Chantel Long, MD
Smoky Hill Family Medicine Residency, Salina, Kansas; Clinical Assistant Professor, Department of Family and Community Medicine, University of Kansas School of Medicine–Wichita, Wichita, Kansas
Condylomata Acuminata; Warts (Verrucae)

Colleen Loo-Gross, MD, MPH
Assistant Professor, Department of Family & Community Medicine, University of Kansas School of Medicine-Wichita, Wichita, Kansas
Amenorrhea

James M. Lyznicki, MS, MPH
Senior Manager, Council on Scientific Affairs, Science Institute, American Dental Association, Chicago, Illinois
Biologic Agents Reference Chart; Toxic Chemical Agents Reference Chart: Symptoms and Treatment

Bahaa S. Malaeb, MD
Associate Professor, Genitourinary Trauma and Reconstructive Surgery, Department of Urology, University of Michigan, Ann Arbor, Michigan
Trauma to the Genitourinary Tract

Uma Malhotra, MD
Department of Medicine, Section of Infectious Diseases, Virginia Mason Medical Center, Seattle, Washington
Ebola Virus Disease

Michael A. Malone, MD
Program Director, Designated Institutional Official, Family Medicine, Tidelands Health-MUSC, Murrells Inlet, South Carolina
Vulvovaginitis

Emily Manlove, MD
Family Medicine, IU Health Southern Indiana Physicians, Bloomington, Indiana
Cough

JoAnn E. Manson, MD, DrPH
Professor of Medicine, Harvard Medical School; Chief, Division of Preventive Medicine, Department of Medicine, Brigham and Women's Hospital, Boston, Massachusetts
Menopause

Meghna P. Mansukhani, MD
Assistant Professor of Family Medicine, Senior Associate Consultant, Center for Sleep Medicine, Mayo Clinic and Foundation, Mayo Clinic College of Medicine, Rochester, Minnesota
Sleep Disorders

Claudio Marcocci, MD
Professor of Endocrinology, Department of Clinical and Experimental Medicine, University of Pisa; Head, Endocrine Unit 2, University Hospital of Pisa, Pisa, Italy
Hyperparathyroidism and Hypoparathyroidism

Curtis E. Margo, MD, MPH
Clinical Associate Professor, Departments of Pathology and Cell Biology, and Ophthalmology, University of South Florida Morsani College of Medicine, Tampa, Florida
Uveitis

Jason E. Marker, MD, MPA
Associate Director, Memorial Hospital Family Medicine Residency; Clinic Director, E. Blair Warner Family Medicine Center, South Bend, Indiana
Neurofibromatosis (Type 1)

Paul Martin, MD
Chief, Gastroenterology and Hepatology, Mandel Chair in Gastroenterology, University of Miami, Miami, Florida
Cirrhosis

Mark A. Matza, MD, MBA
Department of Rheumatology, Massachusetts General Hospital, Boston, Massachusetts
Polymyalgia Pneumatica and Giant Cell Arteritis

Pinckney J. Maxwell IV, MD
Associate Professor of Surgery, Division of Gastrointestinal and Laparoscopic Surgery, Medical University of South Carolina, Charleston, South Carolina
Tumors of the Colon and Rectum

Anthony L. McCall, MD, PhD
James M. Moss Professor of Diabetes in Internal Medicine, Division of Endocrinology and Metabolism, University of Virginia School of Medicine, Charlottesville, Virginia
Diabetes Mellitus in Adults

Christopher McGrew, MD
University of New Mexico Health Sciences Center, Departments of Family and Community Medicine and Orthopedics and Rehabilitation, Sports Medicine Division, Albuquerque, New Mexico
Sports-Related Head Injuries

Christopher C. McGuigan, MB, ChB, MPH
Consultant in Public Health Medicine, Health Protection, NHS Fife, Cameron Hospital, Leven, Fife, United Kingdom
Psittacosis

Michael McGuigan, MD
Medical Director, Long Island Regional Poison and Drug
  Information Center, Winthrop-University Hospital, Mineola,
  New York
Medical Toxicology

Mick S. Meiselman, MD
Director of Advanced Therapeutic Endoscopy, Central Coast
  Gastroenterology, San Luis Obispo, California
Calculous Biliary Disease

Moises Mercado, MD
Director, Experimental Endocrinology Unit, Hospital de
  Especialidades, Centro Medico Nacional Siglo XXI, Institute
  Mexicano del Seguro Social, Mexico City, Mexico
Acromegaly

Ryan Merrell, MD
Neurology, NorthShore University HealthSystem, Evanston,
  Illinois
Brain Tumors

Steven L. Meyers, MD
Vice Chair, Quality and Informatics, Neurology, NorthShore
  University Health System, Evanston, Illinois
Acute Facial Paralysis

Brian J. Miller, MD, PhD, MPH
Professor, Department of Psychiatry, Augusta University,
  Augusta, Georgia
Schizophrenia

Moben Mirza, MD
Associate Professor, Residency Program Director, Division of
  Urologic Oncology, Department of Urology, University of
  Kansas Medical Center, Kansas City, Kansas
Hematuria

Kriti Mishra, MD
Department of Dermatology, University of New Mexico,
  Albuquerque, New Mexico
Fungal Infections of the Skin

Howard C. Mofenson, MD
Professor of Pharmacology and Toxicology, New York College
  of Osteopathic Medicine, Old Westbury, New York;
  Professor of Pediatrics and Emergency Medicine, Stony Brook
  University Medical Center School of Medicine, Stony Brook,
  New York
Medical Toxicology

Kris M. Mogensen, MS
Team Leader Dietitian Specialist, Department of Nutrition,
  Brigham and Women's Hospital, Boston, Massachusetts
Parenteral Nutrition in Adults

Timothy I. Morgenthaler, MD
Associate Professor of Medicine, Pulmonary and Critical Care
  Medicine, Center for Sleep Medicine, Mayo Clinic and
  Foundation, Rochester, Minnesota
Sleep Disorders

Warwick L. Morison, MD
Professor of Dermatology, The Johns Hopkins University,
  Baltimore, Maryland
Sunburn

Rami Mortada, MD
Endocrine Center of Kansas, Wichita, Kansas
Diabetes Insipidus

Scott E. Moser, MD
Associate Dean for Curriculum, Professor of Family and
  Community Medicine, University of Kansas School of
  Medicine–Wichita, Wichita, Kansas
Attention-Deficit/Hyperactivity Disorder

Heather E. Moss, MD, PhD
Assistant Professor, Departments of Ophthalmology &
  Neurology and Neurological Sciences, Stanford University,
  Stanford, California
Optic Neuritis

Ladan Mostaghimi, MD
Dermatologist, University of Wisconsin–Madison, Madison,
  Wisconsin
Psychocutaneous Medicine

Judd W. Moul, MD
James H. Semans, MD Professor of Surgery, Urologic Surgery,
  Duke University, Durham, North Carolina
Benign Prostatic Hyperplasia

Heidi E.K. Mullen, DO
General Surgery, Maricopa Integrated Health System, Phoenix,
  Arizona
Contact Dermatitis

Michael Murphy, MD
Professor of Dermatology, University of Connecticut School
  of Medicine; Attending Dermatopathologist, Department of
  Dermatology, UConn Health, Farmington, Connecticut
Nevi

Diya F. Mutasim, MD
Professor of Dermatology and Pathology, University of
  Cincinnati College of Medicine, Cincinnati, Ohio
Bullous Diseases

Arjun Muthusubramanian, MD, MPH
Department of Family Medicine, University of Virginia,
  Charlottesville, Virginia
Bacterial Pneumonia

Alykhan S. Nagji, MD
Associate Program Director, Cardiothoracic Surgery Residency
  Program, University of Kansas, Kansas City, Kansas
Atelectasis

Moniba Nazeef, MD
Department of Medicine, Division of Hematology/Oncology,
  University of Wisconsin School of Medicine and Public
  Health, UW Carbone Cancer Center, Madison, Wisconsin
Venous Thromboembolism

Donald A. Neff, MD
Assistant Professor, Department of Urology, University of
  Kansas School of Medicine, Kansas City, Kansas
Urinary Tract Infections in the Male

Tara J. Neil, MD
Clinical Associate Professor, Department of Family and Community Medicine, University of Kansas School of Medicine–Wichita, Senior Associate Director, Via Christi Family Medicine Residency, Wichita, Kansas
Postpartum Care

William G. Nelson, MD, PhD
Marion I. Knott Professor of Oncology, Director of the Sidney Kimmel Comprehensive Cancer Center, The Johns Hopkins University School of Medicine, Baltimore, Maryland
Prostate Cancer

David G. Neschis, MD
Clinical Associate Professor of Surgery, University of Maryland School of Medicine, Baltimore, Maryland; Maryland Vascular Center, Glen Burnie, Maryland
Aortic Disease: Aneurysm and Dissection

Theresa Nester, MD
Medical Director of Integrated Transfusion Service Laboratories, Bloodworks Northwest, Seattle, Washington
Blood Component Therapy and Transfusion Reactions

Tam T. Nguyen, MD
Vice Chair, Family Medicine, Washington Township Medical Group, Fremont, California
Papulosquamous Eruptions

Andrea L. Nicol, MD, MSc
Associate Professor, Department of Anesthesiology, University of Kansas School of Medicine, Kansas City, Kansas
Fibromyalgia

Lucybeth Nieves-Arriba, MD
Assistant Professor, Gynecology Oncology, Zimmer Cancer Center, Wilmington, North Carolina
Cancer of the Uterine Cervix

Andrei Novac, MD
Clinical Professor of Psychiatry, University of California–Irvine School of Medicine, Irvine, California
Depressive, Bipolar, and Related Mood Disorders

Enrico M. Novelli, MD
Associate Professor of Medicine, Chief, Section of Benign Hematology, Director, Adult Sickle Cell Program, Department of Medicine, Division of Hematology/Oncology, Vascular Medicine Institute, Pittsburgh, Pennsylvania
Sickle Cell Disease

Lauren Nye, MD
Assistant Professor of Internal Medicine, Division of Medical Oncology, Breast Cancer Prevention and Survivorship Research Center, University of Kansas Medical Center, Kansas City, Kansas
Benign Breast Disease; Breast Cancer

Andrea T. Obi, MD
Section of Vascular Surgery, Department of Surgery, University of Michigan, Ann Arbor, Michigan
Venous Thrombosis

Jeffrey P. Okeson, DMD
Professor and Chief, Division of Orofacial Pain, Program Director, Orofacial Pain, Department of Oral Health Science, University of Kentucky College of Dentistry, Lexington, Kentucky
Temporomandibular Disorders

Carlos R. Oliveira, MD, PhD
Assistant Professor, Yale School of Medicine, Division of Pediatric Infectious Diseases, Yale Child Health Research Center, New Haven, Connecticut
Lyme Disease

Peck Y. Ong, MD
Associate Professor of Clinical Pediatrics, Keck School of Medicine, University of Southern California/Children's Hospital Los Angeles, Los Angeles, California
Atopic Dermatitis

Daniel S. Oram, MD
Clinical Lecturer, Department of Family Medicine, Women's Health Fellow, Department of Obstetrics and Gynecology, University of Michigan Medical School, Ann Arbor, Michigan
Postpartum Depression

Gary D. Overturf, MD
Professor Emeritus, Pediatrics and Pathology, University of New Mexico School of Medicine, Albuquerque, New Mexico
Bacterial Meningitis

Bulent Ozgonenel, MD
Associate Professor in Pediatric Hematology/Oncology, Children's Hospital of Michigan, Wayne State University, Detroit, Michigan
Hemophilia and Related Conditions

Karel Pacak, MD, PhD, DSc
Senior Investigator, Chief, Section on Medical Neuroendocrinology, Head, Developmental Endocrinology, Metabolism, Genetics and Endocrine Oncology Affinity Group, Professor of Medicine, Eunice Kennedy Shriver NICHD, NIH, Bethesda, Maryland
Pheochromocytoma

Jose A. Padin-Rosado, MD
Associate Professor, Department of Neurology, University of New Mexico School of Medicine, Albuquerque, New Mexico
Seizures and Epilepsy in Adolescents and Adults

John E. Pandolfino, MD
Hans Popper Professor of Medicine, Feinberg School of Medicine, Northwestern University, Chicago, Illinois
Dysphagia and Esophageal Obstruction

Yael Paran, MD
Head, the Clinic for Tropical Medicine, Senior Physician, Tel Aviv Sourasky Medical Center, Tel Aviv, Israel
Travel Medicine

Jotam Pasipanodya, MD
Research Scientist, University of Texas Southwestern Medical Center at Dallas, Dallas, Texas
Tuberculosis and Other Mycobacterial Diseases

Pasquale Passarella, MD
Endocrinologist, Assistant Professor of Medicine at Albany
   Medical Center, Albany, New York
Diabetic Ketoacidosis

Simon Patton, MD
Female Pelvic Medicine and Reconstructive Surgery, Via Christi
   Health, Wichita, Kansas
Urinary Incontinence

Gerson O. Penna, MD, PhD
Senior Researcher, Tropical Medicine Center, University of
   Brasilia, Brasilia, Brazil
Leprosy

Maria Lucia Penna, MD, PhD
Professor, Department of Epidemiology and Biostatistics,
   Universidade Federal Fluminense, Rio de Janeiro, Brazil
Leprosy

Allen Perkins, MD, MPH
Professor and Chair, Family Medicine, University of South
   Alabama, Mobile, Alabama
Marine Poisonings, Envenomations, and Trauma

Leah Peterson, MD
Smoky Hill Family Medicine Residency, Salina, Kansas; Clinical
   Assistant Professor, Department of Family and Community
   Medicine, University of Kansas School of Medicine–Wichita,
   Wichita, Kansas
Hypertension in Pregnancy

Georg A. Petroianu, MD, PhD
Professor and Chair, Cellular Biology and Pharmacology,
   College of Medicine–Florida International University, Miami,
   Florida
Hiccups

Vesna M. Petronic-Rosic, MD, MSc, MBA
Professor and Chair, Department of Dermatology, Georgetown
   University School of Medicine; MedStar Washington
   Hospital Center, MedStar Georgetown University Hospital,
   Washington, DC
Melanoma

Hanna Phan, PharmD
Assistant Department Head, Pharmacy Practice & Science,
   Associate Professor, Department of Pediatrics and Pharmacy
   Practice & Science, Associate Research Scientist, Asthma &
   Airway Disease Research Center, Colleges of Pharmacy and
   Medicine, The University of Arizona, Tucson, Arizon
Cystic Fibrosis

Claus A. Pierach, MD
Professor, University of Minnesota Medical School, Minneapolis,
   Minnesota
Porphyrias

Mark Pietroni, MD, MBA
Medical Director, Gloucestershire Hospitals NHS Foundation
   Trust, Gloucester, United Kingdom
Cholera

Susan M. Pollart, MD, MS
Ruth E. Murdaugh Professor, Family Medicine, University of
   Virginia School of Medicine, Charlottesville, Virginia
Asthma in Children

Maria de Andrade Pontes, MD
Dermatology, Technical Director and Coordinator of the
   Research Center, Dona Libânia Dermatology Center,
   Fortaleza, Brazil
Leprosy

Andrew S.T. Porter, DO
Clinical Assistant Professor, Department of Family and
   Community Medicine, University of Kansas School of
   Medicine–Wichita; Director, University of Kansas School of
   Medicine–Wichita Sports Medicine, Wichita, Kansas
Common Sports Injuries

C.R. Powell, MD
Associate Professor, Department of Urology, Indiana University
   School of Medicine–Indianapolis, Indianapolis, Indiana
Prostatitis

Margaret Pusateri, MD
University of New Mexico Health Sciences Center, Department
   of Emergency Medicine, Albuquerque, New Mexico
Sports-Related Head Injuries

Peter S. Rahko, MD
Professor of Medicine, Cardiovascular Medicine Division,
   University of Wisconsin, Madison, Wisconsin
Mitral Valve Prolapse

S. Vincent Rajkumar, MD
Professor of Medicine, Division of Hematology, Mayo Clinic,
   Rochester, Minnesota
Multiple Myeloma

Kalyanakrishnan Ramakrishnan, MD
Professor, Department of Family and Preventive Medicine,
   University of Oklahoma Health Sciences Center, Oklahoma
   City, Oklahoma
Necrotizing Skin and Soft-Tissue Infections

Julio A. Ramirez, MD
Professor of Medicine, University of Louisville School of
   Medicine; Chief, Division of Infectious Diseases, Department
   of Veterans Affairs Medical Center, Louisville, Kentucky
Legionellosis (Legionnaires' Disease and Pontiac Fever)

Matthew A. Rank, MD
Associate Professor of Medicine, Division of Allergy, Asthma,
   and Clinical Immunology, Mayo Clinic Alix School of
   Medicine, Mayo Clinic in Arizona, Scottsdale, Arizona
Asthma in Adolescents and Adults

Didier Raoult, MD, PhD
Unite de recherche sur les maladies infectieuses tropicales,
   Aix-Marseille Universite, Marseille, France
Q Fever

Anita Devi K. Ravindran, MD
Faculty of Medicine, Atma Jaya Catholic University of
   Indonesia, Jakarta, Indonesia
Foodborne Illnesses

Elizabeth Reddy, MD
Assistant Professor of Infectious Disease, Upstate Medical
   University Hospital, Syracuse, New York
Intestinal Parasites

Deon Regis, MD
Family Medicine, Mount Carmel St. Ann's Family Medicine
    Center, Westerville, Ohio
Whooping Cough (Pertussis)

Ian R. Reid, MD
Distinguished Professor of Medicine and Endocrinology,
    University of Auckland, Auckland, New Zealand
Paget's Disease of Bone

Elissa Rennert-May, MD, MSc
Clinical Lecturer, University of Calgary, Alberta Health Services
    Calgary, Calgary, Alberta, Canada
Methicillin-Resistant Staphylococcus aureus

Karl T. Rew, MD
Associate Professor of Family Medicine and Urology, University
    of Michigan Medical School, Ann Arbor, Michigan
Erectile Dysfunction

Mona Rezapour, MD, MHS
Clinical Instructor, Gastroenterology, University of California,
    Los Angeles, Los Angeles, California
Inflammatory Bowel Disease

Amanda Rhyne, MD
Clinical Instructor, University of Kansas School of Medicine,
    Wichita Department of Family and Community Medicine
    Family Medicine Residency Program at Smoky Hill, Salina,
    Kansas
Serum Sickness

Amy Robertson, PharmD
Clinical Assistant Professor, Departments of Pharmacy Practice
    and Family and Community Medicine, University of Kansas
    School of Pharmacy; Clinical Pharmacist, Wesley Family
    Medicine Residency Clinic, Wichita, Kansas
Serum Sickness

Malcolm K. Robinson, MD
Associate Professor of Surgery, Harvard Medical School;
    Associate Chair of Surgery for Clinical Operations, Director,
    Nutrition Support Service, Brigham and Women's Hospital,
    Boston, Massachusetts
Parenteral Nutrition in Adults

William P. Roche, MD
Neuromuscular Division, Emory University, Atlanta, Georgia
    Myasthenia Gravis

Michelle Roett, MD, MPH
Professor and Chair, Department of Family Medicine, MedStar
    Georgetown University Hospital, Georgetown University
    Medical Center, Washington, DC
Ovarian Cancer

Peter G. Rose, MD
Case Western Reserve University School of Medicine; Section
    Head, Gynecologic Oncology, Women's Health Institute,
    Cleveland Clinic, Cleveland, Ohio
Cancer of the Uterine Cervix

Richard N. Rosenthal, MD
Professor of Psychiatry, Icahn School of Medicine at Mount
    Sinai, New York, New York
Alcohol Use Disorder

Alan R. Roth, DO
Chairman, Department of Family Medicine, Ambulatory Care
    and Community Medicine, Chief, Department of Pain and
    Palliative Care Medicine, MediSys Health Network, Flushing
    Hospital Medical Center, Jamaica Hospital Medical Center,
    Queens, New York
Fever

Anne-Michelle Ruha, MD
Vice-Chair, Department of Medical Toxicology, Banner–
    University Medical Center Phoenix; Professor, Departments
    of Internal Medicine and Emergency Medicine, University of
    Arizona College of Medicine–Phoenix, Phoenix, Arizona
Spider Bites and Scorpion Stings

Kristen Rundell, MS, MD
Program Director, Riverside Methodist Family Medicine
    Residency, Riverside Methodist Hospital, Columbus, Ohio
Drug Hypersensitivity Reactions; Mumps

Richard Sadovsky, MD
Associate Professor of Family Medicine, SUNY-Downstate
    Medical Center, Brooklyn, New York
Tinnitus

Heitor de Sá Gonçalves, MD, PhD
Dermatology, Ceara State University, Fortaleza, Brazil
Leprosy

Adnan Said, MD, MS
Associate Professor of Medicine, Gastroenterology, and
    Hepatology, University of Wisconsin School of Medicine
    and Public Health, Chief Gastroenterology and Hepatology,
    Director, Liver Transplant, William S. Middleton VAMC,
    Madison, Wisconsin
Nonalcoholic Fatty Liver Disease

Tomoko Sairenji, MD
Assistant Professor of Family Medicine, University of
    Washington, Seattle, Washington
Bronchitis and Viral Respiratory Infections

Susan L. Samson, MD, PhD
Associate Professor, Baylor College of Medicine, Houston,
    Texas
Hyponatremia

Carlos E. Sanchez, MD
Interventional Cardiology, Structural Heart Disease,
    Cardiovascular Diseases, OhioHealth, Columbus, Ohio
Valvular Heart Disease

Sandeep Sangodkar, DO, MS
Cardiology Specialists Medical Group; Associate Professor
    of Clinical Medicine, University of California, Riverside;
    Riverside, California; Western University of Health Sciences,
    Evanston, Illinois
Hypertrophic Cardiomyopathy

Ravi Sarode, MD
John H. Childers, MD, Professor of Pathology and Internal
    Medicine (Hematology/Oncology), Chief of Pathology and
    Medical Director, USTW Clinical Laboratory Services,
    Director, Division of Transfusion Medicine and Hemostasis,
    UT Southwestern Medical Center, Dallas, Texas
Thrombotic Thrombocytopenic Purpura

J. Terry Saunders, PhD
Assistant Professor of Medical Education in Internal Medicine, University of Virginia School of Medicine, Charlottesville, Virginia
Diabetes Mellitus in Adults

Michael Schatz, MD, MS
Department of Allergy, Kaiser Permanente; Clinical Professor, Department of Medicine, University of California San Diego School of Medicine, San Diego, California
Asthma in Adolescents and Adults

Alex Schevchuck, MD
Assistant Professor, Internal Medicine/Cardiology, University of New Mexico, Albuquerque, New Mexico
Tachycardias

Lawrence R. Schiller, MD
Program Director, Gastroenterology Fellowship, Baylor University Medical Center, Dallas, Texas
Malabsorption

Kim Schoessow, OTD, OTR/L
Assistant Professor of Occupational Therapy, MGH Institute of Health Professions, Boston, Massachusetts
Vision Rehabilitation

Sarina Schrager, MD, MS
Professor of Family Medicine, University of Wisconsin, Madison, Wisconsin
Abnormal Uterine Bleeding

Dan Schuller, MD
Chair and Professor, Department of Internal Medicine–Transmountain, Texas Tech University Health Sciences Center–El Paso, Paul L. Foster School of Medicine, Dallas, Texas
Lung Abscess

Cassie Scripter, MD
Hillside Medical Group, Clinical Assistant Professor of Family and Community Medicine, University of Kansas School of Medicine–Wichita, Wichita, Kansas
Varicella (Chickenpox)

Amy Seery, MD
Assistant Professor, Department of Family and Community Medicine, University of Kansas School of Medicine–Wichita; Associate Director of Pediatrics, Via Christi Family Medicine Residency, Wichita, Kansas
Normal Infant Feeding

Steven A. Seifert, MD
Editor-in-Chief, Clinical Toxicology; Professor of Emergency Medicine, University of New Mexico School of Medicine, Albuquerque, New Mexico
Venomous Snakebite

Jeffery D. Semel, MD
Head, Section of Infectious Diseases, NorthShore University Healthsystem, Evanston, Illinois
Clostridium difficile Colitis

Saeed Kamran Shaffi, MD, MS
Associate Professor, Internal Medicine/Nephrology, University of New Mexico, Albuquerque, New Mexico
Primary Glomerular Diseases

Beejal Shah, MD
Endocrinologist, Bay Pines VA HealthCare System, Bay Pines, Florida
Hyponatremia

Prediman K. Shah, MD, MACC
Shapell and Webb Chair in Clinical Cardiology, Director, Oppenheimer Atherosclerosis Research Center and Atherosclerosis Prevention and Treatment Center, Smidt Heart Institute, Cedars-Sinai Medical Center; Professor of Medicine, University of California, Los Angeles, Cedars-Sinai Medical Center, Los Angeles, California
Acute Myocardial Infarction

Samir S. Shah, MD, MSCE
Professor, Department of Pediatrics, University of Cincinnati College of Medicine; Director, Division of Hospital Medicine, James M. Ewell Endowed Chair, Cincinnati Children's Hospital Medical Center, Cincinnati, Ohio
Viral Meningitis

Shenil Shah, MD
Cardiovascular Medicine, University of Wisconsin School of Medicine and Public Health, Madison, Wisconsin
Mitral Valve Prolapse

Jamile M. Shammo, MD
Professor of Medicine and Pathology, Division of Hematology Oncology and Stem Cell Transplantation, Rush University Medical Center, Chicago, Illinois
Myelodysplastic Syndromes

Eugene D. Shapiro, MD
Professor of Pediatrics (General Pediatrics) and Epidemiology (Microbial Diseases), Vice Chair for Research, Department of Pediatrics, Deputy Director, Investigative Medicine PhD Program, Co-Director of Education, Yale Center for Clinical Investigation, New Haven, Connecticut
Lyme Disease

Ala I. Sharara, MD
Professor, Division of Gastroenterology, American University of Beirut Medical Center, Beirut, Lebanon, Consulting Professor, Duke University Medical Center, Durham, North Carolina
Bleeding Esophageal Varices

John P. Sheehan, MD
Department of Medicine, Division of Hematology/Oncology, University of Wisconsin School of Medicine and Public Health, UW Carbone Cancer Center, Madison, Wisconsin
Venous Thromboembolism

Sable Shew, MD
Department of Urology, Naval Medical Center San Diego, San Diego, California
Urethral Stricture Disease

Abraham Shulman, MD
Professor Emeritus, State University of New York–Downstate Medical Center, Brooklyn, New York
Tinnitus

Karlynn Sievers, MD
Faculty Physician, Family Medicine, St. Mary's Family Medicine Residency, Grand Junction, Colorado
Trigeminal Neuralgia

Hugh Silk, MD, MPH
Professor, Department of Family Medicine & Community Health, UMass Medical School, Learning Communities Mentor, Blackstone House; Part-time Lecturer, Harvard School of Dental Medicine, Boston, Massachusetts; Medical Director, Primary Care Wellness Center/Community Healthlink, Center for Integration of Primary Care and Oral Health, Worcester, Massachusetts
Trigeminal Neuralgia

Aaron Sinclair, MD
Assistant Professor, Department of Family and Community Medicine, University of Kansas School of Medicine–Wichita, Wesley Family Medicine Residency, Wichita, Kansas
Diverticula of the Alimentary Tract

Philip D. Sloane, MD, MPH
Elizabeth and Oscar Goodwin Distinguished Professor, Department of Family Medicine; Co-Director, Program on Aging, Disability, and Long-Term Care, Cecil G. Sheps Center for Health Services Research; University of North Carolina, Chapel Hill, North Carolina
Alzheimer's Disease

Zachary L. Smith, DO
Division of Gastroenterology and Liver Disease, University Hospitals Digestive Health Institute; Assistant Professor of Medicine, Case Western Reserve University School of Medicine, Cleveland, Ohio
Calculous Biliary Disease

William J. Somers, MD
Urology Department, Veteran Affairs Ambulatory Care Center, Columbus, Ohio
Nephrolithiasis

Timothy Sowder, MD
Associate Professor, Department of Anesthesiology, University of Kansas School of Medicine, Kansas City, Kansas
Fibromyalgia

Linda Speer, MD
Professor and Chair, Family Medicine, University of Toledo, Toledo, Ohio
Dysmenorrhea

Abby L. Spencer, MD, MS
Vice Chair of Education–Medicine Institute, Associate Professor of Medicine, Cleveland Clinic Lerner College of Medicine, Cleveland, Ohio
Contraception

Erik Kent St. Louis, MD, MS
Associate Professor, Neurology, Mayo Clinic College of Medicine, Rochester, Minnesota
Sleep Disorders

Todd Stephens, MD
Clinical Assistant Professor, Department of Family and Community Medicine, University of Kansas School of Medicine–Wichita; Associate Director, Via Christi Family Medicine Residency, Wichita, Kansas
Genital Ulcer Disease: Chancroid, Granuloma Inguinale, and Lymphogranuloma

Dennis L. Stevens, MD, PhD
Associate Chief of Staff, Research and Development Service, Veterans Affairs Medical Center, Boise, Idaho
Bacterial Diseases of the Skin

John H. Stone, MD, MPH
Professor of Medicine, Harvard Medical School, The Edward Fox Chair in Medicine; Director, Clinical Rheumatology, Massachusetts General Hospital, Boston, Massachusetts
Polymyalgia Rheumatica and Giant Cell Arteritis

Constantine A. Stratakis, MD, PhD
Head, Section on Endocrinology and Genetics; NICHD, National Institutes of Health, Scientific Director, NICHD, National Institute of Health, Bethesda, Maryland
Cushing's Syndrome

Daniel Stulberg, MD
Professor and Vice Chair of Education, Department of Family and Community Medicine, University of New Mexico School of Medicine, Albuquerque, New Mexico
Premalignant Skin Lesions

Masayoshi Takashima, MD
Chairman, Department of Otolaryngology–Head and Neck Surgery, Houston Methodist Hospital, The Texas Medical Center, Houston, Texas
Obstructive Sleep Apnea

Varun Takyar, MD
Division of Gastrointestinal and Liver Diseases, University of Southern California, Los Angeles, California
Hepatitis A, B, D, and E

Carolina Talhari, MD, PhD
Associate Professor of Dermatology, State University of Amazonas; Dermatologist, Alfredo da Matta Foundation for Dermatology, Manaus, Amazonas, Brazil
Leprosy

Jie Tang, MD
Associate Professor, Division of Kidney Diseases and Hypertension, Albert Medical School, Brown University, Providence, Rhode Island
Hypokalemia and Hyperkalemia

Jessica Tate, MD
Assistant Professor of Neurology, Wake Forest University School of Medicine, Winston-Salem, North Carolina
Parkinson Disease

Joyce M.C. Teng, MD, PhD
Professor of Dermatology and Pediatrics, Stanford University School of Medicine; Lucile Packard Children's Hospital at Stanford, Stanford, California
Urticaria and Angioedema

Joanna Thomson, MD, MPH
Pediatric Hospitalist, Cincinnati Children's Hospital Medical Center; Assistant Professor, Department of Pediatrics, University of Cincinnati College of Medicine, Cincinnati, Ohio
Viral Meningitis

J. Brantley Thrasher, MD
Executive Secretary of the American Board of Urology; Professor Emeritus, Department of Urology, University of Kansas Hospital; University of Kansas Medical Center, Kansas City, Kansas
Hematuria

William Tillett, MBChB, PhD
Consultant Rheumatologist, Royal National Hospital for Rheumatic Diseases; Senior Lecturer, Pharmacy and Pharmacology, University of Bath, Bath, United Kingdom
Psoriatic Arthritis

Kenneth Tobin, DO
Clinical Assistant Professor, Director, Chest Pain Center, University of Michigan, Northville, Michigan
Angina Pectoris

Theodore T. Tsaltas, MD
Tri-Star Summit Medical Center, Hermitage, Tennessee; OB Hospitalist Group, Chattanooga, Tennessee
Uterine Leiomyoma

Arvid E. Underman, MD
Director of Graduate Medical Education, Huntington Hospital, Pasadena, California; Clinical Professor of Medicine and Microbiology, Keck School of Medicine, University of Southern California, Los Angeles, California
Salmonellosis

Mark Unruh, MD, MS
Chair, Department of Internal Medicine, University of New Mexico School of Medicine, Albuquerque, New Mexico
Chronic Kidney Disease

Locke Uppendahl, MD
Obstetrics and Gynecology, Division of Gynecologic Oncology, University of Kansas School of Medicine–Wichita, Wichita, Kansas
Cancer of the Endometrium

Anusha Vallurupalli, MBBS
Assistant Professor of Medicine, Division of Hematologic Malignancies and Cellular Therapeutics, University of Kansas Medical Center, Kansas City, Kansas
Hodgkin Lymphoma; Pernicious Anemia/Megaloblastic Anemia

George Van Buren II, MD
Associate Professor of Surgery, Michael E. DeBakey Department of Surgery, Baylor College of Medicine, Houston, Texas
Acute and Chronic Pancreatitis

David van Duin, MD, PhD
Associate Professor of Medicine, University of North Carolina, Chapel Hill, North Carolina
Histoplasmosis

Daniel J. Van Durme, MD, MPH
Professor and Chair, Family Medicine and Rural Health, Florida State University College of Medicine, Tallahassee, Florida
Acne Vulgaris; Rosacea

Kyle Vincent, MD
Clinical Associate Professor, Department of Surgery, University of Kansas School of Medicine–Wichita, Wichita, Kansas
Gastritis and Peptic Ulcer Disease

Donald C. Vinh, MD
Director, Infectious Disease Susceptibility Program, FRQS Clinician-Scientist, Associate Professor, Department of Medicine, Divisions of Infectious Diseases and Allergy and Clinical Immunology, Departments of Medical Microbiology and Human Genetics, McGill University Health Centre–Research Institute, Montreal, Quebec, Canada
Blastomycosis

K.N. Viswanathan, MD
Professor of Medicine and Tropical Medicine, PK Das Institute of Medical Sciences, Ottapalam, Kerala, India
Foodborne Illnesses

Jatin M. Vyas, MD, PhD
Associate Professor of Medicine, Division of Infectious Disease, Massachusetts General Hospital, Boston, Massachusetts
Rat-Bite Fever

Thomas W. Wakefield, MD
Stanley Professor of Surgery, Section of Vascular Surgery, Department of Surgery, University of Michigan, Ann Arbor, Michigan
Venous Thrombosis

Arnold Wald, MD
Division of Gastroenterology and Hepatology, University of Wisconsin School of Medicine and Public Health, Madison, Wisconsin
Irritable Bowel Syndrome

Ellen R. Wald, MD
Chair, Department of Pediatrics, University of Wisconsin School of Medicine and Public Health, Madison, Wisconsin
Urinary Tract Infections in Infants and Children

Robin A. Walker, MD
Northwest Family Physicians Clinical Assistant Professor, Department of Family and Community Medicine, University of Kansas School of Medicine–Wichita, Wichita, Kansas
Epididymitis and Orchitis

Barry M. Wall, MD
Professor of Medicine, Division of Nephrology, Veterans Affairs Medical Center, University of Tennessee Health Science Center, Memphis, Tennessee
Diabetic Ketoacidosis

Anne Walling, MB, ChB
Professor Emeritus, Department of Family and Community Medicine, University of Kansas School of Medicine–Wichita, Wichita, Kansas
Migraine Headache; Obsessive-Compulsive Disorder

Andrew Wang, MD
Professor of Medicine (Cardiology), Vice Chief for Clinical Affairs, Division of Cardiology, Duke University Medical Center, Durham, North Carolina
Infective Endocarditis

Ernest Wang, MD
Associate Professor of Emergency Medicine, Evanston Hospital, NorthShore University HealthSystem, Evanston, Illinois
Disturbances due to Cold

Jennifer Wang, DO
Assistant Professor, Critical Care Medicine, The Mount Sinai Hospital, New York, New York
Targeted Temperature Management (Therapeutic Hypothermia)

Koji Watanabe, MD, PhD
Staff Doctor, AIDS Clinical Center, National Center for Global Health and Medicine, Tokyo, Japan
Amebiasis

Ruth Weber, MD, MSEd
Clinical Associate Professor, Department of Family and
Community Medicine, Medical University of South Carolina,
Charleston, South Carolina
Pharyngitis

Cheryl Wehler, MD
Assistant Professor, Department of Psychiatry and Behavioral
Sciences, University of Kansas School of Medicine–Wichita,
Wichita, Kansas
Panic Disorder

Jane A. Weida, MD
Associate Professor, College of Community Health Sciences, The
University of Alabama; Interim Department Chair, Family,
Internal and Rural Medicine; Director of Clinical Affairs,
Tuscaloosa, Alabama
Measles (Rubeola)

David N. Weissman, MD
Director, Respiratory Health Division, National Institute
for Occupational Safety and Health, Morgantown,
West Virginia
Pneumoconiosis: Asbestosis and Silicosis

Robert C. Welliver Sr., MD
Children's Hospital Foundation Hobbs-Recknagel Endowed
Chair in Pediatrics, Professor of Pediatrics, Chief, Division
of Pediatric Infectious Diseases, The Children's Hospital at
University of Oklahoma Health Sciences Center, Oklahoma
City, Oklahoma
Viral Respiratory Infections

Rebecca M. Wester, MD
HOMAHA Senior Care, Omaha, Nebraska
Pressure Injury

Ryan P. Westergaard, MD, PhD, MPH
Associate Professor, Departments of Medicine and Population
Health Sciences, University of Wisconsin–Madison, Madison,
Wisconsin
Treatment and Prevention of HIV Infection

Randell Wexler, MD MPH
Professor, Vice Chair, Clinical Services, Department of Family
Medicine, The Ohio State University, Columbus, Ohio
Premature Beats

Brian M. Whitley, MD
Assistant Professor of Surgery, Division of Urology, Duke
University, Raleigh, North Carolina
Benign Prostatic Hyperplasia

Katarzyna Wilamowska, MD, PhD
Department of Family and Community Medicine, University of
New Mexico School of Medicine, Albuquerque, New Mexico
Premalignant Skin Lesions

Kimberly Williams, MD
Assistant Professor, Department of Family and Community
Medicine, University of Kansas School of Medicine–Wichita,
Wichita, Kansas; Program Director, Family Medicine, Smoky
Hill Residency, Salina, Kansas
Otitis Externa

Tracy L. Williams, MD
Associate Professor, Department of Family and Community
Medicine, University of Kansas School of Medicine–Wichita;
Associate Director, Via Christi Family Medicine Residency,
Wichita, Kansas
Chlamydia trachomatis

Boris Winterhoff, MD
Assistant Professor, Obstetrics, Gynecology, and Women's
Health, University of Minnesota, Minneapolis, Minnesota
Cancer of the Endometrium

Jennifer Wipperman, MD, MPH
Associate Professor, Department of Family and Community
Medicine, University of Kansas School of Medicine–Wichita;
Associate Director, Via Christi Family Medicine Residency,
Wichita, Kansas
Dizziness and Vertigo

Robert Wittler, MD
Professor of Pediatrics & Pediatric Infectious Diseases,
University of Kansas School of Medicine–Wichita, Wichita,
Kansas
*Tickborne Rickettsial Diseases (Rocky Mountain Spotted
Fever and Other Spotted Fever Group Rickettsioses,
Ehrlichioses, and Anaplasmosis)*

Gary S. Wood, MD
Professor and Founding Chair, Dean's Chair in Cutaneous
Research, Geneva F. and Sture Johnson Professor Emeritus,
Department of Dermatology, University of Wisconsin–
Madison,
*Cutaneous T-Cell Lymphomas, Including Mycosis Fungoides
and Sézary Syndrome*

Scott Worswick, MD
Associate Clinical Professor of Dermatology, Keck Hospital of
the University of Southern California; Director of Inpatient
Dermatology, Los Angeles County Hospital; Co-Program
Director, USC Dermatology Residency Program, Los Angeles,
California
Stevens-Johnson Syndrome and Toxic Epidermal Necrolysis

Steve W. Wu, MD
Associate Professor, University of Cincinnati College of
Medicine; Assistant Professor, Cincinnati Children's
Hospital Medical Center, Cincinnati, Ohio
Gilles De La Tourette Syndrome

Hadley Wyre, MD
Assistant Professor of Urology, University of Kansas Medical
Center, Kansas City, Kansas
Urethral Stricture Disease

Steven J. Yakubov, MD
John H. McConnell Chair of Advanced Structural Heart
Disease, System Chief, OhioHealth Structural Heart
Disease, Columbus, Ohio
Valvular Heart Disease

Xinghong Yang, PhD
Infectious Diseases and Pathology, University of Florida,
Gainesville, Florida
Brucellosis

Yooni Yi, MD
University of Michigan, Ann Arbor, Michigan
Trauma to the Genitourinary Tract

James A. Yiannias, MD
Associate Professor of Dermatology, Mayo Clinic, Scottsdale, Arizona
Contact Dermatitis

Nata Young, MD
Physician, AnMed Health Family Medicine Center, AnMed Health Oglesby Center, Anderson, South Carolina
Antepartum Care

Mark E. Zafereo, MD
Assistant Professor, Head and Neck Surgery, MD Anderson, Cancer Center, Houston, Texas
Thyroid Cancer

Jane Zuckerman, MD
Royal Free London Travel Health and Immunization Clinic, Royal Free London NHS Foundation Trust; Honorary Senior Lecturer, University College Medical School, London, United Kingdom
Travel Medicine

Preface

Conn's Current Therapy 2020 is the 72nd edition of a text that combines art and science. William Osler stated that "the practice of medicine is an art based on science." Using a format that honors "the method of" our expert clinical authors allows their practical experience to provide therapeutic insight that cannot be obtained from guidelines alone. *Current Therapy* is a vector from which information flows to the clinician so the science can be applied artfully to the patient.

As artificial intelligence (AI) grows, computers will be able to process algorithms, direct guidelines, and interpret diagnostic images much better than humans. As we become smarter in utilizing AI to improve efficiency of care, Alexa, Google, and Siri will inform us about the next drug to use or the severity of the lung nodule on the CT scan. But they won't be able to incorporate the art of medicine, a uniquely human ability, that matches the best therapy with the context of someone's life.

Primary care is the foundation from which value in health care is obtained. It has been estimated that for every $1 invested in primary care, there is a $13 return on investment. Not only does primary care reduce costs, it reduces mortality. For a population of 100,000, adding 10 primary care clinicians has been calculated to extend life by 51.5 days, while adding 10 specialists added 19.2 days.[1] Both generalists and specialists are vitally important to a well-functioning health care system. Value comes when we are able to provide the best care within a medical home that knows the patient best. This reduces unnecessary testing and fragmentation of care while enhancing value-based outcomes. Our goal is to empower the primary care team with information that is current and accurate so they can bring their art to the patient's highest therapeutic need.

Current Therapy uses experts who have researched and developed clinical excellence on their topic of focus to allow you to channel the information and adapt it to your patient's needs. For this reason, *Current Therapy* continues to focus on therapeutics, providing easy to interpret graphics, tables, and boxes that highlight key take-home points. We are also incorporating more electronic links in the text that connect you to apps and prediction tools that will improve ease of practice. We continue to add and delete chapter topics based on what is most prevalent in practice. And as Dr. Conn intended when he published the 1st edition 71 years ago, we are constantly finding new authors to keep the information fresh and timely.

We would like to thank the 425 authors who have contributed to this text and their willingness to share their expertise. This publication could not happen without their dedication to their craft. We are grateful for their willingness to share their wisdom so we can apply it locally in the communities we serve.

With the annual publication schedule of *Current Therapy*, there are significant time pressures and coordinated efforts that require the dedication of an inter-professional team of hard-working individuals. We are grateful to Miriam Chan, PharmD, who checks the accuracy of the pharmaceutical dosing and indications. Charlotta Kryhl, Senior Content Strategist, and Sarah Barth, Publisher, at Elsevier provide unwavering support and guidance. Congratulations to Charlotta who took some time off from this edition to expand her family. A big thanks to Laura Schmidt, our Senior Content Development Manager, who kept us on task and did the majority of the heavy lifting for this edition. Welcome to the team, Laura! And thanks to Kate Mannix, Senior Project Manager, for putting together the final product.

We are eternally grateful to our families for tolerating the late nights, deadlines, and weekend time required to see this product to the finish line.

Finally, we would like to dedicate this edition to Joan Ryan, the Developmental Editor and "central nervous system" of *Current Therapy* for the past 10 years. Joan is a fantastic human being who was able to get the work done, communicate artfully, and have fun in the process. She has retired from Elsevier but not from our hearts. We are very grateful for her years of dedication and support.

David P. Rakel, MD
Rick D. Kellerman, MD

---

[1] Basu S, Berkowitz SA, Phillips RL, et al: Association of primary care physician supply with population mortality in the United States, 2005-2015. *JAMA Internal Medicine*, 2019.

Contents

SECTION 4
Digestive System

SECTION 5
Endocrine and Metabolic Disorders

SECTION 6
Hematology

SECTION 7
Diseases of the Head and Neck

SECTION 8
Infectious Diseases

SECTION 9
Nervous System

Contents

Contents

xxxiii

SECTION 12
Rheumatology and the Musculoskeletal System

SECTION 13
Sexually Transmitted Diseases

SECTION 14
Diseases of the Skin

Contents

xxxv

SECTION 18
Pregnancy and Antepartum Care*

*Section 18 is available online at ExpertConsult.com

SECTION 19
Children's Health

SECTION 20
Physical and Chemical Injuries

Symptomatic Care Pending Diagnosis

CHEST PAIN

Method of
William E Cayley Jr., MD, MDiv

CURRENT DIAGNOSIS

- Initial evaluation of chest pain should include evaluation of clinical stability, a concise history and physical, and a chest x-ray and electrocardiogram (ECG) unless the cause is clearly not life-threatening.
- Chest pain described as exertional, radiating to one or both arms, similar to or worse than prior cardiac chest pain, or associated with nausea, vomiting, or diaphoresis indicates high risk for acute coronary syndrome. ECG identifies ST elevation myocardial infarction (STEMI), and cardiac biomarkers are essential for further evaluation of suspected chest pain in the absence of STEMI.
- The Wells, Geneva, and Pisa clinical prediction rules can help stratify a patient's risk of pulmonary embolism.
- Aortic dissection is an uncommon cause of chest pain, but patients with abrupt or instantaneous chest pain that is ripping, tearing, or stabbing should have evaluation for dissection with chest x-ray, computed tomography (CT), or magnetic resonance imaging.
- Esophageal rupture may be suspected in patients with pain, dyspnea, and shock following a forceful emesis, and prompt imaging with CT or esophagram is essential.
- Patients who have suspected tension pneumothorax and who are clinically stable should have a chest x-ray for confirmation before needle decompression is attempted.

CURRENT THERAPY

- Patients with STEMI require urgent reperfusion, and those with unstable angina or non–ST elevation myocardial infarction require admission for further monitoring and evaluation.
- Most patients with pulmonary embolism require admission for monitoring and anticoagulation, although outpatient treatment may be possible for low-risk patients after initial evaluation and anticoagulation.
- Prompt surgical consultation is required for patients with confirmed or suspected aortic dissection or esophageal rupture.
- Clinically unstable patients with suspected tension pneumothorax need immediate needle decompression.

Epidemiology

Chest pain is the chief complaint in 1% to 2% of all outpatient primary care visits. More than 50% of emergency department (ED) visits for chest pain are due to serious cardiovascular conditions such as acute coronary syndrome (ACS) or pulmonary embolism (PE), but these account for less than 15% of outpatient primary care encounters for chest pain, and up to 15% of chest pain episodes never reach a definitive diagnosis. Other potentially life-threatening etiologies for chest pain include PE, dissecting aortic aneurysm (AA), esophageal rupture, and tension pneumothorax. In outpatient primary care the most common causes of chest pain are musculoskeletal, gastrointestinal, angina due to stable coronary artery disease (CAD), anxiety or other psychiatric conditions, and pulmonary disease.

Initial Assessment

In initial evaluation of chest pain, it is important to obtain a clear history of the onset and evolution of chest pain, especially details such as location, quality, duration, and aggravating or alleviating factors. Initial physical examination should include vital signs, assessment of the patient's overall general condition, and examination of the heart and lungs. If there are any clinical signs of instability (altered mental status, hypotension, marked dyspnea, or other signs of shock) then initial stabilization and diagnosis must both be addressed simultaneously, consistent with current guidelines for emergency cardiovascular care. Unless the history and physical examination suggest an obviously nonthreatening cause of chest discomfort, most adults with chest pain should at least have basic diagnostic testing with an ECG and a chest x-ray. Several clinical prediction rules are available to help confirm or exclude some common causes of chest pain (Box 1).

Diagnosis and Treatment

Acute Coronary Syndrome

ACS includes acute myocardial infarction (MI) (ST-segment elevation and depression, Q wave and non–Q wave) or unstable angina. A review of prospective and retrospective studies correlating specific chest pain characteristics with the likelihood of ACS found that components of the patient history that increase the likelihood of ACS include radiation of pain to the right arm or shoulder, to both arms or shoulders, or to the left arm; or pain associated with exertion, diaphoresis, nausea, or vomiting; or pain described as pressure or as "worse than previous angina or similar to a previous MI." Similarly, components of the history that predicted decreased likelihood of ACS were pleuritic, positional, or sharp chest pain; pain in an inframammary location; or pain not associated with exertion. A physical examination finding of chest pain reproducibility with palpation also decreased the likelihood of ACS. Additional physical examination findings that may be helpful are the presence of hypotension or an S_3 on cardiac auscultation, both of which suggest increased likelihood of ACS. The Marburg Heart Score (MHS) can help exclude CAD in primary care patients with chest pain (most patients with a score of 2 or less will not have CAD), and use of the MHS when evaluating primary care patients with chest pain has been shown to improve clinical diagnostic accuracy. Recent studies have demonstrated that the presence or absence of typical cardiac risk factors (eg, diabetes, hypertension, smoking, high cholesterol, or family history) have little diagnostic value for determining the likelihood of ACS in patients over age 40.

An ECG should be obtained promptly for any patient with suspected ACS. ST-segment elevation in two or more contiguous leads, or presumed new left bundle branch block, is diagnostic of ST segment elevation Type I MI (STEMI) and requires urgent revascularization with thrombolysis or angioplasty at an appropriate facility. Ischemic ST-segment

BOX 1 — Clinical Prediction Rules for Evaluating Patients with Chest Pain*

Acute Coronary Syndrome (ACS)

- Diagnosing cardiac ischemia with Exercise Treadmill Testing: Duke treadmill score: https://www.mdcalc.com/duke-treadmill-score
- What is the risk of a major cardiac event in the next 6 weeks? HEART Score: https://www.mdcalc.com/heart-score-major-cardiac-events.
- What is the risk of ACS in someone with chest pain? Marburg Heart Score: https://www.mdcalc.com/marburg-heart-score-mhs
- Assesses long-term risk in those with ACS: GRACE ACS risk calculator: http://www.outcomes-umassmed.org/grace/
- Estimates mortality for patients with unstable angina and non-ST elevation MI: TIMI risk score: http://www.timi.org/

Pneumonia

- Diehr diagnostic rule for pneumonia in adults with acute cough: http://www.soapnote.org/infectious/diehr-rule/

Pulmonary Embolism

- Geneva score for predicting risk of pulmonary embolism: https://www.mdcalc.com/geneva-score-revised-pulmonary-embolism
- Pisa clinical model for predicting the probability of PE: https://ebmcalc.com/PulmonaryEmbRiskPisaCXR.htm
- Wells scoring system for risk of pulmonary embolism: https://www.mdcalc.com/wells-criteria-pulmonary-embolism

Thoracic Aortic Dissection

- Aortic Dissection Detection Risk Score (ADD-RS): https://www.mdcalc.com/aortic-dissection-detection-risk-score-add-rs

TABLE 1 — Marburg Heart Score

FINDING	POINTS
Woman > 64 years, man > 54 years	1
Known CAD, cerebrovascular disease, or peripheral vascular disease	1
Pain worse with exercise	1
Pain not reproducible with palpation	1
Patient assumes pain is cardiac	1

Abbreviation: CAD = coronary artery disease.
Approximately 97% of patients with a MHS score of 2 or less will not have CAD.
Approximately 23% of patients with a MHS score of 3 or more will have CAD.
Adapted from: Haasenritter J, Bösner S, Vaucher P, Herzig L, Heinzel-Gutenbrunner M, Baum E, Donner-Banzhoff N. Ruling out coronary heart disease in primary care: external validation of a clinical prediction rule. Br J Gen Pract. 2012 Jun;62(599):e415-21. doi: 10.3399/bjgp12X649106. http://www.ncbi.nlm.nih.gov/pmc/articles/PMC3361121/.

depression more than 0.5 mm, dynamic T-wave inversion with chest discomfort, or transient ST-segment elevation of 0.5 mm or more are classified as unstable angina or non-ST segment elevation Type I MI (NSTEMI). However, none of these findings is sensitive enough that its absence can exclude MI, and patients whose chest pain is not low risk still require further assessment for ACS.

In patients with high-risk chest pain who do not have STEMI, elevated cardiac biomarkers distinguish NSTEMI from unstable angina. Cardiac troponins T and I are more sensitive for detecting NSTEMI than creatine kinase (CK) or the MB isoform (CK-MB). High-sensitive troponins will be coming into use with an even greater sensitivity (negative predictive values = 99.5%).

Initial management of NSTEMI includes hospital admission for antiplatelet, antithrombin, and antianginal therapy. Patients with unstable angina should also be hospitalized for observation, and patients with either NSTEMI or unstable angina require risk stratification using the TIMI or GRACE risk scores (see Box 1). Patients with chest pain suspicious for CAD, but no definite initial diagnosis of STEMI or NSTEMI on initial presentation, are often admitted to hospital for overnight observation and serial cardiac biomarker measurements at 6 and 12 hours after symptom onset to "rule out MI." However, use of the HEART, TIMI, or GRACE scores may help determine who is at sufficiently low risk of major adverse cardiac events to allow discharge for close follow-up, and recent evidence suggests that the HEART score may outperform TIMI and GRACE in determining which patients are low risk. (see Box 1).

Patients at low risk for ACS or MI can usually defer further testing unless there are other risk factors in their family or past medical history markedly increasing the likelihood of CAD. Current recommendations are that all other patients with chest pain suggesting CAD should have further noninvasive testing within 7 days; however, a recent study of 4181 patients in an ED chest pain unit found that a reasonable alternative may be to test troponin levels twice over a 6-hour interval, with no stress testing done if both values are normal. Patients who can exercise and who have no left-bundle branch block, preexcitation, or significant resting ST depression on a resting ECG can be evaluated with an exercise stress ECG, and the Duke treadmill score can then be used to further quantify cardiac risk (see Box 1). Patients with baseline ECG abnormalities should have perfusion imaging performed, along with a stress ECG, and patients who cannot exercise may be evaluated with a pharmacologic stress or vasodilator test (e.g., dobutamine [Dobutrex][1] or adenosine [Adenocard]). Patients at high risk for CAD or those with NSTEMI should generally proceed directly to angiography, which allows definitive assessment of coronary artery anatomy.

Pulmonary Embolism

There are no individual symptoms or physical examination findings that reliably diagnose or exclude pulmonary embolism (PE), but three clinical prediction rules have all been validated for use in determining likelihood of PE and therefore whether further testing is needed (Box 1). While the Pisa rule may be the most accurate, it is also the most mathematically complicated and depends on clinical, ECG, and x-ray findings. The Geneva rule requires blood gas and chest x-ray findings. The Wells rule (Table 2) is based on the simplest

TABLE 2 — Simplified Wells Scoring System for Pulmonary Embolism

CLINICAL FINDING	SCORE
Symptoms of deep vein thrombosis (DVT)	3.0
No alternative diagnosis more likely than PE	3.0
Heart rate > 100 bpm	1.5
Immobilization greater than 3 days or surgery in past 4 weeks	1.5
Previous objectively diagnosed DVT or PE	1.5
Hemoptysis	1.0
Malignancy	1.0

Probability of PE: < 2 points = low, 2–6 points = moderate, > 6 points = high.

Abbreviations: DVT = deep vein thrombosis; PE = pulmonary embolism.
Adapted from Miniati M, Bottai M, Monti S. Comparison of 3 clinical models for predicting the probability of pulmonary embolism. Medicine (Baltimore) 2005;84:107–114; Torbicki A, Perrier A, Konstantinides S, et al, ESC Committee for Practice Guidelines (CPG): Guidelines on the diagnosis and management of acute pulmonary embolism. Eur Heart J 2008;29:2276–315. http://eurheartj.oxfordjournals.org/content/29/18/2276.long.

---

[1] Not FDA approved for this indication.

combination of history and examination findings, and a comparison between the Wells and Geneva rules found the Wells rule has a lower failure rate. With the Wells and Geneva prediction rules, the likelihood of PE is approximately 10% in the low-probability category, 30% in the moderate-probability category, and 65% in the high-probability category. Routine tests done for patients with chest pain are not particularly helpful in diagnosing or excluding PE. The chest x-ray may be abnormal, but findings that typically occur with PE (atelectasis, effusion, or elevation of a hemidiaphragm) are nonspecific. ECG signs of right ventricular strain (S wave in lead I, Q wave and inverted T wave in lead III) may be helpful if present, but their absence does not exclude PE. Hypoxia may be present, but up to 20% of patients with PE have a normal alveolar-arterial oxygen gradient.

Additional tests recommended for evaluating patients with suspected PE include D-dimer testing by enzyme-linked immunosorbent assay (ELISA; sensitivity > 95%; specificity, approximately 40%) or latex agglutination (sensitivity 85%–90%), compression ultrasonography, ventilation–perfusion scintigraphy, or computed tomography (CT) angiography. Patients with suspected high-risk PE (i.e., those with shock or hypotension) should have immediate CT angiography and treatment for PE if the CT is positive, although an echocardiographic finding of right ventricular overload may be used to justify treatment for PE in the unstable patient with high clinical suspicion for PE when CT angiography is not available. Patients who have suspected PE and who are not at high risk (i.e., no shock or hypotension) and who have a high clinical probability (based on Wells, Geneva, or Pisa scoring) should also proceed directly to CT, with appropriate treatment if the scan is positive. Patients with low clinical probability of PE (based on one of the validated clinical prediction rules) do not need further D-dimer testing or imaging. Patients with intermediate clinical probability should initially have D-dimer testing; further testing or treatment for PE is unnecessary if the D-dimer is negative, and CT angiography should be performed if the D-dimer is positive.

Anticoagulation, with thrombolysis in high-risk patients, is the foundation of treatment for PE. Patients with shock or hypotension are at high risk and require hemodynamic and respiratory support, thrombolysis, or embolectomy, and then appropriate attention to anticoagulation. Normotensive patients with echocardiographic evidence of right ventricular dysfunction or serologic evidence of myocardial injury (elevated troponins or CK-MB) have intermediate risk and should be admitted for anticoagulation. Normotensive patients who have normal results on echocardiography and testing for myocardial injury are at low risk and often may be discharged early for management at home after initiation of anticoagulation. Anticoagulation for PE should be started at the time of diagnosis with unfractionated heparin, low-molecular-weight heparin, or fondaparinux (Arixtra) and continued for at least 5 days, with simultaneous initiation of oral anticoagulation with warfarin (Coumadin), titrated to maintain an international normalized ratio (INR) between 2.0 and 3.0. The newer anticoagulants dabigatran (Pradaxa), rivaroxaban (Xarelto), or apixaban (Eliquis) may be an option for patients who have difficulty maintaining steady anticoagulation with warfarin.

Thoracic Aortic Dissection

Thoracic aortic dissection is a much less common cause of chest pain; prevalence estimates are 2 to 3.5 cases per 100,000 person-years. Up to 40% of patients die immediately, and 5% to 20% die during or shortly after surgery. Risk factors for acute thoracic aortic dissection include hypertension, presence of a pheochromocytoma, cocaine use, weight lifting, trauma or a rapid deceleration event, coarctation of the aorta, and certain genetic abnormalities. Pain due to acute aortic dissection is perceived as abrupt and severe in 84% to 90% of cases, and more than 50% of patients describe the pain as sharp or stabbing. No physical findings are sensitive or specific for detecting aortic dissection, because approximately equal percentages of patients are hypertensive, normotensive, or have hypotension or shock, and the

most common physical findings (a murmur of aortic insufficiency or a pulse deficit) occur in less than half of patients.

In any patient with severe chest pain that is abrupt or instantaneous in onset or has a ripping, tearing, or stabbing quality, acute thoracic aortic dissection should be suspected. Physical examination should assess for a pulse deficit, a systolic pressure differential between limbs of greater than 20 mm Hg, a focal neurologic deficit, or a new aortic regurgitation murmur. It is also important to ask about a family history of connective tissue disease (including Marfan syndrome), about any family or personal history of aortic dissection or thoracic aneurysm, and about any known aortic valve disease or recent aortic interventions. D-dimer testing has been proposed as a way to screen for aortic dissection, but it is more important to obtain prompt imaging and surgical intervention for those in whom dissection is confirmed. A low-risk Aortic Dissection Detection Risk Score (ADD-RS) can help exclude the diagnosis of aortic dissection, while patients with a high-risk score require further evaluation.

An ECG should be obtained in all patients with suspected aortic dissection to exclude STEMI (which can manifest with similar symptoms). In all low- and intermediate-risk patients, a prompt chest x-ray can help by either confirming an alternative diagnosis or confirming the presence of thoracic aortic disease. High-risk patients should have prompt imaging with CT or magnetic resonance imaging (MRI), and those who are in shock or clinically unstable may be evaluated by bedside transesophageal echocardiography. If thoracic aortic dissection is confirmed on imaging, urgent surgical consultation is required. Medical therapy should be started with intravenous β-blockers. Patients with dissection of the ascending aorta require urgent surgery, whereas those with descending thoracic aortic dissection may be managed medically unless hypotension or other complications develop.

Esophageal Rupture

Esophageal rupture, or Boerhaave's syndrome, has a high mortality rate. Esophageal rupture is rare, and the most common cause is endoscopically induced injury, but it can happen in other settings as well. Common misdiagnoses include perforated ulcer, MI, PE, dissecting aneurysm, and pancreatitis. The "classic" presentation has been described as pain, dyspnea, and shock followed by forceful emesis, but history and physical are commonly nonspecific. Diagnosis most commonly is made by contrast esophagram or CT scan of the chest.

Patients whose rupture is diagnosed less than 48 hours after symptom onset should be treated surgically (especially if sepsis is present) or endoscopically. Those who present more than 48 hours after symptom onset may be considered for conservative treatment with hyperalimentation, antibiotics, and nasogastric suction.

Tension Pneumothorax

Tension pneumothorax is relatively rare among patients presenting with chest pain, but it is potentially life-threatening if not treated properly. Common symptoms and physical findings include chest pain, respiratory distress, decreased ipsilateral air entry, and tachycardia; hypoxia, tracheal deviation, and hypotension are less common.

Emergency needle decompression is usually recommended if tension pneumothorax is suspected, but this is ineffective in some cases and is associated with risks to the patient of pain, bleeding, infection, and cardiac tamponade. However, waiting for radiographic confirmation of the diagnosis is associated with up to a four fold increase in mortality due to delay in decompression of the pneumothorax. Patients most likely to benefit from an immediate attempt at needle decompression are those with an oxygen saturation < 92% while on oxygen, a decreased level of consciousness while on oxygen, a systolic blood pressure less than 90 mm Hg, or a respiratory rate < 10. Patients without these signs of instability may be better managed by waiting for chest imaging to confirm or exclude the presence of a pneumothorax. Although plain chest x-rays have typically been used for diagnosing a pneumothorax, one study has found that pleural ultrasound may have higher sensitivity.

TABLE 3 · Diehr Diagnostic Rule for Pneumonia in Adults with Acute Cough

SIGNS AND SYMPTOMS

FINDING	POINTS
Rhinorrhea	–2
Sore throat	–1
Night sweats	1
Myalgia	1
Sputum all day	1
Respiratory rate > 25	2
Temperature > 100°F	2

Interpretation

Score	Probability of Pneumonia
–3	5
–1	12
0	21
1	30
3	37

Adapted from Cayley Jr WE. Diagnosing the cause of chest pain. Am Fam Physician 2005;72:2012–2021. http://www.aafp.org/afp/2005/1115/p2012.html.

TABLE 4 · Evaluation for Chest Pain from Panic Disorder

ITEM	0	1	2	3	4	5
When you are nervous, how often do you think "I am going to pass out?"		Never	Rarely	Half the time	Usually	Always
During the last 7 days, including today, how much have you been bothered by pains in the chest?		Not at all	A little bit	Moderately	Quite a bit	Extremely
To what degree is your chest pain tiring or exhausting		None	Mild		Moderate	Severe

Adapted from: Dammen T, Ekeberg O, Arnesen H, Friis S. The detection of panic disorder in chest pain patients. Gen Hosp Psychiatry. 1999 Sep-Oct;21(5):323–332. PubMed PMID: 10572773. http://www.ncbi.nlm.nih.gov/pubmed/10572773.
Approximately 76% of patients with a score of 4 or less will not have panic disorder (PD).
Approximately 71% of patients with a score of 5 or more will have PD.

Other Causes of Chest Pain

A patient with chest pain and cough, fever, egophony, or dullness to percussion might have pneumonia, but none of these individual findings are specific enough to confirm the diagnosis. A large study in 1984 developed a decision rule (Table 3) using seven clinical findings to predict the likelihood of pneumonia. Although there is ongoing debate over the reliability of pneumonia diagnosis based solely on history and physical examination and chest x-ray is usually considered the reference standard, a recent Cochrane review found two trials suggesting routine chest radiography does not affect the clinical outcomes in adults and children presenting suggestive of a lower respiratory tract infection. Thus, at least for clinically stable outpatients, treatment for pneumonia based on appropriate clinical findings alone may be reasonable.

Heart failure alone is an uncommon cause of chest pain, but it may accompany ACS or cardiac valve disease. A displaced apical impulse and a prior history of CAD support this diagnosis, and because virtually all patients with heart failure have exertional dyspnea, its absence is very helpful in excluding this diagnosis. An abnormal ECG and cardiomegaly on chest x-ray can increase the likelihood of heart failure among patients with chest pain, and B-natriuretic peptide (BNP) is now commonly used for detecting heart failure in patients presenting with acute dyspnea. One recent study also found that point-of-care ultrasound (POCUS) may have high sensitivity and specificity for diagnosing acute cardiogenic pulmonary edema.

A 3-item questionnaire has been developed specifically to assess for panic disorder among patients with chest pain referred for cardiac evaluation (Table 4), and there is good evidence that psychological interventions such as cognitive behavioral therapy (CBT) and breathing exercises can improve chest pain symptoms for patients with nonspecific chest pain who do not have CAD. However, even in patients with possible panic disorder, further cardiac testing should be done if there are significant cardiac risk factors.

Gastrointestinal disease can cause chest pain, but the history and physical examination are relatively inaccurate for diagnosing or excluding serious gastrointestinal pathology. However, if life-threatening cardiovascular or pulmonary causes of chest pain have been excluded, it is appropriate to try a short course of high dose PPI (omeprazole [Prilosec] 40 mg twice daily[3], lansoprazole [Prevacid] 30 mg daily, or esomeprazole [Nexium] 40 mg twice daily[3]) to evaluate for undiagnosed gastroesophageal reflux disease (GERD) as the cause of chest pain (even for patients without typical GERD symptoms.)

Chest wall pain can usually be diagnosed by history and examination if other etiologies have been excluded, and chest wall pain is more likely if the patient's pain is reproducible by palpation. Measurement of the sedimentation rate is not generally helpful in making the diagnosis, although in unusual situations radiography may be helpful.

References

Cao AM, Choy JP, Mohanakrishnan LN, Bain RF, van Driel ML: Chest radiographs for acute lower respiratory tract infections, Cochrane Database Syst Rev 12, 2013 Dec 26. CD009119.

Cayley Jr WE: Chest pain–tools to improve your in-office evaluation, J Fam Pract 63(5):246–251, 2014 May.

Cayley Jr WE: Diagnosing the cause of chest pain, Am Fam Physician 72:2012–2021, 2005.

de Schipper JP, Pull ter Gunne AF, Oostvogel HJ, van Laarhoven CJ: Spontaneous rupture of the oesophagus: Boerhaave's syndrome in 2008. Literature review and treatment algorithm, Dig Surg 26:1–6, 2009.

Harskamp RE, Laeven SC, Himmelreich JC, et al: Chest pain in general practice: a systematic review of prediction rules, BMJ Open 27;9(2):e027081, 2019.

Hendriksen JM, Geersing GJ, Lucassen WA, et al: Diagnostic prediction models for suspected pulmonary embolism: systematic review and independent external validation in primary care, BMJ 8;351:h4438, 2015.

Hiratzka LF, Bakris GL, Beckman JA, et al: 2010 ACCF/AHA/AATS/ACR/ ASA/SCA/SCAI/SIR/STS/SVM guidelines for the diagnosis and management of patients with Thoracic Aortic Disease: a report of the American College of Cardiology Foundation/American Heart Association Task Force on Practice Guidelines, Circulation 121:e266–e369, 2010. Erratum in Circulation 2010;122(4):e410.

Kisely SR, Campbell LA, Yelland MJ, Paydar A: Psychological interventions for symptomatic management of nonspecific chest pain in patients with normal coronary anatomy, Cochrane Database Syst Rev 30(6):CD004101, 2005.

Leigh-Smith S, Harris T: Tension pneumothorax–time for a re-think? Emerg Med J 22:8–16, 2005.

McConaghy JR, Oza RS: Outpatient diagnosis of acute chest pain in adults, Am Fam Physician 87(3):177–182, 2013 Feb 1.

Nienaber CA, Clough RE: Management of acute aortic dissection, Lancet 385(9970):800–811, 2015.

[3]Exceeds dosage recommended by the manufacturer.

O'Connor RE, Al Ali AS, Brady WJ, Ghaemmaghami CA, Menon V, Welsford M, et al: Part 9: acute coronary syndromes: 2015 American Heart Association guidelines update for cardiopulmonary resuscitation and emergency cardiovascular care, *Circulation* 132(18 Suppl. 2):S483–S500, 2015.

Raja AS, Greenberg JO, Qaseem A, Denberg TD, Fitterman N, Schuur JD: Clinical Guidelines Committee of the American College of Physicians. Evaluation of patients with suspected acute pulmonary embolism: best practice advice from the clinical guidelines committee of the American College of Physicians, *Ann Intern Med* 163(9):701–711, 2015.

Reinhardt SW, Lin CJ, Novak E, Brown DL: Noninvasive Cardiac Testing vs Clinical Evaluation Alone in Acute Chest Pain: A Secondary Analysis of the ROMICAT-II Randomized Clinical Trial, *JAMA Intern Med.* 178(2):212–219, 2018 Feb 1.

Swap CJ, Nagurney JT: Value and limitations of chest pain history in the evaluation of patients with suspected acute coronary syndromes, *JAMA* 294:2623–2629, 2005.

Wong BC: Is proton pump inhibitor testing an effective approach to diagnose gastroesophageal reflux disease in patients with noncardiac chest pain?: a meta-analysis, *Arch Intern Med.*2005 Jun 13;165(11):1222–8.

CONSTIPATION

Method of
Melissa Gaines, MD

CURRENT DIAGNOSIS

- While constipation is a benign process, it is important to recognize signs of a serious condition.
- Classification of normal transit constipation, slow transit constipation, or pelvic floor dysfunction guides therapy.
- Clinical testing has low benefit, but colonoscopy or imaging can assess for organic causes.

CURRENT THERAPY

- Initial therapy includes soluble dietary fiber to improve symptoms in chronic constipation.
- Osmotic laxatives are preferred while using stimulant laxatives as rescue agents.
- Surgery is reserved for pelvic floor dysfunction after optimal therapies have failed.

Epidemiology

Constipation is common, with a prevalence of 1.9% to 27.2%, but the description of symptoms is variable. A thorough history and focused physical examination aids diagnosis. Treatment is directed toward relief of symptoms, alleviation of precipitating factors, and prevention of recurrence. While constipation is a benign process, it is important to recognize concerning signs for a more serious medical condition such as malignancy.

Risk Factors

Vulnerable populations include female, elderly, neurodegenerative disease, low-fiber diet, painful rectal disorders, hypothyroidism, and diabetes mellitus.

Pathophysiology

With aging, there is decreased rectal compliance, diminished rectal sensation, and decreased resting anal pressures, while colonic transit time is preserved. Normal transit constipation is a component of irritable bowel syndrome with normal transit time and stool frequency. Slow transit constipation is a condition with colonic dysmotility resulting from altered enteric nervous system. Defecatory disorders include structural disturbances of the pelvic floor. Pelvic floor dysfunction is the paradoxical contraction of the external anal sphincter and puborectalis muscles during defecation. Secondary causes of constipation are listed in Table 1.

Prevention

Provide an environment of privacy and comfort to allow for natural defecation. Prescribe an adequate fluid and fiber intake with specific amounts that vary depending on the patient's condition. Encourage physical activity, with a low to moderate level of exercise depending on the patient's functional status. Develop a routine for defecation with a prompt response to a call to defecate urgently. Recurrent fecal impaction can be prevented with polyethylene glycol (PEG, MiraLax).

Clinical Manifestations

Patients will complain using qualitative terms of hard stools, a feeling of incomplete voiding, straining, prolonged time for laxation, the need for additional maneuvers, abdominal bloating, and abdominal pain (Table 2). A change in bowel habit differentiates the current complaint from a serious medical condition. Red flags include acute onset, weight loss, abdominal pain or cramping, rectal bleeding, nausea or vomiting, rectal pain, fever, or a change in stool caliber. Infants with abdominal distension and failure to pass meconium within 24 hours indicate Hirschsprung's disease. Patients should be asked if they have had loose stools or bowel incontinence to assess for fecal impaction. A medication review is required (see Table 1). Classification of patients with normal transit constipation, slow transit constipation, or pelvic floor dysfunction/defecatory disorders guides therapy.

Diagnosis

Diagnostic criteria have been established because the symptoms can vary (see Table 2). Conduct a physical examination that includes an assessment of vital signs, weight, volume status, auscultation of bowel sounds, abdominal percussion for tympani, and abdominal palpation for tenderness or mass. A rectal examination can detect resting rectal tone, fecal impaction, anorectal disorders, or rectal mass. Defecatory disorders show an increased resistance to the insertion of the examiner's finger with an impaired relaxation of the sphincter complex and reduced perineal descent during a Valsalva maneuver. Conduct laboratory testing on electrolytes, hemoglobin, thyroid-stimulating hormone, and fecal occult after initial measures fail. Red flag

TABLE 1	Causes of Constipation
Dietary	Low-fiber diet, dementia, depression, anorexia, dehydration
Metabolic	Diabetes mellitus, hypercalcemia, hypokalemia, hypothyroidism, systemic sclerosis
Neurologic	Parkinson's disease, spinal cord disorder, multiple sclerosis, cerebrovascular disease (stroke)
Iatrogenic	Antacids, iron, anticholinergics, antidepressants, antipsychotics, opiates, antiepileptics
Painful anorectal condition	Anal fissure, hemorrhoids, abscess, fistula, pelvic floor dysfunction, malignancy

TABLE 2	Rome III Criteria

More than two present:
- Straining in more than 25% of defecations
- Hard or lumpy stool in more than 25% of defecations
- Sensation of incomplete evacuation
- Sensation of anorectal blockage
- Manual maneuvers
- Fewer than three defecations per week

Loose stools are rare without laxative use

Insufficient criteria for irritable bowel syndrome

Symptoms for 3 months with onset 6 months before diagnosis

		TABLE 3 Drug Dosing and Adverse Effects			
CLASS	**DRUG NAME (BRAND)**	**ADULT DOSING**	**MECHANISM OF ACTION**	**TIME TO ONSET (H)**	**ADVERSE EFFECT**
Fiber	Bran Psyllium (Metamucil) Methylcellulose (Citrucel) Calcium polycarbophil (FiberCon)	1 cup/day 1 tsp 1 tbsp or 1 tab twice daily 2–4 tabs/day	Increase water content and bulk of stool decreasing transit time	Unknown	Bloating excessive gas
Hyperosmolar agent	Sorbitol 70% Lactulose (Chronulac)	15–30 mL twice daily	Disaccharide metabolized by colonic bacteria into acetic acid and short-chain fatty acids	24–48	Sweet tasting, transient abdominal cramps, flatulence
Hyperosmolar agent	PEG-ES (GoLytely,* CoLyte*) PEG (Miralax)	8–32 oz daily 17 g (1 tbsp) qd	Osmotic effect increasing intraluminal fluids	0.5–1	Incontinence
Hyperosmolar agent	Plecanatide (Trulance)	3 mg daily	Osmotic effect increasing intraluminal fluids, increase transit time	Cannot be calculated	Diarrhea
Stimulant	Glycerin suppository Bisacodyl (Dulcolax) Senna (Senokot, Perdiem) Senna/docusate (Peri-Colace) Cascara†	1 daily 10 mg suppository or 5–10 mg PO 3 times a week 2–4 tabs twice daily 20–30 mg/day	Local rectal stimulation, secretory and prokinetic effect	8–12	Degeneration of Meissner's and Auerbach's plexus
Enemas	Mineral oil retention enema Tap water enema Sodium phosphate enema (Fleet)	199–250 mL daily PR 500–1000 mL PR 1 unit PR	Evacuation induced by distended colon and mechanical lavage	6–8 for a mineral oil enema 5–15 min for all other enemas	Mechanical trauma, incontinence, rectal damage
Opioid antagonist	Methylnaltrexone (Relistor)	8–12 mg 1 dose SC every other day as needed for opioid-induced constipation (OIC) with advanced illness. 450 mg PO once daily or 12 mg SC once daily for OIC with chronic non-cancer pain.	Opioid mu receptor antagonist in gut decreasing transit time	4	Diarrhea, intestinal perforation
Opioid antagonist	Naloxegol (Movantik)	12.5–25 mg PO daily	Same as Relistor	6–36	Abdominal pain, opioid withdrawal reported

*Not FDA approved for this indication.
†Available as dietary supplement.

symptoms require imaging with CT of the abdomen and pelvis or endoscopy to diagnose malignancy or fecal impaction. Anorectal testing with manometry and a rectal balloon expulsion test is appropriate for pelvic floor dysfunction or defecatory disorders. Hirschsprung's disease is diagnosed with barium enema, rectal manometry, or a rectal suction biopsy. Colonic transit rates with radiopaque markers (Sitz) on serial abdominal radiographs over 4 to 7 days diagnose slow transit constipation disorders.

Treatment

Nonpharmacologic therapies have limited benefit. Unless there are signs of dehydration, increasing fluid intake is not indicated. Moderate-intensity exercise improves symptoms of irritable bowel syndrome. Probiotics are not beneficial.

There is moderate evidence for pharmacologic agents (Table 3). Normal transit constipation responds to soluble dietary fiber supplements (e.g., psyllium [Metamucil]); however, these should not be used in the case of slow transit constipation or drug-induced constipation. Osmotic agents with PEG (Miralax) or lactulose

(Chronulac) can be dose increased for soft stools. Stimulant laxatives are used as rescue therapy if patients do not have a bowel movement for 2 days.

New classes of drugs to manage constipation include intestinal secretagogues, serotonin 5-HT$_4$ receptor antagonists, and opiate antagonists. Lubiprostone (Amitiza) requires a negative pregnancy test with contraception. Linaclotide (Linzess) is a 14-amino acid peptide similar to heat-stable enterotoxins that cause diarrhea. Lubiprostone and linaclotide are FDA-approved for chronic idiopathic constipation and irritable bowel syndrome with constipation. Plecanatide (Trulance) is an approved drug for chronic idiopathic constipation in adults. It is a guanylate cyclase-C agonist that increases fluid secretion into the upper intestine. Methylnaltrexone (Relistor) and naloxegol (Movantik) are opiate receptor antagonists that can cause laxation in patients on chronic opiate therapy with NNT 5.

Pelvic floor dysfunction or defecatory disorders respond to biofeedback therapy by using manometry and visual or auditory feedback. Patients practice expelling a balloon and improve pelvic floor muscle coordination with Kegel exercises. Surgical intervention with subtotal colectomy with ileorectal anastomosis is indicated for slow transit constipation or defecatory disorders after failure of optimal medical management.

Complications

Fecal impaction a complication and a large bowel obstruction with colonic perforation has high mortality. Pediatric and geriatric patients are most susceptible, with signs and symptoms of fecal incontinence, abdominal pain, abdominal distention, anorexia, weight loss, and delirium. Treatments for adults include a large-volume tap-water enema (500–1000 mL), local anesthetics administered topically with abdominal massage, a colonoscopy, or surgery. The prevention of recurrence requires maintenance bowel regimen with osmotic agents such as PEG (Miralax).

References

Arshad A, Powell C: Easily missed? Hirschsprung's disease, *Br Med J* 345:e5521, 2012.

Bharucha AE, Pemberton JH, Locke GR: American Gastroenterological Association technical review on constipation, *Gastroenterology* 144:218–238, 2013.

Gallagher PF, O'Mahony D, Quigley EM: Management of chronic constipation in the elderly, *Drugs Aging* 25:807–821, 2008.

Higgins PD, Johanson JF: Epidemiology of constipation in North America: A systematic review, *Am J Gastroenterol* 99:750–759, 2004.

Larkin PJ, Sykes NP, Centeno C, et al: The management of constipation in palliative care: Clinical practice recommendations, *Palliat Med* 22:796–807, 2008.

McCallum IJ, Ong S, Mercer-Jones M: Chronic constipation in adults, *Br Med J* 338:b831, 2009.

Nee J, et al: Efficacy of Treatments for Opioid-induced Constipation: A Systemic Review and Meta-Analysis, *Clin Gastroenterol Hepatol*. 2018 Jan 25.

Schoenfeld P, et al: Low-Dose Linaclotide (72μg) for Chronic Idiopathic Constipation: A 12-Week, Randomized, Double-Blind, Placebo-Controlled Trial, *Am J Gastroenterol*, 2018:113-105-114. https://doi.org/10.1038/ajg.2017.230.

Thomas J, Karver S, Cooney GA, et al: Methylnaltrexone for opioid-induced constipation in advanced illness, *N Engl J Med* 358:2332–2343, 2008.

Wald A: Management and prevention of fecal impaction, *Curr Gastroenterol Rep* 10:299–501, 2008.

Gastroenterology, n.d.: *Rome criteria* Available at, http://www.romecriteria.org/, 2006.

Wald A: Constipation: Advances in diagnosis and treatment, *JAMA* 315(2):185–191, 2016 Jan 12.

COUGH

Method of
Emily Manlove, MD

CURRENT DIAGNOSIS

- Acute Cough
  - Noninfectious
    - Chronic obstructive pulmonary disease exacerbation
    - Asthma exacerbation
    - Congestive heart failure exacerbation
    - Pulmonary embolism
  - Infectious
    - Viral rhinosinusitis (the common cold)
    - Acute bacterial sinusitis
    - Acute bronchitis (chest cold)
    - Pneumonia
    - Pertussis (whooping cough)
    - Bronchiolitis (infants)
- Chronic cough
  - First, evaluate/rule out
    - Tobacco smoking and risk for lung cancer
    - Angiotensin-converting enzyme (ACE) inhibitor associated cough

- Next, evaluate for the three most common etiologies
  - Chronic upper airway cough syndrome
  - Cough variant asthma/nonasthmatic eosinophilic bronchitis
  - Gastroesophageal reflux disease
- Last, consider other causes and more advanced testing (bronchoscopy, high-resolution computed tomography [CT] scanning, referral) and consider earlier if history, physical, or chest x-ray suggests an alternative diagnosis
  - Oral pharyngeal dysphagia
  - Lung tumors
  - Interstitial pulmonary diseases
  - Bronchiectasis
  - Occupational and environmental exposures
  - Sarcoidosis
  - Tuberculosis
  - Somatic cough syndrome
  - Tic cough

CURRENT THERAPY

- Acute cough due to viral rhinosinusitis
  - Dextromethorphan (Delsym) 30 mg PO every 6 to 8 hours × 1 week
  - Diphenhydramine (Benadryl) 25 mg PO every 4 hours × 1 week
  - Nasal saline irrigation twice daily × 1 week
- Acute or subacute cough caused by *Bordetella pertussis*
  - Azithromycin (Z-Pak)[1] 500 mg PO on day 1 followed by 250 mg PO daily on days 2 to 5
- Treatment of unexplained chronic cough
  - Multimodality speech pathology therapy
  - Gabapentin (Neurontin) 300 mg PO daily, can be titrated up to a maximum daily dose of 1800 mg a day in two divided doses (off label use)

---

[1]Not FDA approved for this indication.

Acute Cough

Acute cough is a cough that lasts fewer than 3 weeks. It is a common presenting complaint in the primary care physician's office and also in the emergency room. The key goal is to differentiate between those patients whose cough has a benign cause and those who may be at risk for more serious illness. Infectious causes of cough are most common, but noninfectious causes should also be considered. Exacerbations of preexisting pulmonary conditions such as asthma and chronic obstructive pulmonary disease (COPD) can be associated with cough, therefore a thorough medical history should be obtained. Cough can also be associated with decompensated heart failure; in fact, cough is present in 70% of congestive heart failure (CHF) exacerbations. Also, 30% to 40% of patients with acute pulmonary embolism (PE) have a new cough at presentation of symptoms, and the classic signs and symptoms of chest pain, dyspnea, and hypoxia may not always accompany the cough.

Upper respiratory tract infections are a common cause of benign acute cough. The common cold, also known as viral rhinosinusitis, is probably the most common cause of acute cough. The lung exam is normal. If fever is present it is low grade and is only present on the first or second day of illness. Most symptoms begin to resolve by 7 to 10 days, but cigarette smokers may be ill for twice as long. Symptomatic treatment is the mainstay of therapy. First-generation antihistamines combined with a decongestant and naproxen have been proven to reduce the length of cough. Second-generation antihistamines are not effective in the treatment of cough associated with viral rhinosinusitis; it is likely that first-generation antihistamines are effective because of their anticholinergic properties. Other treatments that may be helpful include nasal saline irrigation, nasal glucocorticoids, and nasal decongestants. It is necessary to distinguish viral rhinosinusitis from acute bacterial rhinosinusitis, which may also be associated with cough. Less than 2% of all rhinosinusitis has a bacterial cause. Acute bacterial rhinosinusitis should not be diagnosed in the first week of symptoms unless the patient displays severe symptoms such as high fever. Sinus imaging studies are unlikely to be helpful, as both viral and bacterial sinusitis will have radiologic evidence of inflammation.

It is also necessary to distinguish an acute cough caused by an upper respiratory tract infection and that caused by a lower respiratory tract infection. Furthermore, it is necessary to distinguish between acute bronchitis, which almost always has a viral cause, versus pneumonia, which has a bacterial cause. Both illnesses often have a presenting symptom of cough, which may be productive. If there is any derangement in vital signs or evidence of pulmonary consolidation on the lung exam, a chest x-ray should be performed. Infectious Diseases Society of America (IDSA) guidelines require the presence of consolidation on chest x-ray to diagnose pneumonia. Influenza should also be considered for those patients who have fever and cough during flu season. An elevated procalcitonin level may help guide the physician in his or her decision to prescribe antibiotics. Beta agonists should not be routinely used to alleviate cough in acute viral bronchitis, but may be helpful for the alleviation of wheezing and are more likely to benefit patients with airflow obstruction at baseline.

In pediatric patients, bronchiolitis should be considered as a cause of cough and fever. It is the most common cause of hospitalization in those less than 1 year old. The most recent guidelines recommend abstaining from lab testing (including viral swabs), radiographic imaging, and treatment with beta agonists, epinephrine, or glucocorticoids as these interventions do not change the course of illness. Exclusive breastfeeding for the first 6 months of infancy can decrease the morbidity of respiratory infections. *Bordetella pertussis* can cause severe illness with cough and apnea in infants. However, adults have subtle symptoms and lack the classic "whooping cough" and posttussive emesis seen in children. The physician should have suspicion for pertussis in patients who have a cough lasting longer than 2 weeks and paroxysms of coughing; the cough can last up to 2 months. The diagnosis can be confirmed with polymerase chain reaction (PCR). Antibiotics do not alter the course of illness but reduce the spread of infection; azithromycin (Zithromax)[1] should be given for 3 to 5 days. Vaccination rates remain low. Pregnant women should be vaccinated with each pregnancy and other adults should replace 1 dose of Td at the earliest convenience.

Chronic Cough

A chronic cough is a cough lasting more than 8 weeks. Patients may have a presenting symptom of a cough that has been present for more than 3 but fewer than 8 weeks; this is considered a subacute cough. In this case, the physician should illicit a history of respiratory infection; the patient is likely suffering from a postinfectious cough, which is related to inflammation of the airway epithelium, mucus hypersecretion, and/or increased cough reflex sensitivity. Inhaled corticosteroids may provide some benefit. If there is no history of recent infection, then the cough should be managed as a chronic cough. Chest x-ray can be considered during this time frame, but if no red flags are present (fever, unintended weight loss, night sweats, dysphagia, odynophagia, hemoptysis) the physician and patient together can decide to wait on radiography.

Chronic cough must be approached in a systematic manner, which is more likely to identify the causative agent of the cough and provide alleviation of symptoms. All of the common causes of chronic cough (see later) must be considered, as the associated symptoms and the patient's description of the cough do not alter the diagnostic algorithm. It is important to confirm compliance throughout the treatment course and identify barriers to compliance with the patient. Failure to respond to empiric treatment does not necessarily rule out a diagnosis, as the patient may have two diagnoses. Therefore, it is prudent to continue any partially effective treatment for chronic cough.

First, it must be determined if the patient smokes. If so, the differential diagnosis is altered. The physician must determine if the cough is a simple smoker's cough, chronic bronchitis, or possibly lung cancer; cough is the most common presenting symptom of lung cancer. Smokers are less likely to seek help for a cough and may not see a physician until a more serious problem has advanced. It is possible for a cough to worsen initially after smoking cessation, but a cough persisting more than 1 month after cessation should be investigated. Any change in a smoker's cough, a new cough, and cough with hemoptysis should be investigated. Physicians should consider low dose CT scanning as screening for lung cancer in qualifying smokers. The second factor to rule out in all chronic cough cases is cough induced by an angiotensin-converting enzyme (ACE) inhibitor. All patients with chronic cough should stop taking an ACE inhibitor. The medication is more likely to cause a cough if it was started in the prior year, and the cough should resolve within 1 month after cessation of the ACE inhibitor. The next step to determining the cause of a chronic cough is to rule out the three most common causes of cough. Last, all patients with a cough lasting more than 8 weeks should be evaluated with chest radiography to identify any obvious causative factors.

Upper Airway Cough Syndrome

Upper airway cough syndrome (UACS), previously called postnasal drip syndrome, is likely caused by activation of cough receptors in the hypopharynx or larynx and increased sensitivity of these receptors. It is likely the most common cause of chronic cough. UACS is almost always associated with rhinosinusitis, which can be caused by a number of factors (allergic rhinitis, postinfectious rhinitis, perennial nonallergic rhinitis, rhinitis resulting from chemical irritants, rhinitis medicamentosa, pregnancy-associated rhinitis, bacterial sinusitis, allergic fungal sinusitis, etc.). The patient may complain of frequently needing to clear the throat or a sensation of "dripping" in the back of the throat; however, absence of these symptoms does not rule out UACS, nor does a history of wheezing. Physical exam may reveal mucus in the posterior oropharynx and cobblestoning of the mucosa. If the cause of rhinitis is obvious, it should be specifically treated. Otherwise, a trial of a first-generation antihistamine should be started; improvement should be seen in 2 weeks. If the side effects of this therapy are intolerable, a nasal antihistamine, nasal anticholinergic, or nasal corticosteroid can be used. If the diagnosis of UACS is highly suspected but the patient does not respond to empiric therapy, sinus CT imaging may be necessary to guide diagnosis and treatment.

Cough Variant Asthma and Nonasthmatic Eosinophilic Bronchitis

Cough variant asthma and nonasthmatic eosinophilic bronchitis (NAEB) both primarily present with a cough, and the patient may have few other symptoms. Patients with cough variant asthma will have abnormal spirometry, whereas those with NAEB will not. When spirometry is performed, bronchoprovocation testing with methacholine should be performed as it increases the negative predicative value of the test. If spirometry is negative, the sputum should be evaluated for eosinophils, which are present in both diseases. Both diseases are treated as asthma; an inhaled corticosteroid should be started and long-acting beta agonists and leukotriene receptor antagonists can be considered as adjunctive therapy. A positive response should be expected within 2 weeks.

Gastroesophageal Reflux Disease

Gastroesophageal reflux disease (GERD) is common, but not all patients with GERD have an associated cough; therefore, the

---

[1]Not FDA approved for this indication.

presence of GERD does not ensure that it is the source of the patient's cough. However, those patients whose cough is clearly not caused by UACS, cough variant asthma, or NAEB are very likely to have a GERD-induced cough. Cough can be caused by acidic and nonacidic reflux, so a proton pump inhibitor (PPI) may not always be of benefit. A pH probe can be performed in cases when it is unclear whether reflux is occurring. All patients should utilize lifestyle changes to attenuate reflux, such as smoking cessation, avoidance of alcohol and acidic foods, weight loss, and treatment of sleep apnea. It may take 3 to 6 months of treatment to see improvement in cough. If the patient does not improve and GERD is highly suspected, referral to a surgeon may be necessary for fundoplication.

Other Causes of Chronic Cough

In those patients who still suffer from chronic cough and the above causes have been ruled out, further investigation should be sought. Referral to a pulmonologist may be necessary, in addition to high-resolution CT scanning and bronchoscopy. Causative factors may include oral pharyngeal dysphagia, lung tumors, interstitial pulmonary diseases, bronchiectasis, occupational and environmental exposures, sarcoidosis, and tuberculosis. Somatic cough syndrome (previously referred to as psychogenic cough) and tic cough (previously referred to as habit cough) may be considered in some patients; hypnosis, suggestion therapy, and/or counseling may be beneficial. In patients who remain symptomatic, regardless of known or unknown causes, the diagnosis of "difficult to treat" cough is made. Assessing cough severity and quality of life with validated tools may be beneficial. Options do remain for these patients, including speech language pathology intervention, empiric gabapentin, and/or referral to a cough clinic.

Reference

Irwin RS, French CL, Chang AB, et al: Classification of cough as a symptom in adults and management algorithms: CHEST guideline and expert panel report, *Chest* 153(1):196–209, 2018.

DIZZINESS AND VERTIGO

Method of
Jennifer Wipperman, MD, MPH

CURRENT DIAGNOSIS

- Benign paroxysmal positional vertigo
  - Repeated, brief episodes lasting less than 1 minute
  - Triggered by changes in head position
  - Positive Dix-Hallpike or Supine Roll Test
- Vestibular neuritis
  - Single, severe, constant episode lasting days
  - Subacute onset
  - Positive head impulse test
  - Nystagmus is unilateral and horizontal
- Vestibular migraine
  - Recurrent episodes lasting hours to days
  - Associated with migraine headache
  - Responds to traditional migraine treatment
- Ménière's disease
  - Recurrent episodes of vertigo lasting hours
  - May have hearing loss, tinnitus, or ear fullness
- Red flags for stroke include:
  - Sudden onset
  - Risk factors for stroke
  - Nystagmus with a central pattern
  - Abnormal HINTS exam
  - Additional neurologic signs
  - Inability to walk

CURRENT THERAPY

- Benign paroxysmal positional vertigo
  - The canalith repositioning procedure (Epley maneuver) is the most effective treatment.
  - Avoid vestibular suppressant medications
  - Consider observation with close follow-up if a patient will not tolerate the canalith repositioning procedure or if symptoms are mild
- Vestibular neuritis
  - Brief symptomatic care with benzodiazepines, antiemetics, and antihistamines
  - Early vestibular rehabilitation speeds recovery.
  - Use of corticosteroids is controversial.

The "dizzy" patient is often a frustrating phenomenon in clinical medicine. However, after a careful history and physical examination, most patients can be diagnosed and serious causes excluded. Peripheral causes of vertigo are usually benign and include vestibular neuritis and benign paroxysmal positional vertigo (BPPV). Life-threatening central causes include stroke, demyelinating disease, and an intracranial mass. The first step in evaluating vertigo is differentiating among the four types of dizziness: near syncope or lightheadedness, disequilibrium, psychogenic dizziness, and true vertigo. True vertigo is a false sense of motion, and patients often report that "the room is spinning." This chapter will focus on the two most common causes of episodic vertigo: BPPV and vestibular neuritis.

Epidemiology

Vertigo is a common office complaint. Every year, millions of Americans are evaluated for dizziness in ambulatory care settings, and approximately 50% of these cases are vertigo. BPPV and vestibular neuritis are two of the most common causes of vertigo seen in the office setting.

Risk Factors

BPPV is seven times more likely in individuals over age 60, and it is also more common in women. A history of prior head trauma and other vestibular disorders places patients at risk for BPPV. There are no identified risk factors for vestibular neuritis.

Pathophysiology

BPPV is thought to occur when calcium carbonate debris (otoconia) are dislodged and float freely in the semicircular canals of the inner ear. The posterior canal is most often involved. During head movement, loose otoconia move in the canal and cause a continued sense of motion for a few seconds until they settle. The pathophysiology of vestibular neuritis is uncertain. Limited evidence supports a viral infection, most likely HSV-1, which causes inflammation of the eighth cranial nerve. When hearing loss accompanies vertigo, the condition is called *acute labrynthitis*.

Clinical Manifestations

The history and physical examination are fundamental in the evaluation of vertigo. Key questions include the frequency and duration of attacks, triggers such as positional or pressure changes, prior head trauma, associated neurologic symptoms, hearing loss, and headache. A personal history of diabetes, hypertension, and hyperlipidemia are risk factors for stroke. BPPV, stroke, and migraine can have a familial preponderance. Many medications, including anticonvulsants and antihypertensives, cause dizziness.

BPPV causes brief, recurrent episodes that last less than 1 minute and are brought on by changes in head movement or position. Nausea and vomiting may be associated. Vestibular neuritis usually has a subacute onset over several hours, peaks in intensity for 1 to 2 days, and then gradually subsides over the next few weeks. Symptoms of vertigo are constant, and nausea and vomiting can

TABLE 1 Differentiating Peripheral and Central Causes of Vertigo

	PERIPHERAL CAUSES		CENTRAL CAUSES
	BPPV	**VESTIBULAR NEURITIS**	
History	Brief, recurrent attacks of vertigo lasting less than 1 minute Triggered by positional changes No vertigo between attacks	Subacute onset Constant and severe vertigo lasting days Nausea and vomiting may be severe	Sudden onset Risk factors for stroke May have severe headache
Nystagmus	Up-beating and torsional	Horizontal and unidirectional	Direction changing Pure vertical Pure torsional
Gait	Unaffected between episodes	May veer towards affected side	Unable to walk
Specialized physical examination tests	Positive Dix-Hallpike maneuver Positive supine roll test	Positive head impulse test Visual fixation stops nystagmus	HINTS exam abnormal Visual fixation does not stop nystagmus
Additional neurologic signs	Rare	Rare	Common (e.g., dysarthria, aphasia, incoordination, weakness, or numbness)

Abbreviation: BPPV = benign paroxysmal positional vertigo.

Figure 1 Head impulse test. Top panel shows a positive head impulse test. The examiner moves the patient's head quickly 10 degrees to the side, in this case to the patient's left. A catch-up saccade is observed when the patient looks away and then refixes on the visual target, indicating a peripheral lesion on the left. Lower figure shows a normal head impulse test. The patient maintains visual fixation during head movement. Adapted from Seemungal BM, Bronstein AM. A practical approach to acute vertigo. *Pract Neurol* 2008; 8:211–21.

be severe during the first few days. Patients with vestibular neuritis may have difficulty standing and veer toward the affected side. Although changes in position worsen the vertigo in vestibular neuritis, vertigo is always present at baseline. In BPPV, patients have no vertigo between attacks.

General physical examination should include a thorough cardiovascular, ear, nose, throat, and neurologic examination. The neurologic examination can differentiate between benign (peripheral) and life-threatening (central) causes based on the ability to walk, type of nystagmus, results of the head impulse test, and presence of associated neurologic signs (Table 1).

Patients with vestibular neuritis may have difficulty walking, but the inability to walk is a red flag for a central lesion. Nystagmus is unidirectional (always beats in the same direction) and horizontal in vestibular neuritis, and is suppressed by visual fixation. Having a patient focus on an object in the room will stop the nystagmus, which reappears if a blank sheet of paper is placed a few inches in front of the patient's face. Nystagmus in central causes is not suppressed by visual fixation and may be direction-changing (nystagmus beats to the right when the patient looks right, and beats to the left when the patient looks left) or purely vertical. The head impulse test (Figure 1) is positive in peripheral causes like vestibular neuritis. The examiner holds the patient's head while the patient fixes her eyes on the examiner's nose, and then the examiner quickly moves the patient's head 10 degrees to the right and left. If a saccade (the eyes look away and then re-fixate on the examiner's nose) is found, this indicates a peripheral lesion on the side that the head is turned toward. Central lesions will not cause saccades, and the head impulse test will be negative. HINTS (Head Impulse test, Nystagmus, Test of Skew), which combines three physical examination findings, has been found to have a 97% sensitivity and 99% specificity for a central cause of vertigo in the acute setting and to be more accurate than MRI in the initial 24 hours after symptom onset. If one or more of the tests indicate a central cause, (e.g., a negative head impulse test, direction-changing horizontal nystagmus, or vertical eye misalignment), then the HINTS test is considered positive for a central cause and imaging should be obtained. A negative HINTS exam is an excellent rule-out test for stroke, with a negative likelihood ratio of 0.02.

The Dix-Hallpike maneuver is diagnostic of posterior canal BPPV (Figure 2). The patient should be warned that nausea and vomiting may occur. After the patient is placed in the head-hanging position, there is a 5- to 20-second latency period before the nystagmus and symptoms appear. Both the nystagmus and vertigo will increase in severity and then resolve within 60 seconds. The nystagmus observed is up-beating and torsional. The maneuver should be repeated with the head held to the opposite side. The side that elicits the symptoms and nystagmus diagnoses BPPV in the ipsilateral ear. If both sides elicit symptoms, the patient may have bilateral BPPV. If the test is negative and BPPV is strongly suspected, the patient should lie supine and the examiner can turn the head to each side (supine roll test). This maneuver will cause vertigo and nystagmus in patients with horizontal canal BPPV.

Diagnosis

BPPV and vestibular neuritis are diagnosed clinically. Further diagnostic testing is indicated if the diagnosis is uncertain or a central cause is suspected. Audiometry may be abnormal in Ménière's disease. MRI is the best imaging test for central lesions

Figure 2 Treatment maneuver for posterior canal benign paroxysmal positional vertigo affecting the right ear. To treat the left ear, the procedure is reversed. The drawing of the labyrinth in the center shows the position of the particle as it moves around the posterior semicircular canal (PSC) and into the utricle (UT). The patient is seated upright, with head facing the examiner, who is standing on the right. **A,** The patient is rapidly moved to head-hanging right position (Dix-Hallpike test). This position is maintained until the nystagmus ceases. **B,** The examiner moves to the head of the table, repositioning hands as shown. **C,** The head is rotated quickly to the left with right ear upward. This position is maintained for 30 seconds. **D,** The patient rolls onto the left side while the examiner rapidly rotates the head leftward until the nose is directed toward the floor. This position is then held for 30 seconds. **E,** The patient is rapidly lifted into the sitting position, now facing left. The entire sequence should be repeated until no nystagmus can be elicited. After the maneuver, the patient is instructed to avoid head-hanging positions to prevent the particles from reentering the posterior canal. Reprinted with permission from Rakel RE. *Conn's Current Therapy 1995.* Philadelphia, WB Saunders, 1995, p 839.

because it includes the posterior fossa and is most sensitive for stroke. Vestibular function testing is useful if the diagnosis is unclear or in cases of refractory vertigo. Vestibular function testing evaluates the ocular and vestibular response to position changes and caloric stimulation. Video-oculographic recordings of nystagmus can magnify the eye and allow for repeated viewings for further study. Some patients with BPPV may have additional vestibular disorders causing vertigo that vestibular function testing can elucidate.

Differential Diagnosis
Ménière's disease is suspected in patients with the triad of tinnitus, fluctuating hearing loss, and vertigo. Episodes usually last hours, are disabling, and are recurrent over years, over time leading to permanent dysfunction. Migrainous vertigo features episodes lasting hours to days in patients with other migraine symptoms such as headache, photophobia, phonophobia, or aura. Central lesions such as stroke or intracranial mass are most concerning. Red flags for stroke include sudden onset, risk factors for stroke, associated neurologic signs, inability to walk, positive HINTS exam, severe associated headache, and characteristic nystagmus. Posttraumatic vertigo may occur in patients after head trauma who present with vertigo, tinnitus, and headache. A perilymphatic fistula is rare, but may be suspected in a patient with episodic vertigo after head trauma, heavy lifting, or barotrauma. Pressure changes with sneezing or coughing trigger vertigo attacks. Postural hypotension should be ruled out in all patients. An acoustic neuroma presents with slowly progressive, unilateral sensorineural hearing loss and tinnitus. Many patients may have an unsteady gait, but true vertigo is rare.

Treatment
Posterior canal BPPV is best treated with the *canalith repositioning procedure (CRP)*, also known as the Epley maneuver (Figure 2). Studies have shown the procedure is safe and effective with an odds ratio of 4.2 (95% CI. 2.3-11.4) for symptom resolution. Patients should be warned that nausea or vomiting may occur during the procedure, and may be pretreated with an antiemetic medication. The procedure can be repeated immediately if unsuccessful, and the majority of patients will respond after three attempts. Post-treatment activity restrictions are unnecessary. Horizontal canal BPPV can be treated with the barbeque roll maneuver. Vestibular rehabilitation (VR) is a treatment option for BPPV but is significantly less effective than the canalith repositioning procedure. VR is helpful in patients with chronic, nonspecific dizziness after successful treatment with CRP and for improving gait stability in those with increased fall risk, such as the elderly. Observation is an option if symptoms are mild or if a patient will not tolerate the canalith repositioning procedure or vestibular rehabilitation. However, time to resolution with observation is 1–3 months, and recurrence rates are higher compared to treatment with CRP. Vestibular-suppressant medications such as antihistamines and benzodiazepines are discouraged because they increase fall risk and treatment with CRP is effective. Surgery is rarely needed for BPPV, but may be helpful in refractory cases.

Vestibular neuritis is primarily treated with rest, vestibular suppressant medications, and vestibular rehabilitation. Patients may initially be admitted if symptoms, such as nausea and vomiting, are severe or if stroke is suspected. Treatment with antihistamines (dimenhydrinate [Dramamine][1] 50 mg every 6 hours), antiemetics (promethazine [Phenergan][1] 25 mg every 6 hours), or benzodiazepines (lorazepam [Ativan][1] 1 to 2 mg every 4 hours) may be used to treat severe symptoms. However, these should not be continued for more than 2 to 3 days because they inhibit central compensation. In vestibular neuritis, patients' vertigo improves not due to return of vestibular nerve function, but due to central compensation for the peripheral deficit. Using vestibular suppressants blocks central compensation and lengthens the course of the disease. The use of corticosteroids is controversial. Although studies show that vestibular-function testing improves more quickly in patients treated with corticosteroids, there is conflicting evidence that corticosteroids hasten the recovery of clinical signs and symptoms of vestibular neuritis. A 2011 Cochrane review concluded that there is insufficient evidence to recommend corticosteroids for the treatment of vestibular neuritis. Finally, antiviral medications have not been proven effective for vestibular neuritis.

For patients with vestibular neuritis, vestibular rehabilitation should be started as soon as symptoms improve and a patient can tolerate the exercises. Exercises include balance and gait training as well as coordination of head and eye movements. Vestibular rehabilitation hastens recovery and improves balance, gait, and vision by increasing central compensation for vestibular dysfunction. Exercises may be home-based for compliant patients with mild symptoms, whereas formal referral may be more beneficial for patients with severe symptoms, or for the elderly.

Monitoring
Patients diagnosed with BPPV should be reassessed in 1 month regardless of treatment. Failure to improve warrants further evaluation for other etiologies, including central causes. Similarly, patients with vestibular neuritis should slowly improve over several weeks, and failure to do so suggests alternative diagnoses.

Complications
Patients with BPPV are at increased risk for falls. Thirty percent of elderly patients with BPPV have multiple falls in a year. Thus patients should be assessed for fall risk, functional mobility, and balance. Home safety evaluation and home supervision should be considered. BPPV often recurs, with an estimated rate of 15% per

---

[1]Not FDA approved for this indication.

year. Counseling patients about recurrence can lead to earlier recognition, earlier treatment, and avoidance of falls. Patients with vestibular neuritis are at increased risk for BPPV and Ménière's disease. Vestibular neuritis rarely recurs.

References

Baloh RW: Vestibular neuritis, *N Engl J Med* 348:1027–1032, 2003.
Bhattacharyya N, Gubbels SP, Schwartz SR, et al: Clinical practice guideline: benign paroxysmal positional vertigo (update), *Otolaryngol Head Neck Surg.* 156(3_suppl):S1–S47, 2017.
Chan Y: Differential diagnosis of dizziness, *Otolaryngol Head Neck Surg* 17:200–203, 2009.
Epley JM: The canalith repositioning procedure: for treatment of benign paroxysmal positional vertigo, *Otolaryngol Head Neck Surg* 107:399–404, 1992.
Fishman JM, Burgess C, Waddell A: Corticosteroids for the treatment of idiopathic acute vestibular dysfunction (vestibular neuritis), *Cochran Database Syst Rev 5*, 2011. CD008607. Review.
Hilton MP, Pinder DK: The Epley (canalith repositioning) manoeuvre for benign paroxysmal positional vertigo, *Cochrane Database Syst Rev.* 12, 2014. CD003162.
Kerber KA: Vertigo and dizziness in the emergency department, *Emerg Med Clin North Am* 27:39–50, 2009.
McDonnell MN, Hillier SL: Vestibular rehabilitation for unilateral peripheral vestibular dysfunction, *Cochrane Database Syst Rev.* 1, 2015. CD005397.
Newman-Toker DE, Kerber KA, Hsieh YH, et al: HINTS outperforms ABCD2 to screen for stroke in acute continuous vertigo and dizziness, *Acad Emerg Med* 20(10):986–996, 2013.
Seemungal BM, Bronstein AM: A practical approach to acute vertigo, *Pract Neurol* 8:211–221, 2008.

FATIGUE

Method of
Janet C. Lindemann, MD, MBA

CURRENT DIAGNOSIS

- The clinical evaluation of fatigue begins with a thorough medical and psychosocial history.
- Consider monitoring for a month before beginning a laboratory evaluation, because it usually does not yield a diagnosis. Initial evaluation should include a complete blood count (CBC), electrolytes, glucose, liver and kidney function tests, thyroid function tests, and urinalysis.
- Among the many possible causes of fatigue, the most common include depression, environmental stress, anemia, and diabetes. In many cases, a cause is not determined.

CURRENT THERAPY

- Any underlying cause discovered in the history, examination, or laboratory evaluation should be treated.
- If depression, anxiety, or environmental stress is suspected, early assessment and treatment is important.
- Symptom relief includes exercise, regular sleep habits, family discussion about the impact of fatigue, and a symptom and sleep diary.

Epidemiology

Fatigue or tiredness is a common complaint in the general population, representing the chief complaint in nearly 10% of patients presenting to a primary care physician and reported as a symptom in 21% of all patient encounters. While acute, prolonged, and chronic fatigue are relatively common, chronic fatigue syndrome is relatively rare.

Risk Factors

Risk factors for fatigue in adolescence include having depressive symptoms, being highly sedentary, and, conversely, being highly physically active. In adults, risk factors include age over 65 years, presence of one or more chronic medical conditions, and female gender. Precipitating factors include physical stresses such as infectious mononucleosis and psychological stresses such as job-related problems. Perpetuating factors include physical inactivity, emotional disorders, and disturbances of sleep.

Prevention

Because physical inactivity, psychological stress, and lack of sleep are predisposing and perpetuating factors for fatigue, it is helpful to advise patients about stress reduction, regular exercise, and proper sleep habits.

Clinical Manifestations

Fatigue is characterized by general malaise, vague physical discomfort, and an inability to perform routine activities. Acute fatigue is short-lived and generally attributable to physical exertion or an acute illness. Prolonged fatigue is defined as self-reported, persistent fatigue lasting 1 month or longer, whereas chronic fatigue is defined as similar symptoms lasting 6 months or more.

Diagnosis

The clinical evaluation begins with a thorough medical and psychosocial history. It is important to allow the patient to speak uninterrupted for the first minute or two of the interview, because this often provides pertinent clues. The history should include exploration of all medically unexplained symptoms, inquiry into work and life stressor issues, questions regarding alcohol and other substance use, and the current use of prescription, over-the-counter, and alternative therapies. A mental status examination and screening for depression and anxiety should follow. The Beck Depression Inventory or SIG-E-CAPS mnemonic (Sleep, Interest, Guilt, Energy, Concentration, Appetite, Psychomotor retardation, Suicidal) are useful screening tools. The challenge with the diagnostic workup for fatigue is that most laboratory tests do not yield a significant diagnosis. Repeated studies show that only about 15% of patients in primary care settings will have an organic cause for their fatigue (Harrison, Ponka), and laboratory results affect management in as little as 5% of patients (Rosenthal). The following recommendations for the laboratory investigation of fatigue are adapted from guidelines developed by Dutch, Canadian, and Australian general practice groups (Harrison):

- Consider monitoring for a month after initial presentation, while initiating conservative management.
- CBC, electrolytes, glucose, liver and kidney function tests, thyroid function tests, urinalysis.
- Clues from the history and examination may indicate the need for erythrocyte sedimentation rate, monospot, antinuclear antigen testing, or chest radiography.

Differential Diagnosis

The common causes of fatigue are represented in the mnemonic DEAD TIRED (Box 1). Depression, environmental factors such as lifestyle, anxiety, and anemia are among the most common causes of fatigue. Diabetes and other endocrine disorders, including

BOX 1	Common Causes of Fatigue: DEAD TIRED
D Depression	T Thyroid, Tumors
E Environment/lifestyle	I Infection, Insomnia
A Anxiety, Anemia	R Rheumatologic
D Diabetes/endocrine	E Endocarditis/cardiovascular
	D Drugs (medications or substance abuse)

thyroid disease, should be considered, as well as an undiscovered tumor. Many infections, especially those of viral origin, cause fatigue, as well as insomnia and sleep disorders such as obstructive sleep apnea. Rheumatologic disorders, such as rheumatoid arthritis, systemic lupus erythematosus, and fibromyalgia, are often accompanied by fatigue. Endocarditis, while rare, is a must-not-miss diagnosis, as are other cardiac conditions such as coronary artery disease. Finally, drugs, either prescription or of personal use or abuse, should be considered.

Chronic fatigue syndrome is a specific clinical diagnosis characterized by unexplained persistent or relapsing fatigue, not relieved by rest, that substantially limits daily activity. In addition, there must be at least four of the following: memory or concentration impairment, sore throat, tender cervical or axillary lymph nodes, muscle pain, multijoint pain without swelling or tenderness, new headaches, unrefreshing sleep, or postexertional malaise lasting more than 24 hours.

Treatment
The treatment of fatigue begins with acknowledging the patient's concern and providing reassurance and information about the natural course and most frequent causes of fatigue. Any underlying cause discovered in the history, examination, or laboratory evaluation should be treated. If depression, anxiety, or environmental stress is suspected, early assessment and treatment is important. In fatigue that remains unexplained, therapy should emphasize symptom relief and include exercise, regular sleep habits, family discussion about the impact of fatigue, and a symptom and sleep diary. These same therapies, along with cognitive behavioral therapy, have been shown to have moderate benefit in chronic fatigue syndrome.

Monitoring
Ongoing fatigue can be monitored through a three question assessment:
- Are you experiencing fatigue?
- If so, how severe has it been, on average, during the past week? (0–3 is mild fatigue, 4–6 moderate, and 7–10 severe)
- How does fatigue interfere with your ability to function?

References
Beck A, Ward C, Mendelson M, et al: An inventory for measuring depression, *Arch Gen Psychiatry* 4:561, 1961.
Gialamas A, Beilby JJ, Pratt NL, et al: Investigating tiredness in Australian general practice, *Aust Fam Physician* 32:663, 2003.
Harrison M: Pathology testing in the tired patient: a rational approach, *Aust Fam Physician* 37:908, 2008.
Poluri A, Mores J, Cook DB, et al: Fatigue in the elderly population, *Phys Med Rehabil Clin N Am* 16:91, 2005.
Ponka D, Kirlew M: Top 10 differential diagnoses in family medicine: Fatigue, *Can Fam Physician* 53:892, 2007.
Rosenthal TC, Majeroni BA, Pretorius R, Malik K: Fatigue: An overview, *Am Fam Physician* 78:1173, 2008.
Sharpe M, Wilks D: Fatigue, *BMJ* 325:480, 2002.
Viner RM, Clark C, Taylor SJ, et al: Longitudinal risk factors for persistent fatigue in adolescents, *Arch Pediatr Adolesc Med* 162:469, 2008.

FEVER

Method of
Alan R. Roth, DO and Gina M. Basello, DO

CURRENT DIAGNOSIS

- Numerous endogenous and exogenous factors play a role in determining body temperature. Current standards define *fever* as an oral temperature of ≥100.4 °F (≥38 °C).
- Though temperature varies with measurement technique, in clinical practice, most recommendations refer to oral, rectal, and axillary temperature measurements, with rectal temperature being the standard of care in infants and young children.

- Tympanic thermometers should not be used in young children.
- Fever is not an illness. It is the body's physiologic response to a disease process and has beneficial effects in fighting infection.
- All neonates with a fever should be admitted to the hospital for a full sepsis evaluation. For infants between 1 and 3 months of age, evidence-based guidelines, along with clinical evaluation, determine the diagnostic and therapeutic approach.
- With widespread immunization use, the incidence of bacteremia and bacterial meningitis in young infants has significantly decreased and UTI is now the most prevalent bacterial infection.
- *Fever of unknown origin* (FUO) is defined as a temperature greater than 100.9 °F (38.3 °C) for longer than 3 weeks with no identified cause after 3 days of hospitalization or three outpatient visits.
- FUO requires a systematic, thoughtful, and thorough evaluation based on the age of the patient and the existing clinical evidence, with repeated clinical assessments being essential.
- Hyperthermia is an unregulated, significant elevation of core body temperature above the normal diurnal range due to failure of thermoregulation from a hypothalamic insult, not a pyogenic source, and is considered a medical emergency. It is not synonymous with fever and often requires immediate intervention to avoid deleterious central nervous system (CNS) effects.

CURRENT THERAPY

- Treating a fever significantly increases the patient's level of comfort, activity, and oral feeding and fluid intake, in addition to decreasing the body temperature.
- Multiple randomized, controlled trials reveal that treating fever does not shorten or prolong the overall duration of illness or reduce the occurrence of febrile seizures.
- Many clinical recommendations state that a temperature less than 102.2 °F (39 °C) in healthy children does not require treatment. Antipyretics are known to provide comfort to children and their caregivers.
- Antipyretic treatment for children includes acetaminophen (Tylenol) 10 to 15 mg/kg every 4 to 6 hours or ibuprofen (Advil, Motrin) 10 mg/kg every 6 hours.
- Ibuprofen and acetaminophen have both been shown to reduce fever effectively and safely. Combination therapy has been shown in some studies to have an added benefit in both reduction of temperature and comfort without an increase in side effects, though caution should be taken to avoid dosing errors.
- Antipyretic therapy for adults and adolescents includes acetaminophen 650 to 1000 mg orally (PO) every 6 hours to a maximum of 3 g per day, ibuprofen 200 to 400 mg PO every 6 hours, or aspirin (ASA) 325 to 650 mg every 6 hours as needed (PRN) for fever.
- ASA should not be used in children due to the risk of Reye's syndrome.
- Sponge bathing should be done with tepid water and no alcohol. Recommendation: sponge bathing and other home remedies should not be used as sole treatment.

Fever is one of the most common clinical presentations encountered by primary care physicians and the most common complaint of acute visits for children in the ambulatory or emergency department setting. Fever is a symptom and one of the most reliable signs of illness rather than a disease process itself. Most causes of fever are secondary to acute viral illnesses such as upper respiratory infections (URIs), which account for 50 million visits to primary care providers annually. Less commonly, bacterial infections may cause pharyngitis, otitis, sinusitis, pneumonia, and urinary tract infections (UTIs). A cost-effective, evidence-based approach using clinical protocols, guidelines, and consensus recommendations to the diagnosis and management of febrile illness, including the appropriate use of antibiotic therapy, is the cornerstone of quality medical care for this presentation. Fever produces significant anxiety for patients, parents, and health care providers, which can lead to overtreatment. Typically, fever is transient and only requires treatment to provide patient comfort.

Definitions

The definition of fever is dependent on numerous endogenous and exogenous factors that play a role in determining body temperature, including age, time of day, site, and measuring device, as well as operator variables. Fever is an elevation of body temperature due to the adjustment of the hypothalamic-pituitary set point. This usually occurs in response to a pathologic stimulus. Fever is a beneficial physiologic mechanism that helps to promote an augmented immunologic response.

Despite individual variability, core body temperature is maintained at about 98.6°F (37°C). Diurnal variation results in lower body temperatures in the early morning and a temperature higher in the late afternoon or early evening, which is consistent with what is encountered in clinical practice.

In adults, a morning oral temperature of 98.9°F (37.2°C) or higher, or an evening temperature of 99.9°F (37.7°C) or higher defines a fever. Rectal temperatures are generally considered to be 0.7°F (0.4°C) higher than oral readings.

In infants and young children, rectal temperatures are still considered the standard of care and a rectal temperature greater than 100.4°F (38°C) is considered a fever.

Axillary temperatures of greater than 98.6°F (37°C) are regarded as a fever, though this measurement site is generally considered less accurate. An accurate measurement of body temperature is dependent on site, measuring device, and the clinical skills of the operator. Site selection should be determined by the age of the patient.

Young infants and older adults often have a diminished febrile response due to physiologic factors, thereby warranting the use of other clinical factors to guide diagnosis.

Recent technologic advances, including electronic devices, tympanic membrane scanning, and temporal artery scanning, have replaced the older mercury-in-glass thermometers. These devices offer faster results and minimal inconvenience to the patient and are becoming increasingly reliable. Chemical content or liquid crystal thermometers applied to the skin are neither accurate nor cost-effective.

Hyperthermia is an uncontrolled elevation of core body temperature that exceeds the body's ability to lose heat. In hyperthermia, the setting of the hypothalamic thermoregulatory center is unchanged, in contrast to fever. Hyperthermia requires urgent medical intervention because it could be rapidly fatal and does not respond to antipyretics. Common etiologies include heat stroke, neuromalignant syndrome, serotonin syndrome, malignant hyperthermia, endocrinopathy, and CNS damage.

Classic *fever of unknown origin* (FUO) is defined as a disorder with temperatures ≥100.9°F (38.3°C) that have persisted for at least 3 weeks, with no definitive cause elucidated after initial comprehensive inpatient or outpatient workup. The etiologies of FUO generally fall into four diagnostic categories: infectious, autoimmune or inflammatory, neoplastic, and miscellaneous.

Pathophysiology

Fever occurs as part of an inflammatory response to an inciting stimulus. The response includes the production of various cytokines that ultimately increase the production of prostaglandin E_2 (PGE_2), which resets the hypothalamic thermoregulatory set point at a higher level. Important pyogenic cytokines include interleukin-1 (IL-1), interleukin-6 (IL-6), tumor necrosis factor α (TNF-α), interferon-β (IFN-β), and interferon-γ (IFN-γ).

Risks and Benefits of Fever

Fever is known to enhance the immunologic response while suppressing the growth and replication of bacterial and viral infections. Though often uncomfortable for patients, caregivers, and health care providers, evidence supports the notion that fever is beneficial and ultimately protects against the development of asthma and other allergic disorders. In most instances, fever is not harmful. It does increase cardiac demand and metabolic needs, resulting in the common associated signs and symptoms of tachycardia, tachypnea, shivering, malaise, and diaphoresis.

The use of antipyretic agents has not been shown to either prolong or shorten the duration of illness. Febrile seizures cause significant anxiety for parents. They occur most commonly in children between the ages of 6 months and 6 years. Most febrile seizures are uncomplicated and have not been shown to be associated with significant bacteremia or to lead to the development of seizure disorder in older children. Antipyretic agents have not been shown to decrease the incidence of febrile seizures.

Diagnostic Evaluation of Fever

In most cases, the etiology of a febrile illness is a self-limiting viral infection. From 5% to 10% of fevers may be associated with a more serious bacterial infection such as pneumonia, UTI, bacteremia, meningitis, or bone and joint infections. At times, these conditions may be challenging to distinguish, and a thoughtful, systematic, evidence-based approach to the diagnostic evaluation will be most cost-effective while avoiding the inappropriate use of antibiotics.

All infants less than 28 days old with a fever should be admitted to the hospital for a full sepsis workup and empiric intravenous antibiotic therapy.

Young infants, 1 to 3 months of age, with a febrile illness can be especially challenging. Numerous studies addressing this challenging population have led to the development of multiple guidelines and clinical protocols that utilize risk stratification criteria. The use of these age-specific stratification criteria, along with clinical treatment guidelines, helps guide the clinician in the evaluation of febrile illness. Clinical judgment remains the cornerstone of good clinical care.

With the widespread use of *Haemophilus influenzae* type B (Hib) and pneumococcal vaccinations, the incidence of bacteremic illness has decreased significantly. UTI has emerged as the most prevalent bacterial infection. The increased use of rapid viral testing in the office and emergency department settings may alleviate the need for more invasive testing and antibiotic use because the risk of concurrent bacterial infection has been reported to be negligible.

In this age group, an initial workup that reveals a white blood cell (WBC) count of less than 5000 or greater than 15,000 indicates an increased likelihood of a significant bacterial illness (SBI). Blood cultures, urinalysis, urine culture, and cerebrospinal fluid (CSF) evaluation should then be obtained and accompanied by intravenous antibiotic therapy. Elevated C-reactive protein (CRP) or procalcitonin levels have also been associated with SBI in children with a febrile illness and have shown increased specificity and sensitivity when compared to the WBC count. Incorporating urine concentration when interpreting urine analyses can help in the differentiation of infants at higher risk of UTI.

Children age 3 to 36 months, who appear well and do not have any underlying medical history, require only a comprehensive clinical evaluation and do not warrant antibiotic therapy or diagnostic testing in most instances. Septic or ill-appearing children need a more aggressive evaluation, including complete blood count (CBC), inflammatory markers, urinalysis, urine culture, blood cultures, and a chest x-ray. High-risk children in this age group require empiric antibiotic therapy, and clinical judgment should guide the decision to hospitalize.

Classic FUO is defined as a disorder with temperatures greater than 100.9°F (38.3°C) that has persisted for at least 3 weeks with no clear etiology determined after 3 days of hospital evaluation or three outpatient visits. Common etiologic categories include infectious, neoplastic, inflammatory, and miscellaneous causes, of which drug fever has been shown to be the most prevalent.

The initial approach includes a thorough history, physical examination, and appropriate laboratory testing. The initial choice of imaging should be guided by clinical findings and most commonly includes a chest x-ray and a CAT scan of the abdomen and pelvis. If the etiology remains elusive, positron emission tomography (PET) scanning or invasive diagnostic testing should then be considered.

Differential Diagnosis

Hyperthermia is an unregulated, significant elevation of core body temperature above the normal diurnal range due to failure of thermoregulation from a hypothalamic insult, not a pyogenic source, and is considered a medical emergency. It is not synonymous with fever and often requires immediate intervention to avoid deleterious CNS effects. Since the hypothalamic set point remains unchanged, antipyretics are ineffective in hyperthermia. The most common etiology is the inability to regulate or dissipate excess body heat. Hyperthermia is a medical emergency that requires immediate treatment to prevent excessive morbidity and mortality.

Treatment

Though controversy exists regarding the necessity of lowering fever, antipyretics have been shown to effectively and safely reduce temperature and improve symptoms with minimal side effects. Acetaminophen (Tylenol) is available in many formulations. Dosing should be based on body weight and not age of the patient. The dose is 10 to 15 mg/kg every 4 to 6 hours, not to exceed 3 g daily or 2 g in patients with renal or hepatic impairment. Ibuprofen (Advil, Motrin) is a nonsteroidal antiinflammatory drug (NSAID) that has both antiinflammatory and antipyretic effects. Dosing is 10 mg/kg every 6 to 8 hours in children and 200 to 400 mg every 6 hours in adolescents and adults. Ibuprofen is also available in multiple formulations, including a newer intravenous preparation (ibuprofen [Caldolor]) that may be beneficial in oral-intolerant hospitalized patients. Some studies suggest that ibuprofen may be a more effective antipyretic agent than acetaminophen.

In adults, aspirin (ASA) remains a therapeutic alternative for lowering fever at a dose of 325 to 650 mg every 4 to 6 hours. It should not be used in children with a febrile illness due to the risk of Reye's syndrome.

A combination of acetaminophen and ibuprofen in alternating doses has been shown in some studies to have an added benefit in both reduction of temperature and comfort without an increase in side effects, though caution should be taken to avoid dosing errors.

Nonpharmacologic therapies such as sponge bathing with tepid water and other environmental measures to control temperature, including adjusting room temperatures and sipping cool fluids to avoid dehydration, are used commonly and do provide symptom relief and comfort. These measures should never be used as the sole therapy for fever reduction.

References

Cunha BA: Fever of unknown origin: focused diagnostic approach based on clinical clues from the history, physical examination, and laboratory tests, *Infect Dis Clin North Am* 21:1137–1187, 2007.
Dorney K, Bachur RG: Febrile infant update, *Curr Opin Pediatr* 29:280–285, 2017.
Hernandez D, Nguyen V: Fever in infants <3 months old: what is the current standard? *Pract J Pediatr Emerg Med* 16:1–15, 2011.
Herzog L, Phillips S: Addressing concerns about fever, *Clin Pediatr* 50:383–390, 2011.
Huppler AR, Eickhoff JC, Wald ER: Performance of low-risk criteria in the evaluation of young infants with fever: review of the literature, *Pediatrics* 125:228, 2010.
Jhavier R, Byington C, Klein J, Shapiro E: Management of the non-toxic appearing acutely febrile child: a 21st century approach, *J Pediatr* 159:181–185, 2011.
Makoni M, Mukundan D: Fever, *Curr Opin Pediatr* 22:100–106, 2010.
Roth AR, Basello GM: Fever. In Paulman PM, Harrison JD, Paulman MD, et al, *Signs and Symptoms in Family Medicine*, Philadelphia, 2012, Mosby, pp 317–326.
Roth AR, Basello GM: Approach to the adult patient with fever of unknown origin, *Am Fam Physician* 68:2223–2228, 2003.
Sullivan J, Farrar HC: Clinical report: fever and antipyretic use in children, *Pediatrics* 127:580–587, 2011.
Van den Bruel A, Thompson MJ, Haj-Hassan, et al: Diagnostic value of laboratory tests in identifying serious infections in febrile children; systematic review, *BMJ* 342:382, 2011.

GASEOUSNESS, INDIGESTION, NAUSEA, AND VOMITING

Method of
Justin Bailey, MD

Nausea is a vague, subjective feeling that vomiting (forceful expulsion of gastric contents) is imminent. Dyspepsia (based on ROME III criteria) can include postprandial fullness, early satiety, epigastric pain, burning, and reflux (return of gastric content to the lower esophagus or mouth, accompanied by a sour taste or "heartburn" sensation). Gaseousness can present with a variety of complaints including belching, bloating, abdominal pain, or flatulence.

Epidemiology

Nausea and vomiting (ICD-9 Code 787.01) is one of the top reasons patients see a primary care provider. Infectious diseases causing nausea and vomiting, gastroenteritis, diarrhea, and dehydration are leading causes of death in developing countries, and of sick days and reduction of employee productivity in the United States. Nausea and vomiting postoperatively and during cancer chemotherapy add significant costs, pain, and discomfort to hospital and ambulatory treatment. Dyspepsia occurs in an estimated 25% of the U.S. population every year, many of whom do not seek care. Gaseousness is ubiquitous in the population and is troubling to a small portion.

Risk Factors

Previous gastrointestinal surgery, certain medications, chemotherapeutic regimens, substance abuse, pregnancy, infectious diseases, medical conditions, and central nervous system disorders increase the risk for nausea and vomiting symptoms. Dyspepsia risk is increased significantly with ingestion of NSAIDs, tobacco use, *H. pylori* infection, obesity, anxiety, somatization, neuroticism, depression, and unemployment. Increased upper gastrointestinal gaseousness can be seen with air swallowing from gum chewing and eating quickly as well as consumption of foods that relax the lower esophageal sphincter (e.g., chocolate, fats, mints). Ingestion of lactose, fructose, sorbitol, undigested starches (e.g., bran) and carbonated beverages can all increase the risk of bloating and flatulence.

Pathophysiology

The pathophysiologic regulation of nausea and vomiting is complex and incompletely understood. Multiple neurotransmitters are involved, including acetylcholine, dopamine, histamine, and serotonin. The therapeutic action of antiemetics is often based on blocking the action of these neurotransmitters. Neurologic regulation of nausea and vomiting involves the chemoreceptor triggers in the fourth ventricle, the nucleus tractus solitarius in the medulla, motor nuclei that control the vomiting reflex, and vagal afferent nerves from the GI tract. The sympathetic and parasympathetic nervous systems are involved in conjunction with the smooth muscle cells and the enteric brain within the wall of the stomach and intestine.

The pathophysiology of dyspepsia is unclear, but probably has multiple causes. Delayed gastric motility can occur in up to 30%

TABLE 1 Key Symptoms and Differential Vomiting, Dyspepsia, and Bloating

SYMPTOMS	DIFFERENTIAL
Abdominal Pain ± N/V • RUQ • Epigastric • RLQ • LLQ • Pelvic	Organic etiologies • Cholelithiasis, cholecystitis • Dyspepsia, pancreatitis, GERD, gastritis, MI • Appendicitis • Diverticulitis • PID, ovarian torsion, ectopic pregnancy
Abdominal pain + distention + N/V	Bowel obstruction
Abdominal distention associated with foods (lactose, wheat-based products, bran, legumes)	Lactose intolerance Celiac disease Carbohydrate malabsorption, Oligosaccharide fermentation (legumes)
Vomiting several hours after eating + succussion splash + N/V	Gastric obstruction Gastroparesis
Heartburn ± N/V	GERD, dyspepsia
Early morning + N/V	Pregnancy
Feculent vomiting + N/V	Intestinal obstruction Gastrocolic fistula
Vertigo + nystagmus + N/V	Vestibular neuritis
Dental erosions, parotid gland enlargement, lanugo-like hair, callus on dorsal surface of hands	Bulimia
Positional N/V	Neurogenic

Abbreviations: GERD = gastroesophageal reflux disease; LLQ = left lower quadrant; MI = myocardial infarction; N/V = nausea and vomiting; PID = pelvic inflammatory disease; RLQ = right lower quadrant; RUQ = right upper quadrant.

of patients with dyspepsia. Additionally, decreased gastric compliance can be seen in dyspeptic patients.

Sensations of lower tract gaseousness result from one of three different mechanisms: excess gas production, abnormal intestinal transit, and increased visceral sensitivity. Gas production caused by carbohydrate maldigestion, (e.g., lactose intolerance, poorly absorbed starches) results in bloating and a sensation of fullness. High-fiber diets, celiac disease, and small intestine bacterial overgrowth can increase gas production. Dysmotility associated with diabetes mellitus, scleroderma, amyloidosis, and endocrine disease may result in gastroparesis and chronic intestinal pseudo-obstruction. Additionally, previous Nissen fundoplication, fat intolerance, and various familial conditions may cause dysmotility. Increased visceral sensitivity is thought to be a main cause of pain and fullness in patients with functional bowel disorders such as irritable bowel syndrome (IBS) and functional dyspepsia.

Prevention
Once the diagnosis has been established, appropriate treatment of the underlying cause of the symptoms can be instituted. When the cause of nausea and vomiting is related to medication, the dose can be adjusted or the medication changed as appropriate.

Upper GI bloating and fullness is almost exclusively caused by excess air swallow and can be improved with altering behaviors such as gulping food and gum chewing. Lower GI symptoms can be prevented by avoiding problem foods such as milk products in patients with lactose intolerance.

Clinical Manifestations
Nausea and vomiting are extremely common and are associated with many conditions. Associated symptoms are helpful

in sorting out causes. Many common historical associations are listed in Table 1.

The diagnosis of dyspepsia is based mainly on clinical symptoms. The Rome III criteria are listed in the opening paragraph. Alarm symptoms that should raise suspicions for gastric cancer include unintended weight loss, persistent vomiting, progressive dysphasia, odynophagia, unexplained anemia, iron deficiency, hematemesis, palpable abdominal mass, lymphadenopathy, family history of gastric cancer, previous gastric surgery, or jaundice.

Gaseousness usually presents with abdominal fullness and bloating. Pain associated with the fullness is often relieved with eructation or flatulence (see Table 1).

Diagnosis
The first step in the assessment of patients with abdominal complaints is complete history of the duration of symptoms, the frequency of episodes, work environment, recent travel, household member illness, association of symptoms with certain foods or beverages (i.e., pain relief or worsening with food), and determination of the success or failure of what the patient has tried to alleviate the symptoms, all of which may offer diagnostic clues. Focused inquiries into surgeries, sexual activity, and other elements of a review of symptoms may be helpful. A complete review of medication usage, with particular attention to GI-irritating medications such as NSAIDs and over-the-counter medications, illicit drugs, and herbal products is important. Physical examination and diagnostic work-up can help isolate the cause (Table 2).

In patients with acute (<24 hours) nausea and vomiting, a laboratory workup is often unnecessary. Patients with the most commonly identified acute causes, such as acute gastroenteritis, vestibular neuritis, chemotherapy, medication, and alcohol ingestion, and those who are postoperative, can be started on symptomatic therapy. For persistent symptoms of nausea and vomiting, laboratory workup is guided by the history and physical examination and can include a complete blood count and differential, serum chemistries, renal function, liver function tests, serum protein and albumin, thyroid-stimulating hormone, amylase or lipase, drug screen, and a pregnancy test in women of childbearing age. Imaging should not be routine but should be directed by the history and physical findings as well as pertinent laboratory results. Useful studies may include acute abdominal series (chest x-ray, flat and upright views of the abdomen), abdominal computed tomography (CT), and abdominal ultrasound.

Similarly, in patients with dyspeptic symptoms, laboratory tests should be obtained based on the history and physical examination. Many therapies, such as discontinuing offending medications (e.g., NSAIDs) or acid suppression in patients without alarm symptoms, may be started without a laboratory work-up. Blood count chemistries and *H. pylori* testing can be considered if warranted. Alarm symptoms may warrant further imaging or direct visualization with esophagogastroduodenoscopy (EGD).

In gaseousness and bloating, the most sensitive work-up is the history and physical examination. Further work-up should be directed by initial findings. Patients with alarm symptoms such as weight loss, diarrhea, abdominal pain, distention, and anorexia may benefit from a malabsorption work-up including lactose tolerance test, stool fat, ova and parasites, stool culture, *C. difficile*, acute abdominal series, or EGD. A hydrogen breath test may be beneficial in selected patients to assess the relationship between specific foods and symptoms. Other blood work, tests, and imaging, such as CT, magnetic resonance imaging (MRI), and EGD are guided by availability of testing and the history, examination and laboratory findings.

Differential Diagnosis
Tables 3, 4, and 5 summarize the wide differential diagnosis of nausea and vomiting, dyspepsia, and gaseousness.

TABLE 2 Physical Examination: Nausea, Vomiting, Dyspepsia, and Gaseousness

FINDINGS	POSSIBLE ETIOLOGY
Fever	Infectious
Tachycardia, hypotension	Dehydration, volume depletion, sepsis (infectious), ectopic pregnancy, myocardial infarction, aortic aneurysm
Exophthalmos	Hyperthyroid
Papilledema	Increased intracranial pressure (tumors, subdural hemorrhage)
Bulging tympanic membrane	Otitis media, effusion
Thyromegaly	Hypothyroid
Lymphadenopathy	Infection, malignancy
Dry mucous membranes	Dehydration, volume depletion
Dental erosions	Bulimia
Abdominal distention	Obstruction, ileus, gastroparesis, irritable bowel, hepatic/spleenic flexure syndrome, postoperative gas-bloat syndrome
Absent bowel sounds	Ileus, perforation
Sense of abdominal distention without bloating	Irritable bowel syndrome
Abdominal bloating	Irritable bowel syndrome, obstruction
RUQ abdominal pain/guarding	Cholecysitis, cholelithiasis
RLQ/LLQ abdominal pain/ guarding	Appendicitis (RLQ), ovarian torsion, diverticulitis, ectopic pregnancy
Cervical motion tenderness	Pelvic inflammatory disease, endometriosis
Bladder tenderness	Urinary tract infection
Testicular pain	Torsion, epididymitis
Abnormal rectal examination	Fecal impaction, prostatitis, appendicitis, ovarian tumor, ectopic pregnancy, endometriosis
Delayed cap refill, poor skin turgor	Dehydration
Jaundice	Gallbladder disease, biliary obstruction

Abbreviations: LLQ = left lower quadrant; RLQ = right lower quadrant; RUQ = right upper quadrant.

TABLE 3 Differential Diagnosis for Nausea and Vomiting

Central Nervous System
Multiple sclerosis, tumor, intracranial bleeding, infarction, abscess, meningitis, trauma, labyrinthitis, Ménière's disease, vestibular neuritis, motion sickness
Migraine headaches, seizure disorders

Gastrointestinal Disorders
Appendicitis, gastric bypass, gastroparesis, hepatobiliary disease cholecystitis, hepatitis, neoplasia
Ileus
Crohn's disease, ulcerative colitis
Irritable bowel syndrome
Ischemia: mesenteric, small bowel
Obstruction: scarring/adhesions from previous surgeries, small bowel obstruction, esophageal spasm
Pancreatitis
Peptic ulcer disease: esophagitis, gastritis, gastroesophageal reflux
Peritonitis

Endocrine
Addison's disease, diabetes (ketoacidosis, gastroparesis), hyperthyroidism, hypothyroidism, hyperparathyroidism, hypoparathyroidism, porphyria

Genitourinary
Nephritis, nephrolithiasis, torsion (ovary, testicle), uremia, kidney stone

Infectious Etiologies
Bacterial: *Campylobacter, Salmonella, Shigella,* Enterogenic *E. coli,*
Viral: rotavirus, influenza
Otitis media: bacterial or viral
Sexually transmitted infection: cervicitis, epididymitis, pelvic inflammatory disease, prostatitis, urethritis; multiple organisms including gonorrhea and chlamydia
Urinary tract infection: lower (cystitis) or upper (pyelonephritis)

Pregnancy
Morning sickness, hyperemesis gravidarum, intrauterine and ectopic pregnancies

Psychiatric
Anorexia, anxiety, bulimia, depression

Medication Related
Acetaminophen (Tylenol)
Acyclovir (Zovirax)
Alcohol abuse
Antibiotics: azithromycin (Zithromax), sulfasalazine (Azulfidine), erythromycin, metronidazole (Flagyl), sulfonamides (e.g., sulfamethoxazole-trimethoprim [Bactrim]), tetracycline
Antidepressants: Selective serotonin reuptake inhibitors (SSRIs)
Antihypertensives: β-blockers (atenolol [Tenormin], metoprolol [Lopressor]), calcium channel blockers, diuretics (hydrochlorothiazide)
Chemotherapeutic agents: cisplatinum (Cisplatin [Platinol]), cyclophosphamide (Cytoxan), nitrogen mustard (Mustargen), dacarbazine (DTIC-Dome), methotrexate (Trexall), vinblastine (Velban)
Diabetes treatment: metformin (Glucophage), sulfonylureas
Digoxin (Lanoxin)
Ergotamines: dihydroergotamine (Migranal), methysergide (Sansert)[2]
Ferrous gluconate, ferrous sulfate
Gout treatment: allopurinol (Zylprim)
Hormones: estrogen, progesterone and oral and injected contraceptives
Levodopa (L-dopa), carbidopa (Lodosyn)
Nicotine (patch, gum, smokeless tobacco, cigarette/pipe/cigar)
Nonsteroidal antiinflammatory: aspirin, ibuprofen (Motrin), naproxen (Naprosyn)
Opioids: codeine, heroin, hydrocodone, oxycodone, morphine, burprenorphine/naloxone (Suboxone)
Prednisone
Seizure medications: phenobarbital, phenytoin (Dilantin)
Theophylline (Uniphyl)

[2]Not available in the United States.

Treatment

Antiemetics, hydration, and dietary changes are the first-line treatments for acute episodes of nausea and vomiting. Controlling the symptoms is often all that is necessary in acute, self-limited bouts of nausea and vomiting symptoms. If patients are dehydrated, oral rehydration can be accomplished by encouraging the patient to take small amounts (6 ounces or less) of cool water or electrolyte solutions on a frequent basis. If patients are unable to accomplish this, parenteral rehydration and antiemetics may be warranted.

Table 6 lists the common antiemetics agents, indications, dosages, side effects, and relative cost of medications.

Location of the cause with directed treatment is most effective for gaseousness. If no cause is found, it can be difficult to treat. Avoiding foods that are contributory, such as those containing lactose, fructose, sorbitol, high fiber, and starches, may be all that is necessary. Symptoms associated with increased sensitivity to normal levels of gas (i.e., IBS) can be difficult to treat. Therapeutic relationships, education, and dietary modification are the mainstays of IBS treatment. For moderate to severe symptoms,

TABLE 6 Medications for Nausea and Vomiting—cont'd

DRUG	USE	SIDE EFFECTS	DOSAGE	COST*
Metoclopramide (Reglan)	2nd-line therapy for chemotherapy-induced nausea		10 mg (PO, IM, IV) q6h	10 mg: 30 ct = $6
Trimethobenzamide (Tigan)	Chemotherapy-induced nausea		250 mg PO q6h	30 ct = $65
Butyrophenones: Dopamine antagonists		Sedation, hypotension, extrapyramidal effects, tachycardia, dizziness, QT prolongation and torsades de pointes, neuroleptic malignant syndrome		
Droperidol (Inapsine)			0.625–1.25 mg (IM, IV) q4h	IV and IM only
Haloperidol (Haldol)			0.5–5 mg (PO, IM, IV) q8h	5 mg: 90 ct = $26
Phenothiazines: Dopamine antagonists		Sedation, hypotension, extrapyramidal effects, neuroleptic malignant syndrome, cholestatic jaundice		
Chlorpromazine (Thorazine)	Generalized nausea		10–25 mg (PO, IM, PR) q6h	10 mg: 30 ct = $12
Prochlorperazine (Compazine)	Generalized nausea		10 mg (PO, IM, IV) q6h; 25 mg q12h PR	10 mg: 30 ct = $30
5-Hydroxytryptamine type 3 (5-HT3): Serotonin Antagonists		Fever, constipation, diarrhea, dizziness, sedation, nervousness, altered liver function tests, headache, fatigue		
Dolasetron (Anzemet)	Chemotherapy-induced nausea		100 mg (PO, IV) q24h	100 mg: 5 ct = $360
Granisetron (Kytril)	Chemotherapy-induced nausea		2 mg (PO, IV) q24h	1 mg: 2 ct = $130
Ondansetron (Zofran)	Chemotherapy-induced nausea		4–8 mg (PO, IV) q8-12h)	8 mg: 30 ct = $40
Palonosetron (Aloxi)	Prevention of chemotherapy-induced nausea		0.5 mg PO or 0.25 mg IV ×1	0.25 mg: $406
Neurokinin Receptor Antagonists		Headache, site reaction		
Aprepitant capsule (Emend)	Prevention of postoperative nausea and vomiting (PO)		40 mg PO × 1 prior to anesthesia	40 mg cap #1: $40
Fosaprepitant (Emend)	Prevention of chemotherapy-induced nausea		115 mg IV × 1, 125 mg PO ×1	115 mg: $223
Steroids		GI upset, anxiety, euphoria, flushing, insomnia		
Dexamethasone (Decadron)	Prophylaxis of chemotherapy-related nausea and vomiting		4 mg–10 mg (PO, IM, IV) q6–12h	4 mg: 90 ct = $20
Methylprednisolone (Medrol)			40–100 mg (PO, IM, IV) q24h	8 mg: 25 ct = $25
Cannabinoids		Vertigo, xerostomia, hypotension, dysphoria		
Dronabinol (Marinol)	Chronic or chemotherapy-induced nausea and vomiting		5 mg PO q2-4h; 4–6 per day	5 mg: 30 ct = $1200
Miscellaneous				
Erythromycin SE nausea, abdominal pain	Nausea associated with gastroparesis		250 mg PO q8h × 5–7 d	250 mg: 30 ct = $70
Ginger	Nausea associated with pregnancy		250 mg PO q6h or 1 g qd	250 mg: 60 ct = $8
Pyridoxine (vitamin B6)	Nausea associated with pregnancy (traditionally combined with doxylamine)		10 mg q6h	100 mg: 100 ct = $15

*Cost estimates from www.drugstore.com.

TABLE 7	Medications for Treatment of Gaseousness and Bloating		
MEDICATION	**INDICATION**	**DOSE**	**SIDE EFFECTS/COST**
Rifaximin (Xifaxan)	Bloating (flatulence) from suspected bacterial overgrowth	200 mg PO tid × 7 d	Edema, nausea, dizziness, flatulence 200 mg: 30 ct = $355
Probiotics (multi-component)	Bloating (flatulence)	Varies by preparation	Varies by preparation
Alpha-galactosidase (Bean-o)	Bloating associated with gas-producing foods	300–1200 mg with meals high in fermentable carbs	300 mg: 100 ct = $10
Simethicone	Bloating (flatulence) (indicated but not found to be effective)	80–120 mg qid prn	80 mg: 100 ct = $5
Bismuth subsalicylate	Odor from flatus	525 mg PO qid prn	525 mg: 15 ct = $5
Odor-neutralizing devices (briefs, pillows)	Odor from flatus	prn	Pillows: ~$25 Briefs: ~$20

References

Abraczinskas D: *Intestinal gas and bloating*, Available, http://www.uptodate.com, November, 2013 (accessed 6.24.15).

ACOG Practice Bulletin No. 52: American College of Obstetrics and Gynecology: Nausea and vomiting in pregnancy, *Obstet Gynecol* 103:803–814, 2004.

Bailey J: Effective Management of flatulence, *Am Fam Phys* 79:1098–1100, 2009.

Flake ZA, Scalley RD, Bailey AG: Practical selection of antiemetics, *Am Fam Phys* 69:1169–1174, 2004.

Hasler WL, Chey WD: Nausea and vomiting, *Gastroenterology* 125:1860–1867, 2003.

Kraft R: Nausea and vomiting. In Bope ET, Rakel RE, Kellerman R, editors: *Conn's Current Therapy 2010*, Philadelphia, 2010. Saunders, pp 5–9.

Longstreth GF: *Functional dyspepsia in adults*, Available at http://www.uptodate.com, December 2014 (accessed 6.24.15).

Longstreth GF: *Approach to the patient with dyspepsia*, Available at http://www.uptodate.com, September, 2014 (accessed 6.24.15).

Owings S: Gaseousness and dyspepsia. In Bope ET, Rakel RE, Kellerman R, editors: *Conn's Current Therapy 2010*, Philadelphia, 2010. Saunders, pp 9–11.

Talley NJ, Vakil NB, Moayyedi P: 2005 American Gastroenterological Association technical review on the evaluation of dyspepsia, *Gastroenterology* 125:1756–1780, 2005.

HEADACHE

Method of
R. Michael Gallagher, DO

Interest and understanding of the headache problem have increased during recent years, allowing physicians to help more sufferers. This interest was the result of Food and Drug Administration (FDA) approvals of medications for the treatment of headache and subsequent pharmaceutical company support of medical and community education. Although the more recently approved treatments are for migraines, the overall increase in headache awareness of medical professionals has resulted in help for patients afflicted with all types of headache.

- Headache is a disturbing and sometimes fearsome affliction that has plagued humankind throughout recorded history. It often is debilitating and particularly disturbing to the sufferer because the pain is located in the head, the very center of the body's cognitive and control functions. With its accompanying pain and debilitating symptoms, stress can mount and the headache can become all consuming.
- Headache is experienced by all age groups, from young children to the elderly. It is more common than asthma, diabetes, mental illness, and rheumatoid arthritis. In fact, the World Health Organization identifies severe migraine, along with psychosis and quadriplegia, as "one of the most debilitating chronic conditions."

Although the majority of Americans experience tension-type headaches (TTHAs) at some time in their lives, approximately 30 million experience migraine headache: 13% of women and 6% of men, predominantly in their most productive years between the ages of 13 and 55 years. *One out of every four households are affected by migraine headache.* Prepubescent boys and girls suffer equally; however, boys often outgrow their migraine attacks as they mature, and they are less subjected to hormonal influences. Smaller percentages of people, by comparison, suffer with other chronic headaches, such as cluster headache and chronic daily headache.

- No sure diagnostic tests are available to differentiate headache types. The headache condition can progress or change over time in frequency, severity, and debilitation. Each sufferer can be different and may require a detailed evaluation and individualized treatment plan; more frequent or prolonged attacks often necessitate a more comprehensive treatment plan. Thus, the headache problem can be a challenge for both the sufferer and the clinician.
- During the twentieth century, dramatic advancements were made in medicine. Longevity and quality of life improved for many individuals. Unfortunately, for headache sufferers, most of these advances were for maladies that killed or maimed rather than for non-life-threatening conditions. It was not until the 1960s that even a reasonable preventive medication, propranolol (Inderal), was introduced, and by the 1980s only a handful of medications were available for wide use. Physicians had to improvise with medications and treatments that were originally designated for other medical conditions.

In the late 1980s and 1990s, epidemiologic, psychosocial, and pharmacologic research resulted in an increase in available headache information and treatment possibilities. The development of the triptans, serotonin agonists, brought a new awareness to both physicians and sufferers. Today, seven triptans and two relatively new preventive medications are available. In spite of this, a minority of migraine sufferers use these options, and more than 50% continue to self-treat without benefit of professional care.

In the past, surveys indicated that patients wanted their physician to believe their headache problem was real. They hoped that they would be taken seriously and that the physician would make a sincere attempt to help them. The headache patient has changed. The headache sufferer who seeks treatment today is more knowledgeable and interested in rapid relief and tolerability of medication.

Evaluation and Diagnosis

An accurate diagnosis is essential for effective management of patients with the more commonly encountered headaches. Because no biologic markers or diagnostic tests exist to determine headache type, the history is the single most important element in the evaluation of the headache patient. Various headache types sometimes have similar initial presentations, or patients may suffer with more than one type of headache (e.g., migraine and tension-type headache), which can be confusing at first, but the

TABLE 1 Current Diagnosis

TYPE	SYMPTOMS	FREQUENCY	DURATION
Tension type	Bilateral variable pain	Variable	Hours to days
	Squeezing or band-like	Recognizable cause	
	Tightness of neck and shoulders		
Migraine	Mostly unilateral	1–4/mo	Hours to days
	Throbbing or constant pain	Can be cyclic	
	Nausea, vomiting		
	Photophobia/phonophobia		
	Fluid disturbances		
	Mood changes		
	Incapacitating		
	Can be associated with aura		
Cluster	Unilateral, severe boring or burning pain	Multiple daily or near daily	45–90 min
			Cycles of attacks
	Ipsilateral lacrimation		
	Scleral injection, eyelid droop		
	Rhinorrhea		
	Restlessness		
Chronic daily	Dull, whole headed	Daily	Months
	Variable		

careful history usually differentiates the headache type. In general, little in the way of diagnostic testing is needed unless a physical cause is suspected. Some physicians prefer to perform simple laboratory tests to establish a baseline for medication toleration and monitoring as necessary (Table 1).

- The headache complaint on occasion can be a sign of a more serious medical condition, such as a tumor, infection, or aneurysm. For this reason, the clinician always must be cautious and diligent in establishing an accurate and timely diagnosis. Certain so-called red flags in the history require immediate attention. These include any complex of symptoms or history that does not fit a typical headache type; report of a significant neurologic deficit; significant or prolonged neurologic deficit with aura; late-onset migraine (in a patient older than 30 years); sudden onset of a new head pain without history of similar headaches; changes in headache character; headache associated with elevated temperature; or completely unresponsive attacks in the absence of analgesic or caffeine overuse. When any of these symptoms are present or physical examination reveals significant findings, further diagnostic evaluation with imaging studies and consultation is imperative.

The appropriate headache patient evaluation includes a thorough history; physical examination with special attention to the head and the neurologic, cardiovascular, and musculoskeletal systems; and diagnostic tests when appropriate. The history should include headache onset, location, pain character (e.g., pressure, throb), frequency, duration, associated symptoms, aura or prodrome, triggers, previous treatment, and family history. Certain clues in the history may lean toward the diagnosis of migraine, such as motion sickness; absence of headache during pregnancy; and headache relationship to menses, sun glare, oversleep, fatigue, fasting, foods, or alcohol.

Various diagnostic screening questionnaires and tools have been developed over the years to assist busy clinicians in establishing the diagnosis of migraine. Most are long and cumbersome and do not easily become a part of routine patient evaluation. A simple three-question screener for migraine is helpful for generalist clinicians.

A "yes" answer to all three questions indicates a strong possibility of the migraine diagnosis:
1. Do you experience headaches severe enough to see a physician?
2. Are your headaches accompanied by other symptoms?
3. Are your headaches intermittent (i.e., nondaily)?

Note: This screener should not be substituted for a complete history; it should be used only for screening purposes.

Tension-Type Headache

Tension-type headache (TTHA) is the most common of headaches and first was believed to be caused by sustained muscle contraction of the neck, jaw, scalp, or facial muscles. However, consideration is being given to the possibility that sustained muscle contraction can, in fact, be an epiphenomenon to possible central disturbances rather than a primary process. Evidence suggests that altered levels of serotonin, substance P, and neuropeptide Y in the serum or platelets of patients with TTHA are responsible.

- TTHA is characterized by intermittent or persisting bilateral pain, usually described as a squeezing pressure or a band-like sensation around the head. Most patients experience their symptoms in the frontal, temporal, or occipital areas of the head. Location frequently varies with the attack, and tightness of the neck and shoulders is common. Intensity varies greatly. The attacks can last from hours to days, and in some extreme cases they may last for months. Aura, nausea, photophobia and phonophobia, and incapacitation are not typically associated with TTHA.

Many TTHA sufferers easily recognize the origin of their attacks. TTHA typically results from emotional upset, periods of stress, and major life changes. Anxiousness, poor adaptation skills, and anxiety and depression often are present. Physical causes, such as degenerative joint disease, trauma to the head or neck, awkward neck position, poor posture, temporomandibular joint dysfunction, bruxism, or heavy chewing also can precipitate attacks. Persons older than 50 years are prone to excessive muscle contraction because of arthritis of the neck and jaw, poor posture, or stress. TTHA that is consistently precipitated by tension or pathology of the neck frequently is referred to as a cervicogenic headache. In contrast to migraine headache, TTHA is more likely to begin in later life.

Migraine Headache

Migraine headache is a familial disease characterized by unilateral or bilateral paroxysmal headache lasting hours to days. Adult women experience attacks more than men by a ratio of 3:1. Children and the elderly experience migraine equally. Attacks occur from as infrequently as one or two per year to several times weekly. Associated symptoms usually occur and frequently include throbbing, nausea, vomiting, photophobia, phonophobia, fluid retention, and mood changes.

The two basic types of migraine headache are migraine with aura (previously called classic migraine) and migraine without aura (previously called common migraine). Migraine with aura is preceded by an aura, a transient neurologic symptom that usually is visual, such as scotoma, teichopsia, tunnel vision, or visual field deficit, lasting 5 to 30 minutes. However, aura can manifest as any neurologic deficit. Migraine without aura is more commonly experienced and comes on gradually or is present on awakening from sleep. In some patients, these headaches are associated with a nonspecific prolonged prodrome, such as mood changes, food cravings, or fluid retention hours before the pain.

The underlying cause of migraine headache is not clearly established, and various theories are proposed. Migraine appears to be of genetic origin and to be an inflammatory disease that causes disturbances in serotonin use and activity. Strong evidence indicates that the migrainous attack originates in the central nervous system by stimulation of the locus ceruleus and dorsal raphe nuclei. Resultant changes alter cerebral and extracranial blood flow; activate the trigeminovascular system; and cause vascular dilation, neurogenic inflammation, and pain. Various precipitants are known, and many sufferers report that migraine attacks frequently are associated with menstruation or are triggered by foods containing vasoactive amines, strong odors, too much or too little sleep, sun glare, stress, altitude, weather changes, exertion, or fasting (Boxes 1 and 2).

Some physicians classify migraine according to its precipitant or description (e.g., menstrual migraine, exertional migraine, coital migraine, cervicogenic migraine, cyclic migraine, "painless" or acephalic migraine). When a sufferer experiences headache for 50% of the month, it is referred to as chronic migraine. Regardless, the fundamentals of evaluation and treatment are similar.

Cluster Headache

The cause of cluster headache is unknown, and little credible research is available. Various possibilities or theories are suggested and include, but are not limited to, disturbances in histamine production or use; hypothalamic biorhythm dysfunction; or serotonin and neurotransmitter mechanisms similar to those of migraine. Some authorities consider cluster headache one of the most severe pain conditions known to humankind.

- Cluster headache predominantly affects men, with a male-to-female ratio of 6:1. It occurs in well under 0.5% of the population. Onset later in life (after age 30 years) is common, and patients sometimes report head injury or a traumatic event occurring months before onset. Attacks occur on a daily or near-daily basis for weeks or months at a time and mysteriously disappear for months to years regardless of treatment, only to recur and cycle again. Although nonspecialist physicians only occasionally encounter the patient with cluster headaches, it is important to consider cluster headaches in the differential diagnosis.

BOX 1   Common Migraine Dietary Triggers

- Dairy: ripened cheese (cheddar, brie, camembert), sour cream >½ cup
- Meats: processed lunch meats, hot dogs, sausage, bologna, salami, chicken liver
- Fish: pickled or dried herring
- Grains: sourdough bread
- Fruits: bananas, raisins, figs, avocado, citrus >½ cup
- Vegetables: broad and fava beans, onions, snow peas, garlic
- Other: chocolate, nuts, peanut butter, pickled foods, most Chinese food
- Beverages: most wines and alcohol, caffeine > 200 mg
- Additives: MSG, soy sauce, meat tenderizers, aspartame, sulfites

---

BOX 2   Migraine Triggers

- Altitude
- Alcohol
- Caffeine withdrawal
- Fatigue
- Fluorescent or flickering lights
- Sun glare
- Weather changes
- Stress, stress letdown
- Foods
- Skipping meals
- Smoky environment
- Noisy environment
- Strong odors

The typical patient with a cluster headache experiences relatively brief attacks (45–90 minutes) of horrible unilateral head pain associated with ipsilateral lacrimation, scleral injection, rhinorrhea, or eyelid droop. The hallmark of the syndrome is its associated symptoms and its severe and intense pain. During attacks, most cluster patients move about, trying unsuccessfully to get more comfortable, similar to renal colic; this is in contrast to migraine sufferers, who prefer to lie quietly in a dark quiet room. Few triggers are identified, and alcohol almost always precipitates an attack during a cluster "on" cycle. A rare form of cluster headache, chronic cluster, does not cycle and continues on a daily or *near-daily* basis without cessation.

Chronic Daily Headache

A small percentage of headache sufferers present with chronic daily headache. The majority of these daily headaches are of the tension or migraine type. However, patients may present with daily nonincapacitating generalized headache. These headaches frequently are associated with major life changes (negative or positive), financial or relationship difficulties, and depression or emotional problems.

The assessment of the chronic daily headache patient is similar to other headache syndromes, but may require particular attention to mental health and medication rebounding issues.

Posttraumatic Headache

Posttraumatic headaches are headaches resulting from physical injury to the head. The trauma can be direct or the result of a contra-coux type injury encountered with whiplash or forced movement of the head or neck. The degree of injury and headache is not necessarily related to the degree of trauma. Seemingly minor injuries sometimes can result in significant and prolonged headache, while apparent severe blows to the head sometimes do not result in significant headache.

Complicating the posttraumatic headache can be an associated spasm of shoulder, neck, and scalp muscles or reactive anxiety and depression. Patients with preexisting headaches may experience an increase in severity or frequency of headaches. It is not unusual for there to be a delay in the onset of headache.

It is imperative that the detailed evaluation of the posttraumatic headache patient include psychological and cognitive examination while keeping in mind that presumed trivial injuries can have significant sequela. The more frequent type of headache encountered is of the tension or chronic daily type. Migraine and cluster are reported.

Treatment

The doctor–patient relationship frequently is the key to successful treatment in the headache patient. Although to some this statement seems an obvious truism, its importance cannot be overemphasized.

Patients who experience frequent, near-daily or daily headaches invariably require a comprehensive treatment program that necessitates good communication. Anxious patients sometimes do not comprehend medical explanations or instructions; busy doctors sometimes do not have or take the time to ensure that the patient understands.

The two elements of headache treatment are abortive treatment, directed at attacks once they have begun, and prophylactic treatment, directed at preventing or reducing the frequency or necessarily related to the frequency or the degree of attacks. In general, the abortive approach is used for patients who suffer infrequent attacks and for those who experience breakthrough attacks while undergoing prophylactic therapy.

Prophylactic therapy should be instituted when headaches are frequent, when headaches are unresponsive to abortive medication, or when there are contraindications to abortive medications.

- Headache treatment can include nonpharmacologic measures, such as physical exercise, stretching, stress avoidance, relaxation exercises, biofeedback, manipulation, massage, cold/warm packs or neuromodulation devices. Pharmacologic therapies can include a vast array of medicaments from over-the-counter (OTC) drugs to prescription drugs such as triptans, newly approved monoclonal antibodies (MAbs),other vasoconstrictors, β-blockers, calcium channel blockers, antiepileptic agents, antidepressants, nonsteroidal antiinflammatory drugs (NSAIDs), analgesics, muscle relaxants, anxiolytics, and others.

Treatment, whether prophylactic or abortive, should follow a definite plan incorporating the clinician and the patient into a team focused on reducing the headache frequency, severity, and disability.

As mentioned earlier, impressions and physical findings should be explained to the patient in as much detail as necessary to ensure the patient's complete understanding. The complexity of the headache condition needs to be explained, emphasizing its chronicity, rather than its curability, and that the goal of treatment is disease control.

- The comprehensiveness of the treatment plan depends on the frequency of the patient's attacks. The more frequent and severe the attacks, the more detailed plan may be necessary. Patients experiencing infrequent attacks (e.g., once or twice monthly) may require only an abortive medication and little else. Patients with more frequent attacks may benefit from dietary restrictions, psychosocial intervention, biofeedback relaxation training, manipulation, and physical modality intervention, in addition to medication (Table 2).

TTHA Treatment

TTHA is often associated with emotional stress and muscle strain or tension of the shoulders and neck. Simple self-administered measures, such as stress avoidance, stretching, warm packs, or relaxation techniques, can be helpful in reducing or relieving attacks. More comprehensive professional intervention, such as manual manipulation, physical therapy, local injections, or biofeedback training, is a consideration for more frequent or severe cases. The ultimate goal is to restore normal function of involved muscles.

- Prophylactically, the use of OTC or prescription medications can be considered in addition to nonmedicinal measures for reducing the frequency and duration of attacks. NSAIDs, muscle relaxants, tricyclic antidepressants (TCA), selective serotonin reuptake inhibitors (SSRI), or serotonin-norepinephrine reuptake inhibitors (SNRI), at the lowest effective doses, are more commonly used. Other categories of antidepressants are reported to be effective in some sufferers.
- Daily use of the longer-acting NSAIDs, such as naproxen[1] (Naprosyn) or celecoxib[1] (Celebrex), in the appropriately screened patient over a 2- to 3-week period, can be an effective preventative.

TCAs, such as nortriptyline[1] (Pamelor) or amitriptyline[1] (Elavil), in low doses at night over 1 to 3 months, are frequently effective, especially in patients with anxiety or mild depression. The SSRI drugs, such as fluoxetine[1] (Prozac) or sertraline[1] (Zoloft), or the SNRI drugs such as duloxetine[1] (Cymbalta) or venlafaxine[1] (Effexor), similarly can be useful.

The muscle relaxant cyclobenzaprine[1] (Flexeril), at low doses, with a similar mechanism to the TCAs, can be administered at night for limited periods. Other muscle relaxants occasionally can be helpful. Potential side effects can limit the use of NSAIDs (gastrointestinal irritation) and the TCAs (fatigue and weight gain).

OnabotulinumtoxinA (Botox)[1] reportedly is helpful in the treatment of the tension-type headache, but controlled studies are limited. In this treatment, a diluted solution of botulinum toxin is injected into various muscles of the face, scalp, neck, or shoulders. It is imperative that these injections be administered by physicians skilled in the procedure to avoid complication and adverse events.

- Abortive or symptomatic treatment of TTHA can include simple OTC medications (e.g., aspirin or acetaminophen), NSAIDs (short acting), muscle relaxants, combination analgesics, and, in rare cases, tramadol (Ultram). Limited studies have shown analgesic qualities of riboflavin (vitamin B$_2$)[7] 200 mg is recommended for patients who cannot tolerate NSAID type medications. Caution should be exercised in prescribing potentially habituating drugs. Daily or near-daily use of analgesics, and especially those containing caffeine, can lead to analgesic rebound headache or medication overuse headache, which can compound the patient's headache problem.

Migraine Treatment

Migraineurs are unique individuals, and the effectiveness and tolerance of medications can vary from patient to patient. Medication changes, combinations of medications, and trial and error may be necessary in the early stages of treatment.

- Nonmedicinal measures for migraine sufferers include biofeedback, stress reduction, neuromodulation devices, caffeine and dietary restrictions, regimentation of meals and sleep, rest, exercise, stretching, and avoidance of work or activity overload. Strict limitation of caffeine to less than 200 mg/day is important to prevent caffeine headache (rebound headache) in most patients. Elimination of vasoactive foods, such as chocolate, aged cheese, and processed meats, and avoidance of fasting for more than 4 hours can be helpful for patients with more frequent attacks (see Box 1). Regular exercise and stretching, planned relaxation, regular sleep schedules, and following a healthy lifestyle are frequently included in a comprehensive treatment regimen. In some patients, especially children and adolescents, biofeedback stress reduction or psychotherapeutic intervention may be necessary.
- The more commonly used medications for prophylaxis are β-blockers, calcium channel blockers, antiepileptics (neurostabilizers), and the antidepressants. Treatment should be continued for a 6- to 8-week trial before discontinuation for

HEADACHE TYPE	PRN	PROPHYLAXIS
Tension type	OTC drugs	Stress/trigger avoidance
	NSAIDs	Stretching exercises
	Muscle relaxants	Warm compresses
	Combination analgesics	Relaxation exercises
		Muscle relaxants
		Antidepressants
Migraine	NSAIDs*	Biofeedback
	Triptans*	β-Blockers*
	Ergotamine*	Divalproex ER*
	Dihydroergotamine (DHE)*	Topiramate*
	Isometheptene*	TCA antidepressants
	Combination analgesics Cefaly Unit	Ca channel blockers
	Cerena" (Migraine aura) gammaCore	Cefaly Unit OnabotulinumtoxinA (Botox)†
Cluster	Oxygen	No alcohol
	Triptans	Ca channel blockers
	DHE	Divalproex
	Ergotamine gammaCore	NSAIDs
		Lithium Steroids

TABLE 2 Current Therapy

*FDA indication
†Indicates for chronic migraine
Abbreviations: NSAID = nonsteroidal anti-inflammatory drug; OTC = over-the-counter drug; TCA = tricyclic antidepressant.

[1]Not FDA approved for this indication.
[7]Available as a dietary supplement.

ineffectiveness. The determination of which medication to use depends on comorbidities, interactions with concomitant medications, and tolerability.

β-Blockers such as propranolol and timolol (Blocadren) are nonselective and are approved by the FDA for migraine prevention. Other β-blockers, such as nadolol (Corgard)[1], metoprolol (Lopressor)[1], and atenolol (Tenormin)[1], also can be effective. The mechanism of action in migraine is not wholly understood, but it is thought to involve anxiolytic effects and vascular changes and stabilization. The usual dosage is recommended (e.g., timolol 10–30 mg/day, propranolol 120–160 mg/day), and many consider the nighttime dose the more significant.

Calcium channel antagonists are well tolerated in general and can be effective in many patients. They are believed to alter serotonin release and inhibit platelet serotonin uptake and release within the brain. Verapamil (Calan)[1] is considered the more effective and is commonly recommended to patients. Dosage can vary from 120 to 480 mg/day. Nimodipine (Nimotop)[1] is equally effective but has been rarely used in the United States because of its high cost.

- Antiepileptic medications such as phenytoin (Dilantin)[1] and carbamazepine (Tegretol)[1] have been prescribed for migraine prevention over the years, with mixed results. Their use is now limited with the advent of newer, more easily tolerated agents, such as divalproex sodium (Depakote ER) and topiramate (Topamax, Trokendi XR).
- Divalproex sodium is effective in reducing migraine attacks and is particularly useful in patients with coexisting head injury, seizure disorders, and bipolar disorders. It is thought to improve inhibitory and excitatory amino acid imbalance in the brain. It is best to start with a lower dose and to gradually increase as needed and tolerated. The dosage of 500 to 1000 mg/day is more frequently prescribed. A commonly experienced side effect is sedation, which can sometimes be used to the patient's advantage when anxiolytic effects are needed.
- Topiramate is a preventive medication approved by the FDA for migraine prophylaxis. It has multiple mechanisms of action, but its exact mechanism in migraine headache is unknown.

Its effectiveness is believed to involve sodium ion channel stabilization, calcium ion channels, GABA (γ-aminobutyric acid) receptors, and neuronal membrane stabilization. The average daily dose is variable and ranges from 30 to 100 mg/day. A most unusual side effect of weight loss or appetite suppression can be used to the patient's advantage in preventing weight gain, which frequently accompanies migraine prophylactic medications.

The TCAs can be useful for patients who experience frequent attacks and for those who experience anxiety and depression. The TCAs inhibit synaptic reuptake of serotonin, thereby reducing neuron firing and release of neurotransmitters. Starting with a low dose in the evening and titrating up to efficacy and tolerability is recommended. Significant anticholinergic and sedation effects sometimes limit their use. The SSRIs are reported helpful in some patients, but their use in migraine prevention is limited.

Other medications have been utilized in migraine prophylaxis with varying success. These include NSAIDs, cyproheptadine (Periactin)[1], clonidine (Catapres)[1], phenothiazines, anxiolytics, ergotamine (Ergomar), magnesium[1], feverfew[7], and others.

- In general, prophylactic medications should be taken for 6 to 8 weeks to determine efficacy. If effective, a course of 4 to 6 months is recommended before an attempt is made to discontinue medication.
- OnabotulinumtoxinA (Botox) has been approved by the FDA for the treatment of chronic migraine. Multiple injections to the head and neck can be helpful for patients who experience symptoms for more than 14 days per month and it can be repeated after 3 months. Because this treatment is administered by physicians in headache specialty and pain practices, simultaneous comprehensive treatment measures and medication can contribute to positive patient results. Side effects are

relatively low when injected by experienced physicians; alteration of facial expressions is the most common. Proper administration of the toxin is imperative.

A large meta-analysis of 27 controlled clinical trials concluded that onabotulinumtoxinA injections showed a small to moderate benefit over placebo in patients experiencing chronic migraine and chronic daily headache. Patients with chronic tension type or episodic migraine showed no benefit.

- A trigeminal nerve stimulator, Cefaly device, was approved by the FDA in 2014. The Cefaly head-band apparatus can be self-administered 20 minutes daily to reduce migraine frequency. Experience with this TENS device is limited.
- A variety of abortive treatment options are available for migraine sufferers. Although the triptans (Table 3) have generated much interest and are frequently prescribed, other medications continue to be used, including ergotamine and its derivatives, isometheptene, and NSAIDs. Many of the abortive medications carry significant prescribing limitations that must be taken into consideration. Vasoconstrictor medications are contraindicated in patients with cardiovascular or peripheral vascular disease. NSAIDs should not be used in those with gastrointestinal or bleeding disorders. As with all medications, the clinician must consider appropriate prescribing, contraindications, and side-effect information.
- The vasoconstrictor ergotamine is available in oral, rectal (with caffeine [Cafergot]), and sublingual forms (Ergomar). Ergotamine has a relatively long half-life and duration of action (up to 3 days) and should be used no more frequently than every 4 to 5 days to avoid ergotamine rebound headache. The ergot derivative dihydroergotamine (DHE, Migranal NS) is available for intramuscular, subcutaneous (SC), and intranasal use. Intravenous DHE sometimes is used for intractable migraine (status migrainosus) in emergency departments and inpatient settings. The intranasal form (Migranal) is an effective treatment when administered correctly by the patient. Unfortunately, DHE is not absorbed by the gastrointestinal tract, and unlike other abortive nasal sprays, any swallowed medication will be wasted. DHE has a low headache recurrence rate of approximately 12%. All forms of ergotamine and DHE are more effective when taken early in attacks.

Isometheptene is used in combination with dichloralphenazone and acetaminophen (Midrin). It is slow acting and more effective when taken early in attacks and when used for attacks preceded or

TABLE 3	Triptans		
MEDICATION	**BRAND NAME**	**HALF-LIFE (h)**	**FORM/STRENGTH**
Sumatriptan	Imitrex	1.5	Oral: 25, 50, 100 mg NS: 5, 20 mg Injection: 4, 6 mg
	Treximet		Oral: Sumatriptan 85 mg + naproxen sodium 500 mg
	Zembrace Onzetra Xsail		Injection: 3 mg NS 22 mg
Naratriptan	Amerge	6	Oral: 1, 2.5 mg
Zolmitriptan	Zomig	3	Oral: 2.5, 5 mg MLT: 2.5, 5 mg NS: 2.5, 5 mg
Rizatriptan	Maxalt	2–3	Oral: 5, 10 mg MLT: 5, 10 mg
Almotriptan	Axert	3–4	Oral: 6.25, 12.5 mg
Frovatriptan	Frova	25	Oral: 5 mg
Eletriptan	Relpax	4	Oral: 20, 40 mg

Abbreviations: MLT = oral disintegrating; NS = nasal spray; TD = transdermal.

[1]Not FDA approved for this indication.
[7]Available as a dietary supplement.

accompanied by stress and muscle tension of the neck. Although isometheptene is considered less potent than ergotamine and triptans, it is preferred by many patients whose headaches have features of both migraine and tension type.

At the present time, seven serotonin agonists (triptans) are approved for abortive migraine treatment in the United States (see Table 3). As a category, the triptans are approximately 65% to 70% effective in published clinical trials. Their similarities are greater than their differences, but each triptan is not necessarily effective for all patients, and familiarity with their differences can be helpful to the treating physician. Half-life, onset and duration of action, adverse events, tolerability, recurrence of headache, and routes of administration may vary and allow the physician to match the medication to the individual patient. For example, a slower onset of action and longer-lasting triptan may be appropriate for slow-onset, longer-lasting migraine attacks.

- As with other headache treatments, oral triptan tablets are more effective in the early phases of migraines. It is thought that peripheral sensitization—allodynia—is a sign of later-phase migraine, and treating the attack before this phenomenon occurs is important. When treatment is delayed or the patient awakens with severe migraine, the injection, nasal spray, or rapidly acting triptans may be more beneficial. Although triptans as a group are very effective, recurrence of headache, after initial relief, requiring retreatment is common and can be as high as 40%. The recurrence rate tends to be less with triptans having a longer half-life.

The ergotamines and triptans are contraindicated in patients with ischemic heart disease, uncontrolled hypertension, and cerebrovascular disease. Physicians initially were extremely cautious about recommending triptans to their patients when they were first introduced in the United States. However, significant human exposure to the triptans has shown that myocardial infarction or serious ischemia is rare. Chest pain following triptan use affects a small percentage of patients, and because its significance continues to be unclear, it is recommended that triptan use be held pending cardiac evaluation.

- Sumatriptan (Imitrex, Zembrace, Onzetra), the first triptan approved in the United States, is available in nasal spray (5, 20, 22 mg), SC (3, 4, 6 mg), and oral formulations (25, 50, 100 mg). Its half-life is approximately 1.5 hours, and its duration of action is less than 4 hours. The injectable form produces rapid relief in 70% to 80% of patients, and it appears to be the most effective of all the available triptan forms. Conversely, it appears to cause the most side effects, and for this reason it should be used only for the more severe attacks. The oral forms are more favorable with regard to adverse effects, and their effectiveness is similar to that of other triptans (approximately 65%). Because of sumatriptan's short half-life and duration of action, recurrence of headache is common, necessitating repeat dosing.
- Naratriptan (Amerge) was the first to be approved of the gradual onset, longer-acting triptans. It is available as oral 1 and 2.5 mg tablets and has a half-life of 6 hours. Naratriptan is well tolerated by patients and often is used by patients with slow-onset migraine. Some specialists prescribe daily naratriptan[1] for limited periods for treatment of menstrual or intractable migraine attacks.
- Zolmitriptan (Zomig) is available in 2.5 and 5 mg oral and oral disintegrating tablets (ZMT) and as 2.5 and 5 mg nasal sprays. The efficacy of oral zolmitriptan is approximately 65% and that of the nasal form is 70%. The half-life of oral zolmitriptan is 3 hours, and its duration of action is longer than the nasal form, which improves on the need to remedicate. The nasal spray has a biphasic absorption curve, which accounts for its favorable adverse effect profile over the 5 mg oral tablet.

- Rizatriptan (Maxalt) is available as oral 5 and 10 mg tablets and as an oral disintegrating form (MLT). It's half-life is 2 to 3 hours and it has a favorable one-dose 2-hour response rate. Patients who are undergoing concomitant treatment with propranolol should take the lesser 5 mg rizatriptan dose because of higher resultant rizatriptan plasma levels.
- Almotriptan (Axert) is available in 6.25 and 12.5 mg tablets. It has a half-life of 3.5 hours and, because of a broad Tmax (time of maximal concentration) range of 1.4 to 3.8 hours, a relatively rapid onset of action. Almotriptan has favorable adverse effect and headache recurrence profile. Chest pain symptoms after almotriptan use were similar to placebo in clinical trials.
- Frovatriptan (Frova) is a long-acting triptan available in 2.5 mg oral tablets. It has the longest half-life of 25 hours and a favorable recurrence rate. Frovatriptan is frequently used for treatment of menstrual migraine and for attacks of longer duration. Some specialists prescribe daily frovatriptan for a limited period for menstrual and prolonged migraine attacks.[1]
- Eletriptan (Relpax) was the last triptan to be approved. It is available in 20 and 40 mg oral tablets and has a half-life of nearly 5 hours. Eletriptan has a relatively rapid onset but a longer duration of action and a favorable recurrence rate. In studies, some patients who were unresponsive to other triptans responded to eletriptan.

Various attempts have been made to compare triptans. Head-to-head trials mostly have compared one triptan to sumatriptan. A meta-analysis of 53 clinical trials published in 2001 compared the efficacy, recurrence, duration of action, and tolerability of all available triptans. Almotriptan and eletriptan were rated favorably across the major parameters of onset of action, efficacy, adverse events, and recurrence. In spite of efforts to adjust for variations in protocols and placebo response, specialists reached no clear consensus as to the validity or value of the meta-analysis or the preferability of one triptan over another.

- Newly developed anti-calcium gene related peptide (CGRP) human or humanized monoclonal antibodies (MAb) have demonstrated efficacy for reducing migraine (with and without aura) frequency and reducing the number of symptomatic days. These medications interfere with CGRP activity by blocking CGRP or its receptor and are injected monthly. Generally, MAbs are well tolerated and are injected because of their large molecular size. As of this writing, three MAbs have been approved in the U.S. for adult use (see Table 4). They should not be taken during pregnancy and have not been

TABLE 4	Monoclonal Antibodies		
MEDICATION	BRAND NAME	HALF-LIFE (D)	FORM/ STRENGTH
Erenumab*	Aimovig	28	inj SQ 70 mg
Fremanezumab†	Ajovy	31	inj SQ 225 mg
Galcanezumab‡	Emgality	27	inj SQ 120 mg

*Erenumab (Aimovig) is a fully human MAb that blocks CGRP by binding to its receptors. 70-140 mg is self administered SQ monthly. If 140 mg is to be administered, two consecutive 70-mg SQ injections at different sites is best. As with other MAbs, it is well tolerated, with the most common side effects being injection site inflammation and constipation. Erenumab reaches peak serum concentration at 6 days, and its elimination half life is 28 days.
†Fremanezumab (Ajovy) is a humanized MAb that blocks CGRP by binding to the CGRP ligand. 225 mg is self administered SQ monthly or 675 mg at 3-month intervals. If 675 mg is to be administered, 3 consecutive 225 mg injections at different sites is best. It is well tolerated, and the most common reported side effect is injection site inflammation. Fremanezumab reaches peak serum concentration at 5-7 days and its elimination half life is 31days.
‡Galcanezumab (Emgality) is a humanized MAb that blocks CGRP by binding to the CGRP ligand. A loading dose of 240 mg is self administered SQ initially, followed by 120 mg injections at 3-month intervals.[3] If 240 mg is to be administered, 2 consecutive 120 mg injections at different sites is best. It is well tolerated, and the most common reported side effect is injection site inflammation. Galcanezumab reaches peak serum concentration at 5-7 days and its elimination half life is 27 days.
[3]Exceeds dosage recommended by the manufacturer

[1]Not FDA approved for this indication.

studied in patients over 65. Although well tolerated, significant hypersensitivity reactions are possible. At this time it is thought that triptans and MAbs can be taken concomitantly for migraine attacks.

- NSAIDs frequently are recommended for treatment of acute migraine and can be effective when taken early. Their effects on the physiology of pain, inflammation, and platelets are thought to be the mechanisms responsible. Some physicians recommend taking a NSAID with the first dose of a triptan for added efficacy. Various agents are used, but none of the rapid-acting NSAIDs appears to have significant efficacy superiority. Naproxen sodium 500 mg in combination with sumatriptan 85 mg (Treximet), OTC ibuprofen (Motrin, Advil), and aspirin combination with caffeine and acetaminophen (Excedrin Migraine) are approved by the FDA for treatment of acute migraine.
- Symptomatic treatment of pain may be necessary in patients who do not respond to recommended abortive treatment. Any effective analgesic can be appropriate, provided it is used infrequently and not on a daily or near-daily basis. In general, the more effective analgesics have antiinflammatory and sedative properties.
- Three neuromodulation devices are FDA approved for the treatment of migraine headache. "The Cefaly Unit", a trigeminal nerve stimulator, can be self-administered to the forehead for 20 minutes as needed for acute migraine pain. The "Cerena", a self-administered transcranial magnetic stimulator delivers two consecutive impulses at regular intervals to the occipital area as needed for pain of migraine with aura. A vagus nerve stimulator, "gammaCore", can be self-administered to the neck for pain of migraine. Mild electrical charges are released to stimulate the vagus nerve, which has been shown to be involved in migraine and cluster headache symptoms.

Cluster Headache Treatment

Cluster headache is one of the more unusual pain conditions occasionally encountered by physicians. Pain onset is rapid, and the duration of the attack is brief. For this reason, prophylactic treatment usually is the most practical. Abortive prescriptions frequently are given, but, for the most part, the cluster attack is resolving by the time medication is absorbed.

- Nonmedicinal prophylactic measures are extremely limited. The reduction of cigarette smoking and the addressing of individual stress and hostility during cluster periods should be part of any treatment program. There are no FDA-approved medications for the prophylactic treatment of cluster headache. Numerous medications can be helpful and include the calcium channel blockers verapamil (Calan, Isoptin, Verelan, Covera, Verap)[1] and nimodipine (Nimotop)[1], the neurostabilizers valproate (Depakote)[1] and topiramate (Topamax, Trokendi XR)[1], various NSAIDs, ergotamine[1], lithium (Eskalith)[1], cyproheptadine[1], combination H_1 and H_2 histamine antagonists, and, in extreme cases, short intervals of steroids. The addition of magnesium[7] 500 to 750 mg can be helpful in some sufferers. These medications are used in average therapeutic doses, and combinations of medications are commonly needed. The preventatives should be used during the cluster cycle and discontinued during off-cycle periods.
- Abortive treatment is less preferred for cluster headache, as noted previously. However, inhalation oxygen via facial mask at 6 L/min terminates cluster attacks in 75% to 80% of sufferers within 12 minutes. The vagus nerve stimulator, "gammaCore" mentioned above, can be self-administered to the neck for pain reduction. Other possibilities include sumatriptan[1] SC or nasal spray, zolmitriptan[1] nasal spray, ergotamine[1] sublingual, or DHE-45 injection[1] or nasal spray (Migranal)[1]. The occasional patient reports relief with the oral triptans or potent analgesics. When triptans, ergotamine, or analgesics are used, appropriate prescribing and frequency guidelines should

be followed. In general, with the exception of oxygen, daily as-needed medications should be avoided.

Chronic Daily and Posttraumatic Headache Treatment

The care of patients with chronic daily and posttraumatic headaches is determined by the type or types of headache being experienced. Treatment of each type follows what has been described above. In the patient experiencing posttraumatic headache, frequent follow-up visit monitoring is most appropriate. Extra care should be taken when prescribing medications, especially those that could affect cognitive function and recovery. Often, posttraumatic headache patients benefit with concomitant psychologic and cognitive professional support.

Conclusion

Headache continues to present a challenging problem for clinicians as well as for suffering patients. In spite of recent treatment advances and more public awareness, millions continue to needlessly endure pain and debilitation. Desperate sufferers in a quest for relief sometimes resort to unorthodox therapies or anxiolytics, habituative analgesics, or excessive caffeine that ultimately worsen their headache problems.

At first glance, the headache problem appears complex and difficult when, in actuality, most sufferers experience straightforward, easily diagnosed headaches. The interested generalist or specialist who takes the time to elicit a careful history can establish the headache diagnosis and direct a simple treatment plan that can make a tremendous difference in the headache sufferer's life.

References

Edvinsson L, Hanes K, Warfvinge K, Krause D: CGRP as target of new migraine therapies - successful transition from bench to clinic, *Nat Rev Neurol* 14:338–350, 2018.

Escher CM, Paracka L, Dressler D, Kollewe K: Botulinum toxin in management of chronic migraine: clinical evidence and experience, *Ther Adv in Neurol Disorders* 10(2):127–135, 2017.

Goadsby PJ: Primary headache disorders - five new things, *Neurol Clin Prac* 9(03):233–240, 2019.

Kahriman A, Zhu S: Migraine and tension-type headache, *Semin Neurol* 38(06):608–618, 2018.

Monzani L, Espi-Lopez GV, Zurriaga R, Anderson LL: Manual therapy for tension type headache related to quality of life and work presenteeism: secondary analysis of a randomized controlled trial, *Complement Ther Med* 25:86–91, 2016.

Peters GL: Migraine overview and summary of current and emerging treatment options, *Am J Manag Care* 25:S25–34, 2019.

Robbins MS, et al: Treatment of cluster headache: amer headache society evidence based guidelines, *Headache* 56(7):1093–1106, 2016.

■ HEMATURIA

Method of
Moben Mirza, MD; and J. Brantley Thrasher, MD

CURRENT DIAGNOSIS

- Hematuria is defined as the presence of red blood cells in the urine. Hematuria can be gross (readily visible) or microscopic (detected by dipstick or microscopy). In the adult population, any unexplained hematuria should be presumed to be of malignant origin until proven otherwise. Urologic evaluation of the upper and lower urinary tract is compulsory for patients with gross hematuria. Patients with asymptomatic microscopic hematuria (>3 rbc/hpf) should undergo urologic evaluation once benign causes have been ruled out. The urologic evaluation includes urine analysis, serum creatinine, cystoscopy, and multiphasic computed tomography. Concurrent nephrologic evaluation should occur in select cases.

---

[1]Not FDA approved for this indication.
[7]Available as a dietary supplement.

Epidemiology

Hematuria is a common clinical finding in adults. The prevalence of hematuria ranges from 0.2% to 16%. Prevalence varies based on age, gender, frequency of testing, threshold used to define hematuria, and study group characteristics (Davis et al., 2012). Transient microscopic hematuria may occur in up to 40% of patients; however, persistent microscopic hematuria in greater than three evaluated urine samples is limited to 2% of the population (Masahito, 2010). A wide range of causes can result in hematuria. Transient hematuria may be caused by vigorous exercise, sexual intercourse, mild trauma, menstrual contamination, and instrumentation. Patients with underlying urinary tract disease can have transient or persistent hematuria. The difference between gross and microscopic hematuria is that the chances of finding significant pathology are higher in patients with gross hematuria. For example, approximately 5% of patient with microscopic hematuria in contrast to 40% of patient with gross hematuria are found to have urologic malignancy on evaluation (Khadra et al., 2000). The most common cause of gross hematuria in adults older than age 50 is bladder cancer (Gerber and Brendler, 2011).

Risk Factors

Given the wide range of etiologies for hematuria, the risk factors are dependent on the etiology itself. The most concerning etiology of hematuria is urothelial malignancy. Smoking is the best-established and the most significant risk factor for the development of urothelial malignancies of the kidney, ureter, and bladder.

Pathophysiology

The presence of blood in the urine can be separated into glomerular and nonglomerular origin. Normal urine contains less than three red blood cells per high power field. The kidney does not excrete red blood cells under physiologic conditions. Therefore, presence of blood in the urine is due to pathology at the glomerulus (glomerular hematuria), allowing excretion of red blood cells into the urine or pathology in the urinary tract distal to the glomerulus (nonglomerular hematuria), which results in blood mixing into the already excreted urine. Nonglomerular hematuria can be further divided into medical and surgical disorders. Except for renal tumors, nonglomerular hematuria of medical/renal origin is due to tubulointerstitial, renovascular, or systemic disorders. Surgical nonglomerular hematuria or essential hematuria includes urologic tumors, stones, and urinary tract infections (Gerber and Brendler, 2011).

The urine dipstick commonly used for the detection of blood in the urine is dependent on the peroxidase-like activity of hemoglobin, which catalyzes the reaction and causes oxidation of the chromogen indicator. False positives can occur in states of hemoglobinuria and myoglobinuria, and microscopic examination of the urine for red blood cells can distinguish hematuria. Glomerular hematuria is suggested when dysmorphic erythrocytes, red blood cell casts, and proteinuria are present. Nonglomerular hematuria can be distinguished from glomerular hematuria in the presence of circular erythrocytes and the absence of erythrocyte casts. In the surgical and medical subcategories of nonglomerular hematuria, surgical hematuria is suggested by the absence of significant proteinuria.

Anticoagulation at normal therapeutic levels does not predispose patients to hematuria. Therefore, patients who have hematuria while receiving anticoagulation therapy should undergo evaluation similarly to patients who are not receiving anticoagulation therapy. In fact, super therapeutic anticoagulation may serve to unmask underlying pathology.

Prevention

Hematuria can be caused by a spectrum of causes. Prevention can be achieved by the prevention of what results in the pathologic state. For example, smoking is a modifiable risk factor in urothelial malignancy. Patients who have never smoked are at low risk for bladder cancer. Smoking cessation can also reduce the risk of developing bladder cancer. Liberal fluid intake and balanced sodium and protein intake can help prevent urolithiasis. Urinary tract infections can also be prevented by good voiding habits, facilitation of complete bladder emptying, and use of vaginal estrogen cream[1] in postmenopausal women.

Clinical Manifestations

The presentation of hematuria is often dependent on the cause. Certain characteristics of the presentation can help in the investigation. Is the hematuria gross or microscopic? Is the hematuria associated with pain? Are there any irritative voiding symptoms? Is there a presence of blood clots? Is it related to exercise? Is there any family history? Is there a presence of rash, arthritis, hemoptysis, upper respiratory infection, skin infection? Is there a history of radiation, diabetes, analgesic abuse? Is there a history of smoking or occupational exposures? Table 1 highlights findings in etiologies of hematuria. Patients with bladder cancer generally present with gross painless hematuria.

Diagnosis

The diagnosis and evaluation of hematuria starts with a careful history, physical examination, and microscopic urine analysis. The cause in an adult patient is urologic malignancy until proven otherwise. Some important questions are outlined in the clinical manifestation section. The physical examination should focus on blood pressure, a cardiovascular examination, an abdominal examination, a palpable mass, costovertebral angle tenderness, and a complete genitourinary examination inclusive of a prostate examination in the male and vaginal examination in the female patient. The assessment should help rule out causes such as infection, menstruation, vigorous exercise, medical renal disease, viral illness, trauma, or recent urologic procedures.

The urine should be collected as a midstream sample, and patients should be instructed to discard the initial 10 mL. The sample should be collected in a sterile cup after gently cleaning the urethral meatus with a sterilization towelette. Uncircumcised men should retract the foreskin before collection. Female patients should be asked to spread the labia adequately to allow cleansing of the urethral meatus and avoid introital contamination. The following patients may require catheterization for collection: menstruating women, obese patients, patient with a nonintact urinary tract, and patients who do intermittent catheterization or have an indwelling urinary catheter (Davis et al., 2012). A urine dipstick can be performed in the office setting, but all samples should be sent for microscopic analysis. As mentioned previously, attention should be paid to dysmorphic erythrocytes, red blood cell casts, and the presence of protein. A urine culture should be performed based on the clinical presentation and findings of urine analysis. Urine cytology does need to be performed as part of the standard workup. The laboratory workup should include an evaluation of the serum creatinine (Davis et al., 2012). Additional helpful tests are serum electrolytes and a complete blood count.

Patients with a urinary tract infection should be treated appropriately and should have a urine analysis repeated in 2 to 6 weeks after treatment. Patients with an identified etiology such as urolithiasis should have a reevaluation of urine after the stone has been passed or treated.

A urologic evaluation of the upper and lower urinary tract is compulsory for patients with gross hematuria. Patients with asymptomatic microscopic hematuria (>3 rbc/hpf) should undergo urologic evaluation once benign causes have been ruled out. The urologic evaluation is especially important for patients with high risk factors for urothelial malignancy, such as age >35, irritative voiding symptoms, chemical exposures, smoking history, or history of urologic disorder or malignancy. Urologic evaluation should include a cystoscopy to evaluate the urethra and bladder. Multiphasic computed tomography with and without intravenous contrast should be performed to evaluate the upper tracts.

---

[1] Not FDA approved for this indication.

TABLE 1 Differential Diagnosis and Findings in Etiologies of Hematuria

DIAGNOSIS	FINDINGS	OTHER
Glomerular		
Familial Hematuria	Abnormal urine analysis	Family history
Systemic Lupus Erythematous	Elevated C3, C4, ANA	Rash, arthritis
Goodpasture Syndrome	Microcytic anemia	Hemoptysis, bleeding tendency
Poststreptococcal Glomerulonephritis	Elevated ASO titer, C3	Recent upper respiratory infection, rash
IgA Nephropathy	Normal ASO and C3, renal biopsy positive for IgA, IgG	Related to exercise
Nonglomerular Medical		
Exercise-Induced Hematuria	Abnormal urine analysis	After strenuous exercise
Papillary Necrosis	Gross hematuria, absence of urolithiasis on CT	Flank pain, African American, analgesic abuse, diabetes
Medullary Sponge Kidney, Polycystic Kidney Disease	Abnormal CT	Family history of renal cystic disease
Renovascular Disease	Renal artery embolus, vein thrombus, AV fistula	Atrial fibrillation, dehydration, bruit
Nonglomerular Surgical		
Urinary Tract Infection	Urine dip with LCE, Nit. Positive urine culture, elevated WBC	Dysuria, fever
Urolithiasis (renal, ureteral, or bladder stone)	Demonstrated on imaging such as CT, ultrasound, KUB	Flank pain, pelvic pain, vomiting, infection, renal obstruction
Urologic Tumor (kidney, ureter, bladder, urethra)	Demonstrated on CT, cystoscopy, ureteropy-eloscopy	Constitutional, irritative symptoms, pain if obstruction, blood clots
Enlarged Prostate or Benign Prostatic Hyperplasia	Enlarged prostate on examination or cystoscopy	Irritative and obstructive voiding symptoms
Radiation Cystitis	Generally gross hematuria, friable tissue on cystoscopy	Irritative voiding symptoms, history of pelvic radiation
Urothelial Strictures (ureter or urethra)	Demonstrated on ureteroscopy, pyelography, cystoscopy, or urethrography	Flank pain, renal insufficiency, bladder outlet obstruction

Sufficient imaging phases should be performed. Ideally, a three-phase study including a noncontrast phase (e.g., stone disease), arterial phase (e.g., renal masses), and excretory phase (e.g., ureteral masses) should be performed (Sudakoff et al., 2008). The urologist can determine the appropriate study if contrasted CT cannot be performed because of allergy or renal insufficiency. Concurrent nephrologic evaluation should occur for patients who are suspected to have glomerular causes, and the evaluation may include further serum testing and renal biopsy (Davis et al., 2012).

Differential Diagnosis

The differential diagnosis of hematuria includes glomerular diseases, nonglomerular medical diseases, and nonglomerular surgical diseases. Table 1 shows a differential diagnosis for hematuria. Hematuria is considered to be from a malignant source until proven otherwise.

Therapy, Monitoring, and Complications

Therapy, monitoring, and complications for hematuria are dependent on the etiology. It is important that hematuria not be ignored even when treated empirically. For example, it is important to recheck a urine analysis after a course of antibiotics for a presumed urinary tract infection. Often, the transient nature of hematuria fools clinicians into thinking that an intervention or observation without the appropriate workup is adequate. Unfortunately, this can result in significant morbidity from the progression of disease, especially in the case of urothelial malignancies.

References

Davis R, Jones SJ, Barocas D, et al: Diagnosis, evaluation and follow-up of asymptomatic microscopic hematuria (AMH) in adults. AUA guideline, *J Urol* 188(Suppl 6): 2473, 2012.

Gerber GS, Brendler CB: Evaluation of the urologic patient: History, physical, and urinalysis. In *Wein Campbell-Walsh Urology*, ed 10th, Philadelphia, 2011, Saunders, pp 73–98.

Khadra MH, Pickard RS, Charlton M, et al: A prospective analysis of 1,930 patients with hematuria to evaluate current diagnostic practice, *J Urol* 163:524, 2000.

Masahito J: Evaluation and management of hematuria, *Prim Care* 37:461, 2010.

Sudakoff GS, Dunn DP, Guralnick ML, et al: Multidetector computerized tomography urography as the primary imaging modality for detecting urinary tract neoplasms in patients with asymptomatic hematuria, *J Urol* 179:862, 2008.

HICCUPS

Method of
Georg A. Petroianu, MD, PhD

Mechanistic Description

Hiccup (Latin, *singultus*) is caused by an involuntary, usually repetitive and rhythmic, spasmodic contraction of the diaphragm (or hemidiaphragm) and accessory inspiratory muscles followed shortly (within 35 msec) by the sudden closure of the glottis. The forcefully inspired air meeting a closed glottis causes the typical hiccup sound. Occasional hiccups are generally perceived as being "funny"; however, hiccupping of extended duration can be incapacitating. Its most common direct consequence is esophagitis, due to concomitant relaxation of the lower esophageal sphincter favoring reflux, but extended hiccupping can also lead to wound dehiscence, depression, weight loss, malnutrition, insomnia, and exhaustion. The possibility of developing tardive dyskinesia weighs against the routine use of this drug

Classifications

Most classifications use arbitrary time limits to categorize hiccupping. Generally hiccups lasting less than 1 day are considered transient (acute), those lasting less than 1 week are labeled persistent, and hiccupping for more than 1 week is described as chronic. A simplified categorization draws the line at 48 hours: any hiccupping episode lasting longer is described as chronic. The practical value of these classifications is questionable; by the time the practitioner sees the patient, almost invariably the case involves persistent or chronic hiccup forms requiring drug therapy. The exceptions (in terms of time between appearance and presentation) are hiccup forms presenting immediately postoperatively or in critical care units. Brief episodes of hiccupping, as experienced by the vast majority of people at some point in time, are certainly physiologic. The point of transition to a pathologic form is not well defined. The rule of thumb of hiccup therapy, however, is that the longer the duration of the hiccupping, the less amenable it will be to nonpharmacologic interventions.

Etiologic classifications are also fraught with problems. Hiccup is not a disease, but a symptom. Literally, there is no known disease that has not been associated with hiccups. Although the categories psychogenic, organic, and idiopathic are most commonly used in practice, the situation most commonly encountered is that of hiccup of unknown (idiopathic) origin. In this context, "idiopathic" describes one's inability to demonstrate, rather than the absence of, an organic origin.

Epidemiology

During intrauterine life, hiccups are universally present, their incidence peaking in the third trimester. They can also be seen regularly in the newborn, the frequency of occurrence decreasing slowly over the first year of life. In adults, occasional transient hiccup is also so frequent that it can be viewed as physiologic. Persistent and chronic idiopathic singultus, the pathologic forms, are rare, their prevalence being estimated at 1 in 100,000. Males are almost exclusively affected (the male-to-female patient ratio is approximately 80:1), suggesting a hormone (estrogen) protective effect. The incidence increases with age. The psychogenic form, though less frequent overall by one order of magnitude, is believed to be more prevalent in females, with an even distribution among all age groups; however, data to support this view are almost nonexistent.

Pathophysiology

The universality of hiccups during fetal life begs the question of purposefulness. As early as 1887, it was suggested that hiccups might represent a necessary and vital primitive reflex that would permit intrauterine training of the diaphragm without aspiration of amniotic fluid. During intrapartum and postpartum maturation, higher centers would then suppress this primitive reflex. Immaturity or damage to the central nervous system would favor the persistence or reappearance of the reflex. The putative reflex arch includes autonomic afferent fibers (the majority vagal fibers) from the digestive tract to a putative medullary hiccup center and motor efferent fibers via the phrenic nerve (diaphragm) and other branches of the vagus nerve to the intrinsic muscles of the larynx adducting the vocal cords. In an analogy with the vomiting center, the assumed role of the medullary hiccup center is to coordinate and fine-tune the sequence of events required for hiccupping; it is therefore a "pattern generator." The concept described, though useful for the purpose of designing a quasi-rational treatment protocol for hiccup, is neither proven nor generally accepted.

Another school of thought that questions the assumption that hiccupping is a reflex phenomenon suggests instead a similarity with cardiac arrhythmias: hiccups would therefore be due to arrhythmias of the breathing center. Still other researchers work on the assumption that hiccup is a myoclonic event, or that it represents brainstem seizures. These views are not necessarily mutually exclusive, because hiccup is not primarily a disease but a symptom, possibly representing different pathophysiologies.

Evaluation of the Hiccup Patient

Hiccup is a symptom associated with a multitude of pathologies. The practitioner must take the hiccupping patient seriously, and for the purpose of finding and treating hidden pathology, persistent and chronic hiccups should be investigated. No consensus exists, however, concerning the extent of such investigations. Even the most enthusiastic users of modern imaging technologies will in most cases end up with a working diagnosis of chronic idiopathic singultus. Nonetheless, a detailed history, a thorough physical examination, and basic laboratory and diagnostic procedures are essential.

History

Ask about previous episodes, as well as precipitating and alleviating factors. The patient who describes vomiting as a "cure" for previous hiccup episodes gives a telltale sign that acidity is an etiologic factor, and omeprazole is a drug to consider. If the patient indicates that hyperventilation is a "sure bet" to worsen his or her hiccups, you can assume that drugs lowering the excitability of the nervous system are likely to help. Elucidating present drug consumption (medical and recreational) is essential: aripiprazole (Abilify), benzodiazepines, barbiturates, alcohol, and steroids are well-known hiccup inducers.

Physical Examination

Foreign bodies in the external auditory canal can induce hiccups, so look in the ears. Examine neck, chest, and abdomen, looking for possible sources of irritation (infection, neoplastic processes, or both) to the vagus and phrenic nerves and the diaphragm. Perform a neurologic examination, keeping in mind the association of hiccup with multiple sclerosis and intracranial processes.

Laboratory and Diagnostic Procedures

An upright chest x-ray, together with complete blood count (CBC) with differential, will help exclude neoplastic or infectious disease. An electrocardiogram (ECG) will help exclude pericarditis and malfunctioning pacemakers, and electrolyte and urea determinations will exclude known metabolic causes (hyponatremia and uremia).

To what extent magnetic resonance imaging (MRI), ultrasound scanning, or endoscopic examinations are necessary is a judgment call, and no generalizations are possible; they might occasionally be indicated.

Nonpharmacologic Interventions

A multitude of nonpharmacologic interventions to terminate hiccup belong to the public-domain hiccup "mythology" or have been described in the medical literature as case reports. Though usually effective in terminating bouts of acute hiccup, they are mostly ineffective in cases of hiccupping that has been present for an extended period. The common denominator of these maneuvers (also used to terminate paroxysmal supraventricular tachycardia) is their ability to directly or indirectly increase efferent vagal activity; the increased parasympathetic tone has a limiting effect on hiccupping. Interestingly, estrogens are also considered to be parasympathomimetic, which offers a plausible explanation of why the singultus prevalence in females is much lower than in males.

Pharmacologic Interventions

Probably only a few drugs in the *Physician's Desk Reference* have not been tried in the therapy of singultus, and anyone who looks hard enough at the literature will be able to find anecdotal support for the use of almost any drug. However, prospective controlled studies to support the use of a particular therapy are very few and rare.

Conceptually, all drugs potentially successful in the therapy of chronic hiccups work either by decreasing the input from the gastrointestinal tract to a (putative) hiccup center or by decreasing the excitability of the nervous system and therefore the output from the (putative) hiccup center.

Sedative-Hypnotics

Both benzodiazepine and barbiturate γ-aminobutyric acid receptor type A (GABA$_A$) agonists have been tried for treatment of hiccups. The consensus is that these substances not only are ineffective but can actually worsen the clinical picture, producing a situation similar to the paradoxical excitation seen with the use of sedatives and explained by inhibitory effects on inhibitory centers.

Antiemetics

Following up on the analogy between the vomiting center and hiccup center as pattern generators, "setron"-class antiemetics (5-HT$_3$ receptor antagonists) have been tried, with no success. Anecdotal evidence hints at possible worsening of the hiccup under the influence of ondansetron (Zofran).[1]

Analeptics

The use of analeptics derives from the concept that hiccup is a suppressed primitive reflex. Analeptics potentiate the central suppression. Although some success has been reported with methylphenidate (Ritalin),[1] caffeine produced failure.

Anticonvulsants

Anticonvulsants (phenytoin [Dilantin],[1] carbamazepine [Tegretol],[1] valproate [Depacon][1]) have been used to try to suppress hiccups. Considering the multitude of pharmacodynamic effects of anticonvulsants, it is not surprising that some success was achieved.

Antipsychotics

Historically, chlorpromazine (Thorazine) has been the most widely used drug for treatment of hiccup, and it is the only drug approved by the FDA for the disorder. Aliphatic phenothiazines such as chlorpromazine have strong sedative, hypotensive, and anticholinergic properties and mild to moderate extrapyramidal effects. For hiccup control, results are mixed at best, and in view of the side effects, routine use is not warranted. Haloperidol (Haldol),[1] a butyropherone derivative, has also been used for hiccup control; again, results are mixed at best, and the possibility of developing tardive dyskinesia weighs heavily against the routine use of this drug.

Antidepressants

The tertiary amine tricyclic antidepressant amitriptyline (Elavil)[1] is one of the oldest players in the therapy of hiccup; its use was being suggested in the mid-1960s. As with anticonvulsants, considering the multitude of pharmacodynamic effects of tricyclic antidepressants, it is not surprising that some success was achieved with these drugs. Their effectiveness is not related to their ability to inhibit monoamine uptake, but probably to their sodium channel blocking properties.

Calcium Channel Blockers

Nifedipine (Adalat)[1] is the dihydropyridine derivative most commonly used for hiccup control. Nimodipine (Nimotop)[1] has also been tried for the same purpose. Interestingly, anecdotal reports about the use of calcium for the same purpose also exist.

Sodium Channel Blockers

The local anesthetic class Ib antidysrhythmic lidocaine (Xylocaine)[1] and its oral analogue mexiletine (Mexitil)[1] have been used for hiccup control, with mixed results.

GABA$_B$ Agonists

Among the substances acting on the nervous system, baclofen (Lioresal)[1] has by far the best credentials in the treatment of chronic hiccup. It is one of the very few substances proven in clinical studies (albeit with small patient numbers) to be efficacious. This γ-aminobutyric acid receptor type B (GABA$_B$) agonist, normally used to lower an increased muscle tone (spasticity), has also been shown to suppress hiccups in an animal (cat) hiccup model. GABA$_B$ agonists, by reducing transmitter release, are generally able to depress complex reflexes.

Antacids

Lowering the acidity of the stomach using H$_2$-receptor blockers or proton pump inhibitors conceptually decreases the input from the gastrointestinal tract to the hiccup center. Omeprazole (Prilosec)[1] has been shown in a limited number of trials to be effective in hiccup treatment.

Gastrokinetic Drugs

One of the few reliable methods to induce a physiologic hiccup in humans is rapidly drinking an ice-cold can of beer on a hot summer day. Although it is highly debatable whether it has to be beer, stomach distention by carbon dioxide induces hiccups. Conversely, reducing stomach distention by using a gastrokinetic drug is helpful in alleviating hiccups. The strongest evidence available for the usefulness of a gastrokinetic drug was for cisapride (Propulsid); however, this selective serotonine 5-HT$_4$-receptor agonist was withdrawn from the market because of its propensity to prolong the QT interval and induce torsades de pointes. The available alternative is the related benzamide metoclopramide (Reglan),[1] a mixed dopamine receptor antagonist, 5-HT$_4$-receptor agonist, and cholinesterase inhibitor, with a long tradition in the treatment of hiccups, going back to the late 1960s. The possibility of developing tardive dyskinesia weighs against the routine use of this drug.

Physical Interventions

Phrenic Nerve Destruction

Irreversible surgical destruction of the phrenic nerve cannot be recommended. Even if hiccup relief is achieved after unilateral local anesthetic blockade of the phrenic nerve without serious compromise in respiratory function, the long-term effects of phrenic nerve destruction are unpredictable. Possible effects include both hiccup reappearance—even after bilateral phrenic nerve transection—and deterioration in respiratory function. More recently, diaphragmatic (phrenic) pacing has been described; however, experience is very limited.

Hypercapnia

Rebreathing in a paper bag is a well-known and reliable remedy for hyperventilation tetany. The increase in blood CO$_2$ levels (hypercapnia) thus induced leads to mild acidosis and thus to a liberation of calcium ions from the protein binding. The increase in plasma-free calcium decreases neuronal excitability, thus terminating not only the tetany but possibly also hiccupping. It was suggested that abolishing the venous-arterial CO$_2$ gradient is required for efficacy of the method. A more high-tech version of this is the induction of normoxic hypercapnia in ventilated patients.

Positive End-Expiratory Pressure

Also practicable only in intubated patients is the application of high positive end-expiratory pressure (PEEP), a high-tech version of the Valsalva maneuver.

Nasogastric Tube

Gastric decompression via a nasogastric tube can terminate hiccups.

---

[1]Not FDA approved for this indication.

[1]Not FDA approved for this indication.

Treatment

The treatment algorithm described is based on the assumption that correctable organic causes have been excluded or treated.

We start therapy with omeprazole (Prilosec)[1] 20 to 40 mg orally (PO) daily. If after 7 days no satisfactory change has occurred, baclofen (Lioresal)[1] is introduced. With baclofen, a "start low, go very slow" approach is indicated in order to avoid excessive drowsiness, weakness, and fatigue. The maximum daily dose is 45 mg. Quite often, patients are already on a proton pump inhibitor (PPI) when presenting. In these cases, immediate introduction of baclofen and continuation of the PPI are recommended. In our experience, the time of response to the combination therapy omeprazole plus baclofen is unpredictable; however, all changes that we observed happened within the first 6 months, and the vast majority within the first 6 weeks. If the desired result is achieved, we continue therapy for another 6 months, after which a very cautious weaning from baclofen is attempted. In cases where the combination therapy omeprazole plus baclofen is not (or not entirely) satisfactory, the addition of gabapentin (Neurontin)[1] or pregabalin (Lyrica)[1] "on the top" can be attempted. As with baclofen, with gabapentin or pregabalin a "start low, go slow" approach is indicated, the maximum dose of 400 mg three times daily or pregabalin 100 mg three times daily used in such cases being reached after 3 weeks. An inverse approach with PPI plus gabapentin or pregabalin as initial combination is also possible.

In addition to any pharmacologic therapy, the practitioner must convey to the patient the feeling that he or she understands and appreciates the seriousness of the condition. Compliance with the treatment is required from the patient, who must understand that success can take time. Lifestyle and habit changes are also required. The hiccup patient must limit the size of meals and avoid carbonated beverages and "gas-forming" foods.

The approach presented here represents our experience in the treatment of chronic singultus. The views expressed are neither guidelines nor regulations.

References

Jatzko A, Stegmeier-Petroianu A, Petroianu GA: Alpha-2-delta ligands for singultus (hiccup) treatment: three case reports, *J Pain Symptom Manage* 33:756–760, 2007.

Petroianu G: Idiopathic chronic hiccup (ICH): phrenic nerve block is not the way to go, *Anesthesiology* 89:1284–1285, 1998.

Petroianu G, Hein G, Petroianu A, et al: Idiopathic chronic hiccup: combination therapy with cisapride, omeprazole, and Baclofen, *Clin Ther* 19:1031–1038, 1997.

Petroianu G, Hein G, Petroianu A, et al: ETICS study: empirical therapy of idiopathic chronic singultus, *Z Gastroenterol* 36:559–566, 1998.

Petroianu G, Hein G, Stegmeier-Petroianu A, et al: Gabapentin "add-on therapy" for idiopathic chronic hiccup (ICH), *J Clin Gastroenterol* 30:321–324, 2000.

Petroianu G: Treatment of hiccup by vagal maneuvers, *J Hist Neurosci* 24:123–136, 2015.

[1]Not FDA approved for this indication.

HOARSENESS AND LARYNGITIS

Method of
Lee Akst, MD

CURRENT THERAPY

- Appropriate treatment of voice complaints depends on accurate diagnosis.
- Supportive therapy is all that is necessary for most cases of acute laryngitis associated with viral upper respiratory tract infections.
- Laryngopharyngeal reflux is a common cause of chronic laryngitis, and appropriate therapy often requires twice-daily administration of proton pump inhibitors for at least 2 months.
- Microlaryngeal phonosurgery may be indicated for some patients with benign phonotraumatic lesions.
- Vocal cord medialization can rehabilitate the voice in a patient with unilateral vocal cord paralysis.
- Many patients with dysphonia benefit from voice therapy, alone or in combination with other treatment strategies.

CURRENT DIAGNOSIS

- The general term to describe vocal difficulty is dysphonia. Hoarseness is a specific term for rough voice quality, which is one type of dysphonia. Laryngitis signifies laryngeal inflammation, which is one possible cause of dysphonia.
- An accurate history and physical examination guide the diagnosis of voice complaints. Although many portions of the examination for dysphonia can be done in a general setting, videostroboscopy is often necessary for diagnosis and may be available only in specialized laryngology offices.
- The most common cause of acute hoarseness is viral laryngitis. Symptoms are self-limited and usually resolve within 2 weeks.
- Dysphonia persisting for longer than 2 weeks suggests the possibility of another diagnosis, such as vocal cord paralysis, neoplasm, phonotraumatic lesion, or chronic laryngitis.
- Indications for referral of a patient with voice complaints to an otolaryngologist include dysphonia that persists for longer than 2 weeks, that is of acute onset during voicing, or that is accompanied by other symptoms such as otalgia, dysphagia, or difficulty breathing.

Voice is an essential component of communication. Vocal difficulty is very distressing to patients and can have a negative impact on physical, social, and emotional qualities of life. To understand the pathophysiology, evaluation, and treatment of voice complaints, it is important to understand the anatomy and physiology of normal voice production. Looking first at how good voice quality is achieved makes it readily apparent how alterations in vocal fold vibration, symmetry, or closure can lead to various vocal difficulties.

To aid discussion of voice complaints, clarification of terminology is necessary. Although "hoarseness" is a term that most patients use to describe any type of voice complaint and "laryngitis" is the presumptive explanation that many patients provide for their symptoms, each of these terms has a more precise meaning. Dysphonia is the general term for vocal difficulty. Hoarseness implies a rough or raspy change in voice quality and is one type of dysphonia. Other categories include limited vocal projection, strained vocal effort, and change in pitch—each of which may occur with or without vocal roughness. The term "laryngitis" specifically describes inflammation of the larynx. This inflammation may be acute or chronic, and again it describes some but certainly not all cases of dysphonia. This distinction will be made clear as the evaluation and management of dysphonia are described.

Normal Laryngeal Function

The larynx plays a central role in voice production by serving as a vibrating instrument that turns airflow from the lungs into sound. The sound is shaped into intelligible speech through the resonating and articulating functions of the pharynx and oral cavity. The ability of the larynx to create vibration and serve as a sound source is a function of its complex, layered microanatomy. The deeper layers of the vocal fold include the thyroarytenoid muscle and the vocal ligament, which position the more superficial layers of the superficial lamina propria and epithelium during phonation. Compared with the fibrous nature of the vocal ligament, the superficial lamina propria is a loose gelatinous layer whose pliability allows for voice production.

During inspiration (Figure 1A), the vocal folds are abducted so that air can move past the larynx without resistance. During phonation (Figure 1B), the vocal folds are held in an adducted position while the lungs drive air toward the larynx. Air pressure builds in the subglottis, beneath the vocal folds, until it overcomes the forces of vocal fold closure, pushes past the vocal folds, and generates negative pressure in its wake as it moves past the larynx. A combination of the vocal folds' intrinsic viscoelasticity and the negative pressure created through Bernoulli's effect draws the vocal fold edges back together, allowing subglottic pressure to rebuild and the cycle to repeat. Repeated cycles of opening and closing at the level of the vocal fold edges generate a so-called mucosal wave, which travels from the inferior edge of each vocal fold up across the medial and superior edges (Figure 1C). These waves may repeat hundreds of times each second, depending on pitch. This cycled opening and closing of the vocal folds during phonation imparts pressure waves to the air column that moves the vocal folds, generating sound. The ability of vocal folds to vibrate easily and symmetrically in this very rapid fashion allows for clear, smooth voicing.

Evaluation of Dysphonia

Central to the evaluation of dysphonia is the understanding that any disruption of vocal fold closure, symmetry, or vibration impairs the ability of the vocal folds to generate a clear sound source. Most voice complaints arise from anatomic or functional limitations in glottal closure or mucosal wave formation, although other parts of the respiratory tree are also responsible for components of the voice. General points concerning evaluation of dysphonia are discussed in this section, with specific causes discussed afterward.

History

A careful history can provide many clues that point toward the proper diagnosis in patients with dysphonia. Although many patients offer the complaint of "hoarseness" as a general term, a careful historian distinguishes between complaints related to voice quality, vocal projection, vocal effort or strain, vocal fatigue, and so on. Two questions that can help a patient organize his or her own thoughts related to poor voice are "What abnormal things does your voice do now that it did not do before?" and "What normal things did your voice do before that it no longer can do?" The acuteness of onset, duration, severity, and progression of any complaint should be determined.

The history should also determine what other factors or events might have caused or exacerbated the dysphonia. Recent sources of laryngeal inflammation might include intubation, excessive voice use, or upper respiratory tract infection. Baseline conditions

that foster chronic laryngeal inflammation include environmental allergies, rhinitis, and laryngopharyngeal reflux. Laryngopharyngeal reflux can exist in the absence of heartburn, with reflux-associated inflammation of the larynx and pharynx providing symptoms of globus pharyngeus, throat clearing, nonproductive cough, effortful swallowing, and even mild dysphagia in association with dysphonia.

Concerning the possibility of laryngeal malignancy, any patient with dysphonia should be asked about smoking and alcohol use, because these are risk factors for squamous cell carcinoma. Another important question in distinguishing inflammatory dysphonia from a mass lesion of the vocal fold concerns whether there are any periods of normal voice or the dysphonia is constant—inflammation may wax and wane, but dysphonia associated with mass lesions is usually progressive and unremitting. Finally, the history should elicit other possible head and neck complaints, including dyspnea, stridor, dysphagia, odynophagia, otalgia, sore throat, and pain with speaking (odynophonia). If hoarseness is associated with some of these symptoms for longer than 2 weeks, the suspicion of malignancy is increased.

Physical Examination

The physical examination for patients with dysphonia includes a complete head and neck evaluation with focus on the larynx and laryngeal function. Although much of the head and neck examination can be performed in a general setting, some portions of the laryngeal examination require specialized equipment found only in some otolaryngology offices that specialize in voice care. Routine head and neck evaluation should include systematic examination of the ears, nose, oral cavity, oropharynx, and neck.

Complaint of otalgia in the setting of an unremarkable ear examination suggests a possibility of referred pain from a lesion of the larynx or pharynx, and is concerning for possible malignancy. Edematous and erythematous nasal mucosa suggests rhinitis, with the possibility of postnasal drip contributing to laryngeal inflammation. Tremor of the tongue or palate might suggest neurologic disorder, whereas pharyngeal erythema and exudate suggest possible acute infection. Pachydermia (cobblestoning) of the posterior pharyngeal wall suggests the possibility of laryngopharyngeal reflux. Tenderness with manipulation of the hyoid bone suggests tension of the strap muscles and correlates closely with complaint of odynophonia and the possibility of muscle tension dysphonia. A neck mass might represent either metastatic lymphadenopathy from a laryngeal malignancy or a primary lesion which itself compresses the recurrent laryngeal nerve and causes paralytic dysphonia. Surgical scarring along the neck suggests the possibility that prior thyroid surgery, carotid endarterectomy, or anterior approach to the cervical spine might have led to vocal fold paralysis.

Laryngeal Examination

Beyond a general examination of the head and neck, there should be directed evaluation of the larynx and laryngeal function. The examiner should listen to the voice carefully, because vocal

Figure 1 A, Normal vocal folds in abducted position for inspiration. B, Normal vocal folds in adducted position for phonation. C, Displacement of the vocal fold medial edges creates mucosal wave propagation during phonation and produces voice.

characteristics such as roughness, breathiness, strain, vocal breaks, and diplophonia (pitch instability, with two different pitches present simultaneously) can help guide the differential diagnosis of dysphonia. Visual examination of the larynx has many forms, ranging from mirror examination to flexible fiberoptic laryngoscopy to videostrobolaryngoscopy.

Mirror examination offers an adequate view of the vocal folds in many patients but may be limited by patient tolerance, physician inexperience, and the inherently limited ability of this technique to brightly illuminate the larynx or record the examination for later review. Flexible laryngoscopy is routinely available in almost all otolaryngology offices, is well tolerated by patients, and offers good views of the larynx that can be recorded with appropriate equipment. Mirror examination and flexible laryngoscopy are limited to observation of vocal fold motion and anatomy but cannot observe laryngeal function because they do not visualize vibration of the vocal folds. To examine vocal fold vibration, videostroboscopy uses a strobe light to create the impression of slow-motion analysis of mucosal waves. Stroboscopy is typically available only in selected otolaryngology practices in which laryngologists specialize in the treatment of voice disorders.

Other Testing
Videostroboscopic evaluation, combined with a thorough history and routine physical examination, can establish the diagnosis for almost all patients with voice complaints, but further testing is sometimes indicated. For instance, electromyography is used by some laryngologists for further evaluation of vocal fold paralysis or paresis. More commonly, radiographic studies are used for further evaluation of some voice complaints. Computed tomography (CT) scans are ordered most often in the evaluation of suspected laryngeal neoplasms and for patients with vocal fold paralysis.

In the case of neoplasm, CT scanning is useful to assess the extent of the primary lesion and to evaluate possible metastatic cervical lymphadenopathy. In patients with laryngeal malignancy, chest radiography is also important to assess for pulmonary metastases. For patients with vocal fold paralysis who do not have a clear history of surgical injury of the recurrent laryngeal nerve, a CT scan from skull base to thoracic inlet identifies possible lesions along the course of the recurrent laryngeal nerve. Central problems are less likely, but if they are suspected as a cause of vocal fold paralysis, then magnetic resonance imaging of the brain may be indicated as well.

Types of Dysphonia
Although not comprehensive, the conditions discussed here account for the vast majority of voice complaints. Some patients with voice complaints have more than one condition, and not every patient will fit neatly into a single category. Nevertheless, understanding how each of these conditions creates dysphonia, and knowing which particular history and physical examination findings might be associated with each cause, can help a physician to appropriately diagnose and manage voice complaints.

Acute Laryngitis
Acute laryngitis is the most common cause of hoarseness and dysphonia. It is most often viral in nature, and onset of laryngeal symptoms may be associated with other symptoms of upper respiratory tract infection, including fever, myalgia, sore throat, and rhinorrhea. Viral inflammation of the vocal folds leads to diminished and more effortful vocal fold vibration, yielding a voice characterized by increased effort and a harsh, strained quality with decreased projection. Characteristic findings on laryngoscopy include vocal fold edema and erythema with decreased amplitude of the mucosal wave. Treatment of acute viral laryngitis is supportive, with counseling for hydration, humidification, and mucolytics. Symptoms generally are self-limited and resolve within 2 weeks. During this time, patients should be instructed to use the voice in a comfortable fashion, rather than straining or pushing to get loudness, because pushing behaviors may lead to the development of persistent muscle tension dysphonia.

Bacterial or fungal infections also cause acute laryngitis in rare cases. With appropriate physical findings and in the right clinical setting, antibiotic or antifungal therapy may be used to treat these conditions. Amoxicillin-clavulanate (Augmentin) is often the antibiotic of choice, and fluconazole (Diflucan) is a commonly used antifungal agent.

Chronic Laryngitis
Chronic laryngitis is the nonspecific condition of prolonged laryngeal inflammation; the term itself does not indicate an etiology for the inflammation. Among the many possible sources for this inflammation are mechanical irritation from traumatic coughing or prolonged speaking, chemical irritation from environmental irritants (e.g., smoking, inhaled medications), and irritation from postnasal drip or laryngopharyngeal reflux. More than one cause may exist simultaneously. Issues related to cigarette use, excessive voice use, medication effect, and rhinitis can be identified with careful history taking. Laryngopharyngeal reflux is a very common source of chronic laryngitis. It may manifest with several nonspecific symptoms, such as throat irritation, globus pharyngeus, frequent throat clearing, and nonproductive cough, with or without accompanying heartburn. Because vocal fold inflammation increases with continued mechanical trauma, the hoarseness of chronic laryngitis typically gets worse with prolonged voice use and improves with voice rest. Examination findings in chronic laryngitis include generalized laryngeal edema and erythema, and careful inspection may also reveal interarytenoid hyperplasia, subglottic edema, laryngeal ventricular obliteration, and an increase in thick glottic secretions.

Treatment of chronic laryngitis is tailored to the cause of the inflammation. Vocal hygiene with moderate voice use and instructions to reduce throat clearing and coughing may diminish mechanical irritation, and smoking cessation is recommended to any smoker with laryngeal complaints. Several studies have suggested that an appropriate trial of proton pump inhibitors for treatment of laryngopharyngeal reflux includes twice-daily therapy for at least 2 months, in contrast to the once-daily dosing often used for typical heartburn complaints. Lifestyle counseling to limit consumption of caffeine, carbonation, alcohol, and acidic foods can improve reflux, and attention to hydration and humidification decreases the viscosity of glottic secretions. For patients who are troubled by vocal difficulties associated with chronic laryngitis, referral to a speech–language pathologist for voice therapy can improve compliance with suggested lifestyle changes and help foster vocal improvement.

Vocal Fold Paralysis
The dysphonia in cases of vocal fold paralysis usually relates to poor vocal fold closure (Figure 2). The result is a breathy voice with limited projection and increased vocal effort. The farther

Figure 2 Vocal fold paralysis prevents the right vocal fold from closing to midline and creates dysphonia.

from midline the immobile vocal fold, the more air leaks through the incompetent glottal valve without being turned into sound. Patients whose immobile vocal fold sits in a lateral position may have severely weak and breathy voices, whereas patients whose immobile vocal fold sits near midline may have a perceptually near-normal conversational voice and complain only of mild increase in effort, vocal fatigue, or problems with loud projection. Because of their glottal insufficiency, patients may complain of "running out of air" with prolonged speech. Impaired glottal closure may also decrease airway protection during swallowing, so patients with vocal fold paralysis need to be questioned about aspiration as well. Whereas rehabilitation of poor voice may be elective, patients with increased aspiration risk need prompt therapy.

Evaluation of vocal fold paralysis includes identification of the cause of paralysis. Surgical injury to the recurrent laryngeal nerve accounts for almost half of all cases of unilateral vocal fold paralysis, and cervical or thoracic neoplasm and idiopathic paralysis account for most of the remaining cases. In a patient without a clear surgical history explaining the paralysis, CT scanning from skull base to mediastinum can identify any possible lesions along the course of the recurrent laryngeal nerve. In those patients whose histories suggest other possible causes (e.g., central neurologic injury, Lyme disease), further investigations, such as magnetic resonance imaging of the brain or blood work may be indicated as well. Some physicians perform laryngeal electromyography to help with the prognosis of paralysis or to differentiate neurologic injury from cricoarytenoid joint fixation; however, this study is neither standardized nor routine in many practices. Although flexible laryngoscopy alone may be satisfactory to document vocal fold immobility, stroboscopy can be added to investigate the impact of glottal insufficiency on vocal cord vibration and possible vocal fold flutter.

Treatment of vocal fold paralysis might include any combination of voice therapy, injection laryngoplasty, transcervical medialization laryngoplasty, and laryngeal reinnervation. Depending on the cause of the paralysis, some patients experience gradual recovery with synkinetic reinnervation or recovery of purposeful vocal fold motion over a period of several months. Based on the degree of voice and swallowing handicap, treatment of patients with vocal fold paralysis may be optional rather than necessary. Voice therapy can help teach patients to produce a stronger voice despite the paralysis, but by itself will not help a paralyzed vocal cord to recover motion. Various medialization techniques have been developed to help reposition an immobile vocal fold in the midline, where the contralateral mobile vocal fold can provide for complete glottal closure and lead to improved voice and swallowing. Injection medialization can be performed in the office or in the operating room, with temporary or permanent materials; if recovery of vocal fold motion is thought possible, then temporary injection is preferred. Transcervical medialization is a permanent but reversible surgical technique performed by otolaryngologists that repositions an immobile vocal fold in the midline. Laryngeal reinnervation offers the possibility of midline positioning of the immobile vocal fold with restored tone and bulk of the vocal fold musculature; however, because results may not mature for several months, this technique is less commonly performed than either injection or transcervical medialization.

Phonotraumatic Lesions: Nodules, Polyps, and Cysts

During vibration, vocal folds are subject to the shearing stresses of vibration. Although vocal fold structure is designed to accommodate these stresses in most circumstances, patients with vocal abuse or excessive voice use are at risk for development of lesions as the result of cumulative phonotrauma. Depending on the location and nature of these lesions, they are categorized as nodules, polyps, or cysts.

Vocal fold nodules are areas of fibrovascular scarring that are located just beneath the epithelium, at the level of the basement membrane and superficial lamina propria. They are typically bilateral and symmetrical, sitting at the junction of the anterior one third and the posterior two thirds of each vocal fold. Polyps are typically unilateral lesions that may be edematous or

Figure 3 A large right hemorrhagic polyp, which can impair vocal fold vibration.

fibrous in nature and may contain hemorrhage (Figure 3). They usually are exophytic and extend outward from the vocal fold epithelium, although the fibrous base of a polyp may extend into the superficial lamina propria of a vocal fold. In contrast to an epithelial-based lesion such as a polyp, a vocal fold cyst is a subepithelial encapsulated lesion that sits entirely within the vocal fold; its size may exert a mass effect that deforms the medial edge of the involved vocal fold. These cysts are occasionally noted as congenital lesions in children, but in adults they are more often caused by traumatic occlusion of the ducts of the seromucinous glands within the larynx.

Nodules, polyps, and cysts cause dysphonia by disturbing vocal fold vibration, leading to rough voice quality. These lesions get larger as traumatic voice use accumulates, and vocal roughness usually becomes more severe and more constant as the lesions progress. Because vibration is more easily disturbed at high pitch, performers with these lesions may notice that high pitch is affected first. Effort of phonation often increases, but projection remains intact. Lesions large enough to limit vocal fold closure may also cause a slightly breathy voice quality. Because patients with excessive voice use are at risk for these lesions, a history of social and occupational voice demands is valuable in cases of suspected phonotrauma.

Treatment for these lesions always begins with voice therapy designed to modify the patient's voice use so as to diminish trauma. Voice therapy may be all that is necessary to allow resolution of some early traumatic changes, particularly in the case of edematous nodules. If dysphonia persists despite voice therapy and other conservative measures, surgery may be considered. Surgery with the goal of voice preservation and restoration (phonosurgery) is typically performed by otolaryngologists who specialize in the care of persons with vocal difficulties. The goal of phonosurgery for these lesions is to remove the lesion that impairs vibration while preserving as much of the remaining, pliable superficial lamina propria as possible, so that vocal fold vibration can be restored.

Reinke's Edema

Reinke's edema, also known as polypoid corditis, is a benign swelling of the vocal folds that is most commonly seen in patients with a long-term smoking history. The edema, a reaction to long-term irritation, accumulates within the superficial lamina propria. The edema is most often bilateral and occurs diffusely along the entire length of the vocal fold, rather than being limited to a more discrete area, as is seen with phonotraumatic polyps (Figure 4). As vocal fold mass increases with disease progression, the pitch of the voice decreases, and this is the change in voice most associated with Reinke's edema. A classic presentation of this condition is a female in her fifth or sixth decade of life who provides a long history of smoking and progressive deepening of her voice. In rare circumstances, the vocal folds gradually accumulate enough

Figure 4 Symmetrical polypoid degeneration of the bilateral vocal folds, characteristic of Reinke's edema.

Figure 5 Recurrent respiratory papillomatosis, whose presence along each vocal fold medial edge disrupts sound production.

edema to compromise the airway, so breathing complaints should be evaluated as well.

Because a significant smoking history is also a risk factor for vocal fold leukoplakia and malignancy, good visualization of the vocal folds is necessary to evaluate for other lesions in these patients. If benign edema of the vocal folds is truly the only lesion noted, management depends on the degree to which voice quality is disturbing to the patient or the degree to which the airway is narrowed. Smoking cessation can lead to stabilization of pitch at its current level, and phonosurgery to remove excess vocal fold mass can help lead to normalization of pitch and improve the airway. Phonosurgery may be performed with cold instruments or with the pulsed photoangiolytic lasers, an emerging therapy; in either case, there is a risk of creating a vocal fold scar that might limit vocal fold vibration even as vocal fold contours are improved.

Recurrent Respiratory Papillomatosis
Recurrent respiratory papillomatosis (Figure 5) is a benign laryngeal neoplasm that is caused by the human papilloma virus. It is the most common source of hoarseness in children, although adults also may be affected. As the lesions grow on the laryngeal epithelium, they create hoarseness and sometimes effortful voice by disrupting vocal fold vibration, particularly if the lesions are located along the medial edge of either vocal fold. Large and bulky lesions may lead to airway compromise, and advanced disease may spread throughout the mucosa of the upper aerodigestive tract rather than being limited to the larynx. Although accurate diagnosis depends on histopathologic analysis, a diagnosis of benign papilloma can be suspected from the characteristic appearance of the vascular fronds, which can be seen under magnified visualization in the office or in the operating room.

Treatment of recurrent respiratory papillomatosis is surgery, which is performed with a carbon dioxide laser, microdebrider, cold instruments, or the emerging technology of pulsed potassium titanyl phosphate (KTP) laser. As its name implies, the condition is recurrent: Even though surgery may reduce or remove the papilloma temporarily, the tissue continues to harbor the papilloma virus, and the disease usually grows back. Because repeated surgeries are expected, the goal of any single procedure is to remove as much disease as possible while limiting surgical scarring of the vocal folds. Scarring created as a result of surgery is cumulative, and over time patients develop persistent dysphonia caused as much by repeated surgeries as by recurrence of the disease. An ability to treat epithelial lesions while limiting scarring at the level of the superficial lamina propria is one main advantage of pulsed laser photoangiolysis; that these pulsed laser procedures can be performed in the office as well as the operating room is another. To help limit the need for repeated surgical procedures, adjunct medical therapies such as interferon and cidofovir are sometimes used for treatment of advanced disease.

Vocal Cord Cancer
In 2008, an estimated 12,250 new cases of laryngeal cancer and 3,670 deaths attributable to laryngeal cancer occurred in the United States. The annual incidence of laryngeal cancer is 6.4 cases per 100,000 for men and 1.3 cases per 100,000 for women. Smoking is the single largest risk factor for laryngeal cancer, and excessive alcohol use has a synergistic effect as a risk factor as well. Survival rates for laryngeal cancer depend on the stage of the tumor at the time of diagnosis, which is a function of tumor size and possible tumor spread to the cervical lymph nodes or distant metastatic sites. Cancers that occur on the medial edge of the vocal fold produce dysphonia while still small, and many laryngeal cancers are diagnosed early.

The dysphonia associated with laryngeal cancer is constant, progressive, and unremitting, without the intermittent vocal improvement that may occur in inflammatory conditions. The presence of dysphagia, odynophagia, otalgia, hemoptysis, or unexplained weight loss further increases the index of suspicion for malignancy. Cervical lymphadenopathy is associated with advanced tumors. Diagnosis may be suspected on the basis of laryngeal examination and is confirmed with biopsy. The presence or absence of mucosal waves on the involved vocal fold on videostroboscopic examination can help predict the depth of the lesion. Both a CT scan of the neck and chest radiographs are indicated to assess for tumor size and spread. Early cancers are treated with surgery or radiation therapy, with similar cure rates. Emerging technologies such as pulsed photoangiolytic lasers may allow for surgical treatment of early disease with better preservation of surrounding normal tissue. More advanced tumors are usually treated with a combination of radiation therapy and surgery or chemotherapy.

Leukoplakia, or a raised white plaque on the epithelial surface, is a visual marker for the likely presence of dysplasia or carcinoma in situ. As a very early lesion, vocal fold leukoplakia may manifest with mild dysphonia or may be found incidentally on head and neck examination performed for other reasons. This early disease may take many years before progressing to invasive carcinoma, and recognition of leukoplakia presents an opportunity for early treatment to prevent progression of disease. Pulsed laser photoangiolysis has emerged as a state-of-the-art therapy for treatment of this epithelial lesion with preservation of the underlying vocal fold pliability.

Neurologic Disorders and the Voice
Neurologic conditions that affect the voice usually do so by causing poor coordination of vocal fold motion. Spasmodic

dysphonia, for instance, leads to involuntary spasms that bring the vocal folds either tightly together (adductor spasmodic dysphonia) or apart (abductor spasmodic dysphonia) during phonation. These spasms lead to vocal breaks that are strained or breathy, respectively. Although the cause of spasmodic dysphonia is thought to lie within the central nervous system, the gold standard treatment of botulinum toxin is targeted at the end organ. Injection of botulinum toxin (Botox)[1] into appropriate laryngeal muscles can weaken these muscles and diminish the spasm.

Vocal fold tremor is a neurologic disorder that is distinct from spasmodic dysphonia. Its hallmark is tremulous voice quality caused by tremor of the larynx, which may occur both during phonation and at rest. Vocal fold tremor may exist alone or as part of systemic tremor. Botulinum toxin[1] can decrease the amplitude of the tremor but may exacerbate the loss of projection that many tremor patients also have as a complaint. Medications such as anxiolytics or β-blockers that are used to treat systemic tremor may also improve the voice in patients with vocal fold tremor without worsening hypophonia.

Functional Voice Disorders

Functional dysphonia may exist by itself or in combination with an anatomic or neurologic source of dysphonia. The most common form of functional voice disorder is muscle tension dysphonia, which describes inappropriate hyperfunction of the supraglottic muscles. This hyperfunction often occurs in response to another source of hoarseness, as the patient tries to force out a strained voice with improved projection rather than accept the limited voice quality that may accompany the other disorder. The hyperfunction may then become an entrenched habit separate from the original pathology. In this sense, a classic scenario for muscle tension dysphonia is a patient who strains to speak more loudly during an acute laryngitis episode and whose strained, squeezed voice pattern persists even after the acute laryngitis has resolved. Patients with muscle tension dysphonia may complain of odynophonia as tension in the involved supraglottic muscles leads to muscular pain with prolonged speaking. Once other lesions have been evaluated, the treatment of muscle tension dysphonia is expert voice therapy with an emphasis on decreased hyperfunction.

Presbylaryngis

Presbylaryngis is the term that is used to describe the aging voice. It typically manifests in the seventh or eighth decade but can develop earlier. Acoustically, presbylaryngis results in a characteristic thinned voice, often with decreased projection and increased vocal strain. The condition occurs as cumulative voice use leads to traumatic thinning of the superficial lamina propria, particularly at the mid-cord level. This loss of superficial lamina propria leads to deficiency at the medial edge of each vocal fold, and a spindle-shaped defect in glottal closure may be noticed with close evaluation. Many patients with a complaint of presbylaryngis find that appropriate voice therapy to address breath support and vocal projection leads to satisfactory improvement in the voice without altering the vocal fold anatomy. For those patients who remain unsatisfied with their voice after therapy, vocal fold medialization procedures can restore straight vocal cord edges and may lead to improved projection; however, currently available injectables and implants that address contour defects cannot restore pliability.

Conclusion

Understanding the anatomy and physiology of normal voice production provides a framework through which dysphonia can be evaluated. Application of this knowledge during the history and physical examination guides the diagnosis of hoarseness and allows clinicians to distinguish among conditions as varied as acute laryngitis, benign phonotraumatic lesions, vocal fold paralysis, and laryngeal cancer as part of a differential diagnosis. Videostrobolaryngoscopy allows evaluation of vocal fold function as well as structure and can confirm diagnosis. As with any condition, accurate diagnosis directs appropriate therapy. Because no further evaluation or management is necessary for acute viral laryngitis, many patients with hoarseness require no more than a careful history and physical examination. However, if dysphonia persists for longer than 2 weeks or is accompanied by other laryngopharyngeal symptoms that are not thought to be related to an upper respiratory tract infection, referral should be made to an otolaryngologist for further evaluation.

References

Koufman JA, Aviv JE, Casiano RR, et al: Laryngopharyngeal reflux: Position statement of the committee on speech, voice, and swallowing disorders of the American Academy of Otolaryngology-Head and Neck Surgery, *Otolaryngol Head Neck Surg* 127:32–35, 2002.

Merati AL, Heman-Ackah YD, Abaza M, et al: Common movement disorders affecting the larynx: A report from the neurolaryngology committee of the AAO-HNS, *Otolaryngol Head Neck Surg* 133:654–665, 2005.

Swibel Rosenthal LH, Benninger MS, Deeb RH: Vocal fold immobility: A longitudinal analysis of etiology over 20 years, *Laryngoscope* 117:1864–1870, 2007.

Wilson JA, Deary IJ, Millar A, et al: The quality of life impact of dysphonia, *Clin Otolaryngol* 27:179–182, 2002.

Zeitels SM, Casiano RR, Gardner GM, et al: Management of common voice problems: Committee report, *Otolaryngol Head Neck Surg* 126:333–348, 2002.

Zeitels SM, Healy GB: Laryngology and phonosurgery, *N Engl J Med* 349:882–892, 2003.

PAIN

Method of
Steven A. House, MD

CURRENT DIAGNOSIS

- Always use history and physical examination and consider imaging or laboratory studies to rule out life- or function-threatening pathologies before merely providing symptomatic treatment.

Acute Pain
- Acute pain has a sudden onset, is usually nociceptive (somatic, visceral) in nature, and likely is due to apparent injury or medical condition.
- It can last up to 3 months and can demonstrate hypersympathetic signs of tachycardia, elevated blood pressure, dilated pupils, or diaphoresis.

Chronic Pain
- Chronic pain is usually gradual in onset, lasts more than 3 months, and rarely serves any purpose. It can manifest with hyperalgesia (hurts more than it should) or allodynia (hurts when it should not, e.g., light touch).
- Vegetative symptoms such as depression, fatigue, or anorexia may be present.
- A significant neuropathic component may be present.
- Psychiatric and social or socioeconomic issues may be exacerbating factors.
- Examples can include headaches, low back pain, osteoarthritis, and fibromyalgia.
- While opioids might be appropriate for some conditions or situations, in general, they are proving to be neither as safe nor as effective for chronic, non-cancer pain as had been believed.

Quality
- Quality of the pain (e.g., sharp, dull, radiating, deep, superficial, lancinating, tingling, burning) is an important factor in determining the best management modalities.
- Quality plays a role in ruling in or ruling out severe disease that can require urgent surgical or other interventions rather than analgesics or adjunctive medications or therapies.

---

[1]Not FDA approved for this indication.

Severity
- Severity of the pain can be rated on a variety of scales such as numerical (0 to 5, 0 to 10), analogue (marked on a line with a range from no pain to the worst possible pain), or facial expression (smiles to grimaces, available for children and the elderly or patients with dementia).
- Functional scales (fully satisfactory function to debilitated) may be more helpful in determining the impact of the pain on the person's life.

CURRENT THERAPY

- Acute pain commonly responds to simple analgesics of the nonopioid, opioid, or combination varieties. Rest, ice, compression, and elevation (RICE) are helpful for acute inflammatory conditions and injuries.
- Chronic pain, because of its complexity, often requires multiple modalities. Pharmacologic options include nonopioid, opioid, adjuvant, or homeopathic medications. Nonpharmacologic options include physical therapy, chiropractic care, transcutaneous electrical nerve stimulation (TENS) unit, acupuncture, or surgical or anesthesia interventions.
- Adjuvant medications are drugs that are used for pain but do not have pain treatment as their primary indication, and they are often the most effective agents in neuropathic and/or chronic pain.
- Opioids are sometimes safer for long-term use, but the individual's risk for falls must be considered in the elderly, as opioids can increase this risk, and the risks of overdose and other adverse effects rise with increasing age and duration of exposure. For many chronic conditions such as low back pain, the evidence supporting the use of opioids is lacking, with efficacy often superseded by nonopioid medications. The risk of addiction MUST be considered before starting opioids on any patient. From 1999 to 2017, overdose death rates have increased from 8.2 to 29.1/100,000 in males and from 3.9 to 14.4 in females; 67.8% of the 70,237 drug overdose deaths in 2017 involved opioids, and the rates were highest in the 25 to 54-year-old age range. According to the CDC, nearly 2 million Americans above the age of 12 years abused or were dependent on opioids in 2014.
- Nonsteroidal antiinflammatory drugs (NSAIDs) carry a risk for GI and cardiac complications, especially in the elderly and those with a history of CAD or GI ulcers or gastritis.
- The patient *must* be involved in and cooperative with the treatment plan. Honesty and trust are necessary components of a therapeutic physician-patient relationship.
- Do not underestimate the placebo effect. If the patient feels that a harmless treatment is beneficial, take advantage of it.
- If the patient is not improving adequately, consult a surgeon if the source of pain is an operable condition, or consult a pain specialist if surgical intervention is not appropriate.

Epidemiology

Although estimates vary, approximately 50 million Americans experience chronic pain and incur costs and overall economic impact is estimated as high as $635 billion per year. Pain is the most common symptom that causes patients to pursue medical evaluation and management. The prevalence of several common pain syndromes including headaches, facial pain, abdominal pain, pelvic pain, and low back pain is slightly higher in women than in men because there are gender variations in the perception, coping, and reporting of pain. Pain tends to be undertreated in women,

people of color, children, and the elderly, and it is underreported in nonverbal or cognitively impaired children and adults.

Risk Factors

Traumatic injury is a cause of acute pain and a risk factor for chronic pain. Patients who have mastectomy, laminectomy, thoracotomy, or amputations are at risk for pain syndromes. Chronic musculoskeletal conditions such as arthritis, spinal stenosis, degenerative disk disease, or fibromyalgia; infectious diseases including HIV or varicella zoster; neuropathies from diagnoses such as diabetes, B_{12} deficiency, or multiple sclerosis; treatment with certain chemotherapies or isoniazid (INH) without adequate vitamin B_6; psychiatric disorders such as depression, anxiety, or posttraumatic stress disorder (PTSD), especially as a consequence of domestic violence; or autoimmune disorders including lupus and rheumatoid arthritis can predispose the individual to chronic pain. Although the risk of pain increases with age, pain should not be considered a usual part of aging until it is appropriately evaluated. A motor vehicle accident or work-related injury or other condition where secondary gain is a possibility, especially if there is no apparent injury, raises the consideration of malingering.

Pathophysiology

Injury or potential injury is detected by nociceptors in the peripheral nervous system, and the signal is then transmitted through the dorsal horn of the spinal cord up to the brain for processing. The three primary classes of opioid receptors are the mu, kappa, and delta receptors, which are located in areas throughout the central and peripheral nervous system. Upon binding these receptors, opioids block calcium channels and modulate the nociceptive pathways. The hyperstimulation of chronic pain (often via the N-methyl-D-aspartate [NMDA] receptor and the resultant increase in intracellular calcium are neurotoxic due to lowering the neuronal firing threshold and increasing firing frequency. This neurotoxicity can lead to ongoing pain in the absence of physical insult. Additionally, NMDA receptor activation can increase pre- and post-synaptic substance P while downregulating the mu receptors. This can decrease the efficacy of mu-agonists, as there are fewer receptors to bind. Neuropathic pain can result from chronic pain or from physical or pathophysiologic injury or changes to the nerve, as in diabetic neuropathy or other neuropathies.

Prevention

The best prevention is a safe and healthy lifestyle. The combination of healthy diet and exercise has been demonstrated to improve pain in osteoarthritis better than either intervention alone, and maintaining a healthy weight can help prevent the arthritis in the first place. Smoking and obesity (odds ratio increasing with BMI) have been associated with chronic pain. Relative to people of normal weight, rates of recurring pain were 20% higher in the overweight, 68% greater with class I obesity, 136% more in class II obesity, and 254% more in the morbidly obese.

Regarding safety, wearing seat belts while driving or using appropriate safety equipment at work and during recreational activities can help reduce the severity of injuries should they occur. Proper body mechanics are important as well.

Clinical Manifestations

Manifestations of pain depend on the location and underlying cause. In the acute setting, the patient can have tachycardia, elevated blood pressure, or diaphoresis, whereas chronic pain can manifest with vegetative symptoms of depression, fatigue, anorexia, or insomnia.

Diagnosis

Pain is most commonly a symptom rather than a disease in and of itself, so it behooves the provider to pursue treatable causes, especially red flag conditions, in addition to providing symptomatic treatment. The history regarding onset (shorter or longer than 3 months), exacerbating or remitting factors, quality, radiation, severity, and timing of the pain (constant versus intermittent), in addition to any associated signs or symptoms such as fever, nausea, vomiting, or diarrhea, can help the provider in that regard. The physical examination is a key component in ruling out life- or function-threatening disorders. Is there tenderness, swelling, bruising, erythema, or deformity? Are strength, reflexes, and sensation intact? Does the patient demonstrate a consistent demeanor (grimace or other signs of pain) and gait (antalgic versus normal) when moving from the waiting area to the examination room and out to the parking lot? The choice to use laboratory studies or imaging is determined by the location of the pain and the structures or organs that might be in that area. When determining severity, "What does the pain keep you from doing?" (which uses function as the measure of impairment and treatment efficacy rather than a subjective pain score to guide therapy) may be a much more helpful question than "How bad is your pain?" If function is not improving, that could be considered a treatment failure, and medications and therapy should be adjusted rather than continuing the same regimen.

Differential Diagnosis

The differential diagnosis for all types of pain is far too extensive for the brevity of this chapter, but in addition to the plethora of physical diagnoses to be considered, the provider must consider that chronic fatigue, depression, and domestic abuse can manifest as a chronic pain syndrome.

Treatment

Nonpharmacologic

Physical therapy for chronic pain (for recent-onset low back pain, relief was statistically but not clinically significant as compared to usual care), TENS units, chiropractic care, and regular exercise have shown benefit in certain conditions. Cognitive behavioral therapy (CBT) and mindfulness training improve function more than pain, and CBT, acupuncture, and mind-body therapies (e.g., yoga, tai chi, mindfulness-based stress reduction) provide safer options that may be both beneficial and cost-effective. Surgery may be required, and interventions such as nerve blocks or epidural injections may also be of benefit. Kyphoplasty and vertebroplasty have fallen out of favor. Aerobic exercise and water therapy are helpful for fibromyalgia, but the patient must not overexert because this can exacerbate the pain.

Pharmacologic

Nonopioid Analgesics

Acetaminophen (Tylenol) is generally a safe and effective medication provided the total daily dose for adults remains less than 3 g/day. For osteoarthritis of the hips and knees, acetaminophen provides modest short-term benefit, and it is not generally effective for the management of low back pain. However, due to its relative safety as compared to other medications, it is certainly worth a try. Chronic use can increase the likelihood of transaminase elevations 4-fold, so this is a consideration when patients are using other potentially hepatotoxic medications. There is an IV preparation available, but the only benefit of the IV over the oral preparations is shorter onset of action. Both the absorption and the action of acetaminophen are augmented by caffeine, so caffeine is utilized in multiple over the counter (OTC) and prescription medications (e.g., Excedrin or Fioricet).

Numerous NSAIDs are available, but none has been shown to be superior to another except for the convenience of dosing daily versus every 6 hours. All are generally safe in the acute setting but should be used with caution if needed long term, and they should be avoided altogether for long-term use in the elderly or patients with cardiovascular, renal, or peptic ulcer disease. This caution includes the cyclooxygenase (COX)-2-specific drugs. Naproxen seems to have the best cardiac profile while the COX-2 drugs tend to have the best GI profile. Misoprostol (Cytotec) or proton pump inhibitors can be used for GI prophylaxis.

Topical agents such as diclofenac (Flector 1.3% Patch, Voltaren 1% Gel), menthol, camphor, lidocaine, and capsaicin (Zostrix Cream, Qutenza 8% Patch) are effective in some patients.

Opioids (Table.1)

For patients with inadequate response to the nonopioid analgesics, opioids are an option (see Table 1). However, the proven efficacy for cancer pain and palliative care as well as some acute pain conditions cannot be extrapolated to chronic pain syndromes. The benefits of opioids in some conditions (e.g., chronic low back pain), and the overall safety of opioids have been called into question due to the dramatic increase in opioid abuse and opioid overdose deaths. Recent research has demonstrated a 2- to 3-fold increase in all-cause mortality with chronic opioid use and up to 11-fold increase if using more than 200 mg/day morphine equivalent dose (MED) and/or sustained-release or long-acting (methadone) preparations. Additionally, risk of overdose death is increased to 3.7- to 4.6-fold at doses of 50 to 100 mg/day MED and as high as 9-fold increased risk for MED >100 mg/day as compared to MED of less than 20 mg/day. After exceeding 200 mg/day MED, 1 in 32 dies. These risks are further escalated by co-administration of benzodiazepines or gabapentinoids. A prescription for naltrexone should be considered if the patient is using >50 mg MED per day, and it is highly recommended if using >100 mg MED per day. A useful calculator to calculate MED can be found at http://www.agencymeddirectors.wa.gov/calculator/dosecalculator.htm

According to the CDC, opioids were implicated in 71% of the pharmaceutical overdose deaths in 2013, and 60% were legally prescribed by a single provider. Opioids might be a safer option in the elderly as compared to NSAIDs, but they can increase fall risk. They should be avoided in patients with untreated sleep apnea because of increased risk for complications, especially in combination with benzodiazepines. This risk increases with age with as much as an eightfold increase for those older than 80 years of age. The risk of postoperative respiratory depression also increases with age. The risks of using chronic opioids likely outweigh the benefits in the management of headache, fibromyalgia, and chronic low back pain, according to a 2014 position paper from the American Academy of Neurology.

The risks and the adverse outcomes (abuse, addiction, overdose, and death) related to this class of medications culminated in the release of guidelines with twelve recommendations from the CDC in March 2016 for the prescribing of opioids for chronic pain. A brief summary of the author's recommendations: (1) Nonpharmacologic therapy and nonopioids are preferred for chronic pain. (2) Benefits of opioids on pain and function need to outweigh the risks. Screen for risk of dependence. (3) Establish treatment goals with the patient and discuss plan to discontinue opioids if treatment fails. (4) On initiation, use immediate release rather than ER/LA (extended release, long-acting) preparations. (5) Use the lowest effective dose, and reassess risks if dose is increased, especially if greater than 50 mg MED per day. (See Table 1 for equivalent doses.) (6) Acute pain should be treated acutely; less than 3 days usually but no more than 7 days. (7) Reassess within 1 to 4 weeks of initiation of treatment or dose escalation and at least every 3 months thereafter. Discontinue if benefits do not justify risk. (8) Consider prescribing naloxone if there is concurrent benzodiazepine use, a history of overdose, or MED >50 mg/day. (9) Use state drug monitoring programs at initiation and at least every 3 months. (10) Obtain a urine drug screen at initiation and at least annually. Nothing but the prescribed medications should be present. (Additionally, consider testing periodically for the presence of prescribed NSAIDs and adjuvant medications to assess compliance with the whole treatment plan rather than just the opioid.) (11) Avoid concurrent with benzodiazepines. (12) Offer or arrange evidence-based treatment for patients with opioid use disorder.

In addition to these steps, multiple drugs have been formulated with "abuse-deterrent" properties. Preparations that meet the FDA's Guidance for Industry regarding abuse-deterrent opioids include: OxyContin (oxycodone), Targiniq ER (oxycodone/

TABLE 1	Opioid Analgesics, Equianalgesic Table			
	ADMINISTRATION			
OPIOID	**PARENTERAL**	**ORAL**	**PROPERTIES**	

OPIOID	**PARENTERAL**	**ORAL**	**PROPERTIES**
Buprenorphine			
Butrans transdermal patch: 5, 7.5, 10, 15, 20 µg/h weekly patches Subutex* SL tab and film: 2, 8 mg Buprenex injection: 0.3 mg/mL	0.3 mg (IV) Patch: MED <30 mg/day = 5 µg/h patch 30–80 mg/day = 10 µg/h patch; >80 mg/day: do not use	Oral buprenorphine, with or without naloxone (Suboxone, Subutex) is limited to treatment of opiate addiction Requires training, approval, and new DEA number	Partial agonist Can cause QT prolongation C-III
Codeine			
Tablet: 15, 30, 60 mg Oral solution: 15 mg/5 mL	130 mg	180 mg	Prodrug converted by liver to morphine About 10% of population cannot convert, and some are rapid metabolizers, resulting in increased levels of morphine Ceiling dose is 60 mg/dose
Fentanyl			
Duragesic 72 h patch: 12, 25, 37.5, 50, 62.5, 75, 87.5, 100 µg/h	~100 µg/h	—	Patch for those who cannot swallow Patient *must* have subcutaneous fat, because drug is lipophilic
Actiq or Oralet lozenge: 200, 400, 600, 800, 1200, 1600 µg Fentora buccal tab or Abstral SL tab: 100, 200, 300, 400, 600, 800 µg Subsys sublingual spray: 100, 200, 400, 600, 800 µg/spray. Lazanda nasal: 100, 300, 400 mcg/spray. Fentanyl injection: 50 mcg/mL.	No conversion for lozenges or buccal tabs; various formulations are not bioequivalent, so use caution when switching from one formulation to another; *must* start at lowest dose and titrate	~½ × daily morphine dose, disregarding units, e.g., 200 mg morphine PO/day = 100 µg/h patch	Lozenge or buccal tab for transmucosal use No cheap forms available Buccal formulations *only* indicated for breakthrough cancer pain in the opioid tolerant; can be rapidly fatal in opioid naïve patients.
Hydrocodone			
Tab: 2.5, 5, 7.5, 10 mg with a max of 325 mg APAP per tablet (Norco, Lortab) as of 2014. (Lorcet no longer available) or with 200 mg ibuprofen (Vicoprofen 7.5/200; Ibudone 5/200, 10/200; Reprexain 2.5/200, 5/200, 10/200); Zohydro ER: 10, 15, 20, 30, 40, 50 mg/cap q 12 h; Vantrela ER: 15, 30, 45, 60, 90 mg tab q 12 h; Hysingla ER: 20, 30, 40, 60, 80, 100, 120 mg tabs q 24 h; Solution: with APAP 7.5/325, 10/325 per 15 mL.	N/A	20 mg	C-II as of 2014, so refills and phone orders are no longer allowed. Metabolized to hydromorphone and others
Hydromorphone (Dilaudid)			
Tab: 2, 4, 8 mg Liquid: 1 mg/mL Suppository: 3 mg SR† 24-h tab (Exalgo): 8, 12, 16, 32 mg Injection: 1, 2, 4, 10 mg/mL pre-filled syringes and 1, 2, 4 mg/mL vials.	1.5 mg	7.5 mg	Good alternative to morphine, especially if using SC by continuous infusion (>20 mg/h) Active glucuronide metabolites
Meperidine (Demerol)			
Tab: 50, 100 mg Syrup: 50 mg/5 mL	100 mg	300 mg	Indicated for *acute* use *only* (i.e., <48 h) Contraindicated with MAOI and/or renal disease: neurotoxic metabolite normeperidine can cause seizures and death
Methadone (Dolophine)			
Tab: 5, 10, 40 mg Oral liquid: 1, 2, 10 mg/mL* 40 mg dispersible tab (Methadose)—restricted use in United States, mostly for detox or addiction maintenance dosing		Variable conversion ratios (see Table 2): converted by oral morphine equivalent dose	At least 3 mechanisms: mu agonist, NMDA receptor antagonist, norepinephrine–serotonin reuptake inhibition The longest-acting opioid Cheap: ~ 1¢/mg Can cause QT prolongation Torsades de pointes is more likely with IV dosing STRONGLY consider risks before prescribing. Safety guidelines available from the American Pain Society.

Continued

I Symptomatic Care Pending Diagnosis

	TABLE 1	Opioid Analgesics.—cont'd		

OPIOID	ADMINISTRATION		PROPERTIES
	PARENTERAL	ORAL	
Morphine			
Tab: 15, 30 mg Liquid: 10, 20, or 100 mg/5 mL (Roxanol) SR† 12-h tab (MS Contin): 15, 30, 60, 100, 200 mg SR† 12-h tab (Oramorph SR): 15, 30, 60, 100 mg SR† 24-h cap (Kadian): 10, 20, 30, 50, 60, 80, 100, 200 mg SR† 24-h cap (Avinza): 30, 45, 60, 75, 90, 120 mg SR† cap with naltrexone (Embeda): 20/0.8, 30/1.2, 50/2, 60/2.4, 80/3.2, 100/4 mg Suppository: 5, 10, 20, 30 mg	10 mg	30 mg	Numerous routes; very cheap, readily available; active metabolites, morphine-6-glucuronide 10 × more potent than morphine Avinza and Kadian capsules may be opened and beads sprinkled in applesauce, but the beads should not be crushed Avinza may be opened into apple juice and injected via gastric tube Kadian may be opened into water and given by gastric tube
Oxycodone			
Tab: 5, 10, 15, 20, 30 mg Liquid: 5 mg/5 mL or 20 mg/mL (Oxy-Fast) SR† 12-h tab (generic, OxyContin): 10, 15, 20, 30, 40, 60, 80 mg SR† 12-h w/naltrexone (Troxyca ER caps): 10/1.2, 20/2.4, 30/3.6, 40/4.8, 60/7.2, 80/9.6 mg oxycodone/naltrexone Multiple combinations w/APAP (Percocet, Endocet, Tylox) SR† 12-h w/APAP 7.5/325 (Xartemis XR)	N/A	20 mg	Equal potency but a little more bioavailable than morphine Caution in liver disease: T½ extends up to 4 × normal. Metabolized to oxymorphone: 40 × more potent than oxycodone ER/LA. Opioids require REMS.
Oxymorphone			
Tab: 5, 10 mg (Opana); in opioid-naïve patients, starting dose > 20 mg/day is not recommended	1 mg	10 mg	Potentiated by cimetidine (Tagamet), MAOIs, and other CNS depressants 10% bioavailability Caution with CrCl < 50 or with liver impairment Take 1 h before or 2 h after food (food increases absorption)

*Only approved in the United States for the treatment of opioid dependence.
†Sustained-release formulations should never be crushed.
APAP, Acetaminophen (N-acetyl-*p*-aminophenol); *bid*, two times per day; *CNS*, central nervous system; *CrCl*, creatinine clearance; *IM*, intramuscular; *IV*, intravenous; *MAOI*, monoamine oxidase inhibitor; *MED*, morphine equivalent dose; *NMDA*, N-methyl-D-aspartate; *po*, by mouth; *pr*, per rectum; *prn*, as needed; *qw4h*, every four hours; *q6h*, every 6 hours; *q8h*, every 8 hours; *qAC*, before meals; *qd*, daily; *qHS*, at bedtime; *SC*, subcutaneous; *tid*, three times per day.

naloxone), Embeda (morphine/naltrexone), Hysingla ER (hydrocodone), MorphaBond ER (morphine), Xtampza ER (oxycodone), Troxyca ER (oxycodone/naltrexone), Arymo ER (morphine), Vantrela ER (hydrocodone), and RoxyBond (oxycodone). Unfortunately, there are no generic opioids with FDA-approved abuse-deterrent labeling.

Tramadol (Ultram, ConZip) is a weak mu-agonist and an inhibitor of norepinephrine and serotonin uptake, a quality that gives it a niche in the treatment of neuropathic and radicular pain.[1] It is the only opioid studied for fibromyalgia in a randomized trial. While it was found to be beneficial, this is likely due to its inhibition of serotonin and norepinephrine uptake rather than its weak mu-agonism. A study has demonstrated an increased risk for hypoglycemia, notably in the first 30 days of treatment with tramadol.

Codeine is a prodrug that must be converted to morphine to be effective, and about 10% of the population lacks the cytochrome P450 2D6 enzyme that makes the conversion, resulting in poor analgesic response. Owing to the need for conversion, doses exceeding 60 mg do not increase benefit because the enzyme system is saturated. Avoid prescribing codeine to children, as deaths have been reported, even with the use of age- and weight-appropriate dosages, as a result of the hypermetabolism of codeine to morphine.

Morphine is the prototype for the opioids. It is extremely versatile, it can be given via almost any route, and it is available in multiple dosages and preparations ranging from liquid to daily sustained release. Hydromorphone (Dilaudid, Exalgo) shares similar qualities but is more potent. Hydrocodone is only available in a sustained-release oral form (Zohydro ER, Hysingla ER), and in combination with acetaminophen (Lortab, Norco, Vicodin). It was rescheduled by the DEA to schedule II in 2014. It had been the number-one prescribed medication in the United States for several years until the rescheduling, which led to >20% reduction in prescriptions and >16% reduction in tablets dispensed.

Methadone (Dolophine) is the longest acting of the opioids at a half-life of 23 hours, although the duration of action can be variable. It is active as an NMDA receptor antagonist, inhibits norepinephrine and serotonin uptake, and is an agonist at the mu receptor. Therefore, methadone can be effective when other opioids fail, especially in the case of chronic or neuropathic pain, where the NMDA receptor is more of a factor in pain control. It must be used with caution (Table 2) because it can prolong the QT interval and has an increased dose-dependent risk of respiratory depression as compared to other opioids.

Meperidine (Demerol) is relatively weak compared to morphine and others, and it is limited by poor oral bioavailability, a 48-hour acute pain indication, and the neurotoxicity of one of its metabolites, normeperidine (renally cleared, so it is contraindicated in renal patients). Other opioids are safer and more effective, so its use should be limited.

The mu agonists, other than codeine, meperidine, and tramadol, do not technically have a ceiling dose; however, the dose should be

[1]Not FDA approved for this indication.

TABLE 2 Morphine and Methadone Equivalents

MORPHINE (DAILY REQUIREMENT)	METHADONE EQUIVALENT
<500 mg	5:1
500–1000 mg	10:1
>1000 mg	20:1

Acute pain: methadone = morphine (1:1). Chronic pain: The above conversion is for illustration of the complexity of methadone use. A more detailed table should be referenced before prescribing, and methadone should be used with extreme caution because of the risk for cardiac complications and respiratory depression. Many sources recommend starting at 10% of the calculated equianalgesic dose of methadone.

limited to the lowest effective dose, keeping in mind the possible adverse effects and increased risk of death with higher doses. In the purely palliative or hospice patient, the dosage may be titrated to effect until the pain is relieved or side effects limit the dosage.

The mixed agonist-antagonists such as nalbuphine (Nubain), pentazocine (Talwin), and butorphanol (Stadol) tend to have a higher incidence of hallucination and confusion, and because they are agonists at kappa and delta receptors and antagonists at the mu receptor, they can produce withdrawal symptoms in patients who are routinely taking mu agonists. The partial agonist buprenorphine (Butrans patch, Subutex, Buprenex) is dose limited because it has a maximal effective dose as well as a potential to cause QT prolongation.

Patients who are taking opioids on a chronic basis should use a stimulant laxative such as senna with or without docusate, because fiber and dietary modification are usually inadequate for opioid-induced constipation, and fiber can aggravate the problem. Lubiprostone (Amitiza) can be used for opioid-induced constipation at the 24 mcg twice-daily dose. Naloxegol (Movantik), naldemedine (Symproic), and methylnaltrexone (Relistor) are peripheral rather than central mu antagonists, so they are indicated for managing opioid-induced constipation without negatively impacting pain control. Bisacodyl should not be used chronically due to its potential to damage the myenteric plexus of the gut and cause severe and permanent impairment of colonic motility; however, for PRN use, it can be quite effective with the suppository having quicker onset of action than the tablet.

Adjuvant Drugs

Adjuvant medications are drugs that are useful in the management of pain but do not have pain treatment as an indication. Some adjuvant medications such as duloxetine (Cymbalta) and pregabalin (Lyrica) have received an FDA indication for diabetic peripheral neuropathic pain. Tricyclic antidepressants are useful for chronic pain and they have the benefit, unlike duloxetine, of working at the lowest doses rather than having to titrate to the maximum dose to gain benefit.

Several anticonvulsants have demonstrated efficacy in the management of pain, most notably gabapentin (Neurontin)[1], pregabalin (Lyrica), and carbamazepine (Tegretol)[1]. Others have been tested in trials, but these three have the most evidence to support their use. Gabapentin and pregabalin have the benefit of not requiring monitoring of blood levels or for marrow, liver, or renal toxicities. Gabapentin (Neurontin)[1] has been beneficial using a single dose of 1200 mg preoperatively, notably in combination with celecoxib (Celebrex)[1], in reducing postoperative opioid requirements in mastectomy, laminectomy, and thoracotomy patients. The benefits of the gabapentinoids, a.k.a. α-2-δ-ligand calcium channel blockers, in peripheral neuropathies have been inappropriately extrapolated to pain related to radiculopathy. Significant benefits in lumbar and cervical radiculopathy have not been demonstrated in randomized trials.

Corticosteroids can be beneficial in inflammatory conditions, nerve or spinal cord compression, or increased intracranial pressure due to neoplasms. Any can help, but blood pressure elevations and fluid retention can be problematic in all but dexamethasone (Decadron)[1], which lacks mineralocorticoid activity. Steroids also have the downside of elevating blood glucose and, in long-term use, causing osteoporosis and a host of other problems, including Cushing syndrome.

Muscle relaxants may be beneficial if muscle spasm is a source of pain, but there is insufficient evidence to determine relative efficacy or safety. Of these, two stand out: metaxalone (Skelaxin), which lacks the black-box warning for the operation of heavy equipment, and tizanidine (Zanaflex), which can antagonize α_1 receptors in the spinal cord to provide additional pain relief. In chronic use, the patient will need to be monitored for anemia and leukopenia with metaxalone and for liver abnormalities with tizanidine. Cyclobenzaprine (Flexeril) plus naproxen was not superior to naproxen alone for low back pain.

Calcitonin (Miacalcin)[1] has shown very modest benefit for pain due to osteoporotic vertebral compression fractures, but it shows no benefit for compression fractures due to bone metastasis.

Ziconotide (Prialt) has demonstrated benefit as well as safety for long-term pain management, but it is limited to only intrathecal use owing to gastrointestinal side effects.

Caffeine can modulate pain via action upon adenosine receptors that are involved in nociception. It is found in several over-the-counter analgesics, notably for migraine treatment. Regarding alternative medications, riboflavin,[7] butterbur,[7] and coenzyme Q10 (CoQ10)[7] are effective for migraine prophylaxis. Glucosamine,[7] S-adenosylmethionine (SAM-e)[7], methylsulfonylmethane (MSM),[7] and willow bark[7] are likely effective for arthritic and low-back pain.

Acetyl-L-carnitine (ALC)[7] had demonstrated efficacy in diabetic neuropathy at 2 to 3 g/day. Capsaicin 0.075% cream (Zostrix) and 8% patch (Qutenza) have demonstrated benefit for peripheral neuropathy,[1] post-herpetic neuralgia, and HIV-associated neuropathy.[1]

Numerous medications in multiple drug classes have been studied for fibromyalgia, but many of the trials are small and/or of poor quality. Of these drugs, duloxetine (Cymbalta), pregabalin (Lyrica), and milnacipran (Savella) have received an FDA indication for fibromyalgia; gabapentin (Neurontin)[1], ondansetron (Zofran)[1], and naltrexone (Depade, Revia)[1] demonstrated modest benefit. The greatest benefit seems to be achieved by duloxetine and tricyclic antidepressants.

The use of cannabinoids has become legal in some states; however, their use for the management of pain is somewhat controversial, as the studies evaluating these drugs are often of low to modest quality. A 2015 systematic review and meta-analysis showed mild reductions in pain, but the comparison groups were placebo rather than standard care. Additionally, cannabinoids are not without adverse effects, including impacts on cognition, motivation, reaction time, and psychosis in a 2016 review. Negative impacts could be even greater as unintended consequences of medical and/or recreational use come to light. Isolation of the various compounds such as cannabidiol and β-caryophyllene from others like Δ9-tetrahydrocannabinol (THC) could improve benefit, including oral administration, while limiting adverse physical and psychological effects. The cannabinoids do show some promise, but they need to be studied further and subjected to the same scientific rigor as any other medication in the FDA approval process.

Monitoring

Controlled-substance agreements are beneficial in setting the boundaries for the use of opioid pain relievers (Figure 1). Routine visits are necessary to document ongoing need for and adequate response to the prescribed regimen. Routine drug screening is beneficial for monitoring compliance with the opioid as well as nonopioid medications. However, the provider needs to be aware of the metabolites of the different drugs. Hydromorphone (Dilaudid) and

---

[1]Not FDA approved for this indication.

[1]Not FDA approved for this indication.
[7]Available as a dietary supplement.

Controlled Substances Agreement Template

1. This agreement is provided to prevent misunderstandings about policies regarding medications designated by the DEA as "controlled substances" that you will be taking for pain management or other medical conditions.

2. I understand that my provider is consenting to treat me based on this Agreement.

3. I understand that if I break this Agreement, my provider might stop prescribing these medications, whether by tapering my medication, discontinuing the medication and prescribing another medication to treat the withdrawal symptoms, or discontinuing the medication and referring me to a detoxification program.

4. I will communicate fully and honestly with my provider about the character and intensity of my pain, the effect that my pain has on my daily life and how well the medication is helping to relieve my pain. I will take the medication ONLY as prescribed and for the treatment of my physical pain as opposed to emotional or psychological distress (i.e., to get high).

5. My physician may prescribe other medications (adjuvant medications) or non-pharmacological therapies (physical therapy, TENS unit, etc.) to help with certain aspects of pain such as muscle spasm, burning, tingling or radiating pain. I will comply with this treatment with the same diligence as is expected for my controlled medication.

6. I will not use ANY illegal substances or any legal medication not prescribed to me. Additionally, I understand that alcohol, although legal, should not be used in conjunction with my medication as the combination could be fatal.

7. I will not share, sell or trade my medications with anyone.

8. I will use only one provider and one pharmacy for my medications unless otherwise agreed upon with my provider.

9. I am responsible for my own prescriptions and medications. I will safeguard my written prescription and medications from loss or theft, understanding they will not be replaced. I will secure my medication in a lock box or safe out of the reach of children at all times.

10. I understand that refills of my prescriptions will be made at the time of an office visit or during regular office hours and never during evenings or weekends when the office is closed.

11. I authorize my provider and my pharmacy to cooperate fully with any city, state and/or federal law enforcement agency in the investigation of any possible misuse, sale or other diversion of my medications.

12. I agree to submit to a blood or urine test, if requested by my provider, in order to determine my compliance with my medication program.

13. I understand that the use of these medications may adversely affect my ability to drive, operate machinery or perform certain tasks, and I agree not to attempt these tasks under the influence of medication. Additional risks include low testosterone, depression, sleep disturbances, constipation, respiratory depression, and death.

14. I understand that smoking cessation and a healthy lifestyle can be helpful in achieving control of pain. I will strive toward smoking cessation, a healthy diet, and exercise as my condition allows.

15. I agree to these guidelines, and they have been fully explained to me. All of my questions and concerns regarding treatment have been adequately answered.

I agree to use _____ pharmacy, and only this pharmacy, for my prescriptions for controlled substances.

This Agreement entered on this date: _____

Patient / Parent / Guardian signature:_____

Provider signature:_____

Figure 1 Controlled substances agreement.

oxymorphone (Opana) are metabolites of hydrocodone (Lortab, Norco) and oxycodone (Percocet, Endocet, OxyContin), respectively. All states except Missouri have prescription-monitoring programs that allow providers to monitor for the use of multiple providers and pharmacies to obtain controlled medications. Rules governing the prescribing and use of controlled substances vary among states, so the provider should be knowledgeable of local regulations as well as federal DEA requirements.

Complications

The Centers for Disease Control and Prevention (CDC) reported in 2011 that opioid pain relievers were involved in 73.8% of the 20,044 prescription drug overdose deaths. By 2017, overdose deaths increased to 70,237 with 47,600 (67.8%) involving opioids. Of the 47,600 overdoses, deaths were mostly driven by synthetic opioids other than methadone (i.e., fentanyl, fentanyl analogs, and tramadol [60%], followed by heroin [32.5%], natural and semi-synthetic, for example, hydrocodone and oxycodone [30.5%], and methadone [6.7%]. (Percentages do not equal 100% due to some deaths involving more than one drug.) There are over 130 opioid overdose deaths per day in the United States. From 1999 to 2017, overdose death rates have increased from 8.2 to 29.1/100,000 in males and from 3.9 to 14.4 in females, and the rates were highest in the 25- to 54-year-old age range. Medicaid populations are at greater risk of opioid overdose than non-Medicaid populations, and prescription drug overdose death rates are higher in the more rural and impoverished counties.

In addition to the deaths, there is a significant cost burden of substance abuse treatment admissions, with the 2008 rates being six times the 1999 rate. Nonmedical use of opioids represents up to $78.5 billion in healthcare costs, lost productivity, addiction management, and legal and law enforcement involvement. Drug addiction is very real, and about 15% of patients may be genetically predisposed to addiction; therefore, clinicians should strongly consider this in their risk/benefit analysis before exposing a patient to these powerful medications. About 25% of opioid-managed chronic pain patients misuse the medications, and about 10% develop opioid use disorders. Using a tool such as the Opioid Risk Tool may be helpful in determining the risk of addiction in a particular individual.

Long-term safety of opioids has not been demonstrated, and chronic use has been associated with sleep disorders, adrenal suppression, and hypogonadism (and secondary erectile dysfunction and depression) among other problems.

References

Baratloo A, Rouhipour A, Forouzanfar MM, et al: The role of caffeine in pain management: a brief literature review, *Anesth Pain Med* 6(3):e33193, 2016, Published online March 26, 2016.
Center for Behavioral Health Statistics and Quality (CBHSQ): *2017 National Survey on Drug Use and Health: Detailed Tables*, Rockville, MD, 2018, Substance Abuse and Mental Health Services Administration2018, 05.24.2019 https://www.samhsa.gov/data/nsduh/reports-detailed-tables-2017-NSDUH[Accessed 05.24.19]
Chou R, Peterson K, Helfand M: Comparative efficacy and safety of skeletal muscle relaxants for spasticity and musculoskeletal conditions, *J Pain Sympt Manage* 28:140–175, 2004.
Dowell D, Haegerich TM, Chou R: CDC guideline for prescribing opioids for chronic pain—United States, *JAMA*, March 15, March 15.
Franklin GM: Opioids for chronic noncancer pain: a position paper of the American Academy of Neurology, *Neurology* 83:1277–1284, 2014.
Fritz JM, Magel JS, McFadden M, et al: Early physical therapy vs usual care in patients with recent- onset low back pain: a randomized clinical trial, *JAMA* 314(14):1459–1467, 2015.
Gomes T, Mandani MM, Dhalla IA, Paterson JM, Juurlink DN: Opioid dose and drug-related mortality in patients with nonmalignant pain, *Arch Intern Med* 171(6):686–691, 2011.
Hedegaard H, Minino A, Warner M: *Drug Overdose Deaths in the United States, 1999-2017. NCHS Data Brief, No. 329*, November 2018, 05.24.2019 https://www.cdc.gov/nchs/data/databriefs/db329-h.pdf. .
Jellin JM, Gregory PJ, et al: *Pharmacist's Letter/Prescriber's Letter Natural Medicines Comprehensive Database*, ed 12, Stockton, CA, 2009, Therapeutic Research Faculty2009.
Jones CM, Lurie PG, Throckmorton DC: Effect of US Drug Enforcement Administration's rescheduling of hydrocodone combination analgesic products on opioid analgesic prescribing, *JAMA Intern Med* 176(3):399–402, 2016, https://doi.org/10.1001/jamainternmed.2015.7799.
Machado GC, Maher CG, Ferreira PH, et al: Efficacy and safety of paracetamol for spinal pain and osteoarthritis: systematic review and meta-analysis of randomised placebo controlled trials, *BMJ* 350:h1225, 2014. Accessed 20 April 2019.
Okifuji A, Hare BD: The association between chronic pain and obesity, *Journal of Pain Research* 8:399–408, 2015. https://doi.org/10.2147/JPR.S55598.
Onysko M, Legerski P, Potthoff J, Erlandson E: Targeting neuropathic pain: consider these alternatives, *J Fam Pract* 64(8):470–475, 2015.
Scholl L, Seth P, Kariisa M, Wilson N, Baldwin G. Drug and opioid-involved overdose deaths – United States, 2013-2017. *Morb Mortal Wkly Rep*. ePub: 21 December 2018.
Seth P, Scholl L, Rudd RA, Bacon S: Increases and geographic variations in overdose deaths involving opioids, cocaine, and psychostimulants with abuse potential—United States, 2015-2016, *MMWR Morb Mortal Wkly Rep*. ePub: March 29, ePub: March 29.
Volkow ND, Swanson JM, Evins AE, et al: Effects of cannabis use on human behavior, including cognition, motivation, and psychosis: a review, *JAMA Psychiatry* 73(3):292–297, 2016.
Vowles KE, McEntee ML, Julnes PS, Frohe T, Ney JP, van der Goes DN: Rates of opioid misuse, abuse, and addiction in chronic pain: a systematic review and data synthesis, *Pain* 156(4):569–576, 2015, https://doi.org/10.1097/01.j.pain.0000460357.01998.f1.
Whiting PF, Wolff RF, Deshpande S, et al: Cannabinoids for medical use: a systematic review and meta-analysis, *JAMA* 313(24):2456–2473, 2015.

PALLIATIVE AND END-OF-LIFE CARE

Method of
Steven A. House, MD

CURRENT DIAGNOSIS

- Any symptom can be in the realm of palliative care. Rapid identification and aggressive management of symptoms are important in maintaining the patient's quality of life.
- Palliative care is treatment that is focused on pain and symptom management, as well as quality of life for patients and their families. It can be rendered at any point in the course or treatment of illness, whether that illness is life limiting/threatening or not.
- Hospice is a philosophy and method of care that is completely focused on symptom management, quality of life for patients and families, and the transition at the end of life.

CURRENT THERAPY

- Recommend that all adult patients, regardless of current health status, execute advance directives (living will, power of attorney for healthcare, healthcare surrogate, etc.) to help ensure that their treatment wishes and end-of-life care goals are met.
- For patients with life-threatening (e.g., progressing cancer) or life-limiting (e.g., patients with severe chronic obstructive pulmonary disease [COPD] or heart failure, requiring dialysis, or residing in a nursing home) illness, consider a Physician Order for Life-Sustaining Treatment (POLST) or Medical Order for Scope of Treatment (MOST) form (the name varies by state). These forms are used to convert the salient points of advance directives into medical orders so that they are immediately actionable by nurses or emergency medical services if the situation arises.
- Advance care planning discussions are billable under Medicare: 99497 for the first 30 minutes and 99498 for each additional 30 minutes.
- The best palliative care involves an interdisciplinary approach by physicians, nurses, counselors, chaplains, and others for the optimal management of symptoms (whether the suffering is physical, emotional, spiritual, existential, or practical) and family support.
- Early addition of palliative care to the overall treatment plan can improve survival and quality of life.
- Cancer pain is an indication for opioid therapy because opioids have proven efficacy in this scenario. For detailed information on opioids, see Table 1 in chapter titled "Pain". Multiple modalities may be required for optimal pain control.
- For patients using opioids chronically, initiate a stimulant laxative such as sennosides (Senokot, Ex-Lax) or lubiprostone (Amitiza) as the opioid's companion. Peripheral mu antagonists such as methylnaltrexone (Relistor), naldemedine (Symproic), or naloxegol (Movantik) are indicated for refractory opioid-induced constipation.
- Control nausea because it can contribute to anorexia, weight loss, and functional decline. The antiserotonergic drugs (e.g., ondansetron [Zofran], granisetron [Kytril], palonosetron [Aloxi], dolasetron [Anzemet]) or the combination netupitant/palonosetron (Akynzeo) are superior to the other classes of antiemetics in the settings of chemotherapy administration and postanesthesia. For uncomplicated nausea, prochlorperazine (Compazine) was found to be superior to promethazine (Phenergan).

- Dyspnea can be improved by providing a fan, a cooler room, and a view to the outside and avoiding confined spaces. Opioids, benzodiazepines, and/or other agents, depending on the situation, might be required. Thoracentesis can be palliative when an effusion is the source of dyspnea.
- Delirium must be evaluated for potential causes. Delirium with or without agitation can occur in up to 80% of patients, depending on the underlying condition. Medications are common causes, but pain and multiple other conditions can cause it as well. Medications such as haloperidol (Haldol)[1], chlorpromazine (Thorazine, brand discontinued),[1] or olanzapine (Zyprexa, Zyprexa Zydis)[1] can be helpful in many patients, but haloperidol is by far the cheapest alternative and a good place to start.
- Chlorpromazine is the only medication with the US Food and Drug Administration (FDA) indication for hiccups.
- Feeding tubes do not improve outcomes in late-stage dementia and can contribute to suffering.

[1]Not FDA approved for this indication.

Epidemiology

There are more than 2.5 million deaths in the United States annually. The most recent year for which mortality data are available is 2017, and cardiovascular disease is the top cause of death, followed by all cancers combined, unintentional injuries, chronic obstructive pulmonary disease (COPD), congestive heart failure, cerebrovascular disease, chronic kidney disease, and chronic liver disease, among others. The ranking was unchanged from 2016. Any of these disease processes can have a significant symptom burden that worsens with disease progression.

Life has 100% mortality, so individuals should take the time to plan for it. The consequences of failing to plan for the transition to end-of-life care include increased psychological distress, medical treatments that are inconsistent with individual preferences, increased utilization of healthcare resources that have little therapeutic benefit while being very costly in dollars, as well as quality of life, and a more difficult bereavement for survivors.

Cardiopulmonary resuscitation has poor outcomes under the best of circumstances (~15%), but it is even worse in patients with late-stage cancer, with only approximately 2% surviving to hospital discharge. Outcomes are also poor for the other

TABLE 1	Coanalgesic and Adjuvant Treatments for Pain: Adult Dosages

Nonsteroidal Antiinflammatory Drugs

Celecoxib (Celebrex) 200 mg PO daily or 100–200 mg PO bid; maximum: 400 mg/d
Diclofenac sodium (Voltaren, Voltaren XR) 50–75 mg PO bid; injection (Dyloject) 37.5 mg IV q6h prn; maximum: 150 mg/d; Diclofenac epolamine topical (Flector patch 1.3%); apply 1 patch to most painful area bid
Ibuprofen (Motrin, Advil) 400–800 mg PO tid; maximum: 3200 mg/d
Ketorolac Nasal (Sprix) 15.75 mg/spray
<65 years old and <50 kg: 1 spray in one nostril q6h prn. Maximum: 4 sprays/d ×5 days
<65 years old and ≥50 kg: 1 spray in each nostril q6h prn. Maximum: 8 sprays/d ×5 days
(Toradol, brand discontinued)
10 mg PO q4h prn. Maximum: 40 mg/day ×5 days
Single dose: 30–60 mg IM or 15–30 mg IV
Multiple dose: if <65 years old and >50 kg, 30 mg IM/IV q6h prn. Maximum: 120 mg/d ×5 days
Or if >65 years old or <50 kg, 15 mg IM/IV q6h prn up to 60 mg/d ×5 days
Naproxen (Naprosyn, EC-Naprosyn) 250–500 mg PO bid prn; maximum: 1500 mg/d
Naproxen sodium (Aleve, Anaprox) 220–550 PO q12h prn: maximum: 1650 mg/d

Bisphosphonates—Usually Provide Analgesia Within a Week and Last Up to 3 Months

Pamidronate (Aredia)
Malignant hypercalcemia: 60–90 mg (depending on the severity of hypercalcemia) IV ×1
Osteolytic lesions (multiple myeloma) or bone metastases: 90 mg IV monthly
Zoledronic acid (Zometa)
Malignant hypercalcemia: 4 mg IV ×1
Osteolytic lesions (multiple myeloma) or bone metastases: 4 mg IV q3–4 weeks

Radiopharmaceuticals—usually provide analgesia within 1–2 weeks and lasting 1–6 months. Dosing determined by radiation oncologist.

Antidepressants

Tricyclics
Amitriptyline (Elavil)[1] 25–100 mg qhs. Can increase to 150 mg daily for pain.
Nortriptyline (Pamelor)[1] 25–100 mg qhs. Up to 150 mg/d.
Start low and titrate as needed. Use with caution in the elderly.
Selective norepinephrine reuptake inhibitors—can be used to improve coexisting anxiety and/or depression.
Duloxetine 60 mg/d; >60 mg rarely more effective for pain, but can titrate higher for comorbid anxiety and/or depression if needed
Venlafaxine (Effexor)[1] 37.5–225 mg daily. Start low and titrate.

Antiepileptic Drugs

Gabapentin (Neurontin)[1] 300–1200 mg tid. Maximum: 3600 mg/d. Start 300 mg qhs ×2–3 days, then bid ×2–3 days, then tid. May start with 100 mg qhs in the elderly.
Pregabalin (Lyrica) 50–300 mg bid. Maximum: 600 mg/d. Start low and titrate for effect, using the lowest effective dose.

General Anesthesia/Sedation

Ketamine (Ketalar)[1] 0.1–0.2 mg/min IV (no bolus). This dosage is an adjunct to opioid therapy for severe uncontrolled pain and NOT intended to achieve general anesthesia. However, the clinician should seek assistance from anesthesiology or palliative care specialists. Hospital policies may vary.

[1]Not US Food and Drug Administration approved for this indication.
bid, Two times per day; *IM*, intramuscular; *IV*, intravenous; *q4h*, every four hours; *q6h*, every 6 hours; *q8h*, every 8 hours; *qAC*, before meals; *qd*, daily; *qHS*, at bedtime; *po*, by mouth; *pr*, per rectum; *prn*, as needed; *SC*, subcutaneous; *tid*, three times per day.

noncardiac diseases listed previously and decline further with age and comorbidities.

Risk Factors

Factors associated with worse pain or less symptom control are being female, elderly, or a child and race other than white. Historically, these groups have received less pain medication than white males for very similar diagnoses. These trends should be reversing. Lacking advance directives and failing to have such discussions with family members are related to receiving excessive and/or unbeneficial interventions/treatments.

Pathophysiology

A patient's symptoms can be caused by the underlying disease itself, mechanical encroachment on other organs and structures (e.g., bowel obstruction, neuropathic pain from nerve destruction, bone metastasis), becoming more sedentary or bedbound, medications, and/or tumor necrosis factor, neurokinin-1, and other inflammatory cytokines. Therefore symptoms may have different etiologies and pathophysiology depending on the underlying disease state. Such a review would be far too extensive for this section.

Prevention

Encourage all adult patients, regardless of current health status, to execute advance directives (living will, power of attorney for healthcare, healthcare surrogate, etc.) to help ensure that their treatment wishes and end-of-life care goals are met. These discussions are billable under Medicare using CPT 99497 for the first 30 minutes face to face with patient, family members, and/or surrogate and 99498 for each additional 30 minutes. For patients with life-threatening (e.g., progressing cancer) or life-limiting (e.g., severe COPD or heart failure, dialysis-dependent, or nursing home residents) illness, consider a Physician Order for Life-Sustaining Treatment (POLST) or a Medical Order for Scope of Treatment (MOST) form (forms vary by state). They are used to convert the salient points of advance directives into medical orders so that they are immediately actionable by nurses, emergency medical services, and others if the situation arises.

Ascertain the patient's/family's goals of care, and assess whether those goals are realistic under the circumstances. Evaluate whether a particular intervention will help achieve that goal. For example, if a patient's goal is to take a child on a special vacation, this cannot be achieved if the patient remains in the hospital receiving chemotherapy that is not working. Another example is a nursing home resident with dementia whose family just wants them "to be kept comfortable" but is considering feeding tube placement. Placing a feeding tube in advanced dementia does not improve outcomes and might require physical restraints to keep the patient from removing the tube. Therefore feeding tube placement will negatively impact the goal of comfort.

When maintaining comfort and improving quality of life become the primary goals, assist patients and their families with the transition to hospice care. Hospice is grossly underused, with median and average lengths of service of only 24 days and 71 days, respectively. Referrals are too often made excessively late, with 28% of patients having 7 or fewer days of service; therefore all of the benefits of hospice cannot always be fully realized in such a short time.

Palliative and end-of-life care, like all medical care, needs to be influenced by all four major aspects of medical ethics: autonomy (patient/surrogate has the right to pursue aggressive treatment, as well as to refuse treatment, even if that treatment could be considered life sustaining), beneficence (do "good" for the patient), nonmaleficence ("do no harm"), and justice (appropriate distribution of finite resources to do the most good for the most people). These four ethics can come into conflict at times, especially with the emphasis on autonomy above the other three in the healthcare system in the United States. Hospitals and other medical facilities should have specific policies regarding medical futility, and ethics committees can be helpful in difficult or unusual cases.

Clinical Manifestations

Common symptoms in palliative care include pain, nausea with or without vomiting, dyspnea, delirium, constipation, dysphagia (cannot swallow food, fluids, or medications), and general functional decline (i.e., requiring more assistance with transfers, toileting, and self-care). Anorexia and lack of thirst are very common, notably in the last few hours to days of life, but anorexia can also be a side effect of medications. Intervening with intravenous (IV) fluids or nasogastric feeding can exacerbate symptoms (secretions, dyspnea, pain, nausea) and worsen outcomes. Weight loss is commonly observed. Medications for diabetes and other disorders can often be discontinued at this stage to help avoid side effects, drug interactions, and adverse reactions (e.g., hypoglycemia).

As patients enter the last hours of life, they might experience decreased level of consciousness, agitated delirium, mottling of the extremities beginning distally and moving proximally, changes in breathing (Cheyne-Stokes, rapid and shallow, Kussmaul, or agonal), decreased or absent oral intake, and/or skin cool to touch.

Diagnosis

Diagnosis and prognosis will vary widely depending on the underlying disease processes, but in palliative care, much of the diagnosis (symptom identification) is based on history. Any patient with symptom burden is a candidate for palliative care, whether the symptoms are physical, psychological, spiritual, or existential. The Edmonton Symptom Assessment Scale rates each of 11 different symptoms on a scale of 0 to 3, for a total score of 0 to 33. This scale gives an idea of overall symptom burden. The Karnovsky and Palliative Performance Scales range from 0% (deceased) to 100% (fully functional) rated on ambulation, activity and evidence of disease, self-care, oral intake, and level of consciousness. A score of approximately 40% is often associated with appropriateness for hospice. Hospice eligibility in the United States is solely based on a life expectancy of 6 months or less if the disease progresses on its expected course. The National Hospice and Palliative Care Organization (NHPCO) has devised some prognostic criteria for a variety of diagnoses including dementia, amyotrophic lateral sclerosis (ALS), acquired immune deficiency syndrome (AIDS), congestive heart failure, end-stage liver or kidney disease, COPD, and so on. Although not fully validated, the criteria can help to guide the clinician in discussions with patients/families. "Hospice" is commonly associated with cancer; however, according to the NHPCO, only 27.2% of hospice patients in 2016 suffered from cancer (often referred late, as the median length of stay was only 19 days), followed by 18.7% cardiovascular and 18.0% dementia to round out the top three. There are various prognostic scoring systems for different disease states, and the Palliative Prognosis Score can help to determine the prognosis for patients with terminal cancer. In addition, the American Cancer Society has 5-year survival rates for various stages of numerous cancers on its website.

Differential Diagnosis

Because this chapter discusses management of symptoms for a plethora of different diseases, the differential diagnosis of all symptomatic disease processes is far beyond its scope. However, when assessing various symptoms, treatment options can be selected based on the probable source. Is the pain new or in a new location, or is it in the same area, radiating, or worsening? Are the nausea/vomiting due to chemotherapy, anesthesia, metabolic disorders, bowel obstruction, anxiety, increased intracranial pressure, or something else? Is the constipation opioid induced, due to poor intake, a result of using fiber without adequate fluid intake, or caused by another issue altogether? Is the dyspnea due to pleural effusion (may respond to thoracentesis far better than it would respond to medications), anxiety (could use selective serotonin reuptake inhibitors [SSRIs], hydroxyzine [Vistaril], benzodiazepine, cognitive behavioral therapy), airway obstruction (might use bronchoscopy, suction, or bronchodilators rather than other medications), excessive secretions (could treat with anticholinergic medications such as glycopyrrolate [Robinul] or scopolamine), or other cause?

Therapy

To meet the needs of all forms of suffering (physical, emotional/psychological, spiritual, existential), an interdisciplinary approach using physicians, nurses, chaplains, counselors, social workers, and others is essential. For all patients entering palliative care, and especially hospice care, all of their medications should be evaluated for risk and benefit and then prioritized based on the goals of care. In one study, patients with a life expectancy of less than 1 year taking a statin for primary or secondary prevention were randomized to continue or stop the statin. The average number of days until death was 229 after discontinuation versus 190 for continuation; thus survival and quality of life improved at a lower cost. Consider discontinuing statins, some oral hypoglycemic agents (notably sulfonylureas due to risk of hypoglycemia), or oral anticoagulants such as warfarin (Coumadin), apixaban (Eliquis), or dabigatran (Pradaxa) if risks now outweigh benefits. As the end of life approaches, discontinue other medications that are not essential for symptom control or quality of life, have more risks than benefits, or contribute to symptom burden (e.g., cholinesterase inhibitors) at this advanced stage of the disease.

Clinicians might withhold or withdraw treatments, but they should never withdraw "care." Providers can change from "doing everything possible to cure a patient" to "doing everything possible to maintain comfort and quality of life." This is more than semantics. Consider turning off the defibrillator component of a pacer-defibrillator to avoid unnecessary shocks. The pacer can remain on because it can improve some symptoms while not prolonging life.

Pain

For a detailed review of medications used for pain, especially opioids, see chapter titled "Pain." This section will focus on cancer pain and end-of-life pain.

Pain of All Types

Opioids have demonstrated efficacy for cancer-related pain in numerous clinical trials. Methadone (Dolophine) can be effective when other opioids have failed, but it should be used with caution and by those familiar with its use due to variable pharmacokinetics and an increased risk of respiratory depression as compared to other opioids.

Bone Pain

The bone pain due to metastatic lesions is partly due to prostaglandin release; thus coanalgesics such as nonsteroidal antiinflammatory drugs or adjuvant medications such as corticosteroids, (e.g., dexamethasone[1] or prednisone[1]) can be particularly helpful. Bisphosphonates such as zoledronic acid (Zometa) and pamidronate (Aredia) usually provide analgesia within a week that lasts up to 3 months. Monthly dosing may be required. In addition, radiopharmaceuticals such as strontium-89 (Metastron), samarium-153 (Quadramet), and phosphorus-32 (Phosphocol P-32) may be helpful for cancer-related bone pain, with analgesia usually beginning within 1 to 2 weeks and lasting 2 to 6 months. Their benefit is derived from significant uptake by areas of high bone turnover to provide internal, localized radiation. Radium-223 (Xofigo; indication limited to castration-resistant prostate cancer with bone metastasis) emits alpha radiation rather than the beta radiation of the three aforementioned agents, and it is more selective for metastatic lesions. External-beam radiation treatment (EBRT) achieves pain relief in more than 75% of patients with analgesia beginning in 1 to 2 weeks and lasting 2 to 6 months. The appropriateness and dosing of radiopharmaceuticals and EBRT are determined by a radiation oncologist. The radiation oncologist might choose a single large fraction of EBRT rather than multiple small fractions if survival is expected to be greater than 3 months or if prolonged treatment will present too much hardship (transportation, increased suffering, time off work for caregivers, etc.) on the patient/family.

Neuropathic Pain

Neuropathic pain can have multiple causes, such as nerve invasion/compression, medication toxicities, human immunodeficiency virus (HIV), and complications of diabetes. Adjuvant medications that have proven efficacy, but not necessarily an indication for use by the US Food and Drug Administration (FDA), include antidepressants such as amitriptyline (Elavil)[1], duloxetine (Cymbalta), and venlafaxine (Effexor)[1], anticonvulsants such as pregabalin (Lyrica) and gabapentin (Neurontin)[1], or, for highly refractory cases (due to significant risk, side effects, and/or legality), ketamine (Ketalar)[1] or cannabinoids[1]. Topical agents such as capsaicin (Capzasin-HP, Salonpas Gel Patch Hot) have evidence to support their use in diabetic neuropathy. Highly active antiretroviral therapy can decrease viral load and improve symptoms of AIDS, including those of HIV-related neuropathy.

Visceral Pain

Octreotide (Sandostatin) can be used for the severe abdominal cramping and diarrhea associated with carcinoid tumors (can overproduce serotonin) or VIPomas (overproduce vasoactive intestinal peptide) or off-label for abdominal pain and other symptoms related to malignant bowel obstruction. An interventional radiologist or pain specialist could provide additional options, such as celiac plexus blocks or thoracoscopic splanchnicectomy, for refractory abdominal pain, notably in patients with pancreatic cancer.

Dyspnea

Dyspnea is a sensation of breathlessness, and the only measure is a patient's self-report. It does not correlate well with respiratory rate, blood gas measurements, or pulse oximetry. The potential causes are many, and they should be considered before merely managing the symptom. The cause can determine the therapy. Anxiety can be managed with SSRIs or benzodiazepines. Airway obstruction could be relieved by suction or bronchoscopy. Hypoxemia has numerous causes that would have to be considered, but supplemental oxygen could help. Pleural or pericardial effusions could be drained. Pneumonia can be treated with antibiotics, pulmonary edema can be managed with diuretics and opioids, and pulmonary embolus can respond to anticoagulants. Transfusions can be helpful for dyspnea due to significant anemia (hemoglobin <7 g/dL) resulting from hemorrhage or myelosuppression. Bronchospasm usually responds to inhaled β_2 agonists. If underlying causes are addressed, either by management or recognizing that treatment would not achieve the goals of care, symptom control is appropriate. Opioids can be helpful for symptom management. Nebulized morphine[1] is no better than saline. Excessive secretions can be managed with scopolamine or glycopyrrolate. The latter is preferred in the elderly because it does not cross the blood-brain barrier. For nonpharmacologic interventions, see Box 1.

Nausea/Vomiting

The treatment of nausea and vomiting depends on the underlying cause. For chemotherapy-related nausea/vomiting, the 5HT3 receptor antagonists are far more effective than other classes of antiemetics. The 5HT3 class includes ondansetron (Zofran), granisetron (Sancuso, Sustol), dolasetron (Anzemet), and palonosetron (Aloxi). In addition, there is a combination of netupitant/palonosetron (Akynzeo), which combines a 5HT3 antagonist for acute-phase nausea/vomiting and a substance P/neurokinin-1 receptor antagonist (NK1RA) for the delayed phase, and it should be given with dexamethasone (Decadron)[1]. Its only indication is for prophylaxis of chemotherapy-related nausea/vomiting, especially with highly emetogenic chemotherapy. The combination demonstrated superiority over palonosetron alone.

---

[1]Not FDA approved for this indication.

- Reassure, work to manage anxiety.
- Behavioral approaches: relaxation, distraction, hypnosis.
- Limit the number of people in the room.
- Open window.
- Eliminate environmental irritants.
- Keep line of sight clear to outside.
- Reduce room temperature, but avoid chilling the patient.
- Introduce humidity.
- Reposition, elevate the head of the bed, keep patient turned.
- Educate and support the family.

Rolapitant (Varubi), another NK1RA, has a longer half-life than netupitant, with fewer drug interactions. Aprepitant (Emend) is an NK1RA with fosaprepitant (Emend injection) as its IV alternative. Olanzapine (Zyprexa)[1] was more effective than aprepitant and noninferior to fosaprepitant in the setting of highly emetogenic chemotherapy, whereas it is far more cost-effective than either NK1RA and serves as a better acute antiemetic than metoclopramide (Reglan). Prochlorperazine (Compazine) was found to be superior to promethazine (Phenergan) for uncomplicated nausea/vomiting (Table 2).

Constipation

Constipation is quite common in palliative care, and it is easier to prevent than to treat. It is one of the primary side effects of opioids that does not attenuate with time. For routine constipation, almost any laxative will do. Polyethylene glycol 3350 (MiraLax, GlycoLax) daily with as-needed sennosides (Senokot) or bisacodyl (Dulcolax) is one example of a simple regimen. If the patient is taking medications that have constipation as a side effect, such as anticholinergic medications or calcium channel blockers, they should be discontinued if possible. Opioid-induced constipation is due to the interaction of opioids with the mu receptors in the gut, thus leading to poor motility. It can be prevented for the most part if a stimulant laxative is initiated simultaneously with the opioid. Senna is safe for long-term use, but bisacodyl can damage the myenteric plexus over time. The chloride-channel activator lubiprostone (Amitiza) and the guanylate cyclase activator linaclotide (Linzess)[1] increase intestinal fluid secretion and motility, and the peripheral mu antagonists methylnaltrexone (Relistor) and naloxegol (Movantik) are indicated for use by the FDA to treat refractory opioid-induced constipation. Alvimopan (Entereg)[1] is another peripheral mu antagonist, but its primary indication is for ileus, especially postoperatively. Fiber and bulking agents should be avoided because they can worsen the problem (Table 3).

Anxiety

There are numerous reasons for patients receiving palliative care to be anxious, whether undergoing painful/unpleasant but curative interventions, suffering uncontrolled pain or dyspnea, or progressing toward hospice. Fear and uncertainty about the future are common causes, and they can be related to physical, psychological, social, spiritual, or practical (finances, managing home responsibilities) issues. Excessive alcohol or caffeine use can exacerbate anxiety, which may present with agitation, insomnia, restlessness, sweating, tachycardia, hyperventilation, panic disorder, worry, tension, and/or psychosomatic symptoms. For patients with expectation of cure or longer survival, SSRI or serotonin and norepinephrine reuptake inhibitor (SNRI) antidepressants can be beneficial. Venlafaxine (Effexor ER) has the shortest half-life, and steady state can be reached in 4 to 7 days. Benzodiazepines are helpful for shorter life expectancy, or they can be used until the antidepressants take effect. Diazepam (Valium) has a long duration of action due to numerous active metabolites, but it is slower

in onset, as is clonazepam (Klonopin)[1]. Alprazolam (Xanax) has very rapid onset but short duration of action. Lorazepam (Ativan) strikes a happy medium between speed of onset and duration of action. Counseling and cognitive behavioral therapy are effective, especially in combination with medications.

Delirium

Delirium is a waxing/waning state of confusion that can be characterized by anxiety, disorientation, cognitive dysfunction, and hallucinations. There is also a catatonic variety of delirium. This condition can be caused by many things, but a short list would include constipation/impaction, hypoxemia, infection, electrolyte abnormalities, medications (including benzodiazepines and opioids), and pain. If a cause is identified and corrected but the patient is still symptomatic, haloperidol (Haldol)[1], chlorpromazine (Thorazine)[1], or olanzapine (Zyprexa)[1] can be helpful; however, haloperidol is by far the cheapest alternative and a good place to start. It can be given intravenously or orally, or it can be given subcutaneously (off-label).

Hiccups

Hiccups (singultus) is a common nuisance that can become quite distressing, especially if persistent (>48 hours) or intractable (>1 month). For patients with pain in the chest or abdominal regions, hiccups can make pain difficult to control in addition to being a bothersome symptom that can significantly decrease quality of life. Chlorpromazine, at 25 to 50 mg PO up to four times per day prn, is the only FDA-approved medication for hiccups, but haloperidol[1] is a viable and much cheaper alternative, as is metoclopramide (Reglan)[1]. Gabapentin (Neurontin)[1] and phenytoin (Dilantin)[1] have been used with some success, notably in cases with a central nervous system etiology. Many other medications, including baclofen (Lioresal)[1], have been tried without much success (i.e., some improvement in symptoms but did not eliminate the hiccups). Nonpharmacologic methods (e.g., breath holding, hyperventilation, gargling) are worth trying, but evidence is lacking for any particular intervention.

Monitoring

Patients should be reevaluated routinely for the adequacy of pain and symptom control, as well as for their ability to cope with the underlying disease, symptom burden, and functional decline. The family needs to be assessed for additional stressors and coping mechanisms, as the family's adjustment, or lack thereof, can be detrimental to the patient's condition. If opioids or benzodiazepines are being used, the supply needs to be monitored for any signs of aberrant use by the patient and/or the family and visitors. In addition, patients can be monitored for excessive sedation or respiratory depression, especially when using methadone with or without a benzodiazepine. The FDA has issued a warning regarding coadministration of benzodiazepines and opioids as a cause of worsened respiratory depression, so these patients in particular should be monitored.

Palliative Sedation

For symptoms refractory to all other measures and with a life expectancy of less than 2 weeks, palliative sedation can be considered, after informed consent, without hastening death according to one study.

Physician-Assisted Suicide

Although this practice has been legalized in several states, the American Medical Association's Council on Ethical and Judicial Affairs has determined that physician-assisted suicide (PAS), as opposed to "aid in dying," is the most accurate description of the practice and that the AMA's current policy forbidding PAS should be upheld. Similarly, in 2017 the American College of Physicians (ACP) also determined that PAS is contradictory to the physician's role in the physician–patient relationship. The NHPCO issued a statement opposing all

---

[1]Not FDA approved for this indication.

TABLE 2 Antiemetics

Antipsychotics/Dopamine Antagonists

Chlorpromazine (Thorazine) 10–25 mg PO q4h prn. Can use 25–50 mg IM q3h prn, but change to PO as soon as possible. Also available as 25 mg or 100 mg (can be halved) suppositories that can be given every 6 hours as needed.
Haloperidol (Haldol) 0.5–5 mg PO/IV bid–tid prn (off-label for nausea/vomiting); maximum 100 mg/d, but use lowest effective dose. Good choice when also managing delirium.
Metoclopramide (Reglan) 5–10 mg PO/IV q6h prn
Olanzapine (Zyprexa) 5–10 mg PO daily–bid prn (off-label for nausea/vomiting)
Prochlorperazine (Compazine) 5–10 mg PO/IM/IV q6h prn; maximum 10 mg/dose, 40 mg/d. Suppository, 25 mg PR q12h prn

Antihistamines

Hydroxyzine (Atarax, Vistaril) 25–100 mg PO q6h prn or IM q4h prn
Meclizine (Antivert, Bonine) 25–100 mg/d PO divided bid–tid prn (off-label)
Promethazine (Phenergan) 12.5–25 mg PO/PR/IM/IV q4h prn. Use with caution IV: can cause necrosis and gangrene.

Antiserotonin (5HT3 Antagonists)

Dolasetron (Anzemet) 12.5 mg IV 15 min before ending anesthesia or at onset of postoperative nausea/vomiting; 100 mg PO ×1 within an hour before chemotherapy.
Granisetron (Granisol, Sancuso [transdermal], Sustol [sustained release SC injection]) 2 mg PO ×1 or 1 mg PO q12h ×2 doses given within an hour before chemotherapy. If IV, 10 mcg/kg IV ×1 within 30 min before chemotherapy. Transdermal, apply 1 patch (3.1 mg/24 h) ×1 24 h before chemotherapy and leave on for up to 7 days. If SC, 10 mg SC q 7 days (give with dexamethasone [Decadron][1]).
Ondansetron (Zuplenz, Zofran, Zofran ODT) 8 mg PO q8h for nausea/vomiting; 24 mg PO ×1 30 min before highly emetogenic chemotherapy.
Palonosetron (Aloxi) 0.25 mg IV ×1 or 0.5 mg PO ×1 30 min before chemotherapy.

Antineurokinin (NK1 RA)

Aprepitant (Emend), fosaprepitant (Emend injection) 125 mg PO ×1 day 1 of chemotherapy, then 80 mg PO daily ×2 days. Or 150 mg IV ×1 30 min before chemotherapy.
Netupitant/palonosetron (Akynzeo) 300/0.5 mg, 1 capsule 1 h before highly emetogenic chemotherapy.
Rolapitant (Varubi) 180 mg PO ×1, 1–2 h before chemotherapy.
Netupitant/palonosetron is already a combination, but all NK1RAs should be given with an HT3RA and dexamethasone before highly emetogenic chemotherapy.

Cannabinoid Receptor Agonists

Dronabinol (Marinol, Syndros) 2.5–10 mg PO bid prn. Syndros is available as a 5 mg/mL solution.
Nabilone (Cesamet) 1–2 mg PO bid prn; maximum: 2 mg PO tid
Both drugs are indicated for chemotherapy-related nausea/vomiting refractory to other drugs. Significant psychiatric adverse events are possible.

Unknown Mechanism

Trimethobenzamide (Tigan) 300 mg PO or 200 mg IM q6h prn

[1]Not US Food and Drug Administration approved for this indication.
bid, Two times per day; *IM*, intramuscular; *IV*, intravenous; *q4h*, every four hours; *q6h*, every 6 hours; *q8h*, every 8 hours; *qAC*, before meals; *qd*, daily; *qHS*, at bedtime; *po*, by mouth; *pr*, per rectum; *prn*, as needed; *SC*, subcutaneous; *tid*, three times per day.

TABLE 3 Laxatives

Osmotic

Lactulose (Kristalose) 10 g per 15 mL; 15–30 mL daily or BID, maximum 60 mL/day (40 g/day)
Magnesium citrate (1.745 g/30 mL) 195–300 mL/d PO daily or divided bid; maximum: 300 mL/d
Magnesium hydroxide (milk of magnesia), 400 mg/5 mL; 30–60 mL (2400–4800 mg) PO daily PRN. Maximum 60 mL/day, can be divided 2–4 doses per day.
Polyethylene glycol 3350 (MiraLax), 17 g in 8 oz. liquid PO daily

Stimulant

Bisacodyl (Dulcolax) 5 mg tabs 1–3 PO daily prn or 10 mg suppository PR daily prn
Sennosides (Senna) 8.6 mg tabs; 2–4 tabs PO bid; maximum: 4 tabs PO bid

Secretory

Linaclotide (Linzess)[1] 145 mcg PO daily. Stimulates cGMP production to increase intestinal fluid secretion and motility.
Lubiprostone (Amitiza) 24 mcg PO bid. Activates chloride channel to increase intestinal fluid secretion and motility.
Plecanatide (Trulance)[1] 3 mg PO daily. Stimulates cGMP production to increase intestinal fluid secretion and motility.

Peripheral Mu-Receptor Antagonists

Methylnaltrexone (Relistor) 8–12 mg SC qod prn (or 0.15 mg/kg SC qod prn). Maximum: 1 dose/24 h
Naldemedine (Symproic) 0.2 mg PO daily
Naloxegol (Movantik) 25 mg PO daily

Avoid fiber and bulking agents in patients taking opioids or with limited fluid intake.

[1]Not US Food and Drug Administration approved for this indication.
bid, Two times per day; *IM*, intramuscular; *IV*, intravenous; *q4h*, every four hours; *q6h*, every 6 hours; *q8h*, every 8 hours; *qAC*, before meals; *qd*, daily; *qHS*, at bedtime; *po*, by mouth; *pr*, per rectum; *prn*, as needed; *SC*, subcutaneous; *tid*, three times per day.

forms of "Legally Assisted Death" in November 2018, citing numerous reasons for their rationale. Notable among these is that PAS does not meet the World Health Organization (WHO) definition of palliative care (i.e., "intends to neither hasten nor postpone death"). Conversely, the American Academy of Family Physicians (AAFP) and the American Academy of Hospice and Palliative Medicine (AAHPM) have taken a neutral stance.

Complications

Emergencies do exist within the palliative care and hospice settings. Spinal cord compression, hypercalcemia, superior vena cava syndrome, seizures, airway obstruction, hemorrhage, or acute worsening or crisis in pain or other symptom are examples. Management will depend on the patient's goals of care and stage of illness; however, uncontrolled symptoms should always be addressed. Having dark-colored linens and towels are good to have on hand for patients at risk for hemorrhage, because the blood does not appear as dramatic or traumatic for the patient and family as it would on white or light-colored materials.

References

2017 NHPCO Facts & Figures—NHPCO April 2018. Available at: https://www.nhpco.org/sites/default/files/public/Statistics_Research/2017_Facts_Figures.pdf. [accessed 05.24.2019].
Bath C. ASCO 2014: Stopping statins is safe and can improve quality of life for patients with cancer near the end of life. Available at: http://www.ascopost.com/News/16304. Posted 6/11/14. [accessed 05.24.2019].
Davis MP: New therapies for antiemetic prophylaxis for chemotherapy, *J Community Support Oncol* 14:11–20, 2016.
Dowling R: Bill end-of-life discussion codes correctly, Med Econ March 10, 2016. Available at: http://medicaleconomics.modernmedicine.com/medical-economics/news/how-bill-end-life-discussion-codes-correctly. [accessed 05.20.2019].
Ebell MH: Determining prognosis for patients with terminal cancer, *Am Fam Physician* 72:668–669, 2005.
Farmer C. Fast facts and concepts #81. Management of hiccups. Updated June 2015. Available at: https://www.mypcnow.org/blank-mkw97. [accessed 05.20.2019].
Murphy SL, Xu J, Kochanek KD, Arias E. Mortality in the United States, 2017. NCHS data brief No. 328, November 2018. Available at: https://www.cdc.gov/nchs/data/databriefs/db293.pdf. [accessed 05.30.2018].
NCCN clinical practice guidelines in oncology: *antiemesis, version 1*, National Comprehensive Care Network, 20152015, AE2–6.
Planning the transition to end-of-life care in advanced cancer–health professional version (PDQ). Available at: http://www.cancer.gov/cancertopics/pdq/supportivecare/transitiontoEOLcare/healthprofessional. [accessed 05.20.2019].
Reisfield GM, Wilson GR: Fast facts and concepts #116. Radiopharmaceuticals for painful osseous metastases, Available at: https://www.mypcnow.org/blank-qfwwm. June 2015 [accessed 05.20.2019].
Rutter C, Johnstone C, Weissman DE. Fast facts and concepts #66. Radiation for palliation – part 1. Updated April 2016. Available at: https://www.mypcnow.org/blank-r9t7g. [accessed 05.20.2019].
Rutter C, Johnstone C, Weissman DE: Fast facts and concepts #67. Radiation for palliation – part 2, ed 2. Available at: https://www.mypcnow.org/fast-fact-61-120. [accessed 05.20.2019].
"NHPCO Statement on Legally Accelerated Death." https://www.nhpco.org/sites/default/files/public/communications/Legally_Accelerated_Death_Position_Statement.pdf. [accessed 05.24.2019].
Weinstein E, Arnold R: Fast facts and concepts #113. Bisphosphonates for bone pain, Available at: https://www.mypcnow.org/blank-ux03d; June 2015 [accessed 05.20.2019].

PALPITATIONS

Method of
Rebecca Katzman, MD; and Justin Bailey, MD

CURRENT DIAGNOSIS

- History and physical examination
- Electrocardiogram
- Complete blood count (CBC)
- Thyroid-stimulating hormone (TSH)
- Complete metabolic panel

CURRENT THERAPY

- Dependent on underlying etiology. See Table 7.

Palpitations are the unpleasant sensation or awareness of one's own heartbeat. Patients may feel a racing heart, skipped heartbeats, or pounding in the chest or neck. Palpitations have been described as a "flip-flop" or "fluttering" in the chest. Palpitations may be due to cardiac arrhythmia, nonarrhythmic cardiac disease, drugs, other medical conditions, or psychiatric disease. Cardiac arrhythmias and anxiety account for a majority of cases. Palpitations may be completely benign or a manifestation of a potentially fatal arrhythmia.

Epidemiology

Palpitations (ICD-9-CM 785.1, ICD-10-CM R00.2) are a common presenting complaint in a primary care office or the emergency department. They affect all genders and ages. Up to 16% of patients in general medical settings report palpitations, and up to 18% of cardiology outpatient visits are for cardiac arrhythmias. The most common etiologies are cardiac arrhythmias (43%) and anxiety/psychiatric (31%). In outpatient clinics psychiatric etiologies are slightly more common; in emergency department settings cardiac causes are increasingly likely. The underlying cause of palpitations in 15% of patients cannot be identified.

Nearly 90% of patients who have palpitations have recurrent symptoms of palpitations. Overall, 1-year mortality does not appear to be significantly increased, but patients report a moderate impact on their quality of life.

Although arrhythmias are frequently found to be the underlying cause of palpitations, it is important to note that many patients with arrhythmias do not have any symptoms.

Differential Diagnosis

The differential for palpitations is broad but can generally be broken down into cardiac versus noncardiac causes. Cardiac causes may be further divided into structural or arrhythmic causes. Noncardiac causes include medications and drugs, high-output states, and certain medical conditions. Gastroesophageal reflux or esophageal spasm may present as a brief intermittent episode of tightness or pounding in the chest. See Table 1 for a full listing of causes.

Psychiatric causes may account for up to one-third of presentations; however, it is important to note that psychiatric illness can coexist with cardiac or other medical causes, and palpitations can occur with panic attacks, generalized anxiety, depression, and somatization.

Cardiac arrhythmias often present as palpitations. Nearly any arrhythmia or change from a sinus rhythm can produce this sensation. A less common condition in otherwise healthy patients is inappropriate sinus tachycardia (IST), demonstrated by an elevated resting heart rate, an exaggerated heart rate response to exercise, or both. IST is thought to be due to abnormal autonomic control and response. Long QT syndrome, both congenital/familial and medication-induced, may predispose to ventricular tachyarrhythmias, including the often-fatal Torsades de pointes.

Risk Factors

Structural cardiac disease, including valvular disease, may predispose patients to arrhythmias and palpitations. Table 2 lists symptoms and risk factors that indicate an increased likelihood that palpitations are due to an underlying arrhythmia.

Pathophysiology

An arrhythmia is caused by the disruption of the normal electrical impulse that originates at the sinoatrial node and is conducted to the atrioventricular node, then through the His-Purkinje system to

TABLE 1 Differential Diagnosis for Palpitations

NONCARDIAC		CARDIAC	
Medications		*Arrhythmias*	Atrial fibrillation
Prescription	Digoxin (Lanoxin)		Atrial flutter
	Beta agonists (Albuterol [Proventil])		Benign ectopy (premature ventricular contractions, premature atrial contraction)
	Terbutaline Digitalis (digoxin)		Nonsustained ventricular tachycardia
Over-the-counter	Caffeine		Supraventricular tachyarrhythmias (ex atrioventricular reentrant tachycardia)
	Antihistamines		Inappropriate sinus tachycardia
	Pseudoephedrine (Sudafed)		Long QT syndrome
	Ephedrine, Ephedra[a]		Torsades de pointes
	Atropine		
	Diphenoxylate/atropine [Lomotil]		
Drugs of abuse	Cocaine	*Structural abnormalities*	Mitral regurgitation
	Amphetamines		Aortic insufficiency
	Alcohol		Mitral valve prolapse
	Nicotine		Hypertrophic obstructive cardiomyopathy
Medical causes	Thyrotoxicosis	*Other*	Pericarditis
	Pheochromocytoma		Pacemaker-mediated tachycardia
	Anemia		Vasovagal syncope
	Hypoglycemia		
	Mastocytosis		
	Gastroesophogeal reflux		
	Esophogeal spasm		
High output states	Fever		
	Pregnancy		
	Paget's disease		
	Extra cardiac shunt		
	Exercise		
	Stress		
Psychiatric	*Panic attack*		
	Generalized anxiety		
	Depression		
	Somatization		

[a]Dietary supplement banned by the U.S. FDA.

TABLE 2 Risk Factors for Palpitations

Increased likelihood of underlying arrhythmia
Known structural or valvular cardiac disease
Visible neck pulsations
Palpitations that affect sleep
Palpitations that occur at work
Subjective feeling of irregular heart rate
Duration of palpitations more than 5 min
Male gender
Older age
Decreased likelihood of underlying arrhythmia
Family history of panic disorder
Duration of palpitations less than 5 min

depolarize the ventricles. Disruption may occur anywhere along this pathway. Underlying structural disease, prior ischemia, congenital abnormalities in myocytes, or electrical pathways affect a normal electrical conduction pathway. Palpitations that are due to supraventricular or ventricular tachyarrhythmias often result from sympathetic stimulation and catecholamine surges.

Palpitations involving skipped or premature beats are often a sensation that results from the following episode of systole, when stroke volume is increased secondary to the prolonged length of the preceding diastole and increased ventricular inotropy.

Clinical Assessment

The keys to evaluation are a history and physical, a 12-lead electrocardiogram (ECG), and a basic laboratory evaluation including

TABLE 3	History and Physical Examination Clues to the Etiology of Palpitations

CLUES FROM HISTORY OR EXAMINATION	SUGGESTED DIAGNOSIS
Onset in childhood or adolescence	Accessory pathway rhythms: AV nodal reentrant tachycardia Wolff Parkinson White Idiopathic ventricular tachyarrhythmia
Onset in older adult Description of irregular rate	Atrial fibrillation
Feeling of "fluttering"	Prolonged tachyarrhythmia
Pounding in the neck Exaggerated "a" wave in jugular venous pulse	Atrioventricular dissociations
Midsystolic click followed by late systolic murmur	Mitral valve prolapse
Holosystolic murmur along left sternal border that increases with Valsalva	Hypertrophic obstructive cardiomyopathy Left ventricle outflow tract obstruction
Pale conjunctiva	Anemia
Exophthalmos Goiter	Thyrotoxicosis
Gravid abdomen	Pregnancy

TABLE 4	Medications That Cause QT Prolongation

Cardiac Antiarrhythmics Amiodarone (Cordarone)
  Disopyramide (Norpace)
  Procainamide
  Quinidine
  Sotalol (Betapace)
  Diuretics
  Sympathomimetics
  Vasodilators

Antibiotics Fluoroquinolones
  Macrolides

Psychiatric Phenothiazines Chlorpromazine (Thorazine)
  Promethazine (Phenergan)
  Prochlorperazine (Compazine)
  Fluphenazine (Prolixin)
  Trifluoperazine (Stelazine)
  Selective serotonin reuptake inhibitors
  Tricyclic antidepressants
  Haloperidol (Haldol)

Other Amphetamines
  Anticholinergics
  Antihistamines
  Protease inhibitors
  Methadone (Dolophine)

TABLE 5	ECG Findings Suggestive of Diagnosis of Palpitations

ECG FINDINGS	SUGGESTED DIAGNOSIS
Irregularly irregular rhythm Absent P waves	Atrial fibrillation
Delta wave Short PR interval Widened QRS	Wolff Parkinson White
Short PR	AV nodal reentrant tachycardia
QT interval>460 msec in women, >440 msec in men	Predisposition to ventricular tachyarrhythmias, including Torsades de pointes
Left ventricular enlargement with left atrial abnormality	May be a focus for atrial fibrillation

TABLE 6	Diagnostic Considerations in the Evaluation of Palpitations

FINDINGS	FURTHER EVALUATION
Arrhythmia or predisposition to arrhythmia seen on ECG	Echocardiogram to look for structural heart disease
Palpitations brought on by exertion	Exercise stress test (avoid dobutamine if suspect arrhythmia)
Suspected arrhythmia, but none identified on ECG	Ambulatory cardiac monitoring – Holter monitor (24–48 h) – Continuous loop event recorder – Implantable loop recorder
Associated dizziness, syncope, presyncope	Referral to cardiologist for electrophysiology study
Known cardiac dysfunction, structural or valvular abnormality	Referral to cardiologist for electrophysiology study
Family history of sudden cardiac death	Referral to cardiologist for electrophysiology study

ventricular arrhythmias (see Tables 3 and 4). A physical examination should be performed but may be limited, as clinicians rarely have the opportunity to examine a patient during an episode of palpitations.

Diagnostic Testing

A 12-lead ECG should be performed in all patients. It is appropriate to do limited laboratory evaluation with a complete blood count (CBC), thyroid-stimulating hormone (TSH), and complete metabolic panel (CMP or Chem-14) to identify anemia, thyroid disease, and electrolyte abnormalities that predispose to arrhythmias. Etiology can be determined in 40% of patients from this limited evaluation (see Tables 5 and 6).

Traditionally, ambulatory cardiac monitoring has been done via a Holter monitor. Patients keep a diary of the time and characteristics of their symptoms. This method is appropriate for patients who have daily palpitations. The monitor is worn for 24 to 48 hours. If symptoms are not present during the time the monitor is being worn, the test will be unrevealing. In addition, Holter monitoring may uncover arrhythmias (most commonly benign ectopy) that are unrelated to patient symptoms.

If arrhythmia is suspected in a patient but 24 to 48 hours is insufficient time to record an event, it is recommended that the patient be evaluated with a continuous loop event recorder for

an evaluation of the thyroid gland. Clinicians must identify which patients are more likely to have underlying arrhythmia and require further evaluation. A good clinical history includes age of onset, description of palpitations, frequency, duration, timing, position, and associated symptoms, including dizziness, presyncope, and syncope. The clinical history should include a thorough medication review, including over-the-counter medications, alcohol and tobacco use, and illicit substance use. An increasing number of medications are being found to cause QT prolongation, especially when used in combination, and may predispose the patient to

TABLE 7 Treatment of Specific Causes of Palpitations

CAUSES OF PALPITATIONS	TREATMENT
Due to medication or drug	Stop offending agent
Premature atrial contractions	Decrease caffeine and alcohol Tobacco cessation
Ectopy (PACs)	Beta blockers for prevention of ectopy – *Metoprolol* [Toprol XL][a] 50 mg PO daily – *Atenolol* [Tenormin][a] 50 mg PO daily
Narrow complex SVT	Vagal maneuvers (carotid massage, Valsalva, dive reflex) help during episode
Hospitalized patient with prolonged SVT	*Adenosine* [Adenoscan] 6 mg IV bolus over 1 to 2 s, increased up to 12 mg IV every 1 to 2 min as needed for 2 doses
Atrial fibrillation with rapid ventricular response	*Metoprolol* [Lopressor][a] 2.5 to 5 mg IV bolus over 2 min, repeated at 5 min intervals to a total of 15 mg *Esmolol* [Brevibloc] 0.5 mg/kg IV over 1 min, followed by 50 µg/kg/min continuous infusion with re-bolusing and increasing rate of infusion by 50 µg/kg/min every 4 min up to a maximum infusion rate of 200 µg/kg/min *Verapamil* [Isoptin] 5 to 10 mg IV over 2 to 3 min, repeated every 15 to 30 min as necessary *Diltiazem* [Cardizem], 0.25 mg/kg IV over 2 min with a second bolus of 0.35 mg/kg 15 min later if first dose is tolerated but does not produce desired reduction in heart rate. Diltiazem can then be run as a continuous infusion at a rate of 5 to 15 mg/h
Regular supraventricular tachyarrhythmias, such as WPW or AV nodal reentrant tachycardia	Radiofrequency ablation in electrophysiology laboratory

[a]Not FDA approved for this indication.

2 weeks. These ambulatory monitors record continuously, but only save data from the specific interval when the patient activates the monitor (e.g., 2 min before and after an episode of palpitations). These monitors frequently send information transtelephonically rather than keeping data stored within the device itself. In patients with infrequent palpitations but known severe heart disease, an implantable loop recorder is an option. These monitors are implanted subcutaneously, typically in the left pectoral region, and usually left in place for 1 year. As with other loop event recorders, they save data when activated by the patient and can send information transtelephonically.

Panic disorder or anxiety is a diagnosis of exclusion. A patient with anxiety or other psychiatric illness may have a significant underlying arrhythmia. The catecholamine increase in patients with psychiatric disorder in times of stress or intense emotional experience may be proarrhythmogenic. These patients should undergo evaluation for arrhythmia, especially in the presence of risk factors, before having all of their symptoms attributed to their psychiatric illness.

Patients who have palpitations associated with dizziness, presyncope, or syncope in whom the diagnosis is not apparent should be referred for evaluation by a cardiologist. This sort of palpitation is the kind most likely to be associated with ventricular tachycardia or other serious arrhythmia.

Palpitations may occur more frequently during pregnancy, which is a high-output state. Postpartum cardiomyopathy is a structural disease that is unique to this population. Because pregnant women also have an increased risk of new arrhythmias, including atrial fibrillation, persistent palpitations should be evaluated thoroughly.

Treatment

Treatment should be focused toward the underlying cause of the palpitation.

Discussion of the management of specific causes of palpitations, including anemia, thyrotoxicosis, and hypoglycemia, can be found elsewhere. Chronic management of atrial fibrillation is also beyond the scope of this article.

Table 7 outlines the treatment of specific causes of palpitations. Referral to a cardiologist is appropriate for patients with supraventricular tachyarrhythmias, long QT syndrome, or palpitations associated with syncope/presyncope, as these are more likely to be ventricular arrhythmias.

Patients with potentially malignant ventricular tachyarrhythmias (e.g., frequent premature ventricular depolarizations, up to 3–10 per hour with some repetitive forms) are at increased risk for sudden cardiac death, but there is little evidence that treating with antiarrhythmics decreases mortality; in fact, some evidence suggests that these drugs actually increase mortality via proarrhythmic mechanisms. In these patients, consider a referral to a cardiologist for evaluation for an implantable cardiac defibrillator.

References

Abbott AV: Diagnostic approach to palpitations, *Am Fam Physician* 71:743–750, 2005.
Chan T, Worster A: The clinical diagnosis of arrhythmias in patients presenting with palpitations, *Ann Emerg Med* 57:303–304, 2011.
Crawford MH, Bernstein SJ, Deedwania PC, et al: ACC/AHA guidelines for ambulatory electrocardiography: executive summary and recommendations, *Circulation* 100:886–893, 1999.
Tayal U, Dancy M: Palpitations, *Medicine* 41:118–124, 2013.
Weber BE, Kapoor WN: Evaluation and outcomes of patients with palpitations, *Am J Med* 100:138–148, 1996.
Wexler AK, Pleister A, Raman S: Outpatient approach to palpitations, *Am Fam Physician* 84:63–69, 2011.

PHARYNGITIS

Method of
Ruth Weber, MD, MSEd

CURRENT DIAGNOSIS

- Patients prioritize symptom relief over microbiologic cure.
- Most pharyngitis is viral; microbiologic confirmation is required for group A β-hemolytic streptococcus pharyngitis diagnosis.
- In adults, throat culture is not necessary if rapid antigen detection test is negative.
- Stop presumptive antibiotic therapy if throat culture results are negative for group A β-hemolytic streptococcus.

CURRENT THERAPY

- Penicillin is the drug of choice for group A β-hemolytic streptococcus pharyngitis. A first-generation cephalosporin or macrolide is indicated if the patient is allergic to penicillin.
- Treatment is necessary for 10 days to eradicate group A β-hemolytic streptococcus from the pharynx.
- Amoxicillin can be substituted for penicillin. Patients older than 12 years may be treated with once-daily amoxicillin (Moxatag).
- Patients are not infectious after 24 hours of appropriate antibiotic treatment.

TABLE 1   Pharyngitis: Distribution of Causative Organisms (All Age Groups)

PATHOGEN	PERCENTAGE OF POPULATION
Group A β-hemolytic streptococcus	15–30
Rhinovirus	20
Adenovirus	2–5
Coronavirus	2–5
Coxsackievirus	2–5
Group C β-hemolytic streptococcus	2–5
Herpes simplex virus	2–5
Influenza virus	2–5
Chlamydia trachomatis	< 1
Corynebacterium diphtheriae	< 1
Epstein-Barr virus	< 1
Human immunodeficiency virus	< 1
Arcanobacterium haemolyticum	< 1
Mycoplasma spp.	< 1
Neisseria gonorrhoeae	< 1

Epidemiology

Pharyngitis is common and has substantial medical and societal costs. "Sore throat" accounts for more than 7 million outpatient visits by children annually. The estimated total cost of pharyngitis in children is $540 million per year.

An estimated 30% of childhood pharyngitis is caused by group A β-hemolytic streptococcus (GABHS). In temperate climates, pharyngitis occurs in outbreaks during winter and early spring, predominantly involving children 5 to 15 years of age. GABHS is uncommon in preschool-aged children and in adults. Group C β-hemolytic streptococcus pharyngitis occurs mainly in college students and young adults.

Of other causes of pharyngitis (Table 1), gonococcal pharyngitis is most common in older adolescents and young adults. Transmission is by oral-genital contact. If gonococcal pharyngitis is diagnosed in a prepubertal child, sexual abuse must be considered.

Risk Factors

The major risk factors for GABHS pharyngitis are age and exposure such as in crowded schools or through household contacts. Oral sexual activity is implicated in gonococcal pharyngitis. Swimming pools have been implicated in transmission of group C and D β streptococcal pharyngitis.

Pathophysiology

Pathogenic strains of *Streptococcus pyogenes* can be differentiated by Lancefield antigens and by hemolysis on blood agar. The strain containing group A antigen and displaying β hemolysis causes pharyngitis (GABHS). The M protein is responsible for virulence. The M protein cross-reacts with cardiac myosin and laminin, potentially causing rheumatic heart disease. More than 100 M-protein serotypes have been identified. Some streptococcus strains produce erythrogenic toxins, causing the rash of scarlet fever. Patients develop lifelong immunity to one serotype after infection, but reinfection with a different serotype is possible.

Prevention

GABHS is transmitted by droplet spread. No evidence supports other forms of transmission. Patients and household/close contacts should be educated on minimizing droplet spread to reduce the transmission of GABHS.

Phase I trials have been completed on a multivalent vaccine targeting streptococcus M proteins that cause pharyngitis, invasive disease, and rheumatic fever.

Clinical Manifestations

The type of pharyngitis cannot be identified by history and clinical findings. Microbiologic confirmation is necessary to diagnose GABHS pharyngitis.

Group A β-Hemolytic Streptococcal Pharyngitis

In patients age 3 years to adult, sudden onset of sore throat, pain on swallowing, and fever (101°F–104°F) suggest GABHS pharyngitis. Nausea and vomiting can also occur in school-aged children. Clinical signs can include tonsillar erythema with or without exudate, anterior cervical lymphadenitis, soft palate petechiae, red swollen uvula, and scarletiniform rash. Infants rarely present with exudative pharyngitis but have coryza with excoriation and crusting of the nares. Posttonsillectomy patients with GABHS can have milder symptoms and clinical signs.

Patients with suppurative complications of GABHS have unusually severe symptoms, with neck swelling, drooling, and "hot potato" voice. The clinician must look for peritonsillar abscess and infections in the parapharyngeal and submandibular spaces (Ludwig's angina).

Scarlet Fever

Some strains of GABHS produce a pyogenic exotoxin that causes scarlet fever in susceptible patients. The clinical signs and symptoms are identical to GABHS pharyngitis plus development of the characteristic rash within 24 to 48 hours of symptom onset. The fine, papular, bright red rash blanches with pressure, begins on the neck, and spreads to the extremities and trunk. It is more pronounced in creases and feels rough, with a goose-pimple appearance. The punctate rash spares the face, but patients have flushed cheeks and forehead with pallor around the mouth. The rash fades in 3 to 4 days and is followed by desquamation. After desquamation of an initial white coating, the tongue has a classical strawberry appearance caused by edematous papillae.

Poststreptococcal Glomerulonephritis

Renal symptoms of hypertension, edema, and hematuria can occur 1 to 3 weeks after GABHS pharyngitis. Glomerulonephritis is an autoimmune response to M proteins. It is not preventable by antibiotics.

Viral Pharyngitis

Coryza, hoarseness, cough, diarrhea, viral exanthem, anterior stomatitis, and conjunctivitis can indicate a viral etiology for pharyngitis. Adenovirus infections can cause fever for 7 days, and conjunctivitis can persist for 14 days. Adenoviral outbreaks are often associated with swimming pools.

Enterovirus pharyngitis (coxsackievirus, echovirus, enterovirus) occurs in summer and fall. Fever, cervical adenopathy, and erythema of the tonsils are common, but exudates are rare. Herpangina (Coxsackie virus A/B) manifests with fever and painful papulovesicular lesions in the posterior oropharynx that resolve in 7 days. Hand-foot-and-mouth disease (Coxsackie virus A-16) manifests with painful vesicles and ulcers in the mouth plus painful vesicles on the palms, soles, and occasionally trunk. Lesions resolve in 7 days.

Primary oral herpes simplex infection occurs in young children. It manifests as acute gingivostomatitis, with ulcerating vesicles on the anterior mouth and lips but not on the posterior pharynx. High fever with intense pain is common, and dehydration can occur. Symptoms last for 14 days.

Diagnosis

It is necessary to obtain microbiologic confirmation of infection before treating GABHS pharyngitis. If the clinical symptoms suggest GABHS pharyngitis, a throat culture or rapid antigen detection test (RADT) are indicated. If the clinical symptoms suggest viral pharyngitis, the pretest probability of GABHS infection is low, and a diagnostic test should not be performed.

Several methods for determining the probability of GABHS infection have been proposed. The Centor criteria (for adults) are widely accepted. A score of 1 is given for each of the following characteristics: tonsillar exudate, tender anterior cervical adenopathy, history of fever, and an absence of cough. A score of 3 or more indicates a positive predictive value for GABHS of 40% to 60%. A score of 0 to 1 indicates a positive predictive value for GABHS of 1% to 5%.

Throat culture is the gold standard for diagnosing GABHS infection. The tonsils and the posterior pharynx should be aggressively swabbed. Other areas of the mouth should not be touched when obtaining the culture. The culture should be obtained before beginning antibiotic therapy, because even a single dose of antibiotics can cause the culture to be negative. The swab is plated on a sheep's blood agar plate and incubated. The plate must be read at both 24 and 48 hours of incubation. When done correctly, the throat culture has 90% to 95% sensitivity. Although throat culture is considered the gold standard for diagnosing GABHS infection, it does not differentiate a carrier state from clinical infection.

RADT has high specificity but low sensitivity. The many tests available have different performance characteristics. In children aged 5 to 15, a throat culture should be performed if the RADT test is negative to identify patients who have a false-negative RADT result. In adults, throat culture is not necessary after a negative RADT because of the low incidence of GABHS and extremely low risk of acute rheumatic fever. The use of RADT has allowed clinicians to begin antibiotic therapy early in those with a positive test. This decreases the risk of spread of GABHS, allows earlier return to school or work, and modestly improves clinical signs and symptoms.

Streptococcal antibody testing has no value in the acute diagnosis of GABHS pharyngitis. Testing has some value in confirming prior GABHS infection in patients in whom acute rheumatic fever or acute poststreptococcal glomerulonephritis is suspected. The two antibodies that can be identified are antistreptolysin O (ASO) and antideoxyribonuclease B (ARB). Positive, elevated, or increasing titers are confirmation of recent GABHS infection. ASO titers rise within a week of infection and peak 3 to 6 weeks after infection. ARB titers rise within 1 to 2 weeks of infection and peak at 6 to 8 weeks. In some patients titers remain elevated for prolonged periods; therefore a doubling of the titer in 6 weeks is necessary for diagnosing prior GABHS infection.

Differential Diagnosis

Infectious Mononucleosis
Classically a triad of severe sore throat, lymphadenopathy, and fever (up to 104°F) in 15- to 25-year-olds, mononucleosis begins with a prodrome of chills, sweats, fever, and malaise. Clinical signs include enlarged tonsils; posterior and anterior cervical, axillary and inguinal adenopathy; and hepatosplenomegaly. Approximately 15% of patients present with jaundice and 5% with rash. Patients with mononucleosis who are treated with amoxicillin (Amoxil)[1] often develop a pruritic maculopapular rash. Complete blood count (CBC) shows an absolute lymphocytosis with greater than 10% atypical lymphocytes. Within 2 to 3 weeks, the heterophile antibody test (Mono Spot) becomes positive. The antibody test has a higher false-negative rate in children than in adults. If a false-negative test is suspected, an IgM antibody to viral capsid antigen is indicated to confirm the diagnosis.

Acute Retroviral Syndrome
Primary infection with HIV can manifest as a syndrome of fever, nonexudative pharyngitis, arthralgia, myalgia, and lymphadenopathy. Some 40% to 80% of patients develop a rash. HIV antibodies are negative. Assay for HIV type 1 RNA or p24 antigen is positive.

Neisseria gonorrhea
N. gonorrhea pharyngitis is usually asymptomatic and associated with oral sexual practices. The diagnosis is confirmed by isolating the organism on Thayer-Martin medium. All patients should be screened and treated for coinfection with chlamydia.

Lemierre's Syndrome
Lemierre's syndrome is a rare etiology of severe pharyngitis caused by *Fusobacterium necrophorum*. Infection spreads from the pharynx to include the surrounding tissues, with subsequent thrombophlebitis of the internal jugular vein.

Treatment
A major therapeutic decision is to determine if whether the patient needs an antibiotic in addition to symptomatic treatment.

The goal of treatment of viral pharyngitis is control of symptoms, especially relief of pain. Nonsteroidal antiinflammatory drugs are slightly superior to acetaminophen (Tylenol) for pain relief. No evidence supports the use of Chinese herbs for symptom relief. A single dose of corticosteroids (oral dexamethasone[1] 0.6 mg/kg—maximum dose 10 mg) may provide pain relief, for severe symptoms without serious side effects. The risk of recurrent dosing of corticosteroids has not been determined. Many patients mistakenly believe that antibiotic therapy relieves pain. Ancillary treatment options include rest, adequate fluid intake, and antipyretic medications.

The goals of antibiotic treatment of GABHS pharyngitis are to decrease infectivity and prevent suppurative and other complications, especially acute rheumatic fever. Symptoms generally improve within 3 to 4 days without treatment. Delay of treatment of GABHS pharyngitis for up to 9 days after symptoms begin does not appear to increase the risk of acute rheumatic fever, and a delay of 24 to 48 hours while awaiting culture results does not increase the risk of acute rheumatic fever. Early treatment of GABHS pharyngitis does reduce infectivity, lessens morbidity, and promotes early return to normal activities. Nevertheless, criteria for initiating antibiotics remain controversial.

The choice of antibiotic is determined by the bacteriology of GABHS, clinical efficacy, patient adherence to treatment regimen, adverse effects, and cost. It is not recommended to initiate antibiotics while awaiting throat culture results in children. However, if an antibiotic is started it must be discontinued if the culture is negative.

Penicillin remains the antibiotic of choice for GABHS pharyngitis. GABHS has never shown resistance to penicillin or cephalosporins. Amoxicillin[1] can replace penicillin for treatment. (Liquid amoxicillin has a better taste than liquid penicillin.) In the penicillin-allergic patient, a first-generation cephalosporin or macrolide may be substituted. In some areas of the United States up to 8% of GABHS is resistant to macrolides and less than 1% is resistant to clindamycin (Cleocin). Antibiotics should be given for 10 days to eradicate GABHS from the pharynx. At this time, short-course (≤ 5 days) treatment cannot be recommended, except with azithromycin (Zithromax).

No clear evidence supports antibiotic treatment for group C or group G streptococcal pharyngitis. Treatment might shorten the course of infection. Treatment options are identical to those for GABHS pharyngitis.

Treatment Regimens
- Oral penicillin: PenicillinVK (Veetids)[1]: 40 mg/kg/day (up to adult dose of 1000 mg/day) in divided doses two or three times daily for 10 days.
- Amoxicillin[1]: 50 mg/kg/day (up to adult dose of 1000 mg/day) twice daily for 10 days; the FDA has approved amoxicillin ER tab (Moxatag) for patients older than 12 years at 775 mg once a day.

[1]Not FDA approved for this indication.

- Penicillin G benzathine (Bicillin-LA): Patients weighing less than 27 kg, 600,000 units IM; patients weighing 27 kg or more, 1.2 million units IM once. Penicillin G is used for patients who are unlikely to complete a full 10-day course of oral medication and for those with a personal or family history of rheumatic fever.
- First-generation oral cephalosporin: Cephalexin (Keflex) 25 to 50 mg/kg/day (up to adult dose of 1000 mg/day) twice daily for 10 days. This regimen should be used if the patient is allergic to penicillin; shorter courses are not FDA approved.
- Macrolides should be used if the patient is allergic to penicillin: Erythromycin 20 to 40 mg/kg/day (up to adult dose of 1000 mg/kg/day) in three or four doses for 10 days. Azithromycin (patients older than 6 months): Day 1: 10 mg/kg once (up to adult dose of 500 mg); days 2 to 5: 5 mg/kg once daily (up to adult dose of 250 mg/day). The dose of azithromycin is not established in infants younger than 6 months.

Tetracycline, sulfonamides, and older fluroquinalones are not recommended because of high rates of resistance. All patients should be considered infectious until they have completed 24 hours of antibiotic therapy.

Monitoring

In general, follow-up throat cultures or RADT for patients successfully treated for GABHS pharyngitis (i.e., test for cure) are not necessary. An additional RADT or throat culture is required if symptoms do not abate, symptoms recur, or the patient had previous rheumatic fever.

Patients who have repeated symptomatic episodes of GABHS have either recurrent new infections or are carriers of GABHS, with repeated superimposed viral infections.

GABHS carriers have positive cultures for GABHS without clinical symptoms. Approximately 20% of school-aged children are carriers. GABHS carrier status is suspected if the clinical picture is of viral pharyngitis but the patient has positive RADT or cultures both when symptomatic and when asymptomatic. Carriers do not respond to antibiotics and have no serologic response to ASO and anti-DNA B. These patients do not need to be identified or treated. These patients do not develop rheumatic fever and are not important in the spread of GABHS to others.

Patients with repeated GABHS pharyngitis have a clinical picture of recurrent bacterial pharyngitis. They respond to antibiotics and have negative RADT and culture when they are asymptomatic. They have a serologic response to ASO and anti-DNA B. Prophylactic antibiotics are not recommended for these patients. Tonsillectomy may be considered when infection attack rates do not decrease over time and no other explanation of recurrent infection can be found. Meta-analyses have found inconclusive evidence of benefit from tonsillectomy compared to nonsurgical treatment.

Patients with GABHS pharyngitis who remain symptomatic and continue to have positive cultures should receive a second course of antibiotics, with either the same antimicrobial agent or intramuscular penicillin. If a patient experiences repeated infections and there is concern that the GABHS infection is being spread among close contacts, all close and family contacts should be cultured, and only those who are positive should be treated. Family pets are not reservoirs and do not spread disease.

Mass screening should be considered in outbreaks of GABHS in a closed or semiclosed community or in outbreaks of acute rheumatic fever or poststreptococcal glomerulonephritis.

Non-GABHS pharyngitis (i.e., group C or G β-hemolytic streptococcus) is not associated with rheumatic fever, and no evidence supports treatment or follow-up culture.

Complications

The complications of GABHS pharyngitis can be classified as suppurative and nonsuppurative.

Suppurative complications occur when the infection spreads to cause conditions such as lateral pharyngeal abscess, cervical lymphandenitis, sinusitis, otitis media, retropharyngeal abscess, Lemierre's syndrome, and mastoiditis. Appropriate treatment of GABHS with antibiotics decreases these complications.

Nonsuppurative complications include acute rheumatic fever, acute poststreptococcal glomerulonephritis, and poststreptococcal reactive arthritis. Acute rheumatic fever occurs 2 to 3 weeks after GABHS pharyngitis. It is not seen after GABHS skin infections. Starting antibiotics within 9 days of symptoms can prevent acute rheumatic fever. Acute poststreptococcal glomerulonephritis can occur 10 days after pharyngeal infection and 21 days after skin infection. Antibiotics do not alter the attack rate. Poststreptococcal reactive arthritis is similar to other reactive arthritis, and the attack rate is not altered by antibiotics.

Potential complications from treatment of GABHS pharyngitis include anaphylactic reaction to antibiotics and antibiotic resistance.

References

ESCMID Sore Throat Guideline Group, Pelucchi C, Grigoryan L, et al: Guideline for the management of acute sore throat, *Clin Microbiol Infect* 18(Suppl 1):1–28, 2012. http://www.ncbi.nlm.nih.gov/pubmed/22432746.

Kociolek L, Shulman S: In the clinic pharyngitis, *Ann Intern Med* 157, 2012. ITC3-1–ITC3-16, Downloaded from http://annals.org.

Sadeghirad B, Siemieniuk RA, Brignardello-Petersen R, et al: Cortiosteroids for treatment of sore throat: Systematic Review & meta-analysis of randomized trials, *BMJ* 358, 2017. j3887/doi:10.1136/bmj.j3887.

Shulman ST, Bisno AL, Clegg HW, et al: Clinical practice guideline for the diagnosis and management of group A streptococcal pharyngitis: 2012 update by the Infectious Diseases Society of America, *Clin Infect Dis* 55:e86–e102, 2012.

PRURITUS

Method of
Hassan Bencheqroun, MD

CURRENT DIAGNOSIS

- A careful history and physical examination will reveal a clear exposure, a sick contact, a recent travel, or clues to a systemic disease.
- Antihistamines are effective in treating histamine-mediated pruritus, but they are less effective in mechanisms involving serotonin, leukotrienes, etc.
- Initial testing in the absence of improvement with nonpharmacologic methods or antihistamine should include complete blood counts, thyroid-stimulating hormone, renal and liver panel, human immunodeficiency virus (HIV) test, and chest radiograph.
- Chronic pruritus may precede a systemic illness, especially in older adults. Hodgkin lymphoma is the malignant disease most strongly associated with pruritus and occurs in up to 30% of patients diagnosed with pruritus.

CURRENT THERAPY

- Acute and localized pruritus may resolve with nonpharmacologic methods, such as skin hydration with hypoallergenic, alcohol-free, and fragrance-free moisturizing creams; decreasing the length of showers and baths as well as the temperature of the water; identifying material that may irritate the skin either in jewelry or clothing items; and avoiding scratching.
- Wound care of scratch lesions includes any cellulitic portions.
- First-line pharmacologic treatments may include the use of antihistamine and antipruritic creams. Antipruritic agents may be used as second-line treatments.

> - In the absence of improvement, the management of chronic pruritus should be directed at the underlying cause, or targets on the pruritic cascade-from blockade of intracellular and intercellular signaling pathways in the skin to the modulation of neurotransmission.

Pruritus is defined as an unpleasant sensory perception that causes the desire to scratch. While it shares similarities with pain, the neurophysiology of pruritus is distinct: pain causes withdrawal, whereas pruritus induces the reflex of reaching out and scratching.

Classification

Pruritus can be distinguished as acute or chronic, with the latter defined by the International Forum for the Study of Itch (IFSI) as lasting for 6 or more weeks.

Despite many classifications over the years, there is no uniform, clinically based classification of pruritic diseases to assist in the diagnosis and management of patients with pruritus. The classification chosen for this chapter focuses on clinical signs and distinguishes between the disease with and without primary or secondary skin lesions.

1. Group 1: Pruritus of primary diseased, inflamed skin
2. Group 2: Pruritus of primary nondiseased, noninflamed skin
3. Group 3: Pruritus with chronic secondary scratch lesions

Pathophysiology

The sensation of pruritus stems from a number of different causes. It is generally transmitted through slow-conducting unmyelinated C fibers and free pruriceptive cutaneous nerve endings located superficially in the skin, which appear to be more sensitive to pruritogenic substances than pain receptors. Histamine, neuropeptide substance P, interleukin 31 (mostly in atopic dermatitis), serotonin (a key component in several diseases), bradykinin, mast cell tryptase, and other unknown mediators (e.g., in uremic pruritus, cholestatic pruritus) may be involved in the genesis of pruritus. Impulses are transmitted from the dorsal root ganglion to the spinothalamic tract. Pruritus then generates a spinal reflex response, the scratch, which is as innate as a deep tendon reflex. Other pathogenic mechanisms include neuropathic (e.g., herpes zoster), acute traumatic stress (following burns and skin grafts), chronic puritis increasingly seen in the elderly including paraneoplastic, and immune-mediated (atopic dermatitis). Lastly, opioids are known to modulate the sensation of pruritus, both peripherally and centrally.

Clinical Manifestations

Pruritus is among the most common symptoms in dermatology. While often overlooked, it is in fact rated by patients as the most quality-of-life–altering symptom of the underlying disease. Other associated symptoms depend on the etiology and may include urticarial skin lesions, dry skin, jaundice, and thyroid-related symptoms. Left untreated, itch and its associated scratching increase the risk of chronic skin changes and secondary infection.

Differential Diagnosis

The patient's workup further places him or her in one of the following categories:

1. Primary diseased, inflamed skin
   - *Inflammatory:* Atopic and contact dermatitis, psoriasis, dry skin, drug reactions
   - *Infectious:* Mycotic, bacterial and viral infections, folliculitis, scabies, pediculosis, arthropod reactions, and insect bites
   - *Autoimmune:* Bullous dermatoses, especially dermatitis herpetiformis, bullous pemphigoid, and dermatomyositis
   - *Dermatoses of pregnancy*
   - *Neoplasms:* Cutaneous T-cell-lymphoma (especially erythrodermic variants), cutaneous B-cell lymphoma, leukemic infiltrates of the skin

2. Primary nondiseased, noninflamed skin
   - Endocrine and metabolic diseases: Chronic renal failure, liver diseases/cholestasis, hyperthyroidism, malabsorption, perimenopausal pruritus
   - Infectious diseases: HIV infection, helminthosis, parasitosis
   - Hematologic and lymphoproliferative diseases, iron deficiency, polycythaemia vera, Hodgkin and non-Hodgkin lymphoma
   - Visceral neoplasms of the cervix, prostate, or colon, carcinoid syndrome
   - Pregnancy: Pruritus gravidarum with and without cholestasis
   - Drug-induced pruritus: Opioids, ACE-inhibitors, amiodarone, hydrochlorothiazide, estrogens, simvastatin, hydroxyethyl starch, allopurinol

3. Pruritus with chronic secondary scratch lesions (The underlying origin may be a systemic disease or a skin disease.)
   - Neurogenic origin (without neuronal damage), such as hepatic itch
   - Neuropathic diseases (neuronal damage causes itch)
   - Multiple sclerosis, neoplasms, abscesses, cerebral or spinal infarcts, brachioradial pruritus, postherpetic neuralgia, vulvodynia, small fiber neuropathy
   - Somatoform pruritus (e.g., obsessive-compulsive disorders)

Therapy

- Basic measures to lessen drying of skin: Limit bathing to short, cool showers with soap applied only to oily skin areas. A mild moisturizing cream is preferably applied immediately after bathing to lock in moisture. The patient's home should be humidified, especially during dry, cold winter months. Avoid contact irritants, such as wool, fiberglass, and detergents.
- Topical corticosteroids, oral melatonin[7], and clonidine (Catapres)[1] showed some efficacy in reducing nocturnal itching or improving sleep quality in nocturnal pruritus.
- Many topical and systemic medications are available, but must be chosen according to existing comorbidities, possible interactions and side effects, and patient's compliance. Ultraviolet therapy may be administered in certain cases.
- Nonspecific therapy: A wheal and flare response is a marker of histamine-induced pruritus in patients with urticaria or an allergic dermatitis. These patients benefit from long-acting antihistamines. Concurrent H1 and H2 blockers increase therapeutic effectiveness. Also exercises focused on learning to disengage patient's attention away from pruritus or pain in chronic pruritis improves the symptoms.
- Specific antipruritic therapies target several points in the pruritic cascade—from blockade of intracellular and intercellular signaling pathways in the skin to the modulation of neurotransmission.
- Nemolizumab[5], an anti-IL-31 A receptor monoclonal antibody, was shown in a Phase II trial to induce a decrease of pruritus intensity in active treatment group when compared to placebo in atopic dermatitis patients.
- Neurokinin 1 receptor antagonists such as aprepitant (Emend)[1] showed potential activity in chronic pruritus. Novel derivates with longer half-life time, such as serlopitant[5] or tradipitant[5], are currently investigated in clinical trials.
- Future treatments also include bile acid transport inhibitors, phosphodiesterase-4 inhibitors, and nerve ion channels modulators.
- Treatment specific: Itching gradually recedes as the primary systemic condition improves.

Complications

Pruritus is accompanied by intense scratching. Skin may thicken, displaying lichen simplex chronicus: a localized skin thickening often appearing over the posterior neck, extremities, scrotum, vulva, anus, and buttocks. In prurigo nodularis, a variant of

---

[1] Not FDA approved for this indication.
[5] Investigational drug in the United States.
[7] Available as a dietary supplement.

lichen simplex chronicus, some nodules develop over areas within easy scratching reach, such as the extensor arms and legs. Impetigo may result from superinfected excoriations in patients with atopic dermatitis.

References

Cho YL, Liu HN, Huang TP, Tarng DC: Uremic pruritus: roles of parathyroid hormone and substance P, *J Am Acad Dermatol* 36:538–543, 1997.

Duval A, Dubertret L: Aprepitant as an antipruritic agent? *The New England Journal of Medicine* 361(14):1415–1416, 2009.

Ganesh E, Maxwell LG: Pathophysiology and management of opioid-induced pruritus, *Drugs* 67:2323–2333, 2007.

Ikoma A, Rukwied R, Ständer S, et al: Neurophysiology of pruritus: interaction of itch and pain, *Arch Dermatol* 139:1475–1478, 2003.

Kwa KAA, Pijpe A, Rashaan ZM, Tuinebreijer WE, Breederveld RS, Van Loey NEE: Course and predictors of pruritus following burns: a multilevel analysis, *Acta Derm Venereol* 98:636–640, 2018.

Krajnik M, Zylicz Z: Understanding pruritus in systemic disease, *J Pain Symptom Manage* 21:151–168, 2001.

McEwen MW, Fite EM, Yosipovitch G, Patel T: Drugs on the horizon for chronic pruritus, *Dermatol Clin* 36(3):335–344, 2018 Jul.

Reamy B: A diagnostic approach to pruritus, *Am Fam Physician* 84:195–202, 2011.

Reich A, Misery L, Takamori K: Pruritus: From the bench to the bedside, *Biomed Res Int* 2018:5742753, 2018 May 22.

Ruzicka T, Hanifin JM, Furue M, et al: Anti-interleukin-31 receptor A antibody for atopic dermatitis, *The New England Journal of Medicine* 376(9):826–835, 2017.

Ständer S, Siepmann D, Herrgott I, Sunderkötter C, Luger TA: Targeting the neurokinin receptor 1 with aprepitant: a novel antipruritic strategy, *PLoS ONE* 5(6), Article ID e10968.

Ständer S, Weisshaar E, Mettang T, et al: Clinical classification of itch: a position paper of the International Forum for the Study of Itch, *Acta Derm Venereol* 87:291–294, 2007.

Zirwas MJ, Seraly MP: Pruritus of unknown origin: a retrospective study, *J Am Acad Dermatol* 45:892–896, 2001.

RHINITIS

Method of
Sheryl Beard, MD

CURRENT DIAGNOSIS

- Rhinitis presents as nasal congestion, sneezing, itching, rhinorrhea, and postnasal drainage.
- Patients with palatal and nasal itching should be considered for allergic disease.
- Allergic rhinitis is confirmed by positive skin-prick testing and IgE reactivity.
- Nonallergic rhinitis patients lack allergic evidence for disease.
- Nonallergic rhinitis conditions have multiple presentations.

CURRENT THERAPY

- Avoidance therapy should be first-line treatment for all forms of rhinitis.
- Second generation oral antihistamines have good therapeutic efficacy for allergic rhinitis.
- Intranasal corticosteroids are the mainstay of treatment for nonallergic rhinitis and moderate-to-severe allergic rhinitis.
- Consultation with an allergy specialist should be considered in cases with multiple treatment failures.
- Patients whose allergic rhinitis is uncontrolled on multiple therapies should be considered for immunotherapy.

Introduction

Rhinitis is defined as inflammation of the nasal mucous membranes. Rhinitis presents as nasal congestion, sneezing, itching, rhinorrhea, and postnasal drainage; it can be divided into allergic and nonallergic rhinitis. Mixed rhinitis has components of both allergic and nonallergic disease. Allergic rhinitis is nasal inflammation that is mediated by IgE to environmental allergens. Nonallergic rhinitis is defined by non–IgE-mediated perennial symptoms. Nonallergic rhinitis shares symptoms with allergic rhinitis, but is only distinguishable by negative allergy tests. Nonallergic rhinitis is also known as perennial nonallergic rhinitis, idiopathic rhinitis, and vasomotor rhinitis.

Most research still classifies allergic rhinitis according to its seasonality or its perennial nature. Seasonal allergic rhinitis is commonly caused by pollen allergens; perennial allergic rhinitis is mainly caused by dust mites and animal dander. Allergic rhinitis can be further classified as mild, moderate, or severe. Mild rhinitis is rhinitis that does not impair work, school, daily functioning, or sleep. Moderate to severe rhinitis interferes with activities of daily living, quality of life, and/or sleep. Severe rhinitis is so marked that normal functioning cannot take place without treatment. Episodic allergic rhinitis occurs with sporadic inhalant aeroallergen exposure not typically encountered by the patient's usual indoor and outdoor environments. An example of episodic allergic rhinitis is a child who is allergic to cats but is not normally exposed, but then visits a household with cats and develops symptoms.

The Allergic Rhinitis and its Impact on Asthma Guidelines: Revised 2010 (ARIA) discouraged the use of the terms seasonal and perennial rhinitis in favor of intermittent and persistent rhinitis. Intermittent rhinitis can be defined as nasal symptoms lasting less than 4 weeks' duration and fewer than 4 days per week. Persistent rhinitis is rhinitis lasting more than 4 weeks' duration or more that 4 days per week.

No standard classification exists for nonallergic rhinitis. A variety of conditions present with similar symptoms and are called nonallergic rhinitis. Nonallergic rhinitis includes vasomotor rhinitis, gustatory rhinitis, nonallergic rhinitis with eosinophilia syndrome (NARES), occupational rhinitis, hormonal rhinitis, drug-induced rhinitis, and atrophic rhinitis. Another entity classified in or out of nonallergic rhinitis is infectious rhinitis.

Local allergic rhinitis is a newly defined entity found in nonatopic patients. Local allergic rhinitis is characterized by local inflammatory reactions including local eosinophils and localized IgE in response to aeroallergens. Local allergic rhinitis does not show significant skin-prick testing reactions, and patients have negative systemic IgE reactions to aeroallergens.

Rhinitis may be viewed by some as a trivial disease, but it places a significant financial burden on society. The estimated direct and indirect costs to society of rhinitis were around $11.58 billion in 2002.

Epidemiology/Risk Factors

The National Health and Nutrition Survey (NHANES II and III) suggests that the overall prevalence of IgE sensitivity might be increasing. Of the patients evaluated for rhinitis in the United States, 43% (58 million people) have allergic disease, 23% (19 million people) have nonallergic disease, and 34% (26 million people) have mixed rhinitis. Seventy percent of allergic patients develop the disease in childhood (20 years and younger) as opposed to nonallergic rhinitis patients, 70% of whom develop disease in adulthood. Approximately two thirds of nonallergic rhinitis patients have vasomotor rhinitis, and one-third have NARES. Nonallergic rhinitis has a female predominance.

The prevalence of local allergic rhinitis is largely unknown. In a small study of rhinitis patients, the prevalence of local allergic rhinitis was 25.7%, nonallergic rhinitis was 11.2%, and allergic rhinitis was 63.1%. Local allergic rhinitis is associated with asthma and conjunctivitis, and commonly begins in childhood.

Pathophysiology
Allergic

Allergic rhinitis is the result of an IgE mediated, type I hypersensitivity allergic reaction in response to an inhaled allergen. Allergens are proteins derived from airborne particulate matter, including dust-mite feces, pollens, animal dander, and cockroach particles. Antigen-presenting cells (APCs) engulf allergens in the nose and break them into antigenic peptides. APCs present these peptides to naïve T cells (T_H0). T_H0 cells differentiate once activated, into the T_H2 subtype. The T_H2 lymphocytes generate cytokines that regulate B-lymphocytes and sequester inflammatory cells (including eosinophils).

B-lymphocytes produce IgE. IgE attaches to mast cells and basophils and renders them sensitized. Once sensitized and cells are exposed to allergen, the mast cells and basophils degranulate. Degranulation of these cells releases a host of mediators including histamine and prostaglandin. Histamine stimulates histamine type I (H1) receptors on nerve endings that cause pruritus, sneezing and increased secretions. These symptoms constitute the early-phase response of allergic rhinitis. The early-phase response occurs within minutes of allergen exposure and dissipates within 1 hour.

Eosinophils produce IL-5, which acts to promote activation and survival of other eosinophils. Eosinophils also produce toxic products that damage local mucosal cells. The damage done by these cells is what constitutes the late-phase reaction. The late-phase reaction occurs several hours after allergen exposure and is characterized by nasal congestion.

Nonallergic Rhinitis

The nasal mucosa has two major functions; one is trapping inhaled particles through mucus production and the second is humidifying inhaled air through a complex vascular system. The mucus glands and the vascular system are regulated by the parasympathetic and the adrenergic nervous systems. Sensory nerves are stimulated by irritants in the nose through the use of a sensory receptor called a *nociceptor*. The nociceptive signal generates a neural reflex in the central nervous system (CNS) controlling sympathetic and parasympathetic tone in the nasal mucosa. Parasympathetic stimulation results in mucus production. Sympathetic stimulation causes vasoconstriction, which empties venous cavities. Lack of sympathetic tone causes venous engorgement and nasal congestion.

Symptomatic nonallergic rhinitis is an exaggeration of a normal defensive mechanism. Inflammation in the nose causes an upregulation of this neural activity, resulting in the exaggerated response (also known as neural hyperresponsiveness). Hyperresponsive parasympathetic efferent nerves trigger glandular activation in the nasal mucosa, leading to vasodilation and mucus production. Excessive mucus production anteriorly causes rhinorrhea and posteriorly causes postnasal drip. This hyperresponsiveness can be due to structural or functional components of the nasal mucosa altered through genetic or pathologic factors. The exact mechanisms of nonallergic rhinitis conditions are poorly understood because of their multiple presentations.

Infectious Rhinitis/Rhinosinusitis

Acute sinusitis (rhinosinusitis) most commonly occurs as a complication of viral upper-respiratory infections (URIs). Viral URIs cause nasal mucosal edema, which leads to obstruction of the sinus openings and ciliary impairment. Bacteria proliferate in the stagnant mucus as well as the low–oxygen-tension environment of the sinus cavities. Chronic rhinosinusitis is the result of long-term obstruction and/or dysfunction of the sinuses. Chronic inflammation leads to chronic low-grade infections.

Prevention

Environmental control of allergens can improve the severity of allergic rhinitis and can reduce the need for medications. Environmental control should be thorough if treatment is sought, but the full beneficial effects of the change may take weeks to months. Mild disease can usually be managed with avoidance measures. Complete avoidance of allergen, particularly pollen, is usually not feasible.

Reduction of dust mite allergen exposure can be done in the following ways: remove carpets and soft toys, use covers impermeable to allergen for mattresses and pillows, vacuum beds weekly, and wash bedding at 60 degrees Celsius (140 degrees Fahrenheit). Pet dander avoidance can only be effectively managed by removing the pet and carefully cleaning all carpets, furniture and mattresses.

Clinical Manifestations

If the patient presents with symptoms of palatal itching, nasal itching, ocular symptoms, or sneezing, consideration should be given to an allergic cause.

The presentation of nonallergic rhinitis is dependent on the type of nonallergic rhinitis. Overall, patients with nonallergic rhinitis lack other allergic conditions.

The vasomotor rhinitis patient will present with predominantly nasal obstruction and rhinorrhea. Typically, symptoms are triggered by temperature, exercise, and environmental stimuli (odors, smoke, and dust).

NARES patients generally have more intense symptoms than vasomotor rhinitis or allergic disease patients. NARES patients present with paroxysms of flares to include sneezing, watery rhinorrhea, nasal itching, congestion, and some anosmia. NARES patients have eosinophils on a nasal smear, but lack other allergic evidence by skin-prick testing.

Gustatory rhinitis sufferers complain of nasal congestion and rhinorrhea associated with ingestion of foods and, sometimes, alcoholic beverages.

Nasal crusting, dryness, and fetor are the characteristics of atrophic rhinitis. These findings are due to glandular cell atrophy. Patients will have abnormally wide nasal cavities and may have squamous metaplasia.

Occupational rhinitis patients have components of allergic and nonallergic disease. Patients present with nasal congestion and rhinorrhea triggered by an occupational exposure. Symptoms are present during duty and generally improve away from the work environment. Substances leading to symptoms include irritating chemicals, grain dust, ozone, lab animal antigens, and wood. Often occupational rhinitis co-exists with occupational asthma.

Hormonal rhinitis manifests as nasal congestion during pregnancy or the menstrual cycle. Pregnant women are six times more likely to have rhinitis and sinusitis than nonpregnant women. Rhinitis usually resolves two weeks postdelivery.

Drug-induced rhinitis occurs with certain medications. ACE inhibitors, phosphodiesterase-5 selective inhibitors, alpha-receptor antagonists, and phentolamine are common triggers. Patients present with rhinorrhea and nasal congestion.

Rhinitis medicamentosa is a condition that presents with severe congestion. It is caused by prolonged and repetitive use of topical nasal decongestants. It can also be associated with cocaine use.

Anatomic rhinitis is more likely in patients who present with unilateral nasal symptoms.

Infectious rhinitis presents with sinus tenderness, erythema to the mucosa, postnasal drainage and sometimes periorbital edema.

Diagnosis

The diagnosis of allergic rhinitis, nonallergic rhinitis, and infectious rhinitis is based largely on history and physical examination. Other diagnostic testing can be performed to aid in providing a more definitive diagnosis or to rule out other causes.

Allergic rhinitis is confirmed by IgE reactivity to environmental allergen sensitivity through skin-prick testing. When skin-prick testing is difficult to interpret or if it is not feasible, serum–allergen-specific IgE testing can be used. Nasal smears looking for eosinophils are not recommended for routine use in the diagnosis of allergic rhinitis.

Other testing available for evaluation of rhinitis includes nasal endoscopy, rhinomanometry, and radiologic imaging. Fiberoptic nasal endoscopy is reserved for those with atypical symptoms or an inadequate response to treatment. Rhinomanometry measures airflow obstruction in the upper airway. Rhinomanometry provides an objective measurement of nasal congestion. Rhinomanometry is used to evaluate clinical response to interventions and assess anatomic severity, such as in patients with obstructive sleep apnea. Radiologic imaging, such as computerized tomography (CT) and magnetic resonance imaging (MRI), is used to evaluate anatomic structure. Imaging may not correlate well with nasal function and is expensive.

If a provider suspects a cerebrospinal fluid (CSF) leak, the rhinorrhea can be evaluated for beta transferrin protein, which is present only in CSF.

History

The best diagnostic tool in the evaluation of rhinitis is the history. Information regarding previous evaluation and treatment should be elicited. A positive family history of rhinitis points towards allergic disease. The history of symptoms should include questions regarding congestion; sneezing; rhinorrhea; sore throat; dry throat; cough; itchy, red, or tearing eyes; voice changes; sinus symptoms of drainage; pressure or pain; snoring; ear pain or loss of hearing; and smelling difficulty.

When gathering the details of each symptom, evaluate the onset (such as those in childhood), frequency (episodic versus continual), pattern (seasonality), characteristics of secretions, triggers, severity (to include quality of life evaluation), and associated geographic location or environment (home versus work). Once a trigger is identified, history needs to be gathered even further to evaluate the possibility of modifying the exposure.

Physical Examination

As with any disease process, the physical examination provides clues into the diagnosis. Although the physical examination in rhinitis patients should focus on the nasal mucosa, other body areas should be examined to rule out other processes. For example, the tympanic membranes should be examined for mobility, retraction, erythema, and Eustachian tube dysfunction.

Examination of the eyes in allergic rhinitis might show that the conjunctiva have edema, erythema, and/or cobblestoning. Excessive lacrimation could be another finding. Darkening of the skin of the lower eyelids is prevalent in allergic disease and is also called "allergic shiners."

Allergic and nonallergic nasal mucosa may have a similar appearance. The nasal mucosa may appear boggy with a bluish appearance or be erythematous. Excessive watery-clear mucus might be present. Turbinate hypertrophy is another physical examination finding in rhinitis. Other nasal mucosa findings to look for are nasal polyps, sinusitis, septal deviation, septal perforation, and crusting.

Looking for elongated facies, mouth breathing, and a high arch in the palate may provide a clue to the severity of the nasal obstruction. The tonsils and adenoids should be examined for enlargement. Posterior nasal drainage and cobblestoning in the oropharynx are common findings in rhinitis patients.

The skin examination provides useful information in the patient with rhinitis. Atopic dermatitis or urticaria may be findings associated with allergic disease. The skin should be evaluated for dermatographism. Patients with dermatographism cannot be evaluated for allergic disease using skin-prick testing.

Differential Diagnosis

Many different pathologic conditions can present similarly to rhinitis. Conditions to keep in mind while evaluating and treating a patient for rhinitis include: nasal polyps, ciliary dyskinesia syndrome, anatomic abnormalities such as deviated septum or tumors, nasal turbinate hypertrophy, cerebrospinal fluid rhinorrhea, pharyngonasal reflux, systemic disorders such as Wegener's disease, aspirin intolerance, and other medication side effects.

Treatment

Overall

Current guidelines in treatment of rhinitis do not take cost into consideration. However, the individual treatment goals should be based on factors such as age, route of administration preference (i.e., nasal versus oral), severity, seasonality, side effects, cost, benefit to comorbid conditions, and onset of action. For example, onset of action is an important consideration for an individual who has more episodic symptoms. Also, individual patients respond differently to treatment regimens within a given group.

Avoidance

Due to the lack of high-quality evidence, implementation of avoidance measures is largely based on panel recommendations. In addition, the ubiquitous nature of allergens may limit the effectiveness of the avoidance measures. For dust mites, encasing pillows and bedding in dust mite resistant materials may be beneficial. Pollen is seasonal and can be minimized by keeping the windows closed, using air conditioning, and limiting outdoor exposure. Using particulate filters in the home can also assist in reducing overall allergen load of pollens and dust. Avoiding basements and lowering household humidity may reduce the amount of mold exposure patients receive. Pet avoidance can only be reached by ridding the house of the pet altogether. Other, less-effective measures include limiting exposure of the pet to the house and/or bedroom.

Intranasal Corticosteroid (INS)

Intranasal corticosteroids are first-line treatment for moderate to severe allergic rhinitis and most nonallergic rhinitis conditions. All allergic rhinitis symptoms can be treated with INS. The intranasal corticosteroids budesonide aerosol (Rhinocort Aqua), fluticasone propionate aqueous (Flonase), and beclomethasone aqueous (Beconase AQ) preparations all have a Federal Drug Administration (FDA) treatment indication of nonallergic rhinitis. Intranasal corticosteroid side effects include irritation, bleeding, and perforation of the nasal septum; rarely, local candidiasis is seen with INS use. They are safe to use in pregnancy. No single INS preparation is more efficacious than, or has any relevant difference from, any other. INS has negligible hypothalamic-pituitary-adrenal axis suppression, and systemic burden is clinically insignificant.

Intranasal Anticholinergic (IP)

Ipratropium bromide (Atrovent), a specific intranasal anticholinergic, inhibits parasympathetic function in the nasal mucosa. The parasympathetic blockade reduces the output of secretions from seromucus glands in the nose. Ipratropium can be used in treatment of anterior watery rhinorrhea but has a very limited role in reducing postnasal drip, nasal congestion, or sneezing. Topical ipratropium prior to ingestion of food can be used as pretreatment of gustatory rhinitis and is effective in treatment of the common cold and skier's nose. Side effects of IP include nasal dryness, burning, irritation, stuffy nose, headache, and dry mouth.

Intranasal Antihistamine (INA)

Azelastine (Astelin) is a nasal spray approved by the FDA for allergic and vasomotor rhinitis. Olopatadine (Patanase) intranasal spray has been approved for seasonal allergic rhinitis. INA has faster onset of action than intranasal corticosteroids. INA should be taken twice per day for maximum clinical benefit and may benefit those with nasal congestion. INA does not produce a significant amount of sedation, but side effects include headache, epistaxis, bitter taste, and nasal irritation.

Nasal Cromolyn

Cromolyn (NasalCrom) should be considered for early mild rhinitis, but should not be considered a first-line treatment in allergic rhinitis. Nasal cromolyn can be used prior to allergen exposure for prophylaxis of episodic allergic rhinitis. Cromolyn is mostly void of side effects. Cromolyn inhibits mast cell degranulation and is administered three to four times a day. Cromolyn has very limited usefulness for nonallergic rhinitis conditions.

Nasal Saline

Using nasal saline to irrigate the nasal cavities may remove mucus, enhance ciliary movement, improve sinus opening, and remove allergic and irritant particles. Several devices exist including: the neti pot, a nasally adapted plastic bottle, and a pulse irrigator.

Evidence suggests that hypertonic saline provides modest benefit over isotonic saline, although it might be more irritating.

Topical Decongestants

Topical decongestants reduce congestion, but have no effect on itching, sneezing, or rhinorrhea. Oxymetazoline (Afrin), a common topical decongestant, causes nasal vasoconstriction. Vasoconstriction can cause tissue hypoxemia and inflammation, leading to severe rebound nasal congestion. Topical decongestants are not recommended for continued use because they can cause rhinitis medicamentosa.

Oral Antihistamines

Oral antihistamines block H1 receptors, thereby reducing nasal and palatal itching, rhinorrhea, sneezing, conjunctivitis, and urticaria. Nasal congestion is not treated well with oral antihistamines. First-generation oral antihistamines are poorly selective for H1 receptors. The sedative effects of these antihistamines result from crossing the blood–brain barrier; they have been linked to industrial accidents and contribute to loss of function at work and school. For these reasons, first-generation antihistamines have limited usefulness. Second generation H1 antagonists have excellent evidence for therapeutic efficacy. These medications may have some role in the treatment of nonallergic rhinitis because of their anticholinergic properties, but consideration must be given to these systemic properties, including dry mucous membranes, blurry vision, constipation, tachycardia, and urinary retention. A combination of intranasal corticosteroid treatment with oral antihistamines may be effective for sneezing and rhinorrhea in NARES.

Leukotriene Receptor Antagonists (LTRA)

Leukotriene receptor antagonists were originally studied in the treatment of asthma. The only LTRA approved by the FDA for treatment of allergic rhinitis is montelukast (Singulair). Montelukast is clinically efficacious in both perennial and seasonal allergic rhinitis. Montelukast is approved for children 6 months and older and has a pregnancy category B rating. The oral antihistamine loratadine (Claritin) and montelukast have similar efficacy, and can have additional benefit when used together. Although rare, montelukast has been associated with adverse psychiatric behavior, including suicidality. LTRA have no role in nonallergic rhinitis.

Oral Decongestants

Oral decongestants such as pseudoephedrine reduce nasal congestion. Oral decongestants have a sales restriction in many states. Side effects include insomnia, anorexia, irritability, and palpitations. Blood pressure elevation is rarely a concern in controlled hypertensive patients or in normotensive patients. Oral decongestants should be considered last-line treatment for nonallergic rhinitis conditions.

Systemic Corticosteroids

Few studies are available to support the use of systemic steroids in the treatment of rhinitis. Oral corticosteroids may have a role for severe resistive rhinitis, but not as first-line treatment. Short-term use of 5 to 7 days of oral corticosteroids is the standard, but they should not be used for longer than 3 weeks because of the risk for adverse effects. Oral steroids should be used as first-line treatment for severe nasal polyposis, a subset of anatomic rhinitis. Systemic steroids should not be used in children or pregnant women. Intraturbinate injections of corticosteroids have no role in the treatment of rhinitis. Parenteral corticosteroids are contraindicated because of long-term effects.

Surgery

Surgery can reduce nasal obstruction caused by septal deviation, turbinate hypertrophy, or adenoid hypertrophy. Procedures that can be performed include nasal polypectomy, septoplasty, reductive hypertrophic turbinate surgery, adenoidectomy, and endoscopic sinus surgery. Two nerves can be transected to decrease the parasympathetic nerve supply to the nasal mucosa: the vidian nerve, through endoscopic resection; and the anterior ethmoid nerve, through electrocoagulation, which leads to reduced nasal secretions.

Anti IgE

Omalizumab (Xolair) is a monoclonal antibody available for the treatment of poorly controlled asthma, but it might have a role in the treatment of allergic rhinitis.[1] Omalizumab binds to IgE, hindering its relationship with inflammatory cells. Omalizumab only binds to circulating IgE and not bound IgE. Due to its high cost, reports of anaphylaxis, and its injectable only formulation, omalizumab has a limited role in allergic rhinitis treatment.

Immunotherapy

Allergen extract immunotherapy has been used in the treatment of respiratory allergic disease since 1911, and its efficacy has been documented since the 1970s. The amount of allergen in each immunotherapy dose is slowly increased with each dose until a maintenance phase is reached. Immunotherapy is an effective treatment for allergic rhinitis and is the only treatment proven to alter the course of allergic disease. Debate exists regarding which form of immunotherapy is superior. Contraindications to immunotherapy include beta-blocker use, due to complications in treating anaphylaxis, and uncontrolled underlying diseases, such as uncontrolled asthma.

Subcutaneous immunotherapy uses the injectable form of allergen extract. Adequate treatment usually consists of a 3- to 5-year course of immunotherapy. Subcutaneous immunotherapy is indicated in those patients for whom medications and avoidance measures are inadequate, as well as those with only a few relevant allergens. The inherent risk of subcutaneous immunotherapy is systemic anaphylaxis, therefore it is dosed in the physician's office. The rate of local reactions in subcutaneous immunotherapy is 0.6-58% and systemic reactions is 0.06 to 0.9%. The risk of death is 1 per 2.5 million injections. Subcutaneous immunotherapy is covered by most insurance plans.

Studies for local-route immunotherapy (noninjected), many of which were carried out in Europe, have only been undertaken in adults. Local routes of immunotherapy include sublingual, local nasal, oral, and bronchial. Indications for local-route immunotherapy are the same as those for subcutaneous immunotherapy.

Sublingual immunotherapy was approved by the FDA in April 2014. Sublingual immunotherapy formulations in the United States are low dose compared to those used in Europe, but have limited allergens available. The risk profile is low and therefore can be dosed at home. The rate of local reactions with sublingual immunotherapy is 0.2-97% and systemic reactions is 0.056%. No deaths have been reported with sublingual immunotherapy use. Some medical allergy providers use subcutaneous extracts (aqueous) as sublingual therapy, but this is an off-label use.

Use of local nasal immunotherapy is used mostly in Europe. Oral and bronchial immunotherapy are not supported by evidence.

Monitoring

The provider should consider stepping down treatment when the patients' symptoms have been controlled. The Total Nasal Symptoms Score [TNSS] is a subjective assessment of the patient's specific symptoms, including rhinorrhea, nasal congestion, sneezing, and pruritus, and can be used to assess effectiveness of medications. The Rhinoconjunctivitis Quality of Life Questionnaire can also be used. Consideration for referral to an allergist might be extended to patients who have had a prolonged course, secondary infections, polyps, or other comorbid conditions including chronic sinusitis and asthma, or if immunotherapy is a consideration.

---

[1] Not FDA approved for this indication.

Complications

Rhinitis is associated with multiple complications including fatigue, decline in cognitive function, loss of productivity, headache, and disturbance of sleep. Patients with mild disease may experience these in mild form. Patients with moderate to severe disease may experience these complications in addition to impairment of activities, leisure, and work or school functioning.

References

Brozek J, Bousquet J, Baena-Cagnani C, et al: Allergic rhinitis and its impact on asthma (ARIA) guidelines: 2010 revision, *J Allergy Clin Immunol* 126:466–476, 2010.

Chaaban M, Corey J: Pharmacotherapy of rhinitis and rhinosinusitis, *Facial Plast Surg Clin North Am* 20:61–71, 2012.

Cox L, Compalati E, Canonica W: Will sublingual immunotherapy become an approved treatment method in the United States? *Curr Allergy Asthma Rep* 11:4–6, 2011.

Dykewicz M: Management of rhinitis: guidelines, evidence basis, and systematic clinical approach for what we do, *Immunol Allergy Clin North Am* 31:619–634, 2011.

Greiner A, Meltzer E: Overview of the treatment of allergic rhinitis and nonallergic rhinopathy, *Proc Am Thorac Soc* 8:121–131, 2011.

Rondon C, Campo P, Galindo L, et al: Prevalence and clinic relevance of local allergic rhinitis, *Allergy* 67:1282–1288, 2012, https://doi.org/10.1111/all.12002.

Seidman MD, Schwartz SR, Bonner JR, et al: Clinical practice guideline: allergic rhinitis, *Otolaryngol Head Neck Surg* 152(1 Suppl.):S1–S43, 2015.

Settipane R, Charnock D: Epidemiology of rhinitis: allergic and nonallergic, *Clin Allergy Immunol* 19:23–34, 2007.

Sin B, Togias A: Pathophysiology of allergic and nonallergic rhinitis, *Proc Am Thorac Soc* 8:106–114, 2011.

van Cauwenberge P, Bachert C, Passalacqua G, et al: Consensus statement on the treatment of allergic rhinitis. European Academy of Allergology and Clinical Immunology, *Allergy* 55:116–134, 2000.

Wallace D, Dykewicz M: The diagnosis and management of rhinitis: an updated practice parameter, *J Allergy Clin Immunol* 122:S1–S84, 2008.

Young-Yuen Wu A: Immunotherapy: vaccines for allergic disease, *J Thorac Dis* 4:198–202, 2012.

SPINE PAIN

Method of
David Borenstein, MD; and Federico Balagué, MD

CURRENT DIAGNOSIS

- Most spine pain is mechanical in origin in 95% or more of patients.
- Symptoms of mechanical acute spine pain resolve in most patients in 1 to 8 weeks.
- Most patients with spine pain do not require laboratory tests or radiographs to achieve resolution of their symptom of spine pain.

CURRENT THERAPY

- Localized neck or low back pain
  - Encouragement to remain active out of bed
  - Patient education about the natural history to improvement
  - Reassurance about the incidence of resolution
  - Effective oral drug therapy: NSAIDs, analgesics, muscle relaxants
  - Physical therapy with exercise program
- Radicular pain
  - Encouragement to remain active out of bed
  - Patient education about the potential for improvement
  - Efficacy of oral drug therapy: NSAIDs, analgesics, muscle relaxants, corticosteroids, antiseizure medication, epidural corticosteroid injections
  - Physical therapy: Mackenzie exercises for disk herniation
  - Surgical decompression for cauda equina, motor weakness, or intractable pain

Abbreviation: NSAID = nonsteroidal antiinflammatory drug.

Spine pain is a common symptom that is diagnosed and treated by a wide variety of health care professionals. The interest in this medical problem is not limited to its incidence as a patient problem but also stems from the likelihood of spine pain being experienced by the treating physician as well. The good news about spine pain is that the vast majority of patients (about 90%) improve over 2 months with minimal intervention, but relapses are frequent. The bad news is that the smaller number of patients who develop chronic spine pain use more than the majority of health resources expended on this expensive medical problem. The goal of therapy is to relieve spine pain while it is acute so that chronic pain does not develop.

The axial skeleton may be divided into cervical, thoracic, lumbar, sacral, and coccygeal locations. The lumbar and cervical areas are the most mobile and at greatest risk for damage. These two areas will be the primary subjects of this article.

Epidemiology

Spine pain is the most common musculoskeletal complaint worldwide and produces direct and indirect costs of hundreds of billions of dollars each year in the United States. More than 80% of the world's population at some time during their lives will have an episode of low back pain. An estimated 20% of the US population has back pain every year. Neck pain occurs at a variable rate ranging from 0.055/1000 person-years (disk herniation with radiculopathy) to 213/1000 person-years (self-reported neck pain). Thoracic spine pain is relatively rare compared with the incidence of pain in the other two locations in the axial skeleton.

Persons of all ages develop spine pain. Younger people are at risk for developmental problems (idiopathic scoliosis, spondylolysis, spondylolisthesis), and older patients develop disorders associated with degeneration of spinal structures (osteoarthritis, spinal stenosis).

Risk Factors

Psychosocial factors are stronger predictors of incident low back pain than mechanical factors in adolescent populations. In adults, psychosocial difficulties are risk factors for chronicity more strongly related to outcome than any clinical or mechanical variables. Previous episodes of spine pain are strong predictors of future ones.

Studies of cohorts of twins have shown that nonspecific low back pain is more than 60% genetically determined, and work and leisure-time physical activities play a minor role. Other environmental factors, such as smoking and obesity, have not been shown to be a predictor of the development of spine pain on a consistent basis.

Pathophysiology

Most of the structures of the axial skeleton receive sensory input. The presence of anatomic alterations in these structures is not sufficient to predict the presence of pain. In general, spine pain is referred to as nonspecific because no definite pain generator can be identified. The nociceptive inputs generated by musculoskeletal structures is referred to as *somatic pain*.

In the first few decades of life, muscular sprains and strains of the paraspinous muscles in the lumbar and cervical regions are the most likely source of spinal pain. These muscular injuries occur when lifting in a position that places stress on paraspinous structures. Often the spine is in an awkward position and is mechanically disadvantaged. The subsequent muscle injury results in reflexive muscular contraction that can recruit muscles in the same myotome. Tonic contraction approximates the damaged components of the muscle but results in relative anoxia that causes the production of anaerobic metabolites that stimulate nociceptors. The number of recruited muscles may be extensive, manifested by severe spinal stiffness and limitation of motion. Most of these soft-tissue injuries to the muscle heal spontaneously without any long-term structural alterations.

Simultaneously, as people age, intervertebral disks become flatter as the nucleus pulposus loses its absorbency and the annulus fibrosus fissures and degenerates. The process results in the loss of disk integrity. Degeneration of normal biomechanical and biochemical disk properties results. Biomechanical insufficiency inevitably results in a transfer of stresses posterior to the facet joints and ligaments that are ill suited to assume compressive, tensile, and shear loads. Osteophytes form in response to these abnormal pressures, compromising the space for the neural elements. Disk degeneration itself might not be a painful process until alterations in facet joint alignment result in the onset of articular pain.

Spondylolysis is a developmental abnormality associated with a stress fracture in the growth plate of the pars interarticularis. This abnormality may be discovered as a radiographic abnormality in an asymptomatic patient. An increased risk of low back pain occurs with spondylolisthesis, the abnormality associated with instability of spinal elements in the setting of spondylolysis.

Pain generation in the axial skeleton may be somatic or neuropathic in origin. The joints, ligaments, muscles, fascia, blood vessels, and disks can be the source of localized somatic spine pain. Somatic pain, when it does radiate, tends to be less focused in distribution and exacerbated by specific positions of the spine.

Neuropathic or radicular pain is the sensation generated by damage of neural elements. Intervertebral disk herniation with compression of spinal nerve roots causes neural inflammation resulting in neuropathic and radicular pain. Radicular pain follows the path of the corresponding spinal nerve root. In addition to pain, sensory deficits and muscle weakness can occur, depending on the intensity of the nerve compression. In the setting of chronic low back pain, the role of the central nervous system in mediating persistent symptoms has been highlighted increasingly in the medical literature.

Prevention

Since the turn of the century, adolescents have reported nonspecific spine pain at an incidence similar to that in adult populations. This finding suggests that primary prevention must be given at a very early age to have any chance of efficacy.

Among papers reporting on primary prevention, only exercise has shown effectiveness, with effect sizes ranging from 0.39 to 0.69. Other techniques, such as stress management, shoe inserts, back supports, education, and reduced lifting, were found ineffective.

Clinical Manifestations

The most common symptoms of spinal disorders are regional pain and decreased range of motion associated in a minority of patients with radiating pain. For the majority of patients, pain has mechanical characteristics: Its intensity increases with physical activity, movements, or some postures and decreases with rest. However, it has been demonstrated that nocturnal pain is not uncommon in the absence of serious, specific spinal disorders. The precise topography of pain is often difficult for the patient to describe, and its interpretation is difficult owing to the overlap of the cutaneous projections between adjacent spinal levels and the similarities between dermatomes, myotomes, and sclerotomes.

Diagnosis

The diagnosis of spine pain is based upon the patient's history and physical examination. The history and physical examination should include a description of the pain that is as detailed as possible (e.g., past episodes, precise location, beginning of symptoms, factors increasing or decreasing pain intensity, radiating pain, neurologic symptoms, systemic symptoms), patient's medical history (e.g., past spinal surgery, neoplasia, corticosteroid treatments), and a limited physical examination focused on the posture of the spine, range of motion, muscle contraction, pain on palpation or percussion, and a brief neurologic examination.

Besides the high rate of false-positive results and financial costs, imaging studies have a negative effect on a patient's quality of life. Therefore, unless there is a clear-cut surgical indication or a suspicion of an underlying life-threatening disorder, no imaging studies should be ordered on the first encounter for a patient with acute nonspecific low back or neck pain. Similarly, laboratory testing is not required unless a patient presents with clinical symptoms that suggest a systemic illness (e.g., fever, weight loss).

Differential Diagnosis

A number of guidelines are available in the literature to help a clinician in the diagnosis and treatment of patients with spine pain. The purpose of these approaches is to differentiate the vast majority of patients with mechanical disorders who will improve with noninvasive therapy without the need for radiographic or laboratory investigation from the small minority with a specific cause of spinal pain.

Traditionally, red flags have been used to identify patients with a systemic disorder causing spine pain. The red flags have included questions regarding prior history of cancer, weight loss, prolonged morning stiffness, bladder dysfunction, and bowel dysfunction. The presence of these findings suggests a diagnosis of malignancy, infection, spondyloarthropathy, or cauda equina syndrome, respectively. A study has reported that red-flag disorders occur so infrequently and have so many false-positive findings as not to be helpful in the primary care setting at the initial visit. The one exception was spine pain associated with osteoporotic vertebral compression fractures.

Despite the findings of this one report, clinicians need to be mindful of patients who would be harmed to a significant degree by delayed therapy. The disorders that require expeditious evaluation and treatment are intraabdominal vascular disorders with tearing pain and hemodynamic instability (expanding aortic aneurysm); cauda equina syndrome with bilateral sciatica; saddle anesthesia; bladder or bowel incontinence (lumbar space-occupying compressive lesions); and cervical myelopathy with balance difficulties, autonomic dysfunction, and hyperreflexia with spasticity and Babinski's sign (cervical space-occupying compressive lesions). These disorders require expeditious vessel repair or decompression surgery.

The differential diagnosis of mechanical low back pain (Table 1) and mechanical neck pain (Table 2) includes disorders ranging from muscle strain and herniated disk to scoliosis and whiplash injuries. The age of patients, pain pattern with exacerbating and mitigating factors, tension signs, and findings of plain radiographs can help differentiate among these common causes of spine pain.

Nonspecific is a term used commonly to describe the pain associated with mechanical disorders. On occasion, physicians have confused the use of "nonspecific" as meaning an absence of pathology causing pain associated with mechanical disorders. The "nonspecific" designation refers to the inability to identify the specific pain-generating anatomic structure, not the absence of somatic pain.

Therapy

Many mechanical disorders of the spine are self-limited in duration, with a vast majority of patients improving gradually over time (Box 1). This progression to "natural healing" makes placebo look efficacious in many clinical trials investigating therapies for spine pain. This situation results in evidence-based reviews of spine pain therapies revealing very few categories that have a clinically significant impact on improvement. Nonetheless, physicians need to make therapeutic choices for their patients despite this relative paucity of evidence. Therapy for spine pain includes controlled physical activity, nonsteroidal antiinflammatory drugs (NSAIDs), skeletal muscle relaxants, local and epidural corticosteroid injections, and long-term pain therapy. Surgical intervention is reserved for patients who have surgically correctable abnormalities and who have cauda equina syndrome, increasing motor weakness, spasticity, or intractable pain.

The treatment of an individual patient has to be tailored based on the patient's expectations and preferences. Goals of the treatment should be clearly defined, and the patient should be informed about the expected benefits and side effects of the treatment at the first encounter. A short trial limited to a few days may be a good start.

TABLE 1 Mechanical Low Back Pain

FEATURE	MUSCLE STRAIN	HERNIATED NUCLEUS PULPOSUS	OSTEOARTHRITIS	SPINAL STENOSIS	SPONDYLOLIS-THESIS	SCOLIOSIS
Age (yr)	20–40	30–50	>50	>60	20	30
Pain Pattern						
Location	Back (unilateral)	Back/leg (unilateral)	Back (unilateral)	Leg (bilateral)	Back	Back
Onset	Acute	Acute (previous episodes)	Insidious	Insidious	Insidious	Insidious
Standing	↑	↓	↑	↑	↑	↑
Sitting	↓	↑	↓	↓	↓	↓
Bending	↑	↑	↓	↓	↑	↑
Straight leg	–	+	–	+ (stress)	–	–
Plain radiograph*	–	–	+	+	+	+

Reprinted with permission from Mechanical low back pain. In Borenstein DG, Wiesel SW, Boden SD (eds): Low back and neck pain, 3rd ed. Philadelphia, Saunders, 2004.
*Possibility of seeing the abnormality, not a recommendation to get radiographs.
↑, increased; ↓, decreased; +, present; –, absent.

TABLE 2 Mechanical Neck Pain

FEATURE	NECK STRAIN	HERNIATED NUCLE-US PULPOSUS	OSTEOARTHRITIS	MYELOPATHY	WHIPLASH
Age (yr)	20–40	30–50	>50	>60	30–40
Pain Pattern					
Location	Neck	Neck/arm	Neck	Arm/leg	Neck
Onset	Acute	Acute	Insidious	Insidious	Acute
Flexion	+	+	–	–	+
Extension	–	+/–	+	+	+
Plain radiograph*	–	–	+	+	–

*Possibility of seeing the abnormality, not a recommendation to get radiographs.
+, present; –, absent.
Reprinted with permission from Mechanical neck pain. In Borenstein DG, Wiesel SW, Boden SD (eds): Low back and neck pain, 3rd ed. Philadelphia, Saunders, 2004.

Self-management with education of the patient about maintaining physical activities as tolerated has been encouraged for neck and low back pain. Information on nonpharmacologic pain-management strategies and daily life activities may be provided by health care providers, but patients adhere more to the former than to the latter.

Exercises are slightly effective for pain and function in patients with chronic low back pain. No specific form of exercise is clearly better than others.

The use of manipulative physical techniques in the care of patients with spine pain remains controversial. The absence of clear-cut distinctions between manipulative techniques with or without thrust adds to the confusion when one analyzes the efficacy of manual therapy treatments. Overall there is some clinical trial evidence in favor of spinal manipulation for acute low back pain.

NSAIDs have short-term efficacy for both acute and chronic low back pain; however, the effect sizes are not very large. The efficacy of these drugs for patients with radicular pain has not been evaluated well enough to make general recommendations. No single class of NSAIDs has superiority to another. Cyclooxygenase 2 (COX-2) inhibitors have a better gastrointestinal (GI) safety profile but no greater efficacy. A patient's response cannot be predicted, and a trial-and-error approach is often necessary.

Opiates have not demonstrated any favorable influence in the outcome of low back pain patients. Side effects are quite common and the risk of addiction is real. When these kinds of drugs are effective, the improvement is more important in pain intensity than in terms of function. Muscle relaxants do have some efficacy for acute and chronic low back pain, but the effect size is limited.

Antidepressants are not generally prescribed owing to an inconsistent improvement of patients. For patients with chronic low back pain and depression, an optimized antidepressant treatment shows a better effect on depression than on pain and functional capacity. Duloxetine (Cymbalta), a serotonin and norepinephrine reuptake inhibitor, is approved by the U.S. Food and Drug Administration for the indication of chronic low back pain.

Evidence is lacking to support the prescription of systemic corticosteroids. However, corticosteroids have the advantage of not being toxic to the kidneys. Oral corticosteroids may be considered in patients with radicular pain from a herniated disk or spinal stenosis where epidural injections are relatively contraindicated (chronic warfarin therapy).

Some patients will have persistent neuropathic pain despite surgical decompression or as a result of postsurgical fibrosis. Opioid therapy is ineffective in many patients with chronic neuropathic pain. Antiseizure medicines, such as gabapentin (Neurontin)[1] and pregabalin (Lyrica), have efficacy in peripheral neuropathic pain. These same medicines are prescribed in patients with chronic

---

[1] Not FDA approved for this indication.

BOX 1 — Management of Low Back Pain

BOX 1   Management of Low Back Pain

Acute (3–6 weeks)
First consultation: gather information on core outcome domains
Rule out pain of nonspinal origin
Rule out specific causes (red flags)
No routine imaging
Inform and reassure the patient. Advise to stay active and continue daily activities, if possible, including work
Prescribe analgesia, if necessary. First choice: acetaminophen; second choice: NSAIDs
Consider adding muscle relaxants (short course) or referring for spinal manipulation
Avoid overmedicalizing, especially in patients with favorable outcome
Be aware of yellow flags: inappropriate attitudes and beliefs about back pain, inappropriate pain behavior, emotional problems

Subacute (6–12 weeks)
Reassessment

Bear in mind minimum clinically important difference of core outcome tools
Consider patients' expectations
Consider yellow flags if outcome is not favorable
Reassess regularly by valid outcome tools to evaluate response to treatment
Focus on function
Give priority to active treatments
Consider multidisciplinary program in occupational setting for workers with subacute low back pain and sick leave (>4–8 weeks)

Chronic (3–12 weeks)
Repeat thorough clinical examination
In cases of low impairment and disability, simple evidence-based therapies (e.g., exercises, medication, brief interventions) might be sufficient
In cases of more-severe disability or chronicity, give priority to multidisciplinary approaches (biopsychosocial)

Abbreviation: NSAID = Nonsteroidal antiinflammatory drug.
From Balagué F, Mannion AF, Pellisé F, Cedraschi C. Clinical update: low back pain. Lancet 2007;369(9563):726–728.

---

neuropathic radicular pain with the hope that the mechanisms that work with peripheral neuropathy will also work for spine pain patients. Other medicines including antidepressants (duloxetine [Cymbalta], tricyclic antidepressants) have been tried when other drugs have been ineffective.

Epidural, selective nerve root, or facet joint injections have not shown adequate efficacy to be recommended on a regular basis. However, a limited number (2 or 3) of spinal injections may be attempted for patients with radicular pain who do not improve with oral medication.

Spinal surgery is indicated for disk herniation with radicular compromise, cervical or lumbar spinal stenosis with myelopathy or neurogenic claudication, and unstable spondylolisthesis. Controversy remains, however, concerning the relative benefit of surgical versus medical therapy for radiculopathy. Diskectomy significantly shortens (by about 8 weeks) the acute phase of pain associated with radiculopathy. However, studies with longer follow-up periods have never shown a clear difference between conservative and surgical therapies. Some studies have shown that intensive, multidisciplinary, conservative programs can be compared with surgical fusion procedures for patients with spinal instability.

For the most chronically disabled spine pain patients only, intensive multidisciplinary programs including, among others, physical reconditioning and cognitive-behavioral methods, have shown effectiveness.

Monitoring

From the standpoint of monitoring the efficacy of the treatment, five main dimensions have been recommended to evaluate the outcome of patients with spine pain. The intensity of pain is relevant, but so is the perceived functional capacity, generic health status, work disability, and satisfaction with treatment. Many tools are available for the evaluation of each specific dimension. The clinician who decides to start using any specific tool needs to know, among other information, the minimal clinically meaningful changes for each tool, because differences that may be statistically significant when comparing two groups of patients may be irrelevant at the individual patient level. For example, in terms of intensity of pain, the threshold usually accepted is 3.5 to 4.7 and 2.5 to 4.5 out of 10 for patients with acute and chronic pain, respectively.

Precisely evaluating several domains with specific tools is rather time consuming. However, for busy clinicians, there are brief instruments (core set of measures) with roughly 7 or 8 questions

that include all the previously mentioned dimensions and that have been properly validated.

Complications

The clinician should inform the patient about the possible side effects of therapies as they are initiated. At subsequent visits, specific questions regarding the potential side effects are asked. For example, the presence of hypertension, peripheral edema, and hepatic and renal dysfunction need to be evaluated in patients who are taking chronic NSAID therapy.

In addition, a majority of NSAIDs have potential GI toxicity including mild mucosal irritation, ulcers, and perforations. Hematologic and neurologic toxicity are quite variable depending on the prescribed drug. Cardiovascular toxicity may clearly be an issue, particularly for long-term treatments. The benefit of persistent use of NSAIDs for patients with chronic spine pain needs to be weighed against the increased risk of toxicities.

The use of opiates induces constipation and urinary retention that may be a serious problem for some patients. These drugs can also produce drowsiness, headache, nausea, or vomiting.

Antidepressants also produce drowsiness and anticholinergic symptoms during the first couple of weeks of use. These drugs have specific side effects including tachycardia, weight gain, or sexual problems.

References

Balague F, Mannion AF, Pellise F, Cedraschi C: Seminar on nonspecific low back pain, *Lancet* 379(9814):482–491, 2012.
Bigos SJ, Holland J, Holland C, et al: High-quality controlled trials on preventing episodes of back problems: Systematic literature review in working-age adults, *Spine J* 9(2):147–168, 2009.
Borenstein D: Mechanical low back pain - a rheumatologist's view, *Nat Rev Rheumatol* 9:643–653, 2013.
Briggs AM, Smith AJ, Straker LM, Bragge P: Thoracic spine pain in the general population: Prevalence, incidence and associated factors in children, adolescents and adults. A systematic review, *BMC Musculoskelet Disord* 10:77, 2009.
Chou R, Fu R, Carrino JA, Deyo RA: Imaging strategies for low-back pain: systematic review and meta-analysis, *Lancet* 373(9662):463–472, 2009.
Chou R, Baisden J, Carragee EJ, et al: Surgery for low back pain: A review of the evidence for an American Pain Society Clinical Practice Guideline, *Spine* 34(10):1094–1109, 2009.
Chou R, Deyo R, Friedly J, et al: Nonpharmacoogic therapies for low back pain: A systematic review for an American College of Physicians clinical practice guideline, *Ann Intern Med* 166:493–505, 2017.
Chou R, Deyo R, Firedly J, et al: Systematoic pharmacologic therapies for low back pain: A systematic review for an American College of Physicians clinical practice guideline, *Ann Intern Med* 166:480–492, 2017.
Cohen SP: Epidemiology, diagnosis and treatment of neck pain, *Mayo Clin Proc* 90:284–299, 2015.

Costa Lda C, Maher CG, et al: Prognosis for patients with chronic low back pain: Inception cohort study, *BMJ* 339:b3829, 2009.

Deyo RA, Mirza SK, Turner JA, Martin BI: Overtreating chronic back pain: Time to back off? *J Am Board Fam Med* 22(1):62–68, 2009.

Deyo RA, Mirza SK: Herniated lumbar intervertebral disk, *N Engl J Med* 374:1763–1772, 2016.

Deyo RA, Von Korff M, Duhrkoop D: Opioids for low back pain, *BMJ.* 350G6380.

Enomoto H, Fujikoshi S, Funa J, et al: Assessment of direct analgesic effect of duloxetine for chronic low back pain: post hoc path analysis of double-blind, placebo-controlled studies, *J Pain Res* 10:1357–1368, 2017.

Friedly JL, Comstock BA, Turner JA, et al: A randomized trial of epidural glucocorticoid injections for spinal stenosis, *N Engl J Med* 371:11–21, 2014.

Henschke N, Maher CG, Refshauge KM, et al: Prevalence of and screening for serious spinal pathology in patients presenting to primary care settings with acute low back pain, *Arthritis Rheum* 60(10):3072–3080, 2009.

Hooten WM, Cohen SP: Evaluation and treatment of low back pain: a clnicially focused review for primary care specialists, *Mayo Clin Proc* 90:1699–1718, 2015.

Maher C, Underwood M, Buchbinder R: Non-specific low back pain, *Lancet* 389(10070):736–747, 2017 Feb 18.

Rubinstein SM, de Zoete A, van Middelkoop M, et al: Benefits and harms of spinal manipulative therapy for the treatment of chronic low back pain: systematic review and meta-analysis of randomised controlled trials, *BMJ* 364:I689, 2019 http://dx.doi.org/10.1136/bmjI689.

Steffens D, Maher CG, Pereira, et al: Prevention of low back pain: a systematic review and meta-analysis, *JAMA Intern Med* 176:199–2087, 2016.

Qaseem A, Wilt TJ, McLean RM, et al: Noninvasive treatments for acute, subacute, and chronic low back pain: A clinical practice guideline from the American College of Physicians, *Ann Intern Med* 166:514–530, 2017.

TINNITUS

Method of
Richard Sadovsky, MD; and Abraham Shulman, MD

CURRENT DIAGNOSIS

- Tinnitus is common among those exposed to loud noise, among veterans, and among older adults.
- Tinnitus severity can range from very mild occasional noise awareness to a disruptive sound that can result in depression, cognitive impairment, and even suicide.
- Many people who complain of tinnitus also have a moderate to severe hearing loss.
- Pulsatile and/or unilateral tinnitus may be a sign of cardiovascular disease.
- Children also can have tinnitus, but are even less likely than adults to complain.

CURRENT THERAPY

- No cure exists for tinnitus, although proper diagnosis and management using a team approach can result in some relief.
- Tinnitus intensity and bother are affected by many individual factors beyond the actual volume and frequency of noise, such as patient affect and mental state.
- Cognitive-behavioral therapy and a hearing aid or masking device are the most common successful management tools for tinnitus, although combined treatment including medication offers the best success for patients with severe idiopathic tinnitus.
- Protection should be worn when exposed to loud noise.
- Successful management of troublesome complications, including insomnia, anxiety, and depression, will decrease tinnitus-associated symptom severity in most patients.

Definition and Epidemiology

Tinnitus is a symptom defined as perception of an internally generated sound that usually cannot be heard by others. Modern definitions include the dynamic advances in underlying neurophysiology noting a clinically conscious awareness of aberrant activity in synaptic circuitry that can manifest as an aberrant auditory perception that may increase with time, causing severe disabling symptoms. Perception can be a tonal sensation or ringing or noise-like sound, but can also include more complex sounds (crickets buzzing, pulsing noise), may fluctuate over time, and can be perceived in one or both ears or heard diffusely in the head. Thirty million people in the United States, or 10% of the entire population, note the presence of tinnitus at some time during their lives, with the incidence as high as 26.7% for people 65 to 84 years of age and a peak from ages 60 to 69. There appears to be no gender difference in tinnitus prevalence, although a few studies report a higher incidence among men. Some estimates of tinnitus incidence among older adults are even higher because fear of serious causes of tinnitus can discourage them from mentioning it. Wartime veterans often suffer from tinnitus, making it one of the major causes of disability among veterans. The incidence of tinnitus among children is 13%, with a higher rate among those who have had severe hearing loss.

Half of sufferers are bothered whereas others report no impact on life. Nearly 40% experience tinnitus more than 80% of the time. There is a wide variety of loudness, pitch, temporal variability, and family history of tinnitus among sufferers.

Some experts believe that the severity of tinnitus appears to be correlated with exposure to noise. Forty-four percent report no hearing loss, although it is agreed that most people with tinnitus have hearing loss. Among some, the hearing loss is mild and not noticed, but others report moderate and even profound hearing loss. Most tinnitus is *subjective*, heard only by the patient. *Objective tinnitus* can be heard by the examiner, by a careful stethoscope examination near the patient's ear, head, and/or neck.

Risk Factors/Etiologies (Subjective and Objective Tinnitus)

The most common risk factors for subjective tinnitus include (1) older age and/or hearing loss (presbycusis) and (2) exposure to loud noises (e.g., wartime veterans). Others include the following:

1. Conductive local causes of hearing loss such as cerumen impaction, obstruction of the external auditory canal, middle ear effusion, otosclerosis
2. Sensorineural and neurovascular causes/associated disorders such as loud sounds, Ménière's disease, acoustic neuroma, multiple sclerosis, head trauma, cerebral infarctions, seizures
3. Cardiovascular and hematologic disorders, including hypertension and blood pressure fluctuations, heart disease, arrhythmias, anemia
4. Metabolic disorders, including diabetes, dyslipidemia, hypertriglyceridemia, hypothyroidism or hyperthyroidism, obesity, vitamin B_{12} or zinc deficiency
5. Ototoxic medications such as salicylates, NSAIDs, aminoglycosides, erythromycin, methotrexate, loop diuretics, chloroquine (Aralen), quinine (Qualaquin)
6. Temporomandibular joint disorder
7. Trigger factors, including anxiety, bad news, upper respiratory infections, and any other activities/disorders causing increased arousal mediated by the autonomic nervous system

The most common risk factors for objective tinnitus include (1) vascular abnormalities (e.g., arterial bruits, venous hums, heart murmurs), (2) neurologic disease, and (3) eustachian tube dysfunction (e.g., patulous eustachian tube causing blowing sounds with breathing). Others include glomus tumor and palatomyoclonus (stapedial muscle spasm).

Pathophysiology

The mechanism that produces tinnitus remains unclear. Subjective tinnitus is considered to be sensorineurophysiologic in origin, whereas objective tinnitus is thought to arise from vascular, muscular, or respiratory origins, as well as the temporomandibular joint. Tinnitus may originate peripherally or centrally at any location along the auditory pathway from the cochlear nucleus to the auditory cortex, as well as from other nonauditory central brain structures. Leading theories for auditory pathway tinnitus include the following: (1) sequential injury to outer, then inner cochlear hair cells; (2) repetitive discharge in auditory nerve fibers in the dorsal cochlear nucleus that are stimulated in a continuous cycle; (3) hyperactive spontaneous activity in the auditory nuclei in the inferior colliculus of the brainstem; and (4) less than the usual suppressive activity of the central auditory cortex on peripheral auditory nerve activity. Pathologic changes in neural patterns create a subjective perception of sounds that resembles the pattern of actual sounds. Recent research is demonstrating a common pathway involving three separate neuroanatomic substrates in the central nervous system that are activated in severe idiopathic tinnitus, including sensory, affective (emotion and behavior), and psychomotor centers, meaning that multiple symptoms may occur at the same time.

The reorganization of edge frequencies in the cortical tonotropic map, in which cortical neurons begin to respond preferentially to sound frequencies at the edge of normal hearing, has recently been detected in tinnitus sufferers by neuromagnetic brain imaging. Other researchers using functional magnetic resonance imaging have recently implicated auditory-limbic interactions to explain the etiology of chronic tinnitus. They found moderate hyperactivity on MRI in the primary and posterior auditory cortices of tinnitus patients. However, the greatest degree of hyperactivity was noted in two limbic structures, the nucleus accumbens and the ventromedial prefrontal cortex.

Positron emission tomography (PET) studies predominantly show increased blood flow in several auditory structures, including the medial geniculate nucleus, the primary and secondary auditory cortex, the auditory brainstem, and temporal-parietal association areas. Brain changes can also be seen in nonauditory areas, including the hippocampus, amygdala, and cingulate gyrus.

Prevention

- Limit or avoid exposure to loud noises.
- Wear earplugs or ear defenders. (Tissues and cotton balls are not sufficient because they may become lodged in the ear canal).
- Cut back on alcohol and caffeine.
- Do not smoke (nicotine reduces blood flow to the ear structures).
- Exercise regularly to improve blood flow.
- Maintain healthy weight (tinnitus is more common in obese people).
- Take care of cardiovascular health.
- Avoid ototoxic medications (see Risk Factors above), especially among patients predisposed to ototoxicity such as advanced or very young age, pregnancy, renal or hepatic disease, or history of hearing loss. Monitor hearing when these medications must be used.

Clinical Manifestations

Patients with the symptom of tinnitus may complain of a mild inconsequential ringing, buzzing, hissing, roaring, clicking, or rough sounds, heard from time to time and for short periods of time, to an unbearable, constant noise, which can seriously degrade the patient's ability to function and enjoy life. Tinnitus can be acute or chronic in nature, unilateral or bilateral, nonpulsatile or pulsatile: arterial, venous, or nonvascular. The great majority of patients experience tinnitus without significant associated symptoms, but more than one-fourth of persons with tinnitus are distressed by it. Associated anxiety or depression often leads to more severe tinnitus-associated symptoms and to a greater negative impact on the patient's life. Various questionnaires, including the Tinnitus Handicap Questionnaire and the Tinnitus Severity Index, quantify the effect that tinnitus has on multiple areas in a patient's life.

The potential adverse effects of tinnitus are noted under Complications.

Diagnosis

The primary care office is an appropriate place to initiate the management of tinnitus.

History

Complete medical and psychological history
Tinnitus components
   Sensory
   Affect
   Psychomotor
Any factors that worsen or relieve symptoms
Prior treatment history

Complete physical examination

Concentrate on the following:
   Audiologic
   Neurologic
   Cardiovascular
   Metabolic
   Psychological

Laboratory tests

Thyroid function tests
Vitamin B_{12}
Complete blood count
Fasting glucose
Lipids, including triglycerides
Zinc

The evaluation of the patient with tinnitus begins with a thorough patient history, which involves an attempt to determine the etiologic and/or contributing factors causing ear noise. Certain parameters of the sounds heard can help identify potential etiologies and determine the need for further evaluation and treatment as seen in Box 1. Besides identifying the (sensation) of tinnitus, a review of the patient's affect and psychomotor functioning is an important part of strategizing the total management plan.

In the primary care office, the tinnitus patient should undergo a thorough physical examination with special attention to audiologic (including vertigo), cardiovascular, neurologic, and metabolic systems. A basic otologic examination includes (1) using a stethoscope to identify objective tinnitus, (2) examination of the external canal, (3) basic hearing testing, and (4) specific testing for sensorineural or

---

BOX 1 Useful Tinnitus Parameters for Primary Care Clinicians

1. Sensory perception—directs evaluation
   Subjective
   Objective
2. Level of distress—directs degree of evaluation and management
   Mild (not bothersome)
   Moderate (noticeable)
   Severe (bothersome)
3. Etiology/contributors—directs precision vs general management choices
   Identifiable
   Idiopathic
4. Tinnitus origin (pathways)—directs evaluation and management
   Central (nonauditory system)
   Peripheral (auditory system)
5. Components of tinnitus sensation—directs priority and types of management strategies
   Sensory
   Affective (emotion and behavior)
   Psychomotor
6. Sensory characteristics requiring early consultation with an appropriate specialist
   Unilateral
   Objective
   Sudden onset
   Pulsatile

conductive hearing loss using the Weber and Rinne tests. Thyroid studies, a hematocrit determination, complete blood chemistry, vitamin B_{12}, and lipid profile should be obtained if the patient has any suggestion of a metabolic abnormality. Primary care clinicians can identify many of the parameters that will determine further evaluation and management plans (see Box 1).

The management team evaluation continues with diagnostic audiologic testing, including audio testing, speech discrimination testing, and tympanometry. Other audiologic measurements of tinnitus may include pitch masking, loudness masking, minimum masking level, and residual inhibition.

Further investigation should be dictated by team discussion of potential etiologic/exacerbating factors for the individual patient. Patients with unilateral or pulsatile tinnitus are more likely to have serious underlying disease, such as vascular middle ear tumors, and should be evaluated by an otolaryngologist and possibly a cardiologist or neurologist. Many of these patients also require accompanying computed tomography (CT) angiogram, magnetic resonance imaging (MRI), carotid ultrasound, and perhaps standard angiography.

Differential Diagnosis
Not all sounds of internal origin perceived by the patient are those defined as tinnitus. Patients can also have ear noise caused by auditory hallucinations, as well as benign "transient noise."

Auditory hallucinations can occur in both psychotic and nonpsychotic patients. In a patient who by appropriate evaluation is considered to be psychotic, and more likely schizophrenic, hearing voices or other sounds may be auditory hallucinations. Stress or sleep deprivation can also cause auditory hallucinations in nonpsychotic patients. In a patient who is not sleep deprived or stressed, or drinking large amounts of caffeine-containing beverages, ear noise is more likely to be tinnitus.

Transient noise is defined as a whistling sound accompanied by a sensation of sudden temporary hearing loss. These episodes generally disappear in seconds and occur rarely, whereas tinnitus is generally defined as lasting over 5 minutes and occurring at least twice weekly. They are usually not related to any specific event or activity, often unilateral, and sometimes accompanied by a feeling of ear blockage. Usually, no treatment is necessary beyond patient education.

Management
There is no cure for tinnitus, although a multidisciplinary approach (tinnitus-targeted therapy) with a medico-audiologic approach can partially alleviate associated symptoms. The goal is "control" rather than "treatment." In expert hands, a majority of severely disabled tinnitus patients can get long-term relief with targeted medication and instrumentation.

Tinnitus management includes the following:
1. Eliminate potentially ototoxic medications and/or any precipitating active diseases/disorders (see Risk Factors/Etiologies above).
2. Administer targeted medication based on contributory medical conditions, severity of distress, tinnitus type (cochlear-peripheral or central), and tinnitus components involved (sensory, affective, and/or psychomotor).
3. Use instrumentation such as hearing aids, tinnitus masks, tinnitus retraining including low noise generators, and/or relaxing external sound stimulation with silence avoidance.
4. Provide mental health support, including stress management, biofeedback, reassurance, and relaxation techniques.

No medications have been found to consistently reduce tinnitus symptoms, probably because of the heterogeneity of clinical tinnitus types. Pharmacologic treatment should deal specifically with the component(s) of severe tinnitus being targeted and uses drugs for their FDA-approved purposes to logically manage an individual's tinnitus presentation. The sensory component symptoms among patients with predominantly cochlear-type severe tinnitus (peripheral) can be treated with pentoxifylline (Trental),[1] which can enhance

---

[1]Not FDA approved for this indication.

the oxygen-carrying capacity of the blood. If response is poor, intratympanic drug therapy with a steroid and/or instrumentation can be considered. Sensory symptoms among patients with predominantly central-type severe tinnitus can be offered trial instrumentation or brain scanning. If scanning is positive, neuroprotection using medications such as gabapentin (Neurontin)[1] and clonazepam (Klonopin)[1] may be helpful. The affective component of tinnitus can be pharmacologically managed with psychiatric consultation and may also include gabapentin and/or clonazepam (useful for anxiolytic and antiepileptic effects) or some other anxiolytic. The psychomotor component can sometimes be improved with medications such as papaverine[1] or clopidogrel (Plavix)[1] for cerebrovascular insufficiency and antiseizure drugs for epilepsy. Medications can be used continuously or as needed. There are no set regimens for the pharmacologic management of tinnitus. Because anxiolytics and antidepressants can sometimes cause or worsen tinnitus, close follow-up is important for treatment success. Other potentially contributing conditions and/or distressing symptoms should be appropriately treated.

Patients with severe tinnitus not responding to initial therapies or who are in significant distress should be referred to audiology, dentistry, neurology, physical therapy, and a mental health expert. Audiologist recommendations about masking devices to cover up the constant ringing may be helpful. Pleasant sounds such as TVs, radios, or fans can provide distractions. Sound generators can be worn in the ear to produce stable signal (white noise) and are most effective alone in patients with normal or near-normal hearing. This therapy can be combined with a hearing aid, which is most effective when done by a professional hearing expert with strict protocols. The amplification of ambient sound may also reduce tinnitus. Surgical cochlear implant in the profoundly hard-of-hearing patient can help with hearing issues but can also cause tinnitus for the first time.

Dentists can be helpful by evaluating for temporomandibular joint problems and other habits and recommending dental orthotics and home exercises to reduce clenching and grinding when appropriate. Neurologists can evaluate for vestibular symptoms, pain syndromes, and other cranial disorders. Physical therapists can evaluate the head and neck for biomechanical and posture problems and teach useful exercise techniques. Psychological counseling can improve levels of distress with greater improvement shown in combined cognitive strategies/education interventions. Patients can be taught to pay less attention to symptoms, overcome fear, accept tinnitus as part of life, and keep busy with happy activities. Acceptance and commitment therapy to better understand tinnitus and to look at it more objectively than emotionally may be useful. Careful choices and titrations of anxiolytic, antidepressant, and hypnotic medications reduce some of the affective components of tinnitus. Herbs and dietary supplements are commonly used, but there is no evidence to support their efficacy.

Experimental treatments include transcranial magnetic stimulation, low-level laser therapy, phase-out treatment (individualized sound developed to cancel out tinnitus), neuromonics (customized sound therapy), and tinnitus retraining therapy (remove perception from consciousness). The relationship between the auditory and limbic systems may offer a route of management via limbic stimulation and/or external limbic activation associated with emotional stress or depression. These areas are all under active study.

Monitoring
Patients with tinnitus should be monitored for (1) distress symptoms, (2) adverse effects of symptoms, (3) effectiveness of management plan, and (4) hearing. This can be done using direct questions and annual hearing tests. Scales that have been shown to be particularly useful in monitoring patients with tinnitus include the Tinnitus Handicap Inventory—Screening Version (THI-S), the Patient Health Questionnaire (PHQ-9), the Tinnitus Treatment Monitoring Interview (TOMI), and the Generalized Anxiety Disorder 7 (GAD-7). Although the causal relationship is unclear, suicide risk must be monitored, especially among persons who were at high suicide risk before they developed tinnitus.

Recent data using nuclear imaging hint that patients with severe subjective idiopathic tinnitus may be at high risk for brain

BOX 2 Complications and/or Comorbid Conditions

Affective

Stress

Sleep problems/insomnia—trouble falling asleep, waking up in the middle of the night, worries about getting enough sleep

Depression—restlessness, lack of energy, change in appetite

Anxiety and irritability—worrying, muscle tension and headaches, shortness of breath, rapid pulse, difficulty concentrating

Headaches

Psychomotor

Fatigue

Trouble concentrating, memory problems

Major negative effect on work performance

---

ischemia and neurodegenerative central nervous system disease consistent with senile dementia of the Alzheimer's type. Monitoring mental status in chronic severe tinnitus sufferers may be useful.

Complications

Different people are affected by tinnitus in different ways. For some, it may be simply irritating. For others, it may be more disruptive. Tinnitus primarily affects the ability to concentrate and sleep. Newer theories pointing out the central nervous substrate activation with tinnitus of sensory, affect, and psychomotor centers help explain the complexity and variability of tinnitus comorbidities (Box 2).

References

Baguley D, McFerran D, Hall D: Tinnitus, *Lancet* 382:1600–1607, 2013.

Crummer RW, Hassan GA: Diagnostic approach to tinnitus, *Am Fam Physician* 69:120–126, 2004.

Fioretti A, Eibenstein A, Fusetti M: New trends in tinnitus management, *Open Neurol J* 5:12–17, 2011.

Folmer RL, Martin WH, Shi Y: Tinnitus: questions to reveal the cause, answers to provide relief, *J Fam Pract* 53:532–540, 2004.

Henry JA, Zaugg TL, Myers PJ, et al: A triage guide for tinnitus, *J Fam Pract* 59:389–394, 2010.

Langguth B, Kreuzer PM, Kleinjung T, De Ridder D: Tinnitus: causes and clinical management, *Lancet Neurol* 12:920–930, 2013.

Newman CW, Sandridge SA, Bea SM, et al: Tinnitus: patients do not have to "just live with it", *Cleve Clin J Med* 78:312–319, 2011.

Roberts LE, Eggermont JJ, Caspary DM, et al: Ringing ears: the neuroscience of tinnitus, *J Neurosci* 30:14972–14979, 2010.

Shulman A, Goldstein B: Subjective idiopathic tinnitus and palliative care: a plan for diagnosis and treatment, *Otolaryngol Clin North Am* 42:15–37, 2009.

Shulman A, Goldstein B: Principles of tinnitology: tinnitus diagnosis and treatment a tinnitus-targeted therapy, *Int Tinnitus J* 16:73–85, 2010.

Shulman A, Goldstein B, Strashun A: Central nervous system neurodegeneration and tinnitus: a clinical experience. Part 1: diagnosis, *Int Tinnitus J* 13:118–131, 2007.

Sismanis A: Pulsatile tinnitus, *Otolaryngol Clin North Am* 36:389–402, 2003.

Yew KS: Diagnostic approach to patients with tinnitus, *Am Fam Physician* 89:106–113, 2014.

Diseases of Allergy

ALLERGIC REACTIONS TO INSECT STINGS

Method of
Theodore M. Freeman, MD

CURRENT DIAGNOSIS

- Determine the insect involved by recording circumstances of sting event.
- Determine the type of reaction: usual (expected), large local, or systemic (anaphylaxis).

CURRENT THERAPY

- Treatment for usual reactions
  - H_1-antihistamines, analgesics, cold compresses
  - Discussion of avoidance measures
- Treatment of large local reactions
  - H_1-antihistamines, analgesics, cold compresses
  - Discussion of avoidance measures and possible prescription of epinephrine autoinjectors (e.g., Auvi-Q, EpiPen)
- Treatment of systemic reactions
  - Epinephrine
  - Supplemental therapy, including antihistamines, β-adrenergics, oxygen, intravenous fluids, and perhaps vasopressors
  - Patients on β-blockers may require glucagon (e.g., Glucagon Emergency Kit, GlucaGen HypoKit)
  - Discussion of avoidance measures, medical alert accessories, prescription for epinephrine autoinjectors
  - Referral to allergist-immunologist to evaluate for specific IgE and possible institution of immunotherapy

Most stinging insects belong to the order Hymenoptera. They include species of bees (genus *Apis*, including honey bees and bumblebees), wasps (genus *Polistes*), yellow jackets (genus *Vespula*), hornets (genus *Dolichovespula*), and fire ants (genus *Solenopsis*).

Diagnosis

There are two important historical points to ascertain when seeing a patient with an allergic reaction to a stinging insect. The first is the type of insect that caused the sting. The physician may not rely on the patient's identification. Clues about the type of insect can be obtained from the circumstances of the sting.

Bees are herbivores and not aggressive. Stings from these insects often occur in fields with flowering plants when a barefoot patient steps or accidently sits on them. Bees have a barbed stinger and attached venom sac, which may be left in place after a sting. These should be removed immediately with a scraping motion; any pinching of the sac may inject additional venom.

Yellow jackets are aggressive scavengers and are found wherever food is left in the open. Stings from these insects usually occur in picnic areas or around open garbage containers. Like bees, yellow jackets occasionally leave a stinger in place, so this historical feature is not definitive. Wasps usually are not aggressive, except in defense of their nests. However, they tend to build these nests under the eaves and overhangs of our homes, and people stung by wasps are usually entering or exiting their homes.

Hornets are not as aggressive, except in defense of their nest. Because the nests are built in trees, stings by these insects are rarer.

Fire ants are very aggressive in defense of their nests, which are low mounds built above ground with extensive tunnels beneath the surface. In endemic areas (mostly the southeastern United States), they swarm and attack as a group when disturbed. Patients stung by fire ants are usually outdoors and accidently stand in a mound or disturb a mound while working or playing in their yard or garden. Fire ant workers do not fly. They bite only to get a grip and then sting from the abdomen and inject a toxic alkaloid venom. Because they attack as a group, they are usually seen and clearly identified by the patient. The size of the fire ants means their venom is injected less deeply than that of other hymenoptera, which leads to the usual development of a pseudopustule about 24 hours after a sting. These pseudopustules contain necrotic cellular material but are sterile because fire ant venom has antibiotic properties that can kill bacteria and fungi. The pseudopustules should be left alone; opening and draining them only increases the risk of secondary infection.

The second historical point is the type of reaction by the patient to the sting. The active venom components produce immediate swelling, redness, and tenderness with fairly intense pain at the site of the sting that slowly resolves over several hours. Sometimes, the immediate reaction progresses, and swelling (>10 cm) continues for 1 to 2 days and extends across several contiguous joints away from the site of the sting. This large local reaction may take 5 to 10 days to fully resolve, and it may be difficult to differentiate this from a secondary infection. Large local reactions peak in 1 to 2 days and then slowly recede, whereas secondary infections continue to get worse. Large local reactions do not cause systemic fever or lymphangitis, which should be treated with antibiotics if they occur.

The reaction of most concern is anaphylaxis. Unfortunately, many of the symptoms are similar to those of anxiety, which also may occur in a concerned patient: feelings of impending doom, a rapid heartbeat, shortness of breath, and nausea. Other symptoms that should not be seen in anxiety include a metallic taste, pruritus, and abdominal or uterine cramping. Signs of anaphylaxis include flushing, urticaria, angioedema, vomiting, diarrhea, bronchospasm, hypotension, and shock. Diagnosis of anaphylaxis requires involvement of 2 organ systems out of cutaneous, pulmonary, gastrointestinal or cardiovascular or a drop in blood pressure after a known allergen exposure. Involvement of the upper airway and cardiopulmonary systems is associated with death, and hymenoptera stings are the cause of about 40 deaths per year in the United States. Documentation of the type of reaction is essential for future risk assessment and determination of whether prophylactic therapy should be offered.

The risk for a systemic reaction after hymenoptera sting in the general population is estimated to be 3% to 5%. In patients who have a documented large local reaction to an insect sting or a generalized cutaneous reaction (hives angioedema without other organ system involvement), the risk of systemic reactions increases slightly to about 10%. Patients suffering large local reactions or generalized cutaneous reactions, may be referred to a specialist for specific IgE testing. For patients who have suffered anaphylaxis, the risk of systemic reactions after a sting is 50% to 60%. If a patient has suffered an anaphylactic event after a hymenoptera sting and has specific IgE to that hymenoptera as determined by in vivo (skin testing) or in vitro methods and is then placed on immunotherapy for that insect, the risk of systemic reaction after another sting is only 2% to 3%. Immunotherapy entails the use of specific venom products for each species, with the exception of fire ants. Because of the difficulty in extracting venom from fire ants, the only commercially available product for fire ants is the whole-body extract. Although whole-body extract is not effective therapy for other hymenoptera, it has been shown to be effective for fire ants.

Treatment

Immediate therapy for insect stings depends on the type of reaction. For the expected short-duration local reaction, treatment includes cold compresses; antihistamines, such as diphenhydramine (Benadryl 25–50 mg for adults; 1 mg/kg [up to 50 mg] for children) or cetirizine (Zyrtec 10 mg for adults and children older than 6 years; 5 mg for children younger than 6 years); and analgesics, such as acetaminophen (Tylenol) or ibuprofen (Motrin). Avoidance of future stings may be discussed with the patient. Recommendations include the following:

- Remove wasps' nests from around the home, especially near doorways.
- Avoid areas near open garbage.
- Do not leave open food or drinks during outdoor eating.
- Wear shoes, socks, and work gloves when working in the yard or garden.

Large local reactions may be treated as described for short-duration local reactions, with the addition of a short course (5–7 days) of oral steroids (e.g., Medrol dose pack), especially if there is significant morbidity associated with the site of the reaction. For instance, if a hand or foot is involved, a patient may not be able to write, work, or walk for up to a week. Avoidance measures should be discussed. Epinephrine auto-injectors (e.g., epipen, Epipen Jr, Auvi-Q, and generic autoinjectors [available from Mylan, Teva, Impax]) may be given, depending on the patient's anxiety about future stings. Epinephrine auto-injectors are simple devices with instructions clearly printed on them, but mistakes in usage do occur. The most common include "bouncing" the injector off the leg, which ejects the epinephrine onto the leg instead of delivering it intramuscularly, and putting the thumb over the end of the injector, which if the injector is reversed leads to no delivery of epinephrine and thumb trauma. The auto-injector Auvi-Q provides audible instructions to the user. The FDA has approved a new prefilled, manually injected epinephrine syringe (Symjepi 0.15 mg/0.3 mL) that minimizes delivery errors but requires the patient to push the plunger down physically. Demonstration pens and videos of proper technique may be obtained from the manufacturers (e.g., Adamis/Sandoz, Impax, Kaleo, Mylan, Teva).

The primary treatment of anaphylaxis is epinephrine (1:1000 concentration), with 0.3 to 0.5 mL given intramuscularly in adults or 0.01 mL/kg in children (less than 30 kg) every 5 to 15 minutes as needed. The patient should be placed in a recumbent position with the feet elevated. Supplemental therapy includes antihistamines (i.e., H_1-receptor antagonists); H_2-blockers (e.g., ranitidine [Zantac[1]] 150 mg PO) for cutaneous signs and symptoms; β-adrenergics (e.g., albuterol [Proventil, AccuNeb]) administered by metered-dose inhaler or nebulizer for bronchoconstriction; oxygen for hypoxia; intravenous fluids and possibly vasopressors for hypotension; and intubation for compromise of the upper airway.

In patients who have suffered prior anaphylaxis physicians must avoid the tendency to treat the initial cutaneous-only symptoms with antihistamines alone, because cutaneous signs and symptoms often develop rapidly into life-threatening events. When a patient has a prior history of anaphylaxis to insect stings, the appropriate therapy is epinephrine even if the initial presenting symptoms are cutaneous only. Most anaphylaxis responds quickly to a single dose of epinephrine, although up to 30% of anaphylaxis cases require two or more doses. Because anaphylaxis may be prolonged and last hours and epinephrine has a short duration of action (1 hour), patients should be observed for 4 to 6 hours after the last epinephrine dose. They should remain symptom free during that time before being released from the clinic or emergency department. In 3% to 20% of patients, a biphasic reaction occurs with recurrence of signs and symptoms 4–6 hours (range, 1–72 hours) after the initial reaction. For patients with prolonged or severe reactions, which are more often associated with a recurrence, overnight admission for observation should be considered.

Oral (prednisone 1 mg/kg up to 50 mg daily) or intravenous (methylprednisolone [Solu-Medrol] 1–2 mg/kg every 6 hours) steroids are sometimes given to minimize recurrences. Many patients are on β-blocking agents, which may make patients suffering anaphylaxis refractory to treatment with epinephrine. In this case, glucagon (e.g., GlucaGen HypoKit, Glucagon Emergency Kit[1]) at a dose of 1 to 5 mg (20–30 μg/kg [maximum 1 mg] in children)[3] may be tried intravenously over 5 minutes, followed by infusions (5–15 μg/min)[3] titrated to clinical response. Patients who have suffered anaphylaxis must be given instructions on avoidance of future stings, epinephrine pen autoinjectors, and information on medical alert accessories (e.g., necklaces, bracelets). They should also be referred to an allergist-immunologist to evaluate them for the presence of specific IgE, counseling, and consideration of immunotherapy, which may significantly reduce their future risk.

---

[1] Not FDA approved for this indication.

[3] Exceeds dosage recommended by the manufacturer.

References

An epinephrine prefilled syringe (Symjepi) for anaphylaxis, *The Medical Letter on Drugs and Therapeutics* 61(1566):25–26, 2019.

Freeman TM: Hypersensitivity to hymenoptera stings, *N Engl J Med* 351:1978–1984, 2004.

Freeman TM, Hylander RD, Ortiz AA, Martin MF: Imported fire ant immunotherapy: Effectiveness of whole body extracts, *J Allergy Clin Immunol* 90:210–215, 1992.

Golden DBK, Demain J, Freeman T, et al: Stinging insect hypersensitivity: A practice parameter update 2016, *Ann Allergy Asthma Immunol* 118:28–54, 2017.

Hunt KJ, Valentine MD, Sobotka AK, et al: A controlled trial of immunotherapy in insect hypersensitivity, *N Engl J Med* 299:157–161, 1978.

Sampson HA, Munoz-Furlong A, Campbell RL, et al: Second symposium on the definition and management of anaphylaxis: Summary report—Second National Institute of Allergy and Infectious Disease/Food Allergy and Anaphylaxis Network symposium, *J Allergy Clin Immunol* 117:391–397, 2006.

Schuberth KC, Lichtenstein LM, Kagey-Sobotka A, et al: Epidemiologic study of insect allergy in children. II. Effects of accidental stings in allergic children, *J Pediatr* 102:361–365, 1983.

ANAPHYLAXIS

Method of
Justin Greiwe, MD; and Jonathan A. Bernstein, MD

CURRENT DIAGNOSIS

- There is no universal agreement on the definition of anaphylaxis or the criteria for diagnosis.
- A comprehensive clinical history of the events surrounding the reaction provides the most valuable data along with a detailed review of current medications, recently ingested

- foods and/or drugs, insect stings, and physical activities before or after the event.
- While anaphylaxis remains primarily a clinical diagnosis, measurement of selected biomarkers (most commonly serum tryptase) has been used in research and clinical settings to assist in confirming this reaction.
- Cutaneous or serum-specific immunologic testing should only be performed to confirm or exclude a suspected agent under the supervision of an allergy specialist trained to interpret the meaning of the test results. Random testing to a large panel of foods or other allergens without a specific history has low diagnostic utility.

 CURRENT THERAPY

- Prompt administration of intramuscular epinephrine is the gold-standard first-line medication for the treatment of anaphylaxis. Delay in treatment with epinephrine has been associated with increased morbidity and mortality.
- Patients with severe reactions can have massive fluid shifts that can occur rapidly due to increased vascular permeability which require aggressive fluid resuscitation.
- Additional treatments are considered supportive and include the addition of H1 and H2 antihistamines for itching, urticaria, and gastrointestinal complaints; albuterol for bronchospasm; oxygen; and placing the patient in the Trendelenburg position.
- Corticosteroids are not useful for the acute treatment of anaphylaxis since these medications take 4 to 6 hours to reach maximum effectiveness and there is a lack compelling evidence that corticosteroids reduce anaphylaxis severity or prevent biphasic reactions.

Introduction

Anaphylaxis is an acute, potentially life-threatening multisystem reaction caused by the sudden systemic release of preformed mediators from mast cells and basophils which include histamine, tryptase, chymase, heparin, histamine-releasing factor, and platelet-activating factor (PAF). Cellular activation also stimulates the production of lipid-derived newly formed mediators, such as prostaglandins and cysteinyl leukotrienes. These reactions are frequently, but not always, mediated by an immunologic mechanism involving two or more organs and/or are associated with hypotension or upper respiratory compromise. Other clinical manifestations include flushing, pruritus, urticaria, angioedema, shortness of breath, wheezing, nausea, vomiting, and diarrhea. Risk of death is mainly from cardiovascular collapse or asphyxiation caused by laryngeal edema. Drugs (nonsteroidal antiinflammatory drugs [NSAIDs]/antibiotics), foods, and Hymenoptera venom stings are the most common triggers; however any agent capable of inciting a sudden, systemic degranulation of mast cells can lead to anaphylaxis.

Various organizations have attempted to clarify the definition of anaphylaxis but with no consensus agreement. Experts from the National Institute of Allergy and Infectious Disease (NIAID) and Food Allergy and Anaphylaxis Network (FAAN) met in 2005 and published diagnostic criteria for anaphylaxis. Controversy arose shortly thereafter with the World Allergy Organization (WAO) claiming that the published definition of anaphylaxis might exclude patients with clinical manifestations expressed by a single system only. Subsequent criteria published by Sampson et al. attempted to address this concern by adding single system caveats. Regardless of the continuing debate, the NIAID/FAAN criteria has been validated in real-world emergency room settings, establishing an accurate diagnosis of anaphylaxis with a sensitivity of 96.7% and a specificity of 82.4% (positive predictive value of 68.6%, negative predictive value of 98.4%).

TABLE 1	Comorbidities and Risk Factors for the Development of Anaphylaxis

Age: infants are at risk because manifestations might not be detected; teenagers are at risk because of "risky behavior"; elderly are at risk because of medical comorbidities and increased use of medications such as β-blockers leading to more severe cardiovascular symptoms at presentation

Gender: anaphylaxis is more common overall in females

Drugs: medications may impact severity of symptoms and response to treatment (see Table 2)

Comorbid Conditions: asthma, other respiratory diseases (e.g., chronic obstructive pulmonary disease, interstitial lung disease), cardiovascular disease, mast cell disorder (e.g., systemic mastocytosis)

Route of Administration: oral antigens are less likely to trigger anaphylaxis than parenteral antigens

Geography: prescription rates for self-injectable epinephrine devices are greater in northern than in southern states; living in a rural environment may affect incidence

Atopy: risk factor for anaphylactic and anaphylactoid reactions in general

Exposure History: the longer the interval since previous antigen exposure, the less likely a reaction will occur; previous anaphylactic reaction

Other Factors: active infections (e.g., upper respiratory tract infection, fever), physical exertion, premenstrual status, delayed administration of epinephrine, substance abuse (impairs judgement and can diminish recognition of symptoms), mental illness not well controlled

Epidemiology

The prevalence of anaphylaxis in industrialized countries is estimated to range between 0.05% to 2%; however, rates seem to be increasing. In one study the majority (80.2%) of anaphylaxis cases were triggered by food, principally peanut and tree nut, indicating that increased rates of anaphylaxis might coincide with increasing rates of food allergy worldwide. Given increased prevalence rates, accurate recognition and management of anaphylactic episodes is of the utmost importance as a delay in treatment can lead to increased morbidity and mortality. In this regard, several consensus guidelines, including the American, European, and WAO guidelines, have been published to simplify this task.

Risk Factors

Anaphylactic reactions are becoming increasingly more common with an estimated 1500 fatalities/year caused by anaphylaxis in the United States. Comorbidities and concurrent medications may impact the severity of symptoms and response to treatment in patients experiencing anaphylaxis. Risk factors for the development of anaphylaxis and medications that may impact severity of symptoms and response to treatment are reviewed in Tables 1 and 2. Risk factors for fatal reactions include adolescence, a history of a previous anaphylactic reaction, allergy to peanut or tree nuts, history of asthma, absence of cutaneous symptoms, and delayed administration of epinephrine.

Pathophysiology

Most anaphylactic reactions are mediated by immunoglobulin E (IgE); however not all episodes can be attributed to this mechanism. The term anaphylactoid was coined to describe a clinically similar event defined as a sudden degranulation of mast cells or basophils without the involvement of antibodies like IgE. The WAO attempted to change this terminology in 2003 when they suggested anaphylactic episodes be divided into immunologic (IgE-mediated, IgG-mediated, immune complex/

TABLE 2	Concurrent Medications That May Impact Severity of Symptoms and Response to Treatment

Possibly put patient at risk for more serious, treatment resistant anaphylaxis*

- β-adrenergic blockers
- α-adrenergic blockers
- Angiotensin-converting enzyme (ACE) inhibitors
- Angiotensin II receptor blockers
- Some tricyclic antidepressants (e.g., amitriptyline)
- Monoamine oxidase inhibitors

Potentially affect recognition of anaphylaxis

- Sedatives, hypnotics, antidepressants, ethanol, recreational drugs

Exacerbate anaphylaxis symptoms by causing nonimmunologic mast cell activation

- Ethanol, opiates, nonsteroidal anti-inflammatory drugs

*Evidence of impact for most of these medications are still controversial/debatable, and expert opinion continues to shift with regard to the safety of these medications in anaphylaxis, especially with regard to concurrent use during aeroallergen and venom immunotherapy. A recent systematic review and meta-analysis of studies that assess the influence of β-blockers and ACE inhibitors on anaphylaxis suggest that the quality of evidence showing that the use of these medications increases the severity of anaphylaxis is low owing to differences in the control of confounders arising from the concomitant presence of cardiovascular diseases

complement-mediated mechanisms) and nonimmunologic (anaphylactoid) categories. There is an ongoing debate regarding consensus terminology but the term "anaphylactoid" continues to be used.

Prevention

Avoidance of the confirmed trigger is the best way to prevent recurrence of anaphylaxis. For foods, this means educating patients about reading food labels, informing family and friends about these reactions, and being vigilant about avoiding the food(s) when eating in public establishments. Other triggers are more difficult to avoid such as venomous stinging insects or not possible in the case of idiopathic anaphylaxis (IA). In rare instances, an infection may require treatment with an antibiotic known to cause anaphylaxis in a patient. If there are no equally efficacious alternatives (i.e., penicillin for syphilis), an allergist/immunologist may perform skin testing to penicillin major and if available, minor determinants to confirm the allergy, and if positive, perform penicillin desensitization. This procedure involves relatively rapid administration of increasing amounts of the antibiotic under carefully controlled conditions by trained personnel with emergency therapy readily available until the target dose is reached. Thus desensitization results in tolerance which allows the allergic patient to take the medication without a reaction. Immunologic changes associated with immunotherapy are complicated, but the goal is to induce immune tolerance. The mechanism for inducing tolerance for different antigens is still poorly elucidated but is believed to occur by increasing regulatory T cells resulting in increased production of inhibitory cytokines like interleukin (IL)-10, transforming growth factor β (TGF-β), or both. IL-10 and TGF-β encourage the shift of antibody production from IgE toward the noninflammatory isotypes IgG4 and IgA, respectively. IL-10 is also involved in the reduction of proinflammatory cytokine release from mast cells, eosinophils, and T cells, as well as elicitation of tolerance in T cells by means of selective inhibition of the CD28 costimulatory pathway which effectively reduces lymphoproliferative responses to allergens. There also seems to be a shift in the immune response from a Th2 to a Th1 cytokine profile later in the immunotherapy course possibly mediated by the increased production of IL-12.

Long-term preventive measures include venom immunotherapy for Hymenoptera stinging insects (honey bee, wasp, yellow jacket, yellow hornet, white faced hornet) and food immunotherapy

(oral, sublingual) for IgE-mediated food allergies. It is essential to recognize and manage poorly controlled comorbid conditions such as asthma and other respiratory diseases, cardiovascular disease, mastocytosis, and mast cell activation syndrome that may increase the risk for anaphylaxis. Administration of certain medications such as β-blockers and possibly angiotensin-converting enzyme (ACE) inhibitors (see Table 2) are associated with a greater risk for severe anaphylaxis by interfering with the therapeutic response to epinephrine and should be avoided if possible. This is especially true for the administration of therapeutics that place the patient at increased risk for anaphylaxis such as allergen immunotherapy (i.e., subcutaneous, sublingual, and venom immunotherapy).

Clinical Manifestations

Anaphylaxis is an acute multiorgan system reaction that generally begins within seconds to minutes but can be delayed occurring anywhere from 1 to 24 hours later after exposure to a trigger. The most common organ system involved is the skin or mucous membranes with >90% of patients presenting with some combination of pruritus, urticaria, and/or angioedema and erythema. Anaphylaxis, by nature, is unpredictable and heterogeneous in its presentation so it may be mild and resolve spontaneously or it may be severe and progress to significant respiratory or cardiovascular compromise. To help classify the severity of anaphylactic reactions, the WAO developed a universal 5-stage grading system. It was intended to more accurately assess when epinephrine should be administered during subcutaneous immunotherapy (SCIT), but has since been used to better classify all forms of systemic reactions. Each grade is based on the organ system involved defined as cutaneous, conjunctival, upper respiratory, lower respiratory, gastrointestinal, cardiovascular, or other, and the severity is based on clinical judgement (Table 3).

Anaphylaxis can present as a uniphasic response, biphasic response, or as being refractory to treatment, all of which need to be considered and recognized by the clinician evaluating these patients. Biphasic anaphylaxis is defined as a potentially life-threatening recurrence of symptoms after the resolution of the initial immediate anaphylactic episode without re-exposure to the causative agent. The delayed portion of the biphasic reaction typically occurs within 12 hours but has been reported to occur up to 72 hours after resolution of initial symptoms. Biphasic reactions have been reported to develop in up to 21% of anaphylactic episodes (all ages) and in up to 15% of children. Biphasic reactions seem to be associated with the severity of the initial anaphylactic episode. Rarely, the onset of anaphylaxis will be delayed beginning hours rather than minutes after exposure to the causative agent. This is especially true for red meat allergy, also called mammalian meat allergy or α-gal allergy. This condition is characterized by development of an IgE antibody directed against a mammalian oligosaccharide epitope, galactose-α-1,3-galactose ("α-gal") after a lone star tick bite which contains the α-gal protein. Patients typically do not develop symptoms until several hours (4 to 6 hours or even longer) after eating red meat.

Diagnosis

There is no universal agreement on the definition of anaphylaxis or the criteria for diagnosis. Table 4 summarizes the NIAID/FAAN criteria established in 2005 which continues to be generally accepted today.

While anaphylaxis remains primarily a clinical diagnosis, measurement of selected biomarkers has been used in research and clinical settings to assist in confirming this reaction. Plasma histamine, platelet activating factor, and serum tryptase can be obtained in certain situations; however, there are specific collection timeframes that need to be strictly adhered to for the result to be valid. Serum tryptase is the most commonly used biomarker to distinguish anaphylaxis from other conditions with a similar presentation (i.e., carcinoid syndrome, vasovagal reactions, seizures). Acute elevation of serum tryptase secondary to mast cell degranulation can occur through an IgE-mediated mechanism

TABLE 3 World Allergy Organization Subcutaneous Immunotherapy Systemic Reaction Grading System

Grade 1:

Symptom(s)/sign(s) of 1 organ system present
Cutaneous: generalized pruritus, urticaria, flushing, or sensation of heat or warmth

or

Angioedema (not laryngeal, tongue or uvular)

or

Upper respiratory: rhinitis (e.g., sneezing, rhinorrhea, nasal pruritus, and/or nasal congestion)

or

Throat-clearing (itchy throat)

or

Cough perceived to originate in the upper airway, not the lung, larynx, or trachea

or

Conjunctival: erythema, pruritus, or tearing
Other: nausea, metallic taste, or headache

Grade 2:

Symptom(s)/sign(s) of more than 1 organ system present

or

Lower respiratory: asthma: cough, wheezing, shortness of breath (e.g., less than 40% PEF or FEV1 drop, responding to an inhaled bronchodilator)

or

Gastrointestinal: abdominal cramps, vomiting, or diarrhea

or

Other: uterine cramps

Grade 3:

Lower respiratory: asthma (e.g., 40% PEF or FEV1 drop NOT responding to an inhaled bronchodilator)

or

Upper respiratory: laryngeal, uvula, or tongue edema with or without stridor

Grade 4:

Lower or upper respiratory: respiratory failure with or loss of consciousness

or

Cardiovascular: hypotension with or without loss of consciousness

Grade 5: Death

FEV1, forced expiratory volume in one second; *PEF*, peak expiratory flow.

TABLE 4 Clinical Criteria for Diagnosing Anaphylaxis

Anaphylaxis is highly likely when any one of the following three criteria are fulfilled:

1. Acute onset of an illness (minutes to several hours) with involvement of the skin, mucosal tissue, or both (e.g., generalized hives, pruritus or flushing, swollen lips-tongue-uvula)
   AND AT LEAST ONE OF THE FOLLOWING
   a. Respiratory compromise (e.g., dyspnea, wheeze-bronchospasm, stridor, reduced PEF, hypoxemia)
   b. Reduced BP or associated symptoms of end-organ dysfunction (e.g., hypotonia [collapse], syncope, incontinence)
2. Two or more of the following that occur rapidly after exposure to a likely allergen for that patient (minutes to several hours):
   a. Involvement of the skin-mucosal tissue (e.g., generalized hives, itch-flush, swollen lips-tongue-uvula)
   b. Respiratory compromise (e.g., dyspnea, wheeze-bronchospasm, stridor, reduced PEF, hypoxemia)
   c. Reduced BP or associated symptoms (e.g., hypotonia [collapse], syncope, incontinence)
   d. Persistent gastrointestinal symptoms (e.g., crampy abdominal pain, vomiting)
3. Reduced BP after exposure to known allergen for that patient (minutes to several hours):
   a. Infants and children: low systolic BP (age specific) or greater than 30% decrease in systolic BP*
   b. Adults: systolic BP of less than 90 mm Hg or greater than 30% decrease from that person's baseline

*Low systolic blood pressure for children is defined as less than 70 mm Hg from 1 month to 1 year, less than (70 mm Hg + [2 × age]) from 1 to 10 years, and less than 90 mm Hg from 11 to 17 years.
PEF, Peak expiratory flow; *BP*, blood pressure.

More accurate diagnostic testing can be utilized in some cases when the patient or clinician suspects a specific antigen as the triggering agent. Cutaneous or serum specific immunologic testing should only be performed to confirm or exclude a suspected agent under the supervision of an allergy specialist trained to interpret the meaning of the test results. Random testing to a large panel of foods or other allergens (i.e., venoms) without a specific history has a low diagnostic utility and can result in more questions rather than answers given the high rate of false positive reactions reported, especially for foods. If diagnostic skin testing is performed, it should be delayed for at least 3 to 4 weeks after the event to obtain an accurate test result in order to allow for recovery of skin mast cells. In certain cases there may be no validated cutaneous or in vitro test to detect the potential for an IgE-mediated reaction. In these circumstances, a graded challenge or provocation test can safely be carried out under the supervision of an experienced allergist in a setting that is fully equipped to respond to any potential medical emergency including anaphylaxis. Unlike desensitization, graded challenges do not work by modifying the allergic response to the agent. Therefore patients who tolerate a graded challenge is an indication that they are not allergic to the specific agent administered.

Differential Diagnosis

Anaphylaxis can sometimes be difficult to recognize because it can mimic other conditions and is variable in its presentation. Common conditions that mimic anaphylaxis are included in Table 6.

Therapy (or Treatment)

Prompt administration of intramuscular epinephrine is the gold-standard first-line medication for the treatment of anaphylaxis. Delay in treatment with epinephrine has been associated with increased morbidity and mortality. Epinephrine autoinjectors (EAI [Auvi-Q (kaléo, Richmond, VA), EpiPen Jr, EpiPen (Mylan Inc, Canonsberg, PA)]) are commercially available in three different concentrations in the United States: 0.1 mg (7.5 to 14 kg body weight), 0.15 mg (15 to 30 kg), and 0.3 mg (>30 kg). Epinephrine can be administered intramuscularly (preferred) or

(i.e., venom and drug allergy) or direct degranulation of mast cells through a non-IgE mediated mechanism (i.e., NSAIDs or opiates). Tryptase can rise in serum or plasma as early as 15 minutes after clinical onset of anaphylaxis and should be collected between 30 minutes and 2 hours after symptom-onset if possible. Samples collected before or after this window are less accurate due to diminished sensitivity. Previous studies have questioned the sensitivity of serum tryptase in food-induced reactions; however a recent prospective study suggests that serum tryptase is a valuable tool in food allergic reactions as well and correlates with symptom severity. There is still debate on how serum tryptase can be used effectively in diagnosing anaphylaxis or mast cell activation with different studies quoting different cutoff values. Data on cutoffs specifically for food allergy are even harder to come by (Table 5).

According to this study comparing peak tryptase reaction levels at 2 hours with baseline is essential in correct interpretation, and a rise in tryptase of 30% above baseline is associated with a food allergic reaction. It is important to note that a normal serum tryptase level does not exclude anaphylaxis as the diagnosis.

A comprehensive clinical history of the events surrounding the reaction provides the most valuable data along with a detailed review of current medications, recently ingested foods and/or drugs, insect stings, and physical activities before or after the event. This approach oftentimes uncovers the appropriate trigger; however, in many cases no clear trigger can be identified.

TABLE 5	Proposed Optimal Cutoffs for Tryptase Elevations Signifying Mast Cell Activation or Anaphylaxis	
AUTHOR	**CRITERIA FOR TRYPTASE INCREASE**	**CRITERIA IDENTIFY**
Phadia AB, 2008	Values above 11.4 ng/mL (upper 95th percentile)	Raised tryptase
Valent et al., 2012	20% plus 2 ng/mL over baseline level	Mast cell activation
Enrique et al., 1999	Levels >8.23 ng/mL	Anaphylaxis
Brown et al., 2009	Increase of 2 µg/L	Anaphylaxis
Egner et al, 2016	Threshold increment of 20%	Mast cell mediator release
Wongkaewpothong et al., 2014	Delta tryptase 0.8 µg/L	Anaphylaxis

TABLE 6	Differential Diagnosis of Anaphylaxis
SYSTEM	**DIFFERENTIAL DIAGNOSIS**
Cutaneous	acute generalized urticaria, acute angioedema, ACE inhibitor angioedema, hereditary/acquired angioedema, carcinoid syndrome, postmenopause, Red man syndrome
Cardiac	vasovagal syncope, myocardial infarction, arrhythmia, shock
Respiratory	asthma or COPD exacerbation, vocal cord dysfunction syndrome, laryngospasm, pulmonary embolism, inhaled foreign body (infants/toddlers)
Psychological	panic attacks or acute anxiety, Munchausen syndrome
Other	mastocytosis and mast cell activation syndrome, pheochromocytoma, capillary leak syndrome, scombroid fish ingestion, hypoadrenergic or hyperadrenergic paroxysmal orthostatic tachycardia (POTS)

ACE, Angiotensin-converting enzyme; *COPD*, chronic obstructive pulmonary disorder.

subcutaneously every 5 to 15 minutes but can be given more frequently if deemed appropriate. The recommended adult dose of 1:1000 (1 mg/mL) epinephrine is 0.2 to 0.5 mg (mL), whereas the pediatric dose is 0.01 mg/kg (0.01 mL/kg/dose of 1 mg/mL solution), with a maximum dose of 0.3 mg. If not administered through an autoinjector, the epinephrine dose should be drawn up using a 1 mL syringe and injected intramuscularly into the mid-outer thigh. A higher dose (e.g., 0.5 mL) within the recommended dose range should be considered in patients with severe anaphylaxis.

Patients with severe reactions can have massive fluid shifts that can occur rapidly due to increased vascular permeability which require aggressive fluid resuscitation. Additional treatments are considered supportive and include the addition of H1 and H2 antihistamines for itching, urticaria, and gastrointestinal complaints; albuterol for bronchospasm; oxygen; and placing the patient in the Trendelenburg position. Corticosteroids are not useful for the acute treatment of anaphylaxis since these medications take 4 to 6 hours to reach maximum effectiveness. Despite this, corticosteroids are often used in the emergency treatment of anaphylaxis under the assumption that these medications may be beneficial in preventing biphasic reactions. A comprehensive literature review of 31 studies recently reported that biphasic reactions were more likely to occur in moderate to severe anaphylaxis or when anaphylaxis was not treated with timely epinephrine. Due to the potential adverse effects of corticosteroids and lack of compelling evidence demonstrating an effective role in reducing anaphylaxis severity or preventing biphasic anaphylaxis, the authors do not advocate their routine use for treatment of anaphylaxis. The appropriate observation period after an anaphylactic event often depends on the severity and duration of the initial reaction as well as the patient's response to treatment, previous reaction history, associated comorbidities, and access to medical care. Patients with moderate to severe anaphylaxis should be observed for a minimum of 4 to 8 hours; however, milder presentations can be observed for a shorter time period. All patients

with a history of anaphylaxis should be given a prescription for an EAI along with instructions for self-administration and an allergy action plan specific to their trigger.

Monitoring

The main tenants of anaphylaxis management and prevention are simple in theory but difficult in practice. Complete avoidance of the triggering agent provides protection from future episodes however, accidental exposures can occur, especially for food induced anaphylaxis. Other conditions like IA occur randomly with no known triggers making avoidance impossible. While episodes of IA tend to decline in frequency over time, patients experiencing more frequent attacks often benefit from daily prophylactic treatment with H1 and/or H2 antihistamines, leukotriene receptor antagonist (LTRA), and oral prednisone as needed. In refractory cases omalizumab (Xolair) has been shown to be effective as well[1].

Carrying an EAI at all times provides patients with quick access to life-saving treatment; however, adherence has historically been poor. The predicament of poor adherence to medical treatment is a well-recognized problem; however in anaphylaxis the consequences of nonadherence can be fatal. One study from 2008 demonstrated that 48% of children prescribed an EAI did not have the device available at school, and of those with the medication on site, 78% of the autoinjectors were kept in the nurse's office or by another administrator not in close proximity to the child. Real-world data from a 2018 survey also demonstrated a poor level of adherence in patients and caregivers to anaphylaxis treatment guidelines which recommend carrying more than one EAI at all times. Most (82%) did not carry two EAIs at all times, mainly due to keeping one EAI in another location; 84% respondents said they kept at least one EAI at home; however, few patients and caregivers kept more than one. More than half of the respondents (64%) said they received counseling with an

---

[1]Not FDA approved for this indication.

emphasis on always having one EAI and keeping another in a different location, but only 27% reported counseling that emphasized always having two EAIs available. It is important to recognize that a second epinephrine dose may be required in 16% to 36% of patients; therefore a more concerted effort should be made by physicians to properly educate patients and caregivers on the importance of following standard treatment guidelines. According to a 2018 study, only 26% of milk-allergic children in the U.S. had a current EAI prescription, the lowest reported rate among the top nine food allergies.

While poor patient adherence deserves some of the blame, evidence suggests that prescribers are equally responsible for this omission. Among 208 patients identified with anaphylaxis, 64.4% were seen in the emergency department and discharged home, but only 36.6% were prescribed an EAI, and only 31.3% were referred to an allergy specialist for further evaluation. Another retrospective cross-sectional descriptive study of patients 21 years old or younger who received care for anaphylaxis reported that EAIs were prescribed to only 63%, and referral to an allergist was recommended to only 33%. Both of these studies suggest that emergency department physicians may be missing an important opportunity to empower patients with the ability to self-administer treatment for a recurrent episode and to prevent future anaphylactic reactions by not referring patients for specialized follow-up care. Finally, a comprehensive analysis of 10,184 anaphylaxis incidents using the European anaphylaxis register revealed that in the early 2000s 27.1% of patients with anaphylaxis treated by a health professional received epinephrine while only 14.7% of lay or self-treated cases were treated with an EAI. Progress was tracked over the next decade and epinephrine administration from a health professional almost doubled to 30.6% in 2015–2017 but no significant change was found in the lay emergency respondents group.

Failing to follow published guidelines for the treatment of anaphylaxis is another barrier to timely and appropriate treatment. Oftentimes antihistamines are used as first-line agents in the treatment of an anaphylactic reaction and is the most common reason providers report for not using epinephrine, leaving patients at increased risk for life-threatening sequelae. It should be reiterated that antihistamines have no effect on arresting true anaphylactic reactions and should only be used for symptomatic relief of associated pruritus and urticaria.

Reasons for patients and caregivers not to carry or use their EAIs or to delay administration are multifaceted and complex. Teenagers and young adults are at highest risk of fatal anaphylaxis-related reactions due to delayed epinephrine injection. Cost can be a difficult barrier for patients to overcome either related to having no insurance, high insurance co-pays, and/or deductibles. The cost of the best-known autoinjector, EpiPen, made headline news in recent years when pricing rose to more than $600/2-pak by 2016. Bad press followed by public outcry led the manufacturer to produce a generic version for half the cost. Potential barriers for not carrying an EAI are summarized in Table 7.

Since many patients who have been prescribed an EAI do not routinely carry one, and emergency rooms fail to prescribe them, it is essential that life-saving EAIs be readily available in community spaces and public venues. To improve access to life-saving treatment, there is an increasing effort to distribute nonspecific EAIs to public locations including schools, parks, pools, airports, public venues, and shopping malls. In 2013, President Obama signed the "School Access to Emergency Epinephrine Act," which encouraged, but did not require, all states to adopt stock epinephrine regulations for schools. Several drug companies like Mylan Specialty (EpiPen4Schools) and Kaléo ("Q Your School") are providing free stock EAIs for schools to help improve access to epinephrine in the event a person experiences anaphylaxis in an academic setting. According to a recent EpiPen4Schools survey sponsored by Mylan Specialty, in each academic year, one in every six U.S. schools will have a student or staff member experience

TABLE 7	Reasons for Patients and Caregivers Not to Carry or Use Their Epinephrine Autoinjectors or to Delay Administration

- Never prescribed
- Cost
- Inconvenience
- Lack of perception of need of the medication
  - many do not use device for years so may not think it is essential or forget how to use it properly
- Poor knowledge of appropriate use
- Lack of familiarity with different brands of autoinjectors
- Mistakenly believe EAI might be available for emergency use in many public spaces
- History of mild allergic reaction
  - might think they are not at risk for a potentially fatal reaction
- Emotional/behavioral
  - embarrassment, feeling different
- Having been OK after a past reaction without treatment
- Wait for antihistamine to work
- Rely on other medications
- Don't want to go to the emergency department
- Needle phobia

EAI, Epinephrine autoinjectors.

anaphylaxis. About 1140 episodes of anaphylaxis occurred across 6574 U.S. schools with most (89.5%) incidents involving students. More reactions were seen in high school students, who tend to be at higher risk, and food was the trigger for a majority (60%) of the reactions. Other triggers include environmental, medication, and insect stings or bites; however, 22% of severe reactions were from unknown triggers. EAIs (both stock and personal) were used to treat 77% of anaphylactic events reported. Overall this survey revealed that not only are anaphylactic events a relatively common occurrence in schools, but also that the risk extends beyond those with diagnosed allergies. A quarter of the individuals who experienced anaphylaxis in a school setting had no known allergies. The previously stated data tend to further support the need for stock EAIs in schools, and training for staff on when and how to use them.

With increased availability of epinephrine in public settings there needs to be a focus on increased educational initiatives for the people administering life-saving treatment. Just having epinephrine available does not improve outcomes during an anaphylactic event. Healthcare professionals, first responders, and the general public need to be able to recognize classic anaphylactic symptoms and know how to properly initiate treatment. Unfortunately, when these groups are surveyed, anaphylaxis is still underrecognized and undertreated (Table 8).

Management of Complications

In general, anaphylactic reactions resolve without any major complications. Even though the prevalence rates of anaphylaxis seem to be increasing, fatal outcomes are rare, making up less than 1% of total mortality risk. In older patients, cardiovascular complications like atrial fibrillation and myocardial infarction can arise during anaphylaxis, but these events are also infrequent.

Conclusion

Anaphylaxis is a common medical condition affecting both adult and pediatric populations and its incidence and prevalence continue to increase. Prompt recognition and treatment with epinephrine administered in a timely manner remains the mainstay of treatment for anaphylaxis. Preventive measures including patient education, immunotherapy when appropriate, antigen avoidance, and optimal management of comorbid conditions is important in preventing recurrences. There is a concerning lack of knowledge and preparedness for management of anaphylaxis at all care levels that needs to be better addressed.

TABLE 8 Are Healthcare Professionals and First Responders Able to Appropriately Recognize and Treat Anaphylaxis?

SURVEY	RESULTS
1114 pediatric emergency medicine physicians	• 93.5% correctly identified epinephrine as the treatment of choice for anaphylaxis • 66.9% used the intramuscular (IM) route of administration • 37.4% admitted affected patients for observation • Many discharge patients home after an abbreviated period
468 pediatricians (41%) responded to the survey	• 70% agreed that the clinical scenario was consistent with anaphylaxis • 72% chose to administer epinephrine • 56% of respondents agreed with both the diagnosis of anaphylaxis and treating with epinephrine • 70% did not recognize that a 30-min observation period after anaphylaxis was too short
7822 physicians, allied health, medical students, and other health professionals	• 80% of responders correctly identified the case of anaphylaxis with prominent skin and respiratory symptoms • 55% correctly recognized the case without skin symptoms as anaphylaxis • 23% of responders correctly selected risk factors for anaphylaxis

3537 paramedics	• 98.9% correctly recognized a case of classic anaphylaxis
	• 2.9% correctly identified the atypical presentation
	• 46.2% identified epinephrine as the initial drug of choice
	• 38.9% chose the IM route of administration
	  • 60.5% identified the deltoid as the preferred location
	  • 11.6% correctly identified the thigh
	• ~98% were confident they could recognize and manage anaphylaxis
	  • 39.5% carry EAIs on response vehicles
	• 95.4% were confident they could use an EAI
	  • 36.2% stated that there were contraindications to epinephrine administration in anaphylactic shock

EAI, Epinephrine autoinjectors.

Readings

Brown SGA, Blackman KE, Heddle RJ: Can serum mast cell tryptase help diagnose anaphylaxis? *Emerg Med Australas* 16:120–124, 2004.

Campbell RL, Kelso JM: Anaphylaxis: Acute diagnosis. Walls RM, ed. UpToDate. Waltham, MA: UpToDate Inc. http://www.uptodate.com (Accessed on December 04, 2018.)

Commins SP, Jerath MR, Cox K, et al: Delayed anaphylaxis to alpha-gal, an oligosaccharide in mammalian meat, *Allergol Int* 65:16, 2016.

Dua S, Dowey J, Foley L, et al: Diagnostic value of tryptase in food allergic reactions: a prospective study of 160 adult peanut challenges, *J Allergy Clin Immunol Pract* 6(5):1692–1698, 2018 Sep - Oct.

Egner W, Sargur R, Shrimpton A, et al: 17-year experience in perioperative anaphylaxis 1998-2015: harmonizing optimal detection of mast cell mediator release, *Clin Exp Allergy* 46:1465–1473, 2016.

Enrique E, García-Ortega P, Sotorra O, Gaig P, Richart C: Usefulness of UniCAP-Tryptase fluoroimmunoassay in the diagnosis of anaphylaxis, *Allergy* 54:602–606, 1999.

Grabenhenrich LB, Dölle S, Ruëff F, et al: Epinephrine in severe allergic reactions: the European anaphylaxis register, *J Allergy Clin Immunol Pract* 6(6):1898–1906, 2018 Nov - Dec.

Grossman SL, Baumann BM, Garcia Peña BM, et al: Anaphylaxis knowledge and practice preferences of pediatric emergency medicine physicians: a national survey, *J Pediatr* 163(3):841–846, 2013.

Jacobsen RC, Toy S, Bonham AJ, et al: Anaphylaxis knowledge among paramedics: results of a national survey, *Prehosp Emerg Care* 16(4):527–534, 2012.

Krugman SD, Chiaramonte DR, Matsui EC: Diagnosis and management of food-induced anaphylaxis: a national survey of pediatricians, *Pediatrics* 118(3):e554–e560, 2006.

Lee S, Bellolio MF, Hess EP, et al: Time of onset and predictors of biphasic anaphylactic reactions: a systematic review and meta-analysis, *J Allergy Clin Immunol Pract* 3:408, 2015.

Lieberman P, Nicklas RA, Randolph C, et al: Anaphylaxis--a practice parameter update 2015, *Ann Allergy Asthma Immunol* 115:341, 2015.

Phadia AB: *ImmunoCAP Tryptase. Directions for Use.* Uppsala, Sweden: Phadia AB; 2008.

Simons FE, Frew AJ, Ansotegui IJ, et al: Risk assessment in anaphylaxis: current and future approaches, *J Allergy Clin Immunol* 120(suppl 1):S2–S24, 2007.

Tejedor-Alonso MA, Farias-Aquino E, Pérez-Fernández E, et al: Relationship between anaphylaxis and use of beta-blockers and angiotensin-converting enzyme inhibitors: a systematic review and meta-analysis of observational studies, *J Allergy Clin Immunol Pract* 7(3):879–897, 2019 Mar.

Turner PJ, Jerschow E, Umasunthar T, et al: Fatal anaphylaxis: mortality rate and risk factors, *J Allergy Clin Immunol Pract* 5(5):1169–1178, 2017.

Valent P, Akin C, Arock M, et al: Definitions, criteria and global classification of mast cell disorders with special reference to mast cell activation syndromes: a consensus proposal, *Int Arch Allergy Immunol* 157:215–225, 2012.

Wang J, Young MC, Nowak-Węgrzyn A: International survey of knowledge of food-induced anaphylaxis, *Pediatr Allergy Immunol* 25(7):644–650, 2014.

SERUM SICKNESS

Amy Robertson, PharmD; and Amanda Rhyne, MD

CURRENT DIAGNOSIS

• Identified by: fever, rash, joint pain (in combination or isolated)
• 7–14 days after exposure to offending agent
• Most frequently in the adult female population
• There are no disease defining labs, although complement tests may be elevated

CURRENT THERAPY

• Identify and discontinue offending agent
• Symptomatic relief with analgesics and antihistamines, as needed
• Those with severe disease may be treated with oral or intravenous corticosteroids for 10–14 days
• If symptoms reappear after discontinuation of corticosteroid, reinitiate with a slow taper

Pathophysiology

Serum sickness is classified as a type III delayed immune-complex–mediated hypersensitivity reaction. It was first noted by Von Pirquet in the early 1900s after administration of equine antisera. The mechanism consists of exposure to an antigen (often a large protein) that leads to formation of an antigen-antibody complex. The immune complex load becomes too high to be appropriately excreted from the body, causing deposition in joints, tissues, and vascular endothelium. It also leads to activation of the complement pathway, which prompts mast cell and basophil degranulation with vasoactive amine release. The deposition of immune complexes and release of inflammatory mediators (histamine, serotonin) leads to the common symptoms of urticarial rash, joint pain, and fever.

Serum sickness–like reaction is not as well defined as true serum sickness. It is postulated that a non-protein drug binds to a serum protein to make a complete antigen. The newly formed antigen goes on to become an antigen-antibody complex. These complexes mimic the inflammatory cascade and symptomatic response of a true serum sickness reaction.

Epidemiology

Serum sickness is most common in the adult female population. A systematic review involving 33 cases of rituximab (Rituxan)-induced serum sickness (RISS) showed 76.7% female predominance with a mean age of 39.1 years. The majority of cases occurred in patients with an autoimmune condition, specifically immune thrombocytopenic purpura and Sjogren. Due to a lack of clear diagnostic tools and varying symptoms that can closely mimic a flare of an underlying rheumatologic illness, these reactions are often poorly documented or not identified. A study of Australian snake antivenom showed that the incidence of serum sickness was 29% ($N = 32/109$). Further research will need to be done to determine current incidence with the increasing treatment of rheumatologic disorders with immunologic medications.

Risk Factors

Risk factors for serum sickness include parenteral and cutaneous administration of chemicals, especially those with large molecular weights (e.g., proteins, serum). Heterologous (animal-derived) proteins, in particular, are associated with a high risk for a delayed immune response. Historically, equine-derived antisera and antitoxins were common causes and now includes murine and chimeric monoclonal antibodies such as rituximab (Rituxan) and infliximab (Remicade). Fewer adverse events have been reported with adalimumab (Humira), a humanized monoclonal antibody. Additional risk factors include administration of large doses, repeated dosing, and longer administration times. Patients with autoimmune disorders, circulating histamine-releasing factors, and atopy are also at an increased risk.

Serum sickness–like reactions are associated with a wider variety of molecules, including non-protein medications (e.g., antibiotics), vaccines, allergy extracts, hormones, and enzymes. See Table 1 for a list of agents commonly associated with serum sickness and serum sickness–like reactions.

Clinical Manifestations

Common manifestations of serum sickness include fever, pruritic rash (not involving mucosal membranes), and arthralgia of the metacarpophalangeal joints, knees, wrists, ankles, and shoulders. The timing of these symptoms occurs 7 to 14 days after exposure to the offending agent and can happen more promptly if there has been previous exposure. Urticaria has been reported as the most prominent symptom, present in 90% of cases. In a study of 33 cases of RISS: 78.8% presented with fever, 72.7% with arthralgia, and 69.7% with rash. The triad of fever, rash, and arthralgia were present in 48.5% of the cases. There are many less prominent manifestations of serum sickness, including headache, gastrointestinal (GI) bloating, cramps, diarrhea, and nephropathy.

Diagnosis

Recommended workup includes complete blood count (CBC), erythrocyte sedimentation rate (ESR), C-reactive protein (CRP), urinalysis (UA), and comprehensive metabolic panel (CMP). Although lab work can help to differentiate from other causes, diagnosis is made clinically. Attempts have been made to link serum sickness to elevated levels of rheumatoid factor, complement, and antibody levels without success.

Differential Diagnosis

The differential diagnoses for serum sickness include: serum sickness–like reaction, other hypersensitivity reactions, viral illness,

| TABLE 1 | Medications Associated With Serum Sickness and Serum Sickness–Like Reactions |

Serum Sickness

Heterologous (animal-derived) proteins:
- Antivenom for snake bites: Crotalidae polyvalent immune fab, North and South American snake antivenom (CroFab)
- Chimeric (murine/human) monoclonal antibodies: rituximab (Rituxan), infliximab (Remicade)
- Equine serum heptavalent botulism antitoxin
- Equine-derived antivenom for spider bites
- Equine-derived diphtheria antitoxin
- Murine monoclonal antibodies
- Polyclonal antibodies: equine or rabbit anti-thymocyte globulin (Atgam, Thymoglobulin)

Homologous (human-derived) proteins:
- Anti-D (Rho[D]) immune globulin (RhoGAM)
- Humanized monoclonal antibodies: adalimumab (Humira), omalizumab (Xolair), natalizumab (Tysabri), alemtuzumab (Lemtrada)
- Intravenous immune globulin (Carimune NF, Gamunex-C)

Serum Sickness–like Reactions
- Allopurinol (Zyloprim)
- Antimicrobials
  - Cephalosporins (especially cefaclor [Ceclor])
  - Ciprofloxacin (Cipro)
  - Griseofulvin (Gris-PEG)
  - Isoniazid (Nydrazid, INH)
  - Minocycline (Minocin)
  - Penicillins (Pen-Vee K)
  - Streptomycin (Agri-mycin-17, Agrept)
  - Sulfonamides
- Barbiturates
- Bupropion (Wellbutrin)
- Captopril (Capoten)
- Hydantoins
- Hydralazine (Apresoline)
- Iodides
- Methyldopa (Aldomet)
- Phenytoin (Dilantin)
- Procainamide (Pronestyl, Procan-SR, Procanbid)
- Quinidine (Cardioquine)
- Thiouracils (e.g., methimazole [Tapazole])

rheumatologic disease, tick-borne disease, reactive arthritis, Stevens-Johnson syndrome, rheumatic fever, and lupus.

Treatment

Treatment of serum sickness and serum sickness–like reactions are similar. Discontinuation and avoidance of the offending agent is recommended and usually leads to spontaneous resolution within several weeks. Due to the self-limiting nature and generally mild presentation, treatment is symptom driven. Low-grade fever and/or arthralgias can be treated with analgesics (e.g., acetaminophen [Tylenol]) or nonsteroidal anti-inflammatory drugs. Antihistamines and corticosteroids are commonly used, but there are limited data to support their efficacy. Antihistamines may be used to treat urticarial symptoms. Those with more severe disease (e.g., temperature >38.5°C, severe arthralgias, extensive rashes) can be treated with a short course of corticosteroids (e.g., prednisone [Deltasone] 40 to 60 mg by mouth daily). Generally oral corticosteroids are sufficient, but intravenous agents may be appropriate for some patients (e.g., methylprednisolone [Solu-Medrol] 1 to 2 mg/kg in one or two divided doses intravenously). A systematic review revealed intravenous methylprednisolone (Solu-Medrol) as the most common treatment of RISS. Other treatment options identified were intravenous betamethasone (Celestone Soluspan), intravenous hydrocortisone (Solu-Cortef), oral prednisone (Deltasone), and oral prednisolone (Millipred). This study demonstrated a mean treatment duration of 9 days with complete resolution of symptoms in all cases. Some studies recommend tapering corticosteroids over 2 weeks to avoid rebound symptoms. There are currently no evidence-based guidelines available to guide dosing or duration of therapy.

Plasmapheresis or plasma exchange is another treatment option used to eliminate immune complexes. One study reports the use of plasmapheresis in five patients post–renal transplant who experienced anti-thymocyte globulin-induced serum sickness with no improvement after administration of oral prednisone (Deltasone) 1 mg/kg/d or intravenous prednisolone (Millipred) 2 mg/kg/d. This treatment method is generally reserved for refractory cases that do not respond to corticosteroid therapy due to limited evidence of its safety and efficacy.

References

de Silva HA, Ryan NM, de Silva HJ: Adverse reactions to snake antivenom, and their prevention and treatment, *Br J Clin Pharmacol* 81(3):446–452, 2015.
Erffmeyer JE: Serum sickness, *Ann Allergy* 56:105–109, 1986.
Karmacharya P, Poudel DR, Pathak R, et al: Rituximab-induced serum sickness: a systematic review, *Semin Arthritis Rheum* 45:334–340, 2015.
Lawley TJ, Bielory L, Gascon P, et al: A prospective clinical and immunologic analysis of patients with serum sickness, *N Engl J Med* 311:1407–1413, 1984.
Lin RY: Serum sickness syndrome, *Am Fam Physician* 33(1):157–162, 1986.
Lundquist AL, Chari RS, Wood JH, et al: Serum sickness following rabbit antithymocyte-globulin induction in a liver transplant recipient: case report and literature review, *Liver Transpl* 13:647–650, 2007.
Naguwa SM, Nelson BL: Human serum sickness, *Clin Rev Allergy* 3:117–126, 1985.
Ryan NM, Kearney RT, Brown S, et al: Incidence of serum sickness after the administration of Australian snake antivenom (ASP-22), *Clin Toxicol* 54(1):27–33, 2016.
Solensky R, Khan DA, et al: Drug allergy: an updated practice parameter, *Ann Allergy Clin Immunol* 105:259–273, 2010.
Tatum AJ, Ditto AM, Patterson R: Severe serum sickness-like reaction to oral penicillin drugs: three case reports, *Ann Allergy Asthma Immunol* 86:330–334, 2011.
Tanriover B, Chuang P, Fishbach B, et al: Polyclonal antibody-induced serum sickness in renal transplant recipients: treatment with therapeutic plasma exchange, *Transplantation* 80:279–281, 2005.

DRUG HYPERSENSITIVITY REACTIONS

Method of
Miriam Chan, PharmD; Kristen Rundell, MS, MD; and Ann M. Aring, MD

CURRENT DIAGNOSIS

- Detailed history should include past medical history; current diagnosis; previous and current medication use, including over-the-counter drugs and herbals; duration of the medication use; any similar reactions in the past.
- Physical examination should include vitals, temperature, and skin examination for rash.
- Laboratory testing should be conducted based on symptoms that may include complete blood count (CBC) with differential, eosinophils, sedimentation rate, liver enzymes, international normalized ratio (INR), and diagnostic skin biopsy or testing.

CURRENT THERAPY

- For life-threatening anaphylaxis reaction, start basic life support using pneumonic ACB (airway, compression, breathing) and give epinephrine immediately.
- Discontinue the offending drug if medically possible. Try drug substitution if warranted.
- An alternative option is to reduce the dose or frequency of the drug.
- Start symptomatic treatment based on the type of reaction and the offending medication.
- Some reactions may respond to treatment with antihistamines, H_2 blockers, or steroids.

Epidemiology

Drug hypersensitivity reactions are one of the many different types of adverse drug reactions (ADRs). ADRs are common, yet the more severe reactions have been estimated to cause 3% to 6% of hospital admissions. More than 100,000 deaths annually are caused by serious ADRs, making these reactions one of the leading causes of death in the United States. Early detection of all ADRs can potentially improve patient outcomes and lower health care costs.

Classifications

An ADR is a broad term that refers to any predictable or unpredictable reaction to a medication. A predictable (type A) reaction is dose dependent and is related to the known pharmacologic properties of the drug. Predictable reactions account for about 80% of all ADRs. An example of a type A reaction is gastritis that results from taking nonsteroidal antiinflammatory drugs (NSAIDs). The remaining 20% of ADRs are caused by unpredictable (type B) reactions. Type B reactions occur in susceptible individuals. These are hypersensitivity reactions that are different from the pharmacologic actions of the drug; they are results of interactions between the drug and the individual human immune system. Type B reactions can be further divided into drug intolerance, drug idiosyncrasy, drug allergy (immunologically medicated), and pseudoallergic reactions (anaphylactoid reactions). This chapter will focus on these type B drug hypersensitivity reactions.

Pathophysiology

Several mechanisms may play a role in the underlying etiology of immunologic drug reactions. The Gell and Coombs classification system was the original system to describe four predominant immune mechanisms. These four reaction types are listed as type I reactions (IgE medicated), type II reactions (cytotoxic), type III reactions (immune complex), and type IV reactions (delayed, cell mediated). Table 1 provides a detailed description of this classification. Type I and IV reactions are more common than type II and III reactions. Most drugs cause one type of reaction, whereas certain drugs, such as penicillin, can induce all four types of reactions.

The Gell and Coombs classification has recently been revised to reflect the functional heterogeneity of T cells. Under the new system, type IV reactions are further subclassified into four categories: IVa (macrophage activation), IVb (eosinophils), IVc (CD4+ or CD8+ T cells), and IVd (neutrophils). Nevertheless, many common hypersensitivity reactions cannot be classified in this system because of the lack of knowledge of their immune mechanism or a mixed mechanism.

A new concept of drug interaction with immune receptors has recently been developed by Pichler and colleagues. It is called the *p-i concept* (pharmacologic interaction with immune receptors). In this concept, a drug binds noncovalently to a T-cell receptor and stimulates an immune response, which can cause inflammatory reactions of different types. The stimulation of the T cell is enhanced by the additional interaction with the major histocompatibility complex molecule. This is direct stimulation of memory and effector T cells, and no sensitization is required. The skin has a high concentration of effector memory T cells, which can be rapidly stimulated by antigen penetration. The skin also possesses a dense network of dendritic cells that act as antigen-presenting cells and increase hypersensitivity reactions. As a result, clinical symptoms by p-i drugs may appear more rapidly. Some severe reactions—such as Stevens-Johnson syndrome (SJS), toxic epidermal necrolysis (TEN), the drug rash with eosinophilia and systemic symptoms (DRESS) syndrome, or hypersensitivity syndrome—are believed to be p-i related. Examples are abacavir (Ziagen) hypersensitivity syndrome and SJS/TEN from carbamazepine (Tegretol).

Risk Factors for Hypersensitivity Drug Reactions

The chemical structure and molecular weight of the drug may help predict the type of hypersensitivity reaction. Larger drugs

TABLE 1 Classification of Drug Hypersensitivity Reactions

TYPE	MECHANISM	CLINICAL FEATURES	TIMING OF REACTIONS	EXAMPLES
Type 1 (IgE mediated)	Drug-IgE complex binds to mast cells	Urticaria, angioedema, bronchospasm, pruritus, GI symptoms, anaphylaxis	Immediate (minutes to hours after drug exposure, depending on the route of administration)	β-lactam antibiotic
Type II (cytotoxic)	Specific IgG or IgM antibodies directed at drug-hapten–coated cells	Hemolytic anemia, neutropenia, thrombocytopenia	Variable	Penicillin (hemolytic anemia), heparin (thrombocytopenia)
Type III (immune complex)	Antigen-antibody complexes	Serum sickness, vasculitis, drug fever	1–3 weeks after drug exposure	Penicillin (serum sickness), sulfonamides (vasculitis), azathioprine (drug fever)
Type IV (delayed, cell mediated)	Activation and expansion of drug-specific T cell	Prominent skin findings: Contact dermatitis, morbilliform eruptions	2–7 days after exposure	Topical antihistamine, penicillin, sulfonamides

with greater structural complexity are more likely to be immunogenic. However, drugs with small molecular weight (< 1000 Da) can elicit hypersensitivity reactions by coupling with carrier proteins to form hapten-carrier complexes. Other drug-related factors include the dose, route of administration, duration of treatment, repetitive exposure to the drug, and concurrent illness. Topical and intravenous drug administrations are more likely to cause hypersensitivity reactions than are oral medications.

Patient risk factors include age, female gender, infection with human immunodeficiency virus, atopy, specific genetic polymorphisms, previous drug hypersensitivity reactions, and inherent predisposition to react to multiple unrelated drugs.

Clinical Manifestations

Drug hypersensitivity reactions can manifest in a great variety of clinical symptoms and diseases. While some reactions are mild and often unnoticed, others, such as anaphylaxis, can be severe and even fatal. Dermatologic symptoms are the most common physical manifestation of allergic drug reactions. Drug hypersensitivity reactions can also affect various internal organs, causing diseases such as hepatitis, nephritis, and pneumonitis. The noncutaneous physical findings are generally nonspecific and may not be helpful and even delay the diagnosis and management decisions.

Dermatologic Symptoms

The most common allergic drug reactions affect the skin and can cause a variety of different exanthems. The most common skin reaction is the classic "drug rash," which is a morbilliform eruption originating on the trunk. Other dermatologic symptoms include urticaria, angioedema, acne, bullous eruptions, fixed drug eruptions, erythema multiforme, lupus erythematosus, photosensitivity, psoriasis, purpura, vasculitis, and pruritus. The most severe forms of cutaneous drug reactions are Stevens-Johnson syndrome (SJS), toxic epidermal necrolysis (TEN), and drug rash with eosinophilia and systemic symptoms (DRESS) syndrome.

Stevens-Johnson Syndrome

SJS is a systemic disorder that has cutaneous manifestations. SJS was previously thought to be synonymous with erythema multiforme major. There are now criteria that separate the two disorders. In contrast to erythema multiforme, the target lesions associated with SJS have only two rings. The inner ring may have urticaria, pustules, or necrotic lesions surrounded by macular erythema. It is a T-cell–mediated toxic reaction to the basement membrane of the epidermal cells. There is massive and widespread apoptosis, for which there are several associated cytokines. The recent theories suggest that there are two pathways, one that consists of granule-medicated exocytosis (perforin and granzyme B), and one that consists of Fas-Fas ligand interaction associated apoptosis for the keratinocytes. More recent data suggest that

granulysin, which is a cationic cytolytic protein released by T lymphocytes, may play a role as well.

Interestingly, HLA genotype may predispose patients to SJS or TEN. Those patients with the HLA-B1502 found among the Han Chinese population may be associated with increased risk for developing SJS/TEN and use of carbamazepine.

SJS and TEN are on the same continuum. The definition of epidermal detachment and desquamation of epidermal cells is less than 10% of the body surface area for SJS and more than 30% for TEN. There is an overlapping diagnosis of SJS/TEN for the 10% to 30% category. To help differentiate from other ADRs, there is often a prodromal period in which a patient may have a cough and a fever. The lesions may occur up to 4 weeks after exposure to the drug. In addition, the lesions may be limited to the trunk; however, they more commonly involve the palmar surface of the hands and the dorsum of the feet, as well as the mucous membranes.

The most common drug classes associated with SJS and TENs are sulfonamides, cephalosporins, imidazole agents, and oxicam derivatives. Drugs such as carbamazepine, phenytoin (Dilantin), valproic acid (Depakote), lamotrigine (Lamictal), allopurinol (Zyloprim), nevirapine (Viramune), peramivir (Rapivab), and quinolones have been reported to cause SJS/TEN. In a retrospective chart review of 64 patients who had a diagnosis of SJS/TEN, Miliszewski et al. identified allopurinol as the single most common offending agent (20% of cases). According to the US Food and Drug Administration (FDA) Safety Alerts in 2013, acetaminophen has been associated with SJS, TEN, and acute generalized exanthematous pustulosis (AGEP). The evidence supporting causality primarily comes from a small number of cases reported in the medical literature.

The treatment is immediate cessation of the culprit drug and symptomatic treatment. Glucocorticoids are controversial and depend on the course and extent of the disease.

Toxic Epidermal Necrolysis

As previously stated, TEN is the cell-mediated disorder that involves more than 30% of the body surface. This is the more-severe form of the ADR: the mortality rates may be as high as 50%, mostly from sepsis. Patients are usually admitted to the burn unit for electrolyte and infection management. Glucocorticoids are contraindicated. There have been mixed results using IV immunoglobulin (IVIG)[1] in these patients. The IVIG is believed to inhibit the Fas-Fas ligand, which is the underlying mechanism for the basement membrane separation.

Drug Rash with Eosinophilia and Systemic Symptoms

DRESS syndrome or drug-induced hypersensitivity syndrome (DIHS) is a rare, life-threatening drug-induced reaction with a

_____

[1] Not FDA approved for this indication.

mortality rate of 10%. Therefore it is important to recognize the signs and symptoms early to initiate treatment. Most patients will have fever, lymphadenopathy (75%), eosinophilia, and an erythematous morbilliform rash on the face and body in addition to liver and multiorgan damage. The symptoms can occur 2 to 6 weeks after the drug administration. There are many drugs that can cause DRESS syndrome such as allopurinol, sulfonamides, and psychotropic medications. Based on literature review, DRESS syndrome is increasingly being recognized by psychiatrists. Carbamazepine is the most frequently reported etiology; however, DRESS syndrome is also seen with lamotrigine, phenytoin, valproate, and phenobarbital. The treatment is drug withdrawal, systemic corticosteroids, topical treatment for lesions, and supportive care, often in the ICU or burn unit.

Acute Generalized Exanthematous Pustulosis

Acute generalized exanthematous pustulosis (AGEP) is a rare ADR that presents as a fever and small nonfollicular pustules on a widespread erythematous background. AGEP may closely mimic pustular psoriasis clinically. The presence of acanthuses and papillomatosis and a personal or family history of psoriasis favor a diagnosis of pustular psoriasis. Exposure to medication, especially antibiotics with a short latency from the initiation of the drug, favors AGEP. The eruption usually occurs within 24 hours of the initiation of the drug, and healing occurs quickly after the discontinuation of the drug. Lesions heal within 2 weeks of discontinuation without scarring. The exact mechanism of drug-specific T lymphocytes is unknown, yet IL-3 and IL-8 may be the trigger for neutrophil-activating cytokines in the skin.

Acute Interstitial Nephritis

Acute interstitial nephritis (AIN) is an important cause of acute kidney injury (AKI). More than two thirds of AIN cases are caused by drug hypersensitivity reactions. Drugs most commonly associated with AIN include antibiotics (particularly β-lactam, fluoroquinolones, and rifampicin), NSAIDs, proton pump inhibitors, phenytoin, allopurinol, and 5-aminosalicylates.

The clinical presentation of drug-induced AIN is highly variable and depends on the class of drug involved. Patients with AIN may be asymptomatic with elevation in creatinine or blood urea nitrogen or abnormal urinary sediment. When present, symptoms are nonspecific. The "classic" triad of fever, rash, and eosinophilia is present in less than 5% to 10% of patients. Each individual component of the triad also occurs at various rates.

A diagnosis of AIN should be considered in any patients with unexplained AKI, clinical manifestations of a hypersensitivity reaction, and a history of exposure to any drug associated with AIN. A definitive diagnosis of AIN is established by kidney biopsy. AIN is characterized by interstitial inflammation, tubulitis, edema, and, in some cases, eventual interstitial fibrosis. The precise disease mechanism is unclear, but the presence of T lymphocytes in the inflammatory infiltrate suggests a type IV hypersensitivity response.

Early recognition is crucial as patients can ultimately develop chronic kidney disease. The mainstay of therapy is timely discontinuation of the causative agent. If AIN persists, corticosteroids may be used to improve kidney function. However, available data on corticosteroids are inconclusive, and randomized controlled trials are needed to confirm the benefits of corticosteroids in the treatment of AIN.

Evaluation

Because the history is essential for determining whether a patient is experiencing a drug hypersensitivity reaction, it is important to review all medications and the timeline of exposure. This includes any over-the-counter medications, herbal supplements, or occasional-use medications. Occasional-use medications may include NSAIDs, acetaminophen, cold medications, and so forth. It is important to establish a temporal relationship to the onset of the medication and the initiation of the symptoms. Oftentimes, the medication may have been discontinued before the appearance of the first symptom, so a review of medications from several weeks

before the symptoms is also important. In addition, because the host immune response plays a role in some of the IgE-mediated reactions, it is important to review any immunocompromising chronic or acute illnesses or states that the patient may have or is currently experiencing. This includes HIV, chronic obstructive pulmonary disease (COPD), asthma, chemotherapy, and pregnancy. For some ADRs, HLA type may be important. A patient's known genetic predisposition needs to be taken into account as well. A thorough history will also need to include any organ system or symptom that may be related to the suspected ADR.

A physical examination should augment and help to establish the working diagnosis of the type of ADR and the potentially offending drug. This should include vital signs of temperature, respiratory, and hydration status. The skin examination is important, as are appropriate evaluation and documentation of the type of lesion or lesions present. An examination of the oral mucosa and the conjunctiva of the eye should be done. Any lymphadenopathy, petechiae, or pallor should be noted.

Laboratory testing may be obtained to confirm or rule out a diagnosis. This may include a chest x-ray, CBC with differential, possible skin biopsy, liver function testing, creatinine, and electrolyte testing. A sedimentation rate and CRP testing may also be useful. Although additional autoimmune or antibody testing may be done, caution is suggested. There may not be a high yield on these tests, and they can be quite costly for patients.

Management

Anaphylaxis

Anaphylaxis can be a fatal drug hypersensitivity reaction because of its rapid onset. It is often underrecognized and undertreated because it can mimic other conditions and is variable in its presentation. However, respiratory compromise and cardiovascular collapse are of greatest concern, because they are the most common causes of death. Urticaria and angioedema are the most common manifestations but may be delayed or absent. The more quickly anaphylaxis occurs after exposure to the offending agent, the more likely the reaction is to be severe and potentially life threatening.

Most anaphylaxis episodes are IgE-mediated reactions resulting in a sudden mast cell and basophil degranulation. This sudden release of mediators affects the cutaneous, pulmonary, cardiac, GI, vascular, and neurologic systems. Medications are a common trigger of anaphylaxis in adults. Most cases of IgE-mediated drug anaphylaxis in the United States are due to penicillins and cephalosporins. Antibiotics are also the most common cause of perioperative anaphylaxis because skin eruptions may be missed in patients who are draped during surgery. Some anaphylaxis reactions involve other immunologic mechanisms. Administration of blood products (e.g., IVIG, animal antiserum) can cause an anaphylactoid reaction due, at least in part, to complement activation. Activation of the complement cascade can cause mast cell/basophil degranulation. Anaphylaxis episodes can also occur independently of any immunologic mechanism. Certain drugs, such as opioids, dextrans, and protamine, can cause a direct release of histamine and other mediators from mast cells and basophils. Finally, there are acute systemic reactions without any obvious triggers or mechanisms (idiopathic anaphylaxis).

Anaphylaxis is a clinical diagnosis with a short window of treatment time available. Therefore laboratory testing is limited and may not be of much value. Initially, the patient will describe flushing, pruritus, and a sense of impending doom. Some patients will have dyspnea, dizziness, syncope, or GI symptoms of diarrhea and abdominal cramping. Most patients will have cutaneous symptoms of flushing, urticaria, or angioedema. Some patients will progress to respiratory or cardiovascular complications.

The goal of therapy should be early recognition and treatment with epinephrine to prevent a progression to life-threatening respiratory or cardiovascular failure. The immediate intervention should include stopping the offending drug if possible, epinephrine injection, basic life support, high-flow oxygen, cardiac monitoring, and IV access. Epinephrine is the drug of choice for anaphylaxis. The therapeutic actions of epinephrine include α-1-adrenergic vasoconstrictor effects (decreases mucosal edema, thereby relieving upper airway obstruction, and increases blood pressure to prevent shock), β-1 adrenergic effects (increases rate and force of cardiac contractions), and β-2 effects (increases bronchodilation and decreases the release of mediators of inflammation from mast cells/basophils). Delayed epinephrine administration has been associated with fatalities. Intramuscular epinephrine in the thigh results in high-plasma concentrations and is preferred in the setting of anaphylaxis. The recommended dose of epinephrine is 0.3 mg (1 mg/mL) IM every 5 minutes. Typically, only one or two additional doses are needed. Patients in shock should receive epinephrine by slow IV infusion at 2 to 10 mcg/min with the rate titrated according to response and the presence of continuous hemodynamic monitoring. Patients taking beta-blockers may be resistant to treatment with epinephrine. In this case, glucagon[1] 1 to 5 mg IV over 5 minutes should be administered because its cardiac effects are not mediated through beta-receptors.

Adjunctive therapies for the treatment of anaphylaxis include antihistamines and corticosteroids. Consider an inhaled beta-agonist if wheezing. Diphenhydramine (Benadryl), an H_1 antihistamine, may be given intravenously at the dose of 25 to 50 mg. If an H_2 blocker is considered, give ranitidine (Zantac)[1] 50 mg/20 mL as an IV infusion over 5 minutes. Use of both diphenhydramine and ranitidine is superior to diphenhydramine alone. Corticosteroids are used to prevent a potential late-phase reaction that may occur in up to 23% of adults with anaphylaxis. There is no proven best dose or route of steroid therapy. The most common dosage is prednisone 20 to 60 mg daily for 3 to 5 days.

Angioedema

Angioedema is characterized by a deep dermal, subcutaneous, mucosal swelling. Many patients present with both urticaria and angioedema. Angioedema can progress rapidly from a mild swelling of the oral mucosal to a life-threatening laryngeal edema. With this rapid sequence of events, the most important part of treatment is obtaining and maintaining a patent airway. Epinephrine 0.3 mg IM every 10 minutes should be administered to patients who present with anaphylaxis, respiratory distress, or severe laryngeal edema. Once the airway is patent, the patient should be treated with H_1 antihistamines, H_2 blockers, and steroids. The milder cases may be treated similarly to other allergic reactions. H_1 antihistamines such as diphenhydramine and hydroxyzine (Atarax) are effective in relieving pruritus but can cause significant sedation. Therefore second-generation H_1 antihistamines[1] (loratadine [Claritin], cetirizine [Zyrtec], desloratadine [Clarinex], fexofenadine [Allegra]) are often chosen for outpatient therapy. Doxepin (Sinequan),[1] a tricyclic antidepressant with potent H_1 and H_2 blocker activities, can be used as an alternative to H_1 antihistamines. However, it should not be used as first-line treatment for acute urticaria and angioedema because of its significant side effects of severe sedation, dry mouth, and weight gain. Corticosteroids are used in patients who are not responsive to antihistamines. For most patients, a short course of oral prednisone is adequate.

In drug-induced angioedema, the offending drug should be stopped and avoided. Further trial of the medication is not recommended, because the patient will respond more quickly and with more severe symptoms on reintroduction. The patient should be counseled, and epinephrine 0.3 mg in an auto-injectable device (EpiPen, Auvi-Q) may be prescribed in case of recurrence in the future.

Specific Drugs

Almost all drugs can cause a drug hypersensitivity reaction. However, certain drugs are more frequently associated with specific types of reactions. Some of the more commonly used drugs are discussed here in more detail.

Antibiotics

Penicillin

Penicillin allergy is the most well-known drug allergy and also the most costly ADR. Although most drugs usually have type I and

___
[1]Not FDA approved for this indication.

type IV reactions, penicillin may cause all four types of allergic drug reactions. The rate of penicillin-induced anaphylaxis after intravenous administration is approximately 1 to 2 per 10,000 treated patients.

Only about 10% of patients who report a penicillin drug allergy actually have a true immunologic response. The other 90% are actually able to tolerate penicillin or a cephalosporin. Because of this overreporting, there are several patient safety concerns. These include the antibiotic coverage of an organism not being optimal and an increase in drug resistance, which results in higher health care costs. Therefore it is important to evaluate a patient for true penicillin allergy.

Penicillin skin testing is the best method for diagnosing an IgE-mediated penicillin allergy. A commercially available product, PrePen, contains benzylpenicilloyl polylysine (PPL), which is a major antigenic determinant of penicillin. Minor determinants are metabolic derivatives of penicillin that may also produce an immune response. The current recommendations for penicillin skin testing are to administer both the major determinant (PPL) and the minor determinants (penicillin G). These two tests identify approximately 90% to 97% of the currently allergic patients. Patients with a history of penicillin allergy but negative skin testing to PPL and the minor determinants rarely experience allergic reactions on reexposure. If they should occur, the reactions are mild and self-limiting.

In general, patients who report symptoms consistent with an immediate or type I reaction or are skin-test positive to penicillin should not receive penicillin. Desensitization should be considered if penicillin is the treatment of choice for an infection and no acceptable nonpenicillin alternatives are available. Patients should be desensitized in a hospital setting. Desensitization involves administering incremental doses of oral penicillin every 15 minutes for a total of 4 to 12 hours, after which time the first dose of penicillin is given. An example of a penicillin desensitization protocol is available in the Morbidity and Mortality Weekly Report at https://www.cdc.gov/std/tg2015/pen-allergy.htm.

Penicillin and Cephalosporin Cross-Reactivity

The rate of cross-reactivity between penicillin and cephalosporins has been historically cited to be as high as 10%. Recent data suggest that the rate may be much lower. The degree of cross-reactivity is highest between penicillins and first-generation cephalosporins, which have identical R-group side chains. In this case amoxicillin would be cross-reactive with cefadroxil (Duricef) and cefprozil (Cefzil), whereas ampicillin would be with cefaclor and cephalexin. Because of the differences in the chemical structures, second- and third-generation cephalosporins (cefdinir [Omnicef], cefuroxime [Ceftin], cefpodoxime [Vantin], and ceftriaxone [Rocephin]) are unlikely to be associated with cross-reactivity with penicillin. According to the latest guidelines for acute otitis media from the American Academy of Pediatrics and American Academy of Family Physicians, alternative initial antibiotics in patients with penicillin allergy include cefdinir, cefuroxime, cefpodoxime, or ceftriaxone.

Patients with penicillin allergy who have a negative skin-test result to penicillin (major and minor determinants) may safely receive cephalosporins. Cephalosporin treatment of patients with penicillin allergy who did not have a severe or recent penicillin reaction history shows a reaction rate of 0.1%. Use cephalosporin with caution in patients who report an immediate or accelerated penicillin allergy or those with a positive skin test to penicillin.

Sulfonamides (Sulfa Drugs)

Beside penicillins, sulfonamide antibiotics are the second most common cause of drug-induced allergic reactions. They commonly cause a delayed maculopapular/morbilliform eruption. Acute urticarial reactions (IgE mediated) to sulfamethoxazole (SMX) or trimethoprim (TMP) are relatively infrequent; the incidence of skin rash resulting from SMX-TMP (Bactrim) in healthy subjects is estimated to be 3%. Sulfonamides are also the most common cause of SJS and TEN.

Patients with HIV have the greatest risk of sulfonamide-induced allergic reactions. The typical reaction to SMX-TMP in patients with HIV is a generalized maculopapular eruption that occurs during the second week of treatment and is usually accompanied by pruritus and fever. Because SMX-TMP is the drug of choice for a number of HIV-associated infections such as *Pneumocystis carinii* pneumonia and spontaneous bacterial peritonitis, several methods of desensitization have been devised to administer SMX-TMP to patients with HIV with a history of allergic reaction to the drug.

There are three classes of sulfonamides based on chemical structure: sulfonylarylamines (including sulfa antibiotics), non-sulfonylarylamines, and sulfonamide-moiety-containing drugs. A sulfonylarylamine has a sulfonamide moiety directly attached to a benzene ring with an amine ($-NH_2$) moiety at the N4 position. A nonsulfonylarylamine also has a sulfonamide moiety attached to a benzene ring, but it does not have an amine group at the N4 position. A sulfonamide-moiety–containing drug has a sulfonamide group that is not connected to a benzene ring. Table 2 presents a list of sulfonamide-containing drugs based on their chemical structure.

The N4 amine is critical for the development of delayed reactions to sulfa antibiotics. Given the important chemical differences between drugs containing sulfa antibiotics and sulfa in nonantibiotics, the risk of cross-reactivity is extremely unlikely. A retrospective cohort study by Strom and colleagues showed that approximately 90% of patients with sulfa antibiotic allergy did not have a reaction to a sulfonamide nonantibiotic. Patients with allergic reactions to sulfa antibiotics are also more likely to experience allergic reactions to the other types of sulfonamides, but this is not because of cross-sensitivity. There is no reliable skin test to rule out or confirm sulfa allergy. Some experts recommend

avoiding all classes of sulfonamides in patients with serious reactions such as SJS, TEN, or anaphylaxis to any one sulfonamide.

Most diuretics are sulfonamide derivatives. The only diuretics that are not in this group are the potassium-sparing diuretics (triamterene [Dyrenium], spironolactone [Aldactone], amiloride [Midamor]) and ethacrynic acid (Edecrin). Dapsone is a sulfone that is chemically unrelated to sulfonamides. *It should also be noted that sulfates, sulfur, and sulfites are chemically unrelated to sulfonamides and do not cross-react.*

Angiotensin-Converting Enzyme Inhibitors

Angiotensin-converting enzyme inhibitors (ACEIs) have two major adverse effects: cough and angioedema. The cough is typically dry and nonproductive. The incidence of ACEI-induced cough has been reported to be 5% to 35%. Cough occurs more commonly in women, African-Americans, and Asians. The onset of cough ranges from within hours of the first dose to months after the initiation of therapy. The diagnosis is confirmed by the resolution of cough, usually within 1 to 4 weeks after discontinuation of the ACEI; however, the cough can linger for up to 3 months. The cause for ACEI-induced cough is unclear but might be related to bradykinin, substance P, or another mechanism. Angiotensin II receptor blockers (ARBs) are not associated with an increased incidence of cough and can be used as an alternative to ACEIs. Because the cough may persist for several months after stopping the ACEI, starting the ARB is not a contraindication at this time, yet the cough may persist through the initiation of the new drug.

The incidence of angioedema with ACEIs is approximately 0.1% to 0.7%. With the widespread use of ACEIs, angioedema has become a growing problem. ACEI-induced angioedema is more common in patients who are over age 65, black, or female. Angioedema frequently involves swelling of the face or upper airway and can be life threatening or fatal. It can occur within days, months, or even years after the start of treatment. However, nearly 60% of cases occur within the first week of therapy. ACEIs cause angioedema by direct interference with the degradation of bradykinin, thereby increasing bradykinin levels and leading to increased vascular permeability, inflammation, and activation of nociceptors. Bradykinin is also a prominent mediator in hereditary angioedema. Therefore ACEIs are contraindicated in patients with hereditary angioedema.

ARBs directly inhibit the angiotensin receptor and do not interfere with bradykinin degradation. Theoretically, they can be relatively safe alternatives for patients with a previous history of ACEI-associated angioedema. However, some reports of ARB-induced angioedema have recently been published. The mechanism of how ARBs cause angioedema is unclear. A meta-analysis suggests that for patients who developed angioedema when taking an ACEI, the risk of persistent angioedema when subsequently switched to an ARB is less than 10%. Therefore ARBs may be an alternative only for patients with a high therapeutic need for angiotensin inhibition. ARB treatment should be started with observation. Patients should be educated on the signs of angioedema and provided with proper emergency instructions on how to proceed if angioedema should occur.

The direct renin inhibitor aliskiren (Tekturna) does not alter local or circulating bradykinin and is believed to be an alternative in patients with ACEI- and ARB-related angioedema. However, cases of angioedema have been reported with aliskiren. As with ARBs, renin inhibitors should be used with caution in patients who previously experienced angioedema to ACEIs.

Aspirin and NSAIDs

Aspirin (ASA) and NSAIDs can cause several types of hypersensitivity reactions. The four most-common types of reactions are based on the drug pathways. Aspirin-exacerbated respiratory disease (AERD) is a serious reaction induced by ASA and NSAIDs in patients with asthma and chronic rhinosinusitis. AERD does not fit precisely into a specific type of ADR and is often referred to as a type of pseudo-allergic reaction. AERD affects up to 20% of adults with asthma. It is more common in women. The usual age of onset is around

TABLE 2	Classification of Sulfonamides Based on Chemical Structure

Drug

Sulfonylarylamines

Antibiotics:	*Antiinflammatory:*
Sulfadiazine	Sulfasalazine (Azulfidine)
Sulfamethoxazole	Protease Inhibitors:
Sulfisoxazole	Darunavir (Prezista)
Sulfapyridine	Fosamprenavir (Lexiva)

Nonsulfonylarylamines

Carbonic Anhydrase Inhibitors:	*Sulfonylureas:*
Acetazolamide (Diamox)	Chlorpropamide
Brinzolamide (Azopt)	Glimepiride (Amaryl)
Dorzolamide (Trusopt)	Glipizide (Glucotrol)
Methazolamide (Neptazane)	Glyburide (Diabeta)
Cyclooxygenase 2 (COX-2)	Tolbutamide
Inhibitors:	Tolazamide (Tolinase)
Celecoxib (Celebrex)	Other Agents:
Loop Diuretics:	Mafenide (Sulfamylon)
Bumetanide (Bumex)	Probenecid
Furosemide (Lasix)	Tamsulosin (Flomax)
Torsemide (Demadex)	Tipranavir (Aptivus)
Thiazides Diuretics:	
Chlorothiazide (Diuril)	
Chlorthalidone	
Hydrochlorothiazide	
Indapamide (Lozol)	
Metolazone (Zaroxolyn)	

Sulfonamide-Moiety-Containing Drugs

5-HT Agonists:	*Other Agents:*
Naratriptan (Amerge)	Ibutilide (Corvert)
Sumatriptan (Imitrex)	Simeprevir (Olysio)
	Sotalol (Betapace)
	Topiramate (Topamax)
	Zonisamide (Zonegran)

30 years. The pathophysiology of AERD is related to aberrant arachidonic acid metabolism. Patients with AERD also have increased respiratory tract expression of cysteinyl leukotriene 1 receptor and heightened responsiveness to inhaled leukotriene E_4. Administration of aspirin or an NSAID to these patients leads to inhibition of cyclooxygenase 1 (COX-1), resulting in a decrease in prostaglandin E_2 levels. Prostaglandin E_2 normally inhibits 5-lipooxygenase. As a result of decreased prostaglandin E_2 levels, arachidonic acid is preferentially metabolized in the 5-lipooxygenase pathway, leading to increased production of cysteinyl leukotrienes.

Patients with AERD typically have both rhinoconjunctivitis and bronchospasm within minutes of ingestion of a dose of ASA or NSAID. The bronchospasm can be severe and result in respiratory failure, which may require intubation and mechanical ventilation. Management of patients with AERD involves treatment of the patient's asthma and chronic rhinosinusitis and avoidance of aspirin and NSAIDs. Desensitization is available in cases when the patient has a specific therapeutic need for regular ASA or NSAID therapy. Selective COX-2 inhibitors very rarely cause reactions in patients with AERD and can be taken safely.

The second type of ASA and NSAID hypersensitivity reaction is an exacerbation of urticaria or angioedema in patients with chronic idiopathic urticaria. Approximately 20% to 40% of patients with chronic urticaria may have this drug-induced reaction. The mechanism of this reaction is related to COX-1 inhibition. The exacerbating effects are usually dose dependent. All drugs that inhibit COX-1 cross-react to cause this reaction. Selective COX-2 inhibitors are generally considered safe to take in patients with chronic idiopathic urticaria.

The third type of hypersensitivity reaction is an anaphylactic or immediate urticarial reaction or angioedema appearing soon after the intake of a specific NSAID. Other NSAIDs from other groups or even an NSAID from the same group with a slightly different chemical structure is tolerated by the patient. An IgE-mediated mechanism is implicated only in some instances. The diagnosis is made mainly by exclusion. Further research is needed in this topic.

The fourth type of hypersensitivity reaction is urticaria or angioedema caused by ASA or any NSAID that inhibits COX-1 in patients without chronic urticaria. These reactions may be either drug specific or cross-reactive to other NSAIDs. Rarely, patients may have combined respiratory and cutaneous reactions that cannot be classified into one of the four reaction types described.

Corticosteroids

Corticosteroids are the most frequently used drugs for the treatment of allergic conditions, yet they can also induce hypersensitivity reactions. Most hypersensitivity reactions to steroids can be classified into type I (immediate, IgE-mediated) and type IV (delayed, cell-mediated) mechanisms. Type I reactions are characterized by the presence of urticaria and anaphylaxis. Type IV reactions can be presented as maculopapular exanthema and delayed urticaria.

Allergic contact dermatitis (type IV reaction) caused by topical administration of steroids is the most common type of allergic reaction induced by this class of drugs, occurring at the rate of 3% to 6%. Usually this is seen as a failure to improve or a worsening of an existing dermatitis that is being treated with topical steroid. Keep in mind that the reaction can also be due to other constituents of the creams, such as neomycin or cetostearyl alcohol. The diagnosis can be done using patch testing, which detects more than 90% of allergic patients. The topical steroids most frequently involved are nonfluorinated, such as hydrocortisone and budesonide.

Inhaled and intranasal steroids can induce both local and systemic reactions. Local reactions include contact dermatitis, pruritus, nasal congestion, erythema, and dry cough and are quite often irritant in nature. Systemic reactions include eczematous lesions, particularly on the face, exanthema, and urticaria. The most frequently involved steroid is budesonide. The actual mechanism of this reaction is not clear, but it may be a T-cell–mediated reaction.

Hypersensitivity reactions to systemically administered steroids seldom occur. Most of the data come from case reports. Both immediate and delayed reactions have been described, ranging from urticaria to sudden cardiovascular collapse and death. Most immediate reactions are caused by intravenous methylprednisolone and hydrocortisone. In a few cases, the reactions can be induced by salts, such as succinate, or rarely by certain diluents such as carboxymethylcellulose or metabisulfite. Nonimmediate reactions are mainly mild, such as delayed urticaria or maculopapular exanthema. The drug involved most often is betamethasone.

Cross-reactivity between steroids is difficult to assess. Based on corticosteroid patch test results and their chemical structure, Coopman and colleagues divided the steroids into four groups: A (hydrocortisone type), B (triamcinolone acetonide type), C (betamethasone type), and D (hydrocortisone-17-butyrate type). Group D can be subdivided into D1 and D2 depending on the presence or absence of a C16 methyl substitution and/or halogenations on the C9 of the B ring. Table 3 provides the listing of the four groups. High cross-reactivity exists between corticosteroids in each group, as well as between group D2 and groups A and B, with group D1 exhibiting quite low cross-reactivity with the other groups.

Local Anesthetics

The most common immunologic reaction to local anesthetic is allergic contact dermatitis (type IV). IgE-mediated reactions (type I) to local anesthetics are very rare. Most adverse reactions are due to nonallergic factors such as vasovagal response, anxiety,

TABLE 3	Coopman Classification of Cross-Reactivity in Corticosteroids	
GROUP	**TYPE**	**DRUGS**
A	Hydrocortisone	Hydrocortisone (acetate, succinate, phosphate) Methylprednisolone (acetate, succinate, phosphate) Prednisolone, prednisolone acetate Tixocortol pivalate*
B	Triamcinolone acetonide	Amcinonide (Cyclocort) Budesonide (Pulmicort, Rhinocort, Entocort) Desonide (Desonate, DesOwen) Flunisolide Fluocinolone acetonide (Synalar) Fluocinolone Halcinonide (Halog) Triamcinolone Triamcinolone acetonide (Kenalog)
C	Betamethasone	Betamethasone (Celestone) Desoxymethasone Dexamethasone Paramethasone* Fluocortolone*
D1	Hydrocortisone-17-butyrate	Beclomethasone dipropionate (QVAR) Betamethasone valerate Betamethasone dipropionate Clobethasone 17-butyrate* Clobetasol 17-propyonate (Clobex)
D2	Hydrocortisone-17-butyrate	Fluticasone (Flonase) Mometasone Prednicarbate (Dermatop) Hydrocortisone 17-butyrate (Locoid) Hydrocortisone 17-propionate* Methylprednisolone aceponate*

*Not available in the United States.
From Torres and Canto (2010).

dysrhythmias, and toxic reactions resulting from inadvertent IV epinephrine effects.

Any patient who presents with a history of an allergic reaction to local anesthetics should be carefully evaluated. Skin testing and graded challenge can be performed in patients who present with a history suggestive of a possible IgE-mediated allergic reaction to these drugs. A local anesthetic that does not contain epinephrine or other additives, such as parabens or sulfites, is preferred in this situation.

It is necessary to identify the type of local anesthetics to be used. Local anesthetics are classified as esters or amides based on their chemical structure. Drugs in the esters group include benzocaine (Americaine, Dermoplast, Lanacane, Hurricaine), chloroprocaine, cocaine, procaine (Novocaine), proparacaine (Alcaine, Opthaine), and tetracaine (Tetcaine). Most allergic reactions reported in the literature have been caused by agents in the esters group, which are derivatives of para-aminobenzoic acid (PABA), a known allergen. Cross-reactivity occurs among members of the ester group, but the esters do not cross-react with the amides. Agents in the amides group include bupivacaine (Marcaine), lidocaine, mepivacaine (Polocaine), prilocaine (Citanest), and ropivacaine (Naropin). Amide local anesthetics generally do not cross-react with other amides or with the esters.

Radiocontrast Media

There are two types of radiocontrast media (RCM): ionic high osmolality and nonionic low osmolality. Both of these agents contain iodine. The nonionic RCMs are much more widely used today than the ionic agents.

Allergic reactions to RCM are common and can range from mild to life threatening. Anaphylactoid reactions and severe life-threatening reactions occur in 1% to 3% and 0.22% of patients who receive ionic RCM, respectively. Less than 0.5% and 0.04% of patients who receive nonionic agents have anaphylactoid reactions and severe reactions, respectively. The fatality rate is approximately 1 to 2 per 100,000 procedures, and it is similar for both ionic and nonionic agents. RCM reactions are typically not mediated by IgE antibodies. RCM acts directly on mast cells and basophils, resulting in the release of histamine and other systemic mediators, which cause the anaphylactoid reactions. Patients at greater risk for more serious anaphylactoid reactions include females; those with asthma, heart disease, and a history of previous anaphylactoid reaction to RCM; and those taking beta-blockers. People who have seafood allergy are not at increased risk for reactions to RCM compared with the general population. The pathogenesis of anaphylactoid reactions is also not related to iodine.

Management of patients with previous RCM reactions include the use of a nonionic, low-osmolarity agent and a pretreatment regimen. One common regimen consists of prednisone (50 mg PO at 13, 7, and 1 hour before the procedure), diphenhydramine (50 mg at 1 hour before the procedure), and a histamine H_2-receptor antagonist (1 hour before the procedure). This will significantly reduce the risk for anaphylactoid reaction with reexposure to RCM.

Delayed reactions to RCM occur 1 hour to 1 week after RCM administration. Approximately 2% of patients have delayed reactions to RCM. These reactions are generally mild, self-limited cutaneous eruptions. The mechanism is usually T-cell mediated. Rarely, more serious and life-threatening delayed reactions such as SJS, TEN, and DRESS syndrome have been reported.

Chlorhexidine

Chlorhexidine gluconate is an antiseptic agent. It is commonly available in OTC products as a skin and wound disinfectant (e.g., Betasept, Hibiclens). Hypersensitivity reactions to chlorhexidine include contact dermatitis, pruritus, urticaria, dyspnea, and anaphylaxis. Prescription chlorhexidine gluconate mouthwashes and oral chips used for gum disease contain a warning about the rare but serious allergic reactions in their labels. According to a recent FDA Drug Safety Communication, the number of reports of serious allergic reactions to chlorhexidine-containing products has increased over the last several years. As a result, an anaphylaxis warning is now added to the OTC product labels under Drug Facts.

Several case reports have suggested that some patients with prior exposure to chlorhexidine and patients with chlorhexidine-induced contact dermatitis may be susceptible to anaphylaxis caused by chlorhexidine sensitization. Since chlorhexidine is the standard skin disinfectant used before surgery or invasive procedures, the exposure to the agent becomes more widespread. Even though severe anaphylaxis to chlorhexidine has been estimated to be rare, the actual rate may be higher than reported. Such reports remind clinicians to be vigilant about chlorhexidine as a hidden allergen, especially in surgical patients.

Herbal Supplements

There is a perception that herbal supplements are "natural" and therefore safe. In fact, severe allergic reactions including asthma and anaphylaxis have been well documented in patients using bee pollen products and echinacea. Echinacea is an herb belonging to a group of flowering plants known as Asteraceae. Asteraceae-derived pollens are an important cause of hay fever and asthma. Asteraceae may cause contact allergic dermatitis. Cross-reactivity exists between members of the Asteraceae family, such as ragweed, dandelion, daisy, chamomile, echinacea, feverfew, and milk thistle.

A lack of quality control has been a major concern in the herbal supplement industry. Chinese herbal products may be adulterated with synthetic medications not listed on the label. Contaminated supplements may be a potential risk for systemic contact dermatitis in nickel- and mercury-allergic patients. Because of the widespread use of herbal supplements and the underreporting of adverse events to herbs, all patients should be questioned about the use of herbal supplements when being evaluated for hypersensitivity reactions.

Conclusion

Drug hypersensitivity reactions are common; fortunately, severe and often fatal reactions are not. It is important for the clinician to have a working knowledge of common drug-induced hypersensitive reactions as well as the ability to identify and document common dermatologic findings. With that background knowledge, a thorough history and physical examination should enable the clinician to diagnose the majority of these types of reactions. A timely and appropriate management plan can then be implemented. As always, it is important to educate patients regarding their drug hypersensitivity history and the potential for future reactions.

References

American Academy of Pediatrics: Clinical practice guideline: The diagnosis and management of acute otitis media, *Pediatrics* 131:e964–e969, 2013.

Bommersbach TJ, Lapid MI, Leung JG, et al: Management of psychotropic drug-induced DRESS syndrome: A systematic review, *Mayo Clin Proc* 91(6):787–801, 2016.

CDC: Sexually transmitted disease treatment guidelines 2015, *MMWR* 64(3):149–151, 2015.

Fernando SL: Acute generalized exanthematous pustulosis, *Australas J Dermatol* 53:87–92, 2012.

Harr T, French L: Toxic epidermal necrolysis and Stevens-Johnson syndrome, *Orphanet J Rare Dis* 5:39, 2010. Available at http://www.ojrd.com/content/5/1/39.

Haymore BR, Yoon J, Mikita CP, et al: Risk of angioedema with angiotensin receptor blockers in patients with prior angioedema associated with angiotensin-converting enzyme inhibitors: A meta-analysis, *Ann Allergy Asthma Immunol* 101:495–499, 2008.

Husain Z, Reddy BY, Schwartz RA: DRESS syndrome, part I. Clinical perspectives, *J Am Acad Dermatol* 68:693.e1–693.e14, 2013.

Inomata N: Recent advances in drug-induced angioedema, *Allergol Int* 61:545–557, 2012.

Joint Task Force on Practice Parameters, AAAAI, ACAAI: Drug allergy: An updated practice parameter, *Ann Allergy Asthma Immunol* 105:259–273, 2010.

Khan DA, Solensky R: Drug allergy, *J Allergy Clin Immunol* 125:S126–S137, 2010.

Lieberman P, Nicklas RA, Opperheimer J, et al: The diagnosis and management of anaphylaxis practice parameter: 2010 update, *J Allergy Clin Immunol* 126:477–480, 2010.

Miliszewski MA, Kirchhof MG, Sikora S, et al: Stevens-Johnson syndrome and toxic epidermal necrolysis: An analysis of triggers and implications for improving prevention, *Am J Med* 129(11):1221–1225, 2016.

Moka E, Argyra E, Siafaka I, Vadalouca A: Chlorhexidine: Hypersensitivity and anaphylactic reactions in the perioperative setting, *J Anaesthesiol Clin Pharmacol* 31(2):145–148, 2015.

Murata J, Abe R: Soluble Fas ligand: Is it a critical mediator of toxic epidermal necrolysis and Stevens-Johnson syndrome? *J Invest Dermatol* 127:744–745, 2007.

Perazella MA, Markowitz GS: Drug-induced acute interstitial nephritis, *Nat Rev Nephrol* 6(8):461–470, 2010.

Philips JF, Yates AB, Deshazo RD: Approach to patients with suspected hypersensitivity to local anesthetics, *Am J Med Sci* 334:190–196, 2007.

Pichler WJ: Consequences of drug binding to immune receptors: Immune stimulation following pharmacological interaction with immune receptors (T-cell receptor for antigen or human leukocyte antigen) with altered peptide-human leukocyte antigen or peptide, *Dermatol Sin* 31:181–190, 2013.

Ponka D: Approach to managing patients with sulfa allergy. Use of antibiotic and nonantibiotic sulfonamides, *Can Fam Physician* 52:1434–1438, 2006.

Sharma P, Nagarajan V: Can an ARB be given to patients who have had angioedema on an ACE inhibitor? *Cleve Clin J Med* 80:755–757, 2013.

Torres MJ, Canto G: Hypersensitivity reactions to corticosteroids, *Curr Opin Allergy Clin Immunol* 10:273–279, 2010.

3 Cardiovascular System

ACUTE MYOCARDIAL INFARCTION

Method of
Kuang-Yuh Chyu, MD, PhD; and Prediman K. Shah, MD, MACC

CURRENT DIAGNOSIS

- Patients are encouraged to seek medical evaluation as soon as possible when chest pain or angina-equivalent symptoms occur.
- Early presentation leads to early recognition, diagnosis, and treatment of acute myocardial infarction.
- The diagnosis of acute myocardial infarction relies on detailed history, ECG changes consistent with myocardial ischemia, and elevation of serum biomarkers.
- Although echocardiogram is not essential to diagnose acute myocardial infarction, it is useful in diagnosing complications from acute myocardial infarction and guiding management.

CURRENT THERAPY

- Timely reperfusion of occluded coronary artery is essential in managing STEMI.
- Early reperfusion therapy (PCI or CABG) in NSTEMI patients with high-risk features such as congestive heart failure, dynamic ECG changes, arrhythmia, and refractory angina is beneficial.
- Medical therapy and lifestyle modification strategies are important to reduce long-term atherosclerotic cardiovascular events.

Coronary heart disease (CHD) results from atherosclerotic coronary artery disease (CAD), and its acute manifestation is acute coronary syndrome (ACS). Based on the presenting symptoms, characteristic ECG changes, and cardiac biomarkers, ACS can be further subdivided into unstable angina (USA), non-ST-elevation myocardial infarction (NSTEMI), or ST-elevation myocardial infarction (STEMI). Most patients with ACS have similar underlying pathophysiology: atherosclerotic plaque formation leading to narrowing of coronary arteries with plaque rupture or erosion and superimposed thrombus formation resulting in an acute presentation. A small portion of ACS cases can be due to conditions such as coronary artery spasm, spontaneous coronary artery dissection, coronary embolization, or cocaine use. Stress-induced acute cardiomyopathy, without angiographic signs of severely occlusive disease, can closely simulate atherothrombotic STEMI.

Although the three ACS entities share similar pathophysiology, their presentations vary widely. The initial recognition, diagnostic testing, and management strategies for these entities are similar and applicable to all patients with ACS. Diagnostically, patients with STEMI as a whole reflect a more homogeneous group of patients when compared with patients with USA or NSTEMI,

and patients with STEMI carry the highest risk regarding acute morbidity and mortality. The major difference in managing these three groups of patients lies in the decision for and timing of acute reperfusion of occluded culprit coronary arteries.

In the past three decades, there has been a steady decline in the incidence of STEMI and significant improvement in the outcomes of patients with STEMI with the introduction of early coronary reperfusion strategies; improved adjunctive pharmacologic therapies; adoption of guideline-directed treatments such as lipid lowering, blood pressure control, and diabetes mellitus control; and cigarette smoking cessation to effectively modify risk factors. Currently, the in-hospital mortality of STEMI has reached as low as 7%.

Diagnosis

Electrocardiogram

ECG is the most important diagnostic test to detect STEMI because clinical features, physical examination, and CAD risk factor profile only have modest sensitivity and specificity in diagnosing STEMI. Current guidelines define ST elevation at the J point in at least two continuous leads of 2 mm or greater in men or 1.5 mm or greater in women in leads V2 to V3 and/or 1 mm or greater in other contiguous chest leads or the limb leads in the absence of left ventricular (LV) hypertrophy or left bundle branch block (LBBB). Other ECG abnormalities such as paced rhythm, drug or electrolyte (hyperkalemia) effects, or Brugada syndrome also reduce the sensitivity and specificity of STEMI ECG interpretation.

Some patients present with ECG changes, although not with typical ST elevation, indicating equivalent clinical risk to STEMI, and should be treated as having a true STEMI. These STEMI-equivalent ECG patterns include (1) isolated ST depression in two or more precordial leads (V1 to V4), indicating true posterior wall myocardial infarction (MI); (2) ST depression in multiple leads with ST elevation in aVR, indicating left main or triple-vessel CAD; (3) Wellens sign with symmetrical deep T-wave inversions in anterior precordial leads; (4) hyperacute T wave; and (5) de Winter sign showing ST depression and peaked T waves in the precordial leads. Occasionally, patients with left circumflex artery occlusion can present with a normal or near-normal ECG.

Serum Biomarkers

Serum biomarkers of myocardial necrosis such as cardiac-specific troponins T and I are complementary to diagnosing STEMI. In clinical practice, STEMI is often diagnosed with ECG alone, before the laboratory result of biomarkers is available. The troponin level typically rises 4 to 6 hours after the onset of symptoms and peaks within 12 to 24 hours if reperfusion therapy succeeds in reperfusing the occluded coronary artery and patients present early in the course of STEMI; its level tends to peak after 24 hours if reperfusion therapy fails or in patients who receive no reperfusion therapy. After STEMI, successfully reperfused or not, the troponin level remains elevated for 7 to 10 days. For patients suspected of having recurrent ACS within a week after the index STEMI, given the troponin level remains elevated, creatine kinase (CK) and the MB isoform of CK (CK-MB) levels can be used as biomarkers to establish additional myocardial necrosis from a recurrent event because CK and CK-MB levels usually return to normal 48 to 72 hours after the initial index event.

Imaging

STEMI is commonly accompanied with wall motion abnormalities on echocardiogram, but echocardiogram is not essential to diagnose STEMI. Echocardiogram is extremely useful in managing patients with STEMI, especially when they present with acute complications from STEMI such as acute congestive heart failure, acute mitral regurgitation, free wall or ventricular septal rupture, pericardial effusion, cardiogenic shock, or LV thrombus.

Management of STEMI

The principal concept of managing STEMI is "time is muscle"; hence, it is important for patients to recognize symptoms for early presentation and for the medical community to administer suitable reperfusion therapy in a timely manner.

Prehospital Phase

Current guidelines recommend that patients with STEMI receive reperfusion therapy as soon as possible but within 12 hours of symptom onset to achieve optimal myocardial salvage to reduce mortality and morbidity. In daily clinical practice, a substantial number of patients still present late and miss the golden window of reperfusion. Common reasons for late presentation include (1) patients' lack of knowledge to recognize symptoms, (2) patients' inertia to seek medical care, (3) patients' lack of access to medical care, and (4) atypical symptoms that mislead patients or medical care providers to consider noncardiac problems.

Patients with suspicious myocardial ischemic symptoms are encouraged to call emergency medical services (EMS) immediately for help; this has the following benefits: (1) patients can receive early treatment, (2) patients can receive immediate resuscitation should STEMI complications such as cardiac arrest occur en route to the hospital, and (3) an early prehospital ECG and communication with a hospital capable of percutaneous intervention (PCI) by EMS significantly reduce reperfusion time and improve outcome. A recent Lifeline STEMI Accelerator Study reported only 55% of STEMI patients were transported via EMS. Improving this requires public education to enhance recognition of symptoms, implementation of an efficient EMS system, and infrastructures with standardized treatment algorithms for STEMI.

Initial management by EMS usually includes pain relief by morphine, administration of nitroglycerin,[1] oxygen, and non-enteric-coated aspirin (162 to 325 mg) unless contraindicated. The role of routine oxygen supplementation to patients with STEMI has recently been questioned. A recent randomized clinical trial (Air Versus Oxygen in Myocardial Infarction [AVOID] trial) suggests that supplemental oxygen therapy (8 L/min via face mask) in patients with STEMI without hypoxia (oxygen saturation >94%) may increase early myocardial injury and is associated with larger myocardial infarction size at 6 months.

Once STEMI is identified by a prehospital ECG performed by EMS, an assessment of candidacy for and availability of reperfusion therapy is an important next step of management to ensure immediate reperfusion and administration of its adjunctive therapy to maintain culprit coronary artery patency, limit infarct size and adverse LV remodeling, and improve outcome. To achieve the best outcome from reperfusion therapy, patients with STEMI should receive suitable reperfusion therapy within 12 hours of symptom onset—the earlier the better. Current reperfusion therapy options for STEMI include primary percutaneous coronary intervention (PPCI) or fibrinolysis. PPCI is the treatment of choice for STEMI because it confers a beneficial reduction in mortality and recurrent ischemia when compared with fibrinolysis. Hence, current guidelines recommend EMS to transport patients to a PCI-capable hospital and PPCI as the preferred method of reperfusion therapy with a system goal of less than 90 minutes from first medical contact (FMC) to device time.

---

[1]Not FDA approved for this indication.

| **TABLE 1** | Contraindications and Cautions for Fibrinolytic Therapy in STEMI.* |

Absolute Contraindications

- Any prior ICH
- Known structural cerebral vascular lesion (e.g., arteriovenous malformation)
- Known malignant intracranial neoplasm (primary or metastatic)
- Ischemic stroke within 3 months except acute ischemic stroke within 4.5 h
- Suspected aortic dissection
- Active bleeding or bleeding diathesis (excluding menses)
- Significant closed-head or facial trauma within 3 months
- Intracranial or intraspinal surgery within 2 months
- Severe uncontrolled hypertension (unresponsive to emergency therapy)
- For streptokinase, prior treatment within the previous 6 months

Relative Contraindications

- History of chronic, severe, poorly controlled hypertension
- Significant hypertension on presentation (SBP >180 mm Hg or DBP >110 mm Hg)
- History of prior ischemic stroke >3 months
- Dementia
- Known intracranial pathology not covered in absolute contraindications
- Traumatic or prolonged CPR (>10 min)
- Major surgery (<3 weeks)
- Recent (within 2–4 weeks) internal bleeding
- Noncompressible vascular punctures
- Pregnancy
- Active peptic ulcer
- Oral anticoagulant therapy

CPR, Cardiopulmonary resuscitation; *DBP*, diastolic blood pressure; *ICH*, intracranial hemorrhage; *SBP*, systole blood pressure; *STEMI*, ST-elevation myocardial infarction.
*Viewed as advisory for clinical decision making and may not be all-inclusive or definitive.

Not every hospital is PCI capable. Based on the Nationwide Inpatient Sample database, only 33.7% of hospitals in the United States provided STEMI-related PCI in 2011. If a patient is sent to or arrives at a non-PCI-capable hospital, guidelines recommend transferring that patient to a PCI-capable hospital for PPCI with a system goal of less than 120 minutes from FMC to device time. If there is an anticipated delay of FMC to device time of 120 minutes or more, a fibrinolytic agent can be given within 30 minutes of hospital arrival if the patient has no contraindications for fibrinolysis (Table 1). Prehospital fibrinolysis, administered by EMS with physician supervision, has been shown to be feasible and safe, with a shortened reperfusion time and reduced mortality. Such strategy, however, is not used in the United States.

In clinical practice, sometimes it is not possible to achieve strict time goals because of uncertainty of the initial diagnosis, necessity to treat concomitant comorbidities or complications, patient preference or consent issues, and local factors delaying transport. Therefore, emphasis should be to deliver reperfusion therapy to eligible patients as rapidly as possible.

In-Hospital Reperfusion Strategy
Primary Percutaneous Coronary Intervention
PPCI performed in a high-volume hospital by experienced operators achieves a higher patency rate of infarct-related artery (IRA) and lower rate of recurrent ischemia, reinfarction, hemorrhagic stroke, and death when compared with fibrinolysis. In particular, PPCI has the greatest benefit in high-risk patients such as those with cardiogenic shock. Hence, PPCI is the preferred method of reperfusion whenever possible with the system goal of 90 to 120 minutes.

The reperfusion technique used in PPCI has evolved greatly in the past few decades, from balloon angioplasty, bare-metal stent (BMS), and drug-eluting stent (DES) to bioresorbable vascular scaffolds (BVSs). Compared with balloon angioplasty, BMS used

TABLE 2	Comparison of Fibrinolytic Agents		
	ALTEPLASE (T-PA) (ACTIVASE)	**RETEPLASE (R-PA) (RETAVAS)**	**TENECTEPLASE (TNK-TPA) (TNKASE)**
Dose	Up to 100 mg in 90 min (weight based)	10 U + 10 U IV boluses given 30 min apart	30–50 mg based on weight
Bolus administration	No	Yes	Yes
Antigenic	No	No	No
Allergic reaction	No	No	No
Fibrin specificity	++	++	++++
90 min TIMI 2 or 3 patency rate (%)	73–84	84	85
TIMI 3 flow (%)	54	60	63

Modified from 2013 ACCF/AHA STEMI guideline.

in PPCI confers reduced risk for subsequent target-vessel revascularization but does not reduce the mortality rate. Compared with BMS, DES used in PPCI decreases the restenosis rate and need for reintervention without reduction in reinfarction and death. BVS is a new stent technology, but its role in PPCI has not been well established because data concerning using BVSs in STEMI are insufficient and because of its association with a higher rate of stent thrombosis, especially in the first 30 days after implantation, and late lumen loss when compared with DES.

Fibrinolysis

The currently available intravenous fibrinolytic agents are tenecteplase (TNKase), reteplase (Retavase), and alteplase (Activase) (Table 2). A fibrinolytic agent should be administered to eligible patients without contraindication within 30 minutes of arrival at the emergency department. It is important to evaluate the risk/benefit ratio for each individual patient before administering fibrinolytic therapy because it carries a small but fatal risk of hemorrhage stroke (about 1%). The ideal patient to receive a fibrinolytic agent would be with symptom onset within 1 to 2 hours, low bleeding risk, and age younger than 65 years.

Although fibrinolysis achieves a reasonable patency rate of IRA (see Table 2), a substantial portion of patients fail to achieve successful reperfusion as defined by the following clinical criteria: (1) resolution of chest pain, (2) reduction of >50% of the initial ST-segment elevation pattern on follow-up ECG 60 to 90 minutes after initiation of fibrinolysis, and (3) occurrence of reperfusion arrhythmia (accelerated idioventricular rhythm [AIVR]). If fibrinolysis does not achieve resolution of ST elevation by at least 50% in the worst lead at 60 to 90 minutes, rescue PCI (transfer to PCI-capable hospital if necessary) should be strongly considered.

Percutaneous Intervention After Fibrinolysis

Approximately 40% of STEMI patients who receive fibrinolysis fail to achieve successful reperfusion and require emergent rescue PCI. Other indications for rescue PCI include severe heart failure, cardiogenic shock, persistent chest pain, or electrical instability. Hence, these patients should be transferred to a PCI-capable hospital immediately if fibrinolysis has been administered in a non-PCI capable hospital.

Otherwise, stable patients after successful fibrinolysis can undergo coronary angiography with an intent to revascularize as soon as logistically feasible, ideally between 3 and 24 hours after fibrinolysis (so-called *pharmaco-invasive strategy*). In patients older than 75 years, if a pharmaco-invasive strategy is chosen as

the reperfusion strategy, a fibrinolytic agent at half dose (such as the half dose of tenecteplase used in the STREAM trial) should be used to reduce bleeding risks because patients will receive concomitant antiplatelets and anticoagulants for PCI. A recent EARLY-MYO trial confirmed the efficacy of a pharmaco-invasive strategy using half dose alteplase followed by PCI within 3 to 24 hours was non-inferior to primary PCI in 30-day rates of total death, reinfarction, heart failure, or major bleeding but with a higher rate of minor bleeding. Very early PCI after successful fibrinolysis (<2 to 3 hours) is not recommended.

Facilitated Percutaneous Intervention

This strategy refers to a full dose or partial dose of fibrinolysis plus a glycoprotein IIb/IIIa antagonist or antithrombotic followed by immediate PCI if there is no evidence of reperfusion failure. Current guidelines do not recommend this strategy owing to potential harms such as an increase in ischemic events, bleeding, and mortality.

Patients With STEMI and Multivessel Coronary Artery Disease

About 40% to 65% of patients with STEMI undergoing PPCI for culprit IRA have multivessel CAD. Significant multivessel CAD, if left unrevascularized, is associated with a worse clinical prognosis. For patients with STEMI with cardiogenic shock, conventional paradigm deemed it reasonable to perform multivessel PPCI (or emergency coronary artery bypass grafting [CABG] in selected patients) to achieve as complete a revascularization as possible. However, a recent CULPRIT-SHOCK trial showed that initial revascularization of the culprit vessel only by PCI in patients with acute MI and multivessel ACD with cardiogenic shock resulted in a lower 30-day risk of death or renal-replacement therapy when compared with a strategy of immediate multivessel PCI.

For stable patients, randomized clinical trials have demonstrated the feasibility of performing multivessel PPCI in acute settings. This approach has the following advantages: complete revascularization leading to improved LV function and prognosis, decreased vascular complications from repeated procedures, and reduced length of stay and medical costs. However, the procedure will be longer with potentially higher radiation exposure, higher risk for contrast nephropathy owing to a higher contrast load, risk of compromising viable myocardium supplied by the nonculprit coronary artery owing to procedure complications, and unnecessary stenting to the nonculprit artery without objective evidence of ischemia. The 2015 American College of Cardiology (ACC)/AHA/Society for Cardiovascular Angiography and Interventions (SCAI) focused update on PPCI for patients with STEMI supports multivessel PCI, either at the time of PCI to the STEMI culprit vessel or as a staged procedure in selected hemodynamically stable patients. Interventional cardiologists should integrate clinical data, characteristics of lesions and procedures, clinical risks, and complications from procedures to determine the best timing and strategy to achieve the optimal benefit. The guideline does not endorse routine multivessel PPCI in patients with STEMI and multivessel CAD.

Patients With STEMI Who Present Later Than 12 Hours After Symptom Onset

Patients with STEMI who present between 12 hours and 2 days after symptom onset without unstable symptoms or signs are no longer eligible for fibrinolysis but are still eligible for PPCI to salvage myocardium, which confers the benefit of reduced infarct size when compared with conventional therapy guided by a predischarge symptom-limited exercise test or unplanned PCI guided by clinical instability as demonstrated in the Beyond 12 Hours Reperfusion Alternative Evaluation (BRAVE-2) trial. For patients with STEMI who present more than 48 hours after symptom onset without clinical instability, a strategy of symptom-limited stress test first or coronary

Figure 1 Pathways of managing ST-elevation myocardial infarction *(STEMI)*. *FMC*, First medical contact; *LHC*, Left heart catheterization; *PCI*, percutaneous intervention; *PPCI*, primary percutaneous coronary intervention.

angiography first to delineate high-risk features of coronary anatomy is reasonable with an intent to revascularize high-risk coronary anatomy. If patients are clinically stable without high-risk coronary anatomy noted by angiography and present between 3 and 28 days after symptom onset, PCI to open the occluded IRA does not confer a clinical benefit in reducing mortality, congestive heart failure, or nonfatal myocardial infarction when compared with medical therapy as demonstrated in the Occluded Artery Trial (OAT). Irrespective of time of presentation, patients with STEMI who present with hemodynamic or electrical instability should undergo coronary angiography with an intent to revascularize the jeopardized myocardium as soon as possible.

Figure 1 summarizes current pathways of managing patients with STEMI based on their time of presentation, their clinical status, and availability of reperfusion therapy.

Adjunct Therapy
Antiplatelet Therapy
Aspirin
Unless contraindicated, 162 to 325 mg of aspirin should be administered as a loading dose immediately and continued indefinitely at a dose of at least 81 to 325 mg daily in all patients with STEMI, with 81 mg being the preferred maintenance dose. Patients with a history of aspirin allergy can be given clopidogrel (Plavix) instead.

P2Y$_{12}$ Receptor Inhibitors
Clopidogrel is a second-generation thienopyridine and irreversibly blocks the platelet P2Y$_{12}$ receptor to inhibit platelet activation and aggregation. Current guidelines support the use of clopidogrel during fibrinolysis or PPCI. For patients undergoing

fibrinolytic therapy, a loading dose of 300 mg followed by a maintenance dose of 75 mg daily has been recommended for patients younger than 75 years. For patients older than 75 years, only the maintenance dose of 75 mg should be given. Prasugrel (Effient) and ticagrelor (Brilinta) have not been studied and, hence, are not recommended in the setting of fibrinolysis as reperfusion therapy. For patients undergoing PPCI, depending on whether they are receiving a fibrinolytic agent and the timing of subsequent PCI, a different dosing regimen of clopidogrel may be recommended (Figure 2).

Prasugrel is a third-generation thienopyridine P2Y$_{12}$ receptor inhibitor. It is metabolized to its active form more quickly than clopidogrel and hence confers a more potent effect. In a subset of patients with STEMI in the TRITON-TIMI 38 trial, prasugrel was more efficacious in preventing composite endpoints of cardiovascular (CV) death, myocardial infarction, and stroke when compared to clopidogrel, but it had a higher major bleeding rate. Prasugrel is also contraindicated in patients older than 75 years, with body weight less than 60 kg, or with prior history of stroke or transient ischemic attack.

Ticagrelor is a direct reversible P2Y$_{12}$ receptor inhibitor with a more potent, faster-acting property when compared with clopidogrel or prasugrel. In the pivotal Platelet Inhibition and Patient Outcomes (PLATO) trial, ticagrelor lowered composite CV death, myocardial infarction, and stroke when compared with clopidogrel but with an increase in non-procedure-related bleeding.

Clopidogrel, prasugrel, and ticagrelor require several hours to achieve maximal platelet inhibition. Additionally, in the setting of STEMI, the bioavailability of these oral agents may be hampered by clinical factors such as nausea, vomiting, and cardiogenic shock, leading to poor GI absorption and leaving patients not adequately

Figure 2 Oral regimen of different $P2Y_{12}$ receptor inhibitors based on reperfusion strategies. *PCI*, Percutaneous intervention. (Modified from 2013 ACCF/AHA STEMI guideline.)

protected by platelet inhibition during immediate PPCI. Cangrelor (Kengreal) is a fast-acting, reversible adenosine diphosphate (ADP) receptor inhibitor that is administered intravenously to achieve $P2Y_{12}$ inhibition within 2 minutes. Its plasma half-life is 3 to 6 minutes, and platelet function returns to normal within 60 minutes after discontinuation of infusion. The US Food and Drug Administration (FDA) has approved cangrelor to be used as an adjunct therapy during PCI to reduce repeat coronary revascularization and stent thrombosis in patients who have not been pretreated with an oral $P2Y_{12}$ inhibitor and are not receiving a glycoprotein IIb/IIIa receptor antagonist. How to transition from cangrelor to an oral $P2Y_{12}$ inhibitor after PCI depends on which oral $P2Y_{12}$ inhibitor a patient is being transitioned to. Based on the CHAMPION PHOENIX trial, to transition to clopidogrel, 600 mg clopidogrel loading is necessary immediately after discontinuation of cangrelor infusion. Based on pharmacodynamic data, prasugrel 60 mg should be administered immediately after stopping cangrelor infusion, whereas ticagrelor 180 mg can be given anytime during cangrelor infusion or immediately after infusion ends.

The 2016 ACC/AHA-focused update on duration of dual antiplatelet therapy (DAPT) in patients with CAD recommends at least 12 months of DAPT in patients with ACS (STEMI or NSTEMI) after BMS or DES implantation. Continuation of DAPT beyond 12 months is reasonable in patients who tolerate DAPT, do not have bleeding complications, and are not at high bleeding risk (prior bleeding on DAPT, coagulopathy, or oral anticoagulant use).

Glycoprotein IIb/IIIa Receptor Antagonists

Glycoprotein (GP) IIb/IIIa receptor antagonists include abciximab (ReoPro, a chimeric monoclonal antibody), eptifibatide (Integrilin, a synthetic peptidic inhibitor), and tirofiban (Aggrastat, a nonpeptidic inhibitor). The benefit of intravenous GP IIb/IIIa

receptor antagonists in patients with STEMI was largely established before the era of oral DAPT. With current use of DAPT, contemporary trials fail to show benefit with upstream administration of GP IIb/IIIa receptor antagonists before PPCI with either unfractionated heparin (UFH)[1] or bivalirudin (Angiomax). Current US and European guidelines recommend using GP IIb/IIIa receptor antagonists for bailout situations after a large thrombus burden, no reflow or slow flow, or inadequate $P2Y_{12}$ receptor antagonist loading during PCI.

Anticoagulants

UFH[1], low-molecular-weight heparin with enoxaparin (Lovenox) as prototype, fondaparinux (Arixtra)[1], and bivalirudin (Angiomax) are widely used in reperfusion therapy to limit thrombus propagation, reduce reocclusion and reinfarction, and improve vessel patency unless contraindicated. The choice of individual agent and its dose and duration of use depends on the choice of reperfusion therapy, concomitant use of other antiplatelet agents, and renal function (Table 3).

Given that PPCI is the preferred method of reperfusion and occurs early after presentation, and given physicians' familiarity with UFH, intravenous UFH is the preferred anticoagulant agent for PPCI. In patients with high bleeding risk, bivalirudin with DAPT is a reasonable alternative to UFH (whether the patient was pretreated with UFH) when avoidance of GP IIb/IIIa receptor antagonists is desired during PPCI.

For patients with STEMI who receive fibrinolysis as initial reperfusion therapy, UFH, enoxaparin, and fondaparinux all receive a class I recommendation based on ACC/AHA guidelines. UFH is preferred since a pharmaco-invasive strategy is common or for patients who may need rescue PCI. Bivalirudin may be used

---

[1]Not FDA approved for this indication.

TABLE 3	Dosage of Anticoagulants in Reperfusion Therapy for STEMI	
	REPERFUSION THERAPY	
	FIBRINOLYSIS	**PRIMARY PCI**
Unfractionated Heparin*	• IV bolus of 60 U/kg (maximum 4000 U) followed by an infusion of 12 U/kg/h (maximum 1000 U) initially, adjusted to maintain aPTT at 1.5–2.0 times control (approximately 50–70 s) for 48 h or until revascularization	• With GPI planned, 50–70 U/kg IV bolus, to achieve ACT 200–250 s • Without GPI planned, 70–100 U/kg IV bolus to achieve ACT 250–300 s with HemoTec or 300–350 s with Hemochron
Low-Molecular-Weight Heparin (enoxaparin [Lovenox])	• If age <75 years: 30-mg IV bolus, followed in 15 min by 1 mg/kg subcutaneously every 12 h (maximum 100 mg for the first 2 doses) • If age ≥75 years: no bolus, 0.75 mg/kg subcutaneously every 12 h (maximum 75 mg for the first 2 doses) • Regardless of age, if CrCl <30 mL/min: 1 mg/kg subcutaneously every 24 h • Duration: For the index hospitalization, up to 8 days or until revascularization	No information
Bivalirudin (Angiomax)	No information	• With or without prior heparin: 0.75 mg/kg bolus, 1.75 mg/kg/h infusion to the end of PCI. Additional bolus of 0.3 mg/kg if needed • Reduce infusion to 1 mg/kg/h if estimated CrCl <30 mL/min • Prefer over heparin and GPI in high-risk cases of bleeding
Fondaparinux (Arixtra)*	• Initial dose 2.5 mg IV, then 2.5 mg subcutaneously daily starting the following day, for the index hospitalization up to 8 days or until revascularization • Contraindicated if CrCl <30 mL/min	Not recommended as sole anticoagulant

ACT, Activated clotting time; *aPTT*, activated partial thromboplastin time; *CrCl*, creatinine clearance; *GPI*, glycoprotein IIb/IIIa inhibitors; *PCI*, percutaneous intervention; *STEMI*, ST-elevation myocardial infarction.
*Not FDA approved for this indication.
Modified from 2013 ACCF/AHA STEMI guideline.

after fibrinolysis in patients who develop heparin-induced thrombocytopenia and require continued anticoagulation.

Guideline-Directed Medical Therapy
Beta Blocker

Beta-blocker therapy decreases myocardial oxygen demand and improves myocardial remodeling with the benefits of reducing angina, infarct size, and mortality. Current guidelines recommend initiating oral beta blockers in the first 24 hours in patients with STEMI who are without contraindications such as congestive heart failure, evidence of a low output state, increased risk for cardiogenic shock, heart block, or reactive airway disease. If not given in the first 24 hours owing to contraindications, physicians need to reevaluate patients to determine their subsequent eligibility. Oral beta blockers should be continued for 3 years after MI as recommended by the ACC/AHA secondary prevention guideline, and longer if there are other indications (such as systolic LV dysfunction). Commonly used beta-blocker regimens are (1) metoprolol tartrate (Lopressor) 25 to 50 mg every 6 to 12 hours orally, transitioned over the next 2 to 3 days to twice-daily dosing of metoprolol tartrate or to daily metoprolol succinate (Toprol XL), and then titrated to a daily dose of 200 mg as tolerated, and (2) carvedilol (Coreg)[1] 6.25 mg twice daily, titrated to 25 mg twice daily as tolerated.

Current guidelines recommend intravenous beta blocker only for patients with refractory hypertension or ongoing ischemia without contraindications. Several small randomized clinical trials have suggested that early use of intravenous metoprolol tartrate in selected patients with STEMI with Killip class I to II and no atrioventricular (AV) block before PPCI may reduce infarct size with a higher LV ejection fraction (LVEF) or reduce the incidence of malignant arrhythmia in the acute phase without an excess of adverse events.

Angiotensin-Converting Enzyme Inhibitors or Angiotensin II Receptor Blockers

Angiotensin-converting enzyme inhibitors (ACEIs) and angiotensin II receptor blockers (ARBs) reduce afterload and decrease myocardial remodeling. Either ACEIs or ARBs should be started within 24 hours if there are no contraindications such as worsening renal function, advanced kidney disease, bilateral renal artery stenosis, hyperkalemia, or hypotension. These agents have the largest benefit in patients with anterior STEMI, congestive heart failure, or LVEF less than 40%. ACEIs may be given routinely to all patients without contraindication, whereas ARBs are an alternative for patients intolerant to ACEIs. There is no additional benefit, only more harm if ACEIs and ARBs are given concomitantly.

Commonly used ACEI regimens are (1) captopril 6.25 to 12.5 mg three times per day to start, titrated to 25 to 50 mg three times per day as tolerated; (2) lisinopril (Prinivil) 2.5 to 5 mg/day to start, titrated to 10 mg/day or higher as tolerated; (3) ramipril (Altace) 2.5 mg twice daily to start, titrated to 5 mg twice daily as tolerated; and (4) trandolapril (Mavik) test dose 0.5 mg, titrated up to 4 mg daily as tolerated. A commonly used ARB regimen is valsartan (Diovan) 20 mg twice daily to start, titrated to 160 mg twice daily as tolerated.

HMG CoA Reductase Inhibitors (Statins)

Treatment with statins after ACS lowers the risk of CV mortality, recurrent MI, stroke, and the need for coronary revascularization. Without contraindications, all patients should receive high-intensity statins as early as possible to improve compliance. Although current guidelines do not endorse a specific low-density lipoprotein (LDL) level as a treatment goal, it is recommended to obtain a fasting lipid panel within 24 hours of presentation. A commonly used high-intensity statin regimen is atorvastatin (Lipitor)[1] 40 to 80 mg or rosuvastatin (Crestor)[1] 20 to 40 mg

[1]Not FDA approved for this indication.

[1]Not FDA approved for this indication.

daily as tolerated. Statins need to be used cautiously with drugs metabolized via CYP3A4 and fibrates, with frequent monitoring for myopathy and hepatic toxicity. Statin use needs to be combined with diet and therapeutic lifestyle therapies.

Aldosterone Antagonists

Eplerenone (Inspra) improves myocardial remodeling and may reduce all-cause and CV mortality and rehospitalization. The 2013 ACC/AHA STEMI guideline recommends starting this medication 3 to 14 days after STEMI in eligible patients (creatinine ≤2.5 mg/dL in men and ≤2.0 mg/dL in women, potassium ≤5.0 mEq/L) with heart failure, with LVEF less than 35% to 40%, and already on adequate doses of beta blockers and ACEIs or ARBs. However, earlier administration (<7 days) is preferable to achieve mortality and rehospitalization benefits as suggested by a post hoc analysis of the Eplerenone Post-Acute Myocardial Infarction Heart Failure Efficacy and Survival Study (EPHESUS) trial.

Implantable Cardioverter-Defibrillator

Patients who develop ventricular tachycardia (VT) or fibrillation more than 48 hours after STEMI have the highest risk of sudden cardiac death (SCD) and, hence, are eligible for an implantable cardioverter-defibrillator (ICD) as a secondary prevention measure for SCD. For primary prevention, multiple trials have established the efficacy of prevention of SCD by ICD implantation in patients with LVEF less than 35% and New York Heart Association (NYHA) class II or III symptoms (or LVEF <30% with NYHA class I symptoms) despite optimal medical therapy 40 days after index STEMI and expectation of at least 1-year survival.

Other Medical Therapy
Morphine

Morphine is a time-honored medication used to reduce pain and anxiety, especially in patients with pulmonary edema during acute presentation of STEMI. However, analysis of results from several clinical trials suggests that a morphine/$P2Y_{12}$ inhibitor interaction exists, which could lead to adverse clinical consequences. Several recent pharmacokinetic studies in healthy volunteers have shown that intravenous morphine administration can reduce the level of active metabolites of clopidogrel and delay the maximal inhibition of platelet aggregation. A similar effect of morphine on ticagrelor was also reported. Given the current trend of using oral $P2Y_{12}$ receptor inhibitors before PPCI for STEMI, administration of morphine with $P2Y_{12}$ receptor inhibitors deserves careful consideration. However, routine avoidance of morphine has not been recommended.

Nitrate

Nitroglycerin reduces LV preload, increases coronary blood flow, and relieves chest pain symptoms. However, it plays no role in decreasing myocardial injury from coronary artery occlusion in STEMI. Its use in STEMI is mostly for congestive heart failure, hypertension, or rare cases of coronary spasm. It is contraindicated in patients with hypotension (systolic blood pressure [SBP] <90 mm Hg or SBP >30 mm Hg below baseline), right ventricular infarction from right coronary artery occlusion, or use of phosphodiesterase-5 inhibitors within 24 to 48 hours.

Complications of STEMI
Cardiogenic Shock

Cardiogenic shock is defined as an SBP less than 90 mm Hg for longer than 1 hour that is (1) not responsive to fluid administration alone, (2) secondary to cardiac dysfunction, or (3) associated with signs of hypoperfusion or cardiac index less than 2.2 L/min per m^2 and pulmonary capillary wedge pressure greater than 18 mm Hg. It occurs in fewer than 10% of STEMI patients (2.4% in 1986 GISSI-1 trial; 6.5% in Germany ALKK-PCI registry as reported in 2013).

Almost 75% to 80% of cases of cardiogenic shock are due to severe LV systolic dysfunction; right ventricular infarction,

TABLE 4	Management Measures for Cardiogenic Shock

Immediate Stabilization of Patients to Prevent End-Stage Organ Damage

Maintain adequate mean arterial blood pressure with norepinephrine (Levophed), dopamine, or dobutamine with intraarterial pressure monitoring; norepinephrine preferred over dopamine for less arrhythmogenic effect

Hemodynamic monitoring with Swan-Ganz catheter to guide inotrope or fluid management

Selective use of mechanical circulatory support* if patient cannot be stabilized by previous measures

Early echocardiography to define etiology of cardiogenic shock

Early mechanical ventilation

Management of hemodynamically significant arrhythmia

Fibrinolysis in STEMI if delay to PCI >2 h

Early Coronary Angiography and Revascularization

Early transfer to regional tertiary care hospital for revascularization

Prophylactic IABP placement before transfer

PCI often the treatment of choice

CABG (with correction of mechanical complications if present) in cardiogenic shock if feasible

CABG, Coronary artery bypass grafting; *IABP*, intraaortic balloon pump; *LV*, left ventricular; *PCI*, percutaneous intervention; *STEMI*, ST-elevation myocardial infarction.

*IABP is more readily available; limited experience with other LV assist devices such as Impella and TandemHeart device.

mechanical complications from ventricular septal rupture, acute mitral regurgitation, and free wall rupture leading to tamponade account for the rest. Other uncommon causes of non-cardiogenic shock after STEMI are bleeding, systemic inflammatory response syndrome, infection, bowel ischemia, or iatrogenic (such as due to medication).

Cardiogenic shock due to mechanical complications after STEMI occurs in a bimodal fashion, with most cases occurring within 24 hours. An early echocardiogram is extremely helpful to delineate the etiology of cardiogenic shock to guide subsequent definitive treatment. Cardiogenic shock carries a high in-hospital mortality, approaching 50%, and is higher in patients older than 75 years. These high-mortality patients require immediate stabilization to prevent end-stage organ damage followed by emergency coronary angiography and revascularization (Table 4).

Electrical Complications
Ventricular Arrhythmia

Lethal ventricular arrhythmia, VT or ventricular fibrillation (VF), is the most common cause of out-of-hospital cardiac arrest in STEMI. For hospitalized patients, VT/VF occurs in fewer than 10% of cases in the era of reperfusion therapy, and most cases occur within 48 hours of presentation. VT/VF is often associated with congestive heart failure, cardiogenic shock, or failed reperfusion of an occluded coronary artery. Hence, correction of electrolyte and acid-base disturbance, adequate reperfusion to reduce myocardial ischemia, and treatment of heart failure or shock are important preventive measures. Early administration of beta blockers within 24 hours to patients without contraindications reduces the incidence of VF. If VT/VF occurs, treatment includes immediate defibrillation or cardioversion and an antiarrhythmic agent such as amiodarone (Cordarone). Isolated premature ventricular contractions, nonsustained VT without hemodynamic instability, and AIVR do not generally require specific treatment.

Supraventricular Arrhythmia

Common supraventricular arrhythmias after STEMI include atrial fibrillation, atrial flutter, and sinus tachycardia. They are usually the consequence of or triggered by congestive heart failure, atrial infarction, pericarditis, hypoxia, or other underlying systemic problems (such as chronic obstructive pulmonary disease, bleeding, anemia, or infection). Treatment is directed to the underlying causes. For atrial fibrillation/flutter, physicians should pay special attention to anticoagulation use given the frequent concomitant use of DAPT and antithrombotics and the rate versus rhythm control strategy.

Bradycardia and Heart Block

Sinus bradycardia may occur after inferior STEMI. Because it is generally mediated through increased vagal tone, close monitoring usually suffices. High-grade AV block (second or third degree) can occur after inferior or anterior STEMI, with a worse prognosis after anterior STEMI owing to a greater degree of myocardial injury. High-grade AV block after inferior STEMI usually is transient and with a narrow complex escape rhythm, which subsides within 2 weeks. Occasionally, temporary pacemaker placement may be necessary if bradycardia causes hemodynamic instability. High-grade AV block from anterior STEMI usually requires placement of a prophylactic temporary pacing system because it is commonly associated with hemodynamic instability.

References

Bainey KR, Armstrong PW: Transatlantic comparison of ST-segment elevation myocardial infarction guidelines: Insights from the United States and Europe, *J Am Coll Cardiol* 67(2):216–219, 2016.

Bates ER, Tamis-Holland JE, Bittl JA, et al: PCI strategies in patients with ST-segment elevation myocardial infarction and multivessel coronary artery disease, *J Am Coll Cardiol* 68(10):1066–1081, 2016.

Carville SF, Henderson R, Gray H: The acute management of ST-segment-elevation myocardial infarction, *Clin Med (Lond)* 15(4):362, 2015.

Cassese S, Byrne RA, Ndrepepa G, et al: Everolimus-eluting bioresorbable vascular scaffolds versus everolimus-eluting metallic stents: A meta-analysis of randomized controlled trials, *Lancet* 387(1018):537–544, 2016.

Chandrasekhar J, Mehran R: The ideal anticoagulation strategy in ST-elevation myocardial infarction, *Prog Cardiovasc Dis* 58:247–259, 2015.

Di Pasquale G, Filippini E, Pavesi PC, et al: Complete versus culprit-only revascularization in ST-elevation myocardial infarction and multivessel disease, *Intern Emerg Med* 11(4):499–506, 2016.

Dind A, Allahwala U, Asrress KN, et al: Contemporary management of ST-elevation myocardial infarction, *Heart Lung Circ* 26(2):114–121, 2017.

Ellis SG, Kereiakes DJ, Metzger DC, et al: Everolimus-eluting bioresorbable scaffolds for coronary artery disease, *N Eng J Med* 373(20):1905–1915, 2015.

Hochman JS, Lamas GA, Buller CE, et al: Coronary intervention for persistent occlusion after myocardial infarction, *N Engl J Med* 355:2395–2407, 2006.

Ibanez B, Macaya C, SÆnchez-Brunete V, et al: Effect of early metoprolol on infarct size in ST-segment-elevation myocardial infarction patients undergoing primary percutaneous coronary intervention: the Effect of Metoprolol in Cardioprotection During an Acute Myocardial Infarction (METOCARD-CNIC) trial, *Circulation* 128(14):1495–1503, 2013.

Kragholm K, Lu D, Chiswell K, et al: Improvement in care and outcomes for emergency medical service-transported patients with ST-elevation myocardial infarction (STEMI) with and without prehospital cardiac arrest: A mission:lifeline STEMI accelerator study, *J Am Heart Assoc* 6:e005717, 2017.

Kubica J, Kubica A, Jilma B, et al: Impact of morphine on antiplatelet effects of oral P2Y12 receptor inhibitors, *Int J Cardiol* 215:201–208, 2016.

Pu J, Ding S, Ge H, et al: Efficacy and safety of a pharmaco-invasive strategy with half-dose alteplase versus primary angioplasty in ST-segment-elevation myocardial infarction: EARLY-MYO Trial (Early Routine Catheterization After Alteplase Fibrinolysis Versus Primary PCI in Acute ST-Segment-Elevation Myocardial Infarction), *Circulation* 136:1462–1473, 2017.

Qamar A, Bhatt DL: Current status of data on cangrelor, *Pharmacol Ther* 159:102–109, 2016.

Reed GW, Rossi JE, Cannon CP: Acute myocardial infarction, *Lancet* 389(10065):197–210, 2017.

Roolvink V, IbÆæez B, Ottervanger JP, et al: Early intravenous beta-blockers in patients with ST-segment elevation myocardial infarction before primary percutaneous coronary intervention, *J AM Coll Cardiol* 67(23):2705–2715, 2016.

Schomig A, Mehilli J, Antoniucci D, et al: Mechanical reperfusion in patients with acute myocardial infarction presenting more than 12 hours from symptom onset: A randomized controlled trial, *JAMA* 293(23):2865–2872, 2005.

Serruys PW, Chevalier B, Sotomi Y, et al: Comparison of an everolimus-eluting bioresorbable scaffold with an everolimus- eluting metallic stent for the treatment of coronary artery stenosis (ABSORB II): A 3 year, randomised, controlled, single- blind, multicentre clinical trial, *Lancet* 388(10059):2479–2491, 2016.

Shah RU, Henry TD, Rutten-Ramos S, et al: Increasing percutaneous coronary interventions for ST-segment elevation myocardial infarction in the United States: Progress and opportunity, *JACC Cardiovasc Interv* 8:139–146, 2015.

Thiele H, Akin I, Sandri M, et al: PCI strategies in patients with acute myocardial infarction and cardiogenic shock, *N Engl J Med* 377(25):2419–2432, 2017.

Yadlapati A, Gajjar M, Schimmel DR, et al: Contemporary management of ST-segment elevation myocardial infarction, *Intern Emerg Med* 11(8):1107–1113, 2016.

ANGINA PECTORIS

Method of
Kenneth Tobin, DO; and Kim Eagle, MD

CURRENT DIAGNOSIS

- The clinical diagnosis of angina depends largely on the accurate assessment of a patient's risk factor profile for coronary artery disease and the typicality of the symptom complex.
- The most common symptom of angina pectoris is left-sided chest pain or pressure, with or without associated radiation of pain or pressure to the jaw or left arm, occurring with exertion and relieved with rest or sublingual nitroglycerin.
- Women may present with atypical symptoms such as sharp, nonexertional chest pain, generalized fatigue, shortness of breath, or right-sided chest pain.
- Basic screening tests (e.g., 12-lead electrocardiogram, laboratory data, chest radiograph) are normal in most cases.
- For an initial diagnosis, appropriate noninvasive testing or coronary angiography, or both, is important to define the amount of ischemic myocardium and an overall treatment plan.
- Even when invasive procedures are clinically indicated, aggressive medical therapy with high-dose statins, attainment of appropriate blood pressure levels, smoking cessation, and use of antiplatelet therapy is of paramount importance.
- Patients who have clinical evidence of unstable angina and laboratory evidence of myocardial ischemia most often benefit from early invasive treatment strategies.

CURRENT THERAPY

Stable Angina Pectoris
- Treatment includes β-blockers, nitrates, and calcium channel blockers for symptom control.
- Consider the addition of ranolazine (Ranexa) if symptoms are not adequately controlled.

Aggressive Cholesterol Treatment Based on the American College of Cardiology (ACC)-American Hearth Association (AHA) Blood Cholesterol Guidelines
- Blood pressure management
- Antiplatelet therapy
- Lifestyle modifications:
  - Smoking cessation
  - Exercise prescription
  - Mediterranean, plant-based diet
  - Depression assessment

Unstable Angina
- With positive biomarkers for myocardial ischemia, consider coronary angiography.
- With negative biomarkers for myocardial ischemia, consider noninvasive assessment once symptoms are controlled.
- With a substantial ischemic burden identified, consider coronary angiography.
- With no or minimal ischemia identified, consider increasing medical therapy.
- With persistent symptoms, consider other treatment modalities.

Angina pectoris is defined as cardiac-induced pain that is a direct result of a mismatch between myocardial oxygen supply and demand. The initial presentation of ischemic heart disease is chronic stable angina in approximately 50% of patients; it is estimated that 16.5 million Americans are being diagnosed with this condition. Ischemic heart disease is the leading cause of death in the United States.

Stable angina refers to predictable chest discomfort during various levels of exertional activity that is predictably resolved with rest or administration of sublingual nitroglycerin (Nitrostat). Unstable angina is an acute ischemic event; this diagnosis includes patients with new-onset cardiac chest pain, angina at rest, postmyocardial infarction angina, or an accelerating pattern of previously stable angina. The terms unstable angina and non–Q wave myocardial infarction are often used interchangeably and should be further defined on the basis of myocardial necrosis as measured by serum biomarkers.

The clinical sensation of angina pectoris is caused by stimulation of chemosensitive and mechanosensitive receptors of unmyelinated nerve cells found within cardiac muscle fibers and around the coronary vessels. This stimulation cascade is thought to occur when lactate, serotonin, bradykinin, histamine, reactive oxygen species, and adenosine are released into the coronary circulation during periods of lactic acidosis. Nerve stimulation via the sympathetic ganglia occurs most commonly between the seventh cervical and fourth thoracic portions of the spinal cord. This explains from an anatomic standpoint why the most commonly recognized pain patterns for angina pectoris involve discomfort in the chest, neck, jaw, and left arm.

The most common cause of angina pectoris is coronary atherosclerosis. As plaque is initially deposited within a coronary vessel, there may be no significant internal luminal compromise during the early positive remodeling phase. However, at the point at which this compensatory mechanism fails, internal luminal compromise ensues. As long as the coronary artery segment distal to the stenosis retains the ability to vasodilate in response to increasing blood flow demands, coronary homeostasis is maintained. Once the critical threshold is passed, the blood supply cannot accommodate this demand, and angina may occur. The four major factors that determine myocardial oxygen demand are heart rate, systolic blood pressure, myocardial wall tension, and myocardial contractility.

Clinical Features

For patients with documented coronary artery disease (CAD) who have predictable episodes of classic symptoms, the diagnosis of angina pectoris is straightforward. Most patients are aware of the levels of exertion that typically induce angina symptoms. Most describe a pain or heaviness across their middle chest that may or may not radiate to the jaw or left arm. Some patients deny chest pain symptoms altogether and instead complain of exertional dyspnea or diaphoresis. Environmental situations such as cold exposure, emotional stress, or heavy meals can induce angina. The Canadian Cardiovascular Society and the New York Heart Association classification systems are used to define angina severity. Both systems use a I through IV scale, with mild angina (class I) referring to episodes that occur with extreme exertion and severe angina (class IV) to episodes that occur with minimal or no exertion. These classification systems are useful for risk stratification and for assessing medical therapy efficacy.

There are clear gender differences in the clinical presentations of angina. Pleuritic, musculoskeletal-type pain, nonexertional pain, and nocturnal pains have been reported as anginal equivalents in women. Fatigue is one of the most common presenting symptoms for CAD in women. The key to the diagnosis in men and women lies in a thorough history, which should always include the quality, location, provoking activities, and duration of pain and factors that relieve the pain. Based on a detailed clinical history, the many diagnoses that can masquerade as angina may be eliminated (Table 1).

Diagnostic Testing

A baseline electrocardiogram (ECG) is often one of the initial tests obtained in a patient with the complaint of chest pain. A normal tracing does not exclude the diagnosis of ischemic heart disease. More than 50% of patients with diagnosed angina have a normal ECG at rest. The baseline ECG may, however, show evidence of pathologic Q waves or left ventricular hypertrophy, either of which increases the statistical probability of significant CAD. Baseline laboratory data should include a fasting lipid panel to help define the patient's risk factor profile.

TABLE 1	Differential Diagnosis of Chest Pain

Cardiac ischemia

Angina

Myocardial infarction

Vasospastic angina

Pericarditis

Aortic dissection (new-onset chest pain and new aortic insufficiency noted on auscultation is an aortic dissection until proven otherwise)

Pulmonary embolism

Esophageal spasm

Gastroesophageal reflux disease

Musculoskeletal pain

Biliary colic

Acute pneumonia

Stress testing is an appropriate screening tool for the initial diagnosis of CAD, risk stratification after acute ischemic syndrome, and assessment of treatment efficacy. Whenever feasible, it is more advantageous to obtain an exercise stress test rather than a pharmacologically based study. The additional prognostic data obtained through exercise include blood pressure response, heart rate response, heart rate recovery, metabolic equivalent level attained, and ECG assessment of the ST segment. There are several validated exercise protocols that provide additional risk stratification measures to the test results.

The predictive value of exercise treadmill stress testing ranges from 40% for single-vessel disease to 90% for three-vessel disease. A baseline left bundle branch block, paced rhythm, poorly controlled atrial arrhythmia, or left ventricular hypertrophy with secondary ischemic changes often renders the test inconclusive when assessing for ischemic changes. However, if stress testing is being performed for attainment of hemodynamic responses and achievable metabolic equivalent levels, these baseline ECG abnormalities may be overlooked.

Stress test accuracy is markedly improved by the addition of an imaging modality such as echocardiography or nuclear perfusion scanning. The sensitivity and specificity of stress echocardiography and stress nuclear imaging are 85% to 90%. Stress echocardiography is believed to be more specific, and stress nuclear imaging is thought to be more sensitive. A stress echocardiogram also allows assessment of left ventricular systolic function and valvular function and prediction of right ventricular pressure. In deciding on which stress test to perform, one should rely on the expertise of the testing facility and the individual patient's circumstance.

Risk Factor Management
Hypertension
Hypertension is a commonly occurring, well-established, major cardiovascular risk factor. Initial treatment of hypertension in patients with ischemic heart disease should always include lifestyle management. Appropriate weight loss with a goal of achieving a body mass index <25 kg/m² can improve hypertension control. A reduction in dietary salt intake can also have positive effects on a patient's blood pressure. Following a heart healthy diet and increased physical activity with a structured exercise program are also very important.

Discord has resulted from the publication of several recent hypertension guidelines by various medical societies, as well as the 2014 Evidence-Based Guideline for the Management of High Blood Pressure in Adults Report from the Panel Members Appointed to the Eighth Joint National Committee. It has been shown that cardiovascular risk progressively increases at blood pressures greater than 115/75 mm Hg. A meta-analysis of 61 prospective observational trials of hypertension involving 1 million adults with no known vascular disease at baseline revealed several interesting findings. Patient outcomes were related per decade of age to the usual blood pressure at the start of that decade. For example, from ages 40 to 69 years, for each increase in 20 mm Hg systolic blood pressure, a twofold increase in cardiovascular death rate occurred. These findings were much more pronounced in patients who were between 80 and 89 years old than in the youngest cohort, 40 to 49 years old. Although the relative risk was much higher in the younger group, the absolute risk was greatest among the octogenarians. These increased cardiovascular risks were not confined to subjects with blood pressures greater than 140/90 mm Hg; rather, there was a threshold of risk shown all the way down to 115/75 mm Hg. Even small reductions in blood pressure can have a significant positive impact on cardiovascular disease. Blood pressure reductions of 4 mm Hg systolic and 3 mm Hg diastolic were shown to reduce cardiovascular events by 15% in a cohort of 20,888 patients.

The Heart Outcomes Prevention Evaluation study asked the question whether all patients with atherosclerosis, regardless of blood pressure, should be treated with an angiotensin-converting enzyme inhibitor. Although many subsequent editorials implied that all patients with CAD could benefit from this therapy, a closer look at the data suggests a different interpretation. The mean blood pressure was 139/79 mm Hg, suggesting that a significant portion of the 9297 participants had a baseline blood pressure higher than this value. Compared with placebo, the treatment group had a 22% reduction in the primary outcome composite of myocardial infarction, stroke, or cardiovascular death. A small substudy using 24-hour ambulatory blood pressure monitoring showed blood pressure differences of 11 mm Hg systolic and 4 mm Hg diastolic in the treatment group compared with the placebo group, which may explain the cardiovascular event reductions reported.

The Systolic Blood Pressure Intervention Trial (SPRINT) studied cardiovascular outcomes in patients with increased cardiovascular risk (excluding diabetes) and randomized the more than 9000 participants to either intensive blood pressure control of <120 mm Hg or a standard blood pressure goal of <140 mm Hg. The trial was halted early because of the significant benefits seen in the intensive blood pressure arm. The intensive group had a 25% relative risk reduction for the primary composite endpoint compared to the standard care group. The blood pressure goal for treatment of hypertension in patients at high cardiovascular risk should be <130/80 mm Hg. High cardiovascular risk is defined as a history of clinical cardiovascular (CV) disease (established coronary artery disease, heart failure, or stroke), or an estimated 10-year atherosclerosis CV disease of ≥10%. (One must be careful with aggressive diastolic blood pressure management, as some studies have shown a J-shaped curve relationship between diastolic blood pressures and coronary events.)

Hyperlipidemia

Dyslipidemia is an important risk factor for atherosclerotic cardiovascular disease, and the lowering of low density lipoprotein (LDL)-cholesterol has been shown to correlate with reductions in cardiovascular disease event rates. Previously published cholesterol treatment guidelines recommended achieving less than 70 mg/dL LDL-cholesterol levels in CAD patients. The current guidelines published by the ACC-AHA depart from these specific values, and instead recommend using high-intensity 3-hydroxy-3-methylglutaryl coenzyme reductase inhibitors (statins) to reduce the LDL-cholesterol levels by more than 50%. These agents have been shown to be well tolerated and have positive nonlipid pleiotropic effects, as well as the ability to dramatically lower LDL levels.

Observational evidence suggests that regardless of how cholesterol is lowered, a reduction in atherosclerotic cardiovascular disease will result. However, to achieve meaningful reductions in cardiovascular mortality, the recommended choice for lowering LDL-cholesterol levels among the currently available pharmacology are the statins. These agents have been studied exclusively using fixed-dose combinations and not dose-titrated to achieve various LDL-C levels; therefore currently available data do not support specific LDL target goals.

The Cholesterol Treatment Trialists' meta-analysis, including 90,056 subjects from 14 trials, showed a 12% reduction in all-cause mortality per 38.6 mg/dL (1 mmol/L) reduction in LDL-cholesterol, with a 19% reduction in coronary mortality, a 24% reduction in need for revascularization, a 17% reduction in stroke incidence, and a 21% reduction in any major vascular event during a mean follow-up period of 5 years. These benefits were observed in different age groups, across genders, at different baseline cholesterol levels, and equally among those with and without prior CAD and cardiovascular risk factors.

The Heart Protection Study showed that in patients with established CAD, other atherosclerotic vascular disease, or diabetes, statin therapy reduced cardiovascular events regardless of the baseline LDL-cholesterol level. The trial, which enrolled 20,536 patients aged 40 to 80 years, showed a 24% reduction in major cardiovascular events, a 25% reduction in stroke, and a 13% reduction in overall mortality with statin therapy.

Patients with a recent acute ischemic syndrome were enrolled in the Pravastatin or Atorvastatin Evaluation and Infection Therapy trial, known as Thrombolysis in Myocardial Infarction 22, which compared 80 mg atorvastatin (Lipitor) with 40 mg of pravastatin (Pravachol). The atorvastatin group achieved a median LDL level of 62 mg/dL, compared with 96 mg/dL in the pravastatin group. The relative risk reduction for this reduced LDL level was 16%. A substudy looking at the LDL-cholesterol levels achieved with atorvastatin showed that those subjects achieving a level of 40 to 60 mg/dL had a 22% reduction in events, compared with those achieving a level of 80 to 100 mg/dL. Therefore, it appears that high-dose statin therapy and aggressive LDL-lowering in this patient population lead to reduced cardiovascular events.

The Treating to New Targets trial was the first to compare a more intensely treated group with a less intensely treated group using the same agent. The design of this 10,000-patient study eliminated concerns that outcome differences were induced by dissimilar statin preparations. The mean LDL level achieved was 101 mg/dL with 10 mg atorvastatin, and 77 mg/dL with the 80 mg dose. This LDL reduction was associated with a relative risk reduction of 27% for the primary endpoint of the first major cardiovascular event.

There is an increased risk of myopathy and rhabdomyolysis in patients taking 80 mg simvastatin (Zocor), according to the Study of the Effectiveness of Additional Reductions in Cholesterol and Homocysteine (SEARCH). The US Food and Drug Administration (FDA) has subsequently restricted high-dose simvastatin to patients who have been on this dose for longer than 12 months without evidence of myopathy, and the agency has recommended that new patients should not be started on this particular dose.

To effectively achieve a greater than 50% LDL-cholesterol reduction in CAD patients utilizing currently available pharmacologic agents, the most recent treatment guidelines suggest either atorvastatin 40 to 80 mg or rosuvastatin (Crestor) 20 to 40 mg. In other patient populations that require moderate-intensity statin therapy, there are several statin choices. Because there is no currently available evidence to suggest that nonstatin lipid-altering agents effectively reduce cardiovascular mortality, these medications should not be routinely prescribed.

It is apparent from both primary and secondary prevention lipid trials that achieving lower LDL levels reduces cardiovascular event rates. Because there is no high-quality clinical evidence to support achieving specific LDL levels in patients with diagnosed CAD, high-dose statin therapy should be the mainstay of pharmacologically based therapy, if tolerated.

Although statins are the standard pharmacologic approach for primary and secondary prevention of atherosclerotic cardiovascular disease, as many as 20% of patients may be intolerant. The numbers may be even higher if medication adherence is included. For secondary prevention in patients whose cholesterol levels are not adequately achieved on a statin or other cholesterol-lowering medication, a proprotein convertase subtilisin kexin type 9 (PCSK9) inhibitor is an FDA-approved option. PCSK9 inhibitors can also be considered for those with familial hypercholesterolemia and can be prescribed with or without a statin. The FOURIER Cardiovascular Outcomes trial studied more than 27,000 patients with stable atherosclerotic cardiovascular disease and showed that evolocumab (Repatha) reduced the primary endpoint of atherosclerotic events by 15%, without significant safety differences between treatment groups. Subgroup analyses suggested that greater benefits were seen in patients with longer exposure to evolocumab, recent acute coronary syndrome, multiple myocardial infarctions, multivessel coronary artery disease, peripheral arterial disease, as well as the subgroup who achieved very low low-density lipoprotein-cholesterol levels of below 0.3 mmol/L (10 mg/dL).

Metabolic Syndrome

The combined presence of insulin resistance, hypertension, dyslipidemia, and abdominal obesity define metabolic syndrome. There is debate about whether this is a true syndrome or simply a clustering of cardiovascular risk factors in a particular individual. The key concept is that the concomitant presence of these particular cardiovascular risk factors markedly increases a patient's chances of developing diabetes mellitus and coronary atherosclerosis. The approach to treatment for this syndrome is no different from that for the individual components. Recognition of the components is key to the treatment of this disorder.

Smoking

Cigarette smoking is probably the most important of the identified modifiable cardiovascular risk factors. The incidence of CAD is two to four times higher in smokers than in nonsmokers. The pathophysiologic process that leads to atherosclerosis from smoking stems from induced platelet dysfunction, endothelial dysfunction, smooth muscle cell proliferation, and attenuated high-density lipoprotein cholesterol levels. Smoking cessation must be sought for every CAD patient.

Diet

Lifestyle changes for patients with CAD must incorporate healthy eating habits. The Mediterranean diet has been shown to positively affect cardiovascular disease, and conversely, a diet high in saturated fats has been shown to negatively influence multiple cardiac risk factors. Patients should be encouraged to incorporate high proportions of fruits and vegetables into their diet, along with olive oil and regular servings of fish coupled with a reduced amount of red meats and excess sugar.

Other Lifestyle Changes

Exercise should be encouraged in patients with stable angina, once all appropriate invasive and noninvasive tests have been completed and a stable medical regimen has been established.

Increasing a patient's aerobic capacity can lower the body's oxygen requirement for a given workload, which can lead to increased exercise tolerance and reduced anginal symptoms. Aerobic exercise can improve endothelial function and positively affect baroreflex sensitivity and heart rate variability in patients with CAD.

Endorphins released during exercise are thought to be mood enhancers, as well as effective muscle relaxants. Exercise itself improves sleep patterns. Cortisol levels are reduced with regular exercise, which may attenuate the body's sensation of stress and anxiety. For these reasons, appropriate exercise programs for patients with stable angina have far-reaching positive benefits. Exercise guidelines for CAD patients have been published and should be reviewed before patients begin aggressive secondary prevention efforts.

Major depression affects approximately 25% of people recovering from a myocardial infarction, and another 40% suffer from mild depression. In any given year, one of every three long-term acute ischemic syndrome survivors will develop depression. The Heart and Soul Study examined 1017 patients with stable CAD over a period of 4.8 years. Patients identified with depression were twice as likely to experience recurrent cardiovascular events. Physical inactivity was associated with a 44% greater rate of cardiovascular events. Patients with symptoms of depression were less likely to follow dietary, exercise, and medication recommendations.

Approach to Treatment

Medical Therapy

Medications used to treat angina pectoris and typical dosages are listed in Table 2.

Nitrates

Nitrates provide an exogenous source of nitric oxide, which serves to relax smooth muscle and inhibit platelet aggregation. Nitrates exert their antianginal effect by reducing myocardial oxygen

TABLE 2	Medications Used for the Treatment of Angina Pectoris
NAME	**DOSAGE**
β-Blockers	
Atenolol (Tenormin)	25–200 mg PO qd
Metoprolol tartrate (Lopressor)	25–200 mg bid
Metoprolol succinate (Toprol XL)	25–200 mg qd
Carvedilol (Coreg)[1]	6.25–25 mg PO bid
Carvedilol phosphate (Coreg CR)[1]	20–80 mg PO qd
Propranolol (Inderal)	80–320 mg/d, divided bid or tid
Propranolol (Inderal LA)	80–160 mg PO qd
Labetalol (Trandate, Normodyne)[1]	200–800 mg bid
Nitrates	
Isosorbide dinitrate (Isordil)	10–40 mg PO bid or tid
Isosorbide mononitrate (Imdur)	30–240 mg PO qd
Nitroglycerin (Nitrostat)	0.4 mg SL q5min
Nitroglycerin transdermal (Nitro-Dur)	0.2–0.8 mg/h 12–14 h patch
Calcium Channel Blockers	
Dihydropyridines	
Amlodipine (Norvasc)	2.5–10 mg PO qd
Felodipine (Plendil)[1]	2.5–10 mg PO qd
Nifedipine (Procardia XL)	30–90 mg PO qd
Nondihydropyridines	
Verapamil (Calan)	80–120 mg PO tid
Verapamil (Calan SR)	120–480 mg PO qd
Diltiazem (Cardizem)	360 mg/d PO, divided tid or qid
Diltiazem (Cardizem LA)	180–360 mg PO qd
Other	
Ranolazine (Ranexa)	500 mg twice daily and increase to 1000 mg twice daily as needed, based on clinical symptoms

[1]Not FDA approved for this indication.

demand through coronary and systemic vasodilation. Nitrates are strong venodilators, and in higher doses they can also induce arterial dilation. Reducing the preload through venodilation reduces myocardial oxygen demand. Coronary artery dilatation of stenotic vessels and intracoronary collaterals directly increases myocardial oxygen delivery. Through these mechanisms, nitrates have been shown to prevent recurrent episodes of angina and to increase exercise tolerance.

There are several nitrate preparations; they differ mainly in route of administration, onset of action, and effective half-life. Nitrate tolerance can occur with long-term use of any nitrate preparation and can be avoided by providing a 10- to 12-hour nitrate-free interval. Nitrates should be used with caution in patients with a diagnosis of hypertrophic obstructive cardiomyopathy.

β-Blockers

β-Blockers competitively inhibit catecholamines from binding to β-receptors. Over time, β-blocker therapy leads to an increase in β-receptor density. Because of receptor upregulation, acute β-blocker withdrawal may lead to a transient supersensitivity to catecholamines and subsequent angina or even myocardial infarction. There are three classes of β-receptors. Some β-blockers are receptor specific, and some exert an effect over all three receptors. However, at higher doses, even β-selective agents have cross-reactivity for all β-receptors. β-Blockers reduce myocardial oxygen demand through a negative inotropic effect, a chronotropic effect, and a reduction in left ventricular wall stress.

Several cardioselective β-blockers, including atenolol (Tenormin) and metoprolol (Lopressor), have been shown to be effective antianginals that are fairly well tolerated in patients with underlying bronchospastic disease. Dosing is important for β-blocker efficacy. A study comparing atenolol with placebo showed that all doses from 25 through 200 mg/day were effective in reducing angina, but only the two highest doses led to an increase in exercise tolerance. Certain β-blockers have intrinsic sympathomimetic activity, including pindolol (Visken)[1] and acebutolol (Sectral).[1] Although they may be effective in reducing angina, they should be used with caution in patients with a prior history of myocardial infarction and in those with left ventricular dysfunction, because they may not reduce heart rate or blood pressure at rest.

When β-blockers are used to treat angina, a goal resting heart rate should be between 55 and 60 beats/min. Caution should be used in patients with resting bradycardia and in those with known reactive airway disease. Atenolol is renally excreted and should be used with caution in the elderly and in those with known renal dysfunction.

Calcium Channel Blockers

Calcium channel blockers are classified as either dihydropyridines or nondihydropyridines. The former group includes amlodipine (Norvasc), felodipine (Plendil)[1], nifedipine (Procardia), and nicardipine (Cardene); the latter includes diltiazem (Cardizem) and verapamil (Calan). There are differences among the two subclasses in terms of chronotropic, dromotropic, and inotropic effects.

Calcium channel blockers positively alter myocardial oxygen supply and demand, mainly through direct arterial vasodilatation. The nondihydropyridines also exhibit negative chronotropic and inotropic effects, thus further lowering myocardial oxygen demands.

One of the early quick-release preparations of a dihydropyridine calcium channel blocker, nifedipine, was reported to potentially induce myocardial infarction when used to treat angina. This was most likely due to a rapid drop in afterload leading to reflex adrenergic activation. Sustained-release preparations of nifedipine (Procardia XL), as well as the other dihydropyridines, have been proven safe and effective in patients with cardiovascular disease. Although amlodipine and felodipine are tolerated in patients with left ventricular systolic dysfunction, other calcium channel blockers should be avoided in this patient subset.

Ranolazine (Ranexa)

Ranolazine (Ranexa) is a new and unique antianginal drug approved for the treatment of stable angina. It is a sustained-release preparation that has been approved for patients who remain symptomatic while on standard angina pharmacotherapy. Its mechanism of action may be through reduction of fatty acid oxidation or effects on sodium shifts and intracellular calcium levels. QT prolongation has been reported, but a significant increase in arrhythmias has not been seen. Side effects include dizziness, constipation, and nausea. Dosing is 500 or 1000 mg twice daily, and the major route of metabolism is the cytochrome P 450 system. Ranolazine should be used cautiously in patients who are taking other pharmacologic agents that have the potential to prolong the QT interval, and in patients with liver cirrhosis.

Ivabradine (Corlanor)[1]

Heart rate has a profound effect on diastolic perfusion time and subsequent myocardial oxygen supply. Ninety percent of coronary blood flow occurs in diastole. Therefore, an elevated heart rate may result in myocardial ischemia and angina. Ivabradine (Corlanor) selectively reduces heart rate without affecting inotropic function or coronary vasomotor tone. Ivabradine does not affect central aortic pressure or ventricular repolarization.

Ivabradine is a selective and specific inhibitor of the cardiac pacemaker current (If) that controls the spontaneous diastolic depolarization in the sinus node and regulates heart rate. It is metabolized by both the liver and the gut by oxidation through the cytochrome P450 3A4 (CYP3A4). Although ivabradine has a low affinity for CYP3A4, potent inhibitors and inducers of CYP3A4 may affect its plasma levels. Although nondihydropyridine calcium channel blockers should not be co-administered, other first-line coronary artery disease medications such as β-blockers, renin-angiotensin-aldosterone system inhibitors, aspirin, and HMG-CoA reductase inhibitors can be safely combined. Starting dosage is 5 mg twice daily in patients <75 years old, and 2.5 mg twice daily for patients ≥75 years old. No dosage adjustments are necessary in patients with renal impairment or creatinine clearance >15 mL/min. In patients with moderate hepatic impairment, caution is advised, and ivabradine is contraindicated in patients with severe liver impairment. The maintenance dose is ≤7.5 mg twice daily, with up titration possible after 4 weeks if initial dose is well tolerated, symptoms persist, and heart rate is >60 bpm. Ivabradine is contraindicated in patients with a pre-treatment resting heart rate <70 bpm.

Heart rate reduction triggered by ivabradine appears to be greatest in those patients with highest pre-treatment baseline heart rates. Borer et al. showed that ivabradine improved exercise stress testing variables in a dose-dependent fashion. In this study, ivabradine improved time to 1 mm ST-segment depression as compared to placebo ($P = .016$). In a pooled analysis of 5 randomized, double blind, parallel-group studies of patients with stable angina, ivabradine ≥5 mg/day (maximum dose 7.5 mg/day) resulted in a 14.5% heart rate reduction, a −59.4% change in the number of angina attacks per week, and a −53.7% change in the consumption of nitrates.

There is mounting clinical evidence that ivabradine improves angina symptoms and quality of life (QOL) regardless of age, gender, and pre-treatment angina class. It also appears to improve prognosis and reduce hospitalizations in angina patients with left ventricular systolic dysfunction.

Medication Combinations

Many patients with chronic stable angina require more than one antianginal medication to control their symptoms. Current guidelines recommend β-blockers or calcium channel blockers as initial

---

[1]Not FDA approved for this indication.

[1]Not FDA approved for this indication.

therapy unless otherwise contraindicated, with the addition of nitrates as symptoms dictate. Further medications may be added and individualized to each patient based on their degree of angina and overall clinical response.

However, it is important to recognize medication side effects when deciding which agents to combine. β-Blockers block the atrioventricular (AV) node and exert a portion of their effectiveness through this mechanism. The nondihydropyridine calcium channel blockers also have AV-nodal blocking properties and therefore should be used cautiously with β-blockers, especially in patients with preexisting conduction system disease. The dihydropyridine agents do not have AV-nodal blocking effects and may be a safer choice when used in combination with β-blockers. Nitrates do not have a side-effect profile that raises concerns when they are used with β-blockers or with calcium channel blockers.

Antiplatelet Therapy

The common etiology leading to an acute ischemic syndrome is a platelet-rich clot occurring at the site of a significant coronary artery stenosis, often after a plaque rupture. Antiplatelet medications have been shown to consistently decrease morbidity and mortality in a wide array of cardiovascular disease patients. A meta-analysis suggested that for patients with stable cardiovascular disease, low-dose aspirin therapy (50 to 100 mg daily) is as effective as higher doses (>300 mg). In this patient population, aspirin therapy resulted in a 26% reduction in myocardial infarction; the number of patients needed to treat to prevent a myocardial infarction was 83.

The Antiplatelet Trialists' Collaboration study demonstrated a reduction in myocardial infarction, stroke, and death in high-risk cardiovascular patients treated with antiplatelet therapy. Consensus guidelines recommend indefinite oral aspirin for the secondary prevention of cardiovascular events in all angina patients.

Clopidogrel (Plavix)[1] is an effective alternative to aspirin for the treatment of stable cardiovascular disease in those patients with a true aspirin allergy. However, there are no compelling data to indicate that clopidogrel (or newer agents, such as prasugrel [Effient][1] and ticagrelor [Brilinta][1]) are superior to aspirin in this particular patient population. In patients with unstable angina, dual antiplatelet therapy with aspirin and clopidogrel is recommended.

Invasive Assessment

The decision to pursue an invasive treatment approach differs significantly in patients with chronic stable angina and in those with acute coronary syndromes. Within both groups, accurate risk stratification is the key consideration in choosing who will benefit from coronary angiography and subsequent percutaneous coronary intervention. An invasive strategy in unstable angina patients has been shown to reduce recurrent acute coronary syndrome events consistently in many trials. A routine invasive strategy is recommended for patients with non-ST-segment acute ischemic syndromes who have refractory ischemia, elevated cardiac biomarkers suggesting myocardial necrosis, or new ST-segment depression on ECG monitoring.

In patients with unstable angina, there are significant gender differences in outcomes related to the use of invasive therapy. Both men and women with elevated biomarkers from myocardial necrosis have comparable reductions in rates of death, myocardial infarction, and rehospitalization with invasive treatment strategies. However, in the absence of positive biomarkers, women appear to have potentially negative outcomes with an invasive approach. The current American College of Cardiology and American Heart Association guidelines recommend a conservative approach in such women.

Patients diagnosed with stable angina comprise a vast array of clinical presentations. The two most heated debates in this arena concern the initial choice of medical therapy versus an invasive approach, and when to cross over from a medical treatment plan to an invasive one. The Atorvastatin Versus Revascularization Treatment (AVERT) trial studied the effects of intensive lipid-lowering therapy on ischemic events in a relatively low-risk population of patients with single- or two-vessel disease compared with percutaneous transluminal coronary angioplasty. AVERT randomized 341 patients to medical therapy plus atorvastatin 80 mg or to angioplasty followed by usual medical care (which included the option of statin therapy at the choice of the treating physician). The medical treatment group experienced a 36% reduction in the composite endpoint of ischemic events compared with the angioplasty group. This difference was due primarily to repeated angioplasty, coronary artery bypass grafting, or hospitalization for worsening angina. The primary outcome of this trial from a practical standpoint was that high-dose statin therapy was safe in this patient population and did not increase cardiovascular events, compared with an angioplasty-based treatment plan.

One of the keys in interpreting the available data is recognizing that by the time many of these trials are published, the percutaneous treatment choices are often outdated. Early trials used mainly balloon angioplasty; later trials used early-generation bare metal stents. Equally as important is to determine what the background medical treatment plans were for any particular trial on this subject. Often, lipid therapy was not aggressive, hypertension management was not confirmed to be adequate, and intravenous glycoprotein IIb/IIIa antagonists were either not available or not used as a standard protocol when indicated.

The Clinical Outcomes Utilizing Revascularization and Aggressive Drug Evaluation (COURAGE) trial was designed to address the potential advantages of current medical therapy over a percutaneous approach in patients with demonstrable ischemia but stable CAD. Of the 35,000 patients screened, only 2287 met the study inclusion criteria. All participants of the COURAGE trial underwent a coronary angiography, and patients with high-risk anatomic findings such as severe left main coronary artery stenosis were excluded. The biggest difference in this trial compared with previous studies was that strict guideline-based medical therapy was followed in both groups. In the entire cohort, 85% of subjects were taking a β-blocker, 93% were taking a statin, and 85% were taking aspirin. The final interpretation of the COURAGE trial results was not that medical therapy is superior for all patients with CAD, but that in selected cohorts, aggressive medical therapy is an appropriate first step in the treatment of ischemic heart disease.

It is well accepted that a coronary artery lesion ≥70% is clinically significant. Historically, the interventional cardiologist has relied on visually estimating this value during coronary angiography to determine when a percutaneous intervention is appropriate. However, physiology-guided revascularization has become an established practice in the management of patients with coronary artery disease. Both instantaneous wave free ration (iFR) and fractional flow reserve (FFR) are well-studied techniques that allow assessment of the pressure differences across a coronary artery stenosis.

iFR isolates a specific period in diastole where pressure and flow are linearly related, which is referred to as the wave-free period. During this time, competing forces (waves) that affect period diverge; an iFR value below 0.9 suggests flow restriction (normal value is 1.0). iFR is measured at rest, without the need for pharmacologic vasodilators or stressors.

FFR utilizes a guidewire that is passed through a coronary lesion and allows for measurement of both blood flow and pressure. After direct administration of the hyperemic agent adenosine (Adenocard)[1], the pressure difference across a stenosis is determined. An FFR of ≤0.80 is considered clinically significant.

Physiologic assessment of obstructive coronary artery disease adds clarity to the visual angiogram interpretation, thereby leading to more appropriate coronary interventions.

The ORBITA trial was a 200-patient placebo-controlled randomized trial assessing the efficacy of percutaneous coronary

---

[1] Not FDA approved for this indication.

[1] Not FDA approved for this indication.

intervention (PCI) compared with a placebo sham procedure for the relief of angina in patients with severe (>70%) single-vessel coronary artery disease. Patients were randomized in a 1:1 fashion, and all patients had assessment of their coronary lesion by both FFR and iFR. All patients were assessed by cardiopulmonary exercise testing, symptom questionnaires, and dobutamine stress echocardiography before and six weeks after the procedure.

Compared with placebo, PCI reduced ischemia as assessed by stress echocardiography. However, there was no difference in the primary endpoint of exercise time between the two arms, or statistically significant differences between the two groups with respect to angina frequency. Changes in the Duke treadmill score and exercise time were both numerically higher in the PCI arm, which poses the question of small sample size effects on these outcomes.

Novel Therapies
External Counterpulsation
External counterpulsation is a noninvasive method of increasing coronary blood flow through diastolic augmentation. Large blood pressure cuffs are placed on both legs and thighs and are inflated to a pressure of 300 mm Hg in early diastole (triggered by the patient's ECG), promoting venous return to the heart. The mechanism is unclear but may be related to enhanced endothelial function, improved myocardial perfusion, and possibly placebo effect. Several small studies have suggested a clinical reduction in angina episodes, but no positive mortality benefit has yet been published. A meta-analysis that included 13 observational studies and followed 949 patients with stable angina. Using the CCS classification scheme, there was at least a one-class improvement in 86% of the study population. Contraindications to this treatment include certain aortic valvular diseases, aortic aneurysm, and peripheral vascular disease.

Spinal Cord Stimulation
For patients whose angina is refractory to medical therapy and who are not candidates for revascularization, spinal cord stimulation may be considered. Little intermediate or long-term data are available, but many short-term studies suggest reduced angina episodes. Placement of the device and subsequent stimulation at the C7-T1 level suggests that the mechanism of action is reduced pain sensation.

Acupuncture
Acupuncture has been shown to be of benefit for the relief of both acute and chronic pain in various medical conditions. With respect to patients with documented CAD and symptomatic angina, there are only limited data currently available to recommend this modality.

A recently published randomized trial of treating chronic stable angina patients with acupuncture as an adjunct to standard medical therapy was undertaken in China. It was a small study of 398 relatively healthy angina patients. Those with prior myocardial infarction or a history of congestive heart failure were excluded. Patients were randomized to the following groups; disease-affected meridian (DAM), nonaffected meridian (NAM), sham acupuncture group, and a wait-list group. Treatment was 3 times per week for 4 weeks; each session was for 30 minutes. The greatest reduction of angina episodes occurred in the DAM group as compared to each of the other 3 groups.

This is the largest published clinical trial showing evidence that adding acupuncture to goal-directed medical therapy reduces angina frequency. There were some study limitations that are worth mentioning that may soften the results. Namely, the operators were not blinded to their treatment plans, angina episodes were reduced in the sham and wait-list groups (suggesting a strong placebo-associated effect), and the study population was small.

Other Causes of Angina
Syndrome X
The cardiac syndrome X refers to patients who have normal or near-normal epicardial coronary arteries and episodic chest pain. This disorder is much more common in women and is often seen in patients younger than 50 years of age. The chest pain episodes may last longer than 30 minutes and may have a variable response to sublingual nitrates. Patients with syndrome X often describe typical stress-induced angina. Risk factors include hypertension, diabetes, and hyperlipidemia. Female patients are typically postmenopausal and frequently have stress-induced symptoms and ischemia on stress imaging. They often respond to standard angina medications and typically have a better prognosis than patients with significant epicardial plaque.

Vasospastic or Prinzmetal Angina
The classic definition of Prinzmetal angina is chest pain with documented ST-segment elevation during symptoms or during exercise in the face of angiographically normal or near-normal coronary arteries. Over the years, the definition has expanded to include patients who have classic angina symptoms commonly relieved with nitrates or calcium channel blockers and minimal or no CAD. It has been shown that patients with nonobstructive CAD may be prone to focal artery spasm at the stenosis site; therefore, the previous requirement of normal coronary arteries is not an absolute necessity. Other disease states (e.g., Raynaud phenomenon) can increase a patient's development of coronary artery spasm, as can illicit drug usage (e.g., cocaine). Vasospasm is more common in active smokers. β-Blockers should be used cautiously in these patients because they may exacerbate coronary spasm. Patients with angiographically documented intramyocardial bridging may be prone to focal coronary spasm and subsequent angina pectoris.

Newer Imaging Techniques
Calcium Scoring
Coronary artery calcium scoring is a well-studied imaging modality used to assess a patient's pretest probability of CAD. With respect to evaluation for angina, one must remember that electron-beam computed tomographic (CT) scanning does not offer physiologic data and therefore does not allow determination of myocardial ischemia. This study is most useful in the workup of a low-risk patient with an atypical chest pain syndrome. If such a patient has an elevated calcium score, other studies may be reasonable and further assessment of the patient's cholesterol values should be performed.

Computed Tomographic Coronary Angiography
CT coronary angiography is a noninvasive way to image the coronary arteries. Similar to electron-beam CT, it does not provide physiologic data regarding coronary artery perfusion, but it does provide anatomic information such as the presence and percentage of coronary artery stenosis. Although selected patients with stable or unstable angina may be considered candidates for CT angiography, its main utility is to evaluate patients for chest pain who are otherwise at low risk and have a low pretest probability. Because of the volume of intravenous contrast required by CT angiography, the risk of contrast nephropathy must be considered when contemplating this study.

Summary
The approach to the patient with angina should be based on a global assessment and intensive treatment of all identified cardiovascular risk factors. It is recommended that all patients receive the appropriate dose of statin and antiplatelet therapy. Noninvasive testing is helpful for an initial diagnosis and to guide the decision for a more invasive approach. Familiarity and adherence to current treatment guidelines is of paramount importance. There are important gender differences that should not be overlooked in the clinical presentation of angina and in the approach to optimal therapy.

References
Allan BS, Krumholz HM, SM reviewing The SPRINT Research Group: N Engl J Med 2015 Nov 9 Chobanian AV, N Engl J Med, 2015 Nov 9.
Anderson JL, Adams CD, Antman EM, et al: ACC/AHA 2007 guidelines for the management of patients with unstable angina/non-ST-elevation myocardial infarction: A report of the American College of Cardiology/American Heart Association Task Force on Practice Guidelines, J Am Coll Cardiol 5067:e1–e157, 2007.

Antithrombotic Trialists Collaboration: Collaborative meta-analysis of randomized trials of antiplatelet therapy for prevention of death, myocardial infarction, and stroke in high risk patients, *BMJ* 324:71–86, 2002.

Berger J, Brown D, Becker R, et al: Low-dose aspirin in patients with stable cardiovascular disease: A meta-analysis, *Am J Med* 121:43–49, 2008.

Blood Pressure Lowering Treatment Trialists Collaboration: Effects of different blood pressure lowering regimens on major cardiovascular events: Results of prospectively-designed overviews of randomized trials, *Lancet* 362:1527–1545, 2003.

Boden WE, O'Rourke RA, Teo KK, et al: Optimal medical therapy with or without PCI for stable coronary disease, *N Engl J Med* 35:1503–1516, 2007.

Borer JS, Fox K, Jaillon P, et al: Antianginal and antischemic effects of Ivrabadine, a novel I(f) inhibitor, in stable angina:a randomized, double-blind, multicentered, placebo-controlled trial, *Circulation* 107:817–823, 2003.

Cholesterol Treatment Trialists' Collaborators: Efficacy and safety of cholesterol-lowering treatment: Prospective meta-analysis of data from 90,056 participants in 14 trials of statins, *Lancet* 366:1267–1278, 2005.

De Bruyne B, Fearon WF, Pijls NH, et al: Fractional flow reserve-guided PCI for stable coronary artery disease, *N Engl J Med* 371:1208–1217, 2014.

Fihn SD, Gardin JM, Abrams J, et al: 2012 ACCF/AHA/ACP/AATS/PCNA/SCAI/STS guideline for the diagnosis and management of patients with stable ischemic heart disease: A report of the American College of Cardiology Foundation/American Heart Association Task Force on Practice Guidelines, and the American College of Physicians, American Association for Thoracic Surgery, Preventive Cardiovascular Nurses Association, Society for Cardiovascular Angiography and Interventions, and Society of Thoracic Surgeons, *J Am Coll Cardiol* 60:e44–e164, 2012.

Gibbons RJ, Abrams J, Chatterjee K, et al: ACC/AHA 2007 guideline update for the management of patients with chronic stable angina: A report of the American College of Cardiology/American Heart Association Task Force on Practice Guidelines (Committee to Update the 2002 Guidelines for the Management of Patients with Chronic Stable Angina) Reston, VA, American College of Cardiology, American Heart Association Available at: www.acc.org/qualityandscience/cl inical/guidelines/stable/stable_clean.pdf (accessed August 20, 2014).

Grundy SM, Cleeman JI, Merz NB, et al: Implications of recent clinical trials for the National Cholesterol Education Program Adult Treatment Panel III guidelines, *Circulation* 110:227–239, 2004.

Heart Outcomes Prevention Evaluation Study Investigators: Effects of an angiotensin-converting-enzyme inhibitor, ramipril, on cardiovascular events in high-risk patients, *N Engl J Med* 342:145–153, 2000.

James PA, Oparil S, Carter BL, et al: 2014 evidence-based guideline for the management of high blood pressure in adults: Report from the panel members appointed to the eighth Joint National Committee (JNC 8), *JAMA* 311:507–520, 2014.

Mehta SR, Cannon CP, Fox KA, et al: Routine vs selective invasive strategies in patients with acute coronary syndromes: A collaborative meta-analysis of randomized trials, *JAMA* 293:2908–2917, 2005.

Messerli FH, Mancia G, Conti CR, et al: Dogma disrupted: Can aggressively lowering blood pressure in hypertensive patients with coronary artery disease be dangerous? *Ann Intern Med* 144:884–893, 2006.

Montalescot G, Sechtem U, Achenbach S, et al: Editor's choice: 2013 ESC guidelines on the management of stable coronary artery disease: The Task Force on the management of stable coronary artery disease of the European Society of Cardiology, *Eur Heart J* 34:2949–3003, 2013.

Petraco R, Al-Lamee R, Gotberg M, et al: Real-time use of instantaneous wave-free ratio: results of the ADVISE in-practice: an international, multicenter evaluation of instantaneous wave-free ratio in clinical practice, *Am Heart J* 168:739–748, 2014.

Ray K, Cannon C: Optimal goal for statin therapy use in coronary artery disease, *Curr Opin Cardiol* 20:525–529, 2005.

Sabatine MS, Giugliano RP, Keech AC, et al: Evolocumab and clinical outcomes in patients with cardiovascular disease, *N Engl J Med* 376:1713–1722, 2017.

SEARCH Collaborative Group: Intensive lowering of LDL cholesterol with 80mg versus 20mg simvastatin daily in 12,064 survivors of myocardial infarction: A double-blind randomised trial, *Lancet* 376:1658–1669, 2010.

Stone G, Teirstein P, Rubenstein R, et al: A prospective, multicenter, randomized trial of percutaneous transmyocardial laser revascularization in patients with nonrecanalizable chronic total occlusions, *J Am Coll Cardiol* 39:1581–1587, 2002.

Stone NJ, Robinson J, Lichtenstein AH, et al: 2013 ACC/AHA guideline on the treatment of blood cholesterol to reduce atherosclerotic cardiovascular risk in adults: A report of the American College of Cardiology/American Heart Association Task Force on Practice Guidelines, Circulation .

Tendera M, Borer JS, Tardif JC: Efficacy of I(f) inhibition with Ivabradine in different subpopulations with stable angina pectoris, *Cardiology* 114:116–125, 2009.

Weber MA, Schiffrin EL, White WB, et al: Clinical practice guidelines for the management of hypertension in the community, *J Clin Hypertens* 16:14–26, 2014.

Wenger NK: *Cardiac Rehabilitation: A Guide to Practice in the 21st Century*, New York, 1999, Marcel Dekker.

Whooley MA, Jonge P, Vittinghoff E, et al: Depressive symptoms, health behaviors, and risk of cardiovascular events in patients with coronary heart disease, *JAMA* 300:2379–2388, 2008.

Acupuncture as Adjunctive Therapy for Chronic Stable Angina: A Randomized Clinical Trial.

Zhao L, Li D, Zheng H, et al: *JAMA Intern Med*, 2019 Jul 29.

2017 ACC/AHA/AAPA/ABC/ACPM/AGS/APhA/ASH/ASPC/NMA/PCNA Guideline for the Prevention, Detection, Evaluation, and Management of High Blood Pressure in Adults: A Report of the American College of Cardiology/American Heart Association Task Force on Clinical Practice Guidelines

AORTIC DISEASE: ANEURYSM AND DISSECTION

Method of
David G. Neschis, MD

CURRENT DIAGNOSIS

- Because the majority of patients with abdominal aortic aneurysms are asymptomatic, the majority of abdominal aortic aneurysms are detected on imaging studies performed for other indications.
- Patients older than 50 years who present with abdominal or back pain of unclear etiology should be considered for evaluation of possible abdominal aortic aneurysm.
- Asymptomatic men older than 65 years who have ever smoked are eligible for abdominal aortic aneurysm screening.
- All patients older than 60 years who have a strong family history of abdominal aortic aneurysms should be considered for screening.
- Patients presenting with sudden onset of chest or back pain without clear etiology should be evaluated for dissection.
- Dissection can mimic numerous other conditions.

CURRENT THERAPY

Indications for Repair of Aneurysm
- Fusiform abdominal aortic aneurysms greater than 5.5cm in maximum diameter
- Most saccular aneurysms and pseudoaneurysms
- Thoracic and thoracoabdominal aortic aneurysms of greater than 6cm in maximal diameter
- Aneurysms that are symptomatic or are rapidly enlarging

Indications for Repair of Aortic Dissection
- Dissections involving the ascending aorta
- Dissections involving only the descending aorta are usually managed medically unless complicated by the following: unrelenting pain, end organ ischemia, or significant aneurysmal degeneration to greater than 6cm in maximal diameter

Abdominal Aortic Aneurysms

Epidemiology

A ruptured abdominal aortic aneurysm is a devastating event leading to approximately 15,000 deaths per year, and it is the 13th leading cause of death in the United States. It is the 10th leading cause of death in men. Once rupture occurs, there is an 85% chance of death overall and approximately 50% mortality in the patients who make it to the hospital alive. Clearly, the goal is to identify this life-threatening lesion and repair prior to rupture. Abdominal aortic aneurysms are approximately four times more prevalent in men than in women. The overall incidence in persons older than 60 years is approximately 3% to 4%, with incidence as high as 10% to 12% in an elderly hypertensive population.

Risk Factors

Men are approximately 4 times more likely than women to develop an abdominal aortic aneurysm. Clearly, older persons, particularly those older than 60 years, are at higher risk. Tobacco use is probably the strongest preventable risk factor, with tobacco users being approximately eight times more likely to be affected than nonsmokers. Hypertension is present in approximately 40% of patients with abdominal aortic aneurysms. Family history also plays a significant role. In fact, men who have first-degree female relatives who had aneurysms are approximately 18 times more likely than the general population to develop an abdominal aortic aneurysm. There is also a strong correlation between abdominal aortic aneurysms and other peripheral artery aneurysms. Patients with bilateral popliteal artery aneurysms have an approximately 50% to 60% risk of having an abdominal aortic aneurysm.

Pathophysiology

An aneurysm is a dilatation of a blood vessel that could occur in any blood vessel in the body, even in the veins. Most commonly it is defined as a dilatation of approximately 1.5 to 2 times at that diameter of the adjacent normal vessel.

The definition of a pseudoaneurysm is often misunderstood. The attempt to describe a pseudoaneurysm in terms of the number of layers of the artery wall involved does nothing to help resolve this confusion. A pseudoaneurysm is a walled-off defect in the artery wall. A circular shell of adventitial and surrounding connective tissue contains the blood, preventing free hemorrhage. However, there remains continued flow out and back into the arterial lumen, resulting in a classic to-and-fro pattern on duplex ultrasound. The most common cause of a pseudoaneurysm is iatrogenic, from needle puncture, but it also can be caused by trauma or focal rupture of the artery at the site of an atherosclerotic ulcer.

The etiology of true aneurysms is not clear, although in the past these have been attributed to atherosclerosis. However, it is well known that the majority of patients with abdominal aortic aneurysms do not have associated significant occlusive disease. Biochemical studies have demonstrated decreased quantities of elastin and collagen in the walls of aneurysmal aortas. It is believed that a family of enzymes known as matrix metalloproteinase (MMP), particularly those that have collagenase and elastase activity, are likely involved in development of arterial aneurysms. The propensity for growth and rupture is based on Laplace's law, $T = PR$, where T represents wall tension (or in other words the propensity to rupture), P is the transmitted pressure, and R is the radius. This explains why patients with hypertension and those with larger aneurysms are at higher risk for aortic rupture.

Prevention

Currently the most effective means to prevent aneurysm rupture is early detection and elective repair. Avoidance of smoking and aggressive control of blood pressure would likely be helpful in preventing aneurysmal development and growth. Patients with known abdominal aortic aneurysms that are relatively small and at low risk for rupture are generally serially followed with imaging studies over time. These patients are advised to avoid straining (e.g., heavy lifting), avoid smoking, and keep their blood pressure well controlled.

Investigation is ongoing in efforts to develop a medication that may be helpful in slowing the growth of abdominal aortic aneurysms. It has been known since 1985 that tetracycline antibiotics have activity against MMPs. There had been several animal studies and at least one small human study suggesting that doxycycline (Vibramycin)[1] may be effective at slowing the growth of abdominal aortic aneurysms. Currently, larger human studies are ongoing. At this point, there are no formal recommendations regarding the use of doxycycline for the purpose of slowing aneurysmal growth.

Clinical Manifestations

Approximately 75% of abdominal aortic aneurysms are asymptomatic and discovered incidentally. Unfortunately, physical examination is an unreliable method for detecting aneurysms or determining aneurysm size. In heavier patients it may be simply impossible to adequately palpate the aorta. The majority of aneurysms are incidental findings identified on imaging studies performed for other reasons. Occasionally, an aneurysm is first detected upon operation for another condition.

Unfortunately, when an aneurysm becomes symptomatic, this is usually a sign of impending rupture. Symptoms related to abdominal aortic aneurysms can include abdominal or back pain. The classic triad of findings in the setting of abdominal aortic aneurysm rupture includes abdominal pain, hypotension, and a pulsatile abdominal mass. This triad, however, occurs in only approximately 20% of the patients. Often a high index of suspicion needs to be maintained.

The episode of hypotension associated with aneurysm rupture may be manifested as an episode of syncope or near-syncope before the patient arrives at the hospital. It is quite possible for the patient to have a contained rupture of the abdominal aorta and appear quite stable with a normal blood pressure in the emergency department. Although uncommon, a primary fistula between the aneurysm and gastrointestinal tract can occur and manifest as gastrointestinal bleeding.

Diagnosis

Several imaging modalities are available that can accurately diagnose and measure abdominal aortic aneurysms. Real-time B-mode ultrasound scanning has the advantage of being almost universally available, relatively inexpensive, and essentially risk free. The major disadvantage, however, is that it is technician dependent. Computed tomography (CT) scans can provide a very accurate representation of the aorta in a very short study time (Figures 1 and 2). The use of iodinated contrast is not necessary to obtain a gross size

Figure 1 Large abdominal aortic aneurysm. Notice how the majority of this aneurysm is filled with laminated thrombus. The flow lumen is only mildly dilated, and this aneurysm could be missed on angiography alone.

Figure 2 Classic image of a ruptured abdominal aortic aneurysm, which in this case can be seen even without the use of intravascular contrast. Note the lack of symmetry and obliteration of tissue planes in the retroperitoneum on the left.

measurement of the aorta. The contrast, however, helps delineate the flow lumen more clearly, and it is quite valuable in planning repair. Disadvantages include the use of ionizing radiation and the use of iodinated contrast material. MRI is also accurate in determining the size of the aneurysm; however, study times are longer, equipment is less widely available, and the expense is considerable. Angiography, while excellent for evaluating the status of important aortic branches and for evaluating occlusive disease, is not an accurate study for the purpose of determining maximal diameter of the aneurysm. Often aneurysms are filled with laminated thrombus, and the flow lumen, which was seen on aortography, is not representative of the true aneurysm size.

Treatment

The decision on when to intervene in an abdominal aortic aneurysm is based on a careful analysis of the patient's risk for rupture versus the risk of operative repair. Historically, open repair can be performed with less than 5% in-hospital mortality. Based on historical studies it was estimated that the risk of rupture for an approximately 5-cm aneurysm was about 1% per year, which increased dramatically to 6.6% for aneurysms between 6 and 7 cm. It has been fairly well established for years that aneurysms larger than 5.5 cm are generally recommended for repair and those less than 4 cm are generally observed over time. There remains a gray area for moderate aneurysms in the 4- to 5.5-cm category.

Two large prospective randomized trials were developed to answer this question. These include the United Kingdom Small Aneurysm Trial and the Department of Veterans Affairs Aneurysm Detection and Management (ADAM) trial. Both these studies randomized patients with moderately sized aneurysms to observation versus open repair. Results of both trials were fairly similar. The rupture rate for aneurysms under observation was 0.5% to 1% per year, and neither trial showed a difference in long-term survival. Both studies concluded that it was relatively safe to observe patients with aneurysms less than 5.5 cm in diameter, particularly in men who would be compliant with the follow-up regimen. The diameter of the aneurysm, however, should not be the only data point used for a decision on whether to repair.

Women seem to have a higher rupture rate for a particular aneurysm diameter than men, perhaps because they are starting with smaller aortas to begin with. Patients with COPD may be at higher risk for rupture as well. Saccular or eccentric-shaped aneurysms may also have a higher propensity to rupture and should not be subject to diameter recommendations for fusiform aneurysms (Figures 3 and 4). Additionally, rapidly growing aneurysms—growing at a rate faster than approximately 0.5 cm per year—should be considered for repair.

Once it has been determined that repair is indicated, a number of options are available. Traditional open repair involves a relatively large abdominal incision, cross clamping of the aorta, and replacement of the aneurysmal segment with a graft of polyethylene terephthalate (Dacron) or polytetrafluoroethylene (PTFE; Teflon). Often the iliac arteries are involved, and in these cases a bifurcated graft is placed. Open repair is quite durable and very effective at preventing aneurysm-related deaths. Long-term complications are rare, and patients following open repair generally enjoy 95% freedom from issues related to the repair over the course of their lifetime. Disadvantages, however, include the large incision and an approximate 1-week hospital stay. Recovery to a relatively normal level of function occasionally takes months. In the past, many patients were deemed too old or frail to be expected to undergo open surgery.

Endograft repair has revolutionized the practice of vascular surgery. Using small incisions placed at the groin and performing the procedure under fluoroscopic guidance, devices can now be advanced into the aorta from the femoral artery. Using angiography as a guide, the graft typically is deployed below the renal arteries and effectively excludes the aneurysm from the circulation. Advantages include small incisions and very short hospital stays. Patients are typically discharged on the first or second day after aneurysm repair. Recovery to normal activity is also quite rapid, taking approximately 1 to 2 weeks. Use of this modality has allowed treatment of older and frailer patients who previously were denied treatment due to concerns of operative risk.

Endograft repair, however, is clearly not without its disadvantages. Currently, the durability of endograft repair is unknown,

Figure 3 Axial CT slice and reconstructed images of a saccular abdominal aortic aneurysm. This lesion could also be described as a pseudoaneurysm. For these, treatment is recommended because it is thought that the risk of rupture is higher than for a similarly sized fusiform abdominal aortic aneurysm.

Figure 4 Angiogram of patient in Figure 3, demonstrating aneurysm before and after deployment of an endograft, which successfully excluded the lesion from the circulation.

AT ABD AORTA

ABD AORTA/LAT

and these patients are subject to frequent serial imaging. Also, there is a higher incidence of graft-related complications, which can occur in up to 35% of patients. These include the development of leaks of blood into the aneurysm sac outside the graft device, issues related to graft failure and migration, and graft limb thrombosis. These grafts are also quite expensive.

Two major prospective randomized trials studying traditional open versus endograft repair are often cited. These include the United Kingdom–based EVAR-1 trial (first Endovascular Aneurysm Repair trail) and the Dutch-based DREAM trial (Diabetes REduction Assessment with ramipril and rosiglitazone Medication trial). Both studies randomized patients who were believed to be good risks for open repair to endograft versus traditional open repair. The results of both of these studies were relatively similar in that both studies demonstrated a clear early survival benefit for patients in the endograft group. However, this came at a cost of an increased incidence of graft-related complications in the endograft group and a higher cost for the endograft group. Additionally, at 2 to 4 years, there was no clear difference in long-term survival in either group.

Ultimately, the decision about whether to proceed with open or endograft repair is a decision between surgeon and patient based on the patient's aortic anatomy, overall health, and the patient's and physician's preference. It would appear, however, that older and frail patients with good anatomy should be strongly considered for endograft repair.

Monitoring

Patients with abdominal aortic aneurysms should be evaluated for the presence of femoral and popliteal aneurysms (particularly in men) and for thoracic aortic aneurysms. After open repair, a follow-up CT scan with contrast should be considered approximately 5 years out to evaluate for the integrity of the graft (i.e., pseudoaneurysms), as well as development of new aneurysms. Patients who have undergone endograft repair require more-intensive monitoring. Typical regimens include a contrast-enhanced CT scan approximately 2 weeks after repair, then 6 months after repair, and then based on the perceived stability of the graft, approximately yearly thereafter. Some centers have used duplex ultrasonography for evaluating patients after endograft repair in efforts to reduce the amount of ionizing radiation the patients receive. However, it should be remembered that duplex ultrasound is highly technician dependent, and follow-up of patients with endograft repairs using only duplex ultrasound should be performed in experienced centers.

Thoracic Aortic Aneurysms

Thoracic aortic aneurysms (TAAs) are limited to the chest cavity. Although they are less common than infrarenal abdominal aortic aneurysms, they share similar risk factors. The male-to-female ratio incidence of the TAA is approximately 1:1.

In the past, the threshold for repair was at a diameter greater than 6 cm. This threshold was chosen due to the higher operative risks associated with repair of the thoracic aorta. Now with the availability of endograft, patients with good anatomy are generally recommended for repair at a diameter similar to those for the infrarenal aorta.

Open repair involves performing a thoracotomy and cross-clamping the aorta. Repair in this location is often performed with the addition of extracorporeal bypass to maintain perfusion to the viscera and spinal cord drain performance of the repair. Although the risk of paraplegia in the treatment of infrarenal aortic is exceedingly low, the risk of paraplegia from a repair of an isolated TAA is approximately 6%. Endograft devices for repair of TAA are now widely available and have reduced the incidence of paraplegia to approximately 3%.

Thoracoabdominal Aortic Aneurysms

By definition, thoracoabdominal aortic aneurysms require entrance to both the thoracic and abdominal cavity to perform repair. These lesions are usually true aneurysms of the aorta and should not be confused with dissection. Repair of thoracoabdominal aortic aneurysms is quite complex and carries risks of death and paraplegia as high as 20% in some settings. These procedures are generally performed at larger institutions with considerable experience with this condition. Unfortunately, endograft devices for the repair of thoracoabdominal aortic aneurysms are limited to a handful of centers in the United States.

Thoracic Aortic Dissection

Thoracic aortic dissection is the most common aortic emergency, even more common than ruptured abdominal aortic aneurysm. This potentially fatal condition is rare in patients younger than 50 years and is approximately two times more common in men than women. Patients at risk include patients with a history of connective tissue disorders and patients with severe, poorly controlled hypertension.

An aortic dissection occurs when there is loss of integrity of the intima and blood dissects into the media. Once in the media, there is a natural plane through which dissection is quite easy.

Although there are various classification systems for aortic dissection, the Stanford classification is perhaps the most widely used and

TABLE 1	Dissection: The Great Mimic	
TERRITORY INVOLVED OR AFFECTED BY DISSECTION	**MIMICS**	
Rupture into pericardial sac	Cardiac tamponade	
Dissection through aortic valve	Acute aortic insufficiency	
Dissection occluding coronary arteries	Myocardial infarction	
Involvement of cerebral vessels	Stroke	
Involvement of subclavian arteries	Upper extremity ischemia (cold arm)	
Dissection running down descending thoracic aorta	Severe back pain and paralysis	
Mesenteric artery obstruction	Mesenteric ischemia	
Renal artery obstruction	Oliguria and acute renal failure	
Iliac artery occlusion	Lower extremity ischemia (cold leg)	

the most useful. In this classification, any dissection that involves the ascending aorta, whether it involves the ascending aorta alone or both the ascending and descending thoracoabdominal aorta, are classified as type A. Dissections that do not involve the ascending aorta are classified as type B. This classification is useful because type A dissections require urgent surgery. Type B dissections are typically managed medically unless they are associated with complications such as unremitting pain, aneurysmal expansion, and end-organ ischemia. By convention, aortic dissections that are evaluated within 14 days after the onset of symptoms are considered acute, and those evaluated beyond 14 days are considered chronic.

Helical CAT scanners with the use of contrast are excellent at defining the location and extent of aortic dissection. However, being alert to the potential for this diagnosis requires a high index of suspicion. Aortic dissection can mimic a variety of common conditions based on the extent of the dissection and the aortic branches involved (Table 1). Uncomplicated type B dissections are typically managed medically. This is usually performed in an intensive care setting with the use of intravenous medications to control contractility and, if necessary, hypertension.

In the past, due to the friability of dissected aortic tissue, the results of operative repair for type B dissections have been particularly poor. Currently, endograft repair with the purpose of excluding the entry point of dissection and reestablishing flow to the true lumen is gaining popularity in the treatment of complex dissection. This at times may be supplemented by stenting of affected aortic side branches and fenestration to establish a connection between the true and false lumen to restore perfusion to certain organs. Once the acute phase has passed and medically treated patients are under good hypertensive control, these patients are then converted to an oral medication regimen and transferred out of the intensive care setting. Patients need to be followed up with serial CT imaging after discharge to evaluate for aneurysmal degeneration of the false lumen. This evaluation should occur every 6 months until the patient is stable and then yearly thereafter.

In cases where the total aortic diameter grows to greater than 6 cm, repair for the purpose of preventing rupture is indicated, although this is often technically more complicated than treating a fusiform aneurysm in the absence of a previous dissection. Patients should strictly adhere to their blood pressure medication regimen for life.

References

Blankensteijn JD, de Jong SE, Prinssen M, et al: Two-year outcomes after conventional or endovascular repair of abdominal aortic aneurysms, *N Engl J Med* 352(23):2398–2405, 2005.
Crawford ES, Crawford JL, Safi HJ, et al: Thoracoabdominal aortic aneurysms: Preoperative and intraoperative factors determining immediate and long-term results of operations in 605 patients, *J Vasc Surg* 3(3):389–404, 1986.
Daily PO, Trueblood HW, Stinson EB, et al: Management of acute aortic dissections, *Ann Thorac Surg* 10(3):237–247, 1970.
EVAR Trial Participants: Endovascular aneurysm repair versus open repair in patients with abdominal aortic aneurysm (EVAR trial 1): Randomised controlled trial, *Lancet* 365(9478):2179–2186, 2005.
EVAR Trial Participants: Endovascular aneurysm repair and outcome in patients unfit for open repair of abdominal aortic aneurysm (EVAR trial 2): Randomised controlled trial, *Lancet* 365(9478):2187–2192, 2005.
Lederle FA, Wilson SE, Johnson GR, et al: Immediate repair compared with surveillance of small abdominal aortic aneurysms, *N Engl J Med* 346(19):1437–1444, 2002.
Lee ES, Pickett E, Hedayati N, et al: Implementation of an aortic screening program in clinical practice: Implications for the Screen For Abdominal Aortic Aneurysms Very Efficiently (SAAAVE) Act, *J Vasc Surg* 49(5):1107–1111, 2009.
Nevitt MP, Ballard DJ, Hallett JW Jr: Prognosis of abdominal aortic aneurysms. A population-based study, *N Engl J Med* 321(15):1009–1014, 1989.
Nienaber CA, Rousseau H, Eggebrecht H, et al: Randomized comparison of strategies for type B aortic dissection: The INvestigation of STEnt Grafts in Aortic Dissection (INSTEAD) trial, *Circulation* 120(25):2519–2528, 2009.
Rentschler M, Baxter BT: Pharmacological approaches to prevent abdominal aortic aneurysm enlargement and rupture, *Ann N Y Acad Sci* 1085:39–46, 2006.

ATRIAL FIBRILLATION

Method of
Lin Yee Chen, MD, MS; and Samuel C. Dudley Jr., MD, PhD

CURRENT DIAGNOSIS

- History taking and physical examination for atrial fibrillation (AF) should be focused on determining symptom severity (to decide on treatment strategy), risk of thromboembolic stroke, and associated cardiovascular risk factors.
- Symptoms include palpitations, chest discomfort, shortness of breath, and reduced exercise capacity. Some patients are symptom free.
- Investigations include 12-lead electrocardiogram (ECG) for confirmation; transthoracic echocardiogram to evaluate left atrial size, left ventricular ejection fraction, and rule out valvular abnormalities; and blood tests for thyroid, renal, and hepatic function.

CURRENT THERAPY

- Rate control: Achieve average ventricular rate of less than 110 beats/min by using atrioventricular node (AVN) blockers or catheter ablation of AVN
- Rhythm control: Prevent AF recurrence by using antiarrhythmic drugs or catheter ablation (pulmonary vein isolation)
- Stroke prophylaxis: Risk stratification and stroke prevention by oral anticoagulation or left atrial appendage closure
- Risk factor management or lifestyle modification: Prevent AF by weight management, intensive blood pressure lowering, and exercise training

Epidemiology

AF is the most common sustained arrhythmia in the adult general population. Globally, the estimated number of individuals with AF in 2010 was 33.5 million. Between 1990 and 2010, the global estimated age-adjusted prevalence rate of AF increased from 569.5 to 596.2 per 100,000 men and from 359.9 to 373.1 per 100,000 women. This increase in prevalence was accompanied by a substantial increase in health burden: disability-adjusted life-years increased by 18.8% in men and 18.9% in women from 1990 to 2010. Finally, the lifetime risk for development of AF in adults at age 40 is 1 in 4.

| TABLE 1 | Risk Factors of Atrial Fibrillation |

Cardiovascular risk factors
  Older age
  Male sex
  Diabetes mellitus
  Overweight and obesity
  Hypertension
  Chronic kidney disease
Structural heart disease
  Valvular heart disease
  Cardiomyopathy (dilated, restrictive, and hypertrophic)
  Congenital heart disease
  Coronary heart disease
  Left ventricular diastolic dysfunction
  Left atrial enlargement
  Family history
  Genetics (polygenic and monogenic inheritance)
  Inflammation
  Low serum magnesium
  Heavy alcohol consumption
  Poor cardiorespiratory fitness
  Low physical activity
  Premature atrial contractions or supraventricular ectopy

Risk Factors and Pathophysiology

Table 1 shows the known risk factors of AF; many of these are also risk factors for atherosclerotic disease. Traditional cardiovascular risk factors such as diabetes, hypertension, and obesity can lead to AF via the following pathway: cardiovascular risk factors → left ventricular diastolic dysfunction → structural and functional alterations in the atria (enlargement, impaired function, fibrosis, etc.) → AF. The aforementioned pathway creates the substrate for AF; premature atrial contractions and supraventricular ectopic beats are the trigger for AF. Other pathophysiological pathways include inflammation and increased oxidative stress leading to electrical remodeling, and, consequently, AF.

Clinical Manifestations

Common symptoms of AF include palpitations, irregular heart beat sensation, lightheadedness, dyspnea, chest discomfort, and fatigue. Some patients may have no symptoms at rest but report poor stamina or easy fatigability with physical activity. Other patients, particularly in the elderly, may be asymptomatic.

Diagnosis

The absence of distinct P waves with irregularly irregular RR interval on the ECG are the sine qua non for diagnosing AF. Rhythm documentation can be obtained via the standard 12-lead ECG, Holter monitors that can record up to 48 hours, leadless patch monitors that can record up to 2 weeks, or implantable loop recorders. Newer wearable technologies that can diagnose AF include smart watches and smart phones with specialized apps.

Paroxysmal AF is defined as AF that terminates spontaneously typically in <24 hours and in all cases <7 days. AF that continues for >7 days and requires cardioversion for conversion to sinus rhythm is termed *persistent AF*. Long-standing persistent AF refers to AF that has been continuous for longer than 1 year. Permanent AF refers to a clinical scenario when both patients and physician have decided not to pursue further attempts to maintain sinus rhythm.

Differential Diagnosis

These include other supraventricular arrhythmias such as atrial tachycardia, atrial flutter, long runs of premature atrial contractions, and multifocal atrial tachycardia.

Treatment

Rate Control

The goal of rate control is to prevent excessive ventricular rate response. This is a reasonable treatment strategy given data from randomized controlled trials (RCTs), which did not show any difference in cardiovascular outcomes between rate versus rhythm control strategy.

The AFFIRM (Atrial Fibrillation Follow-up Investigation of Rhythm Management) trial found no difference in mortality or stroke rates between patients assigned to rhythm control or ventricular rate control strategies. Similarly, the RACE (Rate Control versus Electrical Cardioversion for Persistent Atrial Fibrillation) trial found that rate control was not inferior to rhythm control for prevention of death.

The RACE II study showed that lenient ventricular rate control targeting heart rate of lower than 110 beats/min was not inferior to stricter rate control of less than 80 beats/min. Lenient rate control is more convenient and requires fewer outpatient visits and fewer medications.

Other than pharmacologic agents (Table 2), catheter ablation of the AVN is effective in controlling ventricular rate in patients with AF. AVN ablation is indicated if patients fail to achieve adequate ventricular rate control despite maximum doses of AVN blockers.

Rhythm Control

Although AF is associated with an increased risk of stroke and mortality, current evidence indicates that there is no difference in the rates of these cardiovascular outcomes between rhythm and rate control strategy. However, in selected younger patients with paroxysmal AF, rhythm control may be a better approach. Additionally, catheter ablation to maintain sinus rhythm in selected patients with symptomatic AF and heart failure with reduced left ventricular ejection fraction may reduce mortality rate and hospitalization for heart failure. Finally, in patients who continue to have symptoms despite an adequately controlled ventricular rate, rhythm control is an appropriate next step.

Rhythm control can be achieved by the use of antiarrhythmic drugs (Table 3) or catheter ablation. In patients with paroxysmal and persistent AF who have failed at least one antiarrhythmic drug, catheter ablation by pulmonary vein isolation is indicated to maintain sinus rhythm. In persistent AF, the Substrate and Trigger Ablation for Reduction of Atrial Fibrillation Trial Part II (STAR AF II) showed that performing additional linear ablation or ablation targeting complex fractionated electrograms does not improve rhythm control compared with pulmonary vein isolation alone. The optimal approach to ablate persistent AF remains to be defined.

Stroke Prophylaxis

Stroke prevention is a two-staged process: determination of thromboembolic stroke risk and selection of prevention strategy. The most commonly used risk stratification scheme for stroke prevention is the CHA_2DS_2-VASc score https://www.mdcalc.com/cha2ds2-vasc-score-atrial-fibrillation-stroke-risk (Table 4). Oral anticoagulation is recommended for CHA_2DS_2-VASc score ≥2. Oral anticoagulation is recommended for CHA2DS2-VASc score of 2 or greater in men or 3 or greater in women. Aspirin should not be used for stroke prevention in AF.[1]

Oral Anticoagulants

These include vitamin K antagonists (warfarin [Coumadin]) and non-vitamin K oral anticoagulants or novel or direct oral anticoagulants (NOAC, DOAC) (Table 5). Compared with warfarin, NOACs are as effective in preventing thromboembolic stroke in AF. The risk of intracranial hemorrhage from the use of NOACs is 33% to 60% less than warfarin. Other advantages of NOACs over warfarin include fewer interactions with food and obviating the need for international normalized ratio monitoring.

---

[1] Not FDA approved for this indication

TABLE 2   Pharmacologic Agents for Rate Control

DRUG	INTRAVENOUS ADMINISTRATION	USUAL ORAL MAINTENANCE DOSE	MAJOR SIDE EFFECTS
β-Blockers			
Metoprolol (Lopressor)*	2.5–5 mg IV bolus; up to 3 doses	100–200 mg (long-acting) daily	Bradycardia, hypotension, heart block, asthma, heart failure
Atenolol (Tenormin)*	N/A	25–100 mg daily	
Esmolol (Brevibloc)	50–200 µg/kg/min IV	N/A	
Propranolol (Inderal)	1–3 mg IV	10–40 mg TID	
Carvedilol (Coreg)*	N/A	3.125–25 mg BID	
Non-Dihydropyridine Calcium Channel Antagonists			
Verapamil (Calan)	5–10 mg bolus	80 mg TID or up to 360 mg (long-acting) daily	Hypotension, heart block, heart failure
Diltiazem (Cardizem)	0.25–0.35 mg/kg	60 mg TID or up to 360 mg (long-acting) daily	
Digitalis Glycosides			
Digoxin (Lanoxin)	0.25–0.5 mg	0.125–0.25 mg daily	Digitalis toxicity, bradycardia, heart block

*Not FDA approved for this indication.
IV, Intravenous.

TABLE 3   Pharmacologic Agents for Rhythm Control

DRUG	USUAL ORAL MAINTENANCE DOSE	MAJOR SIDE EFFECTS
Flecainide (Tambocor)	50–200 mg BID	Hypotension, atrial flutter with high ventricular rate
Propafenone (Rythmol)	150–300 mg TID	
Propafenone Extended Release (Rythmol SR)	225–425 mg BID	
Sotalol (Betapace)	80–160 mg BID	Bradycardia, hypotension, QT prolongation, torsades de pointes
Dofetilide (Tikosyn)	125–500 µg BID	QT prolongation, torsades de pointes
Amiodarone (Pacerone)*	100–200 mg daily	Hypotension, bradycardia, QT prolongation
Dronedarone (Multaq)	400 mg BID	QT prolongation

*Not FDA approved for atrial fibrillation.

TABLE 4   CHA$_2$DS$_2$-VASc Score

RISK FACTOR	SCORE
Congestive heart failure, LV dysfunction	1
Hypertension	1
Age ≥ 75 years	2
Diabetes mellitus	1
Stroke, TIA, or thromboembolism	2
Vascular disease (MI, PAD, complex aortic plaque)	1
Age 65–74 years	1
Sex category: Female	1

LV, Left ventricular; *MI,* myocardial infarction; *PAD,* peripheral arterial disease; *TIA,* transient ischemic attack.

TABLE 5   Non–Vitamin K Oral Anticoagulants

DIRECT THROMBIN INHIBITOR		
DRUG	USUAL DOSE	COMMENTS
Dabigatran (Pradaxa)	150 mg BID	Reversal agent (Idarucizumab [Praxbind]) FDA-approved; interacts with P-glycoprotein inhibitors and inducers
FACTOR XA INHIBITOR		
Apixaban (Eliquis)	5 mg BID	Interacts with P-glycoprotein and CYP3A4 inhibitors and inducers
Edoxaban (Savaysa)	60 mg once daily	Avoid if CrCl >95 mL/min due to increased rate of stroke
Rivaroxaban (Xarelto)	20 mg once daily	Interacts with P-glycoprotein and CYP3A4 inhibitors and inducers; should be taken with evening meal

Atrial Fibrillation

107

Left Atrial Appendage Closure

The Watchman device is approved by the Food and Drug Administration (FDA) for stroke prevention in AF patients with a contraindication to long-term oral anticoagulation and who are at risk of thromboembolic stroke. Patients, however, must be able to take oral anticoagulants for at least 6 weeks after implantation of the device.

Risk Factor Management and Lifestyle Modification

Recent compelling evidence underscores the importance of a fourth pillar of AF management: Risk factor and lifestyle modifications.

Weight Loss

An RCT showed that weight reduction with intensive risk factor management resulted in a reduction of AF symptom burden and severity and reversal of cardiac remodeling.

Intensive Blood Pressure Lowering

Blood pressure lowering targeting a systolic blood pressure of 120 mm Hg is associated with lower incidence of AF compared with 140 mm Hg.

Exercise Training

A small RCT showed that, compared with nonexercise control patients, high-intensity interval training reduced AF burden and improved atrial contractile function. This time-efficient form of exercise can potentially overcome the lack of time problem—an oft-quoted reason for the poor compliance with regular aerobic exercise.

Complications

Other than thromboembolic stroke, heart failure, and death, AF is also associated with greater cognitive decline and risk of dementia. More recently, AF has been reported to be associated with a higher risk of sudden cardiac death in the general population. Apart from stroke prevention and rate and rhythm control to prevent heart failure, we currently lack effective prevention strategies for dementia and sudden cardiac death.

Special Considerations

Subclinical Atrial Fibrillation

Subclinical AF is commonly detected from interrogation of cardiac implantable electronic devices. Whether subclinical AF poses the same health risks as clinical AF is the subject of much debate and active investigation.

Atrial Fibrillation Burden

A corollary to the problem of subclinical AF is that of AF burden—the amount of AF that a patient has. Studies based on cardiac implantable electronic devices suggest that higher AF burden is associated with higher risk of thromboembolic stroke, but it is unclear whether the risk increases continuously or whether a threshold exists.

References

Abed HS, Wittert GA, Leong DP, et al: Effect of weight reduction and cardiometabolic risk factor management on symptom burden and severity in patients with atrial fibrillation a randomized clinical trial, *JAMA* 310:2050–2060, 2013.

Chen LY, Bigger JT, Hickey KT, et al: Effect of intensive blood pressure lowering on incident atrial fibrillation and p-wave indices in the ACCORD Blood Pressure Trial, *Am J Hypertens* 29:1276–1282, 2016.

Chen LY, Norby FL, Gottesman RF, et al: Association of atrial fibrillation with cognitive decline and dementia over 20 years: the ARIC-NCS (Atherosclerosis Risk in Communities Neurocognitive Study), *J Am Heart Assoc* 7(6).

Chen LY, Sotoodehnia N, Bůžková P, et al: Atrial fibrillation and the risk of sudden cardiac death: the Atherosclerosis Risk in Communities (ARIC) Study and Cardiovascular Health Study (CHS), *JAMA Intern Med* 173:29–35, 2013.

Chugh SS, Havmoeller R, Narayanan K, et al: Worldwide epidemiology of atrial fibrillation: a Global Burden of Disease 2010 Study, *Circulation* 129:837–847, 2014.

January CT, Wann LS, Calkins H, et al: 2019 AHA/ACC/HRS focused update of the 2014 AHA/ACC/HRS guideline for the management of patients with atrial fibrillation: a report of the American College of Cardiology/American Heart Association Task Force on Clinical Practice Guidelines and the Heart Rhythm Society, *Circulation*, 2019. https://doi.org/10.1161/CIR.0000000000000665.

Lloyd-Jones DM, Wang TJ, Leip EP, et al: Lifetime risk for development of atrial fibrillation—The Framingham Heart Study, *Circulation* 110:1042–1046, 2004.

Malmo V, Nes BM, Amundsen BH, et al: Aerobic interval training reduces the burden of atrial fibrillation in the short term a randomized trial, *Circulation* 133:466–473, 2016.

Marrouche NF, Brachmann J, Andresen D, et al: Catheter ablation for atrial fibrillation with heart failure, *N Engl J Med* 378:417–427, 2018.

Okin PM, Hille DA, Larstorp ACK, et al: Effect of lower on-treatment systolic blood pressure on the risk of atrial fibrillation in hypertensive patients, *Hypertension* 66:368–373, 2015.

Van Gelder IC, Groenveld HF, Crijns HJGM, et al: Lenient versus strict rate control in patients with atrial fibrillation, *N Engl J Med* 362:1363–1373, 2010.

Van Gelder IC, Hagens VE, Bosker HA, et al: A comparison of rate control and rhythm control in patients with recurrent persistent atrial fibrillation, *N Engl J Med* 347:1834–1840, 2002.

Verma A, Jiang CY, Betts TR, et al: Approaches to catheter ablation for persistent atrial fibrillation, *N Engl J Med* 372:1812–1822, 2015.

Wyse DG, Waldo AL, DiMarco JP, et al: A comparison of rate control and rhythm control in patients with atrial fibrillation, *N Engl J Med* 347:1825–1833, 2002.

CONGENITAL HEART DISEASE

Method of
Richard A. Lange, MD, MBA; and Joaquin E. Cigarroa, MD

CURRENT DIAGNOSIS

- Examine blood pressures in arms and legs, pulse oximetry, mucous membranes and nail beds, respiratory rate, and peripheral pulses.
- In addition to listening over the precordium for heart sounds and murmurs, palpate for thrills and evidence of right or left chamber enlargement.
- Ancillary testing should include chest radiography, electrocardiography, and echocardiography.
- Consult a cardiologist if the physical examination or ancillary tests suggest congenital heart disease.

CURRENT THERAPY

- All congenital heart disease patients should have long-term follow-up for possible complications.
- Endocarditis prophylaxis is recommended for subjects with:
  - Unrepaired cyanotic congenital heart disease
  - Recently repaired congenital heart disease (<6 months after surgical or percutaneous repair)
  - Repaired congenital heart disease with residual defects
- Closure of defects with large left-to-right shunts (i.e., atrial septal defect, ventricular septal defect, atrioventricular canal, or patent ductus arteriosus) is recommended unless pulmonary vascular obstructive disease is far advanced.
- Patients with bicuspid aortic valves should be monitored for aortic root dilation.
- Pregnancy should be avoided in women with cyanotic congenital heart disease because of high maternal and fetal morbidity and mortality rates.

Congenital heart disease affects 0.4% to 0.9% of live births. Nowadays, most survive to adulthood because of improved diagnosis and treatment. Congenital cardiac defects can be categorized according to the presence or absence of cyanosis (due to right-to-left shunting) and the amount of pulmonary blood flow (Box 1).

BOX 1 Categorization of Congenital Heart Disease

Acyanotic Cardiac Defects
Increased pulmonary blood flow
- Atrial septal defect
- Ventricular septal defect
- Atrioventricular canal defect
- Patent ductus arteriosus

Normal pulmonary blood flow
- Aortic stenosis
- Pulmonic stenosis
- Aortic coarctation

Cyanotic Cardiac Defects
Normal pulmonary blood flow
- Ebstein's anomaly

Decreased pulmonary blood flow
- Tetralogy of Fallot
- Eisenmenger syndrome

Figure 1 Atrial septal defect. Blood from the pulmonary veins enters the left atrium, after which some of it crosses the atrial septal defect into the right atrium and ventricle *(longer arrow)*. Thus left-to-right shunting occurs. (Reprinted with permission from Brickner ME, Hillis LD, Lange RA: Congenital heart disease in adults. First of two parts. N Engl J Med 2000;342:256–263.)

Acyanotic Conditions

Atrial Septal Defect

Atrial septal defect (ASD) occurs in female patients two to three times as often as in male patients. Although most result from spontaneous genetic mutations, some are inherited.

The physiological consequences of ASD result from the shunting of blood from one atrium to the other; the direction and magnitude of shunting are determined by the size of the defect and the relative compliances of the ventricles. A small defect (<0.5 cm in diameter) is associated with a small shunt and no hemodynamic sequelae, whereas a sizable defect (>2 cm in diameter) usually is associated with a large shunt and substantial hemodynamic consequences. In most patients with ASD, the right ventricle is more compliant than the left; as a result, left atrial blood is shunted to the right atrium, causing increased pulmonary blood flow and dilation of the atria, right ventricle, and pulmonary arteries (Figure 1). Eventually, if the right ventricle fails or its compliance declines, the magnitude of left-to-right shunting diminishes.

In a patient with a large ASD, a right ventricular or pulmonary arterial impulse may be palpable, and wide, fixed splitting of the second heart sound is present. A systolic ejection murmur, audible in the second left intercostal space, is caused by increased blood flow across the pulmonic valve; flow across the ASD itself does not produce a murmur.

Because ASDs initially produce no symptoms or striking physical examination findings, they are often undetected for years. Small defects with minimal left-to-right shunting cause no symptoms or hemodynamic abnormalities, so they do not require closure. Even patients with moderate or large ASDs (characterized by a ratio of pulmonary to systemic blood flow of 1.5 or more) often have no symptoms until the third or fourth decade of life. Over the years, the increased blood volume flowing through the right heart chambers usually causes right ventricular dilation and failure. Obstructive pulmonary vascular disease (Eisenmenger syndrome) occurs uncommonly in adults with ASD.

The symptomatic patient with an ASD typically reports fatigue or dyspnea on exertion. Alternatively, the development of supraventricular tachyarrhythmias, right heart failure, paradoxical embolism, or recurrent pulmonary infections might prompt the patient to seek medical attention. Although an occasional patient with an unrepaired ASD survives to an advanced age, those with sizable shunts often die of right ventricular failure or arrhythmias in their 30s or 40s.

Echocardiography can reveal atrial and right ventricular dilation and identify the ASD's location. The sensitivity of echocardiography may be enhanced by injecting microbubbles in solution into a peripheral vein, after which the movement of some of them across the defect into the left atrium can be visualized.

An ASD with a pulmonary-to-systemic flow ratio of 1.5 or more should be closed (surgically or percutaneously) to prevent worsening right ventricular dysfunction. Prophylaxis against infective endocarditis is not recommended for patients with ASD (repaired or unrepaired) unless a concomitant valvular abnormality is present.

Ventricular Septal Defect

Ventricular septal defect (VSD) is the most common congenital cardiac abnormality, with similar incidence in boys and girls. Approximately 25% to 40% of them close spontaneously by 2 years of age.

The physiological consequences of a VSD are determined by the size of the defect and the relative resistances in the systemic and pulmonary vascular beds. A small defect causes little or no functional disturbance, because pulmonary blood flow is only minimally increased. In contrast, a large defect causes substantial left-to-right shunting, because systemic vascular resistance exceeds pulmonary vascular resistance (Figure 2). Over time, however, the pulmonary vascular resistance usually increases, and the magnitude of left-to-right shunting declines. Eventually, the pulmonary vascular resistance equals or exceeds the systemic resistance; the shunting of blood from left to right ceases; and right-to-left shunting begins (e.g., Eisenmenger physiology).

A small, muscular VSD can produce a high-frequency systolic ejection murmur that terminates before the end of systole (when the defect is occluded by contracting heart muscle). With a moderate or large VSD and substantial left-to-right shunting, a holosystolic murmur, loudest at the left sternal border, is audible and is usually accompanied by a palpable thrill. If pulmonary hypertension develops, the holosystolic murmur and thrill diminish in magnitude and eventually disappear as flow through the defect decreases.

Echocardiography is usually performed to confirm the presence and location of the VSD and to delineate the magnitude and direction of shunting. With catheterization, one can determine the magnitude of shunting and the pulmonary vascular resistance.

The natural history of VSD depends on the size of the defect and the pulmonary vascular resistance. Adults with small defects

Figure 2 Ventricular septal defect. When the left ventricle contracts, it ejects some blood into the aorta and some across the ventricular septal defect into the right ventricle and pulmonary artery *(arrow)*, resulting in left-to-right shunting. (Reprinted with permission from Brickner ME, Hillis LD, Lange RA: Congenital heart disease in adults. First of two parts. N Engl J Med 2000;342:256–263.)

Figure 3 Patent ductus arteriosus. Some of the blood from the aorta crosses the ductus arteriosus into the pulmonary artery *(arrows)*, with resultant left-to-right shunting. (Reprinted with permission from Brickner ME, Hillis LD, Lange RA: Congenital heart disease in adults. First of two parts. N Engl J Med 2000;342:256–263.)

and normal pulmonary arterial pressure are generally asymptomatic, and pulmonary vascular disease is unlikely to develop. In contrast, patients with large defects who survive to adulthood usually have left ventricular failure or pulmonary hypertension (or both) with associated right ventricular failure.

Closure of VSDs (surgically or percutaneously) is recommended if the pulmonary vascular obstructive disease is not severe. Prophylaxis against infective endocarditis is recommended for patients with unrepaired VSD and those with a residual shunt despite surgical or percutaneous closure.

Atrioventricular Canal Defect
The endocardial cushions normally fuse to form the tricuspid and mitral valves, as well as the atrial and ventricular septa. Atrioventricular (AV) canal defects are caused by incomplete fusion of the endocardial cushions during embryonic development. They are the most common congenital cardiac abnormality in patients with Down syndrome. Such cushion defects include a spectrum of abnormalities, ranging from ASD with a cleft anterior mitral valve leaflet to a common AV canal defect in which a single AV valve in association with a large ASD and VSD is present.

A common AV canal defect permits substantial left-to-right shunting at both the atrial and ventricular levels, which leads to excessive pulmonary blood flow and resultant pulmonary congestion within months of birth. Eventually, the excessive pulmonary blood flow leads to irreversible pulmonary vascular obstruction (e.g., Eisenmenger physiology).

In the patient with an AV canal defect and left-to-right intracardiac shunting, the physical examination reveals a loud holosystolic murmur audible throughout the precordium. As pulmonary vascular resistance increases, the holosystolic murmur diminishes in intensity and duration, eventually disappearing as flow through the defect decreases.

AV canal defects require surgical repair if the magnitude of pulmonary vascular obstructive disease is not prohibitive. Although such patients might initially benefit from medical treatment with diuretics and afterload reduction, the onset of heart failure symptoms is generally the point at which surgery is considered. Prophylaxis against infective endocarditis is recommended for patients with repaired and unrepaired AV canal defects.

Patent Ductus Arteriosus
The ductus arteriosus connects the descending aorta (just distal to the left subclavian artery) and the left pulmonary artery. In the fetus, it permits pulmonary arterial blood to bypass the unexpanded lungs and to enter the descending aorta for oxygenation in the placenta. Although it normally closes spontaneously soon after birth, it fails to do so in some infants, so that continuous flow from the aorta to the pulmonary artery (i.e., left-to-right shunting) occurs (Figure 3). The incidence of patent ductus arteriosus (PDA) is increased in pregnancies complicated by persistent perinatal hypoxemia or maternal rubella infection as well as among infants born prematurely or at high altitude.

A patient with PDA and a moderate or large shunt has bounding peripheral arterial pulses and a widened pulse pressure. A continuous "machinery" murmur, audible in the second left intercostal space, begins shortly after the first heart sound, peaks in intensity at or immediately after the second heart sound (thereby obscuring it), and diminishes in intensity during diastole. If pulmonary vascular obstruction and hypertension develop, the murmur decreases in duration and intensity and eventually disappears.

With echocardiography, the PDA can usually be visualized, and Doppler studies demonstrate continuous flow in the pulmonary trunk. Catheterization and angiography allow one to quantify the magnitude of shunting and the pulmonary vascular resistance and to visualize the PDA.

The subject with a small PDA has no symptoms attributable to it and a normal life expectancy. However, it is associated with an elevated risk of infective endarteritis. A PDA of moderate size might cause no symptoms during infancy; during childhood or adulthood, fatigue, dyspnea, or palpitations can appear. Additionally, the PDA can become aneurysmal and calcified, with subsequent rupture. Larger shunts can precipitate left ventricular failure. Eventually, pulmonary vascular obstruction can develop; when the pulmonary vascular resistance equals or exceeds the systemic vascular resistance, the direction of shunting reverses.

One third of patients with an unrepaired moderate or large PDA die of heart failure, pulmonary hypertension, or endarteritis by 40 years of age, and two thirds die by 60 years of age. Because of the risk of endarteritis associated with unrepaired PDA (about 0.45% annually after the second decade of life) and the safety of surgical ligation (generally accomplished without cardiopulmonary bypass) or percutaneous closure, even a small PDA should be ligated surgically or occluded percutaneously. Once severe pulmonary vascular obstructive disease develops, ligation or closure is contraindicated.

Aortic Stenosis

A bicuspid aortic valve is found in 2% to 3% of the population and is four times more common in males than in females. The bicuspid valve has a single fused commissure and an eccentrically oriented orifice. Although the deformed valve is not typically stenotic at birth, it is subjected to abnormal hemodynamic stress, which can lead to leaflet thickening and calcification. In many patients, an abnormality of the ascending aortic media is present, predisposing the patient to aortic root dilation. Twenty percent of patients with a bicuspid aortic valve have an associated cardiovascular abnormality, such as PDA or aortic coarctation.

In patients with severe aortic stenosis (AS), the carotid upstroke is usually delayed and diminished. The aortic component of the second heart sound is diminished or absent. A systolic crescendo–decrescendo murmur is audible over the aortic area and often radiates to the neck. As the magnitude of AS worsens, the murmur peaks progressively later in systole.

In most patients, echocardiography with Doppler flow permits an assessment of the severity of AS and of left ventricular systolic function. Cardiac catheterization is performed to assess the severity of AS and to determine if concomitant coronary artery disease is present.

The symptoms of AS are angina pectoris, syncope or near syncope, and those of heart failure (dyspnea). Asymptomatic adults with AS have a normal life expectancy. Once symptoms appear, survival is limited. The median survival is 5 years once angina develops, 3 years once syncope occurs, and 2 years once symptoms of heart failure appear. Therefore patients with symptomatic AS should undergo valve replacement.

Pulmonic Stenosis

Pulmonic stenosis (PS) is the second most common congenital cardiac malformation (after VSD). Although typically an isolated abnormality, it can occur in association with VSD.

The patient with PS is usually asymptomatic, and the condition is identified by auscultation of a loud systolic murmur. When it is severe, dyspnea on exertion or fatigue can occur; less often, patients have retrosternal chest pain or syncope with exertion. Eventually, right ventricular failure can develop, with resultant peripheral edema and abdominal swelling.

In patients with moderate or severe PS, the second heart sound is widely split, with its pulmonic component soft and delayed. A crescendo-decrescendo systolic murmur that increases in intensity with inspiration is audible along the left sternal border. If the valve is pliable, an ejection click often precedes the murmur. On echocardiography, right ventricular hypertrophy is evident; the severity of PS can usually be assessed with measurement of Doppler flow.

Adults with mild PS are usually asymptomatic and do not require a corrective procedure. In contrast, patients with moderate or severe PS should undergo percutaneous balloon dilation.

Aortic Coarctation

Aortic coarctation typically consists of a diaphragm-like ridge extending into the aortic lumen just distal to the left subclavian artery (Figure 4), resulting in an elevated arterial pressure in both arms. Less commonly, the coarctation is located immediately proximal to the left subclavian artery, in which case a difference in arterial pressure is noted between the arms. Extensive collateral arterial circulation to the lower body through the internal thoracic, intercostal, subclavian, and scapular arteries often develops in patients with aortic coarctation. Aortic coarctation, which is two to five times as common in males as in females, can occur in conjunction with gonadal dysgenesis (e.g., Turner's syndrome), bicuspid aortic valve, VSD, or PDA.

Figure 4 Coarctation of the aorta. Coarctation causes obstruction to blood flow in the descending thoracic aorta; the lower body is perfused by collateral vessels from the axillary and internal thoracic arteries through the intercostal arteries. (Reprinted with permission from Brickner ME, Hillis LD, Lange RA: Congenital heart disease in adults. First of two parts. N Engl J Med 2000;342:256–263.)

On physical examination, the arterial pressure is higher in the arms than in the legs, and the femoral arterial pulses are weak and delayed. A harsh systolic ejection murmur may be audible along the left sternal border and in the back, particularly over the coarctation. A systolic murmur, caused by flow through collateral vessels, may be heard in the back.

On chest radiography, increased collateral flow through the intercostal arteries causes notching of the posterior third through eighth ribs. The coarctation may be visible as an indentation of the aorta, and one may see prestenotic and poststenotic aortic dilation, producing the "reversed E" or "3" sign. Computed tomography, magnetic resonance imaging, and contrast aortography provide precise anatomic delineation of the coarctation's location and length.

Most adults with aortic coarctation are asymptomatic. When symptoms are present, they are usually those of hypertension: headache, epistaxis, dizziness, and palpitations. Complications of aortic coarctation include hypertension, left ventricular failure, aortic dissection, premature coronary artery disease, infective endocarditis, and cerebrovascular accidents (due to rupture of an intracerebral aneurysm). Two thirds of patients older than 40 years who have uncorrected aortic coarctation have symptoms of heart failure. Three fourths die by the age of 50 years and 90% by the age of 60 years.

Surgical repair or intraluminal stenting should be considered for patients with a transcoarctation pressure gradient greater than 30 mm Hg, with the choice of procedure influenced by the age of the patient, anatomic considerations of the coarctation, and the presence of concomitant cardiac abnormalities. Persistent hypertension is common despite surgical or percutaneous intervention, and recurrent coarctation or aneurysm formation at the repair site may occur.

Cyanotic Conditions
Ebstein's Anomaly

With Ebstein's anomaly, the tricuspid valve's septal leaflet and often its posterior leaflet are displaced into the right ventricle, and

Figure 5 Ebstein's anomaly. With Ebstein's anomaly, the tricuspid valve is displaced apically, a portion of the right ventricle is atrialized (i.e., located on the atrial side of the tricuspid valve), and the functional right ventricle is small. (Reprinted with permission from Brickner ME, Hillis LD, Lange RA: Congenital heart disease in adults. Second of two parts. N Engl J Med 2000;342:334–342.)

Figure 6 Tetralogy of Fallot. Tetralogy of Fallot is characterized by a large ventricular septal defect, obstruction of the right ventricular outflow tract, right ventricular hypertrophy, and an aorta that overrides the left and right ventricles. With right ventricular outflow tract obstruction, blood is shunted through the ventricular septal defect from right to left *(arrow)*. (Reprinted with permission from Brickner ME, Hillis LD, Lange RA: Congenital heart disease in adults. Second of two parts. N Engl J Med 2000;342:334–342.)

the anterior leaflet is usually malformed and abnormally attached or adherent to the right ventricular free wall. As a result, a portion of the right ventricle is atrialized, in that it is located on the atrial side of the tricuspid valve, and the remaining functional right ventricle is small (Figure 5). The tricuspid valve is usually regurgitant, but it may be stenotic. Eighty percent of patients with Ebstein's anomaly have an interatrial communication (ASD or patent foramen ovale) through which right-to-left shunting of blood can occur.

The severity of the hemodynamic derangements in patients with Ebstein's anomaly depends on the magnitude of displacement and the functional status of the tricuspid valve leaflets. On the one extreme, patients with mild apical displacement of the tricuspid valve leaflets have normal valvular function; on the other extreme, those with severe leaflet displacement or abnormal anterior leaflet attachment, with resultant valvular dysfunction, have an elevated right atrial pressure and right-to-left shunting if an interatrial communication is present.

The clinical presentation of subjects with Ebstein's anomaly ranges from severe right heart failure in the neonate to the absence of symptoms in the adult in whom it is discovered incidentally. Older children with Ebstein's anomaly often come to medical attention because of an incidental murmur, whereas adolescents and adults may be identified because of a supraventricular arrhythmia.

On physical examination, the severity of cyanosis depends on the magnitude of right-to-left shunting. The first and second heart sounds are both widely split, and a third or fourth heart sound is often present, resulting in triple or even quadruple heart sounds. A systolic murmur caused by tricuspid regurgitation is usually present at the left lower sternal border.

Echocardiography is used to assess the presence and magnitude of right atrial dilation, anatomic displacement and distortion of the tricuspid valve leaflets, and the severity of tricuspid regurgitation or stenosis.

Prophylaxis against infective endocarditis is recommended. Patients with symptomatic right heart failure should receive diuretics. Tricuspid valve repair or replacement in conjunction with closure of the interatrial communication is recommended for older patients with severe symptoms despite medical therapy and those with less severe symptoms who have cardiac enlargement.

Tetralogy of Fallot

Tetralogy of Fallot is characterized by a large VSD, an aorta that overrides both ventricles, obstruction to right ventricular outflow (subvalvular, valvular, supravalvular, or in the pulmonary arterial branches), and right ventricular hypertrophy (Figure 6).

Most patients with tetralogy of Fallot have substantial right-to-left shunting through the large VSD because of increased resistance to flow in the right ventricular outflow tract; the magnitude of right ventricular outflow tract obstruction determines the magnitude of shunting. Because the resistance to flow across the right ventricular outflow tract is relatively fixed, changes in systemic vascular resistance affect the magnitude of right-to-left shunting: A decrease in systemic vascular resistance increases right-to-left shunting, whereas an increase in systemic resistance decreases it.

Patients with tetralogy of Fallot typically have cyanosis from birth or beginning in the first year of life. In childhood, they might have sudden hypoxic spells, characterized by tachypnea and hyperpnea, followed by worsening cyanosis and, in some cases, loss of consciousness, seizures, cerebrovascular accidents, and even death. Such spells do not occur in adolescents or adults. Without surgical intervention, most patients die in childhood.

On physical examination, patients with tetralogy of Fallot have cyanosis and digital clubbing. A right ventricular lift or tap is palpable. The second heart sound is single, because its pulmonic component is inaudible. A systolic ejection murmur, audible along the left sternal border, is caused by the obstruction to right ventricular outflow. The intensity and duration of the murmur are inversely related to the severity of right ventricular outflow obstruction; a soft, short murmur suggests that severe obstruction is present.

Laboratory examination reveals arterial oxygen desaturation and compensatory erythrocytosis. Echocardiography can be used

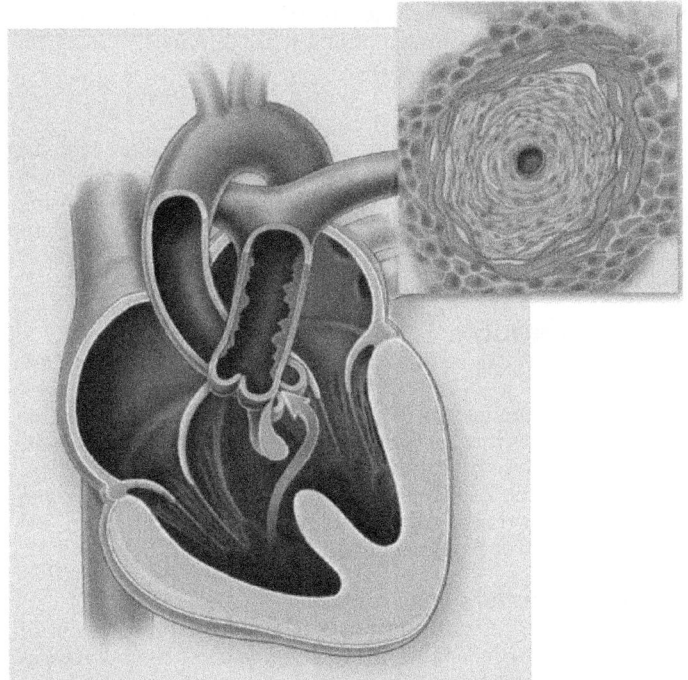

Figure 7 Eisenmenger syndrome. In response to substantial left-to-right shunting, morphologic alterations occur in the small pulmonary arteries and arterioles *(inset)*, leading to pulmonary hypertension and the resultant reversal of the intracardiac shunt *(arrow)*. In the small pulmonary arteries and arterioles, medial hypertrophy, intimal cellular proliferation, and fibrosis lead to narrowing or closure of the vessel lumina. With sustained pulmonary hypertension, extensive atherosclerosis and calcification often develop in the large pulmonary arteries. (Reprinted with permission from Brickner ME, Hillis LD, Lange RA: Congenital heart disease in adults. Second of two parts. N Engl J Med 2000;342:334–42.)

to establish the diagnosis and to assess the location and severity of right ventricular outflow tract obstruction.

Complete surgical repair (closure of the VSD and relief of right ventricular outflow tract obstruction) is recommended to relieve symptoms and to improve survival; it should be performed when patients are very young. Those with tetralogy of Fallot (repaired or unrepaired) are at risk for endocarditis and therefore should receive antibiotic prophylaxis before dental or elective surgical procedures.

Patients with repaired tetralogy of Fallot require careful follow-up, because they can subsequently develop atrial or ventricular arrhythmias, pulmonic regurgitation, right ventricular dysfunction, or recurrent obstruction of the right ventricular outflow tract.

Eisenmenger Syndrome

With substantial left-to-right shunting, the pulmonary vasculature is exposed to increased blood flow under increased pressure, often resulting in pulmonary vascular obstructive disease. As the pulmonary vascular resistance approaches or exceeds systemic resistance, the shunt is reversed (right-to-left shunting develops), and cyanosis appears (Figure 7).

Most patients with Eisenmenger syndrome have impaired exercise tolerance and exertional dyspnea. Palpitations are common and most often result from atrial fibrillation or flutter. As erythrocytosis (due to arterial desaturation) develops, symptoms of hyperviscosity (visual disturbances, fatigue, headache, dizziness, and paresthesias) can appear. Patients with Eisenmenger syndrome can experience hemoptysis, bleeding complications, cerebrovascular accidents, brain abscess, syncope, and sudden death.

Eisenmenger syndrome patients typically have digital clubbing and cyanosis, a right parasternal heave (due to right ventricular hypertrophy), and a prominent pulmonic component of the second heart sound. The murmur caused by a VSD, PDA, or ASD disappears when Eisenmenger syndrome develops.

The chest x-ray reveals normal heart size, prominent central pulmonary arteries, and diminished vascular markings (pruning) of the peripheral vessels. On transthoracic echocardiography, evidence of right ventricular pressure overload and pulmonary hypertension is present. The underlying cardiac defect can usually be visualized, although shunting across the defect may be difficult to demonstrate by Doppler because of the low jet velocity.

Even though patients with Eisenmenger syndrome have severe pulmonary hypertension, they have a favorable long-term survival: 80% at 10 years after diagnosis, 77% at 15 years, and 42% at 25 years. Death is usually sudden, presumably caused by arrhythmias, but some patients die of heart failure, hemoptysis, brain abscess, or stroke.

Phlebotomy with isovolumic replacement should be performed in patients with moderate or severe symptoms of hyperviscosity; it should not be performed in asymptomatic or mildly symptomatic patients regardless of the hematocrit. Repeated phlebotomy can result in iron deficiency, which can worsen the symptoms of hyperviscosity, because iron-deficient erythrocytes are less deformable than iron-replete ones. Anticoagulants and antiplatelet agents should be avoided, because they exacerbate the hemorrhagic diathesis.

Patients with Eisenmenger syndrome should avoid intravascular volume depletion, high altitude, and the use of systemic vasodilators. Because of high maternal and fetal morbidity and mortality, pregnancy should be avoided. Patients with Eisenmenger syndrome who are undergoing noncardiac surgery require meticulous management of anesthesia, with attention to maintenance of systemic vascular resistance, minimization of blood loss and intravascular volume depletion, and prevention of iatrogenic paradoxical embolization. In preparation for noncardiac surgery, prophylactic phlebotomy (usually of 1 to 2 units of blood, with isovolumic replacement) is recommended for patients with a hematocrit greater than 65% to reduce the likelihood of perioperative hemorrhagic and thrombotic complications.

Lung transplantation with repair of the cardiac defect or combined heart–lung transplantation are options for patients with Eisenmenger syndrome who are deemed to have a poor prognosis (as reflected by the presence of syncope, refractory right heart failure, a high New York Heart Association [NYHA] functional class, or severe hypoxemia). Because of the somewhat limited success of transplantation and the reasonably good survival among patients treated medically, careful selection of patients for transplantation is imperative. Although pulmonary vasodilators improve exercise capacity, they have not been proved to improve survival.

References

Brickner ME, Hillis LD, Lange RA: Congenital heart disease in adults. First of two parts, *N Engl J Med* 342:256–263, 2000.

Brickner ME, Hillis LD, Lange RA: Congenital heart disease in adults. Second of two parts, *N Engl J Med* 342:334–342, 2000.

Deanfield J, Thaulow E, Warnes C, et al: Management of grown up congenital heart disease, *Eur Heart J* 24:1035–1084, 2003.

Lange RA, Hillis LD, Vongpatanasin WP, Brickner ME: The Eisenmenger syndrome in adults, *Ann Int Med* 128:745–755, 1998.

Marelli AJ, Mackie AS, Ionescu-Ittu R, et al: Congenital heart disease in the general population: Changing prevalence and age distribution, *Circulation* 115:163–172, 2007.

Warnes CS, Williams RG, Bashore TM, et al: ACC/AHA 2008 Guidelines for the management of adults with congenital heart disease: Executive summary. A report of the American College of Cardiology/American Heart Association Task Force on Practice Guidelines (Writing Committee to Develop Guidelines for the Management of Adults With Congenital Heart Disease), *Circulation* 118:2395–2451, 2008.

CONGESTIVE HEART FAILURE

Method of
Bart L. Cox, MD; and Prasheda Bremjit, MD

CURRENT DIAGNOSIS

- Identify clinical symptoms and signs of heart failure.
- Determine left ventricular ejection fraction with echocardiography.
- Evaluate the potential causes of heart failure.

CURRENT THERAPY

- Beta blockers, angiotensin-converting enzyme (ACE) inhibitors, angiotensin receptor blocking agents (ARB) and angiotensin receptor-neprilysin inhibitors (ARNI) are vital to the management of patients with systolic heart failure.
- Diuretics should be used for the management of congestion and volume overload.
- Therapy for HFpEF (heart failure with preserved ejection fraction) entails management of volume overload with diuretics, treatment of atrial fibrillation, management of hypertension, and coronary revascularization if ischemia is believed to be contributing to symptoms.
- Referral for advanced therapies including left ventricular assist device and heart transplantation should be considered in those patients with refractory or stage D heart failure.

Heart Failure Definition

According to the 2013 heart failure guidelines, "heart failure is a clinical syndrome that occurs as a result of structural or functional impairment of either ventricular filling or ejection of blood." It is a progressive condition that results from an index event that damages the heart muscle or impedes the myocardium from generating force. There are several compensatory mechanisms that are triggered after the decrease in pumping ability of the heart, including the adrenergic nervous system, renin angiotensin system, and the cytokine system. Although these systems may initially limit the damage that is already done, over the long term, activation of these systems leads to secondary end-stage organ damage and worse left ventricular (LV) remodeling. LV remodeling is the way in which the LV shape, size, and function change in response to various different mechanical and neurohormonal factors.

Epidemiology

Heart failure is reported to affect 2% to 3% of the US population. The lifetime risk for development of heart failure is 20% for Americans ≥40 years of age. The prevalence of heart failure increases with age. Patients with a primary diagnosis of heart failure make up >3 million physician visits per year, and the cost of heart failure is significant and was estimated to be $39.2 billion in 2010. There are approximately 5.1 million patients with clinical heart failure in the United States, and the prevalence is increasing with time.

Heart Failure Classification Based on Left Ventricular Ejection Fraction (LVEF)

Heart failure with reduced ejection fraction (HFrEF): signs and symptoms of heart failure with LVEF ≤40%

Heart failure with preserved ejection fraction (HFpEF): signs and symptoms of heart failure with LVEF ≥50%

Heart failure with preserved ejection fraction, borderline (HFpEF, borderline): signs and symptoms of heart failure with LVEF 41% to 49%

Heart failure with preserved ejection fraction, improved (HFpEF, improved): signs and symptoms with current LVEF ≥40% with a previous LVEF <40%

Diagnosis

Three diagnostic schemes for diagnosing heart failure are the Framingham, Boston, and NHANES criteria. The Framingham criteria are one of the most widely used criteria for diagnosing heart failure. Table 1 lists the Framingham major and minor criteria for the diagnosis of heart failure, requiring either two major or one major and two minor criteria.

Functional Capacity

Exercise capacity can be subjectively assessed using the New York Heart Association (NYHA) functional classification and objectively by the 6-minute walk test or cardiopulmonary exercise testing (CPET). All three assessments have prognostic implications. Therapeutic decisions are dependent on NYHA classification. Advanced therapies, such as mechanical circulatory support and orthotopic heart transplantation, require both NYHA functional class and, if appropriate and possible, CPET.

Clinical Manifestions and Diagnosis

Heart failure is a clinical diagnosis. The clinical presentation of a heart failure patient is far more dependent on hemodynamics than on ventricular function. The cardinal symptoms are exercise intolerance due to dyspnea and fatigue and salt and water retention (congestion). Patients may be asymptomatic with severe LV dysfunction (e.g., LVEF 20%) or significantly symptomatic with preserved LVEF.

Elevated left-sided filling pressures give rise to pulmonary congestive symptoms (e.g., orthopnea, paroxysmal nocturnal dyspnea, dyspnea on exertion, nocturnal cough) and physical examination signs (e.g., left-sided S_3 gallop, mitral regurgitant murmur, loud P_2 in the presence of pulmonary hypertension, rales). Increased right-sided filling pressures are responsible for systemic congestive symptoms (e.g., anorexia, early satiety, constipation, right upper quadrant discomfort, weight gain, increased abdominal girth, shoes/jewelry//belt fitting tighter) and signs (e.g., jugular vein distention [JVD], abdominal jugular reflux, right-sided S_3, tricuspid regurgitant murmur, lower-extremity edema, anasarca, ascites, hepatomegaly). Evidence of reduced cardiac output includes a decreased arterial pulse pressure percentage (<25%-30%), cold extremities, exercise intolerance, fatigue, hypotension in response to guideline-directed medical therapy (GDMT), cachexia, mental status changes, and inability to tolerate a regimen of GDMT that was once well tolerated. Decreased exercise capacity is multifactorial and includes deconditioning, pulmonary congestion, skeletal muscle abnormalities, reduced cardiac output, and arrhythmias.

Laboratory and Diagnostic Tests

As stated previously, heart failure is a clinical diagnosis and involves integrating clinical signs and symptoms, laboratory testing, as well as imaging to make the diagnosis. Useful laboratory tests include a complete blood count, urinalysis, complete metabolic count, fasting lipid profile, liver function tests, and thyroid-stimulating hormone. B-type natriuretic peptide (BNP) and N-terminal pro BNP (NTproBNP) are heart failure–specific laboratory tests that can be very helpful in making the diagnosis of heart failure. BNP has 70% sensitivity and 99% specificity, whereas N-terminal proBNP has 99% sensitivity and 85% specificity. BNP is an activated form of proBNP found in the both the atria and ventricles. In volume overload proBNP is released by the ventricles and breaks down into NT-proBNP and BNP. In addition to their utility in diagnosing heart failure, both NT-proBNP and BNP are helpful for prognosis of heart failure.

Twelve-lead electrocardiography (EKG) is an important test to perform in patients with suspected heart failure. Although it is usually abnormal in patients with heart failure, it can be normal in 10% of patients. Abnormalities that can be seen on EKG

TABLE 1	Criteria of CHF*

Major criteria

- Paroxysmal nocturnal dyspnea or orthopnea
- Neck-vein distention
- Rales
- Cardiomegaly
- Acute pulmonary edema
- S$_3$ gallop
- Increased venous pressure (≥16 cm of water)
- Circulation time ≥25 sec
- Hepatojugular reflux

Minor criteria

- Ankle edema
- Night cough
- Dyspnea on exertion
- Hepatomegaly
- Pleural effusion
- Vital capacity ↓1/3 from maximum
- Tachycardia (rate of ≥120/min)

Major or minor criterion

- Weight loss ≥4.5 kg in 5 days in response to treatment

*For establishing a definite diagnosis of congestive heart failure in this study, two major or one major and two minor criteria had to be present concurrently.
From McKee PA, Castelli WP, McNamara PM, et al: The natural history of congestive heart failure: the Framingham Study. *N Engl J Med* 285:1441–1446, 1971.

include ST- and T-wave changes, left ventricular hypertrophy, bundle branch block, and atrial fibrillation. The EKG can be a useful screening test, because a normal EKG is unlikely to be seen in patients with left-sided heart failure.

Echocardiography is vital in terms of noninvasive assessment of left ventricular function and should be performed in all patients with suspected heart failure. Patients who should undergo echocardiography include the following: patients with suspected heart failure, shortness of breath in the presence of a murmur, shortness of breath with atrial fibrillation, and patients at high risk of LV dysfunction.

Therapy
Diuretics

Diuretics are used for symptomatic improvement in patients with pulmonary and systemic congestion arising from elevated left- and right-sided filling pressures, respectively. In volume-overloaded patients, diuretics are used to optimize the filling pressures to eliminate all congestive signs and symptoms while avoiding signs and symptoms of hypovolemia. It is essential to evaluate for orthostatic hypotension in patients treated with diuretics. Additionally, close monitoring of electrolytes and renal function is indicated. Typically the loop diuretics furosemide (Lasix), bumetanide (Bumex), and torsemide (Demadex) are used. Rarely, thiazide and thiazide-like diuretics are effective at maintaining optimal filling pressures. Diuretic efficacy is evaluated by the physical examination demonstrating no edema, no JVD, no hepatomegaly, clear lungs, and absent symptoms of pulmonary congestion (orthopnea, paroxysmal nocturnal dyspnea, nocturnal cough, dyspnea on exertion) and systemic congestion (absence of anorexia, early satiety, abdominal discomfort due to hepatic and enteric congestion). A weight-based scale of diuretics, in which the daily diuretic dose is predicated on the morning weight, may be more effective than a fixed dose irrespective of weight change or increasing congestive signs and symptoms. Usually, a twice-daily regimen is effective for most patients, although a once-daily diuretic strategy can maintain optimal filling pressures in some patients. Adverse effects include hypokalemia, hypomagnesemia, orthostatic hypotension, renal insufficiency, electrolyte disturbance, ototoxicity, and gout.

Renin Angiotensin System Inhibitors
Angiotensin-Converting Enzyme Inhibitors (ACEI)

ACEI improve survival and decrease heart failure hospitalizations in HFrEF patients. The benefit appears to be generalized among all agents in this class. They are used in HFrEF irrespective of NYHA functional capacity. The initial doses are usually small and up-titrated every 2 weeks, with the goal of attaining those doses used in clinical trials demonstrating survival benefit and reducing HF hospitalization as recommended below. Approximately 20% of patients will have a nonproductive cough develop, because ACEI prevents the breakdown of bradykinin. When the cough is noted, it is imperative to distinguish the cough of pulmonary congestion (requiring diuretics) from the ACEI-induced cough (which may require the discontinuance of ACEI therapy). Additional adverse effects include hyperkalemia, renal insufficiency, hypotension, angioedema, rash, and dysgeusia. Starting doses of captopril (Capoten) are 6.25 mg 3 times daily (with a goal of 50 mg 3 times daily), enalapril (Vasotec) 2.5 mg twice daily (with a goal of 10 to 20 mg twice daily), and lisinopril (Prinivil) 2.5 to 5 mg once daily (with a goal of 20 to 40 mg daily). Other ACEI may be used for HFpEF as well. Once initiated, the renal function and potassium should be evaluated 1 to 2 weeks later. Increasing the dose of ACEI has no significant effect on survival but clearly decreases hospitalizations.

Angiotensin Receptor Blockers (ARBS)

Notwithstanding the use of ACEI, angiotensin is synthesized via other pathways. The AT1 receptor is the site of the effects of angiotensin II, and thus antagonism of this receptor yields similar survival and hemodynamic benefits in HFrEF as ACEI. Three ARBs have been evaluated in HFrEF: losartan (Cozaar),[1] candesartan (Atacand), and valsartan (Diovan). Valsartan has also been evaluated in patients after myocardial infarction (MI) with LV dysfunction. One trial did not demonstrate superiority of losartan over captopril, and one trial demonstrated noninferiority to captopril. The combination of an ACEI and ARB may be useful in patients with a contraindication to mineralocorticoid receptor antagonists (MRA), and the simultaneous combination of the triad of ACEI, ARB, and MRA is contraindicated because of the risks of hyperkalemia. Use of an ARB is appropriate in those patients with an intolerable ACEI-induced cough. Although the incidence of angioedema is lower in ARBs than ACEI, crossover has been reported. ARBs and ACEI have similar physiological effects resulting in hypotension, renal insufficiency, and hyperkalemia. Like ACEI, the initiation of an ARB requires a follow-up evaluation of renal function and potassium 1 to 2 weeks afterward. The initial dose of losartan is 25 mg daily (with a goal of 150 g daily), valsartan is 40 to 80 mg twice daily (goal of 160 mg twice daily), and candesartan 4 to 8 mg daily (with a goal of 32 mg daily). Doses should be increased to those used in clinical trials demonstrating benefits unless contraindicated or not tolerated.

Angiotensin Receptor–Neprilysin Inhibitors (ARNI)

Neutral endopeptidases deactivate both vasoconstrictor and vasodilatory substances. Deactivation of angiotensin II is beneficial in HFrEF, but the same enzyme system also deactivates beneficial vasodilatory substances such as natriuretic peptides, substance P, and adrenomedullin. Sacubitril is such a neutral endopeptidase inhibitor. Combining sacubitril with an antagonist of the AT1 receptor (ARB) promotes the benefits of vasodilation by antagonizing the degradation of vasodilatory substances while inhibiting the effects of angiotensin II. The combination of valsartan–sacubitril (Entresto) has been evaluated for safety and efficacy and the sacubitril–valsartan combination is superior to ACEI in improving both cardiovascular (CV) and all-cause mortality while decreasing HF hospitalizations. Sacubitril, like ACEI, may precipitate angioedema, and thus the combination of an ACEI with sacubitril-valsartan is contraindicated; thus, the

---

[1] Not FDA approved for this indication.

ACEI must be discontinued when an ARNI is initiated. At least 36 hours must elapse between the last dose of ACEI and the first dose of ARNI to avoid the increased risk of angioedema inherent to simultaneous ACEI and ARNI use. Because both sacubitril and valsartan have vasodilatory properties, the combination may precipitate hypotension. The diuretic dose may be decreased in response to hypotension. The initial dose of sacubitril-valsartan is 24/26 mg twice daily, and up-titration is recommended every 2 to 4 weeks to 49/51 mg twice daily, and finally to the maximum dose of 97/103 mg twice daily. Follow-up evaluation of renal function and potassium is appropriate 1 to 2 weeks after initiation and up-titration of the ARNI. Both cough and angioedema may be seen with ARNI use. Initiation is indicated in those patients who have been on a stable dose of ACEI or ARB for at least 4 weeks with an LVEF of ≤35% to 40% and NYHA class II or III symptoms.

Beta Blockers

Three beta blockers that improve survival are carvedilol (Coreg), bisoprolol (Zebeta),[1] and metoprolol succinate (not metoprolol tartrate) (Loprol XL). They are to be initiated in euvolemic patients and are usually started simultaneously or shortly after initiation of RAS antagonists. Up-titration may proceed by doubling the dose every 2 to 3 weeks once the current dose is well tolerated. The dose should be increased to attain those doses used in clinical trials demonstrated to prolong survival notwithstanding improvement in symptoms and functional class. The initial dose of carvedilol is 3.125 mg twice daily, 12.5 mg/d of metoprolol succinate, and 1.25 mg/d of bisoprolol. The goal dose of carvedilol is 25 mg twice daily (50 mg twice daily for patients weighing >85 kg), 200 mg once daily of metoprolol succinate, and 10 mg bisoprolol once daily. Evidence-based beta blockers are indicated in HFrEF patients irrespective of NYHA functional class.

Mineralocorticoid Receptor Antagonists (MRA)

Both spironolactone (Aldactone) and eplerenone (Inspra) improve survival and decrease HF hospitalizations in HFrEF patients with functional class NYHA 3-4 (spironolactone) and NYHA 2 (eplerenone) when added to a background of ACE and beta blockers. Contraindications include a serum creatinine >2.5 mg/dL in males, >2.0 mg/dL in females, potassium >5.0, or eGFR <30 mL/min/1.73 m². The starting dose is spironolactone 12.5 to 25 mg/d and eplerenone 25 mg/d with up-titration to 25 to 50 mg/d of spironolactone and 50 mg/d of eplerenone if eGFR is ≥50 mL/min/1.73 m². Hyperkalemia is best avoided by monitoring potassium and renal function 3 and 7 days after initiation, then monthly × 3, then every 3 months thereafter. A change in the dose of diuretic, ACEI, or ARB warrants repeating the monitoring cycle. Additionally, eplerenone improved survival in post-MI patients with LVEF ≤40% with either heart failure at presentation or a history of diabetes mellitus (DM). For male patients, breast tenderness or gynecomastia with spironolactone conversion to eplerenone is appropriate. Use of MRA is appropriate in HFrEF patients with LVEF ≤35% and NYHA functional class II to IV symptoms already treated with an RAS antagonist and beta blocker.

Hydralazine and Isosorbide Dinitrate Combination

Although not a substitute for GDMT RAS inhibitors, this combination demonstrated improved survival when compared with placebo and prazosin (Minipress)[1] and may be used in HFrEF patients in whom renal dysfunction, hypotension, or drug intolerance precludes the use of ACEI/ARB/ARNI. Additionally, this combination prolongs survival in self-described African American patients who remain with NYHA 3-4 symptoms despite the use of beta blockers, MRA, and RAS inhibitors. The starting dose of the combination (BiDil) is a single tablet of 37.5 mg hydralazine/20 mg isosorbide dinitrate 3 times daily and increased to 2 tablets 3 times daily.

Digoxin

Digoxin (Lanoxin) has been demonstrated to reduce heart failure hospitalizations in patients with HFrEF and NYHA 2 and 3 symptoms with no significant effect on mortality. It is indicated in HFrEF patients barring contraindications already treated with ACEI/ARB/ARNI, MRA, and beta blocker and who continue to have symptoms or in patients with severe symptoms while GDMT is being up-titrated. The plasma level should be kept between 0.5 to 0.9 ng/mL. There is no indication for a loading dose, and the usual dose is 0.125 mg daily.

Statins

Although statins have antiinflammatory effects and are indicated in primary and secondary prevention of coronary artery disease, there is no indication to use statins solely for heart failure in the absence of other established indications.

Omega-3 Polyunsaturated Fatty Acids (PUFA)

Omega-3 PUFA[7] have salutary effects on inflammation and have been shown to reduce both all-cause mortality and all-cause mortality and CV hospital admissions as per the GISSI-HF trial. Use of one gram daily of omega-3PUFA is reasonable in both HFrEF and HFpEF patients with NYHA class II-IV to reduce mortality and CV hospitalization.

Anticoagulation

Atrial fibrillation, whether paroxysmal, persistent, or permanent, in the presence of heart failure and one other risk factor for thromboembolism, warrants anticoagulation (INR 2-3 if warfarin is used). It is also reasonable to anticoagulate patients with atrial fibrillation and heart failure without other thromboembolic risks. Direct oral anticoagulants (apixaban [Eliquis], rivaroxaban [Xarelto], or dabigatran [Pradaxa]) may be used as a substitute for warfarin. Barring atrial fibrillation, a prior thromboembolic event, or a cardioembolic source, anticoagulation is not indicated in heart failure.

Devices

Implantable cardiodefibrillators (ICD) and cardiac resynchronization (also known as a biventricular pacemaker) therapy have both been demonstrated to improve survival in appropriate patients. In the setting of left bundle branch block, the right ventricle depolarizes first, precipitating desynchrony between septal activation and the left ventricular free wall. This desynchrony results in deterioration of both LV filling and contraction. Cardiac resynchronization therapy (CRT) involves implanting a pacemaker lead in the RV apex and a lead in the coronary sinus positioned near the base of the LV in the posterolateral branch of the coronary vein, allowing simultaneous activation of both ventricles. This pacemaker-induced synchronization may result in restoration of LV volumes, LVEF, and improved functional class and survival. The primary indication for CRT is a LVEF ≤35%, sinus rhythm with a LBBB (QRS width ≥150 msec), NYHA II-ambulatory IV symptoms despite optimized guideline directed therapy. ICD implantation is indicated for primary prevention in those patients with LVEF <35%, NYHA II and III symptoms despite optimized GDMT, at least 40 days after MI or 90 days after revascularization. In patients with a nonischemic cardiomyopathy, treatment with optimal doses of GDMT are required for 3 to 9 months with reassessment of LV function at that time, demonstrating LVEF ≤35% with NYHA II-III symptoms.

Therapy for HFpEF

Neurohormonal antagonists that are effective in improving survival in patients with HFrEF have not been shown to confer the same benefit in HFpEF patients. The current paradigm of HFpEF is that it is the final common pathway of a systemic proinflammatory state associated with comorbidities leading to LV remodeling

---

[7]Available as dietary supplement.

with resulting signs and symptoms. The clinical presentation of patients with HFpEF is remarkably similar to patients with HFrEF, and differentiation of HFpEF and HFrEF cannot be made by history and physical examination alone. There are currently no data supporting survival-prolonging agents in HFpEF. The treatment of HFpEF is thus aimed at symptomatic improvement by optimizing filling pressures while treating comorbidities. The recommended therapy for HFpEF is use of diuretics in the presence of congestion, control of hypertension per guidelines (e.g., reduce the SBP to <130 mm Hg), treatment of atrial fibrillation in accordance with the latest guidelines, revascularization if ischemia is thought to be significantly contributing to heart failure symptoms, and the use of ACEI, ARB, or beta blockers as first-line therapy to control hypertension. Two agents that appear to decrease HF hospitalizations are candesartan (Atacand) and spironolactone (Aldactone).

Advanced Therapies

For patients with end-stage heart failure, two options exist. The first option is mechanical circulatory support such as a left ventricular assist device or orthotopic heart transplantation. Mechanical circulatory support may be used as a bridge to transplant (bridge to transplantation therapy) or to be used indefinitely in patients ineligible for transplantation (destination therapy). Mechanical circulatory support may also serve as a temporary device in those patients with hemodynamic compromise due to a reversible cause while awaiting myocardial recovery. Transplantation is the final option for patients with end-stage heart failure who have failed to respond or deteriorated despite optimal GDMT, device/surgical/catheter-based therapies barring contraindications.

References

Inamdar AA, Inamdar AC: Heart failure: diagnosis, management and utilization, *J Clin Med* 5(7):62, 2016.
Jackson G, Gibbs CR, Davies MK, et al: ABC of heart failure: pathophysiology, *BMJ* 320(7228):167–170, 2000.
Mann D: *Braunwald's heart disease*, ed 11, Philadelphia, 2015, Elsevier.
McKee PA, Castelli WP, McNamara PM, et al: The natural history of congestive heart failure: the Framingham Study, *N Engl J Med* 285:1441–1446, 1971.
Tavazzi L, Maggioni AP, Marchioli R, et al: Effect of n-3 polyunsaturated fatty acids in patients with chronic heart failure (the GISSI-HF trial): a randomised, double-blind, placebo-controlled trial, *Lancet* 372(9645):1223–1230, 2008.
Yancy CW, Jessup M, Bozkurt B, et al: ACC/AHA/HFSA Focused Update on New Pharmacological Therapy for Heart Failure: An Update of the 2013 ACCF/AHA Guideline for the Management of Heart Failure: A Report of the American College of Cardiology/American Heart Association Task Force on Clinical Practice Guidelines and the Heart Failure Society of America, *Circulation* 134:e282–e293, 2016.
Yancy CW, Jessup M, Bozkurt B, et al: ACCF/AHA Guideline for the Management of Heart Failure. A Report of the American College of Cardiology Foundation/American Heart Association Task Force on Practice Guidelines, *Circulation* 128:e240–e327, 2013.

HEART BLOCK

Method of
Kelley P. Anderson, MD

CURRENT DIAGNOSIS

- Assess risk for heart block in the absence of symptoms or heart block on electrocardiogram (ECG).
  - Review cardiac or systemic disorders associated with cardiac conduction disease (CCD), ECG pattern, family history, maternal antibodies, cardiac interventions, and surgery.
- Evaluate documented asystole or bradycardia due to heart block.
  - Classify heart block: transient, recurrent, progressive, permanent.
  - Grade signs and symptoms: none, mild, severe.
- Evaluate signs or symptoms of possible transient heart block with no documentation.
  - Establish temporal pattern: recent versus remote onset, solitary versus recurrent, daily, weekly, monthly, yearly.
  - Grade signs and symptoms: none, mild, severe.
  - Document rhythm during symptoms: telemetry monitoring, Holter monitor, external loop recorder, implantable recorder.

CURRENT THERAPY

- Methods of heart rate support:
  - Immediate: intravenous catecholamines, atropine, or aminophylline[1]; transcutaneous pacing
  - Short term: transvenous temporary pacing
  - Long term: permanent pacemakers
- Pacemaker configuration:
  - Number of leads: 1, 2, 3, 4
  - Lead locations: right atrial appendage, Bachman's bundle, right ventricular apex, outflow tract, left ventricle, coronary sinus
  - Programming to minimize ventricular pacing: manufacturer dependent

[1]Not FDA approved for this indication.

Heart block refers to block or delay of electrical propagation between the atria and ventricles. It is a form of cardiac conduction disease (CCD), which applies more generally to disorders of electrical impulse formation or propagation anywhere along the cardiac conduction system from the sinus node to the ventricular myocardium. Heart block or CCD may present as a syndrome, as an electrocardiographic (ECG) pattern, or as a mechanism of serious signs and symptoms such as sudden death or syncope. Pacemaker therapy is an effective treatment, but it is associated with significant short- and long-term complications. This underscores the importance of recognizing preventable and reversible causes of heart block for accurate targeting of permanent pacing. Risk stratification of patients with heart block, assessment of the benefits and risks of the therapeutic options, and patient education and guidance are largely in the domain of heart rhythm specialists. However, heart block may be encountered unexpectedly in any patient during any clinical encounter. Furthermore, some patients may require evaluation in the absence of known cardiac disease because of increased risk of CCD, or increased risk of CCD in family members or future children. A basic understanding of heart block may be useful to initiate emergency treatment and to recognize patients who warrant further evaluation or specialist referral.

Epidemiology

The prevalence and incidence of heart block are difficult to establish because they are strongly dependent on the demographic and clinical characteristics of the population sample. The prevalence is higher among the elderly and those with cardiovascular disease. First-degree heart block, defined as prolongation of the PR interval >200 ms on ECG, occurs in the population setting with prevalence of 0.7% to 2% in the young and up to 14% in the elderly. Higher degrees of heart block can be expected to be less common but similarly associated with age and underlying cardiovascular disease. In a study of the Framingham population, the prevalence of first-degree heart block was 1.6% and was associated with an incidence of pacemaker implantation of 59 per 10,000 person-years in persons with a PR interval >200 ms compared to 6 per 10,000 person-years in persons with a PR interval <200 ms. Approximately 36% of the pacemakers were for high-grade atrioventricular (AV) block.

Risk Factors

Patients with genetic or acquired CCD and patients subject to trauma or surgical procedures that can damage the conduction system are at increased risk for developing symptomatic advanced heart block. In the Framingham population, subjects with first-degree AV block had an increased risk of mortality, atrial fibrillation, and pacemaker implantation. However, the vast majority with risk factors never develop symptomatic heart block and have not been shown to benefit from intense monitoring or prophylactic pacemaker placement. The few possible exceptions are discussed below.

Pathophysiology

The function of the cardiac conduction system is to initiate and coordinate cardiac contraction to circulate blood according to physiological needs. Electrical activation is initiated by pacemaker cells of the sinus node regulated by the autonomic nervous system. Unlike conduction in common electrical circuits in which electrons flow along a conductor according to the voltage gradient, electrical activity in cardiac cells propagates from segment to segment of the cell membrane in cardiac myocytes (myocardial cells) and in specialized cardiac conduction cells. Energy-requiring ion pumps maintain an electrochemical gradient across the insulating cell membrane. Electrical activity opens voltage-sensitive ion channels causing regenerative electrical activity as ions shift along their electrochemical gradient. Electrical activity in a single cell excites several adjacent cells via gap junctions. This cascade effect makes it possible for a single cell impulse to spread rapidly throughout the myocardium to enhance synchronous contraction. This also provides a safety mechanism in that each myocardial cell can be activated by many electrical paths. In addition, specialized conduction cells exhibit automaticity (impulse formation). Although normally latent because normal activation inhibits spontaneous discharge, when the normal impulse is blocked, discharges from these subsidiary physiological pacemakers provide vital heart rate support.

Block of electrical activation can occur due to failure of any step in the process, for example, lack of metabolic energy, electrolyte imbalance, inflammatory disruption of the membrane, block of ion channels by drugs, or interference with gap junction function due to infiltration of fibrous tissue (Table 1). Because of the extensive redundancy and interconnectivity and because of the capacity to compensate for injury by electrical and anatomic remodeling, there may be extensive damage before signs or symptoms of heart block occur. Regions of the heart where there are fewer alternative paths for electrical activation, such as proximal portions of the His-Purkinje system where all conducting fibers are confined to a relatively small area, are more vulnerable to complete block. Subsidiary pacemakers sometimes fail to provide adequate rate support when heart block occurs because of preexisting injury.

If the patient survives an episode of heart block, there is a possibility for recovery due to remodeling. However, remodeling can be maladaptive and result in an adverse long-term outcome by further conduction system damage, by left ventricular dysfunction, and by bradycardia-induced ventricular tachyarrhythmias (VTAs). The mechanisms of bradycardia-induced VTAs are not known, but bradyarrhythmias precipitate torsades de pointes, a specific form of VTA, in the presence of drugs that block potassium channels, electrolyte disturbances, certain genetic abnormalities of ion channel function, heart failure, and myocardial hypertrophy. A comprehensive list of drugs that may account for bradyarrhythmia-related ventricular arrhythmias is available at www.torsades.org.

Although there are many potential causes of heart block, the pathophysiology is not known for the vast majority of cases because there are no tests that allow detailed structural or functional examination in patients. By the time of death, morphologic examination may reveal only nonspecific changes such as fibrosis. Instead, most etiologies are inferred by history of recent or past exposures (e.g., trauma or radiation), concomitant disorders (e.g., muscular dystrophy, cardiac sarcoidosis), abnormal test results (e.g., Lyme disease) or family history (e.g., SCN5A sodium channel mutations) (Table 2). Because most etiologies cannot be verified, the clinician must remain open to alternative explanations and accept the likelihood of multiple contributors.

Some patients, usually young, otherwise healthy individuals, present with prolonged asystole due to heart block but have no other detectable abnormalities and have excellent outcomes in the absence of intervention beyond counseling. This suggests that autonomic influences alone can cause prolonged heart block and suppression of subsidiary pacemakers. It is not known whether such responses result from an abnormality or an exaggerated normal reflex. However, the identification of such patients is important because most can be managed without pacemakers.

TABLE 1	Mechanisms of Conduction Disturbances (Examples)

- Prolonged refractory period (vagal activity, drugs, ischemia)
- Sarcolemmal ion gradient disturbances (hyperkalemia, hypokalemia)
- Sodium channel dysfunction (SCN5A mutations, sodium channel blocking drugs such as lidocaine, procainamide, flecainide [Tambocor], amiodarone [Cordarone], and imipramine [Tofranil])
- Calcium channel dysfunction (verapamil [Isoptin], diltiazem [Cardizem], mutations)
- Energy deprivation (ischemia, cyanide)
- Cell dysfunction (inflammation, barotrauma, thermal injury)
- Cell death (apoptosis, ischemic necrosis, inflammatory necrosis, surgical trauma, ablation)
- Congenital structural defects (endocardial cushion defects)
- Gap junction disturbances (fibrosis, edema, inflammation, genetic defects)
- Genetic defects (SCN5A and NKX2.5 mutations)

TABLE 2	Etiologies of Heart Block

- Frequently permanent or progressive (examples)
  - Alcohol septal ablation (acute, delayed)
  - Cardiomyopathies (hypertrophic, idiopathic, mitochondrial)
  - Catheter ablation (atrioventricular nodal reentry, accessory atrioventricular connections)
  - Congenital heart block (neonatal lupus)
  - Congenital heart disease (endocardial cushion defects)
  - Genetic disorders (SCN5A sodium channel mutations, gap junction gene mutations, fatty acid oxidation disorders, PRKAG2 mutations, LMNA gene mutations)
  - Hypertension
  - Idiopathic fibrosis and calcification (Lev's disease, Lenegre's disease)
  - Infectious disorders—destructive (endocarditis)
  - Infiltrative disorders (amyloidosis)
  - Myocardial infarction
  - Neuromyopathic disorders (myotonic dystrophy, Erb's dystrophy, peroneal muscular atrophy)
  - Noninfectious inflammatory disorders (HLA-B27–associated disorder, sarcoidosis)
  - Tumors (mesothelioma, metastatic cancer)
  - Valvular heart disease
- Frequently transient or reversible (examples)
  - Blunt trauma (baseball)
  - Cardiac surgery (valve replacement)
  - Cardiac transplant rejection
  - Central nervous system
  - Drugs (antiarrhythmics, digoxin [Lanoxin], edrophonium [Enlon])
  - Electrolyte disturbances (hyperkalemia)
  - Metabolic disturbances (hypothermia, hypothyroidism)
  - Increased vagal activity
  - Infectious disorders—nondestructive (Lyme disease)
  - Myocardial ischemia
  - Myocarditis (Chagas disease, giant cell myocarditis)
  - Rheumatic fever

Prevention

Prevention of heart block is a challenge for the future. Some instances can be prevented by treatment of inflammatory disorders that cause heart block, such as Lyme disease or cardiac sarcoid. Other individuals who should be identified are those with conditions that place them, their relatives, or their unborn children at risk for heart block. This includes patients and family members with genetic disorders associated with heart block. Genetic testing and counseling may be appropriate in some patients with a family history of CCD. Neonatal lupus syndrome is a rare disorder with a high mortality rate and risk of permanent complete heart block in survivors. This occurs in pregnant women with anti-Ro/SSA or anti-La/SSB antibodies. Some such women have autoimmune disorders such as systemic lupus erythematosus and Sjögren's syndrome, but many are symptom free. Members of this group may benefit from counseling and anticipatory evaluation and treatment of offspring. Although controversial, fetal monitoring of pregnant women with anti-Ro/SSA and/or anti-La/SSB antibodies and treatment of those with signs of fetal conduction system involvement have been recommended. It should be recognized that with current methods the vast majority of heart block events cannot be predicted or prevented, and the vast majority of persons with risk factors never develop symptomatic heart block.

Clinical Manifestations

Most of the symptoms experienced by patients with heart block are common and nonspecific, including syncope, lightheadedness, fatigue, and dyspnea. Asystole or profound bradycardia may cause syncope, death, or other manifestations of hypoperfusion. Rarely, first-degree AV block results in significant symptoms (e.g., fatigue, palpitations, chest fullness), probably due to atrial contraction against a partially closed mitral valve.

Diagnosis

Because various arrhythmias and other cardiac and noncardiac disorders may be responsible for similar symptoms, it is important to identify the cause. An ECG recording of asystole or bradycardia due to heart block at the time of symptoms strongly suggests a causal relationship, but this is usually difficult to accomplish because the symptoms are often transient and infrequent. Absence of arrhythmias at the time of symptoms is also helpful in excluding heart block as the cause. Asymptomatic heart block is not infrequent. Cardiac conduction disturbances are classified by the pattern of ECG complexes. A normal 12-lead ECG lessens the probability of conduction disturbances due to structural changes but it does not eliminate the possibility of transient third-degree block due to reversible functional effects such as intense vagal activity or ischemia. Significant disease of the His bundle may be electrocardiographically silent, but more often concomitant distal disease is evident in the form of fascicular or bundle branch block or a nonspecific intraventricular conduction delay. In a patient with syncope, the presence of bifascicular block raises the possibility of transient third-degree block as the mechanism and of progression to permanent complete block. Most patients with conduction disorders are not symptomatic and do not progress to complete block. However, the combination of right bundle branch block (RBBB) and left posterior fascicle block has a greater tendency to progress to complete block than the more common RBBB and left anterior fascicle block. Nevertheless, conduction disturbances of the His-Purkinje system should not be assumed to be responsible for syncope or cardiac arrest because they are relatively common in patients with cardiovascular disorders that cause syncope or cardiac arrest due to other mechanisms. Conduction disturbances can cause dyssynchronous contraction and result in adverse remodeling. In addition, they can mask or mimic the ECG signs of myocardial infarction. Alternating bundle branch block refers to a changing ECG pattern in which both RBBB and left bundle branch block are observed or when the bifascicular block pattern switches between the anterior and posterior fascicle involvement. This pattern is considered a harbinger of complete block and warrants continuous monitoring and evaluation for permanent pacemaker implantation.

Differential Diagnosis

The challenge in second- and transient third-degree AV block is distinguishing between block in the AV node, which is often functional and reversible, and infranodal block, which often progresses to permanent complete heart block. ECG clues that block is in the AV node include normal QRS duration (<100 ms), type I (Wenckebach) pattern, PR prolongation before blocked impulses and PR shortening after pauses, occurrence during enhanced vagal activity (e.g., sleep), narrow QRS escape complexes, and no factors favoring infranodal block. ECG clues for infranodal block include prolonged QRS duration (≥120 ms), type II pattern, and escape QRS complexes broader than intrinsic complexes. Type II second degree AV block is almost always due to block in the His-Purkinje system. Other second-degree AV block ECG patterns have poor sensitivity and specificity for site of block.

Unsustained polymorphic ventricular tachycardia is an ominous sign in any context and may result from a variety of cardiac, metabolic, and autonomic abnormalities. However, in the presence of heart block it suggests that heart rate support may be necessary to prevent sustained VTA. QT prolongation and postpause U-wave accentuation should be sought as other harbingers of bradycardia-related VTA.

The importance and value of ECG documentation of heart block cannot be overemphasized. ECGs are subject to artifact and may be misleading when standards for acquisition and analysis are not followed. Multiple tracings of suspicious events should be obtained in multiple leads when possible. A 12-lead simultaneous rhythm recording mode is available on most modern ECG machines and should be used when continuous recordings are obtained to document arrhythmias.

Clinicians encounter heart block in three general contexts. For the patient with documented heart block, the clinician selects therapy based, in part, on whether the arrhythmia is permanent or likely to recur. There are currently no tests that provide direct information about the pathologic state of the AV conduction system. Instead, these outcomes must be inferred from functional assessment, that is, from the ECG or electrophysiological testing. Other indirect sources such as coronary angiography, magnetic resonance imaging, nuclear imaging, and myocardial biopsy, as well as a large number of specific laboratory tests, are often helpful for identifying disorders that may be causative or associated with heart block and that may affect the choice of treatment.

Another common context is the patient with symptoms for whom the objective is to verify or exclude heart block as the mechanism by correlating the cardiac rhythm with symptoms. Real-time monitoring (e.g., in-patient telemetry) is used for patients who might require immediate access to drugs or pacing devices to prevent or terminate asystole or bradycardia-dependent VTA. Holter monitoring is useful for patients who have very frequent events (at least 1 every 24 hours), and they are useful for capturing asymptomatic rhythm disturbances. External recorders are applied for a month or longer and are very helpful to associate rhythm abnormalities with symptoms and to rule out a rhythm disorder as the cause of symptoms in patients with at least one event per month. Patients with infrequent events may be candidates for implantable loop recorders, which monitor for greater than a year. Modern monitors will provide a permanent record of arrhythmias on activation by the patient or by a detection algorithm.

Electrophysiological studies allow precise measurements of AV node and His-Purkinje system function and can provide definitive information regarding the site of block if the conduction disturbance occurs during the study. Additional tests have been developed that "stress" the AV conduction system, including rapid atrial and ventricular pacing and administration of drugs such as procainamide and disopyramide (Norpace). The provocation of heart block is assumed to indicate a propensity for spontaneous AV block. Unfortunately, the sensitivity is low and a negative test does not imply a low risk of future episodes. Electrophysiological studies have the additional advantage of providing immediate test results, as well as providing the results of programmed stimulation for provocation of supraventricular and VTAs, which may be included in the differential diagnosis.

Therapy

The object of the evaluation and management for heart block is to prevent death and morbidity by (1) heart rate support in patients with poorly tolerated bradycardia; (2) monitoring and standby heart rate support in patients at high risk for asystole or severe bradycardia; (3) identifying and treating reversible causes of heart block; (4) identifying patients at high risk for sudden death, syncope, or recurrent symptoms; and (5) selecting and implanting the appropriate rate support system as soon as safety permits.

Advanced cardiac life-support guidelines apply to the patient who is unresponsive or severely compromised by heart block. However, heart block is rarely the primary problem. Therefore evaluation and treatment of other disorders should continue while efforts to obtain the appropriate heart rate are underway.

The initial evaluation should include a detailed history and physical examination and review of current and previous ECGs and rhythm strips to determine whether heart block is present or occurred in the past and whether there were symptoms or other evidence of hemodynamic compromise. Basic laboratory tests (electrolytes, metabolic panel, cardiac biomarkers, thyroid function, blood count, and coagulation studies) and basic imaging (chest x-ray and echocardiography) are usually appropriate. The patient should then be stratified for the appropriate level of care: (1) the unstable patient who requires ongoing evaluation and treatment in an intensive care setting, (2) the stable patient at high risk for asystole or complications who needs temporary transvenous pacing or other invasive procedures, (3) the patient at moderate risk who requires continuous monitoring and standby noninvasive heart rate support measures, (4) the patient at low risk who requires rapid but not immediate access to heart rate support measures that hospital monitoring provides, and (5) the patient at low risk who can be evaluated and managed as an outpatient. Additional testing and procedures may be necessary to determine the etiology of heart block and to determine whether there is a significant risk of future adverse events.

Determination of the need for long-term heart rate support, as well as other issues that may affect implantable device selection (e.g., risk for VTAs), should be accomplished as soon as possible because the risk of complications and anxiety associated with temporary heart rate support measures increases over time. Major societies have developed guidelines for implantable rhythm management devices (http://www.cardiosource.org/Science-And-Quality/Practice-Guidelines-and-Quality-Standards.aspx; http://www.escardio.org/guidelines-surveys/esc-guidelines/Pages/GuidelinesList.aspx). The reasons for the selected therapy, including the rationale for any deviation from established guidelines, should be documented and provided to the patient. This will reduce future confusion or misunderstanding about the original rationale for implantation that can affect management of patients with device complications, recalls (safety alerts), and those with a compelling need for device upgrade or explantation.

Patients with acute coronary syndromes require special consideration. The incidence of heart block in patients with myocardial infarction based on creatine phosphokinase as the marker of necrosis is approximately 10%. Although the incidence is probably lower using more sensitive markers such as troponin, heart block is still likely to be associated with increased in-hospital mortality due to larger infarct size. Tachycardia and high blood pressure increase myocardial oxygen consumption. Therefore overcorrection of heart rate and blood pressure should be avoided and ischemia should be relieved by reperfusion as soon as possible. Studies in the prethrombolytic era did not demonstrate a benefit in mortality with prophylactic temporary transvenous pacing, and complications were frequent. The risks of transvenous insertion may be higher in patients requiring administration

TABLE 3	Suggestions for Temporary Pacing in Acute Myocardial Infarction

- Transvenous pacing
  - Asystole or poorly tolerated bradycardia unresponsive to atropine or aminophylline
  - Persistent third-degree AV block
  - Alternating RBBB and LBBB, or RBBB and alternating LAFB and LPFB
  - Bifascicular block, new
  - Second-degree AV block (any type) and QRS >110 ms
  - Any indication listed below at time of cardiac catheterization if performed
- Standby transcutaneous pacing
  - Any indication listed above until transvenous pacing system inserted
  - Transient asystole or poorly tolerated bradycardia
  - Bifascicular block, uncertain time of onset, or old
  - Second-degree AV block (any type) and QRS <110 ms
  - New first-degree AV block

Abbreviations: AV = atrioventricular; LAFB, LPFB=left anterior, left posterior fascicle block; LBBB, RBBB=left, right bundle branch block.

of thrombolytics and other anticoagulants. Catheter-based revascularization methods should be given strong consideration because of established effectiveness, the possible avoidance of thrombolytic drugs, and because transvenous temporary pacing, if needed, is readily and safely accomplished during the procedure. Suggestions for standby temporary pacing (Table 3) should take into consideration the risks of transvenous pacing based on local circumstances (experience, fluoroscopic guidance, insertion site, use of anticoagulants, etc.). Most conduction disturbances associated with myocardial ischemia or infarction resolve quickly but can persist for days or weeks. The need for permanent pacemaker implantation as a consequence of myocardial infarction is rare, and prophylactic pacemaker implantation in high-risk subsets has not been shown to reduce mortality. Guidelines for temporary and permanent pacing in acute myocardial infarction have been published (http://www.cardiosource.org/Science-And-Quality/Practice-Guidelines-and-Quality-Standards.aspx; http://www.escardio.org/guidelines-surveys/esc-guidelines/Pages/GuidelinesList.aspx).

Selection of the correct therapeutic approach balances the risks and benefits of therapy against the risks of heart block for both immediate and long-term management. Catecholamines (dobutamine, dopamine, epinephrine, isoproterenol [Isuprel]) are useful for emergency, temporary, and standby heart rate support. The standby mode is accomplished by a prepared infusion at the bedside. To avoid underdoses or overdoses at the time of sudden symptomatic heart block, the optimal dose can be established in advance by test doses starting at low infusion rates. Atropine (0.5 mg every 3–5 minutes, with a maximum dose of 0.04 mg/kg or total of 3 mg) may be useful for treatment or pretreatment of patients who develop heart block at the level of the AV node in the context of elevated vagal tone (e.g., in association with nausea or endotracheal tube suction). Atropine should be avoided in patients with infranodal AV block because prolonged asystole sometimes occurs due to more frequent His-Purkinje system depolarization from increased sinus rate. Vagal activity inhibits sympathetic activity; therefore, reduction of vagal tone by atropine disinhibits sympathetic activity and may account for the unpredictable effects of atropine on heart rate. Elevations in heart rate after atropine can persist for hours and cannot be readily reversed. Aminophylline[1](2.5–6.3 mg/kg IV) is reported to reverse heart block resistant to atropine and epinephrine by antagonizing adenosine. Stimulation of β-adrenergic receptors increases sinus node and subsidiary pacemaker rates, AV node and His-Purkinje system conduction velocities, and myocardial contractility. The

---

[1] Not FDA approved for this indication.

effective refractory period shortens in most tissue but this effect varies with dose and specific tissue type. Dobutamine[1] (2–40 μg/kg/min) is a useful β-receptor agonist because it increases cardiac output and lowers filling pressures without excessive rise or fall of blood pressure. Dopamine[1] (2–20 μg/kg/min IV) stimulates β1-adrenergic receptors and increases heart rate by enhancing impulse formation and conduction, as well as myocardial contractility. At higher doses (10–20 μg/kg/min) dopamine causes vasoconstriction by α1-receptor stimulation. Isoproterenol (0.02–0.06 mg IV bolus, 0.5–10.0 μg/min IV infusion) stimulates β1- and β2-adrenergic receptors and enhances vasodilation more than the other catecholamines. This can result in unwanted hypotension in some circumstances but it is also less likely to cause a reflex increase in vagal tone than drugs that cause vasoconstriction. Epinephrine (1 mg IV boluses for cardiac arrest, 0.2–1 mg subcutaneously, 0.5–10 μg/min IV) stimulates both α- and β-adrenergic receptors. It is recommended for asystolic cardiac arrest in part because it increases myocardial and cerebral flow. However, the increase of systemic vascular resistance may be detrimental by augmenting metabolic acidosis and decreasing cardiac performance in patients with poor left ventricular function. The suggested dose ranges are broad because the response to β-adrenergic stimulants such as improved AV conduction varies widely and may be affected by β-adrenergic receptor down-regulation in patients with chronic elevations in sympathetic activity such as patients with long-standing heart failure.

Temporary pacing includes primarily transcutaneous and transvenous approaches. Transthoracic, transesophageal, and transgastric approaches are rarely used. Transcutaneous pacing provides noninvasive heart rate support, as well as immediate access to countershock, but it is often so painful that most patients require sedation. For these reasons its principal uses are for short-term pacing during cardiopulmonary resuscitation and standby pacing in patients at risk for bradyarrhythmias. Capture is not achieved in some patients. Therefore users should be ready to continue mechanical cardiopulmonary support and seek alternative methods. If used in standby applications, ventricular capture should be verified in advance. Capture is often difficult to ascertain because transcutaneous stimuli cause large deflections on the ECG, and pectoral muscle stimulation can be confused with a pulse. Capture should be verified by careful ECG analysis at subthreshold and suprathreshold stimulus amplitudes and confirmed by appropriately timed femoral artery pulses, Korotkoff sounds, or arterial pressure waveforms.

Transvenous insertion of an electrode catheter is the method of choice for most patients who require temporary pacing. This approach is reliable and safe when performed by competent staff with strict aseptic technique, fluoroscopic guidance, and appropriate catheters. Small studies suggest that long-term (>5 days) temporary pacing can be accomplished with active-fixation permanent pacemaker leads attached to an external pulse generator (not approved by the US Food and Drug Administration [FDA]). Tunneling the lead may enhance stability and reduce the risk of infection.

Monitoring
Patients with high-grade or symptomatic heart block require close monitoring until the process is reversed by treatment or a pacemaker is implanted. All patients who receive pacemakers require lifelong follow-up by a trained team of physicians, nurses, and ancillary personnel using standard procedures guided by practice guidelines and manufacturer recommendations.

Complications
Catecholamines used to increase heart rate may precipitate tachyarrhythmias by electrophysiological effects mediated by adrenergic receptors or by myocardial ischemia, and they may worsen hemodynamic status. The adverse effects of catecholamines increase with duration of exposure. Ischemia and receptor-mediated electrophysiologic effects occur immediately after administration; changes in gene expression of ion channels begin as early as several hours; and long-term changes such as myocardial hypertrophy, apoptosis, and fibrosis occur within 24 hours and may progress over much longer periods. This suggests that the duration and dose of catecholamine infusions should be minimized. Complications of temporary transvenous pacing include inadequate pacing or sensing thresholds, vascular complications, pneumothorax, myocardial perforation, infection, and dislodgment. Permanent pacemakers are highly effective, safe, and cost-effective with few contraindications. Although the complications are rarely life threatening, they should be carefully considered and acknowledged. Septicemia or endocarditis has been reported in 0.5% of patients. In patients with pacemaker-related endocarditis, the in-hospital mortality rate is reported to be over 7% with a 20-month mortality rate over 25%. The rate of significant complications has been reported to be 3.5%. About 10% of pacemakers will become infected or develop some other type of failure that may require extraction. In a recent series the rate of major complications associated with extraction was 1.4%. There is a long-term continuous risk of infection, thrombosis, and erosion. In young persons there is a periodic need to replace generators and leads. Abandoned leads block venous access and extractions are associated with significant risks. Perhaps of greater consequence is the constant inconvenience of lifelong follow-up, electromagnetic interference, and false alarms from electronic surveillance devices, as well as exclusion from important procedures, such as magnetic resonance imaging of the thorax. Conventional pacing, that is, from the right ventricular apex, is now known to be detrimental and may cause adverse ventricular remodeling, atrial fibrillation, heart failure, and premature death. Although it has been shown that patients with reduced left ventricular function are at greater risk for adverse effects, it is not known how to identify other patients at risk. Strategies for reducing the adverse effects of conventional pacing are under study, and recommendations are evolving. Because the decision for pacemaker implantation includes selection of lead configuration, lead locations, and pacing mode, patient guidance and education are complex.

Conclusions
Heart block remains a challenge because the cellular mechanisms responsible are poorly understood, prediction of symptomatic heart block (who and when) is unreliable, treatments that restore normal conduction do not exist for most conditions, and pacemaker therapy can have significant long-term adverse consequences. Fortunately, current devices and leads are much more reliable than in the past, and remote monitoring has enhanced early detection of problems and has substantially reduced the inconvenience of device monitoring. The newest generation of devices will allow many patients with pacemakers to safely undergo magnetic resonance imaging. Ongoing clinical trials will provide guidance in pacemaker configurations and programming that will minimize adverse effects. In the future, achievements in molecular biology will elucidate mechanisms and produce treatments that will relegate artificial pacemakers to museum pieces.

References
Ackerman MJ, Priori SG, Willems S, et al: HRS/EHRA expert consensus statement on the state of genetic testing for the channelopathies and cardiomyopathies, *Europace* 13:1077, 2011.

Carvalheiras G, Faria R, Braga J, et al: Fetal outcome in autoimmune diseases, *Autoimmun Rev* 11:A520, 2012.

Cheng S, Keyes MJ, Larson MG, et al: Long-term outcomes in individuals with prolonged PR interval or first-degree atrioventricular block, *JAMA* 301:2571, 2009.

Epstein AE, DiMarco JP, Ellenbogen KA, et al: ACC/AHA/HRS 2008 guidelines for device-based therapy of cardiac rhythm abnormalities, *J Am Coll Cardiol* 51:e1, 2008.

Hazinski MF, Samson R, Schexnayder S: Handbook of emergency cardiovascular care for healthcare providers, Dallas, TX: American Heart Association; 2010.

Smits JPP, Velkkamp MW, Wilde AAM: Mechanisms of inherited cardiac conduction disease, *Europace* 7:122, 2005.

Vardas PE, Auriccho A, Blanc JJ, et al: Guidelines for cardiac pacing and cardiac resynchronization therapy, *Eur Heart J* 28:2256, 2007.

HYPERTENSION

Method of
Timothy P. Graham, MD

CURRENT DIAGNOSIS

- Identification of individuals with hypertension is the first step.
- Screening should begin at 18 years of age for the general population.
- Adults with risk factors should be screened annually beginning at 40 years of age.
- Stage 1 hypertension is established at blood pressures of 140 mm Hg systolic and 90 mm Hg diastolic.
- Stage 2 hypertension is established at blood pressures of 160 mm Hg systolic and 100 mm Hg diastolic.
- Secondary causes of hypertension should be explored and identified to optimize treatment.

CURRENT THERAPY

- Initial interventions, regardless of stage, should include lifestyle modifications, including diet and exercise.
- Optimal pharmacologic therapy should be tailored to take into account age, race, and the presence or absence of chronic kidney disease.
- For individuals 60 years of age or older, consider initiation of pharmacotherapy when systolic blood pressure is 150 mm Hg and diastolic blood pressure is 90 mm Hg.
- For individuals younger than 60 years of age but at least 18 years of age, pharmacotherapy should be initiated when systolic blood pressure is 140 mm Hg and diastolic blood pressure is 90 mm Hg.
- First-line agents for nonblack individuals should include thiazide-type diuretics, calcium channel blockers, angiotensin-converting enzyme inhibitors, or angiotensin receptor blockers.
- First-line agents for black individuals should include thiazide-type diuretics or calcium channel blockers.
- Individuals with chronic kidney disease should have therapy that includes angiotensin-converting enzyme inhibitors or angiotensin receptor blockers.

Epidemiology

Hypertension is one of the most common conditions encountered in primary care offices. It affects 33% of individuals over the age of 20 in the United States, which translates to more than 78 million Americans. The most commonly affected individuals are black adults, making up 44% of the total.

In the pediatric population the prevalence of hypertension in the United States is between 1% and 5%, with obese children having the highest prevalence at 11%.

Risk Factors

Diet and Sodium Intake

Diet is a clear target for nonpharmacologic management of hypertension. Diets that are high in sodium and fat can put individuals at risk for suboptimal blood pressure control. Limiting sodium to less than 2400 mg per day confers some health benefit to individuals at risk for hypertension. Limiting even further to 1500 mg or less is more ideal and results in a significant improvement in both systolic and diastolic blood pressure typically. Additionally, putting limits on the consumption of sweets, red meat, and soda, as well as other sugar-sweetened beverages, can help weight reduction and overall health.

Sedentary Lifestyle and Obesity

Lack of physical activity is another important risk factor contributing to poor overall health and obesity. Current recommendations endorse engaging in at least 150 minutes of moderate-intensity activity per week. If patients are unable or unwilling to commit to that level of physical activity, then encouraging any physical activity is prudent, as it will convey at least some health benefit. Participation in physical activity results in absolute reduction in chronic comorbidities including hypertension, stroke, heart disease, diabetes, and metabolic syndrome. Resultant weight loss also results in significant improvement in blood pressure. It is noted that a weight loss of 22 pounds has the potential to reduce systolic blood pressure by 5 to 20 mm Hg.

For children and adolescents, elevated body mass index is the greatest risk factor for the development of hypertension.

Alcohol Intake

Although moderate alcohol intake is thought to actually reduce cardiovascular risk, heavier consumption is a risk factor for hypertension. Limiting alcohol intake to no more than two drinks per day (with "drink" defined as 12 oz. of beer, 5 oz. of wine, or 1 oz. of liquor) for men and no more than one drink per day for women (or lightweight men) is beneficial for overall health.

Smoking

Along with the myriad other reasons that smoking is not a good choice (cancer risk, chronic obstructive pulmonary disease, stroke, coronary artery disease, etc.), it is also a risk factor for hypertension. This is believed to be at least in part due to a resultant increase in sympathetic nervous system activity, which leads to an increase in myocardial oxygen demand. Additionally, smoking is the leading modifiable cause of death in the United States.

Sleep Apnea

Obstructive sleep apnea is a well-known secondary cause of and independent risk factor for hypertension. Statistically, at least half of individuals with sleep apnea also have hypertension.

Age

Age is a nonmodifiable risk factor for cardiovascular disease. Risk is higher in men 55 years of age or older and women 65 years of age or older.

Gender

Gender is another nonmodifiable risk factor. Men are at greater risk for hypertension prior to age 45. After age 45 and until age 64, the risk for men and women is approximately equivalent. At 65 years of age or older, women have a higher hypertensive risk than men.

Race

Black individuals have a higher risk of hypertension than nonblack individuals. Statistics from 2015 demonstrated that in the general population aged 18 and older, approximately 34% of black individuals had hypertension, compared to approximately 24% of white individuals. Native Americans had a slightly higher risk than white individuals at 28%, and Asians had the lowest prevalence at approximately 20%. Hispanic/Latino individuals had a slightly lower prevalence than white individuals at 23%.

Family History

Family history is another nonmodifiable risk factor for cardiovascular disease. Individuals with family history of premature cardiovascular disease (men younger than 45 years of age and women younger than 55 years of age) are at increased risk themselves.

Pathophysiology

The pathophysiology of hypertension is a matter of debate. Essential hypertension, which is defined as hypertension without a clear secondary cause, makes up the majority of cases. Two primary mechanisms have been proposed for essential hypertension: neurogenic and renogenic (or nephrogenic). The neurogenic model suggests that hypertension is the result of a chronic increase in sympathetic nervous system activity. This is in contrast to the renogenic model, which attributes blood pressure increase to renal origins either through decreased renal blood flow or through renal parenchymal disease.

Prevention

Prevention of hypertension involves optimization of modifiable risk factors. Maintaining a healthy body weight, avoiding smoking, and moderating alcohol use are all key factors in minimizing risk. Additionally, engaging in regular, moderate-intensity cardiovascular exercise and eating a healthy diet without excessive sodium or fat can help significantly reduce cardiovascular risk and optimize health. These risk factors were discussed in detail in the preceding section.

Clinical Manifestations

Hypertension may have very few symptoms or none at all. If symptoms are present, they can include headaches, visual changes, dizziness, nausea, or chest pain. Oftentimes, however, there are no symptoms, and individuals can function for years without being diagnosed.

Diagnosis

Screening

As noted previously, hypertension is oftentimes an asymptomatic condition. As such, screening plays a critical role in early detection to minimize the end-organ damage that could result from untreated, long-standing hypertension. The U.S. Preventative Services Task Force (USPSTF) recommends screening for hypertension in adults who are 18 years or older (grade A recommendation). Adults 40 years and older and those with increased risk of hypertension should be screened annually. A review of the existing evidence demonstrated minimal harm in screening and a significant resultant benefit in the form of a reduction in cardiovascular events. Adults 18 to 39 years of age with no additional risk factors should be screened every 3 to 5 years. Recommended screening techniques include measurement of blood pressure in the office setting with either a manual or automatic cuff and ambulatory or home blood pressure measurement. Office measurement should be done with the patient seated and after at least 5 minutes of the patient arriving in the room. Home measurement may be beneficial after the initial screening for confirmation purposes.

For children and adolescents, the USPSTF indicates that the current evidence is insufficient to assess the risk versus benefit of screening in asymptomatic individuals (grade I evidence). The predictive value of childhood hypertension for adult hypertension is modest, with a risk for false-positive readings.

Clinical Diagnosis

Hypertension is classified in two stages based on degree of elevation. In stage 1 hypertension, systolic blood pressure is greater than or equal to 140 mm Hg to 159 mm Hg and diastolic blood pressure is greater than or equal to 90 mm Hg to 99 mm Hg. Stage 2 hypertension is reached when systolic blood pressure is 160 mm Hg or greater and diastolic blood pressure is 100 mm Hg or greater. This classification is important as the approach to treatment differs for each category, as will be discussed later.

Primary (Essential) Hypertension

Primary hypertension encompasses persistent blood pressure elevation without a discernable cause (idiopathic or of unknown cause). The majority of cases of hypertension will have no discernable cause and fall into this category.

Secondary Hypertension

Secondary hypertension is persistent blood pressure elevation that is the result of some other underlying cause. About 10% of all cases of hypertension will fall into this category. If another cause can be identified, in many cases it may be correctable.

Looking for Secondary Causes

Identifying these underlying causes can be a challenge. Using a systematic method of investigating potential etiologies can simplify this process and improve the chances of identifying a source that with treatment can improve outcomes. One such approach is the *ABCDE* mnemonic. The A in this mnemonic stands for *accuracy* (making sure the reading is correct—such as checking the cuff for appropriate sizing and measurement technique—and repeating readings that are obtained on automatic cuffs manually), *apnea* (considering the presence of obstructive sleep apnea, which is a known contributor to difficult-to-control hypertension), and *aldosteronism* (investigating for the presence of primary hyperaldosteronism through urinary potassium excretion and an elevation in plasma aldosterone level to plasma renin activity). B stands for *bruits* (looking for renovascular sources of hypertension/renal artery stenosis, which would often present with renal bruits upon auscultation) and *bad kidneys* (hypertension resulting from renal parenchymal disease). C stands for *catecholamines* (elevation that can contribute to "white coat" hypertension, as well as overproduction with pheochromocytoma or associated with other conditions such as obstructive sleep apnea and acute stress reactions), *coarctation* (of the aorta), and *Cushing syndrome* (with mineralocorticoid effects of excess glucocorticoids in this setting). D represents both *drugs* (including nonsteroidal antiinflammatory drugs, decongestants, estrogens, and immunosuppressive agents, as well as nicotine and alcohol) and *diet* (particularly excess sodium intake). The final letter in the mnemonic, E, stands for *erythropoietin* (high endogenous levels—such as in chronic obstructive pulmonary disease—or exogenous levels) and *endocrine disorders* (hypothyroidism or hyperparathyroidism). Utilizing a methodical and organized approach to considering potential causes of hypertension can assist with maximizing the chances of optimally controlling blood pressure.

Differential Diagnosis

The differential diagnosis for hypertension coincides with the array of potential secondary causes that were noted earlier (see Looking for Secondary Causes section). It is important to rule out potentially treatable secondary causes in the initial phases of hypertension management.

Treatment Approaches

Approaching treatment of a patient with hypertension can be challenging. Many factors need to be considered when making these decisions, including reflection on patient age, race, gender, and comorbidities. Each of these factors can influence what the optimal treatment strategy might be. Figure 1 provides a stepwise strategy to blood pressure management.

Initial treatment should always include lifestyle modification as discussed previously, and this modification needs to be continued throughout the remainder of any management strategies.

In 2014, the Eighth Joint National Committee (JNC 8) released new recommendations regarding the treatment of hypertension. These guidelines were a divergence from the prior JNC 7 recommendations, effectively loosening the goals and the levels at which treatment is initiated. The following is a summary of the eight treatment recommendations from JNC 8. (Please note that the strength of recommendation that is referenced corresponds to the following: grade A—strong recommendation based on evidence; grade B—moderate recommendation based on evidence; grade C—weak recommendation with moderate certainty of a small benefit; grade D—recommendation against; grade E—expert opinion with insufficient or conflicting evidence; grade N—no recommendation for or against).

Figure 1 Algorithm for management of hypertension. *Abbreviations*: ACE = angiotensin-converting enzyme; ARB = angiotensin receptor blocker; DASH = dietary approaches to stop hypertension. (Reprinted with permission from Chobanian AV. Shattuck Lecture. The hypertension paradox—More uncontrolled disease despite improved therapy. *N Engl J Med* 2009;361:878–887.)

Recommendation 1

Individuals aged 60 years or older in the general population should have pharmacologic treatment initiated at a systolic blood pressure level of 150 mm Hg or a diastolic blood pressure of 90 mm Hg with treatment goals of less than 150 mm Hg systolic and less than 90 mm Hg diastolic. (Strength of recommendation: grade A.)

An additional aspect of this recommendation is that if the pharmacologic treatment results in adequate blood pressure reduction and there is no adverse effect on quality of life or patient health, then the treatment can be continued without alteration. (Strength of recommendation: grade E.)

Recommendation 2

Individuals younger than 60 years in the general population should have pharmacologic treatment initiated at a diastolic blood pressure of 90 mm Hg with a treatment goal of less than 90 mm Hg. (Strength of recommendation: grade A for ages 30–59 years, grade E for ages 18–29 years.)

Recommendation 3

Individuals younger than 60 years in the general population should have pharmacologic treatment initiated at a systolic blood pressure of 140 mm Hg with a treatment goal of less than 140 mm Hg. (Strength of recommendation: grade E.)

Recommendation 4

Individuals aged 18 years or older with chronic kidney disease should have pharmacologic treatment initiated at a systolic blood pressure of 140 mm Hg or a diastolic blood pressure of 90 mm Hg with a treatment goal of less than 140 mm Hg systolic and less than 90 mm Hg diastolic. (Strength of recommendation: grade E.)

Recommendation 5

Individuals older than 18 years with diabetes should have pharmacologic treatment initiated at a systolic blood pressure of 140 mm Hg or a diastolic blood pressure of 90 mm Hg with a treatment goal of less than 140 mm Hg systolic and less than 90 mm Hg diastolic. (Strength of recommendation: grade E.)

Recommendation 6

The treatment of nonblack individuals in the general population (including those with diabetes) who require pharmacologic treatment should include thiazide-type diuretics, calcium channel blockers, angiotensin-converting enzyme inhibitors, or angiotensin receptor blockers. (Strength of recommendation: grade B.)

Recommendation 7

The treatment of black individuals (including those with diabetes) should include thiazide-type diuretics or calcium channel blockers. (Strength of recommendation: grade B for general population, grade C for patients with diabetes.)

Recommendation 8

The treatment of individuals older than 18 years with chronic kidney disease should include, either as initial or add-on treatment, angiotensin-converting enzyme inhibitors or angiotensin receptor blockers to improve renal outcomes. (Strength of recommendation: grade B.)

Recommendation 9

The goal of hypertension treatment is to reach and maintain blood pressure goals consistent with the previous recommendations. If goals are not reached within a month of starting pharmacologic treatment, the dose of the initial agent should be increased or a second agent from recommendation 6 should be added. Blood pressure should continue to be assessed until the goal blood pressure is achieved. If blood pressure goals are not achieved with two agents, a third agent should be added.

- Angiotensin-converting enzyme inhibitors (ACEIs) and angiotensin receptor blockers (ARBs) should not be used together.
- If necessary, other classes of agents can be used if more than three agents are required or if there are contraindications to the agents in recommendation 6.
- Referral to a hypertension specialist should be considered for patients whose blood pressure goals cannot be met with the previous strategies or who are more complicated. Strength of recommendation: grade E.

ACC/AHA 2017 Hypertension Guidelines

In late 2017, the American College of Cardiology and the American Heart Association released an updated Hypertension Guideline. This guideline provided a different approach to hypertension management, particularly around blood pressure goals. Hypertension stages have tighter cut points than under the JNC-8 Guidelines. Under the ACC/AHA Guidelines, normal blood pressure is defined as less than 120/80. Blood pressure is considered elevated when systolic blood pressure is in the 120–129 mm Hg range and when diastolic remains under 80 mm Hg. Stage 1 hypertension is defined as systolic blood pressure between 130 and 139 mm Hg and a diastolic blood pressure between 80 and 90 mm Hg. Stage 2 hypertension is defined as blood pressures that are greater than 140/90. This classification is a deviation from the set points within the JNC-8 recommendations.

Nonpharmacologic

For stage I hypertension (140–159/90–99 mm Hg), the first treatment step is to aggressively modify lifestyle. This includes targeting both diet and exercise. These nonpharmacologic strategies should continue even if pharmacologic treatment is found to be necessary. The relative effects of lifestyle modification on blood pressure reduction are noted in Table 1. ACC/AHA Guidelines also recommend lifestyle changes as initial intervention for individuals with stage 1 hypertension without other cardiovascular risk factors and with a ASCVD risk of less than 10%; however, as noted above, the definition of stage 1 hypertension is at a lower blood pressure level (130-139/80-90 mm Hg.)

Diet

Dietary modifications include salt restriction to a level of less than 2400 mg per day but ideally less than 1500 mg per day. Suggested dietary interventions also include the use of the DASH (dietary approaches to stop hypertension) framework. This nutritional framework includes recommendations such as increased consumption of fruits and vegetables, preferential use of complex carbohydrates, and consumption of low-fat dairy products. The DASH diet emphasizes the intake of whole grains, fish, poultry, legumes, nuts, and nontropical vegetable oils. This diet also endorses decreasing higher-fat foods.

Exercise

Current exercise recommendations suggest that engaging in a minimum of 150 minutes of moderate-intensity exercise on a weekly basis confers the greatest health benefits. Exercise at this

TABLE 1 Effect of Lifestyle and Diet Modifications on Systolic Blood Pressure

MODIFICATION	AMOUNT	REDUCTION IN SBP (MM HG)
Dietary sodium restriction	< 30–50 mmol/d	2–8
Moderation of daily alcohol intake	150–200 mL	2–4
Increased physical activity	30 min 3 × per wk	4–9
Reduction in body weight	10 kg or 22 lb	5–10
Adoption of DASH eating plan (high potassium)		8–14

Abbreviations: DASH = dietary approaches to stop hypertension; SBP = systolic blood pressure.

level of intensity reduces the risk of multiple chronic conditions including cardiovascular disease and type 2 diabetes, as well as overall all-cause mortality.

Other Lifestyle Modifications

In addition to diet and exercise, other lifestyle interventions can optimize health. Smoking cessation is an important modifiable risk factor and is the single leading cause of preventable death in the United States. Smoking increases the risk of cardiovascular morbidity and mortality, including myocardial infarction.

Alcohol consumption is another important lifestyle modification that can have a significant impact on overall health. The effects of alcohol consumption, unlike smoking, depend on quantity. It has been shown that at moderate levels of consumption, alcohol can actually decrease blood pressure (defined as no more than two drinks per day for males and no more than one drink per day for females). However, when consumed in greater quantity, alcohol can increase blood pressure, contributing to hypertension. It is emphasized that alcohol consumption should not be promoted in nondrinkers simply for the purpose of decreasing blood pressure.

Stress reduction is another lifestyle change that can have effects on blood pressure control. The mechanism of this reduction is not clear, but it is hypothesized that it may be related to decreasing autonomic nervous system output. Studies suggest that activities such as transcendental meditation can lead to modest blood pressure reduction. As such, inclusion of these activities in patient treatment plans may provide additional nonpharmacologic options.

Patients frequently ask about the utility of dietary supplements or other natural alternatives for blood pressure management. There is some evidence for select supplements in the management of hypertension, although such effects appear to be small. Examples of natural substances that may convey a small benefit include garlic and cocoa. Evidence is lacking for other agents including vitamin C, coenzyme Q10, omega-3 fatty acids, and magnesium.

Pharmacologic

In cases where hypertension is more significant or nonpharmacologic methods have failed to adequately reduce blood pressure, initiation of medications is indicated (Table 2). The selection of an agent or agents is based on a number of factors including race and comorbidities. As noted earlier, JNC 8 provides a stepwise, evidence-based approach to blood pressure management including recommended cut points where pharmacologic intervention is appropriate.

One of the points of emphasis of JNC 8 is that the point of intervention for individuals age 60 years or older is higher than those younger than that age. One should also balance the side effects or risks of medications with the benefits of intervention in this age group. The cut points for individuals with chronic kidney disease and diabetes do not differ from the general population.

TABLE 2	Antihypertensive Classes

Diuretics

GENERIC	BRAND NAME	CLASSIFICATION	MECHANISM OF ACTION	DOSING
Chlorthalidone	Thalitone	Thiazide	Inhibits sodium and chloride reabsorption in distal tubules	25 mg by mouth once daily. May increase to maximum of 100 mg once daily.
Hydrochlorothiazide	Microzide	Thiazide	Inhibits sodium and chloride reabsorption in distal tubules	25 mg by mouth once daily to maximum of 50 mg in single or divided doses.
Metolazone	Zaroxolyn	Thiazide	Inhibits sodium and chloride reabsorption in distal tubules	5–20 mg by mouth once daily.
Triamterene/ hydrochlorothiazide	Dyazide	Potassium-sparing/ thiazide	Inhibits sodium reabsorption in the distal tubules	1–2 capsules by mouth once daily (37.5/25 mg capsules).
Furosemide	Lasix	Loop	Inhibits sodium and chloride reabsorption in the ascending loop of Henle	40 mg twice daily by mouth initially.
Torsemide	Demadex	Loop	Inhibits sodium and chloride reabsorption in the ascending loop of Henle	5 mg once daily by mouth initially. May increase to 10 mg once daily.

Angiotensin-Converting Enzyme (ACE) Inhibitors

Mechanism of action: Suppress the renin-angiotensin-aldosterone system

GENERIC	BRAND NAME	CLASSIFICATION	SPECIAL NOTE	DOSING
Fosinopril	Monopril	ACE inhibitor	Only ACE excreted by both renal and hepatic routes	5 mg by mouth daily initially. May be increased to 40 mg daily.
Captopril	Capoten	ACE inhibitor		Take 1 hour before meals. 25 mg two to three times daily by mouth. May increase to 50 mg two to three times daily by mouth. Maximum 450 mg per day.
Ramipril	Altace	ACE inhibitor		2.5 mg once daily by mouth. May increase to maximum of 20 mg once daily by mouth.
Enalapril	Vasotec	ACE inhibitor		5 mg daily by mouth initially. Typical dose range is 10–40 mg by mouth daily (may be divided doses).
Lisinopril	Prinivil, Zestril	ACE inhibitor		10 mg by mouth daily initial dose. Usual dose range 10–40 mg daily. Doses above 40 mg are not shown to have greater effect.
Quinapril	Accupril	ACE inhibitor		10–20 mg daily by mouth initial dose.

Angiotensin II Receptor Blockers (ARBs)

Mechanism of action: Block binding of angiotensin II to angiotensin I receptors with a resultant inhibition of angiotensin II–mediated vasoconstriction, sodium retention, and release of aldosterone

GENERIC	BRAND NAME	CLASSIFICATION	SPECIAL NOTE	DOSING
Losartan	Cozaar	ARB		50 mg daily by mouth initial dose (25 mg initial dose if also on diuretics). Titrate to a maximum of 100 mg daily.
Valsartan	Diovan	ARB	Adding a diuretic has greater effect than dose increases over 80 mg daily.	80–160 mg daily by mouth initial dose. May titrate to a maximum dose of 320 mg daily.
Olmesartan	Benicar	ARB		20 mg daily by mouth initial dose. May be titrated to 40 mg daily.
Eprosartan	Teveten	ARB		600 mg daily by mouth initial dose. May increase to 800 mg daily maximum dose. Usual range 400–800 mg daily.
Azilsartan	Edarbi	ARB		80 mg once daily by mouth. If on diuretics start at 40 mg once daily.

Beta-Blockers

GENERIC	BRAND NAME	CLASSIFICATION	MECHANISM OF ACTION	DOSING
Atenolol	Tenormin	Beta-1 selective		50 mg once daily by mouth. May increase to maximum of 100 mg once daily

Continued

TABLE 2 Antihypertensive Classes—cont'd

GENERIC	BRAND NAME	CLASSIFICATION	MECHANISM OF ACTION	DOSING
Metoprolol	Lopressor, Toprol XL	Beta-1 selective		Immediate-release formulations: 50–100 mg in single or divided doses. Maximum 450 mg per day.
				Extended-release formulations: 25–100 mg daily in a single dose. Maximum 400 mg per day.
Propranolol	Inderal LA, InnoPran XL	Beta-1 noncardioselective		Immediate-release formulations: 40 mg by mouth twice daily initial dose. Typical dosing 120–240 mg daily. Maximum 640 mg daily. Extended-release formulations: 80 mg once daily initial dose.
				Extended-release formulations: 80 mg once daily initial dose.
Bisoprolol	Zebeta	Beta-1 selective	More beta-1 specific than other beta-blockers	5 mg by mouth once daily initial dose (2.5 mg if patient has bronchospastic disease—i.e., asthma, chronic obstructive pulmonary disease). May titrate to a maximum of 20 mg per day.
Timolol		Beta-1 noncardioselective	CAUTION: Avoid abrupt discontinuation as may exacerbate ischemic heart disease.	10 mg twice daily by mouth initially. May titrate to a maximum of 60 mg per day in divided doses.
Labetalol	Trandate	Alpha and beta antagonist		100 mg twice daily by mouth (initial dose). May titrate in 2–3 days by 100 mg twice-daily increments. Maximum dose 2400 mg per day.

Calcium Channel Blockers

GENERIC	BRAND NAME	CLASSIFICATION	MECHANISM OF ACTION	DOSING
Nifedipine, extended release	Adalat CC, Procardia XL	Dihydropyridine	Binds to L-type calcium channels in sinoatrial (SA) and atrioventricular (AV) node, as well as myocardium and vasculature	30–60 mg by mouth once daily. Maximum 120 mg daily.
Diltiazem, extended release	Cardizem CD, Cardizem LA, Cartia XT, Dilacor XR	Nondihydropyridine	Binds to L-type calcium channels in SA and AV node (primarily), as well as myocardium and vasculature	180–240 mg by mouth per day initially. May titrate after 14 days. Maintenance dosing typically 180–420 mg daily. Maximum dose 480 mg per day.
Verapamil	Calan, Calan SR	Nondihydropyridine	Binds to L-type calcium channels in SA and AV node, as well as myocardium and vasculature	80 mg by mouth every 8 hours initially. Usual dose range: 240–480 mg per day.
Amlodipine	Norvasc	Dihydropyridine	Binds to L-type calcium channels in smooth muscle (vasculature)	5 mg by mouth daily (initially). May increase by 2.5 mg every 1–2 weeks. Maximum 10 mg per day.
Felodipine	Plendil	Dihydropyridine	Binds to L-type calcium channels in smooth muscle (vasculature)	2.5–5 mg by mouth once daily initially. May increase to a maximum of 20 mg by mouth once daily.*

Aldosterone Antagonists

GENERIC	BRAND NAME	CLASSIFICATION	MECHANISM OF ACTION	DOSING
Spironolactone	Aldactone	Selective aldosterone antagonist	Competes with aldosterone receptor sites. Reduces sodium reabsorption	25–100 mg by mouth once daily or divided twice daily (if being used for more than 2 weeks).
Eplerenone	Inspra	Selective aldosterone antagonist	Competes with aldosterone receptor sites. Reduces sodium reabsorption	50 mg by mouth once daily initially. May increase to twice daily if needed. (May cause hyperkalemia if doses exceed 100 mg per day.)

TABLE 2 Antihypertensive Classes—cont'd

Alpha-2 Agonists

Mechanism of action: Stimulate presynaptic aldosterone receptors, decreasing sympathetic nervous activity

GENERIC	BRAND NAME	CLASSIFICATION	MECHANISM OF ACTION	DOSING
Clonidine	Catapres, Catapres-TTS	Centrally acting alpha-2 agonist	Stimulation of alpha-2 adrenoreceptors, reducing sympathetic nervous system output	0.1 mg every 12 hours by mouth. Maximum 2.4 mg per 24 hours. (Usual dose range 0.1–0.2 mg every 12 hours.) If using transdermal formulation, 0.1 mg patch applied once every 7 days. May increase by 0.1 mg to maximum of 0.3 mg per week.
Methyldopa		Centrally acting alpha-2 agonist	Directly affects peripheral sympathetic nerves through stimulation of central alpha-adrenergic receptors	250 mg by mouth every 8–12 hours initially then can increase every 2 days. (Maximum 3 g per day.) Typical maintenance dose is 250–1000 mg by mouth divided every 6–12 hours.

Alpha Blockers

Mechanism of action: Selectively block postsynaptic alpha-1 adrenergic receptors

GENERIC	BRAND NAME	CLASSIFICATION	MECHANISM OF ACTION	DOSING
Prazosin	Minipress	Alpha-1 blocker	Competitive antagonist, reduces vascular resistance	1 mg by mouth every 8–12 hours (initial). Maintenance dose typically 6–15 mg divided every 6–8 hours. Typical maximum 20 mg per day in divided doses (although may increase to 40 mg per day in divided doses in some patients).
Terazosin	Hytrin		Selective competitive inhibitor, decreases vascular resistance	1 mg by mouth at bedtime (initial). Typical maintenance 1–5 mg daily or in divided dose every 12 hours. Maximum 20 mg per day.
Doxazosin	Cardura		Selective postsynaptic alpha-1 receptor inhibitor, vasodilation	1 mg once daily initially, titrate to maximum of 16 mg/day.

*Exceeds dosage recommended by the manufacturer.
Adapted from Medscape. Hypertension Medication. Available at: http://www.emedicine.medscape.com/article/241381-medication. Accessed May 5, 2017.

The choice of agent according to JNC 8 does not differ based on the presence or absence of diabetes, but does differ based on race (see recommendations 6 and 7 earlier). Individuals with chronic kidney disease also should have an ACEI or an ARB included in their treatment regimen (either as a lone agent or an add-on). In practice, decisions will need to be tailored to individual patient needs and also should consider other factors including whether or not the patient is a reproductive-age female (as ACEIs and ARBs are contraindicated in pregnancy). This is where our role as family physicians becomes increasingly important—embracing our ability to look at the whole patient when making treatment decisions.

ACC/AHA recommends the initiation of pharmacologic therapy in adults with high cardiovascular risk or preexisting cardiovascular disease and stage 1 or greater hypertension. Patients with both diabetes and hypertension are also assumed to fall into the high-risk category. Again, the defined level of blood pressure classified as stage 1 hypertension under ACC/AHA (130–139/80–90 mmHg) is lower than the JNC8 criteria as noted above. ACC/AHA also emphasizes the need to balance comorbidities as well as preferences, life expectancy, and clinical judgment when making decisions regarding antihypertensive initiation and titration in older individuals (65 or older.)

Monitoring

Clinical practice guidelines vary in their recommendations regarding optimal monitoring. It is clear that monitoring in the early stage or during periods of treatment change should be more frequent than during times of stability, somewhere between monthly and every 6 weeks. Once the patient is stabilized, periodic monitoring can occur either every 3 to 6 months for everyone or in a more risk-stratified manner, with lower-risk patients being seen every 6 months and higher-risk patients every 3 months.

JNC 8 recommendations, as previously discussed, suggest that patients with hypertension be monitored on at least a monthly basis until goal blood pressure is achieved, with any necessary adjustments being made at these visits.

Complications

Hypertension is often referred to as "the silent killer." This menacing name refers to the fact that this condition often presents without any discernable symptoms, which at times can make treatment compliance challenging. One of the greatest concerns with uncontrolled hypertension is the risk of end-organ damage, which is far-reaching.

Uncontrolled hypertension can lead to serious complications including myocardial infarction, stroke, peripheral artery disease, retinopathy, and renal failure. Given that hypertension is at the same time the most common condition we treat as primary care physicians, the opportunities to circumvent these sources of morbidity and mortality present themselves on a daily basis.

References

Al-Ansary L, et al: A systematic review of recent clinical practice guidelines on the diagnosis, assessment and management of hypertension, PLOS One 8(1):1–18, 2013.

Bie P, Evans R: Normotension, hypertension and body fluid regulation: brain and kidney, Acta Physio 219:288–304, 2017.

Carey, et al: Prevention, detection, evaluation, and management of high blood pressure in adults: synopsis of the 2017 American College of Cardiology/American Heart Association Hypertension Guideline, Ann Intern Med 168(5):351–358, 2018.

Chobanian AV: Guidelines for the management of hypertension, *Med Clin N Am* 101:219–227, 2017.

Garjon J, et al: First-line combination therapy versus firstline monotherapy for primary hypertension (review), *Cochrane Database Syst Rev* 1:CD10316, 2017.

James P, Oparil S, Carter BL, et al: 2014 Evidence-based guideline for the management of high blood pressure in adults: report from the panel members appointed to the Eight Joint National Committee (JNC 8h), *JAMA* 311(5):507–520 2014.

Kallioinen A, Hill A, Horswill MS, et al: Sources of inaccuracy in the measurement of adult patients' resting blood pressure in clinical settings: a systematic review, *J Hypertension* 35:421–441, 2017.

Langan R, Jones K: Common questions about the initial management of hypertension, *Am Fam Physician* 91(3):172–176, 2015.

Leeman L, et al: Hypertensive disorders of pregnancy, *Am Fam Physician* 93(2):121–127, 2016.

Mann S: Redefining beta-blocker use in hypertension: selecting the right beta-blocker and the right patient, *J Am Soc Hypertens* 1–12, 2016.

Onusko E: Diagnosing secondary hypertension, *Am Fam Physician* 67(1):67–74, 2003.

Oza R, Garcellano M: Nonpharmacologic management of hypertension: what works? *Am Fam Physician* 91(11):772–776, 2015.

Quyen N: Screening for high blood pressure in adults, *Am Fam Physician* 93(6):511–512, 2016.

Sexton S: Screening for high blood pressure in adults: recommendation statement, *Am Fam Physician* 93(4):300–302, 2016.

Sexton S: Screening for primary hypertension in children and adolescents: recommendation statemen, *Am Fam Physician* 91(4)2015, A–D.

Springer K: Chlorthalidone vs. hydrochlorothiazide for treatment of hypertension, *Am Fam Physician* 92(11):1015–1016, 2015.

Medscape: Hypertension. Available at: http://emedicine.medscape.com/article/241381. [accessed May 9, 2017].

HYPERTROPHIC CARDIOMYOPATHY

Method of
Sandeep Sangodkar, DO, MS

CURRENT DIAGNOSIS

- Echocardiography is mainstay of clinical diagnosis.
- Cardiac MRI can provide important prognostic information.
- Left ventricular outflow tract pressure and flow measurements have a classic dynamic pattern.
- Left ventricular wall thickness of at least 15 mm.

CURRENT THERAPY

Asymptomatic Disease
- Periodic follow-up to assess symptoms and risk for sudden cardiac death.
- The patient should follow a strategy to modify risk factors for coronary artery disease.
- Patients with concurrent atrial fibrillation should be anticoagulated.

Symptomatic Disease
- β-Blockade or calcium channel blockers are drugs of choice.
- Implantable defibrillator is indicated if the patient has risk factors for sudden cardiac death.
- Surgical myectomy may be undertaken in patients who do not respond to pharmacologic therapy.
- Alcohol ablation may be used in patients who are not candidates for surgery.

Definition

Many names, terms, and acronyms (more than 80) have been used to describe hypertrophic cardiomyopathy (HCM). Common names such as idiopathic hypertrophic, subaortic stenosis and hypertrophic obstructive cardiomyopathy, popular in the literature in the 1960s and 1970s, imply that left ventricular outflow tract (LVOT) obstruction is a required component of the disease, whereas one-third of patients have no obstruction at rest or exertion. The term *HCM*, first used in 1979, encompasses both the obstructive and nonobstructive hemodynamic variants of this disease and is now considered the formal name.

Epidemiology

Although once thought of as a rare entity, HCM is now recognized as a common inherited cardiovascular disease. Epidemiologic studies from various parts of the world report a similar prevalence, thought of as 1 in 500 people, which occurs equally among sexes and ethnic groups. This may, in fact, be underreported because many people with HCM are not clinically diagnosed and achieve normal life expectancy without any HCM-related complications.

Risk Factors

HCM is caused by mutations in genes coding for thin and thick filament proteins of the sarcomere. These mutations are inherited in an autosomal dominant pattern with variable penetrance and expression. At least 11 genes have been identified as responsible for causing HCM, with 70% of successfully genotyped patients found to have mutations in the two most-common genes: β-myosin heavy chain and myosin binding protein C. More than 1500 individual mutations have been identified, which complicates the role of mutational analysis in predicting prognosis for individual patients.

Clinical Manifestations

HCM is seen from pediatric to geriatric populations. A classic description of a murmur suggestive of HCM is a systolic ejection murmur that increases in intensity with valsalva. Most patients with HCM are asymptomatic or only mildly symptomatic, with the most common presenting complaints being dyspnea or chest pain. The most worrisome manifestation is sudden cardiac death owing to ventricular tachyarrhythmia, seen more commonly in younger symptom-free patients. Systolic anterior motion of the mitral valve can cause significant mitral regurgitation. Heart failure with preserved ejection fraction is another manifestation of HCM; however, systolic dysfunction can be present owing to myocardial scarring. In addition, atrial fibrillation is associated with an increased risk of thromboembolism in patients with HCM and anticoagulation must be considered. Most patients with HCM have normal life expectancy without a need for major intervention.

Pathogenesis

The pathophysiology of HCM stems from multiple abnormalities including LVOT obstruction, diastolic dysfunction, mitral regurgitation, cardiac ischemia, and arrhythmias. The peak instantaneous LV outflow gradient is an important factor in determining treatment options. The obstruction was originally thought to be caused by a hypertrophied basal septum that caused ventricular outflow obstruction during systolic contraction. More recently, it is thought mitral valve systolic anterior motion and mitral-septal contact caused by venturi forces on the mitral leaflets and displacement into the outflow tract cause obstruction of LVOT. The increased LV systolic pressure in turn results in elevated diastolic pressures, mitral regurgitation, and, ultimately, decreased cardiac output.

Diagnosis

Clinically, HCM is defined as maximal LV wall thickness of at least 15 mm based on echocardiography. Patients with thickened LV wall and concurrent presence of HCM genetic substrates or family members with pathologic sarcomere mutations are considered to have genotype-positive–phenotype-negative HCM or subclinical HCM. A distinction between HCM and physiologic LV hypertrophy from athletic conditioning must be recognized because the athletic hearts may demonstrate enlargement of the cardiac chambers and thickened septum. The likelihood of clinically significant HCM is determined by identification of sarcomere mutations, marked LV thickness (more than 25 mm), and LVOT obstruction with systolic anterior motion and mitral-septal contact. Provocative testing (exercise or pharmacologic) may elucidate the diagnosis of HCM in symptomatic patients presenting with a normal LVOT gradient at rest. Measurement of outflow gradients by echocardiography and invasive pressures by cardiac catheterization show a characteristic dynamic pattern that can be enhanced by loading conditions.

Imaging

The mainstay of imaging has been held by echocardiography. Transthoracic echocardography is recommended in the initial evaluation of all patients with suspected HCM, as well as family members of those diagnosed with HCM. Transesophageal echocardiography is used for diagnosis as well as intraprocedural guidance of surgical myectomy and alcohol septal ablation.

In recent years, cardiac magnetic resonance imaging (MRI; CMR) has proven to be an increasingly useful modality in the diagnosis and treatment of HCM. Contrast enhanced CMR allows imaging of presumed myocardial fibrosis. Late gadolinium enhancement (LGE) is commonly seen in HCM and an amount >15% of left ventricular mass is associated with a higher risk of sudden cardiac death. An absence of LGE is associated with a lower risk of sudden cardiac death and can often provide reassurance.

Treatment
Asymptomatic Disease

Given that a large subset of HCM patients are symptom free and will achieve normal life expectancy, it is important to educate patients about the disease process, screen family members, and advise them to avoid strenuous activity. Coronary artery disease has an impact on survival and, thus, aggressive modification of risk factors contributing to atherosclerosis (diabetes, hyperlipidemia, and obesity) is recommended. Low-intensity aerobic exercise is reasonable to allow the patient to maintain fitness. Adequate hydration and avoidance of situations leading to vasodilation are encouraged to minimize exacerbation of an existing LVOT obstruction.

Septal reduction therapy is not indicated in a symptom-free patient with any degree of obstruction.

Symptomatic Disease
Pharmacologic Management

β-Blockade is the mainstay of treatment owing to negative inotropic and negative chronotropic effect. Disopyramide (Norpace)[1] may be added to β-blockers for further symptom relief. Verapamil (Calan)[1] or diltiazem (Cardizem)[1] is recommended for those who do not respond or have contraindications to β-blockade. IV phenylephrine (Neo-Synephrine) is recommended for acute hypotension with obstructive HCM in those who do not respond to fluids.

Nifedipine (Procardia)[1] or other dihydropyridine calcium channel blocking agents are potentially harmful owing to their vasodilative effects, which can cause an under-filled LV and worsen LVOT obstruction. Digitalis is potentially harmful in patients without atrial fibrillation. Dopamine, dobutamine[1], norepinephrine (Levophed), and other positive inotropic agents may be harmful for the treatment of acute hypotension. Aldosterone inhibitors have not been shown to impede development or progression of myocardial fibrosis.

For the treatment of atrial fibrillation in HCM, it is recommended to keep a low threshold for initiating prophylactic anticoagulation owing to the higher risk of thromboembolic stroke.

Invasive Therapies

The major septal reduction therapies are surgical myectomy and alcohol ablation. Septal reduction therapy should not be performed in symptom-free adults.

Surgical septal myectomy is considered the most appropriate therapy for eligible patients unresponsive to optimal medical therapy. The most common procedure is a Morrow procedure in which a rectangular trough is created in the basal septum below the aortic valve, which abolishes or reduces the LVOT gradient. Eligible patients include those with severe dyspnea, chest pain, or exertional syncope despite maximal medical therapy. Hemodynamic considerations that determine eligibility consist of an LVOT gradient of at least 50 mm Hg associated with septal hypertrophy and mitral valve systolic anterior motion. Studies have shown that surgical myectomy can reverse heart failure symptoms owing to the fact it permanently removes LVOT obstruction and can reduce mitral regurgitation.

When surgery is contraindicated, alcohol septal ablation can benefit adult patients with HCM and LVOT obstruction. This percutaneous procedure involves injection of ethanol into a major septal perforator coronary artery, with the intent of inducing infarction of the basal septal wall near the anterior leaflet contact point. The effectiveness of alcohol septal ablation is not clear in patients with more than 30 mm of septal hypertrophy, and it should not be performed in patients with disease (coronary artery disease, mitral valve repair) that would need surgical correction regardless. Other downsides of septal ablation include an increased risk of complete heart block requiring pacemaker implantation and an undefined risk of arrythmogenicity owing to scar tissue.

Role of Implantable Devices

Determining which patients with HCM should receive an implantable cardiac defibrillator (ICD) is challenging given the unpredictability of the disease. ICDs are the only treatment to have proven to decrease mortality given their ability to reliably abort life-threating arrhythmias. All patients with HCM need comprehensive sudden cardiac death risk stratification, with strong consideration of ICDs for primary prevention in those with personal history of ventricular fibrillation, sustained ventricular tachycardia, family history of sudden cardiac death, unexplained syncope, abnormal exercise blood pressure response, LGE >15% of LV mass, massive left ventricular hypertrophy (LVH) (>30 mm), or documented nonsustained ventricular tachycardia on Holter monitor. Implantable defibrillators are recommended for secondary prevention in patients with prior cardiac arrest, ventricular fibrillation, or hemodynamically significant ventricular tachycardia (VT). Device-related complications and issues such as inappropriate shocks and multiple generator changes for those patients receiving a device at a young age must also be weighed when considering implantation of ICD. Subcutaneous defibrillators are still largely untested in the HCM population; thus it is recommended to exercise caution when considering this modality.

Participation in Competitive Sports

HCM is a common cause of sudden death in young patients, including competitive athletes. It has been reported that 1/3 of deaths in US high school and college athletes are caused by HCM, which occurs more often in males without previous suspicion of having HCM and African Americans. In the United States, there have been cardiovascular screening initiatives, including history and physical in addition to 12 lead electrocardiograms (ECGs), with limited success. The American College of Cardiology and American Heart Association do not currently recommend a national mandatory cardiovascular screening program.

It is reasonable for HCM patients to engage in low-intensity competitive sports (golf, bowling) and recreational sporting activities. Participation in competitive sports is a modifiable risk factor, and it is recommended that HCM patients avoid participation in intense competitive sports regardless of age, sex, LVOT obstruction, prior septal reduction, or ICD.

Monitoring

The unpredictability of HCM disease makes regular surveillance a necessity. Patient age has been seen as a predictor of HCM-related

---

[1] Not FDA approved for this indication

events, with sudden death events more common in young patients. With a family history of sudden cardiac death, periodic screening by transthoracic echocardiography (every 12 to 18 months) is recommended in children by the age of 12 (or younger if the child has signs of early puberty) or if there are plans for intense sports competition. Repeat transthoracic echocardiography is recommended for any change in clinical status or new cardiovascular event. As recognition of the genetic basis of this disease has improved over time, genetic screening and counseling of all first-degree family members of patients with HCM is now recommended.

Future Research

The perception of HCM has evolved from a rare and deadly condition to a more common and treatable disease. Effective use of ICDs for primary prevention and advances in surgical treatment of obstruction now allow most HCM patients to achieve normal life expectancy. Although significant progress has been made in elucidating the etiology and pathophysiology of HCM, there is much room for advancement. In addition, the relationship between genetics and environmental influences, as well as the management of family members of genotype positive–phenotype negative patients, is still unclear. Although rapid genetic testing to identify those at risk has become more widespread, further understanding of pathogenic mutations is required. Furthermore, advancement in technology will hopefully lead to therapies that can specifically target these pathways.

References

Cannan CR, Reeder GS, Bailey KR, et al: Natural history of hypertrophic cardiomyopathy. A population based study, 1976 through 1990, *Circulation* 92:2488–2495, 1995.
Elliott PM, Anastasakis A, Borger MA, et al: ESC Guidelines on diagnosis and management of hypertrophic cardiomyopathy, *Eur Heart J* 35:2733–2799, 2014.
Gersh BJ, Maron BJ, Bonow RO, et al: 2011 ACCF/AHA guideline for the diagnosis and treatment of hypertrophic cardiomyopathy, *Circulation* 124:e783–e831, 2011.
Marian AJ: Genetic determinants of cardiac hypertrophy, *Curr Opin Cardiol* 23:199–205, 2008.
Marian AJ: Recent advances in genetics and treatment of hypertrophic cardiomyopathy, *Future Cardiol* 1:341–353, 2005.
Maron B, Ommen S, Semsarian C, et al: State of the art review: hypertrophic cardiomyopathy, *JACC* 64(1).
Maron BJ: Hypertrophic cardiomyopathy: A systematic review, *JAMA* 287:1308–1320, 2002.
Robinson, AK: Imaging in Hypertrophic Cardiomyopathy. *JACC* April 24 2018.

INFECTIVE ENDOCARDITIS

Method of
Andrew Wang, MD

CURRENT DIAGNOSIS

- Infective endocarditis (IE) should be considered as a diagnosis in the setting of fever and heart murmur.
- Health care–associated interventions and resulting infections are an increasingly noted cause of IE, changing the epidemiology of this disease.
- Blood cultures show growth in approximately 90% of cases, and multiple sets should be obtained before initiating antibiotics to improve diagnostic yield.
- Echocardiography, particularly transesophageal echocardiography, improves diagnostic sensitivity for infective endocarditis as well as its complications (e.g., intracardiac abscess, fistula).
- The diagnosis of complications, including heart failure, embolic events, and abscess, requires close surveillance, particularly during the first week of therapy, and has adverse prognostic implications.

CURRENT THERAPY

- Empiric antibiotic therapy for *Staphylococcus aureus* should be considered before results of blood cultures are available.
- Prompt initiation of antibiotic therapy is important because the rate of complications, such as embolization, decreases rapidly within several days.
- Multidisciplinary care for the patient with IE should include evaluation by specialists in infectious diseases, cardiology, and cardiothoracic surgery, especially in cases of complicated IE.
- Surgery for IE has not been studied in randomized, controlled trials compared with medical therapy alone. Surgery should be considered for IE complicated by heart failure, embolism, intracardiac abscess, or persistent bacteremia.
- Although stroke due to embolism is not uncommon in IE, data do not suggest a benefit in delaying cardiac surgery after cerebral infarction if surgery is otherwise indicated.

Definition

Infective endocarditis (IE) is a microbial infection of the valves or endocardium of the heart.

Epidemiology and Risk Factors

The incidence of IE varies regionally from 2.6 per 100,000 population reported in France to 11.6 per 100,000 population in urban areas of the United States. This range of incidence has been attributed to differences in predisposing cardiac conditions or risk factors, such as the use of injection drugs. The incidence of IE is also affected by age and sex. The incidence of native valve IE increases with age and exceeds 30 per 100,000 after 30 years of age. The average age of the patient with IE has increased over time, likely related to the decreased prevalence of rheumatic heart disease and increased prevalence of degenerative valvular disease in the aging population. IE is more commonly diagnosed in men, with studies showing male-to-female ratios as high as 9:1.

In earlier eras, streptococcal species were the predominant cause of native valve IE. However, changes in the delivery of health care, with increasing exposure to invasive procedures and devices, and the changing demographics of patients and their risk factors for IE have led to major changes in the microbiologic causes of endocarditis. There is an increasing incidence of health care–associated IE, including nosocomial infection and infection related to ambulatory care, which accounts for approximately 25% of IE cases. For example, in one large multinational study, the International Collaboration on Endocarditis (ICE) registry (N = 2781 patients with definite native or prosthetic endocarditis), 31% of cases were attributable to *Staphylococcus aureus*, 17% to viridans streptococci, 11% to enterococci, 10% to coagulase-negative staphylococci, 12% to other streptococcal species, 2% to the HACEK (*Haemophilus* spp., *Aggregatibacter* spp., *Cardiobacterium hominis*, *Eikenella corrodens*, *Kingella* spp.) group, 2% to non-HACEK gram-negative bacteria, and 2% to fungi. Among those with *S. aureus* endocarditis, health care–associated infection accounted for 39% of cases.

Cardiac conditions predisposing to the development of IE include degenerative valve disease (approximately 40% of cases of mitral IE and 25% of aortic valve IE), presence of prosthetic valves, injection drug use, and rheumatic heart disease.

Pathophysiology

A preexisting valvular or endocardial condition, such as mitral valve prolapse with regurgitation, degenerative aortic valve disease (including bicuspid aortic valve), or congenital heart disease is a major host factor related to IE. Endothelial damage and denudation of the endothelium exposes the underlying basement membrane and fosters platelet and fibrin deposition, a process that occurs spontaneously in persons with valvular heart disease. These deposits are called *nonbacterial thrombotic endocarditis* and form the nidus for vegetation to begin in the setting of bacteremia. The classic lesion of IE, the vegetation, is made up of fibrin, platelets, inflammatory cells, and microorganisms adherent to the endothelium of the heart.

The degree of mechanical stress exerted on the valve might contribute to endothelial denudation and the location of vegetation formation, with left-sided IE more common than right-sided IE. Endocarditis involving the nonvalvular endocardium of the heart similarly occurs at sites of endothelial damage due to mechanical stress, such as the left ventricular outflow tract in patients with hypertrophic obstructive cardiomyopathy and congenital heart defects (ventricular septal defects and patent ductus arteriosus).

The adhesion of bacteria to the denuded endothelium might depend on specific properties of the bacteria. Cell surface characteristics of the organism promote its adherence. For example, the adherence of *S. aureus* to a traumatized animal heart valve has been found to be reduced in the setting of impaired fibronectin binding. Similarly, the ability of bacteria to form biofilm may be associated with their ability to form localized clusters of infections that can make these clusters more resistant to killing by the host immune system and antimicrobial therapy.

With the progressive development of a vegetation, function of the specific heart valve is impaired. Regurgitation or insufficiency of the affected valve most commonly results, leading predominantly to volume overload of the ventricular chamber. In the setting of acute or rapid development of regurgitation, there may be no ventricular adaptation to this volume overload; as a result, acute, severe pulmonary edema and cardiogenic shock may quickly ensue. Less commonly, a large vegetation can result in stenosis of the valve orifice and pressure overload of the proximal or upstream cardiac chamber. As infection extends, destruction of other cardiac tissue, including myocardium and fibrous structures, can occur and result in intracardiac abscess or fistula formation between cardiac chambers.

Prevention

The efficacy of antimicrobial prophylaxis in preventing IE continues to be debated. Current recommendations are generally based on the likelihood of bacteremia occurring as a result of the procedure, the potential for adverse outcome as related to the predisposing cardiac condition, and the level of evidence for antibiotic prophylaxis as effective for the prevention of IE. The American Heart Association has published updated guidelines for IE prophylaxis with a continued trend toward fewer indications for prophylaxis.

Based on an extensive review of published literature and expert consensus, these guidelines have concluded that IE is more likely to result from bacteremia associated with daily activities than with a dental procedure. Antibiotic prophylaxis, even if 100% effective, is estimated to prevent only an extremely small number of cases of IE. These recommendations concluded that antibiotic prophylaxis should not be prescribed solely on the basis of an increased lifetime risk of IE but on the basis of cardiac conditions associated with highest risk of an adverse outcome from IE.

Conditions that warrant IE prophylaxis before dental procedures and procedures on respiratory tract, skin, and musculoskeletal structures are listed in Box 1 and Table 1. The American Heart Association no longer recommends prophylaxis before gastrointestinal or genitourinary procedures solely for the prevention of IE.

Clinical Manifestations and Diagnosis

The diagnosis of IE depends on findings of bacteremia with an organism associated with IE and evidence of endocardial involvement. Because these objective findings may not be sought unless the possibility of IE is considered, careful attention to the patient's history and physical examination is critical to the eventual diagnosis. The clinical presentation of IE is highly variable and can range from chronic fatigue with low-grade fever to acute heart failure due to new, severe valvular regurgitation. Although the virulence of the organism can influence acuity of presentation, the onset of infection is generally followed by the onset of symptoms

---

BOX 1	Prophylaxis Against Infective Endocarditis

High Risk Cardiac Conditions Where Prophylaxis Is Indicated
- Prosthetic heart valve or prosthetic material used for valve repair
- Previous infective endocarditis
- Congenital heart disease including unrepaired cyanotic lesions, palliative shunts or conduits, previous repair with residual defect at site of prosthetic patch or device, and recent repair (<6 months) involving prosthetic device or material
- Cardiac transplant with valve regurgitation due to structurally abnormal valve

Procedures Warranting Prophylaxis for Those at High Risk
- Dental procedures that involve manipulating gingival tissue or the periapical region of teeth
- Dental procedures that involve perforating the oral mucosa
- Respiratory tract procedures, including tonsillectomy, adenoidectomy, or bronchoscopy with biopsy
- Skin or soft tissue procedures
- Cardiac surgery with prosthetic material

TABLE 1	Regimens for Dental Procedure		
REGIMEN	**ANTIBIOTIC AGENT**	**ADULT**	**CHILDREN**
Oral	Amoxicillin	2 g	50 mg/kg
Penicillin allergy	Cephalexin	2 g	50 mg/kg
	or clindamycin	600 mg	20 mg/kg
	or azithromycin or clarithromycin	500 mg	15 mg/kg
Unable to take oral medication	Ampicillin	2 g IM or IV	50 mg/kg IM or IV
Unable to take oral medication plus penicillin allergy	Cefazolin or ceftriaxone	1 g IM or IV	50 mg/kg IM or IV
	or clindamycin	600 mg IM or IV	20 mg/kg IM or IV

Note: The antibiotic agent is administered as single dose 30–60 minutes before the procedure.
Adapted from Bonow RO, Carabello BA, Kanu C, et al: ACC/AHA 2006 guidelines for the management of patients with valvular heart disease: A report of the American College of Cardiology/American Heart Association Task Force on Practice Guidelines (writing committee to revise the 1998 Guidelines for the Management of Patients with Valvular Heart Disease): Developed in collaboration with the Society of Cardiovascular Anesthesiologists: Endorsed by the Society for Cardiovascular Angiography and Interventions and the Society of Thoracic Surgeons. *Circulation* 2006;114(5):e84–e231.

of bacteremia within 2 weeks. Four processes contribute to the clinical presentation of IE: (1) infection on the valve, including local intracardiac complications; (2) septic or aseptic embolization to distant organs; (3) continuous bacteremia, often with metastatic foci of infection; and (4) circulating immune complexes and other immunopathologic factors.

Approximately 85% of patients present with fever, although this finding might not be present in immunosuppressed states and in patients who have previously been on antibiotic therapy. Nonspecific signs and symptoms such as chills, sweats, anorexia, weight loss, malaise, dyspnea, and cough are common but generally occur in less than half of patients with IE. In addition, predisposing conditions or risk factors for the development of IE, including a history of structural heart disease, injection drug use, or recent invasive procedure, should be sought in the patient's history.

Evidence of a *new or changing* regurgitant murmur in the presence of fever of undetermined origin should prompt additional, timely evaluation for possible IE. Because of the lack of ventricular adaptation to acute volume overload and the resulting hemodynamic changes (tachycardia, hypotension), the murmur in acute aortic insufficiency may be poorly audible. Embolic phenomena, a common extracardiac complication of IE, can manifest with localizing symptoms such as focal neurologic deficit due to stroke or left upper abdominal pain due to splenic infarction. The patient should be carefully examined for any peripheral stigmata of IE such as petechiae, splinter hemorrhages, Janeway lesions, Osler nodes, and Roth spots. Many of these findings are immune-mediated yet infrequently present. Although Janeway lesions, Osler nodes, and Roth spots are more specific abnormalities for IE, they can occur in other conditions and their low incidence in cases of proven IE limits their diagnostic utility.

Blood Cultures

Blood cultures are the definitive microbiologic procedure for the diagnosis of IE. Continuous and low-grade bacteremia makes it unnecessary to await fever spikes or chills to obtain blood cultures, and the first two blood cultures yield an etiologic agent in 90% of cases. In patients who have not received antibiotics recently, it is recommended that at least three blood culture sets from separate venipunctures should be obtained over the first 24 hours, which will increase the yield to more than 95% in cases of untreated IE with continuous bacteremia. Each culture media bottle should be inoculated with at least 10 mL of blood to increase the number of colony-forming units per culture. The results of blood cultures should be interpreted based on the specific microorganisms identified as well as the recognized, constant nature of bacteremia in IE.

Other laboratory data may provide clues to the diagnosis yet lack specificity for IE. Hematologic parameters are often abnormal. A normocytic, normochromic anemia (70%–90%), thrombocytopenia (5%–15%), and leukocytosis (30%) are common findings. The erythrocyte sedimentation rate (ESR) and C-reactive protein concentrations are usually elevated.

Echocardiography and Diagnostic Criteria

The diagnosis of IE is based on clinical suspicion derived from signs and symptoms and, most importantly, the demonstration of associated bacteremia. Given the nonspecific nature of findings from history, physical examination, and even blood cultures, the inclusion of echocardiographic findings has improved the sensitivity of diagnostic criteria for this condition (see modified Duke criteria, Box 2).

ECG findings provide specific evidence of IE that include vegetations, evidence of periannular tissue destruction (abscess), aneurysm, fistula, leaflet perforation, and valvular dehiscence.

The diagnostic utility of transthoracic echocardiogram (TTE) for suspected IE is highest in patients with intermediate to high likelihood of this disease (e.g., a patient with a new or changed heart murmur and bacteremia). Hence, TTE should be performed in all patients with suspected IE. However, the diagnostic sensitivity of TTE for the visualization of an intracardiac vegetation

or abscess is limited, ranging from 40% to 80%, and thus the diagnosis of IE cannot be ruled out because of a negative study. The absence of five clinical criteria has been associated with zero probability of a TTE showing evidence of IE: positive blood cultures, presence of central venous access, recent history of injection drug use, presence of prosthetic valve, and vasculitic or embolic phenomena.

Transesophageal echocardiography (TEE) has greater spatial resolution compared with TTE and so is more sensitive than TTE for detecting intracardiac vegetations (sensitivity, 87%; specificity, 95%). As a result, TEE should be performed in patients with a high likelihood of IE and a negative TTE. Although TTE and TEE have been found to have concordant results in approximately half of patients with suspected IE, TEE provides additional diagnostic information in a high percentage of patients, particularly those with prosthetic valves. Specific subsets of patients in whom TEE should be performed, even as the primary imaging modality (without TTE), include patients with prosthetic heart valves and suspected IE and patients with persistent staphylococcal bacteremia without known source or nosocomial infection. In addition, TEE should be performed in patients with IE when paravalvular abscess is suspected.

Other Cardiac Imaging Modalities

Cardiac magnetic resonance imaging with contrast appears promising for detecting paravalvular abscesses, thrombus associated with vegetations, valvular complications, and aortocameral fistulas, although temporal resolution might limit its use for detecting vegetation. Cardiac computed tomography has also been used to detect aortic root abscess. However, clinical experience with these techniques in IE patients is limited, and their sensitivities and specificities in comparison to echocardiography are not well defined. Positron emission tomography–computed tomography (PET-CT) scans have been used to evaluate prosthetic devices, including cardiac implanted electronic devices, for inflammation localized to these devices, and may help differentiate postsurgical changes from active infection.

Routine coronary angiography is recommended in patients older than 55 years and in those at high risk for coronary artery disease before surgery for IE.

Differential Diagnosis

Given the protean manifestations of IE, the differential diagnosis includes a number of systemic conditions: systemic lupus erythematosus, acute rheumatic fever, atrial myxoma, vasculitis, and renal cell carcinoma.

Treatment

Multidisciplinary care of the patient with IE, involving cardiologists, infectious disease specialists, and cardiac surgeons, improves the outcome of IE by optimizing appropriate antibiotic treatment and assessment for surgical indications and operative risk. Antibiotic therapy has improved survival in IE by 70% to 80% and has been shown to reduce the incidence of complications of IE. Detailed descriptions of antibiotic regimens for specific causative organisms are found in guidelines by the American Heart Association (updated in 2015) and the European Society of Cardiology (also updated in 2015). Recommended antimicrobial regimens against typical organisms causing IE are outlined in Table 2. Although the choice of antimicrobial therapy is mainly guided by the infecting organism and its antibiotic susceptibilities, there are three basic principles of antibiotic treatment for the eradication of native valve infection.

First, a prolonged course of antibiotic treatment (4 to 6 weeks) is necessary to eradicate infection because bacterial concentration within vegetations is high and organisms deep within vegetations are inaccessible to phagocytic cells. Repeat sets of blood cultures after antibiotic initiation should be obtained every 24 to 48 hours until the resolution of bacteremia is confirmed. If surgery for IE is performed, completion of the 4- to 6-week course of antibiotic therapy is generally favored to reduce the risk of recurrent IE.

Modified Duke Criteria
Major Criteria
Positive blood cultures
- Typical microbes consistent with IE from two separate blood cultures: viridans streptococci, *Streptococcus bovis*, HACEK group, *Staphylococcus aureus*; community-acquired enterococci in absence of another focus

or

- Microorganisms consistent with IE from persistently positive blood cultures defined as follows: at least two blood cultures drawn more than 12 hours apart, all of three blood cultures, or a majority of positive blood cultures in more than four drawn
- Single positive blood culture for *Coxiella burnetii* or antiphase IgG antibody titer >1:800

Evidence of endocardial involvement
Echo findings of IE, defined as:
- Oscillating intracardiac mass on valve or supporting structure
- Abscess
- New partial dehiscence of prosthetic valve
- New valvular regurgitation

Minor Criteria
- Predisposition: predisposing heart condition or injection drug use
- Fever, temperature >38°C
- Vascular phenomena, major arterial emboli, septic pulmonary infarcts, mycotic aneurysm, intracranial hemorrhage, conjunctival hemorrhage, and Janeway lesions
- Immunologic phenomena: glomerulonephritis, Osler nodes, Roth spots, rheumatoid factor
- Microbiologic evidence: positive blood cultures but does not meet a major criterion as noted previously, or serologic evidence of active infection with organism consistent with causing IE

Case Definitions
Definite Infective Endocarditis
Presence of any pathologic criteria:
- Microorganisms demonstrated by culture or histologic examination of a vegetation, a vegetation that has embolized, or an intracardiac abscess specimen

or

- Pathologic lesions; vegetation or intracardiac abscess confirmed by histologic examination showing active endocarditis

If there are no pathologic criteria, then clinical diagnosis of definite IE:
- Two major criteria

or

- One major and three minor criteria

or

- Five minor criteria

Possible Infective Endocarditis
- One major criterion and one minor criterion
  or
- Three minor criteria

Rejected
- Firm alternative diagnosis explaining evidence of IE
  or
- Resolution of IE syndrome with antibiotic therapy for ≤4 days
  or
- No pathologic evidence of IE at surgery or autopsy, with antibiotic therapy for <4 days
  or
- Does not meet criteria for possible IE, as above.

HACEK, *Haemophilus* spp., *Aggregatibacter* spp., *Cardiobacterium hominis, Eikenella corrodens, Kingella* spp.; IE, infective endocarditis; Ig, immunoglobulin.

Adapted from Li JS, Sexton DJ, Nettles R, et al. Proposed modifications to the Duke criteria for the diagnosis of infective endocarditis. *Clin Infect Dis* 2003;30(4):633–638.

III Cardiovascular System

Second, parenteral administration of antibiotic therapy is necessary to achieve adequate drug levels required to eradicate infection. Parenteral therapy is typically initiated in the hospital setting, and the patient may receive outpatient parenteral treatment for the remaining duration after an initial period of observation to assess for clinical response to therapy (e.g., clearance of bacteremia and absence of complications).

Third, because of the need for prolonged therapy and rising antimicrobial resistance among organisms, combination therapy typically involving a β-lactam and aminoglycoside antibiotic is recommended. Combination therapy has been shown to reduce the duration of bacteremia in *S. aureus* endocarditis, although this more-rapid resolution of bacteremia was not associated with an improved clinical response or outcome. Both antibiotics should be given temporally close together so that maximum synergistic bactericidal effect is obtained. In addition, the dosage and kidney function should be monitored carefully, because combination therapy has been associated with a higher rate of kidney dysfunction.

Complications

IE can progress to the development of various intracardiac and extracardiac complications before or despite effective treatment. Heart failure or pulmonary edema is a common complication, occurring in about one third to one half of patients with IE, and it is the most common indication for urgent surgery. Valvular destruction and the ensuing insufficiency can result in volume overload and heart failure; in rare cases of large vegetations, heart failure may be a result of valvular stenosis. Heart failure complicates aortic valve IE more often than mitral or tricuspid IE, and

can result in the setting of moderate, rather than severe, regurgitation because the left ventricle is unable to compensate for the acute increase in preload and afterload in this condition.

Medical therapy alone is generally insufficient in managing IE complicated by heart failure, particularly in the setting of severe or progressive valvular regurgitation. Surgery should be prompt, and unnecessary delays should be avoided.

Paravalvular abscess complicates 30% to 40% of cases of IE and is a result of invasive infection that generally spreads along contiguous tissue planes, particularly with aortic valve infection. In the International Collaboration on Endocarditis (ICE) cohort, 22% cases of definite aortic valve IE were complicated by a periannular abscess. These patients were more likely to have prosthetic valves and coagulase-negative staphylococcal infection. TEE is the diagnostic test of choice when an abscess is suspected clinically. An abscess is diagnosed by TEE as the visualization of a periannular area of thickening or mass with a heterogeneous echogenic or echolucent appearance. Rarely, antibiotic therapy alone may be used to treat an intracardiac abscess, although this treatment alone is generally reserved for patients who are poor surgical candidates. The vast majority of patients with an intracardiac abscess require cardiac surgery for débridement. In addition, surgery represents the gold standard for the diagnosis of abscess.

Embolic phenomena often complicate the clinical course in IE. Although clinical signs of embolization occur in approximately one third of patients with IE, at least another third of patients have silent embolism. In the majority of cases, embolic events occur before antibiotic therapy is initiated. The most frequent sites of embolic events were the central nervous system (approximately

TABLE 2 Antimicrobial Regimens Against Typical Infective Endocarditis Organisms

ORGANISM	SUSCEPTIBILITY	REGIMEN	DOSAGE	DURATION (WK)
Native Valve				
Streptococcus viridans, Streptococcus bovis	Penicillin	Penicillin	12–18 MU IV per 24 h continuously or in 4–6 equally divided doses	4
		or ceftriaxone	2 g IV or IM per 24 h	4
		or vancomycin	30 mg/kg IV per 24 h in 2 divided doses Max: 2 g/24 h	4
	Penicillin-relative resistance	Penicillin	24 MU IV per 24 h continuously or in 4–6 equally divided doses	4
		or ceftriaxone	2 g IV/IM per 24 h	4
		plus gentamicin	3 mg/kg IV/IM per 24 h in 1 dose	2
		or vancomycin	30 mg/kg IV per 24 h in 2 divided doses (limit 2 g/24 h)	4
Enterococcus spp.	Penicillin	Ampicillin	12 g IV per 24 h in 6 divided doses	4–6
		or penicillin	18–30 MU IV per 24 h continuously or in 6 equally divided doses	4–6
		plus gentamicin	3 mg/kg IV or IM per 24 h in 3 divided doses	2
		or ampicillin	12 g IV per 24 h in 6 divided doses	6
		plus ceftriaxone	2 g IV every 12 h	6
	Penicillin-resistant	Vancomycin	30 mg/kg IV per 24 h in 2 divided doses (limit 2 g/24 h)	
Staphylococcus spp.	Oxacillin	Nafcillin or oxacillin	12 g IV per 24 h in 4–6 divided doses	6
		or cefazolin	3 mg/kg IV/IM per 24 h in 3 equally divided doses	6
			6 g IV per 24 h in 3 divided doses	6
	Oxacillin-resistant	Vancomycin *plus* gentamicin	30 mg/kg IV per 24 h in 2 divided doses (goal: 1 h peak concentration 30–45 µg/mL and trough 10–15 µg/mL)	
Oxacillin-resistant Staphylococcus spp.		Vancomycin	30 mg/kg IV per 24 h in 2 divided doses Goal: 1 h peak concentration 30–45 µg/mL and trough 10–15 µg/mL	6
Prosthetic Valve				
Staphylococcus spp.	Oxacillin-susceptible	Nafcillin or oxacillin	12 g IV per 24 h in 4–6 divided doses	6
		plus gentamicin	3 mg/kg IV or IM per 24 h in 3 divided doses	2
		plus rifampin[1]	900 mg IV or PO per 24 h in 3 divided doses	6
	Oxacillin-resistant	Vancomycin	30 mg/kg IV per 24 h in 2 divided doses Goal: 1 h peak concentration 30–45 µg/mL and trough 10–15 µg/mL	6
		plus gentamicin	3 mg/kg IV or IM per 24 h in 3 divided doses	2
		plus rifampin[1]	900 mg IV or PO per 24 h in 3 divided doses	6

Max, maximum.
[1]Not FDA approved for this indication.

40% of embolic events), lungs (approximately 20%), spleen (20%), peripheral artery (approximately 15%), and kidney (10%).

Factors including vegetation size, mobility, location, and the causative organism have been associated with the likelihood of embolic event. Vegetations larger than 10 mm in greatest diameter are associated with an increased risk of embolization. Causative organisms such as *S. aureus* and *Streptococcus bovis* confer an independent risk of embolization. Embolism also occurs with greater frequency in IE caused by enterococci, fastidious gram-negative organisms (HACEK), and fungi as compared with streptococcal IE. In addition to causing infarction of distal vascular beds, embolic events can result in metastatic sites of infection.

Cerebral embolization occurs in 10% to 35% of cases and is at times complicated by meningitis, brain abscess, or intracerebral hemorrhage. The risk of stroke dramatically decreases with initiation of antibiotic therapy. Findings from the ICE merged database suggested a 65% reduction in stroke incidence by week 2 of initiating antimicrobial therapy. Given the low incidence of embolic event after initiation of antibiotic therapy, routine screening for emboli in patients with IE is not recommended. However, patients with persistent fever or bacteremia or localizing symptoms of possible infarction should undergo computed tomographic imaging with radiographic contrast for the diagnosis of embolic complications.

Embolic events have been found to be an independent predictor of in-hospital death in IE. In patients who experience recurrent embolic events, particularly if they occur after initiation of antibiotic therapy, surgical treatment is indicated. For the prevention of embolic events, surgery may be considered for patients with IE who have residual large (>10 mm), mobile vegetations involving mitral or aortic valve. A recent, small, randomized trial of early surgery for native, left-sided IE has found significant reduction in embolic events in patients treated with earlier surgery.

Surgical Therapy

Surgical intervention for IE may be performed in either the acute or active phase of infection or after the eradication of infection. The optimal timing of surgery in the setting of active IE has not been well evaluated. In patients with serious, life-threatening complications of IE, surgery should be performed emergently. A number of case series have shown that surgery in the active phase of IE can be performed with acceptable risk and without an obvious risk of infecting a prosthetic valve. Surgery during the active phase is generally considered for patients in whom the likelihood of cure of infection with antibiotic therapy alone is low or in whom severe complications have or will likely occur. In contemporary series, surgery is performed in 40% to 50% of patients with IE during the index hospitalization. Surgery after eradication of infection is predominantly performed for adverse hemodynamic effects of valvular regurgitation that results from valve damage.

Indications for surgery in IE are shown in Box 3. A majority of patients with left-sided IE will have an indication for surgery but may be poor candidates for surgery due to hemodynamic instability or other comorbid conditions. Heart failure is the most common indication for urgent surgical intervention, yet even without overt heart failure symptoms, hemodynamic evidence of severe regurgitation (such as premature closure of the mitral valve in severe aortic regurgitation or pulmonary hypertension in severe mitral regurgitation) should also prompt surgical intervention because valvular regurgitation—or rarely, stenosis—is a mechanical complication of IE that will not improve with antimicrobial therapy alone. For mitral valve regurgitation, surgical repair of the native valve without replacing the valve with a prosthesis has been reported in a number of case series. However, the role of repair versus replacement has not been evaluated in controlled studies, and its feasibility will be limited by the extent of infection and valvular damage, as well as the experience of the surgeon. Surgery for IE may be performed with an acceptable operative mortality rate, although urgent or emergent surgery is associated with higher mortality.

Because embolic complications often involve the central nervous system and can worsen neurologic function after cardiopulmonary bypass, the timing of surgery after a cerebral embolic infarct is controversial. A high percentage of patients with left-sided IE may develop asymptomatic brain embolic events if MRI is performed. Studies found that neurologic deterioration did not occur among patients with IE who experienced transient ischemic attacks or asymptomatic emboli, even if surgery was performed acutely. However, patients with recent hemorrhagic strokes may be at risk for extension and deterioration after cardiac surgery. In patients with ischemic stroke with major neurologic deficit or intracranial hemorrhage, it is recommended to delay valve surgery for at least 4 weeks.

Regarding persistent bacteremia as an indication for surgery, it is important to recognize that certain microorganisms, particularly S. aureus, may be associated with prolonged bacteremia (up to 10 days) after initiation of antibiotic therapy. Because of possible difficulty in eradicating infection from prosthetic materials, all cases of prosthetic valve IE should receive surgical consultation. With valve conservation and improved surgical techniques, the surgical mortality rates have declined over time, with recent reported rates in the range of 7% to 14%. In comparison to therapy alone, surgery appears to confer a survival benefit for those patients with major complications of IE, such as heart failure or intracardiac abscess.

Despite the high rate of surgical intervention in IE, the in-hospital mortality rate for native valve IE in the contemporary era remains high at approximately 15% to 20%, and nearly 25% for prosthetic valve IE. Among host factors, older age, female sex, diabetes mellitus, acute physiology (APACHE II) score, elevated white blood cell count, serum creatinine level greater than 2 mg/dL, and lower serum albumin have been associated with worse outcome. Congestive heart failure, paravalvular complication (e.g., abscess formation), infection with virulent organisms (particularly S. aureus), prosthetic valve infection, and absence of surgical intervention are also factors related to higher mortality in IE.

BOX 3 — Indications for Surgical Intervention in Infective Endocarditis

Class I Indications
- Valve dysfunction with heart failure symptoms
- Left-sided IE due to *S. aureus*, fungal, or other highly resistant organism
- IE complicated by heart block, annular or aortic abscess, or destructive penetrating lesions
- Persistent bacteremia or fevers lasting longer than 5 to 7 days after onset of appropriate antimicrobial therapy
- Prosthetic valve endocarditis with relapsing infection
- Complete removal of pacemaker or defibrillator system when evidence of device infection

Class IIa Indications
- Recurrent embolic and persistent vegetation despite appropriate antibiotic therapy
- Complete removal of pacemaker or defibrillator system in patients with IE due to *S. aureus* or fungal organism, or when undergoing valvular surgery for valvular IE

Class IIb Indications
- Native IE with vegetation >10 mm in length, with or without emboli

---

Class I, benefit >>> risk, surgery should be performed; *class IIa*, benefit >> risk, reasonable to perform surgery; *class IIb*, benefit ≥ risk, surgery may be considered, additional studies are needed.
Adapted from Nishimura RA, et al. 2014 AHA/ACC guideline for the management of patients with valvular heart disease: executive summary: a report of the American College of Cardiology/American Heart Association Task Force on Practice Guidelines. *Circulation.* 2014; 129(23):2440–2492.

References

Baddour LM, Wilson WR, Bayer AS, et al: On behalf of the American Heart Association Committee on Rheumatic Fever, Endocarditis, and Kawasaki Disease of the Council on Cardiovascular Disease in the Young, Council on Clinical Cardiology, Council on Cardiovascular Surgery and Anesthesia, and Stroke Council. Infective endocarditis in adults: diagnosis, antimicrobial therapy, and management of complications: a scientific statement for healthcare professionals from the American Heart Association, *Circulation* 132:1435–1486, 2015.

Cahill TJ, et al: Challenges in Infective Endocarditis, *J Am Coll Cardiol* 69(3):325–344, 2017.

Chu VH, Cabell CH, Benjamin Jr. DK, et al: Early predictors of in-hospital death in infective endocarditis, *Circulation* 109(14):1745–1749, 2004.

Fowler Jr. VG, Miro JM, Hoen B, et al: *Staphylococcus aureus* endocarditis: A consequence of medical progress, *JAMA* 293(24):3012–3021, 2005.

Gaca JG, Sheng S, Daneshmand MA, et al: Outcomes for endocarditis surgery in North America: a simplified risk scoring system, *J Thorac Cardiovasc Surg* 141:98–106, 2011.

Habib G, Lancellotti P, Antunes MJ, et al: 2015 ESC Guidelines for the management of infective endocarditis: The Task Force for the Management of Infective Endocarditis of the European Society of Cardiology (ESC). Endorsed by: European Association for Cardio-Thoracic Surgery (EACTS), the European Association of Nuclear Medicine (EANM), *Eur Heart J* 36(44):3075–3128, 2015.

Hasbun R, Vikram HR, Barakat LA, et al: Complicated left-sided native valve endocarditis in adults: Risk classification for mortality, *JAMA* 289(15):1933–1940, 2003.

Hoen B, Alla F, Selton-Suty C, et al: Changing profile of infective endocarditis: Results of a 1-year survey in France, *JAMA* 288(1):75–81, 2002.

Kang DH, Kim YJ, Kim SH, et al: Early surgery versus conventional treatment for infective endocarditis, *N Engl J Med* 366:2466–2473, 2012.

Kiefer T, Park L, Tribouilloy C, et al: Association between valvular surgery and mortality among patients with infective endocarditis complicated by heart failure, *JAMA* 306:2239–2247, 2011.

Li JS, Sexton DJ, Nettles R, et al: Proposed modifications to the Duke criteria for the diagnosis of infective endocarditis, *Clin Infect Dis* 30(4):633–638, 2000.

Moreillon P, Que YA: Infective endocarditis, *Lancet* 363(9403):139–149, 2004.

Nishimura RA, Otto CM, Bonow RO, et al: 2014 AHA/ ACC guideline for the management of patients with valvular heart disease: a report of the American College of Cardiology/American Heart Association Task Force on Practice Guidelines, *J Am Coll Cardiol* 63:e57–185, 2014.

Task Force on the Prevention: Diagnosis, and Treatment of Infective Endocarditis of the European Society of Cardiology; European Society of Clinical Microbiology and Infectious Diseases; International Society of Chemotherapy for Infection and Cancer; ESC Committee for Practice Guidelines: Guidelines on the prevention, diagnosis, and treatment of infective endocarditis (new version 2009): the Task Force on the Prevention, Diagnosis, and Treatment of Infective Endocarditis of the European Society of Cardiology (ESC), *Eur Heart J* 30(19):2369–2413, 2009.

Vikram HR, Buenconsejo J, Hasbun R, et al: Impact of valve surgery on 6-month mortality in adults with complicated, left- sided native valve endocarditis: A propensity analysis, *JAMA* 290(24):3207–3214, 2003.

Wang A, Athan E, Pappas PA, et al: Contemporary clinical profile and outcome of prosthetic valve endocarditis, *JAMA* 297(12):1354–1361, 2007.

MITRAL VALVE PROLAPSE

Method of
Kurt M. Jacobson, MD; Peter S. Rahko, MD; and Shenil Shah, MD

CURRENT DIAGNOSIS

- A midsystolic click with or without a middle- to late-peaking crescendo systolic murmur is the classic auscultatory finding of mitral valve prolapse (MVP).
- Key examination maneuvers can help differentiate MVP from other valvular heart diseases.
- Diagnostic echocardiographic findings of MVP are systolic billowing of the mitral valve leaflets 2 mm above the annulus into the left atrium.
- The presence of significant myxomatous thickening of the valve leaflets (>5 mm) is significant for prognosis.

CURRENT THERAPY

- Patients with physical findings of mitral valve prolapse (MVP) should have an echocardiogram to confirm the diagnosis, determine the severity of prolapse, determine the amount of myxomatous thickening, document the severity (if present) of mitral regurgitation, and determine left ventricular size and function.
- Uncomplicated MVP without significant mitral regurgitation can be evaluated clinically every 3 to 5 years.
- Complicated MVP (associated with significant mitral regurgitation, left ventricular structural changes, pulmonary hypertension, atrial fibrillation, or stroke) should be observed closely with serial clinical evaluation and echocardiography.
- Surgery may be required for complicated MVP associated with severe mitral regurgitation. Repair rather than replacement is the procedure of choice and should be performed at surgical centers experienced with mitral valve repair.
- Recommendations for surgery are the same for MVP as for other forms of chronic severe mitral regurgitation.
- Percutaneous intervention with the MitraClip (Abbott Vascular) is an option in symptomatic patients with moderate to severe or severe mitral regurgitation, prohibitive surgical risk, and acceptable anatomy.

Mitral valve prolapse (MVP) has been known by many names, including floppy valve syndrome, Barlow's syndrome, click/murmur syndrome, myxomatous mitral valve disease, and billowing mitral cusp syndrome. MVP is a common cardiac valvular abnormality characterized by redundant, floppy mitral valve leaflets; it is often detected initially by characteristic nonejection clicks or a middle- to late-peaking crescendo systolic murmur on physical examination.

Prevalence

MVP is the most common congenital cause of mitral regurgitation (MR) in adults and the most common indication for mitral valve surgery in the United States today. Previously, it was one of the most overdiagnosed conditions within cardiology, with suggested prevalence rates ranging from 5% to 15%. With the use of current diagnostic standards, rates are much lower; the overestimation was a consequence of diverse and nonuniformly accepted two-dimensional echocardiographic diagnostic criteria. Freed and colleagues, using the Framingham study population and applying consistent and more stringent echocardiographic diagnostic criteria, demonstrated a much lower prevalence of MVP (approximately 2.4%). The incidence appeared to be similar among men and women. Gender differences do exist, however. Women tend to have a more benign course, whereas men tend to have more advanced myxomatous disease resulting in a greater chance of more severe MR.

Classification

Primary MVP is characterized by idiopathic myxomatous change of the mitral valve leaflets or the chordal structures or both. Secondary MVP is present when underlying conditions such as Marfan's syndrome, Ehlers-Danlos syndrome, osteogenesis imperfecta, or other collagen vascular disorders are evident. Certain congenital cardiac abnormalities, including Ebstein anomaly, aortic coarctation, hypertrophic cardiomyopathy, and ostium secundum atrial septal defects, are also associated with MVP. Familial variants with an autosomal dominant pattern of inheritance have been identified, and work to identify the genes involved is under way. The reported prevalence of MVP in first-degree relatives is between 30% and 50%.

Pathology

Macroscopic and microscopic changes can involve both the anterior and posterior leaflets as well as the chordal structures of the leaflet apparatus. Macroscopically, the surface area of the leaflet is increased, providing the accentuated, billowing appearance of the valve leaflets. Additional notable changes are thickening of the individual leaflets, increased leaflet length, thinning and stretching of the chordae, and increased circumference of the mitral valve annulus. At the microscopic level (Figure 1), normal mitral valves have three well-defined layers, each containing cells and a characteristic composition and configuration of the extracellular matrix: the fibrosa, composed predominantly of collagen fibers densely packed and arranged parallel to the free edge of the leaflet; the centrally located spongiosa, composed of loosely arranged collagen and proteoglycans; and the atrialis, composed of elastic fibers. In myxomatous mitral valves, the spongiosa layer is expanded by loose, amorphous extracellular matrix that has more proteoglycans but less collagen and more fragmented elastic fibers. What collagen is present appears to be disorganized and fragmented, giving the appearance of a haphazard layering of the spongiosa. It is this thickening that produces the classic macroscopic appearance of the myxomatous valve on two-dimensional echocardiography.

Clinical Presentation

Most patients with MVP are asymptomatic and will remain so, testifying to the often benign nature of this disease. Previously, various nonspecific symptoms, including fatigue, dyspnea, palpitations, postural orthostasis, anxiety, and panic attacks, were described as an MVP syndrome when present in association with the characteristic nonejection systolic click or middle- to late-peaking crescendo systolic murmur. Other symptoms, including

Figure 1 Morphologic features of normal mitral valves *(left)* and valves with myxomatous degeneration *(right)*. Myxomatous valves have an abnormal layered architecture: loose collagen in fibrosa, expanded spongiosa strongly positive for proteoglycans, and disrupted elastin in atrialis *(top)*. Movat pentachrome stain (collagen stains yellow, proteoglycans blue-green, and elastin black). (Modified from Rabkin E, Aikawa M, Stone JR, et al: Activated interstitial myofibroblasts express catabolic enzymes and mediate matrix remodeling in myxomatous heart valves. *Circulation* 2001;104:2525.)

chest discomfort, near-syncope, and syncope, have also been described by patients with MVP. However, in a community-based study, the prevalence of various clinical complaints including chest pain, dyspnea, and syncope was no higher in patients with MVP than in those without evidence of MVP, making such findings nonspecific. In a controlled study that compared symptomatic MVP patients with first-degree relatives with and without echocardiographic evidence of MVP, there also was no association of MVP with atypical chest pain, dyspnea, panic attacks, or anxiety. There was, however, a significant association of MVP with physical findings of systolic clicks, systolic murmurs, thoracic bony abnormalities, low body weight, and low blood pressure. Congestive heart failure, atrial fibrillation, stroke or transient ischemic attack, hypertension, diabetes, and hypercholesterolemia are no more likely in patients with MVP than in those without MVP. However, previous retrospective studies suggested a higher incidence of cerebral embolic events, infectious endocarditis, severe MR, and need for mitral valve replacement in patients with classic (complicated) versus nonclassic MVP. Symptoms of poor cardiac reserve, such as reduced exercise tolerance, dyspnea on exertion, and fatigue, may reflect the presence of significant MR and warrant clinical concern.

Diagnosis

Symptoms are not predictive of the presence or absence of MVP. Certain physical and auscultatory characteristics on examination do support the diagnosis of MVP. Patients with MVP more often have a lower body mass index, have a lower waist-to-hip ratio, and are taller. Findings of scoliosis, pectus excavatum, and hyperextensibility are also prevalent among patients with MVP. The classic auscultatory findings include a midsystolic click and a middle- to late-peaking crescendo systolic murmur heard best at the apex. The auscultatory findings are best elicited with the diaphragm of the stethoscope, and they change in relation to the first and second heart sounds (S_1 and S_2) in response to changes in left ventricular (LV) volume. Therefore the patient should be examined in several positions: supine (including lateral decubitus), sitting, standing, and, if possible, squatting. Changes in LV filling and volume affect the degree of prolapse.

The most important and most specific finding on auscultation is the presence of a nonejection midsystolic click or clicks caused by snapping of the valve apparatus as parts of the valve leaflets billow into the atrium during systole. Although these clicks can be heard over the entire precordium, they are best heard at the apex. The click can be misinterpreted as a split S_1, a true S_1 with an S_4, or a true S_1 with an early ejection click from a bicuspid valve. It can be differentiated from an ejection click heard in bicuspid aortic valves by its timing relative to the beginning of the carotid upstroke. Ejection clicks occur as the aortic valve opens and therefore precede

the carotid upstroke, whereas the nonejection clicks of MVP occur afterward. Clicks from atrial septal aneurysms are uncommon but can be difficult to distinguish from those of MVP. Ejection clicks and clicks from atrial septal aneurysms are not altered by changes in loading characteristics, allowing them to be differentiated from clicks of MVP. Often, but not always, a middle- to late-peaking crescendo systolic murmur can be appreciated by itself or after a click. The murmur terminates with closure of the aortic valve (A2). This represents MR, and, in general, the duration of the murmur correlates with the severity of the MR. The earlier in systole the murmur is detected, the more severe the MR. Eventually, with more severe MR, the murmur becomes holosystolic. MVP manifestations on examination vary, and they may not always be reproducible, even in the same patient.

Certain maneuvers can aid in more accurately diagnosing MVP on examination (Figure 2). MVP is very sensitive to LV filling, and subtle changes in auscultatory findings elicited by careful examination maneuvers can be instrumental in separating MVP from other valvular abnormalities. Generally, measures that decrease LV volume or increase contractility produce earlier and more prominent systolic prolapse of the mitral leaflets, causing the systolic click and murmur to move closer to S_1. For example, in the transition from squatting to standing, LV volume is reduced, and the onset of the click and murmur is moved closer to S_1. Conversely, anything that increases LV volume, such as leg-raising, squatting, or slowing the heart rate (increased diastolic filling), delays the onset of the click or murmur and usually diminishes its duration and intensity.

Use of Echocardiography

Two-dimensional echocardiography has proved to be the most accurate noninvasive tool for the diagnosis, assessment, and follow-up of clinically suspected MVP. In fact, physical signs of MVP in an asymptomatic patient are an American College of Cardiology/American Heart Association (ACC/AHA) class I indication for use of echocardiography to make the diagnosis of MVP and assess the severity of MR, leaflet morphology, and ventricular size and function. Once the diagnosis is made, follow-up is determined by the severity of MVP. Routine echocardiographic follow-up of asymptomatic patients with MVP is not recommended unless there are significant findings of MR or LV structural changes. Frequency of follow-up in patients with prolapse and MR is determined by the severity of MR and should be at least annual in patients with severe MR.

Diagnostic criteria for MVP on two-dimensional echocardiography are:
- Billowing of one or both mitral valve leaflets or their prolapse superiorly across the mitral annular plane in the parasternal long-axis view by greater than 2 mm during systole
- The degree of thickening of the leaflets

Figure 2 Auscultative findings with changes in position in patients with mitral valve prolapse (MVP). *Abbreviations:* C = click of MVP; S_1, mitral valve closure; S_2, aortic valve closure. (Modified from Devereux RB, Perloff JK, Reichek N, et al: Mitral valve prolapse. *Circulation* 1976;54[1]:3–14.)

Supine   Sitting   Standing   Squatting

Combined leaflet prolapse of greater than 2 mm and leaflet thickness greater than 5 mm are supportive of classic MVP, whereas prolapse in the absence of increased thickness is considered nonclassic MVP. In addition to more often being associated with the auscultative findings of the click and murmur, the classic form is more commonly associated with increased risk of endocarditis, stroke, progressive MR, and need for mitral valve repair or replacement.

Because the mitral apparatus is saddle-shaped, certain echocardiographic views are more specific than others for determining leaflet prolapse. Most practitioners agree that the parasternal long-axis and apical two-chamber or apical long-axis views are the most accurate for determining prolapse. A finding of prolapse as determined on other views, particularly the apical four-chamber view, is much less specific and frequently leads to a false-positive diagnosis.

Medical Management

Most patients with MVP remain asymptomatic and require no additional management aside from careful observation over time. It is appropriate to provide reassurance that uncomplicated (nonclassic) MVP is a non–life-threatening condition and is unlikely to affect longevity. Periodic clinical evaluation every 3 to 5 years is reasonable. Patients who develop palpitations, lightheadedness, dizziness, or syncope should undergo Holter or event monitoring for detection of arrhythmias. Palpitations are frequently controlled with β-blockers or calcium channel blockers, although the presence of specific arrhythmias may mandate additional therapy. Endocarditis prophylaxis is no longer recommended for patients with MVP unless they have a history of endocarditis or valve replacement. Prophylaxis is recommended for patients who have undergone repair if prosthetic material was used (e.g., in ring repairs). Aspirin or warfarin (Coumadin) therapy may be recommended for certain symptomatic patients with neurologic events who have atrial fibrillation, significant MR, hypertension, or heart failure (Table 1).

Patients with classic (complicated) MVP deserve regular clinical follow-up, particularly if MR is present. These patients are more likely to develop moderate or severe MR over time. Patients with mild to moderate MR and normal LV function should be clinically evaluated at least annually and should undergo echocardiography every second or third year if stable. Patients with severe MR should have an annual echocardiogram and closer clinical follow-up. Those who have severe MR and develop symptoms or impaired LV systolic function require cardiac catheterization and evaluation for mitral valve surgery. Often the valve can be repaired rather than replaced, with a low operative mortality rate and excellent short- and long-term results when performed at experienced centers. Preservation of the native valve allows for lower risks of thrombosis and endocarditis than does prosthetic valve replacement.

Surgical Management

MVP is the most common cause of adult MR requiring mitral valve surgery. Symptoms of heart failure, severity of MR,

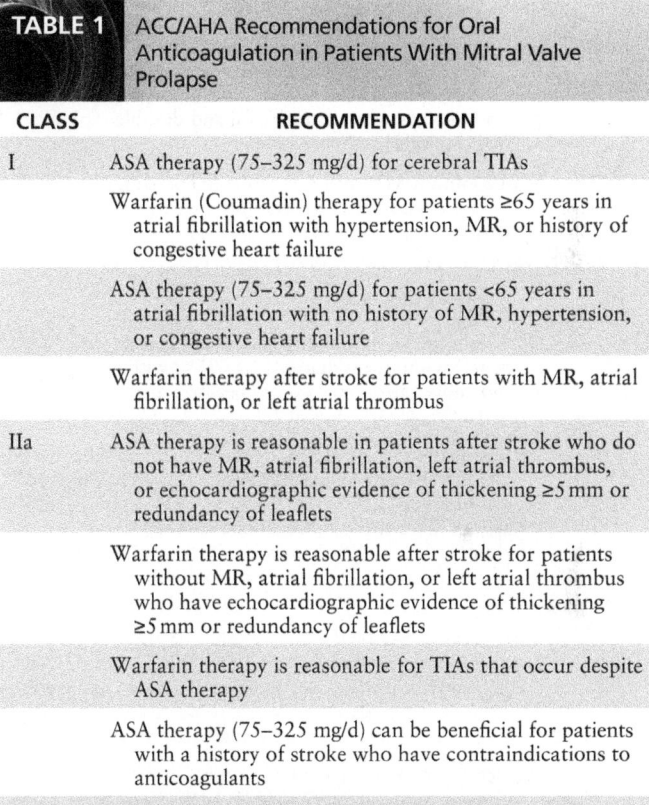

CLASS	RECOMMENDATION
	TABLE 1 ACC/AHA Recommendations for Oral Anticoagulation in Patients With Mitral Valve Prolapse
I	ASA therapy (75–325 mg/d) for cerebral TIAs
	Warfarin (Coumadin) therapy for patients ≥65 years in atrial fibrillation with hypertension, MR, or history of congestive heart failure
	ASA therapy (75–325 mg/d) for patients <65 years in atrial fibrillation with no history of MR, hypertension, or congestive heart failure
	Warfarin therapy after stroke for patients with MR, atrial fibrillation, or left atrial thrombus
IIa	ASA therapy is reasonable in patients after stroke who do not have MR, atrial fibrillation, left atrial thrombus, or echocardiographic evidence of thickening ≥5 mm or redundancy of leaflets
	Warfarin therapy is reasonable after stroke for patients without MR, atrial fibrillation, or left atrial thrombus who have echocardiographic evidence of thickening ≥5 mm or redundancy of leaflets
	Warfarin therapy is reasonable for TIAs that occur despite ASA therapy
	ASA therapy (75–325 mg/d) can be beneficial for patients with a history of stroke who have contraindications to anticoagulants
IIb	ASA therapy (75–325 mg/d) may be considered for patients in sinus rhythm with echocardiographic evidence of complicated MVP

Abbreviations: ACC/AHA = American College of Cardiology/American Heart Association; ASA = aspirin; MR = mitral regurgitation; TIA = transient ischemic attack.
Adapted from Bonow RO, Carabello BA, Chatterjee K, et al: 2008 Focused update incorporated into the ACC/AHA 2006 guidelines for the management of patients with valvular heart disease. *Circulation* 118(15):e523–661, 2008.

presence or absence of atrial fibrillation, LV systolic function, LV end-diastolic and end-systolic volumes, and pulmonary artery pressure (at rest and with exercise) influence the decision to recommend mitral valve surgery. Indications for surgery in patients with MVP and MR mirror those with other forms of nonischemic severe MR. Patient outcomes after mitral valve repair are typically very good, and the surgical risk is lower than for many other forms of cardiac surgery, including mitral valve replacement.

Based on a Cleveland Clinic review of 1072 patients who underwent primary isolated mitral valve repair for MR due to myxomatous disease, the in-hospital mortality rate was 0.3%. The Mayo Clinic reviewed 1173 patients who underwent mitral

CLASS	RECOMMENDATION
TABLE 2	**ACC/AHA Recommendations for Surgery in Patients With Chronic Primary Mitral Valve Regurgitation**
I	Mitral valve (MV) surgery is recommended for symptomatic patients with chronic severe primary MR (stage D) and left ventricular ejection fraction (LVEF) >30%
	MV surgery is recommended for asymptomatic patients with chronic severe primary MR and left ventricular (LV) dysfunction (LVEF 30%-60% and/or left ventricular end-systolic dimension [LVESD] ≥40mm, stage C2)
	MV repair is recommended in preference to mitral valve replacement (MVR) when surgical treatment is indicated for patients with chronic severe primary MR limited to the posterior leaflet
	MV repair is recommended in preference to MVR when surgical treatment is indicated for patients with chronic severe primary MR involving the anterior leaflet or both leaflets when a successful and durable repair can be accomplished
	Concomitant MV repair or replacement is indicated in patients with chronic severe primary MR undergoing cardiac surgery for other indications
IIa	MV repair is reasonable in asymptomatic patients with chronic severe primary MR (stage C1) with preserved LV function (LVEF >60% and LVESD <40mm) in whom the likelihood of a successful and durable repair without residual MR is >95% with an expected mortality rate of <1% when performed at a Heart Valve Center of Excellence
	MV repair is reasonable for asymptomatic patients with chronic severe primary MR (stage C1) and preserved LV function (LVEF >60% and LVESD <40mm) in whom there is a high likelihood of a successful and durable repair with 1) new onset of atrial fibrillation or 2) resting pulmonary hypertension (pulmonary artery systolic arterial pressure >50mm Hg)
	MV repair is reasonable for asymptomatic patients with chronic severe primary MR (stage C1) and preserved LV function (LVEF >60% and LVESD <40mm) with progressive increase in LV size or decrease in ejection fraction on serial imaging studies
	Concomitant MV repair is reasonable in patients with chronic moderate primary MR (stage B) undergoing cardiac surgery for other indications
IIb	MV surgery may be considered in symptomatic patients with chronic severe primary MR and LVEF less than or equal to 30% (stage D)
	MV repair may be considered in patients with rheumatic mitral valve disease when surgical treatment is indicated if a durable and successful repair is likely or if the reliability of long-term anticoagulation management is questionable
	Transcatheter MV repair may be considered for severely symptomatic patients (New York Heart Association class III/IV) with chronic severe primary MR (stage D) who have a reasonable life expectancy but a prohibitive surgical risk because of severe comorbidities and remain symptomatic despite optimal goal directed medical therapy for heart failure
III Harm	MVR should not be performed for treatment of isolated severe primary MR limited to less than one half of the posterior leaflet unless MV repair has been attempted and was unsuccessful

Adapted from 2017 AHA/ACC focused update of the 2014 ACC/AHA guidelines for the management of patients with valvular heart disease. *Circulation* 135(25); e1159–e1195, 2017.

valve repair for MVP from 1980 to 1999, observing mortality rates of 0.7%, 11.3%, and 29.4% at 30 days, 5 years, and 10 years, respectively.

Because of the remarkably low mortality rates associated with MVP repair, some experts advocate earlier rather than later repair of MVP in asymptomatic patients with severe MR and no evidence of LV dysfunction, pulmonary hypertension, or atrial fibrillation. AHA/ACC recommendations for surgery in patients with chronic primary mitral valve regurgitation are shown in Table 2.

Percutaneous Management

In 2013 the FDA approved the MitraClip (Abbott Vascular) for patients with symptomatic degenerative MR who are deemed high risk for mitral valve surgery. The MitraClip technology is based on the Alfieri edge-to-edge repair in which the middle segments of the anterior and posterior leaflet are sutured together to create a double-orifice. It is approved for use in patients with New York Heart Association Class III or IV heart failure despite medical therapy, chronic moderate to severe or severe primary MR, favorable anatomy typically involving the middle segments of the anterior and posterior leaflets, reasonable life expectancy, and prohibitive surgical risk. This approval is based on the results of the Endovascular Valve Edge-to-Edge Repair Study (EVEREST II), which randomized 279 patients to either percutaneous repair or conventional surgery for repair or replacement of the mitral valve with a primary endpoint of freedom from death, from surgery for mitral valve dysfunction, and from grade 3+ or 4+ MR at 12 months. The rates of the combined primary endpoints were 55% in the percutaneous group and 73% in the surgery group (p=0.007). Rates of death (6% and 6%, respectively) and 3+ or 4+ MR (21% and 20%, respectively) were similar in each group. Major adverse events occurred in 15% of patients in the percutaneous repair group versus 48% in the surgery group at 30 days (p<0.001). Although the MitraClip was less effective at reducing MR, it was approved on the bases of its superior safety and similar clinical outcomes.

References

2008 Focused update incorporated into the ACC/AHA 2006 guidelines for the management of patients with valvular heart disease: a report of the American College of Cardiology/American Heart Association Task Force on Practice Guidelines (Writing Committee to Revise the 1998 Guidelines for the Management of Patients With Valvular Heart Disease): endorsed by the Society of Cardiovascular Anesthesiologists, Society for Cardiovascular Angiography and Interventions, and Society of Thoracic Surgeons, *Circulation* 118(15):e523–661, 2008.

Devereux RB, Kramer-Fox R, Brown WT, et al: Relation between clinical features of the mitral prolapse syndrome and echocardiographically documented mitral valve prolapse, *J Am Coll Cardiol* 8:763–772, 1986.

Feldman T, Foster E, Glower DD, et al: Percutaneous repair or surgery for mitral regurgitation, *N Engl J Med* 364(15):1395–1406, 2011.

Flack JM, Kvasnicka JH, Gardin JM, et al: Anthropometric and physiologic correlates of mitral valve prolapse in a biethnic cohort of young adults: the CARDIA study, *Am Heart J* 138:486, 1999.

Freed LA, Benjamin EJ, Levy D, et al: Mitral valve prolapse in the general population: the benign nature of echocardiographic features in the Framingham Heart Study, *J Am Coll Cardiol* 40:1298–1304, 2002.

Freed LA, Levy D, Levine RA, et al: Prevalence and clinical outcome of mitral-valve prolapse, *N Engl J Med* 341:1–7, 1999.

Gillinov AM, Cosgrove DM, Blackstone EH, et al: Durability of mitral valve repair for degenerative disease, *J Thorac Cardiovasc Surg* 116(5):734–743, 1998.

Levy D, Savage D: Prevalence and clinical features of mitral valve prolapse, *Am Heart J* 113:1281–1290, 1987.

Marks AR, Choong CY, Sanfilippo AJ, et al: Identification of high-risk and low-risk subgroups of patients with mitral-valve prolapse, *N Engl J Med* 320:1031–1036, 1989.

Rabkin E, Aikawa M, Stone JR, et al: Activated interstitial myofibroblasts express catabolic enzymes and mediate matrix remodeling in myxomatous heart valves, *Circulation* 104:2525–2532, 2001.

Savage DD, Devereux RB, Garrison RJ, et al: Mitral valve prolapse in the general population: 2. Clinical features: The Framingham Study, *Am Heart J* 106:577–581, 1983.

Savage DD, Garrison RJ, Devereux RB, et al: Mitral valve prolapse in the general population: 1. Epidemiologic features: The Framingham Study, *Am Heart J* 106:571–576, 1983.

Suri RM, Schaff HV, Dearani JA, et al: Survival advantage and improved durability of mitral repair for leaflet prolapse subsets in the current era, *Ann Thorac Surg* 82(3):819–826, 2006.

PERICARDITIS

Method of
Amir Azarbal, MD; and Martin M. LeWinter, MD

CURRENT DIAGNOSIS

- Acute pericarditis is an inflammatory syndrome thought to be caused by a viral infection in most cases. It is diagnosed when 2 of the following are present: (1) typical anterior pleuritic chest pain, (2) pericardial friction rub, (3) electrocardiography (ECG) changes (widespread ST segment elevation or PR depression, and (4) new or worsening pericardial effusion.
- Leukocytosis and an elevated high-sensitivity C-reactive protein or erythrocyte sedimentation rate (ESR) are present in most cases.
- Echocardiography is routinely used to detect pericardial effusion. Cardiac magnetic resonance imaging or computed tomography can be used to support the diagnosis.

CURRENT THERAPY

- Limitation of physical activity and high-dose aspirin[1] or other nonsteroidal antiinflammatory drugs such as ibuprofen (Advil)[1] plus colchicine[1] is the treatment of choice for idiopathic (presumed viral) pericarditis.
- Corticosteroids with gradual taper can be added for recurrences.
- Antiinflammatory drugs such as azathioprine (Imuran),[1] anakinra (Kineret),[1] and human intravenous immunoglobulin (Gammagard)[1] have been used in difficult cases of recurrent pericarditis
- Pericardiectomy is reserved for refractory cases and constrictive pericarditis.

[1]Not FDA approved for this indication.

Anatomy and Functions of the Pericardium

The pericardium consists of 2 layers. A visceral monolayer comprised of mesothelial cells is adherent to the epicardium and reflects over the origin of the great vessels, where it is continuous with the inner layer of the parietal pericardium. The latter is approximately 2 mm thick and comprised mainly of collagen and elastin. The pericardial sac is the space between visceral and parietal layers and normally contains up to 50 mL of serous fluid. The pericardium has several functions, including (1) acting as a barrier to infections, (2) providing a mechanism whereby hydrostatic pressure is exerted on the surface of the heart when gravitational or inertial forces are altered, (3) participating in neuro-humoral responses, and (4) limiting short-term distention and displacement of the heart, facilitating interactions between the cardiac chambers and modulating pressure-volume relationships and cardiac output.

Acute Pericarditis

The main inflammatory pericardial syndromes include acute and recurrent pericarditis and constrictive and effusive-constrictive pericarditis. These can be isolated to the pericardium or be a component of a systemic disease.

Acute pericarditis is the most common pericardial syndrome and is responsible for approximately 5% of emergency room visits for chest pain and 2% of patients presenting with ST elevations on ECG. An in-hospital mortality rate of approximately 1% has been reported. Acute pericarditis is more common in males. Recurrence occurs in 15% to 20% of patients within 18 months after a first episode. Acute pericarditis can also involve

the myocardium and cause myopericarditis, with elevated cardiac injury biomarkers (e.g., troponin I).

Etiology

Almost any disease that affects the pericardium can cause acute pericarditis. Acute pericarditis can also cause pericardial effusion; the incidence is highly dependent on etiology. Infectious etiologies are considered to be responsible for the majority of cases. In developed countries 80% to 90% of cases are idiopathic, that is, no specific cause is detected on routine evaluation. These cases are assumed to be viral in etiology. Bacterial and rarely fungal infections account for a small percentage of cases in the developed world. However, *Mycobacterium tuberculosis* is the most common cause of pericarditis in developing countries. Very rarely, parasitic diseases such as echinococcus and toxoplasma species can cause acute pericarditis.

Autoimmune diseases are another common cause of acute pericarditis. These include systemic autoimmune diseases such as lupus erythematosus (SLE), rheumatoid arthritis, Sjögren syndrome, and scleroderma, as well as vasculitic diseases such as eosinophilic granulomatosis with polyangiitis or allergic granulomatosis (previously named *Churg-Strauss syndrome*), Takayasu disease, and Behçet syndrome. Other autoimmune disorders associated with acute pericarditis are sarcoidosis, familial Mediterranean fever, and inflammatory bowel disease.

Malignancies affecting the pericardium also cause acute pericarditis. Almost all neoplastic pericarditis is caused by secondary metastases from extracardiac tumors, especially lung and breast cancer.

Pericarditis can occur after myocardial infarction (MI), both early (i.e., 2 to 4 days after MI) and late (Dressler syndrome, ≈1 week to 2 months after MI), and after heart surgery. The incidence of post-MI pericarditis has markedly declined because of reperfusion therapy. Trauma such as penetrating and non-penetrating thoracic injury, esophageal perforation, and procedural complications of cardiac procedures (coronary stenting, pacemaker lead insertion, radiofrequency ablation) are all reported. Although these can cause acute cardiac tamponade, acute pericarditis occurs as a late complication within 1 to 2 weeks to as late as 3 months after the initial event. These causes are collectively termed *post-cardiac injury syndromes* and are believed to have an autoinflammatory basis. Acute pericarditis has also been reported as an immune-mediated response to various drugs.

Presentation

The diagnosis of acute pericarditis is made if two of the following are present: (1) typical anterior chest pain, (2) pericardial friction rub, (3) typical ECG changes (widespread ST segment elevation or PR depression, and (4) new or worsening pericardial effusion. In cases with typical chest pain but no other criteria, additional findings that can establish the diagnosis are elevated cardiac injury biomarkers and evidence of pericardial inflammation or thickening based on advanced imaging modalities (cardiac magnetic resonance imaging [cMRI], computed tomography [CT]). An elevation of either high-sensitivity C reactive protein (hsCRP) or the erythrocyte sedimentation (ESR) rate is supportive but not diagnostic.

Chest pain is the most common symptom of acute pericarditis, present in >90% of cases. The pain is typically sharp, located under the sternum or over the left anterior chest, and almost always pleuritic. The trapezius ridge is a classic radiation. The pain is worst supine and improved by sitting forward. Approximately one-third of patients have a pericardial friction rub (a scratchy or squeaking sound at the left sternal border) because of contact between the layers of the pericardium. The friction rub ordinarily has 3 components. Typical ECG changes include ST elevation in all leads except AVR and sometimes V1, as well as PR segment depression. Over time, these changes either simply disappear or go through a phase of ST segment normalization and T-wave inversion before disappearing. Both the friction rub and ECG changes are often evanescent. In cases where it is difficult to establish a diagnosis, repeated auscultation and ECGs can be rewarding. A pericardial effusion has been reported in as many as two-thirds of patients with acute pericarditis. The great majority are small. Sinus tachycardia and low-grade fever are also common. If cardiac tamponade is present, elevated jugular venous pressure, muffled heart sounds, hypotension, and pulsus paradoxus are seen. Other diagnoses that can be confused with acute pericarditis include acute MI, pleuritis, pulmonary embolism, costochondritis, and herpes zoster before appearance of vesicles.

Features accompanying acute pericarditis that indicate an elevated risk (mainly for development of cardiac tamponade) include fever >38.5°C, subacute onset of symptoms, moderate to large pericardial effusion, lack of response to aspirin or nonsteroidal antiinflammatory drugs (NSAIDs), immunosuppression, white blood cell count >13,000/mm^3, anticoagulant therapy, and suspicion of a nonidiopathic/viral cause such as cancer, SLE, or bacterial infection.

Diagnostic Evaluation

Routine evaluation is directed toward identifying patients with or at elevated risk for cardiac tamponade or patients with a nonidiopathic/viral cause. In addition to a careful history, physical examination, and ECG, routine evaluation should include a chest radiograph, CBC, hs-CRP, routine blood chemistries, and an echocardiogram. Echocardiography should be performed in all patients to detect pericardial effusion, which can be hemodynamically significant despite a normal radiographic cardiac silhouette, and to assess cardiac function in cases with myopericarditis. In the vast majority of cases myopericarditis has no long-term prognostic significance.

Clinical Laboratory Data

Leukocytosis and elevated hs-CRP or ESR are present in most cases. The hs-CRP in particular is increased in about 75% of cases and usually normalizes within 1 to 2 weeks. Failure of normalization within this time frame is associated with higher rates of recurrence. In patients with concomitant myocarditis, markers of cardiac injury such as troponin-I are elevated.

ECG

As discussed earlier, typical ECG changes considered to be hallmarks of acute pericarditis include widespread ST segment elevations or PR segment depression (Figure 1). ECG changes are dynamic, and about 60% of patients have the following evolution over time: stage I (PR depression, ST segment elevation), stage II (ST normalization), stage III (T-wave inversion after ST segment normalization), and stage IV (ST-T normalization). These evolutionary changes have no known prognostic significance.

Imaging

The chest radiograph is normal in acute pericarditis unless a moderate- to large-size pericardial effusion or associated pulmonary pathology is present. The echocardiogram is usually normal except for the common presence of small pericardial effusions (Figure 2). In cases with associated myopericarditis, the left ventricular ejection fraction is almost always normal.

Figure 2 Parasternal long-axis view of a transthoracic echocardiogram performed in a patient with acute pericarditis showing small to moderate-sized pericardial effusion (asterisk). Also note a pacemaker lead in the right ventricle (arrow) and associated acoustic shadowing artifact.

Cardiac MRI or CT typically shows pericardial thickening and enhanced gadolinium uptake (Figure 3). Advanced imaging modalities can be used to support the diagnosis of pericarditis in difficult cases.

Treatment

Treatment of common pericardial syndromes is summarized in Table 1. Reliable patients without high-risk features need not be hospitalized. For treatment of an initial episode of acute idiopathic pericarditis, avoidance of physical activity greater than walking at a normal pace is recommended until symptoms resolve and CRP has normalized. Athletes should refrain from competitive sports activities for at least 3 months. NSAIDs plus colchicine[1] is a first-line pharmacologic treatment. We recommend ibuprofen (Advil)[1] 600 to 800 mg by mouth 3 times daily or aspirin[1] 2 to 4 g by mouth daily in divided doses and colchicine[1] 0.6 mg twice daily (0.6 mg once daily for patients <70 kg) until symptoms resolve and CRP normalizes. The NSAID should then be tapered over 1 to 2 weeks and colchicine continued for 3 months from onset of symptoms. All patients should receive a proton pump inhibitor while receiving NSAIDs.

In pregnancy ibuprofen, aspirin >100 mg/day by mouth, and colchicine are contraindicated after 20 weeks' gestation. Corticosteroids are preferred in this circumstance. In addition, colchicine is contraindicated during lactation.

[1] Not FDA approved for this indication.

Figure 1 Electrocardiogram demonstrating typical changes of acute pericarditis. Note the widespread ST segment elevations with concomitant PR segment depression.

Figure 3 Cardiac MRI image in a patient with acute pericarditis after intravenous gadolinium administration. Note late gadolinium enhancement of the pericardium along with pericardial thickening indicating inflammation (asterisk). Other findings are pericardial fat (arrowhead) and trivial pericardial effusion (arrow).

In patients in whom a specific cause for acute pericarditis other than idiopathic/viral has been identified, the treatment should be directed at that cause. Thus, in patients with autoimmune diseases, corticosteroids may be more appropriate as the initial treatment.

Recurrent Pericarditis

Recurrent pericarditis is the most common complication of acute pericarditis and is defined as a repeat episode after a symptom-free interval of at least 4 to 6 weeks. The recurrence rate after an initial episode of acute pericarditis is approximately 15% to 20% and may increase to as much as 50% after a first recurrent episode. Patients with recurrent pericarditis can be severely incapacitated. Certain rare conditions such as familial Mediterranean fever, tumor necrosis factor receptor–associated periodic syndrome, and other periodic fever syndromes are often characterized by bouts of recurrent pericarditis. Inadequate treatment of a first episode (e.g., inadequate drug doses, too short a treatment duration or too rapid discontinuation, or tapering of medications) can be responsible for recurrences

Recurrent pericarditis after an initial bout of idiopathic/viral pericarditis is currently considered to be an autoinflammatory process (as opposed to an autoimmune disease such as SLE). It is hypothesized that, after an initial viral infection, immune system cross-reaction between viral particles and host tissue occurs. A similar mechanism is believed to be operative in the periodic fever syndromes. Of course, pericarditis due to other, specific causes can also recur.

The most feared complication of recurrent pericarditis is constrictive pericarditis. The incidence is high (≤30%) in cases of bacterial pericarditis and low to moderate (<5%) in systemic inflammatory diseases and cancer. In patients with recurrences after an initial bout of viral/idiopathic pericarditis, symptoms almost always eventually resolve, and progression to constrictive pericarditis is very rare (<1%).

The diagnosis of a recurrence is based on the same criteria as for an initial episode (i.e., history, friction rub, ECG findings, and a new or worsening pericardial effusion). Elevated hs-CRP, ESR, and white blood cell count remain useful for monitoring disease activity and response to treatment. More advanced imaging modalities such as CT or cMRI are rarely required to diagnose a recurrence but are useful if there is a concern about development of constriction.

TABLE 1 Treatment Summary of Common Pericardial Syndromes

PERICARDIAL SYNDROME	TREATMENT OVERVIEW	SPECIFIC CONSIDERATIONS
Acute pericarditis	Physical activity restriction *and* NSAIDs *plus* Colchicine[1]	Restriction of physical activity until resolution of symptoms NSAIDs until symptoms resolve and CRP normalizes Colchicine for 2 to 3 months See text for pregnancy and lactation considerations
Recurrent pericarditis	Acute pericarditis treatment *plus* Corticosteroids (in refractory cases) *or* Immunosuppressive therapy (for multiple recurrences) *or* Pericardiectomy (last resort)	Restriction of physical activity until resolution of symptoms NSAIDs until symptoms resolve and CRP normalizes for 1 to 2 weeks with subsequent taper Colchicine[1] for at least 6 months For multiple recurrences, low to moderate doses of corticosteroids until resolution of symptoms and normalization of CRP followed by slow taper Immunosuppressants (anakinra [Kineret],[1] azathioprine [Imuran],[1] intravenous immunoglobulin[1]) for multiple recurrences Pericardiectomy in refractory cases (last resort)
Constrictive pericarditis	Treatment of underlying condition (ie, tuberculosis, inflammation) *or* Pericardiectomy (if chronic and refractory)	In cases of pericardial inflammation, an empiric antiinflammatory regimen may reverse the disease process and obviate the need for pericardiectomy.

[1]Not FDA approved for this indication.

In general, for patients with a recurrence after an index episode of idiopathic/viral pericarditis we recommend that treatment be the same as for the initial episode (i.e., restriction of physical activity, NSAID, and colchicine[1]) until complete resolution of symptoms and normalization of hs-CRP. Some patients are able to manage recurrences by initiating treatment at the very first sign of symptoms. If the response is prompt, the recurrence is converted to a minor illness.

Use of corticosteroids for treatment of recurrent pericarditis should be reserved for cases where the above-mentioned measures have failed, especially if recurrences are frequent and severe and do not respond well to NSAIDs. Unusual patients with an initial episode who do not respond to first-line therapy are also candidates. Corticosteroids usually provide rapid relief of symptoms, and almost all patients respond favorably initially. However, corticosteroids appear to increase the chance of further recurrences, especially when high initial doses are used with rapid tapering. High doses also have a much higher incidence of adverse effects.

[1] Not FDA approved for this indication.

If a decision is made to use corticosteroids, we recommend low to moderate doses (e.g., prednisone[1] 0.25 to 0.5 mg/kg/day or equivalent) usually for about 4 to 8 weeks, followed by gradual tapering (assuming symptom resolution and normalization of hs-CRP) in conjunction with colchicine. NSAIDs may also be included or added later as corticosteroids are tapered. Colchicine should ordinarily be continued for 6 months. During tapering, recurrences typically occur with doses <10 to 15 mg/day dose of prednisone or equivalent. Patients symptom free at this threshold should be treated with smaller subsequent dose decrements at intervals of 2 to 6 weeks. If possible, recurrences occurring during tapering should be treated with NSAID optimization rather than increasing corticosteroids. To prevent side effects of long-term corticosteroid use, specifically bone loss, consideration should be given to supplementary calcium and vitamin D. Bisphosphonates are recommended in all men ≥50 years and postmenopausal women in whom long-term treatment with corticosteroids at a dose of 5.0 to 7.5 mg/day of prednisone or equivalent is required.

In patients with multiple recurrences (≥3 episodes) despite the aforementioned strategies, alternative drugs have been suggested based on case reports, case series, and small randomized trials. These include azathioprine (Imuran),[1] methotrexate (Trexall),[1] and intravenous human immunoglobulin.[1] Recently, the interleukin (IL)-1β antagonist anakinra (Kineret)[1] (1 to 2 mg/kg/day up to 100 mg subcutaneously for several months) has shown considerable promise; other IL-1β antagonists are in development. Finally, as a last resort for refractory cases of recurrent pericarditis, pericardiectomy may be effective.

Constrictive Pericarditis
Etiology
Constrictive pericarditis is a consequence of chronic forms of pericarditis, especially bacterial (20% to 30%), immune-mediated, and neoplastic (2% to 5%) disease. Some cases are idiopathic. Other causes include cardiac injury syndromes, postradiation, uremia, and sarcoidosis. Before the availability of effective antimicrobial therapy, tuberculous pericarditis was the most important cause, but this is now rare in the developed world. In the third world, tuberculosis remains an important cause of pericardial disease in general and constrictive pericarditis in particular, often in association with HIV/AIDs. It is very rare (<1%) for idiopathic/viral pericarditis to result in constrictive pericarditis.

When tuberculosis was the major cause of constrictive pericarditis, cases typically presented as a very chronic disease with the features described below. Heavy pericardial calcification was a classic feature. In contemporary practice, most cases of constrictive pericarditis occur in conjunction with the syndrome of effusive-constrictive pericarditis, where pericardial effusion and constriction coexist in varying combinations.

Presentation and Physical Findings
Patients with constrictive pericarditis present with signs and symptoms of right heart failure, with small cardiac volumes and preserved ejection fraction (EF). (In extreme cases EF may be reduced due to severely impaired filling.) Symptoms include fatigue, peripheral edema, dyspnea, hepatomegaly, pleural effusions, and ascites. On physical examination, the venous pressure is markedly elevated, with an M- or W-shaped waveform caused by rapid atrial pressure descents. There is a paradoxical rise in venous pressure with inspiration (Kussmaul's sign), consistent with impaired filling of the right ventricle. A paradoxical pulse is present in as many as one-third of patients. Auscultation may reveal a pericardial knock, an early diastolic, medium-frequency sound (occurring slightly earlier than a usual third heart sound) that reflects abrupt cessation of rapid filling of the ventricles caused by the constricting pericardium. Atrial fibrillation is very common.

By definition, patients with effusive-constrictive pericarditis have pericardial effusions of variable size, which often contain adhesions and fibrous strands and are sometimes large enough to cause cardiac tamponade. In these cases, the diagnosis of constriction is often made after pericardiocentesis, when right heart filling pressures remain elevated and typical hemodynamic features become apparent.

Diagnostic Tests
The ECG often reveals nonspecific repolarization abnormalities, but there are no specific findings. In effusive-constrictive pericarditis, low-voltage and electrical alternans may be apparent if there is a large effusion. The chest X-ray film may reveal pericardial calcification, but its incidence is now low. Pleural effusions are common.

Major echocardiographic-Doppler findings include small cardiac chambers, a septal "bounce" because of exaggerated septal motion related to increased ventricular interdependence, increased mitral and tricuspid respiratory flow variation, and pericardial thickening and calcification. Interdependence is explained on the basis of a fixed intrapericardial volume, as a result of which when the volume of one ventricle changes (e.g., during respiration), the volume of the other must change reciprocally.

Cardiac catheterization reveals rapid atrial pressure descents, equalization of left- and right-sided filling pressures, increased respiratory variation in LV and RV systolic pressure (also due to ventricular interdependence) and a characteristic "dip and plateau" or "square root" sign evident in the ventricular diastolic pressure.

Cardiac CT and MRI are the best methods for imaging the pericardium. These demonstrate variable increases in pericardial thickness and calcification if present, although rare cases without increased thickness have been reported. Pericardial calcifications can be especially well visualized by cardiac CT and increased ventricular interdependence can be appreciated on real-time cine MR images. Modern cases of constrictive and effusive-constrictive pericarditis often have prominent pericardial inflammation, best imaged by gadolinium uptake during cMRI.

Treatment
Medical management of constrictive pericarditis is symptomatic and supportive, primarily consisting of diuretics to manage signs of right heart failure. It is important to avoid drugs that slow the heart rate, as these patients are critically dependent on heart rate to maintain cardiac output. Ultimately, these patients become refractory to diuretics.

Pericardiectomy has been considered the most definitive treatment for constrictive pericarditis. However, these are often difficult surgeries with high morbidity and mortality rates and delayed benefit. A number of patients are deemed too debilitated for surgery. Postradiation constriction has been considered a specific contraindication. Before pericardiectomy is undertaken, consideration should be given to a trial of an antiinflammatory regimen, especially in idiopathic cases, cases due to systemic inflammatory diseases, and cases due to post-cardiac injury syndromes. High-intensity gadolinium uptake on cardiac MRI in association with pericardial thickening is a signal that such a regimen may be successful, and apparent cures have been reported. Patients with evidence of intense inflammation often have a subacute course and belong in the subset with effusive-constrictive pericarditis. There have been no formal trials of specific antiinflammatory regimens. We favor a course of intermediate-dose prednisone[1] followed by a gradual taper similar to that recommended for recurrent pericarditis, along with colchicine[1] for at least 6 months. In cases of effusive-constrictive pericarditis presenting with cardiac tamponade, a few days of higher-dose prednisone initially may be reasonable. If an antiinflammatory regimen is to be attempted, we recommend committing to at least 2 to 3 months of prednisone treatment before tapering is begun. Reimaging the pericardium to ensure that inflammation has resolved before tapering is helpful.

References

Adler Y, Charron P, Imazio M, et al: 2015 ESC Guidelines for the diagnosis and management of pericardial diseases. Task Force for the Diagnosis and Management of Pericardial Diseases of the European Society of Cardiology (ESC), *G Ital Cardiol (Rome)* 16:702–738, 2015.

Azarbal A, LeWinter MM: Pericardial effusion, *Cardiol Clin* 35:515–524, 2017.

Cantarini L, Lucherini OM, Brucato A, et al: Clues to detect tumor necrosis factor receptor-associated periodic syndrome (TRAPS) among patients with idiopathic recurrent acute pericarditis: results of a multicentre study, *Clin Res Cardiol* 101:525–531, 2012.

Hoit BD: Anatomy and physiology of the pericardium, *Cardiol Clin* 35:481–490, 2017.

Imazio M, Battaglia A, Gaido L, Gaita F: Recurrent pericarditis, *Rev Med Interne* 38:307–311, 2017.

Imazio M, Brucato A, Cemin R, et al: A randomized trial of colchicine for acute pericarditis, *N Engl J Med* 369:1522–1528, 2013.

Imazio M, Brucato A, Cumetti D, et al: Corticosteroids for recurrent pericarditis: high versus low doses: a nonrandomized observation, *Circulation* 118:667–671, 2008.

Imazio M, Gaita F, LeWinter M: Evaluation and treatment of pericarditis: a systematic review, *JAMA* 314:1498–1506, 2015.

Kyto V, Sipila J, Rautava P: Clinical profile and influences on outcomes in patients hospitalized for acute pericarditis, *Circulation* 130:1601–1606, 2014.

LeWinter MM: Clinical practice: acute pericarditis, *N Engl J Med* 371:2410–2416, 2014.

PERIPHERAL ARTERY DISEASE

Method of
Tracie C. Collins, MD, MPH, MHCDS

CURRENT DIAGNOSIS

- Leg pain, fatigue, weakness, or numbness with walking
- Ankle-brachial index is a common initial diagnostic approach

CURRENT THERAPY

- Risk factor control (e.g., tobacco cessation, lipid lowering therapy) is key
- Cilostazol improves walking distance
- Exercise rehabilitation is an important first approach in patients without severe PAD

Overview

Epidemiology and Risk Factors

Peripheral artery disease (PAD) is a prevalent disease affecting 20% to 30% of patients ≥50 years of age, or up to 12 million Americans. The annual age-specific incidence of PAD is 61 per 10,000 men and 54 per 10,000 women aged 65 to 74 years. The most common anatomical sites for PAD are the abdominal aorta and arteries of the lower extremities. The most common etiology of PAD is atherosclerosis, with risk factors that include age 65 years and older, smoking, diabetes mellitus, hypertension, and dyslipidemia.

Pathophysiology

PAD is atherosclerotic plaque build-up sufficient to cause a reduction of blood flow in the abdominal aorta and/or arteries of the lower extremities. The reduced blood flow can lead to exertional leg symptoms. Inflow disease is defined as blockages involving the aortoiliac and femoropopliteal arteries. Outflow disease involves the infrapopliteal (below-the-knee) arteries.

Prevention and Screening Recommendations

Prevention of PAD includes control of atherosclerotic risk factors. The US Preventive Services Task Force on PAD Screening concluded that there is no direct evidence and limited indirect evidence on the benefits of screening for PAD using the ankle-brachial index (ABI) in asymptomatic patients. Furthermore, based on available studies, there is low sensitivity and no evidence of benefit toward health outcomes with screening for asymptomatic PAD.

Clinical Manifestations

Persons with PAD may present without exertional leg symptoms (asymptomatic disease) or with symptoms of leg pain, fatigue, weakness, or numbness with walking (symptomatic disease). Symptomatic disease is categorized as atypical leg pain (pain in legs that is not classic intermittent claudication), classic intermittent claudication (exertional calf pain that resolves within 10 minutes of rest), or critical limb ischemia (ischemic rest pain, ulcers, or gangrene).

Diagnosis

The resting ABI—ratio of systolic blood pressure in the ankle to systolic blood pressure in the arm—is a commonly used, initial diagnostic test for PAD. The ABI exam is conducted by placing a patient in the supine position for 5 minutes with blood pressure cuffs placed just above each brachial artery and at each ankle. A hand-held Doppler is used to measure systolic blood pressures in both brachial arteries and in both ankles (i.e., the dorsalis pedis and posterior tibial arteries). The resting ABI is calculated based on the ratio of the ankle and arm pressures, based on the higher pressure for each ankle and the higher of the arm pressures. In patients with exertional leg symptoms and normal or borderline resting ABI results, exercise treadmill ABI testing is important to objectively measure functional limitations attributable to leg symptoms and PAD. The toe-brachial index provides additional diagnostic information for patients with evidence of arterial stiffness (ABI >1.40). Studies that provide more anatomic detail for patients with PAD who are being considered for invasive intervention include duplex ultrasonography, computed tomography angiography (CTA), or magnetic resonance angiography (MRA).

Ankle-Brachial Index

If the highest systolic blood pressure measured at the posterior tibialis artery is 160 and the highest systolic blood pressure measured on the upper arm is 130, then the ABI is normal at 1.23 (Ankle: 160/Brachial: 130 = 1.23) (Table 1).

Differential Diagnosis

The differential diagnosis for PAD includes spinal stenosis, venous claudication, popliteal artery entrapment syndrome, nerve root compression, or arthritis (Table 2). Additional history including a patient's age, approach to relieve symptoms, and/or joint involvement can help to further delineate the diagnosis. PAD can certainly coexist with other chronic conditions.

Treatment

Risk Factor Control

Control of atherosclerotic risk factors is a key component to reducing systemic ischemic events in persons with PAD (Figure 1). Among persons with PAD, disease severity increases fourfold with heavy smoking and twofold with diabetes mellitus. Current guidelines for PAD management include smoking cessation,

TABLE 1	Ankle-Brachial Index	
ABI	**RISK OF ARTERIAL DISEASE**	**REFER TO VASCULAR SPECIALIST**
1–1.4	Normal	None
0.9–1.0	Borderline	None
0.7–0.89	Some Arterial Disease	Treat Risk Factors
0.5–0.69	Moderate Arterial Disease	Refer
<0.5	Severe Arterial Disease	Refer

TABLE 2   Differential Diagnosis for Symptomatic PAD

CONDITION	LOCATION	CHARACTERISTIC	EFFECT OF EXERCISE	EFFECT OF REST	OTHER CHARACTERISTICS
Venous claudication	Entire leg, worse in calf	Tight, bursting pain	After walking	Slowly subsides	History of iliofemoral deep vein thrombosis; edema; signs of venous stasis
Popliteal artery entrapment syndrome	Calf muscles	Tight, tearing pain	After moderate to vigorous exercise (jogging)	Subsides slowly	Typically heavy muscular athletes
Spinal stenosis	Often bilateral buttocks, posterior leg	Pain and weakness	May mimic claudication	Variable relief but can take a long time to recover	Worse with standing and extending spine
Nerve root compression	Radiates down leg	Sharp lancinating pain	Induced by sitting, standing, or walking	Often present at rest	History of back problems; worse with sitting; relief when supine or sitting
Arthritis (hip, foot, or ankle)	Lateral hip, thigh, foot arch, ankle	Aching discomfort	After variable degree of exercise	Not quickly relieved	Symptoms variable; may be related to activity or present at rest

---

```
┌─────────────────┐         ┌─────────────────┐
│      Limb       │         │  Cardiovascular │
│   improvement   │         │  risk reduction │
└─────────────────┘         └─────────────────┘
```

- Reduce pain
- Improve walking distance
- Reduce limb loss

- Reduce systemic ischemic events

Figure 1 Overall goals for management of peripheral artery disease.

blood pressure <130/80 mm Hg (per the current ACC/AHA guidelines), and glycosylated hemoglobin A1c level of <7%. Furthermore, all patients with PAD should have their serum low-density lipoprotein cholesterol (LDL-C) reduced to <1.8 mmol/L (<70 mg/dL).

Tobacco Cessation

Smoking cessation in patients with PAD reduces the progression of disease including the severity of claudication, occurrence of rest pain, likelihood of amputation, need for revascularization, and failure of arterial bypass grafts.

A highly successful option for smoking cessation is pharmacotherapy. Varenicline (Chantix) is efficacious for smoking cessation at a dose of 1 mg twice per day for 12 weeks. Varenicline is associated with nausea that may resolve with continued use. Use of varenicline may be associated with an increased risk of cardiovascular adverse events. In 2018, in a population-based study conducted in Canada, varenicline use was associated with a 34% higher risk for cardiovascular events in the risk compared with control interval. These findings included persons without a history of cardiovascular disease.

Glycemic Control

Approaches to achieving glucose control include diet, exercise, and medications. Prior clinical trials have demonstrated the value of blood glucose control to prevent micro- but not macrovascular complications (e.g., progression of PAD). Certain minority populations are at higher risk for adverse limb outcomes as compared to non-Hispanic whites. One such outcome is lower extremity amputation. In the Strong Heart Study—an observational cohort study of cardiovascular disease and its risk factors in 13 American Indian communities—and among 1874 individuals without a lower extremity amputation at baseline, 4.4% experienced amputation within 8 years. Longer duration of diabetes mellitus and higher levels of glycosylated hemoglobin were risk factors for this adverse outcome.

Less is known of the benefit of glucose control to reduce adverse limb events in persons with PAD. However, in one retrospective cohort study involving more than 790 veterans with PAD, glucose control in African Americans was associated with a 67% reduced risk for a major limb event (i.e., lower extremity bypass surgery or lower extremity amputation). Thus, there is some evidence that supports aggressive blood glucose lowering to prevent macrovascular complications in PAD.

Caution must be taken with the use of certain drugs for patients with diabetes. Specifically, the use of the sodium-glucose cotransporter-2 (SGLT-2) inhibitor, canagliflozin (Invokana), has been associated with an increased risk for lower extremity amputations, largely toe or metatarsal level, as based on results from two trials of patients with diabetes. Furthermore, in a retrospective cohort study involving 40,000 new users of SGLT-2 inhibitors, users of the SGLT-2 inhibitor were significantly more likely to undergo amputations compared with users of older antidiabetes drugs.

Antiplatelet Therapy

By reducing platelet aggregation, antiplatelet therapy reduces the risk of myocardial infarction and ischemic cerebrovascular accidents. Because of the high burden of coexisting coronary artery disease and cerebrovascular disease in patients with PAD, antiplatelet therapy is an important part of pharmacologic therapy for this disease. In addition, aside from their systemic benefits, antiplatelet agents may reduce poor limb outcomes (i.e., reduced risk for peripheral arterial surgery and an improvement in vascular graft patency). The most common antiplatelet therapies for PAD include aspirin (75 to 325 mg daily) and clopidogrel ([Plavix] 75 mg daily); clopidogrel is an oral P2Y12 inhibitor. Aspirin (ASA) is recommended for patients with asymptomatic PAD with stable cardiovascular disease and without contraindications or a greater risk to harm ratio (e.g., 70 years or older). Clopidogrel or ticagrelor (Brilinta)[1] (also a P2Y12 inhibitor) monotherapy is an option for patients with symptomatic PAD without clinically manifest coronary artery disease (CAD) or cerebrovascular disease. Clopidogrel is more effective than ASA to prevent a major cardiovascular event (MACE) in patients with symptomatic PAD without clinical evidence of CAD or cerebrovascular disease. Ticagrelor (90 mg twice daily) is an acceptable alternative for patients who are poor metabolizers of clopidogrel. For patients with symptomatic PAD and stable cardiovascular disease, ASA (or clopidogrel, if ASA is contraindicated) should be used to prevent MACE. For patients taking ASA who are at high risk of cardiac and ischemic limb events and one year out from a myocardial infarction, the addition of ticagrelor can be

---

[1]Not FDA approved for this indication.

considered to prevent MACE or a major adverse limb event (MALE—defined as acute limb ischemia or major amputation). For patients at high risk for ischemic limb events (prior acute limb ischemia or more severe PAD as defined by an ABI <0.60), vorapaxar (Zontivity 2.08 mg daily), a protease-activated receptor-1 antagonist that inhibits thrombin-induced platelet aggregation, can be added to a regimen of ASA or clopidogrel.

Lipid Lowering Therapy

In patients with PAD and dyslipidemia, statin therapy reduces the incidence of mortality, cardiovascular events, and stroke. High-intensity statin therapy is a guideline recommended therapy for patients with PAD, per the American Heart Association. Based on results from the Heart Protection Study (HPS), there was a 13% to 27% reduction in total mortality, vascular mortality, coronary artery events, or carotid artery events during five years of follow-up among 6748 patients with PAD who were randomized to 40 mg of simvastatin (Zocor) therapy. These findings were independent of the coexistence of coronary artery disease at the time of randomization.

Newer treatment for lipid lowering to be considered after use of statin therapy include the proprotein convertase subtilisin/kexin type 9 (PCSK9) inhibitor evolocumab (Repatha 140 mg every 2 weeks or 420 mg once monthly), which reduced cardiovascular events in patients with PAD. In the Further Cardiovascular Outcomes Research with PCSK9 Inhibition in Subjects with Elevated Risk (FOURIER) trial, 27,564 patients with atherosclerotic disease on statin therapy were randomized to evolocumab versus placebo and followed for a median of 2.2 years. Evolocumab significantly reduced the composite primary endpoint of cardiovascular death, myocardial infarction, stroke, hospital admission for unstable angina, or coronary revascularization in patients with PAD (hazard ratio [HR] 0.79; 95% confidence interval [CI], 0.66 to 0.94; $P = .0098$.

Statin use is also associated with a reduction in adverse limb outcomes. In the Reduction of Atherothrombosis for Continued Health (REACH) registry, statin therapy was associated with a reduction in the combined endpoint of worsening claudication, new critical limb ischemia, lower extremity revascularization, or amputation.

In the FOURIER trial, evolocumab reduced the risk of major adverse limb events (acute limb ischemia, major amputation, or urgent peripheral revascularization for ischemia) in patients with and without PAD.

Hypertension Therapy

Control of blood pressure (<130/80) is another crucial target to reduce the risk for cardiovascular morbidity and mortality in persons with PAD. The management of hypertension in patients with PAD includes lifestyle modifications and drug therapy. Thiazide diuretics are first-line agents. Angiotensin-converting enzyme inhibitors or angiotensin receptor blockers should be used in patients with renal disease or in those with chronic heart failure. Calcium channel blockers can be added for difficult to control hypertension. In the Heart Outcomes Protection Evaluation Study (HOPE), ramipril (Altace) at 10 mg daily significantly reduced cardiovascular events in persons with symptomatic and asymptomatic PAD; most of these patients had increased blood pressure. In the ONTARGET (Ongoing Telmisartan Alone and in Combination with Ramipril Global Endpoint Trial), telmisartan (Micardis), an angiotensin receptor blocker, was noninferior to ramipril for the composite outcome of cardiovascular death, myocardial infarction, stroke, and hospitalization for congestive heart failure. Although there has been concern with the risk for worsening of leg symptoms in persons with PAD who are prescribed β-blockers, this concern has not been validated.

Cilostazol

Cilostazol (Pletal), a phosphodiesterase type-3 with antiplatelet and vasodilator properties, is efficacious for treatment of *symptomatic* PAD (intermittent claudication). Cilostazol inhibits platelet aggregation, vascular smooth muscle proliferation, and causes vasodilatation. Cilostazol improves both pain-free and maximal treadmill walking distance. In a study involving 54 outpatient vascular clinics and 698 patients, cilostazol improved mean maximal walking distance by 54% at six months. Additionally, cilostazol reduces restenosis after superficial femoral artery stenting with self-expandable nitinol stents. The recommended dose is 100 mg twice daily (reduce to 50 mg twice daily for patients concomitantly taking CYP2C19 or CYP3A4 drugs).

Although several physiologic benefits of cilostazol are recognized, its mechanism of action in improving symptoms of intermittent claudication is unknown. As a phosphodiesterase type-3 inhibitor, cilostazol is in the same class of agents as milrinone (Primacor). In patients with heart failure, milrinone is associated with increased mortality. Although cilostazol has fewer cardiac inotropic effects, it has equivalent vasodilating and platelet-inhibiting effects as milrinone and is contraindicated in patients with PAD and heart failure. Cilostazol may offer some benefit toward improving lipid profiles. Rizzo and colleagues reported that cilostazol lowers plasma triglyceride levels and increases high-density lipoprotein cholesterol concentrations.

Exercise Rehabilitation and Revascularization

Walking therapy reduces walking impairment (i.e., walking distance, speed, and/or stair climbing). The exact mechanisms by which walking therapy improves lower limb function in PAD are not clear. One possible mechanism is an improvement in lower limb blood flow and walking economy (i.e., achieving gait stability without compromising walking velocity).

Walking therapy is an excellent yet underutilized component of care for persons with mild to moderately severe symptomatic PAD. Supervised treadmill walking (conducted within a clinical setting with supervision by a trained clinician) improves walking distance in patients with symptomatic PAD. Improvement is initially evident at 12 weeks, with significantly greater improvement at 24 weeks. In a typical regimen, the exercise physiologist coaches the patient to walk until there is moderate pain, to rest, and then to resume walking when pain subsides; this cycle of intermittent walking is continued for a total of 50 minutes. Short-term improvement in maximal distance with supervised treadmill walking can exceed 150%. As of May 2017, the Centers for Medicare and Medicaid has approved coverage for 36 sessions over 12 weeks of supervised exercise therapy for patients with symptomatic PAD who are referred to a cardiac rehab lab (hospital or outpatient) by a physician; the cost is $55 per session with a 20% co-payment, which may be covered by supplemental insurance. An additional 36 sessions may also be covered without a requirement for completion of all sessions within 12 weeks; the Current Procedural Terminology (CPT) is 93668 (under Peripheral Arterial Disease Rehabilitation).

An alternative to supervised walking is a home-based walking program (community-based walking therapy). Gardner and colleagues completed a walking intervention trial that compared home-based walking to supervised walking in patients with PAD. One hundred nineteen patients were randomized and 92 completed the study. At 12 weeks, patients randomized to either home-based or supervised walking improved both their onset to pain ($P < .001$) and peak walking times ($P < .01$). A change in daily average cadence—walking rate as captured in steps per minute—was significantly greater in the home-based walking group ($P < .05$) as compared to the supervised walking or usual care groups. Improvements in walking speed were also noted with a trial in which 145 participants with diabetes mellitus and PAD were randomized to a six-month home-based walking intervention or attention control. Participants randomized to the home-based walking intervention significantly improved their walking speed ($P < .05$) and a quality of life subscale score ($P < .05$). A key challenge to the use of home-based walking is patient adherence to such therapy. Adherence to walking is impacted by several factors including patient knowledge of disease, access to environmentally safe sites, and motivation. A psychosocial mediator for behavior change, self-efficacy, was shown to positively impact home-based walking for persons with diabetes mellitus and PAD.

Vascular Interventions

Aside from noninvasive management, patients with intermittent claudication are often referred from their primary care clinicians (e.g., internists and family medicine physicians) to vascular interventionists for consideration for lower limb revascularization. Many of these patients could be managed with exercise therapy. In patients with symptomatic PAD who have failed maximal medical therapy and exercise programs, or whose symptoms are advanced or deteriorating, lower extremity revascularization (either surgical or, more commonly, endovascular) represent treatment options. Both strategies have demonstrated an improvement in walking performance and relief of symptoms of limb-threatening ischemia.

Similar to supervised exercise therapy, endovascular intervention improves functional outcomes in patients with PAD. The Claudication: Exercise versus Endoluminal Revascularization (CLEVER) trial randomized 111 patients with aortoiliac arterial occlusive disease to one of three treatments: optimal medical care (OMC), OMC plus supervised exercise, and OMC plus stent revascularization. The primary outcome was change in peak walking time at six months. Secondary outcomes included free-living step activity and quality of life. For the primary outcome, participants randomized to supervised exercise therapy and OMC experienced the greatest mean change in peak walking time 5.8 (SD 4.6) minutes. Participants randomized to stent revascularization had a mean change of 3.7 (SD 4.9) minutes and those randomized to OMC had a mean change of 1.2 (SD 2.6) minutes in peak walking time. There were statistically significant differences between the supervised exercise group as compared to the OMC and stent revascularization, $P < .001$ and 0.04, respectively. Interestingly, both treatment groups experienced an improvement in quality of life, but persons randomized to stent revascularization versus supervised exercise therapy experienced the greatest improvement.

Monitoring

Over 5 years, up to 80% of patients with intermittent claudication remain stable and up to 20% worsen, based on data largely involving non-Hispanic whites. Risk factors for disease progression are comparable to those risk factors that increase the risk for PAD. Follow-up should occur at least annually and more frequently, per the severity of PAD.

References

Bonaca MP, Nault P, Giugliano RP, et al: Low-density lipoprotein cholesterol lowering with evolocumab and outcomes in patients with peripheral artery disease: Insights from the FOURIER Trial (Further Cardiovascular Outcomes Research With PCSK9 Inhibition in Subjects With Elevated Risk), *Circulation* 137(4):338–350, 2018.
Collins T, Petersen N, Suarez-Almazor M, et al: The prevalence of peripheral arterial disease in a racially diverse population, *Arch Intern Med* 163:1469–1474, 2003.
Collins TC: PAD: Medical treatment and risk reduction strategies. In Slovut D, Dean S, Jaff M, et al , editors: *Comprehensive Review in Vascular and Endovascular Medicine*, 2012.
Gershon AS, Campitelli MA, Hawken S, et al: Cardiovascular and neuropsychiatric events after varenicline use for smoking cessation, *Am J Respir Crit Care Med* 197(7):913–922, 2018.
Guirguis-Blake JM, Evans CV, Redmond N, et al: Screening for peripheral artery disease using the ankle-brachial index: Updated evidence report and systematic review for the US Preventive Services Task Force, *JAMA* 320(2):184–196, 2018.
Hess CN, Hiatt WR: Antithrombotic therapy for peripheral artery disease in 2018, *JAMA* 319(22):2329–2330, 2018.
Norgren L, Hiatt WR, Dormandy JA, et al: Inter-society consensus for the management of peripheral arterial disease (TASC II), *J Vasc Surg* 45(Suppl S):S5–67, 2007.
Olin JW, White CJ, Armstrong EJ, et al: Peripheral artery disease: Evolving role of exercise, medical therapy, and endovascular options, *J Am Coll Cardiol* 67(11):1338–1357, 2016.
Ostergren J, Sleight P, Dagenais G, et al: Impact of ramipril in patients with evidence of clinical or subclinical peripheral arterial disease, *Eur Heart J* 25(1):17–24, 2004.

PREMATURE BEATS

Method of
Randell Wexler, MD, MPH

CURRENT DIAGNOSIS

- The cause of a premature beat may be either atrial (premature atrial contractions or PAC) or ventricular (premature ventricular contractions or PVC) in origin.
- PACs are most often benign but are associated with increased risk of atrial fibrillation.
- PVCs may be benign, but underlying structural heart disease is not uncommon and must be ruled out with echocardiography.
- PACs and PVCs are most commonly diagnosed by EKG although Holter or event monitoring may be required.
- A heavier PVC burden is associated with increased development of cardiomyopathy and cardiovascular morbidity and mortality.

CURRENT THERAPY

- PACs are treated if their presence causes the patient symptoms and interferes with daily life.
- Beta blockers are most often used for the treatment of symptomatic PACs.
- In patients with underlying structural heart disease, the treatment of PVCs is directed at the underlying cardiac condition.
- Antiarrhythmics show no benefit in treatment of PVCs in patients with cardiomyopathy and should not be used to suppress their presence post myocardial infarction.
- Patients with a PVC burden of > 15% should see an EPS specialist for evaluation and treatment, as there is an increased risk of a significant cardiac arrhythmia.

It is not uncommon for a patient to present to a primary care physician with the complaint of their "heart pounding," "skipping beats," or having "palpitations." Though often the only symptom, patients may also complain of concomitant dizziness, lightheadedness, or frank syncope. The patient may be young or old, have underlying structural heart disease (or not), or risk factors for heart disease such as hypertension. A patient with such a history may be experiencing one of a number of cardiac arrhythmias, although it is not uncommon to find no underlying etiology at all.

Normal electrical propagation in the heart begins with the spontaneous electrical discharge at the sinoatrial node, which is then propagated along the right atrial wall to the atrioventricular node and from there to the ventricles via the His-Purkinje System. Disruption anywhere along this pathway may lead to an arrhythmia, which is defined as a rhythm that is not sinus and is accompanied by an abnormal electrical conduction.

If an arrhythmia is present, it is classified by its anatomic location of origin. Common atrial arrhythmias include atrial fibrillation/flutter, paroxysmal supraventricular tachycardia, and premature atrial contractions (PACs). Ventricular arrhythmias are often designated as premature ventricular contractions (PVCs), ventricular tachycardia, and ventricular fibrillation. Other arrhythmias that are often seen include bradycardia, tachycardia, and first-, second-, and third-degree heart block (complex morphology is normal). This chapter will review arrhythmias commonly referred to as premature beats: PACs, and PVCs.

Premature Atrial Contractions
Epidemiology and Risk Factors
PACs are common and are found in both the general population as well as in those with underlying cardiac disease. Research has established that PACs exist in up to 99% of those over the age of 50 with increasing frequency with each decade of life. It has long been believed that atrial ectopy, especially in a patient with no underlying heart disease, is benign and more of a nuisance than a risk. However, it is now understood that PACs do present an increased risk for atrial fibrillation or ischemic stroke, and although most often benign, are not entirely so.

Underlying structural heart disease (such as mitral valve disease or left ventricular dysfunction) is significantly correlated to the risk of developing PACs. Additional risk factors associated with PACs include: 1) height (potentially due to the relationship between body size and left atrial measurements); 2) those with higher levels of B natriuretic peptide (BNP); as well as 3) those with abnormalities of high-density lipoprotein (HDL) lipid metabolism in which a lower HDL is associated with increased risk of PACs. This inverse relationship has also been reported between PACs and physical activity. The difficulty in determining the clinical significance of PACs is owing to their frequent presence in the population at large.

Pathophysiology
The true etiology of PACs is not well researched and therefore not well understood. Investigation has suggested that normally functioning sino-atrial (SA) and atrio-ventricular (AV) nodes can be impacted by stimuli arising from outside of the atria. It has been proposed that this stimuli leads to reversible nodal remodeling. As a result it has been hypothesized that PACs may occur due to an adversely impacted SA or AV node subsequent to such remodeling. Others have postulated that mechanisms such as reentry and abnormal automaticity initiate PAC transmission but the actual cause is not known.

An electrocardiogram (EKG) provides an electrical account of heart function. Electrical impulses begin in the sinus node and then travel through Bachmann's bundle (the sole specialized atrial conduction system) subsequently diffusing over the atria. The P wave represents atrial electrical activity. A normal P wave as seen on the EKG is smooth and never peaked or sharp. The leads best used to review the P wave are leads II and V1.

A patient may have a left atrial abnormality (LAA), right atrial abnormality (RAA), or both. An LAA abnormality results in prolonged atrial activation times, because left atrial activation is later than right atrial activation. Such abnormalities may result in "notched" P waves because of the spatial separation of the left and right atrial peaks. When a patient has a RAA, the P wave tends to have increased amplitude due to the summation of the two peaks. Whenever possible, P wave abnormalities should be labeled left or right in nature.

A PAC will typically be seen on EKG as an abnormal P wave followed by a normal QRS complex. Morphologically, the P wave will be different than a normal (sinus) P wave. If the site of the PAC origin is near the AV node, it will be inverted, whereas if it is more distal, it will be upright. Should the PAC reach the SA node, the resulting finding on the EKG will be a longer interval between sinus beats, but it is not compensatory in nature. PACs may occur singularly or at regular intervals (every other beat is termed bigeminy) or in a group (two sequential PACs are termed a couplet). In addition, a PAC may be blocked (buried in a T wave) or conducted aberrantly (an atypical electrical configuration).

Prevention and Clinical Manifestations
The majority of PACs are idiopathic unless there is underlying heart disease. Potential non-cardiac causes include tobacco use, alcohol consumption, substance abuse, and coffee. Reducing and/or eliminating these substances can be helpful in preventing symptoms. Additionally, certain medications, supplements, or substances of abuse may cause PACs, and therefore in any patient presenting with the complaint of extra beats, a thorough review of all medications, supplements, and elicit substance use should be undertaken.

Although the vast majority of patients who are found to have PACs incidentally will not experience symptoms, patients presenting with the complaint of PACs may state that they feel that their heart is racing, skipping beats, or fluttering, or that they are experiencing palpitations. Though not common, some patients may experience dizziness.

PACs are now known to be precursors to atrial fibrillation or ischemic stroke. Thus the previous belief that atrial ectopy is benign and more of a nuisance has been shown to be incorrect. In fact, some studies suggest that a single PAC on EKG not only predicts atrial fibrillation but may also be a predictor of fatal outcome.

Diagnosis and Differential Diagnosis
The diagnosis of PACs is often made on EKG, especially if the patient is symptomatic at the time of testing. If the EKG does not demonstrate an etiology, a 24-hour Holter monitor or 30-day event monitor may also be considered. The diagnoses of a PAC can be made if the P wave has a morphology that is different from and occurs earlier in the cardiac cycle than that of a sinus P wave. Many patients experience palpitations in which the EKG evaluation suggests no underlying etiology. Therefore, in addition to electrocardiography, patients with PACs should have baseline labs drawn to include a thyroid stimulating hormone, complete blood count, magnesium and phosphate, and electrolytes. If drug use is a possible etiology, a toxicology screen can be useful.

Differential diagnosis includes other cardiac arrhythmias such as PVCs, atrial fibrillation, atrial flutter, and paroxysmal supraventricular tachycardia. Underlying disorders that may be the cause include underlying anxiety or thyroid and other metabolic disorder, as well as substance abuse.

Treatment and Monitoring
Echocardiography is helpful in determining if the patient has underlying structural heart disease requiring further evaluation and intervention. If the patient has no underlying structural heart disease, then no treatment is necessary, especially if the individual is asymptomatic and the PACs are found incidentally. If the patient does have symptomatic PACs to a degree that they interfere with the patient's quality of life, interventions include the use of beta blockers, and if they fail, a trial type IA, type IC, or type III antiarrhythmic agents may be considered. If the problem is electrophysiological in nature, catheter ablation or pulmonary vein isolation may be helpful.

If the patient has underlying structural heart disease, then treatment is directed at the underlying disorder. Patients with PACs should be educated as to the association of atrial fibrillation or stroke with instructions to notify their physician or seek attention immediately should symptoms occur.

Premature Ventricular Contractions
Epidemiology and Risk Factors
Premature ventricular contractions (PVCs) are a common cardiac finding, with upward of 40% to 75% of apparently healthy people being affected. As with PACs, they tend to increase with age. Underlying cardiovascular disease, especially ischemic heart disease increases one's risk for PVCs. As such, evaluation should be focused on excluding structural heart disease. It should be noted that PVCs are also common in those with inherited channelopathies, so a good family history is also important. PVCs are also common in well-conditioned athlete's due to autonomic tone. Although this may be a normal compensatory mechanism, structural heart disease still needs to be eliminated. PVCs associated with exercise portend increased cardiac mortality.

Pathophysiology
After propagation through the atria, the electrical impulse activates the AV node that serves as the sole pathway for electrical transmission between the atria and the ventricles. The terminal portion of the AV junction becomes the bundle of His that propagates the electrical impulse to the bundle branches, which further

divide into smaller subdivisions eventually connecting to the Purkinje fibers. From the Purkinje fibers, the electrical impulse diffuses synchronously across the ventricles.

PVCs arise from ectopic foci in the ventricle and occur earlier in the cardiac cycle than expected for a sinus beat. They may be generated by increased automaticity, reentry, or triggered activity. Monomorphic PVCs suggest a triggering component whereas polymorphic PVCs tend to suggest an underlying cardiomyopathy. If the patient has no structural heart disease, the focus is likely to be the right ventricular outflow tract, whereas if the patient has structural heart disease, the left ventricle is most likely to be the site of origin.

PVCs are not preceded by a P wave and demonstrate a prolonged QRS (> 120 ms) with a compensatory pause (as opposed to a non-compensatory pause found with PACs). Conflicting ST and T wave changes are also often seen. ST depression and T-wave inversion tends to occur in R-wave dominant leads, whereas ST elevation and an upright T wave occur in S-wave dominated leads. PVCs may be unifocal or multifocal and their morphology may at times resemble right or left bundle branch blocks. If the PVC occurs with every other beat, it is termed bigeminy (or trigeminy if every third, etc.), or if the PVC is paired with another PVC, it is called a couplet. One may also see an R on T phenomenon whereby the PVC occurs at or near the T wave of the previous QRS complex resulting in the R wave of the PVC blending with the T wave of the preceding beat.

Patients with frequent PVCs will often develop subsequent cardiomyopathy, though the etiology is unknown. There is an increased risk in developing cardiomyopathy the longer one is exposed to PVCs. It is suspected this may be due to a less efficient heartbeat with suboptimal cardiac output similar to bradycardia. Risk factors for progression to cardiomyopathy have been inconsistently identified but likely include increasing age, high body mass index, and male gender.

Prevention and Clinical Manifestations

Patients with symptoms caused by PVCs often present with palpitations, dizziness, chest pain, syncope, dyspnea, orthopnea, decreased exercise tolerance, and fatigue. If a patient has a cough of unknown etiology, they should be evaluated for PVCs, as PVCs are noted to produce cough as the only symptom. PVCs have also been associated with dysphagia, especially when intermittent, as well as paroxysmal choking or vomiting. As such, PVCs should be considered if a gastroenterological evaluation is normal, or if symptoms persist despite treatment for an underlying gastrointestinal disorder.

PVCs are associated with a multitude of pathologic cardiac processes including heart failure, myocardial ischemia, left ventricular hypertrophy, idiopathic ventricular tachycardia, and right ventricular dysplasia. On exam patients may present with an irregular pulse or canon A wave. PVCs may also be associated with pulmonary or thyroid disease, the consumption of alcohol, caffeine, and the use of beta agonists. Cocaine, amphetamines, or other illicit drugs may precipitate symptoms as well. Syncope is uncommon with PVCs but, if present, represents a red flag for the presence of malignant arrhythmias.

PVCs are found on 40% to 75% of holter monitor evaluations and 1% of EKGs. They are defined as frequent if they are seen on an EKG, or are present at a rate of more than 30 an hour on event monitoring. In this instance there is a significantly increased cardiovascular risk as well as mortality. In the athlete, sinus bradycardia is common due to enhanced conditioning. This results in a lengthening of the RR interval and is thought to promote the occurrence of PVCs in this population.

The most important prognostic indicator for PVCs is the presence or absence of structural heart disease. Multifocal PVCs are considered to be risk factors for adverse cardiovascular events.

Potential contributors that are amenable to treatment include electrolyte abnormalities, hypoxia, drugs (including prescription as well as illegal), increased adrenergic drive, or ischemia.

Diagnosis and Differential Diagnosis

A 12-lead EKG is the initial test of choice. Echocardiography is necessary in individuals in which structural heart disease is suspected, or if PVC frequency is high (one or more PVCs on EKG, or more than 30 an hour on event monitoring). This is based on the understanding that the likelihood of underlying structural heart disease increases with PVC burden. In addition, if ischemia is suspected or if PVCs are triggered/evident on exertion, cardiovascular exercise stress testing is recommended. Polymorphic PVCs are more commonly seen in those with underlying cardiomyopathy.

Differential diagnosis includes ventricular arrhythmias such as ventricular tachycardia and ventricular fibrillation. Cardiac conditions include left ventricular hypertrophy in the setting of hypertension, myocarditis, acute coronary syndrome, heart failure, congenital heart disease, and hypertrophic cardiomyopathy.

Treatment and Monitoring

PVCs have been demonstrated to be an independent risk factor for cardiovascular mortality in heart failure and are associated with ejection fraction and wall motion abnormalities as well. Patients with a family history of frequent PVCs should be evaluated for inherited channelopathies such as catecholamine urgent polymorphic ventricular tachycardia. In patients with PVCs but without underlying coronary artery disease or structural heart disease, the clinical course is generally benign. It should be recalled, however, that patients with a history of PVCs can develop coronary artery disease or underlying structural heart disease, so periodic reevaluation of cardiac status is warranted.

Treatment for those with symptomatic PVCs may include beta blockers or non-dihydropyridine calcium channel blockers, but treatment is not necessary in asymptomatic patients. Use of anti-arrhythmic medication to treat PVCs has not been shown to benefit patients with cardiomyopathy. In addition, treatment is not indicated following myocardial infarction to suppress PVCs that may be present. If the patient has a large PVC burden, considered to be greater than 15%, referral to an EPS specialist for consultation and possible radiofrequency ablation should be considered.

Premature Junctional Contractions

PJCs are less common than either PACs or PVCs and are rarely seen in the setting of a normal heart. These beats arise from the atrioventricular junction. On EKG they are seen as an aberrant beat with underlying sinus rhythm. The P wave may be absent, inverted, or occur following the associated QRS complex that is morphologically normal. Causes include electrolyte and thyroid abnormalities, underlying lung or cardiac disease, or the use of excessive amounts of caffeine, nicotine, or alcohol. Medication toxicity may also be a cause, with digitalis toxicity being the classic example. If patients are asymptomatic, no treatment is required, though structural heart disease needs to be ruled out. In addition, the patient should be observed over time, as PJCs may be a harbinger of progression to a more serious arrhythmia. In the symptomatic patient, treatment is directed at the underlying cause. Supplemental oxygen may be of benefit.

References

Al-Khatib SM, et al: 2017 AHA/ACC/HRS Guideline for Management of Patients With Ventricular Arrhythmias and the Prevention of Sudden Cardiac Death: A Report of the American College of Cardiology/American Heart Association Task Force on Clinical Practice Guidelines and the Heart Rhythm Society: Developed in Collaboration With the Heart Failure Society of America, *Circulation*. DOI: https://doi.org/10.1161/CIR.0000000000000549. October 30, 2017.

Cohen D, et al: Premature atrial contractions in the general population: frequency and risk factors, *Circulation*, 2012 https://doi.org/10.1161/CirculationAHA.112.112300.

Hancock EW, et al: AHA/ACCF/HRS Recommendations for the Standardization and Interpretation of the Electrocardiogram Part V: Electrocardiogram Changes Associated With Cardiac Chamber Hypertrophy: A Scientific Statement From the American Heart Association Electrocardiography and Arrhythmias Committee, Council on Clinical Cardiology; the American College of Cardiology Foundation; and the Heart Rhythm Society: Endorsed by the International Society for Computerized Electrocardiology, *Circulation* 119:e251-261. https://doi.org/10.1161/CirculationAHA.108.191097.

Giles K, Green MS: Workup and management of patients with frequent premature ventricular contractions, *Candain Journal of Cardiology* 29:1512–1515, 2013.

Lai E, Chung EH: Management of arrhythmias in athletes: atrial fibrillation, premature ventricular contractions, and ventricular tachycardia, *Curr Treat Options Cardio Med* 19:86, 2017. https://doi.org/10.1007/s11936-017-0583-x.

LaPlante L, Benzaquen BS: A review of the potential pathogencity and management of frequent premature ventricular contractions, *PACE* 39:723–730, 2016.

Lin CY, et al: Prognostic significance of premature atrial complexes burden in prediction of long-term outcome, *J Am Heart Assoc* 2015:4e002192. https://doi.org/10.1161/JAHA.115.002192.

Marcus GM, Dewland TA: Premature atrial contractions. A Wolf in Sheep's clothing? *JACC* 66:242–244, 2015.

Nguen KT, et al: Ectopy on a single 12-lead ECG, incident cardiac myopathy, and death in the community, *J am Heart Assoc* 6, 2017:e006028. https://doi.org/10.1161/JAHA.117.006028.

Stroobandt RX, Barold SS, Sinnave AF: *ECG from basics to essentials: step by step.* Wiley Publishers; 2016.

TACHYCARDIAS

Method of
Alex Schevchuck, MD, MS; and Paul Andre, MD

CURRENT DIAGNOSIS

- Tachycardia is defined as cardiac rhythm with heart rate >100 bpm.
- 12-lead EKG and hemodynamic assessment are essential in each patient with tachycardia.
- Sustained arrhythmia is an arrhythmia that lasts for more than 30 s.
- Narrow complex rhythm (QRS ≤120 ms) favors supraventricular origin, whereas wide complex (QRS >120 ms) could be either supraventricular (with aberrant conduction) or ventricular.
- Every patient with tachyarrhythmia should be promptly assessed for hemodynamic instability and presence of symptoms (palpitations, angina, shortness of breath, lightheadedness, presyncope, syncope, volume overload).

CURRENT TREATMENT

- Vagal maneuvers may be useful for diagnosis and treatment of tachyarrhythmia
- DC cardioversion should be considered early if hemodynamic instability is present.
- If uncertain whether arrhythmia is ventricular tachycardia (VT) or supraventricular tachycardia (SVT), VT should be presumed and treated.
- Hemodynamic instability implies medical emergency and culprit tachyarrhythmia should be treated immediately.
- A subspecialty consultation should be considered for each patient with tachyarrhythmia and high-risk features, such as syncope or family history of sudden cardiac death for diagnostic evaluation, treatment recommendations, and risk stratification.

Definition

Tachycardia is defined as a heart rate greater than 100 beats per min (bpm). This can be a normal response by the heart to the stress on the body (such as sinus tachycardia with exercise or sepsis) or a primary cardiac pathologic condition, such as atrioventricular nodal reentry tachycardia (AVNRT) or ventricular tachycardia (VT). Tachycardia present in the setting of an abnormal cardiac rhythm is defined as tachyarrhythmia.

Classification

Tachycardias classify into two major categories: wide complex (QRS duration >120 ms) or narrow-complex (QRS duration ≤120 ms). This classification is key, as wide-complex tachycardias are usually due to an arrhythmia arising from the ventricles, such as monomorphic or polymorphic ventricular tachycardia, which are associated with considerable morbidity and mortality. On the other hand, narrow-complex tachycardias reflect ventricular activation by a competent conduction system below the atrioventricular (AV) node, indicating a source of the arrhythmia above the AV node or within the AV node or bundle of His, and are rarely life threatening.

When the tachyarrhythmia originates in the atria or within the conduction system in the AV node, it is described as a supraventricular tachycardia (SVT).

Wide-complex tachycardias include VT, supraventricular tachycardias with aberrant conduction (i.e., presence of a bundle branch block), and some types of pathway-mediated reciprocating tachycardias discussed separately in the following.

Epidemiology

Based on the Marshfield Epidemiological Study Area (MESA) data, the incidence of SVT in the general population is 35/100,000 person-years and the prevalence is 2.25 per 1000 persons. The mean age of onset in the study was 37 years old and the most likely presenting location was the emergency room.

Prevalence of ventricular arrhythmias is higher in men than in women, increases with age, and is strongly linked to the presence of cardiovascular disease. Fifteen percent to 16% of patients with VT have coronary atherosclerosis and 8% to 9% have hypertension, valvular disease, or nonischemic cardiomyopathy. Only 2% to 3% of patients with VT do not have cardiovascular disease. Five percent to 10% of patients with acute MI demonstrate VT/VF, most of which occurs during the first 48 hours of hospital admission.

Pathophysiology

There are two major mechanisms of supraventricular tachycardias: automaticity and reentry.

Automaticity involves occurrence of one or multiple ectopic foci of depolarization that are located above or within the AV node. Examples of such tachycardias include focal and multifocal atrial tachycardia and junctional tachycardia.

Reentry mechanism utilizes a formation of an electrical circuit that may involve the AV node or accessory pathways. These tachyarrhythmias include atrial flutter, AVNRT, and AV-nodal reciprocating tachycardias (AVRT).

Ventricular tachycardias utilize three major mechanisms: automaticity, triggered activity, and reentry.

Automatic VTs occur from an ectopic focus of depolarization and may originate from either ventricular myocytes or Purkinje fibers. Triggered activity includes early afterdepolarization and delayed afterdepolarization. Early depolarizations occur during the repolarization phase of the membrane, usually in a setting of acquired action potential prolongation (long QT) and serves as a trigger for polymorphic VT or torsades de pointes. Delayed afterdepolarizations occur after a complete cell repolarization and serve as VT triggers in digoxin toxicity, right ventricular outflow tract VT, and catecholaminergic polymorphic VT. Reentry-type VT occurs when an electrical circuit forms around either an anatomic barrier (scar, artificial material in postoperative patients) or an area of a functional block. This mechanism usually results in monomorphic ventricular tachycardia.

Clinical Presentation

Clinical manifestation of tachyarrhythmias may include palpitations or fluttering sensation in the chest and neck, and signs of decreased perfusion, such as hypotension, dizziness, lightheadedness, syncope, hot flushes, altered mentation, and shock. Ventricular tachyarrhythmias in particular may result in acute loss of circulation and sudden cardiac death (SCD). Effects of tachycardia on cardiac output mostly owe to shortened diastole that affects ventricular filling and decreasing preload leading to decreased cardiac output. VTs, in turn, also result in atrioventricular and

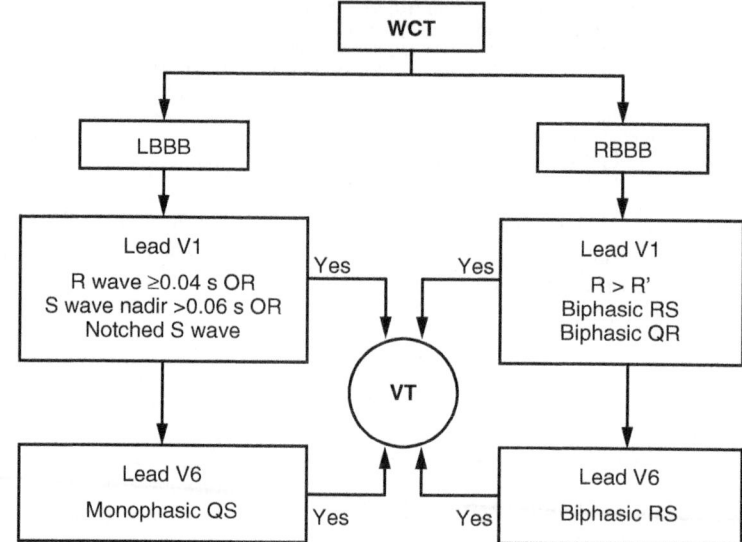

1. Is RS complex present in the precordial leads?

2. Is the longest R-S interval from the onset of the R wave to the deepest part of the S wave greater than 100 ms?

3. Is there AV-dissociation?

4. If none of the above, proceed with morphologic QRS criteria shown on the right

Figure 1 Brugada algorithm for differentiating supraventricular tachycardia from ventricular tachycardia. *LBBB,* Left bundle branch block; *RBBB,* right bundle branch block; *WCT,* wide complex tachycardia.

intraventricular dyssynchrony that may additionally affect cardiac stroke volume and output.

Diagnosis

In the acute setting, prompt and accurate diagnosis of the type of tachycardia is paramount. Every patient with suspected tachyarrhythmia should have a 12-lead electrocardiogram (ECG). Since many tachyarrhythmias may cause hemodynamic compromise, an expedited hemodynamic assessment should be performed (vital signs, oxygen saturation, presence of shock that may manifest as altered mentation or evidence of organ system dysfunction). An unstable patient should be treated emergently with an appropriate antiarrhythmic strategy defined by Advanced Cardiac Life Support (ACLS) algorithms.

History plays an important role in diagnosis of tachycardias. Nature and onset of symptoms, frequency of episodes and possible triggers or predisposing conditions, as well as alleviating factors, should be identified. Past medical history may be helpful in differentiation of different types of tachycardia, such as presence of ischemia or a structural heart disease that may favor VT. History of syncope, specifically if suggesting cardiogenic etiology, may help to identify high-risk patients. Family history of arrhythmias or sudden cardiac death may yield important information regarding familial arrhythmias, such as Wolff-Parkinson-White (WPW) or long-QT interval syndromes.

If the patient has an implanted cardiac device, such as permanent pacemaker or a defibrillator, the device interrogation is diagnostic in most cases, especially if an AV system is present that is capable of tracking both atrial and ventricular electrical activity.

Differential Diagnosis for Narrow Complex Tachycardias

Twelve-lead ECG is the first step in differentiating between different types of narrow-complex tachycardia. Analysis of QRS regularity, axis, atrial activity, baseline and relationships between atrial and ventricular activations, as well as presence of delta-wave (see Figure 4) or preexcitation should be performed.

Identification of atrial activity is key in differentiating between subtypes of SVT. When identification of atrial activity is difficult (as during rapid ventricular rate), vagal maneuvers, carotid sinus pressure or administration of IV adenosine (Adenocard)[1] may assist in diagnosis or potentially terminate the arrhythmia.

Irregular tachyarrhythmia with no identifiable pattern or P waves is diagnostic of atrial fibrillation with rapid ventricular response. Variable baseline that resembles a sawtooth pattern is suggestive of atrial flutter. AV-nodal reentry usually results in a

retrograde P wave that may be hidden within QRS complex or follows QRS immediately (short R-P tachycardia). Atrial tachycardia will have one or more P wave morphologies with 1:1 relationship; however, P wave morphology and axis will be different from sinus P waves. Comparison to prior ECG in sinus rhythm may be particularly helpful in this scenario.

An electrophysiology study is the gold-standard diagnostic approach if the mechanism of tachycardia is unclear from the surface ECG.

Differential Diagnosis for Wide Complex Tachycardias

Because SVT with aberrancy and some types of AVRT (discussed in the following) may result in wide QRS complex, differentiation of such arrhythmia from VT may be challenging even for experts. Orthodromic arrhythmia suggests the electrical impulse travels straight down the normal pathway and antidromic arrhythmia suggests that the impulse travels in the opposite direction.

Atrial activity is typically not affected by the VT (unless retrograde conduction is present), leading to AV disassociation, when P waves have no relationship to the QRS complexes. This may help in differentiating VT from SVT with aberrancy. Fusion and capture beats are other hallmarks of monomorphic VT. Fusion beats occur when atrial activity can conduct through the AV node down the His-Purkinje system and "fuse" with ventricular activity. The resulting QRS complex is a hybrid of the sinus rhythm narrow QRS complex and the widened VT QRS complex. Capture beats occur when atrial activity conducts down the His-Purkinje system and creates a narrow QRS complex, followed by ongoing VT. These findings are very specific for VT, but their absence does not rule it out.

Multiple algorithms have been proposed to assist in differentiating SVT from VT. We will discuss the Brugada algorithm that has excellent sensitivity and specificity (0.978 and 0.965, respectively) for diagnosis of VT. If the answer to any of the following questions is yes, subsequent steps are not necessary and the rhythm is VT (Figure 1).

Specific Tachycardias and Their Treatment
Sinus Tachycardia

Sinus tachycardia is a common narrow-complex tachycardia. It can represent a normal response to stress or a disease process (Table 1). Sinus tachycardia on a 12-lead ECG presents with ventricular rate >100 bpm and sinus P waves that are positive in leads I, II and III, negative in aVR, and biphasic in lead V_1 with a normal PR interval (120 to 200 ms). When compared to an ECG in normal sinus rhythm, the P wave axis and morphology should be unchanged. A syndrome of inappropriate sinus tachycardia is a diagnosis of

---

[1]Not FDA approved for this indication.

TABLE 1	Common Causes of Sinus Tachycardia	
PHYSIOLOGIC CAUSES	**PATHOLOGIC CONDITIONS**	**MEDICATIONS AND SUBSTANCES**
Exercise	Fever	Caffeine
Stress (fight or flight response)	Substance withdrawal	Nicotine
Anxiety	Hyperthyroidism	Atropine
Emotions	Pulmonary embolism	Dobutamine
Pain	Sepsis	Dopamine
	Dehydration	Pseudoephedrine
	Chronic anemia or acute blood loss	Theophylline
	Pheochromocytoma	Cocaine
	Heart failure	Methamphetamine

Figure 2 AV-nodal reentry (short R-P) tachycardia. Retrograde P waves are seen (arrows).

TABLE 2	Doses of Common AV Blocking Agents Used in Acute Setting for SVT Treatment
AGENT	**DOSE**
IV Metoprolol (Lopressor)[1]	2.5–5 mg over 2 min, up to 3 doses
IV Diltiazem (Cardizem)	First dose: 0.25 mg/kg over 2 min, average adult dose, 20 mg; second dose (if first dose is ineffective and tolerated): 0.35 mg/kg in 15–30 min over 2 min, average adult dose is 25 mg
IV Verapamil (Calan)	First dose: 0.075–0.15 mg/kg over 2 min; second dose (if first dose is ineffective and tolerated): 10 mg in 15–30 min over 2 min

[1]Not FDA approved for this indication.

exclusion, when average heart rate exceeds 90 bpm over a 24-hour period and no physiologic or medical cause can be identified.

Atrioventricular-Nodal Reentry Tachycardia

AV-nodal reentry tachycardia results from activation of a dual-pathway conduit (slow and fast) that includes the AV node. This is the most common type of SVT, with a slightly higher prevalence in women. AVNRT manifests as a regular, usually rapid tachycardia with heart rates that may exceed 250 bpm. Patient will usually experience palpitations and symptoms of decreased perfusion, such as lightheadedness, dizziness, hypotension, flushing, etc. Syncope is rare but may occur with very rapid heart rates or in subjects with dehydration or underlying heart disease. A distinguishing symptom of AVNRT is neck palpitations. The mechanism of that is the simultaneous atrial and ventricular systole due to excitation origin located within the AV node, which is located between the atria and ventricles. This results in right atrial contraction against the closed tricuspid valve, forcing blood back into jugular system that is subjectively perceived as palpitations in the neck. Diagnosis of AVNRT is based on a surface electrocardiogram that will classically demonstrate a rapid narrow complex tachycardia with P waves occurring within the QRS complex; therefore, they are not immediately discoverable, but may cause subtle deflection at the terminal portion of the QRS or immediately after the QRS (short R-P tachycardia, Figure 2). Electrophysiology study yields definitive diagnosis by demonstration of a dual-pathway physiology.

In the acute setting, as soon as AVNRT is suspected, termination of the arrhythmia should be attempted. Vagal maneuvers, such as Valsalva, carotid massage, or application of a cold wet towel to the patient's face may be helpful. Adenosine (Adenocard) has been reported to be effective in greater than 95% of patients with AVNRT. If the type of tachyarrhythmia is uncertain, adenosine may also help to make a diagnosis by blocking AV conduction and causing ventricular pause that will unmask the underlying atrial activity, and may reveal arrhythmias, such as atrial tachycardia or atrial flutter. It is important to remember that adenosine has a very short half-life and should be administered as a very rapid IV injection followed by a 20 mL fluid bolus. ACLS recommends the initial dose of 6 mg followed by 12 mg, if no response. The 12-mg dose can be repeated one more time. Patients taking theophylline (adenosine antagonist) may require a higher initial dose (12 mg), whereas patients with a heart transplant or on carbamazepine

(Tegretol) should be given a lower initial dose (3 mg). A 12-lead ECG recording should be performed in a continuous mode while performing this intervention for more accurate rhythm identification. If these measures are ineffective to terminate the arrhythmia, a brief assessment of hemodynamic status must be made. If patient is hemodynamically unstable, a DC cardioversion should be performed, whereas in a stable patient further treatment may include IV beta blockers, IV verapamil (Calan), or IV diltiazem (Cardizem) (Table 2). IV amiodarone (Pacerone)[1] is recommended as the next line of treatment, if all prior measures are ineffective or not feasible. In a stable patient who is not responding to medications, a DC cardioversion should still be performed to restore the sinus rhythm.

Follow-up management of AVNRT should include a specialty consultation for consideration of slow pathway radiofrequency or cryo catheter ablation. The patient may be started on a maintenance oral beta blocker or a nondihydropyridine calcium channel blocker, such as diltiazem or verapamil. An antiarrhythmic medication, such as flecainide (Tambocor), may also be used to control occurrences of tachyarrhythmia; however, ischemic and structural heart disease has to be ruled out before these agents can be used due to their proarrhythmic effects with these conditions.

Pathway-Mediated Tachycardias (Orthodromic AVRT, Antidromic AVRT, WPW Syndrome)

Atrioventricular structures (AV valves and annuli) serve as an insulator, and normally there is no electrical communication between atrial and ventricular myocardium outside the normal conduction system. An accessory pathway is defined as an abnormal extranodal electrical communication between atrial and ventricular myocardium. A pathway that causes ventricular preexcitation pattern on a surface ECG (P-R interval <0.12 and presence of a delta-wave) is called a *manifest* pathway. A pathway that is not detectable on a surface ECG is called *concealed*. Accessory pathways can be located anywhere around AV annuli and may be capable of anterograde, retrograde, or bidirectional conduction. They are responsible for two types of reentry

[1]Not FDA approved for this indication.

tachycardias: *ORT* that utilizes the normal conduction system for anterograde conduction and the accessory pathway for retrograde conduction, and *ART*, that uses the accessory pathway for anterograde conduction and AV node for retrograde conduction.

ORT is the most common type of pathway-mediated SVT and accounts for more than 90% of AVRT cases. Because ORT uses the normal conduction system for ventricular activation, it will demonstrate a normal, narrow QRS morphology, whereas ART leads to direct ventricular activation from pathway-conducting anterograde, which results in a wide-complex QRS morphology (Figure 3).

A WPW syndrome is a bundle of a manifest accessory pathway on a surface ECG in sinus rhythm (preexcitation pattern, Figure 4) and presence of supraventricular tachyarrhythmias.

If a patient with an accessory pathway capable of rapid anterograde conduction develops atrial fibrillation, it may result in a very rapid ventricular response rate and sudden cardiac death. AV blocking agents, such as beta blockers, or calcium channel blockers (CCBs) are contraindicated for treatment of atrial fibrillation in WPW patients, as they suppress the AV node (that competes with accessory pathway for atrioventricular conduction and serves as a rate-control "gate keeper") and further facilitates the conduction down the pathway, increasing the ventricular rate.

Figure 3 Antidromic reciprocating tachycardia. Wide QRS morphology results from ventricular activation via the accessory pathway. P wave is preceding the QRS complex (long R-P).

Figure 4 Manifest accessory pathway in a patient with Wolff-Parkinson-White syndrome. A short PR interval and delta-wave *(arrow)*.

Instead, procainamide (Pronestyl)[1] should be used to suppress voltage-gated sodium channels of the accessory pathway.

Acute management of AVRT should include assessment of the 12-lead ECG for presence of preexcitation. If no preexcitation is present (ORT), the management is similar to AVNRT, as discussed in previous topic. If preexcitation is detected (ART, WPW), AV blocking agents should be avoided or used with caution. DC cardioversion should be considered early, regardless of hemodynamic status.

For ongoing management, all patients with AVRT should undergo a subspecialty consultation for consideration of a catheter ablation procedure. Patients with a manifest accessory (e.g., WPW) pathway should also undergo risk stratification for sudden cardiac death, as soon as diagnosis is made.

Atrial Tachycardias

Atrial tachycardias can be focal or multifocal. Focal atrial tachycardia is usually regular and is characterized by the presence of distinct uniform P waves on the surface ECG. Morphology of these P waves differs from those in sinus rhythm. Multifocal atrial tachycardia will contain three or more different P wave morphologies, and is associated with structural heart disease, pulmonary disease, and pulmonary hypertension.

Treatment of atrial tachycardias may be challenging, with limited utility for antiarrhythmic medications and cardioversion that is often ineffective. AV-nodal blockers and ablation procedures have the most established role in treatment of these conditions.

Junctional Tachycardia

Junctional tachycardia is a rapid narrow QRS complex tachyarrhythmia with rates up to 220 bpm that originates within the AV junction and may be regular or irregular. It is more commonly seen in pediatric populations and occurs rarely in adults. In the acute setting, IV beta blockers, nondihydropyridine CCBs, or procainamide[1] can be used. For chronic suppression, oral beta-blockers, verapamil[1] or diltiazem[1], as well as antiarrhythmic drugs may be effective.

Atrial Flutter

Atrial flutter, also known as *macroreentrant atrial tachycardia*, is a reentry arrhythmia that propagates around the tricuspid valve annulus. It most commonly involves the cavotricuspid isthmus (isthmus-dependent) and may be typical, when the signal travels up the intraatrial septum and down the lateral right atrial wall in a counterclockwise fashion around the annulus when observed from the RV apex (Figure 5, panel A), or reverse typical, or clockwise, traveling down the septum and up the atrial wall (see Figure 5, panel B).

Flutter that does not involve the cavotricuspid isthmus is called atypical, or isthmus independent.

Figure 5 *Panel A:* direction of a typical, counterclockwise activation in atrial flutter. *Panel B:* direction of a reverse typical, clockwise activation in atrial flutter. *IAS,* Intraatrial septum; *IVC,* inferior vena cava; *SVC,* superior vena cava; *TV,* tricuspid valve.

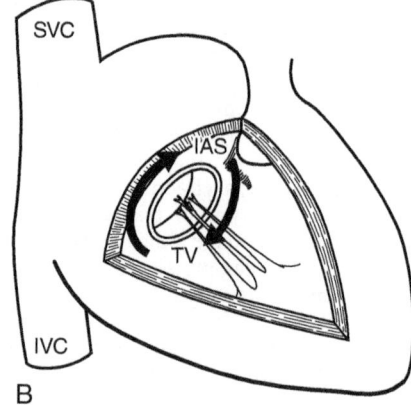

A   B

---

[1] Not FDA approved for this indication.

Macroreentrant arrhythmias create a characteristic pattern on the ECG that resembles the "sawtooth" appearance of the electrical baseline, best seen in the inferior leads (Figure 6).

Counter-clockwise activation creates positive deflection in lead V_1 (signal travels up the septum toward the lead) and negative deflection in the inferior leads, whereas clockwise demonstrates the opposite. Since the reentrant circle utilizes a fairly consistent anatomic path, the cycle length of reentry is around 220 ms, resulting in an atrial waveform rate around 300 bpm. The AV node will attempt to block the portion of atrial activations, resulting in slower ventricular rates. Two-to-one conduction commonly results in a ventricular rate around 150 bpm, whereas variable conduction may lead to an irregular ventricular response, which, however, usually follows identifiable patterns with R-R intervals multiple to the flutter cycle length, or 220 ms (440 ms, 660 ms, etc.). If the tricuspid annulus is dilated or the patient is receiving an antiarrhythmic medication that slows myocardial conduction (for example, flecainide), it may increase the flutter cycle length, decreasing the flutter rate. This may have an important negative implication. Usually, AV node is able to block fast flutter, decreasing the ventricular response to 2:1. However, when the flutter rate is decreased, it allows the AV node to conduct in 1:1 fashion, leading to very rapid ventricular responses that may result in syncope and ventricular fibrillation. If flecainide

Figure 6 Macro-reentrant atrial tachycardia: typical atrial flutter with 2:1 AV-nodal conduction. A variable baseline is seen that resembles a sawtooth pattern. Positive deflections in lead V_1 and negative in lead III *(arrows)* indicate counter-clockwise signal propagation around the tricuspid annulus.

is chosen as an antiarrhythmic therapy to control atrial flutter, it is important to always use it in a combination with an AV blocking agent to avoid 1:1 conduction, in case of a relapse.

Medical treatment of atrial flutter may be challenging, due to weaker ventricular rate responses to AV blocking agents that results in notorious difficulty with the rate-control strategy. One-to-one response should be treated as a medical emergency with a prompt DC cardioversion. For typical flutter, an EP consultation for a radiofrequency catheter ablation procedure should always be considered due to a high success rate and relative simplicity of the procedure. Atypical flutter ablations, however, may be more technically challenging with lower success rates.

Ventricular Tachycardias

Ventricular tachycardia is defined as a cardiac arrhythmia of three or greater beats at a rate of >100 bpm that originates in the ventricles. Sustained VT, just as SVT, is a VT that sustains for >30 seconds. Nonsustained VT terminates spontaneously within 30 seconds after onset.

VT that manifests with uniform beat-to-beat QRS morphology is called *monomorphic* (Figure 7). This type of morphology is more likely to represent structural or functional electrical reentry as the leading mechanism. A common substrate for such arrhythmia is a myocardial scar resulting from chronic ischemic or structural heart disease.

Polymorphic ventricular tachycardia is characterized by the presence of multiform QRS complexes and likely represents unstable myocyte membranes. Such arrhythmia may be seen in multiple conditions, including long-QT syndromes (congenital and acquired). QT should always be assessed as soon as sinus rhythm is restored. When QT prolongation is detected, a reversible cause, such a medication effect or electrolyte abnormality, should be considered and treated. If no cause can be identified, a congenital condition may be suspected.

If polymorphic VT occurs without QT prolongation, acute myocardial ischemia should be considered and promptly evaluated and treated.

Torsades de pointes represents a subtype of polymorphic VT that usually associated with long-QT syndromes and demonstrates a characteristic ECG pattern with rotating QRS axis appearance (Figure 8).

Figure 7 Onset of monomorphic ventricular tachycardia.

25 mm/s

Figure 8 Polymorphic ventricular tachycardia: torsades de pointes in a patient with acute inferior myocardial infarction.

999999999 4/8/2018 11:39:04 PM

V TACH   HR 84

SPO2 97%   ***RATE 84   NBP 89 / 62 (08)23:02

V TACH

Normal QRS complexes

II

III

Figure 9 Artifact masquerading ventricular tachycardia. A diagnosis of wide-complex tachycardia is dismissed by presence of sinus rhythm in lead III.

Of all the arrhythmias seen in clinical practice, ventricular tachycardias are of most concern to practitioners due to the high morbidity and mortality associated with these disorders. Although both subtypes require emergent medical attention, polymorphic VT poses particular danger due to the often rapid deterioration of hemodynamics, loss of circulation, and death. Sustained polymorphic VT should be treated immediately with an unsynchronized DC cardioversion.

The approach to monomorphic VT starts with assessment of hemodynamic stability. Faster ventricular rates (>150 bpm) and underlying structural heart disease may be associated with more rapid hemodynamic decline. ACLS algorithms for specific types of VT must be implemented. Each patient with ventricular tachycardia should undergo a prompt specialty consultation and risk stratification for sudden cardiac death.

Artifact

All providers should be aware of telemetry and ECG artifacts that may masquerade as ventricular arrhythmias. If multi-lead recording is available, all leads should be examined. If sinus rhythm can be found in one or more leads, that indicates the recording is an artifact (Figure 9).

References

Al-Khatib SM, Stevenson WG: AHA/ACC/HRS Guideline for Management of Patients With Ventricular Arrhythmias and the Prevention of Sudden Cardiac Death, 2017.

Aronow WS, Ahn C, Mercando AD, Epstein S, Kronzon I: Prevalence and association of ventricular tachycardia and complex ventricular arrhythmias with new coronary events in older men and women with and without cardiovascular disease, *The Journals of Gerontology Series A: Biological Sciences and Medical Sciences* 57(3):M178–M180, 2002.

Brady WJ, Mattu A, Tabas J, Ferguson JD: The differential diagnosis of wide QRS complex tachycardia, *The American Journal of Emergency Medicine* 35(10):1525–1529, 2017.

Brugada P, Brugada J, Mont L, Smeets JLRM, Andries EW: A new approach to the differential diagnosis of a regular tachycardia with a wide QRS complex, *Circulation* 83(5):1649–1659, 1991.

Low PA, Sandroni P: Postural tachycardia syndrome (POTS). In *Primer on the Autonomic Nervous System*, Academic Press, 2012, pp 517–519.

Meiltz A, Weber R, Halimi F, et al: Permanent form of junctional reciprocating tachycardia in adults: peculiar features and results of radiofrequency catheter ablation, *Europace* 8(1):21–28, 2006.

Orejarena LA, Vidaillet H, DeStefano F, et al: Paroxysmal supraventricular tachycardia in the general population, *Journal of the American College of Cardiology* 31(1):150–157, 1998.

Page RL, et al: 2015 ACC/AHA/HRS guideline for the management of adult patients with supraventricular tachycardia: a report of the American College of Cardiology/American Heart Association Task Force on Clinical Practice Guidelines and the Heart Rhythm Society, *Journal of the American College of Cardiology* 67:13, 2016.

VENOUS THROMBOSIS

Method of
Thomas W. Wakefield, MD; and Andrea T. Obi, MD

CURRENT DIAGNOSIS

- The diagnosis of deep venous thrombosis (DVT) is made with duplex ultrasound imaging and secondarily laboratory testing, because history and physical examination are inaccurate in up to half of cases.
- Although clinical assessment and D-dimer levels are useful to rule out thrombosis, there is no combination of clinical findings and biomarker testing at this time that can rule in the diagnosis.
- Duplex ultrasound imaging is the gold standard for the diagnosis of DVT.
- Spiral computed tomographic (CT) scanning, especially higher-resolution multidetector-row CT imaging, is preferred as the initial imaging test to establish the diagnosis of pulmonary embolism.

CURRENT THERAPY

- Initial preventative therapy includes anticoagulation, compression garments, and ambulation.
- The new direct oral anticoagulants (DOACs) are favored over warfarin for acute VTE treatment and no cancer. Rivaroxaban (Xarelto) and apixaban (Eliquis) are administered as monotherapy whereas dabigatran (Pradaxa) and edoxaban (Savaysa) require a low-molecular-weight heparin (LMWH) bridge.
- LMWH should be administered for at least 5 days, during which time an oral anticoagulant (warfarin, dabigatran, or edoxaban) is begun. If warfarin is used, it should be therapeutic (international normalized ratio 2.0-3.0) for 2 consecutive days before stopping LMWH.

- The duration of anticoagulation depends on a number of factors, including the presence of risk factors for thrombosis, the type of thrombosis (idiopathic or provoked), the number of times thrombosis has occurred and risk factors for bleeding.
- Reduced dose DOACs lessen VTE recurrences more than placebo or aspirin for long-term treatment after VTE.
- Significant iliofemoral DVT may be treated with aggressive pharmocomechanical thrombolysis if a trial of anticoagulation fails to improve moderate to severe symptoms and the patient is ambulatory, has no contraindications to thrombolysis, and places a strong value on reducing the severity of post-thrombotic syndrome (PTS) while accepting the inherent bleeding risk. Pulmonary embolism causing hemodynamic deterioration or right heart strain should be treated with thrombolysis.

Epidemiology

Venous thromboembolism (VTE) includes deep venous thrombosis (DVT) and pulmonary embolism (PE). VTE affects up to 900,000 patients per year and results in 300,000 deaths per year. The incidence has remained constant and may be increasing since the 1980s and increases with age. The annual VTE rate among persons of European ancestry ranges from 104 to 183 per 100,000 person years. Overall VTE incidence may be higher in blacks and lower in Asians and Asian- and Native-Americans. The increasing prevalence of obesity, cancer, and surgery account in part for the persistent VTE incidence. Treatment of an acute VTE appears to be associated with incremental direct medical costs of $12,000 to $15,000 (2014 US dollars) with subsequent complications to increase cumulative costs up to $18,000 to $23,000 per incident case. Sequelae from VTE including recurrent VTE, post-thrombotic syndrome (PTS), ulcers, and varicosities increase the incident cost by an average of 75%. The annual incident cost to the US healthcare system is $7 to $10 billion dollars each year.

Risk Factors

Risk factors for VTE include acquired and genetic factors. Acquired factors include increasing age, malignancy, surgery, immobilization, trauma, oral contraceptives and hormone replacement therapy, pregnancy and the puerperium, neurologic disease, cardiac disease, obesity, sepsis, pneumonia, and inflammatory bowel disease. Genetic factors include antithrombin deficiency, protein C deficiency and protein S deficiency, factor V Leiden, prothrombin 20210A, blood group non-O, abnormalities in fibrinogen and plasminogen, elevated levels of clotting factors (e.g., factors XI, IX, VII, VIII, X, and II), and elevation in plasminogen activator inhibitor-1. When a patient presents with an idiopathic VTE, family history of thrombosis, recurrent thrombosis, or thrombosis in unusual locations, a work-up for hypercoagulability, including testing for the conditions noted in the previous sentence, may be indicated, although even in these situations, testing is controversial. Routine testing for hypercoaguable states in the setting of a provoked DVT is not indicated. Hematologic diseases associated with VTE include heparin-induced thrombocytopenia and thrombosis syndrome, disseminated intravascular coagulation, antiphospholipid antibody syndrome, myeloproliferative disorders, thrombotic thrombocytopenic purpura, and hemolytic uremic syndrome. There are a number of risk prediction scores that have been advanced, the most widely-used being the Caprini risk score (https://www.mdcalc.com/caprini-score-venous-thromboembolism-2005).

Pathophysiology

Although Virchow's triad of stasis, vein injury, and hypercoagulability has defined the events that predispose to DVT formation since the mid-19th century, the understanding today of events that occur at the level of the vein wall and thrombus, including the inflammatory response on thrombogenesis, thrombus resolution and the subsequent changes to the vein wall and venous valves, is increasingly becoming apparent, and may direct therapy in the future.

Diagnosis

Deep Venous Thrombosis

The diagnosis of DVT can be ruled out with a clinical scoring system known as the Wells score (https://www.mdcalc.com/wells-criteria-dvt) and a negative D dimer. Wells has classified patients into a scoring system that emphasizes physical presentation, and the most common physical finding is edema. Characteristics that score points in the Wells system include active cancer, paralysis or paresis, recent plaster/cast immobilization of the lower extremity, being recently bedridden for 3 days or more, localized tenderness along the distribution of the deep venous system, swelling of the entire leg, calf swelling that is at least 3 cm larger on the involved side than on the noninvolved side, pitting edema in the symptomatic leg, collateral superficial veins (nonvaricose), and a history of previous DVT. With extensive proximal iliofemoral DVT there may be significant swelling, cyanosis, and dilated superficial collateral veins. The negative predictive value of a low or intermediate risk patient as stratified by Well's score and a negative D dimer is near 100%. The incidence of DVT over the next 3 months in this patient cohort is 0.0% to 0.6%, suggesting that additional testing is unlikely to improve outcomes.

Duplex ultrasound imaging has become the gold standard for ruling in the diagnosis of DVT. Duplex imaging includes both a B-mode image and Doppler flow pattern. Duplex imaging demonstrates sensitivity and specificity rates greater than 95%. According to the grade criteria for the strength of medical evidence, duplex ultrasound is given a 1B level of evidence, depending on the pretest probability for DVT. Even at the level of the calf, duplex imaging is an acceptable technique in symptomatic patients. Duplex imaging is painless, requires no contrast, can be repeated, and is safe during pregnancy. Duplex imaging also identifies other causes of a patient's symptoms. Other tests available for making the diagnosis include magnetic resonance imaging (MRI) (especially good for assessing central pelvic vein and inferior vena cava [IVC] thrombosis) and spiral computed tomographic (CT) scanning (especially with chest imaging during examination for PE).

A single complete negative duplex scan is accurate enough to withhold anticoagulation with minimal long-term adverse thromboembolic complications. This requires that all venous segments of the leg have been imaged and evaluated. If the duplex scan is indeterminate owing to technical issues or to edema, treatment may be based on factors such as biomarkers, with the duplex repeated in 24 to 72 hours. Combining clinical characteristics with a high-sensitivity D-dimer assay can decrease the number of duplex scans performed in the low risk patient. Although clinical characteristics and D-dimer levels are useful to rule out thrombosis, the converse is not true, and there is no combination of biomarkers and clinical presentation that can rule in the diagnosis. Work is ongoing to establish new biomarkers based on the inflammatory response to DVT. We have data suggesting that a combination of soluble P-selectin and the Wells score can rule in the diagnosis of DVT, whereas D-dimer plus Wells is still the best combination to rule out the diagnosis of DVT.

Conditions that may be confused with DVT include lymphedema, muscle strain, and muscle contusion and systemic problems such as cardiac, renal, or hepatic abnormalities. These systemic problems usually lead to bilateral edema.

Rarely, massive iliofemoral DVT can result in phlegmasia alba dolens (white swollen leg) or phlegmasia cerulean dolens (blue swollen leg). If phlegmasia is not aggressively treated, it can lead to venous gangrene when the arterial inflow becomes obstructed owing to venous hypertension. Alternatively, arterial emboli or spasm can occur and contribute to the pathophysiology. Venous gangrene is often associated with underlying malignancy and is always preceded by phlegmasia cerulea dolens. Venous gangrene is associated with significant rates of amputation and pulmonary embolism and with mortality.

Pulmonary Embolism

The diagnosis of PE historically has involved ventilation-perfusion scanning and pulmonary angiography. However, the most current techniques include spiral CT scanning and MRI, along with assessments of pretest probability and high sensitivity D-dimer measurements Age-adjusted D-dimer measurements may increase the diagnostic usefulness of these measurements. CT scanning demonstrates excellent specificity and sensitivity. Emboli down to the subsegmental level can be identified. The sensitivity for isolated chest CT imaging is increased when clinical analysis is added and when adding lower extremity imaging to the chest scan, although with the introduction of higher resolution multidetector-row CT imaging, the need for lower extremity imaging combined with CT is being questioned. Useful alternate techniques when there are contraindications to CT imaging include MRI and ventilation-perfusion imaging.

In low-risk individuals, a score of 0 on the PE Rule-Out Criteria (https://www.mdcalc.com/perc-rule-pulmonary-embolism) gives confidence that further testing (d-dimer and CT) is not necessary. The PE Rule-Out Criteria include (1) pulse oximetry of 94% or less, (2) heart rate of 100 beats/min or greater, (3) age of 50 years or older, (4) unilateral leg swelling, (5) hemoptysis, (6) recent trauma or surgery, (7) previous PE or DVT, (8) exogenous estrogen use.

Axillary and Subclavian Vein Thrombosis

Thrombosis of the axillary and subclavian veins accounts for less than 5% of all cases of DVT. However, it may be associated with PE in up to 10% to 15% of cases and can be the source of significant disability. Upper extremity DVT may be primary (approximately 20%), such as from thoracic outlet syndrome, effort thrombosis, or idiopathic; or secondary (approximately 80%), such as from catheter-related, cancer-associated, surgery-related, or mediastinal tumors. Primary axillary and subclavian vein thrombosis results from obstruction of the axillary vein in the thoracic outlet from compression by the subclavius muscle and the costoclavicular space, the Paget-Schrötter syndrome, noted especially in muscular athletes. Patients with axillary and subclavian vein thrombosis present with arm pain, edema, and cyanosis. Superficial venous distention may be apparent over the arm, forearm, shoulder, and anterior chest wall.

Upper extremity venous duplex ultrasound scanning is used to make the diagnosis of axillary and subclavian vein thrombosis. A secondary DVT (such as related to a central venous catheter or other risk factor) is treated with anticoagulation alone, with the same recommendation regarding anticoagulant type, dose, and duration. If Paget-Schrötter syndrome is suspected, thrombolysis and phlebography are considered as next interventions. If phlebography is performed, it is important that the patient undergo positional phlebography with the arm abducted to 120 degrees to confirm extrinsic subclavian vein compression at the thoracic outlet once the vein has been cleared of thrombus. Because a cervical rib may be the cause of such obstruction, chest x-ray should be obtained to exclude its presence (although its incidence is quite low). Ultimately, decompression of the thoracic outlet with first rib resection (and cervical rib, if present), is necessary to prevent recurrent DVT.

Treatment

Standard Therapy for Venous Thromboembolism

The traditional treatment of VTE is systemic anticoagulation, which reduces the risk of PE, extension of thrombosis, and thrombus recurrence. Because the recurrence rate for VTE is higher if anticoagulation is not therapeutic in the first 24 hours, immediate anticoagulation should be undertaken. For PE, this usually means anticoagulation followed by testing. For DVT, because duplex imaging is rapidly obtained, usually testing precedes anticoagulation. Recurrent DVT can still occur in up to one third of patients over an 8-year period, even with appropriate anticoagulant therapy.

The first line of therapy in the modern-day treatment of VTE is DOACs. Currently 5 DOACs are FDA approved for the treatment of DVT. These include rivaroxaban (Xarelto) and apixaban (Eliquis) as oral monotherapy (both require a loading dose period, followed by a lower dose) and dabigatran (Pradaxa) and edoxaban (Savaysa), which require a LMWH bridge, and Betrixaban (Bevyxxa) for prophylaxis. Alternatively, LMWH or unfractionated heparin is given for 5 days, during which time oral anticoagulation with vitamin K antagonists (warfarin) is begun as soon as anticoagulation is therapeutic. With warfarin, it is recommended that the international normalized ratio be therapeutic for 2 consecutive days before stopping heparin or LMWH.

The new agents for venous thrombosis treatment and prophylaxis include factor Xa inhibitors and direct thrombin inhibitors. The new oral anticoagulants are favored over warfarin (grade 2B) for acute VTE and no cancer. Dabigatran targets activated factor II (factor IIa), whereas rivaroxaban, apixaban, and edoxaban target activated factor X (factor Xa). Dabigatran etexilate is FDA approved for stroke and systemic embolization prevention in patients with non-valvular atrial fibrillation and for treatment and reduction of DVT and PE in patients who have been treated with a parenteral anticoagulant for 5–10 days.

Rivaroxaban is FDA approved for VTE prophylaxis in patients undergoing hip or knee replacements, for stroke and systemic embolization prevention in patients with nonvalvular atrial fibrillation, and for VTE treatment. The Einstein trial evaluated rivaroxaban compared with standard anticoagulation in the treatment of acute DVT. As monotherapy, rivaroxaban was found statistically noninferior to standard therapy, without increased bleeding. A similar finding with PE has been noted. Apixaban is currently FDA approved for the prevention of complications of nonvalvular atrial fibrillation, for prophylaxis of DVT after hip or knee replacement surgery, for the treatment of DVT/PE, and for the reduction in risk of recurrence of DVT/PE. Edoxaban has been approved for prevention of stroke and non-central-nervous system (CNS) systemic embolism in patients with nonvalvular atrial fibrillation and for treating DVT and PE in patients who have been treated with a parenteral anticoagulant for 5 to 10 days. Betrixaban is indicated for the prophylaxis of VTE in adult patients hospitalized for an acute medical illness who are at risk for thromboembolic complications due to restricted mobility and other risk factors.

When an anticoagulant bridge is required, LMWH is the standard for initial treatment. LMWH is preferred because it is administered subcutaneously, it requires no monitoring (except in certain circumstances such as renal insufficiency or morbid obesity), and it is associated with a lower bleeding potential. Additionally, LMWH demonstrates less direct thrombin inhibition, more factor Xa inhibition, and has anti-inflammatory properties. Compared with standard unfractionated heparin, LMWH has significantly improved bioavailability, less endothelial cell binding and protein binding, and an improved pharmacokinetic profile. The half-life of LMWH is dose independent. LMWH is administered in a weight-based fashion.

Warfarin (Coumadin), when used, should be started after heparinization is therapeutic to prevent warfarin-induced skin necrosis. For standard unfractionated heparin, this requires a therapeutic activated partial thromboplastin time (aPTT); for LMWH, warfarin is administered after an appropriate weight-based dose of LMWH is administered and allowed to circulate. Warfarin causes inhibition of protein C and S before factors II, IX, and X, leading to paradoxical hypercoagulability at the initiation of therapy. The goal for warfarin dosing is an international normalized ratio between 2.0 and 3.0.

Fondaparinux (Arixtra) is the final agent that is approved for the treatment of VTE. It is a synthetic pentasaccharide that has an antithrombin sequence identical to heparin and targets factor Xa. Fondaparinux has been additionally approved for thrombosis prophylaxis in patients with total hip replacement, total knee replacement, and hip fracture; in extended prophylaxis in patients with hip fracture; and in patients undergoing abdominal surgery. It is administered subcutaneously and has a 17-hour half-life. Dosage is based on body weight. It exhibits no endothelial or protein binding and does not produce thrombocytopenia. However, no antidote is readily available. For the treatment of VTE, fondaparinux was found equal to LMWH for DVT, and for PE, it was found equal to standard heparin.

Duration of Treatment

The recommended duration of anticoagulation after a first episode of provoked VTE is 3 months for both proximal (grade 1B evidence) and distal thrombi (if symptomatic, grade 2C evidence). After a second episode of VTE, the usual recommendation is prolonged oral anticoagulation indefinitely (grade 1B), unless the patient is at high bleeding risk (2 or more risk factors, grade 2B) or the patient is very young at the time of presentation. VTE recurrence is increased with homozygous factor V Leiden and prothrombin 20210A mutation, protein C or protein S deficiency, antithrombin deficiency, antiphospholipid antibodies, and cancer until resolved. Long-term oral anticoagulation is usually recommended in these situations. However, heterozygous factor V Leiden and prothrombin 20210A do not carry the same risk as their homozygous counterparts, and the length of oral anticoagulation is shortened for these conditions.

Regarding idiopathic DVT, in those with a low bleeding risk, the recommended length of treatment is extended therapy for more than 3 months (grade 2B evidence), provided the patient is at low or moderate risk of bleeding. Patients at high risk of bleeding should be treated for 3 months (grade 1B) and reevaluated. Additional tools that can aid in the decision making to continue or discontinue anticoagulation include thrombosis risk factors, residual thrombus burden, and coagulation system activation. The HERDOO2 score (https://www.mdcalc.com/herdoo2-rule-discontinuing-anticoagulation-unprovoked-vte) has been suggested as a way for identifying women at low risk of recurrent VTE for whom anticoagulation can be stopped. In addition, there is growing evidence that in certain circumstances, such as active cancer, the use of LMWH is superior to LMWH converted to warfarin for long-term treatment, for at least the first 3 to 6 months (grade 2C evidence). There is now evidence that rivaroxaban and apixaban may be as effective as LMWH in cancer patients, with the convenience of an oral medication. However, due to a slightly increased risk of GI bleeding, DOACs should be restricted to those patients with a non-GI malignancy and low bleeding risk.

Extended therapy is now recommended with low-dose DOACs when the risk-benefit relationship favors continued treatment. Extended rivaroxaban showed a significant decrease in recurrent VTE without a significant increase in major bleeding compared with aspirin for an additional 6 to 12 months of therapy after initial therapy in the Einstein Choice trial. Apixaban as extended treatment of VTE was also investigated. After initial treatment, an additional 12 months of apixaban therapy was compared with placebo. This study revealed a significant decrease in the rate of VTE without an increase in bleeding risk. In patients who cannot continue on DOACs after initial therapy for VTE and who do not have a contraindication, aspirin should be administered to prevent recurrent thrombosis.

Complications

Bleeding is the most common complication of anticoagulation. Risk factors for bleeding while on anticoagulation include age >65, previous bleeding, cancer, renal or liver failure, thrombocytopenia, previous stroke, diabetes, anemia, concurrent antiplatelet therapy, poor anticoagulant control, recent surgery, frequent falls, alcohol abuse, and nonsteroidal antiinflammatory drug use. Presence of zero risk factors (low risk) confers an absolute risk of major bleeding of 0.8% per year. Patients with one risk factor have a risk of 1.6% per year, and those with two or more have a 6.5% risk or higher per year. With standard heparin, bleeding occurs over the first 5 days in approximately 10% of patients. Warfarin is associated with a major bleeding rate of 1% to 2% per year. Even with the new DOACS, bleeding (major plus minor) may occur in 5% to 10% of cases, although the risk of intracerebral bleeding appears to be less than with warfarin. Problems specific to the DOACs include the inability

at the present time to reliably reverse their anticoagulant effects and the difficulty with laboratory monitoring. A monoclonal antibody idarucizumab (Praxbind) for the reversal of dabigatran and a recombinant modified human Factor Xa protein andexanet alfa (Andexxa) for the reversal of Factor Xa inhibitors have been FDA approved. Aripazine (a Factor Xa inhibitor) is under development.

Heparin-induced thrombocytopenia (HIT) occurs in 0.6% to 30% of patients. Although historically morbidity and mortality rates have been high, it has been found that early diagnosis and appropriate treatment have decreased these rates. HIT usually begins 3 to 14 days after unfractionated heparin is begun, although it can occur earlier if the patient has been exposed to heparin in the past. A heparin-dependent antibody binds to platelets, activates them with the release of procoagulant microparticles leading to an increase in thrombocytopenia, and results in both arterial and venous thrombosis. Both bovine and porcine unfractionated heparin and LMWH have been associated with HIT, although the incidence and severity of the thrombosis is less with LMWH. Even small exposures to heparin, such as heparin coating on indwelling catheters, can cause the syndrome. The diagnosis should be suspected with a 50% or greater drop in platelet count, when the platelet count falls below 100,000/μL, or when thrombosis occurs during heparin or LMWH therapy. The enzyme-linked immunosorbent assay detects the antiheparin antibody in the plasma. This test is highly sensitive but poorly specific. The serotonin release assay is used as a confirmatory test, that is more specific but less sensitive than the enzyme-linked immunosorbent assay test.

When the diagnosis is made, heparin must be discontinued. Oral anticoagulation should not be given until an adequate alternative anticoagulant has been established and until the platelet count has normalized. Because LMWHs demonstrate high cross-reactivity with standard heparin antibodies, they cannot be substituted for standard heparin in patients with HIT. Agents that have been FDA approved as alternatives include the direct thrombin inhibitor argatroban. Fondaparinux (Arixtra)[1] has also been found effective for treatment of HIT in most cases, but it is not FDA approved for this indication.

Nonpharmacologic Treatments

The symptoms of swelling and leg fatigue can be controlled after DVT by the use of compression stockings. Additionally, walking with good compression does not increase the risk of PE, whereas it significantly decreases the incidence and severity of the PTS. A recent multicenter randomized trial has suggested that stockings do not prevent development of PTS after a first proximal DVT, and for that reason, the most recent ACCP guidelines suggest not using compression stockings to prevent PTS (grade 2B evidence). It must be remembered that the use of strong compression and early ambulation after DVT treatment can significantly reduce the symptoms of pain and swelling resulting from the DVT, even if the development of PTS is not prevented, and a new study suggests that certain surrogate markers for PTS may be lessened by the application of immediate compression.

Aggressive Therapies for Venous Thromboembolism

The goals of DVT treatment are to prevent extension or recurrence of DVT, prevent pulmonary embolism, and minimize the late sequela of thrombosis, namely chronic venous insufficiency. Standard anticoagulants accomplish the first two goals but not the third goal. The PTS (venous insufficiency related to venous thrombosis) occurs in up to 30% to 50% of patients after DVT and in an even higher percentage of patients with iliofemoral level DVT. It has been hypothesized that reopening the vein will alleviate venous hypertension or prevent PTS. This is known as the "open vein hypothesis." The following evidence suggests more aggressive therapies for extensive thrombosis are indicated: experimentally, prolonged contact of the thrombus with the vein wall increases damage. The thrombus initiates an inflammatory response in the vein wall that can lead to vein wall fibrosis and

---

[1] Not FDA approved for this indication.

valvular dysfunction. The longer a thrombus is in contact with a vein valve, the more chance that valve will no longer function.

Venous thrombectomy has proved superior to anticoagulation over 6 months to 10 years as measured by venous patency and prevention of venous reflux. Catheter-directed thrombolysis has been used in many nonrandomized studies and, in small, randomized trials, was more effective than standard therapy. Quality of life was improved with thrombus removal, and results appear to be optimized further by combining catheter-directed thrombolysis with mechanical devices. These devices include but are not limited to the Angiojet rheolytic catheter, the EKOS ultrasound accelerated catheter, and new larger bore extraction devices (Penumbra and angiovac). With these devices, thrombolysis is hastened, the amount of thrombolytic agent is decreased, and bleeding is thus decreased. Additionally, the use of venous stents for iliac venous obstruction has been shown to decease the incidence of PTS and chronic venous insufficiency.

To more fully elucidate the role of aggressive therapy in proximal iliofemoral venous thrombosis, the ATTRACT trial randomized 692 patients with acute proximal DVT to either anticoagulation alone or anticoagulation plus pharmacomechanical thrombolysis. This study found that more aggressive therapy did not decrease the incidence of PTS but did result in more major bleeding. The severity of the PTS was lessened by the pharmacomechanical thrombolysis, suggesting that more aggressive therapy should be offered to patients with significant iliofemoral venous thrombosis, who do not respond appropriately to a course of anticoagulation.

For PE, evidence exists that thrombolysis is indicated when there is hemodynamic compromise from the embolism. It is controversial whether thrombolysis should be used in situations in which there is no hemodynamic compromise, but there is evidence of right heart dysfunction or there are positive biomarkers.

Inferior Vena Cava Filters

Traditional indications for the use of IVC filters include failure of anticoagulation, a contraindication to anticoagulation, or a complication of anticoagulation. Protection from PE is greater than 95% using cone-shaped, wire-based permanent filters in the IVC. With the success of these filters, indications have expanded to the presence of free-floating thrombus tails, prophylactic use when the risk for anticoagulation is excessive, when the risk of PE is thought to be high, and to allow the use of perioperative epidural anesthesia. IVC filters are not recommended as first-line therapy in patients who are treated with anticoagulants.

IVC filters can be either permanent or retrievable. If a retrievable filter is left, then it becomes a permanent filter; the long-term fate of these filters has yet to be defined adequately in the literature. Thus great efforts should be made to remove retrievable IVC filters when the risk period is over. Most filters are placed in the infrarenal location in the IVC. However, they may be placed in the suprarenal position or in the superior vena cava.

Indications for suprarenal placement include high-lying thrombi, pregnancy or childbearing age, or previous device failure filled with thrombus. Although some have suggested that sepsis is a contraindication to the use of filters, sepsis has not been found to be a contraindication because the trapped material can be sterilized with intravenous antibiotics. Filters may be inserted under x-ray guidance or using ultrasound techniques, either external ultrasound or intravascular ultrasound.

References

Ahmed Z, Hassan S, Salzman GA: Novel oral anticoagulants for venous thromboembolism with special emphasis on risk of hemorrhagic complications and reversal agents, *Current Drug Therapy* 11:3–20, 2016.

Bruinstroop E, Klok FA, Van De Ree MA, et al: Elevated D-dimer levels predict recurrence in patients with idiopathic venous thromboembolism: a meta-analysis, *J Thromb Haemost* 7:611, 2009.

Elsharawy M, Elzayat E: Early results of thrombolysis vs. anticoagulation in iliofemoral venous thrombosis. A randomised clinical trial, *Eur J Vasc Endovasc Surg* 24(3):209, 2002.

Freund Y, Cachanado M, Aubry A, et al: Effect of the pulmonary embolism rule-out criteria on subsequent thromboembolic events among low-risk emergency department patients: The PROPER Randomized Clinical Trial, *JAMA* 319(6):559–566, 2018.

Gross PL, Weitz JI: New anticoagulants for treatment of venous thromboembolism, *Arterioscler Thromb Vasc Biol* 28:380, 2008.

Grosse SD, Nelson RE, Nyarko KA, Richardson LC, Raskob GE: The economic burden of incident venous thromboembolism in the United States: a review of estimated attributable healthcare costs, *Thromb Res* 137:3–10, 2016.

Guyatt GH, Akl EA, Crother M, et al: Executive summary: Antithrombotic therapy and prevention of thrombosis, 9th ed: American College of Chest Physicians' evidence based clinical practice guidelines, *Chest* 141:7S–47S, 2012.

Heit JA, Spencer FA, White RH: The epidemiology of venous thromboembolism, *J Thromb Thrombolysis* 41:3–14, 2016.

Heit JA, Ashrani AA, Crusan DJ, McBane RD, Petterson TM, Bailey KR. Reasons for the persistent incidence of venous thromboembolism, *Thromb Haemost* 117:390–400, 2017.

Hull RD, Pineo GF, Brant R, et al: Home therapy of venous thrombosis with long-term LMWH versus usual care: patient satisfaction and post-thrombotic syndrome, *Am J Med* 122:762, 2009.

Kahn SR, Shapiro S, Wells PS, et al: Compression stockings to prevent post-thrombotic syndrome: a randomized placebo controlled trial, *Lancet* 383:880–888, 2014.

Kearon C, Akl EA, Comerota AJ, et al: Antithombotic therapy and VTE disease. Antithombotic therapy and prevention of thrombosis, 9th ed: American College of Chest Physicians Evidence-Based Clinical Practice Guidelines, *Chest* 141(Suppl): e419S–e494S, 2012.

Kearon C, Aki EA, Ornelas J, et al: Antithrombotic therapy for VTE disease: Chest Guideline and Expert Panel Report, *Chest* 149:315–352, 2016.

Knepper J, Horne D, Obi A, Wakefield TW: A systematic update on the state of novel anticoagulants and a primer on reversal and bridging, *J Vasc Surg Venous Lymphat Disord* 1418–26, 2013.

Kucher N: Deep-vein thrombosis of the upper extremity, *N Engl J Med* 364:861, 2011.

Merli G, Spyropoulos AC, Caprini JA: Use of emerging oral anticoagulants in clinical practice: Translating results from clinical trials to orthopedic and general surgical patient populations, *Ann Surg* 250:219, 2009.

Morillo R, Jimenez D, Aibar MA, et al: DVT management and outcome trends, 2001 to 2014, *Chest* 150:374–383, 2016.

Mismetti P, Laporte S, Pellerin O, et al: Effect of a retrievable inferior vena cava filter plus anticoagulation vs anticoagulation alone on risk of recurrent pulmonary embolism: a randomized clinical trial, *JAMA* 313:1627–1635, 2015.

Neglen P, Hollis KC, Olivier J, et al: Stenting of the venous outflow in chronic venous disease: Long-term stent-related outcome, clinical, and hemodynamic result, *J Vasc Surg* 46:979, 2007.

Palareti G, Cosmi B, Legnani C, et al: D-dimer testing to determine the duration of anticoagulation therapy, *N Engl J Med* 355:1780, 2006.

Righini M, Ebadi HR, Gal GL: Diagnosis of acute pulmonary embolism, *J Thromb Haemost* 15:1251–1261, 2017.

Schulman S: Advances in the management of venous thromboembolism, *Best Prac Res Clin Haematol* 25:361–377, 2012.

Schulman S, Kearon C, Kakkar AK, et al: Dabigatran versus warfarin in the treatment of acute venous thromboembolism, *N Engl J Med* 361(24):2342, 2009.

Stein PD, Fowler SE, Goodman LR, et al: Multidetector computed tomography for acute pulmonary embolism, *N Engl J Med* 354(22):2317, 2006.

Turpie AG, Bauer KA, Eriksson BI, et al: Fondaparinux vs. enoxaparin for the prevention of venous thromboembolism in major orthopedic surgery: a meta-analysis of 4 randomized double-blind studies, *Arch Intern Med* 162(16):1833, 2002.

Vedantham S, Goldhaber SZ, Julian JA, et al: Pharmacomechanical catheter-directed thrombolysis for deep-vein thrombosis, *N Engl J Med* 377:2240–2252, 2017.

Weitz JI, Jaffer IH, Fredenburgh JC: Recent advances in the treatment of venous thromboembolism in the era of the direct oral anticoagulants, *F1000 Research* 6:985, 2017.

Wells PS, Anderson DR, Rodger M, et al: Evaluation of D-dimer in the diagnosis of suspected deep-vein thrombosis, *N Engl J Med* 349(13):1227, 2003.

VALVULAR HEART DISEASE

Carlos E. Sanchez, MD; Steven J. Yakubov, MD; and Arash Arshi, MD

CURRENT DIAGNOSIS

- The diagnosis of severe aortic valve stenosis is based on an integration of clinical symptoms and hemodynamic echocardiographic criteria.
- Classic symptoms of severe aortic stenosis include fatigue, dyspnea on exertion, angina, near syncope or syncope, and congestive heart failure.
- Chronic mitral regurgitation tends to be a slowly progressive disease and symptoms may not be apparent.
- Cardiac imaging, especially echocardiography, is crucial to the management of patients with valvular heart disease.

- Diagnostic echocardiographic findings of severe aortic stenosis are peak aortic valve velocity of greater than or equal to 4 m/s, transaortic mean gradient of greater than or equal to 40 mm Hg, and aortic valve area less than or equal to 1 cm^2 or aortic valve area index of less than or equal to 0.6 cm^2/m^2.
- Echocardiography should be performed to determine the etiology of and characterize the severity of mitral regurgitation.
- Left ventricular size and function should be assessed in patients with mitral regurgitation.

CURRENT THERAPY

- Medical therapy has not been shown to change hemodynamic progression or clinical outcomes in patients with aortic stenosis.
- Reevaluation for early symptoms and transthoracic echocardiography should be performed every 6–12 months in asymptomatic patients with severe aortic stenosis and normal left ventricular systolic function.
- Transcatheter aortic valve replacement is currently approved in patients with severe symptomatic aortic stenosis with any level of surgical risk.
- The etiology of mitral regurgitation dictates its treatment.
- Primary (degenerative) mitral regurgitation typically requires surgical repair or replacement.
- The management of secondary (functional) mitral regurgitation requires treatment of the underlying cardiomyopathy.
- Transcatheter mitral valve repair with MitraClip (Abbott Laboratories, Abbott Park, IL) is currently indicated in secondary mitral regurgitation patients with left ventricular dysfunction who remain symptomatic despite guideline-directed medical therapy.
- The decision-making process in the management of patients with severe aortic stenosis or severe mitral regurgitation is best achieved by a heart team and should include a systematic risk assessment of the patient's comorbidities and estimation of the 30-day cardiac surgical mortality using the Society of Thoracic Surgeons' Predicted Risk of Mortality (STS-PROM) score.

Aortic Stenosis

Aortic stenosis (AS) is the most common form of adult valvular heart disease, becoming more prevalent in the aging population. It is estimated that more than 4% of the U.S. population over age 75 have AS. Aortic valve stenosis is the most common cause of left ventricular (LV) outflow tract obstruction, while less common causes of obstruction may also occur above (supravalvular) or below (subvalvular) the level of the aortic valve and will not be discussed in this chapter.

Etiology

There are three main causes of valvular AS: congenital in origin (which is usually a bicuspid aortic valve), rheumatic valve disease, and degenerative calcification of a normal aortic valve. Congenitally affected aortic valves may be unicuspid or bicuspid and may become stenotic during childhood. In the majority of cases, a congenital bicuspid valve will develop significant calcific stenosis later in life, usually presenting after the fifth decade.

Rheumatic AS is an important cause of aortic valve disease worldwide; however, with the decline of rheumatic fever in developed countries, it is now a rare cause of AS in the United States. Rheumatic valve disease is characterized by commissural fusion, fibrosis, and calcification. Rheumatic AS is also commonly associated with rheumatic involvement of the mitral valve.

Degenerative or calcific AS is now the most common cause of AS in adults in North America. It has been associated with the same risk factors as vascular atherosclerosis including age, smoking, hypertension, diabetes, and hyperlipidemia. Histopathologic data suggest that calcific aortic valve disease is a chronic inflammatory process with lipid deposition and active leaflet calcification leading to restriction of the cusps.

Pathophysiology

In adults with AS, the gradual obstruction of the LV outflow produces a systolic pressure gradient between the left ventricle and aorta. The average time interval of disease progression from nonobstructive valve thickening (aortic sclerosis) to severe AS is 8 years. However, only 16% of individuals with aortic sclerosis will develop any grade of valve obstruction. The average rate of hemodynamic progression once moderate AS is present is an increase in aortic jet velocity of 0.3 m/s per year and mean pressure gradient of 7 mm Hg per year with a decrease in aortic valve area of 0.1 cm^2/year. LV response to chronic pressure overload ultimately leads to concentric wall hypertrophy. This compensatory mechanism helps maintain normal LV contractile function to counteract the gradual increase in afterload at the expense of decreased LV compliance and delayed relaxation resulting in diastolic dysfunction.

Clinical Presentation

The cardinal symptoms of severe AS are angina, syncope, and congestive heart failure. Because symptoms in severe AS may not occur until late in the disease process, usually in the sixth to ninth decades of life, clinicians should obtain a careful history of symptoms during the patient's initial assessment. Particular attention must be directed at early symptoms of fatigue or decreased exercise tolerance as elderly patients may minimize and attribute these symptoms to aging.

Dyspnea on exertion occurs once the pulmonary capillary pressure increases as a result of excessive elevation in LV end-diastolic pressure in a poorly compliant ventricle. Symptoms of angina pectoris in severe AS may occur in a similar manner as in coronary artery disease, with symptoms precipitated by exertion and relieved by rest even in the absence of obstructive epicardial coronary artery disease. Syncope may result from the inability of the heart to increase cardiac output from the stenotic valve in the setting of transient vasodilatation during physical activity, resulting in decreased cerebral perfusion. Other causes of syncope may also be attributable to arrhythmias, either advanced forms of atrioventricular blocks from calcification impinging on the conduction system or tachyarrhythmias causing a sudden decline in cardiac output such as in atrial fibrillation.

Diagnosis and Management

Diagnosis of AS is usually suspected after a systolic ejection murmur is heard during cardiac auscultation. The classic physical findings in patients with severe AS are a loud, late-peaking systolic murmur at the base of the heart radiating to the carotid arteries with a delayed and diminished carotid upstroke (*pulsus parvus et tardus*). The latter physical finding may be masked in elderly patients with stiff, inelastic arterial walls. Distinctively, a normally split-second heart sound is the only reliable physical finding to help exclude the diagnosis of severe AS.

A transthoracic echocardiogram (TTE) is recommended as the initial diagnostic test in the evaluation of patients with aortic valve stenosis to determine hemodynamic severity, LV size and function, and prognosis, and to evaluate timing of valve intervention. Echocardiographic valve hemodynamics define the severity of AS (Table 1). Severe AS is characterized by a peak aortic valve velocity of 4 m/s or higher, transaortic mean gradient of 40 mm Hg or higher, and aortic valve area of less than or equal to 1 cm^2 or aortic valve area index of less than or equal to 0.6 cm^2/m^2. In severe symptomatic patients with low-flow, low-gradient severe

TABLE 1 Echocardiographic Stages of Aortic Valve Stenosis and Frequency of Echocardiograms in Asymptomatic Patients With Aortic Stenosis and Normal Left Ventricular Ejection Fraction

	MAXIMUM AORTIC VELOCITY	MEAN PRESSURE GRADIENT	AORTIC VALVE AREA	TTE FOLLOW-UP IN ASYMP-TOMATIC PATIENTS
Mild aortic stenosis	2.0–2.9 m/s	<20 mm Hg	>1.5 cm^2	Every 3–5 years
Moderate aortic stenosis	3.0–3.9 m/s	20–30 mm Hg	1.0–1.5 cm^2	Every 1–2 years
Severe aortic stenosis	≥4.0 m/s	≥40 mm Hg	≤1.0 cm^2	Every 6–12 months
Very severe aortic stenosis	≥5 m/s	≥60 mm Hg	≤1.0 cm^2	

TTE, Transthoracic echocardiogram.

AS and abnormal LV function (<50%), a dobutamine stress echocardiogram can be used to differentiate between true severe AS and pseudo-severe AS. Low-flow, low-gradient true severe AS is characterized by a severely calcified valve with aortic valve area less than or equal to 1 cm^2 and peak aortic valve velocity less than 4 m/s that increases to 4 m/s or higher with low-dose dobutamine administration. Conversely, in pseudo-severe AS the aortic valve area increases to more than 1 cm^2 and flow normalizes during dobutamine stress echocardiogram.

Patients with asymptomatic AS require frequent monitoring owing to the progressive nature of the disease. The frequency of echocardiograms in asymptomatic patients with AS and normal LV systolic function should be performed every 6 to 12 months for reevaluation in severe AS, every 1 to 2 years for moderate AS, and every 3 to 5 years for mild AS (see Table 1). In seemingly asymptomatic patients with severe AS, exercise testing is safe and helpful to expose symptoms, arrhythmias, or abnormal blood pressure response. Exercise testing should not be performed in symptomatic patients.

Treatment

Indication for intervention in patients with severe AS is dependent on the presence or absence of symptoms, the severity of AS, and LV function. Routine aortic valve replacement in asymptomatic AS is currently not recommended. Importantly, event-free survival at 2 years in asymptomatic patients with severe AS (jet velocity ≥ 4.0 m/s) is 30% to 50%, and as low as 21% in those with very severe AS (jet velocity ≥ 5.0 m/s). Therefore close clinical follow-up to evaluate for early-onset AS symptoms and education regarding the disease course should be performed routinely.

Medical therapy has not been shown to change hemodynamic progression or clinical outcomes in patients with AS. Clinical data have failed to support the use of statins specifically for the prevention of progression of AS. However, all patients with concomitant coronary artery disease or hypercholesterolemia should be treated per established guidelines. Likewise, concurrent hypertension in patients with severe AS is common and should receive appropriate treatment per standard guidelines starting at a low dose and slowly titrating upward with frequent blood pressure monitoring. Although indicated in the treatment of acute heart failure, diuretics should be used with caution to avoid volume depletion, which may result in marked reduction in cardiac output.

Surgical Treatment

Transcatheter aortic valve replacement (TAVR) has expanded rapidly as an alternative to surgical aortic valve replacement (SAVR) since its approval in 2011, with more than 50,000 patients treated in the United States alone. It is currently approved for use in patients with severe symptomatic AS with any level of surgical risk. Recent published clinical trials in low-surgical-risk candidates showed that the risk of death or disabling stroke and new onset atrial fibrillation was lower among the TAVR treated patients compared to SAVR. Additionally,

rehospitalization and hospital length of stay was shorter with TAVR.

Recommendations and timing of intervention for aortic valve stenosis by either SAVR or TAVR are summarized in Table 2. Once the patient with AS is considered to meet an indication for aortic valve replacement, an important component when choosing between SAVR and TAVR is the underlying risk assessment for SAVR. In the United States, the Society of Thoracic Surgeons' Predicted Risk of Mortality (STS-PROM) risk score calculator is the initial step in predicting 30-day mortality for SAVR, with three categories: low risk defined as less than 4%, intermediate risk defined as 4% to 8%, and high risk defined as greater than 8% STS mortality risk. This risk calculator, however, does not include certain comorbid conditions that would also increase the surgical mortality risk such as frailty, porcelain aorta, liver cirrhosis, severe pulmonary hypertension, chest wall abnormalities, and hostile mediastinum. If three or more major organ systems are compromised, with severe frailty, or the morbidity and mortality risk is greater than 50%, the patient is considered prohibitive risk for SAVR. In patients with severe AS and a life expectancy less than 1 year, TAVR or SAVR is considered futile despite successful procedure and it is appropriate to avoid any intervention for severe AS. Hence the risk assessment is a combination of the STS-PROM score, frailty, disability, and major cardiovascular and noncardiovascular comorbidities.

The final treatment decision should be individualized with a risk-benefit assessment by a multidisciplinary heart team (including structural interventional cardiologists, imaging specialists, cardiovascular surgeons, and nursing professionals). The heart team assesses potential procedural outcomes based on the patient's individual procedural risk, comorbidities, goals, expectations, life expectancy, and potential quality-of-life improvement with SAVR or TAVR. The importance of a collaborative and multidisciplinary heart team approach to the evaluation and management of patients with complex AS has been endorsed by professional guidelines to maximize appropriate outcomes.

Once the patient is considered to be a suitable candidate for TAVR, the evaluation of all patients undergoing the procedure should include (1) right and left heart catheterization to assess hemodynamic pressures and presence of coronary disease; and (2) computed tomography of the chest, abdomen, and pelvis to determine preferred vascular access or contraindications to it and aortic annulus dimension for prosthesis sizing (Figure 1).

The currently available TAVR valves approved by the United States Food and Drug Administration (FDA) include the balloon-expandable Edwards Sapien XT and Sapien 3 (Edwards Lifesciences, Irvine, CA), self-expandable Medtronic Evolut R and Evolut PRO systems (Medtronic, Minneapolic, MN), and Lotus Edge (Boston Scientific, Marlborough, MA). The choice of valve mostly depends on anatomic reasons and operator preference and experience.

A series of major procedural cardiovascular complications have been described after TAVR, including paravalvular aortic regurgitation, ischemic strokes, conduction disturbances, cardiac perforation, coronary occlusion, and vascular access complications.

COR	RECOMMENDATION
I	• AVR is recommended for symptomatic patients with severe high-gradient AS who have symptoms by history or on exercise testing • AVR is recommended for asymptomatic patients with severe AS and LVEF <50% • AVR is indicated for patients with severe AS when undergoing other cardiac surgery
IIa	• AVR is reasonable for asymptomatic patients with very severe AS (aortic velocity ≥ 5.0 m/s) and low surgical risk • AVR is reasonable in asymptomatic patients with severe AS and decreased exercise tolerance or an exercise fall in BP • AVR is reasonable in symptomatic patients with low-flow/low-gradient severe AS with reduced LVEF with a low-dose dobutamine stress study that shows an aortic velocity ≥4.0 m/s (or mean pressure gradient ≥40 mm Hg) with a valve area of 1.0 cm² at any dobutamine dose • AVR is reasonable in symptomatic patients who have low-flow/low-gradient severe AS who are normotensive and have an LVEF ≥50% if clinical, hemodynamic, and anatomic data support valve obstruction as the most likely cause of symptoms • AVR is reasonable for patients with moderate AS (aortic velocity 3.0–3.9 m/s) who are undergoing other cardiac surgery
IIb	• AVR may be considered for asymptomatic patients with severe AS and rapid disease progression and low surgical risk

TABLE 2 American College of Cardiology/American Heart Association Recommendations for Timing of Intervention in Patients With Aortic Stenosis

AS, Aortic stenosis; *AVR,* aortic valve replacement by either surgical or transcatheter approach; *BP,* blood pressure; *COR,* class of recommendation; *LVEF,* left ventricular ejection fraction.
Modified from Nishimura RA, Otto CM, Bonow RO, et al. 2014 AHA/ACC guideline for the management of patients with valvular heart disease: a report of the American College of Cardiology/American Heart Association Task Force on Practice Guidelines. *J Am Coll Cardiol.* 2014;63:e57–e185.

Figure 1 Multidetector computed tomography measurements of the aortic valve complex and peripheral vascular assessment. (A) Aortic annulus perimeter, area, and diameter measurement. (B) The maximum sinus of Valsalva diameters. (C) Height of the left coronary artery from the annular base. (D) Reconstructed view of the iliofemoral anatomy. (E) Left subclavian view with measurement obtained (*left* of image).

With the advancement of valve technology and increase in operator experience, the frequency of procedural complications has reduced since the arrival of TAVR procedures. Preprocedure planning by an expert heart team is essential to recognizing and preventing expected complications during and after transcatheter valve implantation.

Currently the optimal antithrombotic regimen following TAVR is daily clopidogrel (Plavix)[1] 75 mg and aspirin[1] 75 to 100 mg for 3 to 6 months followed by daily aspirin alone for life. If there is an indication for chronic anticoagulation, it should follow current guidelines' recommendations for each individual condition (e.g., atrial fibrillation, deep venous thrombosis). The safety of antiplatelet therapy use in conjunction with oral anticoagulation should be individualized based on the patient's bleeding risk.

[1]Not FDA approved for this indication

Mitral Regurgitation

Mitral regurgitation (MR) is a common valvular disease, and pathology in any of the structures of the mitral valve apparatus may lead to dysfunction of the valve. The base of the leaflets of the mitral valve are attached to the annulus, and the leaflets themselves are attached to the papillary muscles of the left ventricle by the chordae tendineae. The mitral valve is an integral part of both the left atrium and left ventricle, and disorders of these structures affect mitral valve function; likewise, disorders of the mitral valve lead to abnormalities of the left atrium and left ventricle.

Etiology

MR can be divided into primary (degenerative) MR and secondary (functional) MR (Figure 2). Primary MR refers to pathology of the mitral valve leaflets and chordae tendineae that results in valve dysfunction. The most common etiology is mitral valve prolapse, where the underlying pathology is myxomatous mitral valve degeneration that results in redundant leaflets, causing prolapse of the leaflets. A myxomatous mitral valve is also prone

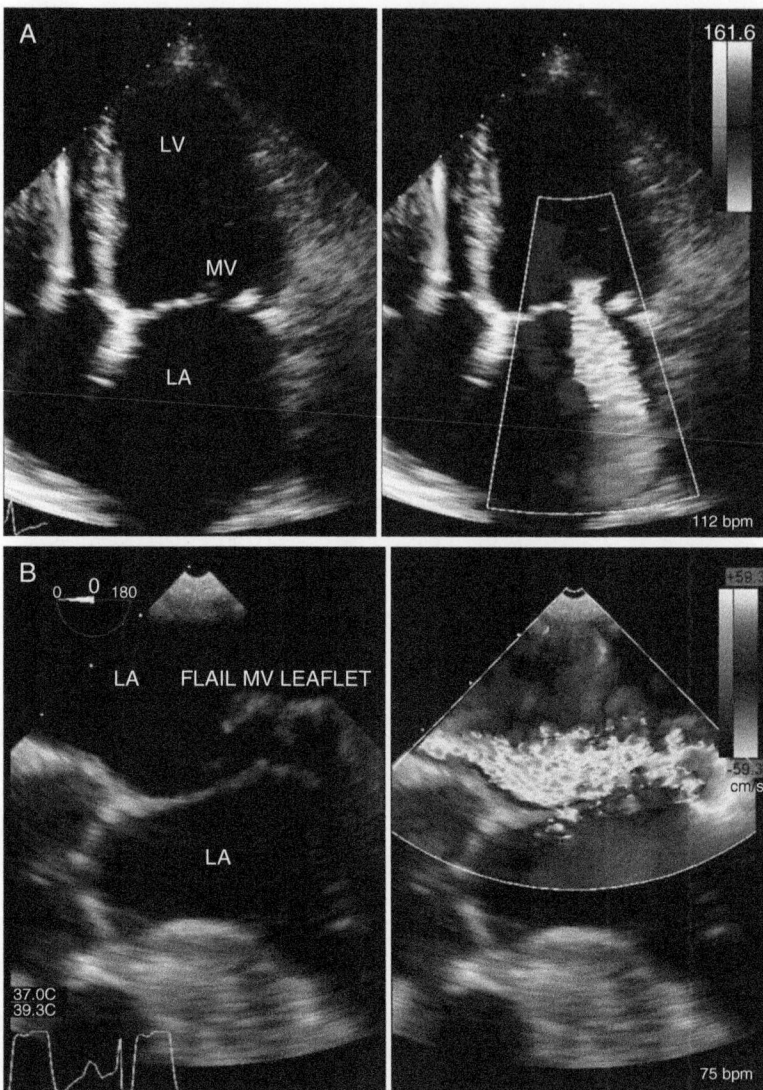

Figure 2 (A) Transthoracic echocardiogram of a patient with a dilated cardiomyopathy with annular dilation resulting in incomplete coaptation of the mitral valve leaflets and severe functional (secondary) mitral regurgitation. The regurgitant jet is central. (B) Transesophageal echocardiogram reveals a markedly myxomatous mitral valve with a large flail segment of the posterior leaflet resulting in severe degenerative (primary) mitral regurgitation. This jet is extremely eccentric. *LA*, Left atrium; *LV*, left ventricle; *MV*, mitral valve.

to rupture of the chordae tendineae, leading to a flail leaflet or segment of a leaflet. Other common etiologies of MR include rheumatic heart disease and endocarditis. Mitral annular calcification may cause mild to moderate MR, but severe regurgitation is uncommon.

In contrast, in secondary MR, the mitral valve itself has a relatively normal structure. Instead, the pathology is an abnormality of the left ventricle. This most commonly occurs after myocardial infarction, with focal wall motion abnormalities and displacement of the papillary muscle causing tethering of the chordae and leaflets, along with dilatation of the mitral valve annulus, resulting in incomplete coaptation of the mitral valve leaflets during systole. Secondary MR may also occur in a dilated cardiomyopathy.

Clinical Manifestations

The clinical presentation of MR is extremely variable and depends largely on the severity of the regurgitation and its acuity. MR tends to be asymptomatic when mild to moderate, but severe MR frequently results in symptoms. Acute MR occurring from papillary muscle rupture complicating an acute myocardial infarction leads to rapid hemodynamic collapse and carries a high risk of mortality. These patients experience pulmonary edema due to the acute volume overload of the left ventricle and left atrium. In contrast, chronic severe MR may have a relatively indolent course,

with some patients reporting few symptoms. While chronic MR typically manifests as congestive heart failure, with exertional dyspnea, orthopnea, and lower extremity edema as the hallmark symptoms, owing to the insidious nature of the disease, patients may not always recognize their symptoms. A detailed history with a specific focus on symptoms of congestive heart failure in addition to fatigue and effort intolerance must be elicited. Atrial fibrillation is a common complication of MR and is associated with worse outcomes.

Diagnosis

Physical examination classically may reveal a soft S1 and a holosystolic murmur at the apex that radiates to the left sternal border or to the axilla. However, the intensity of the murmur does not correlate to the severity of disease, nor does the absence of a murmur reliably rule out severe MR. Physical examination is important to assess the patient's volume status, with pulmonary rales and lower extremity edema suggesting congestive heart failure, and an irregularly irregular rhythm indicative of atrial fibrillation.

Cardiac imaging, in particular echocardiography, is crucial in the evaluation of suspected MR. Transthoracic echocardiography can reveal abnormalities of the mitral valve and provide important information on LV size and function and estimation of pulmonary arterial pressure. Given the orientation of the mitral valve and the limits of transthoracic echocardiography, the severity of MR can be grossly underestimated, particularly if the regurgitant jet is eccentric. Transesophageal echocardiography, especially with the availability of three-dimensional imaging, provides higher-quality images of the mitral valve and allows more precise evaluation of the severity and etiology of MR, and has become the gold-standard test in the evaluation of patients with clinically significant MR. Echocardiography with color Doppler can be used to provide a visual estimate of the severity of regurgitation. The presence of reversal of flow into the pulmonary veins during systole suggests severe regurgitation. Quantitative analysis can also be performed to determine the volume of regurgitation and the orifice of the regurgitant jet. There is currently no single echocardiographic parameter to define severe MR, but integration of multiple qualitative and quantitative measurements is recommended. Accurate assessment of LV dimensions and function is important in patients with chronic severe MR. Methods of determining the LV ejection fraction include visual estimation and volumetric analysis. Owing to the volume of blood exiting the left ventricle through both the mitral and aortic valves during systole, the ejection fraction will be increased. In the presence of severe MR, a normal LV ejection fraction approaches 70%, and LV dysfunction is deemed anything less than 60%. Even what would otherwise be considered a mildly reduced ejection fraction may indicate significant myocardial dysfunction in the presence of MR. Left atrial enlargement as a rule is found in chronic severe MR, and its absence should lead to reconsideration of the diagnosis. Exercise echocardiography can play an important role in patients with MR, especially in those with severe MR who report few symptoms, as it is an objective means to assess functional capacity and can also be used to assess changes in pulmonary pressures with exercise. In patients who have mild MR at rest but severe exertional symptoms, exercise echocardiography can identify ischemic MR with concomitant regional wall motion abnormalities.

Cardiac catheterization is performed in many patients with suspected severe MR. Right heart catheterization with measurement of right atrial, right ventricular, pulmonary arterial, and pulmonary capillary wedge pressures and cardiac outputs can help determine volume status and assess for pulmonary hypertension. Attention should be paid to the pulmonary capillary wedge waveform, with large "v" waves, corresponding to ventricular systole, suggestive of severe MR. Left heart catheterization with selective coronary angiography is recommended to identify concomitant obstructive coronary artery disease. Left ventriculography using contrast is commonly performed, and the presence of contrast in the left atrium suggests MR. However, the clinical utility of left ventriculography is limited with the ready availability of echocardiography. The visual estimation of MR by contrast ventriculography is subjective, and the etiology of valve pathology is unable to be defined precisely. Furthermore, in a patient with congestive heart failure, the contrast load may result in acute decompensation.

Magnetic resonance imaging (MRI) is not currently a routinely used test in the evaluation of severe MR but may provide more reproducible quantification of the regurgitant volume and fraction and more accurate measurements of LV size and function. Given the importance of defining the severity of the MR and abnormalities of LV function in the management of MR, MRI may eventually have a central role in the evaluation of patients and is strongly recommended when echocardiographic data is not satisfactory.

Management and Treatment

The etiology of MR dictates its treatment (Table 3). Primary (degenerative) MR is a mechanical problem of the valve or its apparatus and requires a mechanical solution such as a surgical or percutaneous repair or replacement. Secondary (functional) MR is a problem of the left ventricle and treatment of the underlying ventricular pathology is indicated. Transcatheter mitral valve repair with percutaneous MitraClip (Abbott Laboratories, Abbott Park, IL) in secondary MR is currently indicated in

TABLE 3 Paradigm for Management of Mitral Regurgitation Based on Etiology and Surgical Risk

	PRIMARY (DEGENERATIVE)	SECONDARY (FUNCTIONAL)
Low surgical risk	Surgical repair or replacement	CHF therapy Surgery in selected patients
High surgical risk	Percutaneous repair in selected patients	CHF therapy ± percutaneous mitral valve repair with MitraClip

CHF, Congestive heart failure.

TABLE 4 Indications for Intervention in Severe Primary (Degenerative) Mitral Regurgitation

Symptomatic
Recommended if LVEF >30%
May be considered if LVEF ≤30%

TMVR may be considered if severely symptomatic with reasonable life expectancy but prohibitive surgical risk

Asymptomatic
Recommended if LV dysfunction (LVEF 30%–60% or LVESD <40 mm)
Reasonable if preserved LV function (LVEF >60% and LVESD >40 mm) if >95% chance of successful repair with <1% mortality risk
Reasonable if preserved LV function with new-onset atrial fibrillation or PASP >50 mm Hg if high likelihood of successful repair

LV, Left ventricular; *LVEF*, left ventricular ejection fraction; *LVESD*, left ventricular end-systolic dimension; *PASP*, pulmonary arterial systolic pressure; *TMVR*, transcatheter mitral valve repair.

patients with LV dysfunction who remain symptomatic despite guideline-directed medical therapy.

In patients with acute severe MR, the role of medical therapy is to stabilize the patient until surgery. Afterload reduction is the initial treatment strategy, which allows for greater flow through the aortic valve, thereby increasing cardiac output while diminishing the MR. Afterload reduction may be accomplished with intravenous vasodilators such as sodium nitroprusside (Nitropress)[1] or with an intraaortic balloon pump if the clinical situation requires. The role of medical therapy for chronic severe degenerative MR is less clear, especially in asymptomatic patients with normal LV function. Symptomatic patients with a reduced ejection fraction (<60%) may be treated with heart failure therapy such as angiotensin-converting enzyme (ACE) inhibitors or angiotensin receptor blockers (ARBs), beta-adrenergic blockers, or aldosterone antagonists, in addition to loop diuretics for symptomatic relief while awaiting surgery. Ultimately most patients with severe primary MR will be referred to surgery (Table 4), and valve repair is preferable to replacement provided the anatomy is amenable to repair. If valve replacement is necessary, options include mechanical and bioprosthetic valves. Mechanical valves provide superior hemodynamic results and durability but are prone to thrombus formation and therefore require lifelong anticoagulation with warfarin (Coumadin). If after consultation with a cardiac surgeon the patient is deemed to be at prohibitive risk for surgery, percutaneous mitral valve repair with the MitraClip device is a reasonable alternative. This procedure is performed under general anesthesia with fluoroscopic and transesophageal echocardiographic guidance, and from the femoral vein via transseptal access, a clip is delivered to the regurgitant orifice of the mitral valve, grasping the anterior and posterior leaflets, thereby improving leaflet coaptation.

[1] Not FDA approved for this indication

For patients with secondary MR, the target for treatment is the left ventricle. Medical therapy for the underlying cardiomyopathy is recommended, with administration of ACE inhibitors or ARBs ± neprilysin inhibitors, aldosterone antagonists, and beta-blockers. If indicated, these patients may require cardiac resynchronization therapy. With medical and device therapy, LV remodeling and function may improve, with reduction in the degree of MR. If severe MR persists despite maximally tolerated medical therapy, percutaneous mitral valve repair with the MitraClip device is the only interventional therapy currently approved that significantly reduces mortality and heart failure rehospitalizations at 2 years while improving heart failure symptoms. In patients with ischemic cardiomyopathy secondary to obstructive coronary artery disease with severe secondary MR, surgical revascularization and concomitant mitral valve repair is frequently performed if the surgical risk is not prohibitive.

MR can progress over time, as the volume overload can lead to LV dilation and worsening mitral leaflet coaptation. As the disease process may be slow and without sudden worsening of symptoms, patients will require close follow-up. Mild MR can be followed by serial transthoracic echocardiography every 3 to 5 years, and moderate MR every 1 to 2 years. In patients with asymptomatic severe MR who do not undergo surgery, transthoracic echocardiography should be performed at least annually, with special attention to LV dimensions and function.

References

Cosmi JE, Kort S, Tunick PA, et al: The risk of the development of aortic stenosis in patients with "benign" aortic valve thickening, *Arch Intern Med* 162:2345–2347, 2002.

Dal-Bianco JP, Khandheira BK, Mookadam F, et al: Management of asymptomatic severe aortic stenosis, *J Am Coll Cardiol* 52:1279–1292, 2008.Nkomo VT, Gardin JM, Skelton TN, et al: Burden of valvular heart diseases: a population- based study, *Lancet* 368:1005–1011, 2006.

Feldman T, Foster E, Glower DD, et al: Percutaneous repair or surgery for mitral regurgitation, *N Engl J Med* 364:1395–1406, 2011.

Freeman RV, Otto CM: Spectrum of calcific aortic valve disease: pathogenesis, disease progression, and treatment strategies, *Circulation* 111:3316–3326, 2005.

Ling LH, Enriquez-Sarano M, Seward JB, et al: Early surgery in patients with mitral regurgitation due to flail leaflets: a long-term outcome study, *Circulation* 96:1819–1825, 1997.

Mack MJ, Leon MB, Thourani VH, et al: Transcatheter aortic-valve replacement with balloon expandable valve in low-risk patients, *N Engl J Med*, 2019. https://doi.org/10.1056/NEJMoa1814052.

Nishimura RA, Otto CM, Bonow RO, et al: 2014 AHA/ACC guideline for the management of patients with valvular heart disease: a report of the American College of Cardiology/American Heart Association Task Force on Practice Guidelines, *J Am Coll Cardiol* 63:e57–e185, 2014.

Otto CM, Kumbhani DJ, Alexander KP, et al: 2017 ACC Expert Consensus Decision Pathway for Transcatheter Aortic Valve Replacement in the Management of Adults with Aortic Stenosis, *J Am Coll of Cardiol* 69(10):1313–1346, 2017. https://doi.org/10.1016/j.jacc.2016.12.006.

Peltier M, Trojette F, Enriquez-Sarano M, et al: Relation between cardiovascular risk factors and nonrheumatic severe calcific aortic stenosis among patients with a three-cuspid aortic valve, *Am J Cardiol* 91:97–99, 2003.

Popma JJ, Deeb GM, Yakubov SJ, et al: Transcatheter aortic valve replacement with a self-expanding valve in low-risk patients, *N Engl J Med*, 2019. https://doi.org/10.1056/NEJMoa1816885.

Stone GW, Lindenfeld J, Abraham WT, et al: Transcatheter mitral-valve repair in patients with heart failure, *N Engl J Med* 379:2307–2318, 2018.

Wu AH, Aaronson KD, Bolling SF, et al: Impact of mitral valve annuloplasty on mortality risk in patients with mitral regurgitation and left ventricular systolic dysfunction, *J Am Coll Cardiol* 45:381–387, 2005.

Zilberszac R, Gabriel H, Schemper M, et al: Asymptomatic severe aortic stenosis in the elderly, *J Am Coll Cardiol Img* 10:43–50, 2017.

Digestive System

ACUTE AND CHRONIC PANCREATITIS

Method of
George Van Buren II, MD; and William E. Fisher, MD

CURRENT DIAGNOSIS

- Acute pancreatitis is usually caused by gallstones, and chronic pancreatitis is usually caused by alcohol abuse.
- Other less-common causes of acute and chronic pancreatitis are considered only when gallstones and alcohol are definitively ruled out.
- Pancreatic cancer and chronic pancreatitis can sometimes be difficult to distinguish.

CURRENT THERAPY

- There has been a recent trend toward conservative medical therapy for acute and chronic pancreatitis, reserving surgery for select patients.
- In acute pancreatitis, try to avoid necrosectomy except in the setting of infected necrosis with organ failure.
- Asymptomatic pseudocysts can generally be observed.
- Persistent symptomatic pseudocysts can often be addressed endoscopically.
- Medical therapy for chronic pancreatitis includes pain management, nutrition, diabetes control, and cessation of drinking alcohol and smoking.
- Surgical treatment for chronic pancreatitis currently favors strict patient selection and consideration of various surgical techniques.

Acute Pancreatitis

Acute pancreatitis is an inflammatory disease of the pancreas that is associated with little or no fibrosis of the gland. It can be initiated by several factors including gallstones, alcohol, trauma, and infections, and in some cases it is hereditary (Box 1). Very often, patients with acute pancreatitis develop additional complications such as sepsis, shock, and respiratory and renal failure, resulting in considerable morbidity and mortality.

Epidemiology

The annual incidence of acute pancreatitis is probably about 50 cases per 100,000 population in the United States. Approximately 3000 of these cases are severe enough to lead to death. Studies worldwide have shown a rising but variable incidence of acute pancreatitis, including large increases in incidence in pediatric populations.

Risk Factors

Biliary tract stone disease accounts for 70% to 80% of the cases of acute pancreatitis. Alcoholism accounts for another 10%, and the remaining 10% to 20% is accounted for either by idiopathic disease or by a variety of iatrogenic and miscellaneous causes

---

BOX 1	Common Causes of Acute Pancreatitis Gallstones

Alcoholism
Hereditary
Hypertriglyceridemia
Trauma (including iatrogenic: ERCP or surgery)
Drugs: azathioprine (Imuran), furosemide, mercaptopurine (Purinethol), opiates, pentamidine (Pentam), steroids, sulfasalazine (Azulfidine), sulindac (Clinoril), tetracycline, trimethoprim-sulfamethoxazole (Bactrim), valproic acid (Depakote)
Tumor
Infection (parasitic and viral)
Idiopathic

ERCP, Endoscopic retrograde cholangiopancreatography.

---

including trauma, endoscopy, surgery, drugs, heredity, infection, and toxins. Medications appear to cause less than 5% of all cases of acute pancreatitis. The drugs most strongly associated with the disorder are azathioprine (Imuran), 6-mercaptopurine (Purinethol), didanosine (Videx), valproic acid (Depakote), angiotensin-converting–enzyme inhibitors, and mesalamine (Asacol). It is difficult to determine whether the drug is responsible. Tobacco use has also been heavily linked to pancreatitis. Meta-analysis has shown cigarette smoking to be associated with acute pancreatitis development in a dose-response manner.

Pathophysiology

Pancreatitis begins with the activation of digestive zymogens inside acinar cells, which cause acinar cell injury. Digestive zymogens are co-localized with lysosomal hydrolase, and cathepsin-B catalyzed trypsinogen activation occurs, resulting in acinar cell injury and necrosis. This triggers acinar cell inflammatory events with the secretion of inflammatory mediators. Studies suggest that the ultimate severity of the resulting pancreatitis may be determined by the events that occur subsequent to acinar cell injury. These include inflammatory cell recruitment and activation, as well as generation and release of cytokines, reactive oxygen species, and other chemical mediators of inflammation, ultimately leading to ischemia and necrosis. Early mortality in severe acute pancreatitis is caused by a systemic inflammatory response syndrome with multiorgan failure. If the patient survives this critical early period, a septic complication caused by translocated bacteria, mostly gram-negative microbes from the intestine, leads to infected pancreatic necrosis. Late deaths are caused by infected necrosis, leading to septic shock and multiorgan failure.

Prevention

Gallstones are present in about 15% to 20% of patients older than 60 years, but only a fraction become symptomatic. Although gallstone pancreatitis can rarely be the first symptom of gallstones, most patients have symptoms of cholecystitis before developing pancreatitis. Thus it is important to make early and prompt referral of patients with symptomatic cholelithiasis for laparoscopic cholecystectomy to prevent life-threatening complications such as acute pancreatitis.

Clinical Manifestations

All episodes of acute pancreatitis begin with severe pain, generally following a substantial meal. The pain is usually epigastric, but it can occur anywhere in the abdomen or lower chest. It has been described as penetrating through to the back, and it may be relieved by the patient's leaning forward. It precedes the onset of nausea and vomiting, with retching often continuing after the stomach has emptied. Vomiting does not relieve the pain, which is more intense in necrotizing than in edematous pancreatitis.

On examination the patient may show tachycardia, tachypnea, hypotension, and hyperthermia. The temperature is usually only mildly elevated in uncomplicated pancreatitis. Voluntary and involuntary guarding can be seen over the epigastric region. The bowel sounds are decreased or absent. There are usually no palpable masses. The abdomen may be distended with intraperitoneal fluid. There may be pleural effusion, particularly on the left side. With increasing severity of disease, the intravascular fluid loss may become life-threatening as a result of sequestration of edematous fluid in the retroperitoneum. Hemoconcentration then results in an elevated hematocrit. However, there also may be bleeding into the retroperitoneum or the peritoneal cavity. In some patients (about 1%), the blood from necrotizing pancreatitis can dissect through the soft tissues and manifest as a bluish discoloration around the umbilicus (Cullen sign) or in the flanks (Grey Turner sign). The severe fluid loss can lead to prerenal azotemia, with elevated blood urea nitrogen and creatinine levels. There also may be hyperglycemia, hypoalbuminemia, and hypocalcemia sufficient in some cases to produce tetany.

Diagnosis

The definition of acute pancreatitis is based on the fulfillment of two out of three of the following criteria: clinical (upper abdominal pain), laboratory (serum amylase or lipase >3× upper limit of normal) and/or imaging (computed tomographic [CT], magnetic resonance imaging [MRI], ultrasonography) criteria. Although serum amylase is often elevated in acute pancreatitis, there is no significant correlation between the magnitude of serum amylase elevation and severity of pancreatitis. Other pancreatic enzymes also have been evaluated to improve the diagnostic accuracy of serum measurements. Specificity of these markers ranges from 77% to 96%, the highest being for lipase. Measurements of many digestive enzymes have methodologic limitations and cannot be easily adapted for quantitation in emergency laboratory studies. Because serum levels of lipase remain elevated for a longer time than total or pancreatic amylase, it is the serum indicator of highest probability of the disease.

Abdominal ultrasound examination is the best way to confirm the presence of gallstones in suspected biliary pancreatitis. It also can detect extrapancreatic ductal dilations and reveal pancreatic edema, swelling, and peripancreatic fluid collections. However, in about 20% of patients, the ultrasound examination does not provide satisfactory results because of the presence of bowel gas, which can obscure sonographic imaging of the pancreas.

A CT scan of the pancreas is more commonly used to diagnose pancreatitis. CT scanning is used to distinguish milder (nonnecrotic) forms of the disease from more severe necrotizing or infected pancreatitis, in patients whose clinical presentation raises the suspicion of advanced disease (Figures 1 and 2). Pancreatic protocol CT scan of the abdomen and pelvis is recommended when not limited by renal insufficiency: a tri-phasic thin, multislice CT scan with an arterial, venous, and delayed phase in conjunction with sagittal and coronal views; no oral contrast, instead drink 1000 cc water to opacify the stomach. The scan assesses the degree of pancreatic necrosis, peripancreatic fluid collections, and the surrounding vascular structures. This tri-phasic scan can also help to detect underlying mass lesions.

Magnetic resonance cholangiopancreatography (MRCP) is also of value to assess the pancreatic duct and biliary tree. This can often reveal pancreatic ductal disruption.

Differential Diagnosis

The clinical diagnosis of pancreatitis is one of exclusion. Hyperamylasemia can also occur as a result of conditions not involving

Figure 1 Computed tomographic scan confirming acute edematous pancreatitis.

Figure 2 Computed tomographic scan confirming acute necrotizing, emphysematous pancreatitis.

pancreatitis. The other upper abdominal conditions that can be confused with acute pancreatitis include perforated peptic ulcer and acute cholecystitis, and occasionally a gangrenous small bowel obstruction. Because these conditions often have a fatal outcome without surgery, urgent intervention is indicated in the small number of cases in which doubt persists. A tumor should be considered in a nonalcoholic patient with acute pancreatitis who has no demonstrable biliary tract disease. Approximately 1% to 2% of patients with acute pancreatitis have pancreatic carcinoma, and an episode of acute pancreatitis can be the first clinical manifestation of a periampullary tumor.

Treatment

The severity of acute pancreatitis covers a broad spectrum of illness, ranging from the mild and self-limiting to the life-threatening necrotizing variety. Some cases are so mild they can be treated in an outpatient setting. However, most cases require hospitalization for observation and diagnostic study. A conservative approach has been advocated in the treatment of acute pancreatitis (Box 2). Severity is assessed with imaging results and clinical parameters and is quantitated with scores such as Ranson criteria (Box 3), the Atlanta classification, and the APACHE II (Acute Physiology and Chronic Health Evaluation) score. Severe acute pancreatitis is defined by associated organ dysfunction. The Atlanta classification is based on an international consensus conference held in Atlanta in 1992 and has been updated. APACHE II was designed to measure the severity of disease for adult patients admitted to intensive care units. Though not specific to pancreatitis, APACHE II can be used in an effort to differentiate patients with mild and severe acute pancreatitis. APACHE II scores of 8 points or more correlate with a mortality rate of 11% to 18%.

Upon confirmation of the diagnosis, patients with severe disease should be transferred to the intensive care unit for observation and maximum support. Adequate fluid resuscitation optimizing organ perfusion and oxygenation is essential. The use of prophylactic intravenous antibiotics in the initial stages of severe acute pancreatitis is not proved to be useful. Two randomized, controlled studies failed to show any benefit from antibiotics. Prophylactic antibiotics did not decrease the incidence of infected pancreatic necrosis or lower mortality. Data from these well-designed trials refute prior data from less-rigorous studies suggesting prophylactic antibiotics were useful. Additional studies are required, but there is increasing concern that the prolonged use of potent antibiotics might result in an increased prevalence of fungal infections and possibly increased mortality. Currently, antibiotic therapy should be reserved for treatment of specific infections such as positive blood, sputum, and urine cultures or percutaneous or operative cultures of necrotic tissue.

Randomized clinical trials have also shown a benefit from early nasojejunal feeding compared to total parenteral nutrition. Gastric decompression with a nasogastric tube is selectively used in patients with severe ileus and vomiting but is not necessary in a majority of cases. A debate remains regarding the optimal nutritional management in the majority of pancreatitis patients. There has been a trend toward oral enteric feeding in the less severe cases.

In biliary pancreatitis, the gallbladder must eventually be removed or recurrent acute pancreatitis will occur in 30% to 60% of cases. The timing of the cholecystectomy depends on the severity of the pancreatitis. Usually laparoscopic cholecystectomy is performed during the index admission as soon as the attack of acute pancreatitis has resolved. In more severe cases, the cholecystectomy is delayed and often combined with interventions for late complications of acute pancreatitis. In cases with severe comorbidity, endoscopic sphincterotomy has been considered as an alternative to cholecystectomy. However, if the patient has a postinflammatory fluid collection, bacteria can be introduced during endoscopic retrograde cholangiopancreatography (ERCP), and sphincterotomy should be delayed.

Currently, there is no role for routine early laparotomy and necrosectomy or resection in the setting of acute necrotizing pancreatitis. If the necrotic pancreas becomes infected and the patient fails to respond to conservative treatment, then necrosectomy may be warranted. Patients with infected necrosis are rarely managed conservatively without eventual surgical intervention. However, even in the setting of infected necrosis, there has been consideration for antibiotic therapy until the acute inflammatory response has subsided, if possible, with the view that surgery that is deferred for several weeks is more easily accomplished with one intervention. Patients who suffer from infected necrosis without having clinical signs of sepsis or other systemic complications might not need immediate surgical necrosectomy.

A nonsurgical alternative for the treatment of infected necrosis is percutaneous catheter drainage. This is considered a temporary measure to allow stabilization of the patient so that a safer surgical necrosectomy can be done at a later time. Multiple large drains are required, and patients frequently undergo repeat CT and revision of the drains. Current recommendations are to postpone surgery for as long as possible, usually beyond the second or third week of the disease or later, when necrotic tissue can be easily distinguished from viable pancreas and débridement without major blood loss can be performed. When surgery is performed, tissue-preserving digital necrosectomy is the usual technique rather than a classic surgical resection of the pancreas (Figure 3).

Necrosectomy can be performed by an open anterior approach with closed lavage or with leaving the abdomen open and packing. The packing is replaced at intervals of 24 to 72 hours. Sometimes a left lateral retroperitoneal approach is helpful. Newer approaches are the video-assisted retroperitoneal débridement (VARD). This procedure is a combination of percutaneous drainage and the open lateral retroperitoneal approach. An anterior laparoscopic approach has also been described and mimics the open anterior approach using laparoscopic ports. Surgical necrosectomy is indicated in patients with sepsis caused by infected necrosis and in selected patients with extended sterile necrosis causing severe systemic organ dysfunction and sepsis without a septic focus.

In some cases, the acute inflammatory process can lead to erosion into retroperitoneal vessels, and acute hemorrhage occurs. This acute emergent complication is best managed with immediate angiography to determine the exact site of bleeding and can often be treated with embolization rather than surgery (Figure 4).

Although previously frowned upon, there has been a move toward enteric drainage of all necrotic collections (even when infected) when technically feasible. This can be initiated through either an endoscopic or surgical approach.

Monitoring

Despite a conservative operative approach, endocrine and exocrine insufficiency develop in as many as half of the patients and

Figure 3 Necrotic material débrided from the retroperitoneum in a case of acute necrotizing pancreatitis.

Figure 4 Acute necrotizing pancreatitis. (A) Erosion into the splenic artery as seen on computed tomography. (B) Erosion into the splenic artery as seen on angiogram. (C) This complication of acute pancreatitis is best treated with angiographic embolization.

are determined by the extent of pancreatic necrosis. Therefore patients must be monitored with blood glucose measurements, stabilization of body weight, and proper nutrition.

Complications

The most common complication after successful management of acute pancreatitis is a pseudocyst. The term "pseudocyst" is currently used to broadly categorize most pancreatic and peripancreatic fluid collections (including walled-off pancreatic necrosis [WOPN] and acute peripancreatic fluid collection). The Acute Pancreatitis Classification Working Group recently proposed a revised Atlanta classification that refers to collections within 4 weeks of symptom onset as either acute peripancreatic fluid collections (APFC) or postnecrotic pancreatic fluid collections (PNPFC), depending upon the absence or presence of pancreatic/peripancreatic necrosis, respectively. After 4 weeks of the onset of symptoms, persistent collections with discrete walls are referred to as pseudocyst or WOPN, again depending upon the absence or presence of necrosis, respectively. In addition, these collections are further classified as sterile or infected and the term "pancreatic abscess" has been abolished.

The management of pseudocysts has followed a minimally invasive trend. Most pseudocysts resolve spontaneously, even beyond 6 weeks, so asymptomatic pseudocysts are usually observed (70% of pseudocysts will resolve without intervention). Endoscopic cystogastrostomy is the approach of choice for symptomatic fluid-predominant pseudocysts when there is minimal necrosis. If there is significant necrotic debris or a solid-predominant pseudocyst, surgical drainage with laparoscopic cystogastrostomy is preferred (Figure 5). This can also be performed with the traditional open technique. Cystojejunostomy (laparoscopic or open) is used in cases in which the site of the pseudocyst precludes drainage into the posterior aspect of the stomach.

Chronic Pancreatitis

Chronic pancreatitis is a chronic fibro-inflammatory disease of the pancreas characterized by irreversible morphologic changes that typically are associated with pain or permanent loss of function, or both.

Epidemiology

Population studies suggest a prevalence of chronic pancreatitis that ranges from 5 to 27 persons per 100,000 population, with considerable geographic variation. Autopsy data are difficult to interpret because a number of changes associated with chronic pancreatitis, such as fibrosis, duct ectasia, and acinar atrophy, are also present in asymptomatic elderly patients. Differences in diagnostic criteria, regional nutrition, alcohol consumption, and medical access account for variations in the frequency of the diagnosis, but the overall incidence of the disease has risen

progressively since the 1960s. Chronic pancreatitis in the United States currently results in more than 120,000 outpatient visits and more than 50,000 hospitalizations per year.

Figure 5 Computed tomographic scan showing fluid-predominant (A) and solid-predominant (B) pseudocysts. The former can be treated with endoscopic cystogastrostomy, and the latter is best treated with laparoscopic cystogastrostomy.

Risk Factors

Alcohol consumption and alcohol abuse are associated with chronic pancreatitis in up to 70% of cases. Other major causes include tropical (nutritional) and idiopathic disease, as well as hereditary causes. There is a linear relationship between exposure to alcohol and the development of chronic pancreatitis. The incidence is highest in heavy drinkers (15 drinks/day or 150 g/d). Prolonged alcohol use (four to five drinks daily over a period of more than 5 years) is required for alcohol-associated pancreatitis; the overall lifetime risk of pancreatitis among heavy drinkers is 2% to 5%. The duration of alcohol consumption is definitely associated with the development of pancreatic disease. The onset of disease typically occurs between ages 35 and 40 years, after 16 to 20 years of heavy alcohol consumption. Recurrent episodes of acute pancreatitis are typically followed by chronic symptoms after 4 or 5 years. In most cases, chronic pancreatitis has already developed and the acute clinical presentation represents a flare superimposed on chronic pancreatitis.

Tobacco use has also been heavily linked to pancreatitis. Meta-analysis has shown that both ever and current smokers had higher risks of developing pancreatitis compared with never smokers. This causative relationship was verified by the reduced or eliminated risk after smoking cessation. In comparison with current smokers, the risk of pancreatitis decreased for those who were former smokers.

Pathophysiology

Multiple episodes (or a prolonged course) of pancreatic injury ultimately leading to chronic disease is widely accepted as the pathophysiologic sequence. Abundant data indicate that acute pancreatitis may progress to recurrent acute pancreatitis and then to chronic pancreatitis in a disease continuum. Most investigators believe that alcohol metabolites such as acetaldehyde, combined with oxidant injury, result in local parenchymal injury that is preferentially targeted to the pancreas in predisposed persons. Repeated or severe episodes of toxin-induced injury activate a cascade of cytokines, which in turn induces pancreatic stellate cells to produce collagen and cause fibrosis.

The most common form of chronic pancreatitis is the calcifying type, characterized by the development of intraductal stones; the predominant causative agent is alcohol. Progressive functional impairment can develop from the dilated main pancreatic duct. Furthermore inflammatory enlargement of the pancreatic head may cause local complications such as stenosis of the pancreatic or bile duct, duodenal obstruction, or compression of retropancreatic vessels.

The pain caused by chronic pancreatitis is thought to be due to increased pressure in the pancreatic ducts and tissue, "parenchymal hypertension" from pancreatic ductal obstruction. Neural and perineural inflammation is also thought to be important in pathogenesis of pain in chronic pancreatitis. Neuropeptides released from enteric and afferent neurons and their functional interactions with inflammatory cells might play a key role.

Prevention

Because alcohol is the cause of most cases of chronic pancreatitis, cessation of alcohol consumption is recommended to prevent progression to chronic pancreatitis. Unfortunately, the majority of patients are not able to recover from alcoholism, and relapse is common.

Clinical Manifestations

Symptoms of chronic pancreatitis may be identical to those of acute pancreatitis, typically midepigastric pain penetrating through to the back. Patients with chronic pancreatic pain typically flex their abdomen and either sit or lie with their hips flexed, or lie on their side in a fetal position. Unlike ureteral stone pain or biliary colic, the pain causes the patient to be still. Nausea or vomiting can accompany the pain, but anorexia is the most common associated symptom. Patients with continuous pain can have a complication of chronic pancreatitis, such as an inflammatory mass, a cyst, or even pancreatic cancer. Other patients have intermittent attacks of pain with symptoms similar to those of mild to moderate acute pancreatitis. The pain sometimes is severe and lasts for many hours or several days.

As chronic pancreatitis progresses, endocrine and exocrine insufficiency begin to appear. Patients describe a bulky, foul-smelling, loose (but not watery) stool that may be pale and float on the surface of toilet water. Patients often describe a greasy or oily appearance to the stool or describe an "oil slick" on the water's surface. In severe steatorrhea, an orange, oily stool is often reported. As exocrine deficiency increases, symptoms of steatorrhea are often accompanied by weight loss. Patients might describe a good appetite despite weight loss, or they might have diminished food intake due to abdominal pain. The combination of decreased food intake and malabsorption of nutrients usually results in chronic weight loss. As a result, many patients with severe chronic pancreatitis are below ideal body weight. Usually islet cells are spared early in the disease process despite being surrounded by fibrosis, but eventually the insulin-secreting beta cells are also destroyed, gradually leading to diabetes.

Diagnosis

The diagnosis of chronic pancreatitis depends on the clinical presentation, a limited number of indirect measurements that correlate with pancreatic function, and selected imaging studies. Diagnosis is usually simple in the late stages of the disease because of the presence of structural and functional alterations of the pancreas. Early in the disease, the diagnosis is more difficult. Various classification systems have been developed. The

Figure 6 Computed tomographic scan of a patient with autoimmune pancreatitis and an inflammatory mass in the head of the pancreas. Preoperative diagnosis is not always possible, but surgery should be avoided because this disease often responds to steroid therapy.

Cambridge classification uses imaging tests such as ERCP, CT, and ultrasound to grade severity. The Mayo Clinic system is based on functional as well as imaging results. Tests of pancreatic function include the secretin-cerulein test, Lundh test, fecal excretion of pancreatic enzymes, and quantitation of fecal fat.

Chronic pancreatitis can be classified as calcifying (lithogenic), obstructive, inflammatory, autoimmune, tropical (nutritional), hereditary, or idiopathic. Autoimmune and hereditary pancreatitis have recently been better understood and diagnosed more than before. Autoimmune pancreatitis is associated with fibrosis, a mononuclear cell (lymphocyte, plasma cell, or eosinophil) infiltrate, and an increased titer of one or more autoantibodies. It is usually associated with autoimmune diseases such as Sjögren syndrome. Increased levels of serum β-globulin or immunoglobulin (Ig)G$_4$ are often present, however autoimmune pancreatitis can present without these markers. This disease can be mistaken for chronic pancreatitis, with an inflammatory mass in the head of the pancreas suspicious for pancreatic cancer (Figure 6). Diagnosis is important because steroid therapy is uniformly successful in ameliorating the disease, including any associated bile duct compression.

Hereditary pancreatitis first occurs in adolescence with abdominal pain; patients develop progressive pancreatic dysfunction, and the risk of cancer is greatly increased. The disease follows an autosomal dominant pattern of inheritance with 80% penetrance and variable expression. Recent mutational analysis has revealed a missense mutation resulting in an Arg to His substitution at position 117 of the cationic trypsinogen gene, or *PRSS1*, one of the primary sites for proteolysis of trypsin. This mutation prevents trypsin from being inactivated by itself or other proteases, and it results in persistent and uncontrolled proteolytic activity and autodestruction within the pancreas. Similarly, *PSTI*, also known as *SPINK1*, has been found to have a role in hereditary pancreatitis and some cases of sporadic chronic pancreatitis. *SPINK1* specifically inhibits trypsin action by competitively blocking the active site of the enzyme.

It is likely that many of the "idiopathic" forms of chronic pancreatitis, as well as some patients with the more common forms of the disease, will be found to have a genetic linkage or predisposition.

Differential Diagnosis

There are several clinical conditions from which chronic pancreatitis needs to be distinguished. Other causes of upper abdominal pain, such as peptic ulcer disease, biliary tract disease, mesenteric vascular disease, or malignancy must be excluded. The major difficulty in the differential diagnosis of chronic pancreatitis is distinguishing it from pancreatic ductal adenocarcinoma. Chronic

pancreatitis can closely mimic pancreatic cancer, both clinically and morphologically. In addition, chronic pancreatitis is a risk factor for the development of pancreatic cancer. Although in pancreatic resection specimens this problem may be finally resolved, distinguishing these two diseases preoperatively in small (needle) biopsy specimens is a formidable challenge for the pathologist. Therefore especially in the setting of an inflammatory mass in the head of the pancreas, consideration of pancreatic cancer and surgical referral is important. Workup of these patients should include a pancreatic protocol CT scan, an MRCP, and an endoscopic ultrasound to evaluate the parenchyma and the ducts of the pancreas.

Treatment

Therapy for chronic pancreatitis is aimed at managing associated digestive dysfunction and relieving pain (Box 4). It is important to first address malabsorption, weight loss, and diabetes. When pancreatic exocrine capacity falls below 10% of normal, diarrhea and steatorrhea develop. Lipase deficiency tends to manifest itself before trypsin deficiency, so the presence of steatorrhea may be the first functional sign of pancreatic insufficiency. As pancreatic exocrine function deteriorates further, the secretion of bicarbonate into the duodenum is reduced, which causes duodenal acidification and further impairs nutrient absorption. Frank diabetes is seen initially in about 20% of patients with chronic pancreatitis, and impaired glucose metabolism can be detected in up to 70% of patients.

The medical treatment of chronic or recurrent pain in chronic pancreatitis requires the use of analgesics, a cessation of alcohol use, oral enzyme therapy, and endoscopic stent therapy. Administration of pancreatic enzyme (e.g., Pancrease MT, Pancrelipase, Creon) serves to reverse the effects of pancreatic exocrine insufficiency and might also reduce or alleviate the pain[1] experienced by patients. Interventional procedures to block visceral afferent nerve conduction or to treat obstructions of the main pancreatic duct are also an adjunct to medical treatment. It has been taught that the pain of chronic pancreatitis decreases with increasing duration of the disease, the so-called burn-out phase, where endocrine and exocrine insufficiency occurs and the pain decreases. However, recent studies have called this concept into question, demonstrating continued pain in patients with chronic pancreatitis despite long-standing disease and pancreatic insufficiency. Cessation of alcohol abuse, if possible, causes the pain to stop in about half of the patients.

Pain relief usually requires the use of narcotics, but these should be titrated to achieve pain relief with the lowest effective dose. Opioid addiction is common, and the use of long-acting analgesics by transdermal patch together with oral agents for pain exacerbations slightly reduces the sedative effects of high-dose oral narcotics. Celiac plexus neurolysis has been an effective form of analgesic treatment in patients with pancreatic carcinoma. However, its use in chronic pancreatitis has been disappointing, with about half of the patients deriving a benefit that lasts 6 months or less.

Pancreatic duct stenting is used for treatment of proximal pancreatic duct stenosis, decompression of a pancreatic duct leak,

[1] Not FDA approved for this indication

and drainage of pancreatic pseudocysts that can be catheterized through the main pancreatic duct. Pancreatic duct stones can also be removed endoscopically. Stent therapy in chronic pancreatitis definitely plays a role and can help select patients for successful operative therapy. However, the duration of success with stent therapy for chronic pancreatitis is probably less than with surgical therapy.

There has been significant debate over the years regarding the role and type of surgical therapy in chronic pancreatitis. Progressive functional pancreatic impairment can be delayed by surgical decompression of the dilated main pancreatic duct. Furthermore, inflammatory enlargement of the pancreatic head may cause local complications that require further treatment, such as stenosis of the pancreatic or bile duct, duodenal obstruction, or compression of retropancreatic vessels. Surgery may be superior to conservative or endoscopic treatment in terms of pain relief and preservation of pancreatic function and quality of life. Major pancreatic resections for chronic pancreatitis have a significant complication rate, both early and late. Patients with large duct disease who can have nutrition restored, are working, are not drinking alcohol, and have a supportive family structure fare better with surgical therapies. Failure to carefully select patients for either drainage or resection procedures leads to disappointing results. The surgical management of pancreatic duct stones and stenosis has been shown to be superior to endoscopic treatment in randomized clinical trials. Beger introduced the duodenum-preserving pancreatic head resection (DPPHR) in the early 1980s. Later in the decade, Frey and Smith described the local resection of the pancreatic head with longitudinal pancreaticojejunostomy, which included excavation of the pancreatic head including the ductal structures in continuity with a long ductotomy of the dorsal duct. This operation is basically a hybrid of the Beger and Puestow (Partington-Rochelle modification) procedures and is more popular in the United States (Figures 7 and 8).

Previous randomized prospective studies have compared the Whipple, Beger, and Frey procedures for chronic pancreatitis. Patients who had a Beger procedure had a shorter hospital stay, greater weight gain, less postoperative diabetes, and less exocrine dysfunction than standard Whipple patients over a 3- to 5-year follow-up. Pain control was similar between the two procedures. In a study comparing the pylorus-preserving Whipple to the Frey procedure, there was a lower postoperative complication rate associated with the Frey procedure (19%) compared to the pylorus-preserving Whipple group (53%), and the global quality-of-life scores were better (71% vs. 43%, respectively). Both operations were equally effective in controlling pain over a 2-year follow-up. Operation times, intraoperative blood loss, and transfusion requirements have been shown to be decreased with the Frey and Beger procedures compared to the Whipple procedure. In long-term (>8 years) follow-up, there was no difference between the Beger and Frey procedures in pain relief, pancreatic insufficiency, quality of life, and late mortality. Compared to the Whipple procedure, the Beger and Frey procedures may produce a lower incidence of immediate complications and diabetes but no significant differences in pain relief. Although these limited pancreatic procedures have a lower initial rate of endocrine dysfunction, the long-term risk of diabetes is more related to the progression of the underlying disease than to the effects of operation.

Recent multicenter randomized, controlled, double-blinded, trial compared DPPHR to partial pancreatoduodenectomy with a primary endpoint of quality of life within 24 months after surgery. The results showed that DPPHR was not superior to partial pancreatoduodenectomy in terms of the primary endpoint, long-term postoperative quality of life. With both resection and drainage procedures offering viable options for treatment, patient selection becomes critical in assuring there is clinical improvement postoperatively.

Recent refinements in the methods of harvesting and preserving pancreatic islets, and standardization of the methods by which islets are infused into the portal venous circuit for intrahepatic engraftment,

Figure 7 Computed tomographic scan of a patient with chronic calcific pancreatitis and a massively dilated pancreatic duct. (A) Axial view with calcified pancreatic head. (B) Axial view with dilated pancreatic duct.

have improved the success and rekindled interest in islet autotransplantation for chronic pancreatitis. The ability to recover a sufficient quantity of islets from a sclerotic gland depends on the degree of disease present, so the selection of patients as candidates for autologous islet transplantation is important. As success with autotransplantation increases, patients with nonobstructive, sclerotic pancreatitis may be considered for resection and islet autotransplantation earlier in their course, because end-stage fibrosis bodes poorly for transplant success. Patient selection and surgeon experience play a very large role in the outcomes of autotransplantation.

Monitoring
Chronic pancreatitis is of course a chronic disease, so continued monitoring and maintenance therapy is essential after an acute exacerbation of chronic pancreatitis. Pain control, proper nutrition, and alcohol and smoking cessation must be maintained as an outpatient. The clinician must also be looking for the development of common complications. An annual physical exam and CT or MRI should be considered in this population to assess for the progression of disease.

Complications
Pseudocysts in the setting of chronic pancreatitis are less likely to resolve without intervention. Often, the pancreatic duct and bile duct are compressed, and the compression might need to be addressed at the same time as the pseudocyst. A trend toward minimally invasive management remains appropriate, with

Figure 8 (A) The pancreatic duct is opened to reveal a preoperatively placed pancreatic duct stent. (B) The residual stones removed from the pancreatic duct. (C) In the Frey procedure, the head of the pancreas is cored out in addition to a longitudinal pancreatic ductotomy. The pancreas is drained with a Roux-en-Y limb of jejunum.

endoscopic drainage preferred over laparoscopic cystogastrostomy unless additional procedures are required. Resection of a pseudocyst is sometimes indicated for cysts located in the pancreatic tail, or when a midpancreatic duct disruption has resulted in a distally located pseudocyst. Distal pancreatectomy for removal of a pseudocyst, with or without splenectomy, can be a challenging procedure in the setting of prior pancreatitis. An internal drainage procedure of the communicating duct, or of the pseudocyst itself, should be considered when distal resection is being contemplated.

Pancreatic ascites results from a disrupted pancreatic duct with extravasation of pancreatic fluid that does not become sequestered as a pseudocyst but drains freely into the peritoneal cavity. Occasionally, the pancreatic fluid tracks superiorly into the thorax, causing a pancreatic pleural effusion. Both complications are seen more often in patients with chronic pancreatitis, rather than after acute pancreatitis. Paracentesis or thoracentesis reveals noninfected fluid with a protein level greater than 25 g/L and a markedly elevated amylase level. Paracentesis is critical to differentiate pancreatic from hepatic ascites.

ERCP is most helpful to delineate the location of the pancreatic duct leak and to elucidate the underlying pancreatic ductal anatomy. Pancreatic duct stenting may be considered at the time of ERCP. Paracentesis and antisecretory therapy with the somatostatin analogue octreotide acetate, together with bowel rest and parenteral nutrition, is successful in more than half of patients. Reapposition of serosal surfaces to facilitate closure of the leak is considered a part of therapy, and this is accomplished by complete paracentesis. For pleural effusions, a period of chest tube drainage can facilitate closure of the internal fistula. Surgical therapy is reserved for those who fail to respond to medical treatment.

References

Acute Pancreatitis Classification Working Group: *Revision of the Atlanta Classification of Acute Pancreatitis*, 2010. Available at: http://www.pancreasclub.com/resources/AtlantaClassification.pdf. [accessed 25.08.14].

Beger HG, Matsuno S, Cameron JL: *Diseases of the pancreas: Current surgical therapy*, Berlin, 2008, Springer-Verlag.

Beger HG, Warshaw AL, Buchler MW, et al, editors: *The pancreas: An integrated textbook of basic science, medicine, and surgery*, ed 2nd, Malden, MA, 2008, Blackwell Publishing.

Cunha EF, Rocha Mde S, Pereira FP, et al: Walled-off pancreatic necrosis and other current concepts in the radiological assessment of acute pancreatitis, *Radiol Bras* 47(3):165–175, 2014.

Dellinger EP, Tellado JM, Soto NE, et al: Early antibiotic treatment for severe acute necrotizing pancreatitis: a randomized, double-blind, placebo-controlled study, *Ann Surg* 245:674–683, 2007.

Diener MK, Hüttner FJ, Kieser M, et al: Partial pancreatoduodenectomy versus duodenum-preserving pancreatic head resection in chronic pancreatitis: the multicentre, randomised, controlled, double-blind ChroPac trial, *Lancet* 390(10099):1027–1037, 2017 Sep 9. https://doi.org/10.1016/S0140-6736(17)31960-8.

Fisher WE, Anderson DK, Bell RH, et al: Pancreas. In Brunicardi FC, Andersen DK, Billiar TR, et al, editors: *Schwartz's principles of surgery*, ed 9th, New York, 2010, McGraw-Hill, pp 1167–1243.

Forsmark CE, Vege SS, Wilcox CM: Acute Pancreatitis, *N Engl J Med* 375(20):1972–1981, 2016 Nov 17.

Impact of smoking on the risk of pancreatitis: a systematic review and meta-analysis.

Isenmann R, Runzi M, Kron M, et al: Prophylactic antibiotic treatment in patients with predicted severe acute pancreatitis: a placebo-controlled, double-blind trial, *Gastroenterology* 126:997–1004, 2004.

Working Group IAP/APA Acute Pancreatitis Guidelines: IAP/APA evidence-based **guidelines** for the management of acute **pancreatitis**, *Pancreatology* 13(4 Suppl 2):e1–15, 2013 Jul-Aug. https://doi.org/10.1016/j.pan.2013.07.063.

Ye X, Lu G, Huai J, Ding J: *PLoS One* 10(4):e0124075, 2015 Apr 16, https://doi.org/10.1371/journal.pone.0124075. eCollection 2015.

Zaheer A, Singh VK, Qureshi RO, Fishman EK: The revised Atlanta classification for acute pancreatitis: updates in imaging terminology and guidelines, *Abdom Imaging* 38(1):125–136, 2013.

ACUTE DIARRHEA

Method of
Tate de Leon, MD

CURRENT DIAGNOSIS

History
- Onset, duration, and frequency of diarrhea
- Related symptoms (fever, abdominal pain, nausea, emesis, bloody stool)
- Current medications, including recent antibiotic use
- Recent sick contacts or hospitalizations
- Recent foreign travel
- Exposure to contaminated water source or undercooked meats and seafood
- Immune status

Physical Examination
- Hydration status
- Abdominal examination

Laboratory Testing
- Acute secretory diarrhea: normally not necessary
- Acute bloody diarrhea: complete blood count, stool culture, consider ova and parasite testing and *Clostridium difficile* evaluation

CURRENT THERAPY

- Symptomatic therapy
- Rehydration: enteral versus parenteral
- Antibiotics (depending on duration, severity, and other risk factors)
  - Emperic therapy
    - Adults
      - Fluoroquinolones
        - Ciprofloxacin (Cipro) 500 mg PO twice daily for 3–7 days
        - Levofloxacin (Levaquin)[1] 500 mg PO four times daily for 3–5 days
    - Children
      - Azithromycin (Zithromax)[1] 5–12 mg/kg PO four times daily for 3–5 days
  - C difficile
    - Metronidazole (Flagyl)[1] 500 mg PO every 8 hours for 10–14 days
    - Vancomycin (Vancocin) 125 mg PO every 6 hours for 10 days
- Antidiarrheal medications (if no contraindications such as fever or hematochezia)
  - Loperamide (Imodium) Initial 4 mg PO followed by 2 mg PO with each loose stool. Max 16 mg per day
- Probiotics[2]

[1]Not FDA approved for this indication.
[2]Not available in the United States.

BOX 1　Clinical History of Acute Infectious Diarrhea

- Description of diarrhea
  - Duration
  - Frequency
  - Presence of blood, pus, in stool
  - Symptoms of fever, tenesmus, dehydration
  - Weight loss
- Other gastrointestinal symptoms
  - Anorexia
  - Cramping
  - Emesis
  - Nausea
- Previous episodes with similar symptoms
- Recent antibiotic exposure
- Other medication exposure
  - Anticholinergics
  - Antimotility agents
  - Aspirin (ASA)
  - Proton pump inhibitors
- Recent dietary history
  - Shellfish
  - Undercooked meat (chicken)
  - Unsanitary water
  - Animal or reptile contacts
- Travel history
  - Travel to endemic or epidemic areas
- Sexual history
- Vaccination history
- Contact with institutions, e.g., hospitals, nursing homes, day care facilities
- Employment history
- Immune status
  - Presence of HIV
  - Presence of other congenital or acquired immunodeficiencies

BOX 2　Physical Examination for Acute Infectious Diarrhea

- Vital signs
- Blood pressure (look for postural changes)
- Heart rate (look for postural changes)
- Respiratory rate
- Temperature
- Weight changes (particularly useful to assess effects of rehydration)
- Cardiovascular examination
  - Volume status
- Respiratory examination
- Rule out hyperventilation (compensatory respiratory alkalosis for metabolic acidosis resulting from dehydration and loss of bicarbonate)
- Abdominal examination
- Focal tenderness
- Guarding
- Hepatosplenomegaly
- Consider rectal examination (look for bloody stool)
- Decreased skin turgor
- Lymphadenopathy
- Rashes

Acute diarrhea in the United States is one of the most common diagnoses in general practice. Acute diarrhea can have a functional definition of a greater number of loose stools from normal lasting less than 14 days. If the episode lasts more than 14 days, it is called persistent diarrhea. If the episode lasts for more than 30 days, it is deemed chronic diarrhea. These episodes may be accompanied by nausea, vomiting, abdominal cramping, other systemic symptoms, and malnutrition. The majority of acute diarrhea cases are self-limited and do not need medical intervention. Most often, these cases are caused by infectious agents such as viruses, bacteria, or parasites. Infection is often spread through contaminated food or drinking water or from person-to-person. Pathogens that cause diarrhea are usually transmitted through a fecal–oral route. The main risk factor for this transmission is poor hand hygiene. Other risk factors include improper food preparation, inadequate food refrigeration, and exposure to contaminated water.

Thorough investigation of a patient with acute diarrhea should include a detailed history, physical examination, and laboratory testing when indicated (Boxes 1 and 2). Acute diarrhea can be classified into two subtypes: secretory diarrhea and inflammatory diarrhea. Determining the subtype of the diarrhea is useful for suggesting the etiology and therefore the management of the diarrhea.

Secretory diarrhea is an electrolyte absorption impairment that leads to profuse, watery diarrhea that contains little or no blood or leukocytes. These episodes can last from a few hours to days. The main concern is dehydration and weight loss if oral intake is not continued. Clinical signs of severe dehydration include lethargy or unconsciousness, dry or sunken eyes, dry mouth, decreased skin turgor, and a history of poor or absent fluid intake.

Inflammatory diarrhea is bloody, usually has leukocytes, and produces less volume. The most common causes are *Salmonella*, *Campylobacter*, *Shigella*, *Escherichia coli* O157:H7, and *Entamoeba hystolytica*. The main concerns related to inflammatory diarrhea are intestinal damage, sepsis, and malnutrition. Stool cultures and evaluation for ova and parasites are recommended.

Preventive measures can help reduce the spread of infectious agents. Proper hand hygiene with soap and water, especially after exposure to feces or individuals with acute diarrhea, can help limit the spread of infection. Barrier precautions are an effective adjunct when dealing with the possibility of exposure to feces in a hospital setting. For children, vaccinations have been shown to be effective in reducing rotavirus infections. Furthermore, it is imperative to separate diaper-changing areas from food-preparation areas. Proper sanitization with a bleach-based cleaner is recommended. Proper food handling and storage, along with water purification, are important means to help prevent the spread of infectious agents. Probiotics[2] are finding a home in the prevention and treatment of diarrhea. Initial studies have suggested that probiotics are useful in reducing antibiotic-associated diarrhea. Currently, more studies are needed to confirm their usefulness. Prophylactic antibiotics are usually only reserved for possible exposure to traveler's diarrhea.

Epidemiology

Worldwide, acute diarrhea still accounts for significant morbidity and mortality. The very young, the very old, and the immunocompromised populations are the most adversely affected. Acute infectious diarrhea is more prevalent in developing countries and among travelers to developing countries. Diarrhea is the second leading cause of death worldwide in children under 5 years of age. The World Health Organization estimates that globally, there are over 1.7 billion cases of acute diarrhea each year and attributes 760,000 deaths to it annually. The majority of these deaths are in children who are younger than age 5 and live in developing countries. In the United States, foodborne infectious diarrhea accounts for approximately 325,000 hospitalizations and 5000 deaths each year.

Etiology and Treatment

The precise cause of acute diarrhea is usually not found. Causes can be both infectious and noninfectious. Noninfectious causes can include medications, food allergies, and other gastrointestinal diseases. In general, clinical investigation of acute infectious diarrhea is more useful in identifying consequences of diarrhea, such as dehydration, than it is in revealing the precise etiology. Most cases of diarrhea are likely viral, as indicated by negative stool culture results in most studies. Severe cases of diarrhea tend to be a result of bacterial infection. The most common pathogens for bacteria-induced diarrhea is discussed below. To date, the optimal strategy for obtaining stool cultures has not been ascertained. It is thus reasonable to treat the patient symptomatically for several days before obtaining a stool culture for mild to moderate cases because most cases of diarrhea are self-limited. The clinician should take into consideration individual comorbidities, immune status, the presence of severe or bloody diarrhea, underlying inflammatory bowel disease, and occupation (food handlers, day care employment, etc.) as possible indications for stool evaluation.

Bacteria

Campylobacter

Campylobacter is a common cause of diarrhea in the United States. The pathogen is often spread by consumption of undercooked meat and poultry. Symptoms may present 2 to 5 days after exposure and last up to 1 week. The patient presents with diarrhea (possibly bloody), abdominal pain, nausea, vomiting, and fever. Stool cultures are needed for a definitive diagnosis. Prevention includes thoroughly cooking all meat products, good hand and utensil hygiene before preparing foods, and avoiding unpasteurized milk. The treatment for severe *Campylobacter* diarrhea includes azithromycin (Zithromax)[1] and ciprofloxacin (Cipro), although resistance to fluoroquinolones is growing. Antimicrobial susceptibility testing is required for specific resistance. Positive stool cultures should be reported to the local health department. *Campylobacter* infections have been linked to both rheumatoid arthritis and also Guillain-Barré syndrome.

Clostridium difficile

C difficile is the organism of antibiotic-associated colitis. Antibiotics disrupt the normal flora of the GI tract, which in turn provides a window of opportunity for *C difficile* to produce toxins and flourish. The most frequent antibiotics implicated

are clindamycin (Cleocin), fluoroquinolones, and beta-lactam antibiotics. *C difficile* is treated with oral metronidazole[1] (Flagyl 500 mg PO every 8 hours for 10–14 days) and vancomycin (Vancocin 125 mg PO every 6 hours for 10 days). The diagnosis is confirmed with either polymerase chain reaction (PCR), enzyme immunoassay, or anaerobic culture. Endoscopy and biopsy can also be obtained if there is a high clinical suspicion for *C difficile* with negative laboratory results or if the patient did not respond to antibiotic treatment.

E coli

E coli are a large and versatile group of pathogens that can cause widespread disease and affect multiple organ systems. *E coli* is a part of the normal flora of both human and animal digestive tract. Certain *E coli* strains can cause acute diarrhea. Pathogenic strains include enterotoxigeneic *E coli* (ETEC), enteropathogenic *E coli*, enteroaggregative *E coli*, enteroinvasive *E coli*, diffusely adherent *E coli*, and enterohemorrhagic *E coli* (EHEC may also be referred as Shiga toxin-producing *E coli* or verocytotoxin-producing *E coli*). The two most common and notorious strains are ETEC and EHEC. ETEC is a major cause of traveler's diarrhea and diarrhea in children of developing countries. EHEC has led to high-profile outbreaks of diarrhea as a result of contaminated meats.

ETEC is a type of *E coli* that produces toxins that stimulate the intestines to secrete excessive fluid, thus producing diarrhea. ETEC produces two different toxins: heat-stable toxin and heat-labile toxin. Both types of toxins produce similar illnesses. Contaminated food and water is the usual source of infection. Although stool culture is needed for definitive diagnosis, ETEC infections are usually diagnosed on history and clinical symptoms. Symptoms usually appear after 1 to 2 days after exposure and may last from 5 to 7 days. Most cases of ETEC diarrhea are treated symptomatically with adequate rehydration alone. Oral rehydration salts may be used and purchased over the counter to help address electrolyte losses. Both bismuth compounds (e.g., Pepto-Bismol) and antimotility agents (e.g. loperamide [Imodium]) can help reduce severity of symptoms; they both may prolong the time the body takes to clear the toxin. Antibiotics are reserved for moderate to severe disease. The most common effective antibiotics include fluoroquinolones. Antibiotics can shorten the duration of symptoms but are usually not required.

EHEC is a strain of *E coli* that produces a Shiga toxin. The toxin acts on vascular endothelium of small vessels of multiple organ systems. The toxin causes the breakdown and hemorrhage of the endothelium. When the toxin affects the vascular endothelium of the digestive tract, it causes bloody diarrhea. The pathogen often invades the kidney and lungs. Sequelae of EHEC infection include hemorrhagic diarrhea, hemolytic uremic syndrome, and thrombotic thrombocytopenic purpura. *E coli* O157 is the most common strain of EHEC. The infection is spread via the oral–fecal route, which includes consumption of contaminated food, unpasteurized milk and cheeses, and unsanitary water. Good hand hygiene is imperative. Symptoms usually appear 3 to 4 days after exposure and may last as long as 10 days. Positive stool cultures should be reported to the local health department. Supportive treatment, including rehydration, is the cornerstone of treatment. Antibiotics are contraindicated because of evidence of increased Shiga toxin release and thus increased risk of hemolytic uremic syndrome.

Salmonella

Salmonella is the most common foodborne cause of diarrhea in the United States. It is associated with ingestion of infected poultry, eggs, and milk products. *Salmonella* can also be transmitted from pets, especially reptiles. Stool cultures are required for definitive diagnosis. Fluoroquinolones remain the antibiotic of choice, although sensitivities will guide antibiotic usage.

Shigella

Shigella is the pathogen that causes dysentery and is a major cause of morbidity in developing countries. Dysentery usually presents

---

[1] Not FDA approved for this indication.
[2] Not available in the United States.

as high fever, abdominal cramping, and bloody diarrhea. Positive stool cultures usually warrant treatment with fluoroquinolones.

Vibrio

Vibrio cholera is endemic to developing countries. Symptoms usually present 1 to 3 days after exposure. Symptoms usually include profuse watery diarrhea (rice-water stools), abdominal cramping, and vomiting. Fever is infrequent. Rehydration with appropriate electrolyte replacement is paramount. Antibiotics can be an adjunct to rehydration and include fluoroquinolones and tetracycline at 500 mg PO every 8 hours for 3 days.

Yersinia

Yersinia enterocolitica infections are less common. Symptoms include diarrhea, fever, abdominal pain, and vomiting. Stool cultures are needed to confirm the diagnosis.

Viruses

Viral pathogens are likely responsible for the majority of gastroenteritis in the United States. Given the transient nature and characteristic symptoms, the specificity of the exact virus is not usually obtained. The most common viral etiologies tend to be adenovirus, rotavirus, norovirus, and astrovirus. Rotavirus tends to affect infants and children from 3 to 36 months of age, resulting in a spectrum of disease from asymptomatic shedding to severe gastroenteritis. Vaccination has played an important role in decreasing the cases of rotavirus infections.

Norovirus (i.e., Norwalk virus) is responsible for many high-profile outbreaks in daycare centers, cruise ships, and hospitals. Norovirus can be easily transmitted from person to person, from contact of contaminated surfaces, or from exposure to contaminated food or water. Symptoms present 1 to 3 days after exposure. Symptoms include fever, explosive vomiting, and diarrhea. PCR testing can confirm the diagnosis but is not usually necessary unless there seems to be an outbreak.

Parasite

Entamoeba histolytica, *Cryptosporidium*, *Giardia*, and *Cyclospora* spp. are the most common parasitic or protozoal infections that cause diarrhea. Protozoa infections are even less common. It is usually not cost-effective to evaluate for ova and parasites unless there are specific indications, such as a history of immunocompromise, exposure to daycare centers, or history of exposure to contaminated water. Multiple stool samples are needed if there are concerns of parasite infection resulting from possible intermittent shedding. *E histolytica* can cause amoebic dysentery and lead to bloody diarrhea. Microscopy, antigen testing, and serology are all possible tests for diagnosis. Parasitic infections are usually treated with metronidazole (Flagyl), tinidazole (Tindamax 2 g PO four times daily for 1–3 days) or albendazole[1] (Albenza 400 mg PO four times daily for 5 days).

Traveler's Diarrhea

Traveler's diarrhea is common to individuals from developed countries traveling to developing countries. Episodes can be caused by bacteria, viruses, and parasites. The most common pathogen is *E coli* (ETEC). Travelers should choose their food and water sources carefully. Water purification and avoiding foods prepared with contaminated water is useful. Prolonged or other symptoms such as fever or bloody stool should be further investigated.

Treatment

Fluid and electrolyte replacement are the most important therapies for acute diarrhea. The route of administration depends on the severity of the dehydration. For mild cases of diarrhea in a normally healthy individual, adequate oral intake of juices, soups, and electrolyte-infused water can be sufficient. For severe dehydration, IV fluids or oral rehydration therapy with isotonic electrolyte solutions may be needed. Oral hydration is preferred over IV fluids if possible. IV fluids are more expensive and less practical than oral rehydration. The World Health Organization has a lower-osmolarity oral rehydration solution (ORS), which is very effective in reducing stool volume and the need for switching to IV therapy in children. A number of effective ORSs are also available over the counter, including Pedialyte and Rehydralyte. IV fluids, including normal saline and lactated Ringers solution, are indicated in severe dehydration or in patients who cannot tolerate oral fluid intake.

Antimicrobial agents have a secondary role in treatment of acute diarrhea. Given the fact that most cases of diarrhea are mild, self-limited, and caused by nonbacterial pathogens, antibiotics should be used sparingly. Antibiotic treatment should be used in invasive bacterial infections, traveler's diarrhea, or in patients with immunosuppression. Empirical antibiotics can be appropriate as described above for *Campylobacter* or *C difficile* infections.

Antidiarrheal medications can be useful to help alleviate symptoms in patients with no other contraindications, such as fever or bloody diarrhea. Loperamide (Imodium initial 4 mg PO followed by 2 mg PO with each loose stool, maximum 16 mg per day) decreases intestinal peristalsis and facilitates intestinal absorption. Bismuth (Pepto-Bismol) is less effective. Bismuth produces both antisecretory and antimicrobial effects in the gastrointestinal tract.

References

Centers for Disease Control and Prevention: Division of Foodborne, Waterborne, and Environmental Diseases (DFWED). Available at: http://www.cdc.gov/ncezid/dfwed/a-z.html. Updated April 2013.

Fontaine O, Griffin P, Henao O, et al: Diarrhea, Acute. In Heymann DL, editor: *Control of Communicable Diseases Manual*, ed 19th, Washington, DC, 2008, American Public Health Association, pp 179–194.

Guerrant RL, Van Gilder T, Steiner TS, et al: Practice guidelines for the management of infectious diarrhea, *Clin Infect Dis* 32:331–351, 2001.

Singh SK: Diarhea. In Andreoli TE, Benjamin IJ, Griggs RC, Wing EJ, editors: *Cecil Essentials of Medicine*, ed 8th, Philadelphia, PA, 2010, Saunders, pp 396–400.

Theilman NM, Guerrant RL: Clinical practice. Acute infectious diarrhea, *N Engl J Med* 350:38–47, 2004.

World Health Organization: Diarrheal disease. Available at: http://www.who.int/mediacentre/factsheets/fs330/en/ Updated May 2017.

BLEEDING ESOPHAGEAL VARICES

Method of
Cecilio M. Azar, MD; and Ala I. Sharara, MD

 CURRENT DIAGNOSIS

- Endoscopic screening for esophageal varices is recommended in patients with liver cirrhosis.
- Noninvasive predictors of the presence of large varices, such as splenomegaly and thrombocytopenia, have limited accuracy.
- A combination of clinical and endoscopic findings including the Child-Pugh class, size of varices, and the presence of red wale markings correlates with the risk of first bleeding in patients with cirrhosis.
- Measurement of hepatic venous pressure gradient may be the best indicator of risk and severity of bleeding in patients with varices. It is an invasive test and is not widely available or used routinely in practice.

---

[1] Not FDA approved for this indication.

CURRENT THERAPY

- Nonselective β-blockers and endoscopic band ligation are both effective first-line therapy in the primary prophylaxis of esophageal varices.
- The management of acute variceal hemorrhage consists of prompt resuscitation and correction of coagulation abnormalities, followed by endoscopic and pharmacologic therapy with vasoactive agents. Antibiotic prophylaxis is given to decrease the risk of infection and of rebleeding. Transjugular intrahepatic portosystemic shunt (TIPS) is reserved for refractory, uncontrolled, acute variceal bleeding.
- Strategies for secondary prophylaxis of variceal bleeding include endoscopic band ligation, pharmacologic therapy with nonselective β-blockers with or without nitrates, TIPS, and surgical shunts.
- Comparative cost-effectiveness of secondary prophylaxis strategies is unknown but should take into consideration the cost of failed therapy (e.g., rebleeding, shunt revision) and that of treatment related-complications (e.g., encephalopathy, esophageal stricture).

Epidemiology

Bleeding of esophageal varices is a major complication of portal hypertension, usually in the setting of liver cirrhosis, accounting for 10% to 30% of all cases of upper gastrointestinal hemorrhage. More than any other cause of gastrointestinal bleeding, this complication results in considerable morbidity and mortality, prolonged hospitalization, and increased affiliated costs. Variceal bleeding develops in 25% to 35% of patients with cirrhosis and accounts for up to 90% of upper gastrointestinal bleeding episodes in these patients. About 10% to 30% of these episodes are fatal, and as many as 70% of survivors rebleed following an index variceal hemorrhage. Following such events, the 1-year survival is 34% to 80%, being inversely related to the severity of the underlying liver disease.

Treatment of patients with esophageal varices includes preventing the initial bleeding episode (primary prophylaxis), controlling active variceal hemorrhage, and preventing recurrent bleeding after a first episode (secondary prophylaxis). Data on the optimal management of gastric varices are much more limited, and this topic is not covered in this article.

Pathophysiology

Chronic liver disease leading to cirrhosis is the most common cause of portal hypertension. The level of increased resistance to flow varies with the level of circulatory breach and can be divided into prehepatic, hepatic or sinusoidal, and posthepatic. In cirrhosis, several organ systems are involved in the pathophysiology of portal hypertension. At the splanchnic vascular bed level there is marked vasodilatation and increase in angiogenesis, leading to increase in portal blood flow and formation of collateral circulation, such as gastroesophageal varices, along with decrease in response to vasoconstrictors. At the systemic circulation level, there is an increase in cardiac output, decrease in vascular resistance, and hypervolemia. This hyperkinetic syndrome leads to an effective hypovolemia, with a resultant increase in vasoactive factors to maintain a normal arterial blood pressure.

Varices represent portosystemic collaterals derived from dilatation of preexisting embryonic vascular channels, such as those between the coronary and short gastric veins and the intercostal, esophageal, and azygous veins. In the distal esophagus, over an area extending 2 to 5 cm from the gastroesophageal junction, veins are found more superficially in the lamina propria rather than the submucosa. This results in reduced support from surrounding tissues owing to the predominant intraluminal location of these varices and might explain the predilection for bleeding at this site. The opening and dilation of portosystemic collaterals appears to depend on a threshold portal pressure gradient

(measured as hepatic venous pressure gradient [HVPG]) of 12 mm Hg, below which varices do not form. This pressure gradient is necessary but not sufficient for the development of gastroesophageal varices.

Diagnosis

The current consensus states that every patient with liver cirrhosis should undergo an upper endoscopy to detect gastroesophageal varices. The main aim behind screening for gastroesophageal varices is to identify patients requiring prophylactic treatment or further surveillance. Several invasive and noninvasive procedures help in detecting portal hypertension and can, with variable accuracy, predict the presence of gastroesophageal varices. Unfortunately, none are sensitive enough to replace endoscopy. A recent meta-analysis showed that transient elastography may be a useful screening tool for the detection of significant liver fibrosis and associated portal hypertension, but it is not useful at predicting the presence or size of esophageal varices. Smaller trials have evaluated the usefulness of spleen and liver MR elastography in assessing portal hypertension and varices, but this modality has not yet found its way into clinical practice. The combination of an elastography value below 20 kPa together and a platelet count above 150,000 nearly excludes the presence of esophageal varices requiring treatment. Endoscopic videocapsule is a new modality introduced for visualizing the esophagus; it allows correct identification of varices in 80% of cases but can have poor accuracy in identifying the presence of hypertensive gastropathy and gastric varices.

Not all esophageal varices bleed; hemorrhage occurs in only 30% to 35% of patients with cirrhosis. Variceal rupture is directly related to physical factors such as the radius, thickness, and elastic properties of the vessel in addition to intravariceal and intraluminal pressure and tension. Endoscopic findings that predict a higher risk of bleeding include larger size of varices and the presence of endoscopic red signs (described as red wale markings) on the variceal wall, indicating dilated intraepithelial and subepithelial superficial veins. A combination of clinical and endoscopic findings, including the Child-Pugh class, size of varices, and the presence or absence of red wale markings, was found to correlate highly with the risk of first bleeding in patients with cirrhosis. Hemodynamic parameters examined as predictors of bleeding include HVPG, azygous blood flow, and direct measurement of intravariceal pressure.

HVPG, calculated by the gradient of wedged and free hepatic vein pressure (normal value, 5 mm Hg), is used most often and provides reliable measurement of portal pressure in patients with cirrhosis. The extent of elevation of HVPG may be the best indicator of risk of bleeding, severity of bleeding, and survival. A rise in pressure in a patient with known varices increases the risk of bleeding, and the extent of portal pressure elevation has an inverse relationship to prognosis after hemorrhage has occurred. In general, however, a linear relationship between the degree of portal hypertension and the risk of variceal hemorrhage or formation of varices does not exist, so this technique cannot be used routinely to identify individual patients at high risk for bleeding.

Treatment
Primary Prophylaxis

The natural evolution of gastroesophageal varices without treatment is characterized by an increase in size from small to large varices, which eventually rupture and bleed. The progression rate ranges from 5% to 30% per year. The incidence of bleeding from small esophageal varices is estimated to be 4% per year, and it is as high as 15% per year for medium to large varices. In a randomized, controlled trial, the nonselective β-blocker timolol (Blocadren)[1] failed to reduce the development of varices or variceal bleeding in patients without varices. Adverse events were more common in the timolol group. Therefore, it is not

---

[1] Not FDA approved for this indication.

TABLE 1	Summary of Therapy for Esophageal Varices			
	FIRST-LINE THERAPY	**COMMENTS**	**ALTERNATIVE THERAPY**	**COMMENTS**
Primary prophylaxis*	β-Blockers or band ligation	In advanced cirrhosis, the best therapy is unclear (probably band ligation) Transplantation should be considered for these patients		The effectiveness of combined β-blockers and band ligation is unknown Neither TIPS nor sclerotherapy is recommended for primary prophylaxis
Active variceal bleeding	Somatostatin,[2] octreotide (Sandostatin),[1] vapreotide (Sanvar),[5] or terlipressin (Glypressin)[2]	Vasoconstrictors should be continued for ≥2 days after endoscopic therapy Band ligation is superior to endoscopic sclerotherapy	Balloon tamponade or SEMS (self-expandable metal stent) TIPS	Tamponade is indicated primarily as a temporizing measure if first-line treatment fails TIPS is reserved for refractory or recurrent early bleeding but should also be considered when basal HVPG >20 mm Hg
	plus Endoscopic therapy	Antibiotic prophylaxis should be initiated	Shunt surgery	Surgery is reserved for patients with compensated liver disease in whom TIPS fails or is not technically feasible
Secondary prophylaxis	β-Blockers ± nitrates *or* Band ligation	The combination of band ligation and β-blockers ± nitrates may be more effective than either alone Nitrates alone are not recommended Patients with advanced liver disease are often intolerant of β-blockers	TIPS Shunt surgery	TIPS is best used after failure of first-line therapy or as a bridge to transplantation in patients with advanced liver disease Shunt surgery is reserved for selected patients with compensated cirrhosis in whom TIPS fails or is not feasible

Abbreviations: HVPG = hepatic venous pressure gradient; TIPS = transjugular intrahepatic portosystemic shunt.
[1]Not FDA approved for this indication.
[2]Not available in the United States.
[5]Investigational drug in the United States.
*Upon documentation of varices, variceal hemorrhage occurs in 25%–30% of patients by 2 years. β-Blockers reduce the risk to 15%–18%, and combination β-blockers plus nitrates reduce the risk to 7.5%–10%.

recommended to start β-blockers in patients who do not yet have esophageal varices.

Based on prospective studies of cirrhotic patients with varices identified at endoscopy and of untreated groups in randomized controlled trials, the risk of bleeding from esophageal varices has been estimated at 25% to 35% at 1 year. Therapy for primary prophylaxis against variceal bleeding (prevention of a first variceal bleeding) is summarized in Table 1.

Pharmacologic Therapy

The general objective of pharmacologic therapy for variceal bleeding is to reduce portal pressure and consequently intravariceal pressure. Drugs that reduce portocollateral venous flow (vasoconstrictors) or intrahepatic vascular resistance (vasodilators) have been used and include β-blockers, nitrates, β2-adrenergic blockers, spironolactone (Aldactone),[1] pentoxifylline (Trental),[1] molsidomine (Corvaton),[2] and simvastatin (Zocor).[1] Because varices do not bleed at an HVPG less than 12 mm Hg, reduction to this level is ideal, but substantial reductions in HVPG (i.e., by >20%) are also clinically meaningful.

β-Blockers exert their beneficial effect on portal venous pressure by diminishing splanchnic blood flow and consequently gastroesophageal collateral and azygous blood flow. The effectiveness of β-blockers for primary prophylaxis against variceal bleeding has been demonstrated in several controlled trials. Meta-analyses have revealed a 40% to 50% reduction in bleeding and a trend toward improved survival. The estimated overall response rate is 49%, with bleeding rates of 6% in responders and 32% in nonresponders, with a number needed to treat (NNT) of 10.

The nonselective β-blockers, such as propranolol (Inderal)[1] and nadolol (Corgard),[1] are preferred because of the dual benefit of β1- and β2-receptor blockade. In the absence of HVPG determination, β-blockers are titrated to achieve a reduction in resting heart rate to 55 beats/min or 25% of baseline. Propranolol is generally given as a long-acting preparation and titrated to a maximum dose of 320 mg/day. Nadolol is initiated at 80 mg daily up to a maximum daily dose of 240 mg. Carvedilol (Coreg)[1] is initiated at 6.25 mg daily and increased if tolerated to 12.5 mg/day. Carvedilol is superior to propranolol at reducing portal hypertension although available data do not allow a satisfactory comparison of adverse events. The portal pressure–reducing effects of β-blockers are not predictable; the resultant reduction in heart rate or the measurement of drug blood levels are not good indicators of response to therapy. For example, portal venous pressure is reduced in about 60% to 70% of patients who receive propranolol therapy, but only 10% to 30% of these patients show a substantial response (i.e., >20% reduction). Additionally, approximately 20% to 25%

---

[2] Not available in the United States.

of patients have no measurable decline in portal pressure despite increasing dosage of propranolol. Of note, there is increasing evidence that the use of beta-blockers can be deleterious in patients with decompensated liver cirrhosis and refractory ascites (Sersté) or in patients with spontaneous bacterial peritonitis (Mandorfer).

In addition to β-blockers, a number of vasodilators have been investigated in patients with portal hypertension and in animal models of portal hypertension, most notably isosorbide mononitrate (Imdur).[1] Of note, there is increasing evidence that the use of β-blockers can be deleterious in patients with decompensated liver cirrhosis, refractory ascites, and severe circulatory dysfunction (systolic blood pressure 90 mm Hg, serum sodium <30 meq/fL, or hepatorenal syndrome). The exact mechanism of action of nitrates is unclear but is thought to be mediated primarily by reducing intrahepatic resistance and possibly by splanchnic arterial vasoconstriction induced in response to venous pooling and vasodilation in other regional vascular beds. Monotherapy with nitrates is ineffective in primary prophylaxis and can have detrimental effects, particularly in cirrhotic patients with ascites, and should not be used.

The addition of isosorbide mononitrate to β-blockers, however, has been shown to result in an enhanced reduction in portal pressure in humans. In a randomized, controlled trial involving 42 patients with cirrhosis and esophageal varices, a reduction of greater than 20% in HVPG was documented in only 10% in the propranolol group compared to 50% in the combination therapy group. In patients with Child-Pugh class A and B cirrhosis, the addition of isosorbide mononitrate to nadolol has been shown, in a randomized trial, to result in a greater than 50% additional reduction in variceal bleeding rate when compared with nadolol monotherapy (12% versus 29%). However, a large subsequent double-blind, placebo-controlled study failed to confirm these results. Based on the existing evidence, the combination of β-blockers and isosorbide is not recommended in primary prophylaxis.

Endoscopic Therapy

Endoscopic therapies play a prominent role in treatment of esophageal varices. Endoscopic band ligation (EBL) is the endoscopic procedure of choice in the management of esophageal varices. As of 2010, 16 randomized, controlled trials have compared EBL to β-blockers in the primary prevention of variceal bleeding. These studies suffered from significant heterogeneity, and a large number were published in abstract form. Two meta-analyses of these trials showed a slight advantage of EBL over β-blockers in terms of primary prevention of variceal bleeding, but there were no differences in mortality. A recent Cochrane database systematic review found a beneficial effect of band ligation compared to β-blockers in primary prevention of upper gastrointestinal bleeding in adult patients with esophageal varices. Again, there was no difference in mortality.

β-Blockers are cheaper and much easier to administer but are associated with issues of noncompliance and a higher incidence of adverse events (e.g., hypotension, impotence, insomnia) than EBL. However, most of these side effects are easy to manage and none require hospitalization or result in direct mortality. On the other hand, adverse events related to EBL, such as bleeding from band-related ulcers, albeit infrequent, are more significant, often requiring hospitalization and blood transfusion, and may rarely be associated with death.

According to the Baveno consensus conference, nonselective β-blockers should be considered as a first choice for preventing first variceal bleeding in high-risk patients who have not bled, and EBL should be provided for patients with contraindications or intolerance to β-blockers. The recent guidelines by the American College of Gastroenterology (ACG) and American Association for the Study of Liver Diseases (AASLD) recommend using β-blockers in low-risk patients who have medium to large varices but suggest both EBL and β-blockers for high-risk patients as first-line therapy. The optimal primary prophylaxis in patients with

decompensated cirrhosis remains unclear and is arguably expedited liver transplantation. The combination of pharmacologic plus endoscopic therapy has been investigated in such patients with conflicting results. In one study, EBL plus β-blockers offered no benefit in terms of prevention of first bleeding when compared to EBL alone. In a more recent study, combination therapy significantly reduced the occurrence of the first episode of variceal bleeding and improved bleeding-related survival in a group of cirrhotic patients with high-risk esophageal varices awaiting liver transplantation.

Management of Acute Variceal Hemorrhage

Variceal hemorrhage is usually an acute clinical event characterized by rapid gastrointestinal blood loss manifesting as hematemesis (which can be massive), with or without melena or hematochezia. Hemodynamic instability (tachycardia, hypotension) is common. Although variceal bleeding is common in patients with cirrhosis presenting with acute upper gastrointestinal hemorrhage, other causes of bleeding, such as ulcer disease, must be considered. Urgent initiation of empiric pharmacologic therapy with vasoactive agents is indicated in situations where variceal hemorrhage is likely. Subsequently, direct endoscopic examination is critical to establish an accurate diagnosis and to provide the rationale for immediate and subsequent therapies. The immediate steps in the management of acute variceal bleeding include: volume resuscitation, prevention of complications, ensuring hemostasis, and initiating measures to prevent early and delayed rebleeding.

Patients with variceal hemorrhage and ascites are at increased risk for bacterial infections, particularly spontaneous bacterial peritonitis. This risk appears to be increased in the setting of uncontrolled hemorrhage or as a result of transient bacteremia following endoscopic sclerotherapy or variceal ligation. Short-term systemic antibiotics (e.g., third-generation cephalosporins or fluoroquinolones for 4–10 days) have been shown to decrease the risk of bacterial infections and to reduce rebleeding as well as mortality in cirrhotic patients with gastrointestinal bleeding.

A restrictive transfusion strategy should be used, aiming for a hemoglobin of 7 to 8 gm/dL to avoid volume overexpansion and perpetuation of bleeding. The role of platelet transfusion or fresh frozen plasma administration has not been assessed appropriately. The routine administration of fresh frozen plasma in patients with active variceal bleeding may in fact be detrimental because of the resultant volume expansion and should be discouraged. Hypofibrinogenemia should be treated with cryoprecipitate aiming for levels >100 mg/dL. The use of recombinant activated coagulation factor VII (rFVIIa [Novoseven]),[1] which corrects prothrombin time in cirrhotic patients, has been assessed in two randomized, controlled trials. The first trial showed, in a post hoc analysis, that rFVIIa administration might significantly improve the results of conventional therapy in patients with moderate and advanced liver failure (Child-Pugh B and C) without increasing the incidence of adverse events. A more recent trial tested rVIIa in patients with active bleeding at endoscopy and with a Child-Pugh score 8 points or higher. This trial failed to show a benefit of rVIIa in terms of decreasing the risk of 5-day failure, but it did show improved 6-week mortality. In a small prospective study involving cirrhotic patients with acute variceal bleeding and new portal vein thrombosis identified by positive intra-thrombus enhancement on contrast ultrasonography, the use of low molecular weight heparin after hemostasis is achieved by band ligation was shown to be safe, well tolerated, and effective, with complete recanalization of the portal vein within 2 to 11 days and no recurrence of bleeding.

Pharmacologic Therapy

Pharmacologic therapy can be administered early, requires no special technical expertise, and is thus a desirable first-line option

---

[1]Not FDA approved for this indication.

for managing acute variceal hemorrhage. Drugs that reduce portocollateral venous flow (vasoconstrictors) or intrahepatic vascular resistance (vasodilators) or both have been used to achieve this effect. Vasoconstrictors work by decreasing splanchnic arterial flow, and vasodilators are used in combination with vasoconstrictors to reduce their systemic side effects, but they can also exert an added beneficial effect on intrahepatic resistance (see Table 1).

Vasopressin and Terlipressin. Vasopressin (Pitressin)[1] is a nonselective vasoconstricting agent that causes a reduction of splanchnic blood flow and thereby a reduced portal pressure. Vasopressin, which is associated with severe vascular complications, has been largely replaced by other vasoconstrictors such as its synthetic analogue, triglycyl-lysine vasopressin (terlipressin [Glypressin]).[2] Terlipressin has fewer side effects and a longer biological half-life, allowing its use as a bolus intravenous injection (2 mg every 4 hours for the initial 24 hours, then 1 mg every 4 hours for the next 24–48 hours). Terlipressin has been shown in numerous placebo-controlled trials to control bleeding in about 80% of cases and is the only pharmacologic therapy proven, as of 2010, to reduce mortality from acute variceal hemorrhage. In patients with esophageal variceal bleeding, a 24-hour course of terlipressin was shown to be as effective as a 72-hour course when used as adjunct therapy to successful variceal band ligation. Terlipressin is not currently available in the United States.

Somatostatin, Octreotide, and Vapreotide. Somatostatin,[2] a naturally occurring peptide, and its analogues, octreotide (Sandostatin)[1] and vapreotide (Sanvar),[5] stop variceal hemorrhage in up to 80% of patients and are generally considered equivalent to vasopressin (Pitressin), terlipressin[2] (Glypressin), and endoscopic therapy for the control of acute variceal bleeding. Their precise mechanism of action is unclear but might result from an effect on the release of vasoactive peptides or from reduction of postprandial hyperemia. Somatostatin is used as a continuous intravenous infusion of 250 µg/hour following a 250-µg bolus injection. Octreotide is used as a continuous infusion of 50 µg/hour and does not require a bolus injection. Side effects are minor, including hyperglycemia and mild abdominal cramps. The addition of octreotide or vapreotide to endoscopic sclerotherapy or banding improves control of bleeding and reduces transfusion requirements, with no change in overall mortality. A continuous infusion of octreotide or vapreotide is therefore recommended for 2 to 5 days following emergency endoscopic therapy.

Endoscopy
Endoscopic sclerotherapy stops variceal hemorrhage in 80% to 90% of cases. Its drawbacks include a significant risk of local complications including ulceration, bleeding, stricture, and perforation. Rare systemic complications have been reported including bacteremia with endocarditis, formation of splenic or brain abscesses, and portal vein thrombosis. Randomized trials in patients with acute variceal bleeding have shown that EBL is essentially equivalent to endoscopic sclerotherapy in achieving initial hemostasis with lesser complications. These include superficial ulcerations, transient chest discomfort, and, rarely, stricture formation. Erythromycin infusion before endoscopy[1] in patients with acute variceal bleeding has been shown to significantly improve endoscopic visibility and to shorten the duration of the procedure.

Balloon Tamponade/SEMS
The use of the Sengstaken-Blakemore or Minnesota tube for hemostasis of variceal bleeding is based on the principle of the application of direct pressure on the bleeding varix by an inflatable—esophageal or gastric—balloon fitted on a rubber nasogastric tube. When properly applied, balloon tamponade is successful in achieving immediate hemostasis in almost all cases. However, early rebleeding following balloon decompression is high. Complications of balloon tamponade include esophageal perforation or rupture, aspiration, and asphyxiation from upper airway obstruction. Balloon tamponade or use of SEMS is generally not recommended and should largely be reserved for rescue of cases of hemorrhage uncontrolled by pharmacologic and endoscopic methods and as a temporary bridge to more definitive therapy. Self-expandable metal stents (SEMS) have recently been shown to be effective in controlling severe bleeding.

Transjugular Intrahepatic Portosystemic Shunt
Treatment with a transjugular intrahepatic portosystemic shunt (TIPS) consists of the vascular placement of an expandable metal stent across a tract created between a hepatic vein and a major intrahepatic branch of the portal system. TIPS can be successfully performed in 90% to 100% of patients, resulting in hemodynamic changes similar to a partially decompressive side-to-side portocaval shunt while avoiding the morbidity and mortality associated with a major surgical procedure. TIPS has been shown to be effective in treating refractory, uncontrolled, acute variceal bleeding. Patients with advanced liver disease and multiorgan failure at the time of TIPS have a 30-day mortality that approaches 100%.

Surgery
Surgery is generally considered in the setting of continued hemorrhage or recurrent early rebleeding—uncontrolled by repeated endoscopic or continued pharmacologic therapy—and when TIPS is not available or is not technically feasible. Surgical options include portosystemic shunting or esophageal staple transection alone or with esophagogastric devascularization and splenectomy (Sugiura procedure). Devascularization procedures may be useful in patients who cannot receive a shunt because of splanchnic venous thrombosis. Regardless of the choice of surgical technique, morbidity is high and the 30-day mortality for emergency surgery approaches 80% in some series. Understandably, rescue liver transplantation is not a practical option in patients with uncontrolled variceal hemorrhage.

Secondary Prophylaxis
Variceal hemorrhage recurs in approximately two thirds of patients, most commonly within the first 6 weeks after the initial episode. Patients with advanced liver disease (MELD [model for end-stage liver disease] score ≥18) have an increased risk of early rebleeding and death. Early rebleeding (within the first 5 days) is reduced by the adjuvant use of octreotide[1] or vapreotide[5]—and possibly terlipressin[2] and somatostatin[2]—after initial endoscopic or pharmacologic control of hemorrhage.

The severity of portal hypertension correlates closely with the severity and risk of rebleeding as well as actuarial probability of survival following an index episode. In a cohort of patients presenting with variceal hemorrhage, those with an initial HVPG greater than 20 mm Hg had a 1-year mortality of 64% compared to 20% for patients with lesser elevations in portal pressure. Given the high risk of recurrent hemorrhage and its associated morbidity and mortality, strategies aimed at prevention should be rapidly instituted following the index episode. The choice of preventive therapy should, therefore, take into consideration the efficacy of therapy, the side effects of the selected treatment, the patient's expected survival, and overall cost. Preventive strategies include pharmacologic, endoscopic, and surgical methods and are listed in Table 1. Relative effectiveness of these strategies is shown in Figure 1.

---

[1] Not FDA approved for this indication.
[2] Not available in the United States.
[5] Investigational drug in the United States.

---

[1] Not FDA approved for this indication.
[2] Not available in the United States.
[5] Investigational drug in the United States.

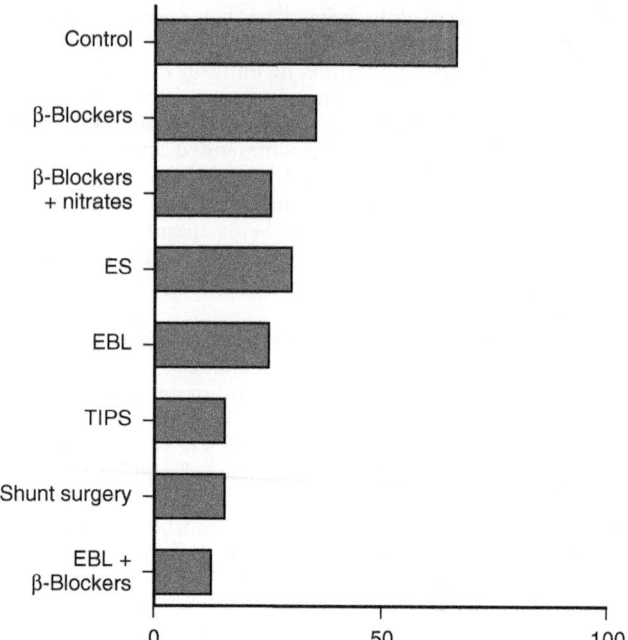

Figure 1 Relative effectiveness of available therapies for preventing recurrent variceal bleeding. The estimates shown are based on the cumulative data available in the literature for recurrent bleeding at 1 year. *Abbreviations:* EBL = endoscopic band ligation; ES = endoscopic sclerotherapy; TIPS = transjugular intrahepatic portosystemic shunt.

Pharmacologic Therapy

Reducing the portal pressure by more than 20% from the baseline value pharmacologically results in a reduction in the cumulative probability of recurrent bleeding from 28% at 1 year, 39% at 2 years, and 66% at 3 years to 4%, 9%, and 9%, respectively. Although adjustment of medical therapy based on portal pressure measurement would be ideal, HVPG determination might not be readily available, and treatment must be adjusted using empiric clinical parameters. Several randomized, controlled trials, including a meta-analysis, have demonstrated that β-blockers prevent rebleeding and prolong survival. The addition of isosorbide mononitrate[1] to β-blockers appears to enhance the protective effect of β-blockers alone for preventing recurrent variceal bleeding but offers no survival advantage and reduces the tolerability of therapy. A recent randomized controlled trial showed that carvedilol[1] is as effective as the combination of nadolol plus isorsobide-5 mononitrate in the prevention of gastroesophageal variceal rebleeding, with fewer severe adverse events and similar survival. Compared with either sclerotherapy or endoscopic band ligation, combination medical therapy is superior in reducing the risk of recurrent bleeding in patients with esophageal variceal hemorrhage, primarily in patients with Child-Pugh class A and B cirrhosis. Notably, in patients who show a significant hemodynamic response to therapy (defined as a reduction in the hepatic venous pressure gradient to <12 mm Hg or >20% of the baseline value), the risk of recurrent bleeding and of death is significantly reduced.

Endoscopy

Endoscopic therapy has been established over the past decade as a therapeutic cornerstone for preventing esophageal variceal rebleeding. Gastric varices, however, are not effectively treated by sclerotherapy or ligation. Patients with recurrent gastric variceal hemorrhage are best treated by *N*-butyl-2-cyanoacrylate injection[1] or by nonendoscopic means such as TIPS. On the other hand, EBL is highly effective at obliterating esophageal varices and is considered the endoscopic therapy of choice for secondary prophylaxis.

Combination modality approaches, usually including an endoscopic and pharmacologic treatment, are pathophysiologically attractive and may be more effective than single therapy. Two randomized, controlled trials have shown that adding β-blockers to EBL reduces the risk of rebleeding and variceal recurrence, suggesting that if EBL is used, it should be used in association with β-blockers. One randomized, controlled trial has evaluated whether EBL could improve the efficacy of the combined administration of nadolol[1] plus isosorbide.[1] In this study, adding band ligation to nadolol plus isosorbide was shown to be superior to nadolol plus isosorbide alone in preventing variceal rebleeding, but there were no significant differences in mortality. The combination of the best endoscopic treatment (EBL) and the best pharmacologic treatment (β-blockers plus isosorbide) may be the best choice in preventing rebleeding but needs further studies for confirmation. Statins improve liver generation of NO and hepatic endothelial dysfunction in experimental models of cirrhosis and may also reduce liver fibrosis. Randomized placebo-controlled trials found that simvastatin[1] decreased HVPG and improved liver perfusion and had an additive effect in patients treated with NSBB, and showed survival benefit in patients with early stages of cirrhosis and variceal bleeding.

Transjugular Intrahepatic Portosystemic Shunt

Transjugular shunting is more effective than endoscopic therapy for preventing variceal rebleeding but offers no survival benefit. The cumulative risk of rebleeding following TIPS placement is 8% to 18% at 1 year. The trade-off, however, is that TIPS is associated with a higher incidence of clinically significant hepatic encephalopathy (new or worsened portosystemic encephalopathy was noted in about 25% of patients after TIPS). Advanced liver disease is the main determinant of poor outcome following TIPS. Consequently, in patients with advanced liver disease, TIPS is best used as a bridge to liver transplantation.

TIPS, using bare stents, has been compared with surgical shunts in two studies (8 mm portocaval H-graft shunt in one and distal splenorenal shunt in the second). Although the first study showed a significantly lower rebleeding rate in the surgical group, the second and larger trial did not find any differences in rebleeding rates, hepatic encephalopathy, or mortality, but it found a significantly higher reintervention rate in the TIPS group. However, the obstruction and reintervention rates are markedly decreased with the recent use of polytetrafluoroethylene (PTFE)-covered stents. According to these data, TIPS using PTFE-covered stents represents the best rescue therapy for failures of medical and endoscopic treatment.

Surgery

Portosystemic shunt surgery is the most effective means by which to reduce portal pressure. Although effective at eradicating varices and preventing rebleeding, nonselective portocaval shunts are associated with a significant incidence of hepatic encephalopathy, portal vein thrombosis, and occasionally liver failure. Commonly used shunts include the distal splenorenal shunt and the low-diameter (mesocaval or portocaval) interposition shunt. Rates of recurrent bleeding are on the order of 10%, with the highest risk of bleeding occurring in the first month after surgery. Devascularization procedures (i.e., esophageal transection and gastroesophageal devascularization) are usually considered in patients who cannot receive shunts because of splanchnic venous thrombosis and should be performed only by experienced surgeons. Surgical therapy has been largely supplanted by TIPS.

Cost-Effectiveness of Available Therapies

Data examining the cost of variceal bleeding and the cost-effectiveness of commonly used therapies are limited. The treatment cost of an episode of variceal bleeding has been estimated at $15,000 to $40,000. The cost-effectiveness of diagnostic methods

---

[5] Investigational drug in the United States.

[1] Not FDA approved for this indication.

used to guide therapy is unclear. For example, HVPG determination, which can accurately predict pharmacologic response to therapy, is an attractive, although invasive, adjunct in the management of patients with variceal bleeding, but its cost-effectiveness remains in question. Further, screening endoscopy for detecting large varices, while recommended, has not been demonstrated to be cost-effective.

There are areas in which management is controversial and not standardized. For example, given the right expertise, secondary prophylaxis with surgical shunts or TIPS may be more effective than medical or endoscopic therapy in Child-Pugh class A patients. On the other hand, patients with advanced cirrhosis are often intolerant of β-blockers—let alone in combination with nitrates—and therefore the use of combination therapy remains controversial in such patients. Arguably, the preferred treatment for such patients is TIPS as a bridge to early liver transplantation.

Therefore, when choosing a specific treatment plan, the clinician must take into consideration the direct costs of health care utilization, as well as the efficacy and morbidity of therapy. The treatment chosen should be tailored to fit the patient's clinical condition while also taking into account the possibility that the patient's liver disease can progress and thus necessitate transplantation. The cost-effectiveness of various treatment modalities should factor in the cost of failed therapy (e.g., rebleeding, shunt revision) and that of treatment-related complications (e.g., encephalopathy, esophageal stricture).

Summary

Esophageal variceal hemorrhage is a common and devastating complication of portal hypertension and is a leading cause of morbidity and mortality in patients with cirrhosis. Because the clinical outcomes are poor once variceal bleeding has occurred, primary prophylaxis with β-blockers or EBL should be considered in high-risk patients. The treatment of acute variceal hemorrhage is aimed at judicious volume resuscitation and ensuring hemostasis with pharmacologic agents and endoscopic techniques as well as prevention of complications, such as infections by the use of prophylactic antibiotics.

A high risk of rebleeding after an index episode mandates the institution of preventive strategies. Wedge pressure-guided medical therapy may be the preferred mode of secondary prophylaxis in patients with Child Pugh class A or B cirrhosis, but is invasive and not widely available. Patients at high risk for rebleeding, including those with decompensated or advanced liver disease, should be considered for TIPS followed by liver transplantation when applicable. Treatment with a combination of methods is pathophysiologically attractive, but the choice of therapy should ultimately be tailored to fit the patient's clinical condition, risk factors, and prognosis, taking into account issues of risk-to-benefit ratio, compliance, and cost.

References

Abraldes JG, Villanueva C, Aracil C, et al: Addition of simvastatin to standard therapy for the prevention of variceal rebleeding does not reduce rebleeding but increases survival in patients with cirrhosis, *Gastroenterology* 2016 Jan 13. Epub ahead of print.

Azam Z, Hamid S, Jafri W, et al: Short course adjuvant terlipressin in acute variceal bleeding: a randomized double blind dummy controlled trial, *J Hepatol* 56:819–824, 2012.

Bambha K, Kim WR, Pedersen R, et al: Predictors of early rebleeding and mortality after acute variceal haemorrhage in patients with cirrhosis, *Gut* 57:814–820, 2008.

de Franchis R, Baveno VIF: Expanding consensus in portal hypertension: report of the Baveno VI Consensus Workshop: stratifying risk and individualizing care for portal hypertension, *J Hepatol* 63(3):743–752, 2015.

Feu F, Garcia-Pagan JC, Bosch J, et al: Relation between portal pressure response to pharmacotherapy and risk of recurrent variceal haemorrhage in patients with cirrhosis, *Lancet* 346:1056–1059, 1995.

Garcia Pagan JC, De Gottardi A, Bosch J: Review article: the modern management of portal hypertension—primary and secondary prophylaxis of variceal bleeding in cirrhotic patients, *Aliment Pharmacol Ther* 28:178–186, 2008.

Garcia-Pagan JC, Feu F, Bosch J, Rodes J: Propranolol compared with propranolol plus isosorbide-5-mononitrate for portal hypertension in cirrhosis. A randomized controlled study, *Ann Intern Med* 114:869–873, 1991.

Gluud LL, Krag A: Banding ligation versus beta-blockers for primary prevention in oesophageal varices in adults, *Cochrane Database Syst Rev* 8, 2012, CD004544.

Laine L, Cook D: Endoscopic ligation compared with sclerotherapy for treatment of esophageal variceal bleeding. A meta-analysis, *Ann Intern Med* 123:280–287, 1995.

Lo GH, Chen WC, Wang HM, Yu HC: Randomized, controlled trial of carvedilol versus nadolol plus isosorbide mononitrate for the prevention of variceal rebleeding, *J Gastroenterol Hepatol* 27(11):1681–1687, 2012.

Mandorfer M, Bota S, Schwabl P, et al: Nonselective β-blockers increase risk for hepatorenal syndrome and death in patients with cirrhosis and spontaneous bacterial peritonitis, *Gastroenterology* 146:1680–1690, 2014.

Maruyama H, Takahashi M, Shimada T, Yokosuka O: Emergency anticoagulation treatment for cirrhosis patients with portal vein thrombosis and acute variceal bleeding, *Scand J Gastroenterol* 47:686–691, 2012.

Merkel C, Marin R, Sacerdoti D, et al: Long-term results of a clinical trial of nadolol with or without isosorbide mononitrate for primary prophylaxis of variceal bleeding in cirrhosis, *Hepatology* 31:324–329, 2000.

Moitinho E, Escorsell A, Bandi JC, et al: Prognostic value of early measurements of portal pressure in acute variceal bleeding, *Gastroenterology* 117:626–631, 1999.

North Italian Endoscopic Club for the Study and Treatment of Esophageal Varices: Prediction of the first variceal hemorrhage in patients with cirrhosis of the liver and esophageal varices: A prospective multicenter study, *N Engl J Med* 319:983–989, 1988.

Northup PG, Caldwell SH: Coagulation in liver disease: A guide for the clinician, *Clin Gastroenterol Hepatol* 11:1064–1074, 2013.

Polio J, Groszmann RJ: Hemodynamic factors involved in the development and rupture of esophageal varices: a pathophysiologic approach to treatment, *Semin Liver Dis* 6:318–331, 1986.

Poynard T, Cales P, Pasta L, et al: β-Adrenergic-antagonist drugs in the prevention of gastrointestinal bleeding in patients with cirrhosis and esophageal varices. An analysis of data and prognostic factors in 589 patients from four randomized clinical trials. Franco-Italian Multicenter Study Group, *N Engl J Med* 324:1532–1538, 1991.

Sersté T, Melot C, Francoz C, et al: Deleterious effects of beta-blockers on survival in patients with cirrhosis and refractory ascites, *Hepatology* 52:1017–1022, 2010.

Sharara AI, Rockey DC: Gastroesophageal variceal hemorrhage, *N Engl J Med* 345:669–681, 2001.

Shi KQ, Fan YC, Pan ZZ, et al: Transient elastography: a meta-analysis of diagnostic accuracy in evaluation of portal hypertension in chronic liver disease, *Liver Int* 33:62–71, 2013.

Sinagra E, Perricone G, D'Amico M, Tiné F, D'Amico G, *Systematic review with meta-analysis: the haemodynamic effects of carvedilol compared with propranolol for portal hypertension in cirrhosis. Aliment Pharmacol Ther* 39:557–568, 2014.

Villanueva C, Minana J, Ortiz J, et al: Endoscopic ligation compared with combined treatment with nadolol and isosorbide mononitrate to prevent recurrent variceal bleeding, *N Engl J Med* 345:647–655, 2001.

CALCULOUS BILIARY DISEASE

Method of
Zachary L. Smith, DO; and Mick S. Meiselman, MD

CURRENT DIAGNOSIS

- True biliary colic is characterized by the abrupt onset and cessation of severe mid-epigastric or, less commonly, right upper quadrant pain.
- Pain commonly starts 1 to 2 hours after eating and can be localized or radiate to the back, right shoulder, or chest.
- The onset of biliary colic commonly occurs during sleep.
- Nausea and vomiting commonly follow the onset of pain.
- Elevations of total and conjugated bilirubin, ALP, and GGT with modest elevations in AST and ALT support a suspected diagnosis of choledocholithiasis.
- A normal serum biochemistry profile has a negative predictive value of 97% for ruling out choledocholithiasis.
- Transabdominal ultrasonography is a useful and cost-effective test for diagnosing cholelithiasis; however, it has significantly lower utility for choledocholithiasis.
- For intermediate-risk patients with suspected choledocholithiasis, examination of the common bile duct with magnetic resonance cholangiopancreatography (MRCP) or endoscopic ultrasonography (EUS) is warranted.

CURRENT THERAPY

- The treatment of choice for symptomatic cholelithiasis is laparoscopic cholecystectomy. Elective laparoscopic cholecystectomy should only be performed for true biliary colic. Vague symptoms such as bloating, dyspepsia, and atypical abdominal pain are not commonly related to gallstone disease and thus are not an indication for gallbladder removal.
- Laparoscopic cholecystectomy should generally take place within 72 hours of presentation for acute cholecystitis in appropriate surgical candidates.
- Laparoscopic cholecystectomy is recommended in pregnant patients with symptomatic cholelithiasis and acute cholecystitis. This is best done by experienced surgeons in the second or early third trimesters.
- Patients who should undergo preoperative ERCP for choledocholithiasis include those with high risk stratification and those deemed intermediate risk in whom a common bile duct stone is identified on MRCP or endoscopic ultrasonography.

Cholelithiasis

Epidemiology

Gallstone disease is common in Western populations, affecting 10% to 15% of adults. It is estimated that 6.3 million men and 14.2 million women in the United States have gallstones. Although the vast majority of patients remain asymptomatic throughout their lifetime, roughly one third develop symptoms or complications.

Pathophysiology

Gallstones can be categorized based on their composition. Of patients with gallstone disease in the Western world, 80% to 90% have cholesterol stones or cholesterol-predominant stones (mixed stones). Pigment gallstones account for the remaining 5% to 10%. Patients with hemolytic disorders are prone to pigment stone formation, and therefore the correspondence with disorders such as sickle cell anemia, hereditary spherocytosis, and Gilbert's syndrome is high.

Risk Factors

Risk factors for gallstone disease include female sex, age greater than 40 years, white, Latin American, and Native American descent, family history, obesity, rapid weight loss, starvation, total parenteral nutrition, bariatric surgery, diabetes mellitus, and hypertriglyceridemia.

Clinical Manifestations

The typical symptomatic presentation of gallstone disease is biliary colic. This is described as severe pain located in the midepigastrium or, less commonly, the right upper quadrant, that begins and ceases abruptly. The pain is typically constant, occurring 1 to 2 hours after a meal, and can either be localized or radiate to the back or right shoulder. Often the onset of pain occurs during sleep. Nausea and vomiting commonly accompany biliary pain, and, as with most surgical entities, pain typically precedes the onset of these symptoms. Biliary colic can also manifest as chest pain and is occasionally mistaken for cardiac angina. Prolonged episodes of pain localized to the right upper quadrant often herald cholecystitis rather than biliary colic. A clinical history containing the cardinal features of biliary colic carries a high diagnostic accuracy.

Diagnosis

Transabdominal ultrasonography is the preferred initial imaging test for cholelithiasis. The sensitivity for detecting the presence of gallstones within the gallbladder lumen on ultrasonography is 97%.

Biliary Sludge

Biliary sludge is often diagnosed on transabdominal ultrasonography. It appears as low-amplitude nonshadowing echoes that layer in dependent portions of the gallbladder. The clinical course of biliary sludge varies from patient to patient. Some patients remain symptom free, and others develop overt biliary colic. A fraction of patients demonstrate resolution of biliary sludge on repeat imaging. Symptomatic biliary sludge should be treated the same as cholelithiasis. Similarly, patients with asymptomatic biliary sludge should be managed expectantly.

Treatment

In patients with symptomatic cholelithiasis, treatment should be aimed at acute pain control and prevention of recurrent episodes. In patients without contraindications, cholecystectomy is the preferred choice for treatment of symptomatic uncomplicated cholelithiasis. This is preferably done via laparoscopy, which offers lower rates of complications and postoperative pain along with better cosmetic results when compared with open cholecystectomy.

Because of the high incidence of cholelithiasis, true biliary colic should be identified before a decision is made to proceed with laparoscopic cholecystectomy. Vague symptoms such as bloating or atypical abdominal pain are not typical of gallstone disease and thus often persist after surgery. In cases of asymptomatic uncomplicated cholelithiasis, elective cholecystectomy is not recommended unless the patient is diabetic or is undergoing an operation such as gastric bypass surgery, after which there is an increased risk of gallstone formation.

There is a very limited role for medical management of gallstone disease. Nonoperative management of symptomatic cholelithiasis involves bile dissolution with ursodeoxycholic acid (Actigall). The use of medical therapy is limited based on poor efficacy and high rates of recurrence and thus should be reserved only rarely for nonsurgical candidates.

Analgesia is an important adjunct in the treatment of symptomatic cholelithiasis. In patients with severe symptoms requiring narcotic pain medication, meperidine (Demerol) is preferred over morphine because it has less effect on the sphincter of Oddi. Nonsteroidal antiinflammatory drugs (NSAIDs) are another mainstay of therapy. Parenterally administered ketorolac (Toradol) is perhaps the most commonly used agent for biliary colic in the acute care setting. Studies have shown that NSAIDs are beneficial in the management of pain due to gallstones, and at least one study has suggested that early administration of NSAIDs might decrease the progression to acute cholecystitis.

Complications

Complications that can potentially arise from cholelithiasis include acute cholecystitis, cholangitis, pancreatitis, obstructive jaundice, and, rarely, gallstone ileus.

Choledocholithiasis

Choledocholithiasis often manifests concomitantly with symptomatic gallstone disease and is a finding in 5% to 10% of patients undergoing laparoscopic cholecystectomy for symptomatic cholelithiasis. The workup for suspected choledocholithiasis combines history, physical examination, laboratory data, and various imaging modalities. If the clinical history and physical examination are suggestive, the clinician should obtain serum liver biochemistry tests including alanine aminotransferase (ALT), aspartate aminotransferase (AST), total and fractionated bilirubin, alkaline phosphatase (ALP), and γ-glutamyl transpetidase (GGT).

The typical pattern of serum biochemistry is one of cholestasis. A conjugated hyperbilirubinemia along with high levels of GGT and ALP are seen often in the setting of modest elevation of the transaminases. ALP is usually elevated out of proportion to the transaminases; however, extreme levels of AST and ALT have been described. Transaminase levels greater than 1000 U/L, although rare in gallstone disease, should not dissuade the clinician from a diagnosis of choledocholithiasis. Serum biochemistries provide the most utility in ruling out common bile duct stones. A normal biochemical profile has a negative predictive value of 97%. Clinical predictors for assessing the likelihood of choledocholithiasis in patients with symptomatic cholelithiasis are listed in Box 1.

BOX 1 — Strategy to Assign Risk of Choledocholithiasis in Patients with Symptomatic Cholelithiasis, Based on Clinical Predictors

Predictors of Choledocholithiasis

High Risk
1. Common bile duct stone on ultrasound, CT scan or MRI
2. Total bilirubin >4 mg/dl *and* dilated common bile duct
3. Ascending cholangitis

Intermediate Risk
1. Other abnormal liver chemistry (e.g. total bilirubin 1-8-3.9 mg/dl, elevated AST, ALT, alkaline phosphatase)
2. Age >55 years
3. Dilated common bile duct on imaging

Low Risk
None of the above are present

From ASGE Standards of Practice Committee Buxbaum JL, Abbas SM, Sultan S, et al. ASGE guideline on the role of endoscopy in the evaluation and management of choledocholithiasis. Gastrointest Endosc. 2019;89(6):1075–1105.e15.

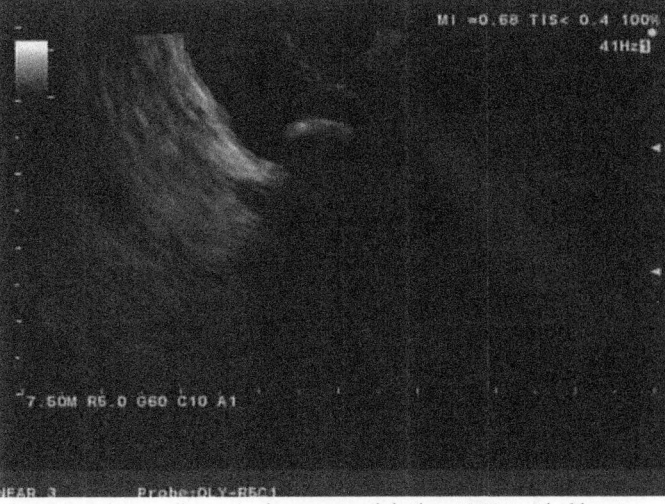

Figure 1 A large gallstone in the common bile duct (CBD) with dilatation of the CBD proximally. The endoscopic ultrasound probe is visualized in the top of the image, and a large cone-shaped shadow is cast distal to the gallstone.

Diagnosis

A variety of modalities are available for diagnosing choledocholithiasis. Perhaps the least expensive and most widely available test is transabdominal ultrasound. Although the sensitivity for cholelithiasis is quite high with transabdominal ultrasound, identifying stones in the common bile duct (Figure 1) is more difficult. Prospective studies have reported sensitivities ranging from 22% to 55% for detecting common bile duct stones; however, in our clinical experience the sensitivity is much lower. Other indirect indicators of choledocholithiasis such as common bile duct dilation (77%–88% sensitivity) can provide additional diagnostic clues. Based on the high false-negative rates for common bile duct stones and dilation, a negative transabdominal ultrasound scan cannot rule out choledocholithiasis. CT scanning has a higher sensitivity for choledocholithiasis than transabdominal ultrasound. Levels of radiation and cost have limited its use as a first-line diagnostic tool.

Three nonsurgical modalities offer true visualization of the common bile duct with comparable sensitivities: Magnetic resonance cholangiopancreatography (MRCP), endoscopic retrograde cholangiopancreatography (ERCP), and endoscopic ultrasonography (EUS). MRCP has a diagnostic sensitivity of 85% to 92% for detecting choledocholithiasis, and, although it is useful for helping determine which intermediate-risk patients would benefit from preoperative ERCP, small and distal common bile duct stones are often missed.

EUS and ERCP are both minimally invasive techniques useful in the diagnosis and management of choledocholithiasis. Owing to the proximity of the extrahepatic bile duct to the proximal duodenum, EUS provides high sensitivity (89%–94%) for detecting common bile duct stones and is especially useful for detecting stones less than 5 mm in diameter. ERCP provides similar diagnostic sensitivity; however, ERCP offers therapeutic capability. Because of the reasonably high risk of complications including pancreatitis (1.3%–15.1%), infection (0.6%–5.0%), gastrointestinal hemorrhage (0.3%–2.0%), and perforation (0.1%–1.1%), ERCP as an initial modality should be reserved for patients who have a high pretest probability for choledocholithiasis and particularly for those with complications such as acute cholangitis or severe pancreatitis.

Research has evaluated the use of ultrasound-guided ERCP with the goal of avoiding unnecessary bile duct cannulation, and reserving its use for therapeutic purposes only. A systematic review from 2009 showed that compared with ERCP alone, the use of EUS avoided unnecessary ERCP in 67.1% of patients in whom no common bile duct stone was identified. As more gastroenterologists become trained in this modality, EUS-guided ERCP might prove to be the preferred diagnostic modality in intermediate-risk patients for the diagnosis and initial therapy of choledocholithiasis.

Treatment

Patients with choledocholithiasis should be treated to avoid recurrent symptoms and development of complications. Stones can be extracted from the common bile duct via ERCP or laparoscopic cholecystectomy with bile duct exploration. Studies have shown similar efficacies without significant differences in morbidity or mortality; however, clinical expertise varies widely with the laparoscopic approach. Ultimately, cholecystectomy should be performed to prevent recurrence in surgical candidates. In patients undergoing laparoscopic cholecystectomy for suspected choledocholithiasis, perioperative management differs based on the risk stratification of the patient (see Box 1). High-risk patients should proceed directly to ERCP before surgery for attempted stone extraction. In intermediate-risk patients, a preoperative MRCP or EUS should be performed, and, if the results are positive, the patient should undergo ERCP as a prelude to surgery. For suspected choledocholithiasis in low-risk patients, surgery should be performed without further imaging of the common bile duct.

Complications

The two most common adverse complications of choledocholithiasis are gallstone pancreatitis and acute cholangitis. Gallstone pancreatitis develops in 3% to 7% of patients with gallstones and is the most common cause of acute pancreatitis in the United States. The diagnosis and management of acute pancreatitis is discussed in a separate chapter.

Acute cholangitis is caused by obstruction and stasis of the biliary tract with complicating bacterial infection. The syndrome is characterized by fever, jaundice, and abdominal pain, also known as Charcot's triad. Patients who develop hypotension and changes in mental status (Reynold's pentad) have a poorer prognosis. Elderly patients often do not demonstrate the classic signs of acute cholangitis, but they can develop a delayed-sepsis–like syndrome, of which hypotension is the most pronounced feature. High biliary pressures promote the translocation of bacteria from the portal circulation into the biliary tree. The most common bacterial organism seen in acute cholangitis is *Escherichia coli* (25%–50%), followed by *Klebsiella, Enterobacter,* and *Enterococcus* species.

Treatment for acute cholangitis should focus on antimicrobial therapy and biliary drainage. Empiric antibiotic regimens should provide adequate activity against gram-negative and anaerobic organisms. Common regimens include monotherapy with ampicillin and sulbactam (Unasyn) or pipercillin and tazobactam

(Zosyn) or combination therapy with a fluoroquinolone plus metronidazole (Flagyl).

Patients without hypotension or mental status changes commonly show initial improvement after empiric antibiotics are administered, and thus biliary drainage can be done nonurgently. In patients demonstrating signs of sepsis or severe infection, emergency biliary drainage via ERCP is warranted. Patients who are not candidates for ERCP may undergo percutaneous transhepatic biliary drainage as an alternative.

Acute Cholecystitis

Acute cholecystitis is a syndrome defined by right upper quadrant pain, fever, and leukocytosis in the setting of gallbladder inflammation. Nausea and vomiting often occur as concurrent symptoms. Patients commonly have a positive Murphy's sign on physical examination, which is defined as abrupt cessation of inspiration on deep palpation of the gallbladder fossa, just beneath the liver edge. Approximately 95% of patients with acute cholecystitis have gallstones. In these instances, cholecystitis is thought to be precipitated by obstruction of the cystic duct and by local irritation of the gallbladder wall. Local inflammation is followed by release of pro-inflammatory prostaglandins. Superimposed bacterial infection might or might not complicate acute cholecystitis. As with cholangitis, the main bacteria responsible for infections during acute cholecystitis are *E. coli* and *Klebsiella, Enterobacter,* and *Enterococcus* species.

Diagnosis

The diagnosis of acute cholecystitis can often be made on physical examination alone. The most common laboratory finding in acute cholecystitis is leukocytosis. Mild elevations in AST and ALT can also be seen. Elevations of bilirubin and ALP are typical of biliary obstruction and are not commonly seen in acute cholecystitis. These abnormalities, if present, should raise suspicion for other conditions such as choledocholithiasis, cholangitis, or Mirizzi's syndrome. Mirizzi's syndrome is a rare cause of obstructive jaundice characterized by an impacted cystic duct stone that causes mass effect and compression of the common bile duct or common hepatic duct.

The initial imaging study of choice for acute cholecystitis is transabdominal ultrasound. Findings suggestive of cholecystitis include cholelithiasis, pericholecystic fluid (Figure 2), and a sonographic Murphy's sign (Figure 3). Thickening of the gallbladder wall supports a diagnosis of acute cholecystitis, but it is a nonspecific finding. Transabdominal ultrasound has a sensitivity of 88% for diagnosing acute cholecystitis. Hepatobiliary cholescintigraphy (HIDA scan) (Figure 4) is recommended if the suspicion of cholecystitis remains after a negative transabdominal ultrasound. MRCP and CT scan are typically not necessary for the diagnosis, although CT scan can be useful if complications from cholecystitis such as perforation are suspected.

Treatment

The treatment for acute cholecystitis involves supportive care, analgesia, antibiotics, and either surgery or percutaneous gallbladder drainage. If treatment is delayed or inadequate, numerous potential complications can result. These include emphysematous or gangrenous cholecystitis and gallbladder perforation. All patients with acute cholecystitis should be admitted to the hospital and given supportive care including intravenous fluids. NSAIDs and opioid analgesics are typically used for pain control.

Although bacterial etiologies complicate less than half of all episodes, empiric antibiotics are commonly administered to patients with acute cholecystitis. Appropriate antibiotic regimens are the same as those used in the setting of acute cholangitis (see the discussion of complications of choledocholithiasis).

In patients who are adequate surgical candidates, cholecystectomy should be performed within 72 hours of initial presentation. Numerous prospective trials and a Cochrane Database review have evaluated early versus delayed (6–12 weeks) cholecystectomy. There is overwhelming consensus that early surgery carries no increase in complications or perioperative morbidity and is associated with

Figure 2 Computed tomography (CT) scan demonstrating acute cholecystitis. The *outline arrow* indicates gallstones within the gallbladder lumen. The two *solid arrows* highlight mural thickening of the gallbladder wall and small amounts of pericholecystic fluid. Image courtesy of Richard M. Gore, MD, Department of Radiology, NorthShore University Health System, Evanston, IL.

Figure 3 Acute cholecystits: ultrasound. Gallbladder (**g**) is distended, with mural thickening *(arrowhead)* and a stone in the gallbladder neck *(arrow)*. Positive sonographic Murphy sign was present.

shorter hospital stays. Furthermore, early laparoscopic cholecystectomy eliminates the risk of recurrent episodes of acute cholecystitis.

Acute Acalculous Cholesystitis

An estimated 5% to 10% of cases of acute cholecystitis develop without the presence of gallstones. Acute acalculous cholecystitis is often seen in the setting of serious medical illness, complicated surgery, severe blunt trauma, and burn injuries. Other conditions such as diabetes mellitus, vasculitis, AIDS, and congestive heart failure have also been implicated as risk factors. Acute acalculous cholecystitis carries major risks of gangrene (50%) and perforation (10%), and mortality ranges from 30% to 50%. Numerous

Figure 4 Hepatobiliary iminodiacetic acid (HIDA) scan demonstrating acute cholecystitis. There is nonfilling of the gallbladder *(outline arrow)*, with isotope noted in the stomach and duodenum *(solid arrows)*. (Image courtesy of Richard M. Gore, MD, Department of Radiology, North-Shore University Health System, Evanston, IL.)

organisms have been associated with acute acalculous cholecystitis, including bacterial, viral, fungal, and parasitic infections.

The diagnosis is difficult. Patients are often critically ill and unable to elicit their symptoms. Transabdominal ultrasound is the best modality to evaluate acute acalculous cholecystitis in the critically ill patient owing to its availability, cost, and ease of performance. Hepatobiliary iminodiacetic acid (HIDA) and computed tomography (CT) scanning can have a role in difficult-to-diagnose acute acalculous cholecystitis and should be considered if ultrasound is nondiagnostic. Whereas false-positive test results can occur, a normal HIDA scan has a high negative predictive value in evaluating acute acalculous cholecystitis.

Because of the high rate of gangrene and perforation, early cholecystectomy should be performed in patients who are surgical candidates. In patients too ill to undergo surgery, biliary drainage with percutaneous cholecystostomy should be considered.

Gangrenous Cholecystitis, Emphysematous Cholecystitis, and Gallbladder Perforation

Gangrenous cholecystitis is most often seen in elderly patients and diabetics along with patients who delay seeking medical treatment for their symptoms. It is the most common complication of acute cholecystitis and carries a high mortality. Emphysematous cholecystitis is caused by gas-forming bacteria that infect the gallbladder. *E coli* and *Clostridium* species are most commonly implicated. Gas in the gallbladder may be seen on imaging, particularly CT or magnetic resonance imaging (MRI). Patients with gangrenous or emphysematous cholecystitis are at an elevated risk for gallbladder perforation. Early empiric antibiotics and cholecystectomy are crucial in the management of these complications to minimize mortality and prevent perforation of the gallbladder, a condition that carries a mortality rate of 42% to 60%.

Gallbladder Disease in Pregnancy

Pregnancy is a major risk factor for cholesterol gallstone formation. Because of anatomic changes secondary to the gravid uterus, biliary colic can be difficult to delineate from other causes of abdominal pain. Pregnant patients often have gallstones on transabdominal ultrasound, and thus a detailed history and physical examination are needed to diagnose a patient's abdominal pain

as biliary. Patients with other symptoms including bloating or dyspepsia should be evaluated for other etiologies.

In pregnant patients with recurrent symptomatic cholelithiasis, laparoscopic cholecystectomy remains the treatment of choice. The second and early third trimesters are the best times to perform cholecystectomy owing to ease and lower rates of complications. Nonsurgical management of gallstones is limited in pregnancy. NSAIDs are generally avoided late in pregnancy owing to the risk of premature closure of the ductus arteriosis, especially after 30 to 32 weeks of gestation.

After appendicitis, acute cholecystitis is the second most common nonobstetric surgical emergency during pregnancy. As with nonpregnant patients, pregnant women with acute cholecystitis should be treated with cholecystectomy in addition to medical management. Early surgery for pregnant patients with acute cholecystitis has been found to decrease relapse rates and hospital readmissions. No differences in maternal or fetal morbidity and mortality have been found in patients treated conservatively versus surgically for acute cholecystitis during pregnancy.

References

Abboud PA, Malet PF, Berlin JA, et al: Predictors of common bile duct stones prior to cholecystectomy: A metaanalysis, *Gastrointest Endosc* 44:450–455, 1996.

Akriviadis EA, Hatzigavriel M, Kapnias D, et al: Treatment of biliary colic with diclofenac: a randomized, double-blind, placebo-controlled study, *Gastroenterology* 113:225–231, 1997.

ASGE Standards of Practice Committee, Buxbaum JL, Abbas fehmi SM, Sultan S, et al: ASGE guideline on the role of endoscopy in the evaluation and management of choledocholithiasis, *Gastrointest Endosc* 89(6):1075–1105.e15, 2019.

Barie PS, Eachempati SR: Acute acalculous cholecystitis, *Gastroenterol Clin North Am* 39:344–357, 2010.

Dhupar R, Smaldone GM, Hamad GG: Is there a benefit to delaying cholecystectomy for symptomatic gallbladder disease during pregnancy? *Surg Endosc* 24:108–112, 2010.

Everhart JE, Khare M, Hill M, Maurer KR: Prevalence and ethnic differences in gallbladder disease in the United States, *Gastroenterology* 117:632–639, 1999.

Freitas ML, Bell RL, Duffy AJ: Choledocholithiasis: Evolving standards for diagnosis and management, *World J Gastroenterol* 12:3162–3167, 2006.

Gore RM, Thakrar KH, Newmark GM, et al: Gallbladder imaging, *Gastroenterol Clin North Am* 39:265–267, 2010.

Gurusamy KS, Samraj K: Early versus late laparoscopic cholecystectomy for acute cholecystitis, *Cochrane Database Syst Rev* 18: CD005440.

Papi C, Catarci M, Ambrosio D, et al: Timing of cholecystectomy for acute calculus cholecystitis: A meta-analysis, *Am J Gastroenterol* 9:147–155, 2004.

CHRONIC DIARRHEA

Method of
André de Leon, MD

CURRENT DIAGNOSIS

History
- Duration, frequency, and timing
- Presence of fever/blood
- Food/medication intake
- Travel history

Physical Examination
- Gastrointestinal examination
- Hydration status
- Digital rectal examination
- Other systems: endocrine, ophthalmologic, skin

Testing
- Fecal occult blood testing
- Stool for ova/parasites, *Clostridium difficile* and other bacteria
- Stool antigen for cryptosporidium, giardia
- Fecal electrolytes (Na, K, Osm)

- Fecal leukocytes
- Erythrocyte sedimentation rate (ESR)
- Complete blood count (CBC)
- Other: iron panel (celiac sprue), TSH (hyperthyroidism), liver function tests (LFTs)
- Colonoscopy with biopsy

 CURRENT THERAPY

- Supportive care and rehydration, if necessary
- Trial of discontinuation of possible offending medication/food (lactose, gluten, sorbitol)
- Dietary modification with increased fiber intake (dietary or supplementation)
- Specific therapy as directed by culture and susceptibilities or biopsy
- Empiric therapy trial with antibiotics
- Empiric trial of probiotics[1] (limited evidence of efficacy in healthy adults with chronic diarrhea)

[1]Not FDA approved for this indication.

Chronic diarrhea has traditionally been defined based on consistency, volume, and frequency of stools. However, recent studies have found that there is considerable variability in definition when using these markers. Therefore the American Gastroenterological Association has released a consensus statement suggesting that chronic diarrhea should be defined as a decrease in fecal consistency lasting for 4 or more weeks.

Epidemiology

Chronic diarrhea is a common cause of mortality in developing countries as well as the second leading cause of overall mortality in children 1 to 59 months old. The prevalence in the general population in developed nations and economic impact of chronic diarrhea has not been well established. This could be related to the variable nature of the studies that have been performed with regard to definition, population characteristics, and overall study design. The American Gastroenterological Association Burden of Illness study estimates that the direct costs of chronic diarrhea are $524 million per year and indirect costs are at least $136 million per year. A meta-analysis of current studies suggest that chronic diarrhea can affect anywhere from 1%–5% of the population.

Classification Based on Etiology

Elucidating the exact cause of chronic diarrhea can be very challenging, as there are several hundred conditions that can be related. Consideration of comorbid symptoms and epidemiologic clues can help in constructing a differential diagnosis. Chronic diarrhea can be evaluated based on two etiologies: functional and organic. The functional chronic diarrhea category includes conditions when abdominal pain accompanies the diarrhea (e.g., irritable bowel syndrome) and when abdominal pain is absent. Organic disorders are conditions that are associated with physiologic, structural, or biochemical abnormalities. Organic disorders are more likely in adults with alarm features such as gastrointestinal (GI) bleeding, fevers, or significant weight loss.

Functional Disorders

Functional diarrhea is characterized by chronic or recurrent diarrhea not explained by structural or biochemical abnormalities. Causes may include physiologic factors (small bowel bacterial overgrowth), psychological factors (stress and anxiety), and dietary factors (carbohydrate malabsorption). Patients with functional diarrhea should not meet criteria for irritable bowel syndrome (IBS) as based on the Rome IV criteria. Patients with functional diarrhea may have abdominal pain and/or bloating, but unlike IBS, these are not predominant symptoms.

Functional Disorders: Irritable Bowel Syndrome
Multiple investigations have shown conflicting data, and no abnormality has been found to be specific for this disorder. The traditional focus has been on alterations in gastrointestinal motility and on visceral hypersensitivity; however, more recent studies have considered the role of inflammation, alterations in fecal flora, and bacterial overgrowth as possible causes. The role of food sensitivity is also being considered as a possible cause. The Rome criteria help to provide a framework for the diagnosis of IBS and emphasize pain. When these criteria are not met, then other etiologies should be considered and evaluated. The Rome criteria emphasize chronic abdominal pain that is relieved by defecation and associated with a change in stool frequency or consistency. Psychological stress also appears to correlate to the diagnosis of IBS. Patients with IBS can experience altered bowel habits with a predominance of diarrhea vs. constipation or alternating between the two (mixed type). IBS can also be postinfectious, following recovery from *Clostidrium difficile* and other bacterial infections.

Organic Disorders
Organic disorders leading to chronic diarrhea are conditions that are associated with structural, physiologic, or biochemical abnormalities. Alarm features such as gastrointestinal (GI) bleeding, fever, significant weight loss, occurrence after 50 years of age, and positive family history of colorectal cancer or inflammatory bowel disease (IBD) are more likely in organic disorders.

Organic Disorders: Fatty/Malabsorptive
Malabsorptive diarrhea is, as the name implies, secondary to impaired absorption along the gut. This can be due to structural abnormalities (gastric bypass, short bowel syndrome, celiac sprue, pancreatic insufficiency), structural abnormalities related to vascular compromise (mesenteric ischemia), or lack of enzymes that aid in digestion (e.g., lactose intolerance). Impaired absorption can also occur secondary to infections such as *Tropheryma whipplei* (Whipple's Disease), *Giardia*, small bowel bacterial overgrowth, and tropical sprue. Medications such as aminoglycoside antibiotics, orlistat (Xenical, Alli), thyroid supplementation, acarbose (Precose), and ticlopidine (Ticlid) can also cause malabsorptive diarrhea.

Organic Disorders: Inflammatory
Inflammation leading to diarrhea is often due to autoimmune, infectious, or neoplastic processes or radiation exposure. Autoimmune processes are felt to play a large role in inflammatory bowel disease (IBD), which often manifests as Crohn disease or ulcerative colitis. Microscopic colitis may also have laboratory findings suggesting an underlying autoimmune disorder. Infections such as *Clostridium difficile*, *Mycobacterium tuberculosis*, *Yersinia*, *Campylobacter*, *Giardia*, *Cryptospordium*, *Amebae*, *Strongyloidedes*, cytomegalovirus, and herpes simplex virus can lead to a diarrhea with associated inflammation of the bowel. Colon cancer (villous adenocarcinoma) and lymphoma can also cause inflammatory diarrhea.

Organic Disorders: Postcholecystectomy
In the absence of a gallbladder, bile acids drain directly and more continuously into the small bowel. This increase may overcome the terminal portion of the ileum's absorptive capacity. The increased bile acids then are allowed to reach the colon, leading to diarrhea (cholerheic diarrhea).

Clinical Manifestations
History. Thorough investigation of a patient complaining of ongoing diarrhea-like features should always include a detailed medical history. A clear understanding of the patient's symptoms

TABLE 1	Medications Commonly Associated with Diarrhea

Antiarrhythmic medications

- Digoxin
- Quinidine

Antibiotic medications

- Aminoglycosides
- Macrolides

Antihypertensive medications

- ACE inhibitors
- Beta blockers

Antiinflammatory medications

- 5-aminosalicylates
- Nonsteroidal antiinflammatory drugs (NSAIDs)

Antiretroviral medications (many)

Chemotherapuetic medications (many)

Dermatologic medications

- Isotretinoin (occasionally causes diarrhea)

Endocrine medications

- Alpha-glucosidase inhibitors (cause diarrhea in ≥20% of patients)
- Biguanides (cause diarrhea in ≥20% of patients)
- Thyroid hormones

Gastrointestinal medications

- Acid-reducing medications
  - H₂-receptor blocker
  - Proton pump inhibitors
- Antacid medications (magnesium containing)

Parasympathetic nervous system medication

- Cholinergic agonists

Psychiatric medications

- Selective serotonin reuptake inhibitors

Respiratory medications

- Xanthine derivative (Theophylline)

Data from Schiller LR, Sellin JH. Sleisenger and Fordtran's Gastrointestinal and Liver Disease: Pathophysiology/Diagnosis/Management. 9th Edition, Philadelphia, 2010, Elsevier; and Soriano M, Vaziri H. Clinical Gastroenterology, Diarrhea: Diagnostic and Therapeutic Advances, New York, 2010, Humana Press, Springer.

is vital: not all complaints may truly be defined as diarrhea but may rather be symptoms related to an interplay between fecal incontinence and stool impaction. A detailed history of travel, food intake, and medication use is essential. This can help direct the early workup and diagnostic testing. Stool frequency, volume, consistency, and timing can aid in categorization; however, they are no longer what define the condition, as noted previously. If considering the diagnosis of irritable bowel syndrome (IBS), use of the Rome IV criteria will be beneficial.

Physical Examination. The physical examination is very important to the workup and diagnosis of chronic diarrhea. Ophthalmologic findings such as episcleritis or exophthalmia can be related to IBD; skin findings such as dermatitis herpetiformis can be related to celiac sprue (seen in 15%–25% of patients with celiac disease). Prominent lymphadenopathy and weight loss can be suggestive of possible infection or malignancy. A thorough abdominal examination should include the evaluation of bowel sounds (hypermotility), skin for scars (surgical cause of diarrhea), tenderness

(infection/inflammation), and masses (neoplasia) and should be followed by a digital rectal examination with fecal occult blood testing. Anoscopy can also be used to detect for ulcerations or fecal impaction, given that seepage around impacted stools can create a picture similar to diarrhea.

Testing for Diagnosis

Serum testing for chronic diarrhea should include a complete blood count (CBC), serum electrolytes, liver function tests, serum albumin, thyroid-stimulating hormone, and erythrocyte sedimentation rate. An iron panel should be performed if indicated based on the results of the CBC. Serum anti-tissue transglutaminase antibody testing may be helpful if symptoms are suggestive of celiac sprue. Stool evaluation may include fecal occult blood testing, fecal leukocytes, stool ova and parasites, stool culture (including *Salmonella*, *Shigella*, and *Campylobacter*), and stool antigen for *Giardia*. Stool testing for *Cryptosporidium* should be considered, especially in the immunocompromised. Stool pH and electrolytes may be helpful, especially when the patient is lactose intolerant. Stool testing for *C. difficile* should be performed if the patient has recently used antibiotics or been hospitalized. If medication abuse is suspected as a possible cause, a stool laxative screen (i.e., stool phenolphthalein test) may be warranted. Diagnostic testing may include a colonoscopy with biopsy.

Treatment

The exact cause of chronic diarrhea can prove elusive, and treatment trials may be warranted. Specific treatment depends on the specific diagnosis. If there is concern about possible bacterial or protozoa infection, an empiric trial of vancomycin (Vancocin), ciprofloxacin (Cipro), or metronidazole (Flagyl) may be warranted. If there is concern for possible medication (Table 1) or food relation to diarrhea, a trial of discontinuation of offending substance/food may be reasonable. The effectiveness of probiotics[7] looks favorable; however, large intervention studies and epidemiologic investigations of long-term probiotic effects on healthy adults are largely missing. At this time, probiotics have been found efficacious in treatment of acute diarrhea, prevention of antibiotic-associated diarrhea, and prevention of traveler's diarrhea. Dietary modification continues to be an important starting point for treatment, with increased intake in bulk-forming agents such as fiber. Treatment of specific disorders such as Crohn's disease and ulcerative colitis are discussed in other chapters.

References

De Vrese M, Marteau PR: Probiotics and prebiotics: Effects on diarrhea, *J Nutr* 137:8035–8115, 2007.

Dellon ES, Ringel Y: Treatment of functional diarrhea, *Curr Treat Options Gastroenterol* 9(4):331–341, 2006.

Everhart JE, editor: Digestive Disease in the United States: Epidemiology and impact. Washington, DC: National Institutes of Health; 1994 NIH Publication No. 94-1447.

Everhart JE, Ruhl CE: Burden of digestive diseases in the United States part II: lower gasteroentestinal diseases, *Gasteroenterology* 136(3):741–754. Epub 2009.

Fine KD, Schiller LR: AGA technical review on the evaluation and management of chronic diarrhea, *Gastroenterology* 116:1464–1486, 1999.

Juckett G, Trivedi R: Evaluation of chronic diarrhea, *Am Fam Physician* 84:1119–1126, 2011.

Peery AF, et al: Burden of Gastrointestinal Disease in the United States: 2012 Update, *Gastroenterology* V143, Issue 5:1179–1187, 2012 e3.

Rodrigo L: Celiac disease, *World J Gastroenterol* 12:6585–6593, 2006.

Schiller LR, et al: Chronic Diarrhea: Diagnosis and Management, *Clinical Gastroenterology and Hepatology* V15(Issue 2):182–193, 2017 e3.

Soriano M, Vaziri H: Clinical Gastroenterology, Diarrhea: Diagnostic and Therapeutic Advances, New York: Humana Press, Springer; 2010.

Thomas PD, Forbes A, Green J, et al: Guidelines for the investigation of chronic diarrhea, 2nd edition, *Gut* 52(Suppl. 5):v1–v15, 2003.

Whitehead WE, Borrud L, Goode PS, et al: Fecal incontinence in U.S. adults: Epidemiology and risk factor, *Gastroenterology* 137:512–517, 2009 e2.

World Health Organization. Children: Reducing mortality, Fact Sheet #178, Available at http://www.who.int/mediacentre/factsheets/fs178/en/ (accessed October 17, 2013).

---

[7] Available as dietary supplement.

CIRRHOSIS

Method of
Andres F. Carrion, MD; and Paul Martin, MD

The term *cirrhosis* is a neologism derived from the Greek *kirrhós*, which describes the yellowish discoloration of the liver during advanced stages of chronic liver disease, and the suffix *–osis*, which denotes a specific condition in medical terminology. Morphologically, cirrhosis reflects the consequences of chronic hepatic necroinflammatory activity with an incomplete and disorganized repair process that results in regenerative nodules and extensive fibrosis replacing normal hepatic parenchyma with disturbance of normal hepatic physiology. Cirrhosis can result from any etiology of chronic liver disease (Table 1). Activation of hepatic stellate cells into myofibroblasts and matrix deposition are key steps in the pathogenesis of cirrhosis.

Epidemiology

The prevalence of cirrhosis varies significantly in different regions of the world and is directly influenced by the epidemiology of individual chronic liver diseases that lead to progressive hepatic fibrosis. The estimated global prevalence of cirrhosis is 4.5% to 9.5%; however, this estimate likely underestimates the real magnitude of disease burden, as a sizeable proportion of asymptomatic individuals remain undiagnosed. Similarly, it is difficult to obtain accurate estimates of mortality related to cirrhosis, but countries in Central and South America and Southern Europe exhibit the highest mortality rates, particularly in males. Epidemiologic trends of cirrhosis have changed considerably over time in many countries, underscoring variations in the incidence and prevalence of specific etiologies of chronic liver disease. For instance, widespread immunization against hepatitis B virus (HBV) has markedly reduced its incidence, prevalence, and associated liver disease including cirrhosis. Alcohol consumption has varied strikingly across different regions of the globe over the past several decades. A steady decline in mortality due to cirrhosis has occurred in some European countries (mainly Mediterranean) as alcohol use has diminished. A similar trend has also been noted in North America; however, hospitalizations for alcoholic hepatitis have increased over the recent past in the United States. In contrast, a significant increase in mortality related to cirrhosis has been noted in some Eastern European countries with increased alcohol consumption. In addition, eradication of hepatitis C virus (HCV) is associated with a reduction in hepatic dysfunction, liver-related and all-cause mortality, complications of cirrhosis such as hepatocellular carcinoma (HCC), and portal hypertension. The impact of highly effective direct-acting antiviral agents against HCV on the epidemiology of cirrhosis and its complications has resulted in a decline in liver transplant listings for HCV. In contrast, the growing prevalence of nonalcoholic fatty liver disease (NAFLD) is reflected in its current prominence as a cause of cirrhosis. NAFLD is anticipated to become the single most frequent cause of chronic liver disease and cirrhosis in the mid- to second half of this century.

Clinical findings

In the absence of hepatic decompensation, the overwhelming majority of individuals with cirrhosis are asymptomatic and may only exhibit subtle clinical findings. Clues to the presence of cirrhosis can include elevated serum aminotransferases and/or bilirubin, decreased albumin, and prolongation of the prothrombin time. Approximately 10% to 17% of individuals with unexplained elevation of aminotransferases have unrecognized cirrhosis. Thrombocytopenia in the absence of a primary hematologic explanation is another clue to the presence of cirrhosis and primarily reflects hypersplenism due to portal hypertension but also diminished production of thrombopoietin, a platelet growth and development factor synthetized by the liver. A platelet count below $160 \times 10/\mu L$ provides the highest diagnostic accuracy for cirrhosis among routine blood tests (sensitivity 74%, specificity 88%, positive likelihood ratio 6.3, negative likelihood ratio 0.29). Thrombocytopenia is also a component of noninvasive scoring systems that predict fibrosis, such as the AST (aspartate aminotransferase) to Platelet Ratio Index (APRI) and Fibrosis-4 (FIB-4).

Physical examination may reveal somewhat diminished liver span by percussion and a firm liver edge on palpation. Splenomegaly is suggested by dullness to percussion in the left upper abdominal quadrant or a palpable spleen tip. Cutaneous signs of cirrhosis include palmar erythema, spider nevi, facial telangiectasia, decreased chest and/or axillary hair, inversion of the normal male pubic hair pattern, Terry nails ("ground glass" appearance of nails with absent lunula), and Muehrcke nails (paired, white, transverse bands separated by normal color). Nail clubbing may also be present in individuals with cirrhosis, particularly in those with hepatopulmonary syndrome. Dupuytren contracture is relatively common in alcoholic cirrhosis but its pathogenesis is not well understood. Palmar erythema due to altered sex hormone metabolism is more evident on the thenar and hypothenar eminences and typically spares the central portion of the palm. Hypogonadism in both sexes and gynecomastia and testicular atrophy in males can be detected, reflecting altered sex hormone metabolism (increased production of androstenedione, enhanced aromatization to estrone, and increased conversion to estradiol). The catabolic effects of advanced cirrhosis often result in marked sarcopenia, which adversely affects quality of life and survival and is also associated with poorer outcomes after liver transplantation.

Various noninvasive methods for evaluation of liver fibrosis are now widely used in clinical practice for staging of hepatic fibrosis and diagnosis of cirrhosis. These include vibration-controlled transient elastography (Fibroscan), acoustic radiation force impulse (ARFI), shear wave and point quantification elastography, and magnetic resonance elastography.

Natural history of cirrhosis and prognostic models

Cirrhosis may be broadly categorized into two distinct clinical phases, regardless of the etiology: compensated and

TABLE 1	Etiologies of Cirrhosis
ETIOLOGY	**EXAMPLES**
Infectious	Hepatitis B Hepatitis C Hepatitis D
Autoimmune and cholestasis	Autoimmune hepatitis Biliary atresia Primary biliary cholangitis Primary sclerosing cholangitis Secondary biliary cirrhosis Secondary sclerosing cholangitis
Toxins	Alcohol Arsenic Drugs
Metabolic	Nonalcoholic steatohepatitis Alpha-1 antitrypsin deficiency Hemochromatosis Wilson disease Glycogen storage diseases Lysosomal storage diseases Galactosemia
Vascular	Cardiac cirrhosis Budd-Chiari syndrome Sinusoidal obstruction syndrome
Granulomatous	Sarcoidosis Tuberculosis Syphilis
Cryptogenic	Unrecognized nonalcoholic fatty liver disease, infections, or drugs

decompensated. Compensated cirrhosis implies the absence of index complications such as jaundice, ascites, hepatic encephalopathy, or gastroesophageal variceal hemorrhage. In contrast, hepatic decompensation indicates an advanced phase of the disease, which is rapidly progressive and characterized by development of one or more complications and diminished hepatocellular function with prolongation of the prothrombin time and hypoalbuminemia. Characterizing cirrhosis as compensated or decompensated is simple and reproducible, and offers useful prognostic information for clinical practice (Table 2).

More precise prognostic models such as the Child Turcotte Pugh (Table 3) and the Model for End-Stage Liver Disease (MELD) are also widely used, the latter being considered the most accurate predictor of short-term mortality for individuals with cirrhosis and serving as the basis for the current organ allocation system in liver transplantation in the United States and elsewhere (calculator available at www.optn.transplant.hrsa.gov). The most recent modification of the MELD score resulted in inclusion of the serum sodium into the formula: MELD-Na. Incorporation of the serum sodium in the MELD formula increases its prognostic accuracy in patients with relatively low scores and hyponatremia.

The specific etiology of cirrhosis may help determine its prognosis. For instance, persistent viremia in individuals with chronic HBV or HCV infection is implicated in the development of decompensated cirrhosis. Effective antiviral therapy can abort progression of chronic viral hepatitis to cirrhosis and decompensation.

Although cirrhosis per se is not an indication for liver transplantation, it is important to identify individuals with cirrhosis who should be considered for liver transplantation. Development of an index complication of cirrhosis such as gastroesophageal variceal hemorrhage, ascites, or hepatic encephalopathy is an indication to refer a patient for liver transplantation and initiate pretransplant evaluation. The MELD score provides objective and reproducible prognostication of short-term survival without liver transplantation (Figure 1), and data from a seminal study showed that liver transplantation is associated with improved survival in individuals with MELD scores greater than 17.

Major complications of cirrhosis
Portal Hypertension
Although portal hypertension can be inferred by clues such as splenomegaly with thrombocytopenia in a patient with cirrhosis, it is defined by a hepatic venous pressure gradient (HVPG) greater than 5 mm Hg. This gradient is calculated by subtracting the measured free hepatic vein pressure from the wedged hepatic venous pressure (a measurement that reflects portal venous pressure by using the same hemodynamic principle as the wedged pulmonary capillary pressure to assess left atrial pressure). Clinically significant portal hypertension typically occurs when the HVPG is 10 mm Hg or greater, at which threshold gastroesophageal varices and ascites occur. Unfortunately, accurate noninvasive measurement of portal pressure is not available, limiting its use in routine clinical practice as it requires passage of a transjugular catheter.

Increased intrahepatic resistance to portal venous flow aggravated by increased splanchnic blood flow in cirrhosis leads to portal hypertension. In addition to cirrhosis, which is the most common cause of portal hypertension in Western countries (hepatic schistosomiasis is the leading cause in areas where this infection is common), other disorders may result in pre- or posthepatic portal hypertension. Portal vein thrombosis is a common cause of prehepatic portal hypertension. Cardiomyopathy, constrictive pericarditis, Budd-Chiari syndrome, and inferior vena cava webs may result in posthepatic portal hypertension. Ascites and gastroesophageal variceal hemorrhage are the two most common complications of portal hypertension in cirrhosis. Less common but clinically significant complications include portal hypertensive gastropathy, hepatic hydrothorax, hepatopulmonary syndrome, portopulmonary hypertension, and hepatorenal syndrome.

Gastroesophageal Variceal Hemorrhage
Portal hypertension leads to formation of multiple portosystemic collaterals, including gastroesophageal varices. Formation of gastroesophageal varices typically occurs when the HVPG is 10 mm Hg or greater, with the risk for variceal hemorrhage increasing once HVPG is greater than 12 mm Hg. Gastroesophageal varices are present in approximately 50% of patients with cirrhosis and are more common in patients with hepatic decompensation (Child-Turcotte-Pugh class C). Variceal hemorrhage is the most dramatic complication of cirrhosis and occurs at a rate of 5% to 15% per year. Risk factors for variceal hemorrhage include larger variceal size, more advanced hepatic decompensation, and presence of vascular "red wale" signs during endoscopic evaluation. Esophageal varices are classified according to their size as small (≤ 5 mm) or large (> 5 mm).

Screening for gastroesophageal varices with esophagogastroduodenoscopy (EGD) is recommended when cirrhosis is suspected. Management strategies for patients with esophageal varices that have not previously bled (primary prophylaxis) are summarized in Table 4.

Management of esophageal varices that have previously bled (secondary prophylaxis) includes a combination of a nonselective beta-blocker with endoscopic variceal ligation (EVL). The dose of the nonselective beta-blocker should be titrated to the maximal tolerated dose (resting heart rate of 55 to 60 beats/minute or 25% decrease from baseline) and EVL should be repeated frequently (every 2 weeks or so) until complete variceal obliteration. Recurrence of esophageal varices may occur following EVL; thus, surveillance EGD is recommended: first EGD performed 3 to 6 months after variceal obliteration and then at 6- to 12-month intervals.

Gastric varices are classified according to relationship with esophageal varices and location (Table 5).

Acute variceal hemorrhage occurs at a yearly rate of 5% to 15% and is associated with high mortality (at least 20% at 6 weeks). Adequate resuscitation is crucial in acute variceal hemorrhage with some additional precautions. Patients with variceal hemorrhage are at high risk for aspiration, and endotracheal intubation for airway protection should be performed prior to endoscopy. Overly aggressive expansion of blood volume should be avoided as it may result in increased portal venous pressure. A target hemoglobin level of between 7 and 9 g/dL is appropriate. Current guidelines recommend against correcting the international normalized ratio (INR) by use of fresh frozen plasma or recombinant factor VIIa, as this has not shown a clear benefit in individuals with acute variceal hemorrhage. There are no data to support or recommend against transfusion of platelets in this clinical scenario. Prophylactic broad-spectrum antibiotics (i.e., intravenous ceftriaxone [Rocephin][1]) reduce bacterial infections, risk of rebleeding, and mortality. Administration of vasoactive drugs such as octreotide (Sandostatin)[1] or terlipressin (Lucassin)[5] result in increased rates of initial endoscopic control of bleeding, reduced 7-day mortality, and lower transfusion requirements. EGD is recommended within 12 hours and EVL is the endoscopic treatment of choice for management of esophageal varices. Balloon tamponade (i.e., Sengstaken Blakemore, Minnesota, or Linton-Nachlas tubes) or esophageal stenting are effective rescue therapies when variceal hemorrhage cannot be controlled with standard endoscopic therapy. The role of transjugular intrahepatic portosystemic shunt (TIPS) has expanded from a salvage intervention for individuals with recurrent variceal hemorrhage following EVL to an early "preemptive" intervention in carefully selected individuals at high-risk for treatment failure (Child-Turcotte-Pugh class B or C but with MELD scores ≤ 13) following EVL, in which case it appears to be superior to beta-blocker plus EVL. Patients who survive an episode of variceal hemorrhage should receive secondary prophylaxis with a combination of a nonselective beta-blocker and repeated EVL until complete obliteration of the varices is achieved. Cyanoacrylate

---

[1] Not US Food and Drug Administration (FDA) approved for this indication.
[5] Investigational drug in the United States.

TABLE 2 Stages of Cirrhosis Based on Clinical Complications and 1-Year Outcome Probabilities

CIRRHOSIS	D'AMICO STAGE	COMPLICATIONS	PROBABILITY OF ADVANCING TO NEXT STAGE	1-YEAR MORTALITY
Compensated	Stage 1	(−) varices (−) ascites	7%	1%
	Stage 2	(+) varices (−) ascites	6.6%	3.4%
Decompensated	Stage 3	(+) ascites (+) varices	7.6%	20%
	Stage 4	(+) variceal hemorrhage (+) ascites	–	57%

From D'Amico G, Garcia-Tsao G, Pagliaro L. Natural history and prognostic indicators of survival in cirrhosis: A systematic review of 118 studies. J Hepatol 2006;44:217–31.

TABLE 3 Child-Turcotte-Pugh Classification

CLINICAL AND LABORATORY CRITERIA	POINTS		
	1	2	3
Albumin (g/dL)	> 3.5	2.8–3.5	< 2.8
Ascites	None	Mild to moderate (diuretic responsive)	Severe (diuretic refractory)
Bilirubin (mg/dL)	< 2	2–3	> 3
Encephalopathy	None	Mild to moderate (grade 1 or 2)	Severe (grade 3 or 4)
Prothrombin time Prolongation in seconds International normalized ratio	< 4 < 1.7	4–6 1.7–2.3	> 6 > 2.3

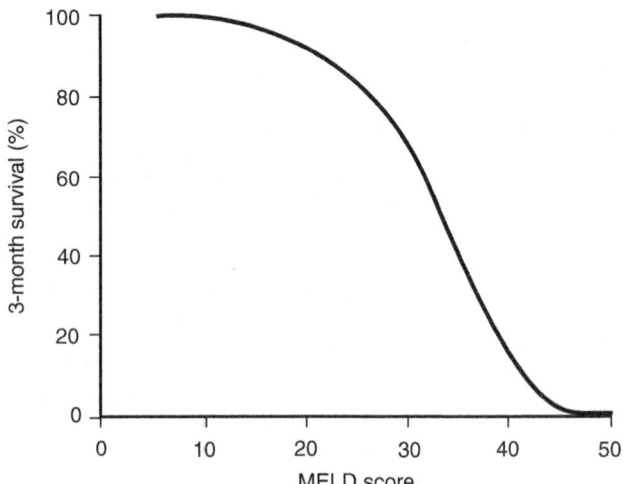

Figure 1 Relationship between Model for End-Stage Liver Disease (MELD) score and survival at 3 months. From *Sleisenger and Fordtran's Gastrointestinal and Liver Disease*, 10th ed., Chapter 97, page 1634. Elsevier; 2016.

injection, TIPS, or balloon occluded transvenous obliteration (BRTO) are the treatments of choice for management of gastric variceal hemorrhage.

Ascites
Ascites denotes pathologic accumulation of fluid in the peritoneal cavity (> 25 mL) and is the most common complication of cirrhosis. Portal hypertension is required for development of cirrhotic

ascites, as individuals with HVPG less than 12 mm Hg do not develop this complication.[16] Importantly, sinusoidal hypertension appears to be a requirement for development of ascites, as prehepatic portal hypertension does not invariably result in development of this complication. Other relevant mechanisms include splanchnic vasodilatation and its consequences such as humorally mediated sodium retention and diminished free-water excretion by the kidneys, hypoproteinemia and reduced oncotic pressure, and disruption of normal lymphatic drainage in the liver due to extensive fibrosis.

Ascites can be demonstrated by physical examination when its volume is greater than 1500 mL, although ultrasonography can detect as little as 100 mL. Clinical signs include flank dullness on percussion, shifting dullness, and, if the amount of ascites present is large, demonstration of a fluid wave. A diagnostic paracentesis is mandatory in the following settings: new-onset ascites, change in clinical status including hospitalization of a patient with previously diagnosed ascites, and suggestion of spontaneous bacterial peritonitis (SBP). The following tests on the fluid are indicated: leukocyte count with differential (purple or lavender top tube with ethylenediaminetetraacetic acid [EDTA]), culture (on two blood culture bottles inoculated at the bedside), total protein, and albumin (red top tube). The appearance of the ascitic fluid may yield important clinical clues (Table 6). The serum-to-ascites albumin gradient (SAAG), obtained by subtracting the ascitic fluid albumin value from the serum albumin value, helps make a distinction between transudative and exudative ascites. A gradient of 1.1 g/dL or greater confirms portal hypertension as the etiology of ascites, whereas a value less than 1.1 g/dL suggests etiologies other than portal hypertension. The absolute number of polymorphonuclear (PMN) cells in the ascitic fluid is an important clue to SBP.

Cirrhotic ascites is unlikely to resolve without specific therapeutic intervention. Management of ascites is centered on sodium restriction rather than free-water restriction; total dietary intake of sodium should be less than 2000 mg (88 mmol) per day and compliance with this intervention can be documented by monitoring urinary sodium concentrations. A sodium-to-potassium concentration ratio of greater than 1 on a random urine sample correlates well with a 24-hour sodium excretion greater than 78 mmol/day and implies compliance with sodium restriction. Nevertheless, dietary restriction of sodium is efficacious in only 10% of patients, and enhanced natriuresis is typically needed to provide adequate control of ascites. Combining diuretics that work at different sites of the nephron is more effective than using a single agent. Aldosterone is upregulated in cirrhosis owing to diminished effective arterial blood volume and consequential increased renin and angiotensin activity, resulting in enhanced renal sodium and free water retention. Spironolactone (Aldactone) competitively inhibits aldosterone-dependent sodium–potassium exchange in the distal convoluted renal tubule and the collecting ducts. The recommended initial dose of spironolactone for patients with ascites due to portal hypertension is

TABLE 4 Recommendations for Primary Prophylaxis Against Esophageal Variceal Hemorrhage

SIZE OF VARICES	RISK OF HEMORRHAGE	SURVEILLANCE INTERVAL	PRIMARY PROPHYLAXIS
No varices	CTP class A	EGD every 2 years if ongoing liver injury (i.e., obesity or alcohol abuse), or every 3 years if liver injury is quiescent (i.e., viral eradication or alcohol abstinence)	None
	CTP class B/C	EGD yearly	None
Small esophageal varices	CTP class A	EGD yearly if ongoing liver injury (i.e., obesity or alcohol abuse), or every 2 years if liver injury is quiescent (i.e., viral eradication or alcohol abstinence)	BB may be used
	CTP class B/C	EGD yearly; if BB are used, repeat EGD unnecessary	BB recommended
Large esophageal varices	CTP class A/B/C	If BB are used, repeat EGD unnecessary; if no BB, repeat EGD for EVL every 2-8 weeks until variceal eradication, then once in 3-6 months, and regularly every 6-12 months	Either BB or EVL recommended

Abbreviations: BB = beta-blocker; CTP = Child-Turcotte-Pugh; EGD = esophagogastroduodenoscopy; EVL = endoscopic variceal ligation. Child-Turcotte-Pugh class obtained by adding points for each variable
Class A: 5–6 points (compensated cirrhosis)
Class B: 7–9 points (decompensated cirrhosis)
Class C: 10–15 points (decompensated cirrhosis)

TABLE 5 Classification of Gastroesophageal and Gastric Varices and Recommendations for Primary Prophylaxis

TYPE OF VARICES	CHARACTERISTICS	PRIMARY PROPHYLAXIS
Gastroesophageal varices type 1 (GOV1)	Extension of esophageal varices along the lesser curvature into the gastric cardia	Similar to esophageal varices
Gastroesophageal varices type 2 (GOV2)	Extension of the esophageal varices along the greater curvature into the gastric fundus	BB can be used, although data not as strong as for esophageal varices
Isolated gastric varices type 1 (IGV1)	Gastric varices localized in the fundus	If high risk, consider BB or cyanoacrylate injection
Isolated gastric varices type 2 (IGV2)	Gastric varices localized in the antrum	No data, consider BB if high risk

Abbreviations: BB = beta-blocker.

TABLE 6 Characteristics of Ascitic Fluid and Differential Diagnosis

FLUID APPEARANCE	DIFFERENTIAL DIAGNOSIS	BIOCHEMICAL HINTS ON FLUID ANALYSIS
Clear	Uncomplicated transudative ascites due to cirrhosis	WBC < 500 cells/µL, PMN < 250 cells/µL, SAAG ≥ 1.1
Turbid/cloudy	Infection	PMN ≥ 250 cells/µL
Bloody	Traumatic paracentesis, hemoperitoneum	RBC > 10,000 cells/µL
Milky	Chylous ascites due to obstruction or trauma of lymphatic vessels or thoracic duct	Triglycerides > 200 md/dL

Abbreviations: PMN = polymorphonuclear cells; SAAG = serum-to-ascites albumin gradient; WBC = white blood cell.

100 mg orally daily. Administration of a loop-acting diuretic such as furosemide (Lasix)[1] is recommended in addition to spironolactone, as it potentiates natriuresis. The recommended initial dose for furosemide is 40 mg orally daily. Further increases in doses of diuretics should be made maintaining this 100/40 ratio to a maximum dose of 400 mg orally daily of spironolactone and 160 mg orally daily of furosemide, as it prevents hypo- or hyperkalemia. Renal function and electrolytes must be monitored regularly, particularly after dose modifications. Tender gynecomastia is an unpleasant side effect of spironolactone, and some patients may need to discontinue it, in which case amiloride (Midamor)[1] (10–40 mg orally daily) can be used. Two outcomes may occur in patients with ascites that is not adequately controlled with diuretics: (1) refractory ascites to maximum diuretic doses and sodium restriction, which typically recurs rapidly following large-volume paracenteses (LVP); and (2) inability to increase diuretic doses owing to symptomatic hypotension or deterioration in renal function as evidenced by increasing serum creatinine levels.

Repeated LVP with removal of more than 5 liters of ascitic fluid per session is a safe and effective intervention to treat refractory ascites; however, mortality within 6 months is 20% once this develops, reflecting the severity of the underlying liver disease, and thus patients should be referred for evaluation for liver transplantation. Continued dietary restriction of sodium is necessary to avoid overly frequent LVP, and continuation of diuretics should be assessed on a case-by-case basis taking into consideration potential benefits and adverse reactions. Expansion of plasma volume for patients undergoing LVP is endorsed by current guidelines and supported by data demonstrating reduced postparacentesis circulatory dysfunction and improved survival. Plasma volume should be expanded with albumin at a dose of 6 to 8 g/liter of ascitic fluid removed during or immediately after LVP.

Insertion of TIPS corrects portal hypertension and offers an attractive alternative for amelioration of refractory ascites in selected patients. TIPS is a minimally invasive technique in which an endovascular stent is used to create an intrahepatic portocaval shunt and has replaced surgical shunts. Transplant-free survival is superior with TIPS compared with repeated LVP. Assessment of systolic and diastolic heart functions is recommended prior to TIPS as significant hemodynamic changes occur following the creation of the portosystemic shunt that can result in post-TIPS heart failure in individuals with underlying systolic or diastolic dysfunction.

The MELD score is a prognostic model that was initially developed to assess risk of death following TIPS placement, and data demonstrate that patients with a MELD score greater than 18

[1] Not FDA approved for this indication.

TABLE 7 Spontaneous Bacterial Peritonitis and Associated Conditions Based on Characteristics of the Ascitic Fluid

CLINICAL ENTITY	POLYMORPHONUCLEAR CELL COUNT	CULTURE RESULTS	ANTIBIOTICS RECOMMENDED
Spontaneous bacterial peritonitis	≥ 250 cells/μL	Positive, single organism	Yes
Culture-negative neutrocytic ascites	≥ 250 cells/μL	Negative	Yes
Monomicrobial nonneutrocytic bacterascites	< 250 cells/μL	Positive, single organism	Yes
Polymicrobial bacterascites	< 250 cells/μL	Positive, multiple organisms	Yes

are at high risk of death; thus TIPS should be avoided in this population. TIPS results in hepatic encephalopathy in a high proportion of patients, but pharmacologic therapy typically provides adequate treatment for this complication.

Spontaneous Bacterial Peritonitis

Cirrhosis and portal hypertension are associated with abnormal intestinal permeability leading to bacterial translocation resulting in SBP. The most commonly isolated microorganisms responsible for SBP are *Escherichia coli* (43%), *Klebsiella pneumoniae* (11%), *Streptococcus pneumoniae* (9%), other streptococcal species (19%), *Enterobacteriaceae* (4%), *Staphylococcus* (3%), and miscellaneous organisms depending on the region of the world (10%). A small-volume diagnostic paracentesis (30–60 mL) rather than LVP (which can increase the risk of hepatorenal syndrome in the setting of SBP) is mandatory for diagnosis of SBP and should be performed prior to administration of antibiotic therapy. Aerobic and anaerobic blood culture bottles should be inoculated at the bedside to avoid contamination and to increase diagnostic yield. Diagnosis of SBP is supported by the presence of 250 PMN/μL or more in the ascitic fluid without an obvious source of infection. Based on the PMN count and the microbiologic analysis of the ascitic fluid, four clinical scenarios summarized in Table 7 may be encountered.

Treatment of SBP is centered on administration of broad-spectrum empiric antibiotics with bactericidal activity against the likely infecting bacteria. Third-generation cephalosporins such as cefotaxime (Claforan) 2 g intravenously every 8 hours or ceftriaxone (Rocephin) 2 g intravenously daily offer appropriate antimicrobial coverage and are initial agents of choice for treatment of SBP. For patients allergic to beta-lactams, alternatives include fluoroquinolones such as levofloxacin (Levaquin),[1] although this agent exhibits less penetration into the ascitic fluid compared with a third-generation cephalosporin.

Current guidelines do not recommend routinely performing a follow-up paracentesis in patients with a typical initial presentation of SBP and when antibiotic therapy results in rapid clinical improvement. Repeat paracentesis, however, may be indicated to document sterility of ascitic fluid and reduction in the PMN count in patients with a slow or absent response to antibiotic therapy or in those with atypical microorganisms on initial culture results.

Plasma volume expansion with albumin is an important adjunct to antibiotic therapy in patients with SBP, as it decreases the incidence of acute kidney injury and reduces mortality. The physiologic effects of intravenous infusion of albumin include increased oncotic pressure with consequential expansion of the effective arterial blood volume, as well as its ability to bind a wide range of endogenous and exogenous ligands including bacterial lipopolysaccharides, reactive oxygen species, nitric oxide and other nitrogen reactive species, and prostaglandins, thus modulating the inflammatory response. Current guidelines recommend a selective approach for administration of intravenous albumin to patients with SBP. Specifically, this therapy should be reserved for high-risk individuals such as those with serum creatinine greater than 1 mg/dL, blood urea nitrogen greater than 30 mL/dL, or total serum bilirubin greater than 4 mg/dL. The recommended

dosage of albumin is 1.5 g/kg of body weight within 6 hours of establishing the diagnosis of SBP and a second dose of 1 g/kg on day 3.

Following an episode of SBP, recurrence occurs in 69% of individuals within 1 year; thus secondary prophylaxis is indicated, and current guidelines recommend long-term use of norfloxacin (Noroxin)[1] 400 mg orally twice daily or trimethoprim/sulfamethoxazole (Bactrim DS)[1] one double-strength tablet orally daily. Risk factors for recurrent SBP include ascitic fluid total protein concentration less than 1 g/dL and gastroesophageal variceal hemorrhage. Recommended antibiotic prophylaxis for patients hospitalized with gastroesophageal variceal hemorrhage include ceftriaxone[1] 1 g intravenously daily; once the patient is able to tolerate oral antibiotics, this may be changed to trimethoprim/sulfamethoxazole[1] one double-strength tablet orally daily, ciprofloxacin (Cipro)[1] 500 mg orally daily, or norfloxacin[1] 400 mg orally twice daily for a total of 7 days of antibiotic therapy. Importantly, some data suggest an increased risk for SBP in patients with cirrhosis and ascites taking proton pump inhibitors; thus unnecessary use of these agents should be avoided. The exact mechanism by which acid suppression increases the risk of SBP in cirrhosis is unclear, but intestinal bacterial overgrowth, increased intestinal permeability, and altered intestinal immune response may play important roles.

Hepatorenal Syndrome

The ominous significance of impaired renal function as a predictor of mortality in patients with cirrhosis is reflected by inclusion of the serum creatinine level in the MELD score. Renal dysfunction is commonly encountered in patients with cirrhosis, particularly in those with hepatic decompensation. Some studies reported acute kidney injury (AKI) in approximately 20% of hospitalized patients with cirrhosis. The differential diagnosis of AKI in patients with cirrhosis is broad and includes common etiologies such as acute tubular necrosis and nephrotoxicity, but specific glomerulopathies associated with HBV and HCV must be considered (i.e., membranous and membranoproliferative glomerulonephritides). In addition, nonalcoholic steatohepatitis is characterized by a high prevalence of type 2 diabetes mellitus and systemic hypertension; thus patients are at increased risk for diabetic and hypertensive nephropathies. Hepatorenal syndrome (HRS) is one of several potential causes of AKI that occurs in patients with cirrhosis and portal hypertension but has also been recognized in patients with acute liver failure. Importantly, HRS is a diagnosis of exclusion, and other etiologies of AKI should be considered. The pathophysiology of HRS includes splanchnic vasodilatation causing a decline in renal perfusion with consequent reductions in the glomerular filtration rate and renal excretion of sodium (typically < 10 mEq/L).

There are two distinct types of HRS depending on the acuity and severity of renal dysfunction. Type I HRS is characterized by rapid deterioration of renal function with at least a twofold increase in serum creatinine to a level greater than 2.5 mg/dL in

---

[1] Not FDA approved for this indication.

less than 2 weeks and is often precipitated by SBP, acute alcoholic hepatitis, or gastrointestinal hemorrhage. Type II HRS is more indolent and is associated with less severe renal impairment, typically resulting in ascites resistant to diuretics. Prognosis also differs significantly for both types of HRS, with the median survival in the absence of liver transplantation being 2 weeks for HRS type I and 6 months for HRS type II.

Discontinuation of all diuretics and nephrotoxic agents is critical in patients with HRS. Plasma volume expansion with administration of intravenous albumin[1] at a dose of 1 g/kg of body weight (up to a maximum of 100 g/day) to increase renal perfusion is recommended. HRS is characterized by absent or minimal proteinuria (< 500 mg/day) and normal urine sediment reflecting the lack of intrinsic renal disease. Renal ultrasonography is also recommended as it provides good assessment for chronic parenchymal changes that may suggest the presence of a chronic underlying renal disease and accurately rules out obstructive nephropathy.

Patients with HRS require either improvement in hepatic function or liver transplantation for renal function to recover. Pharmacotherapy can be used as a bridge to liver transplantation. Based on the pathophysiology of HRS, vasoconstriction with alpha-adrenergic agonists (i.e., midodrine [ProAmatine][1] or norepinephrine [Levophed][1]) or vasopressin analogs (i.e., terlipressin [Lucassin][5]) is the therapy of choice along with plasma volume expansion achieved with intravenous albumin infusion. The use of norepinephrine is reserved for critically ill patients with HRS. Terlipressin is not licensed for use in the United States. The combination of the somatostatin analog octreotide[1] along with oral midodrine and intravenous albumin infusion appears to have beneficial effects based on results from small clinical trials and is currently recommended in the United States for noncritically ill patients with type I HRS. Data from a meta-analysis support the efficacy of vasoconstrictor therapy (terlipressin, octreotide + midodrine, or norepinephrine) in combination with intravenous albumin in reducing short-term mortality in patients with type I HRS. The largest randomized clinical trial to date evaluating terlipressin in combination with albumin versus placebo plus albumin showed no difference in reversal of type I HRS, but the terlipressin group had greater improvement in renal function. Renal replacement therapy may be needed for patients with HRS not responding to pharmacologic therapy awaiting liver transplantation; however, mortality is exceedingly high and hypotensive episodes commonly occur during hemodialysis. Following liver transplantation, renal function improves in approximately 60% of patients with HRS.

Hepatic Encephalopathy

Hepatic encephalopathy (HE) is a clinical syndrome of reversible neuropsychiatric impairment of varying severity. There is continuing controversy about its exact pathogenesis, but gut-derived toxins, including ammonia, are clearly implicated. Features of HE may be subclinical (covert) or clinically evident (overt) and include a wide range of neuropsychiatric signs and symptoms. The prevalence of HE varies depending on the clinical subtype and the severity of liver disease, with cumulative prevalence rates of up to 80% for covert HE and 30% to 40% for overt HE in patients with cirrhosis. Although the West Haven criteria are widely used for grading the severity of HE (Table 8), current guidelines recommend using three additional axes to classify HE based on the etiology, time course, and presence or absence of a precipitating factor (Table 9).

Covert HE is considered preclinical and encompasses minimal HE (features of HE that are only diagnosed by specialized neuropsychiatric testing) and grade 1 HE as per West Haven criteria. In contrast, overt HE is characterized by clinical findings of HE ranging from subtle changes in orientation and presence of asterixis to hepatic coma (grades 2 to 4 per West Haven criteria).

Specialized testing is necessary to establish a diagnosis of covert HE. The psychometric hepatic encephalopathy score is regarded as the gold standard, but additional assessments include the number connection test, computerized tests such as the inhibitory control test, the cognitive drug research battery, and electroencephalogram. These tests, however, are not applicable in routine clinical practice and usually require consultation with a specialist. A smartphone application that evaluates psychomotor speed and cognitive alertness has been developed and validated as a point-of-care screening tool for covert HE: EncephalApp Stroop.

The diagnosis of overt HE is clinical and supported by the presence of a wide spectrum of global neurologic deficits. Severe HE, grades 3 and 4 West Haven criteria, should prompt attention to airway protection, and endotracheal intubation ought to be considered.

There are no laboratory markers that can be accurately used to diagnose overt HE. Blood ammonia levels lack sensitivity and specificity and correlate poorly with the severity of encephalopathy. Furthermore, a normal ammonia level does not preclude the presence of HE, and venous ammonia levels are influenced by several other factors including phlebotomy technique and handling of the blood specimen. Efforts must be directed at identifying potential precipitating factors for HE, such as compliance with treatment of HE, new medications, gastrointestinal bleeding, AKI, electrolyte imbalances, and infections.

Management of covert and overt HE is centered on the use of nonabsorbable disaccharides and antibiotics. Lactulose (Enulose) is the most widely used nonabsorbable disaccharide. Although the exact mechanism responsible for its therapeutic efficacy is still unclear, this agent is degraded by colonic microbiota to short-chain organic acids, resulting in acidification of the intestinal lumen and increased conversion of absorbable ammonia to nonabsorbable ammonium. The starting dosage for lactulose depends on the acuity and severity of HE but must be titrated to achieve two to four soft bowel movements per day. For patients who cannot tolerate oral administration (i.e., high risk for aspiration or coma), lactulose can be administered as an enema (300 mL of lactulose solution 10 g/15 mL in 700 mL of saline or water). The cathartic effects of nonabsorbable disaccharides may result in profuse diarrhea, dehydration, and hypernatremia. Rifaximin (Xifaxan) is a broad-spectrum antibiotic with activity against gram-positive, gram-negative, and anaerobic enteric bacteria that can be used in addition to lactulose for prevention of recurrent episodes of HE. Data from clinical trials show marked reductions in HE-related hospitalization and significant improvements in health-related quality of life in patients treated with a combination of lactulose and rifaximin without an increased rate of adverse events.

The efficacy and safety of other pharmacologic therapies such as probiotics[7], branched-chain amino acids[7], L-ornithine L-aspartate (LOLA)[7], ammonia scavengers, and other laxatives (i.e., polyethylene glycol [MiraLax][1]) need to be further confirmed by clinical trials. Because of concerns about oto- and nephrotoxicity, neomycin is no longer used.

Creation of a portosystemic shunt (now usually with TIPS) for management of complications of portal hypertension is associated with a 13% to 36% incidence of overt HE. Careful patient selection prior to insertion of TIPS and medical therapy with nonabsorbable disaccharides with or without additional rifaximin remain standard therapy; however, despite compliance, approximately 3% to 7% of patients have recurrent or persistent overt HE post-TIPS. For these patients, endovascular techniques aimed at decreasing the size of the shunt should be considered.

Liver transplantation offers definitive therapy for patients with end-stage liver disease, resulting in restoration of hepatic synthetic function and resolution of complications associated with portal hypertension. However, residual cognitive impairments

---

[1] Not FDA approved for this indication.
[5] Investigational drug in the United States.

[1] Not FDA approved for this indication.
[7] Available as a dietary supplement.

TABLE 8 West Haven Criteria for Grading Hepatic Encephalopathy

GRADE	LEVEL OF CONSCIOUSNESS	INTELLECT AND BEHAVIOR	NEUROLOGIC FINDINGS
0	Normal	Normal	Normal examination, abnormal neuropsychiatric testing
1	Mild lack of awareness	Shortened attention span	Impaired addition or subtraction, mild asterixis
2	Lethargy	Mild–moderate disorientation, inappropriate behavior	Severe asterixis, slurred speech
3	Somnolence but arousable	Severe disorientation, inexplicable behavior	Clonus, hyperreflexia, muscular rigidity
4	Coma	Coma	Decerebrate posture

TABLE 9 Classification of Hepatic Encephalopathy Based on Four Different Axes

TYPE OF HEPATIC ENCEPHALOPATHY	GRADE		TIME COURSE	SPONTANEOUS/PRECIPITATED
A (acute liver failure)	MHE	Covert	Episodic (one episode in 6 months)	Spontaneous: no precipitating factor discovered
B (portosystemic bypass)	1	Covert	Recurrent (more than one episode in 6 months)	
	2	Overt	Persistent (no return to normal baseline)	Precipitated by one or more specific factors
C (cirrhosis)	3	Overt		
	4	Overt		

From Patidar KR, Bajaj JS. Covert and overt hepatic encephalopathy: Diagnosis and management. Clin Gastroenterol Hepatol 2015;13:2048–2061.

may persist following liver transplantation, adversely impacting health-related quality of life.

Hepatocellular Carcinoma

Hepatocellular carcinoma (HCC) is the most common primary hepatic malignancy in adults, currently representing the fifth most common cancer and the second leading cause of cancer-related death worldwide. The epidemiology of HCC varies significantly by region and ethnicity. The majority of patients with HCC in Western populations (95%) have underlying cirrhosis (predominantly due to chronic HCV infection, alcoholic liver disease, and nonalcoholic steatohepatitis), thus limiting applicability of surgical resection (see later) as curative therapy. In contrast, only 60% of patients with HCC in Eastern populations have cirrhosis, largely reflecting the high prevalence of chronic HBV infection and its oncogenic potential. Regions of the world with intermediate to high incidence of this malignancy (more than 3 cases per 100,000 persons per year) include Asia, sub-Saharan Africa, and Western Europe. North and South America have been typically considered low-incidence regions; however, over the past two decades there has been a steady increase in the incidence of HCC, particularly in the United States.

Current guidelines endorse implementation of surveillance strategies for early diagnosis of HCC in individuals at risk for this malignancy and recommend the use of ultrasonography every 6 months as the primary surveillance modality. Populations at risk for HCC that benefit from surveillance include individuals with cirrhosis of any etiology, Asian males with chronic HBV over age 40, Asian females with chronic HBV over age 50, patients with chronic HBV and family history of HCC, African/North American blacks with chronic HBV, and individuals with stage 4 primary biliary cholangitis.

HCC can be accurately diagnosed without the need for liver biopsy by contrast-enhanced multiphase cross-sectional imaging modalities such as computed tomography (CT) or magnetic resonance imaging (MRI) based on specific patterns of contrast enhancement of the tumor in relation to the hepatic parenchyma. Key diagnostic characteristics for HCC on CT or MRI are contrast enhancement of the tumor during the early arterial phase and "washout" of contrast from the tumor during the portal venous and delayed phases. Additional features include presence of a capsule and interval growth of the lesion when previous imaging studies are used for comparison. Biopsy of the tumor carries a small risk for tumor seeding in the biopsy-needle tract (approximately 3%) and is rarely required to diagnose HCC owing to high accuracy of CT and MRI. The use of serum alpha-fetoprotein (AFP) has been controversial for routine surveillance owing to its low sensitivity and poor specificity; however, data from a recent meta-analysis suggest that addition of AFP to ultrasound increases the sensitivity of HCC detection. If not previously available, once a focal liver lesion is identified on imaging studies, AFP should be obtained as an additional diagnostic tool. AFP levels greater than 200 ng/mL are highly specific for HCC, and longitudinal follow-up of serum levels permits evaluation of response to therapeutic interventions. Additional serologic markers for HCC include the L3 isoform of AFP (AFP-L3) and des-gamma carboxy prothrombin (DCP); however, further validation of these tests for surveillance of individuals at risk for HCC is still required.

The Barcelona Clinic Liver Cancer (BCLC) staging system can be used to categorize patients with HCC and to assist with therapeutic decisions (Figure 2). Surgical resection of HCC is reserved for patients with a single lesion and no evidence of cirrhosis or portal hypertension. Locoregional therapies include radiofrequency ablation, percutaneous ethanol injection, transarterial chemoembolization, radioembolization, and microwave ablation. These modalities are typically used for patients with early and intermediate stages (BCLC stages A and B, respectively). Liver transplantation is an effective treatment for patients with cirrhosis and HCC within the so-called Milan criteria: a single lesion up to 5 cm or no more than three lesions with the largest one being less than 3 cm, and in the absence of portal venous invasion or metastatic

Figure 2 Barcelona Clinic Liver Cancer (BCLC) staging system for hepatocellular carcinoma (HCC). CLT, cadaveric liver transplantation. LDL, living donor liver transplantation. OS, overall survival. PEI, percutaneous ethanol injection. PST, performance status. RF, radiofrequency ablation. TACE, transarterial chemoembolization. (From EASL–EORTC Clinical Practice Guidelines: Management of hepatocellular carcinoma. *J Hepatol* 2012;56[4]:908–43.

disease. Liver transplantation for HCC within these limits results in long-term survival equivalent to that seen in patients with cirrhosis but no HCC. Under the current organ allocation policy in the United States, patients with HCC within Milan criteria are listed for liver transplantation with their biological MELD score (calculated by the MELD formula and without exception points) for 6 months, after which time they automatically accrue MELD exception points and the score increases to 28, with 10% increments thereafter every 3 months until the maximum score of 34 is reached. MELD exception points are granted to patients with HCC 2 cm or greater in an effort to balance risk of death that is not adequately represented by the degree of hepatic dysfunction. For patients with HCC listed for liver transplantation, the use of locoregional therapies is recommended to prevent tumor progression that may result in dropout from the waiting list. Furthermore, active surveillance is recommended to evaluate for tumor recurrence or progression, development of new lesions, and metastatic disease while awaiting liver transplantation.

Systemic chemotherapeutic agents licensed for use in patients with HCC include sorafenib (Nexavar), regorafenib (Stivarga), nivolumab (Opdivo), and lenvatinib (Lenvima). Sorafenib and lenvatinib are currently recommended for patients with BCLC stage C as first line therapy, and regorafenib and nivolumab are licensed as second line therapies for HCC. Adverse reactions, tolerability, and potential benefits must be carefully weighed and individualized according to overall health and performance status, as well as severity of hepatic dysfunction. The survival benefit of these agents is modest.

Portopulmonary Hypertension

Pulmonary artery hypertension in a patient with established portal hypertension is indicative of portopulmonary hypertension (PPHTN), but other etiologies of pulmonary hypertension must be excluded prior to establishing this diagnosis. The prevalence of PPHTN varies depending on the severity of liver disease and has been reported in 0.7% of patients with cirrhosis but can be as high as 12.5% in patients undergoing evaluation for liver transplantation.

The exact pathophysiology of PPHTN remains enigmatic, but increased exposure to humoral vasoconstrictors in the pulmonary vasculature due to portosystemic shunting and hyperdynamic circulation is among the most widely accepted hypotheses. Histologic findings in the pulmonary vasculature of patients with PPHTN are indistinguishable from those found in idiopathic pulmonary arterial hypertension and include medial hypertrophy with remodeling of the pulmonary artery walls and occasional in situ microthrombosis.

The majority of patients with PPHTN remain largely asymptomatic for extended periods of time. Symptoms associated with PPHTN are similar to those of other types of pulmonary arterial hypertension and include dyspnea on exertion, syncope, chest pain, fatigue, hemoptysis, and orthopnea. Physical examination may demonstrate jugular venous distention and lower extremity edema, the latter typically being out of proportion to the severity of ascites. Cardiopulmonary auscultation usually reveals normal clear breath sounds throughout both lung fields, an accentuated pulmonic component of the second heart sound, and a systolic murmur located along the left sternal border that is accentuated with inspiration (tricuspid regurgitation). Chest radiographs may demonstrate right ventricular enlargement and a prominent pulmonary artery.

The diagnostic workup for PPHTN should begin with transthoracic echocardiography, which provides an estimate of right ventricular and pulmonary arterial pressures and rules out left ventricular dysfunction. An estimated right ventricular systolic pressure greater than 50 mm Hg is typically used as a threshold to obtain more accurate direct hemodynamic measurements through right heart catheterization. Hemodynamic criteria used to diagnose PPHTN include mean pulmonary artery pressure (mPAP) greater than 25 mm Hg, pulmonary capillary wedge pressure less than 15 mm Hg, and pulmonary vascular resistance greater than or equal to 240 dyn·s·cm^{-5} by right heart catheterization.

Pharmacologic therapy has been extrapolated from studies performed in patients with idiopathic pulmonary arterial hypertension and includes endothelin receptor antagonists (bosentan [Tracleer][1] and ambrisentan [Letairis][1]), phosphodiesterase inhibitors (sildenafil [Revatio][1]), and prostacyclin analogs (epoprostenol [Flolan][1] and iloprost [Ventavis][1]).

Survival in PPHTN correlates with the severity of right ventricular dysfunction, and the safety and efficacy of liver transplantation are reliant on the severity of pulmonary arterial hypertension. Liver transplantation may be offered to selected patients with PPHTN but is typically contraindicated in those with mPAP greater than 35 mm Hg despite medical management, particularly if right ventricular dysfunction is present, due to considerable perioperative mortality.

Hepatopulmonary Syndrome

Hepatopulmonary syndrome (HPS) is characterized by hypoxemia due to intrapulmonary vascular dilatations with right-to-left shunting in the setting of cirrhosis and portal hypertension. Although intrapulmonary vasodilatation is encountered in over 50% of patients with cirrhosis undergoing evaluation for liver transplantation, only 15% to 30% have hypoxemia and true HPS. The most widely accepted pathophysiologic mechanism responsible for HPS is increased pulmonary synthesis of nitric oxide. Similar to PPHTN, the majority of patients with HPS are largely asymptomatic.

Clinical manifestations include dyspnea of insidious onset and two characteristic clinical findings: platypnea and orthodeoxia (worsening dyspnea and hypoxemia in upright posture, respectively). Other, more obvious but nonspecific clinical findings include spider angiomata, digital clubbing, and cyanosis. Screening for HPS relies on point-of-care oximetry indicating peripheral arterial oxygen saturation (SpO$_2$) less than 96% at rest and at sea level. Hypoxemia must be confirmed by arterial blood gas analysis demonstrating an arterial partial pressure of oxygen (PaO$_2$) less than 70 mm Hg and a widened alveolar–arterial oxygen gradient greater than or equal to 15 mm Hg ($\geq$ 20 mm Hg for patients 65 years of age or older). Importantly, blood for arterial gas analysis should be obtained with the patient sitting upright, at rest, and breathing ambient air. After establishing a diagnosis of hypoxemia, documentation of pulmonary vascular dilatations with right-to-left blood shunting is necessary. Two-dimensional contrast-enhanced transthoracic echocardiography offers high sensitivity and is widely available. Agitated saline to produce microbubbles is injected intravenously as contrast, and under normal cardiopulmonary physiology the gas bubbles are rapidly seen in the right atrium and ventricle but then diffuse into alveoli during normal flow through the pulmonary capillaries. In patients with HPS, the presence of intrapulmonary right-to-left shunting due to vascular dilatations results in the presence of the microbubbles opacifying the left heart chambers at least three heartbeats after being seen in the right ventricle. Intracardiac right-to-left blood shunting (i.e., atrial or ventricular septal defects, patent foramen ovale) should be suspected if contrast is seen in the left heart within three heartbeats. Radionuclide lung perfusion scintigraphy using technetium-labeled macroaggregated albumin particles (^{99m}Tc-MAA scan) is less sensitive than contrast-enhanced echocardiography for diagnosis of HPS but is more specific and permits accurate quantification of the intrapulmonary shunt fraction, even in the presence of coexisting intrinsic lung disorders. Shunt fractions greater than 6% confirm the diagnosis of HPS in the appropriate clinical setting.

HPS is associated with increased mortality and diminished quality of life compared with patients with cirrhosis but no HPS.

Following the diagnosis of HPS, median survival is 10.6 months; thus patients with HPS should undergo prompt liver transplantation evaluation. Under current organ allocation policies by the United Network for Organ Sharing (UNOS), patients with HPS and PaO$_2$ less than 60 mm Hg are eligible for standard MELD exception score of 22 points at the time of listing, regardless of their calculated (biological) MELD score, and a 10% mortality equivalent increase in points every 3 months. Liver transplantation remains the definitive therapy for HPS based on marked improvement or even resolution of hypoxemia in more than 85% of transplant recipients; however, clinically meaningful changes may be slow and take up to 1 year following transplantation.

Hepatic Hydrothorax

Hepatic hydrothorax is a transudative process leading to accumulation of more than 500 mL of fluid in the pleural space in patients with cirrhosis and portal hypertension in the absence of primary cardiopulmonary disease. Hepatic hydrothorax is thought to result from passage of ascitic fluid from the peritoneal cavity into the pleural spaces (typically on the right in up to 85% of patients) via subcentimeter defects and/or microscopic fenestrations in the tendinous portion of the diaphragm and is facilitated by negative intrathoracic pressure generated during inspiration. Clinical features include dyspnea, nonproductive cough, pleuritic chest pain, and even hypoxemia and hypotension in cases of tension hydrothorax. Fluid analysis demonstrates similar chemical characteristics than ascites: high serum–to–pleural fluid albumin gradient (> 1.1 g/dL) and low total protein concentration (< 2.5 g/dL).

Management of noninfected hepatic hydrothorax follows the same principles as those for ascites: sodium restriction, diuretics, repeated thoracenteses, and placement of TIPS for refractory cases. Importantly, indwelling pleural catheters should be avoided because of the high risk for complications including severe infections that may jeopardize possible liver transplant candidacy in the future.

In patients with fevers and worsening pleuritic chest pain, spontaneous bacterial empyema (SBEM) must to be excluded. Similar to the diagnostic criteria for SBP, a diagnosis of SBEM is established by a PMN count greater than 250 cells/μL and a positive bacterial culture in the absence of a parapneumonic effusion. In cases in which bacterial cultures are negative, a PMN count threshold of greater than 500 cells/μL should be used to diagnose SBEM. Microorganisms responsible for this infection are also similar to those responsible for SBP; thus third-generation cephalosporins remain the antibacterial agents of choice for empiric therapy.

Liver transplantation

Liver transplantation is effective in salvaging patients with acute liver failure (ALF) and decompensated cirrhosis, as well as selected patients with HCC (see earlier), with excellent short- and long-term outcomes. Survival after 1 and 5 years following liver transplantation is approximately 80% to 90% and 60% to 75%, respectively. Cirrhosis per se is not an indication to initiate evaluation for liver transplantation, as it is not associated with survival benefit in patients with low MELD scores. Consequently, patients should be referred for liver transplantation evaluation when the MELD score is 15 or higher or when an index complication of cirrhosis such as ascites or variceal hemorrhage occurs. Organ allocation in the United States and many other countries is based on disease severity as reflected by the MELD score for patients 12 years of age or older and the Pediatric End-Stage Liver Disease (PELD) score for patients younger than 12 years of age (includes international normalized ratio, bilirubin, albumin, and growth failure). The most recent modification of the MELD score now includes serum sodium in the mathematical equation (MELD-Na), as hyponatremia is an independent predictor of mortality in patients with cirrhosis. Some etiologies of cirrhosis result in diminished survival that is not accurately predicted by the MELD score or are associated with extremely poor quality of life; thus MELD exceptions exist. Standardized MELD exception criteria are summarized in Table 10. For patients with complications related to liver disease and associated increased morbidity and mortality

---

[1]Not FDA approved for this indication.

TABLE 10 Medical Conditions That Qualify for Standard MELD Exception Points

CONDITIONS	REMARKS
Hepatocellular carcinoma	T2 lesions (at least 2 cm in diameter) within Milan criteria
Hepatopulmonary syndrome	Pao_2 < 60 mm Hg on ambient air
Portopulmonary hypertension	Mean pulmonary arterial pressure < 35 mm Hg with treatment
Familial amyloid polyneuropathy	Confirmed by DNA analysis and histology
Primary hyperoxaluria	Need simultaneous liver–kidney transplant
Cystic fibrosis	Forced expiratory volume in 1 s (FEV1) < 40%
Hilar cholangiocarcinoma	Stage I or II, liver transplantation center must have a UNOS-approved protocol
Hepatic artery thrombosis	Within 14 days of liver transplantation, not meeting criteria for status 1A

Abbreviations: MELD = Model for End-Stage Liver Disease; UNOS = United Network for Organ Sharing.

TABLE 11 Absolute Contraindications to Liver Transplantation

CONTRAINDICATIONS TO LIVER TRANSPLANTATION
Uncontrolled sepsis
Acquired immunodeficiency syndrome
Active alcohol or substance abuse
Advanced cardiac or pulmonary disease
Intrahepatic cholangiocarcinoma
Hepatic hemangiosarcoma
Hepatocellular carcinoma with metastasis
Extrahepatic malignancy
Anatomic abnormalities that preclude liver transplantation
Lack of social support
Persistent nonadherence to medical care

TABLE 12 Criteria for Status 1A Designation in Patients With Acute Liver Failure

Age >18 years
Life expectancy <7 days without liver transplantation
Onset of encephalopathy within 8 weeks of first symptom of liver disease
Absence of preexisting liver disease
Admission to intensive care unit, and one of the following: • Ventilator dependence • Requirement of renal replacement therapy • International normalized ratio > 2
Fulminant Wilson disease
Primary graft nonfunction
Hepatic artery thrombosis

TABLE 13 Advantages and Disadvantages of Living-Donor Liver Transplantation

ADVANTAGES	DISADVANTAGES
Thorough donor screening process	Only offered in selected liver transplantation centers
Elective timing of liver transplantation permitting optimization of therapies	Donor morbidity and mortality
Diminished wait time with consequent reduction in dropout from the waiting list	Higher risk for biliary complications in the donor and recipient
Minimal cold ischemia time	

not adequately reflected by the MELD score and not qualifying for standard MELD exceptions, additional points may be petitioned by the transplant center to the regional review board on a case-by-case basis with no guarantee that they will be granted. Some examples of conditions that may receive additional MELD points include recurrent bacterial cholangitis in patients with primary sclerosing cholangitis, intractable and debilitating pruritus in patients with primary biliary cholangitis, ascites refractory to maximum-tolerated doses of diuretics, hepatic encephalopathy refractory to medical therapy, and recurrent variceal hemorrhage despite adequate therapy.

Contraindications to liver transplantation continually evolve over time. Relative contraindications are usually associated with suboptimal outcomes following liver transplantation and vary widely across different transplant centers. Absolute contraindications imply that a successful outcome following liver transplantation is unlikely; thus it should not be pursued (Table 11).

ALF is an uncommon but important indication for liver transplantation owing to the high mortality associated with this condition. Although a significant proportion of patients with ALF may have spontaneous recovery, its clinical course is usually unpredictable and early referral for liver transplantation is recommended, regardless of the etiology. Patients with ALF have the highest priority for organ allocation if they meet specific criteria for UNOS status 1A (Table 12).

Evaluation for liver transplantation is a multidisciplinary process carried out over multiple encounters aimed to unveil additional medical, surgical, behavioral, social, and economic issues that may affect liver transplantation candidacy and/or outcomes. Once the patient's candidacy is deemed appropriate, formal listing occurs with UNOS. Blood type (ABO) is the major determinant for organ compatibility, and appropriate size (based on body weight) must be taken into consideration.

Living-donor liver transplantation was developed as an alternative owing to ongoing shortage of deceased-donor organs; however, living donation carries important risks for the donor that must be carefully taken into consideration. The advantages and disadvantages of living-donor liver transplantation are summarized in Table 13.

Additional approaches to try to expand donor organ supply include donation after cardiac death, using grafts from hepatitis B core antibody–positive and hepatitis C–positive donors, and splitting a graft for use in adult and pediatric recipients.

Adequate long-term immunosuppression prevents graft rejection and is currently centered on the use of calcineurin inhibitors (tacrolimus [Prograf] primarily, and less often cyclosporine [Neoral]) with or without concomitant antimetabolite agents such as mycophenolic acid (Myfortic) or its prodrug mycophenolate mofetil (CellCept). Additional agents include inhibitors of the mammalian target of rapamycin (mTOR) such as sirolimus (Rapamune)[1] and everolimus (Zortress).

---

[1] Not FDA approved for this indication.

Long-term care of liver transplant recipients should not by any means focus exclusively on graft function and prevention of rejection, but rather be comprehensive and aimed at maintaining an overall good state of health by instituting preventive health strategies and monitoring for other complications that may ensue, such as diabetes mellitus, hypertension, dyslipidemia, renal dysfunction, obesity, and alcohol relapse, among many others.

References

Ahluwalia V, Wade JB, White MB, et al: Liver transplantation significantly improves global functioning and cerebral processing, *Liver Transplant* 22:1379–1390, 2016.

Angeli P, Volpin R, Gerunda G, et al: Reversal of type 1 hepatorenal syndrome with the administration of midodrine and octreotide, *Hepatology* 29:1690–1697, 1999.

Arguedas MR, Singh H, Faulk DK, et al: Utility of pulse oximetry screening for hepatopulmonary syndrome, *Clin Gastroenterol Hepatol* 5:749–754, 2007.

Arroyo V, Garcia-Martinez R, Salvatella X: Human serum albumin, systemic inflammation, and cirrhosis, *J Hepatol* 61:396–407, 2014.

Bajaj JS, Heuman DM, Sterling RK, et al: Validation of EncephalApp, smartphone-based Stroop test, for the diagnosis of covert hepatic encephalopathy, *Clin Gastroenterol Hepatol* 13:1828–1835, 2015 e1.

Bass NM, Mullen KD, Sanyal A, et al: Rifaximin treatment in hepatic encephalopathy, *N Engl J Med* 362:1071–1081, 2010.

Bernardi M, Caraceni P, Navickis RJ, et al: Albumin infusion in patients undergoing large-volume paracentesis: a meta-analysis of randomized trials, *Hepatology* 55:1172–1181, 2012.

Blachier M, Leleu H, Peck-Radosavljevic M, et al: The burden of liver disease in Europe: a review of available epidemiological data, *J Hepatol* 58:593–608, 2013.

Bureau C, Thabut D, Oberti F, et al: Transjugular intrahepatic portosystemic shunts with covered stents increase transplant-free survival of patients with cirrhosis and recurrent ascites, *Gastroenterology* 152:157–163, 2017.

D'Amico G, Garcia-Tsao G, Pagliaro L: Natural history and prognostic indicators of survival in cirrhosis: a systematic review of 118 studies, *J Hepatol* 44:217–231, 2006.

Dasarathy S, Merli M: Sarcopenia from mechanism to diagnosis and treatment in liver disease, *J Hepatol* 65:1232–1244, 2016.

Escorsell À, Pavel O, Cárdenas A, Morillas R, Llop E, Villanueva C, et al: Esophageal balloon tamponade versus esophageal stent in controlling acute refractory variceal bleeding: a multicenter randomized, controlled trial, *Hepatology* 63:1957–1967, 2016.

Flemming JA, Kim WR, Brosgart CL, et al: Reduction in liver transplant wait-listing in the era of direct-acting antiviral therapy, *Hepatology* 65(3):804–812, 2017.

Garcia-Pagan JC, Caca K, Bureau C, et al: Early use of TIPS in patients with cirrhosis and variceal bleeding, *N Engl J Med* 362:2370–2379, 2010.

Garcia-Pagan JC, Barrufet M, Cardenas A, et al: Management of gastric varices, *Clin Gastroenterol Hepatol* 12:919–928, 2014, e1; quiz e51-2.

Garcia-Tsao G, Sanyal AJ, Grace ND, Carey W: Practice Guidelines Committee of the American Association for the Study of Liver D, Practice Parameters Committee of the American College of G. Prevention and management of gastroesophageal varices and variceal hemorrhage in cirrhosis, *Hepatology* 46:922–938, 2007.

Garcia-Tsao G, Abraldes JG, Berzigotti A, Bosch J: Portal Hypertensive Bleeding in Cirrhosis: Risk Stratification, Diagnosis, and Management: 2016 Practice Guidance by the American Association for the Study of Liver Diseases, *Hepatology* 65:310–335, 2017.

Ge PS, Runyon BA: Serum ammonia level for the evaluation of hepatic encephalopathy, *JAMA* 312:643–644, 2014.

Gines P, Fernandez-Esparrach G, Arroyo V, et al: Pathogenesis of ascites in cirrhosis, *Semin Liver Dis* 17:175–189, 1997.

Gluud LL, Christensen K, Christensen E, et al: Systematic review of randomized trials on vasoconstrictor drugs for hepatorenal syndrome, *Hepatology* 51:576–584, 2010.

Goel GA, Deshpande A, Lopez R, et al: Increased rate of spontaneous bacterial peritonitis among cirrhotic patients receiving pharmacologic acid suppression, *Clin Gastroenterol Hepatol* 10:422–427, 2012.

Grace JA, Angus PW: Hepatopulmonary syndrome: update on recent advances in pathophysiology, investigation, and treatment, *J Gastroenterol Hepatol* 28:213–219, 2013.

Kristina Tzartzeva K, Obi J, Rich NE, Parikh ND, Marrero JA, Yoop A, et al: Surveillance imaging and alpha fetoprotein for early detection of hepatocellular carcinoma in patients with cirrhosis: a meta-analysis, *Gastroenterology* Feb 6, Epub ahead of print.

Krowka MJ, Plevak DJ, Findlay JY, et al: Pulmonary hemodynamics and perioperative cardiopulmonary-related mortality in patients with portopulmonary hypertension undergoing liver transplantation, *Liver Transplant* 6:443–450, 2000.

Kurokawa T, Zheng YW, Ohkohchi N: Novel functions of platelets in the liver, *J Gastroenterol Hepatol* 31:745–751, 2016.

Lim YS, Kim WR: The global impact of hepatic fibrosis and end-stage liver disease, *Clin Liver Dis* 12:733–736, 2008 vii.

Lin ZH, Xin YN, Dong QJ, et al: Performance of the aspartate aminotransferase-to-platelet ratio index for the staging of hepatitis C-related fibrosis: an updated meta-analysis, *Hepatology* 53:726–736, 2011.

Llovet JM, Ricci S, Mazzaferro V, et al: Sorafenib in advanced hepatocellular carcinoma, *N Engl J Med* 359:378–390, 2008.

Marik PE, Wood K, Starzl TE: The course of type 1 hepato-renal syndrome post liver transplantation, *Nephrol Dial Transplant* 21:478–482, 2006.

Mazzaferro V, Regalia E, Doci R, et al: Liver transplantation for the treatment of small hepatocellular carcinomas in patients with cirrhosis, *N Engl J Med* 334:693–699, 1996.

Merion RM, Schaubel DE, Dykstra DM, et al: The survival benefit of liver transplantation, *Am J Transplant* 5:307–313, 2005.

Mullen KD, Sanyal AJ, Bass NM, et al: Rifaximin is safe and well tolerated for long-term maintenance of remission from overt hepatic encephalopathy, *Clin Gastroenterol Hepatol* 12:1390–1397, 2014 e2.

Ohlsson B, Nilsson J, Stenram U, et al: Percutaneous fine-needle aspiration cytology in the diagnosis and management of liver tumours, *Br J Surg* 89:757–762, 2002.

Patidar KR, Bajaj JS: Covert and overt hepatic encephalopathy: diagnosis and management, *Clin Gastroenterol Hepatol* 13:2048–2061, 2015.

Pereira K, Carrion AF, Martin P, et al: Current diagnosis and management of post-transjugular intrahepatic portosystemic shunt refractory hepatic encephalopathy, *Liver Int* 35:2487–2494, 2015.

Runyon BA, Committee APG: Management of adult patients with ascites due to cirrhosis: an update, *Hepatology* 49:2087–2107, 2009.

Runyon BA, Squier S, Borzio M: Translocation of gut bacteria in rats with cirrhosis to mesenteric lymph nodes partially explains the pathogenesis of spontaneous bacterial peritonitis, *J Hepatol* 21:792–796, 1994.

Saab S, Hernandez JC, Chi AC, et al: Oral antibiotic prophylaxis reduces spontaneous bacterial peritonitis occurrence and improves short-term survival in cirrhosis: a meta-analysis, *Am J Gastroenterol* 104:993–1001, 2009, quiz 2.

Salerno F, Merli M, Riggio O, et al: Randomized controlled study of TIPS versus paracentesis plus albumin in cirrhosis with severe ascites, *Hepatology* 40:629–635, 2004.

Sort P, Navasa M, Arroyo V, et al: Effect of intravenous albumin on renal impairment and mortality in patients with cirrhosis and spontaneous bacterial peritonitis, *N Engl J Med* 341:403–409, 1999.

Udell JA, Wang CS, Tinmouth J, et al: Does this patient with liver disease have cirrhosis? *JAMA* 307:832–842, 2012.

Vallet-Pichard A, Mallet V, Nalpas B, et al: FIB-4: An inexpensive and accurate marker of fibrosis in HCV infection. Comparison with liver biopsy and fibrotest, *Hepatology* 46:32–36, 2007.

Villanueva C, Colomo A, Bosch A, et al: Transfusion strategies for acute upper gastrointestinal bleeding, *N Engl J Med* 368:11–21, 2013.

Wang FS, Fan JG, Zhang Z, et al: The global burden of liver disease: the major impact of China, *Hepatology* 60:2099–2108, 2014.

Wells M, Chande N, Adams P, Beaton M, Levstik M, Boyce E, et al: Meta-analysis: vasoactive medications for the management of acute variceal bleeds, *Aliment Pharmacol Ther* 35:1267–1278, 2012.

Williams Jr JW, Simel DL: The rational clinical examination. Does this patient have ascites? How to divine fluid in the abdomen, *JAMA* 267:2645–2648, 1992.

Zaiac MN, Walker A: Nail abnormalities associated with systemic pathologies, *Clin Dermatol* 31:627–649, 2013.

DIVERTICULA OF THE ALIMENTARY TRACT

Method of
Aaron Sinclair, MD

CURRENT DIAGNOSIS

- Endoscopy or barium swallow study may be used in the evaluation of most upper alimentary tract diverticula.
- Symptomatic small intestinal diverticula are difficult to diagnose and require a high index of suspicion and radiographic examination (nuclear medicine scans, capsule endoscopy, or computed tomography scans).
- Diverticulitis of the colon is most accurately identified and the treatment planned with computed tomography of the abdomen and pelvis.
- Diverticulitis of the colon that is slow to resolve may require additional imaging or direct visualization with endoscopy to identify an alternative diagnosis.

CURRENT THERAPY

- Most asymptomatic diverticula are identified incidentally and may only require monitoring.
- Surgical management of symptomatic diverticula may require surgical resection.
- Early in the disease process, uncomplicated diverticulitis of the colon may be managed on an outpatient basis with a conservative no-intervention approach or oral antibiotics.
- Complicated diverticulitis of the colon should be managed in conjunction with a surgeon and in the hospital with intravenous antibiotics.

A diverticulum is an abnormal saccular protrusion from the wall of the alimentary tract. Diverticula may be classified as either true or false. The wall of the alimentary tract is composed of submucosal, mucosal, and muscular layers. A false diverticulum is a protrusion of the submucosa and mucosa through a defect in the muscular wall of the alimentary tract. A true diverticulum is a protrusion of all layers of the alimentary tract wall. Many diverticula are asymptomatic and require no treatment. Some diverticula cause symptoms depending on their anatomic location or associated pathophysiologic complications (e.g., obstruction, infection, inflammation, or bleeding). This chapter categorizes alimentary canal diverticula by their location.

Esophagus
Zenker Diverticulum
Zenker diverticulum is a false diverticulum that develops in the upper posterior esophagus in an area known as Killian triangle, located between the inferior pharyngeal constrictors and the cricopharyngeal muscles. Zenker diverticulum typically presents after age 60 and has a male predominance for reasons that are unclear. It affects only 2 per 100,000 patients per year. Though it can be asymptomatic for years before the development of symptomatology, patients may experience dysphagia, aspiration, and regurgitation of undigested food. The exact cause is unclear, but proposed mechanisms suggest a dysfunction in coordinated swallowing muscle movement and increased intraluminal pressure in the esophagus. There may be an additive component of long-term upper esophageal sphincter irritation from acid reflux.

Diagnosis is primarily made through barium swallow, though small diverticula may be missed (Figure 1). Although endoscopic direct visualization is possible, caution should be exercised owing to the risk of perforation. Small asymptomatic diverticula can be monitored. Zenker diverticulum greater than 2 cm in size, regardless of symptomatology, should be surgically evaluated and repair considered. Methods for closure include endoscopic diverticulostomy and myotomy or traditional surgical resection. However, recent studies seem to favor flexible endoscopic cricopharyngeus myectomy; follow-up has shown no recurrence of diverticula at 19 months. Although most patients (>90%) demonstrate symptom improvement, recurrence rates can be as high as 35%.

Figure 1 Zenker diverticulum. (Image courtesy Gastrolab—The Gastrointestinal Site. http://www.gastrolab.net [Accessed August 25, 2014].)

Traction Diverticulum
Traction diverticula are the only true diverticula of the esophagus. Traction diverticula are rare. Their size tends to stay below 2 cm. Owing to the proposed mechanism of formation, traction diverticula are isolated to the middle third of the esophagus. It is not fully clear how traction diverticula form. One proposed mechanism is related to a precedent pulmonary infection, most commonly tuberculosis or histoplasmosis, with resultant mediastinal lymph node formation. After the active infection subsides, resultant fibrosis and scarring between the tissues surrounding the mediastinal lymph nodes and esophagus occur. Initially, a small diverticulum develops from this fibrosis, which produces "traction" or a lack of mobility. Diverticular progression results when age-related changes from the dysfunction of coordinated swallowing muscle movement and increased intraluminal pressure in the esophagus develop. Surgical management is rarely needed unless these diverticula become symptomatic or complications, such as fistulas, occur.

Epiphrenic Diverticulum
Epiphrenic diverticula are false diverticula of the distal esophagus affecting only 0.015% of the general population. They are thought to arise secondary to mucosal injury from gastroesophageal reflux and muscle dysmotility. They occur within 10 cm of the gastroesophageal junction, and symptoms include dysphagia, spasmodic chest pain, and gastroesophageal reflux. There does not appear to be a correlation with between diverticular size and symptomatology. With progression of diverticular size, obstruction can become a potential complication. Diagnostic measures start with barium swallow and may be followed with additional tests, including endoscopy, 24-hour pH probe, and esophageal manometry.

Management depends on patient symptoms and size of the diverticulum. If small (<5 cm) and asymptomatic, routine clinical and endoscopic surveillance is permissible. However, any symptomatology necessitates surgical evaluation and repair. Surgical options include open resection and laparoscopy. Partial fundoplication may be indicated, depending on the severity of gastroesophageal reflux present as indicated by ancillary testing of a 24-hour pH probe.

Stomach
Gastric Diverticula
Gastric diverticula are rare with an endoscopic incidence of 0.01%. Most are asymptomatic and small (<3 cm). Symptoms may include epigastric pain, dyspepsia, and emesis. Rarely, ulcerations, perforations, or bleeding can occur. Diagnosis involves endoscopy, barium swallow, or contrast-aided computed tomography scan. If symptomatic, typical treatment includes a proton pump inhibitor and monitoring for symptom improvement. Persistent symptoms may necessitate gastrectomy of the diverticulum, especially if concerns about cancer exist.

Small Intestine
Duodenal Diverticula
Diverticula located in the duodenum are relatively common, affecting up to 22% of the general population (Figure 2). Duodenal diverticula may be either true or false diverticula. The most common location is the second portion of the duodenum. The size and position of the diverticula may lead to complications such as obstruction of the sphincter of Oddi and/or impingement of the hepatobiliary tree drainage. This impingement may result in jaundice, right upper quadrant pain, or infection signs/symptoms similar to cholecystitis. Although usually asymptomatic, ulcerative bleeding or perforation may occur on occasion.

Duodenal diverticula may be identified on barium swallow, contrast-enhanced computed tomography, magnetic resonance imaging, or endoscopy. Duodenal diverticula found incidentally do not require treatment. If symptoms arise, endoscopic evaluation and surgical resection should be considered. However, intervention should be considered with caution owing to a high risk (30%) of complications, in particular fistula formation and mortality.

Figure 2 Duodenal diverticulum. (Image courtesy Gastrolab—The Gastrointestinal Site. http://www.gastrolab.net [Accessed August 25, 2014].)

Jejunal and Ileal Diverticula

Jejunal and ileal diverticula occur throughout the length of the small intestine in 1% to 2% of the population. There does not appear to be any statistically significant relationship with morbidity or mortality of these types of diverticula with respect to location, gender, size, number, and so forth. These false diverticula are located predominantly where the blood vessels penetrate the muscular wall of the mesenteric side of the bowel. Most are noted incidentally on radiographic studies, but some manifest with symptoms secondary to bleeding, obstruction, or infection. These symptoms are believed to be due to bacterial overgrowth that may occur within the cavity of the diverticulum. Diagnosis can be made with capsule endoscopy or a small bowel barium contrast follow-through study, although some may be noted on computed tomography with intravenous and oral contrast. Advanced endoscopic procedures such as push enteroscopy and double balloon endoscopy can be utilized to further evaluate symptomatic diverticula.

Asymptomatic jejunal and ileal diverticula should not be resected. Bacterial overgrowth symptoms may respond to antibiotic treatment and intestinal promotility drug therapy. If diverticulitis is seen radiographically, intravenous antibiotics and bowel rest should be initiated. Surgical intervention with small bowel resection is indicated if symptomatic diverticula persist despite conservative management.

Meckel Diverticulum

Meckel diverticulum is a congenital anomaly that occurs owing to incomplete closure of the vitelline duct. This duct typically obliterates during the ninth week of gestational age. Owing to the embryologic origin of the diverticulum, it is almost always located within 2 feet of the ileocecal valve. Meckel diverticulum has a prevalence of 1% to 2% of the population, with a 2:1 male predominance. About 2% of all existing Meckel diverticula will become symptomatic. Symptomatic diverticula most commonly cause nausea, vomiting, and abdominal pain. The sign most commonly associated with Meckel diverticulum is intussusception. This occurs owing to residual fibrous attachments to the umbilicus causing a lead point for the proximal bowel to involute onto the distal bowel. It most commonly presents with bloody mucoid stools, abdominal pain, and vomiting in children under six years of age, most commonly within the first 2 years of life. However, other symptoms may occur if ectopic tissue exists in the diverticulum. Gastric ectopic tissue may cause abdominal pain and bloody stools from ulceration of the underlying ileal tissue. Duodenal and pancreatic tissues have been identified in Meckel diverticulum but are very rare and do not typically cause symptoms.

Diagnosis in adults requires a high level of suspicion and is aided by the use of a technetium 99 m (^{99m}Tc) scan to identify ectopic gastric mucosa in those patients with bleeding and symptoms of ulceration. For children with obstructive signs or symptoms, the diagnosis may be aided by ultrasound and/or computed tomographic scans. Plain film radiographs of the abdomen have low sensitivity and specificity for the diagnosis of intussusception. The sensitivity of the Meckel scan for the pediatric population is 85% to 97% but is much lower in the adult population at 62%. The choice of imaging procedure is dictated by the experience of the radiologic personnel performing the procedure.

Symptomatic Meckel diverticulum should be surgically resected. Up to 90% of intussusception secondary to Meckel diverticulum may be reduced utilizing diagnostic ultrasonography with saline or pneumatic enema. Treatment of Meckel diverticulum largely depends on age and symptomatology because operating on asymptomatic Meckel diverticulum has been shown to have a fivefold increase in complications, such as postoperative bowel obstruction, leaks, ileus, and infection. Many experts have advocated that incidental, asymptomatic Meckel diverticulum should not be resected. Some experts advocate for selective surgical resection of asymptomatic patients with an incidentally noted Meckel diverticulum for the following: healthy young children, healthy adults younger than 50 years of age with palpable abnormalities suggestive of heterotrophic tissue, size longer than 2 cm, or a broad base wider than 2 cm.

Colon
Diverticulosis

The colon is where most diverticula occur in the alimentary tract. Owing to this predominance, this condition is commonly termed *diverticulosis* or *diverticular disease*. Diverticulum of the colon is of the false type. The incidence increases with age. The incidence of left-sided diverticulosis approaches 5% at age 40 and increases to greater than 60% at age 80. Diverticulosis is most commonly located in the sigmoid colon.

The exact pathogenesis of diverticulosis is unclear. The proposed mechanism of colonic diverticular formation places an emphasis on intraluminal pressure buildup. The pressure across the colonic wall increases as the radius of the wall decreases. Accordingly, the radius is the smallest in the sigmoid colon and thus the most likely location of diverticulosis. Normally, pressure is constant throughout the colon. However, as diverticular disease develops, abnormal pressure segmentations occur, resulting in pressure gradient changes in the colon. With increased pressure, the integrity of collagen and elastin in the wall muscle changes, the circular muscles thicken, colonic segments shorten, and the lumen narrows, leading to propagation of the disease. Several risk factors have been associated with the development of diverticular disease: smoking, lack of physical activity, and obesity. By increasing the amount of dietary fiber, it is theorized that the resultant bulking of the stools may decrease the pressure in the colon lumen and prevent diverticular disease progression. Yet, mixed results have been noted on studies of fiber intake and diverticular development and progression of disease. There is no associated risk with the ingestion of caffeine, alcohol, popcorn, seeds, or nuts and the development of diverticulosis, diverticular bleeding, or diverticulitis.

Colonic Diverticular Bleeding

Diverticula tend to develop where an arteriole penetrates the circular muscle layer of the colon. This results in vessels arching over the dome of the diverticulum. This leaves fragile vessels in a vulnerable position of a relatively thin mucosal layer prone to trauma and resultant diverticular bleeding. Bleeding typically manifests as hematochezia—a darkish to bright red bleeding that is typically characterized as brisk and acute in nature. Diverticulosis is attributed to 30% to 50% of all hematochezia. Fifteen percent of patients will experience at least one episode of bleeding in their lifetime, with a recurrent bleeding risk of up to 38%. Most patients presenting with diverticular bleeding are asymptomatic, but some may experience bloating or cramping.

Selection of the diagnostic modality depends largely on the degree of bleeding and the cardiovascular stability of the patient. Endoscopy is the preferred treatment modality for stable patients

Figure 3 Colonoscopy in a patient with hematochezia from the source isolated to a diverticulum (A) and hemostasis noted after placement of two hemoclips (B). (Courtesy Janak Shah.) (From Feldman M. *Sleisenger and Fordtran's Gastrointestinal and Liver Disease.* 9th ed. Philadelphia: Elsevier; Figure 117.8.)

owing to its potential for diagnosis and treatment options. Up to 80% of diverticular bleeding can be isolated with direct endoscopic visualization (Figure 3).

Endoscopic failure to identify or control diverticular bleeding may occur in the patient with massive or intermittent bleeding. Depending on the patient's cardiovascular stability and degree of bleeding, the typical evaluative progression if the site of bleeding is not identified is endoscopy, followed by tagged red blood cell scan, and then angiography. Hemodynamically unstable patients may have a high complication risk from the bowel preparation, sedation, or the procedure. Radionuclide imaging can be considered in unstable patients, nondiagnostic endoscopy, or bleeding recurrence. Radionuclide imaging requires that bleeding be active (at least 0.05 to 0.1 mL/min) to accurately isolate the location of the diverticulum. Radionuclide imaging using technetium (^{99m}Tc) sulfur colloid (shorter half-life, thus utilized for acute bleeding) or ^{99m}Tc pertechnetate (longer half-life more useful for intermittent bleeding)–labeled autologous red blood cells can be used to isolate the location of obscure gastrointestinal bleeding. However, numerous studies have produced highly variable sensitivities (26% to 91%). Many advocate for radionuclide imaging to be used as an ancillary test for directing more definitive treatments such as surgery or angiography-directed therapies. Angiography can be used if bleeding is active (at least 0.5 mL/min) and can isolate the bleeding location with a diagnostic yield of 40% to 78%. Angiography can be combined with embolization and/or vasopressin infusion to achieve hemostasis; however, complications may occur, including bowel infarction and contrast-induced nephrotoxicity.

Diverticulitis

Diverticulosis is largely asymptomatic. Only about 4% will develop inflammation and infection known as diverticulitis. The disease severity and complications occur along a spectrum. The proposed mechanism of diverticulitis may be a blocked diverticulum or trauma-associated mucosal injury. Colonic diverticula become filled with feces and obstruction may occur. With the resultant bacterial overgrowth, expansion of the diverticula occurs. Subsequent vascular compromise and microperforation may occur, leading to localized infection and inflammation. These microperforations are usually sequestered and may lead to small localized abscess formation. This process is generally referred to as uncomplicated diverticulitis. Complicated diverticulitis is classified when a localized abscess or infection infiltrates into adjacent organs or viscera causing macroperforations, fistulas, obstructions, or enlarged abscesses.

The clinical presentation often begins with mild left lower abdominal pain, fever, and leukocytosis. Patients who seek care later in the disease process may present with sepsis or diffuse peritonitis. Initial diagnosis should be accomplished with history, physical examination, radiographic imaging, and laboratory evaluation. Abdominal radiography may indicate severe complications of diverticulitis such as bowel perforation or bowel obstruction. Ultrasonography and magnetic resonance imaging can be used with high levels of sensitivity and specificity in centers with demonstrated expertise. Ultrasonography has sensitivities and specificities of 92% and 90% for the detection of diverticulitis, respectively. With sensitivities and specificities of 94% and 99%, respectively, computed tomography appears to be the imaging test of choice. This is especially true, as an alternative diagnosis was more likely to be identified with computed tomography than with ultrasonography (50% to 100% vs. 33% to 78%). Those patients with a past medical history of diverticulitis may be empirically treated without imaging, although imaging may be needed if no clinical improvement is noted within 48 hours.

Recent data indicate no added benefit with antimicrobial therapy; thus, uncomplicated diverticulitis may be treated without antibiotics and close clinical follow-up. Until further studies are done, many experts recommend that traditional treatment should include supportive care, liquid diet, and antibiotics for uncomplicated diverticulitis. Outpatient management is reasonable if the diagnosis is made early in the disease process. Uncomplicated diverticulitis responds to medical therapy in most cases. Complicated diverticulitis occurs in 25% of all diverticulitis diagnoses, requiring a surgical evaluation and intervention. Optional antibiotic regimens for gram-negative coverage and anaerobic coverage are listed in Table 1. Inpatient management is recommended with any comorbid conditions, immunosuppression, high-grade fever, or leukocytosis and/or for elderly patients. Patient improvement should be seen within 48 hours. Those who do not improve should undergo additional evaluation such as repeat imaging or endoscopy. This is done to evaluate for underlying pathology such as cancer or inflammatory bowel disease, which would change the management strategy.

Follow-up scanning should also be considered for cases of slow-resolving diverticulitis. In the past, up to 10% of computed tomography (CT) scans in which diverticulitis was the primary diagnosis, cancer could not be fully excluded. As CT scanner resolution has improved, newer studies have demonstrated only a small number of underlying cancers or indeterminate findings. A colonoscopy should be performed to evaluate the extent of diverticular disease and to rule out other comorbid pathology in all patients. Colonoscopy is typically recommended 6 weeks after diverticulitis symptoms have resolved. Introduction of stool softeners and a high-fiber diet should begin immediately and continued indefinitely for all patients to help decrease the intraluminal pressure within the colon.

Diverticulitis that is complicated with abscess formation should be evaluated by a surgeon or radiologist for percutaneous

TABLE 1	Antibiotic Therapy for Diverticulitis	
OPTIONAL REGIMENS	**DOSAGE (ADULT)**	
Uncomplicated Diverticulitis		
Outpatient (10–14 days)		
Ciprofloxacin (Cipro) and Metronidazole (Flagyl)	500 mg PO bid 500 mg PO tid	
Amoxicillin-clavulanate (Augmentin)[1]	875 mg PO bid	
Moxifloxacin (Avelox)	400 mg PO daily	
Complicated Diverticulitis		
Inpatient Transitioning to Outpatient (10–14 days total)		
Piperacillin-tazobactam (Zosyn)[1]	3.375–4.5 g IV every 6 h	
Imipenem-cilastatin (Primaxin)	500 mg IV every 6 h	
Levofloxacin (Levaquin)[1] and Metronidazole	500 mg IV every 24 h 500 mg IV every 8 h	
Ceftriaxone (Rocephin) and Metronidazole	1 g IV every 24 h 500 mg IV every 8 h	

[1]Not FDA approved for this indication.
Clindamycin (Cleocin) may be substituted in metronidazole intolerance/allergy.
Antibiotics continued in complicated diverticulitis cases until negative cultures, clinical improvement, or sensitivities obtained on any surgical specimens.
bid, Twice a day; *tid*, three times a day.
Modified from Jacobs DO. Clinical practice: Diverticulitis. *N Engl J Med.* 2007;357:2057–2066.

Figure 4 Diverticulitis. (A) Computed tomography (CT) image demonstrates thickened wall of the sigmoid colon *(arrows)* with stranding in the adjacent fat *(*)* indicative of diverticulitis. Fat stranding refers to abnormally increased attenuation of fat from edema and engorgement of lymphatics. (B) CT image slightly more caudal demonstrates an air-filled abscess cavity *(arrows)* with adjacent thickened sigmoid colon wall. (From McNally PR. GI/Liver Secrets Plus, 4th ed. *Noninvasive Gastrointestinal Imaging: Ultrasound, Computed Tomography, Magnetic Resonance Imaging.* Philadelphia: Mosby Elsevier; 2010, Figure 70–16.)

drainage using computed tomography or ultrasonography (Figure 4). Depending on location, drainage tubes may be placed transanally for drainage. A general recommendation exists for consideration of drainage, preferably with interventional radiology localization, for any abscess measuring greater than 3 to 4 cm.

New research to prevent recurrent diverticulitis with medical management is emerging. Mesalamine (Asacol)[1] and rifaximin (Xifaxan), in combination or separately, may help prevent recurrent episodes of diverticulitis. Probiotics[2] have not been shown to prevent recurrence. Fiber may be used as a beneficial supplement for the prevention of recurrent diverticulitis. Debate exists regarding elective segmental colectomy for patients who have experienced recurrent episodes of diverticulitis. Current recommendations suggest surgical consultation with discussion of the benefits and risks of surgery compared to the risks of recurrent diverticulitis. This discussion should take into account the diverticulitis frequency and severity, the impact on the patient's lifestyle, and the patient's other comorbid conditions. This consultation should at a minimum occur after the fourth recurrence of diverticulitis in patients over age 50. There is insufficient evidence to advise a patient who has experienced fewer than four recurrent cases of diverticulitis or who is younger than age 50 on the benefit of a segmental colectomy.

References

Choi JJ, Ogunjemilusi O, Divino CM: Diagnosis and management of diverticula in the jejunum and ileum, *Am Surg* 79(1):108–110, 2013.

Delavux M: Diverticular disease of the colon in Europe: Epidemiology, impact on citizen health and prevention, *Aliment Pharmacol Ther* 18(Suppl 3):71–74, 2003.

Fry RD, Mahmoud NN, Maron DJ, et al: Colon and rectum. In Townsend Jr CM, Beauchamp D, editors: *Sabiston Textbook of Surgery*, 19th ed, Philadelphia, 2012, Saunders, pp 1309–1314.

Greene CL, McFadden PM, Oh DS, et al: Long-term outcome of the treatment of Zenker's diverticulum, *Ann Thorac Surg* 100:975–978, 2015.

Jacobs DO: Clinical practice, Diverticulitis, *N Engl J Med* 357:2057–2066, 2007.

Janes SE, Meagher A, Frizelle FA: Management of diverticulitis, *BMJ* 332:271–275, 2006.

Kilic A, Schuchert MJ, Awais O, et al: Surgical management of epiphrenic diverticula in the minimally invasive era, *JSLS* 13:160–164, 2009.

Lameris W, van Randen A, Bipat S, et al: Graded compression ultrasonography and computed tomography in acute colonic diverticulitis: Meta-analysis of test accuracy, *Eur Radiol* 18:2498–2511, 2008.

Lin S, Suhocki PV, Ludwig KA, et al: Gastrointestinal bleeding in adult patients with Meckel's diverticulum: The role of technetium 99m pertechnetate scan, *South Med J* 95:1338, 2002.

Maish MS: Esophagus. In Townsend Jr CM, Beauchamp D, editors: *Sabiston Textbook of Surgery*, 19th ed, Philadelphia, 2012, Saunders, pp 1023–1025.

Martinez-Cecilia D, Arjona-Sanchez A, Gomez-Alvarez M, et al: Conservative management of perforated duodenal diverticulum: A case report and review of the literature, *World J Gastroenterol* 14:1949–1951, 2008.

Mohan P, Ananthavadivelu M, Venkataraman J: Gastric diverticulum, *CMAJ* 182:E226, 2010.

Morris AM, Rogenbogen SE, Hardiman KM, et al: Sigmoid diverticulitis: A systematic review, *JAMA* 311:287–297, 2014.

Mulder CJ, Costamagna G, Sakai P: Zenker's diverticulum: Treatment using a flexible endoscope, *Endoscopy* 33:991–997, 2001.

Oukachbi N, Brouzes S: Management of complicated duodenal diverticula, *J Visceral Surg* 150:173–179, 2013.

Park JJ, Wolff BG, Tollefson MK, et al: Meckel diverticulum: The Mayo Clinic experience with 1476 patients (1950– 2002), *Ann Surg* 241:529–533, 2005.

Pang M, Koop A, Brahmbhatt B, et al: Comparison of flexible endoscopic cricopharyngeal meyctomy and myotomy approaches for Zenker diverticulum repair, *Gastroinest Endosc* 89(4):880–886, 2019.

Sartelli M, Catena F, Ansaloni L, et al: WSES Guidelines for the management of acute left sided colonic diverticulitis in the emergency setting, *World J Emerg Surg* 11:37, 2016.

Shabanzadeh DM, Wille-Jørgensen P: Antibiotics for uncomplicated diverticulitis, Nov 14, *Cochrane Database Syst Rev* 11, 2012. https://doi.org/10.1002/146518 58.CD009092.pub2 Art. No.: CD009092.

Shahedi K, Fuller G, Bolus R, et al: Long-term risk of acute diverticulitis among patients with incidental diverticulosis found during colonoscopy, *Clin Gastroenterol Hepatol* 11(12):1609–1613, 2013.

Sinha CK, Pallewatte A, Easty M, et al: Meckel's scan in children: A review of 183 cases referred to two paediatric surgery specialist centres over 18 years, *Pediatr Surg Int* 29:511–517, 2013.

Strate LL: Lower GI, bleeding: Epidemiology and diagnosis, *Gastroenterol Clin North Am* 34:643–664, 2005.

Verdonck J, Morton RP: Systematic review on treatment of Zenker's diverticulum, *Eur Arch Otorhnolaryngol* 272:3095–3107, 2015.

Weizman AV, Nguyen GC: Diverticular disease: epidemiology and management, *Can J Gastroenterol* 25:385–389, 2011.

Young-Fadok TM: Diverticulitis, *N Engl J Med* 379, 2018, 1635-164.

Zani A, Eaton S, Rees CM, et al: Incidentally detected Meckel diverticulum: To resect or not to resect? *Ann Surg* 247:276–281, 2008.

[1]Not US Food and Drug Administration (FDA) approved for this indication.
[2]Available as dietary supplement.

DYSPHAGIA AND ESOPHAGEAL OBSTRUCTION

Method of
Kumar Krishnan, MD; and John E. Pandolfino, MD

CURRENT DIAGNOSIS

- The evaluation of dysphagia begins with a careful history, though additional diagnostic testing is often required.
- Oropharyngeal dysphagia is best initially evaluated with a video fluoroscopoic examination, whereas esophageal dysphagia is best evaluated with endoscopy.
- Esophageal dysphagia with negative endoscopy and biopsy should be evaluated next with esophageal physiological testing (esophageal manometry or endoscopic functional lumen imaging probe EndoFLIP).

CURRENT THERAPY

- Underlying neuromuscular conditions such as amyotrophic lateral sclerosis, myasthenia gravis, or Guillain-Barré syndrome should be treated accordingly.
- Endoscopic therapy with dilation (often multiple) is the mainstay of treating fibrotic esophageal strictures regardless of etiology.
- Achalasia can be treated surgically or with dilation, which are equally effective. Minimally invasive endoscopic therapy for achalasia is promising and may provide a competing approach.

Dysphagia is a symptom generated by the perceived sensation of difficulty or inability to swallow. It ranges in severity from mild difficulty with no associated clinical sequelae, to a complete inability to swallow with aspiration and severe malnutrition. Dysphagia can coexist with and must be distinguished from odynophagia, which is pain when swallowing, with associated swallowing aversion. The etiology of dysphagia is protean and includes two main categories, mechanical obstruction and motor dysfunction.

Epidemiology

Dysphagia is a common condition. A recent investigation surveyed 790 ambulatory patients who were awaiting their annual primary care visit; 22.6% of patients reported dysphagia at least several times per month. Only half of these patients had discussed their symptoms with their physician. Elderly patients and women were more likely to note symptoms of dysphagia.

Pathophysiology

Effective swallowing and transfer of food bolus into the stomach requires multiple steps. These steps can be broadly placed into two phases: the oropharyngeal phase and the esophageal phase. The oropharyngeal phase of swallowing ultimately transforms the hypopharynx from a respiratory organ to a digestive organ. It requires five main coordinated steps to occur: (1) elevation of the soft palate and closure of the nasopharynx, (2) relaxation of the upper esophageal sphincter (UES), (3) traction opening of the UES, (4) closure of the laryngeal vestibule and, hence, airway protection, and (5) propulsion of the food bolus by the tongue and pharyngeal constrictors. This process is a carefully coordinated neuromuscular phenomenon with both autonomic and volitional components.

The esophageal phase of swallowing begins when a food bolus passes through the UES. During swallowing, the rapidity of bolus transit into the stomach is accomplished primarily by gravity. Esophageal peristalsis is a secondary contributor that functions to strip the bolus and clear the esophagus. Primary peristalsis is associated with oropharyngeal swallowing and propagates down through the predominantly striated muscle esophagus via a sequential activation pattern originating from the brainstem. This continues into the smooth muscle esophagus where it also engages the intrinsic enteric nervous system to promote peristalsis through a similar but distinct mechanism. Secondary peristalsis is stimulated by distention of the proximal esophagus and will generate a propagating peristaltic contraction similar to primary peristalsis without a swallow-induced trigger. The strength, propagation velocity, and order of peristaltic contractions can be altered, and this may lead to motor abnormalities associated with dysphagia.

Diagnosis

Dysphagia is never a normal symptom and always requires additional investigation. The first step in the diagnostic evaluation of dysphagia begins with a careful history to distinguish true dysphagia from other associated conditions such as odynophagia and globus sensation. Odynophagia can coexist with dysphagia; however, the predominant symptom is pain during swallowing. Globus is a sensation of a lump in the throat. It is likely a pharyngeal hypersensitivity that may coexist with other esophageal diseases or occur alone as a functional disorder. Unlike dysphagia, the symptoms in globus persist between swallows and may actually improve during the swallow.

After the above conditions have been ruled out, the next step focuses on distinguishing oropharyngeal dysphagia from esophageal dysphagia. Unfortunately, patients have a difficult time communicating their symptoms because localization of the point of perceived obstruction is hampered by poor discriminant capacity and may be masked by compensatory mechanisms. Localization of dysphagia to the throat or sternal notch is unreliable because the point of obstruction may be further down in the body. However, localization in the midchest or below is more reliable that the obstruction is esophageal in origin.

As a result, the most useful and underused test for distinguishing oropharyngeal and esophageal dysphagia focuses on observing the patient swallow sips of water in the office. Often this allows the distinction between oropharyngeal and esophageal dysphagia to become apparent. Patients with oropharyngeal dysphagia will have difficulty almost immediately after initiating a swallow, such as coughing, choking, and nasal regurgitation. Patients who can initiate a swallow without difficulty, but note symptoms soon after the swallow, are likely to have esophageal dysphagia. Furthermore, this exercise may be able to elicit associated odynophagia or regurgitation.

Physical examination plays a minor role in evaluating dysphagia outside of assessing the patient's baseline status to rule out malnutrition and dehydration because this will determine whether an expedited evaluation is required. A careful assessment of the oropharynx and a careful neck examination may unmask a mass lesion, and a neurologic examination should be performed if oropharyngeal dysphagia is suspected. Additionally, a skin examination and assessment of the oropharyngeal mucosa may be helpful in assessing for potential dermatologic diseases that are associated with esophageal dysphagia. Regardless of findings, most patients will ultimately be referred for diagnostic testing, and this is dependent on the anatomic zone of interest—oropharyngeal versus esophageal (Figure 1).

Diagnostic Testing
Oropharyngeal Dysphagia

Once a distinction is made that the patient is experiencing oropharyngeal dysphagia, the next step in the evaluation should be referral for a video fluoroscopic swallowing examination, also known as a modified barium study. Standard upper endoscopy is of limited value given the general inability to evaluate lesions in the hypopharynx and the upper esophageal sphincter. Video fluoroscopic swallow examinations have the added benefit of providing functional information in addition to anatomic information. They differ from a standard fluoroscopic examination (i.e., esophogram) by offering the patient various radiopaque food items of different consistency and are often performed by a speech

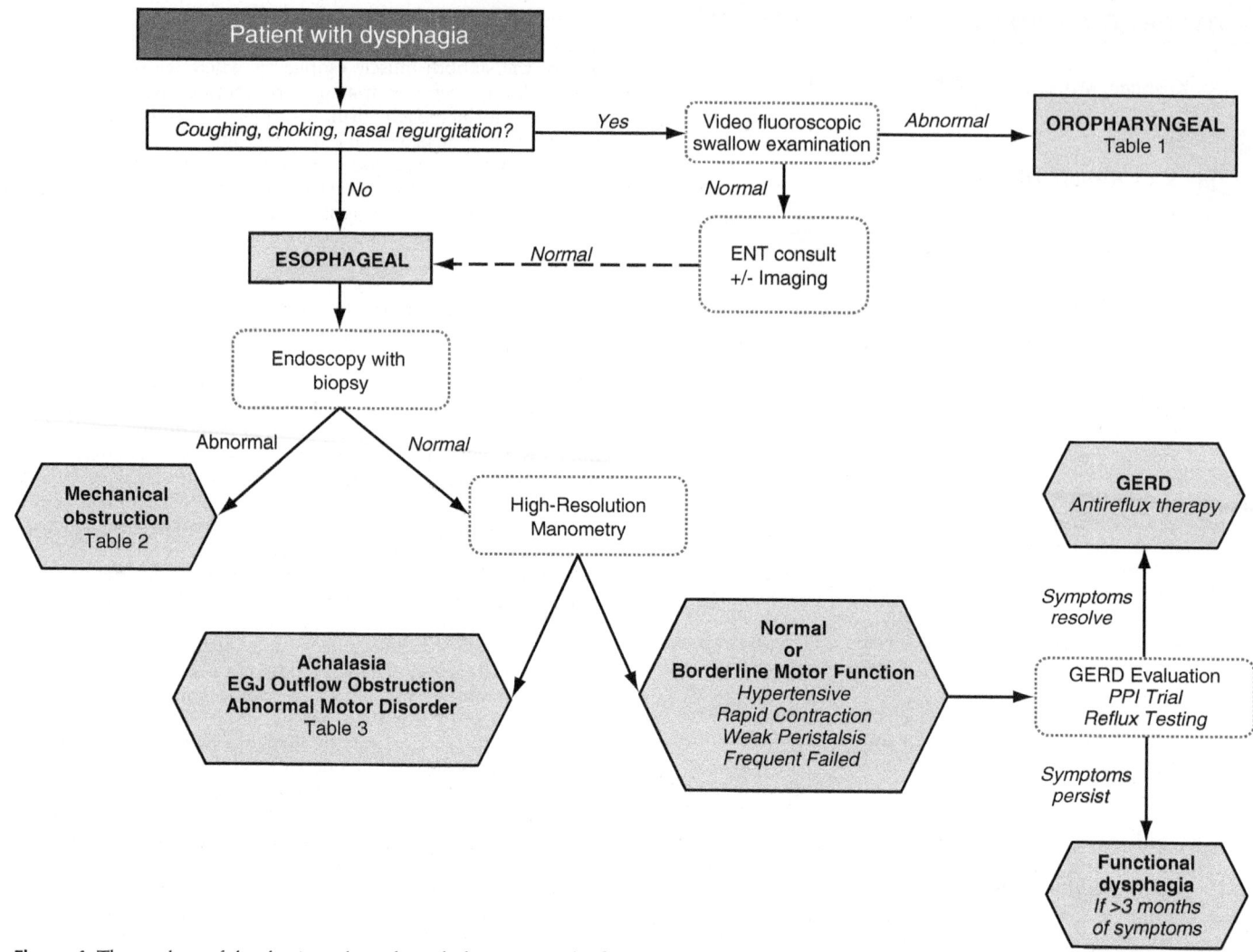

Figure 1 The workup of dysphagia and esophageal obstruction. The first step in the workup of dysphagia focuses on distinguishing oropharyngeal from esophageal dysphagia, which can be done with a history and careful assessment of swallowing during liquid swallows. The workup once this distinction is made is very different. Oropharyngeal dysphagia is typically evaluated by speech pathology and otolaryngology (ENT) based on the results of a video fluoroscopic swallow evaluation. Esophageal dysphagia is evaluated primarily with endoscopy because biopsies and interventions are often required. The primary indication for manometry is to rule out a major motor disorder in patients with a negative endoscopy. Alternatively, the functional lumen imaging probe (FLIP) can be utilized at the time of endoscopy to assess for a primary motor disorder. If a major motor abnormality is not seen on manometry or FLIP, a diagnosis of functional dysphagia should be considered; however, underlying GERD must also be addressed.

pathologist. They can evaluate delay in initiation of pharyngeal swallowing, aspiration of solids and liquids, retrograde flow of ingested bolus, and residual pharyngeal contents.

If there is a suspicion for a malignancy or mechanical obstruction, a referral to otolaryngology is required. Direct laryngoscopy is used to evaluate for anatomic lesions in the nasopharynx and hypopharynx. In addition to anatomic abnormalities, function can be assessed by having the patient drink liquids with the nasal endoscope positioned in the hypopharynx. Oropharyngeal pooling of liquid indicates ineffective hypopharyngeal clearance and can suggest a high aspiration risk. Cross-sectional imaging is often an adjunct to the functional assessment of videoscopic imaging or direct laryngoscopy when an obstruction is noted without a clear lesion noted on direct examination.

Esophageal Dysphagia

If oropharyngeal dysphagia is excluded on history, the evaluation of dysphagia should proceed to upper endoscopy to rule out a mechanical obstruction. Although an esophagram can be used to assess for obstruction, most patients will eventually require endoscopy to obtain biopsies to rule out malignancy or eosinophilic esophagitis. Additionally, endoscopy has the added benefit of being therapeutic in some circumstances, and thus it is more cost-effective to begin the evaluation with endoscopy.

If the endoscopy is negative, the next step is to evaluate for an underlying esophageal motor disorder. This is traditionally done by performing esophageal manometry. Recently, a novel method of assessing esophageal motor function has been developed. The functional lumen imaging probe (FLIP) is a catheter that can be placed at the time of endoscopy. Using a variety of sensors positioned along the length of the probe, it measures diameter and pressure along the esophagus. This information can be used to evaluate for contractility of the esophageal body and esophageal distensibility at the EGJ, thus providing a comprehensive assessment of esophageal motility (Carlson DA AJG). If these studies are negative, a careful evaluation for the presence of gastroesophageal reflux disease (GERD) should be performed and if suspected, the patient may benefit from ambulatory reflux testing or an empiric trial of proton pump inhibitors. Patients with no evidence of obstruction, abnormal esophageal motor function, or evidence of GERD may be classified as having functional dysphagia if the symptoms fulfill the Rome III consensus (onset greater than 6 months before presentation with 3 months of symptoms).

Oropharyngeal Dysphagia
Differential Diagnosis

The etiology of oropharyngeal dysphagia can be broadly separated based on neuromuscular causes and anatomic causes (Table 1). The

TABLE 1 Oropharyngeal Dysphagia

Iatrogenic

- Medication side effects (chemotherapy, neuroleptics, etc.)
- Postsurgical muscular or neurogenic
- Radiation
- Corrosive (pill injury, intentional)

Infectious

- Diphtheria
- Botulism
- Lyme disease
- Syphilis
- Mucositis (herpes, cytomegalovirus, candida, etc.)

Metabolic

- Amyloidosis
- Cushing's syndrome
- Thyrotoxicosis
- Wilson's disease

Myopathic

- Connective tissue disease (overlap syndrome)
- Dermatomyositis
- Myasthenia gravis
- Myotonic dystrophy
- Oculopharyngeal dystrophy
- Polymyositis
- Sarcoidosis
- Paraneoplastic syndromes

Neurologic

- Brainstem tumors
- Head trauma
- Stroke
- Cerebral palsy
- Guillain-Barré syndrome
- Huntington's disease
- Multiple sclerosis
- Polio
- Postpolio syndrome
- Tardive dyskinesia
- Metabolic encephalopathies
- Amyotrophic lateral sclerosis
- Parkinson's disease
- Dementia

Structural

- Cricopharyngeal bar
- Zenker's diverticulum
- Cervical webs
- Oropharyngeal tumors
- Osteophytes and skeletal abnormalities
- Congenital abnormalities (cleft palate, diverticula, pouches, etc.)

most common neurologic cause is cerebrovascular accident (CVA), with an incidence reported between 20% and 80%. CVAs involving the cerebrum, cerebellum, and brainstem can each lead to swallow dysfunction. Cerebral CVA can lead to impairment in mastication and the oral phase of swallowing and can interrupt normal pharyngeal peristalsis. CVA involving the brainstem can lead to disruption of the sensory afferents in the pharynx that help trigger pharyngeal swallow, and can also lead to motor dysfunction of laryngeal elevation, glottic closure, and cricopharyngeal relaxation/opening. Tumors in these areas can also produce similar effects.

A variety of neuromuscular disease can lead to bulbar symptoms, which manifest as dysphagia. This includes myasthenia gravis, amyotrophic lateral sclerosis (ALS), and Guillain-Barré syndrome (GBS). Clinicians need to be able to identify systemic manifestations of these conditions because dysphagia can often be the first manifestation of neuromuscular disorders.

The most common structural abnormalities of the hypopharynx associated with dysphagia are hypopharyngeal diverticula and cricopharyngeal bars. Acquired hypopharyngeal diverticula are most common in men after age 60 and typically present with symptoms of dysphagia, halitosis, post-swallow regurgitation, or even aspiration of material from the pharyngeal pouch. Hypopharyngeal diverticula are the result of a restrictive myopathy associated with diminished compliance of the cricopharyngeus muscle. The treatment of hypopharyngeal diverticula is cricopharyngeal myotomy with or without a diverticulectomy. Good or excellent results can be expected in 80% to 100% of Zenker's patients treated by transcervical myotomy combined with diverticulectomy or diverticulopexy. Small diverticula may spontaneously disappear following myotomy.

Other anatomic causes associated with oropharyngeal dysphagia that should be considered are cervical osteophytes and head and neck cancers. Cervical osteophytes are associated with cervical spine arthritis and may be confused with a cricopharygeal bar because the dysphagia is structural and localized to the area of the upper esophageal sphincter. It is easily differentiated on contrast studies because the cervical osteophyte can be seen impinging on the upper sphincter. Additionally, head and neck lesions of the larynx, tonsil, tongue, oral cavity, vocal cord, and nasopharynx may also impair bolus transit into the esophagus. Rapid weight loss in a patient with oropharyngeal dysphagia warrants further evaluation for malignancy; however, it is often difficult to distinguish weight loss resulting from malignancy from weight loss secondary to dysphagia. Constitutional symptoms (night sweats, fever, etc.) associated with oropharyngeal dysphagia should raise the suspicion for lymphoma.

Management

The management of oropharyngeal dysphagia is dependent on the underlying cause. Neuromuscular conditions such as stroke may respond to speech therapy and rehabilitation. Systemic neuromuscular dysfunction from conditions such as myasthenia gravis, GBS, or ALS will require treatment of the underlying condition. Patients who cannot safely take oral nutrition may need a temporary enteral feeding tube until swallow function is intact.

Management of dysphagia in patients with head and neck cancers requires a multidisciplinary approach and treatment of the underlying malignancy. Some patients are able to take adequate nutrition with dietary modification (soft or full liquid diet) while undergoing therapy. Patients who are losing weight, are dehydrated, or are unable to meet nutritional requirement by dietary modification alone may require enteral nutrition in the form of a gastrostomy tube. Although endoscopic gastrostomy tube placement is typically safe, and routinely performed in patients with head and neck cancer, there are reports of seeding the gastrostomy tube tract with malignant cells from the pharynx. In such circumstances, a direct gastrostomy tube placed by a radiologist may be preferable.

Esophageal Dysphagia

Esophageal dysphagia can be easily separated into mechanical causes and motor abnormalities after upper endoscopy is performed. Mechanical causes can be further separated into malignant and benign causes of dysphagia, and motor disorders can be conceptualized as primary motor abnormalities versus borderline motor abnormalities. Patients who have symptoms in the context of a normal endoscopy (negative biopsies for eosinophilic esophagitis) and no evidence of a primary motor disorder may also have underlying GERD or functional dysphagia (see Figure 1).

Differential Diagnosis: Mechanical Obstruction (Table 2)
Stricture

Fibrotic esophageal strictures are common and can be caused by erosive esophagitis (peptic stricture), radiation therapy, surgical anastomosis, eosinophilic esophagitis, and desquamating lesions (pemphigus, lichen planus, etc.). Peptic strictures are common

TABLE 2	Esophageal Dysphagia (Mechanical)

Mucosal disease
  GERD (peptic stricture)
  Esophageal rings
  Esophageal cancer
  Caustic injury (e.g., lye ingestion, pill esophagitis, sclerotherapy)
  Radiation injury
  Infectious esophagitis
  Eosinophilic esophagitis
  Anastomotic stricture
  Submucosal disease
  Gastrointestinal stromal tumor
  Sarcoidosis
  Invasive carcinoma (primary or secondary)
Mediastinal disease
  Tumors (lymph nodes, lung cancer)
  Infection (histoplasmosis, tuberculosis)
  Vascular compression
  Dysphagia lusoria
  Dysphagia aortica

and are the result of long-standing erosive esophagitis. They typically occur in the distal esophagus. Such patients often have underlying physiologic derangements that favor aggressive reflux (weak lower esophageal sphincter, hiatal hernia, poor esophageal clearance). Postsurgical anastomotic strictures are an unfortunate consequence of surgical therapy for esophageal disease, but these lesions are often amenable to endoscopic therapy.

Eosinophilic Esophagitis

Eosinophilic esophagitis (EoE) requires some focused discussion because its prevalence in patients presenting with dysphagia is increasing. EoE is a condition characterized by marked eosinophilic infiltrate within the esophageal epithelium. This infiltrate results in characteristic endoscopic findings of esophageal rings, furrows, exudate, and eventually stricture formation. The most common symptom in patients with EoE is dysphagia, which often leads to food bolus impaction. Patients are typically young Caucasians and there is a clear male predominance. Atopic conditions are more prevalent in patients with EoE. Patients should initially be treated with proton pump inhibitor (PPI) therapy because there is an overlap between GERD and EoE. Patients with persistent eosinophilia on PPI therapy can be treated by swallowing inhaled formulations of steroids (fluticasone [Flovent],[1] budesonide [Pulmicort][1]) or a food elimination diet (avoid: soy, nuts, wheat, eggs, dairy, seafood) to reduce the inflammatory component of the disease. Additional therapy with dilation will be required in many patients because histologic improvement does not always result in regression of fibrotic strictures. The esophageal body is more prone to fracture in EoE, and deep mucosal tears are often associated with dilation therapy; thus these lesions may require a more gradual and careful dilation protocol.

Rings/Webs

Esophageal webs can exist along the length of the esophagus and lead to dysphagia. The classic triad of proximal esophageal web, iron deficiency anemia, and dysphagia is Plummer-Vinson syndrome. The etiology of this condition is not entirely known; however, it is thought that iron deficiency leads to a decrease in iron-dependent oxidative enzymes, which results in degradation of esophageal tissue, resulting in web formation. Interestingly, iron supplementation alone may result in resolution of symptoms. Whereas Plummer-Vinson syndrome is a rare condition, esophageal webs are relatively common and should prompt an evaluation for caustic pill injury if localized to the transition zone along the aortic impression or distal esophagus. Medications that

can be associated with pill esophagitis include NSAIDs, tetracycline, iron, bisphosphonates, potassium, and quinidine.

Malignancy

Dysphagia is often the presenting symptom in a patient with esophageal cancer. There are two subtypes of mucosal cancer in the esophagus, squamous cell and adenocarcinoma. In general, esophageal cancer has a male predominance and is slightly more prevalent among African Americans. The racial disparity is largely due to squamous cell carcinoma, which has noted a sharp decline since the 1960s. Adenocarcinoma tends to be a disease of white men (SEER database). Squamous cell carcinoma typically occurs in the mid esophagus, whereas adenocarcinoma is localized to the distal esophagus where it is associated with intestinal metaplasia (Barrett's esophagus).

Management for Esophageal Obstruction

Endoscopic dilation therapy is the most common therapeutic intervention for patients with nonmalignant mechanical dysphagia. This can be done with a single, large-diameter dilating balloon or semirigid bougie over a guide wire. There has not been any convincing data to demonstrate superiority of balloon dilators over bougie dilators. In cases of membranous webs or Schatzki rings, the goal of endoscopic therapy is to tear the lesion with a single, large-diameter dilation. In the case of a Schatzki ring, postdilation PPI therapy is associated with decreased recurrence rates.

When treating fibrotic strictures (peptic, anastomotic, radiation, EoE), the goal should be gradual stretching of the stricture. The choice of initial dilation size is based on an estimate of the diameter of the stricture. The extent to which a stricture can be dilated is expressed by the endoscopic axiom of the "rule of threes." This refers to the approach whereby the diameter of the stricture is approximated, and no more than three subsequent dilations are performed at 1-mm intervals once resistance is noted. Although there is no controlled trial for support, this approach is used to minimize the most serious risks of dilation therapy, perforation, and bleeding.

In patients with refractory strictures despite dilation therapy, several therapies have been attempted with variable efficacy. Temporary self-expanding stents have been placed to maintain lumen patency. When placed across a stricture, stents serve two purposes. First, they relieve symptoms of dysphagia by maintaining a patent lumen. In addition, the self-expanding nature of the stent provides ongoing radial force, which gradually stretches the lumen. The main disadvantage of stents is their tendency to migrate. Plastic and biodegradable stents are currently not available, but may be promising in the future.

An alternative endoscopic approach is incisional therapy with an electrocautery knife. This is used to make incisions in the mucosa and fibrotic submucosa. This approach has been best studied in the setting of refractory anastomotic strictures; however, no head-to-head comparisons have been made between incisional therapy and other modalities.

Treatment of malignant etiologies for dysphagia will ultimately depend on the tumor type and extent of disease. Benign tumors and early-stage lesions can be treated with endoscopic resection or surgery. Endoscopic therapy using stents is also an important component of the treatment of malignancy and may be used during the treatment phase of malignant disorders or as a palliative technique for later-stage disease.

Differential Diagnosis: Motility Disorders (Table 3)

Esophageal motor disorders are defined based on patterns of contractile vigor, propagation, and the presence of deglutitive relaxation. Multiple classifications have been proposed; however, a new technique using a more advanced high-resolution manometric system that provides greater detail and accuracy has become available. This classification scheme is based on previous conventional schemes with modifications based on refining disorders into clinically relevant phenotypes.

---

[1]Not FDA approved for this indication.

TABLE 3	Esophageal Dysphagia (Abnormal Motor Function)

Achalasia
EGJ outflow obstruction
Absent peristalsis
Spasm
Jackhammer

Achalasia

The diagnosis of achalasia is made by esophageal manometry and requires two main manometric criteria: (1) inability of the lower esophageal sphincter to relax and (2) absence of peristalsis. Recently achalasia has been subdivided into three different phenotypes using high-resolution manometry, which are associated with varying clinical outcomes. Patients typically describe both solid and liquid dysphagia. Other common symptoms are regurgitation (especially nocturnal), chest pain, and aspiration. Weight loss and malnutrition may be dominant symptoms as the disease progresses. Given that there is no treatment to reverse absent peristalsis, the treatment is focused on improving esophagogastric junction (EGJ) opening by disrupting the poorly relaxing lower esophageal sphincter. This can be accomplished using pneumatic dilation with rigid balloons ranging in size from 3 to 4 cm or surgical myotomy. It appears that the two treatment approaches are associated with good outcomes with surgery having a more durable single intervention success rate and pneumatic dilation typically requiring multiple sessions. Botulinum toxin type A (Botox)[1] injected into the lower esophageal sphincter has been shown to reduce EGJ pressure and improve symptoms; however, this treatment only provides temporary relief and should only be reserved for poor surgical candidates or patients unwilling to undergo surgery or dilation. Occasionally, esophageal dilatation may progress to a point where treatment with pneumatic dilation and myotomy are not adequate and esophagectomy must be performed to prevent severe complications, such as aspiration and severe malnutrition.

Esophagogastric Junction Outflow Obstruction

This pattern of motor disturbance is associated with preserved peristalsis and evidence of high pressures through the EGJ during swallowing. This may be an achalasia variant or could be associated with a subtle obstruction at the distal esophagus not evident on endoscopy. Thus recognition of this pattern should prompt an evaluation for an infiltrating tumor or other potential etiology of obstruction. Treatment is focused on the underlying cause of the obstruction.

Absent Peristalsis

Absent peristalsis is defined as complete absence of contractile activity on all swallows in the context of a normal or low EGJ relaxation pressure. This pattern was previously categorized as scleroderma esophagus if it was found in the context of a hypotensive lower esophageal sphincter; however, this has been abandoned because this pattern may be found in patients with severe GERD without scleroderma. Treatment is focused on aggressive antireflux therapy and lifestyle modifications to reduce dysphagia and caustic injury to the esophagus.

Distal Esophageal Spasm

Distal esophageal spasm is a rare primary motor disorder that may present with dysphagia and chest pain. It is associated with impaired deglutitive inhibition of the esophageal body and results in unopposed activation of the cholinergic intrinsic neurons resulting in premature contractions associated with a rapid contractile velocity. The premature contraction is the most important aspect of this disorder and this has replaced an emphasis on peristaltic velocity because high-resolution manometry has shown that rapid contractions are usually associated with weak contractions. Treatment for this disorder is extremely difficult and focuses on medical management with smooth muscle relaxants, such as calcium channel blockers,[1] nitrates,[1] and 5-phosphodiesterase inhibitors.[1]

Jackhammer

Jackhammer esophagus is an extreme form of nutcracker esophagus associated with contractile vigor not encountered in asymptomatic controls or under normal conditions. Previous definitions for hypertensive esophagus had a significant overlap with data from cohorts of asymptomatic controls, and thus the clinical significance of these disorders was unclear. This pattern is associated with dysphagia and chest pain and is typically treated similar to distal esophageal spasm. This motor pattern can also be seen with distal esophageal obstruction, and this should be considered in the differential diagnosis because it would alter management to focus on the obstruction.

Borderline Motor Abnormalities

Borderline motor abnormalities are those associated with ineffective esophageal motility and mild abnormalities of peristaltic propagation (rapid contraction) or hypertensive contraction. These disorders are not considered to be primary motor disorders, and secondary cause for symptoms, such as GERD and visceral sensitivity, should be considered and treated.

Monitoring

Patients with dysphagia or esophageal obstruction should be monitored for three important complications:
- Evidence of aspiration and nocturnal regurgitation because these can be associated with severe complications, such as chemical pneumonitis and aspiration pneumonia.
- Malnutrition and dehydration because this may prompt more aggressive therapy or consideration of non-oral feeding methods.
- Progressive symptoms because this could lead to progression of the disease and early therapy may avoid the above complications.

Acknowledgment

This work was supported by R01 DK079902 (JEP) from the U.S. National Institutes of Health.

References

Bredenoord AJ, Fox M, Kahrilas PJ, et al: Chicago classification criteria of esophageal motility disorders defined in high resolution esophageal pressure topography, *Neurogastroenterol Motil* 24(Suppl. 1):57–65, 2012.

Cook IJ, Kahrilas PJ: AGA technical review on management of oropharyngeal dysphagia, *Gastroenterology* 116:455–478, 1999.

Drossman DA: The functional gastrointestinal disorders and the Rome III process, *Gastroenterology* 130:1377–1390, 2006.

Egan JV, Baron TH, Adler DG, et al: Esophageal dilation, *Gastrointest Endosc* 63:755–760, 2006.

Francis DL, Katzka DA: Achalasia: update on the disease and its treatment, *Gastroenterology* 139:369–374, 2010.

Liacouras CA, Furuta GT, Hirano I, et al: Eosinophilic esophagitis: updated consensus recommendations for children and adults, *J Allergy Clin Immunol* 128:3–20, 2011. e26; quiz 21–2.

Pandolfino JE, Kahrilas PJ: AGA technical review on the clinical use of esophageal manometry, *Gastroenterology* 128:209–224, 2005.

Pandolfino JE, Kwiatek MA, Nealis T, et al: Achalasia: a new clinically relevant classification by high-resolution manometry, *Gastroenterology* 135:1526–1533, 2008.

Spechler SJ: AGA technical review on treatment of patients with dysphagia caused by benign disorders of the distal esophagus, *Gastroenterology* 117:233–254, 1999.

Wilkins T, Gillies RA, Thomas AM, et al: The prevalence of dysphagia in primary care patients: a HamesNet Research Network study, *J Am Board Fam Med* 20:144–150, 2007.

---

[1]Not FDA approved for this indication.

[1]Not FDA approved for this indication.

NONALCOHOLIC FATTY LIVER DISEASE

Method of
Vladimer Bakhutashvili, MD; and Adnan Said, MD, MS

CURRENT DIAGNOSIS

- Suspected in patients with steatosis noted on imaging or elevated liver enzymes (alanine aminotransferase, aspartate aminotransferase, γ-glutamyl transferase)
- Diagnosis of exclusion
  - Exclude alcohol excess by history (>21 drinks/week for men and 14 units/week for women)
  - Hepatitis C virus antibody, hepatitis B surface antigen
  - Review medications that can cause steatosis (methotrexate [Trexall], tamoxifen [Nolvadex], diltiazem [Cardizem], amiodarone [Pacerone], steroids)
  - Check serum ferritin, iron saturation (hemochromatosis)
  - Check serum ceruloplasmin and unbound copper (Wilson disease)
  - Check autoantibodies (ANA, antismooth muscle antibody) (autoimmune hepatitis)
- Liver biopsy gold standard.
  - Not essential for diagnosis
  - Useful for diagnosis of nonalcoholic steatohepatitis (NASH) and fibrosis
  - Useful in excluding other conditions (if above tests raise suspicion)
- Noninvasive serum tests (more useful for diagnosis or exclusion of advanced fibrosis and potentially in decision of whom to biopsy)
  - Nonalcoholic fatty liver disease fibrosis score
  - FIB-4 index
- Noninvasive imaging tests for diagnosis of steatosis
  - Transient elastography with controlled attenuation parameter score
  - Right upper quadrant ultrasound
  - Magnetic resonance imaging of liver with proton density fat fraction
- Noninvasive imaging tests for diagnosis of fibrosis
  - Transient elastography with FibroScan
  - Magnetic resonance elastography

CURRENT THERAPY

Lifestyle Modifications Mainstay of Therapeutic Plan
- Goal is to lose 7% to 10% of body weight gradually
- Lose no more than 1 to 2 lbs/week

Dietary Modification
- Reduce calories by 30% (500 to 1000 kcal/day)
- Reduce sugars, carbohydrates, fructose-enriched foods, and sugar sweetened beverages
- Reduce consumption of processed foods and saturated fat
- Coffee consumption (>2 cups/day, avoid adding sugar, syrups) has been shown to be beneficial

Exercise
- 150 to 200 minutes per week divided over 3 to 5 days
  - Moderate to vigorous intensity (swimming, biking, jogging, playing tennis, weights)
- Pioglitazone (Actos)[1] can be used for diabetic or nondiabetic NASH but causes weight gain and does not treat fibrosis.
- Vitamin E (800 IU/day)[7] can be used for nondiabetic NASH
- Bariatric surgery can be considered if indicated for morbid obesity, complications of metabolic syndrome

[1]Not FDA approved for this indication.
[7]Available as a dietary supplement.

Nonalcoholic fatty liver disease

Nonalcoholic fatty liver disease (NAFLD) is defined as the presence of hepatic steatosis (hepatic fat accumulation), on imaging or liver biopsy, in the absence of secondary causes for the fat accumulation (such as excessive alcohol consumption, hepatitis C, certain medications). NAFLD is closely associated with metabolic comorbidities, including obesity, diabetes, dyslipidemia, and hypertension, and is the most common cause of chronic liver disease worldwide.

NAFLD comprises a spectrum of disease spanning from isolated steatosis (sometimes called *nonalcoholic fatty liver* or NAFL) to more advanced liver disease such as nonalcoholic steatohepatitis (NASH) (Figure 1). NASH signifies steatosis with inflammation and hepatocyte injury and has a higher likelihood of progress to cirrhosis, liver failure, and occasionally liver cancer. Besides liver disease, NAFLD is also closely associated with cardiovascular disease (CVD) and malignancy.

Epidemiology of NAFLD

The global prevalence of NAFLD is estimated at 25% according to a recent systematic review, with the highest prevalence reported in South America (31%) and the Middle East (32%) followed by Asia (27%), the United States (24%), Europe (23%), and Africa (14%). The largest datasets for these prevalence studies come from North America, Asia, and Europe, with lower numbers from the Middle East, Africa, and South America.

In the United States, the prevalence of NAFLD is highest in Hispanic Americans (22% to 45%), followed by non-Hispanic whites (15% to 33%) and blacks (13% to 24%). A significant contribution to this ethnic difference can be explained by genetic differences, particularly a single nucleotide polymorphism (SNP) in a gene (PNPLA3) that is involved in triglyceride (lipid) hydrolysis in the liver, and the ethnic prevalence that mirrors the ethnic differences in the frequency of NAFLD.

NAFLD prevalence increases with age, with a range from 22% to 30% from age 30 to a peak in the sixth decade. Very few studies report on NAFLD prevalence after age 70. Pediatric NAFLD is on the rise paralleling childhood obesity trends, but population data are scant, with estimated population prevalence of 7% to 8% in the United States. An autopsy study of 742 children (ages 2 to 19) who died of unnatural causes used liver histology as the gold standard and demonstrated a NAFLD prevalence of 9.6% adjusted for age, sex, race, and ethnicity. Pediatric obesity clinic studies have shown NAFLD prevalence of 34.2% in a meta-analysis. Differences in sex prevalence also exist, with some studies reporting the prevalence of NAFLD in men as almost double that of women.

Although the prevalence of alcohol and infectious hepatitis has remained stable, the prevalence of NAFLD has been rising in the global and US adult and pediatric population, growing in parallel with the epidemic of obesity and metabolic syndrome. From 2000 to 2015, the worldwide prevalence of NAFLD progressively increased from 20% to 27%. A recent study using data from the U.S. National Health and Nutrition Examination Survey found that NAFLD prevalence doubled between the survey periods of 1988–1994 and 2005–2008 from 5.5% to 11%.

In higher-risk populations such as patients with diabetes, the prevalence of NAFLD is higher, varying from 33% to 70%. In patients with morbid obesity attending bariatric surgery clinics, the prevalence of NAFLD has been reported at 95%.

Risk Factors for NAFLD

NAFLD is a complex disease that has genetic predispositions and is affected by various environmental factors. The degree of contribution of each of the risk factors requires further study and may vary depending on the region of the world.

NAFLD is regarded as the hepatic manifestation of the metabolic syndrome (presence of at least three of the following: abdominal obesity, hypertriglyceridemia, low high-density lipoprotein levels, hypertension, and high fasting glucose levels). Obesity (defined as waist circumference >102 cm in men or >88 cm in women or simplified to body mass index (BMI)

Figure 1 Histology of NAFLD. (A) Hepatic steatosis. Arrow points to macro-vesicular steatosis in Hepatocytes. (B) NASH. Arrow points to ballooned hepatocytes. Arrowhead points to lobular inflammation. (C) NASH with cirrhosis. Arrow points to fibrosis bands (collagen) trichrome stain.

≥ 30) and diabetes are two of the primary associated risk factors for NAFLD. Underpinning the rising prevalence of these associated conditions and NAFLD are societal and individual trends in unhealthy eating habits (proliferation of high-caloric processed foods and diets with a high content of sugar, corn syrup, and fat) and decreased physical activity levels. The industrialization of food production, as well as deficiencies in neighborhood planning with poor walkability and public transport system availability, are partly to blame for this epidemic. Being overweight in childhood and adolescence, especially weight gain during school years, is a significant risk factor for development of NAFLD by late childhood and adulthood.

Several genetic risk factors have been reported, with nonsynonymous SNPs in two genes in particular, PNPLA3 (patatin-like phospholipase domain-containing protein 3) and TM6SF2 (transmembrane 6 superfamily member 2), being the most consistently validated. The prevalence of the PNPLA3 SNP is highest in the Hispanic population and leads to the higher prevalence of NAFLD in this population. I148M PNPLA3 genetic mutation has consistently been shown to be the most common genetic determinant of NAFLD and correlates with hepatic steatosis, as well as severity of liver disease and risk of cirrhosis and liver cancer in NAFLD.

Heavy alcohol intake and obesity have been shown to act synergistically in increasing the risk of liver disease. The effect of more moderate alcohol consumption on NAFLD is unclear currently and will require more study of cumulative lifetime alcohol consumption. There are population data suggesting that low levels of alcohol use (1 or fewer drinks per day), wine in particular, may be associated with lower risk for development of NAFLD compared with those who drink more or do not drink at all. NASH, which has a higher chance of progression to fibrosis and cirrhosis, is independently associated with diabetes, age, BMI, as well as genetic polymorphisms in PNPLA3.

Pathophysiology of NAFLD

The hallmark finding of NAFLD is accumulation of triglyceride in the cytoplasm of hepatocytes. This is caused by an imbalance between lipid buildup (fatty acid uptake and de novo lipogenesis) and removal (mitochondrial fatty acid oxidation and export as a part of very low-density lipoprotein particles). Further factors contributing to transition from a healthy liver to NAFLD include adipose tissue dysfunction, hepatic insulin resistance, dysbiosis of the gut microbiome, toxic metabolites, and genetic factors (Figure 2).

Along with storage of triglycerides, adipose tissue is involved in the secretion of hormones, cytokines, and chemokines, called *adipokines*. Overnutrition and sedentary lifestyle cause obesity and adipose tissue dysfunction, which likely plays a pivotal role in the development of insulin resistance and NAFLD. Obesity results in excess free fatty acids entering the liver through the portal circulation, which can increase lipid synthesis and gluconeogenesis. Increased levels of circulating free fatty acids also lead to peripheral insulin resistance, along with inflammation and induction of cytokine production, thereby contributing to NAFLD. In NASH, liver cell injury occurs (ballooning hepatocytes, inflammation) along with steatosis and varying degree of fibrosis.

Clinical Manifestations of NAFLD

NAFLD patients are typically symptom free until the condition progresses to cirrhosis. Early in the course of disease, it is often found incidentally on abdominal imaging including ultrasound, computed tomography (CT) or magnetic resonance imaging (MRI) (hepatic steatosis). Hepatomegaly may be the presenting symptom in some patients. Vague right upper abdominal discomfort, malaise, or fatigue can occur in patients with NASH but is very nonspecific.

The other common presentation of NAFLD is with elevation of liver enzymes, with mild to moderate elevations in aspartate aminotransferase (AST) and alanine aminotransferase (ALT). However, even advanced NAFLD can present with normal liver enzyme levels in up to 30% of individuals.

Figure 2 Pathophysiology of NAFLD. An interaction between intestine, adipose tissue and hepatocytes. *Abbreviations:* FFA = free fatty acids; TNF = tumor necrosis factor; IL = interleukin; TLR = toll-like receptor.

Patients with NAFLD frequently have comorbidities including hyperlipidemia, obesity, metabolic syndrome, hypertension, and type 2 diabetes mellitus. Associated conditions also include hypothyroidism, obstructive sleep apnea, and, less commonly, hypopituitarism, hypogonadism, polycystic ovarian syndrome, pancreaticoduodenal resection, and psoriasis among others.

In a community study of more than 7 years of follow-up from Minnesota, patients with NAFLD were shown to have excessive risk of mortality compared to population-based age- and sex-matched control subjects (SMR 1.34, 1.003-1.76). Given the commonality of risk factors for NAFLD and CVD, cardiac disease is the leading cause of death in these patients. A meta-analysis of observational studies also confirmed that the increased risk of CVD is NAFLD (odds ratio [OR] 1.64, 1.26–2.13) and in NASH as well (OR 2.58, 1.78–3.75). Obesity, diabetes, and metabolic syndrome are also risk factors for carcinogenesis, and a multitude of cancers are increased in patients with NAFLD, including liver cancer, breast cancer, kidney cancer, and colon cancer, among others. Liver disease mortality from cirrhosis and liver cancer is the third most common risk of death in these patients.

NAFLD is an increasingly common reason for decompensated cirrhosis and liver cancer. Over their lifetime 5% to 10% of patients with NAFLD progress to cirrhosis. Isolated hepatic steatosis without evidence of hepatocellular injury carries a minimal risk of progression to cirrhosis (<2%). NASH has a higher likelihood of progress to cirrhosis (5% to 12%), liver failure, and occasionally liver cancer. Patients who are older and have type 2 diabetes are at higher risk for progressing to NASH and fibrosis, and in these patients liver disease mortality predominates the clinical picture. Complications of cirrhosis, including variceal hemorrhage, ascites, hepatic encephalopathy and liver failure, can occur.

NAFLD is the second-most common cause of liver transplantation in the United States after chronic hepatitis C and is on track to becoming the most common indication by 2020. In the US general population NAFLD is already the most common reason for developing liver cancer, and the risk of developing liver cancer in patients with NAFLD related cirrhosis is 1% to 2% per year. Hepatocellular cancer (HCC) in NASH, as in most other chronic liver diseases, occurs predominantly in the setting of cirrhosis. Age, obesity, diabetes, and PNPLA3 I148M SNP are risk factors for HCC in these patients. NAFLD associated HCC is the third-most common cause of HCC in the United States, and the incidence of NAFLD-associated HCC is increasing the fastest by a 9% annual incidence rate compared with other causes of HCC.

Diagnosis of NAFLD (Figure 3)

The diagnosis of NAFLD is made by confirming the presence of hepatic steatosis on either imaging or liver biopsy, in the absence of alternative explanations for the steatosis. Diagnosing NAFLD based on elevated liver enzymes alone (without imaging or biopsy) is not recommended. Not *** are elevation of liver enzymes nonspecific, but they are also frequently normal in patients with NAFLD including in those with advanced liver disease.

Alternate causes of steatosis that must be excluded before diagnosing NAFLD include the following:

- Alcohol excess (typically defined as greater than 21 standard drinks of alcohol per week in men and greater than 14 drinks per week in women)
- Hepatitis C infection
- Medications that cause steatosis (amiodarone [Pacerone], tamoxifen [Nolvadex], methotrexate [Trexall], diltiazem [Cardizem], prednisone)
- Hemochromatosis
- Wilson disease

These conditions are easily screened for by history and serologic studies (hepatitis C virus antibody, ferritin and iron saturation, serum ceruloplasmin and copper, and serum autoantibodies).

During serologic workup in patients with suspected NAFLD, it is common to find elevated ferritin, and this is due to NAFLD itself in the majority of cases. In patients with significantly elevated ferritin and transferrin saturation, serum testing for mutations in the hemochromatosis gene (HFE) should be performed, and if there are heterozygous or homozygous mutations in this gene, then a liver biopsy should be performed for iron quantification. It is also common to find autoantibodies in NAFLD that are often elevated in autoimmune hepatitis (ANA > 1:160, Anti-smooth muscle antibody>1:40). These are often epiphenomena, but if the level of liver enzymes is significantly elevated (> 5 fold above normal), then a liver biopsy can be done to exclude autoimmune hepatitis.

NAFLD is usually diagnosed in one of two common scenarios:
Patients with unsuspected hepatic steatosis detected on imaging done for other indications (Ultrasound or CT) or
Patients with unexplained abnormal liver chemistries (liver enzymes). These patients should be assessed for associated metabolic risk factors (obesity, diabetes mellitus, or dyslipidemia).

Evaluation of elevated liver enzymes or Incidental Steatosis on imaging (US, CT, MRI)

Liver-Specific Imaging to Confirm Steatosis
(Liver US, MRI with PDFF, Fibroscan with CAP)

Evaluation for Alternate Causes of Steatosis
(Alcohol Use history (>21 drinks/week for men,
14/week for women
Hepatitis C virus, Ferritin and Iron Saturation, Ceruloplasmin,
Medication history, TSH)

Evaluation for Underlying Metabolic Risk Factors
Obesity(Waist circumference, BMI),
Dyslipidemia (TG>150 and/or HDL<40 men < 50 women),
Insulin resistance or type 2 Diabetes (Fasting blood sugar, HbA1c, fasting insulin, HOMA-IR),
arterial hypertension (>130/85)

Evaluation for Advanced Liver Disease
Imaging findings such as nodular liver , splenomegaly, Fibrosis Scores such as NAFLD
Fibrosis Score or APRI, Fibroscan or MR Elastography

Consider Liver Biopsy
a. if Advanced Fibrosis or Cirrhosis suspected based on above testing,
b. to exclude other causes of liver disease based on prior testing (e.g.elevated iron studies, elevated autoantibodies)
c. to evaluate for NASH prior to pharmacologic therapies OR
d. to confirm steatosis if imaging equivocal

Figure 3 Diagnostic evaluation for suspected NAFLD. *Abbreviations:* US = ultrasound; PDFF = proton density fat fraction; CAP = controlled attenuation parameter; TG = triglyceride; HDL = high-density lipoprotein; HOMA-IR = homeostatic model assessment- insulin resistance; APRI = AST to platelet ratio index.

Routine Screening for NAFLD in high-risk groups attending primary care, diabetes, or obesity clinics is not advised at this time, but there should be a high index of suspicion for NAFLD and NASH in patients with type 2 diabetes. This is primarily due to gaps in our knowledge regarding the natural history of NAFLD and treatment outcomes in NAFLD discovered by screening.

It is essential to emphasize that a diagnosis of NAFLD includes the determination of whether progressive liver disease, NASH, and fibrosis, are present to tailor treatment and monitoring. The state of comorbidities including dyslipidemia, obesity, insulin resistance, diabetes, hypothyroidism, polycystic ovary syndrome, and sleep apnea is important to evaluate at the initial evaluation to recommend specific treatment for these associated disorders.

Role of Liver Biopsy in NAFLD
Currently, the gold standard for establishing a diagnosis of NAFLD and staging fibrosis is liver biopsy. In NAFLD liver histology typically shows steatosis graded as mild (<33% of hepatocytes involved), moderate 33% to 66% or severe (>66% steatosis).

Other findings seen in NASH include lobular inflammation and hepatocyte ballooning indicative of hepatocyte injury, as well as varying degrees of fibrosis from none (stage 0) to cirrhosis (stage 4).

Although liver biopsy is not essential for diagnosing hepatic steatosis, liver biopsy should be considered in patients with NAFLD who are

- At increased risk of having steatohepatitis (NASH) or advanced fibrosis because no serum or radiologic marker thus far can reliably differentiate NASH from isolated steatosis. Thus patients who are older (>50), have long-standing metabolic syndrome, or have noninvasive scores that indicate advanced fibrosis (NAFLD or FIB-4 scores, or elevated liver stiffness measured by imaging techniques such as vibration-controlled transient elastography or MRE) may fall into this category.
- Liver biopsy should also be considered when presence or severity of coexisting chronic liver diseases cannot be excluded without a liver biopsy. This may include patients with serum antibodies in whom coexistent autoimmune hepatitis cannot be excluded or patients with significantly elevated ferritin and iron saturation.

Despite the useful information obtained in some patients with NAFLD, liver biopsy has several limitations, including sampling error and intraobserver and interobserver variability in interpretation. It is costly and invasive and also carries risks including a mortality risk of up to 0.1% after the procedure, pain, intraperitoneal bleeding, bile leaks, and infection. As a result, it is not practical for screening millions of at-risk individuals or for frequent repeated assessments. Noninvasive approaches to diagnosis of NAFLD are thus widely used and include imaging of the liver, liver stiffness testing, and biological marker testing.

Noninvasive Testing in NAFLD
Hepatic Steatosis
Abnormal hepatic steatosis is defined by a liver fat content of $\geq 5\%$. The most accurate noninvasive method to quantify liver fat content is magnetic resonance spectroscopy. However, this modality requires special expertise, is time consuming to perform, and is not readily available clinically. A good alternative is MRI that uses proton density fat fraction (MRI-PDFF), which provides an accurate estimate of liver fat content, as well as spatial imaging of the liver. Conventional ultrasonography remains the most commonly used imaging modality to diagnose hepatic steatosis. It is wide availability and lower in cost than MRI, but it has limited accuracy, especially in obese individuals. It is not sensitive in detecting mild steatosis (<33%) and is also less specific than MRI with fibrosis and iron, also resulting in similar findings.

Transient elastography–based techniques are increasingly used to diagnose steatosis and estimate the degree of hepatic fibrosis. Fat and fibrosis affects shear wave propagation through tissue, and this property can be used to measure liver attenuation (steatosis) and velocity (fibrosis) using a FibroScan machine. This machine uses an ultrasonic probe placed over the skin in the right upper quadrant to produce shear waves of 50 MHz that pass through the liver. Measurements of shear wave attenuation called *controlled attenuation parameter* assess for presence and grade of hepatic steatosis. Controlled attenuation parameter has been shown to be less accurate than MRI-PDFF in diagnosing steatosis, but it is cheaper and is a point-of-care quantitative modality.

Currently there are many widely available serum-based diagnostic panels for NAFLD that use a mix of serum tests and other demographic, anthropometric measures that are combined in single measurements for diagnosis of NAFLD. Examples include fatty liver index (triglycerides, BMI, γ-glutamyl transferase, waist circumference) and NAFLD Liver Fat Score (metabolic syndrome, type 2 diabetes mellitus, fasting insulin, alanine aminotransferase, aspartate aminotransferase). These panels have been found to have sensitivities and specificities in the 70% range and show reasonable accuracy for predicting steatosis. These tests are not as accurate as imaging or biopsy tests and therefore are less often used clinically and more often used as research tools in epidemiologic research.

Assessing Fibrosis
Fibrosis is highly correlated with outcomes in liver disease and a marker of worse outcomes. Fibrosis histologically is categorized (staged) as follows on liver biopsy:

- F0: no fibrosis
- F1: portal fibrosis without septa
- F2: portal fibrosis with few septa, extending outside of portal areas
- F3: bridging fibrosis or numerous septa without cirrhosis
- F4: cirrhosis

F3 and F4 are categorized as advanced fibrosis and F0-F1 are considered none-minimal fibrosis.

Clinical decision aids such as *NAFLD fibrosis score* (https://www.mdcalc.com/nafld-non-alcoholic-fatty-liver-disease-fibrosis-score) (biomarkers evaluated: age, glucose level, BMI, platelet count, albumin, and AST/ALT ratio) or *fibrosis-4 index* (https://www.mdcalc.com/fibrosis-4-fib-4-index-liver-fibrosis((FIB-4- biomarkers measured include age, AST, platelet count, ALT) use a combination of serum and clinical variables to predict the

TABLE 1 Therapy of NAFLD
Assessment of steatosis versus more advanced liver disease (NASH, fibrosis)
Consider pharmacotherapy or investigational agents for more advanced liver disease in addition to lifestyle modifications
Lifestyle modifications aimed at weight loss *Goals* Lose 7% to 10% of body weight Gradual weight loss, no more than 2 lbs per week till at goal *Diet changes* Reduce calories by 30% (750–100 kcal/day), reduce simple sugars, decrease saturated fat, reduce sugar sweetened beverages and foods including fructose enriched foods *Exercise* 150–200 minutes per week spaced over 5 days; moderate to vigorous intensity (e.g., jogging, playing tennis, swimming laps, biking)
Treatment of associated metabolic factors as per best practices *Diabetes* No particular agent proven beneficial as primary treatment for NAFLD although pioglitazone (Actos)[1] may benefit histologic NASH. Causes weight gain Metformin (Glucophage)[1] no proven benefit for NASH Insulin can cause weight gain and insulin resistance associated with NASH *Dyslipidemia* Treat per standard guidelines Statins are safe to use if indicated (except in decompensated cirrhosis)
Pharmacotherapy for NASH *Pioglitazone[1]* Histologic benefits in diabetic and non-diabetic NASH except for fibrosis Can cause weight gain *Vitamin E[7]* Histologic benefits in non-diabetic NASH except for fibrosis Concerns for long term use: small risk in in all-cause mortality, increase risk of prostate cancer
Investigational trials (generally for biopsy proven NASH)

[1]Not FDA approved for this indication.
[7]Available as dietary supplement.

presence of advanced fibrosis or cirrhosis. These tests are most useful in distinguishing patients who may have advanced fibrosis from those without fibrosis and thus may aid in clinical decision making including whether to perform a liver biopsy or make a referral to a liver specialist (in patients with test indicating advanced fibrosis).

Imaging-based techniques such as vibration-controlled transient elastography (FibroScan) or MRI-based elastography can be used to identify those at low or high risk for advanced fibrosis (bridging fibrosis or cirrhosis) with more accuracy than serum-based markers. The drawbacks to these methods include cost and availability (MRE) and limited utility in obesity, ascites, and acute inflammation (FibroScan). However FibroScan is increasingly available and widely used at point of care in liver clinics for fibrosis assessment.

Therapy of NAFLD (Table 1)
Treatment of NAFLD entails treatment of the liver disease, as well as of the associated metabolic syndrome (obesity, diabetes, hyperlipidemia and hypertension).

Lifestyle Modifications in NAFLD
Lifestyle modifications are integral in the treatment of NAFLD at any stage and are the principal intervention for patients with isolated steatosis and NASH without fibrosis. Patients are advised to lose ≥7% of body weight if overweight or obese (3–5% weight loss will improve steatosis, 7–10% is needed to improve histopathologic features of NASH and fibrosis).

This weight loss is best achieved gradually (losing no more than 1 to 2 lbs per week) and sustained through a combination of diet and exercise.

Basic principles of diet include reducing calories (by at least 30% or by 750–1000 kcal/day for an average US adult) and reducing consumption of simple carbohydrates and saturated fat. Reduction of sugar-sweetened beverages and of fructose-enriched food and drinks is recommended. In general, using fresh fruits and vegetable and lean meats and minimizing processed foods is recommended. Although many different diets have been studied and shown to be beneficial (Mediterranean diet), studies have also shown that any diet that follows the basic principle noted above and results in weight loss achieves the benefits of reversing NASH.

Significant alcohol use can exacerbate steatohepatitis, and limiting consumption of alcohol (≤1 drink/day for women and ≤2 drinks/day for men) is recommended.

A preponderance of epidemiologic data also shows that consumption of coffee (2 or more cups) per day is associated with reduced prevalence of NAFLD. If coffee is consumed, it should be caffeinated; addition of sweetened syrups, sugar, and large servings of milk/other calories may negate any beneficial effects.

Recommendations for physical activity include at least 150 to 200 minutes of moderate- to vigorous-intensity physical activity per week (examples are moderate jogging, weight training, sports such as tennis, swimming, or biking). For patients who do not exercise, a gradual buildup to this level is recommended. Limited data suggest that the combination of diet and exercise may be more beneficial than either in isolation.

Pharmacotherapeutics in NAFLD

Currently there are no pharmacologic agents that have an FDA indication specifically for NAFLD or NASH. There are, however, pharmacologic treatments aimed at different components of metabolic syndrome that can be used off label for NAFLD-related liver disease based on controlled trials studies and published guidelines. These agents, when used for NAFLD, should generally be limited to those with biopsy-proven NASH and fibrosis.

Pioglitazone (Actos)[1] is an insulin-sensitizing agent used in diabetes (PPAR Gamma agonist) and can be used to treat patients with and without type 2 diabetes with biopsy-proven NASH. It has been shown to improve histologic changes in NASH, including steatosis, ballooning, and inflammation but not fibrosis. For nondiabetic adults with biopsy-proven NASH, vitamin E[7] administered at a daily dose of 800 IU/day can be used as well and can cause similar histologic improvements as pioglitazone.

It must be noted that trials of these agents in NASH were generally limited to 24 months or less, and longer-term benefits are not known. Consideration to side effects must also be given; pioglitazone can cause weight gain, has been associated with osteoporosis, and has been known to exacerbate heart failure in susceptible individuals. Vitamin E has some concerns regarding increased all-cause mortality, potentially small increased risk of hemorrhagic stroke, and, in a large trial, increased risk of prostate cancer.

Patients with NAFLD are at high risk for cardiovascular morbidity and mortality, and aggressive modification of CVD risk factors should be considered in all patients with NAFLD. Statins can be used to treat dyslipidemia in patients with NAFLD, NASH, and NASH cirrhosis, but they should be avoided in patients with decompensated cirrhosis.

Currently, the following drugs are not recommended as specific treatment for NAFLD because they have shown no specific benefit for NASH: metformin (Glucophage) and GLP-1 agonists are agents that can be used for diabetes, including in patients with NAFLD; however, they have no beneficial effects specifically on NASH, although trials with GLP-1 agonists are ongoing; ursodeoxycholic acid (ursodiol [Actigall])[1] and omega-3 fatty acids[7] (can consider for hypertriglyceridemia concurrent with NAFLD) do not specifically improve NAFLD.

There are numerous pharmacologic agents in phase 1 and phase 2 trials and a few in phase 3 trials for NAFLD. Some of these agents work on glucose or lipid metabolism in the liver, whereas other are antifibrotic or antioxidant. Obeticholic acid (Ocaliva)[1] and elafibranor[5] are two compounds that show promise and are undergoing phase 3 registration trials. More safety and efficacy data are needed before they can be recommended.

Foregut bariatric surgery can be considered in otherwise eligible obese individuals with NAFLD or NASH, although it is not an established option to treat NASH specifically. Case series have shown improvement in histologic markers of NASH in patients after bariatric surgery.

Prevention of NAFLD

Prevention of NAFLD is imperative and is a societal challenge that should focus on reducing obesity and the metabolic syndrome. Early education and focus on healthy nutrition and childhood physical activity are key initiatives, as are neighborhood planning for improving access to healthy foods and healthy spaces.

Monitoring of NAFLD

Patients with NASH, especially those with significant fibrosis, are at the greatest risk for increased progression to cirrhosis and mortality. Patients with NASH and F0 or F1 fibrosis are monitored annually for liver disease progression via blood work (liver enzymes and function tests, platelet counts) and physical examinations. Evaluation of fibrosis progression in these patients through repeat liver biopsy or noninvasive testing such as FibroScan or MR elastography can be done approximately 5 years after diagnosis; however, with high interindividual variation in fibrosis progression, the timeline of testing is tailored to each individual.

For patients with more advanced fibrosis (F2 or higher) at NASH diagnosis, severity of the fibrosis governs the management. Once F3 or F4 fibrosis occurs, the risk of liver-related illness and death increases significantly, making closer follow-up appropriate.

Patients with NASH cirrhosis should be screened for gastroesophageal varices (upper endoscopy) and considered for hepatocellular carcinoma screening (guidelines from the American Association for the Study of Liver Diseases recommend ultrasound of the liver and serum alpha-fetoprotein measurements every 6 months).

References

Chalasani N, Younossi Z, Lavine JE, et al: The diagnosis and management of nonalcoholic fatty liver disease: practice guidance from the American Association for the Study of Liver Diseases, *Hepatology* 67:328–357, 2018.

Diehl AM, Day C: Cause, pathogenesis, and treatment of nonalcoholic steatohepatitis, *N Engl J Med* 377(21):2063–2072, 2017.

Lindenmeyer CC, Mccullough AJ: The natural history of nonalcoholic fatty liver disease-an evolving view, *Clin Liver Dis* 22:11–21, 2018.

Loomba R: Role of imaging-based biomarkers in NAFLD: recent advances in clinical application and future research directions, *J Hepatol* 68:296–304, 2018.

Said A, Akhter A: Meta-analysis of randomized controlled trials of pharmacologic agents in non-alcoholic steatohepatitis, *Ann Hepatol* 16:538–547, 2017.

Tapper EB, Lok AS: Use of liver imaging and biopsy in clinical practice, *N Engl J Med* 377:756–768, 2017.

Tsai E, Lee TP: Diagnosis and evaluation of nonalcoholic fatty liver disease/nonalcoholic steatohepatitis, including noninvasive biomarkers and transient elastography, *Clin Liver Dis* 22:73–92, 2018.

Younossi Z, Anstee QM, Marietti M, et al: Global burden of NAFLD and NASH: trends, predictions, risk factors and prevention, *Nat Rev Gastroenterol Hepatol* 15:11–20, 2018.

Younossi ZM, Loomba R, Anstee QM, et al: Diagnostic modalities for nonalcoholic fatty liver disease (NAFLD), non-alcoholic steatohepatitis (NASH) and associated fibrosis, *Hepatology*, 2017.

---

[1]Not FDA approved for this indication.
[7]Available as a dietary supplement.

[5]Investigational drug in the United States.

GASTRITIS AND PEPTIC ULCER DISEASE

Method of
Kyle Vincent, MD

CURRENT DIAGNOSIS

- Diagnosis of gastritis and peptic ulcer disease (PUD) is based on history of dyspepsia and elimination of other conditions.
- *Helicobacter pylori (H. pylori)* and nonsteroidal anti-inflammatory drugs (NSAIDs) are the most common cause of ulcer disease. Hypersecretory conditions such as Zollinger-Ellison syndrome are rare.
- If testing for *H. pylori* is indicated (test and treat strategy), IgG antibody, urea breath test, and fecal antigen test are available.
- Young patients with no "warning signs" can usually be managed on an outpatient basis without immediate endoscopy.
- Patients older than 55 with bleeding, anemia, loss of more than 10% of body weight, dysphagia, odynophagia, early satiety, history of previous malignancy, lymphadenopathy, abdominal mass, or a previously documented ulcer should undergo upper endoscopy promptly.

CURRENT TREATMENT

- The two principal strategies are empiric treatment or test and treat.
- In areas with an *H. pylori* infection rate of less than 10% a 4–8 week course of proton-pump inhibitors (PPIs) given empirically is appropriate.
- In patients who fail empiric PPI treatment or in areas with an *H. pylori* infection rate of greater than 10%, a test and treat strategy should be employed. A verified noninvasive *H. pylori* test should be used.
- First-line treatment of *H. pylori* consists of a PPI, clarithromycin (Biaxin), and amoxicillin (Amoxil) all taken twice a day for 14 days.
- Test of cure should be undertaken in any patient treated for *H. pylori*.
- NSAIDs should be discontinued or standard dose PPI for ulcer prophylaxis used to treat any dyspepsia.

Epidemiology

An estimated four million Americans have active gastric ulcers with 350,000 new cases diagnosed each year. The lifetime prevalence of this condition is around 10%. The incidence was previously higher in men but is currently equal in men and women. Familial clustering is now believed to result from transmission of *Helicobacter pylori* (*H. pylori*) from person to person or a genetic predisposition to infection with *H. pylori* rather than a genetic predisposition to gastric ulcers.

Risk Factors

Most gastric and duodenal ulcers can be attributed to *H. pylori*, NSAID use, severe physiologic stress, or hypersecretory conditions. In America, 10% of young adults harbor *H. pylori* infections, and this incidence increases with age. Lower socioeconomic status and recent immigration from areas with high rates of infection also increase the incidence of *H. pylori* infection. Hypersecretory conditions such as Zollinger-Ellison syndrome are rare, estimated to be responsible for only 0.1% of all ulcers. These conditions should not be routinely considered except in refractory or recurrent cases or in patients who have multiple ulcers.

Pathophysiology

The low pH of gastric acid is required to kill ingested bacteria and to promote proteolysis and activation of pepsin. Postprandial gastric acid production is stimulated by expression of gastrin from G cells and is inhibited in a negative feedback loop by somatostatin from antral D cells. Contrary to previous beliefs, peptic ulcer disease is not simply due to excessive acid production. Almost all patients with gastric ulcer have normal acid production and only one-third of patients with duodenal ulcer have evidence of increased acid production. The protective mechanisms of the mucosa play an important role in maintaining mucosal integrity.

The gastric and duodenal mucosa forms a gelatinous layer that is impermeable to gastric acid and pepsin. Mucosal blood flow as well as the production of mucus and bicarbonate secretion are largely regulated by E type prostaglandins (PGE). Anything that can disrupt the balance between acid production and the protective barrier has the potential to cause loss of mucosal integrity and tissue exposure to gastric acid and pepsin with subsequent inflammation and potential ulceration.

Two major mechanisms contribute to gastritis and/or ulcer formation. *H. pylori* is a gram-negative curved rod that produces ammonia to control the surrounding pH. Ammonia is toxic to epithelial cells, causing gastritis or duodenitis and damaging mucosal integrity. Many patients with gastritis also have a marked decrease in the number of somatostatin secreting antral D cells, leading to diminished feedback to control acid secretion during gastrin stimulation.

Prevention

The United States Preventative Task Force does not currently recommend routine screening for *H. pylori* in asymptomatic individuals. Prevention is based on avoidance or minimization of risk factors. Long-term NSAID use should be avoided. Prophylactic antisecretory medication should be considered when prolonged NSAID use is necessary. Proton pump inhibitors (PPIs) have better protective efficacy than histamine receptor antagonists (H2RAs) when prolonged NSAID use is necessary. Patients with a previous history of ulcer disease who use steroids or are older than 65 years of age should strongly be considered for prophylaxis with an antisecretory medication. Because of the high risk of gastric ulceration, prophylaxis is recommended for patients experiencing severe physiologic stress such as mechanical ventilation for longer than 48 hours, hypoperfusion, high dose corticosteroids, and large surface area burns (>35% total body surface). Histamine receptor antagonists such as famotidine (Pepcid),[1] cimetidine (Tagamet),[1] and ranitidine (Zantac)[1] or PPIs are recommended. No agent has shown to be clearly superior for prophylaxis in patients on steroids or undergoing physiologic stress.

No immunization against *H. pylori* is currently available but early stage animal trials are in progress.

Clinical Manifestations

Dyspepsia is defined by the American College of Gastroenterology as chronic or recurrent pain or discomfort centered in the upper abdomen. Discomfort is defined as a subjective negative feeling that is not painful. Discomfort can incorporate a variety of symptoms including early satiety or upper abdominal fullness. A thorough history alone is usually sufficient to establish the diagnosis and to differentiate gastritis and peptic ulcers from other common conditions, though gastritis and peptic ulcer disease are difficult to differentiate from each other. Patients with peptic ulcer disease tend to have symptoms more pronounced with food intake. A patient with a duodenal ulcer usually reports increased pain 2-3 hours after a meal; conversely, a patient with a gastric ulcer tends to have pain precipitated or exacerbated by food intake. However, these classical findings are not reliable diagnostic indicators. Physical examination is important to rule out serious complications from peptic ulcer disease. Patient with a rigid abdomen, rebound tenderness, or guarding should be evaluated with imaging and by a surgeon to rule out perforation. The most common physical finding in peptic ulcer disease is tenderness in the epigastrium.

---

[1]Not FDA approved for this indication.

Differential Diagnosis

The differential diagnosis for gastritis and peptic ulcer disease is broad given its nonspecific nature, but can be narrowed down fairly quickly by a good initial history. The differential diagnosis includes gastroesophageal reflux disease (GERD), cardiac disease, gastric cancer, pancreatitis, pancreatic neoplasm, biliary disease including cholelithiasis or cholecystitis, delayed gastric emptying, or bowel ischemia. Patients presenting with a predominant complaint of heartburn or abdominal pain with heartburn more than once per week should be considered to have GERD until proven otherwise. Any symptoms associated with dyspnea or chest pressure should raise concern for a cardiac etiology. Biliary pain often radiates to the right shoulder and is associated with fatty or greasy foods. Patients with pancreatitis usually describe a severe boring type pain in the epigastrium. They may also get relief from leaning forward.

Diagnosis

While most dyspepsia symptoms can be treated on a nonurgent basis, specific "warning signs" should prompt referral or performance of upper endoscopy. These include age 55 or older, bleeding, anemia, loss of more than 10% of body weight, dysphagia, odynophagia, early satiety, history of previous malignancy, lymphadenopathy, abdominal mass, or a previously documented ulcer.

H. pylori testing is a cornerstone of managing dyspepsia. However, most other laboratory studies are usually not helpful in establishing the diagnosis in uncomplicated peptic ulcer disease or gastritis but may be helpful in eliminating other conditions in the differential diagnosis.

Noninvasive Testing

Antibody Test—Serum IgG antibodies are typically present at 21 days after the onset of *H. pylori* infection but can persist long after active infection. Antibody testing has a sensitivity of 85% and specificity of 79%. The positive predictive value is greatly influenced by the prevalence of the organism in the community and therefore it is less useful in areas with lower rates of *H. pylori* infection. The excellent negative predictive value makes IgG testing a good screening test. However, given that the IgG antibodies can persist for up to a year or longer after infection, it is not as helpful in the acute phase.

Urea Breath Test—This test identifies infection through urease activity. The patient ingests urea labeled with either ^{13}C or ^{14}C. In the presence of *H. pylori*, urease activity produces labeled CO_2 that is expired and can be collected and measured. Sensitivities and specificities of this test exceed 95%. It maintains a strong positive and negative predictive value despite the prevalence of *H. pylori*, but the test is not universally available.

Fecal Antigen Test—This assay uses either polyclonal or monoclonal antibodies to identify *H. pylori* antigens in the stool. The sensitivity and specificity exceed 90% in most studies. Like the breath test, it is unaffected by prevalence, however, both tests are affected by previous exposure to bismuth, antibiotics, and PPIs.

Treatment

The treatment of dyspepsia was revolutionized in the 1990s following the discovery of the role of *H. pylori* in pathogenesis. For patients who present with dyspepsia but no "warning signs," two separate and approximately equivalent treatment strategies are recommended. The "test and treat" option recommends using a validated noninvasive test for *H. pylori* and treatment of positive tests. The "empiric" acid suppression option recommends treating with a PPI for 4-8 weeks without testing for *H. pylori*. The test and treat strategy is recommended for populations where the *H. pylori* infection rate is higher than 10%, in patients with active or past PUD, low-grade gastric mucosa-associated lymphoid tissue (MALT) lymphoma, or history of endoscopic resection of early gastric cancer. As the US prevalence varies from 10% to 40% in different communities, either strategy may be appropriate. The test and treat strategy is more appropriate for most urban areas and in communities with a high immigrant population or known high rates of *H. pylori* infection. In populations with low *H. pylori* prevalence, such as high socioeconomic areas, empiric acid suppression is an appropriate first strategy, followed by *H. pylori* testing in those patients who have continued symptoms (Figure 1).

Figure 1 The treatment of dyspepsia.

The recommendations for eradication of *H. pylori* were updated by the American College of Gastroenterology in 2017. Previous regimens had focused on specific PPI medications. This has been replaced with a general recommendation for standard or double dose PPI of choice. There are two key considerations for selection for initial treatment: (1) Is there a penicillin allergy? and (2) Has there been any previous macrolide exposure for any reason? Current first-line treatment is the so-called triple therapy with standard or double dose PPI, clarithromycin (Biaxin), and amoxicillin (Amoxil) for 14 days. This regimen has an eradication rate of 70% to 85%. Studies show no statistical difference between 7- and 10-day treatment regimens; however, there were trends toward higher eradication rates with the longer regimen. In addition, these studies have not been duplicated in the U.S. population where 7-day regimens have shown efficacy rates below 80%. Therefore, regimens less than 10 days are not recommended and 14-day treatment should be considered. In patients who are penicillin allergic, metronidazole (Flagyl)[1] may be substituted for amoxicillin, but resistance rates for metronidazole are more than double those for amoxicillin. Second-line therapy for those with previous macrolide exposure or penicillin allergy is the so-called quadruple therapy. This consists of standard dose PPI, bismuth subcitrate,[2] tetracycline (Sumycin),[1] and metronidazole (Flagyl).[1] Bismuth subcitrate, metronidazole, and tetracycline are available as a combination product, Pylera, which is approved to use with omeprazole for the treatment of patients with *H. pylori* infection and duodenal ulcer disease. There are multiple other regimens with similar eradication rates in European studies that have not been well validated in North America. Nonetheless, they are recommended by the American College of Gastroenterology and can be used for patients who are having difficulty with intolerance to the more common regimens. They are listed in Table 1.

Monitoring

The recommendations for routine testing for eradication of *H. pylori* were updated in 2017. Although strong evidence is lacking, expert consensus supports testing for eradication in most cases. There is clear benefit in testing patients who have persistent symptoms despite the test and treat strategy, any patient with an *H. pylori*–associated ulcer, any patient who has had a resection of any early gastric cancer, or those with an *H. pylori*–associated MALT lymphoma. In these patients, testing should be done no sooner than 4 weeks after the completion of eradication treatment. Patients requiring follow-up endoscopy, such as for an ulcer or MALT lymphoma, should undergo endoscopic testing for eradication. Patients who are not undergoing endoscopy can be tested for eradication with fecal antigen or urea breath testing. The serum antibody test is unreliable for follow-up as it can remain positive for quite some time after successful treatment.

The most common causes of treatment failure are poor compliance with the medications and antibiotic resistance by the organism. Patients should be counseled on the side effects of their regimen and the importance of compliance. About 10% of patients report headaches and diarrhea with PPI use. Clarithromycin (Biaxin) can cause diarrhea, gastrointestinal upset, and altered taste. Similar effects can be seen with amoxicillin and metronidazole. Metronidazole also has disulfiram-like effects if taken with alcohol. Bacterial resistance is relatively rare, with multicenter U.S. data showing resistance rates to be 37% for metronidazole, 10% for clarithromycin, 3.9% for both antibiotics, and 1.4% for amoxicillin. For patients with persistent *H. pylori* infections, a new regimen should be attempted that does not include previously used antibiotics.

[1]Not FDA approved for this indication.
[2]Not available in the United States.

TABLE 1 *H. pylori* Regimens

REGIMEN	ANTIBIOTIC			ANTACID	DURATION
Clarithromycin Triple Therapy	Clarithromycin (Biaxin) 500 mg BID	Amoxicillin (Amoxil) 1 g BID[a]		PPI (Standard or double dose)	14 days[b]
Bismuth Quadruple Therapy[c]	Tetracycline (Sumycin)[1] 500 mg QID	Metronidazole (Flagyl)[1] 500 mg QID	Bismuth subcitrate[2] or subsalicylate (Pepto-Bismol) 300 mg QID	PPI (Standard dose)	10-14 days[b]
Concomitant[c]	Clarithromycin (Biaxin) 500 mg BID	Amoxicillin (Amoxil) 1 g BID	Metronidazole (Flagyl)[1] 500 mg BID	PPI (Standard dose)	10-14 days[b]
Sequential[c]	Amoxicillin (Amoxil) 1 g BID and PPI (Standard dose)	Clarithromycin (Biaxin) 500 mg BID and metronidazole (Flagyl) 500 mg BID and PPI (Standard dose)			5-7 days
Hybrid[c]	Amoxicillin (Amoxil) 1 g BID and PPI (Standard dose)	Amoxicillin (Amoxil) 1 g BID, PPI (Standard dose), clarithromycin (Biaxin) 500 mg BID, and metronidazole (Flagyl)[1] 500 mg BID			5-7 days
Levofloxacin triple[c]	Amoxicillin (Amoxil) 1 g BID	Levofloxacin (Levaquin)[1] 500 mg daily		PPI (Standard dose)	10-14 days[b]
Levofloxacin sequential[c]	Amoxicillin (Amoxil) 1 g BID and PPI (Standard dose)	Amoxicillin (Amoxil) 1 g BID, PPI (Standard dose), levofloxacin 500 mg daily, and metronidazole (Flagyl) 500 mg BID		PPI (Standard or double dose)	5-7 days
LOAD[c]	Levofloxacin (Levaquin) 250 mg daily	Doxycycline (Vibramycin)[1] 100 mg daily	Nitazoxanide (Alinia)[1] 500 mg BID	PPI (Double dose)	7-10 days

[a]In patients with penicillin allergy, metronidazole (Flagyl) 500 mg TID can be substituted, although not FDA approved.
[b]14-day courses should be considered secondary to increased eradication rates.
[c]Not FDA approved for this treatment regimen.
[1]Not FDA approved for this indication.
[2]Not available in the United States.

Patients who continue to have dyspepsia after successful eradication of *H. pylori* or who have persistent symptoms after a negative test and acid suppression should be considered for upper endoscopy.

Complications

Peptic ulcer disease can have severe complications, almost always requiring hospital admission. The most significant complications are gastric bleeding, perforation, or outlet obstruction.

Gastrointestinal bleeding is the most common cause of death in patients with peptic ulcer disease. Most cases of massive hemorrhage are due to erosion of a posterior ulcer into the gastroduodenal artery. Although the most common site of such hemorrhage is proximal to the ligament of Trietz, profuse bleeding can result in bright red blood from the rectum.

Approximately 5% of peptic ulcers cause perforation. This usually occurs anteriorly through the duodenum or lesser curve of the stomach. These patients often present in extremis with fever, tachycardia, dehydration, and abdominal findings of rigidity and rebound due to chemical peritonitis. Free air is commonly present under the diaphragm. Perforation is almost always requires surgical management.

Gastric outlet obstruction can occur acutely due to inflammation from peptic ulcer disease or more chronically secondary to inflammation and healing that lead to scarring and fibrosis of the duodenum. These patients can present with severe hypochloremic hypokalemic alkalosis due to the loss of hydrogen, potassium, and chloride from gastric secretions. Electrolyte derangements must be corrected prior to any attempted surgery. Initial treatment with balloon dilation can be attempted, especially in cases with newly diagnosed *H. pylori*. If the patient is negative for *H. pylori* or has successfully eradicated the organism, the long-term outcomes of dilation do not compare well to surgery.

References

Chey WD, Leontiadis GI, Howden CW, et al: ACG Clinical Guideline: Treatment of Helicobacter pylori infection, *AM J Gastroenterol* 112:112–238, 2017.

Chey WD, Wong BC: The Practice Parameters Committee of the American College of Gastroenterology: American College of Gastroenterology guideline on the management of *Helicobacter pylori* infection, *AM J Gastroenterol* 102:1808–1825, 2007.

Helicobacter pylori and peptic ulcer disease: FDA approved drug regimens. Available at. http://www.cdc.gov/ulcer/keytocure.htm (accessed December 30, 2013).

Mercer DW, Robinson EK: Stomach. In *Sabiston Textbook of Surgery*, ed 18, Philadelphia, 2008, Saunders, pp 1223–1277.

Nordenstedt H, Graham DY, Kramer JR, et al: *Helicobacter pylori*—Negative gastritis prevalence and risk factors, *AM J Gastroenterol* 108:65–71, 2013.

Surgical critical care evidence based-medicine guidelines: Stress ulcer prophylaxis. Available at. http://www.surgicalcriticalcare.net/Guidelines/stress%20ulcer%20prophylaxis%202011.pdf (accessed December 15, 2013).

Talley NJ, Vakil NB: The Practice Parameters Committee of the American College of Gastroenterology: Guideline for the management of dyspepsia, *AM J Gastroenterol* 100:2324–2337, 2005.

GASTROESOPHAGEAL REFLUX DISEASE (GERD)

Method of
Mustafa Abdul-Hussein, MD, MSCR; and Donald O. Castell, MD

Gastroesophageal reflux disease (GERD) is a motility disorder of the lower esophageal sphincter (LES). The definition of this disease has evolved over time, reflecting better understanding of the roles that transient LES relaxations and acid/pepsin contact with esophageal mucosa play, as well as the ability to identify these events. The diagnosis of GERD has changed from identification of a hiatal hernia, to identification of erosive esophagitis, to the currently accepted patient-centered definition: any symptom or injury to esophageal mucosa resulting from reflux of gastric contents into the esophagus. GERD should not be confused with physiologic gastroesophageal reflux, which is not associated with symptoms or esophageal mucosal injury.

The prevalence of GERD is difficult to ascertain, although several studies have indicated it to be as high as 50% of adults in Western countries, with 10% to 18% experiencing heartburn on a daily basis. Studies using health care utilization data may underestimate the prevalence because of self-treatment by individuals in the community, whereas population surveys may overestimate it because of inaccurate assessment of symptoms and absence of objective data. Regardless of the real number, the management of this disease costs more than $10 billion annually in the United States. GERD has been called a disease of white males, although recent data suggest increasing prevalence in Asia and Pacific regions.

Pathophysiology

GERD is a motility disorder of the LES characterized by inappropriate or transient relaxations that allow gastric contents to reflux into the esophagus. The LES is a tonically contracted ring of smooth muscle fibers innervated by the vagus nerve. Vagal stimulation during swallowing produces physiologic LES relaxation and is a likely source for transient LES relaxations. Gastroesophageal reflux occurs most frequently during postprandial periods, at a rate of six reflux episodes per hour, but averages two episodes per hour over the entire day. Increasing frequency of reflux in the postprandial period results from gastric distention after a meal and stimulation of tension receptors in the proximal stomach leading to transient LES relaxations (Box 1). A chronically hypotensive LES is not a major mechanism for GERD in most patients but can be seen in cases of severe erosive esophagitis.

Reflux of acidic gastric contents can lead to injury of the esophageal mucosa, including inflammation, ulceration, stricturing, Barrett's metaplasia, and adenocarcinoma. Peristaltic clearance, tissue resistance, and salivary bicarbonate make up host defense mechanisms that work by clearing reflux and neutralizing the acid residue on the mucosa. Erosive esophagitis or strictures result in the most severe form of GERD, which includes nocturnal reflux with longer acid contact times, decreased salivary production, and lower frequency of swallowing during sleep.

Complications

Acid reflux can lead to significant morbidity if it is not recognized and treated appropriately. Habitual contact of acid and activated pepsin with the stratified squamous epithelium, along with impaired defense mechanisms, results in tissue injury (Box 2). The end result of this process can be ulceration, fibrosis with stricture formation, Barrett's esophagus, or adenocarcinoma. These complications can produce alarm symptoms (Box 3). Patients presenting with alarm symptoms should undergo immediate diagnostic evaluation with an esophagogastroduodenoscopy (EGD).

Erosive Esophagitis

The endoscopic finding of erosive esophagitis is seen in fewer than 50% of patients with heartburn. The severity is stratified

BOX 1	Factors That Modulate Transient Lower Esophageal Sphincter Relaxation

Stimulants
- Gastric distention
- Pharyngeal intubation
- Upright orientation
- Foods (fatty foods, caffeine, alcohol)
- Tobacco

Inhibitors
- Recumbency
- Lateral decubitus (left side)
- Anesthesia
- Sleep

BOX 2 Esophageal Tissue Defense Mechanisms

Preepithelial
- Mucous layer
- Unstirred water layer
- Surface bicarbonate concentration

Epithelial Structures
- Cell membranes
- Intercellular junctional complexes (tight junctions, glycoconjugates/lipid)

Cellular
Epithelial transport (Na^+/H^+ exchanger, Na^+-dependent Cl^-/HCO_3^- exchanger)
- Intracellular and extracellular buffers
- Cell restitution
- Cell replication

Postepithelial
- Blood flow
- Tissue acid-base status

BOX 3 Alarm Symptoms of Gastroesophageal Reflux Disease

Presence of any of the following symptoms requires immediate evaluation:
- Dysphagia
- Odynophagia
- Weight loss
- Spontaneous resolution of GERD symptoms
- Iron deficiency anemia
- Gastrointestinal bleeding

according to the Los Angeles Classification of Esophagitis. Treatment with a proton pump inhibitor (PPI) for 4 to 12 weeks heals erosive esophagitis in 78% to 95% of cases. The healing effect of antisecretory therapy, and particularly PPIs, demonstrates the important role of acid reflux in causing tissue injury. The recurrence rates for erosive esophagitis are high after discontinuation of PPI maintenance therapy (75%–92%), necessitating continuation of gastric acid suppression.

Strictures

Most strictures caused by GERD are peptic in origin and are located at the squamocolumnar junction. Patients with GERD and strictures, compared to those without strictures, are more likely to have a hypotensive LES, abnormal peristalsis, and prolonged acid clearance time. Stricture formation decreases the luminal diameter, resulting in solid food dysphagia. Dysphagia in these patients is often a combination of decreased luminal diameter and dysmotility of the distal esophageal body with low-amplitude peristalsis. Patients with GERD who develop dysphagia should have immediate barium radiography and an endoscopic evaluation.

Barrett's Esophagus

Barrett's esophagus (BE) is a premalignant condition that may evolve into esophageal adenocarcinoma. The histologic abnormality involves intestinal-like metaplasia of the stratified squamous epithelium. Epidemiologic studies show Barrett's to be more common among Caucasians, males, and the elderly (mean age, 60 years). The relative risk of esophageal adenocarcinoma (EAC) in BE patients was thought to be 30- to 125-fold with an incidence of 0.5% per patient year; however, recent population studies have shown a lower incidence of 0.12% to 0.13%. Despite the

prevalent use of PPIs in the treatment of GERD, the incidence of adenocarcinoma has been increasing. Current guidelines encourage endoscopic surveillance for patients with Barrett's esophagus, yet there are sparse data showing the cost-effectiveness or mortality benefit of this strategy.

Adenocarcinoma

Approximately 50% of esophageal cancers are adenocarcinomas. Since the 1970s, the incidence has been rising for reasons that are still unknown. GERD is a risk factor for esophageal adenocarcinoma, and the risk increases with the duration and severity of GERD symptoms. There is a suggestion that cagA strains of *Helicobacter pylori* are protective against development of Barrett's esophagus and adenocarcinoma. The declining incidence of *H. pylori* may be a possible explanation for the rising incidence of adenocarcinoma.

Diagnosis

GERD is largely a clinical diagnosis under the current definition (i.e., any symptom or tissue injury resulting from reflux of gastric contents into the esophagus). Patients with the typical symptoms of heartburn and regurgitation most often associated with meals have a high pretest probability of having GERD. A well-obtained history and symptom questionnaire are usually sufficient to form a presumptive diagnosis and are more cost-effective than ambulatory reflux testing or EGD. An empiric trial of PPI therapy that leads to a significant reduction or resolution of symptoms likely confirms the diagnosis.

The pathophysiology of GERD is much more complex than previously thought. It involves more than acid reflux, because nonacid reflux with a pH greater than 4 can be a common source of symptoms. This entity is unmasked when PPI therapy is found to control gastric acid secretion and impedance-pH testing identifies a temporal relationship between symptoms and episodes of nonacid reflux.

Direct-to-consumer marketing and the availability of over-the-counter PPI medications (e.g., Prilosec OTC) have led to self-treatment of GERD-type symptoms and a consequent change in the type of patients seeking medical care for their symptoms. Patients with typical GERD symptoms that do not completely respond to therapy with PPIs, including over-the-counter and prescription PPIs, warrant a more detailed evaluation of their symptoms. A separate population requiring earlier diagnostic evaluation includes patients with exclusively atypical GERD symptoms such as cough, hoarseness, throat clearing, asthma attacks, and chest pain. Less commonly, patients presenting with signs or symptoms of tissue injury, such as solid food dysphagia, should also be more rigorously tested for GERD (Box 4).

Patients who have symptoms associated with GERD, whether typical or atypical, are frequently treated empirically with PPI therapy. With a lack of discrimination regarding symptom types, this population is very heterogeneous and comprises patients with symptoms that are truly associated with GERD, not at all associated with GERD, and a combination of both. The pretest probability of GERD in this group is diluted, and nonresponders to empiric therapy are numerous. Partial responders and nonresponders to PPI therapy should undergo ambulatory reflux testing using combined multichannel intraluminal impedance (MII)-pH or standard pH. MII-pH catheters measure both esophageal pH changes and impedance changes that occur as an ion-rich refluxate passes a pair of ring electrodes, resulting in a drop in the resistance to a low-voltage current between the electrodes. The change in impedance can detect gastroesophageal reflux regardless of the acid content and can distinguish reflux types as liquid, gas, or mixed.

The goals of ambulatory reflux testing are to determine whether the esophageal acid contact time is abnormal, whether there are an abnormal number of reflux episodes, and whether a relationship between reflux and symptoms exists. The advantage of combined MII-pH is its ability to identify both acid and nonacid reflux, so that testing can be done while the patient is on

Esophageal
Symptomatic Syndromes
- Typical reflux syndrome
- Reflux chest pain syndrome

Syndromes With Tissue Injury
- Reflux esophagitis
- Reflux stricture
- Barrett's esophagus
- Adenocarcinoma

Extraesophageal
Established Association
- Reflux cough
- Reflux laryngitis
- Reflux dental erosions

Proposed Association
- Sinusitis
- Reflux asthma
- Pulmonary fibrosis
- Pharyngitis
- Recurrent otitis media

acid-suppression therapy and the artifact of acidic food or beverage ingestion is eliminated; pH-only testing is affected by both of these conditions. The major disadvantage is that MII-pH testing is less available than conventional pH testing.

EGD is specific for detecting reflux-related tissue injury but is not sensitive, because fewer than 50% of patients with GERD-related heartburn have endoscopic findings of reflux. If erosive esophagitis or Barrett's esophagus is found on endoscopy, aggressive antisecretory therapy with a PPI is warranted.

A barium esophagram is unlikely to add useful diagnostic information in patients with GERD symptoms without dysphagia. It is a useful tool in distinguishing obstructive from nonobstructive dysphagia and may even be more sensitive than EGD in detecting causes of obstructive dysphagia. Achalasia is often mistaken for GERD during the onset of symptoms, and early use of esophagography may help make this diagnosis.

Management

GERD is predominantly a postprandial event involving transient LES relaxations. The primary focus in management of this disease is to eliminate or improve symptoms and prevent tissue injury. In most patients with recurrent GERD symptoms, this can be accomplished by controlling gastric acid secretion with antisecretory therapy. PPIs are the most effective pharmacologic therapy for improving symptoms and preventing tissue injury from acid reflux. Individuals with only occasional heartburn may successfully treat symptoms with a combination of lifestyle modifications and over-the-counter antacids, histamine 2 receptor antagonists, or a PPI.

Patients presenting with typical symptoms and a history consistent with GERD should be given a trial of PPI once daily for at least 4 weeks. A validated GERD symptom assessment questionnaire such as the Reflux Disease Questionnaire should be used as an initial screening tool, because symptom response is the primary outcome measure, and subsequent questionnaire responses are useful in comparison with the initial responses for measuring treatment efficacy. If symptoms have not responded or have responded only partially after this trial, then the dosing or frequency of the PPI should be increased over another 4-week period. If the response is still unsatisfactory, diagnostic testing with ambulatory combined MII-pH or pH-only monitoring is indicated.

PPIs are an effective maintenance therapy for most patients with GERD and may be stepped down or used on demand, but GERD is a chronic condition with a high recurrence rate of symptoms without some form of maintenance therapy. This creates a large population of patients on antisecretory therapy for a disease with a low mortality rate, which raises the question of drug safety. There are insufficient data available that would warrant a recommendation against long-term PPI therapy. Clinical judgment in specific patient populations should be used to determine the optimal PPI regimen.

At present, pharmacologic reflux reduction therapy consists solely of the use of baclofen (Lioresal),[1] which has been shown to reduce transient LES relaxations and associated gastroesophageal reflux. The drawback of this medication is its unwanted side effects, which include somnolence and dizziness, limiting its tolerability and clinical utility as a stand-alone therapy.

Antireflux surgery is another alternative that is effective in limiting GERD symptoms in patients with a positive reflux-symptom relationship. Candidates for surgery include younger patients who do not want to continue chronic PPI therapy and patients with symptomatic nonacid reflux. Today, most antireflux surgery is performed laparoscopically with a 360-degree Nissen fundoplication. The associated mortality rate is small (0.5%–1%), and this approach is preferred to open laparotomy. Traditional predictors for surgical success have included the presence of typical symptoms (heartburn and regurgitation), symptom response to a trial of PPIs, and an abnormal ambulatory pH study. These criteria exclude the important group of patients with atypical symptoms or symptoms related to nonacid reflux. However, such patients should be considered candidates for antireflux surgery if a positive reflux–symptom relationship can be demonstrated.

In recent years, several endoscopic therapeutic procedures have been developed for treatment of GERD. Among these procedures, transoral incisionless fundoplication (TIF) and Stretta are well studied and viable options. Stretta is the delivery of radiofrequency energy to the gastro-esophageal junction (GEJ). Stretta efficacy lays in increasing thickness of LES, decreasing compliance of GEJ without fibrosis, and decreased transient lower esophageal sphincter relaxations. Randomized trials showed improvement in GERD symptoms compared to sham procedure, though follow-up periods in these trials were only 6–12 months. A meta-analysis of 18 studies and 1441 patients concluded that Stretta is safe, well tolerated, effective in GERD symptom relief, and significantly reduces acid exposure to the esophagus, though it did not consistently normalize pH. In a recent meta analysis of 28 studies of 2468 patients with mean follow-up time of 25.4 months, Stretta improved quality-of-life scores and heartburn scores. However, 49% of the patients were still using PPIs at follow-up.

Patients with alarm symptoms and those who are partial responders to PPI therapy should also undergo EGD to aid in determining the cause of the symptoms, such as obstructive dysphagia from peptic strictures, adenocarcinoma, and bleeding esophageal ulcers (which can cause anemia). EGD findings that suggest GERD are a result of acid reflux. However, the incidence of these findings has declined with the use of PPIs.

Nonerosive reflux disease is increasingly common as more patients are converted from acid refluxers to nonacid refluxers with PPI therapy. By definition, these patients have no findings on endoscopy to suggest ongoing GERD. Absence of endoscopic findings does not exclude GERD, however, because tissue injury can occur at the microscopic as well as the macroscopic level. Patients with either erosive esophagitis or nonerosive reflux disease have dilated intercellular spaces on electron microscopy.

As previously discussed, patients with GERD may develop Barrett's esophagus. The metaplastic transformation from normal stratified squamous epithelium to an intestinal-type, columnar-lined epithelium creates a premalignant lesion with a 0.5% per year risk of progression to adenocarcinoma. Screening for Barrett's esophagus remains controversial. There is no evidence that screening results in a mortality benefit due to early detection of esophageal adenocarcinoma. Screening of all patients with GERD

---

[1]Not FDA approved for this indication.

for Barrett's esophagus is clearly not cost-effective, but it is reasonable to target the highest-risk populations, such as Caucasian men older than 50 years of age with chronic reflux symptoms. Current American College of Gastroenterology guidelines recommend surveillance endoscopy in patients with known Barrett's esophagus at intervals determined by the degree of dysplasia. Because there have been no long-term, controlled studies, it is a grade C recommendation.

References

Bonino J, Sharma P: Barrett's esophagus, *Curr Opin Gastroenterol* 21:461–465, 2005.

Castell DO, Richter JE: *The Esophagus*, ed 4, Philadelphia, 2003, Lippincott Williams & Wilkins.

Corley DA, Katz P, Wo JM, et al: Improvement of gastroesophageal reflux symptoms after radiofrequency energy: a randomized, sham-controlled trial, *Gastroenterology*. 125:668–676, 2003.

Fass R, Cahn F, Scotti DJ, et al: Systematic review and meta-analysis of controlled and prospective cohort efficacy studies of endoscopic radiofrequency for treatment of gastroesophageal reflux disease, *Surg Endosc* 31(12):4865–4882.

Frye J, Vaezi M: Extraesophageal GERD, *Gastroenterol Clin North Am* 37:845–858, 2008.

Hila A, Agrawal A, Castell D: Combined multichannel intraluminal impedance and pH esophageal testing compared to pH alone for diagnosing both acid and weakly acidic gastroesophageal reflux, *Clin Gastroenterol and Hepatol* 5:172–177, 2007.

Hvid-Jensen F, Funch-Jensen P, et al: Incidence of adenocarcinoma among patients with Barrett's esophagus, *NEJM* 365:1375–1383, 2011.

Katz PO, Gerson LB, Vela MF: Guidelines for the diagnosis and management of gastroesophageal reflux disease, *Am J Gastroenterol* 108:308–328, 2013.

Mainie I, Tutuian R, Agrawal A, et al: Combined multichannel intraluminal impedance-pH monitoring to select patients with persistent gastro-oesophageal reflux for laparoscopic Nissen fundoplication, *Br J Surg* 93:1483–1487, 2006.

Mainie I, Tutuian R, Castell D: Comparison between the combined analysis and the DeMeester score to predict response to PPI therapy, *J Clin Gastroenterol* 40:602–605, 2006.

Mainie I, Tutuian R, Shay S, et al: Acid and non-acid reflux in patients with persistent symptoms despite acid suppressive therapy: a multicentre study using combined ambulatory impedance-pH monitoring, *Gut* 55:1398–1402, 2006.

Perry KA, Banerjee A, Melvin WS: Radiofrequency energy delivery to the lower esophageal sphincter reduces esophageal acid exposure and improves GERD symptoms: a systematic review and meta-analysis, *Surg Laparosc Endosc Percutan Tech.* 22:283–288, 2012.

Savarino E, Zentilin P, Tutuian R, et al: The role of nonacid reflux in NERD: lessons learned from impedance-pH monitoring in 150 patients off therapy, *Am J Gastroenterol* 103:2685–2693, 2008.

Vakil N: Review article: test and treat or treat and test in reflux disease, *Aliment Pharmacol Ther* 17(Suppl. 2):57–59, 2003.

Vakil N, Van Zanten SV, Kahrilas P, et al: The Montreal definition and classification of gastroesophageal reflux disease: a global evidence-based consensus, *Am J Gastroenterol* 101:1900–1920, 2006.

Verbeek RE, Siersema PD, et al: Surveillance and follow-up strategies in patients with high-grade dysplasia in Barrett's esophagus: a Dutch population-based study, *Am J Gastroenterol* 107:534–542, 2012.

Wang KK, Sampliner RE: Updated guidelines 2008 for the diagnosis, surveillance and therapy of Barrett's esophagus, *Am J Gastroenterol* 103:788–797, 2008.

HEMORRHOIDS, ANAL FISSURE, AND ANORECTAL ABSCESS AND FISTULA

Method of
Mary R. Kwaan, MD, MPH

CURRENT DIAGNOSIS

- While most anorectal complaints are caused by a benign process, it is important to be mindful that the etiology can be a malignancy or other serious medical condition, such as anorectal Crohn disease.
- A thorough, focused history is often the most helpful diagnostic tool for patients with anorectal complaints.
- In patients where no etiology for bleeding is found or where there has been a change in bowel movements, a further diagnostic work-up should be performed.
- Pain is the predominant symptom with anal fissure, thrombosed external hemorrhoids, and anorectal abscess but is not prominently featured with internal hemorrhoids.

CURRENT THERAPY

- External thrombosed hemorrhoids are treated with evacuation in their early development (<72 h) but with expectant, supportive management only in their subacute phase.
- Most internal hemorrhoids can be treated with outpatient treatments, including measures to normalize bowel movements and hemorrhoidal banding or injection therapy.
- Anal fissures are treated conservatively with medical therapy but require operative therapy in a minority of cases.
- Anal fistula repair techniques have variable success rates and may require multiple procedures to treat effectively.

A number of conditions cause anorectal symptoms, but the majority of patients present with a complaint of "hemorrhoids." Most anorectal conditions can be diagnosed with a focused history and physical examination. Treatment is aimed at the relief of symptoms, education of the patient, and prevention of further symptoms. Although most anorectal complaints are caused by a benign process, it is important for clinicians to be mindful that in some cases the etiology can be a malignancy or other serious medical conditions, such as anorectal Crohn disease.

History

A thorough, focused history is often the most helpful diagnostic tool for patients with anorectal complaints. Clinicians should inquire about pain, itching, discharge, extra tissue or a lump, and bleeding. It is particularly important to understand the patient's bowel habits with respect to constipation or diarrhea as well as any change in defecatory habits. Other relevant history items include previous anorectal procedures and related medical conditions such as Crohn disease, malignancy, sexually transmitted diseases, or immunosuppression.

Pain is an important symptom to elicit from patients. In most cases, pain is the predominant symptom with anal fissure, thrombosed external hemorrhoids, and anorectal abscess. Although discomfort from internal hemorrhoids can cause aching, burning, or itching in the setting of tissue prolapse, internal hemorrhoid disease is most often painless. In contrast, external hemorrhoids that are acutely thrombosed cause pain that is acute in onset, severe, and constant. Fissure pain is often described as a tearing sensation or the feeling of "razor blades" during bowel movements that can continue for more than an hour following defecation. Patients with anal fissures might also express a fear of having bowel movements because of pain. Anorectal abscess is often associated with pain, and patients can also present with an acute lump and occasionally a fever. Anal fistula typically is not associated with much pain, rather patients describe irritation or itching, and the most common symptom is drainage.

Anal discharge and difficulty with anorectal hygiene are also common complaints. The discharge associated with prolapsing internal hemorrhoids might contain mucus or small amounts of stool. In contrast, an anorectal fistula or abscess can spontaneously drain with associated purulent and blood-tinged output.

When a patient has bleeding, specific details to inquire about include color (bright red versus dark blood), amount, frequency, and length of time. When no etiology for bleeding is found, further screening should be performed. Patients who are younger than 50 years and who have no other risk factors should undergo flexible sigmoidoscopy. A colonoscopy should be done when patients are 50 years of age or older who have abdominal pain, anemia, change in bowel habits, a family history of polyps or colon cancer, or a personal history of polyps or colon cancer.

Diagnosis

Although the prone jack-knife position allows the greatest exposure, the left lateral decubitus position with the knees up is preferred by patients and usually allows adequate exposure for the anorectal examination. It is critically important to have adequate lighting with a headlight as well as appropriate instrumentation to perform the anoscopy. An adjunctive test that can also be helpful in patients where mucosal (hemorrhoidal) or full-thickness rectal prolapse is suspected is to have patients bear down on the commode and then to examine externally.

The perianal skin is the skin immediately surrounding the anal verge (Figure 1). Perianal inspection includes careful examination of the surrounding skin for excoriation, an external draining orifice in the case of an anorectal fistula, lichenified skin with chronic irritation, other dermatitis, and the presence of perianal lesions. A low-lying anal fistula can be palpated as a fibrotic tract that heads from the external draining site to the anus. The anal verge is the entrance to the anal canal and is defined by the intersphincteric groove. There is frequently a clear demarcation between hair-bearing and nonhair-bearing skin in this location. Careful separation of the anoderm can help to visualize an anal fissure located at the anal verge and extending into the anal canal.

A digital rectal examination is helpful for assessing resting and squeeze anorectal tone, palpating the prostate in men, assessing for rectocele in women, detecting any palpable anorectal lesions, and evaluating for tenderness within the anal canal or at the level of the levator ani muscles at the anorectal ring. Internal hemorrhoids, however, are not usually palpable as they readily compress with digital pressure and are not associated with fibrosis. Anoscopy is used to visually examine the anal canal, which is between 4 and 5 cm in length starting at the anal verge and extending to the top of the anorectal ring (top of external sphincter and levator ani muscles). Within the anal canal is the dentate line, which acts as a landmark anatomically and is located approximately 2 cm from the anal verge. The dentate line represents the transition from squamous epithelial lining of the anus to the columnar epithelial lining of the rectum. Sensation above the dentate line is mediated by autonomic fibers and results in a relative lack of sensation in comparison to the highly sensitive, somatically innervated tissue below the dentate line. The dentate line is also the location of the crypt anal glands from which anorectal abscesses and fistulas originate.

Hemorrhoids

Hemorrhoids are the anal vascular cushions that are present as normal structures in everyone. In the case of internal hemorrhoids, these cushions are arteriovenous channels that have overlying mucosa, submucosal smooth muscle, and supportive fibroelastic connective tissue. It is believed that internal hemorrhoids function by aiding with fine control of fecal continence of liquids and gases. Internal hemorrhoids enlarge and become symptomatic as fixation by submucosal smooth muscle and connective tissue becomes disrupted and loosens. This results in a sliding or prolapsing of the anal canal lining and further engorgement of the internal hemorrhoid tissues. Common exacerbating factors include constipation, diarrhea, aging, and increased abdominal pressure that can occur with chronic straining, pregnancy, heavy lifting, and decreased venous return. Internal hemorrhoids are not palpable on digital rectal examination and instead must be observed on anoscopy. Internal hemorrhoids are typically staged on a scale from I to IV based upon the extent of prolapse (Table 1).

Internal hemorrhoids, when symptomatic, most commonly present with painless bright red bleeding or prolapsing tissue (Figure 2). Patients describe bleeding with or after bowel movements. Other symptoms include itching and leakage of mucus in the setting of tissue prolapse. Pain is rarely a prominent symptom except in the case of mixed hemorrhoid disease, when there is a thrombosed external component, or in the case of grade IV incarcerated hemorrhoids.

The central principles for conservative treatment of internal hemorrhoids and for long-term prevention of worsening symptoms are the normalization of bowel habits and avoidance of straining. Ideal bowel habits include having regular, soft, and formed stool resulting in minimal straining with elimination. An ideal diet should have high fiber content along with sufficient fluid intake. A total of at least 30 g of fiber per day is

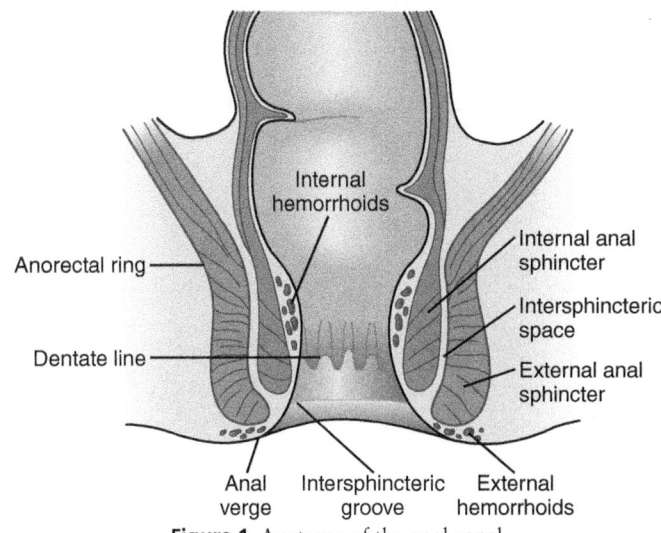

Figure 1 Anatomy of the anal canal.

TABLE 1	Staging of Hemorrhoidal Disease
GRADE	**DESCRIPTION**
I	Protrude only inside the lumen; seen only with the anoscope
II	Protrude during defecation; reduce spontaneously
III	Protrude during defecation; require manual reduction
IV	Permanently prolapsed and irreducible

Figure 2 Prolapsing (grade III) hemorrhoids, with a prominent external component on the right and two sites of recent bleeding seen on the left.

generally recommended. For most patients, this is most easily achieved with the addition of a fiber supplement such as psyllium. Other medical treatment of hemorrhoids includes local anesthetic topical ointments, such as lidocaine gel or ointment, which relieve symptoms but do not improve the hemorrhoids, and steroid ointments, which should only be prescribed for a defined short course for symptoms of itching and irritation. Topical hydrocortisone can thin and atrophy the overlying tissue if used regularly.

Internal hemorrhoids might benefit from further treatment in the setting of persistent prolapse or bleeding. Injection sclerotherapy works through shrinking and scarring the internal hemorrhoid by injecting a sclerosing agent (most commonly 5% phenol

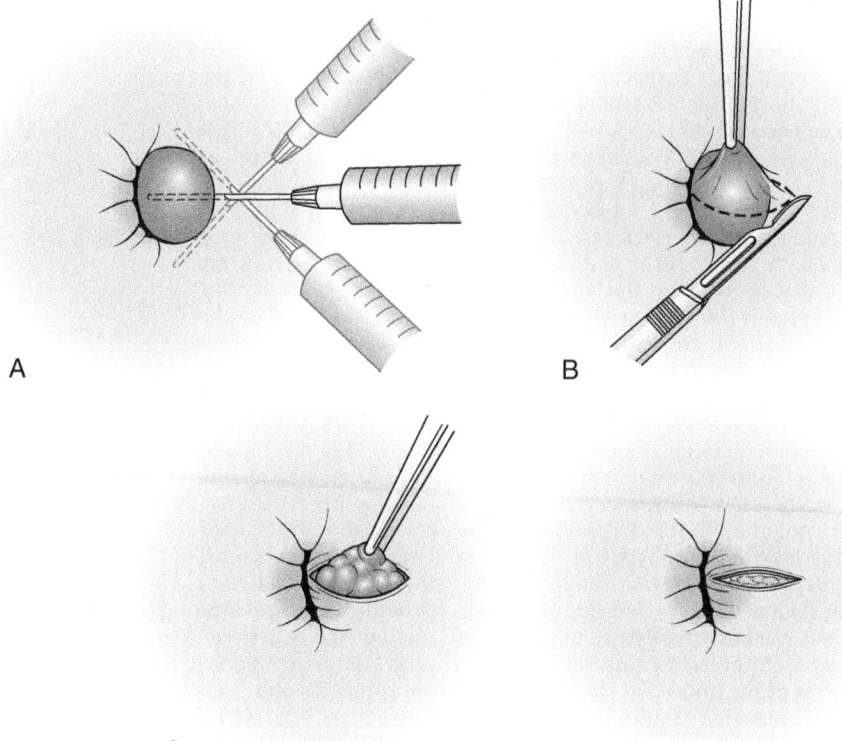

Figure 3 Incision and evacuation of an external thrombosed hemorrhoid. (A) A local anesthetic is injected into the subcutaneous surrounding tissue and at the base of the hemorrhoid. (B) The skin over the hemorrhoid is lifted and a small elliptical excision of skin is made. (C) The thrombotic clot is evacuated. Additional dissection is sometimes needed in the subcutaneous tissue to extract the clot. (D) The appearance of the evacuated area. The incision is left open and the skin heals by secondary intention.

in oil[1] or sodium morrhuate[1]). Alternatively, infrared coagulation may be administered at the apex of the hemorrhoid. Both procedures have moderate effectiveness but are considered less effective than rubber-band ligation, which is widely used in the office setting, with good results.

Rubber-band ligation, an office procedure, requires the use of a rubber-band ligator (either suction type or ligator with clamp) and is performed by placing a rubber band around excess hemorrhoidal tissue at the apex of the hemorrhoid. Rubber-band ligation works by strangulating and cutting off blood flow to the hemorrhoid and by creating a scar that helps to fix tissue into place. The band must be placed well above the dentate line to prevent pain. Most patients experience a sensation of pressure with the procedure. Rarely, this procedure can cause significant pain, bleeding, or a vasovagal reaction. In general, only one or two band applications are performed in the same setting to prevent excessive pain or a vasovagal reaction.

Surgical treatment for hemorrhoidal disease should be considered in patients with grade III or IV internal hemorrhoids. Grade IV hemorrhoids, especially associated with dusky prolapsed rectal mucosa, urinary retention, or significant pain should be evaluated urgently by a surgeon, as necrotic tissue requires operative debridement. Surgery is also a consideration in cases where office procedures and conservative treatment have been ineffective or when internal hemorrhoids are circumferential. In the United States, most hemorrhoidectomies continue to be performed using a closed technique, where the hemorrhoid is excised and the defect sutured closed. More recently, stapled hemorrhoidectomy (sometimes called hemorrhoidopexy) has been introduced. The stapled technique appears to work best in cases where patients have more circumferential disease and is performed by excising the rectal mucosa and disrupting blood flow, thereby shrinking hemorrhoidal tissue and lifting the prolapsing tissue into the anal canal. Although stapled hemorrhoidectomy has been demonstrated to be effective and on average less painful, it does not address external hemorrhoids, costs significantly more, and has been associated with rare but severe complications, including pelvic sepsis, rectal perforation, and rectovaginal fistula.

External hemorrhoids are generally painless, except in the case of thrombosis, and normally appear as more prominent external perianal tissue or painless skin tags. Thrombosed external hemorrhoids, in contrast, are associated with severe pain and a prominent external lump but not with bleeding or fever. On examination, an external thrombosed hemorrhoid appears as a prominent, blue, and firm perianal lump. Patients who present within 72 hours of the onset of symptoms benefit from an excision of the hemorrhoid rather than evacuation of the thrombosed clot (Figure 3). In contrast, patients who present after 72 hours should be treated expectantly with conservative supportive care, including sitz baths, normalization of bowel habits with fiber or stool softener, and pain management. The natural history in these cases is for the thrombosed clot to gradually be reabsorbed within several weeks. In many cases, a residual skin tag is noted by the patient and can interfere with anal hygiene.

Anal Fissure

An anal fissure is a tear in the anoderm extending proximally into the anal canal and initially resulting from a traumatic bowel movement. Fissures typically occur in the setting of constipation or frequent bowel movements. Although most fissures resulting from trauma to the anorectal region will heal, some patients have prolonged symptoms, causing them to seek medical attention. The pathophysiology of anal fissures is still not completely understood but is related to local ischemia caused by hypertonia of the internal sphincter. Most anal fissures are located at the posterior midline; some also occur at the anterior midline (Figure 4). Lateral fissures are rare and can be associated with anal malignancy, anorectal Crohn disease, HIV, syphilis, or tuberculosis. In these cases, a biopsy should be strongly considered to confirm the diagnosis.

Patients who present with anal fissure most often have a tearing pain that is associated with bowel movements and that continues after defecation and bright red bleeding with bowel movements. Physical examination demonstrates a tear in the anoderm with exposed internal sphincter upon separation of the anus. Chronic cases also demonstrate a sentinel tag overlying the distal aspect of the fissure.

Conservative treatment for acute anal fissures includes the normalization of bowel habits to minimize recurrent trauma to the

---

[1] Not FDA approved for this indication.

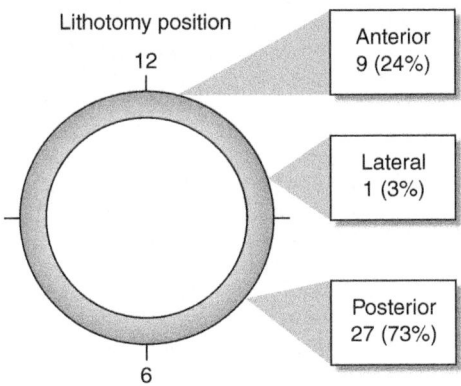

Figure 4 Distribution of the location of anal fissures.

anoderm and sitz baths for comfort. In cases in which the fissure is chronic or unresponsive to conservative treatment, topical therapy to relax the internal sphincter (i.e., a "chemical sphincterotomy") is prescribed. Classically, nitroglycerin ointment (0.2%[1,6] to 0.4% [Rectiv]) has been used but is associated with headaches and lightheadedness. Diltiazem ointment (2%)[1,6] is a commonly used alternative without associated side effects. Either ointment can be applied topically two to three times per day for approximately 8 weeks. Application before bowel movements works best to help with pain on defecation. Reported healing rates are similar and range from 40% to 100%. An alternative agent that can be used for chemical sphincterotomy is botulinum toxin A (Botox)[1], which can be injected in the office or operating room with a single application into the internal sphincter. Although botulinum toxin A appears to be as effective as topical therapy, it is significantly more expensive.

Surgical lateral internal sphincterotomy is the most effective treatment for resolution of anal pain associated with fissures and to expedite healing but is associated with a small risk of fecal incontinence. This procedure is performed in the outpatient setting and should be considered in cases where more-conservative dietary and medical treatments have failed. This procedure can be performed with an open approach (incising mucosa and exposing muscle) or a closed approach (using landmarks and then dividing muscle by feel) and can be full thickness (entire internal sphincter) or tailored (partial thickness and length). Most surgeons perform a tailored sphincterotomy from the level of the top of the fissure distally, with partial division of the internal sphincter muscle to decrease the risk of postoperative fecal incontinence.

Anorectal Abscess and Fistula

Anorectal abscess is most commonly a self-limited process thought to result from obstruction and infection of anal glands located in the crypts along the dentate line. Clinicians should be aware that perianal Crohn disease, trauma, and malignancy can cause anorectal abscess or fistula. Anorectal abscesses typically manifest with acute pain in the perianal area, acutely painful defecation, an indurated painful area, or fever. Most anorectal abscesses manifest with pain and swelling either superficially at the anal verge or deeper within the ischiorectal fossa. These patients have obvious tenderness, induration, or fluctuance on external and/or digital examination. In contrast, patients with intersphincteric abscesses have severe pain but minimal findings on external examination and are only suspected on digital rectal examination.

---

[1] Not FDA approved for this indication.
[6] May be compounded by pharmacists.

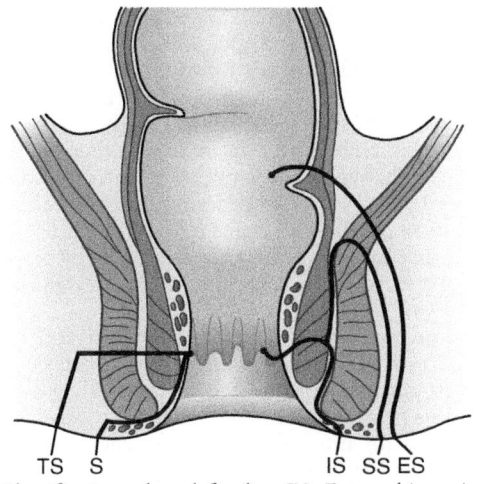

Figure 5 Classification of anal fistulas. *ES*, Extrasphincteric; *IS*, intersphincteric; *S*, superficial; *SS*, suprasphincteric; *TS*, transsphincteric.

The mainstay of therapy is surgical drainage. Superficial abscesses can be drained using local anesthesia, but more-extensive infections typically require general anesthesia. When the abscess is fluctuant and appears easily accessible, an incision and drainage with a local anesthetic can be considered in a motivated patient. Important principles in draining an anorectal abscess include keeping the patient comfortable, using aspiration with a large-bore (14- or 16-gauge) needle to help in the event of difficult localization, using a cruciate incision to ensure adequate drainage, and keeping the incision near the anus to keep any potential fistula tract as short as possible. After the abscess is drained, the area is allowed to heal by secondary intention. Patients are given analgesics and encouraged to take sitz baths. When the abscess is large and extensive, sometimes drainage tubes, débridement, or additional dressing changes are required.

In most patients, drainage of the anorectal abscess is sufficient. However, in one-third of patients, these do not heal and form a fistula with the external opening beyond the anal verge and the internal opening within an infected crypt gland at the dentate line. A recent, small randomized trial suggested that 7 to 10 days of antibiotics after abscess drainage could decrease the risk of fistula formation. Patients developing a fistula can have what appears to be a nearly healed wound but continue to intermittently drain purulent material from the external opening, and some patients continue to have signs and symptoms of infection. The tract of the fistula is most often predicted with Goodsall rule. Goodsall rule states that an anterior fistula follows a radial tract to the internal opening, typically at the anterior midline. In contrast, a posterior fistula follows a curvilinear path to the internal opening at the posterior midline. Anorectal fistulas are defined by their anatomy and path relative to the sphincter muscles and are classified typically as superficial, intersphincteric, transsphincteric, suprasphincteric, and extrasphincteric, as classically described by Parks (Figure 5). In most cases, patients can proceed directly to the operating room for initial definition of the anatomy and placement of a seton (a length of suture or other material that is looped through the fistula), which helps to allow drainage of infection within the tract, prevents recurrent infection, and allows the fistula to mature. Recurrent and complex fistulas may be better defined anatomically with the use of magnetic resonance imaging or endorectal ultrasound.

Superficial, intersphincteric, or low transsphincteric fistulas can be treated with simple fistulotomy, which opens up the fistula tract and allows the tissue to heal by secondary intention. This, however, can result in impaired fecal continence, particularly if the fistula involves a significant amount of sphincter muscle.

Following this, a variety of methods can be used to repair the fistula. One classic technique is the use of a cutting seton, where a taut seton is progressively tightened over several weeks or months to form a scar in place of the fistula and muscle. A cutting seton may be painful, and the scar is associated with impaired continence in some cases. Fibrin glue and fistula plugs have been proposed as a method to repair a fistula, but the recurrence rate with long-term follow-up is high (>85%). Endorectal advancement flaps are the most well-established method to repair an anal fistula. With this technique, the internal orifice is closed, and healthy tissue is brought down over the internal fistula opening to allow the area to heal. This procedure can be technically difficult: failure most commonly results from ischemia of the flap, and repeat flap procedures are often not anatomically feasible owing to scarring and fibrosis. Success rates have been reported between 50% and 80%.

The ligation of intersphincteric fistula tract (LIFT) has been investigated for transsphincteric and suprasphincteric fistulas and shows modest success with the benefit of avoiding any sphincter division. In this procedure, the fistula tract is ligated and partially excised through an intersphincteric approach. Although long-term results are still unknown, reports are favorable (on the order of 60% to 80%) for the short-term success of this technique.

References

Bleier JI, Moloo H, Goldberg SM: Ligation of the intersphincteric fistula tract: An effective new technique for complex fistulas, *Dis Colon Rectum* 53:43–46, 2008.

Davis BR, Lee-Kong SA, Migaly J, Feingold DL, Steele SR: The American Society of Colon and Rectal Surgeons Clinical Practice Guidelines for the Management of Hemorrhoids, *Dis Colon Rectum* 61:284–292, 2018.

Ghahramani L, Minaie MR, Arasteh P, et al: Antibiotic therapy for prevention of fistula in ano after incision and dreainage of simple perianal abscess: A randomized single blind clinical trial, *Surgery* 162:1017–1025, 2017.

Hong KD, Kang S, Kalaskar S, Wexner SD: Ligation of intersphincteric fistula to treat anal fistula: a systematic review and meta-analysis, *Tech Coloproctol* 18:685–691, 2014.

Jayaraman S, Colquhoun PH, Malthaner RA: Stapled versus conventional surgery for hemorrhoids, *Cochrane Database Syst Rev* 4:CD005393, 2006.

Nelson R: Nonsurgical therapy for anal fissure, *Cochrane Database Syst Rev* 4:CD003431, 2006.

Nelson RL: Operative procedures for fissure in ano, *Cochrane Database Syst Rev* 1:CD002199, 2010.

Parks AG, Gordon PH, Hardcastle JD: A classification of fistula-in-ano, *Br J Surg* 63:1–12, 1976.

Shanmugam V, Thaha MA, Rabindranath KS, et al: Rubber band ligation versus excisional haemorrhoidectomy for haemorrhoids, *Cochrane Database Syst Rev* 3:CD005034, 2005.

HEPATITIS A, B, D, AND E

Method of
Varun Takyar, MD and Marc G. Ghany, MD, MHSc

CURRENT DIAGNOSIS

Hepatitis A

- Typical prodromal symptoms are nonspecific (i.e., fever, anorexia, nausea, vomiting, diarrhea, abdominal pain, and weight loss). In about half of patients, prodromal symptoms are followed by icterus (i.e., jaundice, pruritus, and dark urine) lasting 2 weeks.
- Serum aminotransferase levels increase to 10 to 20 times the upper limit of normal during the prodromal phase. Total serum bilirubin rises but rarely exceeds 10 mg/dL during the icteric phase. Biochemical recovery usually occurs within 3 months.
- Acute hepatitis A virus (HAV) infection is diagnosed by the presence of anti-HAV immunoglobulin M (IgM). Anti-HAV IgG appears in the convalescent phase and remains detectable for life. Anti-HAV IgG positivity with the absence of anti-HAV IgM antibodies reflects past exposure or vaccination. The antibody test for HAV usually includes total antibodies (IgM and IgG); thus, diagnosis of acute hepatitis A requires specific anti-HAV IgM testing.

Hepatitis B

- Acute hepatitis B virus (HBV) infection may be asymptomatic or present with nonspecific symptoms of anorexia, nausea, and fever with development of icterus, pruritus, right upper quadrant pain, or, rarely, acute liver failure. Globally, it is a major cause of chronic hepatitis.
- Serum alanine aminotransferase (ALT) levels peak with the onset of symptoms.
- Suspected acute HBV infection is diagnosed by the detection of hepatitis B surface antigen (HBsAg), hepatitis B e-antigen (HBeAg), IgM antibody to hepatitis B core antigen (anti-HBc), and HBV DNA in serum in the appropriate clinical setting. Anti-HBc IgM is detected during acute HBV infection and may be detected during reactivation of chronic HBV infection.
- Chronic infection is defined as the persistence of serum HBsAg for greater than 6 months. If HBsAg is present, serum HBeAg, antibody to hepatitis B e-antigen (anti-HBe), HBV DNA, and serum ALT are used to determine the four phases of chronic infection (immune tolerant, HBeAg-positive and HBeAg-negative immune active, and inactive carrier).

CURRENT THERAPY

Hepatitis A

- Treatment is predominately supportive. Avoid hepatotoxic medications and drugs metabolized by the liver. Acute liver failure with encephalopathy and impaired synthetic function occurs rarely and is more common in patients older than 50 years of age and/or those who have coexisting chronic HBV or hepatitis C virus (HCV) infections.
- Prevention includes administration of the inactivated or attenuated vaccine for children at age 1 year or older and for at-risk populations (e.g., intravenous drug users, travelers to regions with high or intermediate HAV rates, men who have sex with men, patients with chronic liver disease or clotting factor disorders).
- Preexposure passive immunization with pooled human anti-HAV immunoglobulin may be used for those at high or intermediate risk of hepatitis A virus exposure.
- Postexposure passive immunization with pooled human anti-HAV immunoglobulin may be used for close personal contacts of an individual with laboratory-confirmed HAV infection, staff and attendees of child care centers if one or more children and/or staff are diagnosed with HAV infection, and food handlers during a common-source exposure. Concurrent immunization with inactivated or attenuated vaccines for these at-risk contacts is also warranted.

Hepatitis B

- Acute HBV infection in an adult generally only requires supportive care owing to high rates of spontaneous recovery. For people with evidence of acute liver failure, prompt institution of antiviral therapy with a potent nucleos(t)ide analog and referral to a transplant center is recommended. Peginterferon alfa-2a (Pegasys)[1] is contraindicated in persons with acute liver failure.
- Chronic HBV treatment goals are sustained suppression of HBV DNA to prevent the development of cirrhosis, hepatocellular carcinoma, and liver-related mortality. Cure of chronic HBV infection is currently not possible. Treatment recommendations for chronic HBV differ depending on the phase of infection but is generally indicated for immune active HBeAg-positive subjects with confirmed HBV DNA greater than 2000 to 20,000 IU/mL and serum ALT two or more times the upper limit of normal, and for immune active HBeAg-negative patients with HBV DNA greater than or

equal to 2000 IU/mL with serum ALT two or more times the upper limit of normal and patients with liver biopsy–proven moderate to severe inflammation and/or moderate fibrosis. Treatment decisions outside these parameters should be individualized based on the risk for complications (e.g., older age [>40 years], family history of cirrhosis or hepatocellular carcinoma, presence of cirrhosis) and the risk of therapy (e.g., chronic kidney disease, previous treatment history). Four agents are considered first line—peginterferon alfa-2a (Pegasys), entecavir (Baraclude), tenofovir (Viread), and tenofovir alafenamide (Vemlidy)—based on their safety, effectiveness, and low rates of antiviral resistance. Peginterferon is generally recommended for those who prefer a finite course of treatment and who have clinical and laboratory features predictive of a response to peginterferon (high ALT, low HBV DNA, young age, female gender, and HBV genotype A or B). Peginterferon is contraindicated in persons with decompensated cirrhosis, autoimmune illnesses, or active psychiatric illness. Nucleos(t)ide analogs are more potent inhibitors of HBV DNA replication, generally better tolerated than peginterferon, and usually administered long term. The ideal endpoint of treatment is loss of HBsAg, though it is rarely observed with any therapy.

- Prevention includes completion of a two-three–dose HBV vaccination series for all children by 18 months of age with the first dose administered within 24 hours of birth. Infants whose mothers are HBsAg positive or whose HBsAg status is unknown should receive the last dose by 6 months of age.
- Hepatitis B immune globulin (HyperHEP B) and HBV vaccination are recommended at birth for infants whose mothers are HBsAg positive. In mothers with viral loads greater than 200,000 IU/mL, antiviral therapy with tenofovir (Viread), telbivudine (Tyzeka), or lamivudine (Epivir HBV) in the third trimester of pregnancy (gestation weeks 28-32) can be considered.

[1]Not FDA approved for this indication.

Five viruses hepatitis A through E account for the majority of cases of acute and chronic viral hepatitis. Chronic hepatitis is arbitrarily defined as the persistence of elevated serum aminotransferase levels for 6 months or more. Complications of chronic hepatitis (predominantly cirrhosis and hepatocellular carcinoma) account for the majority of morbidity and mortality due to viral hepatitis. Effective vaccines are available for the prevention of hepatitis A, B, and D infections. In addition, safe and effective therapy is available for treatment of chronic hepatitis B and C. Therefore it is important to screen individuals who are at high risk for chronic viral hepatitis to provide them access to care, reduce complications, and offer counseling to prevent transmission of infection.

Hepatitis A Virus

Introduction

HAV is a positive-sense, single-stranded RNA virus of the *Hepatovirus* genus belonging to the Picornaviridae family. Its genome encodes four structural and seven nonstructural proteins. Four genotypes have been identified, but there is only one serotype. Therefore exposure to one HAV genotype confers immunity to all genotypes.

Natural History

HAV is a cause of acute hepatitis and acute liver failure but not chronic hepatitis (Table 1). In ~5% of cases, a prolonged cholestasis lasting more than 3 months may occur, and in ~10% of patients, a relapsing hepatitis has been observed up to 6 months after the acute illness with recrudescence of symptoms and flare of hepatitis. Cases of relapsing hepatitis continue to remain

infectious with fecal shedding of the virus. These atypical presentations of acute hepatitis A should not be mistaken for evolution to chronic hepatitis, as resolution is the rule. Recovery of HAV is associated with development of lifelong immunity.

HAV replication occurs in hepatocytes, and the virus is shed into the intestine via the biliary system. Viral levels peak during the asymptomatic period, and virus shedding continues until around 2 weeks into the icteric phase. HAV is detectable in the blood, but levels are 1000-fold higher in the feces. Children may shed the virus longer than adults.

The incubation period usually lasts 14 to 28 days. This is followed by the onset of symptoms. The presence and severity of symptoms are variable and age related. Generally, more than 70% of adult patients have a symptomatic illness, compared with only 10% of children younger than the age of 10 years. Typical symptoms are nonspecific and include fever, anorexia, nausea, vomiting, diarrhea, abdominal pain, and weight loss. This prodromal phase is followed by an icteric phase in 40% to 70% of patients with jaundice, pruritus, and dark urine. Physical examination findings are usually unremarkable, but hepatomegaly may be observed. Extrahepatic manifestations are uncommon and may include an evanescent rash and arthralgias.

Laboratory studies during the prodromal phase reveal elevated serum aminotransferase levels greater than 10 to 20 times the upper limit of normal. During the icteric phase, total serum bilirubin rises but generally does not exceed 10 mg/dL. In most patients, jaundice lasts 2 weeks and a complete clinical and biochemical recovery can be expected in 2 to 3 months.

Epidemiology

Hepatitis A occurs throughout the world (Figure 1), either sporadically or in epidemics. The prevalence of HAV correlates with the level of sanitation and hygiene of a region. In developing countries, more than 90% of children are infected before the age of 10. In developed countries, including the United States, infection rates are low. Lack of exposure at a young age leads to higher susceptibility in certain high-risk adults including travelers to endemic areas, injection drug users, and men who have sex with men.

In the United States, HAV infection rates have declined by 95% since the introduction of mandatory childhood vaccination in 1995. The overall incidence rate in 2016 was 0.6% per 100,000 persons, representing a 44% increase in cases between 2015 and 2016 due to outbreaks related to imported foods, in homeless persons, and persons who use injection drugs. HAV is spread primarily by the fecal–oral route through the ingestion of contaminated food or water. Humans are the only known reservoir of the virus.

Diagnosis

Serologic testing for antibody to HAV can confirm the diagnosis of acute infection, past exposure, and immunity to the virus. Acute HAV infection is diagnosed by the presence of anti-HAV IgM. Anti-HAV IgG appears in the convalescent phase of infection and remains detectable for life. Past exposure or vaccination confers immunity and is reflected by anti-HAV IgG positivity with the absence of anti-HAV IgM antibodies. The antibody test for HAV usually includes total antibodies (IgM and IgG). Thus, to diagnose acute hepatitis A, it is important to order anti-HAV IgM.

Treatment

Given the self-limiting nature of acute hepatitis A, treatment is predominately supportive. Caution should be taken when using hepatotoxic medications or medications metabolized predominately in the liver. Rarely, acute liver failure with encephalopathy and impaired synthetic function can occur. The patients at highest risk for this complication are generally older than 50 years of age and may have coexisting chronic HBV or HCV infections. Individuals presenting with acute liver failure are more appropriately managed at a liver transplant center.

TABLE 1	Hepatitis A, B, D, and E Characteristics

	HEPATITIS A	HEPATITIS B	HEPATITIS D	HEPATITIS E
Classification	Picornavirus, ssRNA(+)	Hepadnavirus, dsDNA	Deltavirus, ssRNA(-)	Hepevirus, ssRNA(+)
Source	Stool	Blood	Blood	Stool
Transmission	Enteric	Percutaneous/permucosal	Percutaneous/permucosal	Enteric
Acute infections (per 1000/year) in U.S.	125-200	140-320	6-13	unknown
Epidemics	Yes	No	No	Yes
Incubation period range (weeks)	15-45 d	30-180 d	30-180 d	15-60 d
Risk of chronic hepatitis	No	Yes	Yes	Yes
Risk of HCC	No	Yes	Yes	No
Acute Liver Failure	0.10%	0.1-1%	5-20%	1-2%[#]
Prevention	pre-/post-exposure immunization	pre-/post-exposure immunization	pre-/post-exposure immunization	pre-exposure immunization*

Abbreviation: HCC = hepatocellular carcinoma.
*Not available in United States
#Higher in pregnancy at 5-20%

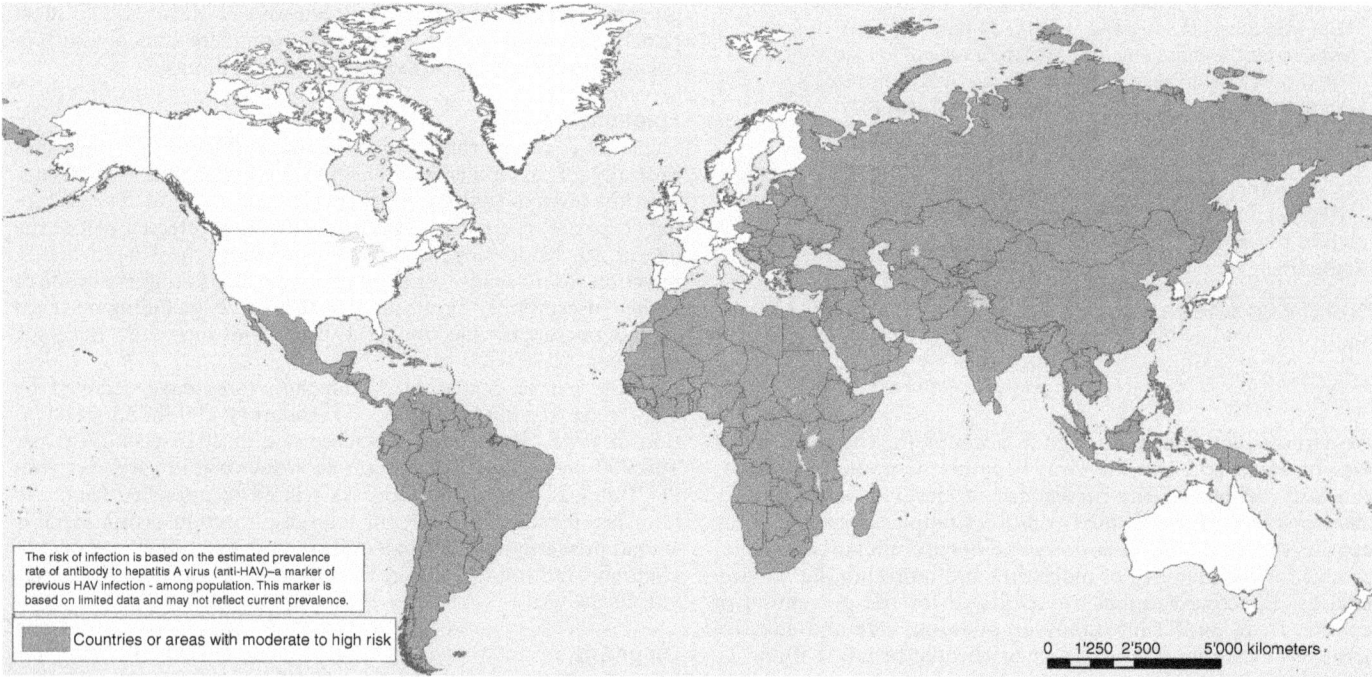

The risk of infection is based on the estimated prevalence rate of antibody to hepatitis A virus (anti-HAV)–a marker of previous HAV infection - among population. This marker is based on limited data and may not reflect current prevalence.

Countries or areas with moderate to high risk

0   1'250 2'500   5'000 kilometers

Figure 1 Global prevalence of hepatitis A and infection risk. Hepatitis A has a worldwide prevalence. Prevalence is related to the regional income, sanitation, and hygiene. High-income areas (e.g., North America, Western Europe, Australia, New Zealand, Japan, the Republic of Korea, and Singapore) have low levels of hepatitis A virus (HAV) endemicity and subsequently a high proportion of susceptible adults. Low-income regions (Sub-Saharan Africa and parts of South Asia) have high endemicity levels and very few susceptible adolescents and adults. Middle-income regions have a mix of intermediate and low endemicity levels.

Prevention

Both inactivated and attenuated vaccines have been licensed against HAV. Inactivated vaccines include HAVRIX (GlaxoSmithKline), VAQTA (Merck), TWINRIX (a combined hepatitis A and B vaccine from GlaxoSmithKline), AVAXIM (Sanofi Pasteur),[2] EPAXAL (Crucell),[2] and HEALIVE (Sinovac).[2] The only live attenuated vaccine is BIOVAC-A (Pukang).[2] The World Health Organization (WHO) recommends routine childhood vaccination for HAV in areas with intermediate infection rates. In the United States, the Advisory Committee on Immunization Practices recommends that all children at age 1 year be vaccinated.

Other at-risk populations for whom vaccination is recommended include intravenous drug users, travelers to regions with high or intermediate HAV rates, men who have sex with men, persons in close contact with new adoptees from countries of high or intermediate hepatitis A endemicity, and patients with chronic liver disease or clotting factor disorders.

Passive immunization with immunoglobulin may also be used for preexposure protection among individuals who are at high or intermediate risk of HAV exposure. Pooled human anti-HAV immunoglobulins (GamaSTAN [IGIM]) decrease the HAV infection risk by 90% for up to 3 months. Passive immunization is also recommended for postexposure protection in cases of close personal contacts to an individual with laboratory-confirmed HAV infection, to staff and attendees of child care centers if one or more

---

[2] Not available in the United States.

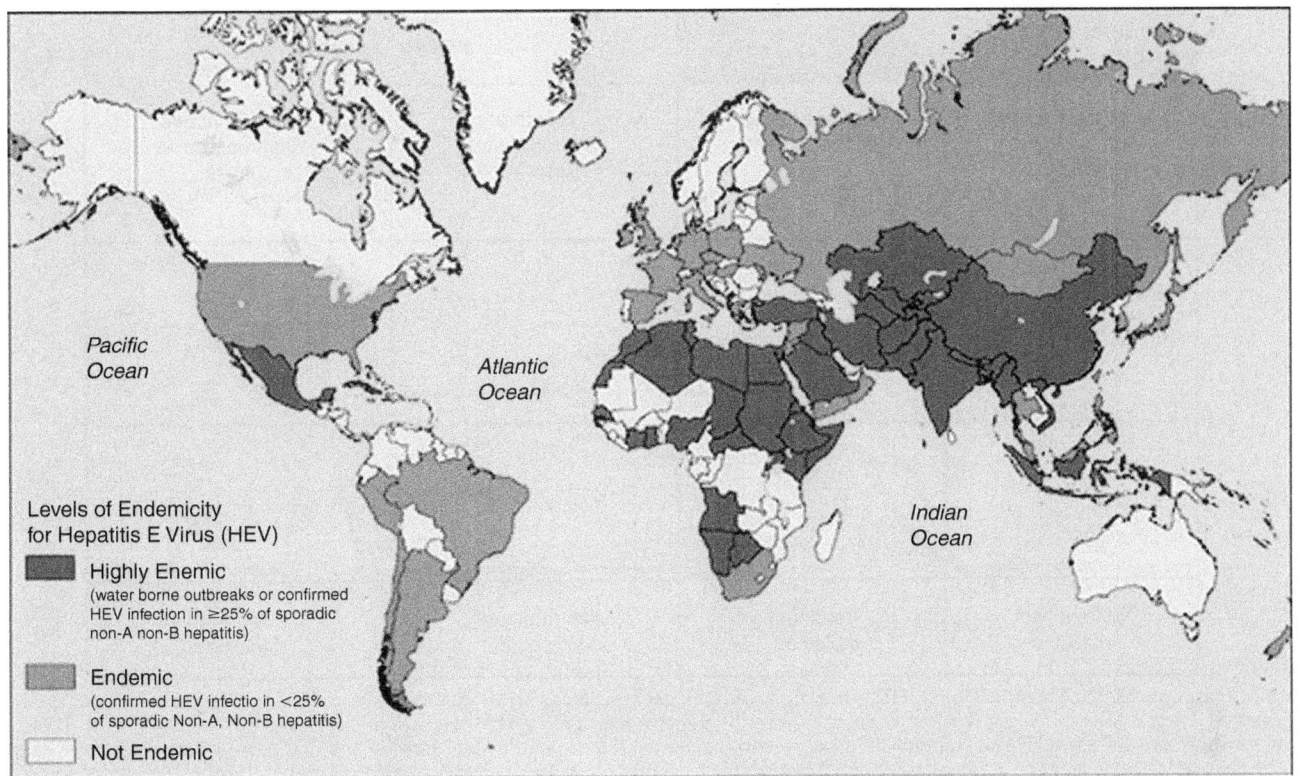

Figure 2 Global prevalence of hepatitis E virus. Hepatitis E is found worldwide. High endemic areas, defined by greater than or equal to 25% prevalence of sporadic non-A, non-B hepatitis, include parts of Central America and Mexico, Africa, the Middle East, and most of Asia. Endemic areas, defined as less than 25% prevalence of sporadic non-A, non-B hepatitis, include the United States, Europe, Russia, and parts of South America. Remaining regions are regarded as nonendemic.

children and/or staff are diagnosed with HAV infection, and to food handlers during a common-source exposure. Concurrent immunization for HAV in these at-risk contacts is also warranted.

Hepatitis E
Introduction
Hepatitis E virus (HEV) is a nonenveloped, single-stranded, positive-sense RNA virus of ~7300 bases in length and the sole member of the Hepeviridae family. Its genome contains three overlapping open reading frames. ORF1 encodes four nonstructural proteins, ORF2 encodes the capsid protein, and ORF3 a protein of unknown function. Four genotypes are known to infect humans, but similar to HAV, only one serotype exists and infection with one strain confers immunity to all others. HEV is likely a zoonosis with multiple nonhuman vectors.

Natural History
HEV is a cause of acute hepatitis and acute liver failure (see Table 1). It can cause chronic hepatitis in immunocompromised individuals. The majority of acute HEV infections are asymptomatic or minimally symptomatic. The incubation period is between 15 and 60 days, and if symptoms arise, they generally consist of anorexia, nausea, vomiting, diarrhea, and abdominal pain. Acute HEV infection rarely causes jaundice, and most symptoms resolve within 6 weeks from onset. A notable exception to the generally favorable outcome is an increased risk of acute liver failure among pregnant women during the second and third trimesters in endemic regions. This leads to a high maternal mortality rate of 15% to 25% and worse maternofetal outcomes in third-trimester infections. Acute HEV infection may also be associated with a lymphocytic destructive cholangitis.

Chronic HEV infection is defined as the presence of HEV RNA in the serum or stool for more than 6 months. It is uncommon and has been observed in solid-organ transplant recipients, HIV-positive subjects, and other immunocompromised hosts. Chronic HEV infection has only been reported with HEV

genotype 3 infections. It is unknown if other HEV genotypes can cause chronic HEV infection. Development of cirrhosis has been described as a consequence of chronic infection.

Epidemiology
HEV is found worldwide and can be divided into three distinct geographical patterns: highly endemic, endemic, and nonendemic (sporadic) (Figure 2). Large waterborne epidemics in highly endemic regions are due to infection with HEV genotypes 1 and 2 in Central America, Africa, and Asia. Sporadic cases of HEV in developed countries (Europe, North America, and Far East Asia) are due to HEV genotypes 3 and 4. The reservoir for autochthonous HEV is unknown but thought to be domestic swine. Sporadic cases may occur in travelers to endemic areas. Interestingly, males are more affected than females in sporadic infections, but this gender bias is not observed during epidemics. HEV is spread by the fecal–oral route, usually through ingestion of contaminated water.

Diagnosis
There are no commercially licensed tests for HEV detection in the United States. Testing is limited to research laboratories and can be obtained through the Centers for Disease Control and Prevention.

The diagnosis of acute HEV is made by detection of anti-HEV IgM in serum or HEV RNA in stool or serum. Anti-HEV IgG has limited utility in diagnosis of HEV infections and may be a serologic marker for past infection. In immunocompromised patients, antibody testing can be falsely negative, making HEV RNA the more reliable marker of acute and chronic infection. Chronic HEV is diagnosed when HEV RNA is present in sera or stool for more than 6 months in suspected cases.

Treatment
Since most acute HEV infections are mild, the treatment is generally supportive. Patients who develop acute liver failure should

HBeAg - positive		HBeAg - negative	
Immune tolerant High replication phase	**Immune active** High replication phase	**Inactive** Low replicative phase	**Immune active** High replicative phase
10^9-10^{10} HBV-DNA (IU/mL)	10^7-10^8	$<10^3$	$>10^5$
ALT			
No treatment indicated	Treatment indicated	No treatment indicated*	Treatment indicated

Figure 3 Phases of chronic hepatitis B virus (HBV) infection. Chronic hepatitis B can be viewed in phases defined by HBeAg status and serum HBV DNA and ALT levels. The initial phase is the immune-tolerant phase, characterized by HBeAg positivity, high HBV DNA level ($> 10^7$ IU/mL), and persistently normal ALT levels. This is seen only in persons who acquire the infection at birth or infancy and that persists for two to three decades of life. The next phase is the immune-active phase, defined by continued HBeAg positivity, high HBV viral load ($> 10^5$ IU/mL), and elevated ALT levels. The next phase is characterized by loss of HBeAg and development of anti-HBe and heralds a transition from a phase of high viral replication to one of low replication. The viral load is typically less than 10^3 IU/mL and serum ALT is normal. This phase is termed the inactive carrier phase. A proportion of individuals develop raised HBV DNA and ALT levels after HBeAg seroconversion. These persons are said to have transitioned to the immune-escape or HBeAg-negative immune-active phase.

be managed at a liver transplant center. The initial approach to management of chronic HEV infection in posttransplant recipients is to reduce the level of immunosuppression. If this is unsuccessful, then off-label use of antiviral therapy with peginterferon (Pegasys)[1] or ribavirin (Rebetol)[1] may be considered. In immunocompromised individuals therapy with peginterferon[1] or ribavirin[1] may be considered.

Prevention

Prevention of hepatitis E relies principally on good sanitation and the availability of clean drinking water. Prevention of transmission in travelers to endemic areas includes avoidance of tap water and consumption of street foods, raw vegetables, or raw or undercooked meats such as pork and seafood. A commercially available vaccine for HEV, HECOLIN[2] (Xiamen Innovax Biotech), has been available in China since 2012.

Hepatitis B
Introduction

HBV is a partially double-stranded DNA virus of ~3200 bases belonging to the Hepadnaviridae family. HBV consists of an outer lipid shell that surrounds a nucleocapsid consisting of the viral DNA and the polymerase. HBV has four overlapping reading frames (core, surface, polymerase, and x), which encode for seven viral proteins. HBsAg is the marker of infection and HBeAg is a marker of high viral replication and infectivity. The virus is classified into 10 major genotypes (A through J) that have a distinct geographical distribution. Four major serotypes have been described. Humans and old world primates (e.g., chimpanzees) are the only known hosts.

Natural History

Hepatitis B virus is a cause of acute hepatitis and acute liver failure (see Table 1). Globally, it is a major cause of chronic hepatitis. Infection with HBV is notable for a long incubation period ranging from 1 to 6 months. The majority (two-thirds) of persons with acute HBV infection are asymptomatic, one-third have an icteric presentation, and less than 1% present with acute liver failure. Symptoms of acute HBV are nonspecific and include anorexia, nausea, pruritus, and right upper quadrant pain. Symptoms usually resolve in ~1 to 3 months. Serum ALT levels peak with the onset of symptoms. The outcome of acute hepatitis B is strongly influenced by age at exposure. Resolution of acute infection occurs in 95% of persons exposed as adults, but chronic infection ensues in more than 90% of persons exposed as infants.

The natural history of chronic HBV infection depends on a complex interplay between the virus and the host immune response. Chronic HBV infection is often viewed in four phases (immune tolerant, HBeAg-positive and HBeAg-negative immune active, and inactive carrier) based on HBeAg status and serum HBV DNA and ALT levels (Figure 3). This classification is useful for providing advice on prognosis and need for treatment. Approximately 25% to 40% of persons with chronic infection will be at risk for development of cirrhosis. The 5-year cumulative incidence of cirrhosis in untreated chronic HBV infection is 8% to 20%. Once cirrhosis develops, the 5-year cumulative incidence of decompensated liver disease (ascites, variceal hemorrhage, hepatic encephalopathy) is approximately 20%, and the annual risk of hepatocellular carcinoma is 2% to 5%. Persons who have resolved chronic infection (cleared HBsAg) should be counseled of the risk for viral reactivation with use of chemotherapy or other immunosuppressive therapies.

Epidemiology

An estimated 2 billion people worldwide have evidence of past HBV infection, and of these an estimated 257 million have

[1] Not FDA approved for this indication.
[2] Not available in the United States.

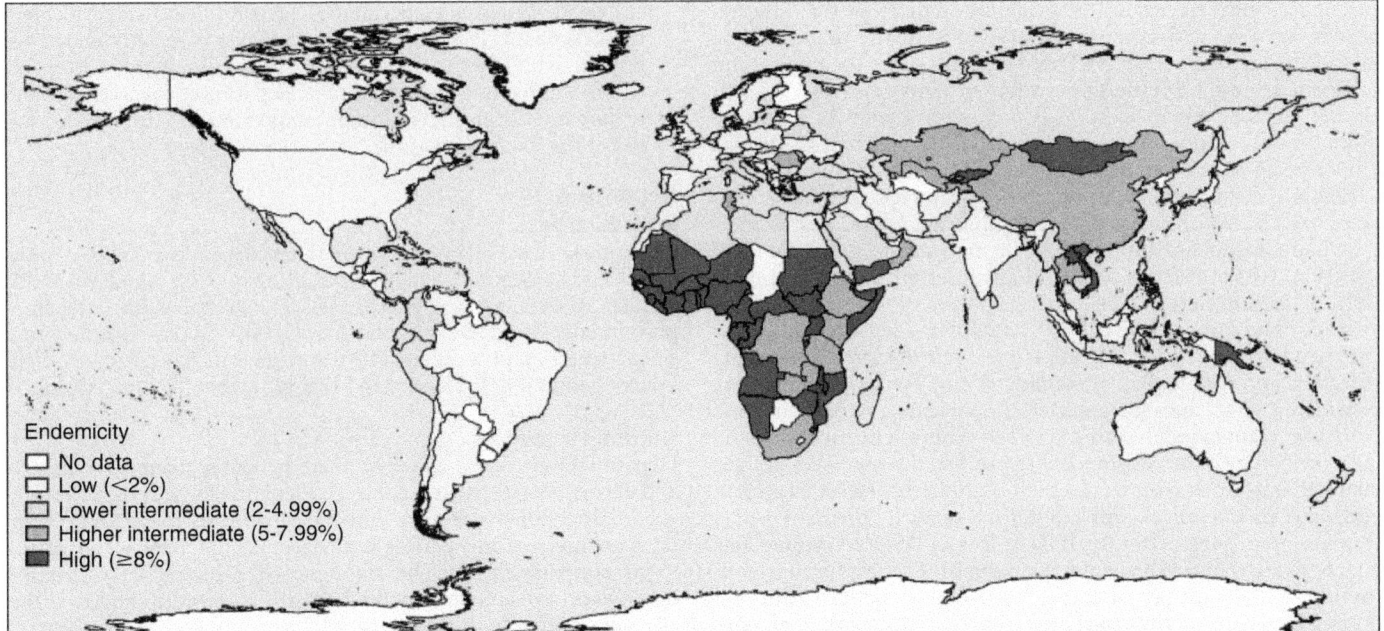

Figure 4 Global prevalence of chronic hepatitis B virus (HBV). Hepatitis B is found worldwide with varying geographical prevalence. High-prevalence areas defined as a prevalence of HBsAg greater than or equal to 8% include West Sub-Saharan Africa and Mongolia. Regions of high intermediate prevalence, defined as HBsAg prevalence of 5% to 7%, include China, Southeast Asia, and the remainder of Sub-Saharan Africa. Regions of low to intermediate prevalence, defined as HBsAg prevalence of 2% to 4%, include the Mediterranean region, India, the Middle East, Australia, and Japan. Regions with low prevalence, defined as HBsAg prevalence of less than or equal to 2%, include North America and Western Europe. Overall, the prevalence of HBV is declining worldwide.

Endemicity
- ☐ No data
- ☐ Low (<2%)
- ☐ Lower intermediate (2-4.99%)
- ▨ Higher intermediate (5-7.99%)
- ▉ High (≥8%)

chronic HBV infection. The prevalence of HBV infection is declining worldwide owing to the availability of an effective vaccine and implementation of successful vaccination programs. The prevalence of HBsAg, the serologic marker of chronic infection, is highest in Sub-Saharan Africa and Central Asia (≥ 8%) (see Figure 4) and lowest (< 2%) in Western Europe, Australia, Canada, and the United States (except Alaska) (Figure 4). HBV is transmitted vertically, sexually, or through percutaneous routes and is more infectious than human immunodeficiency virus or hepatitis C virus. Individuals considered at high risk for acquiring HBV infection should be screened for chronic hepatitis B by testing for HBsAg (Table 2).

Diagnosis

A number of serologic markers (viral antigens and antibodies to the viral antigens) and nucleic acid testing are available to diagnose acute and chronic HBV infection. Cases of suspected acute HBV infection are diagnosed by the detection of HBsAg, HBeAg, IgM anti-HBc, and HBV DNA in serum in the appropriate clinical setting. Although anti-HBc IgM is detected during acute HBV infection, it is not specific for acute hepatitis B and may be seen during reactivation of chronic HBV infection.

Chronic infection is defined as persistence of HBsAg for greater than 6 months in serum. If HBsAg is present, it is advised to check HBeAg, anti-HBe, HBV DNA, and serum ALT to determine the phase of infection.

Treatment

Acute HBV infection in an adult is associated with a high rate of spontaneous recovery, and antiviral treatment is rarely required. Supportive care is advised. For persons with evidence of acute liver failure, prompt institution of antiviral therapy with a potent nucleos(t)ide analog and referral to a transplant center is recommended. Peginterferon alfa-2a (Pegasys)[1] is contraindicated in persons with acute liver failure.

The goals of treatment of chronic HBV are sustained suppression of HBV DNA to prevent the development of cirrhosis,

TABLE 2	Centers for Disease Control and Prevention Guidelines for Hepatitis B Virus (HBV) Screening

Populations recommended or required for routine testing for chronic HBV infections

Persons born in regions of high and intermediate HBV endemicity (HBsAg prevalence ≥ 2%)

U.S.-born persons not vaccinated as infants whose parents were born in regions with high HBV endemicity (≥ 8%)

Injection drug users

Men who have sex with men

Persons with elevated alanine aminotransferase/aspartate aminotransferase of unknown etiology

Donors of blood, plasma, organs, tissues, or semen

Hemodialysis patients

All pregnant women

Persons needing immunosuppressive therapy

Infants born to HBsAg-positive mothers

Household, needle-sharing, or sex contacts of persons known to be HBsAg positive

HIV-positive persons

Persons who are the sources of blood or body fluids for exposures the might require postexposure prophylaxis (e.g., needlestick, sexual assault)

Modified from Centers for Disease Control and Prevention. Recommendations for Identification and Public Health Management of Persons with Chronic Hepatitis B Virus Infection.

hepatocellular carcinoma, and liver-related mortality. Cure of chronic HBV infection is currently not possible because of persistence of covalently closed circular DNA within the hepatocyte nucleus. Treatment recommendations differ among regional

---

[1] Not FDA approved for this indication.

guidelines, but treatment is generally indicated for HBeAg-positive subjects with confirmed HBV DNA greater than 2,000 to 20,000 IU/mL and serum ALT two or more times the upper limit of normal, and for HBeAg-negative patients with HBV DNA greater than or equal to 2000 IU/mL with serum ALT two or more times the upper limit of normal and/or liver biopsy–proven moderate to severe inflammation and/or moderate fibrosis. The decision to treat persons outside these parameters should be individualized based on their risk for complications and risk of therapy. Eight agents are approved for the treatment of chronic HBV infection: two interferon preparations, interferon alfa-2b (Intron A) and peginterferon alfa-2a (Pegasys), and six nucleos(t)ide analogs: lamivudine (Epivir HBV), adefovir (Hepsera), entecavir (Baraclude), telbivudine (Tyzeka), tenofovir disoproxil fumarate (Viread), and tenofovir alafenamide (Vemlidy). Four agents are considered first line—peginterferon, entecavir, tenofovir, and tenofovir alafenamide—based on their safety, effectiveness, and low rates of antiviral resistance. Peginterferon is generally recommended in persons who would prefer a finite course of treatment and who have clinical and laboratory features predictive of a response to peginterferon (high ALT, low HBV DNA, young age, female gender, and HBV genotype A or B). Peginterferon is contraindicated in persons with decompensated cirrhosis, autoimmune illnesses, or active psychiatric illness. Nucleos(t)ide analogs are more potent inhibitors of HBV DNA replication and generally better tolerated than peginterferon. They are usually administered long term. The ideal endpoint of treatment is HBsAg loss, but this is rarely observed with any therapy (< 10% with interferon and after 5 years of therapy with nucleos(t)ide analogs).

Prevention

- Vaccination is the primary method of prevention. An effective vaccine against HBV has been available since 1981. In the United States, the Advisory Committee on Immunization Practices has recommended that all children complete the series of three vaccinations by 18 months of age with the first dose administered within 24 hours of birth. Infants whose mothers are HBsAg positive or whose HBsAg status is unknown should receive the last dose by 6 months of age. Hepatitis B immune globulin (HyperHEP B) and HBV vaccination is recommended at birth for infants whose mothers are HBsAg positive to prevent maternal–infant transmission of HBV. In mothers with viral loads greater than 200,000 IU/mL, antiviral therapy with tenofovir, telbivudine (Tyzeka), or lamivudine (Epivir HBV) in

the third trimester of pregnancy (gestation weeks 28-32) can be considered. Postexposure prophylaxis is recommended for anyone who is exposed to HBV and is considered susceptible to HBV infection and consists of hepatitis B vaccination and/or hepatitis B immune globulin depending on the HBsAg status of the exposure source.

Hepatitis D
Introduction
Hepatitis D virus (HDV) is a viroid that is dependent on HBV for its lifecycle. The genome consists of a negative-sense, single-stranded circular RNA virus of ~1600 bases. The virus has an outer lipoprotein envelope HBsAg derived from HBV and is attached to a single structural protein, the HDV antigen (HDAg). There are eight known genotypes. Immunity to HBV prevents HDV infection.

Natural History
Hepatitis D virus is a cause of acute hepatitis, acute liver failure, and chronic hepatitis (see Table 1). Hepatitis D virus infection can occur either simultaneously with HBV (referred to as coinfection) or as an infection in a patient with chronic HBV infection (referred to as superinfection). The outcome of HBV/HDV coinfection depends on the course of acute hepatitis B infection and is generally self-limiting with a low risk of chronicity (~5%). In contrast, HDV superinfection of a chronic HBV carrier results in chronic HDV infection in more than 90% of cases. Acute liver failure is observed more commonly with coinfection than with superinfection. Chronic HDV infection has a variable course, from an asymptomatic carrier to cirrhosis and decompensated liver disease. In general, HDV infection is associated with more rapid progression to cirrhosis and decompensated liver disease and a higher rate of hepatocellular carcinoma as compared with HBV monoinfection.

Epidemiology
In developed countries, the prevalence of HDV has declined as a consequence of widespread vaccination against hepatitis B. Chronic HDV infection is predominantly seen in intravenous drug users or hemophiliacs requiring frequent transfusions. HDV is prevalent in the Amazon basin, Africa, the Mediterranean basin, Central Asia, Mongolia, and Russia (Figure 5). HDV genotype 1 can be found worldwide, but all other genotypes are restricted to specific geographic areas.

HDV is spread by the same routes as HBV infection and is efficiently transmitted by parenteral and sexual exposure. In contrast

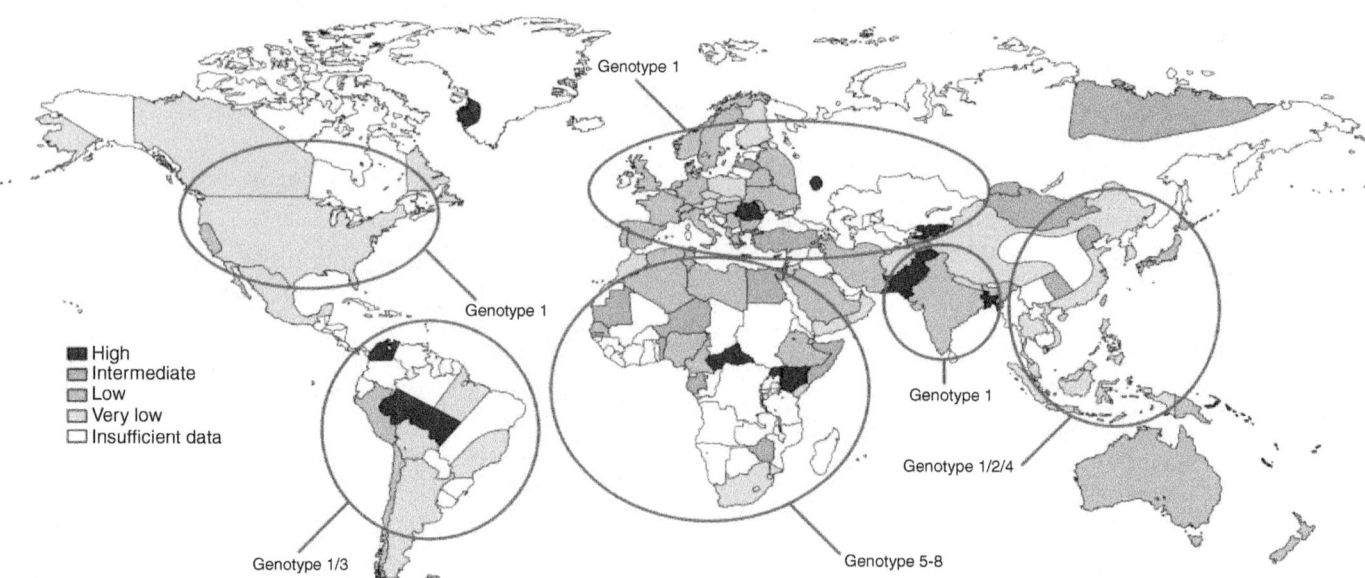

Figure 5 Global prevalence of hepatitis D virus. Hepatitis D is found globally, but prevalence varies among geographic regions. The highest prevalence is observed in Central Africa, Central Asia, and the Amazon. Intermediate-prevalence regions include West Africa and Eastern Europe. Low-prevalence regions include North America, most of Western Europe, and Australia.

to HBV, vertical transmission is not a common mode of transmission. Transmission cannot occur in the absence of HBsAg.

Diagnosis

Testing for hepatitis D should be considered in persons presenting with acute hepatitis B who have additional risk factors for HDV, including a history of injection drug use; persons from endemic regions who present with a severe or protracted hepatitis; patients with chronic hepatitis B who develop an acute hepatitis of undetermined origin; and persons with HBsAg-positive chronic hepatitis B from endemic regions. Total anti-HDV (IgM and IgG) and anti-HDV IgM are the only commercially available assays in the United States. Initial testing for HDV should be with total anti-HDV. Chronic infection should be confirmed by a reverse transcriptase polymerase chain reaction assay for HDV RNA.

Treatment

The goals of treatment are long-term suppression of both HDV and HBV to prevent the development of cirrhosis, hepatocellular carcinoma, and liver-related death. There is no effective treatment for HDV. Interferon alfa (Intron A)[1] has been used for treatment of HDV. The most effective dose and duration of treatment have not been established. Peginterferon alfa-2a (Pegasys)[1] administered for 48 to 72 weeks results in sustained HDV RNA suppression after 6 months off therapy in 17% to 43% of patients. Liver transplantation with the use of hepatitis B immune globulin[1] is an option for patients with decompensated liver disease. Novel agents blocking viral entry and posttranslational prenylation are currently being investigated in clinical studies.

Financial Disclosure: The authors are employees of the U.S. government and have no financial conflicts of interest to disclose.

Acknowledgments: This work is supported by the Intramural Research Program of the National Institute of Diabetes and Digestive and Kidney Diseases, National Institutes of Health.

[1] Not FDA approved for this indication.

References

Hoofnagle JH, Nelson KE, Purcell RH: Hepatitis E, *N Engl J Med* 367(13):1237–1244, 2012.

Hughes SA, Wedemeyer H, Harrison PM: Hepatitis delta virus, *Lancet* 378(9785):73–85, 2011.

Matheny SC, Kingery JE: Hepatitis A, *Am Fam Physician* 86(11):1027–1034, 2012.

Trépo C, Chan HL, Lok A: Hepatitis B virus infection, *Lancet* 384(9959):2053–2063, 2014.

HEPATITIS C

Method of
Arthur Y. Kim, MD

CURRENT DIAGNOSIS

- Hepatitis C virus (HCV) is a common infection in the United States with major morbidity and mortality.
- Incidence of HCV is rising, linked to the opioid epidemic.
- Given the asymptomatic presentation and long period before complications, screening is warranted: undiagnosed persons born between 1945 and 1965 with no previous history of antibody testing, and people who inject drugs (Table 1).
- Diagnosis is made with two-stage testing: initial screening for anti-HCV antibodies followed by HCV RNA testing to confirm the presence of virus.

CURRENT THERAPY

- Novel therapeutic approaches that are safe and highly effective have revolutionized the care of HCV.
- The goal of therapy is cure of virus, which prevents liver-related complications and further transmission.
- Regimens of combination antivirals typically given for 12 weeks can cure over 95% of those living with HCV infection.

The diagnosis, management, and therapeutic approaches for patients living with hepatitis C virus (HCV) have dramatically transformed in recent years. Most people (over 95%) living with HCV infection can be cured after 8 to 12 weeks of safe oral regimens combining antiviral agents. The availability of novel therapies enhances the effectiveness of screening patients for HCV infection who may otherwise be unaware of infection owing to its asymptomatic presentation.

Virology, Pathogenesis, and Natural History

HCV is a single-strand RNA virus whose genome encodes several viral proteins, including nonstructural proteins (NS3/4A, termed protease; NS5A, and NS5B, termed polymerase) that may each be specifically targeted by medications. There are seven known families of virus, commonly known as genotypes 1 through 7, many with subtypes (e.g., genotype 1a or 1b).

After acute infection, in most individuals the virus establishes a chronic lifelong infection characterized by high levels of viremia easily detected in plasma; in a minority, the virus is spontaneously cleared. In the latter scenario, HCV is permanently eradicated as the polymerase is an RNA-RNA polymerase and there is no DNA intermediate to establish latency in the host. Those who achieve clearance of virus, whether spontaneously or via treatment, are susceptible to reinfection if exposed again.

TABLE 1	Recommendations for One-Time Screening.

Persons born between 1945 and 1965, without prior ascertainment of risk

Risk factor-based screening
Risk behaviors
- Injection drug use (current or ever, including those who injected once)
- Intranasal drug use

Risk exposures
- Persons on long-term hemodialysis (ever)
- Persons with percutaneous/parenteral exposures in an unregulated setting
- Healthcare, emergency medical, and public safety workers after needlesticks, sharps, or mucosal exposures to HCV-infected blood
- Children born to HCV-infected women
- Prior recipients of transfusions or organ transplants, including persons who:
- Were notified that they received blood from a donor who later tested positive for HCV infection
- Received a transfusion of blood or blood components or underwent an organ transplant before July 1992
- Received clotting factor concentrates produced before 1987
- Persons who were ever incarcerated

Other considerations
- HIV infection
- Sexually active persons about to start preexposure prophylaxis for HIV
- Unexplained chronic liver disease and/or chronic hepatitis including elevated alanine aminotransferase levels
- Solid-organ donors (deceased and living)
- Pregnant women

HCV, Hepatitis C virus.
Modified from http://hcvguidelines.org.

Both the acute and chronic phases of HCV infection are largely asymptomatic. A minority of those with acute infection may present with nonspecific symptoms such as abdominal pain and malaise, with less than 10% presenting with jaundice. Rarely, those with chronic infection may experience extrahepatic manifestations of HCV infection, such as cryoglobulinemic vasculitis, proteinuria or glomerulonephritis, or lymphoma. Otherwise, alanine transaminase (ALT) levels may be persistently or intermittently elevated but may also be within normal range in up to 20% of infected individuals; thus, ALT is considered an imperfect screening test for HCV.

After establishment of chronic HCV infection, fibrosis occurs at a variable rate and may progress to cirrhosis in about 15% to 20% over a 20-year period. Fibrosis may be accelerated by other liver insults, such as alcohol use, nonalcoholic steatohepatitis, and coinfection with HIV or hepatitis B virus (HBV). Those with HCV-related cirrhosis may experience significant morbidity and mortality from various complications; screening for varices and hepatocellular carcinoma is recommended (see chapter on Cirrhosis).

Epidemiology

HCV is estimated to infect at least 80 million people worldwide. In the United States, it is the leading bloodborne pathogen and infects more than 3 million Americans. The highest-risk groups are those born between 1945 and 1965 (so-called baby boomers), people who inject drugs, and HIV-positive men who have sex with men. In the United States, the incidence reached a peak in the 1970s and 1980s and then steeply declined; in the past decade there has been a resurgence of new incident cases linked to a widespread opioid epidemic.

Owing to the high number of infections that occurred decades ago, a large number of Americans within the baby-boomer cohort are now at risk for unidentified long-standing HCV infection, cirrhosis, and death; at present, the mortality related to HCV exceeds that related to all other notifiable infectious diseases in the United States. HCV remains the leading indication for liver transplantation.

Risk Factors

HCV is most efficiently transmitted via exposure to contaminated blood or its components. In the United States, injection drug use (IDU) is the most common mode of transmission. Nosocomial exposure to contaminated blood or blood products and poorly sterilized or reused contaminated medical equipment remains an important risk, especially if strict universal precautions are not instituted. Mother-to-child transmission is not efficient, as about 5% of children born to HCV-infected women are infected, with higher rates if HIV/HCV coinfection is present. Sexual transmission is considered very rare in the context of heterosexual relationships but does occur at higher rates in men who have sex with men, particularly with HIV and/or practices that result in bloody exposures.

Diagnosis

There are two tests utilized for the diagnosis of HCV infection: testing for anti-HCV antibodies and measuring HCV RNA. The suggested algorithm is initial serologic testing to assess exposure followed by HCV RNA testing to determine current or cleared infection. Currently available anti-HCV testing is highly sensitive (>99%) but may be falsely negative in the earliest stages of infection (typically the first 4 to 12 weeks) or in the setting of immunosuppression (such as dialysis or HIV if CD4 counts are below 200 cells/mm^3). HCV RNA testing may be utilized to confirm current HCV RNA infection after an initial positive anti-HCV test or in settings when anti-HCV may be falsely negative. There are two types of HCV RNA tests: qualitative HCV RNA tests that do not quantify the level of viral replication and quantitative HCV RNA tests. Quantitative testing has improved in recent years and exhibits sensitivity similar to qualitative testing; therefore, it is preferred in most situations.

Those with confirmed current HCV infection (positive HCV RNA) should also be tested for HIV and HBV (the latter typically by HBsAg). Follow-up evaluation includes HCV genotype, which defines therapeutic options. Discovery of advanced fibrosis or cirrhosis may affect the specifics of recommended antiviral regimens but also has prognostic implications. The likelihood of cirrhosis is dependent on various factors, including advancing patient age, duration of infection, and cofactors such as significant alcohol use or HIV. Noninvasive assessment with serologic testing (such as FibroSure) or with novel imaging technologies (such as transient elastography) has largely replaced liver biopsies.

Prevention

Prevention of HCV infection should be targeted to the highest-risk groups. For people who inject drugs, clean injecting equipment, including needles, syringes, and other components of drug preparation, is paramount. Risk reduction should also be achieved after viral clearance to prevent reinfection.

Prevention of fibrosis progression includes minimization or abstinence from regular alcohol use, avoidance of fatty liver, and avoidance of primary infection with or control of coexisting viruses (HIV or HBV). If not immune, vaccines against hepatitis A virus and HBV are recommended. Patients with coexisting substance use disorder should be referred for appropriate care.

Therapy

Antiviral treatments for hepatitis C have been revolutionized with combination regimens of direct-acting antivirals (DAAs). These new drugs are used in combination with the goal to eradicate HCV. Cure is known as a sustained virologic response (SVR), defined as a negative HCV RNA test 12 or more weeks after cessation of therapy. This definition represents a durable cure in the absence of reinfection. Benefits of SVR include a significant reduction in future liver-related events, especially for those with advanced fibrosis or cirrhosis. Additional benefits include abrogation of further HCV transmission, amelioration of extrahepatic manifestations (if present), and improvement in quality of life. Virtually all patients with current HCV infection are candidates for therapy.

Available agents may be classified by the viral protein they target: NS3/4A protease inhibitors: simeprevir, paritaprevir (which requires pharmacologic boosting with ritonavir), glecaprevir and grazoprevir; NS5A inhibitors: daclatasvir, elbasvir, ledipasvir, ombitasvir and pibrentasvir; the NS5A nonnucleoside inhibitor dasabuvir; and the NS5B nucleotide polymerase inhibitor sofosbuvir. Simeprevir (Olysio), daclatasvir (Daklinza), and sofosbuvir (Sovaldi) are available as single agents, but the majority are parts of combination regimens, as described in Table 2. The Infectious Diseases Society of America (IDSA) and American Association for the Study of Liver Diseases (AASLD) maintain guidelines for providers at http://www.hcvguidelines.org, which provides updates with approval of novel agents and as new data become available.

One major consideration in choosing a regimen is the genotype of the virus, although certain regimens can treat all genotypes (termed pan-genotypic). Other potential influences include presence of cirrhosis, the potential for concomitant drug interactions (including those with HIV coinfection on antiretrovirals), prior treatment experience, and adherence to therapy. Certain regimens have been tested for those with advanced renal impairment. Insurance formulary preferences may also dictate the choice. One regimen in particular, elbasvir/grazoprevir (Zepatier), requires testing of genotype 1a virus for resistance-associated substitutions (RASs) that are associated with decreased response; if present, the duration should be increased and ribavirin (Ribasphere) added. In general, almost all patient groups can be offered a regimen with a rate of SVR at or above 95%.

These combinations have favorable safety profiles, with phase III trials reporting very low discontinuation rates. The most common side effects of these regimens are headache and fatigue. At

TABLE 2 · First-Line Combination Antiviral Regimens for Chronic Hepatitis C as of August 2018, Genotypes 1–4

GENOTYPE	COMBINATION	USE OF RIBAVIRIN (RBV)	DURATION (WEEKS)	NOTES
1	Elbasvir 50 mg/grazoprevir 100 mg FDC (Zepatier) once daily	Add RBV and extend to 16 weeks if baseline NS5A RASs present (genotype 1a only)	12–16	Safety in advanced chronic kidney disease; not recommended in decompensated cirrhosis
	Glecaprevir 300 mg/ pibrentasvir 120 mg FDC (Mavyret) once daily	Not proven	8–16	8 weeks for treatment naïve; 12–16 weeks for cirrhosis/ certain treatment experience
	Ledipasvir 90 mg/sofosbuvir 400 mg FDC (Harvoni) once daily	Add RBV if both interferon-experienced and cirrhosis (12 weeks)	8–24	Antacids reduce absorption; 8 weeks consideration only for naïve patients with F0-2 and HCV RNA less than 6M IU/mL
	Sofosbuvir 400 mg/ velpatasvir 100 mg FDC (Epclusa) once daily	Consider in select circumstances	12–24	Antacids reduce absorption
2	Glecaprevir 300 mg/ pibrentasvir 120 mg FDC (Mavyret) once daily	Not proven	8–12	8 weeks for treatment naïve; 12 weeks for cirrhosis/ certain treatment experience
	Sofosbuvir 400 mg/ velpatasvir 100 mg FDC (Epclusa) once daily	Consider in select circumstances	12	Antacids reduce absorption
3	Glecaprevir 300 mg/ pibrentasvir 120 mg FDC (Mavyret) once daily	Not proven	8–16	8 weeks for treatment naïve; 12–16 weeks for cirrhosis/ certain treatment experience
	Sofosbuvir 400 mg/ velpatasvir 100 mg FDC (Epclusa) once daily	Consider in select circumstances	12–24	Antacids reduce absorption
4	Elbasvir 50 mg/grazoprevir 100 mg (Zepatier) once daily	Consider adding RBV for cirrhosis, prior nonresponder	12–16	
	Ledipasvir 90 mg/sofosbuvir 400 mg FDC (Harvoni) once daily	Consider for previous SOF failure	12	
	Glecaprevir 300 mg/ pibrentasvir 120 mg FDC (Mavyret) once daily	Not proven	12	8 weeks for treatment naïve; 12 weeks for cirrhosis/ interferon experienced
	Sofosbuvir 400 mg/ velpatasvir 100 mg FDC (Epclusa) once daily	Consider in select circumstances	12	Antacids reduce absorption

FDC, Fixed-dose combination; *NS5A,* nonstructural protein 5A; *RASs,* resistance-associated substitutions; *RBV,* ribavirin; *SOF,* sofosbuvir.
Daclatasvir may need dose adjustments with certain medications with cytochrome P450 interactions.

times, ribavirin may be added to the regimen, particularly in the cases of relapse after previous treatment and/or cirrhosis (especially if decompensated or previously decompensated).

Drug-drug interactions are also potentially problematic. Sofosbuvir-containing regimens should not be coadministered with amiodarone (Cordarone), owing to reports of symptomatic bradycardia with poor outcomes. Medications may significantly decrease absorption of HCV antivirals, especially rifampin (Rifadin), carbamazepine (Tegretol), oxcarbazepine (Trileptal), and St. John's wort[7]. For the combinations of ledipasvir/sofosbuvir (Harvoni) and sofosbuvir/velpatasvir (Epclusa), care must be taken if coadministered with medications that decrease gastric pH. Involvement of clinical pharmacists may be very useful, along with resources such as the website maintained at the University of Liverpool: http://hep-druginteractions.org.

Monitoring
Compared with previous regimens that were associated with more side effects and complications, current treatments are far more tolerable. Clinical visits or phone calls to monitor for side effects and to promote adherence are often performed monthly while on treatment. A negative HCV RNA at approximately week 4 into therapy confirms adherence. Certain regimens may require more intensive monitoring in the presence of cirrhosis, as cases of decompensation have been reported. Those with active HBV replication who are untreated are at risk for reactivation of this virus once HCV is suppressed, with rare cases of liver failure reported; cotreatment of both viruses or very close monitoring is recommended for this subgroup. Currently, there are no data regarding the use of these agents in pregnancy or breastfeeding.

References
AASLD/IDSA: Hepatitis C guidance: AASLD-IDSA recommendations for testing, managing, and treating adults infected with hepatitis C virus, *Hepatology* 62(3):932–954, 2015.
Edlin BR, Eckhardt BJ, Shu MA, et al: Toward a more accurate estimate of the prevalence of hepatitis C in the United States, *Hepatology* 62(5):1353–1363, 2015.
Kim A: Hepatitis C virus, *Ann Intern Med* 165(5):ITC33–ITC48, 2016.
Ly KN, Hughes EM, Jiles RB, Holmberg SD: Rising mortality associated with hepatitis C virus in the United States, 2003-2013, *Clin Infect Dis* 62(10):1287–1288, 2016.
Suryaprasad AG, White JZ, Xu F, et al: Emerging epidemic of hepatitis C virus infections among young nonurban persons who inject drugs in the United States, 2006-2012, *Clin Infect Dis* 59(10):1411–1419, 2014, 2006-2012.

[7]Available as dietary supplement.

INFLAMMATORY BOWEL DISEASE

Method of

Mona Rezapour, MD, MHS; Danny Avalos, MD; and Oriana M. Damas, MD*,†

Introduction and Epidemiology

Inflammatory bowel disease (IBD) is a chronic relapsing inflammatory disorder of the gastrointestinal (GI) tract that includes Crohn disease (CD) and ulcerative colitis (UC). A subset of patients with IBD have indeterminate colitis (IC), a classification that is determined when clinical features and diagnostic tests do not fit specifically into either CD or UC.

In the United States, about 3 million people have a diagnosis of IBD. Recent epidemiologic studies indicate that although the incidence of IBD in Westernized countries has stabilized, disease burden is expected to continue to rise as the annual prevalence steadily increases. The demographics of the IBD population in the US are also changing. Traditionally a disease that afflicted mainly European whites and the Ashkenazi Jewish population, IBD is now increasingly common among African Americans and Hispanic Americans.

The majority of IBD cases are sporadic. However, a little less than 20% of cases report having a relative with IBD, and this is particularly higher in patients with CD. There is also a higher IBD concordance in patients with CD compared to UC, wherein 2% to 14% of patients with CD report a family history of CD. Previous studies report that first-degree relatives of individuals with IBD have a lifetime risk of developing CD of 5% to 8% and of developing UC of 1.6% to 5.2%. With two affected parents, the risk of developing IBD in offspring increases to as high as 33%. These findings clearly support the influence of underlying genetic susceptibility in IBD development.

There are now more than 200 IBD susceptibility genetic loci associated with IBD risk, with substantial overlap seen between UC and CD. Genome-wide association studies and meta-analyses, thereafter, provide fundamental insights into IBD pathogenesis. Implicated loci are enriched in genes involved in host-microbial interactions and are shared with other complex, immune-mediated diseases. Despite the discovery of these genetic underpinnings, established IBD loci actually explain only a fraction of the variance in disease risk and even less so of disease phenotype. This suggests that other factors, including environmental exposures, likely make larger contributions to pathogenesis and phenotype.

Clinical Features

IBD onset occurs primarily at a young age, between the second and fourth decade of life, although some studies suggest a bimodal distribution with another peak observed in the sixth and seventh decade of life. IBD can be difficult to diagnose because there is no single biomarker that can diagnose IBD. IBD diagnosis is made by a combination of clinical, serologic, radiographic, endoscopic, surgical, and histologic features. Adding further to the complexity is the fact that sometimes symptoms are vague. For example, fatigue, fever, chills, weight loss, failure to thrive in children, and development of extra-intestinal manifestations (EIMs) can at times precede luminal GI symptoms. When IBD is suspected and diarrhea is present, it is imperative that the patient's stool is examined for infectious causes because these can mimic IBD on radiographic imaging and endoscopically. Table 1 describes in detail differences in clinical presentation as well as differences in disease location between UC and CD.

Natural History

Most patients with CD and UC have a chronic, relapsing course. In CD, the natural history of intestinal inflammation can ultimately lead to the development of intestinal complications such as strictures, fistulas, and abscesses (Figure 1). This is particularly true if patients do not receive appropriate timely medical treatment. In many cases, these complications result in need for procedures (such as perianal abscess drainage or seton placements) and surgeries. Similarly, patients with untreated UC may also end up with complications including spontaneous colon perforation or megacolon, in which case a total colectomy is curative. UC patients with longstanding disease are also at risk for colon

---

*The authors disclose no relevant conflicts of interest.

†Funding for Oriana M. Damas was supported by: NIH N3U54MD010722-03S1.

TABLE 1	Clinical Presentation and Differences in Location of Disease Between Ulcerative Colitis and Crohn Disease		
CLINICAL FEATURES	**ULCERATIVE COLITIS**	**CROHN DISEASE**
Bloody diarrhea	++	±
Passage of mucus	++	±
Urgency to have a bowel movement	++	++
Tenesmus	++	±
Abdominal pain	++ (mainly left lower quadrant)	++ (can be diffuse or commonly right lower quadrant)
Weight loss	++	++
Fevers (important to exclude infection)	++	++
Fatigue and exhaustion	++	++
Presence of extra-intestinal manifestations	++	++ (especially in Crohn colitis)
Depression	++	++
Disease Location		
Small bowel involvement	– (never)	± (can be present)
Upper-gastrointestinal tract (proximal to ligament of Treitz)	– (never)	± (can be present)
Fistula presence (enteric, perianal, or entero-vaginal/vesicular or enterocutaneous)	– (never)	± (can be present)
Colonic disease	++ (always)	± (can be present)

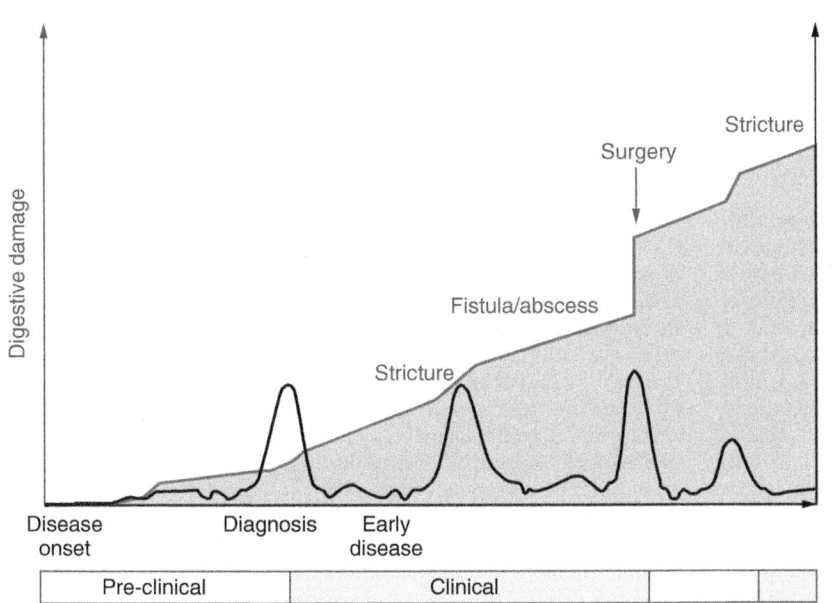

Figure 1 The natural history of Crohn disease if left untreated. (Adapted from Pariente, B, Cosnes J, Danese S, et al. Development of the Crohn's disease digestive damage score, the Lemann score. *Inflamm Bowel Dis* 17(6):1415-1422, 2011.)

Figure 2 Endoscopic images of ulcerative colitis (UC) and Crohn disease (CD). (A) UC with luminal bleeding, loss of vascular pattern, and ulcerations. (B) CD with large deep ulcerations and edema in the terminal ileum.

cancer. Recent studies suggest that progression of disease of both CD and UC is preventable by timely administration of biologic therapy, which can modify the disease course.

Diagnosis

History and Physical

The diagnosis of IBD first starts with a careful clinical assessment, including a detailed history and a thorough physical exam that includes a perianal exam to look for the presence of perianal disease. A family history of IBD in the setting of GI symptoms should also raise clinical suspicion. Based on the clinical exam, the provider can then order a set of diagnostic tests to confirm the diagnosis

Laboratory Testing

It is important to order stool studies if diarrhea is present, to exclude enteric infections, as well as other causes of diarrhea (e.g., pancreatic insufficiency). A stool test to measure inflammation, such as stool fecal calprotectin or lactoferrin, is a noninvasive marker to detect the presence of enteric (mainly colonic) inflammation. These tests are useful for diagnosis and for monitoring of clinical disease activity.

Laboratory results, including presence of iron deficiency anemia, elevated C-reactive protein, and erythrocyte sedimentation rate (ESR), can clue into the diagnosis, although on their own,

they are insufficient to definitely diagnose IBD. IBD-associated antibodies, including antisaccharomyces cerevisiae antibodies (ASCA IgG and IgA), perinuclear antinuclear cytoplasmic antibody (pANCA), antiflagellin (CBir1), antiouter membrane porin C (anti-OmpC), and antipseudomonas fluorescens-associated sequence I2 (anti-I2), can be measured in the blood and can aid in the diagnosis of IBD.

However, it is important to keep in mind that these antibodies can also be present in patients without IBD who have a family history of IBD. In prior studies, serologic markers such as pANCAs detect 40% to 80% of UC patients and the ASCA detect about 68% of CD patients. CD patients can also carry pANCA, as seen in approximately 40% of patients who have Crohn colitis. Therefore, although helpful when positive as they can raise clinical suspicion for either CD or UC on their own, serologic markers are insufficient to diagnose IBD.

Imaging

CT and MRI provide information about the presence of inflammation in the small bowel and can be very useful in the diagnosis of IBD when there is clinical suspicion but no evidence of inflammation on ileocolonoscopy. CT or MR enterography (MRE) provide high contrast resolution that can help define mural and extra-mural complications. MREs are particularly helpful in defining the presence of disease activity in CD and in distinguishing between inflammatory and more complicated CD (such as fistulizing and/or stenotic disease). Pelvic imaging also helps identify the presence of perianal CD such as perianal/perirectal fistulas. An MRI is preferred over CT in patients younger than 17 years of age to prevent long-term exposure to radiation.

Endoscopy and Histology

Colonoscopy with ileal intubation is considered the gold standard for diagnosis of IBD. The endoscopic location and appearance can also help distinguish between CD and UC. Endoscopic hallmarks of CD include patchy areas of inflammation with surrounding normal intervening mucosa, inflammation characterized by edema, nodularity, and ulcerations causing a cobblestone appearance (Figure 2). Endoscopic findings of UC include ulceration, friability, and loss of vascularity starting in the distal rectum and extending proximally in a continuous pattern (see Figure 2). An isolated cecal patch of inflammation can be observed in UC patients with otherwise more distal disease and this should be not be confused as a skip pattern seen in CD. Furthermore, the finding of mild ileal inflammation known as "backwash ileitis" is sometimes seen in UC patients with ileocecal valve inflammation and in the primary sclerosing cholangitis (PSC) patient. Small bowel capsule endoscopy is also helpful in visualizing the small bowel mucosa in patients with a high index of suspicion for small intestinal CD.

Histologic changes seen in CD and UC are distinct from those seen in acute infection and include mucosal separation, distortion and branching of crypts, presence of chronic inflammatory cells in the lamina propria, increase in number of lymphocytes and plasma cells in the crypt bases, and paneth cell metaplasia. In addition, the classical finding of granulomas is only seen in a minority of CD patients and although helpful, is not pathognomonic as they can also be seen in UC.

Extraintestinal Manifestations

EIMs occur in 21% to 36% of IBD patients. Arthropathy is the most common EIM. Some EIMs are associated with disease activity and others are independent of disease activity. EIMs that parallel disease activity include aphthous ulcers and peripheral, dermatologic (erythema nodosum, Figure 3), and ophthalmologic (episcleritis and scleritis) arthropathies. EIMs that do not correlate with luminal inflammation include axial arthropathy (ankylosing spondylitis), hepatobiliary (PSC), and some dermatologic manifestations (such as pyoderma gangrenosum). Although not an EIM, by strict definition, IBD can also result in other extra-luminal disease complications including thromboembolic disease and osteoporosis.

Management of Disease

In IBD, we classify therapy as induction therapy, which controls the inflammation quickly, and as maintenance therapy, which sustains control of inflammation. Figure 4 illustrates currently available inductive and maintenance therapies for IBD. The specific therapy is determined by several disease characteristics including disease location, extent of disease, and disease severity. The goal of therapy is control of inflammation, prevention of complications, and improvement in quality of life. These therapies include corticosteroids, 5-aminosalicylates (5-ASA), immunomodulators, and biologics. Therapeutic drug monitoring (TDM) of biologics is also an important component of therapy. TDM involves checking drug levels and the presence of antibodies to achieve a biologic-specific therapeutic target. TDM as a proactive or a reactive strategy is a topic of ongoing debate and beyond the scope of this chapter.

Medical Therapy

Corticosteroids

Corticosteroids, in particular prednisone, are used in both UC and CD mainly to manage disease flares. In UC, it can also be used for induction of remission in those intolerant to 5-ASAs or those who have failed to respond to 5-ASA treatment. The dose commonly used is 40 mg/day until clinical improvement and then a taper of 5 to 10 mg weekly until 20 mg, at which time a slower taper of 2.5 mg weekly is followed. Methylprednisolone (Solu-Medrol) is an intravenous medication often used in severe disease flares in hospitalized patients in doses from 40 to 60 mg/day. Controlled-release budesonide in the ileum (Entocort EC) and controlled-release budesonide in the colon (UCERIS) also serve as effective short-term corticosteroids with fewer side effects as compared to conventional oral corticosteroids due to their high liver first-pass metabolism and low systemic bioavailability. What limits the use of corticosteroids is their substantial side effect profile that includes psychiatric disturbances, hyperglycemia, impaired wound healing, metabolic bone disease, and ophthalmologic disease. Importantly, steroids, while a convenient oral medication often interpreted as less harmful than biologics, are actually associated with a higher risk of infection than anti-TNFs and do not reliably cause mucosal healing. Steroids are also not effective for maintenance of remission, as they do not alter the natural history of the disease in the same way that biologics can.

Figure 3 Picture of a patient with erythema nodosum, characterized by red/purple, painful lumps present most commonly in the lower extremities. Erythema nodosum is seen more in Crohn disease and its presence parallels active gut inflammation.

Therapeutic pyramid for IBD

Gray drugs are used in mild disease.

Figure 4 Therapeutic algorithm. Patients with milder disease benefit from 5-aminosalicylates (5-ASA) therapies as inductive and maintenance therapies. Other therapies are for moderate-severe disease. *Vedolizumab can be used as inductive therapy, although onset of action can take weeks. 6-MP/AZA, 6-mercaptopurine and azathioprine.

TABLE 2	5-Aminosalicylates Therapies Available in the US for the Treatment of Inflammatory Bowel Disease.						
MEDICATION (BRAND NAME)	**MESALAMINE CONTROLLED-RELEASE (PENTASA)**	**MESALAMINE EXTENDED RELEASE (APRISO)**	**MESALAMINE DELAYED RELEASE (LIALDA)**	**MESALAMINE DELAYED RELEASE (ASACOL HD)**	**SULFASALAZINE (AZULFIDINE)**	**OLSALAZINE (DIPENTUM)**	**BALSALAZIDE (COLAZAL)**
Dosages	*Induction:* 1 g PO 4 times daily	*Maintenance:* 1.5 g PO daily	*Induction:* 4.8 g PO daily *Maintenance:* 2.4 g PO daily	*Induction:* 1.6 g PO 3 times daily	*Induction:* 1 g PO 4 times daily *Maintenance:* 1 g PO twice daily	*Induction*[1]: 1.5–3 g daily *Maintenance:* 500 mg PO twice daily	*Induction:* 2.25 g PO 3 times daily *Maintenance*[1]: 3–6 g PO daily
Location of release	Stomach, Jejunum, Ileum, Colon	Ileum, Colon	Ileum, Colon	Ileum, Colon	Colon	Colon	Colon
Delivery system	Controlled release gradually throughout the GI tract and not pH-dependent	Delayed release and pH-dependent	Delayed release and pH-dependent	Delayed release and pH-dependent	5-ASA linked to Sulfapyridine	Two 5-ASAs joined with one azo bond	One 5-ASA linked to an inert unabsorbed carrier molecule
Drug Monitoring	UA + renal function testing annually	UA + renal function testing annually	UA + renal function testing annually	UA + renal function testing annually	UA + renal function testing annually	UA + renal function testing annually	UA + renal function testing annually

[1]Not FDA approved for this indication.

5-ASAs, 5-Aminosalicylates; *GI,* gastrointestinal; *UA,* urinalysis.

Aminosalicylates

Aminosalicylates are compounds that contain 5-ASAs that exert a topical antiinflammatory effect on the intestinal lining. In UC, both oral and rectal formulations can be used for induction and maintenance of remission in mild-moderate disease. Their effect in CD as induction and maintenance therapy is debatable because they do not have an effect on transmural inflammation and they work mostly in the colon. See Table 2 for specific 5-ASA therapies and their location of action in the colon and/or small bowel. Patients should have yearly renal function and urine analysis testing given the rare but known side effect of acute interstitial nephritis associated with 5-ASA products.

Cytokine Inhibitors
TNF-α-antagonists (Anti-TNFs)

TNF-α-antagonists include infliximab (IFX [Remicade]), adalimumab (ADA [Humira]), certolizumab pegol (CZP [Cimzia]), and golimumab (GOL [Simponi]). They are indicated in moderately to severely active disease and most of them are effective in both UC and CD, although CZP and GOL have only demonstrated clinical efficacy in CD and UC, respectively. There is now evidence that earlier initiation of biologic therapy is more effective for induction of remission, prevention of disease complications, and reduction of steroid use. Early aggressive therapy is also associated with a higher likelihood of achieving mucosal healing, which is associated with the best clinical outcomes. Combination therapy with anti-TNF agents and immunomodulators was shown in the SONIC study to be more effective than monotherapy with anti-TNF or with immunomodulators alone in treatment-naïve patients. This finding we later learned is mainly due to the immunogenicity of anti-TNF agents, wherein introduction of immunomodulators as combination therapy reduces the frequency of antidrug antibody formation in the dual therapy group and promotes higher drug levels. Gastroenterologists starting anti-TNFs ultimately decide the need for dual therapy based on disease severity, but better algorithms for predicting who will do better on which regimen are needed.

TNF-blockers are contraindicated in patients with moderate-to-severe congestive heart failure (New York Heart Association functional class III/IV) and in patients with existing demyelinating diseases. Additionally, relative caution is advised for individuals with a prior lymphoma, known malignancies, a prior history of melanoma, and patients with a family history of demyelinating diseases. Patients should be cautioned about an increased risk of opportunistic infections, lymphoproliferative disorders, and melanoma development in patients who start anti-TNFs. However, mounting evidence suggests that the risk of lymphoproliferative disorders is actually mostly secondary to patients previously exposed to thiopurines. Recent studies show that the risk of non-Hodgkin lymphoma (NHL) is increased fourfold in IBD patients treated with thiopurines. Anti-TNF medications are also associated with an increased risk of NHL of about sixfold (6.1 per 10,000 patient-years); however, all these patients had been treated with immunomodulators previously. This is comparable to the expected rate of NHL in the general population of 1.9 per 10,000 patient-years.

Interleukin-12 and Interleukin-23 Inhibitors

Ustekinumab (Stelara) blocks both interleukin (IL)-12 and IL-23 by binding to the p40 subunit of IL-12 and IL-23, inhibiting their interaction with the IL-12 and IL-23 cell receptor binding complexes. Ustekinumab was found effective for induction of remission and as maintenance therapy for moderate to severe CD in the UNITI trials that incorporated close to 1300 CD patients. Ustekinumab is also now increasingly considered as a first-line therapy for moderate to severe CD due to its rapid onset of action, desirable safety profile, and improved efficacy when used as a first-line agent. Importantly, long-term tolerability and safety trials in both psoriasis and CD have so far reported a favorable safety profile for ustekinumab, including no serious opportunistic infections, injection-site reactions, anaphylaxis, serum sickness-like reaction, or increased rate of malignancies. On post hoc analysis of patients in the UNITI pivotal trials, there was a 1.5-fold increase in inducing fistula response in patients with perianal fistulizing CD. Lastly, the phase 3 UNIFI trial showed that a single IV dose of ustekinumab can induce clinical remission at week 8 in patients with moderate to severe UC who have previously failed conventional or biologic therapy.

Immunomodulators
Calcineurin Inhibitors

Cyclosporine (Neoral, Sandimmune) is effective as salvage therapy in patients with severe steroid-refractory UC and was as effective as IFX in preventing colectomy in this cohort of inpatients. Cyclosporine is not effective in CD. Unfortunately, its safety profile and adverse effects limit its use. These side effects include diarrhea, nausea, vomiting, headache, tremors, hypertension, hepatotoxicity, nephrotoxicity, and neurotoxicity. Cyclosporine can be used in severe or fulminant, steroid-refractory UC, although long-term remission is only improved with the addition of either thiopurines or IFX. It can also be used in severe, steroid-refractory UC patients who have previously failed IFX therapy or have a low albumin level (particularly because low albumin is associated with high clearance of IFX), or as an inpatient bridge to vedolizumab.

Thiopurines

Thiopurines are used in both CD and UC, as either monotherapy or as adjunctive therapy to TNF-blockers. Thiopurines include azathioprine (Imuran)[1], mercaptopurine (6-MP [Purinethol])[1], and thioguanine (6-TG [Tabloid])[1]. Azathioprine is a pro-drug that is metabolized to 6-MP. The metabolic pathway of thiopurines involves three enzymes that convert 6-MP to its two by-products, 6-methylmercaptopurine (6-MMP), 6-thiouric acid, or 6-thioguanine nucleotide (6-TGN). 6-TGN is the therapeutic, targeted pathway. Thiopurine methyltransferase (TPMT) enzyme activity is tested prior to initiation of therapy to determine whether patients can obtain the drug at all and to determine the dosage. Once the drug is initiated, metabolite levels of 6-TGN and of 6-MMP are checked to assess for appropriate treatment efficacy. 6-TGN levels greater than 235 are associated with therapeutic efficacy. In addition, one study showed that 6-TGN levels greater or equal to 125 were sufficient to incur a higher level of anti-TNF in combination therapy. 6-TGN at levels above 400 can lead to myelosuppression and 6-MMP levels above 5700 can lead to hepatotoxicity. For these reasons, patients on thiopurines require more frequent blood monitoring than patients on biologics. Patients should have a hepatic function panel and a CBC checked every 4 months once steady drug dosages and drug levels have been achieved.

Methotrexate

Methotrexate[1] is used in the treatment of CD. It is a folic acid analogue that inhibits dihydrofolate reductase and subsequent folate-dependent synthetic reactions, which suppress inflammation. In CD, intramuscular methotrexate (dose 15 to 25 mg/week) is effective in the maintenance of remission. Oral methotrexate (12.5 to 15 mg/week) is not superior to placebo for maintenance of remission. In addition, methotrexate can be used as adjunctive therapy with anti-TNFs to reduce anti-TNF immunogenicity. Methotrexate is not effective in the treatment of patients with UC. The adverse effects of methotrexate include myelosuppression, alopecia, nausea, vomiting, diarrhea, hepatotoxicity, nephropathy, and neuropathy. Patients should be counseled about alcohol abstinence and contraceptive use.

Agents Targeting Leukocyte Trafficking

Leukocyte trafficking agents are now available for the treatment of severely active UC and CD. Natalizumab (Tysabri), a nonselective anti-α4 integrin antibody, interferes with the systemic trafficking of leukocytes to both vascular cell adhesion molecule-1 and mucosal addressin cell adhesion molecule-1 (MAdCAM-1). It was first approved for use in CD in 2007 when it was shown to have efficacy for induction and maintenance of remission in active CD. However, the risk of progressive multifocal leukoencephalopathy (PML) caused by JC virus has greatly limited its use in practice. Vedolizumab (Entyvio), approved in 2014, is a selective α4β7 integrin inhibitor that binds specifically to peripheral blood lymphocytes and inhibits its adhesion to a gut specific receptor, MAdCAM-1. Therefore it is a gut-specific leukocyte trafficking agent with no cases of PML reported with its use and

with an overall very low systemic toxicity. Vedolizumab has a lower side effect profile, including a lower risk of systemic infections and no reported risk of lymphoproliferative disorders. It is a safer drug to use in conjunction with other immunosuppressants, for example, in patients with transplants who are already immunosuppressed. However, its slower onset of action limits its use in the acute, more urgent, setting.

Small Molecules

Agents Targeting Janus Kinase Family

Tofacitinib (Xeljanz) is the first small molecule approved for the induction and maintenance of remission of moderately to severely active UC. Tofacitinib is an oral, small molecule Janus kinase (JAK) inhibitor that preferentially inhibits *JAK3* and *JAK1*. JAK-STAT pathways regulate signaling of several immune-related mediators including type I interferon and interferon-δ. Inadvertent *JAK1* inhibition by tofacitinib results in higher rate of serious infections including herpes zoster. In addition, in psoriasis and rheumatoid arthritis patients, tofacitinib is associated with an increase in lipid levels, although the significance of this increase in causing cardiovascular events is not seen. Because of the high risk of shingles in patients taking tofacitinib, it is recommended that all patients starting tofacitinib receive the inactivated form of the herpes zoster vaccine, Shingrix, prior to starting therapy.

Pregnancy in Inflammatory Bowel Disease

Pregnancy is possible in patients with IBD. Women with IBD are more likely to have voluntary childlessness due to concerns with heritability of their IBD, risks of congenital abnormalities, and medication side effects and teratogenicity. It is important for patients and providers to know that there is no reduction in fecundity or fertility in women with IBD. This is true in most women with IBD, unless they have previously undergone pelvic surgery, such as in the setting of an ileoanal pouch anastomosis (IPAA) surgery. In this case, reduced rates of fecundity are possible but can be overcome by in vitro fertilization. Women with IBD should undergo disease activity evaluation prior to conception because active disease is the most important determining factor for a healthy, uneventful pregnancy. Patients with active disease during pregnancy are at risk for complications including premature births, low birth weight, babies born too small for gestational age, and of having cesarean deliveries.

In pregnant IBD patients, oral and rectal 5-ASAs, thiopurines, and most biologics should be continued throughout pregnancy to maintain long-term control of inflammation, which is the most influential determinant of a healthy pregnancy. However, medications such as methotrexate, cyclosporine, and allopurinol (Zyloprim)[1] are contraindicated during pregnancy and should be discontinued. Methotrexate should be discontinued in women and men planning to conceive, ideally 3 months prior to conception. Although mesalamines are considered one of the safest drugs during pregnancy, due to a few animal studies, women taking dibutyl phthalate (DBP)-containing 5-ASA (Asacol-HD) should switch to a non-DBP-containing formulation due to potential teratogenicity.

Anti-TNFs can be safely used during pregnancy. It is generally recommended to hold the last dose of an anti-TNF, due to increased placental transfer in the third trimester. That said, many GI providers may choose to continue the therapy based on presence of active inflammation and/or a historically difficult to control IBD. Certolizumab is the only anti-TNF with no placental transfer during pregnancy and can, therefore, be continued without reservations throughout the third trimester.

Several large registries have found that anti-TNFs and thiopurines have an adequate safety profile for the newborn. Studies looking at postnatal outcomes find that babies born of mothers on anti-TNF monotherapy have no increased infection risk during

---

[1] Not FDA approved for this indication

---

[1] Not FDA approved for this indication

the first year of life. However, a small increased risk of immediate postnatal infections was seen in babies born of mothers on dual therapy with anti-TNF and immunomodulators.

Other biologics, when used as monotherapy, show similar safety profiles. Recent trials show that there are no increased safety risks to babies born of mothers treated with vedolizumab during pregnancy. Similarly, data on ustekinumab during pregnancy, largely derived from the rheumatology literature, appear to demonstrate an adequate safety profile. However, the verdict is still out on tofacitinib. So far, observed outcomes of congenital malformations (seen in 1% of patients) and spontaneous abortions (seen in 10.8% of patients) reported in tofacitinib studies mirror the background risks seen in the general population. Nevertheless, due to limited data on tofacitinib during pregnancy, no definitive conclusions or recommendations can be made regarding its use in pregnancy.

Preventive Care in Inflammatory Bowel Disease

IBD is a chronic medical condition associated with an increased risk of complications from influenza, pneumococcal pneumonia, and an increased prevalence of several cancers, including skin cancer. Despite several studies demonstrating this, IBD patients receive less preventive healthcare than other patients with chronic medical conditions. In the following we highlight important health maintenance screening measures for an IBD population. Several checklist resources are available for easy implementation into clinical practice (Figure 5).

Vaccinations

Administration of live vaccines, when deemed appropriate, should be administered to IBD patients off immunosuppression or in patients on low dose immunosuppression. Ideally, these vaccines should be given 4 weeks or less prior to onset of immunosuppression and should be avoided within 2 weeks of initiation of immunosuppression, although vaccinations should never hold off need for urgent treatment of IBD. Low-level immunosuppression includes individuals who have received steroids at a low dose (≤ 20 mg/day) and for a short period of time (<2 weeks), or individuals taking the following medications at low doses: methotrexate ≤0.4 mg/kg/week, azathioprine ≤3.0 mg/kg/day or 6-mercaptopurine ≤1.5 mg/kg/day. Live vaccines such as the measles, mumps, and rubella vaccine (MMR), the yellow fever vaccine, and the live herpes zoster vaccine (Zostavax) are contraindicated in individuals already on immunosuppressive therapy. Fortunately, there is now an inactivated, recombinant herpes zoster vaccine (Shingrix) that is available to patients over the age of 50 and to those anticipating immunosuppression.

IBD patients should receive all age-appropriate vaccinations. Additionally, all IBD patients, irrespective of immunosuppressant medications, should receive the inactivated influenza vaccine annually and the pneumococcal vaccine (PCV13 and PPSV23). The human papilloma virus (HPV) vaccine can also be administered to patients on chronic immunosuppression from age 27 years to 45 years due to recent FDA approval extending the age group.

CCFA Health Maintenance Checklist for Adult IBD Patients

Vaccine-Preventable Illnesses	Which Patients	How Often
Influenza (inactive)	All	Annually
Pneumococcal PCV13	If on/planning immunosuppression	Once[1]
Pneumococcal PPSV23	If on/planning immunosuppression	At baseline, repeat in 5 years
Tdap	All	Every 10 years
HPV	All aged 18-26	Once (3 doses within 6 mos.)
Meningococcal meningitis	All adult patients at risk of meningitis	Once
Hepatitis A	If non-immune	Once (2 doses within 6 mos.)
Hepatitis B	If non-immune	Once (3 doses within 6 mos.)
MMR (live vaccine)	If non-immune[2]	Once (1-2 doses)
Varicella (live vaccine)	If non-immune[2]	Once (1-2 doses within 6 mos.)
Zoster (live vaccine)	All aged > 50 years[3]	Once

Cancer Prevention	Which Patients	How Often
Cervical PAP smear	All on systemic immunosuppression[4]	Annual
Skin screen	All on systemic immunosuppression[4]	Annual
Colonoscopy	All with extensive disease for >8 years	Every 1-3 years

Other Screenings	Which Patients	How Often
DEXA Scan	High risk; women with low BMI, post-menopausal, chronic steroid exposure	At least 2 years apart
PPD or IGRA	Prior to anti-TNF or anti-IL-12/23	Once
Smoking status	All	Annual
Depression check	All	Annual

1. Recommended timing of serial pneumococcal vaccination with both PPSV23 and PCV13 available in ACIP recommendation

2. Patients treated with systemic immunosuppressive therapy (steroids, thiopurines, anti-TNFs) should not receive live (attenuated) vaccines (e.g. measles, mumps, rubella, nasal influenza, varicella, and yellow fever)

3. Patients receiving anti-TNFs, anti-IL-12/23, or >20 mg prednisone should NOT be given the live zoster vaccine. Vaccine can be administered if on methotrexate < 0.4 mg/kg/week, 6-mercaptopurine < 1.5 mg/kg/day or azathioprine <3 mg/kg/day

4. "Systemic immunopsuppression" currently includes azathioprine, mercaptopurine, methotrexate, anti-TNFs, anti-IL-12/23

ADDITIONAL INFORMATION
- ACG
- ACIP
- ACOG
- AGA
- National Cancer Institute
- National Osteoporosis Foundation
- PHQ-9 Depression Survey
- US Preventive Services Task Force (USPSTF) Osteoporosis
- USPSTF Tobacco

The evidence base for this checklist varies from "insufficient to assess benefits" to "moderate net benefits."

Developed by the CCFA Professional Education Committee Sub-Group: Alan Moss MD, Francis Farraye MD, MSc, Glenn Gordon MD, Raluca Vrabie MD • Approved by Committee Chairs: Samir Shah MD, Millie Long MD • V2_January_2017

CROHN'S & COLITIS
FOUNDATION OF AMERICA

Figure 5 Health maintenance checklist. At the time of this print, the inactivated form of the shingles vaccine was not available. This guideline mentions the zoster vaccine, which has now fallen out of favor in our immunosuppressed population. Adapted from the Crohn's and Colitis Foundation (website: http://www.crohnscolitisfoundation.org/science-and-professionals/programs-materials/health-maintenance-checklist.pdf).

Cervical Cancer Screening

Women with IBD on immunosuppressive therapy are at an increased risk of cervical high-grade dysplasia and cancer. Therefore both the American College of Gastroenterology (ACG) and the European Crohn's and Colitis Organization recommend that women with IBD on immunosuppressive therapy should have annual cervical cancer screening.

Melanoma and Nonmelanoma Skin Cancer Screening

IBD increases the risk of melanoma independent of medications. Anti-TNF therapies have also been linked to an increased risk of melanoma. Nonmelanoma squamous cell skin cancer (NMSC) is associated with both current and past use of chronic immunosuppression, specifically thiopurines. In the CESAME study, the hazard ratios for NMSC in IBD who received thiopurines was 5.9 for ongoing treatment and 3.9 for past exposure. Taken altogether, it is, therefore, prudent that all IBD patients undergo evaluation by a dermatologist. Patients on anti-TNFs and on thiopurines should undergo yearly dermatologic examinations.

Depression and Anxiety Screening

IBD patients have an increased prevalence of depression and anxiety disorders, irrespective of their disease severity. In a recent systematic review, about 19% of patients with IBD developed anxiety and 21.2% developed depression. Therefore several recent guidelines now recommend screening patients with IBD for depression and anxiety. Depression and anxiety can be assessed by the Hospital Anxiety and Depression Scale, the Beck Depression inventory (BDI), the Spielberger Anxiety inventory, and the Perceived Stress Questionnaire.

Osteoporosis Screening

The pathogenesis of bone loss in IBD is multifactorial, due to steroid treatment, systemic effects of chronic inflammation, calcium and vitamin D deficiencies, and malnutrition. That said, not all IBD patients need to be screened for osteoporosis. IBD patients should be screened if they report a history of steroids for at least 3 months in a dose of greater than 7.5 mg/day or if they have any non-IBD established risk factors for osteoporosis, such as decreased body mass index, dietary deficiency of vitamin D and calcium, and previous fracture history.

Smoking Cessation Counseling in Inflammatory Bowel Disease Patients

Cigarette smoking is the strongest environmental factor impacting onset and disease course of CD. Cigarettes are associated with an increased need for steroids, development of postsurgical neo-TI strictures, and development of arthropathy. By corollary, smoking is also associated with an increased risk of colon cancer. In UC, cigarette smoking can ameliorate disease inflammation and smoking cessation can result in UC onset and/or flare-up. However, the global adverse effects of cigarette smoking are above any potential therapeutic benefit to smoking in UC.

Colon Cancer Screening and Surveillance

UC patients and CD patients with colitis are at an increased risk for colorectal cancer (CRC). The risk factors for developing CRC are similar in UC and CD and include duration, severity and extent of disease, PSC, and a family history of CRC. This risk is usually seen 8 to 10 years after the diagnosis of pancolitis. Patients with less involvement of the colon, specifically with less than a third of the colon involved, can start screening for colon cancer later, after 15 years of disease. Once screening starts, surveillance should take place every 1 to 2 years as recommended by several task force guidelines. Patients with PSC, however, need to undergo an annual surveillance colonoscopy, irrespective of duration of disease, due to their high risk of colon cancer.

Conclusion

IBD is a chronic, complex disease associated with high morbidity if untreated. In this chapter, we discuss new therapies available that can significantly alter the natural history of disease and improve quality of life. Primary care doctors, at the forefront of care, should be well acquainted with the diagnostic workup of IBD as well as with pertinent preventive health measures that are specific to an immunosuppressed population. We expect that future studies will deliver more patient-specific care models that improve delivery of healthcare, response to treatment, and ultimately IBD outcomes.

References

Beigel F, Steinborn A, Schnitzler F, et al: Risk of malignancies in patients with inflammatory bowel disease treated with thiopurines or anti-TNF alpha antibodies, *Pharmacoepidemiol Drug Saf* 23:735-744, 2014.

D'Haens G, Baert F, van Assche G, et al: Early combined immunosuppression or conventional management in patients with newly diagnosed Crohn's disease: an open randomised trial, *Lancet* 371:660–667, 2008.

Drugs for inflammatory bowel disease, *Med Lett Drugs Ther* 60:107-114, 2018.

Farraye FA, Melmed GY, Lichtenstein GR, et al: ACG clinical guideline: Preventive care in inflammatory bowel disease, *Am J Gastroenterol* 112:241–258, 2017.

Laine L, Kaltenbach T, Barkun A, et al: SCENIC international consensus statement on surveillance and management of dysplasia in inflammatory bowel disease, *Gastrointest Endosc* 81:489–501; e26, 2015.

Lichtenstein GR, Abreu MT, Cohen R, et al: American Gastroenterological Association Institute technical review on corticosteroids, immunomodulators, and infliximab in inflammatory bowel disease, *Gastroenterology* 130:940–987, 2006.

Lichtenstein GR, Loftus EV, Isaacs KL, et al: ACG clinical guideline: Management of Crohn's disease in adults, *Am J Gastroenterol* 113:481–517, 2018.

Luu M, Benzenine E, Doret M, et al: Continuous anti-TNF alpha use throughout pregnancy: possible complications for the mother but not for the fetus. A retrospective cohort on the French National Health Insurance Database (EVASION), *Am J Gastroenterol* 113:1669–1677, 2018.

Mahadevan U, Robinson C, Bernasko N, et al: Inflammatory bowel disease in pregnancy clinical care pathway: A report from the American Gastroenterological Association IBD Parenthood Project Working Group, *Gastroenterology*, 2019.

Rubin DT, Ananthakrishnan AN, Siegel CA, et al: ACG clinical guidelines: ulcerative colitis in adults, *Am J Gastroenterol* 114:384–413, 2019.

INTESTINAL PARASITES

Method of
Elizabeth Reddy, MD; and Tarvinder Gilotra, MD

 CURRENT DIAGNOSIS

Signs and Symptoms
- Watery diarrhea—Most protozoal infections: *Giardia, Blastocystis, Dientamoeba, Cryptosporidium, Cyclospora, Cystoisospora, Microsporidia*
- Dysentery—Most commonly *Entamoeba histolytica*; less commonly *Balantidium coli, Trichuris trichiura* (whipworm)
- Eosinophilia—Throughout chronic infection: *Strongyloides,* schistosomiasis, *Cystoisospora;* usually only in early infection: *Ascaris,* hookworm, whipworm
- Prolonged or severe diarrhea in HIV infection—Spore-forming protozoal infections: *Cryptosporidium, Cyclospora, Cystoisospora, Microsporidia*
- Visible worms passed in stool—*Ascaris,* Taeniasis, *Diphyllobothrium*

Diagnosis of Parasitic Infections
- Stool antigen or nucleic acid amplification assay—*E. histolytica, Giardia, Cryptosporidium*
- Serology*—*Strongyloides,* schistosomiasis
- Stool for ova and parasites—All intestinal parasites. Sensitivity increased with repeat examinations if necessary. Concentration, preservation, and staining improve diagnosis of certain pathogens.

Note: Key features of intestinal parasitic infection may overlap with other conditions, including nonparasitic infections, and extraintestinal parasites.

*Optimal method of diagnosis in returned travelers and immigrants from endemic to nonendemic areas. Does not distinguish between active and resolved infections.

Intestinal parasites are a diverse group of pathogens with local and global significance. Immigration, international adoption, travel, and the frequency of HIV/AIDS and other immune-compromising conditions (e.g., malignancy, organ transplantation) have all contributed to a need for ongoing and increased awareness of parasitic infections in the United States. Persons who reside in chronic care facilities, children in daycare, and persons whose sexual practices increase the likelihood of fecal-oral contact are also at risk for acquiring intestinal parasitic infection.

Globally, intestinal parasites are responsible for an enormous burden of disease. Although these pathogens are rarely fatal, ongoing exposure to intestinal parasites among persons in endemic areas exacerbates malnutrition, carries multiple morbidities, and causes stunting of growth and development in children, all of which have far-reaching consequences.

Patients who present with diarrheal illness (especially prolonged or travel-associated), unexplained eosinophilia, or expulsion of worms should be evaluated for intestinal parasites. In such cases, a careful history should focus on the patient's country of origin, detailed travel and recreational activities, dietary habits and new or unusual food exposures, occupation, sexual history, sick contacts, and risks for or known immunodeficiency. Some specialists advocate obtaining a complete blood count with differential to assess eosinophil count in all international adoptees and immigrants from areas where parasitic infections are common. If eosinophilia is present, antibody testing for schistosomiasis and strongyloidiasis—two chronic parasitic infections with potentially serious consequences—should be performed, and appropriate therapy should be administered if infection is discovered. For key features of common intestinal parasitic infections, see the Current Diagnosis box.

Diagnosis of intestinal parasites has improved recently with the advent of quick, simple, and accurate stool antigen tests for some major pathogens, such as *Entamoeba*, *Giardia* and *Cryptosporidium* species. In addition, multiplex nucleic acid amplification tests (NAATs) are frequently used to detect various bacterial, viral, and parasitic pathogens as a work-up for infectious diarrhea. However, the fecal examination for ova and parasites is still the mainstay of diagnosis in many cases. Whenever possible, stool specimens should be sent to a laboratory with clinical expertise in parasitology, where wet preparation, concentration, or staining can identify most pathogens. Evaluation of fresh specimens and repeated examinations improve diagnostic sensitivity. Key diagnostic points are summarized in the Current Diagnosis box.

This review focuses on basic understanding, recognition, diagnosis and treatment of common intestinal parasites in the United States and throughout the world. Within each section, parasites are listed in order of relative clinical significance.

Protozoa: Amoebae, Flagellates, Ciliates

Entamoeba histolytica

Entamoeba histolytica, the cause of amoebic dysentery and amebic liver abscess, is a worldwide pathogen of major clinical significance. Approximately 10% of the world's population and up to 60% of children in highly endemic areas show serologic evidence of infection, and *E. histolytica* is estimated to cause 100,000 deaths per year globally. In the United States, infection is almost exclusively found among returned travelers, immigrants from endemic areas (especially Mexico and Central and South America), men who have sex with men (MSM), and institutionalized persons. *Entamoeba dispar*, *Entamoeba bangladeshi*, and *Entamoeba moshkovskii* are morphologically indistinguishable from *E. histolytica*. Although these species are usually considered nonpathological species. there have been increasing reports of *E. moshkovskii* infections associated with gastrointestinal symptoms in humans in endemic areas. Other *Entamoeba*, including *Entamoeba hartmanni*, *Entamoeba coli*, *Entamoeba polecki*, and others, can be individually identified on microscopy. Again these organisms are

of uncertain pathogenicity and generally considered as commensal organisms, however, *E. polecki*, *Dientamoeba fragilis*, and *Iodaamopeba bütschlii* have occasionally been associated with diarrheal illness.

E. histolytica exists in two forms, the hardy cyst (infective form) characterized by four nuclei, and the trophozoite (responsible for invasive disease), which has a single nucleus and survives poorly outside the human body. *E. histolytica* infection is acquired by ingestion of cysts in contaminated water or food or by fecal-oral contact. Acquisition of the parasite can result in asymptomatic infection (most common), diarrheal illness, or extraintestinal infection, the latter most commonly manifest as amebic liver abscess. An appropriately robust layer of colonic mucin may be protective against symptomatic infection, whereas trophozoite attachment to the intestinal epithelium results in penetration of the organism into the submucosal layer, where extensive tissue destruction can take place in the form of apoptosis and lysis of cells, hence the name "histolytica."

Symptoms of classic amebic dysentery usually begin insidiously over 1 to 3 weeks after infection. Diarrhea is almost universal and typically consists of numerous small-volume stools that can contain mucus or frank blood, or both. Stools are almost always heme positive if not grossly bloody. Abdominal pain and tenesmus are common; fever is present in approximately 30% of cases. Some patients have a chronic course characterized by weight loss, intermittent loose stools, and abdominal pain. Rare presentations of amebic dysentery include amebomas, which can mimic malignancy, and perianal ulcerations or fistulae. Severe disease can occur in the form of fulminant colitis or toxic megacolon; the latter almost universally requires colectomy. Young age, pregnancy, corticosteroid use, malignancy, malnutrition, and alcoholism predispose to severe infection. Although persons with HIV infection or AIDS can develop invasive disease, *E. histolytica* does not appear to be a common opportunistic infection, and infection is curable in this population.

Amebic liver abscess is the most common extraintestinal complication of *E. histolytica* that traffics to the liver via the portal venous system. Cerebral and ocular amebiasis have also been reported. Amebic liver abscess affects children of both sexes equally, but it is up to 7 to 10 times more common in men, indicating that hormonal milieu likely plays a role. Amebic liver abscess almost always manifests within 3 to 5 months of initial infection, but it can surface years later. Illness is characterized by fever and right upper quadrant abdominal pain that worsens over the course of several days to weeks. Weight loss, jaundice, and cough from diaphragmatic irritation can also occur. Symptoms of dysentery usually are not present, and diarrhea is reported in less than one third of cases. Hepatomegaly and point tenderness over the liver is present in about 50% of cases. Rupture of the abscess can occur into the abdomen or pleuropulmonary space, manifesting as acute abdomen or empyema. Laboratory abnormalities include leukocytosis without eosinophilia, transaminitis, elevated alkaline phosphatase, and elevated sedimentation rate. Abscess is usually identified as a well-circumscribed hypoechoic mass on ultrasound, a low-density mass with enhancing borders on CT, and hypointense on T1 and hyperintense on T2-weighted MRI images. Chest radiograph often demonstrates elevation of the right hemidiaphragm, and pleural effusion may be present. Radionuclide uptake liver scans can help in distinguishing amebic abscesses as "cold" compared to pyogenic abscesses that are usually "hot."

Diagnosis of intestinal *E. histolytica* infection has classically relied on stool microscopy, which remains the only available method in most parts of the world. At least three stool specimens should be examined to improve sensitivity. Cysts visualized in stool cannot differentiate active disease from colonization and cannot distinguish pathogenic from non-pathogenic *Entamoeba*. Presence of trophozoites with ingested red blood cells (hematophagous trophozoites) on stool preparation and/or mobile amebae seen on fresh biopsy material stained with iron hematoxylin and/or Wheatley's trichrome are diagnostic of invasive intestinal amebic disease. Contrary to the common belief, presence of hematophagous trophozoites on stool microscopy is not pathognomonic of *E. histolytica*, as they can be seen with *E. dispar* infections as well.

Diagnosis of *E. histolytica* infection has improved greatly with the advent of antigen tests, now available as enzyme-linked immunosorbent assays (ELISAs), radioimmunoassay, and immunofluorescent probes. The Techlab ELISA antigen test is highly sensitive and specific if used on fresh stool specimens. It becomes positive with onset of symptomatic disease and resolves on treatment of infection. Parasite DNA/RNA polymerase chain reaction (PCR) fecal probes are highly sensitive and can differentiate Entamoeba species but are not yet commercially available.

Aspirate of liver abscess may be necessary to distinguish from pyogenic liver abscess or when empiric therapy fails. Aspirated specimens consist mainly of necrotic hepatocytes ("anchovy paste"), and trophozoites are only seen in less than 20% of cases. Nested multiplex PCR tests on hepatic aspirates might be useful, although sensitivities range from 75% to 100%. As simultaneous colitis and amebic liver abscess are rare, negative stool microscopy and PCR for *E. histolytica* does not preclude amebic liver abscess. In a patient at high risk for amebic liver abscess (e.g., young male immigrants), an adequate response to a trial of antimicrobial therapy can help confirm the diagnosis as well.

Serological testing with indirect hemagglutination assay is highly sensitive in excluding the pathogenic *E. histolytica* infection as antibodies can be detected within 5 to 7 days of infection. Positive serostatus however does not discriminate between acute and past infection. Also, serology can be negative for nonpathogenic strains such as *E. dispar*.

All patients who have confirmed *E. histolytica* infection and reside in nonendemic areas should be treated regardless of whether they are symptomatic, because invasive disease can develop in the future. Asymptomatic cyst passers may be treated with an intraluminal agent alone, such as paromomycin (Humatin) or iodoquinol (Yodoxin).[2] In the United States, the most readily available effective treatment for patients with amebic colitis or liver abscess is metronidazole (Flagyl). It can be given intravenously for patients who are unable to tolerate oral medications. Experts recommend that a course of therapy with an intraluminal agent be given following the completed course of the systemic agent for all cases of invasive *E. histolytica*. See Table 1 for medications and doses.

Giardiasis

Giardia duodenalis, previously known as Giardia lamblia or Giardia intestinalis, is the most commonly identified diarrheal parasitic infection in the United States, with an estimated 100,000 to 2.5 million cases per year. It is globally distributed and found in fresh water throughout mountainous regions of the United States and Canada. The organism is a flagellated aerotolerant anaerobe that exists in a cyst and trophozoite form. Cysts can survive for several weeks in cold water. Contaminated food and water are the most common sources of infection, but the organism can also be passed by person-to-person contact. In the United States, giardiasis is primarily diagnosed among international travelers, persons with recreational water exposure, institutionalized persons and children in daycare, and persons with anal-oral sexual practices.

Illness can result from ingestion of as few as 10 to 25 cysts, which transform into trophozoites in the small intestine and attach to and damage the small bowel wall. Symptomatic disease begins insidiously over approximately 2 weeks in 25% to 50% of persons who ingest *Giardia* cysts. Others become asymptomatic cyst passers (5% to 15%) or have no signs of infection (35% to 50%). Hallmarks of infection are watery diarrhea, bloating,

flatulence, abdominal pain, and weight loss; less commonly, patients have nausea, vomiting, or low-grade fever. Steatorrhea and malabsorption, particularly secondary to *Giardia*-induced lactase deficiency is frequently observed. Chronic *Giardia* infection should be considered in the differential diagnosis for a long-standing diarrheal illness, especially if there is history of exposure to possibly contaminated water. Patients with common variable immune deficiency, X-linked agammaglobulinemia, and IgA deficiency syndromes are at risk for fulminant and sometimes incurable disease, suggesting a significant role for humoral immunity in control of infection. Persons with HIV infection or AIDS usually have similar presentation as in non-HIV patients, can remain asymptomatic, and can be typically cured of infection with standard therapy. However, profound immunosuppression can be associated with more severe, atypical, disseminated and refractory disease requiring combination therapy with quinacrine and metronidazole.

Diagnosis of giardiasis is made by examination of fresh or preserved stool or by stool antigen assays. Stool microscopy can be specific; however, it has low sensitivity because of intermittent shedding of Giardia cysts. Trophozoites may be directly visualized in fresh liquid stool; semiformed and preserved stool are likely to contain only cysts and should be stained with polyvinyl alcohol and/or formalin preparation. Antigen detection assays including immunochromographic assays, direct immunofluorescencent assays, and ELISA assays have higher sensitivity with rapid turnaround time. Many assays are commercially available, including the ImmunoCard STAT! Cryptosporidium/Giardia Rapid Assay (Meridian Bioscience, Cincinnati, Ohio) that tests for both pathogens simultaneously, or multiplex NAAT. Although it is rarely necessary, the diagnosis can sometimes be made on duodenal biopsy.

For details of treatment options, see Table 1. Tinidazole (Tindamax) and Nitazoxanide (Alinia) are now the preferred agents for the initial treatment of giardiasis. Metronidazole (Flagyl)[1] is no longer the first line therapy because of its adverse effects, including metallic taste, nausea, gastrointestinal discomfort, and headache. Patients who fail first-line therapy might have a persistent source of infection (contaminated water source, close contact with an infected person), immune deficiency predisposing to difficult eradication, or persistence of cysts. Once possible sources of reinfection have been investigated and eliminated, relapsed infections should either be re-treated with a longer course of therapy (21 to 28 days) or treated with a different agent. Quinacrine (Atabrine)[2] is reserved for refractory cases but is contraindicated in pregnancy. Paromomycin (Humatin)[1] is an alternative in those with contraindications to other agents such as in pregnancy. Patients who fail more than one course of therapy should undergo immunologic work-up.

Prevention of *Giardia* infection, as with other parasitic infections, involves primarily close attention to personal hygiene, hand washing, and avoidance of ingestion of fresh unfiltered water. Boiling water or use of a 0.2- to 1-μm water filter offers optimal protection against *Giardia* and other parasitic pathogens, although such filters still might not protect against *Cryptosporidium*.

Blastocystis

Blastocystis, formerly considered a yeast, has now been related to *E. histolytica* and is thought to be an anerobic protozoan. The pleomorphic nature and karyotype diversity of this organism, its worldwide distribution, and varying diagnostic techniques have led to challenges in its identification and taxonomy. Although it has a worldwide distribution, its prevalence is higher in developing countries and is most commonly isolated in tropical regions. In temperate regions, *Blastocystis hominis* is detected at a high rate among MSM. It is a commensal of humans and several other animals. It appears to be transmitted via the fecal-oral route, possibly from waterborne sources. *Blastocystis* was long thought

---

[2]Not available in the United States

---

[1]Not FDA approved for this indication.
[2]Not available in the United States.

TABLE 1 Pharmacologic Treatment of Major Protozoan Infections

CLINICAL SITUATION	DRUG	ADULT DOSE	PEDIATRIC DOSE	COMMENTS
Amebiasis				
Entamoeba histolytica				
Asymptomatic	Recommended: Paromomycin* *or* Iodoquinol[†,2]	25–35 mg/kg/d in 3 doses × 7 days 650 mg tid × 20 days	25–35 mg/kg/d in 3 doses × 7 days 30–40 mg/kg/d (max 2 g) in 3 doses × 20 days	
	Alternative: Diloxanide furoate[‡,2]	500 mg tid × 10 days	20 mg/kg/d in 3 doses × 10 days	
Mild to moderate intestinal disease	Recommended: Metronidazole[§] *or* Tinidazole[¶,§]	500–750 mg tid × 7–10 days 2 g once daily × 3 days	35–50 mg/kg/d in 3 doses × 7–10 days ≥3 y: 50 mg/kg once daily (max 2 g) × 3 days	Treatment should be followed by a course of iodoquinol or paromomycin in the dosage used to treat asymptomatic amebiasis.
Severe intestinal or extraintestinal disease	Metronidazole *or* Tinidazole[§]	500–750 mg tid × 7–10 days 2 g once daily × 5 days	35–50 mg/kg/d in 3 doses × 7–10 days ≥3 years: 50 mg/kg once daily (max 2 g) × 5 days	Treatment should be followed by a course of iodoquinol or paromomycin in the dosage used to treat asymptomatic amebiasis.
Balantidiasis				
Balantidium coli				
Symptomatic and asymptomatic disease	Recommended: Tetracycline[¶,‖] Alternatives: Metronidazole[¶] *or* Iodoquinol[¶,†,2]	500 mg qid × 10 days 500–750 mg PO tid × 5 days 650 mg tid × 20 days	40 mg/kg/d (max 2 g) in 4 doses × 10 days 35–50 mg/kg/d in 3 doses × 5 days 30–40 mg/kg/d (max 2 g) in 3 doses × 20 days	
Blastocystis hominis				
Symptomatic disease only				Organism's pathogenicity is uncertain.[¶]
Cryptosporidiosis				
Cryptosporidium				
Immune competent	Nitazoxanide	500 mg bid × 3 days	1–3 y: 100 mg bid × 3 days 4–11 years: 200 mg bid × 3 days ≥12 years: adult dose	FDA approved as a pediatric oral suspension for treating *Cryptosporidium* in immunocompetent children <12 years and for *Giardia*. It might also be effective for mild to moderate amebiasis. Nitazoxanide is available in 500-mg tabs and an oral suspension; it should be taken with food.
HIV-infected	No optimal therapy available			All HIV-infected patients with cryptosporidiosis should receive HAART whenever possible. Nitazoxanide,[¶] paromomycin,[¶] or paromomycin + azithromycin[¶] may have a role in decreasing diarrhea in chronic cases of HIV-infected persons.
Cyclosporiasis				
Cyclospora cayetanensis	Recommended: TMP-SMX (Bactrim, Septra)[¶] Alternative: Ciprofloxacin[¶]	160 mg TMP, 800 mg SMX (1 DS tab) bid × 7–10 days 500 mg PO bid × 7 days	5 mg/kg TMP, 25 mg/kg SMX bid × 7–10 days (No recommended pediatric dose)[¶]	In immunocompetent patients, usually a self-limited illness. Immunosuppressed patients might need higher doses, longer duration (TMP-SMX qid × 10 days, followed by bid × 3 wk) and long-term maintenance.
Dientamoebiasis				
Dientamoeba fragilis Symptomatic disease only	Iodoquinol[¶,†,2] *or*	650 mg tid × 20 days	30–40 mg/kg/d (max 2 g) in 3 doses × 20 days	

Continued

TABLE 1 Pharmacologic Treatment of Major Protozoan Infections—cont'd

CLINICAL SITUATION	DRUG	ADULT DOSE	PEDIATRIC DOSE	COMMENTS
	Paromomycin[1],* or	25–35 mg/kg/d in 3 doses × 7 days	25–35 mg/kg/d in 3 doses × 7 days	
	Metronidazole[1]	500–750 mg tid × 10 days	35–50 mg/kg/d in 3 doses × 10 days	

Giardiasis

Giardia lamblia

CLINICAL SITUATION	DRUG	ADULT DOSE	PEDIATRIC DOSE	COMMENTS
All symptomatic disease and asymptomatic carriage in nonendemic areas	Recommended:			
	Metronidazole[1] or	250 mg tid × 5–7 days	15 mg/kg/d in 3 doses × 5 days	
	Nitazoxanide or	500 mg bid × 3 days	1–3 y: 100 mg bid × 3 days 4–11 years: 200 mg bid × 3 days	
	Tinidazole§	2 g once	50 mg/kg (max 2 g) once	Treatment should be followed by a course of iodoquinol[1,2] or paromomycin in the dosage used to treat asymptomatic amebiasis.
	Alternatives: Quinacrine[2]** or	100 mg tid × 5 days	6 mg/kg/d (max 300 mg/d) tid × 5 days	Albendazole[1], 400 mg daily × 5 days alone or in combination with metronidazole may also be effective. Combination treatment with standard doses of metronidazole and quinacrine × 3 wk is effective for a small number of refractory infections. In one study, nitazoxanide was used successfully in high doses to treat a case of *Giardia* resistant to metronidazole and albendazole.
	Furazolidone[2] or	100 mg qid × 7–10 days	6 mg/kg/d in 4 doses × 10 days	
	Paromomycin[1]	25–35 mg/kg/d in 3 doses × 7 days	25–35 mg/kg/d in 3 doses × 7 days	Nonabsorbed luminal agent; may be useful for treating giardiasis in pregnancy

Cystoisosporiasis

CLINICAL SITUATION	DRUG	ADULT DOSE	PEDIATRIC DOSE	COMMENTS
				In immunocompetent patients, usually a self-limited illness. Immunosuppressed patients might need higher doses, longer duration (TMP-SMX qid × 10 days, followed by bid × 3 wk)[1] and long-term maintenance. For isosporiasis in sulfonamide-sensitive patients, pyrimethamine[1] 50–75 mg qd in divided doses (*plus* leucovorin[1] 10–25 mg/d) is effective.
Cystoisospora belli	Recommended: TMP-SMX[1]	160 mg TMP, 800 mg SMX bid × 7–10 days	5 mg/kg TMP, 25 mg/kg SMX bid × 7–10 days	Ciprofloxacin[1] is an alternative but may not be as effective.

Microsporidiosis

Enterocytozoon bieneusi

CLINICAL SITUATION	DRUG	ADULT DOSE	PEDIATRIC DOSE	COMMENTS
Intestinal disease	Fumagillin+,[2]	60 mg/d PO × 14 days		Oral fumagillin (Sanofi Recherche, Gentilly, France) is effective in treating *E. bieneusi* but is associated with thrombocytopenia and neutropenia. HAART can lead to microbiological and clinical response in HIV-infected patients with microsporidial diarrhea. Octreotide (Sandostatin)[1] has provided symptomatic relief in some patients with large-volume diarrhea.
	Albendazole[1]	400 mg PO bid × 21 days	15 mg/kg/d in 2 doses (max 400 mg/dose)	

TABLE 1 Pharmacologic Treatment of Major Protozoan Infections—cont'd

CLINICAL SITUATION	DRUG	ADULT DOSE	PEDIATRIC DOSE	COMMENTS
Encephalitozoon intestinalis				
Diarrheal or disseminated disease	Albendazole[1]	400 mg bid × 21 days	15 mg/kg/d in 2 doses (max 400 mg/dose)	

[1]Not FDA approved for this indication
[2]Not available in the United States
*Should be taken with meals.
†Should be taken after meals.
‡The drug is not available commercially, but as a service it can be compounded by Panorama Compounding Pharmacy, 6744 Balboa Blvd., Van Nuys, CA 91406 (800-247-9767) or Medical Center Pharmacy, New Haven, CT (203-688-6816).
§A nitroimidazole similar to metronidazole, tinidazole is FDA approved and appears to be as effective and better tolerated than metronidazole. It should be taken with food to minimize GI adverse effects. For children and patients unable to take tablets, a pharmacist may crush the tablets and mix them with cherry syrup. The syrup suspension is good for 7 days at room temperature and must be shaken before use. Ornidazole, a similar drug, is also used outside the United States. Dosing recommendations are only available for children ≥3 years of age.
‖Contraindicated in pregnant and breastfeeding women and children <8 years.
¶Clinical significance of these organisms is controversial; metronidazole[1] 750 mg tid × 10 days, iodoquinol[2] 650 mg tid × 20 days, or TMP-SMX[1] 1 double-strength tab bid × 7 days are effective. Metronidazole resistance may be common. Nitazoxanide[1] is effective in children.
**Should be taken with liquids after a meal.
Adapted from World Health Organization. Drugs for parasitic infections. *Med Lett Drug Ther.* 2010;8(Suppl.).
DS, Double strength; *GI,* gastrointestinal; *HAART,* highly active antiretroviral therapy; *max,* maximum; *tab,* tablet; *TMP-SMX,* trimethoprim-sulfamethoxazole.

to cause only asymptomatic colonization, but there is some evidence to suggest a role in human disease, although this remains controversial. *Blastocystis* has marked morphological variability and has been known to exist in at least four forms: vacuolated, amoeba-like, granular, and cystic, the latter of which is likely to be the infectious form. Ongoing molecular analysis has identified at least 17 subtypes of *B. hominis* (hence now referred to as *Blastocystis* spp., formerly identified as *B. hominis*) with varying degrees of pathogenicity in humans.

As suggested previously, most infections appear to be entirely asymptomatic, and number of organisms does not appear to accurately predict severity of illness. Symptoms consist mainly of watery diarrhea, bloating, flatulence, abdominal cramps, urticaria, and fatigue. There are typically no pathologic findings on colonoscopy and there are no reports of invasive disease. Infection is diagnosed by stool microscopy with the use of a trichrome or hematoxylin-stained preserved specimen. Fecal leucocytes are generally not found. PCR techniques have also developed with excellent sensitivity and are available worldwide. The organism is susceptible in vitro to numerous antimicrobials. Asymptomatic detection does not need treatment. Metronidazole[1] and tinidazole[1] are the preferred agents for treating symptomatic disease. Trimethoprim/sulfamethoxazole (TMP-SMX, Bactrim)[1] and paromomycin[1] are alternative agents with good efficacy; details are listed in Table 1.

Dientamoeba fragilis

D. fragilis was originally classified as an amoeba, but it is more closely related to the flagellates such as *Trichomonas vaginalis*. It is distributed globally, including in the Western nations; however, it is generally more prevalent in the areas of the world with limited public sanitation. *D. fragilis* has only recently been recognized as a clinically significant pathogen, possibly because it is difficult to visualize without specific staining techniques. Illness has commonly been found in travelers and MSM, but it can affect anyone. Some studies suggested a coinfection of *D. fragilis* with *Enterobius vermicularis* as trophozoites were believed to survive in *E. vermicularis* eggs. However, this association has not been consistently demonstrated.

Similar to most other intestinal parasites, *D. fragilis* is now known to exist in both trophozoite and cystic forms, although for a long time, it was only known to have trophozoite phase. Despite its genetic relationship to the flagellates such as *Trichomonas*, *D. fragilis* does not have a flagellum and is immotile. Trophozoites

range in size from 7 to 20 μm and can be binucleate. Cysts and precystic forms have recently been identified from human fecal specimens, suggesting a fecal-oral mode of transmission.

Most patients are asymptomatic; however, numerous case reports and small series describe patients with no other organisms identified to cause their symptoms who improve significantly after treatment and documented clearance of *D. fragilis* from their stool. Illness is typically subacute to chronic, characterized by abdominal pain, watery diarrhea, anorexia, fatigue, and malaise. Unlike most other enteric parasites, *D. fragilis* is associated with marked peripheral eosinophilia and can masquerade as allergic colitis. Diagnosis can be challenging, because the trophozoites are fragile and usually missed on direct microscopy. If *D. fragilis* is suspected, stool should be preserved with polyvinyl alcohol and quickly stained with iron-hematoxylin and trichrome. PCR-based assays are very sensitive and are increasingly being used for diagnosis.

Metronidazole[1] remains the drug of choice and has been efficacious in the eradication of *D. fragilis* with a 10-day course. Other nitroimidazoles such as tinidazole[1] (better tolerated than metronidazole), secnidazole (Solosec)[1] and ornidazole[2] have been tested with good efficacy, but data is limited. Paromomycin[1] appears to be efficacious but is only backed up by limited data. Iodoquinol (Yodoxin)[2] has been successfully used very commonly in the past; however, its availability has now declined. For full treatment information, see Table 1.

Balantidium coli

Balantidium coli is the largest protozoan—and the only ciliate—that infects humans. Balantidiasis is a relatively rare cause of illness and is found primarily in rural agrarian communities in Southeast Asia, Central and South America, and Papua New Guinea. *B. coli* is highly associated with animal farming, in particular, pigs and primates; humans are incidental hosts. The parasite is transmitted by direct contact with animals or on ingestion of water or food contaminated by animal excrement. Persons with malnutrition or immune deficiency are particularly susceptible to infection.

B. coli invades the intestinal mucosa from the terminal ileum to the rectum. About one half of infections are asymptomatic; the other half result in a subacute or chronic diarrheal illness with abdominal cramping, nausea, vomiting, weight loss, and occasional low-grade fever. Fewer than 5% of patients present with

[1]Not FDA approved for this indication.

[1]Not FDA approved for this indication.
[2]Not available in the United States.

severe or even fulminant dysentery, and rare cases of colonic penetration with peritonitis, mesenteric lymphadenitis, or hepatic infection have been reported.

Diagnosis is made by visualization of trophozoites in fresh stool specimens or preserved and permanently stained samples. The trophozoite is relatively large (40 to 200 microns) and ciliated; cysts are difficult to distinguish. It displays a distinct spiraling motility that can be seen under low power. On stained sample, visualization of *B. coli*'s characteristic bean-shaped macronucleus and spiral micronucleus can help confirm the diagnosis. All patients should be treated regardless of symptoms. Tetracycline[1] (Sumycin and others) is the therapy of choice; alternative agents include metronidazole,[1] tinidazole[1] and paromomycin;[1] see Table 1 for dosing information.

Spore-Forming Protozoa and Microsporidia
Cryptosporidiosis
Cryptosporidium is an intracellular pathogen with worldwide distribution that has been increasingly reported in the United States and other countries, including Nordic countries, Denmark, England, and Scotland in the last decade. Humans are most commonly infected by the recently reclassified *Cryptosporidium hominis* (formerly *C. parvum* genotype 1), but *Cryptosporidium parvum* (previously *C. parvum* genotype 2), primarily a bovine pathogen, also causes human disease. *Cryptosporidium* is known to be one of the important parasitic causes of diarrhea globally; however, it is more frequently associated with overcrowded and poor sanitary environments. In Unites States and other developed countries, the incidence is higher in children than adults. *Cryptosporidium* infections have been reported as sporadic outbreaks, diarrhea and malnutrition syndrome in children from developing countries, and chronic and severe illness in immunocompromised hosts (especially with HIV infection). It is primarily a waterborne illness and has caused multiple outbreaks in the United States secondary to recreational water exposure (e.g., swimming pools, water parks). The best-known outbreak occurred from contamination of drinking water supply in Wisconsin in 1993 that was thought to be secondary to runoff from the cattle pastures versus contaminated water from melting ice entering water treatment plants through Lake Michigan. It resulted in 403,000 documented cases of cryptosporidiosis and contributed to the deaths of dozens of persons with advanced HIV infection or malignancy.

Cryptosporidium is a coccidian spore-forming protozoa obligate intracellular parasite with a complex life cycle that matures and reproduces both asexually and sexually entirely within human hosts, thereby enabling infection to occur both from environmental sources and by direct person-to-person contact. Its oocysts, the source of infection on ingestion, are markedly hardy; they can withstand heavy chlorination, survive for months in cold water, and are small enough to occasionally evade even the smallest available water filtration systems. As few as 100 oocysts can cause infection, which results when the parasite penetrates small bowel epithelium and replicates just beneath its surface. Villous flattening and small bowel wall edema are seen on pathologic examination from infected persons.

Cryptosporidium infection can be asymptomatic or manifest as mild diarrhea to severe enteritis with or without biliary involvement. Mild illness is usually is self-limited in 10 to 14 days without treatment in immunocompetent patients, although a substantial percentage of patients report a relapse of symptoms after initial improvement. It can have a protracted course with more severe symptoms in immunocompromised hosts. Fulminant and chronic infection has been frequently reported in those with HIV infection (especially those with CD4 <50), malignancy, and in malnourished children. The incubation period ranges from 3 to 28 days following the ingestion of oocysts and appears to be associated with the number of ingested oocysts. The hallmark of infection is explosive watery diarrhea, which can be so voluminous as to resemble cholera and can cause significant dehydration and electrolyte imbalance. Abdominal discomfort, nausea, vomiting, fever, malaise, and myalgia can also be present, and weight loss is common. Extraintestinal manifestations including biliary tract (cholecystitis, cholangitis, pancreatitis) and lung involvement have been reported, particularly in patients with HIV infection.

Diagnosis of *Cryptosporidium* has improved dramatically in recent years with the advent of antigen tests, which are highly sensitive and specific and can be used on a single sample of fresh stool. The ImmunoCard STAT! Cryptosporidium/Giardia Rapid Assay is useful because it can detect both pathogens. PCR is also available, has more sensitivity than direct microscopy and can differentiate between various genotypes. When such tests are not available, stools submitted for examination should be fixed in formalin and stained for trophozoites or cysts; availability of multiple stool specimens improves the diagnostic sensitivity. Luminal fluid or biopsy specimens obtained during endoscopy can also reveal the organism.

Infection with *Cryptosporidium* is typically a self-limited illness in otherwise healthy persons, but symptoms can be improved, and the course shortened with the antiparasitic nitazoxanide (Alinia). If nitazoxanide is not available or tolerated, paromomycin can be used, although it is not specifically indicated for this infection. *Cryptosporidium* remains an extremely challenging and potentially devastating infection in immunocompromised patients, especially those with HIV and a low CD4 count (counts <200 increase risk of severe illness, and counts <50 markedly increase risk). Although anticryptosporidial therapies in this population have shown very limited efficacy, restoration of immune function with HAART often effects cure. Limited data suggest a trial of nitazoxanide[1] may be reasonable in this circumstance as well. Appropriate supportive measures are also crucial in all patients with *Cryptosporidium*, including fluid and electrolyte replacement; avoiding lactose products is likely to be beneficial during the first 2 weeks after infection as the brush border regenerates. Appropriate treatment doses for nitazoxanide are listed in Table 1.

Prevention of *Cryptosporidium* infection requires a highly developed public water purification system including flocculation, sedimentation, and filtration. Use of 0.2- to 1-μm personal water filters for campers and hikers greatly reduces but does not eliminate risk of infection, whereas boiling water before drinking kills oocysts. Close attention to hygiene and avoidance of fecal–oral contact is the mainstay of prevention in the settings of institutional and community outbreaks. Patients should avoid swimming in public pools for 2 weeks after diarrhea resolution.

Cyclospora Species
Cyclospora cayetanensis is a coccidian with a structure similar to that of *Cryptosporidium*. *C. cayetanensis* is distributed worldwide, most commonly in the tropics and subtropics including Latin America (Guatemala, Peru, Mexico), the Indian subcontinent, and Southeast Asia. Outbreaks in the United States have been associated with the import of contaminated produce, such as raspberries and snow peas from Guatemala in 1996 and 2004, respectively. Similar outbreaks were attributed to contaminated lettuce and basil from Peru, and cilantro and prepackaged salad from Mexico. It has also become increasingly recognized as a cause of infectious diarrhea in returned travelers. Unlike *Cryptosporidium*, *C. cayetanensis* oocysts are shed in the stool as unsporulated oocysts (uninfected) and require few days of humid environment conditions to become sporulated infective oocysts. Hence, the possibility of close person-to-person contact as a means of acquiring the infection is unlikely.

All persons are susceptible to infection, but those with HIV are at risk for more severe and prolonged disease, as seen with cryptosporidiosis and isosporiasis. Symptomatic disease appears to be most common in adults who do not have previous exposure to *Cyclospora*, such as travelers or persons who have relocated to endemic areas. Illness begins about a week after ingestion

---

[1]Not FDA approved for this indication.

of sporulated oocysts and is characterized by watery diarrhea, abdominal cramping, bloating, anorexia, and weight loss. Low-grade fever can occur; marked fatigue is common and can last weeks or even months, and untreated infections can relapse after apparent resolution. Biliary involvement can occur in patients with HIV coinfection, as with cryptosporidiosis. Cyclosporiasis, similar to infection with other coccidians, causes damage to the small bowel epithelium, with resultant crypt flattening, edema, and inflammatory infiltrate. Lactose deficiency can remain for months after initial infection.

Diagnosis is made by stool examination. As with diagnosis of other parasitic infections, multiple stool specimens improve sensitivity. In the case of *Cyclospora*, concentration of the stool specimen also increases yield. If cyclosporiasis is suspected, specific testing should be requested, because the organism exhibits unique properties. Similar to *Cryptosporidium*, organisms can be stained and visualized with Kinyoun acid-fast stain, but they are about two times the size of *Cryptosporidium* (8 to 10 μm in diameter). The cell wall of their oocysts also maintains its autofluorescence under ultraviolet microscopy, which is not the case with *Cryptosporidium*. The commonly used BioFire Film Array multiplex antigen detection test includes *C. cayetanensis*. Various conventional and real-time PCR techniques have been developed with good sensitivity. No serological tests are available yet.

Cyclosporiasis is best treated with trimethoprim-sulfamethoxazole (Bactrim)[1]; nitazoxanide[1] and ciprofloxacin (Cipro)[1] may be effective for patients who have a sulfa allergy. Patients with HIV infection can require longer courses of treatment or chronic suppressive therapy; appropriate antiretroviral therapy is also important in the treatment of severe or relapsing infections. See Table 1 for details.

Cystoisospora Species

Cystoisospora belli, formerly *Isospora belli*, is a large coccidian distributed worldwide; however, infections are more frequent in tropical and subtropical areas. In United States, infections are largely identified in travelers from endemic areas and foreign-born patients with HIV. This is the most common parasitic cause of diarrhea in HIV-infected patients in India. Similar to *Cyclospora*, it requires a period of maturation (sporulation) outside the human body and therefore cannot be spread directly from person to person.

It appears to cause largely asymptomatic or mild infection in the tropical areas to which it is endemic; the exception is among patients coinfected with HIV and particularly those with AIDS, in which it is a very common cause of chronic diarrhea in the Caribbean and Central America. Currently, in wealthy countries, it is found primarily in travelers returning from endemic areas. Illness is typically mild and self-limited, consisting primarily of watery diarrhea. However, some immunocompetent persons can develop a chronic sprue-like syndrome with malabsorption, and those with HIV infection or AIDS often have severe and prolonged diarrhea. *Cystoisospora* can invade to the lamina propria and can cause eosinophilia, which is different from other protozoan infections.

Diagnosis is made by the observation of cysts in stool. As with *Cyclospora* and *Cryptosporidia*, they are usually not detected on routine stool ova and parasite examinations; hence, acid-fast staining or ultraviolet microscopy techniques should be requested for high suspicion. Stool may also contain Charcot–Leiden crystals. No antigen detection tests are yet available. PCR tests have been developed; however, they are not widely available.

Illness is usually self-limited in immunocompetent hosts; hence, antimicrobial therapy is only indicated when symptoms do not resolve spontaneously in 5 to 7 days. Patients with HIV and other immunocompromised patients who are symptomatic should always be treated. Trimethoprim-sulfamethoxazole (Bactrim)[1] is the treatment of choice. Ciprofloxacin (Cipro)[1] or pyrimethamine (Daraprim)[1] may be used in cases of sulfa allergy. Doses are listed in Table 1.

Microsporidiosis

Microsporidia are eukaryotic organisms that have been recently reclassified as fungi based on molecular genotyping. They are distributed globally, and more than 100 genera have been identified, seven of which contain species known to be pathogenic in humans: *Encephalitozoon*, *Enterocytozoon*, *Trachipleistophora*, *Pleistophora*, *Nosema*, *Vittaforma*, and *Microsporidium*. These pathogens cause a wide variety of systemic and focal illnesses throughout the world.

Many immunocompetent patients in wealthy nations exhibit positive serology for certain types of microsporidial infections without a history of disease or travel. Microsporidia are most commonly associated with systemic infection in immunosuppressed persons, particularly those with HIV and a CD4 count of less than 100 or patients with organ transplants. The mode of transmission is not entirely clear, but the pathogen is likely spread both from water sources and possibly from close household contact.

Encephalitozoon intestinalis and *Enterocytozoon bieneusi* are responsible for intestinal microsporidial infections. *E. bieneusi* has been associated with self-limited diarrheal illness; *E. intestinalis* is commonly found in stool specimens throughout the developing world, but its pathogenicity is often not certain. Symptomatic infections, most often in patients coinfected with HIV, typically include a gradual onset of watery diarrhea, which may be worse in the morning and after oral intake. Significant volume and electrolyte depletion can occur, as well as fatigue, anorexia, weight loss, and malabsorption. *E. intestinalis* can disseminate and cause acute abdomen with peritonitis, cholangitis, nephritis, and keratoconjunctivitis, and *E. bieneusi* infection can result in cholangitis and nephritis as well as rhinitis, bronchitis, and wheezing. Other microsporidia are implicated in disseminated disease with a wide variety of extraintestinal manifestations including ocular, pulmonary, cerebral, renal, and muscular both in previously healthy and immunosuppressed hosts.

Diagnosis of microsporidiosis is attained by visualization of spores in stool or in tissue specimens. As suggested by their name, microsporidial spores are much smaller than those produced by spore-forming protozoal infections; most are approximately 1 μm in length and can easily be confused with bacteria or debris on slides. Special staining techniques have been described, but electron microscopy is required for species identification. PCR assays have been increasingly used for highly sensitive identification and speciation indirect immunofluorescence assays (IFA) are also available for *Encephalitozoon spp.* and *E. bieneusi*. Albendazole (Albenza)[1] is the treatment of choice for *E. intestinalis*.

Treatment of *E. bieneusi* is more challenging. Although some response to albendazole has been reported, oral fumagillin[2] may have more efficacy. Unfortunately, it is not currently commercially available in the United States. Use of appropriate antiretroviral therapy is perhaps the most important treatment for patients with HIV infection or AIDS and chronic microsporidial infections. See Table 1 for details of treatment.

Helminths
Nematodes

Nematodes (roundworms) are cylindrical nonsegmented organisms that are found throughout the world both as free-living species and as human and animal pathogens. Nematodes are the most common type of human parasitic infestation, found in approximately one quarter of the world's population; often, susceptible hosts carry multiple different pathogenic nematodes. There are at least 60 species that have been shown to infect humans and 10 times that many that cause disease in other animals, but a few pathogens account for the bulk of human infections, in particular

---

[1]Not FDA approved for this indication.

[1]Not FDA approved for this indication.
[2]Not available in the United States.

Ascaris, hookworm, and whipworm. These three organisms all require a period of maturation outside the human body—typically in warm, moist soil—underscoring the fact that repeated contact with fecally contaminated soil or food and water is necessary to sustain the cycle of infestation. *Strongyloides* and *Enterobius* are unique in that they can both complete their life cycle on or within human hosts and can therefore cause chronic infection and be transmitted directly by close person-to-person contact where there is the possibility of fecal-oral contamination.

Ascaris

Ascaris lumbricoides, the most common human helminthic infection, is estimated to affect 20% to 25% of the world's population. Up to 80% of community members are infected in heavily endemic areas, namely in Africa, Asia, and Central and South America. Cases of *Ascaris* infestation are also seen in rural areas in the southeastern United States. *A. lumbricoides* are white to pinkish worms that range from 10 to 40 cm in length. Transmission in humans occurs most commonly by ingestion of infectious eggs from human or pigs' feces. These are white, oval-shaped bodies with an adherent mucopolysaccharide capsule that clings to multiple surfaces and aids in the transmissibility of the parasite. Eggs are also remarkably durable, capable of surviving up to 6 years in moist soil and are able to weather brief droughts and periods of freezing. Another means of transmission is by ingesting uncooked pig or chicken liver containing *A. suum* larvae.

Fecal contamination of water, food, and environmental surfaces such as doorknobs and countertops provide the means of transmission for *Ascaris*, and recurrent infection occurs as long as living conditions that predispose people to infection remain unchanged. Lack of adequate public sanitation, use of human feces as fertilizer (night soil), and frequent contact with soil or shared contaminated surfaces among close household members are risk factors for infection. Persons who move to environments with improved sanitation typically lose their infection within 2 years as all the adult worms die. Eggs excreted by an infected person must mature outside the human body for approximately 2 weeks. Upon ingestion by a susceptible host, mature eggs hatch in the small intestine and release larvae, which penetrate the intestinal wall and travel through the venous circulation to the lungs, where they are coughed up and swallowed. They then undergo maturation into adult worms in the intestine and produce eggs by 2 to 3 months after initial infection. The eggs are excreted in the feces and mature outside the body to continue the cycle.

Most persons with *Ascaris* infection are asymptomatic. Approximately 15% of infected people have morbidity, which is associated with young age, large burden of worms, coinfection with other intestinal parasites, and genetic predisposition. In children, infection contributes to the malabsorption of protein, fat, and vitamins A and C, and treatment of heavily infected children can improve their nutritional status. *Ascaris* infection can also cause intestinal, pancreatic, or biliary obstruction as a result of worm mass or worm migration. Despite the low incidence of obstructive complications per infected person, the *Ascaris*-related acute abdomen is a significant problem on a global level given the enormous number of people infected. Some patients with intestinal *Ascaris* infection report vague abdominal complaints, such as abdominal discomfort, nausea, vomiting or diarrhea, but these are relatively rare. Pulmonary migration of a large quantity of worms can produce Löeffler syndrome, or eosinophilic pneumonitis.

Diagnosis is easily attained with standard saline stool preparation, and large numbers of eggs are typically seen. Larvae or worms can also sometimes be seen in sputum or stool samples. In cases of intestinal obstruction, worms may be visualized on upper gastrointestinal series, computed tomography, and even ultrasound. Multiplex PCR assays are highly sensitive at identification and quantification but are currently not routinely used. Peripheral eosinophilia with *Ascaris* infection is found only during the larval migratory phase, but not at all times. Chronic eosinophilia in an

at-risk person suggests another parasitic infection, often *Strongyloides*. Sputum eosinophilia and Charcot-Leyden crystals can be seen, although this is common with many parasitic eosinophilic pulmonary infections.

All persons documented to carry *Ascaris* who have migrated to nonendemic areas should be treated to prevent complications in the future; in endemic areas, adults need only be treated if they are symptomatic. Children have been shown to benefit from intermittent anthelminthic therapy in heavily affected areas of the world. For patients with intestinal obstruction, bowel rest and intravenous hydration are usually sufficient to relieve the obstruction, at which time anthelminthic therapy can be administered. In such cases, gastroenterology consultation should be obtained. In rare cases, surgical intervention is required. Treatment of pulmonary infection is controversial; however, most experts recommend steroid therapy for severe infections followed 2 to 3 weeks later (at the time full-grown worms will have migrated to the intestine) by administration of anthelminthic therapy. Strongyloides infection should be ruled out prior to corticosteroid administration as the latter can induce Strongyloides hyperinfection syndrome. The benzimidazoles (mebendazole [Vermox], albendazole [Albenza],[1] and levamisole[2] exhibit excellent activity against *Ascaris*. Ivermectin (Stromectol)[1] and nitazoxanide[1] are suggested as reasonable alternatives. Doses and other options are listed in Table 2. Pregnant women should be treated with pyrantel pamoate (Pin X)[1] as albendazole and mebendazole carry a pregnancy class B label. Pyrantel pamoate is a depolarizing neuromuscular blocking agent that causes paralysis in helminths, preventing them from invading the intestinal wall and eventually resulting in their natural expulsion for the intestinal lumen. Because no consistent teratogenic effects have been demonstrated with albendazole use in late pregnancy, WHO has allowed the use of albendazole to treat mass infections in the second and third trimesters.

Sanitary conditions that allow for proper management of human feces are crucial in control and prevention of *Ascaris* infection; boiling water kills the eggs.

Whipworm (Trichurasis)

Trichuris trichiura has become recognized in recent years as a worldwide pathogen and is frequently found as a coinfection with *A. lumbricoides* as they share a similar scope and environment conditions. Almost 90% of individuals from endemic regions are infected. Sanitary conditions that predispose to ingestion of food and water contaminated with human feces place people at risk for infection.

The adult organism is a small worm about 4 cm in length with a unique whip-like structure that allows its thin tail to become embedded in colonic crypts. Infection is acquired by ingesting *Trichuris* eggs that have undergone embryonation in the soil for 2 to 4 weeks after excretion from a previous host. Larvae emerge from eggs in the intestine and migrate into crypts, where they begin to mature. Egg production begins approximately 3 months later.

Most persons with whipworm carry few worms (~20) and are asymptomatic. As with many other intestinal parasites, children are at greater risk for symptomatic infection, which can cause failure to thrive, anemia, clubbing, inflammatory colitis, and rectal prolapse. Adults with a high worm burden can also experience inflammatory colitis characterized by frequent—often bloody—diarrhea and tenesmus. Infection has been shown to result in the production of tumor necrosis factor (TNF)-α by lamina propria cells in the colon, which can contribute to poor appetite and wasting that can be seen with significant infection.

Diagnosis is made by standard stool microscopy without a need to concentrate stool, because large numbers of eggs are excreted. Whipworm eggs have a characteristic barrel shape with mucous (hyaline) plugs at either end. Worms can also be seen on colonoscopy, or they can be visualized grossly in cases of rectal prolapse. PCR tests are now available with improved but variable sensitivity for species identification. Peripheral eosinophilia may be seen.

---

[1]Not FDA approved for this indication.
[2]Not available in the United States.

CLINICAL SITUATION	DRUG	ADULT DOSE	PEDIATRIC DOSE	COMMENTS
Anisakiasis				
Anisaka spp. or Pseudoterranova decipiens	No recommended medical therapy Surgical or endoscopic removal of worm	—	—	Successful treatment of a patient with Anisakiasis with albendazole[1] has been reported.
Ascariasis				
Ascaris lumbricoides	Albendazole (Albenza)[1],* or Mebendazole[†] (Vermox) or Ivermectin[1],[†] (Stromectol)	400 mg once 100 mg bid × 3 days or 500 mg once 150–200 µg/kg once	400 mg PO once 100 mg bid × 3 days or 500 mg once 150–200 µg/kg once	In heavy infection, therapy may be given for 3 days.
Enterobiasis (Pinworm)				
Enterobius vermicularis	Mebendazole[†] or Albendazole[1],* or Pyrantel pamoate[‡]	100 mg once, repeat in 2 wk 400 mg once, repeat in 2 wk 11 mg/kg base (max 1 g) once; repeat in 2 wk	100 mg once, repeat in 2 wk 400 mg once, repeat in 2 wk 11 mg/kg base (max 1 g) once; repeat in 2 wk	Because all family members are usually infected, treatment of the entire household is recommended.
Hookworm				
Ancylostoma duodenale, Necator americanus	Albendazole[1],* or Mebendazole or Pyrantel pamoate[‡],[1]	400 mg once 100 mg bid × 3 days or 500 mg once 11 mg/kg (max 1 g) × 3 days	400 mg once 100 mg bid × 3 days or 500 mg once 11 mg/kg (max 1 g) × 3 days	
Schistosomiasis				
Schistosoma haematobium, Schistosoma mansoni	Praziquantel[§]	40 mg/kg/d in 2 doses × 1 day	40 mg/kg/d in 2 doses × 1 day	
S. mansoni only	Oxamniquine[‖]	15 mg/kg once	20 mg/kg/d in 2 doses × 1 day	Praziquantel is first line, but oxamniquine may be effective in some patients in whom praziquantel is less effective. Contraindicated in pregnancy
Schistosoma japonicum, Schistosoma mekongi	Praziquantel[§]	60 mg/kg/d in 2 or 3 doses × 1 day	60 mg/kg/d in 3 doses × 1 day	
Strongyloidiasis				
Strongyloides stercoralis	Recommended: Ivermectin[†] Alternative: Albendazole[1],*	200 µg/kg/d × 2 days 400 mg bid × 7 days	200 µg/kg/d × 2 days 400 mg bid × 7 days	In immunocompromised patients or in patients with disseminated disease, it may be necessary to prolong or repeat therapy or use other agents. Veterinary parenteral and enema formulations of ivermectin are used in severely ill patients unable to take oral medications.
Tapeworm				
Taenia solium (intestinal disease), Taenia saginata, Diphyllobothrium latum	Praziquantel[1] or Niclosamide[¶]	— 2 g once	— 50 mg/kg once	Available in the United States only from the manufacturer

Continued

CLINICAL SITUATION	DRUG	ADULT DOSE	PEDIATRIC DOSE	COMMENTS
Trichurasis (Whipworm)				
Trichuris trichiura	Recommended:	100 mg bid × 3 days or 500 mg once	100 mg bid × 3 days or 500 mg once	
	Mebendazole			
	Alternatives: Albendazole[1],* or	400 mg daily × 3 days	400 mg daily × 3 days	
	Ivermectin[†,1]	200 µg/kg daily × 3 days	200 µg/kg daily × 3 days	

[1]Not FDA approved for this indication
[†]Safety of Ivermectin in young children (<15 kg) and pregnant women not yet established. Ivermectin should be taken on an empty stomach with water.
*Should be taken with a fatty meal.
[‡]Limited availability; can be mixed with juice or water to improve palatability.
[§]Should be taken with liquids during a meal.
[||]Limited or no availability in the United States.
[¶]Available in the United States only from the manufacturer. Must be chewed or crushed thoroughly and swallowed with a small amount of water. Limited or no availability in the United States.
Adapted from World Health Organization. Drugs for parasitic infections. *Med Lett Drug Ther.* 2010;8(Suppl.).

Treatment of symptomatic infections can be accomplished with mebendazole (Vermox), albendazole (Albenza),[1] or ivermectin (Stromectal)[1]; see Table 2 for details.

Hookworm (Necator americanus and Ancylostoma duodenale)

Like other helminthic infections, hookworm affects a substantial portion of the world's population, particularly in rural subtropical and tropical communities where human feces is used as a component of fertilizer. Infection results primarily from parasite penetration into the skin; therefore, persons with an agrarian lifestyle and significant soil contact are at greatest risk.

Two species are responsible for the majority of human hookworm: *Necator americanus* and *Ancylostoma duodenale*. *Ancylostoma braziliense*, a canine intestinal pathogen, causes cutaneous larval migrans in humans because the pathogen cannot penetrate the human dermis. Of the two common forms of human hookworm, *N. americanus* is a smaller and less aggressive pathogen with a longer life span than *A. duodenale*. Both parasites are found in warm climates throughout the world; *A. duodenale* exists in smaller pockets in Mediterranean countries, Iran, India, Pakistan, and the Far East, whereas *N. americanus* is widely distributed throughout impoverished rural areas of the tropics in the Americas, Asia, and Africa.

Hookworms are small helminths, between 0.5 and 1 cm in length. Infection results from larval penetration of the skin on contact with contaminated soil. An intensely pruritic, erythematous, papulovesicular rash called *ground itch* can develop at the site of entry. Parasites then enter the venous or lymphatic circulation and travel to the lungs, at which point an urticarial rash with cough can develop. The larvae are swallowed and migrate to the small intestine, where they attach to the bowel wall with teeth or biting plates and take a continuous blood meal by sucking with strong esophageal muscles. As the larvae lodge in the small intestine, peripheral eosinophilia peaks and gastrointestinal discomfort with or without diarrhea can result. Large oral ingestion of *A. duodenale* can cause Wakana syndrome, characterized by cough, shortness of breath, nausea, vomiting, and eosinophilia. The most important clinical manifestation of hookworm infection is iron-deficiency anemia, which can be mild or severe and may be accompanied by the malabsorption of protein in hosts with a heavy burden of disease. Infants and pregnant women can become extremely ill or even die as a result of the anemia.

Hookworm may be difficult to diagnose because light infections often do not produce enough eggs to be readily seen on stool examination; stool should therefore be concentrated if infection is suspected. Eggs do not appear in stool until approximately 2 months after dermal penetration of *N. americanus* and up to 38 weeks from cutaneous entry of *A. duodenale*; hence, patients with pulmonary complaints will not yet have a positive stool examination. Multiplex PCR assays that detect *A. lumbricoides*, *T. trichiura*, and hookworm have a higher sensitivity than direct microscopy, however these are not as widely available yet.

Hookworm infection can be eradicated with benzimidazole antihelminthics; see Table 2 for details. Prevention of hookworm infection, as with other parasites, lies in improved sanitary conditions; wearing shoes is especially important because most infections are acquired through the skin. Mass anthelminthic treatment campaigns have shown some efficacy in reducing disease in children; however, reinfection and concern regarding the development of resistance continue to present significant challenges. Candidate vaccines are currently under investigation.

Strongyloides

Strongyloides stercoralis is a global pathogen that is estimated to affect as many as 100 million people, mostly in tropical regions of the world. In recent years, it has become more commonly recognized in the United States among immigrants as a cause of chronic eosinophilia, as well as symptomatic infection.

Strongyloides infection results when filariform larvae dwelling in fecally contaminated soil penetrate the skin or mucous membranes of a susceptible host. Larvae move to the lungs and subsequently to the trachea, where they are coughed up and swallowed. Females, about 2 cm in length, lodge in the lamina propria of the duodenum and proximal jejunum where they begin to oviposit. Rhabditiform larvae (noninfectious form) emerge from these eggs and either transform into infectious filariform larvae (infectious form) that can repenetrate the intestinal wall (autoinfection; unique to *S. stercolaris* amongst other helminths) or are passed into the feces, at which point they can begin a free-living cycle and reproduce sexually, or can molt directly into an infectious form ready to enter a subsequent susceptible host.

Persons infected with *Strongyloides* are typically asymptomatic. Those who have symptoms might report abdominal discomfort, diarrhea alternating with constipation, or, rarely, blood-tinged stool. Severe intestinal infections can occur and are manifest by chronic watery or mucousy diarrhea. In such cases, colonoscopy reveals excessive bowel wall thickening and copious secretions, or edema (catarrhal enteritis or edematous enteritis). Parasite migration through the dermis can manifest as pathognomonic serpiginous, erythematous, and pruritic patches along the buttocks, perineum, and thighs, known as *larvae currens ("running" larvae)*.

Strongyloides appear to attain a balanced state in their host, with similar numbers of adult worms throughout the many years of infection. During periods of host immunocompromise, in particular in patients taking corticosteroids, *Strongyloides* can enter into a state of rapid autoinfection and rampant reproduction called *hyperinfection syndrome*, which results in devastating

[1]Not FDA approved for this indication.

illness. Persons with HIV infection do not seem to be at particular risk for symptomatic disease or hyperinfection, but hyperinfection has been linked to HTLV-1 infection. *Strongyloides* has also caused hyperinfection in organ transplant patients whose donor had been infected asymptomatically with the parasite. Although it has long been thought that steroid-induced immune compromise was the major trigger for hyperinfection, growing evidence suggests that steroids themselves may be the culprit by directly inducing the accelerated life cycle in the parasite.

The hyperinfection syndrome is characterized by systemic illness with fever, cough, hypoxia, patchy or diffuse pulmonary infiltrates with alveolar microhemorrhages, and dermatitis; it can include myocarditis, hepatitis, splenic abscess, meningitis and cerebral abscess, and endocrine organ involvement. Larvae migrating out of the intestines can drag bacteria with them, resulting in gram-negative or polymicrobial sepsis. The prognosis of *Strongyloides* hyperinfection syndrome is grave, even with highly effective anthelminthic treatment, given the diffuse nature of this disease. However, earlier recognition and intensive supportive care result in cure.

Diagnosis of uncomplicated *Strongyloides* infection in endemic areas can be challenging because few larvae are passed in stool, and numerous examinations may be necessary to detect them. ELISA IgG serologies to filariform larvae are highly sensitive, but positive results cannot distinguish between active and past infections. Moreover, serologies can be falsely negative in immunocompromised hosts. It is, however, the test of choice for persons who have migrated to nonendemic areas, and all persons in this setting should be treated. Ivermectin is the treatment of choice; albendazole[1] has some activity again *S. stercoralis* and can be tried as an alternative; see Table 2 for dosing. During the first days of treatment, patients can experience intense dermal pruritis as parasites die. Eosinophilia and positive ELISA can persist for months, even after effective therapy.

Enterobius vermicularis

Human pinworm infection, caused by the thread-like nematode *E. vermicularis*, is found throughout the world and continues to be diagnosed commonly in the United States, especially in children aged 5 to 10 years. It is the most common helminthic infection in the United States and Europe. Its persistence is likely related to the fact that pinworm does not require a period of maturation outside the human body, and autoinfection or transmission by very close contact sustains the parasite within communities. *E. vermicularis* is at maximum 1 cm long with a tapered tail, and dwells in the cecum, appendix, and adjacent colon. At night, female worms travel to the anus and lay small (25 to 50 μm), double-walled oval eggs in the perianal skin. Within 6 hours, the eggs embryonate within their capsule and are infectious. In scratching the perianal area and subsequently bringing his or her hand to the mouth, the host ingests the embryos, which then hatch in the bowel about 2 months later and continue the cycle of infection. Embryonated eggs can also attach to bedclothes, thereby placing other household members with close contact at risk for infection. In family groups, infection is associated with close living quarters, poor hand washing, and infrequent washing of clothes and sheets. It can also be prevalent amongst institutionalized persons.

Infection is often asymptomatic, but it can cause perianal itching, which helps to facilitate persistent infection by encouraging frequent touching of the perianal area. Rarely, worms migrate into ectopic foci and produce painful genitourinary tract disease with granulomatous inflammation; pinworm infection rarely results in pain that mimics acute appendicitis.

Pinworm infestation is best diagnosed by the classic Scotch tape test, which involves placing and immediately removing a piece of sticky tape firmly across the perianal area early in the morning when the eggs have been deposited. The tape can then be brought into a physician's office or laboratory, where it is placed sticky side down for microscopic examination to detect the eggs. Sensitivity can be increased by examining at least three specimens. Eggs are small (25 × 50 μm) with a characteristic "bean-shaped" appearance. It is also sometimes possible to see the small white female worms directly on the perianal region, although they are so small (8 to 13 mm in length) that they may easily be mistaken for residual bits of toilet paper. Although *E. vermicularis* is susceptible to standard albendazole[1] or mebendazole (see Table 2), pyrantel pamoate is most frequently used in the United States as it is cheap and effective. All household contacts should be empirically treated with the same regimen to avoid reintroducing infection from family members who may be asymptomatically carrying the parasite. Careful laundering of all bedclothes is recommended as well.

Anisakiasis

Anisakiasis is a descriptive term for human infection with parasites of two distinct genera: *Anisakis* and *Pseudoterranova*. Humans are incidental hosts for these roundworms that inhabit multiple species of fish and other marine animals (tuna, mackerel, hake, cod, sardines, and cephalopods) as intermediate hosts, and marine mammals such as whales, seals, sea lions, and walruses as final hosts. Humans acquire the parasite in its larval stage by eating undercooked or raw fish (e.g., sushi, ceviche), and therefore, the condition predominates in cultures where uncooked fish is consumed. Cases are most commonly reported from Japan but are seen throughout the world in other coastal nations and among restaurateurs.

On consumption of fish with anisakid larvae embedded in its musculature, humans can experience immediate symptoms in the form of itching or burning in the throat, which can provoke coughing that expels the parasite. If the parasite is swallowed, the larva attempts to embed in the gastric musculature at the pylorus. This can produce acute, short-lived epigastric abdominal pain and possibly immediate vomiting, at which point the parasite might again be ejected. If the larva does manage to penetrate gastric tissue, it dies because it is incapable of further tissue invasion in humans. An intense inflammatory response to the dead pathogen can then result, with gastric pain, nausea, and occasionally diarrhea with blood or mucus if a gastric ulcerative lesion has resulted. Eosinophilic enterocolitis, ileitis, appendicitis, and focal peritonitis and abscess formation from penetration of larva into the peritoneum are also rarely reported. Bronchosconstriction, angioedema, and anaphylaxis have been described, mimicking seafood allergy. *Pseudoterranova* appears to cause milder symptoms and less tissue invasion, and the worm might simply be vomited several days after initial ingestion and presented to a physician, often by an alarmed patient. Because the vast majority of infections are caused by a single organism, vomiting of the parasite results in a definitive cure and patients can be reassured. Diagnosis in patients with ongoing symptoms related to an embedded parasite is ultimately endoscopic. Effective cure results on endoscopic or surgical removal of the worm. Albendazole[1] as an effective therapy is reported; however, data is limited.

Trematodes
Schistosomiasis

Schistosomes are freshwater pathogens with areas of endemicity in Africa, South America, Southeast Asia, and parts of the Middle East. These small trematodes cause varied, often chronic infections that can carry significant morbidity, although some species cannot invade beyond the dermis in humans and result strictly in cercarial dermatitis or swimmer's itch. There are five species of schistosomes known to cause disease in humans: *Schistosoma haematobium*, found through much of Africa and parts of the Middle East; *Schistosoma mansoni*, also native to Africa and the Middle East as well as Latin America; *Schistosoma japonicum*, present in China, Southeast Asia, and the Philippines;

Schistosoma mekongi, found only in the Mekong River basin in Laos and Cambodia; and *Schistosoma intercalatum*, endemic only in West Africa.

All persons who come in contact with schistosomes are at risk for infection, even with brief exposure to fecally contaminated freshwater in which the intermediate hosts of the pathogen (snails) reside. Frequency and degree of infection tend to be highest in children in endemic areas and then level off in the early teenage years, likely secondary to level of environmental exposure and possibly to host immunity. *S. haematobium* causes disease in the genitourinary system; the others cause intestinal, hepatic, and sometimes pulmonary diseases.

Infection is acquired rapidly on contact with freshwater (including brief swims or by repeated splashing, as can occur during river rafting), when free-living fork-tailed schistosomal larvae (cercariae) penetrate human skin and lose their tail. These schistosomulae can cause intense itching and a papulovesicular, pruritic rash at the site of penetration – swimmer's itch. Invasive schistosomulae then enter the venous bloodstream and reach the liver through portal venules, where they mature into adults. Adult worms then migrate against the portal venous flow to the mesenteric venules of the gut (*S. mansoni, S. japonicum, S. intercalatum, S. mekongi*) and vesical venous plexus (*S. hematobium*), where male and female forms mate for life. Females begin to oviposit, and the resultant inflammatory response to the eggs can cause either acute illness or chronic fibrosis and granulomatous inflammation of the tissues in which they reside.

Acute illness, called *Katayama fever*, is more common among hosts who have not been previously exposed to the organism and can be quite severe, even fatal. Katayama fever begins 3 to 8 weeks after infection, with acute onset of fever, chills, myalgias, cough, urticaria, angioedema, abdominal pain, hepatomegaly, and lymphadenopathy. Eggs might not yet be present in the stool at the time of diagnosis. Chronic schistosomiasis is a slowly progressive illness presenting chiefly with intermittent abdominal pain, diarrhea, and anorexia. Colonic ulceration with gastrointestinal bleeding and iron-deficiency anemia from huge parasitic burden has been described. Hepatosplenic schistosomiasis can be caused by granulomatous inflammation surrounding the eggs, eventually leading to periportal fibrosis (Symmers' pipestem fibrosis), portal hypertension and splenomegaly. Portal hypertension can then lead to portosystemic collateral vessel development, and deposition of eggs in the pulmonary vasculature. Granulomatous inflammation in the pulmonary tissues eventually causes endarteritis, fibrosis, pulmonary hypertension and cor pulmonale. *S. haematobium* infection can manifest as gross or microscopic hematuria, irritative urinary symptoms, and chronic bacterial urinary tract infections; ultimately, ureteral fibrosis, hydronephrosis, and granulomatous genital lesions also can ensue. Neuroschistosomiasis can cause both myelopathy and intracerebral lesions and can have varied presentation including seizures, focal deficits, encephalopathy, and rapidly progressive transverse myelitis.

Diagnosis of schistosomiasis is by observation of eggs in stool (intestinal disease), urine (urinary tract disease), or biopsy specimens, or by serum antibody testing. Concentration of stool may be necessary to detect the pathogen. The eggs of the three most common species of schistosomes can be readily identified microscopically: *S. haematobium* has an inferior spine, *S. mansoni* an inferolateral spine, and *S. japonicum* lacks a spine. Quantification of eggs is important as the parasite burden is proportional to the risk of complications and is usually reported as light (up to 100 eggs/g), moderate (100 to 400 eggs/g), and severe (>400 eggs/g) in stool specimens. Eosinophilia is a hallmark of chronic infection and is a common cause of asymptomatic eosinophilia among immigrants from endemic regions of the world. Serology is useful, particularly in returned travelers with low parasite burden; however, it can be negative in early infection as it takes 6 to 12 weeks after exposure to become positive. It is highly specific but cannot distinguish acute, chronic, or cleared infection. Antigen testing targeting specific schistosomal glycoproteins, circulating cathodic antigen (CCA, genus specific) and circulating anodic antigen (CAA, more specific to *S. mansoni*) is more sensitive than microscopy and can lead to rapid diagnosis, particularly in specimens with low parasite burden. Highly sensitive PCR assays have been developed to be used on blood, stool, and urine specimens. However, these are not as widely available. Histopathology is better than microscopy particularly in ectopic manifestations but is usually not required.

All patients with schistosomiasis should be treated, and those with chronic manifestations might experience significant regression of even late-stage organ-specific disease. Treatment of choice is praziquantel (Biltricide); see Table 2 for details.

Prevention of schistosomiasis involves improving access to treated water and exploration of avenues to eliminate the intermediate snail hosts. Host immunity does appear to occur, and efforts are underway to better understand and induce such immunity in the form of a vaccine.

Cestodes

Taeniasis

Human tapeworm infection has long been implicated in North American oral folklore as a cause of insatiable appetite and excessive weight loss. In reality, despite their impressive size of up to 12 meters, tapeworm infection tends to be minimally symptomatic.

Taenia solium, pork tapeworm, and *Taenia saginata*, beef tapeworm, are the two most common flatworm infections of humans (humans are the only definitive hosts) worldwide and occur in any setting in which raw or undercooked meat is served and where cattle and pigs have access to feed contaminated with human feces. *T. saginata* is still found in areas of North America and Europe, as well as in Central and South America and Africa; *T. solium* is common throughout Mexico, Central and South America, Africa, China, and the Indian subcontinent. Although humans are the definitive hosts for both parasites, *T. solium* is best known for its pathogenicity in the form of cysticercosis. Cysticercosis is not an intestinal parasitic infection.

Domesticated animals acquire infection on ingestion of eggs or gravid proglottids excreted by humans; the eggs mature in their musculature and develop a scolex. When humans consume infected meat, the scolex attaches in the small intestine, and the adult tapeworm develops over approximately 2 months. Adult tapeworms are made up of hundreds to thousands of gravid proglottids and can live for up to 25 years with intermittent shedding in the stool.

Symptoms tend to be mild or absent but can include nausea, abdominal pain, loose stools, anal pruritus, and occasionally weakness or increased appetite, especially in children. Serious illness rarely results when tapeworm proglottids become lodged in the appendix, biliary or pancreatic ducts, or are coughed up and aspirated. Some patients come to medical attention when the worm is noted emerging from the anus or upon extrusion of proglottids in the stool.

Diagnosis of taeniasis can be made upon visualizing the round eggs with hooks and double wall with characteristic striations. However, the species cannot be determined unless its proglottids are examined (*T. saginatum* has 12 or more uterine branches, whereas *T. solium* has < 10). Since the eggs and proglottids are shed intermittently, the sensitivity of microscopy is poor. Serum antibody and antigen tests, as well as stool PCR, have been developed for diagnosis but are not widely used in clinical practice. Eosinophilia and elevated IgE levels may be present. Single-dose praziquantel[1] (see Table 2) is curative in almost all cases, but infectious eggs can still be released in the feces for some time after worm eradication; ingestion of these could result in the subsequent development of cysticercosis, so patients should be counseled to avoid fecal-oral contact.

---

[1]Not FDA approved for this indication.

Proper cooking of meat is the mainstay of prevention; disposal of human waste away from animals would also be effective in interrupting the life cycle.

Diphyllobothriasis

Diphyllobothrium latum (fish tapeworm) is the longest parasite known to infect humans (10 to 12 m). It is found in freshwater lakes in areas of the Americas, Northern Europe, Africa, China, and Japan and has a complex life cycle involving two intermediate hosts: crustaceans and small fish. Humans and other fish-eating mammals are the definitive hosts and acquire the infection upon ingestion of raw fish or roe.

Eggs and proglottids are intermittently shed in human stool that embryonate in the water. Coracidiae hatch from the eggs and are ingested by small crustaceans (the first intermediate hosts). Coracidia mature into procercoid larvae in the crustaceans that are then ingested by the small freshwater fish (the second intermediate host). Procercoid larvae develop into plerocercoid larvae (sparganum) that are then passed onto the large predator fish (later intermediate host), which is then consumed by humans (definitive host). Sparganum develops into the adult worm inside the human intestine.

The mature adult tapeworm attaches within the small intestine, and hosts are usually asymptomatic. Infected persons might complain of increased appetite, nausea, or abdominal discomfort. Many patients present after the passage of portions of the tapeworm in stool, as with taeniasis. In others, diagnosis is incidental on the stool examination done for other purposes or during screening colonoscopy. As with other worms, the parasite occasionally migrates into biliary ducts or causes intestinal obstruction. Attachment of the parasite higher in the intestine competes with the host for vitamin B_{12} absorption and can result in vitamin B_{12} deficiency (pernicious anemia).

Diagnosis is made either by seeing eggs with an operculum (lid-like opening) in an unconcentrated stool or by encountering the adult worm. Proglottids can be differentiated from those in taeniasis by the presence of rosette-shaped uterus. Eosinophilia is present in a minority of cases. Treatment with praziquantel[1] is curative (see Table 2). Vitamin B_{12} supplementation is necessary in cases of severe or symptomatic deficiency, but it will not recur once the tapeworm is eliminated. Prevention involves not ingesting undercooked fish.

---

[1]Not FDA approved for this indication.

References

Abubakar I, Aliyu SH, Hunter PR, Usman NK: Prevention and treatment of cryptosporidiosis in immunocompromised patients, *Cochrane Database Syst Rev* (1), CD004932.

Bethony J, Brooker S, Albonico M, et al: Soil-transmitted helminth infections: Ascariasis, trichiurasis, and hookworm, *Lancet* 367(9521):1521–1532, 2006.

Boggild A, Yohanna S, Keystone J, Kain K: Prospective analysis of parasitic infections in Canadian travelers and immigrants, *J Travel Med* 13:138–144, 2006.

Boulware DR, Stauffer WM, Hendel-Paterson RR, et al: Maltreatment of strongyloides infection: Case series and worldwide physicians-in-training survey, *Am J Med* 120:545.e1–545.e8, 2007.

Concha R, Hartington Jr W, Rogers AI: Intestinal strongyloidiasis: Recognition, management, and determinants of outcome, *J Clin Gastroenterol* 39(3):203–211, 2005.

Drugs for Parasitic Infections: *Treatment Guidelines from the Medical Letter*, 2013, pp e1–e31, 11.

Goodgame RW: Understanding intestinal spore-forming protozoa: Cryptosporidia, microsporidia, isospora, and cyclospora, *Ann Intern Med* 124(4):429–441, 1996.

Guerrant R, Walker D, Weller P, editors: *Tropical Infectious Diseases: Principles, Pathogens, and Practice*, Philadelphia, 1999, Churchill Livingstone.

Huang DB, White AC: An updated review on Cryptosporidium and Giardia, *Gastroenterol Clin North Am* 35:291–314, 2006.

Mandell G, Bennett J, Dolin R, editors: *Mandell, Douglas and Bennett's Principles and Practice of Infectious Diseases*, 5th ed., Philadelphia, 2005, Churchill Livingstone.

Pardo J, Carranza C, Muro A, et al: Helminth-related eosinophilia in African immigrants, Gran Canaria, *Emerg Infect Dis* 12(10):1587–1589, 2006.

Stark D, Beebe N, Marriott D, et al: Dientamoebiasis: Clinical importance and recent advances, *Trends Parasitol* 22(2):92–96, 2006.

IRRITABLE BOWEL SYNDROME

Method of
Arnold Wald, MD

CURRENT DIAGNOSIS

- Fulfilling diagnostic criteria for irritable bowel syndrome (IBS) using Manning or Rome criteria is mandatory but not sufficient, as some organic diseases may also meet these criteria.
- Against the diagnosis of IBS is new onset in old age, a steady progressive course, frequent awakening by abdominal pain or urge to defecate, and weight loss not caused by depression.
- The diagnostic approach to patients with IBS symptoms with no "alarm signs" includes a complete blood count, stool testing for occult blood or calprotectin, C-reactive protein and colonoscopy if patient is age >50 years, has positive stool or blood test results as above, or if there is a poor response to treatment.
- After a diagnosis of IBS is established with confidence, repeated testing is counterproductive unless there is a distinct change in clinical symptoms or new alarm signs develop.

CURRENT THERAPY

- A robust patient–health care provider relationship is perhaps the most important determinant of outcome and reduced health care use in patients with IBS.
- There is significant support for the use of a low-FODMAP (fermentable oligo-, di-, and monosaccharides and polyols) diet in patients with IBS. Gluten restriction is part of this diet and will cover those patients who believe that they are gluten intolerant in the absence of celiac disease.
- Pharmacologic agents can be divided into those for IBS-C or IBS-D or in any patient with IBS to ameliorate abdominal pain. The evidence to support these agents varies in quality and strength, and none is effective in the majority of patients who have been tested.
- Cognitive behavioral therapy (CBT) can be very effective in IBS with unrelenting symptoms but may also be effective for any patient with IBS who exhibits poor stress management.

Introduction and Definitions

Irritable bowel syndrome (IBS) is a chronic functional disorder of the gastrointestinal tract characterized by chronic abdominal pain and altered bowel habits in the absence of an organic disease. In the absence of a biologic disease marker, the diagnosis has traditionally been based on a cluster of symptoms. The earliest was the so-called "Manning criteria," which was based on the presence of three or more characteristic symptoms (Table 1).

Subsequently, there have been various iterations of IBS criteria created by the Rome study groups, which are currently used for research purposes (see Table 1). When evaluating the relevant literature for IBS, it is important to note that various studies have used different criteria, which may result in variable data concerning prevalence and economic costs considerations.

From a clinical standpoint, subtypes of IBS have been defined as follows:
- **IBS with constipation (IBS-C):** Patient reports that abnormal bowel movements are usually constipation (types 1 and 2 in the Bristol Stool Form Scale; BSFS)
- **IBS with diarrhea (IBS-D):** Patient reports that abnormal bowel movements are usually diarrhea (types 6 and 7 in the BSFS)
- **Mixed IBS (IBS-M):** Patient reports that abnormal bowel movements are usually both constipation and diarrhea (more

TABLE 1	Criteria for IBS
Manning Criteria	**Rome III Criteria***
Looser stools with onset of pain	Recurrent abdominal pain or
More frequent bowel movements at onset of pain	discomfort at least 3 days per month in the last 3 months
Visible distension	associated with two or more
Feeling of distension	of the following:
Mucus per rectum	Improvement with defecation
Feeling of incomplete emptying (often)	Onset associated with change in stool frequency
Strict criteria > 3 of above	Onset associated with change in
Less strict criteria > 2 of above	form of Stool

*Criterion fulfilled for the last 3 months with onset of symptoms at least 6 months prior to diagnosis.

than one-fourth of all the abnormal bowel movements are constipation and more than one-fourth are diarrhea) over at least 3 months

- **Unclassified IBS (IBS-U):** Patients who meet diagnostic criteria for IBS but cannot be accurately categorized into one of the other three subtypes

Epidemiology of IBS

Prevalence

There have been numerous surveys concerning the prevalence of IBS in the community. Most of these studies have used accepted diagnostic criteria, and some have used more than one definition within the same population. In one meta-analysis, 23 studies used the Manning criteria, 24 used Rome I criteria, 36 used Rome II criteria, and 5 used Rome III criteria. The prevalence ranged from 5% to 10% (USA, China) to 15% to 20% (Canada, Brazil, Russia). There was little or no data from Africa, Central America, and large parts of South America.

Most studies did not report the predominant stool pattern in IBS. Of the nine that included IBS-U subtypes as well, there was an even distribution, ranging from 22% to 24% mean prevalence for each of the four subgroups. In general, the pooled prevalence was higher in women than in men (14%; range 11%–16% vs. 9%; range 7.3%–10.5%), with significant heterogeneity between studies. There appeared to be no relationship between socioeconomic status in the four studies that reported it and no strong influence of age as well.

It is important to note that the meta-analysis was restricted to studies based on the general population and excluded those based on convenience samples. This makes the data more generalizable to community individuals with IBS.

Causality—a biopsychsocial conceptual model for IBS

The ability to study causality in a disorder with no biologic disease markers is fraught with difficulties. This is certainly the case with IBS as a representative of functional gastrointestinal disorders. Many hypotheses have been advanced and found wanting. The current (and in my opinion most relevant) conceptual model is the biopsychosocial construct, as shown in Figure 1.

Impact on Population Health

Although there is no mortality associated with IBS, symptoms are long lasting, and there are no curative therapies available. As a chronic illness, the economic impact of this disorder is considerable.

In a 2015 survey conducted by the American Gastroenterological Association, IBS patients reported that their symptoms interfered with work productivity on an average of 9 days per month and missed work on average of 2 days per month. Indirect costs (i.e., loss of work and reduced productivity) have been estimated to be up to $20 billion annually in the United States, with an estimated annual cost per patient of $9933 (in 2012 US dollars)

In a study of indirect costs, impairment experienced at work (presenteeism) accounted for approximately 75% of the total

Biopsychosocial Conceptual Model

Figure 1 Predeterminants such as early life experiences, together with psychosocial factors, may interact with altered gut physiology via the brain-gut axis. This concept infers that these factors are bidirectional and mutually interactive and therefore influence both the clinical presentation of the disorder and the clinical outcomes. Among the physiological processes that may lead to GI symptoms are abnormal gut motility, visceral hypersensitivity, immune dysregulation, inflammation and barrier dysfunction, the intestinal microbiome, diet, and the brain-gut axis. No one factor alone accounts for the symptoms of IBS, and all must be considered in the management of affected patients. This becomes apparent when considering treatment approaches (Reprinted with permission from Drossman DA. Functional gastrointestinal disorders: History, pathophysiology, clinical features and Rome IV. *Gastroenterology* 2016; 150:1262-79.). FGID = functional gastrointestinal disorders.

annual indirect costs for respondents with IBS, far in excess of absenteeism from work. Compared with control subjects, IBS respondents missed significantly more work (5.1% vs. 2.9%), experienced higher levels of presenteeism (17.9% vs. 11.3%), and had greater overall work productivity loss (20.7% vs. 13.2%) and higher daily activity impairment.

Direct Health Care Costs

It has been estimated that up to 25% of all visits to gastroenterologists in the United States were for IBS with additional others for other functional GI disorders. This accounted for 3.5 million visits to health care practitioners in 1991 and undoubtedly is much higher today. IBS patients made twice as many health care visits per year as did age-matched control subjects, and 78% of the excess visits were for nongastrointestinal complaints. A subsequent analysis of this phenomenon suggests that comorbidity in IBS may be a consequence of the psychological trait for somatization, defined as the tendency to amplify the intensity and overinterpret the significance of any somatic sensation. This excess comorbidity is the primary determinant of excess health care costs associated with IBS, although it does not apply to all patients with IBS.

Recent attempts to identify factors of high users with IBS have been made, using a conceptual framework for accessing health care services, which holds that a decision to use health care is related to (1) predisposition to use services, (2) ability to use services, and (3) need for services. The important conclusion was that decisions to use health care are influenced not only by symptom-specific factors but by a variety of lifestyle and (most importantly) economic factors such as health insurance coverage.

Evaluation of Patients with Suspected IBS

The diagnosis of IBS should be made based on the clinical history, physical examination, minimal laboratory testing, and colonoscopy or other appropriate tests when clinically indicated. Fulfilling diagnostic criteria is, of course, mandatory but insufficient, because some organic diseases may also meet these criteria. The prevalence of organic disease is lowest in IBS-C and highest in IBS-D, followed by IBS-M; one of the most common considerations would be Crohn's disease. Against the diagnosis of IBS,

TABLE 2	Diagnostic Approach to Patient With IBS Symptoms (No "Alarm Signs")

Complete blood count
Stool for occult blood
Routine colon cancer screening at ages > 50 yrs.

C-Reactive protein (inflammatory marker)
Fecal calprotectin (indicator of inflammation)
Stool for C/S (if CRP/calprotectin positive)
Diagnostic colonoscopy (if poor response to Rx)

Rome IV (2016)

include the new onset in old age, a steady progressive course, frequent awakening by pain or need to defecate, and weight loss not attributed to depression. Additional features that would increase concern about organic disease would include a positive family history of colorectal cancer or inflammatory bowel disease, rectal bleeding, and anemia associated with iron or vitamin B_{12} deficiency.

In the absence of "alarm signs," a consensus diagnostic approach to patients with IBS symptoms is listed in Table 2. This may vary according to clinical circumstances.

Tests of Unproven Value

It is not uncommon to screen patients with IBS for celiac disease based on reports of non-US populations. However, a large US study found no increased prevalence of abnormal serum tests for celiac disease in patients with IBS (n = 492) versus healthy control subjects (n = 458).

A high prevalence of small intestinal bacterial overgrowth (SIBO) has been claimed by some centers leading to the frequent utilization of either lactulose or glucose breath tests. This hypothesis is based on poor methodology and erroneous conclusions. The original studies have not been reproduced by other centers using either similar or better techniques. This has led to the frequent use of expensive antibiotics, which can be effective in some patients with bloating and IBS but not because these patients have SIBO.

Lastly, after a diagnosis of IBS has been established with confidence, repeated testing is counterproductive unless there is a distinct change in clinical symptoms or new alarm signs develop. This is especially so if endoscopy procedures have already been performed.

Treatment of IBS

A validated standardized algorithm for the treatment of IBS does not exist. Treatment therefore depends on the type and severity of symptoms and the nature of associated psychosocial issues in an individual patient. A strong guiding principle is that a robust patient–health care provider relationship is an important determinant of outcome and reduction of health care use. Treatments may generally be divided into dietary and lifestyle modifications, pharmacologic agents, and behavioral therapies, all of which have been validated by randomized and controlled studies.

Dietary Modifications

Fiber supplements are widely recommended for IBS, but a meta-analysis of seven high-quality studies failed to find significant benefit, although some benefits might occur with soluble (psyllium) versus insoluble (bran) fiber in IBS-C. Unfortunately, fiber supplements may exacerbate symptoms such as abdominal bloating and discomfort.

Other dietary interventions such as gluten-free and low-FODMAP (fermentable oligo-, di-, and monosaccharides and polyols) diets have become increasingly popular. Several studies support the benefit of gluten-free diets in a subset of IBS patients in the absence of celiac disease. It remains uncertain whether the clinical benefits are a consequence of gluten withdrawal, elimination of other wheat proteins and highly fermentable short-chain fatty acids, or a placebo effect. Adding a gluten-free diet

to patients who are already on a low-FODMAP diet offers no additional benefits.

There is accumulating evidence from prospective controlled studies that dietary FODMAP restriction is associated with significant symptom improvement in many patients with IBS (Table 3). It appears that restriction of both fructose and fructans is most beneficial. Significant symptom improvement was noted in IBS patients compared to several standard diets in Australia and the United States.

Response to a low-FODMAP diet is usually assessed after about 2 weeks. Responders are then asked to engage in a structured reintroduction of restricted foods to allow the individual to tailor his or her diet. It is optimal to involve a properly trained dietician or nutritionist oversee the care of these patients.

Pharmacologic Agents for IBS

Pharmacologic approaches to IBS may be divided into medications for IBS-C, patients with IBS-D, and for any patient with IBS in order to ameliorate abdominal pain (Table 4).

Most drugs work through different pathophysiological mechanisms. For example, for patients with IBS-C, linaclotide (Linzess), plecanatide (Trulance), and lubiprostone (Amitiza) increase intestinal chloride and water secretion to combat constipation, whereas PEG (polyethylene glycol 3350, Miralax)[1] does so through a hyperosmolar effect. For IBS-D, rifaximin (Xifaxan) is an antibiotic, loperamide (Imodium)[1] is a μ-opioid agonist, alosetron (Lotronex) works through the serotonin 3 receptor, and eluxadoline (Viberzi) has effects on all 3 opioid receptors in the gut (mu, kappa, and delta). Tricyclic agents (TCAs) presumably work via central neurochemical changes, and antispasmodics (dicyclomine [Bentyl], encapsulated oil of peppermint[7]) work largely through peripheral anticholinergic pathways. The large and diverse number of drugs are indicative of the lack of fundamental understanding of IBS. Moreover, few drugs are effective in the majority of IBS patients, and there is no more than a 10% to 15% improvement over placebo in most published studies.

The AGA guidelines for use of pharmacologic agents in IBS incorporated the Grading of Recommendations Assessment, Development and Evaluation (GRADE) methodology and best practices as outlined by the Institute of Medicine. **Recommendations** are either strong or conditional (weak). The **evidence** that provides the basis for recommendation is rated high, moderate, or low quality. Because of the relatively recent release of plecanatide and eluxadoline, these drugs were not incorporated into present guidelines, although they have been approved for use in IBS by the Food and Drug Administration (FDA).

Of the pharmacologic agents for IBS-C, linaclotide received a strong recommendation with high-quality evidence, lubiprostone received a conditional recommendation on moderate-quality evidence, and PEG was given a conditional recommendation based on weak evidence. The first two agents showed modest benefit over placebo, whereas there are no data to support the use of PEG. For all three agents, adverse effects were relatively few, and diarrhea is perhaps the major side effect. Both linaclotide and lubiprostone are costly (as are eluxadoline and plecanatide) and may involve high out-of-pocket expenses for patients.

For IBS-D, both rifaximin and alosetron received conditional recommendations based on moderate quality evidence. The latter is approved by the FDA only for women in whom all other treatments have failed. There is a very small risk (approximately 1 case/1000 patient-years) for ischemic colitis with alosetron. Although loperamide has very low-quality evidence to support its use, it can be very effective if used in a proactive fashion.

The case for TCAs and antispasmodics is based on low-quality evidence, but both agents can be very effective for abdominal pain and, in the case of TCAs, for reducing diarrhea in IBS patients.

---

[1] Not FDA approved for this indication.
[7] Available as a dietary supplement.

TABLE 3	Low-FODMAP Diet		
AVOID OR REDUCE THESE FOODS			
FRUCTOSE	**LACTOSE**	**OLIGOS**	**POLYOLS**
Fruits: Apple, mango, pear, watermelon, juice, dried fruit	Milk: milk from cows/goats/sheep, custard, ice cream, yogurt, eggnog	Vegetables: Beets, broccoli, brussels sprouts, cabbage, fennel, garlic, onion, chicory root	Fruits: Apricot, avocado, blackberry, cherry, nectarine, peach, plum, prune, fig
Other: Asparagus, honey, high fructose corn syrup, molasses	Cheese: Soft, unripened cheese	Other: Barley, beans, chickpeas, couscous, inulin, lentils, pistachios, rye, soy milk, wheat (pasta, bread), veggie burgers	Vegetables: Cauliflower, corn, mushroom, sweet potato Sweeteners: Ending in "ol" (for example: xylitol, sorbitol), isomalt and sucralose (Splenda)

TABLE 4	Pharmacologic Agents for IBS	
INDICATION	**DRUG**	**DOSE**
IBS-C	Linaclotide (Linzess)	72-290 µg/d[3]
	Plecanatide (Trulance)	3 mg/d
	Lubiprostone (Amitiza)	8 µg bid[3]
	PEG-3350 (Miralax)[1]	8.5-17 g/d
IBS-D	Rifaximin (Xifaxan)	550 mg tid × 2 weeks
	Alosetron (Lotronex)[#]	1 mg qd- bid
	Eluxadoline (Viberzi)	75-100 mg bid
	Loperamide (Imodium)[1]	2-16 mg/d
IBS-All	Dicyclomine (Bentyl)	10-20 mg QID
	Desipramine (Norpramin)[1*]	10-100 mg/d

*Alternative TCAs: amitriptyline (Elavil)[1], imipramine (Tofranil)[1], nortriptyline (Pamelor)[1].
#Available only to physicians enrolled in the REMS Program for alosetron.
[1]Not FDA approved for this indication.
[3]Exceeds dosage recommended by the manufacturer.

Behavioral Therapy for IBS

For patients with unrelenting IBS symptoms, cognitive behavioral therapy (CBT) and gut-directed hypnosis have been found to be beneficial. Such therapies should be performed by experienced and well-trained behavioral specialists who are an integral part of the medical team that treats patients with functional GI disorders. The most robust data for efficacy is for CBT. One potential drawback is that these treatments are provider-intensive approaches, but recent studies suggest that CBT can be as effective when given in a shortened course as is the traditional method.

References

Buono JL, Carson RT, Flores NM: Health-related quality of life, work productivity, and indirect costs among patients with irritable bowel syndrome with diarrhea, *Health Qual Life Outcomes* 15:35, 2017.

Drossman DA: Functional gastrointestinal disorders: History, pathophysiology, clinical features and Rome IV, *Gastroenterology* 150:1262–1279, 2016.

Eswaran S, Farida JP, Green J, Miller JD, Chey WD: Nutrition in the management of gastrointestinal diseases and disorders: the evidence for the low FODMAP diet, *Curr Opin Pharmacol* 37:151–157, 2017.

Gudleski GD, Satchidanand N, Dunlap LJ, Tahiliani V, Li X, Keefer L, Lackner JM, IBSOS Outcome Study Research Group: Predictors of medical and mental health care use in patients with irritable bowel syndrome in the United States, *Behav Res Ther* 88:65–75, 2017.

Lovell RM, Ford AC: Global prevalence of and risk factors for irritable bowel syndrome: a meta-analysis, *Clin Gastroenterol Hepatol* 10:712–721, 2012. e4.

Nellesen D, Yee K, Chawla A, Lewis BE, Carson RT: A systematic review of the economic and humanistic burden of illness in irritable bowel syndrome and chronic constipation, *J Manag Care Pharm* 19:755–764, 2013.

Radziwon CD, Lackner JM: Cognitive behavioral therapy for IBS: how useful, how often, and how does it work? *Curr Gastroenterol Rep* 19(10):49, 2017.

Rao SS, Yu S, Fedewa A: Systematic review: dietary fiber and FODMAP restricted diet in the management of constipation and IBS, *Aliment Pharm Ther* 41:1256–1270, 2015.

Skodje GI, Sarna VK, Minelle IH, et al: Fructan, rather than gluten, induces symptoms in patients with self-reported non-celiac gluten sensitivity, *Gastroenterology* 154:529–539, 2018.

Weinberg DS, Smalley W, Heidelbaugh JJ, et al: American Gastroenterological Association Institute Guideline on the Pharmacological Management of Irritable Bowel Syndrome, *Gastroenterology* 147:1146–1148, 2014.

MALABSORPTION

Method of
Lawrence R. Schiller, MD

CURRENT DIAGNOSIS

- Recognize the presence of generalized malabsorption by the combination of typical symptoms: diarrhea, greasy stools, flatulence, weight loss, fatigue, edema.
- Recognize the presence of specific malabsorption by associated symptoms and those symptoms particular to deficiency states of the malabsorbed substance: flatus, diarrhea, anemia, dermatitis, glossitis, neuropathy, paresthesias, tetany, ecchymosis.
- Documentation of generalized malabsorption is best done by stool analysis demonstrating steatorrhea and acid stools (reflecting carbohydrate malabsorption). Diagnosis depends on visualization of the small bowel by endoscopy or radiography and small bowel biopsy. Additional tests may be needed.
- Documentation of specific malabsorption is best done by demonstrating low blood levels of the malabsorbed substance or by tests designed to measure absorption of that substance. Diagnosis depends on studies designed to identify the likely diagnosis for a given situation.

CURRENT THERAPY

- Once a diagnosis is reached, therapy can be directed toward that specific problem:
  - Gluten-free diet for celiac disease
  - Antibiotics for bacterial overgrowth
  - Lactose-free diet for lactase deficiency

Every day the average human being consumes 2000–3000 kcal of food, much of it in the form of polymers or other complex molecules that must be digested and absorbed by the gut. The processes of digestion and absorption are complex and are readily disturbed by pathologic processes. More than 200 conditions have been described that can adversely affect nutrient absorption.

Strictly speaking, *maldigestion* refers to impaired hydrolysis of nutrients, usually due to lack of luminal factors, such as bile acids and pancreatic enzymes, and *malabsorption* refers to impaired mucosal transport. For clinical purposes, "malabsorption" is used to describe both processes.

Malabsorption can be generalized (panmalabsorption) or limited to a specific category of nutrients. Generalized malabsorption is usually due to maldigestion or to extensive mucosal dysfunction. Specific malabsorption occurs when a single transporter is disabled.

The causes of malabsorption can be divided into three categories: impaired luminal hydrolysis, impaired mucosal function (mucosal hydrolysis, uptake, packaging, and excretion), and impaired removal of nutrients from the mucosa (Box 1).

Diagnosis

Symptoms and Signs

Most patients with panmalabsorption have changes in their stools (Box 2). Steatorrhea (excess fat in stools) is characterized by pale color, bulkiness, greasiness, and a tendency to float (probably because of incorporated gas). Occasionally patients with malabsorption present with watery stools due to the osmotic effects of unabsorbed carbohydrates and short-chain fatty acids.

Abdominal distention and excess flatus also commonly occur due to fermentation of unabsorbed carbohydrate by colonic bacteria. This can occur not only with panmalabsorption but also with specific malabsorption of carbohydrate (e.g., lactase deficiency).

Weight loss is typical with severe panmalabsorption, but it might not be very prominent with lesser degrees of malabsorption due to compensatory hyperphagia. Weight loss is most prominent early in the course of the illness, but body weight usually stabilizes as calorie absorption and body weight come into balance again. This is in contrast to illnesses like cancer or tuberculosis that produce continuing weight loss. If a patient with malabsorption has continuing weight loss, inflammatory bowel disease or lymphoma should be considered.

Abdominal pain is usually not present with malabsorption, although some cramping may be associated with diarrhea. Severe pain should bring chronic pancreatitis, Zollinger-Ellison syndrome, lymphoma, Crohn's disease, or mesenteric ischemia to mind.

Constitutional symptoms of fatigue and weakness commonly occur, even early in the course. In contrast, appetite is impaired only late in the course of most malabsorption states. Edema is uncommon until late in the course unless protein-losing enteropathy is present.

Vitamin and mineral deficiencies can lead to several symptoms or signs. Glossitis and cheilosis are common in patients with water-soluble vitamin deficiencies. Florid beriberi, pellagra, and scurvy are not commonly seen unless malabsorption has been particularly severe or long-lasting. Fat-soluble vitamin deficiencies also are unlikely to develop except when malabsorption has been long-standing because of substantial body stores.

Miscellaneous findings occasionally seen in patients with malabsorption can provide clues to the diagnosis. Aphthous ulcers in the mouth may be seen with celiac disease, Behçet's syndrome, or Crohn's disease. Hyperpigmentation is seen in Whipple's disease, and dermatitis herpetiformis (pruritic, blistering skin lesions) is seen in celiac disease. Scleroderma can manifest with tight skin, digital ulceration, nail changes, and Raynaud's phenomenon. Chronic sinusitis, bronchitis, and recurrent pneumonia suggest cystic fibrosis or IgA deficiency. Several systemic diseases can be associated with malabsorption syndrome (Box 3).

Tests

Routine Laboratory Tests

Routine laboratory tests (Box 4) commonly are abnormal in patients with established malabsorption syndrome. Anemia is common but not universal. Iron deficiency anemia may be the only finding in some patients with celiac disease. Microcytic anemia may be present in Whipple's disease (due to occult blood loss) and in lymphomas manifesting with malabsorption. Macrocytic anemia due to folate or vitamin B_{12} deficiency can occur in short bowel syndrome, small bowel bacterial overgrowth, or ileal disease. Lymphopenia may be present in patients with AIDS or lymphangiectasia.

Electrolyte abnormalities may be due to a combination of poor intake and excess loss in stool. Renal function usually is well maintained in malabsorption syndrome, but blood urea nitrogen

---

BOX 1 Causes of Malabsorption or Maldigestion

- Impaired luminal hydrolysis or solublization
  - Bile acid deficiency
  - Impaired mucosal hydrolysis, uptake, or packaging
  - Pancreatic exocrine insufficiency
  - Postgastrectomy syndrome
  - Rapid intestinal transit
  - Small bowel bacterial overgrowth
  - Zollinger-Ellison syndrome
- Brush border or metabolic disorders
  - Abetalipoproteinemia
  - Glucose-galactose malabsorption
  - Lactase deficiency
  - Sucrase-isomaltase deficiency
- Mucosal diseases
  - Amyloidosis
  - Crohn's disease
  - Celiac sprue
  - Collagenous sprue
  - Eosinophilic gastroenteritis
  - Immunoproliferative small intestinal disease (IPSID)
  - Lymphoma
  - Nongranulomatous ulcerative jejunoileitis
  - Olmesartan enteropathy
  - Radiation enteritis
  - Systemic mastocytosis
- Infectious diseases
  - AIDS enteropathy
  - *Mycobacterium avium-intracellulare*
  - Parasitic diseases
  - Small bowel bacterial overgrowth
  - Tropical sprue
  - Whipple's disease
- After intestinal resection
- Chronic mesenteric ischemia
- Impaired removal of nutrients
  - Lymphangiectasia

BOX 2 Symptoms and Signs of Malabsorption or Maldigestion

- Changes in stool characteristics
  - Floating stools
  - Pale, bulky, greasy stools
  - Watery diarrhea
- Increased colonic gas production
  - Abdominal distention
  - Borborygmi
- Vitamin and mineral deficiencies
  - Anemia
  - Cheilosis
  - Glossitis
  - Dermatitis
  - Neuropathy
  - Night blindness
  - Osteomalacia
  - Paresthesia
  - Tetany
- Ecchymosis
- Fatigue, weakness
- Edema
- Weight loss, muscle wasting

BOX 3 — Systemic Diseases Associated with Malabsorption or Maldigestion

Endocrine Diseases
- Addison's disease
- Diabetes mellitus
- Hypoparathyroidism
- Hyperthyroidism, hypothyroidism

Collagen-Vascular and Miscellaneous Diseases
- AIDS
- Amyloidosis
- Scleroderma
- Vasculitis (systemic lupus erythematosus, polyarteritis nodosa)

BOX 4 — Laboratory Tests for Evaluation of Malabsorption or Maldigestion

Complete Blood Count
- Hemoglobin/hematocrit
- Platelet count
- WBC differential count

Biochemistry Tests
- Blood urea nitrogen
- Potassium
- Prothrombin time
- Serum albumin
- Serum calcium
- Serum creatinine

Blood Levels of Potentially Malabsorbed Substances
- Serum iron, vitamin B_{12}, folate, 25-OH vitamin D, carotene

Fat absorption
- Qualitative fecal fat (Sudan stain)
- Quantitative fecal fat (Timed collection)

Protein Absorption and Protein-Losing Enteropathy
- α_1-Antitrypsin clearance
- Fecal nitrogen excretion

Carbohydrate Absorption
- Osmotic gap in stool water
- Quantitative excretion (anthrone)
- Stool pH <5.5
- Stool reducing substances
- D-Xylose absorption test
- Oral glucose, sucrose, and lactose tolerance tests
- Breath hydrogen tests

Vitamin B_{12} Absorption
- Serum B_{12} level

Bile Acid Malabsorption
- ^{14}C-glycocholic acid breath test
- Fecal bile acid excretion
- Serum 7α-hydroxy-4-cholesten-3-one (C4)
- ^{75}SeHCAT retention

Small Bowel Bacterial Overgrowth
- ^{14}C-glycocholic acid breath test
- ^{14}C-xylose breath test
- Glucose breath hydrogen test
- Quantitative culture of jejunal aspirate

Exocrine Pancreatic Insufficiency
- Secretin/CCK test
- Stool elastase or chymotrypsin concentration

Serologic Testing for Celiac Disease
- Anti-tissue transglutaminase antibody (IgA)
- Anti-endomysial antibody (IgA)

Abbreviations: CCK = cholecystokinin; SLE = systemic lupus erythematosus; ^{75}SeHCAT = selenium-75-labeled taurohomocholic acid; WBC = white blood cell.

---

may be low due to poor protein absorption, and serum creatinine concentration may be low due to depletion of muscle mass. Serum calcium levels may be low due to malabsorption, vitamin D deficiency, or intraluminal complexing of calcium by fatty acids. Hypomagnesemia can produce hypocalcemia or hypokalemia that is resistant to intravenous repletion. Serum phosphorus, cholesterol, and triglyceride levels may be reduced due to poor intake or malabsorption. Liver tests may be abnormal due to fatty liver. Serum protein and albumin levels are well preserved in patients with malabsorption unless protein-losing enteropathy or an acute illness is present.

Prothrombin time is normal unless vitamin K malabsorption (typically associated with steatorrhea), anticoagulant therapy, antibiotic therapy, or colectomy is present.

Assays are available for several potentially malabsorbed substances, including iron, vitamin B_{12}, folate, 25-hydroxyvitamin D, and β-carotene. Malabsorption tends to lower blood levels, but substantial body stores of many of these can mitigate the reduction in concentration that otherwise might occur. Thus, the sensitivity and specificity of these assays for malabsorption are poor.

Tests for Malabsorption

Fat Malabsorption. The simplest test for fat malabsorption is a qualitative microscopic examination of stool using a fat-soluble stain, such as Sudan III. The finding of more than five stained droplets per high-power field is abnormal and correlates well with quantitative measurement of fecal fat excretion. The test is subject to false-positive results with some drugs and food additives, such as mineral oil, orlistat, and olestra.

A more precise estimate of fat absorption is obtained by a quantitative analysis of a timed stool collection (48 or 72 hours). During the collection, a diary of dietary intake should be maintained so that fat excretion can be assessed as a percentage of intake. Normal fat excretion is <7% of intake when stool weight is normal, but it can be twice as high due to voluminous diarrhea without indicating defective mucosal transport of fat. Thus, fat excretion must be judged against stool weight. Stool fat concentration (grams of fat per 100 grams of stool) also is of value. Pancreatic exocrine insufficiency is associated with high fecal fat concentration (>10 g/100 g stool) because, unlike hydrolyzed fat, unhydrolyzed fat does not stimulate colonic water and electrolyte secretion that would dilute fecal fat concentration.

Protein Malabsorption. Fecal nitrogen excretion can be employed as a marker of protein malabsorption, but is not often used in clinical medicine because it adds little to the evaluation. If protein-losing enteropathy is suspected, an α_1-antitrypsin clearance study can be done. In this study, fecal excretion of α_1-antitrypsin, a serum protein that is relatively resistant to hydrolysis by luminal enzymes, is divided by serum concentration of α_1-antitrypsin, and the volume of serum leaked into the lumen can be calculated. Values of more than 180 mL/day are associated with hypoalbuminemia.

Carbohydrate Malabsorption. Carbohydrate malabsorption is difficult to measure directly because fermentation of malabsorbed carbohydrate by colonic bacteria reduces the amount of intact carbohydrate that can be recovered in stool. Indirect estimates of carbohydrate malabsorption can be made by examining fecal pH (<5.5 with carbohydrate malabsorption) or fecal osmotic gap (> 100 mOsm/kg with osmotic diarrhea) based on chemical analysis of stool water. Oral carbohydrate tolerance tests may be used to evaluate absorption of sugars, such as lactose or fructose. Following an oral load of a given sugar, blood glucose levels are monitored; failure of blood glucose to increase suggests malabsorption.

Another test for carbohydrate malabsorption is the D-xylose absorption test. In this test, a 25-gram dose of D-xylose is given orally; blood xylose levels are measured 1 and 3 hours later, and urinary excretion of xylose is measured for 5 hours. Failure of blood xylose to rise above 20 mg/dL at 1 hour or above 22.5 mg/dL at 3 hours or failure of urinary excretion to exceed 5 g in 5 hours suggests malabsorption. In addition, because xylose does not require pancreatic enzymes or bile acids for absorption, an abnormal D-xylose test suggests a mucosal problem as the cause for malabsorption. The results of this test can be misleading if the patient is dehydrated or has ascites, if renal function is compromised, or if bacterial overgrowth is present in the upper small bowel.

Breath hydrogen testing is another method to assess carbohydrate absorption. If substrates such as lactose or sucrose are not absorbed in the small intestine, they pass into the colon, where bacterial fermentation produces hydrogen gas. The hydrogen is absorbed into the bloodstream and then is exhaled. The concentration of hydrogen in exhaled breath can be measured easily; a rise of more than 10 to 20 ppm after ingestion of a specific substrate is consistent with malabsorption. False-positive results can be seen in patients with small bowel bacterial overgrowth, and false-negative results can be seen in patients who lack hydrogen-producing flora or who have been on antibiotics recently.

Vitamin B$_{12}$ Malabsorption. Although the Schilling test has been used to measure Vitamin B$_{12}$ absorption, commercial testing kits are no longer available in the United States. Instead, serum B$_{12}$ levels are measured: low levels are consistent with B$_{12}$ malabsorption, but normal levels do not exclude it because B$_{12}$ is stored in the liver and can maintain serum levels for several years.

Bile Acid Malabsorption. Tests for bile acid malabsorption are not widely available in the United States. Direct measurement of bile acid excretion has been used mainly in research studies. Retention of a radioactive taurocholic acid analogue (SeHCAT, selenium-75-labeled taurohomocholic acid) is used in Europe to assess bile acid malabsorption. A breath test using ^{14}C-glycocholic acid has been used for evaluating small bowel bacterial overgrowth, but it may have application for assessing bile acid malabsorption as well. Serum 7α-hydroxy-4-cholesten-3-one (C4) reflects bile acid synthesis; higher levels reflect increased synthesis in patients with bile acid malabsorption.

Small Bowel Bacterial Overgrowth. The gold standard method used to test for small bowel bacterial overgrowth in the upper intestine is quantitative culture of jejunal fluid. The sample can be obtained during endoscopy and sent to the laboratory with instructions to quantitate the aerobic and anaerobic flora. Finding more than 10^5 bacteria per mL confirms bacterial overgrowth. Breath tests using glucose, ^{14}C-xylose, and lactulose also have been described for this purpose.

Pancreatic Exocrine Insufficiency. Tests for pancreatic exocrine insufficiency are not commonly used. The gold standard test is a secretin test. This study requires duodenal intubation, injection of secretin, and measurement of bicarbonate output. Measurement of fecal chymotrypsin or elastase activity is only moderately useful in predicting the presence of exocrine pancreatic insufficiency. For most situations, a therapeutic trial using a high dose of pancreatic enzymes with monitoring of the effect on steatorrhea is the best that can be done.

Evaluation of Suspected Malabsorption

When malabsorption is suspected because of the history, physical findings, and setting, the physician must decide if the malabsorption involves a specific nutrient or represents a generalized process (Figure 1). If the malabsorption seems to be specific, a diet and symptom diary, breath tests using the presumptively malabsorbed substrate, and stool pH to identify acid stools seen with carbohydrate malabsorption are reasonable diagnostic maneuvers.

Suspected generalized malabsorption requires a more intense evaluation. Steatorrhea should be confirmed with either a qualitative fecal fat test (e.g., Sudan stain) or a quantitative stool collection for measurement of fat excretion. If steatorrhea is confirmed,

Figure 1 Flow chart for evaluation of malabsorption or maldigestion. *Abbreviations:* CT = computed tomography; R/O = rule out; SB = small bowel.

the small bowel should be visualized with either capsule endoscopy or radiography (small bowel follow-through examination or computed tomography) and biopsied from above by enteroscopy and from below by colonoscopy. During enteroscopy, an aspirate of small bowel contents can be obtained for quantitative culture to look for small bowel bacterial overgrowth. An alternative method to detect small bowel bacterial overgrowth is breath testing (see earlier). Stool samples also should be examined with microscopy or immunoassay for the presence of parasites that may be associated with malabsorption.

This sequence of evaluation often leads to a specific diagnosis. When it does not, empiric trials of high-dose pancreatic enzyme replacement or low-dose bile acid supplementation can lead to a presumptive diagnosis of pancreatic exocrine insufficiency or bile acid deficiency. Hard endpoints (e.g., quantitative fat excretion) should be used to assess the effectiveness of these empiric trials.

Specific Disorders Associated With Malabsorption
Malabsorption of Specific Nutrients
Disaccharidase Deficiency
Ingested disaccharides such as lactose and sucrose and starch-digestion products such as maltotriose and α-limit dextrins must be hydrolyzed by brush border enzymes into monosaccharides for abosorption by the mucosa. If these brush border enzymes are not active or if the brush border is damaged, malabsorption of the specific carbohydrate substrate results. This can result in gaseousness or osmotic diarrhea when those substrates are ingested. This rarely occurs on a congenital basis, but it commonly occurs as an acquired disorder.

Lactase deficiency is the most common acquired disaccharidase deficiency. Infant mammals all rely on lactose as the carbohydrate source in milk, but lactase activity is shut off after weaning in most species. Most human populations lose lactase activity during adolescence as a normal part of maturation. Members of the northern European gene pool might maintain lactase activity into adult life, but lactase activity declines gradually in many. At some point the amount of lactose ingested might exceed the ability of the remaining enzyme to hydrolyze it, resulting in lactose malabsorption and symptoms. This also can occur with acute conditions such as gastroenteritis that can disturb the mucosa and temporarily reduce lactase activity. Patients might not recognize lactose ingestion as a cause of their problem because they have not had difficulty tolerating lactose in the past. Restriction of lactose in the diet (or use of products that have predigested lactose) mitigates symptoms. Use of exogenous lactase as a tablet may only be partially effective because of incomplete hydrolysis of ingested lactose.

Transport Defects at the Brush Border

Glucose-galactose malabsorption is a rare congenital disorder resulting from an inactive hexose transporter in the brush border. Hydrolysis of lactose is intact, but transport across the apical membrane of the enterocyte fails to occur. Fructose absorption, which is mediated by a different carrier, is unaffected.

In all human beings, the ability to absorb fructose is limited by the availability of carriers in the brush border and may be overwhelmed when excess fructose is ingested. This can occur relatively easily nowadays, because high-fructose corn syrup is used frequently as a sweetener in commercial products such as soda pop. Limiting the amount of fructose ingested will reduce symptoms.

Abetalipoproteinemia is a rare condition that prevents absorption of long-chain fatty acids due to failure to form chylomicrons. Use of medium-chain triglycerides that do not require transport in chylomicrons can bypass this defect.

Pernicious anemia develops when failure to secrete intrinsic factor in the stomach prevents vitamin B_{12} absorption by the ileal mucosa. Parenteral replacement with cyanocobalamin by injection (Cyanoject) or nasal spray (Nascobal) is necessary.

Generalized Malabsorption
Celiac Disease

Celiac disease (also known as celiac sprue) is a disorder in which the mucosa of the small bowel is damaged due to activation of the mucosal immune system by ingestion of gluten, a protein component found in wheat, barley, and rye. People who have HLA-DQ2 or DQ8 are susceptible to this condition because these specific antigen-presenting proteins produce particularly strong reactions by interacting with a unique peptide digestion product of gluten. Tissue transglutaminase, an enzyme produced in the mucosa, is an important cofactor in pathogenesis by amplifying the immunogenicity of gluten peptide fragments and is the target of autoantibodies that are characteristic of this disease. The condition produces generalized malabsorption by destroying the villi of the small intestine, reducing the surface area available for absorption.

In addition to malabsorption syndrome with diarrhea and weight loss, celiac disease can produce a host of nonspecific symptoms, including abdominal pain, fatigue, muscle and joint pains, and headaches and seemingly unrelated problems such as iron deficiency anemia, abnormal liver tests, and osteoporosis. These protean manifestations mean that celiac disease must be considered in the differential diagnosis of many conditions. The clinical course is quite variable, with symptoms coming and going. Symptoms can develop during childhood and produce growth retardation or first become manifest in adulthood.

Testing for celiac disease has been simplified by the development of an assay for anti–tissue transglutaminase antibodies. This test largely supplants measurement of antigluten antibodies, although these remain of some use in evaluating adherence to a gluten-free diet. IgA antibodies are the most useful for diagnosis, but IgA deficiency is common enough that an IgA level should be measured concomitantly.

Although serologic tests have high sensitivity and specificity, the implications of adhering to a gluten-free diet are so extreme that the diagnosis of celiac disease should be confirmed whenever possible by small bowel mucosal biopsy, now obtained routinely by endoscopy. An empiric trial of a gluten-free diet may be difficult to interpret because many persons with gastrointestinal symptoms improve with dietary carbohydrate restriction. Wheat starch is particularly hard to digest; ordinarily 20% of wheat starch is not digested and absorbed by the small bowel, and enters the colon.

Treatment of celiac disease at present involves strict lifetime exclusion of gluten from the diet. This is a difficult regimen that excludes most processed foods. Assistance of a dietitian is most helpful. The prognosis with effective treatment is very good. Symptoms should respond to the diet within weeks; failure to do so should prompt an examination of compliance with the diet or reconsideration of the diagnosis. Failure to respond may be seen when lymphoma or adenocarcinoma complicate the course of celiac disease or in cases of "refractory sprue" or "collagenous sprue," which can have a different autoimmune basis from classic celiac disease and which might respond to immunosuppressive drugs such as corticosteroids or azathioprine (Imuran).[1] Persistent diarrhea may be observed in patients with celiac disease who have concomitant microscopic colitis, another condition that is linked to HLA-DQ2 and HLA-DQ8.

Olmesartan (Benicar) and perhaps other angiotensin II receptor blockers can produce enteropathies resembling celiac disease clinically, but which are not related to gluten ingestion. Diarrhea and malabsorption resolve with discontinuing the medication.

Inflammatory Diseases

Diseases that produce extensive mucosal damage by inflammation cause generalized malabsorption by reduction of mucosal surface area, by promotion of small bowel bacterial overgrowth, by ileal dysfunction, or by development of enteroenteral or enterocolic fistulas. Examples include jejunoileitis due to Crohn's disease, nongranulomatous ulcerative jejunoileitis, radiation enteritis, and chronic mesenteric ischemia. With Crohn's disease, previous resection can add to the problem (see later). Therapy aimed at the underlying process can improve absorption; in some cases (e.g., radiation enteritis), no effective therapy is available for the underlying problem, and symptomatic management is all that is possible. This includes use of antidiarrheal drugs to prolong contact time between luminal contents and the small bowel mucosa, ingestion of a reduced-fat diet to reduce steatorrhea, and use of vitamin and mineral supplements to prevent deficiency states.

Infiltrative Disorders

Several conditions involve infiltration of the intestinal mucosa with cells or extracellular matrix that impede absorption or modify mucosal function by secretion of cytokines and other regulatory substances. These include eosinophilic gastroenteritis, systemic mastocytosis, immunoproliferative small intestinal disease (IPSID), lymphoma, and amyloidosis. These conditions are diagnosed by mucosal biopsy, but special stains might have to be employed to identify the infiltrating cells or matrix accurately.

Treatment of the underlying processes can improve absorption, but it is not uniformly effective. For eosinophilic gastroenteritis, a hypoallergenic (elimination) diet and corticosteroids may be useful. Mild systemic mastocytosis is treated with the mast cell-stabilizer sodium chromoglycate, H_1- and H_2-receptor antagonists, and low-dose aspirin.[1] More advanced disease might respond to interferon or cytotoxic chemotherapy. IPSID initially is treated with antibiotics, because small bowel bacterial overgrowth may be a causative factor. Once malignant change has occurred, it is treated like lymphoma with cytotoxic chemotherapy. Amyloidosis affecting the gut is not amenable to therapy and is usually fatal.

Infectious Diseases

Small Bowel Bacterial Overgrowth. Small bowel overgrowth in the jejunum can produce generalized malabsorption. It can occur whenever the mechanisms that reduce overgrowth are compromised. These situations include achlorhydria or hypochlorhydria, motility disorders of the small intestine (e.g., diabetes mellitus or scleroderma), and anatomic alterations (e.g., diverticulosis, gastrocolic fistula, or blind loops postoperatively). Fat malabsorption is attributed to bacterial deconjugation of bile acid. Bacterial toxins or free fatty acids can produce patchy mucosal damage, leading to less efficient carbohydrate and

---

[1]Not FDA approved for this indication.

protein absorption. Bacteria also can compete with the mucosa for uptake of certain nutrients such as vitamin B_{12}.

Diagnosis of small bowel bacterial overgrowth can be difficult (see earlier). Treatment consists of antibiotic therapy unless a surgically correctable anatomic defect is discovered. Tetracycline is no longer uniformly effective; amoxicillin–clavulanic acid (Augmentin), cephalosporins, ciprofloxacin (Cipro), metronidazole (Flagyl), and rifaximin (Xifaxan)[1] may be employed. Therapy should be given for 1 to 2 weeks initially and then discontinued. It should be restarted when symptoms recur. If this occurs quickly, longer treatment periods should be considered. Continuous antibiotic therapy is needed rarely.

Tropical Sprue. Tropical sprue is a progressive, chronic malabsorptive condition occurring in both the indigenous population and in visitors residing in certain tropical countries for extended periods. The prevalence of tropical sprue seems to be decreasing for uncertain reasons. The disease starts as an acute diarrheal disease that becomes a persistent diarrhea associated with substantial weight loss and typically megaloblastic anemia. Villi become shortened and thickened (partial villous atrophy), but the flat mucosa of celiac disease is not usually present. Enterocytes have disrupted brush borders and can have megaloblastic changes; the submucosa has a chronic inflammatory infiltrate. Intestinal biopsy is required for diagnosis.

Currently, tropical sprue is believed to represent a form of bacterial overgrowth with organisms that secrete enterotoxins. Most patients have evidence of excessive gram-negative bacterial colonization of the jejunum. The declining prevalence of tropical sprue may be due to improved nutrition, better sanitation, or prompt treatment of acute diarrhea with antibiotics. Treatment consists of pharmacologic doses of folic acid (folate) (5 mg daily[3]), injection of cyanocobalamin (if deficient), and antibiotic therapy for 1 to 6 months. Tetracycline 250 mg four times a day or sulfonamide is the treatment of choice. Newer antibiotics have not been tested extensively in this condition. Improvement should be noted after a few weeks. The prognosis with treatment is excellent; without treatment, tropical sprue can be fatal. Recurrence can occur.

Whipple's Disease. Whipple's disease is a rare chronic bacterial infection with multisystem involvement. The small bowel typically is heavily infiltrated with foamy macrophages containing periodic acid–Schiff (PAS)-positive material, distorting the villi. Small bowel biopsy with special stains or electron microscopy or a specific polymerase chain reaction (PCR) is diagnostic. Foamy macrophages and bacteria can be found outside the intestine in lymph nodes, spleen, liver, central nervous system, heart, and synovium. Accordingly, symptoms are protean. The bacterium has been identified as *Tropheryma whippelii*, a relative of *Acinetobacter*. It does not appear to be very contagious, and no direct person-to-person transmission has been demonstrated. Presumably, differences in host resistance allow proliferation within macrophages without clearance of the bacteria.

Whipple's disease occurs mainly in older white men, but women and all ethnic groups are susceptible. Patients can present with malabsorption syndrome or with symptoms related to the extraintestinal disease (arthritis, fever, dementia, headache, or muscle weakness). Gross or occult gastrointestinal bleeding can occur. Protein-losing enteropathy may be present.

Treatment with any of several antibiotics (penicillin, erythromycin, ampicillin, tetracycline, chloramphenicol, or trimethoprim-sulfamethoxazole [TMP-SMX]) produces excellent symptomatic responses within days to weeks, but it should be continued for months to years. Even with protracted courses, relapses are common.

Other Infections. *Mycobacterium avium–intracellulare* is another chronic bacterial infection that can cause malabsorption, particularly in patients with AIDS. Mucosal biopsy with special stains to distinguish it from Whipple's disease is essential. Antibiotic therapy can reduce the intensity of infection; clearance depends on immunologic reconstitution with antiretroviral therapy. Clarithromycin (Biaxin) and ethambutol (Myambutol) are recommended as initial therapy.

Parasitic diseases can produce malabsorption by competing for nutrients and causing mechanical occlusion of the absorptive surface and epithelial damage. Protozoa that may be associated with malabsorption include *Giardia lamblia, Isospora belli, Cryptosporidium,* and *Enterocytozoon bieneusi*. Tapeworms associated with malabsorption include *Taenia saginata* (beef tapeworm), *Hymenolepis nana* (dwarf tapeworm), and *Diphyllobothrium latum* (fish tapeworm).

Giardia lamblia is a cosmopolitan parasite acquired from contaminated water or from another person by fecal-oral transmission. Cysts are relatively hardy, and ingestion of as few as 10 cysts is sufficient to establish infection. Patients with dysgammaglobulinemia (especially IgA deficiency) are likely to become infected. Diagnosis depends on finding the organism (cysts or trophozoites) in stool by microscopy (sensitivity ~50% for a single specimen), or detection of giardia antigens by immunologic testing of stool (sensitivity >90%), multiplex PCR testing (sensitivity >95%), or discovery of the organism on small bowel biopsy.

Therapy consists of a single dose of tinidazole (Tindamax) (2 g), metronidazole (Flagyl)[1] (250 mg three times a day for a week), nitazoxanide (Alinia) (500 mg twice a day for three days), or quinacrine[2] (100 mg three times a day for a week).

Isospora belli and *Cryptosporidium* spp. are coccidia, protozoa that disrupt the epithelium by intracellular invasion *(Isospora)* or by attaching to the brush border, destroying microvilli *(Cryptosporidium)*. Stool examination or small bowel biopsy can identify the organism. *Cryptosporidium* can be discovered by antigen immunoassay or multiplex PCR testing on stool with excellent sensitivity. *Isospora* can be treated with trimethoprim/sulfamethoxazole (TMP-SMX)[1] or furazolidone.[2] *Cryptosporidium* can be treated by nitazoxanide.

Microsporidia are intracellular organisms now believed to be most closely related to fungi and are implicated in diarrhea and malabsorption in patients with AIDS and other immunodeficiency states. Small bowel biopsy can show partial villous atrophy, and electron microscopy displays characteristic changes. Stool examination occasionally is helpful. No treatment is of proven value.

Tapeworms compete with their hosts for nutrients in the lumen. *Diphyllobothrium latum* can produce vitamin B_{12} deficiency. The others can result in more extensive nutritional deficiencies. Diagnosis is based on stool examination, and treatment depends on the particular organism identified.

Luminal Problems Causing Malabsorption

Pancreatic Exocrine Insufficiency. Pancreatic exocrine insufficiency is the most common luminal problem that results in maldigestion. Patients develop symptoms of malabsorption when pancreatic enzyme secretion is reduced by >90%. There are several clinical features that distinguish pancreatic exocrine insufficiency from mucosal disorders, such as celiac disease. When fat is not digested, it is transported through the gastrointestinal tract as intact triglyceride, which can appear as oil in the stool. In contrast, if fat is digested but not absorbed, it is in the form of fatty acids that can produce secretory diarrhea in the colon, resulting in more voluminous, even watery stools. This has two important ramifications: Fecal fat concentration is lower with mucosal disease (typically <9% by weight), and hypocalcemia due to formation of soaps (calcium plus 2 fatty acids) is seen with mucosal disease but not with pancreatic exocrine insufficiency. In addition, patients with mucosal disease tend to have more problems with water-soluble vitamin deficiencies than those with pancreatic exocrine insufficiency. In some patients with pancreatic exocrine insufficiency, carbohydrate malabsorption can produce substantial bloating, flatulence, and watery diarrhea.

---

[3]Exceeds dosage recommended by the manufacturer.

[1]Not FDA approved for this indication.
[2]Not available in the United States.

Tests to document pancreatic exocrine insufficiency are not widely available or are nonspecific (see earlier), and so diagnosis usually hinges on a consistent history, demonstration of anatomic problems in the pancreas (calcification or abnormal ducts), and documentation of a response of steatorrhea to empiric treatment with a large dose of exogenous enzymes.

Bile Acid Deficiency. Bile acid deficiency is a less common cause of maldigestion, and malabsorption in this setting is limited to fat and fat-soluble vitamins. The usual setting is a patient with an extensive ileal resection (see later), but this also occurs in certain cholestatic conditions in which bile acid secretion by the liver is markedly compromised, such as advanced primary biliary cirrhosis, or complete extrahepatic biliary obstruction. As with pancreatic exocrine insufficiency, stools tend to have high fat concentrations (>9% by weight) when bile acid secretion is limited by hepatic or biliary disorders.

Zollinger-Ellison Syndrome. Zollinger-Ellison syndrome produces several abnormalities that can affect absorption. High rates of gastric acid secretion produce persistently low pH in the duodenum, which precipitates bile acid and inactivates pancreatic enzymes. In addition, excess acid can damage the absorptive cells directly.

Postoperative Malabsorption

Substantial malabsorption can result from bariatric or other gastric surgeries. Weight loss can result from inadequate intake due to early satiety or symptoms of dumping syndrome. Malabsorption can result from impaired mechanical disruption of food, mismatching of chyme delivery and enzyme secretion, rapid transit, or small bowel bacterial overgrowth due to loss of the gastric acid barrier. In addition, gastric surgery sometimes brings out latent celiac disease.

Short intestinal resections are well tolerated, but more extensive resections produce diarrhea and malabsorption of variable severity. When these symptoms are associated with weight loss or dehydrating diarrhea, short bowel syndrome is said to exist. In general, nutrient absorptive needs can be met if at least 100 cm of jejunum are preserved, but fluid absorption will be insufficient and diarrhea may be profuse. The process of intestinal adaptation permits improved absorption with time; it depends on exposure of the absorptive surface to nutrients. Absorption of specific substances, such as bile acids or vitamin B_{12}, is reduced permanently by resection of the terminal ileum.

Malabsorption in short bowel syndrome is not due solely to loss of absorptive surface area. Gastric acid hypersecretion, bile acid deficiency, rapid transit (due to loss of the ileal brake), and bacterial overgrowth may be present. These conditions are amenable to treatment and therapy with antisecretory drugs, exogenous bile acids, opiate antidiarrheals, or antibiotics can produce substantial improvement. Injection of teduglutide (Gattex), a glucagon-like peptide-2 intestinal growth factor, or growth hormone in combination with glutamine and a special diet have been approved as treatments for short bowel syndrome; they can reduce the volume of parenteral fluid or nutrients required. Results with small bowel transplantation are improving with the use of better immunosuppressive regimens, and it remains the only cure for select patients with postresection malabsorption.

Attention to nutrition is vital in any patient with malabsorption. If adequate nutrition cannot be maintained by oral intake, nutritional therapy is needed. Because of impaired bowel function, success with enteral nutrition may be impossible; parenteral nutrition may be needed. It is important to distinguish between the need for supplemental fluid and electrolytes and the need for nutrients; total parenteral nutrition is not a good choice for patients who only require fluids and electrolytes.

References

Carroll RE, Benedetti E, Schowalter JP, Buchman AL: Management and complications of short bowel syndrome: an updated review, *Curr Gastroenterol Rep* 18:40, 2016.

Dominguez-Muñoz JE: Diagnosis and treatment of pancreatic exocrine insufficiency, *Curr Opin Gastroenterol* 34:349–354, 2018.

Fassio F, Facioni MS, Guagnini F: Lactose maldigestion, malabsorption, and intolerance: a comprehensive review with a focus on current management and future perspectives, *Nutrients* 10:1599, 2018.

Hujoel IA, Johnson DH, Lebwohl B, et al: Tropheryma whipplei infection (Whipple Disease) in the USA, *Dig Dis Sci* 64:213–223, 2019.

Husby S, Murray JA, Katzka DA: AGA clinical practice update on diagnosis and monitoring of celiac disease—changing utility of serology and histologic measures: expert review, *Gastroenterology* 156:885–889, 2019.

Jansson-Knodell CL, Hujoel IA, Rubio-Tapia A, Murray JA: Not all that flattens villi is celiac disease: a review of enteropathies, *Mayo Clin Proc* 93:509–517, 2018.

Jeejeebhoy KN, Duerksen DR: Malnutrition in gastrointestinal disorders: detection and nutritional assessment, *Gastroenterol Clin North Am* 47:1–22, 2018.

Lebwohl B, Sanders DS, Green PHR: Coeliac disease, *Lancet* 391:70–81, 2018.

Nikaki K, Gupte GL: Assessment of intestinal malabsorption, *Best Pract Res Clin Gastroenterol* 30:225–235, 2016.

Schiller LR, Pardi DS, Sellin JH: Chronic diarrhea: diagnosis and management, *Clin Gastroenterol Hepatol* 15:182–193, 2017.

Vijayvargiya P, Camilleri M: Update on bile acid malabsorption: finally ready for prime time? *Curr Gastroenterol Rep* 20:10, 2018.

PANCREATIC CANCER

Method of
Robert S. Freelove, MD

Epidemiology

Cancer of the exocrine pancreas is the fourth-leading cause of cancer death in both men and women in the United States in spite of being only the 12th-leading cause of cancer. This is primarily because the majority of pancreatic cancers are diagnosed at an advanced stage, with a 5-year survival rate of only 3%. The incidence increases steeply with age but rarely occurs in people younger than 45. It affects men 1.3 times more than women and is seen more in black patients than in other races.

Risk Factors

Risk factors can be divided into hereditary and nonhereditary categories. The defined hereditary syndromes that increase risk include hereditary pancreatitis, Peutz-Jeghers syndrome, hereditary nonpolyposis colon cancer, familial atypical multiple mole melanoma syndrome, and carrying BRCA1, BRCA2, or both genes. Non-O blood types are at increased risk for developing pancreatic cancer. Pancreatic cancer in a first-degree relative also increases risk, although a genetic basis has not been determined. Risk increases significantly with each first-degree relative affected, and familial pancreatic cancer occurs when pancreatic cancer is diagnosed in more than one first-degree relative.

Nonhereditary risk factors include chronic pancreatitis, diabetes mellitus, cigarette smoking, obesity, and physical inactivity; all independently increase the risk of developing pancreatic cancer.

Screening

No effective screening mechanism exists for early diagnosis of pancreatic cancer in asymptomatic adults at average risk. The United States Preventive Services Task Force gives screening for pancreatic cancer a grade D recommendation, recommending specifically against screening symptom-free adults using palpation, ultrasonography, or serologic markers. Although it is believed that adults with significant hereditary risk factors should receive screening, there is no clear guidance on when to initiate screening or the interval at which to perform repeat screening. There is also no strong evidence for which modality to use, although most experts suggest screening should be done with either endoscopic ultrasound scanning or magnetic resonance cholangiopancreatography (MRCP).

Clinical Presentation

Overall, the most common clinical findings at diagnosis are jaundice, vague abdominal pain, weight loss, and hepatomegaly. Other signs and symptoms that can be present include back pain, diarrhea, steatorrhea, vomiting, right upper quadrant or epigastric mass, ascites, weakness, malaise, fatigue, and dark urine. Migratory thrombophlebitis (Trousseau's sign) and presence of a nontender, palpably distended gallbladder (Courvoisier's sign) occur less commonly but are strongly linked to pancreatic cancer when present.

Tumor size and location within the pancreas, as well as existence and location of metastases determine which of those clinical features mentioned above are present. Approximately 70% of pancreatic cancers arise in the head of the pancreas, causing biliary obstruction and leading to jaundice from conjugated hyperbilirubinemia, weight loss, steatorrhea, and dark urine. Another 25% of tumors occur in the body or tail, and the remaining 5% involve the entire pancreas. These tumors are insidious and usually present with only nonspecific findings such as unintentional weight loss, anorexia, fatigue, generalized weakness, nausea, and dyspepsia.

Diagnosis

A thorough history and physical examination are insufficient for diagnosing pancreatic cancer but can raise suspicion and influence further workup. The imaging modality of choice is a triphasic, contrast-enhanced helical computed tomography (CT) scanning of the abdomen and should be the preferred initial imaging test for patients presenting with abdominal pain and weight loss. A transabdominal ultrasound scan may be ordered initially based on the patient's presentation. In those patients strongly suspected of having pancreatic cancer, CT scanning is indicated if the ultrasound scan is negative. Endoscopic ultrasound–guided fine-needle aspiration can usually be used for a histologic diagnosis. There are no specific serologic tests that are helpful in diagnosing pancreatic cancer, but general serologic testing appropriate for the patient's presentation should be undertaken. The serum tumor maker carbohydrate antigen 19-9 (CA 19-9) can be used for monitoring response to treatment but has no diagnostic value.

Staging

Staging of pancreatic cancer can generally be accomplished through CT scanning. Endoscopic ultrasound scanning may provide more information for smaller tumors in the head of the pancreas and in predicting vascular invasion if not clear on CT. If metastasis is strongly suspected but not confirmed by imaging studies, staging laparoscopy can be performed.

Staging of pancreatic cancer categorizes tumors as resectable or unresectable. Extensive vascular involvement, direct invasion into adjacent organs, and distal metastasis all make tumors unresectable.

Treatment

The only potentially curative treatment for pancreatic cancer is surgical resection. Only 15% to 20% of patients diagnosed with pancreatic cancer are candidates for resection, which has a 10% to 30% 5-year survival rate. Factors that influence postresection survival rates include histology, tumor size, adequacy of the resection, and presence of positive lymph nodes. Pancreaticoduodenectomy (Whipple procedure) is still performed on tumors of the head and neck of the pancreas. Variations in surgical technique meant to have less morbidity have not shown a significant difference in outcome. Once plagued with high death rate, the perioperative mortality rate has declined significantly to only 4% as outcomes have improved at centers where surgeons perform a higher volume of procedures. Distal pancreatectomy and splenectomy is performed for resectable lesions in the body or tail of the pancreas. The addition of postoperative adjuvant chemotherapy has been shown to add a few months to survival.

Treatment of unresectable pancreatic cancer may improve survival slightly but is primarily aimed at palliation. There is no curative treatment for unresectable lesions, and treatment decisions must be weighed against patient preferences, symptoms, and goals of care. If a patient with unresectable disease desires treatment, enrollment in a clinical trial of chemotherapeutic agents is preferred. For those not able to be enrolled in a clinical trial, there are chemotherapy protocols for both locally advanced disease and metastatic disease. The choice of which regimen depends on functional status, comorbid conditions, and serum bilirubin levels.

Palliative Care

Given the high mortality and likelihood of developing significant complications, physicians should perform a full assessment of psychological status, end-of-life care wishes, symptom burden, and existing social support systems for all patients with a new diagnosis of pancreatic cancer. Early intervention with palliative services should occur, as evidence shows an improved quality of life and a reduction in aggressiveness of end-of-life care as measured by provision of chemotherapy within 14 days of death, admission to the intensive care unit or hospital near death, and visits to the emergency department. Hospice services should be discussed with patients soon after the diagnosis, and consultation should be made as soon as appropriate to maximize the hospice benefit.

Pain is one of the most common symptoms that needs to be addressed in patients with advanced pancreatic cancer. Opioid analgesics are commonly used, and the type and nature of the pain should be clearly assessed to determine whether adjuvant medications for neuropathic pain could be helpful. Radiation therapy can be beneficial for pain, especially from bony metastases. Celiac plexus neurolysis performed percutaneously, during surgery, or under endoscopic ultrasound guidance can be more effective than pharmacologic therapy and avoids opioid-related complications such as sedation and constipation.

Biliary obstruction and resultant jaundice occurs commonly. Palliation of jaundice is primarily accomplished through endoscopic placement of a bare metal stent because it is less invasive than surgical intervention. However, surgical bypass of the biliary obstruction can be performed if endoscopic intervention is technically impossible. Gastric outlet obstruction also can occur and is treated in similar fashion with either expandable metal stents or surgical bypass.

Weight loss and malnutrition can be severe. In addition to managing gastric outlet and biliary obstruction, physicians must address pancreatic exocrine insufficiency, as it is another significant contributor. Oral pancreatic enzyme replacement should be initiated empirically with doses of 10,000 international units of pancreatic lipase (Creon)[1] taken at the beginning, middle, and end of each meal. High-calorie or calorie-dense diets and nutritional supplements should be recommended over appetite stimulants because the stimulants increase risk for thromboembolic disease.

Patients with pancreatic cancer have a higher incidence of venous thromboembolism (VTE) than other cancers, and patients should know the signs and symptoms. Primary prophylaxis in ambulatory patients is not recommended, but low-molecular-weight heparin prophylaxis should be provided to hospitalized patients who are not at increased risk of bleeding complications. Long-term treatment with low-molecular-weight heparin in patients with pancreatic cancer and VTE has been shown to reduce incidence of VTE with no difference in survival or bleeding outcomes over warfarin (Coumadin). As such, long-term low-molecular-weight heparin should be considered over warfarin as treatment for VTE, especially if the patient is on drugs that affect warfarin metabolism.

References

Balaban EP, Mangu PB, Khorana AA, et al: Locally advanced, unresectable pancreatic cancer: American Society of Clinical Oncology Clinical Practice Guideline, *J Clin Oncol* 34:2654–2668, 2016.

De La Cruz MS, Young AP, Ruffin MT: Diagnosis and management of pancreatic cancer, *Am Fam Phys* 89:626–632, 2014.

Final Recommendation Statement: Pancreatic Cancer: Screening. U.S. Preventive Services Task Force, Dec 2014, https://www.uspreventiveservicestaskforce.org/Page/Document/RecommendationStatementFinal/pancreatic-cancer-screening. Accessed 3/2/2018.

Jang RW, Krzyzanowska MK, Zimmerman C, Taback N, Alibhai SM: Palliative care and the aggressiveness of end-of-life care in patients with advanced pancreatic cancer, *J Natl Cancer Inst* 107(3).

Ryan DP, Hong TS, Bardeesy N: Pancreatic adenocarcinoma, *N Engl J Med* 371:1039–1049, 2014.

Siegel RL, Miller KD, Jemal A: Cancer statistics, 2017, *CA Cancer J Clin* 67:7–30, 2017.

Sohal DP, Mangu PB, Khorana AA, et al: Metastatic pancreatic cancer: American Society of Clinical Oncology Clinical Practice Guideline, *J Clin Oncol* 34:2784–2796, 2016.

[1] Not FDA approved for this indication.

TUMORS OF THE COLON AND RECTUM

Method of
Pinckney J. Maxwell IV, MD; and Gerald A. Isenberg, MD

CURRENT DIAGNOSIS

- Screening of asymptomatic, average-risk patients should begin at 50 years of age.
- Colonoscopy should be performed if any screening test result is positive.
- Colonoscopy should be performed for any patient with signs or symptoms of colorectal cancer.
- Screening of high-risk patients—those with inflammatory bowel disease, familial adenomatous polyposis, or hereditary nonpolyposis colorectal cancer) and those with a significant positive family history—should begin at an earlier age and occur more frequently.

CURRENT THERAPY

- Patients with familial adenomatous polyposis or hereditary nonpolyposis colorectal cancer should undergo early, prophylactic colon resection.
- Colon tumors should be treated with segmental laparoscopic or open resection.
- Chemotherapy is offered for colon cancers with locally advanced, nodal (stage III), or metastatic (stage IV) disease.
- Rectal tumors that are small (<3 cm), involve <25% of the rectal circumference, are superficial (Tis or T1), lack nodal involvement, and have favorable pathologic characteristics should be removed by transanal techniques.
- Rectal tumors that are larger, are locally invasive, or have nodal involvement should be removed by formal open resection, with sphincter preservation if possible.
- Combination chemotherapy and radiation therapy is offered for advanced (stage II), nodal (stage III), or metastatic (stage IV) rectal cancer.
- Postoperative surveillance includes frequent office evaluations, measurements of carcinoembryonic antigen, endoscopy, and imaging.

Background, Epidemiology, and Etiology

Colorectal cancer is the third most common cancer in men and women, after prostate and lung/bronchus cancer in men and breast and lung/bronchus cancer in women. The American Cancer Society estimates that there will be 102,900 new diagnoses of colon cancer and 39,670 new diagnoses of rectal cancer in the United States in 2010. The incidence of colorectal cancer has been decreasing since the mid-1980s, with a more dramatic decrease occuring in the most recent decade. This decrease is likely related to an increase in screening with removal of precancerous polyps. The American Cancer Society expects an estimated 51,370 deaths from colorectal cancer in 2010, accounting for 9% of all cancer deaths. The mortality rate of colorectal cancer has similarly decreased since the mid-1980s, again with a sharper decline in the past decade most likely related to improved screening. Colorectal cancer is a highly treatable and frequently curable malignancy when it is detected early, highlighting the need for better screening.

The development of colorectal cancer is related to a number of factors, including age, diet, activity, environmental exposures, family history, and genetics. Ninety percent of colorectal cancers are diagnosed after the age of 50 years, and fewer than 5% of cases are diagnosed before the age of 40. The peak incidence of diagnosis is in the seventh decade of life. Dietary factors play a role in carcinogenesis. Western diets, containing high fat and low fiber, have been associated with increased rates of colorectal cancer, as has the intake of red or processed meats and alcohol. It is likely that the low-fiber Western diet slows transit time, leading to increased exposure to carcinogens. Activity level also can play a role in carcinogenesis: studies have shown an increase in cancer among those with sedentary jobs and a decreased incidence among those who exercise regularly. Exposure to cigarette smoke increases the risk of colorectal adenomas and cancers. The American Cancer Society Cancer Prevention Study II revealed that 12% of colorectal cancer deaths in the general U.S. population can be attributed to smoking. Family history and genetics also play a significant role in carcinogenesis, because approximately 10% of patients diagnosed have a first-degree relative with colorectal cancer.

Adenomatous Polyps

The progression from normal mucosa to an adenomatous polyp and then to an invasive colorectal cancer proceeds through a well-defined process over many years. Aberrant crypt foci develop into microadenomas and then into adenomatous polyps. Dysplastic cells develop within the polyp, continue to multiply, become a tumor and then break through the subepithelial barrier and invade the layers of the bowel wall, eventually spreading to pericolic tissues or to lymph nodes and distant sites. A number of genes have been implicated in carcinogenesis, including proto-oncogenes (*KRAS, SRC, MYC*), tumor-suppressor genes (*APC, DCC, TP53, MCC, DPC4*), and DNA-mismatch repair genes (*HMSH2, MLH1, PMS1, PMS2, GTBP*). Sporadic colorectal cancers develop as a result of several cumulative genetic insults involving these genes (Figure 1).

Familial Colorectal Cancer Syndromes

Familial adenomatous polyposis (FAP) is an inherited, non–sex-linked, mendelian dominant disease that accounts for approximately 1% of all colorectal cancers. The high penetrance of FAP means that there is a 50% chance of development of colorectal cancer among members of affected families. However, 20% of FAP patients have no family history, and their cases most likely represent new, spontaneous mutations. The disorder is caused by mutations in the tumor-suppressor *APC* gene, which is located on chromosome 5 (5q21–q22), or in the *MUTYH* gene, which is located on chromosome 1 (1p34.3–p32.1). FAP is characterized by the progressive development of hundreds or thousands of adenomatous polyps located throughout the entire colon. The clinical diagnosis is based on histologic confirmation of at least 100 adenomas. All patients eventually develop colorectal cancer. The adenomas typically appear by the mid-twenties, and cancers by the late thirties.

An attenuated form of FAP is recognized in which fewer adenomas (20–100) are identified. Adenomas and cancers develop somewhat later, at average ages of 44 and 56 years, respectively. FAP also exhibits extracolonic manifestations, including gastric, duodenal, and small-bowel polyps; osteomas and desmoid tumors (Gardner's syndrome); eye lesions (congenital hypertrophy of retinal pigment epithelium [CHRPE]); epidermoid cysts; and brain neoplasms (Turcot's syndrome).

Hereditary nonpolyposis colon cancer (HNPCC), also called Lynch syndrome, is an inherited, non–sex-linked, mendelian dominant disease with virtually complete penetrance. HNPCC is caused by a defect in any of a number of DNA-mismatch repair genes (*MLH1, MSH2, MSH6, PMS, PMS2*) that leads to high-level microsatellite instability (MSI-H). A number of criteria have been generated for the diagnosis of HNPCC, including the Amsterdam I and II criteria and the Bethesda guidelines (Box 1). According to the EPICOLON study, the revised Bethesda guidelines are the most discriminating set of clinical parameters for diagnosis of HNPCC.

HNPCC is subdivided into Lynch syndrome types I and II. Lynch type I refers to site-specific nonpolyposis colon cancer, and

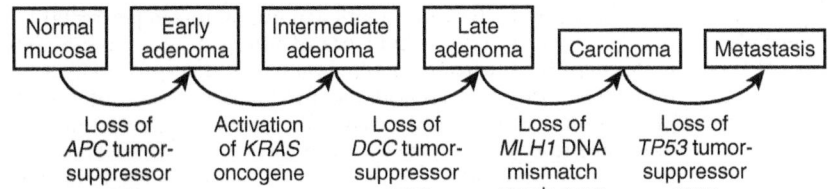

| Normal mucosa | → | Early adenoma | → | Intermediate adenoma | → | Late adenoma | → | Carcinoma | → | Metastasis |

Loss of *APC* tumor-suppressor gene   Activation of *KRAS* oncogene   Loss of *DCC* tumor-suppressor gene   Loss of *MLH1* DNA mismatch repair gene   Loss of *TP53* tumor-suppressor gene

Figure 1 Sequence of progression from adenoma to carcinoma.

BOX 1   Diagnosis of Hereditary Nonpolyposis Colon Cancer (HNPCC)

Amsterdam I Criteria, 1990
- Three or more family members with histologically verified colorectal cancer, one of whom is a first-degree relative (parent, child, sibling) of the other two
- Two successive affected generations
- One or more colon cancers diagnosed before age 50 years
- Familial adenomatous polyposis has been excluded.

Amsterdam II Criteria, 1999
- Three or more family members with histologically verified HNPCC-related cancers (endometrium, ovary, stomach, small intestine, hepatobiliary, upper urinary tract, brain, or skin), one of whom is a first-degree relative (parent, child, sibling) of the other two
- Two successive affected generations
- One or more colon cancers diagnosed before age 50 years
- Familial adenomatous polyposis has been excluded.

Revised Bethesda Guidelines, 2002
- Colorectal cancer diagnosed in a patient who is younger than 50 years of age
- Presence of a synchronous, metachronous colorectal or other HNPCC-related malignancy, regardless of age
- Colorectal cancer with the high-level microsatellite instability (MSI-H) histology diagnosed in a patient who is younger than 60 years of age
  - Presence of carcinoma infiltrating lymphocytes, Crohn's-like lymphocytic reaction, mucinous/signet-ring differentiation, or medullary growth pattern
  - No general consensus based on this age
- Colorectal cancer diagnosed in one or more first-degree relatives with an HNPCC-related neoplasm
  - With one or more neoplasms being diagnosed before age 50 years
- Colorectal cancer diagnosed in two or more first- or second-degree relatives with HNPCC-related malignancies, regardless of age

---

Lynch type II (formerly called familial cancer syndrome) refers to cancers that develop in the colon and related organs such as the endometrium, ovaries, stomach, pancreas, and proximal urinary tract, among others. Lynch syndrome differs from sporadic colorectal cancer in a number of important ways. It has an autosomal dominant inheritance, a predominance of proximal lesions (75% are found in the right colon), an excess of multiple primary colorectal cancers (18%), an early age at onset (average, 44 years), a significantly improved survival rate with right-sided lesions (53% at 5 years, compared with 35% for distal colorectal cancer in family members), and an increased risk for development of metachronous lesions (24%). Patients and family members of those diagnosed with HNPCC or FAP should undergo genetic testing to help improve future diagnosis and treatment options.

Inflammatory Bowel Disease
Both Crohn's disease and ulcerative colitis are associated with an increased risk of colorectal cancer; with the latter conferring approximately double the risk of the former. The duration and severity of Crohn's disease and the duration and extent (left-sided colitis versus pancolitis) of ulcerative colitis contribute to cancer risk in patients with inflammatory bowel disease. Cancer in Crohn's disease typically occurs in a stricture or bypassed segment. Neoplasia in ulcerative colitis does not follow the adenoma-carcinoma development sequence seen in sporadic colorectal cancer, and this has important screening and treatment implications.

Evaluation
Screening Average-Risk Patients
Patients with no personal history of colorectal polyps or cancers, no personal history of inflammatory bowel disease, no symptoms suspicious for colorectal cancer, no family history of colorectal polyps or cancers, and no evidence of a familial or genetic syndrome may be screened as having average risk. The two main categories of screening tests are those that detect adenomatous polyps and cancers (flexible sigmoidoscopy, colonoscopy, double-contrast barium enema, and computed tomographic [CT] colonography) and those that primarily detect cancer (fecal occult blood testing, fecal immunohistochemical testing, and stool DNA testing). The goal of screening is to reduce mortality rates by reducing the incidence of advanced disease. It seems intuitive that tests that detect polyps, the premalignant phase of colorectal cancer, would be preferred to tests that detect only cancers. However, testing for polyps and cancers is usually procedure related, whereas testing for only cancers can be conducted on stool samples alone. Screening with simple stool samples has the potential to more easily increase overall screening.

Regardless of the method used, testing in the average-risk, symptom-patient should begin at age 50 years. A total colonoscopy is required only every 10 years but involves oral bowel preparation and carries a small risk of perforation (approximately 1/1000). A flexible sigmoidoscopy is required every 5 years, in combination with annual fecal occult blood testing. Flexible sigmoidoscopy requires only enemas for preparation and carries a lower risk of perforation. Air-contrast barium enemas may be used for screening every 5 years, but they also require oral bowel preparation and are only diagnostic. CT colonography is an evolving method for screening every 5 years and offers the opportunity for more accessible screening; however, the procedure is limited in regard to identification of polyps smaller than 1 cm, also requires oral bowel prepation, and is only diagnostic. Fecal occult blood testing and fecal immunohistochemical testing are done annually. The interval for stool DNA testing is uncertain, and it tests only for a limited number of mutations. The most complete screening test, which allows removal of any precancerous lesions that are identified, remains the total colonoscopy.

Screening High-Risk Patients
High-risk patients include those with a personal history of colorectal polyps or cancers, a family history of colorectal cancer in a first-degree relative, Crohn's disease or ulcerative colitis, or a personal or family history of FAP or HNPCC. Screening in these patients has been adjusted for changes in incidence and age at onset of neoplasia (Table 1).

Symptoms and Diagnosis
Symptoms of colorectal cancer include bleeding (85%), a change in bowel habits, abdominal pain, malaise, and obstruction. Frequently, anemia is the only sign a patient exhibits. Patients with

symptoms suspicious for colorectal cancer should undergo a colonoscopy. An anorectal source of bleeding should not preclude a complete colonic evaluation.

Management

Preoperative Management

Before operative intervention is undertaken, a complete evaluation should occur, including a careful history and physical examination, routine laboratory testing, and measurement of the level of carcinoembryonic antigen. A complete evaluation of the colon is essential, including colonoscopy with biopsy, or barium enema or CT colonography if colonoscopy is incomplete. Bowel preparation is no longer indicated as a routine preoperative measure for colonic surgery.

Preoperative staging should be undertaken for colorectal cancers. CT scanning of the abdomen and pelvis are indicated to aid in evaluating the extent of localized or metastatic disease and the presence of enlarged lymph nodes. Staging of rectal cancers includes determining the distance from the anal verge, frequently with the use of a rigid proctoscope; the depth of invasion; and the presence of enlarged lymph nodes, using endorectal ultrasound or endoanal coil magnetic resonance imaging. Metastatic disease mandates neoadjuvant chemotherapy in the absence of acute symptoms of obstruction or exsanguination.

Rectal cancers with evidence of local invasion into perirectal fat or adjacent structures or evidence of enlarged metastatic lymph nodes may benefit from neoadjuvant chemotherapy and irradiation. Preoperative staging allows for the application of neoadjuvant therapy in selected candidates, which can downstage and downsize tumors and can decrease rates of local recurrence in rectal cancer. Neoadjuvant therapy can also allow for sphincter-preserving procedures in patients with previously bulky or very low rectal tumors.

Surgery for Colonic Tumors

The primary therapy for tumors of the colon is operative. The basic principles of surgery for colon cancer are the following:

- Exploration: adequate visual, tactile, and potentially intraoperative hepatic ultrasound staging at the time of primary resection
- Removal of the entire cancer with enough proximal and distal bowel to encompass the possibility of submucosal lymphatic tumor spread
- Removal of the regional mesenteric pedicle, including draining lymphatics, based on the predictable lymphatic spread of the disease and the potential for regional mesenteric involvement without concurrent distant involvement
- En bloc resection of involved structures (T4 tumors)

TABLE 1	Screening High-Risk Patients for Colorectal Cancer		
RISK CATEGORY	**AGE TO BEGIN**	**RECOMMENDED TEST**	**COMMENT**
Personal history of <3 adenomas with low-grade dysplasia	5–10 y after the initial polypectomy	Colonoscopy	Examination interval should be based on other clinical factors, such as prior findings, family history, or endoscopist or patient preference.
Personal history of 3–10 adenomas, or 1 adenoma >1 cm, or any adenoma with villous features or high-grade dysplasia	3 y after the initial polypectomy	Colonoscopy	Adenomas require compete excision. If the follow-up is normal, the next examination should be in 5 y. Presence of >10 adenomas should raise suspicion of a familial syndrome.
Personal history of colorectal cancer	1 y after resection	Colonoscopy	Patients should undergo high-quality preoperative clearance. Follow-up after normal examinations should be extended to 3 y and then to 5 y.
Family history of adenomas or cancer in a first-degree relative <60 y of age or in 2 first-degree relatives at any age	Age 40 y, or 10 y before the age at onset of youngest affected family member	Colonoscopy	Every 5 y
Family history of adenomas or cancer in a first-degree relative >60 y of age or in 2 second-degree relatives with cancer	Age 40 y	Colonoscopy	Screening should be initiated at an earlier age. Intervals are based on findings or on the average-risk patient.
FAP or suspected FAP	Age 10–12 y	Annual FS, counseling for genetic testing if showing polyps	Colectomy should be considered for positive genetic testing.
HNPCC or risk for HNPCC	Age 20–25 y, or 10 y before the age at onset of youngest affected family member	Colonoscopy, counseling for genetic testing	Every 1–2 y. Genetic testing should be offered to first-degree relatives of persons with a known DNA-mismatch repair gene defect or with 1 of the first 3 Bethesda criteria.
IBD, Crohn's disease, or chronic UC	8 y after the onset of pancolitis, or 12–15 y after the onset of left-sided colitis	Colonoscopies with random four-quadrant biopsies every 10 cm for dysplasia	Screening should be offered every 1–2 y, and patients are best referred to a center with experience in the surveillance and management of IBD.

Abbreviations: FAP = familial adenomatous polyposis; FS = flexible sigmoidoscopy; HNPCC = hereditary nonpolyposis colorectal cancer; IBD = inflammatory bowel disease.

Segmental colonic resections (right, transverse, left, or sigmoid colectomy) are undertaken based on the tumor location and blood supply with lymphatic drainage, specifically the ileocolic, middle colic, and left colic arteries. These arteries define a convenient anatomic boundary for standard colonic resection and also provide for adequate regional lymph node clearance, because the major draining lymphatics follow these blood vessels in the mesentery. Locally invasive tumors (T4) require en bloc resection of involved structures. Metastatic colonic tumors (M1) may require neoadjuvant chemotherapy before resection or palliation.

Numerous studies have verified that laparoscopic surgery is appropriate, and perhaps preferred, for colon cancer in experienced hands. The landmark Clinical Outcomes of Surgical Therapy (COST) trial in 2004 established that laparoscopic resection is equivalent to open resection for colon cancer.

Surgery for Rectal Tumors

Two approaches for rectal tumors are local excision and formal rectal resection. Local excision is the treatment of choice for a select, small group (3%–5% of all patients diagnosed with rectal cancer). Tumors amenable to transanal excision are small (<3 cm), involve less than 25% of the rectal circumference, are confined to the mucosa or submucosa (Tis or T1), lack nodal involvement by preoperative imaging, and have favorable pathologic characteristics (well or moderately differentiated with no lymphovascular invasion). Tumors in the lower or middle third of the rectum are accessible by simple transanal excision, but tumors of the upper rectum require the use of transanal endoscopic microsurgery (TEMS) techniques for resection. Local excision requires a 1-cm normal margin, but the defect usually does not require closure.

Tumors staged at T2 or greater require a formal resection, the type of which depends on the location of the tumor. Upper and middle rectal tumors can usually be managed with a low or very low anterior resection. Lower rectal tumors frequently require a proctectomy with coloanal anastomosis or an abdominoperineal resection. The goal of resection is to obtain a 5-cm distal margin, but lower tumors can be managed with a 2-cm distal margin. Very low tumors and those involving the sphincter mechanism require an abdominoperineal resection.

Rectal tumors with greater depth of rectal wall invasion (T3), evidence of fixation or local invasion (T4), or evidence of lymph nodal (N1–2) or metastatic (M1) disease mandates neoadjuvant chemoradiation therapy. Proctectomy requires a specimen-appropriate total mesorectal excision. This involves complete excision of all mesorectal tissue located behind the rectum with no carcinoma at the lateral or circumferential margins. The goal is to remove all malignant tissue, so as to reduce or eliminate the possibility of locally recurrent disease.

Locally advanced rectal tumors may preclude an effective or safe resection. Some indications for likely inoperability include extensive pelvic disease, invasion of ileofemoral vessels, extensive lymphatic involvement or significant lower extremity lymphedema, bony involvement, and life expectancy less than 3 to 6 months.

Laparoscopy is being performed for rectal malignancies in advanced centers, and studies are under way to verify the efficacy and safety of laparoscopic rectal resection in comparison with traditional open resection.

Complicated Disease

Colorectal tumors may manifest with complications such as obstruction, perforation, or significant bleeding. These presentations are generally related to more advanced disease and may preclude a complete staging workup or potential neoadjuvant therapy. Unless patients are unstable or critically ill or the tumor is unresectable, the tumor should be appropriately resected. An ostomy is usually performed, whether as an end ostomy or as a proximal loop diversion for a primary anastomosis. Colonic stenting is an attractive option for obstructing lesions as palliation or as a bridge to resection after medical stabilization and staging for potential neoadjuvant therapy.

Surgery for High-Risk Conditions

High-risk conditions for the development of colorectal malignancies include FAP, HNPCC, and chronic ulcerative colitis. Surgical management may be prophylactic or possibly therapeutic after a malignancy has been diagnosed. The mainstay of operative management in FAP and chronic ulcerative colitis is a total proctocolectomy. Reconstructive options include an ileal pouch–anal anastomosis, a continent ileostomy (Kock pouch), or an end ileostomy. A total abdominal colectomy with ileorectal anastomosis may be performed for temporary preservation of rectal function in selected cases of chronic ulcerative colitis with rectal sparing and FAP with few rectal polyps, but this requires aggressive surveillance of the remaining rectal mucosa because of the risk of malignancy. Patients with HNPCC should also undergo subtotal colectomy with ileorectal anastomosis; because of the prevalence of associated gynecological malignancies, a total hysterectomy with bilateral salpingo-oophorectomy should be offered to women as well.

Pathologic Staging and Adjuvant Therapy

Excellent pathologic sampling and review of the operative specimen provide important prognostic and therapeutic information. Current standards recommend that at least 12 lymph nodes be removed for adequate staging of colon cancer. The decision for adjuvant chemotherapy or radiation therapy or both is based on the pathologic staging. This information also provides prognostic information in terms of survival for the patient and family. A number of staging systems have been developed, but the tumor-node-metastasis (TNM) system is the one most commonly used in the United States (Table 2).

Chemotherapy is offered for patients who have colorectal cancers with locally advanced, nodal (stage III), or metastatic (stage IV) disease. The combination of chemotherapy and radiation therapy for advanced rectal cancer (stage II–IV) has decreased local recurrence and increased survival. Numerous protocols are available for treatment, with the standard of care being FOLFOX: oxaliplatin (Eloxatin), 5-fluorouracil (5-FU [Adrucil]), and leucovorin. Elderly patients and those with multiple comorbidities who may not be able to tolerate full-dose chemotherapy may be candidates for capecitabine (Xeloda) or 5-FU and leucovorin. Numerous study protocols are available at specialized centers evaluating other medications. Newer technologies continue to evolve, such as antiangiogenesis agents and immunomodulatory agents.

Metastatic Disease

Surgical therapy is also available for metastatic disease in certain situations. Metastatic liver lesions amenable to resection can be addressed at the time of colon resection or after the patient has healed from colectomy. The lesions could be resected or treated with radiofrequency ablation, a newer technology that allows in situ destruction of liver lesions. Similarly, selected pulmonary metastases can be resected, possibly with the use of minimally invasive thoracoscopic techniques.

Surveillance

Surveillance for colon and rectal cancer is a lifelong process. Patients are seen and examined in the office every 3 months for 2 years, then every 6 months for 3 years, and then yearly for 5 years. Levels of carcinoembryonic antigen are measured at each office visit, but current literature recommends obtaining levels every 3 months for 3 years as a marker for tumor recurrence in stage II–III patients. Colonoscopy should be performed at 1 year postoperatively, assuming a high-quality preoperative study has cleared the rest of the colon. A normal colonoscopy at 1 year postoperatively would allow the next surveillance colonoscopy to be performed 3 years later. If that one is normal, subsequent examinations should be performed every 5 years. After the examination at 1 year postoperatively, the subsequent intervals should be shortened if there is evidence of HNPCC or if additional adenomas are found. As an addition to formal colonoscopies, flexible

TABLE 2	Pathologic Staging Systems for Colorectal Cancer					
PATHOLOGIC FEATURES		STAGE	TNM	DUKES	ASTLER-COLLER	5-YR SURVIVAL (%)
Depth of Invasion						
Lamina propria, muscularis mucosa		0	T0/Tis	A		>90
Submucosa		I	T1	A	B1	
Muscularis propria		I	T2	A	B1	
Subserosa, pericolic fat		II	T3	B	B1	70–85
Adjacent organs, perforation		II	T4	B	B2	55–65
Lymph nodal involvement						
None			N0			
1–3 nodes		III	N1	C	C1, C2	45–55
>3 nodes		III	N2	C	C1, C2	20–30
Distant metastatic disease						
Absent			M0			
Present		IV	M1	D		<5

Abbreviation: TNM = tumor-node-metastasis system.

sigmoidoscopies are performed with each office visit for patients with rectal cancer. Routine imaging utilizing CT scans of the chest, abdomen, and pelvis is performed annually for 3 years in patients with colorectal cancer. Patients with increased or rising CEA levels, as noted by routine surveillance checks, or evidence of recurrent disease, as noted by history and physical examinations or routine surveillance imaging studies, can be evaluated with the use of positron emission tomography (PET), an emerging sensitive test for tumor recurrence.

References

American Cancer Society: *Cancer Facts and Figures 2013*, Atlanta, GA: American Cancer Society; 2013. Available at: http://www.cancer.org/Research/CancerFactsFigures/CancerFactsFigures/cancer-facts-figures-2013 [accessed August 25, 2014].

Beart RW, Steele Jr GD., Menck HR, et al: Management and survival of patients with adenocarcinoma of the colon and rectum: A national survey of the Commission on Cancer, *J Am Coll Surg* 181:225–236, 1995.

Bentrem DJ, Okabe S, Wong WD, et al: T1 Adenocarcinoma of the rectum: Transanal excision or radical surgery? *Ann Surg* 242:472–479, 2005.

Clinical Outcomes of Surgical Therapy Study Group: A comparison of laparoscopically assisted and open colectomy for colon cancer, *N Engl J Med* 350:2050–2059, 2004.

Desch CE, Benson 3rd AB, Somerfield MR, et al: Colorectal cancer surveillance: 2005 update of an American Society of Clinical Oncology Practice Guideline, *J Clin Oncol* 23(33):8512–8519, 2005.

Floyd ND, Saclarides TJ: Transanal endoscopic microsurgical resection of pT1 rectal tumors, *Dis Colon Rectum* 49:164–168, 2005.

Lan Y-T, Lin J-K, Li AF-Y, et al: Metachronous colorectal cancer: Necessity of post-operative colonoscopic surveillance, *Int J Colorectal Dis* 20:121–125, 2005.

Levin B, Lieberman DA, McFarland B, et al: Screening and surveillance for the early detection of colorectal cancer and adenomatous polyps, 2008: A joint guideline from the American Cancer Society, the US Multi-Society Task Force on Colorectal Cancer, and the American College of Radiology. For the American Cancer Society Colorectal Cancer Advisory Group, the US Multi-Society Task Force, and the American College of Radiology Colon Cancer Committee, *Gastroenterology* 134:1570–1595, 2008.

Maetani I, Tada T, Ukita T, et al: Self-expandable metallic stent placement as palliative treatment of obstructed colorectal carcinoma, *J Gastroenterol* 39:334–338, 2004.

Pinol V, Castells A, Andreu M, et al: Accuracy of Revised Bethesda Guidelines, microsatellite instability, and immunohistochemistry for the identification of patients with hereditary nonpolyposis colorectal cancer, *JAMA* 293:1986–1994, 2005.

Rex DK, Kahi CJ, Levin B, et al: Guidelines for colonoscopy surveillance after cancer resection: A consensus update by the American Cancer Society and the US Multi-Society Task Force on Colorectal Cancer, *Gastroenterology* 130:1865–1871, 2006.

Sauer R, Becker H, Hohenberger W, et al: for the German Rectal Cancer Study Group: Preoperative versus postoperative chemoradiotherapy for rectal cancer, *N Engl J Med* 351:1731–1740, 2004.

Stipa F, Chessin DB, Shia J, et al: A pathologic complete response of rectal cancer to preoperative combined-modality therapy results in improved oncological outcome compared with those who achieve no downstaging on the basis of preoperative endorectal ultrasonography, *Ann Surg Oncol* 13(8):1047–1053, 2006.

Winawer SJ, Zauber AG, Fletcher RH, et al: Guidelines for colonoscopy surveillance after polypectomy: A consensus update by the US Multi-Society Task Force on Colorectal Cancer and the American Cancer Society, *CA Cancer J Clin* 56:143–159, 2006.

TUMORS OF THE STOMACH

Method of
Scott A. Hundahl, MD

CURRENT DIAGNOSIS

- Intestinal metaplasia, which predisposes to cancer, results from chronic *Helicobacter pylori* infection.
- In the United States, screening studies are reserved for those with definite risk factors.
- Pretreatment staging drives subsequent treatment and involves endoscopy, endoscopic ultrasound, helical computed tomography, and often laparoscopy or mini-laparotomy.
- Mucosal abnormalities can be largely absent in early gastrointestinal stromal tumors, small carcinoids, and even diffuse-type linitis plastica. Deep endoscopic biopsies are required.

CURRENT THERAPY

Adenocarcinoma
- To ensure complete surgical resection, resection should be customized (e.g., gross margin, use of endoscopic mucosal resection for certain mucosal tumors).
- For tumors beyond mucosal depth, survival is maximized with either computer-guided "low Maruyama Index surgery," or an JGCA-defined "D-2" operation
- Adjuvant therapy options include preoperative chemotherapy (± postoperative treatment), or postoperative chemoradiation

Gastric Adenocarcinoma

Thanks to happy accident rather than specific planning, over the past 80 years, gastric adenocarcinoma has changed from the most-common solid organ malignancy in the United States to a relatively uncommon disease. Worldwide, however, it remains a scourge second only to lung cancer.

Classification and Epidemiology

Several classification schemes exist. Two are commonly used. Bormann's morphologic classification relies on gross characteristics of the tumor. The histologic classification of Lauren, first described by Jarvi and Lauren in 1951, divides gastric adenocarcinomas into intestinal (gland-forming) and diffuse (discohesive) types, based on their microscopic appearance. Several other classification schemes have been proposed, including Broder's classification of differentiation, the World Health Organization (WHO) classification, the Nagayo–Komagome classification, the Ming classification, and the Goseki classification, but none eclipses the Lauren classification.

Epidemiologically, three patterns of disease can be discerned, with *Helicobacter pylori* infection playing an important role in the first two patterns: intestinal-type tumors arising from the lesser curve and distal stomach, related to *H pylori*–associated atrophic gastritis and intestinal metaplasia; diffuse-type tumors involving the body of the stomach, often associated with intense *H pylori*–associated inflammation but not associated with significant intestinal metaplasia; and intestinal-type tumors of the gastroesophageal junction.

In high-incidence regions of the world, such as Japan and Korea, up to two thirds of gastric adenocarcinomas are of the first type and are strongly associated with chronic multifocal atrophic gastritis and intestinal metaplasia from chronic *H pylori* infection. The process usually begins at the antrum–corpus junction along the lesser curvature and predisposes to cancers of the intestinal type occurring in the sixth or seventh decades of life. The second type of gastric adenocarcinoma, also associated with *H pylori*, afflicts younger persons in the fourth and fifth decades of life. The last type, seen in lower-incidence regions of the world such as the United States, is associated with chronic gastroesophageal reflux and Barrett's esophagitis.

Epidemiologists and public health experts estimate that more than 40% of gastric adenocarcinomas worldwide can be attributed to chronic *H pylori* infection. Strains containing the *cagA* gene appear more dangerous. The infection usually starts by the second or third decade, and unless it is successfully treated, it gives rise to chronic inflammation, atrophic gastritis, and eventually intestinal metaplasia, which is a premalignant histologic condition. Dietary factors such as high salt and high nitrates can accentuate this progression as well as the march to cancer. As the condition progresses, acid-producing oxyntic mucosa is progressively wiped out, gastric pH increases, and bacterial overgrowth with non–*H pylori* bacteria is facilitated. The original *H pylori*, which requires an acid environment to thrive, often disappears at this point.

Once intestinal metaplasia is established, dietary factors become particularly important in mitigating the risk of cancer development. Protective factors include intake of vitamin C, fresh fruits and vegetables, and antioxidants. The association of *H pylori* infection with the development of intestinal metaplasia suggests that early detection and elimination of this infection might prevent gastric cancer. Unfortunately, in high-incidence areas, reinfection from contaminated water supply and other sources is common, thus undermining the strategy. Also, in prevention trials to date, benefit appears restricted to the subgroups without preexisting intestinal metaplasia.

Risk Factors

Risk factors other than *H pylori* infection include low socioeconomic status, smoking, a diet deficient in fresh fruits and vegetables or high in salt-preserved high-nitrate foods, previous gastric ulcer, ionizing radiation, family history, and previous gastric resection. Blood group A is associated with higher risk of developing a diffuse-type tumor. Predisposing genetic conditions include Lynch's syndrome (hereditary nonpolyposis colorectal cancer [HNPCC], a condition with microsatellite instability due to deficient DNA repair enzymes), as well as dominantly inherited germline mutations in the E-cadherin gene.

Diagnosis

In Western populations, by the time gastric cancer causes symptoms, the disease is often relatively advanced. In a large National Cancer Data Base survey of US patients, presenting ascribable symptoms included weight loss (62%), abdominal or epigastric pain (52%), nausea (34%), anorexia (32%), early satiety (32%), dysphagia (26%), and melena (18%).

Mass screening combining upper GI series, endoscopy, and serum pepsinogen I/II ratio have proved beneficial in high-incidence areas such as Japan, but they cannot be justified in the United States, where incidence is low. However, for defined risk groups, such as those with established atrophic gastritis and established intestinal metaplasia, strong family history, and those with HNPCC syndrome, surveillance screening should definitely be considered. For those with hereditary E-cadherin mutations associated with gastric cancer, prophylactic total gastrectomy is recommended.

In the United States, diagnosis is usually made by upper endoscopy. One should be aware that diffuse-type cancers manifesting as linitis plastica are often associated with minimal visible mucosal changes, and deep biopsies are often required for establishing the diagnosis. Furthermore, small, early gastric cancers (defined by the Japanese as in-situ and T1 cancers, with or without node involvement) can be associated with particularly subtle mucosal changes, presenting a challenge for even the most experienced endoscopist. Chromo-endoscopy and other sophisticated mucosal imaging techniques have been used to identify such changes but are not yet standard.

Extent-of-disease studies for gastric adenocarcinoma include endoscopic ultrasound (good for estimating depth of tumor and visualizing immediately adjacent nodes), and helical CT scanning, which is good for evaluating extraluminal extent of disease, intraabdominal or mediastinal extension or spread, and liver or lung metastases. Because even high-resolution CT scanning can miss small peritoneal implants, extraregional nodal spread, and small liver metastases, staging laparoscopy or minilaparotomy are valuable adjuncts and should be considered mandatory if any preoperative chemotherapy is considered.

Staging

Eighth Edition American Joint Committee on Cancer/International Union Against Cancer (AJCC/UICC) staging, to be applied to cases diagnosed after January 1, 2018, classifies any tumor whose epicenter is in the proximal 2 cm of the stomach and proximally crosses the esophagogastric junction as an esophageal cancer. Tumors whose epicenter is distal to the proximal 2 cm are deemed a stomach cancer. Gastric cancer staging continues to harmonize the T-category designations with colon sites. T1 tumors, which involve mucosa or submucosa, are now subcategorized T1a or T1b accordingly. T2 tumors involve the muscularis propria. T3 tumors penetrate to subserosal connective tissue without breaching the visceral peritoneum. T4 tumors breach the serosa (T4a) or invade adjacent structures (T4b). Nodal categories specify N1 as reflecting 1 to 2 nodes involved, N2 as 3 to 6 nodes involved, and N3 designating 7 or more nodes involved. In the overall TNM staging matrix, stage IV is now restricted to patients with documented peritoneal (including positive peritoneal washing cytology), distant-organ, or extraregional nodal metastases.

Treatment

Curative treatment of gastric cancer involves, as main therapy, complete negative-margin surgical resection of disease. For select tumors, such resection sometimes follows up-front chemotherapy. For localized in situ and select T1 tumors, endoscopic mucosal resection and minimally invasive techniques have been successfully employed. Unfortunately, most tumors in the United States are discovered at a stage where formal open surgery is required.

To secure a histologically negative mural margin of resection, a gross margin of 2 cm is usually adequate for exophytic, non-infiltrating tumors, and a margin of at least 5 to 6 cm of grossly normal tissue is recommended for ulcerated or infiltrating tumors or diffuse histology. Closest mural margins are generally checked by frozen section at the time of surgery to confirm adequacy of resection. Total gastrectomy is not indicated as a routine procedure, except in diffuse-type tumors involving most of the stomach (linitis plastica), but it is warranted whenever required for a negative-margin resection.

Routine splenectomy in the treatment of gastric cancer, as well as routine distal pancreatectomy (performed in the past to clear splenic nodes), should be avoided unless definitely required for complete resection of visible or palpable disease.

The optimal extent of lymph node dissection in this disease has generated—and continues to generate—international controversy. Although several prospective randomized trials to date in non-Asian populations—none perfect—fail to demonstrate that routine extensive lymphadenectomy increases survival, it has also been shown that insufficient lymphadenectomy definitely compromises survival. A prospective randomized single-institution trial in Taipei has documented survival benefit associated with radical lymph node dissection. The adequacy of lymphadenectomy for a given case can be quantified using the Maruyama Index of Unresected Disease. In both a large US adjuvant chemoradiation trial and in a blinded reanalysis of a large Dutch surgical trial, low Maruyama Index score independently correlates with survival. Moreover, a dose–response effect is seen for the extent of surgical clearance of node groups at risk. Using the Maruyama computer program to predict the extent of nodal spread for a given cancer case before surgery is one way to facilitate a low Maruyama Index operation. A JGCA-defined "D-2" operation will also generate such a result.

Sentinel node biopsy, an established technique in the treatment of other cancers, has largely failed to win support in cancer of the stomach owing to the organ's lymphatic complexity and relatively high reported false-negative rates.

A large North American prospective randomized trial of postoperative adjuvant 5-fluorouracil–based chemoradiation in completely resected gastric cancer revealed a significant increase in disease-free and overall survival with this treatment. The postoperative nature of this trial thwarted implementation of surgical guidelines, and the extent of node dissection for most patients in the trial was suboptimal. Practitioners in some countries, such as Japan, dismiss the necessity of adjuvant postoperative adjuvant chemoradiation with the argument that this is only a salvage technique for inadequate surgery. A separate Korean chemoradiation series has shown benefit even for radically treated cases, however. For patients with good postoperative performance status, good organ function, and adequate nutrition, postoperative adjuvant chemoradiation therapy remains standard in North America for those who received up-front surgery.

A 2006 UK study of preoperative plus postoperative chemotherapy showed improvement in survival over surgery alone. In 2017, a newer chemotherapy regimen, FLOT (5-fluorouracil [Adrucil], leucovorin[1], oxaliplatin[1], and docetaxel [Taxotere]),

used in similar fashion, generated superior survival, and also more pathologic complete responses. FLOT is now considered an established regimen for perioperative chemotherapy. Preoperative chemotherapy is now recommended for localized advanced tumors, especially for those considered borderline resectable.

In Korea, a positive trial of adjuvant perioperative intraperitoneal chemotherapy has been reported. Considerable morbidity and mortality are associated with this adjuvant treatment, however, and it is unlikely it will be implemented without refinement and successful independent duplication of results.

For localized disease deemed not resectable to negative margins, both chemotherapy and chemoradiation have been used to convert such tumors to potentially resectable status. With successful negative-margin resection, some of these patients indeed survive free of disease long term. When localized unresected disease is documented to exist, administering chemoradiation with 5-fluorouracil as a radiation sensitizer can also result in some degree of 5-year survival (per reports, >10%).

Gastrointestinal Stromal Tumors

Gastrointestinal stromal tumors (GISTs) manifest as submucosal spindle cell tumors in the sarcoma family. In contrast to leiomyosarcomas and other spindle cell sarcomas, they express the antigen CD117, and most (>80%) tumors have activating mutations of *c-KIT*. Formerly considered rare, approximately 5000 of these tumors per year are now diagnosed in the United States. Owing to pattern of growth in the gastric wall, deep to the mucosa, early symptoms are unusual, and these tumors often grow to massive size before mucosal ulceration and hemorrhage (or other major symptoms) finally develop. GISTs are classified as sarcomas. Even low-risk GISTs (<5 cm and <1 mitosis per 10 high-power fields) can metastasize, and no GIST can be considered truly benign.

Treatment of localized primary GISTs consists of complete surgical resection, and a 2-cm margin of grossly normal tissue usually accomplishes this. Specific lymph node dissection is not indicated for this histology. Surgical series indicate that approximately 50% of primary gastric tumors metastasize and recur within 5 years. For patients with widespread metastases, generally located in the peritoneal cavity or the liver, first-line therapy is now a well-tolerated oral agent, imatinib mesylate (Gleevec or STI-571) at an initial dose of 400 mg daily, which generates partial responses in more than 50% of cases and stable disease in an additional 25% of cases. Side effects are minimal, and 1-year survival in treated patients is approximately 85%. On the basis of a completed American College of Surgeons Oncology Group (ACOSOG) trial, patients who have all disease completely resected should receive postoperative adjuvant therapy for at least 1 year.

For tumors resistant to imatinib, SU11248, sunitinib malate (Sutent), is now used as effective second-line therapy. Additional targeted biologic agents are under active investigation.

Carcinoid Tumors

The term "carcinoid" is reserved for a low-intermediate grade neuroendocrine tumor. In contrast, high-grade tumors are classified as "neuroendocrine carcinomas." In the stomach, the most common carcinoid (type I) is smaller (<2 cm in size), often multiple, and associated with chronic elevation of gastrin caused by either atrophic gastritis or gastrinoma. Behavior is generally benign, and such tumors have been shown to regress if gastrin levels can be normalized. In contrast, so-called "sporadic carcinoids" are usually >2 cm and unassociated with gastrin elevation. They are often aggressive and can spread to lymph nodes or liver. Complete, negative-margin resection with lymphadenectomy is recommended. When metastatic to the liver or other organs, surgical cytoreduction (or other means of tumor ablation) can offer considerable palliation to those with carcinoid syndrome, and this should always be considered. Octreotide (Sandostatin) therapy is now a palliative mainstay in all patients with carcinoid syndrome.

---

[1]Not FDA approved for this indication.

Gastric Lymphomas

Gastric lymphomas encompass most of the lymphoma subtypes, but low-grade, mucosa-associated B-cell lymphomas (B-cell MALT lymphomas) deserve special mention because they are strongly associated with *H pylori* infection. Indeed, localized cases can be controlled simply by treating the *H pylori* infection. In such cases, molecular studies indicate persistence of the offending lymphoid clone in about one half of cases. However, and, particularly if *H pylori* infection recurs, the lymphoma in such cases returns.

Aggressive, high-grade, diffuse-type B-cell gastric lymphomas, stage IE and IIE, once treated with multimodal therapy, are now treated with chemotherapy alone as the primary treatment, with or without radiotherapy. Surgical intervention is now reserved for emergencies, such as perforation.

For further information on this and other gastrointestinal lymphomas, please see the chapter on lymphoma.

References

Al-Batran SE, Homann N, Schmalenberg H et al., Perioperative chemotherapy with docetaxel, oxaliplatin, and fluorouracil/leucovorin (FLOT) versus epirubicin, cisplatin, and fluorouracil or capecitabine (ECF/ECX) for resectable gastric or gastroesophageal junction (GEJ) adenocarcinoma (FLOT4-AIO): A multicenter, randomized phase 3 trial. J Clin Oncol 2017 35:15_suppl, 4004.

Amin MB, Edge SB, Greene FL, et al., editors. AJCC Cancer Staging Manual. 8th ed. 2017.

Ferrucci PF, Zucca E: Primary gastric lymphoma pathogenesis and treatment: What has changed over the past 10 years? *Br J Haematol* 136(4):521–538, 2007.

Hundahl SA, Macdonald JS, Benedetti J, et al: Surgical treatment variation in a prospective, randomized trial of chemoradiotherapy in gastric cancer: The effect of undertreatment, *Ann Surg Oncol* 9(3):278–286, 2002.

Hundahl SA, Peeters KC, Kranenbarg EK, et al: Improved regional control and survival with "low Maruyama Index" surgery in gastric cancer: Autopsy findings from the Dutch D1-D2 Trial, *Gastric Cancer* 10(2):84–86, 2007.

Macdonald JS, Smalley SR, Benedetti J, et al: Chemoradiotherapy after surgery compared with surgery alone for adenocarcinoma of the stomach or gastroesophageal junction, *N Engl J Med* 345(10):725–730, 2001.

Modlin IM, Kidd M, Latich I, et al: Current status of gastrointestinal carcinoids, *Gastroenterology* 128(6):1717–1751, 2005.

Siehl J, Thiel E: C-kit, GIST, and imatinib. Recent Results, *Cancer Res* 176:145–151, 2007.

5 Endocrine and Metabolic Disorders

ACROMEGALY

Method of
Moises Mercado, MD

CURRENT DIAGNOSIS

Clinical
- Headaches, visual field defects
- Coarse features, increased size of hands (rings) and feet (shoes)
- Thick, oily skin, skin tags, acanthosis nigricans
- Arthralgias, osteoarthritis
- Paresthesias, carpal tunnel syndrome
- Hypertension, arrhythmia, heart failure
- Glucose intolerance, diabetes, hypertriglyceridemia
- Snoring, sleep apnea
- Risk of colon polyps or colon cancer
- Risk of thyroid cancer

Biochemical
- Glucose-suppressed growth hormone >0.4 ng/mL by ultrasensitive assays or >1 ng/mL by old radioimmunoassays
- Elevated age-adjusted insulin-like growth factor 1

Imaging
- Magnetic resonance imaging

CURRENT THERAPY

- If a pituitary surgeon is available: Transsphenoidal surgery for microadenomas, intrasellar macroadenomas, and debulking or decompressing surgery in invasive macroadenomas
- Depot Somatostatin analogues (lanreotide autogel [Somatuline Depot] or octreotide LAR [Sandostatin LAR Depot]) as secondary treatment for patients failing surgery or waiting for radiotherapy effect to occur and as a primary treatment for patients with inaccessible lesions, contraindications for surgery, or preference
- Dopamine agonists: Cabergoline (DOSTINEX)[1] is effective alone or in combination with somatostatin analogues in 15% to 30% of patients
- Growth hormone receptor antagonists: Pegvisomant (Somavert) for patients resistant or intolerant to somatostatin analogues and who have tumors >5 mm from the optic chiasm
- Radiotherapy for patients resistant or intolerant to pharmacologic therapy, with clinically and biochemically active disease and a tumor remnant on MRI

[1]Not FDA approved for this indication.

Acromegaly is a disorder resulting from an excessive secretion of growth hormone (GH), with a prevalence of 40 to 60 cases per million and an annual incidence of 3 to 4 per million.

Physiology, Biochemistry, and Regulation of the GH/IGF-1 Axis

GH secretion is regulated at the hypothalamus (Figure 1). The pulsatile secretion of GH-releasing hormone (GHRH) stimulates somatotroph proliferation and GH gene transcription, whereas somatostatin, which is secreted tonically, inhibits GH synthesis. These two hypothalamic signals result in the pulsatile secretion of pituitary GH, with most pulses occurring during the night. GH is also stimulated by ghrelin, a hypothalamic and gastrointestinal orexigenic hormone that binds specific receptors in the somatotroph known as GH-secretagogue receptors. GH exerts its actions through a specific membrane receptor located predominantly in the liver and cartilage, but ubiquitously present in all tissues. One molecule of GH interacts with two molecules of GH receptor, resulting in functional dimerization and conformational changes that lead to the phosphorylation of several kinases and eventually the interaction with target genes such as the insulin-like growth factor (IGF)-1 gene.

IGF-1 is closely related to proinsulin and circulates in plasma bound to six binding proteins (IGFBPs) that are synthesized and released by the liver. IGFBP3 is the most important of these binding proteins and is also GH dependent; it forms a heterotrimeric complex composed of BP3, IGF-1, and the acid-labile subunit (ALS). IGF-1 is responsible for most of the trophic and growth-promoting effects of GH. Blood levels of IGF-1 are increased during puberty, coinciding with the acceleration of somatic growth, and decline with aging. Malnutrition, poorly controlled type 1 diabetes, hypothyroidism, and liver failure all result in diminished IGF-1 concentrations. IGF-1 is the main player in GH negative feedback regulation and it acts at both the pituitary and the hypothalamic levels. Glucose regulates GH release by increasing (hyperglycemia) or decreasing (hypoglycemia) somatostatin synthesis in the hypothalamus. Exercise and amino acids such as arginine also stimulate GH secretion.

Etiopathogenesis of Growth Hormone–Secreting Tumors

The molecular pathogenesis of pituitary tumors includes the inactivation of tumor suppressor genes, the activation of oncogenes, and the trophic effect of factors such as the hypothalamic releasing hormones. Approximately 40% of GH-producing tumors in whites harbor somatic point mutations of the α subunit stimulatory G protein coupled to the GHRH receptor (GSPα mutations). This molecular alteration causes constitutive activation of the GHRH receptor, resulting in an increased transcription of the GH gene and the promotion of somatotroph proliferation. Acromegalic patients whose tumors harbor GSPα mutations usually have a more benign clinical course and appear to be more susceptible to management with somatostatin analogues. Nonwhite acromegalic populations, including persons of Japanese, Korean, and Mexican heritage, have a much lower prevalence of GSPα mutations.

Other molecular events should be present in GSPα-negative somatotrophinomas. Menin is a protein encoded by a tumor suppressor gene located on the short arm of chromosome 11. Inactivating mutations of menin are the molecular basis of type 1 multiple endocrine neoplasia (MEN1); however, GH-secreting tumors occurring out of this context do not have such genetic abnormalities. Inactivating mutations of other putative tumor-suppressor genes located relatively close to the menin locus have been described in several kindreds with familial acromegaly;

Figure 1 GH is regulated positively by GHRH and negatively by somatostatin. Fifty percent of circulating GH is bound to the GH binding protein, which represents the extracellular portion of the GH receptor. One molecule of GH dimerizes two molecules of GH receptor, and the ensuing signal transduction results in IGF-1 synthesis and secretion, which exerts negative feedback on GH secretion at the hypothalamic and pituitary levels. *Abbreviations:* ALS = acid-labile subunit; GH = growth hormone; GHRH = growth hormone–releasing hormone; IGF = insulin-like growth factor; IGFBP3 = insulin-like growth factor binding protein 3; IRS = insulin receptor S; JAK2 = Janus kinase 2; SRIH = somatostatin; SSTR = somatostatin receptor.

however, they do not seem to play an important oncogenic role in the sporadic form of the disease. Other genetic alterations such as underexpression of GADD 45γ (growth arrest and DNA damage-inducible protein) and overexpression of the securing molecule PTTG (pituitary tumor transforming gene) have also been shown to be involved in the molecular pathogenesis of acromegaly. Although hereditary acromegaly is rare (less than 2% of the cases), familial somatotrophinomas account for 30% of the tumors seen in the syndrome of familial isolated pituitary adenomas. Patients with isolated familial somatotrophinomas are younger and usually have more aggressive tumors than subjects with sporadic acromegaly. Affected members do not show any molecular alterations in the MEN1 gene. However, 15% of 73 tested families harbor inactivating, germline mutations of the AIP (aryl hydrocarbon interacting protein) gene located on chromosome 11q13.3.

In more than 90% of cases, acromegaly is caused by a sporadic pituitary adenoma. In approximately 70% of these patients, these benign epithelial neoplasms are larger than 1 cm in diameter and are known as *macroadenomas*, whereas one-third of the patients harbor lesions smaller than 1 cm or *microadenomas*. One-third of the patients have tumors that cosecrete GH and prolactin (PRL) (mammosomatoroph cell adenomas). Real pituitary GH-secreting carcinomas, with documented metastasis as the irrefutable malignancy criterion, are exceedingly rare. On rare occasions, acromegaly results from GHRH-secreting neuroendocrine tumors, usually located in the lungs, thymus, or endocrine pancreas. In this scenario, the ectopically produced GHRH leads to hyperplasia of the somatotroph, with the consequent excessive production of GH. Even less common are GH-secreting tumors arising in ectopic pituitary tissue, usually located in the sphenoid sinus. A case of GH-secreting lymphoma has been reported.

Clinical Manifestations
Acromegaly develops insidiously over many years. An 8- to 10-year delay in diagnosis has been estimated from the beginning of the first symptom. Clinical characteristics are often attributed to aging. Symptoms and signs can be divided into those resulting from the compressive effects of the pituitary tumor and those that are a consequence of the GH and IGF-1 excess.

Local Tumor Effects
Headache results from an increase in intracranial pressure and from the effects of GH itself; it is usually described as a dull pain that

persists throughout the day. Occasionally, large tumors invading laterally into the cavernous sinuses give rise to cranial nerve syndromes, usually third and sixth. Visual field defects are relatively common with macroadenomas extending superiorly and compressing the optic chiasm. This usually results in different combinations of bitemporal homonymous hemianopia or quadrontopia.

Consequences of the GH/IGF-1 Excess
Skeletal Growth and Skin Changes
A GH excess developing before the pubertal closure of epiphyseal bone leads to an acceleration of linear growth, and this results in gigantism. Once the patient is in adulthood, the GH/IGF-1 excess results in acral enlargement, which is manifested by increases in ring and shoe sizes as well as enlargement of the nose, supraciliary arches, frontal bones, and mandible. There is thickening of soft tissues of the hands and feet; hands are fleshy and bulky and the heel pad is increased. The skin is thickened due to the deposition of glycosaminoglycans and excessive collagen production. Hyperhidrosis and seborrhea occur in 60% of patients; skin tags (previously associated with colon cancer) and acanthosis nigricans are common.

Musculoskeletal System
Generalized arthralgias are present in the majority (80%) of patients. Degenerative osteoarthritis is more common than in the general population. Paresthesias of the hands and feet and a proximal painful myopathy are often reported. Nerve entrapment syndromes such as the carpal tunnel syndrome occur in nearly half of patients.

Cardiovascular System
Arterial hypertension is found in 30% of patients, and when associated with diabetes, it contributes to the increased mortality rate of the disease. Hyperaldosteronism with low renin levels and the resulting sodium retention play an important role in the pathogenesis of hypertension, but other contributors such as an increased sympathetic tone are also present. Echocardiographic findings include left ventricular and septal hypertrophy with varying degrees of diastolic dysfunction. Symptomatic cardiac disease develops in 15% of patients and is usually due to coronary artery disease, heart failure, and arrhythmias. Although the existence of an acromegalic cardiomyopathy is still controversial, there are patients without hypertension and with angiographically normal coronaries, who develop severe congestive heart failure, in whom

histologic evidence of subendocardial, subepicardial, and myocardial fibrosis and necrosis has been documented.

Respiratory Abnormalities
The majority of patients with acromegaly are affected by loud snoring. A significant fraction of these have sleep apnea (with both central and obstructive components) with significant drops in oxygen saturation, which can be complicated by arrhythmias, daytime somnolence, and chronic fatigue.

Abnormalities in Glucose Metabolism
Chronic GH hypersecretion creates a state of insulin resistance, and glucose intolerance has been reported in 30% to 50% of patients with acromegaly; the percentage with fasting hyperglycemia can be close to 30%, depending on the population. Hyperglycemia has correlated with GH concentrations in some studies and with IGF-1 levels in others. Although successful treatment of acromegaly, be it by surgical, pharmacological, or radiotherapeutical interventions, results in significant improvements in metabolic control, the prevalence of diabetes remains higher than in the general population.

Abnormalities in Lipid Metabolism
The classic lipid profile consists of diminished total cholesterol, along with elevated triglyceride concentrations. Intermediate-density lipoprotein (IDL) particles and lipoprotein(a) might also be elevated, and there is a higher percentage of the more atherogenic type II low-density lipoprotein (LDL).

Bone and Calcium Metabolism
Acromegaly is associated with hypercalciuria and hyperphosphatemia. High serum 25-hydroxyvitamin D_3 and urinary levels of hydroxyproline can be found, reflecting a state of increased bone turnover. Cortical bone mineral density is elevated, whereas trabecular bone mass is diminished.

Neoplasia
Retrospective studies suggested that colonic adenomatous polyps and adenocarcinoma were more frequent in acromegalic patients than in the general population. Prospective studies have demonstrated that the risk, albeit smaller than previously thought, is real and probably justifies screening colonoscopy in these patients. Patients with uncontrolled acromegaly have a higher risk of recurrence of premalignant polyps and a higher mortality rate from colon cancer compared with subjects with biochemically controlled disease and the general population. Recently, an increased incidence of well-differentiated thyroid carcinoma has been documented.

Associated Endocrine Abnormalities
A euthyroid goiter is often found but seldom requires specific treatment. Hypopituitarism occurs variably, depending on the size and extension of the tumor and whether the patient has undergone surgery or radiation therapy. Hypogonadotropic hypogonadism is the most common pituitary deficiency, occurring in 20% of patients. A decreased libido is a common presenting complaint in both male and female patients with acromegaly; women often have menstrual and ovulatory disturbances and men complain of impotence.

Although an elevated PRL is common, it does not always reflect cosecretion of this hormone by the somatotrophinoma, but rather an interruption of the descending dopaminergic tone by the tumor compressing the pituitary stalk. Central hypocortisolism and hypothyroidism are less common.

GH-secreting pituitary adenomas are the second, after prolactinomas, pituitary tumor occurring in the context of MEN1 (multiple parathyroid adenomas, pituitary adenoma, and pancreatic islet cell tumors). Acromegaly can also develop in patients with the McCune-Albright syndrome (polyostotic fibrous dysplasia, café au lait spots, and endocrinopathies such as sexual precocity and autonomous thyroid nodules), and occurs in the context of the Carney complex.

Mortality
Life expectancy in patients with acromegaly is decreased by about 10 to 15 years, and the standardized mortality ratio is 1.5 to 2. Most patients die of cardiovascular causes, followed by cerebrovascular events, respiratory abnormalities, and neoplastic diseases. Hormonal control has a definite impact on survival. Lowering serum GH to less than 2.5 ng/mL results in reduction of the mortality rate to levels comparable with the general population. These safe GH levels were obtained using old radioimmunoassays, and there are no equivalent studies using ultrasensitive GH assays. IGF-1 levels have not been as good as GH as independent predictors of mortality. Other factors associated with an increased mortality include advanced age and the presence of hypertension and diabetes. Mortality rate in acromegaly can be reduced to that seen on the general population when patients are treated using a multidisciplinary approach not only aiming at controlling the GH and IGF-1 levels but also focusing on the management of comorbidities.

Biochemical Diagnosis
Due to the pulsatile nature of GH secretion, random determinations of this hormone are not useful in the diagnosis of acromegaly. The gold standard for the diagnosis is the measurement of GH after an oral glucose load of 75 g; current guidelines state that suppression to less than 0.4 ng/mL (using ultrasensitive assays) reliably excludes the diagnosis. Situations associated with decreased suppression of GH by glucose include puberty, pregnancy, use of oral contraceptives, uncontrolled diabetes, and renal and hepatic insufficiency.

IGF-1 levels reflect the integrated concentrations over 24 hours of GH and correlate well with clinical activity. Blood IGF-1 concentrations decrease with age, reflecting the parallel decline of the somatotropic axis. There is a gender difference in IGF-1 (premenopausal women have lower levels than age-matched male subjects). Other conditions that lower IGF-1 levels include malnutrition, uncontrolled diabetes, and hepatic and renal failure. Normal ranges for IGF-1 should be established in each particular center based on age. The determination of other GH-dependent peptides such as IGFBP3 and ALS has not proved to be superior to IGF-1.

Imaging
Pituitary magnetic resonance imaging (MRI) with gadolinium enhancement allows visualization of lesions as small as 2 or 3 mm in diameter. High-resolution computed tomography (CT) is a reasonable alternative, although it is much less sensitive. An ectopic source of GHRH should be suspected when the MRI is completely normal. In these rare cases, serum GHRH should be measured and the ectopic tumor should be sought, usually with high-resolution CT of the chest and abdomen.

Treatment
The decision as to what therapeutic modality should be used has to take into account medical issues (cardiopulmonary comorbidities, size, and extension of the tumor) as well as the local characteristics of the treating center. The latter refers to the availability of pituitary surgeons and radiotherapeutic technologies as well as the economic feasibility of pharmacologic therapy.

Surgery
Transsphenoidal surgery has been the traditional treatment for acromegaly and achieves biochemical cure (achievement of a post-glucose GH <1 ng/mL and normalization of IGF-1) in 80% to 90% of microadenomas. According to the latest published acromegaly consensus, biochemical cure is defined as a glucose-suppressed GH of 0.4 ng/mL as well as a normal age-adjusted IGF-1. Cure rates for macroadenomas are much lower (40%–50%), and invasive lesions have a very slight chance (<10%) of being cured by surgery. Even though surgery often fails to achieve a full biochemical cure, debulking the pituitary adenoma relieves optic chiasm compression and can result in a sufficient decrement of tumor mass (and therefore of GH production) to allow better results with either pharmacologic or radiotherapeutic regimens.

Pharmacologic Therapy

Somatostatin analogues are the most commonly used medical treatment for acromegaly. Somatostatin inhibits GH secretion and somatotroph cell growth via its interaction with five different somatostatin receptor (SSTR) subtypes. The development of long-acting somatostatin analogues such as octreotide (Sandostatin) and lanreotide (Somatuline) overcame the pharmacologic difficulties of native somatostatin (short half-life, rebound GH secretion, and need for IV administration) and resulted in a more potent inhibition of GH secretion. The most commonly used preparations are intramuscular octreotide LAR (long-acting repeatable) (Sandostatin LAR Depot) and subcutaneous lanreotide autogel (Somatuline Depot), which are administered every 4 weeks. Doses of octreotide-LAR range from 10 to 40 mg and those of lanreotide autogel from 60 to 120 mg, both administered every 4 weeks, although in specific patients the interval of injection can be increased to every 6 or even 8 weeks, thus diminishing the cost of therapy. Octreotide and lanreotide have very high affinities for SSTR-2 and to a lesser extent SSTR-5, which are precisely the most commonly expressed somatostatin receptors in GH-secreting adenomas.

When used after surgery has failed, somatostatin analogues can achieve a safe and a normal IGF-1 in 25% to 35% of patients. Primary treatment with somatostatin analogues is increasingly being used in patients with invasive tumors, when cardiopulmonary contraindications are present, and more recently as a result of the patient's or treating physician's preference. In these settings, biochemical success rates (achievement of a GH <2.5 ng/mL and normalization of IGF-1) have ranged between 30% and 80%, and more than 80% report significant relief of symptoms. More recent trials performed in unselected populations reveal that the real success rate lies between 25% and 35%. Tumor shrinkage occurs in 70% of primarily treated patients. Overall, treatment success is directly related to the abundance of SSTR-2 and SSTR-5 in the tumor. Lower pretreatment GH levels are also associated with a better response to somatostatin analogues. Side effects of somatostatin analogues, including nausea, abdominal pain, alopecia, and biliary sludge, occur in 20% of subjects. The currently recommended biochemical targets when treating patients with somatostatin analogues are the achievement of a GH of 1 ng/mL and an IGF-1 level within the normal age-adjusted range patients with somatostatin analogues is 1 ng/mL.

Pegvisomant (Somavert) is a GH mutant that prevents functional dimerization of the GH receptor, thus acting as an antagonist. Its use results in normalization of IGF-1 in more than 70% of patients, while increasing GH levels. Concern about adenoma growth due to the abolition of IGF-1 negative feedback on the tumoral somatotroph prevents its use in patients with very large lesions in close proximity to the optic chiasm. Transient elevations of liver aminotransferases can occur, although this seldom requires drug discontinuation. Pegvisomant does not compromise insulin secretion, as somatostatin analogues do. GH-receptor antagonists are expensive and should not be used as primary treatment; they are currently indicated in patients who are intolerant or have failed somatostatin analogue therapy.

Few patients respond marginally to difficult-to-tolerate large doses of bromocriptine. Newer dopamine agonists, such as cabergoline,[1] are better tolerated and achieve biochemical control in 20% to 30% of patients. Combination treatment with cabergoline and octreotide appears to be promising in cases resistant to somatostatin analogues.

Radiation Therapy

Both external-beam radiotherapy and radiosurgery are indicated in patients with persistent disease and a demonstrable tumor remnant who are either intolerant or resistant to pharmacologic treatment. Biochemical success occurs in 20% to 60% and requires many years to become apparent. Hypopituitarism, involving at least two axes, develops in more than 50% of patients within 10 years. Serious adverse effects such as brain necrosis and optic nerve damage seldom occur with the currently used techniques that minimize radiation to the normal surrounding tissues. With the currently available radiation techniques, radiotherapy is an effective and safe treatment alternative. The two major drawbacks of radiotherapy are the time it takes to achieve biochemical control and the almost unavoidable induction of hypopituitarism.

Novel pharmacologic therapies are being developed, some of which will likely become useful particularly in patients who do not respond to current somatostatin analogues. These include the so-called "universal" somatostatin analogue pasireotide (Signifor LAR), which is capable of interacting not only with the SSTRs 2 and 5, but also with subtypes 1 and 3. Pasireotide seems to be slightly more effective than octreotide in achieving GH and IGF-1 targets; however, its major drawback is the worsening of hyperglycemia. Dopastatin[5] is a recently developed chimeric compound that behaves both as an analog and as a dopamine agonist; clinical trials had to be discontinued at early stages due to lack of efficacy. Oral octreotide, known as octreolin,[5] is a new preparation of octreotide acetate attached to a transient permeability enhancer, which selectively allows the translocation of the somatostatin analog through the paracellular tight junctions. Recently tested in a phase III trial its efficacy is almost equivalent as that of parenteral octreotide but it has not been approved by the FDA.

---

[5] Investigational drug in the United States.

References

Beckers A, Daly AF: The clinical, pathological and genetic features of familial isolated pituitary adenomas, *Eur J Endocrinol* 157:371–382, 2007.

Bevan JS: Clinical review: the antitumoral effects of somatostatin analog therapy in acromegaly, *J Clin Endocrinol Metab* 90:1856–1863, 2005.

Colao A, Ferone D, Marzullo P, Lombardi G: Systemic complications of acromegaly: epidemiology, pathogenesis and management, *Endocr Rev* 25:102–152, 2004.

Espinosa E, Ramirez C, Mercado M: The multimodal treatment of acromegaly: current status and future perspectives, *Endocr Metab Immune Disord Drug Targets* 14:169–181, 2014.

Espinosa-de-Los-Monteros AL, González B, Vargas G, et al: Clinical and biochemical characteristics of acromegalic patients with different abnormalities of glucose metabolism, *Pituitary* 14:231–235, 2011.

Espinosa de los Monteros AL, Gonzalez B, Vargas G, et al: Octreotide LAR treatment of acromegaly in "real life": long term outcome at a tertiary care center, *Pituitary* 18:290–296, 2015.

Espinosa-de-Los-Monteros AL, Sosa E, Cheng S, et al: Biochemical evaluation of disease activity after pituitary surgery in acromegaly: a critical analysis of patients who spontaneously change disease status, *Clin Endocrinol* 64:245–249, 2006.

Freda P: Current concepts in the biochemical assessment of the patient with acromegaly, *Growth Horm IGF Res* 13:171–184, 2003.

Gadelha MR, Kasuki L, Lim DST, Fleseriu M: Systemic complications of acromegaly and the impac of the current treatment landscape: an update, *Endocr Rev* 40:268–332, 2019.

Giustina A, Chanson P, Bronstein MD: A consensus on criteria for cure of acromegaly, *J Clin Endocrinol Metab* 95:3141–3148, 2010.

Giustina A, Chanson P, Kleinberg D, et al: Expert consensus document: a consensus on the medical treatment of acromegaly, *Nat Rev Endocrinol* 10:243–248, 2014.

Gonzalez-Virla B, Vargas-Ortega G, Martinez-Vazquez KB, Espinosa de los Monteros AL, Sosa-Eroza E, López-Felix B, Mendoza-Zubieta V, Mercado M: Effocacy and safety of fractionated conformal radiation therapy in acromegaly: A long-term follow-up study, *Endocrine* 65:386–392, 2019.

Holdaway IM, Rajasoorya RC, Gamble GD: Factors influencing mortality in acromegaly, *J Clin Endocrinol Metab* 89:667–674, 2004.

Kopchick JJ, Parkinson C, Stevens EC, Trainer PJ: Growth hormone receptor antagonists: discovery, development, and use in patients with acromegaly, *Endocr Rev* 23:623–646, 2002.

Mercado M, Espinosa E, Ramirez C: Current status and future directions of pharmacological therapy for acromegaly, *Minerva Endocrinol* 41:351–365, 2016.

Mercado M, Gonzalez B, Vargas G, et al: Successful mortality reduction and of comorbidities in patients with acromegaly followed at a highly specialized multidisciplinary clinic, *J Clin Endocrinol Metab* 99:4438–4446, 2014.

Mercado M, Ramirez-Rentería C: Metabolic complications of acromegaly, *Front Horm Res* 49:20–28, 2018.

Portocarrero-Ortiz LA, Vergara-Lopez A, Vidrio-Velazquez M, et al: The Mexican Acromegaly Registry: clinical and biochemical characteristics at diagnosis and therapeutic outcomes, *J Clin Endocrinol Metab* 101:3997–4004, 2016.

---

[1] Not FDA approved for this indication.

ADRENOCORTICAL INSUFFICIENCY

Method of
Fabienne Langlois, MD; and Maria Fleseriu, MD

CURRENT DIAGNOSIS

- Initial diagnosis of adrenocortical insufficiency (AI) is based in most cases on a morning cortisol level, measured at 8–9 AM in patients with a normal circadian rhythm.
- A morning cortisol level less than 5 μg/dL supports diagnosis, and a value greater than 15 μg/dL effectively rules out AI.
- To confirm diagnosis, especially in cases with intermediate cortisol values, a high-dose (250 μg) cosyntropin (Cortrosyn) stimulation test is suggested with a normal cutoff peak cortisol greater than 18 to 20 μg/dL at 30 or 60 minutes.
- Primary AI is characterized by elevated endogenous adrenocorticotropic hormone (ACTH) levels and absence of mineralocorticoid hormones in addition to glucocorticoid deficiency; antibody screening and/or adrenal imaging is indicated.
- Secondary AI is characterized by an inappropriately normal or low endogenous ACTH level and low cortisol with preserved mineralocorticoid hormones. If exogenous glucocorticoid use is ruled out, magnetic resonance imaging (MRI) of the pituitary sella is appropriate.

CURRENT THERAPY

- Oral hydrocortisone (Cortef) is the preferred form of steroid to attain physiologic replacement. Doses are usually 15 to 20 mg divided into two or three daily doses, with the highest dose in the morning.
- In case of physiologic stress, such as fever, severe infection, or minor surgery, doses should be doubled or tripled (depending on the type of stress or procedure) for the duration of the event.
- In patients with primary AI, fludrocortisone (Florinef), a mineralocorticoid, should be added to the treatment regimen, with a typical dose between 0.05 and 0.1 mg daily.
- For adrenal crisis in patients with known AI, administer hydrocortisone injection (Solu-Cortef) 50 to 100 mg IV every 6 to 8 hours along with generous volumes of saline.
- Patients should wear a medical alert bracelet or necklace and have frequent education regarding AI and treatment and prevention of adrenal crisis.

Epidemiology

Primary AI, also known as Addison disease when of autoimmune cause, has a prevalence of 100 to 140 cases per million persons. More than 90% of primary AI in the developed world is secondary to autoimmune adrenalitis, and it is more common in women. Secondary AI caused by therapeutic glucocorticoid administration is the most prevalent; pituitary tumors and surgeries are other common etiologies.

Risk Factors
Primary Adrenocortical Insufficiency

A personal or family history of autoimmune disease (e.g., type 1 diabetes, Hashimoto disease, vitiligo, pernicious anemia) is a risk factor for autoimmune adrenalitis. Especially in the context of acute AI in the hospital, thrombosis and secondary hemorrhage must be ruled out and the possibility of heparin-induced thrombocytopenia (HIT) must be elicited if the patient is receiving parenteral anticoagulation. Miliary tuberculosis is the most frequent cause of primary AI in developed countries. Infiltration in the context of malignancy is often due to a known plurimetastatic cancer; other infiltrative diseases are rare.

Secondary Adrenocortical Insufficiency

The most prevailing risk factor for secondary AI is prolonged use of exogenous glucocorticoids. Patients taking more than 5 mg of prednisone or equivalent for longer than 3 weeks are at risk for secondary AI. In some patients with glucocorticoid receptor hypersensitivity, even smaller doses of glucocorticoid other than oral (topical, injected, or inhaled) can also suppress the hypothalamo-pituitary-adrenal axis. Immunotherapy-related hypophysitis can be due to blockage of cytotoxic T-lymphocytes antigen-4 (CTLA-4), programmed cell death 1 (PD-1), and/or its ligand (PD-L1), and is rarely reversible. Chronic opioid use can also suppress central ACTH and induce AI.

Patients with a tumor of the hypothalamic–pituitary region or history of treatment of such tumors with surgery and/or radiation are at significant risk. Patient with traumatic brain injury may experience AI in both the acute and/or recovery phase and can be transient or permanent. Other causes, such as autoimmune lymphocytic hypophysitis, are most frequent peripartum, either in the third trimester or postpartum. Sheehan syndrome is rare and characterized by pituitary apoplexy secondary to shock due to severe blood loss during parturition.

Pathophysiology

Primary AI is characterized by a complete destruction of the adrenal cortex, inducing deficits in all hormones: glucocorticoid, mineralocorticoid, and androgens. With loss of cortisol feedback inhibition, ACTH will be markedly elevated. Secondary AI is the result of isolated low glucocorticoid production due a defect at the pituitary or hypothalamus level resulting in low [or inappropriately normal] ACTH. Mineralocorticoid activity is maintained in secondary AI, as it is controlled by the renin-angiotensin-aldosterone system.

Prevention

No clinically practical strategy for preventing primary AI exists. Glucocorticoid-associated secondary AI may be prevented through judicious use of systemic glucocorticoids, with efforts made to limit administration of glucocorticoids to the lowest effective dose for the shortest possible time.

Clinical Manifestations
Primary Adrenocortical Insufficiency

The presentation of primary AI is sometimes dramatic, with a constellation of weakness, fatigue, anorexia, weight loss, nausea, abdominal pain, salt craving, and orthostatic hypotension. Symptoms start as subtle and nonspecific in some patients but may evolve rapidly in adrenal crisis. The skin and buccal mucosa are often hyperpigmented, owing to the effect of excess ACTH on cutaneous melanocortin receptors. Hyponatremia and hyperkalemia (as a result of mineralocorticoid deficiency) are often present.

Secondary Adrenocortical Insufficiency

The presentation of secondary AI is more insidious, with weight loss, fatigue, and malaise as presenting features. This often leads to a delay in diagnosis. Because production of mineralocorticoid is relatively intact in secondary AI, electrolyte abnormalities and hypotension are rarer. Hyperpigmentation is not present, reflecting normal or low ACTH levels. Laboratory abnormalities are less common, but hypoglycemia is occasionally seen, especially with concomitant growth hormone deficiency. Because isolated ACTH deficiency is rare, signs and symptoms of other pituitary hormone abnormalities, such as hyperprolactinemia, central hypogonadism, growth hormone deficiency, or central hypothyroidism, may be present. Secondary AI may be masked by concomitant central hypothyroidism.

Diagnosis

Morning cortisol (within 2 hours of waking up) of 5 μg/dL or less has a relatively high predictive value for AI, and a morning cortisol level greater than 15 μg/dL effectively rules out AI. To confirm the diagnosis of AI, a cortisol stimulation test is performed. Insulin tolerance testing has largely been replaced by stimulation testing with synthetic cosyntropin (ACTH—Cortrosyn, Synacthen). ACTH stimulation testing of cortisol is a reliable method of evaluating the adrenal reserve. In high-dose testing, a cortisol level is checked before and 30 and 60 minutes after 250 μg of IV cosyntropin is administered. A peak cortisol level greater than 18 to 20 μg/dL defines a normal response. Cosyntropin testing should not be used in cases of short-term secondary insufficiency, such as apoplexy or after recent pituitary surgery, because adrenal atrophy must have occurred for the adrenal response to cosyntropin to be blunted. The low-dose (1 μg) test measures cortisol 20 to 30 minutes after cosyntropin administration and may be more sensitive for diagnosis of secondary AI, with cutoff of 16–18 μg/dL. However, the high-dose (250 μg) test remains the standard. One must consider the total serum cortisol as affected by its binding protein, which is elevated by high estrogen levels and could be low in hypoalbuminemia. If the clinical picture is not concordant with the investigation, an endocrinology consult should be sought.

Once diagnosis is confirmed, a low or normal plasma ACTH level indicates secondary AI, although care must be taken with the methodology of the test as some immunoassays for ACTH can give falsely low results if preanalytic precautions are not respected. An elevated ACTH level (more than twofold the upper limit of normal) typically indicates primary AI, and hyperkalemia, high plasma renin, and simultaneously low aldosterone, levels will confirm associated mineralocorticoid deficiency. After the diagnosis of primary versus secondary AI has been established, an etiology should be sought (Boxes 1 and 2). Serology for antiadrenal (21-hydroxylase) antibodies or evidence of other autoimmune diseases is useful in primary AI, given the very large fraction of these patients with autoimmune adrenalitis. Enlarged adrenal glands with high-density areas or calcification on computed tomography can suggest granulomatous disease or neoplasm. Acute hematoma or fluid collections around the adrenals during an acute adrenal crisis can indicate adrenal hemorrhage. Secondary AI is most often associated with chronic glucocorticoid therapy but may be caused by a number of other diseases affecting the hypothalamo-pituitary region. If exogenous steroids have been excluded, MRI and testing of the other pituitary axes are appropriate.

Differential Diagnosis

Because the presentation of AI can be subtle (especially in secondary AI), the differential diagnosis is broad and includes a number of illnesses associated with fatigue, weight loss, and malaise, including occult malignancies, renal or hepatic dysfunction, and endocrinologic electrolyte disturbances. In acute AI crisis, differential diagnosis includes other systemic illnesses associated with orthostatic hypotension and electrolyte abnormalities, including dehydration and distributive and septic shock. Fever can be part of an AI crisis, but one must rule out an infectious process as the precipitating cause.

Treatment

Glucocorticoid replacement is recommended with oral hydrocortisone two or three times daily. One-half to two-thirds of the daily dose is given upon waking, and the dosage is roughly 15 to 20 mg per day (or 10–12 mg/m² body surface area per day), typically 10 or 15 mg in the morning and 5 mg in the afternoon. Once-daily, modified-release hydrocortisone is available in Europe and may better mimic the physiological circadian rhythm of cortisol, but it is not yet available in the United States.

Patients should be instructed to increase this dosage according to physiologic stress, as doses should be doubled or tripled for 3 or more days in case of fever or intercurrent systemic illness. Day-to-day emotional stress does not require an increment in dosing. For surgery, parenteral glucocorticoid doses should be administered according to the level of surgical stress, such as 25 mg for minor stress (e.g., cataract surgery), 50 to 75 mg for moderate

stress (e.g., cholecystectomy), and 100 to 150 mg daily in divided doses for major stress (e.g., heart surgery).

Patients should wear a medical alert bracelet or necklace and should be dispensed hydrocortisone or dexamethasone injection with instructions for home self-administration in case of vomiting and inability to take oral doses. If symptoms do not improve within hours after injection, patients should seek an urgent medical evaluation.

Mineralocorticoid replacement is indicated in most patients with primary AI, and fludrocortisone (Florinef) is the available drug with a typical dose between 0.05 and 0.2 mg once daily.

If a patient with known AI presents in adrenal crisis, hydrocortisone (Solu-Cortef) 150 to 250 mg per day, divided, every 6 to 8 hours is an appropriate initial therapy, with the dose tapered to an appropriate oral dose as the patient's condition improves.

| BOX 1 | Causes of Primary Adrenocortical Insufficiency |

Autoimmune
Isolated
Autoimmune polyglandular syndromes 1 and 2

Infectious
Fungal
  Tuberculosis
  Histoplasmosis
Viral
  Human immunodeficiency virus
  Cytomegalovirus
Parasitic
Syphilis
Rarely bacterial

Bilateral Adrenal Infarction
Hemorrhage
  Anticoagulation
  Sepsis (e.g., meningococcemia)
  Trauma
Thrombosis
  Thrombophilic condition (e.g., antiphospholipid antibody syndrome)
  Heparin-induced thrombocytopenia

Neoplastic
Metastatic cancer
  Breast
  Colon
  Melanoma
  Lymphoma
Non–small cell lung cancer

Drugs
Ketoconazole (Nizoral)
Mitotane (Lysodren)
Etomidate perfusion (Amidate)

Infiltrative Diseases
Hemochromatosis
Primary amyloidosis
Sarcoidosis

Postbilateral Adrenalectomy
For bilateral tumors or intractable Cushing syndrome

Familial or Genetic
Classical congenital adrenal hyperplasia
Adrenoleukodystrophy
Familial glucocorticoid deficiency
Adrenocorticotropic hormone insensitivity syndromes
X-linked adrenal hypoplasia (associated with DAX-1 mutation, may be late-onset)
Triple-A or Allgrove syndrome (alacrymia, achalasia, adrenal insufficiency)

BOX 2 Etiologies of Secondary Adrenocortical Insufficiency

Iatrogenic/Medication
Chronic steroid therapy, most often oral or parenteral, but could also be inhaled, topical, or injected
Chronic opioid therapy
Immunotherapy (CTLA-4 and PD1/PDL-1 inhibitors)

Pituitary Injury
Post-transsphenoidal or transcranial surgery
Radiation to the sella
Infarction (e.g., Sheehan)
Traumatic brain injury

Tumors of the Sella
Pituitary adenoma
Craniopharyngioma
Meningioma
Rathke cleft cyst
Metastatic cancer

Infiltrative Diseases
Sarcoidosis, tuberculosis, or other granulomatous diseases
Lymphocytic hypophysitis
Idiopathic adrenocorticotropic hormone deficiency
Adrenal insufficiency
Associated with cirrhosis
Associated with critical illness

Acknowledgments
The authors thank Justin Moore, MD, the author of the previous chapter version, and Shirley McCartney, PhD, for editorial assistance.

References
Annane D, Pastores SM, Rochwerg B, et al: Guidelines for the Diagnosis and Management of Critical Illness-Related Corticosteroid Insufficiency (CIRCI) in Critically Ill Patients (Part I): Society of Critical Care Medicine (SCCM) and European Society of Intensive Care Medicine (ESICM) 2017, *Crit Care Med* 45:2078–2088, 2017.
Arlt W, Allolio B: Adrenal insufficiency, *Lancet* 361:1881–1893, 2003.
Bancos I, Hahner S, Tomlinson J, Arlt W: Diagnosis and management of adrenal insufficiency, *Lancet Diabetes Endocrinol* 3:216–226, 2015.
Bornstein SR, Allolio B, Arlt W, et al: Diagnosis and treatment of primary adrenal insufficiency: an Endocrine Society clinical practice guideline, *J Clin Endocrinol Metab* 101:364–389, 2016.
Charmandari E, Nicolaides NC, Chrousos GP: Adrenal insufficiency, *Lancet* 383:2152–2167, 2014.
Dillard T, Yedinak CG, Alumkal J, Fleseriu M: Anti-CTLA-4 antibody therapy associated autoimmune hypophysitis: serious immune related adverse events across a spectrum of cancer subtypes, *Pituitary* 13(1):29–38, 2010.
Dorin RI, Qualls CR, Crapo LM: Diagnosis of adrenal insufficiency, *Ann Intern Med* 139:194–204, 2003.
Fleseriu M, Hashim IA, Karavitaki N, et al: Hormonal replacement in hypopituitarism in adults: an Endocrine Society clinical practice guideline, *J Clin Endocrinol Metab* 101:3888–3921, 2016.
Husebye ES, Allolio B, Arlt W, et al: Consensus statement on the diagnosis, treatment and follow-up of patients with primary adrenal insufficiency, *J Intern Med* 275:104–115, 2014.
Isidori AM, Venneri MA, Graziadio C, et al: Effect of once-daily, modified-release hydrocortisone versus standard glucocorticoid therapy on metabolism and innate immunity in patients with adrenal insufficiency (DREAM): a single-blind, randomised controlled trial, *The Lancet Diabetes & Endocrinology* 6:173–185, 2018.
Kazlauskaite R, Evans AT, Villabona CV, et al: Corticotropin tests for hypothalamic-pituitary-adrenal insufficiency: a metaanalysis, *J Clin Endocrinol Metab* 93:4245–4253, 2008.

Aggressive hydration with a saline solute will help increase the intravascular volume, and high-dose glucocorticoids have some mineralocorticoid activity; thus mineralocorticoids are not required in the treatment of acute adrenal crisis.

In critical illness, treatment of AI should not be delayed if diagnosis cannot be established and the patient is unstable. Baseline cortisol and ACTH levels should preferably be drawn prior to initiation of treatment and should be interpreted as a stress value (i.e., should be >18 µg/dL). If in doubt, high-dose stress steroids are administered until testing is complete, and cosyntropin stimulation testing may be delayed until the patient's condition improves because hydrocortisone has to be suspended at least 24 hours before testing. The controversial entity of suboptimal cortisol response during acute stress may be associated with worse outcome, but no consensus exists for its diagnosis and treatment.

Dehydroepiandrosterone (DHEA) use is controversial and not recommended by present guidelines. However, a trial may be warranted in selected cases of women with primary AI and persistent symptoms, including low libido and low energy. DHEA is only available as a dietary supplement.

Monitoring

Patients should be interviewed and examined routinely for indicators of excess glucocorticoid replacement, such as weight gain, striae, facial plethora, osteoporosis, or glucose intolerance, or under replacement if symptoms of AI persist. Cortisol levels and ACTH are not helpful in monitoring glucocorticoid doses. Monitoring of mineralocorticoid status should include volume status, electrolytes, blood pressure, and occasionally serum renin levels. Development of hypertension, edema, or hypokalemia could mandate a dose reduction.

Complications

Adrenal crisis in patients with known AI occurs at a rate of approximately 6 cases per 100 patient-years. Precipitating causes of adrenal crisis are mainly gastrointestinal infection and other infections, with other stressful events (pain, surgery, severe emotional distress, and pregnancy) occurring less commonly. Iatrogenic Cushing syndrome can develop if the dose of glucocorticoid replacement is supraphysiologic over the long term.

CUSHING'S SYNDROME

Method of
Constantine A. Stratakis, MD, PhD

CURRENT DIAGNOSIS

- Cushing's syndrome remains one of the most challenging diagnoses in endocrine medicine.
- Cushing's disease is caused by corticotropin (ACTH)-producing pituitary adenomas (corticotropinomas) and constitutes the most common cause of endogenous Cushing's syndrome, although its prevalence varies across different age groups.
- Growth failure in children, facial plethora and rounded face, central fat deposition, supraclavicular fat accumulation, buffalo hump, purple striae, thin skin, and proximal myopathy are relatively sensitive clinical features of Cushing's syndrome.
- Ectopic ACTH syndrome occasionally has an unusual presentation of rapid onset, severe weakness, and hypokalemia without classic symptoms of Cushing's syndrome.
- A urinary free cortisol test is the most cost-effective and reliable outpatient screening test.
- A 1-mg overnight dexamethasone screening test is less useful and more expensive than the urinary free cortisol test, but it provides a good alternative for patients in whom urinary collection is impossible or unreliable.
- Midnight salivary cortisol levels greater than 3.6 nmol/L (0.13 µg/dL) have a sensitivity and specificity of approximately 95% for the diagnosis of Cushing's syndrome.
- Undetectable ACTH levels (<1 pmol/L or <5 pg/mL) indicate a primary autonomous adrenocortical disease.
- Postcontrast spoiled gradient-recalled acquisition (SPGR) magnetic resonance imaging (MRI) is superior to conventional MRI for the localization of corticotropinomas in children and adults.
- Computed tomography (CT) is used to investigate adrenal disease in patients with ACTH-independent Cushing's syndrome. Usually, conventional MRI is less useful owing to motion artifacts.

CURRENT THERAPY

- The initial therapy of choice for patients with Cushing's disease is transsphenoidal surgery of the pituitary gland to remove the responsible adenoma.
- Transsphenoidal surgery has a success rate greater than 80% in most experienced centers. Lower success rates and higher incidence of relapse are recorded in less-experienced centers.
- Laparoscopic adrenalectomy has become the treatment of choice for benign adrenal lesions with a diameter of less than 6 cm.
- In stages I to III adrenocortical carcinoma, complete tumor resection offers the best chance for cure.
- Mitotane (Lysodren), an adrenolytic agent, is used in the treatment of metastatic adrenocortical carcinoma and also as an adjuvant for tumors with a high risk of recurrence.
- Medical treatment with ketoconazole[1], metyrapone[1], aminoglutethimide (Cytadren)[2], and mitotane[1] may be used to control hypercortisolism in preparation for surgery; medical adrenalectomy may also be used in cases of cyclic Cushing's syndrome.
- Pasireotide (Signifor) and mifepristone (Korlym) may be used for the treatment of Cushing's disease that cannot be cured by surgery and/or irradiation.
- The most effective treatment option for ectopic ACTH syndrome is resection of the tumor. Somatostatin analogues and various chemotherapeutic regimens have been used in the treatment of metastatic tumors.

[1]Not FDA approved for this indication.
[2]Not available in the United States.

Definition and Epidemiology

Cushing's syndrome remains one of the most difficult diagnoses in endocrinology. By definition, Cushing's syndrome is a multisystem disorder that develops in response to glucocorticoid excess. Iatrogenic Cushing's syndrome is common, but endogenous Cushing's syndrome is a rare condition, with an estimated incidence of 0.7 to 2.4 per million population per year. The etiology of Cushing's syndrome may be excessive adrenocorticotropic hormone (ACTH) production from the pituitary gland, ectopic ACTH secretion by nonpituitary tumors, or autonomous cortisol hypersecretion from adrenal hyperplasia or tumors (Table 1). Cushing's disease refers to the subset of Cushing's syndrome cases caused by an ACTH-producing pituitary adenoma. Cushing's disease is the most common cause of spontaneous Cushing's syndrome in almost all ages, including older children and adolescents. Approximately 20% to 30% (with the exception of very young children) of endogenous Cushing's syndrome is caused by primary adrenocortical diseases that are not ACTH-dependent. Cushing's disease and adrenocortical adenomas occur more commonly in women, with a female-to-male ratio of 3–5:1.

Pathophysiology

Cortisol inhibits the biosynthesis and secretion of corticotropin-releasing hormone (CRH) and ACTH in a negative-feedback loop that is tightly controlled. The hallmark of Cushing's syndrome is the absence of suppression of cortisol levels after low-dose dexamethasone (Decadron) administration owing to autonomous ACTH secretion by a tumor or autonomous glucocorticoid production by a primary adrenocortical disease. It is essential to understand that all diagnostic testing in Cushing's syndrome relies on the disturbance of this feedback mechanism, as revealed by dexamethasone, CRH (corticorelin ovine triflutate [Acthrel]), and all related testing.

ACTH-producing pituitary adenomas are microadenomas (<1 cm in diameter) in 80% to 90% of cases. Macroadenomas are rare and often invasive, with extension outside of the sella turcica. Chronic ACTH hypersecretion commonly leads to secondary adrenocortical hyperplasia.

TABLE 1	Etiology of Cushing's Syndrome in Older Children, Adolescents, and Young Adults*
SYNDROME	**% OF TOTAL**
ACTH-dependent	
Cushing's disease	60–70
Ectopic ACTH syndrome	5–10
Ectopic CRH syndrome	<1
ACTH-independent	
Adrenocortical adenoma	10–15
Adrenocortical carcinoma	5
Bilateral adrenocortical disease	5–10

*In infants and younger children, the distribution is different.
Abbreviations: ACTH = adrenocorticotropic hormone; CRH = corticotropin-releasing hormone.

Ectopic ACTH secretion is most often associated with small cell lung carcinoma, which accounts for half of the cases in adult patients with Cushing's syndrome. The ectopic ACTH syndrome causes severe hypokalemia and is usually underdiagnosed in patients during advanced stages of neoplasia. Other tumors causing the syndrome are bronchial, thymic, and pancreatic carcinoids; medullary thyroid carcinoma; pheochromocytoma; or other rare neuroendocrine tumors, especially in pediatric patients.

Adrenocortical tumors are more often adenomas that are usually smaller than 5 cm. Adrenocortical carcinomas are rare but very aggressive neoplasms; they most commonly occur as large nonsecreting abdominal masses at diagnosis, and only rarely does Cushing's syndrome develop.

Up to recently, only two types of primary adrenal hyperplasias that are ACTH-independent and cause Cushing's syndrome were known: primary pigmented nodular adrenocortical disease (PPNAD) and ACTH-independent macronodular adrenocortical hyperplasia, also known as massive macronodular adrenocortical disease.

Table 2 lists no fewer than six types of bilateral adrenocortical hyperplasias. They are divided into two groups of disorders, macronodular and micronodular hyperplasias, on the basis of the size of the associated nodules. In macronodular disorders, the greatest diameter of each nodule exceeds 1 cm; in the micronodular group, nodules are less than 1 cm. Although nodules less than 1 cm can occur in macronodular disease (especially the form associated with McCune-Albright syndrome), and single large tumors may be encountered in PPNAD (especially in older patients), the size criterion has biological relevance, because we rarely see a continuum in the same subject: most patients have either macronodular or micronodular hyperplasia. We use two additional basic characteristics in this classification of bilateral adrenocortical hyperplasias: presence of tumor pigment and status (hyperplasia or atrophy) of the surrounding cortex.

Pigment in adrenocortical lesions is rarely melanin; most of the pigmentation in adrenocortical adenomas and bilateral adrenocortical hyperplasias that produce cortisol is lipofuscin. The accumulation of lipofuscin-like material results from the progressive oxidation of unsaturated fatty acids by oxygen-derived free radicals in lysosomes. Lipofuscin pigmentation appears macroscopically as light brown to occasionally dark brown or even black discoloration of the tumor or hyperplastic tissue. Lipofuscin can be seen with a light microscope, but it is better detected by electron microscopy. Massive macronodular adrenocortical disease is a bilateral disease and may be caused by abnormal hormone receptor expression or activating mutations of $G_s\alpha$, which lead to stimulation of steroidogenesis. About 30% to 50% of the cases may be caused by ARMC5 mutations. Another cause of ACTH-independent Cushing's syndrome is primary pigmented nodular adrenocortical disease, usually associated with a syndrome of cardiac myxomas, lentigines, and schwannomas (Carney's complex).

TABLE 2 Bilateral Adrenal Hyperplasias Causing Cushing's Syndrome

LESION	AGE GROUP	HISTOPATHOLOGY	GENETICS	GENE, LOCUS
Macronodular Hyperplasias (Multiple Nodules >1 cm Each)				
Bilateral macroadenomatous hyperplasia	Middle age	Distinct adenomas (usually 2 or 3) with internodular atrophy	MEN1, FAP, MAS, HLRCS; isolated (AD); other	Menin, *APC,GNAS*, FH, ectopic GPCRs, ARMC5, PRKACA 5
Bilateral macroadenomatous hyperplasia of childhood	Infants, very young children	Distinct adenomas (usually 2 or 3) with internodular atrophy; occasional microadenomas	MAS	*GNAS*
ACTH-independent macronodular adrenocortical hyperplasia, also known as massive macronodular adrenocortical disease	Middle age	Adenomatous hyperplasia (multiple) with internodular hyperplasia of the zona fasciculata	Isolated, AD	Ectopic GPCRs; WISP2 and Wnt-signaling; 17q22-24, other; ARMC5, PRKACA 5
Micronodular Hyperplasias (Multiple Nodules <1 cm Each)				
Isolated primary pigmented nodular adrenocortical disease	Children; young adults	Microadenomatous hyperplasia with (mostly) internodular atrophy and nodular pigment (lipofuscin)	Isolated, AD	*PRKAR1A, PDE11A; PDE8B*; 2p16; PRKACA 5 other
Carney complex–associated primary pigmented nodular adrenocortical disease	Children; young and middle aged adults	Microadenomatous hyperplasia with (mostly) internodular atrophy and (mainly nodular) pigment (lipofuscin)	CNC (AD)	*PRKAR1A*, 2p16; other
Isolated micronodular adrenocortical disease	Mostly children; young adults	Microadenomatous, with hyperplasia of the surrounding zona fasciculata and limited or absent pigment	Isolated, AD; other	*PDE11A, PDE8B*; other; 2p12-p16, other

Abbreviations: ACTH = adrenocorticotropic hormone; AD = autosomal dominant; *APC* = adenomatous polyposis coli gene; cAMP = cyclic adenosine monophosphate; CNC = Carney complex; FAP = familial adenomatous polyposis; FH = fumarate hydratase; *GNAS* = gene coding for the stimulatory subunit alpha of the G-protein (Gsα); GPCR = G-protein-coupled receptor; HLRCS = hereditary leiomyomatosis and renal cancer syndrome; MAS = McCune–Albright syndrome; MEN1 = multiple endocrine neoplasia type 1; *PDE8B* = phosphodiesterase 8B gene; *PDE11A* = phosphodiesterase 11A gene; *PRKAR1A* = protein kinase, cAMP-dependent, regulatory, type I, alpha gene; WISP2 = Wnt1-inducible signaling pathway protein 1; Wnt = wingless-type MMTV integration site family.

Clinical Manifestations

The clinical presentation of Cushing's syndrome is variable and differs in severity (Table 3). Truncal obesity is the most common clinical sign and is usually the initial manifestation in most patients. Growth failure in children is the most reliable sign of Cushing's syndrome, especially when combined with continuing weight gain. Other symptoms include central fat deposition, supraclavicular fat accumulation, buffalo hump, plethora, rounded face, purple striae, thin skin, proximal muscle weakness, hypertension, impaired glucose metabolism, gonadal dysfunction, and hirsutism (see Table 3). Diabetes mellitus and hypertension also develop. Osteoporosis, mood disorders, emotional lability and cognitive deficits are commonly observed. Proximal myopathy is common, especially in older patients. Ectopic ACTH syndrome caused by small cell lung cancer can have an unusual presentation characterized by rapid onset, severe weakness, and associated hypokalemia without classic symptoms of Cushing's syndrome. In contrast, ACTH-secreting carcinoids manifest with typical clinical manifestations.

Diagnosis
Confirmation of the Diagnosis

The initial evaluation should always include a careful clinical history and physical examination. Reliable symptoms and signs of Cushing's syndrome (see Table 3) should be present in any patient who undergoes evaluation for Cushing's syndrome; patients with no reliable symptoms and signs of Cushing's syndrome should not be investigated, as this often leads to unnecessary, extensive, and expensive testing. It is essential to investigate the use of exogenous glucocorticoids and other conditions that may be associated with mild hypercortisolism, such as alcoholism, anorexia nervosa, severe depression, and morbid obesity; these are pseudo-Cushing's states and are often difficult to exclude, especially in older or chronically ill patients.

The first task in the workup of any patient is documentation of hypercortisolism. On an outpatient basis, this is typically done through the urinary free cortisol test. This is the most cost-effective and reliable outpatient screening test. We typically recommend collections over two or three consecutive days so that we avoid errors due to over- or undercollection that are not uncommon with single 24-hour studies. The results of the test need to be corrected for body surface area, as long as total creatinine excretion is normal. A 1-mg overnight dexamethasone test is less useful and more expensive, but it provides a good alternative for patients in whom urinary collection is impossible or unreliable. During these screening tests for hypercortisolism, patients should avoid any activation of the hypothalamic-pituitary-adrenal axis by stress, especially physical. The baseline measurements may be repeated as needed, because cyclic hypercortisolism often precedes overt Cushing's syndrome (Figure 1).

A 24-hour urinary free cortisol excretion of greater than 250 nmol per 24 hours (90 µg/24 hours measured by radioimmunoassay) is highly specific for the diagnosis of hypercortisolism. However, pseudo-Cushing's states are often associated with

TABLE 3	Clinical Manifestations of Cushing's Syndrome
SIGNS AND SYMPTOMS	**INCIDENCE (%)**
Central obesity	97
Plethora	89
Moon facies	89
Decreased libido	86
Atrophic skin and easy bruising	75
Decreased linear growth	70–80
Menstrual irregularities	80
Hypertension	76
Hirsutism	56
Depression or emotional lability	67
Glucose intolerance/diabetes mellitus	70
Purple striae	60
Buffalo hump	54
Osteoporosis	50
Headache	10

abnormal levels of 24-hour urinary free cortisol. Administration of 1 mg dexamethasone (15 µg/kg for children) at 11 PM results in suppression of the hypothalamic-pituitary-adrenal axis in normal persons and a fall in plasma and urinary cortisol levels. At 8 AM, serum cortisol should be less than 50 nmol/L (1.8 µg/dL). Unfortunately, dexamethasone is primarily metabolized by the cytochrome P-450 (CYP) system; several drugs, such as phenobarbital, carbamazepine (Tegretol), and rifampicin (Rifadin), that induce the activity of CYP3A4 can lead to false-positive tests. Oral contraceptives also interfere with serum cortisol levels owing to an increase in corticosteroid-binding globulin and by increasing dexamethasone metabolism. The test can only be interpreted if the serum dexamethasone levels reach the expected range; however, this additional requirement can make the test significantly more cumbersome and expensive.

Once hypercortisolism is suspected by the urinary free cortisol or the overnight dexamethasone test, the patient may undergo testing of the cortisol diurnal rhythm. The lack of circadian rhythm of cortisol is the earliest consistent biochemical abnormality of Cushing's syndrome, even in situations of cyclic or other atypical forms of Cushing's syndrome. Serum or salivary cortisol levels at midnight may be used for this test. Normally, the level of serum cortisol begins to rise at 3 to 4 AM and reaches a peak at 7 to 8 AM, falling during the day. A sleeping midnight serum cortisol level lower than 50 nmol/L (1.8 µg/dL) excludes the diagnosis of Cushing's syndrome, whereas a midnight serum cortisol higher than 207 nmol/L (7.5 µg/dL) is highly suggestive of Cushing's syndrome. This test does require inpatient admission. Salivary cortisol levels have an excellent correlation with serum cortisol levels and offer an easy and convenient outpatient way of evaluating circadian rhythm; saliva is also stable at room temperature (for up to 7 days). Midnight salivary cortisol levels greater than 3.6 nmol/L (0.13 µg/dL) have a sensitivity and specificity of approximately 95% for the diagnosis of Cushing's syndrome (see Figure 1).

After the biochemical confirmation of hypercortisolism, the next step is to investigate the source (see Figure 1). Baseline ACTH plasma levels greater than 2 to 5 pmol/L (>20–25 pg/mL) are diagnostic of ACTH-dependent Cushing's syndrome. On the other hand, undetectable ACTH levels (<1 pmol/L or 5 pg/mL) indicate a primary autonomous adrenocortical disease. Values in between should be further investigated with dynamic testing.

High-Dose Dexamethasone Testing
Oral dexamethasone is administrated as 2 mg every 6 hours for 48 hours or as a single 8 mg (120 µg/kg for children) overnight dose. Urinary and serum cortisol levels are suppressed by more than 50% in most patients with Cushing's disease.

Corticotropin-Releasing Hormone Testing
Synthetic ovine CRH (corticorelin ovine trifluate [Acthrel]), an analogue of human CRH is administered intravenously (100 µg), and plasma ACTH and cortisol levels are measured at 15-minute intervals during the next 60 minutes. Patients with Cushing's disease typically have an increase in ACTH or cortisol level of 35% and 22%, respectively. This test has a sensitivity of approximately 85% for the diagnosis of Cushing's disease, but it is often falsely positive in patients with adrenal, ACTH-independent Cushing's syndrome, who do not have a fully suppressed hypothalamic-pituitary-adrenal axis.

Inferior Petrosal Sinus Sampling
None of the noninvasive tests are 100% accurate in distinguishing pituitary (Cushing's disease) from ectopic sources of ACTH. Inferior petrosal sinus sampling (IPSS) is indicated in all cases where an ACTH-dependent source of hypercortisolism is expected but the diagnosis of Cushing's disease versus an ectopic source remains uncertain. Typically, IPSS is done when the ovine CRH and dexamethasone tests are in disagreement or when the pituitary imaging by magnetic resonance imaging (MRI) is negative. An ACTH gradient of central-to-peripheral ACTH levels of 2 or more suggests Cushing's disease. When ovine CRH, human CRH, or desmopressin (DDAVP) testing is performed during IPSS, the diagnostic accuracy of IPSS increases. After ovine CRH stimulation, a central-to-peripheral ratio of ACTH levels of 3 or more suggest the diagnosis of Cushing's disease with specificity and sensitivity greater than 95%. The test is less useful for suggesting the tumor location (right versus left side of the pituitary gland).

Imaging Studies
Pituitary Magnetic Resonance Imaging
Unfortunately, less than 50% of ACTH-producing pituitary adenomas are detectable with MRI, even with the use of contrast enhancement. Typically, we recommend against obtaining an MRI until ACTH dependency is established, because as many as 20% of the patients have an incidental pituitary microadenoma. To avoid false-negative and false-positive imaging, several centers have sought improved methods for MRI detection of ACTH-producing tumors. Our studies demonstrated that postcontrast spoiled gradient-recalled acquisition (SPGR) MRI in addition to the conventional T1-weighted spin echo was superior to conventional MRI for the diagnostic evaluation of corticotropinomas in both children and adults.

Adrenal Imaging
Computed tomography (CT) and MRI are used to investigate adrenal disease in patients with ACTH-independent Cushing's syndrome. Adrenal tumors larger than 6 cm are highly suspicious for adrenocortical carcinomas. The fat content contributes to the differentiation between benign and malignant adrenal tumors. Measurement of Hounsfield units (HU) in unenhanced CT is of great value in differentiating malignant from benign adrenal lesions. Adrenal lesions with an attenuation value of more than 10 HU in unenhanced CT or an enhancement washout of less than 50% and a delayed attenuation of more than 35 HU (on 10- to 15-min delayed enhanced CT) are suspicious for malignancy. MRI with dynamic gadolinium-enhanced and chemical shift technique is as effective as CT in distinguishing malignant from benign lesions. However, MRI is much less useful for detecting adrenal nodularity owing to motion artifacts. Thus, especially for detecting small unilateral adrenocortical adenomas or bilateral micronodular hyperplasia, we recommend a dedicated (thin-sliced) adrenal CT rather than MRI.

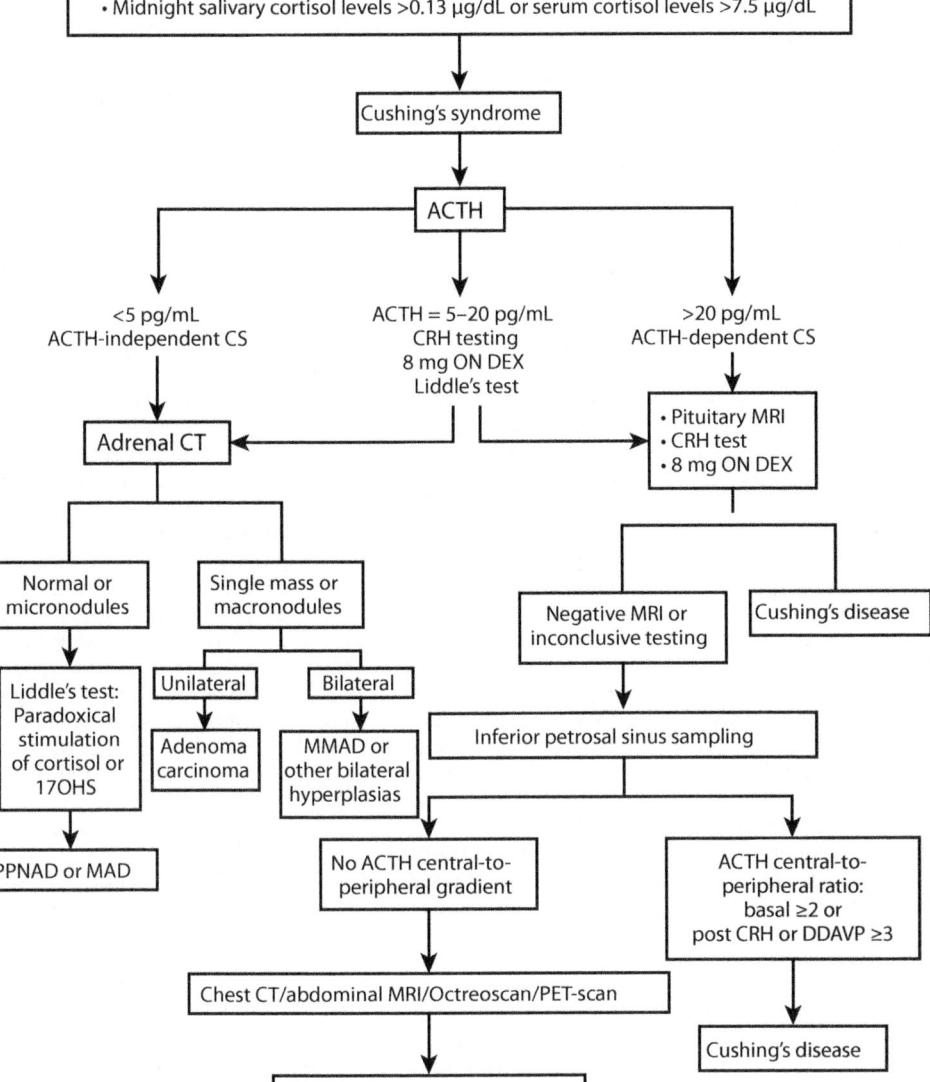

Figure 1 Algorithm for evaluating patients with Cushing's syndrome. *Abbreviations:* ACTH = adrenocorticotropic hormone; CRH = corticotropin-releasing hormone; CS = Cushing's syndrome; CT = computed tomography; DDAVP = desmopressin; DHPLC = denaturing high-performance liquid chromatography; ICMA = immunochemiluminometric assay; MAD = micronodular disease; MMAD = massive macronodular adrenocortical disease; MRI = magnetic resonance imaging; 17OHS = 17-hydroxysteroids; ON DEX = overnight dexamethasone; PET = positron emission tomography; PPNAD = primary pigmented nodular adrenocortical disease; RIA = radioimmunoassay.

Ectopic Adrenocorticotropic Hormone Syndrome

High Resolution Chest-CT 7 and abdominal MRI are the recommended imaging procedures in patients with an IPSS that indicates a nonpituitary ACTH-producing source. Additionally, somatostatin receptor scintigraphy is a useful and complementary tool in the evaluation of patients with ectopic ACTH-dependent Cushing's syndrome. Recent studies have demonstrated a higher sensitivity of somatostatin receptor scintigraphy in comparison to CT or MRI for diagnosing occult ectopic tumors. Additional methods include PET-CT and FDG scans.

Treatment

Untreated chronic hypercortisolism is associated with high morbidity and mortality owing to diabetes mellitus, hypertension, cardiovascular disease, thromboembolism, and suppression of the immune system. Cushing's syndrome should be treated effectively; patients should be closely monitored to rapidly detect recurrent disease.

Treatment of Pituitary Corticotropinomas
Transsphenoidal Pituitary Surgery

The initial therapy of choice for patients with Cushing's disease is transsphenoidal surgery. This procedure is associated with low

mortality and morbidity, but complications can include cerebrospinal fluid leaks, meningitis, hypopituitarism, and venous thromboembolism. The success rate for transsphenoidal surgery varies between 60% and 80%, but in experienced centers can be as high as 90% to 95%. Relapses are rare when surgery is performed in an experienced tertiary care center; it can be as high as 30% in less-experienced centers. Postoperative morning serum cortisol levels of less than 50 nmol/L (2 μg/dL) are highly predictive of remission and a low recurrence rate of less than 10% at 10 years.

After successful transsphenoidal surgery, glucocorticoid replacement therapy (hydrocortisone at 12–15 mg/m²/day; 20–30 mg daily in adults) is mandatory until the hypothalamic-pituitary-adrenal axis recovers from the chronic exposure to glucocorticoid excess; this usually takes place within a year after surgery. For recurrent disease, the choice of second-line therapy remains controversial. Repeat surgery can be successful when residual tumor is detectable on MRI imaging, but it carries a high risk of hypopituitarism. Irradiation is recommended in most cases where a tumor is not seen on MRI.

Radiotherapy

Radiotherapy has been used to suppress pituitary secretion of ACTH, but its success rate is variable (50% in some series).

TABLE 4	Medical Treatment for Hypercortisolism		
MEDICATION	**INITIAL DOSE**	**MAXIMUM DOSE**	**ADVERSE EFFECTS**
Ketoconazole (Nizoral)[1]	100–200 mg bid/tid	1200 mg	Nausea, vomiting, abdominal pain, weakness, hypothyroidism, gynecomastia, hepatotoxicity, hypertriglyceridemia
Metyrapone (Metopirone)[1]	250 mg qid	6000 mg	Headache, alopecia, hirsutism, acne, nausea, abdominal discomfort, hypertension, weakness, leucopenia
Mitotane (Lysodren)[1]	500 mg tid	9000 mg	Nausea, vomiting, anorexia, diarrhea, ataxia, confusion, skin rash, hepatotoxicity
Aminoglutethimide (Cytadren)[2]	250 mg qid	2000 mg/d	Lethargy, nausea, anorexia, hypothyroidism, somnolence

[1]Not FDA approved for this indication.
[2]Not available in the United States.

It can take as long as 5 years for a full effect; hypopituitarism develops in more than 70% of the patients over a period of 10 to 20 years after the therapy is completed. Stereotactic radiosurgery with gamma knife is associated with a more-rapid effect and a lower risk of hypopituitarism, but it has not been extensively studied.

Medical Treatment to Control Secretion of Adrenocorticotropic Hormone

Cushing's disease responds to the dopamine agonist cabergoline (Dostinex)[1] with a normalization of cortisol production in as many as 40% of the cases. The peroxisome proliferator-activated receptor γ (PPAR-γ) agonist rosiglitazone (Avandia)[1] was demonstrated to be effective in animal models, but it was unsuccessful in controlling ACTH oversecretion in patients with Cushing's disease. A new agent, SOM-230 (pasireotide [Signifor]), blocks both type 2 and type 5 somatostatin receptors and reduces ACTH secretion in vitro. Mifepristone (Korlym), a glucocorticoid receptor antagonist, recently became available for patients who failed surgical or irradiation therapies (see also below).

Bilateral Adrenalectomy

Bilateral adrenalectomy offers a definitive treatment that provides immediate control of hypercortisolism, but this surgery should be reserved for patients with Cushing's disease who have failed all other treatments. Bilateral adrenalectomy in active Cushing's disease often leads to Nelson's syndrome, a condition characterized by unabated progression of a corticotropinoma (owing to the lack of negative feedback by cortisol), very high ACTH levels, and high morbidity.

Treatment of Adrenal Disease
Adrenocortical Tumors

For adrenocortical tumors, the recommended treatment is surgical. Laparoscopic adrenalectomy has become the treatment of choice for benign adrenal lesions with a diameter of less than 6 cm. In stages I to III adrenocortical carcinoma, complete tumor removal by a well-trained surgeon offers by far the best chance for cure. Surgery often needs to be extensive, with en bloc resection of invaded organs, and regularly includes lymphadenectomy. Surgery for local recurrences or metastatic disease is accepted as a valuable therapeutic option and was associated with improved survival in retrospective studies. The overall 5-year survival in different series ranged between 16% and 38%. Median survival for metastatic disease (stage IV) at the time of diagnosis is still consistently less than 12 months.

Radiotherapy has been considered ineffective for treatment of adrenocortical cancer, but it can be indicated to control localized disease not amenable to surgery.

Mitotane (o,p′-DDD [Lysodren]) is the only adrenal-specific agent available for treating adrenocortical cancer. Mitotane is indicated in metastatic adrenocortical carcinoma and can also be used as an adjuvant for tumors with a high risk of recurrence. Mitotane exerts a specific cytotoxic effect on adrenocortical cells, leading to focal degeneration of the fascicular and particularly the reticular zone. In most patients, treatment should be initiated with a dose that does not exceed 1.5 g/day; this is then rapidly increased, depending on gastrointestinal symptoms, to 5 to 6 g/day. This high-dose regimen requires measurement of mitotane blood levels 14 days after initiation of therapy. The dose is then adjusted according to the medicine's plasma concentrations (which should be greater than 14 mg/L) and tolerance of the side effects. Because mitotane treatment induces adrenal insufficiency and increases the metabolic clearance of glucocorticoids, glucocorticoid replacement is indicated, often at higher than normal doses owing to increased clearance.

Cytotoxic Chemotherapy

Cytotoxic chemotherapy includes etoposide (VePesid)[1], doxorubicin (Adriamycin)[1], and cisplatin (Platinol)[1], or streptozocin (Zanosar)[1] plus mitotane. Chemotherapy has limited efficacy for advanced adrenocortical cancer and is associated mainly with partial responses.

Bilateral Adrenal Hyperplasias

The treatment of choice for bilateral adrenal hyperplasias associated with ACTH-independent Cushing's syndrome is bilateral adrenalectomy. Patients require lifelong replacement therapy with glucocorticoids and mineralocorticoids, and they should be adequately educated about the risk of acute adrenal insufficiency.

Treatment of Ectopic Corticotropin Syndrome

The choice of treatment for ectopic ACTH syndrome depends on tumor identification, localization, and classification. The most effective treatment option is surgical resection, although this is not always possible in metastatic disease or in the case of occult tumors. Because the ectopic ACTH syndrome is usually severe and occult tumors can become evident at imaging studies only during the follow-up, medical treatment to control hypercortisolism is often necessary. Bilateral adrenalectomy may be an option to be considered when the hypercortisolism cannot be controlled by other treatment options.

Medical Adrenalectomy

Several drugs that inhibit steroid synthesis are often effective for rapidly controlling hypercortisolism in preparation for surgery, after unsuccessful transsphenoidal surgery or removal of an adrenal tumor such as extensive cancer, or while awaiting the full effect of radiotherapy in recurrent Cushing's disease (Table 4).

[1]Not FDA approved for this indication.

[1]Not FDA approved for this indication.

Most experience with inhibitors of steroidogenesis has been with metyrapone (Metopirone)[1] and ketoconazole (Nizoral)[1], two medications that appear to be more effective and better tolerated than aminoglutethimide (Cytadren)[2]. Metyrapone reduces cortisol and aldosterone production by inhibiting 11β-hydroxylation in the adrenal cortex. Ketoconazole is a broad-spectrum antifungal drug, which inhibits c17-20 desmolase, cholesterol side-chain cleavage, and 11β-hydroxylation. Ketoconazole is also associated with inhibition of testosterone biosynthesis and gynecomastia.

RU-486, or mifepristone (Korlym), is an antagonist of the progesterone and glucocorticoid receptors. Unexpectedly, the treatment of Cushing's disease with this glucocorticoid antagonist has been associated with increased ACTH secretion and consequent stimulation of cortisol production. RU-486 may be more useful in ectopic ACTH-producing tumors and in adrenal Cushing's syndrome, but its efficacy and potential side effects when administered chronically are currently unknown.

---

[1]Not FDA approved for this indication.
[2]Not available in the United States.

References

Allolio B, Fassnacht M: Clinical review: Adrenocortical carcinoma: clinical update, *J Clin Endocrinol Metab* 91:2027–2037, 2006.

Assie G, Libe R, Espiard S, et al: ARMC5 mutations in macronodular adrenal hyperplasia with Cushing's syndrome, *N Engl J Med* 369(22):2105–2114, 2013.

Batista D, Courkoutsakis NA, Oldfield EH, et al: Detection of adrenocorticotropin-secreting pituitary adenomas by magnetic resonance imaging in children and adolescents with Cushing disease, *J Clin Endocrinol Metab* 90:5134–5140, 2005.

Batista DL, Riar J, Keil M, Stratakis CA: Diagnostic tests for children who are referred for the investigation of Cushing syndrome, *Pediatrics* 120:e575–e586, 2007.

Bertagna X, Guignat L, Groussin L, Bertherat J: Cushing's disease, *Best Pract Res Clin Endocrinol Metab* 23:607–623, 2009.

Biller BM, Grossman AB, Stewart PM, et al: Treatment of adrenocorticotropin-dependent Cushing's syndrome: a consensus statement, *J Clin Endocrinol Metab* 93:2454–2462, 2008.

Boscaro M, Arnaldi G: Approach to the patient with possible Cushing's syndrome, *J Clin Endocrinol Metab* 94:3121–3131, 2009.

Feelders RA, Hofland LJ: Medical treatment of Cushing's disease, *J Clin Endocrinol Metab* 98(2):425–438, 2013.

Newell-Price J, Trainer P, Besser M, Grossman A: The diagnosis and differential diagnosis of Cushing's syndrome and pseudo-Cushing's states, *Endocr Rev* 19:647–672, 1998.

Terzolo M, Angeli A, Fassnacht M, et al: Adjuvant mitotane treatment for adrenocortical carcinoma, *N Engl J Med* 356:2372–2380, 2007.

DIABETES INSIPIDUS

Method of
Rami Mortada, MD

CURRENT DIAGNOSIS

- Diabetes insipidus (DI) is a disorder of excess urine production (i.e., "diabetes") that is dilute and tasteless (i.e., "insipidus"). DI contrasts with the concentrated and sweet urine in diabetes mellitus.
- Patients with DI present with polyuria and polydipsia; urine output is usually more than 40 mL/kg/day or more than 3 L/day.
- There are three subtypes of DI:
  - Central DI: due to relative or absolute lack of vasopressin
  - Nephrogenic DI: due to partial or total resistance to the renal antidiuretic effects of vasopressin
  - Dipsogenic DI (also called primary polydipsia): where polyuria is secondary to excessive, inappropriate fluid intake
- Initial labs should include plasma sodium and urine osmolality. Under normal physiologic conditions, the urine osmolality is less than 300 mOsm/L, but if the patient does not have sufficient fluid intake, the urine osmolality can be higher.

- The diagnosis is confirmed by examining urine output and osmolality. It can be followed by an assessment of renal response to the synthetic arginine vasopressin (AVP) analogue desmopressin (DDAVP).
- In primary polydipsia, urine concentration is normal in response to dehydration.
- In central DI, urine concentration does not increase appropriately with dehydration, but does respond to desmopressin (DDAVP). After dehydration in central DI, urine osmolality remains <300 mOsm/kg, and plasma osmolality is >290 mOsm/kg. Urine osmolality rises to >750 mOsm/kg after desmopressin.
- In nephrogenic DI, urine concentration does not increase appropriately with either dehydration or exogenous desmopressin.

CURRENT THERAPY

- The treatment goal is to control polyuria and ensure electrolyte stability.
- In Central DI:
  - The mild form might not require treatment.
  - Significant polyuria can be treated with desmopressin in divided doses: nasal spray 5 to 100 µg/day; tablets 100 to 1000 µg/day; or parenterally 0.1 to 2.0 µg/day.
  - Overtreatment can cause hyponatremia.
- In Nephrogenic DI:
  - Urine output should not be expected to normalize after DDAVP administration.
  - Correct the culprit cause (hypercalcemia or lithium [Eskalith, Lithobid] cessation).
  - Follow a low-sodium, low-protein diet, as tolerated.
  - Hydrochlorothiazide[1] 25 to 50 mg/day may be taken either alone or in combination with indomethacin (Indocin) 25 to 50 mg twice daily.
  - Symptoms may respond partly to high-dose desmopressin (e.g., 4 mcg IM twice daily).
- Primary polydipsia is treated by limiting an excessive fluid intake.

[1]Not FDA approved for this indication.

Physiology of Antidiuretic Hormone

Arginine vasopressin (AVP), also known as antidiuretic hormone (ADH), is a neurohypophysial hormone. It is a peptide hormone that promotes water retention by increasing the permeability of the kidney's collecting duct and distal convoluted tubule to water. It also increases peripheral vascular resistance, which in turn increases arterial blood pressure. In the clinical setting, the terms AVP, ADH, and vasopressin are used interchangeably.

Vasopressin is considered the main hormone involved in the regulation of water homeostasis and osmolality. The regulation and synthesis of vasopressin is under the influence of two systems: osmotic and pressure/volume status. In the case of osmoregulation, a small increase in plasma osmolality produces a parallel increase in vasopressin secretion; a small decrease in plasma osmolality causes a parallel drop in vasopressin.

Vasopressin is one among other hormones and systems that are involved in the regulation of volume and blood pressure. Other factors influence vasopressin production. For example, glucocorticoids inhibit secretion, whereas nausea and vomiting have a stimulatory effect.

Pathophysiology of Diabetes Insipidus

The kidneys exercise one of their urine-concentrating abilities by promoting water retention. If the concentration of vasopressin is decreased, polyuria occurs and diluted urine is excreted. A decrease in total body water results in an increase in the plasma osmolality. If the physiologic response is intact, thirst is stimulated, which leads to an increase in water consumption and the correction of plasma osmolarity. Therefore, unless there is a dysregulation in the thirst mechanisms or water consumption is limited due to a lack of availability (e.g., decreased level of consciousness, immobility, or physical restraints) severe dehydration does not develop.

Clinical Causes

There are three subtypes of diabetes insipidus (DI).

- DI secondary to excess water intake (primary polydipsia)

    Primary polydipsia is a disorder characterized by inappropriate excess fluid intake due to a disordered thirst sensation seen mostly in patients with psychiatric illnesses. A central defect in thirst regulation plays an important role in the pathogenesis of primary polydipsia. Such patients continue drinking even if the plasma osmolality falls below normal. It is not easy to achieve or maintain a low plasma osmolality because vasopressin secretion will normally be suppressed by the fall in plasma osmolality, resulting in rapid excretion of the excess water. If vasopressin regulation is intact, primary polydipsia should not lead to clinically important disturbances in the plasma sodium concentration unless hyposmolar fluid intake overwhelms the kidneys' ability to excrete excess water. Thus the serum sodium concentration is usually normal or slightly reduced in primary polydipsia. These patients may be asymptomatic or present with complaints of polydipsia and polyuria. In rare circumstances where water intake exceeds the kidneys' ability to excrete the water load of about 500 mL/hour, symptomatic severe hyponatremia might result in severe psychosis. Psychosis from hyponatremia in primary polydipsia is most commonly seen in institutionalized patients or in individuals attempting to dilute their urine to avoid a positive urine drug test.

- DI secondary to a decrease in or absence of vasopressin secretion (central DI)

    Central DI may be caused by genetic anomalies of the vasopressin gene (Table 1). Familial neurohypophyseal DI is characterized by the onset of DI with polyuria and polydipsia in childhood or early adulthood. The most common MRI finding in familial neurohypophyseal DI is the progressive disappearance of the posterior pituitary bright spot in children. The normal pituitary bright spot seen on unenhanced T_1-weighted MRI is thought to result from the T_1-shortening effect of the vasopressin stored in the posterior pituitary. The disappearance of the bright spot corresponds to the disappearance of vasopressin stores in the posterior pituitary. Wolfram's syndrome is a rare autosomal recessive syndrome manifested by DI, diabetes mellitus, optic atrophy, and deafness.

    Central DI may be caused by mass lesions of the neurohypophysis, such as craniopharyngiomas, and primary germ cell tumors in childhood. DI can be the initial presentation. MRI often shows a thickened pituitary stalk and may show a hypothalamic mass. Metastasis to the pituitary usually is found with widespread metastatic disease and is twice as likely to involve the posterior pituitary than the anterior pituitary. DI can be associated with pituitary infiltration associated with lymphomas and leukemias.

    In granulomatous disease that affects the hypothalamic-pituitary axis, there is usually clear evidence of disease elsewhere in the body. MRI shows an absence of the pituitary bright spot and widening of the hypothalamic-pituitary stalk. Lymphocytic infundibuloneurohypophysitis is a new, well-recognized cause of autoimmune DI, characterized by MRI appearance of a thickened hypothalamic-pituitary stalk and large posterior pituitary gland mimicking a pituitary tumor. Pituitary abscess is a rare cause of pituitary mass and DI. In situations where the cause is not easily diagnosed, an autoimmune process should be suspected. In some patients, the cause is idiopathic.

TABLE 1	Central Diabetes Insipidus (DI) Etiologies
Idiopathic	Unknown etiology
Genetic	Familial neurohypophyseal DI, Wolfram's syndrome (autosomal recessive)
Mass effect	Craniopharyngiomas, primary germ cell tumors, metastatic tumors
Infiltrative diseases	Lymphoma, leukemia, sarcoidosis, amyloidosis
Autoimmune	Lymphocytic infundibuloneurohypophysitis
Trauma	Motor vehicle accident, closed head trauma
Surgical	Surgical intervention at the pituitary region

Central DI may be caused by surgery or trauma to the pituitary region. Vasopressin is normally secreted after any kind of surgical stress, and secretion is more pronounced after surgery to the pituitary region. Only a small percentage of patients undergoing pituitary surgery have permanent DI. A triphasic DI can occur after complete hypothalamic-pituitary stalk transection. The first phase is polyuric and appears within the first 24 hours after surgery. It is thought to be secondary to axonal shock with a resultant inability to release prefabricated vasopressin. The second phase is antidiuretic and starts on about day 6, after stalk injury. It is thought to be secondary to the unregulated release of vasopressin stores. The third phase, also polyuric, starts about day 12, after vasopressin stores have been depleted. It may result in permanent or partial DI or resolve to clinically asymptomatic disease.

The same patterns of DI that occur after pituitary surgery can be seen in patients who experience a closed head trauma. Three-quarters of traumatic induced DI are secondary to motor vehicle accidents. Trauma is usually severe and causes unconsciousness. There is a high association of anterior pituitary deficiency in association with DI induced by head trauma, so the possibility of central hypocortisolism should be considered and treated immediately. DI is reported in 50% to 90% of patients with brain death.

- DI secondary to the lack of renal response to vasopressin (nephrogenic DI)

    Genetic anomalies resulting in a lack of renal response to vasopressin are caused by either a mutation in the V2 receptors or a mutation of the aquaporin 2 water channels gene. The majority of the cases are X-linked recessive disorders in males. Newborns present with polyuria, vomiting, constipation, and failure to thrive. Symptoms usually occur within the first week of life.

    Acquired nephrogenic DI can be caused by a kidney disease that distorts the architecture of the kidney and impairs its urine-concentrating ability (e.g., polycystic kidney disease, sickle cell disease). Decreased function of vasopressin or downregulation of aquaporin 2 channels can be caused by hypokalemia, hypercalcemia, and relief of bilateral urinary tract obstruction. Drugs such as lithium (the most common cause of drug-induced nephrogenic DI) and demeclocycline (used clinically to treat a syndrome of inappropriate ADH secretion) may cause nephrogenic DI.

Clinical Manifestations

Patients with central DI typically present with polyuria, nocturia, and polydipsia. The serum sodium concentration in untreated central DI is often in the high normal range, which provides the ongoing stimulation of thirst that replaces urinary water losses. Moderate to severe hypernatremia can develop when thirst is impaired or if there is a lack of access to free water, such as the postoperative period in patients with unrecognized DI or infants with DI. For uncertain pathophysiologic reasons, patients with central DI may develop decreased bone

TABLE 2 Values Before and After Water Restriction

	INITIAL PLASMA OSMOLALITY	INITIAL PLASMA SODIUM	POSTTEST URINE/PLASMA OSMOLALITY	POSTTEST URINE/PLASMA OSMOLALITY+ADH
Normal	NL	NL	>1	>1
Central DI	High (high NL)	High (high NL)	<1	>1
Nephrogenic DI	High (high NL)	High (high NL)	<1	<1
Primary polydipsia	Low (low NL)	Low (low NL)	>1	>1

mineral density at the lumbar spine and femoral neck, even if treated with desmopressin.

Nephrogenic DI in its mild form can be asymptomatic. Patients with moderate to severe nephrogenic DI, as with central DI, typically present with polyuria, nocturia, and polydipsia.

Primary polydipsia is the result of an abnormal compulsion to drink water. This disorder is most often seen in middle-aged women and in patients with psychiatric illnesses. The excessive water intake initially drives the excessive urination.

Diagnosis

Polyuria must be distinguished from simple urinary frequency in the absence of excess urine volume. The initial diagnostic approach should be to confirm polyuria, defined as greater than 30 mL/kg or 3 L/day, with a urine osmolality measuring less than 300 mOsm/L. Simple metabolic causes such as hyperglycemia, uremia, and hypercalcemia should be excluded. A definitive diagnosis of DI requires testing of vasopressin production and action in response to osmolar stress. All forms of DI may be partial or complete. In primary polydipsia, the plasma sodium, blood urea nitrogen (BUN), and uric acid are relatively low. In other forms of DI, the plasma sodium and uric acid are relatively high and the BUN is relatively low.

Central DI usually has an abrupt onset resulting from destruction of more than 80% of vasopressin-secreting hypothalamic neurons. The etiology of polyuria is not always evident after history and laboratory tests are completed. In that case, a water restriction test (e.g., dehydration test or water deprivation test) is completed. The water deprivation test is an indirect assessment of the AVP axis, measuring renal concentrating capacity in response to dehydration. It can be followed by assessment of the renal response to the synthetic AVP analogue desmopressin to determine whether any defect identified in urine-concentrating ability can be corrected with AVP-replacement. Office testing is acceptable unless the patient cannot be watched closely. No food or water is allowed. The patient is watched for signs of dehydration and surreptitious water drinking. Baseline measurements include weight, plasma osmolality, sodium, BUN, glucose, and urine volume and osmolality. Weight, plasma osmolality, and urine osmolality are measured hourly. The test is ended if urine osmolality has not increased to more than 300 mOsm/kg for 3 consecutive hours, plasma osmolality has reached 295 to 300 mOsm/kg, or the patient has lost 3% to 5% of body weight. All initial measurements are repeated at the end of the water restriction test. Then, 5 units of aqueous AVP (Pitressin) is administered or 2 µg of desmopressin is given subcutaneously and the plasma osmolality, sodium, BUN, glucose, and urine volume and osmolality are measured at 30, 60, and 120 minutes.

In primary polydipsia, urine concentration is normal in response to dehydration (Table 2).

In central DI, urine concentration does not increase appropriately with dehydration, but responds to desmopressin. Urine osmolality remains <300 mOsm/kg, accompanied by plasma osmolality >290 mOsm/kg after dehydration, and urine osmolality rising to >750 mOsm/kg after desmopressin administration.

In nephrogenic DI, urine concentration does not increase appropriately with either dehydration or exogenous desmopressin.

In practice, many results are indeterminate. If central DI is suspected, but the water deprivation test data are inconclusive, a

TABLE 3 Treatment Options for Diabetes Insipidus

Central DI	Divide doses of two to three times per day:
	Desmopressin nasal spray 5–100 µg/day
	Desmopressin tablets 0.1–1 mg/day
	Desmopressin injection 0.1–2 µg/day
Nephrogenic DI	Low-salt, low-protein diet
	HCTZ[1] 25 mg one to two times per day
	Indomethacin[1] 25–50 mg bid
	Amiloride[1] 5–10 mg bid
Primary polydipsia	Water restriction to less than 1.5 L/day

[1]Not FDA approved for this indication.

reasonable approach is a therapeutic trial of 10 to 20 µg intranasal desmopressin per day with close monitoring of plasma sodium. If the diagnosis is confirmed, pituitary function testing and cranial MRI should follow.

Treatment

The treatment goal is to improve polyuria and polydipsia symptoms while attempting to treat the etiologic factors (Table 3). This is achieved by appropriate correction of dehydration, if present, and replacing vasopressin or augmenting its effect on the target tissue.

Mild forms of central DI may not require pharmacologic treatment. Desmopressin effectively treats polyuria and polydipsia. Desmopressin comes in different forms, and dosages usually need to be divided.

Hyponatremia from plasma dilution can be avoided by skipping treatment for a short period on a regular basis (e.g., on Sunday). No second dose of desmopressin should be given unless the patient has urine output after the first dose.

Nephrogenic DI may respond to the removal of the offending agent (e.g., lithium) or correction of the underlying electrolyte disturbance (e.g., hypercalcemia or hypokalemia). Drug-induced nephrogenic DI, however, may persist after discontinuation of the drug.

Patients should be instructed to eat a low-sodium, low-protein diet, resulting in a decrease in urine output secondary to the drop in solute excretion. If symptomatic polyuria persists, hydrochlorothiazide[1] can be started. Hydrochlorothiazide presumably acts by inducing mild hypovolemia that induces an increase in proximal sodium and water reabsorption, thereby diminishing water delivery to the vasopressin-sensitive sites in the collecting tubules and reducing the urine output. Indomethacin (Indocin[1]) is an add-on medication if there is not enough response. Given that prostaglandins antagonize the action of vasopressin, indomethacin inhibits renal prostaglandin synthesis and subsequently decreases urine output.

Amiloride (Midamor)[1] might be more effective for lithium-induced nephrogenic DI. This drug closes the sodium channels in the luminal membrane of the collecting tubule cells. These

[1]Not FDA approved for this indication.

channels constitute the mechanism by which filtered lithium normally enters the collecting tubule cells and interferes with the collecting tubule response to ADH.

The approach to primary polydipsia treatment is reduction in fluid intake. Desmopressin treatment should be avoided due to the risk of hyponatremia.

Monitoring

Primary polydipsia is the most challenging of all types of DI to treat. It requires a multidisciplinary approach that frequently demands medical and psychiatric involvement.

In central DI, patients will require frequent follow-up to adjust desmopressin dosing. Once stable, patients can be seen less frequently to assess symptom control and to check plasma sodium levels to avoid overtreatment resulting in hyponatremia.

In nephrogenic DI, after the precipitating agent has been withdrawn, follow-up is needed to assess the reversibility of polyuria. If acquired nephrogenic DI becomes irreversible, patients might require prolonged pharmacological treatment. In both central and nephrogenic DI, the patient is advised to wear a medical alert bracelet stating the disease and the potential complications.

Acknowledgment

I would like to thank K. James Kallail, PhD, for his contribution to the final editing of this chapter.

References

Bockenhauer D, Bichet DG: Inherited secondary nephrogenic diabetes insipidus: Concentrating on humans, *Am J Physiol Renal Physiol* 304:F1037–F1042, 2013.

Crowley RK, Sherlock M, Agha A, et al: Clinical insights into adipsic diabetes insipidus: A large case series, *Clin Endocrinol (Oxf)* 66:475–482, 2007.

Fujiwara TM, Bichet DG: Molecular biology of hereditary diabetes insipidus, *J Am Soc Nephrol* 16:2836–2846, 2005.

Hannon MJ, Sherlock M, Thompson CJ: Pituitary dysfunction following traumatic brain injury or subarachnoid haemorrhage, *Best Pract Res Clin Endocrinol Metab* 25:783–798, 2011.

Monnens L, Jonkman A, Thomas C: Response to indomethacin and hydrochlorothiazide in nephrogenic diabetes insipidus, *Clin Sci (Lond)* 66:709–715, 1984.

Oiso Y, Robertson GL, Nørgaard JP, Juul KV: Clinical review: Treatment of neurohypophyseal diabetes insipidus, *J Clin Endocrinol Metab* 98:3958–3967, 2013.

Vande Walle J, Stockner M, Raes A, Nørgaard JP: Desmopressin 30 years in clinical use: A safety review, *Curr Drug Saf* 2:232–238, 2007.

DIABETIC KETOACIDOSIS

Method of
Aidar R. Gosmanov, MD, PhD, DMSc; Pasquale Passarella, MD; and Barry M. Wall, MD

CURRENT DIAGNOSIS

- Initial evaluation includes physical examination and comprehensive metabolic panel, serum osmolality, serum ketones and β-hydroxybutyrate, complete blood count, urinalysis, urine ketones, and arterial blood gases.
- Search for precipitating causes. Omission of insulin, underlying medical illness, cardiovascular events, gastrointestinal disorders, recent surgery, stress, medications, eating disorders, psychological stress, insulin pump malfunction, and infection are potential causes; white blood cell count greater than 25,000 suggests presence of infection.
- β-Hydroxybutyrate of 3.8 mmol/L or greater in adults indicates presence of diabetic ketoacidosis (DKA), even if serum ketones are negative.
- Patients with severe chronic kidney disease (CKD) require careful evaluation of acid-base status.

CURRENT THERAPY

- Start intravenous fluids early before insulin therapy.
- Potassium level should be more than 3.3 mEq/L before insulin therapy is initiated. Supplement potassium intravenously if needed.
- Initiate continuous insulin infusion at 0.14 U/kg/h and measure bedside glucose every 1 h to adjust the insulin infusion rate.
- Avoid hypoglycemia during the insulin infusion by initiating dextrose-containing fluids and/or reducing the insulin infusion rate until DKA is resolved.
- Transition to subcutaneous insulin only when DKA resolution is established.

Epidemiology

There were 168,000 hospital discharges for diabetic ketoacidosis (DKA) in 2014 in the United States, compared to 140,000 in 2009 and 80,000 in 1988. The in-hospital fatality rates declined consistently from 2009 to 2014 from 1.1% to 0.4%, although mortality remains high in developing countries. In 2005, the direct and indirect annual cost of DKA hospitalization was $2.4 billion.

Risk Factors

Omission of insulin is the most common precipitant of DKA. Infections, acute medical illnesses involving the cardiovascular system (myocardial infarction, stroke) and gastrointestinal tract (bleeding, pancreatitis), diseases of the endocrine axis (acromegaly and Cushing syndrome), and stress from recent surgical procedures can contribute to the development of DKA by causing dehydration, increase in insulin counterregulatory hormones, and worsening of peripheral insulin resistance. Medications such as diuretics, β-blockers, corticosteroids, second-generation antipsychotics, and anticonvulsants can affect carbohydrate metabolism and volume status and can, therefore, precipitate DKA. Other factors that can contribute to DKA include psychological problems, eating disorders, insulin pump malfunction, lower socioeconomic status, and drug abuse. It is now recognized that new-onset type 2 diabetes mellitus can manifest with DKA. These patients are obese, mostly African American or Hispanic, and extremely insulin resistant on presentation. Recently, the use of sodium-glucose cotransporter 2 (SGLT-2) inhibitors has been implicated in the development of DKA in patients with both type 1 and type 2 diabetes. The immune checkpoint inhibitors (ICI) used in patients with advanced malignancy can cause DKA de novo in patients without a prior history of diabetes. The DKA risk is significantly more common with use of programmed cell death protein 1 inhibitors such as nivolumab (Opdivo) compared to cytotoxic T-lymphocyte associated antigen 4 inhibitors such as ipilimumab (Yervoy).

Pathophysiology

Insulin deficiency, increased insulin counterregulatory hormones (cortisol, glucagon, growth hormone, and catecholamines), and peripheral insulin resistance lead to hyperglycemia, dehydration, ketosis, and electrolyte imbalance, which underlie the pathophysiology of DKA. The hyperglycemia of DKA evolves through accelerated gluconeogenesis, glycogenolysis, and decreased glucose utilization, all due to absolute insulin deficiency. Owing to increased lipolysis and decreased lipogenesis, abundant free fatty acids are converted to ketone bodies: acetoacetate and β-hydroxybutyrate (β-OHB). Hyperglycemia-induced osmotic diuresis, if not accompanied by sufficient oral fluid intake, leads to dehydration, hyperosmolarity, electrolyte loss, and subsequent decrease in glomerular filtration.

With a decline in a renal function, glycosuria diminishes, and hyperglycemia worsens. With impaired insulin action and hyperosmolar hyperglycemia, potassium uptake by skeletal muscle is markedly diminished, which, along with hyperosmolarity-mediated efflux of potassium from cells, results in intracellular potassium depletion. Potassium is lost via osmotic diuresis, causing profound total body potassium deficiency. Therefore DKA patients can present with a broad range of serum potassium concentrations. A "normal" plasma potassium concentration still indicates that potassium stores in the body are severely diminished and the institution of insulin therapy and correction of hyperglycemia will result in hypokalemia.

On average, patients with DKA have the following deficit of water and key electrolytes: water 100 mL/kg, sodium 7 to 10 mEq/kg, potassium 3 to 5 mEq/kg, and phosphorus 1 mmol/kg.

Clinical Manifestations

Polyuria, polydipsia, weight loss, vomiting, and abdominal pain usually are present in patients with DKA. Abdominal pain can be closely associated with acidosis and resolves with treatment. Physical examination findings such as hypotension, tachycardia, poor skin turgor, and weakness support the clinical diagnosis of dehydration in DKA. Mental status changes can occur in DKA and are likely related to the degree of acidosis and hyperosmolarity. A search for symptoms of precipitating causes such as infection, vascular events, or existing drug abuse should be initiated in the emergency department. Patients with hyperglycemic crises can be hypothermic because of peripheral vasodilation and decreased utilization of metabolic substrates.

Diagnosis

Diagnostic criteria for DKA include blood glucose higher than 250 mg/dL, arterial pH 7.30 or less, bicarbonate level 18 mEq/L or less, and adjusted for albumin anion gap greater than 10 to 12. Therefore initial laboratory evaluation should include a comprehensive metabolic panel and arterial blood gases. Positive serum and urine ketones can further support the diagnosis of DKA but are not required. In early DKA, acetoacetate concentration is low, but it is a major substrate for ketone measurement by many laboratories; therefore ketone measurement in serum by usual laboratory techniques has a high specificity but low sensitivity for the diagnosis of DKA. Conversely, β-OHB is an early and abundant ketoacid that can first signal development of DKA, but its measurement requires the use of a specific assay that is different from ketone measurement. β-OHB of 3.8 mmol/L or higher was shown to be highly sensitive and specific for DKA diagnosis.

In patients with chronic kidney disease stage 4 or 5, the diagnosis of DKA is challenging because of the presence of chronic metabolic acidosis and the possibility of mixed acid-base disorders on presentation with DKA. An anion gap greater than 20 supports the diagnosis of DKA in such patients.

Differential Diagnosis

Hyperglycemic hyperosmolar state is usually not associated with ketosis, but mixed hyperglycemic hyperosmolar state and DKA can occur. Clinical scenarios that may be accompanied by acidosis are described in Table 1. Pregnancy, starvation, and alcoholic ketoacidosis are not characterized by hyperglycemia greater than 250 mg/dL. With hypotension or a history of metformin (Glucophage) use, lactic acidosis should be suspected. Ingestion of methanol, isopropyl alcohol, and paraldehyde[2] can also alter the anion gap and/or osmolality but are not associated with hyperglycemia.

Treatment

The therapeutic goals of management include optimization of volume status, hyperglycemia and ketoacidosis, electrolyte abnormalities, and potential precipitating factors. DKA management workflow is presented in Figure 1. The efficiency of early DKA therapy can be improved by clustering key diagnostic and therapeutic steps in one protocol that is easy to understand by both nursing staff and physicians. Table 2 provides one example of such a DKA care bundle. Given the complexity of the condition

---

management, provision of a single care bundle/order set allows the fundamentals of DKA treatment to be delivered safely and efficiently while giving the providers guidance on tackling unanticipated issues during DKA care. Special considerations should be given to patients with congestive heart failure and chronic kidney disease (CKD). These patients tend to retain fluids; therefore caution should be exercised during volume resuscitation in these patient groups.

Bicarbonate therapy is not indicated in mild and moderate forms of DKA because metabolic acidosis should correct with insulin therapy. The use of bicarbonate in severe DKA is controversial owing to a lack of prospective randomized studies. It is thought that the administration of bicarbonate actually results in peripheral hypoxemia, worsened hypokalemia, paradoxical central nervous system acidosis, cerebral edema in children and young adults, and an increase in intracellular acidosis. Because severe acidosis is associated with worse clinical outcomes and can lead to an impairment in sensorium and a deterioration of myocardial contractility, bicarbonate therapy may be indicated if the pH is 6.9 or less. Therefore the infusion of 100 mmol (2 ampoules) of bicarbonate in 400 mL of sterile water mixed with 20 mEq potassium chloride over 2 hours and repeating the infusion until the pH is greater than 7.0 can be recommended pending the results of prospective trials.

A whole-body phosphate deficit in DKA can average 1 mmol/kg. Insulin therapy during DKA will further lower serum phosphate concentration. Prospective randomized studies have failed to show any beneficial effect of phosphate replacement on the clinical outcome in DKA. However, a careful phosphate replacement is sometimes indicated in patients with serum phosphate concentration less than 1.0 mg/dL and in those with cardiac dysfunction, anemia, or respiratory depression who have a serum phosphate level between 1.0 and 2.0 mg/dL. An initial replacement strategy may include infusion of potassium phosphate at the rate of 0.1 to 0.2 mmol/kg over 6 hours, depending on the degree of phosphate deficit (1 mL potassium phosphate solution for intravenous use contains 3 mmol phosphorous and 4.4 mEq potassium). Overzealous phosphate replacement can result in hypocalcemia; therefore close monitoring of phosphorous and calcium levels is recommended. Patients who have renal insufficiency or hypocalcemia might need less-aggressive phosphate replacement.

When DKA is resolved, and independent of the patient's ability to tolerate oral intake, transition to subcutaneous insulin must be initiated. Patients are given intermediate neutral protamine Hagedorn (NPH) or long-acting insulin (detemir [Levemir], glargine [Lantus]) 2 hours before termination of intravenous insulin to allow sufficient time for the injected insulin to start working (Table 3). Once the patient can eat, we recommend the addition of short- or rapid-acting insulin for prandial glycemic coverage (see Table 3). This is the basal-bolus insulin regimen and provides physiologic replacement of insulin. It is common to see transition from intravenous to subcutaneous insulin using sliding-scale insulin only. This strategy as a sole approach should be discouraged because it cannot provide the necessary insulin requirement in patients recovering from hyperglycemic crisis and beta-cell failure.

If the patient used insulin prior to admission, the same dosage can be restarted in the hospital. Insulin-naïve patients require insulin at a total dose of 0.5 to 0.8 U/kg/day divided as 50% basal insulin and 50% as prandial insulin before each meal. Initially, after DKA resolution and given the possibility of fluctuating oral intake, the use of once-daily long-acting insulin such as glargine or detemir to provide basal insulin coverage is encouraged. Long-acting insulin glargine U300 (Toujeo) and insulin degludec (Tresiba), which were approved by the FDA in 2015, as well as biosimilar insulin glargine (Basaglar), which was approved in 2016, have not been studied in hospitalized patients treated for DKA and, therefore, cannot be recommended for subcutaneous administration immediately following DKA resolution. For patients who are not able to adhere to or afford multiple daily insulin injections, conversion of inpatient basal-bolus

---

[2]Not available in the United States

TABLE 1 Laboratory Evaluation of Metabolic Causes of Acidosis

LAB VALUE	DKA	STARVATION KETOSIS	LACTIC ACIDOSIS	UREMIC ACIDOSIS	ALCOHOL KETOSIS	SALICYLATE POISONING	METHANOL OR ETHYLENE GLYCOL POISONING
pH	↓	Normal	↓	Mild ↓	↑↓	↑↓*	↓
Plasma glucose	↑	Normal	Normal	Normal	↓ or normal	Normal or ↓	Normal
Plasma ketones†	↑↑	Slight ↑	Normal	Normal	↑	Normal	Normal
Anion gap	↑	Slight ↑	↑	Slight ↑	↑	↑	↑
Osmolality	↑	Normal	Normal	↑ or normal	Normal	Normal	↑↑
Other	—	—	Lactate ↑	BUN ↑	—	Serum level +	Serum level +

*Respiratory alkalosis or metabolic acidosis.
†Acetest and Ketostix (Bayer, Leverkusen, Germany) measure acetoacetic acid only; thus, misleadingly low values may be obtained because the majority of "ketone bodies" are β-hydroxybutyrate.
BUN, Blood urea nitrogen; *DKA,* diabetic ketoacidosis.

WORKFLOW OF MANAGEMENT OF ADULT DKA

Figure 1 Diabetic ketoacidosis management protocol. *BG,* Blood glucose.

insulin regimen before discharge to split-mix insulin preparation (Humulin 70/30, Novolin 70/30, Humalog mix 75/25, Novolog mix 70/30) twice a day that contains a mixture of intermediate-acting insulin NPH and short-acting insulin formulations such as regular (Humulin R, Novolin R), aspart (Novolog), or lispro (Humalog) can be considered. Finger-stick glucose measurements before each meal and at night should be taken after discontinuation of intravenous insulin to correct for possible fluctuations in insulin needs while in the hospital.

Monitoring

Serial measurements—every 2 to 4 hours—of metabolic parameters are required to monitor therapy and then confirm the resolution of DKA. DKA is considered resolved when plasma glucose is less than 200 to 250 mg/dL, serum bicarbonate concentration is 15 mEq/L or higher, venous blood pH is greater than 7.3, and anion gap 12 or less. In general, resolution of hyperglycemia,

normalization of bicarbonate level, and closure of the anion gap is sufficient to stop insulin infusion. The anion gap is calculated by subtracting the sum of Cl⁻ and HCO₃⁺ from measured (not corrected) Na⁺ concentration and can improve even before the restoration of serum bicarbonate owing to hyperchloremia from normal saline infusion. Venous pH is adequate for assessing the degree of acidosis, with consideration that it is 0.02 to 0.03 lower than arterial blood. If plasma glucose is less than 200 mg/dL but bicarbonate and pH are not normalized, insulin infusion must be continued, and dextrose-containing intravenous fluids started. The latter approach will continue to suppress ketogenesis and prevent hypoglycemia.

Complications

Hypoglycemia is the most common complication and can be prevented by the timely adjustment of insulin dosage and frequent monitoring of blood glucose levels. Hypoglycemia is defined as

TABLE 2	Diabetic Ketoacidosis Order Set

Allergies: ☐ NKDA or ☐ Other (specify):

Baseline Labs:
☐ CBC w/ Diff, CMP, Magnesium, Phosphorus, ABG, Serum Ketones, Fingerstick Blood Glucose, Hemoglobin A1c
☐ Urinalysis ☐ Troponins q6h ×3 ☐ β-hydroxybutyrate ☐ Other (specify):

Follow-up Labs:
☐ Fingerstick Blood Glucose q1h ☐ BMP, Magnesium, Phosphorus q2h ☐ VBG q____h
☐ BMP, Magnesium, Phosphorus q4h ☐ Other (specify):

Consults: ☐ Endocrinology ☐ Diabetes Education

Nursing: ☐ Strict I + O

PHASE I: INITIAL MANAGEMENT
Initial Potassium Replacement for baseline potassium <3.3mmol/L
☐ Potassium Chloride_____mEq IVPB (infuse at 10mEq/h)

Initial Fluid Replacement
☐ 2 L bolus 0.9% NaCl at 500 mL/h OR ☐_____L bolus 0.9%NaCl at_____mL/h (specify)

Insulin Therapy:
Do NOT start insulin infusion until K+ > 3.3 mmol/L
☐ Regular Human Insulin Continuous Infusion: (specify below)
☐ 0.14 units/kg/h (_____units/h)
☐ 0.05 units/kg/h (_____units/h) (if end-stage renal disease)

PHASE 2: USE UNTIL BLOOD GLUCOSE <250 mg/dL for the FIRST TIME during insulin therapy

BLOOD GLUCOSE (MG/DL)	INSULIN INFUSION RATE (ROUND UP TO NEAREST WHOLE NUMBER)		FLUID THERAPY
<100	See PHASE 3		
100–250	Decrease current infusion rate by half, MOVE to PHASE 3		D5 ½ NS + KCl 20 mEq/L at 200 mL/h
>250 AND: a) Glucose dropped by less than 50 mg/dL in 1 h b) Glucose dropped by 50–100 mg/dL in 1 h c) Glucose dropped by over 100 mg/dL in 1 h	a) Maintain current infusion rate and CALL MD for additional bolus (0.1 units/kg) b) Maintain current infusion rate c) Decrease current infusion rate by half		½ NS + KCl 20 mEq/L at 200 mL/h

PHASE 3: USE FOR ALL BLOOD GLUCOSE READINGS AFTER PHASE 2, or if blood glucose is <100 mg/dL at any time

BLOOD GLUCOSE (MG/DL)	INSULIN INFUSION RATE (ROUND UP TO NEAREST WHOLE NUMBER)	FLUID THERAPY
<70	1. HOLD insulin infusion and give 1 amp D50W IV 2. NOTIFY MD and check fingerstick blood glucose every 15 min until glucose >70, then every 1 h until glucose >100 3. RESTART insulin at half the previous rate when glucose >100	D5 ½ NS + KCl 20 mEq/L at 200 mL/h
70–100	1. HOLD insulin infusion and give ½ amp D50W IV 2. NOTIFY MD and recheck BG in 15 min 3. RESTART insulin at half the previous rate when glucose >100	D5 ½ NS + KCl 20 mEq/L at 200 mL/h
101–200	• If current rate ≥2 units/h, decrease rate by half • If current rate <2 units/h, continue current rate	D5 ½ NS + KCl 20 mEq/L at 200 mL/h
201–250	Maintain current infusion rate	D5 ½ NS + KCl 20 mEq/L at 200mL/h
> 250	Return to PHASE 2	

ABG, Arterial blood gas; *BMP*, basic metabolic profile; *CBC*, complete blood count; *CMP*, comprehensive metabolic panel; *IVPB*, intravenously per bag; *NKDA*, no known drug allergies; *VBG*, venous blood gas.

any blood glucose level below 70 mg/dL. If DKA is not resolved and blood glucose level is below 200 to 250 mg/dL, decreases in insulin infusion rate and/or addition of 5% or 10% dextrose to current intravenous fluids may be implemented (see Figure 1). For patients in whom DKA is resolved, strategies to manage hypoglycemia depend on whether the patient is able to eat or not. For patients who are able to drink or eat, ingestion of 15 to 20 g of carbohydrates—for example, four glucose tablets or 6 oz orange or apple juice or "regular" soft drink—is advised. In patients who are allowed nothing by mouth, are unable to swallow, or have an altered level of consciousness, administer 25 mL 50% dextrose IV or give 1 mg glucagon IM if no IV access is present. Blood glucose should be rechecked in 15 minutes; only if the glucose level is less than 80 mg/dL should these steps be repeated.

Non–anion-gap hyperchloremic acidosis occurs from urinary loss of ketoanions, which are needed for bicarbonate regeneration, and preferential reabsorption of chloride in proximal renal tubules secondary to intensive administration of chloride-containing fluids and low plasma bicarbonate. The acidosis usually resolves and should not affect the treatment course. Cerebral edema has been reported in young adult patients. This condition is manifested by the appearance of headache, lethargy, papillary changes, or seizures. Mortality is up to 70%. Mannitol (Osmitrol) infusion and mechanical ventilation should be used to treat this condition. Rhabdomyolysis is another possible complication resulting from hyperosmolality and hypoperfusion. Pulmonary edema can develop from excessive fluid replacement in patients with CKD or congestive heart failure.

TABLE 3	Pharmacokinetics and Pharmacodynamics of Subcutaneous Insulin Preparations				
INSULIN	**ONSET OF ACTION**	**TIME TO PEAK**	**DURATION**	**TIMING OF DOSE**
Regular (Humulin R, Novolin R)	30–60 min	2–3 h	8–10 h	30–45 min before meal
Aspart (Novolog)	5–15 min	30–90 min	4–6 h	15 min before meal
Ultra-rapid Aspart (Fiasp)	2.5 min	63 min	5–7 h	Within 0–20 min after meal start
Glulisine (Apidra)	15 min	30–90 min	5.3 h	15 min before meal
Lispro (Humalog)	5–15 min	30–90 min	4–6 h	15 min before meal
NPH (Humulin N and Novolin N)	2–4 h	4–10 h	12–18 h	Twice a day
Detemir (Levemir)	2 h	No peak	12–24 h	Once or twice a day
Glargine (Lantus)	2 h	No peak	20–24 h	Once a day
Glargine (Basaglar)	2 h	No peak	20–24 h	Once a day
Glargine U-300 (Toujeo)	6 h	No peak	24–36 h	Once a day
Degludec (Tresiba)	1 h	No peak	42 h	Once a day

Prevention

Discharge planning should include diabetes education, selection of an appropriate insulin regimen that the patient can understand and afford, and preparation of set of supplies for the initial insulin administration at home. Many cases of DKA can be prevented by better access to medical care, proper education, and effective communication with a healthcare provider during an intercurrent illness.

Sick-day management should be reviewed periodically with all patients. It should include specific information on when to contact the healthcare provider, blood glucose goals and the use of supplemental short- or rapid-acting insulin during illness, insulin use during fever and infection, and initiation of an easily digestible liquid diet containing carbohydrates and salt. Most importantly, the patient should be advised to never discontinue insulin and to seek professional advice early in the course of the illness. The patient or family member must be able to accurately measure and record insulin administered, blood glucose, and blood β-hydroxybutyrate with a point-of-care device when blood glucose is higher than 300 mg/dL. Recent studies demonstrated that β-OHB testing in outpatient setting is more effective than urine acetoacetate testing in preventing DKA, which may reduce the costs of care of patients with insulin-dependent diabetes.

Because of the significant cost of repeated admissions for DKA, resources should be directed toward educating primary care providers and school personnel so that they can identify signs and symptoms of uncontrolled diabetes earlier.

References

Cardoso L, Vicente N, Rodrigues D, et al: Controversies in the management of hyperglycaemic emergencies in adults with diabetes, *Metabolism* 68:43–54, 2017.
Centers for Disease Control and Prevention: Diabetes data and trends: diabetes complications. Available at https://www.cdc.gov/diabetes/pdfs/data/statistics/national-diabetes-statistics-report.pdf (accessed January 26, 2018).
Fadini GP, Bonora BM, Avogaro A: SGLT2 inhibitors and diabetic ketoacidosis: data from the FDA Adverse Event Reporting System, *Diabetologia* 60:1385–1389, 2017.
Hirsch IB: Insulin analogues, *N Engl J Med* 352:174–183, 2005.
Kamel KS, Halperin ML: Acid-base problems in diabetic ketoacidosis, *N Engl J Med* 372:546–554, 2015.
Kitabchi AE, Umpierrez GE, Fisher JN, et al: Thirty years of personal experience in hyperglycemic crises: diabetic ketoacidosis and hyperglycemic hyperosmolar state, *J Clin Endocrinol Metab* 93:1541–1552, 2008.
Kitabchi AE, Umpierrez GE, Miles JM, et al: Hyperglycemic crises in adult patients with diabetes, *Diabetes Care* 32:1335–1343, 2009.
Kitabchi AE, Umpierrez GE, Murphy MB, et al: Hyperglycemic crises in adult patients with diabetes: a consensus statement from the American Diabetes Association, *Diabetes Care* 29:2739–2748, 2006.
Sheikh-Ali M, Karon BS, Basu A, et al: Can serum beta-hydroxybutyrate be used to diagnose diabetic ketoacidosis? *Diabetes Care* 31:643–647, 2008.
Stamatouli AM, Quandt Z, Perdigoto AL, et al: Collateral damage: insulin-dependent diabetes induced with checkpoint inhibitors, *Diabetes* 67(8):1471–1480, 2018 Aug.
Tzamaloukas AH, Ing TS, Siamopoulos KC, et al: Pathophysiology and management of fluid and electrolyte disturbances in patients on chronic dialysis with severe hyperglycemia, *Semin Dial* 21:431–439, 2008.
Umpierrez GE, Smiley D, Kitabchi AE: Narrative review: ketosis-prone type 2 diabetes mellitus, *Ann Intern Med* 144:350–357, 2006.
Vellanki P, Umpierrez GE: Increasing hospitalizations for DKA: a need for prevention programs, *Diabetes Care* 41(9):1839–1841, 2018.

DIABETES MELLITUS IN ADULTS

Method of
Anthony L. McCall, MD, PhD; J. Terry Saunders, PhD; Niyaz Gosmanov, MD; and Albina Gosmanova, MD

CURRENT DIAGNOSIS

- Screening for diabetes should be done in high-risk populations, especially:
  - Those with prediabetes, signs of insulin resistance (e.g., acanthosis nigricans), or the metabolic syndrome.
  - High-risk ethnic groups (e.g., Native American, Latino American, African American).
  - History of gestational diabetes or polycystic ovary disease.
- Patients might present with atypical symptoms.
- Most diabetes is type 2 in adults, but type 1 does occur in adults, and delayed diagnosis is common.
- Cardiovascular risk should be aggressively screened for and treated.
- Complications should be documented and tracked.
- Check fasting lipids or, if inconvenient, get nonfasting lipids focused on cardiovascular risk using a calculator.
- Check renal function and albuminuria yearly.
- Have a low threshold for stress testing, with imaging for all patients who have symptoms of ischemia or clinical equivalents.
- Refer for yearly eye examinations by an eye professional.
- Check feet for sensation, deformity, and circulation at regular visits.
- All patients should receive an ongoing educational assessment and training in self-management and self-monitoring of blood glucose in both class and individual settings.
- Take a diet history; this is especially important for patients on insulin.
- Get a baseline HbA1c and repeat two to four times per year (twice yearly, if at glycemic goal).

CURRENT THERAPY

- Diabetes requires nutrition and behavioral self-management counseling, as well as drug therapy.
  - Individualize goals for every patient (for glycemia, lipids, blood pressure): Base individualization on age, quality of life, life expectancy, motivation, complications, diabetes duration, hypoglycemia risk.
  - Involve patient and caregivers in the decision making.
- Repeatedly encourage healthy eating and an active lifestyle.
- Prediabetes diagnosis represents an opportunity for behavioral and drug interventions.
- Metformin (Glucophage) is usually the first drug therapy.
- Don't expect one drug to do the job for very poorly controlled glycemia, especially if HgbA1c is greater than 9% or greater than 2% above the target.
- Dual defects (insulin resistance and secretion) should be addressed in most patients.
- Very insulin-resistant patients might need a dual insulin resistance strategy.
- Therapy goals for both HbA1c and self-monitored blood glucose can be achieved in most patients.
- Cardiovascular risk reduction therapy is a very high priority—statins and blood pressure control are best.
- Consider use of new American College of Cardiology (ACC)/ American Heart Association (AHA) Omnibus cardiovascular disease risk calculator for when to start statin therapy.
- When patients have not met goals on two or three oral agents as therapy, basal insulin is often the most appropriate choice, particularly when patients are not near glycemic goals.
- For oral agent therapy, add—don't switch—unless side effects require it.
- When adding basal insulin, initially continue oral agent therapies.
- Threatening patients with insulin therapy is counterproductive.
- Follow the 3F rule: *Fix the fasting glucose first*, especially in patients with poor glycemic control. As control improves, pay attention to postmeal sugar levels.
- Prompt recognition of the need for meal-time insulin is critical to achieve glycemic goals.
- Usually start with a single-meal insulin dose for the largest meal.
- Balance meal and basal insulin; check postmeal BG.

Epidemiology

The Centers for Disease Control and Prevention (CDC) estimated that in 2015 the prevalence of diabetes in the United States was 30.3 million, affecting 9.4% of the US population. Diabetes is diagnosed in 23.1 million persons and undiagnosed in 7.2 million. Type 2 diabetes mellitus (T2DM) is 90% to 95% of prevalent diabetes, and type 1 diabetes (T1DM) is about 3% to 4%. There are few persons with secondary or monogenic forms of diabetes, such as *maturity-onset diabetes of the young*. About 84 million people above the age of 20 years in the United States are thought to have prediabetes.

The focus of this chapter is T2DM because it is the most prevalent form and continues to increase in prevalence in the United States and worldwide. A few comments are made on adult T1DM. This chapter emphasizes both lifestyle and pharmacologic treatments. Although prediabetes may not require drug therapy, it represents an important opportunity to prevent or delay onset of diabetes and initiate critical lifestyle changes.

Diagnosis and Classification of Diabetes and Prediabetes
Diagnosis
Most diabetes is diagnosed by random or fasting glucose (Table 1). Symptoms should be present (e.g., thirst, frequent urination) if random glucose criteria are used, but, surprisingly, many people with diabetes are relatively symptom free. In the elderly, cognitive changes can occur, and atypical symptoms such as prostatism or genital or skinfold yeast infections can suggest the diagnosis. The American Diabetes Association (ADA) screening recommendations suggest screening every 3 years starting at age 45 for the general population, but they suggest earlier and more frequent screening in those at high risk. Elevated HbA1c when 6.5% or higher can be used for screening and diagnosis of diabetes.

Patients from diabetes-prone ethnic groups (e.g., Latin Americans, African Americans, Native Americans, Asian Americans) or with a strong family history, polycystic ovary syndrome, or gestational diabetes should have early and frequent screenings. High-risk persons include those with prediabetes (impaired glucose tolerance, impaired fasting glucose) or who meet the National Cholesterol Education Program criteria for the metabolic syndrome or its individual components (dyslipidemia, hypertension, central obesity, and prediabetes). Despite the limitations of the metabolic syndrome as a diagnostic tool, it does not reduce the importance of fully documenting and treating coexisting cardiometabolic risk factors in those with or at risk for T2DM in a targeted manner (Box 1). Teach patients and clinicians about these risks and encourage the overweight and sedentary to adopt a healthier lifestyle. Effective intervention programs, such as the Diabetes Prevention Project, provide strong support for effectiveness of lifestyle modification in prevention of type 2 diabetes.

Classification
The classification of diabetes into its two most prominent types (T1DM and T2DM) seems straightforward in theory, but in practice is increasingly confusing as more Americans become overweight. Although T1DM patients were traditionally described as being lean, a significant proportion of the group is overweight and some have characteristics of metabolic syndrome. About 80% to 90% of persons with T2DM are overweight or have metabolic syndrome characteristics, but some are leaner and more active and do not have features of the metabolic syndrome. C-peptide measurements are not very helpful for those who are difficult to classify but measuring three antibodies—including IA-2 (islet cell antigen 512), anti-GAD$_{65}$ (glutamic acid decarboxylase), and antiinsulin antibodies in high titers—can clarify a diagnosis of latent autoimmune diabetes. Younger age at onset, lean body habitus, severe loss of glycemic control with or without ketonemia, and weight loss all suggest insulin deficiency but might not be definitive.

Pathophysiology
The primary causes of most adult diabetes are insulin resistance and lack of compensatory insulin secretion. Abnormalities in incretin hormone physiology may also underlie early pathophysiology, although deficiency of glucagon-like peptide-1 (GLP-1) is probably not the simple explanation. Insulin resistance is typically long-standing and begins at a young age because of heredity combined with environmental causes (sedentary lifestyle and calorie overconsumption with resultant overweight). Insulin secretory defects usually start about 10 years before diagnosis, and no therapy is proven so far to prevent progressive loss of insulin secretion, although consistent lifestyle modifications, involving diet and exercise, can help slow down the process and reduce rates of conversion of prediabetes to clinically apparent diabetes. Long-standing insulin resistance is associated with dyslipidemia, central obesity, and hypertension, which suggests a shared etiology of diabetes and metabolic derangements.

Cardiovascular Risk Management
Cardiovascular (CV) risk management in diabetes starts at the time of diagnosis and includes lifestyle counseling and education. It is paramount that patients understand the intimate and direct links among diabetes, glycemic control, and cardiovascular disease (CVD). Drug interventions are ultimately needed for glycemia, lipid risks, and blood pressure in most patients. Women have higher relative risk and similar overall risk as men and are often undertreated. Specific recommended targets of therapy for

TABLE 1   Diagnosis and Classification of Diabetes and Prediabetes

DIAGNOSIS	GLUCOSE TEST	DIAGNOSTIC LEVEL	COMMENTS
Diabetes	Random	≥ 200 mg/dL	Plus classic symptoms*
Diabetes	Fasting	≥ 126 mg/dL	8-h fast; need confirmation
Diabetes	Postglucose load (75 g in nonpregnant adults)	≥ 200 mg/dL at 2 h	Need confirmation
Diabetes	HbA1c†	6.5%	NGS standardized lab
Prediabetes	IFG Fasting	≥ 100 mg/dL	Decreased insulin secretion
Prediabetes	IGT Postglucose load (75 g)	140–199 mg/dL at 2 h	Increased insulin resistance
Prediabetes	HbA1c	5.7%–6.4%	NGS standardized lab

IFG, Impaired fasting glucose; *IGT*, impaired glucose tolerance.
*Polyuria, polydipsia, unexplained weight loss.
†NGS nationally standardized lab method.

BOX 1   Summary of Goals for Treatment

Lifestyle
Medical Nutrition Therapy (individualized)
- Appropriate calories for weight, 5%–10% weight loss for obese patients
- Low saturated and trans fats, substitute with healthy fats
- Moderate, consistent carbohydrates (whole grains, vegetables, fruits with low glycemic effects)
- Foods that can reduce postmeal sugar surges (low glycemic index and load)
- Healthy fats and proteins (decreased saturated and trans fats, increased monosaturated fat; reduced consumption of animal protein)

Activity
- Consistent, regular activity tailored to complications and safety (ECG or stress test may be needed before starting an exercise program)

Glycemia: It Is Critical That These Goals Are Individualized*
- Best possible without frequent or severe hypoglycemia
- HbA1c <7% generally; 6% or less if possible in selected patients early in disease course; 7%–8% may be appropriate in those with shortened lifespan

Self-Monitored Blood Glucose
- Preprandial 80–130†
- Postprandial (1–2 h) <180 minimal; <140 ideal

Lipids
- All DM patients with overt ASCVD should be on high intensity statins
- DM patients <40 or >75 years old with CVD risk‡
- DM patients 40–70 years old with CVD risk consider high intensity statins
- DM patients >40 without CVD risk statins are not recommended
- Blood Pressure§
- Systolic <140 mm Hg
- Diastolic <90 mm Hg

---

*See ADA guidelines for factors.
†80 mg/dL is too low for patients with high risk of hypoglycemia. 110 ideally; 20 to 30 mg/dL higher is acceptable for high-risk for hypoglycemia patients or those with hypoglycemia unawareness.
‡CVD risk factors include low-density lipoprotein cholesterol ≥100 mg/dL (2.6 mmol/L), high blood pressure, smoking, and overweight and obesity consider medium-intensity to high-intensity statins.
§More-aggressive BP goals may be appropriate for individual patients if tolerated well and there are no increases in risk of side effects. Relaxed criteria based on age, comorbidities, long duration of diabetes, behavioral, motivational criteria, and others.
ACS, Acute coronary syndrome, *ASCVD,* atherosclerotic cardiovascular disease; *CVD,* cardiovascular disease; *DM,* diabetes mellitus.

diabetes in glycemia, blood pressure, dyslipidemia, and lifestyle are shown in Box 1. Latest guidelines incorporate the use of diabetes drugs with known CV benefit. For adults with type 2 diabetes and heart disease, the ADA recommends that, after lifestyle management and metformin, healthcare providers should prescribe medications proven to improve heart health by prevention of major acute cardiac event, related hospitalizations, and death.

Documenting and Monitoring Complications

Patients should have a thorough examination and evaluation for complications at the time of diabetes diagnosis. About half of patients with newly diagnosed T2DM have established chronic complications, indicating delayed recognition of this disorder.

Neuropathy and circulatory signs and symptoms on foot examination should be assessed. Risk of ulcer and amputation can be gauged by 10-g Semmes-Weinstein monofilaments that test for severe neuropathy and attendant risk of ulceration. Retina examinations should be done by skilled eye professionals likely to pick up significant eye disease. High-risk patients (poor glycemic control, established retinopathy, especially if preproliferative or worse) should be referred promptly to an eye specialist. Pregnancy counseling should be given to all women of childbearing age with diabetes. Albumin-to-creatinine ratio in the urine should be assessed and kidney function (serum creatinine, estimated glomerular filtration rate [eGFR], and blood urea nitrogen) should be tracked yearly. Many drugs for diabetes are dosed based on kidney function, so it may be appropriate to track eGFR closely (e.g., every 3 to 6 months) when it is abnormal.

Home glucose monitoring should be taught to patients so they understand the effects of food, stress, acute intercurrent illness, and exercise on glycemic patterns. Diabetes education in both individual and group settings should be arranged for all patients, preferably by a diabetes educator. Diabetes is unique in being a self-managed condition where patient knowledge and skills are critical to avoiding complications. Moreover, behavioral management is critical to success in diabetes care.

Treatment
Behavioral Self-Management

Self-management of behavioral factors, including eating, physical activity, and psychological stress, is essential to good diabetes self-care. Ideally, professional support for behavioral self-management should be a coordinated, multidisciplinary effort involving expertise appropriate to a given patient from the areas of nutrition, nursing, physical activity, and behavioral counseling. The provider should develop basic behavior change skills and refer to appropriate multidisciplinary and community-based resources.

Quick, one-shot interventions seldom change long-standing patterns of behavior. Initial sessions should be scheduled close together (1 to 2 weeks), then further apart as the patient gains momentum and confidence. If multiple one-on-one sessions are impossible, other options such as group meetings, telephone support, or e-mail messaging should be considered.

Behavior change interventions should be highly individualized and specific. General advice about diet and exercise does not address the life experience or problems of a given patient and is often perceived as insensitive or unhelpful. Arriving at individualized objectives for behavior change can be accomplished using a simple three-step process composed of initial assessment, setting behavioral objectives, and follow-up and reassessment. Basic principles of the process of setting behavioral objectives can be summed up by the mnemonic SMART (specific, measurable, achievable, relevant, and time-oriented).

Initial Assessment

Initial assessment includes identifying salient features of social and family history that can affect efforts to change behavior. A nutrition assessment should be performed, including an appraisal of usual food intake, the patient's perception of problem eating behavior, and weight history. A physical activity assessment should also be conducted, focusing on past and current physical activity, preferences, perceived barriers, and general attitudes. Readiness to make changes in behavior should be assessed by asking how important a patient thinks it is to change a given area of behavior and how confident she or he is that she or he can succeed in making changes (on a scale of 1 to 10). Discussion of specific objectives for behavioral change should occur in areas where the patient indicates a definite readiness to begin. Finally, ask patients about current levels and sources of stress. Because depression is common with diabetes, patients should be screened for possible depression.

Behavioral Objectives

Setting behavioral objectives is initiated and facilitated by the provider, but the patient is responsible for selecting his or her own behavioral objectives. Objectives should be FIRM: *few* (1 to 3 at a time is plenty), *i*ndividualized to the patient's specific behavioral challenges, *r*ealistic (beware of trying to make big strides quickly), and *m*easurable (weight, waist circumference, exercise capacity). The patient should be encouraged to keep a daily record of progress on each objective. For those with access, phone and computer-based applications enhance the ease and accuracy of tracking. The primary focus of provider-patient discussions of progress should be on behavioral objectives, not outcomes.

Accurate knowledge of current behavior is key to setting behavioral objectives for nutrition and exercise. Obtaining a 3-day food record (2 workdays and 1 nonworkday) and a baseline for activity (we generally use a week of daily steps measured with a pedometer) provide a solid baseline for setting objectives.

A modest reduction in caloric consumption of around 250 to 500 kcal/day and moderate physical activity on the order of at least 150 minutes a week are the recommended approaches to weight loss. Reducing calories through decreased food consumption is more effective for weight loss than increasing energy expenditure through physical activity. Box 2 contains a checklist of healthy eating behaviors that can be used to stimulate patients' thinking about areas in which they might like to make changes. Note that an irregular pattern of eating often underlies unhealthy food choices. For example, staying up late encourages late-night snacking, which in turn can suppress interest in eating breakfast. Eating tends to be deferred to the afternoon or evening, perpetuating the cycle.

Physical activity plays an important role in weight maintenance. Higher levels of activity (200 min/week) may be required to prevent long-term weight regain. Box 3 lists ways that patients can become more active. It is worth repeating that the point of these and other suggestions is not to direct patients but to expand their thinking about what might work for them.

Follow-up and Reassessment

Follow-up and reassessment occur during each return visit, after a period of patient efforts to carry out mutually agreed on behavioral objectives. Reassessment focuses on the behavioral records kept by

---

| BOX 2 | Checklist of Healthy Eating Behaviors |

✓ Eat meals and snacks at set times to promote health.
Examples:
- I will eat breakfast within 1 h of getting up.
- I will not skip meals.
- Other:..
....

✓ Eat healthy carbohydrates.
Examples:
- I will avoid regular soft drinks and choose water or diet soft drinks instead.
- I will eat 5–7 servings of fruits and vegetables every day.
- I will choose whole-grain breads and cereals.
- Other:..
....

✓ Decrease serving sizes.
Examples:
- I will keep a record of the food I eat and drink.
- I will know what counts as a serving size.
- When I am eating out, I will share or split an entrée and eat a salad.
- Other:..
....

✓ Eat less fat and choose healthy fats.
Examples:
- I will bake, broil, roast, grill, or boil instead of fry food.
- I will have a meatless meal at least once a week.
- I will choose fried or high-fat foods no more than once a week.
- I will drink fat-free or low-fat milk.
- I will use healthy oils (olive oil, canola oil) and buy tub margarine.
- Other:..
....

✓ Make other healthy choices.
Examples:
- I will drink plenty of fluids (at least 8 glasses of water or low-calorie fluid per day).
- I will limit how much alcohol I drink. (Women should drink no more than 1 alcoholic drink per day. Men should drink no more than 2 alcoholic drinks per day.)
- Other:..
....

Unpublished source: Virginia Center for Diabetes Professional Education, University of Virginia; Virginia Diabetes Council.

---

patients as well as on their verbal reports of difficulties and successes. Praise and encouragement are the order of the day. Efforts to initiate behavior change are highly responsive to external positive reinforcement, and the patient will need maximum external reinforcement until new behavior becomes self-sustaining. After review and discussion of patient records, new behavioral objectives or incremental changes in existing objectives are selected by mutual agreement, with the patient taking the lead.

A modest weight loss of 5% to 10% has a positive impact on CV risk factors and progression of diabetes. Reassure patients that medical goals for weight loss are achievable and worth the effort.

When discussing changes in eating with patients, distinguish dieting from gradual behavioral changes that result in a lasting pattern of healthy eating. Diets are impermanent and run the risk of large weight losses followed by even larger weight gains. Gradual behavioral changes offer the possibility of permanent lifestyle changes.

Prohibiting or demonizing foods is counterproductive. It leads patients to think of food in moral extremes (e.g., "sugar is bad for my diabetes") rather than along a continuum of nutritional benefit and blood glucose control with emphasis on moderation. Food

BOX 3   Checklist for Physical Activity

✓ Do something that you enjoy.
   Examples:
- I will take the stairs.
- I will park my car farther away and walk.
- I will walk.
- I will swim or do water exercises.
- I will ride a bike.
- I will use an exercise video.
- I will do yoga.
- Other:..
     ....

✓ How often?
   Examples:
   ☐ Every day
   ☐ 3×/week
   ☐ 5×/week
   ☐ ....
✓ How long?
   Examples:
   ☐ 10 min
   ☐ 15 min
   ☐ 20 min
   ☐ 30 min
   ☐ 60 min
   ☐ ___ min
✓ Limit inactivity.
   Examples:
- I will watch no more than 1 h of television per day.
- I will spend no more than 2 h per day on the computer.
- Other:..
     ....

Unpublished source: Virginia Center for Diabetes Professional Education, University of Virginia; Virginia Diabetes Council.

BOX 4   Examples of Coping Behaviors

- Talk about how you feel to people you trust.
- Decide one small way to change your mood or old habit and do it.
- Write down 10 good things about your life and think about and appreciate them.
- Organize your day with a "To Do" list.
- Learn how to relax through yoga, meditation, biofeedback, tai chi, deep breathing, or visual imagery.
- Take 30 min each day to relax through music, yoga, bath, writing, etc.
- Take time to have fun every day by exploring a new interest, watching a funny movie, going shopping, playing with a pet, etc.
- Get in touch with your spiritual side to help you feel better about yourself.
- Keep a stress diary to see what triggers your stress and discover better ways to react.
- Exercise every day to help you focus your energy on a more positive path.
- Keep your sleep cycle as regular as possible.
- Develop a favorite hobby.
- Other:................. ....

Unpublished source: Virginia Center for Diabetes Professional Education, University of Virginia; Virginia Diabetes Council.

prohibition also casts the provider as withholding and overly controlling. These traps can be avoided by exploring very small changes that are not perceived as significant losses with periods of consolidation of the acquired knowledge and experience.

Current nutrition therapy recommendations emphasize a flexible, individualized approach to macronutrient distribution and a carbohydrate-counting meal-planning approach for individuals with T1DM. Patients should be encouraged to emphasize vegetables, fruits, whole grains, legumes, and dairy products as preferred sources of carbohydrate. Recommendations for achieving consistent, appropriate carbohydrate intake at meals are based on controlling postprandial blood glucose (<180 mg/dL 1 to 2 hours after beginning a meal). Carbohydrate counting and blood glucose pattern management are complicated and time-consuming to teach. Referral to a dietitian for medical nutrition therapy or nutrition education through an ADA-recognized diabetes patient education program is recommended.

Stress reduction is important in controlling blood glucose and can also play a role by helping patients achieve a mental focus on their behavior-management efforts. We encourage patients to sit calmly for a period of 5 to 10 minutes each day, focusing on slow deep breathing and muscle relaxation. Activities such as yoga or tai chi also reduce stress and support awareness of body and mind. Box 4 contains suggestions for coping behaviors that may be useful to patients in dealing with stress.

Use of weight-loss medications should be considered to either "jump-start" weight loss or for the maintenance of achieved results.

Pharmacologic Therapy
Overview
Optimal glycemia goals must be individualized but may be generally defined as a hemoglobin A1c (HgbA1c) less than 7% (see Table 1) as recommended by the ADA. Preprandial capillary blood glucose should be 80 to 130 mg/dL and postprandially at the peak (typically about 2 hours after meals) should be generally less than 180 mg/dL. Individualizing glycemic goals should be based on several factors including duration of diabetes, age, life expectancy, comorbid conditions such as known CVD, advanced microvascular complications, hypoglycemia unawareness, and other individual patient considerations. Both HgbA1c and capillary blood glucose concentrations should be individualized to reduce the risk of hypoglycemia. A summary of other goals is provided in Box 1.

Eventually, most patients with T2DM require drug treatment, often using multiple agents (combination therapy). Progressive insulin secretory loss probably is the primary explanation for the need to advance treatment. A resultant general rule with all therapies is *add, don't switch*, but it is important to remember that lifestyle modification should always be part of the therapy if possible. Table 2 lists major types of pharmacotherapeutic interventions with their usual hemoglobin (Hb) A1c lowering, balance of preprandial versus postprandial effects, and some comments on their actions and side effects. Table 3 lists classes of drugs, commonly used agents, and typical doses.

In 2018, the ADA and European Association for the Study of Diabetes (EASD) updated the Consensus Report on Management of Hyperglycemia in T2DM. It is now becoming a common practice to initiate behavioral self-management with and sometimes without medication. Metformin is the first medication usually started unless there are contraindications or intolerance. Commonly, ineffective early attempts by physicians to change behavior (e.g., giving general advice) lead to abandonment of this therapy. Referral to an ADA-recognized diabetes education program is a more efficacious alternative. A second oral medication may be initiated if patients cannot achieve glycemic goals. Commonly, we favor insulin secretagogues, especially glimepiride (Amaryl) or extended-release glipizide (Glucotrol XL), for their relatively low risk of hypoglycemia, convenient once-daily dosing, and low expense, or an oral incretin drug. An alternative treatment strategy for heavier, more insulin-resistant patients is use of a thiazolidinedione (TZD), pioglitazone, effectively a dual insulin resistance strategy (see TZDs).

More reliably effective is the use of basal insulin treatment as a second agent to achieve control, although it is less accepted

DRUG TYPE	HBA1C LOWERING (%)	EFFECT ON GLYCEMIA		ACTIONS	SIDE EFFECTS/COMMENT
		PREPRANDIAL	POSTPRANDIAL		
SU and non-SU secretagogues	1.5–2.0*	++	+†	Direct and indirect secretagogue	Hypoglycemia, weight gain, rash
Biguanides	1.5–2.0*	+++	0	↓ hepatic glucose release, weight neutral	Adjust dose for CKD,‡ lactic acidosis (rare)
Thiazolidinediones	0.5–1.5	+++	0	↑ insulin sensitivity in muscle, fat	Edema, CHF, fractures
GLP-1 agonists	0.8–1.5	+	++	Strong GLP-1 effects, ↑ insulin, ↓ glucagon, ↓ stomach emptying	Nausea, vomiting, weight loss§
DPP-4 inhibitors	0.6–0.8	+	++	Moderate GLP-1 effects, ↑ insulin, ↓ glucagon	Weight neutral
Colesevelam (bile acid sequestrant)	0.4–0.8	+	+	Mechanisms of action uncertain	Constipation, hypertriglyceridemia
SGLT inhibitors Canagliflozin, Dapagliflozin, Empagliflozin, Ertugliflozin	0.5–1.0	+	+	↓ renal tubule reabsorption of glucose	Altered kidney function, hypotension, UTI, *Candida* in groin
Pramlintide (amylin agonist)	0.5–0.7	0–+	++	↓ glucagon, slow stomach emptying	Hypoglycemia, GI upset
Basal insulin	1.5–2.5	+++	0*	↓ hepatic glucose output, ↑ muscle glucose disposal	Hypoglycemia, weight gain
Meal insulin	1.0–2.0	0–+	++	↓ hepatic glucose output, ↑ muscle glucose disposal	Hypoglycemia, weight gain

CHF, Congestive heart failure; *CKD*, chronic kidney disease; *GI*, gastrointestinal; *UTI*, urinary tract infection.
*Older drugs may be less effective in well-controlled patients.
†Rapid-acting secretagogues may have less fasting and more early postprandial effects.
‡Metformin dosing: Adjust for CKD stage 3a (45 to 60 eGFR); watch closely but continue, and in 3b (30 to 44 eGFR), reduce dose to ½ usual or less and check eGFR every 3 months.
§Although risk of pancreatitis exists, unclear if increased. Risk of pancreatic cancer not proven and based on controversial data.

by many patients. Insulin initiation should be preceded by an open discussion of the patient's attitudes, beliefs, and possible fears regarding insulin. Insulin therapy should never be used as a threat or possible negative consequence for failure to carry out behavioral management. Many patients associate insulin with serious diabetes complications and mortality. A positive attitude about the value of insulin therapy and its natural presence and essential role in the body, along with reassurance that insulin can prolong life and improve its quality, can help reduce initial fears enough to begin. Availability of many noninsulin medications has often moved insulin to later in the sequence, but it can be used at any time.

In-clinic demonstrations of injection technique using saline is also useful in overcoming fear of injections and increasing acceptance. Improvement in blood glucose control with insulin generally makes patients feel better, which further reinforces its perceived value. Use of insulin pens may further increase acceptance of insulin treatment, patient convenience, and dosing accuracy.

It should be noted that an alternative algorithm for glycemic control therapy is proposed by the American College of Endocrinology (ACE). A patient-centered approach with emphasis on safely achieving goals and including patient choices and preferences is increasingly emphasized in both ADA and AACE guidelines.

Oral Agents

Secretagogues. These drugs enhance insulin secretion. There are first- and second-generation oral sulfonylureas; the latter are most commonly used. They are inexpensive, are moderately effective, and often can be dosed once daily. First-generation agents such as tolbutamide, chlorpropamide (Diabinese), and tolazamide (Tolinase) are less often used than the second-generation agents glyburide (DiaBeta, Glynase), glipizide (Glucotrol), and glimepiride (Amaryl). Glyburide should not generally be used in elderly patients or those with renal disease due to hypoglycemia risk.

The dose-response characteristics of sulfonylureas suggest that one-half the approved maximum dose achieves maximum HbA1c lowering, typically 1 to 1.5 percentage points (the latter with poorer baseline control). If the patient is not at goal with half-maximum doses, it is more effective to add a second agent than to raise the dose. Common side effects include hypoglycemia, weight gain of about 2 kg, and, more rarely, hematologic or skin reactions.

Shorter-acting Secretagogues. The glinides (repaglinide [Prandin] and nateglinide [Starlix]) are more expensive and should be considered for patients who are sulfonylurea-allergic, erratic in eating, or at high risk for hypoglycemia between meals and at nighttime.

Biguanides. Metformin is the only available agent in this class. It is useful in both obese and normal-weight patients with T2DM. HbA1c lowering is typically about 1.5 percentage points in monotherapy or in combination therapy. Maximum efficacy is achieved with 2000 mg daily. The sustained-release preparation will last 24 hours if given with the evening meal.

Metformin's hypoglycemic mechanism is primarily by reduction of liver glucose production, probably through effects on adenosine monophosphate-activated protein kinase, a fuel sensor enzyme, and partially through effects on glucagon. It is cleared by the kidney, and the risk of lactic acidosis, a rare side effect

TABLE 3 Dosing Used for Noninsulin Agents

AGENT	DOSE
Thiazolidinediones	
Pioglitazone (Actos)	15, 30, 45 mg
Rosiglitazone* (Avandia)	2, 4, 8 mg
α-Glucosidase Inhibitors	
Acarbose (Preset)	25, 50, 100 mg ac
Miglitol (Glyset)	25, 50 mg ac
Biguanides	
Metformin IR (Glucophage)	500, 850, 1000 mg†
Metformin ER	500, 750, 1000 mg
Glinides	
Nateglinide (Starlix)	60–120 mg ac
Repaglinide (Prandin)	0.5–4 mg ac
Sulfonylureas (Second Generation)	
Glipizide IR (Glucotrol)	2.5–20 mg
Glipizide ER (Glucotrol XL)	2.5–10 mg
Glimepiride (Amaryl)	1–4 mg
Glyburide (Glynase)	1.25–10, 1.5–6 mg
Incretins	
Exenatide (Byetta)	5, 10 µg
Exenatide QW Bydureon	2.0 mg
Liraglutide (Victoza)	0.6. 1.2, 1.8 mg
Dulaglutide (Trulicity)	0.75, 1.5 mg
Lixisenatide (Adlyxin)	10, 20 µg
DPP-4	
Sitagliptin (Januvia)	100, 50, 25 mg§
Saxagliptin (Onglyza)	5, 2.5 mg§
Linagliptin (Tradjenta)	5 mg
Alogliptin (Nesina)	25, 12.5, 6.25 mg§
Amylin Agonist	
Pramlintide (Symlin)	15, 30, 45, 60, 90, 120 µg¶
Bile Acid Sequestrant	
Colesevelam (Welchol)	1875–3750 mg
Dopamine Agonist	
Bromocriptine (Cycloset)	0.8–4.8 mg¶¶
SGLT-2 Inhibitor	
Canagliflozin** (Invokana)	100, 300 mg
Dapagliflozin** (Farxiga)	5, 10 mg
Empagliflozin** (Jardiance)	10, 25 mg
Ertugliflozin** (Steglatro)	5, 15 mg

*Restriction on use lifted as CVD risk not clearly increased.
†Also available as a liquid preparation 500 mg/5 mL.
‡Powder reconstitutes in the pen before use with twist.
§Dose adjusted for renal function.
¶Pens come in range for type 1 (15 to 60 µg) and type 2 (60 to 120 µg).
¶¶Take with food within 2 h of awakening.
**All SGLT2 drugs use lower doses with moderate renal dysfunction and are contraindicated in severe renal dysfunction.

(1:30,000 patient-years) with a 50% mortality rate, may be increased in renal dysfunction. The original FDA guidelines suggesting serum creatinine should be less than 1.4 mg/dL in women and less than 1.5 mg/dL in men have recently been supplanted by a more practical approach to use eGFR, which should be assessed in all patients, for decision making about continuation of the drug. Full doses of metformin appear safe down to eGFR of 45 mL/min, with routine checking of eGFR every 3 to 6 months. Once eGFR falls to the 30 and 44 mL/min range, the metformin dose should be reduced to 1000 mg or less, and eGFR should be checked every 3 months. There may be an increased lactic acidosis risk in patients with congestive heart failure (CHF) or respiratory insufficiency, especially during exacerbations of these conditions with hypoxia and activation of anaerobic glycolysis. Intravascular contrast administration should prompt holding the drug for 24 to 48 hours until renal function is confirmed to be adequate. Gastrointestinal (GI) side effects are common initially and are dose-dependent but wane; they can require gradual titration and are often ameliorated by postprandial administration. Sustained-release preparations have fewer GI side effects. Weight gain is less with this drug than with many others for diabetes, and in fact, the use of metformin might contribute to a loss of 3 to 4 lbs of weight. The United Kingdom Prospective Diabetes Study found that risk of myocardial infarction (MI) and death was reduced among metformin users, making it a first choice for pharmacotherapy in most patients.

Thiazolidinediones. Two TZDs are used, namely pioglitazone (Actos) and rosiglitazone (Avandia). TZDs increase the sensitivity of muscle tissue and fat to the action of insulin via the peroxisome proliferator-activated receptor gamma mechanism. HbA1c lowering varies, dependent on the degree of insulin resistance (i.e., central adiposity) and levels of endogenous insulin secretion, duration of clinical diabetes, use of secretagogues, or use of insulin.

TZDs can precipitate edema, weight gain caused by redistribution of fat (from central to peripheral location), and occasionally CHF, even absent a prior heart failure history. It is thus wise to track weight in all patients and limit gains to 5 or 6 lbs. TZDs are contraindicated in patients with heart failure; however, they have been shown to significantly reduce ischemic risk (e.g., stroke or MI) in individuals with high insulin resistance, prediabetes, and history of transient ischemic attack or stroke as was demonstrated in the recently published IRIS Trial with pioglitazones. As a class, TZDs are associated with an increase in fractures in women, which suggests avoiding this medication in patients with high risk for osteoporosis or fragility fractures. The use of pioglitazone is associated with a slightly higher risk of bladder cancer. Sales of rosiglitazone in the United States were restricted by the FDA between 2011 and 2013 due to concerns about an increase in heart attacks and death. These restrictions were lifted in 2013.

Incretins. Incretins are gut hormones that enhance food-induced insulin secretion. Incretin drugs either are receptor agonists (e.g., exenatide) for GLP-1, perhaps the most important incretin, or they enhance endogenous levels for both GLP-1 and gastrointestinal insulinotropic polypeptide (GIP).

Exenatide is available as immediate release (Byetta) given twice daily and in once-weekly extended release (Bydureon). There are two GLP-1 receptor agonists, liraglutide (Victoza) and lixisenatide (Adlyxin), with once-daily dosing. Other agonists, dulaglutide (Trulicity) and semaglutide (Ozempic), are approved by the FDA; they are given once weekly. These incretin agonists increase meal insulin, decrease meal hyperglucagonemia, decrease rate of stomach emptying, and suppress appetite, which may cause a moderate weight loss. They work rapidly on injection. Substantial GI side effects including nausea, vomiting, and diarrhea are experienced by approximately 25% of patients. Despite this, many patients favor them, probably because the side effects generally wane within weeks and there can be moderate weight loss, especially in significantly overweight patients. Typically, exenatide (Byetta) is given in doses of 5 µg twice daily at meals, advancing after a month to 10 µg twice daily. Liraglutide is usually started at 0.6 mg once daily and advanced to 1.2 and then 1.8 mg as needed and tolerated. Patients might report that nausea is more tolerable if they have a little food in their stomach at the time of dosing. Pancreatitis may rarely occur (case reports). Exenatide in a sustained-release once-weekly preparation (Bydureon) is embedded into microspheres that permit slow release. To deliver the medication, injections require a somewhat larger needle (23 gauge) that is short and well tolerated, although somewhat more frequent site reactions and immunogenicity occur with this formulation. Adaptation to nausea seems quicker in longer-acting preparations (once daily or weekly) than in immediate-release exenatide.

Because incretin drugs all have a glucose-dependent insulin secretion and glucagon suppression, there is little risk for hypoglycemia used alone or when they are combined with metformin and TZDs; in contrast, hypoglycemia is increased when combined with sulfonylureas or with insulin therapy. HbA1c lowering with exenatide has been 0.8 to 1.5 percentage points, and although albiglutide (Tanzeum)[2] is similar to exenatide, liraglutide, dulaglutide, or sustained-release exenatide have similar or slightly more efficacy in lowering HbA1c but equal weight effects. Concerns are raised about pancreatitis risk and pancreatic dysplasia, but these remain inconclusive and controversial. Risk of C-cell hyperplasia or medullary thyroid cancer prevents these drugs from use in patients with that disorder.

Dipeptidyl Peptidase-4 Inhibitors. Dipeptidyl peptidase-4 (DPP-4) is the enzyme that normally rapidly degrades the incretins GLP-1 and GIP to inactive proteolytic products. Inhibitors of DPP-4 have been shown to enhance GLP-1 and GIP levels to high physiologic levels and thereby reduce HbA1c concentrations, typically about 0.6 to 0.8 percentage points. Four drugs, sitagliptin (Januvia), saxagliptin (Onglyza), linagliptin (Tradjenta), and alogliptin (Nesina), are approved in the US and appear to be similarly effective in recommended doses (see Table 3). Sitagliptin (standard dose 100 mg/day) and alogliptin (standard dose 25 mg/day) are excreted by the kidneys and thus should be given in lower doses (50 mg/day for sitagliptin and 12.5 mg/day for alogliptin) for those with moderate renal insufficiency (eGFR 30 to 45 mL/min/1.73 m^2 for sitagliptin and 30 to 59 for alogliptin) and further reduced (25 mg/day and 6.25 mg/day, respectively) for those with severe renal dysfunction (eGFR <30 mL/min/1.73 m^2). Saxagliptin is reduced from 5 mg/day to 2.5 mg/day in moderate renal insufficiency (eGFR <45), whereas linagliptin does not need dose adjustment with kidney disease. All have similar actions and probably potential side effects, including pancreatitis. These drugs are available in combination pills with metformin and some with SGLT2 inhibitors.

Because DPP-4 inhibitors are oral, they may be preferred to the injectable incretins. The side effects for these drugs are relatively minor, and these drugs cause little nausea, vomiting, or diarrhea. They appear to be weight neutral. Rare but serious allergic reactions such as angioedema and Stevens-Johnson syndrome have been reported in a few patients. Pancreatitis has been observed with this class of drugs in post-marketing analysis and is very rare. Joint pain is a new uncommon side effect.

Amylin Agonists. Insulin is cosecreted with another beta cell hormone called *amylin*. The effects of amylin appear to be to help lower glycemia, reduce excess glucagon levels, curb appetite, and possibly reduce the rate of gastric emptying. A synthetic analogue of amylin, pramlintide (Symlin), is available as an injectable agent for treating both T1DM and T2DM as an adjunct to insulin. It lowers HbA1c about 0.5 to 0.7 percentage point. It also appears to have some effects of weight loss, typically around 1 to 2 kg. Its action primarily controls glucose postprandially. Nausea and vomiting can occur in patients with either T2DM or T1DM but are worse in patients with T1DM who require lower doses at first (≤ 15 µg with meals) and slower titration. Those with T2DM usually start with 60 µg and can usually advance to 90 to 120 µg at meals.

Bile Acid Sequestrants. Colesevelam hydrochloride (Welchol), in either single (3.75 g [6 tablets]) or divided doses (twice daily; 1.875 g [3 tablets]), reduces hyperglycemia compared with placebo in patients with T2DM. A1c reductions range from 0.4% to 0.8% when used alone, with metformin, with sulfonylureas, and when used with insulin and other oral agents. Although this drug has already been approved for treatment of hyperlipidemia, it is now also FDA approved for T2DM. It has the potential, however, to increase triglycerides, and thus baseline fasting lipid values should be obtained and tracked, especially in patients with hypertriglyceridemia—use is not recommended when baseline triglycerides exceed 250 mg/dL. There is little justification for its use

alone or with TZDs, but it may be appropriate for some patients with T2DM not at goal on other therapies.

Dopamine Receptor Agonists. Bromocriptine (Cycloset), a dopamine receptor agonist in a rapid-release formulation, is a relatively new addition to antidiabetes medications. Although its mechanism of action is not precisely clear, the drug will reduce premeal and postmeal blood sugars without changing insulin levels, which suggests a benefit to insulin action, perhaps through mediation of central nervous system mechanisms. Its side effects are somewhat similar to those of the bromocriptine used for pituitary disease. Nausea is a common initial side effect. Its efficacy is moderate, with HbA1c reductions of 0.5% or slightly more. Its preliminary data suggest a favorable CV safety profile associated with its use, which is reassuring. Usual starting doses are 0.8 mg once daily in the morning; gradual increase may occur at weekly intervals in 0.8 mg increments as tolerated (usual dose: 1.6 to 4.8 mg once daily; maximum dose: 4.8 mg/day).

SGLT-2 Inhibitors. Four approved drugs are available: canagliflozin (Invokana), dapagliflozin (Farxiga), empagliflozin (Jardiance), and ertugliflozin (Steglatro). They act as inhibitors of sodium glucose transporters, which lead to urinary glucose reabsorption blockade, shifting the glucose reabsorption threshold to low-normal range, resulting in substantial glucosuria (causing on average 80 to 120 g of glucose loss per day). This drug is effective in lowering HbA1c to ≥1% with a relatively low risk of hypoglycemia when used alone or with other drugs such as metformin, but they may cause hypoglycemia when combined with insulin or insulin secretagogues such as sulfonylureas. These drugs may have favorable effects on blood pressure, partly from diuretic effects, and may cause postural hypotension if volume is allowed to get depleted. In monotherapy with these drugs, average HbA1c reductions of 0.5% to 0.8% may be seen, although it is dependent on the initial HbA1c level. Added to metformin, the reduction is 0.5% to 0.75%. Additional benefits may include weight loss of 1.2 to 3.3 kg and a modest reduction in systolic blood pressure of 4 to 9 mm Hg, but postural hypotension symptoms or acute kidney injury may occur. Urinary infections are more common but are treatable. *Candida* vulvovaginitis and balanitis are more common with SGLT-2 inhibitors. Assess renal function before initiating a SGLT-2 inhibitor and periodically thereafter. The usual starting dose is the lowest dose shown in Table 3 once daily before the first meal. For canagliflozin, the dose may be advanced if needed for improving glucose control but only if the eGFR is ≥60 mL/min/1.73 m^2. If the eGFR is between 45 and 60, canagliflozin should not be advanced beyond 100 mg/day, and if the eGFR is persistently less than 45, the drug should not be used. For dapagliflozin and empagliflozin, the dose can be increased if needed but they should not be used when the eGFR is less than 45. Ertugliflozin should not be initiated or continued in patients with an eGFR less than 60. Frequent monitoring of eGFR is recommended with values less than 60. These drugs should be used with caution in the event of significant renal dysfunction and should not be used in advanced liver or kidney dysfunction (eGFR <30). Rarely, ketoacidosis can occur when used with insulin.

The recent hallmark trial, EMPA-REG OUTCOME, demonstrated that empagliflozin reduced the primary major adverse cardiac event endpoints (CV death, nonfatal MI, nonfatal stroke) by 14% in patients with T2DM with a high risk for or prior history of CVD. This beneficial effect was driven by a 38% reduction in CV mortality with no significant decrease in nonfatal MI or stroke. The drug also caused a 35% reduction in hospitalization for heart failure without affecting hospitalization for unstable angina. Although SGLT-2 inhibitors exert multiple metabolic benefits (e.g., decreases in HbA1c, body weight, and blood pressure, and an increase in HDL cholesterol), all of which could reduce CVD risk, it is unlikely that the reduction in CV mortality can be fully explained by these factors. More likely, a combination of positive hemodynamic effects is enhanced by changes in intrarenal blood flow dynamics, contributing to the reduction in CV mortality and heart failure hospitalization. This subject is currently being intensively investigated. Impact of the study results was significant enough that it led to a new ADA recommendation: in patients with established atherosclerotic CVD on metformin, empagliflozin is a preferred add-on agent to reduce major adverse CV events. Empagliflozin has recently received FDA approval for this indication.

Insulin

Barriers to Insulin Use. Insulin deficiency underlies the genesis of both T1DM and T2DM. Progression of therapy to use of insulin, typically with oral agents in T2DM, also seems predicated on progressive loss of insulin secretion. Nonetheless, it is often started too late, and patients often are in very poor control when this is done. Reluctance by patients and physicians alike might underlie this. Physicians should understand that exogenous insulin in T2DM is needed, does not negatively alter life quality, and is more likely to achieve therapeutic targets. Moreover, exogenous insulin does not worsen insulin resistance, does not cause excess CVD, and has a low frequency of severe hypoglycemia, especially when used relatively early in the disease. Table 4 lists common insulin preparations and some notes about kinetics and timing.

Starting Insulin: Use of Basal Insulin in Type 2 Diabetes. How should insulin be started? Practitioners should use temporary insulin for patients whose glycemia is initially poorly controlled or when patients temporarily have worse control due to illness or medications, such as glucocorticoids. It is unwise to use insulin as a threat because it creates a sense of personal failure and dread of insulin use. When therapy progresses but there is failure to achieve glycemic goals after one or two oral medications, use of basal insulin is often the best way to achieve euglycemia, especially if patients are much more than 1 percentage point from HbA1c goal (<7%).

The Treat-to-Target Trial offers a good example of how to initiate insulin therapy. In this study, as often in our practice, patients started with a basal insulin either with NPH insulin or insulin glargine (Lantus). Most patients (~60%) attained HbA1$_c$ ≤7% with either type of insulin. However, with glargine, nearly 25% more patients attained this target without documented nocturnal hypoglycemia. Moreover, rates of other categories of symptomatic hypoglycemia were 21% to 48% lower with glargine.

TABLE 4 Insulin Preparations.

INSULIN TYPE	PHARMACOKINETICS			COMMENTS
	ONSET (H)	PEAK (H)	DURATION (H)	
Basal Insulins				
NPH (Humulin N, Novolin N)	0.5	4–10	18	Kinetics are dose dependent Peak effects exert meal action Dose at breakfast, bedtime, supper*
Glargine U-100† (Lantus, Basaglar)	2–4	Little peak	24*	Dose can be given at any time of day if consistent
Glargine U-300 (Toujeo)‡	3–4	No peak	30 +	Dose at any time but consistently
Detemir† (Levemir)	2–3	Little peak		Kinetics are dose dependent Dose at breakfast, bedtime, supper*
U-500 regular insulin (Humulin R U-500)	1–3 h	3–6 h	8–10	Kinetics are dose dependent, even though they are similar to NPH
	Approximately 2 h	No peak	>40 h	
Insulin Degludec† (Tresiba U-100, U-200)	2 h	No peak	Up to 40	No risk of "stacking"; can be preferred in those who might be skipping doses
Meal Insulins				
Regular (Humulin R, Novolin R)	0.25–0.5	2–3	5–8	Give 30 min before meals Do not use at bedtime
Lispro (Humalog U-100, U-200, Admelog)	0.1–0.2	1.5–2.0	4	Dose up to 20 min before mealtime or immediately after
Aspart (Novolog, Fiasp)§	0.1–0.2	1.5–2.0	4	Dose up to 20 min before mealtime or immediately after
Glulisine (Apidra)	0.1–0.2	1.5–2.0	4	Dose up to 20 min before mealtime or immediately after
Mixed Preparations				
NPH/regular (Humulin 70/30, Novolin 70/30)	70/30 dual kinetics based on components			Dosing ½ h before meals Should not be dosed at bedtime
Lispro/NPH Lispro (Humalog 75/25)	75/25 dual kinetics based on components			Dosing at mealtime; should not be dosed at bedtime
Lispro/NPH Lispro Humalog 50/50)	50/50 dual kinetics based on components			Dosing at mealtime, should not be dosed at bedtime
Aspart/NPHAspart (NovoLog 70/30)	70/30 dual kinetics based on components			Dosing at mealtime; should not be dosed at bedtime

NPH, Neutral protamine Hagedorn.
*Bedtime dosing may be preferred for some patients, especially those on low doses.
†Should not be mixed with other insulins or used in the same syringe that other insulin has been in.
‡Advance dose no faster than every 3 to 4 days, slightly higher doses may be needed compared with U-100 insulin glargine.
§Formulated with niacinamide for faster absorption.

Insulin detemir (Levemir) represents another long-acting insulin analogue option to be used similarly. Insulin is instituted as 10 U once daily, commonly in the evening near bedtime, followed by weekly increases of between 2 and 8 units depending on proximity to glucose goals, focusing on the fasting glucose.

This strategy is sometimes called the *fix the fasting first* rule. Average doses in that study were around 45 to 50 units for patients whose body mass index was about 31 kg/m². An alternative initial dosing might be 0.2 U/kg body weight, but whatever the starting dose, a forced titration guided by patient self-monitoring with clear communication of target fasting glucose (90 to 130 mg/dL), size of increment (or decrement in case of hypoglycemia; usually 10% to 20% of dose), and frequency of change (every 3 to 7 days) is necessary to get most patients to overall glycemic (HbA1c) goal. This strategy is referred to as *pattern management*. The intent is to use monitoring to adjust the insulin dose likely to affect the fasting glucose for basal insulin therapy. NPH and detemir usually can be used once daily, typically at bedtime. Patients using glargine may choose any time of the day as long as it is reasonably consistent, usually within the hour of a 24-hour day cycle. In some patients, twice-daily NPH or detemir is used if daytime insulin levels are deemed insufficient. The new U-300 insulin glargine (Toujeo) may be helpful in reduction of overnight hypoglycemia, as it has a flatter kinetic profile and longer duration of action.

When and How to Add Meal Insulin. At some point, basal insulin therapy alone may be insufficient for glycemic control for T2DM patients. Usually, this is a consideration in patients whose HbA1c values are 9% to 9.5% or where the fasting goal is met but HbA1c or daytime glycemia remains elevated. The need for meal insulin is particularly likely to occur with larger meals, such as supper. Diagnostically, what is important is to have patients check either both before and after large meals or, if they are unwilling to check frequently, simply check about 2 to 3 hours after meals. Self-monitored glucose values that exceed even minimum postprandial glycemic guidelines (<180 mg/dL) indicate the need for meal insulin. A common mistake made in practice is to treat fasting hyperglycemia only with increases in basal insulin, when in some patients the cause is overeating or lack of meal insulin coverage from the previous evening. This can be discerned by observing the pattern of glycemia, with lows often between meals or overnight and highs occurring after meals or at bedtime.

Fixed-Ratio Combined Insulins

A commonly used strategy to use fixed-ratio combination short-acting (either regular or rapid analogue) insulin combined with intermediate insulin (NPH or neutral protamine modified rapid analogue that mimics NPH timing) is being replaced by basal-bolus regimens. However, for the purposes of compliance, fixed-ratio combination preparations are still used and include {70/30} NPH and regular insulin, {75/25} neutral protamine lispro and lispro insulin (Humalog), and {70/30} neutral protamine aspart and aspart insulin (Novolog). These combination products have the advantage of being able to achieve glycemic improvement conveniently (i.e., simple twice-daily injection regimen) in T2DM patients whose conditions otherwise are poorly controlled (HbA1c of 9.5% or more). These preparations also offer the advantage of greater dosing accuracy, especially when used with insulin pens. Important to the success of these formulations is consistent eating and carbohydrate intake with meals. Unfortunately, when such consistency is not attainable, patterns of glycemia can be erratic, and hypoglycemia can be significantly increased. Patients who skip meals are poor candidates for combination product therapy and should either switch to individual dosing of an insulin mixture or, even safer, use a basal-bolus insulin regimen.

Fixed-Ratio Combinations of Long-Acting Insulin With GLP-1 agonists

In 2016, the FDA approved two new fixed-ratio combinations of insulin and a GLP-1 agonist: Soliqua (glargine/lixisenatide) and Xultophy (degludec/liraglutide). These products can be considered as an option before starting basal-bolus insulin therapy. Both preparations are indicated after failure of one shot (either insulin or GLP-1 agonist) in combination with oral hypoglycemic agents to achieve the target. Slow up-titration of the combination has significantly improved tolerability, offset insulin therapy–associated weight gain, and resulted in a substantially higher portion of T2DM patients achieving glycemic goals with no additional risk of hypoglycemia.

Adults With T1DM

A significant minority of patients with a diagnosis of T2DM actually have a late onset of T1DM and typical autoimmunity (IA-2 antibodies, GAD-65 antibodies, and insulin antibodies), also known as *LADA* (latent autoimmune diabetes of adults). The diagnosis should certainly be suspected in patients for whom combination oral agent therapy rapidly fails. Nonobese body habitus, marked weight loss, extremely elevated glucose values, or a family or personal history of autoimmune disease (e.g., Hashimoto or Graves thyroid problems) should lead to diagnostic evaluation for such signs of autoimmunity.

Patients with T1DM need combined mealtime and basal insulin therapy. Although it is tempting to do so in a convenient fashion with combined preparations, such as those with analogue fixed ratios, it usually is far preferable to use a better basal insulin, such as glargine or detemir combined with a rapid-acting analogue (separately injected) before meals. Sometimes an insulin pump is the best way for patients who have frequent hypoglycemia or marked variability to achieve good glycemic control safely. Patients with T1DM should preferably be seen by an endocrine specialist or other practitioner with extensive experience in T1DM management. Ready access to diabetes educators is an important key to success with both T1DM and T2DM.

Adults With T2DM

Many patients with T2DM eventually need mealtime insulin. For those on basal insulin alone, incretin mimetics[1] can be successfully used for mealtime control because they effectively lower prandial hyperglycemia. If exenatide is used, then additional injections will be required at the two major meals of the day. If using an incretin-enhancer drug such as sitagliptin, injections are not required. This approach is useful with incretin agonists exenatide or liraglutide in patients who need to lose weight, who gain considerable weight with meal insulin, or who experience poor control despite attempts to regulate meal glycemia with short-acting insulins. Recent studies suggest possible benefit of combining long-acting basal insulins with incretin receptor agonists.

---

[1] Not FDA approved for this indication.

References

Abdul-Ghani M, Del Prato S, Chilton R, DeFronzo RA: SGLT2 inhibitors and cardiovascular risk: lessons learned from the EMPA-REG OUTCOME Study, *Diabetes Care* 39:717–725, 2016.

Accord Study Group: Effects of intensive blood-pressure control in type 2 diabetes mellitus, *N Engl J Med* 362:1575–1585, 2010.

American Diabetes Association: Facilitating behavior change: key strategies for empowering your patients, Available at: http://www.facilitatingbehaviorchange.org/2009.

American Diabetes Association: Summary of revisions: standards of medical care in diabetes—2018, *Diabetes Care* 41(Suppl 1):S4–S6, 2018.

American Diabetes Association: *Releases: standards of medical care in diabetes, with notable new recommendations for people with cardiovascular disease and diabetes [news release]*, 2018, ADA's website Available at: http://www.diabetes.org/newsroom/press-releases/2017/american-diabetes-association-2018-release-standards-of-medical-care-in-diabetes.html.

Aroda VR, Rosenstock J, Wysham C, et al: Efficacy and safety of lixilan, a titratable fixed-ratio combination of insulin glargine plus lixisenatide in type 2 diabetes inadequately controlled on basal insulin and metformin: the LixiLan-L Randomized Trial, *Diabetes Care* 39:1972–1980, 2016.

Centers for Disease Control and Prevention: *National Diabetes Statistics Report*, Atlanta, GA, 2017, US Department of Health and Human Services, 2017.

Cifu AS, Davis AM: Prevention: detection, evaluation, and management of high blood pressure in adults, *JAMA* 318:2132–2134, 2017.

Diabetes Prevention Program Research Group: The Diabetes Prevention Program (DPP): Description of lifestyle intervention, *Diabetes Care* 25:2165–2171, 2002.

Fox CS, Golden SH, Anderson C, et al: Update on prevention of cardiovascular disease in adults with type 2 diabetes mellitus in light of recent evidence: a scientific statement from the American Heart Association and the American Diabetes Association, *Diabetes Care* 38:1777–1803, 2015.

Garber AJ, Abrahamson MJ, Barzilay JI, et al: American Association of Clinical Endocrinologists' comprehensive diabetes management algorithm 2013 consensus statement—executive summary, *Endocrinol Pract* 19:536–557, 2013.

Grundy SM, Cleeman JI, Daniels SR, et al: Diagnosis and management of the metabolic syndrome. An American Heart Association/National Heart, Lung, and Blood Institute Scientific Statement. Executive summary, *Circulation* 112:2735–2752, 2005.

Harja E, Lord J, Skyler JS: An analysis of characteristics of subjects examined for incretin effects on pancreatic pathology, *Diabetes Technol Ther* 15:609–618, 2013.

Inzucchi SE, Bergenstal RM, Buse JB, et al: Management of hyperglycaemia in type 2 diabetes, 2015: a patient-centred approach. Update to a position statement of the American Diabetes Association and the European Association for the Study of Diabetes, *Diabetologia* 58:429–442, 2015.

Jonassen I, Havelund S, Hoeg-Jensen T, et al: Design of the novel protraction mechanism of insulin degludec, an ultra-long- acting basal insulin, *Pharm Res* 29:2104, 2012.

Kahn R, Buse J, Ferrannini E, Stern M: The metabolic syndrome: Time for a critical appraisal. Joint statement from the American Diabetes Association and the European Association for the Study of Diabetes, *Diabetes Care* 8:2289–2304, 2005.

Kernan WN, Viscoli CM, Furie KL, et al: for the IRIS Trial Investigators. Pioglitazone after ischemic stroke or transient ischemic attack, *N Engl J Med* 374:1321–1331, 2016.

Knowler WC, Barrett-Connor E, Fowler SE, et al: Reduction in the incidence of type 2 diabetes with lifestyle intervention or metformin, *N Engl J Med* 346:393–403, 2002.

Linjawi S, Bode BW, Chaykin LB, et al: The efficacy of IDegLira (insulin degludec/liraglutide combination) in adults with type 2 diabetes inadequately controlled with a GLP-1 receptor agonist and oral therapy: DUAL III Randomized Clinical Trial, *Diabetes Ther* 8:101–114, 2017.

Lipska KJ, Bailey CJ, Inzucchi SF: Use of metformin in the setting of mild-to-moderate renal insufficiency, *Diabetes Care* 34:1431–1437, 2011.

Monnier L, Lapinski H, Colette C: Contributions of fasting and postprandial plasma glucose increments to the overall diurnal hyperglycemia of type 2 diabetic patients: variations with increasing levels of HbA1c, *Diabetes Care* 26:881–885, 2003.

Nesto RW, Bell D, Bonow RO, et al: Thiazolidinedione use, fluid retention, and congestive heart failure: a consensus statement from the American Heart Association and American Diabetes Association, *Diabetes Care* 27:256–263, 2004.

Riddle MC, Rosenstock J, Gerich J: The treat-to-target trial: randomized addition of glargine or human NPH insulin to oral therapy of type 2 diabetic patients, *Diabetes Care* 26:3080–3086, 2003.

Stone NJ, Robinson JG, Lichtenstein AH, et al: ACC/AHA guideline on the treatment of blood cholesterol to reduce atherosclerotic cardiovascular risk in adults: a report of the American College of Cardiology/American Heart Association Task Force on Practice Guidelines, *Circulation* 129(25 Suppl. 2):S1–45, 2013, 2014.

Tuomilehto J, Lindstrom J, Eriksson J, et al: Finnish Diabetes Prevention Study Group. Prevention of type 2 diabetes mellitus by changes in lifestyle among subjects with impaired glucose tolerance, *N Engl J Med* 344:1343–1350, 2001.

GOUT AND HYPERURICEMIA

Method of
Saima Chohan, MD

CURRENT DIAGNOSIS

- Gout is the most common inflammatory arthritis in men and is increasing in prevalence.
- A definitive diagnosis of gout requires demonstration of monosodium urate crystals in synovial fluid or tophi.
- Gouty arthritis often begins in the lower extremity joints.
- Septic arthritis, rheumatoid arthritis, and calcium pyrophosphate disease (pseudogout) can mimic gout and should be ruled out.

CURRENT THERAPY

- The goals of successful gout treatment include terminating the acute attack, preventing intermittent attacks, and undertaking long-term therapy to avoid chronic arthritis.
- Indications for chronic treatment of gout include frequent attacks, recurrent arthritis, and kidney disease.
- A serum urate level of <6.0 mg/dL is the goal when using urate-lowering therapy.
- Nonpharmacologic treatment includes lifestyle modification and dietary changes.
- The mainstay of urate-lowering therapies remains xanthine oxidase inhibition.

Epidemiology

Gout, or monosodium urate crystal deposition disease, is the most common inflammatory arthritis of men and is an increasingly common problem among postmenopausal women. It is a chronic disorder, affecting more than 5 million people in the United States and increasing in both prevalence and incidence, especially in persons older than 65 years. Gout is often accompanied by serious comorbid disorders (hypertension, cardiovascular disease, chronic kidney disease, and all of the component features of the metabolic syndrome) and is managed in primary care practice in about 90% of affected persons. Therefore identifying risk factors, optimizing diagnosis, and choosing the appropriate treatment for gout are important skills for a wide array of caregivers.

Pathophysiology and Risk Factors

Uric acid is the end product of purine metabolism in humans. Hyperuricemia, a serum urate concentration exceeding urate solubility (6.8 mg/dL), is an invariable accompaniment of gout, although serum uric acid levels might not be elevated during an acute attack. Hyperuricemia predisposes affected persons to urate crystal formation and deposition, which lead to the inflammatory responses underlying the symptoms of gout. Thus treatment of gout is aimed at reducing and maintaining serum urate concentration at subsaturating levels, usually set at less than 6.0 mg/dL.

Hyperuricemia

Risk factors for hyperuricemia include obesity, hypertension, hyperlipidemia, insulin resistance, renal insufficiency, and use of diuretics. Diets rich in certain foods are also associated with increased risk for gout. Many studies with large patient cohorts have demonstrated a relationship between hyperuricemia and hypertension, cardiovascular and peripheral vascular disease, chronic kidney disease, and diabetes mellitus. The association of hyperuricemia and metabolic syndrome has also been shown in children and adolescents. Interventional trials of asymptomatic patients with hyperuricemia and high cardiovascular risk must be performed before such treatment can be advocated.

Diagnosis

Acute gout is characterized by an abrupt onset of joint pain, erythema, and swelling, usually of one joint, but less commonly of more than one. The arthritis most often occurs first in a lower extremity joint, especially the first metatarsophalangeal (MTP) joint at the base of the great toe. The predilection for this site is thought to be secondary to cooler acral temperature or repeated trauma and pressure on this joint.

The gold standard for diagnosis of gout is the demonstration of monosodium urate crystals by polarized light microscopy, either in joint fluid aspirated during an acute attack or between attacks, or from material aspirated from suspected tophi. To aspirate the first MTP joint, the joint is first identified by palpating the space at the base of the metacarpal on the dorsal aspect while flexing and extending the toe. The needle is then inserted perpendicularly into the joint space to avoid the extensor hallucis tendon. Synovial fluid from affected joints should immediately be examined under polarized microscopy to confirm the diagnosis of needle-shaped crystals with negative birefringence. If polarized microscopy is unavailable, then fluid should be promptly sent in a sterile tube for crystal confirmation to an appropriate laboratory.

Unfortunately, the equipment and analytical expertise necessary to make this diagnosis are not widely available to primary care physicians. As a result, the diagnosis of acute gout is commonly made on clinical grounds, using the 2015 American College of Rheumatology and the European League Against Rheumatism classification criteria. These diagnostic guidelines use a point system and emphasize the presence of signs of inflammation (redness, tenderness, and loss of joint function), abrupt onset, monoarticular involvement, occurrence in the first MTP joint, presence of tophi, and radiographic findings.

The initial symptoms and signs of gout often occur after many years of asymptomatic hyperuricemia. In untreated or

Figure 1 Intradermal urate deposit (tophus). (Reprinted with permission from Mandell BF: Gout and crystal deposition disease. In Weisman MH, Weinblatt ME, Louie JS, Van Vollenhoven R (eds): Targeted Treatment of the Rheumatic Diseases. Philadelphia, Saunders, 2010, 293–302).

BOX 1   Indications for Urate-Lowering Therapy

- Frequent and disabling gouty attacks, often defined as two or three flares annually, although this is not evidence based; the decision to treat is based on both number of flares and the consequent disability resulting from flares
- Chronic gouty disease: clinically or radiographically evident joint erosions
- Tophaceous deposits: subcutaneous or intraosseous
- Gout with renal insufficiency
- Recurrent kidney stones
- Urate nephropathy
- Urinary uric acid excretion exceeding 1100 mg/d (6.5 mmol), when determined in men younger than 25 years or in premenopausal women

inadequately treated patients, the course of the disease often involves acute attacks at increasing frequency, with shortening of asymptomatic periods (called intercritical gout) and, ultimately, development of chronic joint disease (gouty arthropathy) and tophi (masses of urate crystals in a chronic inflammatory matrix) in bone, joints, skin, and even solid organs (Figure 1).

Indications for Treatment

Early in gout, patients might have attacks that are separated by years and manageable over the course of a few days with antiinflammatory medications and adjuncts such as joint rest and application of ice. Over time, the attacks usually become more frequent, prolonged, and disabling, eventually requiring long-term urate-lowering treatment aimed at preventing urate crystal deposition and eventually abolishing acute flares and resolving tophi. Indications for urate-lowering (antihyperuricemic) therapy are listed in Box 1.

Treatment

Acute Gout

Gouty arthritis occurs suddenly, and attacks are often very painful and disabling. Patients describe acute onset of exquisite pain, swelling, erythema, and inability to bear weight on the afflicted joint. Occasionally, patients have constitutional symptoms including fever and chills, with an elevation of sedimentation rate and white blood cell count. To terminate an attack, nonsteroidal anti-inflammatory drugs (NSAIDs), colchicine (Colcrys), or corticosteroids can be offered. If given at full antiinflammatory dosage, NSAIDs have a rapid onset and are quite efficacious in relieving pain and shortening the duration of an attack. The utility of this class of drugs may be limited by renal insufficiency, cardiovascular risk factors, and gastrointestinal bleeding. Although indomethacin (Indocin), sulindac (Clinoril), and naproxen (Naprosyn) are all FDA approved for treating acute attacks of gout, nearly every drug in this class and the selective cyclooxygenase (COX) 2 inhibitors also have considerable efficacy. High-dose

salicylate therapy lowers serum uric acid by interfering in renal urate transport; low-dose aspirin[1] has the opposite effect, but it is often continued in gout patients because of its overriding importance in managing coronary artery disease.

Oral colchicine has been used to treat gout for many years as an unproven drug with no FDA dosage recommendations or prescribing information. In July 2009, however, the FDA approved Colcrys, a single-ingredient colchicine product, for the first day of treatment of acute gout attacks at a low-dose regimen of 1.2 mg followed by 0.6 mg in 1 hour (total 1.8 mg). With this regimen, colchicine can be used to abort an attack if taken immediately after the development of the first symptom of gout flare. Higher colchicine doses (0.6 mg every hour, until symptoms improve or until gastrointestinal symptoms of diarrhea, nausea, or vomiting develop, for a total of 4.8 mg over 6 hours)[3] have traditionally been recommended. A randomized, placebo-controlled trial comparing the low-dose and high-dose regimens showed both approaches had equivalent efficacy in pain relief at 24 hours (compared with placebo). However, adverse gastrointestinal events were significantly less common with the low-dose regimen. In subjects warranting additional flare treatment, continued use of colchicine 0.6 mg twice daily (reducing to once daily as the flare subsides) is appropriate in persons with normal renal and hepatic function. Oral colchicine is now available in generic and two branded versions (Colcrys, Mitigare).

Gastrointestinal symptoms are generally the first clinical signs of colchicine toxicity in patients with normal renal and hepatic function. More serious toxicities do occur and include neuromyopathy, aplastic anemia, and worsening renal and hepatic function. Care should be used in patients with renal or hepatic impairment, and because of potentially serious drug-drug interactions, colchicine should be avoided in patients receiving cyclosporine (Neoral), clarithromycin (Biaxin), verapamil (Calan), and amlodipine (Norvasc). Intravenous colchicine is not available in Europe. The FDA has stopped the marketing of unapproved injectable colchicine products in the United States and discourages the compounding of IV colchicine because of reports of preparation errors causing deaths.

Corticosteroids provide a safe alternative for patients with contraindications to NSAIDs or colchicine. For isolated monoarticular attacks, especially of medium or large joints, aspiration of joint fluid and intraarticular injection with triamcinolone acetonide (Kenalog) 20 to 40 mg can quickly terminate an attack. For polyarticular attacks or attacks in smaller joints, systemic corticosteroids (oral or intramuscular) may be used. Oral prednisone starting at 20 mg twice daily with a taper over 10 to 14 days is very effective. Patients can have rebound attacks if oral steroids are terminated too quickly, and thus methylprednisolone (Medrol) dose packs should be

---

[1]Not FDA approved for this indication.
[3]Exceeds dosage recommended by the manufacturer.

avoided. If intramuscular injection is used, a single dose of triamcinolone 40 mg may be used.

There is interest in agents blocking the action of interleukin 1 (IL-1), a cytokine thought to play a major role in initiating and sustaining acute gouty inflammation. Anakinra (Kineret)[1] and canakinumab (Ilaris)[1] are potent injectable IL-1 inhibitors, and studies are ongoing to assess the utility of these agents to mitigate acute attacks. In 2013 canakinumab became the first biologic agent approved for acute gout in Europe. It was approved by the European Medicines Agency for symptomatic treatment of adult patients with frequent gouty arthritis attacks in whom NSAIDs and colchicine are contraindicated, are not tolerated, or do not provide an adequate response and in whom repeated courses of corticosteroids are not appropriate. Rilonacept (Arcalyst)[1], which is also in this class, was declined approval for gout by the FDA in 2012 because of concerns about long-term safety.

Intercritical Gout

After an attack subsides, management is directed at preventing recurrent attacks. During acute attacks of gout, normal serum urate concentration is reported in up to 40% of affected patients, and thus it is not an accurate reflection of the true urate pool. Confirmation of hyperuricemia is best achieved either before the resolution of an attack or 2 to 4 weeks after it, to achieve an accurate serum urate concentration. There is a generalizable correlation between the serum urate level and risk for recurrent attack.

Prophylaxis of future attacks during early urate-lowering therapy can consist of colchicine at doses of 0.6 mg once or twice a day (based on renal function) or NSAIDs. If chronic NSAIDs are used, acid-reducing medications such as proton pump inhibitors or histamine-2 blockers may be used for patients at risk for gastrointestinal bleeding.

Long-Term Urate-Lowering (Antihyperuricemic) Therapy

The aim of urate-lowering therapy is to reduce and maintain serum urate at concentrations below those at which extracellular fluids are saturated with monosodium urate. In general, an ultimate serum urate concentration of less than 6.0 mg/dL is advised. Urate lowering can be achieved either by increasing urinary excretion or by decreasing production of urate.

Nonpharmacologic urate-lowering treatment begins with lifestyle changes. Diet and weight loss must be addressed. Obesity and weight gain are risk factors for gout, and weight loss has been shown to decrease the risk of gout. A purine-restricted diet has often been recommended to patients but is often unpalatable and impractical. Reduction in alcohol intake, namely beer and liquor, can effectively reduce urate levels. Similarly, reduced intake of red meat and shellfish also lowers the risk of recurrent gouty attacks. Studies have shown an increased frequency of attacks in patients who consume fruit juices and soft drinks containing high-fructose corn syrup, an ingredient not found in diet drinks.

Once the decision is made to institute serum urate-lowering therapy, the duration of treatment is indefinite and must be long-term to be effective. The majority of patients with gout and tophaceous disease will continue to have attacks if therapy is discontinued, and thus education is a key part of the treatment plan. Patients should be instructed that, with initiation of any urate-lowering therapy, they will be at increased risk for a flareup and thus must continue regular use of prophylactic agents as outlined above. At least 80% to 95% of cases of hyperuricemia and gout are attributable to impaired urate excretion, which is reflected in diminished urate clearance or fractional excretion of uric acid but not usually in low daily urine uric acid excretion. In practice, 24-hour urine collections are rarely performed. Patients are preferentially treated with xanthine oxidase inhibitors because of the easier dosing schedule and because many patients have contraindications to uricosurics such as renal insufficiency and kidney stones.

Uricosurics

Relative to medications aimed at urate synthesis, uricosurics are relegated to second-line treatment of patients with elevated urate burden or tophaceous disease. The most commonly used uricosuric agent in the United States is probenecid. This is a very effective drug that concentrates and promotes urinary excretion of urate. Its utility is limited in patients with renal insufficiency, and probenecid is not recommended as first-line therapy in patients with nephrolithiasis or uric acid overexcretion. The maintenance dose of probenecid required to achieve and maintain serum urate concentration at less than 6.0 mg/dL is 0.5 to 3 g/day[3], administered in 2 or 3 daily doses. Once goal serum urate concentration is achieved with a uricosuric agent, the risk of uric acid calculi is diminished, because urinary uric acid excretion becomes normal.

Lesinurad (Zurampic) is another uricosuric agent; it is an inhibitor of renal transport proteins and was FDA approved in 2016. It is used at a dose of 200 mg/day in combination with a xanthine oxidase inhibitor, including allopurinol (Zyloprim) or febuxostat (Uloric). In 2017, the FDA approved Duzallo, a combination product of lesinurad 200 mg and allopurinol 300 mg, one tablet in the morning for hyperuricemia. Duzallo is also available in lesinurad 200 mg and allopurinol 200 mg tablet for patients with renal impairment. This drug has a boxed warning regarding the risk of acute renal failure.

Other drugs found to have uricosuric effects include fenofibrate (Tricor)[1], a fibric acid derivative used to treat hyperlipidemia, and the antihypertensives losartan (Cozaar)[1] and amlodipine (Norvasc)[1]. These agents have mild uricosuric properties and may be useful adjuncts to urate-lowering therapy. Skim milk ingestion has been shown to lower serum urate levels through uricosuric effects. Lower urate levels have also been seen in patients who consume coffee, but the mechanism of action is unknown.

Xanthine Oxidase Inhibitors

Allopurinol (Zyloprim) and febuxostat (Uloric) are the only FDA-approved xanthine oxidase inhibitors for the treatment of gout. Allopurinol, introduced in 1966, is approved in doses of 100 to 800 mg/day. More than 90% of patients with gout treated with urate-lowering medication in the United States are given allopurinol, but dosages of more than 300 mg/day are infrequently employed, and often patients do not achieve serum urate concentrations of 6.0 mg/dL or less. Appropriate use of allopurinol is limited for several reasons. There are genuine concerns about allopurinol drug interactions, gastrointestinal intolerance, rashes (ranging from mild to life-threatening), and the rare but sometimes fatal hypersensitivity syndrome. Allopurinol should be avoided with the immunosuppressives azathioprine (Imuran) and 6-mercaptopurine (Purinethol) because it can increase the risk of bone marrow toxicity, because these medications are partially metabolized by xanthine oxidase. Allopurinol should not be taken with ampicillin owing to increased risk of rash.

Effective dosing of allopurinol is often not achieved because of compliance with published but recently disputed recommendations for allopurinol dose reduction in states of renal impairment. Allopurinol should be initiated at 100 mg daily in patients with creatinine clearance of 40 mL/min or greater, and it should be titrated in 100-mg increments every 2 to 4 weeks, with the endpoint of dosing determined by achievement of serum urate concentration of 6.0 mg/dL or less.

The FDA approved febuxostat (Uloric) in 2009. Unlike allopurinol, this is a nonpurine analogue and selective xanthine oxidase inhibitor that is not incorporated into purine nucleotides and does not appear to affect pyrimidine metabolism. Febuxostat is primarily metabolized by oxidation and glucuronidation in the liver, with little renal excretion of drug; this contrasts with the renal elimination of oxypurinol, the main allopurinol metabolite. The recommended

---

[1]Not FDA approved for this indication.

[1]Not FDA approved for this indication.
[3]Exceeds dosage recommended by the manufacturer.

starting dose of febuxostat is 40 mg daily, with an increase to 80 mg daily if serum urate concentrations do not reach goal urate levels in 2 weeks in patients with normal renal function. In Europe, higher dosages (80–120 mg daily)[3] have received approval, and studies have affirmed the efficacy and safety of dosing in this range. In the FOCUS trial, a 5-year study of efficacy and safety, febuxostat was shown to have durable maintenance of serum urate concentration at 6.0 mg/dL or less, nearly complete elimination of gouty flares, and resolution of baseline tophi in subjects. An advantage of febuxostat over allopurinol is that it can safely be taken by patients with creatinine clearance greater than 30 mL/min.

Pegloticase

Pegloticase (pegylated porcine recombinant uricase, Krystexxa) was granted FDA approval in 2010 for treatment of refractory gout. Humans lack the enzyme uricase, which converts uric acid to allantoin, a more soluble purine degradation product. Replacement of this missing enzyme allows direct conversion of urate to allantoin, with eventual depletion of increased body urate pools and control of disease, including resolution of tophi. Recombinant uricase therapy profoundly lowers serum urate concentration, as was demonstrated in two large trials. Pegloticase is approved at a dosage of 8 mg intravenously every 2 weeks.

Potential New Therapies

A number of other novel agents with new therapeutic targets for the treatment of acute and chronic gout are under investigation.

---

[3]Exceeds dosage recommended by the manufacturer.

References

Becker MA, Chohan S: We can make gout management more successful now, *Curr Opin Rheumatol* 20:167–172, 2008.

Dalbeth N, Stamp L: Allopurinol dosing in renal impairment: Walking the tightrope between adequate urate lowering and adverse events, *Semin Dial* 20:391–395, 2007.

Neogi T, Jansen T, Dalbeth N, et al: 2015 Gout Classification Criteria: An American College of Rheumatology/European League Against Rheumatism Collaborative Initiative, *Arthr Rheum* 67:2557–2568, 2015.

Schumacher HR, Becker MA, Lloyd E, et al: Febuxostat in the treatment of gout: 5-year findings of the FOCUS efficacy and safety study, *Rheumatology* 48:188–194, 2009.

Stamp L, O'Donnell JL, Zhang M, et al: Using allopurinol above the dose based on creatinine clearance is effective and safe in patients with chronic gout, including those with renal impairment, *Arthritis Rheum* 63:412–421, 2011.

Sundy JS, Becker MA, Baraf HS, et al: Reduction of plasma urate levels following treatment with multiple doses of pegloticase (polyethylene glycol–conjugated uricase) in patients with treatment-failure gout. Results of a phase II randomized study, *Arthritis Rheum* 58:2882–2891, 2008.

Terkeltaub R, Furst DE, Bennett K, et al: High versus low dosing of oral colchicine for early acute gout flare, *Arthritis Rheum* 62:1060–1068, 2010.

Zhu Y, Pandya BJ, Choi HK: Comorbidities of gout and hyperuricemia in the US general population: NHANES 2007-2008, *Am J Med* 125:679–687, 2012.

HYPERALDOSTERONISM

Method of
Ruchi Gaba, MD; Jongoh Kim, MD; and Lawrence Chan, MD

CURRENT DIAGNOSIS

- Hyperaldosteronism may be suspected in patients with severe, resistant, or early-onset hypertension and hypertensive patients with family history, hypokalemia, adrenal mass, and obstructive sleep apnea. Evaluation begins with measurement of morning plasma aldosterone concentration (PAC in ng/dL) and plasma renin activity (PRA in ng/mL/h) in a sodium- and potassium-repleted state and off of significantly interfering medications (spironolactone [Aldactone], eplerenone [Inspra], amiloride [Midamor], triamterene [Dyrenium], potassium-wasting diuretics, and licorice-derived products[7]) for at least 4 weeks.

- Elevated PRA and PAC suggest secondary hyperaldosteronism; suppressed PRA and PAC suggest conditions mimicking hyperaldosteronism; suppressed PRA but elevated PAC suggests primary hyperaldosteronism (screening positive if PAC/PRA ratio >20 to 40 and PAC >5 to 10 ng/dL).

- Positive screening of primary hyperaldosteronism should be confirmed with one of the following tests: IV saline suppression, oral salt loading, fludrocortisone (Florinef)[1]suppression, or captopril (Capoten)[1] challenge test (may skip if spontaneous hypokalemia, renin below the detection limit, and PAC >20 ng/dL).

- Once primary hyperaldosteronism is biochemically confirmed, computed tomography (CT) of the adrenal glands is recommended to exclude adrenocortical carcinoma and help subtype primary hyperaldosteronism.

- If surgical treatment is considered, adrenal vein sampling is indicated to differentiate unilateral versus bilateral lesions (may skip if the patient is <35 years with spontaneous hypokalemia, PAC >30 ng/dL, and unilateral adenoma). A cortisol-corrected aldosterone ratio from the high to the low side greater than 4:1 with cosyntropin (Cortrosyn) stimulation confirms unilateral aldosterone excess.

---

[7]Available as a dietary supplement.
[1]Not FDA approved for this indication.

CURRENT THERAPY

- Laparoscopic adrenalectomy is recommended for unilateral disease. Otherwise, medical treatment with a mineralocorticoid receptor antagonist (MRA; spironolactone [Aldactone] as the primary agent and eplerenone [Inspra] as an alternative) is recommended.

- Spironolactone: 12.5 to 25 mg/day titrated to a maximum dose of 400 mg/day to achieve normal blood pressure and normokalemia. Side effects include increased serum creatinine, hyperkalemia, gynecomastia, and menstrual irregularities.

- Eplerenone: 25 mg once or twice daily titrated to a maximum dose of 100 mg/day to achieve normal blood pressure and normokalemia. Side effects include increased creatinine, hyperkalemia, hypertriglyceridemia, increased liver enzymes, headache, and fatigue.

- Amiloride (Midamor)[1] or triamterene (Dyrenium)[1] (epithelial sodium channel antagonists) can be used in those who cannot tolerate MRAs or are still hypertensive/hypokalemic while on MRAs. Other antihypertensive agents are also added if necessary to control hypertension.

---

[1]Not FDA approved for this indication.

Introduction

Hyperaldosteronism is a state of excessive aldosterone secretion. Primary hyperaldosteronism occurs due to autonomous hypersecretion of aldosterone relative to suppressed plasma renin, whereas secondary hyperaldosteronism occurs due to activation of the renin-angiotensin-aldosterone system (RAAS). Primary hyperaldosteronism is the most common cause of secondary hypertension, and recent reports suggest that 5% to 20% of hypertensive patients have primary hyperaldosteronism (as opposed to less than 1%, as previously reported). Secondary hyperaldosteronism includes two different categories; one is compensatory activation of the RAAS due to decreased effective circulating volume, as in congestive heart failure and liver cirrhosis; the other is overactivity of the RAAS accompanied by hypertension, as in renovascular hypertension. There are also several conditions that mimic aldosterone excess through various

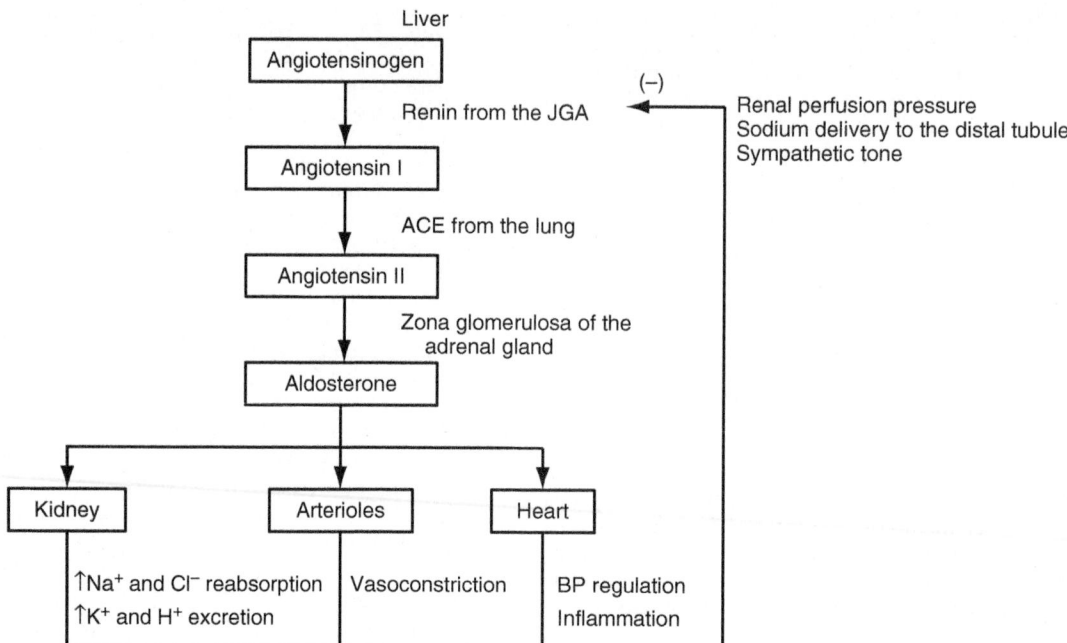

Figure 1 The renin-angiotensin-aldosterone system (RAAS). *ACE,* Angiotensin-converting enzyme; *BP,* blood pressure; *JGA,* juxtaglomerular apparatus.

mechanisms that present with hypertension and other metabolic perturbations. Except for the compensatory activation of the RAAS, these conditions cause secondary hypertension with or without other metabolic consequences, such as hypokalemia and metabolic alkalosis, which bring them to medical attention. This chapter covers the current approaches to hyperaldosteronism for patients suspected of having hypertension secondary to excess aldosterone production.

Pathophysiology

Aldosterone is a steroid hormone produced by the zona glomerulosa in the adrenal gland and contributes to volume and potassium homeostasis via its action primarily on the principal cells in the collecting tubule of the kidney. The main stimuli of aldosterone secretion are angiotensin II and hyperkalemia, which increase synthesis and activity of aldosterone synthase mediated by calcium signaling. Angiotensin II releases calcium from the endoplasmic reticulum, whereas both angiotensin II and hyperkalemia depolarize membrane potential and open voltage gated calcium channels. Therefore changes in genes regulating ionic homeostasis and membrane potential can affect aldosterone secretion. Aldosterone and angiotensin II are part of the RAAS; plasma renin from the juxtaglomerular apparatus converts angiotensinogen to angiotensin I, and angiotensin-converting enzyme (ACE) converts angiotensin I to angiotensin II. Subsequently, angiotensin II stimulates secretion of aldosterone. Renin secretion is controlled by renal artery pressure, sodium delivery to the distal nephron, and sympathetic activation (via β1). Increased effective arterial circulating volume from the action of aldosterone decreases renin secretion by negative feedback (Figure 1). Other minor factors involved in aldosterone secretion are adrenocorticotropic hormone and hyponatremia (which increase aldosterone secretion) and atrial natriuretic peptide (which decreases aldosterone secretion).

Aldosterone binds to the nuclear mineralocorticoid receptors. Activation of the mineralocorticoid receptors upregulates the basolateral Na$^+$/K$^+$ pumps and the epithelial sodium channels (ENaC), leading to increased reabsorption of Na$^+$ and Cl$^-$ and secretion of K$^+$ and H$^+$. The mineralocorticoid receptors can also be activated by other hormones with mineralocorticoid activity. Cortisol is able to bind to the mineralocorticoid receptors with similar affinity as aldosterone but normally is converted to inactive cortisone by 11β hydroxysteroid dehydrogenase 2 (11β HSD2). Mutations/inhibition of 11β HSD2 or very high cortisol

levels above the capacity of 11β HSD2, as in Cushing syndrome (particularly ectopic Cushing syndrome), and glucocorticoid resistance can cause activation of the mineralocorticoid receptors. Aldosterone precursors such as deoxycorticosterone have a weak mineralocorticoid effect but can cause features of hyperaldosteronism when they are present at very high levels as in some forms of congenital adrenal hyperplasias (11β hydroxylase deficiency or 17α hydroxylase deficiency) or deoxycorticosterone-secreting tumors. In addition, activating mutations of the ENaCs also cause increased sodium absorption and hypertension mimicking hyperaldosteronism (Liddle syndrome).

Clinical Manifestations

Primary hyperaldosteronism usually presents with normokalemic hypertension. Hypokalemia is present only in 9% to 37% of cases and may indicate more severe cases. Patients with primary hyperaldosteronism usually do not develop severe volume overload or edema because of aldosterone escape possibly related to atrial natriuretic peptide, pressure natriuresis, or decreased sodium absorption at other nephron segments. Metabolic alkalosis, mild hypernatremia (due to reset osmostat from volume expansion), and hypomagnesemia may be observed. Glomerular filtration rate and urinary albumin excretion can be elevated independent of systemic hypertension. Target organ (heart and kidney) damage and cardiovascular-related morbidity and mortality are higher in primary hyperaldosteronism than in essential hypertension with similar degrees of blood pressure (BP) elevation. Secondary hyperaldosteronism (when it is not from hypovolemia) and other conditions mimicking hyperaldosteronism can present with similar features as primary hyperaldosteronism plus specific manifestations for each disease entity. Depending on the mechanism of disease, more severe volume overload and pulmonary edema may be found (e.g., renovascular hypertension) because aldosterone escape may not work.

Evaluation
Screening

Hyperaldosteronism may be suspected based on severe (BP >150/100 on three separate occasions) or resistant hypertension (uncontrolled BP despite use of three conventional antihypertensive agents including a diuretic, or well-controlled BP in the presence of four or more antihypertensive agents), early-onset hypertension without known risk factors, and

Groups Indicated for Case Detection With Relatively High Prevalence of Primary Hyperaldosteronism

- Sustained blood pressure >150/100 mm Hg on three different occasions
- Drug-resistant hypertension (>140/90 mm Hg despite three medications including a diuretic)
- Hypertension and hypokalemia (spontaneous or diuretic-induced)
- Hypertension and family history of early-onset hypertension or cerebrovascular accident at a young age (<40 years)
- Hypertension with adrenal incidentaloma
- Hypertensive first-degree relatives of primary hyperaldosteronism patients
- Hypertension with obstructive sleep apnea

hypertension with other features such as family history of hyperaldosteronism, early-onset hypertension, cerebrovascular accident at a young age, hypokalemia, adrenal mass, and obstructive sleep apnea. Currently there is no evidence-guided screening strategy. Some experts believe that routine screening for primary hyperaldosteronism is warranted in newly diagnosed hypertension considering its high prevalence, whereas others recommend that targeted screening is more appropriate, such as the Endocrine Society guidelines for primary hyperaldosteronism in 2016 (Box 1).

When a decision is made to screen for excessive mineralocorticoid effect, one should first examine the plasma renin and aldosterone levels; that is, plasma renin activity (PRA, ng/mL/h) and plasma aldosterone concentration (PAC, ng/dL). It is important to note that several factors can affect PRA and PAC, such as age, medications, time of day, diet (salt intake), posture, method of blood collection, level of potassium, and level of creatinine (Table 1). Diuretics (both potassium sparing and wasting) and mineralocorticoid antagonists can have a significant effect on PRA and PAC. Angiotensin-converting enzyme inhibitors/angiotensin receptor blockers (ACEI/ARB) and dihydropyridine calcium channel blockers can affect PRA and PAC modestly. Ideally, all medications and other factors that may affect PRA and PAC should be removed; unfortunately, it is not always practical and safe to do this because of the possibility of uncontrolled hypertension. If necessary, antihypertensive agents that affect PRA and PAC only minimally such as slow-release verapamil (Calan SR), hydralazine (Apresoline), prazosin (Minipress), doxazosin (Cardura), or terazosin (Hytrin) can be used. The Endocrine Society 2016 guidelines recommend certain caveats that optimize the chance for obtaining more easily interpretable PRA and PAC results (Box 2).

Patterns of PRA and PAC help differentiate among primary hyperaldosteronism, secondary hyperaldosteronism, and conditions mimicking hyperaldosteronism. Differential diagnoses according to different patterns of PRA and PAC are listed in Box 3. If both PRA and PAC are high, further investigation for causes of secondary hyperaldosteronism should follow. If both PRA and PAC are suppressed, further investigation for conditions that mimic hyperaldosteronism is indicated. Suppressed PRA and elevated PAC suggest primary hyperaldosteronism, and aldosterone renin ratio (ARR) should be calculated; ARR above 20 to 40 is considered screening positive for primary hyperaldosteronism. PAC greater than 15 ng/dL was recommended by some investigators to avoid false-positive ARR from very low renin level, but in many cases PAC can be less than 15 ng/dL, though this occurs more commonly in bilateral adrenal hyperplasia (BAH) than in aldosterone-producing adenoma. PAC should at least be above the level considered positive for confirmatory tests (5 to 10 ng/dL). Confirmatory tests should follow to avoid false positives. Diagnostic flow and subsequent management of hyperaldosteronism are summarized in Figure 2. Of note, there is no consensus on cutoff values for PRA, PAC, or ARR. In addition, PRA and PAC

are often obtained in a less-than-optimal condition. Therefore it is important to understand how PRA and PAC can be affected by various factors. For example, if ARR is positive while on medications that decrease PAC or increase PRA (thus decreasing ARR), ARR off this medication will be clearly positive. Screening tests should be repeated if results are inconclusive or if PA is strongly suspected but the initial screening tests are negative.

Confirmatory Tests of Primary Hyperaldosteronism

The positive screening test should be followed by one or more confirmatory tests to avoid false positives. The confirmatory tests are designed to physiologically suppress aldosterone levels that would normally occur in the absence of primary hyperaldosteronism. However, some experts believe that some aldosterone-producing lesions are not completely independent of the RAAS, and confirmatory suppression tests can give false-negative results. Other experts think that confirmatory tests are not necessary for those with obvious clinical/biochemical features. Those with spontaneous hypokalemia, renin level below the detection level plus PAC greater than 20 ng/dL may not need further confirmatory tests. Furthermore, there is no gold-standard confirmatory. Therefore factors such as cost, accessibility, feasibility, patient compliance, local expertise, and accuracy of assay should be taken into consideration in selecting confirmatory tests. The Endocrine Society guidelines in 2016 state that any of the following four confirmatory tests can be used: oral salt loading test, saline suppression test, fludrocortisone (Florinef)[1] suppression test, and captopril (Capoten)[1] challenge test (Table 2).

Subtype Classification of Primary Hyperaldosteronism

Once primary hyperaldosteronism is biochemically confirmed, subtype classification follows to guide treatment. Lateralization of the source of excessive aldosterone production is crucial as the next step, as unilateral lesions such as aldosterone-producing adenomas (APAs) can be treated surgically; in contrast, bilateral lesions such as BAHs are treated medically. Aldosterone-producing carcinoma is rare but should be ruled out. In this regard, CT of the adrenal glands should be done first to rule out aldosterone-producing carcinoma and obtain anatomic information. However, imaging studies are usually not reliable enough to lateralize lesions. If surgical treatment is considered, adrenal vein sampling (AVS) should be performed. Young patients (<20 years of age) and those with family history of primary hyperaldosteronism or strokes at young age (less than 40 years) should have genetic testing for glucocorticoid remediable aldosteronism (GRA) or familial hyperaldosteronism type 1 (FH-1), which is caused by the hybrid gene of 11β hydroxylase and aldosterone synthase (increased aldosterone synthesis by adrenocorticotropic hormone). In very young patients, *KCNJ5* germline mutations, causing familial hyperaldosteronism type III, should be tested. Familial hyperaldosteronism type II is clinically indistinguishable from nonfamilial hyperaldosteronism, and its molecular basis has not been identified.

Imaging

CT/MRI scans of the adrenal glands provide one of five conclusions: normal adrenal glands, unilateral macroadenomas (>1 cm), minimal unilateral adrenal limb thickening, unilateral microadenomas (≤1 cm), and bilateral macroadenomas and/or microadenomas. APAs are typically smaller than 2 cm, and BAHs exhibit either normal or nodular changes. Aldosterone-producing adrenal carcinomas are almost always larger than 4 cm in diameter and have imaging characteristics suspicious for malignancy. However, there are limitations; small APAs may be missed, hyperplasia may be misread as adenomas, and nonfunctional tumors are radiologically indistinguishable from APAs. Although several studies suggested imaging criteria for different subtypes, no study has conclusively established specific criteria that differentiate

---

[1]Not FDA approved for this indication.

TABLE 1	Medical Factors That May Affect Aldosterone and Renin Measurement		
	EFFECT ON ALDOSTERONE	**EFFECT ON RENIN**	**EFFECT ON ALDOSTERONE–RENIN RATIO**
Medications			
β-Blocker	↓	↓↓	↑
Central α$_2$ agonists (clonidine [Catapres], α-methyldopa [Aldomet])	↓	↓↓	↑
NSAIDs	↓	↓↓	↑
K$^+$ wasting diuretics	→↑	↑↑	↓
K$^+$ sparing diuretics	↑	↑↑	↓
ACE inhibitors	↓	↑↑	↓
Angiotensin II receptor blockers	↓	↑↑	↓
Dihydropyridine Ca^{2+} blockers	→↓	↑	↓
Renin inhibitors	↓	↓ plasma renin activity ↑ direct renin concentration	↑ ↓
Potassium Status			
Hypokalemia	↓	→↑	↓
Potassium loading	↑	→↓	↑
Dietary Sodium			
Sodium restricted	↑	↑↑	↓
Sodium loaded	↓	↓↓	↑
Others			
Advanced age	↓	↓↓	↑
Renal impairment	→	↓	↑
Oral contraceptives*	↑	↑ plasma renin activity ↓ direct renin concentration	→ ↑
Pregnancy	↑	↑↑	↓
Renovascular hypertension	↑	↑↑	↓
Malignant hypertension	↑	↑↑	↓

NSAIDs, Nonsteroidal antiinflammatory drugs.
*Premenopausal women have higher aldosterone level during the luteal phase and lower renin level throughout the cycle than men. False positive ARR during the luteal phase was reported when direct renin concentration was used.

among different subtypes of primary hyperaldosteronism. In fact, CT accurately lateralizes in only about 50% to 70% of cases, and there is no evidence that MRI is superior to CT for subtype classification. Therefore AVS is required to differentiate unilateral from bilateral lesions if surgical resection is being pursued. Patients younger than 35 years with marked hyperaldosteronism with spontaneous hypokalemia and PAC greater than 30 ng/dL and solitary unilateral adenoma may not need AVS, because nonfunctioning tumors are uncommon in this young age group.

Adrenal Vein Sampling

Aldosterone levels are measured from adrenal venous blood samples (Box 4) obtained through adrenal vein cannulation to distinguish between unilateral and bilateral lesions. Unilateral lesions are associated with a marked increase in PAC on the side of the tumor (and suppressed PAC on the other side), whereas bilateral lesions have little difference between the two sides. AVS should be performed only by experienced physicians in part because recognition and successful cannulation of the right adrenal vein especially can be challenging. Complications of AVS include

adrenal hemorrhage, adrenal infarction, adrenal vein perforation, and adrenal vein thrombosis, which occur only rarely (<2.5%) in the hands of a physician skilled in the procedure.

The use of cosyntropin (Cortrosyn) stimulation to minimize stress-induced fluctuation in aldosterone level is controversial, and some believe that it has no effect on AVS accuracy. If cosyntropin is not used, then AVS should be done in the morning after overnight recumbency to avoid postural aldosterone changes and reflect circadian aldosterone secretion.

In reality, different centers use different techniques, protocols, and interpretation criteria. The Endocrine Society guidelines in 2016 provide interpretation criteria with and without cosyntropin use. The first step for interpretation is to determine whether the procedure was done correctly. The adrenal vein-to-IVC cortisol ratio should be greater than 5:1 with cosyntropin given and greater than 3:1 without cosyntropin. If the ratio is significantly lower than these values, improper cannulation is implied. Next, divide the PAC values for the right and left adrenal veins by their respective cortisol values to correct the dilutional effect of the inferior phrenic vein flow into the left adrenal vein; this is termed

BOX 2 — Approach to Measure Plasma Renin Activity and Plasma Aldosterone Concentration

- Correct hypokalemia to 4 mmol/L.
- Liberalize sodium intake.
- Withdraw the following agents that markedly affect PRA and PAC for at least 4 weeks: spironolactone (Aldactone), eplerenone (Inspra), amiloride (Midamor), triamterene (Dyrenium), potassium-wasting diuretic, and products from licorice.[7]
- If not diagnostic and hypertension can be controlled with relatively noninterfering medications, withdraw the following agents for at least 2 weeks: β-blockers, central α_2 agonists (clonidine [Catapres], methyldopa [Aldomet]), NSAIDs, ACEIs/ARBs, renin inhibitors, and dihydropyridine calcium channel antagonists.
- If necessary, start other antihypertensive agents that have fewer effects on ARR: slow-release verapamil (Calan-SR), hydralazine (Apresoline) (with verapamil to prevent reflex tachycardia), prazosin (Minipress), doxazosin (Cardura), and terazosin (Hytrin).
- Obtain blood for PRA and PAC mid-morning after the patient has been up for at least 2 h and seated for 5–15 min.
- Establish use of estrogen products and menstrual cycles. Premenopausal females have higher ARR than men, especially during the luteal phase. False-positive ARR was reported during the luteal phase and from the use of estrogen products when direct renin concentration was used.

[7]Available as dietary supplement.
ARB, Angiotensin receptor blockers; *ARR*, aldosterone renin ratio; *NSAIDs*, nonsteroidal anti-inflammatory drugs; *PAC*, plasma aldosterone concentration; *PRA*, plasma renin activity.

BOX 3 — Differential Diagnoses According to Plasma Renin Activity and Plasma Aldosterone Concentration

Causes of Primary Hyperaldosteronism: ↓ PRA and ↑ PAC (>5–10 ng/dL); ARR >20–40
- Most Common
  - Aldosterone-producing adenoma
  - Bilateral adrenal hyperplasia or idiopathic hyperaldosteronism
- Less common
  - Unilateral hyperplasia or primary adrenal hyperplasia
  - Familial hyperaldosteronism type 1 or glucocorticoid remediable aldosteronism
  - Familial hyperaldosteronism type 2
  - Aldosterone-producing adrenocortical carcinoma
  - Ectopic aldosterone-secreting tumor (ovary, kidney)
  - Multiple endocrine neoplasia type 1

Causes of Secondary Hyperaldosteronism: ↑ PRA and ↑ PAC; ARR ≈ 10
- Renovascular hypertension
- Diuretic use
- Renin-secreting tumor
- Malignant hypertension
- Coarctation of the aorta

Causes of Conditions That Mimic Mineralocorticoid Excess: ↓ PRA and ↓ PAC
- Congenital adrenal hyperplasia
- Exogenous mineralocorticoid
- Deoxycorticosterone-producing tumor
- Cushing syndrome
- 11β HSD2 deficiency
- Altered aldosterone metabolism
- Liddle syndrome
- Glucocorticoid resistance

ARR, Aldosterone-renin ratio; *PAC*, plasma aldosterone concentration; *PRA*, plasma renin activity.

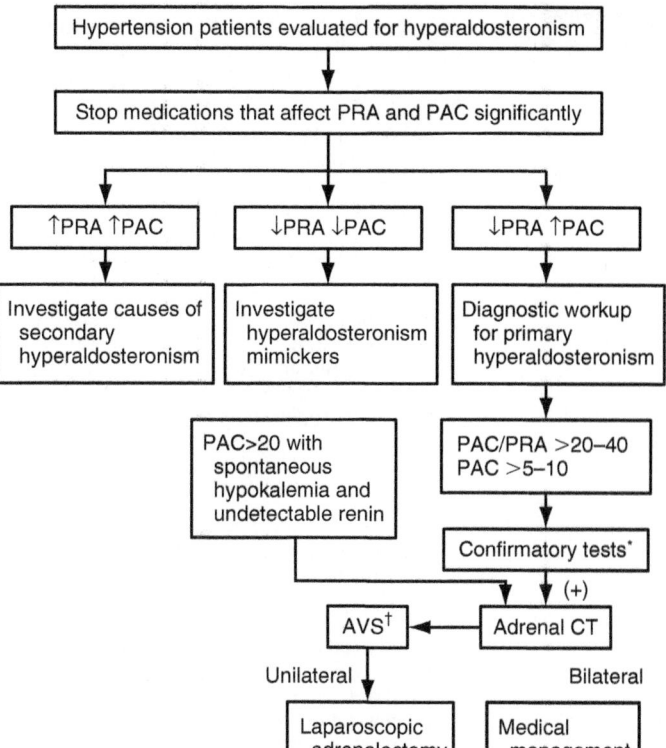

Figure 2 Evaluation of hyperaldosteronism. *AVS*, Adrenal vein sampling; *CT*, computed tomography; *PAC*, plasma aldosterone concentration in ng/dL; *PRA*, plasma renin activity in ng/mL/h. *May skip if spontaneous hypokalemia, renin level below the detection limit, and PAC >20 ng/dL. †If surgical treatment is pursued. May skip if <35 years old, spontaneous hypokalemia, PAC >30 ng/dL, and unilateral adenoma.

the *cortisol-corrected aldosterone* (A/C). If cosyntropin is used, an A/C ratio of the high to the low side of greater than 4:1 indicates unilateral aldosterone hypersecretion, whereas an A/C ratio of less than 3:1 suggests bilateral aldosterone hypersecretion. These cutoffs were reported to have sensitivity of 95% and specificity of 100% for unilateral lesions. If the A/C ratio is between 3:1 and 4:1, the results of AVS should be interpreted in the context of CT, clinical findings, and other tests. Without cosyntropin, an A/C ratio of the high to the low side of greater than 2 or an A/C ratio of the high side to the periphery greater than 2.5 plus an A/C ratio of the low side to the periphery of less than 1 (suppressed contralateral aldosterone secretion) is consistent with unilateral aldosterone excess.

Ancillary Tests

Clinical findings and other ancillary tests may help differentiate unilateral APAs from BAHs. BAHs will respond with increase in plasma aldosterone to postural stimulation, whereas APAs will not. Plasma 18-hydroxycorticosterone level tends to be higher in APAs as compared with BAHs. Iodocholesterol scintigraphy may be able to show functional correlation of anatomic abnormalities (but is not available at most centers). APA-specific tracers such as (11)C-Metomidate for positron emission tomography may be useful. Interpretation criteria of these tests are listed in Table 3. Patients with APAs tend to be younger (<40 years), predominantly female, very hypertensive with marked hypokalemia (<3 mmol/L), and tend to have a very high PAC (>25 mg/dL) compared with those with BAHs.

Treatment

Treatment of secondary hyperaldosteronism and conditions mimicking hyperaldosteronism depends on their etiology. Treatment of primary hyperaldosteronism is discussed here. The goals of treatment of primary hyperaldosteronism are (1)

TABLE 2 Protocols and Interpretation of Recommended Confirmatory Tests

	PROTOCOL	INTERPRETATION	REMARKS
Oral sodium loading test	1. Place the patient on a high-sodium diet (> 200 mmol/day) for 3 days. 2. Replace potassium to compensate for the kaliuresis induced by the high-sodium diet. 3. Collect a 24-h urine on the third day for determination of aldosterone, sodium, and creatinine; adequate if the urine sodium >200 mmol/24 h	Confirmed if the 24-h urine aldosterone is > 12 mcg (33.3 nmol) to 14 mcg (38.8 nmol). Ruled out if the 24-h urine aldosterone is <10 mcg (27.7 nmol). The test is equivocal if the value falls in between	Do not perform this test in patients with severe uncontrolled hypertension, renal failure, cardiac failure/arrhythmias, or severe hypokalemia
IV saline infusion test*	1. Place the patient supine 1 h before drawing blood for morning baseline fasting levels of renin, aldosterone, cortisol, and potassium 2. Infuse 2 L of 0.9% NaCl over 4 h, keeping the patient supine. Monitor blood pressure and heart rate 3. After 4 h, draw blood for measurement of renin, aldosterone, cortisol, and potassium	Confirmed if the PAC is >10 ng/dL (277 pmol/L). Ruled out if the PAC is <5 ng/dL (139 pmol/L). If the PAC falls between these values, the test is equivocal	Do not perform this test in patients with severe uncontrolled hypertension, renal failure, cardiac failure/arrhythmias, or severe hypokalemia
Fludrocortisone[1] suppression test	1. Give 0.1 mg fludrocortisone every 6 h for 4 days, with the potassium level checked every 6 h to be sure that it is greater than 4 mmol/L 2. Encourage a liberal sodium diet to keep urinary sodium excretion greater than 3 mmol/kg/day 3. On day 4, draw blood for an upright 7 a.m. plasma cortisol level and 10 a.m. plasma aldosterone, renin, and cortisol levels	Confirmed if the 10 a.m. PAC is >6 ng/dL, as long as PRA is <1 ng/mL/h and the plasma cortisol at 10 a.m. is less than at 7 a.m. (to exclude the ACTH effect)	The test may require hospitalization. Risks include severe hypokalemia, QT changes, worsening of left ventricular function, hypertension, and frequent phlebotomy
Captopril[1] challenge test	1. Give 25–50 mg captopril after the patient has been sitting or standing for 1 h. The patient remains seated throughout the test. 2. Draw blood for measurement of plasma renin, aldosterone, and cortisol at time 0, at 1 h, and at 2 h	Normally, captopril suppresses PAC by more than 30% from baseline. Confirmed if there is no suppression of PAC and PRA remains suppressed. The false-negative rate for this test is high because suppression occurs in more than 30% of cases. A slight decrease in aldosterone can suggest bilateral adrenal hyperplasia	

*The patient may be seated for 30 minutes before and during the infusion to improve sensitivity and PAC greater than 6 ng/dL (170 pmol/L) confirms primary hyperaldosteronism.
[1]Not FDA approved for this indication.
ACTH, Adrenocorticotropic hormone; *PAC*, plasma aldosterone concentration; *PRA*, plasma renin activity.

normalization of the serum potassium in hypokalemic patients, (2) normalization of the BP, and (3) reversal of the effects of hyperaldosteronism on the cardiovascular system. When a small group of patients were followed after treatment with adrenalectomy or mineralocorticoid receptor antagonists (MRAs), left ventricular mass was reduced (faster with adrenalectomy than MRAs), increase in carotid intima-media thickness and arterial stiffness was reversed, glomerular filtration rate and urinary albumin secretion decreased and became similar to that in essential hypertension, and excessive cardiovascular risk compared to essential hypertension disappeared. Cardiovascular complications were rather related to age, duration of hypertension, and smoking. In addition, there was an improvement in the quality of life at 3 months, which was sustained at 6 months. Therefore timely diagnosis and treatment is essential. For unilateral lesions, surgical resection of the affected adrenal gland is recommended mainly to obviate the need for prolonged medical treatment and side effects. For bilateral lesions, medical treatment is recommended because surgical risk outweighs benefits. BP control per se does not reduce risk of cardiovascular complications unless renin activity is restored to normal (>1 ng/mL/h), which can be accomplished by salt restriction or increasing the dose of the MRA. MRAs are a key component of medical treatment and used as a preoperative measure or maintenance treatment (GRA should be treated with the lowest dose of glucocorticoid that can normalize BP and potassium levels rather than MRAs). A low-sodium diet (sodium <100 mEq/day = 2.3 g/day or salt 6 g/day) is also important, because left ventricular hypertrophy is associated with urine sodium

---

BOX 4 Adrenal Vein Sampling

- After both adrenal veins have been cannulated, draw baseline samples for PRA, PAC, ACTH, and cortisol from the peripheral such as cubital or iliac, right adrenal vein, and left adrenal vein.
- Inject 250 mcg of cosyntropin (Cortrosyn) after cannulation, or infuse 50 mcg cosyntropin per hour beginning 30 min before adrenal vein cannulation. This reduces stress-related fluctuations in aldosterone and cortisol values and augments the biochemical gradients. (This step is controversial.)
- Draw blood for aldosterone and cortisol levels at 5, 15, and 30 min from the peripheral site and from each adrenal vein.

ACTH, Adrenocorticotropic hormone; *PAC*, plasma aldosterone concentration; *PRA*, plasma renin activity.

excretion in primary hyperaldosteronism but not in essential hypertension. Other lifestyle changes include aerobic exercise, smoking cessation, and weight loss.

Unilateral Hypersecretion

Adrenalectomy, usually laparoscopic, is recommended. After adrenalectomy, BP improves in all patients (maximal improvement in 1 to 6 months, sometime continues to fall up to 1 year), but 30% to 60% of patients have persistent hypertension. BP and potassium level should be controlled before surgery. MRAs such as

TEST	FINDINGS
TABLE 3 Interpretation of Dynamic Testing	
Screening Test	
PAC/PRA ratio	Positive if >20–40 with PAC >5–10 ng/dL
Confirmatory Tests	
Oral sodium loading test	Positive if 24-h urine aldosterone excretion is >12–14 mcg
Saline infusion test	Positive if PAC after infusion is >10 ng/dL
Fludrocortisone[1] suppression test	Positive if upright PAC is >6 ng/dL on day 4 at 10 a.m.
Captopril[1] challenge test	Positive if PAC does not decrease by 30% and PRA remains suppressed
AVS	
With cosyntropin stimulation	A/C ratio (the high to the low side) >4:1 → unilateral aldosterone excess A/C ratio 3:1–4:1 → unclear A/C ratio <3:1 → bilateral aldosterone excess
Without cosyntropin stimulation	A/C ratio from the high to the low side >2:1 → unilateral aldosterone excess A/C ratio from the high side to the periphery >2.5 and A/C ratio from the contralateral side to the periphery <1 → unilateral aldosterone excess
If Equivocal AVS	
Postural stimulation test	PAC falls or fails to rise by 30%: consistent with APAs PAC increases by at least 33%: consistent with BAHs
Recumbent 18-hydroxycorticosterone	>100 ng/dL is consistent with APAs
NP-59 iodocholesterol scintigraphy	Unilateral early uptake (<5 days): consistent with unilateral aldosterone excess Bilateral early uptake (<5 days): consistent with bilateral aldosterone excess Negative scan does not rule out either etiology
(11)C-Metomidate positron emission tomography	Preliminary data showed (11)C-Metomidate uptake in APA

[1]Not FDA approved for this indication.

A/C ratio, Cortisol-corrected aldosterone ratio; *APA,* aldosterone-producing adenomas; *AVS,* adrenal vein sampling; *BAH,* bilateral adrenal hyperplasia; *PAC,* plasma aldosterone concentration; *PRA,* plasma renin activity.

spironolactone (Aldactone) and eplerenone (Inspra)[1] can be used to control BP in patients awaiting adrenalectomy and also to prevent postoperative hypoaldosteronism. Postoperatively, normal saline is given to maintain volume status, MRAs and potassium supplements are discontinued, and antihypertensive medications may be reduced. To confirm biochemical cure, PAC and PRA should be checked shortly after the operation though renin levels might not change immediately. Risk factors for persistent hypertension after adrenalectomy include older age, duration of hypertension (>5 years), use of two or more antihypertensive agents preoperatively, BP higher than 165/100 mm Hg, low ARR preoperatively, low

[1]Not FDA approved for this indication.

urine aldosterone, poor response to spironolactone preoperatively, family history of more than one first-degree relative with hypertension, and elevated serum creatinine level.

Bilateral Hypersecretion

MRAs and/or ENaC antagonists combined with other antihypertensives are used. One study showed that spironolactone had stronger antihypertensive effect than eplerenone, but there is insufficient evidence to choose one medication over another. Subtotal adrenalectomy has been tried, but only a minority of patients have responded with significant BP improvement. Unilateral adrenalectomy, however, may help selected patients by debulking aldosterone-producing tissues.

Spironolactone is the most widely used MRA. It is very effective in decreasing BP. The medication is initiated at 12.5 to 25 mg/day and can be titrated to 400 mg/day, with most patients requiring at least 200 mg/day. Potassium should be maintained at normal levels without use of potassium supplements. Use of spironolactone can be limited by side effects; antiandrogenic effects can cause gynecomastia in men and progesterone effect can cause menstrual irregularities in women. There are drug interactions to consider; spironolactone increases the half-life of digoxin (Lanoxin) and salicylates, and other NSAIDs may decrease the effectiveness of spironolactone. Serum potassium and creatinine should be closely monitored for the first 4 to 6 weeks, in particular for those with renal insufficiency or diabetes. Spironolactone is not recommended if creatinine clearance is less than 30 mL/min.

Eplerenone[1] is a competitive and selective antagonist of the aldosterone receptors. It has a lower binding affinity to androgen and progesterone receptors than spironolactone. This leads to fewer side effects. Eplerenone is 25% to 50% less potent in antagonizing the aldosterone receptors than spironolactone. Eplerenone has a short half-life and should be taken twice daily. Dosing is started at 25 mg twice daily, with a maximum dose of 100 mg/day. Again, serum potassium and creatinine should be closely monitored for the first 4 to 6 weeks in particular for those with renal insufficiency or diabetes. Other adverse effects include hypertriglyceridemia, increased liver enzymes, headache, and fatigue. Eplerenone is contraindicated if serum potassium is greater than 5.5 mEq/L at initiation, if creatinine clearance is less than 30 mL/min, or if there is concomitant use of strong CYP3A4 inhibitors such as ketoconazole (Nizoral) and itraconazole (Sporanox).

ENaC antagonists, amiloride (Midamor)[1] and triamterene (Dyrenium)[1], can be used in patients who cannot tolerate MRAs or are still hypertensive/hypokalemic while on MRAs. Amiloride is prescribed at 10 to 20 mg/day in divided doses. Side effects include dizziness, fatigue, and impotence. Triamterene is dosed at 100 to 300 mg/day in divided doses, and its side effects are mainly dizziness and nausea. Addition of thiazide diuretics can help control BP by relieving volume overload. If BP remains uncontrolled, other antihypertensive agents such as ACEIs/ARBs or calcium channel blockers may be used.

[1]Not FDA approved for this indication.

References

Born-Frontsberg E, Reincke M, Rump LC, et al: Cardiovascular and cerebrovascular comorbidities of hypokalemic and normokalemic primary aldosteronism: results of the German Conn's registry, *J Clin Endocrinol Metab* 94:1125–1130, 2009.

Catena C, Colussi G, Lapenna R, et al: Long-term cardiac effects of adrenalectomy or mineralocorticoid antagonists in patients with primary aldosteronism, *Hypertension* 50:911–918, 2007.

Catena C, Colussi GL, Nadalini E, et al: Cardiovascular outcomes in patients with primary aldosteronism after treatment, *Arch Intern Med* 168:80–85, 2008.

Funder JW: Primary aldosteronism and cardiovascular risk, before and after treatment, *Lancet Diabetes Endocrinol* 6:5–7, 2018.

Funder JW, Carey RM, Mantero F, et al: The management of primary aldosteronism: case detection, diagnosis, and treatment: an endocrine society clinical guideline, *J Clin Endocrinol Metab* 101:1889–1916, 2016.

Gordon RD, Gomez-Sanchez CE, Hamlet SM, et al: Angiotensin-responsive aldosterone-producing adenoma masquerades as idiopathic hyperaldosteronism (IHA: adrenal hyperplasia) or low-renin essential hypertension, *J Hypertens* 5:S103–S106, 1987.

Hundemer GL, Curhan GC, Yozamp N, et al: Cardiometabolic outcomes and mortality in medically treated primary aldosteronism: a restrospective cohort study, *Lancet Diabetes Endocrinol* 6:51–59, 2018.

Kempers MJ, Lenders JW, van Outheusden L, et al: Systematic review: diagnostic procedures to differentiate unilateral from bilateral adrenal abnormality in primary aldosteronism, *Ann Intern Med* 151:329–337, 2009.

Mulatero P, Bertello C, Rossato D, et al: Roles of clinical criteria, computed tomography scan, and adrenal vein sampling in differential diagnosis of primary aldosteronism subtypes, *J Clin Endocrinol Metab* 93:1366–1371, 2008.

Parthasarathy HK, Menard J, White WB, et al: A double-blind, randomized study comparing the antihypertensive effect of eplerenone and spironolactone in patients with hypertension and evidence of primary aldosteronism, *J Hypertens* 29:980, 2011.

Pimenta E, Gordon RD, Ahmed AH, et al: Cardiac dimensions are largely determined by dietary salt in patients with primary aldosteronism: results of a case-control study, *J Clin Endocrinol Metab* 96:2813–2820, 2011.

Reincke M, Fischer E, Gerum S, et al: Observational study mortality in treated primary aldosteronism: the German Conn's registry, *Hypertension* 60:618–624, 2012.

Rossi GP: A comprehensive review of the clinical aspects of primary aldosteronism, *Nat Rev Endocrinol* 7:485–495, 2011.

Rossi GP, Barisa M, Allolio B, et al: The adrenal vein sampling international study (AVIS) for identifying the major subtypes of primary aldosteronism, *J Clin Endocrinol Metab* 97:1606–1614, 2012.

Rossi GP, Bernini G, Caliumi C, et al: A prospective study of the prevalence of primary aldosteronism in 1,125 hypertensive patients, *J Am Coll Cardiol* 48:2293–2300, 2006.

Rossi GP, Seccia TM, Pessina AC: Adrenal gland: a diagnostic algorithm—the holy grail of primary aldosteronism, *Nat Rev Endocrinol* 7:697–699, 2011.

Sawka AM, Young WF, Thompson GB, et al: Primary aldosteronism: factors associated with normalization of blood pressure after surgery, *Ann Intern Med* 135:258–261, 2001.

Sechi LA, Novello M, Lapenna R, et al: Long-term renal outcomes in patients with primary aldosteronism, *JAMA* 295:2638–2645, 2006.

Stowasser M: Update in primary aldosteronism, *J Clin Endocrinol Metab* 100:1–10, 2015.

Sukor N, Gordon RD, Ku YK, et al: Role of unilateral adrenalectomy in bilateral primary aldosteronism: a 22-year single center experience, *J Clin Endocrinol Metab* 94:2437–2445, 2009.

Zennaro MC, Boulkroun S, Fernandes-Rosa F: An update on novel mechanisms of primary aldosteronism, *J Endocrinol* 224:R63–R77, 2015.

HYPERLIPIDEMIA

Method of
Xiaoming Jia, MD; Mandeep Bajaj, MD; and Lawrence Chan, MD

CURRENT DIAGNOSIS

- Hyperlipidemia is diagnosed based on the fasting lipid profile in the context of global cardiovascular risk. The exception is when the triglyceride level is greater than 500 mg/dL because of substantial risk of pancreatitis.
- Secondary causes of hyperlipidemia, such as hypothyroidism, alcoholism, uncontrolled diabetes mellitus, kidney disorders, pregnancy, and medications, should be thoroughly investigated and treated if diagnosed.
- Possibility of familial hyperlipidemia based on the lipid profile, family history, and physical examination should be considered because cardiovascular risk can be underestimated and treatment can be challenging.

CURRENT THERAPY

- Therapy should be guided by goals of treatment based on estimated cardiovascular risk unless triglyceride level >500 mg/L, in which case lowering triglycerides to prevent acute pancreatitis is a priority.
- Low-density lipoprotein (LDL) cholesterol is a primary goal followed by non-high-density lipoprotein (HDL) cholesterol as a secondary goal. Triglycerides have also emerged as a target to further reduce residual cardiovascular risk in select patients with high cardiovascular risk.

- Therapeutic lifestyle changes should be initiated in everyone with lipid parameters above their target. Therapeutic lifestyle changes are also recommended for those with very high, high, or moderately high cardiovascular risk.
- Pharmacologic agents should be added if therapeutic lifestyle changes are not successful. Pharmacologic agents can be considered from the beginning for those with very high, high, or moderately high cardiovascular risk.
- Statin therapy is preferred if tolerated, and the intensity of therapy to use should be dictated by the degree of cardiovascular risk.
- Statins are the treatment of choice for their proven effects on cardiovascular outcomes. Other agents can be added based on response to statins and other targets such as high triglycerides.
- All other cardiovascular risk factors should be treated aggressively at the same time.

Hyperlipidemia is a condition of elevated serum lipids and lipoproteins. Hyperlipidemia is associated with an increased risk of atherosclerotic cardiovascular disease (ASCVD) and, if the triglyceride level is greater than 500 mg/dL, pancreatitis. Unless the triglyceride level is greater than 500 mg/dL, the primary goal of management of hyperlipidemia is to decrease the risk of ASCVD. ASCVD as defined by the *2018 Multisociety Guideline on the Management of Blood Cholesterol* encompasses acute coronary syndrome, history of myocardial infarction, stable or unstable angina or coronary or other arterial revascularization, stroke, transient ischemic attack, or peripheral arterial disease including aortic aneurysm, all of atherosclerotic origin. In this regard, appropriate treatment of hyperlipidemia is essential in patients with established cardiovascular disease (secondary prevention), whereas detection and treatment of hyperlipidemia are guided by the risk of ASCVD in patients without known clinical ASCVD (primary prevention).

The prevalence of hyperlipidemia varies with the definition of hyperlipidemia and the population studied. The percentage of US adults with a total cholesterol level of 240 mg/dL or higher declined from 19% to 14% in men and from 21% to 15% in women from 1988 to 2008. This may be in part due to increased use of lipid-lowering medications, from 3.4% to 15.5%. However, major risk factors for cardiovascular disease actually have become more common: the prevalence of obesity (BMI ≥ 30 kg/m²) increased from 19.9% to 31.6% in men and from 25.2% to 34.1% in women, and the prevalence of diabetes increased from 5.5% to 11.1% in men and from 4.6% to 6.3% in women over this period. Therefore optimal treatment of hyperlipidemia to reduce cardiovascular risk is of paramount importance.

Various societies and professional organizations have published clinical guidelines for hyperlipidemia. The approach used in this chapter is mostly based on the *2013 ACC/AHA Guideline on the Treatment of Blood Cholesterol to Reduce Atherosclerotic Cardiovascular Risk in Adults: A Report of the American College of Cardiology/American Heart Association Task Force on Practice Guidelines* and the *2018 Multisociety Guideline on the Management of Blood Cholesterol*. The 2013 American College of Cardiology/American Heart Association guideline represents a substantial departure from previous guidelines in that it emphasizes the use of statins of appropriate strength according to the estimated cardiovascular risk without specific low-density lipoprotein (LDL) cholesterol targets. The 2016 European Society of Cardiology and European Atherosclerosis Society (ESC/EAS) Guidelines for the Management of Dyslipidaemias will also be integrated in the sections on Evaluation and Treatment.

Pathophysiology

Lipids have two main points of entry into the circulation: the gut (exogenous pathway) and the liver (endogenous pathway). The exogenous and endogenous pathways are interconnected by

Figure 1 Overview of exogenous and endogenous pathways of lipid metabolism. *CM,* chylomicrons; *HDL,* high-density lipoproteins; *IDL,* intermediate-density lipoproteins; *LDL,* low-density lipoproteins; *VLDL,* very-low-density lipoproteins.

intermediate pathways (reverse cholesterol transport pathway and others). These pathways are outlined in Figure 1.

Exogenous Pathway

Lipids in food are emulsified by bile acids and then hydrolyzed into fatty acids and cholesterol by pancreatic lipases in the intestinal lumen. Inside the intestinal cells, fatty acids and cholesterol are re-esterified and then packaged with apolipoprotein (Apo) B48 into chylomicrons. Chylomicrons are secreted into the intestinal lymph and delivered to the systemic circulation. At peripheral tissues, triglycerides are hydrolyzed by lipoprotein lipase with Apo CII acting as a cofactor. Released free fatty acids are then taken up for further metabolism or storage. Chylomicron remnants are taken up by the liver via the chylomicron remnant receptors.

Endogenous Pathway

The endogenous pathway begins in the liver with the synthesis of triglyceride-rich very-low-density lipoproteins (VLDLs). Microsomal triglyceride transfer protein facilitates the transfer of lipids onto Apo B100 and stabilizes the protein for secretion as VLDLs. VLDLs, as chylomicrons, undergo lipolysis by lipoprotein lipase, releasing free fatty acids, generating smaller particles called intermediate-density lipoproteins (IDLs, also known as VLDL remnants). IDLs are either removed by the liver or further processed into cholesterol-rich LDLs. LDLs are taken up into the liver or other cells via LDL receptors, a process regulated by cellular cholesterol requirement. Macrophages in the arterial wall can also take up LDLs via the scavenger receptors and become foam cells. Foamy macrophages play a key role in the development of atherosclerosis. Recent research has further suggested that the precursors of macrophages, monocytes, can also uptake lipoprotein particles in circulation and transform into foamy monocytes, which may also play a role in atherogenesis.

Reverse Cholesterol Transport

High-density lipoproteins (HDLs) are the major lipoproteins involved in the transport of cholesterol from peripheral tissues back to the liver. HDLs are synthesized by both the hepatocytes and the enterocytes in the form of small discoidal particles containing Apo AI and phospholipids. HDLs acquire additional lipids and apolipoproteins from triglyceride-depleted chylomicrons and VLDL remnants. HDLs remove free cholesterol from tissues with the help of Apo AI and esterify it with lecithin cholesterol acyltransferase. Cholesteryl esters are then transferred to Apo B 100-containing lipoproteins (VLDLs, IDLs, and LDLs) by cholesteryl ester transfer protein (CETP). HDLs can also be taken up directly by the liver class B type I scavenger receptors (SR-BI).

Plasma Lipids and Atherosclerosis

Multiple studies have shown that total cholesterol and LDL cholesterol levels contribute to cardiovascular disease risk and that lowering of total cholesterol and LDL cholesterol levels reduces the risk. Non-HDL cholesterol (i.e., total cholesterol – HDL cholesterol = VLDL + IDL + LDL cholesterol) reflects total atherogenic lipoprotein burden and may be a better risk indicator than LDL cholesterol, especially in people with combined hyperlipidemia, diabetes, metabolic syndrome, and chronic kidney disease. Table 1 shows the classification of lipid profile.

TABLE 1	Classification of LDL, Total, and HDL Cholesterol and Triglycerides (mg/dL)
LDL Cholesterol (mg/dL)	
<100	Optimal
100–129	Near optimal/above optimal
130–159	Borderline high
160–189	High
≥190	Very high
Total Cholesterol (mg/dL)	
<200	Desirable
200–239	Borderline high
≥240	High
HDL Cholesterol (mg/dL)	
<40	Low
≥60	High
Triglycerides (mg/dL)	
<150	Normal
150–199	Borderline high
200–499	High
≥500	Very high

Based on the NCEP/ATPIII.
HDL, high-density lipoprotein; *LDL,* low-density lipoprotein; *NCEP/ATP III,* National Cholesterol Education Program Adult Treatment Panel III guidelines.

Recent Mendelian randomization studies have suggested that triglyceride-rich lipoproteins (TRLs), including chylomicrons, VLDLs, and their remnants, also have a causal relationship with ASCVD. Therefore not only does hypertriglyceridemia represent an independent cardiovascular risk marker, it is also a significant risk factor and a target for therapy. Not surprisingly, the development of treatments targeting triglyceride pathways is an area of immense interest in the last few years. It is significant that Mendelian randomization studies suggest that HDL cholesterol does not have a causal relationship with ASCVD. Moreover, medications that increase HDL cholesterol (i.e., niacin and CETP inhibitors) have largely failed to show efficacy in ASCVD risk reduction in randomized clinical trials. Therefore, although HDL cholesterol was shown to be inversely associated with cardiovascular risk, the mechanism of the relationship between HDL cholesterol and ASCVD is not fully understood. Importantly, ASCVD cannot be viewed as a disease caused solely by a lipid disorder; rather, it is the result of a complex interplay between dyslipidemia, metabolic derangements, inflammation, and endothelial dysfunction. For instance, even mildly elevated triglycerides (>150 mg/dL) can suggest metabolic syndrome, an important risk factor for cardiovascular disease. Meanwhile, chronic systemic inflammation was shown to accelerate atherogenesis, and therapies that target inflammation have been demonstrated in clinical trials to reduce the risk for ASCVD.

Evaluation

Global Cardiovascular Risk Assessment

Risk assessment is an integral part in the evaluation of patients with hyperlipidemia. Contemporary guidelines from the United States provide detailed algorithms for risk stratification. The 2013 and 2018 cholesterol guidelines identified four subgroups of patients for whom the benefits of statin therapy outweigh the risk. Secondary prevention patients are automatically considered to be at high risk for recurrent ASCVD events and, thus, would necessitate initiation of lipid lowering therapy. In the 2018 Multisociety guideline, secondary prevention patients may be further stratified into those at very high risk, and those at not very high risk, for ASCVD, based on the presence or absence of high-risk features. The value of further delineating risk among secondary prevention patients was in part to facilitate the evidence-based use of newer nonstatin therapies (i.e., ezetimibe [Zetia][1] and PCSK9 inhibitors).

Among primary prevention patients, a history of diabetes mellitus, or significantly elevated LDL cholesterol (≥190 mg/dL or 4.9 mmol/L) signifying a likely genetic cause of hypercholesterolemia (i.e., familial hypercholesterolemia), automatically warrants initiation of lipid lowering therapy. In primary prevention patients with hyperlipidemia but without these two high-risk features, a global cardiovascular risk score can be used to further stratify a patient. Global risk scores estimate 10-year cardiovascular risk, which combines the effects of well-known risk factors, using one of several risk-calculation tools. Individual tools have been developed based on large epidemiology studies examining a limited number of available risk factors. Traditional risk factors such as age, sex, cigarette smoking, cholesterol, diabetes, and blood pressure are able to predict 80% to 90% of the cardiovascular events in people 40 years or older. However, these tools may not accurately estimate cardiovascular risk in individuals with unaccounted risk factors or those with demographics distinct from the populations used to derive the risk scores. The risk score most commonly used (and endorsed by guidelines) in the United States is the Pooled Cohort Equation (PCE). The PCE is used to estimate a 10-year risk for ASCVD for men and women aged 40 to 79 years, who are white or black race, incorporating age, sex, race, HDL and total cholesterol, diabetes, hypertension, and smoking status (http://tools.cardiosource.org/ASCVD-Risk-Estimator). The 2018 Multisociety guidelines recommend the initiation of statin therapy in patients with intermediate (≥7.5% to <20%) and high (≥20%) 10-year ASCVD risk, with consideration of statins even in select patients with borderline 10-year risk (5% to <7.5%). Of note, the risk stratification used by the European guideline is similar to that used by the American guideline. Although patients with a history of clinical ASCVD and those with high-risk comorbidities (i.e., diabetes mellitus, significant chronic kidney disease) are also classified as higher risk, the risk assessment score used is different. The Systematic COronary Risk Evaluation (SCORE), used in the ESC/EAS Guidelines for the Management of Dyslipidemias, incorporates similar risk factors and predicts fatal cardiovascular events (www.heartscore.org).

Finally, further risk assessment for subclinical coronary atherosclerosis via the measurement of coronary calcium by computer tomography (calcium score) has also been incorporated into the most current guidelines. With the rapid advancement of cardiovascular imaging technologies, further refinement of risk assessment that incorporates calcium score or other imaging modalities will likely play a significant role in future clinical practice.

Measurement of Lipid Profiles

Lipid profiles should be measured as a part of global risk assessment, and the frequency of checkup is determined by age, sex, and risk factors for cardiovascular disease. In patients on lipid lowering therapy, a lipid panel should be performed after the initiation or dose change in therapy; it should also be performed periodically in patients on stable therapy to assess treatment efficacy and medication adherence.

A fasting lipid profile (fasting for 9 to 12 hours) is recommended to ensure the most precise lipid assessment, specifically triglycerides (subsequently LDL cholesterol if calculated using the Friedewald equation). Nonfasting lipid profile provides an accurate measurement of other lipids, including total cholesterol, HDL cholesterol, Apo B, and Apo AI. Recent studies showed that differences in triglyceride levels according to fasting time were small. Therefore lipid values from nonfasting samples should not be ignored.

LDL cholesterol can either be calculated or measured directly. The standard method used to derive LDL cholesterol from other components of the lipid panel is the Friedewald equation (LDL cholesterol = total cholesterol – HDL cholesterol – triglycerides/5). This equation should be used with appropriate caution: fasting state samples should be used; it becomes less accurate if triglycerides >200 mg/dL; it becomes invalid with triglycerides >400 mg/dL; LDL cholesterol can be underestimated at levels <70 mg/dL.

Apolipoproteins, including Apo B and Apo AI, may also be measured. The Apo B level (Apo B100) reflects the number of atherogenic lipoprotein particles. Apo B level and Apo B/Apo AI ratio are as good as traditional lipid profiles and are especially useful in certain situations such as combined hyperlipidemia, metabolic syndrome, diabetes, and chronic kidney disease. In patients with history of premature ASCVD, recurrent ASCVD events despite optimal therapy, and those with a strong family history of premature ASCVD, a measurement of lipoprotein (a) [Lp(a)] may be considered.

Other medical conditions may also affect lipid profiles. Secondary causes include hypothyroidism, nephrotic syndrome, dysgammaglobulinemia, use of progestin (especially those with androgenic activity), cholestasis, use of protease inhibitors, chronic kidney disease, uncontrolled diabetes, obesity, excessive alcohol intake, use of thiazide or β-blockers, use of corticosteroids, use of oral estrogen (not transdermal), and pregnancy. These conditions should be detected and treated, if appropriate, to improve control of hyperlipidemia.

Family history of premature cardiovascular disease and hyperlipidemia and physical findings such as xanthomas, xanthelasmas, and premature arcus cornealis may suggest familial hypercholesterolemia. As the risk for ASCVD associated with very elevated levels of atherogenic lipoproteins begins to accumulate very early in life, patients with familial hypercholesterolemia should be treated aggressively.

Treatment
Overview

Treatment is primarily aimed at lowering LDL cholesterol level, which has been shown to decrease the risk of cardiovascular disease in numerous randomized clinical trials. In clinical scenarios where the triglyceride level is >500 mg/dL, triglycerides should be lowered immediately to prevent acute pancreatitis. Every reduction of LDL cholesterol of 1 mmol/L (~40 mg/dL) is associated with ~20% reduction in cardiovascular risk. The absolute risk reduction by lowering LDL cholesterol is proportional to the global cardiovascular risk.

It should be noted that the American guidelines have shifted away from hard LDL cholesterol targets. The treatment goals and approaches according to the 2018 cholesterol guidelines are summarized in Table 2. Briefly, high-risk patients are recommended to be started on a high-intensity statin with a goal LDL cholesterol reduction of ≥50%. In high-risk patients who cannot tolerate high-intensity statins and in intermediate risk patients, a moderate-intensity statin is recommended with a goal of LDL-C reduction of 30% to 49%. In secondary prevention patients who are determined to be at very high risk, additional validated nonstatin medications (ezetimibe and PCSK9 inhibitors) may be considered if LDL cholesterol remains ≥70 mg/dL on maximally tolerated therapy. At the time of the writing of this chapter, the Europeans, as reflected by the 2016 ESC/EAS guidelines, have maintained hard LDL cholesterol targets based on patient risk, as presented in Table 3.

As a first line, therapeutic lifestyle changes should be initiated when LDL cholesterol is above the target range. People with very high, high, or moderately high risk should also start making therapeutic lifestyle changes regardless of their LDL cholesterol level. Medications may be added at the same time as therapeutic lifestyle changes for these patients. If medications are indicated, statin is preferred because of proven efficacy that has been consistently shown in multiple clinical trials. The intensity of treatment is dictated by the patient's risk profile, ability to tolerate therapy as well as patient preference. Generally, response to treatment by a lipid panel and appropriate safety laboratory measures should

---

[1] Not FDA approved for this indication

TABLE 2 Risk Groups and Treatment Goals (2018 Multisociety Blood Cholesterol Guideline)

	RISK CATEGORY	RECOMMENDED STATIN THERAPY TO INITIATE	NONSTATIN THERAPY
Secondary Prevention	Very high risk*	High-intensity statin (Goal LDL cholesterol reduction of ≥50%).	If LDL cholesterol ≥70 mg/dL on maximally tolerated statin then adding ezetimibe or a PCSK9 inhibitor should be considered. Ezetimibe should be tried first, given cost effectiveness.
	Not very high risk	High-intensity statin (Goal LDL cholesterol reduction of ≥50%).	If LDL cholesterol ≥70 mg/dL on maximally tolerated statin then may consider adding ezetimibe.
Primary Prevention	LDL cholesterol ≥190 mg/dL	High-intensity statin (Goal LDL cholesterol reduction of ≥50%).	If LDL cholesterol reduction of ≥50% was not achieved or if an LDL cholesterol level remains above 100 mg/dL on maximally tolerated statin, may consider ezetimibe and then a PCSK9 inhibitor if needed.
	Diabetes mellitus	Moderate-intensity statin (Goal LDL cholesterol reduction of 30% to 49%). In patients with multiple other ASCVD risk factors, high-intensity statin may be considered.	Reasonable to add ezetimibe to maximally tolerated statin therapy to reduce LDL cholesterol by ≥50%.
	High risk (10 years ASCVD risk[†] ≥20%)	High-intensity statin	Reasonable to add ezetimibe to maximally tolerated statin therapy to reduce LDL cholesterol by ≥50%.
	Intermediate risk (10 year ASCVD risk ≥7.5% to <20%)	If risk enhancers[‡] present or if CAC score elevated, should initiate moderate intensity statin.	In patients with multiple additional ASCVD risk factors. Reasonable to add ezetimibe to maximally tolerated statin therapy to reduce LDL cholesterol by ≥50%.
	Borderline risk (10 year ASCVD risk 5% to <7.5%)	If risk enhancers present, then may consider moderate intensity statin.	
	Low risk (10 years ASCVD risk <5%)		

*Very high risk defined by a history of multiple major ASCVD events or at least 1 major ASCVD event plus multiple high-risk conditions (age ≥65 years, heterozygous familial hypercholesterolemia, history of coronary bypass surgery or percutaneous coronary intervention outside of the major ASCVD events, diabetes mellitus, hypertension, chronic kidney disease, current smoking, persistently elevated LDL cholesterol ≥100 mg/dL despite maximally tolerated statin and ezetimibe, or history of congestive heart failure).

[†]10 year ASCVD risk as estimated by the Pooled Cohort Equation.

[‡]Risk enhancers include family history of premature ASCVD, chronic kidney disease, metabolic syndrome, inflammatory disease, conditions specific to women (i.e., pre-eclampsia, premature menopause), ethnicity (i.e., South Asian ancestry), persistently elevated LDL cholesterol ≥160 mg/dL, persistently elevated triglycerides (≥175 mg/dL), high sensitivity C-reactive protein ≥2.0 mg/L, lipoprotein (a) >50 mg/dL or 125 nmol/L, apolipoprotein B ≥130 mg/dL, ankle-brachial index <0.9.

ASCVD, atherosclerotic cardiovascular disease; *CAC,* calcium; *LDL,* low density lipoprotein; *PCSK9,* proprotein convertase subtilisin/kexin type 9.

TABLE 3 LDL Cholesterol and Apo B Goals in the ESC/EAS Guideline*

	GOAL	
	LDL CHOLESTEROL (MG/DL)	APO B (MG/DL)
Very high risk: established cardiovascular disease, diabetes plus major cardiovascular risk factor(s), severe CKD (GFR <30 mL/min/1.73 m²), or 10 year fatal CVD risk ≥10%	70 or > 50% reduction if baseline 70–135	80
High risk: markedly uncontrolled risk factor(s), diabetes, moderate CKD (GFR 30–59 mL/min/1.73 m²), or 10 years fatal CVD risk 5%–10%	100 or >50% reduction if baseline 100–200	100

*10-year risk calculation using Systematic COronary Risk Evaluation (SCORE).

Apo B, apolipoprotein B; *CKD,* chronic kidney disease; *CVD,* cardiovascular disease; *GFR,* glomerular filtration rate; *LDL,* low density lipoprotein.

be assessed 4 to 12 weeks after treatment initiation or change. Once under control, lipid panels and clinical laboratory safety profiles can be monitored every 3 to 12 months.

Therapeutic Lifestyle Changes

All patients with hyperlipidemia should be counseled on lifestyle modifications. Dietary modification to limit intake of lipids is an essential component, given that the main source of lipids is exogenous dietary fat. Saturated fatty acids and trans-unsaturated fatty acids increase LDL cholesterol, whereas dietary fibers decrease LDL cholesterol. Carbohydrates do not affect LDL cholesterol but increase triglycerides and decrease HDL cholesterol, particularly if they have a high glycemic index. Intake of fructose, a component of sucrose, increases triglycerides and decreases HDL cholesterol. Body weight reduction, increasing physical activity,

and avoidance of a sedentary lifestyle have a small effect on LDL cholesterol, but they reduce triglycerides, increase HDL cholesterol, and are associated with improved cardiovascular outcome. Alcohol intake has an adverse effect on triglycerides and should be avoided.

Individual patients will need different approaches based on their cardiovascular risk and lipid profiles. Generally, total dietary fat is recommended to constitute 25% to 35% of the total calorie intake mainly as mono- or poly-unsaturated fat, limiting saturated fat <7% and trans fat <1% of the total calorie intake. Therapeutic lifestyle changes include diets with emphasis on vegetables, fruits, whole grains, low-fat dairy products, poultry, fish, legumes, nontropical vegetable oils, and nuts as well as limited intake of sweets, sugar-sweetened beverages, and red meats; further reduction of saturated fat (<5% to 6% of the total

TABLE 4 Major Drugs for Management of Hyperlipidemia

AGENT	STARTING DAILY DOSAGE	DOSAGE RANGE	MECHANISM	SIDE EFFECTS
Statins				
Lovastatin (Mevacor)	20 mg	10–80 mg	Decreased cholesterol synthesis, increased hepatic LDL receptors, decreased VLDL release	Myalgias, arthralgias, high liver enzymes, dyspepsia
Pravastatin (Pravachol)	40 mg	10–80 mg		
Simvastatin (Zocor)	20–40 mg	5–80 mg		
Fluvastatin (Lescol)	40 mg	20–80 mg		
Atorvastatin (Lipitor)	10–20 mg	10–80 mg		
Rosuvastatin (Crestor)	10 mg	5–40 mg		
Pitavastatin (Livalo)	2 mg	2–4 mg		
Cholesterol Absorption Inhibitors				
Ezetimibe (Zetia)	10 mg	10 mg	Deceased intestinal cholesterol absorption	High liver enzymes
Combination Therapies (single pill)				
Ezetimibe/Simvastatin (Vytorin)	10/20 mg	10/10–10/80 mg		
PCSK9 Inhibiting Monoclonal Antibodies (subcutaneous)				
Alirocumab (Praluent)	75 mg every 2 weeks	75–150 mg every 2 weeks	Increased hepatic LDL receptors	Injection site reactions, nasopharyngitis, upper respiratory tract infection, influenza, back pain
Evolocumab (Repatha)		140 mg every 2 weeks or 420 mg monthly		
Bile Acid Sequestrants				
Cholestyramine (Questran)	8–16 g	4–24 g	Increased bile acid excretion, increased LDL receptors	Bloating, constipation, elevated triglycerides
Colestipol (Colestid)	2 g	2–16 g		
Colesevelam (Welchol)	3.75 g	3.75 g		
Fibrates				
Fenofibrate (Tricor)	48–145 mg	48–145 mg	Increased LPL activity, decreased VLDL synthesis	Dyspepsia, myalgia, gallstones, high liver enzymes
Gemfibrozil (Lopid)	1200 mg	1200 mg		
Fenofibric acid (Trilipix)	45–135 mg	45–135 mg		
Niacin				
Immediate release	250 mg	250–3000 mg	Decreased VLDL synthesis	Flushing, high glucose, uric acid, high liver enzymes
Extended release (Niaspan)	500 mg	500–2000 mg		
Omega-3 Fatty Acid Prescriptions				
Icosapent ethyl (Vascepa)	4 g	4 g		Arthralgia, atrial fibrillation, lower extremity edema*
Omega-3 fatty acid ethyl esters (Lovaza)	4 g	4 g		Eructation, dyspepsia, and taste perversion

*The on-label side-effect profile of icosapent ethyl includes arthralgia. Increased rates of atrial fibrillation and lower extremity edema were reported in the REDUCE-IT trial. However, at the time of the writing of this chapter, the use of icosapent ethyl in patients meeting REDUCE-IT entry criteria would be considered off-label use.
LDL, low-density lipoprotein; LPL, lipoprotein lipase; TG, triglycerides; VLDL, very–low-density lipoprotein.

caloric intake) and trans fat; weight reduction; and increased regular physical activity. The amount of cholesterol intake is not well correlated with LDL cholesterol level and there is no recommended limit for intake. Management of other risk factors such as smoking cessation and controlling blood pressure in hypertensive patients and blood glucose in diabetics is also very important.

Pharmacologic Agents
The currently available lipid-lowering agents can be classified based on their mechanism of action. Statins (3-hydroxy-3-methylglutaryl coenzyme A [HMG-CoA] reductase inhibitors), ezetimibe (Zetia), PCSK9 (proprotein convertase subtilisin/kexin type 9) inhibitors, and bile acid sequestrants are used primarily to reduce LDL cholesterol. Fibrates, niacin, and omega-3 fatty acid prescriptions are used primarily for the treatment of hypertriglyceridemia. These classes of agents differ with regard to degree and type of lipid lowering, and agents within the same group may differ in efficacy and side effects. Conventional dosing regimens and common adverse effects are summarized in Table 4. Expected changes in lipid profiles are shown in Table 5. The choice of drug depends on the specific lipid abnormalities, patient's tolerability to the medication, and concurrent medical conditions. In general, statins are the most effective drugs to lower cardiovascular risk and are the treatment of choice when medications are indicated based on the global cardiovascular risk. If the treatment goal is not achieved

TABLE 5	Metabolic Effects of Each Lipid-Lowering Drug Class		
	LDL CHOLESTEROL	HDL CHOLESTEROL	TRIGLYCERIDES
Statins	↓ 21%–55%	↑ 2%–10%	↓ 6%–30%
Fibric acids	↓ 20%–25%	↑ 6%–18%	↓ 20%–35%
Niacin	↓ 10%–25%	↑ 10%–35%	↓ 20%–30%
Bile acid sequestrants	↓ 15%–25%		May ↑
Cholesterol absorption inhibitors	↓ 10%–18%		
PCSK9 inhibitors	↓ 39%–62%	↑ 4%–7%	↓ 12%–17%

Adapted from lipoprotein management in patients with cardiometabolic risk, consensus statement from the American College of Cardiology Foundation and the American Diabetes Association (ACC/ADA) (2008), and American Association of Clinical Endocrinologists' (AACE) guidelines for management of dyslipidemia and prevention of atherosclerosis (2012).

TABLE 6	Equipotency and Percentage Reduction in Total Cholesterol According to the Different Types and Doses of Statins				
REDUCTION IN TOTAL CHOLESTEROL (%)	PRAVASTATIN (PRAVACHOL), mg	FLUVASTATIN (LESCOL), mg	SIMVASTATIN (ZOCOR),* mg	ATORVASTATIN (LIPITOR), mg	ROSUVASTATIN (CRESTOR), mg
6–15	5	10	-	-	-
15–17	10	20	5	2.5	-
22	20	40	10	5	-
27	40†	80†	20†	10†	5†
32	80†		40†	20†	10†
37		-	(80)	40‡	20‡
42	-	-	-	80‡	40‡

*See the text for the FDA warning.
†Moderate-intensity statins (reduction of low-density lipoprotein (LDL) cholesterol 30%–50%).
‡High-intensity statins (reduction of LDL cholesterol >50%).
Modified from Penning-van Beest FJA, Termorshuizen F, Goettsch WG, et al. Adherence to evidence-based statin guidelines reduces the risk of hospitalizations for acute myocardial infarction by 40%: a cohort study. *Eur Heart J.* 2007;28:154–159.

by statins or statins are not tolerated, other validated nonstatin therapies (ezetimibe and PCSK9 inhibitors) may be considered, followed by other agents such as bile acid sequestrants. If the primary goal is to lower triglycerides, fibrates, omega-3 fatty acids, or niacin may be more effective.

Statins

Statins are usually the first drug of choice in patients with high cholesterol levels to reduce cardiovascular risk and have been validated in multiple randomized controlled trials and their meta-analyses. Furthermore, risk reduction was apparent in a wide range of patients in both primary and secondary prevention, in men, women, smokers, patients with diabetes, as well as those with hypertension. In general, statins result in a high degree of LDL cholesterol reduction. The approximate equipotent dosages of various statins and their cholesterol-lowering effects are listed in Table 6. The 2013 and 2018 cholesterol guideline recommends moderate- or high-intensity statins (see Table 6) based on the global risk. Statins inhibit HMG-CoA reductase, the rate-limiting enzyme in cholesterol biosynthesis. By blocking cholesterol biosynthesis, statins upregulate the LDL receptor on the hepatocytes and increase clearance of IDL and LDL. In addition to their direct effects on lipid metabolism, statins have been reported to have pleiotropic effects (e.g., reduced formation of reactive oxygen species, inhibition of platelet reactivity, and decreased vasoconstriction).

Statins are usually well tolerated. Potential common side effects include myopathy, fatigue, headaches, and nonspecific gastrointestinal symptoms such as dyspepsia. Elevation of liver enzymes occurs in less than 1%. There is also a small but significant association with increase in risk of developing diabetes. Myopathy is one of the most common causes for cessation of statins. Myalgia can occur in about 10% to 20% of patients, which is much more

often than reported in the clinical trials. The risk of rhabdomyolysis, however, is very low (0.1 to 0.2 per 1000 person-years). Risk for myopathy is increased in patients with advanced age, female sex, small body habitus, hypothyroidism, alcoholism, medical conditions (particularly liver or kidney disease), major surgery, excessive physical activity, history of myopathy, family history of myopathy, high-dose statins, and interacting medications or food such as grapefruit juice (>1 L/day). Simvastatin (Zocor), lovastatin (Mevacor), and atorvastatin (Lipitor) are primarily metabolized through CYP3A4, which is inhibited by protease inhibitors, cyclosporine (Neoral, Sandimmune), amiodarone (Cordarone, Pacerone), nondihydropyridine calcium channel blockers, fibrates, and other agents. Pravastatin (Pravachol) is metabolized by the kidney, not by the P450 system. Fluvastatin (Lescol) and rosuvastatin (Crestor) are primarily metabolized through CYP2C9. Pitavastatin (Livalo) is marginally metabolized by CYP2C9 and to a lesser extent by CYP2C8. Simvastatin and lovastatin should be avoided in patients receiving protease inhibitors. Statin dosage should be reduced in patients taking cyclosporine. Because of significant risk of myopathy and rhabdomyolysis related to high-dose simvastatin, the FDA recommends that 80 mg/day should not be used. The FDA further recommends that the dose be limited to 20 mg if the patient is also taking amiodarone, amlodipine (Norvasc), or ranolazine (Ranexa), and to 10 mg/day if taking diltiazem (Cardizem), dronedarone (Multaq), or verapamil (Calan). Addition of fibrates increases the risk of myopathy; in patients on a statin, fenofibrate (Tricor) is preferred, whereas gemfibrozil (Lopid), which has a much higher risk of rhabdomyolysis, is contraindicated. Symptoms of statin myopathy are heaviness, stiffness, cramping associated with weakness during exertion, and tendon-associated pain. Location of symptoms can be at the thighs, at the calves, or generalized. Symptoms can be very nonspecific, and differentiating statin-related myopathy from other causes is not easy. Therefore baseline symptoms, physical examination, and assessment of creatinine kinase level before the initiation of statins can be very helpful. Further decisions regarding stopping, dose reduction, or switching medications can be made based on the severity of symptoms, level of creatinine kinase elevation, and presence of rhabdomyolysis. In patients who develop myopathy while on simvastatin or atorvastatin, if the decision is to continue treatment with a statin, one option is to cautiously switch them to pravastatin, fluvastatin, or rosuvastatin, which are less prone to cause myopathy. Alternatively, lower statin dosing or less frequent dosing may be considered. For instance, rosuvastatin has a long duration of action and can be taken once every other day or weekly[1] if necessary. Theoretically, coenzyme Q10[7] may help manage statin-induced myopathy, but there is insufficient data to support its use. For patients who cannot tolerate statins, other agents should be used, starting with validated nonstatin agents.

Ezetimibe

Ezetimibe (Zetia) is the first in a new class of pharmaceutical agents that primarily targets the cholesterol transport protein Niemann-Pick C1-like 1 protein in the intestine. Ezetimibe is an efficacious and cost-effective add-on agent in people taking a statin, if the LDL cholesterol goal is not achieved or high doses of statin cannot be tolerated. Ezetimibe was shown to modestly decrease LDL cholesterol and cardiovascular events when added to simvastatin in high-risk patients in the Improved Reduction of Outcomes: Vytorin Efficacy International Trial (IMPROVE-IT) study. Moreover, ezetimibe has become a generic prescription in the United States and its safety profile is well characterized. Elevated liver enzymes have been reported but the risk of hepatotoxicity seems to be not different from that of placebo.

PCSK9 Inhibitors

The PCSK9 (proprotein convertase subtilisin/kexin type 9) protein plays a major role in regulating the number of LDL receptors at the cell surface, including on hepatocytes. Binding of the LDL receptor by PCSK9 leads to the destruction of the LDL receptor. Therefore interference with the binding capacity of PCSK9 to LDL receptor or silencing the expression of the PCSK9 gene allows more LDL receptors to recycle to the cell surface effecting the removal of more of the circulating plasma LDL. Over a decade ago, individuals with gain-of-function mutations of the PCSK9 gene were found to underlie a rare form of autosomal dominant hypercholesterolemia. Subsequently, individuals with loss-of-function mutations were found to have very low LDL cholesterol levels and were protected from coronary heart disease (CHD). These discoveries led to the development of monoclonal antibodies directed against PCSK9 as a novel cholesterol-lowering agent.

Two human monoclonal antibodies against PCSK9, alirocumab (Praluent) and evolocumab (Repatha), have been approved by the FDA. Both are given by subcutaneous injection. In the Further Cardiovascular Outcomes Research With PCSK9 Inhibition in Subjects With Elevated Risk (FOURIER) trial, evolocumab was found to significantly reduce the risk for ASCVD events in patients with clinical ASCVD and LDL-C ≥70 mg/dL or a non–HDL-C level ≥100 mg/dL, who were receiving optimized lipid-lowering using high-intensity statin or at least atorvastatin 20 mg with or without ezetimibe. Similarly, in the Evaluation of Cardiovascular Outcomes After an Acute Coronary Syndrome During Treatment With Alirocumab (ODYSSEY OUTCOMES) trial, alirocumab was shown to significantly reduce the risk for ASCVD events in patients with recent acute coronary syndrome, who had a LDL-C ≥70 mg/dL, a non–HDL-C ≥100 mg/dL, or an apolipoprotein B level ≥80 mg/dL and were receiving statin therapy at a high-intensity dose or at the maximum tolerated dose. Taking into account the results, inclusion criteria, and secondary analyses from these trials, the 2018 Multisociety guidelines recommended

the consideration of PCSK9 inhibitors in secondary prevention patients, especially those at very high risk, whose LDL cholesterol remains above 70 mg/dL or non-HDL cholesterol remains above 100 mg/dL on maximally tolerated statin therapy. Both alirocumab and evolocumab are also indicated for heterozygous familial hypercholesterolemia. Evolocumab is also indicated for homozygous familial hypercholesterolemia as an adjunct to other LDL-lowering therapies.

PCSK9 inhibitors are powerful LDL cholesterol lowering agents and enable reduction of LDL cholesterol by up to ~60% as a single agent or an adjunct therapy. Moreover, the absolute level of LDL cholesterol achieved may be as low as <25 mg/dL. There have been concerns regarding the potential adverse effects that may occur at such low LDL cholesterol levels, such as neurocognitive side effects. However, results from these trials and their sub-analyses have not shown a significant signal, although more long-term follow-up analysis is needed. Common side effects associated with PCSK9 inhibitors include injection site reactions, nasopharyngitis, upper respiratory tract infection, influenza, and back pain.

Currently, a significant hurdle to more widespread use of PCSK9 inhibitors is their high cost. Multiple cost-effective analyses have concluded that PCSK9 inhibitors are not yet cost effective. In 2018, the price of evolocumab was reduced by 60% by its manufacturer. Further studies will be needed to assess whether PCSK9 inhibitors are cost effective with this price reduction.

Bile Acid Sequestrants

Bile acid sequestrants have been in clinical use for many decades. These agents promote fecal excretion of bile acids. The liver responds with increased integration of cholesterol into bile acid synthesis to maintain a stable bile acid pool. The consequent decrease in cholesterol in the liver leads to upregulation of the LDL receptor and enhanced LDL clearance from the plasma. HMG-CoA synthase activity can increase, so combination therapy with statins would be synergistic, especially in patients with a suboptimal response. Available agents are cholestyramine (Questran), colestipol (Colestid), and colesevelam (Welchol). Most side effects involve the gastrointestinal tract, with constipation and bloating being the most common. These agents may interfere with the absorption of warfarin, phenobarbital, levothyroxine (Synthroid), and digoxin (Lanoxin), among other medications. Patients on multiple medications should be advised to take bile acid sequestrants 1 hour before or 4 hours after taking the other medications. These agents can also cause elevation of triglyceride level. As they are not systemically absorbed, the bile acid sequestrants may be the preferred agents when systemic absorption is to be avoided, such as during pregnancy or lactation.

Fibrates

The effect of fibrates on cardiovascular outcomes is not as favorable as with statins. However, fibrates can be useful in subsets of patients with high triglycerides and low-HDL cholesterol. Recently, the Action to Control Cardiovascular Risk in Diabetes (ACCORD) lipid trial showed that addition of fenofibrate to simvastatin in type 2 diabetic patients with cardiovascular risk factors did not improve cardiovascular outcomes, although there was a trend for better outcomes in a subgroup with triglycerides greater than 204 mg/dL and HDL cholesterol less than 34 mg/dL. Fibrates have multiple favorable metabolic effects including activation of peroxisome proliferator-activated receptor-α (contributing to the regulation of both lipid and carbohydrate metabolism), stimulation of lipoprotein lipase (increasing triglyceride hydrolysis), and downregulation of Apo CIII (improving lipoprotein remnant clearance as Apo CIII inhibits lipoprotein lipase). An enhanced VLDL-to-LDL conversion may lead to mild LDL cholesterol elevation in some patients. This effect may decrease over weeks, as the LDL receptors are upregulated. Fibrates are generally well tolerated. The most common side effect is dyspepsia. Other side effects include myopathy and hepatic enzyme elevation, particularly when fibrates are added to statins. The use of gemfibrozil (Lopid) should be avoided in patients on statin therapy due to increased

---

[1] Not FDA approved for this indication
[7] Available as a dietary supplement

risk for muscle-related adverse events. Fibrates increase the risk of gallstones, and patients on warfarin (Coumadin) may need dose adjustment. Monitoring of liver enzymes is recommended, at baseline and within 3 months and then periodically. Creatinine level can be increased through unclear mechanisms.

Niacin

Niacin or nicotinic acid effectively decreases the hepatic production of VLDL and thus, LDL cholesterol levels, and raises HDL cholesterol levels by reducing cholesterol transfer from HDL to Apo B-containing lipoproteins and HDL clearance by the liver. Niacin is also the most potent agent currently available to reduce the level of Lp(a); however, this effect on the reduction of cardiovascular events in patients with elevated Lp(a) is not known. Several trials showed the effect of niacin in preventing cardiovascular disease; however, the benefit of adding niacin to statins has not been proved. Niacin did not improve cardiovascular risk when added to simvastatin in patients with high risk for cardiovascular disease in the Atherothrombosis Intervention in Metabolic Syndrome with Low HDL/High Triglycerides: Impact on Global Health Outcomes (AIM-HIGH) study and the Heart Protection Study 2–Treatment of HDL to Reduce the Incidence of Vascular Events (HPS2-Thrive) study. There were excess adverse events and trends toward signs of harm among the niacin groups. The FDA has recently withdrawn the approval for the coadministration of niacin extended-release tablets (Niaspan) with statins. The most common side effect of niacin is flushing. This can be avoided or minimized by initiating therapy with a low dose of niacin, taking an aspirin 1 hour before niacin, avoiding hot foods or beverages at the time the niacin is taken, or switching to extended-release forms (Niaspan). Hepatotoxicity can occur at any time. Immediate-release forms are less likely to cause hepatotoxicity than sustained-release forms (Slo-Niacin). Extended-release forms can minimally elevate transaminases but significant hepatotoxicity is rare. They can, however, also cause dose-dependent reversible thrombocytopenia, which can be insidious and severe. When switching to different forms, it is recommended that one should start with low doses and titrate up to achieve desired response. Liver function tests should be monitored regularly, at baseline and every 3 months for the first year and then periodically. Other side effects include pruritus, increased uric acid levels, and hyperglycemia.

Omega-3 Fatty Acid Prescriptions

Highly purified omega-3 fatty acid preparations containing either a mixture of eicosapentaenoic acid (EPA) and docosahexaenoic acid (DHA) (Lovaza) or EPA alone (Vascepa) are effective agents used in the treatment of hypertriglyceridemia, the first FDA approved indication for these agents. Omega-3 fatty acids are polyunsaturated fatty acids (PUFA) and are essential in humans. A significant proportion of omega fatty acids is consumed in the diet. Major dietary sources of omega-3 fatty acids include nuts, vegetable oils, flax seeds, and leafy vegetables as well as fish and fish oil. EPA and DHA are the two major types of marine-derived omega-3 fatty acids. The mechanism by which omega-3 fatty acids lower triglycerides is incompletely understood.

Multiple clinical trials have been examining the efficacy of omega-3 fatty acid in improving cardiovascular outcome. Although trials using lower doses of EPA-DHA mixtures (≤1 g total daily) have shown inconsistent results, findings from recent trials assessing higher doses of pure EPA have been more favorable.

Purified EPA was first shown in the Japan Eicosapentaenoic acid (EPA) Lipid Intervention Study (JELIS) trial to significantly reduce risk for major coronary events in patients with hypercholesterolemia. Subsequently, the Reduction of Cardiovascular Events With Icosapent Ethyl–Intervention Trial (REDUCE-IT) study, a large, randomized controlled trial, assessed the efficacy and safety of purified EPA ethyl ester, icosapent ethyl (Vascepa) in secondary prevention and high-risk primary prevention patients with reasonably controlled LDL cholesterol but elevated triglycerides. The REDUCE-IT trial showed that treatment with icosapent ethyl was associated with a significant reduction in ASCVD events. In secondary analyses, icosapent ethyl has also been shown to reduce the risk for total ischemic events (first plus subsequent events). Results from REDUCE-IT suggest that in addition to LDL cholesterol lowering, high-risk patients with elevated triglycerides will likely benefit from icosapent ethyl. It is unknown whether higher doses of EPA-DHA mixtures may have similar efficacy as purified EPA; however, the relevant trial is underway. Lastly, the overall rates of adverse events were not significantly different between the treatment and control arms of REDUCE-IT. However, there were increased rates of atrial fibrillation and peripheral edema associated with patients taking icosapent ethyl observed in the trial.

References

ESC/EAS Guidelines for the management of dyslipidaemias, *Eur Heart J* 37:2999–3058, 2016.

Bhatt DL, Steg PG, Miller M, et al: Cardiovascular risk reduction with icosapent ethyl for hypertriglyceridemia, *N Engl J Med* 380(1):11–22, 2019.

Bhatt DL, Steg PG, Miller M, et al: Effects of icosapent ethyl on total ischemic events: from REDUCE-IT, *J Am Coll Cardiol*, 2019.

Brunzell JD, Davidson M, Furberg CD: Lipoprotein management in patients with cardiometabolic risk: consensus conference report from the ADA and the ACC foundation, *J Am Coll Cardiol* 51:1512–1524, 2008.

Carroll MD, Kit BK, Lacher DA, et al: Trends in lipids and lipoproteins in U.S. adults, 1988–2010, *JAMA* 308:1545–1554, 2012.

Dullaart RP: PCSK9 Inhibition to reduce cardiovascular events, *N Engl J Med* 376:1713–1722, 2017.

Eckel RH, Jakicic JM, Ard JD, et al: 2013 ACC/AHA guideline on lifestyle management to reduce cardiovascular risk: a report of the American College of Cardiology/American Heart Association task force on practice guidelines, *J Am Coll Cardiol* 63:2960–2984, 2014.

Everett BM, Smith RJ, Hiatt WR: Reducing LDL with PCSK9 inhibitors — the clinical benefit of lipid drugs, *N Eng J Med* 373:1588–1591, 2015.

Ginsberg HN, Elam MB, Lovato LC, et al: Effects of combination lipid therapy in type 2 diabetes mellitus, *N Engl J Med* 362:1563–1574, 2010.

Greenland P, Alpert JS, Beller GA, et al: 2010 ACCF/AHA guideline for assessment of cardiovascular risk in asymptomatic adults: a report of the American College of Cardiology Foundation/American Heart Association Task Force on Practice Guidelines developed in collaboration with the American Society of Echocardiography, American Society of Nuclear Cardiology, Society of Atherosclerosis Imaging and Prevention, Society for Cardiovascular Angiography and Interventions, Society of Cardiovascular Computed Tomography, and Society for Cardiovascular Magnetic Resonance, *J Am Coll Cardiol* 56:e50–e103, 2010.

Grundy SM, Cleeman JI, Merz CNB, et al: Implications of recent clinical trials for the national cholesterol education program adult treatment panel III guidelines, *Circulation* 110:227–239, 2004.

Grundy SM, Stone NJ, Bailey AL, et al: AHA/ACC/AACVPR/AAPA/ABC/ACPM/ADA/AGS/APhA/ASPC/NLA/PCNA Guideline on the Management of Blood Cholesterol: Executive Summary: a report of the American College of Cardiology/American Heart Association Task Force on Clinical Practice Guidelines, *J Am Coll Cardiol* (18):39033–39038, 2018. pii: S0735-1097.

Hlatky MA, Kazi DS: PCSK9 inhibitors: economics and policy, *J Am Coll Cardiol* 70(21):2677–2687, 2017.

Huffman MD, Capewell S, Ning H, et al: Cardiovascular health behavior and health factor changes (1988–2008) and projections to 2020: results from the National Health and Nutrition Examination Surveys (NHANES), *Circulation* 125:2595–2602, 2012.

IMPROVE-IT Investigators: Ezetimibe added to statin therapy after acute coronary syndromes, *N Eng J Med* 372:2387–2397, 2015.

Jellinger PS, Smith DA, Mehta AE, et al: American Association of Clinical Endocrinologists' guidelines for management of hyperlipidemia and prevention of atherosclerosis, *EndocrPract* 18:1–78, 2012.

Joy TR, Hegele RA: Narrative review: statin-related myopathy, *Ann Intern Med* 150:858–868, 2009.

Kazi DS, Moran AE, Coxson PG, et al: Cost-effectiveness of PCSK9 inhibitor therapy in patients with heterozygous familial hypercholesterolemia or atherosclerotic cardiovascular disease, *JAMA* 316(7):743–753, 2016.

Keaney JF, Curfman GD, Jarcho JA: A pragmatic view of the new cholesterol treatment guidelines, *N Engl J Med* 370:275–278, 2014.

Lloyd-Jones DM, Morris PB, Ballantyne CM, et al: 2017 Focused update of the 2016 ACC expert consensus decision pathway on the role of non-statin therapies for LDL-cholesterol lowering in the management of atherosclerotic cardiovascular disease risk: a report of the American Colelge of Cardiology Task Force Expert Consensus Decision Pathways, *J Am Coll Cardiol* 70:1785–1822, 2017.

Musunuru K, Kathiresan S: Surprises from genetic analyses of lipid risk factors for atherosclerosis, *Circ Res* 118(4):579–585, 2016.

O'Connell C, Horwood K, Nadamuni M: Correction of refractory thrombocytopenia and anemia following withdrawal of extended release niacin, *Am J Hematol* 91(7):E318, 2016.

Otvos JD, Collins D, Freedman DS, et al: Low-density lipoprotein and high-density lipoprotein particle subclasses predict coronary events and are favorably changed by gemfibrozil therapy in the Veterans Affairs High-Density Lipoprotein Intervention Trial, *Circulation* 113:1556–1563, 2006.

Penning-van Beest FJA, Termorshuizen F, Goettsch WG, et al: Adherence to evidence-based statin guidelines reduces the risk of hospitalizations for acute myocardial infarction by 40%: a cohort study, *Eur Heart J* 28:154–159, 2007.

Phan BAP, Dayspring TD, Toth PP: Ezetimibe therapy: mechanism of action and clinical update, *Vasc Health Risk Manag* 8:415–427, 2012.

Reiner Z, Catapano AL, De Backer G, et al: ESC/EAS guidelines for the management of dyslipidaemias: the task force for the management of dyslipidaemias of the European Society of Cardiology (ESC) and the European Atherosclerosis Society (EAS), *Eur Heart J* 32:1769–1818, 2011.

Ridker PM, Cook NR: Statins: new American guidelines for prevention of cardiovascular disease, *Lancet* 382:1762–1765, 2013.

Robinson JG, Farnier M, Krempf M, et al: Efficacy and safety of alirocumab in reducing lipids and cardiovascular events, *N Eng J Med* 372:1489–1499, 2015.

Robinson JG, Rosenson RS, Farnier M, et al: Safety of very low low-density lipoprotein cholesterol levels with alirocumab, *Journal Amn Coll Cardiol* 69(5):471–482, 2017.

Sabatine MS, Giugliano RP, Keech AC, et al: Evolocumab and clinical outcomes in patients with cardiovascular disease, *N Engl J Med* 376(18):1713–1722, 2017.

Sabatine MS, Giugliano RP, Wiviott SD, et al: Efficacy and safety of evolocumab in reducing lipids and cardiovascular events, *N Engl J Med* 372:1500–1509, 2015.

Schwartz GG, Steg PG, Szarek M, et al: Alirocumab and cardiovascular outcomes after acute coronary syndrome, *N Engl J Med* 379(22):2097–2107, 2018.

Stone NJ, Robinson J, Lichtenstein AH, et al: ACC/AHA guideline on the treatment of blood cholesterol to reduce atherosclerotic cardiovascular risk in adults: a report of the American College of Cardiology/American Heart Association task force on practice guidelines, *J Am Coll Cardiol* 63:2889–2934, 2014.

Tall AR, Rader DJ: Trials and tribulations of CETP inhibitors, *Circ Res* 122(1):106–112, 2018.

The HPS2-THRIVE Collaborative Group: Effects of extended-release niacin with laropiprant in high-risk patients, *N Eng J Med* 371:203–212, 2014.

The AIM-HIGH Investigators: Niacin in patients with low HDL cholesterol levels receiving intensive statin therapy, *N Engl J Med* 365:2255–2267, 2011.

Third report of the National Cholesterol Education Program (NCEP) expert panel on detection, evaluation, and treatment of high blood cholesterol in adults (Adult treatment panel III) final report, *Circulation* 106:3143–3421, 2002.

Tsimikas S: A test in context: lipoprotein(a): diagnosis, prognosis, controversies, and emerging therapies, *J Am Coll Cardiol* 69(6):692–711, 2017.

Wu H, Ballantyne CM: Dyslipidaemia: PCSK9 inhibitors and foamy monocytes in familial hypercholesterolaemia, *Nat Rev Cardiol* 14(7):385–386, 2017.

Xu L, Perrard XD, Perrard JL, et al: Foamy monocytes form early and contribute to nascent atherosclerosis in mice with hypercholesterolemia, *Arterioscler Thromb Vasc Biol* 35:1787–1797, 2015.

Yokoyama M, Origasa H, Matsuzaki M, et al: Effects of eicosapentaenoic acid on major coronary events in hypercholesterolaemic patients (JELIS): a randomised open-label, blinded endpoint analysis, *Lancet* 369(9567):1090–1098, 2007.

HYPERPARATHYROIDISM AND HYPOPARATHYROIDISM

Method of
Claudio Marcocci, MD

CURRENT DIAGNOSIS

Primary Hyperparathyroidism

- Third most common endocrine disorder and most common cause of hypercalcemia in the general population.
- Diagnosis based on confirmed hypercalcemia (total calcium [albumin corrected] or ionized calcium) associated with elevated or inappropriately normal serum parathyroid hormone level.
- Hypercalcemia on routine blood testing or in postmenopausal women investigated for osteoporosis is typically the first clue to the diagnosis.
- Mainly occurs as a solitary disease (90%) but may be part of hereditary syndromes.
- Genetic causes should be searched for in young patients.

Secondary Hyperparathyroidism

- Secondary hyperparathyroidism defines any condition in which the increased PTH secretion occurs as a normal physiologic response, often mediated by a decrease of serum calcium.
- Vitamin D deficiency, as a result of inadequate nutritional intake/sun exposure, malabsorption, liver diseases, or chronic renal failure, is the most common cause.
- At variance with primary hyperparathyroidism, secondary hyperparathyroidism is characterized by low or, more often, low-normal serum calcium and decreased urinary calcium excretion.

Hypoparathyroidism

- Rare disorder.
- Inadvertent removal or damage to the parathyroid gland during thyroid surgery and, much less frequently, autoimmune destruction are the most common causes.
- Diagnosis based on low serum calcium along with undetectable or inappropriately low serum parathyroid hormone level.

CURRENT THERAPY

Primary Hyperparathyroidism

- Parathyroidectomy is the only definitive therapy.
- Surgery should be considered in all cases and recommended in symptomatic patients and in those who, albeit asymptomatic, meet the surgical criteria.
- Surveillance without surgery can be considered in asymptomatic patients who do not meet the surgical criteria.
- Patients followed without surgery should be replete with vitamin D and calcium intake should not be restricted.
- Medical treatment can be considered in selected cases: antiresorptive therapy to increase bone mineral density and cinacalcet (Sensipar) to lower serum calcium.

Hypoparathyroidism

- Severe hypocalcemia is a medical emergency and treatment with intravenous calcium should be promptly instituted and maintained for 24 to 48 hours; oral therapy with calcium and active vitamin D metabolites should be started as soon as practical.
- The goal of chronic treatment is to maintain serum calcium in the low-normal range, avoiding hypocalcemic symptoms and long-term complications.
- Chronic conventional therapy is based on adequate calcium intake (calcium supplement needed in most cases) and active vitamin D metabolites.
- Recombinant full-length parathyroid hormone 1-84 (Natpara) has been approved by the U.S. Food and Drug Administration for patients not controlled with conventional therapy.
- An individualized approach is necessary to optimize patient care. Lifelong monitoring is needed to decrease the risk of complications.

Primary Hyperparathyroidism

Epidemiology

Primary hyperparathyroidism (PHPT) is currently the third most common endocrine disorder and the most frequent cause of hypercalcemia in the general population.

The disease was considered rare until the early 1970s, when its incidence in the United States rose dramatically following the introduction of serum calcium in the multichannel autoanalyzer. The incidence varies according to geographic areas and assessment measures; recent data in the United States indicate an incidence of 79.6 per 100,000 person-years in women and 35.6 per 100,000 person-years in men of all races, with the highest rate among blacks. The incidence peaks in the sixth decade of life. The prevalence ranges between 1 and 7 cases per 1000 adults. Most cases occur in women (with a female-to-male ratio of 3:1), but there is no sex difference before the age of 45 years. PHPT is rare in children and adolescents.

Pathogenesis

PHPT mainly occurs as a solitary disease (90%) but may be part of hereditary syndromes (e.g., multiple endocrine neoplasia [MEN] types 1, 2A, and 4; hyperparathyroidism–jaw tumor syndrome [HPT-JT], and familial isolated hyperparathyroidism [FIPH]) (Table 1). A single, benign adenoma is found in 80% to 85% of cases, multigland involvement in 15% to 20%, and parathyroid

TABLE 1	Hereditary Forms of PHPT and Related Involved Gene	
DISORDER	**GENE**	**PATTERN OF INHERITANCE**
Multiple endocrine neoplasia type 1	MEN1	Autosomal dominant
Multiple endocrine neoplasia type 2A	RET	Autosomal dominant
Multiple endocrine neoplasia type 4	CDKN1B	Autosomal dominant
Hyperparathyroidism–jaw tumor syndrome	CDC73	Autosomal dominant
Familial isolated hyperparathyroidism	MEN1, CDC73, CASR, CDKN1B	Autosomal dominant
Familial hypocalciuric hypercalcemia type 1	CASR	Autosomal dominant
Familial hypocalciuric hypercalcemia type 2	GNA11	Autosomal dominant
Familial hypocalciuric hypercalcemia type 3	AP2S1	Autosomal dominant
Neonatal severe hyperparathyroidism	CASR	Autosomal recessive

Abbreviations: AP2S1 = Adaptor-related protein complex 2 sigma 1 subunit CASR = calcium-sensing receptor; CDC73 = cell division cycle 73; CDKN1B = cyclin-dependent kinase inhibitor 1B; GNA11 = G protein subunit alpha 11; MEN1 = multiple endocrine neoplasia type 1; PHPT = primary hyperparathyroidism; RET = rearranged during transfection.

carcinoma in less than 1%. Multigland involvement is more common in hereditary cases, particularly MEN1. In the absence of local infiltration or metastases, the diagnosis of parathyroid carcinoma may be difficult at histology. Genetic studies (DCD73 gene mutations) and immunohistochemical studies (loss of parafibromin [the protein encoded by the CDC73 gene] expression) may help in equivocal cases. Predisposing factors are external neck irradiation in childhood and long-term lithium therapy.

PHPT is characterized by excessive parathyroid hormone (PTH) secretion from one or more parathyroid glands, due to the loss of the homeostatic control of PTH synthesis and secretion. Extracellular ionized calcium (Ca^{2+}_o) is the main regulator of PTH secretion. Ca^{2+}_o interacts with the Ca^{2+}-sensing receptor (CaSR) present on the surface of parathyroid cells; there is an inverse sigmoidal relationship between Ca^{2+}_o concentration and PTH release. In adenomas hypercalcemia is due to the loss of normal sensitivity of the parathyroid cell to the inhibitory action of Ca^{2+}_o, whereas in parathyroid hyperplasia the increased number of parathyroid cells, which have a normal sensitivity to the inhibitory action of Ca^{2+}_o, causes hypercalcemia. Serum phosphate, 1,25-dihydroxyvitamin D (1,25(OH)$_2$D), and fibroblast growth factor 23 (FGF23) are also involved in the control of PTH secretion.

Although major progress has been made in the last two decades, the molecular basis of PHPT is still unclear in the majority of cases. The clonality of most parathyroid tumors suggests a defect in the pathways that control parathyroid cell proliferation or the expression of PTH. The genes involved are listed in Table 1. Germline mutations are often found in hereditary forms. On the other hand, somatic mutations may occur in sporadic cases, even though germline mutations have also been described in apparently sporadic cases.

Clinical Presentation
In recent years the clinical presentation of PHPT in Western countries has changed from a symptomatic disease, characterized by hypercalcemia and renal (nephrolithiasis and nephrocalcinosis)

and skeletal (osteitis fibrosa cystica, fragility fractures) manifestations, to one with subtle and nonspecific clinical manifestations (asymptomatic PHPT). Nephrolithiasis remains the most common classic clinical manifestation (15%–20%), and silent stones are frequently detected at ultrasound. Bone mineral density (BMD) is reduced particularly at sites rich in cortical bone (one-third distal radius). Studies using peripheral high-resolution quantitative computed tomography (CT) has shown involvement of both cortical and trabecular sites, the latter confirmed by the trabecular bone score (TBS) at the lumbar spine. An increased rate of vertebral and nonvertebral fractures has also been documented. Nonclassical manifestations, including subtle cardiovascular abnormalities and psychological and cognitive symptoms, have also been reported.

A new variant of PHPT (normocalcemic PHPT) has recently been identified, namely patients with increased serum PTH levels in the absence of hypercalcemia (also by measurement of ionized calcium) or other causes of secondary hyperparathyroidism. This condition, called normocalcemic PHPT, has been typically recognized in persons evaluated for low BMD, in whom PTH was measured even in the absence of hypercalcemia. In some cases this new phenotype may represent an early phase of classical hypercalcemic PHPT, when PTH elevation precedes the occurrence of hypercalcemia.

Evaluation and Diagnosis
The finding of hypercalcemia on routine blood testing or in postmenopausal women investigated for osteoporosis is typically the first clue to the diagnosis of PHPT. Hypercalcemia should be confirmed in repeated testing, preferably evaluating albumin-corrected total calcium (measured total calcium in mg/dL + [0.8 × (4.0 − serum albumin in g/dL)]) or ionized calcium. The next diagnostic step is the measurement of serum PTH. An elevated (or unexpectedly normal) serum PTH in the face of hypercalcemia is virtually diagnostic of PHPT. Serum phosphate is normal or in the low-normal range in mild PHPT and low in severe cases. A low or undetectable PTH level in a hypercalcemic patient rules out the diagnosis of PHPT. The most common cause of PTH-independent hypercalcemia is malignancy, where hypercalcemia is due to the secretion by the tumor of PTH-related peptide, a molecule that shares with PTH the amino-terminal active part but does not cross-react in the PTH assay, or osteolytic lytic bone metastases. Urinary calcium should also be measured. If hypercalciuria is greater than 400 mg per day, a more extended evaluation of the stone risk profile should be performed. Urinary calcium measurement is also useful to exclude familial hypocalciuric hypercalcemia (FHH), which is suggested by the finding of the calcium-to-creatinine clearance ratio of less than 0.01.

A hereditary form of PHPT, accounting for 5% to 10% of cases, should be sought in patients younger than 30 years at diagnosis, with a family history of hypercalcemia and/or neuroendocrine tumors (see Table 1). In this setting serum calcium should be measured in first-degree relatives and genetic tests performed. Parathyroid cancer should be suspected in individuals, especially males, with marked hypercalcemia, a palpable neck mass, and serum PTH concentration 3 to 10 times the upper normal value.

Renal ultrasound should be performed in all patients, even in those with no history of nephrolithiasis, since recent studies have shown that silent kidney stones are common in patients with asymptomatic PHPT. Routine BMD testing by dual-energy x-ray absorptiometry (DXA) at the lumbar spine, hip, and distal forearm is also an essential component of the evaluation. BMD is typically low at the one-third distal radius, a site of enriched cortical bone, but a few patients may show predominant cancellous bone involvement, as documented by vertebral osteopenia or osteoporosis. The involvement of the trabecular compartment is also confirmed by the TBS at the lumbar spine. Vertebral imaging by x-ray or DXA (vertebral fracture assessment, VFA) should also be routinely performed to detect silent vertebral deformities since vertebral fracture risk is increased in asymptomatic patients.

Neck imaging (ultrasound and sestamibi scanning) has no value in the diagnosis of PHPT, but it is a useful tool for localizing the abnormal parathyroid gland in patients selected for parathyroidectomy (PTx). Sestamibi has the advantage of localizing the ectopic parathyroid gland outside the neck. The 4D computerized tomography protocol has emerged as a useful tool.

Treatment

The aim of treatment is to remove all hyperfunctioning parathyroid tissue, resolve biochemical abnormalities, improve BMD, and decrease the risk of nephrolithiasis and fractures.

Surgical Treatment

Parathyroid surgery represents the only definitive cure of PHPT. Successful PTx normalizes serum calcium and PTH, improves BMD, and decreases the risk of nephrolithiasis and fragility fractures. Patients selected for surgery should be referred to an experienced parathyroid surgeon. A focused, minimally invasive approach, guided by imaging studies associated with intraoperative monitoring of serum PTH, is the preferred surgical procedure in sporadic PHPT. In experienced hands the rate of surgical cure reaches 95% to 98% with a negligible rate of surgical complications. In hereditary cases the surgical approach (bilateral neck exploration by classical cervicotomy) may differ, since multigland involvement is common. An *en bloc* resection of the parathyroid lesion together with the ipsilateral thyroid lobe with clear gross margins and the adjacent structures is recommended when parathyroid carcinoma is suspected. Particular attention should be paid to avoid seeding of neoplastic parathyroid cells. Surgery should be considered for any patient with a confirmed diagnosis of PHPT and recommended in those with symptomatic disease.

Patients with mild hypercalcemia (serum calcium < 12 mg/dL [3 mmol/L]) can proceed directly to surgery. When serum calcium is higher, preoperative treatment with saline infusion eventually followed by loop diuretics, intravenous bisphosphonates, denosumab (Prolia, Xgeva)[1], or cinacalcet (Sensipar) may be considered to reduce serum calcium levels and decrease the risk of complications, particularly cardiac arrhythmias, which are associated with more severe hypercalcemia.

Surgery is also a reasonable option for patients with asymptomatic PHPT. International guidelines provide guidance to select patients who should be referred for surgery or followed without surgery. The most recent revised (2013) guidelines for surgery or monitoring are reported in Table 2. These guidelines are largely consistent with the previous ones and recommend PTx for all patients with symptomatic PHPT and asymptomatic patients who meet one or more of the indicated criteria. The new indications for surgery in asymptomatic patients include (1) the presence of silent vertebral fractures detected by x-ray, CT, magnetic resonance imaging (MRI), or vertebral fracture assessment (VFA) by DXA; and (2) a 24-hour urinary calcium excretion greater than 400 mg/dL, increased stone risk (evaluated by urinary stone risk profile), and subclinical kidney stone or nephrocalcinosis detected by x-ray, ultrasound, and CT. According to the guidelines, about 60% of patients with asymptomatic PHPT meet the criteria for surgery. As mentioned before, patients with mild PHPT may have subtle cardiovascular abnormalities and complain of psychological and cognitive symptoms. It is unclear whether and to what extent these abnormalities are reversible after successful PTx; for the time being they are not considered indications for surgery. Nonetheless, surgery could be considered in a middle-aged patient in whom asymptomatic PHPT is associated with increased cardiovascular risk (metabolic syndrome, hypertension, ischemic heart disease) if the surgical risk is low.

Randomized clinical trials have also shown that patients with sporadic asymptomatic PHPT who do not meet the surgical criteria may benefit from surgery, not only because it normalizes serum calcium and PTH, but also because it improves BMD and quality of life (QoL). On the other hand, surgery could be

TABLE 2   Guidelines for Surgery for Patients With Asymptomatic PHPT and Monitoring for Those Followed Without Surgery

PARAMETER	GUIDELINES FOR SURGERY	GUIDELINES FOR MONITORING
Serum calcium	> 1 mg/dL (0.25 mmol/L) above the upper normal limit	Annually
Skeletal	• BMD by DXA: T-score < –2.5 at lumbar spine, femoral neck, total hip, or distal one-third radius • Vertebral fractures by x-ray, CT, MRI, or VFA	• BMD by DXA every 1–2 years at lumbar spine, total hip, or distal one-third radius • Spine x-ray of VFA when clinically indicated (e.g., back pain or height loss)

Renal	• Creatinine clearance < 60 mL/min
	• Daily urinary calcium excretion > 400 mg and increased stone risk by the urinary biochemical stone risk profile
	• Nephrolithiasis or nephrocalcinosis by x-ray, ultrasound, or CT
		• Serum creatinine annually
		• If renal stone suspected:
		  • 24-h urinary biochemical stone risk profile
		  • Renal imaging by x-ray, ultrasound, or CT

Age	< 50 years	-

Abbreviations: BMD = bone mineral density; CT = computed tomography; DXA = dual x-ray absorptiometry; MRI = magnetic resonance imaging; PHPT = primary hyperparathyroidism; VFA = vertebral fracture assessment.
Modified from Bilezikian et al. Guidelines for the management of asymptomatic primary hyperparathyroidism: Summary statement from the fourth international workshop. *J Clin Endocrinol Metab* 99:3561, 2014.

postponed in hereditary cases with mild hypercalcemia, because multigland disease, occasionally with asynchronous involvement of the various parathyroid glands, is not uncommon and carries an increased risk of surgical complications and recurrence/persistence of PHPT.

Therefore individual counseling addressing the benefits and risks of PTx is mandatory, and the preference of the patients should be taken into account. It is well known that parathyroid surgery, when performed by skilled neck surgeons, is safe, cost-effective, and associated with low perioperative morbidity. On the other hand, it is important to recognize that PTx, particularly if performed by inexperienced surgeons, may be associated with complications that could be invalidating and not acceptable for a patient with mild disease and a good QoL. In this regard, the choice of surgery may be reconsidered in a patient with asymptomatic PHPT in whom parathyroid surgery was initially advised or selected by the patient when preoperative imaging studies are negative. Indeed, in this setting the patient may feel uncomfortable undergoing a blind neck exploration, a surgical procedure more extensive than the minimally invasive approach and carrying the greatest risk of complications.

Nonsurgical Management

As mentioned before, many patients with PHPT do not meet the criteria for surgery. These patients, as well as those who decline surgery or have contraindications to surgery, need to be monitored.

Monitoring. Randomized clinical studies have shown stability over a short period of observation (up to 2 years) in patients with asymptomatic PHPT followed without surgery and benefits in those who underwent PTx even if they did not meet the criteria for surgery. The extension up to 5 years of one of these randomized studies has shown a more frequent occurrence of a vertebral fracture in patients belonging to the observation group than in

---

[1]Not FDA approved for this indication.

TABLE 3	Classification of Hypoparathyroidism*

Congenital

- Isolated
  - Defective PTH biosynthesis (*PTH*) ^
  - Abnormal development of parathyroid glands (*GCMB, GCM2, GATA3*)
  - Autosomal dominant hypocalcemia
    - Type 1 (*CASR*)
    - Type 2 (*GNA11*)
- Associated with additional features or organ defects
  - Autoimmune
    - Isolated
    - Polyglandular syndrome type 1 (*AIRE*)
  - Di George syndrome (*TBX1*)
  - Sanjad-Sakati/Kenny-Caffey type 2 (*TBCE*)
  - Kenny-Caffey type 2 (*FAM111A*)
  - Mitochondrial DNA mutations
- Defective action of PTH
  - Pseudohypoparathyroidism
    - Type 1a (*GNAS*)
    - Type 1b (*STX16, GNAS*; in sporadic form paternal UPD)
    - Type 1c (*GNAS*)
    - Type 2 (not yet identified)

Acquired

- Destruction or removal of the parathyroid glands
  - Postoperative (neck surgery)
  - Radiation induced
  - Infiltration of the parathyroid glands (metastatic, granulomatous)
  - Deposition of heavy metals (iron, copper)
- Reversible impairment or PTH secretion or action
  - Severe magnesium deficiency
  - Hypermagnesemia (e.g., due to tocolytic therapy)
- CaSR-stimulating antibodies

Mutated genes are indicated in parentheses.

Abbreviations: AIRE = autoimmune regulatory; CASR = calcium-sensing receptor; FAM111A = family with sequence similarity 111 member A; GATA3 = GATA-binding protein 3; GCM2 = glial cell missing homolog 2; GCMB = glial cell missing gene; GNA11 = G protein subunit alpha 11; GNAS = GNAS complex locus; PTH = parathyroid hormone; STX16 = syntaxin 16; TBCE = tubulin folding cofactor E; TBX1 = T-Box1; UPD = uniparental disomy.

those cured by PTx. Long-term observational studies indicate that the disease remains stable in the majority for up to 8 to 9 years, but more than one-third of patients show a progression of the disease.

Calcium intake should not be restricted, and an intake appropriate for age and sex as in the general population (preferably with food) should be recommended (Table 3). Vitamin D–depleted patients should be supplemented with daily doses of 800 to 1000 IU of vitamin D; weekly or monthly doses calculated on this daily dose can also be used. A serum level of 25(OH)D greater than 20 ng/mL should be reached, and the attainment of a higher target (> 30 ng/mL) is suggested by some guidelines.

General principles for monitoring are reported in Table 2. Serum calcium and creatinine (estimated glomerular filtration rate [eGFR]) should be measured annually and BMD at the lumbar spine, total hip, and distal forearm measured every 1 to 2 years. Vertebral morphometry (by x-ray or VFA) should be performed when clinically indicated (back pain, height loss). Finally, 24-hour urinary collection for biochemical stone risk profile and renal imaging (x-ray, ultrasound, or CT) should be performed if there is a suspicion of renal stones.

Parathyroid surgery should be recommended in patients who are followed without surgery in the following instances: (1) serum calcium concentration greater than 1 mg/dL above the upper normal limit; (2) creatinine clearance less than 60 mL/min; (3) detection of nephrocalcinosis or kidney stones; (4) BMD T-score at any site less than −2.5 or the finding of a significant (greater than the least significant change as defined by the International Society for Clinical Densitometry) decrease of BMD, even if the T-score

is not less than −2.5; and (5) clinical fractures or morphometric vertebral fractures, even if asymptomatic.

Medical Treatment. No medical treatment is currently available to cure PHPT. Therefore when PTx is indicated and there are no contraindications for surgery, medical treatment should not be considered a valuable alternative option. Medical treatment may be considered for patients who have contraindications to surgery or are unwilling to undergo PTx, as well as for those who have failed surgery. Treatment should be guided by the aim of therapy.

Calcimimetics. If the aim of treatment is to reduce serum calcium, the calcimimetic cinacalcet (Sensipar) can be effective. The serum calcium typically declines over a few weeks and may normalize in most patients with moderate hypercalcemia. In addition, cinacalcet increases serum phosphate and only slightly reduces PTH concentration, but has no effect on BMD. The beneficial effects are sustained over time as long as the drug is used. Adverse events are dose related: modest and transient when low doses of cinacalcet are used (up to 30 mg twice daily), but rather frequent, particularly gastrointestinal, symptoms, occasionally severe enough to require treatment withdrawal, when higher doses are employed. The use of cinacalcet has been approved by the US Food and Drug administration (FDA) for the treatment of severe hypercalcemia in patients with PHPT who are unable to undergo PTx, and by the European Medical Agency (EMA) for the reduction of hypercalcemia in patients with PHPT, for whom PTx would be indicated on the basis of serum calcium levels (as defined by relevant guidelines), but in whom surgery is not clinically appropriate or contraindicated. As clearly stated, the EMA indications leave more room for the use of cinacalcet.

Cinacalcet should not be used as an initial treatment or in patients who do not meet the approved criteria for its prescription. The long-term safety of cinacalcet has not been established. Moreover, the rather high cost is another important limit for its long-term use.

Bisphosphonates. If the aim is to increase BMD, antiresorptive therapy can be considered. Alendronate (Fosamax) is the bisphosphonate that has been more extensively used and shown to be effective in reducing bone turnover markers and increasing BMD. Over a short period of time, its effectiveness in increasing BMD is comparable to that observed after successful PTx. No effect has been shown on serum calcium and PTH levels.

Combined Therapy With Cinacalcet and Bisphosphonates. As mentioned before, cinacalcet is effective in the control of hypercalcemia but has no effect on BMD. Conversely, bisphosphonates increase BMD, with no effect on serum calcium. Limited data indicate that combination therapy is associated with both the calcium-lowering effect of cinacalcet and the skeletal advantage of bisphosphonates. Therefore if a patient has a low BMD and serum calcium concentration appropriate for the use of cinacalcet, combined therapy could be of benefit.

Pregnancy and Lactation

PHPT may be diagnosed during pregnancy by the finding of hypercalcemia on routine blood testing. There are some distinctive features that should be considered in the evaluation and management: (1) pregnancy is associated with hemodilution and occasionally hypoalbuminemia, and therefore it would be preferable to measure ionized calcium; (2) the hereditary form should be sought because of the young age of pregnant women; and (3) women with mild elevation of calcium should be managed conservatively, mostly by hydration—in the case of worsening of hypercalcemia PTx in the second trimester and cinacalcet[1] may be considered.

Secondary Hyperparathyroidism

Secondary hyperparathyroidism (SHPT) defines any condition in which the increased PTH secretion occurs as a normal physiologic response, often mediated by a decrease of serum calcium.

---

[1]Not FDA approved for this indication.

Vitamin D deficiency, as a result of inadequate nutritional intake/sun exposure, malabsorption, liver diseases, or chronic renal failure, is the most common cause. Other, less common causes include vitamin D resistance (Fanconi syndrome, vitamin D receptor defects), PTH resistance (pseudohypoparathyroidism, hypomagnesemia), drugs (calcium chelators, inhibitors of bone resorption, and drugs that interfere with vitamin D metabolism [phenytoin and ketoconazole]), acute pancreatitis, and osteoblastic metastases (prostate and breast cancer).

SHPT should always be considered and ruled out before making the diagnosis of normocalcemic PHPT. At variance with PHPT, SHPT is characterized by low or, more often, low-normal serum calcium and decreased urinary calcium excretion. An elevation of serum phosphate levels can be a clue to pseudohypoparathyroidism.

A prolonged stimulation of PTH synthesis and secretion, as may occur in end-stage renal failure and severe gastrointestinal diseases, may lead to the emergence of an autonomous clone of parathyroid cells into a single gland, leading to hypercalcemia (tertiary hyperparathyroidism).

Hypoparathyrodism

Hypoparathyroidism (HypoPT) is the clinical spectrum caused by insufficient production of PTH by the parathyroid glands. The major distinguishing feature is hypocalcemia, resulting from inadequate mobilization of calcium from bone and reabsorption of calcium at the distal tubule, and decreased activity of renal 1α-hydroxylase and therefore generation of calcitriol; as a consequence, the intestinal calcium absorption will be reduced.

Epidemiology

HypoPT is a rare condition designated in both the United States and Europe as an orphan disease. The estimated prevalence is 37 and 24 per 100,000 inhabitants in the United States and Europe, respectively.

Pathogenesis

HypoPT can be congenital or acquired (Table 3).

Congenital HypoPT is usually hereditary and may be isolated or combined with organ defects. The autoimmune is the most common form and may be either isolated or part of the autoimmune polyglandular syndrome type 1 (APS1). The other forms are much more rare.

Acquired HypoPT is much more common than the congenital counterpart. Bilateral neck surgery for thyroid or parathyroid disorders is the most common cause. Postoperative HypoPT can be transient (caused by reversible parathyroid ischemia and resolving within a few weeks) or chronic/permanent (caused by irreversible parathyroid damage such as ischemia, electric scalpel damage, or, rarely, inadvertent removal of parathyroid glands). Its rate largely depends on the experience of the surgeon and the extent of the neck surgery.

Clinical Presentation

The clinical manifestations of HypoPT are largely related to the level of serum calcium and the speed of its fall and may range from asymptomatic cases, when hypocalcemia is mild (corrected calcium ≥ 7.0 mg/dL [1.75 mmol/L]), to a severe, life-threating condition that requires hospital admission and intensive treatment. In mild cases signs related to neuromuscular irritability, namely the Chvostek sign (twitching and/or contracture of the facial muscles produced by tapping on the facial nerve just anterior to the ear and just below the zygomatic bone) and Trousseau sign (carpal spasm evoked by inflating a sphygmomanometer cuff above systolic blood pressure for several minutes), may be present at physical examination. Moderate to severe hypocalcemia (corrected calcium < 7.0 mg/dL [1.75 mmol/L]) is usually symptomatic, even though there is no strict relationship between the severity of symptoms and the degree of hypocalcemia. In patients with postoperative HypoPT, symptoms usually appear on the first postoperative day, but in some cases hypocalcemia may become clinically manifest even after 3 to 4 days. Classical manifestations include paresthesias, carpopedal spasm, tetany, seizures, positive Chvostek and Trousseau signs, and prolongation of the QT interval on electrocardiography. Papilledema and subcapsular cataract can be present. Pseudohypoparathyroidism is a group of genetic disorders caused by end-organ resistance to the action of PTH. Patients with the type 1a variant have a typical phenotype (Albright hereditary osteodystrophy), characterized by short stature, shortened fourth and fifth metacarpals, rounded face, and mild intellectual deficiency. Other endocrine glands, including the thyroid and the gonads, may be dysfunctional. This clinical and endocrine phenotype is also typical of patients with type 1c. Patients with type 1b have PTH resistance and in some cases partial resistance to thyroid-stimulating hormone (TSH) and mild brachydactyly. Patients with the type 2 variant have PTH resistance in the absence of the aforementioned clinical phenotype.

Evaluation and Diagnosis

The finding of low albumin-corrected serum calcium, high serum phosphate, and inappropriately low or undetectable serum PTH confirms the diagnosis of HypoPT. A recent neck surgery strongly suggests the postoperative form. A family history of hypocalcemia suggests a genetic cause. Coexistence of other autoimmune endocrinopathies (i.e., adrenal insufficiency) or candidiasis prompts consideration of APS1. Immunodeficiency and the presence of other congenital organ defects point to DiGeorge syndrome. Genetic testing may be warranted to confirm the diagnosis of this and other genetic forms. Magnesium should also be measured because magnesium deficiency impairs the secretion of PTH and its action in target tissues. Urinary calcium is usually low because of the low filtered calcium. The 24-hour calcium-to-creatinine clearance ratio is increased in patients with the activating mutation of *CaSR*. A biochemical profile of low serum calcium and high phosphate levels, together with high serum PTH, in the absence of vitamin D deficiency, reflects the PTH-resistant state, and suggests a case of pseudohypoparathyroidism.

Treatment

The goal is to control symptoms of hypocalcemia and improve QoL while avoiding side effects and complications. The target serum calcium concentration is in the lower part of the normal range. Treatment relies on the administration of calcium (oral [dietary or supplements] or intravenous), active vitamin D metabolites, magnesium, and, where available, recombinant human PTH$_{1-84}$ (Natpara). Thiazide diuretics may help reduce hypercalciuria; a low-phosphate diet and phosphate binders may help control hypophosphatemia and lower the calcium–phosphate product.

Acute Hypoparathyroidism

Acute hypocalcemia typically follows neck surgery and may be favored by a low vitamin D status and magnesium deficiency that, when present, should be corrected before surgery. In patients with high risk (total thyroidectomy, repeated thyroid surgery), perioperative administration of calcitriol (Rocaltrol) decreases the incidence of postoperative hypocalcemia and shortens the hospital stay.

Mild Hypocalcemia. In mild hypocalcemia (corrected calcium ≥ 7.0 mg/dL [1.75 mmol/L]), oral calcium supplements (usually calcium carbonate, 1–3 grams daily in divided doses) alone or combined with active vitamin D metabolites should be administered. Calcitriol is typically initiated at an initial dose of 0.5 to 1.0 μg twice daily; equivalent doses of 1α-calcifediol[2] (1.0–2.0 μg) may also be used (see later [Chronic Hypoparathyroidism, Conventional Therapy] for more details on calcium and active vitamin D therapy) (Table 4). Serum calcium is checked weekly until optimal levels are reached.

---

[2]Not available in the United States.

TABLE 4 Calcium Preparation and Vitamin D Metabolites in the Management of Hypocalcemia

Calcium

AGENT	FORMULATION AND DOSE	COMMENTS
Calcium gluconate	One ampule of 10% calcium gluconate contains 93 mg; preferably diluted in 5% dextrose	Tissue necrosis may be caused by elemental calcium; preferably diluted in 5% dextrose extravasation in the adjacent subcutaneous space
Calcium salts		
Calcium carbonate	40% elemental calcium by weight: 1 g calcium carbonate contains 400 mg elemental calcium	Best absorbed with meals in an acidic environment; constipation is a common side effect
Calcium citrate	21% elemental calcium by weight, 1 g calcium citrate contains 210 mg elemental calcium	Well absorbed independent of meal and acid environment; in patients with atrophic gastritis or taking proton pump inhibitors

Vitamin D Metabolites

MEDICATION	TYPICAL DAILY DOSE	TIME TO ONSET OF ACTION	TIME TO OFFSET OF ACTION
Calcitriol [1,25(OH)$_2$D]$_3$ (Rocaltrol)	0.25–2.0 μg once or twice	1–2 days	2–3 days
Alfacalcidol* [1α(OH)D]*	0.5–4 μg once	1–2 days	5–7 days
Dihydrotachysterol*,†	0.3–1.0 mg once	4–7 days	7–21 days
Vitamin D$_2$ (ergocalciferol) (Drisdol) or vitamin D$_3$ (cholecalciferol)‡	25,000–200,000 IU	10–14 days	14–75 days

*Not available in the United States.
†This compound is rapidly activated in the liver to 25(OH) dihydrotachysterol.
‡These compounds could be used in a setting where active vitamin D metabolites are not available and/or are too expensive.
Modified from Shoback D: Clinical practice. Hypoparathyroidism. *N Engl J Med* 2008;359:391–403, 2008.

Moderate to Severe Hypocalcemia. Patients with moderate to severe hypocalcemia (corrected calcium <7.0 mg/dL [1.75 mmol/L]) are usually admitted to the hospital and treated with IV calcium until an oral regimen can be started. One to two ampules of 10% calcium gluconate diluted in 50 to 100 mL of 5% dextrose should be infused over a period of 10 to 20 minutes with electrocardiographic and clinical monitoring. The calcium infusion will raise the serum calcium concentration for no more than 2 to 4 hours; thus this initial treatment should be followed by a continuous infusion (50–100 mL/h) of a solution containing 1 mg/mL of elemental calcium (11 ampules of 10% calcium gluconate added to 5% dextrose in a final volume of 1 liter). The rate should be adjusted according to corrected serum calcium level, which should be measured initially every 1 to 2 hours and subsequently every 4 to 6 hours, and maintained at the lower limit of the normal range, while the patient is asymptomatic. This calcium infusion protocol maintained for 8 to 10 hours will raise serum calcium by approximately 2 mg/dL. Oral administration of active vitamin D metabolites and calcium should be started as soon as practical. Calcitriol is typically initiated at a dose of 0.5 to 1.0 μg twice daily; oral calcium (1–3 g daily in divided doses) is also added.

If hypocalcemia is due to magnesium deficiency, the previous protocol should be applied while magnesium is being replaced by administering IV magnesium sulfate (initial dose 2 g as a 10% solution over 10–20 minutes, followed by 1 g/h in 100 mL) until a normal serum level of magnesium is reached. The only administration of magnesium will be unable to correct hypocalcemia because hypomagnesemia inhibits the secretion of PTH, and consequently the renal activation of 25OHD and induces a peripheral resistance to the action of PTH.

The rate of calcium infusion should be increased if symptoms of hypocalcemia recur. The IV infusion should be slowly tapered and discontinued when an effective regimen of oral calcium and active vitamin D is reached (up to 24–48 hours or longer) and stable desired serum calcium levels are obtained.

Chronic Hypoparathyroidism

The goal of therapy is to maintain serum calcium in the low-normal range, avoid hypocalcemic symptoms and long-term complications, and improve QoL. An individualized approach is

necessary to optimize patient care. Guidelines for the management of chronic HypoPT have only recently been developed by the European Society of Endocrinology, the American Association of Clinical Endocrinologists, the American College of Endocrinology, and a panel of international experts.

Conventional Therapy. An adequate calcium intake from dietary sources (mainly dairy products) should be recommended, but calcium supplements (1–3 g daily in divided doses) are needed in almost all adult patients. Calcium carbonate is generally preferred because fewer pills per day are needed. Calcium carbonate requires an acidic gastric environment to be absorbed and should be taken with meals. Its bioavailability decreases in patients with atrophic gastritis or taking proton pump inhibitors. In these circumstances, calcium citrate, which is well absorbed independent of meal and acid environments, should be preferred. Calcium citrate might also be a preferred option for patients who complain of gastrointestinal side effects using calcium carbonate or who prefer to take calcium supplements outside mealtimes. Calcium carbonate and calcium citrate interfere with levothyroxine absorption; therefore thyroidectomized patients should be advised to take levothyroxine well apart from calcium supplements.

Prior to the availability of synthetic active vitamin D metabolites, supraphysiologic doses (25,000–200,000 IU daily) of either cholecalciferol (vitamin D$_3$) or ergocalciferol (vitamin D$_2$) were used. Nowadays, active 1α-hydroxylated vitamin D metabolites are preferred because patients with HypoPT have impaired renal activation of 25-hydroxivitamin D. Calcitriol (Rocaltrol) and alfacalcidol (One-Alpha)[2] have a similar time of onset, but the latter has a longer time of offset (5–7 vs. 2–3 days). Calcitriol is more potent (about 50%) than alfacalcidol when compared in terms of the calcemic effect. The daily dose of calcitriol in adults ranges between 0.25 and 2.0 μg, equal to 0.5 to 4 μg of alfacalcidol. Weight-based dosing (0.01–0.04 μg per kg peer day), eventually associated with calcium supplements (20–40 mg per kg per day) should be used in infants and young children. Adult doses should be used in older children. Another active vitamin D analog, dihydrotachysterol, is also available in some countries. Where active vitamin D metabolites are not available or too expensive, large

---

[2]Not available in the United States.

doses of parent vitamin D can still be used, but attention should be paid to the risk of vitamin D toxicity.

A low vitamin D status is not uncommon in patients with HypoPT, and vitamin D–deficient patients treated with active vitamin D metabolites should be supplemented with vitamin D_2 or D_3, because active vitamin D metabolites do not correct hypovitaminosis D.

Active vitamin D metabolites stimulate intestinal absorption of phosphate, which may cause hyperphosphatemia and an increased calcium–phosphate product, with the risk of soft tissue calcification. In this setting the intake of phosphate-rich foods should be reduced and the daily dose of calcium supplements increased, since calcium binds phosphate.

Hypercalciuria ($\geq$ 250 mg [6.25 mmol] in women or $\geq$ 300 mg [7.5 mmol] in men or > 4 mg [0.1 mmol]/kg body weight in both sexes) is a common feature in patients with chronic HypoPT, because of the lack of PTH-dependent renal tubular reabsorption of calcium. In such instances a low-sodium diet should be advised either alone or combined with the administration of a thiazide diuretic that decreases renal calcium excretion. The combination of thiazide with amiloride[1] may further lower urinary calcium excretion and decrease the risk of hypokalemia. Thiazide diuretics are not advised in autosomal dominant hypocalcemia, a condition caused by mutations of the CaSR. Magnesium deficiency, when present, should also be corrected.

Lifelong monitoring is needed in patients with chronic HypoPTH. No study has evaluated how to best monitor these patients. The target serum calcium concentration is within the low-normal range, with no symptoms of hypocalcemia. In some patients a higher serum calcium level is needed to be symptom-free. A baseline renal imaging should be obtained. The recently published guidelines of the European Society of Endocrinology suggest measuring ionized or albumin-corrected total calcium, magnesium, and creatinine (eGFR) and 24-hour urinary calcium excretion every 3 to 6 months and performing renal imaging when patients have symptoms of nephrolithiasis or increasing serum levels of creatinine. Biochemical monitoring should be performed weekly or every other week when changing the daily dose of calcium or active vitamin D metabolites or introducing a new drug. It is important to note that serum calcium may fluctuate once the therapeutic regimen has been stabilized. Several comorbidities (e.g., gastrointestinal disease, diarrhea, immobilization) and drugs (loop and thiazide diuretics, systemic glucocorticoids, proton pump inhibitors, antiresorptive drugs, cardiac glycosides, and chemotherapeutics) may interfere with calcium homeostasis, and therefore patients should be periodically asked about their occurrence or use.

Conventional therapy only partially restores calcium homeostasis, and patients with chronic HypoPT have a reduced QoL and an increased risk of comorbidities, which include nephrocalcinosis, nephrolithiasis, impaired renal function, neuropsychiatric diseases, muscle stiffness and pain, infections, and seizures. An increased rate of intracerebral calcifications and cataracts has been documented in nonsurgical HypoPT. Bone mineral content is increased in patients with chronic HypoPT, but cancellous bone microarchitecture is abnormal.

Parathyroid Hormone. Until recently, HypoPT was the only major hormonal insufficiency state not treated with the missing hormone. The development of the recombinant human N-terminal 1-34 fragment (rhPTH$_{1-34}$) and the full-length 1-84 (rhPTH$_{1-84}$) molecule has stimulated several studies on its use as replacement therapy, which led to the approval by the Food and Drug Administration of rhPTH$_{1-84}$ (Natpara) for the management of chronic HypoPT.

The official recommendation is to consider rhPTH$_{1-84}$ therapy "only in patients who cannot be well-controlled on calcium and active forms of vitamin D and for whom the potential benefits are considered to outweigh the potential risk." Treatment should be started with subcutaneous administration in the thigh of 50 µg once daily, while reducing by 50% the daily dose of active vitamin D if serum calcium is greater than 7.5 mg/dL (1.875 mmol/L). Serum calcium should be monitored every 3 to 7 days and the daily dose of rhPTH$_{1-84}$ titrated every 4 weeks, aiming to reduce the daily calcium supplements to 500 mg and discontinue active vitamin D therapy while maintaining the serum calcium in the low-normal range. Afterward, serum calcium should be monitored every 3 to 6 months. Hypercalcemia has been reported in some cases, but a careful adjustment of the daily dose may decrease this risk. A "black box" in the official recommendation highlights the potential risk of osteosarcoma (studies in rats have shown that both rhPTH$_{1-34}$ and rhPTH$_{1-84}$ can cause osteosarcoma). However, there is no evidence that individuals treated with either PTH molecules are at increased risk for osteosarcoma. The safety and efficacy of rhPTH$_{1-84}$ in pediatric patients have not been established.

The FDA and the European Medical Agency approval for using rhPTH$_{1-84}$ in patients with HypoPT leaves room for decision making in individual cases. The guidelines recently elaborated by a panel of international experts suggest considering the use of rhPTH$_{1-84}$ therapy, where available, in any patient with chronic HypoPT of any etiology, except in patients with autosomal dominant hypocalcemia.

Pregnancy and Lactation

There are limited data to inform treatment strategies in chronic HypoPT in pregnancy and lactation. The guidelines of the European Society of Endocrinology suggest the use of active vitamin D metabolites and oral calcium as in nonpregnant women. Frequent monitoring (every 2–3 weeks) of serum calcium, possibly ionized calcium, is recommended. No studies have addressed the use of rhPTH$_{1-84}$ therapy in pregnant women. The FDA suggests that it should be used "only if the potential benefit justifies the potential risk to the fetus."

References

Arnold A, Levine A: Molecular basis of primary hyperparathyroidism. In Bilezikan JP, et al, editor: *The Parathyroids, Basic and Clincial Concept*, London, 2015, Academic Press, pp 279–296.

Bilezikian JP, Bandeira L, Khan A, et al: Hyperparathyrodism, *Lancet* 1:168178, 2018.

Bilezikian JP, Brandi ML, Eastell R, et al: Guidelines for the management of asymptomatic primary hyperparathyroidism: summary statement from the fourth international workshop, *J Clin Endocrinol Metab* 99:3561–3569, 2014.

Bilezikian JP, Cusano NE, Khan AA, et al: Primary hyperparathyroidism, *Nat Rev Dis Primers* 2:16033, 2016.

Bilezikian JP, Khan A, Potts Jr JT, et al: Hypoparathyroidism in the adult: epidemiology, diagnosis, pathophysiology, target-organ involvement, treatment, and challenges for future research, *J Bone Miner Res* 26:2317–2337, 2011.

Bollerslev J, Rejnmark L, Marcocci C, et al: European Society of Endocrinology Clinical Guideline: treatment of chronic hypoparathyroidism in adults, *Eur J Endocrinol* 173:G1–G20, 2015.

Brandi ML, Bilezikian JP, Shoback D, et al: Management of hypoparathyroidism: summary statement and guidelines, *J Clin Endocrinol Metab* 101:2273–2283, 2016.

Cetani F, Marcocci C: Parathyroid carcinoma. In Bilezikian JP, editor: *The Parathyroids. Basic and Clincial Concepts*, London, 2015, Academic Press, pp 409–422.

Cusano NE, Silverberg SJ, Bilezikian JP: Normocalcemic primary hyperparathyroidism, *J Clin Densitom* 16:33–39, 2013.

EMA/CHMP/124164/2017 Media and Public Relations, 2017: http://www.ema.europa.eu/docs/en_GB/document_library/Press_release/2017/02/WC500222215.pdf.

Khan AA, Koch C, Van Uum SHM, et al: Standards of care for hypoparathyroidism in adults, *Eur J Endocrinol* EJE-18-0609.R1. doi:10.1530/EJE-18-0609. [Epub ahead of print], 2018.

Mannstadt M, Bilezikian JP, Thakker RV, et al: Hypoparathyroidism, *Nat Rev Dis Primers* 3:17055, 2017. http://www.ema.europa.eu/docs/en_GB/document_library/Press_release/2017/02/WC500222215.pdf.

Mannstadt M, Clarke BL, Vokes T, et al: Efficacy and safety of recombinant human parathyroid hormone (1-84) in hypoparathyroidism (REPLACE): a double-blind, placebo-controlled, randomised, phase 3 study, *Lancet Diabetes Endocrinol* 1:275–283, 2013.

Marcocci C, Bollerslev J, Khan AA, Shoback DM: Medical management of primary hyperparathyroidism: proceedings of the fourth international workshop on the management of asymptomatic primary hyperparathyroidism, *J Clin Endocrinol Metab* 99:3607–3618, 2014.

Marcocci C, Cetani F: Clinical practice, *Primary hyperparathyroidism*, *N Engl J Med* 365:2389–2397, 2011.

NATPARA: Shire-NPS Pharmaceuticals, Inc, 2015: [package insert]. In https://www.accessdata.fda.gov/drugsatfda_docs/label/2015/125511s000lbl.pdf.

---

[1]Not FDA approved for this indication.

Rubin MR, Bilezikian JP, McMahon DJ, et al: The natural history of primary hyperparathyroidism with or without parathyroid surgery after 15 years, *J Clin Endocrinol Metab* 93:3462–3470, 2008.

Shoback D: Clinical practice. Hypoparathyroidism, *N Engl J Med* 359:391–403, 2008.

Shoback DM, Bilezikian JP, Costa AG, et al: Presentation of hypoparathyroidism: etiologies and clinical features, *J Clin Endocrinol Metab* 101:2300–2312, 2016.

Udelsman R, Akerstrom G, Biagini C, et al: The surgical management of asymptomatic primary hyperparathyroidism: proceedings of the fourth international workshop, *J Clin Endocrinol Metab* 99:3595–3606, 2014.

Vignali E, Viccica G, Diacinti D, et al: Morphometric vertebral fractures in postmenopausal women with primary hyperparathyroidism, *J Clin Endocrinol Metab* 94:2306–2312, 2009.

HYPERPROLACTINEMIA

Method of
Ming Li, MD, PhD; and Lawrence Chan, MD

CURRENT DIAGNOSIS

- Hyperprolactinemia is diagnosed by biochemical tests based on two-site immunoassay, which can be confounded by extreme hyperprolactinemia (hook effect) and biologically inactive macroprolactinemia.
- Hyperprolactinemia can be caused by physiological, pharmacological, or pathological conditions; careful clinical, laboratory, and radiology evaluations are required to identify its underlying cause.
- The most common causes of hyperprolactinemia include medications, prolactinoma, and other pituitary and hypothalamic/pituitary stalk diseases.
- Clinical features of hyperprolactinemia include galactorrhea, menstrual abnormalities (in women), impotence (in men), infertility, and osteoporosis.
- Patients with prolactinoma may also have local compression symptoms including headache, visual disturbance, and hypopituitarism.
- Pituitary magnetic resonance imaging (MRI) is the imaging method of choice for diagnosing prolactinoma and other sellar/parasellar lesions.

CURRENT THERAPY

- For secondary hyperprolactinemia, treatment should be directed at correcting underlying causes.
- Treatment goals for prolactinoma are relief of symptoms and the long-term effects of hyperprolactinemia, and of tumor mass effects.
- The dopamine agonists cabergoline (Dostinex) and bromocriptine (Parlodel) are effective in normalizing the prolactin level and shrinking the tumor in patients with prolactinoma.
- Surgery and radiotherapy of prolactinoma are reserved for patients resistant to or intolerant of medical therapy.
- Temozolomide (Temodar)[1] monotherapy is the first-line chemotherapy for aggressive or malignant prolactinomas after failing standard treatments.

[1]Not FDA approved for this indication.

Biochemistry and Physiology of Prolactin

Prolactin is a polypeptide hormone produced by pituitary lactotroph cells. It is also produced locally in a variety of extrapituitary tissues such as mammary glands, decidua, gonads, brain, liver, fat, pancreas, and the immune system, along with its receptors. Prolactin is highly pleiotropic in terms of its functions. Many of its actions collectively support puerperal lactation. Prolactin displays considerable sequence homology to growth hormone (GH) and placental lactogen. The prolactin and GH receptors both belong to the class I cytokine/hematopoietic receptor superfamily. Prolactin is responsible for maturation of the mammary glands during pregnancy, but it plays only a minor role for pubertal mammary development, which requires GH instead. It appears not to be an essential hormone for non-childbearing individuals. Rare patients deficient for either prolactin or its receptor are largely healthy despite difficulty with fertility and lactation.

Prolactin circulates mainly as a 23-kDa 199-aa polypeptide. Several of its cleavage products exist in blood, which may have functions unrelated to lactation; for example, one 16-kDa cleavage product of prolactin displays antiangiogenic and prothrombotic properties, and has been implicated in the development of preeclampsia and peripartum cardiomyopathy. Several forms of prolactin aggregate, known as macroprolactins, also exist in circulation at lower levels. They are formed either by covalent bonding of prolactin monomers or by their nucleating around autoimmune IgG. These macroprolactins are not biologically active in vivo and have a prolonged half-life. At times they can build up in the circulation to a level high enough to cause diagnostic difficulties.

Among the major pituitary hormones, prolactin is unique for its predominantly negative mode of regulation by the hypothalamus. It does not have a known hypothalamus-derived releasing hormone. Instead, lactotrophs are under tonic inhibition by dopamine secreted from hypothalamic neurons. Increase in prolactin output is mostly mediated by withdrawing dopaminergic control in response to environmental cues, such as physical activity, stress, and nipple stimuli (Figure 1). Under experimental and pathological conditions, several factors, including thyrotropin-releasing hormone (TRH), vasoactive intestinal peptide (VIP), oxytocin, and vasopressin, have been shown to increase prolactin secretion, but these peptides appear to play only minor and insignificant roles for the physiological regulation of prolactin.

Estrogen is the main driver of prolactin secretion during pregnancy. Stimulated by persistently elevated estrogen, lactotrophs grow in number and size. By term the pituitary gland can reach 2 to 3 times its normal size, and prolactin levels increase some 20-fold. Along with placental hormones such as estrogen, progesterone, and placental lactogen, prolactin drives the maturation of the mammary glands. Lactation starts after parturition, when estrogen withdraws from the circulation. Frequent infant suckling maintains physiological hyperprolactinemia, which is important for sustained milk production. In addition, hyperprolactinemia during this critical period provides a natural though unreliable way of contraception. This is achieved by suppression of the hypothalamus–pituitary–gonad axis. Hyperprolactinemic hypogonadism and parathyroid hormone related peptide (PTHrP) secreted from mammary epithelial cells help mobilize skeletal calcium store in support of milk production. Through its receptors in liver, intestine, fat, and pancreas prolactin also adjusts maternal nutrient metabolism for optimal milk output. In the brain, prolactin modifies parental behavior toward closer infant attendance (see Figure 1).

Pathophysiology of Hyperprolactinemia

Physiological hyperprolactinemia as occurs during pregnancy and nursing is essential for child raising through the actions of prolactin in target organs discussed above. Similar changes in these organs under the influence of persistent pathological hyperprolactinemia in the absence of pregnancy and lactation, however, are inappropriate and could lead to a variety of undesired long-term consequences.

Mammary Glands

One common symptom of persistent hyperprolactinemia is galactorrhea, that is, milk production not associated with childbirth or breast-feeding. As puerperal lactation normally ends within 6 months after delivery or weaning, any milk production beyond this point is also considered galactorrhea. Since maturation of

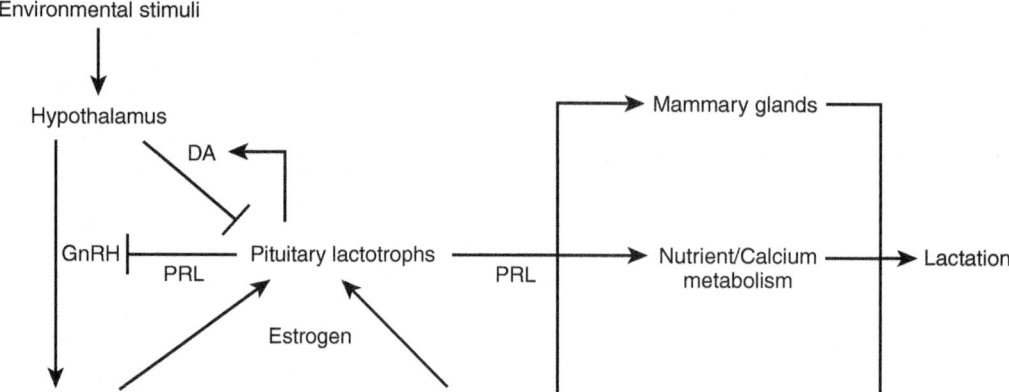

Figure 1 Physiology of prolactin and its regulation. At baseline, prolactin production and secretion are under tonic inhibition by dopamine released from hypothalamic neurons. The hypothalamus controls prolactin production by altering output of dopamine after integrating environmental stimuli and changes in hormonal homeostasis. Prolactin increases hypothalamic dopamine output, providing a negative feedback regulatory loop. Estrogen stimulates prolactin synthesis and secretion during pregnancy. Prolactin supports puerperal lactation via its action on the mammary glands, nutrient/calcium metabolism, and brain. Unlike most other anterior pituitary hormones, feedback regulation of prolactin secretion does not occur via factors produced by a peripheral endocrine target organ. Prolactin also suppresses hypothalamic-pituitary-gonadal axis by inhibiting GnRH release. *Abbreviations:* DA = dopamine; GnRH = gonadotropin releasing hormone; PRL = prolactin.

mammary glands is completed during pregnancy, galactorrhea typically happens in women between 20 to 35 years of age with previous childbirths. It also occurs in nulligravid women, postmenopausal women, and men, although less frequently.

Prolactin is a known mitogen for mammary epithelial cells, and concern has been raised regarding its potential role in the pathogenesis of breast cancer. In a large prospective study by the Women's Health Initiative (WHI), there was evidence of a significant increase in breast cancer incidence in postmenopausal women with high normal prolactin levels, which is within the highest quartile of the normal range compared with those in the lowest quartile. On the other hand, increased breast cancer risk has not been observed in patients with overt hyperprolactinemia. In fact, early parity and lactation history are strong protective factors against breast cancer. Further research is required to resolve these seemingly discrepant observations.

Female Reproductive System
Persistent hyperprolactinemia significantly diminishes the pulsatile release of gonadotropin-releasing hormone (GnRH). As GnRH neurons do not themselves express prolactin receptors, prolactin exerts its effects on their afferent neurons instead by suppression of secretion of kisspeptin, a potent secretagogue for GnRH. Prolactin receptors are also found in the gonads, and prolactin has been reported to inhibit folliculogenesis and estrogen production in the ovary directly. However, this likely has only a limited contribution to infertility and hypogonadism associated with hyperprolactinemia, for the hypothalamus-pituitary-gonad axis can be reactivated by administration of GnRH or kisspeptin, with return of ovulation and fertility in subjects with hyperprolactinemia.

Male Reproductive System
As in women, hyperprolactinemia causes secondary hypogonadism and infertility in men by suppression of GnRH pulses and a decrease in luteinizing hormone (LH) and follicle-stimulating hormone (FSH) levels. Patients often have low or low normal testosterone levels, as well as abnormal sperm counts and morphology in semen analysis. Patients usually seek medical attention for diminished libido and impotence. The central nervous system (CNS) actions of prolactin are likely partly responsible for these symptoms, as restoration of testosterone level alone is often inadequate for symptom relief, which occurs only when prolactin levels also return to normal.

Adrenal Glands
Prolactin stimulates the synthesis of androgen in the zona reticularis of the adrenal cortex. Mild elevations in serum levels of adrenal androgens, for example dehydroepiandrosterone (DHEA) and dehydroepiandrosterone sulfate (DHEA-S), are seen in approximately 50% of women with hyperprolactinemia. Symptoms of clinical hyperandrogenism such as hirsutism and acne are rare in these patients. When present, they are almost always associated with a concurrent increase in testosterone level. Elevation of adrenal androgens in hyperprolactinemia may contribute to the suppression of GnRH release in the hypothalamus and secondary hypogonadism.

Skeletal System
Premenopausal women with hyperprolactinemia have lower bone density and approximately a 4.5 times higher risk for osteoporotic fractures. Hypogonadism associated with hyperprolactinemia is the main cause of bone loss, whereas restoration of sex hormones with either hormonal replacement or correction of hyperprolactinemia improves bone density. Bone density is preserved in women with hyperprolactinemia who continue to have regular menses. Nonetheless, not all studies showed a clear correlation between the degree of bone loss and duration of amenorrhea or levels of sex hormones suggesting involvement of additional processes. For example, the levels of parathyroid hormone–related protein (PTHrP) were found to be significantly higher in patients with hyperprolactinemia, and correlated well with bone density measurements. Correction of hyperprolactinemia by dopamine agonists was shown to normalize PTHrP levels.

Etiology of Hyperprolactinemia
Any conditions that affect production or clearance of prolactin can lead to hyperprolactinemia (Table 1). Physiological hyperprolactinemia is transient and adaptive, whereas persistent hyperprolactinemia from pharmacological and pathological causes is often symptomatic with undesired long-term consequences. Pituitary adenomas over producing prolactin (prolactinomas) are the most important cause of pathological hyperprolactinemia. In addition to the elevated prolactin levels, prolactinomas also produce pathological local mass effects. Secondary hyperprolactinemia is most commonly related to disruption of dopaminergic control of lactotrophs, secondary to the use of dopamine antagonists or hypothalamic and pituitary stalk lesions.

Epidemiology and Natural History of Prolactinoma
Prolactinoma is the most common type of pituitary adenoma, contributing to approximately 40–50% of pituitary tumor cases. Prolactinomas are categorized according to size into

TABLE 1 Causes of Hyperprolactinemia

PHYSIOLOGICAL

Pregnancy

Lactation and breast stimulation

Neonatal period

Physical activity

Stress

Sexual intercourse

PHARMACOLOGICAL

Dopamine antagonists—antipsychotics and antiemetics

Tricyclic antidepressants

Selective serotonin reuptake inhibitors (SSRI)

Antihistamines (H2)

Verapamil (Calan)

Protease inhibitors

Dopamine synthesis inhibitors

PATHOLOGICAL

PITUITARY DISEASES

Prolactinoma

Plurihormonal adenomas

Lymphocytic hypophysitis

Empty sella syndrome

Macroadenoma with or without suprasellar extension

Idiopathic hyperprolactinemia

HYPOTHALAMIC/PITUITARY STALK DISEASES

Tumors: meningioma, craniopharyngioma, germinoma, metastasis, etc.

Granulomas

Infiltrative diseases

Irradiation

Trauma

NEUROGENIC: chest wall lesions, spinal cord lesions, herpes zoster, and epileptic seizure

PARANEOPLASTIC SYNDROME

SYSTEMIC DISEASES

End-stage renal disease

Cirrhosis

Adrenal insufficiency

Pseudocyesis

Adapted from Bronstein, 2016; Melmed et al., 2017.

microprolactinomas (under 1 cm) and macroprolactinomas (larger than 1 cm). Clinically these two conditions behave very differently and can be considered as separate entities. In general, macroprolactinomas tend to grow progressively and are often locally invasive; they are also generally more resistant to treatment and have a higher risk of recurrence. On the other hand, microprolactinomas rarely progress in size (~ 7% of cases) and have a good chance (~ 15% of cases) of going into remission on their own.

The prevalence of prolactinoma has been estimated to be 500 cases per million and incidence about 27 cases per million per year based on survey of asymptomatic populations. In autopsy series, however, lactotroph neoplasms staining positive for prolactin are much more common, being found in approximately 5% of the subjects. They are predominantly microadenomas. Only a small fraction of these small lactotroph neoplasms develop overt hyperprolactinemia by escaping tonic dopaminergic suppression from the hypothalamus, presumably via down-regulation of dopamine D2 receptor-mediated signaling pathway and/or bypassing the portal system for blood supply. Microprolactinomas predominantly affect women of childbearing age, with a female-to-male ratio of approximately 20:1. Macroprolactinoma, on the other hand, shows no sex predilection. Neoplastic transformation of lactotroph involves accumulation of genetic and epigenetic events. The best-understood candidate genes involved include the pituitary tumor transforming gene (PTTG) and the heparin-binding secretory transforming gene (HST). PTTG expression is positively regulated by estrogen.

Most prolactinomas occur sporadically. The vast majority of prolactinomas are benign, although they can be locally invasive. Malignant prolactinomas, as defined by the presence of extrapituitary metastases, are extremely rare. Familial cases, such as those associated with multiple endocrine neoplasia I (MEN-I) and familial isolated pituitary adenoma (FIPA), typically occur at a younger age and are more often macroprolactinomas that are locally invasive.

Clinical Manifestations

Clinical manifestations of prolactinomas fall under two categories: systemic effects of hyperprolactinemia, and local compression symptoms.

Symptoms of Hyperprolactinemia

Persistent hyperprolactinemia inappropriately recapitulates symptoms associated with normal pregnancy and nursing. In extreme cases, hyperprolactinemia has been associated with delusions of pregnancy in susceptible individuals, for example some women on psychotropic medications.

Menstrual abnormalities and infertility are the most common symptoms associated with hyperprolactinemia in women of childbearing age. These symptoms may be masked by use of oral contraceptive pills, which often delays diagnosis. The mildest cases include women presenting with infertility caused by shortened luteal phase despite preserved regular menses. As the degree of hypogonadism worsens, patients experience menstrual irregularities ranging from anovulatory cycles to oligomenorrhea and amenorrhea. Patients with amenorrhea may also experience psychological stresses and other menopausal symptoms like vaginal dryness and dyspareunia. Of note, high prolactin levels may sometimes mask vasomotor symptoms of menopausal and perimenopausal women with prolactinoma, who may develop hot flashes once they are successfully treated with dopamine agonists.

Galactorrhea occurs in up to 80% of cases of hyperprolactinemia. This will need to be differentiated from nipple discharges of other causes, especially those from breast neoplasms. Further evaluation with breast imaging and cytology is indicated when the discharge is unilateral, bloody, or associated with a breast mass. Galactorrhea is by definition milk-like in appearance, and when in doubt, Sudan Black B staining showing fat globules is confirmatory. Although considered a classic sign and symptom for hyperprolactinemia, galactorrhea per se is a poor predictor for hyperprolactinemia in the absence of additional symptoms, for it can be seen in about 10% of healthy women of childbearing age. If amenorrhea is present at the same time, the patient should be assumed to harbor a prolactinoma unless proven otherwise. The degree of galactorrhea is quite variable, from barely expressible to bothersome bra stain and copious free flow, and does not necessarily reflect the severity of hyperprolactinemia. In fact, the majority of patients with galactorrhea and normal menses have normal prolactin levels. On the other hand, in some patients with extremely high levels of prolactin, galactorrhea could be masked by severe hypogonadism.

Men with hyperprolactinemia mainly present with impotence and diminished libido, which is not always corrected with testosterone replacement. As noted in the section on pathophysiology, these symptoms are not all caused by hypogonadism but may involve the central effects of prolactin. Other symptoms and signs of hypogonadism, such as loss of body hair and muscle bulk, are less common. Infertility could also occur with decrease in sperm count and morphology, although hyperprolactinemia is only present in approximately 5% of male patients seeking treatment for infertility.

For both male and female patients, persistent hypogonadism from hyperprolactinemia leads to osteoporosis and increased risk of fracture. This could be effectively treated with either sex hormone replacement or dopamine agonists.

Mass Effects of Prolactinomas

Headache is the most common neurological symptom caused by pituitary tumors. It can occur even with microadenomas presumably caused by dural stretch. More severe headache results from larger tumors, especially those with extrasellar invasion, and occasionally from apoplexy.

Visual disturbance typically only happens with macroadenomas with suprasellar extension impinging on the optic chiasm leading to loss of visual acuity and visual field defects. The typical pattern of visual field defect is bitemporal hemianopsia, which usually starts from the upper field and progresses downward as the tumor impinges upward from below. Ophthalmoparesis typically happens in the setting of apoplexy and only rarely results from parasellar invasion of the cavernous sinus and impingement of cranial nerves III, IV, or VI.

By compressing the rest of the pituitary gland, including the stalk, prolactinoma can cause deficiencies of other anterior pituitary hormones including GH, thyroid-stimulating hormone (TSH), and adrenocorticotropic hormone (ACTH), in addition to hypogonadism from the hyperprolactinemia. The degree of the risk is proportional to tumor size.

CSF rhinorrhea occurs when a macroprolactinoma invades inferiorly into the sphenoid sinus. Other rare compressive symptoms from giant prolactinomas include epilepsy (temporal lobe involvement), exophthalmos, and hydrocephalus. Life- and vision-threatening emergencies could arise from apoplexy and CNS infection.

Laboratory Evaluation

Prolactin Assay and Pitfalls

Hyperprolactinemia is diagnosed by individual measurements of serum prolactin levels. Patients should be well rested, as physical activity stimulates prolactin secretion, but fasting is not needed. Dynamic tests such as TRH stimulation do not appear to add to diagnostic value and are not recommended. The level of prolactin may provide valuable diagnostic clues. Secondary hyperprolactinemia rarely exceeds 150 ng/mL. On the other hand, a prolactin level of greater than 100 ng/mL is highly suggestive, and severe hyperprolactinemia of greater than 500 ng/mL is virtually diagnostic for prolactinoma. On rare occasions, secondary hyperprolactinemia can produce prolactin levels in the prolactinoma range. For example, risperidone (Risperdal)-induced hyperprolactinemia could be as high as 250 to 500 ng/mL, and patients with end-stage renal disease who are on antipsychotics or antiemetics can have prolactin levels greater than 1000 ng/mL. The size of the prolactinoma shows a rough correlation with the serum prolactin level. Patients with microprolactinomas usually have prolactin levels in the range of 50 to 300 ng/mL, whereas those with macroprolactinomas have levels of 200 to 5000 ng/mL.

Most clinical laboratories measure prolactin using a two-site immunoassay. A capture antibody first affixes prolactin in the sample to a solid matrix. Subsequently a second signal antibody is attached to the now immobilized prolactin. The signal antibody is engineered to carry either a radioisotope or a chemiluminescent enzyme to provide a readout. The assay is accurate within its designed linear range, which is typically under 10,000 ng/mL. Beyond this level both capture and signal antibodies

could be saturated preventing the signal antibody to attach. As a result, signal outputs will be falsely diminished. This phenomenon, known as the hook effect, produces a falsely low reading that could lead to the misdiagnosis of a macroprolactinoma as a nonfunctioning pituitary tumor. This artifact can be circumvented by repeating the assay with a 100-fold diluted sample. Many laboratories also opt for an additional washout step to eliminate excess prolactin before adding the signal antibody, preempting the artifact.

Macroprolactinemia is another potential diagnostic pitfall masquerading as true hyperprolactinemia. Macroprolactins are biologically inactive prolactin aggregates that could accumulate in blood to a high level. Macroprolactinemia does not cause any morbidities but could contribute to analytical difficulties as the antibodies used in prolactin assays cross-react with macroprolactins. Most laboratories rely on polyethylene glycol (PEG) precipitation to determine the proportion of macroprolactins and the true concentration of monomeric prolactin. Up to 25% of monomeric prolactin can be also precipitated by PEG, potentially masking true hyperprolactinemia. Therefore patients with macroprolactinemia may still need to be further evaluated if clinical suspicion is high for true hyperprolactinemia.

Other Supporting Laboratory Tests

After confirming hyperprolactinemia, a simple chemistry panel may reveal or suggest the underlying cause such as chronic kidney disease and cirrhosis. A pregnancy test (beta human chorionic gonadotropin [βhCG] level) is essential for women of childbearing age, and hypothyroidism needs to be ruled out with a TSH assay. Both pregnancy and hypothyroidism may have presenting symptoms of sellar mass and hyperprolactinemia and therefore be mistaken for prolactinoma.

For established prolactinoma cases it is important to also assess other pituitary axes. Up to 20% of GH-secreting tumors cosecrete prolactin, and IGF-1 level is an essential screening test for these cases. If hypogonadism is suspected, levels of LH, FSH, and sex hormones (testosterone or estrogen) should be obtained. Screening for central hypothyroidism and secondary adrenal insufficiency should be done with TSH, free thyroxine (T4), and morning cortisol levels, respectively, for patients with pituitary tumors larger than 6 mm.

Neuroimaging

Pituitary imaging should be considered for all patients with unexplained significant hyperprolactinemia, especially if there are signs or symptoms of local compression. MRI with and without gadolinium contrast with dedicated pituitary protocol is the test of choice. Compared with other modalities MRI provides superior soft tissue contrast revealing the tumor's inner structure and its relationship to surrounding tissues, including cavernous sinus, pituitary stalk, and optic chiasm. Computed tomography (CT) scan still has a role for patients with metal implants or other contraindications for MRI, and is especially useful for revealing bony erosions and tissue calcification; its use is limited by suboptimal soft tissue contrast and exposure to ionizing radiation.

Visual Field Testing

A formal visual field test with a perimeter is recommended when suprasellar extension of a pituitary adenoma brings it close to the optic chiasm. Improvement or worsening in visual field often precedes imaging evidence of tumor shrinkage or expansion during treatment. Therefore visual field testing is an excellent monitoring tool for patients under treatment for macroadenoma and visual impairment.

Diagnosis

Prolactin testing is usually prompted by suggestive signs and symptoms of hyperprolactinemia such as menstrual abnormalities, infertility, and galactorrhea. A careful history, including medication use, physical examination, and routine laboratory evaluation (see preceding sections), is invaluable for uncovering

Figure 2 Diagnostic algorithm for hyperprolactinemia. If hyperprolactinemia occurs in the absence of relevant clinical symptoms and signs, one should rule out macroprolactinemia by PEG precipitation. When hyperprolactinemia is confirmed, pregnancy should be ruled out with a βhCG test. In the absence of pregnancy, if the PRL level is higher than 100 ng/dl, the pretest probability for a prolactinoma is high enough to justify a pituitary MRI scan, even if potential secondary causes exist. Regardless of prolactin levels, secondary causes should be carefully evaluated with medication history, physical examination, and laboratory tests such as thyroid function tests and chemistry panel, and appropriately treated. If hyperprolactinemia remains unexplained or persists despite correction of other contributing factors, a pituitary MRI is in order. Patients with negative sellar findings have idiopathic hyperprolactinemia. Patients with sellar mass may have either prolactinoma or pseudoprolactinoma. The latter is suggested by a discordant prolactin level less than 150 ng/mL for a large sellar, or a parasellar mass greater than 1 cm, after hook effect has been ruled out. *Abbreviations:* βhCG = β human chorionic gonadotropin; MRI = magnetic resonance imaging; PEG = polyethylene glycol; PRL = prolactin.

secondary causes. Pituitary imaging should be performed when no other underlying causes are found especially if the levels of prolactin are higher than 100 ng/mL. A diagnostic algorithm shown in Figure 2 provides a framework for a structured and cost-effective workup of hyperprolactinemia.

Differential Diagnosis

An exhaustive list of etiologies has been provided in Table 1. A few entities deserve additional comments.

Drug-induced hyperprolactinemia is common and at times may produce serum prolactin levels matching those in patients with prolactinoma (see prior section on laboratory evaluation). A more typical range of prolactin level is 25 to 100 ng/mL for drug-induced hyperprolactinemia. It is not always possible to correlate in time the initiation of the culprit drug with the onset of symptoms, or rise of prolactin levels. The way to confirm medication-related hyperprolactinemia is to discontinue the putative offending agent(s) for three days before repeating a prolactin assay. Some medications may require a longer period of abstinence, and in such cases the level of prolactin can be retested later if the second value is reduced but still elevated. Before discontinuing psychotropic medications, one should consult with the prescribing psychiatrist to prevent worsening of the patient's mental symptoms.

Pseudoprolactinoma refers to a nonfunctioning sellar or suprasellar mass associated with hyperprolactinemia caused by stalk disruption. The prolactin level is seldom above 150 ng/mL. However, before making such a diagnosis, one must exclude hook effect with a 100-fold diluted sample. Prolactin levels are typically normalized within several days after initiation of dopamine agonists, as lactotrophs are still sensitive to dopamine, but local compressive symptoms do not improve. In contrast, patients with true macroprolactinoma experience more gradual decrease in prolactin levels after they are put on dopamine agonists, but they could expect improvement in compressive symptoms within 12 hours to days, and imaging evidence of tumor shrinkage in weeks.

Polycystic ovary syndrome (PCOS) and hyperprolactinemia are among the most common causes of menstrual irregularities and infertility, and affect women of similar ages. PCOS has also been associated with hyperprolactinemia. However, multiple studies have shown that the prevalence of hyperprolactinemia in women with PCOS is not significantly higher than that of matched populations. Although mild elevations of DHEA-S or DHEA are common in patients with hyperprolactinemia, hirsutism is rare, and when present is always associated with an increase in testosterone level, likely reflecting possible coexisting PCOS. Therefore the presence of hyperprolactinemia in patients with PCOS or hirsutism warrants additional evaluation.

Management of Secondary Hyperprolactinemia

Treatment of secondary hyperprolactinemia should focus on correcting the underlying conditions, for example treating hypothyroidism, and resection of nonfunctioning pituitary tumors. For drug-induced hyperprolactinemia, the responsible medications should be removed or replaced with alternatives. Newer antipsychotics such as aripiprazole (Abilify) may be used in place of older agents such as risperidone (Risperdal) because they have better metabolic/hormonal profiles. For irreversible conditions such as end-stage renal disease, hyperprolactinemia can be effectively controlled with dopamine agonists. Ectopic prolactin secretion, which occurs in paraneoplastic syndrome, is a rare exception where dopamine agonists are ineffective, because extrapituitary production of prolactin is driven by alternative promoters, which do not respond to dopamine. Asymptomatic patients with modest hyperprolactinemia may not need treatment, however, and sex hormone replacement may be adequate for correcting hypogonadism if fertility is not desired.

Management of Prolactinoma

The goals for managing prolactinomas are twofold: treating symptomatic hyperprolactinemia, and relief of tumor mass effects. Treatment thus needs to be tailored to the patient's unique clinical picture and the desired outcome. Mass effects are not a concern for microprolactinomas, whereas for patients with giant prolactinomas (defined as >4 cm or >2 cm of suprasellar extension) and extreme hyperprolactinemia, normalization of prolactin levels is less likely, and treatment should focus on reversal or minimization of mass effects. The following are appropriate options in specific settings.

Observation

Active surveillance is appropriate for patients with microprolactinoma who are asymptomatic or not troubled by galactorrhea, especially if fertility is not a concern. As long as regular menses are preserved, they seem to be spared from any long-term consequences from hyperprolactinemia. Bone mineral density appears to be preserved in these patients. It is noteworthy that a significant fraction of patients may have tumor resolution during surveillance without treatment. Tumor expansion is a rare event, and serial measurements of serum prolactin level are effective for monitoring interval tumor growth. Pituitary imaging is indicated when there is significant increase in prolactin level or emergence of local compression symptoms.

Hormonal Replacement

For patients with microprolactinoma bothered only by symptoms related to hypogonadism including menstrual abnormalities, sexual dysfunction, and osteoporosis, but who no longer desire fertility, hormonal replacement is a valid alternative to dopamine agonists, especially when the latter are not tolerated or are contraindicated. This can be achieved with oral contraceptive pills in premenopausal women, or testosterone in men. This approach compares favorably to dopamine agonists in terms of cost and side effects. Patients may experience slight increases in prolactin level, but tumor progression has not been associated with use of oral contraceptive pills for up to 2 years. It would be prudent to use lower doses of estradiol (≤ 30 µg/day) and closely monitor patients for prolactin level and tumor growth.

Dopamine Agonists

Medical treatment with dopamine agonists has replaced surgery as the first-line treatment for prolactinomas, with excellent efficacy in achieving treatment goals and minimal risk. The therapeutic effects of dopamine agonists are mediated by dopamine D2 receptors in tumor cells, which inhibit prolactin synthesis and secretion, slow cell proliferation, and reduce tumor vascularity. Normalization of prolactin levels and reduction of tumor size can be expected in the majority of patients. A small fraction of prolactinomas is resistant to dopamine agonists, as defined by failure in normalizing prolactin level, reduction in tumor size by 50%, or restoration of gonadal function with standard doses. In general, microprolactinomas are more sensitive to dopamine agonists than macroprolactinomas are, and men are more likely to be drug resistant than are women. Rapid responders experience significant improvement of visual symptoms within 24–72 hours; some of them may develop complications resulting from the rapid receding of macroprolactinomas (uncorking), e.g., pituitary apoplexy, optic chiasm herniation, and/or CSF leak. For most patients, however, progressive reduction of tumor size occurs over the course of months to years, though some patients may never experience tumor shrinkage despite normalization of prolactin levels at the highest tolerated doses.

Patients with microprolactinoma may discontinue treatment upon menopause because their treatment goal has been fulfilled. Patients with macroprolactinoma, on the other hand, may require life-long treatment to prevent tumor regrowth. A meta-analysis showed that a small fraction of patients may enter long-term remission after discontinuing dopamine agonists (21% for microprolactinomas and 16% for macroprolactinomas). The odds are significantly improved if patients have been treated for at least

2 years and tumor size reduced by $\geq 50\%$. The 2011 Endocrine Society practice guidelines suggest that tapering or discontinuing dopamine agonists may be attempted in patients who have been treated for at least 2 years and experienced complete biochemical and radiographic resolution. The risk for recurrence after drug discontinuation is related to the size of adenoma at the time of the diagnosis. For tumors larger than 2 cm, especially giant prolactinomas, tapering the dopamine agonists to a lower maintenance dose for life-long treatment after achieving maximal tumor reduction would be a better strategy for these patients. Tapering or withdrawal of dopamine agonists should be followed by close surveillance of prolactin levels and pituitary MRI when prolactin level increases, especially during the first year.

Three dopamine agonists are currently used for treating hyperprolactinemia, including bromocriptine (Parlodel), cabergoline (Dostinex), and quinagolide (available only in Europe). Bromocriptine was the first dopamine agonist available, and it has the best established safety record. It is still the only dopamine agonist approved by the Food and Drug Administration (FDA) to be used in pregnancy, when indicated. Cabergoline is a more specific agonist of the D2 dopamine receptor, and is superior in many respects to bromocriptine, for example, because of dosing convenience, tolerability, and treatment efficacy. Many patients not controlled with bromocriptine may achieve normal prolactin levels after switching to cabergoline, which has become the drug of choice for cases not involving pregnancy. The safety data for cabergoline are not as extensive as those for bromocriptine. Common side effects for this class of drugs include nausea, orthostatic hypotension, fatigue, mental fogginess, and, less frequently, nasal stuffiness, Raynaud phenomenon, constipation, depression, and psychosis. Nausea is more common in patients taking bromocriptine; for these patients the intravaginal route[1] can be tried. Patients receiving higher doses of cabergoline are at risk of developing cardiac valvulopathy. This has so far been a concern for patients with Parkinson's disease, who may require much higher doses. However, the life-long exposure to high cumulative doses in patients with resistant prolactinoma is considerable, and regular echocardiogram surveillance is recommended for patients taking doses higher than 2 mg/week. Dosing regimens for bromocriptine and cabergoline are listed in Table 2. In general, patients should be started on the lowest doses and titrated upward monthly based on the serum prolactin level until treatment goals are reached.

Surgery

With the availability of the second-generation dopamine agonists, surgery is mostly reserved for the following situations: (1) patients intolerant of, or resistant to, dopamine agonists; (2) women with macroprolactinoma who are planning for conception, to forestall tumor expansion during pregnancy; (3) pituitary apoplexy threatening neurological and visual functions if not managed urgently. Transsphenoidal tumor resection is the standard surgical approach. Perioperative mortality and morbidity are low in the hands of experienced pituitary surgeons in high-volume centers. Major surgical complications include visual loss, CNS infection, stroke, and oculomotor palsy. Craniotomy is occasionally needed for masses with extrasellar extensions that may be inaccessible by the transsphenoidal route, with higher risk for complications. Postoperatively patients need to be monitored for signs of diabetes insipidus and secondary adrenal insufficiency, which may be transient or permanent.

---

[1]Not FDA approved for this indication.

TABLE 2	Use of Dopamine Agonists in Hyperprolactinemia			
	ROUTE	DOSING FREQUENCY	STARTING DOSE	USUAL DOSE RANGE
Bromocriptine	PO intravaginal[1]	Twice a day	1.25 mg after dinner or before bed for 1 week, then twice a day	2.5–10 mg/day
Cabergoline	PO	Once to twice a week	0.25 mg twice a week or 0.5 mg once a week	0.5–2 mg/week

[1]Not FDA approved for this indication.

Radiotherapy

Radiotherapy is inadequate as a primary treatment for prolactinoma, as its efficacy is poor and latency long. It is also associated with long-term complications including permanent hypopituitarism, cerebrovascular accidents, and secondary intracranial malignancies. Currently it is reserved mostly for patients with aggressive and malignant prolactinomas failing medical/surgical treatment. Stereotactic radiosurgery is preferred over conventional fractionated radiotherapy for more convenient dosing, better efficacy, and lower rate of complications. However, radiosurgery should not be attempted for tumors in close proximity to the visual apparatus (less than 5 mm of clearance), as it is associated with an unacceptably high rate of vision loss.

Management of Prolactinoma During Pregnancy

Mild hyperprolactinemia is part of normal pregnancy, and there are concerns for the safe use of dopamine agonists in pregnant women. There is convincing evidence that as long as bromocriptine is withdrawn within a week after confirmation of pregnancy, obstetric outcome is not altered. Less robust data to date suggest that continuing bromocriptine treatment till term is also safe. Despite its longer half-life, as long as cabergoline is discontinued in early pregnancy, it also has not been found to be associated with adverse outcomes. Until there is incontrovertible evidence for the absolute safety of these dopamine agonists, however, it is prudent to discontinue these drugs as soon as pregnancy is confirmed. Given its shorter half-life and established safety record, bromocriptine is the preferred agent for fertility induction in women with hyperprolactinemia, although cabergoline would also be acceptable if bromocriptine is not tolerated. The major indication to treat prolactinomas medically during pregnancy is the concern for tumor expansion. Such risk is negligible for microprolactinomas. For patients with macroprolactinoma, however, symptomatic tumor expansion during pregnancy can occur in up to about 30% of cases. This risk can be significantly reduced if the patient has been treated with a dopamine agonist for at least a year with evidence of tumor shrinkage, or has undergone pituitary surgery or radiotherapy prior to pregnancy. Until these conditions are met, women of childbearing age with macroprolactinomas should be advised to take nonhormonal contraceptive measures. For patients who fail to achieve tumor shrinkage with dopamine agonists or cannot tolerate them, prophylactic surgery prior to pregnancy may be considered, after careful discussion with the patient on surgical risks and the possibility of permanent hypopituitarism, which further impairs fertility. The Endocrine Society practice guidelines recommend against measurement of serum prolactin levels during pregnancy. Instead the patient should be followed clinically for any signs or symptoms of tumor expansion. MRI without gadolinium and visual field testing should be done when clinical suspicion arises. If tumor expansion is confirmed, the patient should be reinitiated on bromocriptine. Debulking surgery is reserved for patients failing or not tolerating medical treatment. Lactation usually does not cause tumor progression, and patients are encouraged to breastfeed their infants with close surveillance. They should not take either bromocriptine or cabergoline, however, as both are secreted in the milk.

Management of Resistant and Malignant Prolactinoma

Several other treatment options are available for patients who fail the highest tolerated doses of dopamine agonists, surgery, and radiation. A small fraction of these patients have malignant prolactinoma, which is defined by extrapituitary metastasis; histopathologically, malignant prolactinomas can appear very similar to aggressive prolactinomas. An alkylating agent, temozolomide (Temodar)[1], has been successfully used in the treatment of aggressive pituitary adenoma and pituitary carcinoma. Monotherapy with temozolomide has been established as the first-line chemotherapy for these conditions, following documented tumor growth despite standard therapies. Selective estrogen receptor modulators (SERMs), including raloxifene (Evista)[1] and tamoxifen (Nolvadex)[1], have been found to be useful adjuncts that can reduce prolactin level and inhibit tumor growth.

References

Ahuja N, Moorhead S, Lloyd AJ, Cole AJ: Antipsychotic-induced hyperprolactinemia and delusion of pregnancy, *Psychosomatics* 49:163–167, 2008.

Bernard V, Young J, Chanson P, Binart N: New insights in prolactin: pathological implications, *Nat Rev Endocrinol* 11:265–275, 2015.

Bronstein MD: Disorders of prolactin secretion and prolactinomas. In Jameson JL, De Groot LJ, editors: *Endocrinology: Adult and Pediatric*, 7th ed., Philadelphia, 2016, Elsevier.

Chanson P, Maiter D: Prolactinoma. In Molmed S, editor: *The Pituitary*, 4th ed., San Diego, 2017, Elsevier.

Ciccarelli A, Daly AF, Beckers A: The epidemiology of prolactinomas, *Pituitary* 8:3–6, 2005.

Dekkers OM Lagro J, Burman P, Jorgensen JO, Romijn JA, Pereira AM: Recurrence of hyperprolactinemia after withdrawal of dopamine agonists: systematic review and meta-analysis, *J Clin Endocrinol Metab* 95:43–51, 2010.

Filho RB, Domingues L, Naves L, et al: Polycystic ovary syndrome and hyperprolactinemia are distinct entities, *Gynecol Endocrinol* 23:267–272, 2007.

Glezer A, Bronstein MD: Prolactinomas, cabergoline, and pregnancy, *Endocrine* 47:64–69, 2014.

Grattan DR: 60 years of neuroendocrinology: the hypothalamo-prolactin axis, *J Endocrinol* 226:T101–T122, 2015.

Horseman ND, Gregerson KA: Prolactin. In Jameson JL, De Groot LJ, editors: *Endocrinology: Adult and Pediatric*, 7th ed., Philadelphia, 2016, Elsevier.

Huang W, Molitch ME: Evaluation and management of galactorrhea, *Am Fam Physician* 85:1073–1080, 2012.

Melmed S, Casanueva FF, Hoffman AR, et al: Diagnosis and treatment of hyperprolactinemia: an Endocrine Society clinical practice guideline, *J Clin Endocrinol Metab* 96:273–288, 2011.

Melmed S, Kleinberg D: Pituitary masses and tumors. In Melmed S, et al, editors. Williams Textbook of Endocrinology, 13th ed., Philadelphia, 2016, Elsevier.

Miyai K, Ichihara K, Kondo K, Mori S: Asymptomatic hyperprolactinaemia and prolactinoma in the general population: mass screening by paired assays of serum prolactin, *Clin Endocrinol (Oxf)* 25:549–554, 1986.

Molitch ME: Drugs and prolactin, *Pituitary* 11:209–218, 2008.

Raverot G, Burman P, McCormack A, et al: European Society of Endocrinology Clinical Practice Guidelines for the management of aggressive pituitary tumors and carcinomas, *Eur J Endocrinol* 178:G1–G24, 2018.

Samson SL, Hamrahian AH, Ezzat S: American Association of Clinical Endocrinologists, American College of Endocrinology disease state clinical review: clinical relevance of macroprolactin in the absence or presence of true hyperprolactinemia, *Endocr Pract* 21:1427–1435, 2015.

Schlechte J, Dolan K, Sherman B, et al: The natural history of untreated hyperprolactinemia: a prospective analysis, *J Clin Endocrinol Metab* 68:412–418, 1989.

Stiegler C, Leb G, Kleinert R, et al: Plasma levels of parathyroid hormone-related peptide are elevated in hyperprolactinemia and correlated to bone density status, *J Bone Miner Res* 10:751–759, 1995.

Testa G, Vegetti W, Motta T, et al: Two-year treatment with oral contraceptives in hyperprolactinemic patients, *Contraception* 58:69–73, 1998.

Vartej P, Poiana C, Vartej I: Effects of hyperprolactinemia on osteoporotic fracture risk in premenopausal women, *Gynecol Endocrinol* 15:43–47, 2001.

HYPERTHYROIDISM

Method of
William J. Hueston, MD

CURRENT DIAGNOSIS

- Hyperthyroidism or thyrotoxicosis is most often caused by Graves' disease, toxic nodular goiter (Plummer's disease), or acute thyroiditis.
- Common symptoms in hyperthyroidism are tachycardia, elevated systolic blood pressure, tremor, and anxiety. Patients with Graves' disease also might exhibit exophthalmos. In contrast, elderly patients can present with apathetic hyperthyroidism, which can be confused with hypothyroidism.
- Hyperthyroidism should be suspected in all patients who present with atrial fibrillation, palpitations, panic disorder, or unexplained tremors.
- Thyroid storm is an acute, life-threatening condition usually occurring in patients with undiagnosed or untreated hyperthyroidism placed under physiologic stress.
- An elevated free T_4, usually with a low thyroid-stimulating hormone is the hallmark of hyperthyroidism, and anti–thyroid-stimulating hormone antibodies can help identify Graves' disease.

- Ultimately, a thyroid scan and uptake are usually necessary to differentiate the cause of hyperthyroidism.
- Subclinical hyperthyroidism is an uncommon finding of uncertain long-term clinical significance but treatment for patients over 65 with cardiac disease or osteoporosis should be considered.

CURRENT THERAPY

- In patients with Graves' disease or autonomous thyroid nodules (toxic nodular goiter), short-term treatment includes thyroid suppression medications (such as methimazole [Tapazole]) and β-blockers (such as propranolol [Inderal][1]). Long-term management with radioiodine thyroid gland ablation is often pursued once symptoms are controlled.
- Patients with acute thyroiditis might need transient β-blockade but can often be managed expectantly until symptoms abate and thyroid hormone levels normalize. A small number of patients (~10%) have persistent hypothyroidism after an episode of illness.
- Thyroid storm is a medical emergency that requires close monitoring along with an antithyroid drug, β-blockers, corticosteroids, and iodine-potassium solution (Lugol's solution).

[1]Not FDA approved for this indication.

Epidemiology

Hyperthyroidism is relatively uncommon and usually caused by three conditions: Graves' disease, toxic nodular goiter, or acute thyroiditis. Graves' disease is the most common cause of hyperthyroidism in the United States and usually affects younger patients from the teens to the 40s. Like other autoimmune diseases, women are at higher risk (seven to eight times) than men. Toxic nodular goiter accounts for 15% to 30% of hyperthyroid diagnoses. It usually occurs after age 50 years, is more common in women, and follows several decades of multinodular thyroid disease. A less-common cause is administration of amiodarone. Amiodarone is about one third iodine and can cause hyperthyroidism either through iodine-induced thyroid damage or from increased thyroxine synthesis owing to excessive iodine.

Subclinical hyperthyroidism, defined as an abnormally low TSH but normal free thyroxine (T$_4$) and triiodothyronine (T$_3$) affects 1% to 2% of the population. This condition is most common with mild forms of hyperthyroidism but also can be observed transiently in thyroiditis. Subclinical hyperthyroidism is more common in individuals over age 70 and those with iodine-deficient diets.

Risk Factors

There are no known environmental or reversible risk factors for any of the causes of hyperthyroidism. Graves' disease is associated with a specific human leukocyte antigen (HLA) region on chromosome 6 (CTLA 4).

Pathophysiology

The most common causes of hyperthyroidism are shown in Box 1.

Graves' disease is an autoimmune disorder caused by antibodies against thyroid-stimulating hormone (TSH) receptors on the thyroid gland. Graves' disease is associated with many other autoimmune diseases, including pernicious anemia, vitiligo, type 1 diabetes mellitus, autoimmune adrenal disease, Sjögren's syndrome, rheumatoid arthritis, and lupus. As with these other disorders, the etiology is unknown.

Toxic nodular goiter, also known as Plummer's disease, results from the development of autonomous thyroid adenoma. Patients who develop a toxic nodular goiter usually have a long history of

---

BOX 1 Conditions Causing Hyperthyroidism

Graves' disease
Autonomous thyroid nodule (toxic nodular goiter)
Acute thyroiditis
- Hashimoto's thyroiditis
- Subacute granulomatous thyroiditis (de Quervain's thyroiditis)
- Subacute lymphocytic thyroiditis (silent or painless thyroiditis)
- Suppurative thyroiditis (bacterial infection of thyroid)
Excessive exogenous thyroid use
- Over-replacement after thyroid ablation or for hypothyroidism
- Thyroxine (Synthroid) abuse for weight loss
Iodine overconsumption
Amiodarone administration

---

many other nodules that spontaneously burn out over time, but then develop a single large nodule (usually 2.5 cm or greater) that continues to produce thyroid hormone in such large quantities that patients become hyperthyroid. No clear cause is known for the development of the nodules.

Acute thyroiditis can also produce hyperthyroidism. Several different conditions can cause thyroiditis (see Box 1). The inflammation resulting in thyroiditis is thought to be related to subacute viral infections or autoimmune reactions; suppurative thyroiditis is a rare bacterial thyroid infection, usually caused by *Staphylococcus aureus*. During the acute period of thyroid inflammation, damage to the gland leads to the release of stored thyroxine from thyroid lakes, producing hyperthyroidism. However, after the initial release of thyroid hormone from the stored lakes, damage to the gland inhibits production of new thyroxine. After the initial surge in thyroid hormone levels, thyroxine levels drop, often to levels that can result in transient hypothyroidism. Most patients return to the euthyroid state after the thyroid gland heals, but about 10% of patients with acute thyroiditis remain chronically hypothyroid.

Other, less common causes of hyperthyroidism include excessive exogenous administration of thyroid medications. This is most commonly the result of over-replacement of thyroxine (Levoxyl, Synthroid) in patients with hypothyroidism, but it may be intentional for weight loss. Because thyroxine and triiodothyronine (T$_3$) are highly protein bound, over-replacement is most common if patients experience hypoproteinemia, such as in nephrotic syndrome, cirrhosis, or malnutrition.

Excessive iodine consumption, referred to as the Jod-Basedow effect, can also lead to thyrotoxicosis. The source of the iodine may include iatrogenic sources such as iodine-containing medications or radiologic contrast agents.

Several other medications, such as amiodarone (Cordarone), lithium, and interferon α (Intron A) also can cause thyrotoxicosis by causing drug-induced thyroiditis.

Prevention

There are no known strategies to prevent hyperthyroidism. For patients with hypothyroidism, annual monitoring of TSH levels is recommended to ensure that patients receive the appropriate replacement dose and not over-replacement.

Clinical Manifestations

Patients with hyperthyroidism complain of a variety of symptoms that can include anxiety, tachycardia, wide-pulse pressure hypertension, palpitations, fine tremor, weight loss, heat intolerance, and, particularly in the elderly, confusion or delirium. Patients with Graves' disease also have ophthalmopathy characterized by lid retraction and exophthalmoses that can lead to optic nerve damage. In contrast, older patients can have few of the classic signs of hyperthyroidism and instead might complain of fatigue or weakness (apathetic hyperthyroidism), unexplained delirium, weight loss, heart failure, or isolated atrial fibrillation.

Some patients have a rapid escalation of symptom severity (thyroid storm) that is life-threatening if not identified and treated promptly. These patients usually have underlying thyrotoxicosis from Graves' disease complicated by a secondary physiological stressor such as infection, surgery, or trauma. This is a medical emergency and needs immediate attention, including hospitalization with close observation.

On physical examination, patients with hyperthyroidism due to Graves' disease or thyroiditis might have a diffusely enlarged and mildly tender thyroid gland. In suppurative thyroiditis, the thyroid gland is red, hot, and very tender and accompanied by a fever and other systemic signs of severe infection. Patients with toxic nodular goiter can have palpable nodules in their thyroid gland and often have a single palpable nodule.

Diagnosis

Hyperthyroidism is diagnosed by finding an elevation in the free thyroxine (T_4) level accompanied by a low TSH level. Patients with Graves' disease often have positive anti–thyroid receptor antibody titers. Only anti-thyroglobulin receptor antibody testing is helpful because it can help differentiate Graves' disease from other causes. No other anti-thyroid tests are clinically indicated. Once the thyroid level abnormalities are found, a definitive diagnosis of the cause for the hyperthyroidism is needed to select the appropriate treatment strategy.

Other conditions can produce a depressed TSH but normal free T_4 levels. These include T_3 toxicosis and subclinical hyperthyroidism. T_3 toxicosis refers to situations where triiodothyronine (T_3) is produced in excess rather than thyroxine (T_4); this can occur in any of the conditions that can cause hyperthyroidism, as well as in surreptitious triiodothyronine (Cytomel) ingestion.

Thyroid scanning and radiolabel uptake are usually necessary to differentiate the causes of hyperthyroidism. Thyroid scanning and uptake rely on the thyroid gland to concentrate radioactive molecules, such as iodine-131 (^{131}I) or technetium. Because of the risk of thyroid storm with iodine administration, patients should be treated with antithyroid drugs for 2 to 8 weeks before a scan and the drugs should be stopped at least 4 days before the test. Patients with Graves' disease show increases in uptake and diffuse distribution of the tracer throughout the thyroid gland. Patients with toxic nodular goiter also have increased uptake, but the isotope is concentrated in a one or a few focal areas, with the remainder of the thyroid gland suppressed. In contrast, patients with thyroiditis have decreased uptake of the radiolabel and a washed-out or mottled distribution on scanning.

Differential Diagnosis

Symptoms of hyperthyroidism also occur in patients with panic disorder and other anxiety conditions. These patients can have sinus tachycardia, tremor, and nervousness that mimic hyperthyroidism.

Treatment

Treatment depends on the cause of the hyperthyroidism (Table 1). In Graves' disease, immediate goals of treatment include reducing thyroid hormone production and blocking the peripheral effects of the excessive thyroid hormone. About 30% to 60% of patients, mostly adolescents, enter remission spontaneously, and the remission may be permanent. Remission rates are highest for those with a small goiter, no ophthalmopathy, thyroglobulin levels less than 50 µg/mL, and thyroxine levels less than 20 µg/dL. Signs of remission include a decreased ratio of T_3 to T_4, lower thyroid-stimulating thyroglobulin levels, and decreased radioactive iodine uptake on rescanning. When remissions do occur, it is usually within a year of starting antithyroid medications.

For those who do not undergo spontaneous remission, which includes most adults, consideration should be given to thyroid

TABLE 1	Treatment Strategies for Hyperthyroidism	
TREATMENT	**DRUG**	**DOSAGE**
Graves' Disease and Toxic Nodular Goiter		
Thyroid hormone suppression	Methimazole Propylthiouracil	Initial: 30–40 mg/d Maintenance: 5–15 mg/d Initial: 300–400 mg/d Maintenance: 100–300 mg/d
β-Blockade	Propranolol[1] Metoprolol (Lopressor)[1]	10 mg qid 50–100 mg bid
Thyroid gland removal	Radioactive iodine ablation Thyroidectomy	
Acute Thyroiditis		
β-Blockade transiently May need thyroid replacement long term		
Thyroid Storm		
Thyroid hormone suppression	Propylthiouracil	300–400 mg/d
β-Blockade	Propranolol[1]	1 mg/min IV to max 10 mg[3]
Iodine	Lugol's solution	1–2 gtt mixed in water tid
Cardiac and fluid monitoring	Dexamethasone (Decadron)[1]	2 mg q6h

[1]Not FDA approved for this indication.
[3]Exceeds dosage recommended by the manufacturer.

gland ablation to permanently treat this condition. Although the dosage can be calculated to attempt to leave patients euthyroid, permanent hypothyroidism occurs in about half of all patients treated with radioactive iodine ablation.

The initial approach to toxic nodular goiter is similar to that for symptom control, but thyroid ablation should be recommended routinely because remissions are very rare.

Thyroid gland production of hormone can be reduced rapidly with either methimazole (Tapazole) or propylthiouracil. For treatment of Graves' disease, methimazole is the preferred treatment and has the advantage of less frequent dosing, which improves compliance. Propylthiouracil is an alternative that is recommended for women in the first trimester of pregnancy and patients who cannot tolerate methimazole. However, the FDA issued a black box warning about the use of propylthiouracil in 2010 because of liver toxicity; physicians should be aware of this and use propylthiouracil only when methimazole is not suitable. With both drugs, clinicians need to be aware of drug-associated agranulocytosis, which can result in life-threatening bacterial infections. In patients on either of these medications who develop a sore throat, fever, or other signs of infection, a white blood cell count should be done immediately to ensure that they are not neuropenic. Additionally, antithyroid drugs are associated with drug-induced lupus syndromes and other forms of vasculitis.

In addition to reducing production of thyroid hormone, initial therapy for patients with Graves' disease and toxic nodular goiter should include a β-blocker to reduce the tachycardia, tremor, hypertension, and anxiety. A β-blocker that crosses the blood-brain barrier, such as propranalol (Inderal)[1] or metoprolol (Lopressor)[1], is the best choice in this situation because these also

[1]Not FDA approved for this indication.

reduce the central nervous system effects such as anxiety, as well as the vascular problems caused by thyroid hormones.

Thyroid storm requires immediate attention and should be managed in the hospital setting, especially in older patients where tachycardia and hypertension can lead to cardiac instability. Prompt administration of β-blockers and propylthiouracil along with cardiac monitoring for dysrhythmias and appropriate fluid management are essential for managing this life-threatening condition. Once antithyroid drugs have been administered, iodine-potassium solution (Lugol's solution) at a dose of 1 or 2 drops three times a day should be administered, which will further reduce thyroid hormone production and reduce peripheral conversion of T_4 to T_3. Finally, corticosteroids also have been shown to rapidly reduce thyroid hormone levels in thyroid storm.

For long-term management, thyroid ablation with radioactive iodine (sodium iodide, ^{131}I) can restore patients to a permanent euthyroid state. However, radioactive iodine thyroid ablation often results in destruction of more thyroid than optimal, causing hypothyroidism. Radioactive iodine thyroid ablation is contraindicated in pregnancy. For patients in whom radioactive iodine is either contraindicated or not acceptable, thyroidectomy is an option. Thyroidectomy almost always results in permanent hypothyroidism, as well as having other risks inherent in surgery including hypoparathyroidism and recurrent laryngeal nerve damage.

In patients with hyperthyroidism associated with acute thyroiditis, symptoms often resolve by the time the evaluation is complete. In the interim, symptoms can be managed with β-blockers. β-Blocker therapy can be discontinued fairly rapidly (2 to 3 weeks) after the initial onset of symptoms.

Indications for the treatment of subclinical hyperthyroidism are less clear. Based on recommendations of the American Thyroid Association, patients with a persistently low TSH who are over age 65 or who have underlying cardiac disease or osteoporosis should be considered for treatment. The treatment strategy should be directed at the presumed cause of the condition and may include antithyroid medication for suspected Graves' disease or thyroid ablation for toxic nodular goiter or a solitary autonomous nodule.

Monitoring

In patients on antithyroid drugs, thyroid hormone levels should be monitored frequently until they reach a stable euthyroid state. Any change in the patient's underlying health, especially changes that could alter protein levels, should prompt reevaluation. In addition, patients who have thyroid ablation need follow-up testing of TSH and free T_4 levels to ensure that sufficient thyroid tissue has been destroyed to reverse their hyperthyroidism but not make them hypothyroid. This should be done 6 to 8 weeks following ablation therapy.

Complications

Complications of hyperthyroidism include acute and chronic conditions. Acutely, the most concerning complications are cardiac dysrhythmias, especially atrial fibrillation. Chronically, excessive thyroxine is associated with cardiomyopathy and osteoporosis. In patients with ophthalmopathy, untreated Graves' disease can lead to progressive vision loss and blindness.

Hyperthyroidism in pregnancy, even when adequately treated, has been shown to be an independent risk factor for cesarean section but not for any additional pregnancy complications. Some patients with existing hyperthyroidism may experience transient increases in free T_4 levels during pregnancy that can be associated with hyperemesis gravidarum. Assessing free T_4 levels in pregnant patients who have hyperthyroidism and develop hyperemesis may be useful.

References

Cooper DS: Antithyroid drugs for the treatment of hyperthyroidism caused by Graves' disease, *Endocrinol Metab Clin North Am* 27:225–247, 1998.
Kharlip J, Cooper DS: Recent developments in hyperthyroidism, *Lancet* 373:1930–1932, 2009.
Lazarus JH: Hyperthyroidism, *Lancet* 349:339–343, 1997.
Nayak B, Hodak SP: Hyperthyroidism, *Endocrinol Metab Clin North Am* 36(3):617–656, 2007.
Zimmerman D, Lteif AN: Thyroxicosis in children, *Endocrinol Metab Clin North Am* 27:109–126, 1998.
Donangelo I, Suh SY: Subclinical hyperthyroidism: When to consider treatment, *Amer Family Phys* 95:710–716, 2017.

HYPOKALEMIA AND HYPERKALEMIA

Method of
Jie Tang, MD

CURRENT DIAGNOSIS

- The "initial approach" to the evaluation of dyskalemia is to determine if it is secondary to transcellular shifts (in vitro or in vivo) of potassium (K), or a result of a true change in total body K.
- A thorough history and physical will provide useful information regarding the causes of hypokalemia and hyperkalemia, especially in cases of low or high intake of K, and transcellular shifts.
- Key steps in the diagnostic approach to hypokalemia include assessments of urinary K excretion and acid-base status.
- Key steps in the diagnostic approach to hyperkalemia include assessments of renal function and aldosterone activity.

CURRENT THERAPY

- For both hypokalemia and hyperkalemia, it is critical to assess the underlying transcellular K shift, given the risk of rebound hyperkalemia after K repletion or hypokalemia after K restriction and removal.
- In cases of severe dyskalemia, close cardiac monitoring is needed.
- The aggressiveness of therapy for dyskalemia is directly related to the rapidity with which the condition has developed, the absolute level of serum K, and the clinical evidence of toxicity.
- In severe or symptomatic cases of hypokalemia, both intravenous and oral K repletion are often needed.
- In severe or symptomatic cases of hyperkalemia, supported by ECG abnormalities, both immediate temporizing measures and definitive therapy for K removal are necessary.

Epidemiology

Hypokalemia is defined as a serum K level of 3.5 mmol/L or lower. It is a common electrolyte disorder encountered in clinical practice. According to one study, serum K < 3.6 mmol/L was found in up to 20% of hospitalized patients. The majority of these patients had serum K concentrations between 3.0 and 3.5 mmol/L, but as many as 25% had values < 3.0 mmol/L. Even mild or moderate hypokalemia increases the risks of morbidity and mortality in patients with cardiovascular disease.

Hyperkalemia is defined as a serum K of 5.5 mmol/L or higher. The prevalence among hospitalized patients not yet on dialysis was reported to be about 3.3%, and among them, up to 10% had significant hyperkalemia (≥ 6.0 mmol/L). Hyperkalemia also carries a significantly increased risk of mortality.

Risk Factors

People most at risk for hypokalemia are those who are malnourished, with poor oral intake; those who use certain medications, such as diuretics; and those who have uncontrolled vomiting or diarrhea. People most at risk for hyperkalemia are those with reduced kidney function, those who have a history of diabetes mellitus, or those who take certain medications, such as angiotensin-converting enzyme inhibitors.

Pathophysiology

K is the most abundant cation in the human body. It regulates intracellular enzyme function and helps determine neuromuscular and cardiovascular tissue excitability. The total body store is approximately 55 mmol/kg of body weight. Over 98% of total body K is located in the intracellular fluid (primarily in muscle), and less than 2% in the extracellular fluid. A typical western diet provides 40 to 120 mmol of K per day. Tight control of the serum K is primarily accomplished by the kidney, where ~95% of body K is excreted. Under normal circumstances, K losses in stool and sweat are small. In addition, the interplay of several hormonal systems (insulin, catecholamine), serum tonicity, and the internal acid-base environment contribute to the exchange of K between the extracellular fluid and intracellular fluid, which helps keep the serum K concentration tightly controlled.

Hypokalemia occurs when there is a significant intracellular K shift or a reduced total body K store from poor intake, or excessive renal or extrarenal loss, whereas hyperkalemia develops when there is a significant extracellular shift, high body K load, or ineffective K elimination (aldosterone resistance/deficiency or reduced renal function).

Prevention

For patients at risk for hypokalemia, adequate dietary K intake is essential. Additional K supplements may be needed for patients taking high doses of diuretics (especially thiazide diuretics) or experiencing prolonged vomiting or diarrhea. For patients with hyperkalemia and severe kidney dysfunction, dietary K restriction is critical in maintaining body K balance. Sometimes, the empirical use of K exchange resin is needed to prevent hyperkalemia. Lastly, medications that contribute to hypokalemia or hyperkalemia should be avoided if possible.

Clinical Manifestations

Mild hypokalemia (serum K 3.0–3.5 mmol/L) is usually well tolerated. Moderate hypokalemia (serum K 2.5–3.0 mmol/L) may cause nonspecific symptoms, such as fatigue, weakness, muscle cramps, and constipation. When the serum K drops to < 2.5 mmol/L, muscle necrosis and flaccid paralysis with eventual respiratory failure may occur. K depletion also causes supraventricular and ventricular arrhythmias, especially in patients on digitalis therapy. Although severe hypokalemia is more likely to cause complications, even minimal decreases in serum or total body K can be arrhythmogenic in patients with underlying heart disease or who are receiving digitalis therapy. Lastly, increases in systolic and diastolic blood pressures can occur in patients with hypokalemia while they are on a liberal salt diet. Overall, the likelihood of symptoms tends to correlate with the rapidity of the decrease in serum K.

As with hypokalemia, patients with hyperkalemia may present with nonspecific complaints such as fatigue and malaise. But the predominant manifestations in more severe hyperkalemia are neuromuscular and cardiac. Neuromuscular symptoms range from muscle weakness to paralysis. Cardiac arrhythmias, including asystole, ventricular tachycardia or fibrillation, and pulseless electrical activity, can also occur in severe hyperkalemia.

Diagnosis

Figures 1 and 2 illustrate the diagnostic approaches to hypokalemia and hyperkalemia. It is important to assess for pseudodyskalemia (in vitro shift of K) and dyskalemia from in vivo transcellular shift of K, because neither is associated with disturbances in total body K balance. Although cellular shift of K and changes in total body K occur as isolated problems, they frequently coexist. In hypokalemia, the assessment of renal K excretion is a key step in the initial diagnostic evaluation, followed by the assessment of acid-base status. In hyperkalemia, medical history and laboratory testing can help identify altered K distribution, reduced urinary K excretion or an excessive K load from exogenous intake or transcellular leakage. Under normal circumstances, high K intake alone is not sufficient to lead to significant hyperkalemia unless there are other risk factors present such as reduced aldosterone action, or significant loss of kidney function.

Measurement of the trans-tubular potassium gradient (TTKG) has been widely used as a diagnostic tool in both conditions. However, recent evidence suggests that the assumption inherent in the calculation of the TTKG lacks validity. Therefore I no longer use TTKG in the clinical assessment of patients with dyskalemia.

Differential Diagnosis

Figures 1 and 2 outline a diagnostic approach, including differential diagnosis, for hyperkalemia and hypokalemia.

Therapy

The treatment of hypokalemia depends on the underlying cause, the degree of K depletion, and the risk of K depletion to the patient. In general, hypokalemia secondary to cell shift is managed by treating underlying conditions. For example, hypokalemia in the setting of catecholamine increases, as in chest pain syndromes, is managed with appropriate treatments for the pain. However, when cell-shift hypokalemia is associated with life-threatening conditions such as paresis, paralysis, or hypokalemia in the setting of myocardial infarction, the administration of K is indicated. With K depletion, replacement therapy depends on the estimated degree of decreases in total body K. For example, decreases in total body K accompanied by a fall in serum K from 3.5 to 3.0 mmol/L are associated with a K deficit of 150 to 200 mmol. Decreases in serum K from 3 to 2 mmol/L are associated with 200- to 400-mmol additional decreases in total body K. K can be administered intravenously, but in limited quantities (10 mEq/h into a peripheral vein; 15–20 mEq/h into a central vein). Larger K requirements can only be accomplished by oral therapy or with dialysis.

The treatment of hyperkalemia depends on the presence or absence of ECG and neuromuscular abnormalities. In the absence of symptoms or ECG abnormalities, hyperkalemia is treated conservatively—for example, by decreasing dietary K or withdrawing offending drugs. In the presence of ECG abnormalities or symptoms, the goal of therapy is to stabilize cell membranes. First-line therapy includes calcium gluconate, 10 to 30 mL IV as a 10% solution (onset of action 1 or 2 min). Although the mechanism remains undefined, calcium "stabilizes" the cardiac membranes. Other therapies include 8.4% IV sodium bicarbonate,[1] 50 to 150 mEq (onset 15–30 min), and rapid-acting insulin[1] 5 to 10 units intravenously (onset 5–10 min). Insulin increases the activity of the Na-K-ATPase pump in skeletal muscle and drives K into cells. Glucose 50%, 25 g intravenously, is given simultaneously with insulin to prevent hypoglycemia. Albuterol inhalation solution 0.5%,[1] 20 mg in 4 mL normal saline by nebulizer (onset 15–30 min), also activates the Na-K-ATPase and drives K into cells. K driven intracellularly generally begins to move extracellularly again after approximately 6 hours, increasing the serum K concentration. Therefore therapy to remove K from the body should be started simultaneously. Reductions in total body K may be achieved through a K exchange resin. The primary K resin used is sodium polystyrene sulfonate (Kayexalate). One gram of this medication binds approximately 1 mEq of K and releases 1 to 2 mEq of sodium back into the circulation. This medication may be given orally (onset 2 hours) or by enema with sorbitol to induce diarrhea (onset 30–60 minutes). If renal function is adequate, volume expansion with simultaneous diuresis can be attempted. Finally, hemodialysis is very effective in removing excess K.

---

[1] Not FDA approved for this indication.

Figure 1 The diagnostic approach to hypokalemia. *Abbreviations:* ACS = acute coronary syndrome; ATN = acute tubular necrosis; DKA = diabetic ketoacidosis; FEK = fractional excretion of K; GI = gastrointestinal; Met = metabolic; RTA = renal tubular acidosis.

Figure diagram

```
Hyperkalemia (Serum K ≥5.5 mmol/L)
```

No further workup ◄—Yes— Pseudohyperkalemia —— Severe leukocytosis

Severe thrombocytosis

Tissue breakdown/cell lysis
- Rhabdomyolysis
- Massive hemolysis
- Resolving hematoma
- Trauma
- Tumor lysis

High K load —— History and Physical, corresponding tests —Transcellular shift—

Low endogenous insulin/catecholamines

Acidosis

Hyperglycemia

Hyperkalemic periodic paralysis

Medications:
- Mannitol
- Beta-blockers
- Succinylcholine
- Somatostatin
- Octreotide
- Digitalis

1. Acute renal failure or Advanced CKD (GFR<20ml/min)*
2. Reduced renal tubular flow from low sodium
3. Reduced effective renal blood flow

—— Reduced renal K excretion ——

Other medications:
1. Collecting tubule Na/K ATPase blockade
   - Cyclosporin
   - Tacrolimus
2. ENAC blockade
   - Amiloride
   - Triamterene
   - Trimethoprim
   - Pentamidine

—— TTKG<5 ——

Primary hypoaldosteronism

Secondary hypoaldosteronism
1. Renin deficiency/resistance
   - Diabetes mellitus
   - RTA-4
   - Multiple myeloma
   - Meds: β blocker; direct renin inhibitor; NSAIDS
2. Aldosterone deficiency/resistance
   - Addison's disease
   - RTA-4
   - Renal tubulointerstitial disease
   - Hereditary diseases: Gordon's syndrome, pseudohypo-aldosteronism type 1
   - Medications: ACEI/ARB; Heparin; Spironolactone; Eplerenone

Figure 2 The diagnostic approach to hyperkalemia. *Hyperkalemia may occur with higher GFR if K load is excessive. *Abbreviations:* ACEI = angiotensin-converting enzyme inhibitor; ARB = angiotensin receptor blocker; ENAC = epithelial sodium channel; GFR = glomerular filtration rate; NSAIDS = non-steroidal anti-inflammatory drugs; RTA = renal tubular acidosis.

Monitoring

Treatment for severe or symptomatic dyskalemia requires close cardiac monitoring and frequent laboratory testing to prevent over-correction. If insulin and glucose are used in patients with hyperkalemia, blood sugars should be monitored for approximately 6 hours to identify and treat hypoglycemia from the insulin.

Complications

Complications from dyskalemia include cardiac arrhythmias, neuromuscular events, and, rarely, death. There are potential treatment-related complications if pseudodyskalemia or dyskalemia from in vivo transcellular shift are not recognized.

References

Paice BJ, Paterson KR, Onyanga-Omara F, et al: Record linkage study of hypokalaemia in hospitalized patients, *Postgrad Med J* 62:187–191, 1986.
Gennari FJ: Hypokalemia, *N Engl J Med* 339:451–458, 1998.
Stevens MS, Dunlay RW: Hyperkalemia in hospitalized patients, *Int Urol Nephrol* 32:177–180, 2000.
Krishna GG, Kapoor SC: Potassium depletion exacerbates essential hypertension, *Ann Intern Med* 115:77–83, 1991.

HYPONATREMIA

Method of
Beejal Shah, MD; and Susan L. Samson, MD, PhD

CURRENT DIAGNOSIS

- Perform a thorough history and physical examination with focus on the accurate assessment of volume status, neurologic symptoms and signs, current medications, and concurrent illnesses.
- Classify the hyponatremia as hypovolemic, euvolemic, or hypervolemic.
- Determine whether the hyponatremia is acute or chronic, based on the history and the clinical manifestations.
- Order the key laboratory tests, including a basic metabolic panel (serum sodium, glucose, blood urea nitrogen, and creatinine), plasma osmolality, urine osmolality, and urine sodium.

- Severe and symptomatic hyponatremia should be treated with hypertonic saline (3%) at 1 to 2 mL/kg per hour. Neurologic status and serum sodium should be monitored every 2 to 4 hours. The objective is to raise sodium by 2 mEq/L per hour (or to >125 mEq/L) until deleterious neurologic symptoms improve. After this, the rate of infusion should be titrated to increase the serum sodium by 0.5 to 1.0 mEq/L per hour, with a maximum increase of 10 to 12 mEq/L over 24 hours and no more than 18 mEq/L over 48 hours, to avoid precipitating osmotic demyelination.
- As a general rule, the treatment of hyponatremia should be adjusted so that the serum sodium increases by 0.5 to 1.0 mEq/L per hour with a maximum increase of 10 to 12 mEq/L over 24 hours and no more than 18 mEq/L over 48 hours. Acute hyponatremia (<48 hours) may be treated more rapidly than chronic hyponatremia if dictated by neurologic findings. Treat SIADH with fluid restriction, medications, or observation; rule out adrenal insufficiency and hypothyroidism.
- Most cases of euvolemic hyponatremia are caused by the syndrome of inappropriate antidiuretic hormone (SIADH), which usually can be managed with fluid restriction, salt tablets, and demeclocycline (Declomycin)[1] in refractory cases.
- Discontinue thiazide diuretics in all cases of hypoosmolar hyponatremia.
- Hypovolemic and hypervolemic hyponatremia require therapy to correct the underlying cause (e.g., heart failure) and restore status to euvolemia.
- Vasopressin receptor antagonists (vaptans) are approved for short term management of euvolemic and hypovolemic hyponatremia. The same parameters apply for rate of sodium correction and monitoring as in conventional therapy.

[1]Not FDA approved for this indication.

Homeostasis maintains the concentration of sodium in the serum between 138 and 142 mEq/L (normal, 135–145 mEq/L) despite variations in water intake. Hyponatremia is defined as a serum sodium concentration of less than 135 mEq/L. It is one of the most common electrolyte abnormalities found in the inpatient setting, occurring in up to 2.5% of patients, and it is a significant marker for mortality, associated with a 60-fold higher risk of death. It is not clear whether hyponatremia itself is the cause of a more adverse prognosis or whether it echoes the degree of stress caused by illness. In the outpatient setting, chronic hyponatremia is most prevalent among the elderly and nursing home residents. The approach to management of hyponatremia is highly dependent on the underlying process. Establishing the correct etiology is critical, because inappropriate treatment can worsen hyponatremia. Therapy must be administered judiciously because of the risk of severe neurologic sequelae, including central nervous system demyelination. However, with a systematic approach to the differential diagnosis of hyponatremia, the correct diagnosis can be made and therapy initiated.

Clinical Presentation
Acute hyponatremia is defined as hyponatremia of less than 48 hours in duration. Mild symptoms include headache, nausea, vomiting, confusion, and weakness, which usually occur with a sodium level of less than 129 mEq/L. More severe neurologic manifestations—seizure and coma—are seen usually below a threshold of 120 mEq/L, although there currently is no evidence-based critical sodium level above which neurologic sequelae do not occur. The neurologic manifestations of acute or recurrent symptomatic hyponatremia can be delayed, so continued monitoring is important.

In contrast, patients with chronic hyponatremia more often are asymptomatic or have blunted symptoms. In elderly patients with mild chronic hyponatremia, subtle neurocognitive manifestations can occur, with decreased balance, lowered reaction speed, memory loss, and directed gait. Mild hypoosmolar hyponatremia is not independently associated with increased morbidity and mortality. Even so, the underlying etiology needs to be determined because of the potential for other factors (e.g., new medications, dehydration, occult illness) to contribute to the development of more severe hyponatremia with its potential for neurologic injury.

Regulation of Water Balance
Approximately two thirds of total body water is contained in the intracellular fluid (ICF) and one third as extracellular fluid (ECF). Plasma osmolality is tightly regulated between 280 and 290 mOsm/kg and reflects the osmolality of the ECF. A change in plasma osmolality results in a shift of total body water between the ECF and the ICF to maintain their osmolar equivalence. Because sodium is the major osmole in the ECF, hyponatremia most often is a manifestation of decreased osmolality, so-called hypoosmolar or hypotonic hyponatremia.

Renal Handling of Water
The major osmoregulatory hormone is arginine vasopressin, also called antidiuretic hormone, which is synthesized in the paraventricular and supraoptic nuclei of the hypothalamus. It is transported along axons to the posterior pituitary, where it is processed and stored in vesicles. Vasopressin secretion is regulated by osmotic and nonosmotic stimuli. Secretion occurs with a 1% to 2% rise in osmolality (>288 mOsm/kg), as detected by receptors in the anterolateral walls of the hypothalamus adjacent to the third ventricle. Vasopressin secretion is inhibited when the plasma osmolality is lower than 280 mOsm/kg. The major nonosmotic stimulus is a decrease in effective circulating volume, which is detected by baroreceptors in the aortic arch and carotid sinuses. Although this mechanism requires a large drop (10%–15%) in blood pressure, the secretory response is more robust than for increases in osmolality. As such, acutely lowered blood pressure can override the inhibitory signal of low osmolality because of the need to maintain perfusion. Other physiologic nonosmotic stimuli include catecholamines and angiotensin II, but there is a long list of hormones and pharmacologic agents that induce or repress vasopressin secretion (Table 1).

The renal site of action of vasopressin is the V_2 receptors on the basolateral membrane of collecting duct cells in the distal nephron. The hormone-receptor interaction initiates intracellular signaling via cyclic adenosine monophosphate–dependent pathways, resulting in translocation of cytoplasmic aquaporin-2 channels to the surface of the collecting duct luminal membrane. These channels allow movement of water back into the cell for later reabsorption into the circulation. This results in a net concentration of urine and decreased plasma osmolality.

Renal Handling of Sodium
In addition to renal water handling, sodium reabsorption and excretion are important for maintenance of water homeostasis. The renin-angiotensin-aldosterone system is activated by reduced arterial perfusion pressure sensed by the juxtaglomerular apparatus of the afferent renal arteriole. Reduced arteriole effective volume (low or perceived) is sensed by the juxtaglomerular apparatus, which secretes renin, activating the renin-angiotensin system. This cascade of events ultimately stimulates aldosterone secretion, which acts at the distal nephron to cause reabsorption of filtered sodium via Na^+,K^+-adenosine triphosphatase (ATPase)–dependent sodium channels.

Central Nervous System Response to Hyponatremia/Hypoosmolality
Osmolar equivalence between the ECF and ICF is closely maintained by shifts in water between the two compartments. The major symptoms and signs of hyponatremia are neurologic in nature and are a clinical manifestation of swelling of the cells in the central nervous system, which results in cerebral edema.

TABLE 1	Molecules That Regulate Vasopressin Secretion
STIMULATE VASOPRESSIN RELEASE	**INHIBIT VASOPRESSIN RELEASE**
Hormones and Neurotransmitters	
Acetylcholine (nicotinic)	Atrial natriuretic peptide
Histamine (H₁)	γ-Aminobutyric acid
Dopamine (D₁ and D₂)	Opioids (κ receptors)
Glutamine	
Aspartate	
Cholecystokinin	
Neuropeptide Y	
Substance P	
Vasoactive inhibitory peptide	
Prostaglandin	
Angiotensin II	
Pharmacologic Agents	
Vincristine (Oncovin)	Ethanol
Cyclophosphamide (Cytoxan)	Phenytoin (Dilantin)
Tricyclic antidepressants	Low-dose morphine
Selective serotonin reuptake inhibitors	Glucocorticoids Fluphenazine (Prolixin)
Nicotine	Haloperidol (Haldol)
Adrenaline (epinephrine)	Promethazine (Phenergan)
High-dose morphine	Butorphanol (Stadol)

Figure 1 The differential diagnosis of hypoosmolar hyponatremia. *Abbreviations:* RTA = renal tubular acidosis; SIADH = syndrome of inappropriate antidiuretic hormone.

The most devastating consequence is herniation due to anatomic limitations on brain volume within the confines of the skull. Premenopausal women are at the highest risk for brain injury from hyponatremia.

A major compensatory mechanism in the central nervous system is the extrusion from the cells of intracellular solutes, which prevents further water influx. In the first few hours, inorganic ions (potassium, sodium, chloride) move out of the cell. After a few days of persistent hypoosmolality, the cells further compensate by extruding organic osmoles (glutamate, taurine, inositol). The clinician must be aware of this protective adaptation, because it necessitates a slower time course of correction during treatment. A rapid rise in plasma osmolality from aggressive treatment causes water to rapidly shift out of the cells, resulting in demyelination of neurons. In the past, this was termed pontine demyelinosis, but it has also been reported for extrapontine neurons and is now referred to as osmotic demyelination. The sequelae are permanent and devastating. There is clinical progression from lethargy to a change in affect, to mutism and dysarthria, and finally to spastic quadriparesis and pseudobulbar palsy.

Classification and Differential Diagnosis of Hyponatremia

Initial evaluation of hyponatremia requires a systematic and sequential approach. First, a thorough history and physical examination are required. It is important to identify any history of brain injury, stroke, mental illness, or chronic illness and the patient's current medication usage. On examination, special attention should be paid to mental status and neurologic abnormalities; manifestations of cardiac, hepatic, or renal disease; and signs of adrenal insufficiency or hypothyroidism. From the assessment of volume status, the hyponatremia should be classified as hypervolemic, euvolemic, or hypovolemic; each of these conditions leads in a different direction for diagnosis and treatment of the underlying cause (Figures 1 and 2). Finally, it should be

determined whether the hyponatremia is acute (<48 hours) or chronic, because this can determine the time course of treatment.

For the laboratory work-up, essential basic tests are the serum sodium and potassium levels, renal function tests with blood urea nitrogen (BUN) and creatinine, and liver function tests. It is likely that these tests have already been performed, motivating the assessment of hyponatremia. After this, the plasma osmolality (P_{Osm}), urine osmolality (U_{Osm}), and urine sodium concentration are key diagnostic tests. P_{Osm} is directly measured in the laboratory and also can be calculated. Calculated osmolality is the sum of the concentrations of the known major osmoles—sodium and glucose—in the ECF and the BUN:

$$P_{Osm} = (2 \times Na) + (glucose) + (BUN)$$

The calculation is done in SI units. For sodium, mEq/L is the same as the SI unit, mmol/L; if glucose and BUN values were reported in mg/dL, they must be divided by 18 and 2.8, respectively, to convert to SI units (mmol/L). The directly measured osmolality should be within 10 to 12 mOsm/kg of the calculated value; an increased osmolar gap compared with the calculated value points toward the presence of additional osmoles in the plasma that are causing hypertonicity.

Because hyponatremia usually is a reflection of plasma osmolality, most patients also have a low P_{Osm}, and the clinician often can proceed to the differential diagnosis of hypoosmolar (or hypotonic) hyponatremia after excluding pseudohyponatremia (which usually has normal osmolality) and hyperosmolar hyponatremia. Pseudohyponatremia can occur if the plasma lipid or protein content is greatly increased in the plasma (usually to >6%–8% of volume), as in extreme hypertriglyceridemia and paraprotein disorders. These extra components decrease the aqueous portion of the plasma volume and thereby interfere with the laboratory measurement of sodium by dilutional, indirect methods such as flame photometry. Most laboratories now use direct measurement of sodium to avoid this problem.

Hyperosmolar hyponatremia can occur if there are additional osmoles present that cause water movement from the ICF into the ECF, resulting in ECF expansion and dilutional hyponatremia. Overall, the total body water and total body sodium are unchanged in this situation. An important clinical example occurs with hyperglycemia, and the reported sodium value should be corrected for high glucose by the clinician by adding 1.6 mEq/L to the measured Na for every 100 mg/dL rise in glucose above 200

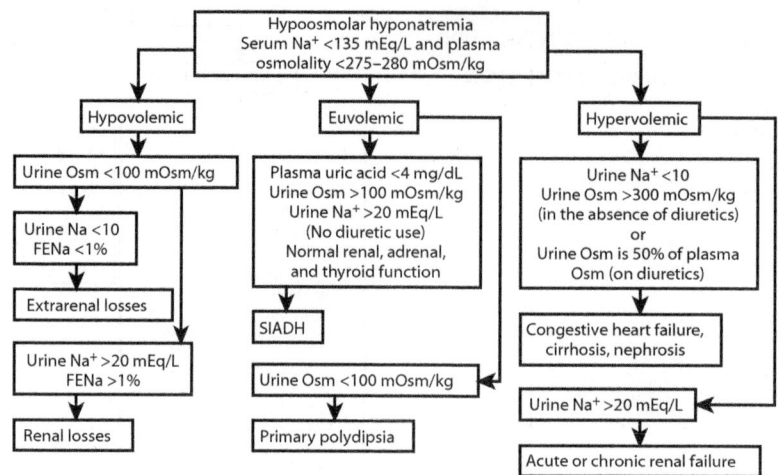

Figure 2 Laboratory findings in hypoosmolar hyponatremia. *Abbreviations:* FENa = fractional excretion of sodium; Osm = osmoles; SIADH = syndrome of inappropriate antidiuretic hormone.

mg/dL. Because glucose is included in the calculation of osmolality, there will be no significant osmolar gap.

Other osmotically active solutes encountered clinically are mannitol, which is used to manage increased intracranial pressure, and glycine, which is used for irrigation in urologic procedures. Mannitol and glycine are retained in the ECF and are not part of the calculated osmolality, so their presence results in an osmolar gap. High levels of alcohol or ethylene glycol also increase the osmolality, but these substances are so quickly metabolized that an osmolar gap may not be apparent by the time testing is performed.

Once pseudohyponatremia and hypertonicity have been ruled out, the diagnosis is narrowed to hypoosmolar hyponatremia. The combined physical examination and laboratory results allow classification of the patient as having hypervolemic hyponatremia with excess total body sodium, hypovolemic hyponatremia with a deficit of total body sodium, or euvolemic hyponatremia with near-normal total body sodium.

Hypovolemic Hyponatremia

The causes of hypovolemic hyponatremia can be classified as extrarenal or renal (see Figure 1). Signs of volume contraction are apparent on examination, including poor skin turgor, skin tenting (forehead), decreased or undetectable jugular venous pressure, dry mucous membranes, and orthostatic changes in blood pressure and pulse rate. If the volume status is not completely clear from the examination, laboratory values can be helpful (see Figure 2), but they need to be interpreted in the context of renal function tests. If the urine osmolality is less than maximally concentrated (<500 mOsm/kg), an infusion of 0.5 to 1 L of isotonic saline over 24 to 48 hours may help with differentiation. With hypovolemia, the sodium will begin to correct and the patient should improve clinically. Conversely, if the patient is actually euvolemic, such as with syndrome of inappropriate antidiuretic hormone (SIADH), discussed later, the serum sodium level will remain constant or decrease due to retention of free water with a concomitant increase in urinary sodium.

Extrarenal causes of hyponatremia include gastrointestinal losses and third-space losses such as in severe burns and pancreatitis. In the volume-depleted state, with intact renal function, the urine sodium is low (<10 mEq/L), reflecting a normal response by the kidney to maximally reabsorb sodium in response to volume depletion.

The renal causes of hypovolemic hyponatremia involve the inappropriate loss of sodium into the urine, and this is reflected by a urine sodium concentration of greater than 20 mEq/L.

Thiazide diuretics cause renal sodium loss, so the urine sodium is high. However, they also impair the kidney's diluting capacity, decreasing free water excretion and concentrating the urine. Only certain patients may be susceptible to hyponatremia while on thiazides. These patients may have an abnormally sensitive thirst response to the mild hypovolemia induced by the diuretics, causing increased water intake. Elderly women are the most susceptible, and hyponatremia can occur within days after initiation of thiazide therapy. Additional laboratory results reveal hypokalemia and a metabolic alkalosis. It is appropriate to stop the diuretic and restore potassium levels and volume status. Patients often have a recurrence of hyponatremia if rechallenged with thiazides. Loop diuretics, such as furosemide, are a less frequent cause of hyponatremia, which occurs only after long-term therapy.

In the absence of diuretic use, a urine sodium concentration greater than 20 mEq/L with hypovolemia is evidence for underlying renal pathology. Patients with salt-wasting nephropathy, from a number of causes (see Figure 1), usually have significant renal failure, with a creatinine value in the range of 3 to 4 mg/dL. Because of the large net sodium loss, this condition is treated with salt tablets. Renal tubular acidosis causes bicarbonaturia, which requires a compensatory excretion of urinary cations, mainly Na^+ and K^+, to maintain electroneutrality. Similarly, excretion of ketones into the urine also demands additional electrolyte losses in spite of ECF volume depletion, leading to a loss of sodium.

Cerebral salt wasting (CSW), although it could be considered an extrarenal cause, also involves the renal loss of sodium (>20 mEq/L). The biochemical presentation is very similar to that of SIADH, but the diagnosis of CSW is restricted to cases involving extreme central nervous system pathology. CSW is most commonly associated with subarachnoid hemorrhage but also has been reported with stroke, brain trauma, infection, metastases and after neurosurgery. Onset of CSW is usually within the first 10 days after the neurologic event.

CSW may be a protective mechanism against increased intracranial pressure. The proposed pathophysiologic mechanism of CSW is controversial, but one hypothesis is that the initiating event is a primary natriuresis, with renal loss of sodium, caused by the secretion of natriuretic peptides. Clinical studies have found both increased brain natriuretic peptide and increased atrial natriuretic peptide in neurosurgical patients with hyponatremia. Both hormones are vasodilators that increase the glomerular filtration rate while suppressing the renin-angiotensin system. This increases renal sodium losses, as well as water excretion, resulting in volume depletion. Vasopressin levels rise in response to low volume, so that it becomes biochemically difficult to differentiate CSW from SIADH, with a urine sodium level greater than 20 mEq/L, low uric acid, and high urine osmolality. It is helpful if CSW patients have signs of volume depletion in combination with the laboratory results. Also, the hyponatremia of CSW responds to normal saline, whereas SIADH worsens with normal saline. CSW is relatively rare in most case series, and it is important to rule out other causes for natriuresis.

Hypervolemic Hyponatremia

There are a variety of causes of hypervolemic hyponatremia (see Figure 1), all of which are a result of decreased effective circulating volume. To correct this imbalance, the ECF expands, leading to fluid retention and hyponatremia. In spite of the increased total body water and low serum sodium on testing, all of these patients have some degree of total body sodium excess. In many cases, volume overload is clinically evident from the presence of subcutaneous edema, ascites, elevated jugular venous pressure, or pulmonary edema.

In congestive heart failure (CHF), patients can develop hyponatremia with only 2 to 3 L of fluid intake per day despite normal renal function. The decreased filling pressures and cardiac output of CHF are perceived as volume depletion, detected by the baroreceptors. This stimulates vasopressin secretion, overriding the signal of low osmolality detected by the hypothalamic osmoreceptors. This lack of inhibition of vasopressin secretion is believed to be the most important contributing factor to the development of hyponatremia. In addition, decreased right atrial pressures result in inhibition of secretion of atrial natriuretic peptide, contributing to the water and sodium gain. With the low perfusion pressure, there is a decrease in the glomerular filtration rate, which is sensed by the juxtaglomerular apparatus, causing neurohumoral activation of the renin-angiotensin system and sympathetic nervous system. This leads to increased circulating levels of catecholamines, angiotensin II, and aldosterone, further stimulating tubular sodium and water reabsorption. In the absence of diuretics, the urine sodium level is very low (<10 mEq/L) in patients with CHF because of activation of the renin-angiotensin-aldosterone system and maximal tubular reabsorption of sodium. Also, there is less than maximally dilute urine (usually >300 mOsm/kg) in the absence of diuretic therapy. An elevated brain natriuretic peptide concentration helps to confirm the hypervolemia.

A similar mechanism is at work in cirrhotic patients, in whom the incidence of hyponatremia is even higher and is a strong predictor of poor outcome. In cirrhosis, low albumin results in third-spacing and decreased effective circulating volume. In addition, portal hypertension leads to splanchnic vasodilation, which also decreases the effective circulating volume. This serves to activate vasopressin secretion and the renin-angiotensin-aldosterone system.

Hyponatremia is less common in acute and chronic renal failure, but it can occur with a significant decrease in glomerular filtration rate accompanied by severe hypoalbuminemia. Interpretation of the laboratory results may be confounded by a high urine sodium concentration (>20 mEq/L) that reflects the concomitant presence of tubular dysfunction. Hyponatremia can develop in stage IV or V renal failure when fluid intake is in excess of 3 L/day.

Euvolemic Hyponatremia

Euvolemic hyponatremia is caused by impaired excretion of free water by the kidney. The differential diagnosis is more limited (see Figure 1) and the majority of cases are due to SIADH (Table 2). However, this often is a diagnosis of exclusion, and hypothyroidism and adrenal insufficiency must be ruled out clinically or biochemically in patients with euvolemic hyponatremia.

Hypothyroidism leads to reduced glomerular filtration rate and decreased flow to the distal nephron, causing maximal reabsorption of water to maintain arterial volume. Hypothyroidism has to be severe to cause hyponatremia and usually is obvious on examination. However, in the elderly population, apathetic hypothyroidism may be difficult to diagnose. Hypothyroidism can be confirmed by the presence of a high level of thyroid-stimulating

TABLE 2	Causes of SIADH		
CNS DISORDERS	**PULMONARY DISORDERS**	**MEDICATIONS/DRUGS**	**OTHER**

Mass lesions
  Tumors
  CNS abscess Intracranial
  hemorrhage or hematoma
	Viral/bacterial pneumonia
	Positive-pressure ventilation
	Bronchogenic carcinoma (small cell)
	Acute respiratory failure
		Vasopressin analogues
		  (Desmopressin [DDAVP])
		NSAIDs
		Tricyclic antidepressants
			Pain
			Nausea
			AIDS
			Prolonged exercise

Stroke	COPD	Phenothiazines	Idiopathic
CNS infections or inflammatory diseases	Tuberculosis	Butyrophenones	Acute intermittent porphyria
Spinal cord lesions	Aspergillosis	SSRIs	
Acute psychosis	Pulmonary abscess	Morphine	
Pituitary stalk lesions		Opiates	
Hydrocephalus		Chlorpropamide (Diabinese)	
Dementia		Clofibrate (Atromid-S)[2]	
Guillain-Barré syndrome		Cyclophosphamide (Cytoxan)	
Head trauma		Vincristine (Oncovin)	
		Nicotine	
		Tolbutamide (Orinase)	
		Barbiturates	
		Acetaminophen (Tylenol)	
		ACE inhibitors	
		Carbamazepine (Tegretol)	
		Omeprazole (Prilosec)	
		MDMA (Ecstasy)	

[2]Not available in the United States.

Abbreviations: ACE = angiotensin-converting enzyme; AIDS = acquired immunodeficiency syndrome; CNS = central nervous system; COPD = chronic obstructive pulmonary disease; DDAVP = 1-deamino, 8-D arginine-vasopressin; MDMA = methylenedioxymethamphetamine; NSAIDs = nonsteroidal antiinflammatory drugs; SSRIs = selective serotonin reuptake inhibitors.

hormone and a low level of free T_4 (thyroxine). Treatment involves thyroid hormone replacement and supportive care.

In primary adrenal insufficiency (Addison's disease), the concomitant aldosterone deficiency results in hyponatremia combined with hyperkalemia, prerenal azotemia, a urine sodium concentration greater than 20 mEq/L, and a urine potassium level lower than 20 mEq/L. In secondary or central adrenal insufficiency, the adrenal zona glomerulosa remains intact for the secretion of aldosterone. However, glucocorticoid deficiency still causes impaired water excretion, which can lead to dilutional hyponatremia. Vasopressin release may be stimulated by the nausea, vomiting, and orthostatic hypotension that occurs with adrenal insufficiency. Finally, corticosteroids normally inhibit vasopressin release, so their deficiency leads to enhanced vasopressin release, causing retention of free water that further contributes to the hyponatremia. The appropriate diagnostic test is a 250-µg ACTH (cosyntropin, Cortrosyn) stimulation test, although an extremely low 8 AM cortisol level (<3 µg/dL) can be diagnostic. Treatment consists of glucocorticoid replacement.

Syndrome of Inappropriate Antidiuretic Hormone

SIADH is the most common cause of euvolemic hypoosmolar hyponatremia. Edema, ascites, and orthostasis are absent, and thyroid, adrenal, and renal functions are normal. Recent diuretic use should be ruled out. The primary event is the release of vasopressin, which results in water retention. The increased intravascular volume stimulates a natriuresis, which actually is appropriate, but the resulting loss of sodium compounds the hyponatremia. There is an extensive list of causes of SIADH, usually involving pulmonary or central nervous system pathology (see Table 2). A number of medications also are known to stimulate vasopressin release or to potentiate its antidiuretic properties at the level of the kidney (see Tables 1 and 2).

The diagnosis of SIADH is suggested by a low P_{Osm} (<280 mOsm/kg) with a high U_{Osm} (>100 mOsm/kg), confirming water retention and an inappropriately concentrated urine. A spot urine sodium level will be greater than 20 mEq/L, and usually greater than 30 mEq/L. Other helpful laboratory findings include low plasma uric acid (<4 mg/dL), which has a positive predictive value of 73% to 100% for SIADH in this setting. In complicated cases confounded by use of diuretics, the fractional excretion of uric acid has a positive predictive value of 100% for SIADH when the calculated excretion is greater than 12%.

Reset osmostat can be considered a form of SIADH, but the hyponatremia is usually chronic, mild, and asymptomatic. Vasopressin release continues to be regulated, but at a lower threshold of plasma osmolality. The thirst threshold may be altered as well. Interventions to raise the sodium usually have short-lived effects, and the sodium resets at its previous value over time. Therefore, treatment is not recommended if the sodium level is stable and the patient is asymptomatic. A physiologic example of reset osmostat is seen in pregnancy, when the normal sodium range is lowered by 5 mEq/L.

Other Causes of Euvolemic Hypoosmolar Hyponatremia

Primary or psychogenic polydipsia should be considered in patients presenting with hyponatremia and a history of psychiatric illness and treatment. Almost 6% to 7% of psychiatric inpatients are at risk for hyponatremia from increased water intake. The polydipsia may be related to a lowered osmolar threshold for thirst, below the threshold of suppression of vasopressin secretion. This can be further complicated by the side effect of dry mouth caused by many psychiatric medications, which compounds the increased thirst and water intake. Because the kidney is capable of excreting up to 15 to 20 L/day of dilute urine, the fact that hyponatremia develops in these patients may point toward an additional and inappropriate increase in vasopressin release or sensitivity. These patients are clinically euvolemic because of renal excretion of the excess water and have otherwise normal laboratory results except for a dilute urine (<100 mOsm/kg), which is caused by vasopressin suppression and helps differentiate primary polydipsia from SIADH. However, some patients

have mildly concentrated urine (>100 mOsm/kg), in which case the psychiatric history helps with the diagnosis.

Exercise-induced hyponatremia (e.g., from marathon running) is a form of euvolemic hypoosmolar hyponatremia primarily caused by retention of water relative to fluid lost via sweating or renal excretion. Vasopressin levels are inappropriately increased during exercise-induced hyponatremia. Most importantly, it is an acute hyponatremia, developing in less than 24 hours, and should be treated accordingly.

Vasopressin levels also may be inappropriately high, secondary to pain or the use of NSAIDs, which remove prostaglandin inhibition of vasopressin release. Low solute intake combined with high fluid intake also can cause hyponatremia, as with beer potomania or a low-protein "tea and toast" diet in elderly patients. In both cases, the lack of solute in the urine does not allow retention of water in the filtrate, so the excess water is not excreted.

Hyponatremia also is common after pituitary surgery (transsphenoidal or by craniotomy) and may be a result of damage to the hypothalamic-pituitary tract that causes release of preformed vasopressin from damaged neurons. Often, hyponatremia occurs as the second phase of the classic triphasic response: transient diabetes insipidus, transient SIADH, followed by permanent diabetes insipidus. Hyponatremia can be delayed up to 1 week postoperatively, and sodium should be monitored during the second week as well. Contributions by central adrenal insufficiency and hypothyroidism also are considerations after pituitary surgery, although with these conditions there will be obvious clinical manifestations in addition to the hyponatremia.

Management

The major considerations for choosing the type and time course of treatment for hyponatremia are the duration of hyponatremia (acute or chronic) and the presence of neurologic signs and symptoms, especially severe manifestations such as altered mental status or seizure (see Table 2). Treatment options for hyponatremia include fluid restriction, saline infusion (hypertonic or isotonic), vasopressin receptor antagonists and demeclocycline (Declomycin).[1] Also, treatment of the underlying abnormality, such as CHF or salt wasting, and correction of volume status are important for hypovolemic or hypervolemic patients. Autocorrection may occur after initiation of therapy, especially in cases of hypovolemia, adrenal insufficiency, or thiazide use. Once treatment is started, the contribution of the nonosmotic stimulation of vasopressin secretion is removed, and the patient is able to raise the sodium level by 2 mEq/L per hour over 12 hours.

Acute Severe Symptomatic Hyponatremia

Acute severe hyponatremia is defined as a rapid fall in sodium in less than 48 hours to less than 120 mEq/L. Under these circumstances, most patients develop neurologic symptoms because of the rapid fluid shifts between the ECF and the ICF in the brain. If left untreated, it can result in irreversible neurologic damage and death. Because of the acute drop in sodium, initial rapid correction is acceptable and should not lead to osmotic demyelination. Treatment is aimed at raising the sodium enough to resolve the neurologic signs and symptoms. The goal is to raise the serum sodium by 1 to 2 mEq/L per hour or to greater than 125 mEq/L until symptoms resolve. Hypovolemic patients will respond to infusion of isotonic saline (normal saline 0.9%), especially if the urine sodium concentration is less than 30 mEq/L. If the neurologic findings are severe, hypertonic saline (3%) may be infused at rate of 1 to 2 mL/kg per hour, or even up to 4 to 6 mL/kg per hour if the imbalance is life-threatening. A loop diuretic can be combined with the saline to enhance solute-free water excretion. In exercise-induced hyponatremia, hypertonic (3%) saline is the preferred treatment to prevent cerebral edema due to water shifting into the brain along the osmotic gradient. A hypertonic (3%) saline 100 mL bolus can be given to promptly to decrease

---

[1] Not FDA approved for this indication.

Parameters for acute or chronic hyponatremia:
Do not increase serum Na by more than 9 mEq in 24 hours and 18 mEq in 48 hours

Symptomatic hyponatremia with severe neurologic symptoms (acute <48 hrs or chronic >48 hrs)
1. Correct serum Na at a rate of 1–2 mEq/l per hour (for 2 to 4 hours) until symptoms have resolved
2. Correct Na at a rate of less than 9 mEq/24 h

Acute hyponatremia symptoms
1. Correct at rate of 0.5 to 1 mEq/L per hour to a maximum of 9 mEq/24 h

Chronic hyponatremia with mild symptoms or asymptomatic
1. Correct at a rate of 0.5 mEq/L per hour with fluid restriction
2. Treat underlying etiology

Calculation of the rate of infusion of saline to correct hyponatremia
1. Change in serum sodium per liter infusate

$$(\Delta Na/L) = \frac{Infusate\ [sodium] - Serum\ [sodium]}{TBW + 1}$$

2. Amount of infusate (in L) required in 24 hours

$$L = \frac{desired\ change\ in\ sodium\ (\Delta Na)\ over\ 24\ hrs}{\Delta Na/L\ (from\ 1)}$$

3. Rate of infusate to raise serum Na by desired amount

$$ml/hr = \frac{L\ (from\ 2) \times 1000\ mL/L}{24\ hr}$$

4. (Simplified) Hypertonic saline infused at 1–2 mL/kg per hour

Monitoring:
1. Monitor frequently for clinical improvement or worsening of symptoms
2. If on hypertonic saline or severely symptomatic check sodium q2–4 hrs.
3. If undergoing treatment but asymptomatic, check sodium q6–12 h.

Infusate	Infusate [Na] (mmol/L)
5% sodium chloride in water	855
3% sodium chloride in water	513
Isotonic saline (0.9%)	154
Ringer's lactate solution	130
0.45% sodium chloride in water	77
0.2% sodium chloride in water	34
5% dextrose in water	0

Total Body Water (TBW) is equal to 60% of body weight in young adult men and 50% in young adult women. Older patients have less TBW. In elderly males, TBW is equal to 50% of body weight and in elderly females it is 45%.

Figure 3 Treatment of hyponatremia. *Abbreviation:* TBW = total body water.

the osmotic gradient, which is promoting water entry into cells. Thereafter, in the inpatient setting, hypertonic (3%) saline infusion should be continued to promote correction of hyponatremia. Sodium levels should be monitored every 2 to 4 hours in patients undergoing hypertonic infusion. Once symptoms resolve, the rate of correction should be reduced to 0.5 to 1 mEq/hr, and the total rise in sodium should not exceed 18 mEq in 48 hours. No benefit has been observed for faster rates of correction of hyponatremia, whether acute or chronic. Useful formulas to determine the rate of infusion for fluids are provided in Figure 3. The formulas can only estimate the rate of correction, and sodium should be measured frequently.

Chronic Hyponatremia
Chronic hyponatremia is defined as a gradual fall in sodium over more than 48 hours. By this time, the brain has begun to compensate for hypoosmolality by extrusion of solutes. However, the patient is at risk of osmotic demyelination if hyponatremia is treated too aggressively. If the duration of hyponatremia is unknown, the recommendation is to assume that it is chronic. However, as with acute hyponatremia, severe neurologic symptoms and signs need to be treated with hypertonic saline until they resolve, after which the rate of correction can be slowed to 0.5 to 1 mEq/L per hour. Most cases of osmotic demyelination occur with correction rates of greater than 12 mEq/L in 24 hours, but there are cases reported with increases of 9 or 10 mEq/day. Asymptomatic hyponatremia can be treated with an infusion of isotonic saline calculated to raise the sodium by 0.5 to 1 mEq/hour. If the patient has a dilute urine (<200 mOsm/kg), water restriction may be sufficient.

Syndrome of Inappropriate Antidiuretic Hormone
The mainstays of treatment of SIADH are fluid restriction and treatment of the underlying cause. Mild SIADH usually can be controlled with fluid restriction alone.

In most cases of SIADH, the degree of fluid restriction required can be calculated. It is dependent on three factors: the daily osmolar load, the minimum U_{Osm}, and the patient's maximum urine volume. A typical diet has a daily osmolar load of 10 mOsm/kg of body weight. For a 70-kg person, this would be 700 mOsm/day. With SIADH, the urine osmolality is held constant for that particular patient, as revealed by a spot U_{Osm}. If the U_{Osm} is 500 mOsm/

kg and the solute load is 700 mOsm, the fluid load has to be less than 700/500 or 1.4 L/day just to maintain the serum sodium level. Fluid intake above this amount will cause the sodium to decrease.

When needed, salt tablets (sodium chloride tablet 1-3 g taken once to three times daily) can help to make up for renal loss of sodium in SIADH. With symptoms and severe hyponatremia, short-term use of hypertonic saline may also be instituted to restore sodium to the ECF compartment. Loop diuretics (e.g., furosemide [Lasix]) can increase free water clearance when given with solute (e.g., hypertonic saline or salt tablets). In refractory cases, demeclocycline (300–600 mg PO twice daily)[1] can be used. Demeclocycline (Declomycin) antagonizes the actions of vasopressin by inhibiting formation of cyclic adenosine monophosphate in the collecting duct. Long-term use is limited by the side effect of photosensitivity and by nephrotoxicity in patients with underlying liver disease. Vasopressin receptor antagonists also are important adjunct treatments (see later discussion). A less commonly used treatment is urea (powder or capsules),[1,6] which causes an osmotic diuresis and increased free water excretion. Preclinical data support that urea may decrease osmotic demyelination.

Cerebral Salt Wasting
Management of CSW involves treatment of the underlying neurologic problem, as well as volume replacement. CSW often is difficult to differentiate biochemically from SIADH, but the rise in vasopressin in CSW is secondary to volume depletion. As a result, CSW responds to volume replacement with isotonic saline, suppressing release of vasopressin, whereas SIADH worsens with this therapy. The recommended correction rate is 0.7 to 1.0 mEq/L per hour, with a maximum of 9 mEq per 24 hours. Salt tablets may also be given to replete total body sodium. Fludrocortisone (Florinef 0.05 to 0.1 mg every 12 hours), an aldosterone receptor agonist, is a third-line treatment to encourage volume expansion and sodium retention, but the potassium concentration and blood pressure should be monitored. Fluid restriction is inappropriate for CSW and should be avoided, especially in patients with subarachnoid hemorrhage, because volume depletion can exacerbate cerebral vasospasm and cause infarction. The duration of CSW is usually 3 to 5 weeks.

---

[1]Not FDA approved for this indication.
[6]May be compounded by pharmacists.

Vasopressin Receptor Antagonists

Vasopressin receptor antagonists, or vaptans, are a treatment option for clinically significant euvolemic hyponatremia defined as a serum Na <125 mEq/L or if hyponatremia is symptomatic and resistant to correction with standard therapy. Vaptans also can be used for asymptomatic hypervolemic hyponatremia, but the benefit must clearly outweigh the risk, and the patient should be refractory to standard therapy. There are currently two FDA-approved vaptans, conivaptan (Vaprisol) and tolvaptan (Samsca). Conivaptan is a dual V_{1a}/V_2 arginine vasopressin receptor antagonist and tolvaptan is a selective V_2 arginine vasopressor receptor antagonist with about 29 times the affinity to the V_2 receptor compared to conivaptan. The primary action of both medications is to block the binding of vasopressin to its receptors in the distal nephron which leads to a decrease in translocation of the aquaporin-2 channels to the apical membrane of the collecting duct in the renal tubule. As a result, vaptans cause an increase in excretion of solute-free water resulting in a rise in serum sodium.

Conivaptan is an IV formulation approved for inpatient hospital use for euvolemic and hypervolemic hyponatremia. It is contraindicated for hypovolemic hyponatremia, euvolemic or hypervolemic hyponatremia with moderate to severe central nervous system (CNS) symptoms, and hypervolemic hyponatremia due to cirrhosis. Conivaptan should be used very cautiously in patients with hypervolemic hyponatremia due to heart failure because safety data are limited and efficacy has not been clearly established. Conivaptan is not recommended in those with severe renal impairment CrCl < 30 mL/min. Conivaptan is given intravenously with a bolus of 20 mg over 30 minutes in 100 mL of 5% dextrose in water (D5W) followed by a continuous infusion of 20 mg conivaptan diluted in 250 mL of D5W over 24 hours. After the initial day of treatment, conivaptan can be continued for an additional 1 to 3 days. Sodium is monitored every 2 to 4 hours and the dose may be titrated to 40 mg per 24 hours to obtain an increase in sodium of 0.5 to 1.0 mEq/L per hour. In clinical trials, the average rise in serum Na after 4 days of therapy is about 6 mEq/L. During conivaptan treatment, fluid restriction can be liberal or is not required. Close monitoring of the rate of sodium rise, neurologic status, and hemodynamic stability are required and treatment should be discontinued or resumed at a reduced dose if clinically indicated. The most common side effects of conivaptan are infusion site reactions and to a lesser degree headache, hypotension, nausea, constipation, and postural hypotension.

Tolvaptan is an oral V_2 receptor antagonist that carries the same indications for use as conivaptan. Tolvaptan should be initiated only in the hospital setting for careful monitoring of potassium and the rate of Na rise, and then can be used in the outpatient setting. The starting dose is 15 mg once daily and can be titrated to 60 mg daily after the initial 24 hours. Patients should not be on fluid restriction for the first 24 hours of tolvaptan therapy and be advised to drink based on thirst. Tolvaptan carries a risk of serious liver injury. The FDA recommends that tolvaptan should not be used for durations longer than 30 days or in any patient with underlying liver disease. Monitoring parameters are equivalent to conivaptan the drug should be stopped promptly in patients with abnormal liver tests or symptoms of hepatotoxicity. In clinical studies, the average rise in serum Na after 4 days of therapy is 4.2 mEq/L and 5.5 mEq/L after 30 days of therapy. The vaptans are a substrate and potent inhibitor of cytochrome P-450 3A4 isoenzyme (CYP3A4). Prior to initiation of therapy drug-drug interactions should be reviewed with the pharmacists and vaptans are contraindicated with other CYP3A4 inhibitors.

Summary

Hyponatremia is a common electrolyte abnormality and is usually caused by decreased plasma osmolality. Accurate assessment of volume status is a key to determining the underlying cause and choosing the correct treatment approach. The biggest risk of hyponatremia and its treatment is the possibility of severe neurologic sequelae, including fatal cerebral edema and osmotic demyelination. Therefore more aggressive initial treatment is needed in patients with neurologic manifestations (hypertonic saline), but a more conservative approach (e.g., fluid restriction) is needed for less symptomatic patients. Vasopressin antagonists are additional tools for the treatment of euvolemic or hypervolemic hyponatremia refractory to more conservative measures.

References

Androgué HJ: Consequences of inadequate management of hyponatremia, *Am J Nephrol* 25:240–249, 2005.

Cerdà-Esteve M, Cuadrado-Godia E, Chillaron JJ, et al: Cerebral salt wasting syndrome: Review, *Eur J Intern Med* 19:249–254, 2008.

Dineen R, Thompson CJ, Sherlock M: Hyponatremia presentations and management, *Clin Med (Lond)* 17:263–269, 2017.

Ellison DH, Berl T: Clinical practice: The syndrome of inappropriate antidiuresis, *N Engl J Med* 356:2064–2072, 2007.

Fenske W, Störk S, Koschker A: Value of fractional uric acid excretion in differential diagnosis of hyponatremia patients on diuretics, *J Clin Endocrinol Metab* 93:2991–2997, 2008.

Gankam Kengne F, Decauz G: Hyponatremia and the Brain, *Kidney Int Rep* 3:24–35, 2018.

Hew-Butler T, Rosner MH, et al: Statement of the Third International Exercise-Induced Hyponatremia Consensus Development Conference, *Clin J Sport Med.* 25:303–320, 2015.

Hoom EJ, Zieste R: Diagnosis and treatment of hyponatremia: Compilation of the guidelines, *J Am Soc Nephrol* 28:1340–1349, 2017.

Jovanovich AJ, Berl T: Where vaptans do and do not fit in the treatment of hyponatremia, *Kidney Int* 83:563–567, 2013.

Sterns RH, Silver AM, Hix JK: Urea for hyponatremia? *Kidney Int* 87:268–270, 2015.

HYPOPITUITARISM

Method of
Vanessa Ho, MD

CURRENT DIAGNOSIS

- Symptoms can be vague. Having heightened awareness is key to making an early diagnosis with resultant proper treatment.
- The diagnosis of hypopituitarism is based on a combination of brain imaging studies and demonstration of insufficiency of one or more pituitary hormones.
- Always confirm the diagnosis before initiating treatment.

CURRENT THERAPY

- Primary treatment of hypopituitarism is cortisol replacement.
- Treatment for hypopituitarism can be an emergency in severe cases because cortisol is responsible for supporting peripheral vascular function.
- Use higher doses of cortisol in cases of stress such as illnesses or high-risk surgeries to aid in proper recovery.

Epidemiology

In one study published in 2001 comprising a population of 146,000 in northwestern Spain, the prevalence of hypopituitarism is as high as 45.5 cases per 100,000 individuals. The incidence is estimated to be 4.2 per 100,000 per year. About 50% of patients had 3 to 5 pituitary hormonal deficiencies, with luteinizing hormone/follicle-stimulating hormone (LH/FSH) being the most prevalent. Patients with tumor-induced hypopituitarism showed a tendency to suffer growth hormone (GH) deficiency more frequently than those resulting from nontumor causes.

Risk Factors

The most common cause of hypopituitarism is pituitary tumors (61%), followed by nonpituitary tumors (9%) (Table 1). Thirty

TABLE 1	Causes of Hypopituitarism

Pituitary and nonpituitary tumors

Pituitary surgery

Pituitary radiation

Inflammatory disease—lymphocytic hypophysitis, sarcoidosis, hemochromatosis, histiocytosis X

Infectious disease—tuberculosis, syphilis

Infarction—Sheehan's syndrome, also referred to as postpartum hypopituitarism, is attributed to infarction of the pituitary gland caused by hypovolemia from obstetric hemorrhage

Pituitary apoplexy—a potentially life-threatening syndrome that occurs as a result of hemorrhage, infarction, or hemorrhagic infarction within a pituitary tumor

Genetic diseases—multiple endocrine neoplasia-1 (MEN-1) is the most common; additional genetic problems are caused by pit-1 mutation

Traumatic brain injury

Stroke—both ischemic stroke and subarachnoid hemorrhage

Suppression of hypothalamic-pituitary axis by chronic exogenous steroid use

percent of cases are caused by nontumors. Nontumor causes include inflammatory diseases such as lymphocytic hypophysitis, sarcoidosis, hemochromatosis, and histiocytosis X. Infectious causes include tuberculosis and syphilis. Over the last few years, awareness and detection rates of hypopituitarism after traumatic brain injury (TBI) and subarachnoid hemorrhage (SAH) have steadily increased. Various studies have shown that cases of hypopituitarism resulting from postradiotherapy radiation damage are also on the rise. With radiation doses of 30 to 50 Gy, the incidence of GH deficiency can reach 50% to 100%; long-term gonadotropin, TSH, and ACTH deficiencies occur in 20% to 30%, 3% to 9%, and 3% to 6% of patients, respectively. With higher dose cranial irradiation (>60 Gy), or after conventional irradiation for pituitary tumors (30–50 Gy), multiple hormonal deficiencies occur in 30% to 60% after 10 years of follow-up.

Some degree of hypopituitarism is found in 35% to 40% of patients who have suffered TBI. A rule of three-quarters can be applied clinically for hypopituitarism after TBI: three-quarters of cases are male <40 years of age, three-quarters of cases occur after road traffic accidents, and three-quarters of cases manifest within 1 year.

Hypopituitarism has been observed in 19% of patients with ischemic stroke and 47% of patients with SAH, presenting as an isolated deficiency in most cases. Major risk factors for developing hypopituitarism after ischemic stroke include certain clinical conditions, such as preexisting diabetes mellitus and medical complications during hospitalization. Patients with Alberta Stroke Programme early CT scores of 7 or less have a poorer prognosis and a higher risk of developing hypopituitarism after an ischemic stroke compared with those with a score greater than 7.

Chronic exogenous steroid use is also a known cause of hypopituitarism. In one study published in 2009, Dr. Lansang and colleagues presented cases of hypopituitarism followed by multiple intraarticular and epidural injections of steroids.

Pathophysiology
The pituitary gland is a pea-sized endocrine gland that sits at the base of the brain. Often referred to as the "master gland," the pituitary gland synthesizes and releases various hormones that affect several organs throughout the body (Figure 1). It is composed of two functionally distinct structures that differ in embryologic development and anatomy: the adenohypophysis (anterior pituitary) and the neurohypophysis (posterior pituitary). The anterior pituitary is responsible for GH, prolatin, adrenocorticotropic hormone (ACTH), thyroid-stimulating hormone (TSH), lutein (LH), and follicular-stimulating hormone (FSH). The posterior pituitary is responsible for vasopressin and oxytocin.

Therefore any damage to the pituitary gland can cause an array of symptoms ranging from generalized weakness, generalized fatigue, low blood pressure, electrolyte abnormalities, mental confusion, and even disorientation.

Prevention
In most cases, the condition is not preventable. Awareness can lead to early detection and proper treatment. As little as 7.5 mg of prednisone/prednisolone (Millipred) or 0.75 mg of dexamethasone (Decadron) daily for more than 3 weeks can suppress the HPA axis. This suppression may last for months after the exogenous steroid is stopped. Therefore, to reduce the risk of developing suppression of the HPA axis, we recommend the use of steroids for the shortest time possible and in the smallest dose possible, and to taper down the steroids slowly if used for longer than 2 weeks.

Clinical Manifestation
Signs and symptoms of hypopituitarism vary, depending on which pituitary hormones are deficient and how severe the deficiency is. They may include
- ACTH deficiency—generalized fatigue, generalized weakness, failure to thrive, tachycardia, hypotension, electrolyte abnormalities, confusion, and even disorientation
- TSH deficiency—fatigue, weight gain, cold intolerance
- Gonadotropin deficiency—decreased sex drive, infertility, hot flashes, irregular or no periods, inability to produce milk
- GH deficiency—failure to thrive and short stature in children; most adults are asymptomatic, but some may experience fatigue and weakness
- Anti-diuretic hormone (ADH) deficiency—polyuria, polydipsia, electrolyte abnormalities

Diagnosis
The diagnosis of hypopituitarism is based on a combination of high clinical suspicion, brain imaging studies, and demonstration of insufficiency of one or more pituitary hormones (Figure 2).
A. Corticotropin
1. Total cortisol level:
   Normally, cortisol levels rise during the early morning hours and are highest at about 7 AM. They drop very low in the evening and during the early phase of sleep. Therefore cortisol level should be measured early morning and no later than 9 AM. The normal level is between 4.0 and 22.0 µg/dL. An early-morning serum cortisol level ≤3 µg/dL is abnormal. The next step is to repeat the test for confirmation and at the same time check a serum ACTH level to establish the diagnosis. A low or normal ACTH level is sufficient to make a diagnosis of hypopituitarism versus a high ACTH level that suggests a diagnosis of primary adrenal insufficiency. If the cortisol level is borderline between 4.0 and 10.0 µg/dL, an ACTH stimulation test should be performed to confirm the diagnosis.
2. ACTH stimulation tests:
- Metyrapone response test—or 11-Deoxycortisol (Compound S) test. The metyrapone test is used to evaluate inhibition of cortisol production with metyrapone (Metopirone) and a resultant increase of ACTH in response to the drop of cortisol. Metyrapone blocks cortisol production by inhibiting 11β-hydroxylase. The drop in cortisol stimulates ACTH secretion, which in turn increases plasma 11-deoxycortisol levels. The long version involves 24-hour inpatient admission because of the risk of hypotension. The short version involves the administration of a single dose of metyrapone at midnight and the measurement of serum cortisol in the morning. However, the inhibition of cortisol production may be partial, leading to a partial ACTH response and an inconclusive test result.

Hypothalamus

Pituitary portal system

Anterior pituitary

Posterior pituitary

Growth hormone (GH)

Bones, tissues

Gonadotropins (FSH and LH)

Ovaries, testes

Thyroid stimulating hormone (TSH)

Thyroid gland

Prolactin (PRL)

Mammary glands

Adrenocorticotropic hormone (ACTH)

Adrenal cortex

Oxytocin (OT)

Smooth muscle in uterus

Oxytocin (OT)

Mammary glands

Antidiuretic hormone (ADH)

Kidney tubules

Figure 1 The pituitary gland.

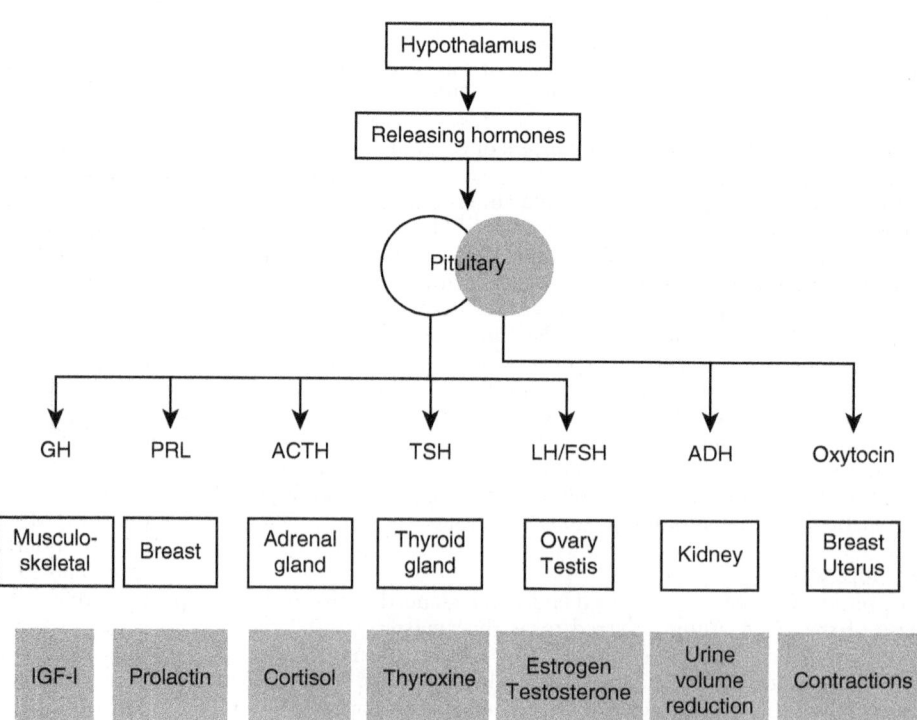

Figure 2 The diagnosis of hypopituitarism.

To conduct the metapyrone response test, metyrapone (30 mg/kg, maximum dose 3000 mg) is administered at midnight usually with a snack. The plasma cortisol and 11-deoxycortisol are measured the next morning between 8:00 and 9:00 AM. A plasma cortisol less than 220 nmol/L indicates adequate inhibition of 11β-hydroxylase. In patients with an intact hypothalamo-pituitary-adrenal (HPA) axis, CRH and ACTH levels rise as a response to the falling cortisol levels. This results in an increase of the steroid precursors in the pathway, including 11-deoxycortisol. Therefore, if the ACTH level rises and 11-deoxycortisol levels do not rise and remain less than 7 μg/dL, it is highly suggestive of impaired adrenal insufficiency. If neither ACTH or 11-deoxycortisol rise, it is highly suggestive of an impaired HPA axis at either the pituitary or hypothalamus.

- Cosyntropin (Cortrosyn) stimulation test—or ACTH stimulation test, is more appropriate than the metapyrone test to perform in an outpatient setting. It involves administering 0.25 mg of cosyntropin (Cortrosyn) to patients and measuring the serum cortisol level 60 minutes later. A 60-minute cortisol level of less than 18 μg/dL is suggestive of abnormal pituitary response or hypopituitarism.

B. Thyrotropin—Patients who have pituitary or hypothalamic diseases may have secondary hypothyroidism. In primary hypothyroidism caused by thyroid gland disorders, the TSH level will be high. In pituitary or hypothalamic disease, the TSH level will be low. Thus it is important to measure not only TSH but also "total T4" and "T3 uptake" or "free T4" levels to make the diagnosis.

C. Gonadotropins—Patients who have pituitary or hypothalamic diseases may have secondary hypogonadism. The characteristics of secondary hypogonadism are a low estrogen level in women or a low testosterone level in men and low or normal FSH and LH. On the contrary, primary hypogonadism caused by ovarian or testicular failure would result in low estrogen or testosterone levels and likely elevated FSH and LH.

D. GH—A measurement of basal serum GH concentration is not reliable. A diagnosis of GH deficiency is based on "serum IGF-1 concentration." A concentration lower than the age-specific normal level confirms the diagnosis of GH deficiency. Alternatively, a provocative test of GH secretion such as the arginine-GHRH test can be performed. Suboptimal increases in the serum GH concentration (less than 4.1 ng/mL) confirm the diagnosis of GH deficiency.

Differential Diagnosis

The differential diagnoses of hypopituitarism consist of isolated primary organ failure and deficiencies such as adrenal insufficiency, thyroid gland disorders, and primary ovarian or testicular failure.

Hypopituitarism may manifest several years after radiation exposure and in chronic Sheehan's syndrome. In acute pituitary failure, as in Sheehan's syndrome, the ACTH stimulation test may be normal because the adrenal glands are not atrophied in the acute setting; adrenal atrophy may require at least 3 months to develop. For many women, the symptoms of Sheehan's syndrome, such as fatigue, are nonspecific and often attributed to other things. It is possible for a woman to be symptom-free with Sheehan's syndrome. A woman might not realize that she has Sheehan's syndrome until she requires treatment for thyroid or adrenal insufficiency. Some women unknowingly live for years with pituitary insufficiency, then go into adrenal crisis triggered by extreme physical stressors, such as severe infection or surgery.

Treatment

Hypopituitarism can be an emergency in severe cases because of the risk of vascular collapse because cortisol is necessary for the maintenance of peripheral vascular function. Less severe cases can cause persistent hypotension and tachycardia.

The primary treatment of hypopituitarism is cortisol replacement. However, should the workup reveal other hormone deficiencies, replacement therapy for other hormones is indicated.

A. Corticosteroids
1. Oral hydrocortisone (Cortef) 15 to 25 mg a day in divided doses is the preferred treatment, because those doses are similar to physiologic daily production rates. Some patients, however, may need a higher or lower dose depending on the degree of severity. The problem with current hydrocortisone replacement regimens is that they are fixed doses given two to three times daily. Current regimens do not reflect the normal circadian pattern of physiological cortisol concentrations, which rise highest in the morning, to an intermediate level in the afternoon, and to low levels in the evening, with a cortisol-free interval at night. The current replacement regimens inevitably result in temporary over- or underreplacement and therefore result in a poor quality of life and increased mortality. Recent effort has studied sustained-release once-a-day hydrocortisone therapy versus a thrice-daily, weight-related dosing regimen. Plenadren is a recently licensed modified-release formulation of hydrocortisone that provides the potential for once-daily dosing. Plenadren provides cortisol concentrations in the afternoon but not in the evening; it does not provide an overnight rise in cortisol concentrations, such that patients have a long period of low cortisol concentrations from late afternoon to when they take their next morning dose. A pilot Chronocort[2] formulation demonstrated delayed release and an overnight rise in cortisol after about 4 hours of administering 30 mg at 10 PM. Pharmacokinetic modeling of Chronocort suggested that giving a 20-mg dose at 10 PM and a 10-mg dose at 7 PM could replicate the normal physiologic cortisol rhythm. Both are currently approved to be used in Europe and are in Phase 2 clinical trials in the United States.
2. Some authorities suggest prednisone or dexamethasone because of their longer duration of action. They can be given once a day, versus hydrocortisone, which is administered two to three times a day.
3. Patients may need a higher dose of hydrocortisone in times of illnesses or other stresses. Before planned surgeries, high-dose hydrocortisone (Solu Cortef) as stress doses for 1 to 3 days allows faster recovery (Table 2).

B. Thyroid deficiency—Thyroid deficiency from hypopituitarism is treated with T3 and T4 in a fashion similar to the treatment of primary hypothyroidism. However, treatment of secondary hypothyroidism should not be administered until adrenal function is restored and found to be normal. Treatment of the hypothyroidism alone may suppress other hormones produced by the pituitary gland and worsen the severity of other deficiencies. Similarly, TSH cannot be used as a guide for thyroid replacement in hypopituitarism; dose adjustment should be based on free T3 and free T4 levels instead.

C. Sex hormone deficiency—This includes testosterone, estrogen, and progesterone. The decision to initiate hormone therapy should be individualized. Risks and benefits should be discussed with patients extensively.

D. GH deficiency—GH replacement is now available as somatropin injections (Accretropin, Genotropin, Humatrope). GH is indicated for treatment of pediatric patients who have growth failure or for treatment of short stature associated with Turner syndrome in pediatric patients whose epiphyses are not closed. GH is not indicated for treatment of adult onset deficiency.

Monitoring

Periodic serum cortisol levels are used to assess treatment adequacy and make adjustments as needed. Most studies use cortisol levels taken approximately 4 hours after the morning cortisol

---

[2]Not available in the United States.

TABLE 2	Recommended Perioperative Hydrocortisone Dosage for Patients on Long-Term Steroid Therapy*	
SURGICAL RISKS	**EXAMPLES**	**RECOMMENDATIONS**
Minor surgery	Endoscopy, colonoscopy, inguinal herniography	Take the usual morning dose. Then take 25 mg/day for 1 day starting before surgery
Moderate surgery	Total joint replacement	Take the usual morning dose. Then take 50–75 mg/day for 1–2 days
Major surgery	Cardiopulmonary bypass	Take the usual morning dose. Then take 100–150 mg/day for 2–3 days

From Shawn (2012).
*Based on the recommendations of Salem M, Tainsh RE Jr, Bromberg J, Loriaux DL, Chernow B. Perioperative glucocorticoid coverage: A reassessment 42 years after emergence of a problem. Ann Surg 1994; 219:416-425.

dose. The challenge of measuring serum cortisol levels is that cortisol sensitivity and concentrations vary between individuals. The total daily hydrocortisone dose should be based on the patient's clinical symptoms, not just cortisol level alone.

Complications

Most of the complications of hypopituitarism are caused by a failure to diagnose the condition. Having a high clinical suspicion is the key, especially after significant traumatic events such as cardiac arrests, acute emergency surgeries, or severe motor vehicle accidents. Inadequate replacement of hormone therapy can lead to persistent symptoms, whereas excessive replacement of hormones can lead to other conditions, such as Cushing's syndrome.

References

Regal M, Páramo C, Sierra SM, et al: Prevalence and incidence of hypopituitarism in an adult Caucasian population in northwestern Spain, *Clin Endocrinol (Oxf)* 55:735–740, 2001.
Darzy KH, Shalet SM: Hypopituitarism following radiotherapy revisited, *Endocr Dev* 15:1–24, 2009.
Garg MK: Hypopituitarism following external cranial irradiation for extrasellar tumors, *Indian J Endocrinol Metab* 11:3–9, 2007.
Popovic V, Aimaretti G, Casanueva FF, et al: Hypopituitarism following traumatic brain injury, *Growth Horm IGF Res* 15:177–184, 2005.
Benvenga S, Campenní A, Ruggeri RM, et al: Clinical review 113: Hypopituitarism secondary to head trauma, *J Clin Endocrinol Metab* 85:1353–1361, 2000.
Bondanelli M, Ambrosio MR, Zatelli MC, et al: Prevalence of hypopituitarism in patients with cerebrovascular diseases, *J Endocrinol Invest* 31:16–20, 2008.
Lansang MC, Farmer T, Kennedy L: Diagnosing the unrecognized systemic absorption of intra-articular and epidural steroid injections, *Endocr Pract* 15:225–228, 2009.
Zepf B: Adrenal insufficiency in a cute severe illness, *Am Fam Physician* 68:1416–1420, 2003.
Lennernäs H, Skrtic S, Johannsson G: Replacement therapy of oral hydrocortisone in adrenal insufficiency: The influence of gastrointestinal factors, *Expert Opin Drug Metab Toxicol* 4:749–758, 2008, https://doi.org/10.1517/17425255.4.6.749.
Shaw M: When is perioperative 'steroid coverage' necessary? *Cleve Clin J Med* 69:9–11, 2002.

HYPOTHYROIDISM

Method of
William J. Hueston, MD

CURRENT DIAGNOSIS

- Hypothyroidism is more common in women as they age.
- The signs and symptoms of hypothyroidism are nonspecific and can mimic other diseases found in the elderly, so clinicians need to have a high index of suspicion.
- The key diagnostic test is to find a low free T_4. The presence of an elevated TSH indicates primary hypothyroidism, and a low TSH indicates secondary hypothyroidism.
- There is insufficient evidence for screening for hypothyroidism in asymptomatic adults.

CURRENT THERAPY

- Thyroxine replacement with L-thyroxine (Synthroid, Levoxyl) is the treatment for hypothyroidism. Medication should be titrated to normalize the thyroid-stimulating hormone (TSH) level, which is usually achieved at an overall dose of 100 to 150 μg.
- Initial dosing for those with potential cardiac disease should be started low (25–50 μg/day) and advanced slowly every 6 to 8 weeks.
- Partial substitution of triiodothyronine (Cytomel) for thyroxine should be reserved for elderly patients with persistent neurocognitive dysfunction despite normalization of their TSH.
- Patients who have subclinical hypothyroidism with a TSH >10.0 should be considered for treatment. Patients with a TSH lower than this do not require therapy.

Epidemiology

Hypothyroidism is second only to diabetes in the prevalence of endocrine disorders in adults in the United States. Hypothyroidism occurs in up to 18/1000 population, with women outnumbering men by approximately 10:1. Rates of hypothyroidism increase dramatically with age, so that about 2% to 3% of all older women have hypothyroidism, and the prevalence is up to 5% in nursing home populations.

The prevalence of subclinical hypothyroidism, defined as an elevated TSH in the presence of normal free thyroxine (T_4) and triiodothyronine (T_3) levels increases with advancing age. Women, individuals over 65, and those from European heritage are at higher risk for subclinical hypothyroidism.

Risk Factors

Thyroid conditions are more common in patients who have a family history of thyroid disorders. In addition, hypothyroidism, as well as thyroid cancers, are more common in patients who had neck irradiation in childhood. However, most cases of hypothyroidism occur in people who have no risk factors.

Pathophysiology

Several conditions can lead to hypothyroidism (Box 1). Two categories, hypothyroidism after thyroiditis and iatrogenic hypothyroidism secondary to treatment of Graves' disease, account for the overwhelming majority of cases of hypothyroidism in the United States.

The most common non-iatrogenic condition causing hypothyroidism in the United States is Hashimoto's thyroiditis. Most idiopathic hypothyroidism also represents Hashimoto's thyroiditis that has followed an indolent course. Hashimoto's thyroiditis, also called chronic lymphocytic thyroiditis, is the most common of the inflammatory thyroid disorders and the most common cause of goiter in the United States. The prevalence of Hashimoto's thyroiditis has been increasing dramatically since the 1960s in the United States, but the cause for this rise is unknown. In patients with acute thyroiditis, either subacute granulomatous (also known as de Quervain's) and subacute lymphocytic (also known as silent or painless), transient hypothyroidism is common after an acute attack, and 10% of these patients also develop long-term hypothyroidism.

Another common cause of hypothyroidism is a medical intervention to treat Graves' disease or thyroidectomy for chronic fibrocytic thyroiditis (Riedel's struma). Radioactive iodine ablation of the thyroid for Graves' disease often results in underproduction of thyroxine in the remaining tissue, necessitating thyroid replacement.

A third uncommon cause of hypothyroidism that should not be overlooked is secondary hypothyroidism due to hypothalamic or pituitary dysfunction. These conditions are seen primarily in patients who have received intracranial irradiation or surgical removal of a pituitary adenoma.

Finally, a variety of other conditions including infiltration of the thyroid (amyloidosis, sarcoidosis), iodine deficiency, or medications (such as amiodarone [Cordarone] or interferon) can cause hypothyroidism.

Prevention
There are no known interventions to prevent hypothyroidism. According to their 2015 analysis, the US Preventive Services Task Force found insufficient evidence to support early detection through routine screening of asymptomatic persons.

Clinical Manifestations
Individual who have hypothyroidism can present with a variety of symptoms, many of which are not specific. Consequently, clinicians must have a high index of suspicion for hypothyroidism when patients come in with any one or combination of the symptoms that could signal hypothyroidism.

Symptoms of hypothyroidism include lethargy, weight gain, hair loss, dry skin, constipation, poor concentration, trouble thinking or forgetfulness, and depression (Box 2). In older patients, hypothyroidism easily can be confused with Alzheimer's disease or other conditions that cause dementia. Patients who present with depression also should have their thyroid function assessed.

The thyroid examination in most patients with hypothyroidism is completely normal. Patients might have a painless goiter; tenderness in the thyroid is generally a sign of active inflammation consistent with acute thyroiditis. Once the thyroid inflammation has subsided, thyroid function might return to normal. Other physical findings that can occur with hypothyroidism include low blood pressure, bradycardia, nonpitting edema, generalized hair loss especially along the outer third of the eyebrows, dry skin, and a lag in the relaxation phase of reflexes that can be assessed most easily in the ankle jerk reflexes.

Finally, there is an association between hypothyroidism and obstructive sleep apnea although it is unclear if this is a causal relationship.

Subclinical hypothyroidism usually has no, or very subtle clinical symptoms which could be explained by other conditions. The primary finding in subclinical hypothyroidism is the abnormal laboratory values. Subclinical hypothyroidism in pregnancy is associated with increases in pregnancy loss, premature rupture of membranes, and neonatal death, but limited evidence does not show a reduction in these risks with thyroid supplementation during pregnancy.

Diagnosis
The diagnosis of hypothyroidism is based on finding a low free thyroxine (T_4) level, usually with an elevation in the thyroid stimulating hormone (TSH) levels. For patients with hypothyroidism due to pituitary dysfunction, also called secondary hypothyroidism, both the free T_4 and the TSH levels are low.

One situation where clinicians need to be wary is evaluating thyroid status in patients who are severely ill. During times of acute physiological stress, patients may have mildly elevated TSH levels that suggest hypothyroidism but are, in fact, euthyroid. This condition, called euthyroid sick syndrome, does not

---

BOX 1 Conditions Causing Hypothyroidism

Thyroiditis
Hashimoto's thyroiditis
Subacute granulomatous thyroiditis (de Quervain's thyroiditis)
Subacute lymphocytic thyroiditis (silent or painless thyroiditis)

Iatrogenic Hypothyroidism
Radioactive iodine treatment of Graves' disease
Thyroidectomy

Secondary Hypothyroidism (Pituitary Dysfunction)
Pituitary surgery
Intercranial radiation
Congenital panhypopituitarism

Other Causes
Infiltratative diseases (sarcoidosis, amyloidosis, hemochromatosis)
Drugs (lithium, interferon, amiodarone [Cordarone])
Iodine deficiency

BOX 2 Symptoms and Signs of Hypothyroidism

Common Symptoms
Lethargy
Weight gain
Constipation
Slowed mentation, forgetfulness
Depression
Hair loss
Dry skin
Neck enlargement or goiter

Physical Examination Findings
Goiter
Low blood pressure and slow pulse
Hair thinning or loss
Dry skin
Confusion
Depressed affect
Non-pitting edema

---

require treatment with thyroid replacement and resolves within a few weeks of recovery, but it may be difficult to distinguish from preexisting or new-onset hypothyroidism. Clinicians need to use other clinical symptoms to try to differentiate euthyroid sick syndrome from hypothyroidism. Even though it does not require treatment, the presence of euthyroid sick syndrome in a critically ill patient is a poor prognostic sign.

In contrast to hyperthyroidism, there is no role for thyroid scans or iodine uptake testing in patients with hypothyroidism. The only exception to this is when the clinician identifies a mass on physical examination. In that situation, scanning or other imaging is essential to determine the malignancy potential of the mass.

Differential Diagnosis
The differential diagnosis for hypothyroidism is broad and depends on the primary complaints given by patients. For patients with slowed mentation, depressed affect, or confusion, clinicians should suspect depression. Patients with lethargy and a slow pulse and low blood pressure might have adrenal insufficiency. Patients with constipation need to have colonic obstruction from a mass considered as well. In the elderly, common drugs that can cause depression (such as centrally acting antihypertensive agents), bradycardia (such as β-blockers or calcium channel blockers), constipation (calcium channel blockers), hair loss, or confusion also should be considered.

In patients with pituitary failure, other pituitary hormones are likely to be deficient as well, so clinicians should look for evidence of adrenal and gonadotropic failure.

Treatment

The treatment for hypothyroidism is thyroxine replacement (Synthroid, Levoxyl). The usual dose required to achieve full replacement is between 100 µg and 150 µg, although patients who are treated with radioactive iodine and have some remaining thyroid activity might require lower doses. For patients with known heart disease or at risk for heart problems, doses should be initiated at 25 to 50 µg with increases of 25 µg every 4 to 6 weeks guided by TSH levels. Young patients who are at low risk for cardiac problems can be started at doses of 100 µg.

In choosing an agent to use for thyroid replacement, there is good evidence that generic substitutes are just as effective as brand-name drugs. A detailed study examining the metabolic effectiveness of a variety of generic drugs compared with a brand-name medication demonstrated no clinical or subclinical differences among preparations. So even though clinicians often hear that they should use a brand-name drug to maintain the stability of the replacement dose, this is not supported by the evidence.

One area of uncertainty is whether the addition of triiodothyronine (T_3, Cytomel) adds additional benefit to thyroid replacement with thyroxine. In some studies with elderly patients, subjects with continued neurocognitive dysfunction benefited from the addition of T_3 at a dose of 125 µg, with a concomitant decrease in the T_4 dose of 50 µg. However, subsequent studies of younger patients (aged 29–44 years) failed to find any benefits of partial T_3 substitution. Furthermore, studies of patients on doses of T_4 adequate to restore TSH levels to normal have been found to have normal T_3 levels. At this time, routine use of T_3 cannot be recommended; however, for selected elderly patients who have lingering confusion, depression, or slow mentation on adequate doses of T_4, a trial of T_3 partial substitution might be tried. Both the American Thyroid Association and European Thyroid Association recommend a trial of combination therapy for patients who are using single therapy with thyroxine alone who are persistently dissatisfied with their therapy.

Another situation where there is controversy is the use of thyroid replacement in patients with a mildly elevated TSH and a normal free T_4. This condition, called subacute hypothyroidism or mild hypothyroidism, is more common in white elderly women. Some studies have shown clinical improvement in symptoms when low doses of T_4 are given to these patients, although the patient populations tend to be those with preexisting thyroid disease (such as Graves' disease), and studies have had only a small number of patients. While an expert panel has suggested using the TSH level as an indication for therapy, a systematic review and meta-analysis showed no improvement in quality of life or thyroid-related symptoms in patients with subclinical hypothyroidism who received levothyroxine supplementation.

When the TSH is <7, almost half of all patients will revert to normal within 2 years. Patients with a TSH <10 do not require any therapy unless there are other individual patient risk factors such as existing cardiac disease or cognitive symptoms. Treatment is reasonable in those with a TSH level of 10.0 because these patients may be most symptomatic and have a progression to overt hypothyroidism of 5%.

Monitoring

In general, once a patient receives a full replacement dose of T_4 (usually between 100 and 150 µg) and has a TSH consistently in the normal range, there is little likelihood that their thyroid requirement will change over time. Although many advocate annual retesting of TSH to ensure patients are euthyroid, there is no evidence to show this is necessary.

Some conditions do warrant closer monitoring of the TSH level. Because T_4 and T_3 are highly protein bound, any conditions where a patient's serum protein status changes should prompt additional testing. This includes conditions that lower serum protein levels, such as liver disease, nephrotic syndrome, or malnutrition, as well as those where serum proteins are increased, such as pregnancy or initiation of estrogen therapy. Because patients' dietary protein usually decreases with advancing age, older patients whose diet declines can also require monitoring and a lowering of their T_4 dose over time.

Patients with subclinical hypothyroidism also might benefit from annual retesting of their free T_4 levels. Approximately 10% of patients with subacute hypothyroidism progress to hypothyroidism within 3 years of diagnosis. Because of this, yearly testing is recommended. Also, 50% of patients with subacute hypothyroidism have positive anti-thyroid antibodies; however, routine testing for these is not recommended.

Complications

Most of the complications of hypothyroidism are associated with undertreatment or overtreatment. Patients with inadequately treated hypothyroidism are at higher risk for cardiac disease. On the other hand, over-replacement of thyroxine increases the risk of both atrial fibrillation and osteoporosis.

In addition, Hashimoto's thyroiditis is associated with other endocrine autoimmune diseases such as Addison's disease and pernicious anemia. Clinicians should be aware of these associations and not overlook new endocrine disorders that might have clinical features similar to hypothyroidism.

Finally, patients with Hashimoto's hypothyroidism also are at higher risk for the future development of lymphoma. Clinicians should educate patients about the need to have newly enlarged lymph nodes evaluated and be aggressive about evaluating symptoms or signs consistent with the development of a lymphoma.

References

Bunevicius R, Kazanavicius G, Zalinkevicius R, Prange AJ: Effects of thyroxine as compared with thyroxine plus triiodothyronine in patients with hypothyroidism, *N Engl J Med* 340:424–429, 1999.

Dong BJ, Hauck WW, Gambertoglio JG, et al: Bioequivalence of generic and brand-name levothyroxine products in the treatment of hypothyroidism, *JAMA* 277:1205–1213, 1997.

Feller M, Snel M, Moutzouri E, et al: Association of thyroid hormone therapy with quality of life and thyroid-related symptoms in patients with subclinical hypothyroidism: A systematic review and meta-analysis, *JAMA* 320:1349–1359, 2018.

Helfand M, Crapo LM: Screening for thyroid disease, *Ann Intern Med* 112:840–849, 1990.

Peeters RP: Subclinical hypothyroidism, *New Engl J Med* 376:2556–2565, 2017.

Sawin CT, Chopra D, Azizi F, et al: The aging thyroid. Increased prevalence of elevated serum thyrotropin levels in the elderly, *JAMA* 242:1386–1388, 1979.

Surks MI, Ortiz E, Daniels GH, et al: Subclinical thyroid disease: Scientific review and guidelines for diagnosis and management, *JAMA* 291(2):228–238, 2004.

U.S. Preventive Services Task Force: Screening for thyroid disease: Available at http://www.ahrq.gov/clinic/uspstf/uspsthyr.htm [accessed July 11, 2015].

OBESITY

Method of
Ana L. Creo, MD and Seema Kumar, MD

CURRENT DIAGNOSIS

- Body mass index (BMI) is calculated as weight in kilograms divided by height in meters squared (kg/m^2). BMI is currently the preferred method for determining whether a patient is obese.
- Patients with a BMI of 30 or greater are considered obese; those with a BMI between 25 and 29.9 are considered overweight. For Asians, overweight is a BMI between 23 and 24.9 kg/m^2 and obesity a BMI greater than 25 kg/m^2.
- Abdominal circumference should also be measured to assess for abdominal obesity.
- A waist circumference of greater than 102 cm (40 inches) in men or greater than 88 cm (35 inches) in women is considered indicative of abdominal obesity. A waist circumference of greater than 80 cm in Asian females and greater than 90 cm in Asian males is considered abnormal.

- Treatment of patients with obesity requires a multidisciplinary team approach.
- Lifestyle modifications, including dietary changes and increased physical activity, remain first-line treatment for patients with obesity.
- Adjuvant pharmacotherapy may be considered for patients with a BMI greater than 30 kg/m² or a BMI of 27 to 30 kg/m² with concomitant weight-related complications.
- Bariatric surgery should be considered for patients with a BMI of 40 kg/m² or greater and for those with a BMI of 35 kg/m² or greater who have significant comorbidities such as severe diabetes, sleep apnea, or joint disease after nonsurgical weight loss attempts have failed.

Epidemiology

Obesity is a complex disease that represents a growing epidemic in the United States and worldwide. During 2015–2016, the prevalence of obesity in the United States was 39.8% and affected about 93.3 million adults. According to the National Health and Nutrition Examination Survey (NHANES), 38% of men and 41.5% of women were obese. There are disparities in the prevalence of obesity between ethnic groups, with Hispanic and non-Hispanic black adults having a higher prevalence of obesity than non-Hispanic white and non-Hispanic Asian adults.

The American Medical Association has officially classified obesity as a disease due to its association with several comorbidities and increased mortality.

Diagnosis

Obesity is a condition marked by the accumulation of excess body fat. The body mass index (BMI) is the most practical way to evaluate the degree of excess weight. It is calculated from the weight (in kilograms) and the square of the height (in meters), as follows:

$$BMI = \frac{Weight}{Height^2}$$

The World Health Organization (WHO) and National Institutes of Health (NIH) define overweight as a BMI between 25 and 29.9 kg/m² and obesity as a BMI equal to or greater than 30 kg/m² (Table 1). These guidelines apply to whites, Hispanics, and blacks. Because Asians can have higher percentage of body fat at a lower BMI, overweight for this particular ethnic group is a BMI between 23 and 24.9 kg/m², and obesity is a BMI equal to or greater than 25 kg/m². The BMI correlates with percentage of body fat and body fat mass, as well as with mortality. The BMI may, however, overestimate the degree of body fat in athletes. However, for a given BMI, the degree of body fatness tends to be higher in women compared with men, and it is higher in older compared with younger people. The relationship between BMI and mortality appears to form a J- or U-shaped curve, with the lowest mortality rate seen in those with a BMI of about 25 kg/m² (Figure 1).

Because people with abdominal (central) adiposity are more likely to develop many of the health conditions associated with obesity, waist circumference is an important adjuvant measurement to obtain when screening for obesity. Waist circumference is measured at the level of the top of the iliac crest with the measuring tape snug against the skin. In adults with a BMI of 25 to 34.9 kg/m², a waist circumference greater than 102 cm (40 inches) for men and 88 cm (35 inches) for women is associated with a greater risk of hypertension, type 2 diabetes, dyslipidemia, and coronary heart disease (CHD; see Table 1). In patients with a BMI ≥ 35 kg/m², measurement of waist circumference is less helpful because it adds little to the predictive power of the disease risk classification of BMI; almost all individuals with this BMI also have an abnormal waist circumference. More precise measurement of abdominal fat can be made with abdominal computed tomography or magnetic resonance imaging (MRI). Alternative methods to assess body composition and degree of fatness include measurements of skinfold thickness, hydrostatic weighing, bioelectric impedance, and scanning by dual-energy x-ray absorptiometry. These methods require specialized equipment and trained personnel and are not used routinely in clinical practice.

Etiology and Pathophysiology

Obesity is a complex, multifactorial disease characterized by excessive caloric consumption and inadequate caloric expenditure. Many factors, including genetic and environmental influences, can contribute to the development of obesity. However, personal decisions regarding food choices, portion sizes, and level of activity also contribute to body size.

When evaluating a patient with obesity, it is important to rule out disorders such as Cushing syndrome and hypothyroidism. Because many medications promote weight gain, including several antipsychotics, antidepressants, antiepileptics, sulfonylureas, and steroids (Table 2), it is prudent to obtain a complete medication history from any patient who is being evaluated for obesity. Single-gene mutations (e.g., in the melanocortin 4 receptor gene and leptin gene) and congenital syndromes (e.g., Prader-Willi, Bardet-Biedel, Cohen) typically cause early-onset obesity before 5 years of age.

TABLE 1 Classification of Overweight and Obesity by Body Mass Index, Waist Circumference, and Associated Health Risk

CLASSIFICATION	BMI (kg/m²)	DISEASE RISK*	
		WAIST ≤102 CM (≤40 IN) IN MEN OR ≤88 CM (≤35 IN) IN WOMEN	WAIST >102 CM (>40 IN) IN MEN OR >88 CM (>35 IN) IN WOMEN
Underweight	<18.5	—	—
Normal†	18.5–24.9	—	—
Overweight	25.0–29.9	Increased	High
Obesity—class I	30.0–34.9	High	Very high
Obesity—class II	35.0–39.9	Very high	Very high
Extreme obesity—class III	>40	Extremely high	Extremely high

*Disease risk for type 2 diabetes, hypertension, and cardiovascular disease relative to normal weight and waist circumference.
†Increased waist circumference can also be a marker for increased risk even in persons of normal weight.
Reproduced from Clinical guidelines on the identification, evaluation, and treatment of overweight and obesity in adults: The evidence report. National Institutes of Health. *Obes Res.* 1998;6(Suppl 2):51S–209S.

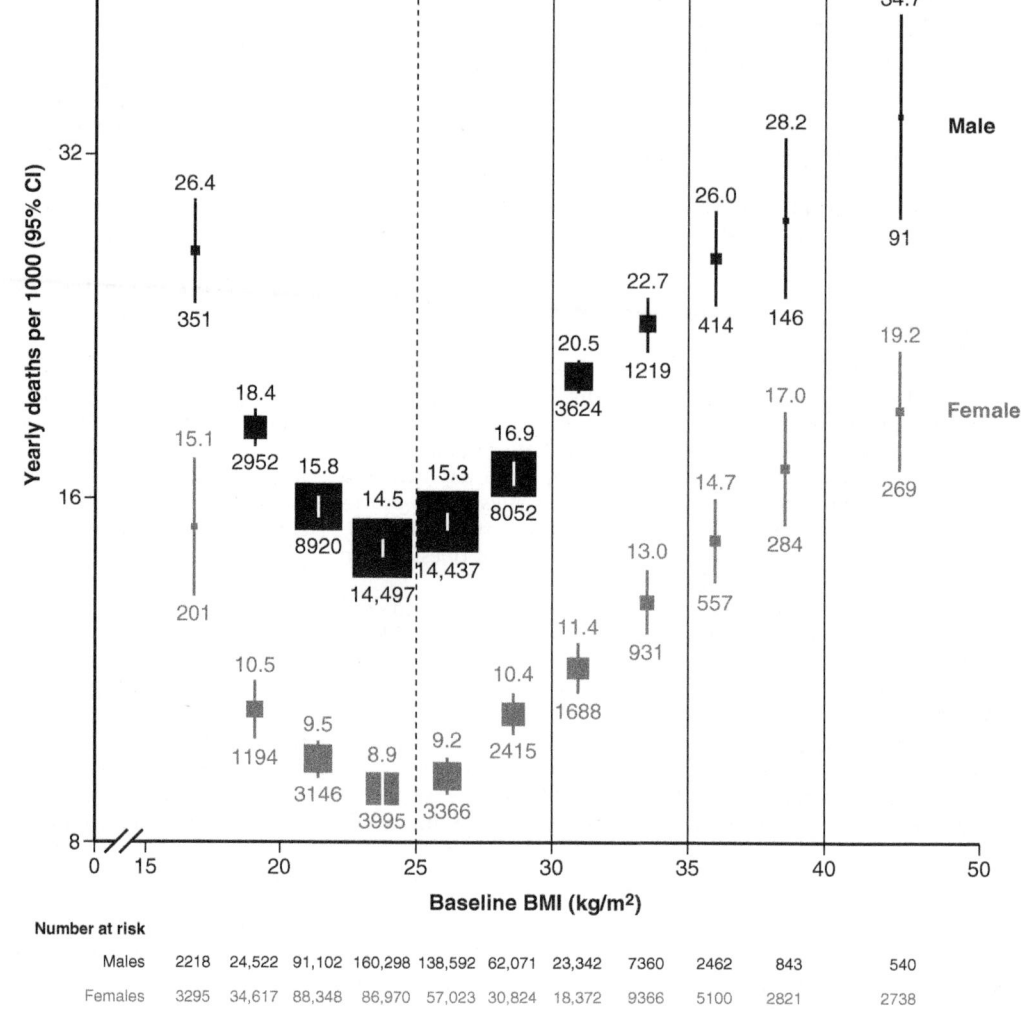

Figure 1 All-cause mortality versus body mass index *(BMI)* for each sex in the range of 15 to 50 kg/m² (excluding the first 5 years of follow-up). (From Whitlock G, Lewington S, Sherliker P, et al. Body-mass index and cause-specific mortality in 900,000 adults: Collaborative analyses of 57 prospective studies. *Lancet.* 2009;373:1083–1096.)

Number at risk

Males	2218	24,522	91,102	160,298	138,592	62,071	23,342	7360	2462	843	540
Females	3295	34,617	88,348	86,970	57,023	30,824	18,372	9366	5100	2821	2738

Associated Comorbidities

Obesity is associated with a variety of other medical conditions that can increase morbidity and mortality. Comorbidities associated with obesity include metabolic syndrome and insulin resistance, type 2 diabetes, dyslipidemia, hypertension, coronary artery disease, degenerative joint disease, nonalcoholic fatty liver disease (NAFLD), and obstructive sleep apnea.

Insulin Resistance and Metabolic Syndrome

Insulin resistance is defined as a subnormal response to endogenous insulin. This results in pancreatic B-cell compensation with hypersecretion of insulin. Insulin resistance leads to various components of the metabolic syndrome, including low high density lipoprotein (HDL) cholesterol, high triglycerides, elevated blood pressure, and hyperglycemia. Patients may also manifest acanthosis nigricans and skin tags.

Type 2 Diabetes

The increasing prevalence of obesity has also resulted in an increasing prevalence of type 2 diabetes. More than 80% of type 2 diabetes can be attributed to obesity, but other factors, such as family history, are also involved. Criteria for the diagnosis of type 2 diabetes include a fasting glucose level greater than 125 mg/dL or glucose levels greater than 200 mg/dL during a 2-hour oral glucose tolerance test.

Hypertension

Hypertension is a common chronic disease, and it has been estimated that obesity is a major risk factor for hypertension. Hypertension is associated with an increased risk for stroke, myocardial infarction, heart failure, and kidney disease. Even a modest weight loss (5% to 10% of initial weight) can lead to a significant fall in blood pressure and, often, decreased need for antihypertensive medications.

Dyslipidemia

A variety of blood lipid abnormalities are seen frequently in obese patients. These include elevated levels of total cholesterol, low density lipoprotein (LDL) cholesterol, and triglycerides, and decreased levels of HDL cholesterol. Patients with central adiposity are at particularly high risk for the development of hypertriglyceridemia and low HDL. Screening for dyslipidemia should be done with a fasting lipid profile. However, if the testing opportunity is nonfasting, the total cholesterol and HDL values can still be measured.

TABLE 2	Drugs That Cause Weight Gain and Some Alternatives	
CATEGORY	DRUGS THAT CAUSE WEIGHT GAIN	POSSIBLE ALTERNATIVES
Antipsychotics		
Conventional	Thioridazine (Mellaril)	Haloperidol (Haldol)
Atypical	Olanzapine (Zyprexa), clozapine (Clozaril), quetiapine (Seroquel), risperidone (Risperdal)	Ziprasidone (Geodon), aripiprazole (Abilify)
Lithium	Lithium carbonate (Eskalith)	
Antidepressants		
Tricyclics	Amitriptyline (Elavil), clomipramine (Anafranil), doxepin (Sinequan), imipramine (Tofranil), nortriptyline (Pamelor)	Protriptyline (Vivactil)
Selective serotonin reuptake inhibitors	Paroxetine (Paxil)	Other SSRIs
Other	Mirtazapine (Remeron)	Bupropion (Wellbutrin), nefazodone (Serzone)
Anticonvulsant drugs	Valproate (Depakene), carbamazepine (Tegretol), gabapentin (Neurontin)	Topiramate (Topamax), lamotrigine (Lamictal), zonisamide (Zonegran)
Antidiabetic drugs	Insulin, sulfonylureas, metiglinide, thiazolidinediones	Metformin (Glucophage), alpha-glucosidase inhibitors
Serotonin and histamine antagonist	Pizotifen[2]	
Antihistamines	Cyproheptidine (Periactin)	
Beta-adrenergic blockers	Propranolol (Inderal), atenolol (Tenormin), metoprolol (Lopressor)	
Steroid hormones	Glucocorticoids	
	Progestins: megestrol acetate (Megace), medroxyprogesterone acetate (Provera)	

Copyright ©2001 George A Bray, MD. Reproduced with permission.
[2]Not available in the United States.

Coronary Heart Disease

Comorbidities associated with obesity such as hypertension, insulin resistance, type 2 diabetes, and dyslipidemia lead to increased risk of cardiovascular disease in obese adults. Obesity is also associated with increased risk of CHD, heart failure, cardiovascular mortality, and all-cause mortality.

Respiratory Abnormalities

Obstructive sleep apnea is the most important respiratory problem associated with obesity. It is often underrecognized and inadequately treated. Patients may present with snoring, apneic episodes, excessive daytime somnolence, fatigue, irritability, and erectile dysfunction. Consequent nocturnal hypoxemia may result in arrhythmias, pulmonary hypertension, and right-sided heart failure. Treatment includes weight loss and use of continuous positive airway pressure at night. Other alterations in pulmonary function that may occur, include higher residual lung volume associated with increased abdominal pressure on the diaphragm, decreased lung compliance and increased chest wall impedance, ventilation-perfusion abnormalities, reduced strength and endurance of respiratory muscles, depressed ventilatory drive, and bronchospasm.

Gastroesophageal Disease

Obesity is associated with an increased risk of gastroesophageal reflux disease symptoms, as well as erosive esophagitis, esophageal adenocarcinoma, and gastric carcinoma. It has been suggested that increased intragastric pressure and relaxation of the lower esophageal sphincter from gastric compression from surrounding adiposity contribute to the reflux rather than the type of diet consumed.

Hepatobiliary Disease

Obesity increases the risk of cholelithiasis and of NAFLD. The spectrum of NAFLD ranges from steatosis with mild disruption of the liver architecture by fat to steatohepatitis with varying degrees of fibrosis and cirrhosis. Increased liver transaminase levels and findings of steatosis on ultrasonography are both suggestive of NAFLD in obese patients. However, the definitive diagnosis remains histologic.

Osteoarthritis

The incidence of osteoarthritis is increased in obese subjects. Osteoarthritis commonly develops in the knees and ankles but can also affect nonweight-bearing joints. Weight loss results in decreased risk of osteoarthritis.

Cancer

For both men and women, increased BMI is associated with increased mortality from several cancers, such as those of the esophagus, colon and rectum, liver, gallbladder, pancreas, and kidney, as well as non-Hodgkin lymphoma and multiple myeloma. In addition, obese men are at increased risk of death from stomach and prostate cancer, and obese women are at increased risk of death from cancers of the breast, uterus, cervix, and ovary.

Psychosocial Function

Obese subjects often are subjected to discrimination in education, employment, and healthcare. Overweight women have been noted to have lower household incomes and higher rates of household poverty than women who were not overweight, independent of their baseline socioeconomic status and aptitude test scores. Depression has also been seen in association with severe obesity, particularly in younger patients and in women.

Economic Consequences of Obesity

Overweight and obesity and their associated health problems have a significant economic impact on the healthcare system. Healthcare costs are higher in obese subjects compared with their normal-weight counterparts. The higher costs are predominantly explained by the presence of CHD, hypertension, and diabetes.

Treatment

Patients must undergo a detailed history and physical examination before a treatment plan is initiated. Secondary causes of obesity, such as Cushing syndrome and hypothyroidism, should be considered in the evaluation. A complete medication history is crucial to determining whether any medications may have promoted weight gain.

Laboratory studies should be directed at ruling out secondary causes in selected patients and ruling out comorbidities (fasting glucose, lipid profile, and liver function tests). It is important that practitioners assess each patient's willingness to change and expectations for weight loss. Treatment should be based on the patient's BMI, risk factors, and willingness to lose weight. Patients who are in the precontemplative phase (i.e., in the early stages of thinking about it) are not likely to be successful despite appropriate counseling. Healthcare providers must enforce the idea that even a modest weight loss improves complications associated with obesity.

Treatment of obesity requires a multidisciplinary team approach. Lifestyle modifications, including dietary change and increased physical activity, represent first-line treatment for patients with obesity. Pharmacotherapy and bariatric surgery may be used as adjuvant therapies in certain patients.

The goal of treatment is to prevent the complications of obesity. The initial target goal of weight loss therapy is to decrease body weight by 5% to 10%. Once this target is achieved, further weight loss can be attempted if indicated. The rationales for this initial goal of moderate weight loss are that:

- It can decrease the severity of obesity-associated risk factors.
- It can set the stage for further weight loss, if indicated.
- It is realistic and can be achieved and maintained over time.

A reasonable timeline for a 5% to 10% reduction in body weight is 6 months of therapy. A period of weight maintenance should then occur. Further weight loss may be considered if the initial goal is achieved and then maintained for at least 6 months. It is important to inform patients that it is preferable to maintain a moderate amount of weight loss over time than to lose more weight but later regain it.

Behavior Modification

Behavior modification is an integral part of any weight loss program. Motivational interviewing (MI) is a client-centered, collaborative decision-making approach that is helpful in facilitating lifestyle modifications. MI helps the healthcare provider provide nonjudgmental feedback to patients, allowing for patients' resistance to change and encouraging patients to develop their own arguments for engaging in health behavior change.

The goal of behavioral therapy is to help patients make long-term changes in their eating behavior by modifying and monitoring their food intake, increasing their physical activity, and controlling cues and stimuli in the environment that trigger eating. Maintaining food diaries and activity records for self-monitoring are key elements in any successful behavioral weight loss program. Stimulus control is considered a key element in a behavioral program. It focuses on gaining control over the environmental factors that activate eating, and eliminating or modifying the environmental factors that facilitate overeating.

This requires the availability of trained personnel such as psychologists and therapists. The behavioral strategies taught are aimed at decreasing caloric intake and increasing physical activity in the long term.

Dietary Therapy

The goal of dietary therapy, therefore, is to reduce the total number of calories consumed. A principal determinant of weight loss appears to be the degree of adherence to the diet, irrespective of the particular macronutrient composition. Recent data suggest that the so-called Mediterranean diet and low-carbohydrate diets may represent effective alternatives to the low-fat diet for weight loss. Thus the macronutrient mix of the diet should be based on patient preferences to improve long-term adherence. Often patients revert to their previous habit of eating and can regain the weight that was lost. Diets that incorporate the patient's preference and culture to find the optimal mix of macronutrients will have the best chance of success.

Approximately 22 kcal/kg is required to maintain a kilogram of body weight in a normal adult. Thus the expected or calculated energy expenditure for a woman weighing 100 kg is approximately 2200 kcal/day. The variability of ± 20% could give energy needs as high as 2620 kcal/day or as low as 1860 kcal/day. An average deficit of 500 kcal/day should result in an initial weight loss of approximately 0.5 kg/week (1 lb/week). However, after 3 to 6 months of weight loss, energy expenditure adaptations occur, which slow the body weight response to a given change in energy intake, thereby diminishing ongoing weight loss.

Patients should be counseled to avoid unnecessary calories from alcohol and sugary beverages such as soda and juice.

Very-low-calorie diets contain less than 800 kcal/day and are usually administered in the form of liquid supplements. Although these diets do produce significant and rapid weight loss, results are difficult to maintain in the long term. These diets require close monitoring by a healthcare professional. Side effects associated with very-low-calorie diets include fatigue, constipation, hair loss, and gallstones. These diets are strictly contraindicated in children and in pregnant and lactating women and are generally reserved for patients who require rapid weight loss for a specific purpose such as surgery.

Physical Activity

Physical activity is an integral component of therapy for obese patients and is most important in the prevention of weight regain. Physical activity also decreases the risks for cardiovascular disease and type 2 diabetes. Sedentary obese patients need to start their exercise program slowly and may require supervision from a healthcare professional. Initially, patients may be encouraged to increase their activities of daily living. For example, it may be suggested that they take the stairs instead of the elevator or that they park farther away from work or shopping. The intensity and duration of exercise should be increased gradually over time, with a goal of achieving 30 minutes of moderate-intensity activity on most days of the week to improve health (150 minutes/week) and 60 minutes of exercise of most days of the week to control body weight.

Ideally, adults should also perform muscle-strengthening exercises on 2 or more days per week. Patients should be encouraged to choose activities that they enjoy and to build these activities into their daily schedule. Sedentary activities, such as watching television, sitting in front of a computer screen, and playing video games, should be discouraged.

Pharmacotherapy

Pharmacotherapy (Table 3) is usually reserved for patients with a BMI greater than 30 kg/m² without complications or a BMI greater than 27 to 30 kg/m² with concomitant weight-related complications. These patients should have failed to achieve weight loss goals through diet and exercise alone. Pharmacotherapy must be used in conjunction with a program that includes dietary changes and physical activity.

The success may be measured by the degree of weight loss and improvement in associated risk factors. Weight loss should be more than 5% below baseline to be considered effective. A weight loss of 5% to 10% can significantly reduce the baseline risk factors for diabetes and cardiovascular disease and improvement in baseline risk factors after weight loss is an important criterion in the determination of whether to continue therapy.

Orlistat (Xenical) is recommended as the first-line drug for patients with dyslipidemia or diabetes; however, its use is often limited due to gastrointestinal side effects. Orlistat is an inhibitor of pancreatic lipases that causes weight loss by limiting fat

TABLE 3	Drugs Approved by the US Food and Drug Administration for Treatment of Obesity	
DRUG	**DOSAGE**	**ADVERSE SIDE EFFECTS**
Pancreatic Lipase Inhibitor Approved for Long-Term Use		
Orlistat (Xenical)	120 mg tid before meals	Cramps, flatulence, diarrhea, oily spotting
Appetite Suppressants Approved for Long-Term Use		
Serotonin agonist Lorcaserin hydrochloride (Belviq)	10 mg bid	Headache, dizziness, nausea, nasopharyngitis
GLP-1 analog approved for weight loss		
Liraglutide (Saxenda)	0.6 mg subQ qd (doses escalated weekly with a max of 3 mg)	Nausea, vomiting, diarrhea, constipation, hypoglycemia
Combination Drugs		
Naltrexone/Bupropion (Contrave)	Week 1: one tablet (8 mg naltrexone/90 mg bupropion) once daily Week 2: one tablet twice daily Week 3: two tablets in the am, one in the pm Week 4: two tablets twice daily	Nausea, headache, constipation, dizziness, and a dry mouth
Phentermine/topiramate (Qsymia)	7.5 mg/46 mg/day*	Dry mouth, tachycardia, depression, anxiety
Noradrenergic Drugs Approved for Short-Term Use		
Phentermine (Adipex-P)	Immediate release: 15–37.5 mg/day	Increase in blood pressure or in heart rate, insomnia, nervousness Dry mouth, constipation Abuse potential due to amphetamine-like effects
Phentermine resin (Ionamin)[2]	Slow-release resin 15–30 mg/day	
Diethylpropion (Tenuate)	Immediate release: 25 mg tid Controlled release: 75 mg every morning	Same
Benzphetamine (Didrex)	25–50 mg tid	Same
Phendimetrazine (Bontril PDM)	17.5–70 mg tid Extended release: 105 mg/day	Same

*Maintenance dose.
[2]Not available in the United States.

absorption. The recommended dose for adults is 120 mg PO three times daily with meals. A lower dose of 60 mg preparation (Alli) is available over the counter in the United States and several other countries. Orlistat has been shown to be effective for weight loss and prevention of weight regain. In a meta-analysis of 12 trials that included patients with and without diabetes and reported data with 12-month outcomes, patients randomly assigned to orlistat plus a behavioral intervention lost 5 to 10 kg (8% of baseline weight) compared with 3 to 6 kg in the control group (placebo plus behavioral intervention), for a mean placebo-subtracted difference of 3 kg. Weight loss was maintained with up to 24 to 36 months of orlistat treatment. Orlistat has also been shown to result in improved metabolic outcomes such as delay in development of type 2 diabetes in those that have impaired fasting glucose and improvement in blood pressure in hypertensive patients and in serum total and LDL cholesterol levels. Side effects associated with orlistat are mostly gastrointestinal and include cramping, flatus, fecal incontinence, oily spotting, and flatus with discharge. These side effects tend to decrease over time as patients learn to restrict their dietary intake to less than 30% fat. Severe cases of liver damage have been reported in patients taking orlistat. Orlistat may also interfere with the absorption of fat-soluble vitamins, so the use of a daily multivitamin supplement at bedtime is recommended.

Lorcaserin hydrochloride (Belviq) is a serotonin 2C receptor agonist that causes weight loss by causing appetite suppression. It appears to have fewer adverse effects than orlistat, although long-term safety data are limited. The recommended dosage is 10 mg twice daily. Lorcaserin should be discontinued if patients do not lose 5% of their body weight in 12 weeks. The efficacy of lorcaserin appears similar to that of orlistat (mean difference in weight loss between active and placebo-treated groups approximately 3 to 4 kg). Common side effects include nausea, headache, dizziness, nasopharyngitis, and fatigue. Lorcaserin may increase the risk of symptomatic hypoglycemia in patients with type 2 diabetes on oral agents, necessitating a reduction in the dose of diabetes medications. Lorcaserin should not be used in individuals with creatinine clearance less than 30 mL/min. It is contraindicated during pregnancy. In addition, lorcaserin should not be used with other serotonergic drugs (e.g., selective serotonin reuptake inhibitors, selective serotonin-norepinephrine reuptake inhibitors, bupropion [Wellbutrin], tricyclic antidepressants, and monamine oxidase inhibitors) because of the theoretical potential for serotonin syndrome.

Qsymia is a combination of phentermine (Adipex-P), an appetite suppressant, and topiramate (Topamax), a medication used to treat epilepsy and migraine. The initial dose of Qsymia (phentermine/topiramate) is 3.75/23 mg for 14 days, followed by 7.5/46 mg thereafter. If after 12 weeks, a 3% loss in body weight is not achieved, the dose can be increased to 11.25/69 mg for 14 days, and then to 15/92 mg daily. If an individual does not lose 5% of body weight after 12 weeks on the highest dose, Qsymia (phentermine/topiramate) should be discontinued gradually, as abrupt withdrawal of topiramate can cause seizures. Qsymia is contraindicated during pregnancy due to an increased risk of orofacial clefts in infants exposed to the combination drug during the first trimester of pregnancy. Women of child-bearing age should have a pregnancy test before starting this drug and monthly thereafter.

It is also contraindicated in patients with glaucoma, hyperthyroidism, and individuals who have taken monoamine oxidase inhibitors within 14 days. Clinicians who prescribe Qsymia (phentermine/topiramate) are encouraged to enroll in a risk evaluation and mitigation strategy, which includes an online or print formal training module detailing safety information. Pharmacies that dispense Qsymia also require a specific certification and must provide patients with a medication guide and brochure each time the drug is dispensed, detailing the risks of birth defects.

Side effects for Qsymia include tachycardia, paresthesias, dizziness, altered taste sensation, insomnia, and constipation. Qsymia is not recommended in patients with cardiovascular disease (hypertension or CHD) and may be considered for obese postmenopausal women and men without cardiovascular disease, particularly those who do not tolerate orlistat or lorcaserin.

Contrave, a combination of bupropion, an antidepressant/anorexiant with naltrexone, an opioid-receptor antagonist was approved by the US Food and Drug Administration in September 2014 as an adjunct to diet and exercise in patients with BMI ≥30 kg/m² (or ≥27 kg/m² with comorbidities). The initial dose is one tablet (8 mg of naltrexone and 90 mg of bupropion) daily. After 1 week, the dose is increased to one tablet twice daily, and by week 4 to two tablets twice daily. If after 12 weeks the patient has not lost at least 5% of baseline body weight, the drug should be discontinued because benefit is unlikely. Contraindications include concomitant use of other bupropion-containing products, long-term opioid use, uncontrolled hypertension, eating disorder, seizure disorders, and use within 14 days of taking monoamine oxidase inhibitors. Side effects for Contrave (bupropion-naltrexone) include nausea, headache, constipation, insomnia vomiting, constipation, dizziness, and dry mouth.

Liraglutide (Saxenda) is a long-acting glucagon-like polypeptide-1 (GLP-1) receptor agonist that is recommended for long-term weight management in conjunction with reduced-calorie diet and physical activity. It is recommended for patients with BMI ≥30 kg/m² or ≥27 kg/m² if one weight-related comorbidity is present. Liraglutide is administered subcutaneously in the abdomen, thigh, or upper arm once daily. The initial dose is 0.6 mg daily for 1 week. The dose can be increased at weekly intervals (1.2, 1.8, 2.4 mg) to the recommended dose of 3 mg. If after 16 weeks a patient has not lost at least 4% of baseline body weight, liraglutide should be discontinued, because it is unlikely the patient will achieve clinically meaningful weight loss with continued treatment. Liraglutide is contraindicated in those with a personal history or family history of medullary thyroid cancer or multiple endocrine neoplasia type 2 or 2B. Side effects for liraglutide include headache, nausea, vomiting, diarrhea, and constipation, which tend to be dose-related. Hypoglycemia can occur in nondiabetics but at a lower frequency than type 2 diabetics.

Several sympathomimetic drugs (phentermine, benzphetamine [Didrex], diethylpropion [Tenuate], and phendimetrazine [Bontril PDM]) are approved for the short-term (up to 12 weeks) treatment of obesity. These drugs can increase blood pressure and have a potential for abuse and therefore are contraindicated in patients with CHD, hypertension, or hyperthyroidism, or in patients with a history of drug abuse.

The most recent prescription aid in weight management to be approved by the Food and Drug Administration is Plenity (Gelesis100), a hydrogel capsule made of cellulose and citric acid. It is approved for adults with a BMI of 25 to 40 kg/m² when used in conjunction with diet and exercise. The recommended dose is three capsules 20 to 30 minutes before lunch and dinner. The capsules release thousands of nonaggregating particles that rapidly absorb water in the stomach, creating small individual gel pieces with the elasticity of plant-based foods without the caloric value. The gel pieces contribute to a sensation of fullness and reduced hunger by increasing the volume and elasticity of the stomach and small intestine contents. In a randomized clinical trial, the most common side effects reported were gastrointestinal symptoms.

Vagal blockade devices are available in the United States for the treatment of adults with a BMI of 40 to 45 kg/m² or of 35 to 39.9 kg/m², with at least one obesity-related comorbidity (e.g., type 2 diabetes) who have failed a supervised weight management program within the past 5 years. The abdominal vagal nerve controls gastric emptying and signals the satiety center in the brain. Electric stimulation of the abdominal vagal nerve from the subcutaneously implanted device blocks vagal nerve conduction between the brain and the stomach, thereby reducing hunger. However, the specific mechanism for weight loss is unknown. Implantation of the device involves laparoscopically placing one lead on the anterior vagal trunk and the other on the posterior intraabdominal vagal trunk. Adverse events include pain at the neuroregulator site, vomiting, surgical complications, nausea, heartburn, belching, and dysphagia. Implantation of the device is contraindicated in patients at high risk for surgical complications, patients with other permanent implanted devices (e.g., heart pacemaker, implanted defibrillator, neurostimulator), or patients likely to need MRI procedures.

Bariatric Surgery

Bariatric surgery should be considered for patients with a BMI greater than 40 kg/m² or a BMI greater than 35 kg/m² with significant comorbid conditions. Patients should be well informed and motivated and have failed a trial of nonsurgical weight loss. They should also be of acceptable risk for surgery. Contraindications to bariatric surgery include untreated major depression or psychosis, binge eating disorders, active drug or alcohol abuse, and the inability to comply with nutritional requirements including lifelong vitamin supplementation. A comprehensive preoperative evaluation and close extended follow-up after surgery are required. Bariatric surgery has been shown to result in a significant and sustained weight loss, as well as resolution of many obesity-related complications, in most patients. Patients may lose more than 60% of their excess weight after bariatric surgery. There is increasing interest in the role of bariatric surgery as a treatment for type 2 diabetes in obese patients who have a BMI less than 35 kg/m². Several unblinded trials comparing bariatric surgery with medical therapy for type 2 diabetes have demonstrated significantly greater improvements in blood glucose control in patients who underwent bariatric surgery.

Bariatric procedures can be divided into three types: restrictive procedures, which decrease gastric volume and limit food intake; malabsorptive procedures, which alter digestion of food and decrease the effectiveness of nutrient absorption; and mixed procedures, which have components of both restriction and malabsorption. Currently, the most common procedures performed in the United States are the laparoscopic Roux-en-Y gastric bypass (RYGB) and the sleeve gastrectomy (Figure 2).

Roux-en-Y Gastric Bypass

The RYGB is characterized by a small (<30 mL) proximal gastric pouch that is divided and separated from the distal stomach and anastomosed to a Roux limb of small bowel, 75 to 150 cm in length. It is the most commonly performed bariatric procedure and involves the creation of a small pouch at the superior portion of the stomach. The pouch is then connected to the jejunum, bypassing the duodenum, where the majority of calories are absorbed. The mortality rate associated with gastric bypass is low (<1%), but patients can have significant postoperative complications, including pulmonary emboli, deep vein thromboses, leaks from the gastrointestinal tract, gastric remnant distention, stomal stenosis, ulcers, gallstones, and hernias. Patients are required to take lifelong vitamin and mineral supplementation because absorption of iron, vitamin B₁₂/folate, and others are affected.

Laparoscopic Sleeve Gastrectomy

Laparoscopic sleeve gastrectomy (LSG) has emerged as a single-stage bariatric procedure. It is a restrictive, nonreversible procedure involving removal of about 85% of the stomach so that the remainder takes the shape of a tube or sleeve. Recent studies have shown that LSG has equivalent results to other procedures. There is durability of results 5 to 9 years after the procedure, but there are no long-term data beyond this. Gastric-sleeve dilatations and staple-line leaks are the most common complications. LSG involves no foreign body, needs no invasive adjustments, and avoids malabsorption of many micronutrients.

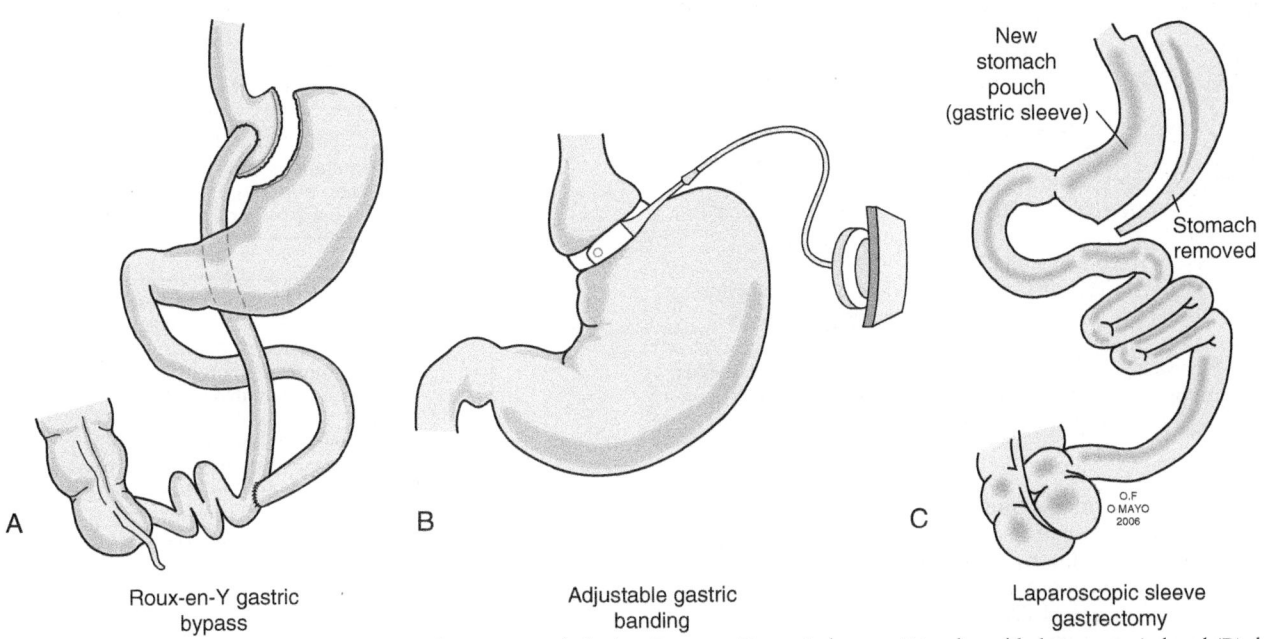

Figure 2 Techniques commonly used for the surgical treatment of obesity: Roux-en-Y gastric bypass (A), adjustable laparoscopic band (B), laparoscopic sleeve gastrectomy (C).

Biliopancreatic Diversion With Duodenal Switch

The biliopancreatic diversion with duodenal switch (BPD/DS) is a less-commonly performed bariatric procedure that is generally recommended for individuals with a BMI greater than 50. This procedure entails two major steps. The first step is sleeve gastrectomy, in which about 80% of the stomach is removed. The second step bypasses the majority of the intestine by connecting the end portion of the intestine to the duodenum near the stomach. It is a restrictive as well as malabsorptive procedure.

The BPD/DS is usually performed as a single procedure; however, in certain circumstances, the procedure may be performed in two stages, with the intestinal bypass being performed after some weight loss has been achieved initially with sleeve gastrectomy. The BPD/DS leads to greater weight loss in comparison to the RYGB or LSG but is associated with greater risk of malnutrition and vitamin deficiencies.

Intragastric Balloon

Intragastric balloon devices are approved to treat obesity in adults with a BMI ≥ 30 kg/m² who have failed previous weight loss attempts. The balloon promotes sensation of satiety and therefore, because the weight loss mechanism is primarily restrictive, the success is dependent on patient's adherence to lifestyle modifications. Adults with a BMI ≥40 kg/m² or a BMI ≥35 kg/m² with one or more comorbidities who qualify for bariatric surgery, but refuse or lack access to bariatric surgery, may also be considered for the balloon. The intragastric balloon IBD may serve as a bridging therapy in the extremely obese patient who is not a bariatric surgical candidate due to excessive anesthesia risk.

Several intragastric balloons are available, and these differ in their volume, means of insertion and removal, duration in stomach, and adjustability. Common initial symptoms include nausea, vomiting, reflux, and abdominal pain. These symptoms tend to diminish in most patients. Total weight loss is intermediate between bariatric surgery and medical measures including drugs and lifestyle modifications.

Aspiration Therapy

Aspiration therapy is approved by the US Food and Drug Administration for patients with a BMI between 35 and 55 who failed to achieve weight loss with nonsurgical therapy. Aspiration therapy induces weight loss by removing a portion of the ingested calories after each meal via a modified percutaneous endoscopic gastrostomy tube system. The patient is instructed to drain the stomach

contents 20 to 30 minutes after each meal. There is a lack of long-term data on the efficacy of the aspiration therapy.

In conclusion, obesity is a growing public health problem that has significant short- and long-term consequences. Lifestyle modification with or without adjuvant therapies should be used to achieve a goal of modest weight loss. With modest weight loss, patients experience a decreased risk of mortality and improvement of obesity-related complications.

References

Bray GA, Ryan DH: Medical therapy for the patient with obesity, *Circulation* 125:1695–1703, 2012.

Jensen MD, Ryan DH, Donato KA, et al: 2013 AHA/ACC/TOS guideline for the management of overweight and obesity in adults: A report of the American College of Cardiology/ American Heart Association Task Force on Practice Guidelines and The Obesity Society, *Obesity* 21.

Mechanick JI, Youdim A, Jones DB, et al: Clinical practice guidelines for the perioperative nutritional, metabolic, and nonsurgical support of the bariatric surgery patient—2013 update: Cosponsored by American Association of Clinical Endocrinologists, The Obesity Society, and American Society for Metabolic & Bariatric Surgery, *Endocr Pract* 19:337–372, 2013.

Sacks FM, Bray GA, Carey VJ, et al: Comparison of weight-loss diets with different compositions of fat, protein, and carbohydrates, *N Engl J Med* 360:859, 2009.

The Practical Guide: Identification, Evaluation, and Treatment of Overweight and Obesity in Adults. Available at: http://www.nhlbi.nih.gov/guidelines/obesity/prctgd_c.pdf.

PARENTERAL NUTRITION IN ADULTS

Method of
Kris M. Mogensen, MS and Malcolm K. Robinson, MD

 CURRENT DIAGNOSIS

- Reserve parenteral nutrition (PN) for patients with intestinal dysfunction or failure.
- Reserve PN for conditions such as short-bowel syndrome, severe malabsorption, ileus or intestinal dysmotility, intractable vomiting, and severe diarrhea.
- Always reevaluate the need for PN and work toward a transition to enteral nutrition, or an oral diet, if possible, to limit complications associated with PN.

CURRENT THERAPY

- Correct electrolyte abnormalities and hyperglycemia prior to the initiation of PN.
- Start with no more than 150 to 200 g dextrose on the first day of PN; start with 100 to 150 g dextrose for patients with diabetes or patients at risk for the refeeding syndrome.
- Advance PN by 100 to 150 g dextrose daily until the goal is achieved.
- Maintain blood glucose <180 mg/dL.
- Monitor electrolytes, including phosphate and magnesium, until stable; the frequency of lab monitoring can be decreased based on stability.
- Monitor closely for complications associated with PN: electrolyte abnormalities, hyper/hypoglycemia, PN-associated liver disease, and central line infections.

Since the inception of parenteral nutrition (PN) in the 1960s, the science of PN has matured in a number of ways. The initial excitement of being able to feed basic nutrients, vitamins, and trace elements intravenously has been tempered by the realization that indiscriminant use of PN can be harmful. Although PN can still be lifesaving, it is imperative that it be used judiciously and only as long as necessary. This chapter discusses the current use of PN in adult patients.

Indications and Contraindications

Enteral nutrition (EN) is the preferred method of nutrition support, primarily because it is associated with fewer infectious and metabolic complications. However, total PN (TPN), which is the provision of all nutrient requirements intravenously, may be indicated when feeding through the gastrointestinal (GI) tract is not possible. PN may be appropriately initiated in those who cannot receive enteral nourishment and are malnourished or at risk for developing malnourishment. Malnourishment can be defined as unintentional loss of more than 10% of usual body weight or greater than 7 to 10 days of inadequate nutrient intake. The body stores of well-nourished persons are generally sufficient to provide the essential nutrients, resist infection, promote wound healing, and support other necessary physiologic functions for this time period. In patients who are anticipated not to be able to receive adequate EN for longer than 10 days, it is not necessary to wait 10 days before initiating PN. This may include patients with short-bowel syndrome and others who are expected to have prolonged GI dysfunction.

According to the American Society for Parenteral and Enteral Nutrition (ASPEN) guidelines, EN is contraindicated in conditions such as diffuse peritonitis, intestinal obstruction, early stages of short-bowel syndrome, intractable vomiting, paralytic ileus, severe GI bleeding, and severe diarrhea and malabsorption syndromes. Other relative contraindications to EN include severe pancreatitis and enterocutaneous fistulas, although depending on the clinical circumstances, EN may be indicated. PN and EN may be provided concomitantly, although in patients who are critically ill, PN should not be started until all strategies to maximize enteral feeding (such as the use of postpyloric feeding tubes and motility agents) have been attempted. PN support is unlikely to benefit a patient who will be able to take EN within 4 or 5 days after the onset of illness or who has a relatively minor injury (Figure 1).

There are four key steps to consider before initiating PN, including assessing nutritional status, determining energy needs, evaluating GI function, and estimating the length of time a patient will require PN (Box 1).

Assessment of Nutritional Status

Nutrient depletion is associated with increased morbidity and mortality, and the prevalence of malnutrition in hospitalized

Consider nutritional support if any are present:
Patient has been without nutrition for 7 d.
Expected duration of illness is >10 d.
Patient is malnourished (unintentional weight loss of >10% body weight).

↓

Initiate nutritional support only if tissue perfusion is adequate and PO₂, PCO₂, electrolytes, and acid-base balance are near normal.

↓

Is there a contraindication to enteral feeding, such as:
Diffuse peritonitis
Intestinal obstruction
Early stages of short bowel syndrome
Intractable vomiting
Paralytic ileus
Severe gastrointestinal bleeding
Severe diarrhea and malabsorption syndromes

No → Administer enteral nutrition
Yes → Administer parenteral nutrition

Enteral nutrition tolerated
Enteral nutrition not tolerated or partially tolerated

Figure 1 Determining route of feeding.

BOX 1 Decision-Making Steps When Initiating Parenteral Nutrition

Assess the patient's nutritional status. Nutrition support (PN or EN) should not be initiated in well-nourished patients unless they have received a suboptimal diet for more than 7 d.

Determine whether the patient has extreme energy needs (hypermetabolism) that warrant the early use of nutrition support (PN and/or EN) within 7 d of injury or illness. These are typically critically ill patients who have suffered severe burns or trauma.

Evaluate the function of the GI tract; if it is intact and can be used safely, PN should be avoided. PN support is indicated until enteral access is established and the patient can meet nutrient needs via tube feedings.

Estimate how long the patient will require PN support. If GI function is expected to return within 5 d, there is no known benefit of initiating PN.

Abbreviations: EN = enteral nutrition; GI = gastrointestinal; PN = parenteral nutrition.

patients is approximately 50%. Therefore it is imperative to identify patients who have or are at risk for developing protein-energy malnutrition or specific nutrient deficiencies. A patient's risk of developing malnutrition-related medical complications needs to be quantified, and it is necessary to monitor the adequacy of nutritional therapy.

Nutrition assessment begins with a thorough history and physical examination in conjunction with select laboratory tests aimed at detecting specific nutrient deficiencies in patients who are at high risk for future abnormalities. The nutrition assessment should establish whether the patient will need maintenance therapy or nutrition repletion and should assess the status of the patient's GI tract, especially if nutrition support will be required.

A thorough history includes an assessment of recent weight changes, dietary habits, GI symptoms, and changes in exercise tolerance or physical abilities that would indicate functional capacity deficiencies. The physical examination includes inspecting for a loss of subcutaneous fat and muscle wasting, which indicate a loss of body energy and protein stores; edema and ascites, which can also indicate altered energy demands or decreased energy intake; and signs of vitamin and mineral deficits such as dermatitis, glossitis, cheilosis, neuromuscular irritability, and coarse, easily pluckable hair.

Several laboratory measurements have been used as nutritional biomarkers to aid the nutritional assessment. The serum proteins prealbumin, transferrin, and retinol-binding protein have a rapid turnover rate and short half-lives and therefore may be used as indicators of recent nutritional intake. However, these proteins are affected by the metabolic responses to stress and illness, as well as other conditions, including iron status (transferrin) and renal status (retinol-binding protein, prealbumin). This can limit their usefulness during acute illness states.

Prealbumin is least affected by fluctuations in hydration status and by liver and renal function compared with other plasma proteins. However, prealbumin levels drop in acute inflammatory conditions during which the liver switches to acute-phase protein production and decreases prealbumin synthesis. A rise in C-reactive protein, a protein synthesized by the liver as part of the acute-phase response, indicates inflammatory states. Thus C-reactive protein, when measured along with prealbumin, can help differentiate a low prealbumin due to nutritional inadequacy versus low prealbumin due to an acute-phase response.

The serum albumin concentration has traditionally been used as an indicator of nutritional status. Although it is a good preoperative predictor of outcome for patients undergoing surgery, it is affected by too many variables in the acute care setting to make it a reliable marker of nutritional status under such conditions or in the immediate postoperative period.

A simple and practical index of malnutrition is the degree of weight loss. Unintentional weight loss of greater than 10% within the previous 6 months indicates protein-energy malnutrition and is a good prognosticator of clinical outcome. Weight can also be compared with an ideal or desirable weight, or an index of body weight relative to height. The body mass index (BMI), reported as weight in kilograms divided by height in meters squared, is the best known such index and can be used to detect both undernutrition and overnutrition. This index is independent of height, and the same standards apply to both men and women. A BMI of 18.5 to 25 kg/m² is considered normal, 25 to 29.9 kg/m² is considered overweight, and greater than 30 kg/m² is considered obese. Patients with a normal or high BMI can still have nutrient deficiencies and therefore can be malnourished if they have recently lost a significant amount of weight. In addition, a BMI of 18 kg/m² or less in an adult indicates moderate malnutrition and a BMI less than 15 kg/m² is associated with increased morbidity.

Another practical tool for evaluating nutritional status is the subjective global assessment (SGA) that encompasses historical, symptomatic, and physical parameters. The SGA technique determines whether nutrient assimilation has been restricted because of decreased food intake, maldigestion, or malabsorption; whether any effects of malnutrition on organ function and body composition have occurred; and whether the patient's disease process influences nutrient requirements. The findings of the history and physical examination are subjectively weighted to rank patients as being well nourished, moderately malnourished, or severely malnourished and are used to predict their risk for medical complications (Box 2).

BOX 2 — Subjective Global Assessment

Select the appropriate category with a checkmark, or enter a numeric value where indicated by #.

History
- Weight change
  Overall loss in past 6 mo: amount=# _____ kg; % loss =# _____
  Change in past 2 wk: _____ increase, _____ no change, _____ decrease
- Dietary intake change (relative to normal)
  _____ No change
  _____ Change duration=# _____ wk.
  _____ Type: _____ suboptimal solid diet, _____ full liquid diet, _____ hypocaloric liquids, _____ starvation
- Gastrointestinal symptoms (that persisted for >2 wk)
  _____ None, _____ nausea, _____ vomiting, _____ diarrhea, _____ anorexia
- Functional capacity
  _____ No dysfunction (e.g., full capacity)
  _____ Dysfunction duration=# _____ wk
  _____ Type: _____ working suboptimally, _____ ambulatory, _____ bedridden
- Disease and its relation to nutritional requirements
  Primary diagnosis (specify): _____
  Metabolic demand (stress): _____ no stress, _____ low stress, _____ moderate stress, _____ high stress

Physical (for each trait specify: 0 = normal, 1+ = mild, 2+ = moderate, 3+ = severe)
_____ Loss of subcutaneous fat (triceps, chest)
_____ Muscle wasting (quadriceps, deltoids)
_____ Ankle edema
_____ Sacral edema
_____ Ascites

SGA Rating (select one)
_____ A=Well nourished
_____ B=Moderately (or suspected of being) malnourished
_____ C=Severely malnourished

Reprinted with permission from Detsky AS; McLauglin JR, Baker JP, et al: What is subjective global assessment of nutritional status? JPEN 1987;11:8–13.

Estimating Nutritional Requirements

Historically, TPN often provided nutrients in excess of actual requirements. This was based on the assumption that patients requiring nutritional intervention were severely depleted and required aggressive repletion; hence, the misnomer "hyperalimentation." Overfeeding is associated with increased carbon dioxide production and difficulty weaning from a ventilator as well as metabolic complications, such as hyperglycemia, which can lead to increased infection, morbidity, and mortality. Thus nutritional support should be titrated to match actual metabolic requirements.

In addition, there are times when *underfeeding* calories may be necessary and beneficial. In such cases, this is referred to as "permissive" underfeeding to distinguish it from underfeeding that occurs due to the unintentional inadequate delivery of nutrients. For example, permissive underfeeding may be appropriate for some critically ill obese patients who are receiving adequate protein. Such permissive underfeeding for critically ill obese individuals is now the recommendation of ASPEN and the Society of Critical Care Medicine (SCCM).

Energy Requirements

There are four components of daily energy requirement. The first is the basal metabolic rate (BMR), which is the amount of energy expended under complete rest shortly after awakening and in a fasting state (12–14 hours). BMR varies with age, sex, and body size; correlates roughly with body surface area;

and is proportional to lean tissue mass. This relationship holds true even among persons of different ages and sexes. Resting metabolic rate or resting energy expenditure (REE) represents the amount of energy expended 2 hours after a meal under conditions of rest and thermal neutrality. However, although it is often used synonymously with BMR, the REE is typically 10% higher.

The second component of daily energy expenditure is the thermic effect of exercise or the energy used in physical activity. The contribution of this component increases markedly during intense muscular work, and admission to a hospital generally results in a marked decrease in physical activity. Hospital activity in ambulatory patients accounts for a 20% to 30% increase in BMR. Critically ill patients who are on a ventilator generally have low activity levels (BMR increases by only 5%–10%) because the ventilator performs the work of breathing, and they are not ambulatory.

The third component of energy expenditure is diet-induced thermogenesis, the increase in BMR that follows food intake. The digestion and metabolism of exogenous nutrients, whether delivered to the gut or vein, result in an increase in metabolic rate. The magnitude of the thermic effect of food varies depending on the amount and composition of the diet and accounts for approximately 10% of daily energy expenditure.

Finally, acute illness adds an additional stress factor to the daily energy expenditure and correlates with disease severity. For example, a patient's metabolic rate increases by 10% to 30% after a major fracture, from 20% to 60% with severe infection, and from 40% to 110% with a severe third-degree burn. In addition, fever accelerates chemical reactions, and the BMR rises approximately 10% for each degree Celsius increase in temperature. Alternatively, cooling of febrile patients produces a reduction in BMR of approximately 10% per degree Celsius.

The first step of estimating energy requirements is to estimate the BMR. This is usually accomplished using one of several predictive equations. The most commonly used method is based on the predictive equations reported by Harris and Benedict in 1919. The Harris-Benedict equations are as follows:

$$BMR\ (men) = 66.47 + 13.75\ (W) + 5.0\ (H) - 6.76\ (A)$$

$$BMR\ (women) = 655.1 + 9.56\ (W) + 1.85\ (H) - 4.68\ (A)$$

where W is weight in kg, H is height in cm, and A is age in years.

After the BMR is calculated, it is adjusted for the level of stress induced by injury or the disease process (Figure 2) and activity level. Activity factors for hospitalized patients are 1.0 to 1.1 for intubated patients, 1.2 for patients confined to bed, and 1.3 for patients out of bed. Therefore the patient's energy requirements (total energy expenditure [TEE]) are finally calculated:

$$TEE = BMR \times Activity\ factor \times Stress\ factor$$

The thermic effect of feeding is generally not included in the calculation of energy requirements for hospitalized patients.

Alternatively, some clinicians estimate energy requirements based on actual body weight. Thus 20 to 25 kilocalories (kcal)/kg is administered to the critically ill intubated patient, and 30 kcal/kg is given to nonventilated patients in whom excessive energy intake is not a major concern.

Predicting energy expenditure in obese patients can be difficult because using predictive formulas with actual body weight can lead to high TEE and potentially to overfeeding. A factor of 18 to 21 kcal/kg has been validated in obese patients, and the Harris-Benedict equation using the average of actual and ideal weight and a stress factor of 1.3 predicts REE in acutely ill obese patients with a BMI of 30 to 50 kg/m².

Indirect calorimetry is a more precise, clinically practical, and individualized method to determine energy expenditure, particularly in patients in whom estimating requirements through

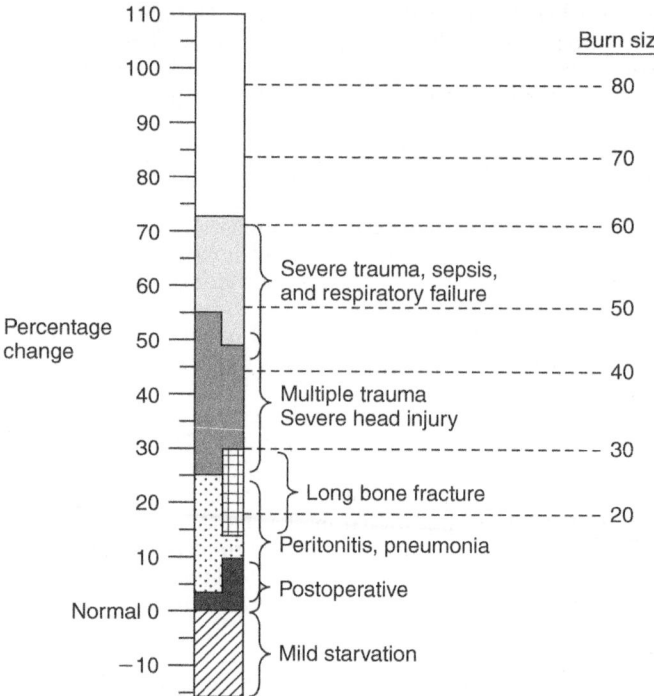

Figure 2 Percentage change in metabolic rate due to injury. Adapted from Wilmore DW: The Metabolic Management of the Critically Ill, New York, Plenum Medical Books, 1977.

predictive equations are difficult, such as those who continue to lose weight despite what appears to be an adequate caloric intake, who are critically ill, or who have rapidly changing energy needs.

Indirect calorimetry measures changes in oxygen consumption and carbon dioxide production to calculate the REE. Including a stress factor to account for injury is not necessary with indirect calorimetry because the measured energy expenditure accounts for the effects of disease state, stress, and trauma. However, the measurement occurs at rest, and therefore an activity factor of 1.0 to 1.3, depending on whether the patient is intubated, bedridden, or ambulatory, must be applied.

Nutrient Requirements

The recommended daily protein allowance for most healthy persons who are not hospitalized is 0.8 g/kg, or about 60 to 70 g of protein each day. The stressed, critically ill patient generally needs a higher dose of protein in the range of 1.0 to 1.5 g/kg/d. For most patients, providing protein beyond 1.5 g/kg/d is not beneficial. In fact, providing excess protein does not enhance uptake and can lead to increased ureagenesis, which can cause renal injury in some patients.

The calorie-to-nitrogen ratio for most PN solutions is typically about 150:1, with an acceptable range of 100:1 to 180:1. Nitrogen content is used as a marker for protein, and, hence, the two terms are used interchangeably. Usually, 6.25 g of protein is equal to 1.0 g of nitrogen. The conversion factor is slightly higher (6.4) for PN solutions, such as those with higher concentrations of crystalline amino acids.

Vitamin and mineral requirements are altered in certain disease states due to increased losses, greater use, or both. Guidelines for parenteral vitamin and trace elements, developed by the Nutrition Advisory Group of the American Medical Association, were approved by the US Food and Drug Administration (FDA) in 1979 and amended in 2000 (Table 1).

Composition of Central and Peripheral Venous Solutions

Central venous access is required for providing TPN because of the hypertonicity of the formulas infused (1900 mOsm/kg). The

TABLE 1	Recommended Daily Doses of Parenteral Vitamins and Trace Elements

MICRONUTRIENT	PARENTERAL DOSE
Vitamins	
Vitamin A	3300 IU
Vitamin D	200 IU
Vitamin E	10 IU
Vitamin K	150 µg
Ascorbic acid (vitamin C)	200 µg
Folic acid	600 µg
Niacin	40 mg
Riboflavin (vitamin B$_2$)	3.6 mg
Thiamine (vitamin B$_1$)	6 mg
Pyridoxine (vitamin B$_6$)	6 mg
Cyanocobalamin (vitamin B$_{12}$)	5 µg
Pantothenic acid	15 mg
Biotin	60 µg
Trace Elements	
Zinc	2.5–5 mg
Copper	0.3–0.5 mg
Chromium	10–15 µg
Manganese	60–100 µg
Selenium	20–60 µg

Data from American Medical Association, Department of Foods and Nutrition: Multivitamin preparations for parenteral use. A statement by the Nutrition Advisory Group, JPEN J Parenter Enteral Nutr 1979;3:258–62; Food and Drug Administration: Parenteral multivitamin products: Drugs for human use: Drug efficacy study implementation: Amendment, Federal Register 2000;65(77):21200–21201.

TABLE 2	Central Vs. Peripheral Parenteral Nutrition

PROPERTY	CENTRAL NUTRITION	PERIPHERAL NUTRITION
Daily calories	2000–3000	1000–1500
Protein	Variable	56–87 g
Volume of fluid required (mL)	1000–3000	2000–3500
Duration of therapy (d)	>7	5–7
Route of administration	Dedicated central venous catheter	Peripheral vein or multiuse central catheter
Substrate profile	55%–60% carbohydrate	30% carbohydrate
	15%–20% protein	20% protein
	25% fat	50% fat
Osmolarity (mOsm/L)	~2000	~600–900

infusion of a hypertonic solution into a peripheral vein, known as *peripheral parenteral nutrition* (PPN), can result in thrombophlebitis and venous sclerosis unless the PN is drastically diluted to lower the tonicity. To minimize the hypertonicity of PPN solutions, dextrose is limited to 5% to 10%, and amino acids are limited to 2.5% to 3.5%. Lipids are isotonic and therefore provide a significant portion of the caloric substrate of PPN formulas.

Central venous solutions, which are prepared by the hospital's pharmacy, typically combine carbohydrate in the form of dextrose, protein as crystalline amino acids, and lipids from polyunsaturated long-chain triglycerides such as soybean oil or a safflower/soybean oil emulsion. Vitamins, electrolytes, and trace elements are added to the formulation as needed. Typical substrate profiles of carbohydrate, protein, and lipids in central PN are shown in Table 2. A usual PN prescription administers 1 to 2 L of a solution each day. Administration of 500 mL of a 20% fat emulsion 1 day each week is sufficient to prevent essential fatty acid deficiency. Alternatively, if additional calories from lipids are needed on a daily basis, they can be administered as a separate infusion or most commonly as part of the mixture of dextrose and amino acids, a technique known as *triple mix* or *three-in-one*.

Including lipid injectable emulsion into a parenteral admixture changes the conventional nutritional solution into an emulsion. Various electrolytes and micronutrients can adversely influence emulsion stability, and therefore their concentration in three-in-one solutions is limited to prevent "cracking" of the PN solution, in which microscopic or macroscopic precipitates are formed. The higher the cation valence, the greater the destabilizing influence to the emulsifier. Therefore trivalent cations such as ferric ion (iron dextran) are more disruptive than divalent cations such as calcium or magnesium ions, which are more disruptive than monovalent cations such as sodium or potassium. No concentration of iron dextran is safe in triple-mix formulations. In-line filtration is necessary for all PN solutions, including triple-mix solutions, because it is impossible to visually detect precipitates until they are grossly incompatible and unsafe for infusion.

Once the basic solution is created, electrolytes are added as needed (Table 3). Sodium or potassium salts are given as chloride or acetate depending on the patient's requirements. Normally, equal amounts of chloride and acetate are provided. However, if chloride losses from the body are increased, which can occur in patients who have nasogastric tubes, then most of the salts should be given as chloride. Similarly, more acetate should be given to patients when additional base is required because acetate generates bicarbonate when it is metabolized. Sodium bicarbonate is incompatible with PN solutions and cannot be added to the mixture. Phosphate may be given as the sodium or potassium salt. Lipid injectable emulsions contain an additional 15 mmol/L of phosphate.

Commercially available preparations of fat-soluble and water-soluble vitamins, minerals, and trace elements are added to the nutrient mix unless they are contraindicated. Adequate thiamine is essential for patients receiving PN and can be provided separately. Vitamin K is now a component of standard IV multivitamin preparations; vitamin preparations without vitamin K are also available for those patients who may need a vitamin K restriction (e.g., patients on warfarin). Trace element preparations that include zinc, copper, manganese, and chromium are added to the PN solution in amounts consistent with the American Medical Association guidelines (see Table 1). Manganese accumulation can be toxic, and overexposure can lead to progressive neurodegenerative damage. Manganese is usually supplied in the PN solution at a daily dose of 0.5 mg as part of a multiple trace element additive. Because manganese is primarily eliminated via biliary excretion, patients with biliary obstruction or cholestasis can accumulate potentially toxic levels of manganese. Hence, manganese should be removed from the PN of patients with hyperbilirubinemia. Higher doses, 10 to 15 mg/d, of zinc are provided to patients with excessive GI losses.

Iron is not a part of commercial additive preparations because it is incompatible with triple-mix solutions and can cause

TABLE 3	Electrolyte Concentrations in Parenteral Nutrition		
ELECTROLYTE	RECOMMENDED CENTRAL PN DOSES	RECOMMENDED PERIPHERAL PN DOSES	USUAL RANGE OF DOSES
Potassium (mEq/L)	30	30	0–120 (CVC) 0–80 (PV)
Sodium (mEq/L)	30	30	0–150
Phosphate (mmol/L)	15	5	0–20
Magnesium (mEq/L)	5	5	0–16
Calcium (mEq/L) (as gluconate)	4.7	4.7	0–10
Chloride (mEq/L)	50	50	0–150
Acetate (mEq/L)	40	40	0–100

Abbreviations: CVC=central venous catheter; PN=parenteral nutrition; PV=peripheral vein.

anaphylactic reactions when it is given intravenously. Patients who need this trace element should receive it orally or by injection. Iron is not given to patients who are critically ill because hyperferremia can increase bacterial virulence, alter polymorphonuclear cell function, and increase host susceptibility to infection.

PPN is less commonly used than central PN and can be disadvantageous. Because of the low concentration of dextrose, greater volumes (typically >2 L/d) are required to provide sufficient calories, which might not be feasible in fluid-restricted patients. PPN generally does not approximate a patient's energy needs because PPN provides only 1000 to 1500 kcal/d, and a large percentage of the calories (60%) are derived from fat. High-fat infusions are undesirable because they are associated with impaired reticuloendothelial system function and are potentially immunosuppressive. There is no evidence that lipid injectable emulsions improve outcomes or significantly decrease nitrogen losses. Generally, PPN should be avoided unless it is combined with enteral feeding in patients who cannot tolerate full enteral feeding, patients who cannot get a central venous catheter, or patients with low body weights in whom PPN can meet at least two-thirds of estimated needs.

Administration and Venous Access

Typically, central PN solutions are administered into the superior vena cava. Access to this vein can be achieved by cannulation of the subclavian or internal jugular veins. Peripherally inserted central venous catheters (PICCs), typically inserted via an antecubital vein and advanced into the superior vena cava, are the most commonly used central venous access devices for providing PN. PICC placement offers the advantage of central venous access, while avoiding the risks associated with accessing the subclavian or jugular veins, such as hemothorax, pneumothorax, and arterial injury.

Tunneled catheters or catheters with indwelling ports should be considered for patients who will need prolonged central venous nutrition (e.g., >6 weeks). Patients who will be using their catheters solely for daily central PN and who require home IV feeding may be best served by a tunneled catheter rather than an indwelling port. Tunneled catheters may be more easily manipulated and cared for, which can minimize the risk of infection.

Inserting a dedicated line for infusing hypertonic solutions requires strict aseptic technique and maximal barrier protection: hat, mask, gown, and gloves must be worn. The position of the catheter tip in the superior vena cava is confirmed by chest x-ray before any concentrated solutions are administered. Once the position of the tip has been confirmed, the line should be used exclusively for administering the hypertonic nutrient solution.

Multiple-lumen central venous catheters are most commonly used. Although at least one lumen is dedicated to the infusion of the PN solutions, the other(s) may be used for monitoring, blood drawing, or medication. The rate of catheter sepsis associated with multiple-port catheters may be the same as or slightly greater than the rate associated with the use of single-port catheters. However, multiple-port PICCs are used to infuse PN solutions for a shorter time, which can minimize their inherent risk. Multiple-port catheters should be carefully maintained, including dressing changes, maintaining the dedicated lumen, careful handling of the other lumens, and removing the catheter as soon as it is no longer needed.

Infusion and Patient Monitoring

It is advisable to start with 1 L of central PN and increase the volume as needed, depending on the patient's metabolic stability. Blood glucose levels should be closely monitored and maintained at <180 mg/dL, tissue perfusion should be adequate, and Po_2, Pco_2, electrolytes (especially potassium, phosphate, and magnesium) and acid-base balance should be near normal before starting or advancing to the goal solution. The solutions should be administered using a volumetric pump set at a constant rate. It is important not to modify the infusion rate during any given day to try to compensate for excess or inadequate administration of the PN solution, such as when the PN solution arrives later than expected. A cyclic schedule (10–16 h/d) for patients requiring long-term PN can be initiated once the patient is metabolically stable. In situations when the central PN solution must be suddenly discontinued, a 10% dextrose solution may be given at the same infusion rate as was used for the PN unless the patient is severely hyperglycemic. PN solutions may be administered at one-half the infusion rate to patients who are undergoing surgical procedures because circulating glucose and electrolyte levels are easier to control.

In addition to hyperglycemia, metabolic complications include hyper- and hypophosphatemia, hyper- and hypokalemia, hyper- and hypomagnesemia, and hyper- and hypocalcemia. Thus it is important to monitor the patient's serum electrolytes closely, especially when initiating TPN. Once the patient has stabilized on the individual nutritional prescription, serum chemistries should be obtained at least twice weekly to measure chloride, CO_2, potassium, sodium, blood urea nitrogen, creatinine, calcium, and phosphate levels and once weekly for a full profile that includes liver function, magnesium, and triglyceride levels. Stable home PN patients may have less frequent chemistry monitoring, typically starting with once per week monitoring, then decreasing to twice per month and then monthly, depending on overall stability and clinical status.

Patients with Special Needs
Glucose Intolerance

Hyperglycemia is the most common metabolic complication related to PN, and glucose regulation may be especially difficult in patients who have diabetes mellitus or who develop insulin resistance in response to severe stress or infection. Control of blood glucose levels is important for all patients who receive PN because uncontrolled hyperglycemia may be associated with complications such as fluid and electrolyte disturbances and increased infection risk due to impairment of host defenses, including decreased polymorphonuclear leukocyte mobilization, chemotaxis, and phagocytic activity. Intensive insulin therapy, maintaining blood glucose concentrations between 80 and 110 mg/dL, was once considered standard practice for critically ill patients. However, other studies have demonstrated significant morbidity and mortality with this approach. For critically ill patients, a target blood glucose of 110 to 150 mg/dL is preferred, and for ambulatory patients, a target blood glucose of 140 to 180 mg/dL is recommended.

Patients with difficult glycemic control may best be managed by continuous insulin infusion, which is safe, effective, and more timely than subcutaneous insulin therapy. Hypoglycemia that occurs during this type of infusion generally is short lived and more easily corrected than hypoglycemia resulting from subcutaneous insulin administration. A separate IV insulin infusion can be used rather than adding incremental doses of insulin to the PN bag every 24 hours in patients for whom glycemic control is difficult. Many intensive care units (ICUs) have an insulin drip infusion protocol in which there are frequent checks of serum glucose and adjustments of the insulin infusion drip (e.g., every 1–2 hours) to maintain target glucose levels. The conventional approach of using sliding scale insulin to cover high blood glucose levels may be unsafe and ineffective, and repetitive doses of subcutaneous insulin in the edematous patient can have a cumulative effect leading to prolonged hypoglycemia. In addition, adjusting insulin in the PN bag every 24 hours might not achieve the desired rapid correction of hyperglycemia deemed appropriate based on the literature, which indicates worse outcomes for those with poor glucose control.

Abrupt discontinuation of PN can lead to hypoglycemia and should be avoided. Instead, it is recommended to decrease the PN infusion rate by one-half for the last hour of infusion prior to discontinuation to prevent rebound hypoglycemia.

Pancreatitis

Most cases of pancreatitis are mild, and nutritional support is not needed. However, 10% to 20% of patients with pancreatitis develop severe disease that results in a hypermetabolic, hyperdynamic, systemic inflammatory response syndrome that creates a highly catabolic stress state. In an evidence-based report evaluating nutrition support in acute pancreatitis patients, EN delivered to the small intestine (distal to the ligament of Treitz) is preferred over PN; EN patients are less likely to suffer from multiorgan failure, systemic infections, and death.

Initiation of PN should be delayed in patients with acute pancreatitis who cannot tolerate EN even though they might eventually require PN. Providing PN within 24 hours of admission has been shown to worsen outcome, and providing PN after resuscitation and abatement of the acute inflammatory process appears to improve outcome compared with standard therapy. Consequently, if EN is not feasible, the initiation of PN should be delayed for at least 5 days after admission to the hospital, when the peak period of inflammation has abated.

Acute Kidney Injury and Chronic Kidney Disease

Acute kidney injury (AKI) is associated with severe nutritional deficits. Most patients with AKI are catabolic and have energy requirements 50% to 100% greater than resting requirements, likely the result of other coexisting conditions such as sepsis, trauma, and burns. Energy is provided to patients with AKI in sufficient quantities to minimize protein degradation, generally in the range of 25 to 35 kcal/kg/day. Lipid injectable emulsions can be used as a source of concentrated energy in patients who require a fluid restriction.

Protein loss is accelerated and protein synthesis is impaired in patients with AKI. Loss of amino acids in the dialysate and renal replacement therapies add to the protein deficit and increase individual protein needs. Approximately 10 to 12 g of amino acids are lost with each dialysis therapy, depending on the type of dialyzer membrane, blood flow rate, and dialyzer reuse procedure, and approximately 10 to 16 g/day of amino acids are lost through continuous renal replacement therapies (CRRT). The provision of protein at 1.0 to 1.4 g/kg/day and 1.5 to 2.5 g/kg/day is recommended for AKI patients receiving hemodialysis and CRRT, respectively.

Protein is provided with a standard solution containing both essential and nonessential amino acids. Although some data suggest essential amino acids alone may be beneficial compared to a mixture of both essential and nonessential amino acids, the efficacy of using essential amino acid solutions remains uncertain. The goal is to provide adequate protein while treating the patient aggressively with dialysis to prevent the accumulation of nitrogenous waste products.

Fluid and electrolyte balance are often impaired in patients with AKI. The amount of fluid from the PN might need to be adjusted daily, depending on the phase of AKI, whether the patient is receiving dialysis, and whether dialysis is continuous or intermittent. Serum potassium and phosphate levels typically rise in patients with AKI until dialysis is initiated, at which time levels might drop, especially with the provision of PN. Potassium, phosphate, and magnesium levels need close monitoring and adjusting to correct imbalances. Acetate salts of potassium or sodium can be administered to help correct a metabolic acidosis.

Standard doses of the water-soluble vitamins and additional folic acid (1 mg/day total) and pyridoxine (vitamin B_6) (10 mg/day) might need to be added to the solution for patients who are being dialyzed because these vitamins are lost from the body in the dialysate bath. Thiamine losses are increased with CRRT and repletion (100 mg/day) must be provided for patients receiving this therapy. The dose of vitamin C might need to be restricted to 100 mg/day to prevent oxalate deposits. However, additional vitamin C (250 mg/day) should be provided to patients receiving CRRT. The supplementation of fat-soluble vitamins is usually not required, especially in patients who also are eating, because excretion of fat-soluble vitamins is reduced in renal failure. For example, serum vitamin A levels may be elevated in ARF due to enhanced hepatic release of retinol and retinol-binding protein, decreased renal catabolism, and decreased degradation of vitamin A transport protein by the kidneys. Vitamin D levels may be decreased because of impaired activation of 1,25-dihydroxycholecalciferol in the kidneys. In anuric patients, trace elements may be withheld from the PN solution; however, for prolonged PN, trace elements and fat-soluble vitamins should be monitored and replaced accordingly.

Patients with chronic kidney disease (CKD) also have nutritional deficits due to anorexia, amino acid losses into the dialysate, concurrent illness, metabolic acidosis, and endocrine disorders. However, unlike those suffering from AKI, patients with CKD have normal energy requirements. Protein intake generally is restricted in predialysis patients to 0.6 g/kg/day or 0.75 g/kg/day if the patient is malnourished. Protein is required in higher amounts in patients on dialysis, depending on the type of dialysis: 1.2 g/kg/day for hemodialysis; 1.2 to 1.5 g/kg/day for peritoneal dialysis. Predialysis patients who become acutely ill should be given protein 1.2 to 1.5 g/kg/day even if this precipitates the need for dialysis. Starvation from insufficient calories or protein in the patient with renal dysfunction increases the risk of nutritionally related complications and should be avoided in the severely ill patient regardless of the potential need for dialysis.

Intradialytic PN is the provision of IV amino acids, carbohydrates, and fat directly into the venous drip chamber of the hemodialysis unit during treatment. It is a method of providing additional calories and protein in malnourished chronic hemodialysis patients. It is associated with significant increases in body weight and serum albumin in patients with end stage renal disease. However, intradialytic PN is expensive and the benefits have not been fully elucidated. A typical solution contains about

1100 kcal and 50 g of protein, which is provided three times per week with hemodialysis. For example, intradialytic PN provides a patient with energy and protein requirements of 2500 kcal and 70 g of protein/day, respectively, only 20% of the weekly calorie and 30% of the weekly protein needs. Thus, intradialytic PN is reserved for patients with CRF who cannot ingest sufficient nutrients by mouth and who are not candidates for nutritional support via EN or PN due to GI intolerance or venous access problems or for other reasons. Appropriate use of intradialytic PN should be limited to a very small fraction of people who are on hemodialysis.

Hepatic Dysfunction and Liver Failure

Hepatic dysfunction is associated with a variety of abnormalities including metabolic abnormalities, malabsorption, maldigestion, anorexia, and early satiety due to ascites. Dietary restrictions also can contribute to malnutrition.

Protein intake in patients with stable chronic liver disease depends on the patient's nutritional status and protein tolerance. Nutritionally depleted patients can require as much protein as 1.5 g/kg estimated dry weight. In a minority of patients who have protein-sensitive hepatic encephalopathy, protein intake might need to be decreased to 0.5 to 0.7 g/kg/day and gradually increased to 1.0 to 1.5 g/kg/day, as tolerated. These patients have deranged plasma amino acid profiles, with increased concentrations of aromatic amino acids (phenylalanine, tyrosine, and tryptophan) and methionine and decreased branched-chain amino acids (leucine, isoleucine, and valine). Randomized, controlled trials that provided parenteral or enteral formulas enriched with branched-chain amino acids have been inconsistent and have had results including no benefit, improved morbidity, no change in mortality, and improvement in encephalopathy. These specialty products should be reserved for patients with disabling encephalopathy who do not tolerate standard proteins and have not responded to other therapies, such as lactulose or neomycin administration.

Energy requirements are difficult to predict in patients with liver failure. Whereas most patients have a normal metabolic rate, up to one-third may be hypermetabolic. Although providing 25 to 30 kcal/kg/day is a guideline for providing energy needs, basing requirements on indirect calorimetry is often recommended.

Fluid restriction due to ascites and edema often necessitates increasing the dextrose concentration in the PN so as to maintain sufficient calories in a restricted volume. Sodium is reduced in the formula because liver-failure patients excrete nearly sodium-free urine. Vitamin and mineral deficiencies often occur as a result of suboptimal nutrient intake, decreased absorption, decreased storage, and in some cases alcohol use, which decreases thiamine (vitamin B_1) and folate absorption. Copper and manganese may be contraindicated because a major route of excretion for these substances is the biliary system. Zinc deficiency is common in cirrhotic patients, and supplementation of this mineral may be necessary, especially if there are excessive GI losses.

Acute Respiratory Distress Syndrome

Patients with protein-calorie malnutrition have an increased incidence of pneumonia, respiratory failure, and acute respiratory distress syndrome (ARDS). Nutritional support is indicated in patients with ARDS, and underfeeding and overfeeding can be detrimental to pulmonary function.

Overfeeding calories, and particularly glucose, can lead to increased minute ventilation, increased dead space, and increased carbon dioxide production and ultimately to difficulty weaning from a ventilator. Hypercapnia from increased carbon dioxide production is the result of glucose combustion causing more carbon dioxide production and excess calories triggering lipogenesis. A healthy person increases ventilation in response to increased calories and thus avoids hypercapnia. However, patients with compromised ventilatory status might not be able to compensate with increased ventilation and can develop respiratory distress, acute respiratory failure, and difficulty weaning from mechanical ventilation. Thus, the use of indirect calorimetry measurements to determine energy expenditure is imperative in patients with ARDS.

Critically Ill Obese Patients

Obesity is a growing problem worldwide, and management of critically ill obese patients poses many challenges. These patients are at risk for hyperglycemia, hyperlipidemia, and hypercapnea, all of which can be exacerbated by metabolic changes associated with critical illness. As with any critically ill patient, obese patients will preferentially use protein and carbohydrate for energy and cannot effectively draw upon adipose tissue for energy. These patients require nutrition support to minimize loss of lean body mass.

The concept of "hypocaloric feeding" has emerged as the preferred way to feed critically ill obese patients. Energy delivery is restricted to approximately 60% to 70% of estimated energy requirements and protein delivery is high (typically >2 g/kg ideal body weight [IBW]). This is to avoid hyperglycemia, hyperlipidemia, and hypercapnea while providing the protein required to spare lean body mass and support recovery. Small-scale studies employing this feeding method have demonstrated that patients can achieve positive nitrogen balance; one study found decreased ICU length of stay, decreased antibiotic days, and a trend toward decreased mechanical ventilation days.

Energy and protein delivery for critically ill obese patients is guided by BMI. The ASPEN-SCCM guidelines recommend providing 11 to 14 kcal/kg actual weight or 22 to 25 kcal/kg IBW for patients with a BMI >30 kg/m². In comparing these recommendations to our experience with measuring REE in this population, we have found that this should be refined further by BMI. For patients with a BMI of 30 to 50 kg/m², 11 to 14 kcal/kg closely represented 60% to 70% of measured REE. For patients with a BMI >50 kg/m², 22 to 25 kcal/kg IBW represents 60% to 70% of measured REE. For protein delivery, ASPEN and SCCM recommend protein provision of ≥2 g/kg IBW for patients with class I and class II obesity (BMI of 30 to 35 kg/m² and 35 to 40 kg/m², respectively) and for patients with class III obesity (BMI >40 kg/m²) protein provision should be ≥2.5 g/kg IBW.

Other Conditions and Nutritional Treatments

The catabolic response to major surgery, trauma, burn, and sepsis is characterized by a net breakdown of body protein stores to provide substrates for gluconeogenesis and acute-phase protein synthesis. Adequate nutrition can attenuate whole-body catabolism but rarely, if ever, prevents or reverses the loss of lean body mass during the acute phase of injury. Several strategies to prevent the loss of lean body mass have been investigated, including growth hormone, growth factors, and conditionally essential amino acids, such as glutamine.

Growth hormone is a potent anabolic agent, and administration to humans increases the rate of wound healing, decreases rates of wound infection, and decreases the catabolism and muscle wasting of critical illness. However, a large European trial found increased morbidity and mortality in patients with prolonged critical illness who received high doses of growth hormone. Thus, the use of growth hormone in patients who are in the acute phase of critical illness is not recommended.

Alternative anabolic agents such as oxandrolone (Oxandrin)[1] and testosterone[1] are being pursued to induce positive nitrogen balance and enhance wound healing in critically ill patients. These anabolic steroid hormones increase protein synthesis and can reduce the rate of protein breakdown. In a study of patients with alcoholic hepatitis, administration of oxandrolone was associated with lower mortality compared with patients receiving placebo. The patients receiving oxandrolone had improvements in the severity of their liver injury and the degree of malnutrition. Several studies have demonstrated a benefit of oxandrolone use in the burn patient population. Other anabolic steroid hormones,

[1] Not FDA approved for this indication.

such as methandienone[2] and nandrolone decanoate (Deca Durabolin),[2] have been shown to increase protein anabolism and nitrogen balance in hospitalized patients.

Growth factors should be reserved for patients with major burns and documented impaired healing; patients who have large wounds or enterocutaneous fistulae and who have impaired healing; and patients with muscle wasting and weakness associated with AIDS; other failure to thrive conditions; and, in general, patients who have not responded to aggressive nutritional support but whose underlying disease processes are controlled. Growth factors have not been shown to decrease length of time on a respiratory in ICU patients. In fact, such factors can increase ventilator time and worsen outcome.

Glutamine-supplemented PN solutions administered to trauma or stressed patients can improve overall nitrogen balance, enhance muscle protein synthesis, improve intestinal nutrient absorption, decrease gut permeability, improve immune function, and decrease hospital stays and costs in some patient populations. A review of 14 randomized trials in surgical and critically ill patients found that glutamine supplementation was associated with reduced mortality, lower rates of infectious complications, and a decreased hospital stay. The greatest benefit was in patients receiving high-dose (>0.29 g/kg/day) parenteral glutamine.

However, a recent randomized trial of glutamine and antioxidant micronutrient supplementation in critically ill patients showed a trend toward increased 28-day mortality and significant in-hospital and 6-month mortality in patients receiving glutamine supplementation. There were limitations in this study in that baseline glutamine levels were not checked for all patients; in a subset of 66 patients with plasma glutamine levels evaluated, all had normal levels at baseline. This suggests that glutamine supplementation may not be appropriate for all critically ill patients. In addition, patients received approximately 50% of goal energy requirements and approximately 45% of goal protein delivery from glutamine. The total amount of glutamine given in this study was significantly higher than the dose of glutamine usually recommended. This raises the possibility that there is an optimal "therapeutic window" for glutamine administration: giving too little glutamine may not be efficacious and giving too much may be toxic. Further study is required before a definitive recommendation can be given based on this study alone.

Patients with intestinal dysfunction requiring PN, such as those with short-bowel syndrome or mucosal damage following chemotherapy and/or irradiation, might benefit from glutamine-containing PN. Glutamine-containing PN might also be beneficial in patients with immunodeficiency syndromes, including AIDS, immune-system dysfunction associated with critical illness, and bone marrow transplantation; patients with severe catabolic illness, such as major burns; patients with multiple trauma; and patients with other diseases associated with a prolonged ICU stay. Glutamine-supplemented solutions should not yet be considered routine care and should not be used in patients with significant renal insufficiency or in patients with significant hepatic failure. A recent ASPEN position paper summarizes recommendations for use of both enteral and IV glutamine.

Common Complications and Management
Catheter Sepsis
Central venous catheter-related bloodstream infection ranges from 3% to 20% in hospitalized patients and is the most common complication of central venous catheters. The migration of microorganisms along the external surface of the catheter is likely the most common cause, followed by intraluminal contamination from manipulation of the catheter hub or IV connectors. The most common organisms associated with catheter-related bloodstream infections include *Staphylococcus epidermidis*, *Staphylococcus aureus*, *Enterococcus* spp., *Candida albicans*, and *Enterobacter* spp. as well as resistant

strains such as methicillin-resistant *S. aureus* and vancomycin-resistant enterococci. Primary catheter sepsis occurs when there are signs and symptoms of infection and the indwelling catheter is the only anatomic focus of infection. Secondary catheter infections are associated with another focus or multiple infectious foci that cause bacteremia and seed the catheter.

Management of patients with catheter infection depends on their clinical condition. With extremely ill patients with high fevers who are hypotensive or who have local signs of infection around the catheter site, the catheter should be removed, its tip cultured, and peripheral and central venous blood cultures obtained. In catheter-related bloodstream infection, the organisms that grow from the catheter tip are the same those identified in the peripheral blood culture, and typically more than 10^3 organisms are grown from cultures of the catheter tip.

Specific therapy should be initiated against the primary source in patients in whom a source of infection, other than the catheter tip, is present. Peripheral blood cultures should be obtained and blood cultures should not be taken from the central venous catheter port dedicated for PN because this increases the risk of contaminating the line. If the infection resolves, central venous feedings can be continued. If a secondary source is not identified and the symptoms persist, the catheter should be removed and its tip should be cultured. If the culture of the catheter tip returns positive or if the index of suspicion is high, appropriate antibiotic therapy is initiated. Central venous feeding can be resumed, maintaining euglyemia.

Occasionally, the situation arises in which a site of infection, other than the catheter, is identified, but signs and symptoms persist despite what is assumed to be adequate therapy. Again, if blood cultures are positive, the safest course of action may be to remove the catheter. If peripheral blood cultures are negative, the catheter may be changed over a guidewire and the catheter tip cultured to determine if it was contaminated. Central venous feedings may be continued during this interval if the patient is stable. If the catheter tip returns positive, a new catheter should be inserted at a different site. Changing the central venous catheter over a guidewire can also facilitate the diagnosis of primary catheter infections. Changing the site of catheter location, rather than guidewire exchange, is recommended in patients in whom infection is suspected.

Other Complications
Common complications, their etiologies, and treatments are outlined in Table 4. Prolonged administration of PN can result in altered hepatic function and changes in liver pathologic conditions that can lead to liver failure. One to 2 weeks after initiating PN, transaminases may be elevated, but this often resolves without any change in the composition of PN or rate of administration. However, in patients receiving long-term PN (>20 days), prolonged elevations of alkaline phosphatase followed by elevated levels of serum transaminases can occur, even after therapy is discontinued.

Serum levels of alkaline phosphatase and bilirubin initially remain normal, but they rise in many patients who receive long-term PN. Patients who do not receive lipids in the PN solution have more frequent and severe hepatic abnormalities, most likely due to higher carbohydrate loads. Excess glucose increases insulin secretion, which stimulates hepatic lipogenesis and results in hepatic fat accumulation. Fatty infiltration is the initial histopathologic change; it is readily reversible and might not be accompanied by altered liver function tests.

Longer PN therapy may be associated with cholestasis, cholelithiasis, steatosis, and steatohepatitis and can progress to active chronic hepatitis, fibrosis, and eventual cirrhosis. The management of PN-related liver dysfunction is summarized in Box 3.

---

[2] Not available in the United States.

TABLE 4 Possible Etiologies and Treatment of Common Complications of Central Parenteral Nutrition

PROBLEM	POSSIBLE ETIOLOGY	TREATMENT
Glucose		
Hyperglycemia, glycosuria, hyperosmolar nonketotic dehydration, or coma	Excessive dose or rate of infusion, inadequate insulin production, steroid administration, infection	Decrease the amount of glucose given, increase insulin, administer a portion of calories as fat
Diabetic ketoacidosis	Inadequate endogenous insulin production and/or inadequate insulin therapy	Give insulin Decrease glucose intake
Rebound hypoglycemia	Persistent endogenous insulin production by islet cells after long-term high-carbohydrate infusion	Give 5%–10% glucose before parenteral infusion is discontinued
Hypercarbia	Carbohydrate load exceeds the ability to increase minute ventilation and excrete excess CO_2	Limit glucose dose to 5 mg/kg/min Give greater percentage of total caloric needs as fat (up to 30%–40%)
Fat		
Hypertriglyceridemia	Rapid infusion	Decrease rate of PN infusion
	Decreased clearance	Allow clearance (~12 h) before testing blood
Essential fatty acid deficiency	Inadequate essential fatty acid administration	Administer essential fatty acids in doses of 4%–7% of total calories
Amino Acids		
Hyperchloremia metabolic acidosis	Excessive chloride content of amino acid solutions	Administer Na^+ and K^+ as acetate salts
Prerenal azotemia	Excessive amino acids with inadequate caloric supplementation	Reduce amino acids Increase the amount of glucose calories
Miscellaneous		
Hypophosphatemia	Inadequate phosphorus administration with redistribution into tissues	Give 15 mmol phosphate/1000 IV kcal Evaluate antacid and Ca^{2+} administration
Hypomagnesemia	Inadequate administration relative to increased losses (diarrhea, diuresis, medications)	Administer Mg^{2+} (15–20 mEq/1000 kcal)
Hypermagnesemia	Excessive administration; renal failure	Decrease Mg^{2+} supplementation
Hypokalemia	Inadequate K^+ intake relative to increased needs for anabolism; diuresis	Increase K^+ supplementation
Hyperkalemia	Excessive K^+ administration, especially in metabolic acidosis; renal decompensation	Reduce or stop exogenous K^+ If ECG changes are present, treat with calcium gluconate, insulin, diuretics, and/or Kayexalate
Hypocalcemia	Inadequate Ca^{2+} administration; reciprocal response to phosphorus repletion without simultaneous calcium infusion	Increase Ca^{2+} dose
Hypercalcemia	Excessive Ca^{2+} administration; excessive vitamin D administration	Decrease Ca^{2+} and/or vitamin D administration
Elevated liver transaminases or serum alkaline phosphatase and bilirubin	Enzyme induction secondary to amino acid imbalances or overfeeding	Reevaluate nutritional prescription Cycle TPN Avoid overfeeding calories Consider administering carnitine

Abbreviations: ECG=electrocardiogram; PN=parenteral nutrition; TPN=total parenteral nutrition.

BOX 3 Management of Parenteral Nutrition-Related Liver Dysfunction

Have the patient eat, if possible.
Avoid administering large amounts of glucose or protein calories.
Supply IV fat emulsions (up to 30% of total calories).
Cycle the parenteral nutrition, infusing for 10–12 h/d.
Reevaluate energy needs; reduce energy delivery if liver dysfunction persists.

Complications are minimized and nutritional therapy maximized when the care of patients who require specialized nutritional support is supervised by a nutrition support team. Ideally, the nutrition support team consists of a pharmacist, dietitian, nurse, and physician.

References

Al-Omran M, Albalawi ZH, Tashkandi MF, Al-Ansary LA: Enteral versus parenteral nutrition in acute pancreatitis, *Cochrane Database Syst Rev* 2010, https://doi.org/10.1002/14651858.CD002837.pub2. CD002837.

A.S.P.E.N. Board of Directors: Guidelines for the use of parenteral and enteral nutrition in adult and pediatric patients, *JPEN J Parenter Enteral Nutr* 26:1SA–138SA, 2002.

Ayers P, Adams S, Boullata J, et al: A.S.P.E.N. parenteral nutrition safety consensus recommendations, *JPEN J Parenter Enteral Nutr* 38:296–333, 2014.

Bistrian BR, McCowen KC: Nutritional and metabolic support in the adult intensive care unit: Key controversies, *Crit Care Med* 34:1525–1531, 2006.

Boullata JI, Gilbert K, Sacks G, et al: A.S.P.E.N. Clinical guidelines: Parenteral nutrition ordering, order review, compounding, labeling, and dispensing, *JPEN J Parenter Enteral Nutr* 38(3):334–377, 2014.

Butler SO, Btaiche IF, Alaniz C: Relationship between hyperglycemia and infection in critically ill patients, *Pharmacotherapy* 25:963–976, 2005.

Heyland DK, Dhaliwal R, Suchner U, Berger MM: Antioxidant nutrients: A systematic review of trace elements and vitamins in the critically ill patient, *Intensive Care Med* 31:327–337, 2005.

Heyland D, Muscedere J, Wischmeyer PE, et al: A randomized trial of glutamine and antioxidants in critically ill patients, *N Engl J Med* 368:1489–1497, 2013.

Li Y, Tang X, Zhang J, Wu T: Nutritional support for acute kidney injury, *Cochrane Database Syst Rev* 2010. https://doi.org/10.002/14651858.CD005426.pub2, CD005426.

McClave SA, Chang W-K, Dhaliwal R, Heyland DK: Nutrition support in acute pancreatitis: A systematic review of the literature, *JPEN J Parenter Enteral Nutr* 30:143–156, 2006.

McClave SA, Taylor BE, Martindale RG, et al: Guidelines for the provision of nutrition support therapy in the adult critically ill patient: Society of Critical Care Medicine (SCCM) and American Society for Parenteral and Enteral Nutrition (ASPEN), *JPEN J Parenter Enteral Nutr.* 40:159–211, 2016 Erratum in: JPEN J Parenter Enteral Nutr 2016;40:1200.

McMahon MM, Nystrom E, Braunschweig C, et al: A.S.P.E.N. Clinical guidelines: Nutrition support of adult patients with hyperglycemia, *JPEN J Parenter Enteral Nutr* 37:26–36, 2013.

O'Grady NP, Alexander M, Burns LA, et al: Guidelines for the prevention of intravascular catheter-related infections, *Clin Infect Dis* 52:e162–e193, 2011. Also available at http://www.cdc.gov/hicpac/BSI/BSI-guidelines-2011.html accessed December 5, 2013.

Vanek VW, Matarese LE, Robinson M, et al: A.S.P.E.N. Position paper: Parenteral nutrition glutamine supplementation, *JPEN J Parenter Enteral Nutr* 26:479–494, 2011.

Worthington P, Balint J, Bechtold M, et al: When is parenteral nutrition appropriate? *JEPN J Parenter Enteral Nutr.* 41:324–377, 2017.

PHEOCHROMOCYTOMA

Method of
Melissa K. Gonzales, BS; and Karel Pacak, MD, PhD, DSc

CURRENT DIAGNOSIS

- Hypertension is the most common clinical sign.
- A triad of headaches, palpitations, and sweating (sometimes associated with paleness), with or without hypertension, indicates the possibility of a pheochromocytoma.
- Biochemical diagnosis of pheochromocytoma should be based on the determination of plasma free or urine fractionated metanephrines.
- Localization of pheochromocytomas should consist of anatomic imaging, preferably computed tomography (CT) or magnetic resonance imaging (MRI), followed by specific functional imaging using positron emission tomography (PET).
- If a pheochromocytoma gene panel is not available, a cost-effective alternative is genetic screening guided by family history, clinical features, and a biochemical phenotype, which should be performed on most patients. The identification of a causative mutation should lead to presymptomatic genetic testing in a patient's relatives.

CURRENT THERAPY

- The optimal therapy for a pheochromocytoma is prompt surgical removal of the tumor.
- At least 1 to 2 weeks before the operation, there should be adequate control of blood pressure using mainly α-adrenoceptor blockers and if tachyarrhythmia is present, β-adrenoceptor blockers; less commonly, calcium channel blockers and metyrosine (Demser) may be used if indicated.
- For most pheochromocytomas, laparoscopy is the procedure of choice.

- Adrenal cortex–sparing surgery should be advocated in all patients with hereditary (except *SDHB* gene mutation) and bilateral adrenal pheochromocytomas, if feasible.
- Clinical follow-up should be lifelong, especially in cases of an underlying germline mutation or with a large primary tumor greater than 4 to 5 cm, which has a higher likelihood to develop a metastasis.
- Management of metastatic tumors requires a multidisciplinary approach, in which pharmacologic treatment, targeted radiotherapy, chemotherapy, and surgery play an important role.

The 2017 WHO classification of endocrine tumors defines pheochromocytoma* as a tumor of chromaffin cells that arises in the adrenal medulla. Pheochromocytomas arise exclusively in the adrenal glands, whereas functionally similar tumors arising in extra-adrenal paraganglia are classified as paragangliomas. Pheochromocytomas and paragangliomas are characterized by the synthesis, metabolism, storage, and usually, but not always, secretion of catecholamines, metanephrines, and/or methoxytyramine.

Parasympathetic paragangliomas are mainly located along cranial and vagus nerves. Glomus or carotid body tumors, for example—head and neck paragangliomas—can be locally invasive but rarely develop metastases and usually do not secrete norepinephrine/normetanephrine but up to 70% secrete dopamine/methoxytyramine.

Sympathetic paragangliomas mainly arise in the abdomen from chromaffin tissue neighboring or inside sympathetic ganglia. Less often, they originate from the pelvis and infrequently from the mediastinum (2%) and neck (1%). In the abdomen, they often derive from the organ of Zuckerkandl, a collection of chromaffin tissue around the origin of the inferior mesenteric artery (Figure 1).

Epidemiology

Pheochromocytomas can occur at any age, including in childhood, but most often they are detected in the fourth and fifth decades. There is no gender preference. In Western countries the prevalence of pheochromocytoma is estimated between 1:6500 and 1:2500, with an annual incidence of 3 to 8 cases per 1 million per year in the general population, although autopsies show a higher incidence. The pheochromocytoma-to-paraganglioma ratio is 0.80 to 0.20. About 35% are familial, and 3% to 50% are malignant, depending on their genetic background.

Genetics

There are no lifestyle-related risk factors that increase the risk of pheochromocytoma. However, understanding of the role of genetics has dramatically increased over the last several years. Up to 35% of pheochromocytomas are hereditary, and a significant number of patients (approximately 20%) with apparently sporadic tumors carry a germline mutation. Thus gene mutations are the largest risk factor involved in the development of pheochromocytoma.

At present, at least 23 well-known susceptibility genes have been discovered that fall into two categories: major susceptibility genes and minor susceptibility genes. Major susceptibility genes represent 85% to 90% of all hereditary tumors: the *VHL* gene, which causes von Hippel–Lindau syndrome; the *RET* gene, for multiple endocrine neoplasia (MEN) types 2A and 2B; the *NF1* gene in neurofibromatosis type 1; and the *SDHB* and *SDHD* genes in familial paraganglioma syndromes. Minor susceptibility genes include *SDHA, SDHC, SDHAF2, FH, MAX, TMEM127, PHD1, PHD2, IDH1, KIF1Bβ, HIF2A (EPAS1), MDH2, DNMT3A,* and *DLST,* which represent 10% to 15% of hereditary tumors. Thirty to 35% of pheochromocytomas can have somatic mutations in

---

*For the purpose of this chapter, the term *pheochromocytoma* also refers to paraganglioma unless otherwise specified.

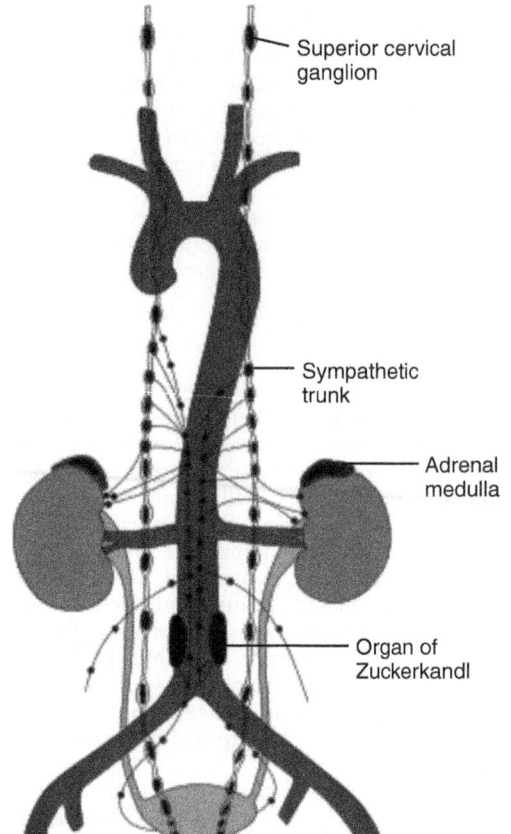

Figure 1 Anatomic distribution of chromaffin tissue. Adapted from Lack E. Tumors of the adrenal gland and extra-adrenal paraganglia. In *Armed Forces Institute of Pathology: Atlas of Tumor Pathology*. Washington, DC: Armed Forces Institute of Pathology; 1997:261–267.

Labels on figure: Superior cervical ganglion; Sympathetic trunk; Adrenal medulla; Organ of Zuckerkandl

also associated with other types of tumors, and early diagnosis improves the prognosis of these patients. If a genetic syndrome can be established by genetic diagnosis, patient management can be individually tailored based on the specific characteristics of the syndrome.

Presymptomatic genetic testing in minors can raise ethical and legal issues, partly owing to the potential emotional impact of the results and the difficulty of obtaining individual informed consent for the testing of minors. To address these issues, the criteria for proper genetic testing should include several steps (Box 2). The advent of next-generation sequencing methods has the potential to decrease the cost of sequencing and enable all patients with pheochromocytoma to be screened as described previously.

Clinical Manifestations

The signs and symptoms of pheochromocytoma are mostly the result of the hemodynamic and metabolic actions of the often inconsistent and disorderly secreted catecholamines on α- and β-adrenoceptors. Most symptoms are nonspecific, including dyspnea, nausea, weakness, weight loss, visual disturbances, arrhythmias, and anxiety or nervousness, but when a triad of headaches, palpitations, and sweating (sometimes with paleness) is accompanied by hypertension, pheochromocytoma should immediately be suspected. The typical episodic symptoms of catecholamine secretion seen in patients (e.g., palpitations, sweating, headache) may be caused by manipulation of the tumor, endoscopy, anesthesia, ingestion of food or beverages that contain tyramine, and certain medications such as current antidepressants. However, very often these symptoms occur spontaneously. Often, many patients exhibit no symptoms or only minor ones. The diagnosis can, therefore, be easily missed. This is especially true in elderly patients.

Pheochromocytoma can also be discovered during preventive screening, as a result of signs and symptoms related to a mass effect of the tumor, and as incidental findings during imaging studies.

The primary clinical indicators for the diagnosis of pheochromocytoma are summarized in Box 3.

Differential Diagnosis

Pheochromocytoma is often referred to as "the great mimic," because it has signs and symptoms that are common in numerous other clinical conditions. As a result, this often leads to the misdiagnosis of pheochromocytoma. Consideration should be given to other conditions that are associated with sympathomedullary activation (e.g., hyperadrenergic hypertension, renovascular hypertension, panic disorders, pseudopheochromocytoma, temporal epilepsy, and some other neuroendocrine tumors that may release vasoactive substances), because they mimic pheochromocytoma most closely. This overlap can be excluded by a normal response to the clonidine suppression test.

Biochemical Diagnosis

Missing a pheochromocytoma can have a fatal outcome. Therefore tests with high sensitivity are needed to safely exclude a pheochromocytoma without using expensive and unnecessary biochemical follow-up or imaging studies.

Pheochromocytomas can secrete all, none, or any combination of catecholamines (epinephrine, norepinephrine, dopamine). After multiple studies at the National Institutes of Health (NIH), measurement of plasma free metanephrines (the O-methylated metabolites of parent catecholamines), which represent metabolism of catecholamines, but not their secretion, showed superior combined diagnostic sensitivity (98%) and specificity (92%) over all other tests. Analysis of free metanephrines and methoxytyramine in plasma is currently the method of choice to both detect and exclude the disease. In addition, 24-hour urine collections may be used and are considered a good alternative to plasma tests when these tests are not available. The decision to rule out pheochromocytoma should be based on normal values of these tests, respecting for age-adjusted reference ranges.

any of the aforementioned genes. The list of susceptibility genes is constantly growing, with recently reported genes having a very low incidence; therefore some of their characteristics have not yet been fully elucidated. We expect more genes to be reported in connection with familial pheochromocytoma, but their relevance must be confirmed. The characteristics of hereditary tumors are described in Table 1.

Pheochromocytomas can occur as part of several syndromes, which are associated with additional clinical conditions (Box 1). A recently described Pacak-Zhuang syndrome connects novel mutations in the gene-encoding hypoxia-inducible factor 2α (HIF2A or EPAS1) with paraganglioma, polycythemia, somatostatinoma, and retinal abnormalities. Other rare syndromes that include pheochromocytomas are Carney triad and Carney-Stratakis syndrome, which are characterized by gastrointestinal stromal tumors and paragangliomas in an SDH gene cluster carrier or due to hypermethylation of the *SDHC* promoter. It is well established that renal cell carcinomas are also related to SDH gene cluster mutations.

Genetic counseling is recommended for all patients with pheochromocytoma, but it would be neither appropriate nor cost-effective to test for each disease-causing gene in every patient with a pheochromocytoma. Currently, a pheochromocytoma gene panel and exome sequencing are the preferred methods for testing about 23 pheochromocytoma susceptibility genes. However, in some countries where these modalities are not available or too costly, an algorithm that takes family history, clinical characteristics, and a biochemical phenotype into consideration is shown in Figure 2. In cases of confirmation of a hereditary disorder, one should offer specific genetic tests and genetic counseling to the patient's family members. Disease screening should be offered to presymptomatic relatives who have a diagnosed mutation, especially because familial syndromes are

TABLE 1 Characteristics of Known Hereditary Pheochromocytomas

SYNDROME	MUTATION	GENE	PROTEIN FUNCTION	PENETRANCE	BILATERAL	MALIGNANT	PHEO OR PGL	PEAK AGE (Y)	BIOCHEMICAL PHENOTYPE
MEN2	10q11.2	RET	Receptor tyrosine kinase	~50%	50%–80%	Rarely malignant	Mainly PHEO	40	Adrenergic
VHL	3p25-26	VHL	von Hippel-Lindau protein/ E3 ubiquitin protein ligase	10%–30%	50%	5%	Mainly PHEO	30	Noradrenergic
NF-1	17q11	NF-1	Neurofibromatosis-related protein	1%–2%	16%	~10%	Mainly PHEO	50*	Adrenergic
PGL5	5p15	SDHA	Catalytic flavoprotein; A subunit of SDH	Has not been studied consistently	Has not been studied consistently	0%–14%	Mainly PGL	40	Noradrenergic and/ or dopaminergic; sometimes silent
PGL4	1p36	SDHB	Catalytic iron-sulfur protein; B subunit of SDH	80%–100% (by age 70 years)†	Rarely	31%–71%	Mainly PGL	30	Noradrenergic and/or dopaminergic; often silent as HNPGL
PGL3	1q21	SDHC	Membrane-spanning protein; C subunit of SDH	Has not been studied consistently	Has not been studied consistently	Rarely malignant	Mainly PGL	38	Noradrenergic and/or dopaminergic; often silent as HNPGL
PGL1	11q23	SDHD	Membrane-spanning subunit; D subunit of SDH	90% if paternally transmitted (by age 70 years)†	Has not been studied consistently	5%	Mainly PGL	35–40	Noradrenergic and/or dopaminergic; often silent as HNPGL
PGL2	11q12.2	SDHAF2/ SDHD5	Assembly factor for SDHA	~100% if paternally transmitted		Malignancy was not reported	Only PGL reported	30–40	Has not been studied consistently
	2q11.2	TMEM127	Transmembrane protein	Has not been studied consistently	33%	<5%	Mainly PHEO	43	Mixed adrenergic and noradrenergic
	14q23	MAX	bHLHLZ transcription factor	Has not been studied consistently (probably paternal transmission only)	67%	~25%	Mainly PHEO	32	Mixed adrenergic and noradrenergic

Note: An adrenergic phenotype represents either an increase only in metanephrine or both metanephrine and normetanephrine; a noradrenergic phenotype represents an increase only in normetanephrine; a mixed phenotype represents an increase in both metanephrine and normetanephrine. *bHLHLZ,* Basic helix-loop-helix leucine zipper; *HNPGL,* head and neck paraganglioma; *MEN,* multiple endocrine neoplasia; *NF,* neurofibromatosis; *PGL,* paraganglioma; *SDH,* succinate dehydrogenase; *VHL,* von Hippel-Lindau.

*Seldom seen in children.

†Our unpublished observations show lower penetrance.

BOX 1 Main Clinical Features of Syndromes Associated With Pheochromocytoma

von Hippel–Lindau Syndrome
Type 1 (No Pheochromocytoma)
Renal cell cysts and carcinomas
Retinal and CNS hemangioblastomas
Pancreatic neoplasms and cysts
Endolymphatic sac tumors
Epididymal cystadenomas

Type 2 (with Pheochromocytoma)
Type 2A: Retinal and CNS hemangioblastomas
• Pheochromocytomas
• Endolymphatic sac tumors
• Epididymal cystadenomas
Type 2B: Renal cell cysts and carcinomas
• Retinal and CNS hemangioblastomas
• Pancreatic neoplasms and cysts
• Pheochromocytomas
• Endolymphatic sac tumors
• Epididymal cystadenomas
Type 2 C: Pheochromocytomas only

Multiple Endocrine Neoplasia Type 2
Type 2A (medullary thyroid carcinoma)
• Pheochromocytomas
• Hyperparathyroidism
• Cutaneous lichen amyloidosis
Type 2B (medullary thyroid carcinoma)
• Pheochromocytomas
• Multiple neuromas
• Marfanoid habitus
FMTC: Familial medullary thyroid carcinoma only.

Neurofibromatosis Type 1
Multiple benign neurofibromas on skin and mucosa
Café au lait skin spots
Iris Lisch nodules
Learning disabilities
Skeletal abnormalities
Vascular disease
CNS tumors
Malignant peripheral nerve sheath tumors
Pheochromocytomas

Paraganglioma Syndromes
Head and neck tumors
• Carotid-body tumors
• Vagal, jugular, and tympanic paragangliomas
Abdominal and/or thoracic paragangliomas
Pheochromocytomas
Renal cell carcinoma (SDHB)
Gastrointestinal stromal tumor (SDHB and SDHD)
Carney-Stratakis syndrome
Carney triad
Pituitary adenoma (SDHx)
Pacak-Zhuang syndrome
Polycythemia

CNS, Central nervous system; *SDH,* succinate dehydrogenase.
Adapted from Lenders JW, Eisenhofer G, Mannelli M, et al. Phaeochromocytoma. *Lancet.* 2005;366:665–675.

The conditions under which blood samples are collected can be crucial to the reliability and interpretations of test results. The optimal circumstances are noted in Box 4. Besides these conditions, numerous foods and medications can cause direct or indirect interference in the measurement of catecholamines and metanephrines. This should be kept in mind when interpreting a positive test result. Any antidepressants, particularly tricyclic ones, α-methyldopa (Aldomet), mesalamine (Pentasa)/sulfasalazine (Azulfidine), phenoxybenzamine (Dibenzyline), acetaminophen, monoamine oxidase inhibitors, sympathomimetics, levodopa, cocaine, and other drugs interfere with test results. The effects of these medications on metanephrine levels are summarized in Table 2. Patients with chronic kidney disease, particularly those on dialysis, commonly have elevated plasma metanephrines (but usually not more than 3 to 4× above the upper reference limit [URL]), even in the absence of pheochromocytoma. The use of liquid chromatography tandem mass spectrometry (LCMS/MS) is the recommended detection method, because it can remove potentially interfering substances. It is also faster, cheaper, and more specific than other techniques.

Besides the initial biochemical tests, which can exclude the disease, follow-up tests are required to establish the diagnosis. This is necessary because although the initial tests are specific, the diagnosis of pheochromocytoma is so rare that there are many false-positive results. Options for biochemical follow-up testing are repeated plasma or urinary metanephrine tests, additional sampling for plasma free or urinary fractionated catecholamines, and the clonidine (Catapres) suppression test. Biochemical follow-up testing is not necessary for patients with increases above four times the URL of plasma free metanephrines, which are almost always diagnostic for the presence of pheochromocytoma, unless they are on antidepressants, which can falsely produce results with very highly elevated levels. The previously used glucagon stimulation test should be abandoned, because this test is insufficiently sensitive and can lead to hypertensive complications.

With the increasing proportion of familial tumors, it is important to highlight their different catecholamine profiles. The biochemical profile of a tumor can help guide genetic testing, as reflected in the genetic testing algorithm depicted in Figure 2. Biochemical measurements can also help identify metastatic tumors; a recent study introduced the O-methylated metabolite of dopamine, plasma methoxytyramine, as an accurate biomarker for discriminating between patients with and without metastases. Several previous studies suggested that increased dopamine could have prognostic significance for metastatic pheochromocytomas, but later, methoxytyramine was shown to be a more sensitive biomarker of a tumor's dopamine production than either plasma or urinary dopamine.

Based on these findings, an algorithm for biochemical diagnosis was designed and is shown in Figure 3.

Localization of Pheochromocytoma

Imaging studies to locate pheochromocytoma should be initiated once there is clear biochemical evidence. For optimal results, anatomic imaging studies such as computed tomography (CT) or magnetic resonance imaging (MRI) should be combined with high-specificity functional imaging studies. CT rather than MRI was suggested as the first-choice imaging modality because of its excellent spatial resolution of the thorax, abdomen, and pelvis. The use of MRI (T2-weighted) is recommended in patients with metastatic pheochromocytoma for the detection of skull base and neck paragangliomas in patients with surgical clips, in patients with an allergy to CT contrast and for patients in whom radiation exposure should be limited (children, pregnant women, patients with known germline mutations, and those with recent excessive radiation exposure).

Initial imaging should be focused on the adrenals. Negative imaging of the adrenals should be followed by CT or MRI scans of the abdomen and pelvis, where paragangliomas are most commonly located. If these scans are negative, chest and neck images should be obtained. Ultrasound is not recommended to localize pheochromocytoma. Exceptions include children and pregnant women when MRI is not available. Recently, there have been some suggestions to use rapid sequence MRI without contrast, but larger and more definitive studies are needed to validate this approach for accuracy to detect this tumor, especially metastatic lesions.

After anatomic imaging, which lacks the specificity to indisputably identify a mass as a pheochromocytoma, functional imaging

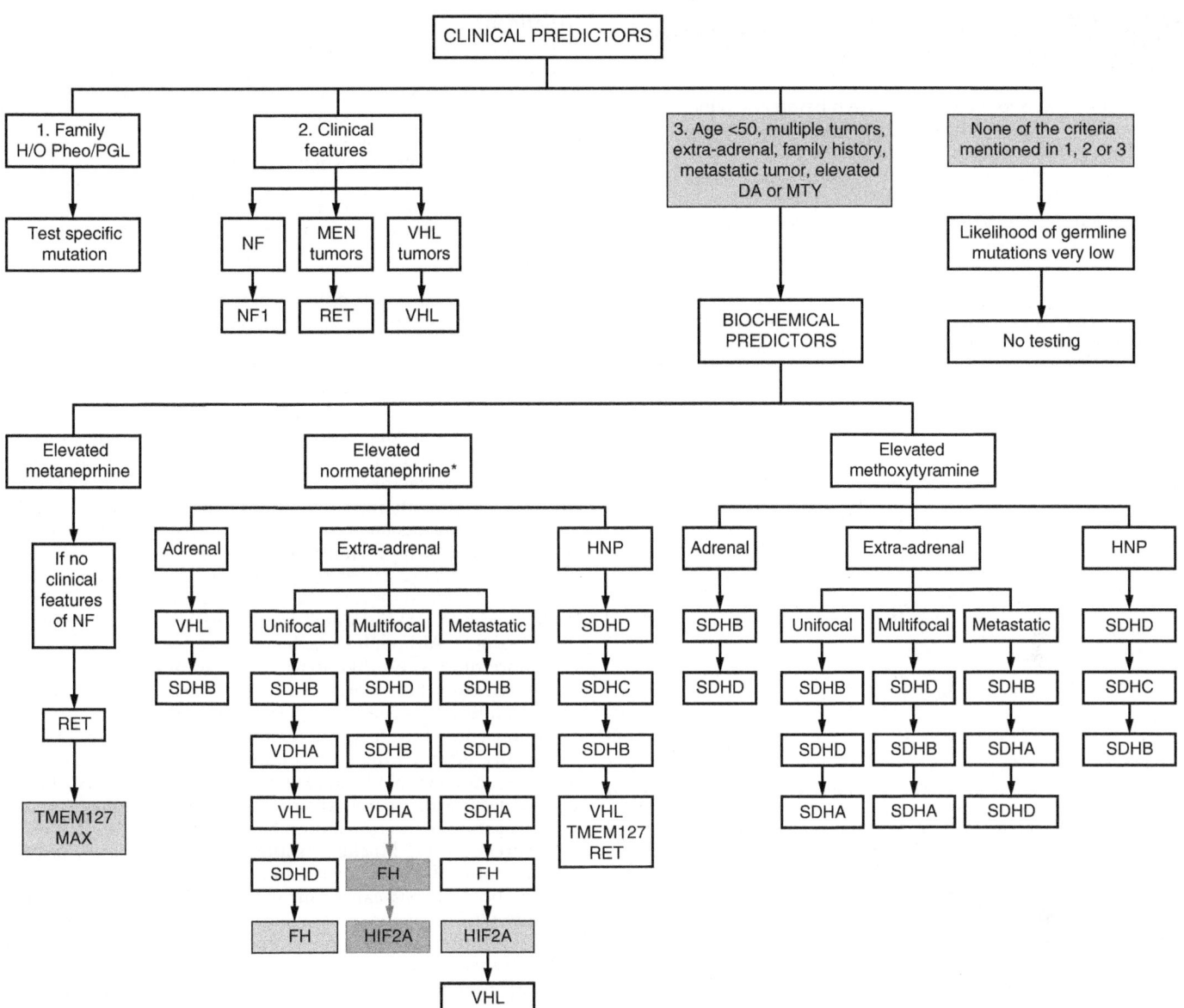

Figure 2 Suggested algorithm for genetic analysis in patients affected by pheochromocytoma or paraganglioma. If both normetanephrine and methoxytyramine are elevated, follow the algorithm for methoxytyramine. If both normetanephrine and metanephrine are elevated, follow the algorithm for metanephrine. *SDHAF2* mutation screening should be considered in patients who suffer exclusively from head and neck paragangliomas and who have familial antecedents, multiple tumors, or a very young age of onset and in whom the *SDHB/C/D* genes have been shown to be negative for mutations. In patients older than 50 years with benign adrenal tumors and no family history, consider *TMEM127* testing. *In a patient with elevated normetanephrine in whom clinical features and investigations do not clearly indicate which gene to test, perform immunohistochemistry before proceeding with testing. *DA*, Dopamine; *FH*, fumarate hydratase; *HIF2A*, hypoxia-inducible factor 2A; *HNP*, head and neck paraganglioma; *H/O*, history of; *MEN*, multiple endocrine neoplasia; *MTY*, methoxytyramine; *NF*, neurofibromatosis; *VHL*, von Hippel-Lindau. (Adapted from Karasek D, Shah U, Frysak Z, et al. An update on the genetics of pheochromocytoma. *J Hum Hypertens.* 2012 May 31 27(3):141–147, 2013. doi: https://doi.org/10.1038/jhh.2012.20.)

BOX 2 Criteria for Proper Genetic Testing in Minors

Decision should be made by both parents after appropriate consultation with a geneticist.

Parents should be advised about how to inform their child about the hereditary disease and the reason for genetic testing.

The discussion of the most appropriate time for testing for each child should take into account the potential medical benefits and the minor's schedule (school schedule, birthdays, etc.).

Periods of medical examinations or hospitalization for the carrier parent should be avoided where possible.

Adapted from Lahlou-Laforet K, Consoli SM, Jeunemaitre X, Gimenez-Roqueplo AP. Presymptomatic genetic testing in minors at risk of paraganglioma and pheochromocytoma: our experience of oncogenetic multidisciplinary consultation. *Horm Metab Res.* 2012;44:354–358.

BOX 3 Patients Who Should Be Evaluated for Pheochromocytoma or Paraganglioma

Anyone with a triad of headaches, sweating, and tachycardia, whether or not the subject has hypertension.

Anyone with a known mutation of one of the susceptibility genes or a family history of pheochromocytoma and paraganglioma.

Anyone with an incidental adrenal mass.

Anyone whose blood pressure is poorly responsive to standard therapy.

Anyone who has had hypertension, tachycardia, or arrhythmia in response to anesthesia, surgery, or medications known to precipitate symptoms in patients with pheochromocytoma and paraganglioma.

BOX 4 Optimal Conditions for Blood Collection of Plasma Free Metanephrines or Catecholamines

Patient is supine for at least 15–20 min before sampling.
Samples are collected through a previously inserted IV to avoid stress associated with the needle stick.
Patient has abstained from nicotine, alcohol, and vigorous exercise for at least 12 h.
Patient has fasted overnight before blood sampling.

TABLE 2 Medications That Interfere With Testing of Fractionated Plasma or Urinary Metanephrines

MEDICATION	METANEPHRINE	NORMETANEPHRINE
Acetaminophen*	—	↑↑↑
α-Methyldopa*	—	↑↑
Tricyclic antidepressants	—	↑↑
Mesalamine*/ sulfasalazine*	—	↑↑
Phenoxybenzamine	—	↑
Monoamine oxidase inhibitors†	↑↑	↑↑
Sympathomimetics†	↑	↑
Cocaine†	—	↑↑
Levodopa*,‡	↑↑	↑

*Whether these drugs interfere with the measurement or elevate fractionated plasma or urinary metanephrines depends on the assay and should be withdrawn 5 days before testing. Drug interference is not an issue when mass spectrometry–based assays are used.
†Monoamine oxidase inhibitors, sympathomimetics, and cocaine can increase catecholamines (thereby metanephrines through peripheral conversion).
‡Levodopa elevates dopamine and thereby methoxytyramine (its measured metabolite), which elevates metanephrine and normetanephrine using non–mass spectrometry-based assays.
From Hannah-Shmouni F, Pacak K, Stratakis CA. Metanephrines for evaluating palpitations and flushing. *JAMA*. 2017 Jul 25 318(4):385–386. https://doi.org/10.1001/jama.2017.5926.
Symbols: ↑↑, clear increase (≥threefold above the upper limit depending on the dose and duration of administration); ↑, mild increase (<threefold above the upper limit); —, no increase.

methods can confirm a tumor as a pheochromocytoma. Functional imaging also detects most cases of metastatic and multifocal disease. They include ¹²³I-MIBG scintigraphy, PET, and somatostatin receptor modality, at present ⁶⁸Ga-DOTATATE PET/CT. PET scanning is preferred for comprehensive localization of metastatic disease. The most commonly used radiopharmaceuticals in PET scanning are currently ¹⁸F-3,4-dihydroxyphenylalanine (¹⁸F-FDOPA), ¹⁸F-fluorodeoxyglucose (¹⁸F-FDG), and recently ⁶⁸Ga-DOTATATE PET/CT. Different circumstances require different radiopharmaceuticals (Figure 4). The ¹⁸F-FDOPA PET/CT is recommended as the imaging modality for head and neck paragangliomas, if ⁶⁸Ga-DOTATATE PET/CT is not available. ⁶⁸Ga-DOTATATE PET/CT or ¹⁸F-FDG PET/CT is recommended for metastatic pheochromocytomas. The use of ¹²³I-MIBG scintigraphy in patients with known metastatic pheochromocytoma should be limited to the evaluation of whether a patient qualifies for ¹³¹I-MIBG treatment. A combined PET/MRI scan has been introduced and might represent a novel advantageous imaging modality.

The algorithm described in Figure 4 provides the basis for diagnostic localization of pheochromocytoma.

If all tests return negative, it is advised to repeat noninvasive localization after 2 to 6 months.

Treatment

The optimal therapy for a pheochromocytoma is prompt surgical removal of the tumor, because an unresected tumor represents a time bomb waiting to explode with a lethal hypertensive crisis. In patients with extensive or metastatic disease, surgery can reduce the hormone secretion and prevent critical anatomic complications, such as urinary tract or cord compression or cardiac obstruction. Safe surgical removal requires the efforts of a team made up of an internist, an anesthesiologist, and a surgeon, preferably in a center experienced with this demanding surgery.

Medical Therapy and Preparation for Surgery

The goal of preoperative medical treatment is to control hypertension, maintain stable blood pressure during surgery, minimize adverse effects during anesthesia, and reduce other clinical signs and symptoms caused by high plasma levels of catecholamines.

As soon as the diagnosis is made, blood pressure should be adequately treated for at least 2 weeks before the operation. With satisfactory pretreatment, perioperative mortality has fallen to less than 3%. α-Adrenergic blockade is the basis of medical management and preoperative preparation. The most commonly used nonselective α-adrenoceptor blocker is phenoxybenzamine (Dibenzyline), which is also used for nonhypertensive patients. Other possibilities include α-blocking agents such as prazosin (Minipress), terazosin (Hytrin), and doxazosin (Cardura). Although these have a shorter duration of action and more often cause hypotension when initially administered for preoperative blood-pressure control, postoperative hypotension is more often seen with phenoxybenzamine. In addition to α-adrenoceptor blockers, one can use β-adrenoceptor blockers (especially when cardiac tachy- and other arrhythmias occur) and calcium-channel blockers such as nicardipine (Cardene). α-Methyl-L-tyrosine or metyrosine (Demser) has limited use as a premedication. Diuretics should be avoided.

β-Adrenoceptor blockers should never be used until α-adrenoceptor blockers have been administered for at least 2 to 3 days, because this can result in severe hypertensive crisis in patients with pheochromocytoma, which is believed to result from inhibition of β₂-adrenoceptor–mediated vasodilation (in the presence of catecholamine stimulation of incomplete α-adrenoceptor blockage). It might be presumed that cardioselective β₁-adrenoceptor–blocking drugs might be administered without adverse effect. Indeed, almost all adverse reactions to β-adrenoceptor blockers in pheochromocytoma patients have involved nonselective β-adrenoceptor blockers. Therefore cardioselective β-adrenoceptor blockers, such as atenolol (Tenormin), esmolol (Brevibloc), and metoprolol, (Lopressor) are favored over nonselective blockers for the management of patients with pheochromocytoma. Nevertheless, because of incomplete specificity and likelihood of some actions on β₂-adrenoceptors, even β-adrenoceptor blockers deemed to be cardioselective should only be administered to patients with pheochromocytoma once there is adequate control of blood pressure by α-adrenoceptor blockade or other means. In patients with persistent tachyarrhythmia, newly introduced drugs, such as ivabradine (Corlanor)[1], can be used.

Patients can be recommended a salt- and fluid-rich diet. A proposed algorithm for preoperative treatment is given in Figure 5.

Operative and Postoperative Management

After extensive preoperative preparation, surgery should be performed by an experienced surgical and anesthesiology team.

To ensure adequate preoperative preparation, several criteria have been proposed. First, targeted blood pressure should be below {140/90} mm Hg for at least 24 hours. Orthostatic hypotension should be present, but not below {80/45} mm Hg. In some cases, Doppler or conventional echocardiography are

---

[1]Not FDA approved for this indication.

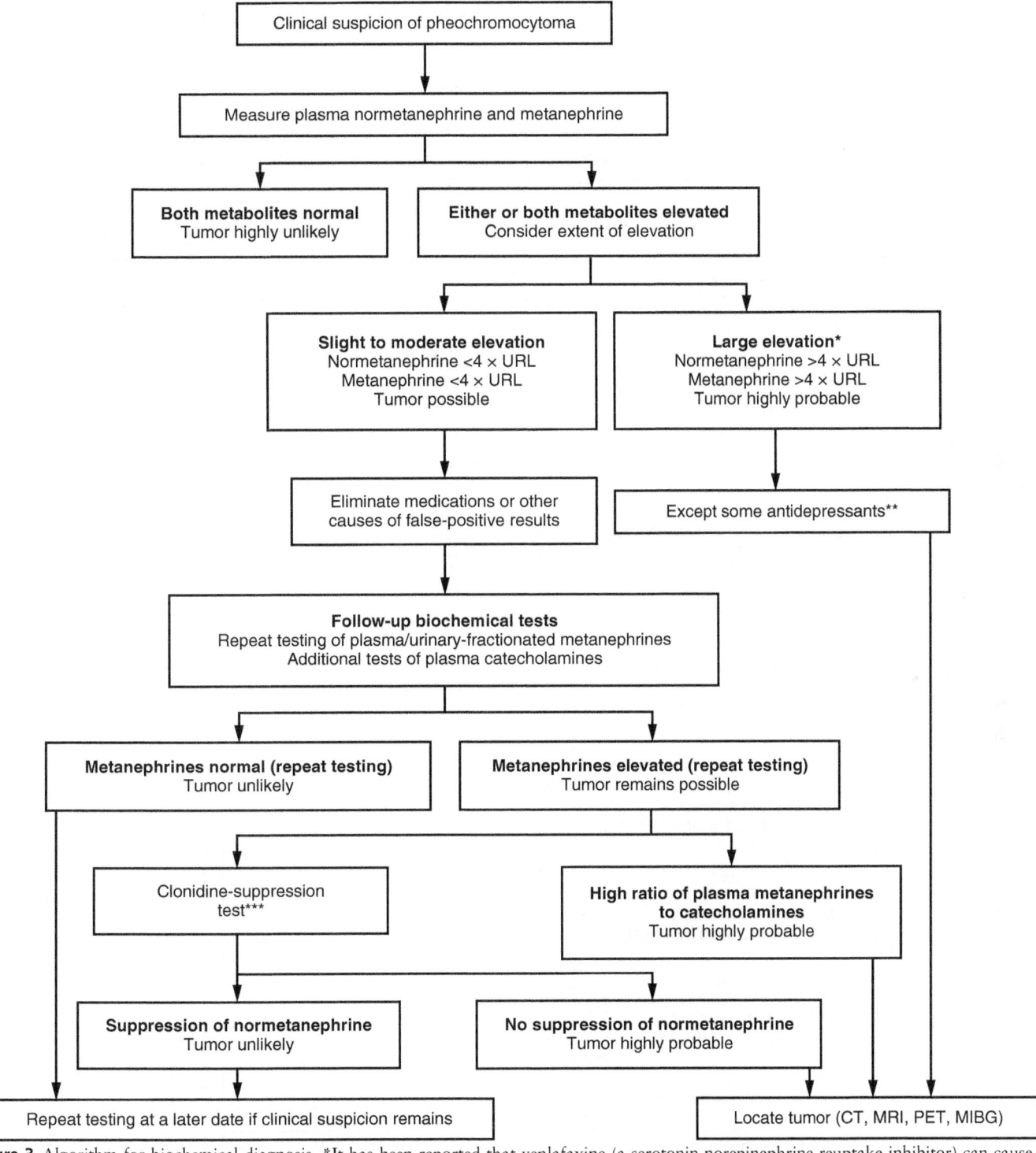

Figure 3 Algorithm for biochemical diagnosis. *It has been reported that venlafaxine (a serotonin-norepinephrine reuptake inhibitor) can cause an increase of more than four times the URL of normetanephrine. **Some antidepressants, especially those with a combination of norepinephrine and serotonin reuptake inhibition, can elevate plasma normetanephrine levels to four times above the URL. ***This test can only be predictive for normetanephrine and/or norepinephrine secreting tumors. *MIBG,* Meta-iodobenzylguanidine; *MRI,* magnetic resonance imaging; *PET,* positron emission tomography; *URL,* upper reference limit.

Figure 4 Recommended imaging studies for the localization of pheochromocytoma. *CT*, Computed tomography; ^{18}F-*FDG*, ^{18}F-fluorodeoxyglucose; ^{18}F-*FDOPA*, ^{18}F-3,4-dihydroxyphenylalanine; *HNPGL*, head and neck paraganglioma; *MIBG*, metaiodobenzylguanidine; *MRI*, magnetic resonance imaging; *PET*, positron emission tomography; *SSA*, somatostatin analogues.

Figure 5 Current recommended preoperative treatment algorithms in patients with pheochromocytoma. *BP*, Blood pressure; *HR*, heart rate. (Adapted from Pacak K. Preoperative management of the pheochromocytoma patient. *J Clin Endocrinol Metab*. 2007;92:4069–4079.)

indicated in addition to ECG to detect the presence of cardiomyopathy or coronary artery disease. In patients with a large left adrenal pheochromocytoma, splenectomy is likely; therefore vaccinations against *Streptococcus pneumoniae*, *Haemophilus influenzae*, and *Neisseria meningitidis* should be given preoperatively.

An experienced anesthesiologist should be aware of potential catecholamine release either as a side effect of the drugs used or as a result of tumor manipulation during the surgery.

A minimally invasive approach is the accepted standard for small, noninvasive, nonmetastatic pheochromocytomas and retroperitoneal paragangliomas, because of its significant postoperative benefits. Locoregional invasion is difficult to establish preoperatively; therefore it has been recommended that potentially invasive tumors should be initially explored by laparoscopy or retroperitoneoscopy followed by conversion to open surgery in cases of critical adhesion. To prevent permanent glucocorticoid deficiency in patients with bilateral pheochromocytomas, adrenal cortex–sparing surgery is advocated (except in *SDHB*-related pheochromocytoma). There are multiple potential hazardous events and situations involved in surgery, including anesthesia induction, tumor manipulation, hypotension, and hypoglycemia. The treatment of hypotension with pressor agents is not recommended, especially when long-acting β-adrenoceptor blockers or metyrosine have been used; these paralyze the vascular bed in a dilated state. Instead, volume replacement is the treatment of choice.

Postoperative hypertension can indicate incomplete tumor resection. However, during the first 24 hours after surgery, hypertension is most likely attributed to pain, volume overload, or autonomic instability, all of which are treated symptomatically. If hypertension persists, any attempts to collect specimens for biochemical evidence of an incompletely resected tumor should be delayed for at least 5 to 7 days after surgery to ensure that the large increases in both plasma and urinary catecholamines produced by surgery have dissipated.

Close monitoring of blood glucose in the postoperative period is recommended, because its level can be decreased due to decreased glucose production and increased glucose utilization in the absence of the previous catecholamine excess and persistence of α-adrenoceptor blockers.

If the patient is hypotensive, hemorrhage should be excluded first; however, the most likely cause of hypotension is the prolonged effect of the α-adrenoceptor blockers in the presence of reduced plasma catecholamine levels.

Hypertensive Crisis

The most dangerous complication of pheochromocytoma is the occurrence of a hypertensive crisis. A hypertensive crisis can manifest as a severe headache, visual disturbances, acute myocardial infarction, congestive heart failure, or a cerebrovascular accident. It is treated with an intravenous bolus of 5 mg of phentolamine (Regitine), a reversible nonselective α-adrenergic antagonist. Phentolamine has a very short half-life; therefore the same dose can be repeated every 2 minutes until hypertension is adequately controlled, or it can also be given as a continuous infusion. Continuous intravenous infusion of sodium nitroprusside (Nitropress) or labetalol (Trandate) are also options to control hypertension. Calcium-channel blockers such as nicardipine (Cardene) can also be used, administered intravenously at a starting dose of 5 mg/h, increasing by 2.5 mg/h every 5 minutes to a maximum of 15 mg/h until the hypertensive crisis has subsided and blood pressure control is regained. Lower doses can be used based on blood pressure and heart rate values based on continuous monitoring.

Malignant Pheochromocytoma

Malignant pheochromocytoma is established only by the presence of metastases at sites where chromaffin cells are normally absent, which is only in lymph nodes or bones based on the current 2017 WHO definition. Paragangliomas are malignant more commonly than pheochromocytomas (25% vs. 7%).

Pheochromocytoma metastasizes via hematogenous or lymphatic routes, and the most common metastatic sites are lymph nodes, bones, lung, and liver. About one half of malignant tumors are found at original presentation, and the other half develop at a median interval of 5.6 years, but they can be delayed up to 24 years. Based on the localization of the metastatic lesions, there are short-term and long-term survivors.

Up to 50% of malignant pheochromocytomas develop because of a germline mutation. *SDHB* mutations with the presence of pheochromocytoma represent about 70% or even more of the risk of malignancy (both in children and adults). Currently, there are several other independent factors of malignancy, including extra-adrenal localization (paragangliomas), the size of the primary tumor (larger than 5 cm), and high norepinephrine and/or dopamine/methoxamine. Particularly owing to the substantial amounts of methoxytyramine produced by a significant portion of metastatic pheochromocytomas, this measurement should also offer utility in patient management as a surrogate biomarker to assess tumor burden, disease progression, and response to treatment.

Malignant disease is often complicated by clinical manifestations of catecholamine excess and is invariably fatal. The 5-year survival probability after the diagnosis of the first metastasis is reported to be 36% in *SDHB* carriers and 67% in the absence of this mutation.

Successful management of malignant pheochromocytoma requires a multidisciplinary approach, where pharmacologic treatment, targeted radiotherapy, chemotherapy, and surgery can all play a part. Although external beam radiation has been used for inoperable tumors or for symptom palliation, especially in the treatment of bone lesions, surgical debulking is considered the mainstay of palliative treatment. About 30% of patients receiving CVD (cyclophosphamide [Cytoxan][1], vincristine [Oncovin][1], and dacarbazine [DTIC-Dome][1]) exhibit clinical benefits; this number is much higher in patients with *SDHB*-related malignant tumors (70% to 80%). Limited documented experience with other chemotherapeutic regimes is available. Radiolabeled somatostatin analogues can be used as an alternative option (for example, lutetium [Lu] 177 dotatate [LUTATHERA][1]). More recently, a type of high specific activity ^{131}I-MIBG therapy known as ^{131}I-Iobenguane (Azedra) has received US Food and Drug Administration (FDA) approval and can also be used as a treatment option if a patient's tumors are avid on ^{123}I-MIBG scintigraphy. Nowadays, a lot is expected from the novel molecular targeted therapies. In fact, some therapies have already been tested in clinical settings with new possible targets emerging, especially in *HIF* genes, the mTOR pathway, Hsp90, and immune cells. Individualized treatment should be performed with the intention to cure limited disease and achieve palliation for advanced disease. Figure 6 shows a proposed algorithm for the treatment of metastatic pheochromocytoma.

Prognosis and Monitoring

The long-term survival of patients after successful removal of a benign pheochromocytoma is essentially the same as that of age-adjusted normal subjects. Findings from a large study with a long-term follow-up showed a recurrence rate of 17%, with half the patients showing signs of malignant disease. Recurrences occur more often in patients with extra-adrenal disease and in patients with a hereditary disorder. At least 25% of patients remain hypertensive after treatment, but this is usually easily controlled with medication.

Clinical follow-up should be lifelong for all patients, but especially in those with an underlying hereditary disorder. The frequency of checkups, once a year or more often, and the kind of diagnostic measurements, only biochemical tests or also imaging studies, should depend on the characteristics of the pheochromocytoma. Follow-up must be more intensive in patients with hereditary and malignant pheochromocytoma.

---

[1]Not FDA approved for this indication.

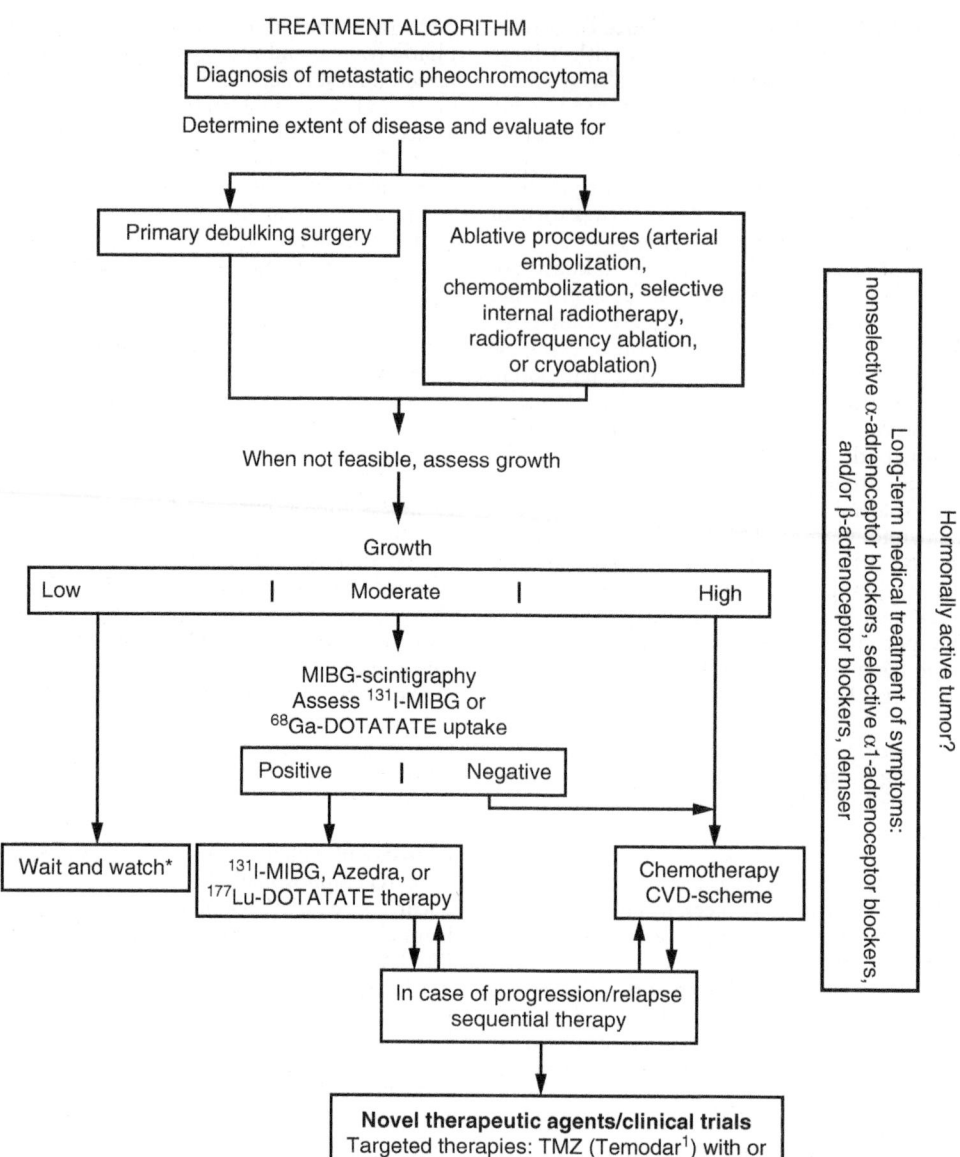

TREATMENT ALGORITHM

Figure 6 Treatment algorithm for metastatic pheochromocytoma. Asterisk indicates that the risk of side effects from therapy exceeds the chance of benefit. *CVD*, Cyclophosphamide, vincristine, and dacarbazine [chemotherapy]; *JR11*, [nat]Ga-NODAGA-JR11; *MIBG*, metaiodobenzylguanidine; *mTOR*, mammalian target of rapamycin; *PARP*, poly ADP ribose polymerase; *TMZ*, temozolomide. Adapted from Adjallé R, Plouin PF, Pacak K, et al. Treatment of malignant pheochromocytoma. *Horm Metab Res.* 2009;41:687–896.

References

Adjalle R, Plouin PF, Pacak K, Lehnert H: Treatment of malignant pheochromocytoma, *Horm Metab Res* 41:687–696, 2009.

Amar L, Baudin E, Burnichon N, et al: Succinate dehydrogenase B gene mutations predict survival in patients with malignant pheochromocytomas or paragangliomas, *J Clin Endocrinol Metab* 92:3822–3828, 2007.

Ayala-Ramirez M, Feng L, Habra MA, et al: Clinical benefits of systemic chemotherapy for patients with metastatic pheochromocytomas or sympathetic extra-adrenal paragangliomas: Insights from the largest single-institutional experience, *Cancer* 118:2804–2812, 2012.

Bayley JP, Kunst HP, Cascon A, et al: *SDHAF2* mutations in familial and sporadic paraganglioma and phaeochromocytoma, *Lancet Oncol* 11:366–372, 2010.

Baysal BE: Screening: Correlation of genotype and phenotype in paraganglioma, *Nat Rev Endocrinol* 5:594–595, 2009.

Bjorklund P, Pacak K, Crona J: Precision medicine in pheochromocytoma and paraganglioma: current and future concepts, *Journal of Internal Medicine* 280(6):559–573, 2016.

Castinetti F, Kroiss A, Kumar R, Pacak K, Taieb D: 15 years of paraganglioma: Imaging and imaging-based treatment of pheochromocytoma and paraganglioma, *Endocr Relat Cancer* 22(4):T135–T145, 2015.

Eisenhofer G, Lenders JW, Siegert G, et al: Plasma methoxytyramine: A novel biomarker of metastatic pheochromocytoma and paraganglioma in relation to established risk factors of tumour size, location and *SDHB* mutation status, *Eur J Cancer* 48:1739–1749, 2012.

Eisenhofer G, Rivers G, Rosas AL, et al: Adverse drug reactions in patients with phaeochromocytoma: Incidence, prevention and management, *Drug Saf* 30:1031–1062, 2007.

Fishbein L, Nathanson KL: Pheochromocytoma and paraganglioma: Understanding the complexities of the genetic background, *Cancer Genet* 205:1–11, 2012.

Gimenez-Roqueplo AP, Dahia PL, Robledo M: An update on the genetics of paraganglioma, pheochromocytoma, and associated hereditary syndromes, *Horm Metab Res* 44:328–333, 2012.

Gimm O, DeMicco C, Perren A, et al: Malignant pheochromocytomas and paragangliomas: a diagnostic challenge, *Langenbecks Arch Surg* 397:155–177, 2012.

Hanna-Shmouni F, Pacak K, Stratakis CA: Metanephrines for evaluating palpitations and flushing, *JAMA* 318(4):385–386, 2017.

Karasek D, Shah U, Frysak Z, et al: An update on the genetics of pheochromocytoma, *J Hum Hypertens* 27(3):141–147, 2013.

King KS, Prodanov T, Kantorovich V, et al: Metastatic pheochromocytoma/paraganglioma related to primary tumor development in childhood or adolescence: Significant link to *SDHB* mutations, *J Clin Oncol* 29:4137–4142, 2011.

Lenders JW, Duh QY, Eisenhofer G, et al: Pheochromocytoma and paraganglioma: an endocrine society clinical practice guideline, *J Clin Endocrinol Metabol* 99(6):1915–1942, 2014.

Lenders JW, Eisenhofer G, Mannelli M, Pacak K: Phaeochromocytoma, *Lancet* 366:665–675, 2005.

Lenders JW, Pacak K, Huynh TT, et al: Low sensitivity of glucagon provocative testing for diagnosis of pheochromocytoma, *J Clin Endocrinol Metab* 95:238–245, 2010.

Mannelli M, Castellano M, Schiavi F, et al: Clinically guided genetic screening in a large cohort of Italian patients with pheochromocytomas and/or functional or nonfunctional paragangliomas, *J Clin Endocrinol Metabol* 94:1541–1547, 2009.

Mannelli M, Dralle H, Lenders JW: Perioperative management of pheochromocytoma/paraganglioma: Is there a state of the art? *Horm Metab Res* 44:373–378, 2012.

Martucci VL, Pacak K: Pheochromocytoma and paraganglioma: diagnosis, genetics, management, and treatment, *Curr Prob Cancer* 38(1):7–41, 2014.

Neary NM, King KS, Pacak K: Drugs and pheochromocytoma—don't be fooled by every elevated metanephrine, *N Engl J Med* 364:2268–2270, 2011.

Neumann HP, Bausch B, McWhinney SR, et al: Germ-line mutations in nonsyndromic pheochromocytoma, *N Engl J Med* 346:1459–1466, 2002.

Pacak K: Preoperative management of the pheochromocytoma patient, *J Clin Endocrinol Metab* 92:4069–4079, 2007.

Pacak K, Eisenhofer G, Ahlman H, et al: Pheochromocytoma: Recommendations for clinical practice from the First International Symposium, October 2005, *Nat Clin Pract Endocrinol Metab* 3:92–102, 2007.

Pacak K, Eisenhofer G, Goldstein DS: Functional imaging of endocrine tumors: Role of positron emission tomography, *Endocr Rev* 25(4):568–580, 2004.

Pasini B, McWhinney SR, Bei T, et al: Clinical and molecular genetics of patients with the Carney–Stratakis syndrome and germline mutations of the genes coding for the succinate dehydrogenase subunits SDHB, SDHC, and SDHD, *Eur J Hum Genet* 16:79–88, 2008.

Renard J, Clerici T, Licker M, Triponez F: Pheochromocytoma and abdominal paraganglioma, *J Visc Surg* 148:e409–416, 2011.

Timmers HJ, Chen CC, Carrasquillo JA, et al: Staging and functional characterization of pheochromocytoma and paraganglioma by ^{18}F-fluorodeoxyglucose (^{18}F-FDG) positron emission tomography, *J Natl Cancer Inst* 104:700–708, 2012.

Timmers HJ, Gimenez-Roqueplo AP, Mannelli M, Pacak K: Clinical aspects of SDHx-related pheochromocytoma and paraganglioma, *Endocr Relat Cancer* 16:391–400, 2009.

Welander J, Soderkvist P, Gimm O: Genetics and clinical characteristics of hereditary pheochromocytomas and paragangliomas, *Endocr Relat Cancer* 18:R253–R276, 2011.

Zhuang Z, et al: Somatic Hif-2α gain-of-function mutations in paraganglioma with polycythemia, *N Engl J Med* 367:922–930, 2012.

THYROID CANCER

Method of
Faisal I. Ahmad, MD; and Mark E. Zafereo, MD

CURRENT DIAGNOSIS

- Thyroid nodules are typically recognized when a physician or patient palpates a central neck mass, or they are discovered incidentally on imaging studies performed for other reasons.
- Ninety-five percent of thyroid nodules are benign, and thyroid ultrasound is the best overall imaging study to evaluate characteristics of thyroid nodules and to determine which nodules may require fine-needle aspiration biopsy.
- Ultrasound-guided fine-needle aspiration biopsy is often performed at the time of thyroid ultrasound for thyroid nodules that have suspicious sonographic features.
- Fine-needle aspiration histopathology can aid in diagnosis of thyroid cancer, but fine-needle aspiration cytology reports often fall into an indeterminate thyroid lesion/neoplasm category.
- Thyroid cancer does not typically affect thyroid hormone levels, but thyroid-stimulating hormone (TSH) should be measured in the work-up of a thyroid nodule to assess thyroid function prior to consideration of thyroid surgery.
- Medullary thyroid carcinoma (MTC) is a rare type of thyroid cancer that can be diagnosed by fine-needle aspiration biopsy and/or elevated serum calcitonin and carcinoembryonic antigen (CEA) levels in the presence of a thyroid mass.
- Twenty percent of MTC is hereditary and associated with autosomal dominant mutations in the RET proto-oncogene (multiple endocrine neoplasia [MEN] syndrome); therefore all patients with MTC should undergo RET genetic testing and evaluation for pheochromocytoma prior to surgery.
- Anaplastic thyroid carcinoma is a rare and extremely aggressive form of thyroid cancer that presents as a very rapidly growing thyroid mass.

CURRENT THERAPY

- Observation with follow-up ultrasound is the most appropriate treatment recommendation for thyroid nodules that are suspected to be benign unless the patient is having compressive symptoms related to a large benign thyroid tumor or goiter.
- Thyroid nodules that are indeterminate for malignancy on fine-needle aspiration biopsy may be treated with short-term observation, thyroid lobectomy, or total thyroidectomy.
- Micropapillary thyroid carcinomas (tumors <1 cm) can be treated with short-term observation, thyroid lobectomy, or total thyroidectomy, depending on patient age and preference.
- Well-differentiated thyroid cancers (papillary and follicular thyroid cancers) may be treated with thyroid lobectomy or total thyroidectomy, with or without central compartment lymph node dissection.
- For patients with intermediate- or high-risk well-differentiated thyroid cancers who undergo total thyroidectomy, radioactive iodine and thyroid hormone suppression may be considered following surgery.
- Total thyroidectomy with central compartment dissection is the recommended treatment for patients with medullary thyroid cancer.
- Postoperative external beam radiation therapy is rarely indicated for patients with well-differentiated thyroid cancer or medullary thyroid cancer unless disease is significantly invasive.
- Cytotoxic chemotherapy is not effective for well-differentiated thyroid cancer, but select molecular targeted therapies have been approved by the US Food and Drug Administration (FDA) for patients with progressive systemic disease.
- Anaplastic thyroid cancer is the most aggressive type of thyroid cancer, characterized by rapid growth and distant metastases. However, recent discoveries of tumor BRAF mutations in almost 50% of anaplastic thyroid cancer patients, coupled with rapid response to combined BRAF and MEK inhibition, have led to FDA approval of combined BRAF and MEK inhibitor therapy for BRAF-mutated anaplastic thyroid cancer.

Epidemiology

Thyroid nodules are very common, affecting approximately 20% of the population. The vast majority (approximately 95%) of thyroid nodules are benign. The incidence of thyroid nodules increases with age, and thyroid nodules are more common in females. The clinical importance of thyroid nodules lies in the need to exclude thyroid cancer, present in 5% to 10% of thyroid nodules. Thyroid cancer represents the most rapidly increasing cancer (>5% increase per year in both men and women) in the United States and the most common endocrine malignancy. Thyroid cancer is more common in females, representing the fifth most common malignancy in women in the United States (5% of estimated cancer diagnoses in females in 2018), and is also relatively more common in young adults, representing 15% of overall US cancer diagnoses among persons aged 20 to 34 years. However, the increasing incidence of thyroid cancer in the United States is largely attributed to higher rates of detection with increasing use of imaging such as neck ultrasonography. A study estimated that almost one-half of papillary thyroid cancers diagnosed in women and men younger than 50 years old in the United States may be clinically irrelevant. Fortunately, thyroid cancer is most often an indolent malignancy, and many patients with thyroid cancer can live unknowingly with disease for years or even decades. Despite increased incidence, mortality from thyroid cancer remains very low (approximately 5%). Patients who die of thyroid cancer most often present with aggressive histopathology, high tumor burden, and distant metastases.

TABLE 1	Classification, Genetics, and Incidence of Thyroid Cancers.				
TYPE OF THYROID CANCER	CELL TYPE	DIFFERENTIATED?	COMMON GENETIC MUTATIONS	ESTIMATED % OF CASES
Papillary	Follicular	Yes	*TKR, BRAF*	80
Follicular	Follicular	Yes	*RAS, PAX8-PPARG*	15
Hurthle cell	Follicular	Yes	–	2*
Poorly differentiated	Follicular	No	*RAS, TP53*	1
Anaplastic	Follicular	No	*TP53, BRAF, RAS*	1
Medullary	Parafollicular (C cell)	No	*RET*	3

RAS, Renin-angiotensin system; *TKR*, tyrosine kinase receptor.
*Included among follicular thyroid cancers.

Risk Factors

Ninety-five percent of thyroid cancers are not associated with any known risk factor. History of ionizing radiation to the thyroid is the only known environmental factor associated with increased risk of thyroid cancer, but this risk factor accounts for less than 1% of thyroid malignancies. Only 5% to 10% of patients with nonmedullary differentiated thyroid cancer have a familial occurrence, and well-differentiated thyroid cancer is generally not considered familial (familial follicular cell–derived differentiated thyroid cancer) unless three or more first-degree relatives are affected. Therefore routine screening for thyroid cancer with thyroid ultrasound is not recommended unless the patient has a specific genetic syndrome that may be associated with differentiated thyroid cancer, such as phosphate and tensin homolog hamartoma tumor syndrome (PTEN), Cowden disease, familial adenomatous polyposis (FAP), or Carney complex. On the other hand, approximately 20% of patients with medullary thyroid carcinoma (MTC) have multiple endocrine neoplasia (MEN) types 2A and 2B hereditary syndromes; therefore patients with MTC should routinely undergo genetic testing.

Pathophysiology

The thyroid gland has two distinct hormone-producing cell types from which tumors arise: follicular cells and neuroendocrine parafollicular C cells. The follicular cells secrete thyroid hormone and are the origin of five types of thyroid cancer: papillary thyroid cancer, follicular thyroid cancer, Hurthle cell thyroid cancer, poorly differentiated thyroid cancer, and anaplastic thyroid cancer. MTC, on the other hand, arises from the calcitonin-secreting parafollicular C cells (Table 1).

Differentiated Thyroid Cancers

Papillary and follicular cancers are collectively referred to as differentiated thyroid cancers, indicating cells that maintain a microscopic appearance more similar to normal thyroid tissue. Differentiated thyroid cancer collectively makes up 95% of thyroid cancer. Papillary thyroid cancer is the most prevalent thyroid cancer subtype, and 70% have genetic alterations causing activation of the mitogen-activated protein kinase (MAPK) pathway. The MAPK pathway is most typically initiated by activation of the tyrosine kinase receptor. Activation of the MAPK pathway often leads to oncogenic conversion of *BRAF*, which is the most common genetic event in papillary thyroid cancer. Therefore tyrosine kinase and *BRAF* inhibition represent two foci of targeted drug therapy for rare cases of advanced and/or metastatic differentiated thyroid cancer. The two most common genetic mutations associated with follicular thyroid cancer are renin-angiotensin system (RAS) and paired box 8/peroxisome proliferator-activated receptor gamma (PAX8-PPARG) mutations.

Hurthle cell carcinomas are considered variants of differentiated follicular thyroid cancer that are distinguished by an accumulation of Hurthle cells. Thyroid Hurthle cells (also called oncocytic cells) are characterized by abundant eosinophilic granular cytoplasm as a result of accumulation of altered mitochondria. This phenomena of Hurthle cell change in the thyroid occurs in inflammatory disorders such as thyroiditis and Graves disease, and the notation of Hurthle cells is, therefore, common with fine-needle aspiration biopsies in which there is associated thyroiditis. The proliferation of oncocytes also may give rise to hyperplastic and neoplastic nodules termed Hurthle cell neoplasms.

Dedifferentiated Thyroid Cancers

Dedifferentiated thyroid cancers are very rare and include poorly differentiated and anaplastic thyroid cancers. Many tumors with poorly differentiated and anaplastic thyroid carcinoma exhibit areas or separate foci of papillary or follicular carcinoma, suggesting that these tumors may arise from preexisting well-differentiated tumors. Poorly differentiated thyroid cancers include tumors with solid/trabecular/insular growth patterns, absence of typical nuclear features of papillary thyroid carcinoma, high mitotic figures, and extensive tumor necrosis. Anaplastic thyroid cancers are similarly thought to derive from a terminal dedifferentiation of carcinoma of the thyroid follicular cell, often with loss of p53 and other genetic mutations. Histopathologically, anaplastic thyroid cancers appear as necrotic and hemorrhagic tumors with cytologic anaplasia showing bizarre tumor cells, high mitotic rate, and significant angioinvasion. Dedifferentiated thyroid cancers exhibit rapid growth, high rates of distant metastases, and overall poor prognosis; anaplastic thyroid carcinomas are almost uniformly fatal.

Medullary Thyroid Cancers

MTCs originate from the neuroendocrine parafollicular C cells of the thyroid gland. Approximately 20% of MTC is hereditary, associated with germline mutations in the RET proto-oncogene, leading to MEN. Ninety-five percent of hereditary MTC is related to *MEN type 2a* (50% incidence parathyroid hyperplasia, 100% incidence MTC, and 33% incidence pheochromocytoma), whereas approximately 5% results from *MEN2b* (85% incidence MTC, 50% incidence pheochromocytoma, 80% incidence marfanoid body habitus, 100% incidence mucosal neuromas). Approximately 50% of patients with sporadic MTC have somatic *RET* mutations. The M918T mutation portends the worst prognosis in both hereditary and sporadic MTC.

Clinical Manifestations

The diagnosis of thyroid cancer is often made after incidental discovery of a nonpalpable thyroid nodule on radiology scans performed for unrelated reasons (e.g., computed tomography [CT] of the neck in the emergency room for a young woman in an automobile accident, or screening carotid ultrasound for an elderly woman with atherosclerosis). Some patients may undergo thyroid ultrasound after self-palpating a thyroid nodule or neck mass, or after their primary care physician palpates a thyroid nodule on routine physical examination. Patients with larger thyroid cancers may have presenting symptoms of hoarseness (caused by recurrent laryngeal nerve paralysis), dysphagia (caused by esophageal compression or invasion), difficulty breathing, or pain.

Patients with advanced medullary thyroid cancer can have diarrhea, Cushing syndrome, or facial flushing because of high serum levels of calcitonin and other hormonally active peptides. However, the vast majority of small thyroid cancers are asymptomatic.

Diagnosis

Serum thyroid-stimulating hormone (TSH) should be measured in the evaluation of a thyroid nodule because, rarely, thyroid nodules can be hyperfunctioning. If serum TSH is subnormal in the presence of a thyroid nodule, a radionuclide thyroid scan may be considered; "hot" nodules (i.e., those with uptake greater than the surrounding thyroid tissue) very rarely represent malignancy and do not require cytologic evaluation.

All patients with thyroid nodules should be evaluated with thyroid ultrasound. Ultrasound-guided fine-needle aspiration biopsy is the "gold standard" in diagnosis of thyroid neoplasia. However, not all thyroid nodules require biopsy. The vast majority of thyroid cancers are solid, and purely cystic nodules are very rarely malignant. Nodules greater than 1 cm with suspicious sonographic features (e.g., solid nodules with irregular margins, microcalcifications, and/or increased central internal vascularity) are recommended for biopsy, but nodules less than 1 cm are rarely recommended for biopsy. Incidental thyroid nodules that are discovered as fluorodeoxyglucose-avid on positron emission tomography (PET) imaging ("PET incidentalomas") are recommended to undergo fine-needle aspiration biopsy because PET-avid nodules have approximately 40% malignancy risk.

Thyroid cytologic classification is according to the criteria and terminology of the Bethesda system and includes the following general diagnostic categories (with associated malignancy risk): nondiagnostic (20% risk), benign (2% risk), follicular lesion (5% to 10% risk), follicular neoplasm (15% to 20% risk), atypical cells of undetermined significance (25% risk), suspicious for malignancy (90% risk), and malignant (99% risk). Papillary thyroid carcinoma can be diagnosed cytologically based on atypical nuclear features such as nuclear grooves and nuclear inclusions. In contrast to papillary thyroid carcinomas, follicular and Hurthle cell carcinomas can rarely be diagnosed on fine-needle aspiration biopsy, because the diagnostic criterion for diagnosis of malignancy requires demonstration of capsular or vascular invasion. Nondiagnostic fine-needle aspiration biopsies fail to meet criteria for cytologic analysis, and repeat biopsy is recommended. Thyroid fine-needle aspirations that fall into the indeterminate category (follicular lesion, follicular neoplasm, atypical cells of undetermined significance) may be further evaluated with molecular testing by one of several commercially available gene expression classifier tests (e.g., Afirma) or individual mutational analysis (e.g., *BRAF*).

If thyroid cytology is suspicious for MTC, serum calcitonin and carcinoembryonic antigen (CEA) should be measured. Although CEA may be elevated with a number of malignancies, calcitonin is more specific to MTC, and calcitonin can rarely be elevated in association with other conditions. Patients with MTC should undergo genetic testing prior to surgery to rule out hereditary MTC because a coexisting pheochromocytoma has the potential to cause hypertensive crisis during thyroid surgery. Often patients with hereditary MTC with associated pheochromocytoma will undergo resection of the pheochromocytoma before their thyroid surgery.

Treatment
Differentiated Thyroid Cancer
Initial Management

Treatment algorithms for nondiagnostic, benign, indeterminate, and differentiated malignant thyroid nodules are illustrated in Box 1. For patients with indeterminate thyroid nodules a molecular gene expression classifier test or individual mutational analysis may be considered to further characterize preoperative risk of malignancy. Determination of observation versus thyroid lobectomy must primarily take into account patient preference after discussion of risks, implications, and benefits of both approaches.

BOX 1 Management of Thyroid Neoplasms and Cancers Based on Fine-Needle Aspiration Cytology.

Nondiagnostic
- Repeat ultrasound-guided fine-needle aspiration biopsy in 3 months
- If repeat biopsy nondiagnostic: Observation (with initial follow-up ultrasound 3–6 months) or thyroid lobectomy

Benign
- Observation, may repeat ultrasound in 12 months

Indeterminate (follicular lesion *or* follicular neoplasm *or* atypical cells of undetermined significance)
- Observation (with initial follow-up ultrasound 3–6 months) or thyroid lobectomy
  - May consider gene expression classifier test

Suspicious or malignant differentiated thyroid cancer
- Thyroid lobectomy *or* total thyroidectomy with possible central compartment lymph node dissection
  - Observation may be considered for older patients with intrathyroidal micropapillary (<1 cm) carcinomas
  - Thyroid hormone suppression and radioactive iodine may be considered postoperatively if total thyroidectomy performed

Medullary thyroid cancer
- Total thyroidectomy with central compartment dissection
  - Measure serum calcitonin/carcinoembryonic antigen and perform genetic testing (rule out multiple endocrine neoplasia type 2 with associated pheochromocytoma) preoperatively

---

Differentiated thyroid cancer is generally treated with surgery, with the exception of intrathyroidal micropapillary carcinomas (tumors <1 cm), which may be observed with follow-up ultrasound, especially in older patients. With micropapillary thyroid carcinoma, risk of rapid growth is low, and many of these lesions demonstrate relatively little growth over the course of 5- or 10-year follow-up.

For tumors between 1 and 4 cm, thyroid lobectomy may be considered in the absence of central compartment lymphadenopathy; total thyroidectomy is recommended for tumors greater than 4 cm. Central compartment (i.e., level VI paratracheal) lymph node dissection should be performed for patients with lymph node metastases and may be performed electively for patients with larger tumors because of the risk of occult lymph node metastases. Intraoperative frozen section evaluation of central compartment lymph nodes may also be useful to guide the decision regarding central compartment lymph node dissection. Patients with lateral neck (most commonly levels II, III, IV, and VB) lymph node metastases should undergo selective comprehensive lateral neck dissection of aforementioned compartments. Single node plucking or "berry-picking" is not recommended because this increases potential morbidity with any subsequent surgery to remove remaining lymph nodes.

Following total thyroidectomy patients with well-differentiated thyroid cancer are recommended for thyroid hormone suppression (suppression of TSH) because TSH is a trophic hormone that stimulates growth of thyroid follicular cells. In addition, patients with distant metastases and/or higher risk tumors may be considered for postoperative radioactive iodine therapy. Postoperative external beam radiation therapy is very rarely indicated for well-differentiated thyroid cancer but is only indicated with particularly aggressive and invasive disease in patients who would not be candidates for future revision surgery (e.g., laryngotracheal invasion, or esophageal invasion). Traditional cytotoxic chemotherapeutic agents are ineffective for well-differentiated thyroid cancer, but select targeted molecular therapies may be considered for patients with progressive and/or symptomatic disease.

Sorafenib and lenvatinib are two small molecule kinase inhibitors that have been approved by the US Food and Drug Administration for advanced and/or metastatic thyroid cancer refractory to radioactive iodine.

Long-Term Management

Approximately 25% of patients undergoing thyroid lobectomy will require thyroid hormone replacement, in addition to all patients undergoing total thyroidectomy. These patients require follow-up to check thyroid function tests and also surveillance testing to detect potential recurrent differentiated thyroid cancer. Depending on prognostic variables, up to 30% of patients with well-differentiated thyroid cancer may develop recurrence over the course of several decades following initial therapy. Thyroid/cervical ultrasound and serum thyroglobulin measurement (for patients who have had total thyroidectomy) are the two primary methods of long-term follow-up for patients with history of well-differentiated thyroid cancer. Whole body diagnostic radioactive iodine scans are less sensitive for detecting recurrent disease but can be useful for localizing disease in the presence of detectable/rising thyroglobulin in the absence of thyroid bed/neck disease (as assessed by ultrasound or CT imaging) or in select high-risk patients whose serum thyroglobulin is unreliable for detection of thyroid disease because of the presence of thyroglobulin antibodies. Serum thyroglobulin can be measured while the patient is on thyroid hormone, or under conditions of stimulation, either by thyroid hormone withdrawal, or administration of recombinant TSH. Stimulated thyroglobulin is more sensitive for detecting residual thyroid tissue and/or recurrent disease.

Ultrasound-guided fine-needle aspiration biopsy can be performed for recurrent thyroid bed or lateral neck nodules/lymph nodes. Small burden recurrent locoregional or distant disease may be monitored for a period of time, because the majority of well-differentiated thyroid cancer is slow growing and asymptomatic in the absence of large tumor burden. Alternatively, surgery may be performed for larger recurrent nodules/lymph nodes, and radioactive iodine and/or targeted molecular therapy may be considered for progressive distant disease.

Medullary Thyroid Cancer
Initial Management

As with differentiated thyroid cancer, surgery is the mainstay of treatment for medullary thyroid cancer. Infants and children with hereditary MTC diagnosed on genetic testing require special consideration; patients with intermediate risk mutations may be recommended for prophylactic thyroidectomy by 5 years of age, whereas patients with MEN2b and high-risk mutations may be recommended for prophylactic thyroidectomy in the first year of life.

Occult cervical lymph node metastases with MTC are common; therefore total thyroidectomy and bilateral central compartment paratracheal lymph node dissection is the generally recommended surgery. For patients with evidence of lateral neck disease on preoperative imaging, a systematic unilateral or bilateral selective or modified radical neck dissection should be performed, preserving important neurovascular structures unless they are invaded with disease. Most commonly cervical levels II, III, IV, and VB are dissected, although patients may rarely have metastases to other levels of the lateral neck. For patients without preoperative lateral neck disease, observation of the lateral neck is appropriate because these patients can undergo subsequent lateral neck surgery if they were to later develop lateral neck metastases. However, some surgeons recommend elective unilateral or bilateral lateral neck dissection at the time of the thyroid surgery for patients with serum calcitonin greater than 20 (elective unilateral dissection) or 200 (elective bilateral dissection).

External beam radiation therapy is only indicated postoperatively for patients with particularly aggressive and invasive disease who would not be candidates for future revision surgery (e.g., laryngotracheal invasion or esophageal invasion). Because medullary thyroid cancer is not a follicular neoplasm, there is no indication for thyroid hormone suppression postoperatively. Patients should be managed with appropriate thyroid hormone supplementation so that their TSH is maintained in the euthyroid range. Radioactive iodine is not indicated in the postoperative treatment of medullary thyroid cancer because parafollicular C cells (and thereby medullary thyroid cancer cells) do not take up radioactive iodine.

Long-Term Management

Measurement of serum calcitonin and CEA is the primary method of surveillance for recurrence and/or distant metastases, and should be measured approximately 3 months postoperatively and at regular intervals thereafter. Rising tumor markers should prompt further evaluation with cross-sectional imaging of the neck, chest, and abdomen, in addition to consideration of bone scan. Higher levels of calcitonin (>1000) are associated with distant metastases, and shorter calcitonin doubling time has been associated with overall poorer prognosis.

Medullary thyroid cancers have variable growth rates, and locoregionally recurrent and distant disease may be monitored in the absence of significant progression or symptoms. Patients with progressive or symptomatic recurrent and/or distant disease may be treated surgically (for patients with operable locoregional recurrence) or with systemic targeted molecular therapy. Vandetanib and cabozantinib are tyrosine kinase inhibitors with activity against RET and vascular endothelial growth factor receptor (VEGFR) with FDA approval for use in advanced medullary thyroid cancer. Patients with symptomatic diarrhea resulting from markedly elevated serum calcitonin should be treated with antimotility agents such as loperamide, diphenoxylate/atropine, or codeine.

Anaplastic Thyroid Cancer

Because of rapid growth (doubling time often measured in weeks) and frequent distant metastases, the historical median survival following diagnosis for patients with anaplastic thyroid cancer has been 3 to 6 months. Patients with anaplastic thyroid cancer often have rapid onset of speech, swallowing, and breathing difficulties, and the decision for a tracheotomy in these patients is based on discussion of risks and implications with the patient. Anaplastic cancers confined to the thyroid gland are rare, but surgery and postoperative chemoradiation therapy can be effective to control disease in this very select group of anaplastic thyroid cancer patients. Unfortunately, the vast majority of patients with anaplastic thyroid cancer present with massive tumor burden beyond the thyroid gland and/or distant metastases, and upfront surgery is generally not effective to control disease in these situations. Historically, these patients have been treated palliatively with radiation, chemotherapy, or both; or they have elected for supportive/hospice care.

However, over the past several years, there have been significant advancements in the treatment of patients with anaplastic thyroid cancer based on tumor mutation status. It has been discovered that almost 50% of patients with anaplastic thyroid cancer have *BRAF* tumor mutations. Anaplastic and poorly differentiated thyroid cancers with *BRAF* mutations often respond rapidly to targeted systemic therapy with *BRAF* inhibitors. Patients with *BRAF*-mutated anaplastic thyroid cancer treated with combination *BRAF* and *MEK* inhibitors have demonstrated improved survival, leading to the FDA approval of combination *BRAF* and *MEK* inhibitor therapy for this disease in 2018. Although *BRAF*-mutated anaplastic thyroid cancer patients can have rapid and dramatic responses to combined *BRAF/MEK* inhibitor therapy, these tumors generally become resistant to this therapy within 1 year. Therefore current clinical trials are studying immunotherapy as a means to prolong treatment response and survival in patients with *BRAF*-mutated anaplastic thyroid cancer.

Complications

Because thyroid cancer is generally treated surgically, operative treatment complications are most common. Significant care must be taken to identify and preserve the bilateral recurrent laryngeal nerves during thyroid surgery; injury to unilateral or bilateral recurrent laryngeal nerves may result in temporary or permanent postoperative hoarseness (unilateral paralysis) or breathing difficulty (bilateral paralysis). Patients with a bilateral vocal cord paralysis may require a temporary or permanent tracheostomy tube. Permanent unilateral recurrent laryngeal nerve paralysis occurs following 1% to 2% of thyroid surgeries.

A second postoperative complication associated with total thyroidectomy is hypocalcemia related to hypoparathyroidism. Care must be taken during thyroid surgery to preserve the bilateral superior and inferior parathyroid glands along with their respective vascular pedicle. Although one normal-functioning parathyroid gland is generally considered sufficient for long-term parathyroid function, many patients become temporarily hypoparathyroid, and hypocalcemic when multiple parathyroid glands are removed and/or devascularized during thyroid and central compartment surgery. Because the inferior parathyroid gland is usually interspersed with central compartment lymph nodes, this gland is often devascularized with central compartment surgery. Any devascularized parathyroid gland should be reimplanted, generally in an adjacent muscle such as the sternothyroid or sternocleidomastoid muscle. Patients who undergo total thyroidectomy should have their calcium and/or parathyroid hormone level checked in the immediate postoperative period prior to discharge. If calcium and/or parathyroid hormone level is low, an appropriate calcium replacement protocol should be initiated. Most postoperative hypocalcemia and hypoparathyroidism are temporary, with permanent hypoparathyroidism occurring in approximately 3% of thyroid surgery.

Patients who undergo lateral neck surgery in association with thyroid surgery have additional risks of neurovascular injury, which includes shoulder weakness (cranial nerve 11 injury), tongue weakness (cranial nerve 12 injury), lower lip weakness (marginal mandibular nerve injury), and chyle leak.

Risks of radioactive iodine include sialadenitis, dry mouth, and altered taste. There are also rare reports of second cancers that may be associated with cumulative high doses of radioactive iodine. Women who are nursing or pregnant should not receive radioactive iodine, and patients are recommended that close contact with others, especially children, should be avoided for several days following administration of radioactive iodine.

Conclusion

Thyroid nodules are very common, and 95% are benign. The gold standard for evaluation of a thyroid nodule is ultrasound-guided fine-needle aspiration biopsy. Benign and many indeterminate nodules may be observed, although thyroid cancer is generally treated with surgery. Most well-differentiated thyroid cancers (papillary and follicular) have good prognosis with surgery (either thyroid lobectomy or total thyroidectomy), and some patients are recommended for postoperative radioactive iodine and thyroid hormone suppression. Medullary thyroid cancer is typically treated with total thyroidectomy and central compartment lymph node dissection. Approximately 20% of MTCs are hereditary, associated with MEN2, and mutation in the RET proto-oncogene; patients with medullary thyroid cancer should, therefore, undergo genetic testing prior to surgery. Postoperative radiation therapy is rarely indicated for well-differentiated or medullary thyroid cancers unless the disease is particularly aggressive and invasive. Anaplastic thyroid cancer is the most aggressive type of thyroid cancer, with historical median survival of 3 to 6 months. However, discoveries of tumor *BRAF* mutations in almost 50% of these patients, coupled with rapid response to combined *BRAF* and *MEK* inhibition, have led to FDA approval of combined *BRAF* and *MEK* inhibitor therapy for *BRAF*-mutated anaplastic thyroid cancer. Because *BRAF*-mutated tumors ultimately become resistance to these drugs, current clinical trials are studying immunotherapy, surgery, radiation, and cytotoxic chemotherapy as adjuvant treatment strategies in this disease.

References

Cabanillas ME, Ferrarotto R, Garden AS, et al: Neoadjuvant BRAF- and immune-directed therapy for anaplastic thyroid carcinoma, *Thyroid* 28:945–951, 2018.

Francis GL, Waguespack SG, Bauer AJ, et al: Management guidelines for children with thyroid nodules and differentiated thyroid cancer: the American Thyroid Association Guidelines Task Force on Pediatric Thyroid Cancer, *Thyroid* 25:716–759, 2015.
Haughen BR, Alexander EK, Bible KC, et al: 2015 American Thyroid Association management guidelines for adult patients with thyroid nodules and differentiated thyroid cancer: The American Thyroid Association Guidelines Task Force on Thyroid Nodules and Differentiated Thyroid Cancer, *Thyroid* 26:1–133, 2016.
Maniakas A, Davies L, Zafereo ME: Thyroid disease around the world, *Otolaryngol Clin North Am* 51:631–642, 2018.
NCCN Clinical Practice Guidelines in Oncology: Thyroid Carcinoma, *Version 1*, 2018, Available at: NCCN.org. Accessed 18 July 2018.
O'Grady TJ, Gates MA, Boscoe FP: Thyroid cancer incidence attributable to over-diagnosis in the United States 1981–2011, *Int J Cancer* 137:2664–2673, 2015.
Pena I, Clayman GL, Grubbs EG, et al: Management of the lateral neck compartment in patients with sporadic medullary thyroid cancer, *Head Neck* 40:79–85, 2018.
Randolph GW: Surgery of the thyroid and parathyroid glands. In Randolph GW, editor: *2nd ed.*, Philadelphia, 2013, Saunders.
Rao SN, Zafereo ME, Dadu R, et al: Patterns of treatment failure in anaplastic thyroid carcinoma, *Thyroid* 27:672–681, 2017.
Siegel RL, Miller KD, Jemal A: Cancer statistics, 2018, *CA Cancer J Clin* 68:7–30, 2018.
Wells Jr SA, Asa SL, Dralle H, et al: Revised American Thyroid Association guidelines for the management of medullary thyroid carcinoma: The American Thyroid Association Guidelines Task Force on Medullary Thyroid Carcinoma, *Thyroid* 25:567–610, 2015.

THYROIDITIS

Method of
Leigh M. Eck, MD

CURRENT DIAGNOSIS

- Thyroiditis is a term used to describe a diverse group of disorders associated with thyroid inflammation.
- Thyroiditis can be associated with a euthyroid state, thyrotoxicosis, or hypothyroidism.
- The clinical presentation of thyroiditis will direct the evaluation with useful testing to include measurement of thyroid hormone levels, thyroid antibody testing, white blood cell count, erythrocyte sedimentation rate, thyroid scintigraphy, and thyroid ultrasound.

CURRENT THERAPY

- Abnormalities of thyroid hormone levels resulting from thyroiditis may be transient and require no or only short-term therapy.
- If symptomatic thyrotoxicosis is present, beta-blocker therapy should be initiated.
- Thyroiditis associated with persistent hypothyroidism is managed with synthetic thyroxine (T4, Levoxyl, Synthroid).
- Thyroid pain associated with subacute thyroiditis is managed with a nonsteroidal antiinflammatory drug or, if ineffective, glucocorticoid therapy.
- Acute suppurative thyroiditis requires immediate parenteral antibiotic therapy as well as surgical drainage, if indicated.

Thyroiditis is a term used to describe a diverse group of disorders characterized by inflammation of the thyroid gland (Table 1). Presentation of thyroiditis is variable depending on the etiology. The most common thyroid disorder in the United States, Hashimoto's thyroiditis, most often presents with hypothyroidism. Other forms of thyroiditis may present with thyrotoxicosis because of inflammation in the thyroid gland resulting in the release of stored hormone. Painful thyroiditis is seen with subacute, suppurative

TABLE 1 Causes of Thyroiditis

Autoimmune thyroiditis: Hashimoto's thyroiditis, postpartum thyroiditis, silent thyroiditis

Subacute thyroiditis, also known as de Quervain's thyroiditis or subacute granulomatous thyroiditis

Suppurative thyroiditis, also known as infectious thyroiditis or pyrogenic thyroiditis

Riedel's thyroiditis, also known as fibrous thyroiditis

Therapy induced thyroiditis: amiodarone (Cordarone), interferon-alpha, interleukin-2, lithium, tyrosine kinase inhibitors, radioactive iodine, checkpoint inhibitor immunotherapy

and radiation-induced thyroiditis, while other variants are most often painless.

Epidemiology

The most common cause of hypothyroidism in iodine-sufficient areas of the world is *Hashimoto's thyroiditis,* also known as *chronic autoimmune thyroiditis.* Elevated serum antithyroid peroxidase antibody concentrations are found in ~ 5% of adults and ~ 15% of older women; overt hypothyroidism is seen in up to 2% of the population. A variant of chronic autoimmune thyroiditis, *postpartum thyroiditis,* is a destructive thyroiditis induced by an autoimmune mechanism that occurs within 1 year of parturition. Postpartum thyroiditis occurs in up to 10% of women in the United States. *Silent thyroiditis* is indistinguishable from postpartum thyroiditis, with the exception of lack of temporal relationship to pregnancy. Silent thyroiditis may account for about 1% of all cases of thyrotoxicosis. Many medications are associated with an alteration in thyroid function testing; however, only a few are known to provoke an autoimmune or destructive inflammatory thyroiditis, including amiodarone (Cordarone), lithium, interferon alfa, interleukin-2, tyrosine kinase inhibitors, and checkpoint inhibitor immunotherapy. *Riedel's thyroiditis* is a progressive fibrosis of the thyroid gland with a prevalence of only 0.05% among patients with thyroid disease requiring surgery. *Subacute thyroiditis* is the most common cause of thyroid pain. It occurs in up to 5% of patients with clinical thyroid disease. *Suppurative thyroiditis,* most commonly caused by bacterial infection, is rare because of the thyroid gland's encapsulation, high iodine content, rich blood supply, and extensive lymphatic drainage. *Radiation-induced thyroiditis* occurs in approximately 1% of patients who receive radioactive iodine therapy for hyperthyroidism.

Risk Factors

Hashimoto's thyroiditis is more common in women, particularly older women. Hashimoto's thyroiditis is associated with several gene polymorphisms, suggesting a role for genetic susceptibility. Subacute thyroiditis frequently follows an upper respiratory tract infection, with its incidence highest in summer. Suppurative thyroiditis is most likely to occur in patients with preexisting thyroid disease, those with congenital anomalies such as pyriform sinus fistula, and those who are immunosuppressed.

Pathophysiology

Hashimoto's thyroiditis, postpartum thyroiditis, and silent thyroiditis all have an autoimmune basis. The antithyroid immune response begins with activation of thyroid antigen-specific helper T cells. Once helper T cells are activated, they induce B cells to secrete thyroid antibodies; thyroid antibodies most frequently measured are those directed against thyroid peroxidase and against thyroglobulin. The mechanism for autoimmune destruction of the thyroid likely involves both cellular immunity and humoral immunity. Riedel's thyroiditis is the local involvement of the thyroid in a systemic disease, multifocal fibrosclerosis; the etiology of Riedel's thyroiditis is not known. Although a viral cause of subacute thyroiditis has been proposed, clear evidence for this proposed etiology

is lacking. Suppurative thyroiditis is most often associated with a bacterial pathogen; however, fungal, mycobacterial, or parasitic infections may also be the cause. Although rare, radiation-induced thyroiditis may occur following the treatment of hyperthyroidism with radioactive iodine because of radiation-induced injury and necrosis of thyroid follicular cells and associated inflammation.

Clinical Manifestations

A symmetrical, painless goiter is frequently the initial finding in Hashimoto's thyroiditis. The usual course of Hashimoto's thyroiditis is gradual loss of thyroid function. Among patients with this disorder who have subclinical hypothyroidism, overt hypothyroidism occurs at a rate of about 5% per year. The classic presentation of postpartum thyroiditis occurs in only approximately 30% of afflicted women, with the characteristic sequence of hyperthyroidism, followed by hypothyroidism, and then recovery. Persistent hypothyroidism is seen in up to 30% of women following an episode of postpartum thyroiditis. Silent thyroiditis is marked by a similar characteristic sequence of thyroid hormone dysfunction. However, it is not temporally associated with pregnancy; 20% will have residual hypothyroidism. *Medication-induced thyroiditis* is variable in its presentation. Amiodarone (Cordarone), rich in iodine, is associated with hypothyroidism and hyperthyroidism; type 2 amiodarone-induced thyrotoxicosis is due to a destructive thyroiditis process. Lithium is more commonly associated with hypothyroidism. Interferon-alfa and interleukin-2 can cause both permanent and transient hypothyroidism likely related to the ability of these substances to induce or exacerbate thyroid autoimmune disease. Riedel's thyroiditis presents with neck discomfort or tightness, dysphagia, hoarseness, and a diffuse goiter that is hard, fixed, and often not clearly separable from the adjacent tissues. Generally, patients are euthyroid, and their antithyroid antibody concentrations are often high. Subacute thyroiditis manifests with a prodrome of myalgias, pharyngitis, low-grade fever, and fatigue with subsequent fever and neck pain, and up to 50% of patients have symptoms of thyrotoxicosis. Patients with suppurative thyroiditis are usually acutely ill with fever, dysphagia, dysphonia, anterior neck pain with erythema, and a tender thyroid mass. Radiation-induced thyroiditis presents 5 to 10 days following radioactive iodine treatment with neck pain and tenderness. In addition, there can be a transient exacerbation of hyperthyroidism.

Diagnosis and Differential Diagnosis

The diagnostic approach to suspected thyroiditis can be focused based on an association with thyroid pain and circulating thyroid hormone status (Figure 1). Hashimoto's thyroiditis is diagnosed when a goiter is found on examination with a subsequently noted elevation of thyroid antibodies or when subclinical or overt hypothyroidism is detected with associated elevated thyroid antibodies. Screening for postpartum thyroiditis with a measurement of TSH and free thyroxine should be undertaken in women presenting with symptoms of thyroid dysfunction in the postpartum period. If hyperthyroidism is present, thyroid scintigraphy (if not contraindicated, e.g., breastfeeding) or measurement of thyroid-stimulating immunoglobulins is helpful in the differentiation of postpartum thyroiditis from Graves' disease. The diagnostic approach to silent thyroiditis is similar. The laboratory hallmark of subacute thyroiditis is a markedly elevated erythrocyte sedimentation rate; the leukocyte count is normal or slightly elevated. Thyrotoxicosis may be present; if so, thyroid scintigraphy will reveal a low iodine uptake state. Thyroid antibody testing is typically normal. Thyroid ultrasound reveals a hypoechogenic gland with low to normal vascularity. Suppurative thyroiditis is typically associated with normal thyroid function. Leukocyte counts and erythrocyte sedimentation rates are elevated. Fine-needle aspiration with Gram stain and culture is the diagnostic test of choice. Radiation-induced thyroiditis should be considered if a temporal relationship to radioactive iodine treatment is present. If there is an exacerbation of hyperthyroidism immediately following radiation treatment for the same, consideration of radiation-induced thyroiditis due to the release of preformed thyroid

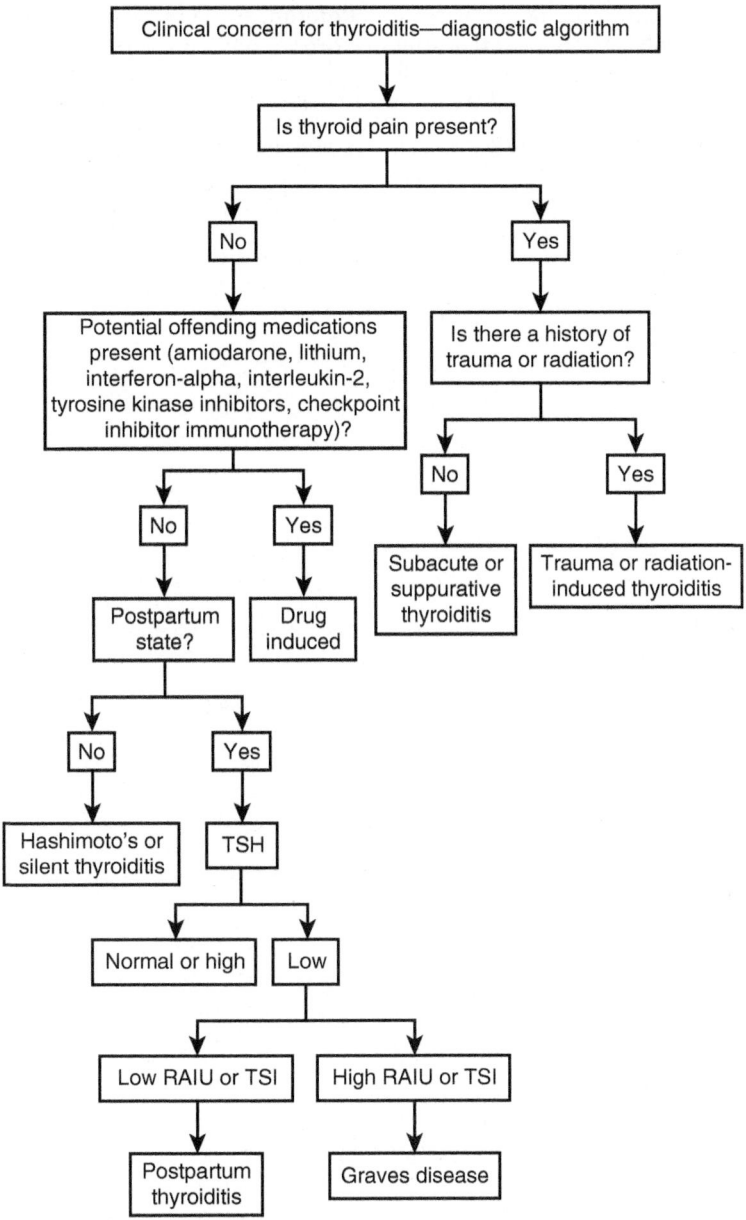

Figure 1 Clinical concern for thyroiditis—diagnostic algorithm. *Abbreviations:* RAIU = radioactive iodine uptake; TSI = thyroid-stimulating immunoglobulins.

hormone associated with destruction of follicular cells should be considered as an etiology of thyrotoxicosis in addition to the underlying disease process.

Treatment

Once overt hypothyroidism is present in the patient with Hashimoto's thyroiditis, treatment with synthetic L-thyroxine (Levoxyl, Synthroid) therapy is indicated. The average replacement dose of thyroxine in adults is approximately 1.6 mcg/kg body weight per day. Adjustment of dosage is undertaken every 6 weeks until a euthyroid status is achieved. The majority of women with postpartum thyroiditis will not need treatment during either the hyperthyroid or hypothyroid phase. If symptomatic hyperthyroidism is present, beta-blocker therapy can be used; antithyroid medications have no utility in the management of postpartum thyroiditis. Women with symptomatic hypothyroidism should be treated with synthetic thyroxine therapy; in asymptomatic women, initiation of thyroxine therapy should be considered if TSH is >10 mU/L. Management of silent thyroiditis is the same as that for postpartum thyroiditis. Symptoms associated with Riedel's thyroiditis may be relieved with prednisone; a small case series associated improvement and even resolution of the process

with tamoxifen (Nolvadex)[1] therapy. Surgery is indicated in Riedel's thyroiditis if compressive symptoms are present. The goal of therapy in subacute thyroiditis is to provide symptom relief. Nonsteroidal antiinflammatory medications are often adequate to control pain; if insufficient, glucocorticoid therapy should be initiated. Beta-blockade therapy can ameliorate symptoms of thyrotoxicosis if indicated. Suppurative thyroiditis is managed with appropriate antibiotics and drainage of any abscess; the disease may prove fatal if diagnosis and treatment are delayed. Pain associated with radiation-induced thyroiditis can be managed with nonsteroidal antiinflammatory therapy or, if ineffective, a short course of glucocorticoid therapy. Radiation-induced thyroiditis is a self-limited process and will resolve spontaneously within days to weeks.

Monitoring

In the patient with Hashimoto's thyroiditis with a euthyroid state, routine TSH testing should be undertaken given the risk of development of overt hypothyroidism at 5% per year. Any woman who has had postpartum thyroiditis should be monitored

[1]Not FDA approved for this indication.

very closely for thyroid dysfunction with future pregnancies, as reoccurrence is likely. For women who have fully recovered from postpartum thyroiditis, yearly TSH measurements should be considered because of underlying chronic autoimmune thyroiditis and risk for overt hypothyroidism. Although overall recurrence rates for silent thyroiditis have not been well established, a similar monitoring plan is warranted for this variant of chronic autoimmune thyroiditis. Subacute thyroiditis recurs in only about 2% of patients. Routine monitoring following resolution of process has not been defined.

References

Bogazzi F, Bartalena L, Martino E: Approach to the patient with amiodarone-induced thyrotoxicosis, *J Clin Endocrinol Metab* 95:2529–2535, 2010.

Cooper DS, Ladenson PW: The thyroid gland. 2011. In Gardner DG, Shoback D, editors: *Greenspan's Basic & Clinical Endocrinology*, 9th ed., New York, 2011, McGraw-Hill. (Available at http://accessmedicine.mhmedical.com/content.aspx?bookid¼380&Sectionid¼39744047 [accessed January 23, 2014].

De Groot L, Abalovich M, Alexander ED, et al: Management of thyroid dysfunction during pregnancy and postpartum: an Endocrine Society clinical practice guideline, *J Clin Endocrinol Metab* 97:2543–2565, 2012.

Pearce EN, Farwell AP, Braverman LE: Thyroiditis, *N Engl J Med* 348:2646–2655, 2003.

Samuels MH: Subacute, silent and postpartum thyroiditis, *Med Clin North Am* 96:223–233, 2012.

Hematology

ACUTE LEUKEMIA IN ADULTS

Method of
William Blum, MD; and Clara Bloomfield, MD

CURRENT DIAGNOSIS

- Diagnosis of acute leukemia is made based on the presence of myeloid (acute myeloid leukemia; AML) or lymphoid (T- or B-cell acute lymphoblastic leukemia; ALL) blasts in blood and/or bone marrow. Acute leukemia may uncommonly have ambiguous lineage or mixed phenotype.
- Medical history-taking should identify risk factors such as prior exposure to chemotherapy for other malignancies, antecedent hematologic disorders, familial hematologic disorders, or other inherited genetic disorders (e.g., Down syndrome, others).
- Clinical examination should identify extramedullary sites of involvement such as meninges/central nervous system (CNS), active infection, hemorrhage, or disseminated intravascular coagulation.
- AML requires the presence of ≥20% blasts in blood or marrow, except in selected subsets of disease with specific cytogenetic aberrations associated with more favorable clinical outcomes, which do not require ≥20% blasts. These favorable subsets are t(8;21)(q22;q22), inv(16)(p13q22) or t(16;16)(p13;q22), or t(15;17)(q22;q12). Testing for additional cytogenetic and molecular aberrations is critical for diagnosis, prognosis, and therapy.
- Acute promyelocytic leukemia (APL) with *PML-RARA* gene fusion, detected by genetic methods or cytogenetics showing t(15;17), is a unique entity requiring different therapy; APL has a favorable prognosis.
- ALL is subcategorized based on B-lymphocyte or T-lymphocyte lineage. For B-ALL (also in mixed phenotype acute leukemia), identification of the Philadelphia chromosome t(9;22)(q34.1;q11.2) or its *BCR-ABL1* gene fusion is essential for proper diagnosis and treatment. As with AML, testing for an established group of other specific chromosomal and molecular aberrations is standard.

CURRENT THERAPY

- AML is typically treated with intensive initial therapy (induction) followed by repetitive cycles of intensive post-remission therapy (consolidation). Induction chemotherapy most commonly consists of anthracycline plus cytarabine (Cytosar). Several acceptable postremission approaches are used; often, these are repetitive high-dose cytarabine based regimens.
- APL is uniquely treated with all-*trans*-retinoic acid (tretinoin [Vesanoid]) and arsenic trioxide (Trisenox), instead of chemotherapy, though cases with high presenting white blood cell count may require chemotherapy for cytoreduction.

- ALL is treated with multidrug regimens for induction and postremission therapies. Postremission therapies include further intensification cycles and prolonged lower-dose maintenance therapy. CNS-directed therapy is a critical component of treatment, even in patients without clear involvement. Most acute leukemias of ambiguous lineage are treated with ALL-type regimens, although clinical outcomes are poor.
- The use of pediatric ALL regimens in adolescents and young adults has improved outcomes.
- Older patients or those with medical infirmities may require less intensive treatment regimens; because of more resistant disease and also higher toxicities, such patients fare worse than younger patients.
- Because of high relapse risks, allogeneic hematopoietic stem cell transplantation (alloHCT) in first remission is an important consideration for all eligible patients with AML, except those with favorable-risk disease. High-risk older patients with ALL are also offered early transplantation. All patients who relapse should be considered for transplantation if remission is again achieved.
- Several subsets of acute leukemia can be treated by new, effective therapies that target specific aberrant signaling or enzymatic activities, or which are directed to unique biologic targets of disease. Most important among these are the use of tyrosine kinase inhibitors in acute leukemia (typically ALL) with *BCR-ABL1*.
- Advances in immunology have rapidly and dramatically improved the options for treatment, especially for those with relapsed B-ALL. Novel antibody constructs and genetically engineered autologous cellular products directed to eliminate B-lymphocytes can induce durable remissions in B-ALL.

Epidemiology

The incidence of AML in the United States is 4.2 per 100,000 per year, with an estimated 21,380 new cases in 2017, according to data from the National Institutes of Health. AML accounts for about 1.3% of all new cancer cases and 31% of all new leukemia cases, according to the American Cancer Society. AML is far more common than ALL in adult patients. Although AML affects all age groups, the incidence increases with advancing age, presenting at a median age of 67 years. ALL has a bimodal distribution across ages, with a peak in early childhood and a second peak around the age of 70 years.

Risk Factors

Most cases of acute leukemia in adults have no established cause. Genetic predisposition, drugs, and radiation have been associated with the development of acute leukemia, particularly AML. Several rare genetic syndromes have increased risk for development of acute leukemia, including Down syndrome, Fanconi anemia, Bloom syndrome, neurofibromatosis type I, and ataxia telangiectasia. AML with germline predisposition represents an uncommon but important subset of disease. Germline mutations associated with increased risk of developing a myeloid neoplasm include *CEBPA, DDX41, RUNX1, ANKRD26, ETV6,* and *GATA2.* Down syndrome-associated AML and ALL have increased risk of toxicity with standard chemotherapy and require dose adjustment (and expert management).

Anticancer drugs are the leading cause of therapy-associated AML. Alkylating agent–associated leukemias typically occur 4 to 6 years after exposure; affected individuals often have multilineage dysplasia and monosomy/aberrations in chromosomes 5 and 7. Topoisomerase II inhibitor-associated leukemias typically occur with shorter latency, 1 to 3 years after exposure; affected individuals often have AML with monocytic features and aberrations involving chromosome 11q23.

Pathophysiology

Acute leukemias are hematologic malignancies arising from hematopoietic progenitor (stem) cells in the bone marrow. Clonal immature cells accumulate in the blood, bone marrow, and occasionally, in the extramedullary tissues. These malignant cells divide and proliferate, but they do not differentiate into functional cells (i.e., neutrophils, lymphocytes, others). Patients with acute leukemia are immunocompromised and have impaired oxygen-carrying capacity (anemia) and bleeding diathesis (because of thrombocytopenia or disrupted coagulation).

Patients experience complications directly from the accumulation of abnormal immature blasts or indirectly from the reduction in functional hematopoietic cells in the marrow and blood. Leukemic involvement of the bone marrow often results in pancytopenia—patients may present with cytopenias in all hematopoietic cell lineages. Patients typically require transfusions of red blood cells and platelets and are at risk of life-threatening infectious complications because of neutropenia. Most patients with acute leukemia die from infection or, less frequently, hemorrhage.

Patients with morphologically similar acute leukemias may experience vastly different clinical outcomes. Increasingly, this is understood by karyotyping or genetic sequencing studies that demonstrate marked heterogeneity in the cytogenetic and mutational profiles among patients with acute leukemia. It is clear that morphology and cytochemical staining alone to establish diagnosis does little to explain the pathophysiology of these varied hematologic cancers. Genetic sequencing studies demonstrate common dysregulation of several critical cellular pathways but also a myriad of genetic differences that occur only in small (or very small/unique) subsets. In adults, most cases of AML ultimately arise in the backdrop of a limited number of mutations that accumulate with advancing age. As noted earlier, cases with a clear cause, such as germline predisposition or drug exposure, are rare. The Cancer Genome Atlas (cancergenome.nih.gov) and other databases have shown that up to 5% to 6% of healthy individuals over 70 years of age have blood cells with potentially "premalignant" mutations that are associated with clonal expansion. There appear to be a variety of "final insults" that transform these expanded clones to AML. However, how all these genetic aberrations contribute to leukemic transformation remains incompletely understood. Although the number of mutations/cell in AML is relatively few (median of 13 mutations) compared with other cancers (e.g., melanoma and non-small cell lung cancer may have several hundred mutations/cell), great heterogeneity exists in the mutations identified between individual patients with AML. The same can be said of ALL. Indeed, dramatic differences in mutations/genetic signatures have been observed between patients with childhood, adolescent, young adult, and older adult ALL, respectively.

Great heterogeneity exists not just between patients with different types of acute leukemia but within each individual patient. Each patient has several leukemic clones and subclones that have slightly different mutational profiles. The presence of genetically different clones and subclones helps explain why a patient may achieve remission but then experience relapse with more resistant disease, since sensitive clones are eliminated by chemotherapy, whereas surviving clones are more resistant to subsequent treatment. Furthermore, clones that persist after treatment may emerge with additional novel mutations.

Clinical Manifestations

Patients with any type of acute leukemia present with similar symptoms. Most have vague symptoms that are consequences of pancytopenia. Typically, the onset of illness is no more than 3 months before diagnosis, unless the leukemia is associated with an antecedent hematologic disorder. Fatigue is common as are anorexia and weight loss. Fever or infection is also common but not universal at presentation. Patients may have evidence of abnormal hemostasis (bleeding, easy bruising). Bone pain, lymphadenopathy, nonspecific cough, headache, and diaphoresis (excessive sweating) may also occur. Bone pain, typically vaguely localized to the pelvis or back, is frequent. Patients with ALL (as compared with AML) are more likely to have lymphadenopathy, splenomegaly, or other sites of extramedullary involvement, such as the testicles or CNS. However, involvement at any of these sites is not exclusive to ALL; their presence is not diagnostic of that type. Rarely, patients present with primary symptoms caused by extramedullary leukemia. Extramedullary disease in AML is known as a myeloid sarcoma (also called a *granulocytic sarcoma* or *chloroma*). This is a tumor mass consisting of myeloid blasts and is most commonly seen in the skin, lymph node, gastrointestinal tract, soft tissue, or testis. Patients who present with isolated myeloid sarcoma typically develop blood or marrow involvement quickly thereafter; such patients thus require systemic (not solely surgical or local radiation) treatment. CNS involvement at initial presentation (headache, cranial nerve palsies) is uncommon. Patients with ALL, however, have increased risk of CNS disease and should thus be given intrathecal chemotherapy as prophylaxis, even without such symptoms (or detectable CNS involvement).

Severe hemorrhagic complications are relatively infrequent at presentation but are most commonly encountered in APL. Recognition of this risk at the time of initial presentation is critical, as replacement of fibrinogen or plasma may be lifesaving. Patients with APL often present with disseminated intravascular coagulation (DIC)-associated hemorrhage and may have intracranial hemorrhage or bleeding at other sites. Thrombosis is a less frequent but well-recognized feature of APL. Bleeding associated with coagulopathy may also occur in monocytic AML and with extreme degrees of leukocytosis or thrombocytopenia in other acute leukemias. Retinal hemorrhage caused by thrombocytopenia and extreme leukocytosis is detected in approximately 15% of patients.

Laboratory parameters are quite variable with any type of acute leukemia. Although many patients present with leukocytosis and high levels of circulating blasts, it is important to note that presenting with low white blood cell (WBC) counts or even no circulating blasts is not rare. Typically, though, review of the peripheral blood smear identifies the classic blast—fine, lacy chromatin, with one or more nucleoli, and a high nucleus-to-cytoplasm ratio that is characteristic of immature cells. The presence in blasts of abnormal rod-shaped granules called *Auer rods* on light microscopy indicates a diagnosis of AML.

Anemia is observed at diagnosis in nearly all patients but is not severe. Decreased erythropoiesis often results in a reduced reticulocyte (immature red blood cell) count, and red blood cell survival may be shortened through accelerated destruction. Most patients also present with at least mild thrombocytopenia (below the normal lower limit value of 150,000/μL).

Diagnosis

When acute leukemia is clinically suspected, in addition to morphologic and flow cytometric analyses, cytogenetic and genetic tests are mandatory to aid rapid diagnosis, assess prognosis, and inform the best approach to treatment. That said, clinical features also remain important. These include a history of antecedent hematologic disorder or prior chemotherapy, advanced age, and a strong family history of acute leukemia or related hematologic disorder (all favoring AML); all of these have an adverse prognosis. In ALL, high WBC at presentation (>100,000/μL for B-ALL and >30,000/μL for T-ALL) and T-cell phenotype have an adverse prognosis.

Initial assessments should evaluate cardiovascular, pulmonary, hepatic, and renal systems; patients should also be evaluated and

TABLE 1	2017 European LeukemiaNet Risk Stratification by Genetics for Acute Myeloid Leukemia*

RISK CATEGORY†	GENETIC ABNORMALITY
Favorable	$t(8;21)(q22;q22)$; *RUNX1-RUNX1T1* inv(16)(p13.1q22) or $t(16;16)(p13.1;q22)$; *CBFB-MYH11* Mutated *NPM1* without *FLT3*-ITD or with *FLT3*-ITD^low‡ Biallelic mutated *CEBPA*
Intermediate	Mutated *NPM1* and *FLT3*-ITD^high‡ Wild type *NPM1* without *FLT3*-ITD or with *FLT3*-ITD^low‡ (w/o adverse-risk genetic lesions) $t(9;11)(p21.3;q23.3)$; *MLLT3-KMT2A*§ Cytogenetic abnormalities not classified as favorable or adverse
Adverse	$t(6;9)(p23;q34.1)$; *DEK-NUP214* $t(v;11q23.3)$; *KMT2A* rearranged $t(9;22)(q34.1;q11.2)$; *BCR-ABL1* inv(3)(q21.3q26.2) or $t(3;3)(q21.3;q26.2)$; *GATA2,MECOM(EVI1)* -5 or del(5q); -7; -17/abn(17p) Complex karyotype,¶¶ monosomal karyotype¶ Wild type *NPM1* and *FLT3*-ITD^high‡ Mutated *RUNX1*** Mutated *ASXL1*** Mutated *TP53*††

*This table excludes acute promyelocytic leukemia. Frequencies, response rates, and outcome measures should be reported by risk category and, if sufficient numbers are available, by specific genetic lesions indicated.

†Prognostic impact of a marker is treatment-dependent and may change with new therapies.

‡Low, low allelic ratio (<0.5); high, high allelic ratio (>0.5); semi-quantitative assessment of *FLT3*-ITD allelic ratio (using DNA fragment analysis) is determined as ratio of the area under the curve (AUC) "*FLT3*-ITD" divided by AUC "*FLT3*-wild type"; recent studies indicate that acute myeloid leukemia with *NPM1* mutation and *FLT3*-ITD low allelic ratio may also have a more favorable prognosis and patients should not routinely be assigned to allogeneic hematopoietic-cell transplantation.

§The presence of $t(9;11)(p21.3;q23.3)$ takes precedence over rare, concurrent adverse-risk gene mutations.

¶¶Three or more unrelated chromosome abnormalities in the absence of one of the World Health Organization–designated recurring translocations or inversions, i.e., $t(8;21)$, inv(16) or $t(16;16)$, $t(9;11)$, $t(v;11)(v;q23.3)$, $t(6;9)$, inv(3) or $t(3;3)$; AML with *BCR-ABL1*.

¶Defined by the presence of one single monosomy (excluding loss of X or Y) in association with at least one additional monosomy or structural chromosome abnormality (excluding core-binding factor AML).

**These markers should not be used as an adverse prognostic marker if they co-occur with favorable-risk AML subtypes.

††*TP53* mutations are significantly associated with AML with complex and monosomal karyotype.

Adapted from Döhner H, Estey E, Grimwade D et al. Diagnosis and management of AML in adults: 2017 ELN recommendations from an international expert panel. *Blood* 2017;129:424–447.

treated for infection or DIC. Preparation for transfusion of blood or platelets requires blood type and crossmatch to be determined, and human leukocyte antigen (HLA) testing is required early in the treatment course (before chemotherapy) in consideration of future alloHCT. Cytogenetic analysis typically requires bone marrow. Genetic testing (from blood or marrow) continues to evolve and is critical for successful diagnosis, prognosis, and therapy.

The diagnosis of AML is based on a finding of at least 20% myeloid blasts by histology, cytochemistry, or flow cytometry. However, this 20% threshold is not required for the diagnosis if any of the following recurrent cytogenetic abnormalities is present: $t(15;17)$, $t(8;21)$, inv(16), or $t(16;16)$. Myeloid blasts stain positive for myeloperoxidase; by flow cytometry, myeloid blasts are typically positive for CD13 and CD33. A prognostic schema developed by the European LeukemiaNet assigns prognostic risk based on cytogenetic and genetic features of disease (Table 1). Some morphologic features associate with specific cytogenetic or molecular findings such as $t(15;17)$ and APL, or dysplastic eosinophils and inv(16) or $t(16;16)$. The expression of B-cell markers (CD19, PAX5, cytoplasmic CD79a) is not infrequent in $t(8;21)$.

The diagnosis of ALL likewise requires at least 20% lymphoid blasts. By immunohistochemical methods, lymphoid blasts stain positive for terminal deoxynucleotidyl transferase (TdT); by flow, lymphoid blasts are typically positive for CD10, CD19, CD22, CD20 (variable), for B-ALL and CD3, CD7, CD4, and CD8 for T-ALL.

Patients may uncommonly present with acute leukemia of ambiguous lineage (undifferentiated or mixed phenotype). However, more common are AML cases that express an aberrant B- or T-cell marker (e.g., CD7 on myeloid blasts); this is called an aberrant immunophenotype. Likewise, B-ALL may aberrantly express CD13 or CD33.

Molecular testing is an important component of diagnosis. For AML, molecular testing should include assessment of *FLT3* (with allelic ratio), *NPM1*, *CEBPA* (bi-allelic), *IDH1*, *IDH2*, *RUNX1*, *ASXL1*, and *TP53*. For ALL, testing is equally complex but is still evolving in terms of commercial availability for important molecular analyses. Critical to the initial assessment of ALL is testing for the *BCR-ABL1* fusion by molecular methods that are widely available; tyrosine kinase inhibitors (TKIs) targeting this lesion are now an important part of treatment. Likewise, testing by interphase fluorescence in situ hybridization for the major recurrent cytogenetic abnormalities seen in ALL, including *ETV6-RUNX1*, *TCF3-PBX1*, and *KMT2A* rearrangements, among others, is mandatory. Although not yet widely available, testing in B-ALL for the "*BCR-ABL1*-like" genetic signature identifies a subset of patients with adverse prognosis but potential responsiveness to TKI therapies. *BCR-ABL1*-like disease as a subset has several common genetic features including disruption of B-lymphoid transcription factors including *IKZF1*, *CRLF2*, *JAK2*, and others. Diagnostic testing guidelines for both AML and ALL are delineated and annually updated by the National Comprehensive Cancer Network (NCCN.org).

Cytogenetic analysis should be performed on the bone marrow aspirate taken at diagnosis in any patient suspected to have acute leukemia. Prognosis is determined on the presence of structural or numeric chromosomal abnormalities and is then more fully informed by additional genetic testing. Broadly speaking, patients with AML with $t(15;17)$, known as APL, as described earlier, have an excellent prognosis, with 80% to 90% cured. Patients with $t(8;21)$ or inv(16) also have a favorable prognosis. Patients with no cytogenetic abnormalities (cytogenetically normal AML; CN-AML) have an intermediate prognosis. Patients with a complex karyotype, $t(6;9)$, inv(3) or –7 (absence of chromosome 7), respectively, have an adverse prognosis with few cures, particularly in older patients. Genetic testing provides valuable additional information, especially in CN-AML. Favorable-genetic risk is observed in those with *NPM1* mutations without a high allelic ratio of *FLT3* internal tandem duplications (*FLT3*-ITD) and also in those with bi-allelic *CEBPA* mutations. Conversely, *TP53* mutations (often, but not exclusively, observed in the setting of complex karyotype) are associated with adverse risk. *IDH2* and *IDH1* mutations may contribute to prognostication but, more importantly, identify patients who are likely to respond to novel therapies that target these aberrant pathways.

Cytogenetic testing for ALL allows classification into several groups, including, for example, *BCR-ABL1* fusion disease. This fusion, known cytogenetically as $t(9;22)$ and colloquially referred to as the Philadelphia (Ph) chromosome (based on the city where it was originally identified) has a poor prognosis. However, the incorporation into multiagent regimens of TKIs that target the aberrantly active kinase has improved clinical outcomes. Other important ALL subsets include *KMT2A* rearrangements at chromosome 11q23 (with various translocation partners but often chromosome 4 in B-ALL). Both *BCR-ABL1* and *KMT2A* aberrant ALL are associated with unfavorable prognosis. Many other subsets of ALL exist in the World Health Organization (WHO) classification. Favorable-risk is seen in patients with B-ALL with

$t(12;21)(p13.2;q22.1)$; the *ETV6-RUNX1* fusion. T-ALL is characterized by activation mutations in *NOTCH1* (present in about 60% of cases) and deregulation of a number of transcription factors; immunophenotyping showing an early T-cell precursor (ETP) phenotype (low expression of CD1a, CD8, CD5) has been associated with adverse prognosis.

Historically, the diagnosis and classification of acute leukemia was based on the French-American-British morphologic and cytochemical criteria, which assigned patients with AML to 1 of 8 groups, designated M0–M7. Likewise, ALL was classified into L1, L2, and L3 groups. These categories, while still in the vernacular on the clinical wards, are practically obsolete. Diagnosis and classification is based instead on the complex morphologic, flow, cytogenetic, and molecular characterization schemas outlined by the WHO for myeloid neoplasms and acute leukemia.

Differential Diagnosis

The differential diagnosis for acute leukemia includes many bone marrow disorders that present with pancytopenia. However, the presence of excess blasts in the blood or marrow limits the diagnosis to AML, ALL, or acute leukemia of ambiguous lineage. For patients without circulating blasts in the blood, highest in the differential diagnosis of pancytopenia are other hematologic cancers with marrow infiltration or bone marrow failure syndromes such as aplastic anemia. Advanced myeloproliferative disorders with bone marrow fibrosis can also present similarly, occasionally with rare circulating blasts. Rarely, the pancytopenia caused by the displacement of hemopoietic bone marrow tissue by fibrosis, tumor, or granuloma (called myelophthisis) mimics acute leukemia (but without blasts). Examples include solid organ cancers with extensive marrow involvement and granulomatous disease such as tuberculosis. However, essentially only acute leukemia is the appropriate diagnosis in patients with high-level circulating blasts visualized on light microscopy.

Treatment of Acute Myeloid Leukemia

Treatment of the newly diagnosed adult patient with AML is usually divided into two phases: (1) induction and (2) consolidation (i.e., postremission management). The aim of induction chemotherapy is complete remission (CR), defined as fewer than 5% blasts on a bone marrow aspirate, with recovery of blood counts (absolute neutrophil count >1000/µL AND platelet count >100,000/µL). At CR, additional defining criteria include absent circulating blasts and no detectable extramedullary disease. Achievement of CR (or failure to do so) is the best predictor for long-term clinical outcome. The definition of CR is further refined based on the detection of measurable residual disease (MRD) by cytogenetic or molecular testing. Marrow response *without* full blood count recovery meets lesser response definitions, but not CR; patients with such responses have outcomes inferior to those with CR. Blood count recovery occurs approximately 4 weeks after initiating intensive induction chemotherapy. CR is achieved in 60% to 90% of younger patients (depending on molecular risk), and in approximately 40% to 60% of older patients (>60 years). Notably, for older patients, this estimate is from the subset limited to those who are actually offered intensive therapy; many older patients are not treated intensively (or at all) due to medical comorbidites. Such patients would likely fare even worse than the estimates provided if offered intensive treatment. Long-term survival estimates are approximately 60% for younger patients with favorable-risk disease (see Table 1), 40% for intermediate-risk disease, and 20% for adverse-risk disease. Older patients do poorly in each group; indeed, for older patients with adverse-risk disease, there are very few long-term survivors.

Induction and consolidation therapies are chosen based on the patient's age, overall fitness, and cytogenetic/molecular risk. Intensive induction therapy is the norm in younger patients (<60 years). In older patients, the benefit of intensive therapy is more controversial in all but favorable-risk patients; novel approaches for selecting patients predicted to be responsive to treatment and new therapies remain under investigation. Notably, large datasets have demonstrated that even more infirm older patients with AML benefit from treatment, as compared with only palliative care.

Standard induction therapy for AML consists of cytarabine (cytosine arabinoside, AraC; Cytosar), 100 to 200 mg/m² per day administered as a continuous infusion for 7 days, and daunorubicin (Cerubidine), 60 to 90 mg/m² per day for 3 days, commonly known as the 7 + 3 schedule. Idarubicin (Idamycin; 12 mg/m²/day) is equivalent to daunorubicin. Resistant disease is more frequent in older patients and those with prior hematologic disorders, therapy-related AML, or cytogenetic and genetic abnormalities that adversely impact clinical outcome (which are more frequent in older patients). In older patients, the long-term outcome is generally poor due to a higher frequency of resistant disease plus an increased rate of treatment-related mortality. As an alternative to intensive induction, unfit or adverse-risk older patients may instead receive lower-intensity therapy with a hypomethylating agent (such as decitabine [Dacogen][1] or azacytidine [Vidaza][1]). For patients older than 75 years or those who are not candidates for intensive therapy, FDA recently approved venetoclax (Venclexta) in combination with hypomethylating agent therapy. Emerging data show that the combination of a hypomethylating agent with the BCL-2 antagonist venetoclax significantly improves response rates compared to a hypomethylating agent alone; survival results are also impressive but need confirmation and longer follow up. All older patients should be considered for clinical trials, but older patients in adverse-risk groups should ideally be offered investigational approaches whenever available.

Induction of first CR (CR1) is critical to long-term survival in AML. However, without further therapy, virtually all patients in CR will eventually relapse. Patients are estimated to have 10^{12} leukemic cells at diagnosis, which intensive induction chemotherapy reduces by 4 to 5 orders of magnitude. Although this reduces the disease burden by 99.9%, approximately 10^8 residual leukemic cells still remain after successful induction therapy. These residual cells may not be measured at all or may only be measured by sensitive techniques such as multiparameter flow cytometry or quantitative reverse transcriptase polymerase chain reaction (RT-PCR). They cannot be detected by morphology alone. Thus, postremission therapy is designed to eradicate residual (typically undetectable) leukemic cells to prevent relapse and prolong survival. As for induction, the type of postremission therapy in AML is selected for each individual patient based on age, fitness, and cytogenetic/molecular risk.

Postremission treatment options include chemotherapy or transplantation. The choice between consolidation with chemotherapy or transplantation is complex and based on age, risk, and practical considerations. In younger patients receiving chemotherapy, postremission therapy with intermediate/high-dose cytarabine for 2 to 4 cycles is standard practice. It is clear that alloHCT is the best relapse prevention strategy currently available for AML. However, the benefit of alloHCT in relapse risk reduction is offset somewhat by increased morbidity and mortality from complications including graft-versus-host disease. Given that relapsed AML is typically resistant to chemotherapy, alloHCT in CR1 is a favored strategy for patients at high risk for relapse. Transplantation is generally recommended for physically fit patients age <75 years who do not have favorable-risk disease and who have a suitable donor. Donors are typically HLA-matched (related or unrelated) or, increasingly, haploidentical (half-matched sibling, parent, or child). Prognostic factors help select the appropriate postremission therapy in patients in CR1. Generally speaking, patients with favorable-risk AML in CR1 are treated with chemotherapy alone; patients with adverse-risk disease should proceed to alloHCT at CR1 if possible. The decision for alloHCT versus chemotherapy in CR1 for intermediate-risk patients remains in debate.

---

[1]Not FDA approved for this indication.

APL is uniquely treated with all-*trans*-retinoic acid (tretinoin [Vesanoid]) and arsenic trioxide (Trisenox), instead of chemotherapy, although cases with high presenting WBC count (>10,000/μL) may require chemotherapy for cytoreduction. Cases with high WBC count are at increased risk for fatal hemorrhage and other complications. Low-risk patients (WBC <10,000/μL) have virtually nonexistent frequency of resistant disease. Patients with APL require expert management to address complications of DIC and hemorrhage and the so-called APL syndrome (formerly differentiation syndrome, retinoic acid syndrome). APL syndrome is marked by rising WBC count, fever, hypoxia, shortness of breath, and fluid accumulation, occurring 1 to 18 days after treatment initiation. It is common, especially in higher WBC presentations, and requires urgent therapy consisting of steroids, diuresis, and possibly cytoreduction.

Treatment of Acute Lymphoblastic Leukemia

Standard chemotherapy treatment of ALL is of much more extended duration and regimen complexity than that of AML. However, the same general principles apply—achievement of CR1 with initial therapy is the critical first step for long-term survival. Postremission therapy in ALL is broken into different segments of various intensity, including interim maintenance, delayed intensification, and prolonged (24 months) maintenance. CNS-directed therapy (systemic chemotherapy with intrathecal chemotherapy, or cranial radiotherapy) is an important mandatory feature of ALL treatment. Generally, treatment approaches include variations on a five-drug induction combination of cyclophosphamide (Cytoxan), prednisone[1] or dexamethasone[1] (Decadron), anthracycline (doxorubicin [Adriamycin]; or daunorubicin [Cerubidine]), PEGylated asparaginase (Oncaspar), and vincristine (Oncovin). The principle of therapy is continuous exposure to multiple chemotherapy agents with non-overlapping resistance mechanisms; all ALL regimens use alternating chemotherapy regimens given over extended time. Additional agents include methotrexate, cytarabine, 6-mercaptopurine (Purinethol), and others. Examples of treatment strategies are the BFM (Berlin-Frankfurt-Munster) approach and the hyper-CVAD regimen.

Unfortunately, although children with B-ALL have favorable long-term survival in the 80% to 90% range, adults fare far worse. Estimated long-term survival rates for adults with ALL are only 30% to 40%. Encouraging data have come from recent cooperative group studies: adolescents and young adults (age 16 to 40 years) treated with "pediatric-inspired" regimens have outcomes far better than those treated with "adult" regimens. Pediatric regimens have a greater focus on less myelotoxic therapies such as PEGylated asparaginase, vincristine, and steroids. Unfortunately, older adults (>40 years) have difficulty tolerating such approaches.

As noted previously, the identification of the Ph chromosome *t*(9;22) or the *BCR-ABL1* fusion is a very important part of the initial diagnosis of B-ALL or mixed-phenotype acute leukemia. The introduction of TKI for Ph + patients into multiagent induction and postremission treatment has dramatically improved outcomes and is now standard. Whether Ph + B-ALL should have mandatory alloHCT in CR1 is now controversial. Imatinib (Gleevec) is a standard TKI; second- or third-generation TKI such as dasatinib (Sprycel), nilotinib (Tasigna)[1], or ponatinib (Iclusig) are also commonly used for Ph + acute leukemia.

Additional advances to traditional approaches over the last 5 years include the use of CD20 monoclonal antibodies (rituximab [Rituxan]) for patients with B-ALL whose lymphoid blasts express this surface marker, and nelarabine (Arranon) in T-ALL. Nelarabine is a purine analogue with increased activity in T-lymphoid blasts and 30% response rates in the relapsed setting; it is being incorporated into front-line multiagent trials. AlloHCT in adult ALL is more controversial than in AML, although most offer alloHCT in CR1 for high-risk disease.

Figure 1 Chimeric antigen receptor (CAR) T cells. (Reprinted with permission from Lim WA, June CH. The principles of engineering immune cells to treat cancer. *Cell* 2017;168:724–740.)

Immune-Based Therapies in Acute Leukemia

Beyond the use of alloHCT, recent years have seen remarkable progress in immunologic therapies for acute leukemia. The US Food and Drug Administration recently approved exciting engineered cellular therapies for relapsed malignancies of B-lymphocytes: chimeric antigen receptor (CAR) T-cells that target CD19 (in B-ALL and non-Hodgkin's lymphoma). In these cases, autologous B-cells are collected by apheresis from the patient, genetically engineered ex vivo to target CD19, then infused back into the patient to treat CD19 + malignancy (typically after some type of lymphodepleting therapy). In the process, CD19 + normal B-cells are also eliminated. High response rates and long-term remissions have been reported in patients with ALL with highly refractory disease using CAR T-cell therapy; complete response rates in the range of 70% to 90% have been observed in CD19 + cancers: ALL, chronic lymphocytic leukemia, and diffuse large B-cell lymphoma (Figure 1). Challenges of CAR T-cells include issues with uncontrolled immune cell activation, killing of normal CD19 + B-cells, and resistance due to loss of CD19 expression on leukemic cells. Whether CAR retargeting can be successfully applied to other hematologic targets beyond CD19 remains to be seen.

Several novel antibodies have also recently been approved. Inotuzumab ozogamicin (Besponsa; targeting CD22 in B-ALL) and gemtuzumab ozogamicin (Mylotarg; targeting CD33 in AML) are antibody–drug conjugates that deliver the toxin calicheamicin to lymphoid or myeloid blasts, respectively. Blinatumomab (Blincyto) is a CD3-CD19 bi-specific antibody.

Monitoring

Measurement of residual disease is an important component of management in acute leukemia. It is not surprising that initial responsiveness to chemotherapy is a useful predictor for long-term outcome. Lack of early clearance of blasts (by day 7 to 14) has adverse prognostic value (especially in ALL). Persistence of abnormal karyotype after induction among patients in CR is also associated with poor clinical outcomes. For patients in morphologic CR, measurement of MRD is an emerging standard (ALL) and research (AML) area. More sensitive methods of MRD measurement beyond light microscopy and cytogenetics are increasingly used to aid decisionmaking. Examples of sensitive MRD assessment include immunophenotyping to detect minute populations of blasts or quantitative RT-PCR to detect leukemia-associated molecular abnormalities. Particularly in

---

[1] Not FDA approved for this indication.

B-ALL, early clearance of MRD is favorable. In ALL and in APL, MRD assessment is a very useful and reliable tool to assess prognosis, detect early relapse, and direct the initiation of additional therapy.

Management of Complications

The treatment of acute leukemia involves repeated cycles of myelotoxic or immunosuppressive chemotherapy, requiring intensive supportive care. The emergence of multidrug-resistant organisms is a growing concern. In addition, invasive fungal infections are associated with early death. Standard infection precautions include reverse isolation, air filtration, and prophylactic antimicrobials. Recommendations on the latter are best tailored based on institutional antibiograms.

Transfusion of red blood cells and platelets is a common and necessary part of treatment. Blood products should ideally be leukodepleted (done by the American Red Cross in the United States) to reduce the risk of febrile transfusion reaction and alloimmunization. Particularly in ALL, it is clear that the management of complications, yet still proceeding with the on-time administration of subsequent therapy, improves outcomes.

References

Arber DA, Orazi A, Hasserjian R, et al: The 2016 revision to the World Health Organization classification of myeloid neoplasms and acute leukemia, *Blood* 127:2391–2405, 2016.

Brown AL, Churpek JE, Malcovati L, et al: Recognition of familial myeloid neoplasia in adults, *Semin Hematol* 54:60–68, 2017.

Ding L, Ley TJ, Larson DE, et al: Clonal evolution in relapsed acute myeloid leukemia revealed by whole-genome sequencing, *Nature* 481:506–510, 2012.

Döhner H, Estey E, Grimwade D, et al: Diagnosis and management of AML in adults: 2017 ELN recommendations from an international expert panel, *Blood* 129:424–447, 2017.

Iacobucci I, Mullighan CG: Genetic basis of acute lymphoblastic leukemia, *J Clin Oncol* 35:975–983, 2017.

Lim WA, June CH: The principles of engineering immune cells to treat cancer, *Cell* 168:724–740, 2017.

Maude SL, Frey N, Shaw PA, et al: Chimeric antigen receptor T cells for sustained remissions in leukemia, *N Engl J Med* 371:1507–1517, 2014.

National Comprehensive Cancer Network (NCCN): Clinical practices guidelines in oncology, Available at NCCN.org [Accessed February 2018].

Papaemmanuil E, Gerstung M, Bullinger L, et al: Genomic classification and prognosis in acute myeloid leukemia, *N Engl J Med* 374:2209–2221, 2016.

TCGA Research Network, Ley TJ, Miller C, et al: Genomic and epigenomic landscapes of adult de novo acute myeloid leukemia, *N Engl J Med* 368:2059–2074, 2013.

Welch JS, Ley TJ, Link DC, et al: The origin and evolution of mutations in acute myeloid leukemia, *Cell* 150:264–278, 2012.

BLOOD COMPONENT THERAPY AND TRANSFUSION REACTIONS

Method of
Theresa Nester, MD

CURRENT DIAGNOSIS

- Fever greater than 1°C rise during or within 4 hours after transfusion should prompt evaluation of the patient and consideration of a transfusion reaction.
- Fever and pain are the most common manifestations of an acute hemolytic transfusion reaction.
- The point of the transfusion reaction laboratory investigation is to evaluate for hemolysis, either intravascular or extravascular. The majority of reactions are negative for hemolysis.
- The differential diagnosis of a transfusion reaction with respiratory symptoms includes febrile nonhemolytic and circulatory overload (common), allergic or anaphylactic reaction, transfusion-related acute lung injury, acute hemolytic reaction, and bacterial contamination (rare).

CURRENT THERAPY

- The decision to transfuse red blood cells to a patient should depend more on the clinical state of the patient than on an absolute trigger for hemoglobin or hematocrit.
- A transfusion trigger of less than 7 g/dL is recommended for hospitalized adult patients who are hemodynamically stable, including critically ill patients. A transfusion trigger of 8 g/dL is recommended for patients undergoing orthopedic or cardiac surgery, as well as those with preexisting cardiovascular disease.
- For severe autoimmune hemolytic anemia, maintenance of hemoglobin at greater than 4 g/dL in younger patients and greater than 6 g/dL in older patients or patients with cardiovascular disease is appropriate.
- Platelets are not typically indicated in thrombotic thrombocytopenic purpura, autoimmune thrombocytopenic purpura (ITP), and heparin-induced thrombocytopenia (HIT) unless the patient has significant bleeding.
- Currently available coagulation tests are not very useful for predicting bleeding in patients with end-stage liver disease. These patients establish a new equilibrium between coagulation, anticoagulation, and fibrinolysis that results in relatively less bleeding than predicted by the international normalized ratio.
- The goal during massive transfusion scenarios should be to prevent marked acidosis, hypothermia, and coagulopathy. The latter is often achieved with replacement of coagulation factors using plasma or cryoprecipitate within the first hour of the resuscitation.
- Cryoprecipitate is useful as a source of concentrated fibrinogen. In a patient who is actively bleeding and has a fibrinogen less than 100 mg/dL, cryoprecipitate is indicated.
- Fibrinogen concentrates are available for select patient populations.

Therapeutic Use of Blood Components

The community blood supply depends on two types of donors: whole blood donors and apheresis donors. Units of whole blood are centrifuged and then separated into components within a closed system. Using apheresis techniques, individual components of whole blood can be collected. Citrate is used to keep blood components from clotting.

The decision to transfuse blood to a patient should always include a consideration of the risks versus the benefits. Risks of transfusion-transmitted diseases are small with current testing standards. Transfusion reactions do occur; the most common ones are not life-threatening unless the patient cannot tolerate tachycardia or hypertension. Rarely, a patient experiences a life-threatening reaction. Thus it is important to ensure that the need for the blood component outweighs the risks. Additionally, in a bleeding patient, it is important to check coagulation parameters (platelet count, prothrombin time [PT], international normalized ratio [INR], activated partial thromboplastin time [aPTT], fibrinogen) in addition to hematocrit (Hct) to ensure that the component that will best address the bleeding is being used.

Red Blood Cells
Indications

Red blood cells should be given to increase oxygen-carrying capacity. The hemoglobin (Hb) and Hct levels alone should not be used to determine the need for transfusion; instead, the patient's clinical picture should drive the decision to transfuse. The patient's intravascular volume status, cardiopulmonary function, and baseline vital signs in the presence of anemia should all be considered. When anemia has persisted over weeks and months, large volume transfusion is often not indicated because compensatory mechanisms have had time to work.

Transfusion Triggers

The most recent clinical practice guideline from AABB (formerly known as the American Association of Blood Banks) has the following recommendations: in hospitalized adult patients who are hemodynamically stable, including critically ill patients, a transfusion threshold of 7 g/dL is acceptable. In patients undergoing orthopedic or cardiac surgery, and those with preexisting cardiovascular disease, a transfusion threshold of 8 g/dL is recommended. The recommendations do not apply to patients with acute coronary syndrome, severe thrombocytopenia, or chronic transfusion dependent anemia, because of insufficient evidence.

Dosage

One unit of packed red blood cells will increase the hemoglobin by 1 g/dL and hematocrit by 3% in the patient who is not bleeding or experiencing hemolysis (Table 1).

Autoimmune Hemolytic Anemia
Special Situation

When the autoantibody responsible for autoimmune hemolytic anemia reacts at body temperature, all red blood cell units can appear incompatible. This is because the antibody binds to an epitope common to all red blood cells, such as the band 3 protein. The clinician needs to decide when to transfuse the (apparently) incompatible units. In a patient who has never received a transfusion or been pregnant, there is little possibility of red blood cell alloantibodies in circulation, and the chance of hemolysis (beyond that being caused by the autoantibody) is low. For the patient who has received a transfusion or who has been pregnant in the past, the risk that a circulating red blood cell alloantibody is present and is being masked by the autoantibody is higher; special studies are available to reduce the risk of an alloantibody being overlooked. The transfusion trigger depends on whether the anemia is acute or chronic. For acute severe anemia, maintenance of hemoglobin at greater than 4 g/dL in younger patients and greater than 6 g/dL in older patients or patients with cardiovascular disease is appropriate.

Platelets

Platelets are required as part of normal clotting. The first stage of clot formation is development of a platelet plug over the site of endothelial injury.

Indications

The indications for platelet transfusion may be divided into prevention of bleeding and treatment of bleeding in the setting of thrombocytopenia or platelet dysfunction.

Transfusion Triggers

Prevention of Bleeding. In a stable patient with normal platelet function, transfusion is appropriate if the platelet count is less than 10,000/μL. One randomized, controlled trial has shown that transfusion at platelet counts of 5000/μL to 10,000/μL prevents bleeding in the stable patient. In a stable patient with other hemostatic abnormalities (e.g., on anticoagulation), transfusion is appropriate with a platelet count less than 50,000/μL.

Before a planned invasive procedure such as open lung biopsy, transfusion is appropriate with a platelet count of <50,000/μL. For lumbar puncture, consensus guidelines suggest that a platelet count of 50,000/μL is appropriate, although there are a few large studies suggesting that counts between 20,000 and 50,000/μL may be adequate. A patient undergoing major surgery should receive platelets if the count is less than 50,000 to 100,000/μL. The transfusion should take place as close to the procedure as possible so the platelets remain in circulation while the procedure is occurring.

Treatment of Bleeding. Platelets may be transfused with a major hemorrhage (e.g., gastrointestinal or genitourinary) and a platelet count less than 30,000 to 50,000/μL. For bleeding with major surgery or trauma, transfusion is appropriate for counts less than 80,000/μL. For bleeding into critical areas (e.g., central nervous system bleeding or diffuse alveolar hemorrhage), platelets may be given for counts less than 100,000/μL.

Dosage

Dosage is determined on the basis of the baseline platelet count, desired platelet count, and estimated blood volume. For a 70-kg patient, 3×10^{11} platelets (four to six units of pooled whole blood platelets or one unit of apheresis platelets) increases platelet count by approximately 30,000 to 50,000/μL in the absence of alloimmunization or excessive consumption. For prophylactic therapy, lower dosages have been shown to be as effective as higher dosages in the prevention of bleeding.

Out of ABO Group Platelet Transfusion

Because platelets can only be stored for a maximum of 7 days following collection, and the community platelet supply is collected from volunteer donors, a platelet product that is identical to the patient's ABO type might not be available (Table 2 and Box 1). Thus it may be necessary to infuse a small volume of incompatible plasma (suspending the platelets) to the patient. There is therefore a small risk of hemolysis of the patient's red blood cells if the iso-agglutinin (anti-A or anti-B) titer in the donated plasma is high. Studies of healthy blood donors indicate that these antibody titers are typically low and do not precipitate hemolysis. Transfusion services often have policies that limit the amount of incompatible plasma a patient has received with platelet transfusion. Alternatively, some centers measure the antibody titer in the donated product and give high-titer products only to patients whose red blood cells lack the corresponding ABO antigen.

TABLE 1	Component Therapy: Dosage and Expected Increment		
COMPONENT	**DOSE**	**EXPECTED INCREMENT**	**AVERAGE VOLUME**
Red blood cells	1 unit	Hct 3%, Hb 1 g/dL	250 mL
Whole blood platelets	1 unit	Platelet count increased by 5000–10,000/μL	50 mL/unit (1 pool of 6 = 300 mL)
Apheresis platelet	1 unit	Platelet count increased by 20,000–60,000/μL	300 mL/unit
Plasma	10 mL/kg	Factor levels increased by 20%	300 mL/unit
Cryoprecipitate	1 unit	Fibrinogen increased by 5 mg/dL	15 mL/unit
Prepooled cryoprecipitate	1 6-unit pool	Fibrinogen increased by 45 mg/dL	120 mL/pool

Abbreviations: Hb = hemoglobin; Hct = hematocrit.

TABLE 2	ABO Compatibility*		
PATIENT'S ABO	**ANTIBODIES IN CIRCULATION**	**COMPATIBLE PACKED RED BLOOD CELLS**	**COMPATIBLE PLASMA**
O	anti-A, anti-B	O	O, A, B, AB
A	anti-B	O or A	A or AB
B	anti-A	O or B	B or AB
AB	None	O, A, B, AB	AB

*For platelet compatibility, see text.

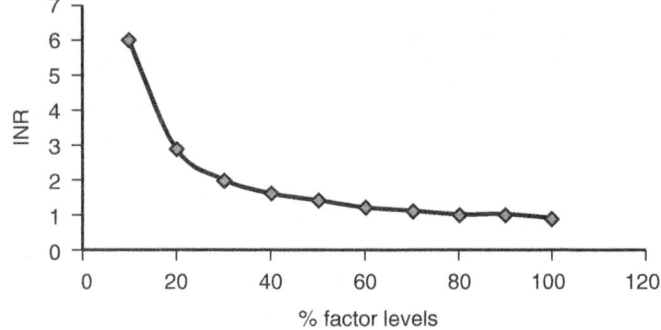

Figure 1 American Association of Blood Banks international normalized ratio (INR) compared with percentage factor levels. Reprinted with permission from Nester T, AuBuchon J: Hemotherapy decisions and their outcomes. In Roback JD (ed): AAB Technical Manual, 17th ed. Bethesda, MD, American Association of Blood Banks, 2011, p 592.

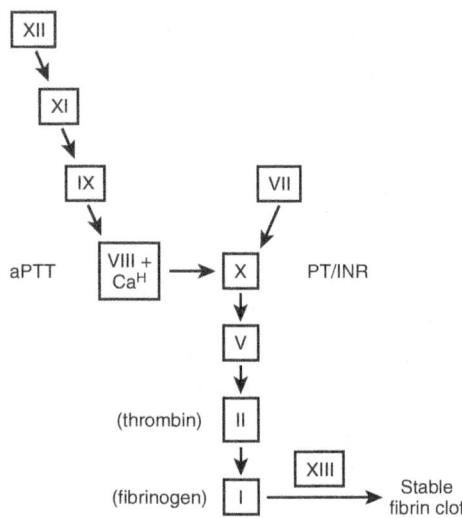

Figure 2 Coagulation cascade.

<table>
<tr><td>**BOX 1**</td><td>Rh(D) compatibility</td></tr>
</table>

Rh(D) negative patients should receive Rh negative red blood cells and platelet units.*†

Rh(D) positive patients can receive Rh positive or Rh negative red blood cells and platelet units.

Rh compatibility does not apply to acellular components (plasma and cryoprecipitate).

Only 15% of blood donors are Rh negative.

---

*In times of shortage, it becomes necessary to preserve the Rh(D) negative red blood cell inventory for females of childbearing potential (< 50 years old).
†Platelet components contain very few red blood cells; Rho(D) immune globulin (RhoGAM) may be administered if prevention of anti-D formation is deemed appropriate. Consult with a transfusion medicine physician if further discussion is needed.

Unresponsiveness to Platelet Transfusion

A number of clinical factors can result in a patient's less-than-optimal response to platelet transfusion. In addition to consumption, some of these factors include splenomegaly, fever, and antifungal therapy. Patients who have been sensitized to foreign human leukocyte antigens through prior pregnancy or transfusion can also have a poor response to platelet transfusion. Transfusion medicine consultation regarding the evaluation of refractoriness to platelet transfusion may be indicated.

Special Situations

Uremia. Patients who are dialysis dependent might have an acquired platelet defect as a result of the uremic environment. Transfusion of platelets into this environment will render the transfused platelets dysfunctional. Thus if optimal platelet function is desired, dialysis should be performed frequently. Consider performing dialysis without heparin if the patient is actively bleeding.

Purpura and Thrombocytopenia. In patients with autoimmune thrombocytopenic purpura (ITP), thrombotic thrombocytopenic purpura (TTP), or heparin-induced thrombocytopenia (HIT), platelet transfusion is not indicated unless the patient has significant bleeding. Other therapies, such as steroid administration for ITP and plasma exchange for TTP, should be initiated to address the condition.

Plasma

Plasma contains all of the coagulation proteins needed for clot formation, as well as all of the fibrinolytic proteins that prevent systemic thrombosis. There are currently several kinds of plasma, such as fresh frozen, FP24, thawed, and liquid. All contain hemostatic levels of coagulation factors as long as they are stored appropriately. The effect of plasma transfusion on the PT and INR is 4 to 6 hours, owing to the short half-life of coagulation factor VII. Thus other, longer-lasting means of restoring coagulation factors, such as vitamin K administration, should be undertaken.

When replacing coagulation factors with plasma, it is not necessary to have 100% factor replacement as the goal. Hemostasis is typically able to occur if circulating coagulation factor levels are between 40% and 50%. It is important to understand that the relationship between the INR and the percentage factor level is a logarithmic, rather than a linear, relationship (Figure 1). Thus whether the INR is 9 or 1.8, the initial dosage of plasma should be 10 to 20 mL/kg, with recheck of the laboratory values a few minutes after infusion. The more prolonged the INR, the more significant the impact of the dose on the INR.

Transfusion Triggers

For bleeding or imminent surgery that cannot be corrected in a timely manner by vitamin K administration, use plasma to correct an INR greater than 1.8 to 2.0. The exception is patients with end-stage liver disease (see later).

Dosage

At a dosage of 10 mL/kg, each unit has an average of 300 mL (3–5 units in a 70-kg adult). This dosage should increase circulating coagulation factors by 20% immediately after infusion.

Special Situations

Liver Disease. The INR is a less useful test in patients with end-stage liver disease. The destruction of liver tissue leads to decreased production of coagulation and fibrinolytic proteins such that a new balance is established. Patients with end-stage liver disease have been shown to have normal levels of circulating thrombin and reduced levels of certain anticoagulant proteins (e.g., protein C), which could explain why they do not bleed as often as predicted with the elevation in INR. Thus the prophylactic use of plasma to correct a mildly prolonged laboratory value in the absence of bleeding is not indicated. It will lead to unnecessary plasma infusion, and the risk of volume overload and transfusion reactions outweighs the benefit in these patients.

Massive Transfusion. In trauma patients, patients with ruptured aortic aneurysms, and patients with other arterial bleeding, massive transfusion may be necessary. The basic principles of such a scenario include taking steps early into the resuscitation to prevent the patient from becoming too cold, acidotic, or coagulopathic to reverse the situation. Some plasma (and cryoprecipitate, if the fibrinogen is very low) should be infused early into the resuscitation to help prevent coagulopathy. Red blood cells and plasma should be infused through a blood warmer, if possible.

Isolated Prolonged aPTT. Other than a deficiency in coagulation factor XI, bear in mind that the differential of an isolated prolonged aPTT includes entities that do not typically require plasma (refer to Figure 2). Hemophilia A, hemophilia B, and von Willebrand disease are no longer treated by plasma but can require factor concentrates to prevent bleeding. Systemic administration of heparin must be reversed by protamine, if fast reversal is desired. Note that plasma transfusion will not reverse the effect of heparin. One of the most common causes of a prolonged aPTT is a lupus anticoagulant; this is an antibody directed against phospholipids that typically leads to thrombosis rather than hemorrhage.

Intracranial Hemorrhage or Life-Threatening Bleeding. Reversal of anticoagulation in the setting of intracranial hemorrhage or life-threatening bleeding depends on the anticoagulant. For patients taking warfarin (Coumadin), refer to Box 2.

Prothrombin complex concentrates (PCCs) may be used to replenish factors II, VII, IX, and X rapidly. For reversal of dabigatran (Pradaxa), a direct oral anticoagulant (DOAC), idarucizumab (Praxbind) is approved by the Food and Drug Administration (FDA) as a reversal agent. KCentra is a 4-factor PCC that has been FDA approved to treat life-threatening hemorrhage in adult patients on warfarin. For reversal of apixaban (Eliquis) and rivaroxaban (Xarelto) in life-threatening bleeding, andexanet alfa (Andexxa) is available.

Cryoprecipitate

Cryoprecipitate contains fibrinogen, coagulation factors VIII and XIII, and von Willebrand factor. The most common current use is as a source of concentrated fibrinogen. It may also be used to treat hemorrhage in the rare patient with factor XIII deficiency.

Indications

Clinical scenarios that increase probability for low fibrinogen include any clinical situation where disseminated intravascular coagulation (DIC) may be present. These include obstetric bleeding, trauma involving head injury or crush injury, and sepsis. Clinical events that can lead to an isolated decrease in serum fibrinogen concentration include administration of L-asparaginase (Elspar) and surgeries that disrupt bladder or salivary gland endothelium. Fibrinogen concentrates are available for patients who will not accept cryoprecipitate.

Transfusion Triggers

Transfusion is appropriate in patients with low serum fibrinogen, typically less than 100 mg/dL. In cases of massive transfusion, a trigger of 150 mg/dL is considered practical, so that the patient becomes less coagulopathic in the time that it takes to draw and review new laboratory values. New evidence indicates that a fibrinogen level of less than 300 mg/dL predicts severe postpartum hemorrhage, as a normal postpartum fibrinogen level is in the 600 mg/dL range. Because component therapy aims to replete coagulation factors to hemostatic (rather than completely normal) levels, consensus guidelines suggest maintaining a fibrinogen level greater than 200 mg/dL during a postpartum hemorrhage.

Dosage

Dosage depends on the type of cryoprecipitate available. If the product requires resuspension in saline before pooling, then one unit (average 15 mL volume) will increase fibrinogen by 5 mg/dL. If the product has been pooled in plasma before freezing, then one unit will increase fibrinogen by 7 to 8 mg/dL; a six-unit pool will increase fibrinogen by 45 mg/dL. Check with the transfusion service laboratory regarding which product is available and the expected increment.

Special Situation

DIC is a state where fibrinogen is consumed at a faster rate than other circulating coagulation factors. This is because DIC is typically a thrombin-generating process (thrombin cleaves fibrinogen into fibrin for clot formation). Thus, although all coagulation factors are being consumed in DIC, timely repletion of fibrinogen by use of cryoprecipitate can result in more-timely cessation of bleeding in a patient with active DIC. The target value is fibrinogen at least 100 mg/dL. If the PT and INR are still prolonged with fibrinogen greater than 100 mg/dL, administration of plasma will replete other coagulation factors being consumed.

Transfusion Reactions

Reactions to transfusion are relatively common; life-threatening reactions are rare (Tables 3 and 4).

Because fever is a feature of both common and dangerous reactions, a transfusion reaction evaluation should be initiated with fever greater than 1°C above patient's baseline temperature at the start of the transfusion. The infusion of product should cease, at least until the laboratory results are known and the

---

BOX 2	Guidelines for Correction of Excessive Warfarin Anticoagulation

INR Higher than Therapeutic but <5, No Significant Bleeding
Lower anticoagulant dosage.
Temporarily discontinue drug, if necessary.

INR >5 but <9, No Significant Bleeding
Omit 1 or 2 doses, monitor INR, resume when INR is in therapeutic range.
Alternative if patient is at increased risk of hemorrhage:
• Omit 1 dose
• Give 1–2.5 mg vitamin K orally.
For rapid reversal before urgent surgery:
• Give 2–4 mg vitamin K orally.
• Give 1–2 mg at 24 hours if INR remains elevated.

INR >9, No Significant Bleeding
Omit warfarin; give 2.5–5.0 mg vitamin K orally.
Closely monitor INR; give additional vitamin K, if necessary.
Resume warfarin at lower dose when INR is within therapeutic range.

Serious Bleeding at Any Elevation of INR
Omit warfarin.
Give 10 mg vitamin K by slow IV infusion.
Supplement with plasma or prothrombin complex concentrate depending on urgency of correction.
Vitamin K infusions may be repeated every 12 hours.

Life-Threatening Hemorrhage
Omit warfarin.
Give prothrombin complex concentrate with 10 mg vitamin K by slow IV infusion.
Repeat as necessary, depending on INR.

Abbreviation: INR = international normalized ratio.
From Nester T, AuBuchon J: Hemotherapy decisions and their outcomes. In Roback JD (ed): AABB Technical Manual, 17th ed. Bethesda, MD, American Association of Blood Banks, 2011, p 571–616.

TABLE 3	Transfusion Reactions
MOST-COMMON REACTIONS	**INCIDENCE**
Allergic reaction of mild severity	1:33 to 1:100
Febrile nonhemolytic reaction	1:100 to 1:1000 with leukocyte reduction
Transfusion-related circulatory overload	< 1:100
MOST DANGEROUS REACTIONS	**INCIDENCE**
Acute hemolytic reaction	1:38,000 to 1:70,000
Anaphylactic reaction	1:20,000 to 1:50,000
Transfusion-related acute lung injury	1:1200 to 1:190,000
Bacterial contamination of red cell unit with gram-negative organisms	1:1,000,000

TABLE 4 Transfusion Reactions with Respiratory Symptoms

REACTION	CLASSIC SIGNS	RELATIVE FREQUENCY	ACUTE MANAGEMENT (TRANSFUSION STOPPED IN ALL CASES)
Febrile nonhemolytic reaction	Transient tachypnea in the presence of rigors and fever	Common	Antipyretic ± meperidine (Demerol)[1]
Circulatory overload	Hypoxia Crackles in lower lung fields Increased BP Chest radiograph consistent with volume overload	Common	Diuresis
Allergic reaction of moderate severity	Wheezes Possible perioral or periorbital edema Possible hives	Uncommon	IV antihistamines and possibly epinephrine (Adrenalin)
Allergic reaction of marked severity	Wheezes, swollen lips, tongue, uvula Stridor or other signs of airway compromise Very decreased BP	Rare	Epinephrine IV fluids and airway management Bronchodilators and glucagon (GlucaGen)[1] for patient on β-blockers
Transfusion-related acute lung injury	Tachypnea and hypoxia during or within 6 of transfusion Persisting for several hours Chest radiograph consistent with bilateral white out	Rare	Respiratory support of noncardiogenic pulmonary edema
Acute hemolytic reaction	Red urine and red serum Hypotension and diffuse oozing may be present Tachypnea (10% of patients)	Rare	Supportive (possibly ICU) care Administration of crystalloid solution Blood component therapy if DIC is present
Bacterial contamination with Gram-negative organism	Very decreased BP Fever Nausea, vomiting Possible tachypnea	Rare	Intensive care for support of Gram-negative sepsis

Abbreviations: BP = blood pressure; DIC = disseminated intravascular coagulation; ICU = intensive care unit.
[1]Not FDA approved for this indication.

patient has responded to treatment. The main point of the laboratory investigation is to evaluate the plasma for abnormal (usually red) color in an effort to detect intravascular hemolysis as quickly as possible. If the clerical check and hemolysis direct antiglobulin tests are negative, one might consider restarting the transfusion with careful surveillance of the patient. A direct antiglobulin test is performed to detect the presence of antibody coating red blood cells in circulation; a positive result could indicate extravascular hemolysis, which is not as dangerous as intravascular hemolysis.

Most-Common Reactions
Febrile Nonhemolytic Reaction
Presentation. A febrile nonhemolytic transfusion reaction manifests as fever greater than a 1°C rise above the patient's baseline, often accompanied by rigors. Hypertension, tachypnea, and transient decrease in oxygen saturation can also occur until the symptoms are treated. Evidence of hemolysis will be absent on laboratory evaluation. These reactions can manifest during or 2 to 3 hours after the transfusion.

Pathophysiology. Cytokines produced by white blood cells present in cellular blood components (red blood cell and platelet units) are responsible for the clinical presentation. Platelets also secrete cytokines; thus leukoreduction of platelet units might not be successful in preventing the reaction.

Acute Management. Administration of an antipyretic is the routine treatment; meperidine (Demerol)[1] may be required to address severe rigors. Slow IV push of 25 mg as a first dose is

recommended; an additional 25-mg dose can be given 10 to 15 minutes later if rigors persist.

Prevention with Future Transfusion. Antipyretic may be administered prior to transfusion. Ordering leukoreduced red blood cells and platelets (if the hospital inventory is not entirely composed of leukoreduced components) is also a preventive measure. For recurring reactions with platelets, volume reduction of the component can reduce the incidence.

Allergic Reaction of Mild Severity
Presentation. Urticaria or flushing occurs during a transfusion. Evidence of hemolysis is absent on laboratory evaluation.

Pathophysiology. Allergic reactions are immunoglobulin (Ig) E-mediated reactions against some allergen in the donor plasma. Because all blood components have some amount of plasma, it is possible to experience an allergic reaction with any blood product.

Acute Management. Slowing the infusion rate may be all that is required to alleviate the reaction. Antihistamine administration also addresses the symptoms.

Prevention with Future Transfusion. A reaction of this type may be a one-time event. For patients with recurrent reactions, transfusing the blood product more slowly (maximum of transfusion over 4 hours), or premedication with antihistamines will reduce the incidence.

Transfusion Associated Circulatory Overload (TACO)
Presentation. The patient has respiratory distress, typically during the transfusion, and increase in blood pressure unless cardiac decompensation occurs. Tachycardia, tachypnea, and decrease in

[1]Not FDA approved for this indication.

oxygen saturation are often present. Jugular venous distension may be seen. Radiographic findings include pleural effusions, perihilar edema, and increased vascular pedicle width.

Pathophysiology. The reaction results in cardiogenic pulmonary edema.

Acute Management. Diuretic should be administered. Supplemental oxygen may be required temporarily to improve oxygen saturation.

Prevention with Future Transfusion. Slowing the infusion rate with a maximum time of transfusion over 4 hours can prevent the reaction. Diuretic administration may be necessary in patients with poor heart function.

Most-Dangerous Reactions
Acute Hemolytic Transfusion Reaction (AHTR)

Presentation. The most common signs include fever with or without rigors and pain. The more commonly reported sites of pain include flank, back, chest, or abdomen. Nausea and vomiting and dyspnea can also occur. In more severe presentations, hemodynamic instability is present, accompanied by oozing from line sites or petechial hemorrhage if DIC is occurring. Red or cola-colored urine is another manifestation of an acute hemolytic transfusion reaction and represents overwhelming of the renal capacity to recirculate free heme.

Pathophysiology. Red blood cells have proteins and carbohydrates on the cell surface that are antigenic. These epitopes are categorized into blood groups based on structure and sharing of a parent protein. A patient who lacks particular epitopes can develop antibodies through pregnancy or transfusion. Such red blood cell alloantibodies then lyse transfused red blood cells that possess the cognate antigen. When time allows for pretransfusion testing, the antibodies are identified, and antigen-negative units are provided. The ABO blood group system is unusual in that almost all patients older than 4 months have naturally occurring antibodies to the A and B antigens that they did not inherit. These antibodies are capable of activating complement and causing intravascular lysis when bound to their cognate antigen. Thus it is of utmost importance to avoid transfusing red blood cells against the ABO antibody in circulation. Refer to the ABO compatibility table (see Table 1).

Acute Management. Management is largely supportive. The end result of intravascular hemolysis and activation of the complement cascade can be shock, uncontrolled bleeding secondary to DIC, and renal failure. Therefore prompt infusion of intravenous crystalloid solutions are indicated to maintain blood pressure and renal perfusion. The goal for urine flow rate should be more than 1 mL/kg per hour. Coagulation laboratory values should be obtained to determine whether DIC is present; if so, component therapy to reverse the DIC is indicated. If the reaction is severe, intensive care is appropriate, because cardiac monitoring and mechanical ventilation may be necessary to support the patient.

Prevention with Future Transfusion. An acute hemolytic reaction is one of the most feared complications of transfusion. It is also often one of the most preventable. Great care should be given to the pretransfusion blood sample draw, comparing the label to the patient's unique identifiers, and labeling the tube at the patient's bedside as soon as the blood is in the tube. Just before transfusion, the unit label attached to the blood product should be compared with the patient's armband to ensure that the product is intended for this particular patient. To prevent intravascular hemolysis from antibodies directed against non-ABO antigens, pretransfusion testing (antibody screen or crossmatch) should be done in advance of the need for red cell transfusion for any patient whose clinical situation indicates a likelihood of needing blood. The exception is a patient who is hemodynamically unstable because of acute red blood cell loss, where uncrossmatched red blood cells are indicated. If the patient's identity is known, a call to the hospital transfusion service in this situation is warranted; explain that the patient needs uncrossmatched red blood cells and ask if there are transfusion records that indicate a need for antigen-negative units.

Allergic Reaction of Marked Severity (Anaphylaxis)

Presentation. Significant drop in blood pressure occurs, typically early into the transfusion. Wheezes, difficulty breathing, and stridor may be present. Tongue or facial edema and hives may be observed.

Pathophysiology. Anaphylaxis is an IgE-mediated reaction against an allergen in the donor plasma. In a patient with absolute IgA deficiency, naturally occurring anti-IgA can precipitate this reaction on binding IgA in the plasma. Anti-haptoglobin antibodies can also induce a severe reaction.

Acute Management. Airway and blood pressure support should be provided with the patient recumbent and the lower extremities elevated. The treatment of choice is epinephrine (Adrenalin) 1 mg/mL, also labeled as 1:1000 or 0.1%, using an adult dosage of 0.3 to 0.5 mg per single dose, typically administered intramuscularly to the mid-quadriceps area. If symptoms persist, the dose may be repeated every 5 to 15 minutes for a maximum of three times, unless palpitations, tremors, or extreme anxiousness occurs. Supplemental oxygen should be administered and the airway maintained. Intravenous fluid administration is also recommended. Bronchodilators such as albuterol can be given as adjunctive treatment for bronchospasm that does not appear to respond to epinephrine. For patients on β-blockers, the addition of intravenous glucagon[1] (GlucaGen) 1 to 5 mg administered over 5 minutes, followed by infusion of 5 to 15 μg/minute, may be required. The addition of glucocorticoids can help prevent the biphasic reaction that occurs in some patients.

Prevention with Future Transfusion. Slow administration with careful observation of any transfusion is required. Premedication with intravenous antihistamines is appropriate. Steroids may be administered, although their effectiveness has not been confirmed through controlled trials. Epinephrine should be available at the bedside. For severe allergic reactions, a discussion with the transfusion service physician regarding washed components is appropriate.

Transfusion-Related Acute Lung Injury

Presentation. The signs of transfusion-related acute lung injury (TRALI) are difficulty breathing, tachypnea, and hypoxia during or within 6 hours of a transfusion of any blood component. Ideally, signs of underlying lung disease or circulatory overload are absent. Chest radiograph may show diffuse bilateral opacities (white-out). Diuretic administration does not result in improvement. The hypoxemia can progress to the point that the patient requires mechanical ventilation, and thus the patient should be closely monitored while the reaction is occurring.

Pathophysiology. The factors that result in TRALI are not entirely known. In a portion of cases, antibodies against white blood cell antigens are present in donor plasma. These antibodies are believed to bind the cognate antigens on the patient's white blood cells, leading to degranulation and a capillary leak syndrome involving the lungs. Other theories regarding the pathophysiology of TRALI exist. One such theory implicates biologically active substances such as lipids and cytokines in the stored blood products. These substances are believed to prime the patient's granulocytes and activate pulmonary endothelium, setting the stage for an additional trigger to cause acute lung injury. Regardless of the cause of TRALI, the end result is an increase in pulmonary vascular permeability and noncardiogenic pulmonary edema. The estimated mortality rate from TRALI is 5% to 8%.

Acute Management. Management consists of supportive care, with particular regard to respiratory support. With adequate supportive care, the process most often reverses over 48 to 96 hours.

Prevention with Future Transfusion. Marked respiratory compromise is occasionally due to white blood cell antibodies in the patient, which bind cognate antigens in the donated red blood cells or platelet unit ("reverse TRALI"). In these cases, leukoreduction of cellular blood products may reduce the severity of subsequent transfusions, although solid evidence to support this is lacking. For TRALI caused by white blood cell antibodies in

---

[1]Not FDA approved for this indication.

the donated product, there are no preventive measures for the clinician to take. The majority of US blood suppliers provide plasma from only male donors, in an effort to reduce the incidence of TRALI caused by multiparous women with white blood cell antibodies.

Bacterial Contamination of a Blood Component

Presentation. The most-common presentation includes fever and rigors, nausea and vomiting, and possible onset of moderate hypotension during or after a platelet transfusion. Rarely, presentation includes signs of overt septic shock, including marked hypotension, typically early into the transfusion of a red blood cell or platelet component. Bacterial contamination of plasma or cryoprecipitate is extremely rare.

Pathophysiology. The most-common organisms to contaminate a platelet product are gram-positive organisms such as *Staphylococcus epidermidis*. These organisms are thought to be introduced into the collection bag via a skin plug that results from phlebotomy using a large-gauge needle when sterilization of the phlebotomy site has been ineffective.

The most common organisms to contaminate a red blood cell unit are gram-negative, endotoxin-producing organisms such as *Yersinia enterocolitica*. This organism is introduced into the blood product as a result of asymptomatic bacteremia in the donor, from sources such as the gastrointestinal tract. The donor-screening questionnaire and vital sign assessment at the time of donation help to make collection from such a donor a very rare event. Transfusion of a bacterially contaminated red blood cell unit is most often a fatal event. It is important to remember that platelets can also be contaminated by the same gram-negative, endotoxin-producing organisms; in this case, signs of septic shock may be manifest.

Acute Management. Blood cultures from the patient should be drawn, and then prompt intravenous antibiotic administration should begin. Supportive care including inotropic agents and close nursing attention may be required.

Prevention with Future Transfusion. Bacterial contamination is associated with a donor product, and thus preventive measures for the patient do not apply. Blood suppliers perform bacterial detection tests on platelet components, and transfusion services have strict policies related to visual inspection of all blood products before they are issued to a patient-care area. However, these measures are not completely effective. The FDA recently approved pathogen inactivation technology for platelets, which may further lower the risk.

Other Reactions

Delayed Hemolytic Transfusion Reaction

Presentation. The main finding with a delayed hemolytic transfusion reaction is usually an unexplained decrease in hematocrit within 2 to 7 days after transfusion. The patient often remains symptom free unless the decline in hemoglobin is poorly tolerated. Jaundice can occur, and laboratory values consistent with hemolysis may be positive (elevated indirect bilirubin, elevated lactate dehydrogenase, decreased haptoglobin). Rarely, signs of intravascular hemolysis can occur.

Pathophysiology. The most common source of this reaction is a red blood cell alloantibody that the patient developed with prior transfusion or pregnancy; the antibody titer wanes over time such that pretransfusion testing does not detect the antibody. A unit of red blood cells positive for the cognate antigen is then transfused, and within a few days the patient's memory B cell response produces the antibody again. Transfused cells are then cleared, most often by an extravascular mechanism.

Acute Management. Most transfusion services have a policy to notify the clinician that a serologic delayed hemolytic transfusion reaction is present on testing a new plasma sample from the patient. If the patient's hematocrit has declined, it may be useful to determine a clinical correlation by obtaining the laboratory values just described. This is of particular importance when the distinction between hemolysis and bleeding will lead to different management strategies for the patient. Although extravascular

clearance of hemoglobin is fairly well tolerated by the kidneys, the conservative approach is to increase renal perfusion with intravenous crystalloid solutions if possible.

Prevention with Future Transfusion. For a patient who routinely receives care through one hospital system, the transfusion service will keep a record of the red blood cell alloantibody and provide antigen-negative cells for transfusion. The prevention, then, is to plan ahead for transfusion when possible, so that fully compatible units can be provided. Uncrossmatched red blood cells may be positive for the cognate antigen.

Allergic Reaction of Moderate Severity

Presentation. The patient has labile blood pressure, either hyper- or hypotension, accompanied by at least one of the following: throat scratchiness, respiratory wheezes, or perioral or periorbital edema. Hives may be present. Gastrointestinal symptoms such as crampy abdominal pain may also be present.

Pathophysiology. This is an IgE-mediated reaction against an allergen in the plasma of the donated product.

Acute Management. Treatment is administration of intravenous antihistamines. If the respiratory component does not resolve, consider epinephrine administration and treat similarly to anaphylaxis (see previous section).

Prevention with Future Transfusion. Slower infusion of blood products can reduce further episodes of this type of reaction. If the patient is atopic, intravenous antihistamines may be administered as a premedication. If the patient requires chronic transfusion and experiences this type of reaction on a repeated basis, discussion with the transfusion service regarding washed components may be warranted.

Hypotensive Transfusion Reaction

Presentation. The patient has isolated hypotension (drop in systolic BP greater than 30 but less than 80 mm Hg) that responds quickly to cessation of the transfusion. The reaction classically occurs within the first 15 minutes of infusion of the blood product.

Pathophysiology. Pathophysiology is unclear. Some research indicates that the patient may have slower ability to metabolize bradykinin compared to other individuals.

Acute Management. Stop the transfusion.

Prevention with Future Transfusion. Prevention is unclear. In the author's experience, rate of infusion has a role. Slower infusion may help to prevent this type of reaction.

Transfusion Associated Dyspnea

Presentation. Mild respiratory distress that occurs within 24 hours of cessation of transfusion.

Pathophysiology. Pathophysiology is unclear.

Acute Management and Prevention with future transfusion. Management is supportive and prevention is unclear.

References

Abdel-Wahab OI, Healy B, Dzik WH: Effect of fresh-frozen plasma transfusion on prothrombin time and bleeding in patients with mild coagulation abnormalities, *Transfusion* 46:1279–1285, 2006.

Carson JL, Guyatt G, Heddle NM, et al: Clinical practice guidelines from the AABB: Red cell transfusion thresholds and storage, *JAMA* 316(19):2025–2035, 2016.

Carson JL, Stanworth SJ, Alexander JH, et al: Clinical trials evaluating red blood cell transfusion thresholds: An updated systematic review and with additional focus on patients with cardiovascular disease, *Am Heart J* 200:96-101, 2018.

Cuker A, Burnett A, Triller D, et al: Reversal of direct oral anticoagulants: Guidance from the anticoagulation forum, *Am J Hem*, epub ahead of print, 2019.

Cushman M, Lim W, Zakai NA: *2011 Clinical Practice Guide on Anticoagulant Dosing and Management of Anticoagulant-Associated Bleeding Complications in Adults*, Washington, DC, 2014, American Society of Hematology.

Kaufman RM, et al: Platelet transfusion: A clinical practice guideline from the AABB, *Ann Internal Med* 162(3):205–213, 2015.

Lisman T, Porte RJ: Rebalanced hemostasis in patients with liver disease: Evidence and clinical consequences, *Blood* 116:878–885, 2010.

Nester T, Jain S, Poisson J: *Hemotherapy decisions and their outcomes. AABB Technical Manual*, 18th ed, Bethesda, MD, 2014, AABB Press.

Savage WJ, Hod EA: Noninfectious complications of blood transfusion. In Fung MK, editor: *AABB Technical Manual*, ed 19th, Bethesda, MD, 2017, American Association of Blood Banks, pp 569–599.

Tummula R, et al: Specific antidotes against direct oral anticoagulants: A comprehensive review of clinical trials, *Int J Cardiol* 214:292–298, 2016.

CHRONIC LEUKEMIAS

Method of
Katarzyna Jamieson, MD

CURRENT DIAGNOSIS

Chronic Myelogenous Leukemia
- Clinical symptoms
  - Constitutional symptoms
  - Splenomegaly (abdominal discomfort, early satiety)
- Laboratory parameters
  - Increased white blood cell count, commonly >100,000/µL, with differential counts showing granulocytes in all stages of differentiation, and two peaks involving neutrophils and myelocytes
  - Absolute basophilia
- Genetic parameters
  - Demonstration of *bcr-abl* by standard cytogenetic analysis, fluorescent in situ hybridization, or polymerase chain reaction

Chronic Lymphocytic Leukemia
- Clinical symptoms
  - B symptoms (fever, night sweats, and weight loss)
  - Lymphadenopathy and organomegaly
  - Recurrent infections
- Laboratory parameters
  - Increased white blood cell count with absolute lymphocytosis
  - Anemia, thrombocytopenia
- Immunophenotypic analysis (flow cytometry)
  - Demonstration of monoclonal population of light chain–restricted mature B lymphocytes expressing CD19, CD20 (dim), and CD23 and coexpressing pan-T cell antigen CD5

CURRENT THERAPY

Chronic Myelogenous Leukemia: Chronic Phase
- Initial therapy
  - Imatinib mesylate (Gleevec) 400–600 mg daily
  - Dasatinib (Sprycel)
  - Nilotinib (Tasigna)
- Second-line therapy:
  - Imatinib mesylate 800 mg daily
  - Dasatinib (Sprycel)
  - Nilotinib (Tasigna)
  - Bosutinib (Bosulif)
  - Ponatinib (Iclusig)
  - Omacetaxine (Synribo)
- High risk for failure:
  - Allogeneic stem cell transplantation

Chronic Lymphocytic Leukemia
- Chemotherapy drugs
  - Fludarabine (Fludara)
  - Deoxycoformycin (Pentostatin [Nipent])
  - Cyclophosphamide (Cytoxan)
  - Chlorambucil (Leukeran)
  - Bendamustine (Treanda)
- Targeted therapy drugs
  - Idelalisib (Zydelig)
  - Ibrutinib (Imbruvica)
- Immunotherapy (monoclonal antibodies):
  - Rituximab (Rituxan)
  - Alemtuzumab (Campath)
  - Ofatumumab (Arzerra)
  - Obinutuzumab (Gazyva)

Chronic Myelogenous Leukemia

Chronic myelogenous leukemia (CML) is a chronic myeloproliferative disorder defined by the presence of a chimeric gene, *bcr-abl*, encoded by translocation between chromosomes 9 and 22, the Philadelphia chromosome. Discovered in 1960, the Philadelphia chromosome was the first chromosomal abnormality implicated in carcinogenesis. This was followed by decades of unraveling of leukemogenic process, which culminated in a development of the *bcr-abl* inhibitor imatinib mesylate (Gleevec). As a result, in 2001 CML became the first human neoplasm in which the rationally designed therapeutic agent to target a carcinogenic pathway demonstrated great clinical efficacy.

Epidemiology and Risk Factors
CML accounts for 7% to 15% of all cases of leukemia in adults. The median age at diagnosis is 45 to 55 years. The disease is extremely rare in children and the overall incidence increases with age. There is slight male predominance, with a male-to-female ratio of 1.4 to 1.0. There is no association with geographic distribution or race. The etiology of CML is unknown. High-dose radiation exposure is the only well-established environmental risk factor. No genetic predisposition is thought to play any role in pathogenesis of CML.

Pathogenesis
bcr-abl is created by a reciprocal translocation of genetic material between the long arm of chromosome 9 (containing the proto-oncogene *c-abl*) and the long arm of chromosome 22 (containing the *bcr* gene). This is the Philadelphia chromosome, and it is correctly annotated t(9;22)(q34.1;q11.21). The translocation results in constitutive upregulation of tyrosine kinase activity of *abl*, which triggers downstream transduction pathways of a signaling cascade of oncogenic events.

The natural course of CML is one of inevitable progression from an initial chronic phase to a more-aggressive accelerated phase and eventually to a rapidly fatal myeloid or lymphoid blast phase. It is thought that the transformation proceeds as a consequence of the accumulation of additional molecular changes in genetically unstable *bcr-abl*–containing cells. Supportive of this hypothesis, up to 80% of patients with advanced CML have secondary cytogenetic abnormalities.

Clinical and Laboratory Characteristics
CML is a clonal myeloproliferative disorder that develops through accumulation of maturing cells of myeloid, erythroid, and megakaryocytic origin. CML has a biphasic or triphasic clinical course. Patients usually present in the initial chronic phase, exhibiting a cluster of specific clinical and laboratory features (listed in the Current Diagnosis box). More than half of patients with CML diagnosed in the chronic phase are asymptomatic, and the diagnosis is established following the incidental discovery of elevated white blood cell (WBC) count on a routine screening test.

The median time to the development of terminal blast phase is 3 to 6 years. The disease typically progresses through slow evolution into an accelerated phase and then blast phase, but it can transform rapidly directly into the blast phase. The detection of a change in the pace of the disease may be difficult and therefore definitions of accelerated phase vary and are imprecise. The blast phase is defined by the presence of extramedullary disease or at least 30% blasts or blasts and promyelocytes in the bone marrow or peripheral blood. Leukemic cells in blast phase are characterized by arrested maturation, and they proliferate rapidly, similar to acute leukemia cells. The symptoms of blast phase are also those typically seen in acute leukemia.

Diagnosis
The diagnosis of CML can be usually made with reasonable certainty based on the results of peripheral blood cell counts and examination of the peripheral blood smear (see the Current Diagnosis box). The detection of the Philadelphia chromosome or *bcr-abl* by cytogenetic analysis, fluorescent in situ hybridization

(FISH), or polymerase chain reaction (PCR) confirms the diagnosis: all patients positive for the Philadelphia chromosome by standard cytogenetic analysis will have a *bcr-abl* fusion gene detectable by FISH or PCR; however, in approximately 5% of patients with *bcr-abl* detectable by FISH or PCR, the Philadelphia chromosome could not be appreciated by standard cytogenetics. The bone marrow biopsy is usually not necessary for diagnosis but should be performed for staging purposes in all patients with newly diagnosed CML.

Differential Diagnosis

At presentation, the differential diagnosis of CML usually involves distinction from leukemoid reaction. Among hematologic malignancies, CML may be difficult to differentiate from other myeloproliferative disorders (essential thrombocytosis, polycythemia vera, and mutagenic myeloid metaplasia), chronic neutrophilic leukemia, chronic myelomonocytic leukemia, juvenile chronic myeloid leukemia, and eosinophilic leukemia. In most cases, the detection of *bcr-abl* is sufficient to make the distinction. However, the differentiation between CML presenting in lymphoid-blast phase and Philadelphia chromosome–positive acute lymphoblastic leukemia might not be possible.

Prognosis

Before the effective therapies became available, the expected median survival of patients with CML was 39 to 47 months, with less than 20% surviving longer than 8 years. Allogeneic stem cell transplantation (SCT) and interferon (IFN) alfa-2b (Intron-A)[1] or INF alfa 2a (Roferon-A) in the 1990s improved median survival to 60 to 65 months. However, the availability of tyrosine kinase inhibitors (TKIs) in 2000s transformed CML into a chronic disease associated with near-normal life expectancy: The 8-year update of the IRIS trial (International Randomized Study of Interferon and STI-571) reported 85% overall survival and 93% survival in patients with only CML-related deaths. At this time, it is still unclear if TKIs are capable of curing CML; and continuation of therapy to maintain the remission is generally considered the standard of care. However, the increasing body of evidence suggests that as many as 30% of imatinib-treated patients who stopped the treatment after 2 years or more of undetectable minimal residual disease by conventional PCR may be able to sustain their remission off treatment. Patients who are suboptimal responders, who are poor responders, or whose disease is refractory to imatinib have poorer prognosis than patients who met expected response criteria (Table 1). The Sokal prognostic score, originally derived from 800 patients treated in the early 1960s and 1970s, still helps to identify patients who are at high risk for failure in the era of TKI.

Definitions of Response and Monitoring of Therapeutic Efficacy

The goal of CML therapy is the maximum possible reduction of leukemia burden. The status of the response is routinely evaluated by peripheral blood counts, cytogenetic analysis and FISH, and real-time quantitative PCR (RQ-PCR). The uniform criteria for hematologic, cytogenetic, and molecular responses have been developed to guide therapy and facilitate meaningful analysis of efficacy data across clinical trials (Tables 1 and 2). Close follow-up of response is critically important to predict when other therapies, such as alternative TKIs or transplantation, should be considered. Selective testing for bcr-abl kinase domain mutations is recommended for all patients who fail to respond to the first-line agent.

Treatment
Chronic Phase

Throughout most of the 20th century CML was considered incurable. The principal options for treating CML included busulfan (Myleran, Busulfex) or hydroxyurea (Hydrea). Such therapy, although successful in alleviating symptoms, did not alter the natural course of the disease. Introduction of allogeneic SCT in 1980s for the first time offered CML patients a prospect of cure. However, the high treatment-related morbidity and mortality associated with this procedure greatly limited its use to patients who were young and fit and for whom an HLA-identical donor could be identified. The alternative was treatment with IFN alfa 2b (Intron-A)[1] or IFN alfa 2a (Roferon-A), which offered prolongation of survival but generally only to a minority of patients who could tolerate it.

First-Line Therapy. In 2001, imatinib mesylate (Gleevec), the first selective bcr-abl tyrosine kinase inhibitor, was introduced into clinical practice. The trial that established imatinib as the treatment of choice for newly diagnosed CML in the chronic phase was the International Randomized Study of Interferon

---

[1] Not FDA approved for this indication.

[1] Not FDA approved for this indication.

TABLE 1	European Leukemia-Net Response Definitions for any TKI First Line, and Second Line in Case of Intolerance, All Patients (CP, AP, BP)		
TIME AFTER DIAGNOSIS	**FAILURE**		**WARNING/SUBOPTIMAL**
Baseline			High risk Major route CCA/Ph+
3 mo	No CHR Ph+ >95%		BCR-ABL*>10% Ph+ 36–95%
6 mo	BCR-ABL >10% Ph+ >35%		BCR-ABL* 1–10% Ph+ 1–35%
12 mo	BCR-ABL*>1% Ph+ >0%		BCR-ABL* 0.1–1%
Then and at any time	Loss of CHR, CCyR or MMR Mutations** CCA/Ph+		CCA/Ph– (–7, or 7q–)

Abbreviations: CCgR = complete cytogenetic response; MMR = major molecular response; PCgR = partial cytogenetic response; Ph = Philadelphia chromosome. Major route CCA/Ph+ are clonal cytogenetic abnormalities in Ph+ cells: +8, 2nd Ph+ CCA/Ph+ are trisomy 8, [+der(22)t(9;22)(q34;q11)], isochromosome 17\[i(17)(q10)], trisomy 19, and ider(22)(q10)t(9;22)(q34;q11)

Reprinted with permission from Baccarani M, Deininger MW, Rosti G, et al: European LeukemiaNet recommendations for the management of chronic myeloid leukemia. *Blood* 122(6):872–884, 2013. http://www.leukemia-net.org/content/leukemias/cml/recommendations/e8078/infoboxContent10260/PocketCard_UPDATE2013_10-5x165_final.pdf (accessed 20.8.2014).

*IS International Scale

**Confirmed by two consecutive tests, of which one is ≥1%

TABLE 2 European LeukemiaNet Definitions and Monitoring Recommendations

HEMATOLOGIC RESPONSE	CYTOGENIC RESPONSE	MOLECULAR RESPONSE
Definitions		
Complete: Platelet count <450 × 10⁹/L WBC count <10 × 10⁹/L Differential without immature granulocytes and with <5% basophils Nonpalpable spleen	Complete: Ph+ 0% Partial: Ph+ <35% Minor: Ph+ 36–65% None: Ph+ >95%	Complete: transcript nonquantifiable and nondetectable Major: ≤0.10
Monitoring		
Check every 2 wk until complete response achieved and confirmed, then every 3 mo unless otherwise required	Check at 3 and 6 mo, then every 6 mo until complete response achieved and confirmed; thereafter every 12 mo if molecular monitoring cannot be ensured; check always for occurrence of treatment failure or unexplained cytopenia	Check every 3 mo until major response is achieved; conduct mutational analysis in case of failure, suboptimal response, or increase in transcript level

Abbreviations: Ph = Philadelphia chromosome; WBC = white blood cell.
Reprinted with permission from Baccarani M, Saglio G, Goldman J, et al: Evolving concepts in the management of chronic myeloid leukemia: Recommendations from an expert panel on behalf of the European LeukemiaNet. *Blood* 108:1809–1820, 2006; Baccarani M, Cortes J, Pane F, et al: Chronic myeloid leukemia: an update of concepts and management recommendations of European LeukemiaNet. *J Clin Oncol* 27:6041–6051, 2009.

Alpha Versus STI571 (IRIS). Between June 2000 and January 2001 IRIS accrued and randomized 1106 patients to imatinib 400 mg daily versus what was then the standard of care, interferon alfa plus subcutaneous cytarabine (Cytosar). After a median of 5 years, 382 of the 553 patients (69%) randomized to imatinib were still receiving it. The estimated progression-free survival was 83% and overall survival was 89%. The responding patients whose disease did not progress in any way in their first 3 years were unlikely to relapse and unlikely to suffer from late-onset side effects.

The recommended dose of imatinib for patients with CML in the chronic phase is 400 mg orally once daily. The drug is well tolerated by the majority of patients; the most common side effects are nausea, vomiting, edema (fluid retention), muscle cramps, skin rash, diarrhea, heartburn, and headache. Hematologic toxicity is quite common, particularly in patients with advanced CML, and the package insert contains exact guidelines for its management. Occasional severe hepatotoxicity has been reported.

Most patients with CML in the chronic phase today achieve and maintain excellent disease control with imatinib and seem to enjoy near-normal survival and quality of life. Given that continuation of TKI in a majority of patients seems necessary to maintain the remission, adherence to therapy is crucial and has recently become an avid focus of clinical investigations.

Since introduction of imatinib, three more second-generation TKIs have been developed and approved for treatment of CML: dasatinib (Sprycel), nilotinib (Tasigna) and bosutinib (Bosulif). All three have been studied extensively and demonstrated efficacy in the setting of imatinib failure. Dasatinib and nilotinib have subsequently been studied and received Food and Drug Administration (FDA) approval for use as first-line agents. Phase III studies comparing dasatinib (DASISION) or nilotinib (ENESTnd) to imatinib as initial therapy for CML in the chronic phase demonstrated faster and deeper responses; however, a longer follow-up will be required to determine if this is going to translate into clinically significant long-term benefits such as improved survival. At this time the choice of a front line TKI is often determined by the patient's tolerance of the drug, as each of the TKIs has some unique and non-overlapping toxicities. Bosutinib has not yet been approved in the first-line setting. A randomized study comparing bosutinib to imatinib (BELA) in newly diagnosed patients indicated comparable response rates but higher rate of gastrointestinal toxicity associated with bosutinib. Neutropenia, musculoskeletal events, and edema were less frequent.

A fourth-generation TKI, ponatinib (Iclusig), is the newest agent of this class granted accelerated FDA approval after demonstrating high levels of response rates on the PACE trial in heavily pretreated patients, including those carrying the T315I mutation. Soon after its approval ponatinib received a black box warning in highlighting the increased risk of serious vascular events and hepatic toxicity. More recently an increased risk of serious complications associated with the long-term use of the other second-generation TKI have also been reported, emphasizing the relative safety of the first drug in this class, namely imatinib.

The long-term follow-up of patients in the IRIS trial indicates that despite the favorable toxicity profile and efficacy, as many as 30% of patients will eventually fail imatinib therapy. Patients who are intolerant to first-line TKIs should be offered, and may be able to tolerate and respond to, other TKIs. Consensus recommends that patients who fail imatinib by progression or relapse should be screened for other medications that could affect metabolism and thus compromise the clinical efficacy of TKIs, for compliance and for *abl* mutations. More than 50 mutations in *bcr-abl* have been described, detection of which may help guide selection of second-line TKI therapy. Younger and otherwise fit patients should be evaluated for an allogeneic SCT.

Other Therapeutic Options. Patients who fail imatinib and/or second-generation TKI have particularly poor prognoses. Those who are not transplant candidates may be treated with omacetaxine (Synribo), which has recently been approved for patients resistant and/or intolerant to two or more tyrosine kinase inhibitors.

Advanced Phase

Imatinib mesylate is indicated for advanced CML in accelerated phase and blast phase. The recommended dosages are higher: 600 mg daily for CML accelerated phase and 800 mg daily for CML in the blast phase. Patients who satisfy criteria for acceleration are a heterogeneous group, because the disease biologically varies from slightly more advanced than late chronic phase to verging on blast phase. Up to 80% of patients achieve a hematologic remission, and approximately 40% achieve a complete cytogenetic response, which is considered a prerequisite to long-term survival. All second- and third-generation TKIs are approved for treatment of advanced CML: dasatinib at 140 mg once daily (or 70 mg twice daily), nilotinib at 400 mg twice daily, bosutinib 500 to 600 mg once daily, and ponatinib 45 mg once daily. Patients who progress to the accelerated phase on the first-line TKI should be screened for *bcr-abl* mutations. In general the likelihood of response to a second-line TKI is 30% to 40%, and the identification of a mutation and selection of the second-line agent accordingly may improve those odds. Ponatinib is the only TKI with significant activity in CML associated with *T315I* mutation. Once the maximum response has been realized, patients who are suitable transplant candidates are offered an allogeneic stem cell transplantation.

Patients presenting in blast phase require a more-aggressive approach and are generally treated with a combination of TKI and chemotherapy or with a second-generation tyrosine kinase inhibitor with or without chemotherapy. Patients who achieve responses are immediately evaluated for an allogeneic SCT. The outcome of allogeneic SCT in advanced CML is much worse than in the chronic phase, but a minority of patients can definitely be cured.

Allogeneic Stem Cell Transplantation
The curative potential of allogeneic SCT is well established, and transplantation remains the widely accepted regimen for patients who failed imatinib. Historically, in the pre-imatinib era the allogeneic SCT has been reported to produce long-term survival between 50% and 60%—and even as high as 80% for larger, more experienced centers—in patients who underwent transplantation in the chronic phase.

Chronic Lymphocytic Leukemia
CLL has historically been considered an indolent disease of older patients. The general approach to treatment was conservative and the few therapies available were only marginally effective; since the 1990s, new treatments, namely purine analogues and monoclonal antibodies, started to change the face of this disease. Intensive research over the past several years provided greatly improved insight into the pathogenesis of CLL and led to the development of several targeted treatment approaches that will likely dramatically change the way we treat CLL. The availability of novel agents that are less toxic and more effective has rekindled hope that treatments with higher curative potential can be developed.

Epidemiology and Risk Factors
The median age at diagnosis is 70 years. The incidence is higher in men, and the male-to-female ratio is 1.7:1. It is the most common leukemia in the Western world; it is rare is Asian people and remains rare in people of Japanese origin who live in Hawaii, suggesting a genetic rather than environmental predisposition. An increased risk of developing the disease has been described in first-degree relatives of patients with CLL.

Pathogenesis
CLL develops by progressive accumulation of genetically altered mature lymphocytes in the blood, bone marrow, and lymphoid tissue. The CLL cell of origin is a B cell arrested in its pathway of differentiation, intermediate between a pre-B cell and mature B cell. One of the most important genetic parameters defining clinical behavior and prognosis is the mutation status of the variable segments of immunoglobulin heavy chain *VH* gene: CLL with unmutated *VH* shows an unfavorable course with rapid progression, whereas CLL with mutated *VH* typically shows slow progression and long survival.

FISH detects genetic aberrations in more than 80% of patients with CLL. The FISH CLL panel typically includes probes for 13q, 11q, 17p, and 6q deletions and for 12q duplication. The most common abnormality is deletion of 13q, which occurs in more than 50% of patients. Persons showing 13q14 abnormalities have a relatively benign disease that usually manifests as stable or slowly progressive isolated lymphocytosis. Trisomy 12 is associated with atypical morphology and progressive disease. Deletions of bands 11q22-q23 are associated with extensive lymph node involvement, aggressive disease, and shorter survival. Deletion of 17p results in loss of function of *p53* and is associated with a particularly poor prognosis.

Clinical Manifestations
The clinical features of CLL are variable and depend on the stage of the disease. Up to 30% of patients with CLL are asymptomatic, and the diagnosis is established following the incidental discovery of leukocytosis and/or absolute lymphocytosis on routine screening tests. The remaining patients present with lymphadenopathy, splenomegaly, or B symptoms (fever, night sweats, and weight loss), alone or in combination. Anemia and thrombocytopenia are considered late signs of the disease but can be present at the time of diagnosis. Due to their immunocompromised state, patients can present with recurrent or persistent infections.

Diagnosis
The diagnosis of CLL requires demonstration of absolute lymphocytosis of greater than 5000/mL and an immunophenotypic evidence of monoclonal population of mature B cells expressing CD19, CD20 (dim), and CD23 and coexpressing pan–T-cell antigen CD5. The malignant cells express low density of monoclonal surface immunoglobulin (IgM or IgD) with either κ or λ light chain. Patients are evaluated and grouped prognostically based on physical examination and complete blood count. The bone marrow biopsy and computed tomography scans are not required for diagnosis but may be indicated based on symptoms.

Differential Diagnosis
The immunophenotypic profile of CLL is quite characteristic, but at times it has to be differentiated from other low-grade lymphoproliferative disorders: hairy cell leukemia, prolymphocytic leukemia, (splenic) marginal zone lymphoma, and lymphoplasmacytic lymphoma. Most importantly, CLL needs to be differentiated from mantle cell lymphoma, which also coexpresses CD5 but is characteristically CD23 negative and cycline D1 positive by immunohistochemical staining.

Prognosis
The natural history of CLL is extremely variable, with survival times ranging from 2 to 20 (or more) years. Clinical staging using the Rai or Binet system provides a good estimate of prognosis but is not very reliable in an individual patient; for example, among patients presenting with early clinical stage disease, up to 30% never progress and eventually die of causes unrelated to CLL, and another 30% progress much more rapidly than expected. A number of additional prognostic factors are considered in estimating prognosis in an individual case: clinical characteristics such as age, sex, and performance status; laboratory parameters reflecting the tumor burden or disease activity such as lymphocyte count, lactate dehydrogenase (LDH), bone marrow infiltration pattern, or lymphocyte doubling time; serum markers such as soluble CD23 and β_2-microglobulin; and genetic markers such as genetic aberrations (see earlier), the *VH* mutation status, or its surrogate markers (CD38, ZAP-70).

Treatment
Early alkylating drug-based treatment strategies in CLL offered control of symptoms but little impact on the natural course of the disease. The introduction of purine analogues in the 1980s represented definite progress but it was not until they were combined with monoclonal antibodies that deeper and more meaningful remissions were experienced. The analysis of historical series suggests that immunotherapeutic regimens offer a modest prolongation of survival. The BCR pathway kinase inhibitors approved in the past few years are certainly very promising in this regard. However at present, short of allogeneic stem cell transplant, CLL is still considered incurable. Asymptomatic patients with CLL are followed expectantly. The treatment is initiated upon progression of the disease or appearance of symptoms such as rapid lymphocyte doubling time, bulky lymphadenopathy or organomegaly, disease-related B symptoms, and autoimmune or nonautoimmune cytopenias. CLL is quite sensitive to many chemo- and immunotherapeutic agents. However, remissions are rarely durable. The disease follows a remitting and relapsing pattern, and most patients receive at least a few different regimens throughout the course of their disease.

First-Line Therapy
The first-line treatment usually consists of the purine analogue fludarabine (Fludara)-based chemotherapy in combination with

the anti-CD20 monoclonal antibody rituximab (Rituxan). FR (fludarabine and rituximab) and FCR (fludarabine, cyclophosphamide [Cytoxan], and rituximab) are the chemoimmunotherapy combinations used most commonly. The overall response rates for these regimens are, respectively, 90% and 95%. FCR offers a higher complete remission rate of 70% versus 47% for FR; however, FR offers a more acceptable toxicity profile. Median overall survival with each of these regimens seems comparable: approximately 5 years. FCR may be particularly effective in CLL associated with del(11q). However, in general the choice between the regimens is made based on the patient's characteristics and the goals of therapy. The treatment cycles are administered every 28 days for up to 6 cycles.

Other treatment options used in the newly diagnosed progressive disease setting include PCR (deoxycoformycin [Pentostatin (Nipent)],[1] cyclophosphamide, and rituximab); bendamustine (Treanda); the anti-CD25 antibody alemtuzumab (Campath); or chlorambucil (Leukeran). Deoxycoformycin is another purine analogue, and the PCR regimen offers an alternative to FCR. The fludarabine-based regimens are only marginally effective in high-risk disease defined by the presence of del(17p). Patients with del-(17p) either do not respond to initial treatment or relapse soon after achieving remission. Therefore, other therapies, including investigational therapies, are often offered in this setting. Alemtuzumab is the only FDA-approved agent that has demonstrated activity in cells lacking *p53* function, as seen in patients with deletion of chromosome 17p.

Bendamustine (Treanda) is an alkylating agent approved for treatment of CLL in March 2008. Based on the results of a randomized trial, like fludarabine, it offers a higher response rate and progression-free survival in comparison to single agent chlorambucil. The toxicity of bendamustine seems intermediate between that of fludarabine and chlorambucil. In the past few years the combination of bendamustine and rituximab (BR) has become an acceptable alternative for patients who are unable to tolerate fludarabine due to co-morbid conditions or due to age. Many older patients too frail to tolerate either fludarabine or bendamustine could still be treated with chlorambucil combined with a novel anti-CD20 antibody either obinutuzumab (Gazyva) or ofatumumab (Arzerra). Both antibodies have been approved for this indication based on greater improvement in response rates and progression-free survival demonstrated in randomized trials. The initial results of those trials also suggest a benefit in overall survival.

Other Therapeutic Options

Relapsed disease occurs in a patient who achieved at least a partial remission that lasted more than 6 months after completion of treatment. Many of those patients can be re-treated successfully with the same medications or can be switched to an alternative strategy. Specifically, it has been demonstrated that patients initially treated with fludarabine often achieve another durable response upon re-treatment. Whether patients treated with fludarabine-containing combination regimens or other newer therapies such as alemtuzumab or bendamustine will respond to re-treatment equally well is not yet known.

Patients who fail to achieve at least a partial remission or whose disease progresses within 6 months from completion of treatment have refractory disease, which is associated with a poor prognosis. Patients refractory to fludarabine historically had expected median survival of 48 weeks and only an 11% likelihood of responding to other therapies, which included alkylating drugs, other purine analogues, high-dose steroids, or monoclonal antibodies (rituximab, alemtuzumab, ofatumumab). The year 2014 was remarkable for FDA approval of two novel agents for treatment of relapsed/refractory CLL. Ibrutinib (Imbruvica) is an oral BTK inhibitor. A randomized trial in relapsed/refractory CLL confirmed a superior response rate and survival when

compared with ofatumumab. The drug produces a rapid and sustained decrease in lymphadenopathy coupled by lymphocytosis. Idelalisib (Zydelig) is an oral inhibitor of PI3K kinase, which in combination with rituximab was shown to have a superior therapeutic activity over rituximab. A phase III randomized trial was stopped prematurely after it demonstrated improved response rate and improved survival over rituximab alone.

Both drugs can be taken by mouth and are well tolerated. Interestingly both drugs generally induce only partial remission, yet, they translate to prolongation of survival. Furthermore it appears that continuation of the drugs is necessary to maintain remissions.

At this time it is still unclear what role these new drugs will play in treatment of CLL.

Patients are encouraged to participate in clinical trials. Those who are potential transplant candidates are considered for an allogeneic stem cell transplant.

Allogeneic stem cell transplantation remains the only potentially curative treatment modality. Unfortunately, data on the use of allogeneic stem cell transplantation are limited to small case series. Allogeneic stem cell transplantation is associated with considerable treatment-related morbidity and mortality and is usually not considered until definitive evidence of poor prognosis.

Complications

Major complications of CLL include cytopenias and immune dysfunction. Anemia and thrombocytopenia can result from direct infiltration of the bone marrow and hypersplenism, in which case response to treatment usually results in improvement. Splenectomy obtained either surgically or via splenic irradiation is clinically useful in patients with splenomegaly and profound cytopenias unresponsive to chemotherapy. Autoimmune hemolytic anemia and thrombocytopenia seen in a significant percentage of patients often respond to steroids. Danazol,[1] high-dose intravenous immunoglobulin (IVIg) (Gammagard),[1] cyclosporine (Neoral),[1] and rituximab[1] have all also been used in this setting.

Infections are the major cause of mortality in CLL. They result from hypogammaglobulinemia, impaired T-cell function, and neutropenia. Patients with repeat major bacterial infections are candidates for treatment with high-dose IVIg.[1] Patients treated with purine analogues and alemtuzumab are at high risk for opportunistic infections by herpes simplex virus and herpes zoster virus, *Listeria monocytogenes*, *Pneumocystis jiroveci*, and cytomegalovirus and should be offered prophylaxis with acyclovir (Zovirax),[1] trimethoprim-sulfamethoxazole (Bactrim), or aerosolized pentamidine (NebuPent) and antifungal agents. Patients receiving alemtuzumab should be monitored for cytomegalovirus reactivation or disease.

Patients with CLL have been reported to have a higher risk of developing other hematologic and solid malignancies. It is unknown how much of this increased risk is due to the underlying disease and accompanying chronic immunosuppression and how much is due to the treatments given. In 5% to 10% of patients with CLL, the disease transforms into an aggressive large-cell lymphoma (Richter's transformation) or prolymphocytic leukemia.

References

Baccarani M, Deininger MW, Rosti G, et al: European LeukemiaNet recommendations for the management of chronic myeloid leukemia, *Blood* 122(6):872–884, 2013.

Byrd JC, Rai K, Peterson BL, et al: Addition of rituximab to fludarabine may prolong progression-free survival and overall survival in patients with previously untreated chronic lymphocytic leukemia: an updated retrospective comparative analysis of CALGB 9712 and CALGB 9011, *Blood* 105:49–53, 2005.

Deininger MW, O'Brien SG, Ford JM, Druker BJ: Practical management of patients with chronic myeloid leukemia receiving imatinib, *J Clin Oncol* 21:1637–1647, 2003.

Druker BJ, Guilhot F, O'Brien SG, et al: Five-year follow-up of patients receiving imatinib for chronic myeloid leukemia, *N Engl J Med* 355:2408–2417, 2006.

Goldman JM: Initial treatment for patients with CML, *Am Soc Hematol Educ Program* 453–460, 2009.

Hallek M: Chronic lymphocytic leukemia: 2013 update on diagnosis, risk stratification and treatment, *Am J Hematol* 88(9):803–816, 2013.

Hallek M: Signaling the end of chronic lymphocytic leukemia: new frontline treatment strategies, *Blood* 122(23):3723–3734, 2013.

---

[1] Not FDA approved for this indication.

---

[1] Not FDA approved for this indication.

Kantarjian H, Shah NP, Hochhaus A, et al: Dasatinib versus imatinib in newly diagnosed chronic-phase chronic myeloid leukemia, *N Engl J Med* 363:2260–2270, 2010.

Keating MJ, Chiorazzi N, Messmer B, et al: Biology and treatment of chronic lymphocytic leukemia, *Hematology Am Soc Hematol Educ Program* 153–175, 2003.

Lee SJ: Chronic myelogenous leukaemia, *Br J Haematol* 111:993–1009, 2000.

Lozanski G, Heerema NA, Flinn IW, et al: Alemtuzumab is an effective therapy for chronic lymphocytic leukemia with *p53* mutations and deletions, *Blood* 103:3278–3281, 2004.

Saglio G, Kim DW, Issaragrisil S, et al: Nilotinib versus imatinib for newly diagnosed chronic myeloid leukemia, *N Engl J Med* 362:2251–2259, 2010.

Sokal risk score calculator. Available at http://www.mdcalc.com/sokal-index-for-cml (accessed July 19, 2016).

Tam CS, O'Brien S, Wierda W, et al: Long-term results of the fludarabine, cyclophosphamide, and rituximab regimen as initial therapy of chronic lymphocytic leukemia, *Blood* 112:975–980, 2008.

DISSEMINATED INTRAVASCULAR COAGULATION

Method of
Kenneth Byrd, DO

CURRENT DIAGNOSIS

- Disseminated intravascular coagulation (DIC) is an abnormal activation of the coagulation system that is caused by predisposing conditions such as sepsis, malignancy, and trauma.
- Clinical manifestations include organ injury due to microvascular thrombosis and less commonly macrovascular thrombosis. DIC can alternatively present with severe bleeding.
- Laboratory findings include thrombocytopenia, elevated D-dimer, elevated international normalized ratio (INR) and partial thromboplastin time (PTT), and sometimes decreased fibrinogen.
- The International Society on Thrombosis and Haemostasis (ISTH) scoring system predicts overt DIC if score ≥5.

CURRENT TREATMENT

- Aggressive and prompt treatment of the underlying condition causing DIC is paramount.
- If the patient is bleeding or undergoing a procedure, aggressive transfusion support with platelets and fresh frozen plasma (FFP) or cryoprecipitate is often advised.
- Unless the patient is bleeding or undergoing a procedure, FFP or cryoprecipitate is usually not indicated, and platelets are only transfused if less than 20×10⁹/L. The major exception is acute promyelocytic leukemia (APL).
- Prophylactic low molecular weight heparin (LMWH) is often indicated in DIC.
- Therapeutic heparin/LMWH is rarely indicated in DIC unless there is clear evidence of a severe prothrombotic state.
- No other treatments are routinely used for DIC, including antithrombin, activated protein C, antifibrinolytics, and thrombomodulin. However, the role of these agents continues to be evaluated.

Introduction

Disseminated intravascular coagulation (DIC) is a complex and often life-threatening manifestation of an acquired disease process. This process stimulates a strong procoagulant cascade that leads to thromboses throughout the vasculature. A risk of hemorrhage often follows due to a depletion of platelets, consumption of coagulation factors, and accelerated plasmin formation.

Epidemiology

DIC has been reported in approximately 10% to 20% of critical care admissions. It is an independent predictor of mortality, and when DIC accompanies sepsis there is a two-fold increased risk of mortality versus sepsis alone. Mortality rates vary based on the scoring system used but can be as high as 46%. The mortality rate appears to correlate with the severity of laboratory abnormalities at diagnosis.

Pathophysiology

DIC is primarily a coagulation dysfunction due to excessive procoagulant activity. The overactivation is multifactorial but is primarily due to the generation of excessive thrombin, which is mediated by the extrinsic pathway involving tissue factor and factor VIIa. Thrombin excess leads to increased platelet aggregation and thrombotic occlusion of small and midsize vessels with fibrin. Vascular occlusion leads to the derangement of oxygen supply and tissue demand, which can compromise multiple organs. This effect is compounded by defects in inhibitors of coagulation as well as fibrinolytic suppression. Antithrombin activity is diminished due to increased consumption, degradation, and impaired synthesis. Likewise, protein C, tissue factor-pathway inhibitor (TFPI), and thrombomodulin activity are decreased in part due to excess inflammatory cytokines. Fibrinolytic suppression occurs in many instances of DIC due to an increase in plasminogen activator inhibitor-1 (PAI-1), which is the principal inhibitor of the fibrinolytic system.

The excessive activation of the coagulation pathway subsequently leads to the depletion of platelets and clotting factors. However, the cause of bleeding in DIC is multifactorial, including consumption of clotting factors, thrombocytopenia, platelet dysfunction, endothelial damage, and fibrin degradation products (FDPs) causing a feedback anticoagulant effect.

Clinical Manifestations

The manifestations of DIC are often obscured by the underlying causative etiology. Many times, the diagnosis of DIC is solely laboratory based without any clear clinical manifestations. At other times, DIC may be overtly symptomatic. Recently, it has been suggested that DIC could be divided into clinical subtypes that include asymptomatic, bleeding, and organ failure types. The presentation depends on whether there is a predominance of thrombosis from excessive thrombin activation or bleeding from consumptive coagulopathy.

Overall, the incidence of major bleeding in DIC is 5% to 12%. DIC that presents with acute bleeding is most commonly seen in acute leukemia, obstetric disorders, and trauma. Typical hemorrhagic features of DIC include bleeding from venipuncture sites or indwelling catheters, generalized ecchymosis that develops spontaneously or with minimal trauma, bleeding from mucous membranes, unexpected and major bleeding from around drain sites or tracheostomies, and concealed hemorrhage in serous cavities such as retroperitoneal hemorrhage.

Thrombotic organ failure type of DIC is most commonly seen with sepsis. The incidence of organ involvement secondary to thrombosis is 10% to 40%. This occurs due to thromboses in small and midsize vessels. Many organs can be involved, but it is most commonly seen in the kidneys, lungs, liver, and brain. This can manifest as respiratory distress syndrome, acute kidney injury, confusion, and seizures. The skin can also be involved and present as purpura fulminans or acral ischemia. Macrovascular thrombosis such as venous thromboembolism may present as a later manifestation.

Diagnosis

Making the diagnosis of DIC starts with identifying an underlying associated disease state. Table 1 lists the known risk factors for DIC. Once this is established, the diagnosis entails a combination of laboratory values along with an analysis of the clinical presentation. The difficulty with diagnosing DIC is that there is no gold standard and no pathognomonic test. There have been several scoring systems developed for DIC to assist in standardizing the diagnosis. The most commonly utilized is the International Society on Thrombosis and Haemostasis (ISTH) scoring system,

TABLE 1	Risk Factors for Disseminated Intravascular Coagulation (Incidence of Disseminated Intravascular Coagulation Per Etiology)

- Sepsis (35%)
  - Most commonly bacterial
- Severe trauma (up to 50%)
  - Most commonly brain injury or burns
- Malignancy
  - Metastatic cancer (up to 20%)
  - Acute leukemia (15%)
  - Acute promyelocytic leukemia (90%)
- Obstetrical
  - Placental abruption
  - Amniotic fluid embolism
  - Postpartum hemorrhage
  - Acute fatty liver of pregnancy
- Vascular malformations
  - Kasabach-Merritt syndrome
  - Large aortic aneurysms
  - Other large vascular malformations
- Severe immunologic reaction
  - Acute hemolytic transfusion reaction
  - Anaphylaxis
- Heat stroke
- Postcardiopulmonary resuscitation

TABLE 2	International Society on Thrombosis and Haemostasis Scoring System

Platelet count × 10⁹/L
- ≥100 = 0
- <100 = 1
- <50 = 2

Fibrin marker levels (D-dimer, fibrin degradation products)
- No increase = 0
- Moderate increase (>ULN but <5× ULN) = 2
- Strong increase (≥5× ULN) = 3

Prothrombin time
- <3 s (*INR <1.3) = 0
- ≥3 but <6 s (*INR 1.3–1.5) = 1
- ≥6 s (*INR ≥ 1.6) = 2

Fibrinogen
- >100 mg/dL = 0
- ≤100 mg/dL = 1

*Assuming the International Survey Index value of the thromboplastin reagents used is close to 1
- A score of ≥5 points is compatible with overt DIC
- The scoring system is only appropriate in patients with an underlying disorder that can be associated with DIC
- If the score if <5 and DIC is still suspected, then consider repeating labs in 1–2 days

DIC, Disseminated intravascular coagulation; ULN, upper limits of normal.

which was originally devised in 2001 and has been subsequently validated. The scoring system is outlined in Table 2. A score of ≥5 verifies overt DIC. A score of less than 5 could indicate a lack of DIC or nonovert DIC (i.e., subtle and compensated hemostatic dysfunction). The ISTH scoring system has a sensitivity of 93% and a specificity of 98%. Most other available scoring systems are more sensitive but less specific for DIC. Importantly, if DIC is suspected but not confirmed, then labs should be repeated to assess trends.

The decreased platelet count in DIC is due to excessive thrombin activation and is almost always less than 100 × 10⁹/L and often trending down. A normal platelet count without a downward trend would essentially rule out DIC. The INR and PTT are often elevated due to consumption of coagulation factors but can be normal in up to 50% of cases. The vast majority of DIC is also marked by an increase in fibrin markers due to increased

fibrinolysis. Traditionally, FDPs were used but have largely been replaced by D-dimer. Fibrinogen is often low but can be normal as it is also an acute phase reactant. It is only rarely severely diminished. A low level of fibrinogen usually reflects the late, severe consumptive stage of DIC.

Thromboelastography (TEG) and rotational thromboelastometry (ROTEM) testing have been evaluated to assess overall coagulation, including platelet function as well as clot dissolving potential. TEG has demonstrated good correlation with clinically important organ dysfunction and survival, although its advantage over usual coagulation assays has not yet been confirmed. The role of these two modalities in DIC is still unclear.

DIC often presents with a small population of schistocytes. If the red blood cell population is greater than 10% schistocytes, then an alternative diagnosis is more likely (i.e., TTP). Of note, a low ADAMTS-13 can be seen in DIC but is certainly not specific. There is also frequently a reduction in antithrombin and protein C. These tests are not done routinely and are likely not as sensitive as the ISTH scoring system. Finally, factor VIII can be low in DIC due to consumption, but it can also be elevated at times as it is an acute phase reactant.

The differential diagnosis of DIC is explained in Table 3.

Therapy

The foundation of treatment for DIC is to treat the underlying disorder. If the underlying disorder is reversed, then DIC typically resolves.

During active DIC there may be a need for transfusion support. It is important to note that the following transfusion recommendations are mostly based on low quality evidence, including expert opinion. In the presence of bleeding, platelet transfusions should be given to keep platelet count greater than 30 to 50 × 10⁹/L. Similarly, in the setting of invasive procedures, platelets should be maintained greater than 20 to 50 × 10⁹/L, depending on the risk of the procedure. Importantly, in the absence of bleeding or procedure, platelets should be transfused only if platelet count is less than 20 × 10⁹/L (a range of 10 to 30 × 10⁹/L has been proposed by various sources). The exception to this threshold would be acute promyelocytic leukemia (APL), in which platelets should be maintained greater than 30 to 50 × 10⁹/L even in the absence of bleeding (less commonly some sources maintain a greater than 20 × 10⁹/L threshold).

A similar approach to the replacement of factors is indicated. If the patient is bleeding or undergoing a high risk procedure and fibrinogen is less than 150 mg/dL or PT/PTT is greater than 1.5 upper limits of normal (ULN), then fresh frozen plasma (FFP) or cryoprecipitate is recommended. Keep in mind the FFP contains all factors of the soluble coagulation system, while cryoprecipitate contains a concentrated subset of plasma factors including fibrinogen, factor VIII, von Willebrand factor, and factor XIII. The choice between FFP and cryoprecipitate is made on a case-by-case basis and can often be influenced by fluid status. The recommended dose of FFP is 15 to 30 mL/kg and cryoprecipitate is 5 to 10 units. A less frequently used option is 2 g of fibrinogen concentrate. Factor replacement is not indicated in the absence of bleeding or procedure. An exception to this threshold is APL, in which factor replacement could be considered if fibrinogen less than 100 to 150 mg/dL, even in the absence of bleeding.

In addition to transfusion support and treatment of the underlying etiology, heparin[1] can be considered in a few circumstances. Most importantly, guidelines recommend prophylactic dose LMWH in the absence of bleeding as long as platelet count is greater than 20 to 30 × 10⁹/L, INR greater than 1.5, and fibrinogen greater than 100 mg/dL. This is especially vital in prothrombotic DIC (i.e., solid malignancy, sepsis). An exception to the general use of LMWH prophylaxis is in hyperfibrinolytic DIC (i.e., APL and prostate cancer), in which more caution is advised with heparin use. Therapeutic heparin is uncommonly advised in DIC, but it can be considered in prothrombotic DIC, as evidenced by

---

[1]Not FDA approved for this indication

TABLE 3 Differential Diagnosis of Disseminated Intravascular Coagulation

DISEASE	SIMILARITIES	DIFFERENCES	COMMENTS
Liver disease	Low plt; prolonged PT/PTT; low fibrinogen; increased FDP (less elevation with liver disease)	No schistocytes in liver disease and sometimes in DIC; worsening labs in DIC and more stable in liver disease	Factor VIII not very helpful for differentiation. Normal or elevated in liver disease (not synthesized in liver). However, as an acute phase reactant, often normal or elevated in DIC
Thrombotic microangiopathy (TMA)	Low plt; increased FDP (less elevation with TMA); ADAMTS can be low in DIC, but much lower in TMA	MAHA in TMA; Normal PT/PTT and fibrinogen in TMA; numerous schistocytes common in TMA, but not DIC	Extremely low plt with normal PT/PTT is common in TMA but unusual in DIC; TMA includes TTP and HUS
Heparin-induced thrombocytopenia (HIT)	Low plt, increased FDP	Normal PT/PTT in HIT; low fibrinogen unusual in HIT	Plt <20 × 10⁹/L is uncommon in HIT
Catastrophic antiphospholipid syndrome (CAPS)	Low plt; increased FDP; PTT elevation (false elevation of PTT commonly due to LA)	Normal PT often screen in CAPS; lab diagnosis of APLS	Normal plt often seen in CAPS and severe thrombocytopenia is rare; microvascular thromboses in both; macrovascular thrombosis is a more common initial presentation of CAPS than DIC
Hemophagocytic lymphohistiocytosis (HLH)	Low plt; prolonged clotting screen; low fibrinogen; increased FDP	HLH with very high ferritin, TGs, organomegaly, and often hemophagocytosis	

APLS, Antiphospholipid antibody syndrome; *DIC*, disseminated intravascular coagulation; *FDP*, fibrin degradation products; *LA*, lupus anticoagulant; *MAHA*, microangiopathic hemolytic anemia; *plt*, platelet count; *PT*, prothrombin time; *PTT*, partial thromboplastin time; *TG*, triglycerides; *TTP*, thrombotic thrombocytopenic purpura.

thromboembolism, purpura fulminans, or acral ischemia. As heparin can partially inhibit activation of the coagulation, it would make sense that it could help offset DIC. In small studies, heparin has shown beneficial effects on coagulation parameters. However, improvement in clinically important outcomes in DIC has not been clearly demonstrated.

Other therapies that have been studied in the treatment of DIC include antithrombin concentrate (AT [Thrombate III]),[1] activated protein C (APC), recombinant thrombomodulin, and antifibrinolytics. Currently, these agents are rarely, if ever, indicated for use. AT and APC have been extensively studied in the setting of sepsis. One of the issues in assessing the benefit of AT and APC is that many clinical trials assess the general sepsis population and do not limit analysis to those specifically with DIC. For AT, there has been no significant reduction in mortality in these studies. However, there is a suggestion that there may be significant benefit in the subset of patients with severe sepsis and DIC. This requires prospective validation. APC has also shown promise at times, including improvement in mortality in an early randomized controlled trial (RCT). However, subsequent studies showed an increased risk of serious bleeding and lack of survival benefit. Therefore, the FDA advised to stop using APC for DIC in 2011.

Caution is advised with the use of antifibrinolytics in DIC. Since the excessive fibrin deposition appears in part to be due to insufficient fibrinolysis, further inhibition of the fibrinolytic system would clearly not be appropriate. This is especially the case in sepsis, but there are a few exceptions to this. Antifibrinolytics can be considered in hyperfibrinolytic DIC (i.e., APL or prostate cancer) only in the setting of life threatening bleeding. The other exception is in acute trauma. A large RCT showed that early use of antifibrinolytics in trauma was beneficial. However, once the acute phase has passed, further thrombin generation eventually predominates, and the balance is tipped toward thrombosis.

Recombinant soluble thrombomodulin continues to be actively evaluated and shows some potential. A 2013 RCT of thrombomodulin versus placebo in sepsis with DIC showed improvement in coagulation parameters. There was a trend towards mortality benefit with thrombomodulin, but this was not statistically proven. There was an updated systematic review in 2019 continuing to show only a nonsignificant trend towards mortality benefit with thrombomodulin. There is an ongoing phase III trial in patients with severe sepsis and coagulopathy.

Finally, it is worth mentioning that a Cochrane review evaluated recombinant factor VIIa (NovoSeven)[1] and concluded that it does not have proven efficacy in DIC and that there is an increased risk of arterial thrombotic events. Its use is not advised.

References

Bakhtiari K, Meijers JC, de Jonge E, Levi M: Prospective validation of the International Society of Thrombosis and Haemostasis scoring system for disseminated intravascular coagulation, *Crit Care Med* 32(12):2416–2421, 2004.

Bernard GR, Vincent JL, Laterre PF, et al: Efficacy and safety of recombinant human activated protein C for severe sepsis, *N Engl J Med* 344(10):699–709, 2001.

Gando S, Levi M, Toh CH: Disseminated intravascular coagulation, *Nat Rev Dis Primers* 2:16037, 2016.

Levi M: Pathogenesis and diagnosis of disseminated intravascular coagulation, *Int J Lab Hematol* 40:15–20, 2018.

Levi M, Scully M: How I treat disseminated intravascular coagulation, *Blood* 131(8):845–854, 2018.

Sanz MA, Grimwade D, Tallman MS, et al: Management of acute promyelocytic leukemia: recommendations from an expert panel on behalf of the European Leukemianet, *Blood* 113(9):1875–1891, 2009.

Squizzato A, Hunt BJ, Kinasewitz GT, et al: Supportive management strategies for disseminated intravascular coagulation, *ThrombHaemost* 116(05):896–904, 2016.

Vincent JL, Ramesh MK, Ernest D, et al: A randomized, double-blind, placebo-controlled, Phase 2b study to evaluate the safety and efficacy of recombinant human soluble thrombomodulin, ART-123, in patients with sepsis and suspected disseminated intravascular coagulation, *Crit Care Med* 41(9):2069–2079, 2013.

Wada H, Thachil J, Di Nisio M, et al: Guidance for diagnosis and treatment of disseminated intravascular coagulation from harmonization of the recommendations from three guidelines, *J ThrombHaemost* 11(4):761–767, 2013.

Warren BL, Eid A, Singer P, et al: High-dose antithrombin III in severe sepsis: a randomized controlled trial, *JAMA* 286(15):1869–1878, 2001.

---

[1]Not FDA approved for this indication

HEMOCHROMATOSIS

Method of
Paul C. Adams, MD

CURRENT DIAGNOSIS

- Consider the diagnosis in patients with Northern European ancestry.
- Initial testing is transferrin saturation or unsaturated iron binding capacity and serum ferritin.
- Secondary testing is the C282Y genetic test.
- More than 90% of typical hemochromatosis patients are homozygotes for the C282Y mutation.
- If genetic testing is not typical, reassess the diagnosis and consider secondary iron overload related to cirrhosis, alcoholism, viral hepatitis, or an iron-loading anemia.
- A number of other hemochromatosis genetic mutations are relevant to only a minority of patients.
- Not all patients need a liver biopsy.
- Siblings are at highest risk in a family study.

CURRENT THERAPY

- Iron overload from hemochromatosis is treated by the weekly removal of 500 mL of blood until the serum ferritin is in the low-normal range of approximately 50 µg/L.
- Some but not all patients require maintenance therapy with three to four phlebotomies per year. In some countries, this can be a voluntary blood donation.
- Excess alcohol, high doses of vitamin C, and iron supplementation should be avoided, but strict dietary restrictions are not recommended.
- Siblings and children of patients should be tested for hemochromatosis with transferrin saturation, ferritin, and genetic testing.

Hemochromatosis is the most common genetic disease in populations of European ancestry. The diagnosis can be elusive because of the nonspecific nature of the symptoms. With the discovery of the hemochromatosis gene (*HFE*) in 1996 came new insights into the pathogenesis of the disease and new diagnostic strategies.

A fundamental issue that arose after the discovery of the *HFE* gene is whether the disease hemochromatosis should be defined strictly on phenotypic criteria such as the degree of iron overload (i.e., transferrin saturation, ferritin, liver biopsy, hepatic iron concentration, iron removed by venesection therapy), or whether the condition should be defined as a familial disease in Europeans most commonly associated with the C282Y mutation of the *HFE* gene and varying degrees of iron overload. Because the genetic test has been increasingly used as a diagnostic tool, most studies now use a combination of phenotypic and genotypic criteria for the diagnosis of hemochromatosis.

Clinical Features

Although hemochromatosis is often classified as a liver disease, it should be emphasized that it is a systemic genetic disease with multisystem involvement. The liver is central in both diagnosis and prognosis. Hepatomegaly remains one of the more common physical signs in hemochromatosis, but it is not always present in the young, asymptomatic homozygote. In a study of 717 homozygotes from Australia, 8% of men and 1.7% of women had cirrhosis of the liver at the time of diagnosis. The prevalence of cirrhosis in asymptomatic or screened patients is much lower. It is likely that there are factors other than iron overload that contribute to cirrhosis

in hemochromatosis. These can include the effects of alcohol or comodifying genes. The effect of iron depletion therapy is usually stabilization of the liver disease, and fibrosis improves with repeat liver biopsy after iron depletion. This accounts for the relatively small number of C282Y homozygotes that require liver transplantation. The other common clinical manifestations are arthralgias, pigmentation, congestive heart failure, impotence, and fatigue. Several large population studies failed to demonstrate an increase in diabetes compared with a control population. A population-based study estimated that only 28% of male and 1% of female C282Y homozygotes will develop symptoms of iron overload.

Diagnosis

A paradox of genetic hemochromatosis is that the disease is underdiagnosed in the general population and overdiagnosed in patients with secondary iron overload.

Preliminary population studies using genetic testing demonstrate a prevalence of homozygotes of approximately 1:227 among whites. The fact that many physicians consider hemochromatosis to be rare implies either a lack of penetrance of the gene (nonexpressing homozygote) or a large number of patients who remain undiagnosed in the community.

Diagnosis
Transferrin Saturation
Previous studies had suggested that transferrin saturation would be a good screening test and diagnostic test for hemochromatosis.

The sensitivity of transferrin saturation in population-screening studies designed to detect C282Y homozygotes (genotypic case definition) was only approximately 75%, and transferrin saturation can be in the normal range in young female homozygotes. A large biologic variation in transferrin saturation within an individual patient has also been reported.

Serum Ferritin
The relationship between serum ferritin and total body iron stores was clearly established by strong correlations with hepatic iron concentration and the amount of iron removed by venesection. However, ferritin can be elevated secondary to chronic inflammation and histiocytic neoplasms. A major diagnostic dilemma in the past was whether the serum ferritin concentration was related to hemochromatosis or to another underlying liver disease, such as alcoholic liver disease, chronic viral hepatitis, or nonalcoholic steatohepatitis. It is likely that most of these difficult cases can now be resolved by genetic testing.

Liver Biopsy
Liver biopsy was previously the gold-standard diagnostic test for hemochromatosis; however, it has shifted from a major diagnostic tool to a method of estimating prognosis and concomitant disease. The need for liver biopsy seems less clear now in the young, asymptomatic C282Y homozygote in whom there is a low clinical suspicion of cirrhosis based on history, physical examination, and liver biochemistry. A large study conducted in France and Canada suggested that C282Y homozygotes with a serum ferritin concentration of less than 1000 µg/L, a normal aspartate transaminase (AST) concentration, and no hepatomegaly have a very low risk of cirrhosis. C282Y homozygotes with a ferritin level greater than 1000 µg/L, an elevated AST, and a platelet count of less than 200,000/mm^3 have an 80% chance of having cirrhosis. Hepatic elastography is another noninvasive tool to assess liver fibrosis in hemochromatosis.

Patients with cirrhosis have a 5.5-fold relative risk of death compared with noncirrhotic hemochromatosis patients. Cirrhotic patients are also at increased risk of hepatocellular carcinoma. Liver biopsy is considered in typical C282Y homozygotes with liver dysfunction and in potentially iron-overloaded patients without the typical C282Y mutation. Simple C282Y heterozygotes, compound heterozygotes (C282Y/H63D), H63D homozygotes, and patients with other risk factors (e.g., alcohol abuse, chronic viral hepatitis) who have moderate to severe iron overload (ferritin > 1000 µg/L) may be considered for liver biopsy.

Since the introduction of genetic testing, hepatic iron concentration and hepatic iron index have become less useful in the diagnosis of hemochromatosis.

Genetic Testing

A major advance stemming from the discovery of the hemochromatosis gene is the use of a diagnostic genetic test. Most studies report that more than 90% of typical hemochromatosis patients were homozygotes for the C282Y mutation. A second minor mutation, H63D, was also described in the original report. Compound heterozygotes (C282Y/H63D) and, less commonly, H63D homozygotes, resemble C282Y homozygotes with mild to moderate iron overload. Genetic mutations involving ferroportin, hemojuvelin, transferrin receptor 2, ceruloplasmin, and hepcidin are associated with iron overload. It is likely that, as more mutations are found, they will be relevant to only a minority of patients. Commercial tests are rarely available for these rare genetic mutations.

Some patients with clinical pictures indistinguishable from genetic hemochromatosis are negative for the C282Y mutation. Most of these cases appear to be isolated, although a few cases of familial iron overload with negative C282Y testing have been reported. A negative C282Y test should alert the physician to question the diagnosis of genetic hemochromatosis and to reconsider secondary iron overload related to cirrhosis, alcoholism, viral hepatitis, or an iron-loading anemia. If no other risk factors are found, the patient should begin phlebotomy treatment, similar to any other hemochromatosis patient.

The interpretation of the genetic test in several settings is shown in Box 1. Genetic discrimination is a concern, given the widespread use of genetic testing, but discrimination has been rarely reported in screening studies. In the case of hemochromatosis, the advantages of early diagnosis of a treatable disease outweigh the disadvantages of genetic discrimination.

Family Studies

Once the proband case is identified and confirmed with the genetic test for the C282Y mutation, family testing is imperative. Siblings have approximately one in four chance of carrying the gene and should be screened with the genetic test (C282Y and H63D mutation), transferrin saturation, and serum ferritin. A cost-effective strategy now possible with genetic testing is to test the spouse for the C282Y mutation to assess the risk in the children. If the spouse is not a C282Y heterozygote or homozygote, the children will be obligate heterozygotes, assuming paternity and excluding another gene or mutation causing hemochromatosis. This strategy is particularly advantageous if the children are geographically separated or in different health care systems.

Treatment

The treatment of hemochromatosis continues to use the medieval therapy of periodic bleeding. Blood is removed, with the patient in the reclining position over 15 to 30 minutes. Initial treatment consists of the weekly removal of 500 mL of blood. A hemoglobin test is done before each phlebotomy. If the hemoglobin concentration has decreased to less than 10 g/dL, the phlebotomy schedule is modified to 500 mL every 2 weeks. Phlebotomies are continued until the serum ferritin concentration is approximately 50 µg/L. Serum ferritin levels are drawn monthly in patients with significant iron overload and increased to weekly as the ferritin decreases to < 200 µg/L. The concomitant administration of a salt-containing sport beverage (e.g., Gatorade) is a simple method of maintaining plasma volume during the phlebotomy.

Maintenance phlebotomies after iron depletion, consisting of three to four phlebotomies per year, are performed in most patients, although the rate of iron reaccumulation is highly variable. Maintenance therapy is initiated when the serum ferritin rises from 50 µg/L to > 300 µg/L. The transferrin saturation remains elevated in many treated patients and does not normalize unless the patient becomes iron deficient. In some countries, patients with mild iron abnormalities are encouraged to become voluntary blood donors.

Chelation therapy[1] is not recommended for hemochromatosis. Patients are advised to avoid oral iron therapy and alcohol abuse, but there are no dietary restrictions. Patient support groups have been concerned by the practice of iron fortification of foods, but much of this iron is in an inexpensive form with poor bioavailability.

Hemochromatosis is a common and often underdiagnosed disease. Early diagnosis and treatment result in an excellent long-term prognosis. The development of a diagnostic genetic test has improved the feasibility of the goal of prevention of morbidity and mortality from hemochromatosis.

---

[1]Not FDA approved for this indication.

BOX 1 — Interpretation of Genetic Testing for Hemochromatosis

"C282Y Homozygote"
This is the classic genetic pattern seen in more than 90% of typical cases. Expression of disease ranges from no evidence of iron overload to massive iron overload with organ dysfunction. Siblings have a one in four chance of being affected and should have genetic testing. For children to be affected, the other parent must be at least a heterozygote. If iron studies are normal, false-positive genetic testing or a nonexpressing homozygotic state should be considered

"C282Y/H63D Compound Heterozygote"
This patient carries two copies of the minor mutation. Most patients with this genetic pattern have normal iron studies. A small percentage have mild to moderate iron overload. Severe iron overload is usually seen in the setting of another concomitant risk factor (e.g., alcoholism, viral hepatitis)

"C282Y Heterozygote"
This patient carries one copy of the major mutation. This pattern is seen in approximately 10% of the white population and is usually associated with normal iron studies. In rare cases, the results of iron studies are high, in the range expected in a homozygote rather than a heterozygote. These patients may carry an unknown hemochromatosis mutation, and liver biopsy is helpful to determine the need for phlebotomy therapy

"H63D Homozygote"
Most patients with this genotype will have normal iron studies. A small percentage have mild to moderate iron overload. Severe iron overload is usually seen in the setting of another concomitant risk factor (e.g., alcoholism, viral hepatitis)

"H63D Heterozygote"
This patient carries one copy of the minor mutation. This pattern is seen in approximately 20% of the white population and is usually associated with normal iron studies. This pattern is so common in the general population that the presence of iron overload can be related to another risk factor. Liver biopsy is required to determine the cause of the iron overload and the need for treatment in these cases

"No HFE Mutations"
If iron overload is present without any mutations in the hemochromatosis gene (HFE), a careful history for other risk factors must be reviewed, and liver biopsy can be useful to determine the cause of the iron overload and the need for treatment. Most of these are isolated, nonfamilial cases. There are cases described involving genetic mutations in ferroportin, hemojuvelin, transferrin receptor 2, ceruloplasmin, and hepcidin genes. Genetic tests for these mutations are not widely available

References

Adams PC, Reboussin DM, Barton JC, et al: Hemochromatosis and iron overload screening (HEIRS) study: Screening in a racially diverse of primary care population, *N Engl J Med* 352:1769–1778, 2005a .

Adams PC: Hemochromatosis case definition: Out of focus, *Nat Clin Pract Gastroenterol Hepatol* 3:178–179, 2006.

Adams PC, Barton JC: How I treat hemochromatosis, *Blood* 116:317–325, 2010.

Allen KJ, Gurrin LC, Constantine CC, et al: Iron-overload-related disease in *HFE* hereditary hemochromatosis, *N Engl J Med* 358:221–230, 2008.

Bacon BR, Adams PC, Kowdley K, et al: Diagnosis and management of hemochromatosis: AASLD practice guidelines, *Hepatology* 54:328–343, 2011.

Beaton M, Guyader D, Deugnier Y, et al: Non-invasive prediction of cirrhosis in C282Y-linked hemochromatosis, *Hepatology* 36:673–678, 2002.

Brissot P, Pietrangelo A, Adams PC, de Graaf B, McLaren C, Loreal O. Nature Reviews Disease Primers: Haemochromatosis; 2018; (in press).

Falize L, Guillygomarch A, Perrin M, et al: Reversibility of hepatic fibrosis in treated hemochromatosis: A study of 36 cases, *Hepatology* 44:472–477, 2006.

Gordeuk V, Lovato L, Vitolins M, et al: Relationship between dietary iron intake and serum ferritin concentration in *HFE* homozygotes, *Can J Gastroenterol* 26:345–349, 2012.

Ong SY, Gurrin LC, Dolling L, et al: Reduction of body iron in HFE-related haemochromatosis and moderate iron overload: a multicentre, participant-blinded, randomised controlled trial. Lancet Haematol 4:e607-e614, 2017.

HEMOLYTIC ANEMIAS

Method of
Thomas G. DeLoughery, MD

CURRENT DIAGNOSES

- Suspect hemolysis when anemia is accompanied by signs of red cell breakdown—high low-density lipoprotein and indirect bilirubin with a low haptoglobin.
- The reticulocyte count is often high.
- A positive direct antibody test confirms the diagnosis of autoimmune hemolytic anemia in the presence of hemolysis.
- In patient with non-immune hemolysis, specific testing is required to make the diagnosis.

At the most basic level, hemolytic anemias are caused by red blood cell destruction. This destruction can be due to factors either intrinsic or extrinsic to the red blood cell. The pace of the hemolysis can vary from being only detectible by laboratory abnormalities to fulminant acute severe anemia. A useful way to think about hemolytic anemias is to divide them into hereditary disorders and acquired disorders (Table 1). Defects in any part of the red blood cell lead to inherited disorders, whereas acquired disorders are caused by immune-related processes and other etiologies extrinsic to the red blood cell.

Pathophysiology
Congenital
The major components of the red blood cell are the membrane, hemoglobin, and enzymes; therefore the three major classes of hereditary hemolytic anemias are due to defects in any of these three red blood cell components.

Hereditary spherocytosis is the most common hemolytic anemia caused by membrane defects. This condition is caused by mutations in the proteins that make up the red blood cell skeleton, which leads to an unstable membrane. The red blood cells in hereditary spherocytosis initially have a normal biconcave disc structure, but after repeated passage through the spleen, they gradually lose portions of the membrane and become more spherical as they age (a process known as *splenic conditioning*). These spherocytes are less deformable and because of that are ultimately trapped and destroyed in the spleen. Less common anemias due to membrane defects are hereditary elliptocytosis and pyropoikilocytosis. In elliptocytosis the skeletal defects are not as profound, so the clinical presentation is usually milder. Most patients with pyropoikilocytosis are homozygous for mutations that cause

TABLE 1	Hemolytic Anemia: Classification of Common Causes

Congenital

Membrane Defects

Hereditary Spherocytosis
Hereditary Elliptocytosis
Hereditary Pyropoikilocytosis

Enzymatic Defects

G-6-PD Deficiency
Pyruvate Kinase Deficiency

Hemoglobin Defects

Sickle Cell Disease
Unstable Hemoglobins

Acquired

Autoimmune

Warm Antibody IgG
Cold Antibody IgM
Drug-Induced
Paroxysmal Nocturnal Hemoglobinuria

Mechanical

Microangiopathic
Toxins
Parasites

elliptocytosis and have very unstable red blood cell membranes; often fragments of red blood cells are seen in the circulation.

The most common red blood cell enzyme defect is glucose-6-phosphate dehydrogenase (G6PD) deficiency. An adequate supply of reduced glutathione (GSH) is necessary to protect the erythrocyte from oxidative damage. G6PD catalyzes the conversion of glucose-6-phosphate to 6-phosphogluconate, in the process reducing NADP to NADPH. NADPH is necessary for the conversion of glutathione (GSSG) to reduced GSH. The erythrocyte does not have any other source of NADPH and so is dependent solely on this pathway for reducing power. When G6PD is deficient, this leads to decreased NADPH, which leads to decreased GSH. When the red blood cell undergoes oxidative stress, this lack of reducing power results in damage of red blood cell proteins, especially hemoglobin. These damaged proteins can aggregate, causing membrane damage and red blood cell destruction as the crystalized proteins are removed by the spleen.

Pyruvate kinase deficiency is a hemolytic anemia caused by an enzymatic defect in the glycolytic pathway. Pyruvate kinase catalyzes conversion of phosphoenolpyruvate to pyruvate, generating ATP in the same reaction. Deficiency of pyruvate kinase results in decreased levels of erythrocyte ATP. Lack of ATP results in a leaky cell membrane and loss of water and potassium. This leads to cellular dehydration and rigid, nondeformable cells, which are susceptible to destruction within the spleen.

By far the most common hereditary hemolytic hemoglobin defect is sickle cell anemia. The abnormal hemoglobin protein forms long polymers that disrupt red blood cell integrity. There are also very rare defects in hemoglobin that can cause unstable molecules that can crystallize and lead to hemolysis—most often due to splenic removal of damaged proteins.

Acquired
Autoimmune hemolytic anemias (AIHA) can be mediated by either anti-red blood cell immunoglobulin G (IgG) or immunoglobulin M (IgM) antibodies. In IgG-mediated disease, the antibody binds to red blood cell membrane proteins. The antibody-coated red blood cells are then phagocytized by macrophages found primarily in the spleen, leading to hemolysis.

In IgM-mediated hemolysis ("cold agglutinin disease"), the antibody binds to the red blood cell most often in the periphery of the body. The "cold" appellation comes from the fact that the antibody binds more strongly when below body temperature. Most commonly, complement is fixed only through C3, and then the C3-coated red blood cells are taken up by the macrophages. In rare patients the IgM can fix complement rapidly, leading to intravascular hemolysis by formation of the end product of complement the membrane attack complex.

Rare patients can develop immune hemolysis induced by medication. There have been three mechanisms proposed for drug AIHA. The hapten mechanism is most often associated with the use of high-dose penicillin. High doses of penicillin lead to drug incorporation into the red blood cell membrane by binding to proteins. Another mechanism is the formation of an immune complex of drug, antibody, and red blood cell membrane, which leads to hemolysis. Finally, patients taking certain drugs such as methyldopa will develop a positive direct antibody (DAT) after 6 months of therapy and hemolysis, which is indistinguishable from warm antibody AIHA.

In paroxysmal nocturnal hemoglobinuria (PNH), red blood cells lack the regulatory membrane proteins that inhibit activated complement proteins. These proteins include membrane inhibitor of reactive lysis (CD59) and decay-accelerating factor (CD55). The molecular defect in PNH is a mutation of the phosphatidyl inositol glycan complementation group A gene located on the X-chromosome. This enzyme is required for synthesis of glycosyl phosphatidylinositol (GPI)–linked proteins. Cells derived from the PNH stem cells are deficient in all proteins that are linked to the membrane by a GPI-molecule, including those that inactivate complement. Normally there is baseline activation of complement; it is believed that one of the functions of red blood cells is inactivation of these active complement proteins. When activated complement binds PNH red blood cells instead of being destroyed, the resulting membrane attack complex leads to lysis of the red blood cell.

Microangiopathic hemolytic anemias (MAHA) result from destruction of circulating red cells. Although MAHA is commonly associated with thrombotic microangiopathies such as thrombotic thrombocytopenia purpura (TTP) and hemolytic uremic syndrome (HUS), there are many other possible associated disease states. For example, patients with malignant hypertension can have very severe hemolysis due to increased shearing of red blood cells traversing damaged glomeruli. There may also be associated thrombocytopenia, which can lead to concern that TTP may be present. Hemolysis associated with malignant hypertension resolves rapidly with control of the blood pressure. Scleroderma renal crisis is often accompanied by a MAHA due to both severe hypertension and renal damage.

Cardiac valvular disease can lead to a MAHA. This is seen most commonly after mitral valve repair if there is a small defect at the site where the valve ring is sewn in. Ventricular contraction leads to a small resurgent jet, which results in a high-shear situation in the jet and red blood cell destruction. In some cases, this can result in severe hemolysis and a transfusion-dependent anemia.

Ventricular assist devices (VAD) to support heart failure patients can also lead to hemolysis. This is blood flowing through the device being subjected to high shear rates. Most patients have low levels of hemolysis, but with VAD thrombosis there is an abrupt increase in hemolysis due to higher shear forces; a rising LDH is an indication to look for VAD thrombosis.

Along with MAHA, there are several other syndromes that may cause mechanical damage to the red blood cells. Clostridium infections can lead to hemolysis by direct damage to red blood cell membranes. The bacteria secrete an alpha-toxin that has phospholipase activity and leads to the red blood cell membrane literally dissolving—which causes the hemoglobin to leak out of the cells. In some cases this can be so severe that the measured hemoglobin may equal the hematocrit. Empty red blood cell "ghosts" may be seen on the smear.

TABLE 2	Drugs That May Precipitate a Hemolytic Crisis With G6PD Deficiency
Acetanilide (Antifebrin)[4]	
Dapsone	
Furazolidone[2]	
Isobutyl Nitrate[4]	
Methylene Blue	
Nalidixic acid[2]	
Naphthalene	
Nitrofurantoin (Macrobid)	
Pamaquine[2]	
Phenazopyridine (Pyridium)	
Phenylhydrazine	
Primaquine	
Quinolones	
Sulfacetamide	
Sulfamethoxazole	
Sulfanilamide	
Sulfapyridine	

[2]Not available in the United States.
[4]Not yet approved for use in the United States.

Wilson's disease may cause episodes of hemolysis along with the neurologic and hepatic disease. This is caused by large amounts of hepatic copper entering the circulation and inducing an oxidative hemolysis. The smear can show spherocytes and "bite cell." The hemolysis is often transient because it is related to high levels of copper in the serum.

Spur cell anemia is a hemolytic process seen in patients with end-stage liver disease. The lipid metabolism alterations induced by severe liver disease lead to cholesterol crystal formation in the red cell membrane. These crystals are removed by the spleen and can lead to both hemolysis and deformed red cells—"spur cells."

Prevention

There are a few supportive steps in patients with hemolysis. Although most food is supplemented with folate, high red cell turn over can increase the need for this vitamin. Patients with hemolysis are often supplemented with folic acid 1 mg daily.[1]

A key preventive measure for those with G6PD deficiency is avoiding agents that can lead to oxidative stress of red cells. The most complete list of medications found at https://www.g6pd.org/ and common medications are listed in Table 2. Some rarer red blood cell enzymatic or hemoglobin defects are also sensitive to oxidative stress, so these medications should be avoided in those disease also.

Clinical Manifestations
Inherited

The severity of congenital hemolytic anemia varies tremendously. Some children are very symptomatic right after birth, whereas older patients may only present with mild anemia and subtle laboratory findings. A common presentation is a burst of hemolysis with oxidative or other stressors. Hereditary hemolytic anemias are often more severe right after birth, and severity may decrease with age. Patients with congenital anemia can present with extrahematologic problems. Given that the serum bilirubin is increased and more bilirubin is excreted in the bile, they may present with

[1]Not FDA approved for this indication.

pigmented gallstones. Patients can present with gallbladder disease in their teens or twenties, and this should raise the suspicion of hemolytic anemia. These patients may be more prone to skin ulcers around the ankle, which may not heal well.

Classically patients with congenital hemolytic anemias can develop three types of crises. The first is the "hemolytic crisis." When patients develop fevers or encounter other stresses, the rate of hemolysis may increase, and any inflammation can suppress erythropoiesis, leading to severe anemia. The second type of crisis is the "megaloblastic crisis" where patients become folic acid deficient because of the high folate demand associated with increased red blood cell production. With mass supplementation of folate in the food supply, this incidence has fallen. The final crisis is the "aplastic crisis" where red blood cell production is temporarily compromised and the reticulocyte count plummets. This is most commonly found with infections with parvovirus B-19. The infection clears in most patients within 1 week, but patients often require transfusion support during this time.

Hereditary spherocytosis is most prevalent in northern European populations and occurs with a frequency of approximately 1 in 5000. Most cases (75%) show an autosomal dominant pattern of inheritance. The remainder is due to autosomal recessive inheritance and new mutations. Common clinical features of hereditary spherocytosis include anemia, jaundice, reticulocytosis, splenomegaly, and microspherocytes. Anemia later in life is variable and usually mild. Complications include hemolytic crises, leg ulcers, and gallstones.

With hereditary elliptocytosis, most patients are symptom free, and the frequent finding of elliptocytes on the blood smear is of no clinical consequence. However, approximately 10% to 15% of patients have significant hemolysis and may develop anemia. Mild hereditary elliptocytosis is inherited in an autosomal dominant fashion. The incidence is higher in African and Asian populations because of its beneficial impact on malarial infection. Patients with pyropoikilocytosis have severe hemolysis.

G6PD deficiency is the most common enzyme defect in humans and affects an estimated 600 million people worldwide. G6PD deficiency is transmitted as an X-linked recessive condition. Hundreds of G6PD variants have been identified. Enzymatic activity varies from normal with no clinical consequences to severe deficiency resulting in chronic hemolysis and shortened red blood cell life span, even in the absence of stressors. The two most common variants are the G6PD A variant, which has moderate enzyme deficiency (10%-15% activity), and the G6PD Mediterranean mutation, which has almost no detectable enzyme activity. Despite this, patients with G6PD Mediterranean have a nearly normal erythrocyte life span except under conditions of metabolic or oxidative stress.

The classic presentation of hemolysis with G6PD deficiency is with oxidant stress. For example, certain medications such as sulfonamides can lead to increased oxidative stress. Patients with G6PD deficiency cannot generate enough reducing power to overcome this stress, which leads to oxidative damage to proteins, especially hemoglobin. The patient presents with fulminant hemolysis that can lead to a severe anemia. Because of membrane damage, the blood smear can show spherocytes and "bite cells"—red blood cells with defects caused by splenic conditioning. Treatment is removing the offending agent and is otherwise supportive. A unique presentation is "favism." After patient eats fava beans, an overwhelming hemolysis develops. This can be idiosyncratic and occur even in patients who have safely eaten the beans in the past.

Pyruvate kinase deficiency is inherited as an autosomal recessive condition. Anemia is variable and may range from a presentation in early infancy requiring transfusions to fully compensated hemolysis presenting with jaundice alone. Many patients have moderate anemia, jaundice, and splenomegaly. Patients with this disorder are also susceptible to the crises identified above. Splenectomy may be helpful in severe cases, but response is variable.

Acquired

AIHA patients who have IgG as the offending antibody are said to have warm antibody AIHA. The name warm comes from the fact that the antibody reacts best at body temperature. The incidence varies by series but is about 1 in 100,000 patients per year, and women are affected more often than men.

Warm AIHA can complicate several diseases. Lupus patients can develop warm AIHA as part of their disease complex. Of malignancies, that with the strongest association with AIHA is chronic lymphocytic leukemia (CLL). Series show that 5% to 10% of patients with CLL will have warm AIHA. The disease can appear concurrently with CLL or may develop during the course of the disease.

A rare but important variant of warm AIHA is Evan's syndrome. This is the combination of AIHA and immune thrombocytopenia. One to three percent of AIHA is the Evan's variant. The immune thrombocytopenia can precede, occur concurrently, or develop after the AIHA. The diagnosis of Evan's syndrome should raise the concern of underlying disorders. In pediatric and young adult patients, immunodeficiencies such as autoimmune lymphoproliferative disease needs to be considered. In older patients, Evan's syndrome is often associated with T-cell lymphomas.

In rare patients with warm AIHA, IgA or IgM antibodies are implicated. Patients with IgM AIHA often have a severe course with a fatal outcome. Patients' plasma may show spontaneous hemolysis and agglutination. The DAT may not be strongly positive or show C3 reactivity. The clinical clues are C3 reactivity with no cold agglutinins and severe hemolysis, sometimes with intravascular hemolysis.

In cold agglutinin disease, in addition to hemolysis, patients often note symptoms related to agglutination of red blood cells in the peripheral circulation. For example, acrocyanosis will be noted in cold weather. Rare patients will have abdominal pain when eating cold food due to ischemia related to agglutination of red blood cells in the viscera. Some patients with cold agglutinins can have an exacerbation of their hemolysis with cold exposure.

In young patients, cold AIHA is often post-infectious (such as from viral and mycoplasma infections), and the course is self-limited. The hemolysis usually starts 2 to 3 weeks after the illness and will last for 4 to 6 weeks. In older patients, the etiology in more than 90% of cases is a B-cell lymphoproliferative disorder, usually with monoclonal kappa B-cells. The most commonly seen are marginal zone lymphoma, small lymphocytic lymphoma, and lymphoplasmacytic lymphoma.

A unique cold AIHA is paroxysmal cold hemoglobinuria (PCH). This AIHA is most often post-viral affecting children; in the past it complicated any stage of syphilis. The antibody is IgG directed against the P antigen on the RBC. Binding is best in the "cold," but then complement is activated at body temperature. Because this antibody can fix complement, hemolysis can be rapid and severe, leading to extreme anemia.

Drug-induced AIHA is a rare drug reaction with a lower incidence than drug-related immune thrombocytopenia. The rate of severe drug-related AIHA is estimated at 1 in 1 million, but less severe cases may be missed. Most patients will have positive DAT without signs of hemolysis, although rare patients will have relentless hemolysis resulting in death. With hapten-related AIHA, very few patients will have hemolysis, and in those cases the hemolysis will resolve a few days after discontinuation of the offending drug. With immune complex disease, most often the patient will only have a positive DAT, but rare patients on exposure or reexposure will have life-threatening hemolysis. The onset of this hemolysis is rapid, with signs of acute illness and intravascular hemolysis. The classic associated drug is quinine, but many other drugs have been implicated.

A virulent form of immune complex hemolysis is associated with both disseminated intravascular coagulation and brisk hemolysis. Patients who receive certain second- and third-generation cephalosporins (especially cefotetan [Cefotan] and ceftriaxone [Rocephin]) have developed this syndrome. The clinical symptoms start 7 to 10 days after receiving the drug—often the patient has only received the antibiotic for surgical prophylaxis. Warm DAT hemolysis with an acute hematocrit drop, hypotension, and disseminated intravascular coagulation develop. The patients are often believed to have sepsis and are then often reexposed to the cephalosporin, resulting in worsening of the clinical status. The outcome is often fatal because of massive hemolysis and thrombosis.

Hemolysis caused by methyldopa is indistinguishable from warm AIHA, which is consistent with the notion that methyldopa induces an autoimmune hemolytic anemia. The hemolysis often resolves rapidly after stopping the methyldopa, although the Coombs test result may remain positive for months. This type of drug-induced hemolytic anemia has been reported with levodopa, procainamide (Pronestyl), and chlorpromazine (Thorazine).

In MAHA, the course of the presentation is dictated by the underlying cause. In valvular hemolysis, the onset of hemolysis is soon after the cardiac procedure and may require transfusion support. With VAD hemolysis, most patients have only mild hemolysis, but with pump thrombosis, the hemolysis can be severe. Patients with spur cell anemia have findings of severe liver disease—high INRs and bilirubin (mean of 9.5 mg/dL). Spur cell hemolysis is associated with an ominous prognosis and average survival of a few months.

PNH is characterized by episodes of hemolysis and a propensity for thrombosis and pancytopenia. Often patients can have PNH for years before the diagnosis is made. The hemolysis can range from being well compensated to transfusion dependence. Patients with PNH often have severe thrombophilia; the leading cause of morbidity and death (before the release of effective therapy) has been thrombosis. The cause of the hypercoagulable state is unknown, but complement-activated platelets have been implicated.

Diagnosis

There are two steps in the diagnosis of hemolytic anemia—first determining the presence of hemolysis, and then finding the cause. Hemolysis is demonstrated by evidence of both red blood cell breakdown as well as the compensatory increase in red blood cell production this stimulates. When red blood cells undergo hemolysis, their contents, mostly hemoglobin and the enzyme LDH, are released. Hemoglobin is by haptoglobin, and the heme moiety is broken down, first to bilirubin and then to urobilinogen, which is excreted in the urine.

The following tests are performed to investigate hemolysis:

LDH: Lactate dehydrogenase is an enzyme found in high concentration in the red blood cell; hemolysis releases this enzyme into the plasma. Most patients with hemolysis will have an elevated LDH level, making this a sensitive test. However, many other processes, including liver disease, pneumonia, and more, will also increase the serum LDH.

Serum bilirubin: Heme is broken down to produce bilirubin. Initially unconjugated, the bilirubin is delivered to the liver where it is conjugated and excreted into the bile. In hemolysis the unconjugated ("indirect bilirubin") is increased as opposed to liver disease, where the conjugated ("direct bilirubin") is increased. If a patient has coexisting liver disease with an elevated direct bilirubin, this test is not reliable.

Serum haptoglobin: Haptoglobin binds free serum hemoglobin and is taken up by the liver. Haptoglobin usually falls to very low levels in hemolysis. It's important to remember that haptoglobin is also an acute-phase reactant that can rise with systemic disease or inflammation. However, patients with advanced liver disease will have low haptoglobin due to a lack of synthesis, and up to 2% of the population may congenitally lack haptoglobin.

Hemoglobinemia: If the hemolysis is very rapid, the amount of free hemoglobin that is released will overwhelm haptoglobin and lead to the presence of free hemoglobin in the plasma. This can be crudely quantified by examining the plasma. Even minute amounts of free hemoglobin will turn the plasma pink. In fulminant hemolysis, the serum will be cola colored.

Urine hemosiderin: When hemoglobin is excreted by the kidney, the iron is deposited in the tubules. When the tubule cells are sloughed off, they will appear in the urine. The urine can be stained for iron, and, if positive, this is another sign of hemolysis. This is a later sign because it takes a week for enough iron-laden tubule cells to be excreted in detectable quantities.

Mean corpuscular volume (MCV): The MCV may be larger in hemolysis for several reasons. The size of reticulocytes is larger than normal red blood cells, so a brisk reticulocytosis will have a higher MCV. In cold agglutinin disease, the aggregation of red blood cells will falsely increase the MCV. Finally, hemolysis can lead to folate deficiency and a rise in MCV.

Reticulocyte count: With hemolysis the breakdown of red blood cells is accompanied by an increase in the reticulocyte count as marrow tries to compensate. The reticulocyte percentage needs to be adjusted for the hematocrit—a correct value of above 1.5% is considered raised. Recently, automated complete blood count machines have taken advantage of the fact that reticulocytes will absorb certain stains, and these machines can directly measure the reticulocyte count via flow cytometry.

This results in an "absolute" reticulocyte count. This does not have to be corrected for hematocrit, and levels about 90,000/μL are consider elevated. However, the reticulocyte count can also be increased in blood loss or in patients who have other causes of anemia (such as treated iron deficiency). In addition, as many of 25% of patients with AIHA will never have elevated reticulocyte counts for reasons such as nutritional deficiency, autoimmune destruction of red blood cell precursors, or lack of erythropoietin.

The blood smear provides vital information (Table 3). The finding of abnormal red blood cell shapes can be a clue to autoimmune hemolysis or red blood cell membrane defects. For example, spherocytes are seen in autoimmune hemolytic anemia, heredity spherocytosis, Wilson's disease, clostridial sepsis, and severe burns. Schistocytes are a sign of microangiopathic hemolytic anemia and should prompt concerns for such disease processes as thrombotic thrombocytopenia purpura, vavular hemolysis, VAD, march hemoglobinuria, among many examples.

In hereditary spherocytosis, the blood smear suggests the diagnosis. Confirmation is by demonstrating an increased osmotic fragility, although direct genetic screening for the molecular defects is becoming more common. The blood smear is also critical for diagnosing hereditary elliptocytosis and hereditary pyropoikilocytosis, although there is an increasing role for genetic diagnosis. Patients with hereditary pyropoikilocytosis are usually

---

TABLE 3 Typical Blood Smear Findings in Hemolysis

Bite Cells

Oxidative Hemolytic Anemia Such as G6PD Deficiency

Elliptocytes

Heredity Elliptocytosis
Schistocytes
Thrombotic Thrombocytopenic Purpura, Valvular Hemolysis,

Spherocytes:

Hereditary Spherocytosis, Autoimmune Hemolytic Anemia, Wilson's Disease, Burns

Spur Cells:

Severe Liver Disease

homozygous or compound heterozygous for one of the mutations causing mild hereditary elliptocytosis.

Diagnosis of G6PD deficiency is made by measuring enzyme activity. This is best done after the hemolytic episode is over, because reticulocytes have higher G6PD levels and can lead to falsely normal enzyme activity levels.

AIHA demonstrate either IgG or complement on the red blood cell. This is done by the "direct antibody" or "Coombs test." IgG bound to red blood cells will not agglutinate them. However, if IgM that is directed against IgG or C3 is added, the red blood cells will agglutinate, proving that there is IgG or C3 on the red blood cell membrane. The finding of a positive DAT in the setting of a hemolytic anemia is diagnostic of AIHA.

There are several pitfalls to the DAT. One is that a positive DAT can be found in 1 in 1000 patients in the normal population and up to several percent of ailing patients, especially those with elevated gamma globulin such as patients with liver disease or HIV. Administration of IVIG can also create a false-positive DAT. Conversely, patients can have AIHA with a negative DAT. Some patients have a low amount of IgG binding the red blood cell, which is below the detection limit of the DAT reagents. Other patients can have IgA or "warm" IgM as the cause of the AIHA. Specialty laboratories can test for these possibilities. The diagnosis of DAT-negative AIHA should be made with caution, and other causes of hemolysis-like hereditary spherocytosis or PNH should be excluded.

The DAT in patients with cold AIHA will show cells coated with C3. The blood smear will often show agglutination of the blood, and if the blood cools before being analyzed, the agglutination will interfere with the analysis. Titers of cold agglutinin can range from 1 in 1000 to 1 in >1 million. The autoantibodies are most often directed against the I/i antigen system, with 90% against I. The I specificity is typical with primary cold agglutinin disease and also following mycoplasma infection. The i-specific antigen is most typical of Epstein-Barr and cytomegalovirus infections.

In PCH the DAT is often weakly positive but can be negative. The diagnostic test is the Donath-Landsteiner test. This complex test is performed by incubating samples in three temperature ranges: one at 0°C to 4°C, one set at 37°C, and one incubated first at 0°C to 4°C and then 37°C. The diagnosis of PCH is made if only the third tube shows hemolysis.

For many patients, the first clue to drug-associated AIHA is the finding of a positive DAT in a patient taking a suspect drug (Table 4). Specialty laboratories such as Wisconsin Blood Center or the L.A. Red Cross can perform in vitro studies of drug interactions that can produce a certain diagnosis.

For PNH, the diagnosis had been based on an in vitro demonstration of increased sensitivity of red blood cells to complement lysis. Currently, flow cytometry is performed to examine cells for the absence of GPI-anchored proteins (CD55 or CD59 on red cells, other GPI-anchored proteins on white blood cells). In patients with microangiopathy the smear will show abundant schistocytes with a marked elevated LDH.

Therapy

Splenectomy is curative for most cases of hereditary spherocytosis but is reserved for patients with severe symptoms. For patients with hereditary pyropoikilocytosis, splenectomy can also be useful.

Most patients with G6PD deficiency require no special management beyond the avoidance of provocative medications and food. Highly symptomatic patients with pyruvate kinase deficiency may respond to splenectomy, and in clinical trials a small molecule agent that can increase enzyme activity.

Initial management of warm AIHA is prednisone starting at 1 mg/kg daily. It can take up to 3 weeks to see a response. Once the hematocrit is >30%, the prednisone is slowly tapered. Eighty percent of patients will respond to steroids, but the steroids can be fully tapered off in only 30%. For patients who can be maintained on 10 mg or less of steroids daily, this maybe the most reasonable long-term therapy.

TABLE 4	Drugs Implicated in Autoimmune Hemolytic Anemia

Most Common

Cefotetan (Cefotan)
Ceftriaxone (Rocephin)
Piperacillin (Pipracil)
Fludarabine (Fludara)

Other Implicated Drugs

Acetaminophen
Amphotericin B
Beta-lactams (any)
Carboplatin (Paraplatin)
Cephalosporins (any)
Chlorpromazine (Thorazine)
Chlorpropamide (Diabinese)
Cimetidine (Tagamet)
Ciprofloxacin (Cipro)
Diclofenac (Voltaren)
Doxycycline
Enalapril (Vasotec)
Erythromycin
Isoniazid
Levodopa
Melphalan (Alkeran)
Methyldopa
Nonsteroidal Antiinflammatory Agents
Omeprazole (Prilosec)
Oxaliplatin (Eloxatin)
Probenecid
Procainamide
Quinidine
Quinine
Rifampin
Sulfa drugs
Teniposide (Vumon)
Tetracycline
Thiazides
Thiopental (Pentothal)
Tolbutamide (Orinase)
Tricyclic Antidepressants

Current data show that adding rituximab (Rituxan)[1] to steroids for warm AIHA will improve overall response and should be considered early in most patients. These responses appear to be durable, and for relapses, repeating treatment is effective. It is important to remember that, for most patients, the response to rituximab is a gradual one over months; one should not expect a rapid response. Most studies have used the "traditional" 375 mg/m^2 dosing weekly for 4 weeks, and another option is 1000 mg repeated once 14 days apart.

Splenectomy is now reserved for patients with warm AIHA who do not respond to steroids or rituximab. Reported response rates in the literature range from 50% to 80%, with 50% to 60% remaining in remission. Timing of the procedure is a balance between allowing time for the steroids to work and the risk of toxicity of steroids. A patient who is at low risk for surgery and has either refractory disease or an inability to be weaned from high doses of steroids should have splenectomy considered early.

For patients who do not respond to either splenectomy or rituximab, the therapy is less certain. Although intravenous immune globulin is a standard therapy for immune thrombocytopenia, response rates are low in warm AIHA. Numerous therapies have been reported in small series, but there is no clear approach. Options include the following:

- Azathioprine (Imuran)[1] 75-150 mg/day
- Cyclophosphamide (Cytoxan)[1] 1000 mg monthly bolus IV
- Mycophenolate (CellCept)[1] 500-1000 mg bid
- Cyclosporine (Neoral)[1] 5 mg/kg daily divided in two doses
- Danazol (Danocrine)[1] 200 mg tid

---

[1]Not FDA approved for this indication.

Our approach has been to use mycophenolate for patients who require high doses of steroids or need transfusions. Patients needing lower doses of steroids may be good candidates for danazol to help wean them off steroids.

The sparse literature on Evan's syndrome suggests it can be more refractory to standard therapy, with response rates to splenectomy being in the 50% range. In patients with lymphoma, antineoplastic therapy is crucial. Data are accumulating for patients with autoimmune lymphoproliferative disease: mycophenolate or sirolimus (Rapamune)[1] starting at 2 mg/m² may be effective for splenectomy or rituximab failures.

The importance of diagnosing cold AIHA and differentiating it from warm AIHA is the fact that standard therapy for warm disease steroids is ineffective. Because C3-coated red blood cells are taken up through the reticulo-endothelial system, especially in the liver, as well as the spleen, splenectomy is an ineffective therapy.

Simple measures to help with cold AIHA should be used. Patients should be kept in a warm environment and should try to avoid the cold. If transfusions are needed, they should be infused via blood warmers to prevent hemolysis. In rare patients with severe hemolysis, plasma exchange can be considered. Given the culprit antibody is IgM—mostly intravascular—use of plasma exchange can slow the hemolysis to give time for other therapies to take effect.

Therapy of cold AIHA remains difficult. Currently the drug of choice is rituximab.[1] Response can be seen in 45% to 75% of patients but is almost always a partial response; retreatment is often necessary. As with other autoimmune hematologic diseases, there can be a delay in response. There are data to support adding either fludarabine (Fludara)[1] or bendamustine (Treanda)[1] 90 mg/m² to rituximab. The response rates are higher, but so are the complications of therapy. Although more toxic, this combination can be considered in patients with aggressive disease.

For most patients with drug-induced AIHA, stopping the offending drug is sufficient. It is doubtful that steroids or other autoimmune-directed therapy is effective. For patients with the DIC-hemolysis syndrome, there are anecdotes that plasma exchange may be helpful. Therapy for patients with positive DAT without signs of hemolysis is uncertain. If the drug is essential, then the patient can be observed. If the patient has hemolysis, the drug needs to be discontinued and the patient observed for signs of end-stage organ damage.

Transfusions can be very difficult in AIHA. The presence of the autoantibody can interfere with typing of the blood and almost always interferes with the cross-match, because this final step consists of mixing the patient's serum with donor red blood cells. In most patients with AIHA the autoantibodies will react with any donor cells, rendering a negative cross-match impossible. Without the cross-match the concern is that underlying alloantibodies can be missed, which can lead to transfusion reactions.

Some of these concerns may be allayed by remembering that patients who have never been transfused or pregnant will rarely have alloantibodies. Second, a patient who has undergone transfusion in the remote past may have an amnestic antibody response but not an immediate hemolytic reaction.

When a patient is first suspected of having AIHA, a generous sample of blood should be given to the transfusion service. This will allow for adequate testing of the sample. Second, many centers will test the blood not only for blood groups ABO and D but will also perform full Rh typing and check for Kidd, Duffy, and Kell status. This can allow transfusion of phenotypically matched blood to lessen the risk of alloantibody formation.

One difficult issue is timing of transfusion. Clinicians are often hesitant to transfuse patients with AIHA due to fear of reactions. But in frail patients with severe anemia—especially elderly patients or those with heart disease—transfusion can be lifesaving.

Because in some cases it can take hours to screen for alloantibodies, it is often preferable to transfuse patients with severe anemia while carefully observing for reactions.

The treatment for PNH is the complement inhibitor eculizumab (Soliris), a humanized monoclonal antibody that targets complement protein C5, thereby preventing assembly of the terminal complement complex during complement activation. In studies, treatment with eculizumab has been shown to reduce hemolysis, as well as improve anemia, fatigue, and quality of life in patients with PNH. In addition, eculizumab has demonstrated efficacy in reducing thrombosis. Just approved is ravulizumab (Ultomiris), another anti-C5 monoclonal antibody that needs infusion only every 8 weeks instead of every 2 weeks (eculizumab).

Management of Complications

The most concerning complication of splenectomy is overwhelming post-splenectomy infection. In adults, the spleen appears to play a minimal role in immunity except for defense from certain encapsulated organisms. Patients will often present with disseminated intravascular coagulation and will rapidly progress to purpura fulminans. Approximately 40% to 50% of patients will die of sepsis even when detected early. The overall lifetime risk may be as high as 1 in 500. The organism most commonly found in these cases is *Streptococcus pneumoniae*, which is reported in more than 50% of cases. *Neisseria meningitidis* and *Haemophilus influenzae* have also been implicated in many cases.

Patients who have undergone splenectomy need to be warned about the risk of overwhelming post-splenectomy infection and instructed to report to the emergency department immediately if they develop a fever greater than 101° or shaking chills. Once in the emergency department, blood cultures should be rapidly obtained and the patient started on antibiotic coverage with agents that cover encapsulated organisms. Patients who are planning to have or are being considered for a splenectomy should be vaccinated for pneumococcal, meningococcal, and H influenza infections. If patients are planning to be treated with rituximab first, they should also be vaccinated because after receiving rituximab, they will not be able to mount an immune response.

The major side effects of rituximab are infusion reactions—often worse with the first dose. These can be controlled with antihistamines, steroids, and, for severe rigors, meperidine (Demerol).[1] Rare patients can develop neutropenia (about 1 in 500) that appears to be autoimmune in nature. Infections appear to be only minimally increased with the use of rituximab. One group at higher risk are patients who are chronic carriers of hepatitis B. These patients may have reactivation of the virus that can be fatal in some cases; patients being considered for rituximab need to be screened for hepatitis B. Progressive multifocal leukoencephalopathy is a very rare risk that is more common in cancer patients and heavily immunosuppressed patients. The overall risk is unknown but is less than 1 in 50,000.

Eculizumab and ravulizumab are well tolerated, except for a risk of meningococcal infection estimated at 1 in 500 risk. All patients receiving this agent should be vaccinated and need to report to the emergency department with any sign of infection.

References

Berentsen S: Cold agglutinin disease, *Hematology Am Soc Hematol Educ Program* 2016:226–231, 2016.

Cappellini MD, Fiorelli G: Glucose-6-phosphate dehydrogenase deficiency, *Lancet* 371(9606):64–74, 2008.

Go RS, Winters JL, Kay NE: How I treat autoimmune hemolytic anemia, *Blood* 129:2971–2979, 2017.

Haley K: Congenital hemolytic anemia, *Med Clin North Am* 101:361–374, 2017.

Hill A, DeZern AE, Kinoshita T, Brodsky RA: Paroxysmal nocturnal haemoglobinuria, *Nat Rev Dis Primers* 3:17028, 2017.

Liebman HA, Weitz IC: Autoimmune Hemolytic Anemia, *Med Clin North Am* 101:351–359, 2017.

---

[1]Not FDA approved for this indication.

[1]Not FDA approved for this indication.

HEMOPHILIA AND RELATED CONDITIONS

Method of
Meera Chitlur, MD; Bulent Ozgonenel, MD; and Roshni Kulkarni, MD

CURRENT DIAGNOSIS

- The hemophilias and von Willebrand disease (vWD) account for 80% to 85% of inherited bleeding disorders. Hemophilia A and B are X-linked, whereas vWD and rare bleeding disorders (RBDs) are autosomal disorders.
- The diagnosis of hemophilia and other inherited bleeding disorders should be confirmed by specific laboratory assays, because screening tests such as prothrombin time (PT) and activated partial thromboplastin time (aPTT) may be normal. Plasma levels of deficient factor determine clinical severity and management.
- Major complications associated with hemophilia are inhibitor development, hemarthrosis, and intracranial hemorrhage. Hemarthrosis is the most common and debilitating complication, and central nervous system bleeding is the most common cause of mortality in hemophilia. Mucosal bleeding and menorrhagia are the most common manifestations of vWD. Bleeding manifestations of RBDs are mild, although homozygotes can present with severe disease.
- Newborns have normal levels of factor VIII; therefore the diagnosis of hemophilia A can be established at birth. Vacuum delivery should be avoided to prevent head bleeds.
- Women and adolescents with menorrhagia and no underlying pathology should be investigated for a bleeding disorder.

CURRENT THERAPY

- Currently there is a paradigm shift in the treatment of hemophilia. In addition to the traditional plasma derived and recombinant concentrates, the new extended half life recombinant products have reduced the treatment burden by reducing the frequency of intravenous injections. Novel, subcutaneously administered, nonfactor replacement therapy with prolonged hemostatic efficiency has been a game changer for patients both with or without inhibitors. Gene therapy is on the horizon, offering a promise of cure. Even for von Willebrand disease (vWD) and rare bleeding disorders (RBDs; such as deficiencies of factors FVII, XI, XIII, X, fibrinogen), replacement factor concentrates are currently available. Early and effective treatment and prophylaxis can prevent bleeding episodes, including repeated hemarthrosis and joint destruction in persons with hemophilia. Patients should be tested annually for the presence of inhibitors. Cryoprecipitate is not recommended for the treatment of hemophilia because of concerns regarding transmission of bloodborne pathogens.
- For mild and moderate hemophilia A and vWD, the use of desmopressin (DDAVP) coupled with antifibrinolytics can obviate the use of concentrates. Continued vigilance should be implemented for inhibitory antibodies and new and emerging bloodborne pathogens.
- All patients with inherited bleeding disorders should be immunized against hepatitis A and B and followed in close collaboration with the local hemophilia treatment center (http://www2a.cdc.gov/ncbddd/htcweb/index.asp). The National Hemophilia Foundation's (www.hemophilia.org) Medical and Scientific Advisory Committee (MASAC) guidelines for updated recommendations and product choice should be followed.

Hemophilia A and Hemophilia B

Hemophilia is an X-linked congenital bleeding disorder caused by a deficiency of factor VIII (hemophilia A) or factor IX (hemophilia B). Hemophilia A is the most common severe bleeding disorder and affects 1 in 5000 males in the United States; hemophilia B occurs in 1 in 30,000 males.

Pathophysiology

The *factor VIII* gene is one of the largest genes and spans 186 kb of genomic DNA at Xq28. Intron 22 of the *factor VIII* gene is particularly large and is, therefore, susceptible to inversion mutations. Inversions of this intron account for 50% of all severe hemophilia A cases, and inversions of other introns, deletions, point mutations, and insertions account for the remainder.

Hepatic and reticuloendothelial cells are presumed sites of factor VIII synthesis. Factor VIII is synthesized as a single chain polypeptide with three A domains (A1, A2, and A3), a large central B domain, and two C domains (Figure 1). The binding sites for vWF, thrombin, and factor Xa are on the C2 domain, and factor IXa binding sites are on the A2 and A3 domains. The B domain can be deleted without any consequences. vWF protects factor VIII from proteolytic degradation in the plasma and concentrates it at the site of injury.

The factor IX gene is 34 kb long and located at Xq26. It is a vitamin K–dependent serine protease composed of 415 amino acids. It is synthesized in the liver and its plasma concentration is approximately 50 times that of factor VIII. Gene deletions and point mutations result in hemophilia B.

Role of Factors VIII and IX in Coagulation

Factor VIII circulates bound to vWF. It is a cofactor for factor IX and is essential for factor X activation. In the classic coagulation cascade, activation of the intrinsic or extrinsic pathway of coagulation results in sufficient thrombin generation. The fact that bleeding still occurs in hemophilia despite an intact extrinsic pathway has led to the revised cell-based model of coagulation.

The revised pathway incorporates all coagulation factors into a single pathway initiated by FVII and tissue factor. The contact factors (XI, XII, kallikrein, and high-molecular-weight [HMW] kininogen) are not essential but serve as a backup. Following injury, encrypted tissue factor is exposed and forms a complex with factor VIIa. The tissue factor–factor VIIa complex activates factor IX to IXa (which moves to the platelet surface) and factor X to Xa. This generates small amounts of thrombin that activates platelets, converts platelet factor V to Va and factor XI to XIa, and releases factor VIII from vWF and activates it. The factor XIa activates plasma factor IX to IXa on the platelet surface, which together with factor VIIIa forms the tenase complex (factor VIIIa/IXa) that converts large amounts of factor X to Xa. Factor Xa forms a prothrombinase complex with FVa and converts large amounts of prothrombin to thrombin, called *thrombin burst*. This results in the conversion of sufficient fibrinogen to fibrin to form a stable clot. (Animations are available at the Foundation of Women and Girls with Blood Disorders (www.fwgbd.org and www.reddymed.com).

In hemophilia, lack of factor VIII or IX produces a profound abnormality. Factor Xa generated by FVIIa and tissue factor is insufficient because this pathway is inhibited by tissue factor pathway inhibitor (TFPI) as part of a negative feedback, and factors VIII and IX, which are required for amplifying the production of Xa, are absent. The primary platelet plug formation and initiation phases of coagulation are normal. Any clot that is formed (from the initiation phase) is friable and porous.

Clinical Features

The diagnosis of hemophilia is often made following a bleeding episode or because of a family history; however, 50% of cases have no family history. Based on the plasma levels of factor VIII or IX (normal levels are 50% to 150%) that correlate with severity and predict bleeding risk, hemophilia is classified

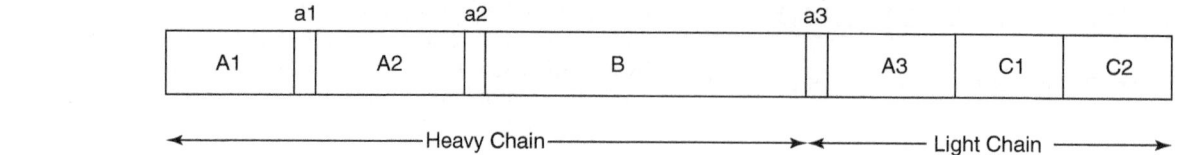

Figure 1 Factor VIII protein structure.

TABLE 1	Hemophilia Severity and Clinical Manifestations.		
CHARACTERISTICS	**SEVERE (50%–70%)**	**MODERATE (10%)**	**MILD (30%–40%)**
Factor VIII or IX activity (normal 50%–150%)	<1%	1%–5%	>5%
Age of diagnosis	At birth to 2 year	Childhood or adolescence	Adolescence or adult
Bleeding patterns	2–4/month	4–6/year	Rare
Clinical manifestations	Hemarthroses, muscle, central nervous system, gastrointestinal bleeding, hematuria	Bleeding into joints or muscle following minor trauma, surgical procedure, dental bleeding Rarely spontaneous	Surgical procedures (including dental) and major trauma

as mild (>5%), moderate (1% to 5%), and severe (<1%) (Table 1). Approximately 65% of persons with hemophilia have severe disease, 15% have moderate disease, and 20% have mild disease. Most cases of severe disease manifest by 4 years of age; moderate or mild disease is diagnosed later and often following bleeding secondary to trauma or surgery.

Hemophilia can be diagnosed in the first trimester, using chorionic villus sampling and gene analysis. In the second trimester, fetal blood sampling can be performed. Prenatal diagnosis to determine fetal gender can aid in the management of pregnancy and delivery.

The hallmark of severe hemophilia is hemarthrosis, or bleeding into the joint, that can occur spontaneously or with minimal trauma. The immediate effects of a joint bleed are excruciating pain, swelling, warmth, and muscle spasms, and the long-term effects of recurrent hemarthrosis is the hemophilic arthropathy, which is characterized by synovial thickening, chronic inflammation. Repeated hemorrhage results in a target joint. Knees, elbows, ankles, hips, and shoulders are commonly affected. Disuse atrophy of surrounding muscles leads to further joint instability. Limitation of joint range of motion due to hemarthrosis often correlates positively with older age, nonwhite race, and increased body mass index, and it adversely affects quality of life.

Muscle hematomas, another characteristic site of bleeding, can lead to compartment syndrome, with eventual fibrosis and peripheral nerve damage. Iliopsoas bleeds manifest with pain and flexion deformity. Gastrointestinal bleeding and hematuria occur less often.

Central nervous system (CNS) hemorrhage is a rare but serious complication with a 10% recurrence rate and is the leading cause of mortality in hemophiliacs. Although most newborns with severe hemophilia experience an uneventful course following vaginal delivery, vacuum extraction is associated with an increased CNS bleeding risk. The incidence of intracranial hemorrhage in newborns with hemophilia is 1% to 4%.

Diagnosis

Hemophilia A and B are clinically indistinguishable, and specific factor assays are the only way to differentiate and confirm the diagnosis. Both should be differentiated from vWD. The prothrombin time (PT), platelet function analysis (PFA)-100, and fibrinogen activity are normal. (PFA, a platelet-function screening test, replaces bleeding time, because the bleeding time has low sensitivity and specificity and is operator dependent.) The activated partial thromboplastin time (aPTT) is prolonged when the factor levels are less than 30%. Table 2 shows the characteristics and differences between the hemophilias and vWD.

Female carriers may be asymptomatic except for those with extreme lyonization resulting in low factor VIII or IX levels. However, some carriers may experience bleeding episodes (such as heavy menstrual bleeding, postpartum hemorrhage, joint bleeding, etc.) even with levels of FVIII or IX in the 40% range. Factor VIII levels increase throughout pregnancy and drop to prepregnancy levels following delivery, but factor IX levels remain constant throughout pregnancy.

Treatment

The treatment for hemophilia consists of replacement therapy with intravenous factor VIII or factor IX concentrates produced by purification of donor plasma (plasma derived) (e.g., factor VIII: Hemofil M, Monoclate-P; factor IX: AlphaNine SD, Mononine) or in cell culture bioreactors (recombinant) (e.g., factor VIII: Afstyla, Helixate FS; factor IX: BeneFix, Rixubis). Careful screening of donors combined with heat treatment and viral inactivation methods have made plasma-derived products safer. Plasma-derived and recombinant products appear to have equivalent clinical efficacy. Cryoprecipitate is no longer recommended because of concerns regarding pathogen safety.

Treatment administered only during bleeding symptoms is known as *episodic therapy*, and periodic administration of factor concentrates to prevent bleeding is known as *prophylactic therapy*. Response to treatment is more effective when it is administered early. Although prophylaxis prevents the development of joint disease, the high cost of factor replacement coupled with the need for venous access makes it expensive and difficult and out of reach for patients in the developing world.

The goal of treatment is to raise factor levels to approximately 30% or more for minor bleeds (hematomas or joint bleeds) and 100% for major bleeds (CNS or surgery). Giving 1 U/kg of factor concentrate raises plasma factor VIII levels by 2% and factor IX levels by 1.5% (except with the recombinant factor IX product, where it increases by 0.8%). The half-life of factor VIII is 8 to 12 hours, and that of factor IX is up to 24 hours with standard factor products.

Factor concentrates can also be given by continuous infusion (3 to 4 U/kg/h). The bolus dose varies from 25 to 50 U/kg depending on the severity, site, and type of bleeding and is dosed to the available vial size because of the cost of the products. Table 3 lists the dosing schedule for various types of bleeds.

For short-term therapy (before dental procedures and minor bleeding episodes), the synthetic vasopressin analog desmopressin acetate (DDAVP [Stimate]) is useful in mild hemophilia A and vWD. It increases plasma concentrations of coagulation factor VIII and vWF threefold to fivefold by releasing the endothelial

CHARACTERISTIC	HEMOPHILIA A	HEMOPHILIA B	von WILLEBRAND DISEASE
Incidence	1:5000	1:30,000	1%–3% of US population
Abnormality	Factor VIII deficiency	Factor IX deficiency	vWF (qualitative and quantitative defect)
Inheritance	X-linked, affects males Gene at the tip of X chromosome	X-linked, affects males Gene at the tip of X chromosome	Autosomal dominant (gene: chromosome 12) Some are recessive or compound heterozygotes
Production site	Unknown, liver endothelium	Liver (vitamin K dependent)	Megakaryocytes and endothelial cells
Function	Cofactor; forms tenase complex with factor IX and activates factor X, leading to thrombin burst that results in conversion of large amounts of fibrinogen to fibrin	Serine protease (inactive form: zymogen) activated by factor XI or VIIa; forms a tenase complex with factor VIII and activates factor X	Platelet adhesion to site of injury or damaged endothelium Protects factor VIII from proteolysis
Classification (normal levels 50%–150%)	Mild (>5%) Moderate (1%–5%) Severe (<1%)	Mild (>5%) Moderate (1%–5%) Severe (<1%)	Type 1 Type 2 (2A, 2B, 2M, 2N) Type 3
Clinical presentation	Positive family history (30% new mutation) Hemarthroses, hematomas, hematuria, intracranial hemorrhage, gastrointestinal hemorrhage, etc.	Positive family history (30% new mutation) Milder disease, although identical hemorrhage sites as hemophilia A	Positive family history Mucocutaneous bleeding (epistaxis, menorrhagia, postdental bleeding, gastrointestinal bleeding in adults) Type 3 can manifest as hemophilia A
PFA, bleeding time	Normal	Normal	May be prolonged
PT	Normal	Normal	Normal
aPTT	Prolonged	Prolonged	Prolonged or normal
Factor VIII assay	Decreased or absent	Normal	Decreased or normal (absent type 3)
Factor IX assay	Normal	Decreased or absent	Normal
vWF:Ag	Normal	Normal	Decreased or absent (type 3)
vWF:RCo	Normal	Normal	Decreased or abnormal
vWF multimers	Normal	Normal	Abnormal in types 1, 2A, 2B; absent in type 3
Specific treatment	Recombinant factor VIII (preferred) Pathogen-safe plasma-derived concentrates DDAVP for mild cases	Recombinant factor IX Pathogen-safe plasma-derived concentrates DDAVP ineffective	DDAVP (intranasal or intravenous) VWF concentrates (pathogen-safe plasma derived or recombinant vWF)
Inhibitor patients	Immune tolerance, recombinant factor Vlla, APCC	Immune tolerance, recombinant factor Vlla	Inhibitors are rare
Adjunct therapy	Antifibrinolytics	Antifibrinolytics	Hormonal therapy (Oral contraceptives), antifibrinolytics

APCC, Activated prothrombin complex concentrates; aPTT, activated partial thromboplastin time; DDAVP, desmopressin; PFA, platelet function analyzer; PT, prothrombin time; RCo, ristocetin cofactor; vWF, von Willebrand factor; vWF:Ag, von Willebrand factor antigen.

stores. A DDAVP trial to determine response is helpful in selecting patients who might benefit from such therapy. For hemostatic purposes, intravenous (0.3 µg/kg in 50 mL of normal saline infused over 15 to 30 minutes) or intranasal dose (150 µg) can be used. The intranasal dose is 15 times larger than that recommended for diabetes insipidus. A multidose intranasal spray formulation (Stimate nasal spray) delivers 150 µg per spray. The recommended dosage is one spray for patients who weigh less than 50 kg and two sprays (one in each nostril) for those who weigh more than 50 kg. Desmopressin is ineffective in hemophilia B or severe hemophilia A. Aspirin and aspirin-containing compounds should be avoided in persons with bleeding disorders because they interfere with platelet function and can exacerbate bleeding.

Antifibrinolytics such as ε-aminocaproic acid (Amicar) and tranexamic acid (Cyklokapron or Lysteda) are used as adjunct therapies and in mild hemophilia and can decrease the need for factor concentrates. The recommended dosage for ε-aminocaproic

TABLE 3	Treatment of Bleeding Episodes and Desired Plasma Levels in Hemophilias A and B.				
TYPE OF BLEEDING	DESIRED FACTOR LEVEL (%)	FACTOR VIII DOSE (U/kg)	FACTOR IX DOSE (U/kg)	DURATION OF TREATMENT (DAYS)	COMMENTS (DOSE FACTOR TO THE CLOSEST)
Persistent or profuse epistaxis Oral mucosal bleeding (including tongue and mouth lacerations)	20–30	10–15	20–30	1–2	Local pressure, antifibrinolytics, fibrin glue for local control, Nosebleed QR for epistaxis Sedation in small children with tongue laceration
Dental procedures	30–50	15–25	30–50	1 hour before procedure	Antifibrinolytics for 7–10 days
Acute hemarthrosis, intramuscular hematomas	30–60	15–50	30–60	1–3	Use lower doses if treated early. Nonweight bearing on affected joint
Physical therapy	30–50	15–25	30–50	Treat before PT	Consider synovectomy (surgical, radioisotope or chemical) for target joints
Life-threatening bleeding such as intracranial hemorrhage, major surgery, and trauma	80–100	40–50	80–100	10–14 days	Bolus dose followed by continuous infusion (3–4 U/kg/h); may switch to bolus before discharge
Gastrointestinal bleeding	30–50	15–25	30–50	2–3	May use oral antifibrinolytics
Persistent painless gross hematuria	30–50	15–25	30–50	1–2	Increase PO or IV fluids with low-dose antifibrinolytics; Risk of clotting in the urinary tract with factor replacement

IV, Intravenous; *PO*, per os (orally); *PT*, physical therapy.

acid is 75 to 100 mg/kg/doseintravenously or orally every 4 to 6 hours (maximum 30 g/24 hours). The recommended dosage for tranexamic acid is 10 mg/kg/dose intravenously or 25 mg/kg body weight orally, three times daily.

For prophylaxis, factor VIII 25 to 40 U/kg administered every other day or factor IX 25 to 40 U/kg twice weekly (because of the longer half-life of factor IX) is aimed at preventing joint disease. Prophylaxis may begin at 1 to 2 years of age and is continued life-long. Self-infusion before any planned strenuous activity is recommended. Because of the complications of central venous catheters (infections, thrombosis, and mechanical), use of a peripheral vein is encouraged.

Extended half-life (EHL) factor products have increased the half-lives by 1.5-fold in the case of factor VIII and 2.4- to 4.8-fold in the case of factor IX products. EHL factor products have been developed with an aim to decrease the frequency of infusions and improve quality of life for patients with hemophilia, achieved through PEGylation or fusion of the factor protein to the Fc fragment of an immunoglobulin or albumin. The first of these EHL products were approved by the US Food and Drug Administration (FDA) in 2014: factor IX (recombinant), Fc fusion protein (Alprolix) for use in patients with hemophilia B, and Factor VIII (recombinant), Fc fusion protein (Eloctate) for use in patients with hemophilia A. Subsequently, PEGylated recombinant factor VIII (Adynovate, Takeda Pharmaceuticals, approved 2015) and PEGylated recombinant factor IX (Rebinyn, Novo Nordisk–approved in 2017 but not for prophylaxis) and recombinant albumin fusion Factor IX (Idelvion, CSL Behring) have been approved for use in PWH.

Novel Therapies for the Treatment of Hemophilia

In recent years, the field of hemophilia treatment has seen dramatic changes. Treatment options that do not target replacement of the missing factor are currently being tested. Factor VIII mimetics such as the bispecific factor IXa- and factor X–directed antibody Emicizumab (Hemlibra) (see later), products targeting the endogenous anticoagulants, such as small interfering RNA (siRNA)

targeting antithrombin (Fitusiran [Alnylam Pharmaceuticals])[5], anti-TFPI antibody (e.g., Concizumab [Novo Nordisk][5]), and products targeting the anticoagulant effect of activated prothrombin complex (APC) are being studied. The advantages are that these products provide the benefits of prophylaxis and can be given subcutaneously, eliminating the need for intravenous injection. More data are needed regarding the safety and efficacy of these medications.

Gene therapy offers promise of a cure and trials of gene therapy for both hemophilia A and B are currently in process. Two gene therapy trials for hemophilia B had shown subtherapeutic or transient expression of factor IX. In December 2011, Nathwani and colleagues reported that a single injection of FIX-expressing adeno-associated virus (AAV) vector was effective in treating patients with hemophilia B for more than a year. Since this breakthrough, there have been more successful gene therapy trials that are currently going on for the treatment of both hemophilia A and B. The trials have incorporated modifications of promoters, transgenes and AAV serotypes, and lentiviral vectors. This has been a significant breakthrough in the treatment of hemophilia.

Complications of Treatment

One of the most serious complications of hemophilia treatment is the development of inhibitors or neutralizing antibodies (immunoglobulin [Ig]G) that inhibit the function of substituted factor VIII and factor IX. Five to 10% of all hemophiliacs and up to 30% of patients with severe hemophilia A develop inhibitors. The incidence of inhibitors in hemophilia B is lower (1%–3%). Most factor VIII inhibitors arise after a median exposure of 9 to 12 days in patients with severe hemophilia A. They can be transient or permanent and should be suspected if a patient fails to respond to an appropriate dose of clotting factor concentrate. Inhibitors can exacerbate bleeding episodes and hemophilic arthropathy.

Inhibitor levels, measured using Bethesda units (BU), are classified as high titer (>5 BU) or low titer (<5 BU). In patients with

---

[5] Investigational drug in the United States.

low-titer inhibitors, higher than normal doses of factor VIII or IX may be used to treat bleeding. For those with high-titer inhibitors, agents that bypass factor VIII or factor IX are used. These include recombinant activated factor VII and, in the case of hemophilia A, activated prothrombin complex concentrates (APCCs) or recombinant porcine factor VIII (currently in prelicensure clinical trials). Immune tolerance induction, a long-term approach designed to eradicate inhibitors, is effective in 70% to 85% of patients with severe hemophilia A; the most important predictor of success of immune tolerance induction is an inhibitor titer of less than 10 BU at the start of immune tolerance induction.

A novel treatment for hemophilia A with inhibitors is emicizumab (also called ACE910, marketed as Hemlibra), a chimeric humanized antibody that triggers and propagates thrombin generation by binding to both factor IX and factor X. By binding to these coagulation factors, the antibody mimics the function of factor VIII. The medication can be given as weekly subcutaneous doses; therefore it is a preferred regimen in young children. Emicizumab has shown success in preventing bleeding complications in patients with severe hemophilia A with inhibitors. Emicizumab was approved by the FDA initially for the treatment of hemophilia A with inhibitors in 2017, but this approval was extended to hemophilia A without inhibitors in 2018. Emicizumab can be administered subcutaneously once a week, every 2 weeks or every 4 weeks, and all these regimens have been found to be equally effective. In general, emicizumab has been warmly embraced by patients with hemophilia as its treatment regimen does not require intravenous dosing and the dose frequency is much easier to manage than prophylaxis with conventional factor VIII products. Emicizumab/Hemlibra treatment is safe by itself, but thrombotic microangiopathy and thrombotic complications have been observed in individuals receiving concomitant high doses of APCC for management of breakthrough bleeds while on Emicizumab (>100U/kg of FEIBA for >24 hours). Hence it is recommended that rFVIIa (NovoSeven RT) be used as the first line of treatment for management of breakthrough bleeds in inhibitor patients on Emicizumab (Medical and Scientific Advisory Committee [MASAC] document #255).

Although inhibitors are rare in hemophilia B, they can result in anaphylaxis with exposure to factor IX–containing products. Immune tolerance regimens are associated with nephrotic syndrome and are successful in eradicating the inhibitor only in 40% of cases.

Another important complication of treatment is the transmission of bloodborne pathogens such as hepatitis B and C viruses and human immunodeficiency virus (HIV). In the 1970s, lyophilized plasma factor concentrates of low purity resulted in the transmission of HIV, causing the deaths of many hemophiliacs. Currently, donor screening for pathogens coupled with viral attenuation by heat or solvent detergent technology make these products pathogen safe. However, nonenveloped viruses (parvovirus and hepatitis A) and prions can resist inactivation and can be potentially transmitted.

Patients with bleeding disorders should be encouraged to attend the comprehensive hemophilia treatment centers (HTCs), where they are educated, trained to self-infuse and calculate dosage, maintain treatment logs, and call for serious bleeding episodes. The mortality rate among patients who receive care at HTCs is lower than among those who do not: 28.1% versus 38.3%, respectively. At the HTCs, hemovigilance for bloodborne and emerging pathogens was maintained through participation in the Centers for Disease Control and Prevention (CDC) Universal Data Collection (UDC) project. The grant cycle of the UDC was completed in 2012, and a new surveillance instrument is currently in use (Community Counts) that incorporates collecting information on comorbidities and complications of bleeding disorders in this population. Routine vaccination against hepatitis A and B is recommended.

von Willebrand Disease

vWD is an inherited (autosomal dominant) bleeding disorder caused by deficiency or dysfunction of vWF, a plasma protein that mediates platelet adhesion at the site of vascular injury and prevents degradation of factor VIII. A defect in vWF results in bleeding by impairing platelet adhesion or by decreasing factor VIII.

vWF is synthesized in endothelial cells and undergoes dimerization and multimerization, forming low-, intermediate-, and HMW multimers. The HMW multimers are most effective in promoting platelet aggregation and adhesion. Circulating HMW multimers are cleaved by the protease ADAMTS13, which is deficient in patients with thrombotic thrombocytopenic purpura.

vWD is the most common bleeding disorder, affecting 1% or more of the population. It occurs worldwide and affects all races. vWD is classified into three major categories: partial quantitative deficiency (type 1), qualitative deficiency (type 2), and total deficiency (type 3). There are several different variants of type 2 vWD: 2A, 2B, 2N, and 2M based on the phenotype. Approximately 75% of patients have type 1 vWD.

Clinical Presentation

Mucous membrane–type bleeding (e.g., menorrhagia, epistaxis) and excessive bruising are characteristic clinical features in vWD. Bleeding manifestations vary considerably, and in some cases the diagnosis is not suspected until excessive bleeding occurs with a surgical procedure or trauma. Although excessive menstrual bleeding may be the initial manifestation, it takes 16 years for a diagnosis of bleeding disorder. It is for this reason that the American College of Obstetrics and Gynecology recommended screening for hemostatic disorders in all adolescents and women presenting with menorrhagia and no pathology and before hysterectomy for menorrhagia. In infants or small children with type 3 (severe) vWD, excessive bruising and even joint bleeding (due to very low levels of factor VIII) can mimic hemophilia A.

Diagnosis

Laboratory evaluation for vWD requires several assays to quantitate vWF and characterize its structure and function. Many variables affect vWF assay results, including the patient's ABO blood type. Persons of blood group AB have 60% to 70% higher vWF levels than those of blood group O. Thus some laboratories interpret vWF levels referenced to specific normal ranges for blood types.

Clinical conditions and disorders with elevated vWF levels include pregnancy (third trimester), collagen vascular disorders, postoperative period, liver disease, and disseminated intravascular coagulation. Low levels are seen in hypothyroidism and the first 4 days of the menstrual cycle.

Symptoms are modified by medications like aspirin or nonsteroidal antiinflammatory drugs (NSAIDs), which can exacerbate the bleeding; oral contraceptives can decrease the bleeding in women with vWD by increasing vWF levels. vWF levels in African-American women are 15% higher than in white women. Clinical symptoms and family history are important for establishing the diagnosis of vWD, and a single test is sometimes not sufficient to rule out the diagnosis.

Initial work-up should include a complete blood count, aPTT, PT, fibrinogen level, or thrombin time. These tests do not rule out vWD but help rule out thrombocytopenia or factor deficiency as the cause for bleeding. The closure times on the PFA-100, which has replaced the bleeding time as a screening test in some centers, may be prolonged. The aPTT in vWD is only abnormal when factor VIII is sufficiently reduced.

Specific tests for vWD include ristocetin cofactor assay, a factor VIII activity, and vWF antigen (vWF Ag) assay. The ristocetin cofactor activity measures induced binding of vWF to platelet glycoprotein Ib and is the best functional assay of vWF activity. Multimer analysis is done by agarose gel electrophoresis using anti-vWF polyclonal antibody and is available at reference laboratories. Collagen binding assay and genotyping, especially for type 2 vWD, are new tests available to assist with the diagnosis.

In type 1 vWD, the vWF is subnormal in amount, with normal multimer structure. Those with types 2A and 2B vWD lack the

TABLE 4	Clinical Variants of von Willebrand Disease.				
TYPE	**FACTOR VIII**	**vWF AG**	**RISOTCETIN COFACTOR**	**RIPA**	**MULTIMER**
1	↓	↓	↓	↓ or normal	Normal
2A	↓ or normal	↓↓	↓	↓↓	Large and intermediate multimers absent
2B	↓ or normal	↓↓	↓ or normal	↓ to low dose	Large multimers absent
2M	Variably ↓	Variably ↓	↓	Variably ↓	Normal
2N	↓↓	Normal	Normal	Normal	Normal
3	↓↓↓↓	↓↓↓↓	↓↓↓↓	None	Absent
Platelet type	↓ or normal	↓ or normal	↓	↓ to low dose	Large multimers absent

Ag, Antigen; *RIPA*, ristocetin-induced platelet aggregation; *vWF*, von Willebrand factor.

HMW multimers. In type 2B, the vWF has a heightened affinity for platelets, often resulting in some degree of thrombocytopenia from platelet aggregation. A useful laboratory test for type 2B is the low-dose ristocetin-induced platelet aggregation (RIPA) assay.

In type 3 (severe) vWD, the affected person has inherited a gene for type 1 vWD from each parent, resulting in very low levels (3%) of vWF (and low factor VIII, because there is no vWF to protect factor VIII from proteolytic degradation). Less commonly, a person with type 3 is doubly heterozygous. Table 4 provides a quick overview of the laboratory findings in the different variants of vWD.

Treatment
In type 1 vWD (with subnormal levels of normally functioning vWF), the treatment of choice is DDAVP, which causes a rapid release of vWF from storage sites. It can be given intravenously or by the intranasal route. The recommended dose for IV use is 0.3 µg/kg, given in saline over 10 minutes. Most persons with type 1 VWD have a twofold to fourfold increase in plasma levels of vWF within 15 to 30 minutes following infusion. The IV route is often used for surgical coverage or for a severe bleeding episode requiring hospitalization. When necessary, repeat doses may be given at 12- to 24-hour intervals. Tachyphylaxis is less commonly seen in vWD patients than in hemophilia patients. It is important to monitor free water intake following DDAVP administration because it can cause hyponatremia and seizures.

The concentrated form of desmopressin for intranasal use (Stimate Nasal Spray) may be used. The recommended dosage is one 150-µg spray for patients who weigh less than 50 kg and two sprays (one in each nostril) for those who weigh more than 50 kg. Some young women with menorrhagia have benefited from its use at the onset of menses, with a second dose after 24 hours. Others have used it approximately 45 minutes before invasive dental procedures, with good results.

In the type 2 variants (vWF produced is abnormal), desmopressin can cause an increase in abnormal vWF. Although some persons with type 2A might respond, desmopressin is seldom useful in type 2 and might even be contraindicated (as in type 2B, where it can exacerbate the thrombocytopenia).

In type 3 vWD, desmopressin is ineffective because there is no vWF to be released from storage sites. For type 3 patients and in persons with type 1 vWD who do not respond adequately to desmopressin, an intermediate-purity plasma-derived concentrate rich in the hemostatically effective HMW multimers of vWF (such as Humate P) should be used to treat moderately severe or severe bleeding episodes and for before surgery. Prophylaxis with vWF concentrates is effective in reducing the bleeding episodes and joint disease in severe vWD. There is also a new recombinant vWF concentrate (Vonvendi) currently approved for use only in adults.

As in hemophilia, antifibrinolytics are an effective adjunctive treatment for invasive dental procedures or other bleeding in the oropharyngeal cavity. These may be effective even when used alone in some vWD women with menorrhagia. For epistaxis, Nosebleed QR, a hydrophilic powder, can help.

Special Situations
Pregnancy
vWF (and factor VIII) levels increase during the third trimester of pregnancy, and women with type 1 vWD have a decrease in bruising or other bleeding symptoms. However, those with type 2 vWD (abnormal vWF) and type 3 (no vWF) have no change in the bleeding tendency. Even in type 1 vWD, vWF levels fall following delivery, so treatment (with IV desmopressin or Humate P) may be needed.

Acquired von Willebrand Disease
Acquired vWD occurs in persons who do not have a lifelong bleeding disorder. Conditions associated with acquired vWD include underlying autoimmune disease (lymphoproliferative disorders, myeloproliferative disorders, or plasma cell dyscrasias), valvular and congenital heart disease, Wilms tumor, chronic renal failure, and hypothyroidism. The mechanism of acquired vWD is unknown. Medications such as valproic acid can also cause vWD. Removal of the underlying condition often corrects the vWF. Desmopressin, Humate P, recombinant factor VIIa, or plasma exchange may be tried, if necessary, to treat bleeding.

Polymorphisms in the von Willebrand Disease Molecule
Individuals with exon 28 D1472H polymorphism of the vWF molecule may have disproportionately low ristocetin cofactor activity along with normal or near-normal levels of vWF antigen. Such individuals may falsely be diagnosed with type 2A vWD, whereas the polymorphism merely affects in vitro interaction with ristocetin without compromising the in vivo function of the vWF molecule.

Rare Bleeding Disorders
The RBDs account for 3% to 5% of inherited coagulation deficiencies, other than factor VIII, factor IX, or VWF deficiencies. They are autosomal recessive and affect both sexes. The prevalence of RBDs ranges from 1:500,000 to 1:2,000,000. Bleeding manifestations are restricted to persons who are homozygotes or compound heterozygotes. RBDs are common in countries such as Iran, where consanguineous marriages are customary. Ashkenazi Jews are particularly affected by factor XI deficiency. Deficiency of factor XII is a risk factor for thrombosis but not for bleeding. Most cases of RBDs are identified by abnormal screening tests coupled with specific factor assays.

Factor concentrates (recombinant or plasma derived) are available for some of the deficiencies such as FVII, X (Coagadex), XIII (Tretten, Corifact), XI (in Europe), and fibrinogen concentrate (Fibryga, RiaSTAP). The advantages of concentrates are pathogen safety and small volume. The use of antifibrinolytics and fibrin glue as adjunct therapy for bleeding manifestations is encouraged. Table 5 lists the inheritance, frequency, manifestations, and treatments of the RBDs.

	TABLE 5	Rare Bleeding Disorders: Inheritance, Clinical Features, and Treatment.					
FACTOR	**PREVA-LENCE**	**TYPE**	**INHERI-TANCE**	**MANIFESTATION AND DIAGNOSIS**	**TREATMENT**	**HEMOSTAT-IC LEVELS**	**HALF-LIFE**
Factor I	1:1,000,000	Afibrinogenemia Dysfibrinogenemia Hypofibrinogenemia	AR AD AD	Mild bleeding CNS, umbilical, joint bleeding Recurrent miscarriage PT, aPTT, TT prolonged Low FI levels Paradoxical thrombosis	FFP 15–20 mL/kg Cryoprecipitate 1 bag/5–10 kg Fibrinogen concentrate (RiaSTAP) Treatment q3–5d	50 mg^{-1} g/dL	2–5 days
Factor II	1:2,000,000	Type I: hypoprothrombinemia Type II: dysprothrombinemia	AR AR	Hematomas, hemarthroses, menorrhagia CNS, umbilical, postpartum hemorrhage PT abnormal	FFP, PCC 20–30 U/kg for prophylaxis or treatment	20%–30%	3–4 days
Factor V	1:1,000,000	Parahemophilia, labile factor, proaccelerin, Owren disease	AR	Mucosal bleeding, postpartum hemorrhage, CNS bleeding Platelet factor V deficiency more reflective of bleeding potential Prolonged PT, aPTT Normal TT	FFP Platelet transfusions Antiplatelet antibodies can develop with repeated platelet transfusions	15%–20%	36 hour
Factor VII	1:500,000	Proconvertin or stable factor	AR	Menorrhagia; mucosal, muscle, intracranial bleeds (15%–60%); hemarthrosis Prolonged PT Normal aPTT, TT, FI, liver functions	Recombinant factor VIIa (NovoSeven), 15–30 µg/kg q2h for major bleeds FFP, PCC 20–30 U/kg for prophylaxis or treatment Plasma-derived factor VII concentrates[2,*]	15%–20%	4–6 hour
Factor X	1:1,000,000		AR	Menorrhagia; umbilical, joint, mucosal, muscle, intracranial bleeding Prolonged PT, aPTT	FFP, PCCs 20–30 U/kg Pd FX (Coagadex)	15%–20%	24–48 hour
Factor XI (common in Ashkenazi Jews)	1:1,000,000		AR	Posttraumatic bleeding, menorrhagia Prolonged aPTT Normal PT	Hemoleven,* FFP 15–20 mL/kg Inhibitors can occur	15%–20%	
Factor XIII	1:2,000,000		AR	Intracranial, joint, umbilical bleeding Delayed wound healing Recurrent miscarriages PT, aPTT normal ↓ FXIII assay	Factor XIII concentrate (Cortifact) 40 IU/kg q28d to maintain trough level of 5%–20% FFP 15–20 mL/kg Tretten, a recombinant FXIII-A subunit concentrate 35 units/kg /month for prophylaxis. Use in patients with FXIII A subunit deficiency Cryoprecipitate 1 bag/5–10 kg q3–4wk	2%–5%	11–14 days
Combined factor V and VIII	1:2,000,000			Mucosal bleeding Prolonged PT, aPTT (disproportionately)	Factor VIII concentrates and FFP	15%–20%	

Continued

TABLE 5 Rare Bleeding Disorders: Inheritance, Clinical Features, and Treatment.—cont'd

FACTOR	PREVA-LENCE	TYPE	INHERI-TANCE	MANIFESTATION AND DIAGNOSIS	TREATMENT	HEMOSTAT-IC LEVELS	HALF-LIFE
Vitamin K–dependent multiple deficiencies	1:2,000,000			Umbilical stump, intracranial, postsurgical bleeding Skeletal abnormalities Hearing loss	Oral vitamin K, FFP, PCC	15%–20%	

AD, autosomal dominant; *aPTT*, activated partial thromboplastin time; *AR*, autosomal recessive; *CNS*, central nervous system; *FFP*, fresh frozen plasma; *FI*, fibrinogen; *PCC*, prothrombin complex concentrate; *PT*, prothrombin time; *TT*, thrombin time.
[2]Not available in the United States.
*Available in Europe.

References

Arnold WD, Hilgartner MW: Hemophilic arthropathy. Current concepts of pathogenesis and management, *J Bone Joint Surg Am* 59(3):287–305, 1977.

Bolton-Maggs PH, Pasi KJ: Haemophilias A and B, *Lancet* 361(9371):1801–1809, 2003.

Franchini M, Mannucci PM: Non-factor replacement therapy for haemophilia: a current update, *Blood Transfus* 14:1–5, 2018.

Gill JC, Wilson AD, Endres-Brooks J, Montgomery RR: Loss of the largest von Willebrand factor multimers from the plasma of patients with congenital cardiac defects, *Blood* 67(3):758–761, 1986.

Hoffman M, Monroe 3rd DM: A cell-based model of hemostasis, *Thromb Haemost* 85(6):958–965, 2001.

Miller CH, Dilley AB, Drews C, et al: Changes in von Willebrand factor and factor VIII levels during the menstrual cycle, *Thromb Haemost* 87(6):1082–1083, 2002.

Miller CH, Dilley A, Richardson L, et al: Population differences in von Willebrand factor levels affect the diagnosis of von Willebrand disease in African-American women, *Am J Hematol* 67(2):125–129, 2001.

Mulder K, Llinas A: The target joint, *Haemophilia* 10(Suppl. 4):152–156, 2004.

National Hemophilia Foundation Medical and Scientific Advisory Council (MASAC): *MASAC recommendations concerning the treatment of hemophilia and other bleeding disorders.* 2008 , Available at http://www.hemophilia.org/Researchers-Healthcare-Providers/Medical-and-Scientific-Advisory-Council-MASAC/MASAC-Recommendations. Accessed 5 August 2015.

Pabinger-Fasching I: Pipe S: Innovations in coagulation: improved options for treatment of hemophilia A and B, *Thromb Res* 131(2):S1, 2013.

Pierce GF, Lillicrap D, Pipe SW, Vandendriessche T: Gene therapy, bioengineered clotting factors and novel technologies for hemophilia treatment, *J Thromb Haemost* 5(5):901–906, 2007.

Shapiro A: Development of long-acting recombinant FVIII and FIX Fc fusion proteins for the management of hemophilia, *Expert Opin Biol Ther* 13(9):1287–1297, 2013.

Soucie JM, Nuss R, Evatt B, et al: Mortality among males with hemophilia; Relations with source of medical care. The Hemophilia Surveillance System Project Investigators, *Blood* 96(2):437–442, 2000.

Veldman A, Hoffman M, Ehrenforth S: New insights into the coagulation system and implications for new therapeutic options with recombinant factor VIIa, *Curr Med Chem* 10(10):797–811, 2003.

Warrier I, Ewenstein BM, Koerper MA, et al: Factor IX inhibitors and anaphylaxis in hemophilia B, *J Pediatr Hematol Oncol* 19(1):23–27, 1997.

Weyand AC, Pipe SW: New therapies for hemophilia, *Blood* 133(5):389–398, 2019 Jan 31.

Flood VH, Gill JC, Morateck PA, et al: Common VWF exon 28 polymorphisms in African Americans affecting the VWF activity assay by ristocetin cofactor, *Blood* 116(2):280–286, 2010 Jul 15.

HODGKIN LYMPHOMA

Method of
Anusha Vallurupalli, MBBS

CURRENT DIAGNOSIS

- Typically presents as painless cervical or mediastinal lymphadenopathy.
- "B" symptoms (fevers, drenching night sweats, and weight loss >10% of body weight) may be present.
- Tissue diagnosis is made by identifying Reed Sternberg cells on either excisional (preferable) or incisional biopsy. Fine needle aspiration (FNA) is never adequate and should be avoided.

CURRENT THERAPY

- Limited-stage disease (stages I to IIA) with favorable risk factors, termed "early favorable" can be treated with combined modality therapy, (Adriamycin, bleomycin, vinblastine, and dubarbazine [ABVD]), for 2 cycles followed by 20 Gy involved-field radiation.
- Limited-stage disease (I to IIA) with unfavorable risk factors, termed "early unfavorable," may be treated with either combined-modality therapy, 4 cycles of ABVD followed by 30 Gy involved-field radiotherapy, or with 6 cycles of ABVD alone. Decisions about therapy should be decided in a multidisciplinary setting and are usually based on patient age and sex, disease bulk, and area of involved field radiation.
- Advanced-stage disease (IIB to IV) can now be treated with either ABVD or A +AVD for 6 cycles.
- Clinical trials should always be considered for the treatment of disease at any stage, if available.

Epidemiology

There were 8500 estimated new cases of Hodgkin lymphoma (HL) in 2018 with 1050 deaths according to the SEER database. 86.6% patients who underwent treatment were surviving at 5 years between 2008 and 2014. There has been a downward trend in new cases and deaths due to HL over the last 10 years. The median age at diagnosis is 39 years and there is a bimodal age distribution with the highest risk in the age group of 20 to 34 years.

Pathology

HL is classified broadly into classical Hodgkin lymphoma (CHL) or nodular lymphocyte predominant Hodgkin lymphoma (NLPHL) based on the WHO classification system. CHL is the most common type, accounting for 95% of the cases. There are four distinctive histologic subtypes of CHL, Nodular Sclerosis (NS), Mixed Cellularity (MC), Lymphocyte Rich (LR), and Lymphocyte depleted (LD) with NS being the most common subtype.

Pathologically, CHL is characterized by the presence of definitive "Reed Sternberg" (RS) cells, which express CD30 and CD15 on their cell surface. NLPHL, on the other hand, is characterized by "popcorn cells" that express CD20 and CD45 on the cell surface.

Risk Factors

Most cases of CHL are sporadic with no clear risk factors. NS is the most common subtype in United States and developed countries. MC and LR are more common in developing countries and are associated with prior Epstein Barr Virus (EBV) infection. HIV infection is associated with a 5 to 10 times higher risk due to immune suppression and associated EBV infection. The incidence of HL in HIV patients may be increasing in the era of antiretroviral therapy. Increased risk is also seen in other acquired or congenital immunodeficiencies.

There is also increased risk of CHL in families with an index case. According to a Nordic study, there is a threefold increase over the general population risk and the risk is the highest in siblings. Familial risk varies by subtypes and is the highest in the LR subtype.

Clinical Presentation

Painless lymphadenopathy either in the neck (75%) or mediastinal lymph nodes (60%) is the most common presentation for CHL, whereas NLPHL usually presents with painless peripheral lymphadenopathy. "B" symptoms, which include fever higher than 38°C, unintentional weight loss of more than 10% of body weight over 6 months, and drenching night sweats can be present and are often considered unfavorable risk factors. Patients may present with local symptoms from bulky lymphadenopathy such as dyspnea, chest pressure or cough due to mediastinal masses, and neck discomfort and trouble swallowing from cervical lymphadenopathy. Prolonged dyspnea, cough, or chest pressure should be evaluated with appropriate imaging in a young patient when CHL is a consideration in the differential diagnosis. Pruritus can also be seen in some patients and often improves with the treatment of CHL.

Spleen involvement can be seen in 20% of cases and is considered as nodal involvement in CHL. Other extra nodal involvement (e.g., bone marrow, lungs, liver, and bone) is uncommon and is usually associated with advanced unfavorable disease with a poor prognosis. CNS involvement is extremely rare.

Initial lab testing may not show any major abnormalities in early stage and favorable risk patients. The Erythrocyte Sedimentation Rate (ESR) is prognostic in CHL and should be performed at diagnosis in all patients. Anemia, lymphopenia, leukocytosis, and hypoalbuminemia may be seen on labs in advanced and unfavorable risk patients and are a result of cytokine response.

Diagnosis

Adequate tissue sampling is essential in the diagnosis of any lymphoma and is even more indispensable in HL. CHL is characterized by background inflammatory cells, which include polyclonal reactive lymphocytes, neutrophils, and eosinophils with the actual malignant RS cells configuring only 1% to 2% of the total cellularity. As a result, diagnosis is often missed on FNA, which is considered a very insensitive diagnostic methodology. Excisional biopsy is preferable and in cases where it is not possible, multiple core needle biopsies or mediastinoscopic biopsies can be considered, based on the location.

On Haemotoxylin and eosin (H&E) staining of the biopsy, the classic presentation for CHL is a rich inflammatory background interspersed with positive CD15 and CD30 RS cells. RS cells are typically large with bilobed eosinophilic nucleoli and abundant cytoplasm. Mononuclear variants also occur. On immunohistochemistry, RS cells are usually negative for the panlymphoid marker CD45 and the B-cell marker CD20. The presence of RS cells will rule out other conditions in the differential diagnosis, including Non-Hodgkin lymphoma, autoimmune diseases, and infections. The NS subtype also presents with dense bands of fibrosis on H&E staining.

NLPHL is also characterized by atypical malignant cells amidst a polyclonal inflammatory microenvironment composed primarily of small lymphocytes in large nodular meshworks of follicular dendritic cells. The "popcorn" cells characteristic of NLPHL express CD20 and CD45, rather than CD15 an CD30, which is the major pathologic differentiating factor from CHL.

Staging and Risk Prognostication

Staging starts with a thorough history and physical exam. "B" symptoms, pruritus, fatigue, alcohol intolerance, and decrease in performance status may all be noted on the history. Careful palpation and measurements of lymph nodes and spleen as well as documentation of extra nodal involvement are important and can be followed after the initiation of treatment for a clinical response assessment.

TABLE 1	Staging Hodgkin Disease
STAGE	**DEFINITION**
I	Confined to single lymph-node region*
II	Involvement of multiple lymph-node regions on a same side of diaphragm
III	Involvement of nodal regions on both sides of the diaphragm
IV	Extensive involvement of extranodal site(s)
Sub Classification	
A	Absence of "B" symptoms
B	Presence of "B" symptoms
Modifiers	
E	Localized focus of extranodal disease or localized extension of nodal disease into an extranodal site.
S	Splenic involvement (the spleen is considered a nodal site in Hodgkin lymphoma)
X (Cotswold modifier)	Bulky disease (>10 cm or >0.33 of the maximal intrathoracic diameter for mediastinal mass per NCCN guidelines)

*Lymph node regions include: right cervical (including cervical, supraclavicular, occipital, and preauricular lymph nodes), left cervical, right axillary, left axillary, right infraclavicular, left infraclavicular, mediastinal, hilar, periaortic, mesenteric, right pelvic, left pelvic, right inguinal femoral, and left inguinal femoral.

NCCN, National Comprehensive Cancer Network.

The Ann Arbor classification is used for staging. CHL is broadly divided into four stages based on the spread of the lymphoma. Stage I disease is confined to a single lymph-node region, while Stage II is the involvement of multiple lymph-node regions on the same side of the diaphragm, Stage III has involvement of nodal regions on both sides of the diaphragm and Stage IV has extensive involvement of an extranodal site or sites. Each stage is subdivided into "A" and "B" depending on the presence or absence of B symptoms. The Cotswold classification includes an "X" category for bulky disease (Table 1).

Radiographic staging is performed with CT scans in conjunction with PET scanning at diagnosis and repeated after two cycles of chemotherapy and at the end of treatment (EOT). Positron emission tomography–computed tomography (PET-CT) imaging leads to a change in staging in 10% to 30% of patients, more often upstaging. Bone marrow aspirate/biopsy is no longer required for the routine evaluation of patients with HL due to the high sensitivity of PET scan. CNS staging with lumbar puncture (LP) and MRI of the brain is only done if there is a high suspicion based on symptoms and physical examination. Routine staging laparotomy and bilateral bone marrow biopsies are no longer performed.

Laboratory evaluation includes a complete blood count with differential, complete metabolic profile, including albumin, ESR, and baseline HIV testing. Due to the routine use of anthracyclines, an echocardiogram or multigated acquisition scan (MUGA; also called equilibrium radionuclide angiogram) is necessary prior to initiation of chemotherapy to assess left ventricular ejection fraction. Pulmonary function testing is performed and a detailed tobacco smoking history should be obtained due to the use of bleomycin. A pregnancy test should be performed on all women of childbearing age prior to the initiation of therapy. Fertility counseling is recommended for age appropriate patients even though the infertility risk is low (2% to 10%) with the ABVD regimen. The risk of infertility is higher with other regimens such as bleomycin, etoposide, doxorubicin hydrochloride (Adriamycin), cyclophosphamide, vincristine (Oncovin), procarbazine, and prednisone (BEACOPP).

Regardless of the stage, CHL is highly curable and 86.6% patients were alive at 5 years following treatment. Therefore, it is highly important to diagnose and treat patients appropriately and to monitor for long-term complications in survivors. Staging and risk prognostication are essential in deciding the appropriate treatment regimen. Age greater than 50, bulky disease more than 10 cm, elevated ESR, presence of "B" symptoms, involvement of greater than three nodal groups, and bulky mediastinal mass greater than 0.33 (maximum width of the mass/maximum intrathoracic diameter) are all unfavorable factors in limited stage disease (Stage I to II). In advanced-stage CHL, the international prognostic score is generated using seven adverse risk factors, which include male sex, age greater than 45 years, stage IV disease, serum albumin of less than 4 g per deciliter, a hemoglobin level of less than 10.5 g per deciliter, leukocytosis (a white-cell count of at least 15,000 per cubic millimeter), and lymphocytopenia (a lymphocyte count of less than 600 per cubic millimeter, a count that was less than 8% of the white-cell count, or both). The score predicted the rate of freedom from progression of disease with 42% survival in patients with a score of 5 or higher.

Treatment

Stage I to IIA constitutes limited stage disease and Stage IIB to IV constitutes advanced disease.

Limited Stage Classical Hodgkin Lymphoma

Combined modality treatment using a combination of radiotherapy (RT) and chemotherapy is the treatment of choice for early stage limited disease with favorable risk factors. Various trials over decades have established the role of combined modality treatment with RT alone or chemotherapy alone being the comparator arms.

The HD 10 trial investigated the reduction of number of cycles of doxorubicin (Adriamycin,[1] bleomycin, vinblastine, and dubarbazine [ABVD]) and the dose of involved field radiation (IFRT) in patients with no unfavorable risk factors. One thousand three hundred and seventy patients were randomized into four different groups. Early stage favorable risk factor patients who received 2 cycles of ABVD followed by 20 Gy IFRT had similar 5 year overall survival (OS) as the patients who received 4 cycles of ABVD followed by 30 Gy IFRT. ABVD for 2 cycles followed by 20 Gy IFRT is now the standard of care for Stage IA to IIA disease with favorable risk patients. Four cycles of ABVD followed by 30 Gy of IFRT or 6 cycles of ABVD is recommended for limited stage (stage I to IIA) disease with unfavorable risk factors or bulky disease. Stanford V and BEACOPP (bleomycin, etoposide [Toposar],[1] Adriamycin,[1] cyclophosphamide, vincristine [Oncovin], procarbazine [Matulane], and prednisone) regimens are considered alternate treatment options and generally yield similar excellent results with 5 year OS rates of 90% to 95%. ABVD is the most commonly used regimen due to greater tolerability and less cumulative dosage of anthracyclines.

Advanced-Stage Classical Hodgkin Lymphoma

Advanced-stage CHL (Ann Arbor stages IIB to IV) used to be a fatal disease until the development of the MOPP (mechlorethamine, vincristine [Oncovin], procarbazine, and prednisone) regimen in the 1960s. ABVD for 6 to 8 months was compared to MOPP in a randomized landmark clinical trial and ABVD was found to be equally or more effective and was associated with less toxicity. ABVD is administered on days 1 and 15 of a 28-day cycle for 6 total cycles. Modern outcomes with ABVD for advanced-stage disease produced 5-year freedom from progression and OS of 78% and 90%, respectively. Combined modality treatment with IFRT is considered in patients with bulky disease for tumor consolidation or in patients with an incomplete response to chemotherapy.

Alternative regimens include escalated BEACOPP and Stanford V. Neither of these regimens improved OS when compared to ABVD and were associated with increased treatment-related toxicity. Most recently, brentuximab vedotin (BV) (Adcetris) in combination with an Adriamycin, vinblastine, and dacarbazine (A+AVD) regimen has been approved in the United States for advanced stage CHL based on the phase III randomized ECHELON-1 study. This regimen had a 4.9 percentage-point lower combined risk of progression, death, or noncomplete response when compared with the use of subsequent anticancer therapy at 2 years in comparison to ABVD with a tolerable safety profile. The modified end point is considered a caveat for this study and long-term survival data for this study is still pending. Both ABVD and A+AVD are reasonable first line options in patients with Stage III and IV disease and should be chosen based on the patient's age, financial status, and preference and comorbidities. There are not enough data at this time to recommend A+AVD over ABVD. There are ongoing clinical trials evaluating the efficacy and tolerability of combination regimens with BV and checkpoint blockade (nivolumab [Opdivo]) in front line settings. As of now, ABVD is still the preferred regimen in United States with ongoing debate in regard to alternative regimens.

Relapsed/Refractory Classical Hodgkin Lymphoma

CHL carries an overall excellent prognosis and approximately 85% of patients are cured. However, approximately 15% of patients do relapse or have primary refractory disease and will require salvage treatment. Prognosis, especially in patients with refractory disease or who relapse within 12 months of treatment, has historically been poor with conventional salvage chemotherapy. However, with the advent of targeted therapy and checkpoint blockade, response rates and OS rates for this group have improved significantly. Currently, conventional salvage chemotherapy followed by autologous stem cell transplant, which offers a 50% cure rate, remains the second line option.

BV maintenance is offered starting 30 to 45 days after stem cell transplant for a total of 16 cycles, 3 weeks apart based on phase III randomized AETHERA trial data. Patients randomized to receive brentuximab consolidation had significantly improved progression-free survival of 43 months, compared with 24 months in placebo-treated patients. There are ongoing clinical trials evaluating newer agents in second-line settings and enrollment in clinical trials is preferable for these patients. Patients who relapse after autologous stem cell transplant are usually considered for allogeneic stem cell transplant after they have demonstrated a response with next line options.

BV is a monoclonal antibody that is active against CD30 bound to the microtubule toxin monomethyl auristatin E (MMAE). BV has been FDA approved for third-line treatment after a pivotal phase II study resulted in an ORR of 75% and CR of 34% compared to single agent treatment. BV is administered every 3 weeks by intravenous infusion at a dose of 1.8 mg/kg. BV is now also used in combination with Bendamustine (Bendeka)[1], which, in multiple single institutional retrospective data, showed improved response rates of around 92% compared to BV alone.

Mostly recently, immunotherapy with checkpoint blockade has been studied in CHL after identification of 9p24.1 amplification, which results in universal overexpression of programmed death-1(PD-1) ligands. Nivolumab and pembrolizumab (Keytruda), which are both PD-1 inhibitors, have been studied in phase II studies and have shown overall response rates of around 69% and 67%, respectively. Nivolumab is FDA approved for patients who have relapsed after autologous stem cell transplant and have failed BV. Pembrolizumab is approved for patients who have failed BV. Further studies are evaluating the role of combination treatments with these agents. There are also ongoing clinical trials evaluating newer treatment options such as CD30 engineered CAR T cells.

Treatment of Nodular Lymphocyte-Predominant Hodgkin Lymphoma

Nodular lymphocyte-predominant Hodgkin lymphoma (NLPHL) is typically an indolent disease and presents with early stage disease in peripheral nodal locations. Early stage patients are treated with IFRT alone with excellent response rates. Ten year OS is

95% in these patients. Advanced-stage NLPHL is relatively uncommon and can be treated with either single agent rituximab (Rituxan),[1] due to CD20 positivity on malignant cells, or combination chemotherapeutic regimens such as ABVD and RCHOP (rituximab, cyclophosphamide, hydroxydaunomycin [doxorubicin], Oncovin, and prednisone), depending on the extent of disease and patient comorbidities.

Response Assessment

End-of-treatment (EOT) assessment is more accurate with PET-CT imaging. The Deauville score, which is a 5-point scoring system, is used to assess responses with PET scan imaging. A score of 1, 2, or 3 is considered a complete metabolic response. There is no indication for routine surveillance scans after the EOT assessment. A score of 4 or 5 is considered a suboptimal response and may require a change of treatment plan. Interim PET scanning after two cycles of ABVD therapy has prognostic significance. However, the significance of interim PET scanning with newer combination regimens has not been validated.

Complications and Long-Term Monitoring

CHL is a curable cancer. Short- and long-term complications from treatment require close monitoring, especially given the young age of presentation in most patients. Most short-term side effects are fatigue, nausea, emesis, constipation, increased risk of infections, and peripheral neuropathy. Patients need long-term cardiac monitoring due to the risk of congestive heart failure with anthracyclines and combination IFRT, and the risk of coronary artery disease with IFRT. Bleomycin can cause long-term pulmonary toxicity and patients should be monitored while on active treatment. Prompt discontinuation of bleomycin is warranted if there is any suspicion of pulmonary complications. There is a long-term risk of secondary malignancies and myelodysplastic syndrome in patients treated for HL.

Patients should undergo regular cancer screenings. Yearly complete blood count is warranted. Thyroid evaluation once a year is recommended for patients who have received neck or superior mediastinal IFRT. Mammography is recommended for women starting 8 years after IFRT to mediastinum.

---

[1] Not FDA approved for this indication.

References

Advani RH, Hoppe RT, Baer D, et al: Efficacy of abbreviated Stanford V chemotherapy and involved-field radiotherapy in early-stage Hodgkin lymphoma: mature results of the G4 trial, *Ann Oncol* 34:1044–1048, 2013.

Armand P, Engert A, Younes A, et al: Nivolumab for relapsed/refractory classic hodgkin lymphoma after failure of autologous hematopoietic cell transplantation: extended follow-up of the multicohort single-arm Phase II CheckMate 205 Trial, *J Clin Oncol* 36(14):1428–1439, 2018 May 10.

Canellos GP, Anderson JR, et al: Chemotherapy of advanced Hodgkin's Disease with MOPP, ABVD, or MOPP alternating with ABVD, *N Engl J Med* 327:1478–1484, 1992.

Chen RC, Chin MS, Ng AK, et al: Early-stage, lymphocyte-predominant Hodgkin's lymphoma: patient outcomes from a large, single-institution series with long follow-up, *J Clin Oncol* 28:136–141, 2010.

Cheson BD, Fisher RI, Barrington SF, et al: Recommendations for initial evaluation, staging, and response assessment of hodgkin and non-Hodgkin lymphoma: the Lugano classification, *J Clin Oncol* 32(27):3059–3067, 2014 Sep 20.

Connors JM, Jurczak W, Straus DJ, et al: Brentuximab vedotin with chemotherapy for stage III or IV Hodgkin's lymphoma, *N Engl J Med* 378:331–344, 2018.

Eichenauer DA, Fuchs M, Pluetschow A, et al: Phase 2 study of rituximab in newly diagnosed stage IA nodular lymphocyte-predominant Hodgkin lymphoma: a report from the German Hodgkin Study Group, *Blood* 118:4363–4365, 2011.

Engert A, Plutschow A, Eich HT, et al: Reduced treatment intensity in patients with early-stage Hodgkin's lymphoma, *N Engl J Med* 363:640–652, 2010.

Gallamini A, Hutchings M, Rigacci L, et al: Early interim 2-[18 F]fluoro-2-deoxy-Dglucose positron emission tomography is prognostically superior to international prognostic score in advanced-stage Hodgkin's lymphoma: a report from a joint Italian-Danish study, *J Clin Oncol* 25:3746–3752, 2007.

Hasenclever D, Diehl V: A prognostic score for advanced Hodgkin's disease. International Prognostic Factors Project on Advanced Hodgkin's Disease, *N Engl J Med* 339(21):1506–1514, 1998 Nov 19.

Jacobson CA, Abramson JS: HIV-associated Hodgkin's lymphoma: prognosis and therapy in the era of cART, *Adv Hematol* 2012:507257, 2012.

Kharazmi E, Fallah M, Pukkala E, et al: Risk of familial classical Hodgkin lymphoma by relationship, histology, age, and sex: a joint study from five Nordic countries, *Blood* 126(17):1990–1995, 2015 Oct 22.

LaCasce AS, Bociek RG, Sawas A, et al: Brentuximab vedotin plus bendamustine: a highly active first salvage regimen for relapsed or refractory Hodgkin lymphoma, *Blood* 11:815183, 2018.

Meyer RM, Gospodarowicz MK, Connors JM, et al: ABVD alone versus radiation-based therapy in limited-stage Hodgkin's lymphoma, *N Engl J Med* 366:399–408, 2012.

Moskowitz CH, Nademanee A, et al: Brentuximab vedotin as consolidation therapy after autologous stem-cell transplantation in patients with Hodgkin's lymphoma at risk of relapse or progression (AETHERA): a randomised, double-blind, placebo-controlled, phase 3 trial, *Lancet* 385(9980):1853–1862, 2015 May 9.

Moskowitz CH, Zinzani PL, Fanale MA, et al: Pembrolizumab in relapsed/refractory classical Hodgkin lymphoma: primary end point analysis of the Phase 2 Keynote-087 Study, *Blood* 128:1107, 2016.

Younes A, Gopal AK, Smith SE, et al: Results of a pivotal phase II study of brentuximab vedotin for patients with relapsed or refractory Hodgkin's lymphoma, *J Clin Oncol* 30(18):2183–2189, 2012 Jun 20.

IRON DEFICIENCY ANEMIA

Method of
Susan Evans, MD

CURRENT DIAGNOSIS

- The presence of symptoms and signs depends on the degree of iron deficiency, the time course of the development of iron deficiency, and the overall physiologic state of the patient. Patients may be asymptomatic. Signs and symptoms are more likely if anemia and/or hemodynamic instability are present.
- Symptoms include fatigue, poor exercise tolerance, weakness, headache, pica, dyspnea, dizziness, vertigo, and angina pectoris.
- Signs include pallor, dry and rough skin, brittle nails, defects of the nail bed (koilonychias), atrophy of the lingual papillae, and cheilosis.
- Systolic heart murmur if anemia is present
- Neonates: delayed growth and development
- Adolescents: learning and behavior problems
- Blood loss is the most common cause of iron deficiency
- Iron deficiency is the most common cause of anemia

Laboratory Findings
- Decreased iron on bone marrow aspirate is the gold standard but is rarely used
- Low serum hemoglobin to diagnose anemia
- Low mean corpuscular hemoglobin: late finding
- Low mean corpuscular volume: late finding
- Low serum iron
- High serum iron-binding capacity
- Low percent transferrin saturation (TSAT)
- Low serum ferritin, but may be normal in the presence of inflammation

CURRENT THERAPY

Oral Replacement
- Ferrous sulfate (or another equivalent iron preparation) 325 mg (65 mg elemental iron) three times daily.
- Avoid taking with meals to increase absorption.

Parenteral Replacement
- Recommended when blood loss exceeds the ability to replace orally, in the context of malabsorption and if oral iron is not tolerated
  - Ferric carboxymaltose (Ferinject and Injectafer)
  - Ferric gluconate (Ferrlecit)
  - Ferumoxytol (Feraheme)
  - Iron sucrose (Venofer)

Epidemiology

Anemia affects more than one-third of the world's population, or 2 billion people. Iron deficiency continues to be the most common cause of anemia. Iron deficiency is the only micronutrient deficiency that remains a significant problem in both developing and developed countries. Iron deficiency refers to a decrease in iron stores below a normal level and can cause fatigue even without anemia. In the case of iron deficiency without anemia, iron stores are still adequate for erythropoiesis. Iron deficiency anemia is a more serious condition in which there is not enough erythroid iron available, leading to anemia. Worldwide levels of iron deficiency are estimated to be twice that of iron deficiency anemia.

Risk Factors

Risk factors for iron deficiency anemia include age, socioeconomic status, gender, diet, disease, and medical treatment. Several groups of people are at an increased risk of iron deficiency based on age or their stage in life. Infants and children ages 0 to 5 years old are at risk for iron deficiency because of their rapid rate of growth, which necessitates increased iron stores. Adolescent girls and women of child bearing age are also at risk due to iron loss through menstruation. During pregnancy, a woman's iron needs triple because of the expansion of red cell mass, the placenta, and the growth of the fetus. Elderly people are also at risk for iron deficiency for a number of reasons, including inadequate diet, poor absorption due to disease or antacid medicines, or as a complication of chronic disease.

Dietary causes of iron deficiency anemia include lack of access to or preference against eating a diet including iron rich foods. While 90% of iron in the body is recycled every day, dietary iron is essential for replacing lost iron, which is mainly excreted in bile. Iron supplementation of common foods such as breads and rice in the United States decreases the risk of dietary iron deficiency. Iron is found naturally in both animal products such as meat and in plant based foods such as green leafy vegetables, sweet potatoes, and legumes. As long as they eat a healthy and well-balanced diet, vegetarians and vegans have not been shown to be at an increased risk for iron deficiency; such diets have many other health benefits.

Any illness or therapy that leads to decreased iron absorption or blood loss may cause iron deficiency. Common causes of blood loss include gastrointestinal diseases such as cancer, inflammatory bowel disease, and ulcer disease. Taking aspirin, nonsteroidal anti-inflammatory drugs (NSAIDs), or anticoagulants also increases the risk of gastrointestinal blood loss. Iron absorption is decreased in the context of celiac disease, post gastric bypass surgery, and *Helicobacter pylori* infection. Chronic diseases associated with iron deficiency include chronic kidney disease, rheumatoid arthritis, cancer, obesity, and chronic heart failure. There are also medical treatments that may cause iron deficiency such as antacid medicines, which decrease iron absorption, dialysis that causes blood loss, and erythropoietin therapy that depletes iron stores through increased erythropoiesis. Frequent phlebotomy, including repetitive blood donation or treatment for polycythemia or hemochromatosis, decrease iron stores. Rarely, there may be a genetic cause for iron deficiency anemia such as iron-refractory iron deficiency anemia.

Pathophysiology

Iron in the body can be broken down into two main types: functional iron and storage iron. Functional iron plays many essential roles in the human body. It is found in hemoglobin, which carries oxygen from the lungs to body tissues, and in muscles as myoglobin, which helps with oxygen use and storage. Iron plays a role in enzymatic reactions, DNA synthesis, mitochondrial energy generation, and cell proliferation. Storage iron is found in ferritin, hemosiderin, and transferrin. Iron homeostasis is very important to the body and is regulated through the diet, gastrointestinal absorption, and the recycling of the iron in red blood cells. Total body iron stores are about 3.5 g for men and 2.5 g for women. Approximately 20 to 25 mg of iron is needed daily for red cell production and body processes. Dietary absorption of iron is limited to about 1 to 2 mg/day; the daily requirement is produced through the recycling of iron in used red blood cells by macrophages.

Dietary iron is found in two forms. Heme iron (Fe^{2+}) is found in animal products such as meat, poultry and seafood and is more easily absorbed than plant-based iron. Nonheme iron (Fe^{3+}) is found in plant sources such as beans and lentils, baked potatoes, dark green leafy vegetables, tofu, and cashews. Dietary iron is also found in iron fortified breakfast cereals and enriched breads. Adding foods high in vitamin C to a meal with nonheme iron can increase iron absorption. There are other foods that inhibit the absorption of iron, including polyphenols found in some vegetables, tannins found in tea, and calcium found in dairy products. Dietary iron absorption takes place almost exclusively in the duodenum and upper jejunum.

The recycling of iron from used red blood cells provides about 90% of body iron and is essential for maintaining normal iron levels in the body. Hepcidin, a peptide hormone mainly synthesized in the liver, controls the process of iron absorption and recycling. When serum iron levels are high, hepcidin levels increase in response, which leads to breakdown of the iron transporter called ferroportin. A decrease in ferroportin leaves more iron inside macrophages, enterocytes, and hepatocytes, and the serum iron level decreases. When serum iron levels drop, expression of hepcidin should decrease as well. However, inflammation and infection can cause hepcidin to increase inappropriately; this is one of the ways in which chronic disease contributes to iron deficiency.

Prevention

Prevention plays a large role in the treatment of iron deficiency anemia worldwide and includes both dietary interventions and supplementation. A food-based approach to prevention would include encouraging patients to eat more iron rich foods such as meats and dark green leafy vegetables. A list of iron rich foods is found in Table 1. Heme iron, found in animal sources, is easily absorbed; however, the absorption of nonheme iron from plant sources is affected by the foods with which they are eaten. Foods that can inhibit the absorption of iron include the tannins in tea and coffee and the calcium found in milk. It is best to eat these foods separately from iron rich foods to increase iron absorption. Nonheme iron absorption can also be increased by accompanying foods such as when it is eaten with a heme iron food such as meat

TABLE 1	Iron Rich Foods
IRON TYPE	**DIETARY SOURCES**
Heme Iron	Beef
	Chicken
	Fish
	Organ Meats
	Oysters
Nonheme Iron	Dark Green Leafy Vegetables
	Beans
	Lentils
	Tofu
	Baked Potato
	Cashews
	Fortified Cereals, Breads and Pasta

or with vitamin C in the form of fruit, orange juice, or broccoli. Encouraging iron fortified foods, which in the United States include cereals, rice, pasta, and bread, is another effective way to prevent deficiency. There are some cases when the risk of developing iron deficiency is so high that supplementation with an oral iron supplement is recommended. The World Health Organization recommends universal supplementation for low-birth-weight infants with 2 mg/kg daily from age 2 months to 23 months. They also recommend universal supplementation for pregnant women with 60 mg iron per day. While supplementation for pregnant women is common practice in the United States, the US Preventive Services Task Force states that there is insufficient evidence to show that these practices help prevent adverse maternal health and birth outcomes. According to the US Preventive Services Task Force, evidence is also insufficient to recommend screening children age 6 months to 2 years of age for iron deficiency anemia in the United States.

Clinical Manifestations

Patients with iron deficiency may be asymptomatic. The presence of symptoms and signs of iron deficiency depend on the degree of deficiency, the time course of the development of iron deficiency, and the overall physiologic state of the patient. Common symptoms of iron deficiency include fatigue, weakness, irritability, poor concentration, exercise intolerance, dry mouth, headache, and restless leg syndrome. Severe iron deficiency can cause pica, a craving to eat substances such as ice, dirt, clay, or paint. Signs of iron deficiency include pallor and a systolic heart murmur if anemia is present, hair loss, atrophy of lingual papillae, and nail changes such as koilonychias.

Diagnosis

Normal hemoglobin levels depend on age, gender, pregnancy status, altitude, and smoking, but in general, an adult male is considered anemic with a hemoglobin level less than 13 g/mL and an adult female at less than 12 g/mL. Iron deficiency may be present with or without anemia; therefore, measuring hemoglobin level is neither a sensitive nor a specific test for iron deficiency. Absolute iron deficiency occurs when the amount of total body iron is low. Functional iron deficiency occurs when there is not enough iron available to meet the demand of body tissues and processes because iron is sequestered either in macrophages or the reticulo-endothelial system.

Diagnosing iron deficiency is not straightforward because serum ferritin level, which is often used as a screening test, is affected by gender, age, inflammation, infection, and chronic diseases such as liver disease and cancer. While a serum ferritin concentration less than 12 μg/L makes iron deficiency very likely, a person with inflammation or chronic disease may have iron deficiency at much higher ferritin levels. Increasing the cutoff for normal ferritin concentration to 30 μg/L has been shown to increase sensitivity for iron deficiency, and an even higher cutoff of 100 μg is recommended by some specialty societies. For this reason, utilizing more than one iron status indicator to make the diagnosis is important. A low iron level (<50 μg/dL) and an elevated total iron binding capacity (TIBC >450 μg/dL) also support the diagnosis of iron deficiency. Other supporting labs include a drop in transferrin saturation (TSAT) to less than 16% or less than 20% if inflammation or disease is present. Low mean corpuscular volume (MCV) may be another sign of iron deficiency, but this is generally a late finding, so MCV may be in the normal range. Low MCV can also be seen in thalassemia. Low mean corpuscular hemoglobin concentration (MCHC) is another late finding in iron deficiency. Decreased iron seen on bone marrow aspiration is still considered the gold standard for diagnosing iron deficiency, but it is rarely done due to both cost and patient discomfort. A new test being developed to diagnose iron deficiency measures the level of serum soluble transferrin receptors (sTfR), which increase in the context of iron deficiency and are not affected by inflammation. A drawback for the test is that the sTfR level may be elevated in those with hemolytic anemia or chronic lymphocytic leukemia as well as in those using recombinant human erythropoietin.

Differential Diagnosis

The differential diagnosis of iron deficiency includes causes of fatigue and exercise intolerance such as hypothyroidism, electrolyte disturbances due to diuretic therapy, left ventricular dysfunction, chronic lung disease, malignancies, or liver disease.

Anemia of chronic disease can mimic iron deficiency anemia and may be found concurrently in the same patient. A low MCV on blood count can also be a sign of thalassemia.

Treatment

The goal of treatment is to replace iron so that hemoglobin levels normalize, and iron stores are replenished. Treatment of iron deficiency must take into consideration the type of patient being treated and the source and amount of iron deficit or blood loss. Patients who are severely anemic and hemodynamically unstable may be candidates for blood transfusion. For people in groups that are at high risk for iron deficiency, such as infants, toddlers, adolescents, and menstruating women, it is reasonable to start with oral supplementation with iron and only proceed with further work up if that is unsuccessful. However, in patients at low risk for iron deficiency, such as men and post-menopausal women, it is important to determine the underlying cause of iron deficiency. Blood loss is the most common cause of iron deficiency, so this work-up includes evaluation for a source of bleeding. Urinalysis and heme-occult testing are preliminary tests, and upper and lower endoscopy is needed to evaluate for gastrointestinal pathology including cancer, colitis, or celiac disease. If those tests are inconclusive, consider proceeding to video capsule endoscopy to further evaluate the small intestine. Heavy gynecologic bleeding may require further evaluation and treatment. Persistent blood noted on urinalysis would warrant referral to urology for further testing.

Oral iron supplementation continues to be the first line treatment for iron deficiency anemia. Common forms include ferrous sulfate (Feosol), ferrous gluconate (Fergon), and ferrous fumarate (Ferro-Sequels). A typical dose of ferrous sulfate is 325 mg, which is 65 mg elemental iron, three times daily. Iron is best absorbed when taken between meals however, this can also worsen side effects. It is best to take iron separate from acid reducing medicines and foods that inhibit iron absorption. Common side effects of oral iron include diarrhea, nausea, epigastric discomfort, and constipation. Side effects can be lessened by taking iron with food, taking smaller doses, or changing to ferrous gluconate 325 mg (35 mg elemental iron).

Parenteral iron may be indicated when oral therapy is unsuccessful due to malabsorption, when oral iron is not tolerated, or when the rate of absorption with oral supplementation is insufficient due to the rate of blood loss. New forms of parenteral iron are safer and less likely to cause hypersensitivity reactions than older high-molecular weight iron dextran.[2] The dose of IV iron needed can be calculated with the following formula: body weight in kilograms x 2.3 x hemoglobin deficiency (target hemoglobin level—patient hemoglobin level). Add another 500 to 1000 mg iron to replace low iron stores. Parenteral iron preparations licensed for use in the United States include iron sucrose (Venofer), ferumoxytol (Feraheme), ferric carboxymaltose (Ferinject and Injectafer), and ferric gluconate (Ferrlecit). A common dose for iron sucrose is 200 mg IV over 2 to 5 minutes, which is often repeated 5 times or until the target dose of iron is reached. Ferumoxytol has a usual dose of 510 mg IV infusion over at least 15 minutes which can be repeated 3 to 5 days after the initial dose. For patients who weigh ≥50 kg, the dose of ferric carboxymaltose is 750 mg IV over 15 to 30 minutes, and this can be repeated 7 days after the first dose. Ferric gluconate is generally used for patients on dialysis, and the typical dose is 125 mg IV over 10 minutes or IV infusion over 60 minutes per dialysis session.

Monitoring

The earliest marker for successful iron replacement is an increase in the reticulocyte count, which occurs within 5 to 10 days of initiation of iron replacement. Darkening of stools after 2 or 3 days of starting oral iron replacement is a reliable marker of compliance. A hemoglobin increase of 2 g/dL is considered an appropriate response to oral iron replacement. Reaching a serum ferritin level of 100 μg/L will ensure good iron stores in nearly all patients. Once iron deficiency has been corrected, a complete blood count and labs to evaluate iron stores should be checked monthly for 3 months and then every 3 months for a year. If iron levels are not maintained, then further work up is indicated to discover the cause.

Management of Complications

If properly treated, iron deficiency has few complications in adults. Untreated iron deficiency in infants and small children can lead to cognitive development and growth deficits. Treating iron deficiency without identifying the source and cause of blood loss could result in a delay or failure to diagnose gastrointestinal malignancies or other serious clinical problems.

Plummer–Vinson syndrome is a rare clinical condition characterized by a triad of iron deficiency anemia, post-cricoid esophageal webs, and dysphagia. The pathogenesis of Plummer-Vinson syndrome remains unclear, though iron and other nutritional deficiencies, genetic predisposition, and autoimmunity have all been implicated in the formation of the webs. Treatment includes the correction of iron deficiency and endoscopic dilation of the esophageal webs to relieve dysphagia.

References

Auerbach M, Adamson JW: How we diagnose and treat iron deficiency anemia, *Am J Hematol* 91(1):31–38, 2016 Jan.

Bermejo F, Garcia-Lopez S: A guide to diagnosis of iron deficiency and iron deficiency anemia in digestive diseases, *World J Gastroenterol* 15(37):4638–4643, 2009 Oct 7.

Camaschella C: Iron-deficiency anemia, *N Engl J Med* 372(19):1832–1843, 2015 May 7.

Centers for Disease Control. Recommendation to Prevent and Control Iron Deficiency in the United States. Available at https://www.cdc.gov/MMWR/preview/mmwrhtml/00051880.htm. [Accessed April 16, 2019].

Craig WJ, Mangels AR, American Dietetic Association: Position of the American Dietetic Association: vegetarian diets, *J Am Diet Assoc* 109(7):1266–1282, 2009 Jul.

Engebretsen KV, Blom-Hogestol IK, Hewitt S, et al: Anemia following Roux-en-Y gastric bypass for morbid obesity; a 5-year follow-up study, *Scand J Gastroenterol* 53(8):917–922, 2018 Aug.

Lopez A, Cacoub P, Macdougall IC, Peyrin-Biroulet L: Iron deficiency anaemia, *Lancet* 387(10021):907–916, 2016 Feb 27.

Parrott J, Frank L, Rabena R, Craggs-Dino L, Isom KA, Greiman L: American Society for Metabolic and Bariatric Surgery Integrated Health Nutritional Guidelines for the Surgical Weight Loss Patient 2016 Update: Micronutrients, *Surg Obes Relat Dis* 13(5):727–741, 2017 May.

Peyrin-Biroulet L, Williet N, Cacoub P: Guidelines on the diagnosis and treatment of iron deficiency across indications: a systematic review, *Am J Clin Nutr* 102(6):1585–1594, 2015 Dec.

World Health Organization/UNICEF/UNU: Iron Deficiency Anaemia: Assessment, Prevention, and Control. A guide for Programme Managers, Geneva, Switzerland, 2001, World Health Organization. Available at https://www.who.int/nutrition/publications/en/ida_assessment_prevention_control.pdf. [Accessed 17 April 2019].

MULTIPLE MYELOMA

Method of
S. Vincent Rajkumar, MD; and Robert A. Kyle, MD

CURRENT DIAGNOSIS

- Malignant clonal plasma cell disorder
- Characterized by presence of a monoclonal immunoglobulin in the serum or urine in most patients
- Typical manifestations include anemia, osteolytic bone lesions, and renal failure
- Initial work-up should include a bone marrow aspiration and biopsy with fluorescent in situ hybridization studies to determine molecular cytogenetic typ0065
- Standard risk: trisomies (hyperdiploidy), t(11;14), and t(6;14)
- High risk: del(17p), gain 1q, t(4;14), (t14;16) or t(14;20)

CURRENT THERAPY

- Do not begin treatment until symptomatic multiple myeloma develops (CRAB: calcium elevated, renal failure, anemia, bone lesions) or other myeloma defining events are present. Patients with high risk smoldering multiple myeloma are candidates for preventive therapy with lenalidomide (Revimid) or lenalidomide plus dexamethasone (Decadron)[1] (Rd)
- Decide whether an autologous stem cell transplant is feasible. If it is, one must avoid melphalan (Alkeran) therapy as initial treatment.
- Initial therapy typically consists of a triplet regimen such as lenalidomide (Revlimid), bortezomib (Velcade), and dexamethasone[1] (VRd)
- Patients who are candidates for autologous stem cell transplantation should collect stem cells after 3 to 4 cycles of induction. After collection, patients proceed to either early transplantation, or resume initial therapy and postpone transplant until relapse. After transplant and after initial therapy for approximately 12 months in patients who delay transplant, patients should receive maintenance therapy.
- Patients who are not stem cell transplant candidates receive initial therapy for a duration of approximately 12 months followed by maintenance. Frail patients can be treated with the doublet regimen of Rd, in which case therapy is continued until progression if tolerated.
- Relapsed or refractory myeloma should be treated with one of the active drugs given alone or in combination. Active agents include thalidomide, lenalidomide, bortezomib, carfilzomib (Kyprolis), pomalidomide (Pomalyst), daratumumab (Darzalex), ixazomib (Ninlaro), elotuzumab (Empliciti), panobinostat (Farydak), corticosteroids, anthracyclines, and alkylators.

[1]Not FDA approved for this indication.

Multiple myeloma is characterized by the neoplastic proliferation of clonal plasma cells. It is typically associated with a monoclonal (M) protein in the serum and/or urine.

Epidemiology

In the United States, multiple myeloma constitutes 1% of all malignant diseases and slightly more than 10% of hematologic malignancies. The annual incidence is 4 to 5 per 100,000; the incidence in African Americans is twice that in whites. The apparent recent increase in rates is probably caused by increased availability and use of medical facilities and improved diagnostic techniques, particularly in the older population. The median age at diagnosis is approximately 70 years.

Risk Factors

The cause of multiple myeloma is unclear. Exposure to radiation might play a role. Persons in agricultural occupations who are exposed to pesticides, herbicides, or fungicides have an increased risk of multiple myeloma. Benzene and petroleum products, hair dyes, engine exhaust, furniture worker products, obesity, and chronic immune stimulation have also been reported as risk factors. The risk of developing multiple myeloma is higher for patients with a first-degree relative with the disease. Clusters of two or more first-degree relatives or identical twins have been recognized.

Clinical Manifestations

Weakness, fatigue, bone pain, recurrent infections, and symptoms of hypercalcemia or renal insufficiency should alert the physician to the possibility of multiple myeloma. Anemia is present in 70% of patients at the time of diagnosis. An M protein is found in the serum or urine in more than 97% of patients with multiple myeloma by immunofixation studies and the serum free light chain (FLC) assay. Lytic lesions, osteoporosis, or fractures are present at diagnosis in 80% of patients and are best detected by whole body low-dose computed tomography (CT) or positron emission tomography (PET)/CT. Magnetic resonance imaging (MRI) and PET/CT are also helpful in patients who have skeletal pain but no abnormality on radiographs or when there are other clinical concerns about the extent of the disease. Conventional radiography is less sensitive and is no longer recommended. Hypercalcemia is present in 15% of patients, and the serum creatinine value is 2 mg/dL or greater in almost 20% of patients at diagnosis.

Diagnosis

If multiple myeloma is suspected, the patient should have, in addition to a complete history and physical examination:

- Determination of values for hemoglobin, leukocytes with differential count, platelets, serum creatinine, calcium, and uric acid
- A radiographic survey of bones, including humeri and femurs using low-dose whole body CT or PET-CT.
- Serum protein electrophoresis with immunofixation
- Quantitation of immunoglobulins (Igs), serum FLC assay
- Bone marrow aspirate and biopsy
- Routine urinalysis
- Electrophoresis and immunofixation of an adequately concentrated aliquot from a 24-hour urine specimen
- Fluorescence in situ hybridization (FISH)
- Measurement of β_2-microglobulin, C-reactive protein, and lactate dehydrogenase

Box 1 lists the International Myeloma Working Group updated criteria for diagnosis of myeloma and related disorders. Metastatic carcinoma, lymphoma, leukemia, and connective tissue disorders can resemble multiple myeloma and must be considered in the differential diagnosis. Patients with multiple myeloma must be differentiated from those with monoclonal gammopathy of undetermined significance (MGUS) and smoldering (asymptomatic) multiple myeloma (SMM). Patients with MGUS and low-risk SMM may remain stable for long periods and not require treatment (see Box 1). Patients with high-risk SMM (any two or more of the following: >20% bone marrow plasma cells, >2g/dL serum M protein, >20 serum FLC ratio) should be considered for lenalidomide (Revlimid) or lenalidomide plus dexamethasone (Decadron)[1] as preventive therapy.

Treatment

Patients with symptomatic multiple myeloma may be classified as having high-risk or standard-risk disease. High-risk disease is defined as the presence of del(17p), gain 1q, t(4;14), t(14;16), or t(14;20) with FISH. Detection of p53 mutations by sequencing is also considered a cytogenetic high-risk factor. The presence of two high-risk cytogenetic abnormalities is considered "double-hit" myeloma; and the presence of three high-risk abnormalities is considered triple-hit myeloma. Lactate dehydrogenase, circulating plasma cells, and β_2-microglobulin levels are additional important risk factors. Approximately 15% to 20% of patients with symptomatic multiple myeloma have high-risk disease.

Initially, patients are classified into those eligible for an autologous stem cell transplant (SCT) versus those not eligible. An autologous SCT adds approximately 1 year of survival on average when compared with patients treated with conventional-dose chemotherapy alone.

Eligibility for autologous SCT in multiple myeloma varies from country to country. In the United States, decisions are made on a patient-by-patient basis depending on the physiologic age rather than the chronologic age. In most institutions, patients older than 70 years or with serum creatinine greater than 2.5 mg/dL, Eastern Cooperative Oncology Group (ECOG) performance status of 3 or 4, or New York Heart Association (NYHA) functional

BOX 1 International Myeloma Working Group Diagnostic Criteria.

Monoclonal Gammopathy of Undetermined Significance
- Serum M protein <3 g/dL
- Clonal bone marrow–plasma cells <10%
- Absence of end-organ damage (CRAB) attributable to a plasma cell proliferative disorder

Smoldering Multiple Myeloma
- Serum M protein ≥3 g/dL and/or clonal bone marrow–plasma cells 10%–60%
- Absence of myeloma defining events or amyloidosis

Multiple Myeloma
- Presence of clonal bone marrow plasma cells 10% or greater or biopsy-proven plasmacytoma
- Presence of end-organ damage (CRAB) thought to be related to a plasma cell proliferative disorder or other myeloma defining event (clonal bone marrow plasma cells 60% or higher, serum free light chain ratio 100 or more provided involved free light chain level is 100 mg/L or more, more than one focal lesion on magnetic resonance imaging)

CRAB, Calcium elevated, renal failure, anemia, bone lesions; *M*, monoclonal.
Derived from Rajkumar SV, Dimopoulos MA, Palumbo A, et al. International Myeloma Working Group updated criteria for the diagnosis of multiple myeloma. *Lancet Oncol.* 2014;15:e538–e548.

status class III or IV are considered ineligible for autologous SCT. Although patients with kidney failure may have an autologous SCT, the morbidity and mortality are higher.

Initial Therapy for Transplant-Eligible Patients

The approach to treatment of newly diagnosed myeloma in patients eligible for stem cell transplantation is summarized in Figure 1A. Bortezomib (Velcade), lenalidomide (Revlimid), dexamethasone (Decadon)[1] (VRD) is the preferred standard initial therapy for multiple myeloma. In a randomized trial conducted by the Southwest Oncology Group, VRD was superior to lenalidomide plus dexamethasone (Rd) in terms of progression-free survival (PFS) and overall survival (OS). Bortezomib and dexamethasone are typically administered once weekly. In the VRD regimen lenalidomide is given at a dose of 25 mg daily on days 1 to 14 of a 21-day cycle. Bortezomib should be given using the once-weekly schedule to reduce the risk of peripheral neuropathy. It is also preferable to administer bortezomib subcutaneously to diminish the risk of neuropathy. An alternative to VRD is daratumumab (Darzalex), lenalidomide, dexamethasone (DRD). For patients who are initiated on DRD, all three drugs are continued until progression, with daratumumab administered once-monthly after the first 6 months of therapy. The addition of daratumumab (Darzalex) to VTD (Velcade, thalidomide, dexamethasone) has shown better response rates and PFS compared with VTD, but more data on OS are needed before this approach can be recommended. Further data from randomized trials on the addition of daratumumab to the current standard of VRD is also needed. Bortezomib plus cyclophosphamide (Cytoxan) 300 mg/m² orally once weekly plus dexamethasone 40 mg once weekly (VCD) is an option for patients presenting with acute renal failure. If lenalidomide is not available, an alternative for initial therapy is bortezomib, thalidomide (Thalomid), and dexamethasone (VTD). For high-risk patients less than 65 years of age, carfilzomib (Kyprolis), lenalidomide, dexamethasone (KRD) or daratumumab plus VRD can be considered as alternatives. In all regimens, it is preferable to administer dexamethasone at a dose no greater than 40 mg per week unless there is need for urgent cytoreduction as in patients with acute renal failure and cast nephropathy.

Figure 1 Approach to the treatment of newly diagnosed myeloma in patients eligible for stem cell transplantation (A) and approach to the treatment of newly diagnosed myeloma in patients not eligible for stem cell transplantation (B). *ASCT,* Autologous stem cell transplantation; *DRD,* daratumumab, lenalidomide, dexamethasone; *KRD,* carfilzomib, lenalidomide, dexamethasone; *VRD,* bortezomib, lenalidomide, dexamethasone. (Modified from Rajkumar SV. Multiple myeloma: 2016 update on diagnosis, risk-stratification, and management. *Am J Hematol.* 2016;91:720–734.)

Autologous Stem Cell Transplantation

Following 3 to 4 months of induction therapy with one of the initial regimens, one must collect the stem cells in patients eligible for transplantation. The stem cells must be collected before the patient is exposed to prolonged therapy, especially melphalan (Alkeran). Granulocyte colony-stimulating factor (G-CSF, Neupogen) with or without cyclophosphamide (Cytoxan) is used for mobilizing stem cells. G-CSF plus cyclophosphamide is preferred in patients who are treated with lenalidomide plus dexamethasone induction, who are older than 65 years, or who have received such therapy for over 4 months. Plerixafor (Mozobil) may also be used for mobilization of hematopoietic stem cells. It is advisable to collect 6×10^6 CD34+ cells/kg, which is sufficient for two transplants in patients below 65 years of age.

The timing of autologous SCT takes into account the patient's wishes, and it may be done early (when the patient recovers from stem cell collection) or delayed until relapse. There is no difference in OS among patients who receive an autologous SCT immediately following collection of stem cells and those who receive it at first relapse. In general, we prefer an early transplant because this provides a better quality of life and time without therapy.

Melphalan 200 mg/m² is the preferred conditioning regimen[3] for autologous SCT. Tandem transplantation is not recommended for most patients. An exception would be young patients (below 65 years of age) with high-risk multiple myeloma, in whom such an approach can be considered on a case-by-case basis.

The mortality rate with autologous SCT is approximately 1%. Unfortunately, multiple myeloma is not eradicated, and the autologous peripheral stem cells are contaminated by myeloma cells or their precursors.

Bone marrow transplantation from an identical twin donor (syngeneic) is the treatment of choice if such a donor is available. Results are superior to allogeneic transplantation.

Maintenance Therapy Following Autologous Stem Cell Transplantation

Randomized trials have tested the value of lenalidomide as maintenance therapy following stem cell transplantation. An OS benefit has been observed in a meta-analysis of three trials. This benefit appears to be mainly restricted to standard-risk patients. An increased risk of second cancers has been noted with lenalidomide maintenance and further follow-up is needed. In another randomized trial improved OS with bortezomib maintenance has been reported, but it is not clear whether the benefit is due to the maintenance therapy or differences in induction therapy between the two groups. We recommend lenalidomide maintenance for

standard-risk patients following autologous SCT, and following approximately 12 months of initial therapy in patients not eligible for SCT and in patients who delay SCT. In high-risk patients, we recommend bortezomib-based maintenance.

Allogeneic Transplantation

Allogeneic bone marrow transplantation (myeloablative and non-myeloablative) has been tested in myeloma, but treatment-related mortality is high and graft-versus-host disease is a troublesome problem. Furthermore, only a small proportion of patients with multiple myeloma are eligible. Allogeneic transplantation is currently not recommended for routine use outside of a clinical trial. An exception to this are young patients with high-risk disease in first relapse after autologous transplantation who are willing to assume the high treatment-related mortality associated with allogeneic SCT.

Initial Therapy for Patients Who Are Ineligible for Autologous Stem Cell Transplantation

The initial therapy for patients not eligible for transplantation now resembles that of transplant-eligible patients. The current approach to treatment of newly diagnosed myeloma in patients not eligible for stem cell transplantation is summarized in Figure 1B. Currently, we prefer VRD as initial therapy. An alternative that has been recently approved for initial therapy in the United States is DRD. Other options include VCD and VTD. For frail patients, the doublet regimen of Rd can be used.

We continue the initial chemotherapy regimen for approximately 12 months followed usually by lenalidomide maintenance in standard-risk patients and bortezomib-based maintenance in high-risk patients.

Relapsed or Refractory Multiple Myeloma

Almost all patients with multiple myeloma who survive eventually relapse. If relapse occurs more than 6 months after treatment is discontinued, the initial chemotherapy regimen should be reinstituted. Most patients respond again, but the duration and quality of response are usually inferior to the initial response. Recently, several new drugs have been approved for the treatment of multiple myeloma including pomalidomide (Pomalyst), carfilzomib (Kyprolis), daratumumab (Darzalex), elotuzumab (Empliciti), panobinostat (Farydak), and ixazomib (Ninlaro).

Thalidomide

Thalidomide (Thalomid) is usually instituted in a dose of 50 to 100 mg daily and, if necessary, escalated to 200 mg daily if tolerated. It is most often used in combinations such as VTD. Side effects include sedation, fatigue, constipation, rash, deep venous thrombosis (DVT), edema, bradycardia, and hypothyroidism. Virtually all patients develop a sensorimotor peripheral neuropathy. The

---

[3]Exceeds dosage recommended by the manufacturer.

use of thalidomide in pregnancy is contraindicated, and the System for Thalidomide Education and Prescribing Safety (STEPS) program must be followed to prevent teratogenic effects.

Bortezomib

Bortezomib (Velcade) is a proteasome inhibitor that produces a response rate of approximately 35% in patients with relapsed or refractory myeloma. It is most often used in combinations such as VRD, VCD, or VTD to maximize response rates. The most troublesome side effect is peripheral neuropathy, which can occur in 35% to 40% of patients. The neuropathy is often painful but does improve in most patients after discontinuing bortezomib. The risk of neuropathy can be greatly reduced by using bortezomib in a once-weekly subcutaneous schedule.

Lenalidomide

Lenalidomide (Revlimid) as a single-agent produces an objective response in approximately 30% of patients with relapsed or refractory multiple myeloma. The major side effects are cytopenias, and the dose needs to be modified accordingly. The combination of lenalidomide plus low-dose dexamethasone (Rd) is the backbone of several myeloma treatment regimens.

Carfilzomib

Carfilzomib (Kyprolis) is a new proteasome inhibitor approved for the therapy of patients with multiple myeloma who have received at least two prior therapies, including both an immunomodulatory agent and bortezomib, and have disease progression on or within 60 days of the completion of the last therapy. Carfilzomib needs to be administered intravenously twice weekly. In a recent randomized trial, the combination of carfilzomib, lenalidomide, and dexamethasone (KRD) was found to have superior response rate, PFS, and OS compared with Rd.

Pomalidomide

Pomalidomide (Pomalyst) is an analog of lenalidomide and thalidomide. It has shown significant clinical activity in patients who are refractory to both bortezomib and lenalidomide (dual refractory). It is approved for patients with multiple myeloma who received at least two prior therapies, including both lenalidomide and bortezomib, and have disease progression on or within 60 days of the completion of the last therapy. It is administered orally at a dose of 2 to 4 mg daily for 21 days every 28 days. The major side effects are cytopenias and fatigue.

Panobinostat

Panobinostat (Farydak) is a pan-deacetylase inhibitor that is approved for the treatment of multiple myeloma in patients who have received at least two prior therapies, including both an immunomodulatory agent and bortezomib. It is administered orally at a starting dose of 20 mg three times a week for 2 weeks every 3 weeks. It is given in combination with bortezomib and dexamethasone. It is associated with severe diarrhea in approximately 25% of patients, so use must be restricted to younger patients in good performance status who have failed other treatments but are not yet refractory to bortezomib. If the drug is used, the dose must preferably be lower than the approved label dose, and the dose of bortezomib and dexamethasone must also be reduced to a once-weekly schedule. The drug approval carries a black box warning concerning cardiac arrhythmias and severe diarrhea.

Elotuzumab

Elotuzumab (Empliciti) is a monoclonal antibody that is approved for the treatment of relapsed myeloma. It targets the signaling lymphocytic activation molecule F7 (SLAMF7). In a randomized trial of 646 patients, elotuzumab plus Rd was superior to Rd, median PFS 19.4 months versus 14.9 months, respectively (*P* < .001).

Daratumumab

Daratumumab (Darzalex) is a monoclonal antibody that is approved for the treatment of relapsed myeloma. It targets CD38, a molecule universally expressed on myeloma cells. Daratumumab has a response rate of approximately 30% in heavily pretreated patients. Two randomized trials have found improvement in PFS with the addition of daratumumab to Rd and bortezomib-dexamethasone, respectively.

Ixazomib

Ixazomib (Ninlaro) is an oral proteasome inhibitor approved for the treatment of relapsed myeloma. It is a boronic acid derivative similar to bortezomib. It is administered once weekly orally. Compared with bortezomib, it has a lower risk of peripheral neuropathy.

Other New Drugs

New drugs that are in clinical trials include new proteasome inhibitors (marizomib[5], oprozomib[5], and dinaciclib[5]). Selinexor (Xpovio) has recently received US Food and Drug Administration (FDA) approval to use in combination with dexamethasone for patients with relapsed or refractory multiple myeloma. Chimeric antigen receptor (CAR) T-cell therapy targeting B-cell maturation antigen (BCMA) and anti-BCMA monoclonal antibody therapy have also shown significant progress in clinical trials.

Supportive Therapy

Radiotherapy

Palliative radiation in a dose of 20 to 30 Gy should be limited to patients who have disabling pain and a well-defined focal process that has not responded to chemotherapy. Analgesics in combination with chemotherapy usually can control the pain. This approach is preferred to local radiation because pain often occurs at another site, and local radiation does not benefit the patient with systemic disease. In addition, the myelosuppressive effects of radiotherapy and chemotherapy are cumulative and can restrict future therapy. Radiation is required for spinal cord compression from plasmacytoma. Postsurgical radiation after stabilization of fractures or impending fractures is rarely needed.

Hypercalcemia

Hypercalcemia must be suspected if the patient has anorexia, nausea, vomiting, polyuria, increased constipation, weakness, confusion, stupor, or coma. If it is untreated, renal insufficiency usually develops. Hydration, preferably with isotonic saline and prednisone (25 mg orally four times daily), is effective in many patients with mild to moderate hypercalcemia (calcium < 13 mg/dL). If more-severe hypercalcemia occurs, zoledronic acid (Zometa) at a dose of 4 mg intravenously over 15 minutes or pamidronate (Aredia) 90 mg given intravenously over at least 2 hours is indicated. Calcitonin (Miacalcin) may be used if rapid reduction of calcium levels is needed. Hemodialysis may be necessary for extremely severe hypercalcemia. The dosage of prednisone must be reduced and discontinued as soon as possible.

Renal Insufficiency

Approximately 20% of patients with multiple myeloma have a serum creatinine level of 2.0 mg/dL or more at diagnosis. Myeloma kidney (cast nephropathy) and hypercalcemia are the two major causes. Myeloma kidney is characterized by the presence of large, waxy, laminated casts in the distal and collecting tubules. Some light chains are very nephrotoxic, but no specific amino acid sequence of the nephrotoxic light chain has been identified.

Dehydration, infection, nonsteroidal antiinflammatory agents, and radiographic contrast media can contribute to acute kidney failure. Hyperuricemia or amyloid deposition can produce renal insufficiency. Nephrotic syndrome rarely occurs in multiple myeloma unless amyloidosis is present.

Maintenance of a high fluid intake producing 3 L of urine per 24 hours is important for preventing kidney failure in patients

---

[5]Investigational drug in the United States.

with Bence Jones proteinuria. If hyperuricemia occurs, allopurinol (Zyloprim) in doses of 300 mg daily provides effective therapy.

Acute kidney failure should be treated promptly with appropriate fluid and electrolyte replacement. Patients with kidney failure should be treated with either VCD or VTD to reduce the tumor mass as quickly as possible. A trial of plasmapheresis is reasonable in an attempt to prevent chronic dialysis. Hemodialysis and peritoneal dialysis are equally effective and are necessary for patients with symptomatic azotemia.

Anemia

Almost every patient with multiple myeloma eventually becomes anemic. Increased plasma volume from the osmotic effect of the M protein can produce hypervolemia and can spuriously lower the hemoglobin and hematocrit values. Patients with significant symptoms should be considered for red blood cell transfusion. If a transfusion is indicated, irradiated leukocyte-reduced red cells are preferred.

In patients with newly diagnosed myeloma, induction chemotherapy is often associated with a prompt improvement in hemoglobin levels, so it is better to avoid the use of erythropoietin. Erythropoietin (Epogen) should be seriously considered in relapsed patients receiving chemotherapy who have a persistent, symptomatic hemoglobin level of 10 g/dL or less.

Erythropoietin reduces the transfusion requirement and increases hemoglobin concentration in more than half of patients. Those with low serum erythropoietin values are more likely to respond. Most physicians proceed with a trial of erythropoietin 150 U/kg three times weekly or 40,000 U once a week. Darbepoetin, a long-lasting erythropoietin (Aranesp), may be given weekly or biweekly. Erythropoietin should be discontinued when the hemoglobin reaches 11 g/dL.

Skeletal Lesions

Bone lesions manifested by pain and fractures are a major problem. A skeletal radiographic survey should be repeated at 6-month intervals or sooner if pain develops. Patients should be encouraged to be as active as possible because confinement to bed increases demineralization of the skeleton. Trauma must be avoided because even mild stress can result in a fracture. Fixation of long bone fractures or impending fractures with an intramedullary rod and methyl methacrylate gives excellent results.

All patients with multiple myeloma who have lytic lesions, pathologic fractures, or severe osteopenia should receive an intravenous bisphosphonate. Pamidronate (Aredia) 90 mg intravenously over 2 hours every 4 weeks or zoledronic acid (Zometa) 4 mg intravenously over 15 minutes every 4 weeks are equally efficacious. The dosage of bisphosphonates should be reduced with renal insufficiency. Because renal insufficiency or nephrotic-range proteinuria can occur, serum creatinine and 24-hour urine protein monitoring is necessary. One should seriously consider stopping the intravenous bisphosphonate in patients who have responsive or stable disease after 2 years of therapy. In other patients, we recommend reducing the dose to once every 3 months. A randomized trial has found that denosumab (Xgeva), a monoclonal antibody targeting RANKL, may be as effective in reducing skeletal events as zoledronic acid and may be an option for selected patients with significant renal impairment.

Bisphosphonates should be resumed upon relapse with new-onset skeletal-related events. Osteonecrosis of the jaw can occur in patients receiving bisphosphonates. Although the relationship is unclear, it is essential to obtain a complete dental evaluation and perform preventive dental treatment before beginning bisphosphonates. The patient should practice good oral hygiene during therapy. Invasive procedures (especially dental extractions) should be avoided during bisphosphonate therapy. Osteonecrosis of the jaw should be managed conservatively.

Vertebroplasty or kyphoplasty may be helpful for patients with an acute compression fracture of the spine. Both have been associated with pain relief. Results appear to be better when the procedure is performed shortly after the compression fracture. Leakage of the methyl methacrylate is a potential adverse event. A choice between vertebroplasty and kyphoplasty depends on the expertise of the physician performing the procedure.

Infections

Bacterial infections are more common in patients with myeloma than in the general population. All patients should receive pneumococcal and influenza immunizations despite their suboptimal antibody response. Substantial fever is an indication for appropriate cultures, chest radiography, and consideration of antibiotic therapy. The greatest risk for infection is during the first 3 months after chemotherapy is initiated, and prophylactic antibiotics (levofloxacin [Levaquin] or cotrimoxazole [Bactrim]) should be considered during this period. Antiviral prophylaxis (acyclovir [Zovirax] 400 mg twice daily or valacyclovir [Valtrex] 500 mg once daily) should be given to all patients receiving bortezomib because of the increased risk of herpes zoster. Intravenous immunoglobulin (IVIg, Gammagard)[1] may be helpful in selected patients who have recurrent serious infections despite the use of prophylactic antibiotics. It is inconvenient, associated with side effects, and very expensive. Consequently, few of our patients receive IVIg.

Hyperviscosity Syndrome

Symptoms of hyperviscosity can include oronasal bleeding, gastrointestinal bleeding, blurred vision, neurologic symptoms, or congestive heart failure. Most patients have symptoms when the serum viscosity measurement is more than 4 cP, but the relationship between serum viscosity and clinical manifestations is not precise. The decision to perform plasmapheresis, which promptly relieves the symptoms of hyperviscosity, should be made on clinical grounds rather than serum viscosity levels. Hyperviscosity is more common in IgA myeloma than in IgG myeloma.

Extradural Myeloma (Cord Compression)

The possibility of cord compression must be considered if weakness of the legs or difficulty in voiding or defecating occurs. The sudden onset of severe radicular pain or severe back pain with neurologic symptoms suggests compression of the spinal cord. MRI or CT of the entire spine must be performed immediately. Radiation therapy in a dose of approximately 30 Gy is beneficial in about one half of patients. Dexamethasone (Decadron)[1] should be administered in addition to radiation therapy. Surgical decompression is necessary only if the neurologic deficit does not improve.

Venous Thromboembolism

Patients with multiple myeloma have an increased risk of venous thromboembolism. This is due to the malignancy itself, as well as therapy with lenalidomide, thalidomide, or pomalidomide. All patients receiving lenalidomide (or thalidomide or pomalidomide) need DVT prophylaxis with aspirin[1] (81 mg or 325 mg daily) or full-dose warfarin (Coumadin)[1] or low-molecular-weight heparin.[1]

Emotional Support

All patients with multiple myeloma need substantial and continuing emotional support. The physician's approach must be positive in emphasizing the potential benefits of therapy. It is reassuring for patients to know that some survive for 10 years or more. It is vital that the physician caring for patients with multiple myeloma has the interest and capacity for dealing with incurable disease over the span of years with assurance, sympathy, and resourcefulness.

---

[1]Not FDA approved for this indication.

References

Anderson K, Ismaila N, Flynn PJ, et al: Role of bone-modifying agents in multiple myeloma: American Society of Clinical Oncology Clinical Practice Guideline Update, *J Clin Oncol*, 2018 Jan 17, JCO2017766402. Available at: https://doi.org/10.1200/ JCO.2017.76.6402. [Epub ahead of print].

Attal M, Lauwers-Cances V, Marit G, et al: Lenalidomide maintenance after stem-cell transplantation for multiple myeloma, *N Engl J Med* 366:1782–1791, 2012.

Dimopoulos MA, Oriol A, Nahi H, et al: Daratumumab, lenalidomide, and dexamethasone for multiple myeloma, *N Engl J Med* 375(14):1319–1331, 2016.

Durie BGM, et al: Bortezomib with lenalidomide and dexamethasone versus lenalidomide and dexamethasone alone in patients with newly diagnosed myeloma without intent for immediate autologous stem-cell transplant (SWOG S0777): a randomised, open-label, phase 3 trial, *Lancet* 389(10068):519–527, 2017.

Facon T, Kumar S, Piesner T, et al: Daratumumab plus lenalidomide and dexamethasone for untreated myeloma, *N Engl J Med* 380(22):2104–2115, 2019.

Krishnan A, Pasquini MC, Logan B, et al: Autologous haemopoietic stem-cell transplantation followed by allogeneic or autologous haemopoietic stem-cell transplantation in patients with multiple myeloma (BMT CTN 0102): a phase 3 biological assignment trial, *Lancet Oncol* 12:1195–1203, 2011.

Kyle RA, Rajkumar SV: Epidemiology of the plasma-cell disorders, *Best Pract Res Clin Haematol* 20:637–664, 2007.

Lonial S, Dimopoulos M, Palumbo A, et al: Elotuzumab therapy for relapsed or refractory multiple myeloma, *N Engl J Med* 373:621–631, 2015.

McCarthy PL, Owzar K, Hofmeister CC, et al: Lenalidomide after stem-cell transplantation for multiple myeloma, *N Engl J Med* 366:1770–1781, 2012.

Mikhael JR, Dingli D, Roy V, et al: Management of newly diagnosed symptomatic multiple myeloma: updated Mayo stratification of myeloma and risk-adapted therapy (mSMART) consensus guidelines 2013, *Mayo Clin Proc* 88:360–376, 2013.

Moreau P, Attal MA, Hulin C, et al: Bortezomib, thalidomide, and dexamethasone with or without daratumumab before and after autologous stem-cell transplantation for newly diagnosed multiple myeloma (CASSIOPEIA): a randomised, open-label, phase 3 study, *Lancet* 394(10192):29–38, 2019.

Moreau P, Masszi T, Grzasko N, et al: Oral ixazomib, lenalidomide, and dexamethasone for multiple myeloma, *N Engl J Med* 374(17):1621–1634, 2016.

Palumbo A, Chanan-Khan A, Weisel K, et al: Daratumumab, bortezomib, and dexamethasone for multiple myeloma, *N Engl J Med* 375(8):754–766, 2016.

Raje N, Terpos E, Willenbacher W, et al: Denosumab versus zoledronic acid in bone disease treatment of newly diagnosed multiple myeloma: an international, double-blind, double-dummy, randomised, controlled, phase 3 study, *Lancet Oncol* Feb 8. pii: S1470-2045(18)30072-X. Available at: https://doi.org/10.1016/S1470-2045(18)30072-X.

Rajkumar SV, Jacobus S, Callander NS, et al: Lenalidomide plus high-dose dexamethasone versus lenalidomide plus low- dose dexamethasone as initial therapy for newly diagnosed multiple myeloma: an open-label randomised controlled trial, *Lancet Oncol* 11:29–37, 2010.

Rajkumar SV, et al: International Myeloma Working Group updated criteria for the diagnosis of multiple myeloma, *Lancet Oncol* 15:e538–e548, 2014.

San Miguel J, Weisel K, Moreau P, et al: Pomalidomide plus low-dose dexamethasone versus high-dose dexamethasone alone for patients with relapsed and refractory multiple myeloma (MM-003): a randomised, open-label, phase 3 trial, *Lancet Oncol* 14:1055–1066, 2013.

Sonneveld P, Schmidt-Wolf IGH, van der Holt B, et al: Bortezomib induction and maintenance treatment in patients with newly diagnosed multiple myeloma: results of the randomized phase III HOVON-65/ GMMG-HD4 trial, *J Clin Oncol* 30:2946–2955, 2012.

Stewart AK, et al: Carfilzomib, lenalidomide, and dexamethasone for relapsed multiple myeloma, *N Engl J Med* 372(2):142–152, 2015.

MYELODYSPLASTIC SYNDROMES

Method of
Jamile M. Shammo, MD

CURRENT DIAGNOSIS

- Myelodysplastic syndromes are diseases of the elderly.
- Chronic unexplained cytopenias should be evaluated to rule out myelodysplastic syndromes.
- Bone marrow biopsy with cytogenetic testing is necessary to make the diagnosis.
- The international prognostic scoring system (IPSS) is an important tool for risk stratification and choice of therapy.

CURRENT THERAPY

- Myelodysplastic syndromes are broadly divided into two therapeutic categories per the IPSS: low-risk disease (encompassing low and intermediate-1 risk groups), and high-risk disease (encompassing Intermediate-2 and high risk groups).
- The IPSS-R defines 5 prognostic groups (very low, low, intermediate, high, and very high risk). Treatment options are also dependent on risk category.
- Patients with low-risk disease should receive supportive care and hematopoietic growth factors; those with deletion 5q abnormality should be treated with lenalidomide (Revlimid).
- Patients with high-risk disease should be treated with a hypomethylating agent and should be considered for allogeneic stem cell transplantation.

Epidemiology

The myelodysplastic syndromes (MDS) represent a group of heterogeneous clonal stem cell disorders that affect the elderly. The reported annual incidence of approximately 4.4 per 100,000 of the general United States population is highest among whites and non-Hispanics. The onset of MDS before the age of 50 years is rare; the incidence rises with age such that in patients older than 70 years, the incidence exceeds 45 per 100,000 persons. Men are nearly twice as likely to be affected as women (5.8 vs 3.3 per 100,000 per year).

Risk Factors

De novo or primary MDS refers to cases in which no prior toxic exposure can be documented. Therapy-related MDS, on the other hand, occurs in patients who have been previously treated with either chemotherapy, radiotherapy or both. Median onset of therapy-related MDS varies with the agents used and is usually 2 to 5 years after initial exposure or chemotherapy.

Tobacco use and occupational exposure to solvents and agricultural chemicals have also been associated with the development of MDS. A minority of MDS cases might have evolved from an antecedent hematologic disorder such as aplastic anemia or paroxysmal nocturnal hemoglobinuria. Several rare and inherited genetic disorders have been associated with a higher risk of developing MDS, such as Fanconi anemia, dyskeratosis congenita, Diamond-Blackfan syndrome, and Shwachman-Diamond syndrome.

Pathophysiology

A variety of pathophysiological processes has been described in association with MDS, resulting in ineffective hematopoiesis and peripheral cytopenias. These processes include excessive apoptosis of myeloid progenitors, abnormal responses to cytokines and growth factors, epigenetic aberrations resulting in gene silencing, chromosomal abnormalities, and a defective bone marrow microenvironment. Recently, several somatic point mutations affecting multiple genes have been identified in up to 50% of MDS patients. However, the initiating event remains is unknown.

Clinical Manifestations

Some patients with MDS are symptom free, but the majority present with peripheral blood cytopenias, of which anemia is the most common. Patients might complain of fatigue, weakness, and exercise intolerance. Those with significant neutropenia and thrombocytopenia can present with infections or bleeding. Systemic symptoms are less common but, when present, can herald disease progression. Similarly, the presence of Sweet's syndrome (acute febrile neutrophilic dermatosis) can herald transformation to acute leukemia. Organomegaly and lymphadenopathy are uncommon. Infection is the cause of death in approximately

20% to 35% of cases. Transformation to acute leukemia occurs in about 30% of all patients.

Diagnosis

The diagnosis of MDS can be challenging, because its clinical and pathologic characteristics can overlap with other disorders such as aplastic anemia, myeloproliferative neoplasms, and acute leukemia.

A thorough history and physical examination should be performed on every patient with one or more peripheral blood cytopenias, along with basic laboratory tests such as iron studies, vitamin B_{12}, and folic acid levels. However, many disorders can cause pancytopenia; therefore consideration for a hematology referral should be entertained for the evaluation of pancytopenia or persistent otherwise-unexplained cytopenias, in which case a bone marrow biopsy may be necessary.

The diagnosis of MDS requires an evaluation of the peripheral blood smear, a bone marrow biopsy and aspirate to ascertain the presence of myeloid dysplasia; iron stains, which are necessary for the detection of ring sideroblasts; and cytogenetic studies to detect abnormal clones. Bone marrow dysplasia involving at least 10% of the cells of a specific myeloid lineage is the hallmark of MDS. Conventional karyotyping can detect cytogenetic abnormalities in 50% of patients with de novo MDS and in 95% of patients with therapy-related MDS. The presence of certain cytogenetic abnormalities can aid in making the diagnosis of MDS, particularly when dysplastic features are not prominent. It should be noted that the presence of +8, -Y, or del(20q) is not considered to be MDS-defining in that setting.

Recently, next-generation sequencing (NGS) has allowed for the identification of point mutations in the majority of patients with MDS. These mutations involve genes encoding for splicing factors, epigenetic modifiers, and transcription factors among others. NGS is increasingly utilized in this patient population to assist in making the diagnosis (.SF3B1 in MDS-RS), or to provide important prognostic information (TP53 in del 5 MDS).

Differential Diagnosis

MDS should be distinguished from a broad number of disorders including megaloblastic anemia, aplastic anemia, large granular lymphocyte leukemia, myelofibrosis, copper deficiency, and HIV infection, which can cause anemia and dysplastic features in the bone marrow. Exposure to certain drugs and toxins can result in marrow dysplasia. These include mycophenolate mofetil (Cellcept), ganciclovir (Cytovene), lead, and excess zinc. Such changes are reversible once the offending agent is discontinued. The diagnosis of MDS can be made by performing a bone marrow biopsy to detect dysplasia and rule out other disorders that can also cause pancytopenia. Every effort should be made to rule out other reactive causes of dysplasia prior to making a diagnosis of MDS.

Classification and Risk Stratification

Since 1982, there have been various proposals for the classification and risk stratification of MDS. The French-American-British (FAB) classification scheme was the first attempt developed to address the broad range of morphologic features and clinical outcomes in MDS. It identified five subtypes based on morphology and percentage of marrow blasts: refractory anemia (RA), refractory anemia with ringed sideroblasts (RARS), refractory anemia with excess blasts (RAEB), refractory anemia with excess blasts in transformation (RAEB-t), and chronic myelomonocytic leukemia (CMML). This classification allowed MDS to be separated into distinct subsets relative to survival and acute leukemia evolution.

The World Health Organization (WHO) revised the FAB system to further refine MDS subsets by adding a category of refractory cytopenia with multilineage dysplasia, recognizing 5q-deletion syndrome as a separate clinical and pathologic entity, and lowering the blast percentage from 30% to 20% to

diagnose acute myelogenous leukemia (AML). The WHO system was revised in 2008 and again in 2016. The most recent revision eliminated reference to refractory anemia and modified the terminology to identify 6 general MDS categories based on presence of single or multilineage dysplasia, ring sideroblasts, blast percentage and del(5q) (Table 1).

The International Prognostic Scoring System (IPSS) was introduced in 1997 to address the variability in prognosis within FAB subtypes. It predicts survival and risk of evolution to acute leukemia. The IPSS is calculated by adding scores assigned to three variables: blast cell count, cytogenetics, and number of cytopenias (Table 2). The IPSS was revised in 2012 (IPSS-R) to incorporate 5 cytogenetic categories and to account for the depth of cytopenias in MDS (Table 3). The IPSS/IPSS-R are widely used to predict the prognosis and clinical behavior of patients with various forms of MDS and to guide choice of therapy.

Treatment

A variety of therapeutic options exist for the treatment of MDS patients spanning the spectrum from supportive care to allogeneic stem cell transplantation. Choice of therapy should take into account the patient's age, comorbidities, and the IPSS/IPSS-R score.

The treating physician should consider the ultimate goal of therapy and whether it is intended to cure, extend survival, or merely palliate symptoms. In the first decade of the 21st century, several novel therapeutic options for MDS have emerged. Clinical trials evaluating novel agents are being conducted to help identify effective agents for patients who have relapsed or failed to respond to standard therapies.

Supportive Care

Supportive care has been the cornerstone of MDS therapy for decades; it includes red blood cell transfusion for symptomatic anemia, platelet transfusion to reduce the risk of or to treat bleeding, and use of hematopoietic growth factors such as erythropoiesis stimulating agents (ESA) and colony-stimulating factors such as granulocyte colony-stimulating factor (G-CSF) (Filgrastim [Neupogen]) and granulocyte-macrophage colony-stimulating factor (GM-CSF) (Sargramostim [Leukine]).[1]

There are two currently available ESAs: a recombinant human erythropoietin (rhu-EPO; epoetin alfa [Epogen, Procrit]) and a super-sialylated form of EPO (darbepoetin alfa [Aranesp]). These are considered the standard of care for the treatment of anemia in patients with low-risk MDS. A predictive model for response to such treatment has been developed by the Nordic MDS study group to guide patient selection. In general, patients with a serum EPO level less than 500 mU/mL and low transfusion burden are likely to respond by improving their hemoglobin level and reducing their need for transfusions.

Immunomodulatory Drugs

The novel class of immunomodulatory drugs includes thalidomide (Thalomid)[1] and lenalidomide (Revlimid). Thalidomide was investigated initially with some success in patients with low-risk disease. However, its use was compromised because of poor tolerability. Lenalidomide has been approved for the treatment of patients with low-risk MDS who harbor deletion 5q abnormality, because it was shown in clinical trials to result in transfusion independence in about two thirds of such patients.

Hypomethylating Agents

Currently, two hypomethylating agents are approved for the treatment of MDS: 5-azacitidine (Vidaza) and decitabine (Dacogen). These agents are cytosine analogues known to inhibit and deplete DNA methyltransferase, which adds a methyl group to

---

[1] Not FDA approved for this indication.

TABLE 1 WHO 2008 Classification of Myelodysplastic Syndromes

DISEASE	BLOOD FINDINGS	BONE MARROW FINDINGS
Refractory cytopenias with unilineage dysplasia (RCUD) Refractory anemia (RA) Refractory neutropenia (RN) Refractory thrombocytopenia (RT)	Unicytopenia or bicytopenia* No or rare blasts (<1%)[†]	Unilineage dysplasia: ≥10% of the cells in one myeloid lineage <5% blasts <15% of erythroid precursors are ring sideroblasts
Refractory anemia with ring sideroblasts (RARS)	Anemia No blasts	>15% of erythroid precursors are ring sideroblasts Erythroid dysplasia only <5% blasts
Refractory cytopenia with multilineage dysplasia (RCMD)	Cytopenia(s) No or rare blasts (<1%)[†] No Auer rods <10⁹/L monocytes	Dysplasia in ≥10% of the cells in ≥2 myeloid lineages (neutrophils, erythroid precursors, megakaryocytes) <5% blasts in marrow No Auer rods ±15% ring sideroblasts
Refractory anemia with excess blasts-1 (RAEB-1)	Cytopenia(s) <5% blasts[†] No Auer rods <10⁹/L monocytes	Unilineage or multilineage dysplasia 5 5%–9% blasts No Auer rods
Refractory anemia with excess blasts-2 (RAEB-2)	Cytopenia(s) 5%–19% blasts ±Auer rods[‡] <10⁹/L monocytes	Unilineage or multilineage dysplasia 10%–19% blasts ±Auer rods[‡]
Myelodysplastic syndrome, unclassified (MDS-U)	Cytopenias ≤1% blasts[†]	Unequivocal dysplasia in <10% of cells in one or more myeloid cell lines when accompanied by a cytogenetic abnormally considered as presumptive evidence for a diagnosis of MDS <5% blasts
MDS associated with isolated del(5q)	Anemia Usually normal or increased platelet count No or rare blasts (<1%)	Normal to increased megakaryocytes with hypolobated nuclei <5% blasts Isolated del(5q) cytogenetic abnormality No Auer rods

*Bicytopenia is occasionally observed. Cases with pancytopenia should be classified as MDS-U.
[†]If the marrow myeloblast percentage is <5% but there are 2%–4% myeloblasts in the blood, the diagnostic classification is RAEB-1. Cases of RCUD and RCMD with 1% myeloblasts in the blood should be classified as MDS-U.
[‡]Cases with Auer rods and <5% myeloblasts in the blood and <10% in the marrow should be classified as RAEB-2.

TABLE 2 International Prognostic Scoring System (IPSS) for MDS

	SCORE VALUE				
PROGNOSTIC VARIABLE	0	0.5	1.0	1.5	2.0
Marrow blasts (%)	<5	5–10	11–20	—	21–30
Karyotype*	Good	Intermediate		Poor	
Cytopenia[†]	0/1	2/3			

*Cytogenetics: Good = normal, -Y alone, del(5q) alone, del(20q) alone; Poor = complex (≥3 abnormalities) or chromosome 7 anomalies; Intermediate = other abnormalities. This excludes karyotypes t(8;21), inv16 and t(15;17), which are considered to be AML, not MDS.
[†]Cytopenias: neutrophil count <1800/µL, platelets <100,000/µL, Hb <10 g/dL.

TABLE 3 Survival and Progression by IPSS Risk Category

RISK CATEGORY	% IPSS POP.	OVERALL SCORE	MEDIAN SURVIVAL (Y) IN THE ABSENCE OF THERAPY	25% AML PROGRESSION (Y) IN THE ABSENCE OF THERAPY
Low	33	0	5.7	9.4
Intermediate 1	38	0.5–1.0	3.5	3.3
Intermediate 2	22	1.5–2.0	1.2	1.1
High	7	≥2.5	0.4	0.2

Abbreviation: IPSS = International Prognostic Scoring System.

cytosine residues in newly formed DNA, resulting in the formation of a hypomethylated DNA in vitro. The exact mechanism of action in vivo has not yet been identified.

Results of randomized clinical trials comparing these agents to best supportive care in patients with MDS have demonstrated a statistically significant improvement in response rate and hematologic improvement. It has been shown for the first time that treatment with 5-azacitidine was reported to result in prolongation of survival in patients with Int-2 and high-risk. Both drugs have myelosuppressive properties and comparable response rates.

Immunosuppressive Therapy

Immunosuppressive therapy with antithymocyte globulin (Thymoglobulin)[1] or cyclosporine (Neoral)[1] (or both) was evaluated in several clinical trials and was shown to result in durable hematological responses in a subset of MDS patients, specifically, younger patients with low-risk disease, hypocellular marrows, PNH clone, human leukocyte antigen (HLA)-DR 15 phenotype, and low transfusion need.

Hematopoietic Stem Cell Transplantation

Allogeneic stem cell transplantation is the only curative therapy for MDS patients; this option is feasible for a small subset: typically, younger patients with good performance status and an available HLA-matched donor. Approximately 40% of patients can be cured with this modality. The recent introduction of reduced-intensity conditioning regimens and nonmyeloablative transplants has resulted in expanding the age limit for performing the procedure, reducing transplant-related complications and mortality. However it has been associated with a higher risk of relapse. Because stem cell transplantation is associated with a high rate of treatment-related death—estimated at 39% at 1 year—and the development of acute and chronic graft versus host disease, such treatment is recommended to patients with high-risk disease. Patients with low-risk MDS may be considered for transplant at disease progression.

Conclusion and Future Direction

MDS is a chronic disease characterized by features reminiscent of bone marrow failure states with a variable propensity for leukemic evolution. It is curable only by allogeneic stem cell transplantation, which is feasible in only a small subset of patients. For all others, the treatment goal is aimed at improving quality of life and prolonging survival. A variety of ongoing clinical trials are evaluating novel agents and combinations of drugs to further optimize the outcome of patients with this disease. Meanwhile, a great deal of research is focused on understanding the molecular underpinning of this disease to enhance our understanding of the biology of this heterogenous disorder.

References

Arber DA, Orazi A, Hasserjian R, et al: The 2016 revision to the World Health Organization (WHO) classification of myeloid neoplasms and acute leukemia, *Blood* 127:2391–2405, 2016.
Bejar R, Stevenson K, Abdel-Wahab O, et al: Clinical effect of point mutations in myelodysplastic syndromes, *NEJM* 364:2496–2506, 2011.
Bennett JM, Catovsky D, Daniel MT, et al: Proposals for the classification of the myelodysplastic syndromes, *Br J Haematol* 51:189–199, 1982.
Brunning RD, Porwit A, Orazi A, et al: Myelodysplastic syndromes/neoplasms. In Swerdlow S, Campo E, Lee Harris N, et al, editors: *WHO Classification of Tumors of Hematopoietic and Lymphoid Tissues*, ed 4th, Lyon, France, 2008, IARC, p 88–103pp.
Cutler CS, Lee SJ, Greenberg P, et al: A decision analysis of allogeneic bone marrow transplantation for the myelodysplastic syndromes: Delayed transplantation for low-risk myelodysplasia is associated with improved outcome, *Blood* 104(2):579–585, 2004.
Fenaux P, Mufti GJ, Hellstrom-Lindberg E, et al: Efficacy of azacitidine compared with that of conventional care regimens in the treatment of higher-risk myelodysplastic syndromes: A randomized, open-label, phase III study, *Lancet Oncol* 10:223–232, 2009.
Godley LA, Larson RA: Therapy-related myeloid leukemia, *Semin Oncol* 35:418–429, 2008.
Greenberg PL: The smoldering myeloid leukemic states: Clinical and biologic features, *Blood* 61:1035–1044, 1983.
Greenberg P, Cox C, LeBeau MM, et al: International scoring system for evaluating prognosis in myelodysplastic syndromes, *Blood* 89:2079–2088, 1997.
Greenberg PL, Tuechler H, Schanz J, et al: Revised International Prognostic Scoring System (IPSS-R) for myelodysplastic syndromes, *Blood* 120:2454–2465, 2012.
Hellstrom-Lindberg E, Negrin R, Stein R, et al: Erythroid response to treatment with G-CSF plus erythropoietin for the anaemia of patients with myelodysplastic syndromes: Proposal for a predictive model, *Br J Haematol* 99(2):344–351, 1997.
Kantarjian H, Issa JP, Rosenfeld CS, et al: Decitabine improves patient outcomes in myelodysplastic syndromes: Results of a phase III randomized study, *Cancer* 106(8):1794–1803, 2006.
List A, Dewald G, Bennett J, et al: Lenalidomide in the myelodysplastic syndrome with chromosome 5q deletion, *N Engl J Med* 355(14):1456–1465, 2006.
Ma X, Does M, Raza A, Mayne ST: Myelodysplastic syndromes: Incidence and survival in the United States, *Cancer* 109(8):1536–1542, 2007.
Martino R, Iacobelli S, Brand R, et al: Retrospective comparison of reduced-intensity conditioning and conventional high- dose conditioning for allogeneic hematopoietic stem cell transplantation using HLA-identical sibling donors in myelodysplastic syndromes, *Blood* 108:836–846, 2006.
Molldrem J, Leifer E, Bahceci E, et al: Antithymocyte globulin for treatment of the bone marrow failure associated with myelodysplastic syndromes, *Ann Intern Med* 137(3):156–163, 2002.
Nisse C, Lorthois C, Dorp V, et al: Exposure to occupational and environmental factors in myelodysplastic syndromes: Preliminary results of a case-control study, *Leukemia* 9:693–699, 1995.
Owen C, Barnett M, Fitzgibbon J: Familial myelodysplasia and acute myeloid leukaemia—a review, *Br J Haematol* 140:123–132, 2008.
Rollison DE, Howlader N, Smith MT, et al: Epidemiology of myelodysplastic syndromes and chronic myeloproliferative disorders in the United States, 2001–2004 using data from the NAACCR and SEER programs, *Blood* 112:45–52, 2008.
Silverman LR, Demakos EP, Peterson BL, et al: Randomized controlled trial of azacitidine in patients with the myelodysplastic syndrome: A study of the Cancer and Leukemia Group B, *J Clin Oncol* 20(10):2429–2440, 2002.
Soppi E, Nousiainen T, Seppa A, Lahtinen R: Acute febrile neutrophilic dermatosis (Sweet's syndrome) in association with myelodysplastic syndromes: A report of three cases and a review of the literature, *Br J Haematol* 73(1):43–47, 1989.
Tefferi A, Vardiman JW: Myelodysplastic syndromes, *N Engl J Med* 361(19):1872–1885, 2009.
Vardiman JW, Harris NL, Brunning RD: The World Health Organization (WHO) classification of myeloid neoplasms, *Blood* 100:2292–2302, 2002.

NON-HODGKIN LYMPHOMA

Method of
Andrew M. Evens, DO, MSc

 CURRENT DIAGNOSIS

- The etiology of non-Hodgkin lymphoma (NHL) is not known, although several risk factors and conditions are associated with an increased risk of developing lymphoma, including congenital immunosuppression conditions (ataxia-telangiectasia, Wiskott-Aldrich syndrome, and X-linked lymphoproliferative syndrome), acquired immunodeficiency states (e.g., human immunodeficiency virus [HIV] and after solid organ transplantation), viruses (e.g., human T-lymphotropic virus [HTLV]-1 and hepatitis C virus), and autoimmune disorders (e.g., Sjögren syndrome, celiac sprue, and systemic lupus erythematosus).
- Patients most commonly present clinically with enlarged lymph nodes, splenomegaly, and bone marrow involvement, but they may also present with other extranodal disease sites (e.g., stomach, skin, liver, bone, brain).
- NHL has many different clinicopathologic subtypes—more than 80 types are included in the World Health Organization's classification of lymphoid neoplasms. The natural history and prognosis of these vary greatly from indolent and slow-growing types (over many years) to highly aggressive (within weeks) types.
- Excisional lymph node resection is the gold standard procedure in establishing the precise NHL histology. Expert hematopathology review incorporating morphologic, immunophenotypic, and genetic features is essential for an accurate diagnosis.

- Indolent lymphomas are low-grade and represent slow-growing non-Hodgkin lymphoma (NHL) that may remain stable with low tumor burden not warranting therapy for several years. The disease is highly responsive to treatment with a variety of treatment options (remission rates exceeding 90% with combined rituximab/chemotherapy), although the clinical course is characterized by repetitive relapses. Outside of early-stage disease and therapy with allogeneic stem cell transplantation, low-grade NHLs are not curable.

- Transformation of follicular lymphoma to a high-grade NHL occurs in 30%–35%, or 2%–3% of patients each year; it is less common in other indolent subtypes. Transformation is typically heralded by an aggressive change in the patient's clinical condition.

- Diffuse large B-cell lymphoma (DLBCL), the most common aggressive NHL, is curable in all stages in the majority of patients with rituximab (Rituxan)-based chemotherapy. A variety of primary extranodal DLBCL clinical subtypes warrant specialized therapy, such as primary central nervous system lymphoma.

- Long-term survivors are at increased risk for second cancers. The highest relative risk of developing a secondary malignancy occurs more than 21 to 30 years after original diagnosis. Patients who received an anthracycline (e.g., doxorubicin [Adriamycin]) as part of therapy are at a long-term increased risk for cardiovascular disease.

The term *malignant lymphoma* was originally introduced by Billroth in 1871 to describe neoplasms of lymphoid tissue. Generally speaking, lymphomas are neoplasms of the immune system. Traditionally, lymphomas are divided into Hodgkin lymphoma (HL) and non-Hodgkin lymphoma (NHL).

There are many different clinicopathologic subtypes of NHL (>60). By cell of origin, the majority of NHLs are of B-cell origin (85% to 90%); T-cell NHLs account for 10% to 15% of lymphomas in the United States, whereas natural killer cell or histiocytic lymphomas are rare (<1%).

NHLs manifest most commonly clinically with involvement of lymph nodes, spleen, and bone marrow, but they can involve other extranodal sites (stomach, skin, liver, bone, brain, etc.). Peripheral blood involvement uncommonly occurs (leukemic phase of lymphoma). The natural history and prognosis vary greatly among the different subtypes of NHL, from indolent subtypes that are often slow-growing (i.e., therapy not warranted for years) to very aggressive and rapidly fatal types (within weeks) if not treated. Most NHL subtypes are highly treatable with initial remission rates greater than 90% to 95% using combined rituximab/chemotherapy; however, indolent NHLs are generally incurable, whereas the goal of treating most aggressive NHLs is cure.

Epidemiology

Currently, NHL represents approximately 5% of all cancer diagnoses, being the seventh most common cancer in women and men. Estimates from the American Cancer Society indicate that in 2019 approximately 74,200 new cases of NHL will be diagnosed in the United States and approximately 19,970 people will die of the disease. In addition, there are approximately 900,000 people living with NHL in the United States.

Geographic Distribution

The incidence of NHL varies throughout the world, in general being more common in developed countries, with rates in the United States of more than 15 per 100,000 compared with 1.2 per 100,000 in China. In the United States, the incidence rates of NHL more than doubled between 1975 and 1995, representing one of the largest increases of any cancer. The increases have been more pronounced in whites, males, the elderly, and those

with NHL diagnosed at extranodal sites. Similar findings have been reported in other developed countries. The incidence rates of NHL began to stabilize in the late 1990s, although the temporal trends vary by histologic subtype, as well as by race and sex (Figure 1). Some of the increase may be related to improved diagnostic techniques and access to medical care and the increased risk of NHL attributable to HIV infection. However, additional factors are likely responsible for this unexpected increase in incidence.

Age

Overall, NHL incidence rises exponentially with increasing age. In persons older than 65 years, the incidence is 90.9 per 100,000 population compared with 7.1 per 100,000 population for persons aged 20 to 49 years. Except for high-grade lymphoblastic and Burkitt lymphomas (the most common types of NHL seen in children and young adults), the median age at presentation for most subtypes of NHL exceeds 60 years.

Race and Ethnicity

Incidence varies by race and ethnicity, with whites overall having a higher risk than African Americans and Asian Americans (incidence rates increased 50% to 60% in whites compared with blacks). Most NHL subtypes are more common in whites than in blacks; however, peripheral T-cell lymphoma, mycosis fungoides, and Sézary syndrome occur more often in blacks than in whites.

Etiology and Risk Factors

Chromosomal Translocations and Molecular Rearrangements

Nonrandom chromosomal and molecular rearrangements play an important role in the pathogenesis of many lymphomas and often correlate with histology and immunophenotype. These chromosomal changes often result in oncogenic gene products; for example, t(11;14)(q13;q32) translocation results in overexpression of *bcl-1* (cyclin D1) in mantle cell lymphoma (MCL), while translocation with 8q24 leads to c-*myc* overexpression in nearly all Burkitt lymphomas and in 10% to 15% of patients with diffuse large B-cell lymphoma (DLBCL). Research to discover more information regarding the prognostic and pathogenic importance of these oncogenes continues, although they are currently used primarily in clinical practice for diagnostic purposes. In addition, these genes serve as potential targets for novel therapeutics.

Environmental Factors

Environmental factors may also play a role in the development of NHL, including particular occupations (e.g., chemists, painters, mechanics, machinists) and chemicals (solvents and pesticides). Patients who receive chemotherapy or radiation therapy for any indication are also at increased risk for developing NHL as a secondary cancer as discussed later.

Viruses

Several viruses have been implicated in the pathogenesis of NHL, including Epstein-Barr virus, human T-lymphotropic virus 1 (HTLV-1), Kaposi sarcoma–associated herpesvirus (KSHV, also known as human herpesvirus 8 [HHV-8]), and hepatitis C virus (HCV). Meta-analyses have shown 13% to 15% seroprevalence of HCV in certain geographic regions among persons with B-cell NHL. Furthermore, HCV infection is associated with the development of clonal B-cell expansions and certain subtypes of NHL, particularly in the setting of essential (type II) mixed cryoglobulinemia. HTLV-1 is a human retrovirus that establishes a latent infection through reverse transcription in activated T-helper cells. A minority (5%) of carriers will develop adult T-cell leukemia lymphoma. KSHV-like DNA sequences are often detected in primary effusion lymphomas in patients with human immunodeficiency virus (HIV) infection and in those with multicentric (plasma cell variant) Castleman disease.

Bacterial Infections

Gastric mucosa-associated lymphoid tissue (MALT) lymphoma is seen most often, but not exclusively, in association with

Figure 1 Surveillance, epidemiology, and end results (SEER) observed incidence, SEER delay adjusted incidence, and US death rates for non-Hodgkin lymphoma, by race and sex.

Source: SEER 9 areas and US mortality files (national center for health statistics, CDC).
aRates are age-adjusted to the 2000 US Std population (19 age groups - census P25-1103).
Regression lines and APCs are calculated using the joinpoint regression program version 4.3.0.0. April 2016, National cancer institute.
The APC is the annual percent change for the regression line segments. The APC shown on the graph is for the most recent trend.
*The APC is significantly different from zero P < .05.

Helicobacter pylori infection. Infection with *Borrelia burgdorferi* has been detected in approximately 35% of patients with primary cutaneous B-cell lymphoma in Scotland. Studies indicate that *Campylobacter jejuni* and immunoproliferative small intestinal disease are related. European reports have noted an association between infection with *Chlamydia psittaci* and ocular adnexal lymphoma. The infection was found to be highly specific and does not reflect a subclinical infection among the general population. Furthermore, remission of NHL to antibiotics has been reported. Attempts to confirm this association in the Western hemisphere have been unsuccessful.

Immunodeficiency
Patients with congenital conditions of immunosuppression are at increased risk of NHL. These conditions include ataxia-telangiectasia; Wiskott-Aldrich syndrome; X-linked lymphoproliferative syndrome; severe combined immunodeficiency; acquired immunodeficiency states, such as HIV infection; and iatrogenic immunosuppression. Relative risk of NHL is increased 150- to 250-fold among patients with acquired immunodeficiency syndrome (AIDS); patients usually develop high-grade NHLs, such as Burkitt lymphoma or DLBCL. The incidence of posttransplantation lymphoproliferative disorders (PTLDs) after solid organ transplantation ranges from 1% to 3% in kidney transplant recipients to 10% to 12% in heart and multiorgan transplant recipients, the latter who require more potent immunosuppressive therapy.

Autoimmunity
An increased incidence of gastrointestinal lymphomas is seen in patients with celiac (nontropical) sprue and inflammatory bowel disease, particularly Crohn disease. An aberrant clonal intraepithelial T-cell population can be found in up to 75% of patients with refractory celiac sprue before overt T-cell lymphoma develops. Sjögren disease is associated with a sixfold increased risk of NHL overall with risk varying in part on severity of disease (5 to 200 times); moreover, the risk specifically of parotid marginal zone lymphoma is increased 1000-fold. In addition, systemic lupus erythematosus and rheumatoid arthritis have been associated with a slightly increased risk of B-cell lymphoma.

Genetic Susceptibility
Several studies have implicated a role for genetic variants in the risk of NHL, including genes that influence DNA integrity and methylation, genes that alter B-cell survival and growth, and genes that involve innate immunity, oxidative stress, and xenobiotic metabolism.

Signs and Symptoms
Fever, weight loss, and night sweats, referred to as B symptoms, are more common in advanced and aggressive subtype NHLs, but they may be present at all stages and in any histologic subtype.

Low-Grade or Indolent Lymphomas
Painless, slowly progressive peripheral adenopathy is the most common clinical presentation in patients with low-grade lymphomas. Patients sometimes report a history of waxing and waning adenopathy before seeking medical attention. Spontaneous regression of enlarged lymph nodes can occur, which may cause a low-grade lymphoma to be confused with an infectious condition. Primary extranodal involvement and B symptoms are uncommon

at presentation; however, both are more common in advanced or end-stage disease and in particular indolent NHL subtypes (e.g., gastric MALT and nongastric extranodal MALT). Bone marrow is frequently involved, sometimes in association with cytopenias. Splenomegaly is seen in approximately 40% of patients, but the spleen is rarely the only involved site besides the specific subtype of splenic marginal zone lymphoma.

High-Grade or Aggressive Lymphomas

The clinical presentation of high-grade lymphomas is more varied. Although the majority of patients present with adenopathy, more than one-third present with extranodal involvement alone or with adenopathy, the most common sites being the gastrointestinal tract (including Waldeyer ring), skin, bone marrow, sinuses, genitourinary tract, bone, and central nervous system. B symptoms are more common, occurring in approximately 30% to 40% of patients. Lymphoblastic lymphoma often manifests with an anterior superior mediastinal mass, superior vena cava syndrome, and leptomeningeal disease. American patients with Burkitt lymphoma often present with a large abdominal mass and symptoms of bowel obstruction. In addition, certain histologic NHL subtypes manifest with symptoms unique to that particular lymphoma subtype; for example, angioimmunoblastic T-cell lymphoma (AITL) in addition to lymphadenopathy presents with disease features including organomegaly, skin rash, pleural effusions, arthritis, eosinophilia, and varied immunologic abnormalities such as positive Coombs test, cold agglutins, hemolytic anemia, antinuclear antibodies, and polyclonal hypergammaglobulinemia.

Screening

No effective methods are currently available for screening patients or populations for NHL.

Diagnosis

A definitive diagnosis can be made only by biopsy of pathologic lymph nodes or tumor tissue. It is critical in most cases to perform an *excisional* lymph node resection to avoid false-negative results and inaccurate histologic classification; fine-needle aspirations or core biopsies are often insufficient for diagnostic purposes. When clinical circumstances make surgical biopsy of involved lymph nodes or extranodal sites prohibitive, a core biopsy obtained under computed tomography (CT) or ultrasonographic guidance may suffice, but it often requires the integration of histologic examination and immunophenotypic and molecular studies for accurate diagnosis. A formal review by an expert hematopathologist is mandatory. In addition to morphologic review and immunostaining of tissue, other studies such as detailed cellular immunophenotyping and genotyping for relevant oncogenes are often needed to complete the diagnosis.

In addition to a detailed history and physical examination, baseline staging studies are warranted. These consist of blood tests (complete blood count with differential, complete metabolic panel including liver function tests, and lactate dehydrogenase), CT of chest, abdomen, and pelvis, and bilateral bone marrow biopsy and aspirate (Box 1). For aggressive NHL histologies, functional imaging is advocated (i.e., fluorodeoxyglucose [^{18}F] positron emission tomography [FDG-PET]), as is assessment of ejection fraction in anticipation of anthracycline-based chemotherapy. Testing for history of hepatitis B virus (HBV) is recommended, especially before starting anti-CD20 antibody therapy; evidence suggests that anti-CD20 antibody therapy (e.g., rituximab [Rituxan]) increases the risk of HBV reactivation above the known rate of chemotherapy-associated reactivation. HIV serology should be obtained in patients with relevant risk factors, especially for DLBCL and Burkitt lymphoma. HTLV-1 serology is recommended in patients who present with cutaneous T-cell lymphoma lesions, especially if they have hypercalcemia.

Examination of cerebrospinal fluid and consideration of intrathecal chemotherapy prophylaxis are applicable for patients with DLBCL with bone marrow, epidural, testicular, paranasal sinus, breast, or multiple extranodal sites (especially when

---

in conjunction with elevated lactate dehydrogenase). Testing is mandatory for high-grade lymphoblastic lymphoma and Burkitt lymphoma and its variants and primary central nervous system lymphoma if there is no evidence of increased intracranial pressure. Upper gastrointestinal endoscopy or gastrointestinal series with small bowel follow-through is recommended in patients with head and neck involvement (tonsil, base of tongue, nasopharynx) and those with primary gastrointestinal disease. MCL is associated with a high incidence of occult gastrointestinal involvement. In addition, magnetic resonance imaging (MRI) of the complete craniospinal axis and ocular examination is advocated with any brain or leptomeningeal disease involvement to rule out multifocal disease.

Classification

The 1965 Rappaport Classification of malignant lymphomas was based solely on architecture and cytology. Since then, with the help of advanced cellular and genetic technologies, numerous new unique NHL entities have emerged. The World Health Organization (WHO) classification was revised in 2016, which continues to emphasize immunophenotyping, genotyping, and clinical features (Table 1). Another way to group the many different lymphoma histologies is by clinical presentation and prognosis (Table 2).

Prognosis

International Prognostic Index

The International Prognostic Index (IPI) was developed as a prognostic factor model for aggressive NHLs treated with doxorubicin-containing regimens (Box 2). In the pre-rituximab era, persons with no risk factors or one risk factor had a predicted 5-year overall survival rate of 73%, compared with 26% for high-risk patients with four or five risk factors. In the post-rituximab era, the survival rates have improved (see Box 2). A variant of the IPI is also useful in predicting outcome in patients with follicular low-grade lymphoma (FLIPI) or MCL (MIPI) and in patients who have relapsed or refractory large B-cell lymphoma.

MATURE B-CELL NEOPLASMS

Chronic lymphocytic leukemia/small lymphocytic lymphoma

Monoclonal B-cell lymphocytosis*

B-cell prolymphocytic leukemia

Splenic marginal zone lymphoma

Hairy cell leukemia

Splenic B-cell lymphoma/leukemia, unclassifiable

Splenic diffuse red pulp small B-cell lymphoma

Hairy cell leukemia-variant

Lymphoplasmacytic lymphoma

Waldenström macroglobulinemia

Monoclonal gammopathy of undetermined significance (MGUS), IgM*

μ heavy-chain disease

γ heavy-chain disease

α heavy-chain disease

Monoclonal gammopathy of undetermined significance (MGUS), IgG/A*

Plasma cell myeloma

Solitary plasmacytoma of bone

Extraosseous plasmacytoma

Monoclonal immunoglobulin deposition diseases*

Extranodal marginal zone lymphoma of mucosa-associated lymphoid tissue (MALT lymphoma)

Nodal marginal zone lymphoma

Pediatric nodal marginal zone lymphoma

Follicular lymphoma

In situ follicular neoplasia*

Duodenal-type follicular lymphoma*

Pediatric-type follicular lymphoma*

Large B-cell lymphoma with IRF4 rearrangement

Primary cutaneous follicle center lymphoma

Mantle cell lymphoma

In situ Mantle cell neoplasia*

Diffuse large B-cell lymphoma (DLBCL), NOS

Germinal center B-cell type*

Activated B-cell type*

T-cell/histiocyte-rich large B-cell lymphoma

Primary DLBCL of the central nervous system (CNS)

Primary cutaneous DLBCL, leg type

EBV+ DLBCL, NOS*

EBV + mucocutaneous ulcer

DLBCL associated with chronic inflammation

Lymphomatoid granulomatosis

Primary mediastinal (thymic) large B-cell lymphoma

Intravascular large B-cell lymphoma

ALK+ large B-cell lymphoma

Plasmablastic lymphoma

Primary effusion lymphoma

HHV8 + DLBCL, NOS

Burkitt lymphoma

Burkitt-like lymphoma with 11q aberration

High-grade B-cell lymphoma, with *MYC* and *BCL2* and/or *BCL6* rearrangements*

High-grade B-cell lymphoma, NOS*

B-cell lymphoma, unclassifiable, with features intermediate between DLBCL and classical Hodgkin lymphoma

MATURE T AND NK NEOPLASMS

T-cell prolymphocytic leukemia

T-cell large granular lymphocytic leukemia

Chronic lymphoproliferative disorder of NK cells

Aggressive NK-cell leukemia

Systemic EBV+ T-cell lymphoma of childhood*

Hydroa vacciniforme–like lymphoproliferative disorder*

Adult T-cell leukemia/lymphoma

Extranodal NK-/T-cell lymphoma, nasal type

Enteropathy-associated T-cell lymphoma

Monomorphic epitheliotropic intestinal T-cell lymphoma*

Indolent T-cell lymphoproliferative disorder of the GI tract

Hepatosplenic T-cell lymphoma

Subcutaneous panniculitis-like T-cell lymphoma

Mycosis fungoides

Sézary syndrome

Primary cutaneous CD30+ T-cell lymphoproliferative disorders

Lymphomatoid papulosis

Primary cutaneous anaplastic large cell lymphoma

Primary cutaneous γδ T-cell lymphoma

Primary cutaneous CD8 + aggressive epidermotropic cytotoxic T-cell lymphoma

Primary cutaneous acral CD8 + T-cell lymphoma

Primary cutaneous CD4 + small/medium T-cell lymphoproliferative disorder

Peripheral T-cell lymphoma, NOS

Angioimmunoblastic T-cell lymphoma

Follicular T-cell lymphoma

Nodal peripheral T-cell lymphoma with TFH phenotype

Anaplastic large-cell lymphoma, ALK+

Anaplastic large-cell lymphoma, ALK-*

Breast implant–associated anaplastic large-cell lymphoma

HODGKIN LYMPHOMA

Nodular lymphocyte predominant Hodgkin lymphoma

Classical Hodgkin lymphoma

Nodular sclerosis classical Hodgkin lymphoma

Continued

TABLE 1	2016 WHO Classification of Mature Lymphoid, Histiocytic, and Dendritic Neoplasms—cont'd

Lymphocyte-rich classical Hodgkin lymphoma

Mixed cellularity classical Hodgkin lymphoma

Lymphocyte-depleted classical Hodgkin lymphoma

POSTTRANSPLANT LYMPHOPROLIFERATIVE DISORDERS (PTLD)

Plasmacytic hyperplasia PTLD

Infectious mononucleosis PTLD

Florid follicular hyperplasia PTLD*

Polymorphic PTLD

Monomorphic PTLD (B- and T-/NK-cell types)

Classical Hodgkin lymphoma PTLD

HISTIOCYTIC AND DENDRITIC CELL NEOPLASMS

Histiocytic sarcoma

Langerhans cell histiocytosis

Langerhans cell sarcoma

Indeterminate dendritic cell tumor

Interdigitating dendritic cell sarcoma

Follicular dendritic cell sarcoma

Fibroblastic reticular cell tumor

Disseminated juvenile xanthogranuloma

Erdheim-Chester disease*

*Changes from the 2008 classification.
Provisional entities are listed in italics.
From Swerdlow SH, Campo E, Pileri SA, et al. The 2016 revision of the World Health Organization classification of lymphoid neoplasms. *Blood.* 2016;127:2375–2390.

Molecular Profiling

DNA microarray technology for gene expression profiling has identified distinct prognostic subgroups in many NHL subtypes including DLBCL and follicular NHL. Patients with germinal center B-like DLBCL have an improved overall survival compared with other molecular profiles. Studies in follicular NHL have identified gene expression signatures that also predicted survival. Interestingly, the genes that defined the prognostic signatures were not expressed in the tumor cells but were expressed by the nonmalignant tumor-infiltrating cells—primarily T cells, macrophages, and dendritic cells.

Treatment

The therapeutic approach for NHL differs for each clinicopathologic subtype. Chemotherapy remains an important modality. However, in some instances, radiation therapy or, rarely, surgical resection plays a role. Biologic approaches, including monoclonal antibodies and antibody-drug conjugates have shown significant activity and are now incorporated into many treatment paradigms. In addition, other novel therapeutics targeting the cell surface of lymphoma cells or varied transcription factors continue to be incorporated into treatment paradigms. Autologous and allogeneic stem cell transplantation are mostly reserved for patients with recurrent or refractory disease, although there are some subtypes where consolidative autologous transplantation after frontline therapy is considered (e.g., MCL and peripheral T-cell lymphomas).

Indolent B-Cell Non-Hodgkin Lymphomas

Indolent lymphomas are low-grade and represent slow-growing NHLs that may be stable with low tumor burden that may not

TABLE 2	Clinical Prognostic Classification of Adult Immunocompetent Non-Hodgkin Lymphomas

LYMPHOMA TYPE	PERCENTAGE OF ALL NON-HODGKIN LYMPHOMAS
Indolent or Low-Grade Non-Hodgkin Lymphomas	
Follicular lymphoma	20–25
Small lymphocytic lymphoma	7
MALT-type marginal zone lymphoma	7
Nodal-type marginal zone lymphoma	<2
Lymphoplasmacytic lymphoma	<2
Aggressive or High-Grade Non-Hodgkin Lymphomas	
Diffuse large B-cell lymphoma	30–35
T-cell lymphomas: peripheral or systemic (multiple subtypes)	10–12
Mantle cell lymphoma	6
Lymphoblastic lymphoma	<2
Burkitt lymphoma	<1

Subtypes are listed in order of most to least common.
MALT, Mucosa-associated lymphoid tissue.

BOX 2	Enhanced International Prognostic Index Risk Factors and Associated Approximate Cure Rates for Diffuse Large B-Cell Lymphoma

Factors/Scoring
Age, years
>40 to ≤60: 1
>60 to ≤75: 2
>75: 3
Lactate dehydrogenase (LDH), normalized
>1 to ≤3: 1
>3: 2
Ann Arbor stage III-IV: 1
Extranodal disease*: 1
Performance status ≥2: 1

Five-Year Progression-Free Survival Rates Based on Score at Diagnosis
Score 0–1: 91%
Score 2–3: 74%
Score 4–5: 51%
Score ≥ 6: 30%

*Disease in bone marrow, central nervous system, liver/GI tract, or lung.

warrant therapy for several years. The disease is responsive to treatment (remission rates greater than 90% with combined rituximab/chemotherapy), although the clinical course is characterized by repetitive relapses. Outside of early-stage disease and therapy with an allogeneic stem cell transplant, low-grade NHLs are not curable. The median survival of patients with advanced-stage follicular lymphoma in the pre-rituximab era was 9 to 10 years, although that is significantly longer now (approximately 16 to 18 years). Transformation to a high-grade NHL occurs in 30% to 35% (2% to 3% of patients each year) of follicular lymphoma patients (less common in other indolent subtypes) and is typically heralded by an aggressive change in the patient's clinical condition (e.g., B symptoms, rapidly rising lactate dehydrogenase [LDH]).

General Principles

Only a minority of patients present with early-stage disease (i.e., stage I or II). Low-dose involved field radiotherapy is a valid treatment option for these patients (especially stage I and not central sites of disease), and associated 20-year disease-free survival rates are greater than 50%. Treatment for patients with advanced-stage disease ranges from observation (i.e., watchful waiting) to anti-CD20 monoclonal antibody therapy (rituximab [Rituxan] or obinutuzumab [Gazyva]) with or without chemotherapy. Treatment choice depends in part on tumor burden and the patient's individual disease characteristics and baseline functional status. Treatment with frontline anti-CD20 monoclonal antibody with chemotherapy (outpatient therapy given once every 3 to 4 weeks typically for 6 to 8 cycles) followed by two years of maintenance therapy with anti-CD20 monoclonal antibody for patients with high tumor burden is associated with median progression-free survival rates of approximately 9 to 10 years.

Treatment options for relapsed indolent lymphoma include repeating rituximab with or without a different chemotherapy regimen, radioimmunotherapy, oral lenalidomide (Revlimid) immunomodulatory therapy, or stem cell transplantation. There is a small subset of follicular lymphoma patients who experience early progression to first line therapy (i.e., within 2 years), and survival rates are significantly inferior with conventional therapies. Autologous stem cell transplantation is an option for patients with relapsed disease, especially early progressors, although an improvement in overall survival is debated. Allogeneic stem cell transplantation is a potential curative modality for patients with relapsed or refractory disease, although patient selection is critical owing to potential morbidity and mortality related to this therapeutic option.

Special Considerations

Localized gastric MALT lymphoma cases often may be managed with therapy for *H. pylori* infection; radiation is typically reserved for failure to eradicate *H. pylori*. Patients with lymphoplasmacytic lymphoma (Waldenström macroglobulinemia) can present clinically with hyperviscosity or cryoglobulinemia, which may be managed acutely with plasmapheresis, but ultimately systemic therapy similar to that for other indolent NHLs is warranted. More recently, the Bruton tyrosine kinase (BTK) inhibitor, ibrutinib (Imbruvica), was US Food and Drug Administration (FDA) approved for the treatment of relapsed or refractory marginal zone lymphoma patients who require systemic therapy after at least one anti-CD20–based therapy.

Aggressive or High-Grade Non-Hodgkin Lymphomas

High-grade B- and T-cell NHLs are typically aggressive lymphomas that are fatal in weeks to a few months if not treated. However, many of these NHLs are curable with multiagent chemotherapy.

General Principles

DLBCL, the most common aggressive NHL, is curable in all stages in the majority of patients (60% to 70%). A key to treatment is anti-CD20 monoclonal antibody combined with anthracycline-based chemotherapy: rituximab-CHOP (R-CHOP) (cyclophosphamide, doxorubicin, vincristine, prednisone). The number of treatment cycles depends on stage of disease and response to treatment. Standard therapy for advanced-stage disease is six R-CHOP cycles, whereas patients with early-stage disease may receive three or four cycles followed by involved field radiation. There are emerging data regarding the prognostic importance of *MYC* rearrangement (from tumor testing) as a single finding and especially in conjunction with *BCL-2* and/or *BCL6* (i.e., double or triple hit) by molecular studies as well as with immunohistochemical staining. Outcomes with R-CHOP for DLBCL patients with a molecular double hit (e.g., presence of MYC and BCL-2 rearrangements) are modest; more intensive and novel therapeutic options should be considered. Therapy for relapsed DLBCL typically includes abbreviated salvage non–cross-resistant

chemotherapy followed by autologous stem cell transplantation for patients who have chemotherapy-sensitive disease, which is curative in approximately 35% to 45% of patients.

MCL is a B-cell NHL with initial high remission rates (>90% to 95%), but it has more modest long-term outcomes, and it is difficult to cure. With standard chemotherapy regimens (e.g., R-CHOP), the median progression-free survival rates are only 18 to 20 months. With more-intensive chemotherapy regimens (e.g., R-hyperCVAD/R-MA [rituximab, cyclophosphamide, vincristine, doxorubicin, dexamethasone/rituximab, methotrexate]), 5-year progression-free survival rates are near 70%. Some groups use induction therapy with aggressive high-dose cytarabine[1] (Cytosar-U)-based chemotherapy followed by consolidative autologous stem cell transplantation in first remission. As noted later, there has been the integration of several novel therapeutic agents into the treatment paradigm of MCL.

Burkitt lymphoma and related high-grade NHLs (e.g., lymphoblastic lymphomas) are often rapidly growing malignancies with a doubling time of 24 hours. Prompt initiation of therapy, including aggressive supportive care measures, is often warranted. With aggressive chemotherapy regimens, including prophylactic intrathecal chemotherapy, the majority of Burkitt patients younger than age 40 years are cured (>70% to 80%). In addition, there are data showing high efficacy using lower-intensity treatment consisting of infused etoposide (Toposar)[1], doxorubicin, and cyclophosphamide with vincristine, prednisone, and rituximab (EPOCH-R) for patients with lower risk, untreated Burkitt lymphoma, including HIV related.

Systemic (i.e., noncutaneous) peripheral T-cell lymphomas (PTCLs) are mostly aggressive malignancies. They are treatable; however, cure rates are lower compared with most aggressive B-cell NHLs. Standard therapy had consisted of CHOP-based chemotherapy with or without autologous SCT in first remission as consolidation. Recently published data from the ECHELON-2 trial combining the antibody drug conjugate, brentuximab vedotin (Adcetris), with cyclophosphamide, doxorubin, and prednisone (CHP) chemotherapy versus standard CHOP for untreated CD30+ PTCLs was associated with significantly improved progression-free survival (PFS) and overall survival (OS). This regimen (i.e., brentuximab vedotin + CHP) was subsequently FDA approved for this indication. Several additional novel targeted agents have also been FDA approved over the past several years for the treatment of T-cell NHL (see later).

Special Considerations

There are several clinical subtypes of DLBCL that present as primary extranodal manifestations such as primary testicular DLBCL and primary gastric DLBCL. If these lymphomas are localized, treatment typically consists of abbreviated cycles (3 to 4) of R-CHOP followed by involved field radiation. In addition, intrathecal chemotherapy prophylaxis is warranted for testicular DLBCL given the predilection of central nervous system (CNS) involvement.

Primary central nervous system lymphoma is typically DLBCL; high-dose methotrexate chemotherapy is a key component of therapy.

A long-standing therapeutic maneuver for solid organ transplant–related PTLDs has been reduction of immunosuppression, although, using this approach alone, mortality rates have ranged from 50% to 60% in most series. Recent evidence with use of initial rituximab-based therapy suggests significantly improved outcomes in the modern era.

The majority of AIDS-related NHLs are aggressive or high-grade types: DLBCL or Burkitt lymphoma. Similar therapy as immunocompetent NHL is often recommended. Response to therapy, including cure rate, has improved significantly with better control of opportunistic infections and highly active antiretroviral therapy (HAART).

---

[1] Not FDA approved for this indication.

Mycosis fungoides and Sézary syndrome are cutaneous T-cell lymphomas that initially might show eczematous lesions. It is often difficult to establish diagnosis, but eventually the lesions develop into plaques and tumors. Lymph nodes, spleen, and visceral organs may be involved. Sézary syndrome is a variant of mycosis fungoides and shows peripheral blood involvement; patients usually have diffuse erythroderma. Skin-targeted modalities for treatment of early-stage mycosis fungoides include psoralens with ultraviolet A light (PUVA), narrowband-ultraviolet light, skin electron-beam radiation, and topical steroids, retinoids, carmustine (BiCNU), and nitrogen mustard (Mustargen).[1] Treatment goals in advanced stages are to reduce tumor burden and to relieve symptoms. Treatment options also include monochemotherapy or polychemotherapy including CHOP, extracorporeal photopheresis, interferons, retinoids, monoclonal antibodies, recombinant toxins, histone deacetylase inhibitors, and most recently, the antibody drug conjugate, brentuximab vedotin (Adcetris).

During therapy for aggressive/high-grade NHLs, attention should be paid to preventing tumor lysis syndrome. Measures to prevent this complication include aggressive hydration, allopurinol (Zyloprim), alkalinization of the urine, and frequent monitoring of electrolytes, uric acid, and creatinine. Rasburicase (Elitek), a recombinant urate oxidase enzyme, is an expensive but potent agent for treating hyperuricemia.

Novel Treatment Options and Modalities

Many new agents targeting specific molecular targets have become available for the treatment of lymphoma. Novel agents in lymphoma include bortezomib (Velcade) and lenalidomide (Revlimid), which are FDA approved for relapsed or refractory MCL (and lenalidomide for relapsed follicular lymphoma), and histone deacetylase inhibitors, which are approved for cutaneous T-cell lymphoma and peripheral T-cell NHLs as well. In addition, bortezomib is FDA approved for untreated MCL patients in combination with immunochemotherapy. Other new agents which are FDA approved for the treatment of patients with chronic lymphocytic leukemia (CLL), including in higher-risk patient populations (e.g., p53 mutated), are idelalisib (Zydeliq), an inhibitor of PI3K delta; the BTK inhibitor ibrutinib (Imbruvica), which is also FDA approved for patients with CLL and MCL; and venetoclax (Venclexta), a BH3 mimetic acting as an inhibitor of BCL2. There are several recently published and a number of ongoing clinical studies to evaluate the optimal sequence and varied combinations for patients with CLL, especially vis-à-vis harnessing frontline targeted therapeutics.

The BTK inhibitor acalabrutinib (Calquence) is FDA approved for relapsed or refractory MCL patients who have received at least one prior therapy. Two other PI3K inhibitors (i.e., copanlisib [Aliqopa] and duvelisib [Copiktra]) are approved for adult patients with relapsed or refractor follicular lymphoma. New anti-CD20 antibodies have also been approved for the treatment of CLL (e.g., obinutuzumab (Gazyva) and antibody drug conjugates, such as brentuximab vedotin (Adcetris), which is FDA approved for relapsed anaplastic (T-cell) large-cell lymphoma. These novel therapeutic agents are mostly FDA approved for patients with relapsed or refractory disease; however, there are a multitude of ongoing studies in the frontline/untreated setting and in varied sequences and combinations.

There is also great excitement in the continued application of new immunotherapy approaches in NHL such as via checkpoint inhibitors (e.g., programmed death-1 (PD-1) inhibitors) as well as chimeric antigen receptor (CAR) T-cell therapy, which involve removal of T cells from patients followed by bioengineered CARs (e.g., CD19) that facilitate T-cell expansion and antigen/tumor recognition when re-infused into the patient. Axicabtagene ciloleucel (Yescarta) and tisagenlecleucel (Kymriah) are anti-CD19 CAR T-cell therapies FDA approved for patients with relapsed or refractory DLBCL. Overall response rates range from 50% to 72%, with complete remission rates of 32% to 51%. Furthermore,

25% to 35% of patients appear to experience longer term disease remission. There are a multitude of other CAR T-cell constructs being studies across several lymphoma subtypes.

Follow-Up of Long-Term Survivors
Relapse

Among patients with aggressive lymphomas, such as DLBCL, most recurrences are seen within the first 2 years after the completion of therapy, although later relapses occur uncommonly. Physical examination and laboratory testing at 2- to 3-month intervals and follow-up CT scans at 6-month intervals for the first 2 years after diagnosis are recommended; however, there is ongoing debate regarding the impact that postsurveillance scans have on disease outcomes. Detection of recurrent disease is important in part because these patients may be candidates for potentially curative therapy (e.g., stem cell transplantation). Patients with advanced low-grade NHL are at a constant risk for relapse, as discussed before.

Secondary Malignancies

Long-term NHL survivors are at an increased risk for second cancers. In general, the risk is increased with history of radiation use, but it is also seen with chemotherapy. In a survey of 28,131 Dutch registry patients with NHL who survived 2 years or longer, significant excesses of second cancers were seen for nearly all solid tumors as well as acute myelogenous leukemia (AML) and HL. The standardized incidence ratio (SIR) for solid tumors after NHL was 1.65. The SIRs for solid tumors are increased for up to 30 years after NHL diagnosis, with the highest relative risk of developing a secondary malignancy occurring more than 21 to 30 years after original diagnosis.

Late Treatment Complications

There has been more selective use of radiation as part of therapy for NHL. Thus the risk of certain radiation-induced complications has been reduced in patients treated more recently. Nevertheless, the risk still exists. Transplant recipients are at increased risk for secondary myelodysplasia and AML, regardless of whether they received radiation. All chemotherapy agents may cause long-term morbidity; in particular, patients who received an anthracycline (e.g., doxorubicin [Adriamycin]) are at a long-term increased risk of cardiovascular disease. Among Dutch and Belgian NHL patients treated with at least six cycles of doxorubicin-based chemotherapy, cumulative incidence of cardiovascular disease was 12% at 5 years and 22% at 10 years. Risk of coronary artery disease matched that of the general population; however, risk of chronic heart failure was significantly increased (SIR, 5.4), as was stroke (SIR, 1.8). Risk factors associated with excess risk included younger age at start of NHL treatment (<55 years), preexisting hypertension, any salvage treatment, and use of radiotherapy; risk relating to radiotherapy was dose dependent. Continued studies are needed to develop optimal secondary prevention strategies.

References

Burger JA, et al: Ibrutinib as initial therapy for patients with chronic lymphocytic leukemia, N Engl J Med 373(25):2425–2437, 2015 Dec 17.

Dunleavy K, Pittaluga S, Shovlin M, et al: Low-intensity therapy in adults with Burkitt's lymphoma, N Engl J Med 369(20):1915–1925, 2013.

Fischer K, Al-Sawaf O, Bahlo J, et al: Venetoclax and obinutuzumab in patients with CLL and coexisting conditions, N Engl J Med 380(23):2225–2236, 2019 Jun 6.

Gopal AK, Kahl BS, de Vos S, et al: PI3Kδ inhibition by idelalisib in patients with relapsed indolent lymphoma, N Engl J Med 370(11):1008–1018, 2014.

Hemminki K, Lenner P, Sundquist J, Bermejo JL: Risk of subsequent solid tumors after non-Hodgkin's lymphoma: Effect of diagnostic age and time since diagnosis, J Clin Oncol 26(11):1850–1857, 2008.

Horwitz S, O'Connor OA, Pro B, et al: Brentuximab vedotin with chemotherapy for CD30-positive peripheral T-cell lymphoma (ECHELON-2): a global, double-blind, randomised, phase 3 trial, Lancet 393(10168):229–240, 2019 Jan 19.

Marcus R, Davies A, Ando K, et al: Obinutuzumab for the first-line treatment of follicular lymphoma, N Engl J Med 377(14):1331–1344, 2017 Oct 5.

Morton LM, Curtis RE, Linet MS, et al: Second malignancy risks after non-Hodgkin's lymphoma and chronic lymphocytic leukemia: differences by lymphoma subtype, J Clin Oncol 28:4935–4944, 2010.

Moser EC, Noordijk EM, van Leeuwen FE, et al: Long-term risk of cardiovascular disease after treatment for aggressive non-Hodgkin lymphoma, Blood 107:2912–2919, 2006.

---

[1] Not FDA approved for this indication.

Neelapu SS, Locke FL, Bartlett NL, et al: Axicabtagene ciloleucel CAR T-Cell therapy in refractory large B-Cell lymphoma, *N Engl J Med* 377(26):2531–2544, 2017 Dec 28.

Prince HM, Kim YH, Horwitz SM, et al: Brentuximab vedotin or physician's choice in CD30-positive cutaneous T-cell lymphoma (ALCANZA): an international, open-label, randomised, phase 3, multicentre trial, *Lancet* 390(10094):555–566, 2017 Aug 5.

Roberts AW, et al: Targeting BCL2 with Venetoclax in relapsed chronic lymphocytic leukemia, *N Engl J Med* 374(4):311–322, 2016 Jan 28.

Schuster SJ, Bishop MR, Tam CS: Tisagenlecleucel in adult relapsed or refractory diffuse large B-Cell lymphoma, *N Engl J Med* 380(1):45–56, 2019 Jan 3.

Shanafelt TD, Wang XV, Kay NE, et al: Ibrutinib-rituximab or chemoimmunotherapy for chronic lymphocytic leukemia, *N Engl J Med* 381(5):432–443, 2019 Aug 1.

Swerdlow SH, Campo E, Pileri SA, et al: The 2016 revision of the World Health Organization classification of lymphoidneoplasms, *Blood* 127(20):2375–2390, 2016 May 19.

Trappe RU, et al: Response to rituximab induction is a predictive marker in B-cell post-transplant lymphoproliferative disorder and allows successful stratification into rituximab or R-CHOP consolidation in an international, prospective, multicenter Phase II trial, *J Clin Oncol.*

Wang ML, Rule S, Martin P, et al: Targeting BTK with ibrutinib in relapsed or refractory mantle-cell lymphoma, *N Engl J Med* 369(6):507–516, 2013.

Woyach JA, Ruppert AS, Heerema NA, et al: Ibrutinib regimens versus chemoimmunotherapy in older patients with untreated CLL, *N Engl J Med* 379(26):2517–2528, 2018 Dec 27.

Zhou Z, Sehn LH, Rademaker AW, et al: An enhanced International Prognostic Index (NCCN-IPI) for patients with diffuse large B-cell lymphoma treated in the rituximab era, *Blood* 123(6):837–842, 2014.

PERNICIOUS ANEMIA/MEGALOBLASTIC ANEMIA

Method of
Anusha Vallurupalli, MBBS

CURRENT DIAGNOSIS

- Megaloblastic anemia is defined as macrocytic anemia with large, structurally and functionally abnormal red blood cells in the bone marrow and peripheral blood and is most commonly associated with folate or B12 deficiencies.
- In adults, folate deficiency is most commonly due to inadequate dietary intake. Vitamin B12 deficiency is mainly due to cobalamin malabsorption from food due to pernicious anemia, an autoimmune disorder, and gastrointestinal malabsorption.
- Megaloblastic anemia often presents with macrocytosis and hypersegmented neutrophils on peripheral smear.

CURRENT TREATMENT

- Prompt recognition and diagnosis are essential to prevent both short-term and long-term complications.
- Recognition of the underlying etiology for megaloblastic anemia is essential for a long-term treatment plan.
- Vitamin B12 deficiency can be treated with both oral and parenteral therapy and the route and duration of treatment is usually based on underlying etiology.
- If vitamin B12 deficiency is untreated, folate repletion will correct the megaloblastic anemia but not the associated neuropathic changes that occur with B12 deficiency.
- Folate replacement is generally accomplished through the oral route.
- Preventive B12 and folate dosing is warranted in certain high risk patients.
- Both B12 and folate replacements are generally well tolerated.

Introduction

Anemia is one of the most common hematologic disorders encountered on a regular basis in various clinical settings. In 2010, the global prevalence of anemia was 32.9%; that is, more than 2.2 billion people were affected. The World Health Organization (WHO) defines anemia as a hemoglobin (Hb) count of less than 13 g/L in men, less than 12 g/L in nonpregnant women, and less than 11 g/L in pregnant women and the elderly. A Hb of less than 10 g/L in any patient should trigger an evaluation. The etiology of anemia is oftentimes multifactorial, especially in elderly patients. In elderly patients, anemia can exacerbate comorbid cardiac complications such as cardiac ischemia and congestive heart failure. Most of the causes of anemia, especially nutritional causes, can usually be treated efficiently. Therefore, the cause of anemia should be identified and treated promptly to decrease the risk of complications.

Megaloblastic anemia, in general, is defined as macrocytic anemia with large, structurally and functionally abnormal red blood cells in the bone marrow and peripheral blood. Hypersegmented neutrophils are also commonly seen on the peripheral smear. The mean corpuscular volume (MCV) is elevated. Megaloblastic anemia is most commonly associated with nutritional deficiencies, specifically B12 and folate. In most cases, diagnosis is made by blood testing.

Epidemiology

The incidence and prevalence of anemia is highly variable and depends on age, sex, ethnicity, country of origin, socioeconomic status, and multifactorial comorbid conditions.

A retrospective study of 1784 randomly selected older adults living at home found macrocytosis in 6.3% of men and 3.3% of women. Folate and B12 deficiencies are the most common causes of megaloblastic anemia. Folate and B12 nutritional deficiencies are often easily treated.

Etiology
Folate Deficiency

Deficiency of folate is the most common cause of megaloblastic anemia. Folate is abundant in green leafy vegetables and approximately 60% of dietary folate is absorbed in the small intestine. However, folate is not stored in the body for a long duration and needs to be constantly replaced. Body stores of folate only last for approximately 6 months. Other causes include malabsorption and factors affecting folate metabolism (Table 1).

Vitamin B12 Deficiency

Deficiency of vitamin B12 can occur due to insufficient capture of the vitamin B12 from dietary sources because of inadequate intake, as seen in vegetarians and vegans or in patients who are malnourished. Malabsorption, as seen in patients with pernicious anemia, atrophic gastritis, or following gastric surgery, is another major cause (Table 2).

Pernicious Anemia

Pernicious anemia is characterized by malabsorption of B12 due to a deficiency of intrinsic factor. It is often associated with other co-existing autoimmune disorders such as celiac disease, Hashimoto thyroiditis, and Sjögren syndrome. Pernicious anemia is usually diagnosed by checking for intrinsic factor antibodies in the blood or by biopsy-proven immune atrophic gastritis. Intrinsic factor neutralizing antibodies are found in the setting of atrophic immune gastritis. *Helicobacter pylori*-related atrophic gastritis is in the differential and, if there is a clinical suspicion, should be evaluated by gastric biopsy. Intrinsic factor antibodies should not be checked after parenteral B12 administration for at least 2 weeks, as it will result in a false negative result.

Clinical Manifestations

Symptoms of anemia and laboratory findings (Table 3) from folate deficiency and B12 deficiency are essentially indistinguishable. B12 deficiency can manifest without anemia and is also characterized by neuropsychiatric symptoms (Table 4). The cause

TABLE 1	Causes of Folate Deficiency

Dietary Deficiency

Malabsorption due to abnormalities of the jejunum
- Celiac disease
- Jejunal resection
- Tropical sprue

Drug-induced malabsorption
- Sulfasalazine (Azulfidine)

Increased requirement
- Pregnancy
- Prematurity
- Chronic hemolytic anemias (sickle cell anemia and autoimmune hemolytic anemias)
- Malignant diseases
- Chronic inflammatory disease

Increased loss
- Some skin diseases
- Long-term dialysis

Acquired abnormality of folate metabolism: dihydrofolate reductase inhibitors (methotrexate and sulfamethoxazole/trimethoprim [Bactrim])

Complex or uncertain mechanism
- Ethanol abuse (some cases)
- Anticonvulsant drugs (some cases)
- Oral contraceptive drugs, glutethimide, and cycloserine

Inherited abnormalities of folate absorption and metabolism
- Hereditary folate malabsorption
- Glutamate formiminotransferase-cyclodeaminase deficiency

Adapted from Wickramasinghe SN. Diagnosis of megaloblastic anemias. *Blood Rev.* 2006;20(6):299–318.

TABLE 2	Causes of B12 Deficiency

Dietary Deficiency

Impaired release of B_{12} from food—food cobalamin malabsorption

Inadequate secretion of intrinsic factor
- Pernicious anemia
- Total or partial gastrectomy
- Congenital intrinsic factor deficiency
- Congenitally abnormal intrinsic factor

Impaired release of B_{12} from B_{12}–R binder complex
- Pancreatic insufficiency
- Zollinger-Ellison syndrome

Diversion of dietary B_{12}
- Abnormal intestinal bacterial flora—jejunal diverticula, small intestinal strictures, and stagnant intestinal loops (blind loop syndrome)
- Fish tapeworm infestation

Malabsorption due to abnormalities in the terminal ileum
- Ileal resection
- Crohn disease
- Chronic tropical sprue
- Other acquired diseases
- Imerslund-Gräsbeck syndrome (selective malabsorption with proteinuria)

Drug-induced malabsorption (amino salicylic acid, neomycin, colchicine, slow-release potassium chloride, metformin, phenformin, biguanides, and cholestyramine)

Inactivation of methyl cobalamin by nitrous oxide

Inherited abnormalities of B_{12} transport or intracellular B_{12} metabolism
- Deficiency or abnormality of transcobalamin II
- Defective methyl cobalamin synthesis (hyper homocysteinemia)
- Defective synthesis of both methyl cobalamin and adenosyl cobalamin (hyper homocysteinemia and methylmalonic acidemia)

Adapted from Wickramasinghe SN. Diagnosis of megaloblastic anemias. *Blood Rev.* 2006;20(6):299–318.

of neurological symptoms is thought to be secondary to the role that vitamin B12 plays in neuronal myelination, although the exact mechanism is not known.

Diagnosis

The diagnosis of pernicious anemia is based on laboratory testing (see Table 3). Complete blood count with differential, peripheral blood smear, complete metabolic profile including total and indirect bilirubin, lactate dehydrogenase, and serum folate and B12 levels are all included in the initial diagnostic testing. Methylmalonic acid (MMA) and homocysteine levels in indeterminate situations where the B12 or folate serum levels are borderline low may be helpful. MMA levels are increased in B12 deficiency, whereas MMA levels are normal in folate deficiency. Homocysteine levels are increased in both folate and B12 deficiencies. There may be fluctuations in MMA and homocysteine levels due to underlying concurrent conditions such as renal insufficiency (increased MMA levels), methylmalonic aciduria (increased MMA levels) and hereditary homocystinemia (increased homocysteine levels), and additional bacterial overgrowth in the small intestine (increased MMA levels), in addition to other rare conditions. Intrinsic factor antibody testing should be ordered prior to initiation of parenteral B12 replacement in patients with pernicious anemia.

Bone marrow aspiration and biopsy are not routinely recommended and should be reserved for cases in which there is persistent anemia despite replacement of both B12 and folate with resultant normalized levels. Patients with pernicious anemia should be evaluated for underlying gastric cancer with esophagogastroduodenoscopy. A systematic meta-analysis of 27 studies revealed a pooled gastric cancer incidence rate in patients with pernicious anemia of 0.3/100 person-years and an estimated sevenfold relative risk of gastric cancer.

Differential Diagnosis

The differential diagnosis for macrocytic anemia includes anemia related to chronic alcohol use (with or without liver disease),

TABLE 3	Laboratory Findings in Megaloblastic Anemia

Common for both B12 and folate deficiencies:
- Macrocytosis with elevated MCV, often greater than 100
- Megaloblasts and hypersegmented neutrophils on peripheral smear
- Anemia
- Elevated homocysteine levels

Specific for B12 deficiency:
- Elevated MMA levels
- Elevated LDH, indirect bilirubin, and low haptoglobin in the setting of intravascular hemolysis, which can be seen in severe B12 deficiency.
- Positive intrinsic factor antibodies in patients with pernicious anemia.

LDH, Lactate dehydrogenase; *MCV*, mean corpuscular volume; *MMA*, methylmalonic acid.

thyroid failure, and myelodysplastic syndromes (Table 5). Symptoms of copper deficiency can mimic B12 deficiency, can occasionally present with macrocytosis and should be ruled out with serum copper level testing if the patient does not respond to B12 supplementation.

Prevention

Providing food sources with nutrients rich in folic acid and/or B12 is best for preventing megaloblastic anemia. Therapeutic supplementation may be necessary, especially for the very old. The Institute of Medicine (United States) Standing Committee on the Scientific Evaluation of Dietary Reference Intakes has

TABLE 4 Signs and Symptoms of B12 Deficiency

Neurological Symptoms/Signs
- Dysesthesia and hypoesthesia
- Subacute combined degeneration presenting with ataxia, decreased proprioception, and vibratory sensation
- Extrapyramidal signs (e.g., dystonia, dysarthria, and rigidity)
- Abnormal deep tendon reflexes
- Ataxia or positive Romberg test

Gastrointestinal Symptoms/Signs
- Glossitis
- Abdominal pain
- Dyspepsia likely related to atrophic gastritis or *H. pylori* infection

Psychiatric Symptoms
- Depression or mood impairment
- Psychosis
- Dementia

Rare Manifestations
- Skin hyperpigmentation
- Grey hair

Anemia Symptoms
- Fatigue
- Palpitations
- Exertional dyspnea
- Chest pain
- lightheadedness

TABLE 5 Differential Diagnosis of Macrocytic Anemia

- Chronic alcohol abuse
- Myelodysplastic syndromes
- Hypothyroidism
- Chronic lung disease with hypoxia
- Heavy smoking
- Chronic liver disease
- Chronic hemolytic anemia
- Therapy with certain anticonvulsant drugs
- Myeloma (some cases)
- Hypoplastic and aplastic anemia
- Physiologic
- Normal neonates
- Normal pregnancy (some cases)

Adapted from Wickramasinghe SN. Diagnosis of megaloblastic anemias. *Blood Rev.* 2006;20(6):299–318.

recommended fortification of cereals with multiple B vitamins, including B12. Prophylactic folate treatment should be administered to patients with increased requirements such as those with chronic hemolytic anemias and women who are pregnant. Preventive therapeutic replacement should be offered to all patients who have undergone bariatric gastric surgery or patients with compromised small intestine absorption due to various causes.

Treatment
General Principles
All patients who are identified as having B12 deficiency and/or folate deficiency should be treated. Replacement of the nutrients usually corrects the anemia. Blood transfusions are generally reserved for emergency situations such as severe symptomatic anemia and in patients with cardiac complications (i.e., chest pain, heart failure) associated with anemia. Oral replacement is generally well tolerated and is the first line treatment of choice. Parenteral replacement, especially for B12 deficiency, should be considered in patients with severe B12 deficiency who present with symptomatic anemia, severe neurologic symptoms, pernicious anemia, as well as in patients who are at risk for malabsorption and in women who are pregnant. Replacement with oral folate in a patient with undiagnosed B12 deficiency will improve the anemia but will not reverse the neurological symptoms.

The underlying cause for B12 deficiency and/or folate deficiency should be identified and treated. The duration of therapy depends on the underlying cause of the deficiency. Lifelong replacement is recommended for patients with irreversible causes (e.g., gastric bypass surgery and pernicious anemia). Short term treatment is recommended for patients with reversible causes (e.g., drug induced, reversible causes of malabsorption, inadequate dietary intake, and alcoholism). Both B12 and folate are water soluble vitamins and do not generally cause any major adverse effects.

Treatment of B12 Deficiency
Vitamin B12 is available in oral, sublingual, intramuscular (IM), subcutaneous (SC), and intranasal formulations. Cyanocobalamin is the most available formulation in United States. The oral formulation is generally effective in patients with a reversible cause and is administered at a dosage of 1000 μg daily for at least 1 month followed by either continuation of the same dose for maintenance or the dose can be decreased to 100 to 500 μg daily in patients with mild reversible deficiencies. The parenteral formulation is preferably administered IM at a dose of 1000 μg daily for 1 week followed by 1000 μg once a week for 1 month. The maintenance dose for IM or parenteral deep SC injection is 1000 μg monthly and indefinitely, depending on the etiology. Patients are usually taught to self-administer the injections to minimize the inconvenience of travel, improve compliance, and decrease costs.

Treatment of Folate Deficiency
The replacement dose for folic acid varies between 1 and 5 mg/day. Usually, therapy is continued for at least 3 to 6 months, provided that the underlying causes of the deficiency have been corrected.

Complications and Long-Term Monitoring
Patients with undiagnosed megaloblastic anemia can develop severe anemia and cardiac comorbidities. Neuropsychiatric changes can become irreversible if the B12 deficiency is not treated promptly. Patients may also develop long-term complications from undiagnosed underlying etiologies.

There is no need for frequent monitoring of B12 and folate levels once the underlying cause of the deficiency has been identified and appropriate treatment has been started.

References
Carmel R, Agrawal YP: Failures of cobalamin assays in pernicious anemia, *N Engl J Med* 367:385–386, 2012.
Green R: Vitamin B12 deficiency from the perspective of a practicing hematologist, *Blood* 129:2603–2611, 2017.
Inelmen EM, D'Alessio M, Gatto MR, et al: Descriptive analysis of the prevalence of anemia in a randomly selected sample of elderly people living at home: some results of an Italian multicentric study, *Aging (Milano)* 6:81–89, 1994.
Kassebaum NJ, Jasrasaria R, Naghavi M, et al: A systematic analysis of global anemia burden from 1990 to 2000, *Blood* 123:615–624, 2014.
Lahner E, Capasso M, et al: Incidence of cancer (other than gastric cancer) in pernicious anemia: A systematic review with meta-analysis, *Digestive and Liver Disease* 50(8):780–786, 2018.
Wazir SM, Ghobrial I: Copper deficiency, a new triad: anemia, leucopenia, and myeloneuropathy, *J Community Hosp Intern Med Perspect* 7(4):265–268, 2017 Oct.
Wang H, Li L, Qin LL, et al: Oral vitamin B12 versus intramuscular vitamin B12 for vitamin B12 deficiency, *Cochrane Database Syst Rev* 3:CD004655, 2018.
Wickramasinghe SN: Diagnosis of megaloblastic anemias, *Blood Reviews* 20(6):299–318, 2006.

PLATELET-MEDIATED BLEEDING DISORDERS

Method of
Eric H. Kraut, MD

CURRENT DIAGNOSIS

- Platelet-mediated bleeding disorders commonly present with bleeding from mucosal surfaces or skin. Bleeding caused by reduced platelet counts may present with petechiae or purpura, whereas abnormalities of function are more likely to present with bleeding after injury or menstruation.
- Evaluation of platelet function used to be measured by the bleeding time. However, it is now more commonly evaluated by the PFA-100 or platelet aggregation studies.

- Thrombocytopenia is most commonly caused by deficient production of platelets from the bone marrow, decreased platelet survival in the circulation, or sequestration of platelets by an enlarged spleen.
- Patients may bleed after trauma at platelet counts under 50,000/μL and develop petechiae or purpura at platelet counts under 20,000/μL, but they usually do not have severe bleeding unless platelet counts drop below 10,000/μL
- The most common causes of new thrombocytopenia in the hospitalized patient are drugs or infection, whereas the usual cause of new platelet function abnormalities are medications.
- Patients in the hospital and placed on heparin should have their platelet counts monitored, and a reduction of 50% should be evaluated for heparin-induced thrombocytopenia.
- Immune thrombocytopenic purpura (ITP) usually presents in outpatients as new-onset mucocutaneous bleeding associated with only a reduced platelet count or unexplained asymptomatic isolated thrombocytopenia.
- Drugs that inhibit platelet activation and aggregation, such as aspirin, clopidogrel (Plavix), and dipyridamole (Persantine) can lead to significant bleeding, especially after surgery or procedures. This effect may last for 7 to 10 days.
- Patients presenting with a lifetime history of easy bruising and or heavy menses should have careful evaluation of their bleeding history and family history of bleeding. If positive, studies to rule out Von Willebrand disease or hereditary disorders of platelet granules such as storage pool disorder should be done.

CURRENT THERAPY

- Patients with severe thrombocytopenia (platelet counts <10,000/μL) that is due to impaired production are at risk of severe bleeding and should be considered for platelet transfusions. The benefit of transfusing platelets when the platelet count reaches this level and the patient is not bleeding has been demonstrated as reducing bleeding in some patients in a recent study.
- Standard practice for platelet transfusions is to maintain platelet counts above 50,000/μL for patients with gastrointestinal bleeding and 75,000-100,000/μL for neurosurgical procedures. Platelet transfusions should be considered for certain other invasive procedures.
- Patients with immune thrombocytopenia should not receive platelet transfusions unless they are having significant bleeding since response to platelet transfusion occurs in less than 10% of patients and is short lasting.
- Patients with ITP who have no bleeding and platelet counts > 30,000/μL can be followed without treatment since the risk of bleeding is low.
- In patients with ITP and thrombocytopenia less than 10,000/μL, initial treatment with high doses of corticosteroids in combination with IVIG (Gamunex) induces a rapid rise in platelets, usually within 24 hours.
- Current treatment for patients with ITP who fail prednisone treatment include splenectomy, rituximab (Rituxan),[1] or thrombopoietin agonists (romiplostim [Nplate] or eltrombopag [Promacta]).
- Patients with chronic renal failure can develop severe bleeding diathesis, which appears to be multifactorial including platelet dysfunction. Dialysis can reduce bleeding but not completely correct it. Other treatment that may help include desmopressin (DDAVP),[1] tranexamic acid (Lysteda),[1] and synthetic erythropoietin (Epogen).[1]
- Patients with drug induced platelet dysfunction who may need to undergo surgery or who are bleeding may require platelet transfusions.

- Patients with inherited platelet disorders and mild bleeding can be treated with desmopressin (DDAVP) but if severe may require platelet transfusions.

[1]Not FDA approved for this indication.

Platelets Role in Hemostasis

Platelets are small non-nucleated blood cells that are derived from bone marrow megakaryocytes. Their production is controlled by the hormone thrombopoietin produced in the liver, and they survive in the circulation for 8 to 10 days. On blood vessel injury, they form a seal or plug at the site of injury to limit bleeding. This initial event, termed *primary hemostasis*, occurs after endothelial injury when the subendothelial surface is exposed to circulating blood. Platelets are drawn to the site via von Willebrand factor (vWF), which, in combination with other proteins including fibrillar collagen, fibronectin and laminin, leads to platelet adhesion. After platelets adhere to the vessel wall, they are activated, undergo a shape change and release products from their granules. These platelet granule products, including ADP and thromboxane A_2, further potentiate this process. Fibrinogen then binds to platelets via GPIIb/IIIa on the platelet surface causing firm platelet aggregation. The platelet secretory release reaction and aggregation recruits other platelets forming a firm hemostatic plug. Platelets also support the coagulation phase by interacting with circulating clotting factors and providing a surface for generation of thrombin. Secondary hemostasis occurs and thrombin-mediated fibrin mesh stabilizes the platelet plug.

Clinical Manifestations

The hallmark of platelet-mediated bleeding disorders is mucocutaneous bleeding such as nose bleeds, prolonged bleeding after tooth extractions, and heavy menstrual bleeding. When the platelet count drops below 30,000/μL, one may also see petechiae or purpuric lesions, especially on lower extremities.

Quantitative Platelet Disorders (Thrombocytopenia)

Primary hemostasis depends on an adequate number of platelets to prevent bleeding. A significant reduction in platelets or thrombocytopenia is usually defined as <100,000/μL. However, bleeding usually does not occur until the platelet count drops much lower. For example, spontaneous bleeding may only occur only when the platelet count is <20,000/μL and severe life-threatening bleeding occurs only <10,000/μL. Thrombocytopenia can develop due to inadequate platelet production from the bone marrow, reduced platelet survival in the circulation, or sequestration of platelets in the spleen. Differentiating the cause requires evaluation of the patients associated medical problems, physical findings, drug history, blood chemistry analysis, and possibly bone-marrow sampling.

Decreased platelet production is often the result of chemotherapeutic drugs for cancer, some antibiotics and antivirals (Table 1), or radiation therapy. These drugs may cause bone-marrow injury including damage to the megakaryocytes. Complete recovery may occur after stopping the offending agent. One common agent that can induce thrombocytopenia is alcohol. Thrombocytopenia associated with reduction in the white blood cell count and or red blood cell count should alert physicians to the possibility of a bone marrow disorder such as forms of leukemia or aplastic anemia. In cases where the cause is not evident, a bone marrow biopsy may be necessary to demonstrate whether there is a malignancy that may require urgent treatment.

Patients with reduced platelet production can often be observed without intervention depending on the severity of the thrombocytopenia, presence of bleeding, or the need to perform invasive procedures. Guidelines for transfusion of platelets to prevent bleeding (prophylactic transfusion) have changed in the last few years. With evidence that severe bleeding may not occur in most patients until the platelet count is below 10,000/μL, limited

CATEGORY	IMPLICATED IN SEVERAL REPORTS
Heparin	Unfractionated and LMWH
Cinchona alkaloids	Quinidine, quinine
Platelet inhibitors	Abciximab (RepPro), eptifibatide (Integrilin), tirofiban (Aggrastat)
Antirheumatic agents	Gold salts
Antimicrobial agents	Linezolid (Zyvox), rifampin, sulfonamides, vancomycin
Sedative and anticonvulsants	Valproic acid, phenytoin, carbamazepine
Histamine receptor antagonists	Cimetidine
Diuretic agents	Chlorothiazide
Analgesic agents	Acetaminophen, naproxen, diclofenac
Chemotherapy agents	Oxaliplatin (Eloxatin), fludarabine (Fludara), and others

TABLE 1 Drugs Commonly Implicated as Causes of Drug-Induced Thrombocytopenia

platelet resources, and potential for development of alloimmunization to platelets, transfusions are not usually given unless sustained platelet counts are below 10,000/μL. When platelets are transfused it is appropriate to measure the response with a platelet count 1 hour post-transfusion. The platelet count should rise 30,000 to 40,000/μL for the usual four-pack of platelet transfusion. Patients requiring frequent transfusions may require single-donor apheresis or HLA-matched platelets to obtain a good response.

Thrombocytopenia Resulting from Increased Platelet Destruction

Normally, platelets live in the circulation for 10 days, and the bone marrow replenishes them at the same rate that they are destroyed. Platelet survival may be altered by both nonimmune and immune processes. Severe infections will often lead to increased platelet destruction, and the platelet count returns to normal when the infection is adequately treated. Consumption of platelets also can occur in association with microangiopathic hemolytic anemia, as seen in disseminated intravascular coagulation (DIC) and thrombotic thrombocytopenic purpura and hemolytic uremic syndrome (TTP/HUS). It is important to review the blood smear to document fragmented red blood cells and evaluate coagulation parameters to help differentiate DIC from TTP/HUS and other causes of consumption. TTP/HUS may require specific and urgent treatment to prevent life-threatening complications. Platelet transfusions are not usually given for TTP because there are reports of patients deteriorating after transfusions.

Immune-mediated platelet destruction is seen in response to several common drugs, including the sulfonamides and vancomycin. The characteristic pattern of immune-mediated platelet destruction is a sharp drop in the platelet count 7 to 10 days after starting the drug. The platelet count may drop to ≤5000/μL. Recognition is important because significant bleeding may occur, and the platelet count will only improve after discontinuation of the drug. Glycoprotein IIa/IIIb inhibitors, which are often used after cardiac stent placement, may cause a dramatic drop in the platelet count to as low as 1000/μL within hours of administration. This is important to recognize because this is one case where platelet transfusions may be necessary to prevent severe bleeding and it can be easily confused with other causes of low platelet counts.

Heparin-induced thrombocytopenia (HIT) is a unique drug reaction for several reasons. First, although thrombocytopenia is the initial sign of this entity, the major and feared complication is arterial and venous thromboses. It appears to affect 4% to 5%

of patients exposed to unfractionated heparin and about 0.5% of patients exposed to low-molecular-weight heparin. Those at highest risk are female surgical patients who receive a minimum of 4 days of either type of heparin. The classic pattern is exposure to heparin at any dose with development of antibodies to heparin at day 4 and a 50% reduction in platelet count by day 6. The antibodies responsible are to the heparin–platelet factor 4 complex (IgG-PF4). A suspicious clinical pattern and a high antibody titer measured by an enzyme-linked immunosorbent assay are often diagnostic. Patients suspected of having HIT are at a high risk of thromboembolic disease within the first 24 hours of the drop in platelet count, and the heparin should be immediately stopped. However, despite the reduced platelet count, bleeding is unusual. Patients should be placed on an alternative anticoagulant, usually a direct thrombin inhibitor. The platelet count takes about 2 weeks to return to normal, and warfarin (Coumadin) should not be started until the platelet count returns to normal to avoid warfarin-associated necrosis. By reducing protein C and protein S, warfarin creates a temporary hypercoagulable state and places the patient at risk for warfarin-associated necrosis during the time when patients are most susceptible to thrombosis from HIT.

Immune thrombocytopenic purpura (ITP), previously termed *idiopathic thrombocytopenic purpura* affects 1 to 3 people per 100,000, but is probably the most common cause of severe isolated thrombocytopenia seen in the outpatient setting. It affects all ages, although ITP in childhood has a unique natural history. Childhood ITP is often associated with viral illness, is commonly transient, and may not need treatment. In adults, 40% of patients may have protracted or recurrent episodes of ITP, and the majority of patients need treatment. It was demonstrated in the 1950s that ITP is caused by circulating antiplatelet antibodies, and, like many autoimmune diseases, it is more common in women. When ITP presents in association with other diseases such as systemic lupus erythematosus or chronic lymphatic leukemia, or in patients with HIV, management of the underlying disease is important. The clinical presentation of ITP depends on the degree of thrombocytopenia. Mild thrombocytopenia of 20,000 to 80,000/μL is often asymptomatic, whereas platelet counts under 20,000/μL may present with mucocutaneous bleeding and diffuse petechiae and purpura. Thrombocytopenia, an otherwise normal blood count and peripheral blood smear without evidence of splenomegaly in a patient with no other illness helps make a tentative diagnosis. A bone marrow biopsy is no longer considered necessary to confirm the diagnosis.

Treatment of ITP has changed over the last several years, and initial treatment after the diagnosis requires evaluation of the platelet count, whether it is increasing or decreasing, and the presence or absence of bleeding. Patients who have counts above 20,000/μL without bleeding and who are not in need of an invasive procedure can be observed without intervention. Patients with counts between 10,000 and 20,000/μL may be started on oral prednisone at 1 mg/kg. Patients with severe thrombocytopenia less than 10,000/μL and those who are bleeding can receive high-dose dexamethasone (Decadron) at 40 mg daily for 4 days and IVIG (Gamunex). There is usually a response to treatment within 24 hours. Although usually not helpful or required, about 10% of patients will have a response to platelet transfusion, and this can be considered for patients presenting with low platelet counts and bleeding. Refractory or recurrent ITP is a common problem in these patients, and recommendations for treatment include splenectomy, rituximab (Rituxan), or thrombopoietin agonists. The choice of which to use depends on the patient and his or her clinical condition.

Thrombocytopenia Due to Hypersplenism

The platelet mass is distributed 70% in the circulation and 30% in the spleen. Enlargement of the spleen and/or alteration of blood flow in portal hypertension may increase platelet sequestration in the spleen and reduce the platelet count in the peripheral blood circulation. Patients' counts rarely drop below 20,000/μL. Thus, thrombocytopenia caused by hypersplenism does not usually need

Qualitative Platelet Function Disorders

Acquired Qualitative Platelet Function Disorders

Acquired disorders of platelet function are commonly seen, because platelets are the target of medications used to prevent arterial and cardiac stent thrombosis. Spontaneous bleeding is not common, but bleeding resulting from trauma or surgery can be a significant clinical problem. Because many patients may be on multiple antiplatelet agents or anticoagulants at the same time, the risk of bleeding needs to be recognized. Acquired qualitative disorders of platelet function may be due to drugs, hematologic diseases, or medical illnesses.

Drugs are the most common cause of acquired platelet dysfunction with differing risks of bleeding due to different targets. Aspirin causes irreversible acetylation of cyclooxygenase I (COX-1) and inhibits generation of prostaglandin A2. Although it is considered a weak antiplatelet agent with up to 25% resistance, aspirin increases the risk of bleeding in otherwise normal patients. Major bleeding was seen in up to 3.7% of patients and, when aspirin is used in combination with other antiplatelet agents or in patients with underlying bleeding disorders, the bleeding risk is higher. Clopidogrel (Plavix) is a thienopyridine prodrug, and the active metabolite irreversibly inhibits the surface receptor $P2Y_{12}$ on platelets. In clinical trials the risk of major bleeding in patients taking clopidogrel was similar to what is described with aspirin. Clopidogrel may significantly increase bleeding after surgery. GPIIb/IIIa receptor antagonists used after cardiac stent placement inhibit platelet aggregation and can induce severe thrombocytopenia.

Malignancies of the bone marrow may produce abnormally functioning platelets or alter platelet function by affecting vWF. The myeloproliferative and myelodysplastic disorders may produce platelets with reduced numbers of granules and may have associated increased risk of gastrointestinal bleeding and bleeding after invasive procedures. Acquired von Willebrand disease an infrequent cause of abnormal bleeding, can be seen in patients with lymphoproliferative disease, multiple myeloma, and Waldenström macroglobulinemia.

Systemic illness can alter platelets and increase the bleeding risk. Acute and chronic renal failure are common causes of platelet-function abnormalities. In uremia, hemorrhagic complications include upper gastrointestinal bleeding, pericardial bleeding, and intracranial bleeding. Bleeding in renal failure is believed to be multifactorial and includes impaired release of platelet granules, decreased prostaglandin formation, vWF dysfunction, and presence of severe anemia. Effective treatment includes improvement of the anemia with erythropoietin (Epogen)[1] or desmopressin (DDAVP)[1] or conjugated estrogens (Premarin).[1]

Hereditary Qualitative Platelet Function Disorders

Inherited abnormalities of platelet function are infrequent disorders that give rise to bleeding of varying severity. Inherited abnormalities of platelet function are often classified according to the type of genetic defect. Bernard-Soulier syndrome (BSS) is a severe bleeding disorder with autosomal recessive inheritance characterized by thrombocytopenia, decreased platelet adhesion, reduced platelet survival, and giant platelets on blood smear. Patients with BSS have defects in the GPIb-IX-V complex leading to reduced binding to vWF. Glanzmann thrombasthenia is an autosomal recessive disorder with defects of integrin αIIbβ3, a receptor on activated platelets that normally binds platelets during aggregation. Platelet aggregation to ADP and thrombin is abnormal. Patients with BSS and Glanzmann thrombasthenia who need treatment require platelet transfusions.

Hereditary disorders of platelet secretion are common reasons patients present to clinicians for evaluation of mucocutaneous bleeding. Defects in platelet dense granules (δ storage pool disease) are suspected in patients with bleeding and a negative workup for von Willebrand disease. Diagnosis is made by platelet electron microscopy and or platelet aggregation studies. Granule deficiency associated with abnormalities of other lysosome-related organelles may lead to specific phenotypes such as Hermansky-Pudlak and Chediak Higashi disease. Gray platelet syndrome (GPS), or alpha granule deficiency, is an autosomal recessive disorder with mild bleeding. GPS patients may also be thrombocytopenic. Treatment for bleeding or in preparation for surgery includes desmopressin (DDAVP)[1] or platelet transfusions.

---

[1]Not FDA approved for this indication.

References

Aster RH, Curtis BR, McFarland JG, Bougie DW: Drug-induced immune thrombocytopenia: pathogenesis, diagnosis, and management, *J Thromb Haemost* 7:911–918, 2009.

Barbour T, Johnson S, Cohney S, Hughes P: Thrombotic microangiopathy and associated renal disorders, *Nephrol Dial Transplant* 27:2673–2685, 2012.

Cuker A, Gimotty PA, Crowther MA, Warkentin TE: Predictive value of the 4Ts scoring system for heparin-induced thrombocytopenia: a systematic review and meta-analysis, *Blood* 120:4160–4167, 2012.

Estcourt L, Stanworth S, Doree C, et al: Prophylactic platelet transfusion in prevention of bleeding in patients with hematologic disorders and stem cell transplantation, *Cochrane Database Syst Rev 5*, 2012. May 16, https://doi.org/10.1002/14651858.CD004269.pub. CD004269.

Hedges SJ, Dehoney SB, Hooper JS, et al: Evidence-based treatment recommendations for uremic bleeding, *Nat Clin Pract Nephrol* 3:138–153, 2007.

Jackson S: Arterial thrombosis: insidious, unpredictable, and deadly, *Nat Med* 17:1423–1436, 2011.

Lakshamanan S, Cuker A: Contemporary management of immune thrombocytopenic purpura in adults, *J Thromb Haemost* 10:1988–1998, 2012.

Nurden A, Nurden P: Advances in our understanding of the molecular basis of disorders of platelet function, *J Thromb Haemost Suppl* 1:76–91, 2011.

Provan D, Stasi R, Newland AC, et al: International consensus report on the investigation and management of primary immune thrombocytopenia, *Blood* 115:168–186, 2010.

Stanworth SJ, et al: Risk of bleeding and use of platelet transfusions in patients with hematologic malignancies: recurrent event analysis, *Haematol* 100(6):740–747, 2015.

Tsantes AE, Nikolopoulos GK, Tsirigotis P, et al: Direct evidence for normalization of platelet function resulting from platelet count reduction in essential thrombocytosis, *Blood Coagul Fibrinolysis* 22:457–462, 2011.

Warkentin AE, Donadni MP, Spencer FA, et al: Bleeding risk in randomized controlled trials comparing warfarin and aspirin: a systemic review and meta-analysis, *J Thromb Haemost* 10:512–520, 2012.

Zucker ML, Hagedorn CH, Murphy CA, et al: Mechanism of thrombocytopenia in chronic hepatitis C as evaluated by the immature platelet fraction, *Int J Lab Hematol* 34:525–532, 2012.

POLYCYTHEMIA VERA

Method of
Peter R. Duggan, MD; and Sonia Cerquozzi, MD

CURRENT DIAGNOSIS

- Polycythemia vera (PV) should be considered when there is persistent elevation of hemoglobin (> 165 g/L in men and > 160 g/L in women) or hematocrit (> 49% in men and > 48% in women).
- *JAK2V617F* mutation testing and erythropoietin levels should be performed when PV is suspected.
- Bone marrow biopsy and aspiration may be necessary in some cases to confirm the diagnosis of PV and to distinguish PV from other myeloproliferative neoplasms (MPNs).
- PV is highly likely when *JAK2V617F* mutation is present and erythropoietin level is subnormal. When *JAK2V617F* mutation is seen with normal erythropoietin level, PV is possible; bone marrow biopsy is recommended to differentiate PV from other MPNs. When *JAK2V617F* is normal and erythropoietin is

low, consider *JAK2* exon 12 mutational analysis or alternative diagnosis of congenital polycythemia. Wildtype *JAK2V617F* with normal or high erythropoietin level makes PV very unlikely, and patients should be investigated for secondary causes of polycythemia.

- Investigations for secondary polycythemia that may be indicated include:
  - Chest x-ray
  - Pulse oximetry
  - Arterial blood gas including carboxyhemoglobin and methemoglobin levels
  - Kidney and liver function tests
  - Abdominal imaging studies (ultrasound or computed tomography [CT] scan)
  - Oxyhemoglobin dissociation curve
  - Sleep studies

CURRENT THERAPY

- All patients should be treated with phlebotomy and/or cytoreductive therapy to target hematocrit less than 45%.
- Low-dose aspirin[1] (acetylsalicylic acid [ASA]) should be used in *all patients* without a contraindication.
- In *high-risk* patients with PV (age > 60 years and/or history of thrombosis), cytoreductive therapy should be used in combination with ASA.
- Alkylating agents should be avoided as cytoreductive therapy owing to the risk of acute leukemia.
- Conventional cardiovascular risk factors (diabetes, hypertension, hyperlipidemia) should be aggressively managed, and cigarette smoking should be discouraged.
- Thromboembolic events should be managed according to accepted management guidelines. Thromboprophylaxis should be used after surgery and in other high-risk situations.

[1]Not US Food and Drug Administration (FDA) approved for this indication.

Polycythemia vera is a clonal stem cell disorder characterized by an increase in red cell production independent of the stimulation by erythropoietin. PV is the most common of the chronic myeloproliferative neoplasms (MPNs), occurring in approximately 2 to 3 people per 100,000 annually. The median age at diagnosis is 70 years, and it is rare in patients younger than 40 years.

A mutation of the tyrosine kinase Janus kinase 2 (*JAK2*) is consistently found in PV. This sheds some light on the pathogenesis of the disease and is useful in the diagnosis of PV and other MPNs. A single acquired mutation (*V617F*) of the gene for the JH-2 domain of *JAK2* can be found in 90% to 95% of patients with PV. The JH-2 domain functions to inhibit *JAK2* activity. In normal erythropoiesis, binding of erythropoietin to its receptor lifts this inhibition and allows *JAK2* stimulation of cell division and differentiation. In mutated *JAK2*, this inhibitory function is absent, leading to constitutive activity of the tyrosine kinase. This mutation is also present in about half of patients with essential thrombocytosis and primary myelofibrosis. The small number of patients with PV who are negative for the common *JAK2V617F* mutation have another functionally similar mutation within *exon 12*.

Presentation

Many patients with PV are asymptomatic, and PV is diagnosed after the incidental finding of an elevated hemoglobin or hematocrit on routine complete blood count. Splenomegaly is present in 30% to 40% of patients. Up to half of patients experience nonspecific symptoms such as weight loss, sweating, headache, fatigue, epigastric discomfort, visual disturbances, and dizziness.

Many of these symptoms are likely caused by decreased blood flow due to an increased blood viscosity from polycythemia.

Generalized pruritus is often described, often after a warm bath or shower (aquagenic pruritus). Although the cause of this is unknown, it is thought to be due to the degranulation of increased numbers of mast cells in the skin of patients, releasing histamine and other inflammatory mediators. However, the symptom responds poorly to antihistamines, and it does not always resolve with treatment of PV.

Venous and arterial thromboembolic events are a major cause of morbidity and mortality in PV. Thrombosis at presentation occurs in up to 40% of patients. Ischemic stroke, transient ischemic attack, and myocardial infarction are common, especially among elderly patients. These, along with deep venous thrombosis and pulmonary embolus, are the most common thrombotic events and often result in serious morbidity, disability, and even death. Thrombotic events that are considered unusual in the general population, such as Budd-Chiari syndrome; portal, mesenteric, and other abdominal vein thrombosis; and cerebral venous thrombosis, occur more commonly among patients with PV. The possibility of an underlying MPN should be considered when a patient presents with such an event.

PV can manifest with symptoms of peripheral vascular disease. Patients with erythromelalgia describe a painful burning sensation of the hands and feet; pallor, erythema, or cyanosis of the extremities; and sometimes cutaneous ulceration. Erythromelalgia results from microvascular thrombosis and ischemia due to platelet activation and aggregation and responds well to platelet reduction and antiplatelet agents such as aspirin (ASA).[1]

Almost all patients with PV are iron deficient at diagnosis, even before the onset of therapeutic phlebotomy. Other manifestations of PV include acute gouty arthritis, peptic ulcer disease, erosive gastritis, and hypertension.

Diagnosis and Differential Diagnosis

The 2016 World Health Organization (WHO) diagnostic criteria for PV are shown in Box 1. The *JAK2V617F* mutation is present in about 95% of cases of PV. Erythropoietin level is decreased in more than 90% and is rarely elevated. Few patients with PV carry a mutation of exon 12 (~4%) of the *JAK2* gene instead of the more common *JAK2V617F* mutation. A *JAK2* mutation can also be found in about half of patients with essential thrombocytosis and primary myelofibrosis.

Leukocytosis and thrombocytosis are present in the majority of cases of PV. Red cell mass is increased. A nuclear medicine study measuring red cell mass and plasma volume is rarely required with the availability of *JAK2* testing, but it may be useful when relative polycythemia is suspected. Bone marrow biopsy and aspiration are not often needed for a diagnosis of PV but have been included as a major criterion within the revised WHO classification. Bone marrow examination can be important for diagnosing PV in the rare cases where *JAK2* is negative and to differentiate PV from other *JAK2*-positive MPNs when the distinction cannot be made based on peripheral blood counts.

Erythrocytosis can occur as a result of a number of other conditions in the absence of PV (Box 2). A careful history and physical examination with selected investigations can usually distinguish PV from secondary polycythemia and relative polycythemia (see Current Diagnosis). In relative (apparent, spurious) polycythemia, there is usually only a modest increase in the hematocrit, because of a decrease in plasma volume rather than a true increase in red cell mass. Thrombocytosis, leukocytosis, and splenomegaly should be absent. Causes include smoking, dehydration, and use of diuretics, and it is also described in middle-aged, obese, hypertensive men (Gaisböck syndrome).

Red cell mass can be elevated owing to increased stimulation of erythropoiesis by high levels of erythropoietin. Erythropoietin can be increased as an appropriate response to chronic hypoxia (sleep

[1]Not FDA approved for this indication.

BOX 1 | 2016 World Health Organization Diagnostic Criteria for Polycythemia Vera

Diagnosis requires three major criteria or first two major criteria and minor criterion.*

Major Criteria

1. Hemoglobin > 165 g/L in men, 160 g/L in women,

   or

   Hematocrit > 49% in men, > 48% in women,

   or

   Other evidence of increased red cell volume[†]
2. Bone marrow biopsy: hypercellular for age with trilineage growth (panmyelosis)
3. Presence of *JAK2V617F* or *JAK2* exon 12 mutation

Minor Criterion

1. Subnormal serum erythropoietin level

---

*Bone marrow biopsy may not be required in sustained erythrocytosis—hemoglobin > 185 g/L (hematocrit > 55.5%) in men or > 165 g/L (hematocrit > 49.5%) in women— if major criterion 3 and minor criterion are present.

[†] > 25% above mean normal predicted value.

BOX 2 | Differential Diagnosis of Polycythemia

Normal Red Cell Mass
Relative polycythemia
Gaisböck syndrome

Elevated Red Cell Mass
Primary Polycythemia
Polycythemia vera

Secondary Polycythemia
- Congenital EPO receptor mutations
- Chuvash polycythemia
- High-affinity hemoglobin
Appropriately elevated EPO (hypoxia driven)
- Chronic hypoxic lung disease
- Cardiac shunts or cyanotic heart disease
- Sleep apnea
- Methemoglobinemia
- High altitude
- Chronic carbon monoxide poisoning
- Cigarette smoking
- Renal artery stenosis
Inappropriately elevated EPO
- Renal cell carcinoma
- Hepatocellular carcinoma
- Hemangioblastoma
- Uterine fibroids
Other causes:
- EPO (Epogen) administration
- Androgens (testosterone)
- Kidney transplant

Abbreviation: EPO = erythropoietin.

apnea, right-to-left cardiac shunts, chronic lung disease, high altitude, smoking, methemoglobinemia), and it can be inappropriately elevated owing to erythropoietin-secreting tumors (renal cell carcinoma, hepatocellular carcinoma, cerebellar hemangioma, uterine fibroids) or decreased kidney perfusion (renal artery stenosis). Familial causes of polycythemia include high-affinity hemoglobins, erythropoietin receptor mutations, and Chuvash polycythemia. Polycythemia occurs in 10% to 15% of patients following kidney transplantation, and this may be due to erythropoietin secretion by the native kidneys or increased sensitivity to erythropoietin. Polycythemia can be drug induced, such as with the use of performance-enhancing drugs (erythropoietin [Epogen], androgens) in athletes and testosterone replacement in men.

Prognosis

Patients with PV have a reduced life expectancy compared with the general population, with a median survival of approximately 14 years, or 24 years if younger than age 60 at diagnosis.

Despite therapy, thrombosis remains an important cause of mortality. Cardiac disease, ischemic stroke, pulmonary embolus, and other thrombotic events account for 40% of deaths among patients with PV. Nonfatal thrombosis is common, occurring in almost 4% of patients annually. Age and a history of prior thromboembolic events are independent risk factors for thrombosis and can be used to predict a patient's risk of future events (Box 3). Low-risk patients are younger than 60 years and have no history of thrombosis. They experience new events at a rate of 2% per year. For patients older than 60 years or with a past history of thrombosis, this rate is 5% annually, but it can be as high as 11% when both risk factors are present.

The contribution of other cardiovascular risk factors (smoking, diabetes, hypertension, hyperlipidemia) to thrombotic risk in PV has been studied, with inconclusive results. However, because these are major contributors to the development of cardiovascular disease in the general population, they should also be considered when assessing risk in patients with PV. Leukocytosis (white blood cell count > 15 × 10^9/L) has been associated with a higher risk of arterial thrombosis.

Conversely, the risk of major hemorrhage is low, with fatal bleeding responsible for less than 5% of all deaths. However, there is considerable excess mortality from malignancy, in particular transformation to a myelodysplastic syndrome, myelofibrosis, or acute leukemia. The rate of leukemic transformation is less than 10% at 20 years. Risk factors for leukemic transformation include advanced age, leukocytosis, and abnormal karyotype. Approximately 10% of patients transform to

BOX 3 | Thrombotic Risk in Polycythemia Vera

Low Risk
Age < 60 years and no history of thrombosis

High Risk
Age ≥ 60 years and/or history of thrombosis

myelofibrosis (post-PV myelofibrosis). Risk factors for post-PV myelofibrosis include leukocytosis and *JAK2V617F* allele burden of greater than 50%.

Treatment

The goals of treatment in PV are to lower the risk of thrombosis while minimizing toxicity. This is achieved by a combination of phlebotomy, aspirin,[1] and hydroxyurea (Hydrea)[1] or other cytoreductive agents. The use of these therapies can be individualized based on a patient's risk of developing future thromboembolic events. Risk stratification (Box 3) aims at identifying patients with PV at higher risk of thrombotic events who require cytoreductive therapy. Because cerebrovascular and cardiovascular disease are among the main causes of morbidity and mortality for these patients, careful attention should be paid to the management of conventional cardiovascular risk factors. Hypertension, diabetes, and hyperlipidemia should be controlled with standard measures based on current guidelines, and patients should be encouraged to stop smoking. As the hematocrit increases in PV, there is a dramatic increase in blood viscosity. Phlebotomy is the fastest, most effective way to normalize a patient's hematocrit, and it should be initiated immediately in those with newly diagnosed PV. Blood volume should be reduced as rapidly as possible. Usually, 500 mL

---

[1] Not FDA approved for this indication.

of blood is removed every 1 or 2 days until the hematocrit is less than 45%. The frequency of phlebotomy or volume of blood removed can be decreased in elderly patients, those with cardiovascular disease, or others who do not tolerate this schedule. The optimal target in patients with PV is to maintain a hematocrit less than 45% to lower the risk of major thrombotic events and death from cardiovascular causes. Regular phlebotomy eventually results in iron deficiency, at which point most patients' phlebotomy needs decrease dramatically. Iron replacement should be avoided.

Aspirin

Previous studies did not support the routine use of aspirin to prevent thrombosis in PV. However, high doses of aspirin were used in these early studies, resulting in excess bleeding in the treatment arm. The results of a recent large randomized trial show that low-dose aspirin (100 mg/day) reduces major thrombotic events (nonfatal myocardial infarction, nonfatal stroke, pulmonary embolism, major venous thrombosis). This was accomplished without an increase in bleeding risk. Although there was a trend suggesting more minor bleeding events in those receiving aspirin, the rates of major bleeding were identical for those receiving aspirin or placebo. The benefit from aspirin was seen, even though this study included many low-risk patients without a prior history of thromboembolism. Low-dose aspirin (75–100 mg daily)[1] should be started in all patients without a contraindication to the drug (history of bleeding or intolerance). Because of the risk of bleeding from acquired von Willebrand disease that can occur with extreme thrombocytosis, aspirin should be held when platelets are more than 1500×10^9/L until the count can be lowered by cytoreduction.

Cytoreductive Therapy

Cytoreductive therapy is recommended for high-risk patients with PV (Box 3). Hydroxyurea (HU)[1] is the cytoreductive agent most commonly used to treat PV. Hydroxyurea can safely control blood counts and decreases spleen size in PV and other MPNs. Randomized data are limited, but hydroxyurea also appears to reduce thrombotic complications. A starting dosage of 15 to 20 mg/kg daily (1000–1500 mg daily) is used. Occasional phlebotomy is still required to maintain hematocrit less than 45%, but the frequency usually decreases. Myelosuppression is the main toxicity. The lowest dosage that provides therapeutic effect should be used, and excess myelosuppression should be avoided. The dosage can be titrated to ensure that the white cell count remains higher than 3.0×10^9/L, neutrophils are higher than 2.0×10^9/L, and platelets are in the normal range.

Hydroxyurea has been associated with leg ulcers and other skin changes, especially after long-term use. There is growing evidence that hydroxyurea does not contribute to the excess rates of acute leukemia seen in PV; rates are no different than in those treated with phlebotomy alone. However, transformation is clearly associated with the use of other chemotherapeutic agents such as chlorambucil (Leukeran)[1], busulfan (Myleran)[1], and pipobroman (Vercyte),[2] accounting for one-third of the deaths among patients with PV treated with these agents. The use of these agents should be avoided. Hydroxyurea resistance can occur in up to 11% of patients and is associated with increased risk of death. Both hydroxyurea resistance and intolerance are defined according to the European Leukemia Net (ELN) criteria.

Interferon-α2b (IFN-α2) (Intron A)[1] is an alternative treatment option in the setting of hydroxyurea resistance and/or intolerance and often is considered in young patients with PV. IFN-αb is available in both short-acting and controlled-release (pegylated) formulations. IFN-α is commonly administered subcutaneously with a starting dose of 3 million units daily, or pegylated IFN-α (Peg-Intron)[1] is given at 45 to 90 μg weekly. Studies have shown its efficacy in controlling blood counts in addition to achieving complete hematologic and molecular responses. The inconvenience of its administration and its side effects including mood disturbances and flulike illness make it a less desirable therapy. Controlled studies are comparing hydroxyurea with pegylated forms of IFN-α. At present, both are first-line cytoreductive treatment options with recommendations that IFN-α be used in females with childbearing potential.

JAK Inhibitors

Ruxolitinib (Jakafi), a *JAK1/2* inhibitor, was originally approved in patients with myelofibrosis, including myelofibrosis evolving[1] from PV. There was a significant reduction in spleen size and constitutional symptoms in almost half of these patients. In the phase III RESPONSE trial, ruxolitinib illustrated its effectiveness in controlling hematocrit (< 45%), reducing spleen size (≥ 35%), and improving symptoms in patients with PV who had hydroxyurea intolerance or resistance, resulting in its approval as a second-line cytoreductive agent in PV. The most common side effects are anemia and thrombocytopenia.

Other Treatment Issues

Hyperuricemia is common in myeloproliferative neoplasms and occasionally results in kidney stones or gout. Allopurinol (Zyloprim) 300 mg daily can be used to reduce uric acid levels in patients with these complications. For those with intractable pruritus, several agents have been used with variable success. Some patients respond to aspirin,[1] hydroxyurea[1], cimetidine (Tagamet)[1], cyproheptadine (Periactin)[1], and paroxetine (Paxil)[1] 20 mg daily. Both IFN-α[1] and ruxolitinib have been successful in the majority of cases.

Less than 60% of pregnancies occurring in patients with PV are successful. First-trimester fetal loss is the most common complication, and third-trimester fetal loss, preterm birth, and intrauterine growth restriction are also common. Phlebotomy should be used to keep the hematocrit at less than 45%. Interferon-α2b[1] is recommended for those requiring cytoreductive therapy during pregnancy; other cytoreductive agents are contraindicated owing to possible teratogenic effects. There is some evidence that the use of low-dose aspirin[1] throughout pregnancy improves live birth rate. It is recommended that prophylactic low-molecular-weight heparin (LMWH) be used for 6 weeks postpartum.

Surgery in patients with PV has a high risk of both operative bleeding and postoperative thromboembolism. Elective surgeries should be delayed until cytoreductive measures and phlebotomy can be used to achieve good control of blood counts. Aspirin should be held for 1 week before surgery to reduce the risk of hemorrhage. LMWH should be given after surgery to prevent deep venous thrombosis. Mechanical compression stockings are an option for patients with bleeding that prevents the use of anticoagulation. When thromboembolic events do occur, treatment should be according to current management guidelines. Venous thromboembolism is treated with LMWH and warfarin (Coumadin). Indefinite anticoagulation should be considered because of the high risk of recurrent events. Low-dose aspirin is indicated in those with a history of arterial events such as stroke and myocardial infarction.

---

[1]Not FDA approved for this indication.

References

Arber DA, Orazi A, Hasserjian R, et al: The 2016 revision to the World Health Organization classification of myeloid neoplasms and acute leukemia, *Blood* 127(20):2391–2405, 2016.

Barosi G, Birgegard G, Finazzi G, et al: A unified definition of clinical resistance and intolerance to hydroxycarbamide in polycythemia vera and primary myelofibrosis: results of a European LeukemiaNet (ELN) consensus process, *Br J Haematol* 148:961–963, 2010.

Finazzi G, Caruso V, Marchioli R, et al: for the ECLAP Investigators: Acute leukemia in polycythemia vera: an analysis of 1638 patients enrolled in a prospective observational study, *Blood* 105(7):2664–2670, 2005.

Kiladjian JJ, Cassinat B, Chevret S, et al: Pegylated interferon-alfa-2a induces complete hematologic and molecular responses with low toxicity in polycythemia vera, *Blood* 112:3065–3072, 2008.

Landolfi R, Marchioli R, Kutti J, et al: Efficacy and safety of low-dose aspirin in polycythemia vera, *N Engl J Med* 350:114–124, 2004.

Marchioli R, Finazzi G, Landolfi R, et al: Vascular and neoplastic risk in a large cohort of patients with polycythemia vera, *J Clin Oncol* 23(10):2224–2232, 2005.

Marchioli R, Finazzi G, Specchia G, et al: Cardiovascular events and intensity of treatment in polycythemia vera, *N Engl J Med* 368:22–33, 2013.

Passamonti F: How I treat polycythemia vera, *Blood* 120(2):275–284, 2012.

Passamonti F, Rumi E, Caramella M, et al: A dynamic prognostic model to predict survival in post-polycythemia vera myelofibrosis, *Blood* 111(7):3383–3387, 2008.

---

[1]Not FDA approved for this indication.
[2]Not available in the United States.

Quintas-Cardama A, Kantarjian H, Manshouri T, et al: Pegylated interferon alfa-2a yields high rates of hematologic and molecular response in patients with advanced essential thrombocythemia and polycythemia vera, *J Clin Oncol* 27:5418–5424, 2009.

Tefferi A, Barbui T: Polycythemia vera and essential thrombocythemia: 2015 update on diagnosis, risk-stratification and management, *Am J Hematol* 90(2):163–173, 2015.

Tefferi A, Guglielmelli P, Larson DR, et al: Long-term survival and blast transformation in molecularly annotated essential thrombocythemia, polycythemia vera, and myelofibrosis, *Blood* 124(16):2507–2513, 2014.

Tefferi A, Rumi E, Finazzi G, et al: Survival and prognosis among 1545 patients with contemporary polycythemia vera: an international study, *Leukemia* 27:1874–1881, 2013.

Vannucchi AM, Kiladjian JJ, Griesshammer M, et al: Ruxolitinib versus standard therapy for the treatment of polycythemia vera, *N Engl J Med* 372:426–435, 2015.

PORPHYRIAS

Method of
Claus A. Pierach, MD

CURRENT DIAGNOSIS

- There is not just one porphyria; there are at least six types (and a few very rare ones because of homozygosity and dual porphyrias).
- There is not one single test covering all porphyrias. For suspected acute porphyria, screening for excessive porphobilinogen in the urine is the test of choice.
- If cutaneous porphyria is in the differential diagnosis, quantitative measurements of porphyrins in urine and stool are recommended.
- Family studies and genetic counseling are always indicated in these hereditary diseases.

CURRENT THERAPY

- Prophylaxis is mandatory and depends on the type of porphyria.
- Abstinence from alcohol is always indicated.
- The drug list should be respected in the acute porphyrias.
- Glucose therapy for the acute attack has been superseded by the more effective, definitive treatment with hematin (hemin, Panhematin), to be instituted as soon as possible once the diagnosis has been ascertained.

The *porphyrias* present a group of mostly inherited diseases where disturbances along the biosynthetic pathway to heme lead to accumulations of metabolic intermediaries. Porphyria cutanea tarda usually occurs without discernible inheritance; it can also be induced by chemicals. All steps of heme synthesis are enzymatically regulated, and all porphyrias are a result of specific impasses along these transitions. Not all enzymatic defects result in clinically relevant or recognizable disease manifestations in every patient. On the one hand, the severity of the enzymatic defect plays a role. On the other, some poorly understood revealing or unveiling cofactors are operational; enzyme cofactors are likely contributing as well. The prevalence of the porphyrias is not known and fluctuates in different parts of the world; for example, variegate porphyria is most common in South Africa, whereas porphyria cutanea tarda is the most common porphyria in the United States.

The porphyrias can be divided between neurovisceral (acute) and cutaneous manifestations. Two types, the very rare delta-aminolevulinic acid-dehydratase deficiency porphyria and acute intermittent porphyria (AIP), have only neurologic symptoms (acute attacks and possibly chronic manifestations). Hereditary coproporphyria and variegate porphyria can have both neurologic and dermatologic signs and symptoms. Congenital erythropoietic porphyria, porphyria cutanea tarda, and erythropoietic protoporphyria exhibit only skin lesions but can be complicated by other problems, such as anemia or hepatic insufficiency.

Heme Synthesis

Succinyl coenzyme-A and glycine are the initial building blocks, subsequently transformed through eight enzymatic steps to the end product, heme, in itself essential not only for hemoglobin but also for other hemoproteins such as cytochromes, myoglobin, and other enzymes including catalase, nitric oxide synthase, and tryptophan pyrrolase. Heme synthesis happens in all cells but mostly in the liver and in the bone marrow. It is controlled by heme through feedback inhibition of the first step, delta-aminolevulinic acid synthase. Figure 1 shows the various steps, intermediaries, and resulting porphyrias. Porphyrins and their precursors, delta-aminolevulinic acid (ALA) and porphobilinogen (PBG), are only generated during heme synthesis and not during heme catabolism toward bilirubin.

Specific enzymatic defects result in specific patterns of heme precursors and are of high diagnostic value when determining the type of porphyria. The ultimate step in ruling in or out if a person has the genetic defect for a specific porphyria is DNA testing, currently offered by the Mount Sinai Genetic Testing Laboratory (porphyria@mssm.edu). However, these specific tests are not necessary in the clinical evaluation of a patient in whom porphyria is suspected. Here, quick and simple tests are sufficient. The excretory pattern of heme precursors is influenced by their water solubility, which decreases toward heme; ALA and PBG are highly water soluble and measured in urine, whereas protoporphyrin is so hydrophobic that it is only excreted in stool and not in urine.

There is no single test that can reveal all types of porphyrias. The porphyric symptomatology can differ from type to type, and there is considerable overlap among the various porphyrias. For this reason, highly specific and sensitive laboratory tests are necessary. All porphyrias with acute manifestations manifest with similar attacks and respond to similar treatment, but they exhibit different biochemical patterns according to their specific enzyme defect. A clinically useful grouping splits the porphyrias between acute (neurovisceral) and cutaneous.

The Acute Porphyrias

There are four types of acute porphyria to consider:
- The very rare ALA-dehydratase deficiency porphyria is inherited in an autosomal recessive fashion.
- AIP, an autosomal dominant disorder, is the most common of the acute porphyrias (except in South Africa where variegate porphyria is more common).
- Hereditary coproporphyria, an autosomal dominant disease, is commonly misdiagnosed because coproporphyrin is often moderately and nonspecifically increased in many disorders.
- Variegate porphyria is autosomal dominant and probably the mildest of the acute porphyrias.

All acute porphyrias are sensitive to a multitude of drugs and circumstances (a short list is included in Box 1). Hereditary coproporphyria and variegate porphyria can also have skin lesions resembling porphyria cutanea tarda. Skin lesions and acute attacks can happen at the same time or one after the other, or only one manifestation may ever be present in a given patient.

Diagnosis

Diagnosis of the porphyric attack hinges mainly on a keen sense of suspicion. Any inexplicable symptom complex involving abdominal pain, tachycardia, and psychological findings should be suspect for porphyria. However, no clinical presentation can be called *porphyric* without biochemical support. Small deviations from the narrow normal range for heme precursors are fairly common and nonspecific. PBG or ALA must be markedly elevated, at least fivefold above the normal range, and, if not, porphyria is an unlikely explanation for a patient's acute symptoms.

Enzyme	Substrate	Porphyria
	Glycine and succinyl CoA	
ALA synthase		
	Delta-aminolevulinic acid (ALA)	
ALA dehydrase		ALA D deficiency porphyria
	Porphobilinogen (PBG)	
PBG deaminase		Acute intermittent porphyria
	Uroporphyrinogen (URO) I	
URO III cosynthase		Günther's disease
	URO III	
URO decarboxylase		Porphyria cutanea tarda
	Coproporphyrinogen (COPRO)	
COPRO oxidase		Coproporphyria
	Protoporphyrinogen (PROTO)	
PROTO oxidase		Variegate porphyria
	Protoporphyrin	
Ferrochelatase		Erythropoietic protoporphyria
	Heme	

Figure 1 Heme biosynthetic pathway. Enzymes that have defects or deficiencies that cause the various porphyrias are listed on the left side, heme and precursors are in the middle, and the resulting[2] porphyrias are on the right side. *Abbreviation:* CoA = coenzyme A.

Older screening mechanisms such as the Watson-Schwartz test and the Hoesch test have been replaced by easier, more specific, semiquantitative tests such as the Trace PBG kit (Thermo Fisher Scientific), but they still rely on the color reaction with Ehrlich's aldehyde. This or a similar test must be available in all emergency departments and in all acute care hospitals. A *random* urine sample is sufficient for the initial diagnostic evaluation, and if it is positive it must be later followed up by more-detailed tests such as quantitative measurements of porphyrins and precursors in a 24-hour urine collection. Fecal porphyrin measurements may also be called for. Enzyme measurements and genetic testing are rarely indicated, but they are used when more routine tests fail. Because the porphyrias are almost always hereditary, family studies are highly appropriate. The proper interpretation of any test result is best done in the context of available clinical information.

Clinical Presentation

Clinical presentations of porphyric attacks vary so much that the term *the little imitator* has been used. Not all signs or symptoms are always present, but severe and poorly localized abdominal pain and unexplained tachycardia are so prevalent that their absence further complicates the diagnosis of an acute porphyric attack. The genesis of the attack is not well understood, but acutely increased demand for heme and production of toxic intermediary products are considered to be the culprit. Increased demand for heme and increased production of intermediary products can be due to a wide variety of circumstances, from drugs through hormones (premenstrual phase) to stress, infection, fasting, and

starvation. However, most carriers of the genetic defect for an acute porphyria remain symptom free all their lives. Some have only one or two attacks, and only a few suffer from many attacks.

The clinical picture with pain, fast heart rate, and neurovisceral symptoms can be complicated by, at times, severe hyponatremia, heralding seizures with therapeutic dilemmas (see Box 1) and respiratory paralysis necessitating ventilatory support. Death is rare nowadays, especially when the diagnosis is made early. The recovery is usually complete, but at times it is prolonged, up to 1 year after a severe attack.

Superb nursing care, initially preferable in an intensive care unit, is necessary, and meticulous attention has to be paid to *all* problems. Dehydration from vomiting is common, and ileus and urinary retention are not infrequent; hyponatremia occurs in approximately half of the porphyric attacks. Muscle strength must be tested frequently. Twice-daily measurement of vital capacity helps to assess the necessity for respiratory assistance. High blood pressure and tachycardia deserve careful attention and, if appropriate, cautious treatment with a β-blocker. A negative caloric balance must be avoided, and, if present initially, it is best treated with carbohydrates (if necessary, intravenously with glucose, up to 300 g/day), and then later with a balanced diet.

Treatment

Therapy must always start with a careful look at the drugs recently taken by the patient. It is best to discontinue as many drugs as possible, especially those deemed unsafe (see Box 1). Appropriate lists of safe and unsafe drugs in porphyria are readily available from websites (www.porphyriafoundation.com and www.porphyria-europe.com). An infection must be diligently searched for and treated at once. Seizure precautions are especially indicated if hyponatremia is found. Analgesics should be adequately dispensed; opiates are often necessary in fairly large doses.

Specific therapy was introduced a generation ago in the form of hematin (hemin, Panhematin), available from Lundbeck Inc. (847-282-1000 or www.lundbeckinc.com). This has largely replaced glucose (300 g/day), which had the main advantages of availability, relatively low cost, and the possibility of curbing an early or mild attack.

But one must not wait for quick improvement in a patient's condition and should at once take steps to obtain the definitive medication, hematin. This represents the equivalent to the end product, heme, and exerts its beneficial effect through repression of the deranged, and in the porphyric attack, markedly activated pathway to heme. It is still unclear whether the quick suppression of potentially toxic heme precursors (in 1–2 days) or a postulated replenishment of an assumed heme deficiency is the effective mechanism. *Early* administration of hematin is strongly advocated because the course of a porphyric attack is unpredictable, and a point of no return can unfortunately be reached quickly. Thus the infusion of hematin must start as soon as possible.

A daily dose of 2 to 4 mg/kg body weight is recommended for up to 4 days. Longer treatment periods are of questionable value but may be tried in severe cases for up to 2 weeks. The infusion must be strictly intravenous and with ample flushing because hematin can cause thrombosis and phlebitis. Because it is a procoagulant and anticoagulant, frequent measurements of coagulation parameters are advisable. Anticoagulants such as warfarin (Coumadin) should if possible be avoided. Admixture of 5% human serum albumin (Albuminar-5) has been advocated to stabilize the final hematin solution and to lessen side effects. Hematin is available in many countries as heme arginate (Normosang).[2]

A beneficial clinical effect can be expected in 1 to 2 days, accompanied by a decrease in all heme precursors, most notably ALA and PBG. Many patients have received many treatment courses with hematin without apparent loss of effectiveness.

[2]Not available in the United States.

BOX 1 — Short List of Safe and Unsafe Drugs in the Acute Porphyrias*

Safe

- Acetaminophen (Tylenol)
- Aspirin
- Atropine
- Bromides
- Cimetidine (Tagamet)
- Erythropoietin (Epogen, Procrit)
- Gabapentin (Neurontin)
- Glucocorticoids
- Insulin
- Narcotic analgesics
- Penicillins
- Phenothiazine
- Ranitidine (Zantac)
- Streptomycin
- Digoxin (Lanoxin)
- Labetalol (Trandate), propranolol (Inderal)
- Paraldehyde[2]
- Bupivacaine (Marcaine)
- Chloral hydrate
- Tetracycline
- Vitamins

Unsafe

- Alcohol
- Barbiturates
- Carbamazepine (Tegretol)
- Carisoprodol (Soma)
- Clonazepam (Klonopin)
- Danazol (Danocrine)
- Diclofenac (Voltaren)
- Ergotamines
- Estrogens, progesterones
- Ethchlorvynol (Placidyl)[2]
- Glutethimide (Doriden)
- Griseofulvin (Grifulvin)
- Mephenytoin (Mesantoin), phenytoin (Dilantin)
- Meprobamate (Equanil)
- Methyprylon (Noludar)[2]
- Metoclopramide (Reglan)
- Primidone (Mysoline)
- Pyrazinamide
- Pyrazolone
- Rifampin (Rifadin)
- Sulfonamides
- Valproic acid (Depakene)

[2]Not available in the United States.
*Drug not listed cannot be considered safe or unsafe.

Prophylactic use of hematin can be helpful in the treatment of women with frequent premenstrual exacerbations of their acute porphyria. Hematin should never be given as a diagnostic test to see if unexplained symptoms reminiscent of porphyria lessen. The diagnosis of a porphyric attack must be as quick, precise, and certain as possible, especially in new cases.

Partial liver transplantation has been successfully undertaken and found to be curative in patients with unrelenting porphyric attacks.

Prophylaxis of porphyric attacks is of great importance and can be accomplished to a large extent by avoidance of unsafe drugs, by stable caloric intake, and by prompt attention to intercurrent illnesses. It is a difficult decision if unsafe drugs have to be administered for a vital indication such as seizures. Here, consultation with an expert in porphyria is strongly advised.

The Cutaneous Porphyrias

The symptomatology of cutaneous porphyrias is mainly photosensitivity, often combined with skin fragility and blisters. All of these findings occur because of porphyrin toxicity, resulting in cutaneous light absorption at the wavelength of 400 to 410 nm and subsequent formation of damaging reactive oxygen species. Thus two therapeutic approaches are plausible: decrease of porphyrins and protection of the skin from sunlight. The usual sunscreens are, however, ineffective, and reflective agents containing zinc or titanium, although better, are less popular because of their appearance.

In three porphyrias—porphyria cutanea tarda, hereditary coproporphyria, and variegate porphyria—the skin lesions are rather similar, but erythropoietic protoporphyria and congenital erythropoietic porphyria can lead to very painful nonblistering skin lesions, and, in congenital erythropoietic porphyria, even to mutilations.

Porphyria Cutanea Tarda

Porphyria cutanea tarda is the most common porphyria and occurs because of uroporphyrinogen-decarboxylase deficiency and accumulation of mostly uroporphyrin. It can be inherited autosomal dominantly but more often occurs sporadically. It can also be due to toxins such as halogenated aromatic hydrocarbons.

The most prominent skin manifestations are seen on the dorsa of the hands and on the face, consisting of blisters filled with mostly clear fluid; shallow, slow-healing ulcers; whitish plaques; and tiny inclusion bodies, *milia.* Hypertrichosis and hyperpigmentation are often seen.

Unveiling factors promote the manifestation of the disease and consist mainly of liver disease, often due to alcohol. Hepatitis, often type C, and HIV infections are also common revealers. The drug list (see Box 1) is *not* applicable to the cutaneous porphyrias. The diagnosis is easily suspected at inspection and confirmed by measurement of urinary uroporphyrin excretion, typically manifold increased above the normal range.

There are two treatment options with different principles but rather similar effectiveness. Repeat phlebotomies of 350 to 450 mL at 1- to 2-week intervals are performed and followed by hemoglobin and ferritin measurements. Overt anemia should be avoided. Ferritin usually reaches the lower end of the normal range after approximately 8 to 10 phlebotomies, and clinical remission can be expected after approximately half a year. Remission can be long lasting, especially when unveiling factors are avoided; total abstinence from alcohol is advocated. Patients should not take iron-enriched vitamins because iron plays a critical role in porphyria cutanea tarda.

If phlebotomies are contraindicated (due to anemia or pulmonary or cardiac disease) or are very inconvenient, low-dose chloroquine (Aralen)[1] (125 mg twice weekly) can be given orally. This flushes porphyrins from the liver and can be continued until remission is reached. In such low doses, the drug is virtually free from side effects.

Patients on chronic dialysis can develop porphyria cutanea tarda and also *pseudoporphyria.* Here, plasma porphyrin measurements establish the correct diagnosis. Patients with porphyria cutanea tarda and end-stage renal disease respond well to erythropoietin (Epogen, Procrit)[1], probably via iron depletion through incorporation of iron into hemoglobin. Pseudoporphyria is also seen as a side effect of many drugs, mostly nonsteroidal antiinflammatory drugs and diuretics. Although it is phenotypically identical to porphyria cutanea tarda, pseudoporphyria does not respond to phlebotomies or chloroquine.

Patients with porphyria cutanea tarda have a much higher incidence of hepatocellular carcinoma and should be checked twice annually with hepatic imaging and measurement of alpha fetoprotein.

[1]Not FDA approved for this indication.

Congenital Erythropoietic Porphyria (Günther Disease)

Congenital erythropoietic porphyria (Günther disease), a rare autosomal recessive disorder, is usually apparent shortly after birth when brick-colored urine in diapers is observed because of excessive amounts of uroporphyrin (even more impressive under UV light). This porphyria and the rare homozygous porphyria cutanea tarda, hepatoerythropoietic porphyria, can be progressive and severely mutilating. Therapy is limited to sun protection and blood transfusion if hemolytic anemia is present.

Erythropoietic Protoporphyria

Erythropoietic protoporphyria is an autosomal dominant disorder due to a deficiency of ferrochelatase, the last enzyme in heme biosynthesis. Urinary porphyrins are normal, but protoporphyrin is markedly elevated in red cells and in stool. These patients suffer from instantly painful sun sensitivity, followed by edema and wrinkles in the thickened, light-exposed skin. In contrast to porphyria cutanea tarda, blisters are not seen here. Approximately one fifth of these patients develop progressive liver disease secondary to hepatic accumulation of protoporphyrin. Liver transplantation can become necessary.

Therapy is often beneficial with oral β-carotene[1] (up to 400 mg/day for adults). This leads to a harmless slight orange-yellow discoloration of the skin and often effective sun protection. Ideally, the β-carotene dose should be adjusted to a plasma level between 11 and 15 mmol/L.

---

[1]Not FDA approved for this indication.

References

American Porphyria Foundation Home page. Available at: http://www.porphyriafoundation.com (accessed April 24, 2019).

Anderson KE, Bonkovsky HL, Bloomer JR, Shedlofsky SI: Reconstitution of hematin for intravenous infusion, *Ann Intern Med* 144:537–538, 2006.

Anderson KE, Bloomer JR, Bonkovsky HL, et al: Recommendations for the diagnosis and treatment of the acute porphyrias, *Ann Intern Med* 142:439–450, 2005.

Anderson KE, Sassa S, Bishop DF, et al: Disorders of heme biosynthesis: X-linked sideroblastic anemia and the porphyrias. In Scriver CR, Beaudet AL, Sly WS, et al, editors: *The Molecular and Metabolic Bases of Inherited Disease*, 8th ed., vol. 1, New York, 2001, McGraw-Hill, pp 2961–3062.

Badminton MN, Elder GH: Management of acute and cutaneous porphyrias, *Int J Clin Pract* 56:272–278, 2002.

Balwani M, Desnick RJ: The porphyrias: advances in diagnosis and treatment, *Blood* 120(23):4496–4504, 2012. https://doi.org/10.1182/blood-2012-05-423186 Epub 2012 Jul 12. Review. Erratum in: Blood. 2013;122(17):3090.

Bissell DM, Anderson KE, Bonkovsky HL: Porphyria, *N Engl J Med* 377(9):862–872, 2017.

Chemmanur AT, Bonkovsky HL: Hepatic porphyrias: Diagnosis and management, *Clin Liver Dis* 8:807–838, 2004.

European Porphyria Network. Home page. Available at: https://porphyria.eu/en/content/home (accessed April 24, 2019).

Kauppinen R: Porphyrias, *Lancet* 365:241–252, 2005.

Puy H, Gouya L, Deybach JC: Porphyrias, *Lancet* 375:924–937, 2010.

Yasuda M, Chen B, Desnick RJ: Recent advances on porphyria genetics: Inheritance, penetrance, & molecular heterogeneity, including new modifying/causative genes, *Mol Genet Metab* S1096–7192(18)30645–0, 2018.

SICKLE CELL DISEASE

Method of

Enrico M. Novelli, MD; Mark T. Gladwin, MD; and Lakshmanan Krishnamurti, MD

CURRENT DIAGNOSIS

- Sickle cell disease (SCD) is diagnosed by neonatal screening in the United States.
- Persons with congenital hemolytic anemia should be tested for SCD by hemoglobin electrophoresis regardless of their ethnic background.
- Infection with parvovirus B19 should be suspected in children presenting with acute anemia and reticulocytopenia.

- Human leukocyte antigen (HLA) class I and II testing should be performed in all patients with SCD and unaffected siblings to identify candidates for hematopoietic stem cell transplant.
- Transcranial Doppler screening for primary prevention of stroke is indicated in children with homozygous SCD.
- Acute chest syndrome is diagnosed in patients presenting with fever, hypoxemia, and a radiographic pulmonary infiltrate.
- Screening for kidney disease should be performed by obtaining a spot urine sample for microalbuminuria
- Screening for iron overload by ferritin, quantitative liver magnetic resonance imaging (MRI), cardiac MRI, or liver biopsy is indicated in all patients who have received more than 10 lifetime transfusions.
- Pulmonary hypertension screening by transthoracic echocardiogram is indicated in all patients with homozygous SCD.

CURRENT THERAPY

- All children with sickle cell disease (SCD) should receive penicillin prophylaxis.
- High fever should be treated empirically with coverage for *Streptococcus pneumoniae* pending results of blood cultures.
- Children with high transcranial Doppler velocity need to be placed on a chronic transfusion regimen to keep the hemoglobin (Hb) S less than 30%.
- Painful vasoocclusive episodes warrant prompt treatment with an individualized intravenous opiate regimen, as well as supportive care and incentive spirometry.
- Preoperative transfusion should aim at a target hemoglobin level of 10 g/dL regardless of the HbS percentage and is indicated in all patients with SCD undergoing major surgery.
- Therapy with hydroxyurea (Droxia, Siklos) is indicated in all patients at all ages with HbSS disease and HbSβ-thalassemia, and in patients with HbSC with a severe phenotype on a case-by-case basis.
- Erythropoietin-stimulating agents can be used in conjunction with hydroxyurea to prevent or ameliorate reticulocytopenia and in patients with underlying renal insufficiency.
- Iron chelation is indicated in all patients with findings of iron overload.
- Treatment of acute chest syndrome includes parenteral antibiotics to cover atypical microorganisms and transfusion, with exchange transfusion reserved for the most severe cases.
- Patients with pulmonary hypertension should receive optimal hematologic care (maximal hydroxyurea and/or chronic transfusion therapy) and specific therapy for pulmonary hypertension in severe cases, with coordination and referral to a pulmonary hypertension specialist.
- Stem cell transplantation should be offered to all patients who have a matched donor and display a severe phenotype.

Epidemiology

Sickle cell disease (SCD) affects 70,000 to 100,000 persons in the United States and millions worldwide. The hemoglobin S (HbS) mutation arose in West-Central Africa approximately 7300 years ago and then propagated to vast tropical and subtropical areas due to the selective pressure of malaria infection. It is predominantly found in persons of African, Mediterranean, Arab, or Indian ancestry. In the United States, approximately 1 in 15 African Americans harbors the HbS (sickle hemoglobin) mutation and 1 in 400 is affected by the disease. Most patients with SCD in the United States are homozygous for HbS (SS), with heterozygous HbSC being the second most common abnormality. Conversely, in Mediterranean countries, HbS/β-thalassemia is the most common SCD syndrome, and in the Arab peninsula HbSS in combination with hereditary persistence of fetal hemoglobin (HPFH) is particularly prevalent.

Pathophysiology

SCD consists of a group of inherited hemoglobinopathies characterized by a qualitatively abnormal hemoglobin molecule that affects the structure and integrity of the red blood cells (RBCs). SCD is an autosomal recessive disease due to homozygosity for HbS, characterized by a single base substitution in the β-globin gene of the hemoglobin tetramer, leading to an amino acid substitution (valine to glutamic acid), or coinheritance of HbS with other abnormal hemoglobins such as hemoglobin C, D, E, and O or β-thalassemia.

HbS is less soluble than normal hemoglobin (HbA) in the deoxygenated state and polymerizes when sickle RBCs are exposed to hypoxic conditions in the microcirculation. In the classic pathophysiologic explanation of SCD, sickled RBCs containing HbS polymers are less deformable and remain trapped in the microcirculation, causing end-organ ischemia and necrosis. Compounding this mechanism, more recent literature has emphasized the role of cellular adhesion, abnormal cytokine levels, ischemia-reperfusion injury, oxidative damage, sterile inflammation, and an abnormal endothelial milieu (Figures 1 and 2). HbS polymers also lead to deformity and fragility of the RBC membrane, with resulting intravascular and extravascular hemolysis.

Patients with SCD suffer from severe chronic hemolytic anemia and acute episodes of RBC trapping and destruction in the microvasculature (vasoocclusive episodes). Vasoocclusive episodes are the hallmark of SCD and are characterized by more intense episodic vasoocclusion, often with increasing hemolysis, and are due to exogenous or endogenous factors that acutely alter the rheologic properties of the RBCs. The main determinants of RBC sickling and vasoocclusion are hypoxemia, RBC dehydration, RBC concentration, high HbS relative to fetal hemoglobin (HbF), and blood viscosity; these can occur in a multitude of clinical settings. Most common clinical inciting events leading to vasoocclusive episodes are dehydration due to inadequate replacement of fluid losses, thermal changes, surgical stress, exposure to low oxygen tension, infections, and psychological stressors.

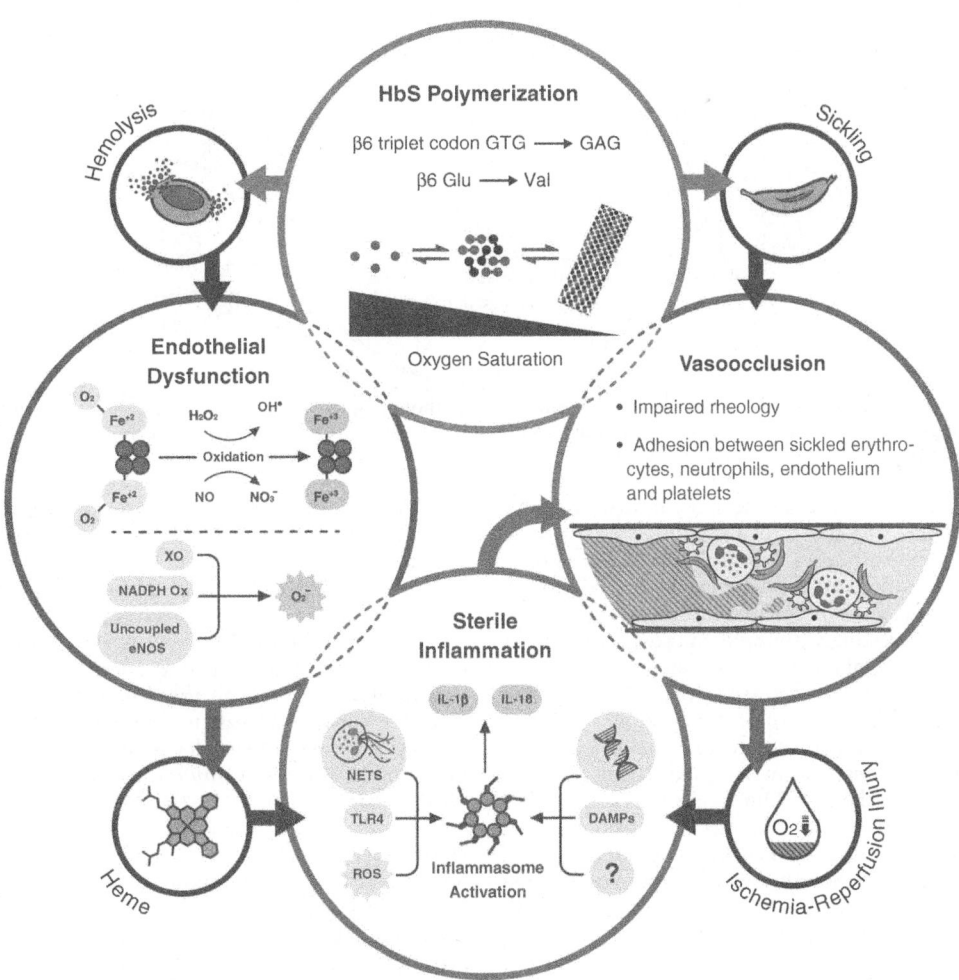

Figure 1 Molecular pathophysiology of SCD. A mutation in the β-globin gene leads to substitution of valine for glutamic acid at the 6th position in the β-globin chain. Following deoxygenation, the mutated hemoglobin (HbS) molecules polymerize to form bundles (top circle). The polymer bundles result in erythrocyte sickling (clockwise), which results in impaired rheology of the blood and aggregation of sickle erythrocytes with neutrophils, platelets and endothelial cells to promote stasis of blood flow referred to as "vaso-occlusion" (right circle). Vaso-occlusion promotes ischemia-reperfusion (I-R) injury (clockwise). Hb polymer bundles (top circle) also promote hemolysis or lysis of erythrocytes (counter-clockwise) that releases cell free Hb into the circulation. Oxygenated Hb (Fe2+) promotes endothelial dysfunction (left circle) by depleting endothelial nitric oxide (NO) reserves to form nitrate (NO3-) and methemoglobin. Alternatively, Hb can also react with H_2O_2 through the Fenton reaction to form hydroxyl free radical (OH·) and methemoglobin (Fe3+). Also, NADPH oxidase (NADPH ox), Xanthine oxidase (XO) and uncoupled endothelial NO synthase (eNOS) generate oxygen free radicals to promote endothelial dysfunction. Methemoglobin (Fe3+) degrades to release cell free heme (counter-clockwise), which is a major eDAMP. Reactive oxygen species (ROS) generation, toll-like-receptor-4 (TLR4) activation, neutrophil extracellular traps (NETs) generation, release of tissue or cell derived DAMPs, DNA and other unknown factors (?) triggered by cell free heme or I-R injury can contribute to sterile inflammation by activating inflammasome pathway in vascular and inflammatory cells to release IL-1β (bottom circle). Finally, sterile inflammation further promotes vaso-occlusion through a feed-back loop by promoting adhesiveness of neutrophils, platelets and endothelial cells. (From Sundd et al. Pathophysiology of sickle cell disease. *Annual Review of Pathology: Mechanisms of Disease* 14:263-292, 2019.)

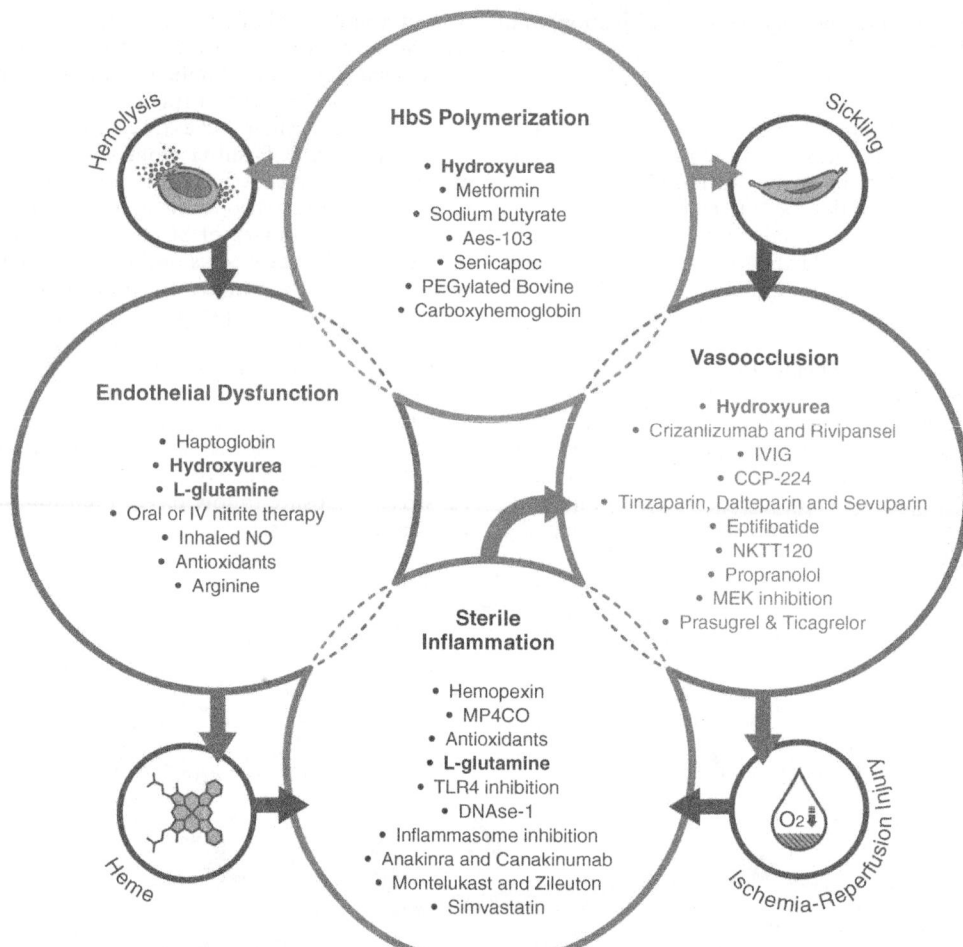

HbS Polymerization

- **Hydroxyurea**
- Metformin
- Sodium butyrate
- Aes-103
- Senicapoc
- PEGylated Bovine
- Carboxyhemoglobin

Hemolysis

Sickling

Endothelial Dysfunction

- Haptoglobin
- **Hydroxyurea**
- **L-glutamine**
- Oral or IV nitrite therapy
- Inhaled NO
- Antioxidants
- Arginine

Vasoocclusion

- **Hydroxyurea**
- Crizanlizumab and Rivipansel
- IVIG
- CCP-224
- Tinzaparin, Dalteparin and Sevuparin
- Eptifibatide
- NKTT120
- Propranolol
- MEK inhibition
- Prasugrel & Ticagrelor

Sterile Inflammation

- Hemopexin
- MP4CO
- Antioxidants
- **L-glutamine**
- TLR4 inhibition
- DNAse-1
- Inflammasome inhibition
- Anakinra and Canakinumab
- Montelukast and Zileuton
- Simvastatin

Heme

Ischemia-Reperfusion Injury

Figure 2 FDA approved and experimental therapies targeting the molecular pathobiology of sickle cell disease. The FDA approved drugs are in bold. (From Sundd et al. Pathophysiology of sickle cell disease, *Annual Review of Pathology: Mechanisms of Disease* 14:263-292, 2019.)

Epidemiologic studies indicate that the risk of vasoocclusive episodes and acute chest syndrome is related to high steady-state hemoglobin levels, leukocytosis, and low HbF levels. These findings are consistent with pathogenic mechanisms of altered red cell rheology, higher viscosity, HbS polymerization, and inflammatory cellular adhesion. Interestingly, the epidemiologic risk factors associated with chronic vascular complications such as pulmonary hypertension (PH), cutaneous leg ulceration, priapism, systemic systolic hypertension, renal failure with proteinuria, and possibly stroke are different and include a low steady-state hemoglobin level, increased hemolytic intensity, iron overload, and markers of low nitric oxide (NO) bioavailability. One hypothesis is that SCD is driven by two overlapping but different mechanisms of disease: on one hand, vasoocclusion causes vasoocclusive episodes and acute chest syndrome, and on the other hand, hemolytic anemia leads to endothelial dysfunction and chronic vasculopathy. Both are caused fundamentally by HbS polymerization.

Prevention

See "Evidence-Based Management of Sickle Cell Disease: Expert Panel Report, 2014" at http://www.nhlbi.nih.gov/health-pro/guidelines/sickle-cell-disease-guidelines for detailed, consensus guidelines on prevention and treatment.

Bacterial Infections

Before the antibiotic era, most patients with SCD succumbed to bacterial sepsis from encapsulated organisms. A landmark multicenter, randomized, double-blind, placebo-controlled clinical trial of prophylaxis with oral penicillin in children with sickle cell anemia published in 1986 showed that bacterial prophylaxis started at birth reduced by approximately 80% the incidence of infection in the penicillin group, as compared with the group given placebo. This study became the foundation for universal screening of SCD. Results of the Penicillin Prophylaxis in Sickle Cell Study II (PROPS 2) trial show that prophylaxis can be safely discontinued at age 5 years as long as there is no history of prior serious pneumococcal infection or surgical splenectomy and in the setting of appropriate comprehensive care. All children should also receive both the 13-valent pneumococcal conjugate (Prevnar 13) and 23-valent pneumococcal polysaccharide (Pneumovax) vaccines, and adults should receive Pneumovax. Vaccinations for *Haemophilus influenzae* and *Neisseria meningitidis* are also indicated.

Neurologic Events

Stroke is a devastating complication of SCD and affects predominantly children with HbSS and abnormal transcranial Doppler (TCD) results. Silent cerebral infarcts are magnetic resonance imaging (MRI)-detectable abnormalities that also carry a high risk of morbidity, including overt stroke and cognitive impairment. There is conclusive evidence that chronic transfusions are effective in the primary and secondary prevention of both overt and silent strokes in SCD. The first landmark trial (STOP) published in 1995 showed that the first stroke can be prevented by placing children with abnormal TCD on prophylactic monthly transfusions with a target HbS of less than 30%. Transfusions were later found to also have a beneficial effect on reducing the incidence of the recurrence of silent cerebral infarcts, as shown by the SIT trial. The importance of continuing transfusions for more than 30 months was underscored by the STOP 2 trial, where TCD abnormalities recurred and the incidence of silent cerebral infarctions on MRI was

TABLE 1	Severity of the Main Sickle Cell Syndromes	
GENOTYPE	CLINICAL SEVERITY	HEMOGLOBIN (G/DL)
HbSS	Usually marked	6–10
HbS-β^0-thalassemia	Moderate to marked	6–10
HbS-β^+-thalassemia	Mild to moderate	9–12
HbSC	Mild to moderate	10–15
HbSS-HPFH	Mild	

HbSC, Heterozygous phenotype; *HbSS*, homozygous phenotype; *HPFH*, hereditary persistence of fetal hemoglobin.

higher in the transfusion-halted group. The enthusiasm over the beneficial effects of transfusions was tempered by the concerns about the side effects of long-term, possibly indefinite use of this therapeutic strategy. Therefore there has been an interest in exploring whether hydroxyurea (Droxia, Siklos) could represent an alternative to transfusion in high-risk children. Specifically, the SWiTCH trial explored the hypothesis that hydroxyurea and phlebotomy could maintain an acceptable stroke recurrence rate and significantly reduce the hepatic iron burden as compared with a prophylactic chronic transfusion regimen. Unfortunately, the trial was terminated early because of a significantly higher stroke recurrence rate in the hydroxyurea arm compared with the transfusion arm, with equivalent hepatic iron burden in both groups. Thus the issue of when, if ever, it is safe to discontinue transfusions for the secondary prevention of stroke is still unknown. Conversely, as shown by the results of the TWiTCH trial, another study halted prematurely by the National Institutes of Health, hydroxyurea is not inferior to chronic transfusions in lowering TCD velocities in children at high risk but without a history of stroke, thereby suggesting that this drug may be equally effective in the primary prevention of neurologic complications.

Clinical Manifestations

Multiple genetic and epigenetic factors affect the SCD phenotype. Patients homozygous for HbS (SS) or compound heterozygous for HbS and a nonfunctional β^0-thalassemia allele tend to display the most severe manifestations. On the other end of the spectrum, HPFH, particularly common in Saudi Arabia, or coinheritance of β-thalassemia mitigates the phenotype. Although the net effect of high HbF levels on the phenotype of SCD is beneficial, coinheritance of one or two α-thalassemia alleles has a more complex effect. α-Thalassemia is present in approximately 30% of patients with SCD and is associated with higher hemoglobin, lower mean corpuscular volume (MCV), and decreased rate of hemolysis. These effects are protective toward stroke and leg ulcers but lead to increased rates of vasoocclusive episodes, osteonecrosis, and acute chest syndrome because of increased blood viscosity related to the higher hemoglobin level. Patients with HbSC and HbS/β^+-thalassemia have an intermediate severity phenotype (Table 1). Haplotypes of polymorphic sites in the β-globin gene cluster in chromosome 11 have been associated with different disease severity and rates of complications. Other yet unidentified genetic factors predispose certain patients to develop a particularly severe hemolysis with brisk reticulocytosis and a high rate of specific complications that include leg ulcers, priapism, and PH.

Hematology

This section describes the main clinical manifestations of SCD in each organ system (Figure 3 and Table 2).

Baseline or Steady-State Hematologic Abnormalities

Chronic intravascular and extravascular hemolysis causes a chronic anemia of moderate to severe intensity in HbSS and HbS/β^0-thalassemia, with a hemoglobin range of 6 to 9 g/dL. In HbSC and HbS/β^+-thalassemia, the anemia may be mild or absent.

The anemia of SCD is usually normocytic in HbSS, with anisocytosis and poikilocytosis and a population of small dehydrated dense cells, irreversibly sickled cells, numerous reticulocytes, and schistocytes. Reticulocytosis is common but not compensatory, and nucleated RBCs are seen in acute exacerbations of the anemia such as in splenic or hepatic sequestration. Baseline leukocytosis with neutrophilia is also common and is a poor prognostic sign associated with acute chest syndrome in adults and frequent vasoocclusive episodes in children. Preclinical studies have shown that leukocytes are not simply a marker of disease activity and acute phase but also have a direct pathogenic role in cellular adhesion and vasoocclusion. The platelet count is commonly elevated in SCD, particularly in patients who are autosplenectomized as a result of repeated splenic infarction, and platelet activation is increased. In the subset of patients with HbSC and HbS/β^+-thalassemia who retain a functional spleen and develop splenomegaly, features of hypersplenism may instead be observed with resulting mild pancytopenia.

Hematologic Indices During Vasoocclusive Episodes

In acute vasoocclusive episodes the total Hb decreases as a result of hemolysis (by 1.6 g/dL in acute chest syndrome). The lactate dehydrogenase (LDH), reticulocyte count, and other markers of hemolysis such as aspartate transaminase (AST) and indirect bilirubin are elevated in steady state, and in many—but not all—patients are further increased during vasoocclusive episodes. Haptoglobin levels are chronically depressed in SCD and typically not measurable, even in steady state, in patients with HbS homozygosity. In patients with HbSC, vasoocclusive episodes may be due to increased blood viscosity and RBC sickling, and worsening hemolysis might not be readily appreciated.

Splenic sequestration crises occur mostly in childhood and are characterized by anemia disproportionate to the degree of hemolysis, reticulocytosis, and acute splenomegaly. Splenic sequestration and repeated episodes of splenic infarction eventually lead to autosplenectomy, although some patients develop splenomegaly. Splenic infarction usually manifests with left upper-quadrant pain and may be massive, involving more than 50% of the splenic tissue.

In severe vasoocclusive episodes, massive bone marrow infarction can also occur. In these instances, the peripheral blood smear reveals a leukoerythroblastic picture with immature neutrophilic forms, nucleated RBCs, and teardrop cells. Fat emboli syndrome, a life-threatening complication of vasoocclusive episodes, can then develop as bone marrow fat embolizes to peripheral capillary beds, leading to multiorgan failure.

Red Blood Cell Alloimmunization

RBC alloimmunization is a common complication of transfusional therapy in SCD and occurs in approximately 30% of patients. It is primarily due to the disparate expression of RBC antigens in African Americans as compared with the donor pool, which is mostly composed of whites. Alloimmunization complicates RBC matching and leads to delayed hemolytic transfusion reactions. Alloantigens that become undetectable by indirect Coombs test 2 months after exposure to mismatched blood have the potential to result in future false-negative cross-matching results. A subset of heavily alloimmunized patients with SCD undergoes life-threatening hemolytic reactions upon exposure to mismatched RBC units. In these hyperhemolytic crises, there is intense hemolysis of transfused and nontransfused RBCs and acute anemia. Treatment of hyperhemolytic crises is empirical and includes erythropoietin-stimulating agents (ESAs), parenteral steroids, and intravenous immunoglobulins (Gammagard).[1]

Iron Overload

Hemosiderosis is the other major complication of transfusional therapy in SCD and is characterized by iron deposition in the

---

[1] Not FDA approved for this indication.

Figure 3 Acute and chronic complications of sickle cell disease.

TABLE 2	Landmark Randomized Clinical Trials in Sickle Cell Disease	
YEAR OF PUBLICATION	**TITLE**	**MAIN FINDINGS**
1986	Prophylaxis with oral penicillin in children with sickle cell anemia: A randomized trial	84% reduction in incidence of infection and no deaths from pneumococcal septicemia in the penicillin group
1995	Multicenter Study of Hydroxyurea in Sickle Cell Anemia (MSH)	Reduced incidence of painful crises, ACS, and transfusion in the hydroxyurea group Survival benefit in follow-up study
1995	Preoperative Transfusion in Sickle Cell Disease Study	A conservative transfusion regimen was as effective as an aggressive regimen in preventing perioperative complications in patients with sickle cell anemia
1996	Multicenter investigation of bone marrow transplantation for sickle cell disease	HCT is safe in SCD with survival and event-free survival at 4 years of 91% and 73% and can lead to cure
1998	Stroke Prevention Trial in Sickle Cell Anemia (STOP)	Transfusion reduces the risk of a first stroke by 92% in children with sickle cell anemia who have abnormal results on transcranial Doppler ultrasonography
2005	Optimizing Primary Stroke Prevention in Sickle Cell Anemia (STOP 2)	Discontinuation of transfusion for the prevention of stroke in children with sickle cell disease results in a high rate of reversion to abnormal blood-flow velocities on Doppler studies and stroke
2009	Improving the Results of Bone Marrow Transplantation for Patients with Severe Congenital Anemias	Nine of 10 adults who received nonmyeloablative allogeneic hematopoietic stem cell transplantation for severe sickle cell disease achieved stable, mixed donor–recipient chimerism and reversal of the sickle cell phenotype, without acute or chronic GVHD.
2011	Pediatric Hydroxyurea Phase III Clinical Trial (BABY HUG)	Children ages 9–18 months randomized to receive hydroxyurea irrespective of disease severity for 2 y had decreased pain episodes, dactylitis, ACS, hospitalization, leukocyte count, and transfusion and increased hemoglobin as compared with children receiving placebo.
2014	Silent Infarct Trial (SIT)	Children with silent cerebral infarcts and normal TCD velocity who were randomized to chronic transfusion therapy had a 58% relative risk reduction in the recurrence of silent cerebral infarct or stroke as compared to those in the observation arm.

ACS, Acute chest syndrome; *GVHD,* graft-versus-host disease; *HCT,* hematopoietic cell transplantation; *SCD,* sickle cell disease; *TCD,* transcranial Doppler; *VOE,* vasooc-clusive crisis.

heart, liver, and endocrine glands, leading to organ failure and significant morbidity and mortality. It commonly occurs in patients who have received more than 10 lifetime transfusions or more than 20 packed RBC units. Liver biopsy is the "gold standard" for diagnosis, but it is an invasive and uncomfortable procedure. Hepatic and myocardial iron quantitation by MRI is supplanting liver biopsy as the preferred test to diagnose iron overload and monitor therapy with iron chelators, although when this is not available diagnosis often rests on the finding of an elevated ferritin and transferrin saturation in the appropriate clinical setting.

Hemostatic Activation and Thrombosis
Numerous studies have shown that arterial and venous thrombosis are common in SCD and include pulmonary embolism, in situ pulmonary thrombosis, and stroke. In SCD, alterations at all levels of the hemostatic system have been described: patients with SCD exhibit increased basal and stimulated platelet activation, increased markers of thrombin generation and fibrinolysis, increased tissue factor activity, and increased von Willebrand factor (vWF) antigen and thrombogenic ultralarge vWF multimers with depressed ADAMTS13 activity. Interestingly, hemostatic activation is amplified during vasoocclusive episodes, as shown by increases in multiple markers of thrombosis as compared with steady state, suggesting a link between hemolysis and thrombosis.

Neurology
Ischemic stroke is common in SCD, with the highest incidence between 2 and 5 years of age. Patients may develop overt stroke

from large vessel occlusion (5% to 8% of patients with HbSS) or silent infarcts from focal ischemia detectable by MRI without symptoms of acute stroke (20% to 35% of patients with HbSS). The pathophysiology of stroke in SCD is unclear, although genetic factors and an unbalance between oxygen demand and supply have been postulated. Multiple epidemiologic studies have shown that the risk factors for ischemic stroke in adult patients include HbSS genotype, severity of anemia, systolic hypertension, male gender, and increasing age. Patients with repeated strokes are at risk for development of anatomic abnormalities and Moyamoya pattern of vascularization, which predisposes to both ischemic and hemorrhagic stroke later in life. The highest incidence of intracerebral hemorrhages occurs in patients older than 20 years.

Both overt and silent strokes have a negative impact on IQ and cause cognitive impairment measurable by psychometric testing. Children and adults with SCD can develop cognitive impairment and subtle signs of accelerated brain aging and vascular dementia even in the absence of focal ischemia by MRI, with a low hematocrit being a predictor of neuropsychological dysfunction. These abnormalities are probably due to chronic and diffuse, as opposed to focal, cerebral anoxia and may be unmasked by psychometric testing.

Ophthalmology

Retinal abnormalities are common in SCD and are often asymptomatic until the occurrence of ophthalmologic emergencies. Retinal disease is due to arteriolar occlusion, with subsequent vascular proliferation, neovascularization, retinal hemorrhage (stage IV), and detachment (stage V). Patients with HbSC are more prone to retinal complications, possibly as a result of increased blood viscosity.

Nephrology

Renal abnormalities are common in SCD and manifest primarily as hematuria, proteinuria, and renal tubular acidosis. Hematuria is usually due to papillary necrosis and is an acute finding that requires supportive care and carries a good prognosis. Rarely, gross hematuria requires urologic consultation. Tubular functional defects include an inability to concentrate the urine (hyposthenuria) and renal tubular acidosis. Hyposthenuria often manifests with enuresis in childhood, and it is clinically relevant because it predisposes patients to an increased risk of dehydration. Renal tubular acidosis similar to type IV renal tubular acidosis is a common finding in SCD and may lead to hyperkalemia, an important consideration in patients already predisposed to hyperkalemia with intravascular hemolysis and whenever therapy with angiotensin-converting enzyme inhibitors is entertained.

Hyperphosphatemia and hyperuricemia are also often observed in SCD. Microalbuminuria may be detected in early adulthood and tends to progress to nephrotic range proteinuria. Focal segmental glomerulosclerosis is the most common glomerular abnormality and it is probably due to glomerular sickling and infarction. There are currently no approved therapies to prevent progression to end-stage renal disease, which occurs in up to 20% of patients and at a median age of 37 years. Renal replacement therapy is often needed in older adults with SCD. Serum creatinine and 24-hour creatinine clearance are not adequate for screening and monitoring of progression of kidney disease, because tubular secretion of creatinine is preserved and glomerular hyperfiltration is common in SCD, leading to a relatively low creatinine and a high glomerular filtration rate even in patients with underlying kidney impairment. Testing for microalbuminuria, plasma cystatin C levels, and hemoglobinuria may instead be used as screening tools for chronic kidney disease.

Leg Ulcers

Leg ulcers occur in 10% to 20% of patients with HbSS and have been associated with a chronically high hemolytic rate. They are usually located over the malleolar areas and are exquisitely painful, debilitating, disfiguring, and nonhealing. Vascular and plastic surgery consultations are recommended and aim at excluding local vascular problems that can complicate management of the ulcers and at providing prompt débridement and skin grafting. Although hydroxyurea is associated with development of leg ulcers in patients with myeloproliferative disorders, there is no such link with leg ulcers in SCD. Although wound healing may be impaired with hydroxyurea use, patients who develop an increase in fetal hemoglobin and have reduced sickling as a result of hydroxyurea therapy might have a net benefit in terms of tissue oxygenation and perfusion. Transfusional therapy, including exchange transfusional therapy, topical nitrates[1], and nutritional zinc[7] or L-arginine[7] supplementation, have shown benefit in anecdotal reports, but the evidence is inconclusive.

Gastroenterology

Nausea, vomiting, and dyspepsia in SCD are related to delayed gastric emptying and gastrointestinal motility disorders, autonomic neuropathy, or medical therapy. Opiates are often responsible for acute nausea and vomiting, whereas other medications such as hydroxyurea and deferasirox (Exjade) are occasionally responsible for chronic symptoms. Gastroparesis may be due to damage of the microvasculature of autonomic nerves (vasa vasorum) from repeated episodes of sickling.

The liver may be episodically affected by hepatic sequestration crises, heralded by direct hyperbilirubinemia, right upper quadrant pain from distention of the hepatic capsule, acute anemia, and reticulocytosis or by sinusoidal vasoocclusion leading to severe episodes of intrahepatic cholestasis. Supportive therapy and transfusions are indicated for hepatic vasoocclusive complications. Exchange transfusion may be the preferred modality for hepatic sequestration with the goal of preventing erythrocytosis once the pooled RBCs are released back into the circulation. Elevation of liver injury tests may be drug induced (hydroxyurea, deferasirox) but also related to hepatic sickling, particularly if it occurs during a vasoocclusive episode.

Infectious Disease

Patients homozygous for HbSS develop functional asplenia during childhood. This is due to repeated episodes of splenic infarction leading to fibrosis and autosplenectomy. As a result, children are susceptible to overwhelming bacterial sepsis from encapsulated organisms such as *Streptococcus pneumoniae*, *H. influenzae*, and *N. meningitidis*. High pediatric mortality from sepsis was therefore common before a landmark study published in 1986 demonstrated the benefit of penicillin prophylaxis instituted at birth. Vaccination for encapsulated organisms is also standard of care in children and adults. In spite of preventive measures, the incidence of life-threatening bacterial infections is increased in SCD, and high fever should be treated empirically as in splenectomized patients, with coverage for penicillin-resistant *S. pneumoniae* pending blood culture results. Patients with indwelling venous catheters are at risk of catheter-related bacteremia.

Viral infections with bone marrow–tropic viruses such as Epstein-Barr virus, cytomegalovirus, and predominantly parvovirus B19 place patients at risk for myelosuppression, which can further worsen chronic anemia. In children, infections with parvovirus B19 are responsible for transient red cell aplasia and severe aplastic crises, characterized by acute anemia and reticulocytopenia due to intramarrow destruction of erythroid precursors. Treatment of these episodes includes transfusion and intravenous immunoglobulins[1], besides supportive measures.

Pulmonology

A subset of patients with vasoocclusive episodes develop acute chest syndrome, the major pulmonary complication of SCD. Acute chest syndrome is a lung injury syndrome defined by fever, pleuritic chest pain, oxygen desaturation, and multilobar radiographic infiltrates associated with severe vasoocclusive episodes, infection, and bone marrow fat embolization (Figure 4). It usually develops 2 to

---

[1] Not FDA approved for this indication.
[7] Available as dietary supplement.

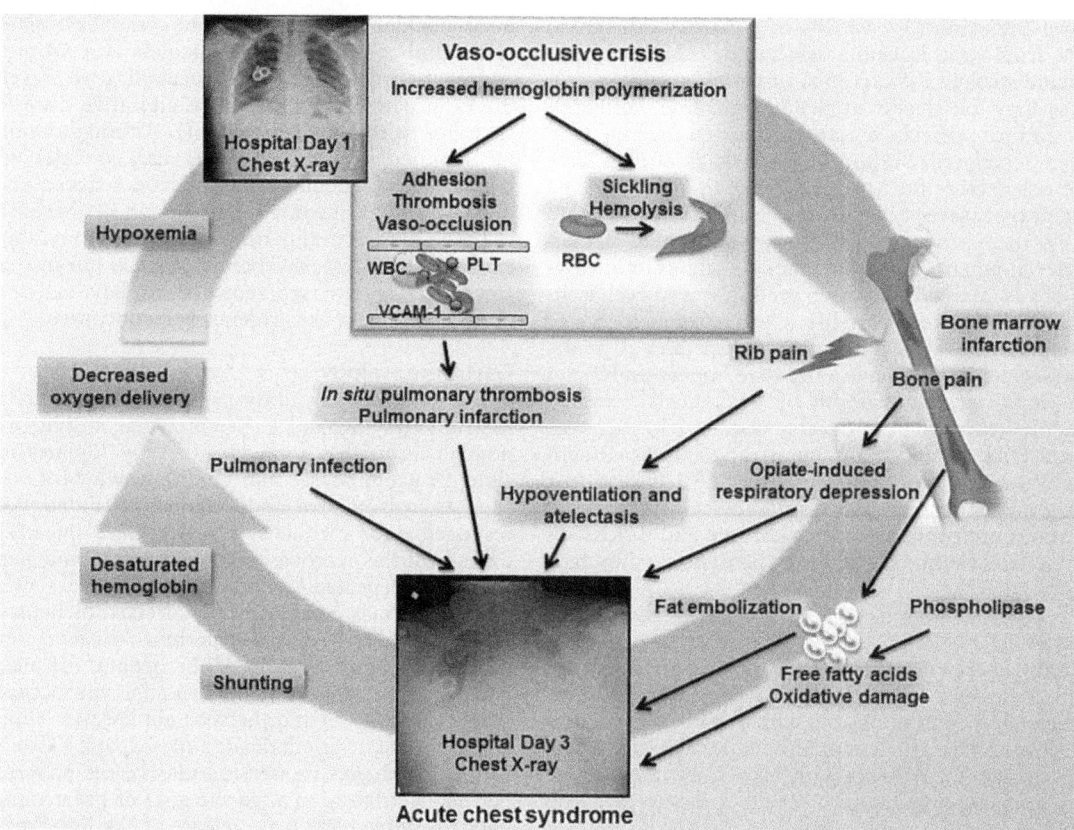

Figure 4 Vicious cycle of acute chest syndrome (ACS). Vasoocclusive crises are characterized by increased intraerythrocytic polymerization of deoxygenated hemoglobin S, leading to red blood cell sickling, cellular hyperadhesion, hemolysis, and vasoocclusion in the microvasculature. These processes are responsible for acute pain (pain crisis) and bone marrow necrosis. ACS typically occurs in a subset of patients 2 to 3 days after hospitalization for a vasoocclusive episode, and radiographically may present as new multilobar, basilar infiltrates on a chest x-ray. Fat embolization from the necrotic marrow is a recognized cause of ACS and is diagnosed by identifying lipid-laden macrophages in the bronchoalveolar lavage. However, pulmonary infection is the most common trigger of ACS and may be superimposed over existing pulmonary infarction. Hypoventilation and molecular pathogens such as reactive oxygen species from ischemia-reperfusion injury and by-products of hemolysis may also play a role in inducing or exacerbating lung injury. Finally, in situ pulmonary thrombosis has been frequently identified as a comorbid condition in patients with ACS and may be caused by endothelial and hemostatic activation. As a result of lung injury, ventilation-perfusion mismatches and shunting ensues, with subsequent hemoglobin desaturation and hypoxemia. Tissue hypoxia in turn triggers further hemoglobin S polymerization and sickling in a vicious cycle.

3 days after hospitalization for vasoocclusive episodes and is often misdiagnosed as nosocomial pneumonia or aspiration pneumonia, particularly because it displays a predilection for the lower lobe of the lungs. Although pneumonia often accompanies acute chest syndrome, proper diagnosis is important because acute chest syndrome warrants simple or exchange transfusion in addition to antibiotic therapy and supportive measures. Common infectious pathogens identified in cases of acute chest syndrome include *Chlamydia pneumoniae, Mycoplasma pneumoniae,* and *Legionella pneumophila,* thus dictating inclusion of a macrolide in the antibiotic cocktail. Pulmonary embolism with resulting infarct is also in the differential diagnosis of acute chest syndrome and may occur concurrently in 17% of patients. If not recognized and treated promptly, acute chest syndrome leads to pulmonary failure and carries a high mortality.

Airway hyperreactivity is common in children with SCD and needs to be actively diagnosed and aggressively treated because it is associated with worse SCD outcomes. Children with chronic respiratory symptoms should be tested for bronchial hyperresponsiveness.

Chronic complications of SCD include pulmonary fibrosis and PH. PH is an emergent complication of SCD and is associated with a high morbidity and mortality. Multiple epidemiologic studies have shown that a high baseline hemolysis rate, low hemoglobin, increasing age, a history of leg ulcers, liver dysfunction, iron overload, and kidney failure are risk factors for the development of PH. Three epidemiologic studies and a randomized clinical trial have shown that an elevated tricuspid regurgitant jet velocity (TRV) measured by Doppler echocardiography is a common occurrence in SCD with 30% of the patients having a TRV of 2.5 m/s (2 standard deviations [SDs] above the normal mean) or higher, and 10%

of the patients having a TRV of 3.0 m/s (3 SDs above the normal mean) or higher. These have proven to be valuable cutoff values, as a TRV of less than 2.5 m/s, when combined with an N-terminal pro B-type natriuretic peptide (NT-proBNP) value less than 160 has a high negative predictive value for PH. A TRV of 3.0 m/s or higher confers a positive predictive value for having PH by right heart catheterization (RHC) of 60% to 75% and a relative risk for death of 10.6. Controversy exists on the significance of an intermediate TRV value of 2.5 to 2.9 m/s, because it is unclear how accurately it predicts RHC-diagnosed PH. In three subsequent studies, patients with intermediate or high TRV values had a prevalence of PH by RHC ranging from 25% to 65% depending on what specific cutoff value was used as the criteria to perform an RHC (2.5 vs. 2.8) and on whether patients with evidence of end-organ damage were included or excluded. However, it is worrisome that regardless of the prevalence of PH, patients with an intermediate TRV are as a whole at increased risk of death (relative risk 4.4). One screening approach is to consider RHC in all patients with TRV of 3.0 or higher and in patients with intermediate TRV values of 2.5 to 2.9 m/s if the NT-proBNP is greater than 160 pg/mL or the 6-minute walk is less than 333 m or there is a high clinical pretest probability of having PH (mosaic perfusion pattern on computed tomography [CT] scan, low diffusing capacity of the lung for carbon monoxide (DLCO), significant dyspnea on exertion, etc.). It is likely that intermediate TRV values will need to be combined with other measures of right ventricular function and functional capacity such as NT-proBNP, and 6-minute walk to derive a highly predictive composite biomarker of PH. All studies have been concordant on the high risk of death conferred by PH in SCD whether measured by echocardiography, NT-proBNP, or RHC. Noninvasive transthoracic Doppler echocardiography is recommended by the American Thoracic Society as a screening test in homozygous SCD due to its safety, low cost, and availability. However, the definitive diagnosis of PH requires a confirmatory RHC.

RHC studies of patients with SCD and PH reveal a hyperdynamic state similar to the hemodynamics characteristic of portopulmonary hypertension. It is increasingly clear that pulmonary pressures rise acutely in vasoocclusive episodes and even more during acute chest syndrome. This suggests that acute PH and right heart dysfunction represent a major comorbidity during acute chest syndrome, and right heart failure should be considered in patients presenting with acute chest syndrome.

Cardiology
Similar to other conditions with chronic anemia, SCD is associated with a hyperdynamic state, low peripheral vascular resistance, and normal blood pressure or hypotension. In this setting, even mild elevation of the blood pressure can indicate relative hypertension and represent a risk factor for stroke. Because there are no studies on the treatment of hypertension in SCD, general guidelines on antihypertensive therapy are applied.

Coronary artery disease is rarely observed in SCD, although many patients complain of chest pain during vasoocclusive episodes. In these instances, the usual work-up for acute coronary syndrome is recommended. It is possible that myocardial microvascular occlusions are the predominant ischemic event in SCD.

Left-sided heart disease in SCD is primarily due to diastolic dysfunction (present in approximately 13% of patients), although systolic dysfunction and mitral or aortic valvular disease (2% of patients) can also occur. The presence of diastolic dysfunction alone in SCD patients is an independent risk factor for mortality. Patients with both pulmonary vascular disease and echocardiographic evidence of diastolic dysfunction are at a particularly high risk for death (odds ratio, 12.0; 95% confidence interval [CI], 3.8 to 38.1; $P < .001$).

Cardiac dysfunction is a late complication and the major cause of death in patients with iron overload. Heart failure and conduction defects are the most common abnormalities and warrant emergent iron chelation treatment. Among the iron chelators, deferiprone (Ferriprox) appears to be particularly apt at reducing cardiac iron content. Chelators may be used in combination for cases of severe cardiac decompensation from hemosiderosis.

Methadone (Dolophine) is associated with a risk of QTc prolongation, which carries a risk of arrhythmias and sudden death, particularly in the setting of PH and iron overload. Frequent electrocardiographic (ECG) monitoring, as well as dosage reduction or discontinuation, are warranted in this group, particularly if the QTc is greater than 500 ms.

Endocrinology
Iron overload is a common cause of endocrinopathy in SCD and thalassemia, with the hypophysis, gonads, and thyroid glands being particularly affected. Patients with iron overload should therefore undergo screening for endocrine dysfunction as it is mandated in thalassemia.

However, patients with SCD are at risk for specific endocrine problems regardless of their iron status. Delayed growth and puberty are relatively common, presenting in females with delayed age of menarche by 2 to 3 years and in males with small testicular size and hypospermia. Likely pathogenic factors include increased catabolism, chronic hypoxemia, hospitalizations with prolonged immobility, ischemic insults during vasoocclusive episodes, and chronic use of opiates.

Priapism
Priapism is the most common urogenital complication in patients with the HbSS genotype. It is a sustained, painful erection in the absence of sexual stimulation from occlusion of the penile blood return. It is defined as stuttering if it lasts from minutes to less than 3 hours and as prolonged if it lasts more than 3 hours. The latter is considered a urologic emergency because of the risk of permanent fibrosis and impotence and requires a urologic consultation. Pseudoephedrine (Sudafed[1]) may lead to detumescence in nonemergency settings, whereas aspiration of the corpus cavernosum is required in the emergency setting and is performed under conscious sedation and local anesthesia. This is usually accompanied by installation of epinephrine. Other supportive measures, such as intravenous fluids and parenteral opiates, are usually indicated.

Penile shunts are used as a last resort to prevent further episodes of priapism by increasing the cavernous blood flow using native vessels or by creating an arteriovenous shunt. They invariably result in erectile dysfunction, which can be ameliorated by implantation of an inflatable penile prosthesis. There are data showing that sildenafil (Viagra)[1] therapy can prevent priapism by altering vascular smooth muscle tone through inhibition of phosphodiesterase 2 activity.

Diagnosis
The diagnosis of SCD rests on the hemoglobin electrophoresis or high-performance liquid chromatography (HPLC), which allows detection of most hemoglobin variants. In patients with microcytosis α-globin gene sequencing may reveal coinheritance of an α-thalassemia trait.

Neonatal Screening
Children with SCD have an increased susceptibility to bacteremia due to *S. pneumoniae,* which can occur as early as 4 months of age and carries a case fatality rate as high as 30%. Acute splenic sequestration crises also contribute to mortality in infancy. Diagnosis by newborn screening and immediate entry into programs of comprehensive care, including the provision of effective pneumococcal prophylaxis, can reach infants who might otherwise be lost to the healthcare system and has been demonstrated to decrease morbidity and improve survival. Currently, newborn screening and follow-up of SCD are carried out in all 50 states in the United States, as well as in most developed countries, and initiatives are under way to introduce universal newborn screening in most sub-Saharan African countries.

Late Diagnoses and Misdiagnoses
Rarely, patients who were born before the adoption of universal screening or who were lost at the time of follow-up of positive neonatal screening results are only diagnosed late in life. This occasionally occurs in patients with HbSC who might have normal hemoglobin and hematocrit and a mild disease phenotype. Alternatively, the disease may be misdiagnosed as iron deficiency in patients with HbS/β+-thalassemia on account of their microcytosis, which places them at risk of futile and potentially harmful prolonged trials of iron supplementation. Patients who have a low HbS level (< 40%) due to recent transfusion or who have only mildly decreased hemoglobin (HbSC or HbS/β+-thalassemia) may receive an erroneous diagnosis of sickle cell trait (carrier state).

Treatment
From the original description of SCD in 1910 to the 1970s, there was no efficacious therapy for SCD, and most patients died within the first 2 decades of life, with infectious complications being responsible for the majority of pediatric fatalities. Several preventive and pharmacologic milestones since then, and the realization that care has to occur in a multidisciplinary setting, have profoundly affected the natural history of the disease (Table 3). Median age at death in resource-rich countries was 42 years in male patients and 48 years in female patients with HbSS, according to data from the Cooperative Study of Sickle Cell Disease in the 1980s (a prehydroxyurea setting), thereby still lagging approximately 2 to 3 decades behind that of the general African-American population. The following sections summarize the therapeutic approach to the most important complications of SCD.

---

[1] Not FDA approved for this indication.

TABLE 3 Manifestations of Sickle Cell Disease With Key Prevention and Treatment Strategies

MANIFESTATION	PREVENTION	TREATMENT
Pneumococcal sepsis	Penicillin, Prevnar/Pneumovax vaccination	Antibiotic therapy for penicillin-resistant *Streptococcus pneumoniae*
Splenic or liver sequestration	—	Exchange transfusion
Painful vasoocclusive episode	Hydroxyurea (Droxia), prevention of exposure to triggers	Intravenous fluids, parenteral opiates, supplemental oxygen
Acute chest syndrome	Incentive spirometry during VOE, hydroxyurea	Transfusion, broad-spectrum antibiotics with atypical coverage
Iron overload	Optimization of transfusion therapy	Iron chelation with deferasirox (Exjade) or deferoxamine (Desferal)
RBC alloimmunization	Transfusion with leukoreduced RBCs	—
CVA	Chronic transfusion in children with high transcranial Doppler velocity	Exchange transfusion and thrombolytics in selected cases
Pulmonary hypertension	Hydroxyurea?, treatment of predisposing conditions such as obstructive sleep apnea, hypoxemia, thromboembolism	Hydroxyurea, chronic transfusion therapy, specific therapy
Kidney disease	Antihypertensive therapy?, hydroxyurea?, ACE inhibitors?	ACE inhibitors?, renal replacement therapy, kidney transplant
Priapism	Hydroxyurea?	Pseudoephedrine (Sudafed)[1], aspiration of corpus cavernosum, sildenafil (Viagra)[1]
Leg ulcers	Hydroxyurea?, chronic transfusion?	Surgical débridement, surgical grafting

[1]Not FDA approved for this indication.

ACE, Angiotensin-converting enzyme; *CVA*, cerebrovascular accident; *RBCs*, red blood cells; *TCD*, transcranial Doppler; *VOE*, vasoocclusive episode (crisis).

Vasoocclusive Episodes

Acute pain from vasoocclusive episodes in SCD is extremely intense, affects both children and adults, and is due to ischemia or necrosis of the vascular beds. Most patients report severe pain in the bones and joints of the extremities, as well as lower back, although acute ischemia and pain can affect unusual sites such as the mandibular area. Infants and young children may experience dactylitis, a painful swelling of the hands from bone marrow infarct in the small bones of the digits. Occasionally, adults may also experience the typical signs of inflammation, such as edema, warmth, and erythema in an affected limb, but a paucity or absence of signs is the norm. Imaging studies such as MRI, positron emission tomography (PET), and bone scan can reveal signs of acute bone marrow infarction in a painful bony area, but they are not routinely used in the work-up of a pain episode, unless osteomyelitis or septic arthritis are suspected.

Intravenous opiates are the mainstay of treatment of a pain episode. Even in opiate-naïve patients with SCD, opioid dosages often exceed those required for other indications. For instance, doses of intravenous hydromorphone (Dilaudid) of 1 to 2 mg are typical in adult patients. However, most patients, are on an oral pain regimen at home and have a history of multiple admissions for vasoocclusive episodes. In these cases, individualized care based on prior effective regimens and the patient's own perception of the intensity of pain are recommended. After an attempt at controlling the pain with three or four closely spaced opiate boluses is made, patients who are in persistent discomfort or have evidence of underlying complications triggering the vasoocclusive episode should be admitted and ideally placed on patient controlled analgesia. Nonsteroidal antiinflammatory drugs such as ketorolac (Toradol) have fallen out of favor due to their risks in patients with renal disease and their questionable efficacy. The American Pain Society and the National Heart, Lung and Blood Institute (NHLBI) have published guidelines for the treatment of acute and chronic pain in SCD, followed by other institutions in the past decade.

Common obstacles to prompt and effective care in SCD are the health professional's fear of overdosing the patient, as well as misconceptions about addiction and pseudoaddiction. In general, healthcare professionals tend to overestimate the prevalence of opioid use disorder in SCD and tend to undertreat patients significantly, leading to patients' frustration and anger when their pain demands are not met (pseudoaddiction).

Nonpharmacologic therapies such as biofeedback, relaxation, and localized heat may be effective and should be incorporated into the management of pain episodes whenever possible. Care for vasoocclusive episodes should also include management of possible precipitating factors: dehydration and hypovolemia should be corrected with hypotonic crystalloids, and an infection work-up should be initiated in patients with fever, hypoxemia, or leukocytosis above baseline. Antiemetics and antipruritus therapy are also usually required.

Prior experiences in multiple institutions have shown that a dedicated facility for effective and rapid management of uncomplicated vasoocclusive episodes reduces hospitalizations and length of stay and facilitates integration of care—psychological, socioeconomic, and nutritional—in a multidisciplinary approach. This experience is the basis of the concept of the day hospital in SCD and relies on the need to provide prompt assessment and treatment of pain, safe dose titration to relief, monitoring of adverse effects, and adequate disposition (emergency department, inpatient admission, home) in a clinical environment familiar with SCD and the individual patient.

Chronic Pain

Chronic pain is common, and a study using pain diaries compiled by patients shows that most patients with SCD experience pain on an almost daily basis (PiSCES study). Orthopedic problems such as avascular necrosis (AVN) are common and tend to develop early in patients with HbSS disease, thus exposing patients to a lifetime of pain. There is an increasing realization that central sensitization and opiate-induced hyperalgesia also play a significant role in chronic pain in SCD. Unfortunately, there is a dearth of safe and effective strategies to manage chronic pain in SCD. At times, short-acting and long-acting opiates are required to empower the patient to manage pain at home and minimize use of the emergency department. Drugs for neuropathic pain, such as gabapentin (Neurontin)[1], may also be used in combination with

[1]Not FDA approved for this indication.

opiates because neuropathic pain may develop as a result of tissue ischemia and necrosis.

Patients who have successfully transitioned from pediatric to adult care, have a good support system, and are distracted by their work or school schedules tend to cope better and require less pharmacologic support.

Because analgesic care is life-long, consultation with pain specialists is often valuable, particularly in patients for whom more-sophisticated pain regimens are needed. For instance, the mu-opioid receptor partial agonist buprenorphine (Buprenex, Butrans), opioid rotation, and methadone used as analgesic can help to reduce the total opiate requirements. Several States in the United States have approved the use of marijuana for medical purposes for several conditions including SCD. Although controlled studies on the benefits and risks of medical marijuana in SCD are lacking, studies in sickle mice and anecdotal reports hold promise. Urine toxicology screens and written "opiate agreements" are indicated in patients receiving opiates to ensure adherence with the therapy and to minimize the risk of use of illicit substances, particularly at a time of heightened surveillance for opiate abuse in the United States.

Transfusional Therapy

In SCD, the benefits of transfusion in terms of improved hemodynamics and oxygenation need to be balanced with the risks of iron overload, alloimmunization, transfusion reactions, and viral transmission of infectious agents. Leuko-reduced, sickle-negative RBCs with extended phenotypic matching for Rh Cc, Ee, and Kell, which account for 80% of detected antibodies, are required. By using extended phenotypic matching, the rate of alloimmunization decreased from 3% to 0.5% per unit, and the rate of delayed hemolytic transfusion reactions decreased by 90% in the STOP study. In previously immunized patients, a full RBC match also inclusive of matching for the Duffy, Kidd, and S antigens is recommended. Indications for transfusion include hemoglobin less than 5 g/dL or less than 6 g/dL with symptoms and any severe complication such as stroke, aplastic anemia, splenic or hepatic sequestration, or acute chest syndrome.

Prophylactic transfusions have been considered standard of care before surgery (with the exclusion of minor procedures such as intravenous port placement); the benefit of preoperative transfusions in preventing SCD-related complications in HbSS patients has also been confirmed in a small randomized clinical trial (the TAPS study). As to the type of transfusion strategy to be used, a clinical trial published in 1995 showed that a conservative prophylactic transfusion regimen to achieve a target hemoglobin of 10 g/dL and any HbS value was as effective as an aggressive regimen to achieve a hemoglobin of 10 g/dL and a target HbS value of less than 30% in preventing postsurgical complications such as acute chest syndrome.

Exchange transfusion (erythrocytapheresis with RBC exchange) is usually reserved for the most severe complications, which include acute chest syndrome with impending pulmonary failure, acute stroke and its prevention in children, multiorgan failure, and sepsis. Box 1 summarizes the main indications for simple and exchange transfusion in SCD, as well as the areas of uncertainty.

Iron Chelation

Patients who have received more than 10 transfusions or 20 units of packed RBCs should be screened for iron overload. Most authorities recommend initiation of iron chelation based on a ferritin level consistently greater than 1000 ng/mL, based on data from the thalassemia literature, although liver iron quantitation by MRI or biopsy should be obtained, when available, prior to therapy and to monitor its effectiveness. In the United States, the oral chelating agents deferasirox (Exjade) and deferiprone (Ferriprox) and the parenteral deferoxamine (Desferal) are available and should be administered until the ferritin level is less than 500 ng/mL for three consecutive measurements. Patients on iron chelation with deferasirox and deferoxamine require monitoring of hepatic, renal, auditory, and visual toxicity, and particular caution has to be exercised in the setting of renal disease, because

| BOX 1 | Indications for Transfusion |

No Indication
Chronic steady-state anemia
Uncomplicated painful episode
Infections
Minor surgery without general anesthesia
Aseptic necrosis of hip or shoulder
Uncomplicated pregnancy

Unclear Indication
Intractable or frequent painful episodes
Leg ulcers
Before receiving intravenous contrast dye
Complicated pregnancy
Cerebrovascular accident in adults
Chronic organ failure

Simple Transfusion
Symptomatic anemia
• High output cardiac failure
• Dyspnea
• Angina
• Central nervous system dysfunction
Sudden decrease in hemoglobin
• Aplastic crisis
• Acute splenic sequestration
Severe anemia (hemoglobin ~5 g/dL) with fatigue or dyspnea
Preparation for surgery with general anesthesia

Exchange Transfusion
Acute cerebrovascular accident
Multiple organ system failure
Acute chest syndrome
Hepatic sequestration
Retinal surgery

transient, reversible increases in serum creatinine and rare instances of irreversible acute kidney injury have been reported in patients with underlying renal insufficiency. Deferiprone has been associated with agranulocytosis and neutropenia, mandating close monitoring of the absolute neutrophil count during therapy.

Erythropoietic Stimulating Agents

Although a brisk reticulocytic response is common in SCD, patients who develop renal failure or aplastic crises or who receive therapy with hydroxyurea may experience a relative or absolute reticulocytopenia (<100,000 reticulocytes/mL) and a worsening of their baseline anemia. In these situations, therapy with ESAs may be beneficial.

Because of bone marrow expansion in patients with HbSS, higher starting doses of erythropoietin (Epogen, (Epogen, Procrit)[1] than in patients without SCD may be considered. For darbepoetin (Aranesp)[1], a reasonable starting dose is 100 to 200 µg/weekly or every 2 weeks. ESAs can be titrated by 20% to 25% increases in dose per week in patients who do not respond adequately. Weekly monitoring of hematocrit is essential to avoid overdosage and relative erythrocytosis, which can lead to hyperviscosity and vasoocclusive episodes.

Nutritional Considerations

Malnutrition, growth retardation, and stunting with findings of low lean and fat body mass are highly prevalent in children and adolescents with SCD, due to their increased caloric demands and a hypermetabolic state. Macronutrient and micronutrient deficiencies are common, and nutritional counseling is warranted. Hypovitaminosis D and low bone mineral density are also prevalent in children and adults. Folic acid[1] is indicated

[1] Not FDA approved for this indication.

at the dose of 1 mg daily as in other hemolytic diseases, particularly where folate nutritional supplementation programs are absent. Strategies aimed at decreasing iron intake and absorption should be implemented early. There is also growing interest in antioxidant nutraceuticals, particularly in light of the clinical trial showing beneficial effects with L-glutamine (Endari) in SCD; however, evidence on other substances remains limited. The small subset of patients who are overweight or obese is at risk for exacerbating or precipitating common orthopedic problems in SCD such as AVN of the femoral head and its resulting disability. These patients should also receive targeted nutritional counseling.

Hydroxyurea

Since the pediatric hematologist Janet Watson suggested in 1948 that the paucity of sickle cells in the peripheral blood of newborns was due to the presence of increased HbF, there has been interest in developing therapies to modulate the hemoglobin switch from fetal to newborn life and prolong HbF production. Several antineoplastic agents, including 5-azacytidine (Vidaza)[1] and hydroxyurea, became the focus of attention after they were found to increase HbF levels in nonhuman primates and individuals with SCD.

The landmark Multicenter Study of Hydroxyurea in Sickle Cell Disease (MSH) showed that the incidence of painful crises was reduced from a median of 4.5 per year to 2.5 per year in hydroxyurea-treated patients with SCD. The rates of acute chest syndrome and blood transfusion were also reduced significantly. A follow-up for up to 9 years of 233 of the original 299 subjects showed a 40% reduction in mortality among those who received hydroxyurea. This study led to the approval of hydroxyurea (Droxia, Siklos) as the first disease-modifying therapy in adults with SCD. More recent studies showed that hydroxyurea is safe and effective in children and adults with SCD. The recently concluded BABY HUG study showed that children 9 to 18 months with HbSS disease randomized to receive 2 years of hydroxyurea therapy, irrespective of the disease severity, had less dactylitis and fewer pain episodes, hospitalizations, and transfusions than children receiving placebo.

On the molecular and cellular levels, the benefits of hydroxyurea are mostly related to increased intracellular HbF, which prevents the formation of HbS polymers and sickling. In addition to this mechanism, some patients on hydroxyurea who do not adequately increase their HbF levels also display clinical benefits, suggesting that hydroxyurea might have other beneficial rheologic properties.

Although the MSH study only included patients with HbSS, its findings traditionally have been extrapolated to other sickle cell syndromes such as HbSC and HbS/β-thalassemia. A report from Greece, where S/β-thalassemia is highly prevalent, has confirmed that hydroxyurea similarly reduces complications and mortality in patients with HbS/β[0]-thalassemia, with a nonsignificant benefit also observed in HbS/β[+] thalassemia. Existing guidelines also recommend hydroxyurea in patients with HbSC disease, but there is still no high-level evidence to support this practice.

Hydroxyurea has been indicated at a dosage of 15 mg/kg (7.5 mg/kg in patients with renal disease) in patients with frequent pain episodes, history of acute chest syndrome, other severe vasoocclusive episodes, or severe symptomatic anemia, although another sensible approach is to prescribe it to all patients with HbSS regardless of their phenotype. End points are less pain, increase in HbF to 15% to 20%, increased hemoglobin level to 7 to 9 g/dL in severely anemic patients, improved well-being, and acceptable myelotoxicity. The dosage can be increased by 500 mg every other day every 8 weeks to a maximum of 35 mg/kg if no toxicity is encountered. Considering the potential myelotoxicity, hepatotoxicity, and nephrotoxicity of this medication, laboratory monitoring needs to be performed every 2 weeks at the time of initiation or escalation and monthly during maintenance therapy. Laboratory studies should include a complete blood cell (CBC)

[1] Not FDA approved for this indication.

Start therapy if one or more of the following conditions are present:
- frequent pain episodes
- history of acute chest syndrome
- other severe VOE
- severe symptomatic anemia

Starting dose: 15 mg/kg or 7.5 mg/kg if the patient has kidney disease

Endpoints:
- less pain
- increase in HbF to 15%–20%
- increased hemoglobin level to 7–9 g/dL
- improved well-being
- acceptable myelotoxicity

Dose escalation: increase dose by 500 mg every other day every 8 weeks if no toxicity encountered to a maximum of 35 mg/kg

Lab monitoring:
- At time of initiation or escalation: check CBC/differential/reticulocyte count every 2 weeks; serum chemistries every 2–4 weeks, percent HbF every 6–8 weeks
- During maintenance: check CBC/differential/reticulocyte count chemistries monthly, percent HbF every 3 months

Criteria to hold:
- ANC <2000
- Hb <9.0 g/dL and reticulocyte count <80,000 (alternatively start Epo)
- Platelet count <80,000
- Raising creatinine
- 2-fold elevation of AST or ALT over baseline
- 2 months prior to planned conception/pregnancy

Figure 5 Protocol for hydroxyurea treatment.

count, differential and reticulocyte count, and serum chemistries. Measurements of HbF can be performed every 3 months. An elevated MCV is a marker of adherence to the therapy.

Criteria for holding hydroxyurea are listed in Figure 5. Patients need to be counseled on the teratogenic potential, as demonstrated in animal studies, as well as the risks of infertility and leukemogenesis, although a growing body of evidence shows that these risks may have been overestimated in patients with SCD.

Other side effects that can affect compliance include, but are not limited to, weight gain, alopecia, skin and nail hyperpigmentation (melanonychia), nausea and vomiting, and mucosal ulcerations. Because of the toxicity concerns, as well as factors intrinsic to long-term preventive therapy, hydroxyurea therapy has had low effectiveness in spite of high efficacy, with underprescribing by healthcare professionals and poor patient compliance being major obstacles to its widespread adoption.

Therapy of Pulmonary Hypertension

Because evidence-based guidelines for managing PH in patients with SCD are not available, recommendations are based upon the pulmonary arterial hypertension literature, case reports, small open-label studies, and expert opinion. For patients with mild PH (tricuspid regurgitant velocity [TRV], 2.5 to 2.9 m/s), it is important to identify and treat risk factors associated with PH such as rest, exercise or nocturnal hypoxemia, sleep apnea, pulmonary thromboembolic disease, restrictive lung disease or fibrosis, left ventricular systolic and diastolic dysfunction, severe anemia, and iron overload. These patients may benefit from aggressive SCD management, including optimization of hydroxyurea dosage and initiation of a chronic transfusion program in those who do not tolerate or respond poorly to hydroxyurea. Consultation with a pulmonologist or cardiologist experienced in PH is also recommended.

For patients with TRV 3 m/s or more, we recommend following the guidelines for TRV 2.5 to 2.9 m/s. In addition, RHC is necessary to confirm diagnosis and to directly assess left ventricular diastolic and systolic function. We would consider specific therapy with selective pulmonary vasodilator and remodeling drugs if the patient has pulmonary arterial hypertension defined by RHC and exercise limitation defined by a low 6-minute walk distance.

Figure 6 Spectrum of immunosuppression and myelosuppression in preparative regimens in hematopoietic stem cell transplantation (HCT) in sickle cell disease (SCD). Most preparative regimens for HCT in SCD have used a backbone of busulfan (BU) (Busulfex)[a] and cyclophosphamide (CY) (Cytoxan)[1]. Additional immunosuppressive agents include equine antithymocyte globulin (Atgam)[1] or leporine antithymocyte globulin (Thymoglobulin) (ATG)[1], antilymphocyte globulin, total lymphoid irradiation (TLI) or total body irradiation (TBI), fludarabine (Flu) (Fludara)[1], and alemtuzumab (Campath)[1]. Attempts to reduce the intensity of preparative regimens for patients with SCD have been based on one of two approaches. The first is the use of reduced-intensity conditioning regimens to produce less myeloablation. These require donor marrow infusion for hematopoietic recovery. The second is the use of nonmyeloablative regimens, which do not eradicate host hematopoiesis and allow hematopoietic recovery even without donor stem cell infusion. (Adapted with permission from Krishnamurti L. Hematopoietic cell transplantation: a curative option for sickle cell disease. *Pediatr Hematol Oncol.* 2007;24:569–575.)

US Food and Drug Administration (FDA)-approved drugs for primary pulmonary arterial hypertension include the endothelin receptor antagonists (bosentan [Tracleer] and ambrisentan [Letairis]), prostaglandin-based therapy (epoprostenol [Flolan], treprostinil [Remodulin, Tyvaso, Orenitram], and iloprost [Ventavis]), the phosphodiesterase-5 inhibitors (sildenafil [Revatio]), and riociguat (Adempas), the first member of a new class of drugs, the soluble guanylate cyclase (sGC) stimulators. No published randomized studies in the SCD population exist for any of these agents, although a multicenter placebo-controlled trial of sildenafil for PH of SCD was stopped early because of an unexpected increase in hospitalizations for vasoocclusive crisis in the treatment group receiving sildenafil.

Anticoagulation is indicated in patients who have evidence of pulmonary thromboembolic complications and is supported by evidence of benefit in other populations with PH.

Hematopoietic Stem Cell Transplantation

Despite improvement of supportive care in SCD, life expectancy remains lower than for those not affected. In addition, quality of life for patients with SCD is usually significantly impaired. Although hydroxyurea can decrease acute complications of SCD such as vasoocclusive episodes and acute chest syndrome, no satisfactory measures exist to prevent the development of irreversible organ damage in adults. Furthermore, therapy with hydroxyurea is lifelong, and only 20% to 30% of eligible patients are prescribed or actually take the drug.

Currently, allogeneic hematopoietic stem cell transplantation (HCT) remains the only curative treatment. Indications for HCT have been empirically determined from prognostic factors derived from studies of the natural history of SCD. The most common indications for which patients with SCD have undergone HCT are a history of stroke, recurrent acute chest syndrome, or frequent vasoocclusive episodes.

Allogeneic HCT after myeloablative therapy has been performed in hundreds of pediatric and numerous adult patients with SCD. The backbone of the preparative regimens have consisted of busulfan (Busulfex)[1] 14 to 16 mg/kg and cyclophosphamide (Cytoxan)[1] 200 mg/kg. Additional immunosuppressive agents used have included antithymocyte globulin (Atgam)[1], rabbit antithymocyte globulin (Thymoglobulin)[1], antilymphocyte globulin, or total lymphoid irradiation (Figure 6). Cyclosporine A (Neoral)[1], alone or with mercaptopurine (Purinethol)[1] or methotrexate[1], has been used for posttransplant graft-versus-host disease prophylaxis.

The outcome of HCT for patients with SCD from matched siblings is excellent. Of 1000 recipients of human leukocyte antigen (HLA)-identical sibling transplants performed between 1986 and 2013 and reported to the European Blood and Marrow Transplant, Eurocord, and the Center for International Blood and Marrow Transplant Research, the 5-year event-free and overall survival were 91.4% (95% CI 89.6% to 93.3%) and 92.9% (95% CI 91.1% to 94.6%), respectively. Event-free survival was lower with increasing age at transplantation (hazard ratio [HR] 1.09; $P < .001$) and higher for transplantations performed after 2006 (HR 0.95, $P = .013$). Twenty-three patients experienced graft failure; 70 patients (7%) died, the most common cause of death being infection. Stabilization or reversal of organ damage from SCD has been documented after HCT. In patients who have stable donor engraftment, complications related to SCD resolve, and there are no further episodes of pain, stroke, or acute chest syndrome. Patients who successfully receive allografts do not experience sickle-related central nervous system complications and have evidence of stabilization of central nervous system disease by cerebral MRI. However, the impact of successful HCT on reversal of cerebral vasculopathy has been variable. Current research is focused on improving the applicability of HCT to a greater proportion of patients with SCD by the development of novel conditioning regimens minimizing myeloablation (see Figure 6), the use of novel sources of hematopoietic stem cells such as umbilical cord blood, extending HCT to adult recipients and alternate donors such as matched unrelated donors and haploidentical donors. The aim of these studies is to develop safe and effective alternatives for patients without matched sibling donors, thus increasing the applicability of curative therapy for SCD.

New and Experimental Therapies

The last few years have witnessed a flourishing of new therapeutic approaches for SCD. One new drug has received FDA approval and has been incorporated in the clinical practice across the United States and several are in the pipeline or being reviewed in accelerated approval pathways by the FDA. Several decades of preclinical research in sickle mouse models are finally bearing fruit with pathologic pathways identified in sickle mice being harnessed for the development of molecular targeted biologicals. Finally, gene therapy is currently on the horizon with several gene therapy and gene editing approached being developed simultaneously.

Antioxidant Strategies

In 2018, pharmacologic *L*-glutamine (Endari) received FDA approval as the second disease-modifying drug in SCD. A

---

[1] Not FDA approved for this indication.

randomized, phase III multicenter trial showed that patients in the *L*-glutamine group had significantly fewer pain crises and hospitalizations than those in the placebo group. Of note, two-thirds of the patients in both arms received concomitant hydroxyurea. Reassuringly, the drug had relatively mild side effects including nausea and fatigue. *L*-glutamine presumably acts by reducing oxidant stress in the sickle RBCs, although its effects on major disease parameters such as hemolysis are unclear.

Modulation of Cellular Adhesion

Adhesive interactions between RBCs, white blood cells, and platelets, and between cells and endothelium are implicated in the pathogenesis of vasoocclusive episodes. Recently, several compounds have been developed to target specific adhesion molecules such as E-selectin and P-selectin. This is a particularly promising area of research that has yielded two compounds in advanced phases of development. The P-selectin inhibitor crizanlizumab[5] has shown significant reduction of the rate of crises per year and longer median time to the first crisis and second crisis when given as intravenous prophylaxis in a double-blind, randomized, phase II clinical trial. As in the case of *L*-glutamine, crizanlizumab was used with and without concurrent hydroxyurea therapy. The pan-selectin inhibitor rivipansel has shown similar promising results and is currently undergoing phase III testing.

Modulation of Hemoglobin Oxygen Affinity

Deoxygenation of HbS leads to polymerization, sickling, and hemolysis. Thus strategies aimed at increasing the oxygen affinity of HbS may be beneficial. Once-daily oral GBT440-007[5] (currently voxelotor) showed improvement in hemoglobin and reduction in daily pain in adolescents and adults with SCD by increasing hemoglobin oxygen affinity and decreasing HbS polymerization and sickling, and a phase III study is currently under way.

Modulation of Nitric Oxide

NO is an active biogas and a free radical species that mediates arterial relaxation, cellular adhesion to endothelium, hemostasis, and blood viscosity. In SCD, NO bioactivity is reduced as a result of decreased production due to endothelial perturbation and NO scavenging by cell-free hemoglobin generated during intravascular hemolysis. Dietary supplementation with *L*-arginine, a precursor of NO, and delivery of exogenous NO or NO bioactivity to the microvasculature in SCD, should promote dilatation of the terminal arterioles where obstruction to flow and tissue damage occurs, improvement of lung ventilation and perfusion is matching, decrease in pulmonary artery pressures, and inhibition of platelet aggregation and cellular adhesion. Although two recent clinical trials on *L*-arginine supplementation and inhaled NO (DeNOVO trial) for vasoocclusive episodes failed to show a clinical benefit, optimization of timing and dosing and novel strategies to target the NO pathway might lead to valuable NO therapeutics in the future.

Gene Therapy

The ultimate cure for SCD, gene therapy, is finally on the horizon. A French group first reported that a patient had been successfully treated with lentiviral-mediated insertion of an anti-sickling β-globin gene into autologous stem cells. The transduced cells were then transplanted into the patient who has since experienced long-term remission from SCD. Subsequently, in a clinical trial at the National Institutes of Health (NIH), several patients were treated with autologous hematopoietic stem cells transduced with a lentiviral vector that encodes for a nonsickling hemoglobin with very promising results. Other gene therapy approaches have targeted fetal hemoglobin induction and have harnessed the CRISPR-Cas9 gene editing technology.

Surgical Issues

Preoperative patient optimization includes prophylactic transfusion, close monitoring of pulse oximetry, adequate analgesia

based on the patient's opiate tolerance, and monitoring for sickle cell–related complications.

AVN of the femoral heads, and more rarely of the humeral heads, is the most common orthopedic problem in SCD. Surgery is usually deferred until the pain and disability from AVN become intolerable and usually involves total hip or shoulder arthroplasty. This is usually a more involved procedure than in the general population on account of the altered bone anatomy in SCD. Patients with bone marrow expansion may experience thinning of the cortical bone and prosthetic instability, whereas some may suffer from the opposite problem of obliteration of the medullary shaft by sclerotic bone in response to multiple necrotic events.

Patients with SCD tend to develop pigmented gallstones and cholelithiasis. Cholecystectomy is performed in patients with SCD with cholelithiasis, right upper quadrant pain, and a positive hepatobiliary iminodiacetic acid (HIDA) scan. In SCD, the rate of intraoperative complications is higher and so is the rate of reversion from laparoscopic to open cholecystectomy.

Splenectomy has been reserved for patients with massive splenic infarction (>50% of the spleen volume); intractable, recurrent splenic pain; and splenic abscess in the setting of splenic infarction. It is important to limit splenectomy to these few specific circumstances, because overwhelming sepsis and acute PH have been reported in the postsplenectomy period in SCD.

Kidney transplantation has been successfully performed in patients with SCD on chronic renal replacement therapy, although survival at 7 years is lower than in African Americans without SCD (67% vs. 83%). This difference is mostly due to vasoocclusive complications in the transplanted kidney, possibly exacerbated by the higher hematocrit in the postoperative period from resumption of endogenous erythropoietin production and increased blood viscosity. It is therefore critical to closely monitor ESA therapy in the posttransplantation period to prevent overdosing and relative erythrocytosis. A chronic transfusion program to prevent intrarenal sickling and maximization of hydroxyurea therapy should also be entertained, although its benefits need to be balanced against the risk of HLA alloimmunization and rejection. Combined solid organ and HCT protocols are being developed to overcome these complications. Recently, lung transplantation has been successfully performed in a SCD patient with severe pulmonary arterial hypertension and pulmonary venoocclusive disease.

References

Adams RJ, Brambilla D: Discontinuing prophylactic transfusions used to prevent stroke in sickle cell disease, *N Engl J Med* 353:2769–2778, 2005.

Adams RJ, Brambilla DJ, Granger S, et al: Stroke and conversion to high risk in children screened with transcranial Doppler ultrasound during the STOP study, *Blood* 103:3689–3694, 2004.

Ataga KI, et al: Crizanlizumab for the prevention of pain crises in sickle cell disease, *N Engl J Med* 376:429–439, 2017.

Bunn HF: Pathogenesis and treatment of sickle cell disease, *N Engl J Med* 337:762–769, 1997.

Charache S, Terrin ML, Moore RD, et al: Effect of hydroxyurea on the frequency of painful crises in sickle cell anemia. Investigators of the Multicenter Study of Hydroxyurea in Sickle Cell Anemia, *N Engl J Med* 332:1317–1322, 1995.

DeBaun MR, et al: Controlled trial of transfusions for silent cerebral infarcts in sickle cell anemia, *N Engl J Med* 371(8):699–710, 2014.

Falletta JM, Woods GM, Verter JI, et al: Discontinuing penicillin prophylaxis in children with sickle cell anemia. Prophylactic Penicillin Study II, *J Pediatr* 127:685–690, 1995.

Gaston MH, Verter JI, Woods G, et al: Prophylaxis with oral penicillin in children with sickle cell anemia. A randomized trial, *N Engl J Med* 314:1593–1599, 1986.

Gladwin MT, Sachdev V: Cardiovascular abnormalities in sickle cell disease, *J Am Coll Cardiol* 59:1123–1133, 2012.

Gladwin MT, Sachdev V, Jison ML, et al: Pulmonary hypertension as a risk factor for death in patients with sickle cell disease, *N Engl J Med* 350:886–895, 2004.

Gladwin MT, Vichinsky E: Pulmonary complications of sickle cell disease, *N Engl J Med* 359:2254–2265, 2008.

Gluckman E, Cappelli B, Bernaudin F, et al: Sickle cell disease: An international survey of results of HLA-identical sibling hematopoietic stem cell transplantation, *Blood*.

Hoppe CC, Inati AC, Brown C, et al: Initial results from a cohort in a phase 2a study (GBT440-007) evaluating adolescents with sickle cell disease treated with multiple doses of GBT440, a HbS polymerization inhibitor, *Blood* 130.

Howard J, Malfroy M, Llewelyn C, et al: The Transfusion Alternatives Preoperatively in Sickle Cell Disease (TAPS) study: A randomised, controlled, multicentre clinical trial, *Lancet* 381:930–938, 2013.

---

[5] Investigational drug in the United States.

Hsieh MM, Fitzhugh CD, Weitzel RP, et al: Nonmyeloablative HLA-matched sibling allogeneic hematopoietic stem cell transplantation for severe sickle cell phenotype, *JAMA* 312(1):48–56, 2014.

Jeong GK, Ruchelsman DE, Jazrawi LM, Jaffe WL: Total hip arthroplasty in sickle cell hemoglobinopathies, *J Am Acad Orthop Surg* 13:208–217, 2005.

Krishnamurti L, Kharbanda S, Biernacki MA, et al: Stable long-term donor engraftment following reduced-intensity hematopoietic cell transplantation for sickle cell disease, *Biol Blood Marrow Transplant* 14:1270–1278, 2008.

Lee MT, Piomelli S, Granger S, et al: Stroke Prevention Trial in Sickle Cell Anemia (STOP): Extended follow-up and final results, *Blood* 108:847–852, 2006.

Little JA, McGowan VR, Kato GJ, et al: Combination erythropoietin-hydroxyurea therapy in sickle cell disease: Experience from the National Institutes of Health and a literature review, *Haematologica* 91:1076–1083, 2006.

Mehari A, Alam S, Tian X, et al: Hemodynamic predictors of mortality in adults with sickle cell disease, *Am J Respir Crit Care Med* 187:840–847, 2013.

Merkel KH, Ginsberg PL, Parker JC, Post MJ: Cerebrovascular disease in sickle cell anemia: A clinical, pathological and radiological correlation, *Stroke* 9:45–52, 1978.

Morris CR, Kato GJ, Poljakovic M, et al: Dysregulated arginine metabolism, hemolysis-associated pulmonary hypertension, and mortality in sickle cell disease, *JAMA* 294:81–90, 2005.

Noguchi CT, Rodgers GP, Serjeant G, Schechter AN: Levels of fetal hemoglobin necessary for treatment of sickle cell disease, *N Engl J Med* 318:96–99, 1988.

Novelli EM, Huynh C, Gladwin MT, et al: Pulmonary embolism in sickle cell disease: A case-control study, *J Thrombosis and Hemostasis* 10:760–766, 2012.

Ohene-Frempong K, Weiner SJ, Sleeper LA, et al: Cerebrovascular accidents in sickle cell disease: Rates and risk factors, *Blood* 91:288–294, 1998.

Niihara Y, et al: A phase 3 trial of l-glutamine in sickle cell disease, *N Engl J Med* 379:226–235, 2018.

Platt OS: The acute chest syndrome of sickle cell disease, *N Engl J Med* 342:1904–1907, 2000.

Platt OS, Brambilla DJ, Rosse WF, et al: Mortality in sickle cell disease. Life expectancy and risk factors for early death, *N Engl J Med* 330:1639–1644, 1994.

Platt OS, Thorington BD, Brambilla DJ, et al: Pain in sickle cell disease. Rates and risk factors, *N Engl J Med* 325:11–16, 1991.

Reiter CD, Wang X, Tanus-Santos JE, et al: Cell-free hemoglobin limits nitric oxide bioavailability in sickle-cell disease, *Nat Med* 8:1383–1389, 2002.

Ribeil J, et al: Gene therapy in a patient with sickle cell disease, *N Engl J Med* 376:848–855, 2017.

Scheinman JI: Sickle cell disease and the kidney, *Nat Clin Pract Nephrol* 5:78–88, 2009.

Smiley D, Dagogo-Jack S, Umpierrez G: Therapy insight: Metabolic and endocrine disorders in sickle cell disease, *Nat Clin Pract Endocrinol Metab* 4:102–109, 2008.

Steinberg MH: Management of sickle cell disease, *N Engl J Med* 340:1021–1030, 1999.

Steinberg MH, Barton F, Castro O, et al: Effect of hydroxyurea on mortality and morbidity in adult sickle cell anemia: Risks and benefits up to 9 years of treatment, *JAMA* 289:1645–1651, 2003.

Telen MJ, Wun T, McCavit TL, et al: Randomized phase 2 study of GMI-1070 in SCD: Reduction in time to resolution of vaso-occlusive events and decreased opioid use, *Blood* 125:2656–2664, 2015.

Vichinsky EP, Neumayr LD, Earles AN, et al: Causes and outcomes of the acute chest syndrome in sickle cell disease, *N Engl J Med* 342:1855–1865, 2000.

Walters MC, Patience M, Leisenring W, et al: Bone marrow transplantation for sickle cell disease, *N Engl J Med* 335:369–376, 1996.

Walters MC, Storb R, Patience M, et al: Impact of bone marrow transplantation for symptomatic sickle cell disease: An interim report. Multicenter investigation of bone marrow transplantation for sickle cell disease, *Blood* 95:1918–1924, 2000.

Yawn BP, et al: Management of sickle cell disease: Summary of the 2014 evidence-based report by expert panel members, *JAMA* 312(10):1033–1048, 2014.

THALASSEMIA

Method of

Sarah A. Holstein, MD, PhD; and Raymond J. Hohl, MD, PhD

CURRENT DIAGNOSIS

- Complete blood count: anemia (very severe in β-thalassemia major, mild in β-thalassemia minor and α-thalassemia trait), low mean corpuscular volume, variable leukocytosis, thrombocytopenia (secondary to splenomegaly) or thrombocythemia (after splenectomy)
- Peripheral blood smear: hypochromia, microcytosis, anisocytosis, poikilocytosis, target cells, Heinz bodies, nucleated red blood cells
- Evidence of hemolytic anemia: indirect hyperbilirubinemia, elevated lactate dehydrogenase, decreased haptoglobin

- Hemoglobin electrophoresis pattern:
  β-Thalassemia minor: elevated HbA2 ($\alpha_2\delta_2$)
  β-Thalassemia intermedia: elevated HbA2, elevated HbF ($\alpha_2\gamma_2$), and decreased HbA ($\alpha_2\beta_2$)
  β-Thalassemia major: absence of HbA, markedly elevated HbF, and elevated HbA2
  α-Thalassemia trait: normal
  Hemoglobin H disease: decreased HbA, presence of HbH (β_4) and HbBart (γ_4)
  Hemoglobin Barts hydrops fetalis: HbBart, absence of HbA, HbA2, and HbF
- Timing of symptomatic disease:
  β-Thalassemia minor: asymptomatic
  β-Thalassemia intermedia: variable
  β-Thalassemia major: within first year of life
  α-Thalassemia trait: asymptomatic
  Hemoglobin H disease: symptomatic at time of birth
  Hemoglobin Barts hydrops fetalis: death during gestation

CURRENT THERAPY

- Chronic packed red blood cell transfusions for β-thalassemia major (1–3 units of packed leukoreduced erythrocytes every 3–5 weeks) with a target hemoglobin concentration of 9 to 10.5 g/dL; variable transfusion needs for β-thalassemia intermedia and hemoglobin H disease
- Splenectomy with antibiotic prophylaxis and vaccination
- Iron chelation: deferoxamine (Desferal), or deferasirox (Exjade); deferiprone (Ferriprox)
- Osteoporosis management: calcium with vitamin D supplementation; bisphosphonates
- Allogeneic hematopoietic cell transplantation for β-thalassemia major

Globin Gene Arrangements

Thalassemia syndromes encompass a spectrum of hemoglobin disorders that arise from impaired production of globin chains. The genes that encode globins are located in two clusters: the β gene cluster on chromosome 11 and the α gene cluster on chromosome 16 (Figure 1). The β gene cluster includes the adult globin genes (β and δ) as well as the fetal Aγ and Gγ genes and the embryonic ε gene. The arrangement of the 5′ to 3′ sequence of these genes parallels the order of their developmental expression. Functional hemoglobin is a tetramer that includes two α and two β globin units. The α gene cluster includes two fetal/adult α genes (α1 and α2) and the embryonic ζ genes. In the embryo, three hemoglobins are found ($\zeta_2\varepsilon_2$, $\alpha_2\varepsilon_2$, and $\zeta_2\gamma_2$). Fetal hemoglobin (HbF) is composed of two α chains and two γ chains ($\alpha_2\gamma_2$). In adults, the predominant hemoglobin is hemoglobin A (HbA), consisting of two α chains and two β chains ($\alpha_2\beta_2$) (see Figure 1). Hemoglobin A2, consisting of two α chains and two δ chains ($\alpha_2\delta_2$), is a normal variant in adults and typically represents less than 3% of the total hemoglobin (see Figure 1).

In β-thalassemia, there is diminished production of β globin genes, resulting in an excess of α globin chains. Conversely, in α-thalassemia there is impaired production of α globin genes, resulting in an excess of β globin chains. This imbalance of globin production is variable, and the degree of accumulation of unpaired globin chains is directly related to the severity of the disease phenotype. The genetic basis of thalassemia is heterogeneous, and several hundred mutations have been identified. These mutations may affect any level of globin gene expression, including arrangement of the globin gene complex, gene deletion, splicing, transcription, translation, and protein stability. In general, β-thalassemia occurs as a result of mutations, whereas α-thalassemia occurs as a result of gene deletion.

It has been estimated that there are 270 million carriers of thalassemia in the world, including 80 million β-thalassemia carriers. The frequency of β-thalassemia carriers is highest in the malarial tropical and subtropical regions of Asia, the Mediterranean, and the Middle East. The term thalassemia, derived from Greek, refers to the Mediterranean Sea. This distribution is secondary to the selective advantage of heterozygotes against malaria. β-Thalassemia is subdivided into major, intermedia, and minor types (Table 1). α-Thalassemia is classified into four syndromes: α-thalassemia trait 2 (loss of one α globin gene [αα/α–]); α-thalassemia trait 1, also referred to as α-thalassemia minor (loss of two α globin genes [αα/–– or α–/α–]); hemoglobin H (HbH) disease (loss of three alleles [α–/––]); and hemoglobin Barts hydrops fetalis (loss of all four α globin loci [––/––]).

Pathophysiology

The clinical manifestations of thalassemia and their severity are a consequence of the relative excess of unpaired globin chains. In particular, excess α globin chains are unstable and insoluble and therefore precipitate inside the red blood cell (RBC). These inclusions (precipitated hemoglobin) may be visualized as Heinz bodies. The accumulation of α globin chains leads to a variety of insults to the erythrocyte, including changes in membrane deformability and increased fragility. Free β chains are more soluble than free α chains and are able to form a homotetramer (HbH). The hallmark of thalassemia is an anemia that is a consequence of both increased destruction (i.e., hemolysis) and decreased production (i.e., ineffective erythropoiesis). The bone marrow typically displays erythroid hyperplasia.

Oxidant injury is closely linked with the pathology of thalassemia. Under normal conditions, a small amount of methemoglobin (Fe^{3+}) is formed via oxidation and can then be reduced back to hemoglobin (Fe^{2+}). However, isolated globin chains can be oxidized to hemichromes, some forms of which are irreversibly oxidized. The hemichromes can then generate reactive oxygen species, which can oxidize membrane components, leading to cell injury. There is an increase in membrane rigidity in β-thalassemia, and this appears to be secondary to the binding of partially oxidized α globin chains to components of the membrane skeleton. Increased membrane rigidity in turn leads to decreased membrane deformability and increased destruction. In α-thalassemia, HbH has a left-shifted oxygen disassociation curve and therefore does not readily transport oxygen. HbH erythrocytes have increased rigidity, which is thought to be secondary to interactions between excess β globin chains and the membrane. Unlike with β-thalassemia, HbH erythrocytes have increased membrane stability. Inclusion bodies have been identified in HbH cells, and there appears to be a correlation between RBC age and solubility of HbH. As cells age, the amount of soluble HbH decreases, and the level of inclusions increases.

It has also been recognized that there is increased phagocytosis of thalassemia RBCs compared with in normal controls. The etiology is not completely understood, but it may be a consequence of reduction in surface levels of sialic acid, increase in surface immunoglobulin G binding, and changes in phosphatidylserine localization.

Despite the pronounced hemolysis and marrow erythroid hyperplasia, patients with thalassemia generally do not display the compensatory reticulocytosis that is indicative of the other basis for anemia, ineffective erythropoiesis. Accumulation of α chain aggregates is thought to lead to death of erythrocyte precursors. Furthermore, abnormal assembly of membrane proteins in erythroid precursors has been demonstrated.

Iron overload is one of the primary causes of morbidity. Even without transfusion, the long-standing anemia, however mild, leads to increased iron absorption in the gut and eventual chronic iron overload. Excessive iron deposition causes devastating damage to multiple organs, particularly affecting the heart, liver, and endocrine organs.

Chromosome 11: Beta globin gene cluster

Chromosome 16: Alpha globin gene cluster

Figure 1 Representation of the β and α globin gene clusters. Also shown are the globin tetramers produced during embryonic development.

472

TABLE 1	Summary of Hematologic and Clinical Features of the Thalassemias		
TYPE	**HEMATOLOGIC FINDINGS**	**HEMOGLOBIN ELECTROPHORESIS PATTERN**	**CLINICAL FEATURES**
β-Thalassemia major	Severe anemia, microcytosis, hypochromia, target cells, nucleated RBCs	Absence of HbA, markedly elevated HbF, elevated HbA2	Splenomegaly, jaundice, skeletal abnormalities, abnormal facies; transfusion dependent
β-Thalassemia intermedia	Mild to moderate anemia, microcytosis, hypochromia	Elevated HbA2, elevated HbF, decreased HbA	Splenomegaly; variable transfusion dependence
β-Thalassemia minor	Mild anemia, microcytosis, target cells	Elevated HbA2	None
Hemoglobin Barts hydrops fetalis	Severe anemia, anisopoikilocytosis, hypochromia, nucleated RBCs	HbBart; absence of HbA, HbA2, and HbF	Death during gestation; fetus with massive hepatosplenomegaly, generalized edema
Hemoglobin H disease	Moderately severe anemia, anisopoikilocytosis, microcytosis, Heinz bodies	Decreased HbA; HbH and HbBart present	Splenomegaly, jaundice; generally transfusion-dependent
α-Thalassemia trait 1	Mild anemia, hypochromia, microcytosis, target cells	Normal	None
α-Thalassemia trait 2	Normal	Normal	None

Abbreviations: Hb = hemoglobin; RBCs = red blood cells.

β-Thalassemia Major

Symptoms of β-thalassemia major are not present at birth, because HbF ($\alpha_2\gamma_2$) is present. However, as HbF levels decline over the first year, the signs and symptoms of severe hemolytic anemia begin to manifest. Affected individuals display hepatosplenomegaly from expansion of the reticuloendothelial system, as well as extramedullary hematopoiesis, pallor, growth retardation, and abnormal skeletal development. If left untreated, 80% of children with β-thalassemia major will die before the age of 5 years.

Laboratory Features

Thalassemia major is characterized by a severe microcytic anemia. Hemoglobin levels may be as low as 3 to 4 g/dL. The peripheral blood smear is markedly abnormal and is notable for hypochromia, microcytosis, anisocytosis, poikilocytosis, target cells, and tear drop cells. Routine stains show the presence of precipitated α globin chains as Heinz bodies. The reticulocyte count is often low. The white blood cell count is often high but may be artifactually elevated as a consequence of automated inclusion of high numbers of circulating nucleated RBCs. The platelet count is typically normal, but progressive hypersplenism can result in decreased platelet counts. Patients who have undergone splenectomy often have increased white blood cell and platelet counts. Iron studies reveal elevated serum iron, transferrin saturation, and ferritin. Consistent with hemolysis and ineffective erythropoiesis, indirect bilirubin and lactate dehydrogenase levels are increased, and haptoglobin levels are low.

Clinical Features

Unique to β-thalassemia major is the development of extramedullary erythropoiesis. This may be so severe that the masses of bone marrow lead to broken bones and spinal cord compression. Sites of involvement include the sinuses and the thoracic and pelvic cavities. The expansion of the erythroid bone marrow can lead to a number of skeletal changes. In particular, characteristic changes in the facial bones and skull result in frontal bossing, overgrowth of the maxillae, and malocclusion. This has sometimes been referred to as chipmunk facies. Other bones are also affected, and premature fusion of the epiphyses results in shortened limbs. Compression fractures of the spine may occur. Even if the disease is managed appropriately with transfusions and iron chelation, patients will still suffer from osteopenia and osteoporosis. Possible mechanisms include changes secondary to hypogonadism or increased bone resorption secondary to vitamin D deficiency.

Hepatomegaly and splenomegaly, secondary to extramedullary erythropoiesis and RBC destruction, are prominent. Injury to Kupffer cells and hepatocytes from chronic overload leads to fibrosis and end-stage liver disease. Hepatic iron overload is probably caused in part by comparatively high levels of transferrin receptors. Iron overload, and perhaps other factors, increase susceptibility to viral hepatitis. Laboratory studies show indirect hyperbilirubinemia, hypergammaglobulinemia, and elevated liver markers. The chronic hemolysis leads to formation of bilirubin gallstones, although cholecystitis or cholangitis is not common. Splenic dysfunction results in immune dysfunction. The shortened erythrocyte survival time leaves patients susceptible to aplastic crisis induced by parvovirus B19 infection. Extramedullary hematopoiesis may also affect the kidneys, and patients often have large kidneys. Rapid cell turnover leads to hyperuricemia, and children may develop gouty nephropathy.

A number of endocrine abnormalities are commonly seen in β-thalassemia major, including hypogonadism, growth failure, diabetes, and hypothyroidism. These abnormalities occur even in chronically transfused patients and may be in part related to iron overload. Endocrine glands, like liver and heart, have high levels of transferrin-receptor and therefore are more susceptible to iron overload. The typical growth pattern for a child with β-thalassemia major is relatively normal until the age of 9 to 10 years. After that time, the growth velocity slows, and the pubertal growth spurt is either absent or reduced. Although secretion of growth hormone does not appear to be altered in thalassemic patients, a reduction in peak amplitude and nocturnal levels of growth hormone has been observed. Amenorrhea is quite common, with 50% of girls presenting with primary amenorrhea. Secondary amenorrhea also develops, particularly in patients who do not receive regular chelation therapy. In males, impotence and azoospermia is common. Primary hypothyroidism typically appears during the second decade of life. The prevalence of diabetes mellitus and impaired glucose intolerance has been estimated at 4% to 20%. Unlike type 1 diabetes mellitus, diabetes associated with thalassemia is rarely complicated by diabetic ketoacidosis. The risk of diabetic retinopathy is lower, but the risk of diabetic nephropathy is higher. Patients with a high ferritin level (above 1800 µg/L) experience a faster progression to hypothyroidism, hypogonadism, and other endocrinopathies.

Thalassemic patients suffer from extensive cardiac abnormalities. Chronic anemia causes cardiac dilation. Although long-term transfusion can help prevent cardiac dilation, the resulting iron overload leads to cardiac hemosiderosis. Pericarditis, ventricular and supraventricular arrhythmias, and end-stage cardiomyopathy can develop. Ventricular arrhythmia is a common cause of death. Patients may also develop pulmonary hypertension. The degree of iron overload in the heart has traditionally been assessed by cardiac biopsy, but cardiac magnetic resonance imaging (MRI) is increasingly being used.

Vitamin and mineral deficiencies may occur. Folic acid deficiency may develop in patients, presumably as a consequence of increased cell turnover. Although the cause is unknown, patients with β-thalassemia major often have very low serum zinc levels. Serum levels of vitamin E and vitamin C may also be low.

Management of β-Thalassemia Major

Transfusion

The key intervention for the management of β-thalassemia major is chronic transfusion therapy. In particular, during the first decade of life, regular transfusion results in improvements in hepatosplenomegaly, skeletal abnormalities, and cardiac dilation. Patients typically require 1 to 3 units of packed RBCs every 3 to 5 weeks. The optimal target total hemoglobin level has yet to be determined. Alloimmunization does occur, and some blood centers try to leukodeplete their products, match donors by ethnicity, and limit the donor pool for any particular patient. Although the risk of blood-borne infections is now quite small, regular transfusion of blood products still carries a risk for infections such as HIV and hepatitis C.

Splenectomy

The general indication for splenectomy is an increase of more than 50% in the RBC transfusion requirement over the period of 1 year. Splenectomy may initially yield a decrease in the RBC transfusion requirement. It has been noted that thalassemia patients are at higher risk for infection after splenectomy than are those patients splenectomized for other reasons. The bacteria that most frequently cause infections in these patients include *Streptococcus pneumoniae*, *Haemophilus influenzae*, *Neisseria meningitidis*, *Klebsiella*, *Escherichia coli*, and *Staphylococcus aureus*. The increased susceptibility to infection compared with other splenectomized patients is thought to be a result of greater immune dysfunction secondary to iron overload. In particular, it has been reported that iron-overloaded macrophages lose the ability to kill intracellular pathogens. Antibiotic prophylaxis with penicillin, amoxicillin, or erythromycin is recommended for children up to age 16 years. In addition, patients should receive immunizations, including the pneumococcal, influenza, and *Haemophilus influenzae* vaccines.

Iron Chelation Therapy

Because of increased iron absorption and long-term transfusion therapy, iron overload develops. As noted earlier, iron overload causes damage to multiple organs. Because iron is poorly excreted, removal must be accomplished by phlebotomy (not an option in thalassemic patients) or by chelation therapy. Historically, deferoxamine (Desferal) has been the most widely used chelator. This agent may be administered subcutaneously, intramuscularly, or intravenously. The dosing for chronic iron overload is 20 to 40 mg/kg/day SQ or 500 to 1000 mg/day IM + 2 g IV per unit transfused blood. The IV-only route is indicated for patients with cardiovascular collapse. Multiple studies have shown that deferoxamine therapy improves long-term survival. In addition, intensive therapy with deferoxamine has been shown to improve cardiac function in patients with severe iron overload. However, compliance with daily injections has been a particular problem, and, unless regular therapy is given, iron will reaccumulate.

Deferiprone (Ferriprox) was the first orally active chelator to be introduced. It is given three times daily (total of 75 mg/kg/day). Studies have indicated that deferiprone may be as effective as deferoxamine in lowering iron levels. A recent Cochrane Review concluded that deferiprone is indicated in the treatment of iron overload in thalassemia major if deferoxamine therapy is contraindicated or inadequate. Agranulocytosis associated with deferiprone has been reported, and, because of this risk, the drug is currently not available in the United States except through the FDA Treatment Use Program. Deferiprone is available in Europe and Asia. There has also been interest in combined therapy with deferiprone and deferoxamine, and one study showed that the combination was more effective in removing cardiac and hepatic iron but did not further improve cardiac function.

Deferasirox (Exjade) is the first orally active agent approved for use in the United States. Its longer half-life in comparison to deferiprone allows this drug to be given once daily (total of 20–40 mg/kg/day). A phase III trial comparing deferasirox to deferoxamine in patients with thalassemia revealed similar decreases in liver iron concentrations. Side effects include gastrointestinal complaints (abdominal pain, nausea, vomiting, diarrhea) and skin rash. There have been postmarketing reports of acute renal failure, hepatic failure, and cytopenias. It is recommended that serum creatinine, ferritin, and alanine aminotransferase be monitored monthly during therapy. A prospective, randomized study comparing deferipronre and deferoxamine vs deferipronre and deferasirox in 96 patients with β-thalassemia major demonstrated that both regimens reduced iron overload. However, the latter regimen was found to be superior with respect to improving cardiac iron, patient compliance, and patient satisfaction.

The gold standard for measurement of liver iron concentration has been liver biopsy with iron measurement by atomic absorption spectrometry. More recently, there has been increasing use of MRI technology to measure liver iron levels. In general, iron content determined by MRI methodology correlates with liver iron concentration determined by biopsy. However, the precision of liver MRI measurement appears to be dependent on iron levels, liver fibrosis, and calibration. Hepatic iron concentration has also been measured using a superconducting quantum interference device (SQUID), although reported consistency has varied and widespread use of this technique has been limited by expense and complexity.

Management of Osteoporosis

Even with calcium and vitamin D supplementation, iron chelation, transfusion therapy, and hormonal therapy, bone loss continues to be a significant problem for thalassemia patients. Recently, there has been interest in the use of bisphosphonates. This class of drugs, which includes clodronate (Bonefos),[2] alendronate (Fosamax), pamidronate (Aredia), zoledronate (Zometa), and neridronate (Nerixia)[2], inhibit osteoclastic bone resorption and have found extensive use in the management of Paget's disease, osteoporosis, and skeletal metastases. Small studies performed in thalassemia patients have failed to show benefit with clodronate 100 mg IM every 10 days or 300 mg IV every 3 weeks. A very small study using alendronate (Fosamax)[1] 10 mg PO daily revealed an increase in bone mineral density only at the femoral level. Conversely, in a study involving pamidronate (Aredia)[1] 30 or 60 mg IV every month, there was an increase in bone density only at the lumbar level. The most promising results have been achieved with the most potent member of the class, zoledronate. Several trials demonstrated that zoledronate (Zometa)[1] 4 mg IV every 3 or 4 months results in significant improvement in femoral and lumbar bone mineral density and reduces bony pain. The largest randomized trial involved 118 β-thalassemia patients who received calcium plus vitamin D with or without neridronate (given every 90 days). At 6 and 12 months, there was increased bone mineral density as well as decreased back pain and analgesic use in the neridronate arm. Larger, long-term trials are necessary before this agent finds widespread use in the management of thalassemia-induced osteoporosis.

Hematopoietic Cell Transplantation

Hematopoietic cell transplantation is the only curative strategy for patients with hemoglobinopathies. Patients are assigned to a risk class (Pesaro class) based on adherence to regular iron chelation therapy, presence or absence of hepatomegaly, and presence or absence of portal fibrosis. Those children with no or little hepatomegaly, no portal fibrosis, and regular iron chelation therapy (class I) have a better than 90% chance of cure, whereas those with both hepatomegaly and portal fibrosis (class III) have long-term survival rates of about 60% in older studies. More recent reports indicate that class III survival has improved to 90%.

The use of human leukocyte antigen (HLA)-identical sibling donors has been preferred, because the use of HLA-mismatched donors has produced inferior results and is associated with increased graft rejection, graft-versus-host disease, and infection. However, it is estimated that only one-third of patients will have a matched donor. The use of unrelated donors has been explored, and initial studies showed poorer outcomes. However, more recent data suggest that matched unrelated donors might be a viable option if a suitable sibling donor is lacking, thanks to improved donor selection and transplantation techniques. The use of partially HLA-matched unrelated cord blood has been reported, although 4 of 9 children did not engraft.

Another emerging technique is the use of reduced-intensity conditioning regimens, although long-term success has yet to be achieved. However, no randomized controlled studies have been performed evaluating the role of transplant in thalassemia patients.

Gene Therapy

Globin gene therapy, achieved through manipulation of autologous stem cells, is an attractive alternative to allogeneic transplantation. There are three major scientific hurdles that must be overcome: design of vectors that yield therapeutic levels of globin gene expression, ability to isolate and transduce autologous stem cells, and development of transplantation conditions that will permit host repopulation. In addition, the safety of viral and nonviral transfections is an issue. Initial studies involved ex vivo transduction of autologous hematopoietic stem cells with a lentiviral vector carrying the transgene. This gene therapy has been administered intravenously or via intra-bone injection following a myeloablative conditioning regimen. Many of the patients treated to date have achieved transfusion independence, and thus far no unusual toxicities have been observed. Another approach that is currently under investigation involves the use of genome editing techniques such as CRISPR.

Pharmacologic Induction of Fetal Hemoglobin

Induction of HbF expression has been proposed as a therapeutic strategy. For β-thalassemia, induced γ globin gene expression would be predicted to decrease globin chain imbalance by complexing with free α chains. Hydroxyurea (Hydrea)[1] is an antimetabolite thought to interfere with DNA synthesis. It is well established in the management of sickle cell disease, where it has been shown to increase levels of HbF. The use of hydroxyurea in β-thalassemia is much less well established. In the United States, hydroxyurea has been approved for use in sickle cell disease but not for thalassemia. Studies published elsewhere in the world have generally shown improvements in hemoglobin

---

[1]Not FDA approved for this indication.
[2]Not available in the United States.

---

[1]Not FDA approved for this indication.

VI Hematology

levels in thalassemia intermedia patients, with some patients becoming transfusion independent. A recent meta-analysis on the use of hydroxyurea in patients with transfusion dependent β-thalassemia concluded that this agent might offer some benefit but that double-blinded placebo-controlled studies are lacking.

5-Azacytidine (azacitidine [Vidaza]),[1] an inhibitor of DNA methyltransferase, has been shown to induce HbF. However, concerns regarding long-term use have prevented further evaluation in thalassemia. Decitabine (Dacogen),[1] an analogue of 5-azacytidine, has been shown to increase HbF levels in patients with sickle cell disease refractory to hydroxyurea. A small pilot study of low-dose decitabine in β-thalassemia intermedia patients demonstrated an increase in total hemoglobin and hemoglobin F levels. Butyrate,[5] an inhibitor of histone deacetylases, is another agent capable of inducing HbF. However, butyrate and its derivatives (arginine butyrate,[5] sodium isobutyramide,[5] and sodium phenylbutyrate [Buphenyl][1]) have failed to show significant clinical benefit in thalassemia patients. Therefore, at this time, no agent has been approved for use in thalassemia patients. A number of hypotheses have been proposed to explain the lack of success of inducers of HbF in thalassemia: there is simply too little γ globin production to significantly affect globin chain balance; these agents decrease expression of partially active β-thalassemia genes; these agents increase expression of α-globin genes; chronic transfusions appear to reduce HbF levels; and these agents suppress erythropoiesis.

Novel Agents Targeting Ineffective Erythropoiesis
An alternative strategy that is being investigated involves the targeting of ineffective erythropoiesis. Janus kinase 2 (JAK2) plays a key role in erythropoiesis, and there is interest in the potential use of JAK2 inhibitors in thalassemia. A phase II study with ruxolitinib (Jakafi)[1] showed a trend toward reduction in transfusions as well as a reduction in spleen size. Luspatercept (ACE-536)[5] and sotatercept (ACE-011)[5] are activin receptor trap ligands that were developed to treat postmenopausal osteoporosis but were noted to increase Hb levels. Initial phase 2 studies with these agents in thalassemia patients revealed reductions in transfusion burden, increase in Hb, and reduction in liver iron levels. A phase 3 study comparing luspatercept plus best supportive care to placebo plus best supportive care is underway.

Antioxidants
Oxidative damage is believed to be an important cause of tissue damage, and there has been interest in the use of antioxidants in thalassemia patients. A variety of substances have been investigated, including ascorbate,[1] vitamin E,[1] N-acetylcysteine (Mucomyst),[1] flavonoids, and indicaxanthin.[5] A variety of antioxidant effects have been observed in vitro with these agents, but none have been shown to improve anemia in patients with thalassemia.

β-Thalassemia Intermedia
Given the underlying genetic heterogeneity, it is not surprising that the clinical manifestations of β-thalassemia intermedia are also quite varied. Some patients with more mild forms of β-thalassemia intermedia do not require long-term transfusion therapy. There is not a clear consensus about when long-term transfusion should be initiated. Factors that are considered for children include growth patterns, spleen size, and bone development. Transfusion may be necessary during infection-induced aplastic crises. In some instances, transfusions are begun in childhood to help with growth and then discontinued after puberty. Some adults gradually become more anemic and eventually require transfusion. Some authors have argued that starting transfusions early in life is advantageous, because the prevalence of alloimmunization appears to increase if transfusion is started after the first few years of life.

Splenomegaly usually develops in all patients, including those who do not require transfusion. With progression of splenomegaly and the accompanying sequestration and hemolysis, there is usually worsening of anemia, to the point at which transfusions may be required. Most patients achieve transfusion independence after splenectomy. Gallstones may develop, and a prophylactic cholecystectomy is sometimes performed at the same time as the splenectomy. As with β-thalassemia major patients, intermedia patients are at increased risk for infection and should be appropriately vaccinated.

For reasons that are not entirely clear, there is an increased risk of thromboembolic complications in intermedia patients compared with thalassemia major patients. An Italian study reported that 10% of thalassemia intermedia and 4% of thalassemia major patients experienced a thromboembolic event. Another study reported that thromboembolism occurred four times more frequently in patients with intermedia versus major disease. This report noted that venous events were more common in the thalassemia intermedia population, whereas arterial events were more common in the thalassemia major population. An even higher rate of venous thrombotic events (29%) was reported in a population of splenectomized patients with thalassemia intermedia. It has been suggested that exposed anionic phospholipids on the surface of damaged RBCs may induce a procoagulant effect. There is no consensus regarding the prophylactic use of antiplatelet agents or anticoagulants in this population.

Patients with thalassemia intermedia may develop iron overload, although it is less severe than in patients with thalassemia major. Even those that are not regularly transfused may develop a degree of iron overload, because there is increased iron absorption. Iron overload may be managed with the iron chelating agents as described earlier. Cardiac toxicity, including congestive heart failure, valvular problems, and pulmonary hypertension (leading to secondary right-sided heart failure), resulting from iron overload is not infrequent in the thalassemia intermedia population.

Bone abnormalities and osteoporosis may develop in thalassemia intermedia patients. In a North American study, the prevalence of fractures in these patients was 12%. Leg ulcers involving the medial malleolus are common and are often difficult to treat. Hypogonadism, hypothyroidism, and diabetes may occur, with frequency related to the severity of anemia and iron overload. Pseudoxanthoma elasticum, a syndrome consisting of skin lesions, angioid streaks in the retina, calcified retinal walls, and aortic valve disease, is more common in thalassemia intermedia than in thalassemia major. Currently, no effective therapy exists, although it has been reported that aluminum hydroxide (Alternagel)[1] reduces skin calcification.

β-Thalassemia Minor
Most patients with β-thalassemia minor are asymptomatic. However, they have an abnormal complete blood count that may sometimes lead to the misdiagnosis of iron deficiency. Although these patients have a microcytic anemia, it is much less severe than in patients with β-thalassemia major. In general, the hematocrit is greater than 30%. The mean corpuscular volume is typically less than 75 fL and the RBC distribution width index is normal, in contrast to iron deficiency, in which the degree of microcytosis is less and the distribution width index is usually increased. The peripheral blood smear shows the presence of target cells. Hemoglobin electrophoresis typically reveals an increase in HbA2. The normal anemia experienced during pregnancy may sometimes be exacerbated in patients with β-thalassemia minor, necessitating transfusion. Otherwise, no long-term effects of β-thalassemia minor have been described, and no interventions are required.

α-Thalassemia
Laboratory and Clinical Features
Patients with α-thalassemia trait 2 are symptom free and have normal laboratory values, including complete blood count, peripheral smear, and hemoglobin electrophoresis. Individuals with α-thalassemia trait 1 are symptom free, and the disease resembles β-thalassemia minor. The peripheral smear shows a hypochromic microcytic anemia with the presence of target cells. Hemoglobin electrophoresis is normal.

---

[1]Not FDA approved for this indication.
[5]Investigational drug in the United States.

---

[1]Not FDA approved for this indication.

HbH disease does produce symptoms. Unlike β-thalassemia major, in which HbF production protects the fetus, individuals with HbH disease develop hemolytic anemia during gestation and are symptomatic at birth. This is because α globin production is required for HbF ($\alpha_2\gamma_2$). As with β-thalassemia major, patients with HbH disease suffer from the consequences of chronic hemolytic anemia, although the severity is somewhat less. The transfusion requirements for HbH patients resemble those for patients with β-thalassemia intermedia, with transfusion support initiated in the second and third decades of life. These patients also develop iron overload, necessitating treatment with chelation therapy.

Hydrops fetalis with hemoglobin Barts is usually fatal in utero. The utter lack of α globin chain production results in absence of HbF. Hemoglobin Barts, a homotetramer consisting of four γ globin genes, is unable to deliver oxygen to tissues. Severe tissue hypoxia develops, leading to widespread tissue ischemia. High cardiac output failure leads to massive edema (hydrops). In most cases, death occurs in the third trimester or late second trimester. There have been reports of live births after intrauterine transfusion, but survival beyond the perinatal period is exceedingly rare. Prenatal diagnosis of hemoglobin Barts hydrops fetalis may be achieved through DNA-based testing using amniocytes from amniocentesis or chorionic villi sampling. Noninvasive testing is under development, including methods that isolate circulating fetal DNA in maternal peripheral blood.

Management

Patients with α-thalassemia 2 and 1 traits do not require treatment. The management of HbH disease is similar to that described for β-thalassemia.

References

Asadov C, Alimirzoeva Z, Mammadova T, et al: β-Thalassemia intermedia: a comprehensive overview and novel approaches, *Int J Hematol* epub ahead of print. 2018.
Bayanzay K, Khan R: Meta-analysis on effectiveness of hydroxyurea to treat transfusion-dependent beta-thalassemia, *Hematology* 20(8):469–476, 2015.
Bhardawj A, Swe KM, Sinha NK, Osunkwo I: Treatment for osteoporosis in people with β-thalassaemia, *Cochrane Database Syst Rev* 3:CD010429, 2016.
Cappelini MD, Motta I: New therapeutic targets in transfusion-dependent and –independent thalassemia, *Hematology Am Soc Hematol Educ Program* 2017(1):278–283, 2017.
Delvecchio M, Cavallo L: Growth and endocrine function in thalassemia major in childhood and adolescence, *J Endocrinol Invest* 33(1):61–68, 2010.
Jagannath VA, Fedorowicz Z, Al Hajeri A, et al: Hematopoietic stem cell transplantation for people with β-thalassaemia major, *Cochrane Database Syst Rev* 10:2014, CD008708.
Marsella M, Borgna-Pignatti C: Transfusional iron overload and iron chelation therapy in thalassemia major and sickle cell disease, *Hematol Oncol Clin North Am* 28:703–727, 2014.
Porter J: Beyond transfusion therapy: new therapies in thalassemia including drugs, alternate donor transplant, and gene therapy, *Hematology Am Soc Hematol Educ Program* 2018(1):361–370, 2018.
Saliba AN, Harb AR, Taher AT: Iron chelation therapy in transfusion-dependent thalassemia patients: current strategies and future directions, *J Blood Med* 6:197–209, 2015.
Taher AT, Weatherall DJ, Cappellini MD: Thalassemia, *Lancet* 391(10116):155–167, 2018.

THROMBOTIC THROMBOCYTOPENIC PURPURA

Method of
Ravi Sarode, MD

CURRENT DIAGNOSIS

- The diagnosis based on unexplained microangiopathic hemolytic anemia (MAHA) and thrombocytopenia in the absence of oliguric renal failure is sufficient to initiate emergent plasma exchange (PLEX) for suspected diagnosis of autoimmune acquired thrombotic thrombocytopenic purpura (TTP).

- These laboratory tests are recommended for patient evaluation:
  - Complete blood count (shows anemia and decreased platelet count, usually <30,000/uL).
  - Peripheral blood smear (shows schistocytes/fragmented red blood cells, a hallmark of thrombotic microangiopathy [TMA]).
  - Reticulocyte count (is elevated).
  - Haptoglobin (is usually undetectable in TTP).
  - Lactate dehydrogenase (LDH) (usually more than twice the upper limit of normal in TTP).
  - Blood urea nitrogen, serum creatinine (determines nonoliguric renal insufficiency, serum creatinine <2.5 mg/dL).
  - Liver function tests, including direct and indirect bilirubin.
  - Troponin—some patients have ischemic cardiac injury
  - Plasma ADAMTS13 activity (<10% is diagnostic of TTP) and inhibitor level (usually detected in 90% of cases of TTP).
  - Prothrombin time, partial thromboplastin time, fibrinogen, and d-dimers (to rule out disseminated intravascular coagulation (DIC).
  - Direct antiglobulin test (to rule out autoimmune hemolytic anemia).
  - Urinalysis.

CURRENT THERAPY

- Daily plasma exchange (PLEX) using plasma as a replacement fluid (1–1.5 total body plasma volume) until platelet count is greater than 150,000/μL for 2 days, then may taper PLEX to three times a week, then twice a week, and then once a week. Discontinue when platelets remain greater than 150,000/μL.
- Prednisone 1 mg/kg/day taper *pari passu* with PLEX.
- Rituximab (Rituxan)[1] (either 100 mg fixed dose or 375 mg/m² weekly × 4) or upfront in the first week once diagnosis of autoimmune TTP is confirmed (reduces length of stay, exacerbation, and number of PLEX).
- Plasma (10–15 mL/kg) or cryoprecipitate (one dose = 10 units of pooled cryoprecipitate) infusion if PLEX will be delayed >6 h.
- Caplacizumab (Cablivi), a nanobody that interferes with binding of von Willebrand factor to GPIb domain on platelets and disrupts pathophysiology of the disease in severe presentations or refractory cases to prevent deaths and reduce number of PLEX.
- Exacerbation or relapsing TTP.
  - Rituximab (Rituxan)[1] (100 fixed dose or 375 mg/m²) weekly for 2 to 4 weeks.
  - Cyclosporine (Neoral)[1] (2–3 mg/kg/day up to 6 months).
  - Vincristine (Oncovin)[1] (1.4 mg/m² once a week for 4 weeks).
  - Bortezomib (Velcade)[1] (1.3 mg/m² 1–2 cycles or 1 mg fixed dose weekly × 4).
  - Splenectomy as a last resort.

[1]Not FDA approved for this indication.

Thrombotic thrombocytopenic purpura (TTP) is a rare (1 to 2 cases/million) but life-threatening thrombotic microangiopathy (TMA) disorder characterized by the presence of microthrombi in microcirculation of various organs, including the brain, kidneys, heart, and abdominal viscera. Microthrombi consist of platelets and von Willebrand factor (VWF), resulting in microangiopathic hemolytic anemia (MAHA) and thrombocytopenia. MAHA refers to the fragmentation of red blood cells (schistocytes) during their passage through partially occluded arterioles and capillaries by microthrombi. TTP diagnosis requires a high degree of suspicion because a delay in initiating PLEX, the current standard of care, could result in a poor response or fatal outcome. In the past, diagnosis of TTP was made based on a pentad that included MAHA, thrombocytopenia, neurologic involvement, renal affection, and fever. This pentad was found in patients who had died of TTP indicating advanced disease; therefore one should not wait for development of a pentad, which could delay TTP diagnosis with a potentially fatal outcome. Currently, unexplained MAHA and thrombocytopenia in the absence of oliguric renal failure are sufficient to make a working diagnosis of TTP and initiate emergent PLEX. Patients may present with only severe thrombocytopenia and/or with warm autoimmune hemolytic anemia and be managed as nonresponding immune thrombocytopenia/Evans syndrome; however, after a few days they may develop MAHA, establishing a TTP diagnosis. Similarly, a young patient may rarely present with unexplained ischemic stroke without hematologic features and later develop hematologic features.

Pathophysiology

In congenital TTP (Upshaw Shulman syndrome), ultra large (UL) multimers of VWF were detected during remission and were absent during relapse. Later, a VWF-cleaving protease (ADAMTS13, *a disintegrin and metalloproteinase with thrombospondin 1 motif, 13th member of the family*) was identified that was responsible for cleaving UL multimers secreted from endothelium into normal-sized VWF multimers seen in normal plasma. This cleavage occurs under high shear rate flow conditions in smaller blood vessels where the UL-VWF undergoes unfolding, exposing the cleavage site for ADAMTS13. ADAMTS13 is severely deficient (<10%) in patients with both congenital and acquired (autoimmune) TTP. Persistence of UL-VWF multimers in microcirculation results in unfolding of the molecule, enabling it to bind to platelets at GPIb, producing platelet-VWF microthrombi in capillaries and arterioles that cause end-organ ischemic damage (Figure 1). Elevated lactate dehydrogenase (LDH) reflects not only MAHA but also tissue damage; hence, very high LDH reflects more severe disease.

Classification

TTP can be divided into (1) a congenital form resulting from a genetic defect in the ADAMTS13 gene and (2) an acquired form owing to an autoantibody against the ADAMTS13 enzyme

Figure 1 During normal hemostasis, ADAMTS13 enzyme cleaves ultralarge multimers of von Willebrand factor *(VWF)* in normal sizes and prevents formation of platelet—VWF aggregates under high shear rates; however, in the absence of ADAMTS13 owing to congenital deficiency or autoantibodies, VWF persist as ultralarge multimers that unfold under high shear rates in small blood vessels and induce VWF-platelet microthrombi in various organs causing ischemic damage. *ADAMTS13*, A disintegrin and metalloproteinase with thrombospondin motif 1, 13th member of the family; *TTP*, thrombotic thrombocytopenic purpura.

Figure 2 Classification of thrombotic thrombocytopenic purpura. *Ab*, Antibody; *ADAMTS13*, a disintegrin and metalloproteinase with thrombospondin motif 1, 13th member of the family; *HUS*, hemolytic uremic syndrome; *MAHA*, microangiopathic hemolytic anemia; *PLEX*, plasma exchange; *TMA*, thrombotic microangiopathy; *TTP*, thrombotic thrombocytopenic purpura.

(Figure 2). Congenital TTP can present in the neonatal period, early childhood, or later in life when it is usually associated with an inciting trigger in the form of pregnancy, severe infection, surgery, or other stress. Acquired TTP is usually idiopathic without underlying disorder or secondary when associated with an underlying autoimmune disorder such as systemic lupus erythematosus (SLE), HIV, the use of ticlopidine, etc. Other clinical conditions that present with MAHA and thrombocytopenia with nonsevere ADAMTS13 deficiency are grouped under a broader term called TMA.

Clinical Presentation

Autoimmune TTP is a disease of young adults (20 to 50 years, female:male [F:M] ratio 2:1), with the majority being African Americans. In the emergency department, most patients present with an acute onset of vague, anemia-like symptoms (malaise, fatigue, weakness) and thrombocytopenia (petechiae, gum bleed). Detailed evaluation reveals the onset of these symptoms several days before presentation. Up to 70% to 80% of patients have some neurologic features including severe headaches, visual disturbances, focal neurologic deficits, transient ischemic attack, memory deficits, unusual behavior, confusion, seizures, paraparesis, stupor, and coma. Mild renal insufficiency is seen in <50% and fever in <15%. Owing to the generalized nature of the disease, any organ system could be affected and ischemic insult to the heart is not uncommon.

Diagnosis

Unexplained MAHA and thrombocytopenia constitute the diagnostic features and are associated with elevated LDH, reticulocytosis, undetectable haptoglobin, elevated bilirubin, and nonoliguric renal insufficiency in some patients. A severe deficiency of ADAMTS13 (<10% activity with a detectable inhibitor in up to 90% of patients) confirms the diagnosis. Because this test is usually sent to a reference laboratory, this measurement is unavailable in most hospitals at the time of clinical diagnosis. Therefore, based on

the initial clinical and laboratory features, PLEX should be initiated emergently because a delay could increase not only morbidity but also mortality. A sample for ADAMTS13 must be drawn before initiating PLEX or plasma/cryoprecipitate infusion to avoid measuring enzyme from transfused products. ADAMTS13 is a stable enzyme; if a sample for ADAMTS13 could not be drawn before plasma therapy, a routine coagulation test sample may be used. In congenital TTP, there is persistent severe deficiency of ADAMTS13 (without an inhibitor) associated with ADAMTS13 gene defect; however, this diagnosis is at times made difficult because many patients, especially children and young adults, are often misdiagnosed as immune thrombocytopenia, anemia of unknown origin, or Hemolysis Elevated Liver enzymes and Low Platelets (HELLP) syndrome in pregnancy.

Differential Diagnosis

The differential diagnosis of TTP includes clinical conditions that present with MAHA and thrombocytopenia but without severe ADAMTS13 deficiency, that is, TMA. These conditions include hematopoietic stem cell transplantation, drug toxicities (mitomycin, clopidogrel [Plavix], cyclosporine A [Neoral], etc.), malignant hypertension (usually mild to moderate thrombocytopenia), HELLP syndrome with severe preeclampsia, mechanical cardiac devices (for example, left ventricular assist devices, intraaortic balloon pumps, and mechanical heart valves), disseminated intravascular coagulation (DIC), vasculitis, and both diarrhea-associated and atypical hemolytic uremic syndrome (HUS).

Treatment

PLEX is the standard of care therapy. Its use has reduced mortality from more than 90% to less than 20%. Ideally, it should be initiated within 4 to 6 hours of suspected diagnosis. The patient's plasma (which contains autoantibody) is selectively removed during PLEX (1.0 to 1.5 plasma volume processed) and replaced with donor plasma containing ADAMTS13. Neurologic symptoms usually disappear within 24 to 48 hours.

The platelet count is the most useful laboratory parameter to assess response. Complete clinical response, defined as normalization of platelet count for at least 2 days with near normal LDH, is generally achieved with seven to nine daily PLEX in most patients. Thereafter, a gradual taper—that is, PLEX every other day in the first week, twice in the next week, and once in the third week—may be performed. Given the autoimmune nature of the disease, glucocorticoid therapy is often given from the beginning. Approximately 30% to 50% of patients will have exacerbation of the disease (worsening of clinical or laboratory features after initial response) or relapses (recurrence of the disease 30 days after discontinuation of PLEX). Such patients require additional PLEX and other immunomodulatory therapies, e.g., rituximab (Rituxan),[1] cyclosporine (Neoral),[1] vincristine (Oncovin),[1] bortezomib (Velcade),[1] or splenectomy as a last resort. Recently, early rituximab use within the first week has been shown to reduce length of stay, exacerbation/relapse, and number of PLEXs. Preliminary data also suggest that a low, fixed-dose rituximab of 100 mg weekly × 4 has a similar clinical response to that of 375 mg/m^2 weekly × 4 but has benefits of reduced cost, infusion time, and side effects. A dialysis-type catheter is required for PLEX and can be placed with ultrasound guidance in patients with platelet counts as low as 10,000/μL. With the exception of a life-threatening bleed, platelet transfusion is contraindicated in TTP because it is a thrombotic disorder of platelet consumption, and transfused platelets may worsen the condition (appearance of new neurologic symptoms, myocardial infarction, etc.). If initiation of PLEX is likely to be delayed, either plasma or cryoprecipitate can be infused temporarily to supplement ADAMTS13. Caplacizumab (Cablivi), a nanobody that interferes with binding of A1 domain of VWF with GPIb/IX/V receptors on platelets, has been approved for the treatment of TTP by the US Food and Drug Administration (FDA). A randomized clinical trial showed that caplacizumab, given once as a bolus (10 mg) followed by daily subcutaneous injections (10 mg) up to 30 days post-PLEX, had a slightly faster platelet count normalization, reduced number of PLEXs, and exacerbation and possibly deaths but higher relapses compared to the placebo. It seems caplacizumab can definitely benefit severe and refractory TTP and may be tailored based on frequent ADAMTS13 testing during the treatment course. Congenital TPP is treated with plasma infusions (10 to 15 mL/kg); however, cryoprecipitate and intermediate purity FVIII concentrate that contain adequate ADAMTS13 have been used successfully to avoid volume overload in susceptible patients. Recently, a recombinant ADAMTS13 has shown very promising results in a phase 1 clinical trial in congenital TTP. Most fatalities occur during the first few days of diagnosis, probably because of the severity of the disease or delay in the initiation of PLEX.

Monitoring

Considering the relatively high frequency of cardiac involvement, cardiac monitoring should initially be performed. Although PLEX is an otherwise safe procedure, complications related to catheter infection and line thrombosis are not uncommon and should be identified as soon as possible to avoid exacerbation of the disease. Exacerbation of TTP is often related to an infection. There is increasing awareness of delayed long-term psychologic and psychosocial effects in up to 50% patients, and a careful follow-up is recommended to identify and manage these issues.

Prognosis

Although PLEX has reduced TTP mortality in the last 2 decades, most deaths occur within 24 to 48 hours of presentation and are caused by the delay in the administration of PLEX for a variety of reasons, including a delay in diagnosis or line placement or nonavailability of PLEX at the institution. After one PLEX, survival rates can increase above 90%. Importantly, no clinical and laboratory parameter exists to predict outcome or relapse. ADAMTS13 can be used during follow-up to detect early subclinical relapse (drop in activity <30%) without hematological changes and preemptive rituxaban[1] has been used to prevent overt relapses.

References

Fujimura Y, Matsumoto M, Isonishi A, et al: Natural history of Upshaw-Schulman syndrome based on ADAMTS13 gene analysis in Japan, *J Thromb Haemost* 9(Suppl 1):283–301, 2011.

Rock GA, Shumak KH, Buskard NA, et al: Comparison of plasma exchange with plasma infusion in the treatment of thrombotic thrombocytopenic purpura. Canadian Apheresis Study Group, *N Engl J Med* 325:393–397, 1991.

Sarode R, Bandarenko N, Brecher ME, et al: Thrombotic thrombocytopenic purpura: 2012 American Society for Apheresis (ASFA) consensus conference on classification, diagnosis, management, and future research, *J Clin Apheresis* 9:148–167, 2014.

Shah N, Rutherford C, Matevosyan K, et al: Role of ADAMTS13 in the management of thrombotic microangiopathies including thrombotic thrombocytopenic purpura (TTP), *Br J Haematol* 163:514–519, 2013.

Tsai HM: Thrombotic thrombocytopenic purpura and atypical hemolytic uremic syndrome—an update, *Hematol Oncol Clin North Am* 27:565–584, 2013.

---

[1]Not FDA approved for this indication.

[1]Not FDA approved for this indication.

7 Diseases of the Head and Neck

DRY EYE DISEASE

Method of
John N. Dorsch, MD

CURRENT DIAGNOSIS

- Signs and symptoms of dry eye disease are nonspecific and may not correlate well with severity of disease.
- There is no single diagnostic test to confirm the diagnosis of dry eye disease.

CURRENT THERAPY

- Artificial tears may help to palliate symptoms by lubricating the ocular surface, but preservatives in some products may complicate dry eye disease when used frequently.
- Patients with severe symptoms (especially visual disturbance or eye pain) should be referred to an ophthalmologist.

Introduction

The Tear Film and Ocular Surface Society (TFOS) have defined dry eye disease (DED) as "a multifactorial disease of the tears and ocular surface characterized by a loss of homeostasis of the tear film, and accompanied by ocular symptoms, in which tear film instability and hyperosmolarity, ocular surface inflammation and damage, and neuro-sensory abnormalities play etiological role."[1] Tear film with an inadequate amount of aqueous and/or lipid component is said to be unstable (i.e., tear film instability), leading to premature evaporation and break-up of tears. Tear instability leads to a loss of lubrication and protection of the ocular surface, which can cause impaired vision. Tear production, proper tear film composition, loss of tears through the nasolacrimal system, and evaporation all contribute to tear film homeostasis. An imbalance in tear film homeostasis causes damage to the ocular surface.

DED is composed of two subtypes: aqueous-deficient dry eye (ADDE) and evaporative dry eye (EDE). Common etiologies of ADDE and EDE are listed in Box 1. Clinically the signs and symptoms of each subtype are identical, but it is important to make an accurate diagnosis to optimize treatment. Despite different underlying causes of ADDE and EDE, inflammation of the ocular surface from hyperosmolarity of tears is the common denominator of DED. Normal tear film is composed of an inner aqueous layer (secreted by the lacrimal glands) and an outer lipid layer (secreted by the Meibomian glands). Dispersed throughout normal tear film are mucin (protein) particles (secreted by goblet cells of the cornea and conjunctivae) that function as a lubricant between the globe and eyelids. ADDE is caused by a deficiency in production of the aqueous portion of the tear film by the lacrimal glands, and EDE is caused by deficiency in production of the lipid layer of tear film by the meibomian glands. Deficiency

[1] Not FDA approved for this indication.

of the lipid layer of tear film causes evaporation of tears, leading to tear film instability, hyperosmolarity, and ocular surface inflammation.

Epidemiology

The prevalence of DED has increased in recent years due to the aging of the population and the increased use of certain medications that cause DED. It is estimated that as much as 30% of the population older than the age of 50 has some form of DED. One study showed that the majority of patients with DED had varying combinations of ADDE *and* EDE, with meibomian gland dysfunction (MGD) as the most common etiology of EDE.

Risk Factors

Aging is believed to be the most common cause of DED. Decreases in androgens play a significant role in lacrimal dysfunction. Estrogen-only hormone replacement treatment (HRT) is a risk factor for DED. MGD, eyelid abnormalities, loss of sensitivity of the cornea from LASIK and contact lens wear, medications, and systemic diseases (e.g., Sjögren syndrome, rheumatoid arthritis, systemic lupus erythematosus, Graves disease, diabetes mellitus) are common causes of DED. Environmental conditions, such as low humidity, extremes in temperature, smoking, and low-blink rate from looking at screens of computers, television, and phones for prolonged periods, cause evaporation of tear film and are significant risk factors for DED.

Pathophysiology

Factors that cause instability of tear film (see Risk Factors, earlier) lead to hyperosmolarity of the tear film. Hyperosmolarity can induce ocular surface damage and initiate an inflammatory cascade with the release of cytokines and other immune mediators on the ocular surface, perpetuating further surface damage. This phenomenon is termed the "Vicious Circle" of DED (Figure 1). Hyperosmolarity of the tear film can also lead to inflammatory changes and obstruction in the meibomian glands, known as the MGD "vicious circle," also depicted in Figure 1.

Prevention

Avoidance of tobacco smoke, temperature extremes, prolonged viewing of screens, and avoidance of certain medications (listed later, under Treatment) may help to prevent DED in some patients.

Clinical Manifestations of Dry Eye Disease

Symptoms and signs of DED are listed in Box 2. In moderate-to-severe forms, DED can be a debilitating disease leading to poor quality of life. DED is highly correlated with depression, anxiety, and sleep disorders.

Diagnosis

The presence of symptoms alone is not sufficient to make a diagnosis of DED, because they are often nonspecific and may not be accompanied by ocular surface changes. Several validated patient questionnaires have been developed that show good correlation with the presence of DED. Although there is no single test that makes a definitive diagnosis of DED, various diagnostic tests performed by eye disease professionals are helpful in making the diagnosis and in guiding treatment. The Schirmer test (more specific for ADDE) is fairly easy to perform but has poor reproducibility and may cause reflex tear secretion. The Tear Breakup Test (TBUT) is a test for tear film stability. After a complete blink, the time to the first break-up of the tear film is measured while viewing through a slit lamp. The normal range for the TBUT is 20 to 30 seconds; a TBUT of less than 10 seconds is pathologic.

Tear film osmolarity does not distinguish between ADDE and EDE but appears to be the most specific test for making the diagnosis of DED and correlates with the severity of DED. Tear film osmolarity greater than 308 mOsm/L is indicative of mild DED, and greater than 312 mOsm/L is indicative of moderate-to-severe DED. A number of new imaging techniques appear to be promising in the diagnosis of DED. Some of these include interferometry, optical coherence tomography (OCT), meibomian gland imaging, and thermography. In recent years, it has been discovered that the levels of matrix metalloprotein-9 (MMP-9) are elevated in the tears of patients with DED. MMP-9 testing is currently available in the clinics of eye disease professionals and appears to be a specific biomarker of DED. Materials used in diagnostic tests for differentiation of ADDE from EDE are expensive and not practical for use in primary care settings.

Differential Diagnosis

The differential diagnosis of DED includes blepharitis (which may coexist with DED), ocular allergies, and viral conjunctivitis.

Treatment

DED is a chronic and progressive disease, and no cure is known. Treatment of DED is aimed at increasing tear production, decreasing tear evaporation, and/or reducing tear resorption. If a patient is taking antihistamines, β-blockers, antispasmodics, diuretics, tricyclic antidepressants, isotretinoin, or psychotropic medications, or is on hormone replacement therapy, discontinuation of those medications should be considered if feasible. The

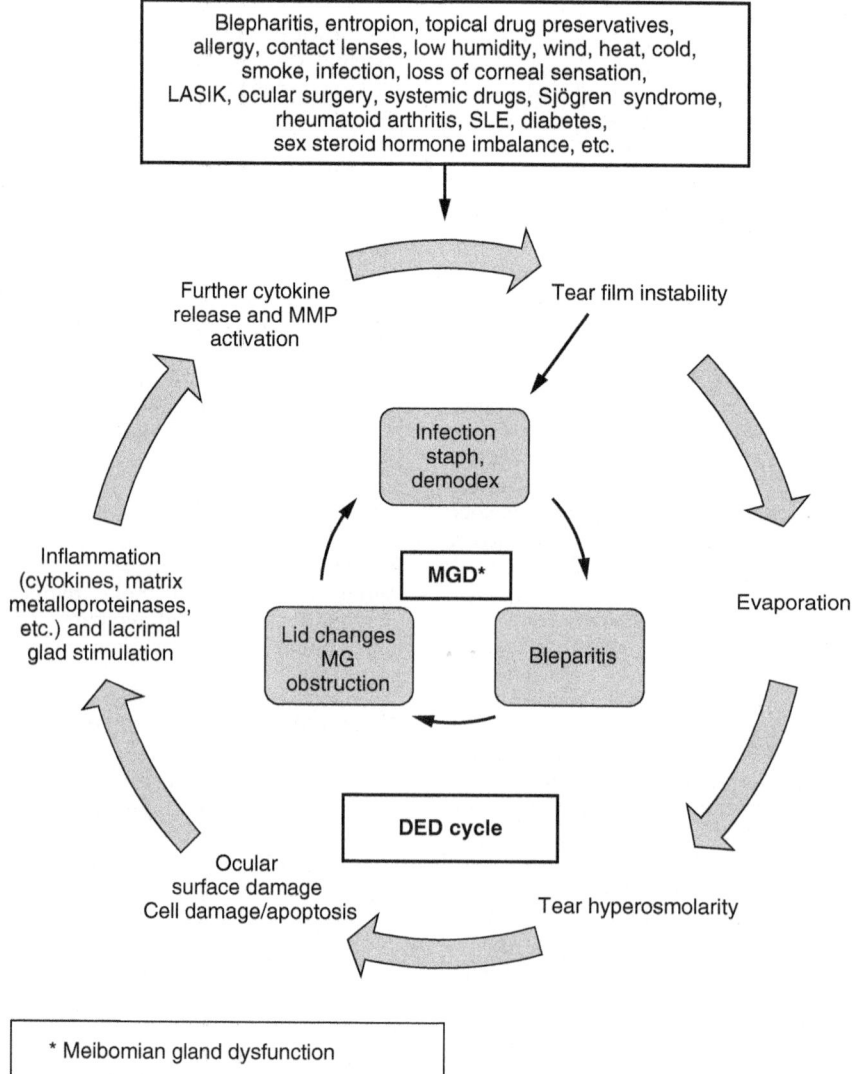

Figure 1 Dry eye disease *(DED)* "Vicious Circle." *MGD*, Meibomian gland dysfunction; *MMP*, matrix metalloprotein; *SLE*, systemic lupus erythematosus.

BOX 2 Symptoms and Signs of Dry Eye Disease

Symptoms	Signs
Dryness	Conjunctival injection (usually symmetric)
Redness	Excessive tearing (paradoxical)
General irritation of eyes	Blepharitis (lid margin redness)
Gritty sensation in eyes (later in day)	Malposition of eyelids (entropion, ectropion)
Burning sensation in eyes	Reduced blink rate
Foreign body sensation in eyes	Visual impairment
Light sensitivity	Scant, white, stringy discharge
Blurred vision	

BOX 3 Artificial Tears Preparations

For Mild DED: contain preservatives; low-to-moderate viscosity

Name	Vehicle	Cost per Month
Blink Tears (AMO)	PEG	$14
GenTeal (Novartis)	HPMC	$13
Liquifilm Tears (Allergan)	PVA	$20-30
Refresh Optive (Allergan)	CMC	$12-20
Systane (Alcon)	PEG + PG + HP-Guar	$13
Refresh Optive Advanced	CMC + Glycerin + Polysorbate	$20
Soothe XP-Xtra Protection (B&L)	Mineral oil	$12-14
Systane Balance (Alcon)	PEG + oil microemulsion	$9-15
Optrex Spray (Reckitt Benckiser)	*Hamamelis virginiana*	$15

For Moderate DED: No preservatives; low-to-moderate viscosity

Name	Vehicle	Cost per Month
Bion Tears (Adv. Vision Research)	HPMC + Dextran	$15–30
Hylo-Fresh (AFT Pharm)	HA	$22–30
Refresh (Allergan)	PVA + Povidone	$23
Refresh Plus (Allergan)	CMC	$15–21
Tears Naturale Free (Alcon)	HPMC + Dextran	$15
TheraTears (Akorn)	CMC	$12

For Severe DED: No preservatives; moderate-to-high viscosity

Name	Vehicle	Cost per Month
Celluvisc (Allergan)	CMC	$13–26
Hylo-Forte (AFT Pharm)	HA	$25
Duratears Ointment (Alcon)	Liquid Paraffin + Wool Fat	$13
Polyvisc (Alcon)	Liquid Paraffin + Wool Fat	$5
GenTeal PM Ointment (Novartis)	Mineral Oil + Petrolatum	$10

Artificial Tears with Lipids for Meibomian Gland Dysfunction

Name	Cost per Month
Refresh Endura	$26
Tears Again	$36–66
Liposic	$12
Refresh Optive Mega-3	$17
Refresh Plus	$11–21

CMC, carboxymethylcellulose; *HP-Guar*, hydroxypropyl guar; *HPMC*, hydroxymethylcellulose; *PEG*, Polyethylene glycol; *PG*, propylene glycol; *PVA*, polyvinyl alcohol.

use of humidifiers in homes and workplaces with low relative humidity may be helpful. Patients who work in proximity to outlet vents for furnaces and air conditioners should be moved away from them. People who smoke should be strongly urged to quit. Patients who work in dusty or smoky conditions should wear goggles. Moisture chambers can be added to eyeglasses to prevent evaporative loss of tears. Patients who look at screens for long periods of time should take more breaks and consciously blink more often to spread the tear film over the corneal surface.

As more proinflammatory mediators are identified in the vicious circle of DED, there are more potential targets at which to direct therapy. Artificial tears help to "break the (vicious) cycle" of inflammation and corneal damage by increasing tear film stability, relieving symptoms, and moisturizing the ocular surface.

Box 3 lists a number of OTC artificial tears preparations, relative cost, and indications for use. Artificial tears with preservatives can be toxic to corneal epithelium when used more than four times daily (QID). For moderate-to-severe DED, artificial drops without preservatives should be used. Drops with higher viscosity are generally used for treatment of more severe DED. Patients with MGD should be tried on artificial tears with lipids. Autologous serum eyedrops contain natural epitheliotropic growth factors and may be helpful in severe DED.

Various antiinflammatory treatments may be used to break the cycle as well. Topical corticosteroids, used for periods of 2 to 4 weeks, often improve symptoms and surface damage. Long-term use of topical steroids can cause cataracts, increased intraocular pressure, and increase the risk of opportunistic infection. Topical cyclosporine A (Restasis) is an immunosuppressant that reduces production of cytokines. Tacrolimus eye drops[5] is an immunosuppressant that may be used in patients who do not tolerate cyclosporine A. Lifitegrast (Xiidra) inhibits T-cell migration into tissues and is approved by the US. Food and Drug Administration (FDA) for treatment of DED. Lubricin, a naturally occurring lubricant, is under investigation as a potential treatment for DED. Tetracyclines[1] and azithromycin[1], in addition to their antibacterial effects, reduce synthesis of MMP-9, interleukins, tumor necrosis factor (TNF), and other inflammatory mediators. They are often used in the treatment of chronic blepharitis and MGB. Dietary intake of essential fatty acids (omega-3 and omega-6)[7] appears to help in the maintenance of ocular surface homeostasis in patients with MGD. Punctal occlusion and surgical approaches may be appropriate for severe DED. For patients with MGD, in-office physical treatments such as LipiFlow and Intense Pulsed Light have proven safe and effective for EDE. Neurostimulation of the lacrimal nerve appears to be a promising treatment for ADDE.

All of the aforementioned treatments are typically prescribed and monitored by eye disease professionals. Primary care physicians can educate patients on environmental issues mentioned earlier, smoking cessation, second-hand smoke avoidance, trying to reduce medication use when appropriate, and eyelid hygiene (heat and massage), as shown in Box 4. Eyelid hygiene consists of scrubbing the eyelids with baby shampoo mixed with water and using hot packs for at least 4 to 5 minutes at least twice a day, followed by pressure on the eyelids to express meibum.

Complications

Inflammation and damage to the ocular surface can lead to visual disturbance and poor quality of life.

[1] Not FDA approved for this indication.
[5] Investigational drug in the United States.
[7] Available as dietary supplement.

| BOX 4 | Primary Care Interventions for Patients With Dry Eye Disease |

Avoid smoke, low humidity, extreme heat or cold

Get moisture chambers for glasses to preserve moisture

Stop medications if possible: estrogen replacement, antihistamines, antidepressants, anxiolytics

Increase dietary intake of omega-3 essential fatty acids

Eyelid hygiene:

1. Eyelid scrubs

2. Mechanical scrubs and mechanical meibomian gland expression

3. Warming for minimum of 4 minutes once or twice daily, followed by moderate-to-firm massage of the eyelids to express meibum

Recommend artificial tears: avoid products with preservatives if used more than QID

Take more frequent breaks from looking at computer monitors and other screens

Consciously blink more often

Monitoring

Patients with typical symptoms of DED should be referred to an eye disease professional for accurate diagnosis. Other than eyelid hygiene and initiating artificial tears, most treatment for DED is initiated by eye disease professionals.

Conclusions

DED is a multifactorial disease caused by tear film instability, hyperosmolarity, and ocular surface damage that can result in discomfort and visual impairment. As the inflammatory cycle of DED becomes better understood, it is likely that more targeted treatments will become available. Even though much of the treatment of DED is directed by eye disease professionals, primary care physicians need to be aware of its symptoms and signs so patients receive the treatment they need.

References

Ayaki M, et al: High prevalence of sleep and mood disorders in dry eye patients: survey of 1,000 eye clinic visitors, *Neuropsychiatric Disease and Treatment* 11:889–894, 2015.

Bron AJ, et al: Rethinking dry eye disease: a perspective on clinical implications, *The Ocular Surface* 12(2S):S1–31, 2014.

Chan T, et al: Advances in dry eye imaging: the present and beyond, *Br J Ophthalmol* 102:295–301, 2018.

Craig J, et al: TFOS DEWS II Definition and Classification Report, *The Ocular Surface* 15:276–283, 2017.

Downie L, Keller P: A pragmatic approach to the management of dry eye disease: evidence into practice, *Optometry and Vision Science* 92(9):957–966, 2015.

Jones L, et al: TFOS DEWS II management and therapy report, *The Ocular Surface* 15:575–628, 2017.

Kashlouli M, et al: Oral azithromycin versus doxycycline in meibomian gland dysfunction: a randomised double-masked open-label clinical trial, *Br J Ophthalmol* 99:199–204, 2015.

Kossler AL, et al: Neurostimulation of the lacrimal nerve for enhanced tear production, *Ophthalmic Plast Reconstr Surg* 31(2):145–151, 2015 Mar-Apr.

Lane S, et al: A new system, the lipiflow, for the treatment of meibomian gland dysfunction, *Cornea Apr* 31(4):396–404, 2012.

Lemp M, et al: Distribution of aqueous-deficient and evaporative dry eye in a clinic-based patient cohort: a retrospective study, *Cornea May* 31(5):472–478, 2012.

Lin H, Yiu S: Dry eye disease: a review of diagnostic approaches and treatments, *Saudi Journal of Ophthalmology* 28:173–181, 2014.

McDonald M, et al: Treatment outcomes in the dry eye amniotic membrane (DREAM) study, *Clinical Ophthalmology* 12:677–681, 2018.

Messmer EM: The pathophysiology, diagnosis, and treatment of dry eye disease, *Dtsch Arztebl Int* 112:71–82, 2015, Available at: https://doi.org/10.3238/arztebl.2015.0071.

O'Brien P, Collum L: Dry eye: diagnosis and current treatment strategies, *Current Allergy and Asthma Reports* 4:314–319, 2004.

Pan Q, et al: Autologous serum eye drops for dry eye (Review), *The Cochrane Library* Issue 8, 2013.

Sambursky R, et al: Sensitivity and specificity of a point-of-care matrix metalloproteinase 9 immunoassay for diagnosing inflammation related to dry eye, *JAMA Ophthalmol* 131(1):24–28, 2013.

Samson M, et al: Characterization of full-length recombinant human proteoglycan 4 as an ocular surface boundary lubricant, *Experimental Eye Research* 127:14–19, 2014.

Stevenson W, et al: Dry eye disease: an immune-mediated ocular surface disorder, *Arch Ophthalmol* 130(1):90–100, 2012 January.

GLAUCOMA

Method of
Albert P. Lin, MD; and Kristin Schmid Biggerstaff, MD

CURRENT DIAGNOSIS

Primary Open Angle Glaucoma

- Primary open angle glaucoma is an irreversible optic neuropathy typically associated with elevated intraocular pressure.
- Primary open angle glaucoma is the most common form of glaucoma and is projected to affect more than three million Americans in 2020. It is more common in African Americans (6% to 7%), Asians (2% to 3%), and Hispanics (2%) and less common in whites (1%). It is more common in older adults: 1 to 2% in 50-year-olds compared with 6% to 12% in 80-year-olds.
- Primary open angle glaucoma is diagnosed by a complete ophthalmic examination, including dilated stereoscopic optic nerve examination and formal visual field.
- Untreated primary open angle glaucoma can lead to slow irreversible loss of vision and blindness. Other common causes of slow and progressive vision loss in older adults include cataracts, macular degeneration, and diabetic retinopathy.

Acute Angle Closure Glaucoma

- Pupillary block in susceptible patients leads to block of aqueous drainage and sudden and extreme rise of intraocular pressure. Acute angle closure can damage the optic nerve, resulting in acute angle closure glaucoma.
- About 0.5% to 1.0% of US adults are at risk for acute angle closure. It is more common in Inuits and Asians and rare in African Americans. The risk of acute angle closure increases with age. It is also more common in hyperopes.
- Patients can present with blurry vision, red eye, pain, headache, nausea, or vomiting. Acute angle closure is sometimes misdiagnosed as migraines or gastrointestinal illnesses. Patients with conjunctivitis, keratitis, uveitis, and corneal abrasion can also present with the same symptoms.
- Peripheral iridotomy prevents acute angle closure in susceptible patients. High intraocular pressure can result in irreversible damage of the optic nerve within hours, making acute angle closure one of the true ophthalmic emergencies.

CURRENT THERAPY

Primary Open Angle Glaucoma

- Topical eye drops, including β-blockers, selective α_2 agonists, carbonic anhydrase inhibitors, prostaglandin analogues, and rho kinase inhibitors, can be used to reduce intraocular pressure.
- Oral carbonic anhydrase inhibitors are typically used in recalcitrant cases until surgery can be performed.
- Laser trabeculoplasty may be used as first-line or adjunct therapy.
- Glaucoma surgery, including trabeculectomy, tube shunt, and cyclodestruction, may be performed if goal intraocular pressure cannot be reached with medical therapy or in nonadherent patients.

Acute Angle Glaucoma

- All glaucoma eye drops are used to reduce intraocular pressure.
- Oral and intravenous medications are added sequentially to reduce intraocular pressure as needed.

- Laser iridotomy can be performed as prophylactic treatment or acutely to break the pupillary block if the patient is unresponsive to medical intervention.
- Emergency glaucoma incisional surgery is performed if the patient is unresponsive to all other treatments.

Glaucoma is an optic neuropathy with characteristic optic nerve head appearance: narrowing of the neuroretinal rim. The optic nerve is a collection of more than 1 million axons from the retinal ganglion cells. The anterior 1-mm portion of the optic nerve within the globe is referred to as the *optic disk* or simply the disk. When the disk is examined with direct or indirect ophthalmoscopy, a cup, or a physiologic empty space, is observed centrally. The remainder of the disk, which has a yellow-orange appearance, contains the axons and is referred to as the *neuroretinal rim*. The area of the cup compared to the entire disk is the cup-to-disk ratio, which is normally less than 0.4 (Figure 1A). When patients develop glaucoma, axons are lost from the neuroretinal rim and the size of the cup increases in relation to the disk. Narrowing of the neuroretinal rim and increased cup-to-disk ratio are the hallmarks of glaucomatous optic neuropathy (see Figure 1B).

Glaucoma can result in significant and irreversible loss of vision and is one of the leading causes of blindness in the United States. Early in the disease state, glaucoma is asymptomatic; it is sometimes called "the sneak thief of sight." As the disease progresses, the patient develops decreased peripheral vision and eventually loss of the central vision.

Glaucoma is typically associated with increased intraocular pressure (IOP), but it is possible to have normal-tension or low-tension glaucoma. Glaucoma treatment is focused on the reduction of IOP to prevent or slow optic nerve damage and preserve visual function.

Glaucoma is classified in many ways, and it is most useful to approach it clinically based on the status of the angle, the area between the cornea and iris where aqueous humor exits the globe through the trabecular network. We further discuss primary open angle glaucoma, the most common form of glaucoma in the United States, and the management of acute angle closure, one of the true ophthalmic emergencies.

Primary Open Angle Glaucoma

Glaucoma is one of the leading causes of blindness in older adults, especially in patients of African American descent. Vision loss from glaucoma is irreversible, and the treatment goal is to reduce IOP, slow disease progression, and preserve visual function during the patient's lifetime. Glaucoma is a slowly progressive disease, and progression to blindness often takes more than 10 years, even in untreated patients. Given its slow progression

and the fact that central vision loss occurs in late disease, most patients do well with early diagnosis and treatment. Treatment is more difficult in late disease because the rate of disease progression and visual deterioration is accelerated, sometimes despite good control of IOP.

Due to the early asymptomatic nature of the disease, the patient's adherence to and persistence with treatment is often less than optimal. Studies have shown patients who obtain glaucoma information from physicians other than their ophthalmologists have a higher rate of medication adherence. Ophthalmologists have the options to use treatment modalities such as laser and surgery to obtain pressure control and decrease or eliminate the need for medication use.

The American Academy of Ophthalmology recommends asymptomatic patients older than 40 years be referred for ophthalmic evaluation once every several years for early detection of glaucoma and other chronic eye diseases. However, the US Preventive Services Task Force found insufficient evidence to recommend for or against screening for glaucoma in adults. Risks, benefits, and cost effectiveness of screening are beyond the scope of this chapter, but symptomatic patients or patients at high risk for glaucoma (African American ethnicity and family history) might benefit from ophthalmology consultation. It is possible to diagnose glaucoma by direct ophthalmoscopy, but this is not a substitute for binocular assessment of the disk through dilated pupils and formal visual field testing. If glaucoma is suspected or diagnosed, primary care visits should include inquiries regarding glaucoma medication use, medication side effects, and the time of last eye examination. Primary care physicians can improve glaucoma outcome by promoting adherence to medication and follow-up. Glaucoma patients need to follow up with their ophthalmologists at least annually, and in severe cases every 3 months, for intraocular pressure checks.

Treatment
Topical Glaucoma Medications

Topical glaucoma medications are administered once or twice daily. Patients should look up, pull down their lower eye lid, drop the medication on the inferior conjunctival cul-de-sac, and keep their eyes closed for 5 minutes. Applying gentle pressure next to the bridge of the nose to occlude the puncta can improve absorption of the medication. Medication bottle caps are color-coded by their class, and patients can usually identify their eye drops by color. Glaucoma medications are not subject to first-pass effect through the liver and can sometimes have significant systemic side effects, especially the β-blockers. Topical glaucoma medications are described later and summarized in Table 1.

Prostaglandin Analogues. Latanoprost (Xalatan), travoprost (Travatan), and bimatoprost (Lumigan) are prostaglandin

Figure 1 Disk appearance. (A) Normal disk. Cup-to-disk ratio is less than 0.4. (B) Glaucoma. Increased cup-to-disk ratio and narrow neuroretinal rim superiorly and inferiorly *(arrows)*.

TABLE 1 Topical Glaucoma Medications: Carbonic Anhydrase Inhibitors

CLASS	β-BLOCKER	SELECTIVE α₂ AGONIST	CARBONIC ANHYDRASE INHIBITOR	PROSTAGLANDIN ANALOGUE	RHO KINASE INHIBITOR	COMBINATION
Medication	Timolol (Timoptic) βxolol (Betoptic) Levobunolol (Betagan)	Brimonidine (Alphagan)	Dorzolamide (Trusopt) Brinzolamide (Azopt)	Latanoprost (Xalatan) Travoprost (Travatan) Bimatoprost (Lumigan) Latanoprostene bunod (Vyzulta)	Netarsudil (Rhopressa)	Timolol/Dorzolamide (Cosopt) Timolol/Brimonidine (Combigan) Brimonidine/ Brinzolamide (Simbrinza)
Dosing	bid or qd	bid	bid	qhs	qd	bid or tid
Cap color	Yellow	Purple	Orange	Teal	White	Blue or light green (Simbrinza)
Side effects	Bradycardia, COPD, and asthma exacerbation	Allergic conjunctivitis, dry mouth, and fatigue in elderly	Stinging and bitter taste	Hyperemia, lash growth, and increased pigmentation	Hyperemia	See individual components

COPD, Chronic obstructive pulmonary disease.

TABLE 2 Oral and Intravenous Glaucoma Medications

	ACETAZOLAMIDE (DIAMOX)	METHAZOLAMIDE (NEPTAZANE)	MANNITOL (OSMITROL)	GLYCERIN 50%[1]
Class	CAI	CAI	Hyperosmotic	Hyperosmotic
Dosage	250 or 500 mg bid	25 mg or 50 mg bid	1 g/kg in 30 min	1 g/kg once
Route	PO or IV	PO	IV	PO
Side effects	Bitter taste, indigestion, paresthesia, tinnitus, polyuria, kidney stones, hypokalemia, aplastic anemia, and sulfa allergy		Polyuria, dehydration Exacerbate CHF and diabetes (glycerin)	

[1]Not FDA approved for this indication.
CAI, Carbonic anhydrase inhibitor; CHF, congestive heart failure

analogues and are color-coded by teal caps. They are administered once at bedtime but may be administered once at any time during the day to promote adherence. They decrease IOP by increasing uveoscleral outflow. Latanoprostene bunod (Vyzulta) is converted into latanoprost and nitric oxide inside the eye and decreases IOP by promoting aqueous outflow through both the uveoscleral and trabecular meshwork pathways. It is considered a prostaglandin analogue with an additional mechanism of action. Side effects are primarily local and include increased conjunctival hyperemia, increased lash growth, and possible irreversible increase in periocular and iris pigmentation.

β-Blockers. Timolol (Betimol, Istalol, Timoptic), levobunolol (Betagan), and betaxolol (Betoptic) are color-coded by yellow caps. They are administered once or twice daily and decrease IOP by decreasing aqueous production. Side effects include bradycardia, exacerbation of chronic obstructive pulmonary disease (COPD) and asthma, impotence, and decreased serum high-density lipoprotein (HDL) cholesterol. Physicians need to be aware that a topical β-blocker is a potential cause of acute changes in cardiovascular or pulmonary status. There are several reported incidents of death following the use of topical β-blockers mostly due to exacerbation of asthma.

Selective α₂ Agonists. Brimonidine (Alphagan) and apraclonidine (Iopidine) belong to the class of selective α₂ receptor agonists, and brimonidine is more commonly prescribed; it is color-coded by purple caps. It is administered twice daily and decreases IOP by decreasing aqueous production. Allergic conjunctivitis has been reported in up to 25% of patients. Rarely, it causes dry mouth and chronic fatigue and drowsiness in the elderly.

Carbonic Anhydrase Inhibitors. Dorzolamide (Trusopt) and brinzolamide (Azopt) are color-coded by orange caps and are sulfa-based medications. They are administered twice daily and decrease IOP by decreasing aqueous production. This class of medication has minimal systemic side effects. However, some patients complain about transient stinging and a bitter taste in the mouth after administration. These side effects, if tolerable, are not indications for discontinuing therapy.

Rho Kinase Inhibitors. Netarsudil (Rhopressa) affects actin and myosin contraction and decreases IOP by increasing aqueous outflow through the trabecular meshwork. It is color coded white and administered once daily. Conjunctival hyperemia is reported in up to 50% of the patients. Ophthalmologists have also observed pinpoint conjunctival hemorrhages and corneal verticillata (lipid deposits on the corneal epithelium) because these observations are asymptomatic and generally not reported by the patients. Compared to other medications, rho kinase inhibitor has a unique mechanism of action and is considered to be an excellent adjunct medication to lower IOP when other medications are already in use.

Combined Topical Medications. Timolol and dorzolamide (Cosopt) and timolol and brimonidine (Combigan) are color-coded by blue caps. Brimonidine and brinzolamide (Simbrinza) are color-coded by a light green cap. Combined medications decrease exposure to preservatives and can decrease irritation and problems with dry eyes. Adherence might also be improved.

Oral Carbonic Anhydrase Inhibitors
Oral carbonic anhydrase inhibitors include acetazolamide (Diamox), 250 mg or 500 mg given twice daily, and

Figure 2 Acute angle closure patient with red eye and mid-dilated and nonreactive pupil.

methazolamide (Neptazane), 25 mg or 50 mg given twice daily. They are sulfa-based medications and decrease IOP by decreasing aqueous production. Oral carbonic anhydrase inhibitors are not commonly used today because effective topical medications are available. They are typically used on a short-term basis to achieve IOP control in acute or refractory cases. Side effects can include aplastic anemia, kidney stones, bitter taste, indigestion, paresthesia of the extremities, tinnitus, and polyuria. Clinicians need to consider the possibility of hypokalemia when patients take other diuretics to control blood pressure (Table 2). Acetazolamide may also be given intravenously.

Laser Trabeculoplasty

Argon or selective laser trabeculoplasty can be used to increase aqueous outflow. Laser trabeculoplasty is noninvasive and safe, and it can be performed in the office in less than 10 minutes. Compared to surgery, IOP reduction is limited, up to 25% as primary treatment, but less as an adjunct modality. It is ineffective or less effective in some patients with light trabecular meshwork pigmentation. The effect of laser decreases over time but may be repeated in the case of selective laser trabeculoplasty.

Surgery

The most commonly performed glaucoma surgeries are trabeculectomy, tube shunt, and cyclodestruction. Trabeculectomy and tube shunt are procedures that create an opening in the sclera to increase aqueous outflow. Cyclodestruction destroys the ciliary body and decreases aqueous production. The procedure can be transscleral or endoscopic; the endoscopic method is typically done at the time of cataract surgery. Alternative surgical methods such as deep sclerectomy, Trabectome, canaloplasty, iStent, Kahook dual blade, and Hydrus are performed at the time of cataract surgery to minimize the invasiveness and potential complications associated with traditional glaucoma surgery. However, these minimally invasive glaucoma surgeries (MIGS) are not as effective at lowering the IOP.

Visual Impairment and Blindness

Patients who are visually impaired (Snellen vision of <20/40) or legally blind (Snellen vision of <20/200 or visual field of <20 degrees) may have significantly decreased mobility and ability to function. Continued glaucoma treatment is still important in these patients because even maintenance of count-finger vision can allow the patients some degree of independence. Low-vision devices and services, including high-contrast video magnifiers, audiobooks, eccentric viewers, and mobility training, can allow patients maximal use of their residual vision and improve their confidence and quality of life.

Acute Angle Closure Glaucoma

Pupillary block in susceptible patients blocks aqueous drainage and leads to sudden and extreme rise of intraocular pressure.

Acute angle closure can damage the optic nerve, resulting in acute angle closure glaucoma.

About 0.5% to 1.0% of US adults are at risk for acute angle closure. It is more common in Inuits and Asians and rare in African Americans. The risk of acute angle closure increases with age. It is also more common in hyperopes (farsightedness).

Mechanism of Acute Angle Closure: Pupillary Block

After aqueous is produced in the ciliary body in the posterior chamber, it travels through the pupil and exits the anterior chamber through the trabecular meshwork located between the iris and the cornea. Pupillary block occurs when the iris contacts the lens and obstructs the flow of aqueous through the pupil. Increased posterior chamber pressure displaces the iris anteriorly against the trabecular meshwork and stops aqueous outflow.

Patients at risk for acute angle closure have narrow occludable angles. These patients have smaller eyes, allowing the lens to contact the iris to initiate papillary block. The distance between the iris and the lens is the shortest when the pupil is mid-dilated. Therefore, patients who present with acute angle closure might have a history of dim light exposure (movies) or use of medications with anticholinergic properties (antihistamines, decongestants, antispasmodics). High IOP causes iris and corneal endothelial cell dysfunction, resulting in nonreactive pupil and hazy cornea, respectively. High IOP also results in inflammation and red eye, as well as severe pain, nausea, and vomiting (Figure 2). Elevated IOP can damage the optic nerve within hours, and acute angle closure needs to be treated on an emergency basis to prevent permanent loss of vision.

Diagnosis

Patients with acute angle closure can present with blurry vision, red eye, pain, headache, nausea, or vomiting. History can include hyperopia, onset after exposure to a dim environment, or taking anticholinergic medications. Examination findings include decreased vision, conjunctival hyperemia, mid-dilated, nonreactive pupil with or without an afferent papillary defect, and increased IOP (by palpation or tonometry). Acute angle closure is sometimes misdiagnosed as migraines or gastrointestinal illness. Patients with conjunctivitis, keratitis, uveitis, and corneal abrasion can also present with the same symptoms.

Treatment

If acute angle closure is suspected, an emergent referral to ophthalmology is indicated. If an ophthalmologist is not immediately available, the goal will be to medically control the IOP as soon as possible. One drop of topical aqueous suppressant—β-blocker, selective α2 agonist, or carbonic anhydrase inhibitor—should be administered (timolol, brimonidine, and dorzolamide) (see Table 1). The maximum dose of oral or intravenous carbonic anhydrase inhibitor is given: acetazolamide 500 mg or methazolamide 50 mg (see Table 2). The patient is placed in the supine position to allow the lens and iris to fall posteriorly. The patient is reassessed in 30 minutes, and if the condition is not improved, topical drops are repeated. If there is no improvement after another 30 minutes, a hyperosmotic, oral glycerin[1] 1 g/kg or intravenous mannitol (Osmitrol) 1 g/kg over 30 minutes, is administered. Hyperosmotics may be contraindicated in patients with congestive heart failure, and glycerin can cause severe hyperglycemia in diabetic patients.

An ophthalmologist can break the pupillary block by medically lowering the IOP or by performing anterior chamber paracentesis, compression gonioscopy, laser peripheral iridotomy, and, in recalcitrant cases, emergent trabeculectomy. Once the pressure is controlled, it is important to perform an iridotomy in both eyes to prevent future episodes. Patients with patent iridotomies may safely take anticholinergic medications.

---

[1]Not FDA approved for this indication.

References

Allingham RR, Damji KF, Freedman S, et al: *Shield's Textbook of Glaucoma*, ed 5th, Philadelphia, 2005, Lippincott Williams & Wilkins, pp 155–190.

American Academy of Ophthalmology: Available at: Practice guidelines. Preferred practice patterns. Primary angle closure. http://www.aao.org/preferred-practice-pattern/primary-angle-closure-ppp–october-2010, October 2010. Accessed 10 July 2015.

American Academy of Ophthalmology: Practice guidelines. Preferred practice patterns. Primary open-angle glaucoma, September 2005. Available at: http://www.aao.org/preferred-practice-pattern/primary-openangle-glaucoma-ppp–october-2010 October 2010 [accessed July 10, 2105].

Congdon N, O'Colmain B, Klaver CC, et al: Eye Diseases Prevalence Research Group; Causes and prevalence of visual impairment among adults in the United States, *Arch Ophthalmol* 122:477–485, 2004.

Friedman DS, Wolfs RC, O'Colmain BJ, et al: Eye Diseases Prevalence Research Group: Prevalence of open-angle glaucoma among adults in the United States, *Arch Ophthalmol* 122(4):532–538, 2004.

Lin AP, Orengo-Nania S, Braun UK: PCP's role in chronic open-angle glaucoma, *Geriatrics* 64:20–28, 2009.

Nordstrom BL, Friedman DS, Mozaffari E, et al: Persistence and adherence with topical glaucoma therapy, *Am J Ophthalmol* 140:598–606, 2005.

Schwartz GF, Quigley HA: Adherence and persistence with glaucoma therapy, *Surv Ophthalmol* 54:S57–S68, 2008.

US Preventive Services Task Force: Screening for glaucoma, Available at: http://www.us preventiveservicestaskforce.org/Page/Topic/recommendation-summary/glaucoma-screening; March, 2005 October 2013 [accessed July 10, 2015].

MÉNIÈRE'S DISEASE

Method of
Terry D. Fife, MD

CURRENT DIAGNOSIS

- Ménière's disease is characterized by recurrent attacks of severe vertigo, nausea, and vomiting typically lasting 1 to 6 hours.
- Ménière's disease causes tinnitus on the side of the affected ear; the tinnitus can change in pitch and loudness during attacks of vertigo.
- Attacks of vertigo are associated with reduced or muffled hearing on the side of the affected ear.
- Fluctuating unilateral hearing loss and low-frequency hearing loss on the side of the affected ear is characteristic.

CURRENT THERAPY

- Initial therapy includes a sodium-restricted diet (preferably <1500 mg of sodium daily) and a diuretic agent (e.g., thiazide diuretics).
- Betahistine,[1] a medication widely used in Europe that may be obtained at compounding pharmacies in the United States, may be helpful in selected patients at a dosage 16 to 24 mg three times daily though some authors have recommended even higher dosages.
- Transtympanic infusion of gentamicin[1] or corticosteroids and endolymphatic sac surgery may be considered as minimally invasive options in patients with serviceable hearing. Gentamicin poses a moderate risk of inducing hearing loss.
- Vestibular nerve sectioning is highly effective in stopping vertigo attacks with a reasonably low risk of causing further hearing loss, but it is a more invasive procedure.
- Labyrinthectomy is highly effective in stopping vertigo attacks but causes complete hearing loss, so it is only an option for patients who have already lost all useful hearing.

Patients who have undergone procedures that cause acute loss of vestibular function often have vertigo for a while after the surgery; the vertigo improves more quickly with vestibular rehabilitative therapy.[1]

---

[1]Not FDA approved for this indication.

Ménière's disease is a disorder of the inner ear that results in recurrent, spontaneous episodes of vertigo, hearing loss, ear fullness, and tinnitus affecting the same ear. The hearing loss often fluctuates early in Ménière's disease, but fluctuating hearing is not always present. Eventually permanent hearing loss occurs, affecting the low frequencies initially but ultimately affecting all frequencies.

Epidemiology

The reported prevalence of Ménière's disease varies from about 50 to 200 per 100,000. Females are somewhat more prone to Meniere's disease than males, with a female/male ratio of about 1.9:1.

Risk Factors

Possible risk factors for later development of Ménière's syndrome include autoimmune disorders, migraine, syphilitic otitis and viral infection of the inner ear, head trauma, and a family history of Ménière's disease.

Pathophysiology

The underlying mechanism is generally thought to be due to endolymphatic hydrops, a type of swelling of the endolymphatic compartment that ultimately leads to permanent damage of the inner ear structures. Possible reasons for this periodic swelling of the endolymph compartment include mechanical obstruction of endolymph flow or at least dysregulation of the electrochemical membrane potential between endolymph and perilymph compartments.

Endolymphatic hydrops appears to be the mechanism for a number of conditions that can lead to Ménière's syndrome. When no primary cause is identified, the idiopathic form of the syndrome is called Ménière's disease. When an underlying cause is found, it is referred to as Ménière's syndrome or secondary Ménière's or secondary endolymphatic hydrops. Secondary Ménière's syndrome can result from delayed endolymphatic hydrops in which symptoms come on years after a prior disorder or viral injury of the labyrinth, syphilitic otitis, autoimmune inner ear disease, and trauma.

Prevention

There is no known way of preventing the development of Ménière's disease because it occurs in many people with no risk factors.

Clinical Manifestations

Ménière's disease can manifest with periodic unilateral (or, less commonly, bilateral) hearing loss or isolated attacks of vertigo. Not uncommonly, Ménière's disease has both elements present at its onset, but the vertigo is usually the symptom that gets the most attention. Vertigo usually lasts 1 to 6 hours but can last as little as 30 minutes or as long as all day. Patients prone to motion sickness often report that their dizziness lasts longer because the aftereffect of vertigo lingers longer in those who are motion sensitive. Vertigo attacks in Ménière's disease are often quite severe and generally render patients unable to move around owing to the vertigo, nausea, and recurrent vomiting.

The hearing loss is usually unilateral, and patients might notice fluctuation in hearing accompanied by ear fullness and a low-pitched roaring tinnitus either before or coincident with the vertigo. If audiometry can be performed during this time, low-frequency (250–1000 Hz) hearing loss may be documented and might improve after the attack ceases. This signature fluctuating low-frequency sensorineural hearing loss is very helpful (Figure 1) when found, but getting patients with vertigo attacks in for testing while they are in the acute stage of vertigo is usually not feasible.

Occasionally, patients with Ménière's have sudden random drop attacks in which they abruptly fall without loss of consciousness. These spells, referred to as otolithic crises of Tumarkin, can lead to serious injury and should prompt aggressive treatment.

RIGHT-SIDED MÉNIÈRE'S DISEASE

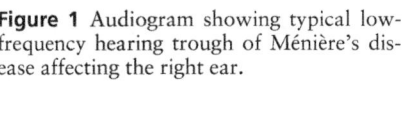

The mechanism is presumed to be related to sudden mechanical deformation or sudden neural discharges related to the otolith structures of the inner ear. Because there is no specific treatment for Tumarkin crises, treatment entails the standard treatments for Ménière's disease in general.

As Ménière's disease progresses, usually over months to years, permanent low-frequency hearing loss develops that gives way to hearing loss at all frequencies. Eventually, the patient can lose all or most hearing on the affected side. Meanwhile, with each vertigo attack, some vestibular function is lost, and so as vertigo attacks continue, vestibular loss ensues, often paralleling the hearing loss. Ménière's occasionally burns out, meaning that enough vestibular function has been lost that acute hydrops no longer produces vertigo. Patients might report less severe dizziness or just a vague feeling of unsteadiness. This usually indicates advanced Ménière's, and unilateral hearing and vestibular loss should be expected.

Bilateral Ménière's disease is present at the time of initial diagnosis in about 10% of cases and by 10 years of symptoms, about 35% have bilateral involvement. Bilateral Ménière's disease has treatment implications because treating one side alone will be unlikely to stop the vertigo attacks, which could be emanating from the untreated side. Surgical treatment of both sides is also problematic because it could leave the patient with bilateral hearing loss, vestibular loss, or both.

Diagnosis

The diagnosis of Ménière's disease is made clinically based on unilateral hearing loss, tinnitus, ear fullness, and episodic vertigo typically lasting 1 to 6 hours. The criteria for definite, probable, and possible Ménière's disease are listed in Box 1. Several recent studies using three-dimensional fluid-attenuated inversion recovery (3D-FLAIR) 24 hours after administration of bilateral intratympanic gadolinium (Gd) injection and similar techniques have demonstrated abnormalities consistent with endolymphatic hydrops. MRI at this point, however, is not yet established as useful in affirming the diagnosis of Ménière's disease.

Differential Diagnosis

Vestibular neuritis causes a single attack of vertigo, sometimes with acute hearing loss (labyrinthitis), but it can usually be distinguished from Ménière's disease because vestibular neuritis has a lifetime recurrence rate of only 2%, whereas Ménière's vertigo attacks recur multiple times and cause fluctuating and gradual decline in hearing.

| **BOX 1** | Diagnostic Criteria for Ménière's Disease |

Definite Ménière's Disease
- Two or more spontaneous (non-positional) episodes of vertigo, each lasting 20 minutes to 12 hours
- Audiometrically documented low- to medium-frequency sensorineural hearing loss in the affected ear on at least one occasion before, during, or after one of the episodes of vertigo.
- Fluctuating hearing, tinnitus or ear fullness in the affected ear.
- Not better accounted for by another vestibular diagnosis.

Probable Ménière's Disease
- Two or more episodes of vertigo or dizziness, each lasting 20 minutes to 24 hours
- Fluctuating hearing, tinnitus or ear fullness in the affected ear.
- Not better accounted for by another vestibular diagnosis.

(From Lopez-Escamez JA, et al. Diagnostic criteria for Ménière's disease. J Vestib Res. 2015;25(1):1–7.)

When a patient reports episodic vertigo attacks in the absence of unilateral tinnitus, ear fullness, and hearing loss, one must be cautious in diagnosing Ménière's disease because vestibular migraine (basilar-type migraine) can produce a similar pattern. Diagnostic criteria have been published for vestibular migraine (Lempert, 2013).

Benign paroxysmal positional vertigo causes brief recurrent spells of spinning without hearing loss, so it is rarely confused with Ménière's disease.

Vertebrobasilar insufficiency can cause isolated vertigo, but the duration is usually only several minutes and without hearing loss, whereas Ménière's attacks last hours and are associated with unilateral auditory symptoms.

Acoustic neuroma (vestibular schwannoma) typically leads to slowly progressive unilateral sensorineural hearing loss, but vertigo is infrequently a prominent feature because patients compensate gradually as their vestibular function wanes due to compressive effects of the tumor.

Fluctuating unilateral hearing loss, ear fullness, and tinnitus can occur without vertigo and is referred to as cochlear hydrops. Such symptoms can precede the development of vertigo but may be treated as Ménière's nonetheless. Lermoyez's syndrome refers to transiently improved hearing and tinnitus during attacks of vertigo. More commonly, however, hearing declines around and during vertigo spells.

Treatment
Medical Management
Treatment of Ménière's disease is mainly aimed at preventing the vertigo attacks, but no treatments are known that reliably restore or arrest hearing loss or tinnitus. It is presumed that if attacks of vertigo, ear fullness, fluctuating hearing, and tinnitus are all stopped, hearing should stabilize, but this is still a supposition. The management of Ménière's is hierarchical, starting with a low-sodium diet and a diuretic and proceeding to more-invasive or destructive surgical procedures only when initial medical treatment fails. When a patient has very frequent vertigo attacks and is disabled, more-aggressive treatment may be considered sooner.

Dietary sodium should be restricted to 1000 to 1500 mg daily. The average person consumes about 4000 mg daily, and the maximum recommended daily intake of sodium is 2300 mg. Because more than 70% of the daily sodium comes from processed foods, this dietary restriction generally requires more than simply stopping the use of table salt, which generally accounts for only about 10% of daily sodium intake for most people.

A diuretic is usually added to the sodium restriction. The most commonly prescribed diuretic is hydrochlorothiazide 25 mg combined with triamterene 37.5 mg (Dyazide)[1] because this combination usually obviates the need for potassium supplementation. Acetazolamide (Diamox)[1] 125 to 250 mg bid or furosemide (Lasix)[1] 10 to 20 mg daily are also options. Patients with severe sulfa allergy can use low-dose ethacrynic acid (Edecrin)[1] 12.5 to 25 mg daily.

An acute attack of vertigo from Ménière's disease can be managed with vestibular suppressants such as dimenhydrinate (Dramamine)[1] 50 mg, meclizine (Antivert) 25 to 50 mg, diazepam (Valium)[2] 2 to 5 mg, or promethazine (Phenergen)[1] 12.5 to 50 mg. Scopolamine in patch form (Transderm-Scōp)[1] is too slow to be useful because it takes hours to be absorbed transdermally. Scopace (oral scopolamine) has been discontinued and is no longer being manufactured in the United States. Scopolamine tablets[1] may be available in certain compounding pharmacies. Nausea can additionally be managed with prochlorperazine (Compazine) 10 mg orally or 25 mg by suppository, with oral or sublingual ondansetron (Zofran)[1] 4 to 8 mg, or with other antiemetics. Generally, the vertigo attacks subside in several hours even without treatment.

Betahistine (Serc)[2] may also be helpful in Ménière's, although it is not commonly used in the United States. The role of betahistine is not firmly established, although it is widely prescribed for vertigo throughout the world. Betahistine may be helpful when successful medical management with diet and diuretics has helped but is inadequate to stop attacks. Betahistine is a vasodilator, a modest H_1 histamine agonist, and a powerful H_3 histamine receptor antagonist. Its method of action in Ménière's is unknown, though it increases blood flow and might also influence endolymphatic fluid regulation and receptors in the endolymphatic sac. Doses of betahistine may start at 8 mg PO three times daily and may be increased to 32 mg three times daily. It is available outside the United States in the form of Serc® and Vertin® (Trade-marks of Abbott Products). Betahistine may be made within the United States at compounding pharmacies with a physician prescription[1] and may also be imported from outside the United States for individual use. Side effects are few, though occasionally patients report some headache. Betahistine is not histamine, and we have not found it to cause or aggravate urticaria.

Oral corticosteroids are often used but rarely seem effective except in cases of bilateral Ménière's resulting from autoimmune inner ear disease (AIED). Oral corticosteroids rarely seem to be effective in typical Ménière's disease.

Ménière's attacks have been said to be triggered by caffeine, chocolate, stress, visual stimuli, and dropping barometric pressure. Such triggers should be avoided when possible, but strong associations with these triggers can also occur in migrainous vertigo. Vestibular rehabilitative therapy is not generally helpful in Ménière's because most vertigo attacks remit and the patients have few vestibular symptoms between attacks. However, when vestibular loss has occurred and the patient appears to have not compensated well for it, vestibular rehabilitation can be helpful.

Bilateral Ménière's Disease
The estimated incidence of bilateral Ménière's disease varies in the literature but is estimated to occur in about 15% of cases and bilateral involvement increases over time. The possibility of bilateral involvement weighs on the decision making for any procedures that sacrifice hearing or vestibular function because it leaves the patient with only one functioning labyrinth.

Serviceability of Hearing
Serviceable hearing is residual hearing that can be useful to the patient by wearing hearing aids. In general, because hearing loss is permanent, one should avoid sacrificing any serviceable hearing.

Injections and Surgical Treatments
Patients who continue to have disabling vertigo despite a low-salt diet, diuretics, and possibly betahistine are considered to have failed conservative medical therapy. The next step in treatment depends on the age, health status, and residual hearing and vestibular function of the patient and also on the surgeon's opinion and experience with the various options. If spells are infrequent, symptomatic management of vertigo attacks may be the best option. Table 1 outlines some of the additional interventional options.

Intratympanic Gentamicin
Transtympanic gentamicin (Garamycin)[1] administration has become increasingly used as an effective treatment of Ménière's disease. This is partly due to the ease of administration of gentamicin and its relative safety. Gentamicin is a commonly used aminoglycoside antimicrobial agent with activity against gram-negative bacteria that also happens to be ototoxic. It damages hair cells of the labyrinth and preferentially affects hair cells of the vestibular neuroepithelium over that of the cochlea. Even so, transtympanic administration still has some risk of causing hearing loss. Gentamicin is administered by injecting a small amount (usually about 0.5 mL) of gentamicin sulfate (80 mg/2 mL) solution through the tympanic membrane into the middle ear space. To avoid rapid drainage through the eustachian tube, the injection is done with the patient supine and kept in that position for an hour or so to allow the gentamicin to absorb through the round window into the inner ear. There are many protocols, but commonly an injection is given once, and additional injections can be considered every 3 to 4 weeks until improvement in vertigo attacks is realized. Studies suggest that intratympanic gentamicin is an effective treatment for vertigo complaints in Ménière's disease but there is some risk of hearing loss.

Endolymphatic Sac Surgery
Another option for patients with residual functional hearing is endolymphatic sac shunt or decompression. This procedure eliminates vertigo in 50% to 75% of those treated. Nevertheless, its

---

[1] Not FDA approved for this indication.
[2] Not available in the United States.

---

[1] Not FDA approved for this indication.

TABLE 1 Procedures Used in the Management of Ménière's Disease

METHOD	TECHNIQUE	ADVANTAGES	DISADVANTAGES
Procedures Intended to Spare Serviceable Hearing			
Meniett device	Applies repetitive low-pressure pulses of air with the aim of enhancing endolymph drainage	Minimally invasive; no significant side effects and no risk of hearing loss	Requires tympanostomy tube placement; usually not covered by insurance; rate of effectiveness still unclear
Intratympatic corticosteroids	Injection of steroid through the tympanic membrane to the middle ear to be absorbed in the inner ear	Minimally invasive, few side effects	Effectiveness unclear when compared to placebo
Intratympanic gentamicin (Garamycin)[1]	Injection of gentamicin through the tympanic membrane to the middle ear to be absorbed in the inner ear	Simple office-based procedure, low risk profile	Number of injections is unpredictable; some risk of hearing loss
Endolymphatic mastoid shunt	Placing a shunt from the endolymphatic sac to the mastoid air cells	Effective in 50%–75% of cases; low risk of hearing loss; day procedure	Vertigo can recur; effectiveness depends on surgical experience and technique
Vestibular neurectomy	Surgical sectioning of the vestibular part of cranial nerve VIII, sparing the auditory part of the nerve	Highly effective in eliminating vertigo attacks	Requires general anesthesia; risk of facial weakness, hearing loss
Procedures Expected to Eliminate Residual Hearing			
Labyrinthectomy or cochleosacculotomy	Several methods of removing all or part of the labyrinth	Highly effective in stopping vertigo attacks	Inevitable complete hearing loss

[1]Not FDA approved for this indication.

effectiveness compared with placebo has remained a point of contention based on a number of studies. It has been suggested that the procedure's effectiveness depends on the operative technique and experience of the surgeon.

Intratympanic Steroids
Sometimes, a trial of intratympanic corticosteroids may be tried, although its effectiveness in controlled trials is still not compelling. Even so, a trial of corticosteroids administered in this manner poses little risk.

Vestibular Neurectomy
The most definitive procedure for stopping vertigo attacks in Ménière's when the goal is to preserve hearing is vestibular neurectomy. This procedure involves craniotomy and severing the vestibular nerve while preserving the cochlear nerve. This procedure requires overnight hospitalization and general anesthesia, and it does pose some risk to facial nerve function and hearing on the affected side.

Labyrinthectomy
For patients who have unilateral Ménière's disease and no serviceable hearing, labyrinthectomy is a commonly used procedure. This procedure entails the removal of the membranous labyrinth and is highly effective in stopping recurrent vertigo attacks from that ear. In elderly patients or those who are poor surgical candidates, a more limited transtympanic cochleosacculotomy may be performed.

Meniett Treatment
The Meniett device is a portable, low-frequency, pressure-wave delivery system that administers a wave of pressure of about 12 cm H_2O to the middle ear via a tympanostomy tube for about 0.6 seconds pulsed at 6 Hz for 5 minutes about three to five times daily. Quality randomized trials demonstrating the effectiveness of this treatment are few, and in at least one recent trial it was not better than patients treated medically. This method has few risks and only requires myringotomy and a pressure equalization tube. A practical limitation is the cost of the device, which is not often paid for by many health insurance companies.

Monitoring
Following patients with Ménière's disease should include monitoring of the frequency and severity of vertigo spells and the fluctuation in hearing, ear fullness, and tinnitus. Periodic audiometry is probably the most sensitive measure of stabilization of the condition. Vestibular testing may be considered when changes might alter the treatment strategy. Brain imaging is only helpful in excluding other disorders, but does not yet have a role in the management of Ménière's disease.

Complications
Known complications include the progression of unilateral and occasionally bilateral hearing and vestibular function. There may also be complications associated with some of the treatments as described earlier. Owing to the unpredictability of the vertigo attacks, many patients avoid certain activities and might even develop agoraphobic features because the attacks are so severe and disruptive. In most cases, these avoidance behaviors improve if Ménière's disease can be controlled.

Conclusion
The management of Ménière's disease is still part art and part science. Treatment options are many, but patients should be reassured that, in most cases, something can be offered to help improve their vertigo and quality of life.

References
Russo FY, Nguyen Y, De Seta D, et al: Meniett device in meniere disease: Randomized, double-blind, placebo-controlled multicenter trial, *Laryngoscope* 127:470–475, 2017.

Lempert T: Vestibular migraine, *Semin Neurol* 33:212–218, 2013.

Lopez-Escamez JA, et al: Diagnostic criteria for Ménière's disease, *J Vestib Res* 25(1):1–7, 2015.

Nevoux J, Franco-Vidal V, Bouccara D, et al: Diagnostic and therapeutic strategy in Ménière's disease. Guidelines of the French Otorhinolaryngology-Head and Neck Surgery Society (SFORL), *Eur Ann Otorhinolaryngol Head Neck Dis*, 134(6):441–444, 2017.

Phillips JS, Westerberg B: Intratympanic steroids for Ménière's disease or syndrome, *Cochrane Database Syst Rev*(7), 2011. https://doi.org/10.1002/14651858.CD008514.pub2. CD008514.

Pullens B, van Benthem PP: Intratympanic gentamicin for Ménière's disease or syndrome, *Cochrane Database Syst Rev*(3), 2011. https://doi.org/10.1002/14651858.CD008234.pub2. CD008234.

Pullens B, Verschuur HP, van Benthem PP: Surgery for Ménière's disease, *Cochrane Database Syst Rev* 28(2), 2013. CD005395.

OTITIS EXTERNA

Method of
Kimberly Williams, MD

CURRENT DIAGNOSIS

- Pain, itching, or fullness of the ear
- Tenderness of tragus, pinna, or both
- Onset <48 h
- Physical examination findings of erythema, edema, ± drainage and debris

CURRENT THERAPY

- Aural toilet
- Topical antimicrobials
- Analgesic treatment

Otitis externa is an inflammation of the ear canal and can be either acute or chronic. It is often called swimmer's ear.

Epidemiology

Acute otitis externa is a common problem seen in the primary care office. The annual incidence falls between 1:100 and 1:250 with a lifetime incidence approaching 10%. Peak incidence is in children 7 to 12 years old. It does appear to have a genetic link, because it occurs more often in people with blood group type A. Chronic otitis externa affects 3% to 5% of the population.

Risk Factors

Otitis externa is more common in warmer climates with high humidity. Increased water exposure, especially from swimming, places a person at higher risk. Other risk factors include debris from dermatologic conditions such as psoriasis, trauma due to use of hearing aids and ear plugs and abrasions from cleaning of the ear canal. Cerumen helps prevent microbial growth by providing an acidic pH; when cerumen is removed in cleaning, an environment ready for microbial growth is set up.

Pathophysiology

Approximately 95% of acute otitis externa is due to bacterial infection (Figure 1). The other 5% can be attributed to fungal infections or, less commonly, herpes zoster. Fungal infection is more common in chronic otitis externa. Of the bacterial infections, 20% to 60% are due to *Pseudomonas aeruginosa. Staphylococcus aureus* is the next major causative organism. Gram-negative organisms account for 2% to 3% of bacterial infections.

Prevention

Prevention is aimed at avoiding water accumulation and retention in the ear canal. Using ear plugs while swimming and using a hair dryer to dry the ear canal after water exposure can be beneficial. The use of acidifying eardrops, such as acetic acid 2% (Vosol), before and after swimming can also help prevent otitis externa. Other preventive measures include stopping the removal of cerumen and avoiding trauma to the ear canal. Finally, proper treatment of dermatologic conditions such as eczema and psoriasis can help reduce debris that can be a risk factor for infection.

Clinical Manifestations

Otitis externa usually develops rapidly over 1 to 2 days. Most patients complain of a feeling of ear pain, fullness, or itching. Hearing loss may be another symptom. Key physical examination findings include tenderness on palpation of the tragus, discomfort with traction on the pinna, edema of the ear canal, and erythema

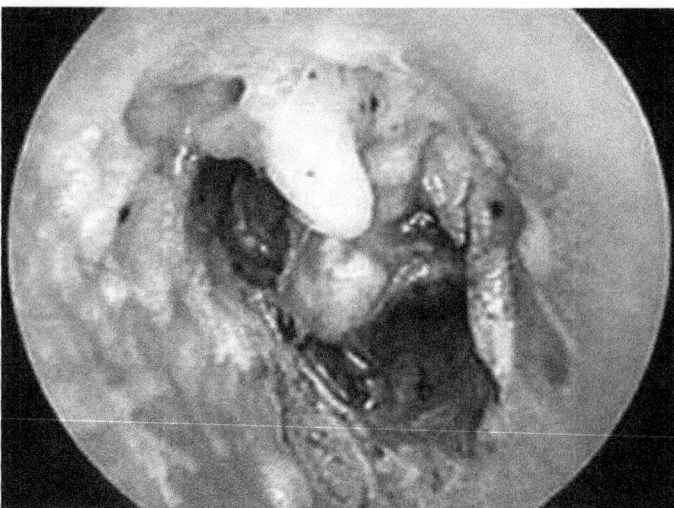

Figure 1 Acute otitis externa with the canal somewhat narrowed from edema and obstructed by desquamating epithelium, soft cerumen, and purulent discharge; this must be removed to visualize the tympanic membrane and to allow ototopical therapy to penetrate to all the superficially infected areas of the canal skin. (Reprinted with permission from Osguthorpe JD, Nielsen DR. Otitis externa: review and clinical update. *Am Family Physician.* 2006;76:9.)

of the canal. Pain may be out of proportion to examination findings. Regional lymphadenitis and cellulitis of the pinna and adjacent skin can also be present.

Diagnosis

The diagnosis of otitis externa is made clinically by history and physical examination. The history should be positive for otalgia, itching, or sense of fullness. The exam should be positive for tenderness if the tragus is palpated or if the pinna is pulled up and out. If the cause is bacterial, purulent drainage is usually present. Otoscopy will show diffuse canal edema, usually present with erythema. Often there will be copious amounts of debris. Debris should be cleared to visualize the tympanic membrane. There should be good mobility of the tympanic membrane and the tympanometry curve will be normal unless there is concomitant acute otitis media.

Differential Diagnosis

Middle ear disease should be distinguished from external disease by ensuring that the tympanic membrane is normal. Acute otitis media with perforation of the tympanic membrane may result in purulent middle ear secretions into the external ear canal. Contact dermatitis of the ear canal can mimic otitis externa, and a thorough history of exposure to metals such as nickel and copper, chemicals such as new soaps, topical antibiotics, detergents, cosmetics, and other irritants should be obtained. Fungal infection of the ear canal can mimic bacterial otitis externa. Fungus tends to infect the medial portion of the ear canal and has spores and filaments that can be seen both macroscopically and microscopically. Also in the differential are carcinoma of the external auditory canal, which mimics chronic infection; herpes, which is rare and forms vesicles on the outer ear canal; and radiation therapy.

Therapy

Topical therapy is the treatment of choice in mild to moderate disease in healthy patients. The choice of topical agent is based on cost, ease of administration, and risk of side effects (Table 1). Topical aminoglycoside and fluoroquinolone antibiotics have a response rate of more than 70%. If there is a perforation of the tympanic membrane, ciprofloxacin topical solutions are preferred because of the risk of ototoxicity from aminoglycosides and neomycin. Using a topical steroid in conjunction with topical antibiotic therapy has been shown to shorten duration of ear pain. Duration of topical therapy should be 7 to 10 days.

TABLE 1	Topical Otic Preparations for Treatment of Otitis Externa.			
ACTIVE DRUGE	**BRAND NAME**	**DOSING**	**COMMENTS**
Acetic acid 2% solution with steroid	Vosol HC, Acetasol HC	q4–6h	Can sting/local irritation
Ciprofloxacin/hydrocortisone	Cipro HC	q12h	Approved if tympanic membrane is perforated
Ciprofloxacin/dexamethasone	Ciprodex	q12h	Approved if tympanic membrane is perforated
Neomycin, polymyxin B, hydrocortisone	Cortisporin Otic	q6h	Neomycin can cause local irritation, ototoxic potential
Ofloxacin	Floxin Otic	q24h	Can cause local irritation
Tobramycin[1]	Tobrex	q6h	Minimally irritating, ophthalmic preparation, ototoxic potential
Gentamycin[1]	Garamycin	q6h	Ophthalmic preparation, ototoxic potential

[1]Not FDA approved for this indication.

Clotrimazole 1%[1] may be used for superficial fungal infections of the ear canal.

For the topical therapy to be effective, it must be delivered to the tissue of the ear canal. First, the canal must be cleared of debris. This can be done in the physician's office under direct visualization or with lavage of the ear canal using saline or hydrogen peroxide warmed to body temperature. The patient should then be instructed on the proper delivery of the eardrops. Eardrops are administered more effectively if another person delivers the drops. The patient should lie on his or her side with the affected ear up, and drops should be placed in the ear canal until it is filled. The patient should remain on his or her side for 3 to 5 minutes. If greater than 50% of the canal is edematous, a wick made of cellulose material should be placed to facilitate delivery of the drops. The wick may fall out or can be removed by either patient or clinician once the edema has resolved.

Systemic therapy should be used in patients who are immune compromised, including those with diabetes, and in patients with surrounding cellulitis. The systemic therapy chosen should be effective against pseudomonas.

Adequate pain control is another important factor in the treatment of otitis externa. Often this can be achieved with nonsteroidal antiinflammatory medications, but opioid analgesics may be necessary, especially to remove debris. Analgesics should be used early in treatment of the disease.

Monitoring

Patients should respond to therapy in 48 to 72 hours. If therapy fails, the clinician should evaluate adherence to therapy and ability of the drug to be delivered properly. Alternative diagnoses should be considered, including fungal infections, dermatitis, foreign bodies, and middle ear disease with perforation of the tympanic membrane. If the infection has spread outside of the ear canal, systemic therapy should be started.

Complications

One complication of simple otitis externa is malignant otitis externa, an invasive infection of the external auditory canal causing osteomyelitis of the temporal bone. It most commonly occurs in elderly diabetic patients or the immunocompromised. Complications include meningitis, dural sinus thrombosis, cranial abscess, and cranial nerve neuropathy including facial nerve paralysis. Diagnosis may require computed tomography and cultures. Treatment includes systemic antipseudomonal antibiotics and surgical débridement. Contact dermatitis from the topical antimicrobials prescribed for otitis externa may also complicate treatment. This is due to a delayed-type hypersensitivity reaction to one or more of the components of the topical therapy. Neomycin is the most common cause, but hypersensitivity reactions can also occur from other agents including preservatives and fragrances. The reaction is characterized by pruritus, edema, and inflammation of the skin in the auditory canal. It can spread beyond the canal to the pinna and even the skin of the neck. This is treated with topical steroids and by stopping the offending agent.

OTITIS MEDIA

Method of
Gretchen M. Irwin, MD, MBA

CURRENT DIAGNOSIS

- History of acute onset of symptoms
- Middle ear effusion
  - Bulging tympanic membrane
  - Limited mobility of tympanic membrane or air fluid level visible behind tympanic membrane
- Middle ear inflammation
  - Erythema of tympanic membrane or distinct otalgia

CURRENT THERAPY

- Watchful Waiting—appropriate for children:
  - i. Greater than 2 years of age with nonsevere illness
  - ii. Greater than 6 months of age with uncertain diagnosis and nonsevere illness
  - iii. Greater than 2 years of age with severe illness, but uncertain diagnosis
  - Need close follow-up in 48 hours
  - Consider delayed prescription
- Antibiotics
  - First line should be amoxicillin (Amoxil) 80 to 90 mg/kg/day[3]
  - Treat 10 days if child less than 6 years of age, 5 to 7 days if greater than 6 years of age
  - Follow-up if not improving in 48 hours
- Analgesia
  - Acetaminophen (Tylenol), ibuprofen (Motrin, Advil)
  - Benzocaine in combination with antipyrine (Allergen, Auroguard), benzocaine with antipyrine and acetic acid (Auralgan)

---

[1] Not US Food and Drug Administration approved for this indication.

- Antihistamines and decongestants are of no benefit
- Surgery—consider tympanostomy tubes when:
  i. First AOM episode at less than 6 months of age and child with 2 or more episodes in 6 months or 3 in 24 months
  ii. First AOM episode at more than 12 months of age and child with 3 episodes in 6 months, 5 episodes in 12 months or 7 episodes in 24 months

[3]Exceeds dosage recommended by the manufacturer.

Epidemiology

Acute otitis media (AOM) is a common condition of childhood, with one in four children having at least one episode of AOM by age 10. In fact, 86% of children will have at least one episode of AOM within the first year of life. Younger children are more likely to be affected, with peak incidence noted between ages 6 and 20 months likely because of the relative immaturity of the immune system and eustachian tube function. On average, 5 billion dollars are spent per year on office visits, lost productivity, and diminished parental quality of life due to AOM infections. As a result, research has focused on effective strategies both to prevent episodes of AOM and also to efficiently treat episodes that do occur.

Risk Factors

Identifying children at risk for AOM has been an important strategy to attempt to limit instances of AOM. Unfortunately, many of the risk factors associated with AOM are not modifiable, including male sex, Native American ethnicity, presence of siblings within the home, and a family history of recurrent AOM. Additional risk factors include low socioeconomic status, premature birth, attendance at out-of-home daycare, lack of breastfeeding, and history of poor maternal health during pregnancy. Limited studies have suggested that interventions such as avoiding supine feeding or bottle propping, reducing pacifier use after the first 6 months of life, and eliminating passive tobacco exposure can help to reduce incidence; however, the evidence in which these interventions demonstrate clear impact is limited. Public health programs that encourage breastfeeding and optimal maternal health during pregnancy, as well as those focused on reducing tobacco use, have perhaps the best opportunity to impact AOM incidence rates.

Not only are these identified risk factors for any episode of AOM, but children with these characteristics are also more likely to have recurrent AOM. Although many children will be affected in their lifetimes, those with recurrent disease are most at risk of complications leading to morbidity or mortality. Other risk factors specifically for recurrent AOM include an early onset of first episode and low parental education.

Pathophysiology

AOM has classically been associated with three bacteria; namely, Streptococcus pneumoniae, Moraxalla catarrhalis, and Haemophillus influenzae. Using data derived from middle-ear fluid analysis, M catarrhalis is responsible for only 3% to 20% of AOM, whereas pneumoniae and H influenzae are more common contributors at 25% to 50% and 15% to 30%, respectively.

The bacteria responsible for AOM become pathogenic in the setting of eustachian tube dysfunction. A relative obstruction of the eustachian tube develops most commonly secondary to secretions from an antecedent viral upper respiratory infection or allergies, but may result from neuromuscular conditions or abnormal anatomy. Such relative obstruction creates a negative pressure within the middle ear leading to serous effusion and secondary infection of this collection of interstitial fluid. Thus prevention of AOM is aimed at both reducing the presence of pathogenic bacteria and preventing upper respiratory infections that may create eustachian tube dysfunction.

Prevention

The successes of immunization programs in virtually eliminating childhood illnesses such as measles, polio, and varicella have led to great interest in the development of vaccines capable of eradicating the causative agents of AOM. Immunizations targeting the specific bacteria most commonly associated with AOM have had mixed success, however.

For example, although the serotypes contained in the 7-valent pneumococcal conjugate vaccine (PCV, Prevnar) are responsible for approximately 66% of pneumococcal-related AOM, only moderate effectiveness has been noted in reducing AOM incidence among vaccinated children. After the introduction of the 7-valent PCV into practice in February of 2000, AOM incidence decreased only 6% to 7% among vaccinated children. The 9-valent and 11-valent PCVs[2] have been shown to result in a risk reduction of S pneumoniae isolates in children with AOM of 17% and 34%, respectively. An increase in serotype 19A has been noted that is not covered in the 7-, 9-, or 11- valent PCVs[2] but is included in the new 13-valent PCV (Prevnar 13). The 13-valent PCV was incorporated into the recommended childhood immunization schedule in February 2010. The effect of this change on AOM rates will be interesting to observe.

Although the ability of the vaccine to prevent AOM episodes may be relatively small, recurrent disease has decreased 23% whereas the need for tympanostomy tubes has decreased nearly 25% in vaccinated children. Hence, the power of the vaccine may be in preventing recurrent disease requiring surgical intervention rather than in prevention of any AOM episodes.

Similar vaccines are in development for H influenzae and M catarrhalis as causative agents of AOM. The current H influenzae b vaccine, or Hib, has had little impact on AOM, because less than 5% of episodes are caused by the type b strain of Haemophilius. Instead non-typeable H influenzae is a much more common cause of AOM.

Although the vaccines targeting specific bacteria that have been shown to cause AOM have been successful, so too has the influenza vaccine been shown to impact the course of AOM. In several studies, children who received seasonal influenza vaccine (Fluzone) were found to have fewer episodes of AOM than unvaccinated children. Furthermore, those who did have an AOM episode were found to use fewer antibiotics and have shorter duration of middle-ear effusion compared with unvaccinated counterparts.

With evidence that reducing incidence of viral influenza may reduce the occurrence of secondary AOM, several other interventions aimed at reducing viral upper respiratory infection incidence have been studied for their impact on AOM rates. The use of zinc[7] and propolis[7] as agents to prevent viral upper respiratory infections, for instance, has been shown to have mixed benefit in reducing AOM in children. In multiple studies, zinc has been well tolerated with no contraindications to use identified. Zinc as a single agent has been shown to prevent AOM only when used in children under age 5 who are also malnourished. However, when combined with propolis, zinc was shown to be effective at reducing AOM episodes for children with a history of recurrent AOM. Of note, in several trials zinc did not reduce upper respiratory infection rates; rather, rates of secondary AOM alone were decreased. Although not necessarily effective as a preventive measure for all children, zinc and propolis may be an option for children with recurrent infection.

Similarly, probiotics[7] added to infant formula have been shown to be beneficial for some children. Although breastfeeding as compared to formula supplementation has been shown to be most beneficial in preventing AOM, infant formulas supplemented with Lactobacillus rhamnosus GG and Bifidobacterium lactis Bb-12 (Enfamil Premium, Nestle Good Start) were shown to reduce incidence of AOM over the first 7 months and the first 1 year. Children who received placebo formula had an incidence

---

[2] Not available in the United States.
[7] Available as a dietary supplement.

of AOM of 50% in the first 7 months, whereas children who received the probiotic-supplemented formula had an incidence of only 22%.

Dietary supplementation to limit AOM is not limited to infant formulas, however. Xylitol[7], a polyol sugar alcohol found in birch plants, plums, strawberries, and raspberries, has been demonstrated in several studies to be effective at preventing both dental caries and AOM, although its dosage forms make administration difficult. Xylitol is available as a chewing gum, which raises concern as a choking hazard in young children. Similarly, in its oral syrup form, xylitol must be administered five times daily to be effective. Studies of thrice-daily dosing have not been able to demonstrate the same preventive effect as dosing five times daily despite a consistent total daily dose of 10 grams per day. Furthermore, emerging evidence suggests that xylitol must be given daily to remain effective at reducing AOM episodes, because prophylaxis only during winter months or use only during upper respiratory tract infections is ineffective. Of note, children who have already received tympanostomy tubes receive no prevention benefit from xylitol administration. Research is ongoing to increase physician awareness of xylitol as a possible prophylactic measure because current studies suggest less than one half of US physicians are aware of xylitol and less than one fourth discuss or recommend its use to patients.

Echinacea[7] and osteopathic manipulation have also been cited as potential prophylactic treatments, particularly for children at high risk of recurrence. However, little evidence exists that either are effective. In fact, one large study demonstrated an increased risk of AOM with Echinacea use during an upper respiratory tract infection episode and no benefit to manipulation treatment. Ongoing studies are examining the use of these modalities.

Clinical Manifestations
AOM presents with a rapid onset of symptoms that may include fever, chills, ear pain, or ear pulling. In fact, ear pulling and ear rubbing have been demonstrated to be quite sensitive for the diagnosis of AOM in the setting of a history consistent with AOM and middle ear effusion. Often, symptoms may be preceded by upper respiratory symptoms such as rhinorrhea, cough, or congestion. Children who have had tympanostomy tubes placed will likely have a far different presentation, with fever and pain being quite unlikely; rather, a thin, yellow or milky discharge may be the only sign that AOM is present.

Diagnosis
The 2013 update of the guidelines of the American Academy of Pediatrics for the diagnosis and treatment of AOM acknowledged that no gold standard exists for the clinical diagnosis of AOM. History and physical examination should be consistent with rapid onset of inflammation in the middle ear. Both pneumatic otoscopy and tympanometry may be useful in the diagnosis of AOM. Tympanic membranes should be evaluated for position, mobility, color, and degree of translucency using pneumatic otoscopy to assess for presence of middle ear effusion or inflammation. Moderate to severe bulging of the tympanic membrane, new onset of otorrhea without other cause, or mild bulging of the tympanic membrane with intense erythema or ear pain should prompt diagnosis of AOM. Furthermore, tympanomtry may be useful in determining whether an effusion is present if the diagnosis is otherwise unclear.

One concern of physicians has been accurately diagnosing middle ear inflammation after a child has been vigorously crying. A study of 125 healthy children, age less than 30 months, assessed the impact of crying on tympanic membrane color by performing otoscopy both before and after administering at least two immunizations. While crying can cause a pinkening of the tympanic membrane, it should disappear when the child quiets and should be less intense than what is observed with inflammation. True middle ear inflammation results in an angry, red eardrum, not the milder, pink flush seen with vigorous crying. The presence of effusion should also help to support a diagnosis of inflammation.

Differential Diagnosis
Otitis media with effusion is often misdiagnosed as an episode of AOM. Like AOM, OME is common, with 2.2 million episodes annually representing an estimated cost of 4 billion dollars. OME can also occur with a viral upper respiratory infection and may follow or precede an episode of AOM. OME differs from AOM, however, because fluid may be present in the middle ear with OME, but there are no signs of acute infection.

Although OME is not associated with acute infection, it is nonetheless critical to diagnose, because research has demonstrated that chronic OME is associated with hearing loss and subsequent developmental delay. In fact, OME in infancy has been shown to be associated with, on average, a 7-point reduction in IQ at age 7.

The cornerstone of treatment for OME is observation for 2 to 3 months to allow the effusion to clear. Avoidance of allergens and tobacco exposure that may worsen eustachian tube dysfunction is also important. Decongestants and antihistamines are not effective. If an effusion does not clear within 2 months, a single course of amoxicillin (Amoxil) or penicillin may be given.

Audiometry should be performed in all children with OME for longer than 3 months or, in the setting of language delay, learning problems or suspected hearing loss in a child with OME. If the effusion persists, or if a child has multiple episodes of OME or has hearing or learning difficulties as a result of OME, surgical intervention should be considered.

Initial surgical intervention for children with persistent OME should be myringotomy with placement of tympanostomy tubes. Tonsillectomy and myringotomy alone are not indicated for treatment of OME. However, adenoidectomy may have a role, particularly in children ages 4 to 8 years. Current recommendations include adenoidectomy only if repeat surgery for OME is needed. However, emerging evidence suggests adenoidectomy may decrease the need for surgical retreatment, reduce ongoing hearing loss, and be of benefit during initial surgery for older children.

Treatment
The treatment of AOM has been controversial in recent years. Because it is the most common childhood bacterial infection for which antibiotics are prescribed worldwide, debate continues about both the most effective regimen and appropriate time to treat AOM. On average, 2.8 billion dollars are spent per year on antibiotics for episodes of AOM, yet emerging evidence suggests that watchful waiting is appropriate for some children. Judicious use of antibiotic therapy remains key in the prevention of morbidity and mortality associated with otitis media but is not an appropriate therapy for every child. All children require analgesia of some type, as well as close, scheduled follow-up, but use of observation or antibiotic varies with severity of illness and age of the child. Treatment options are summarized in Table 1.

Treatment Options: Observation
For some children with AOM, observation has been shown to be an appropriate therapy that avoids the possible side effects of antibiotics, with low risk of complications developing from an untreated otitis media. Evidence suggests that 78% of AOM episodes will spontaneously resolve within the first few days of infection. In fact, for every 100 otherwise healthy at-risk children with AOM, 80 will improve within 3 days without antibiotic therapy. If the same 100 children were all treated with amoxicillin or ampicillin, 92 would improve, although 3 to 10 would develop a rash and 5 to 10 would develop diarrhea. Thus, in a typical family medicine practice, 16 children with AOM would need to be treated with antibiotics to prevent 1 child from experiencing ongoing otalgia, whereas 1 of every 24 children treated will experience harm related to therapy. Hence, the use of antibiotics is not without risk. Multiple studies have demonstrated that even in children as young as 2 months of age, many will improve without antibiotic therapy, and delaying antibiotics may prevent undesirable side effects without exposing the child to undue risk. No studies have demonstrated a resurgence of either mastoiditis or meningitis with implementation of watchful waiting for AOM.

TABLE 1	Treatment Options for Acute Otitis Media					
	AOM WITH OTORRHEA		**AOM WITHOUT OTORRHEA**		**AOM WITH SEVERE SYMPTOMS***	
AGE OF CHILD	**UNILATERAL**	**BILATERAL**	**UNILATERAL**	**BILATERAL**	**UNILATERAL**	**BILATERAL**
6 months to 2 years	Antibiotics	Antibiotics	Antibiotics or observation	Antibiotics	Antibiotics	Antibiotics
>2 years	Antibiotics	Antibiotics	Antibiotics or observation	Antibiotics or observation	Antibiotics	Antibiotics

*Severe symptoms include toxic-appearing child, persistent otalgia for >48 hours, temperature >39°C in past 48 hours, or uncertain access to follow-up.

If observation is chosen as a management strategy for AOM, it is important to re-evaluate the child in 48 to 72 hours to ensure that they are improving and that a rescue antibiotic is prescribed if symptoms are not resolving. Delayed prescriptions are one strategy that has been effective at reducing antibiotic use, maintaining parental satisfaction, and improving healthcare efficiency.

Physicians are often concerned that parental satisfaction will decrease if watchful waiting for an episode of AOM is recommended. Interestingly, satisfaction has been tied to the receipt of an antibiotic prescription, though not necessarily the administration of antibiotics to the child. Declines in satisfaction are noted when parents are advised to return to care in 2 to 3 days if the child is not improving while undergoing watchful waiting. By offering a delayed prescription, the parent can avoid the difficulties associated with needing to be re-seen if the child fails to improve, and parental satisfaction is maintained even if the child never receives any medication. Parents should be educated that up to one third of children who initially are treated with observation will eventually need antibiotic therapy. Although this suggests up to two thirds of children can avoid unnecessary antibiotics, parents should be aware that many children will go on to need antibiotic therapy. Clearly, however, not every child is a candidate for observation therapy.

Treatment Options: Antibiotic Therapy

Antibiotic therapy may be associated with less duration of pain, less analgesic use, and less absence for both children and parents from school and work, respectively. The American Academy of Pediatrics and the American Academy of Family Physicians in a joint position statement have recommended that, when a decision is made to use antibiotics, amoxicillin (Amoxil) be given as a first-line agent at a dose of 80 to 90 mg/kg/day.[3] For penicillin-allergic children, cefdinir (Omnicef), cefpodoxime (Vantin), or cefuroxime (Ceftin) may be used. Although the cross-reactivity of cephalosporins and penicillins is likely lower than previously believed, if concern exists about treating a child with a cephalosporin, clindamycin (30–40mg/kg/day) may be used. Macrolide antibiotics may have limited efficacy. Ceftriaxone (Rocephin) may be used as a single dose for a child unable to tolerate oral medications.

Although amoxicillin continues to be the preferred first-line agent, 30% to 70% of S pneumoniae strains have become penicillin and macrolide resistant whereas 20% to 40% of H influenzae has beta-lacatamase–producing capabilities. Given the various resistance patterns of organisms, a child who fails to improve on amoxicillin should receive amoxicillin with clavulanate (Augmentin) or ceftriaxone as second-line therapy. Clindamycin (Cleocin) or tympanocentesis to identify a causative organism may also be considered.

Current evidence continues to suggest that a 10-day course is optimal for children younger than age 2 years. Less benefit to longer-duration therapy is noted in older children, and therefore a shorter 5- to 7-day course is recommended for those older than 2 years.

If a child has a perforation of the tympanic membrane, treatment considerations may be slightly different. Oral antibiotics continue to be recommended if perforation is a result of the AOM episode; however, if a child has an episode of AOM with tympanostomy tubes in place, topical 0.3% ciprofloxacin/0.1% dexamethasone (Ciprodex Otic) should be added to oral amoxicillin. See Table 2 for antibiotic dosing recommendations.

Regardless of the decision to implement watchful waiting or antibiotic therapy, any child with AOM should be expected to improve within 48 to 72 hours. If improvement is not occurring, the child should be re-evaluated.

Treatment Options: Surgery

For some children, AOM will not be an isolated event. Instead, they will have recurrent infections and require multiple antibiotic courses throughout a year, prompting consideration of tympanostomy tube placement. Currently, referral for evaluation for tympanostomy tubes is recommended when a child has had three or more episodes of AOM within a 6-month period or more than four episodes within a 12-month period. Some have argued, however, that this recommendation should be considered within the context of the child's age at first presentation. A child who has the first episode of AOM before 6 months of age is likely to go on to have many more episodes. Ultimately, they will likely meet the criteria for myringotomy and thus may warrant a more aggressive approach from the outset. Conversely, a child who presents with a first episode of AOM as an older child is less likely to have recurrent episodes and can therefore be treated in a more conservative manner.

Using an age-stratified approach, children who experience a first episode of AOM prior to 6 months of age should receive tympanostomy tubes if they have two episodes in a 6- or 12-month time period or three episodes in 24 months. Similarly, children who have a first episode of AOM after 1 year of age should receive tympanostomy tubes only if they have three episodes within 6 months, five within 12 months, or seven within 24 months.

Referral may also occur if a child has a history of AOM associated with meningitis, facial nerve paralysis, coalescent mastoiditis, or brain abscess. Tympanostomy tubes are also often placed due to prolonged OME resulting in hearing loss and language delay. Myringotomy without tube placement may be considered for either diagnosis of an infection that has not responded to numerous antibiotics or for relief of severe otalgia.

AOM episodes will continue to occur despite tympanostomy tube placement. However, episodes will likely be less severe, of shorter duration, and less frequent. In addition to ongoing AOM episodes, tympanostomy tubes can be problematic if they become clogged. New studies in animal models suggest that applying colchicine[1] in the external ear may prevent this complication.

Treatment Options: Analgesia

Regardless of a decision to pursue watchful waiting or antibiotics, analgesics are an important component in the treatment of AOM. Multiple homeopathic interventions and home remedies including application of heat, ice, or mineral oil (Min-O-Ear)[1] have been used for pain control, although no studies exist to verify their effectiveness. Acetaminophen (Tylenol), ibuprofen (Motrin), narcotics, and tympanostomy have all been

---

[3] Exceeds dosage recommended by the manufacturer.

[1] Not FDA approved for this indication.

TABLE 2 Antibiotic Selection for Specific Patient Populations

	ANTIBIOTIC OF CHOICE	DOSE (mg/kg/day)	ROUTE	DURATION OF THERAPY
AOM in child older than 2 years	Amoxicillin (Amoxil)	80–90[3]	PO	5–7 days
AOM in child younger than 2 years	Amoxicillin	80–90[3]	PO	10 days
AOM in child with allergy to penicillin	Cefdinir (Omnicef)	14	PO	10 days
	Cefpodoxime (Vantin)	10	PO	5 days
	Cefuroxime (Ceftin)	30	PO	10 days
AOM with inability to tolerate oral medications	Ceftriaxone (Rocephin)	50	IV/IM	1 day
AOM with amoxicillin failure	Amoxicillin with clavulanate (Augmentin)	90 of amoxicillin and 6.4 of clavulanate[3]	PO	10 days
	Ceftriaxone (Rocephin)	50	IV/IM	3 days[3]
AOM with amoxicillin/ clavulanate failure	Ceftriaxone (Rocephin)	50	IV/IM	3 days[3]
AOM with ceftriaxone failure and tympanocentesis not available	Clindamycin (Cleocin)[1]	30–40[3]	PO	10 days
Perforated tympanic membrane	Amoxicillin	80–90[3]	PO	10 days
Tympanostomy tube in place	Amoxicillin and topical 0.3% ciprofloxacin/0.1% dexamethasone (Ciprodex Otic)	80–90 8 drops	PO Topical bid	10 days 7 days

[1]Not FDA approved for this indication.
[3]Exceeds dosage recommended by the manufacturer.
Abbreviation: AOM = acute otitis media.

demonstrated to be effective at reducing pain. However, the side effects of altered mental status, gastrointestinal upset, and respiratory depression with narcotics, as well as the skill needed to perform tympanostomy, limit the usefulness of these interventions in primary care practice. Topical medications may help avoid the systemic effects of oral medication. Antipyrine and benzocaine are the only topical analgesics available in the United States. Topical benzocaine has been demonstrated to have minimal side effects and in patients older than 5 years of age may offer more relief than acetaminophen alone. Benzocaine is available in combination with antipyrine (Allergen Ear Drops, Auroguard Otic). Benzocaine is also available with antipyrine and acetic acid (Auralgan) but may be expensive. In other countries, antipyrine, also known as phenazone, is available in combination with procaine and is effective.

Antihistamines have often been prescribed, as have decongestants, in an attempt to reduce the fluid volume in the middle ear and hence provide relief. Unfortunately, use of antihistamines and decongestants has been shown to result in a fivefold to eightfold increase in the risk of side effects with no benefits, including no decreased time to cure, no prevention of surgery or complications, and no increased symptom resolution. Therefore antihistamines and decongestants have not been routinely recommended.

Conclusion

AOM continues to be one of the most costly and common childhood illnesses in developed nations throughout the world. Successful management of this condition requires much more than choosing amoxicillin at an appropriate dose and duration or appropriately timing a surgical referral. Vigilant attention to modifying risk factors when possible, promoting immunization, and limiting the spread of viral illnesses has been shown to prevent AOM instances. Furthermore, adherence to diagnostic criteria to attempt to accurately distinguish between AOM and OME, as well as implementing observation when appropriate, can significantly reduce antibiotic usage, thereby minimizing side effects for patients and opportunity to develop resistance in pathogens.

RED EYE

Method of
John N. Dorsch, MD

CURRENT DIAGNOSIS

- Patients with traumatic injury to the eye, loss of vision, extreme pain not explained by pathology, keratitis, suspected uveitis or glaucoma, chemical injury, or nonhealing corneal abrasion should be referred to an ophthalmologist.
- Bacterial, viral, and allergic conjunctivitis can often be distinguished by the type of ocular discharge present.
- Subconjunctival hemorrhage can occur from trauma, from increased intrathoracic pressure, from anticoagulants, or idiopathically.

CURRENT THERAPY

- Do not use eye patches in patients with corneal abrasions.
- Do not use topical anesthetics for the eye outside a clinic or hospital setting, because corneal toxicity can occur.
- Patients with corneal abrasions should be reexamined the following day.
- Patients with corneal abrasions from extended-wear contact lenses often become colonized with *Pseudomonas aeruginosa* and should be treated with appropriate antibiotics (quinolones).

In the primary care office, the most common causes of red eye are conjunctivitis, subconjunctival hemorrhage, and foreign body causing corneal abrasions. Other common causes of red eye include blepharitis and hordeolum. Less common but serious causes of red eye include viral keratitis, uveitis, scleritis, and angle-closure glaucoma. Other usually less serious causes of red eye include episcleritis, pingueculum, and pterygium. All primary care physicians should have expertise in recognizing and treating the common causes of red eye and should recognize and refer patients with higher-stakes diagnoses (Boxes 1 and 2).

Physical Examination

Always check visual acuity in any patient with an eye complaint. Fluorescein strips (Flu-Glo, Fluorets), topical anesthetic drops, and cobalt blue light are used to examine the cornea for abrasions, keratitis, and ulceration. Cotton-tipped applicators are used to evert the upper eyelid and look for a foreign body.

Pupillary reaction is often affected by angle closure glaucoma and uveitis, but it is rarely affected by conjunctivitis, blepharitis, and corneal disorders. The pupil may be irregular in the patient with uveitis.

Patients with uveitis often have pain in the closed affected eye when a bright light is shined in the normal eye or with convergence of the eyes. This is due to consensual reflex of the pupils to light and accommodation.

The diagnosis of conjunctivitis is made by pulling the lower eyelid down with the examiner's finger. If the bulbar or palpebral conjunctivae are inflamed (i.e., hyperemic, edematous, discharge), conjunctivitis is present. Palpable preauricular nodes may be present with viral conjunctivitis and chlamydial conjunctivitis.

Conjunctivitis

Conjunctivitis is the most common cause of red eye encountered by primary care providers. Among the etiologies of conjunctivitis, viral conjunctivitis is the most common. Although patients with conjunctivitis might have some minor irritation of the eyes, they usually do not complain of pain in the eye or loss of vision. Ocular discharge is generally considered to be an important diagnostic feature of conjunctivitis (Table 1). Although much has been written about characterizing conjunctivitis by the nature of the discharge, one meta-analysis failed to find evidence of the diagnostic usefulness of clinical signs or symptoms in distinguishing bacterial conjunctivitis from viral conjunctivitis.

Viral Conjunctivitis

Viral conjunctivitis is often seen in epidemics and is most commonly caused by members of the Adenovirus family. Typically, viral conjunctivitis starts in one eye and spreads to the other eye a few days later. The conjunctivae appear red and swollen, with copious watery discharge (Figure 1). The natural course of viral conjunctivitis is self-limiting, lasting 10 to 14 days. Tender preauricular lymph nodes, when present, indicate the presence of viral or chlamydial conjunctivitis. Management should be directed at scrupulous hygiene. Patients must be informed that their infection is highly contagious. They should avoid close contact with other persons (e.g., towels, direct contact, swimming pools) for 2 weeks and wash hands frequently to prevent the spread of their infection. Topical antibiotics have been prescribed to try to prevent bacterial superinfection, but there is no good evidence that they have any significant impact. Symptomatic treatment with cold compresses and topical vasoconstrictors may be helpful. Conjunctivitis has very recently (end of 2015) been reported in patients with Zika virus.

Bacterial Conjunctivitis

Bacterial conjunctivitis typically starts abruptly in one eye and spreads to the other eye in 1 to 2 days. Usually a purulent discharge is present that persists throughout the day. A variety of gram-positive and gram-negative organisms cause bacterial conjunctivitis, but the most common causes are *Staphylococcus aureus*, *Streptococcus pneumoniae*, and *Haemophilus pneumoniae*. Treatment of bacterial conjunctivitis is usually empiric, but conjunctival scraping for smears and cultures should be done in infants, immunocompromised patients, and patients with hyperacute conjunctivitis in which *Neisseria gonorrhoeae* or *Chlamydia trachomatis* infection is suspected. Treatment of bacterial conjunctivitis (excluding gonococcal or chlamydial

---

BOX 1 Approach to the Patient with Red Eye

The following questions are often helpful in making the diagnosis in patients with red eyes.

- *Is one eye or are both eyes involved?* Infections, allergy, and systemic illness are more likely to cause bilateral eye involvement.
- *Does the patient have intense eye pain?* If yes, likely diagnoses include acute angle closure glaucoma, uveitis, scleritis, keratitis, foreign body, or corneal abrasion.
- *Does the patient have a foreign body sensation?* If so, consider corneal abrasion, trauma, dry eye, keratitis, and other corneal disorders.
- *Is there a discharge?* If it is *very* copious and purulent, consider gonococcal conjunctivitis. If it is discolored and purulent, consider bacterial conjunctivitis. Copious watery discharge is typical of viral conjunctivitis. Stringy, mucoid discharge is typical of allergic or chlamydial conjunctivitis.
- *Do the eyes itch?* If so, consider blepharitis or allergy in the differential.
- *Are the eyelids swollen?* Consider allergy or infection.
- *Do the eyelids have lumps?* Hordeolum and chalazion should be considered.
- *Do the eyes burn?* Consider blepharitis or dry eye.
- *Is the eye redness recurrent?* Consider herpes keratitis, uveitis, and allergic conjunctivitis.
- *Does the patient have photophobia?* Corneal problems (abrasions, keratitis) and uveitis should be considered.
- *Is there loss of vision?* Consider corneal ulcer, uveitis, and angle closure glaucoma.
- *Is the patient using ocular medications?* Prolonged use of neomycin and sulfa ophthalmic medications can cause sensitization and redness of the eyes.

BOX 2 Red Eye

Common Causes
- Conjunctivitis: bacterial, viral, allergic
- Subconjunctival hemorrhage
- Corneal abrasion
- Blepharitis

Less Common Causes
Less Serious
- Episcleritis
- Pingueculum
- Pterygium

More Serious
- Viral keratitis
- Uveitis
- Scleritis
- Angle closure glaucoma

---

conjunctivitis) usually consists of a topical antibiotic used four times a day (Table 2). Topical antibiotics are usually prescribed for 5 to 7 days, and resolution of conjunctivitis is expected within that time.

Hyperacute bacterial conjunctivitis has an abrupt onset, copious purulent discharge, and rapid progression, and it is usually associated with gonococcal infection in a sexually active patient. Chemosis (edema of the conjunctivae) may be present.

Chlamydial conjunctivitis is acquired through exposure to infected secretions from the genital tract, either direct or indirect. The infection is usually unilateral (at least initially), and often there is involvement of the preauricular node on the ipsilateral side. Gonococcal and chlamydial infections are treated systemically (Box 3).

TABLE 1 Conjunctivitis

TYPE	COURSE	CHARACTERISTICS	DISCHARGE
Bacterial	Starts in one eye, often spreads to other eye		Purulent
Allergic	Accompanies allergic rhinitis	Itchy eyes	Mucus
Viral	Usually bilateral	Very red eyes	Watery

Figure 1 Viral conjunctivitis. Reproduced with permission from the University of Michigan Kellogg Eye Center, http://www.kellogg.umich.edu.

Conjunctivitis of the Newborn
Chlamydial conjunctivitis is the most common cause of infectious conjunctivitis of the newborn in the United States. Onset of conjunctivitis is 3 to 10 days after birth, but it has been reported as late as 2 months after birth. *Chlamydia trachomatis* infection can also cause pneumonia, otitis media, proctitis, and vulvovaginitis in infants. Treatment consists of erythromycin (EryPed Drops) orally 50 mg/kg/day in four divided doses for 14 days. Erythromycin ointment (Ilotycin 0.5%) or tetracycline ointment[2] given shortly after delivery is effective in preventing chlamydial conjunctivitis but not systemic chlamydial infections.

Gonococcal conjunctivitis of the newborn is a hyperacute infection that occurs 2 to 4 days after birth. It can cause corneal ulceration and loss of vision. Gonococcal conjunctivitis can be prevented with silver nitrate drops[2] or erythromycin (Ilotycin) or tetracycline ointment[2] administered shortly after delivery. Silver nitrate commonly causes a self-limited chemical conjunctivitis, which can delay visual bonding of the infant to the parents in the first few hours of life. Therapy of gonococcal conjunctivitis of the newborn consists of IV penicillin G[1] given four times a day for 7 days or ceftriaxone (Rocephin) IV or IM once a day for 7 days or gentamicin (Garamycin)[1] IM given twice a day for 7 days.

Conjunctivitis–Otitis Media Syndrome
Conjunctivitis–otitis media syndrome is a common condition in which children with otitis media also have purulent bilateral ocular discharge. It responds to treatment of otitis media; no topical treatment of conjunctivitis is required.

Methicillin-Resistant *Staphylococcus Aureus* Conjunctivitis
Increasing numbers of cases of bacterial conjunctivitis are caused by methicillin-resistant *S. aureus* (MRSA). MRSA conjunctivitis manifests as bacterial conjunctivitis resistant to conventional therapy and is treated with the same drugs used to treat MRSA in other parts of the body (Doxycycline [Vibramycin],[1] vancomycin [Vancocin], sulfamethoxazole-trimethoprim [Bactrim][1]). Cultures should be obtained when MRSA is suspected.

Allergic Conjunctivitis
Allergic conjunctivitis is an immunoglobulin E (IgE)-mediated condition characterized by bilateral eye involvement, itchy eyes, and mucoid discharge. *Seasonal* conjunctivitis is caused by exposure to common allergens (e.g., pollens, dander) and usually accompanies allergic rhinitis. *Perennial* allergic conjunctivitis is similar to seasonal allergic conjunctivitis, but the symptoms are usually less severe. Patients are usually treated with a systemic antihistamine.

TABLE 2 Topical Antibiotics Used to Treat Bacterial Conjunctivitis

DRUG	DOSAGE
Bacitracin (Ak-Tracin, Bacticin) ointment	Apply 0.5 inch in eye q3–4h
Ciprofloxacin (Ciloxan) 0.3% ophthalmic solution	1–2 gtt in eye q15min × 6h, then q30min × 18h, then q1h × 1 d, then q4h × 12 d[3]
Gatifloxacin (Zymaxid) 0.5% ophthalmic solution	1 gtt in eye q2h up to 8 ×/day on Day1, then 1 gtt 2–4 ×/day on Day 2–7
Gentamicin (Gentak, Gentasol) 0.3% ophthalmic solution or ointment	Ointment: 0.5 inch applied to eye 2–3 times per day Solution: 1–2 gtt in eye q4h
Levofloxacin (Quixin) 0.5% ophthalmic solution	1–2 gtt in eye q2h × 2 d while awake, then q4h while awake × 5 d
Moxifloxacin (Vigamox) 0.5% ophthalmic solution	1 gt in eye tid × 7 d
Neomycin/polymyxin B/ gramicidin (Neosporin) ophthalmic solution	1–2 gtt in eye q4h × 7–10 d
Ofloxacin (Ocuflox) 0.3% ophthalmic solution	1–2 gtt in eye q2–4h × 2 d, then 1–2 gtt in eye qid × 5 d
Polymyxin B and trimethoprim (Polytrim) ophthalmic solution	1 gt in eye q3h × 7–10 d
Sulfacetamide (Isopto Cetamide, Ocusulf-10, Sodium Sulamyd, Sulf-10, AK-Sulf) 10% ophthalmic solution, ointment	Ointment: 0.5-inch ribbon in eye q3–4h and qhs × 7 d Solution: 1–2 gtt in eye q2–3h × 7–10 d
Tobramycin (AK-Tob, Tobrex) 0.3% ophthalmic solution	1–2 gtt in eye q4h

[3]Exceeds dosage recommended by the manufacturer.

BOX 3 Treatment of Chlamydial and Gonococcal Conjunctivitis

Chlamydial Conjunctivitis
- Erythromycin (Ery-Tab)[1] 250 mg PO qid × 14 d

or
- Doxycycline (Vibramycin) 100 mg PO bid × 14 d
- Treat partners

Gonococcal Conjunctivitis
- Ceftriaxone (Recephin 1 g IM)

[1] Not FDA approved for this indication.

[1]Not FDA approved for this indication.
[2]Not available in the United States.

TABLE 3 Topical Medications for Allergic Conjunctivitis

GENERIC NAME	BRAND NAME(S)	DOSING	MODE OF ACTION
Azelastine 0.05% solution	Optivar	1 gt in eye(s) bid	H$_1$-antagonist, mast cell inhibitor
Cromolyn 4% solution	Crolom, generic	1–2 gtt in eye(s) 4–6 times per day	Mast cell inhibitor
Emedastine 0.05% solution	Emadine	1 gt in eye(s) qid	H$_1$-antagonist
Epinastine 0.05% solution	Elestat	1 gt in eye(s) bid	H$_1$- and H$_2$-antagonist, mast cell inhibitor
Ketorolac 0.5% solution	Acular	1 gt in eye(s) qid up to 1 wk	NSAID
Diclofenac 0.1% solution[1]	Voltaren ophthalmic	1 gt in eye(s) qid × 2 wk	NSAID
Lodoxamide 0.1% solution	Alomide	1–2 gtt in eye(s) qid up to 3 mo	Mast cell inhibitor
Loteprednol 0.2% susp.	Alrex	1 gt in eye(s) qd	Corticosteroid
Naphazoline/pheniramine (solution)	Naphcon-A (OTC) Opcon-A (OTC) Visine-A (OTC)	1–2 gtt in eye(s) qd-qid prn	Antihistamine, decongestant
Nedrocomil 2% solution	Alocril	1–2 gtt in eye(s) bid	H$_1$-antagonist, mast cell inhibitor
Olopatadine 0.1% solution	Patanol	1 gt in eye(s) bid	H$_1$-antagonist, mast cell inhibitor
Olopatadine 0.2% solution	Pataday	1 gt in eye(s) qd	Mast cell inhibitor

[1]Not FDA approved for this indication.
Abbreviation: NSAID = nonsteroidal antiinflammatory drug.

Ophthalmic (topical) medications include antihistamine or decongestants, mast cell inhibitors, nonsteroidal antiinflammatory drugs (NSAIDs), H$_1$-antagonists, and various combinations of these (Table 3). Milder cases can be treated with a decongestant-antihistamine combination for about 2 weeks. Moderate to more severe cases can require longer use of these medications or the addition of systemic antihistamines or mast cell inhibitors. Some patients require topical corticosteroids or cyclosporine (Restasis)[1] for severe allergic conjunctivitis, but these should be evaluated by an ophthalmologist because of potential complications of therapy.

Subconjunctival Hemorrhage

In subconjunctival hemorrhage, the redness of the eye is localized and sharply circumscribed, and the underlying sclera is not visible (Figure 2). Conjunctivitis is not present, and there is no discharge. There is typically no pain or visual change. Subconjunctival hemorrhage may be spontaneous, but it can also result from trauma, hypertension, bleeding disorders, or increased intrathoracic pressure (e.g., straining, coughing, retching). No treatment is necessary, but investigation may be warranted if the etiology is in question or the hemorrhage is recurrent. Referral to an ophthalmologist should be considered if the subconjunctival hemorrhage is from trauma or has not resolved within 2 to 3 weeks.

Corneal Abrasion

Corneal abrasions typically result from scratching of the corneal epithelium due to trauma, but they can also occur from extended-wear contact lenses. Patients with corneal abrasions present with pain, excessive tearing from the involved eye, photophobia, a foreign-body sensation (like having sand in the eye), and blurry vision.

Corneal abrasions are identified by staining the cornea with fluorescein and examining under cobalt blue light (Figure 3). The eye should also be examined carefully to check for foreign bodies. Topical anesthetic is administered to make the patient comfortable during the examination, but continued use can cause corneal damage.

Management of corneal abrasions consists of pain relief and prevention of infection. Pain can be relieved with topical NSAIDs such as ketorolac (Acular)[1] and Diclofenac (Voltaren),[1] oral

[1]Not FDA approved for this indication.

Figure 2 Subconjunctival hemorrhage. Reprinted with permission from American Academy of Ophthalmology: Managing the Red Eye. Eye Care Skills for the Primary Care Physician Series. San Francisco: American Academy of Ophthalmology, 2001.

Figure 3 Corneal abrasion with fluorescein stain with cobalt blue light. Reprinted with permission from American Academy of Ophthalmology: Managing the Red Eye. Eye Care Skills for the Primary Care Physician Series. San Francisco: American Academy of Ophthalmology, 2001.

over-the-counter analgesics, and occasionally oral narcotics. Topical antibiotics are usually prescribed to prevent infection. Antibiotic ointments are lubricating and soothing to the eye, making them a good option for traumatic corneal abrasions. Topical ophthalmic antibiotic ointments commonly used are bacitracin (Bacticin), erythromycin (Ilotycin), and gentamicin (Gentak).

TABLE 4	Blepharitis		
TYPE	SITE OF ORIGIN	CLINICAL CHARACTERISTICS	TREATMENT
Staphylococcal	Accessory glands of eyelids	Erythema and induration of eyelid; crusting; discharge; loss of eyelashes	Warm compresses Baby shampoo scrubs Erythromycin ointment (Ilotycin)
Seborrheic	Meibomian glands	More chronic, scaling	Warm compresses Baby shampoo scrubs Oral tetracycline for resistant cases

Figure 4 Staphylococcal blepharitis. Reprinted with permission from American Academy of Ophthalmology: Managing the Red Eye. Eye Care Skills for the Primary Care Physician Series. San Francisco: American Academy of Ophthalmology, 2001.

Figure 5 Seborrheic blepharitis. Reprinted with permission from American Academy of Ophthalmology: Managing the Red Eye. Eye Care Skills for the Primary Care Physician Series. San Francisco: American Academy of Ophthalmology, 2001.

In patients who have corneal abrasions from contact lens overwear, eyes are commonly colonized with *Pseudomonas aeruginosa*. These patients should be treated with topical antibiotics such as ciprofloxacin (Ciloxan) or ofloxacin (Ocuflux) solutions.

Patching of the eye, though a common practice of the past, has not shown evidence of benefit in recent studies. It was found that eye patching can actually cause harm, so this practice is no longer recommended.

Infrequently, patients have traumatic uveitis accompanying corneal abrasion. Traumatic uveitis usually causes significantly more pain than a corneal abrasion, and, if uveitis is suspected, the patient should be evaluated by an ophthalmologist.

Patients with corneal abrasions should be reexamined in 24 hours. Corneal abrasions typically should be healed or greatly improved in 24 hours. If the abrasion is not completely healed after 24 hours, the patient should be examined again in 2 or 3 days. Referral should be considered if any worsening occurs or if the abrasion does not heal within 5 days. Corneal abrasions can be prevented by using protective eyewear.

Figure 6 Hordeolum. Reprinted with permission from American Academy of Ophthalmology: Managing the Red Eye. Eye Care Skills for the Primary Care Physician Series. San Francisco: American Academy of Ophthalmology, 2001.

Other Causes of Red Eye

Other causes of red eye are somewhat less common.

Blepharitis

Blepharitides are inflammatory conditions of the eyelid caused by infection or obstruction of eyelid glands (Table 4). Blepharitis may be accompanied by conjunctivitis. Staphylococcal blepharitis arises from the accessory glands to the eyelashes and causes discharge from the eyelid, often associated with erythema, induration, loss of eyelashes, and crusting of the eyelid (Figure 4). This is treated with hot, moist packs to the eyes, baby shampoo scrubs (3 oz. water and 3 drops baby shampoo used on a washcloth bid), and erythromycin ointment (Ilotycin) at bedtime. Seborrheic blepharitis, a more chronic form of blepharitis, arises from the meibomian glands and causes scaling of the eyelids (Figure 5). Seborrheic blepharitis is often associated with skin disorders such as rosacea, eczema, and seborrheic dermatitis. This is treated with hot, moist packs and baby shampoo scrubs. Resistant cases are treated with oral tetracycline (Sumycin) (or one of its derivatives).

Hordeolum (Stye)

A hordeolum is an acute, painful mass of the eyelid that is caused by inflammation of the glands (Figure 6). It does not usually cause the eye to become red as well. Warm compresses to the eyelid four times a day for 3 to 5 minutes typically causes resolution within 1 week. Because they arise from the same glands, hordeola and blepharitis commonly occur together.

Episcleritis

Episcleritis is a self-limited inflammation of the episcleral vessels and is believed to be autoimmune. It has a rapid onset and usually minimal discomfort. Redness is most often confined to a sector of the eye. Episcleritis usually resolves in 7 to 10 days. Recurrence is not uncommon. Oral NSAID drugs may be prescribed, but treatment is usually not necessary.

Scleritis

Scleritis is, fortunately, much less common than episcleritis. Patients with scleritis experience intense inflammation and deep eye pain. Scleritis is commonly associated with rheumatoid arthritis and inflammatory bowel disease. The patient should be promptly referred to an ophthalmologist if scleritis is suspected.

Acute Angle Closure Glaucoma

Acute angle closure glaucoma is characterized by acute ocular pain and is often accompanied by vomiting, blurred vision, acute photophobia, pupils unreactive to light, and circumcorneal redness (ciliary flush). Treatment of glaucoma with pilocarpine (Isopto Carpine), topical timolol (Timoptic), and acetazolamide (Diamox) should be started, and the patient should be given an urgent referral to an ophthalmologist.

Anterior Uveitis

Uveitis is the inflammation of the iris and ciliary muscle, often associated with autoimmune disease. Trauma can also cause uveitis. Signs of uveitis include ocular pain, ciliary flush, and occasionally irregularity of the pupil. Prompt referral should be arranged for a patient in whom uveitis is suspected.

In general, referral to an ophthalmologist should strongly be considered for:

- Traumatic injury to the eye
- Loss of vision
- Extreme eye pain not explained by pathology
- Keratitis
- Suspected uveitis or glaucoma
- Chemical injury (especially alkali)
- Corneal abrasion not healing

References

American Optometric Association: *Optometric clinical practice guideline: Care of the patient with anterior uveitis*, June 23, 1994. Revised March 1999. PDF available at www.aoa.org/documents/CPG-7.pdf. June 23, 1994 [accessed July 10, 2015].

Arbour JD, Brunette I, Boisjoly HM, et al: Should we patch corneal abrasions? *Arch Ophthalmol* 115(3):313–317, 1997.

Au YK, Henkind P: Pain elicited by consensual pupillary reflex: a diagnostic test for acute iritis, *Lancet* 2:1254–1255, 1981.

Avdic E, Cosgrove SE: Management and control strategies for community-associated methicillin-resistant *Staphylococcus aureus*, *Expert Opin Pharmacother* 9(9):1463–1479, 2008.

Boder F, Marchant C, et al: Bacterial etiology of conjunctivitis-otitis media syndrome, *Pediatrics* 76:26–28, 1985.

Bradford CA: *Basic Ophthalmology*, ed 8, San Francisco, 2004, American Academy of Ophthalmology.

Centers for Disease Control and Prevention. Zika Virus. Symptoms, diagnosis, and treatment. Available at www.cdc.gov/zika/symptoms. Accessed Feb. 3, 2016.

De Toledo AR, Chandler JW: Conjunctivitis of the newborn, *Infect Dis Clin North Am* 6(4):807–813, 1992.

Frith P, Gray R, MacLennan S, et al: *The Eye in Clinical Practice*, Oxford, 1994, Blackwell Scientific.

Jackson WB: Blepharitis: Current strategies for diagnosis and treatment, *Can J Ophthalmol* 43(2):170–179, 2008.

Liebowitz HM: The red eye, *N Engl J Med* 343(5):345–351, 2000.

Patterson J, Fetzer D, Krall J, et al: Eye patch treatment for the pain of corneal abrasion, *South Med J* 89(2):227–229, 1996.

Prochazka AV: Diagnosis and treatment of red eye, *Primary Care Case Reviews* 4:23–31, 2001.

Rietveld RP, van Weert H, Riet G, Bindels P: Diagnostic impact of signs and symptoms in acute infectious conjunctivitis: Systematic literature search, *BMJ* 327(4):789, 2003.

Tarabishy A, Jeng B: Bacterial conjunctivitis: A review for internists, *Cleve Clin J Med* 75(7):507–512, 2008.

Talbot EM: A simple test to diagnose iritis, *BMJ* 295:812–813, 1987.

Trobe JD: *The Physician's Guide to Eye Care*, ed 2, San Francisco, 2001, Foundation of the American Academy of Ophthalmology.

Wilson SA, Last A: Management of corneal abrasion, *Am Fam Physician* 70:123–130, 2004.

Wong AH, Barg SS, Leung AK: Seasonal and perennial allergic conjunctivitis, *Recent Pat Inflamm Allergy Drug Disc* 3(2):118–127, 2009.

RHINOSINUSITIS

Method of
Ann M. Aring, MD

CURRENT DIAGNOSIS

- Because inflammation of the sinuses rarely occurs without concurrent inflammation of the nasal mucosa, rhinosinusitis is a more accurate term for what is commonly called sinusitis.
- Most cases of sinusitis are caused by viral infections associated with the common cold. Viral rhinosinusitis improves in 7 to 10 days.
- Four signs and symptoms with a high likelihood ratio for acute bacterial sinusitis are double sickening, purulent rhinorrhea, erythrocyte sedimentation rate (ESR) >10mm, and purulent secretion in the nasal cavity. A combination of at least three of these four symptoms and signs has a specificity of 0.81 and sensitivity of 0.66 for acute bacterial rhinosinusitis.
- Acute rhinosinusitis lasts up to 4 weeks, subacute rhinosinusitis lasts from 4 to 12 weeks, and chronic rhinosinusitis lasts 12 weeks or longer. Recurrent acute rhinosinusitis is defined as four or more episodes per year with complete resolution between episodes.
- Radiographic imaging in a patient with acute rhinosinusitis is not recommended unless a complication or an alternative diagnosis is suspected. Computed tomography of the sinuses without contrast media is the imaging method of choice.

CURRENT THERAPY

- Mild rhinosinusitis symptoms of less than 7 days' duration can be managed with supportive care including analgesics, saline nasal irrigation, and intranasal corticosteroids.
- Antibiotic therapy is recommended for patients with sinusitis symptoms that do not improve within 7 to 10 days or that worsen at any time.
- First-line antibiotics include amoxicillin with or without clavulanate.
- Macrolides and trimethoprim sulfamethoxazole (Bactrim) are not recommended for empiric therapy owing to high rates of resistance among *Streptococcus pneumoniae* and *Haemophilus influenzae*.
- For adults allergic to penicillin, doxycycline may be used as an alternative regimen for initial empiric therapy for bacterial rhinosinusitis. According to a recent US Food and Drug Administration (FDA) safety alert, fluoroquinolones such as levofloxacin (Levaquin) and moxifloxacin (Avelox) should be reserved for patients who do not have other treatment options.
- In adults with confirmed acute rhinosinusitis, more than 70% will clinically improve after 2 weeks with or without antibiotic therapy.
- Antibiotic use increases the absolute cure rate by 5% compared with placebo at 7 to 15 days.

Epidemiology of Acute Rhinosinusitis and Predisposing Factors

Each year in the United States, rhinosinusitis affects one in seven adults and is diagnosed in 31 million patients. Rhinosinusitis is the fifth most common diagnosis for which antibiotics are prescribed. Rhinosinusitis has a higher frequency in the winter months and lower frequency in the summer and autumn months.

Predisposing Factors

Predisposing factors for acute rhinosinusitis include viral upper respiratory infections and allergic rhinitis. Anatomic malformations including polyps, deviated nasal septum, foreign bodies, and tumors can also predispose to acute rhinosinusitis.

Pathogenesis and Etiology of Rhinosinusitis

Most cases of acute rhinosinusitis are caused by viral infections associated with the common cold. The most common viruses in acute viral rhinosinusitis are rhinovirus, adenovirus, influenza virus, and parainfluenza virus. Mucosal edema occurs with the viral infection with subsequent obstruction of the sinus ostia. In addition, viral and bacterial infections impair the cilia, which help transport the mucus. The ostia obstruction and slowed mucus transport cause stagnation of secretions and lowered oxygen tension within the sinuses. This environment is an excellent culture medium for both viruses and bacteria and the infectious particles grow rapidly. The body responds with an inflammatory reaction. Polymorphonuclear leukocytes are mobilized, which results in pus formation. The most common bacteria found in acute community-acquired bacterial rhinosinusitis are S pneumoniae, H influenzae, Staphylococcus aureus, and Moraxella catarrhalis. Acute adult rhinosinusitis most commonly involves the maxillary and ethmoid sinuses. More than one of the paranasal sinuses can be affected.

Diagnosis of Acute Rhinosinusitis

Diagnosis of acute bacterial rhinosinusitis requires that symptoms persist for longer than 10 days or worsen after 5 to 7 days. Four signs and symptoms with a high likelihood ratio for acute bacterial sinusitis are double sickening, purulent rhinorrhea, ESR > 10 mm, and purulent secretion in the nasal cavity. A combination of at least three of these four symptoms and signs has a specificity of 0.81 and sensitivity of 0.66 for acute bacterial rhinosinusitis. Table 1 lists the sensitivity, specificity, likelihood ratio, and odds ratio of criteria used to diagnose acute rhinosinusitis. If resistant pathogens are suspected or if the patient's immune system is compromised, bacterial culture of the secretions may be used for diagnosis and to direct therapy.

Imaging

For uncomplicated acute rhinosinusitis, radiographic imaging is not recommended. Plain sinus radiography shows air–fluid levels in patients with both viral and bacterial rhinosinusitis. Sinus computed tomography should not be used for routine evaluation of acute bacterial rhinosinusitis. However, sinus computed tomography without contrast media can be used to identify suspected complications and define anatomic abnormalities.

Differential Diagnosis

The signs and symptoms of acute bacterial rhinosinusitis and prolonged viral upper respiratory infection are similar, which can lead to overdiagnosis of acute bacterial rhinosinusitis. Other conditions that mimic bacterial rhinosinusitis are migraine headache, tension headache, trigeminal neuralgia, and temporomandibular joint disorders.

Treatment of Acute Rhinosinusitis
Symptomatic Treatment

Mild rhinosinusitis symptoms less than 7 days in duration can be managed with supportive care including analgesics, saline nasal irrigation, and intranasal corticosteroids. There are no randomized controlled trials that evaluate the effectiveness of decongestants in patients with sinusitis. Nasal saline is used to soften viscous secretions and improve mucociliary clearance. The mechanical cleansing of the nasal cavity with saline has been shown to benefit patients with rhinosinusitis. Most studies of intranasal corticosteroids are industry sponsored. A 2013

TABLE 1	Signs and Symptoms of Acute Bacterial Rhinosinusitis			
SIGN/SYMPTOM	SENSITIVITY (%)	SPECIFICITY (%)	LR +	ODDS RATIO
Symptoms after upper respiratory tract infection	99	8	1.1	2.1
Facial pain on bending forward	90	22	1.2	0.9
Nasal congestion	90	14	1.0	1.1
Purulent rhinorrhea	89	42	1.5	1.6
Bilateral facial pain, pressure, or fullness	78	32	1.2	1.4
Double sickening	72	65	2.1	*
Previous sinusitis	57	38	0.9	0.4
Upper teeth pain	50	50	1.0	1.2
Unilateral facial pain, pressure, or fullness	46	73	1.7	1.9

Abbreviation: LR = Likelihood ratio.
*No data given in reference.

Cochrane review found that patients receiving intranasal corticosteroids were more likely to experience symptom improvement after 15 to 21 days compared with those receiving placebo (73% vs. 66.4%; $p<.05$; number needed to treat [NNT]=15). Antihistamines should not be used for symptomatic relief of acute rhinosinusitis, except in patients with a history of allergic rhinitis.

Antibiotic Treatment

Antibiotic therapy is recommended for patients with sinusitis symptoms that do not improve within 7 to 10 days or that worsen at any time. Amoxicillin with or without clavulanate is recommended as the first-line antibiotic in adults with acute bacterial rhinosinusitis. "High-dose" amoxicillin-clavulanate (Augmentin XR) is recommended for patients with high risk of S pneumoniae resistance, recent antibiotic use, or treatment failure. Macrolides and trimethoprim sulfamethoxazole are not recommended for empiric therapy owing to high rates of resistance among S pneumoniae and H influenzae. Fluoroquinolones are not recommended as first-line antibiotics because they do not demonstrate benefit over beta-lactam antibiotics and are associated with a variety of adverse effects. According to a recent FDA safety alert, fluoroquinolones should be reserved for patients who do not have other treatment options.

Complications and Referral

Complications of acute bacterial rhinosinusitis are estimated to occur in 1 in 1000 cases. Patients with acute bacterial rhinosinusitis who present with visual symptoms (diplopia, decreased visual acuity, disconjugate gaze, difficulty opening the eye), severe headache, somnolence, or high fever should be evaluated with emergency computed tomography with contrast. Sinonasal cancers are uncommon in the United States, with an annual incidence of less than 1 in 100,000 patients. However, cancer should be included in the differential diagnosis. Referral to an otolaryngologist is needed if symptoms persist or progress after maximal medical therapy when computed tomography shows evidence of sinus disease. Table 2 summarizes indications for subspecialist referral in a patient with acute bacterial rhinosinusitis.

TABLE 2	Indications for Subspecialist Referral for Acute Bacterial Rhinosinusitis

Anatomic defects causing obstruction

Complications such as orbital involvement, altered mental status, meningitis, cavernous sinus thrombosis, intracranial abscess, Pott's puffy tumor (osteomyelitis of front bone)

Evaluation of immunotherapy for allergic rhinitis

Frequent recurrences (3–4 episodes per year)

Fungal sinusitis, granulomatous disease, or possible neoplasm

Immunocompromised host

Nosocomial infection

Severe infection with persistent fever >102°F or 39°C

Treatment failure after extended antibiotic courses

Unusual or resistant bacteria

From Aring AM, Chan MM. Current concepts in adult acute rhinosinusitis. Am Fam Physician 2016;94[2]:97–105.

References

Aring AM, Chan MM: Current concepts in adult acute rhinosinusitis, *Am Fam Physician* 94(2):97–105, 2016.

Chow AW, Benninger MS, Brook I, et al: IDSA clinical practice guideline for acute bacterial rhinosinusitis in children and adults, *Clin Infect Dis* 54(8):e72–112, 2012. Epub 2012 Mar 20.

Cornelius RS, Martin J: Wippold, FJ 2nd, et al. ACR appropriateness criteria sinonasal disease, *J Am Coll Radiol* 10(4):241–246, 2013.

DeSutter AI, Lemiengre M, Campbell H: Antihistamines for the common cold, *Cochrane Database Syst Rev*: CD009345, 2015.

Hayward G, Heneghan C, Perera R, Thompson M: Intranasal corticosteroids in management of acute sinusitis: A systematic review and meta-analysis, *Ann Fam Med* 10:241–249, 2012, https://doi.org/10.1370/afm.1338.

King D, Mitchell B, Williams CP, Spurling GKP: Saline nasal irrigation for acute upper respiratory tract infections, Cochrane Database of Syst Rev 4, 2015. https://doi.org/10.1002/14651858.CD006821.pub3.

Lindbaek M, Hjortdahl P, Johnsen U: Use of symptoms, signs, and blood tests to diagnose acute sinus infections in primary care: Comparison with computer tomography, *Fam Med* 23:183–188, 1996.

Rosenfeld RM, Piccirillo JF, Chadrasekhar SS, et al: Clinical practice guideline (update): Adult sinusitis, *Otolaryngol Head Neck Surg* 152(2S):S1–39, 2015.

U.S. Food and Drug Administration. FDA Drug Safety Communication: FDA updates warnings for oral and injectable fluoroquinolone antibiotics due to disabling side effects. Available at http://www.fda.gov/Drugs/DrugSafety/ucm511530.htm [accessed January 28, 2017].

Young J, De Sutter A, Merenstein D, et al: Antibiotics for adults with clinically diagnosed acute rhinosinusitis: A meta-analysis of individual patient data, *Lancet* 371:908–914, 2008.

Zalmanovici Trestioreanu A, Yaphe J: Intranasal steroids for acute sinusitis, *Cochrane Database Syst Rev* 12, 2013.

TEMPOROMANDIBULAR DISORDERS

Method of
Jeffrey P. Okeson, DMD

Temporomandibular disorder (TMD) is a collective term that includes a number of clinical complaints involving the muscles of mastication, the temporomandibular joints (TMJs) and associated orofacial structures. Other commonly used terms are Costen's syndrome, TMJ dysfunction, and craniomandibular disorders. TMDs are a major cause of nondental pain in the orofacial region and are considered a subclassification of musculoskeletal disorders. In many TMD patients the most common complaint is not with the TMJs but rather the muscles of mastication. Therefore the terms *TMJ dysfunction* or *TMJ disorder* are actually inappropriate for many of these complaints. It is for this reason that the American Dental Association adopted the term *temporomandibular disorder*.

Signs and symptoms associated with TMDs are a common source of pain complaints in the head and orofacial structures.

BOX 1	Common Primary and Secondary Symptoms Associated with Temporomandibular Disorders

Primary Symptoms
Facial muscle pain
Preauricular (TMJ) pain
TMJ sounds: jaw clicking, popping, catching, locking
Limited mouth opening
Increased pain associated with chewing

Secondary Symptoms
Earache
Headache
Neckache

Abbreviation: TMJ = temporomandibular joint.

These complaints can be associated with general joint problems and somatization. Approximately 50% of patients suffering with TMDs do not first consult with a dentist but seek advice for the problem from a physician. The family physician should be able to appropriately diagnose many TMDs. In many instances the physician can provide valuable information and simple therapies that will reduce the patient's TMD symptoms. In other instances, it is appropriate to refer the patient to a dentist for additional evaluation and treatment.

Epidemiology

Cross-sectional population-based studies reveal that 40% to 75% of adult populations have at least one sign of TMJ dysfunction (e.g., jaw movement abnormalities, joint noise, tenderness on palpation), and approximately 33% have at least one symptom (e.g., face pain, joint pain). Many of these signs and symptoms are not troublesome for the patient, and only 3% to 7% of the population seeks any advice or care. Although in the general population women seem to have only a slightly greater incidence of TMD symptoms, women seek care for TMD more often than men at a ratio ranging from 3:1 to 9:1. For many patients TMDs are self-limiting or are associated with symptoms that fluctuate over time without evidence of progression. Even though many of these disorders are self-limiting, the health care provider can provide conservative therapies that will minimize the patient's painful experience.

Signs and Symptoms

The primary signs and symptoms associated with TMD originate from the masticatory structures and are associated with jaw function (Box 1). Pain during opening of the mouth or during chewing is common. Some persons even report difficulty speaking or singing. Patients often report pain in the preauricular areas, face, or temples. TMJ sounds are often described as clicking, popping, grating, or crepitus and can produce locking of the jaw during opening or closing. Patients commonly report painful jaw muscles, and, on occasion, they even report a sudden change in their bite coincident with the onset of the painful condition.

It is important to appreciate that pain associated with most TMDs is increased with jaw function. Because this is a condition of the musculoskeletal structures, function of these structures generally increases the pain. When a patient's pain complaint is not influenced by jaw function, other sources of orofacial pain should be suspected.

The spectrum of TMD often includes commonly associated complaints such as headache, neckache, or earache. These associated complaints are often referred pains and must be differentiated from primary pains. As a general rule, referred pains associated with TMDs are increased with any activity that provokes the TMD pain. Therefore, if the patient reports that the headache is aggravated by jaw function, it could very well represent a secondary pain related to the TMD. Likewise, if the secondary symptom is unaffected by jaw use, one should question its relationship to the TMD and suspect two separate pain conditions. Pain or dysfunction due to non-musculoskeletal causes such as otolaryngologic, neurologic, vascular, neoplastic, or infectious disease in the orofacial region is not considered a primary TMD even though musculoskeletal pain may be present. However, TMDs often coexist with other craniofacial and orofacial pain disorders.

Anatomy and Pathophysiology

The TMJ is formed by the mandibular condyle fitting into the mandibular fossa of the temporal bone. The movement of this joint is quite complex as it allows hinging movement in one plane and at the same time allows gliding movements in another plane.

Separating these two bones from direct articulation is the articular disk. The articular disk is composed of dense fibrous connective tissue devoid of any blood vessels or nerve fibers. The articular disk is attached posteriorly to a region of loose connective tissue that is highly vascularized and well innervated, known as the retrodiscal tissue. The anterior region of the disk is attached to the superior lateral pterygoid muscle.

The movement of the mandible is accomplished by four pairs of muscles called the muscles of mastication: the masseter, temporalis, medial pterygoid, and lateral pterygoid. Although not considered to be muscles of mastication, the digastric muscles also play an important role in mandibular function. The masseter, temporalis, and medial pterygoid muscles elevate the mandible and therefore provide the major forces used for chewing and other jaw functions. The inferior lateral pterygoid muscles provide protrusive movement of the mandible, and the digastric muscles serve to depress the mandible (open the mouth).

When discussing the pathophysiology of TMD, one needs to consider two main categories: joint pathophysiology and muscle pathophysiology. Because etiologic considerations and treatment strategies are different for these conditions, they are presented separately.

Pathophysiology of Intracapsular TMJ Pain Disorders

Several common arthritic conditions such as rheumatoid arthritis, traumatic arthritis, hyperuricemia, and psoriatic arthritis can affect the TMJ. These conditions, however, are not nearly as common as local osteoarthritis. As with most other joints, osteoarthritis results from overloading the articular surface of the joint, thus breaking down the dense fibrocartilage articular surface and ultimately affecting the subarticular bone. In the TMJ, this overloading commonly occurs as a result of an alteration in the morphology and position of the articular disc. In the healthy TMJ, the disc maintains its position on the condyle during movement because of its morphology (i.e., the thicker anterior and posterior borders) and interarticular pressure maintained by the elevator muscles. If, however, the morphology of the disc is altered and the discal ligaments become elongated, the disk can be displaced from its normal position between the condyle and fossa. If the disc is displaced, normal opening and closing of the mouth can result in an unusual translatory movement between the condyle and the disc, which is felt as a click or pop. Disc displacements that result in joint sounds might or might not be painful. When pain is present it is believed to be related to either loading forces applied to the highly vascularized retrodiscal tissues or a general inflammatory response of the surrounding soft tissues (capsulitis or synovitis).

Pathophysiology of Masticatory Muscle Pain Disorders

The muscles of mastication are a very common source of TMD pain. Understanding the pathophysiology of muscle pain, however, is very complex and still not well understood. The simple explanation of muscle spasm does not account for most TMD muscle pain complaints. It appears that a better explanation would include a central nervous system effect on the muscle that results in an increase in peripheral nociceptive activity originating from the muscle tissue itself. This explanation more accurately accounts for the high levels of emotional stress that are commonly associated with TMD muscle pain complaints. In other words, an increase in emotional stress activates the autonomic nervous system, which in turn seems to be associated with changes in muscle nociception.

These masticatory muscle pain conditions are further complicated when one considers the unique masticatory muscle activity known as bruxism. Bruxism is the subconscious, often rhythmic, grinding or gnashing of the teeth. This type of muscle activity is considered to be parafunctional and can also occur as a simple static loading of the teeth known as clenching. This activity commonly occurs while sleeping but can also be present during the day. These parafunctional activities alone can represent a significant source of masticatory muscle pain, and certainly bruxism in the presence of central nervous system–induced muscle pain can further accentuate the patient's muscle pain complaints.

Etiology

Because TMD represents a group of disorders, any of several etiologies may be associated. Problems arising from intracapsular conditions (clicking, popping, catching, locking) may be associated with various types of trauma. Gross trauma, such as a blow to the chin, can immediately alter ligamentous structures of the joint, leading to joint sounds. Trauma can also be associated with a subtler injury such as stretching, twisting or compressing forces during eating, yawning, yelling, or prolonged mouth opening.

When the patient's chief complaint is muscle pain, etiologic factors other than trauma should be considered. Masticatory muscle pain disorders have etiologic considerations similar to other muscle pain disorders of the neck and back. Emotional stress seems to play a significant role for many patients. This can explain why patients often report that their painful symptoms fluctuate greatly over time.

Although most TMD patients do not have a major psychiatric disorder, psychological factors can certainly enhance the pain condition. The clinician needs to consider such factors as anxiety, depression, secondary gain, somatization, and hypochondriasis. Psychosocial factors can predispose certain people to TMD and can also perpetuate TMD once symptoms have become established. A careful consideration of psychosocial factors is therefore important in the evaluation and treatment of every TMD patient.

TMDs have a few unique etiologic factors that differentiate them from other musculoskeletal disorders. One such factor is the occlusal relationship of the teeth. Traditionally it was thought that malocclusion was the primary etiologic factor responsible for TMD. Recent investigations, however, do not support this concept. Still, in certain instances occlusal instability of the teeth can contribute to a TMD. This may be true in patients with or without teeth. Poorly fitting dental prostheses can also contribute to occlusal instability. The occlusal condition should especially be suspected if the pain problem began with a change in the patient's occlusion (e.g., following a dental appointment).

History and Examination

All patients reporting pain in the orofacial structures should be screened for TMD. This can be accomplished with a brief history and physical examination. The screening questions and examination are performed to rule in or out the possibility of a TMD. If a positive response is found, a more extensive history and examination is indicated. Box 2 lists questions that should be asked during a screening assessment for TMD. Any positive response should be followed by additional clarifying questions.

Patients experiencing orofacial pain should also be briefly examined for any clinical signs associated with TMD. The clinician can easily palpate a few sites to assess tenderness or pain, as well as assess for jaw mobility. The masseter muscles can be palpated bilaterally while asking the patient to report any pain or tenderness. The same assessment should be made for the temporal regions, as well as the preauricular (TMJ) areas. While the examiner's hands are over the preauricular areas, the patient should repeatedly open and close the mouth. The presence of joint sounds should be noted along with whether these sounds are associated with joint pain.

BOX 2	Recommended Screening Questionnaire for Temporomandibular Disorder

All patients reporting pain in the orofacial region should be screened for TMD with a questionnaire that includes these questions. The decision to complete a comprehensive history and clinical examination depends on the number of positive responses and the apparent seriousness of the problem for the patient. A positive response to any question may be sufficient to warrant a comprehensive examination if it is of concern to the patient or viewed as clinically significant by the physician.

1. Do you have difficulty, pain, or both when opening your mouth, for instance when yawning?
2. Does your jaw get stuck or locked or go out?
3. Do you have difficulty, pain, or both when chewing, talking, or using your jaws?
4. Are you aware of noises in the jaw joints?
5. Do your jaws regularly feel stiff, tight, or tired?
6. Do you have pain in or about the ears, temples, or cheeks?
7. Do you have frequent headaches, neckaches, or toothaches?
8. Have you had a recent injury to your head, neck, or jaw?
9. Have you been aware of any recent changes in your bite?
10. Have you been previously treated for unexplained facial pain or a jaw joint problem?

Abbreviation: TMD = temporomandibular disorder.

BOX 3	Recommended Screening Examination Procedures for Temporomandibular Disorder

All patients with face pain should be briefly screened for TMD using this or a similar cursory clinical examination. The need for a comprehensive history and clinical examination depends on the number of positive findings and the clinical significance of each finding.

1. Palpate for pain or tenderness in the masseter and temporalis muscles.
2. Palpate for pain or tenderness in the preauricular (TMJ) areas.
3. Measure the range of mouth opening. Note any incoordination in the movements.
4. Auscultate and palpate for TMJ sounds (i.e., clicking or crepitus).
5. Note excessive occlusal wear, excessive tooth mobility, buccal mucosal ridging, or lateral tongue scalloping.
6. Inspect symmetry and alignment of the face, jaws, and dental arches.

Abbreviation: TMJ = temporomandibular joint.

A simple measurement of mouth opening should be made. This can be accomplished by placing a millimeter ruler on the lower anterior teeth and asking the patient to open as wide as possible. The distance should be measured between the maxillary and mandibular anterior teeth. It is generally accepted that less than 40 mm is a restricted mouth opening.

It is also helpful to inspect the teeth for significant wear, mobility, or decay that may be related to the pain condition. The clinician should examine the buccal mucosa for ridging and the lateral aspect of the tongue for scalloping. These are often signs of clenching and bruxism. A general inspection for symmetry and alignment of the face, jaws, and dental arches may also be helpful. A summary of this screening examination is shown in Box 3.

Treatment

Most recent studies suggest that TMDs are generally self-limiting, and symptoms often fluctuate over time. Understanding this natural course does not mean these conditions should be ignored. TMD can be a very painful condition leading to a significant decrease in the patient's quality of life. Understanding the natural course of TMD does suggest, however, that therapy might not need to be very aggressive. In general, initial therapy should begin very conservatively and only escalate when therapy fails to relieve the symptoms.

When the physician identifies a patient with a TMD, he or she has two options. The physician can elect to treat the patient or refer the patient to a dentist who specializes in TMD for further evaluation and treatment. The decision to refer the patient should be based on whether the patient needs any unique care provided only in a dental office. The following are some indications for referral to a dentist:

- History of trauma to the face related to the onset of the pain condition
- The presence of significant TMJ sounds during function
- A feeling of jaw catching or locking during mouth opening
- The report of a sudden change in the occlusal contacts of the teeth
- The presence of significant occlusal instability
- Significant findings related to the teeth (e.g., tooth mobility, tooth sensitivity, tooth decay, tooth wear)

- Significant pain in the jaws or masticatory muscles upon awakening
- The presence of an orofacial pain condition that is aggravated by jaw function and has been present for more than several months

The specific therapy for a TMD varies according to the precise type of disorder identified. In other words, masticatory muscle pain is managed somewhat differently than intracapsular pain. Generally, however, the initial therapy for any type of TMD should be directed toward the relief of pain and the improvement of function. This initial conservative therapy can be divided into three general types: patient education, pharmacologic therapy, and physical therapy.

Patient Education

It is very important that patients have an appreciation for the factors that may be associated with their disorder, as well as the natural course of the disorder. Patients should be reassured and if necessary, convinced by appropriate tests, that they are not suffering from a malignancy. Properly educated patients can contribute greatly to their own treatment. For example, knowing that emotional stress is an influencing factor in many TMDs can help the patient understand the reason for daily fluctuations of pain intensity. Attention should be directed toward changing the patient's response to stress or, when possible, reducing exposure to stressful conditions. Patients with pain during chewing should be told to begin a softer diet, chew slower, and eat smaller bites. As a general rule the patient should be told "if it hurts, don't do it." Continued pain can contribute to the cycling of pain and should always be avoided. The patient should be instructed to let the jaw muscles relax, maintaining the teeth apart. This will discourage clenching activities and minimize loading of the teeth and joints.

When pain is associated with a clicking TM joint, the patient should be informed of the biomechanics of the joint. This information often allows the patient to select functional activities that are less traumatic to the joint structures. For example, some patients may report that the pain and clicking are less when they chew on a particular side of the mouth. When this occurs, they should be encouraged to continue this type of chewing.

Pharmacologic Therapy

Pharmacologic therapy can be an effective adjunct in managing symptoms associated with TMDs. Patients should be aware that medication alone will not likely solve or cure the problem. Medication, however, in conjunction with appropriate physical therapy and definitive treatment, does offer the most complete approach to many TMD problems. Mild analgesics are often helpful for many TMDs. Control of pain is not only appreciated by the patient but also reduces the likelihood of other complicating pain disorders such as muscle co-contraction, referred pain, and central sensitization.

Nonsteroidal antiinflammatory drugs (NSAIDs) are very helpful with many TMDs. Included in this category are aspirin, acetaminophen (Tylenol), and ibuprofen. Ibuprofen (Motrin, Advil, Nuprin) is often very effective in reducing musculoskeletal pains. A dosage of 600 to 800 mg three times a day for 3 to 5 days commonly reduces pain and stops the cyclic effects of the deep pain input. For patients with gastrointestinal issues, short-term use of a cyclooxygenase-2 (COX-2) inhibitor such as celecoxib (Celebrex) can also be useful.

Physical Therapy

In many patients with TMD, symptoms are relieved with very simple physical therapy methods. Simple instructions for the use of moist heat or cold can be very helpful. Surface heat can be applied by laying a hot, moist towel over the symptomatic area. A hot water bottle wrapped inside the towel will help maintain the heat. This combination should remain in place for 10 to 15 minutes, not to exceed 30 minutes. An electric heating pad may be used, but care should be taken not to leave it on the face too long. Patients should be discouraged from using the heating pad while sleeping because prolonged use is likely.

Like thermotherapy, coolant therapy can provide a simple and often effective method of reducing pain. Ice should be applied directly to the symptomatic joint or muscles and moved in a circular motion without pressure to the tissues. The patient will initially experience an uncomfortable feeling that will quickly turn into a burning sensation. Continued icing will result in a mild aching and then numbness. When numbness begins the ice should be removed. The ice should not be left on the tissues for longer than 5 minutes. After a period of warming a second cold application may be desirable.

The physician should be aware that many TMDs respond to the use of orthopedic appliances such as occlusal appliances, bite guards, and splints. These appliances are made by the dentist and are custom fabricated for each patient. Several types of appliances are available. Each is specific for the type of TMD present. The dentist should be consulted for this type of therapy.

Other Therapeutic Considerations

Sometimes TMDs become chronic and, as with other chronic pain conditions, might then be best managed by a multidisciplinary approach. If the patient reports a long history of TMD complaints, the physician should consider referring the patient to a dentist associated with a team of therapists, such as a psychologist, a physical therapist, and even a chronic pain physician. Generally, patients with chronic TMD are not managed well by the simple initial therapies discussed in this chapter. Often other factors, such as mechanical conditions within the TMJs or psychological factors, need to be addressed. The physician who attempts to manage these conditions in the private practice setting can become very frustrated with the results. It is therefore recommended that if the patient's history suggests chronicity or if initial therapy fails to reduce the patient's symptoms, referral is indicated.

References

de Leeuw RE: *Orofacial Pain: Guidelines for Assessment, Diagnosis, and Management*, ed 5, Chicago 2013, Quintessence.

Okeson JP: *Management of Temporomandibular Disorders and Occlusion*, ed 8, St. Louis, 2019, Elsevier.

Okeson JP: *Bell's Orofacial Pains*, ed 7, Chicago, 2014, Quintessence.

Scrivani SJ, Keith DA, Kaban LB: Temporomandibular disorders, *N Engl J Med* 359(25):2693–2705, 2008.

UVEITIS

Method of
Curtis E. Margo, MD, MPH; and Lynn E. Harman, MD

CURRENT DIAGNOSIS

- Uveitis is classified by anatomic location and etiology.
- Most forms of uveitis are due to infectious or immune-mediated disease.
- Drug-induced uveitis and masquerade disorders (neoplasms) must be excluded in diagnostic evaluations.
- Patients with first-time uveitis should have a medical history, physical examination, and basic laboratory studies, with the possible exception of adults who have a single episode of mild anterior uveitis that responds to therapy and who have no systemic signs or symptoms.
- Diagnostic evaluation must differentiate infectious from noninfectious uveitis.
- Patients who are immunosuppressed are at higher risk of infectious uveitis and their clinical presentations may be atypical.
- Uveitis in children is uncommon and deserves a thorough medical evaluation at initial presentation.
- Uveitis is managed optimally through a collaborative multidisciplinary approach.

CURRENT THERAPY

- Eradication of infection is the primary objective in infectious uveitis but may require judicious use of local antiinflammatory agents to mitigate structural and functional damage to intraocular tissues.
- The goal of therapy in noninfectious uveitis is to suppress and eliminate inflammation, achieving lasting remission through the stepwise implementation of therapy.
- First-time anterior uveitis in adults with negative medical history and review of systems can be treated with topical corticosteroids and cycloplegic agents and careful clinical monitoring.
- Corticosteroids can be delivered topically, through periocular and intravitreal injection, via sustained release devices implanted in the eye, and systemically.
- Immunomodulating therapy using alkylating agents, antimetabolites, biologic response modulators, or inhibitors of T-lymphocyte signaling are indicated for uveitis not responsive to systemic corticosteroids.
- A thorough history, physical examination, and select laboratory studies are required before initiating immunomodulating therapy.

Current Diagnosis

Uveitis describes a heterogeneous group of disorders that have in common inflammation of the uveal tract (i.e., iris, ciliary body, and choroid). Symptoms are nonspecific, usually involving various combinations of blurred vision, ocular discomfort, intolerance to light, and floaters. Onset may be sudden or insidious. Children may have no symptoms. The essential signs of uveitis are the presence of inflammatory cells in the aqueous humor and/or vitreous gel. Sufficient magnification with a slit lamp is required to confidently detect these inflammatory cells and not avoid confusion with suspended red blood cells or pigment epithelial cells. Although the uveal tract is the conceptual epicenter of uveal inflammation, there is spillover inflammation in the aqueous humor and vitreous gel, the two anatomic locations used to quantify the severity of inflammation and to monitor response to therapy. Grading schemes for recording the severity of anterior chamber and vitreous inflammatory cell density and protein content (flare) have been published by the Standardization of Uveitis Nomenclature (SUN) Classification Working Group.

Clinical Features and Diagnosis

The anatomic classification of intraocular inflammation into anterior, intermediate, and posterior uveitis and panuveitis guides the diagnostic work-up toward the determination of etiology. When the anterior chamber is the principle site of inflammation, the terms iritis or iridocyclitis are often used. When the vitreous is the primary focus of inflammation, the term intermediate uveitis is preferred, but posterior cyclitis or vitritis are commonly used synonyms. Pars planitis falls within the category of intermediate uveitis and is characterized by a layering of inflammatory cells over the pars plana and anterior retina called a "snowbank lesion." Posterior uveitis embraces diverse conditions that are anatomically characterized by terms such as chorioretinitis, retinochoroiditis, or neuroretinitis.

Most cases of uveitis are caused by infection or immune-mediated disease. A substantial proportion of immune-mediated disease is a manifestation of systemic disease. Arriving at a diagnosis of infectious or noninfectious uveitis requires exclusion of drug-induced uveitis and so-called masquerade disorders (usually neoplasms) that mimic uveal inflammation. Most idiopathic forms of uveitis are localized immune-mediated disease whose pathogenesis is not yet understood. A number of immune-mediated uveitides have overlapping features with infectious disease. For instance, syphilis and Lyme disease have been mistaken for several of the uveal white dot syndromes (see later). Tuberculosis can resemble serpiginous choroiditis. The diagnostic evaluation for persons with noninfectious uveitis and no known systemic disorders involves a complete history, review of systems, physical examination, and select laboratory tests. The optimal use of laboratory testing in this setting is unresolved.

The anatomic categories of posterior uveitis and panuveitis vastly expand the number of potential diagnoses. The pattern and distribution of inflammatory lesions of the choroid, retina, and optic nerve, along with a host of other clinical findings (e.g., vascular or perivascular involvement, severity of overlying inflammation, color and shape of choroidal and retinal lesions, etc.) are critical to narrowing the differential diagnosis. The importance of pattern recognition in the diagnosis of posterior uveitis and panuveitis cannot be overstated. Toxoplasma chorioretinitis, the most common form of posterior uveitis, can usually be confidently diagnosed by clinical ophthalmoscopic appearance of a yellow-white retina with overlying vitreal inflammation adjacent to a hyperpigmented chorioretinal scar. On the other hand, the disorders belonging to the so-called white dot syndromes (acute posterior multifocal placoid pigment epitheliopathy, multifocal chorioretinitis with panuveitis, punctate inner choroidopathy, multiple evanescent white dot syndrome, and birdshot chorioretinopathy) require special studies such as fluorescein angiography and optic coherence tomography to elucidate. Most of these disorders, and a few others such as Vogt-Koyanagi-Harada disease and sympathetic ophthalmia, are clinically defined syndromes. Laboratory studies in this context are used to exclude conditions that could possibly mimic their appearance.

Uveitis occurs in children substantially less often than adults. Although a majority of the same infectious and noninfectious etiologies that occur in adults also affect children, juvenile idiopathic arthritis has a relatively unique clinical presentation in young patients. All four subtypes of juvenile idiopathic arthritis are associated with anterior uveitis, but the pauciarticular category may present with anterior chamber inflammation and advanced band keratopathy with few or no symptoms. This degree of incongruity in symptoms and clinical findings on slit lamp examination is unusual in adults.

Current Therapy

The heterogeneous nature of uveitis limits the generalizability of a universal therapeutic algorithm. When the cause of uveitis is infection, the goal of therapy is to eradicate the infectious organism while controlling inflammation during the process. For noninfectious uveitis, the goal of therapy is to suppress and eliminate inflammation and to achieve lasting remission. This is approached through the stepwise implementation of therapeutic agents, beginning with an agent that has a satisfactory safety profile and can suppress inflammation. The severity and pattern of inflammation at presentation and the perceived risks to vision and ocular integrity guide the initial selection of therapy. Timing of treatment escalation and transition to noncorticosteroid therapy are decisions based on multiple factors, including the patient's general medical health. Simultaneous therapies, particularly local and systemic antiinflammatory agents, are commonly used. Multidisciplinary management is ideally suited to combine the expertise needed to track the ocular response to treatment and to prescribe and monitor many of the systemic mediations.

Anterior Uveitis

Anterior uveitis, the most common subset of uveitis, is usually noninfectious. A minority of cases are attributed to viruses, most often herpes simplex virus (HSV), varicella zoster virus (VZV), and cytomegalovirus (CMV). Clinical manifestations of viral anterior uveitis depend on the immune status of the patient. Once appropriate diagnostic evaluation is complete and viral anterior uveitis is suspected or established for HSV or VZV, therapy with oral acyclovir (Zovirax),[1] valacyclovir (Valtrex),[1] and famciclovir (Famvir)[1] is started. Following clinical resolution of inflammation, maintenance therapy with an oral antiviral drug for HSV should be considered. Anterior uveitis due to CMV is treated with intravenous ganciclovir (Cytovene).[1] Maintenance therapy with topical ganciclovir (Zirgan)[1] or oral valganciclovir (Valcyte)[1] should be considered. Duration of maintenance therapies for viral anterior uveitis has not been subject to rigorous study.

The vast majority of anterior uveitis is noninfectious, for which the mainstay of treatment is topical corticosteroids with cycloplegics (Table 1). There are nearly 20 different preparations of topical corticosteroid (e.g., dexamethasone sodium phosphate 0.1% solution; prednisolone acetate 1.0% suspension [Pred Forte]) that come in suspension or solution (and some as ointment) and in different concentrations. Dose and duration of use is tailored to the clinical setting.

Topical nonsteroidal antiinflammatory agents (e.g., diclofenac 0.1% [Voltaren][1]; ketorolac 0.4% [Acular][1]; flurbiprofen 0.03% [Ocufen][1]) are less effective than topical corticosteroids in controlling the inflammation of anterior uveitis. Their use in combination with topical corticosteroids may be additive.

Topical cycloplegics provide pain relief, and the mydriasis they produce reduces the risk of iridolenticular scarring. The selection of a long-acting (e.g., atropine sulfate 1% [Isopto Atropine] twice daily) versus short-acting cycloplegic agent (e.g., cyclopentolate hydrochloride 0.5% to 1.0% [Cyclogyl] two or three times a day) is based on clinical features such as severity of inflammation, presence of synechial scarring, age of patient, ability to take topical medications, etc. Duration of action varies from 1 to 2 weeks for topical atropine to approximately half a day for cyclopentolate.

Noninfectious anterior uveitis is commonly associated with surgical trauma and accidental blunt trauma (concussive injury). They are usually effectively managed with tapering regimens of topical corticosteroids and cycloplegics.

Oral prednisone (1 mg/kg/day) may be needed for severe or recalcitrant anterior uveitis. Strategies for therapeutic escalation beyond oral corticosteroids parallel that of intermediate or posterior uveitis.

---

[1]Not FDA approved for this indication.

TABLE 1	Topical Medications for Anterior Uveitis		
DRUG NAME (TRADE NAMES)		**FORMULATION**	**STARTING DOSE SCHEDULE***
Topical Corticosteroids			
Dexamethasone (Decadron phosphate [Maxidex])		0.1% suspension; 0.1% solution; 0.05% ointment[2]	4 times per day
Difluprednate (Durezol)		0.05% emulsion	4 times per day
Fluorometholine alcohol (Flarex, FML)		0.1 and 0.25% suspensions; 0.1% ointment	2–4 times per day; 1 to 3 times per day
Loteprednol etabonate (Lotemax)		0.5% suspension	4 times per day
Leteprednol etabonate (Alrex)		0.2% suspension[1]	3 times per day
Prednisolone acetate (Pred Forte, Econopred Plus; AK-Tate)		1.0% suspension	4 times per day
Prednisolone sodium phosphate (Inflamase Forte; AK-Pred)		1.0% solution	4 times per day
Prednisolone acetate (Pred Mild; Econopred)		0.12% suspension	4 times per day
Topical Cycloplegic Agents			
Atropine sulfate (Isopto atropine)		1.0%	Once or twice a day
Cyclopentolate hydrochloride (Cyclogel)[1]		0.5% and 1.0%	Twice a day
Homatropine hydrobromide (Isopto homatropine)		2.0%–5.0%	Once or twice a day
Scopolamine hydrobromide (Isopto hyoscine)		0.25%	Once or twice a day
Tropicamide (Mydriacyl)[1]		0.5% and 1.0%	2–3 times a day
Topical Nonsteroidal Antiinflammatory Medications			
Bromfenac (BromSite; Prolensa; Xibrom)[1]		0.075%–0.09% solution	Once or twice daily
Diclofenac (Voltaren)[1]		0.1% solution	2 times per day
Flurbiprofen (Ocufen)[1]		0.03% solution	2 times per day
Ketorolac (Acular LS; Acular)[1]		0.4%–0.5%	3 times per day
Nepafenac (Ilevro; Nevanac)[1]		0.1%–0.3% suspension	3 times per day

*More frequent use of corticosteroids dictated by severity of inflammation then tapered based on clinical response.
[1]Not FDA approved for this indication.
[2]Not available in the United States.

Although topical corticosteroids and cycloplegics do not play a primary role in intermediate and posterior uveitis, they are used as adjuvant therapies for comfort and to minimize the formation of peripheral and posterior synechiae.

Intermediate Uveitis

Intermediate uveitis, characterized by inflammatory cells in vitreous, peripheral retina, and pars plana, can be associated with systemic disorders such as multiple sclerosis, sarcoidosis, syphilis, toxocariasis (in children), and Lyme disease. Vitritis is also a presenting sign of endogenous endophthalmitis and can be mimicked by primary vitreoretinal lymphoma. Once infection, drug-related uveitis, and masquerading conditions are excluded, the approach to therapy for noninfectious forms of intermediate uveitis is similar to the stepladder approach (described later) that typically begins with oral corticosteroids. For pars planitis recalcitrant to medical therapy, options include peripheral ablation of the snowbank lesion with indirect laser photocoagulation and pars plana vitrectomy. Their effectiveness has not been rigorously tested in clinical trials.

Periocular injections of depot corticosteroids (40 mg triamcinolone acetonide [1 mL of 40 mg/mL Kenalog-40][1]) delivers medication closer to the site of inflammation and may be used as a bridge to oral steroid therapy or to reduce the dose of oral steroids. Intravitreal corticosteroid injection through the pars plana (4 mg triamcinolone acetonide suspension [0.1 mL 40 mg/mL Kenalog-40[1]; Triesence]) is often tried before moving to immune modulator therapy. The risk of endophthalmitis and the need for repeat injections are drawbacks.

[1]Not FDA approved for this indication.

Posterior Uveitis and Panuveitis

The general diagnostic approach to posterior uveitis and panuveitis begins by excluding infection and drug-induced uveitis and not overlooking the possibility of a masquerade condition. The optimal strategy for laboratory testing to identify a culpable systemic disorder responsible for noninfectious uveitis is a matter of debate. Many posterior and pan uveitides are clinically defined syndromes. For example, Behçet disease, multifocal choroiditis with panuveitis, acute posterior multifocal placoid pigment epitheliopathy, serpiginous choroiditis, punctate inner choroidopathy, multiple evanescent white dot syndrome, Vogt-Koyanagi-Harada disease, and sympathetic ophthalmia are diagnoses based on clinical findings (e.g., ophthalmoscopy, fluorescein angiography, optical coherence tomography, etc.). These syndromes have no confirmatory laboratory tests, other than several with strong human leukocyte antigen (HLA) haplotype associations (e.g., Behçet disease [HLA-B51]; birdshot chorioretinopathy [HLS-A29]).

Management of inflammation associated with noninfectious posterior uveitis requires systemic medications. Most clinicians initiate oral corticosteroids, understanding that high-dose long-term use is associated with serious and predictable side effects. The risk of systemic side effects may be reduced with judicious use of periocular or intravitreal corticosteroid injections, but those routines of administration also have their own potential adverse effects and complications. These range from elevated intraocular pressure and glaucoma to infectious endophthalmitis. A sustained-release corticosteroid implant is another option. Corticosteroids are embedded to either a biodegradable or nonbiodegradable vehicle to achieve sustained release. The implants are injected into the vitreous or

TABLE 2	Treatment of Infectious Uveitis

DIAGNOSIS	INFECTIOUS ORGANISM(S)	TREATMENT	COMMENT
Acute retinal necrosis	Herpes zoster virus (HZV) Herpes simplex virus (HSV) I and II	Acyclovir (Zovirax)[1] 13 mg/kg/dose divided every 8 h IV for 7 days, followed by 800 mg po 5 times/day for 3–4 months; or, Famciclovir (Famvir)[1] 500 mg po q8h; or Valacyclovir (Valtrex)[1] 1000–2000 mg po q8h for induction Ganciclovir (Cytovene)[1] 500 mg IV q12h; maintenance: (duration varies with response) Valganciclovir (Valcyte)[1] 900 mg po BID for 3 weeks then 450 mg po BID Ganciclovir[1] 1000 mg po TID	Adjuvant intravitreal injection options: Ganciclovir (200–2000 µg/0.1 mL)[6] Foscarnet (Foscavir)[1] (1.2–2.4 mg/0.1 mL)[6]; Possible role for prednisone (0.5–2.0 mg/kg/day po for up to 6–8 weeks)
Anterior uveitis, viral	HSV HZV Cytomegalovirus (CMV)	Valacyclovir[1] 500 mg po TID Acyclovir[1] 400 mg po × 5/day 4 weeks Valacyclovir[1] 1 g po TID Acyclovir[1] 800 mg po × 5/day 5–6 weeks Famciclovir[1] 500 mg po TID 5–6 weeks Ganciclovir[1] 5 mg/kg IV BID 2–3 weeks Valganciclovir[1] 900 mg po BID × 6 weeks, then 450 mg po BID × 6 weeks	Topical corticosteroids and cycloplegic recommended. Alternative options include an intravitreal ganciclovir (2 mg/0.05 mL)[6]. After active infection eradicated, consider maintenance therapy for HSV and CMV
Cat-scratch disease	Bartonella henselae	Doxycycline (Vibramycin)[1] 100 mg po BID, or Azithromycin (Zithromax)[1] 500 mg po day 1; 250 mg po days 2 through 5	Children: Azithromycin 10 mg/kg po day 1; 5 mg/kg po days 2 through 5
Cytomegalovirus retinitis	Cytomegalovirus	Immune reconstitution; ganciclovir 5 mg/kg/day IV BID for 2–3 weeks followed by maintenance 5 mg/kg/day po Cidofovir (Vistide)[1] 5 mg/kg/week IV for 2 weeks then 5 mg/kg every 2 weeks	Immune reconstitution targets cause of immune compromise. Various maintenance regiments (e.g., oral valganciclovir 900 mg/day)
Diffuse unilateral subacute neuroretinitis (DUSN)	Possible larva of Baylisascaris procyonis, Toxocara canis	Photocoagulation of intraretinal nematode	Destruction of intraretinal larva may preserve vision.
Lyme disease	Borrelia burgdorferi	Doxycycline[1] 100 mg po BID × 21 days (adults) Amoxicillin[1] 50 mg/kg po in divided doses × 14–21 days (children)	Alternative: cefuroxime axetil (Ceftin) 500 mg po BID × 14–21 days
Metastatic endophthalmitis (endogenous)	Numerous blood-borne bacteria and fungi	Sepsis treatment protocol; antibiotic selections based on cultures and sensitivities	Role and timing of intravitreal antibiotics and of vitrectomy less well defined
Onchocerciasis	Onchocerca volvulus	Ivermectin (Stromectol) 150 µg/kg single oral dose; repeat at 6 months for the life span of adult worm	Corticosteroids to control ocular inflammation; route of administration depends of site of inflammation
Syphilis	Treponema pallidum	Aqueous penicillin G 18–24 million units, IV q4h for 10–14 days	Ocular syphilis is considered a subset of neurosyphilis
Toxocariasis	Toxocara canis or Toxocara catis	Prednisone 1–2 mg/kg/day po; timing of antihelminthic therapy unresolved.	Laser ablation and vitrectomy depending on stage of disease. Intraocular larval death incites considerable inflammation
Toxoplasmosis	Toxoplasma gondii	Pyrimethamine (Daraprim): loading dose 50–100 mg po; treatment dose 25–50 mg/day po; and sulfadiazine: loading dose 2–4 g po; treatment dose 1.0 g po QID, and prednisone (0.5–1.0 mg/kg/day po) Trimethoprim-sulfamethoxazole (Bactrim DS)[1] 160 mg/80 mg po BID, plus above regimen of prednisone	Modify doses if pregnant or immune compromised.
Tuberculosis	Mycobacterium tuberculosis	Isoniazid (INH) 300 mg po; Rifampin (RIF [Rifadin]) 450 mg (<50 kg) po, 600 mg (>50 kg) po; pyrazinamide 1.5 g (<50 kg) po, 2.0 g (>50 kg) po; and ethambutol (Myambutol) 15 mg/kg po—all qd for 2 months	After sensitivities established, INH and RIF or rifapentine (Priftin) alone daily for 4 months. Follow recommendations for first line therapy for active tuberculosis

[1]Not FDA approved for this indication.
[6]May be compounded by pharmacists.
BID, Twice a day; *IV*, intravenous; *po*, by mouth; *TID*, three times a day.

TABLE 3 Immune Modulator Therapy for Uveitis

GENERIC (TRADE) NAME	DOSE (ROUTE)*	COMMENT/INDICATIONS[†]
Alkylating Agents		
Chlorambucil (Leukeran)[1]	0.15 mg/kg/day po	Behçet disease; juvenile idiopathic arthritis; pars planitis; sympathetic ophthalmia
Cyclophosphamide (Cytoxan)[1]	1–3 mg/kg/day po 15 mg/kg IV at 2, 4, 7, 10 weeks…up to 9 pulses	Sclerouveitis; sympathetic ophthalmia
Antimetabolites		
Azathioprine (Imuran)[1]	1–1.5 mg/kg/day po can increase to 2.5 mg/kg/day	Severe anterior uveitis; panuveitis, juvenile idiopathic arthritis; pars planitis, sarcoidosis; sympathetic uveitis; Vogt-Koyanagi-Harada disease (VKH)
Methotrexate (Folex, Mexate, and Rheumatrex)[1]	7.5–15 mg/week po	Anterior, intermediate, and posterior uveitis; juvenile idiopathic arthritis; sympathetic uveitis
Mycophenolate mofetil (Cellcept)[1]; Mycophenolate sodium (Myfortic)[1]	Cellcept: 1–2 g po in divided doses; Myfortic: 1 g po bid × 6 or more months	Anterior, intermediate, and posterior uveitis
Calcinernin Inhibitors		
Cyclosporine (Neoral, Sandimmune, SangCya)[1]	2.5–5 mg/kg/day po divided doses	Often given with prednisone 10–20 mg/day; Behçet disease; birdshot chorioretinopathy; pan uveitis; posterior uveitis; sarcoidosis; sclerouveitis; sympathetic uveitis; VKH
Tacrolimus (Prograf, Astagraf XL, Hecoria, Envasus XR)[1]	0.15–0.3 mg/kg/day po	Behçet disease; birdshot chorioretinopathy; posterior uveitis
Biologic Response Modifier Tumor Necrosis Factor (TNF)-α inhibitor		
Adalimumab (Humira)	40 mg subcutaneous injection every other week	Anterior, intermediate and posterior uveitis; juvenile idiopathic arthritis; sarcoidosis[‡]
Etanercept (Enbrel)[1]	25 mg subcutaneous injection × 2/week	May increase risk of anterior uveitis in ankylosing spondylitis
Infliximab (Remicade)[1]	3–5 mg/kg/day IV weeks 0, 2, and 6	Behçet disease; anterior uveitis; juvenile idiopathic arthritis; sarcoidosis
Biologic Response Modifier Interleukin-1 Inhibitor		

*Therapeutic regimens used in clinical studies with the same medications have differed in loading dose and maintenance dose.
[†]Indications refer to reported success at controlling or eliminating inflammation as a single or as a steroid-sparing agent.
[1]Not US Food and Drug Administration (FDA) approved for this indication.
[2]Not available in the United States.
bid, Twice a day; *po*, by mouth; *tid*, three times a day.

surgically fixed to the sclera. Dexamethasone (Ozurdex, 0.7 mg) has a delivery span of 6 months, and fluocinolone acetonide (Iluvien 0.19 mg[1]; Retisert 0.59 mg; Yutiq 0.18 mg) 18 to 36 months.

The optimal time to transition to noncorticosteroid immunomodulatory therapy is not well defined. The guidelines for treatment escalation are also imprecise, relying on clinical judgment, individual patient input, and shared decision making. Immunomodulatory therapy for the treatment of uveitis falls into four drug categories: antimetabolites, inhibitors of T-lymphocyte signaling, biologic response modifiers, and alkylating agents (Table 3). Their judicious use has been shown to reduce or eliminate the need for systemic corticosteroids, improve long-term visual prognosis, and reduce ocular complications from inflammation. Meaningful clinical responses should occur within 3 months of initiating therapy. Following achieved clinical end points, drugs can be carefully tapered over 24 months. A thorough history, physical examination, and select laboratory tests and imaging studies should be completed prior to initiation of therapy.

The most commonly used antimetabolites for the treatment of noninfectious uveitis are methotrexate (Rheumatrex),[1] azathioprine (Imuran),[1] and mycophenolate mofetil (Cellcept).[1] Oral methotrexate, 7.5 to 15 mg once per week with daily folic acid[1] 1 mg, can be increased to 20 to 25 mg/week based on clinical response. Intravenous methotrexate (100 to 200 mg weekly) can be tried for persons with gastrointestinal intolerance. Intravitreal injection of 400 μg/0.1 mL has been used for refractory inflammation. Oral azathioprine is begun at 1 mg/kg/day. Depending on clinical response, it can be incrementally increased to 2.5 mg/kg/day. Mycophenolate mofetil is started at 1 to 2 g orally per day in divided doses up to 3 g/day. The manifold side effects of antimetabolites necessitate close clinical monitoring.

Most experience in treating noninfectious uveitis with inhibitors of T-lymphocyte signaling, or calcineurin inhibitors, is with cyclosporine (Sandimmune)[1]. Given 2.5 to 5 mg/kg/day in divided doses, cyclosporine can cause nephrotoxicity, bone marrow suppression, and hypertension.

Alkylating agents used to treat noninfectious uveitis include cyclophosphamide (Cytoxan)[1] and chlorambucil (Leukeran)[1]. These immunomodulating drugs are titrated to keep white blood cell counts in the range of 3000 to 4500 cells per cubic millimeter. Chlorambucil is started at 0.15 mg/kg/day and cyclophosphamide at 1 to 3 mg/kg/day. Regular monitoring for bone marrow suppression and opportunistic infection is needed for both drugs. Risks of hemorrhagic cystitis with cyclophosphamide may be reduced by consuming generous amounts of water daily.

Biologic response modifiers, or "biologics," have expanded the therapeutic arsenal for treating advanced or severe noninfectious uveitis. This family of medications consists of antibodies directed against key cytokines in the immune response pathway. Most experience in treating noninfectious uveitis has been with tumor necrosis factor-α (TNF-α) inhibitors (infliximab [Remicade][1] and adalimumab [Humira]). Although other biologics have been used

[1]Not FDA approved for this indication.

to treat advanced or severe noninfectious uveitis, their equivalence or superiority to the drugs already mentioned are under study. Etanercept (Embrel)[1] may increase the risk of anterior uveitis in persons with ankylosing spondylitis.

Infliximab (Remicade) is given as a subcutaneous injection beginning with two loading doses of 3 to 5 mg/kg each given 2 weeks apart. Injections are then continued at 4-week intervals. Based on clinical response, dose can be gradually increased to 10 mg/kg. Side effects include infection from latent activation of tuberculosis or hepatitis, drug-induced autoimmune disease, and demyelinating disease. There is also a small risk of increased overall cancer mortality when compared with a nonimmunosuppressed population of patients. Adalimumab (Humira) is given subcutaneously starting at 40 mg/kg every 2 weeks. Children are usually started at half this dose. Its adverse risk profile is similar to that of infliximab.

Other biologics used to treat noninfectious uveitis such as anti-CD20 monoclonal antibody (Rituximab [Rituxan][1]) have less established positions in the stepwise implementation of therapy. Interferon alfa-2a (Roferon-A)[1], known for its antiviral and antineoplastic effects, has been used to treat Behçet disease with persistent macular edema. It is given as a subcutaneous injection of 3 to 9 million international units daily for a week then tapered over 3 to 6 months. Interferon alfa-2a is associated with flu-like symptoms and depression, which may limit patient acceptance.

Complications of Uveitis

Chronic uveitis gives rise to a variety of ocular complications such as secondary glaucoma, macular edema, corneal dysfunction, neovascularization of the iris, angle, and retina, retinal tears and detachments, cyclitic membrane formation, and uveal effusion, as well as other conditions. These ocular complications are typically approached by controlling or eliminating ocular inflammation and managing the structural/functional problems according to standards guidelines.

Disease-Specific Recommendations

Strength of recommendations for disease-specific noncorticosteroid immunomodulatory therapy is constrained by the relative lack of prospective clinical trials, drug-to-drug comparison trials, studies that have included patients with diverse forms of uveitis, and the small size of studies. Given these limitations, the strength of recommendations is tempered by a level of evidence for most drugs of 2B or lower on the Oxford Centre for Evidence-Based Medicine level of evidence scale. Mycophenolate preparations[1], azathioprine[1], methotrexate[1], cyclophosphamide[1], cyclosporine[1], sirolimus (Rapamune)[1], infliximab[1], adalimumab, and etanercept[1] have demonstrated varying degrees of success in controlling inflammation, improving visual outcome, and reducing corticosteroid use in severe anterior, intermediate, and posterior uveitis and in panuveitis. Control of inflammation and improved visual acuity in Vogt-Koyanagi-Harada disease have been achieved with systemic methotrexate[1], azathioprine[1], mycophenolate preparations[1], infliximab[1], adalimumab[1], and interferon alfa-2a[1]. The uveitis of Beçhet disease, juvenile idiopathic arthritis, pars planitis, and sympathetic ophthalmia responds to chlorambucil[1]. Mycophenolate preparations[1] have had success in various forms of anterior, intermediate, and posterior uveitis. The inflammation of Beçhet disease has been controlled with azathioprine[1], infliximab[1], adalimumab[1], rituximab[1], and interferon alfa-2a[1]. Sarcoid uveitis has responded to infliximab[1] and adalimumab[1]. The systemic disease of juvenile idiopathic arthritis has been successfully managed with methotrexate, cyclosporine[1], mycophenolate mofetil[1], azathioprine[1], and TNF-α inhibitors adalimumab and infliximab[1]. Therapeutic vitrectomy and/or laser ablation has been used in different forms of noninfectious uveitis, but evidence of long-term effectiveness is sparse.

---

[1]Not FDA approved for this indication.

Systemic Drug Use in Pregnancy and in Children

Because the teratogenic potential of many immunosuppressive drugs is incompletely understood, it may be prudent to discuss contraception when they are administered to women. The largely unknown teratogenic effects of immunosuppressive agents in men should also be considered. Although prednisone is well tolerated during pregnancy, its use should be carefully comanaged with an obstetrician.

The effects of immunosuppressive drugs are less well studied in children than adults. Children on immunosuppressive agents should not receive live virus vaccine for 3 months after immunosuppressive use has ended. This would include high-dose corticosteroids. The impact of immunosuppressive drugs and systemic corticosteroids on growth and collateral effects on social development is not inconsequential. Osteoporosis, adrenal suppression, and heightened susceptibility to infections related to cell-mediated immunity are among the side effects that require monitoring in children. Calcium supplements and vitamin D may be beneficial in some circumstances.

References

Dick AD, Rosenbaum JT, Al-Dhibi HA, et al: Guidance on noncorticosteroid systemic immunomodulatory therapy in noninfectious uveitis. Fundamentals of Care for UveitiS (FOCUS) Initiative, *Ophthalmology* 125:757–773, 2018.

Foster CS, Kothari S, Anesi SD, et al: The Ocular Immunology and Uveitis Foundation preferred practice patterns of uveitis management, *Surv Ophthalmol* 61:1–17, 2016.

Jabs DA, Nussenblatt RB, Rosenbaum JT: Standardization of Uveitis Nomenclature (SUN) Work Group. Standardization of uveitis nomenclature for reporting clinical data. Results of the First International Workshop, *Am J Ophthalmol* 140:509–516, 2005.

Jap A, Soon-Phaik C: Viral anterior uveitis. Diagnosis and management, *Focal Points* 34(5):1–18, 2016, Available at https://store.aao.org/clinical-education/product-line/focal-points.html. [Accessed 21 October 2018].

Levy-Clarke G, Jabs DA, Read RW, et al: Expert panel recommendations for the use of anti-tumor necrosis factor biologic agents in patients with ocular inflammatory disorders, *Ophthalmology* 121:785–796, 2014, e783.

London NJS, Garg SJ, Moorthy MS, et al: Drug-induced uveitis, *Focal Points* 33(5):1–10, 2015. Available at https://store.aao.org/clinical-education/product-line/focal-points.html. [Accessed 21 October 2018].

Lower CY, Lima BR: Pediatric uveitis, *Focal Points* 32(3):1–11, 2014. Available at https://store.aao.org/clinical-education/product-line/focal-points.html. [Accessed 21 October 2018].

Schwartzman S: Advancements in the management of uveitis, *Best Prac Research Clin Rheum* 30:304–316, 2016.

Wakefield D, McCluskey P, Wildner G, et al: Inflammatory eye disease: pretreatment assessment of patients prior to commencing immunosuppressive and biologic therapy: recommendations from an expert committee, *Autoimmun Rev* 16:213–222, 2017.

Yeh S, Suhler ER, Moorly RS, et al: Biologic response modifiers in uveitis, *Focal Points* 30(3):1–16, 2012. Available at https://store.aao.org/clinical-education/product-line/focal-points.html. [Accessed 21 October 2018].

VISION REHABILITATION

Method of
August Colenbrander, MD; Donald C. Fletcher, MD; and Kim Schoessow, OTD, OTR/L

Vision rehabilitation refers to the multidisciplinary effort of assisting those with various degrees of vision loss in coping with the *consequences* of that loss. To describe vision rehabilitation, the nature of vision itself must be understood.

Vision is the major source of information about our environment. The eyes alone contribute as much information to the brain as all other organs combined. It is not surprising therefore that many people fear loss of vision almost as much as loss of life.

Most people will state that "We see with our eyes." On closer examination, this is not true. An isolated eyeball cannot produce any vision; our brain, however, can produce exquisite visual imagery in our dreams, without any input from the eyes.

The visual process goes through three distinct stages. Each stage comes with its own specific problems.

- First is the *optical stage*, where the refractive media of the eye deliver an image to the retina. Familiar problems in this area include refractive errors and cataracts.

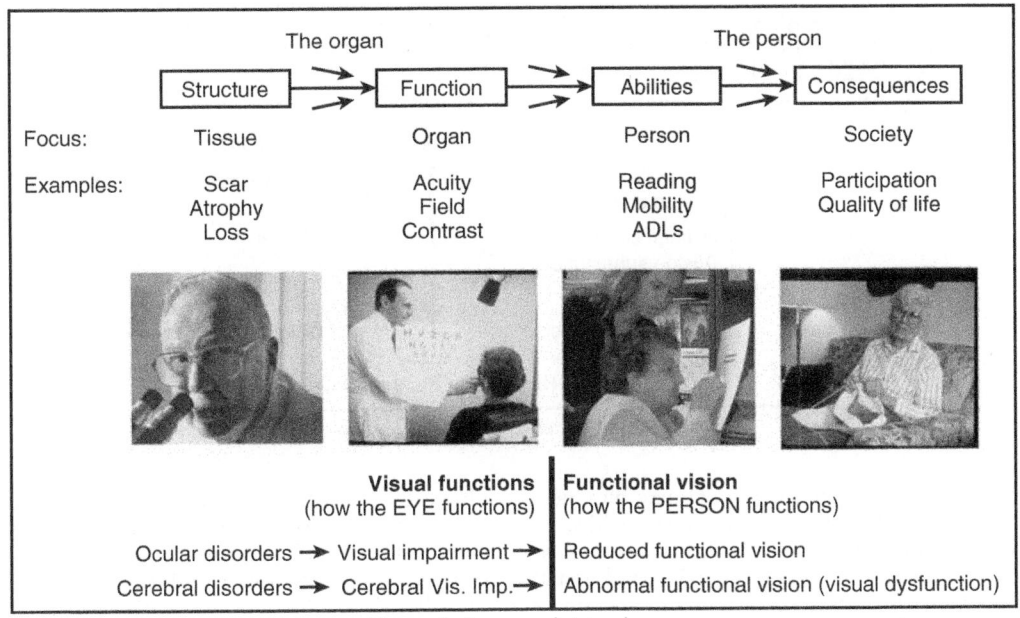

Figure 1 Aspects of vision loss.

- Second is the *receptor stage*, where the optical image is translated into neural impulses. Age-related macular degeneration (AMD) is a significant problem of the receptor stage, which is becoming increasingly common as the population ages.
- Third are various stages of *neural processing*, initially in the inner retina, then in the visual cortex, and finally in higher cortical centers, where the visual input gives rise to visual perception and to visually guided behaviors, actions, and interactions.

The most common visual problems vary for different ages. Today, brain-damage-related vision problems (cerebral visual impairment or CVI) are the most prevalent cause of visual impairment in *infants and young children*. Given that vision is so important for normal development, vision loss in infants constitutes a developmental emergency and should be detected and addressed as early as possible. When a child does not smile back at the mother, the mother may be inclined to leave the baby in its crib instead of holding him or her to provide extra tactile stimulation to compensate for missing visual stimulation.

At *school age* and later, visual health is critical because reading becomes important for academic development. For *adults*, vision is important for maintaining independence in activities of daily living (ADL) and development of vocational skills. For *seniors*, vision loss may exacerbate other age-related dysfunctions. Studies of the elderly have shown correlations between visual impairment and depression, falls, and reduced longevity. In all of these instances, early detection and early intervention are essential; the primary care physician plays a crucial role in this respect.

Four Aspects of Vision Loss

Vision is a complex phenomenon.

A convenient framework for discussing the various impacts of vision loss is to consider four aspects of visual functioning (Figure 1). First to consider is how various external causes may result in *structural changes* to the eyes and the visual pathways. For this aspect, the focus is on the tissue; an ocular pathologist is needed to describe the pathologic condition. However, structural changes alone do not determine how well the eyes actually function. Clinicians need to measure *organ function*, such as visual acuity, visual field, and contrast sensitivity.

Yet even knowing how the eyes function does not tell us how the person functions. In other words, the *abilities* of the person to perform tasks, such as reading, mobility, face recognition, and ADL, must be considered. Occupational therapists (OTs) and other rehabilitation professionals work with patients to teach them how residual vision can be used most effectively. OTs also

assess the person in a societal context. For example, do the visual changes have an impact on the person's *participation* in society, on his or her ability to perform necessary tasks, and on general satisfaction with one's quality of life? It is clear that to cover all aspects of vision rehabilitation, a team approach is necessary, and that the patient must be part of that team.

A single activity of daily living may cover several of the above aspects. When reading, the aspect of minimum print size falls under organ function (retinal resolution). Reading speed (words/minute) and reading endurance (hours/day) define abilities of the person; reading endurance may be poor, even if reading acuity is adequate. Reading enjoyment, finally, falls under the aspect of quality of life.

It is helpful to draw a line between the organ side of Figure 1 on the left and the person side on the right. On the left side of the diagram, we discuss *visual functions*, which describe how the eyes function. On the right side, we speak of *functional vision*, which describes how the person functions in vision-related activities. Medical specialists are well versed in dealing with the left side of the diagram. Yet, the ultimate goal of all interventions is to improve the patient's quality of life. It is the function of vision rehabilitation to make sure that "eye" doctors become "people" doctors by extending their interest to the right side of the diagram as well.

Comprehensive Vision Rehabilitation

Considering all of these aspects, comprehensive vision rehabilitation involves much more than the patient's performance on a letter chart and requires teamwork by different professionals who specialize in different aspects of vision loss. All vision loss starts with some medical condition. So, primary care physicians are well positioned to coordinate team activities. Primary care physicians need to be aware of what other team members can contribute and should know where to locate vision rehabilitation resources and to make appropriate referrals.

Figure 2 illustrates that comprehensive vision rehabilitation involves much more than does the traditional low vision care offered in the past.

Low vision is a term used to describe individuals who suffer from a visual impairment that cannot be eliminated with refractive correction, yet are not blind. Individuals who suffer from low vision may benefit from vision enhancement, vision substitution, and vision assistance as well as from honing of coping skills.

Low vision is distinct from blindness (i.e., no vision). Blindness differs from low vision in that in blindness, the emphasis of rehabilitation is entirely on vision substitution. Patients with severe

Figure 2 Comprehensive vision rehabilitation.

or profound low vision may combine the use of some blindness rehabilitation skills with some low vision rehabilitation skills.

Vision enhancement, which is the traditional focus of low vision care, is primarily oriented at improving residual visual function through visual aids, including a wide range of magnification devices. Additionally, enhancement of contrast, illumination, and filters need to be explored.

Vision substitution expands the options for rehabilitation by optimizing the use of other senses. This can range from using simple tactile markings to sense the position of a stove dial to devices such as talking books, a long cane for travel, and Braille for reading. Vision enhancement and vision substitution are not mutually exclusive. A patient may use a magnifier to read price tags and may prefer talking books for recreational reading. A patient with retinitis pigmentosa, which causes reduced night vision, may have normal mobility in the daytime and need a cane at night. Digital audio books may have Braille labels.

Vision assistance. A special form of vision substitution involves using the eyes of others. Family members, caregivers, and office personnel should be familiar with *sighted guide* techniques to effectively assist visually impaired patients with minimal embarrassment. *Guide dogs* are also a possibility. Using a guide dog requires training of the patient as well as of the dog, so that they can work as a team. Dog users must also demonstrate mastery of long cane travel skills.

Coping skills. How different patients will accept visual aids may differ greatly. It is important to recognize that vision loss often causes a reactive depression. On the one hand, a depressed patient will be less receptive to rehabilitative suggestions. On the other hand, demonstration of rehabilitative success can be a powerful tool to lift a reactive depression and to motivate the patient for further success. It has been shown that the teaching of problem-solving skills may improve the effectiveness of vision rehabilitation.

Many professionals may be involved in vision rehabilitation. Technicians may prescribe magnifiers, rehabilitation workers may teach daily living skills, and psychologists may address depression. Acceptance of the work of these professionals will be improved if the trusted primary care physician is credited with making the referrals.

Beyond the factors that directly involve the patient, the environment must also be considered.

The *human environment* is important. As patients go through the stages of adaptation, a supportive home environment is essential. As patients are counseled, it is important to include spouses, children, or significant others to make sure that they understand the condition, know what can be expected, and know how to support the patient. Answering family and caregiver questions directly is often better than leaving this to the patient, who initially may not have absorbed everything that was said. An overprotective environment, which deprives patients of opportunities to do things for themselves, can be as detrimental as an overdemanding one that puts too much emphasis on the patient's shortcomings. The same holds true for the work or school environment or for social groups.

Initially, patients often feel isolated and believe that they are the only ones experiencing these problems. *Peer support groups* can be helpful; in these groups, patients can experience how others are dealing with similar problems.

Finally, the *physical environment* needs to be considered. An uncluttered environment, where things have a defined, fixed place, is helpful because it reduces the need for searching. Good general illumination and task lighting often help, because at higher illumination levels retinal cells that are damaged but not dead can still contribute to vision. Good contrast is important: do not serve milk in a white Styrofoam cup; mark the edges of steps and stairs. The triangles and circles on men's and women's bathrooms are designed to be visible for those with very low vision; Braille labels in elevators are useful for people who are totally blind.

How Blind Is Blind?

The most common visual function test is the letter chart, developed by Snellen in 1862. That test determines how large a letter, or other symbol, must be to be recognized by the patient. That size is then compared to the size recognized by a standard observer. If the magnification requirement is 2 ×, visual acuity is said to be 1/2; if it is 5 ×, visual acuity is said to be 1/5, etc. That fraction can be recorded in different ways; in the United States, it is customary to use 20 as the denominator (1/2 = 20/40, 1/5 = 20/100); in the British Commonwealth, 6 is used as the denominator (6/12, 6/30); in Europe, decimal fractions are common (0.5, 0.2).

Those calculations are simple; unfortunately, the terminology used to describe various ranges of vision loss is confusing. Figure 3 shows progressively degraded pictures with examples of the terminology used to describe different definitions of visual impairment. The visual acuity level represented by each picture can be determined from the number of lines that are readable on the low vision letter chart.

The first picture shows the visual acuity level that is labeled as "low vision" by the World Health Organization (WHO). Although the bottom lines of the letter chart cannot be read, the appearance of the room is near normal. The next picture shows what the U.S. Social Security Administration considers "statutory blindness" for its programs. It is clear that this is far from actual blindness. Other U.S. programs use a different definition for "legal blindness," and the WHO does not consider a person "blind" until he or she has reached the status of the last picture. At that level, reading even the special letter chart is not possible, but one can still navigate the room. Even this level of visual impairment does not constitute actual blindness.

The widespread use of the word "blindness" is unfortunate, because it cannot be used with modifiers. One is either blind or sighted; one cannot be "a little bit blind." This black-and-white thinking has hampered the acceptance of vision rehabilitation. Terms such as vision loss or visual impairment are preferred because they can be used with modifiers, including mild, moderate, severe, profound, and total vision loss. Although "legal

Figure 3 Ranges of vision loss.

blindness" and "severe vision loss" (ICD-9-CM) have the same definition, there is a big difference between telling a patient "You are legally blind" and "You have a severe visual impairment." The first statement might be followed by "I am sorry, there is nothing more we can do for your eyes"; the second statement leads to the question "What can be done to help you cope with this problem?"

Vision Rehabilitation Techniques and Devices
Having considered the general outlines of vision rehabilitation, some details of rehabilitative interventions can be discussed. Primary care physicians should know what vision rehabilitation techniques are available.

Optical Problems
The most commonly encountered visual problems are those involving the optical system of the eye.

Refractive errors are the easiest visual problems to deal with. Refractive errors can be corrected with glasses or contact lenses, and for those who hate glasses, by refractive surgery. Even if there are other causes of vision loss, determining the best refractive correction is still important.

Uncorrected refractive error is a major cause of visual impairment worldwide. In developed countries, the question may be why people do not avail themselves of the solutions that are available. In developing countries, availability of and accessibility to eye care and to the means for correcting refractive errors often do not exist. Providing these is a matter of infrastructure, not of individual health care.

Opacities disrupt visual image formation. Cataracts are the most familiar opacity; they can be removed by surgery. Other opacities of a temporary or permanent nature may occur in the cornea, in the anterior chamber, or in the vitreous cavity. Corneal and conjunctival infections may cause corneal scarring, as is the case in trachoma; this condition does not exist in the developed world anymore but is a major cause of blindness worldwide.

Letter chart acuity is a good way to measure optical problems. It should be understood, however, that letter chart acuity only measures the function of the retina where the letter read is projected. Even for a patient with 20/200 acuity, this area of the retina is less than 1° in diameter. For optical problems this does not matter, because foveal defocus predicts equal defocus in all other areas of the retina.

Magnification is the primary way to compensate for reduced acuity. One way to provide magnification is to bring print closer to the eye. For the elderly, this requires reading glasses with extra power. Alternatively, large print may be helpful. Larger print on medicine labels, as required in several states, can reduce medication errors by the elderly, who often take several medications. Handheld magnifiers are another option; many have built-in LED illumination that provides more light. Video-magnifiers with a table-mounted large screen are ideal for prolonged reading; they can enhance contrast and brightness, while some devices can even read the text out loud. Tablets and smartphone apps can provide similar advantages in a portable form, as can an increasing number of portable electronic magnifiers that can provide not only magnification, but also contrast enhancement.

Retinal Problems
While primitive forms of cataract surgery have existed for centuries, the study of retinal disorders has only been possible since the invention of the ophthalmoscope in 1851. The ability to effectively treat some retinal disorders is even more recent. Important retinal disorders include the following.

AMD is the most frequent diagnosis encountered in any low vision rehabilitation service. Because the condition is age related, its frequency will increase in the future as our population ages. This has caused profound changes in the nature of low vision care. Until the mid-20th century, most low vision care was provided by special education teachers serving young students in schools for the blind. Today, the majority of low vision patients are seniors. This has resulted in a significant influx of OTs into the field with skills in addressing multiple geriatric impairments. Yet, the needs of seniors to be served still outstrip the available services.

Given that macular degeneration affects central vision and the ability to read, most patients will ultimately seek rehabilitation help. However, if only one eye is affected, AMD may go unnoticed. The patient may only complain when the second eye starts to deteriorate; at that point, the damage in the first eye may be beyond repair. Therefore it is useful to ask patients to alternately cover one eye to see whether there is any vision difference between the eyes. If there is, this is a reason for referral.

Glaucoma is another age-related condition. Glaucoma often goes undetected because it causes loss of peripheral vision and affects central vision only in the late stages. Therefore glaucoma must be sought out, primarily by measuring the intraocular pressure.

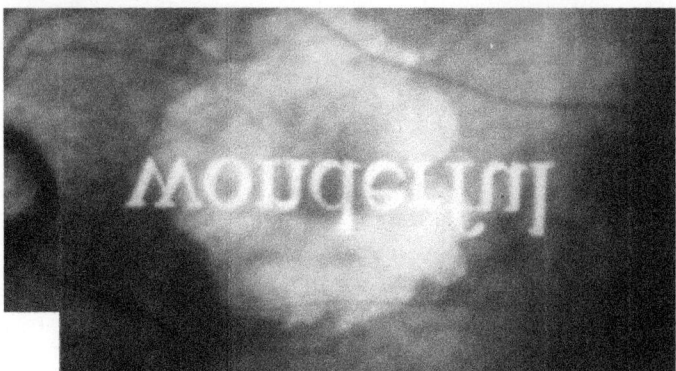

Figure 4 Ring scotoma.

Diabetic retinopathy is not limited to seniors. As the incidence of diabetes is rising worldwide, so is the incidence of diabetic retinopathy. Even if treated with photocoagulation, it will cause scattered blind spots throughout the visual field.

There are many other hereditary and nonhereditary retinal conditions that may cause vision loss, but they occur in small numbers. They all require the help of vision rehabilitation professionals to help patients cope effectively.

Scotomata. Whatever the cause, retinal conditions will generally cause localized blind spots (scotomata). Therefore when retinal damage is suspected, visual acuity alone is no longer a sufficient descriptor of visual impairment, because the retinal area where the chart letter is projected does not predict anything about other retinal areas. In addition to letter chart acuity, the condition of the visual field and the presence of blind spots (scotomata) must be considered (Figure 4).

Figure 4 shows a retinal image, where a word is projected across a ring scotoma that leaves only a small central island of vision. This patient will be able to recognize the central letter but will not be able to read the word. Clinicians must be careful when providing such patients with magnification, because too much magnification will mean that fewer letters fit into the central area. This example also makes it clear that when retinal involvement is suspected, a reading test may be more informative than a letter chart test, given that reading requires a larger retinal area.

Neural Processing Problems

As stated earlier, the most important stages of the visual process take place after the retinal receptors have translated the optical image into neural impulses.

The first transformations take place in the *inner retina*. Here, the input from 100 M receptors in each eye is preprocessed and compressed for transmission through 1 M nerve fibers in each optic nerve. The optic nerve fibers do not simply transmit a pixel-by-pixel image, as does a digital camera. Different retinal ganglion cells probably transmit different aspects of the image, such as edges (contrast enhancement), movement, color, brightness, etc. These separate "movies" are transmitted in parallel. At a later stage of neural processing, the different aspects of the image are combined again into a single visual perception.

In the *visual cortex*, the visual information is further analyzed for shapes and contours. Interestingly, at the first synaptic station in the lateral geniculate nucleus, only 20% of the incoming connections come from the optic nerves; the other 80% come from other cortical centers and probably contribute to filtering based on attention and other factors.

In *higher cortical centers*, the visual information is further processed. Here, the flow of information is no longer strictly visual because it is combined with information from other senses. This results in identification and recognition of objects through comparison to stored concepts (through the ventral stream to the temporal lobe of the brain) and in spatial location of an object (through the dorsal stream to the parietal lobe of the brain), which then result in voluntary or involuntary visually guided action.

Our knowledge of these processes is still relatively new. It has been greatly helped by new modalities for neural and retinal imaging. Today, neural processing problems are increasingly recognized in all age groups.

In young children, CVI is now recognized as the most frequent cause of visual perceptual problems. CVI is often caused by perinatal ischemia, which may cause cortical as well as subcortical changes (periventricular leucomalacia). Because this ischemia is not localized, impairments are often not limited to the visual system. Schools for the blind have increasingly developed into schools for the multiply handicapped.

In contact sports, the results of repeated subclinical injuries are now recognized.

In veterans, traumatic brain injuries may cause problems that may be hard to define. Often visual interpretation and decision making are impaired; oculomotor system problems are often found. Traffic accidents may cause similar damage.

In the elderly, strokes may cause more localized problems and agnosias for specific tasks. In all of these cases, the term *visual impairment* may be used when visual acuity and/or visual field are impaired. The term *visual dysfunction* may be more appropriate when the visual input to the brain is normal but the processing of this information is not.

Patient-Centered Functional Priorities

Vision problems affect all aspects of a patient's life. It is no longer sufficient for clinicians to determine that *nothing more can be done* about the *causes* of vision loss, because *much more can be done* about the *consequences* of vision impairment.

To determine the range of services that may be appropriate for an individual with vision impairment, the American Academy of Ophthalmology recommends consideration of the following functional priority areas:

- *Reading*—for many patients, this is their foremost concern.
- *Activities of Daily Living (ADL)*—even though reading may be the most prominent complaint, most people spend the larger part of their day performing a variety of other vision-dependent activities for self-care and home management.
- *Safety*—are people at risk for falls? How do they cross the street? Do they drive?
- *Community participation*—can the individual still participate in community events, including religious gatherings?
- *Physical, cognitive, and psychosocial well-being*—because many patients with vision loss are elderly, this is an important aspect that should not be overlooked. If cognitive problems exist, it may affect the recommendations to be made.

Based on these considerations, patient-centered priorities can be set and specific rehabilitation goals formulated that reflect the patient's needs and desires.

References

American Academy of Ophthalmology (2013). Preferred practice pattern for vision rehabilitation. Available at http://one.aao.org/preferred-practice-pattern/vision-rehabilitation-ppp-2013.

Bourne RA, et al: Magnitude, temporal trends, and projections of the global prevalence of blindness and distance and near vision impairment: a systematic review and meta-analysis, *The Lancet, Global Health*, September 2017 5(9), Pages e888–e897.

Brunnstrom G, Sorensen S, Alsterstad K, Sjostrand J: Quality of light and quality of life—the effect of lighting adaptation among people with low vision, *Ophthalmic Physiol Opt* 24:274–280, 2004.

Cimarolli VR, Boerner K: Social support and well-being in adults who are visually impaired, *J Vis Impair Blind* 99:521–534, 2005.

Cimarolli VR, Reinhardt JP, Horowitz A: Perceived overprotection: support gone bad? *J Gerontol B Psychol Sci Soc Sci* 61:S18–S23, 2006.

Colenbrander A: Measuring vision and vision loss. In Tasman W, Jaeger EA, editors: *Duane's Ophthalmology. Vol. 5*, Philadelphia, 2013, Lippincott Williams & Wilkins.

Colenbrander A: Towards the development of a classification of vision-related functioning—a potential framework. In Dutton GH, Bax M, editors: *Visual Impairment in Children Due to Damage to the Brain*, London, 2010, Mac Keith Press.

Faul MD, Xu L, Wald MM, et al: *Traumatic brain injury in the United States: emergency department visits, hospitalizations, and deaths, 2002-2006*, Atlanta (GA), 2010, Centers for Disease Control and Prevention, National Center for Injury Prevention and Control.

Fletcher DC, Schuchard RA: Preferred retinal loci relationship to macular scotomas in a low-vision population, *Ophthalmology* 104:632–638, 1997.

Fletcher DC, Schuchard RA, Watson G: Relative locations of macular scotomas near the PRL: effect on low vision reading, *J Rehabil Res Dev* 36:356–364, 1999.

Haymes SA, Lee SA: Effects of task lighting on visual function in age-related macular degeneration, *Ophthalmic Physiol Opt* 26:169–179, 2006.

Moore JE, Giesen JM, Weber JM, Crews JE: Functional outcomes reported by consumers of the independent living program for older individuals who are blind, *J Visual Impair Blind* 95:403–417, 2001.

Schoessow KA: Shifting from compensation to participation: a model for occupational therapy in low vision, *Br J Occup Ther* 73:160–169, 2010.

Additional Website Sources

The AFB website (www.AFB.org) has information for all age groups, including a section on aging.

The MDsupport website (www.MDsupport.org) specializes in support and documentation for AMD patients and care givers.

The Lighthouse Guild International in New York (www.lighthouse.org) offers extensive resources for all forms of vision loss.

These websites contain links to many more websites with additional information and often can provide information about local resources.

Infectious Diseases

AMEBIASIS

Method of
Koji Watanabe, MD, PhD

CURRENT DIAGNOSIS (SEE ALSO BOX 1)

- Amebiasis is transmitted by the ingestion of fecally contaminated water or food and by high-risk sexual behaviors (men who have sex with men [MSM] or oral–anal sexual contact).
- Although self-limiting mild to moderate colitis is the most common disease presentation, various severe illnesses (liver abscess, peritonitis, pleurisy, and pericarditis) can also occur.
- Diagnostic value of microscopic stool or abscess ova and parasite examination (O&P) is low. Antigen detection in stool for intestinal amebiasis and in serum for amebic liver abscess (ALA) shows high sensitivity. Serology shows high sensitivity but cannot distinguish current infection from past infection, and it is ideally used in conjunction with fecal antigen detection or polymerase chain reaction (PCR).

CURRENT THERAPY (SEE ALSO BOX 2)

- Infected individuals who are asymptomatic should be treated with a luminal agent (e.g., paromomycin), because they can be a source of new infection and can develop invasive amebiasis after long-term asymptomatic infection.
- Mild to severe colitis and extraintestinal disease require initial treatment with a tissue-active agent (e.g., metronidazole) followed by a luminal agent.
- Reinfection can occur frequently in endemic settings. The clinician should discuss methods to prevent re-exposure to *Entamoeba histolytica* with treated patients.

Epidemiology and Risk Factors for Acquisition

Amebiasis is transmitted by oral ingestion of the transmissible cyst form of *Entamoeba histolytica* in human stools. Transmission occurs by the ingestion of fecally contaminated food and water, mainly in developing countries. It also transmits directly from human to human by sexual contact or in institutions for the cognitively impaired. Food- or water-borne infection occurs in settings of poor sanitation. It is estimated to be the second most common cause of parasite infection–related mortality worldwide, accounting for 40,000 to 70,000 deaths annually. In developed countries, people who travel to or immigrate from developing countries are at higher risk for this parasitic disease. In the United States, amebiasis is the second most common cause of diarrhea in returning travelers. However, over that last two decades amebic infection has been increasingly reported as a sexually transmitted infection in East Asian developed countries and Australia. In one report from Taiwan, men who have sex with men (MSM) and people engaging in oral–anal sex were more likely to be seropositive for *E. histolytica*. While older studies from the United States have shown that amebiasis in MSM was due to nonpathogenic

Entamoeba dispar, more recently MSM was shown to be an independent risk factor for amebiasis-related mortality. Also, *E. histolytica* infection has been reported as a common comorbidity among HIV-infected MSM or as a sexually transmitted infection in developed European countries. It is important for primary care physicians to take detailed histories of sexual behavior as well as travel whenever amebiasis is suspected.

Pathophysiology and Susceptible Host Factors to Invasive Diseases

E. histolytica has two different forms: the tissue-invasive "trophozoite form" and the infectious "cyst form," which is responsible for transmission. Cysts are notable for environmental stability, demonstrating considerable resistance to chlorination and desiccation, with several outbreaks resulting from the contamination of drinking water. Once cysts are ingested, excystation occurs at the terminal ileum or large intestine, forming motile trophozoites. Trophozoites bind to the mucous layer and the underlying intestinal epithelial cells via a parasite Gal/GalNAc lectin. Blockade of activity of the Gal/Gal lectin prevents contact-dependent cytolysis. Moreover, it has been shown that antilectin IgA in stool or breast milk has a protective effect against future acquisition of amebic infection in cohort studies. These results indicate that the Gal/GalNAc lectin plays a crucial role in amebic infection.

Host factors are also important for susceptibility to amebiasis. Amebiasis is more common in malnourished children, and the nutritional hormone leptin is protective, with a single nucleotide mutation of leptin receptor being the predominant genetic factor controlling amebiasis susceptibility in Bangladeshi children. Amebic liver abscess (ALA) is 10 times more common in men than in women and is uncommon in children. Also, the very young or old, malnourished people, pregnant women, and patients using corticosteroids are at increased risk of severe amebiasis.

Clinical Manifestations and Complications of Amebiasis

Asymptomatic self-limiting infection is the most common disease form of amebiasis. Up to 80% to 90% of people exposed to cysts have no or mild symptoms and clear the infection spontaneously. However, asymptomatic infection persists for a long time in some individuals who are reported as asymptomatic cyst passers or as fecal occult blood–positive, which is incidentally diagnosed by colonoscopy. These asymptomatically infected individuals can be a source of a new infection in the community. Also, some develop symptomatic invasive diseases after long-term latent infection.

Symptomatic intestinal amebiasis (amebic colitis) generally has a subacute onset. Usually it takes 1 to 3 weeks from disease onset to make a diagnosis. Abdominal symptoms range from mild diarrhea to severe dysentery with abdominal pain, diarrhea, and bloody stools. Weight loss and fever are common but not universal symptoms. Intestinal fistula or perforation of the large intestine, resulting in peritonitis, is a rare but life-threatening complication of intestinal amebiasis. Toxic megacolon also can be caused by amebiasis. Amebic colitis sometimes mimics acute appendicitis. In this situation, appendectomy without amebicidal treatment may result in severe postoperative complications, such as abdominal sepsis, gastrointestinal fistula, or hemorrhage. Periodic acid–Schiff (PAS) stain, or ideally, immunoperoxidase with anti-*E. histolytica* antibodies, in addition to routine hematoxylin

BOX 1 — Sensitivity of Tests for Diagnosis of Amebiasis.*

Test	Colitis	Liver Abscess
Microscopy (stool)	25%–60%	10%–40%
Stool antigen detection (e.g., *E. histolytica* II enzyme-linked immunosorbent assay (ELISA)	80%	40%
Serum antigen detection	65%	>95%
Microscopy (abscess fluid)	N/A	<20%
Real time polymerase chain reaction	>95%	>95%
Serologic testing (indirect hemagglutination)		
Acute	70%	70%–80%
Convalescent	>90%	>90%
Histopathology by biopsy	45%	N/A

*Before the initiation of therapy.
Modified from Mandell G, Bennett JE, Dolin R, et al. *Mandell, Douglas, and Bennett's Principles and Practice of Infectious Diseases*. 7th ed. Philadelphia: Elsevier Saunders; 2009.

BOX 2 — Treatment Recommendations for Amebiasis in Adults.

Asymptomatically Infected Individuals
Paromomycin (Humatin) 30 mg/kg/d PO tid × 5–10 days
or
Iodoquinol (Yodoxin)[2] 650 mg PO tid × 20 days

Mild to Severe Intestinal and Extraintestinal Disease
Metronidazole (Flagyl)* 750 mg PO tid × 10 days
or
Tinidazole (Tindamax) 2 g PO once daily × 5 days
Followed by
Paromomycin[1] 30 mg/kg/d PO tid × 5–10 days
or
Iodoquinol 650 mg PO tid × 20 days

*Use of intravenous form of metronidazole (500mg q8h) is limited to patients who cannot take oral medications.
[1]Not FDA approved for this indication.
[2]Not available in the United States.
Modified from Mandell G, Bennett JE, Dolin R, Blaser MJ. *Mandell, Douglas, and Bennett's Principles and Practice of Infectious Diseases*. 7th ed. Philadelphia: Elsevier Saunders; 2009.

and eosin (H&E) stain can help to identify the parasite by the histopathology. Thus, intestinal amebiasis sometimes presents as severe and complicated clinical illnesses.

E. histolytica infection also may have extraintestinal dissemination. Liver abscess is the most common form of extraintestinal amebiasis. Patients usually present with 1 to 2 weeks of fever with or without right upper quadrant abdominal pain. Other common symptoms may include cough, sweating, malaise, weight loss, anorexia, and hiccough. Two-thirds of patients lack intestinal symptoms. Physical examination reveals hepatomegaly and tenderness over the liver in approximately half of cases. Complications can occur by direct invasion of trophozoites or the indirect effect of inflammation. Up to10% of patients with ALA have accompanying thoracic amebiasis (pleuritic and pleural effusion). Pericarditis is the next most common form of extraintestinal amebiasis; it may result from rupture of a liver abscess in the left lobe or through extension of pleural amebiasis. Cerebral amebic abscesses are a rare form of extraintestinal amebiasis; they usually accompany other metastatic lesions, such as liver abscesses and thoracic amebiasis.

Thus, amebiasis can have various clinical presentations. The diagnosis can be very difficult to make in severe cases and in atypical clinical presentations because of secondary bacterial infection at the site of amebic invasion.

Diagnosis

Sensitivity of each diagnostic test is shown in Box 1. Although microscopic stool ova and parasite examination (O&P) is frequently used in many countries including the United States, it has low sensitivity. Identification of trophozoites by microscope in aspirated fluid from amebic abscess is more challenging because trophozoites are present only at the edge of the abscess. Moreover, microscopic examination cannot distinguish pathogenic *E. histolytica* from nonpathogenic *E. dispar* or *Entamoeba moshkovskii* by shape.

Currently, the combination of antigen detection in stool and/or sera and serologic testing is the best diagnostic pathway. Antigen detection in feces by the TechLab *E. histolytica* II enzyme-linked immunosorbent assay (ELISA) is rapid to perform (<2 hours) and can distinguish *E. histolytica* from *E. dispar* and *E. moshkovskii*. These antigen tests have highly sensitive diagnostic value for amebic colitis (70% to 95%), whereas sensitivity is relatively low for asymptomatic carrier (20% to 70%). In one report,

when used on patients' sera, ELISA showed high sensitivity in ALA cases but only before metronidazole treatment began. Real-time polymerase chain reaction (PCR) in stool is superior in sensitivity to stool antigen detection, but is still technically complex for diagnostic use in clinical settings. Serologic tests are sensitive (approximately 90% during the convalescent phase) and noninvasive diagnostic tools for amebiasis. Antibodies are detectable in 70% or more of patients within 5 to 7 days of acute infection and persist for years after treatment. Therefore, a negative serologic result is helpful for exclusion of disease, whereas a positive result cannot distinguish between present and previous infection.

Histopathologic examination using biopsy or resected samples is sometimes useful for the diagnosis of intestinal amebiasis. As mentioned, PAS stain in addition to H&E can increase sensitivity in detection of *Entamoeba*. However, identification of *Entamoeba* in biopsy specimens is often challenging. About half of cases with gross ulcerative lesions in the large intestine, in which *E. histolytica* was proven by PCR, had a negative result on histopathology.

Therapy

Recommended treatment regimens are shown in Box 2. Therapy for invasive infection differs from therapy for noninvasive infection. Noninvasive infections (treatment for asymptomatically infected individuals) require treatment with luminal-active agents: paromomycin (Humatin) is currently recommended because of its high potency in asymptomatic cyst passers.

For symptomatic patients, tissue-active agents should be administered before luminal-active agents. Most patients with mild to moderate colitis and uncomplicated liver abscess respond to treatment with tissue-active agents, such as metronidazole (Flagyl) and tinidazole (Tindamax). Tinidazole has the advantage of less frequent dosing than metronidazole. Treatment with tissue-active agents should be followed by luminal-active agents because parasites persist in the intestine in up to 40% to 60% of patients who receive tissue-active agents. Broad-spectrum antibiotics and/or surgical treatment should be added to tissue-active agents in patients with fulminant colitis in which perforation and peritonitis or bacteremia are suspected. Therapeutic needle aspiration or catheter drainage is not routinely required for uncomplicated liver abscesses. Those interventions in addition to medical treatment are recommended if there is clinical deterioration or lack of response to initial medical treatment, or if alternative diagnoses need to be excluded. Also, some reports suggest that clinicians should consider those interventions for patients with a high risk of abscess rupture, as defined by a cavity with a diameter of more than 5 cm or by the presence of lesions in the left lobe, although these criteria were not conclusive in case-control studies.

Symptoms (diarrhea, dysentery, fever, pain, and tenderness) and laboratory markers (white blood cell counts, red blood cell counts, and C-reactive protein) rapidly improve after effective treatment even in patients with extraintestinal lesions. In contrast, radiologic findings, such as abscess size, often remain unchanged for months after completion of treatment.

Monitoring After Treatment and Disease Prevention

Although routine monitoring after treating amebiasis is not recommended, it is well known that reinfection frequently occurs in endemic situations, including both water- or food-borne infections and sexually transmitted infections. In developed countries, in order to prevent reinfection, it is important for the primary physician to inform patients of behaviors that will place them at risk for acquisition of the cyst and how to avoid them, such as avoiding nonsterilized water or food in developing countries, unsafe homosexual contact, and oral–anal sexual contact. In developing countries, more than 1 billion people still have no access to safe food and water, resulting in the urgent need for an effective vaccine. Induction of acquired mucosal immunity is the current goal for vaccine development. Although there is currently no vaccine in human clinical trials, a vaccine containing the naïve or recombinant Gal/GalNAc lectin of *E. histolytica* has strong immunogenicity and protective effect against amebic colitis and liver abscess in animal models. Continuous effort will be needed to develop an effective vaccine to save the lives of affected people in endemic areas.

References

Barwick RS, Uzicanin A, Lareau S, et al: Outbreak of amebiasis in Tbilisi, Republic of Georgia 1998, *Am J Trop Med Hyg* 67:623–631, 2002.
Blessmann J, Tannich E: Treatment of asymptomatic intestinal *Entamoeba histolytica* infection, *N Engl J Med* 347:184, 2002.
Chavez-Tapia NC, Hernandez-Calleros J, Tellez-Avila FI, et al: Image-guided percutaneous procedure plus metronidazole versus metronidazole alone for uncomplicated amoebic liver abscess, *Cochrane Database Syst Rev* CD004886, 2009.
Duggal P, Guo X, Haque R, et al: A mutation in the leptin receptor is associated with *Entamoeba histolytica* infection in children, *J Clin Invest* 121:1191–1198, 2011.
Gunther J, Shafir S, Bristow B, et al: Short report: amebiasis-related mortality among United States residents, 1990–2007, *Am J Trop Med Hyg* 85:1038–1040, 2011.
Haque R, Mollah NU, Ali IK, et al: Diagnosis of amebic liver abscess and intestinal infection with the TechLab *Entamoeba histolytica* II antigen detection and antibody tests, *J Clin Microbiol* 38:3235–3239, 2000.
Hung CC, Chang SY, Ji DD: Entamoeba histolytica infection in men who have sex with men, *Lancet Infect Dis* 12:729–736, 2012.
Hung CC, Wu PY, Chang SY, et al: Amebiasis among persons who sought voluntary counseling and testing for human immunodeficiency virus infection: a case-control study, *Am J Trop Med Hyg* 84:65–69, 2011.
Kobayashi T, Watanabe K, Yano H, et al: Underestimated Amoebic appendicitis among hiv-1-infected individuals in Japan, *J Clin Microbiol* 55:313–320, 2016.
Korpe PS, Liu Y, Siddique A, et al: Breast milk parasite-specific antibodies and protection from amebiasis and cryptosporidiosis in Bangladeshi infants: a prospective cohort study, *Clin Infect Dis* 56:988–992, 2013.
Leder K, Weller PF: Intestinal and extraintestinal *Entamoeba* histolytica amebiasis. UpToDate. Available at: http://www.uptodate.com/contents/search. Accessed 22 April 2019.
Petri Jr WA, Haque R: *Entamoeba* species, including amebic colitis and liver abscess. In Bennett JE, Dolin R, Blaser MJ, editors: *Mandell, Douglas, and Bennett's principles and practice of infectious diseases*, ed 8th, Philadelphia, 2015, Elsevier Saunders, pp 3047–3058.
Saidin S, Othman N, Noordin R: Update on laboratory diagnosis of amoebiasis, *Eur J Clin Microbiol Infect Dis* 38:15–38, 2019.

ANTHRAX

Method of
Shingo Chihara, MD

CURRENT DIAGNOSIS

Cutaneous Anthrax
- Incubation period of 1 to 7 days from exposure to cattle
- Painless or pruritic lesion progresses to ulcer and eschar

- Significant swelling
- Gram stain and culture of lesion

Gastrointestinal
- Incubation period of 1 to 6 days after consumption of raw or undercooked meat
- Nonspecific symptoms followed by abdominal pain, ascites
- Diarrhea uncommon
- Obtain blood culture and ascitic fluid for culture and Gram stain

Inhalational
- Incubation period of 1 to 7 days (up to 43 days)
- Biphasic: fever, malaise, myalgia followed by dyspnea
- Widened mediastinum seen on chest x-ray and computed tomography (CT) of chest
- Blood cultures turn positive in most

Injection
- Injection drug use
- Significant swelling seen; eschar rare

CURRENT THERAPY

Systemic Anthrax With Possible/Confirmed Meningitis
- Ciprofloxacin (Cipro) 400 mg IV every 8 hours or levofloxacin (Levaquin) 750 mg IV every 24 hours or moxifloxacin (Avelox)[1] 400 mg IV every 24 hours
  plus
- Meropenem (Merrem)[1] 2 g IV every 8 hours or imipenem/cilastatin (Primaxin)[1] 1 g IV every 6 hours or doripenem (Doribax)[1] 500 mg IV every 8 hours
- If penicillin-susceptible strains, then penicillin G 4 million units IV every 4 hours or ampicillin[1] 3 g IV every 6 hours could be an alternative to carbapenems
  plus
- Linezolid (Zyvox)[1] 600 mg IV every 12 hours or clindamycin (Cleocin) 900 mg IV every 8 hours or rifampin (Rifadin) 600 mg IV every 12 hours or chloramphenicol 1 g every 6 to 8 hours

Systemic Anthrax When Meningitis Has Been Excluded
- Ciprofloxacin 400 mg IV every 8 hours or levofloxacin 750 mg IV every 24 hours or moxifloxacin[1] 400 mg IV every 24 hours
  or
- Meropenem[1] 2 g IV every 8 hours or imipenem/cilastatin[1] 1 g IV every 6 hours or doripenem[1] 500 mg IV every 8 hours
  or
- Vancomycin (Vancocin)[1] 60 mg/kg/day IV divided every 8 hours (goal trough 15–20 μg/mL)
  or
- If penicillin-susceptible strains, then penicillin G 4 million units IV every 4 hours or ampicillin[1] 3 g IV every 6 hours
  plus
- Clindamycin[1] 900 mg IV every 8 hours or linezolid[1] 600 mg IV every 12 hours
  or
- Doxycycline 200 mg IV×1, then 100 mg IV every 12 hours, or rifampin[1] 600 mg IV every 12 hours

Oral Treatment for Cutaneous Anthrax Without Systemic Involvement
- One of the agents below for 7 to 10 days in naturally-acquired cases and for 60 days in bioterrorism-associated cases
- Ciprofloxacin 500 mg PO every 12 hours
- Doxycycline 100 mg PO every 12 hours
- Levofloxacin 750 mg PO daily
- Moxifloxacin[1] 400 mg PO daily
- Clindamycin[1] 600 mg PO every 8 hours
- If penicillin-susceptible strain
- Amoxicillin[1] 1 g PO every 8 hours
- Penicillin VK 500 mg PO every 6 hours

[1]Not FDA approved for this indication.

Anthrax has been described for centuries and the name is derived from Greek for "burnt coal" owing to eschar formation from cutaneous anthrax. Anthrax is rarely seen in developed countries, including the United States, but it is important to be aware of this condition because of its potential as a bioterrorism agent. When anthrax is suspected, the clinician needs to contact the local or state health department immediately. Anthrax has historical significance because it was the agent used in Koch's postulate during the 19th century when Koch proved that *Bacillus anthracis* is responsible for anthrax in cattle.

Background

B. anthracis is the bacterium responsible for anthrax. It forms spores that can survive in soil for years. It is hyperendemic in the Middle East and in sub-Saharan Africa. Systemic anthrax is primarily a disease of grazing animals. In naturally-acquired anthrax, humans are accidentally infected from exposure to the animal or its products.

Epidemiology

Since the mid-20th century, there has been a precipitous decline in anthrax owing to animal and human vaccines, improvement in factory hygiene, sterilization procedures for imported animal products, and increased use of alternatives to animal hides or hair. Cutaneous anthrax comprises over 95% of naturally-acquired human anthrax and there are an estimated 2000 cases annually. Between 1900 and 2001 there were 18 cases of inhalational anthrax in the United States, of which 16 were fatal. Over the last decade, there have been several cases of inhalational and cutaneous anthrax related to African drum makers. In late 2001, there were 22 cases of anthrax in the United States from spores delivered in the mail, of which five were fatal. In 1979, accidental release of dried anthrax spores from a biologic weapons facility in Sverdlovsk in the former Soviet Union resulted in 68 deaths from inhalation anthrax.

Pathophysiology

B. anthracis is a gram-positive, encapsulated, spore forming, nonhemolytic, nonmotile rod-shaped bacterium. Infection with anthrax requires three components: the edema factor, the lethal factor, and protective antigen. The edema factor combines with protective antigen and becomes edema toxin, which causes edema and impairment of the immune system. The lethal factor combines with protective antigen and becomes lethal toxin, which causes lysis of macrophages. For cutaneous anthrax, these exotoxins result in extensive edema and tissue necrosis locally. In inhalation anthrax, spores that reach the alveoli or alveolar ducts are phagocytized by the alveolar macrophage and transported to the mediastinal lymph nodes where they replicate and cause hemorrhagic mediastinitis. With gastrointestinal tract infection, *B. anthracis* is transported from the gastrointestinal tract to mesenteric lymph nodes where they multiply and cause mesenteric lymphadenitis, ascites, and sepsis.

Clinical Manifestations

There are four distinct clinical presentations: cutaneous, inhalation, gastrointestinal tract, and injection anthrax, depending on the site of entry. Meningitis is a devastating complication that could occur with any of the four infections.

Cutaneous Anthrax

Cutaneous anthrax is the most common form and seen in developing countries as a result of contact with infected animals or animal products such as wool, hair, or hides. Spores invade through either skin abrasions or hair follicles. Subsequently, they germinate and multiply. The incubation period is commonly 5 to 7 days with range of 1 to 19 days. The lesions appear in exposed areas such as head, neck, forearms, and hands and begin as a small, painless papule. They are pruritic at times and form blisters. Subsequently, they evolve into painless necrotic ulcers with a black, depressed eschar with extensive edema and lymphadenopathy.

Inhalation Anthrax

Inhalation anthrax occurs when spores are aerosolized while working with contaminated animal products or when they are released intentionally in bioterrorism. The incubation period is 1 to 7 days but could be as long as 43 days. The course of disease is usually biphasic. Initially, nonspecific symptoms such as fever, malaise, and myalgia are present, resembling influenza. These symptoms last for several days before the bacteremic phase starts. The manifestations include rapidly, fulminant progressive respiratory symptoms such as severe dyspnea, as well as hypoxemia and shock. Once in this phase, the patient dies within a few days despite support in the intensive care unit. Therefore it is important to suspect anthrax in the prodromal phase, which is difficult owing to its rarity and lack of specific symptoms. Widening of the mediastinum on a chest x-ray may be helpful in establishing the diagnosis. This finding was seen in 7 out of 10 cases of inhalation anthrax from 2001. Hilar abnormalities, pulmonary infiltrates, or consolidation and pleural effusion may be seen.

Gastrointestinal Tract Anthrax

Gastrointestinal tract anthrax occurs after ingestion of raw or undercooked meat from an animal infected with anthrax. Gastrointestinal infection is relatively common and has been reported from mouth to ascending colon. The incubation period is 1 to 6 days. Initially, nonspecific symptoms such as asthenia, headache, low-grade fever, facial flushing and conjunctival injection occur. They are followed by abdominal pain, abdominal distention from ascites, nausea, and vomiting. Diarrhea occurs less frequently. As the disease progresses, abdominal pain becomes severe and findings of hypotension and intravascular depletion are seen. When the infection occurs in the oropharynx, necrotic ulcers with pseudomembranes cause pain and edema.

Injection Anthrax

An outbreak of injection anthrax was described in 2009. It was reported in Scotland among injection heroin users. Among the 47 confirmed cases, typical eschar formation seen in cutaneous anthrax was not seen in all but one case. Prominent edema was seen in most patients and some developed compartment syndrome.

Meningitis

Meningitis is a complication seen with all forms of anthrax. About half of patients with inhalation anthrax develop hemorrhagic meningitis. Symptoms such as altered mental status, seizures, cranial nerve palsies, and myoclonus may be seen. When anthrax is suspected, lumbar puncture should be done on presentation unless there are contraindications.

Diagnosis

When diagnosis of anthrax is suspected, the provider must notify the local department of health and the clinical microbiology laboratory. There has been reported transmission of anthrax to laboratory personnel handling *B. anthracis* and specimen handling in biosafety level 3 facilities is recommended. Because the genus *Bacillus* is part of the normal skin flora, it is crucial for the microbiology laboratory to distinguish *B. anthracis* from other non-*anthracis* species of *Bacillus*. Conventional culture and staining are used for distinction. *B. anthracis* is nonmotile and nonhemolytic and those characteristics are used to distinguish it from non-*anthracis* species of *Bacillus*. Most microbiology laboratories have the ability to make a presumptive identification of an organism, and the identification is confirmed by a reference laboratory.

Specimen Collection

When collecting clinical specimens for suspected anthrax, proper personal protective equipment such as disposable gloves, disposable aprons, and boots, should be used. When there is any potential of aerosolization of spores, then face shields and respirators are recommended. Hand washing with soap and water will reduce the endospore contamination of the skin, but alcohol handrubs are not effective against these endospores. For cutaneous anthrax, the edge of the eschar should be lifted, and two specimens of vesicular fluid should be collected by rotating a swab. One swab will be used for culture and Gram stain while the other would be used for polymerase chain reaction (PCR). Punch biopsy of the cutaneous lesion is an alternative. When inhalational anthrax is suspected, blood cultures must be obtained prior to use of antibiotics. If pleural fluid is present, then thoracentesis should be performed for Gram stain, culture, and PCR. For alimentary tract anthrax, blood cultures must be obtained. If there are oral lesions, then specimens could be collected with swabs similar to a cutaneous lesion. If ascites is present, then paracentesis should be performed for Gram stain, culture and PCR. For meningitis, cerebrospinal fluid (CSF) should be collected for culture, Gram stain and PCR.

There are unique findings observed in routine laboratories with systemic anthrax. Marked hemoconcentration may be seen in the complete blood count, and the initial white blood cell count is frequently within normal limits. In chemistry, decreased sodium, increased blood urea nitrogen, mild transaminitis and hypoalbuminemia are seen. Inflammatory markers such as erythrocyte sedimentation rate and C-reactive protein are elevated in most cases except in cases of injection anthrax, when C-reactive protein is low.

Treatment

Supportive Care

Hospitalization is required for all patients with systemic infections. Only uncomplicated cutaneous anthrax could be treated on an outpatient basis. Close monitoring is warranted because the patient status may deteriorate rapidly. Hemodynamic support should be given, including fluids, vasopressors, blood products, and invasive hemodynamic monitoring. Mechanical ventilation may be needed because of respiratory distress, airway protection for altered mental status, or for airway edema. Adjunctive corticosteroids may be indicated in four situations: patients with history of endocrine or corticosteroid therapy; edema of head or neck; anthrax meningitis; or vasopressor-resistant shock. Pleural fluid and ascites should be drained aggressively. Surgery is indicated in certain situations. Surgery for cutaneous anthrax has led to dissemination and poor outcome. Therefore, in cutaneous anthrax, indication for surgery is limited to tracheotomy for airway obstruction and surgery for compartment syndrome. In gastrointestinal anthrax, surgery might be considered for complications such as bowel ischemia or infarct and perforation. In injection anthrax, removal of necrotic nidus would help reduce the toxin and spore reservoir.

Antimicrobial Treatment for Systemic Disease with Possible Meningitis

At least three intravenous antibiotics with good penetration to the central nervous system are recommended. At least one drug should have bactericidal activity, and at least one drug should inhibit protein synthesis. These should be continued for at least 2 weeks or until clinically stable, whichever is longer. The fluoroquinolone class is bactericidal, has good penetration to the central nervous system, and has no reported resistance by *B. anthracis*. Intravenous ciprofloxacin (Cipro) is the primary bactericidal component in the treatment of systemic disease. Levofloxacin (Levaquin) and moxifloxacin (Avelox)[1] are considered to be alternatives. The carbapenem class has good central nervous system penetration, and meropenem (Merrem)[1] is the preferred second antibiotic in treatment of systemic disease with possible meningitis. Imipenem/cilastatin (Primaxin)[1] and doripenem (Doribax)[1] are considered alternatives. Penicillin G or ampicillin[1] could be used in place of carbapenems when the isolate is known to have a minimum inhibitory concentration (MIC) of less than $0.125\,\mu g/mL$. As for protein synthesis inhibitor, linezolid (Zyvox)[1] is preferred because it provides good central nervous system penetration. If there is

contraindication to linezolid use such as drug–drug interaction or myelosuppression, then clindamycin (Cleocin)[1] is the alternative. When both linezolid and clindamycin cannot be used, rifampin (Rifadin)[1] could be used for synergistic effect in combination with the bactericidal drugs. Chloramphenicol is another antibiotic that is a protein synthesis inhibitor. It could be used if linezolid, clindamycin, and rifampin are unavailable. Doxycycline (Vibramycin) is an inhibitor of protein synthesis but does not adequately penetrate the central nervous system. Therefore doxycycline should not be used when meningitis is not ruled out. If the patient had been exposed to aerosolized spores, then the patient should be transitioned to oral antibiotics after completion of initial intravenous combination therapy to prevent relapse from spores.

Antimicrobial Treatment for Systemic Disease when Meningitis is Ruled Out

At least two antimicrobial agents are recommended for systemic anthrax without meningitis. At least one should be bactericidal and at least one should be a protein synthesis inhibitor. This combination should be administered intravenously for at least 2 weeks or until clinically stable, whichever is longer. For penicillin-susceptible strains, penicillin G is considered equivalent to ciprofloxacin. Vancomycin (Vancocin)[1] is an acceptable alternative bactericidal agent. Clindamycin[1] and linezolid[1] are equivalent first choices for protein synthesis inhibitors. Doxycycline is an alternative agent. If the patient had been exposed to aerosolized spores, then the patient should be transitioned to oral antibiotics after completion of initial intravenous combination therapy to prevent relapse from spores.

Treatment for Cutaneous Anthrax without Systemic Involvement

A single oral antibiotic is adequate to treat cutaneous anthrax without systemic involvement. Fluoroquinolones and doxycycline are considered first-line agents. Clindamycin[1] is a second-line agent when first-line agents are unavailable or contraindicated. Penicillin or amoxicillin[1] may be used if the isolate is found to be sensitive in vitro. It is important to give an adequate dose because resistance may develop when underdosed.

Antitoxins

There are three antitoxins in the Centers for Disease Control and Prevention (CDC) Strategic National stockpile: raxibacumab, obiltoxaximab, and anthrax immune globulin intravenous (AIGIV). These agents are not readily available to the public. They inhibit binding of protective antigen to the anthrax toxin receptor and translocation of lethal factor and edema factor into cells. There are human and animal data from the pre-antibiotic era that suggest that there is lower mortality in those who received the antitoxin in cutaneous anthrax compared with those who did not. Whether this agent should be given for systemic anthrax is controversial owing to lack of data. Because the mortality rate with systemic anthrax is high whereas the complication of antitoxin treatment is low, the potential benefit from antitoxins outweighs the potential risk from the antitoxins in systemic anthrax. This agent should be given in addition to appropriate antibiotics when systemic anthrax is suspected.

Pregnancy

Overall management is similar to that in the nonpregnant patient. In pregnancy, ciprofloxacin is preferred over doxycycline for both treatment and prevention. Newer fluoroquinolones such as levofloxacin and moxifloxacin[1] are not preferred because embryo toxicity has been observed in animal studies. This was not seen with ciprofloxacin. Transplacental transmission of anthrax is known to occur. Ciprofloxacin, levofloxacin, meropenem,[1] ampicillin,[1] penicillin, clindamycin,[1] and rifampin[1] are known to have adequate concentration in the placenta and at least one agent should be used with treatment.

---

[1]Not FDA approved for this indication.

---

[1]Not FDA approved for this indication.

Prognosis

Uncomplicated cutaneous anthrax has a mortality rate of less than 2% with treatment. Injection anthrax has a mortality rate of 28%, and gastrointestinal anthrax has a mortality rate of 40%. Inhalational anthrax has mortality of 45% despite antibiotics and modern intensive care. Meningitis from anthrax is almost always fatal.

Prevention

Postexposure prophylaxis should be started as soon as possible after exposure. Sixty days of antibiotics for immediate protection and a three-dose series of Anthrax Vaccine Adsorbed (AVA, BioThrax) for long-term protection are recommended by the United States Advisory Committee on Immunization Practices. Ciprofloxacin and doxycycline are recommended as first-line antibiotic therapy for postexposure prophylaxis and are FDA-approved for this indication. Alternative agents include levofloxacin, moxifloxacin, amoxicillin, or penicillin VK (if sensitive); and clindamycin. AVA should be administered at diagnosis and at 2 and 4 weeks. AVA is not FDA-approved for postexposure prophylaxis.

References

Anthrax. Available at http://www.cdc.gov/anthrax/ [accessed 31.01.15].

Hendricks KA, Wright ME, Shadomy SV, et al: Centers for disease control and prevention expert panel meetings on prevention and treatment of anthrax in adults, *Emerg Infect Dis* 20, 2014. https://doi.org/10.3201/eid2002.130687.

Knox D, Murray G, Millar M, et al: Subcutaneous anthrax in three intravenous drug users, *J Bone Joint Surg* 93:414–417, 2011.

Logan NA, Hoffmaster AR, Shadomy SV, Stauffer KE: In Versalovic J, editor: *Manual of clinical microbiology*, 10th ed., Washington DC, 2011, ASM Press, pp 381–402.

Meaney-Delman D, Zotti ME, Creanga AA, et al: Special considerations for prophylaxis for and treatment of anthrax in pregnant and postpartum women, *Emerg Infect Dis* 20, 2014. https://doi.org/10.3201/eid2002.130611.

Ruoff KL, Clarridge J, Bernard K: In Garcia LS, editor: *Clinical microbiology procedures handbook*, ed 3rd, Washington DC, 2010, ASM Press. 3.18.1.

Singh K: Laboratory-acquired infections, *Clin Infect Dis* 49:142–147, 2009.

BABESIOSIS

Method of
Cheston B. Cunha, MD; and Burke A. Cunha, MD

CURRENT DIAGNOSIS

- Suspect babesiosis in patients from Ixodes tick-endemic areas who present with a malaria-like illness (MLI) with fever, chills, headache, fatigue, and malaise.
- Clinically, babesiosis usually presents as an acute febrile illness with high fevers (>102 °F), relative bradycardia, and shaking chills accompanied by fatigue and myalgias.
- Myalgias may suggest an influenza-like illness (ILI).
- Severe headaches may suggest an alternate diagnosis, e.g., meningitis.
- Some patients with babesiosis may be short of breath and may go on to develop acute respiratory distress syndrome (ARDS).
- Consider babesiosis for unexplained fevers following blood transfusion.
- In prolonged fevers that meet the definition of fever of unknown origin (FUO), consider babesiosis in patients from endemic areas.
- With babesiosis, there are usually no localizing signs except for splenomegaly. Importantly, no rash is present. If rash is present, consider an alternate diagnosis.
- In babesiosis, nonspecific laboratory test results, considered together, are helpful in excluding or narrowing diagnostic possibilities.

- Common nonspecific laboratory findings of babesiosis include a normal/slightly decreased white blood cell count, relative lymphopenia, atypical lymphocytes, thrombocytopenia, elevated total bilirubin, and high lactate dehydrogenase levels. Sera are mildly elevated.
- The erythrocyte sedimentation rate is usually highly elevated (>90 mm/h) as are serum ferritin levels.
- Definitive babesiosis diagnosis is by peripheral blood smears (thick and thin); thick smears are best for the detection of babesia and thin smears are best to assess the degree of parasitemia.
- In normal hosts, the degree of parasitemia is usually low (1%–5%), but high in compromised hosts (>10%). Severe babesiosis may occur in asplenic individuals (Howell-Jolly bodies reflect the degree of splenic dysfunction), the immunosuppressed, the elderly, and those with coinfections, e.g., ehrlichiosis, Lyme disease.
- If present, babesiosis is diagnosed by peripheral stained blood smears demonstrating the characteristic (but uncommon) "Maltese cross" in tetrads (four merozoites).
- In nonmalarious areas, babesiosis may be diagnosed by demonstrating intraerythrocytic ring forms on the peripheral smear.
- Babesiosis, like malaria, has intracellular ring forms, but babesiosis, unlike malaria, has no intracellular pigment (hemozoin).
- Alternatively, *Babesia microti* serology in the Northeastern United States is diagnostic if IgM titers are highly elevated (>1:64).
- Polymerase chain reaction to detect Babesia is more sensitive than blood smear review. It is particularly useful in patients with a low level of parasitemia.

CURRENT THERAPY

- Preferred therapy is atovaquone (Mepron)[1] plus azithromycin (Zithromax).[1]
- Alternatively, clindamycin (Cleocin)[1] plus quinine[1] may be used.
- In addition to antibabesia therapy, exchange transfusion may be lifesaving in severe cases.
- For severe cases, continue therapy until degree of parasitemia is <5%.
- Recurrent or persistent babesiosis should be treated for >2 weeks after resolution of parasitemia.
- Doxycycline is not effective in babesiosis.
- Coinfection with other tick-borne pathogens is rare, but possible.

[1]Not FDA approved for this indication.

Epidemiology

Babesiosis is a tick-borne zoonosis that clinically presents as a malaria-like illness (MLI). There are many *Babesia* species, but only five are pathogenic in humans. The geographic distribution of babesiosis mimics that of hard-bodied *Ixodes dammini* (*I. scapularis*) ticks and their vertebrate hosts, e.g., dogs, cats, cattle, and rodents. The primary reservoir for babesiosis in the Northeastern United States is the white-footed mouse (*I. dammini* nymphs) and the white-tailed deer (*I. dammini* adults). Sporadic cases of babesiosis also occur in states with the tick vector/vertebrate hosts. Babesiosis may also be acquired by blood/blood product transfusions.

Clinical Features

In the Northeastern United States, babesiosis is usually *B. microti* and clinically manifests as an MLI. Babesiosis may be asymptomatic (IgG seropositive) or a mild, self-limited influenza-like illness (ILI). The incubation period for naturally acquired babesiosis is 1 to 6 weeks and 6 to 9 weeks for transfusion-acquired babesiosis. Clinical presentations in normal hosts are subacute with fever, fatigue, headache, malaise, and anorexia often mimicking Epstein-Barr virus infectious mononucleosis (with false-positive Monospot test results). Babesiosis presenting in patients with prolonged fevers of unknown origins (FUOs) and anorexia/weight loss may mimic a lymphoreticular malignancy. Presentation may be acute in those with impaired splenic function, those on immunosuppressives, or the elderly. Babesiosis may be viewed clinically as the "malaria of Long Island/Nantucket" as it presents with many malarial features, e.g., fever, chills, headache, sweats, myalgias. Excluding epidemiologic considerations, babesiosis differs in geographic distribution from malaria. Clinically, babesiosis differs from malaria in two important aspects. The clinical hallmarks of malaria are acute onset, intermittent fevers, and the classic "malaria paroxysm." Babesia reproduce by asynchronous asexual budding, which is clinically manifest as constant/nonintermittent fever. With malaria, fevers are intermittent with fever periodicity related to the *Plasmodium* species. Only *P. falciparum* has no fever periodicity and like babesiosis has no hepatic phase. Malaria and babesiosis both have extraerythrocytic ring forms, but babesiosis has two distinct morphologic features: extracellular merozoites (tetrads), known as "Maltese crosses," and no extraerythrocytic pigment, which malaria does have.

Unless the liver or spleen is enlarged, the physical features in babesiosis are limited to the fever. The fever curve of babesiosis is remittent without periodicity; fever is between 102 °F and 105 °F and accompanied by relative bradycardia. Rash is not a feature. When babesiosis is suspected, the presence of a rash is either indicative of coinfection, e.g., Lyme disease, or an alternative cause, e.g., viral or drug exanthem. Babesiosis should not be in the differential diagnosis of Rocky Mountain spotted fever with rash on the wrists/ankles. Babesiosis may clinically resemble ehrlichiosis. Peripheral blood smears are the best way to differentiate babesiosis from ehrlichiosis. Nonspecific laboratory abnormalities in babesiosis include normal/decreased white blood cell (WBC) count (leukopenia). Relative lymphopenia is usually present. Atypical lymphocytes are frequently present in the peripheral smear. Thrombocytopenia is a constant finding. The erythrocyte sedimentation rate (ESR) is highly elevated (usually >90 mm/h and often >100 mm/h) as is C-reactive protein (CRP). Since the pathophysiology of babesiosis is that of an acute hemolytic anemia, like malaria, intravascular hemolysis in babesiosis is manifested by increased lactate dehydrogenase (LDH)/total bilirubin. Increased LDH and total bilirubin are the most sensitive indicators of the degree of intravascular hemolysis in babesiosis. The hemoglobin/hematocrit is decreased later in more severe cases. Ferritin levels are highly elevated and prolonged (higher/longer) than would occur with acute-phase ferritin elevations. Since babesiosis impairs T cell function, as in malaria, serum protein electrophoresis often shows polyclonal gammopathy reflecting compensatory B cell hyperactivity. Serum transaminases are mildly elevated, but alkaline phosphatase is unelevated. Cold agglutinins are not a feature of babesiosis. In patients with decreased/absent splenic function, Howell-Jolly bodies are present in the peripheral smear. The number of Howell-Jolly bodies present is inversely proportional to the degree of splenic dysfunction.

Diagnosis of babesiosis is microscopic or serologic. Like malaria, babesiosis may be diagnosed on Giemsa stained blood smears. If malaria is not a diagnostic consideration (geographic distribution, blood transfusion), the presence of intraerythrocytic ring forms is diagnostic. Less common, but more specific, are pathognomonic tetrads (Maltese crosses) of babesiosis in peripheral smears. Also, unlike malaria, there is no extraerythrocytic pigment in babesiosis. Alternatively, elevated IgM *Babesia* species titers are diagnostic.

Therapy

The preferred therapy of babesiosis consists of 7 days combination therapy of azithromycin (Zithromax)[1] plus atovaquone (Mepron).[1] Alternatively, clindamycin (Cleocin)[1] plus quinine[1] for 7 days may be used (Table 1).

Treatment failure may occur in those with impaired T cell function, e.g., patients with HIV or with decreased splenic function. In such cases, exchange transfusion may be lifesaving.

TABLE 1	Babesiosis
PREFERRED THERAPY	**ALTERNATE THERAPY**
Azithromycin (Zithromax)[1] 500 mg PO×1, then 250 mg PO q24h×7 days **plus** Atovaquone suspension (Mepron)[1] 750 mg PO q12h×7 days	Clindamycin (Cleocin)[1] 600 mg PO q8h×7 days **plus** Quinine[1] 650 mg PO q8h×7 days

From Cunha BA, editor. Antibiotic Essentials. 12th ed. Sudbury, MA: Jones & Bartlett; 2013, p. 253–268.
[1]Not FDA approved for this indication.

References

Bonoan JT, Johnson DH, Cunha BA: Life-threatening babesiosis in an asplenic patient treated with exchange transfusion, azithromycin and atovaquone, *Heart Lung* 27:424–428, 1998.

Cunha BA, Raza M, Schmidt A: Highly elevated serum ferritin levels are a diagnostic marker in babesiosis, *Clin Infect Dis* 60:827–829, 2015.

Cunha BA, Mickail N, Laguerre M: Babesiosis mimicking Epstein Barr Virus (EBV) infectious mononucleosis: another cause of false positive Monospot test, *J Infect* 62:531–532, 2012.

Cunha BA, Cohen YZ, McDermott B: Fever of unknown origin (FUO) due to babesiosis in an immunocompetent host, *Heart Lung* 37:481–484, 2008.

Cunha BA, Nausheen S, Szalsa D: Pulmonary complications of Babesiosis: case report and literature review, *Eur J Clin Microbiol Infect Dis* 26:505–508, 2007.

Cunha BA, Crean J, Rosenbaum G: Lipid abnormalities in babesiosis, *Am J Med* 15:758–759, 2000.

Cunha CB: Infectious diseases differential diagnosis. In Cunha BA, editor: *Antibiotic Essentials*, ed 12th, Sudbury, MA, 2013, Jones & Bartlett, pp 474–506.

Hildebrandt A, Gray JS, Hunfeld KP: Human babesiosis in Europe: what clinicians need to know, *Infection* 41:1057–1072, 2013.

Kim N, Rosenbaum GS, Cunha BA: Relative bradycardia and lymphopenia in patients with babesiosis, *Clin Infect Dis* 26:1218–1219, 1998.

Krause PJ, Daily J, Telford SR, et al: Shared features in the pathology of babesiosis and malaria, *Trends Parasitol* 23:605–610, 2007.

Larkin JM: Ticks and tick-related illness, *Med Health RI* 91:209–211, 2008.

Leiby DA: Transfusion-transmitted Babesia spp: bull's-eye on Babesia microti, *Clin Microbiol Rev* 24:14–28, 2011.

Merch K, Holmaas G, Frolander PS, et al: Severe human Babesia divergens infection in Norway, *Int J Infect Dis* 23:37–38, 2014.

Nathavitharana RR, Mitty JA: Diseases from North America: focus on tick-borne infections, *Clin Med* 15:74–77, 2015.

Panduranga V, Kumar A: Severe babesiosis presenting as acute respiratory distress syndrome in an immunocompetent patient, *Conn Med* 78:289–291, 2014.

Rosenbaum GS, Johnson DH, Cunha BA: Atypical lymphocytosis in babesiosis, *Clin Infect Dis* 20:203–204, 1995.

Sharon KP, Krause PJ: Babesiosis. In Cunha BA, editor: *Tickborne infectious diseases diagnosis and management*, New York, 2007, Information Healthcare, pp 111–120.

Usmani-Brown S, Halperin JJ, Krause PJ: Neurological manifestations of human babesiosis, *Handb Clin Neurol* 114:199–203, 2013.

Wudhikarn K, Perry EH, Kemperman M, et al: Transfusion-transmitted babesiosis in an immunocompromised patient: a case report and review, *Am J Med* 124:800–805, 2011.

[1] Not FDA approved for this indication.

BACTERIAL MENINGITIS

Method of
Gary D. Overturf, MD

CURRENT DIAGNOSIS

- Patient age and epidemiology:
  - Clinical symptoms: Fever, headache, meningeal signs
  - CSF examination: High opening pressure (>300 mm Hg)
  - Elevated white blood cell count (>10–>5000)
  - >60% polymorphonuclear cells
- Low CSF glucose (<40 mg/dL or <50% serum glucose)
- High CSF protein (>50–>1.0 g/dL)
- Bacteria present on Gram stain of CSF

Abbreviation: CSF = cerebrospinal fluid.

CURRENT THERAPY

- Neonates <2 mo
  - Group B streptococcal infection: cefotaxime (Claforan) or ampicillin
  - Gram-negative rods, other than *Pseudomonas*: cefotaxime
  - *Pseudomonas*: cefepime (Maxipime), ceftazidime (Fortaz), or meropenem (Merrem)
  - *Listeria*: Ampicillin + gentamicin (Garamycin)
- Children >2 mo
  - Empirical for unknown etiology: cefotaxime or ceftriaxone (Rocephin)
  - *Streptococcus pneumoniae*: cefotaxime or ceftriaxone
  - *Haemophilus influenzae*: cefotaxime or ceftriaxone
  - *Neisseria meningitidis*: ampicillin or cefotaxime
- Older children and adults
  - Empirical for unknown etiology: cefotaxime or ceftriaxone
  - *S. pneumoniae*: cefotaxime or ceftriaxone
  - *N. meningitidis*: ampicillin or cefotaxime
  - Gram negative, postoperative, or *Staphylococcus aureus* (see Tables 1–4)
  - Add vancomycin if at risk for infection with resistant pneumococcus

Acute bacterial meningitis occurs in all age groups, but predominantly in children younger than 2 years and the elderly (older than 60 years). With the introduction of effective protein conjugate vaccines for *Haemophilus* and pneumococcal infection, the incidence of bacterial meningitis is rapidly declining in children, and adults are now the major population affected. Bacterial meningitis is a medical emergency requiring rapid and decisive action to prevent death or neurologic sequelae. Since the introduction of chloramphenicol (Chloromycetin) in the early 1950s, the mortality rate has remained between 5% and 40%, depending on the age of the patient and the etiology. Of the survivors, 10% to 30% suffer permanent neurologic deficits. Prognosis is affected by the timeliness of therapy, the age of the patient, and the etiology. Presumptive diagnosis and administration of therapy are critical.

Diagnosis

Acute bacterial meningitis must be considered in the differential diagnosis of persons of any age presenting with fever and headache or signs of meningeal irritation or acute central nervous system dysfunction. Presentations can be subtle at the extremes of age or in patients who have received partially effective antibiotic therapy. The diagnosis of bacterial meningitis requires the examination of the cerebrospinal fluid (CSF), which must be performed as expeditiously as possible. Studies indicate that lumbar puncture may be safely performed on patients who have normal mental status or are without focal neurologic signs or papilledema; clinical impressions are predictive of the computed tomography (CT) findings. If there are signs or symptoms suggesting the presence of an intracranial mass (e.g., tumor, cerebral hematoma, or brain abscess), blood cultures should be obtained and empirical antibiotics should be administered prior to the performance of a CT scan.

Characteristically, the CSF findings in bacterial meningitis include a cell count of greater than 500 to 5000 white blood cells (WBCs) per mm^3 with a predominance of neutrophils, a protein concentration of greater than 150 mg/mL, and a low glucose (e.g., less than 35–40 mg/dL). No single value is absolute, and a single value may be normal in up to a third of the cases. The Gram-stained sediment of centrifuged CSF is the critical examination leading to a specific diagnosis. In patients who have not received antibiotics capable of reaching the CSF, the Gram stain is positive in 80% to 90% of culture-confirmed cases. In persons previously treated with antibiotics (e.g., β-lactam antibiotics, tetracycline, fluoroquinolones), the frequency of positive Gram stains is much reduced (e.g., 60% to 70%), but the cells, cell type, protein, and glucose concentrations are not significantly affected. CSF antigen tests are not reliable, and variable negative and positive predictive values direct against relying on the use of such tests. Clinical judgment is paramount, and antibiotics should be given in situations of ambiguous results of the CSF examination.

Antibiotic Selection

The outcome of bacterial meningitis is closely related to the timely use of antibiotics. Hypotension, seizures, an altered mental status, and hypoglycorrhachia at the time of initial antibiotic administration are predictive of higher case fatality and neurologic sequelae. Because prompt administration of antibiotics is critical, the choice of antibiotics must be made before results of the CSF cultures are known. If organisms are seen on Gram stain, therapy

TABLE 1 Cerebrospinal Fluid Gram Stain Morphology and Antibiotic Recommendations

MORPHOLOGY	POSSIBLE OR PROBABLE PATHOGENS	TREATMENT OPTIONS	ALTERNATIVE THERAPIES
Gram-positive cocci, short chains or pairs	*Streptococcus pneumoniae, Streptococcus agalactiae* (group B streptococci)	Ceftriaxone (Rocephin) or cefotaxime (Claforan) plus vancomycin (Vancocin)	Chloramphenicol (Chloromycetin)
Gram-positive cocci, clusters; or gram-positive bacilli	*Staphylococcus aureus, Listeria monocytogenes*	Vancomycin, ampicillin plus gentamicin (Garamycin)	Nafcillin (Unipen) or Oxacillin, trimethoprim-sulfamethoxazole (Bactrim)
Gram-negative diplococci	*Neisseria meningitidis*	Ceftriaxone or cefotaxime	Ampicillin, Penicillin G, or chloramphenicol
Gram-negative coccobacilli	*Haemophilus influenzae*	Ceftriaxone or cefotaxime	Chloramphenicol
Gram-negative bacilli	*Escherichia coli, Klebsiella* species, *Pseudomonas aeruginosa*	Cefepime (Maxipime) or ceftazidime (Fortaz)	Imipenem (Primaxin) or meropenem (Merrem)

TABLE 2 Antibiotic Recommendations for Bacterial Meningitis Acquired in the Community, by Age Group and Probable Pathogen

AGE GROUP	PROBABLE PATHOGENS	EMPIRICAL THERAPY
Neonate <1 mo	Group B streptococcus; *E. coli*, or other gram-negative enteric rod; occasionally *L. monocytogenes*	Ampicillin plus cefotaxime (Claforan)
Infants 1–3 mo	*H. influenzae, N. meningitidis, S. pneumoniae*, Group B streptococci	Ceftriaxone (Rocephin) or cefotaxime (Claforan)
Children 3 mo–7 y and older children and adults 7–50 y	*H. influenzae, S. pneumoniae, N. meningitidis*	Ceftriaxone or cefotaxime plus vancomycin (Vancocin)
Older adults >50 y	*S. pneumoniae, N. meningitidis, L. monocytogenes*	Ceftriaxone plus ampicillin

TABLE 3 Antibiotic Recommendations for Presumed Bacterial Meningitis in Persons with Special Risks

CONDITION OR RISK FACTOR	COMMON PATHOGENS	ANTIBIOTIC RECOMMENDATIONS
Impaired immunity (e.g., HIV, early complement deficiency, agammaglobulinemia)	*L. monocytogenes, S. pneumoniae, H. influenzae*	Ampicillin plus ceftriaxone (Rocephin) or cefotaxime (Claforan)
Closed head trauma with CSF leak	*S. pneumoniae, H. influenzae*	Ceftriaxone or cefotaxime plus vancomycin (Vancocin)
Asplenia	*S. pneumoniae, H. influenzae*	Ceftriaxone or cefotaxime plus vancomycin
Terminal complement deficiency	*N. meningitidis*	Ceftriaxone or cefotaxime
Neurosurgical procedures	*S. aureus*	Vancomycin plus ceftriaxone or cefotaxime
CSF shunt infections	Coagulase-negative staphylococci, Gram-negative bacilli	
Elderly patients (>65 y)	*S. pneumoniae, L. monocytogenes*	Ceftriaxone or cefotaxime plus vancomycin
Recurrent bacterial meningitis (see CSF leak)	*S. pneumoniae*	Ceftriaxone or cefotaxime plus vancomycin
Alcoholic patients	*S. pneumoniae* and Gram-negative bacilli	Ceftriaxone or cefotaxime plus vancomycin

Abbreviation: CSF = cerebrospinal fluid.

TABLE 4 Antibiotic Doses for Adults and Children for Treatment of Bacterial Meningitis

ANTIBIOTIC	DAILY ADULT DOSE	DAILY PEDIATRIC DOSE	DOSE INTERVAL
Ampicillin	12 g	200–400 mg/kg	4–6 h
Cefotaxime (Claforan)	12 g	200–300 mg/kg	4–6 h
Ceftriaxone (Rocephin)	4 g	100 mg/kg	12 h
Ceftazidime (Fortaz)	6 g	150–200 mg/kg	8 h
Cefepime (Maxipime)	6 g	100–150 mg/kg	8 h
Meropenem (Merrem)	6 g	120 mg/kg	8 h
Nafcillin (Unipen)	12 g	200 mg/kg	4–6 h
Penicillin G	24 million U	250,000 units/kg	4 h
Vancomycin (Vancocin)	2 g	60 mg/kg	12 h

Adapted from Bradley JS, Nelson JD: 2002–2003 Nelson's Pocket Book of Pediatric Antimicrobial Therapy, 15th ed. Philadelphia, Lippincott Williams & Wilkins, 2002; Gilbert DN, Moellering RC, Sande MA. The Sanford Guide to Antimicrobial Therapy 2005. Hyde Park, Antimicrobial Therapy Inc., 2005.

may be directed by the probable bacterial etiology (Table 1). In the event the CSF Gram stain fails to reveal a possible pathogen, empirical antibiotic therapy should be begun based on the age of the patient for those persons who have acquired their infection in the community (Table 2). For those persons who are members of special risk groups, empirical therapy should be based on the likely etiology (Table 3). Once the CSF cultures are completed, therapy can be modified according to results of the culture and sensitivity data.

Antibiotics used in bacterial meningitis should be rapidly bactericidal and achieve high concentrations in the CSF. Antibiotics should be given in maximal doses (Table 4). Because the bactericidal activity of antibiotics in CSF is dose dependent, the fractional CSF-to-serum ratio is very small. Finally, the use of combinations of antibiotics should be minimized to avoid antagonizing the bactericidal activity.

Special Considerations for Antibiotic Therapy

During the past two decades, resistance to penicillin and some third-generation cephalosporins (e.g., ceftriaxone [Rocephin], cefotaxime [Claforan]) has steadily increased among strains of *Streptococcus pneumoniae*. Currently, approximately 30% to 50% of isolates are either intermediately (inhibitory concentration, 0.1–1.0 µg/mL) or fully (inhibitory concentration more than

2.0 µg/mL) resistant to Penicillin G and ampicillin. Resistance to ceftriaxone (Rocephin) and cefotaxime (Claforan) may occur as well in 10% to 15% of strains. Vancomycin (Vancocin) is recommended in those regimens for meningitis when pneumococci are considered. However, higher maximal doses are required for vancomycin because of its relatively poor penetration into the CSF. In general, lumbar puncture with CSF culture should be repeated in 48 hours in those cases where vancomycin therapy is the primary drug because of demonstrated penicillin or cephalosporin resistance.

Meningitis caused by gram-negative bacilli such as *Pseudomonas aeruginosa, Escherichia coli,* or *Enterobacter cloacae* should be treated with a cephalosporin with an extended spectrum of Gram-negative activity, such as ceftazidime (Fortaz) or cefepime (Maxipime). A carbapenem, such as imipenem (Primaxin) or meropenem (Merrem), can also be used for antibiotic-resistant gram-negative enteric and pseudomonas meningitis. Meropenem is associated with less risk of drug-induced seizures and may be a better choice for bacterial meningitis.

Patients with ventriculoatrial and ventriculoperitoneal shunt–associated meningitis and ventriculitis usually require removal of the shunt for cure, as well as the administration of antibiotics to clear the infection. Certain patients with infections caused by organisms of reduced virulence, such as coagulase-negative staphylococci, or those with exquisitely antibiotic-susceptible infections, can be treated with a trial of antibiotics alone.

Because of the extreme sensitivity of *Neisseria meningitidis* to antibiotics, uncomplicated meningitis may be treated with as little as 5 to 7 days of antibiotics. Pneumococcal meningitis may be treated with 10 to 14 days of antibiotics, and haemophilus infections are treated successfully with 7 to 10 days of antibiotics. Gram-negative meningitis was treated in the past with 3 weeks of aminoglycosides, but current experience with newer extended-spectrum cephalosporins (ceftriaxone, cefotaxime, carbapenems) suggests that 2 weeks of therapy is often sufficient in neonates as well as in some elderly patients and postoperative infections.

All patients with bacterial meningitis should be monitored carefully throughout the treatment period. Infectious disease consultation is recommended for most infections of the central nervous system. Repeated lumbar punctures are not routinely recommended for patients with fully susceptible bacterial isolates or in those who show good response to therapy. Repeated sampling of the CSF with lumbar puncture or, when appropriate, shunt or ventricular reservoir puncture should be performed in those with known resistant bacterial isolates, in patients who have an inadequate response, in those patients who deteriorate on therapy, or in those for whom clinical response may correlate poorly with the microbiologic response (shunt infections, neonates, and elderly patients).

Adjunctive Therapy

Corticosteroids reduce the incidence of permanent neurologic sequelae in children with bacterial meningitis, particularly when caused by *Haemophilus influenza* type b. Data in support of steroids in either pneumococcal or meningococcal infections are less robust. Dexamethasone (Decadron[1]), 0.15 mg/kg every 6 hours for the first 2 to 4 days of treatment, was evaluated in children older than 2 months with bacterial meningitis. The first dose of dexamethasone should be given before, at the start, or no later than 12 hours after beginning antibiotics.

Use of corticosteroids in adults is more controversial. Although doses of dexamethasone are recommended by some experts for adults with bacterial meningitis, its efficacy in adult meningitis has not been evaluated in a well-designed prospective trial. A recent study in adults found that corticosteroids significantly reduced the risk for unfavorable outcomes, particularly in patients with pneumococcal meningitis. There has been concern that the anti-inflammatory properties of dexamethasone may decrease the

penetration of antibiotics, especially vancomycin, into the CSF. One study in children did not show this to be the case. Dexamethasone[1] should be administered in adults with proven or suspected pneumococcal meningitis, but only if it can be given prior to the first dose of antibiotics in a dose of 10 mg every 6 hours for 4 days. In patients with meningitis caused by *S. pneumoniae* highly resistant to penicillin (minimum inhibitory concentration [MIC] >2.0 µg/mL) or cephalosporins (MIC >4.0 µg/mL), vancomycin should not be used as a single agent if corticosteroids are used. The addition of rifampin (Rifadin[1]) is often recommended in these situations.

Chemoprophylaxis for Bacterial Meningitis

Prophylactic antibiotics are recommended in case of meningitis caused by *Neisseria meningitidis* and *H. influenzae* type b. Prophylaxis is provided to eliminate the carriage of organisms among contacts and prevent spread to hosts susceptible to invasive disease. In cases of meningococcal meningitis, prophylaxis is indicated only for those with household or intimate contact with the index case. Administration of prophylaxis to large groups (e.g., college students, schoolchildren, or preschool classes) requires a special assessment and a recommendation of local or regional health departments. Chemoprophylaxis is not necessary for casual contacts or medical personnel unless there is a direct exposure to respiratory secretions. The recommended dose of rifampin (Rifadin) is 10 mg/kg (600 maximal, adults) twice a day for 2 days; ciprofloxacin (Cipro[1]), 500 mg as single dose, is also effective for adults. Third-generation cephalosporins used in treatment of the index case of meningitis are sufficient to eliminate carriage of the organism.

Chemoprophylaxis for *H. influenzae* type b is recommended for all household contacts of an index case if one of the contacts is an unvaccinated child younger than 4 years. If the index case is treated with ceftriaxone (Rocephin) or cefotaxime (Claforan), prophylaxis is not required, but if treated with ampicillin or chloramphenicol (Chloromycetin), prophylaxis is recommended to eliminate carriage. The recommended regimen for prophylaxis is rifampin,[1] 20 mg/kg (or 600 mg in adults) once a day for 4 days. With the near elimination of invasive infections caused by *H. influenzae* type b with the use of routine immunization of children with conjugate haemophilus vaccines, *H. influenzae* types A, F, and (rarely) other serotypes have emerged, and the use of prophylaxis is not recommended in these situations because sufficient data are not available to support its efficacy, nor has spread within contacts been documented.

Vaccines for Bacterial Meningitis

The universal recommendation for the use of protein-polysaccharide conjugate *H. influenzae* type b (HIB) vaccines in 1987 reduced the incidence of bacterial meningitis by this organism by greater than 97%. Three HIB vaccines (PedvaxHIB, ActHIB, HibTITER), licensed in the United States, are routinely given to children in dosage schedules employing three to four doses by 12 to 18 months of age (see www.cdc.gov).

A pneumococcal protein-polysaccharide conjugate vaccine (Prevnar) licensed in 2000 is routinely recommended for children and has markedly reduced the incidence of invasive infections with seven serotypes of pneumococci in children. This vaccine is also recommended for children at high risk of pneumococcal infections (e.g., HIV infection, asplenia, sickle cell disease, and others). A new Prevnar 13 with thirteen serotypes is now recommended to replace Prevnar 7 for routine use and is also recommended for persons over 50 years of age with high-risk conditions. The full recommendations for the use of this vacccine alone and in combination with the polysaccharide vaccine (Pneumovax 23) are available from the CDC. A pneumococcal polysaccharide vaccine (Pneumovax 23) is recommended for adults older than 65 years or for those over 50 years with risk factors (e.g., alcoholism, diabetes or other metabolic or

---

[1] Not FDA approved for this indication.

VIII Infectious Diseases

528

renal disease, chronic pulmonary or cardiac disease). A polysaccharide conjugate vaccine (Prevnar) has been recently approved for limited adult use in high-risk patients; please see recommendations for use in adults and children at www.vaccines.gov. Although clear evidence for prevention of bacterial meningitis is lacking, evidence supports its efficacy against invasive pneumococcal diseases, many of which are the preceding infections leading to bacteremia and meningitis.

Three vaccines are available in the United States for prevention of meningococcal disease. All available vaccines provide protection against four serotypes: A, C, Y, and 1-135. Either of two protein-conjugate vaccines (Menactra and Menveo) are currently recommended for routine administration to all children at 11 to 12 years of age with a repeated dose at 5 years after the first dose. These vaccines are also recommended for persons at high risk for meningococcal disease (e.g., those with complement deficiencies, or asplenia, as well as microbiology technologists or travelers and workers in endemic areas) as early as 9 months of age, to be repeated at 12 months (Menactra) or equal to those who are 2 years of age or older (Menactra and Menveo) up to 55 years of age. It is recommended that younger patients at high risk be given a two-dose primary series and that all high-risk persons be given a second dose at 3 to 5 years depending upon risk and age at first dose (see the package inserts for dosing details). In addition, a single polysaccharide vaccine (Menomune) remains available for high-risk persons over 55 years of age.

References

Anderson EJ, Yogev LR: A rational approach to the management of ventricular shunt infections, *Pediatric Infect Dis J* 24:557–558, 2005.
Andes DR, Craig WA: Pharmacokinetics and pharmacodynamics of antibiotics in meningitis, *Infect Dis Clin North Am* 13(2):595–618, 1999.
Centers for Disease Control and Prevention: Use of 13-valent pneumococcal conjugate vaccine and 23 valent pneumococcal polysaccharide vaccine among children aged 6–18 years with immunocompromising conditions, *MMWR* 61:816–819, 2012.
Centers for Disease Control and Prevention: Use of 13-valent pneumococcal conjugate vaccine and 23 valent pneumococcal polysaccharide vaccine for adults with immunocompromising conditions. Recommendations of the Advisory Committee on Immunization Practices (ACIP), *MMWR* 62:521–524, 2013.
De Gans J, van de Beek D: Dexamethasone in adults with bacterial meningitis, *N Engl J Med* 347:1549–1564, 2002.
Gray LD, Fedorko DP: Laboratory diagnosis of bacterial meningitis, *Clin Microbiol Rev* 5:130–145, 1992.
Hussein AS, Shafran SD: Acute bacterial meningitis in adults: A 12-year review, *Medicine (Baltimore)* 79:360–368, 2000.
Klein JO: Bacterial sepsis and meningitis. In Remington JS, Klein JO, editors: *Infectious Diseases of the Fetus and Newborn Infant*, ed 5th, Philadelphia, 2002, WB Saunders, pp 943–998.
Klinger G, Chin C-Y, Beyene J, et al: Predicting the outcome of neonatal bacterial meningitis, *Pediatrics* 106:477–482, 2000.
Odio CM, Faingezicht I, Paris M, et al: The beneficial effects of early dexamethasone administration in infants and children with bacterial meningitis, *N Engl J Med* 324:1525–1531, 1991.
Ronan A, Hogg GG, Klug CL: Cerebrospinal fluid shunt infections in children, *Pediatr Infect Dis J* 14:782–786, 1995.
Schuchat A, Robinson K, Wenger JD, et al: Bacterial meningitis in the United States in 1995, *N Engl J Med* 337:970–976, 1997.
Unhanand M, Mustapha MM, McCracken GH, et al: Gram-negative enteric bacillary meningitis: A twenty-one year experience, *J Pediatr* 122:15–17, 1993.
Van de Beek D, de Gans J, Spanjaard L, et al: Clinical features and prognostic factors in adults with bacterial meningitis, *N Engl J Med* 351:1849–1858, 2004.

BRUCELLOSIS

Method of
Xinghong Yang, PhD

CURRENT DIAGNOSIS

- The diagnosis of brucellosis relies on the serologic reaction of antibodies to *Brucella's* lipopolysaccharide (LPS) located on the cell surface of smooth *Brucella melitensis, Brucella abortus,* and *Brucella suis.*
- Although the rough species, *Brucella canis,* does not have an intact LPS layer, its detection requires the antigens specifically prepared from *B. canis.*
- Rose Bengal test is regularly used to diagnose infection with smooth *Brucella* spp.
- When patients with brucellosis symptoms test negative by Rose Bengal test, the microagglutination test and 2-mercaptoethanol rapid slide agglutination test are used to determine whether the patient is infected with rough *Brucella* spp.

CURRENT THERAPY

- Three aspects of therapy are critical when using antibiotics to treat brucellosis:
  - The antibiotics must be able to penetrate macrophages to take effect because *Brucella* spp. are intracellular pathogens and normally reside within professional and nonprofessional phagocytes.
  - Multiple antibiotics are typically used to minimize relapses commonly seen when only a single antibiotic is used.
  - In complicated cases, in addition to antibiotic treatment, surgical intervention may be required to remove infected tissues.

Brucellosis is an ancient disease recorded by the Romans more than 2000 years ago. Since *Brucella* was identified as the cause of brucellosis in sick soldiers in 1887 by Sir David Bruce, brucellosis has been defined as an emerging disease. *Brucella* is a zoonotic bacterial pathogen, causing approximately 500,000 new cases annually worldwide. Although rarely fatal (<5% mortality rate), it causes an undulating fever leading to a dramatic decrease in the quality of life. Its incubation time can vary between 1 and 8 weeks, and often infection is asymptomatic; however, serious complications can lead to disability or death. Because no human vaccine is available, antibiotic therapy is the only option for treatment.

A total of ten *Brucella* species have been identified to date (Table 1). Four of these—*Brucella melitensis, Brucella abortus, Brucella suis,* and *Brucella canis*—commonly cause human brucellosis, and their genomes have been sequenced.

Epidemiology

Wildlife and domesticated animals can serve as natural reservoirs for *Brucella* spp. Humans acquire brucellae by exposure to contaminated foods or aerosols or by direct contact. Often contaminated or unpasteurized animal products, such as milk, soft cheese, and butter are consumed, causing oral exposure. *Brucella* spp. can spread via contaminated aerosols or by aerosolization of contaminated animal by-products, resulting in lung infection. *Brucella* can also infect by direct contact of skin cuts or abrasions with sick animals or their products and enter into the blood or lymphatic system and, regardless of route, produce infection, causing a bacteremia. Among the three routes, food ingestion and aerosol inhalation can result in brucellosis. Aerosolized brucellae can be used as a bioweapon because the dosage required for infecting 50% of the population is as little as 1885 colony-forming units (CFUs).

Currently, brucellosis is endemic to Latin America, Africa, the Mediterranean rim, the Middle East, and Central Asia. To prevent human infection, animal immunization campaigns were adopted by many countries, including the United States and the former Soviet Union. The campaigns successfully curbed animal infection and consequently reduced human infection in these areas. When the programs were stopped, the incidence of brucellosis rapidly increased. Thus maintenance of animal immunization programs is essential for protecting humans from infection.

TABLE 1	Brucella Species, Preferred Animal Hosts, and Human Infection Potential		
SPECIES	**HOST ANIMALS OR RESERVOIR**	**HUMAN INFECTION?***
B. melitensis	Goats, sheep, camels	Yes
B. abortus	Cows, bison, camels, yaks	Yes
B. suis	Pigs, wild hares, caribou, reindeer, wild rodents	Yes
B. canis	Dogs	Yes
B. cetaceae	Seals, harbor porpoises	Yes
B. inopinata	Unknown	Yes
B. microti	Common voles, red foxes, soil	Unknown
B. neotomae	Rodents	No
B. ovis	Sheep	No
B. pinnipedialis	Minke whales, dolphins	No

*"Yes" and "no" mean Brucella spp. are able or unable to infect humans, respectively; "unknown" indicates that it is not confirmed whether Brucella spp. are able to infect humans.

Although transmission of brucellae among humans occurs rarely, several cases have been reported. It may be disseminated via sexual contact, milking, and organ transplantation. B. melitensis is the most commonly isolated species from brucellosis patients, followed in descending order by B. abortus, B. suis, and B. canis. B. melitensis and B. abortus can cause acute brucellosis and display the most severe symptoms, which can lead to complications. B. suis can cause extended duration of illness and results in suppurating lesions in infected tissues. Patients with B. canis infections display mild to moderate illness and rarely develop complications.

Risk Factors

The susceptible population includes those who live or travel in the endemic areas, particularly veterinarians, microbiologists, and those who work with or process livestock. The current animal vaccines are all infectious to human, and consequently veterinarians who administer these vaccines are at high risk for being infected. Microbiologists or laboratory workers also can acquire brucellosis through close contact, and indeed laboratory outbreaks are frequently reported. Thus Brucella is also considered an occupational disease or a laboratory-acquired disease.

Pathophysiology

Brucella can be phagocytized by nonprofessional and professional phagocytic cells to establish an intracellular replication niche. Once inside host cells, brucellae stay in early-formed phagosomes, where they prevent phagosomes from fusing with late-formed endosomes and lysosomes and survive intracellularly. Antibiotics must be able to penetrate the host cell membrane to kill brucellae or inhibit their growth.

Brucella uses numerous mechanisms to evade detection by the immune system. Unlike LPS from other gram-negative bacteria, Brucella LPS does not trigger an inflammatory response or activate the alternative complement system, so it helps brucellae avoid recognition. Brucella's LPS endows brucellae with a phenotype highly resistant to cationic bactericidal peptides. The intracellular brucellae do not cause cell death in macrophages or apoptosis in respiratory epithelial cells. Thus the LPS reduces the chances of exposure to the immune system, which aids brucellae survival and meanwhile diminishes the stimulation of the host immune system. Brucella inhibits the macrophage response to interferon-γ (IFN-γ), a critical cytokine for stimulating innate and adaptive

TABLE 2	Symptom Pattern of Human Brucellosis
SYMPTOMS	**PERCENT***
Fever	93
Chills	82
Sweats	87
Aches	91
Lack of energy	95
Joint and back pain	86
Arthritis	40
Spinal tenderness	48
Headache	81
Loss of appetite	78
Weight loss	65
Constipation	47
Abdominal pain	45
Diarrhea	7
Cough	24
Testicular pain, epididymoorchitis	21[†]
Rash	14
Sleep disturbance	37
Ill appearance	25
Pallor	22
Lymphadenopathy	32
Splenomegaly	25
Hepatomegaly	19
Jaundice	1
Central nervous system disorder	4
Cardiac murmur	3
Pneumonia	1

Data from Corbel MJ: Brucellosis in humans and animals. Geneva, World Health Organization, 2006.
*Percentage based on 500 patients.
†Percentage based on 290 male patients.

immunity. Additionally, to maintain vigorous intracellular survival and replication, brucellae equip their outer membranes with phosphatidylcholine and synthesize cyclic β-1,2-glucans to preclude fusion between phagosome and lysosome.

Diagnosis

Accurate diagnosis of brucellosis is always a challenge because brucellosis exhibits symptoms similar to numerous other febrile illnesses (Table 2). In many patients, the symptoms are mild and moderate; thus in a number of cases the diagnosis might not be even considered.

Isolation of brucellae from blood, bone marrow, urine, cerebrospinal fluid, or joint aspirate serves as the gold standard for diagnosing brucellosis. However, under many circumstances, brucellae cannot be cultured from patients' samples. The rate of blood culture positivity ranges from 16% to 90%. Hence, other indices are used to identify brucellosis. Testing for antibodies against Brucella is commonly used. Brucella agglutination titer of 1:160 is considered a clear diagnostic index as long as the patient presents signs and symptoms of the disease. Recommended tests are the Rose Bengal test, the serum agglutination test alone or with 2-mercaptoethanol or dithiothreitol reduction, Coombs' antiglobulin, the complement-fixation test, and the enzyme-linked immunosorbent assay (ELISA). The results of a combination of tests such as the serum agglutination test and Coombs' antiglobulin can be used to assess the stage of evolution of the disease at the time of diagnosis. In the blood sample, infection may also be associated with low levels of red and white blood cells, low platelets, and elevated liver function. A biopsy of body tissues can also assist in making the diagnosis because patients can experience bone marrow hypoplasia or liver fibrosis and cirrhosis.

Depending on the patient's symptoms and severity of the illness, an investigation may be undertaken. Examinations may include computed tomography (CT) scan or magnetic resonance imaging (MRI) to identify signs of inflammation or abscesses in the brain or other tissues. Electrocardiogram (ECG) may be performed to investigate heart infection or damage, and x-rays can show bone and joint deformations.

Differential Diagnosis

Because human brucellosis mimics the symptoms of many other diseases, disease complications vary from patient to patient, and the latency time between exposure and the occurrence of symptoms is irregular and relatively long, making the differential diagnosis tedious and difficult. Therefore, before diagnosis, answers to three questions can help narrow the focus to brucellosis:

- Did the patient have direct contact with large or small ruminants, their carcasses, or their products?
- Did the patient consume unpasteurized dairy products?
- Does the patient live in or travel to areas where brucellae are endemic in humans or epidemic in animals?

In spite of the difficulties in diagnosing brucellosis, some clinical features can still be used to distinguish brucellosis from other infectious diseases. If left untreated, fever of brucellosis displays an undulating pattern. In about 50% of patients, the fever of brucellosis is associated with musculoskeletal symptoms; however, these symptoms are rarely observed in typhoid and malaria fevers.

In patients with hepatosplenomegaly or lymphadenopathy, the differential diagnosis includes glandular fever–like illnesses, such as cytomegalovirus (CMV) infection, Epstein-Barr virus (EBV) infection, HIV infection, toxoplasmosis, and tuberculosis (TB). CMV patients can develop antibodies to the virus. Also, in the active infection phase, CMV can be detected from the blood, saliva, urine, or other body tissues. These indices can be used to differentiate CMV infection from the brucellosis. EBV patients have an elevated white blood cell count, an increased total number of lymphocytes, and greater than 10% atypical lymphocytes, but brucellosis patients usually show a decrease in the white blood cell count.

HIV infection can induce antibodies against HIV, and virologic tests can detect HIV antigens or RNA. HIV infection can be further confirmed by a supplemental antibody test, such as Western blot and indirect immunofluorescence assay. Brucellosis patients' sera do not display any reaction in these tests. For toxoplasmosis patients, serum immunoglobulin (Ig)G and IgM titers can be used to detect whether the patient is infected by Toxoplasma.

For TB patients, a skin test or a special TB blood test can be used for diagnosis, and other tests such as chest x-ray and a sample of sputum coughed up from deep in the lungs may be used for confirmation. In patients with osteomyelitis or septic arthritis, the most important alternative diagnosis is TB.

In patients with acute epididymoorchitis, the differential diagnosis includes mumps and surgical problems, such as torsion. For mumps patients, buccal swab specimens are collected for viral detection via culturing virus in cell lines or using real-time polymerase chain reaction (RT-PCR) to detect mumps viral RNA. For testicular torsion in men, an ultrasound examination of the spermatic cord can provide valuable information regarding whether the patient requires emergency surgery.

Treatment

To date, the only option for treating brucellosis is by means of antibiotics. However, in cases of complications, such as heart brucellosis and spinal brucellosis, antibiotic treatment in combination with surgical intervention may be needed. Antibiotics commonly used are doxycycline (Vibramycin), rifampin (Rifadin),[1] streptomycin, cotrimoxazole (TMP-SMX [Bactrim]),[1] and gentamicin (Garamycin)[1] (Table 3). Regimens of a combination of 2 or 3 antibiotics are recommended to reduce the unacceptably high relapse rates with monotherapy. Antibiotic regimens vary and depend on the patient's age, the severity of the disease, pregnancy, cost of the medicine, and availability of the medicine.

Doxycycline combined with rifampin[1] for a full 6-week course is a commonly used therapy recommended by the World Health Organization. It is considered the most effective regimen, particularly when combined with an aminoglycoside. In patients with spondylitis or sacroiliitis, doxycycline plus streptomycin is an effective combination. For pediatric patients older than 8 years, doxycycline plus gentamicin[1] is the recommended therapy. For children younger than 8 years, trimethoprim-sulfamethoxazole (TMP-SMX) therapy for 3 weeks followed by a 5-day course of gentamicin[1] is most effective. TMP-SMX[1] is also effective in treating pregnant women, either as a single agent or in combination with rifampin[1] or gentamicin[1] (see Table 3).

Once brucellosis is diagnosed, immediate therapy is critical because it can alleviate symptoms and also prevent the development of complications. Nevertheless, even when treatment is executed according to the doctor's prescription, rates of relapse can still reach up to 5% to 10%. Depending on the severity or complications of the illness and the treatment time applied, the recovery time can last from several weeks to several months.

Monitoring

After antibiotic therapy is initiated, patients are periodically monitored by doctors to evaluate whether the therapeutic regimen is effective and whether relapse occurs. Because relapse is indicated by the recurrence of a positive blood culture result during the posttherapy period or signs and symptoms of brucellosis infection, routine examination of the patient includes serum culture for Brucella organism and assessment for brucellosis symptoms after the treatment phase. In addition to monitoring brucellosis symptoms, both doctors and patients should monitor any adverse effects of medication. For instance, adverse reactions to TMP-SMX occur in 50% to 100% of patients with AIDS compared with about 14% of patients without AIDS. Up to 57% of AIDS patients treated with TMP-SMX[1] require a change in therapy owing to the adverse effects.

Generally, brucellosis patients should be followed up clinically for up to 2 years to detect relapse. Patients should be monitored for regaining of body weight. IgG antibody should be checked by serum agglutination test for levels that remain in the diagnostic range for more than 2 years. Complement fixation titers should fall to normal within 1 year of treatment. Relapse should respond to a prolonged course of the same therapy originally used.

Complications

Brucellae are transported into the lymphatic system and can replicate in spleen, liver, kidney, breast tissue, and joints to cause both localized and systemic infections. Infection of the reproductive system can cause fetal abortion. Owing to the low virulence, low toxicity, and multiple mechanisms to protect them from the immune system, brucellae can survive and reproduce in nearly any tissues or organs. At 1 year after infection, the disease can develop into chronic brucellosis that can further cause one or multiple complications in one organ or the whole body.

There are seven major types of complications from Brucella infection.

- Endocarditis: Brucellae can infect the heart's inner lining, which can destroy the heart valves and, if left untreated, will lead to death of the patient.
- Meningitis and encephalitis: Brucellae can infect the central nervous system to cause an inflammation of the brain, the membranes surrounding the brain, and the spinal cord. This is fatal if the patient is not treated in time.

---

[1] Not FDA approved for this indication.

TABLE 3 Treatment for Brucellosis

MEDICATION	ADULT DOSAGE	DOSAGE ADJUSTMENT			ADVERSE EFFECTS
		PEDIATRIC DOSAGE	RENAL FAILURE	HEPATIC INSUFFICIENCY	
Doxycycline (Vibramycin)	100 mg PO q12h	2.2–4.4 mg/kg[3] PO div q12h (>8 y)	No change	No change	Dizziness, headache, photosensitivity, nausea, diarrhea, hemolytic anemia, hepatotoxicity
Rifampin (Rifadin)[1]	600–900 mg PO qd	20 mg/kg PO qd (do not exceed 600 mg qd)	No change	Moderate: caution Severe: avoid	Heartburn, epigastric distress, anorexia, nausea, flatulence, cramps, liver dysfunction, jaundice
Streptomycin	15 mg/kg IM q24h or 1 g IM qd × 2–3 wk	20–40 mg/kg IM qd (do not exceed 1 g/d)	Necessary	No change	Nausea, vomiting, vertigo, face paresthesias, rash, fever, urticaria, angioedema, eosinophilia
Trimethoprim-sulfamethoxazole (TMP-SMX) (Bactrim)[1]	1 DS tab PO q12h (160 mg TMP/800 mg SMX)	8–12 mg/kg TMP PO given in divided doses q12h	Necessary Avoid use in CrCl <15 mL/min	No change	Nausea, vomiting, anorexia, rash, urticaria
Gentamicin (Garamycin)[1]	2 mg/kg[3] IM/IV q8h or 5 mg/kg IM/IV q24h[1] or 240 mg q24h	2.5 mg/kg q8–12h IM/IV	Necessary	No change	Nephrotoxicity, dizziness, vertigo, tinnitus, hearing loss, numbness, skin tingling, muscle twitching, convulsions

Abbreviations: CrCl = creatinine clearance; DS = double strength.
[1]Not FDA approved for this indication.
[3]Exceeds dosage recommended by the manufacturer.

- Arthritis: Osteoarthritis caused by *Brucella* infection is typically associated with pain, stiffness, and swelling of the joints, such as the knees, hips, ankles, wrists, spine, shoulder, elbow, sternoclavicular, and small joints. Spondylitis caused by brucellae is characterized by joint inflammation between the vertebrae bones of the spine or between the spine and pelvis. Spondylitis is difficult to treat and can cause lasting damage. These osteoarticular complications are the clinical forms most commonly observed.
- Epididymitis and epididymoorchitis: Brucellae can infect the epididymis to cause swelling and pain of the testicle.
- Cutaneous complications: Brucellae can infect skin to cause lesions, rashes, nodules, erythema nodosum, papules, petechiae, and purpura.
- Respiratory complications: Inhalation of brucellae can result in lung infection, which can lead to pneumonia, bronchopneumonia, pleural effusion with a predominance of monocytic or lymphocytic infiltrates, and paroxysmal dry cough.
- Hematologic complications: Aspartate aminotransferase (AST) or alanine aminotransferase (ALT) levels can be elevated and are associated with pain in the right upper quadrant or jaundice.

Complications are common in brucellosis patients. Young patients tend to have cutaneous, hematologic, and respiratory complications. Adult patients tend toward osteoarticular and cardiac complications. Middle-aged patients tend to develop genitourinary, neurologic, and gastrointestinal complications.

Prevention

Maintaining hygienic habits is very important for avoiding *Brucella* infection. These include consuming only pasteurized milk and cheese. Meat must be cooked thoroughly before consumption. In these regards, education is beneficial for preventing infection by this pathogen. People who handle animals or animal products should wear personal protective equipment, including glasses, rubber gloves, and clothing to protect skin and eyes from exposure or direct contact. Laboratory workers should use a Biosafety Level 3 (BSL-3) facility to handle the *Brucella* organisms and work according to the laboratory's standard operating procedures. Animal immunization programs must be maintained all over the world to cut off the transmission chain from livestock to humans. In addition, primary care physicians should be familiar with the clinical and laboratory findings of brucellosis symptoms and complications.

References

Centers for Disease Control and Prevention: *Sexually Transmitted Diseases Treatment Guidelines, 2010: Epididymitis,* 2012. Available at http://www.cdc.gov/std/treatment/2010/epididymitis.htm (accessed 07.09.15).

Corbel MJ: *Brucellosis in humans and animals,* Geneva, 2006, World Health Organization.

Dokuzoguz B, Nurcan Baykam N: Brucellosis. In Bope ET, Kellerman RD, Rakel RE, editors: *Conn's Current Therapy 2011,* Philadelphia, 2011, Saunders, pp 74–78.

Gür A, Geyik MF, Dikici B, et al: Complications of brucellosis in different age groups: A study of 283 cases in southeastern Anatolia of Turkey, *Yonsei Med J* 44:33–44, 2003.

Harrison's Practice. Answers on Demand. Brucellosis, 2012. Available at. http://www.harrisonspractice.com. (Accessed 8.11.16).

Joint WHO/FAO Expert Committee on Brucellosis: Sixth report, *World Health Organ Tech Rep Ser* 740:1–132, 1986.

Mayo Clinic. Brucellosis: Complications, 2012. Available at http://www.mayoclinic.com/health/brucellosis/DS00837/DSECTION=complications. 2012 [accessed 07.09.15].

Pappas G, Akritidis N, Bosilkovski M, et al: Brucellosis, *N Engl J Med* 352:2325–2336, 2005.

Pappas G, Bosilkovski M, Akritidis N, et al: Brucellosis and the respiratory system, *Clin Infect Dis* 37:e95–399, 2003.

Skalsky K, Yahav D, Bishara J, et al: Treatment of human brucellosis: Systematic review and meta-analysis of randomised controlled trials, *BMJ* 336:701–704, 2008.

Yang X, Skyberg JA, Cao L, et al: Progress in Brucella vaccine development, *Front Biol* 8:60–77, 2013, https://doi.org/10.1007/s11515-012-1196-0.

CAMPYLOBACTER

Method of
R. Gregory Juckett, MD, MPH

CURRENT DIAGNOSIS

- *Campylobacter jejuni* and *Campylobacter coli* are the leading causes of childhood and traveler's diarrhea worldwide.
- Raw or undercooked poultry (or cross-contamination with poultry juices) is the best-known source of infection.
- Infection is characterized by abrupt onset of crampy abdominal pain, nausea, and profuse diarrhea or dysentery.
- A prodrome of high fever and myalgias precedes diarrheal illness in one third of cases.
- *Campylobacter* gastroenteritis can mimic acute appendicitis and inflammatory bowel disease.
- Late complications of *Campylobacter* infection include reactive arthritis and Guillain-Barré syndrome 1 to 2 weeks after diarrhea.

CURRENT THERAPY

- Antibiotics are not essential for most healthy patients because the illness is self-limited.
- Azithromycin (Zithromax)[1] 500 mg daily×3 days (pediatric dosage, 10 mg/kg/day) is effective if given early in the course (less than 5% resistance).
- Quinolone antibiotics have been effective, but resistance is developing, particularly in South and Southeast Asia owing to the use of quinolones in poultry feed.
- Prevention entails reducing *Campylobacter* colonization of poultry and using proper food-handling techniques. Vaccination may be possible in the future.

[1]Not FDA approved for this indication.

Epidemiology

Campylobacter enteritis is one of the most common forms of bacterial diarrhea in the world and the most common food-related illness in North America. Most cases (95%) are caused by *Campylobacter jejuni*, a commensal gram-negative bacteria found in the gut of animals, particularly poultry. The related *Campylobacter coli* causes a clinically identical but much less common (5%) infection. Children in developing countries are usually infected before age 2 years.

Foodborne outbreaks affect adults in developed counties, as well as travelers to developing nations. *Campylobacter* is a common cause of traveler's diarrhea, and 13% of US *Campylobacter* infections are acquired abroad. Most infections are due to cross-contamination of food with raw poultry (unwashed cutting boards) or from drinking unpasteurized milk or contaminated water. Infections increase in spring and peak during the summer months. The typical incubation period is 3 to 4 days (range, 1–8 days), with the illness lasting up to a week. After recovery, the bacteria are excreted in the feces for several weeks and may be transmitted by improper hand washing, although person-to-person transmission is unusual.

Risk Factors

Anyone exposed to improperly prepared food, unpasteurized milk, or unchlorinated water is at risk. Improperly cooked poultry or food contaminated by raw poultry is the most common source. Contact with infected pets is a common cause of childhood exposure. A 17-state outbreak of multidrug-resistant *Campylobacter* was linked to pet store puppies in 2017. (Reference www.cdc.gov/Campylobacter/outbreaks/puppies-9-17/index.html posted 1/30/18 (accessed 2/13/18). Elderly, immunocompromised, or very young patients are at additional risk for prolonged symptoms, invasive disease, and hospitalization. Proton-pump inhibitors, by reducing protective stomach acid, appear to increase the risk of campylobacteriosis and other bacterial enteritides.

Pathophysiology

Campylobacter infection starts in the small intestine (jejunum, ileum) and spreads to the colon. Symptoms can begin with enteritis (profuse watery stools) or with frank colitis (bloody stools). Colitis thus can mimic inflammatory bowel disease or appendicitis. Inflammatory bowel disease may be excluded by colon biopsies, which demonstrate acute but not chronic inflammatory change.

Prevention

Proper food-handling techniques are the best means of prevention. Poultry products should be cooked until an internal temperature of 165°F is reached and all juices run clear. Hands must be washed with soap after contact with raw poultry or animal feces and after using the rest room. Cross-contamination should be avoided by careful disinfection of countertops and utensils after preparing meats or, better yet, using entirely separate surfaces. Only one drop of poultry juice (<500 organisms) is sufficient to cause disease. Although not currently feasible, *Campylobacter* vaccination has been proposed for prevention.

Clinical Manifestations

Campylobacter enteritis typically manifests as sudden onset of cramping, nausea, vomiting, and diarrhea, often indistinguishable from other bacterial diarrheas. Most cases are self-limited, with recovery in 3 to 4 days. About a third of patients experience a febrile prodrome, with myalgias occurring for about a day before onset of diarrheal illness. Dysenteric (bloody) stools are common (15%) and imply more-invasive disease. Like *Yersinia*, *Campylobacter* infection can mimic acute appendicitis (ileocecitis), especially if this occurs in the absence of significant diarrhea. Computed tomography or ultrasound scanning in bacterial pseudoappendicitis usually documents mesenteric adenitis, and surgery can be avoided. In young children, seizures can occur before the onset of diarrhea and fever, and dysenteric illness (50%) is more common.

Diagnosis

Most cases are diagnosed by stool culture in the setting of acute diarrhea and crampy abdominal pain. On microscopic examination, *C jejuni* is a gram-negative, spiral-shaped rod with a single polar flagellum at one or both ends. It can be isolated in culture media containing cephalothin, to which it is usually resistant. Darkfield microscopic stool examination is occasionally attempted for early diagnosis, but this is not very sensitive. Polymerase chain reaction analysis of stool samples is a very promising diagnostic approach, although it is not yet available in many laboratories. Later diagnosis, subsequent to resolution of diarrhea, requires serologic testing.

Differential Diagnosis

Campylobacter infections are clinically indistinguishable from other bacterial enteritides such as salmonellosis and shigellosis. All of these produce fever, cramps, diarrhea, and dysentery. However, *Campylobacter* colitis is more likely to mimic inflammatory bowel disease and appendicitis and later to cause Guillain-Barré syndrome.

Treatment

Most cases of *Campylobacter* infection are mild and self-limited, and antibiotics are not required. If antibiotics are to be used, they are most effective if given early to high-risk patients, because delayed treatment (e.g., after positive stool culture results) is less likely to affect outcome. First-line choices include macrolides,

Campylobacter

Acute and Chronic *Campylobacter* Complications

Acute Complications
Acute colitis, dysentery
Cholecystitis
Pseudoappendicitis (mesenteric adenitis)
Peritonitis
Pericarditis (chest pain)
Postinfectious irritable bowel syndrome

Chronic Complications
Inflammatory bowel disease (possible contributor)
Guillain-Barré syndrome (1:1000 cases)
Reactive arthritis

such as azithromycin (<5% resistance), or fluoroquinolones, such as ciprofloxacin (Cipro). Azithromycin (Zithromax)[1] is preferred for traveler's diarrhea acquired in South and Southeast Asia, where quinolone-resistant *Campylobacter* is common. Azithromycin has supplanted erythromycin (Ery-Tab)[1] because it is better tolerated and has fewer gastrointestinal side effects. Rarely, intravenous aminoglycosides or carbapenems are necessary in very ill patients unable to take oral medication.

Unfortunately, quinolone resistance is not limited to Asia. Resistance has also increased in the United States. The widespread practice of using antibiotics, especially fluoroquinolones (enrofloxacin [Baytril]),[2] as additives to chicken feed has resulted in increasing quinolone resistance in *Campylobacter* strains found in poultry, the major source of infection. The Foodborne Diseases Active Surveillance Network (FoodNet) of the Centers for Disease Control and Prevention (CDC) found that 40% of US poultry products were contaminated with *Campylobacter*, and 10% of these strains were ciprofloxacin resistant. Although fluoroquinolones were removed from US animal feed in 2005, they continue to be used overseas. A newer strategy involves supplementing poultry feed with bacteriocins, nontoxic antimicrobial peptides, to reduce *Campylobacter* colonization. Irradiation of poultry meat might also be effective.

Empiric self-treatment of traveler's diarrhea is intended to shorten the duration of symptoms and involves immediate ciprofloxacin (Cipro) or azithromycin (Zithromax)[1] at the onset of diarrheal illness. One or two doses of antibiotics are usually sufficient to abort symptoms, and prolonged treatment is usually unnecessary. Loperamide (Imodium) might help control diarrhea in adults, but it should be avoided in dysenteric illness and in young children.

Complications

Campylobacter complications can occur either acutely or after the illness. Acute complications include cholecystitis, pseudoappendicitis, peritonitis, sepsis, and chest pain (pericarditis) (Box 1). Rashes, such as vasculitis or erythema nodosum, can occur. Rarely, focal extraintestinal infections such as septic arthritis or osteitis develop. Childhood complications include meningitis and encephalopathy, and dysenteric illness in infants occasionally mimics intussusception. *Campylobacter* can provoke postinfectious irritable bowel syndrome and is suspected of contributing to inflammatory bowel disease by damaging the intestinal epithelium, leading to chronic inflammation.

Late-term complications include Guillain-Barré syndrome and reactive arthritis. About 1 in 1000 *Campylobacter* infections is complicated by Guillain-Barré syndrome, which occurs several weeks after infection and carries a worse prognosis when associated with *Campylobacter*. As much as 30% to 40% of all Guillain-Barré syndrome has been attributed to *Campylobacter* infection, and even subclinical cases have been associated by later serologic testing.

Reactive arthritis after *Campylobacter* infection is common and also appears unrelated to the severity of the preceding diarrhea. Swelling and arthralgia in the hands, wrists, knees, or ankles develops 1 to 2 weeks after diarrhea and can persist for weeks to months. Nonsteroidal antiinflammatory drugs are usually helpful, and complete recovery is the rule.

References

Centers for Disease Control and Prevention: *Campylobacter: General information*, Available at http://www.cdc.gov/nczved/divisions/dfbmd/diseases/campylobacter/, 2014 [accessed July 9, 2015].

Gupta A, Nelson JM, Barrett TJ, et al: Antimicrobial resistance among *Campylobacter* strains, United States, 1997–2001, *Emerg Infect Dis* 10:1102–1109, 2004.

Kalischuk L, Buret A: A role for *Campylobacter jejuni*–induced enteritis in inflammatory bowel disease? *Am J Physiol Gastrointest Liver Physiol* 298:G1–9, 2010.

Nachamkin I, Allos BM, Ho T: *Campylobacter* species and Guillain-Barré syndrome, *Clin Microbiol Rev* 11:555–567, 1998.

Neal KR, Scott HM, Slack RC, Logan RF: Omeprazole as a risk factor for *Campylobacter* gastroenteritis: Case control study, *BMJ* 312:414–415, 1996.

Neal KR, Wright JM: Reactive arthritis–like symptoms following gastroenteritis—an increased risk with severe *Campylobacter* infection, *Int J Med Microbiol* 291:110, 2001.

Nelson JM, Chiller TM, Powers JH, Angulo FJ: Fluoroquinolone-resistant *Campylobacter* species and the withdrawal of fluoroquinolones from use in poultry: A public health success story, *Clin Infect Dis* 44:977–980, 2007.

Nelson JM, Smith KE, Vugia DJ, et al: Prolonged diarrhea due to ciprofloxacin-resistant *Campylobacter* infection, *J Infect Dis* 190:1150–1157, 2004.

Skirrow MB, Blaser MJ: Campylobacter jejuni. In Blaser MJ, Smith PD, Radin JI, et al: *Infections of the Gastrointestinal Tract*, ed 2nd, Philadelphia, 2002, Lippincott Williams & Wilkins. p. 719–739.

Svetich E, Stern N: Bacteriocins to control *Campylobacter* spp. in poultry—a review, *Poult Sci* 89:1763–1768, 2010.

Ternhag A, Asikainen T, Giesecke J, Ekdahl K: A meta-analysis on the effects of antibiotic treatment on duration of symptoms caused by infection with *Campylobacter* species, *Clin Infect Dis* 44:696–700, 2007.

Tribble DR, Sanders JW, Pang LW, et al: Traveler's diarrhea in Thailand: Randomized, double-blind trial comparing single-dose and 3-day azithromycin-based regimens with a 3-day levofloxacin regimen, *Clin Infect Dis* 44:338–346, 2007.

CAT SCRATCH DISEASE

Method of
Ronen Ben-Ami, MD

CURRENT DIAGNOSIS

- The combination of a compatible clinical syndrome of regional lymphadenopathy with a primary inoculation lesion and cat contact is highly suggestive of cat scratch disease.
- Results of *Bartonella henselae* serology are helpful in confirming the diagnosis; however, up to 20% of patients remain seronegative throughout their disease.
- Detection of *B. henselae* DNA by polymerase chain reaction from pus obtained by needle aspiration or lymph node biopsy is a highly sensitive diagnostic modality and may be particularly useful in seronegative patients.

CURRENT THERAPY

- Typical cat scratch disease is a self-limited disease; therefore, systemic antimicrobials are not routinely indicated in immunocompetent patients with uncomplicated cat scratch disease.
- Indications for antimicrobial therapy include an immunocompromised host, endocarditis, retinitis, and other atypical syndromes.
- Treatment may also be considered for patients who have typical cat scratch disease and who have extensive or bulky lymphadenopathy and are highly symptomatic.
- Suppurative lymph nodes should be drained by large-bore needle aspiration.

Cat scratch disease is a worldwide zoonotic infection caused by *Bartonella henselae*, an intracellular, pleomorphic, gram-negative

---

[1] Not FDA approved for this indication.
[2] Not available in the United States.

bacillus. Other *Bartonella* species have rarely been implicated. The disease typically manifests as benign regional lymphadenopathy, but atypical disease can involve almost any organ system and is associated with significant morbidity.

Epidemiology

B. henselae infection is widespread among domestic cats and other felids worldwide, and serologic studies indicate a higher prevalence in warm, humid climates. Transmission among cats occurs via an arthropod vector, the cat flea *Ctenocephalides felis*. *B. henselae* bacteremia is detected at higher rates in feral than in domesticated cats and in kittens compared to adult cats, explaining the higher infectivity of these animals. Cats infected with *B. henselae* are asymptomatic. Transmission to humans occurs via a scratch, bite, or lick; contamination of cat scratches by flea feces may enhance *Bartonella* transmission.

Cat scratch disease has been estimated to occur in the United States at a rate approaching 10 per 100,000 people. There is some seasonality, with incidence peaking between September and January. Although traditionally considered a disease of childhood, epidemiologic surveys have found a similar incidence of cat scratch disease in adults, and 6% of patients are aged 60 years or older. Cat contact is the most important risk factor: almost all patients are cat owners or were otherwise exposed to cats, and approximately half can recall a recent bite or scratch, most commonly by a kitten.

Clinical Manifestations

Cat scratch disease is divided into two clinical syndromes. Typical cat scratch disease is a subacute, self-limited regional lymphadenopathy and constitutes 80% to 90% of cases. Atypical cat scratch disease encompasses Parinaud oculoglandular syndrome and other clinical entities with systemic extranodal involvement. Bacillary angiomatosis and bacillary peliosis are manifestations of *B. henselae* infection in immunocompromised persons and are not discussed here.

Typical Cat Scratch Disease

A primary skin lesion, usually a papule or pustule, appears at the site of inoculation 3 to 10 days after cat contact and persists for 1 to 3 weeks. Regional lymphadenopathy develops within 1 to 7 weeks and resolves spontaneously after 2 to 4 months. The primary lesion is still present in approximately two thirds of patients when they present for evaluation of lymphadenopathy. The most commonly involved lymph nodes are, in descending order of frequency, axillary and epitrochlear nodes, head and neck nodes, and femoral and inguinal nodes. One third of patients develop lymphadenopathy at multiple sites. Lymph nodes are often painful and red; suppuration occurs in 10% of nodes. Mild constitutional symptoms, including low-grade fever and malaise, are noted in about half the cases. Rash, night sweats, anorexia, and weight loss are uncommon. Infection results in lifelong immunity.

Atypical Cat Scratch Disease

Parinaud oculoglandular syndrome, the most common form of atypical cat scratch disease, is a specific type of regional lymphadenopathy that occurs following conjunctival inoculation of *B. henselae*. The syndrome includes granulomatous conjunctivitis and preauricular lymphadenopathy. Endocarditis and encephalitis represent severe forms of *B. henselae* infection and are more common in elderly patients. Encephalitis manifests with various degrees of altered mental status, agitation, headache, and seizures. Cerebrospinal fluid lymphocytic pleocytosis occurs in only one third of cases, and brain-imaging studies usually fail to show any abnormalities. Neuroretinitis manifests as sudden unilateral loss of visual acuity. The diagnosis is suspected on the basis of typical findings on fundoscopic examination: papilledema and macular exudates in a star-like configuration; however, these findings are not pathognomonic of cat scratch disease. Other infrequent manifestations are self-limited granulomatous hepatitis and splenitis and osteoarticular disease. Prolonged fever of unknown origin has been described in children and adolescents.

Diagnosis

A compatible clinical syndrome in a person with a positive history of cat exposure suggests cat scratch disease. The diagnosis is most commonly confirmed with specific serologic assays. Immunofluorescence and enzyme immunoassays are comparably sensitive, although cross-reactivity can occur with other organisms such as *Chlamydia* species, *Coxiella burnetii*, and non-*henselae* *Bartonella* species. A single, elevated titer of immunoglobulin (Ig) M or IgG in the acute phase or a fourfold increase of IgG in convalescent serum supports the diagnosis.

Biopsy and histopathologic examination of lymph nodes are usually performed only when malignancy is suspected, and necrotizing granulomas are typically observed. The pleomorphic gram-negative bacilli are best visualized with the Warthin-Starry stain; however, the sensitivity of this method is too low to be clinically useful. Similarly, culture lacks sensitivity and requires prolonged incubation, making it impractical for routine use.

Polymerase chain reaction assays for the detection of *B. henselae* in pus aspirated from suppurative lymph nodes or primary skin lesions is highly sensitive and specific, and it can be performed with a rapid turnaround time; however, these assays are not widely available in most clinical microbiology laboratories.

Differential Diagnosis

Cat scratch disease should be differentiated from other infectious and noninfectious causes of regional lymphadenopathy. Importantly, lymphoma and solid tumors with metastases to lymph nodes may be confused with cat scratch disease. Malignancy should be suspected in patients who have marked constitutional symptoms, who are seronegative, or whose lymphadenopathy fails to resolve spontaneously after more than 6 months. Unlike cat scratch disease, pyogenic lymphadenitis manifests with rapid progression, high-grade fever, and a septic-appearing patient. Mycobacterial infection, syphilis, bubonic plague, tularemia, histoplasmosis, and sporotrichosis should be considered based on the presence of specific risk factors and endemic exposures. *Bartonella* endocarditis must be differentiated from other causes of culture-negative endocarditis, specifically Q fever and brucellosis.

Treatment

Because of the self-limiting course of typical cat scratch disease, patients usually require only observation and reassurance of its benign nature. The goals of therapy are alleviation of symptoms in patients with bulky lymphadenopathy and drainage of suppurating lymph nodes to prevent spontaneous formation of chronic sinus tracts. If drug treatment is initiated, azithromycin (Zithromax)[1] is the agent of choice based on a small, randomized placebo-controlled study that showed more rapid resolution of lymphadenopathy in the azithromycin arm, as determined by ultrasound. Suppurative nodes should be drained by large-bore needle aspiration. Incisional drainage is best avoided because it can promote sinus tract formation.

Atypical cat scratch disease syndromes usually require treatment, but there are scant data to support specific regimens, and treatment duration is not well defined. For patients with endocarditis, treatment with an aminoglycoside for at least 14 days is associated with a higher likelihood of recovery and survival. Uncontrolled data suggests that for patients with neuroretinitis, treatment with antibiotics and corticosteroids is associated with better visual outcomes than treatment with antibiotics alone (Table 1).

Prevention

Flea control in domestic cats can reduce the likelihood of *Bartonella* bacteremia and transmission to humans. Bites and scratches should be promptly rinsed. Human immunodeficiency virus (HIV)-infected patients and other immunocompromised persons should be cautioned about the risks of cat exposure because they are susceptible to disseminated visceral *B. henselae* infection, as well as other zoonotic infections such as toxoplasmosis.

---

[1]Not FDA approved for this indication.

TABLE 1 Antibiotic Treatment Regimens for Cat Scratch Disease

CLINICAL SYNDROME	FIRST CHOICE	SECOND CHOICE	COMMENTS
Typical cat scratch disease	Not indicated*	Azithromycin (Zithromax)[1] 500 mg PO on day 1, then 250 mg PO × 4 days	Drain suppurative nodes using large-bore aspiration
Endocarditis	Gentamicin (Garamycin)[1] 1 mg/kg IV q8h × > 14 days plus doxycycline (Vibramycin) 100 mg IV/PO bid × 6 week	Doxycycline 100 mg PO bid plus rifampicin (Rifadin)[1] 300 mg PO bid × 6 week	Some experts recommend extending oral doxycycline treatment × 3–6 months Surgical valve excision may be required
Neuroretinitis	Doxycycline 100 mg PO bid plus rifampicin[1] 300 mg PO bid × 4–6 week	NA	Spontaneous resolution is the rule; the utility of treatment remains unproven
Other atypical cat scratch disease	As for neuroretinitis	NA	Treatment duration should be individualized

*Treatment may be considered for patients with bulky or extensive lymphadenopathy and for immunocompromised patients.
[1]Not FDA approved for this indication.
NA, Not available.

References

Ben-Ami R, Ephros M, Avidor B, et al: Cat-scratch disease in elderly patients, *Clin Infect Dis* 41:969–974, 2005.

Giladi M, Kletter Y, Avidor B, et al: Enzyme immunoassay for the diagnosis of cat-scratch disease defined by polymerase chain reaction, *Clin Infect Dis* 33:1852–1858, 2001.

Habot-Wilner Z, Trivizki O, Goldstein M, et al: Cat-scratch disease: ocular manifestations and treatment outcome, *Acta Ophthalmol* 96(4):e524–e532, 2018.

Hansmann Y, DeMartino S, Piemont Y, et al: Diagnosis of cat scratch disease with detection of *Bartonella henselae* by PCR: A study of patients with lymph node enlargement, *J Clin Microbiol* 43:3800–3806, 2005.

Jackson LA, Perkins BA, Wenger JD: Cat scratch disease in the United States: An analysis of three national databases, *Am J Public Health* 83:1707–1711, 1993.

Jacobs RF, Schutze GE: *Bartonella henselae* as a cause of prolonged fever and fever of unknown origin in children, *Clin Infect Dis* 26:80–84, 1998.

Raoult D, Fournier PE, Vandenesch F, et al: Outcome and treatment of *Bartonella* endocarditis, *Arch Intern Med* 163:226–230, 2003.

Rolain JM, Brouqui P, Koehler JE, et al: Recommendations for treatment of human infections caused by *Bartonella* species, *Antimicrob Agents Chemother* 48:1921–1933, 2004.

Zangwill KM, Hamilton DH, Perkins BA, et al: Cat scratch disease in Connecticut. Epidemiology, risk factors, and evaluation of a new diagnostic test, *N Engl J Med* 329:8–13, 1993.

CHIKUNGUNYA

Method of
Scott Kellermann, MD, MPH; and Rick D. Kellerman, MD

CURRENT DIAGNOSIS

- Clinically, chikungunya is a diagnosis of exclusion, particularly when laboratory testing is not available. Accurate diagnosis depends on the patient's clinical symptoms and the epidemiology of endemic disease.
- Acute symptoms include incapacitating relapsing bilateral symmetrical polyarthralgia accompanied by high fever, headache, backache, and fatigue. Some may have a pruritic maculopapular rash at onset.
- Chronic symptoms include episodic incapacitating symmetrical polyarthralgia. Many have long-term asthenia and depression.
- Virus isolation provides definitive diagnosis.
- Immunoglobulin M antibody levels peak 3 to 5 weeks after the onset of illness and persist for approximately 2 months.
- Paired acute-phase and convalescent-phase antibody sampling may be required for diagnosis.

CURRENT THERAPY

- Medical treatment is primarily supportive.

The word "chikungunya" is a derivation of the Kimakonde (a Mozambique dialect) word "kungunyala" meaning "to become desiccated or contorted." In the Democratic Republic of the Congo, it is called "buka-buka," translated as "broken-broken," reflecting the incapacitating arthralgias that are common manifestations of Chikungunya fever.

Epidemiology

Chikungunya, first diagnosed in Tanganyika in 1952, is found in a large percentage of countries in Africa, Asia, and Southeast Asia and is prevalent in India. Dense human populations and lack of herd immunity likely contribute to the explosive nature of chikungunya epidemics in many regions. In India during 2006, more than 1,500,000 cases of chikungunya were reported, with *Aedes aegypti* implicated as the vector. Prior to 2006, chikungunya virus disease was rarely identified in travelers returning to the United States. From 2006 to 2013, an average of 28 people per year in the United States tested positive for recent chikungunya virus infection. In 2014, there was a large uptick in chikungunya, with 2811 cases reported in US states, with all but 12 infections acquired outside of the continental United States. These 12 cases were locally transmitted in Florida. In 2015, 896 cases were reported, with only one locally transmitted in Texas. In 2016, the case reports dropped to 248, all in returning travelers, and in 2017 there were 156 chikungunya virus disease cases reported from 28 states, all occurring in travelers returning from affected areas. No locally transmitted cases have been reported in the United States since 2015.

It is believed that chikungunya virus originated in Africa and migrated to Asia 200 years ago. Evidence derived from molecular genetics suggests it evolved around 1700; the first recorded outbreak of this disease was probably in 1779.

Interestingly, some medical historians believe that a pandemic of chikungunya occurred in the western hemisphere in the 1800s but was diagnosed as dengue fever. The 21st-century researchers who have examined the accounts of this pandemic now speculate that it was caused by chikungunya because the cases exhibited severe joint arthritis, which is more indicative of chikungunya than dengue. The virus then disappeared from the Americas until it reemerged during the last decade. Chikungunya epidemics appear suddenly and unpredictably and proceed explosively.

Risk factors

Individuals at the highest risk of contracting chikungunya and suffering from more-severe symptoms are those who have chronic arthritis, underlying chronic medical conditions, those over the age of 65 years, and pregnant women. Travelers who spend extended periods of time in endemic areas are at greater risk. These include missionaries, humanitarian aid workers, and those who frequently work outdoors. Mother-to-child transmission of chikungunya virus is frequent in the event of intrapartum maternal viremia and can often lead to severe neonatal complications.

Pathophysiology

Chikungunya is an arthropod transmitted disease caused by a single-stranded RNA arbovirus. As with dengue fever and yellow fever, chikungunya cycles from mosquito to human to mosquito. The mosquito *Aedes aegypti* is the usual vector for transmission of chikungunya. *Aedes albopictus*, the Asian tiger mosquito, is also a vector. Both species are found in the southeastern United States and limited parts of the southwest. The *Aedes albopictus* species survives further north into the Mid-Atlantic states and into the lower Midwest. The risk of person-to-mosquito transmission is highest during the viremic first week of illness. Birds, cattle, monkeys, and other vertebrates may serve as reservoirs. Chikungunya can be transmitted during childbirth, but there are no reported cases of transmission during breastfeeding. Theoretically, chikungunya can be transferred via blood transfusion, but there have been no reported cases. Previous infection will convey permanent immunity.

Prevention

There is no current vaccine. The best preventive measures are wearing permethrin-treated, bite-proof long sleeves and trousers and using a mosquito repellant such as 30% DEET, 20% oil of lemon eucalyptus, or 30% picaridin. Screening windows and doors has only a limited effect, because most contacts between the *Aedes* mosquitoes and humans occur outside.

Standing water, a breeding ground for mosquitoes, should be drained. *Aedes aegypti* breeding sites are associated with human habitation and are seemingly innocuous (i.e., flower vases, water storage vessels and birdbaths). Customary blood handling procedures are recommended.

If a Chikungunya epidemic were to occur in the United States, the standard public health measures of avoidance and mosquito control would be major lines of defense. To prevent local spread, the patient diagnosed with chikungunya should use mosquito repellant for 1 week after onset of fever.

Clinical Manifestations

Chikungunya virus infection should be considered in patients with acute onset of fever and polyarthralgia, especially in travelers who have recently returned from areas with endemic chikungunya. The incubation period of the chikungunya virus ranges from 1 to 12 days, most typically 3 to 7 days. Seventy two percent to 97% of those infected develop symptoms. Clinical onset is abrupt. The hallmarks of chikungunya are erratic, relapsing, and incapacitating polyarthralgia accompanied by high fever, backache, headache, and fatigue. Polyarthralgia is reported in 87% to 98% of cases and represents the most characteristic symptom. The joint pain is mostly polyarticular, bilateral, and symmetrical and occurs mainly in peripheral joints (wrists, ankles, and phalanges) and some large joints (shoulders, elbows and knees). Joint swelling is less frequent, occurring in 25% to 42% of cases. Typically, the fever lasts for 2 days and then will defervesce abruptly. Headache and an extreme degree of prostration may persist for a variable period, usually about 5 to 7 days. Rare symptoms include uveitis, retinitis, myocarditis, hepatitis, nephritis, hemorrhage, and neurologic problems such as myelitis, meningoencephalitis, Guillain-Barré syndrome, and cranial nerve palsies.

In 40% to 50% of cases, skin involvement is present consisting of a pruritic maculopapular rash, predominantly on the thorax, localized petechia, and facial edema. Though rarely affected, children may exhibit a bullous rash with pronounced sloughing. The case fatality ratio is approximately 1 per 1000, with most deaths occurring in newborns, the elderly, and the infirm.

Diagnosis

The instructions for serum diagnostic testing are found on the Centers for Disease Control and Prevention's website (http://www.cdc.gov/chikungunya/hc/diagnostic.html). The virus may be cultured within the first 3 days of illness. Virus isolation provides the most definitive diagnosis but requires 1 to 2 weeks for completion and must be processed in a biosafety level 3 laboratory. Chikungunya viral RNA may be identifiable in the serum during the first 8 days of illness because chikungunya virus antibodies usually develop by the end of the first week of illness. IgM antibody levels peak 3 to 5 weeks after the onset of illness and persist for approximately 2 months. In some cases, paired acute-phase and convalescent-phase antibody sampling may be required for accurate diagnosis. False-positive results may occur due to infection from closely related viruses.

A complete blood count may show lymphopenia and thrombocytopenia. Liver enzymes may elevate, and the serum creatinine might also increase. Radiologic findings are normal, and biologic markers of inflammation are normal or modestly elevated.

In many parts of the world, chikungunya is a clinical diagnosis of exclusion, particularly when laboratory testing is not readily available. The probability of accurate clinical diagnosis depends on the epidemiology of endemic diseases and the patient's clinical symptoms.

Differential Diagnosis

The differential diagnosis for chikungunya includes influenza, malaria, rickettsia, and a multitude of viruses, especially dengue fever. Dengue and chikungunya viruses are transmitted by the same mosquitoes, may have similar clinical features, and can occasionally coinfect the same individual. Clinically differentiating chikungunya from dengue may be difficult, however; in chikungunya the onset of fever is typically more abrupt and shorter lived, with severe arthralgia, rash, and lymphopenia more prevalent, whereas infection with dengue is more likely to present with neutropenia, thrombocytopenia, hemorrhage, shock, and death. Seasonally, chikungunya is more likely to be seen in the summer months when *Aedes* mosquitos proliferate.

Treatment

Medical treatment is primarily supportive. The use of antiviral agents is unproven. It is generally recommended that acetaminophen and, once dengue has been excluded, nonsteroidal antiinflammatory drugs and corticosteroids are useful for the treatment of joint pain. During the first week of the illness, those infected with chikungunya should be protected from further mosquito exposure to reduce the risk of local transmission.

Monitoring

Suspected chikungunya cases should be reported immediately to state or local health departments to facilitate diagnosis and mitigate the risk of local transmission.

Complications

Over the 3 years after the 2006 La Reunion outbreak, 60% of patients experienced continued symptoms of arthralgia, typically episodic, symmetrical (90%), highly incapacitating (77%), and polyarthralgias (70%). Local swelling, asthenia, and depression were common long-term complaints. Age >35 years and the presence of joint pain 4 months after the disease onset were risk factors for long-term arthralgia. Chikungunya is one of the agents researched as a potential biologic weapon.

References

Centers for Disease Control and Prevention: Chikungunya: atypical and severe disease manifestations. http://www.cdc.gov/chikungunya/pdfs/Chikungunya-atypical-severe-disease_Healthcare-provider-factsheet-10-07-2014.pdf.
Centers for Disease Control and Prevention: Chikungunya virus. http://www.cdc.gov/chikungunya/. Accessed May 25, 2019.

Centers for Disease Control and Prevention: Chikungunya virus in the United States, https://www.cdc.gov/chikungunya/geo/united-states.html.

Centers for Disease Control and Prevention: Infectious Diseases Related to Travel-chikungunya, https://wwwnc.cdc.gov/travel/yellowbook/2018/infectious-diseases-related-to-travel/chikungunya.

Cerny T, Schwarz M, Schwarz U: The range of neurological complications in Chikungunya fever, *Neurocrit Care* 27:447–457, 2017.

Couderc T, Khandoudi N, Grandadam M: Prophylaxis and therapy for Chikungunya virus infection, *J Infect Dis* 200:516–523, 2009.

Gerardin P, Barau G, Michault A: Multidisciplinary prospective study of mother-to-child chikungunya virus infections on the island of La Reunion, https://journals.plos.org/plosmedicine/article/file?id=10.1371/journal.pmed.0050060&type=printable.

Mohan A, Kiran DHN, Manohar IC, Kumar DP: Epidemiology, clinical manifestations, and diagnosis of chikungunya fever: lessons learned from the re-emerging epidemic, *Indian J Dermatol* 55:54–63, 2010.

Morens DM, Fauci AS: Perspective: Chikungunya at the door—Déjà vu all over again? *N Engl J Med* 371:885–887, 2014.

Morrison TE: Reemergence of Chikungunya virus, *J Virol* 88:11644–11647, 2014.

Pialoux G, Gaüzère B-A, Jauréguiberry S, Strobel M: Chikungunya, an epidemic arbovirus, *Lancet Infect Dis* 7:319–327, 2007.

Ramful D, Carbonnier M, Pasquet M: Mother-to-child transmission of Chikungunya virus infection, *Pediatr Infect Dis J* 26:811–815, 2007.

Schilte C, Staikovsky F, Couderc T: Chikungunya virus-associated long-term arthralgia: a 36-month prospective longitudinal study, *PLoS Negl Trop Dis* 7(3):e2137, 2013.

Schwameis M, Buchtele N, Wadowski PP: Chikungunya vaccines in development, *Hum Vaccin Immunother* 12:716–731, 2016.

Staples JE, Fischer M: Perspective: Chikungunya virus in the Americas—what a vector-borne pathogen can do, *N Engl J Med* 371:887–889, 2014.

Taksandel A, Vilhekar KY: Neonatal Chikungunya infection, *J Prevent Infect Control* 1:8, 2015.

Thiberville SD, Moyen N, Dupuis-Maguiraga L: Chikungunya fever: epidemiology, clinical syndrome, pathogenesis and therapy, *Antiviral Res*, 99. 2013, pp 345–370.

World Health Organization. Chikungunya. https://www.who.int/en/news-room/fact-sheets/detail/chikungunya. Accessed May 25, 2019.

CHOLERA

Method of
Mark Pietroni, MD, MBA

Cholera affects about 3 million people per year and kills approximately 100,000. It can kill within hours of the onset of symptoms, and even today the impact of an outbreak of cholera can be catastrophic in locations in which the water and sanitation infrastructure is weak, especially in crisis or war situations. The 21st century has already seen large-scale cholera epidemics in Haiti, Zimbabwe, Pakistan and Yemen, as well as many smaller outbreaks in countries and areas in which cholera is endemic. When cholera is untreated, mortality can be as high as 60% to 70%, but even in epidemics, with appropriate management and well-run diarrhea treatment centers, mortality can be reduced to well below 1%.

Oral rehydration therapy (ORT) is now the mainstay of treatment (Table 1). Developed in the 1960s in Dhaka, Bangladesh, ORT was used to great effect during the Bangladesh Liberation War of 1971. Cholera broke out in the refugee camps outside Calcutta, and the medical services ran out of intravenous fluid. ORT was not accepted as routine therapy by the medical profession at that time. The courageous decision to treat people with ORT saved thousands of lives and convinced the world of the effectiveness of ORT in the management of cholera.

Pathophysiology

Cholera is caused by a gram-negative, comma-shaped bacterium called *Vibrio cholerae*. Clinical disease is caused by two serogroups: *V. cholerae* O1 (which has two biotypes: classical and El Tor) and *V. cholerae* O139. Humans are the only known natural host, and asymptomatic human carriage is rare. *V. cholerae* is rapidly killed by boiling water, but it can lie dormant for months in blue-green algae, crustaceans, and copepods in brackish water, especially in estuaries. The Ganges delta provides an ideal habitat and is believed to be the place cholera first emerged.

Human infection is caused by ingestion of contaminated food or drink or from poor hand hygiene in epidemic situations. Relative or absolute achlorhydria facilitates passage through the stomach. Proliferation occurs in the small intestine, where a number of toxins are released. This results in massive secretion of isotonic fluid into the gut. The fluid passes out of the anus full of vibrios to perpetuate the cycle of transmission. Killing the host does not appear to interrupt this cycle!

The cholera toxin is secreted only by the O1 and O139 serogroups. It has two subunits: A (active) and B (binding). Subunit B binds to receptors in the small intestine and subunit A activates adenylate cyclase. This causes the active secretion of a number of ions into the gut, which drags water by osmosis and also blocks the reabsorption of sodium from the gut. The net result is a massive loss of water, sodium chloride, and bicarbonate. This cannot be replaced by drinking a sodium solution because sodium reabsorption is blocked. However, the addition of glucose to a solution of sodium activates a sodium–glucose co-transporter; sodium is absorbed and water follows by osmosis. This is the basis of oral rehydration therapy for diarrhea today.

Clinical Presentation and Diagnosis

Cholera manifests as an acute watery diarrhea without blood in the stool or (usually) abdominal cramps. The majority of cases are clinically indistinguishable from other causes of watery diarrhea. About 10%-20% will develop dehydration but most require only oral rehydration fluid as treatment. However, some will progress to classic or severe cholera.

TABLE 1	Composition (mEq/L) of Common Solutions Used for Rehydration						
SOLUTION	**NA+**	**K+**	**CL−**	**HCO₃⁻**	**CITRATE**	**CA2+**	**GLUCOSE OR CARBOHYDRATE**
Intravenous Solution							
Normal saline	154	—	154	—	—	—	—
Ringer's lactate	130	4	111	28	—	3	—
Ringer's lactate + D₅	130	4	109	28	—	3	278
Cholera saline (Dhaka solution)	133	13	98	48	—	—	140
Oral Solution							
Standard ORS	90	20	80	—	10	—	75
Hypo-osmolar ORS	75	20	65	—	10	—	75
ReSoMal*	45	40	76	—	7	—	125

Abbreviations: D_5 = 5% dextrose; ORS = oral rehydration solution; ReSoMal = reduced osmolarity ORS for malnourished children.
Reprinted with permission from Harris JB, Pietroni M: Approach to the child with acute diarrhea in developing countries. UpToDate. Available at http://www.uptodate.com/contents/approach-to-the-child-with-acute-diarrhea-in-developing-countries (accessed August 11, 2016).
*Also contains Mg 6 mmol/L, Zn 300 μmol/L, Cu 45 μmol/L.

The classic picture is of the rapid onset of profuse watery diarrhea (rice-water stool) and vomiting, which is painless and can result in circulatory collapse within hours without effective treatment. The history is usually less than 24 hours, although it may be longer if the patient is taking oral rehydration solution. Abdominal cramps can occur. Fever is absent. Patients usually remain alert, but severe electrolyte abnormalities such as hypoglycemia and hyponatremia can cause a reduced level of consciousness or convulsions, especially in children. Acidosis is often severe and results in tachypnea, which is commonly misdiagnosed as pneumonia. Patients should be reassessed for the presence or absence of pneumonia 1 to 2 hours after adequate rehydration. The diagnosis of cholera can be confirmed by the presence of rapidly motile vibrios detected by dark-field microscopy or by stool or rectal swab culture. However, the classic history, appearance of the stool, and rapid presentation mean that the diagnosis is usually clinical.

Treatment

A clinical syndrome of acute watery diarrhea (three or more watery stools in the last 24 hours) of short duration (24–48 hours) with or without vomiting associated with dehydration in anyone older than 2 years in an endemic or epidemic situation should be treated as cholera. Children younger than 2 years may be managed in the same way, but other diagnoses such as rotavirus should be considered. The mainstay of management (whatever the causative organism) is appropriate early rehydration, and time should not be wasted worrying about investigations or which antibiotic to use (Figure 1).

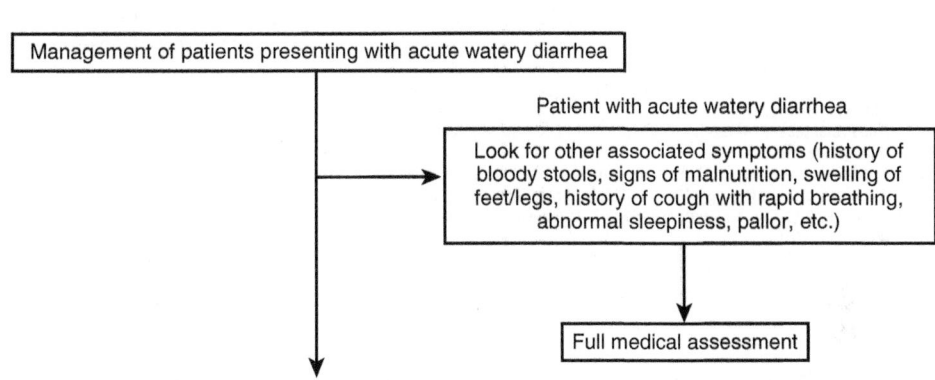

Assess	Condition	Normal	Irritable/less active*	Lethargic/comatose*
	Eyes	Normal	Sunken	Sunken
	Tongue	Normal	Dry	Dry
	Thirst	Normal	Thirsty (drinks eagerly)	Unable to drink*
	Skin pinch	Normal	Goes back slowly*	Goes back very slowly*
	Radial pulse	Normal	Reduced*	Uncountable or absent*
Diagnosis		No sign of dehydration	If at least 2 signs, including one (*) sign, are present, diagnose *some dehydration*	If some dehydration plus one of the (*) signs are present, diagnose *severe dehydration*
Management		A	B	C

A. No sign of dehydration—ORS
- 50 mL ORS per kg body weight *plus* ongoing losses
- Send patient home with 4 packets of ORS
- Continue feeding, including breast milk for infants and young children

B. Some dehydration—ORS
- 80 mL ORS per kg body weight over 4–6 hours plus ongoing losses
- Observe patient for 6–12 hours
- Continue feeding, including breastmilk for infants and young children
- Reassess patient and dehydration status hourly.
- In case of frequent vomiting (>3 times in 1 hour): Treat with IV fluid

C. Severe dehydration—Start IV fluid immediately (100 mL/kg)
IV solution containing sodium, potassium, chloride and bicarbonate (e.g., Ringer's Lactate)

    Children <1 year or malnourished
       30 mL/kg in first 1 hour
       70 mL/kg in next 5 hours

    Adults and children >1 year
       30 mL/kg in first 1/2 hour
       70 mL/kg in next 2 1/2 hours

- Encourage the patient to take ORS as soon as he/she is able to drink
- Antibiotic, if needed, after rehydration
- Zinc[1] 20 mg/day for 10 days in children 6 months to 5 years old, 10 mg/day for 10 days in children under 6 months

Figure 1 Quick identification of cholera cases can be made using a standard case definition. During an outbreak, cholera should be suspected in any patient who is older than 2 years, is attending a health facility, and has a history of acute watery diarrhea (passage of at least three stools in the last 24 hours) of a short duration (less than 24 hours), with or without vomiting, and with signs of dehydration. (Flow chart modified from International Centre for Diarrhoeal Disease Research, Bangladesh (ICDDR,B) internal treatment protocol.) *Abbreviation:* ORS = oral rehydration solution.

BOX 1 Fluids for Patients without Signs of Dehydration

Acceptable
Oral rehydration solution (optimal for both repletion and maintenance)
Salted drinks (salted rice water or salted yogurt drink)
Broth or soup (salted vegetable or meat soup)
Water
Rice water
Coconut water (unsweetened)
Weak tea (unsweetened)
Fresh fruit juice (unsweetened)

Unacceptable
Carbonated beverages
Sweetened juices
Coffee
Medicinal teas or infusions

Fluids containing salt should be encouraged. Unacceptable fluids include carbonated beverages and sweetened juices; the sugar in these fluids may worsen diarrhea. Coffee and medicinal teas or infusions are also unacceptable since they can have diuretic and purgative effects.
Reprinted with permission from Harris JB, Pietroni M: Approach to the child with acute diarrhea in developing countries. UpToDate. Available at http://www.uptodate.com/contents/approach-to-the-child-with-acute-diarrhea-in-developing-countries (accessed August 11, 2016).

BOX 2 Antibiotics in Cholera

Antibiotics should be given to all patients with severe dehydration. Choice of antibiotic depends on local sensitivity pattern.

First-Line Drug (If Susceptibility Report Is Not Available)
Adults
Azithromycin (Zithromax)[1] 1 g (500 mg × 2) PO as a single dose after correcting severe dehydration

Children
Azithromycin[1] 20 mg/kg PO as a single dose after correction of dehydration and cessation of vomiting (if any)

Second-Line Drug (Not Recommended for Children < 5 Years or Pregnant Women)
Adults
Ciprofloxacin (Cipro)[1] 1 g (500 mg × 2) PO as a single dose after correction of severe dehydration

Children
Ciprofloxacin[1] 20 mg/kg PO as a single dose after correction of dehydration and cessation of vomiting (if any)

Third-Line Drugs
Doxycycline (Vibramycin) 300 mg as a single dose after food (not in children or pregnant women)

[1] Not FDA approved for this indication.

Figure 2 Cholera cot.

The initial assessment should be brief but must:
• Confirm the diagnosis of acute watery diarrhea
• Assess the level of dehydration
• Assess the presence or absence of malnutrition
• Recognize any other comorbidities

Accurate assessment and rapid, appropriate treatment of dehydration is critical to the management of cholera. A simple scoring system based on five clinical signs is sufficient and can accurately predict patients with 5% to 10% (some) dehydration and greater than 10% (severe) dehydration. Common mistakes include over-reliance on individual clinical signs and giving too little intravenous fluid during the initial phase and too much during the recovery phase. Patients with less than 5% (no) dehydration and 5% to 10% (some) dehydration can be managed with oral rehydration alone (Box 1) unless there is a reduced level of consciousness or inability to take fluids by mouth. Those with 5% to 10% (some) dehydration must be reassessed every 1 to 2 hours to make sure that hydration is improving.

Patients with severe dehydration require an immediate intravenous fluid bolus of 100 mL/kg given over 3 hours with one third in the first 30 minutes (double the duration in children who are younger than 1 year and have malnutrition). If possible, the intravenous fluid should contain sodium, potassium, and bicarbonate—Ringer's lactate or cholera saline—but normal saline with 5 to 10 mmol/L of potassium may also be used. Oral rehydration should start at the same time. Once the intravenous fluid bolus has finished, further intravenous fluids are usually not required.

Patients are best managed using a cholera cot, especially in an epidemic situation. The cholera cot is a bed (or sometimes a chair) covered with a nonabsorbent sheet with a hole that allows the passage of stool and urine directly to a bucket under the bed (Figure 2). The sheets and bucket should be replaced three times a day and between patients. They may be washed, sterilized, and reused. Patients do not need to use a toilet (which can be several times an hour), linen is not soiled, and body fluids are prevented from running on the floor. This system enables adequate infection control to be maintained with limited resources.

After an initial assessment has been made and fluids started, a fuller clinical assessment can take place. Patients with significant comorbidities can require individually tailored treatment plans.

Antibiotics reduce the length of stay and fluid requirement in patients with severe dehydration due to cholera (Box 2). A single dose is sufficient, but this should be repeated if the dose is vomited back. The choice of antibiotic should be guided by local sensitivities where these are available. If not, a single dose of azithromycin (Zithromax)[1] 1 g in adults and 20 mg/day for 10 days in children 6 months to 5 years old, 10 mg/day for 10 days in children under 6 months. All children between 6 months and 5 years of age should receive zinc[1] 20 mg/day for 10 days because this reduces subsequent mortality and further episodes of diarrhea.

Recovery from cholera is rapid, and mortality is extremely low if the dehydration is treated appropriately. The Cholera Hospital run by the International Centre for Diarrhoeal Disease Research, Bangladesh (ICDDR,B), in Dhaka treats around 120,000 patients a year. The average length of stay is 16 hours, and the mortality rate is zero.

[1] Not FDA approved for this indication.

Prevention

Because the transmission of cholera is feco-oral, cholera can be prevented by good hand hygiene and by providing safe drinking water and appropriate sanitation. Standard food and hygiene precautions should be followed by people travelling in endemic areas (e.g., eat only boiled or fried foods; drink only boiled or bottled water). The FDA recently approved a single-dose live oral cholera vaccine, called Vaxchora in the United States. Vaxchora is indicated for adults 18–64 years old who are traveling to an area of active cholera. Two other oral inactivated cholera vaccines, Dukoral and ShanChol, are not available in the United States. These two cholera vaccines provide around 60% to 80% efficacy for 6 months. They are not recommended for the occasional traveler or tourist but may be given to people working in high-risk situations, such as aid workers in a cholera outbreak. The World Health Organization recommends the use of oral cholera vaccine in endemic areas as part of disease control programmes and maintains a global cholera vaccine stockpile for use in epidemic situations.

References

Updated global burden of cholera in endemic countries. Ali M, Nelson AR, Lopez AL, Sack D: *PLoS Negl Trop Dis* 9(6):e0003832, 2015 https://doi.org/10.1371/journal.pntd.0003832.

Alam NH, Ashraf H: Treatment of infectious diarrhea in children, *Paediatr Drugs* 5:151–165, 2003.

Harris, J.B & Pietroni, M.A.C Approach to the child with acute diarrhea in resource limited countries. In: UpToDate, Calderwood, S.B. & Bloom, A. (Eds), UpToDate, Waltham, MA, 2017.

Roy SK, Tomkins AM, Akramuzzaman SM, et al: Randomised controlled trial of zinc supplementation in malnourished Bangladeshi children with acute diarrhea, *Arch Dis Child* 77:196–200, 1997.

Saha D, Karim MM, Khan WA, et al: Single-dose azithromycin for the treatment of cholera in adults, *N Engl J Med* 354:2452–2462, 2006.

UNICEF Cholera Toolkit www.unicef.org/cholera_toolkit/ especially Chapter 8: Case management and infection control in health facilities and treatment sites pp 110–135. Accessed 10/3/2018.

MYALGIC ENCEPHALOMYELITIS/CHRONIC FATIGUE SYNDROME

Stephen J. Gluckman, MD

Myalgic encephalomyelitis/chronic fatigue syndrome (ME/CFS) is an often-misunderstood syndrome that should not be confused with malingering or hypochondriasis. Patients with ME/CFS are truly suffering from their often-disabling symptoms. It is impossible to successfully treat a patient with ME/CFS unless the clinician believes the patient is genuinely symptomatic. ME/CFS also should not be confused with the isolated symptoms of fatigue. Fatigue is a common patient complaint, whereas ME/CFS has a much lower prevalence.

Definition

ME/CFS is not a new disease; the syndrome has been described since at least the mid-1700s. However, since that time it has been mistakenly ascribed to a number of incorrect pathologic and infectious causes. In the past it has been called febricula, neurasthenia, effort syndrome, DeCosta syndrome, myalgic encephalitis, chronic brucellosis, chronic Lyme disease, chronic Epstein–Barr syndrome, total allergy syndrome, chronic candidiasis, and multiple chemical sensitivity syndrome. More recently it has been falsely attributed to infection with xenotropic murine leukemia virus–related virus (XMRV) and related retroviruses, such as murine leukemia virus (MLV). None of these possible causes has proved to be correct.

In 1988, in an attempt to be descriptive rather than to attribute an incorrect etiology to the disease, the term *chronic fatigue syndrome* was coined. Therefore the name is relatively new but the syndrome is not. The disease is chronic and fatigue is a cardinal feature, but it is more than being chronically tired. It is a syndrome that includes

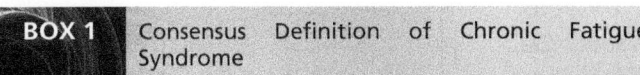

BOX 1   Consensus Definition of Chronic Fatigue Syndrome

Chronic fatigue syndrome is a clinically evaluated, unexplained, persistent or relapsing chronic fatigue (lasting more than 6 months) that is of new or definite onset (has not been lifelong); is not the result of ongoing exertion; is not substantially alleviated by rest; and results in substantial reduction in previous levels of occupational, educational, social, or personal activities.

Four or more of the following symptoms are concurrently present for more than 6 months:
- Impaired memory or concentration
- Multijoint pain
- Muscle pain
- New headaches
- Postexertional malaise
- Sore throat
- Tender cervical or axillary lymph nodes
- Unrefreshing sleep

Exclusionary Clinical Diagnoses
- Any active medical condition that could explain the chronic fatigue
- Any previously diagnosed medical condition whose resolution has not been documented beyond reasonable clinical doubt and whose continued activity can explain the chronic fatiguing illness
- Psychotic major depression, bipolar affective disorder, schizophrenia, delusional disorders, dementias, anorexia nervosa, bulimia nervosa
- Alcohol or other substance abuse within 2 years before the onset of the chronic fatigue and at any time afterward

Adapted from Fukuda K, Straus SE, Hickie I, et al. The chronic fatigue syndrome: a comprehensive approach to its definition and study. *Ann Intern Med.* 1994;121:953–959.

---

a number of additional symptoms as noted in Box 1, the working case definition was published by the Centers for Disease Control and Prevention and then modified in 1992 by the National Institute of Allergy and Infectious Diseases. In March 2015 the Institute of Medicine (IOM) issued an extensive and thorough review of the topic. As a result of this review they proposed a name change to Systemic Exertion Intolerance Disease (SEID). This comprehensive report has three major themes: (1) ME/CFS has acquired a great deal of negative connotation with associated misunderstanding and prejudice. The name change to SEID is an attempt to disconnect this disease from past misunderstandings. However, this name change has not caught on. (2) The criteria for diagnosis were greatly simplified with emphasis on the major features (Box 2). (3) By using the term "disease" and with the ample reference support in the document the IOM unequivocally underscores the very real nature of this malady. The IOM report is by far the most thorough examination of the topic and it unequivocally supports the validity of this disease.

One note of caution: This case definition is an epidemiologic tool and not a strict clinical tool. It is useful for studying the disease. However, some patients do not completely fit this definition but ME/CFS can nonetheless be diagnosed by a knowledgeable clinician.

Because some immune abnormalities are often seen in these patients, some people have called this "chronic fatigue and immune dysregulation syndrome." The immune abnormalities seen in ME/CFS patients are mild and differ from patient to patient. Most significantly, these patients are not immunosuppressed.

It has been noted that many of the symptoms of fibromyalgia overlap with ME/CFS, and some clinicians consider fibromyalgia and ME/CFS to be different aspects of the same disease because both often include pain and fatigue. These different names for the same syndrome can be confusing to patients and clinicians, and when managing patients with ME/CFS it is important to explain this to them.

Diagnosis: Requires that the patient have the following three symptoms:

- A substantial reduction or impairment in the ability to engage in pre-illness levels of occupational, educational, social, or personal activities that persists for more than 6 months and is accompanied by fatigue, which is often profound, is of new or definite onset (not lifelong), is not the result of ongoing excessive exertion, and is not substantially alleviated by rest.
- Postexertional malaise
- Unrefreshing sleep
  At least one of the two following manifestations is also required:
- Cognitive impairment
- Orthostatic intolerance

CFS, Chronic fatigue syndrome; *SEID,* systemic exertion intolerance disease.

Epidemiology

Although chronic fatigue is an extremely common symptom, ME/CFS is not. The former has been noted to have a prevalence of 10% to 25% in a number of studies. However, the point prevalence of ME/CFS has been estimated to be in the range of 0.1%. ME/CFS is overrepresented in young and middle-aged women, but it has been described in men and women and in all age groups.

Pathophysiology

The cause of ME/CFS is unknown. Much effort has gone into trying to discern an infectious, endocrine, immune, or psychiatric cause, but to date none has been proved. Studies have shown a link between ME/CFS and the presence of certain genes that mediate immune and stress responses. The findings suggest that difficulty managing stress may be linked to the development of ME/CFS. They also suggest that there is not a single cause of ME/CFS, but that there may be a number of stress-related triggers (physical or emotional) in those with a genetic predisposition. This is consistent with the typical course, in which a previously healthy person develops an acute illness that resolves but initiates ME/CFS.

Clinical Features and Diagnosis

Although there is, as yet, no diagnostic test, the history, physical examination, and laboratory testing are generally very characteristic and allow a clinician to confidently make the diagnosis. The typical story is one of a previously highly functioning person who develops an acute illness or other stressor. The acute problem resolves; however, from that time on, symptoms of ME/CFS are triggered. Despite often-profound symptoms, physical examination is persistently normal, as is laboratory testing. Symptoms are exacerbated by physical activity. The pre-ME/CFS medical history of the patient is not one of multiple medical problems. Affected patients are typically high functioning persons who are struck down with this disease. Features to emphasize in addition to the case definition noted in Box 1 include those noted in Box 3.

In a patient with a typical story and examination, laboratory testing should be limited (Box 4). Testing for diseases with a low pretest likelihood runs the serious risk of false-positive results. This can result in further testing, diagnostic confusion, and unnecessary treatments. Specifically, the signs and symptoms of ME/CFS are not those of systemic lupus, Lyme disease, cytomegalovirus, bartonellosis, ehrlichiosis, or babesiosis among others. Serologic testing for these diagnoses is not helpful and can be harmful if the presence of antibodies results in the initiation of unwarranted medications. For similar reasons, neuroimaging without objective clinical findings is not indicated. Although abnormalities can be found, they are nonspecific and of no clinical utility. Tilt-table

testing seems to be abnormal in many patients with ME/CFS; however, testing is expensive and uncomfortable, and abnormal results do not alter the management. Of course, if history, physical examination, and initial laboratory testing do reveal abnormalities, further laboratory evaluation should be undertaken to elucidate the cause of the aberration(s).

Treatment

There is no established cure for ME/CFS, but patients should be counseled that a number of things can be done to manage this often-disabling illness (Box 5). These can be divided into things the clinician should do and things the patient should do.

Things the Clinician Should Do

To successfully manage ME/CFS, a clinician must believe that the patient is truly symptomatic. Patients with ME/CFS are not malingering. Because they often appear well and have consistently normal objective testing, they often become very defensive about their limitations. They are sensitive to the validity of their symptoms. Not only are they suffering, but also they are blamed for it. Many patients with ME/CFS are partially or totally disabled. Their outward healthy appearance belies the internal sense of ill health. It is common for relatives and colleagues to believe they are malingering. A vicious cycle of frustration, anger, and depression commonly ensues.

As part of establishing the validity of the diagnosis a clinician should review the history of ME/CFS, emphasizing that this is not a new disease but was originally described centuries ago.

For successful management, a clinician should give the patient enough time, specifically inquire about other diagnoses the patient is concerned about, and explain why they are not correct. The clinician should see the patient at regular intervals.

Make sure that the patient has reasonable expectations. Most patients with ME/CFS have not had previous chronic illnesses or significant prolonged limitations. It is often necessary to review the information about ME/CFS with the patient's family and to emphasize that this disabling illness is not volitional.

Although it is generally wise to avoid a discussion about whether the origin of ME/CFS is psychiatric or organic, depression is an expected consequence of any chronic illness. Depression has specific treatments, and it should be aggressively diagnosed and treated. The patient should be told that successful management of depression will help him or her cope with ME/CFS.

If a sleep disturbance exists, it also should be aggressively managed—if necessary by a sleep specialist. Sleep deprivation makes other symptoms more difficult to deal with.

Chronic pain is very enervating. If pain is prominent, that also should be aggressively managed, often by a pain specialist.

It is important for the clinician to be cautious about ascribing all of a patient's symptoms to ME/CFS. Such patients are, of course, not protected from getting additional illnesses. Each symptom should be considered on its own before defaulting it to ME/CFS.

Complementary therapies must be discussed or the patient might get the impression that the clinician is not comfortable in considering them; this can partially undermine the clinician–patient relationship. Although all are of unproved benefit and often undetermined risk, "complementary" therapies that are not dangerous—such as acupuncture—or expensive, are reasonable to consider.

Things the Patient Should Do

Of the 350 studies that have looked at treatment options for ME/CFS, only cognitive behavioral therapy and graded exercise therapy have been shown to be of possible benefit. In cognitive behavioral therapy, the patient undergoes a series of 1-hour sessions designed to alter beliefs and behaviors that might delay recovery. Although exercise can exacerbate symptoms, deconditioning will also do so. Limiting activity can worsen weakness and depression. The risk of exacerbating symptoms can be reduced by cautiously setting less-ambitious activity/exercise goals. Because many patients with ME/CFS were particularly active before the onset of their illness and are impatient to get their former lives

BOX 3 — Frequent Features of Chronic Fatigue Syndrome

- Sudden onset of fatigue after a relatively common illness or other stressor
- Previously active and healthy person
- Symptoms very sensitive to exacerbation by physical activity
- Normal physical examination and laboratory testing
- Altered sleep
- "Foggy" thought processes
- Lack of progression to organ failure or any significant objective organ abnormality
- Joint and muscle aching without physical evidence of inflammation
- Feverish feeling (sustained elevated temperatures [>37.4°C] should prompt a search for an alternative diagnosis, because the chronic fatigue syndrome patient is not truly febrile)
- Diffuse aching that is not well localized to joints or muscles, but without erythema, effusion, or limitation of motion
- Muscles that are easily fatigued (however, strength is normal, as are biopsies and electromyograms)
- Occasional mild cervical and/or axillary lymphadenitis (painful lymph nodes [lymphadenia] are a common complaint, but this is not a true lymphadenopathy)

BOX 4 — Diagnostic Testing

Tests to Perform
- Complete blood count
- Comprehensive chemistry screen
- Thyroid-stimulating hormone
- Perhaps: Cortrosyn stimulation test, sleep study
- Additional testing *only* with specific clinical indications

Do Not Routinely Do
- ANA
- Serology for CMV, EBV, *Bartonella, Babesia, Ehrlichia, Anaplasma*
- MRI, SPECT, or PET scans
- Tilt-table testing

ANA, Antinuclear antibody test; *CMV,* cytomegalovirus; *EBV,* Epstein–Barr virus; *MRI,* magnetic resonance imaging; *PET,* positron emission tomography; *SPECT,* single-photon–emission computed tomography.

BOX 5 — Therapy of Chronic Fatigue Syndrome

- Educate the patient and his or her support system about the diagnosis of chronic fatigue syndrome. Emphasize the validity of the diagnosis and of the patient's symptoms. Make sure there is an understanding about expectations.
- Aggressively manage specific symptoms of sleep disturbance, pain, and depression.
- Consider cognitive behavioral therapy.
- Emphasize the need for gradual, graded exercise. Give the patient a specific "prescription" for this.
- Avoid the temptation to prescribe antimicrobials, corticosteroids, or other medications with no proven benefit and the potential to do harm.
- Discuss the pros and cons of using unstudied, expensive, or potentially dangerous "alternative therapies."

---

back, they often need strict guidelines to try to prevent overdoing exercise while at the same time getting a clear prescription to exercise. The exercise prescription should be individualized based on the degree of impairment, but it is wise to initially set goals on the low side to avoid exacerbating symptoms.

As part of the management of ME/CFS patients, their families, and, when appropriate, their employers need to reframe their expectations. ME/CFS patients have a chronic, disabling illness. Families and others need to come to some understanding that patients cannot do all that they were able to do before the onset of ME/CFS and that patients cannot "will" the disease away any more than they could will away a more visible disability.

Things that Should Not Be Done

There are many suggested remedies for ME/CFS. Most are either unstudied or disproved. In particular, treatments that are expensive or potentially harmful should be avoided. There is no role for antimicrobial therapy. There is no role for antiviral therapy, including treatment for retroviruses. There is no role for intravenous immunoglobulin, corticosteroids, special diets, or vitamin treatments.

Prognosis

The likelihood for complete recovery from ME/CFS is only fair. The disease tends to wax and wane over time, but in only a minority of patients does it completely resolve. If sustained improvement occurs, it is generally over several years. Several features have been associated with a poorer prognosis, including age older than 38 years, more than eight symptoms, duration longer than 1.5 years, less than 16 years of formal education, a history of a dysthymic disorder, and a sustained belief that the disease is due to a physical cause.

Monitoring

Despite the lack of very effective treatment, many patients benefit from regular monitoring of their condition. Knowing they have scheduled visits minimizes the number of crises and emergency visits and allows the patient to reconnect with a validating physician. Follow-up on a quarterly basis is a reasonable interval.

References

Bouquet J, Gardy JL, Brown S, et al: RNA-seq analysis of gene expression, viral pathogen, and B-cell/T-cell receptor signatures in complex chronic disease, *Clin Infect Dis* 64:476, 2017.

Clark MR, Katon W, Russo J, et al: Chronic fatigue: Risk factors for symptom persistence in a 212-year follow-up study, *Am J Med* 98:187–195, 1995.

Fulcher KY, White PD: Randomised controlled trial of graded exercise in patients with the chronic fatigue syndrome, *BMJ* 314:1647–1652, 1997.

Goertzel BN, Pennachin C, de Souza Coelho L, et al: Combinations of single nucleotide polymorphisms in neuroendocrine effector and receptor genes predict chronic fatigue syndrome, *Pharmacogenomics* 7:475–483, 2006.

Goldenberg DL, Simms RW, Geiger A, et al: High frequency of fibromyalgia in patients with chronic fatigue seen in a primary care practice, *Arthritis Rheum* 33:381–387, 1990.

Green CR, Cowan P, Elk R, et al: National Institutes of Health Pathways to Prevention Workshop: Advancing the research on myalgic encephalomyelitis/chronic fatigue syndrome, *Ann Intern Med* 162:860, 2015.

Haney E, Smith ME, McDonagh M, et al: Diagnostic methods for myalgic encephalomyelitis/chronic fatigue syndrome: a systematic review for a National Institutes of Health Pathways to Prevention Workshop, *Ann Intern Med* 162:834, 2015.

IOM (Institute of Medicine): *Beyond Myalgic Encephalomyelitis/Chronic Fatigue Syndrome: Redefining an Illness*, Washington, DC, 2015, The National Academies Press. http://www.iom.edu/mecfs. Accessed 12 February 2015.

Lightfoot Jr RW, Luft BJ, Rahn DW, et al: Empiric parenteral antibiotic treatment of patients with fibromyalgia and fatigue and a positive serologic result for Lyme disease. A cost-effectiveness analysis, *Ann Intern Med* 119:503–509, 1993.

Schwartz RB, Garada BM, Komaroff AL, et al: Detection of intracranial abnormalities in patients with chronic fatigue syndrome: Comparison of MR imaging and SPECT, *Am J Roentgenol* 162:935–941, 1994.

Wessely S, Chalder T, Hirsch S, et al: The prevalence and morbidity of chronic fatigue and chronic fatigue syndrome: A prospective primary care study, *Am J Public Health* 87:1449–1455, 1997.

White PD, Goldsmith KA, Johnson AL, et al: Comparison of adaptive pacing therapy, cognitive behaviour therapy, graded exercise therapy, and specialist medical care for chronic fatigue syndrome (PACE): A randomised trial, *Lancet* 377:823–836, 2011.

EBOLA VIRUS DISEASE

Method of
Uma Malhotra, MD

CURRENT DIAGNOSIS

- Detection of viral RNA in the blood by reverse transcriptase-polymerase chain reaction (RT-PCR) beginning 3 days after the onset of symptoms.
- Repeat testing may be necessary for patients with illness duration shorter than 3 days.
- Details on specimen collection and handling can be found on the Centers for Disease Control and Prevention (CDC), and World Health Organization (WHO) websites.

CURRENT THERAPY

- Intensive fluid management to correct volume losses and electrolyte abnormalities.
- Aggressive use of antiemetics, antidiarrheals, and rehydration solutions.
- Respiratory and hemodynamic support.
- Blood products for management of coagulopathy.
- Evaluate and treat any concomitant infections.
- There are no approved antiviral therapies. However, a number of experimental treatments, including monoclonal antibodies, convalescent serum, small-molecule antivirals, and short interfering RNAs are available.
- Strict infection control measures, with contact and droplet precautions, must be used.
- Personnel trained in the correct use of personal protective equipment (PPE) should care for the patients.

Filoviridae, derived from the Latin word "filum," meaning thread-like, is a family of viruses with a filamentous structure that can cause severe hemorrhagic fever and fulminant septic shock. Filoviruses have been divided into two genera: Ebola-like viruses with five species—*Zaire, Sudan, Ivory Coast, Bundibugyo,* and *Reston*; and Marburg-like viruses with a single species—*Marburg*, which has caused outbreaks in Central Africa. Using paleoviruses (genomic fossils) found in mammals, we can extrapolate that the viruses probably diverged several thousand years ago, and that the family itself is at least tens of millions of years old.

Epidemiology

Of the five Ebola virus species only four—*Zaire, Sudan, Ivory Coast,* and *Bundibugyo*—cause disease in humans. Since its first recognition in 1976, *Zaire ebolavirus* has caused multiple outbreaks in Central Africa. It is the causative agent of the 2014 West African epidemic, with an initial estimated case fatality rate as high as 70%, although as the epidemic evolved, lower fatality rates in the range of 30% to 40% were observed. The 2014 epidemic began in Guinea, when a 2-year-old child became infected in late 2013, and *Zaire ebolavirus* subsequently spread to Liberia, Sierra Leone, Nigeria, Senegal, and Mali. The epidemic resulted in over 28,000 cases and 11,000 deaths, with more than 800 infections occurring in health care workers. Outbreaks due to the Zaire species continue to occur, with an ongoing outbreak in the Democratic Republic of the Congo (DRC). This outbreak is the largest to occur in the DRC and the second largest in the history of the disease after the 2014-2016 outbreak in West Africa. *Sudan* virus has been associated with a case-fatality rate of approximately 50% in four epidemics, which occurred in Sudan and Uganda between 1970 and 2004. *Ivory Coast* virus has been

identified as the cause of illness in one person following exposure during a necropsy on a chimpanzee found dead in the Tai Forest. *Bundibugyo* virus, most closely related to the Ivory Coast species, emerged in Uganda in 2007, causing an outbreak with a case fatality rate of approximately 30%. *Reston* virus, discovered after an outbreak of lethal infection in macaques imported into the United States in 1989, is maintained in animal reservoirs in the Philippines.

Risk Factors/Transmission

Outbreaks generally begin when an individual becomes infected through contact with the tissue or body fluids of an infected animal. The virus then spreads to others who come into contact with the infected individual's blood, skin, or other body fluids. Prior to the 2014 epidemic in West Africa, outbreaks occurred in remote regions with low population density and were controlled within short periods. However, the recent epidemic has shown that movement of infected individuals facilitates the extensive and rapid spread of the virus.

Transmission occurs most commonly through direct contact of broken skin or mucous membranes with virus-containing body fluids from an infected person, the most infectious being blood, feces, and vomit. During the early phase of illness, the level of virus in the blood is typically quite low, but then increases rapidly to very high levels in advanced stages of the illness, when patients become highly infectious. In fact, corpses of persons who die from Ebola are highly infectious, and ritual washing of bodies at funerals has played a significant role in the spread of infection. The virus has also been detected in urine, semen, saliva, breast milk, tears, and sweat, and can persist in some of these fluids much longer than in blood. To prevent sexual transmission the WHO recommends that men either abstain from sex, or use condoms for three months after onset of symptoms. Ebola virus may also be transmitted though contact with contaminated surfaces where the virus can remain infectious from hours to days.

Transmission to health care workers may occur when appropriate PPE is not used, especially when caring for severely ill patients in advanced stages of illness. During the 2014 outbreak in West Africa, a large number of health care workers became infected. In Sierra Leone, the incidence of confirmed cases at the peak of the epidemic was about 100-fold higher in health care workers than in the general population. Several factors have contributed to the high rates of infections among health providers, including failure to recognize infection among patients and corpses, limited availability and training in the use of appropriate PPE, and inadequate management of contaminated waste and burial of corpses. Although there is no evidence of respiratory transmission, the virus is highly infectious when released in laboratory experiments as a small-particle aerosol, and therefore health care workers may be at risk if exposed to aerosols generated during procedures.

Human infection can occur through contact with infected wild animals during hunting, butchering, and preparing meat, with several episodes having occurred following contact with infected gorillas or chimpanzees. To prevent infection, food products should be properly cooked to inactivate the virus, and basic hygiene measures should be followed. Direct transmission of virus infection from bats to wild primates or humans has not been proven, although Ebola RNA sequences and antibodies have been detected in bats in Central Africa. Bats likely form a major reservoir.

Pathophysiology

Ebolavirus is a negative-sense, single-stranded RNA virus resembling rhabdoviruses and paramyxoviruses in its genome organization and replication mechanisms. The tubular virions contain the nucleocapsid surrounded by an outer envelope, which is derived from the host cell membrane and studded with viral glycoprotein spikes. The virions attach to host cell receptors through the spikes and are then endocytosed into vesicles. Initially, productive infection occurs primarily in dendritic cells, monocytes, and macrophages, resulting in impaired interferon production and release of proinflammatory cytokines, which have secondary effects on innate and adaptive immune responses, inflammation, and vascular integrity. Neutrophils are activated, with resultant degranulation, and lymphocytes undergo apoptosis. The virus then spreads to regional lymph nodes, resulting in further rounds of replication, followed by dissemination to the liver, spleen, thymus, and other lymphoid tissues.

When the virus infects cells, it hijacks the cell and forces it to become a virus-producing factory, churning out new copies of the virus, which results in a loss of cellular function and eventual cell death by apoptosis. As the disease progresses, there is extensive tissue necrosis accompanied by a systemic inflammatory response induced by the release of various cytokines, chemokines, and proinflammatory mediators, as well as a severe coagulopathy triggered by the release of tissue factors. This systemic inflammatory response may contribute to gastrointestinal dysfunction, and ultimately there is a multisystem failure caused by the damage to vascular and coagulation systems.

Clinical Manifestations and Laboratory Findings

Patients with Ebola virus disease (EVD) typically have an abrupt onset of symptoms 5 to 10 days after exposure, with a range of 2 to 21 days. The first phase of the illness is characterized by high fever, chills, headaches, myalgia, and malaise. The second phase is marked by gastrointestinal symptoms, which develop by day 3 to 5, and includes watery diarrhea, nausea, vomiting, and abdominal pain. Patients may also develop chest pain, hiccups, shortness of breath, conjunctival injection, and rash. The rash is usually diffuse erythematous, maculopapular, involving the face, neck, trunk, and arms. Respiratory symptoms such as cough are rare. Common neurologic symptoms include delirium, manifested by confusion, slowed cognition, or agitation, and less frequently, seizures.

The final phase, beginning in the second week, is marked by either progression to shock and death or gradual recovery. Fatal disease is characterized by development of multisystem failure usually as a consequence of massive fluid losses that lead to shock, loss of consciousness, and renal failure. Major bleeding, typically hemorrhage from the gastrointestinal tract, is infrequent and seen in less than 5% during the terminal phase of illness. Patients who survive begin to improve during the second week of illness, with a prolonged convalescence marked by weakness and fatigue. About half of the survivors are plagued by chronic debilitating joint pain and a quarter experience eye problems. The virus can persist in the eye for months, leading to uveitis, cataracts, and sometimes blindness. The prevalence of uveitis, unlike other causes, continues to increase until at least two years after symptom onset, with about 33% of the patients affected by that point.

During acute illness patients typically develop leukopenia, lymphopenia, thrombocytopenia, serum transaminase elevations, and proteinuria. They may develop renal insufficiency and electrolyte disturbances as a result of the gastrointestinal losses. Severe cases develop coagulation abnormalities with prolonged prothrombin and partial thromboplastin times, and elevated fibrin degradation products, consistent with disseminated intravascular coagulation.

Diagnosis

The approach to evaluating patients depends on whether or not appropriate signs and symptoms are evident, and if an exposure occurred within 21 days prior to the onset of symptoms. Infection control precautions must be used for all symptomatic patients with an identifiable risk for EVD. All symptomatic patients should be isolated in a single room with a private bathroom, and implementation of contact and droplet precautions. Only essential personnel who are well trained in the use of PPE should interact with the patient. Phlebotomy and laboratory testing should be limited to essential tests. Both the CDC and the WHO have provided detailed recommendations for approach to the evaluation of persons who may have been exposed to the virus.

Rapid diagnostic tests are the most commonly used tests for diagnosis. Viral RNA is generally detectable by RT-PCR in the blood 3 days after the onset of symptoms. Repeat testing may be necessary for patients with illness duration shorter than 3 days. A negative RT-PCR test greater than or equal to 72 hours after the onset of symptoms rules out EVD. Details on specimen collection and handling can be found on the CDC website. For clinicians outside the United States, the WHO has issued guidance for the collection and shipment of specimens from patients with suspected disease.

Differential Diagnosis

Acute onset of febrile illness in a person who lives or has recently been in West or Central Africa may be caused by a variety of local infectious diseases, which must be considered in the differential diagnosis. **Malaria** may have similar findings and might occur concurrently. Examination of blood smears and rapid antigen tests are typically used to diagnose malaria. **Typhoid** is characterized by fever and abdominal pain, and diagnosed by blood cultures.

Patients with **Lassa fever** may develop a severe clinical syndrome resembling EVD and progress to fatal shock. The illness is restricted to West Africa, where it is transmitted through exposure to the aerosolized excretions of rodents, and diagnosed by RT-PCR testing and/or serology. Clinical manifestations of **Marburg virus disease** are similar to EVD, and cases have been identified in Central Africa. The diagnosis is made by RT-PCR. Patients with **influenza** may have a similar initial presentation, but respiratory signs and symptoms are prominent.

Therapy

Good supportive care can significantly improve the chances of recovery from EVD. Mortality rates have been as low as 18% among those cared for in the US and Europe, receiving careful fluid and electrolyte management, nutritional support, and critical care. Large volumes of intravenous fluids and electrolytes are often needed to correct dehydration and electrolyte abnormalities resulting from gastrointestinal losses. Supportive care is required for complications such as shock, hypoxia, hemorrhage, and multiorgan failure. Patients may develop secondary bacterial infections, which may require concurrent management with antimicrobials. Infection prevention and control measures are critical; all bodily fluids and tissues must be considered potentially infectious. The illness is associated with high rates of pregnancy-associated hemorrhage and fetal death. The Centers for Disease Control and Prevention and the American College of Obstetrics and Gynecology have issued recommendations for the care of pregnant women with EVD. However, there are no definitive data to recommend cesarean section versus vaginal delivery or the preferred timing for delivery.

No FDA-approved antiviral drugs or therapeutic vaccines are available, although several are currently in various stages of testing. Antiviral nucleoside analog favipiravir (T-705, Avigan)[5] has been used in patients with EVD. Favipiravir inhibits the replication of a wide range of RNA viruses, including influenza, and has been evaluated in small trials, but the studies have not demonstrated a definitive efficacy. ZMapp (a combination of humanized monoclonal antibodies)[5] was evaluated in a small randomized controlled trial, but due to the small size of the trial, efficacy could not be conclusively demonstrated. Plasma from patients who have recovered from the disease was used to treat patients during the 2014 outbreak, but no clinical trials have been conducted to date. Clinicians may contact the CDC's Emergency Operations Center for additional information on use of experimental therapeutics for treatment of EVD.

Long-Term Follow-up

The WHO suggests close follow-up of patients after hospital discharge for the first year. A suggested schedule is first follow-up 2 weeks after discharge, then monthly for 6 months, and then every

[5] Investigational drug in the United States.

three 3 months to complete 1 year. Survivors with ocular findings require follow-up to assess for cataracts. Semen testing should be done at follow-up visits until negative for Ebola virus RNA. If semen testing is unavailable, then WHO recommends that men practice safe sex for 12 months from onset of illness.

If patients develop fever, then they should be assessed for relapse, while also being evaluated for other causes of infection. Development of uveitis and meningitis may suggest relapse. Spinal fluid analysis should be done when meningitis is suspected, even if the blood tests are negative for Ebola virus RNA.

Prevention

There is no FDA-approved vaccine available for Ebola, although several vaccines are in various stages of development, and some have shown efficacy against virus challenge in laboratory primates. A vesicular stomatitis virus-based vaccine expressing a surface glycoprotein of *Zaire Ebolavirus* (rVSV-ZEBOV) is a promising candidate that was rapidly escalated into efficacy trials in Africa. In August 2015, the *Lancet* published an interim analysis showing that rVSV-ZEBOV appears to provide 100% protection against the virus. The trial was carried out in Guinea and used a "ring" design in which contacts of infected people are vaccinated, as are any subsequent contacts of those people.

Recommendations for travelers to an area affected by an Ebola outbreak or those residing in such an area are as follows:

- Practice careful hand hygiene and avoid contact with an infected person's blood or body fluids, including personal items that may have come in contact with blood and body fluids.
- Avoid unprotected contact with the body of a deceased person who was infected with EVD.
- Avoid contact with bats and nonhuman primates, including blood, bodily fluids, and tissues from these animals.
- Monitor health for 21 days after return from an Ebola endemic region, and seek medical care immediately if any symptoms develop.

Health care workers at risk for exposure to Ebola must wear PPE and notify appropriate health officials at their institutions if they have unprotected contact with the blood or bodily fluids of a person infected with EVD. Finally institutions must have proper infection control and sterilization measures in place for handling of biohazardous materials. Clinicians may contact the CDC for additional information on use of experimental therapeutics and vaccines for prophylaxis following a high-risk occupational exposure to Ebola virus.

Monitoring

Local authorities may have specific regulations for management of asymptomatic individuals with Ebola virus exposure. This includes self-monitoring versus direct observation by a health official, and the need for quarantine. In general, asymptomatic persons who have had an exposure should be monitored for 21 days after the last known exposure, and should immediately report the development of fever or other clinical manifestations suggestive of EVD to the health authorities.

References

Bah EI, Lamah MC, Fletcher T, et al: Clinical presentation of patients with Ebola virus disease in Conakry, Guinea, *N Engl J Med* 372:40–47, 2015.
Chertow DS, Kleine C, Edwards JK, et al: Ebola virus disease in West Africa—clinical manifestations and management, *N Engl J Med* 371:2054–2057, 2014.
Henao-Restrepo AM: Longini IM, Egger M, et al: Efficacy and effectiveness of an rVSV-vectored vaccine expressing Ebola surface glycoprotein: interim results from the Guinea ring vaccination cluster-randomised trial, *Lancet* S0140-6736(15):61117–61125, 2015.
Schieffelin JS, Shaffer JG, Goba A, et al: Clinical illness and outcomes in patients with Ebola in Sierra Leone, *N Engl J Med* 371:2092–2100, 2014.
United States Centers for Disease Control and Prevention (CDC). Ebola (Ebola virus disease). Available at http://www.cdc.gov/vhf/ebola/.
WHO Ebola Response Team: Ebola virus disease in West Africa—the first 9 months of the epidemic and forward projections, *N Engl J Med* 371:1481–1495, 2014.
World Health Organization (WHO). Ebola. Available at http://www.who.int/csr/disease/ebola/en/.

FOODBORNE ILLNESSES

Method of
Anita Devi K. Ravindran, MD; and K.N. Viswanathan, MD

CURRENT DIAGNOSIS

- Infective foodborne illnesses are innumerable and are caused by various microorganisms. Some microorganisms are established agents, several others are emerging pathogens, and the pathogenicity of the remainder is still under speculation.
- Classification of these illnesses is best done according to their incubation periods, the symptoms they produce, or both.
- Nausea and vomiting predominate in illnesses with short incubation periods caused by preformed toxins, whereas diarrhea predominates in those with long incubation periods caused by toxins produced in the intestine.
- Undercooked charcuterie, meat, poultry, and seafood account for a majority of foodborne illness, but dairy products, salads, pastries, fruits, and vegetables can also cause illness.
- Contaminated water acts as a vehicle in almost all instances.

CURRENT THERAPY

- The majority of infective foodborne illnesses with symptoms confined to the gastrointestinal tract, although apparently alarming, are self-limiting and need only supportive measures including replacement of water and electrolytes.
- Antimicrobial agents are indicated only in certain patients, including those with systemic illnesses, extremes of age, immunocompromised and malnourished states, and severe life-threatening illness.
- Antitoxin is useful in botulism poisoning.
- Vaccines are available against *Vibrio cholerae*, *Salmonella typhi*, hepatitis A virus, and rotavirus, but their effectiveness and cost-effectiveness are debatable.

The Centers for Disease Control and Prevention (CDC) estimates that each year roughly one in six Americans (about 48 million people) gets sick from foodborne illnesses; 128,000 are hospitalized, and 3000 die. These figures are higher in developing nations, and many cases are not brought to light because they occur in remote villages. The 2011 estimates provide the most accurate picture of infective foodborne illnesses, of which bacteria, viruses, and parasites account for the majority. Processing of ready-to-eat foods increases the risk of acquiring foodborne illness because of increased food handling, leading to introduction and growth of pathogens. Increased international travel and migration have also resulted in a greater risk because travelers are at high risk for developing foodborne gastroenteritis caused by pathogens to which they have not been exposed at home.

Classification of Foodborne Illnesses

Agents causing foodborne diseases may be classified in several ways. The most common scheme is a taxonomic combined with a classification based on mode of action (Tables 1 to 3).

Bacteria

Aeromonas Species

Species of *Aeromonas* are ubiquitous and autochthonous in aquatic environments, more so after the tsunami that followed the Indonesian earthquake in December 2004. These aeromonads share many biochemical characteristics with members of the Enterobacteriaceae. The mesophilic species *Aeromonas caviae*, *Aeromonas hydrophila*, and *Aeromonas veronii* are principally associated with gastroenteritis; *A. caviae* particularly infects children younger than 3 years.

TABLE 1 Classification of Foodborne Illnesses

SIGNS AND SYMPTOMS OR MECHANISM	PATHOGENS
Based on Symptoms and Duration of Onset	
Nausea and vomiting within 6 h	*Staphylococcus aureus, Bacillus cereus*
Abdominal cramps and diarrhea within 8–16 h	*Clostridium perfringens, Bacillus cereus*
Fever, abdominal cramps, and diarrhea within 16–48 h	*Salmonella, Shigella, Vibrio parahemolyticus,* enteroinvasive *Escherichia coli, Campylobacter jejuni*
Abdominal cramps and watery diarrhea within 16–72 h	Enterotoxigenic *E. coli, Vibrio cholerae* O1, O139 Bengal, *Vibrio parahemolyticus,* NAG (nonagglutinable) vibrios, *Norovirus*
Fever and abdominal cramps within 16–48 h	*Yersinia enterocolitica*
Bloody diarrhea without fever within 72–120 h	Enterohemorrhagic *E. coli* O157:H7
Nausea, vomiting, diarrhea, and paralysis within 18–36 h	*Clostridium botulinum*
Based on Pathogenesis	
Food intoxications resulting from the ingestion of preformed bacterial toxins	*Staphylococcus aureus, Bacillus cereus, Clostridium botulinum, Clostridium perfringens*
Food intoxications caused by noninvasive bacteria that secrete toxins while adhering to the intestinal wall	Enterotoxigenic *E. coli, Vibrio cholerae, Campylobacter jejuni*
Food intoxications that follow an intracellular invasion of intestinal epithelial cells	*Shigella, Salmonella*
Diseases caused by bacteria that enter the bloodstream via the intestinal tract	*Salmonella typhi, Listeria monocytogenes*
Based on Toxin Production	
The organisms responsible produce two major types of toxins, or they may be invasive, with no toxin production.	
Secretory toxins are enterotoxins produced by microbes that colonize the intestines in large numbers by attaching to the mucosal epithelial cells without invasion of mucosa, and, hence, there is no fever or other systemic symptoms as a result of lack of inflammatory response. Massive quantities of fluid and electrolytes are lost into the large bowel as its reabsorbing capacity is exceeded by the hypersecretion of isotonic fluid produced by the enterotoxins.	*Vibrio cholerae,* enterotoxigenic *E. coli, Shigella dysenteriae, Salmonella typhimurium*
Cytotoxins are those that destroy the epithelial cells of the mucosa.	*Shigella dysenteriae* elaborating Shiga toxin, causing destructive colitis, enterohemorrhagic *E. coli,* producing a similar toxin causing hemorrhagic colitis and hemolytic uremic syndrome (HUS), and *Vibrio parahemolyticus)* *Clostridium perfringens,* which produces a secretory enterotoxin, also has a cytotoxic action.
Secretory toxins, cytotoxins, and/or neurotoxins that are preformed are ingested directly in food.	*Bacillus cereus, Staphylococcus aureus, Clostridium botulinum*
Certain invasive microbes produce systemic symptoms such as fever, headache, and myalgia, in addition to gastrointestinal symptoms.	Salmonellosis typhoid fever, shigellosis, and brucellosis

Transmission is documented as occurring from a contaminated piped water source, as seen in community-based outbreaks, especially among children. The probability of occurrence of *Aeromonas* infection increased significantly when the mean seasonal temperature exceeded 14°C (57°F), and this was exacerbated where the mean free chlorine concentration fell below 0.1 mg/L.

Aeromonas species are potential food-poisoning agents. *A. hydrophila* is psychrotrophic and has been associated with spoilage of refrigerated animal products including chicken, beef, pork, lamb, fish, oysters, crab, and milk.

The incubation period for *Aeromonas*-associated traveler's diarrhea is 1 to 2 days. It usually causes a sporadic illness. Usually a mild to moderate but self-limiting diarrhea occurs, but it can be severe enough in children to require hospitalization. *Aeromonas* gastroenteritis can occur as a nondescript enteritis, as a more-severe form accompanied by bloody stools, as the etiologic agent of a subacute or chronic intestinal syndrome, as an extremely rare cause of cholera-like disease, or in association with episodic traveler's diarrhea. By far the most common presentation of *Aeromonas* gastroenteritis is watery enteritis. The most serious complication resulting from *Aeromonas* gastroenteritis is hemolytic uremic syndrome.

Pathogenesis
Mesophilic *Aeromonas* spp. can express a range of virulence factors, including attachment mechanisms and production of a number of toxins. Toxins include aerolysin (a pore-forming cytolysin that attaches to cell membrane, leading to leakage of cytoplasmic contents) and a cytotonic enterotoxin with activity similar to that of cholera toxin. Strains of *A. hydrophila* produce lectins and adhesins, which enable adherence to epithelial surfaces and gut mucosa.

Laboratory Diagnosis
Samples are best transported using Cary-Blair medium. *Aeromonas* forms a bull's-eye–like colony on the selective medium cefsulodin irgasan novobiocin (CIN) agar owing to fermentation of D-mannitol. Ampicillin blood agar has an

TABLE 2 Common Organisms Implicated in Infective Foodborne Illness

ETIOLOGIC AGENT	USUAL INCUBATION PERIOD	SYMPTOMS	DURATION OF SYMPTOMS	COMMON VEHICLES
Upper Gastrointestinal Tract Symptoms (Nausea, Vomiting) Occur First or Predominate				
Staphylococcus aureus (preformed toxin)	1–6 h	Sudden onset of severe nausea and vomiting Abdominal cramps, diarrhea, and fever may be present	24–48 h	Unrefrigerated or improperly refrigerated meat, potato and egg salads, cream pastries
Bacillus cereus (preformed toxin)	1–6 h	Sudden onset of severe nausea and vomiting Diarrhea may be present	24 h	Improperly refrigerated cooked or fried rice, meat
Lower Gastrointestinal Tract Symptoms (Abdominal Cramps, Diarrhea) Occur First or Predominate				
Bacillus cereus (diarrheal toxin)	10–16 h	Abdominal cramps, watery diarrhea, nausea	24–48 h	Meat, stew, gravy, vanilla sauce
Clostridium perfringens (toxin)	8–16 h	Watery diarrhea, nausea, abdominal cramps; fever is rare	24–48 h	Meat, poultry, gravy, dried or precooked foods, time- and/or temperature-abused food
Vibrio cholerae	2 h to 5 d	Rice-water purging diarrhea leading to dehydration, shock, acidosis, renal failure, abdominal pain Cholera sicca is a severe form; patient dies before diarrhea is manifest; ileus and abdominal bloating result	2–7 d	Sewage-contaminated water Seafood: fish, shellfish, crabs, oysters, clams Contaminated rice, millet gruel, vegetables
Vibrio parahaemolyticus	12–24 h	Watery diarrhea, abdominal cramps, nausea, vomiting Neurologic symptoms can occur, as with *Clostridium botulinum* and *Trichinella spiralis*	2–5 d	Raw or undercooked seafood
Shigella	1–4 d	Abdominal cramps, fever, diarrhea Stool might contain blood and mucus	4–7 d	Food or water contaminated with fecal matter Ready-to-eat food touched by infected food worker
Salmonella (not *typhi*)	1–3 d	Diarrhea, fever, abdominal cramps, vomiting	4–7 d	Contaminated eggs, unpasteurized milk or juice, cheese, contaminated raw fruits and vegetables
Enterotoxigenic *Escherichia coli*	1–3 d	Watery diarrhea, abdominal cramps, some vomiting	3–7 d (or longer)	Food or water contaminated with human feces
Shiga toxin–producing *E. coli*, including *E. coli* O157:H7	2–6 d	Severe diarrhea that is often bloody; abdominal pain and vomiting Usually little or no fever	5–10 d	Undercooked beef, especially hamburger, unpasteurized milk and juice, raw fruit and vegetables (e.g., sprouts), salami (rarely), contaminated water
Campylobacter jejuni	2–5 d	Diarrhea, cramps, fever, vomiting Diarrhea may be bloody	2–10 d	Raw and undercooked poultry, unpasteurized milk, contaminated milk
Vibrio vulnificus	1–7 d	Vomiting, diarrhea, abdominal pain Fever, bleeding within the skin, ulcers requiring surgical removal Can be fatal to people with liver disease or weakened immune systems	2–8 d	Undercooked or raw seafood, especially oysters
Yersinia enterocolitica	3–7 d	Appendicitis-like symptoms: diarrhea, vomiting, fever, abdominal pain	Can remit and relapse over weeks to 1 mo	Drinking water, food contaminated with human fecal matter
Cyclospora	7–10 d	Diarrhea (usually watery), loss of appetite, weight loss, stomach cramps, nausea, vomiting, fatigue	Can remit and relapse over weeks to 1 mo	Fresh herbs and produce (e.g., raspberries, basil, lettuce)
Giardia lamblia (beaver fever)	7–10 d	Diarrhea (acute or chronic), stomach cramps, flatulence, weight loss, malabsorption, developmental delay	Days to weeks	Drinking water, food contaminated with human fecal matter
Entamoeba histolytica	1–4 wk	Intestinal: diarrhea, fever, abdominal pain, dysentery, colitis, bowel perforation, ameboma Extraintestinal amebiasis: liver abscess with anchovy-sauce pus, spread to viscera, lungs, and brain	Days to weeks	Drinking water Food contaminated with human fecal matter

ETIOLOGIC AGENT	USUAL INCUBA-TION PERIOD	SYMPTOMS	DURATION OF SYMPTOMS	COMMON VEHICLES
Both Upper and Lower Gastrointestinal Tract Symptoms				
Rotavirus	18–36 h	Acute onset of fever and vomiting followed 12–24 h later by frequent watery stools	3–7 d	Contaminated drinking water, food, fomites
Norovirus and other caliciviruses	12–48 h	Nausea, vomiting, cramping, diarrhea, fever, myalgia, some headache Diarrhea is more prevalent in adults; vomiting is more prevalent in children	12–60 h	Food (including shellfish) or water contaminated with human fecal matter Ready-to-eat food touched by an infected food worker
Generalized Symptoms				
Listeria monocytogenes	9–48 h or GI symptoms; 2–6 wk for invasive disease	Fever, muscle aches, nausea or diarrhea Pregnant women can have mild flulike illness, and infection can lead to premature delivery or stillbirth Elderly and immunocompromised patients can have bacteremia or meningitis	Variable	Fresh soft cheese, unpasteurized milk, ready-to-eat deli meat, hot dogs
Balatidium coli	4–5 d	Mostly asymptomatic Chronic diarrhea, occasional dysentery, nausea, foul breath, colitis, abdominal pain, weight loss, deep intestinal ulcerations, possible perforation of the intestine, pneumonia-like illness	Variable	Water contaminated with pig feces
Salmonella typhi	8–14 d	Fever, anorexia, lethargy, malaise, headache, rose spots, constipation or diarrhea, hepatosplenomegaly	4–6 wk	Contaminated water; contaminated food, mainly via food handlers; shellfish from polluted water
Ascoris lumbricoides	4–16 d	Nausea, abdominal pain, intestinal obstruction, malnutrition, Loeffler's syndrome (cough, pneumonitis, eosinophilia), biliary colic, colangitis, pancreatitis, appendicitis	Variable (chronic)	Soil-contaminated raw food, food handlers, water
Trichinella spiralis	1–2 wk	Asymptomatic or chronic diarrhea, abdominal pain Allergy leading to rash, periorbital edema, vasculitis, intramural thrombi Weakness of jaw, biceps, diaphragm, intercostals Eosinophilia, subconjunctival, splinter hemorrhages Muscle penetration: myalgia, orbital pain, diplopia Chronic phase: neurologic symptoms	Variable Acute phase: 1–3 wk	Raw or undercooked meat of pig, horse, wild boar, bush pig, warthog, bear
Infective cysticerci of *Taenia solium* (pork tape worm)	2 months on average	Seizures, vasculitis, focal neurologic deficits, intracranial hypertension, hydrocephalus, mental changes, encephalitis and Brun's syndrome (intermittent obstruction of cerebral aqueduct), myosists, vasculitis	Highly variable	Undercooked charcuterie (pork), contaminated raw vegetables, salads, water
Hepatitis A	15–50 d	Diarrhea, dark urine, jaundice, flulike symptoms, fever, headache, nausea, aversion to food, vomiting, abdominal pain; distaste for cigarettes	Variable: 2 wk to 3 mo	Food (including shellfish) or water contaminated with human fecal matter Inadequately cooked clams, oysters, mussels, cockles Contaminated lettuce, slush beverages, frozen strawberries and salad items Ready-to-eat foods touched by an infected food worker
Brucella species	1–8 wk	Flulike illness; undulating fever, malaise, arthralgia, anorexia, hepatosplenomegaly, pleurisy, nausea, vomiting, diarrhea, new onset of increased desire to sleep after lunch	Variable	Unpasteurized dairy products, undercooked meat, bone marrow Contact with laboratory cultures and tissue samples Accidental injection of live brucellosis vaccine

Continued

ETIOLOGIC AGENT	USUAL INCUBATION PERIOD	SYMPTOMS	DURATION OF SYMPTOMS	COMMON VEHICLES
Hepatitis E	3–8 wk	Prodrome: anorexia, nausea, vomiting, arthralgia, myalgia, weight loss, dehydration, abdominal pain Icteric phase: jaundice, pruritus, light-colored stool Urticaria, diarrhea, malaise	Variable (several weeks)	Fecally contaminated drinking water and food Raw and undercooked shellfish incriminated in sporadic outbreaks Possibly zoonotic spread
Microsporidium: Encephalitozoon, Pleistophora, Nosema, Vittaforma, Trachipleistophora, Brachiola, Microsporidium, Enterocytozoon	Unknown	Watery or bloody or unspecified diarrhea, abdominal discomfort, cramps, flatulence, weight loss, loss of appetite, wasting syndrome, subfebrile temperatures Extraintestinal: pneumonitis, myositis, keratoconjunctivitis, seizures, nephritis, cholangiopathy	Variable; self-limiting (1–2 wk) in immunocompetent patients	Contaminated water, food, or inhalation

Abbreviation: GI=gastrointestinal.

advantage over CIN agar in that hemolytic colonies can readily be tested for oxidase. *Aeromonas* species produce hemolysis on sheep blood agar.

Treatment

In *Aeromonas* infections, ciprofloxacin (Cipro)[1] 500 mg PO or 400 mg IV twice daily is the antimicrobial treatment of choice. Piperacillin-tazobactam (Zosyn)[1] 4.5 g IV three times daily or ceftazidime (Fortaz)[1] 2 g IV daily may be added in severe infections. The organism is also susceptible to aminoglycosides and carbapenems. Resistance is now becoming a problem because *Aeromonas* can produce β-lactamases and carbapenemases. Therefore it is preferable to initiate therapy with a fluoroquinolone when the organism is isolated.

Bacillus cereus

Bacillus cereus is found abundantly in the environment and vegetation. It is known to produce two forms of food poisoning, emetic and diarrheal. The emetic (short-incubation) type of illness is associated with contaminated fried rice that is not refrigerated. The organism is present in uncooked rice, and the spores survive boiling. The illness is usually self-limiting, with recovery in a day. It is mediated by a heat-stable, preformed enterotoxin resembling that of *Staphylococcus aureus*. The first major outbreak of *Bacillus cereus* food poisoning was in 1971 in England. The diarrheal (long-incubation) type of illness is produced by a heat-labile diarrheal enterotoxin formed in the intestine, which activates adenylate cyclase, causing intestinal fluid secretion, similar to *Escherichia coli* LT toxin and the toxin of *Clostridium perfringens*.

Pathogenesis

During the slow cooling of cooked rice, spores germinate and vegetative bacteria multiply; then they sporulate again. Sporulation is also associated with toxin production. The toxin is heat stable and can easily withstand the temperatures used to cook fried rice.

Laboratory Diagnosis

The disease is diagnosed by the isolation of *B. cereus* from the incriminated food (emetic type) or from stool and food (diarrheal type). Isolation from stools alone is not sufficient because gastrointestinal colonization with *B. cereus* occurs in many persons.

Treatment

B. cereus food poisoning may be symptomatically managed with replacement of fluids and electrolytes. Antimicrobials have no role in treatment. *B. cereus* is also known to produce a variety of ocular and systemic infections such as meningitis, osteomyelitis, pneumonia, and endocarditis. These are usually not foodborne, and it is in this situation that vancomycin (Vancocin)[1] becomes the drug of choice, with clindamycin (Cleocin)[1] and carbapenems being the alternative drugs, both being used along with aminoglycosides for synergistic action.

Campylobacter jejuni

Campylobacter jejuni are harbored in the reproductive and alimentary tracts of some animals. Other than gastrointestinal symptoms, the patient has malaise and headache. The organism may be shed in the patient's stool for up to 2 months. Bacteremia is observed in a small minority of cases. The disease is usually self-limiting. Guillain-Barré syndrome and Reiter's syndrome are recognized sequelae.

Pathogenesis

As few as 500 organisms can cause enteritis. The organism is invasive but generally less so than *Shigella*. *Campylobacter* produces adenylate cyclase–activating toxins resembling *E. coli* LT and cholera toxin.

Laboratory Diagnosis

The feces may be inoculated in enrichment medium or on selective media such as Campy-BAP or Skirrow's medium.

Treatment

Indications for antibiotic therapy in *C. jejuni* infections are prolonged fever, severe diarrhea, dysentery, and persistent symptoms for more than a week. Therapy of *Campylobacter* infection with ciprofloxacin (Cipro 500 mg orally twice daily for 7 days) early in the course of the illness shortens its duration. Unfortunately, this has led to the emergence of fluoroquinolone-resistant *Campylobacter* infections. Erythromycin eradicates carriage of susceptible *C. jejuni* and might shorten the duration of illness if given early in the disease. Erythromycin (Ery-Tab)[1] 250 mg PO four times daily is the drug of choice in *Campylobacter* enteritis. Azithromycin (Zithromax)[1] is also useful and has the advantage of shorter duration of therapy.

Gentamicin (Garamycin), carbapenems, amoxicillin-clavulanate (Augmentin),[1] and chloramphenicol[1] are useful in systemic infections. The usual duration of treatment is 2 weeks. The therapy is prolonged in immunocompromised persons and in patients with endovascular infections.

[1]Not FDA approved for this indication.

[1]Not FDA approved for this indication.

TABLE 3	Rare and Emerging Infections			
ETIOLOGIC AGENT	USUAL INCUBA- TION PERIOD	SYMPTOMS	DURATION OF SYMP- TOMS	COMMON VEHICLES
Bacillus subtilis	10 min to 14 h (average, 2.5 h)	Vomiting, diarrhea, abdominal cramps, nausea, headache, flushing, sweating	1.5–8 h	Sausage rolls, meat pasties, turkey stuffing, chicken stuffing, pizza, whole-grain bread, steak pie, pork sandwiches
Cyanobacteria: *Microcystic aeuroginosa, Anabaena circinalis, Anabaena flosaquae, Aphanizomenon flosaquae, Cylindrospermopsis racibarskii*	3–6 h	Diarrhea, vomiting, allergic reactions, breathing difficulty, dizziness, tingling and numbness, liver and kidney toxicity	8–16 h	Drinking water from untreated surface sources, inhaling aerosols from jet-skis and boats, consuming dietary supplements contaminated by microcystin
Anisakis	Few hours to days	Gastric: abdominal pain, nausea, vomiting Allergic: urticaria, anaphylaxis Intestinal: ileus, perforation, peritonitis, stenosis	2 wk	Raw, lightly pickled, or salted marine fish: Mackerel, squid, horse mackerel, salmon, bonito Squid, cuttlefish Sushi, sashimi
Astrovirus	1–4 d	Watery diarrhea (especially in children), vomiting, fever, anorexia, abdominal pain	3–4 d	Sewage-polluted water and food
Pleisomonas shigelloides	5 d	Diarrhea with blood and mucus, abdominal pain, headache, nausea, chills, fever, vomiting	1–7 d	Contaminated water used for drinking or rinsing foods to be eaten raw Contaminated raw shellfish, salted fish, crabs, oysters
Cyclospora	7 d	Frequent watery diarrhea, weight loss, abdominal pain, bloating, flatulence, vomiting, nausea, low-grade fever, fatigue, malabsorption, cholecystitis	1–4 wk Relapse is common	Fecally contaminated fresh raspberries, snow peas, mesclun
Iosospora belli	8–11 d	Diarrhea, steatorrhea, headache, fever, malaise, abdominal pain, vomiting, dehydration, weight loss Mesenteric lymph node, liver, spleen involvement	Variable; runs a chronic course in immunocompromised patients	Contaminated food and water
Edwardisella tarda	Not defined	Nausea, vomiting, diarrhea, dysentery, colitis, wound infections, septicemia	Variable: 1–2 wk or longer	Fecal contamination of food, water, raw fish
Citrobacter species	Not defined	Diarrhea, hemolytic uremic syndrome, thrombocytopenic purpura		Meat and milk Parsley (in green butter) from organic gardens using pig manure
Arizona	Not defined	Diarrhea		Cream pie, chocolate eclairs, custard, eggs, chicken, turkey
Achromobacter xylosoxidans	Not defined	Abdominal pain, diarrhea, headache, vomiting		Raw milk, spoiled canned food, contaminated well water

Clostridium botulinum

Clostridum botulinum is widely distributed in soil, in sediments of lakes and ponds, and in decaying vegetation. *C. botulinum* elaborates the most potent toxin known in humans. When the toxin is ingested, paralysis occurs, often requiring prolonged artificial ventilation. Common signs and symptoms include vomiting, thirst, dry mouth, constipation, ocular palsies, dysphagia, dysarthria, bulbar paralysis, and death due to respiratory paralysis. Coma or delirium occurs in some. Infants present with lethargy, poor feeding, loss of head control, and sometimes sudden infant death syndrome (SIDS).

The incriminated foods are corn syrup, home-canned or bottled meat, fruits, fish, vegetables, herb-infused oils, and cheese sauce. Infant botulism is associated with consumption of honey; honey should not be given to infants younger than 1 year.

Pathogenesis

Not all strains of *C. botulinum* produce botulinum toxin. Toxigenic types of the organism, designated A, B, C1, D, E, F, and G, produce immunologically distinct forms of botulinum toxin. Lysogenic phages encode toxin C and D serotypes.

Foodborne botulism is not an infection but an intoxication because it results from the ingestion of foods that contain the preformed clostridial toxin. If contaminated food has been insufficiently heated or canned improperly, the spores can germinate and produce botulinum toxin. The toxin is released only after cell lysis and death. The toxin resists digestion and is absorbed by the upper gastrointestinal tract and enters the blood. The toxin blocks release of acetylcholine by binding to receptors at synapses and neuromuscular junctions and causes flaccid paralysis.

Laboratory Diagnosis

Spoilage of food or swelling of cans or presence of bubbles inside the can indicate growth of *C. botulinum*. Food is homogenized in broth and inoculated in Robertson cooked meat medium and blood agar or egg-yolk agar, which is incubated anaerobically for 3 to 5 days at 37°C. The toxin can be demonstrated by injecting the extract of food or culture into mice or guinea pigs intraperitoneally.

Treatment

Hospitalization in an intensive care unit with immediate administration of botulinum antitoxin is vital in the management of botulism. The antitoxin neutralizes only toxin molecules unbound to nerve endings and does not reverse the paralysis. It should be given within 24 hours after the diagnosis is made. Penicillin is the antimicrobial of choice. Intubation and mechanical ventilation are needed for respiratory failure. If swallowing difficulty persists, intravenous fluids or alimentation should be given through a nasogastric tube.

Clostridium perfringens

C. perfringens is heat resistant and elaborates two toxins that can induce specific pathology in the human intestinal tract. It is the third leading cause of foodborne illnesses in United States, after norovirus and *B. cereus*. It is present abundantly in the environment, vegetation, sewage, and animal feces.

Human diseases caused by this organism are the more common *C. perfringens* type A food poisoning and the less common, but more serious, *C. perfringens* type C food poisoning producing necrotic enteritis. Necrotic enteritis is characterized by vomiting, severe abdominal pain, and bloody diarrhea. The incubation period is 2 to 5 days. Progression to necrosis of the jejunum and death occur.

Pathogenesis

Spores in food can survive cooking and then germinate when the food is improperly stored. When these vegetative cells form endospores in the intestine, they release enterotoxins. Food poisoning is mainly caused by type A strains, which produce alpha and theta toxins. The toxins result in excessive fluid accumulation in the intestinal lumen.

Laboratory Diagnosis

Because the bacterium is present normally in intestines, isolation from feces might not be sufficient to implicate it as the cause of the illness. Similarly, isolation from food, except in large numbers (>10^9/g), might not be significant. The homogenized food is diluted and plated on selective medium, as well as Robertson cooked meat medium, and subjected to anaerobic incubation. The isolated bacteria must be shown to produce enterotoxin.

Treatment

Food poisoning due to *Clostridium perfringens* is managed conservatively with hydration and replacement of electrolytes. *C. perfringens* is susceptible to benzylpenicillin (penicillin G), which may be useful in managing severe infections (1 mU IV every 4 hours). Vancomycin,[1] clindamycin,[1] cefoxitin (Mefoxin), and metronidazole (Flagyl) are alternatives. *C. perfringens* type C toxoid vaccine[2] (two doses, 4 months apart) is preventive in pigbel.

Cronobacter sakazakii

Cronobacter sakazakii causes neonatal meningitis or necrotizing enterocolitis and bacteremia, which results in an alarming mortality rate. Surviving patients sometimes develop ventriculitis and cerebral abscess. *C. sakazakii* has been isolated from infant formulas.

Enterobacter species are generally resistant to the cephalosporins, except cefepime (Maxipime),[1] but are responsive

to carbenicillin (Geocillin),[1] piperacillin (Pipracil),[1] ticarcillin (Ticar),[1] amikacin (Amikin),[1] and tigecycline (Tygacil).[1]

Enterohemorrhagic Escherichia coli

Many serogroups of *E. coli*, including O4, O26, O45, O91, O111, O145, and O157, are pathogenic, but the most common pathogenic serotype is O157:H7. Cattle are the main sources of infection; most cases are associated with the consumption of undercooked beef burgers and similar foods from restaurants and delicatessens.

Pathogenesis

Enterohemorrhagic *E. coli* (EHEC) strains can produce one or more types of cytotoxins, which are collectively referred to as Shiga-like toxins because they are antigenically and functionally similar to Shiga toxin produced by *Shigella dysenteriae*. (Shiga-like toxins were previously known as verotoxins.) The toxins provoke cell secretion and kill colonic epithelial cells, causing hemorrhagic colitis and hemolytic-uremic syndrome (HUS), leading occasionally to disseminated intravascular coagulation (DIC). A fibrin layer forms in the glomerular capillary bed, and acute renal failure occurs due to DIC. These are most likely to occur in children, elderly patients, and pregnant women. The young recover fully, but at times dialysis is warranted.

Laboratory Diagnosis

Laboratory diagnosis is performed by culturing the feces on McConkey's agar or sorbitol McConkey's agar. Strains can then be identified by serotyping using specific antisera. Shiga-like toxins can be detected by enzyme-linked immunosorbent assay (ELISA), and genes coding for them can be detected by DNA hybridization techniques.

Treatment

Hydration with electrolyte replacement is the mainstay of treatment in *E. coli* O157:H7 infection, and patients should be monitored closely and constantly for the development of HUS, which requires management in an intensive care setting with blood transfusion and dialysis. Although dysentery is self-limiting, the use of rifaximin (Xifaxan), a nonabsorbable agent, is recommended in those who are increasingly susceptible to infections. In the absence of dysentery, early institution of drugs like ciprofloxacin (Cipro) or azithromycin (Zithromax),[1] especially in traveler's diarrhea, decreases the duration of illness.

Enterotoxigenic Escherichia Coli

Enterotoxigenic *E. coli* (ETEC) is now ubiquitous in nature. Wild animals and cattle act as reservoirs of the organism. *E. coli* is carried normally in the intestine of humans and animals. Some specific serotypes harbor plasmids that code for toxin production. This bacterium is responsible for a majority of traveler's diarrhea. The disease is self-limiting and resolves in a few days.

Pathogenesis

The bacteria colonize the gastrointestinal tract by means of fimbriae, attaching to specific receptors on enterocytes of the proximal small intestine. Enterotoxins produced by ETEC include the LT (heat-labile) toxin and the ST (heat-stable) toxins. LTs are similar to cholera toxin in structure and mode of action, consisting of A and B subunits. The B (binding) subunit of LTs binds to specific ganglioside receptors (GM1) on the epithelial cells of the small intestine, and facilitates the entry of the A (activating) subunit, which activates adenylate cyclase. Stimulation of adenylate cyclase causes an increased production of cyclic adenosine monophosphate (cAMP), which leads to hypersecretion of water and electrolytes into the lumen and inhibition of sodium reabsorption.

Laboratory Diagnosis

The sample of feces is cultured on McConkey's agar. The ETEC stains are indistinguishable from the resident *E. coli* by biochemical tests. These strains are differentiated from nontoxigenic *E. coli* present in the bowel by a variety of in vitro immunochemical,

---

[1]Not FDA approved for this indication.
[2]Not available in the United States.

tissue culture, or DNA hybridization tests designed to detect either the toxins or the genes that encode for these toxins. With the availability of a gene probe method, foods can be analyzed directly for the presence of ETEC in about 3 days. LTs can be detected by ligated rabbit ileal loop test and by observing morphologic changes in Chinese hamster ovary cells and Y1 adrenal cells. ELISA, immunodiffusion, and coagglutination are also used in diagnosis.

Listeria monocytogenes

Listeria monocytogenes is quite hardy and resists the deleterious effects of freezing, drying, and heat remarkably well for a bacterium that does not form spores. It is capable of growing at 3°C and multiplies in refrigerated foods.

Pathogenesis

L. monocytogenes invades the gastrointestinal epithelium. Once the bacterium enters the host's monocytes, macrophages, or neutrophils, it is bloodborne and can grow. Its presence in phagocytes also permits access to the brain and transplacental migration to the fetus in pregnant women. Granulomatosis infantisepticum is a feature of listeriosis. The pathogenesis of *L. monocytogenes* centers on its ability to survive and multiply in phagocytic host cells.

Laboratory Diagnosis

The diagnosis of listeriosis is most commonly made by isolation of *L. monocytogenes* from a normally sterile site. β-Hemolytic colonies, which test negative for catalase, hydrolyze hippurate, and have a positive cAMP reaction, form on blood agar. Serologic testing is not useful in diagnosing acute invasive disease, but it can be useful in detecting asymptomatic disease and gastroenteritis in an outbreak or in other epidemiologic investigations. Stool testing is not commercially available.

Treatment

Ampicillin[1] (2 g IV every 4 hours) is the drug of choice in *Listeria monocytogenes* infections. Aminoglycosides are added for synergistic effect. Trimethoprim-sulfamethoxazole (TMP-SMX)[1] (Bactrim, 20 mg of trimethoprim/day IV every 6 hours) is an alternative for patients allergic to penicillin. Ampicillin and TMP-SMX may be used in combination. Vancomycin (Vancocin),[1] linezolid (Zyvox),[1] carbapenems, macrolides, and tetracyclines are also effective. Cephalosporins are ineffective in the treatment of listeriosis and should not be used. The duration of therapy is highly variable depending on the clinical situation and is 14 days for bacteremia, 21 days for meningitis, 42 days for endocarditis, and 56 days for neurologic infections. Patients whose disease is promptly diagnosed and treated recover fully, but permanent neurologic sequelae are common in patients with cerebral illnesses. Consuming only pasteurized dairy products and fully cooked meats, meticulously cleaning utensils, and thoroughly washing fresh vegetables before cooking will prevent foodborne listerial infections. Pregnant women and others at risk should avoid soft cheeses and thoroughly reheated ready-to-serve and charcuterie foods.

Nontyphoidal Salmonellosis

Nontyphoidal salmonellosis consists of several causative organisms classified under the family Enterobacteriaceae; one such organism is *Salmonella enteritidis*. It does not occur normally in humans, but several animals act as reservoirs.

The diarrhea may be watery, with greenish, foul-smelling stools. This may be preceded by headache and chills. Other findings include prostration, muscle weakness, and moderate fever.

Pathogenesis

The organism penetrates and passes through the epithelial cells lining the terminal ileum. Multiplication of bacteria in lamina propria produces inflammatory mediators, recruits neutrophils, and triggers inflammation. Release of lipopolysaccharides and prostaglandins causes fever and also loss of water and electrolytes into the lumen of the intestine, resulting in diarrhea.

Laboratory Diagnosis

Culture in selenite F broth and then subculture on deoxycholate citrate agar isolates the organisms. Plates are incubated at 37°C overnight, and growth is identified by biochemical and slide agglutination tests.

Treatment

The antibiotics recommended for gastroenteritis due to nontyphoidal salmonellosis are ciprofloxacin (Cipro)[1] 500 mg PO twice daily, and ceftriaxone (Rocephin) 2 g IV daily, for 3 to 7 days. Amoxicillin (Amoxil)[1] and TMP-SMX[1] are also effective. Therapy is prolonged in bacteremia, endocarditis, or meningitis.

Shigella Species

Shigella species belong to the family Enterobacteriaceae. Bacillary dysentery is caused by *Shigella flexneri*, *Shigella boydii*, *Shigella dysenteriae*, and *Shigella sonnei*. *S. flexneri* is most common in developing countries where hygiene is poor and clean drinking water is unavailable; *S. sonnei* is most common in developed countries. The watery diarrhea that is present initially becomes bloody after a day or two owing to spread of infection from the ileum to the colon. The illness is caused by exotoxin acting in the small bowel.

Extraintestinal manifestations are recognized, including HUS, Reiter's syndrome, meningitis, Ekiri syndrome (reported in Japanese children and consisting of a triad of encephalopathy due to cerebral edema, bizarre posturing, and fatty degeneration of liver), vaginitis, lung infections, and keratoconjunctivitis. Toxic megacolon, pneumatosis coli, perforation, and rectal prolapse are recognized complications.

Tossed salads, chicken, and shellfish are the commonly incriminated foods. Person-to-person spread by anal intercourse or oral sex also occurs. Prepared food acts as a vehicle of transmission. Spread of infection is also linked to flies.

Children are at high risk during the weaning period, and increasing age is associated with decreased prevalence and severity. Children in daycare centers, persons in custodial institutions, migrant workers, and travelers to developing countries are also at high risk.

Pathogenesis

The virulence factor is a smooth lipopolysaccharide cell wall antigen, which is responsible for the invasive features, and the Shiga toxin, which is both cytotoxic and neurotoxic. Shigellae survive the gastric acidity and invade and multiply within the colonic epithelial cells, causing cell death and mucosal ulcers, and spread laterally to involve adjacent cells but rarely invade the bloodstream.

Laboratory Diagnosis

Shigellosis can be correctly diagnosed in most patients on the basis of fresh blood in stool. Neutrophils in fecal smears strongly suggest infection. Any clinical diagnosis should be confirmed by cultivation of the etiologic agent from stools. Cary-Blair medium is the transport medium of choice, and MacConkey agar or deoxycholate citrate agar (DCA) as well as a highly selective medium such as xylose-lysin deoxycholate (XLD), Hektoen enteric (HE), or Salmonella-Shigella (SS) agar are also used.

Treatment

Ciprofloxacin (Cipro, 500 mg PO twice daily for 3 days) is the antibiotic of choice for shigellosis. Alternative agents are pivmecillinam (Selexid),[2] ceftriaxone (Rocephin),[1] and azithromycin (Zithromax).[1]

---

[1]Not FDA approved for this indication.

---

[1]Not FDA approved for this indication.
[2]Not available in the United States.

Staphylococcus aureus

A notable incident of staphylococcal food poisoning occurred in February 1975 when 196 of 344 passengers and one flight attendant aboard a jet from Tokyo to Copenhagen via Anchorage contacted a gastrointestinal illness characterized by nausea, vomiting, and abdominal cramps. The flight attendant and 142 passengers were hospitalized. Symptoms developed shortly after a ham and omelet breakfast had been served. *S. aureus* was incriminated as the offending agent and ham as the vehicle of the outbreak. The source was traced to a cook with pustules on his fingers.

S. aureus is ubiquitous in the environment. Only strains that produce enterotoxin cause food poisoning. Food is usually contaminated by infected food handlers.

Pathogenesis

If food is stored for some time at room temperature, the organism can multiply in the food and produce enterotoxin. Most food poisonings are caused by enterotoxin A, and the isolates commonly belong to phage type III. These are heat stable, and ingestion of as little as 23 μg of enterotoxin can induce symptoms. The toxin acts on the receptors in the gut, and sensory stimulus is carried to the vomiting center in the brain by vagus and sympathetic nerves.

Because the ingested food contains preformed toxin, the incubation period is very short. In severe illness, profound hypotension occurs. Death is known to occur at extremes of age and in the malnourished.

Laboratory Diagnosis

The presence of a large number of *S. aureus* in food can indicate poor handling or sanitation; however, it is not sufficient evidence to incriminate the food as the cause of food poisoning.

Staphylococcal food poisoning can be diagnosed if staphylococci are isolated in large numbers from the food and their toxins are demonstrated in the food or if the isolated *S. aureus* is shown to produce enterotoxins. Dilutions of food may be plated on Baird-Parker agar or mannitol salt agar. Enterotoxin may be detected and identified by gel diffusion.

Treatment

Therapy is mainly supportive. Antibiotics have no role in the treatment because they are not antitoxins. Intravenous fluids and electrolyte replacement are imperative in the severely dehydrated patient.

Yersinia Species

The *Yersinia* species that cause food poisoning are commonly *Yersinia enterocolitica* and rarely *Yersinia pseudotuberculosis*. Pigs and other wild or domestic animals are the hosts, and humans are usually infected by the oral route. Serogroups that predominate in human illness are O:3, O:5, O:8, and O:9.

Yersiniosis is common in children and occurs most often in winter. *Y. enterocolitica* is associated with terminal ileitis and *Y. pseudotuberculosis* with mesenteric adenitis, but both organisms can cause mesenteric adenitis and symptoms that cause a clinical picture resembling appendicitis, resulting in surgical removal of a normal appendix. Rarer strains of *Y. enterocolitica* are likely to cause systemic infections, especially in patients with diabetes or in iron overload states. In Japan, a form of vasculitis, called Izumi fever, occurs, and in Russia a scarlet fever–like illness has been reported.

Pathogenesis

Yersinia organisms can survive and grow during refrigerated storage. Strains that cause human yersiniosis carry a plasmid that is associated with a number of virulence traits. Ingested bacteria adhere and invade M cells or epithelial cells.

Laboratory Diagnosis

Suspect food is homogenized in phosphate-buffered saline and inoculated into selenite F broth and held at 4°C for 6 weeks. The broth is subcultured at weekly intervals on deoxycholate citrate (DCA) or *Yersinia*-selective agar plates. This is termed *cold-enrichment technique.*

Treatment

Antibiotics are not recommended for gastroenteritis caused by *Yersinia enterocolitica* and the less-common *Yersinia pseudotuberculosis*, but bacteremia and extraintestinal infections require treatment with ciprofloxacin[1] (500 mg PO or 400 mg IV twice daily for 2 weeks). Third-generation cephalosporins (cefotaxime[1] [Claforan]), amoxicillin[1] (Amoxil), TMP-SMX[1] (Bactrim), amoxicillin-clavulanate[1] (Augmentin), carbapenems, and gentamicin (Garamycin) are also effective agents in therapy.

Viruses

Noroviruses

Noroviruses (formerly called Norwalk or Norwalk-like viruses and small round structured viruses [SRSV]) and sapoviruses belong to the family Caliciviridae and are the most common cause of gastroenteritis. They account for about 90% of epidemic nonbacterial outbreaks of gastroenteritis around the world. Norovirus infection often affects people during the winter months and is therefore sometimes called winter vomiting disease; however, people may be affected at any time of the year. After a norovirus infection, immunity lasts only for 14 weeks and is incomplete. Persons with blood group O are more susceptible to infection, whereas those with groups B and AB are partially protected. Norovirus infection outbreaks more commonly occur in closed or semiclosed communities, such as prisons, dormitories, cruise ships, schools, long-term care facilities, and overnight camps—places where infection can spread rapidly from human to human or through tainted food and surfaces. Infection outbreaks can also result from food handled by an infected person.

Outbreaks have often been linked to consumption of cold foods, including salads, sandwiches, and bakery products. Salad dressing, cake icing, and oysters from contaminated waters have also been implicated in gastroenteritis outbreaks. Weight loss, lethargy, low-grade fever, headache, and (rarely) ageusia occur. Vomiting is more likely with infections caused by norovirus than sapovirus.

Pathogenesis

Norovirus strains that infect humans are found in genogroups I, II, and IV. GII.4 strains are more commonly associated with person-to-person transmission, and GI strains are identified more commonly in shellfish-associated outbreaks.

Noroviruses were shown to differentially bind to histo-blood group antigens, and the binding pattern correlates with susceptibility to infection and illness. A number of enzymes are important in the synthesis of histo-blood group antigens, including fucosyl transferase-2 (FUT-2, secretor enzyme), FUT-3 (Lewis enzyme), and the A and B enzymes. The glycan produced by FUT-2 H type 1, serves as a viral receptor for noroviruses.

Laboratory Diagnosis

The virus can be recovered from the infected person's stool and vomitus during illness for about 2 weeks. Electron microscopy and reverse-transcriptase polymerase chain reaction (RT-PCR) antigen-detection assays are performed on stool samples. Serologic assays are not available for clinical use. However, infection can be diagnosed by identifying a fourfold or greater increase in antibody titer between acute and convalescent sera using norovirus virus-like particles as antigen.

Treatment

There is no specific treatment for norovirus infection. Hydration is generally adequate for most patients. In developing countries, oral rehydration therapy is the treatment of choice. Effective hand washing, careful food processing, and education of food handlers

---

[1]Not FDA approved for this indication.

along with chlorination of water are important preventive measures. A vaccine for norovirus is in clinical trials.

Rotavirus

Among the seven rotavirus species (A to G), rotavirus A, B, and C can cause disease in humans. Rotavirus A is the most common and is the major cause of waterborne outbreaks in humans. Infections are referred to as infantile diarrhea, winter diarrhea, or acute viral gastroenteritis. Children 6 months to 2 years of age, premature infants, the elderly, and the immunocompromised are particularly prone to more-severe symptoms caused by infection with group A rotavirus. Rotavirus can survive in water for days to weeks, depending on water quality and temperature. Waterborne outbreaks are most common, followed by spread by fomites. Rotaviruses infect intestinal enterocytes; diarrhea may be caused by malabsorption secondary to the destruction of enterocytes, villus ischemia and activation of the enteric nervous system, and intestinal secretion stimulated by the action of rotavirus nonstructural protein 4 (NSP4), a novel enterotoxin and secretory agonist with pleiotropic properties.

Outbreaks caused by group B rotavirus, also called adult diarrhea rotavirus, have also been reported in the elderly and adults. Such infections are rare and usually subclinical. Group C rotavirus has been associated with rare and sporadic cases of diarrhea in children in many countries. Subclinical infection to severe gastroenteritis leading to life-threatening dehydration can occur. The illness has an abrupt onset, with vomiting often preceding the onset of diarrhea. Up to one third of patients have fever of about 39°C. The stools are characteristically watery and only occasionally contain red or white cells. Symptoms generally resolve in a week.

Respiratory and neurologic features in children have been reported. Rotavirus infection has been associated with other clinical conditions including sudden infant death syndrome (SIDS), necrotizing enterocolitis, Kawasaki's disease, and type 1 diabetes.

Laboratory Diagnosis

Electron microscopy, direct antigen detection assays (ELISA, immunochromatography, latex agglutination), and nucleic acid detection (e.g., RT-PCR, polyacrylamide gel electrophoresis [PAGE]), are used mainly in epidemiologic studies during outbreaks.

Treatment

Dehydration due to group A rotavirus infection is treated with early institution of oral and intravenous fluids. The role of probiotics,[7] bismuth subsalicylate (Pepto Bismol),[1] inhibitors of enkephalinase, and nitazoxanide (Alinia)[1] are not clearly defined. Antimicrobials and antimotility agents should be avoided. A marked fall in deaths from childhood diarrhea following introduction of rotavirus vaccines (Rotarix, RotaTeq) has been reported from various parts of the world, and surveillance information has not revealed an association of any serious adverse reactions with the vaccine.

Other Pathogens
Cryptosporidium

Transmission of Cryptosporidium is usually by the fecal-oral route, often through food and water contaminated by livestock mammal feces. Persons most likely to be infected by Cryptosporidium parvum are infants and young children in daycare centers; those whose drinking water is unfiltered and untreated; those involved in farming practices such as lambing, calving, and muck-spreading; people engaging in anal sexual practices; patients in a hospital setting (from other infected patients or health care workers); veterinarians; and travelers.

Pathogenesis

Cryptosporidium spp. are believed to be noninvasive. Malabsorption resulting from the intestinal damage caused by prolonged protozoal infection can be fatal. Although host cells are damaged in cryptosporidiosis, the means by which the organism causes damage is not known. Mechanical destruction and the effects of toxins, enzymes, or immune-mediated mechanisms, working alone or together, may be instrumental. In the immunocompromised, the illness is much more debilitating, with cholera-like diarrhea.

Laboratory Diagnosis

Traditionally, cryptosporidiosis is diagnosed by microscopic observation of developmental stages of the organism in an intestinal biopsy specimen. Oocysts can be recovered from stool samples by formalin-concentration techniques, staining with a modified Ziehl-Neelsen acid-fast stain. Serologic tests (ELISA, immunofluorescence antibody, PCR) are of added value.

Treatment

Nitazoxanide (Alinia, 500 mg PO twice daily for 3 days) is recommended with antiretrovirals for HIV-positive patients. Fluid replacement and antidiarrheal agents are also given.

Trichinosis

Trichinosis is due to Trichinella spiralis infection, commonly as a result of consuming improperly cooked pork. The parasite lodges in the extraocular muscles, deltoid, biceps, intercostals, diaphragm, tongue, or masseter and produces severe weakness with pain, fever, and cough along with splinter hemorrhages and eosinophilia.

Moderate T. spiralis infection is treated with mebendazole (Vermox 200–400 mg PO three times daily for 3 days) or albendazole[1] (Albenza 400 mg PO twice daily for 7–14 days). For severe infections, prednisone is added in a dose of 1 mg/kg/day for 5 days.

Neurocysticercosis

Neurocysticercosis is caused by Taenia saginata infection, commonly as a result of consuming improperly cooked pork or contaminated raw vegetables and water. The parasite lodges in the central nervous system and skeletal muscle and presents as intracranial calcifications and ring-enhancing lesions on radioimaging studies. Other than leukocytosis, eosinophilia, and raised erythrocyte sedimentation rate, antibodies to species-specific antigens of T. solium can be detected by immunosorbent assay and complement fixation-tests. Treatment is aimed at controlling seizures and relief of hydrocephalus. Albendazole (15 mg/kg/day for 8–28 days) or praziquantel (50–100 mg/kg/day in three divided doses for a month) are given for parenchymal cysticerci with glucocorticoids to suppress the inflammatory response around the dying parasites. Surgery may be required to reduce intracranial pressure.

Dinoflagellate toxins

Dinoflagellates, a very large and diverse group of eukaryotic algae in the marine ecosystem, are the major group producing toxins that impact humans. Dinoflagellate toxins are structurally and functionally diverse, and many present unique biological activities. Five major seafood poisoning syndromes caused by toxins have been identified from the dinoflagellates (Table 4): paralytic shellfish poisoning (PSP), neurotoxic shellfish poisoning (NSP), amnesic shellfish poisoning (ASP), diarrheic shellfish poisoning (DSP) and ciguatera fish poisoning (CFP). Symptoms include allergic manifestations, neurologic including paresthesia of the extremities, headache, ataxia, vertigo, cranial nerve palsies, and paralysis of respiratory muscles as well as gastrointestinal. Symptomatic treatment and antihistamines are the mainstay of treatment.

---

[1]Not FDA approved for this indication.
[7]Available as dietary supplement.

---

[1]Not FDA approved for this indication.

TABLE 4	Seafood Poisoning Caused by Neurotoxins Identified from Marine Dinoflagellate Species			
TYPE OF POISONING	**TOXINS**	**SOURCES OF TOXINS**	**PRIMARY VECTOR**	**ACTION TARGET**
PSP	Saxitoxins and gonyautoxins	*Alexandrium* spp., *Gymnodinium* spp., *Pyrodinium* spp.	Shellfish	Voltage-gated sodium channel 1
NSP	Brevetoxins	*Kerenia brevis, Chatonella marina, C. antiqua, Fibrocapsa japonica, Heterosigma akashiwo*	Shellfish	Voltage-gated sodium channel 5
	Yessotoxins	*Protoceratium reticulatum, Lingulodinium polyedrum Gonyaulax spinifera*	Shellfish	Voltage-gated calcium/sodium channel?
CFP	Ciguatoxins	*Gambierdiscus toxicus*	Coral reef fish	Voltage-gated sodium channel 5
CFP	Maitotoxins	*Gambierdiscus toxicus*	Coral reef fish	Voltage-gated calcium channel
AZP	Azaspiracids	*Protoperidinium crassipes*	Shellfish	Voltage-gated calcium channel
Palytoxin poisoning	Palytoxins	*Ostrepsis siamensis*	Shellfish	$Na_+K_+ATPase$

Tetrodotoxin poisoning

It is a neurotoxin concentrated in the skin and viscera of puffer fish, and other fishes of the order Tetraodontiformes and in some amphibian, octopus, and shellfish species. Human poisonings occur when the flesh or organs of the fish are improperly prepared and eaten. Tetrodotoxin acts by blocking the conduction of nerve impulses along nerve fibers and axons and interferes with the transmission of signals from nerves to muscles. Onset of symptoms usually is 30–40 minutes but may be as short as 10 minutes; it includes lethargy, paraesthesia, emesis, ataxia, weakness, and dysphagia; ascending paralysis occurs in severe cases with high mortality (1-2 mg is lethal). Management is symptomatic.

Group B Sreptococcus (GBS)

GBS bacteria is found in 15%–30% of adult human intestines and urinary tract. Rarely implicated in infections of skin, joints, heart and brain, a recent outbreak of food-borne illness caused by the Type III GBS ST283 strain was reported in Singapore during the period of January–July 2015. It is the largest of its kind and first association to food-borne transmission of GBS to people via consumption of "yusheng-style" raw fresh water fish. The primary case presented with giddiness and suffered bouts of vomiting and diarrhea. Further studies are ongoing to establish the link between increase in cases of Group B streptococcus (GBS) infection to consumption of raw fish. Treatment is symptomatic.

Newer Trends in Foodborne Illness

New or unusual pathogens and food hazards are identified in course of investigating outbreaks. In 2011, a novel outbreak of sprout-associated illness caused by a strain of *Escherichia coli* O104:H4 was reported from Germany and France. This enteroaggregative and Shiga toxin-producing strain caused severe illness leading to HUS and death. In 2008, an outbreak following consumption of chicken caused by *Arcobacter butzleri* (found in poultry) was reported from Wisconsin. The calcivirus Sapovirus is emerging as the likely cause of oyster-associated foodborne outbreaks in Japan. New and unsuspected food vehicles are also being identified that had not been previously recognized as problematic (Box 2).

Changing patterns of disease presentation have seen important foodborne challenges emerging. Chagas disease is emerging as a foodborne infection linked to fresh, unpasteurized acai and guava juice. Infected triatomid insects present in fruits are implicated. Outbreaks of Nipah virus encephalitis in Bangladesh and India have been linked to drinking of palm sap, toddy, and well water contaminated with urine of feeding giant fruit bats, the vector of Nipah virus.

More syndromes and other systemic disease presentations are being linked to foodborne infection. The feco-oral transmission

BOX 1	Miscellaneous Organisms Implicated in Foodborne and Waterborne Illnesses

Adenovirus 40, 41
Bacillus anthracis
Bacillus mycoides
Burkholderia cepacia
Burkholderia pseudomallei
Clostridium bifermentans
Corynebacterium diphtheriae
Coxiella burnetii
Dientamoeba fragilis
Enterococcus faecalis, E. faecium
Erysipelothrix rhusiopathiae
Franciccella tularensis
Klebsiella spp.
Leptospira spp.
Mycobacterium bovis
Parvovirus B
Pediococcus
Pestivirus
Picobirnavirus
Proteus spp.
Pseudomonas aeruginosa
Pseudomonas cocovenanans
Reovirus
Streptobacillus moniliformis
Taenia solium, T. saginata
Torovirus
Toxoplasma gondii

of pathogens leading to other systemic manifestation include *Campylobacter* sp. (Guillain-Barre syndrome, irritable bowel syndrome), *Toxoplasma gondii* (behavior changes and neuropsychiatric manifestations) and *Salmonella choleraesuis* (aortitis). Foodborne outbreak of Group G streptococci (GGS) pharyngitis in a school dormitory in Japan (2016) presented with sore throat and fever in a majority; implicated food was a broccoli salad.

Miscellaneous

Many other organisms are implicated in foodborne and waterborne illnesses (Box 1). Some are discussed elsewhere in this book. Amebiasis, brucellosis, cholera, hepatitis A and E, giardiasis, typhoid fever, and other foodborne intestinal nematodes and cestodes are covered in the infectious diseases section of this text and are not covered in this section.

Bagged spinach
Carrot juice
Peanut butter
Broccoli powder on a snack food
Dry dog food
Frozen potpies
Canned chilli sauce
Hot peppers
White and black pepper
Raw cookie dough (likely the flour)
Hazelnuts
Fenugreek sprouts
Papayas
Pine nuts
Raw scrapped tuna

Reprinted from Braden C, Tauxe R: Emerging trends in foodborne diseases, *Inf Dis Clinics N Am* 27:517-533, 2013.

References

Baker AC, Goddard VJ, Davy J, et al: The identification of a diagnostic marker to detect freshwater cyanophages of filamentous cyanobacteria, *Appl Environ Microbiol* 72:5713–5719, 2003.

Braden CR, Tauxe RV: Emerging trends in foodborne diseases, *Infect Dis Clin North Am* 27(3):517–533, 2013

Centers for Disease Control and Prevention: *A–Z index for foodborne illness*, 2012. http://www.cdc.gov/foodsafety/diseases/. 2012 [accessed August 11, 2016].

Centers for Disease Control and Prevention: Available at: *CDC Estimates of Foodborne Illness in the United States*, 2012. Available at: http://www.cdc.gov/foodborneburden/PDFs/FACTSHEET_A_FINDINGS.pdf. 2012 [accessed August 11, 2016].

Centre for Disease Control and Prevention. The National Institute for Occupational Safety and Health (NIOSH) Emergency Response Safety and Health Database; Category Index: Biotoxins, http://www.cdc.gov/niosh/ershdb/emergencyresponse card_29750019.html. August 11, 2016.

Center for Disease Control and Prevention: Tetrodotoxin Poisoning Associated with Eating Puffer Fish Transported from Japan — California, 1996, *Morb Mortal Wkly Rep* 45(19), 1996.

Gamarra RM. Food poisoning- Clinical presentation. Drugs and Diseases, Medscape. updated June 26, 2015, http://emedicine.medscape.com/article/175569-clinical#b5. [Accessed August 11, 2016].

Hajmeer MN, Fung DYC: Other bacteria. In: Riemann H, Cliver DO, editors: *Foodborne Infections and Intoxications*, 3rd ed, New York, 2006, Academic Press, pp 341–363.

Hale TL, Keusch GT: Shigella, 1996: In Baron S, editor: *Medical Microbiology*, 4th ed, Galveston, 1996, TX: University of Texas Medical Branch at Galveston. PMID: 21413252 (PubMed). Available at: http://www.ncbi.nlm.nih.gov/books/NBK7627 (accessed August 11, 2016).

Hedberg CW, Osterholm MT: Outbreaks of food-borne and waterborne viral gastroenteritis, *Clin Microbio Rev* 6:199–210, 1993.

Janda JM, Abbott SL: The genus Aeromonas: Taxonomy, pathogenicity, and infection, *Clin Microbiol Rev* 23:35–73, 2010.

Juranek DD: Cryptosporidiosis: Sources of infection and guidelines for prevention, *Clin Infect Dis* 21:S57–61, 1995.

Ministry of Health, Singapore, National Environment Agency, Agri-food & Veterinary Authority of Singapore 24 July 2015. Update on Investigation into Group B Streptococcus Cases, https://www.moh.gov.sg/content/moh_web/home/pressRoom/pressRoomItemRelease/2015/update-on-investigation-into-group-b-streptococcus-cases.html. [Accessed August 11, 2016].

Nataro JP, Kaper JB: Diarrheagenic Escherichia coli, *Clin Microbiol Rev* 11:142–201, 1998.

Niyogi SK: Shigellosis, *J Microbiol* 43:133–143, 2005.

Ortega YR, Sanchez R: Update on Cyclospora cayetanensis, a food-borne and waterborne parasite, *Clin Microbiol Rev* 23:218–234, 2010.

Parashar UD, Bresee JS, Gentsch JR, Glass RI: Synopses: Rotavirus, *Emerg Infect Dis* 4:561–570, 1998.

Sodha SV, Griffin PM, Hughes JM: Foodborne disease. In Mandell GL, Bennett JE, Dolin R, editors: *Principles and Practice of Infectious Diseases*, 7th ed, Philadelphia, 2009, Churchill Livingstone, pp 1413–1427.

University of Maryland: *Chemical Ecology: Tetrodotoxin- Mode of action*, 2001. http://www.life.umd.edu/grad/mlfsc/zctsim/ionchannel.html.

Wang D-Z: Neurotoxins from Marine Dinoflagellates: A Brief Review, *Marine Drugs* 6(2):349–371, 2008. https://doi.org/10.3390/md20080016.

Yamaguchi T, Kawahara R, et al: Foodborne outbreak of group G streptococcal pharyngitis in a school dormitory in Osaka, Japan, *J Clin Microbiol* 56(5):e01884–17, 2018. https://doi.org/10.1128/JCM.01884-17.

GIARDIASIS

Method of
Rodney D. Adam, MD

CURRENT DIAGNOSIS

- Giardiasis is the most common intestinal protozoan infection worldwide.
- Most cases result from exposure to contaminated drinking or recreational water.
- The clinical manifestations range from asymptomatic to chronic diarrhea with malabsorption and weight loss.
- The diagnosis can be established by stool microscopy or by immunoassays of fecal specimens.
- Occasionally, the trophozoites can be found in duodenal specimens when fecal assays are negative.
- Serologic testing plays no role in the diagnosis.
- Irritable bowel symptoms are very common after successful treatment of giardiasis.

CURRENT THERAPY

- The treatment of choice is metronidazole (Flagyl)[1] or tinidazole (Tindamax); tinidazole can be given as a single dose.
- Albendazole (Albenza)[1] and nitazoxanide (Alinia) are alternative agents.
- Paromomycin,[1] a poorly absorbed aminoglycoside, is commonly recommended during early pregnancy when other agents are avoided.
- True drug resistance has not been documented, but refractory or recurrent cases can be treated by two drugs: a nitroimidazole combined with quinacrine (Atabrine)[2] or albendazole.[1]

[1]Not FDA approved for this indication.
[2]Not available in the United States.

Background

Giardia lamblia (syn. *Giardia intestinalis*, *Giardia duodenalis*) was initially described by Leeuwenhoek in the seventeenth century while doing a microscopic examination of his own diarrheal feces. However, *G. lamblia* was not widely accepted as a human pathogen until the 1960s, when a number of outbreaks were reported in travelers to endemic areas. The presumed source of infection in these cases was contaminated drinking water. Subsequently, *Giardia* has become the most commonly identified parasitic cause of diarrhea, and, along with *Cryptosporidium* species, is among the most commonly identified parasitic causes of waterborne diarrheal disease.

Organism

Giardia species are members of the diplomonad (two bodies) group of flagellated protozoans. The life cycle consists of the environmentally resistant cyst, which infects its host on ingestion. It is oval in shape, is about 8 μm × 12 μm in size and contains four nuclei. It excysts into pear-shaped trophozoites in the proximal small intestine that are about 10 to 12 μm by 5 × 7 μm in size. Two symmetrically placed nuclei are in the body of the trophozoites and four pairs of flagella aid with motility. A ventral concave disk uses primarily mechanical means to attach to the intestinal wall of the host. While still in the small intestine, some of the trophozoites then encyst into the cyst form, which is passed in the feces to continue the cycle of infection. The *Giardia* species are all parasitic and were initially assigned to species on the basis of host of origin. However, in 1952, they were divided into three species [*Giardia agilis*, amphibians; *Giardia muris*, rodents; *G. duodenalis* (*G. lamblia*), mammals and birds] that could easily be distinguished on the basis of morphologic appearance of the trophozoites. Subsequently, the *G. lamblia* morphologic group has been divided into additional species based on differences that can be seen at the ultrastructural or molecular level. Of the organisms that remain assigned to *G. lamblia*, all are found in mammals but are divided into eight genotypes or assemblages (A through H) on the basis of molecular differences with varying host specificities. Only genotypes A and B have been found in humans. It is likely that at least some of these eight genotypes will eventually be assigned to separate species.

Epidemiology

Giardiasis is the most commonly diagnosed human protozoan infection and is one of the most commonly identified forms of gastroenteritis. Most cases occur from ingestion of contaminated water or by human-to-human transmission through the fecal–oral route. Thus the epidemiology of human infections can be understood by examining these mechanisms of transmission. In the United States, most cases are sporadic and occur more often in the summer, probably reflecting infection from recreational water exposure. Infections were more commonly reported in children from ages 1 to 9 years, especially those younger than 4 years of age. In general, the incidence is higher in the northern states, perhaps because cysts survive longer in cool, moist environments (Figure 1).

Direct human-to-human transmission by the fecal oral route also occurs, leading to the higher prevalence found in children in daycare centers. The occasional reports of food-borne transmission most likely occurred because of food being contaminated by infected food handlers.

The greater incidence in children could reflect an increased use of recreational water facilities, daycare exposure, or increased susceptibility to symptomatic disease. The epidemiology of giardiasis in the United States is similar to that found in other developed countries located in temperate regions. However, in developing regions with inadequate availability of purified water, the epidemiology is very different. For example, in a shantytown near Lima, Peru, children were almost universally infected by the age of 2 years, and when treated, they were rapidly reinfected, but there were no symptoms that could clearly be correlated with their infections. Perhaps an outbreak at a ski resort town in the United States can explain these different epidemiologic patterns. In this water-borne outbreak, tourists were disproportionately affected despite drinking from the same water source as the local residents. The conclusion was that the local residents had repeatedly been exposed to water contaminated by *Giardia* cysts and were less susceptible to symptomatic disease.

The degree of zoonotic transmission of giardiasis remains controversial. Human acquisition of infection from dogs or cats has not been well documented, and usually the *Giardia* genotypes found in cats or dogs are distinct from those found in humans (A and B), even in regions where both are endemic. However, genotypes A and B have sometimes been identified in dogs or other animals, so the question is not totally resolved. On the other hand, beavers have been implicated as a source of contaminated water leading to human infections.

Risk Factors

People with hypogammaglobulinemia, and possibly those with IgA deficiency, are at increased risk for prolonged giardiasis. In animal models, deficiency in cell-mediated immunity (CMI) has been associated with increased risk, but in humans the increased risk has not been associated with defects in CMI.

Pathogenesis

Infection is initiated by the ingestion of as few as 10 cysts. After passage through the acidic environment of the stomach, each cyst excysts into two trophozoites in the proximal small intestine.

However, gastric acidity is not required, and people with achlorhydria or who are treated with suppressors of gastric acid remain vulnerable to giardiasis. The trophozoites replicate in the proximal small intestine, where they attach to the intestinal mucosa by their ventral disks. The attachment appears to occur by mechanical means facilitated by the suction generated by the ventral disk and the four pairs of flagella as they provide motility. Although the trophozoites attach to the intestinal wall and leave imprints after separating from the wall, there is no well-documented evidence of invasion, either of the intestinal wall or at extraintestinal sites. Toxins have not been identified as causes of diarrhea. Thus the current evidence suggests that the symptoms result from the immune response to the trophozoite. The host–parasite interaction leads to enterocyte apoptosis, epithelial barrier disruption, and CD8 lymphocyte activation that leads to microvillous shortening, leading to the malabsorption that is a hallmark of the infection. The trophozoites are coated with a cysteine-rich protein encoded by one of a family of related genes, and expression can be switched from one to another, perhaps contributing to the chronicity of the infection.

Prevention

The strategies for prevention should be determined by the most prevalent risk factors in specific situations. For travelers to endemic regions, the major risk is from the ingestion of contaminated water. Therefore drinking water should be purified by boiling for 1 minute or by filtration through a pore size of < 1 μm. Halogenization with iodine or chlorine requires a prolonged contact time (hours) to inactivate cysts and is not recommended. In daycare centers and for food handlers, the best preventive measure is effective hand washing. In addition, children or workers who are infected should be treated.

Clinical Features

Most people with giardiasis are symptom free, but the percentages range from rates of diarrhea no higher than background among children in some highly endemic regions to attack rates of nearly 100% in visitors to endemic regions. Symptomatic patients typically present for evaluation only after several days or even weeks of illness because of the subacute onset. The symptoms of giardiasis typically develop after an incubation period of 1 to 2 weeks and consist of diarrhea that is characterized by loose, foul-smelling stools and abdominal discomfort described as cramping or bloating (Table 1). Fatigue is very common, but fever is unusual and, when present, is mild and occurs only within the first few days. Malabsorption and weight loss are often present. The majority of cases resolve within several weeks, but occasionally the symptoms will last for months in the absence of treatment. Relapse is relatively uncommon after effective treatment.

Diagnosis

The gold standard of diagnosis has been the microscopic evaluation of three separate fecal samples, including concentrated specimens for cysts or, less commonly, trophozoites. The identification of trophozoites is nearly always associated with symptomatic infection, but cysts may be found in symptom-free persons. Because of the challenges in obtaining three fecal specimens and the interobserver variability in skill at identifying *Giardia* cysts, antigen detection tests have come into widespread use. The enzyme immunoassays are more commonly used and have high degrees of sensitivity and specificity. A direct fluorescent assay is slightly more sensitive than the enzyme immunoassays and can also detect *Cryptosporidium* species, but it requires the availability of fluorescent microscopy. PCR tests have also been described but are not widely available. Some patients have negative workups of stool samples, but *Giardia* trophozoites can be detected in duodenal contents with the string test. The patient swallows a capsule on a string, which is left in situ for 4 hours to overnight. The string is then removed and examined microscopically for trophozoites. Alternatively, endoscopy with sampling of duodenal contents and duodenal biopsy can be used. Endoscopy has the

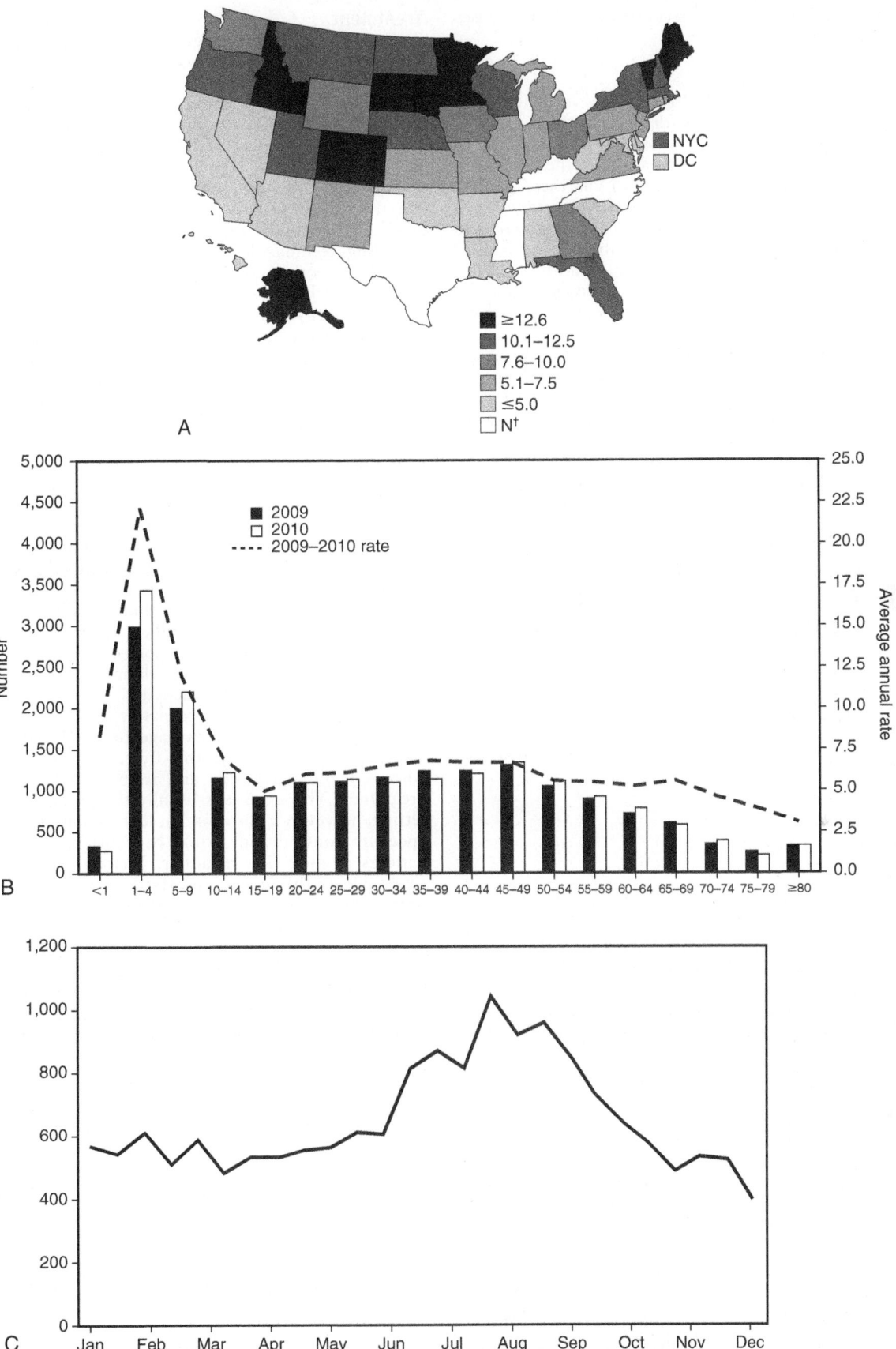

Figure 1 Incidence of giardiasis in the United States, 2011–2012. Information is collected through the National Notifiable Diseases Surveillance System (NNDSS). **A,** Incidence rate (cases per 100,000 population) of giardiasis, by reporting jurisdiction—National Notifiable Diseases Surveillance System, United States, 2012. **B,** Average annual incidence rate (cases per 100,000 population) of giardiasis, by sex and age group—National Notifiable Diseases Surveillance System, United States, 2011–2012. **C,** Number (cases per 100,000 population) of giardiasis case reports, by date of symptom onset—National Notifiable Diseases Surveillance System, United States, 2011–2012. (From Painter, J.E., Gargano, J.W., Collier, S.A., Yoder, J.S., Centers for Disease, C., and Prevention (2015). Giardiasis surveillance—United States, 2011-2012. Morb Mortal Wkly Rep Surveill Summ *64 Suppl 3*, 15–25).

added advantage of being able to detect other possible diagnoses, such as celiac disease or tropical sprue.

Differential Diagnosis

The diagnosis of giardiasis should be suspected in patients presenting with prolonged (>5–7 days) diarrhea without blood in the stools and no fever. In patients presenting relatively early in the course of illness, the major considerations in the differential diagnosis are other infectious etiologies of diarrhea, particularly *Campylobacter jejuni*, *Salmonella*, *Cryptosporidium*, and *Cyclospora cayetanensis*. Thus patients presenting with compatible symptoms should have stool samples submitted for culture and for microscopic examination for ova and parasites (O and P). Watery diarrhea is uncommon, and bloody stools are not seen with giardiasis; thus these findings should prompt the search for other etiologies.

For patients presenting with more prolonged symptoms, a number of noninfectious illnesses should be added to the differential diagnosis. Irritable bowel syndrome and lactose intolerance are among the more common etiologies and should be considered in patients presenting with diarrhea but no weight loss. Gluten enteropathy, tropical sprue, and, rarely, Whipple's disease are among the noninfectious etiologies of diarrhea accompanied by weight loss.

Treatment

Patients with symptomatic giardiasis should be treated. The criteria for treatment of patients with asymptomatic giardiasis are not well defined, but in general, patients in regions with low prevalence or linked with outbreaks should be treated. On the other hand, in settings where the prevalence is high and recurrence rates are high, there is probably no value to treating asymptomatic infection.

The most commonly used agents for treatment of giardiasis are the nitroimidazoles. Metronidazole (Flagyl)[1] and tinidazole (Tindamax) are available in the United States, and others, including secnidazole (Secnil)[2] and ornidazole (Tiberal)[2], are available in other countries (Table 2). These agents are completely absorbed from the gastrointestinal tract and are inactivated primarily by hepatic metabolism. Metronidazole has been available in the United States for decades and has generally been considered the drug of choice for treatment of giardiasis in most situations. More recently, tinidazole has become available and is the only agent available in the United States with a high degree of efficacy when given as a single dose. Metronidazole is mutagenic in bacterial assays and showed some carcinogenic activity in an animal model. However, carcinogenicity in humans has not been documented. Serious adverse reactions to the nitroimidazoles are rare, but nausea and a metallic taste are common and may decrease the compliance of patients with metronidazole. The problem with noncompliance can be addressed by the use of tinidazole or the other agents that can be given as a single dose.

Albendazole (Albenza)[1] is a tubulin inhibitor that was introduced as a broad-spectrum antihelminthic, but it also has good activity against *Giardia* trophozoites. It is generally well tolerated and in areas with endemic helminth infections has the added advantage of antihelminthic activity.

The first trimester of pregnancy poses a special problem because none of the agents have been adequately studied or approved for use during this time. Paromomycin[1] is a nonabsorbed aminoglycoside and is expected to be safe during pregnancy. Therefore it is usually the preferred choice in that setting; however, it is somewhat less effective than other agents. Specialty consultation should be considered for treatment of patients in their first trimester. Metronidazole is used extensively during the second and third trimesters for other indications; thus it can be considered the drug of choice for those patients. Albendazole is known to be teratogenic and should be avoided during pregnancy.

Nitazoxanide (Alinia) has been approved in the United States for treatment of giardiasis (and cryptosporidiosis) and is very well

---

TABLE 1 Symptoms of Giardiasis*

SYMPTOM	AVERAGE (%)
Diarrhea	95
Abdominal cramps	70
Weakness or malaise	70
Nausea	60
Weight loss	50
Anorexia (decreased appetite)	50
Abdominal distention (bloating/distension)	50
Flatulence	50
Vomiting	30
Fever	20

From Hunter 2017; Giardiasis by R. Adam.
*The table includes the approximate frequency of the signs and symptoms reported in six studies of symptomatic giardiasis, but it is important to note that there is substantial variability of symptoms among studies.

[1] Not FDA approved for this indication.
[2] Not available in the United States.

TABLE 2 Treatment of Giardiasis

DRUG	DOSE		FREQUENCY	DURATION	EFFICACY (%)
	ADULT	PEDIATRIC*			
Metronidazole[1] (Flagyl)	250 mg	5 mg/kg	tid	5–7 days	90–100
Tinidazole (Tindamax)	2 gm	50 mg/kg	Single dose	Single dose	90–100
Quinacrine[2,6] (Atabrine)	100 mg	2 mg/kg	tid	5–7 days	80–100
Furazolidone[2,6] (Furoxone)	100 mg	1.5 mg/kg	qid	10 days	80–94
Paromomycin[1] (Humatin)	500 mg	8-10 mg/kg	tid	10 days	55–90
Albendazole[1] (Albenza)	400 mg qd	15 mg/kg	Daily	5 days	90–100
Nitazoxanide (Alinia)	500 mg bid	7.5 mg/kg	bid	3 days	70–80

*The adult dose is the maximum pediatric dose.
[1] Not FDA approved for this indication.
[2] Not available in the United States.
[6] May be compounded by pharmacists.

tolerated. However, the somewhat lower efficacy compared with nitroimidazoles and albendazole, along with the requirement for twice daily dosing, limits its role.

Quinacrine (Atabrine)[2] was one of the first effective treatments for giardiasis but has fallen into disfavor because of toxicity. Nausea and vomiting are common, and toxic psychosis is occasionally seen.

Treatment failures are not uncommon but may or may not be due to true drug resistance because in vitro cultures are not routinely performed, and in vitro testing is not standardized. When treatment failure occurs, the patient may respond to the same or an alternative drug. Treatment-refractory cases have been treated successfully with a combination of metronidazole[1] plus quinacrine[2] or albendazole.[1] The most common reason for persistence of symptoms after treatment is due to post-giardiasis irritable bowel syndrome, which can occur in up to 25% of patients. Thus it is important to re-evaluate stool specimens from patients with symptoms that persist after therapy.

Diet
Lactose intolerance is quite common while patients have giardiasis and potentially for months thereafter, so lactose ingestion should be moderated or eliminated as needed.

References

Adam RD: Biology of *Giardia lamblia*, *Clin Microbiol Rev* 14:447–475, 2001.
Adam RD: Giardiasis. In Magill AJ, Ryan ET, Hill D, Solomon T, editors: *Hunter's Tropical Medicine and Emerging Infectious Disease*, Philadelphia, 2013, Elsevier, pp 668–672.
Cooper MA, Sterling CR, Gilman RH, et al: Molecular analysis of household transmission of *Giardia lamblia* in a region of high endemicity in Peru, *J Infect Dis* 202:1713–1721, 2010.
Cotton JA, Beatty JK, Buret AG: Host parasite interactions and pathophysiology in *Giardia* infections, *Int J Parasitol* 41:925–933, 2011.
Hanevik K, Dizdar V, Langeland N, Hausken T: Development of functional gastrointestinal disorders after *Giardia lamblia* infection, *BMC Gastroenterol* 9:27, 2009.
Lengerich EJ, Addiss DG, Juranek DD: Severe giardiasis in the United States, *Clin Infect Dis* 18:760–763, 1994.
Morrison HG, McArthur AG, Gillin FD, et al: Genomic minimalism in the early diverging intestinal parasite *Giardia lamblia*, *Science* 317:1921–1926, 2007.
Nash TE, Ohl CA, Thomas E, et al: Treatment of patients with refractory giardiasis, *Clin Infect Dis* 33:22–28, 2001.
Rossignol JF: *Cryptosporidium* and *Giardia*: treatment options and prospects for new drugs, *Exp Parasitol* 124:45–53, 2010.
Adam EA, Yoder JS, Gould LH, Hlavsa MC, Gargano JW: Giardiasis outbreaks in the United States, 1971-2011, *Epidemiology & Infection* 144:2790–2801, 2016.

TREATMENT AND PREVENTION OF HIV INFECTION

Method of
Allison K. Cormier, MD; Tyler K. Liebenstein, PharmD; and Ryan P. Westergaard, MD, PhD, MPH

CURRENT DIAGNOSIS

- National guidelines recommend universal screening for HIV infection for all adult and adolescent patients in all healthcare settings after notification that testing will be done, unless the patient specifically declines (opt-out testing). Patients with behavioral risk factors, sexually transmitted diseases, or tuberculosis should be screened annually.
- Revised HIV testing algorithms reflect the increased sensitivity of newer diagnostic assays during early infection, such as fourth-generation HIV-1/2 antigen/antibody combination immunoassays.
- Acute HIV infection is recognized as a variable syndrome including fever, pharyngitis, rash, and arthralgias. As many as half of patients may be asymptomatic during seroconversion and early infection.

CURRENT THERAPY

- Combination antiretroviral therapy (ART) should be offered to all patients with HIV infection, regardless of CD4+ cell count.
- Initial ART regimens preferred for most patients include a combination of two nucleoside analogue reverse transcriptase inhibitors (NRTIs) and an integrase strand transfer inhibitor (INSTI), which are often co-formulated into single-tablet preparations that can be administered once daily.
- While antiretroviral treatment decisions are often made by providers with specialized training, all providers caring for people living with HIV should be aware of the risk of antiretroviral drug interactions, particularly those involving the pharmacokinetic enhancing agents ritonavir (Norvir) and cobicistat (Tybost).
- Since 2014, co-formulated emtricitabine-tenofovir disoproxil fumarate (Truvada) has been approved for daily oral administration for preexposure prophylaxis (PrEP) as an HIV prevention strategy for people at elevated risk of HIV transmission.

Introduction
Remarkable advances in therapeutics, leading to the development of antiretroviral therapy (ART), have transformed HIV infection from an almost universally fatal illness to a chronic disease that can be managed over decades with an enlarging repertoire of treatment options. Further developments in ART have also provided opportunities for preventing HIV infection in high-risk individuals. This chapter provides an overview of the current understanding of HIV pathogenesis, epidemiology, and reviews guidelines for the initial evaluation and long-term management of HIV infection in adult patients.

Pathophysiology
HIV is an enveloped, single-stranded RNA virus belonging to the family Retroviridae. It was recognized as the causative agent of AIDS within 3 years after the initial description of the syndrome in 1981, and ongoing characterization of its molecular biology has provided the identification of multiple targets for drug development. Two human immunodeficiency viruses exist: HIV-1 and HIV-2. HIV-1 has worldwide distribution, accounts for most infections outside western Africa, and is the focus of this chapter.

HIV-2 infection is endemic in West Africa and has limited spread outside this area. It should be considered in infections in patients of West African origin or those who have had sexual contact or shared needles with people of West African origin. HIV-2 generally has a longer asymptomatic stage, lower plasma HIV-2 viral loads, and overall lower mortality rate. Approximately 25% to 30% of patients with HIV-2 not receiving ART will have HIV-2 RNA levels below the rate of detection and some will also have clinical progression and CD4 cell count decline. HIV-2 can progress to AIDS over time. HIV-1 and HIV-2 coinfection may occur and should be a consideration in patients from HIV-2 high-prevalence areas. Patients diagnosed with HIV-2 infection should be managed by an HIV specialist.

Genetic heterogeneity of HIV-1 is reflected in categorization of the virus into three groups (M, O, and N) and several clades (e.g., B, C, D, AE, and CRF01_AE), some of which have overlapping geographic distribution around the world. Subtype C is prevalent in southern and eastern Africa, China, India, South Asia, and Brazil and accounts for 50% of HIV subtypes, whereas subtype B, the most common subtype in the United States, accounts for 12%.

The HIV viral genome is encoded in single-stranded RNA, packaged in core protein structures, and surrounded by a lipid bilayer envelope that is derived from the cell membrane of the host cell as the virus buds from the cell surface after replication.

This outer viral membrane contains HIV-specific glycoproteins, including gp120 and gp41, which facilitate attachment and entry into host cells through interaction with the cell surface receptor, CD4, and coreceptors CCR5 and CXCR4. CD4+ helper T lymphocytes are the predominant host cell affected by HIV; this molecular tropism explains the immune system destruction manifested in chronic HIV infection and provides the rationale for clinical staging of HIV infection using CD4+ T-cell counts. After host cell entry, the key enzyme responsible for viral replication is reverse transcriptase, an RNA-dependent DNA polymerase that is packaged within the virion core. This enzyme facilitates conversion of the HIV genome into a double-stranded DNA intermediate molecule. The second key enzymatic step is integration of this intermediate nucleic acid product into the host genome, which is facilitated by the viral protein integrase. Protein synthesis with packaging of new viral particles ensues, utilizing an HIV-specific protease. The integrase inhibitor class of drugs acts by blocking this step of integration.

Natural History

Within 1 to 4 weeks after the initial HIV infection, seroconversion may be accompanied by a nonspecific, self-limited illness, often referred to as the acute retroviral syndrome. This illness has variable manifestations but may include fever, malaise, myalgias, arthralgias, generalized lymphadenopathy, pharyngitis, and rash. The associated rash may be maculopapular, urticarial, or roseola-like. An illness resembling acute infectious mononucleosis syndrome, similar to that caused by Epstein-Barr virus or cytomegalovirus (CMV), and aseptic meningitis have been described. Diagnosis of acute HIV infection requires a high index of suspicion, which does not commonly occur unless the patient reports a recent history of a high-risk exposure.

During the acute phase of infection, high levels of viremia are present (often exceeding 10 million copies/mL) as HIV becomes widely disseminated throughout the body and the host defenses begin to counteract circulating virus through cell-mediated and humoral (antibody-mediated) immune mechanisms. Antibodies against HIV usually become detectable between 2 and 4 months after infection. The initial, high-level viremia plateaus and then begins a decline as neutralizing antibodies are established. Ongoing replication is partially controlled by the immune response, resulting in a steady-state level of viremia. This virologic level differs from patient to patient and is one of the determinants of the rate of disease progression. A small number of HIV-infected persons are able to control viral replication to levels below the limit of detection, and they tend to have a more benign course of disease. In these patients, designated "elite suppressors" by researchers, HIV replication continues to occur, and HIV RNA can be isolated from latently infected cells by means of specialized laboratory techniques.

After the establishment of HIV infection and seroconversion, a period of asymptomatic infection ensues, during which patients are free of evidence of immune suppression and opportunistic infections (OIs) are uncommon. This phase of clinical latency lasts a median of 8 to 10 years, based on observational studies from the pre-ART era. Ongoing viral replication leads to gradual decline in CD4 counts.

The symptomatic stage of HIV infection can begin at any time after infection, but clinical manifestations become more likely as the CD4 count falls farther below the normal range of 800 to 1200 cells/mm³. For example, *Pneumocystis jirovecii* (formerly *Pneumocystis carinii*) pneumonia (PJP) usually occurs in patients with a CD4 count of less than 200 cells/mm³ or a percentage of less than 10%. CMV retinitis occurs almost exclusively in patients with a CD4 count of less than 50 cells/mm³ or a percentage of less than 5%. Mucocutaneous candidiasis (oral thrush), herpes zoster, HIV-associated nephropathy, peripheral neuropathy, tuberculosis, and community-acquired bacterial pneumonia occur with increased frequency at earlier stages of infection and are less reliably predicted by CD4+ cell measurement.

Diagnosis

The current recommended testing algorithm incorporates fourth-generation antigen/antibody combination HIV-1/2 immunoassay with a confirmatory HIV-1/HIV-2 antibody differentiation immunoassay. The fourth-generation assay detects both HIV-1 and HIV-2 antibodies and HIV p24 antigen. It has increased sensitivity due to its ability to diagnose acute/early infection, as HIV p24 antigen is detected before seroconversion has occurred. If the fourth-generation combination assay is positive, the HIV-1 and HIV-2 antibody differentiation immunoassay both confirms the positive result and determines if the patient is infected with HIV-1 or HIV-2. If the fourth-generation assay is positive but the confirmatory antibody differentiation immunoassay is indeterminate or negative, a plasma HIV RNA level should be obtained.

In facilities where fourth-generation testing is not available, a two-step approach is utilized via enzyme-linked immunosorbent assay (ELISA) to detect HIV antibodies with subsequent confirmation using HIV-1/HIV-2 differentiation assay. ELISA detects HIV IgM and IgG antibodies as early as 3 weeks after virus exposure. This modality has excellent sensitivity and specificity for diagnosing chronic HIV infection; however, diagnosis may be missed in patients with early HIV infection who have not yet had seroconversion. If concern exists for acute/early HIV infection, plasma HIV RNA can be assessed.

Uncommonly, false-negative and false-positive tests occur. False-negative screening tests can occur with ELISA-only testing during acute/early HIV infection. This occurs less often using the fourth-generation antigen/antibody assay, which is more sensitive in detecting early HIV infection by identifying the p24 antigen. False-positive screening test results can occur for several non-HIV reasons, including cross-reaction from alloantibodies in pregnant females, autoantibodies from autoimmune diseases or malignancy, and the influenza vaccine. False-positive results in both screening and confirmatory testing are exceptionally uncommon.

Indeterminate test results occur when the initial screening test is positive and subsequent confirmatory testing is indeterminate or negative. In the event of a positive fourth-generation antigen/antibody test and negative HIV differentiation assay, the detection of p24 antigen would yield a positive result but the differentiation assay would be negative, as no antibody is present. In all patients with indeterminate test results, a plasma HIV RNA should be obtained, as viremia is present prior to antibody seroconversion. A detectable plasma HIV RNA level is diagnostic of HIV infection. If HIV RNA is negative, the patient should be reassured that HIV infection is unlikely. A repeat screening test can be repeated after 3 months for further reassurance. If the patient had a recent high-risk exposure, another plasma HIV RNA can be performed in 1 to 2 weeks. All patients with indeterminate testing should be counseled to avoid activities with potential to transmit HIV to others until evaluation is completed.

Consent

HIV screening should be voluntary and pursued only after discussion with the patient regarding testing. In the United States, written consent is no longer obligatory in any state, but individual states may have policies regarding documentation of the consent process and related counseling. Confidentiality, access to post-testing counseling, and services to support prompt linkage to HIV care for patients with positive results are important resources in HIV testing settings.

Screening

Early detection of HIV infection and subsequent initiation of ART can dramatically reduce morbidity and mortality of affected patients. A relatively normal life span is obtainable in patients in the United States who are diagnosed early in their infection and successfully treated. It also can reduce the transmission of HIV. One-time testing is recommended for patients without high-risk factors for HIV exposure in patients 13 to 75 years of age. Pregnant women should be screened for HIV early in their pregnancy, even if they have been screened during prior pregnancies.

TABLE 1	Preferred Initial Antiretroviral Medication Regimens for Most Patients.		
GENERIC NAME (TRADE NAME) AND RECOMMENDED ADULT DOSING	**SINGLE TABLET REGIMEN?**	**IMPORTANT POINTS**	
INSTI + 2 NRTIs			
Bictegravir/emtricitabine/tenofovir alafenamide (Biktarvy) 50/200/25 mg–1 tablet by mouth once daily	Yes	Bictegravir has been shown to raise serum creatinine from baseline by a median 0.1 mg/dL due to inhibition of creatinine secretion, not a true reduction in GFR	
Dolutegravir/abacavir/lamivudine (Triumeq) 50/600/300 mg–1 tablet by mouth once daily	Yes	Dolutegravir has been shown to raise serum creatinine from baseline by a mean of 0.1 mg/dL due to inhibition of creatinine secretion, not a true reduction in GFR. Dolutegravir has a drug interaction with metformin (maximum daily metformin dose is 1000 mg) Must be confirmed HLA-B*5701 negative before starting to avoid abacavir hypersensitivity reaction	
Dolutegravir (Tivicay) 50 mg–1 tablet by mouth once daily PLUS Tenofovir alafenamide/emtricitabine (Descovy) 25/200 mg–1 tablet by mouth once daily OR Tenofovir disoproxil fumarate/emtricitabine (Truvada) 300/200 mg–1 tablet by mouth once daily	No	Dolutegravir has been shown to raise serum creatinine from baseline by a mean of 0.1 mg/dL due to inhibition of creatinine secretion, not a true reduction in GFR. Dolutegravir has a drug interaction with metformin (maximum daily metformin dose is 1000 mg) Descovy generally preferred over Truvada due to fewer bone and kidney toxicities	
Raltegravir (Isentress HD) 600 mg–2 tablets by mouth once daily OR Raltegravir (Isentress) 400 mg–1 tablet by mouth twice daily PLUS Tenofovir alafenamide/emtricitabine (Descovy) 25/200 mg–1 tablet by mouth once daily OR Tenofovir disoproxil fumarate/emtricitabine (Truvada) 300/200 mg–1 tablet by mouth once daily	No	Isentress HD generally preferred over Isentress due to once daily dosing Descovy generally preferred over Truvada due to fewer bone and kidney toxicities	

GFR, glomerular filtration rate; HLA, human leukocyte antigen.
Biktarvy (package insert). Foster City, CA. Gilead Sciences, Inc.; 2018.
Tivicay (package insert). Research Triangle Park, NC: ViiV Healthcare; 2013.
Adapted from Panel on Antiretroviral Guidelines for Adults and Adolescents. Guidelines for the Use of Antiretroviral Agents in Adults and Adolescents Living with HIV. Department of Health and Human Services. Available at http://aidsinfo.nih.gov/contentfiles/lvguidelines/AdultandAdolescentGL.pdf. Section accessed April 18, 2019 (Table 6).

In patients with elevated risk of HIV exposure, more frequent testing is recommended. Men who have sex with men, with sexual partners who have HIV, or those with unknown serostatus may benefit from HIV screening at least every 6 months. This is especially important in patients aged 13 to 24 years, as this demographic has experienced the highest rate of new infections in recent years. Other high-risk groups include patients who use injection drugs and sex workers.

Approach to the Patient With HIV Infection

HIV patient care is an ever-changing field, with routinely updated professional guidelines and new medications. The quality of care received by patients with HIV has been shown to correlate with the healthcare provider's experience and comfort in treating these patients. Referral to an HIV specialist is recommended for new HIV diagnoses, complications of HIV or antiretroviral drugs, and for treatment failure.

All patients with HIV should have a comprehensive history, physical examination, and laboratory evaluation when establishing care. This baseline evaluation can help establish and define the patient's goals and plan of care. In a patient who has already established treatment with ART and presents for initial evaluation with a new healthcare provider, it is important to document their complete antiretroviral history and drug resistance testing results, if available.

Patients with HIV are often faced with many medical, psychiatric, and social issues. These are best addressed through a patient-centered, multidisciplinary approach. In a patient with a new diagnosis of HIV, it is important to counsel the patient regarding HIV infection and assess their understanding of the disease and its transmission. They should also be assessed for readiness to initiate ART, potential high-risk behaviors, mental illness, substance abuse, social support, medical comorbidities, and/or economic factors, as these are potential issues that may impair adherence to ART.

Antiretroviral Therapy

There are currently six major classes of antiretroviral medications used to treat patients with HIV. Though there are dozens of medications available, only a small selection of agents is currently preferred as initial treatment regimens (Table 1). For most patients, ART includes a combination of two nucleoside analogue reverse transcriptase inhibitors (NRTIs) plus a third medication from a different class.

When to Initiate Antiretroviral Therapy

Combination ART first became available in the mid-1990s and provided life-saving therapy for millions of patients suffering from HIV and AIDS. While the early ART regimens were effective in helping patients with AIDS recover, they were also associated with many toxicities and side effects. In 2006, the US Department of Health and Human Services, the International AIDS Society—USA, and the British HIV Society recommended CD4 counts of 200 cells/mm^3 as the threshold for initiating ART treatment in asymptomatic patients. In the last decade, the paradigm has shifted toward earlier initiation of ART based on accumulating evidence for the beneficial effects of treatment initiation earlier in the course of infection. Antiretroviral therapies have advanced significantly since their conception, consisting of multiple drug classes, fewer toxicities, less pill burden, and overall improved tolerance. Failure to suppress viral loads on these medications is more likely to be due to therapy nonadherence than medication failure.

HIV patients are now achieving normal life spans, and non–AIDS defining illnesses are becoming more prominent.

Cardiovascular, renal, and hepatic disease complications are lower in patients who started ART at higher CD4 thresholds (>350 cells/mm³). Earlier initiation of ART is also associated with reduced risk of transmission and improved immune restoration.

Current Recommendations for Antiretroviral Therapy

ART should be offered to all patients with HIV infection, regardless of CD4 count. The goal of ART is to prevent morbidity, mortality, and transmission associated with HIV. This is accomplished by maximally inhibiting HIV replication to achieve an undetectable HIV viral load. Based on guidelines from the US Department of Health and Human Services, integrase strand transfer inhibitor (INSTI)-based regimens are currently the first-line recommendation as initial therapy for most patients with HIV based on high rates of virologic suppression and tolerability demonstrated in large clinical trials. Nonnucleoside reverse transcriptase (NNRTI)—and protease inhibitor (PI)-based regimens are recommended in certain clinical situations (Table 2). Monotherapy with any antiretroviral drug is not recommended due to increased risk of drug resistance and therapy failure.

Selection of an Antiretroviral Regimen

ART regimens should be individualized based on a regimen's side effect profile, pill burden, potential drug interactions, virologic efficacy, cost, and resistance test results. Before starting ART in any patient with HIV, the following factors must be considered:
- Pretreatment HIV RNA level
- Pretreatment CD4 count
- HIV genotypic drug resistance testing results
- HLA-B*5701 status (if planning to use abacavir-based ART regimen)
- A patient's individual preference
- Anticipated medication adherence

Other factors that are important to consider when choosing an initial regimen include the patient's medical comorbidities (cardiovascular, renal, psychiatric disease), pregnancy or the potential to become pregnant, and coinfections with tuberculosis, hepatitis C virus, and hepatitis B virus (HBV).

The currently recommended ART for treatment-naïve patients usually includes two NRTIs, abacavir/lamivudine (ABC/3TC, [Epzicom]), or either tenofovir alafenamide/emtricitabine (TAF/FTC, [Descovy]) or tenofovir disoproxil fumarate (TDF/FTC, [Truvada]), plus an agent from one of the following classes: INSTI, NNRTI, or a PK-enhanced PI. These recommendations are based on regimens that are well tolerated, have convenient dosing, and provide excellent virologic suppression.

The NRTI combinations of ABC/3TC, TAF/FTC, and TDF/FTC are available as fixed-dose combination tablets. The 3TC and FTC components have few adverse effects. The main differences between these combinations involve ABC, TAF, and TDF. The advantages of TAF and TDF include activity against HBV, and HLA-B*5701 testing is not required prior to use. TDF has some association with lower lipid levels when compared to TAF, but also may cause decline in renal function and reduced bone mineral density. TAF is associated with less bone and kidney toxicity and its use is preferred in patients with underlying bone and kidney disease or those at risk for these conditions. The advantage of ABC is that it has less bone mineral loss and less nephrotoxicity than TDF and does not require dose adjustment in patients with renal insufficiency. Potential drawbacks to ABC include an observed association with cardiovascular events in some studies and a hypersensitivity syndrome, necessitating screening for HLA-B*5701 prior to treatment initiation.

Once the combination NRTI backbone has been chosen, a third drug from either the INSTI, PI, or NNRTI drug classes must be added to the regimen. Current recommendations for most treatment-naïve HIV patients favor the INSTI class due to its high efficacy, fewer side effects, and no significant CYP3A4-associated drug interactions.

Darunavir (DRV, [Prezista])-based regimens may still be preferred in certain patients with difficulty maintaining medication adherence, and a high genetic barrier to resistance is favored or in a situation when ART should be initiated prior to receipt of resistance test results. Darunavir boosted with ritonavir (Norvir) (DRV/r) has a low rate of transmitted PI resistance, high genetic barrier to resistance, and a low rate of treatment-emergent resistance. Dolutegravir (DTG, [Tivicay]) is also a consideration for patients in whom it is necessary to initiate ART prior to resistance testing results due to its high barrier of resistance.

NNRTI-based regimens include efavirenz (EFV, [Sustiva]), rilpivirine (RPV, [Edurant]), or doravirine (DOR, [Pifeltro]) and may be appropriate choices in certain patients with good medication adherence. These medications have a low genetic barrier to resistance. EFV has minimal PK interactions with rifamycins, which makes it an excellent option in patients requiring treatment for tuberculosis. EFV has a high rate of central nervous system-related side effects, which lowers its overall tolerability for some patients. RPV has fewer side effects than EFV, but its virologic efficacy is reduced in patients with high baseline HIV RNA and low CD4 counts.

Monitoring Response to Antiretroviral Therapy

HIV disease progression and response to ART can be monitored via CD4 T lymphocyte (CD4) cell count and HIV RNA (viral load). CD4 count should be measured prior to initiation of ART and provides information regarding the patient's immune function and risk of OI. Recommendations for monitoring viral load and CD4 count are shown in Table 3.

CD4 counts can be highly variable, and significant change is only considered with 30% difference in absolute count or an increase or decrease in CD4 percentage by 3 percentage points. CD4 cell recovery is most rapid in the first 3 months after initiating ART, later followed by more gradual increases. For most patients on ART, adequate response is considered as an increase in CD4 count in the range of 50 to 150 cells/mm³ during the first year of treatment. Subsequent increases may average 50 to 100 cells/mm³ per year until a steady-state level is reached. Peripheral blood CD4 cell counts in most HIV patients will continue to increase over a decade as long as viral suppression is maintained. Most individuals will eventually recover CD4 counts within the normal range (>500 cells/mm³). For approximately 15% to 20% of patients, especially those that initiate ART at very low CD4 counts (<200 cells/mm³), low CD4 counts may persist, which is associated with increased morbidity and mortality. These patients should be evaluated for reversible causes of CD4 cell lymphopenia, including offending medications, untreated coinfections, and underlying malignancy. In patients with appropriate virologic suppression, the addition of more antiretroviral agents or transitioning to a different ART regimen has not been demonstrated to improve CD4 cell recovery.

CD4 counts should be repeated 3 months after ART initiation to monitor immune reconstitution and can be monitored in many patients at 3-to-6 month intervals for the first 2 years of ART. In virally suppressed patients with consistent CD4 counts between 300 and 500 cells/mm³ for at least 2 years, CD4 can be checked annually. While ART is recommended for all patients with HIV, patients who remain untreated should have CD4 counts monitored every 3 to 6 months to assess for the need for OI prophylaxis.

Viral load functions as a marker for ART response and should be monitored at initiation of therapy and regularly thereafter. Pre-treatment viral load can also provide useful information regarding selection of an initial ART. Commercially available HIV-1 RNA assays do not detect HIV-2 viral load. Decreases in viral load following ART initiation are associated with a reduction in risk of disease progression to AIDS or death. Optimal viral suppression is defined as a viral load persistently below the level of detection. Low-level viremia refers to a patient with confirmed detectable HIV RNA less than 200 copies/mL. This may be detected using real-time polymerase chain reaction (PCR) assays and may be predictive of developing viral rebound. Viral rebound, or virologic failure, is considered to occur when a patient with

GENERIC NAME (TRADE NAME) AND RECOMMENDED ADULT DOSING	SINGLE TABLET REGIMEN?	IMPORTANT POINTS
INSTI + 2 NRTIs		
Elvitegravir/cobicistat/tenofovir alafenamide/emtricitabine (Genvoya) 150/150/10/200 mg—1 tablet by mouth once daily OR Elvitegravir/cobicistat/tenofovir disoproxil fumarate/emtricitabine (Stribild) 150/150/300/200 mg—1 tablet by mouth once daily	Yes	Genvoya generally preferred over Stribild due to fewer bone and kidney toxicities Drug interactions with other medications are prevalent with both products due to cobicistat, a CYP3A4 inhibitor
Raltegravir (Isentress HD) 600 mg—2 tablets by mouth once daily OR Raltegravir (Isentress) 400 mg—1 tablet by mouth twice daily PLUS Abacavir/Lamivudine (Epzicom) 600/300 mg—1 tablet by mouth once daily	No	Isentress HD generally preferred over Isentress due to once daily dosing. Must be confirmed HLA-B*5701 negative before starting to avoid abacavir hypersensitivity reaction
NNRTI + 2 NRTIs		
Rilpivirine/tenofovir alafenamide/emtricitabine (Odefsey) 25/25/200 mg—1 tablet by mouth once daily OR Rilpivirine/tenofovir disoproxil fumarate/emtricitabine (Complera) 25/300/200 mg—1 tablet by mouth once daily	Yes	Rilpivirine should only be used if HIV RNA <100,000 copies/mL and CD4 >200 cells/mm^3 Odefsey generally preferred over Complera due to fewer bone and kidney toxicities PPIs contraindicated with rilpivirine. H2 blockers may be used once daily but must be spaced 12 hours apart from rilpivirine. Should be taken with food
Doravirine/tenofovir disoproxil fumarate/lamivudine (Delstrigo) 100/300/300 mg—1 tablet by mouth once daily OR Doravirine (Pifeltro) 100 mg—1 tablet by mouth once daily PLUS Tenofovir alafenamide/emtricitabine (Descovy) 25/200 mg—1 tablet by mouth once daily	Yes, for Delstrigo	May be taken with or without food. Doravirine does not have any restrictions with acid-suppressive medications
Efavirenz/tenofovir disoproxil fumarate/emtricitabine (Atripla) 600/300/200 mg—1 tablet by mouth once daily	Yes	High rates of neuropsychiatric adverse effects (e.g., vivid dreams, depression, suicidal ideation)
PK-Enhanced PI + 2 NRTIs		
Darunavir/cobicistat/emtricitabine/tenofovir alafenamide (Symtuza) 800/150/200/10 mg—1 tablet by mouth once daily OR Darunavir/cobicistat (Prezcobix) 800/150 mg—1 tablet by mouth once daily OR Darunavir (Prezista) 800 mg—1 tablet by mouth once daily + Ritonavir (Norvir) 100 mg—1 tablet by mouth once daily PLUS Tenofovir alafenamide/emtricitabine (Descovy) 25/200 mg—1 tablet by mouth once daily OR Tenofovir disoproxil fumarate/emtricitabine (Truvada) 300/200 mg—1 tablet by mouth once daily OR Abacavir/Lamivudine (Epzicom) 600/300 mg—1 tablet by mouth once daily	Yes, for Symtuza	Prezcobix generally preferred over the combination of Prezista and Norvir due to single tablet and potentially fewer GI side effects and drug interactions Drug interactions with other medications are prevalent with both cobicistat and ritonavir due to CYP3A4 inhibition. Ritonavir also inhibits and induces several other CYP enzymes. Careful attention should be given to manage drug interactions Descovy generally preferred over Truvada due to fewer bone and kidney toxicities. If using Epzicom, must be confirmed HLA-B*5701 negative before starting to avoid abacavir hypersensitivity reaction
Atazanavir/cobicistat (Evotaz) 300/150 mg—1 tablet by mouth once daily OR Atazanavir (Reyataz) 300 mg—1 tablet by mouth once daily + Ritonavir (Norvir) 100 mg—1 tablet by mouth once daily PLUS Tenofovir alafenamide/emtricitabine (Descovy) 25/200 mg—1 tablet by mouth once daily OR Tenofovir disoproxil fumarate/emtricitabine (Truvada) 300/200 mg—1 tablet by mouth once daily	No	Darunavir-containing regimens generally preferred over atazanavir-containing regimens Atazanavir is known to increase serum bilirubin. This generally does not require further workup if patient is asymptomatic Evotaz generally preferred over the combination of Reyataz and Norvir due to single tablet and potentially fewer GI side effects and drug interactions Drug interactions with other medications are prevalent with both cobicistat and ritonavir due to CYP3A4 inhibition. Ritonavir also inhibits and induces several other CYP enzymes. Careful attention should be given to manage drug interactions Descovy generally preferred over Truvada due to fewer bone and kidney toxicities

CYP3A4, Cytochrome P450 3A4; H2, histamine H2 receptor; HLA, human leukocyte antigen; INSTI, integrase strand transfer inhibitor; NNRTI, nonnucleoside reverse transcriptase inhibitor; NRTI, nucleoside reverse transcriptase inhibitor; PI, protease inhibitor; PPI, proton pump inhibitor.
Adapted from Panel on Antiretroviral Guidelines for Adults and Adolescents. Guidelines for the Use of Antiretroviral Agents in Adults and Adolescents Living with HIV. Department of Health and Human Services. Available at http://aidsinfo.nih.gov/contentfiles/lvguidelines/AdultandAdolescentGL.pdf. Section accessed April 18, 2019 (Table 6).

TABLE 3	Recommendations on the Indications and Frequency of Viral Load and CD4 Count.		
CLINICAL SCENARIO	**VIRAL LOAD MONITORING**		**CD4 COUNT MONITORING**
Before initiating ART	At entry into care If ART initiation is deferred, repeat before initiating ART. In patients not initiating ART, repeat testing is optional		At entry into care If ART is deferred, every 3–6 months
After initiating ART	Preferably within 2–4 weeks (and no later than 8 weeks) after initiation of ART; thereafter, every 4–8 weeks until viral load (VL) is suppressed		3 months after initiation of ART
After modifying ART because of drug toxicities or for regimen simplification in a patient with viral suppression	4–8 weeks after modification of ART to confirm effectiveness of new regimen		Monitor according to prior CD4 count and duration on ART, as outlined below.
After modifying ART because of virologic failure	Preferably within 2–4 weeks (and no later than 8 weeks) after modification; thereafter, every 4–8 weeks until viral load is suppressed. If viral suppression is not possible, repeat viral load every 3 months or more frequently if indicated		Every 3–6 months
During the first 2 years of ART	Every 3–4 months		Every 3–6 months
After 2 years of ART (VL consistently suppressed, CD4 consistently 300–500 cells/mm^3) After 2 years of ART (VL consistently suppressed, CD4 consistently >500 cells/mm^3)	Can extend to every 6 months for patients with consistent viral suppression for greater than or equal to 2 years		Every 12 months Optional
While on ART with detectable viremia (VL repeatedly >200 copies/mL)	Every 3 months or more frequently if clinically indicated		Every 3–6 months
Change in clinical status	Every 3 months		Perform CD4 count and repeat as clinically indicated

ART, Antiretroviral therapy; *VL,* viral load Adapted from Panel on Antiretroviral Guidelines for Adults and Adolescents. *Guidelines for the Use of Antiretroviral Agents in Adults and Adolescents Living with HIV.* Department of Health and Human Services.

confirmed virologic suppression has HIV RNA greater than or equal to 1000 copies/mL. If virologic suppression occurs and the patient is found to have a single isolated detectable HIV RNA level with return to virologic suppression in subsequent tests, this is referred to as a virologic blip. This is not usually associated with virologic failure, and they do not require a change in ART. Acute illness, stress, and recent immunizations are a few potential causes of virologic blips. A repeat viral load can be rechecked in 3 months to confirm return to appropriate viral suppression.

If a patient has a very high HIV viral load at the time of ART initiation, it may take several weeks for a measurable virologic response to occur. Certain ART regimens may also have slower rates of virologic suppression than others. A patient who has received ART for at least 24 weeks and has not yet had documented virologic suppression should be evaluated for antiretroviral drug resistance.

Treatment Failure

Patients receiving ART who do not achieve HIV RNA levels below the lower limit of detection or who are shown to have sustained virologic rebound are at risk for developing resistance mutations to their current ART regimen, especially at HIV RNA levels greater than 500 copies/mL. Virologic failure has a strong association with suboptimal medication adherence and drug intolerance/toxicity leading to self-discontinuation of ART.

Some factors that may increase the risk of ART nonadherence include active substance use, neurocognitive impairment, and mental health disorders. Unstable housing and other socioeconomic and psychosocial factors can make ART adherence particularly difficult. The patient's inability to afford the medication may lead to intermittent adherence or nonadherence. Some patients will stop taking ART due to adverse effects of their regimen. Others may not be able to adhere to a high pill burden or frequency of dosing.

Less common causes of treatment failure include existing or newly developed drug resistance. Patients with HIV-2 or HIV-1/ HIV-2 coinfection can have innate resistance to certain ART regimens. Others may have adverse drug–drug interactions with other medications, suboptimal virologic potency, or error in their medication prescription.

If a patient is experiencing virologic failure, it is important to determine the cause because there is potential for choosing a subsequent therapy regimen that promotes better adherence. Management of a patient experiencing treatment failure is often complex and benefits from consultation with an HIV specialist.

Drug Resistance and Resistance Testing

Two types of resistance assays exist to assess viral strains and direct treatment strategies: genotypic and phenotypic. These assays provide useful information regarding resistance to NRTIs, NNRTIs, PIs, and INSTIs. In some settings, INSTI resistance tests must be ordered separately. In patients with newly diagnosed HIV infection, resistance testing can guide therapy selection to optimize virologic response. Genotypic assays detect drug resistance mutations by sequencing reverse transcriptase, protease, and integrase genes. Interpreting these test results requires knowledge of the mutations selected by different antivirals and the potential for cross-resistance to other drugs. Clinical trials have shown that consulting with HIV specialists regarding drug resistance interpretation improves virologic outcomes.

Adverse Drug Reactions and Drug-Drug Interactions

Adverse drug reactions to ART are common, especially when first initiating therapy. Generally, reactions such as nausea, fatigue, and headache often resolve within 1 to 2 weeks of starting ART. Severe or persistent adverse drug reactions should prompt consideration of change to a different agent. Each ART drug class has different characteristic adverse drug reactions. Additionally, each individual ART agent carries its own characteristic adverse drug reactions (Table 4). As drug therapies have evolved and new medications discovered, preferred agents have been updated to avoid those

TABLE 4	Monitoring Recommendations for Antiretroviral Toxicity of Selected Drugs.	
DRUG	**TOXICITY**	**MONITORING**
NRTIs		
Abacavir (Ziagen)	Liver Abacavir hypersensitivity syndrome	LFTs Screening for HLA-B*5701 (should be confirmed negative prior to abacavir initiation) Symptoms of abacavir hypersensitivity may include fever, rash, nausea, vomiting, diarrhea, abdominal pain, malaise, fatigue, or respiratory symptoms such as sore throat, cough, or shortness of breath
Emtricitabine (Emtriva)	Minimal toxicity Liver Hyperpigmentation/skin discoloration	Serum creatinine LFTs Hepatitis B (prior to initiation of therapy) Severe acute exacerbation of hepatitis may occur in patients with HBV/HIV coinfection who discontinue emtricitabine. In patients where discontinuation of tenofovir is necessary, ensure an agent active against HBV is administered
Lamivudine (Epivir)	Minimal toxicity Liver	Serum creatinine LFTs Hepatitis B (prior to initiation of therapy) Severe acute exacerbation of hepatitis may occur in patients with HBV/HIV coinfection who discontinue lamivudine. In patients where discontinuation of tenofovir is necessary, ensure an agent active against HBV is administered
Tenofovir (disoproxil fumarate [Viread], alafenamide [Vemlidy])	Renal toxicity (tubulopathy) Decreases in bone mineral density Liver	Serum creatinine Urine glucose and protein (prior to initiation and as clinically indicated during therapy) Serum phosphorus (in patients with chronic kidney disease) Bone mineral density testing (if history of bone fracture or risk factors for bone loss) LFTs Hepatitis B (prior to initiation of therapy) Tenofovir alafenamide (Vemlidy) is associated with lower rates of bone and kidney toxicity compared to tenofovir disoproxil fumarate Severe acute exacerbation of hepatitis may occur in patients with HBV/HIV coinfection who discontinue tenofovir. In patients where discontinuation of tenofovir is necessary, ensure an agent active against HBV is administered
NNRTIs		
Efavirenz (Sustiva)	Rash Neuropsychiatric symptoms Hyperlipidemia Hepatotoxicity QT interval prolongation	LFTs Lipid panel (prior to therapy periodically during) Signs and symptoms of neuropsychiatric effects (e.g., vivid dreams, depression, suicidal ideation)
Rilpivirine (Edurant)	Rash Depression, insomnia, headache Hepatotoxicity QT interval prolongation	LFTs Lipid panel
PIs		
All	GI intolerance, nausea, vomiting, diarrhea Hyperglycemia Insulin resistance Hepatotoxicity Fat maldistribution Hyperlipidemia	Serum glucose LFTs (at baseline and as clinically indicated thereafter)
Atazanavir (Reyataz)	Indirect hyperbilirubinemia	Bilirubin
Darunavir (Prezista)	Skin rash	Darunavir contains a sulfonamide moiety; Stevens-Johnson syndrome, toxic epidermal necrolysis, acute generalized exanthematous pustulosis, and erythema have been reported. Risk of cross-reactivity between darunavir and sulfonamide medications is very low. However, use caution in patients with severe sulfonamide allergies

Continued

TABLE 4	Monitoring Recommendations for Antiretroviral Toxicity of Selected Drugs.—cont'd	
DRUG	**TOXICITY**	**MONITORING**
INSTIs		
All	INSTIs typically well tolerated for most patients GI intolerance Insomnia Headache Depression and suicidal ideation (rare, usually in patients with pre-existing psychiatric conditions) CPK elevation, muscle weakness, and rhabdomyolysis (primarily reported with raltegravir [Isentress])	LFTs Serum creatinine (dolutegravir [Tivicay] and bictegravir) CPK (if signs of muscle toxicity)

CPK, Creatinine phosphokinase; *GI,* gastrointestinal; *HBV,* hepatitis B virus; *HIV,* human immunodeficiency virus; *HLA,* human leukocyte antigen; *INSTI,* integrase strand transfer inhibitor; *LFT,* liver function test; *NNRTI,* nonnucleoside reverse transcriptase inhibitor; *NRTI,* nucleoside reverse transcriptase inhibitor; *PI,* protease inhibitor. Table is not all inclusive.
Adapted from Panel on Antiretroviral Guidelines for Adults and Adolescents. Guidelines for the Use of Antiretroviral Agents in Adults and Adolescents Living with HIV. Department of Health and Human Services. Available at http://aidsinfo.nih.gov/contentfiles/lvguidelines/AdultandAdolescentGL.pdf. Section accessed April 18, 2019 (Appendix B, Tables 1–4).

that tended to cause more frequent and severe adverse effects. For example, older agents in the NRTI class (e.g., stavudine [Zerit] and didanosine [Videx]) were commonly associated with hepatic steatosis, lipodystrophy, and insulin resistance. Newer generation NRTIs, which have much lower rates of these serious adverse effects, have largely supplanted the use of these older drugs.

All providers caring for patients who receive ART should be aware of the possibility of antiretroviral drug-drug interactions. The use of the pharmacokinetic enhancing agents, ritonavir (Norvir) and cobicistat (Tybost), in many combination ART regimens can pose serious risks to patients receiving other drugs metabolized through the cytochrome P450 pathway, including numerous anticoagulant drugs and synthetic glucocorticoids. When prescribing or altering one or more drugs in an ART regimen, the potential for drug interactions must be explored. It is critical to carefully review the patient's other medications for potential interactions. If multiple drugs with similar or conflicting metabolic pathways are prescribed, healthcare providers should carefully monitor for appropriate therapeutic efficacy and concentration-related toxicities.

Viral Hepatitis Coinfection

Approximately 5% to 10% of patients with HIV in the United States have coinfection with chronic HBV. Disease progression to cirrhosis, end-stage liver disease, and hepatocellular carcinoma is more rapid in these patients. Some antiretroviral toxicities and complications may be attributed to flares of HBV after initiation or discontinuation of ART.

FTC, 3TC, TDF, and TAF are approved for treatment of HIV and are also active against HBV. Discontinuation of these drugs can potentially cause significant hepatic damage due to reactivation of HBV. The anti-HBV drug entecavir (Baraclude) has activity against HIV. When entecavir is used to treat HBV in patients with HBV/HIV coinfection who are not taking ART, the drug can select for M184V mutation, resulting in HIV resistance to 3TC and FTC. When 3TC is the only active drug used to treat HBV in coinfected patients, 3TC resistance develops in approximately 40% to 90% of patients after 2 to 4 years on 3TC monotherapy.

Before ART is initiated, all patients who test positive for HBV surface Ag (HBsAg) should also be tested for HBV DNA using a quantitative assay. This test should be repeated every 3 to 6 months to ensure effective HBV suppression. In patients with HBV/HIV coinfection, immune reconstitution following initiation of treatment for HIV, HBV, or both can be associated with elevated transaminases.

Complications

Diagnosis and Management of Opportunistic Infections (OI)

The widespread availability and use of ART has significantly reduced OI-related mortality in persons with HIV infection. OIs continue to cause considerable morbidity and mortality, however, due to the increasing number of undiagnosed cases of HIV and those with known HIV infection but who are not on ART or unable to maintain adherence to ART.

Pneumocystis pneumonia (PJP) is an infection caused by a ubiquitous fungus, *P. jirovecii.* Most cases occur in patients with an advanced compromised immune system (CD4 count <100 cells/mm³). The most common manifestations are dyspnea, fever, nonproductive cough, and chest discomfort. Onset of symptoms is usually subacute and progressive over days to weeks. Mild cases may present with normal pulmonary physical exam findings at rest but develop dyspnea, tachycardia, and rales with exertion. Hypoxemia is often present to varying severity. Lab findings are consistent with lactate dehydrogenase levels greater than 500 mg/dL and elevated serum 1,3 β-d-glucan. Chest radiography may show diffuse, bilateral, ground-glass interstitial infiltrates, but chest radiography can appear unremarkable in patients with early disease. In patients with normal chest plain films, computed tomography (CT) of the chest can show underlying abnormalities consistent with PJP. HIV-infected patients, including pregnant women and those on ART, should receive PJP chemoprophylaxis if they have CD4 counts less than 200 cells/mm³. Patients receiving pyrimethamine (Daraprim)-sulfadiazine for treatment or suppression of toxoplasmosis do not require additional prophylaxis for PJP. Trimethoprim-sulfamethoxazole (TMP-SMX, [Bactrim]) is the first-line prophylactic agent at one double-strength tablet daily (which also confers prophylaxis against toxoplasmosis[1]) or three times weekly. In those who cannot tolerate TMP-SMX, alternative prophylactic options include dapsone[1], dapsone plus pyrimethamine[1] plus leucovorin[1], aerosolized pentamidine (Nebupent), and atovaquone (Mepron).

Toxoplasma gondii is a protozoan infection and is associated with reactivation of latent tissue cysts. Patients at greatest risk have CD4 counts less than 50 cells/μL. Clinical disease is rare in patients with CD4 counts greater than 200 cells/μL. In patients with AIDS, the typical presentation of infection is focal encephalitis including headache, confusion, focal motor weakness, and fever. In the absence of treatment, disease progression may lead to seizures, coma, and death. CT and MRI of the brain may show multiple contrast-enhancing lesions within the gray matter of the cortex or basal ganglia, often with associated edema. HIV-infected patients with toxoplasma encephalitis are usually seropositive for toxoplasma IgG antibodies. Definitive diagnosis requires the combination of clinical presentation, identification of one or more mass lesions via CT or MRI, and detection of the organism in a sample, with brain biopsy being the most preferred

---

[1] Not FDA approved for this indication.

method. Therapy of choice includes pyrimethamine plus sulfadiazine plus leucovorin[1].

Disseminated *Mycobacterium avium* Complex (MAC) disease typically occurs in patients with CD4 counts less than 50 cells/mm³. Other factors associated with increased susceptibility to MAC disease include HIV RNA levels greater than 100,000 copies/mL, previous OIs, and previous colonization of the respiratory or gastrointestinal tract with MAC. In HIV-infected patients with AIDS who are not on ART, MAC disease usually presents as a disseminated, multiorgan infection. Symptoms may be minimal at first but may include fever, night sweats, weight loss, diarrhea, fatigue, and nonspecific abdominal pain. Lab abnormalities may include anemia out of proportion for that expected from HIV alone and an increase in liver alkaline phosphatase. Physical exam or imaging may note nonspecific hepatomegaly, lymphadenopathy, and/or splenomegaly. Diagnosis is based on a combination of clinical symptoms and the isolation of MAC from cultures obtained from blood, lymph nodes, bone marrow, or other sterile sites. Initial treatment should consist of at least two antimycobacterial medications in an effort to prevent the development of resistance. Infectious disease specialists should be consulted regarding treatment. MAC isolates should be tested for susceptibility to clarithromycin (Biaxin) and azithromycin (Zithromax).

Cryptococcus neoformans meningitis occurs more commonly in patients with CD4 counts less than 100 cells/µL. It can present as a subacute or acute meningoencephalitis associated with fever, headache, and malaise. Classic meningeal symptoms may be absent. Disseminated disease is usually present when diagnosed in a patient with HIV infection and can involve virtually any organ. Diagnosis of meningitis via cerebral spinal fluid (CSF) often demonstrates elevated opening pressure, elevated protein, low-to-normal glucose, and lymphocytic pleocytosis. Numerous yeast forms may be visualized on Gram stain or India ink preparations of CSF. CSF cryptococcal antigen (CrAg) is often positive. Serum CrAg may be positive in both meningeal and nonmeningeal involving infections and its presence can be detected weeks to months prior to the onset of symptoms. A positive serum CrAg should proceed to lumbar puncture to rule out meningeal disease. Treatment of cryptococcosis occurs in three stages: induction, consolidation, and maintenance therapy.

CMV disease can cause disseminated and localized end-organ damage in HIV-infected patients with suppressed immune states with CD4 counts less than 50 cells/mm.³ Clinical disease is usually the result of reactivation of latent infection. Risk factors include not receiving or failing to respond to ART, previous OIs, high level of CMV viremia, and high HIV viral load (>100,000 copies/mL). Retinitis is the most common clinical manifestation of CMV end-organ disease and is often unilateral but can progress to bilateral if therapy or immune recovery are not pursued. Retinitis may present with floaters, scotomata, or peripheral visual field defects. Colitis is another manifestation of CMV disease and may be associated with weight loss, abdominal pain, significant diarrhea, and malaise. Hemorrhage and bowel perforation can be life-threatening. CMV viremia can be measured via PCR and is usually present in end-organ disease.

Mucocutaneous candidiasis of the oropharynx and esophagus occurs commonly in HIV-infected patients and is often an indication of underlying immune suppression (CD4 count <200 cells/mm³). Oropharyngeal candidiasis is usually painless and affects the oropharyngeal mucosa and tongue surface. Esophageal candidiasis may be associated with retrosternal discomfort and odynophagia. Oropharyngeal candidiasis is usually diagnosed clinically. Diagnosis of esophageal candidiasis is made based on symptoms, response to therapy, or visualization of mucosal lesions on examination.

Many treatment guidelines recommend initiating ART within 2 weeks for most diagnosed OI. In patients with cryptococcal meningitis and possible tuberculous meningitis, ART should be deferred due to the risks of serious immune reconstitution

syndrome outweighing the benefits of ART. In patients with AIDS-associated OI for which no effective therapy exists (e.g., progressive multifocal leukoencephalopathy, cryptosporidiosis, and microsporidiosis), improvement in immune function with ART can potentially improve disease outcomes.

Neurologic

Both central nervous system disease and peripheral nerve abnormalities are common in advanced AIDS. HIV infection can directly cause distal sensory neuropathy, which may manifest as dysesthesia or hypersensitivity, decreased reflexes, and chronic neuropathic pain. Inflammatory demyelinating polyneuropathy (e.g., Guillain-Barré syndrome), which has known associations with some enteric pathogens and causes ascending motor weakness, typically without sensory involvement. CMV infection may cause polyradiculopathy, transverse myelitis, and encephalitis/ventriculitis in patients with CD4 counts lower than 50 cells/mm³. CMV end-organ disease, including retinitis (a vision-threatening condition), requires prompt diagnosis and initiation of appropriate anti-CMV therapy.

Focal central nervous system lesions can arise from infectious and malignant conditions. Cerebral toxoplasmosis usually occurs in patients with prior exposure to *T. gondii* who develop reactivation disease when the CD4 count is lower than 100 cells/mm³. The main differential diagnosis for one or several enhancing brain lesions includes toxoplasmosis and primary central nervous system lymphoma (PCNSL). PCNSL is associated with Epstein-Barr virus, and detection of nucleic acid for Epstein-Barr virus in cerebrospinal fluid carries a high specificity for this condition in the proper radiographic context. Progressive multifocal leukoencephalopathy (PML), a rare and potentially devastating demyelinating condition, is caused by reactivation of JC virus and can manifest as focal neurologic deficit, seizures, or cognitive dysfunction. *Cryptococcus neoformans* is a common cause of meningitis in AIDS patients and may manifest with central nervous system mass lesions, pulmonary disease, or gastrointestinal disease. Worldwide, tuberculosis accounts for a large proportion of HIV-associated meningitis; less commonly, it can manifest as single or multiple focal lesions (tuberculomas). Neurosyphilis should be considered in patients with unexplained neurologic disease and sexual risk factors.

Respiratory Complications

Respiratory illnesses are among the most common causes of morbidity in HIV-infected patients. Community-acquired bacterial pneumonia occurs at a significantly higher rate in HIV-infected compared with HIV-noninfected patients, regardless of CD4 count, and is one of the most common reasons for hospitalization. *P. jirovecii* (formerly *Pneumocystis carinii*) pneumonia (PCP) manifests with fever, cough, and dyspnea. Findings on physical examination and chest radiography can be variable, making the diagnosis difficult in the absence of high clinical suspicion. Elevated lactate dehydrogenase and oxygen desaturation with ambulation can be diagnostic clues. More than 90% of cases occur among patients with CD4 counts lower than 200 cells/mm³. The diagnosis is established by visualization of organisms in induced sputum (sensitivity, 50% to 90%) or in bronchoalveolar lavage specimens (sensitivity, 90% to 99%), most commonly with the use of immunofluorescent staining.

The risk of reactivation of latent TB is increased 100-fold in patients with HIV infection. Patients with HIV infection who are latently infected have a 10% annual risk of developing symptomatic tuberculosis, compared with a 10% lifetime risk among the general population. The risk of reactivation increases with decreasing CD4 count, and patients with counts lower than 350 cells/mm³ are more likely to have atypical radiographic presentations, including middle- and lower-lobe infiltrates without cavitation. Patients with low CD4 counts are more likely to have extrapulmonary tuberculosis. Diagnostic approaches to tuberculosis in patients with HIV infection are similar to those in patients without it. Tuberculin skin testing can be used to diagnose latent tuberculosis infection, although the recommended cutoff for a

---

[1] Not FDA approved for this indication.

positive test is 5 mm of induration. Treatment of coinfection with *Mycobacterium tuberculosis* and HIV requires consultation with experienced clinicians and pharmacists because of extensive drug–drug interactions among antiretroviral drugs and rifamycins.

Gastrointestinal Complications

Oropharyngeal candidiasis (thrush) commonly manifests as white plaques on the tongue, palate, or buccal mucosa that are painless and are easily scraped off. Although thrush is typically uncomplicated and easily treatable with topical preparations such as nystatin (Mycostatin) and clotrimazole (Mycelex troches), in the proper clinical setting it can alert the clinician to the presence of esophageal candidiasis. Esophageal involvement should be suspected in patients with dysphagia and odynophagia; retrosternal chest pain may also be present. Thrush is usually present but is not required for the diagnosis, which is often made on clinical grounds rather than being confirmed with endoscopy. Patients with esophageal candidiasis typically respond after several days of treatment, and 7 to 14 days of antifungal therapy is usually sufficient. For cases not responsive to empiric treatment for candidiasis, referral for endoscopy should be considered. Esophagitis caused by CMV or herpes simplex virus requires a histopathologic diagnosis.

Acute diarrhea, defined as three or more loose or watery stools per day for 3 to 10 days, is common among patients with HIV infection, and more than 1000 different enteric pathogens have been described. Data from a large cohort indicate that the most common pathogens isolated are *Clostridium difficile*, *Shigella* spp., *Campylobacter jejuni*, *Salmonella* spp., *Staphylococcus aureus*, and MAC. Culture of the stool can yield a microbiologic diagnosis in many cases, particularly for acute diarrheal illnesses caused by *Campylobacter*, *Yersinia*, *Salmonella*, and *Shigella* species. Infection with *C. difficile*, the most common bacterial enteric pathogen in the United States for both HIV-infected and HIV-uninfected persons, is diagnosed in most settings by detection of cytotoxin in the stool by enzyme immunoassay (EIA) or PCR, although the more laborious tissue culture is considered the gold standard. Enteric viruses are present in 15% to 30% of HIV-infected persons with acute diarrhea. Definitive diagnosis is not feasible in most clinical laboratories; viral enteritis should be suspected in the setting of community outbreaks because of the high transmissibility of viral pathogens. Treatment is supportive with fluid resuscitation and antimotility agents.

Chronic diarrhea (duration 30 days) was a common manifestation of advanced-stage AIDS in the pre-HAART era. Most pathogens that cause acute gastroenteritis can also cause chronic symptoms. Pathogens that should be suspected in cases of chronic watery diarrhea include protozoa such as *Cryptosporidium parvum*, *Isospora belli*, and *Microsporidia* spp. These entities are self-limited in the absence of severe immunosuppression. In advanced HIV infection, pathogen-specific antimicrobial therapy is infrequently effective, and symptoms commonly do not improve without immune reconstitution in response to ART. *Giardia lamblia* causes watery diarrhea, abdominal bloating, and occasionally malabsorption syndrome, and can occur at any CD4 count. CMV infection can affect any segment of the gastrointestinal tract and is a common cause of chronic diarrhea. Diagnosis of gastrointestinal CMV disease is difficult without biopsy. Detection of CMV viremia with PCR does not correlate well with presence of CMV disease in HIV-infected patients, and CMV can be undetectable in serum in patients with extensive gastrointestinal disease.

Other Conditions

ART has dramatically increased the survival of individuals living with HIV, and the HIV elderly population is expanding. There are few clinical trials or studies systematically focused on this cohort. Older adults with HIV may develop comorbidities that can complicate their HIV management. ART-related CD4 cell recovery in older patients has been observed to be slower and with lower magnitude than in younger patients. Hepatic and renal functions

decrease as the body ages and may lead to impaired drug elimination and increased drug exposure in older patients.

Immune Reconstitution Inflammatory Syndrome

Immune reconstitution inflammatory syndrome (IRIS) is a collection of inflammatory disorders often associated with paradoxical worsening of preexisting infectious diseases after initiation of ART. IRIS is usually accompanied by an increase in CD4 count and can occur at any CD4 count. It usually occurs between the first 4 to 8 weeks after initiation of ART. Clinical features are often associated with the type and location of the preexisting OI and can be localized or systemic. Patients should continue on ART and should receive treatment for the underlying OI as quickly as possible. If the patient's presentation involves paradoxical worsening of a previously diagnosed OI that is already receiving treatment, OI therapy should also be continued. Disseminated MAC accounts for up to one-third of the cases of IRIS in the United States. Other important causes of IRIS are tuberculosis, CMV infection, viral hepatitis, and candida infections.

Management of HIV in Pregnancy and Women of Childbearing Potential

HIV in Pregnant Women

All pregnant women with HIV should be on ART regardless of their immunologic or virologic status in order to improve the patient's health and prevent transmission of HIV to the fetus. Increased perinatal transmission risk exists in pregnant women experiencing early HIV infection and high-level viremia. All pregnant women with newly diagnosed HIV infection should start ART as soon as possible to prevent perinatal HIV transmission. The goal of ART is to achieve and sustain viral suppression throughout the pregnancy. In a pregnant woman with newly diagnosed HIV, ART should be initiated as soon as possible. Resistance testing should be performed prior to initiating ART, but therapy may be started before receiving resistance testing results. ART regimen can be modified at a later date once resistance testing results are available.

In a patient already taking a regimen containing efavirenz (EFV, [Sustiva]) who presents for prenatal care during the first trimester and has virologic suppression, EFV can be continued. The risk of fetal neural tube defects is limited to the first 5 to 6 weeks of pregnancy, and pregnancy is often not recognized before weeks 4 to 6. Unnecessary changes to a patient's ART regimen during pregnancy may result in loss of viral suppression with increased risk of perinatal transmission.

In a pregnant patient with an HIV RNA viral load greater than or equal to 1000 copies/mL (or viral load is unknown) near delivery, IV infusion of zidovudine (Retrovir) during labor is recommended regardless of the patient's antepartum ART regimen or resistance profile. Maternal ART should be continued following delivery. Following delivery, the patient should continue to follow up with their HIV care provider as recommended for nonpregnant adults.

Maternal adherence to ART reduces but does not completely eliminate the risk of transmission of HIV in breast milk. Postnatal HIV transmission can occur despite maternal ART adherence, and patients should be counseled to avoid breastfeeding. There have also been reports of mother-to-child transmission of HIV via mothers pre-masticating food and feeding it to their infants.

Preexposure Prophylaxis of HIV Infection

Globally, up to 2 million new HIV infections occur per year. It is estimated that up to 50,000 new HIV infections occur annually in the United States. The highest incidence of new HIV infection occurs in men who have sex with men (MSM), especially young African-American males. For uninfected patients with a high risk of HIV acquisition, preexposure prophylaxis (PrEP) is an evidence-based method for preventing infections in those at risk. Since 2012, tenofovir disoproxil fumarate-emtricitabine (TDF-FTC, [Truvada]) has been approved for PrEP and is at least

TABLE 5	Preexposure Prophylaxis.		
	MEN WHO HAVE SEX WITH MEN	**HETEROSEXUAL WOMEN AND MEN**	**INJECTION DRUG USERS**
Detecting substantial risk of acquiring HIV infection	HIV-positive sexual partner Recent bacterial STI High number of sex partners History of inconsistent or no condom use Commercial sex work	HIV-positive sexual partner Recent bacterial STI High number of sex partners History of inconsistent or no condom use Commercial sex work In high-prevalence area or network	HIV-positive injection partner Sharing injection equipment
Clinical eligibility	Documented negative HIV test result before prescribing PrEP No signs/symptoms of acute HIV infection Normal renal function; no contraindicated medications Documented hepatitis B infection and vaccination status		
Prescription	Daily, continuing, oral doses of FTC/TDF (Truvada), ≤90 day supply		
Other services	Follow-up visits at least every 3 months to provide the following: HIV test, medication adherence counseling, behavioral risk reduction support, side-effect assessment, STI symptom assessment At 3 months and every 6 months thereafter, assess renal function Every 6 months, test for bacterial STIs		
	Do oral/rectal STI testing	For women, assess pregnancy intent Pregnancy test every 3 months	Access to clean syringes/needles and drug treatment services

STI, Sexually transmitted infection.
Preexposure Prophylaxis for the Prevention of HIV Infection in the Unites States—2014 Clinical Practice Guideline. US Public Health Service. Available at https://www.cdc
.gov/hiv/guidelines/preventing.html. Accessed April 18, 2019 (Table 1).

90% effective in reducing risk of HIV transmission. Efficacy is dependent on medication adherence.

Daily oral PrEP is recommended as one HIV prevention option for people who are sexually active with men, adult heterosexually active men and women who are at increased risk of acquiring HIV infection, and adult injection drug users at increased risk of acquiring HIV infection (Table 5). PrEP therapy should be discussed with heterosexually active women and men with sexual partners known to have HIV infection to prevent virus transmission during conception and pregnancy.

Prior to initiating PrEP, it is important to obtain a detailed sexual and drug use history to identify patients likely to benefit from PrEP. Pertinent information includes frequency of condom use, penile-anal or penile-vaginal sex, number of sex partners, HIV serostatus of sex partner(s), drug use during sex, and history of sexually transmitted infections (STIs). It is important to determine sexual practices with a patient's main sexual partner, casual partners, and whether they have any anonymous partners. A drug history over the prior 6 months should be obtained and include injection drug use and sharing of needles. The 2014 PrEP guidelines published by the US Public Health Service recommend the following questions to initiate these discussions with patients regarding their behaviors in the previous 6 months:

- Have you had sex with men, women, or both?
- (if men or both sexes) How many men/women have you had sex with?
- How many times did you have vaginal sex when neither you nor your partner wore a condom?
- How many times did you have receptive anal sex (you were the bottom) with a man who was not wearing a condom?
- How many of your male sex partners were HIV positive?
- (if any positive) With these HIV-positive male partners, how many times did you have insertive anal sex (you were the top)/vaginal sex without wearing a condom?
- Have you used methamphetamines (such as crystal meth or speed)?
- Do you have a history of STIs?

Patients screened for PrEP must be screened for common bacterial STIs including serologic testing for syphilis and nucleic acid amplification tests for gonorrhea and chlamydia. This includes swabs of the oropharynx in patients who participate in oral sex and anal swabs for recipients of anal intercourse. Screening for trichomonas and bacterial vaginosis are not required prior to initiating PrEP, as they do not have a strong correlation with HIV coinfection.

Plasma HIV testing with fourth-generation antigen/antibody test should be obtained to confirm that the patient does not have undiagnosed HIV infection. Additional HIV RNA testing should be performed in patients with signs or symptoms of acute HIV infection in the last 4 weeks, those with indeterminate antigen/antibody test results, and patients with high-risk HIV exposure in the preceding 4 weeks.

TDF-FTC is generally tolerated well by most patients; however, screening for those at increased risk of adverse effects should be performed prior to PrEP initiation. TDF is associated with acute and chronic kidney disease in HIV-infected patients. Its safety in patients without HIV and eGFR less than 60 mL/min/1.73 m² has not been documented. Serum creatinine should be measured as PrEP is not recommended for patients with estimated glomerular filtration rate less than 60 mL/min/1.73 m². No alternative PrEP regimens have been approved for patients with decreased kidney function at this time. In patients without reduced kidney function but have risk factors for developing renal disease, urinalysis to document baseline proteinuria can be obtained for monitoring purposes.

Screening for undiagnosed hepatitis B infection should be performed via hepatitis B surface antigen, hepatitis B core antibody, and hepatitis B surface antibody. If the patient's serology shows nonimmunity, vaccination against HBV should be pursued, as individuals engaging in high-risk sexual and drug-use behaviors have an increased risk of HBV infection. If the patient's serology reveals chronic HBV, it must be determined whether the patient requires HBV treatment. TDF is a first-line treatment choice for chronic HBV and can be used for PrEP and treatment of chronic HBV. In those with chronic HBV who do not require HBV treatment, there is a low risk of HBV flare if TDF is discontinued.

TDF is also associated with decreased bone density; therefore patients considering PrEP should be screened for osteoporosis risk factors. The greatest amount of bone loss has been associated with the first 6 months of treatment. In patients with known osteopenia or osteoporosis, the risk of acquiring HIV versus further bone loss must be considered. If PrEP is pursued in these patients, a baseline dual-energy x-ray absorptiometry (DXA) scan should be obtained prior to PrEP initiation if a recent test is not available. Repeat DXA testing on TDF therapy should be considered on a case-by-case basis as no guidelines for monitoring have been defined.

Females with childbearing potential should be screened for pregnancy. TDF and FTC are felt to be safe in pregnancy (category B), although some concerns have been raised regarding fetal bone development with TDF use. In patients who are pregnant, the risk of acquiring HIV must be considered against the risk of using antiretroviral medication during pregnancy. Limited data is available regarding PrEP efficacy during pregnancy.

Initiating Preexposure Prophylaxis

The combination tablet of TDF-FTC (Truvada) should be taken once daily for a duration of as long as the infection risk continues. It should be dispensed as a 90-day supply and renewed at each 3-month clinic follow-up. Condom use is encouraged while using PrEP. For patients not willing to use condoms consistently, CDC recommends condom use to prevent acquisition of HIV (and other STIs) for the first 7 days after starting PrEP if engaging in receptive anal sex and 21 days if engaging in receptive vaginal sex. Common side effects of once-daily TDF-FTC include nausea and vomiting. These symptoms usually improve and resolve within the first 4 weeks of use.

Some patients who only have discrete periods of high-risk HIV exposure may not wish to take PrEP at all times. In this situation, PrEP should be initiated at least 1 week prior to high-risk sexual activity for male patients and 3 weeks for female patients. After the period of high-risk behavior ends, PrEP should be continued for at least 1 month. This information is based on pharmacokinetic data and not clinical trials.

Preexposure Prophylaxis Monitoring AND Follow-Up

Patients on PrEP should have routine follow-up with their prescribing medical provider. The first follow-up should occur 1 month after initiating PreP and every 3 months thereafter. More frequent follow-up should occur for patients with exposures or symptoms of STIs or medication side effects.

Every 3 months, patients should be screened for HIV infection with fourth-generation antigen/antibody testing, screened for symptoms of acute HIV infection, pregnancy testing, screened for STIs appropriate for recent sexual behaviors, assessed for medication adherence as well as sexual and drug use behaviors. Serum creatinine should be monitored after the first 3 months of PrEP and can be monitored at least every 3 months thereafter in patients with risk factors for kidney disease and every 6 months for patients without kidney disease. Appropriate counseling should be provided to encourage medication adherence and reduce high-risk sexual and drug use behaviors.

Postexposure Prophylaxis of HIV Infection

The most effective means for preventing HIV infection includes preventing exposure. In the event that an isolated occupational, sexual, or injection drug-related exposure occurs, postexposure prophylaxis can be utilized as a second line of defense against HIV acquisition.

Occupational Exposure

Healthcare personnel include all paid and unpaid persons working in a healthcare setting with potential for exposure to infectious materials such as bodily fluids, contaminated medical supplies, or environmental surfaces. In the occupational setting, prevention of exposures to blood and bodily fluids from infected sources is the key to preventing occupationally acquired HIV infection. The overall risk of becoming infected with HIV after inadvertent exposure to body fluids from an HIV-infected patient is low. It is estimated that the average risk for HIV transmission following percutaneous exposure to HIV-infected blood is 0.3%

and after mucous membrane exposure is 0.09%. The average risk of HIV transmission following nonintact skin exposure has not been defined; however, it is estimated to be lower than mucous membrane exposure. Healthcare personnel at the highest risk are those who received an accidental inoculation containing blood from a known HIV-infected source.

Initial Laboratory Evaluation

All patients initiating PEP after potential HIV exposure should be tested for HIV antigens and antibodies at baseline prior to PEP initiation. If baseline HIV testing indicates existing HIV infection, PEP should not be initiated. Repeat HIV testing should be performed at 4 to 6 weeks and 3 months following the exposure to determine if HIV infection has occurred. Administration of PEP should not be delayed while awaiting the results of HIV testing and can be discontinued if the source patient is found to not have HIV infection. PEP is most effective when taken as soon as possible following exposure.

Initiating PEP/Choosing Appropriate PEP Therapy

Post-exposure prophylaxis (PEP) is most effective when initiated as soon as possible following the exposure incident. If PEP is delayed, the effectiveness of therapy may be significantly reduced if initiated 72 hours or more following exposure. Initiating therapy after 72 hours might still be considered if the exposure is proven to be of an extremely high risk of transmission.

The current recommendation for PEP therapy is FTC plus TDF (which can be dispensed as a fixed-dose combination tablet, [Truvada]) plus raltegravir (RAL, [Isentress]) for 4 weeks. Overall, this regimen has acceptable tolerability, convenient dosing, and minimal drug interactions. In patients with significant underlying renal disease, an acceptable PEP alternative is zidovudine plus lamivudine (Combivir)[1] in addition to RAL.

PEP regimens include three (occasionally more) antiretroviral medications. Due to the potential for medication-related side effects, it is important to choose a PEP regimen with a lower toxicity profile to improve patient tolerance and encourage completion of PEP therapy.

HIV PEP should be offered to pregnant or breastfeeding healthcare providers based on the same criteria as any other provider with a similar exposure. Risk of HIV transmission from mother to child during acute HIV infection is increased during pregnancy and breastfeeding.

---

[1]Not FDA approved for this indication.

Additional Resources Regarding PEP Are Available:

PEPline at http://www.nccc.ucsf.edu/about_nccc/pepline; (888)-448-4911

References

Baeten JM, Donnell D, Ndase P, et al: Antiretroviral prophylaxis for HIV prevention in heterosexual men and women, N Engl J Med 367(5):399–410, 2012.

Centers for Disease Control and Prevention. HIV Surveillance Report: Estimated HIV Incidence and Prevalence in the United States 2010–2015; vol 23.

Centers for Disease Control and Prevention: HIV Surveillance report: Diagnoses of HIV Infection in the United States and Dependent Areas, vol 28. 2016.

Dominguez KL, Smith DK, Thomas V, et al: Updated guidelines for antiretroviral postexposure prophylaxis after sexual, injection drug use, or other nonoccupational exposure to HIV-United States, Centers for Disease Control and Prevention, U.S. Department of Health and Human Services, April 18, 2016.

Grant RM, Lama JR, Anderson PL, et al: Preexposure chemoprophylaxis for HIV prevention in men who have sex with men, N Engl J Med 363(27):2587–2599, 2010.

Guidelines for the prevention and treatment of opportunistic infections in HIV-infected adults and adolescents. June 17, 2013.

Kuhar DT, Henderson DK, Struble KA, et al: Updated US Public Health Service guidelines for the management of occupational exposures to Human Immunodeficiency Virus and recommendations for postexposure prophylaxis, Infection Control and Hospital Epidemiology 34(9), 2013.

Global UNAIDS: AIDS update. Available at: http://www.unaids.org/sites/default/files/media_asset/global-AIDS-update-2016_en.pdf, 2016.

US Public Health Service. Preexposure prophylaxis for the prevention of HIV infection in the United States—2014.

INFECTIOUS MONONUCLEOSIS

Method of
Ben Z. Katz, MD

CURRENT DIAGNOSIS

- The classic triad of acute infectious mononucleosis consists of fever, lymphadenopathy, and pharyngitis.
- The diagnosis of infectious mononucleosis is usually based on the clinical picture, the presence of at least 10% atypical lymphocytes in the peripheral blood, and positive heterophil serology (monospot test).

CURRENT THERAPY

- In most patients, infectious mononucleosis is self-limited and requires only symptomatic treatment.
- Steroids and antiviral therapy have no place in the therapy of uncomplicated acute infectious mononucleosis in healthy persons.

Epidemiology and Risk Factors

One must distinguish between the epidemiology of Epstein-Barr virus (EBV) infection and that of infectious mononucleosis (IM), the most common symptomatic manifestation of primary EBV infection. Almost all adults have been infected with EBV. The symptomatology of primary EBV infection varies with the infected person's age at the time, with younger children usually having inapparent or mild infections. In developing countries and in lower socioeconomic groups in industrialized nations, up to 90% of children acquire primary EBV infection by 6 years of age, and IM frequently never develops. In contrast, in higher socioeconomic groups, only 40% to 50% of adolescents have previously experienced EBV infection. From 10% to 20% of susceptible adolescents and adults contract EBV every year thereafter, with IM developing in about half of these patients.

Pathophysiology

Saliva is the main vehicle for transmission of EBV, a double-stranded DNA herpesvirus. Transmission usually requires direct and prolonged contact with infected oropharyngeal secretions, with salivary exchange being the main mode of transmission. The infection begins with viral replication in oropharyngeal epithelial cells and then spreads to local B lymphocytes, which then disseminate throughout the reticuloendothelial system and induce vigorous T- and NK-cell responses and neutralizing antibodies. The atypical lymphocytes that are produced are mainly suppressor T cells directed against EBV-infected B cells.

It is thought that most of the clinical manifestations of IM are due to these T- and NK-cell responses, which might explain why young children, whose immune responses are incompletely developed, are often asymptomatic with primary EBV infection. It is also possible that viral load determines symptomatology, and, because young adults likely spread more virus via salivary exchange than toddlers, young adults are more likely to be symptomatic. All EBV-seropositive persons shed virus intermittently throughout their lives. EBV may rarely be spread via blood transfusion or transplantation.

Clinical Manifestations

IM is usually an acute, self-limited, benign lymphoproliferative disease. EBV is responsible for nearly all heterophil-positive and most heterophil-negative cases. Other causes of heterophil-negative mononucleosis include cytomegalovirus, toxoplasmosis, hepatitis A and B, adenovirus, HIV, rubella, and human herpesvirus 6.

The classic triad of IM consists of fever, lymphadenopathy, and pharyngitis. Other typical findings include lymphocytosis with atypical lymphocytes and the presence of heterophil antibodies. After a 4- to 6-week incubation period, the illness begins with a 3- to 5-day prodrome of malaise, headache, and fatigue, typically followed in about half of the cases by onset of the triad. Additional symptoms can include anorexia, nausea, vomiting, periorbital or facial edema, and generalized lymphadenopathy, which is usually symmetrical. Splenomegaly occurs by the second or third week of illness in about half of all cases; rarely, splenic rupture can occur, which very rarely may be fatal. Hepatomegaly occurs in 10% to 15%, with hepatitis occurring in about 5% of cases. Up to 20% of patients have a rash that may be erythematous, maculopapular, morbilliform, scarlatiniform, or urticarial, especially if ampicillin or one of its derivatives has been given. Other symptoms can include arthritis and jaundice.

IM is a self-limited disease in nearly all patients. Median illness duration is 16 days.

Diagnosis

The diagnosis is usually based on the clinical picture, atypical lymphocytosis, and positive heterophil serology. Most adolescents and young adults with IM have most or all of these features, as well as an elevated white blood cell count with a relative lymphocytosis. Atypical lymphocytes generally represent more than 9% to 10% of the white blood cell count. Many infected persons also have mild thrombocytopenia and elevated hepatocellular enzymes. Heterophil antibody positivity is usually measured as a positive monospot test. If IM is suspected and heterophil antibodies are negative, specific titers for EBV, including viral capsid antigen (VCA) IgM and IgG, early antigen (EA), and Epstein–Barr nuclear antigen (EBNA), should be obtained, as well as serologic testing for cytomegalovirus (CMV) and toxoplasmosis. Acute EBV infection is characterized by the presence of IgM and IgG VCA antibodies and EA antibodies and the absence of EBNA antibodies.

Differential Diagnosis

If liver chemistry values are markedly elevated and antibodies against EBV, CMV, and toxoplasmosis are unrevealing, serology for hepatitis A, B, and C should be measured. If risk factors are present, HIV antibodies should be checked. A throat culture is indicated in patients with pharyngitis or tonsillitis because the tonsillitis of acute IM can be indistinguishable from that of group A streptococcal pharyngitis.

Treatment

In most patients, IM is self-limited and requires only symptomatic treatment, including bed rest, acetaminophen (Tylenol, 10–15 mg/kg every 4–6 hours), aspirin (10–15 mg/kg every 4–6 hours), or nonsteroidal antiinflammatory agents such as ibuprofen (Advil, 5–10 mg/kg every 6–8 hours). Saline gargles can be useful in treating a sore throat. In severe cases, meperidine (Demerol, 1–1.5 mg/kg every 3–4 hours) may be required.

Although a short, tapering course of corticosteroid therapy (e.g., a Medrol Dosepak[1]) is often prescribed, there is little evidence for its clinical efficacy, and caution is warranted. Infection is ultimately self-limited in nearly all cases, and rare reports of neurologic or septicemic complications after steroid use have appeared. Long-term immune responses following steroid use appear to be normal. Corticosteroid therapy should, however, be considered for the treatment of severe cases of IM associated with hemolysis, respiratory embarrassment, or thrombocytopenic purpura. The use of corticosteroids in atypical or antibody-negative cases is inappropriate because the diagnosis of lymphoma can then be confounded.

---

[1] Not FDA approved for this indication.

Parenteral administration of acyclovir[1] (Zovirax, 10–20 mg/kg IV every 8 hours) to patients with acute IM secondary to EBV reduces the level of oropharyngeal viral replication; however, replication returns to the previously high levels after cessation of treatment, little or no reduction is seen in the number of EBV-infected B cells in the peripheral circulation, and the drug has little or no effect on the clinical course. Acyclovir administered in high doses orally (20 mg/kg, maximum dose of 800 mg qid for 5 days) is also ineffective. Antiviral therapy is therefore not recommended for acute IM in a normal host.

In immunosuppressed or severely ill patients, however, specific therapy has a role in many cases. For example, etoposide (VePesid)[1], a drug that reduces macrophage activation, is often used in cases of infection-associated hemophagocytic syndrome. In posttransplant lymphoproliferative disorders, first-line therapy is often a reduction in immunosuppression; other options include rituximab[1] (Rituxan, 375 mg/m[2] IV weekly for 4 weeks). Oral leukoplakia in patients with AIDS responds to oral acyclovir[1] (20 mg/kg, maximum dose of 800 mg qid for 20 days), whereas a tapering course of steroids (as recommended earlier) may be used for lymphocytic interstitial pneumonitis (see below).

Monitoring

Quarantine is not indicated. Ampicillin and related drugs should be avoided when treating secondary bacterial complications because of their association with rash in persons with IM. Contact sports should be avoided as long as splenomegaly is still evident because of the rare possibility of splenic rupture, which usually occurs within 3 weeks of onset of IM but has been reported as late as 7 weeks into the illness.

Complications

Complications of acute IM can be neurologic (seizures, cranial nerve palsies, aseptic meningitis, encephalitis, optic neuritis, transverse myelitis, infectious polyneuritis [Guillain-Barré syndrome], psychosis, Alice in Wonderland syndrome, or acute cerebellar ataxia), hematologic (hemolytic or aplastic anemia, thrombocytopenic purpura, agranulocytosis, or agammaglobulinemia), cardiac (pericarditis or myocarditis), pulmonary (cough or atypical pneumonia), renal (glomerulonephritis, acute kidney failure, or acute interstitial nephritis), or ophthalmologic (conjunctivitis) in nature. In about 10% of adolescents and young adults, fatigue can persist for 6 months or longer, and many of these patients meet the criteria for chronic fatigue syndrome.

Rare patients have very high titers of EBV antibodies, and a chronic active EBV infection associated with unusual clinical manifestations such as uveitis or lymphoma can occur. EBV is also associated with lymphoproliferative disorders in persons with underlying abnormal immune systems. These include X-linked lymphoproliferative syndrome, in which affected males usually die of acute EBV infection, and the related infection-associated hemophagocytic syndrome, which is most commonly (about 75% of the time) triggered by EBV and seems to be due to an overly exuberant macrophage response to EBV-infected lymphocytes. Transplant recipients can acquire EBV-associated lymphoproliferative disease that can range from an asymptomatic infection to fatal IM or lymphoma. Finally, although not seen much anymore due to combination antiretroviral therapy, patients with AIDS are susceptible to several serious complications of EBV infection, including lymphocytic interstitial pneumonitis, oral leukoplakia, leiomyosarcoma, and lymphoma.

References

Candy B, Hotopf M: Steroids for symptom control in infectious mononucleosis, *Cochrane Database Syst Rev*(3), 2006. CD004402.
Cohen JI, Jaffe ES, Dale JK, et al: Characterization and treatment of chronic active Epstein–Barr virus disease: A 28-year experience in the United States, *Blood* 117:5835–5849, 2011.
Katz BZ: Commentary on "Steroids for symptom control in infectious mononucleosis (Review)" by B Candy and M Hotopf, *Evid Based Child Health* 7:447–449, 2012.
Katz BZ, Shiraishi Y, Mears CJ, et al: Chronic fatigue syndrome following infectious mononucleosis in adolescents, *Pediatrics* 124:189–193, 2009.
Odumade OA, Hogquist KA, Balfour HH Jr : Progress and problems in understanding and managing primary Epstein- Barr virus infections, *Clin Microbiol Rev* 24(1):193–209, 2011.
Rouphael N, Talati NJ, Vaughan C, et al: Infections associated with haemophagocytic syndrome, *Lancet Infect Dis* 7:814–822, 2007.
Soltys K, Green M: Posttransplant lymphoproliferative disease, *Pediatr Infect Dis J* 24:1107–1108, 2005.

INFLUENZA

Method of
Jeffrey A. Linder, MD, MPH

CURRENT DIAGNOSIS

- Influenza should be considered in any patient with respiratory symptoms between October and May in North America.
- The single most important piece of information when considering a diagnosis of influenza is the community prevalence of influenza.
- During outbreaks, sudden onset of fever and cough has a positive predictive value of about 85%.
- Rapid testing should be done with molecular tests (e.g., reverse transcriptase polymerase chain reaction [RT-PCR]), which have a high sensitivity and specificity.

CURRENT THERAPY

- The influenza vaccine is the best means of preventing influenza. The inactivated influenza vaccine is recommended for all persons age 6 months and older.
- The antivirals zanamivir (Relenza) and oseltamivir (Tamiflu) can be used for prophylaxis of influenza in unimmunized patients, in close contacts of infected patients, and during institutional outbreaks of influenza.
- Early antiviral treatment should not be delayed and should be used for patients who are hospitalized; have severe, complicated, or progressive illness; or are at higher risk for complications.
- Antivirals may be prescribed within 48 hours of symptom onset for outpatients not at higher risk for influenza complications.

Influenza is a highly contagious viral infection that should be considered in any patient with respiratory symptoms between October and May in North America. Influenza infects 5% to 20% of the population of the United States in a typical year, sickens 3% to 11% of Americans, and is responsible for up to 431,000 hospitalizations and 51,000 deaths per year. Influenza can range in severity from mild illness to life-threatening disease. Those at highest risk of hospitalization, death, or complications from influenza are children younger than 2 years old, adults older than 65 years, people of any age who have underlying medical conditions or immune compromise, and pregnant women.

Information about influenza changes rapidly. To care optimally for patients with influenza-like illness during the influenza season, clinicians need to keep abreast of updated recommendations and the current prevalence of influenza in their community. The influenza vaccine remains the best means of reducing the incidence, severity, and complications from influenza, but antiviral medications and symptomatic treatments have an important role in the prevention and treatment of influenza (Box 1).

Microbiology

There are two types of influenza viruses, A and B. Influenza A is separated into subtypes based on two surface antigens: hemagglutinin (H) and neuraminidase (N). The predominant

BOX 1 | Influenza Vaccine Recommendations.

- All persons aged ≥6 months should be vaccinated annually
- Vaccination efforts should prioritize people at higher risk of influenza complications:
  - Age 6 months to 5 years
  - Age ≥50 years
  - Chronic pulmonary (including asthma), cardiovascular (except hypertension), renal, hepatic, neurologic, hematologic, or metabolic (including diabetes mellitus) disorders
  - Immunosuppressed
  - Pregnant during the influenza season
  - Age 6 months to 18 years old receiving long-term aspirin therapy and who therefore might be at risk for Reye syndrome
  - Residents of nursing homes and other long-term care facilities
  - American Indians/Alaska Natives
  - Morbidly obese (body mass index ≥40)
- Vaccination efforts should also prioritize those likely to transmit influenza to higher risk people:
  - Healthcare personnel
  - Household contacts and caregivers of children aged <5 years and adults aged ≥50 years, with particular emphasis on vaccinating contacts of children aged <6 months
  - Household contacts and caregivers of persons with medical conditions that put them at higher risk for severe complications from influenza

circulating strains of influenza in recent decades have been influenza A (H1N1), influenza A (H3N2), and influenza B. Influenza A (H3N2) subtypes generally cause more severe influenza and are associated with higher mortality than other types. Influenza viruses undergo slight genetic changes from year to year, termed *antigenic drift*. Major changes in surface glycoproteins are termed *antigenic shift* and can result in severe pandemic influenza in a nonimmune population, which happened with an antigenically novel influenza A (H1N1) virus in 2009. Because of antigenic drift, and because immunity to a given type or subtype of influenza provides limited cross-immunity to other types and subtypes, the influenza vaccine needs to be reformulated and administered most years.

Patients contract influenza by being exposed to large-sized respiratory droplets from an infected person or contact with surfaces harboring influenza virus. Influenza has a latency of 1 to 4 days before the onset of symptoms. Adults are infectious from the day before symptom onset through approximately day 7 of illness, but immunosuppressed adults and children shed the virus for longer periods. Symptoms generally last from 7 to 14 days.

Several novel, highly pathogenic respiratory viruses—avian influenza A (H5N1), avian influenza A (H7N9), and Middle East respiratory syndrome coronavirus (MERS-CoV)—have mortality rates ranging from 35% to 55%. Collectively there have been more than 4800 human cases. These pathogens, if they acquire the ability to be highly transmissible between humans, have the potential to cause pandemic respiratory disease.

Prevention

Influenza vaccination is between 20% and 90% effective in preventing influenza or complications of influenza. Influenza vaccination is highly cost-effective and can even be cost-saving in high-risk groups. Influenza vaccination is less effective in younger children, in adults older than 65 years, in adults with comorbid conditions, and when there is a poor match between the influenza vaccine and circulating influenza. The Centers for Disease Control and Prevention (CDC) Advisory Committee on Immunization Practices puts out annual recommendations and supplementary updates on the prevention and treatment of influenza

(www.cdc.gov/flu). The Advisory Committee on Immunization Practices recommends vaccinating all persons 6 months of age and older.

At present, there are four commonly administered, recommended types of influenza vaccine: trivalent inactivated influenza vaccine (IIV3), quadrivalent inactivated influenza vaccine (IIV4), quadrivalent recombinant influenza vaccine (RIV4), and quadrivalent live attenuated influenza vaccine (LAIV4). The IIV4 (Afluria Quadrivalent, Fluarix Quadrivalent, Flucelvax Quadrivalent, FluLaval Quadrivalent, Fluzone Quadrivalent), IIV3 (Afluria), and RIV4 (Flublok Quadrivalent) vaccines are administered as an intramuscular injection.

Different products are approved for administration in different lower age limits. A high-dose IIV3 (Fluzone High-Dose) and an adjuvanted IIV3 (Fluad) are available for patients aged 65 years or older, who are less likely to respond immunologically to standard inactivated influenza vaccine (IIV). The main adverse effect of the IIV is soreness at the injection site. Patients often report a mild immune response of fever, malaise, myalgia, and headache that can last for 1 to 2 days, but rates of most of these symptoms are no different from those in patients who receive placebo injection. IIV, RIV4, or LAIV4 can be administered to people with an egg allergy of any severity.

Allergic reactions to egg proteins or other vaccine components (e.g., antibiotics and inactivating compounds) include hives, angioedema, asthma, and anaphylaxis. For patients with egg allergy who have only hives, any otherwise appropriate IIV or RIV can be administered. For patients with more severe reactions to egg or who received treatment for an allergic reaction can also receive any recommended IIV or RIV in an inpatient or outpatient medical setting and observed for at least 15 minutes by a clinician able to recognize and manage severe allergic reactions. The recombinant influenza vaccine (RIV4; FluBlok Quadrivalent) is considered egg free. Cell culture–based IIV (ccIIV4; Flucelvax Quadravalent) could be egg-derived and contain egg protein. Patients who have had severe allergic reaction to influenza vaccine should not receive the vaccine.

Vaccination should be deferred in patients with acute febrile illness, but patients with more moderate illness can be vaccinated. Guillain-Barré syndrome was associated with the 1976 swine flu vaccine, but there is no consistent evidence that modern influenza vaccines are associated with Guillain-Barré syndrome.

The LAIV4 (FluMist Quadrivalent) is administered as a nasal spray and is approved for patients ages 2 to 49 years. The LAIV4 is contraindicated in children aged 2 to 4 years with recurrent wheezing or asthma; children who are receiving aspirin or aspirin-containing products; patients with comorbid conditions or immunosuppression; pregnant women; and family members or close contacts of severely immunosuppressed patients, who require a protected environment (e.g., hematopoietic stem cell transplant recipients). The LAIV4 should not be administered to those with severe nasal congestion. Adverse effects of the LAIV4 include runny nose, nasal congestion, headache, sore throat, chills, and tiredness, although these are only slightly more common than in patients receiving placebo. Those receiving the LAIV4 should avoid contact with severely immunosuppressed persons for 7 days.

Patients should be vaccinated in the fall when the seasonal vaccine becomes available, even as early as August. In the event of vaccine shortages, higher-risk patients should receive priority (see Box 1). Patients should continue to be vaccinated until February and beyond because in the majority of recent influenza seasons the peak has been February or later. Children 6 months to 8 years of age who have not been previously immunized against influenza should be given two doses separated by at least 4 weeks.

Evaluation
Community Prevalence of Influenza

In caring for a patient with suspected influenza, the single most important piece of data is the community prevalence of influenza among patients with influenza-like illness. This ranges from near 0% during summer months to approximately 30% during a typical influenza seasonal peak. The prevalence may be higher during a particularly severe outbreak. Clinicians can check the local prevalence of influenza among patients with influenza-like illness through the CDC (www.cdc.gov/flu) and their state department of public health.

History and Physical Examination

Beyond the local prevalence of influenza, the diagnosis of influenza rests on the patient's history. All methods of diagnosing influenza—symptom complexes, clinician judgment, and testing—generally are highly specific but have poor sensitivity. Thus it is important to consider a diagnosis of influenza in any patient with respiratory symptoms during influenza season. Influenza is classically described as the very sudden onset of fever, headache, sore throat, myalgias, cough, and nasal symptoms. Children can also have otitis media, nausea, and vomiting. In differentiating influenza from nonspecific upper respiratory tract infections, it is most useful to consider the circulating prevalence of influenza, the abruptness of onset, and the severity of symptoms.

Certain symptom complexes have been shown in trials of antiviral treatment to strongly suggest influenza. For example, in an area with circulating influenza, the acute onset of cough and fever can have a positive predictive value as high as 85%. Other studies have shown that clinician judgment performed as well as or better than hard-and-fast symptom complexes or rapid testing.

The physical examination in influenza primarily serves to identify the severity of influenza, complications, and worsening of underlying medical conditions. Clinicians should record vital signs and perform examinations of the ears, nose, sinuses, throat, neck, lungs, and heart for all patients suspected of having influenza.

Testing

Testing is not required to make a diagnosis of clinical influenza. Treatment for patients at high risk for influenza complications should not wait for test results. However, testing may help inform antiviral use, antibiotic prescribing, site-of-care decisions, and infection control measures. Specimens (nasopharyngeal swab, nasal swab, nasal wash, or nasal aspirate, depending on the particular test) should ideally be collected within 3 to 4 days of symptom onset.

Molecular assays such as reverse transcriptase polymerase chain reaction (RT-PCR) testing are highly sensitive (90% to 95%) and specific. Some can produce results in 15 to 45 minutes, and some can differentiate influenza types and subtypes. RT-PCR should be considered for hospitalized patients, institutional outbreaks, or other situations when clinicians are concerned about false-negative rapid test results. Other nucleic acid amplification tests, which can differentiate influenza from other respiratory pathogens, are becoming more available. The CDC recommends that all hospitalized patients with suspected influenza be tested with a high-sensitivity, high-specificity molecular assay.

Rapid influenza diagnostic tests (RIDTs) are much less sensitive (50% to 70%) and somewhat less specific (90%) than molecular tests. Negative results do not exclude the possibility of influenza, especially if the circulating prevalence of influenza is high (>30%). Some RIDTs can distinguish influenza A from influenza B and can provide a point-of-care result in less than 15 minutes.

In the event of a high prevalence of influenza or a high risk of complications from influenza, empiric antiviral treatment is indicated. Testing may be particularly helpful for hospitalized patients to rule out a need for antibiotics, but antiinfluenza treatment should not be withheld solely on the basis of a negative test result. Chest radiography, cultures, and blood tests are not routinely indicated, but they should be obtained for patients with suspected pneumonia or to identify other suspected complications.

Complications

Complications of influenza include primary complications, suppurative complications, and worsening of comorbid conditions. Primary complications of influenza include viral pneumonia, which is a feared complication and is likely a main cause of death in pandemic influenza. Other, less common primary complications of influenza include myositis and rhabdomyolysis, Reye syndrome, myocarditis, pericarditis, toxic shock syndrome, and central nervous system disease (e.g., encephalitis, transverse myelitis, and aseptic meningitis). Children can have a severe course with influenza, including signs and symptoms of sepsis along with febrile seizures. Suppurative complications of influenza include bacterial pneumonia, otitis media, and sinusitis. Influenza can cause worsening of comorbid conditions such as asthma, chronic obstructive pulmonary disease, congestive heart failure, and chronic kidney disease.

Chemoprophylaxis

Antiviral medications can be used to prevent influenza in patients who did not receive the influenza vaccine, cannot receive the influenza vaccine, received the vaccine in the prior 2 weeks (before reliable immunity develops), or in the event of poor matching between vaccine and circulating influenza strains (Table 1). Chemoprophylaxis should also be considered for close contacts of patients with confirmed influenza or for patients with immune deficiency who are unlikely to respond to the influenza vaccine but who are at high risk for having complications from influenza (see Box 1).

Amantadine (Symmetrel) and rimantadine (Flumadine) are not recommended for chemoprophylaxis or treatment because of a high prevalence of resistant influenza A strains. The neuraminidase inhibitors oseltamivir (Tamiflu), and zanamivir (Relenza) are approximately 80% effective in preventing influenza in household contacts of persons with influenza, and more than 90% effective in preventing influenza in institutional settings. Chemoprophylaxis should be taken for 7 days after last known exposure. For hospital or long-term care facility outbreaks, chemoprophylaxis should be taken and for a minimum of 2 weeks or until 1 week after the end of the outbreak. For patients allergic to or unable to respond to the vaccine, chemoprophylaxis should be used for the duration of circulating influenza. The IIV can be given to patients receiving chemoprophylaxis. The LAIV should not be given from 2 days before to 14 days after taking an antiviral medication. Patients who receive the LAIV in this window should be revaccinated at a later date.

Treatment

The influenza vaccine is the best means of reducing influenza-related morbidity and mortality, but its limitations include production problems, low vaccination rates, and variable effectiveness. Given these limitations, there is an important role in management for influenza-specific antiviral medications (see Table 1). Antiviral medications reduce the duration of influenza symptoms by approximately 1 day, reduce complications requiring antibiotics by 30% to 50%, might decrease hospitalizations, decreases mortality among hospitalized patients, and are cost-effective. Early antiviral treatment, which should not wait for test results, starting up to 5 days after symptom onset can reduce complications for patients who are hospitalized; have severe, complicated, or progressive illness; or are at higher risk for complications (see Box 1). For outpatients not at higher risk for complications, antiviral treatment must be started within 48 hours of symptom onset.

Oseltamivir (Tamiflu) is taken as a capsule or oral suspension. The dose of oseltamivir should be reduced in patients with renal disease. Adverse effects of oseltamivir include nausea, vomiting, and perhaps behavioral changes. Oseltamivir, oral or enterically administered, is the drug of choice for hospitalized patients and those with severe illness. Zanamivir (Relenza) is taken as an oral inhaled powder and is not recommended for patients with underlying lung or heart disease. Adverse effects of zanamivir include worsening of underlying lung disease and allergic reactions. Amantadine and rimantadine are not recommended because of a high prevalence of resistant influenza A strains.

TABLE 1 Antiviral Agents for the Treatment and Prophylaxis of Influenza.

ANTIVIRAL AGENT	TREATMENT*		PROPHYLAXIS†		COMMENTS
	CHILDREN	ADULTS	CHILDREN	ADULTS	
Oseltamivir (Tamiflu)	Any age‡ Dose for 5 days bid: <1 year: 3 mg/kg per dose; ≤15 kg: 30 mg; 16–23 kg: 45 mg; 24–40 kg: 60 mg; >40 kg: 75 mg	75 mg PO bid for 5 days	3 months to 1 year: 3 mg/kg/day‡ Dose qd: ≤15 kg: 30 mg; 16–23 kg: 45 mg; 24–40 kg: 60 mg; >40 kg: 75 mg	75 mg PO qd	For patients with creatinine clearance < 30 mL/min, oseltamivir adult dosing should be reduced to 30 mg qd for treatment and to 30 mg qod for prophylaxis
Zanamivir (Relenza)	Approved for children ≥7 years; 10 mg (2 inhalations) bid for 5 days	10 mg (2 inhalations) bid for 5 days	Approved for children ≥5 years; 10 mg (2 inhalations) qd	10 mg (2 inhalations) qd	Avoid in patients with chronic lung disease (e.g., asthma, chronic obstructive pulmonary disease)
Peramivir (Rapivab)	2–12 years: One 12-mg/kg dose, up to 600 mg maximum IV over minimum 15 min	≥13 years: One 600-mg IV dose over a minimum of 15 min	NA	NA	For patients with creatinine clearance 30–49 mL/min, the dose should be reduced to 200 mg; For patients with creatinine clearance 10–29 mL/min, the dose should be reduced to 100 mg
Baloxavir (Xofluza)	≥12 years and older weighing at least 40 kg: one 40-mg dose	40 to <80 kg: one 40-mg dose; ≥80 kg: one 80-mg dose	NA	NA	For patients within 2 days of illness onset. Avoid in pregnant women or breastfeeding mothers

*Suspected or confirmed influenza among persons with severe influenza or for persons at higher risk for influenza complications up to 5 days after symptom onset. For outpatients not at higher risk for influenza complications, treatment should be started within 48 hours of symptom onset.

†Prophylaxis should be given for 7 days after last known exposure and for institutional outbreaks for at least 2 weeks or until 1 week after the end of the outbreak.

‡Oseltamivir is approved by the US Food and Drug Administration for treatment in children 14 days and older and prophylaxis in children 1 year and older. Treatment in children <14 days old and prophylaxis in children <1 year old is recommended by the Centers for Disease Control and Prevention and the American Academy of Pediatrics.

IV, Intravenous; *NA*, not approved; *PO*, per os (orally).

Adapted from Centers for Disease Control and Prevention. Influenza Antiviral Medications: Summary for Clinicians. Available at http://www.cdc.gov/flu/professionals/antivirals/ (accessed July 24, 2019).

Peramivir (Rapivab), an intravenous neuraminidase inhibitor, was approved in the United State in December 2014 for patients within 48 hours of symptom onset. Peramivir has been associated with diarrhea, rashes including Stevens-Johnson syndrome, and neuropsychiatric changes.

Baloxavir (Xofluza), a cap-dependent endonuclease inhibitor, is active against both influenza A and B. Baloxavir has been associated with diarrhea. It has the advantage of requiring only one dose.

Antibiotics are generally not necessary, but they should be prescribed to treat suppurative complications of influenza. Antitussives such as guaifenesin with codeine (Robitussin AC) help coughing patients to sleep at night. β-Agonists, such as albuterol (Proventil)[1], can help patients with cough, especially if there is wheezing on examination. Analgesics and antipyretics such as acetaminophen (Tylenol) and ibuprofen (Motrin) reduce fever and generally help patients to feel better. Patients should be encouraged to rest and drink plenty of fluids.

Patients with suspected influenza should minimize contact with others to avoid spreading the infection. Use of face masks and hand hygiene can reduce the transmission of influenza.

References

Centers for Disease Control and Prevention: Influenza (Flu): information for health professionals, Available at: http://www.cdc.gov/flu/professionals/index.htm. Accessed 23 July 2019.

Ebell MH, Afonso AM, Gonzales R, et al: Development and validation of a clinical decision rule for the diagnosis of influenza, *J Am Board Fam Med* 25:55–62, 2012.

Falsey AR, Murata Y, Walsh EE: Impact of rapid diagnosis on management of adults hospitalized with influenza, *Arch Intern Med* 167:354–360, 2007.

Grohskopf LA, Sokolow LZ, Broder KR, et al: Prevention and control of seasonal influenza with vaccines: recommendations of the Advisory Committee on Immunization Practices—United States, 2018–19 Influenza Season, *MMWR Recomm Rep* 67(No. RR-3):1–20, 2018. Available at: https://doi.org/10.15585/mmwr.rr6703a1.

Tokars JI, Olsen SJ, Reed C: Seasonal incidence of symptomatic influenza in the United States, *Clin Infect Dis* 66:1511–1518, 2018.

LEISHMANIASIS

Method of
Luigi Gradoni, PhD

CURRENT DIAGNOSIS

- Infected tissues must be sampled for microscopy demonstration of *Leishmania* organisms in Giemsa-stained impression smears or cultures. Polymerase chain reaction (PCR) detection of *Leishmania* DNA increases diagnostic sensitivity.
- Different tissue samplings are performed depending on the clinical form of leishmaniasis: For visceral leishmaniasis, aspirate or biopsy specimens are obtained from spleen, bone marrow, the liver, or enlarged lymph nodes. For cutaneous and mucocutaneous leishmaniasis, the material is obtained by skin lesion scraping or biopsy.
- Serology is useful when the diagnosis of visceral leishmaniasis proves difficult with other methods.

[1] Not US Food and Drug Administration approved for this indication.

CURRENT THERAPY

- The therapy of leishmaniasis relies on a limited number of drugs, most of which are old and relatively toxic. Systemic drug administration requires hospitalization and monitoring of the patient.
- The pentavalent antimony (Sb) drugs sodium stibogluconate (Pentostam)[10] and meglumine antimoniate (Glucantime)[2] are equivalent and used in all clinical forms of leishmaniasis. Dosage is Sb 20 mg/kg/day IM for 21 to 28 days. In cases of uncomplicated cutaneous leishmaniasis, use intralesional administration intermittently over 20 to 30 days.
- Liposomal amphotericin B (Ambisome) is the gold standard for treating visceral leishmaniasis. Dosage: Total dose of 18 to 21 mg/kg IV using one of the following schedules: 3 mg/kg/day on days 1 to 5 and 10; 3 mg/kg on days 1 to 5, day 14, and day 21; 10 mg/kg/day for 2 days.
- Amphotericin B desoxycholate (Fungizone) is used in visceral leishmaniasis[1] and mucocutaneous leishmaniasis. Dosage is 0.5 mg/kg IV every other day for 14 days.
- Other parenteral drugs: Pentamidine isethionate (Pentam 300)[1] is used to treat some forms of New World cutaneous leishmaniasis; dosage is 2 mg/kg IM every other day for 7 days. Paromomycin (aminosidine) sulfate[2] is used for Indian visceral leishmaniasis; dosage is 11 mg/kg/day IM for 21 days.
- Miltefosine (Impavido)[5] is recommended for visceral leishmaniasis therapy in India and Ethiopia and for cutaneous leishmaniasis therapy in Colombia and Bolivia. Dosage is 2.5 mg/kg/day (not exceeding 100 mg/day) PO for 28 days.

[1]Not FDA approved for this indication.
[2]Not available in the United States.
[5]Investigational drug in the United States.
[10]Available in the United States from the Centers for Disease Control and Prevention.

Epidemiology

Leishmaniases are diseases caused by members of the genus *Leishmania*, protozoan parasites infecting numerous mammal species, including humans. The flagellated forms (promastigotes) are transmitted by the bite of phlebotomine sand flies and multiply as aflagellated forms (amastigotes) within cells of the mononuclear phagocyte system. The diseases range over the intertropical zones of America and Africa and extend into temperate regions of Latin America, Southern Europe, and Asia. About 20 named *Leishmania* species and subspecies are pathogenic for humans, and 30 sand fly species are proven vectors. Each parasite species circulates in natural foci of infection where susceptible phlebotomines and mammals coexist. The epidemiology and clinical manifestations of the diseases are largely diverse, being usually grouped into two main entities: zoonotic leishmaniases, where domestic or wild animal reservoirs are involved in the transmission cycle and humans play a role of accidental host, and anthroponotic leishmaniases, where humans are the sole reservoir and source of the vector's infection.

Visceral leishmaniasis (VL) is caused by *Leishmania donovani* in the Indian subcontinent and East Africa (anthroponotic entity) and by *L. infantum (L. chagasi)* in the Mediterranean basin, parts of Central Asia, and Latin America (a zoonotic entity with domestic dogs acting as the main reservoir host). Several species of *Leishmania* cause cutaneous leishmaniasis (CL) or mucocutaneous (MCL) leishmaniasis. The most common are *L. major* (rural zoonotic entity) and *L. tropica* (urban anthroponotic entity) in the Old World and *L. mexicana, L. braziliensis, L. amazonensis, L. panamensis, L. guyanensis,* and *L. peruviana* (sylvatic zoonotic entities) in the New World.

Globally, 80 Old World and 21 New World countries are endemic for human leishmaniasis, with an estimated yearly incidence of 0.7 million to 1.2 million cases of CL forms and 0.2 million to 0.4 million cases of VL forms. Overall estimated prevalence is 12 million people with a disability-adjusted life years burden of 860,000 for men and 1.2 million for women. The disease affects the poorest people in the poorest countries: 72 are developing countries, of which 13 are among the least developed. The incidence is not uniformly distributed in endemic areas: 90% of CL cases are found in only seven countries (Afghanistan, Algeria, Brazil, Iran, Peru, Saudi Arabia, and Syria), whereas 90% of VL cases occur in rural and suburban areas of five countries (Bangladesh, India, Nepal, Sudan, and Brazil). These figures, however, must be regarded as underestimates; currently, it appears that the global incidence of human leishmaniases is higher than before, owing to environmental and human behavioral factors contributing to the changing landscape of these diseases.

Risk Factors

Risk factors for leishmaniasis are primarily associated with geographically and temporally defined human exposure to phlebotomine vectors. In the Old World, colonization and urbanization of desert areas have been identified as the major risk factor for outbreaks of zoonotic CL. Tourists and military personnel are often exposed to *L. major* or *L. tropica* infections in rural or urban endemic settings of North African and Middle Eastern countries. In the New World, the colonization of the primary forest associated with activities of deforestation, road building, mining, and tourism is responsible for the domestication of sylvatic cycles of CL and MCL agents. Increase in density and geographic range of phlebotomine vectors resulting from climate changes, together with the increased mobility of infected pet dogs, has been identified as a cause of northward spreading of zoonotic VL in Europe.

Individual risk factors play a major role in VL disease. Most of the *L. donovani* and *L. infantum* infections are asymptomatic or subclinical in well-nourished immunocompetent persons. Malnourished persons, infants younger than 2 years, and severely immunosuppressed adults are at high risk for acute VL when exposed to infection. Before the era of HAART (highly active antiretroviral therapy), the AIDS epidemics in southern Europe caused more than 2000 HIV and VL co-infection cases among men aged 39 years on average. Other conditions have been reported that influence the clinical outcome of VL, such as immunosuppressive therapies after organ transplantation, corticosteroid and anti–tumor necrosis factor α (TNF-α) treatments for immunologic disorders, hematologic neoplasia, and chronic conditions of hepatic cirrhosis. However, most acute VL episodes in adults remain unexplained. Other factors associated with impaired immune response to *Leishmania* (e.g., genetic factors) are probably involved.

Pathophysiology

Ingestion of metacyclic promastigotes inoculated by the vector in the skin is mediated by several types of receptors found in resident macrophages, monocytes, neutrophils, and dendritic cells. *Leishmania* lipophosphoglycan, the most abundant surface glycoconjugate, is the main factor of virulence. Once in the cell phagolysosome, amastigotes survive from hydrolase activity through pH acidification while selectively inhibiting production of reactive oxygen species. Multiplication of parasites, infection of new cells, and dissemination to tissues are contrasted by the host's inflammatory and specific immune responses. Even in most susceptible natural mammal hosts, most infections are efficiently controlled, giving rise to asymptomatic latent infections. Leishmaniases have typical immunologic polarity: Cure or control are associated with robust cellular immune responses driven by production of interleukin (IL) 12, whereas acute or chronic diseases are characterized by the absence of such responses and the presence of high levels of nonprotective serum antibodies, a condition often associated with high levels of IL-10 production. In spite of this polarity, analysis of cytokine patterns in tissues reveals a less-polar situation, as both T_H1 and T_H2 cytokines were found to be secreted in specimens from tissues infected with CL, MCL, and VL.

Prevention

There are no human vaccines available for the immune protection against leishmaniasis. Promising data on safety and immunogenicity have been provided for the only *Leishmania* candidate vaccine under development, consisting of the recombinant polyprotein antigen LEISH-F1 with MPL-SE as adjuvant. Preventive measures are thus limited to the individual protection from sand fly bites or to community protection through reservoir control. Individual protection is through the use of repellents or insecticide-impregnated nets. Reservoir control measures are largely diverse, depending on the epidemiologic entity of leishmaniasis. Examples related to zoonotic entities with synanthropic reservoir hosts are the destruction of rodent populations around human dwellings (e.g., to control zoonotic CL due to *L. major*) and the fight against canine infections through the mass use of topical insecticides or drug treatments (e.g., to control zoonotic VL due to *L. infantum*). Early diagnosis and treatment of human cases is the main control measure against anthroponotic entities of VL (*L. donovani*) and CL (*L. tropica*).

Clinical Manifestations

Visceral Disease

VL, also known as kala-azar, results from the multiplication of *Leishmania* in the phagocytes of the reticuloendothelial system. In endemic settings, the ratio of incident asymptomatic infections to incident clinical cases varies from 4:1 to 50:1 depending on the epidemiologic type (anthroponotic VL is normally more virulent) and the poverty of the affected country. Classic VL manifests as pallor, fever, and hard splenomegaly; hepatomegaly is less common. Laboratory findings document pancytopenia and hypergammaglobulinemia. The clinical incubation period ranges from 3 weeks (exceptional) to more than 2 years, but 4 to 6 months is average. Patients report a history of fever resistant to antibiotics; on physical examination, the spleen is typically appreciated 5 to 15 cm below the left costal margin. Symptomatic VL is 100% fatal when left untreated.

Cutaneous Disease

CL results from multiplication of *Leishmania* in the phagocytes of the skin. In the classic course of the disease, lesions appear first as papules, advance slowly to nodules or ulcers, and then spontaneously heal with scarring over months to years. The clinical incubation period ranges from 1 week (exceptional) to several months; lesions caused by *L. major* and *L. mexicana* tend to evolve and resolve quickly, whereas those caused by *L. braziliensis*, *L. tropica*, and dermotropic strains of *L. infantum* can have longer periods of incubation and spontaneous healing.

Mucosal Disease

MCL results from parasitic metastasis in the nasal mucosal that eventually extends to the oropharynx and larynx. It can develop from CL lesions caused by *L. braziliensis* and *L. panamensis*. Typically, MCL evolves slowly (3 years on average) and does not heal spontaneously.

Diagnosis

The standard diagnosis method for all forms of leishmaniasis is still the microscopy demonstration of *Leishmania* organisms in Giemsa-stained impression smears or cultures from samples of infected tissues. In general, sensitivity increases when both staining and culture are performed. Polymerase chain reaction (PCR) detection of *Leishmania* DNA on samples further increases the diagnostic sensitivity and also might allow species identification by target DNA sequencing or restriction fragment length polymorphism analysis.

Different tissue samplings must be performed depending on the clinical form of leishmaniasis. For VL, aspirate or biopsy specimens are obtained from the spleen, bone marrow, the liver, or enlarged lymph nodes. Higher diagnostic yields are obtained with spleen aspirates (more than 98%), although bone marrow aspirates (80% to 98% of yield) are usually preferred. For CL and MCL, material is obtained by scraping tissue juice from a nodular lesion or from the edge of an ulcer or by taking punch biopsies of inflamed tissue. Diagnostic yields of about 80% are obtained with impression

smears and cultures during the first half of the natural course of the lesion. After that, standard parasitologic diagnosis becomes more difficult and PCR remains the only reliable method.

Serology is useful when the diagnosis of VL proves difficult with other methods. Commercially available dipstick tests using recombinant antigen K39 can be used in decisions for or against treatment. Negative serology results are common in CL and MCL, as well as in VL when patients are severely immunosuppressed.

Differential Diagnosis

Visceral Disease

The differential diagnosis depends on the local disease pattern associated with endemic areas. In many of them it includes chronic malaria, disseminated histoplasmosis, hepatosplenic schistosomiasis, typhoid fever, brucellosis, tuberculosis, endocarditis, relapsing fever, and African trypanosomiasis. Other cosmopolitan diseases include syphilis, lymphomas, chronic myeloid leukemia, sarcoidosis, malignant histiocytosis, and liver cirrhosis.

Cutaneous Disease

A typical history of CL—an inflammatory, slowly developing, and painless skin lesion associated with recent exposure to sand fly bites—can strongly support a clinical diagnosis of disease. However, there is an extensive differential diagnosis, which includes acute or chronic forms of CL. For the former, insect bites, furuncular myiasis, and bacterial tropical ulcers are the most common; for the latter, keloid, lupus vulgaris, discoid lupus erythematosus, and sarcoidosis.

Treatment

The therapy of leishmaniasis relies on a limited number of drugs, most of which are old and relatively toxic compounds. Systemic drug administration requires hospitalizing and monitoring the patient.

Pentavalent Antimonials

Organic salts of pentavalent antimony (Sb) are still the mainstay therapy for all clinical forms of leishmaniasis. Two preparations are available that are equal in efficacy and toxicity when used in equivalent Sb doses: sodium stibogluconate (Pentostam),[10] available in English-speaking countries, and meglumine antimoniate (Glucantime),[2] available in Southern Europe and Latin America. The recommended dosage of Sb is 20 mg/kg/day for 21 to 28 days, given intramuscularly or intravenously. Treatment should be prolonged for 40 to 60 days in areas with documented Sb-resistant VL (e.g., in Bihar State, India). The drugs can be administered intralesionally in cases of uncomplicated CL, intermittently over 20 to 30 days. Systemic toxicity caused by the antimonials relates to the total dose administered and includes anorexia, pancreatitis, and changes on electrocardiography (e.g., prolongation of the QT interval), which can precede dangerous arrhythmias.

Amphotericin B Drugs

Liposomal amphotericin B (Ambisome) is the current gold standard for VL treatment, being highly effective and nontoxic. However, the high cost of the drug precludes its use in developing countries where leishmaniasis is endemic. Liposomal amphotericin B is given intravenously at the total dose of 18 to 21 mg/kg, with various treatment schedules similarly effective: 3 mg/kg/day on days 1 to 5 and 10; 3 mg/kg on days 1 to 5, 14, and 21; or 10 mg/kg/day for 2 days.

Amphotericin B desoxycholate (Fungizone) is a relatively toxic compound used in Sb-resistant VL[1] and MCL, administered intravenously at the low dosage of 0.5 mg/kg every other day for 14 days. Doses in excess of 1 mg/kg/day commonly result in

---

[1]Not FDA approved for this indication.

[2]Not available in the United States.

[10]Available in the United States from the Centers for Disease Control and Prevention.

severe infusion-related side effects (fever, chills, and bone pain) and delayed side effects (toxic renal effects).

Other Parenteral Drugs

Other parenteral drugs include old second-line drugs whose use is limited. Pentamidine isethionate (Pentam 300)[1] is a toxic compound used to treat some forms of New World CL resistant to Sb therapy and is given intramuscularly at the low dose of 2 mg/kg every other day for 7 days. Treatment in excess of this dosage can result in common side effects such as myalgias, nausea, headache, and hypoglycemia. Paromomycin (aminosidine) sulfate injection[2] (manufactured by Gland Pharma, India, on behalf of Institute of One World Health) is an old aminoglycoside that is being reevaluated as a first-line drug for Indian VL. It is given intramuscularly at the dose of 11 mg base per kg per day for 21 days. Elevation of alanine aminotranferease (ALT) and aspartate aminotransferase (AST) liver enzymes is usually seen during therapy.

Miltefosine, the First Oral Drug for Leishmaniasis

Miltefosine (Impavido)[5] is a hexadecylphosphocholine originally developed as an anticancer agent. It is the first recognized oral treatment for leishmaniasis and is available in Germany and India. So far, it is recommended for VL therapy in India and Ethiopia and for CL therapy in Colombia and Bolivia. The drug is administered at 2.5 mg/kg/day (not exceeding 100 mg/day) for 28 days. Miltefosine administration does not require the patient to be hospitalized for monitoring. Mild gastrointestinal toxicity may be common. The drug is contraindicated in pregnancy.

Monitoring

In VL patients, fever recedes by day 3 to 5 of treatment, and well-being returns by the first week. Hematologic indices start to improve during the second week. Hemoglobin, serum albumin, and body weight are the most useful indicators of progress. The spleen tends to normalize 1 to 2 months after the end of therapy, although it can take up to 1 year to regress completely. Parasitologic assessment of cure is not normally necessary. Relapses can occur after apparent clinical cure from 2 to 8 months after treatment has been discontinued.

In CL patients, clinical response to drugs is rapid, but complete reepithelialization of lesions is observed in only one third of patients by the end of 3- to 4-week treatment courses.

References

Alvar J, Aparicio P, Aseffa A, et al: The relationship between leishmaniasis and AIDS: The second 10 years, *Clin Microbiol Rev* 21:334–359, 2008.

Alvar J, Vélez ID, Bern C, et al: Leishmaniasis worldwide and global estimates of its incidence, PLoS One 7:e35671, 2012.

Aronson N, Herwaldt BL, Libman L, et al: Diagnosis and treatment of leishmaniasis: clinical practice guidelines by the Infectious Diseases Society of America (IDSA) and the American Society of Tropical Medicine and Hygiene (ASTMH), *Clin Infect Dis* 63:e202–e264, 2016.

Berman JJ: Treatment of leishmaniasis with miltefosine: 2008 status, *Expert Opin Drug Metab Toxicol* 4:1209–1216, 2008.

Bern C, Adler-Moore J, Berenguer J, et al: Liposomal amphotericin B for the treatment of visceral leishmaniasis, *Clin Infect Dis* 43:917–924, 2006.

Bhattacharya SK, Sinha PK, Sundar S, et al: Phase 4 trial of miltefosine for the treatment of Indian visceral leishmaniasis, *J Infect Dis* 196:591–668, 2007.

Chappuis F, Sundar S, Hailu A, et al: Visceral leishmaniasis: what are the needs for diagnosis, treatment and control? *Nat Rev Microbiol* 5:873–882, 2007.

González U, Pinart M, Rengifo-Pardo M, et al: Interventions for cutaneous and mucocutaneous leishmaniasis, *Cochrane Database Syst Rev*(2), 2009. CD004834.

Gradoni L, Soteriadou K, Louzir H, et al: Drug regimens for visceral leishmaniasis in Mediterranean countries, *Trop Med Int Health* 13:1272, 2008.

Gramiccia M, Gradoni L: The current status of zoonotic leishmaniases and approaches to disease control, *Int J Parasitol* 35:1169–1180, 2005.

Sundar S, Agrawal N, Arora R, et al: Short-course paromomycin treatment of visceral leishmaniasis in India: 14-day vs 21-day treatment, *Clin Infect Dis* 49:914–918, 2009.

[5]Investigational drug in the United States.

LEPROSY

Method of
Gerson O. Penna, MD, PhD; Maria Araci de Andrade Pontes, MD, PhD; Carolina Talhari, MD, PhD; Heitor de Sá Gonçalves, MD, PhD and Maria Lucia Penna, MD, PhD

CURRENT DIAGNOSIS

- Contact of susceptible person with untreated leprosy cases; travel to or residence in a leprosy-endemic country.
- Skin lesion(s) with altered sensation.
- Thickened or enlarged peripheral nerve, with sensory loss and/or weakness in the muscles supplied by the nerve.
- Presence of acid-fast bacilli in a slit skin smear.
- Skin biopsy with the presence of acid-fast bacilli or typical lesions, thereby aiding disease classification

CURRENT THERAPY

Paucibacillary Leprosy (6 months)
Adult (50–70 kg)
- Dapsone: 100 mg daily
- Rifampin (Rifadin)[1]: 600 mg once a month under supervision

Child (under 10 years)
- Dapsone: 1 mg/kg/day
- Rifampin[1]: 10 mg/kg once a month under supervision

Multibacillary Leprosy (12 months)
Adult (50–70 kg)
- Dapsone: 100 mg daily
- Rifampin[1]: 600 mg once a month under supervision
- Clofazimine (Lamprene)[5]: 50 mg daily and 300 mg once a month under supervision

Child (under 10 years)
- Dapsone: 1 mg/kg/day
- Rifampin[1]: 10 mg/kg once a month under supervision
- Clofazimine: 1 mg/kg/day

[1]Not FDA approved for this indication.
[5]Investigational drug in the United States.

Epidemiology

Leprosy is a chronic disease caused by *Mycobacterium leprae* that affects skin and nerves, often resulting in physical disabilities. The disease has been found around the world, showing that transmission occurs regardless of climate.

Disease transmission has ceased in nearly all developed nations, most likely because of better nutrition and socioeconomic development. Currently, new autochthonous cases are found in all tropical countries, with India and Brazil having the highest number of cases annually. Some insular countries located in the Pacific and Indian Oceans have the highest rates of new case detection, indicating a high risk of transmission.

In the Gulf region of the United States, mostly in the states of Louisiana and Texas, native cases are still diagnosed. There are armadillos *(Dasypus novemcinctus)* in the area that have been infected with strains of *M. leprae* found also in autochthonous human cases. This suggests that leprosy might be a regional zoonosis, even though *M. leprae* was introduced into the Americas by Europeans and Africans. There are also records of *M. leprae* infection in armadillos in Central and South America. Furthermore, cases in African chimpanzees raise the possibility that these animals could be helping to maintain leprosy transmission in Africa.

The mechanisms of leprosy transmission are not well known because there is no easy way to diagnose infection. It is presumed that in endemic areas, infection is much more frequent than actual disease onset. The incubation period can vary from a few months to more than 10 years, with an average of 2 to 5 years for paucibacillary (PB) and 5 to 10 years for multibacillary (MB).

It is known that MB cases excrete large numbers of viable bacilli through nasal mucus, suggesting that transmission may be by respiratory route and, in fact, this is believed to be the main source of transmission. Because *M. leprae* can be eliminated from ulcerated skin lesions, breast milk, urine and feces, and remains viable in the environment for many days, especially in humid climates, it is possible to theorize the existence of many different forms of transmission. The role of insects as vectors of bacilli is arguable.

Leprosy cases are not uniformly distributed in a community but tend to form clusters within different geographic regions, villages, or groups of domiciles. In most countries, cases are more common among men, and the 15- to 29-year-old age group tends to present the highest risk of disease. In areas where transmission is declining, the incidence tends to be higher among the elderly, affecting those who lived during a period with a higher risk of infection.

Until recently, *M. leprae* was the only agent responsible for leprosy until, in 2008, a new species called *Mycobacterium lepromatosis* sp. was described in Mexico as responsible for a diffuse form of the disease associated with increased morbidity and mortality. However, the clinical significance of this new entity, both in magnitude and in distribution, as well as particularities of the immune response to this pathogen, are not well known.

Risk Factors

In endemic areas, the main risk factors are a history of household contact with leprosy cases and low socioeconomic standing. It is estimated that home contacts of MB patients show a 5- to 10-times increased risk of becoming ill; PB case contacts present a 2- to 3- times increased risk, when compared to a group with no history of home exposure. In general, the increased risk between contacts reflects the proximity of these individuals, inside the house, with the potential source of infection. Also important is the sharing of other factors by household members, such as genetic markers, behavior, diet, intercurrent infections, and contextual aspects related to socioeconomic and environmental conditions.

An important fact in leprosy is that, even when living for a long time and in the same house with an untreated MB patient, most people do not get sick. It is estimated that 90% of the population have natural defenses against *M. leprae*. Today, there is evidence that susceptibility and resistance to *M. leprae* are genetically determined. The low frequency of genetically determined susceptibility may be the cause of the wide difference between infection and disease that is believed to exist.

Prevention

Vaccination with bacille Calmette-Guerin (BCG)[1] reduces the risk of leprosy, with studies showing a variable efficacy of 20% to 80%. The revaccination of household contacts also provides protection, especially against the MB forms of the disease.

Chemoprophylaxis of contacts or high-risk groups with a single dose of rifampin (Rifadin)[1] has been shown to be effective for a period of 2 years. However, although the chemoprophylaxis trials reported a benefit, the relatively short duration of protection indicates functional limitations.

Combined strategies, including the integration of rapid diagnostic tests to facilitate the detection of early or asymptomatic leprosy cases, as well as both chemoprophylaxis and immunization, is suggested as an active control strategy with a great potential of reducing the incidence of leprosy.

---

[1] Not FDA approved for this indication.

Improving socioeconomic conditions in the general population in endemic areas is also a very effective strategy for disease control. This can be seen when comparing the current epidemiologic situation in the Hawaiian Islands with Micronesia or the Marshall Islands, where leprosy continues with a high incidence rate.

Pathophysiology

M. leprae is an intercellular microorganism with a particular tropism for skin and peripheral nerve cells. It cannot be cultivated in vitro, but can be inoculated in mouse footpads and armadillos, although growth is quite slow. Active *M. leprae* infection is characterized by a wide clinical range, varying from a disease in which few bacilli are present in the body to one in which a high bacterial load is found in skin lesions.

Upon entering the organism, *M. leprae*, through its PAMPS (molecular patterns associated with pathogens), is recognized by pattern recognition receptors (PRRs) expressed in antigen-presenting cells (APCs), mainly dendritic cells (DCs), macrophages, monocytes, fibroblasts, and Schwann cells. Thus, the innate immune response of the host is initiated, in which the bacilli can be eliminated with a local inflammatory response, avoiding the disease, or, when this does not occur, the innate immunity can, according to the pattern of cytokines produced by APCs, regulate the response of host adaptive immunity.

In the adaptive immunity, the bacilli multiply within macrophages, enter the lymph stream and bloodstream, reach the regional lymph nodes, and from there move on to the organs of the mononuclear phagocyte system. The mycobacterial antigens are then processed and presented by APCs that can be Langerhans cells, DCs, or others from the monocyte-macrophage system that induce the hapten-protein conjugates to link the HLA-DR class II molecules to the CD4 þ lymphocytes. In those individuals where there is stimulation of the T-helper 1 cell response, these lymphocytes will produce interferon (IFN)-gamma cytokines, tumor necrosis factor (α-TNF), interleukin-2 (IL2), IL17, IL1-β, and IL12 that will promote the differentiation of macrophages in epithelioid cells that will undergo a fusion process resulting in giant cells. This inflammatory response will be sufficient to reduce *M. leprae* in the tuberculoid form of leprosy. In the presence of massive tissue infiltration by CD4 T lymphocytes, large production of these cytokines occurs along with the chemokine CXCL-10, leading to edema and tissue inflammation of the leprosy type 1 reaction. On the other hand, the production of TNF-α and IFN-γ by Schwann cells will lead to neural damage, which is also more significant in the type 1 reaction.

On the other hand, in the presence of stimulation of the TH2 sub-population of T lymphocytes (TLs), these will produce the cytokines IL4, IL5, IL6, IL13, TNF-α, and IL10 and TGF-β, these two produced by regulatory T lymphocytes (T-reg). The TGF-β, IL4, and IL10 are suppressors of macrophage activation, leading to an insufficient immune cell response to combat the level of *M. leprae* proliferation within the macrophages. This characterizes the more infectious forms of the disease at the lepromatous end of the spectrum. The cytokines IL4, IL5, IL6, and IL13 activate plasma cells and B lymphocytes, which together with complement activation, will form the immunocomplexes that will trigger leprosy type 2 reactions.

Clinical Manifestations

Due to the complexity of the parasite-host relation and the variable efficacy of the host's cellular immune response, the clinical manifestations of the disease cross a wide spectrum. This can vary from an isolated nerve lesion or a single skin patch to a systemic disease with the presence of nodules or tubercles, generally on the face. The disease can affect several organs beyond skin and nerves, including eyes, testicles, and kidneys.

Ridley and Jopling, in 1966, proposed a case classification system that takes into consideration clinical, bacteriologic, histopathologic, and immunologic parameters: tuberculoid, borderline-tuberculoid, borderline-borderline, borderline-lepromatous, and lepromatous. Indeterminate leprosy can be considered the

Figure 1 Indeterminate leprosy.

Figure 2 Tuberculoid leprosy in child.

first clinical manifestation of the disease. It can be cured spontaneously or evolve into one of the other clinical forms.

Indeterminate Leprosy

This is characterized by one or more hypochromic macules with imprecise borders and reduced thermal sensitivity, although pain and tactile sensation may be preserved (Figure 1). These may occur as areas of sensory disturbance with no alteration in skin color, sweat glands, or hair growth. Any alteration in nerve function is preliminary and, therefore, there are no physical disabilities described with this classification. Bacilloscopic readings are negative.

Tuberculoid Leprosy

This type is characterized by erythematous or hypochromic skin lesions with clear, raised borders (Figure 2). These are limited in number with an asymmetrical distribution and altered thermal sensation. Pain and tactile sensation may also be altered. Reduced perspiration and restricted partial or full alopecia may also be seen. Nerves can be affected intensively but this usually only happens to a few. Slit skin smear results are negative.

Among children, tuberculoid leprosy lesions may have the appearance of nodules or tubercles, generally only one on the face, named nodular benign leprosy of childhood. Although these lesions tend to regress spontaneously, treatment should continue as per standard ethical practice.

Borderline-Tuberculoid Leprosy

This form is characterized by lesions similar to those seen at the tuberculoid end of the spectrum, although more numerous. In general, there are more than five lesions with a diameter of 10 cm or more, less clearly defined borders, and containing possible satellite lesions (Figure 3). These lesions tend to be more symmetrical and several nerves may be affected. However, most patients with this disease type will still have a negative bacilloscopy.

Borderline-Borderline Leprosy

This is a relatively rare variation, given that it commonly evolves quickly toward the lepromatous pole, often spurred on by reaction episodes. There are usually many foveal lesions (infiltrated plaques with expanding outer borders and well-defined inner borders with apparently normal skin in the middle) (Figure 4). Generally, nerves are intensively affected, and skin smears are almost always positive.

Borderline-Lepromatous (Virchowian) Leprosy

A wide number of lesions are present with a range of possible clinical manifestations (infiltrations, papules, plaques, foveae, and nodules) that are common to the lepromatous form. However,

with this type there is a tendency to see some delimitation between the lesions and areas of healthy skin. Bacilloscopy is positive with a high bacterial load.

Lepromatous (Virchowian) Leprosy

Lepromatous leprosy (LL) has the highest bacterial burden of human bacterial infections. Extensive lesions tend to be symmetrical, erythematous, infiltrated, and without clear delineation from normal skin areas. Simple lesions evolve to become papules, tubercles, and nodules that can eventually ulcerate and that are especially full of bacilli (Figure 5). There is diffuse infiltration of the face, with auricular appendages affected in the vast majority of cases and bilateral madarosis also common. Hands and feet may also be infiltrated or showing signs of xerodermia.

LL is a systemic disease that can affect, when patients are not treated properly and opportunely, the liver, spleen, adrenal glands, lymph nodes, eyes, and nose. Nasal obstruction can be present with little or no response to vasoconstrictors. Often the nasal cavities will be affected, and the oropharynges will be full of nasal secretion highly abundant in bacilli. Subsequent nasal dryness can lead to secondary ulceration and infection with possible perforation and destruction of the nasal septum, resulting in what is commonly referred to as saddle nose. With olfactory bulb dysfunction, anosmia will often be the outcome.

Lesions to the palate, lips, gum, and uvula can further compromise the pharynx, nasopharynx, and tonsils. The eyes may show erythema, dryness, dacryocystitis, lagophthalmos, and/or diminished sensation in the cornea. Likewise, iritis and iridocyclitis may be present, so proper intervention is necessary to ensure prevention of early onset of blindness.

The testes may also be directly affected by bacilli, as witnessed by atrophy of the testicular parenchyma and diffuse fibrosis with eventual sterility and alteration of sexual function. When secondary amyloidosis is present, renal insufficiency may result.

Variations of Lepromatous Leprosy

Histoid Lepromatous Leprosy (or Wade's Lepromatous). This form of leprosy is rare. Nodular lesions are present, well defined, and of varying sizes. These may be round or oval with a reddish or pink color. These lesions contain a large number of bacilli and are normally associated with sulfone resistance. Histiocytes with a spongy appearance are present under histologic analysis.

Diffuse Lepromatous Leprosy. Described by Lucio, Alvarado, and Latapi, this is a diffuse form of LL, also called "beautiful" leprosy because this form confers a pinkish and healthy appearance to the skin. It is more frequently seen in Mexico and is characterized by the diffuse infiltration of the skin, altered sensation that starts in the hands and feet, loss of eyebrows, and telangiectasias in the face and torso. Recently a mycobacterium was isolated in cases of diffuse lepromatous leprosy (DLL) with Lucio phenomenon, whose DNA cannot be amplified using usual *M. leprae* primers. As a result, a new species has been proposed

Figure 3 Borderline-tuberculoid leprosy

Figure 4 Borderline-borderline leprosy.

Figure 5 Lepromatous (Virchowian) leprosy.

under the name *M. lepromatosis*, but many specialists do not yet accept that this is a separate microorganism.

Pure Neural Leprosy. This type presents only nerve lesions without any cutaneous patches. The most common nerves affected are the ulnar, tibial, and fibular. The radial, median, facial, trigeminal, and auricular nerves, among others, may also be damaged.

Neuropatic pain is often present spontaneously or when the nerve is palpated, either with or without thickening of the nerve. This can evolve to sensory loss, paresthesia, or muscular atrophy in the corresponding area, in addition to autonomic dysfunction and nerve abscess.

Leprosy Diagnosis

The patient is examined to locate any possible skin lesions with diminished sensation and/or areas of sensory alteration that may be due to compromised peripheral nerves. Lighting must be adequate, and it is important to observe the entire body surface moving from head to toe. Where there are possible signs of disease, thermal, pain, and tactile sensation testing should be done, also looking for areas of alopecia and/or anhidrosis. It must be noted if there is any type of physical disability.

Bacilloscopy consists of the collection and examination of skin smears taken from a suspected lesion, both earlobes, and both elbows, and helps to classify a patient as PB with a negative examination result or MB when positive.

The bacilloscopic results will generally be negative in the indeterminate, tuberculoid, and borderline-tuberculoid forms, which are considered the PB group. Similarly, they tend to be positive for the lepromatous (Virchowian), borderline-lepromatous, and borderline-borderline, which are MB group.

Ideally, the bacilloscopic reading should be expressed quantitatively as a bacteriologic index (BI) so that it is possible to monitor the patient's progress during treatment. In patients with positive bacilloscopy at the time of diagnosis, it is recommended to repeat it at the end of therapy. Smear microscopy is important for differential diagnoses between reactions and relapse.

The histologic examination of a skin biopsy also helps to provide a more precise disease classification and can help to confirm diagnosis in cases that are bacilloscopy negative. In the indeterminate leprosy (HI), there is a nonspecific inflammatory infiltrate, consisting of lymphocytes and sometimes histiocytes, around superficial and deep vessels, affecting the cutaneous appendages, especially the neural fillets. The tuberculoid leprosy (HT) and borderline-tuberculoid leprosy (HBT) forms are characterized histologically by the presence of granulomas-histiocytes, which differentiate into epithelioid cells, giant cells, and lymphocytes, located around vessels, cutaneous appendages, and nervous fillets. Bacillus research is almost always negative. In HBV and HV forms, the inflammatory infiltrate is characterized by the predominance of foamy or vacuolated histiocytes, with large numbers of bacilli, isolated or grouped in structures called *globias*.

In regions with limited access to laboratory resources, clinical diagnosis is sufficient to warrant the beginning of the standard leprosy treatment regimen, keeping in mind that this is the only dermatologic disease with altered sensation in lesions. The World Health Organization (WHO) suggests the classification of cases as either PB or MB based on the number of skin lesions, with MB cases having five or more such patches.

Available serologic testing does not show sufficient accuracy for disease diagnosis or infection. A recent meta-analysis using a fixed model to estimate OR for the association of phenol-glycolipid-1 antigen (PGL-1) positivity and clinical leprosy demonstrated that PGL-1 appears not to be a useful test in the decision of which contacts should receive chemoprophylaxis.

Real-time polymerase chain reaction is available for leprosy and can act as a means of confirmation for diagnosis of PB cases.

TABLE 1	Main Differential Diagnosis by Leprosy Forms	
INDETERMINATE LEPROSY	**TUBERCULOID AND BORDERLINE-TUBER-CULOID LEPROSY**	**BORDERLINE-BORDERLINE, BORDERLINE-LEP-ROMATOUS, AND LEPROMATOUS LEPROSY**
S S Eczematidis (Pityriasis Alba)	Seborrheic dermatitis	Erythema nodosum
Seborrheic dermatitis	Dermatofitosis	Diffuse (anergic) cutaneous leishmaniasis
Localized scleroderma (morphea)	Granuloma annulare	Cutaneous and mucosal leishmaniasis
Residual hypochromia and achromia	Cutaneous leishmaniasis	Systemic lupus erythematous and other rheumatologic diseases
Pityriasis versicolor	Discoid lupus erythematous	Neurofibromatosis (von Recklinghausen disease)
Vitiligo	Pityriasis rosea Gibert	Pityriasis rosea Gibert
Hypochromic nevus	Psoriasis	Congenital syphilis, secondary syphilis, tertiary syphilis
	Sarcoidosis	Cutaneous lymphoma (Mycosis fungoides)
	Secondary syphilis	
	Cutaneous tuberculosis	

Differential Diagnosis

Differential diagnoses of leprosy include a variety of dermatologic conditions, given the wide range of clinical manifestations in leprosy. The sensory loss symptomatic of leprosy can also be difficult to determine in children and in other diseases that produce changes in the normal skin characteristics (Table 1).

Treatment

Leprosy treatment, like tuberculosis treatment, must deal with bacillar resistance and persistence. Single-drug therapy selects drug-resistant bacilli and should be avoided. Therapy duration has, as a target, the reduction of the number of persistent bacilli that could lead to relapses.

Standard multidrug therapy (MDT) with dapsone, rifampin (Rifadin)[1], and clofazimine[5] for 12 months for MB cases and 6-month MDT with dapsone and rifampin for PB cases has dramatically changed the prognosis for leprosy patients. However, the evidence is rather weak on the efficacy of this drug regimen, especially regarding the necessary length of time for treatment, both in terms of the proportion of relapse cases and other outcomes, such as physical disability. The use of rifampin once a month was determined for financial reasons, and there is no study comparing this schedule with daily use. For this reason, research on new drugs and treatment regimens continues.

Shorter regimens were used but had shown high relapse rates: daily doses of rifampin and ofloxacin (Floxin)[1] for 4 weeks; single-dose course of rifampin, ofloxacin, and minocycline (Minocin)[1] for single-lesion patients.

Fluoroquinolones (pefloxacin,[2] ofloxacin, and moxifloxacin [Avelox][1]), macrolides (clarithromycin [Biaxin][1]), and tetracycline (minocycline) are effective against *M. leprae*. Only rifampin, its derivative rifapentine (Priftin)[1], and moxifloxacin are bactericidal drugs; all others are bacteriostatic.

In cases of intolerance or resistance to dapsone, this can be removed from the drug regimen, and for PB patients, clofazimine is used instead. For MB patients, in these cases, minocycline or ofloxacin can be used instead of dapsone, without alteration in treatment duration. Where similar intolerance or resistance is related to rifampin, this should be substituted with a daily dose of 400 mg of ofloxacin. This alternate course lasts 6 months for PB cases and 24 months for MB.

For those who cannot take either dapsone or rifampin, PB patients can be treated with ofloxacin (400 mg/day) or minocycline (100 mg/day), and clofazimine (50 mg/day) in self-administered doses for 6 months. Similarly, MB patients can use ofloxacin plus minocycline plus clofazimine during the first 6 months of treatment (intensive phase), followed by 18 months with daily doses of ofloxacin or minocycline and clofazimine (maintenance phase).

Perspectives on the Use of a Uniform Treatment for All Forms, Regardless of Clinical or Laboratory Classification

Despite the success of MDT, the complexity for the operationalization of the scheme throughout the health system, the prolonged treatment time, and the difficulty of patient adherence reinforce the need for shorter regimens that can be easily implemented in primary care. Since 2002, the WHO recommended clinical studies to investigate the viability of a uniform treatment (U-MDT) for all leprosy cases, regardless of classification, with 6 months' duration.

Several studies developed in India, China, Bangladesh, and Brazil, with different designs, achieved promising results, showing that the reduction in the duration of treatment did not increase relapse rates, reaction frequency, or neural damage. The Brazilian study also demonstrated no statistical differences in BI decline, between regular MDT and U-MDT. Moreover, the same study showed that U-MDT reduced *M. leprae*-specific antibodies during and after treatment.

Thus, the results of the study conducted in Brazil, the first randomized and controlled study on U-MDT, together with the results from three previous studies performed in China, India, and Bangladesh, support the premise that U-MDT is an acceptable option to be adopted in endemic countries to treat leprosy patients in the field worldwide. The proposed U-MDT (daily intake of dapsone plus clofazimine and monthly rifampicin for 6 months) is recommended for both PB and MB leprosy patients, regardless of classification criteria.

Leprosy Reactions and Control

Over the course of this chronic disease, around 30% of the patients develop acute inflammatory episodes called leprosy reactions. These reactions can occur before diagnosis, as well as during or after MDT treatment. They are commonly grouped into (a) type 1 (reversal) reactions (T1Rs) resulting from vigorous cell-mediated immune response; and (b) type 2 reactions (T2Rs), the clinical manifestation of which is frequently erythematous nodosum leprosum (ENL) that comes about mainly from immunocomplex deposits. In patients with borderline-borderline and borderline-lepromatous leprosy, it is possible to have both reaction types simultaneously. There is also Lucio phenomenon, which is an immune system response with important clinical manifestations. Its physiopathology is not well understood, with abundant infection of *M. leprae* in endothelium, which can lead to thrombosis

---

[1]Not FDA approved for this indication.
[5]Investigational drug in the United States.
[2]Not available in the United States.

in the most superficial vases from immunocomplex deposits with hemorrhaging and cutaneous infarction.

In the literature, a robust positive association has been demonstrated between bacterial load and the frequency of leprosy reactions. A reaction can be set off by various factors, such as pregnancy, childbirth, vaccinations, puberty, intercurrent infections, stress (physical, psychological, or surgical), use of potassium iodate/iodide (SSKI), and immune reconstruction inflammatory syndrome (IRIS) linked to anti-retroviral and/or immune-based therapies.

Those patients who experience leprosy reactions during MDT treatment should continue taking their regimen without modification while also beginning a specific and concurrent treatment for the appropriate reaction type.

Type 1 Reaction or Reversal Reaction

Clinically speaking, lesions become more erythematous and infiltrated, and those with previously diminished sensation can become more sensitive to touch. Desquamation may occur and some lesions may even ulcerate. New lesions can erupt along with edema in the hands, feet, and face, as well general systemic symptoms. These reactions can last for years in some patients. It is important to begin an immediate intervention, given that neuritis is the most common, serious, and potentially disabling clinical manifestation of T1R.

The drug of choice for T1R treatment is prednisone (or prednisolone [Millipred]) with a dosage of 1 to 2 mg/kg/day for at least 12 weeks, at which point it can be tapered off until discontinuing medication around the 24th week.

Alternative drugs in type 1 reaction:

Azathioprine (Imuran)[1]: 1 to 2 mg/kg/day, until reaction control.
Cyclosporine (Neoral, Sandimmune)[1]: 5 to 8 mg/kg/day, until reaction control.
Clofazimine[5]: 300 mg to 30 days.
200 mg to 30 days.
100 mg to 30 days.

Type 2 Reaction

This occurs in MB patients, and ENL is the most frequent clinical manifestation of T2Rs. Other variations of T2R are polymorphic erythema and vasculitis.

Clinically, ENL is a systemic condition with the eruption of painful and often symmetrical erythematous nodules on the arms and legs. When deeper, these nodules are more easily palpated than the more visible ones but will often ulcerate. Neuritis is frequent, although it is less aggressive than seen in T1Rs. The systemic impact can produce edema, myalgia, fever, malaise, asthenia, weight loss, cephalalgia, iritis, episcleritis, iridocyclitis, glaucoma, epistaxis, arthralgia, and orchiepididymitis with testicular atrophy, glomerulonephritis, chronic renal insufficiency, hepatosplenomegaly, and amyloidosis.

The most common medication used for ENL is thalidomide (Thalomid) in variable dosage, from 100 to 400 mg/day, depending on the severity of the reaction. The distribution of thalidomide is restricted in some countries due to its teratogenic effects. For this reason, it should be given under strict supervision with proper medical, ethical, and legal measures in place.

For ENL associated with neuritis, iritis, orchitis, and/or hand-foot reactions, or in women of childbearing age, a course of corticosteroids should be given (prednisone at 1 to 2 mg/kg/day).

In chronic cases and those that are nonresponsive to treatment, it is possible to administer clofazimine along with steroids at the initial dosage of 100 mg three times per day for a maximum of 12 weeks. This should be reduced to 100 mg twice daily for another 12 weeks and finally 100 mg/day for 12 to 24 weeks. Cyclosporine (Neoral, Sandimmune)[1] may also offer some benefit to the patient with serious ENL, as can the association of azathioprine (Imuran),[1] methotrexate[1], and corticosteroids.

[1] Not FDA approved for this indication.
[5] Investigational drug in the United States.

TABLE 2	Differences Between Reaction Type 1 and Relapse
REVERSAL REACTION	**RELAPSE**
Generally occurs during course of multidrug therapy or within 6 months of treatment completion	Occurs at least 2 years after treatment completion
Sudden and unexpected onset	Slow and insidious onset
Can be accompanied by fever and malaise	In general, no systemic symptoms present
Old lesions become erythematous, shiny, and infiltrated	Old lesions may present erythematous edges
In general, many new lesions	Few new lesions
There may be ulceration of the reaction lesions	Ulceration may occur on arms and legs in addition to the lesions
Regression with desquamation	No desquamation present
Can quickly affect several nerve trunks, with presence of pain, sensory alteration, and decreased motor function	May affect a single nerve and functional alterations often take place very slowly
Excellent response to corticosteroid therapy	Does not respond well to corticosteroid therapy
Bacteriologic index stable or falls	Bacteriologic index rises

Alternative drugs in type 2 reaction:

Azathioprine[1]: 1 to 2 mg / kg / day, until reaction control.
Cyclosporine[1]: 5 to 8 mg/kg/day, until reaction control.
Methotrexate[1]: 15 mg (IM/SC or PO)/week, until reaction control.
Pentoxifylline: (Trental)[1] 1200 mg/day, until reaction control.
Clofazimine[5]: 300 mg to 30 days.
200 mg to 30 days.
100 mg to 30 days.

Lucio Phenomenon

Lucio phenomenon can occur in forms of LL. The skin lesions can be discrete and limited in number, pinkish or cyanotic, often very painful, and potentially necrotizing and ulcerative. This condition can lead to death. Treatment is based on a course of corticosteroid therapy appropriate for each patient.

Differential Diagnosis Between Relapse and Reaction

Relapse rates are very low whereas reactions are quite frequent, even after completing treatment. Table 2 shows the main differences between reaction type 1 and type 2 relapse. Recently, *M. leprae* whole genome sequencing technique was used to discriminate between cases of relapse and reinfection.

Complications

Leprosy complications are the result of permanent nerve damage. Lesions to the large nerve trunks, such as the ulnar, median, and tibial, cause motor and sensory loss leading to disabilities such as claw hand and footdrop.

The absence of sensation in the hands, soles of the feet, and cornea leaves these areas predisposed to common wounds and pressure ulcers. This reality demands that patients take specific care to avoid ulcers and detect them as soon as possible to prevent secondary infection. In addition, corneal ulcers can result in blindness.

[1] Not FDA approved for this indication.
[5] Investigational drug in the United States.

Acknowledgment

We thank Dr. Anna Maria Salles for the patient's pictures.

References

Becx-Bleumink M: Relapses among leprosy patients treated with multidrug therapy: experience in the leprosy control program of the All Africa Leprosy and Rehabilitation Training Center (ALERT) in Ethiopia; practical difficulties with diagnosing relapses; operational procedures and criteria for diagnosing relapses, *Int J Lepr Other Mycobact Dis* 60:421–435, 1992.

Butlin CR, Pahan D, Maug AKJ, et al: Outcome of 6 months MBMDT in MB patients in Bangladesh- preliminary results, *Lepr Rev* 87, 2016, 171–82.

Cruz RCDS, Bührer-Sékula S, Penna GO, et al: Clinical trial for uniform multidrug therapy for leprosy patients in Brazil (U-MDT/CT-BR): adverse effects approach, *An Bras Dermatol* 93:377–384, 2018.

Cruz RCDS, Bührer-Sékula S, Penna MLF, Penna GO, Talhari S: Leprosy: current situation, clinical and laboratory aspects, treatment history and perspective of the uniform multidrug therapy for all patients, *An Bras Dermatol* 92(6):761–773, 2017.

da Silva Rocha A, Cunha Dos Santos AA, Pignataro P, et al: Genotyping of Mycobacterium leprae from Brazilian leprosy patients suggests the occurrence of reinfection or of bacterial population shift during disease relapse, *J Med Microbiol* 60:1441–1446, 2011.

Ferreira IP, Buhrer-Sékula S, De Oliveira MR, et al: Patient profile and treatment satisfaction of Brazilian leprosy patients in a clinical trial of uniform six-month multidrug therapy (U-MDT/CT-BR), *Lepr Rev* 85(4):267–274, 2014 Dec.

Fine PE: Leprosy: the epidemiology of a slow bacterium, *Epidemiol Rev* 4:161–188, 1982.

Gelber RH, Grosset J: The chemotherapy of leprosy: an interpretive history, *Lepr Rev* 83:221–240, 2012.

Gillis TP, Scollard DM, Lockwood DN: What is the evidence that the putative Myco- bacterium lepromatosis species causes diffuse lepromatous leprosy? *Lepr Rev* 82:205–209, 2011.

Gonçalves H de S, Pontes MA, Bührer-Sékula S, et al: Brazilian clinical trial of uniform multidrug therapy for leprosy patients: the correlation between clinical disease types and adverse effect, *Mem Inst Oswaldo Cruz* 107(Suppl 1):74–78, 2012 Dec.

Guerra JG, Penna GO, Castro LCM: Eritema Nodoso Hansênico: atualização clínica e terapêutica, *Erythema Nodosum Leprosum: clinical and therapeutic up-date An Bras Dermatol* 77:389–407, 2002.

Han XY, Sizer KC, Velarde-Félix JS, et al: The leprosy agents Mycobacterium lepromatosis and Mycobacterium leprae in Mexico, *Int J Dermatol* 51:952–959, 2012.

Hungria EM, Bührer-Sékula S, Oliveira RM, et al: Mycobacterium leprae-specific antibodies in multibacillary leprosy patients decrease during and after treatment with either the regular 12 doses multidrug therapy (MDT) or the uniform 6 doses MDT, *Front Immunol* 9:915, 2018.

Hungria EM, Bührer-Sékula S, de Oliveira RM, et al: Leprosy reactions: The predictive value of Mycobacterium leprae-specific serology evaluated in a Brazilian cohort of leprosy patients (U-MDT/CT-BR), *PLoS Negl Trop Dis* 11(2):e0005396, 2017 Feb 21.

Hungria EM, Oliveira RM, Penna GO, et al: Can baseline ML Flow test results predict leprosy reactions? An investigation in a cohort of patients enrolled in the uniform multidrug therapy clinical trial for leprosy patients in Brazil, *Infect Dis Poverty* 5(1):110–120, 2016 Dec 6.

International Federation of Anti-Leprosy Associations: Available at http://www.ilep.org.uk/about-ilep/. [Accessed 9 July 2015].

Kroger A, Pannikar V, Htoon MT, et al: International open trial of uniform multidrug therapy regimen for 6 months for all types of leprosy patients: rationale, design and preliminary results, *Trop Med Int Health* 13:594–602, 2008.

Lockwood DN, Shetty V, Penna GO: Hazards of setting targets to eliminate disease: lessons from the leprosy elimination campaign, *BMJ* 348:1136, 2014.

Moura RS, Penna GO, Cardoso LP, et al: Description of leprosy classification at baseline among patients enrolled at the uniform multidrug therapy clinical trial for leprosy patients in Brazil, *Am J Trop Med Hyg* 92(6):1280–1284, 2015 Jun.

Moura RS, Penna GO, Fujiwara T, et al: Evaluation of a rapid serological test for leprosy classification using human serum albumin as the antigen carrier, *Journal of Immunological Methods* 412:35–41, 2014.

Nery JS, Pereira SM, Rasella D, et al: Effect of the Brazilian conditional cash transfer and primary health care programs on the new case detection rate of leprosy, *PLoS Neglected Tropical Diseases* 8:e3357–e3360, 2014.

Pedrosa VL, Dias LC, Galban E, et al: Leprosy among schoolchildren in the Amazon region: A cross-sectional study of active search and possible source of infection by contact tracing, *PLoS Negl Trop Dis* 12:e0006261, 2018.

Penna GO, Bührer-Sékula S, Kerr LRS, et al: Uniform multidrug therapy for leprosy patients in Brazil (U-MDT/CT-BR): Results of an open label, randomized and controlled clinical trial, among multibacillary patients, *PLoS Negl Trop Dis* 11:e0005725, 2017.

Penna GO, Pontes MA, Cruz R, et al: A clinical trial for uniform multidrug therapy for leprosy patients in Brazil: rationale and design, *Mem Inst Oswaldo Cruz* 107(Suppl 1):22–27, 2012 Dec.

Penna ML, Bührer-Sékula S, Pontes MA, et al: Primary results of clinical trial for uniform multidrug therapy for leprosy patients in Brazil (U-MDT/CT-BR): reactions frequency in multibacillary patients, *Lepr Rev* 83(3):308–319, 2012 Sep.

Penna ML, Bührer-Sékula S, Pontes MA, et al: Results from the clinical trial of uniform multidrug therapy for leprosy patients in Brazil (U-MDT/CT-BR): decrease in bacteriological index, *Lepr Rev* 85(4):262–266, 2014 Dec.

Penna ML, Penna GO: Leprosy frequency in the world, 1999–2010, *Mem Inst Oswaldo Cruz* 107(Suppl. 1):3–12, 2012.

Penna ML, Penna GO, Iglesias PC, et al: Anti-PGL-1 positivity as a risk marker for the development of leprosy among contacts of leprosy cases: systematic review and metaanalysis, *PLoS Neglected Tropical Diseases* 10:e0004703, 2016.

Santos SD, Penna GO, Costa MCN, et al: Leprosy in children and adolescents under 15 years old in an urban centre in Brazil, *Memórias do Instituto Oswaldo Cruz* 111:359–364, 2016.

Shen J, Yan L, Yu M, et al: Six years' follow-up of multibacillary leprosy patients treated with uniform multi-drug therapy in China, *Int J Dermatol* 54:315–318, 2015.

Stefani MMA, Avanzi C, Bührer-Sékula S, et al: Whole genome sequencing distinguishes between relapse and reinfection in recurrent leprosy cases, *PLoS Negl Trop Dis* 11(6):e0005598, 2017 Jun 15.

Talhari S, Gontijo B, Vale ECS, Marques SA: Editorial - New perspectives for the treatment of Hansen's disease, *An Bras Dermatol* 92(6):760, 2017.

Talhari C, Mira MT, Massone C, et al: Leprosy and HIV coinfection: a clinical, pathological, immunological, and therapeutic study of a cohort from a Brazilian referral center for infectious diseases, *J Infect Dis* 202:345–354, 2010.

Talhari C, Talhari S, Penna GO: Clinical aspects of leprosy, *Clinics in Dermatology* 33:26–37, 2015.

Talhari S, Neves RG, Penna GO, Oliveira MLWR: *Hansemase*, 4th ed., Manaus, 2006, Grafica tropical.

Truman RW, Singh P, Sharma R, et al: Probable zoonotic leprosy in the southern United States, *N Engl J Med* 364:1626–1633, 2011.

Van Brakel W, Cross H, Declercq E, et al: Review of leprosy research evidence (2002–2009) and implications for current policy and practice, *Lepr Rev* 81:228–275, 2010.

Van Veen NH, Lockwood DN, Van Brakel WH, et al: *Interventions for Erythema Nodosum Leprosum (Review)*, Cochrane Collaboration, Hoboken, NJ, 2012, John Wiley & Sons, p 53.

WHO Expert Committee on Leprosy. World Health Organ Tech Rep Ser., 968:1–61.

WHO, editor: *Global Leprosy Strategy 2016 - 2020: Accelerating Towards a Leprosy-Free World*, WHO, 2016.

LYME DISEASE

Method of
Carlos R. Oliveira, MD, PhD; and Eugene D. Shapiro, MD

CURRENT DIAGNOSIS

- Lyme disease, caused by the spirochete *Borrelia burgdorferi*, is the most common vector-borne infection in both the United States and Europe.
- Early localized Lyme disease is a clinical diagnosis that is based on the presence of a single erythema migrans rash. The rash presents as an expanding circular macule that is often uniformly erythematous but occasionally can have central clearing that gives it the appearance of a target lesion. Erythema migrans usually appears 7 to 14 days after a tick bite (although the bite often is not recognized). If untreated, it persists for about 3 to 4 weeks.
- Early disseminated Lyme disease can present as multiple erythema migrans, cranial nerve palsy, lymphocytic meningitis, radiculomyelitis (Bannwarth syndrome), or carditis.
- Arthritis is the primary manifestation of late Lyme disease. Typically it is an oligoarthritis that most often involves a single knee.
- Patients with no objective signs but only nonspecific symptoms (e.g., arthralgia, myalgia, fatigue, or perceived cognitive difficulties) are highly unlikely to have active Lyme disease as the cause regardless of the result of antibody tests.
- Antibody test results for Lyme disease are usually negative in patients with erythema migrans (single or multiple); therefore testing for antibody generally is only indicated for patients with non-cutaneous manifestations of Lyme disease.
- The IgG antibody test has good sensitivity for patients with Lyme disease ≥4 weeks after initial infection.
- Tests for antibodies to *B burgdorferi* should use a two-tier procedure, first with a sensitive quantitative test, usually either a whole-cell or C-6 peptide enzyme-linked immunosorbent assay (ELISA); if that result is either positive or equivocal, a more specific test, the Western immunoblot, is done to con-

firm a positive test result. The presence of antibodies against at least either 2 (for IgM) or 5 (for IgG) proteins of *B burgdorferi* is required for the immunoblot result to be considered positive.

- In patients with symptoms present for 4-6 weeks or longer, Lyme disease should not be diagnosed based on a positive IgM antibody result alone.
- Sensitivity of PCR assays of both blood and CSF are poor because concentrations of *B burgdorferi* in these fluids are low.
- Once serum antibodies to *B burgdorferi* develop, both IgG and IgM antibodies may persist for decades despite adequate treatment; therefore elevated concentrations of antibodies in serum do not necessarily indicate active infection.

 CURRENT THERAPY

- An oral course of doxycycline (Vibramycin)[1] for 10 days or of amoxicillin (Amoxil)[1] or cefuroxime axetil (Ceftin) for 14 days is highly effective for treating early localized Lyme disease.
- A 14-day course of the same antimicrobials also is highly effective in treating multiple erythema migrans and other manifestations of early disseminated Lyme disease, although patients with Lyme meningitis or complete atrioventricular block should be treated either parenterally with ceftriaxone (Rocephin)[1] or cefotaxime (Claforan)[1] or, in some instances, orally with doxycycline.[1]
- A 28-day course of an oral regimen is recommended for the treatment of Lyme arthritis.
- Doxycycline (Vibramycin) is contraindicated in women who are pregnant or are breastfeeding.
- The most effective preventive measure is avoidance of tick-infested areas. If exposure is unavoidable, visual inspection and prompt removal of embedded ticks, use of tick repellents with N, N-diethyl-3-methylbenzamide (DEET), and use of protective clothing have all been found to be modestly effective.
- An infected tick generally must be attached for 36 to 72 hours or longer for there to be a substantial risk of transmission of *B burgdorferi*. If a tick that has been embedded for at least 36 hours is removed, a single dose of doxycycline (Vibramycin) 8.8 mg/kg, maximum 200 mg,[1] given within 72 hours of removing the engorged tick, can be effective in preventing Lyme disease.
- Multiple or prolonged courses of antibiotics have not been shown to be effective and are not recommended for patients with only chronic, subjective symptoms after completing appropriate antibiotic treatment for Lyme disease.

[1]Not FDA approved for this indication.

Epidemiology and Ecology

Lyme arthritis was first described in 1977 when an unusual cluster of children with arthritis in Lyme, Connecticut, was reported. Soon after, Willy Burgdorfer identified the causative bacterial agent, a spirochete that was later named *Borrelia burgdorferi*, in *Ixodes scapularis*, the deer tick. Lyme disease, the most common vector-borne illness in both the United States and Europe, is transmitted by hard-bodied ticks of the *Ixodes* genus. In the United States, *Ixodes scapularis* (in the East and upper Midwest) and *Ixodes pacificus*, the Western black-legged tick (on the Pacific coast), can be vectors of Lyme disease. More than 90% of all cases in the United States occur in nine states: Connecticut, Maryland, Massachusetts, Minnesota, New Jersey, New York, Pennsylvania, Rhode Island, and Wisconsin. In Europe and in Asia, *Ixodes ricinus* (the sheep tick) and *Ixodes perscultatus* (the tiaga tick) can transmit *B burgdorferi*. *Ixodes* ticks feed once in each of the three stages of their 2-year life cycle: larva, nymph, and adult. There are a number of

genomospecies of *Borrelia burgdorferi* sensu lato that cause Lyme disease. In the United States, Lyme disease is almost exclusively caused by *B burgdorferi* sensu stricto, whereas in Europe and in Asia, *Borrelia afzelii* and *Borrelia garinii*, in addition to *B burgdorferi* sensu stricto, are the major causes of Lyme disease.

Lyme disease is a zoonosis. The primary reservoir for *B burgdorferi* are small mammals, such as mice and chipmunks, although birds and other mammals, such as foxes and coyotes, can also serve as reservoirs of the organism. Deer are not a competent reservoir for *B burgdorferi*, but they are important for supporting the life cycle of the deer tick. Ticks are uninfected when they hatch. They can become infected after they feed on an infected animal. The bacteria live in the midgut of the tick, which must remain attached to a host for 36 to 48 hours or longer for the spirochete to travel to the salivary glands so it can be injected into the host. Although ticks may become infected at any stage of the life cycle, nymphs are more likely to transmit the organism. This is because their small size (<2 mm) makes them more difficult to detect than adult ticks and because the organism can be transmitted more rapidly from an infected nymph than from an infected adult tick. Consequently, nymphal ticks are less likely than are adult ticks to be removed before the organism can be transmitted. The most important risk factor for Lyme disease is exposure to ticks in an area in which the disease is endemic. Most cases of Lyme disease occur in the spring and summer, which correlates with peak activity of nymphal ticks and with frequent outdoor activity of humans.

Pathophysiology

The pathogenesis of Lyme disease is predominantly driven by the host immune response to the spirochete. During the first stage of infection, after transfer of the organism to the skin, inflammation ensues that leads to an erythematous lesion at the site of inoculation. The spirochete does not produce toxins; however, it can disseminate via the bloodstream or through the lymph vessels. After dissemination, the spirochete can adhere to distal tissues, and an immune-mediated inflammatory reaction at these sites leads to the characteristic clinical manifestations of Lyme disease.

Prevention

No vaccine is currently available to prevent Lyme disease in humans. The most effective preventive measure is avoidance of tick-infested areas. Tick repellents that contain N, N-diethyl-3-methylbenzamide (DEET) and the use of protective clothing (long sleeves and pants) have been found to be modestly effective at preventing Lyme disease. If exposure is unavoidable, frequent visual inspection with prompt removal of ticks is recommended. In endemic areas, if a nymphal or adult *Ixodes* tick is removed that is partially engorged (has been attached for at least 36 hours), a single dose of doxycycline (Vibramycin)[1] administered within 72 hours of removing the tick can be effective in preventing Lyme disease.

Clinical Manifestations

The clinical manifestations of Lyme disease can be divided into three stages: early localized disease, early disseminated disease, and late disease. About two-thirds of patients with Lyme disease in the United States have early localized disease, which is characterized by a single erythema migrans (EM) rash at the site of the tick bite (although the tick bite is recognized in only a minority of cases). The rash starts as an erythematous macule or papule and then expands as an annular macule that is often uniformly erythematous (about two-thirds of cases of EM), although it can have central clearing that gives it the appearance of a classic target lesion. EM usually appears 7 to 14 days (range 3–30 days) after the tick bite and, if untreated, may expand to an average of 15 cm in diameter before resolving after 2 to 4 weeks or longer. The rash may be asymptomatic or it may be accompanied by systemic symptoms such as fever, malaise, headache, stiff neck, myalgia, or arthralgia.

The second most common manifestation of Lyme disease is multiple EM, which accounts for 15% to 23% of the reported cases in

[1]Not FDA approved for this indication.

the United States. Multiple EM, a manifestation of early disseminated Lyme disease, occurs when the spirochete disseminates via the bloodstream and presents as multiple erythematous round or ovoid macules that are usually smaller than most single EM lesions and are often accompanied by fever and other systemic symptoms. Other manifestations of early disseminated Lyme disease include cranial nerve palsy (especially facial palsy), lymphocytic meningitis, radiculomyelitis, and carditis. Cranial nerve palsies, especially facial nerve palsy, occur more commonly in children and account for approximately 3% to 5% of all cases of Lyme disease. In most cases, facial nerve palsy resolves within 4 to 8 weeks usually leaving minor, if any, obvious residua. Lyme meningitis occurs less frequently (1% to 2% of cases) and typically has a subacute presentation similar to, though often of longer duration, than that of enteroviral meningitis. There is a mononuclear pleocytosis in cerebrospinal fluid. Increased intracranial pressure with papilledema is not uncommon. Neurologic involvement in Lyme disease is more common in Europe and in Asia, presumably because local strains of the bacteria are more neurotropic. Carditis, which is found in fewer than 1% of cases, typically causes various degrees of heart block, which usually is asymptomatic and may be detected only with an electrocardiogram, but may manifest as syncope, dyspnea, or dizziness due to complete heart block. Sudden death due to Lyme carditis has been reported but is very rare.

Arthritis is the main manifestation of late Lyme disease, and in North America accounts for approximately 6% to 8% of reported cases. Lyme arthritis typically is an oligoarthritis that involves a single knee about 90% of the time. Symptoms of arthritis develop 2 to 6 months after the tick bite and present with objective signs of inflammation of the joint. Arthritis typically resolves 2 to 6 weeks after appropriate treatment, although it may persist or recur in 10% to 20% of treated patients.

In Europe and in Asia, uncommon manifestations of Lyme disease include borrelial lymphocytoma, a painless nodule commonly located on the ear, breast, or scrotum; and acrodermatitis chronica atrophicans, a chronic fibrosing skin lesion typically found on the extensor surfaces of the extremities.

Diagnosis

Early localized Lyme disease is a clinical diagnosis based on a history of potential exposure to ticks in an endemic area and the presence of the characteristic EM rash. Antibodies to the organism typically appear 3 to 4 weeks after the initial infection. Consequently, serologic tests are not indicated in patients with EM because most will not have detectable antibodies. Although more patients with multiple erythema migrans may be seropositive at the time of presentation, a majority will still be seronegative early on. Moreover, detectable antibodies may never develop in patients who are treated early in their courses. In patients with extracutaneous manifestations of Lyme disease, serologic testing is useful in making a diagnosis. Tests for antibodies to *B burgdorferi* should use a two-tier procedure, in which a sensitive quantitative test, usually an enzyme-linked immunosorbent assay (ELISA) against either "whole cell" or C6 peptide antigens of the bacteria, is performed. If the result of the quantitative test is either positive or equivocal, a Western immunoblot is done to confirm the specificity of the result. As with most infections, once they develop, elevated concentrations of both IgM and IgG antibodies may persist for decades in symptom-free patients who have been cured of Lyme disease. A positive test result is evidence of prior exposure to the organism and is not evidence of active infection. In addition, false-positive antibody test results are common, especially in patients with a low prior probability of Lyme disease, such as those with chronic nonspecific symptoms such as arthralgia, myalgia, or fatigue, who do not have concomitant objective findings associated with Lyme disease. False-positive IgM test results are especially common. A diagnosis of Lyme disease should rarely be based on a positive IgM test result alone, especially in patients who have had symptoms for a month or longer.

Polymerase chain reaction (PCR) assays can detect the organism in skin biopsies, CSF, blood, or synovial fluid. However, because concentrations of the organism are low in both the blood and the CSF, sensitivity of PCR assays of these fluids is poor. Because the rash is so characteristic and because virtually all patients with Lyme arthritis will have a positive result for IgG antibodies to *B burgdorferi*, such assays rarely are needed to make a diagnosis. The organism can be cultured using special media, but sensitivity generally is poor, and it takes weeks for the organism to grow.

Differential Diagnosis

The differential diagnosis of Lyme disease depends on the clinical stage of the illness. Single EM may be confused with ringworm, cellulitis, nummular eczema, granuloma annulare or insect bites. Southern tick–associated rash illness (STARI) manifests in a rash identical to EM. However, it occurs at the site of a bite from the lone star tick (*Amblyomma americanum*) and is most common in the south-central United States. The cause of STARI is unknown, but, unlike with Lyme disease, it is not associated with significant extracutaneous manifestations. Multiple EM may look very similar to erythema multiforme. Lymphocytic meningitis occurs with numerous viral infections, most commonly enterovirus. There are many other causes of carditis, including a number of viruses, as well as rheumatologic diseases such as lupus and rheumatic fever. There is substantial variation in how Lyme arthritis presents. Most often it is a subacute arthritis that may mimic rheumatoid arthritis or other more chronic arthritides, with <50,000 white blood cells/mL in the synovial fluid. However, it can present acutely and may mimic acute bacterial arthritis (like that due to *Staphylococcus aureus*), with >100,000 white blood cells/mL in synovial fluid.

Relapse Versus Reinfection

Resistance of *B burgdorferi* to recommended antimicrobials has not been reported. First-line antimicrobial therapy for Lyme disease is highly efficacious, and bacteriologic treatment failures are very rare. In a study of patients with two or more episodes of EM that occurred years apart, it was shown that the episodes were caused by different strains of bacteria, indicating that reinfection, rather than persistence of the original organism, was the cause of repeated episodes of EM. Reinfection rarely occurs in patients with late Lyme disease, indicating that most such patients are immune. On the other hand, patients with early Lyme disease who are treated may become reinfected from a new tick bite, presumably because the organism was killed before a protective immune response could occur. Persistent or recurrent arthritis does occur in 10% to 20% of patients with Lyme arthritis. So-called antibiotic-refractory arthritis occurs when frank arthritis persists despite two or more courses of antimicrobial treatment. This may be due to either an autoimmune process or slow clearance of antigens of dead organisms. There is no evidence that the cause is failure of the antibiotic to kill the organisms.

Post-Treatment Lyme Disease Syndrome and "Chronic" Lyme Disease

A small minority of patients with Lyme disease who have completed appropriate treatment may continue to have nonspecific symptoms, such as fatigue, arthralgia, myalgia, or perceived cognitive difficulties, for weeks or months after completing treatment. These have been termed *post-treatment Lyme disease symptoms* and, if they persist for 6 months or longer and are disabling, they are referred to as *post-treatment Lyme disease syndrome* (PTLDS). It is not clear whether the frequency or the nature of these symptoms in patients with PTLDS is greater than that among the general population. In addition, several placebo-controlled, randomized clinical trials of prolonged courses (6 weeks or longer) of intensive antimicrobial treatment (e.g., with ceftriaxone) in patients with PTLDS have found there was virtually no benefit and substantial risk of adverse side effects of this treatment. Consequently, the Infectious Diseases Society of America, the American Academy of Pediatrics, the American Academy of Neurology, the American College of Rheumatology, and expert professional societies from many European countries do not

TABLE 1 Antimicrobials Recommended to Treat Lyme Disease

MANIFESTATION	FIRST-LINE AGENTS	ALTERNATIVE AGENTS	DURATION
Single or multiple erythema migrans, cranial nerve palsy, carditis that is asymptomatic or for which the patient is not hospitalized	Doxycycline (Vibramycin)[1] 4.4 mg/kg/day in 2 divided doses (maximum 100 mg/dose)	Azithromycin (Zithromax)[1] 10 mg/kg/day in 1 dose (maximum 500 mg/dose)	14 days; for single EM, 10-days of doxycycline or 7–10 days of azithromycin is effective
	Amoxicillin (Amoxil)[1] 50 mg/kg per day in 3 divided doses (maximum 500 mg/dose)	Clarithromycin (Biaxin)[1] 7.5 mg/kg in 2 divided doses (maximum 500 mg/dose)	
	Cefuroxime axetil (Ceftin) 30 mg/kg PO in 2 divided doses (maximum 500 mg/dose)	Erythromiin (E.E.S.)[1] 12.5 mg/kg in 4 divided doses (maximum 500 mg/dose)	
Severe carditis, meningitis,* radiculomyelitis	Ceftriaxone (Rocephin)[1] 50–75 mg/kg IV in 1 dose (maximum 2 g/dose)	Cefotaxime (Claforan)[1] 150–200 mg/kg/day IV in 3 divided doses (maximum 2 g/dose) Penicillin G (Pfizerpen)[1] 200,000-400,000 U/kg/day in 6 divided doses (maximum 4 million U/dose)	14 days; for severe carditis and for meningitis, an oral agent may be used to complete a course of treatment after substantial clinical improvement
Lyme arthritis[†]	Same oral agents used for EM	Same oral agents used EM	28 days

[1]Not FDA approved for this indication.
*Some experts treat Lyme meningitis with doxycycline (Vibramycin)[1], administered orally, 4.4 mg/kg/day in 2 divided doses (maximum 100 mg/dose), for 14 days.
[†]Patients with persistent or recurrent arthritis 4 weeks after completing treatment may receive either a second 4-week course of treatment orally or 2 weeks of treatment with a parenterally administered antimicrobial listed above.

recommend prolonged treatment with antimicrobials in patients with PTLDS. These patients are distinguished from patients with so-called "chronic" Lyme disease, who have complaints similar to those with PTLDS but who do not have evidence of ever having had Lyme disease. Of course, prolonged antimicrobial treatment is not indicated for these patients, who might better be described as having medically unexplained symptoms.

Chemoprophylaxis
A single dose of doxycycline (Vibramycin; 8.8 mg/kg, maximum 200 mg)[1] taken within 72 hours of a deer tick bite was effective in preventing Lyme disease. However, because the risk of Lyme disease after a recognized tick bite is low, prophylaxis generally is not recommended routinely, but only for those at higher risk, such as someone in an endemic area who removes an engorged nymphal stage deer tick.

Treatment
Antimicrobial treatment of Lyme disease is highly effective and complications are rare (Table 1). The recommendations for treatment are summarized in the table. Antimicrobials that are highly effective and are considered first-line agents to treat Lyme disease orally include doxycycline (Vibramycin)[1], amoxicillin (Amoxil)[1] and cefuroxime axetil (Ceftin). Amoxicillin (Amoxil) is the preferred agent for women who are either pregnant or breastfeeding. Because the risk of staining of teeth is low, use of doxycycline for ≤21 days of treatment in children <8 years of age is now considered acceptable. Doxycycline (Vibramycin) is the preferred oral agent due to its good activity against other tick-borne illnesses such as human granulocytic anaplasmosis. Although macrolides such as azithromycin (Zithromax),[1] clarithromycin (Biaxin),[1] and erythromycin (EES)[1] are effective for treating early Lyme disease, they may not be as effective as the first-line agents. When parenteral treatment is indicated, ceftriaxone (Rocephin)[1] is the preferred agent because of once-a-day dosing. Alternative antimicrobials such as cefotaxime (Claforan)[1] and penicillin G (Pfizerpen-G)[1] also are highly effective, although penicillin G is rarely used because of frequent dosing due to its short half-life.

For patients with single EM, a 10-day course of doxycycline or a 14-day course of either amoxicillin or cefuroxime is recommended. For multiple EM, cranial nerve palsy (without apparent meningitis) or carditis that is asymptomatic and for which the patient is not hospitalized, a 14-day course of an oral antimicrobial is recommended. For complicated carditis (complete heart block) and for meningitis, a 14-day course of a parental agent is recommended, although there is evidence that 14 days of doxycycline orally may be adequate for treating meningitis. Some experts complete a course of initial parenteral treatment with oral therapy after the patient has improved clinically. Patients with Lyme meningitis should be carefully evaluated for increased intracranial pressure which, if present, should be managed appropriately. There is no evidence that steroids are beneficial for patients with facial palsy due to Lyme disease. For treatment of Lyme arthritis, a 28-day course of an oral antimicrobial is recommended. Nonsteroidal antiinflammatory drugs may be effective for treating the pain and inflammation associated with Lyme arthritis.

References

Centers for Disease Control. Lyme disease: *Data and statistics*. Available at https://www.cdc.gov/lyme/stats/index.html [Accessed April 10, 2018]

Feder HM Jr, Johnson BJB, O'Connell S, et al: A critical appraisal of "chronic lyme disease." *N Engl J Med* 357:1422–1430, 2007.

Hatcher S, Arroll B: Assessment and management of medically unexplained symptoms, *BMJ* 336:1124–1128, 2008.

Klempner MS, Hu LT, Evans J, et al: Two controlled trials of antibiotic treatment in patients with persistent symptoms and a history of Lyme disease, *N Engl J Med* 345:85–92, 2001.

Lantos PM: Chronic Lyme disease: the controversies and the science, *Expert Rev Anti Infect Ther* 9:787–797, 2011.

Ljøstad U, Skogvoll E, Eikeland R, et al: Oral doxycycline versus intravenous ceftriaxone for European Lyme neuroborreliosis: a multicentre, non-inferiority, double-blind, randomised trial, *Lancet Neurol* 7:690–695, 2008.

Nadelman RB, Nowakowski J, Fish D, et al: Tick bite study group: prophylaxis with a single-dose doxycycline for the prevention of Lyme disease after an Ixodes scapularis tick bite, *N Engl J Med* 345:79–84, 2001.

Shapiro ED: Clinical practice: Lyme disease, *N Engl J Med* 370:1724–1731, 2014.

Steere AC, Strle F, Wormser GP, et al: Lyme borreliosis, *Nat Rev Dis Primers* 2:1–18, 2016.

Wormser GP, Dattwyler RJ, Shapiro ED, et al: The clinical assessment, treatment, and prevention of Lyme disease, human granulocytic anaplasmosis, and babesiosis: clinical practice guidelines by the Infectious Diseases Society of America, *Clin Infect Dis* 43:1089–1011, 2006.

[1] Not FDA approved for this indication.

MALARIA

Method of
Lawrence M. Gibbs, MD, MSEd and Dustin A. Creech, MD

CURRENT DIAGNOSIS

History
- Does the patient have a fever? Any other flulike symptoms (chills, sweats, headache, muscle aches, nausea, and/or vomiting)?
- Did the patient travel to a malaria-endemic area? And, how long did the travel precede symptom onset?
- What *Plasmodia* species are known to be present in the area(s) of travel and what corresponding drug-resistance patterns are present?
- Did the patient use appropriate prophylaxis for the region and adequate personal protective measures during travel?

Diagnosis
- Thick and thin blood smears are required for detection, *Plasmodium* speciation, and parasite density determination.
- Use of rapid diagnostic tests for quick detection must be followed by blood smears to confirm diagnosis and monitor parasite density.
- Be mindful of severe disease signs including acidosis, acute respiratory distress, altered consciousness, high parasite density (>5%), hyperbilirubinemia, hypotension, renal impairment, seizures, and severe anemia.

CURRENT THERAPY

- Develop treatment plan based on prompt laboratory confirmation of *Plasmodium* species and drug-resistance patterns of *Plasmodium* species in known area(s) of travel.
- If severe disease is a concern, parenteral artesunate[10] should be used, where available, or quinidine, and the patient should be monitored in an intensive care setting providing supportive care as needed.
- For uncomplicated disease, consider hospital admission for likely *P. falciparum* infection.
  - Administer oral therapies (i.e., artemisinin-based combination therapies or chloroquine) based on resistance patterns in area of travel.
  - To prevent relapse, prescribe primaquine to all with a normal glucose-6-phosphate dehydrogenase (G6PD) status and travel to areas having known *P. vivax* and *P. ovale*.[1]

[1]Not FDA approved for this indication.
[10]Available in the United States from the Centers for Disease Control and Prevention.

Malaria is a potentially fatal parasitic disease caused by intraerythrocytic protozoa of the genus *Plasmodium* and is transmitted to humans primarily via female *Anopheles* mosquito bites. Often considered by many the most important parasitic disease affecting human beings, in 2015 it accounted for over 200 million infections and an estimated 438,000 deaths worldwide, mainly in young children, and it remains a focus of international concern. Thankfully, in the past 15 years, due in part to substantial increases in donor funding (i.e., The Global Fund, World Bank, UNICEF, and United States Agency for International Development) advances in treatment and control measures, and increased enthusiasm for elimination, there has been a significant drop in the infection and mortality rates associated with this disease by 18% and 48%, respectively. Interestingly we have witnessed a very gradual increase in the number of malaria cases in the United States largely due to more tourism to malaria-endemic locations, especially Africa. In 2012, a total of 1687 malaria cases were reported in the United States, which, though somewhat lower than the year prior when reported malaria cases were at a 40-year high, represents an overall upward trend.

By far, the majority of patients developing malaria in the United States are infected during travel to other countries. Whether or not preventive measures were appropriately used, health-care workers should have a high index of suspicion for malaria in the returning traveler with fever and other flulike symptoms. Since cases are rare in North America, misdiagnosis is not uncommon. Clinicians, therefore, must consider malaria in the differential for any febrile illness in an individual who has traveled to an area of known malaria transmission in the past several months or in those with fever of unknown origin regardless of travel history. Since untreated malaria infections can lead to anemia, pulmonary edema, renal failure, coma, and even death, prompt diagnosis and treatment are essential.

Epidemiology

According to the 2015 World Health Organization (WHO) World Malaria Report, 3.2 billion people were considered at risk for malaria and 97 countries reported active transmission (see Figure 1). Though 80% of cases and fatalities are accounted for in 15 sub-Saharan African countries, Asia and Central and South America also have significant disease burden with Europe and the Middle East accounting for a smaller portion of cases. *P. falciparum* is the most prevalent form of malaria in Africa and is responsible for more deaths worldwide than other *Plasmodia* species, and 70% of fatalities are in patients under 5 years of age. Though *P. falciparum* is encountered outside Africa, *P. vivax* is often more prevalent across much of Asia and Central and South America and transmission rates are more frequently low and seasonal. Meanwhile, rates of transmission are much higher across sub-Saharan Africa and parts of Oceania, where *P. falciparum* predominates. *P. vivax* is responsible for most relapsing malarial disease, though *P. ovale* is also responsible but to a lesser extent.

In endemic areas of high, stable transmission, partial immunity can develop after many years of repeat exposure to infectious mosquito bites, and young children often show resistance to severe forms of the disease by the age of 5. By adolescence they also often become resistant to more uncomplicated forms of the disease. Though resistant to clinical malaria, rarely will one become completely resistant to actual infection. In areas of unstable or seasonal transmission (i.e., sub-Sahel region of Africa), transmission can be intense but is isolated to rainy periods and full protective immunity does not develop so symptomatic disease may occur across all ages.

There are also varying drug-resistance patterns that greatly affect prevention, treatment, and mortality. Resistance to antimalarial medications continues to be an important consideration when considering treatment, especially *P. falciparum* infection. By the 1970s, *P. falciparum* chloroquine resistance had been confirmed on every continent where malaria was endemic, and currently only the Caribbean, areas of Central America west of the Panama Canal, and a few Middle Eastern countries show sensitive strains. *P. vivax* has also shown resistance to chloroquine in areas of Indonesia and Papua New Guinea. Mefloquine, too, is currently no longer recommended to treat *P. falciparum* infections originating from Southeast Asia due to increasing levels of resistance, and even artesunate and its partner drugs are showing signs of decreased effectiveness across the Mekong Region in Southeast Asia. When in doubt, clinicians should use the Centers for Disease Control and Prevention's (CDC) online interactive malaria map (http://www.cdc.gov/malaria/map/) or Malaria-by-Country tables (http://www.cdc.gov/malaria/travelers/country_table/a.html) to quickly view the types of *Plasmodium* present and resistance characteristics found in the patient's area of travel.

Risk Factors for Transmission

Risk factors for malaria include both individual risk and environmental conditions that increase transmission rates. Anyone traveling to or living in a malaria-endemic area is at risk for transmission. Children, elderly, pregnant women, and HIV/AIDS patients are at higher risk than the general population. HIV-related immunosuppression, especially, may lead to more severe manifestations of malaria. Because of lack of partial immunity, travelers to endemic regions also have a higher risk of transmission. Also, given the known reductions that can occur via the use of personal protective measures (i.e., insecticide-treated bed nets and insect repellents) and chemoprophylaxis, individuals without access to or noncompliant with these measures are at increased risk. Malaria can also be transferred from mother to baby across the placenta (congenital malaria) or during birth. Though rare, there are some cases of malaria transmission during blood transfusion as well as organ transplantation.

At the population level, there are many conditions that increase transmission as well, most of which relate to effects on any of the 30 or so *Anopheles* species linked to malaria transmission. The rainy season allows for eggs of *Anopheles* mosquitoes to be laid in water more readily and larvae to develop more easily. Transmission is also higher in regions with longer mosquito lifespans and in areas where humans are the choice blood meal over other animals. In addition, elevation, temperature, and humidity of a region all contribute to transmission efficiency of malaria.

Etiology and the Parasite's Life Cycle

There are five species of *Plasmodium* indicated in human malarial disease: *P. falciparum*, *P. vivax*, *P. ovale*, *P. malariae*, and *P. knowlesi*. *P. knowlesi* classically was identified as a simian disease; however, it has become an appreciable cause of malaria in humans in Southeast Asia. The life cycle (Figure 2) of the malaria parasite differs slightly among *Plasmodium* species and these differences explain how species present differently. For instance, the time from initial infection to symptom presentation varies across species. *P. knowlesi* incubation is from 9 to 12 days and *P. falciparum* is often 9 to 14 days, while *P. vivax* ranges from 12 to 17 days and *P. ovale* from 16 to 18 days. *P. malariae* is the most variable with ranges from 18 to 40 or more days.

Regardless of species, the life cycle starts when an infected female *Anopheles* mosquito takes a human blood meal, injecting anywhere from 10 to 100 *Plasmodium* sporozoites into the host. The sporozoites travel to the liver, invading hepatic cells where they then replicate and each divides forming 10,000 to more than 30,000 merozoites (haploid cells). The species determines how quickly this happens and how many merozoites are formed. In the liver, *P. vivax* and *P. ovale* produce another form, called hypnozoites, which remain in the liver for an extended time and are responsible for relapsing illness, sometimes months to even years after initial infection. The merozoites enter circulation and invade red blood cells (RBCs) (asexual replication). Once inside RBCs, the merozoites develop into schizonts, rupture, and more merozoites are released into the bloodstream to invade RBCs. Depending on the species, this cycle can repeat anywhere from 24 to 72 hours. Typically, the number of merozoites in the bloodstream is proportional to disease severity for a given species. However, this is not always the case as sometimes severe disease is seen even in small numbers of infected RBCs, especially in the case of *P. falciparum*. Some merozoites develop into male and female gametocytes entering a sexual stage. Gametocytes enter into the bloodstream where an *Anopheles* mosquito partakes of a blood meal, ingesting the gametocytes, and then these gametocytes develop into gametes in the mosquito midgut. Male and female gametocytes sexually reproduce to form oocysts, which then grow and release sporozoites. The sporozoites travel to the salivary gland and with a subsequent human bite, complete the transmission cycle.

It is worth noting that all *Plasmodium* species may cause recrudescence, which happens when treatment is suboptimal and parasite clearance incomplete. In these cases, patients may show symptoms of infection months to years after initial infection. Patient immunosuppression also furthers this risk. In endemic areas, recurrent *P. falciparum* and *P. vivax* malaria can have pronounced negative effects in children affecting growth, development and schooling.

Clinical Manifestations

The most common presentation of malaria is fever after travel to an endemic area. Fever and chills are the chief complaint in 96% of patients, followed by headaches and muscle aches in 79%

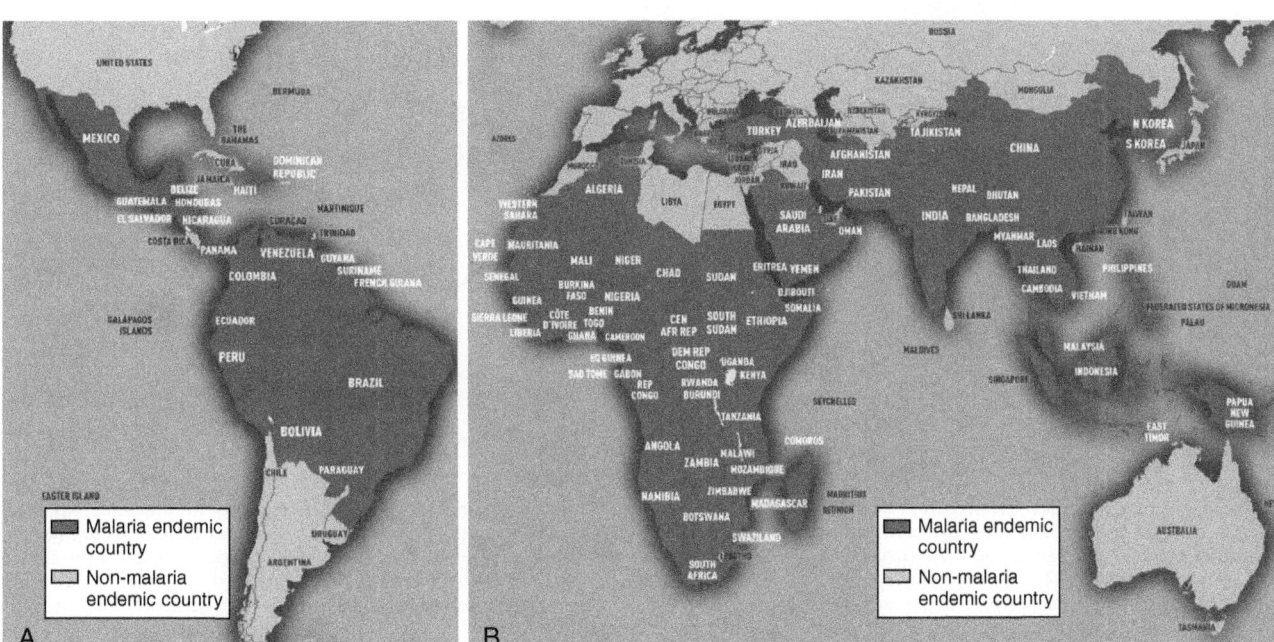

Figure 1 Malaria-endemic countries in the (**A**) Western and (**B**) Eastern Hemispheres. Transmission occurs across most of Africa, Central and South America, and Southern and Southeast Asia, as well as parts of the Caribbean, Eastern Europe, and the South Pacific. Countries are shaded completely even if the area of endemicity is only in a small area of the country. Adapted from Centers for Disease Control and Prevention. CDC Health Information for International Travel 2016. New York: Oxford University Press; 2016. Public Domain.

and 60%, respectively. The classic "paroxysm" of symptoms includes chills for minutes to hours, followed by high fevers when RBCs rupture and merozoites are released, and then sweating and fever breaking. However, the paroxysm is often not present. Also, *P. falciparum* tends to cause a continual fever with spikes as opposed to the cyclical nature of the other species; therefore, absence of paroxysm should not be used to rule out malaria. General malaise, weakness, fatigue, and muscle aches are common. Less common, are palpable liver and/or spleen, nausea and vomiting, abdominal pain, and diarrhea. More severe cases can present with jaundice, confusion, orthostatic hypotension, or seizures depending on the type of malaria and severity.

Most patients will develop anemia and splenomegaly as the spleen acts to remove both infected and noninfected RBCs from the bloodstream. Thrombocytopenia will occur in most patients as well, along with elevations in aspartate aminotransferase and alanine transaminase. Acute kidney injury is common, especially

in more severe malaria. *P. falciparum* and *P. knowlesi* typically cause higher parasitemia than *P. vivax*, *P. ovale*, and *P. malariae* because the former two are less selective in their invasion of RBCs. Infection can quickly lead to severe disease and death if not treated promptly, and so rapid, correct diagnosis can greatly improve survival probability.

P. falciparum causes more severe disease and death than the other species. The parasite causes RBCs to develop "knobs," which express PfEMP1, proteins regulating adhesion to endothelium of capillaries and postcapillary venules. The RBCs are also more rigid. The combination of adhesion to endothelium and rigid RBCs obstructs the vessels, also known as sequestration. Sequestration is implicated in severe disease and leads to metabolism of glucose locally, local tissue factor recruitment, edema, and ultimately end organ damage.

Sequestration in brain tissues is better described, but it is thought to occur in lung tissue as well. Sequestration is thought to

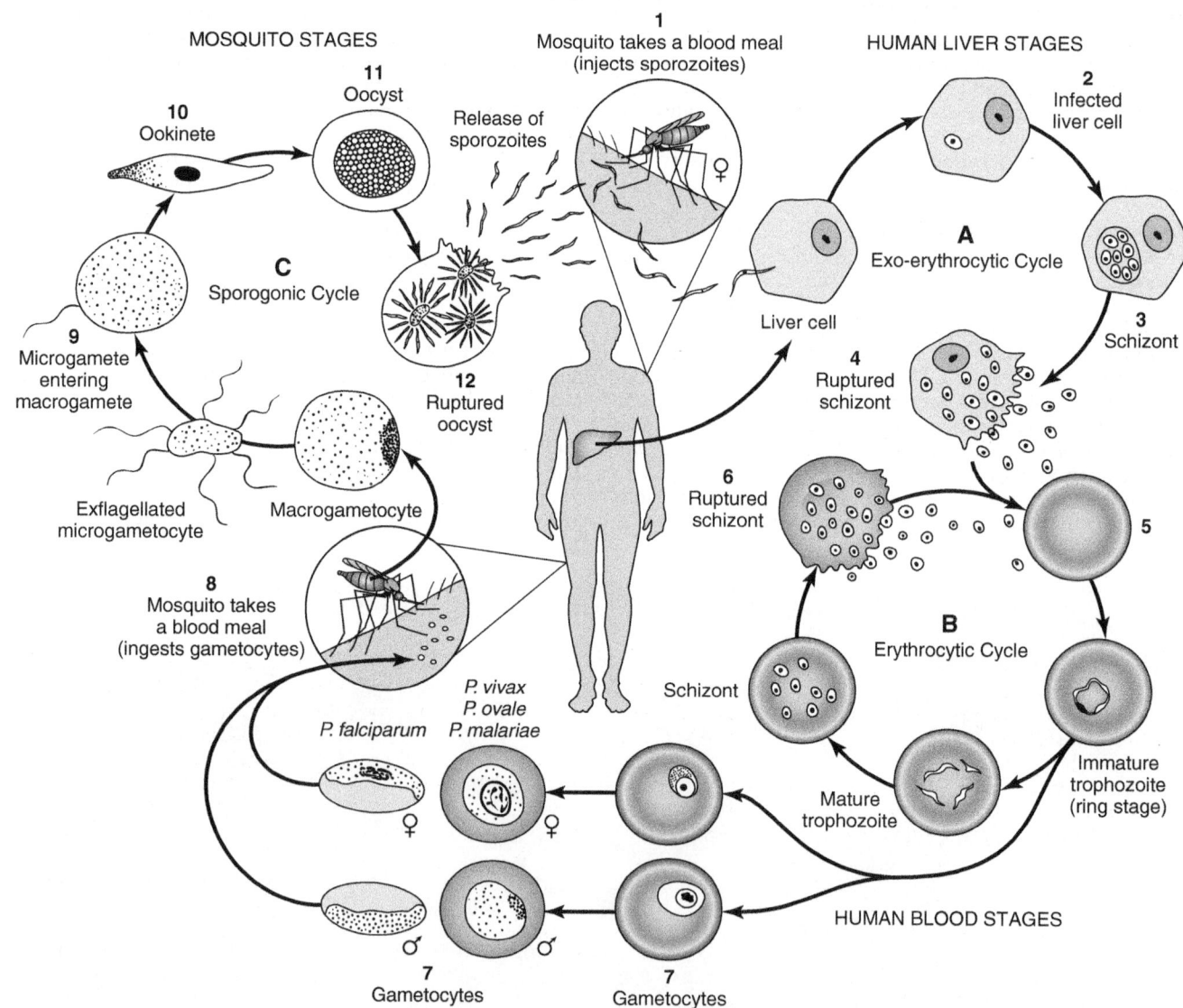

Figure 2 The malaria parasite life cycle involves two hosts. During a blood meal, a malaria-infected female *Anopheles* mosquito inoculates sporozoites into the human host (1). Sporozoites infect liver cells (2) and mature into schizonts (3), which rupture and release merozoites (4). (In *Plasmodium vivax* and *Plasmodium ovale*, a dormant stage [hypnozoites] can persist in the liver and cause relapses by invading the bloodstream weeks to years later.) After initial replication in the liver via exoerythrocytic cycle or tissue schizogony (A), the parasites undergo asexual multiplication in erythrocytes via erythrocytic cycle or blood schizogony (B). Merozoites infect red blood cells (5). The ring stage trophozoites mature into schizonts, which rupture, releasing merozoites (6). Some parasites differentiate into sexual erythrocytic stages (gametocytes) (7). Blood stage parasites are responsible for the clinical manifestations of the disease. The gametocytes, male (microgametocytes) and female (macrogametocytes), are ingested by an *Anopheles* mosquito during a blood meal (8). The parasites' multiplication in the mosquito is known as the sporogonic cycle (C). While in the mosquito's stomach, the microgametes penetrate the macrogametes, generating zygotes (9). The zygotes in turn become motile and elongated (ookinetes) (10) and invade the midgut wall of the mosquito, where they develop into oocysts (11). The oocysts grow, rupture, and release sporozoites (12), which make their way to the mosquito's salivary glands. Inoculation of the sporozoites (1) into a new human host perpetuates the malaria life cycle.

increase intracranial blood pressure. Interestingly cerebral edema is frequently seen in children, but not in adults radiographically. Cerebral edema, seizures, coma, and death can be immediate sequelae of *P. falciparum*. While adult survivors typically do not have lasting neurologic effects, 3% to 15% of children survivors have lasting neurological deficits from *P. falciparum* infection. Cerebral palsy, learning disability, language deficits, and epilepsy are some of the lasting effects in children survivors of *P. falciparum*.

Cerebral malaria, severe anemia, pulmonary edema, and renal failure are examples of end organ failure that can result and quickly lead to severe morbidity and death if not treated correctly and rapidly. Although *P. falciparum* is the prominent cause of severe malaria and death, other species of *Plasmodium* can also develop complications and lead to death if not adequately diagnosed and treated.

Outside of Africa, *P. vivax* accounts for roughly half of all malaria cases and, though often having a much lower case-fatality rate than *P. falciparum*, it still may cause a debilitating febrile illness with progressive anemia and, sometimes causes severe disease including symptoms of thrombocytopenia and acute pulmonary edema. Less common symptoms can include cerebral malaria, pancytopenia, jaundice, splenic rupture, acute renal failure, and shock. Prompt management of these severe cases and treatment in a manner similar to *P. falciparum* infection are recommended.

Chronic malaria infection, characterized by low-level parasitemia, may lead to a variety of complications. For instance, recurrent *P. vivax* infections or relapses may lead to hyperactive malarial splenomegaly that leads to significant anemia, hypersplenism, and hypergammaglobulinemia. Meanwhile, persistent *P. malariae* infection has been linked to risk for nephrotic syndrome in parts of Africa.

Diagnosis

Correctly diagnosing malaria and identifying *Plasmodium* species quickly is paramount to appropriate timely treatment, and testing should be done whether or not an appropriate chemoprophylaxis regimen was followed. Unfortunately, malaria may mimic many diseases due to its common symptom profile, especially high fevers. Other causes of fever including more common bacterial and viral illnesses (i.e., bacterial meningitis, influenza, and acute hepatitis) and tropical diseases such as dengue fever, chikungunya, rickettsial infections, typhoid, and trypanosomiasis, must be considered.

Together, thick and thin smear microscopy are still considered the gold standard for malaria diagnosis, and they are best performed by experienced personnel without delay on any patient presenting with fever and travel to endemic areas. These tests help to answer three questions: Is there malaria present? What species is present? And, what percentage of RBCs are infected?

The general process of microcopy is described here, but strict protocols should be followed to give reliable and reproducible results. Blood is sampled through finger stick or venipuncture, and the thick smear is air dried and not fixed; therefore, hemolysis occurs. Thick smears are more sensitive at identifying infection, as they concentrate parasites, and may also help estimate parasite concentration. However, hemolysis during preparation makes it difficult to identify species-level characteristics using thick smear microscopy. The thin smear is fixed with air drying and methanol and, since RBCs remain intact, can reveal the species of *Plasmodium* present and the percentage of RBCs infected, which serves as a marker for parasitemia and eventually treatment effectiveness. Both slides are stained, typically with Giemsa (pH of 7.2) and slides should be examined under 1000× oil immersion for at least 20 minutes and 200 high-powered fields before reporting as negative. Negative smears should be repeated every 8 to 12 hours until malaria can be ruled out confidently as symptoms may precede parasitemia. The CDC recommends confirming the diagnosis before treating for

malaria; however, with symptoms of suspected severe malaria, it may be appropriate to treat before diagnosis to start treatment rapidly. For further information including slide preparation and diagnostic assistance, clinicians may refer to the CDC's Laboratory Identification of Parasitic Diseases website: http://www.cdc.gov/dpdx/malaria/dx.html.

In addition to direct microscopy, other diagnostic tests are available, such as rapid diagnostic tests (RDTs), polymerase chain reaction (PCR), and serology. Where available, RDTs are immunochromatographic tests that use a dipstick or cassette format and detect specific *Plasmodium* antigens using a single drop of blood. Current RDTs can target the histidine-rich protein 2 of *P. falciparum* (PfHRP2), a panmalarial *Plasmodium* aldolase (PMA), and parasite specific lactate dehydrogenase (pLDH). Often they specifically are designed to target *P. falciparum*, *P. vivax*, or nonspecific *Plasmodium*, and they offer a rapid way (5 to 20 minutes) to test for the presence of *Plasmodium* without the need for a laboratory, electricity, special equipment, or even highly experienced personnel. Though not as sensitive in instances of low parasitemia (<100 to 200 parasites/µL), RDTs have documented sensitivities and specificities reaching up to 95% and 99%, respectively. As they do not give information on parasitemia levels and false-negative results are possible, thick and thin smears should still be performed to confirm or rule out diagnosis and determine level of parasitemia.

PCR, a molecular method based on DNA amplification, may also be used for diagnosis and offers the most accurate method of parasite detection. PCR is less prone to observer error than is microscopy and more sensitive at low levels of parasitemia. As PCR becomes more widespread, it may offer a promising alternative for diagnosis and speciation, but currently it is not widely available due to logistical constraints and the need for well-equipped laboratories and specially trained technicians. It remains an important research tool detecting drug resistance mutations and offering a secondary means of species confirmation. Likewise, a variety of serologic tests can be performed by some laboratories (i.e., CDC reference laboratories) to assess past malaria experience, but not current malaria infection.

Antimalarial Medications

A variety of malaria chemotherapy treatment and prophylaxis options are available, each with their risks, benefits, and availability issues. Treatment options will be dictated not only by drug availability but also location of disease acquisition, infecting species, resistance patterns, and symptom severity (Table 1).

Current antimalarial medications attack the *Plasmodium* organism at various stages in its life cycle. Those that kill malaria parasites when they have been released into the bloodstream during the asexual, erythrocytic cycle are referred to as blood schizonticides. Meanwhile, tissue schizonticides kill parasites during the exoerythrocytic cycle of infection in the liver and also may prevent relapse in certain species. Some medications also have activity against gametocytes. Though not affecting the patient's clinical response, these gametocidal medications do decrease the probability of disease transmission to another person.

Chloroquine phosphate (Aralen) is one of the older drugs still used, and along with its sister medication, hydroxychloroquine sulfate (Plaquenil), is used in the prevention and treatment of malaria. These blood schizonticides are active against all *Plasmodium* species and have gametocidal activity against *P. vivax*, *P. ovale*, *P. malariae*, and *P. knowlesi*. These medications are no longer recommended for prophylaxis against *P. falciparum* (except in some parts of Central America), but can be used to prevent *P. vivax* infections. Chloroquine remains the treatment of choice for all susceptible *Plasmodium* strains; however, growing resistance limits its worldwide use, especially in malaria-endemic areas. It is safe to use in children as well as pregnant women. Response

TABLE 1	Drug Recommendations for Treatment by Malaria Type
DIAGNOSIS	**DRUG**
Uncomplicated, chloroquine-sensitive *P. falciparum*	Chloroquine phosphate or hydroxychloroquine
Uncomplicated, chloroquine-resistant *P. falciparum* or species/ resistance unknown	Artemisinin-combination therapy[1] or atovaquone/proguanil or quinine sulfate[7] + one of the following: doxycycline,[2,3] tetracycline,[2,3] clindamycin,[2] or mefloquine[4]
Uncomplicated, chloroquine-sensitive *P. malariae* or *P. knowlesi*	Chloroquine phosphate or hydroxychloroquine
Uncomplicated, chloroquine-sensitive *P. vivax* or *P. ovale*	Chloroquine phosphate+primaquine phosphate[5] or hydroxychloroquine+primaquine phosphate[5]
Uncomplicated, chloroquine-resistant *P. vivax*	Atovaquone/proguanil plus primaquine phosphate[5] or artemisinin-combination therapy[1] + primaquine phosphate[5] or quinine sulfate[7] + one of the following: doxycycline,[2,3] tetracycline,[2,3] or clindamycin[2] + primaquine phosphate[5] or mefloquine[4] + primaquine phosphate[5]
Chloroquine-sensitive malaria during pregnancy	Chloroquine phosphate or hydroxychloroquine or mefloquine[4]
Chloroquine-resistant malaria during pregnancy	Quinine sulfate[7] + clindamycin[2] or mefloquine[4]
Severe malaria	Quinidine gluconate[7] + one of the following: doxycycline,[2,3] tetracycline,[2,3] or clindamycin[2] or artesunate[6] followed by one of the following: artemisinin-combination therapy,[1] atovaquone/proguanil, doxycycline[2,3] (or clindamycin[2] in pregnant women), or mefloquine[4]

[1]Artemisinin-combination therapy; see Table 2.
[2]Not FDA approved for this indication.
[3]Avoid in patients under 8 years old.
[4]Not recommended for infections acquired in Southeast Asia.
[5]Normal glucose-6-phosphate dehydrogenase levels should be confirmed before starting Primaquine.
[6]Contact CDC for information and to obtain.
[7]For infections acquired in Southeast Asia, quinine treatment should continue for 7 days. For infections acquired elsewhere, quinine treatment should continue for 3 days.

to treatment in pregnant women should be monitored closely, especially during second and third trimesters where serum drug concentrations may be lower. Major side effects include gastrointestinal (GI) upset, headache, dizziness, insomnia, vision changes, and pruritus. Long-term use can lead to ototoxicity, retinopathy, and peripheral neuropathy.

Atovaquone/proguanil (Malarone) is a combination drug effective against both blood and tissue schizonts. The combination is indicated for malaria prophylaxis in all areas and may be used for treatment of uncomplicated chloroquine-resistant malarial infections in travelers outside endemic areas or for combination treatment with artesunate[10] or primaquine.[1] It is seldom used in endemic areas due to emergence of resistance to

[1]Not FDA approved for this indication.
[10]Available in the United States from the Centers for Disease Control and Prevention.

the atovaquone component. The medication is considered safe in children weighing more than 5 kg per WHO (U.S. Food & Drug Administration [FDA] sets 11 kg as the weight minimum). WHO does regard the drug as safe during pregnancy due to no evidence of adverse effects associated with its use in pregnant women. The combination medication is generally well tolerated. Headache, cough, and GI upset are the most frequent side effects in both adults and children. Rarely, dizziness, oral ulcerations, and elevated liver function study results can occur. It is contraindicated in those with severe renal impairment due to increased pancytopenia risk.

Artemisinin derivatives are plant-based compounds derived from the Chinese quinghaosu plant (*Artemisia annua*) whose components are active against blood schizonts and gametocytes. They also lead to much shorter parasite clearance times than other treatments. Artemisinin and its derivatives (artesunate,[10] artemether,[2] and dihydroartemisinin[2]) are highly effective at treating uncomplicated and severe *P. falciparum* infections and preparations are available in oral, rectal, and intravenous formulations. Artemisinin-based combination therapies (ACTs) are increasingly considered standard of care for treatment of uncomplicated falciparum malaria in malaria-endemic areas.

ACT involves administering a combination drug over at least 3 days (7 days for Southeast Asia *P. falciparum*), which allows for more effective blood schizonticidal activity since the individual components have different actions and targets, as well as reducing potential selection for drug-resistant parasites. Currently five ACT options are approved by stringent regulatory authorities or the WHO: artemether+lumefantrine (Coartem; the only FDA-approved treatment), artesunate+amodiaquine (Coarsucam,[2] European Medicines Agency-approved), artesunate+mefloquine (Artequin,[2] WHO prequalified), artesunate+sulfadoxine-pyrimethamine (Arsuamoon[2]+Fansidar,[2] WHO prequalified), and dihydroartemisinin+piperaquine (Eurartesim,[2] European Medicines Agency-approved). Cure rates for all of these preparations exceed 95% based on clinical trial data.

Serious side effects from ACTs have not been reported in humans, but they are still not recommended during the first trimester of pregnancy due to lack of definitive safety data. Generally well-tolerated, common side effects include GI upset, dizziness, headache, neutropenia, and elevated liver enzymes. Although there are minor differences in the oral absorption, bioavailability, and tolerability of the different artemisinin derivatives, there is no evidence that these differences are clinically significant in currently available formulations.

For severe malaria, though artemisinin derivatives may be used alone to initiate therapy (i.e., IV artesunate[10]), another antimalarial medication with a different mode of action should be added as soon as possible. Parenteral artesunate has been available in the United States since 2007 under an investigational protocol. The CDC will provide it to hospitals upon request and on an emergency basis when a patient has severe malaria, a high parasite burden, inability to take oral medicines, lack of access to or failure of IV quinidine, or a contraindication to using quinidine. To enroll a patient in the protocol, clinicians should not hesitate to contact the CDC's Malaria Hotline (770-488-7788 or toll-free at 855-856-4713) from 9 am to 5 pm Eastern Time, or outside of regular hours, physicians should call 770-488-7100 and request the CDC Malaria Branch's on-call physician.

Quinine sulfate (Qualaquin) and quinidine gluconate (parenteral form) are blood schizonticides effective at killing erythrocytic stages of all *Plasmodium* species, and show gametocidal activity against *P. vivax*, *P. ovale*, and *P. malariae*. Currently, IV quinidine is the only FDA-approved treatment for severe malaria

[2]Not available in the United States.
[10]Available in the United States from the Centers for Disease Control and Prevention.

TABLE 2	Medications and Dosing	
MEDICATION	**ADULT DOSING**	**PEDIATRIC DOSING**
Artesunate*	2.4 mg/kg IV push at 0, 12, 24, and 48 hours	<20 kg: 3.0 mg/kg IV push at 0, 12, 24, and 48 hours >20 kg: same as adult dosing
Artemether-lumefantrine[†]	1 tablet=20 mg artemether and 120 mg lumefantrine. A 3-day treatment schedule with a total of 6 oral doses is recommended for both adult and pediatric patients based on weight. Initial dose at 0 hour, second dose 8 hours later, then 1 dose PO bid for the next 2 days. 5 to <15 kg: 1 tablet/dose 15 to <25 kg: 2 tablets/dose 25 to <35 kg: 3 tablets/dose ≥35 kg: 4 tablets/dose	
Atovaquone/proguanil[1]	Adult tab=250 mg/100 mg. 4 tabs PO daily as a single dose for 3 consecutive days	Pediatric tablets=62.5/25 mg. 5 to 8 kg: 2 peds tabs PO qd×3 days 9 to 10 kg: 3 peds tabs PO qd×3 days 11 to 20 kg: 1 adult tab PO qd×3 days 21 to 30 kg: 2 adult tabs PO qd×3 days 31 to 40 kg: 3 adult tabs PO qd×3 days >40 kg: 4 adult tabs PO qd×3 days
Chloroquine phosphate	600 mg base (=1000 mg salt). PO immediately, followed by 300 mg base (=500 mg salt) PO at 6, 24, and 48 hours	10 mg base/kg PO immediately, followed by 5 mg base/kg PO at 6, 24, and 48 hours
Clindamycin	7-day treatment course recommended for adult and pediatric patients both based on weight. Switch to PO clindamycin as soon as patient can take oral medication. IV dosing: 10 mg base/kg loading dose IV followed by 5 mg base/kg IV every 8 hours (avoid rapid administration) PO dosing: 20 mg base/kg/day tid	
Doxycycline[2]	100 mg PO/IV every 12 hours for 7 days	≥8 years of age: 2.2 mg/kg PO/IV every 12 hours up to adult dose of 100 mg/dose for 7 days
Hydroxychloroquine	620 mg base (=800 mg salt). PO immediately, followed by 310 mg base (=400 mg salt) PO at 6, 24, and 48 hours	10 mg base/kg PO immediately, followed by 5 mg base/kg PO at 6, 24, and 48 hours
Mefloquine[3,4]	684 mg base (=750 mg salt). PO as initial dose, followed by 456 mg base (=500 mg salt). PO given 6-12 hours after initial dose.	13.7 mg base/kg (=15 mg salt/kg). PO as initial dose, followed by 9.1 mg base/kg (=10 mg salt/kg). PO given 6–12 hours after initial dose.
Primaquine phosphate[5]	30 mg base (52.6 mg salt)[8] PO, daily for 14 days after departure from the malarious area	0.5 mg/kg base (0.8 mg/kg salt, off-label dosing for children) up to adult dose PO, daily for 14 days after departure from the malarious area
Quinidine gluconate[6]	6.25 mg base/kg (=10 mg salt/kg) loading dose IV over 1–2 hours, then 0.0125 mg base/kg/min (=0.02 mg salt/kg/min) continuous infusion for at least 24 hours. Or 15 mg base/kg (=24 mg salt/kg) loading dose IV infused over 4 hours, followed by 7.5 mg base/kg (=12 mg salt/kg) infused over 4 hours every 8 hours, starting 8 hours after the loading dose. Once parasite density is <1% and patient can take PO medication, complete treatment with PO quinine.	
Quinine sulfate	542 mg base (=650 mg salt). PO every 8 hours×3 or 7 days	8.3 mg base/kg (=10 mg salt/kg). PO every 8 hours×3 or 7 days
Tetracycline[2,7]	250 mg PO every 6 hours×7 days	≥8 years of age: 25 mg/kg/day PO divided every 6 hours×7 days

*Available in United States through Centers for Disease Control and Prevention.
[†]Only FDA-approved artemisinin-combination therapy.
[1]Contraindicated if severe renal impairment (creatinine clearance <30 mL/min). Not recommended for children <5 kg and pregnant women.
[2]Contraindicated in children <8 years of age and pregnant women.
[3]Contraindicated in people allergic to mefloquine or related compounds (quinine, quinidine) and in people with depression, a recent history of depression, generalized anxiety disorder, psychosis, schizophrenia, other major psychiatric disorders, or seizures. Not recommended for persons with cardiac conduction abnormalities.
[4]Currently category B in pregnancy (FDA), recommended as option for treatment and prophylaxis in all trimesters.
[5]Contraindicated in G6PD deficiency. Also contraindicated during pregnancy and lactation, unless infant has normal G6PD level.
[6]Do not give loading dose if patients have received >40 mg/kg quinine in previous 48 hours or received mefloquine within prior 12 hours; loading dose should not be given. Requires continuous cardiac monitoring.
[7]Not FDA approved for this indication.
[8]Exceeds dosage recommended by the manufacturer.

in the United States. Quinine may be used in the treatment of uncomplicated malaria, particularly during the first trimester of pregnancy, or in cases when an effective ACT is not available. Quinine has a narrow therapeutic index and many potential side effects. Potential cardiotoxic effects include conduction disturbances like QT prolongation, angina, and hypotension leading to cardiac arrest. It is, therefore, recommended that IV quinidine be administered under close telemetry monitoring. More common side effects include symptoms of tinnitus, hearing impairment, nausea, headache, dizziness, dysphoria, and sometimes disturbed vision. More severe issues at higher required doses or increased treatment duration include vertigo, vomiting, diarrhea, and marked auditory and visual loss. An important side effect of quinine seen mostly in children, pregnant women, and the elderly is hyperinsulinemic hypoglycemia. Treatment for major side effects is mostly supportive, with particular attention to maintenance of blood pressure, glucose and renal function and to treating any arrhythmias. For infection acquired outside of Southeast Asia, treatment course with quinidine may be shortened from 7 to 3 days when combining treatment with doxycycline,[1] tetracycline,[1] or clindamycin.[1]

Tetracyclines (i.e., doxycycline and tetracycline) are blood schizonticides effective against the erythrocytic stages of all *Plasmodium*. Doxycycline (Vibramycin) is effective in the prophylaxis against *P. falciparum*, including chloroquine- and mefloquine-resistant strains. Tetracyclines may be combined with quinine or quinidine to treat chloroquine-resistant *P. falciparum* and *P. vivax* infections. They should never be used as monotherapy and both are contraindicated in pregnancy and in children less than 8 years old due to possible interference with bone growth. Common side effects for these medications are GI upset, which can be lessened by ensuring it is taken with food, dry mouth, stomatitis, sun hypersensitivity, candida vaginitis, dysphagia, and esophageal irritation. To reduce esophageal problems, doxycycline should always be administered with a full glass of water.

Clindamycin (Cleocin)[1] is another blood schizonticide of all *Plasmodium* species. It may be used in combination therapy with artesunate or quinine for severe or uncomplicated malaria, but never as monotherapy. Clindamycin is often used when tetracyclines are contraindicated. It is generally well tolerated in its oral form. Major side effects include GI upset (especially diarrhea) and skin rashes. Close monitoring is recommended in the elderly, neonates, and individuals with liver disease.

Mefloquine (Lariam) is a long-acting blood schizonticide effective at killing the erythrocytic stages of all *Plasmodium* species. Structurally related to quinine, it is used as prophylaxis against malaria caused by all *Plasmodium* species, and also combined with artesunate to treat *P. falciparum* infections. It is generally thought to be safe during pregnancy, and is well tolerated when given in combination with artesunate for the treatment of uncomplicated *P. falciparum* malaria. It is also effective as a once-weekly prophylactic medication. Though generally well-tolerated, common side effects include GI disturbances, anxiety, irritability, dizziness, paranoia, depression, hallucinations, and sometimes violence in patients who were treated for malaria or taking mefloquine for long-term prophylaxis. Side effects frequently abate once the medication is discontinued. Use of mefloquine for malaria prophylaxis is not recommended for those for whom sudden dizziness or confusion could be hazardous, especially pilots and drivers. Travelers taking mefloquine are advised to stop taking the medication should any neurologic symptoms develop. Mefloquine is contraindicated to use as follow-up therapy for patients after cerebral malaria and should also not be used for prophylaxis in patients with known cardiac conduction disorders, epilepsy, depression or anxiety, psychosis, schizophrenia, or other major psychiatric disorder. It should also never be used in combination with quinine or quinidine. Due to the neuropsychiatric side effects of mefloquine, it is often not considered as first-line for prophylaxis or treatment.

Primaquine sulfate is effective at eradicating both the exoerythrocytic forms (hypnozoites) and the sexual stages of malaria parasites (gametocytes). It is used for radical cure of *P. vivax* and *P. ovale*[1] malaria, primary prophylaxis for destinations where *P. vivax* is the main species, as well as for terminal prophylaxis (presumptive antirelapse therapy) targeting parasites that may remain dormant in the liver, in *P. vivax* and *P. ovale* infections. Both antirelapse therapy and radical cure treatment should be for 14 days—started the first day the patient has left the malarious area—and used in conjunction with a malaria schizonticide. Often it is well tolerated but may cause GI upset that improves when taking the medication with food. Most importantly, primaquine can cause hemolytic anemia in individuals who are deficient in glucose-6-phosphate dehydrogenase (G6PD), so normal G6PD levels must be ensured before starting primaquine. Patients should discontinue primaquine if they pass red or black urine, or have symptomatic anemia. Primaquine is also contraindicated during pregnancy and during breastfeeding unless the infant's G6PD status is known.

In addition to the medications mentioned above, several other antimalarials may be encountered in malaria-endemic areas that are not approved for use by the FDA due to poor efficacy or unwelcome side-effect profiles (e.g., individual components of ACTs like amodiaquine [Camoquin][2] and sulfadoxine-pyrimethamine,[2] or halofantrine [Halfan][2]). Therefore, travelers and physicians counseling patients should be aware of those medications approved by the regulatory authorities in their respective countries.

For travelers, authenticity of medications must also be ensured. Unfortunately, the quality of medications commercially available in malaria-endemic countries can vary greatly. While appearing to be genuine, counterfeit medications may have little to no active ingredient or may contain ingredients not indicated on their label. If travelers have to purchase medications outside of their home country, they need to scrutinize medication packaging for printing errors and signs of tampering. The color, consistency, odor, and taste of the medication may also alert one to counterfeit medication. The Medicines Quality Database (MQDB) through the U.S. Pharmacopeial Convention is one resource available to investigate medicine quality in countries throughout the world (see http://www.usp.org/global-health-programs/promoting-quality-medicines-pqmusaid/medicines-quality-database-mqdb).

Treatment

Unless there is clinical concern for severe disease or prompt laboratory diagnosis is unobtainable, malaria treatment should be initiated once the diagnosis is established by laboratory testing. Upon confirmation of the diagnosis, treatment management should be based on the identity of infecting *Plasmodium* species, the patient's clinical status and level of parasitemia, prior use of antimalarials, and the geographic area where the infection was likely acquired.

If identification reveals the presence of *P. falciparum* malaria or *Plasmodium* species remains uncertain, patients should be hospitalized and monitored closely for possible development of severe malaria symptoms and complications. When clinical and laboratory data support low severity, it is safe to treat patients in the outpatient setting with oral therapy. Should symptoms become more severe, though, as described below, the patient should be started on parenteral therapy and admitted to intensive care. As a default, clinicians should always treat those with malaria where the infecting species is unknown as if they had a chloroquine-resistant *P. falciparum* infection until proven otherwise. Routine serial blood monitoring for parasite density using blood smears will also help modify therapy as needed. Clinicians must be mindful, though, that increases in parasite density within the first 24 hours of treatment may represent normal release of parasite from RBCs and not worsening infection, especially when the patient's symptoms are improving with current therapy. Monitoring should continue until blood smears are negative and alternative treatments need to be considered if the patient's symptoms are not improving and parasite density is not decreasing.

Detailed treatment information regarding dosing and frequency may be found in Tables 1–3.

Chloroquine-Sensitive Plasmodium (*P. falciparum, P. knowlesi, P. malariae, P. ovale,* and *P. vivax*)

Oral chloroquine phosphate is the recommended treatment for all sensitive malaria strains. Confirmed infections with *P. ovale, P. malariae,* and *P. knowlesi* are generally sensitive to chloroquine and treatment should not be delayed, especially for *P. knowlesi*, which has the capacity to increase parasitemia rapidly and become very severe. For *P. falciparum* and *vivax* infections, chloroquine may be indicated if the confirmed geographic area of exposure has no known chloroquine resistance. In addition, for all *P. ovale* and *vivax* infections, patients with normal G6PD activity require primaquine therapy for 14 days to reduce potential relapse.

---

[1] Not FDA approved for this indication.

[2] Not available in the United States.

| TABLE 3 | Artemisinin Combination Therapies (ACTs)*[1] |
MEDICATION	ADULT AND PEDIATRIC DOSING (BY BODY WEIGHT)
Artemether+lumefantrine[2,3]	Artemether+lumefantrine (mg) bid for 3 days: 5 to <15 kg: 20+120 15 to <25 kg: 40+240 25 to <35 kg: 60+360 >35 kg: 80+480
Artesunate+amodiaquine[4,†]	Artesunate+amodiaquine (mg) daily for 3 days: 4.5 to <9 kg: 25+67.5 9 to <18 kg: 50+135 18 to <36 kg: 100+270 >36 kg: 200+540
Artesunate+mefloquine[5,†]	Artesunate+mefloquine (mg) daily for 3 days: 5 to <9 kg: 25+55 9 to <18 kg: 50+110 18 to <30 kg: 100+220 >30 kg: 200+440
Artesunate+sulfadoxine/pyrimethamine[6,†]	Artesunate (mg) daily for 3 days+sulfadoxine/pyrimethamine (mg) single dose day 1: 5 to <10 kg: 25+250/12.5 10 to <25 kg: 50+500/25 25 to <50 kg: 100+1000/50 >50 kg: 200+1500/75
Dihydroartemesinin+piperaquine[7,†]	Dihydroartemesinin+piperaquine (mg) daily for 3 days: 5 to <8 kg: 20+160 8 to <11 kg: 30+240 11 to <17 kg: 40+320 17 to <25 kg: 60+480 25 to <36 kg: 80+640 36 to <60 kg: 120+960 60 to <80 kg: 160+1280 >80 kg: 200+1600

*Recommended therapies per WHO.
†Not available in the United States.
[1]Artemisinins and their partner medicines above should not be used alone for treatment, only in a combination.
[2]Only ACT that is approved for use by U.S. FDA.
[3]Absorption of lumefantrine is enhanced by coadministration with fat.
[4]In patients with HIV, concomitant use of zidovudine, efavirenz, or cotrimoxazole should be avoided.
[5]Contraindicated in people allergic to mefloquine or related compounds (quinine, quinidine) and in people with depression, a recent history of depression, generalized anxiety disorder, psychosis, schizophrenia, other major psychiatric disorders, or seizures. Not recommended for persons with cardiac conduction abnormalities.
[6]Only ACT that it is not available as a fixed-dose combination.
[7]High-fat meals should be avoided as they significantly accelerate the absorption of piperaquine.
Lack of resolution of malaria symptoms or recurrence within 4 weeks of treatment are considered treatment failures and a different ACT should be tried.

Chloroquine-Resistant *P. falciparum*

In the case of *P. falciparum* infection from areas with known chloroquine resistance, several options are available. Where available, artemisinin-based combination therapies (ACTs) are considered the standard of care, but other agents may also be used (see Table 3). In the United States four different treatment options are available: atovaquone-proguanil, artemether-lumefantrine, quinine sulfate combined with doxycycline,[1] tetracycline,[1] or clindamycin,[1] or mefloquine. Due to neuropsychiatric side effects, mefloquin should be considered only when other options are not available or contraindicated. It should also not be used when

the *P. falciparum* strain was acquired in Southeast Asia due to increased resistance to mefloquine in that region.

Chloroquine-Resistant *P. vivax*

Though mostly sensitive to chloroquine, *P. vivax* infections acquired in Indonesia and Papua New Guinea often show resistance. Common treatment regimens for chloroquine-resistant strains include atovaquone-proguanil, quinine sulfate[1] combined with doxycycline[1] or tetracycline,[1] or mefloquine. There is also very good evidence to support using ACTs, where available, for treatment of both chloroquine-resistant and chloroquine-sensitive strains. As mentioned before, all *P. vivax*-infected patients should also receive primaquine therapy for 14 days to eradicate any hypnozoite forms.

Severe Malaria

Severe disease is likely in those patients with a positive blood smear or a concerning exposure history who also exhibit at least one of the following: impaired consciousness or coma, severe normocytic anemia, renal failure, pulmonary edema, acute respiratory distress syndrome, circulatory shock, disseminated intravascular coagulation, spontaneous bleeding, acidosis, hemoglobinuria, jaundice, seizures, and parasitemia of over 5%. Mortality risk increases with increasing numbers of the signs/symptoms especially when signs of acidosis, vital organ dysfunction, or high parasite count are present. Immediate point of care testing, where available, should always include measures of hematocrit, parasite count, and blood glucose. The mortality rate for patients with untreated severe malaria (particularly cerebral malaria) is almost 100%. Fortunately, with prompt effective treatment and supportive care, mortality may fall to 10%.

Any patient considered to be at increased risk should receive the highest level of care available (e.g., intensive care unit) and parenteral antimalarial drug treatment (artesunate or quinidine) should be started without delay. Adults and children with severe malaria (including infants, pregnant women in all trimesters, and lactating women) should be treated with IV or IM artesunate for at least 24 hours where available. As soon as oral therapy can be tolerated after the initial 24 hours of parenteral therapy, treatment with 3 days of an ACT should continue (7 days if likely acquired from Southeast Asia). When IM and IV forms are not available, rectal administration of artesunate (10 mg/kg body weight) in young children (<6 years) in prereferral settings has also proven to be a life-saving adjuvant before arrival at a facility for further care. When quinidine is used, as it most frequently would be in the United States, parenteral therapy (to include IV doxycycline[1] or clindamycin[1]) should be given for a minimum of 24 hours and then switched to oral treatment once tolerated after that. When an ACT is not available for follow-on treatment, artesunate+clindamycin,[1] artesunate+doxycycline,[1] quinine+clindamycin, quinine+doxycycline, or atovaquone-proguanil can be used.

Regarding general monitoring and supportive care, fluid requirements should be assessed individually and signs of shock quickly addressed. Adults with severe malaria are very vulnerable to fluid overload and pulmonary edema, while children are more likely to be dehydrated. Severe malaria can be associated with rapid development of anemia, as erythrocytes are hemolyzed and/or removed from the circulation by the spleen. Ideally, fresh, cross-matched blood should be available for transfusion when hematocrit levels fall to below 15% in children or 20% in adults. Cardiac monitoring is also essential, especially when using quinidine, which is known to cause conduction abnormalities at the loading dosages required for initial treatment. Of note, after artesunate treatment in hyperparasitemic nonimmune travelers, it is common for delayed hemolysis to occur after a week, and so such patients need to be followed for these changes. Given the potential clinical overlap between malaria and sepsis, especially in children, blood cultures should always be taken and empiric

---

[1]Not FDA approved for this indication.

[1]Not FDA approved for this indication.

antibiotic treatment should be started along with antimalarial therapy until bacterial infection can be ruled out. Additionally, though incorporated into some older recommendations, both the CDC and WHO no longer recommend using exchange transfusions or prophylactic anticonvulsants as adjunct treatment in severe malaria as the data do not support any mortality benefit.

Clinicians with questions about effective treatment (or diagnosis) should consult with an infectious disease specialist or a physician with specialized training in travel or tropical medicine. If no such local avenues are available, clinicians should not hesitate to contact the CDC's Malaria Hotline (referenced previously).

Treatment in Pregnancy

Pregnancy complicates the treatment strategy as it affects both the mother and her fetus. Infections, especially with *P. falciparum*, can increase susceptibility to severe disease and risk of developing anemia, while increasing fetal risk for low birth weight and prematurity in addition to miscarriage. Symptoms of pregnant patients may also be more muted in high-transmission areas than for those in low-transmission areas despite the adverse effects on fetal growth. Congenital malaria must be considered when infants born to mothers with acute malaria infection show signs of fever, anemia, or failure to thrive during the first few months of birth. In most cases, treatment of newborns or infants should proceed if symptoms are present and infection status is confirmed. While remaining vigilant, providers must also educate mothers about symptoms and the importance of quick follow-up should they develop. Of note, congenitally acquired malaria in infants does not involve a liver stage so primaquine is not needed.

As pregnant women are largely excluded from many clinical trials, safety and efficacy data are lacking for them, especially during the first trimester. Nevertheless, a number of recommendations have been made from available data regarding treatment of pregnant women. During the first trimester, current guidelines list chloroquine, quinine, clindamycin, and proguanil[2] as safe. Additionally, review of available data has moved the FDA to list mefloquine as a pregnancy Category B medication showing no increase in birth defects or fetal loss throughout pregnancy. Though some prospective data do support its use early in pregnancy, WHO only recommends ACTs in the first trimester if it is the only treatment available, in cases of severe malaria where IV artesunate is indicated, if treatment with quinine plus clindamycin[1] fails, or if uncertainty of compliance with a 7-day treatment exists (quinine is only needed for 3 days if infection was acquired outside Southeast Asia).

After the first trimester, several artemisinin derivatives, alone or in combination with other antimalarials, have been evaluated as safe and efficacious in second and third trimester pregnancy. Therefore, the WHO recommends that ACTs be used during the second and third trimester of pregnancy where the choice of ACT is governed by local efficacy (most recommended are artemether-lumefantrine, artesunate-amodiaquine,[2] artesunate-mefloquine,[2] and artesunate-sulfadoxine-pyrimethamine[2]). For those with *P. malariae*, *P. vivax*, *P. ovale*, or chloroquine-sensitive *P. falciparum* malaria, chloroquine treatment, the same as for nonpregnant patients, should be instituted.

Primaquine phosphate for treatment of *P. vivax* or *P. ovale*[1] hypnozoites should not be given during pregnancy. If *P. vivax* or *P. ovale* infections are confirmed, pregnant patients should be maintained on weekly chloroquine prophylaxis for the duration of their pregnancy, 300 mg base (=500 mg salt) orally once per week. Primaquine therapy can be initiated after delivery in those patients with known normal G6PD levels. Due to possible breast milk excretion of primaquine, it should not be used by nursing women unless infants have known normal G6PD levels.

For severe malaria cases, parenteral antimalarial drugs should be given to pregnant women in full doses without delay regardless of trimester. IM artemether may be used if artesunate is unavailable; otherwise parenteral quinine should be started immediately until artesunate is obtained. Pulmonary edema and hypoglycemia are commonly seen, the latter especially when quinine is used, so patients should be monitored carefully.

Treatment of the Pediatric Patient

Delay in treating *P. falciparum* malaria in infants and young children can have fatal consequences, particularly for more severe infections. The vast majority of malaria cases and deaths in the world, especially Africa, occur in young children. Fortunately, many antimalarial drugs have included children in clinical trials. Therefore, treatment recommendations are not just based on extrapolated data. Recommendations are consistent with those for adult patients but require appropriate dosage changes based on patient weight, and the dosage should never exceed the adult dose.

Chloroquine may be used for any chloroquine-sensitive malaria strains and, where available, artemisinin derivatives (artemether-lumefantrine being the most studied) are considered safe and very well tolerated and represent first-line treatment for chloroquine-resistant *P. falciparum*. Alternatively, quinine sulfate and quinidine may be given in combination with clindamycin[1] in those areas with poorer access to artemisinin derivatives. Atovaquone-proguanil may also be considered in this group as well as mefloquine, but only if no other options are available for the latter. Of note, for small infants weighing less than 5 kg, the WHO does recommend treatment with ACT at the same target dose as for children weighing 5 kg or more. No modifications are currently warranted in those suffering malnutrition; however, their response to treatment should be monitored closely. Regarding treatment combinations with tetracycline[1] or doxycycline,[1] these drugs should only be used with extreme prejudice in those under 8 years of age and only when other treatments are not available or not tolerated and the benefits are judged to outweigh the risks. Also, primaquine should only be given to those children with known normal levels of G6PD.

Prevention

Preventive measures are important to ensure protection against malaria. Limiting exposure to the mosquito disease vector, *Anopheles* species, as well as taking appropriate drug prophylaxis measures are key components in preventing malaria in both travelers and those living in malaria-endemic locations.

The *Anopheles* mosquito is primarily a nocturnal feeder so protecting oneself during the periods from dusk to dawn is essential to avoid possible infection. In this effort, remaining indoors or within well-screened areas, wearing clothing of a tight mesh that covers most of the body, using bed nets, ideally treated with insecticide, and using insecticide sprays on clothing and/or the body especially during evening and nighttime hours are all key. Spraying indoor areas with insecticides also adds protection. Certainly some of the malaria mortality reductions seen worldwide directly relate to the efforts in malaria-endemic areas to increase access to insecticide-treated bed nets and improved efforts in indoor residual spraying.

Several commercial insecticides and insect repellents are available. For clothing and bed nets, pyrethroids (i.e., permethrin) are typically used and fairly effective at protecting against mosquitoes, though some reports warn of developing resistance. Using insect repellents, too, greatly minimizes *Anopheles* exposure. Currently, DEET (diethylmethyl-toluamide) is most frequently used and is known to be safe for all age groups including infants down to 2 months old. Concentrations above 25% are often recommended and individuals should remember to reapply repellent at a minimum of every 8 hours. In addition to DEET, picaradin (e.g., Natrapel 8 Hour Insect Repellent and Sawyer Premium 20% Picaradin Spray) products and IR3535 or ethyl butylacetylamino-propionate (e.g., Avon Skin-So-Soft Bug Guard Plus and Sawyer Insect and Sun Spray) are also recommended by both the CDC and WHO. Meanwhile, oil of lemon eucalyptus (e.g., Repel and Off!) is only recommended by the CDC for those repellents

---

[1] Not FDA approved for this indication.
[2] Not available in the United States.

receiving U.S. Environmental Protection Agency approval. Travelers should always remember that when using topical skin repellents, they should be applied after any sunscreen is applied to exposed skin surfaces.

Chemoprophylaxis measures are also an important preventive medicine concern. For travelers and at-risk groups living in endemic areas, there are a number of recommended chemoprophylaxis regimens currently available (see Table 4). Key to all of these is taking an agent before, during, and after travel to a malaria-endemic area. One must ensure that the prophylactic agent is present in the bloodstream before any potential exposure.

When in doubt, clinicians may use the CDC's online interactive malaria map or Malaria-by-Country tables (both referenced previously) to quickly view the types of *Plasmodium* present and resistance characteristics found in the patient's area of travel. In combination with the patient's individual medical history, age, medications, and travel duration, this information can be used by the clinician to treat the patient appropriately. Additionally, pregnant women who choose to travel to a malaria-endemic area must be aware that malaria severity is often increased during pregnancy. Personal protective measures and steadfast use of chemoprophylaxis (e.g., mefloquine or hydroxychloroquine) are key.

TABLE 4 Recommendations for Malaria Chemoprophylaxis

MEDICATION	USE	ADULT DOSING	PEDIATRIC DOSING	COMMENTS
Atovaquone/proguanil[1]	Prophylaxis, all areas	Adult tab=250 mg/100 mg. 1 tab daily	Pediatric tablets=62.5 mg/25 mg. 5–8 kg: 1/2 pediatric tab daily >8–10 kg: 3/4 pediatric tab daily >10–20 kg: 1 pediatric tab daily >20–30 kg: 2 pediatric tabs daily >30–40 kg: 3 pediatric tabs daily >40 kg: 1 adult tab daily	Begin 1–2 days before travel to malarious areas. Take at same time every day while in malarious area and for 7 days after leaving such areas. Take with food or milk. Pharmacist may be needed to prepare some partial tablet dosing.
Chloroquine phosphate	Prophylaxis, areas with chloroquine-sensitive malaria	300 mg base (500 mg salt) PO, once/week	5 mg/kg base (8.3 mg/kg salt) PO, once/week, up to maximum adult dose of 300 mg base	Begin 1–2 weeks before travel to malarious areas. Take weekly on same day of the week while in malarious area and for 4 weeks after leaving. Can exacerbate psoriasis.
Doxycycline[2]	Prophylaxis, all areas	100 mg PO, daily	≥8 years of age: 2.2 mg/kg up to adult dose of 100 mg/day	Begin 1–2 days before travel to malarious areas. Take at same time every day while in malarious area and for 4 weeks after leaving.
Hydroxychloroquine	An alternative to chloroquine. Prophylaxis, areas with chloroquine-sensitive malaria	310 mg base (400 mg salt) PO, once/week	5 mg/kg base (6.5 mg/kg salt) PO, once/week, up to a maximum adult dose of 310 mg base	Begin 1–2 weeks before travel to malarious areas. Take weekly on the same day of the week while in the malarious area and for 4 weeks after leaving.
Mefloquine[3,4]	Prophylaxis, areas with mefloquine-sensitive malaria	228 mg base (250 mg salt) PO, once/week	≤9 kg: 4.6 mg/kg base (5 mg/kg salt) PO, once/week >9–19 kg: 1/4 tablet once/week >19–30 kg: 1/2 tablet once/week >30–45 kg: 3/4 tablet once/week >45 kg: 1 tablet once/week	Begin 2 weeks before travel to malarious areas. Take weekly on the same day of the week while in malarious area and for 4 weeks after leaving. Use with caution in persons with psychiatric disturbances or a history of depression.
Primaquine phosphate[5,7]	Prophylaxis, areas with *P. vivax* only for short duration	30 mg base (52.6 mg salt)[8] PO, daily	0.5 mg/kg base (0.8 mg/kg salt)[7] up to adult dose PO, daily	Begin 1–2 days before travel to malarious areas. Take daily at same time each day while in malarious area and for 7 days after leaving such areas.
Primaquine phosphate[5]	Used for presumptive antirelapse therapy (terminal prophylaxis) to decrease relapse risk of *P. vivax* and *P. ovale*	30 mg base (52.6 mg salt)[8] PO, daily for 14 days after departure from the malarious area	0.5 mg/kg base (0.8 mg/kg salt)[7] up to adult dose PO, daily for 14 days after departure from the malarious area	Indicated for people who have had prolonged exposure to *P. vivax, P. ovale*, or both. Take daily for 14 days starting first day of departure from malarious area.

TABLE 4 Recommendations for Malaria Chemoprophylaxis—cont'd

MEDICATION	USE	ADULT DOSING	PEDIATRIC DOSING	COMMENTS
Sulfadoxine/ pyrimethamine[6,9]	Intermittent preventive treatment in pregnant women (first or second pregnancy) and in infants (<12 months) in African locations with moderate-high malaria transmission	Give weight-based dose to pregnant women and infants of at least 25/1.25 (25–70/1.25–3.5) mg/kg body weight. 5 to <10 kg: 250/12.5 mg 10 to <25 kg: 500/25 mg 25 to <50 kg: 1000/50 mg >50 kg: 1500/75 mg		Provide to pregnant women as part of antenatal care starting in the second trimester and dosed at least 1 month apart (ensuring at least 3 doses are received). Give to infants (<12 months of age) at the time of the second and third rounds of vaccination against diphtheria, tetanus and pertussis and vaccination against measles.

[1]Contraindicated in severe renal impairment (creatinine clearance <30 mL/min). Not recommended for children <5 kg and pregnant women.
[2]Contraindicated in children <8 years of age and pregnant women.
[3]Contraindicated in people allergic to mefloquine or related compounds (quinine, quinidine) and in people with depression, a recent history of depression, generalized anxiety disorder, psychosis, schizophrenia, other major psychiatric disorders, or seizures. Not recommended for persons with cardiac conduction abnormalities.
[4]Currently Category B in pregnancy (FDA), recommended as option for treatment and prophylaxis in all trimesters.
[5]Contraindicated in G6PD deficiency. Also contraindicated during pregnancy and lactation, unless infant has normal G6PD level.
[6]Dosing based on fixed-dose combination tablets of 500 mg sulfadoxine/25 mg pyrimethamine.
[7]Not FDA approved for this indication.
[8]Exceeds dosage recommended by the manufacturer.
[9]Not available in the United States.

The WHO does encourage intermittent preventive treatment with sulfadoxine-pyrimethamine (SP-IPT)[2] for pregnant women living in endemic areas and for infants. For pregnant women during their first or second pregnancy living in endemic areas in Africa with moderate to high *P. falciparum* transmission, intermittent pregnancy treatment of malaria with SP-IPTp is recommended. Dosing should start in the second trimester and doses should be given at each antenatal visit at least 1 month apart. In addition, as a prophylactic in pediatric patients living in areas of higher malaria transmission in Africa, the WHO recommends providing intermittent preventive treatment with SP-IPTi to infants (<12 months of age) at the time of the second and third rounds of vaccination against diphtheria, tetanus, and pertussis (DTP) and vaccination against measles. Similarly, in areas with seasonal malaria transmission in the sub-Sahel region of Africa, seasonal malaria chemoprevention with monthly amodiaquine[2]+SP is recommended for all children less than 6 years old during each transmission season.

There is no malaria vaccine currently on the market, but RTS,S/AS01 is a candidate vaccine with somewhat promising Phase III trial data in pediatric patients. Consisting of three initial monthly doses and a booster 18 months after the third dose, over a 48-month period it showed efficacy against clinical malaria of up to 39% and against severe malaria of 31.5%. This represented an estimated number of averted clinical malaria cases in pediatric patients on the order of 1774 per 1000 children in those receiving the booster dose. Although certainly representing another worthwhile tool in combating malaria, the extent to which the protection demonstrated can be replicated in the context of a routine health-care system remains uncertain. Similarly, in an effort to combat *P. vivax* infection, Phase III data on tafenoquine, a long-acting primaquine derivative, have shown good activity against all stages of the *P. vivax* life cycle and may be developed for the radical cure of acute *P. vivax* malaria in combination with chloroquine. It may also potentially treat *P. vivax* hypnozoites with a single dose instead of the current 14-day protocol for primaquine.

Note

The views expressed here are those of the authors and do not reflect the official policy or position of the U.S. Air Force, the Department of Defense, or the U.S. government.

[2]Not available in the United States.

References

Abba K, Kirkham AJ, Olliaro PL, et al: Rapid diagnostic tests for diagnosing uncomplicated non-falciparum or *Plasmodium vivax* malaria in endemic countries (online), *Cochrane Database Syst Rev* 2014(12):CD011431, 2014. Available at: http://onlinelibrary.wiley.com/doi/10.1002/14651858.CD011431/full (accessed 14.11.15).

Centers for Disease Control and Prevention: *Treatment of Malaria (guidelines for clinicians)*, 2013a: Available at: http://www.cdc.gov/malaria/resources/pdf/clinic alguidance.pdf (accessed 14.11.15).

Centers for Disease Control and Prevention: *Guidelines for Malaria treatment in the United States*, 2013b: Available at: http://www.cdc.gov/malaria/resources/pdf/tre atmenttable.pdf (accessed 14.11.15).

Cullen KA, Arguin PM: Surveillance summaries: malaria surveillance—United States, 2012, *Morb Mortal Wkly Rep* 63(SS12):1, 2014.

Navy and Marine Corps Public Health Center: *Pocket Guide to Malaria Prevention and Control*, Portsmouth, VA, 2011, US Navy and Marine Corps Public Health Center.

RTS,S Clinical Trials Partnership: Efficacy and safety of RTS,S/AS01 malaria vaccine with or without a booster dose in infants and children in Africa: final results of a phase 3, individually randomized, controlled trial, *Lancet* 386:31, 2015.

Visser BJ, van Vugt M, Grobusch MP: Malaria: an update on current chemotherapy, *Expert Opin Pharmacother* 15:2219, 2014.

Wells TNC, van Huijsduijnen RH, Van Voorhis WC: Malaria medicines: a glass half full? *Nat Rev Drug Discov* 14:424, 2015.

White NJ, Pukrittayakamee S, Hien TT, et al: Malaria, *Lancet* 383:723, 2014.

World Health Organization: *Guidelines for the treatment of malaria*, 3rd ed., Geneva, 2015a, WHO.

World Health Organization: *World Malaria Report – 2015*, Geneva, 2015b, WHO.

MEASLES (RUBEOLA)

Method of
Jane A. Weida, MD

CURRENT DIAGNOSIS

- Highly contagious viral illness with a prodrome of high fever, cough, conjunctivitis, and coryza.
- Pathognomonic enanthem (Koplik spots—small white lesions) may appear on buccal mucosa
- Incubation period of about 10 days to the onset of fever and about 14 days to the onset of rash
- Red maculopapular rash beginning on face and becoming generalized
- History of exposure, particularly history of travel to endemic areas, or in non-immunized individuals

Epidemiology

Measles caused millions of deaths worldwide each year before measles vaccines were introduced. In the decade before the first measles vaccine was licensed in 1963, there were about 549,000 measles cases and 495 deaths annually. It is estimated that the actual incidence was much higher, possibly 3 to 4 million.

Measles was declared eliminated from the United States in 2000, but outbreaks have occurred since then, with a resurgence in 2019. As of May 3, 2019, there were 764 reported cases in 2019 in 23 states, the largest outbreak since 1994.

Most people who get measles are unvaccinated. Travelers with measles continue to bring the disease to the United States. Measles can spread when it reaches an area where groups of people are unvaccinated, including areas where immunity dips below 95%.

Measles continues to be a major problem in many regions of the world. Due to increased worldwide measles vaccination, from 2000 to 2017, annual reported measles cases decreased by 83% and the annual estimated measles deaths decreased by 80%. Despite this, measles caused approximately 109,000 deaths in 2017.

Risk Factors

Being unvaccinated is the largest risk factor for measles in the United States. Infants who have lost maternal immunity but who are too young to be immunized are at higher risk, as are individuals with vitamin A deficiency. Travel to international areas where measles is more common or where there is an outbreak also increases the risk of contracting measles. If measles is suspected in a patient, a careful travel history should be obtained.

Pathophysiology

Measles is caused by an RNA respiratory virus, of the family *Paramyxoviridae* and genus *Morbillivirus*. It is one of the most highly contagious of the communicable diseases. The virus spreads from person to person via respiratory droplets from coughing or sneezing or via direct contact. Patients are usually contagious from about 4 days before to about 4 days after the rash appears. The fact that the disease is contagious before the onset of symptoms makes quarantining difficult. The incubation period is generally 10 days before the prodrome and 14 days before the onset of the rash, but it may vary from 6 to 21 days.

The virus triggers an aggressive immune response. This leads to a suppression of the immune response to other pathogens, which makes the individual susceptible to secondary infections. This immune suppression can last for a few weeks to a few months, but in some cases, it may last for 2 to 3 years.

Once a measles infection is successfully cleared, the person gains lifelong immunity provided they remain immunocompetent. Infants are protected by maternal antibodies, for about 1 month in the case of an immunized mother and for about 4 months in the case of a mother who had a prior measles infection.

Prevention

The best way to prevent measles is with measles vaccination. The Centers for Disease Control and Prevention (CDC) recommends measles-mumps-rubella (MMR) vaccination at ages 12 to 15 months, with the second dose at 4 to 6 years of age. Two doses are more than 99% effective. Students at post-high school institutions who are not immune to measles should have two doses of MMR vaccine at least 28 days apart. Adults born in or after 1957 who do not have evidence of immunity should receive at least one dose of MMR vaccine. The vaccine should not be given to pregnant women or immunocompromised individuals.

International travelers should be protected against measles. Infants who are traveling who are aged 6 to 11 months should receive one dose of MMR vaccine. Children aged 12 months of age and older should have documentation of two doses of MMR vaccine, at least 28 days apart. Teenagers and adults born during or after 1957 without evidence of immunity should have two documented doses of MMR vaccine.

Despite the importance of measles prevention, some parents refuse to vaccinate their children. A study published in the UK in 1998 claimed to find a link between autism and MMR vaccine. The study was later proven to be erroneous and fraudulent, and subsequent studies have consistently shown that there is no link between vaccines and autism. It is vital for clinicians to continue to educate parents about how vitally important MMR vaccination is, particularly given the recent increase of measles cases.

Clinical Signs and Symptoms

Measles generally presents with a prodrome that includes high fever, malaise, anorexia, conjunctivitis, coryza, and non-productive cough. Fever may reach over 40°C. Conjunctivitis may include redness, swelling, photophobia, and discharge. Koplik spots, which are small white spots on the buccal mucosa, are pathognomonic, but they are not always present.

The measles rash is erythematous and maculopapular. It usually appears first on the face and behind the ears and then spreads to the trunk and extremities. The rash lasts for 3 to 7 days. Recovery begins soon after the rash appears.

Diagnosis

Measles is usually diagnosed clinically, based on the presenting signs, vaccination history, and travel/exposure history. Clinical diagnosis can be difficult when the incidence of measles is low. The World Health Organization clinical case definition for measles is a person with fever and maculopapular rash and at least one of the symptoms of cough, coryza, or conjunctivitis.

Laboratory findings include leukopenia, unless there is a secondary bacterial infection, thrombocytopenia, and proteinuria. The most commonly used serologic test used is virus-specific immuoglobulin M (IgM) in serum or oral fluid. IgM antibodies may not be detectable until 4 or more days after the rash appears. Viral cultures may also be obtained as may nasopharyngeal swabs for detection by polymerase chain reaction.

In the United States, measles is a reportable illness. Suspected cases should be reported to the local health department immediately. The CDC recommends that serologic and viral specimens be collected in suspected cases of measles; clinicians can contact their local laboratories to find out which specimens to collect.

Differential Diagnosis

Measles may easily be mistaken for other upper viral respiratory illnesses during the prodromal stage. While Koplik spots are pathognomonic, they are easy to overlook. Once the rash appears, it may be mistaken for other illnesses, including erythema infectiosum, infectious mononucleosis, enterovirus, Kawasaki disease, chikungunya, Rocky Mountain spotted fever, rubella, and scarlet fever.

Treatment

No specific antiviral treatment is available for measles. Treatment is supportive, including rest, adequate fluids, and antipyretics. Patients should be kept at bedrest until they are afebrile. Prompt recognition and treatment of secondary bacterial infections is essential. The World Health Organization recommends administration of vitamin A[1] to all those with measles. The CDC

---

[1]Not FDA approved for this indication.

recommends treatment of children with severe cases of measles, such as those who are hospitalized, with vitamin A.[1] It is given immediately when the disease is diagnosed and then repeated the following day.

Monitoring

Most measles patients do not need hospitalization. For those who do, both standard precautions and respiratory precautions should be initiated. Respiratory precautions should continue for 4 days after onset of rash for healthy children and for the duration of the illness in immunocompromised patients.

For those who have been exposed to measles and are not immune, MMR should be administered within 72 hours of exposure or immunoglobulin (GamaSTAN) administered within 6 days of exposure.

Complications

Complications of measles can occur in up to 40% of patients; complications are highest in the very young, the very old, and those who are malnourished. Often the complications affect the respiratory tract, with pneumonia being the leading cause of death associated with measles. Pneumonia may be caused by a secondary bacterial or viral infection or by the measles virus itself. Otitis media is another common complication. Gastrointestinal complications include diarrhea and stomatitis. Measles keratoconjunctivitis is a common complication, especially in children with vitamin A deficiency.

Rarely, measles can cause severe central nervous system (CNS) complications. About 1 in 1000 cases of measles results in postmeasles encephalomyelitis, leading to fever, seizures, and neurologic abnormalities. Measles causes about 1 to 2 deaths per 1000 due to respiratory or neurologic complications. Subacute sclerosing panencephalitis is a rare delayed neurologic complication of measles, occurring in about 1 in 10,000 to 100,000 patients. This fatal complication causes seizures and progressive intellectual and behavioral deterioration about 7 to 10 years following a measles infection.

References

Bester J: Measles and measles vaccination a review, *JAMA Pediatr* 170(12):1209–1215, 2016.
Centers for Disease Control and Prevention: Measles Cases and Outbreaks. Available at: https://www.cdc.gov/measles/cases-outbreaks.html. [Accessed 12 May 2019].
Centers for Disease Control and Prevention: Measles for Healthcare Professionals. Available at: https://www.cdc.gov/measles/hcp/index.html. [Accessed 12 May 2019].
Centers for Disease Control and Prevention: Progress Toward Regional Measles Elimination – Worldwide, 2000-2017. Available at: https://www.cdc.gov/mmwr/volumes/67/wr/mm6747a6.htm. [Accessed 12 May 2019].
Measles: In Kimberlin DW, Brady MT, Jackson MA, Long SS, editors: *Red Book: 2018 Report of the Committee on Infectious Diseases*, 31st ed., Itasca, IL, 2018, American Academy of Pediatrics, pp 537–550.
Moss W: Measles, *Lancet* 390:2490–2502, 2017.
Moss W, Griffin D: Measles, *Lancet* 379:153–164, 2012.
Shandera WX, Dandachi D: Viral & rickettsial infections: Measles. In Papadakis MA, McPhee SJ, editors: *Current Medical Diagnosis and Treatment 2019*, 58th ed., New York, 2019, McGraw Hill Education, pp 1391–1394.

METHICILLIN-RESISTANT *STAPHYLOCOCCUS AUREUS*

Method of
Elissa Rennert-May, MD, MSc; and John M. Conly, MD

CURRENT DIAGNOSIS

- Healthcare-associated methicillin-resistant *Staphylococcus aureus* (HA-MRSA) is endemic in many hospital settings. The strains are polyclonal, resistant to many non–β-lactam antimicrobials, and typically cause pneumonia, line-related infection, surgical site infection, bacteremia, and infrequently skin and soft tissue infections.
- Strains of community-associated MRSA (CA-MRSA) have risen exponentially over the past two decades. The strains are clonal, sensitive to many non–β-lactam antimicrobials, harbor multiple virulence factors, and typically cause pyogenic skin and soft tissue infections and occasionally severe necrotizing pneumonia, fasciitis, and multifocal osteomyelitis.
- HA-MRSA infections typically affect patients with multiple comorbidities in the healthcare setting, but CA-MRSA typically affects previously healthy persons.
- It can be difficult to differentiate infectious syndromes due to β-hemolytic streptococci versus CA-MRSA.

CURRENT THERAPY

- Methicillin-resistant *Staphylococcus aureus* (MRSA) strains harbor resistance to the β-lactam antimicrobials, including oxacillin, dicloxacillin, cloxacillin[2], nafcillin, methicillin[1], and first-, second-, and third-generation cephalosporins[1].
- Healthcare-associated MRSA (HA-MRSA) strains are typically resistant to macrolides, clindamycin (Cleocin), aminoglycosides, and quinolones (with the exception of delafloxacin [Baxdela]) and are variably resistant to tetracycline and trimethoprim-sulfamethoxazole (Bactrim). They are sensitive to vancomycin (Vancocin) and the lipoglycopeptides, fusidic acid[2], rifampin (Rifadin)[1], the oxazolidinones linezolid (Zyvox) and tedizolid (Sivextro), daptomycin (Cubicin), ceftaroline (Teflaro), and ceftobiprole (Zevtera)[2].
- Community-associated MRSA (CA-MRSA) strains are resistant to macrolides and quinolones (with the exception of delafloxacin [Baxdela]) but usually sensitive to aminoglycosides such as gentamicin (Garamycin), clindamycin, and trimethoprim-sulfamethoxazole (Bactrim)[1], in addition to vancomycin (Vancocin), the lipoglycopeptides, fusidic acid[2], rifampin (Rifadin)[1], the oxazolidinones linezolid (Zyvox) and tedizolid (Sivextro), daptomycin (Cubicin), ceftaroline (Teflaro), and ceftobiprole (Zevtera)[2].
- Empiric antimicrobial therapy should be guided by the clinical presentation, and when full sensitivities are available, the antimicrobials may be tailored accordingly.

[1]Not FDA approved for this indication.
[2]Not available in the United States.

Epidemiology

Staphylococcus aureus is one of the most frequently encountered bacteria causing human infections and may be considered as either methicillin-sensitive *S. aureus* (MSSA) or methicillin-resistant *S. aureus* (MRSA). MRSA was first described in 1961 and is resistant not only to the traditional antistaphylococcal β-lactam antibiotics (methicillin[2], nafcillin, oxacillin, cloxacillin[2], and dicloxacillin) but also other important β-lactam antibiotics, including the first- to fourth-generation cephalosporins and the carbapenem family, thus eliminating an important class of antibiotics from the clinician's armamentarium. The only β-lactams that have activity against MRSA are the recently approved advanced-generation cephalosporin agents ceftaroline (Teflaro) and ceftobiprole (Zevtera)[2].

MRSA strains acquired in the hospital or other healthcare settings have traditionally been referred to as healthcare-associated MRSA (HA-MRSA), whereas community-associated MRSA

[2]Not available in the United States.

TABLE 1 General Features Differentiating HA- and CA-MRSA*

CHARACTERISTIC	HA-MRSA	CA-MRSA
Drug resistance to non–β-lactams	Multiresistance	Pauciresistance
Pathogenicity islands	Few	Multiple
Age predilection	Older	Younger
Comorbidities	Multiple	None
Traditional risk factors	Healthcare contact, prolonged hospital stay, poor hand hygiene, contaminated equipment, invasive procedures, medical devices, recent antibiotic use	Crowded community environment, lack of cleanliness, loss of skin integrity, intravenous drug user, homelessness, incarceration, aboriginal, HIV+, contact sports, athletes, military, chronic skin disorder, veterinary worker

*Features are generalizations only given the appearance of community strains replacing traditional hospital strains in the health care setting and the appearance of typical HA strains in the community setting.

CA, Community-associated; HA, healthcare-associated; HIV, human immunodeficiency virus; MRSA, methicillin-resistant Staphylococcus aureus.

The "5 Cs" for Transmission of CA-MRSA

- **C**rowding
- **C**ontact with skin
- **C**ompromised skin
- **C**ontaminated personal care items
- **C**leanliness lack

Figure 1 The five Cs implicated in transmission of community-associated methicillin-resistant S. aureus. (Adapted from the US Centers for Disease Control and Prevention.)

(CA-MRSA) has referred to isolates acquired in the community setting and in the absence of traditional hospital or healthcare exposures for at least 1 year (overnight stays in an acute care or long-term care facility, surgery, dialysis, or presence of a central venous catheter). Recently the term *community-onset HA-MRSA* has been used to describe the occurrence of MRSA infection in the setting of the presence of a healthcare exposure within the past year. MRSA has been recognized as a healthcare-associated pathogen since the 1970s and became endemic in hospitals in many countries, including the United States, United Kingdom, and many European countries over the next two decades, with exceptions being Denmark, the Netherlands, Scandinavia, and Canada. For several decades, MRSA was typically considered a hospital pathogen. Novel and virulent MRSA strains arising in the community and not associated with any traditional healthcare exposure risks were first encountered in the late 1990s in the United States, Australia, and some European countries and have since risen explosively on a global basis to become the predominant clone of *S. aureus* associated with community infections. Methicillin resistance among community isolates of *S. aureus* has been reported as high as 75% in some US communities. More recently livestock-associated MRSA (LA-MRSA) has been reported on a global basis, and transmission of these strains from swine, cattle, and horses has been implicated as a source of human infections, particularly in farmers, abattoir workers, and veterinarians.

Specific genetic and molecular distinctions initially distinguished the HA- and CA-MRSA strains (Table 1) and have been used to characterize MRSA strains as likely of community or healthcare origin. The HA-MRSA strains were found to harbor large staphylococcal cassette chromosome (SCCmec) types known as SCCmec types I, II, or III; to have multidrug resistance to non–β-lactam antimicrobials; to have the absence of specific virulence characteristics such as carriage of the Panton-Valentine Leukocidin *(PVL)* gene; and to have varying multilocus sequence types (ST5, ST239,

ST 247, ST250). On the other hand, the CA-MRSA strains have been found to harbor SCCmec types IV, V, and more recently VI to XIII have been described; to have paucidrug resistance to non–β-lactam antimicrobials; to have the presence of specific virulence characteristics such as carriage of the *PVL* gene, and to have multilocus sequence types ST1, ST8, and ST80. LA-MRSA strains often are nontypeable or harbor SCCmec V, have high rates of tetracycline resistance, carry multiple virulence factors, and are most often multilocus sequence types ST398 or ST9. However, over the past few years, healthcare-associated strains have moved into the community and likewise community strains have spread rapidly within hospitals, and the original distinctions between CA-MRSA and HA-MRSA from an epidemiologic perspective have become increasingly blurred. The point of transmission of MRSA is not always possible to identify with certainty, making the classification of CA and HA strains increasingly imprecise.

Risk Factors

The risk factors for HA-MRSA may be viewed from the perspective of the healthcare environment and patient-specific risk factors. A major risk factor for acquiring HA-MRSA is exposure to a healthcare setting and particularly in hospital or other institutional settings where the prevalence of carriage of MRSA among patients is high. Additional risk factors in the healthcare environment include poor hand hygiene practices among hospital employees, contaminated bedside equipment and surfaces, overcrowding, and reduced healthcare worker-to-patient ratios. Patient risk factors (see Table 1) include aging, multiple comorbidities, receipt of antibiotics within the preceding 3 months, prolonged duration of hospital stay, admission to a long-term care facility or hospital in the previous year, invasive procedures, and the presence of indwelling catheters or other devices. Initial risk groups for CA-MRSA were injection drug users, homeless populations, incarcerated persons, and indigenous peoples. The Centers for Disease Control and Prevention have suggested the five Cs (Figure 1 and Table 2) as contributing factors implicated in the transmission among these groups. The initial risk groups have currently expanded (Table 3) to include men who have sex with men (MSM), athletes (especially those involved in team and contact sports), military personnel, those with a prior history of abscesses, individuals with chronic skin disorders, individuals with recent antibiotic receipt, underserved urban populations, individuals who have contact with colonized pets or livestock, and veterinary workers. In the drug-using and underserved urban populations, prevalence and social networking studies have identified hospices, shooting galleries, and crack houses as key sites in which CA-MRSA transmission may occur. Recent outbreaks have been reported in hospital nurseries, daycare settings, nursing home workers, schools, and college dormitories. Sexual transmission has been reported, but it may reflect close skin-to-skin genital contact rather than a true sexually transmitted pathogen.

TABLE 2 Risk Factor Associations Reported for CA-MRSA Infections

RISK CATEGORIES	FACTOR	DETAILS FROM REPORTS
High-risk populations	Younger and older age	Age distribution in CA-MRSA younger than HA-MRSA
		High rate of CA-MRSA in children under 2 years
		CA-MRSA more common in children compared to adults
		Outbreaks in hospital nurseries
		Outbreaks in nursing homes with elderly residents
	Indigenous populations: Native or Aboriginal or African American	Aboriginal communities in midwestern United States, Canada, and Australia
		Alaskan natives
		More common in African Americans
	Athletes (predominantly contact sports)	Outbreaks on football teams
		Outbreaks on wrestling team
		Other competitive sports
	Injection (intravenous) drug users (IVDUs)	San Francisco IVDUs
		Canadian report of USA300 strain outbreak
	Men who have sex with men (MSM)	CA-MRSA described in HIV+ population of MSM
	HIV+ individuals	Risk associated with overlapping social networks, intravenous drug use, hemodialysis, and CD4 counts <200 reported as independent risks
	Military personnel	3% of US Army soldiers colonized
	Inmates of correctional facilities	Reports of outbreaks in US prisons
		Two outbreaks (total 10 inmates) in Canada
	Students in elementary schools and college dormitories	Reports of outbreaks in schools and college dormitories
Previous positive MRSA cultures	MRSA carriage	Colonized soldiers more likely to get CA-MRSA disease
	Past MRSA infection	Prior abscess risk factor for CA-MRSA
Medical history	Chronic skin disorder	Dermatologic condition most common underlying medical disorder for CA-MRSA infection
		Classroom contact of index CA-MRSA case had chronic dermatitis
	Recurrent or recent antibiotic use	Antibiotic use associated with CA-MRSA infection in rural Alaska
Environmental	Homelessness and living in shelters	Medically underserved populations at higher risk of CA-MRSA
		Reports of USA300 strain outbreak involving individuals living in shelters or homeless
	Overcrowding	Close contact implicated in jail outbreaks
	Contact with colonized pet	Neonatal intensive care unit transmission
	Veterinary workers and family members	Family dog source of recurrent infection
		Veterinarians working with horses and livestock
		Family members of animal care workers
		Small animal veterinarians
		Swine farmers

CA, Community-associated; HA, healthcare-associated; HIV, human immunodeficiency virus; MRSA, methicillin-resistant *Staphylococcus aureus*.
Adapted from Barton-Forbes M, Hawkes M, Moore D, et al. Guidelines for the prevention and management of community associated methicillin resistant *Staphylococcus aureus* (CA-MRSA): a perspective for Canadian Health Care Practitioners. *Can J Infect Dis Med Microbiol.* 2006;17(suppl C):1B–24B.

TABLE 3 Principles of Empiric Treatment of Minor Skin and Soft Tissue Infections (Folliculitis, Furuncles, Small Abscesses Without Cellulitis, Impetigo, Secondarily Infected Lesions Such as Eczema, Ulcers, or Wounds) Where the Etiology Is Unknown But May Include MRSA as a Possibility

Recommendations
One or more of the following measures may be employed:
- Local therapy using hot soaks, elevation, and dressings as appropriate
- Incision and drainage of furuncles or small abscesses without antimicrobial therapy
- Topical 2% mupirocin ointment (Bactroban) or fusidic acid[2] for impetigo and secondarily infected lesions if local strains are likely sensitive
- Topical antiseptics may be considered
- Antimicrobial therapy is recommended in addition to local measures if one or more of the following is present: multiple sites of infection, evidence of progression, clinical evidence of systemic symptoms and signs, presence of comorbidities, extremes of age, immunosuppression, septic phlebitis, or difficult site for incision and drainage.
- In follow-up, routine screening for colonization of the nares or other body sites is not recommended.

[2]Not available in the United States.
MRSA, Methicillin-resistant *Staphylococcus aureus*.

CA-MRSA has now become endemic in the general population in many communities, and the elderly and the very young seem to have a predilection for infection, especially if other risk factors are present. Risk groups for LA-MRSA include farmers, their family members and farm hands who are engaged in livestock production (especially swine and cattle), abattoir workers, veterinarians, and veterinary assistants. Recent transmission of strains of LA-MRSA has been reported in the hospital setting as well.

Pathophysiology

The resistance to the antistaphylococcal β-lactam antibiotics in MRSA strains is imparted by the presence of an altered configuration for a specific penicillin-binding protein (PBP) known as PBP2a in the cell wall of staphylococci. Normally the PBPs would act as a site for the attachment of the active moieties of the β-lactam agent, which then would inhibit further cell wall assembly. The alteration in the configuration of PBP2a occurs as the result of the presence of the SCC*mec* gene in *S. aureus*, which confers resistance to the β-lactam antibiotics. The origins of the *mec* gene and its insertion into the SCC*mec* element are not known with certainty. Once the MRSA strains acquired resistance to the antistaphylococcal β-lactam antibiotics in the healthcare setting, it is not difficult to appreciate how it emerged as a predominant pathogen in the hospital setting over the years, with increasing acuity of illness in the patient populations and increased use of broad-spectrum antimicrobials.

The appearance and rapid spread of CA-MRSA with the clinical impression of more virulent and lethal infections than what had been seen with traditional HA-MRSA strains may be explained by several factors. The SCC*mec* IV genetic element is very widely distributed among *S. aureus* isolates, which may explain its appearance in multiple settings globally, and these strains appear to have more rapid growth rates than typical HA-MRSA strains, larger numbers of virulence factors, pathogenicity islands, and higher levels of expression of the virulence factors produced. Recently α-type phenol-soluble modulins were described in strains of CA-MRSA, which are produced at very high levels and are potent lysins of neutrophils. High levels of α-toxin production by these strains, which act as pore-forming toxins for multiple cell types, may also contribute to their virulence. The vast majority of CA-MRSA strains also produce the genes for PVL and it functions as a dermonecrotic factor in skin lesions, a potent cell lysin in high concentrations, and a potent inflammatory mediator in lower concentrations. However, there is controversy about the role of PVL as a single predominant virulence factor, because strains of CA-MRSA that have this gene knocked out have demonstrated no difference in pathogenicity in both vertebrate and invertebrate animal models and in human settings when the PVL is not present.

Prevention

Controlling the spread of HA-, CA-, or LA-MRSA from an infected or colonized person to others in the hospital, family, or community is a key goal of prevention. In the hospital setting, strict adherence to hand hygiene, application of barrier precautions (gloves, gowns, and private rooms) for patients colonized or infected with MRSA, environmental and equipment cleaning, and antimicrobial stewardship are the key preventive strategies. Active surveillance cultures to identify colonized patients and decolonization may be effective in selected settings, but its general application is controversial. In the community setting, practicing hygienic measures including good personal hygiene, consistent hand hygiene, ensuring all draining skin and soft tissue lesions have adequate dressings, not sharing potentially contaminated personal articles, and keeping the household environment hygienic are important. Public health organizations may also contribute to the prevention of CA-MRSA by instituting education programs targeting healthcare providers and individuals in high-risk groups in the community, and by promoting appropriate antimicrobial use. In sports settings, in addition to the basic hygienic measures mentioned previously, avoidance of sharing of towels and other personal items, showering after every practice or tournament, cleaning of communal showering and bathing areas, and cleaning or laundering of equipment after each use are also important.

Clinical Manifestations

The specific clinical infections associated with MRSA parallel those associated with MSSA. Almost any body site, organ, or appendage may be affected by infections due to *S. aureus*, but there are specific predilections associated with HA- and CA-MRSA. In the hospital or other healthcare setting, the most commonly encountered sites of infection include pneumonia, line-related infection, surgical site infection, bacteremia, and less often skin and soft tissue infections. In the community setting, the most common sites (>80%) are skin and soft tissue infections (furuncles, cellulitis, and soft tissue abscesses) and less commonly severely invasive infections such as necrotizing pneumonia, necrotizing fasciitis, multifocal osteomyelitis/septic arthritis, epidural abscess, pelvic septic thrombophlebitis, and bacteremia with toxic shock syndrome. The skin and soft tissue infections often affect young previously healthy patients and are characteristically very painful and pyogenic with an initial black eschar that patients presume was a "spider bite" as the initiating process.

Diagnosis

The diagnosis of MRSA infections is based on the clinical presentation and the isolation of the causative organism from purulent discharge, sputum, or urine, or from specimens obtained from normally sterile body fluids (joint fluid, abscess or tissue aspirates, and blood). The organism appears on Gram stain as a gram-positive organism in clusters and is usually seen in association with neutrophils and may be either intracellular or extracellular. The organism is very hardy and grows readily on typical media in the microbiology laboratory within 24 to 48 hours. Some laboratories are using rapid agglutination tests to detect the PBP2a protein or polymerase chain reaction (PCR)-based techniques to provide same-day or next-day identification. In settings where no cultures have been obtained or in the setting of toxic shock syndrome where cultures are often negative, the diagnosis may be difficult and only suspected based on a typical clinical presentation.

Treatment

MRSA strains harbor resistance to the β-lactam antimicrobials, including oxacillin, dicloxacillin, cloxacillin[2], nafcillin, methicillin[2], and first-, second-, and third-generation cephalosporins. The new advanced-generation cephalosporin antimicrobiasl ceftaroline (Teflaro) and ceftobiprole (Zevtera)[2] have activity against MRSA strains. The majority of HA-MRSA strains are resistant to macrolides, clindamycin (Cleocin), aminoglycosides, and quinolones (with the exception of delafloxacin [Baxdela]) and are variably resistant to tetracycline and trimethoprim-sulfamethoxazole (Bactrim)[1], depending on local epidemiologic patterns. They are sensitive to vancomycin (Vancocin) and the lipoglycopeptides such as dalbavancin (Dalvance), telavancin (Vibativ), and oritavancin (Orbactiv) and usually sensitive to fusidic acid[2], rifampin (Rifadin)[1], the oxazolidinones linezolid (Zyvox) and tedizolid (Sivextro), and daptomycin (Cubicin). For hospitalized patients where *S. aureus* is considered a possible etiology of any major infectious syndrome, it should be considered as methicillin-resistant until proven otherwise. Empiric choices of vancomycin or lipoglycopeptides such as dalbavancin (Dalvance), telavancin (Vibativ) or oritavancin (Orbitaciv), linezolid (Zyvox) or tedizolid (Sivextro), daptomycin (Cubicin) or advanced-generation cephalosproins such as ceftaroline (Teflaro) or ceftobiprole (Zevtera)[2] should be considered as appropriate to the presenting syndrome. CA-MRSA strains are resistant to macrolides and often quinolones (with the exception of delafloxacin [Baxdela]) but usually are sensitive to aminoglycosides such as gentamicin (Garamycin), clindamycin, and trimethoprim-sulfamethoxazole (Bactrim)[1], but the resistance patterns vary depending on local resistance patterns. In addition, these strains are sensitive to vancomycin (Vancocin) and the lipoglycopeptides, fusidic acid[2], rifampin (Rifadin)[1], linezolid (Zyvox), daptomycin (Cubicin), ceftaroline (Teflaro), and ceftobiprole (Zevtera)[2]. LA-MRSA strains are almost always resistant to tetracyclines; often resistant to quinolones, macrolides, and clindamycin, and variably resistant to aminoglycosides and trimethoprim-sulfamethoxazole. In addition, these strains are sensitive to vancomycin (Vancocin) and the lipoglycopeptides, fusidic acid[2], rifampin (Rifadin)[1], the oxazolidinones linezolid (Zyvox) and tedizolid (Sivextro), daptomycin (Cubicin), ceftaroline (Teflaro) and ceftobiprole (Zevtera)[2]. Treatment guidelines for MRSA with a focus on the ambulatory setting have been published in Canada, the United Kingdom, and the United States, and provide both empiric choices for common infectious presentations of unknown etiology and definitive treatment once an etiology of MRSA is known. The treatment options for both empiric and definitive use where MRSA is considered or proven are presented in Tables 3 through 6 and represent a

---

[1]Not FDA approved for this indication.
[2]Not available in the United States

TABLE 4	Principles of Empiric Treatment of Non–Life-Threatening Skin and Soft Tissue Infections Other Than Minor Skin Infections Where the Etiology Is Unknown But May Include MRSA as a Possibility

Recommendations
- Antibiotic choice should be based on the severity of illness at presentation, clinical judgment, and regional susceptibility patterns of strains
- Empiric therapy for CA-MRSA and β-hemolytic streptococci is recommended*

*The IDSA guideline suggests to differentiate purulent and nonpurulent cellulitis and reserve empiric therapy for β-hemolytic streptococci only in nonpurulent cellulitis but acknowledges it is an area of controversy. The UK and Canadian guidelines explicitly recommend coverage for β-hemolytic streptococci and do not differentiate cellulitis into different types.
CA, Community-associated; IDSA, Infectious Diseases Society of America; MRSA, methicillin-resistant *Staphylococcus aureus.*

TABLE 5	Principles of Empiric Treatment of Life-Threatening Infections Where the Etiology Is Unknown But May Include MRSA as a Possibility

Recommendations
- Include MRSA coverage, regardless of prevalence rates of CA-MRSA in the community
- Include an agent effective against MSSA until susceptibility results become available

CA, Community-associated; MRSA, methicillin-resistant *Staphylococcus aureus*; MSSA, methicillin-sensitive *Staphylococcus aureus.*

TABLE 6	Guidelines for the Management of MRSA Infections

CLINICAL DISEASE	KEY FEATURES	MANAGEMENT PRINCIPLES	ANTIMICROBIAL CHOICES AND COMMENTS*
Skin and Soft Tissue Infection (SSTI)			
Localized lesion	Infected scratches and minor wounds Insect bites Furuncles Small abscesses Absence of systemic illness	Culture selectively[†] No antibiotic therapy recommended *Exceptions: multiple sites of infection, evidence of progression, systemic symptoms and signs, presence of comorbidities, extremes of age, immunosuppression, septic phlebitis, or difficult site for incision and drainage: antimicrobial therapy is recommended in addition to local measures* Cover draining lesions Emphasize personal hygiene Close follow-up Return if worsening	Generally not indicated, although some evidence exists for treatment with clindamycin PO or trimethoprim-sulfamethoxazole (Bactrim)[1] PO, in conjunction with incision and drainage for small simple abscesses Topical antibacterial (e.g., mupirocin [Bactroban] or fusidic ointment[2]) therapy may be considered Systemic antimicrobial therapy indicated if one or more of the following: multiple sites of infection, evidence of progression, systemic symptoms and signs, presence of comorbidities, extremes of age, immunosuppression, septic phlebitis, or difficult site for incision and drainage
Cellulitis (not extensive) or multiple abscesses with minimal or no associated systemic features for oral treatment consideration	Classic features of rubor, dolor, calor, and swelling suggesting cellulitis with or without associated drainage or exudate	Culture site (if purulent or drainage) Drainage of abscess or needle aspiration Oral therapy in older child and adult Appropriate infection control measures Imaging for extent and complications as appropriate Close follow-up Return if worsening	*Empiric:* Include coverage for β-hemolytic streptococci[¶] Clindamycin (Cleocin) 300–450 mg tid-qid PO for adults and 30–40 mg/kg/day[3] ÷ q6–8h PO for children TMP-SMX (Bactrim)[1] 1–2 DS tab bid PO for adults and 8–12 mg/kg/day (of TMP) ÷ q12h PO for children PLUS coverage for β-hemolytic streptococci (e.g., amoxicillin, cephalexin [Keflex]) Doxycycline (Vibramycin) 100 mg bid PO for adults and 4.4 mg/kg/day mg/kg/day ÷ q12h PO for children** PLUS coverage for β-hemolytic streptococci (e.g., amoxicillin, cephalexin) Delafloxacin (Baxdela) 450 mg bid PO for adults *Comment:* Recently became the first fluoroquinolone approved by the FDA for MRSA SSTI Linezolid (Zyvox) 600 mg bid PO for adults and 30 mg/kg/day ÷ q8h PO for children, not to exceed 600 mg/dose; for children older than 12 years of age 600 mg bid PO *Comment:* Linezolid is more expensive than the other options and may not always be readily available depending on the setting *Comment:* If parenteral therapy considered, see choices for severe SSTI Tedizolid (Sivextro) 200 mg PO/IV once daily for 6 days; safety and efficacy have not been established for children *Proven MRSA:* As above, based on sensitivity testing If parenteral therapy necessary, see choices for SSTI with systemic features

TABLE 6 Guidelines for the Management of MRSA Infections—cont'd

CLINICAL DISEASE	KEY FEATURES	MANAGEMENT PRINCIPLES	ANTIMICROBIAL CHOICES AND COMMENTS*
Cellulitis (severe or rapidly spreading or extensive) or complicated SSTI (deep soft tissue infection, surgical or traumatic wound infection, large or multiple abscesses, or infected ulcers and burns) and/or associated systemic features for parenteral treatment consideration	Classic features of rubor, dolor, calor, and swelling suggesting cellulitis with or without associated drainage or exudate with systemic features of fever, chills, malaise, prostration	Culture (blood if febrile, site if purulent) Hospitalize as appropriate Drainage of abscess or needle aspiration Parenteral therapy Imaging for extent and complications as appropriate Appropriate infection control measures Consultation as indicated	*Empiric:* Include coverage for β-hemolytic streptococci[¶] Vancomycin (Vancocin) 15–20 mg/kg/dose q8–12h IV for adults and 40–60[3] mg/kg/day ÷ q6h IV for children *Proven MRSA:* Based on sensitivity testing Vancomycin 15–20 mg/kg/dose q8–12h IV for adults and 40–60[3] mg/kg/day ÷ q6h IV for children Clindamycin 600–900 mg q8h IV/IM for adults and 30–40 mg/kg/day[3] ÷ q6–8h IV for children Linezolid 600 mg q12h PO/IV for adults and 30 mg/kg/day ÷ q8h PO/IV for children, not to exceed 600 mg/dose; for children older than 12 years of age 600 mg bid PO/IV Tedizolid (Sivextro) 200 mg PO/IV once daily for 6 days; safety and efficacy have not been established for children Ceftaroline (Teflaro) 600 mg IV q12h for adults; safety and efficacy have not been established for children Daptomycin (Cubicin) 4 mg/kg/dose once daily IV for adults and under investigation in children Dalbavancin (Dalvance) 1000 mg IV followed by 500 mg IV 1 week later for adults; safety and efficacy not established in children Telavancin (Vibativ) 10 mg/kg/dose IV once daily Oritavancin (Orbactiv), given as a single 1200 mg 3-hour infusion; not approved for children Delafloxacin (Baxdela) 300 mg bid IV *Comment:* Linezolid, tedizolid, daptomycin, ceftaroline, ceftobiprole,[2] dalbavancin, oritavancin and telavancin are more expensive than the other options and may not always be readily available depending on the setting
Necrotizing fasciitis (NF)	Clinically indistinguishable from group A streptococcus NF disease Extreme toxicity High complication rate	Cultures (blood, tissue) Imaging for extent and complications Surgical débridement Consultation as indicated Parenteral therapy Infection control measures	*Empiric:* Include coverage for β-hemolytic streptococci Vancomycin 15–20 mg/kg/dose q8–12h IV for adults and 40–60[3] mg/kg/day ÷ q6h IV for children Clindamycin 600–900 mg q8h IV/IM for adults and 30–40 mg/kg/day[3] ÷ q6–8h IV for children *Proven MRSA:* Based on sensitivity testing Vancomycin 15–20 mg/kg/dose q8–12h IV for adults and 40–60[3] mg/kg/day ÷ q6h IV for children Clindamycin 600–900 mg q8h IV/IM for adults and 30–40 mg/kg/day[3] ÷ q6–8h IV for children Linezolid 600 mg q12h PO/IV for adults and 30 mg/kg/day ÷ q8h PO/IV for children, not to exceed 600 mg/dose; for children older than 12 years of age 600 mg bid PO/IV TMP/SMX[1] 8–12 mg/kg/day (of TMP) ÷ q8–12h IV for adults and 8–12 mg/kg/day (of TMP) ÷ q6h IV for children *Comments:* Adjuncts such as IVIG (Gamunex)[1] may be considered in severe cases with septic shock Few data available for the use of TMP-SMX in this indication

Musculoskeletal Infection (MSI)

CLINICAL DISEASE	KEY FEATURES	MANAGEMENT PRINCIPLES	ANTIMICROBIAL CHOICES AND COMMENTS*
Osteomyelitis/septic arthritis	Preceding trauma Tendency for multifocal involvement Disease in adjacent muscle not uncommon Progression to chronic osteomyelitis possible May be complicated by deep venous thrombosis	Cultures (blood, bone, and tissue) Imaging for extent and complications Involve surgical team (early débridement and drainage) Consultation as indicated Parenteral therapy Consider combination therapy for severe cases or if slow to respond Infection control measures Look for other infected sites (imaging)	*Empiric:* Vancomycin 15–20 mg/kg/dose q8–12h IV for adults and 40–60[3] mg/kg/day ÷ q6h IV for children Clindamycin 600–900 mg q8h IV/IM for adults and 30–40 mg/kg/day[3] ÷ q6–8h IV for children Linezolid[1] 600 mg q12h PO/IV for adults and 30 mg/kg/day ÷ q8h PO/IV for children, not to exceed 600 mg/dose; for children older than 12 years of age 600 mg bid PO/IV Daptomycin[1] 6 mg/kg/dose once daily IV for adults and 6–10 mg/kg once daily for children TMP/SMX[1] 8–12 mg/kg/day (of TMP) ÷ q8–12h IV for adults and 8–12 mg/kg/day (of TMP) ÷ q6h IV for children *Comments:* Linezolid and daptomycin are more expensive than the other options and may not always be readily available depending on the setting Few data available for the use of TMP-SMX in these indications for children *Proven MRSA:* As above, based on sensitivity testing Addition of rifampin (Rifadin)[1] may be considered for osteomyelitis

Continued

TABLE 6 Guidelines for the Management of MRSA Infections—cont'd

CLINICAL DISEASE	KEY FEATURES	MANAGEMENT PRINCIPLES	ANTIMICROBIAL CHOICES AND COMMENTS*
Pyomyositis	May be extensive Tendency for multifocal involvement	Cultures (blood, tissue) Imaging for extent and complications Surgical drainage Consultation as indicated Parenteral therapy Infection control measures	

Respiratory Tract Infection (RTI)

CLINICAL DISEASE	KEY FEATURES	MANAGEMENT PRINCIPLES	ANTIMICROBIAL CHOICES AND COMMENTS*
Pneumonia	Influenza-like prodrome, hemoptysis, fever, shock, leukopenia, pneumatoceles, multifocal abscesses, consolidation, frequent empyema, respiratory failure, and high mortality	Cultures (blood, pleural fluid, sputum) Imaging for extent and complications Consultation as indicated Intensive care unit as appropriate Infection control measures Combination parenteral therapy Chest tube drainage for empyema	*Empiric:* Vancomycin 15–20 mg/kg/dose q8–12h IV for adults and 40–60[3] mg/kg/day ÷ q6h IV for children Linezolid 600 mg q12h PO/IV for adults and 30 mg/kg/day ÷ q8h PO/IV for children, not to exceed 600 mg/dose; for children older than 12 years of age 600 mg bid PO/IV Clindamycin 600–900 mg q8h IV/IM for adults and 30–40 mg/kg/day[3] ÷ q6–8h IV for children TMP/SMX[1] 8–12 mg/kg/day (of TMP) ÷ q8–12h IV for adults and 8–12 mg/kg/day (of TMP) ÷ q6h IV for children Telavancin (Vibativ) 10 mg/kg/dose IV once daily for adults for hospital or ventilator acquired pneumonia Ceftaroline (Teflaro) 600 mg IV q12h for adults with community-acquired pneumonia; safety and efficacy have not been established for children Ceftobiprole (Zevtera)[2] 500 mg IV q8h for adults with community-acquired and hospital-acquired pneumonia; safety and efficacy have not been established for children *Comment:* Daptomycin not indicated because it is inactivated by lung surfactant *Proven MRSA:* As above, based on sensitivity testing

Other

CLINICAL DISEASE	KEY FEATURES	MANAGEMENT PRINCIPLES	ANTIMICROBIAL CHOICES AND COMMENTS*
Sepsis syndrome Bacteremia Native valve endocarditis	Shock Multiple-organ failure May have purpura fulminans Associated SSTI, MSI, and RTI May be complicated by Waterhouse-Friedrichsen syndrome High mortality	Blood cultures Culture any pus or fluid collection Look for primary or secondary focus Imaging for identification of source including echocardiography Consultation as indicated ICU care Imaging: look for occult abscesses, bone infection, or endocarditis Involve surgery and other specialists as needed Infection control measures Parenteral, multidrug therapy Prolonged therapy for endovascular source infections	*Empiric:* Vancomycin 15–20 mg/kg/dose q8–12h IV for adults and 40–60[3] mg/kg/day ÷ q6h IV for children Daptomycin 6 mg/kg/dose once daily IV for adults and 4–10[3] mg/kg/dose once daily for children[1] *Comments:* Doses of daptomycin of up to 10 mg/kg/dose[3] once daily have been used in adults in this indication Some recommendations have included linezolid in this setting at the doses described above *Proven MRSA:* As above, based on sensitivity testing. *Comment:* New IDSA guidelines for the treatment of *S. aureus* bacteremia are anticipated for summer 2020

*Choice of antimicrobial therapy depends on local susceptibility patterns.

†Patients with risk factors, as a part of an outbreak investigation, patients with slowly responding or recurrent lesions.

¶The IDSA guideline suggests to differentiate purulent and nonpurulent cellulitis and reserve empiric therapy for β-hemolytic streptococci only in nonpurulent cellulitis but acknowledges it is an area of controversy. The UK and Canadian guidelines explicitly recommend empiric coverage for β-hemolytic streptococci and do not differentiate cellulitis into different types. A recent randomized controlled trial in the United States found no significant difference in efficacy between clindamycin and trimethoprim-sulfamethoxazole when used for treatment of uncomplicated skin and soft tissue infections, which were thought to be secondary to either β-hemolytic streptococci or *S. aureus*. Another recent placebo-controlled trial in the United States found that clindamycin or trimethoprim-sulfamethoxazole in conjunction with incision and drainage improved outcomes in patients with simple small abscesses (<5 cm) compared with incision and drainage alone.

[1]Not FDA approved for this indication. Dosing has varied in published reports and specific dosing guidelines are not available.

[2]Not available in the United States.

[3]Exceeds dosage recommended by the manufacturer.

**Not recommended for pediatric patients younger than 8 years of age or in pregnancy.

ICU, Intensive care unit; *IDSA,* Infectious Diseases Society of America; *IVIG,* intravenous immunoglobulin; *MRSA,* methicillin-resistant *Staphylococcus aureus*; *TMP-SMX,* trimethoprim-sulfamethoxazole.

constellation of the various guidelines that have been published. A recent study compared the use of vancomycin versus daptomycin plus ceftaroline for MRSA bacteremia, but the trial was halted due to increased mortality in the vancomycin monotherapy arm.

References

Barton-Forbes M, Hawkes M, Moore D, et al: Guidelines for the prevention and management of community associated methicillin resistant *Staphylococcus aureus* (CA-MRSA): a perspective for Canadian Health Care Practitioners, *Can J Infect Dis Med Microbiol* 17(Suppl. C):1B–24B, 2006.

Chambers HF, Deleo FR: Waves of resistance: *Staphylococcus aureus* in the antibiotic era, *Nat Rev Microbiol* 7:629–641, 2009. https://doi.org/10.1038/nrmicro2200.

Daum RS, Miller LG, Immergluck L: A placebo-controlled trial of antibiotics for smaller skin abscesses, *N Engl J Med* 376(26):2545–2555, 2017.

David MZ, Daum RS: Community-associated methicillin resistant *Staphylococcus aureus:* epidemiology and clinical consequences of an emerging epidemic, *Clin Microbiol Rev* 23:616–687, 2010. https://doi.org/10.1128/CMR.00081-09.

Fluit AC: Livestock-associated Staphylococcus aureus, *Clin Microbiol Infect* 18:735–744, 2012. https://doi.org/10.1111/j.1469-0691.2012.03846.x.

Geriak M, Haddad F, Khulood R, et al: Clinical data on daptomycin plus ceftaroline versus standard of care monotherapy in the treatment of methicillin-resistant Staphylococcus aureus bacteremia, *Antimicrob Agents Chemother*, 2019. https://doi.org/10.1128/AAC.02483-18.

Gorwitz RJ, Jernigan DB, Powers JH, et al: *Strategies for clinical management of MRSA in the community: summary of an experts' meeting convened by the Cent-*

ers for Disease Control and Prevention, 2006: 2006. Available at www.cdc.gov/ncidod/dhqp/pdf/ar/CAMRSA_ExpMtgStrategies.pdf (accessed 02.01.2013).

Gould FK, Brindle R, Chadwick PR, et al: Guidelines (2008) for the prophylaxis and treatment of methicillin resistant *Staphylococcus aureus* (MRSA) infections in the United Kingdom, *J Antimicrob Chemother* 63:849–861, 2009. https://doi.org/10.1093/jac/dkp065.

Kaplan SL, Hulten KG, Gonzalez BE, et al: Three-year surveillance of community-acquired *Staphylococcus aureus* infections in children, *Clin Infect Dis* 40:1785–1791, 2005.

Klevens RM, Morrison MA, Nadle J, et al: Invasive methicillin resistant *Staphylococcus aureus* infections in the United States, *JAMA* 298:1763–1771, 2007.

Kock R, Becker K, Cookson B, et al: Methicillin resistant *Staphylococcus aureus* (MRSA): burden of disease and control challenges in Europe, *Euro Surveill* 15:19688, 2010.

Lakhundi S, Zhang K: Methicillin-resistant Staphylococcus aureus: molecular characterization, evolution, and epidemiology, *Clin Microbiol Rev* 31, 2018, e00020-18. https://doi.org/ 10.1128/CMR.00020-18.

Liu C, Bayer A, Cosgrove SE, et al: Clinical practice guidelines by the Infectious Diseases Society of America for the treatment of methicillin resistant *Staphylococcus aureus* infections in adults and children: executive summary, *Clin Infect Dis* 52:285–292, 2011. https://doi.org/10.1093/cid/cir034.

Miller LG, Daum RS, Creech CB, et al: Clindamycin versus trimethoprim-sulfamethoxazole for uncomplicated skin infections, *N Engl J Med* 372(12):1093–1103, 2015.

Muto CA, Jernigan JA, Ostrowsky BE, et al: SHEA guideline for preventing nosocomial transmission of multidrug-resistant strains of *Staphylococcus aureus* and enterococcus, *Infect Control Hosp Epidemiol* 24:362–386, 2003.

Nathwani D, Morgan M, Masterton RG, et al: Guidelines for UK practice for the diagnosis and management of methicillin resistant *Staphylococcus aureus* (MRSA) infections presenting in the community, *J Antimicrob Chemother* 61:976–994, 2008. https://doi.org/10.1093/jac/dkn096.

MUMPS

Method of
Kristen Rundell, MS, MD

CURRENT DIAGNOSIS

- Parotitis (swelling of the parotid salivary glands): unilateral or bilateral
- Fever
- Headache
- Malaise
- Myalgias
- Anorexia
- Increased serum amylase

CURRENT THERAPY

- Supportive care
- Warm or cold packs on the parotid
- Analgesics and/or antipyretics (such as acetaminophen [Tylenol] or ibuprofen [Motrin])
- IV fluids or hospitalization for cases of pancreatitis, meningitis, or severe orchitis

Epidemiology

Mumps is an extremely contagious, self-limiting virus that had disease rates of 99% until the vaccine was introduced in 1967. Since that time, the yearly disease rate is less than 1 percent. For the United States and Finland, mumps is almost eradicated. For the rest of the world, mumps is still endemic as a result of a vaccination rate of only 61%.

Pathophysiology

Mumps is a single-stranded RNA virus and a member of the *Paramyxovirus* genus. It is transmitted through respiratory secretions, saliva, and contact with contaminated fomites.

Prevention

With the high rate of transmission and no antiviral therapy, prevention for mumps relies on community immunity as a result of high vaccine rates. There are two formulations of the mumps vaccine currently available in the United States: the measles-mumps-rubella vaccine (MMR) and the measles-mumps-rubella-varicella vaccine (MMRV, ProQuad). The dosing schedule for children calls for the first dose at age greater than 12 months to 15 months, and the second dose for children greater than 4 years to 6 years of age. For infants aged 6 through 11 months who are traveling internationally, a single MMR vaccine is recommended. These children should be revaccinated with 2 doses of MMR vaccine with the first dose at ages 12 months to 15 months and the second dose at ages 4 years to 6 years. During an epidemic, a single dose for adults born before 1957 is recommended and may be required by some health care professionals. The first dose gives approximately 80% immunity. Persons receiving both doses may still get the mumps virus if there is outbreak or if they travel to an endemic area. To avoid exposure or contraction of the disease during travel, it is suggested that travelers wash hands frequently and use alcohol-based sanitizers to decrease the contraction or spread of disease.

The vaccine is contraindicated for patients who are pregnant or planning to conceive in the 28 days after vaccination. Vaccine administration is also contraindicated for those who have a severe anaphylactic reaction to the vaccine or one of the components, and those individuals who are severely immunocompromised.

Clinical Manifestations

The incubation period for the mumps virus is 16 to 18 days. At the onset of the illness, patients may develop acute viral infection symptoms of fever, headache, and malaise. The parotitis, swelling of the parotid gland, is the diagnostic hallmark of the mumps virus. This is caused by the infection and inflammation of the parotid ductal epithelium. The swelling may last up to 10 days. Close to 30% of persons may not have this symptom and may be only mildly symptomatic.

Diagnosis

Diagnosis is made by the history and the constellation of symptoms and physical findings. It is difficult to use IgM to determine active infection, because the response may be short in duration, delayed, or even absent. PCR testing is available and requires early sampling.

Differential Diagnosis

Viral infections such as parainfluenza (also in the paramyxovirus genus) coxsackievirus, influenza A, Epstein-Barr, adenovirus, HIV, and cytomegalovirus may present with similar symptoms as mumps. There are also noninfectious etiologies of parotitis, which include salivary stones or tumors, sarcoid, Sjögren's syndrome, and thiazide diuretics.

Therapy (or Treatment)

Treatment for mumps virus is largely supportive. For complicated cases of pancreatitis, meningitis, encephalitis, and orchitis, patient may need to be hospitalized for additional care. The additional care usually includes fever reduction, analgesia, fluid resuscitation, and treatment of secondary bacterial infections.

Monitoring

For persons with active mumps, it is suggested that they be isolated from school or work for 5 days after the onset of symptoms. Shedding of virus usually occurs 4 days prior to the onset of symptoms. For this reason, it is difficult to slow down outbreaks of the disease. The last outbreak in the United States was in 2010.

Complications

Complications from mumps are rare. In children, pancreatitis and hearing loss are the sensorineural complications most often diagnosed. For adolescents and adults the complications are more common and usually more severe. These include aseptic meningitis; orchitis in males, which rarely leads to sterility; oophoritis in females; pancreatitis; and arthritis. Even more uncommon are Guillain–Barré/ascending polyradiculitis, transverse myelitis, facial palsy, interstitial nephritis, and myocardial involvement.

Mumps in pregnancy has been associated with increased fetal loss. There are no known teratogenic effects.

References

American Academy of Pediatrics: Mumps. In Pickering LK, Baker CJ, Kimberlin DW, Long SS, editors: *Red Book: 2009 Report of the committee on Infectious Diseases*, 28th ed, Elk Gove Village IL, 2009, American Academy of Pediatrics, pp 468–472.

Centers for Disease Control and Prevention (CDC): Exposure to mumps during air travel—United States, April 2006, *MMWR Morb Mortal Wkly Rep* 55(401), 2006.

Dayan GH, Rubin S: Mumps outbreaks in vaccinated population: are available mumps vaccines effective enough to prevent an outbreak? *Clin Infect Dis* 47:1458, 2008.

Kleiman MB: Mumps virus. In Lenette EH, editor: *Laboratory Diagnosis of Viral Infections*, ed 2nd, New York, 1992, Marcel Dekker, p. 549.

Kutty PK, Barskey AE, Gallagher KM: *Mumps, Infectious Diseases Related to Travel*, 2012, CDC Yellowbook (chapter 3).

Wharton M, Cochi SLK, William S: Measles, mumps and rubella vaccines, *Infect Dis Clin North Am* 4:47, 1990 www.cdc.gov/travel/yellowbook.

NECROTIZING SKIN AND SOFT-TISSUE INFECTIONS

Method of
Kalyanakrishnan Ramakrishnan, MD

CURRENT DIAGNOSIS

- Physical examination of the affected area may detect:
  - Exquisite pain and tenderness out of proportion to local signs of infection.
  - Cutaneous anesthesia, firm woody subcutaneous tissue, edema, and tenderness extending outside involved skin margins, hemorrhage or bullae of the overlying skin, and soft tissue crepitus.
  - Laboratory Risk Indicator for Necrotizing Fasciitis (LRINEC) score is useful in diagnosing necrotizing fasciitis. Imaging (computed tomography [CT] or magnetic resonance imaging [MRI] in adults; ultrasonography [US] in children) is usually confirmatory. Imaging should not delay surgery if indicated based on suspicion.

CURRENT TREATMENT

- Empiric high-dose intravenous polymicrobial antibiotics and surgical debridement remain the cornerstones of initial management of necrotizing skin and soft-tissue infections. Organism-specific antibiotics continued until resolution of infection and debridement complete (usually 7–14 days).

Epidemiology

Necrotizing skin and soft tissue infections are rare with an estimated annual incidence of 1000 cases in the United States. These infections may be polymicrobial or monomicrobial. Polymicrobial infections are more common (70%–80%) and generally caused by synergistic activity of aerobes and anaerobes originating from the bowel or genitourinary tracts. They are more prevalent among older and immunocompromised patients, individuals with significant comorbidities, and those with underlying abdominal pathology. These infections typically involve the trunk and perineal regions, and follow penetrating abdominal injuries or surgery,

genital or perianal sepsis, or decubitus ulcers. They have a more indolent course and thus are easier to diagnose. Monomicrobial infections (20%–30%) frequently follow minor trauma and are usually caused by group A streptococcus (GAS), occasionally with methicillin-resistant *Staphylococcus aureus* (MRSA), or by clostridia. They are more aggressive, involve the extremities and occur more often in younger healthy individuals. Type 3 infections follow exposure to contaminated fresh or warm seawater or ingestion of raw seafood; organisms responsible include *Aeromonas hydrophila*, *Vibrio vulnificus*, *Mycobacterium marinum*, *Pasteurella multocida*, *Haemophilus* and *Klebsiella* species. Type 4 (fungal) infections generally follow burns or major trauma. Both types 3 and 4 infections are rare, progress rapidly, and have a high mortality rate, especially in immune-suppressed patients.

Risk Factors

Cardiopulmonary disease, debility, diabetes mellitus, hepatorenal disease, immunocompromised states, obesity, arteriovenous/lymphatic insufficiency, and senescence all increase risk of skin and soft tissue infections by reducing tissue vascularity and oxygenation, increasing fluid stasis and risk of trauma, and decreasing ability to counter infections. Diabetes mellitus and hepatic cirrhosis favor polymicrobial infections due to staphylococcus and streptococcus species, anerobes, and gram-negative bacilli. Neutropenia, intravenous drug use, and hot tub exposure promote pseudomonas infection. Human and animal bites cause infections with oral flora, staphylococci, *Pasteurella multocida*, and anerobes. Poor sanitation and soil contamination propagate clostridial infections. Postoperative infections typically follow wound contamination with microorganisms from the patient during surgery.

Pathophysiology

Necrotizing skin and soft tissue infections advance rapidly, breaking down and traversing anatomic barriers, initiating extensive destruction of the subcutaneous tissue, fascia, and muscle and damaging the neurovascular bundle, thrombosing the subcutaneous vessels, and causing overlying skin necrosis. Most infections follow a rift in the protective cutaneous barrier due to trauma or increased tissue tension. Necrotizing fasciitis may also result from blunt injuries (bruise, muscle strain) and, occasionally vascular or lymphatic spread from a distant focus of infection. Various toxins expressed by the organisms (GAS and clostridia) display local and systemic effects (platelet aggregation and thrombosis, decreasing phagocytosis, neutrophil function and vascular tone, myocardial inhibition) triggering the systemic inflammatory response syndrome (SIRS) and multiple organ failure.

Prevention

Preserving cutaneous integrity prevents infection. Abrasions and lacerations should be washed with antibacterial solutions, foreign bodies should be removed, and dead/devitalized tissue excised to minimize infection risk. Preoperative skin cleansing with chlorhexidine/alcohol (Hibiclens) or povidone iodine diminishes rates of superficial and deep incisional infections. Intranasal 2% mupirocin ointment (Bactroban) twice daily with chlorhexidine total body wash daily for 5 days in nasal carriers of staphylococcus reduces hospital-acquired deep surgical–site infections, as does administering antibiotics (aminopenicillins, a second- or third-generation cephalosporin) 60 minutes before incision, sterile surgical technique, minimal tissue handling, and minimally invasive surgery.

Clinical Manifestations

Features of inflammation (redness, warmth, swelling, pain) and loss of function characterize necrotizing skin and soft tissue infections. Altered mental status, anorexia, diaphoresis, fatigue, fever, hypotension, nausea, and tachycardia suggest systemic spread. The extremities, trunk, or anogenital regions are usually involved. Induration denotes cutaneous involvement. Patients with necrotizing fasciitis have severe pain disproportionate to the physical findings and rapid progression of infection. Examination reveals cutaneous anesthesia, firm and woody subcutaneous tissue, edema and tenderness extending beyond involved skin, hemorrhage or bullae of the overlying skin, and crepitus (indicates soft tissue gas; seen especially with gas-forming organisms such as clostridia). Tense edema and bullae have high specificity and positive predictive value for necrotizing fasciitis. Fournier gangrene is a form of polymicrobial necrotizing soft-tissue infection involving the loose groin and genital skin, where subcutaneous vessel thrombosis causes extensive tissue loss.

Diagnosis

Diagnosis is based on a strong clinical suspicion followed by confirmatory laboratory and imaging studies (if time permits), and surgery. Leukocytosis with a marked left shift, elevated C-reactive protein, elevated serum creatinine and creatine phosphokinase (denotes muscle injury), and low serum bicarbonate (suggests acidosis) signify severe infection. The LRINEC score uses six different laboratory parameters (hemoglobin, white blood cell count, C-reactive protein, glucose, creatinine, sodium) to predict risk of necrotizing fasciitis (score ≥ 6 suggestive, ≥ 8 strongly predictive). White blood cell count (< 15,000 mm³) and serum sodium (> 135 mmol/L) levels alone are useful in ruling out necrotizing fasciitis (99% negative predictive value). Gram stains and cultures of aspirates or tissue biopsies, and blood cultures are valuable for detecting the infecting organisms and systemic spread; contamination may yield false-positive results. Biopsy or debridement typically demonstrates swollen gray soft tissue with undermining of the overlying skin, a brownish and odorous exudate and non-contractile muscle. Imaging (plain x-rays, ultrasonography [US], computed tomography [CT], magnetic resonance imaging [MRI]) may show edema or thickening, fluid collections or free air in the soft tissues. US, CT and MRI are highly sensitive (MRI highest) in detecting deep soft tissue involvement characteristic of necrotizing fasciitis; specificity is lower. US is sufficient in children, whose tissues are thin enough to allow adequate evaluation on imaging. Imaging should not delay debridement, if considered necessary.

Therapy

Patients with necrotizing skin and soft-tissue infections typically require in-hospital management, because many have underlying unstable comorbid illnesses, systemic sepsis, severe dehydration and acidosis, muscle breakdown, and organ dysfunction. Initial resuscitation may require airway and oxygen support, large-volume rehydration, and invasive monitoring. High-dose intravenous (IV) broad-spectrum antibiotics effective against the usually infecting polymicrobial spectrum of pathogens are commenced, followed by early and aggressive debridement of all necrotic tissue. IV antibiotics are maintained until the patient is afebrile for 48 to 72 hours and tolerates oral intake, debridement is completed and culture results are available. For polymicrobial necrotizing fasciitis acceptable antimicrobial choices include vancomycin plus piperacillin/tazobactam (Zosyn), a carbapenem (meropenem [Merrem], ertapenem [Invanz] or imipenem-cilastatin [Primaxin]), or cefotaxime (Claforan) with metronidazole (Flagyl) or clindamycin (Cleocin). Streptococcal and clostridial infections are treated with penicillin G and clindamycin. Antibiotic options in methicillin-susceptible S. aureus infections include nafcillin oxacillin or cefazolin. Options for methicillin-resistant S. aureus (MRSA) infections and in penicillin-allergic patients include vancomycin, daptomycin (Cubicin), or linezolid (Zyvox). Antibiotic doses are modified in children. Recommended duration is 7 to 14 days; longer as needed. Doxycycline combined with ciprofloxacin (Cipro) treats Vibria vulnificus infection. Ceftriaxone (Rocephin) or cefotaxime combined with doxycycline is useful in aeromonos infections. Doxycycline is contraindicated in children (< 8 years), as is ciprofloxacin (< 17 years), unless the infection is considered life-threatening. Fungal infections respond well to fluconazole (Diflucan), voriconazole (Vfend) or amphotericin B; the antifungals usually continued for 2 weeks after resolution of symptoms. Debridement/drainage is repeated until all diseased tissue or collections are eliminated and healing begins. Wound vacuum dressings help remove drainage and encourage formation of healing granulation tissue. The tissue defect heals by secondary intention or may require skin grafting or flap closure. Hyperbaric oxygen (3–4 daily treatments at 2–3 atmosphere pressure for 30–90 minutes each) is useful, especially in clostridium-related synergistic infections. Adding intravenous immunoglobulin[1] 0.5–2 g/kg daily for 3 days has shown some success, and is an option in critically ill hemodynamically unstable patients not responding to conventional measures, especially in those with streptococcal toxic shock syndrome. Fournier gangrene is managed along the same principles as above.

Monitoring

Patients in shock or with acute respiratory distress syndrome, SIRS, or multi-organ failure are best managed in an intensive care unit and often require invasive monitoring, cardiorespiratory and renal support, and occasionally, endotracheal intubation.

Complications

Significant disfigurement, limb loss, respiratory and renal failure, and mortality (14%–50%) may eventuate despite timely and appropriate treatment; the mortality influenced by age, extent of infection, degree of biochemical/acid-base imbalance, presence of comorbidities, and treatment delay.

---

[1] Not FDA approved for this indication.

References

Kaafarani HMA, King DR: Necrotizing skin and soft tissue infections, Surg Clin North Am 94:155–163, 2014.
Hakkarainen TW, Kopari NM, Pham TN, Evans HL: Necrotizing soft tissue infections: review and current concepts in treatment, systems of care and outcomes, Curr Probl Surg 51:344–362, 2014.
Morgan MS: Diagnosis and management of necrotizing fasciitis: a multiparametric approach, J Hosp Infect 75:249–257, 2010.
Stevens DL, Bisno AL, Chambers HF, et al: Practice guidelines for the diagnosis and management of skin and soft tissue infections: 2014 update by the Infectious Diseases Society of America, Clin Infect Dis 59:e10–e52, 2014.
Ramakrishnan K, Salinas RC, Agudelo Higuita NI: Skin and soft tissue infections, Am Fam Physician 92:474–483, 2015.

OSTEOMYELITIS

Method of
George D. Harris, MD, MS

CURRENT DIAGNOSIS (FIGURE 1)

- A bone biopsy remains the gold standard when diagnosing osteomyelitis.
- All patients should have blood cultures performed.
- No one imaging modality is routinely recommended to diagnose osteomyelitis.
- Plain film radiography should always be the initial study and can be diagnostic if positive.
- Magnetic resonance imaging (MRI) can detect acute osteomyelitis as early as 3 days.

CURRENT THERAPY

- The most important factor in any treatment is identification of the organism.
- The optimal duration of antibiotic therapy remains undefined, with most authorities recommending treatment for about 6 weeks.
- Hematogenous osteomyelitis is usually monomicrobial, whereas contiguous infections are usually polymicrobial.

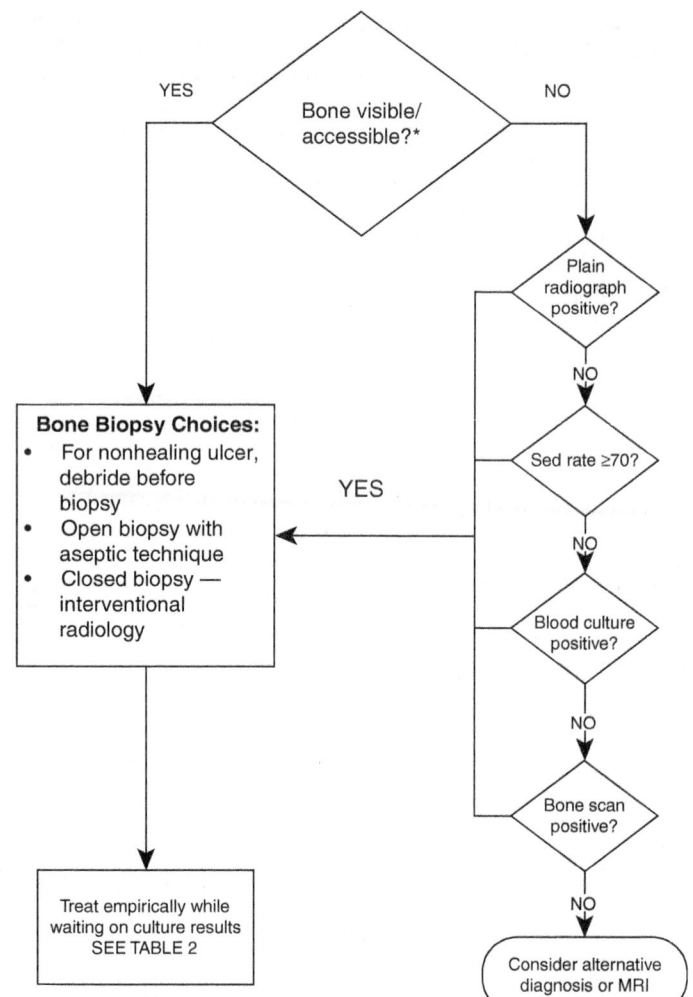

* Some advocate doing plain radiograph, CBC, sed rate, and blood cultures as part of the initial evaluation of osteomyelitis

Figure 1 Algorithm for treatment of suspected osteomyelitis. (Courtesy Edward T. Bope.)

TABLE 1	Cierny-Mader Classification System	
FEATURE	**EXAMPLES**	
Anatomic type	Stage 1: Medullary osteomyelitis	
	Stage 2: Superficial osteomyelitis	
	Stage 3: Localized osteomyelitis	
	Stage 4: Diffuse osteomyelitis	
Physiologic class	A: Normal (healthy) host	
	B: Compromised host	
	B_S: Systemically compromised	
	B_L: Locally compromised	
	C: Treatment worse than disease	
Factors affecting host status		
Systemic	Malnutrition	
	Renal and hepatic failure	
	Diabetes mellitus	
	Chronic hypoxia	
	Immune disease	
	Malignancy	
	Extremes of age	
	Immunosuppression	
Local	Chronic lymphedema	
	Venous stasis	
	Major vessel compromise	
	Arteritis	
	Extensive scarring	
	Radiation fibrosis	
	Small-vessel disease	
	Neuropathy	
	Tobacco use	

Osteomyelitis is an inflammation of the bone as a result of a bacterial infection, resulting in acute or chronic inflammation caused mainly by a bacterial infection. It can primarily occur by hematogenous spread, contiguous spread to the bone from adjacent tissues, or direct inoculation usually from trauma or surgery. Patients usually complain of pain, swelling, and tenderness over the affected area of bone.

Osteomyelitis has changed over the years from a primarily hematogenous disease with high mortality to one of high morbidity as a result of infection from contiguous or direct inoculation, especially in those with diabetes mellitus and/or peripheral vascular disease.

Contiguous or local extension may occur from spread from adjacent structures or direct implantation of organisms as seen in cases of trauma, placement of internal fixation devices for fracture repair, or other surgical procedures. Direct inoculation osteomyelitis tends to involve multiple organisms and results in more clinical localized manifestations than infections from hematogenous spread, where the osteomyelitis is usually monomicrobial. Hematogenous osteomyelitis most commonly involves the vertebrae, with the lumbar spine most commonly affected, and is also more common in infants and children, involving metaphysis of their long bones.

There are several methods used to classify osteomyelitis, separating the illness into acute or chronic types; into hematogenous or contiguous types; and according to the mode of transmission—local extension from adjacent structures or direct implantation of organisms as seen in cases of trauma or surgical procedures.

The Cierny-Mader system assigns the patient to one of several groups based on the anatomy of the infection and health of the host, risk factors such as patients with peripheral arterial obstructive disease or diabetes mellitus and tobacco use. Patients are further stratified according to systemic and local factors that may influence disease progression or healing, such as diabetes and the extremes of age. In patients with diabetes, osteomyelitis is most commonly caused by overlying lower limb cellulitis. In the nondiabetic adult patient, vertebral osteomyelitis is most common.

The Cierny-Mader classification allows the clinician to use tested treatment protocols, including chemotherapy, surgery, and adjunctive therapies, that are most effective for a specific class of disease and for the host status. The Cierny-Mader system divides the patients into four anatomic groups. Stage 1, or medullary osteomyelitis, is confined to the endosteum of the bone and is often hematogenous. State 2, or superficial osteomyelitis, is localized to the surface of the bone. This is a true contiguous lesion. Stage 3, or localized osteomyelitis, involves cortical sequestration or cavitation, or both, and is a full-thickness lesion that extends into the medullary region. Stage 4, or diffuse osteomyelitis, involves the hard and soft tissues ("through and through"), and it requires surgical debridement of the affected bone to remove all the infected tissue.

For treatment to be successful, the patient must be physiologically able to heal any wounds, defend against contamination or infection, and tolerate the stress of treatment. The hosts are classified as A, B, or C, depending on the ability to resist infections. Those with good immunity are classified as an A host, whereas a B host is compromised locally (B_L) or systemically (B_S); Table 1 shows the physiologic classifications. The final class assigns a C rating to patients whose treatment is more detrimental than the disability from the disease. These patients may require suppressive or no treatment. The clinical stages are adjusted during the course of therapy as conditions change, allowing adjustment of the treatment protocol to optimize therapy.

A much simpler system described by Waldvogel classifies the patient by duration (i.e., acute or chronic) and the mechanism of inoculation (i.e., hematogenous or contiguous). Contiguous infections are further classified as those with or without vascular insufficiency. However, this classification does not provide guidance for specific surgical or antibiotic therapy.

Epidemiology

Acute hematogenous osteomyelitis is usually seen in male children of lower socioeconomic class before the age of 2 years or between 8 and 12 years. There may be some genetic influences. Aboriginal children in Western Australia are known to suffer from acute hematogenous osteomyelitis at a rate nearly four times that of Western European children living in the same neighborhood. An acute infection will progress to chronic osteomyelitis if it is not treated.

Chronic osteomyelitis is usually the result of direct inoculation (e.g., trauma, surgery). Its epidemiology is less clearly described, except in diabetic foot infections.

Kremers et al., in a population-based study, described trends in the incidence of osteomyelitis over a four-decade period from 1969 to 2009. The study demonstrated that the incidence of osteomyelitis has increased over time and is generally higher in males than in females, and that the incidence rates remained relatively stable among children and young adults (< 50 years old). However, the incidence has almost tripled among the elderly, driven significantly by an increase in diabetes-related cases.

Because chronic infection can persist for life, it is important to have early identification and treatment to ensure the best possible outcome.

Pathogenesis

The presence of bacteria in an open wound is not sufficient to cause infection. It is the compromised blood supply of traumatized tissue leading to necrosis and subsequent bacterial adherence that promotes the infection. Trauma can delay the inflammatory response to bacteria, depress cell-mediated immunity, and impair chemotaxis, superoxide production, and the microbial killing capacity of polymorphonuclear neutrophils (PMNs). Osteomyelitis usually involves the metaphysis, which is well vascularized and has significant bone growth.

In acute osteomyelitis, signs or symptoms are usually abrupt. Local infection is characterized by edema, vascular congestion, and small-vessel thrombosis. This leads to increased pressure within the intramedullary canal, allowing extravasation through the Havers and Volkmann canals to the periosteum. In children, the periosteum is usually more flexible and easier to detect radiographically; in adults, the bone matrix is more firmly attached to the periosteum. Untreated, the suppurative infection can reach adjacent soft tissue, leading to a cellulitis. The presence of a Brodie or intraosseous abscess without extravasation into surrounding tissue is classified as subacute pyogenic osteomyelitis. The resulting infection can lead to sequestration involving large areas of bone destruction and dead bone, with reactive bone formation leading ultimately to chronic osteomyelitis.

Chronic osteomyelitis is usually polymicrobial and is characterized by the presence of necrotic bone, new bone growth, and exudation of polymorphonuclear leukocytes, plasma cells, and other infection-fighting cells. The involucrum (i.e., layer of reactive competent bone that covers dead bone) is often dotted with tracts that allow pus to pass into surrounding tissue or to form a sinus tract to the skin surface. These sinus tracts are often contaminated with numerous organisms that do not reflect those found with direct sampling. This repetitive process of bone loss and growth and the involucrum explains why chronic osteomyelitis is difficult to eradicate with antibiotics alone. The antibiotics cannot penetrate avascular areas.

Etiology
Children

In children of all ages, the most common bacterial pathogen is *Staphylococcus aureus*, followed by *Streptococcus pneumoniae* and *Kingella kingae*. However, age and chronic illness allow other organisms to flourish; *Salmonella* and pneumococcal disease (*S. pneumoniae*) are common in patients with sickle cell disease. *Pasteurella multocida*, *Streptococcus* species, and anaerobes often are identified after animal or human bites. In children, most cases arise hematogenously and are characteristically seen in the metaphysis of long bones (i.e., femur, tibia, and humerus), accounting for 68% of childhood infections.

The exact mechanism is unclear, but it is thought that the extensive branching of the nutrient-rich arteries at the metaphyses of the long bones leads to sluggish blood flow and ultimate bacterial seeding. Possible routes include the formation of small hematomas in the metaphysis, allowing microbial seeding after transient bacteremia; penetrating injuries or surgical manipulation, causing direct inoculation of bacteria into bone; and local invasion from a contiguous focus of infection.

Adults

Most infections in adults arise by direct inoculation from sources such as trauma, prosthetic joints, open fractures, and diabetic foot infections. The most common organisms remain *Staphylococcus aureus*, coagulase-negative staphylococci, and aerobic gram-negative bacilli.

Other organisms to consider include streptococci, enterococci, *Pseudomonas aeruginosa*, *Escherichia coli*, and *Serratia marcescens*. Most contiguous, related infections are polymicrobial.

Clinical Manifestations

The severity of the signs and symptoms depends on the location of the infection, the patient's age, and any comorbidities. Patients may experience many, few, or no symptoms. Classically, acute osteomyelitis presents with marked pain, erythema, tenderness, and swelling. Fever and leukocytosis are also common.

The probe-to-bone test with a sterile blunt metal tool should be included in the initial assessment of all patients with diabetes with infected pedal ulcers. The probe-to-bone test may be used in the emergency department, the inpatient hospital setting, or the outpatient primary care clinic as a screening test to assess for diabetic foot osteomyelitis. A positive result consists of detection of a hard, gritty surface through the ulcerated skin surface.

The probe-to-bone test along with other diagnostic tests (such as radiographic imaging or bone biopsy) can assist in the therapeutic decision-making process.

Vertebral osteomyelitis can occur either by hematogenous spread, direct inoculation from trauma or spinal surgery, or contiguous spread from adjacent soft tissue infection. Over 50% of cases are due to *S. aureus*. The most common presentation is back or neck pain, with or without fever, with noted local tenderness to percussion over the involved posterior spinous processes.

Vertebral osteomyelitis often causes severe pain, fever, and disability, whereas osteomyelitis of the foot rarely causes pain. An epidural abscess causes pain and neurologic deficits, whereas vertebral osteomyelitis without abscess formation has no neurologic deficits.

Children often present with systemic symptoms (e.g., fever, weight loss, pain). Pseudoparalysis may be the only sign in a newborn, but toddlers often exhibit pain, fever, erythema, edema, or warmth, or they may suddenly stop walking. In contrast, patients with chronic osteomyelitis may exhibit localized signs and symptoms, including nonhealing ulcers, purulence from sinus tracts, soft tissue edema and pain, abscesses, erythema, pain, and fatigue. Generalized signs and symptoms may be seen early in the disease, but they are unlikely in the later or chronic stages.

Leukocytosis is less common with chronic osteomyelitis, but there is usually an elevated erythrocyte sedimentation rate and C-reactive protein.

Blood cultures are most likely positive with hematogenous infection and with vertebral osteomyelitis.

Magnetic resonance imaging (MRI) is the most sensitive radiographic technique, but the infection is confirmed by biopsy of the infected intervertebral disc space or vertebral bone. The antimicrobial therapy should be withheld until a microbiologic diagnosis is confirmed unless there is neurologic compromise and/or sepsis present; in patients with negative culture results, empiric treatment is warranted based on the most likely organisms to cause infection. Treatment is usually for a minimum duration of 6 weeks, but the duration should be based on the individual patient's circumstances. In 2015, the Infectious Diseases Society of America (IDSA) issued new guidelines on vertebral osteomyelitis, and these should be used for treatment and management.

Diagnosis
Laboratory Tests
A bone biopsy remains the gold standard when diagnosing osteomyelitis. However, there is a high false-negative rate, and the negative predictive value is close to 65%, mainly owing to the organism's patchy distribution. No specific laboratory test can be recommended. However, if osteomyelitis is suspected based on clinical history and physical findings, plain radiographs of the involved site should be ordered along with laboratory testing (acute-phase reactants, e.g., erythrocyte sedimentation rate [ESR], C-reactive protein [CRP], leukocyte count with a differential count). These labs can strongly suggest (positive predictive value of 100%) osteomyelitis if the ESR value is greater than 70 mm/h in the absence of an inflamed ulcer. However, these tests lack specificity, and it may take several days to demonstrate significantly elevated levels. Bone biopsy (open being preferred over a percutaneous approach) should be performed for pathogen identification and in cases when the diagnosis of osteomyelitis is uncertain but suspected. All patients should have blood cultures performed. A positive blood culture with a suspicious physical finding can suggest a bone infection, but only one half of the cases have a positive test result. Blood cultures, like bone biopsies, can be affected by recent antibiotic exposure. However, patients receiving antibiotics prior to the bone biopsy still may have a reasonable microbiologic yield, because areas of infection also have associated bony infarction or ischemia.

Radiology
There is no one imaging modality routinely recommended to diagnose osteomyelitis, so diagnosis often requires more than one technique. Plain film radiography should always be the initial study, and the result can be diagnostic if positive. However, changes (usually along the metaphysis) typically require at least 1 to 2 weeks to be seen radiographically.

Positron emission tomography (PET) is the most specific and sensitive of imaging techniques, but its high cost and lack of availability make it impractical for most clinicians. The best choice for imaging depends on the age of the patient, duration of symptoms, suspected location of infection (if known), and concurrent or previous medical conditions.

Plain radiographs are the most available, least expensive, and easiest to obtain, but they lack sensitivity (43%–75%), and a negative result does not exclude the diagnosis. However, they have reasonable specificity (75%–83%), and a positive finding can confirm the diagnosis or provide clues to alternative pathology, such as a tumor. Bony changes can take between 10 and 21 days to become visible on plain films; however, soft tissue changes can be seen in as little as 3 days. The soft tissue changes are especially important in neonates and children because focal soft tissue swelling around the bony metaphysis may be the first sign of bone involvement.

Radionuclide imaging (i.e., triple-phase bone scan, leukocyte scintigraphy, and PET) is a preferred method of advanced imaging, and it has several advantages compared with other techniques. Young children often complete the examination without sedation, and prosthetic joints do not produce the artifact commonly seen

on MRI and computed tomography (CT) scans. Positive results can be seen 24 to 48 hours after onset of symptoms, and a negative examination result effectively rules out osteomyelitis.

The triple-phase bone scan (technetium 99 m diphosphonate) is often the examination of choice (sensitivity of 73%–100%), and it can distinguish between cellulitis and osteomyelitis when complications are absent. However, the sensitivity decreases dramatically when other conditions are present (i.e., trauma, diabetes, or recent surgery), and it has been reported to be as low as 38%. Bone scans usually lack the specificity (25%–90%) of other modalities, fail to provide detailed pictures of complex anatomy, and can be influenced by poor circulation. The examination may take up to 24 hours to complete and often requires the patient to make many trips to the facility. In the early phase, uptake is greatest in areas of acute inflammation. In the next phase, uptake occurs in areas of soft tissue inflammation, and in the late (delayed) phase, uptake remains in the presence of osteomyelitis.

Leukocyte scintigraphy using gallium 67 has a higher specificity (80%–90%) than triple-phase scanning (67%) in the peripheral skeleton, but it decreases to 25% when looking at the axial skeleton. Leukocyte scintigraphy is the preferred method when evaluating patients with previous joint replacements, diabetes, or trauma.

MRI can detect acute osteomyelitis as early as 3 days. It is nearly as sensitive (82%–100%) and specific (75%–96%) as radionuclide studies. MRI allows tracking of disease progress and response to treatment. MRI can be used to date osteomyelitis. Some patients with osteomyelitis are treated and later develop another episode. The MRI can distinguish whether the second episode is a new infection or a recurrence of the previous infection. It also provides detailed visualization of complex anatomy and critical structures, allowing surgeons to map any planned surgical intervention.

CT is rarely used for osteomyelitis, except when sequestered bone is suspected or for interventional procedures. Sinography can be used to map sinus tracts with fluoroscopy or combined with CT. Ultrasound is sometimes used in children and can be helpful in differentiating acute from chronic infections. It provides guidance during drainage, aspirations, or biopsies of the affected bone, and it is a noninvasive method to monitor soft tissue involvement in chronic illness.

Treatment
The Cierny-Mader classification system provides a straightforward algorithm for treatment. However, surgical debridement of necrotic tissue and proper antimicrobial therapy according to the identification of the causative organism and its susceptibilities remain the most important factors in any treatment.

Antibiotic Therapy
Unlike chronic infections, acute infections require hospitalization for initiation of therapy and supportive care. Serial examinations should be undertaken to assess the success of treatment and monitor for systemic signs or symptoms. Cultures of blood and bone should be obtained to guide therapy. Laboratory studies can be followed, but other than CRP levels, they fail to provide significant data. The CRP value can be expected to decrease 24 to 48 hours after initiation of appropriate antibiotic therapy. A lack of response may indicate inappropriate therapy or an occult abscess, and the physician should reconsider surgery if previously delayed.

The medical literature remains inconclusive about the antibiotic treatment of osteomyelitis, especially when trying to determine the best agents, route, or duration of antibiotic therapy.

Initial treatment should cover for methicillin-resistant (MRSA) and methicillin-sensitive S. aureus (MSSA) until cultures are completed with susceptibilities.

Although the optimal duration of antibiotic therapy remains undefined, most authorities recommend treatment for usually at least 6 weeks (Table 2). After the infection is under control, the physician may switch the patient to an oral antibiotic for 3 to 12 months (i.e., a fluoroquinolone with or without rifampin

TABLE 2	Antibiotics for Osteomyelitis	
ORGANISM	**PREFERRED DRUG**	**ALTERNATIVE DRUGS**
Methicillin-sensitive Staphylococcus aureus	Nafcillin (Unipen) 2 g IV or IM q4h	Cefazolin, oxacillin, vancomycin, clindamycin, Trimethoprim-sulfamethoxazole (Bactrim)* 4 mg/kg of the <u>trimethoprim</u> component twice daily) with rifampin (Rifadin) 600 mg once daily.*
Methicillin-resistant *S. aureus*	Vancomycin (Vancocin) 30 to 40 mg/kg IV every 24 hours in two or three divided doses; not to exceed 2 g/dose	Trimethoprim-sulfamethoxazole (Bactrim)* 4 mg/kg of the <u>trimethoprim</u> component twice daily) with rifampin (Rifadin) 600 mg once daily.*
Streptococcus pneumoniae, group A β-hemolytic streptococci	Penicillin G (Pfizerpen)* 2 million units IV q4h	Cefazolin, vancomycin, clindamycin
Enterococci, *Haemophilus influenzae* β-lactamase negative	Cefotaxime (Claforan) 2 g q6h	Trimethoprim-sulfamethoxazole, ceftriaxone
H. influenzae β-lactamase positive, *Klebsiella pneumoniae*	Ceftriaxone (Rocephin) 2 g q24h	Trimethoprim-sulfamethoxazole, ciprofloxacin, piperacillin (Pipracil), imipenem (Primaxin)
Escherichia coli	Cefazolin (Ancef) 2 g q8h	Ciprofloxacin, ceftriaxone, imipenem
Pseudomonas aeruginosa	Ciprofloxacin (Cipro) 400 mg q8h[3]	Piperacillin plus aminoglycoside, aztreonam (Azactam)*
Salmonella	Choose ampicillin, ceftriaxone, imipenem (Primaxin), or ciprofloxacin, depending on sensitivities	
Bacteroides spp.	Clindamycin (Cleocin) 600 mg q6h	Imipenem, metronidazole (Flagyl)
Serratia marcescens	Ceftriaxone (Rocephin) 2 g q24h	Imipenem, trimethoprim-sulfamethoxazole, ciprofloxacin

*Not FDA approved for this indication.
[3]Exceeds dosage recommended by the manufacturer.
(Modified from Cohen J, Powderly WG, editors. *Infectious Diseases.* 2nd ed. St. Louis: Mosby; 2003.)

[Rifadin][1]). However, treatment can be as short as 3 weeks for uncomplicated, acute, hematogenous osteomyelitis. Management can include oral preparations after a short parenteral course, provided the drug has high bioavailability and the organism is susceptible. A microbiologic diagnosis (preferably by bone biopsy) is essential so that the choice of antibiotic accounts for the specific organism, the host status, and the least toxic medication for the individual. Hematogenous osteomyelitis is usually monomicrobial, whereas contiguous infections are usually polymicrobial and may include *Pseudomonas* in certain populations. For this population, fluoroquinolones are an excellent choice.

For MSSA, nafcillin (Unipen) or a first- or second-generation cephalosporin, cefazolin, can be implemented. For MRSA, vancomycin (Vancocin) is recommended. For an anaerobic infection, clindamycin (Cleocin) is a good choice.

Surgery

Bones can heal in the presence of active infection. However, in the presence of obvious signs of infection, such as an abscess or Cierny-Mader stage 3 or 4 disease, acute surgical debridement and irrigation are warranted. The goals of surgery include drainage, debridement, and stabilization. After successful debridement and stabilization, antibiotic therapy is initiated and continued until adequate healing has occurred, usually in 6 weeks. If debridement is unsuccessful, inert substances must be completely removed and tissue debrided. Antibiotics should be placed in contact with the bone using a polymethylmethacrylate antibiotic (PMMA) bead chain or other biodegradable delivery system to achieve higher local antibiotic concentrations. The site needs to be stabilized with an external fixator, and staged reconstruction should be initiated.

References

Berbari EF, Kanj SS, Kowalski TJ, et al: Executive summary: 2015 Infectious Diseases Society of America (IDSA) clinical practice guidelines for the diagnosis and treatment of native vertebral osteomyelitis in adults, *Clin Infect Dis* 61:859–863, 2015.

[1]Not FDA approved for this indication.

Berendt A, Norden C: Acute and chronic osteomyelitis. In Cohen J, Powderly WG, editors: *Infectious Diseases*, 2nd ed., St. Louis, Mosby; 2003.
Cierny 3rd G, Mader JT, Penninck JJ: A clinical staging system for adult osteomyelitis, *Clin Orthop Relat Res.* 414:7–24, 2003.
Kaplan S: Osteomyelitis in children, *Infect Dis Clin N Am.* 19:787–797, 2005.
Kremers HM, Nwojo ME, Ransom JE, et al: Trends in the epidemiology of osteomyelitis: a population-based study, 1969 to 2009, *J Bone Joint Surg Am.* 97:837–845, 2015.
Krogstad P: Osteomyelitis and septic arthritis. In Feigin RD, Cherry JD, Demmler GJ, et al, editors: *Textbook of Pediatric Infectious Diseases*, 5th ed, Philadelphia, Saunders; 2004.
Lam K, van Asten SA, Nguyen T, et al: Diagnostic accuracy of probe to bone to detect osteomyelitis in the diabetic foot: a systematic review, *Clin Infect Dis.* 63(7):944–948, 2016.
Lampe RM: Osteomyelitis. In Behrman RE, Kliegman RM, Jenson HB, Stanton BF, editors: *Nelson Textbook of Pediatrics*, 18th ed., Philadelphia, Saunders; 2007.
Lazzarini L, Lipsky BA, Mader JT: Antibiotic treatment of osteomyelitis: what have we learned from 30 years of clinical trials? *Int J Infect Dis.* 9:127–138, 2005.
Lipsky B, Weigelt J, Gupta V, et al: Skin, soft tissue, bone, and joint infections in hospitalized patients: epidemiology and microbiological, clinical, and economic outcomes, *Infect Control Hosp Epidemiol.* 28:1290–1298, 2007.
Pineda C, Vargas A, Vargas-Rodríguez A: Imaging of osteomyelitis: current concepts, *Infect Dis Clin North Am.* 20:789–825, 2006.
Ziran BH: Osteomyelitis, *J Trauma* 62(Suppl. 6):S59–S60, 2007.

PLAGUE

Method of
Nelson Iván Agudelo Higuita, MD; and Douglas A. Drevets, MD

CURRENT DIAGNOSIS

- Plague should be suspected when a person develops abrupt onset of fever, lymphadenopathy, or sepsis and there is history of a flea bite or possible exposure to an infected animal or person.
- *Yersinia pestis* is an aerobic gram-negative coccobacilli that exhibits bipolar staining with Giemsa, Wright's, and Wayson stains.
- Automated diagnostic systems may misidentify *Y. pestis* as other organism.

CURRENT THERAPY

- Timely and appropriate management is imperative for a good outcome.
- Despite their toxicities, aminoglycosides are the treatment agents of choice.
- Respiratory droplet precautions should be instituted when pneumonic plague is suspected.
- Postexposure prophylaxis is indicated for close contacts.

Historical descriptions indicate that *Yersinia pestis* probably caused Justinian's Plague (AD 541), which led into the first plague pandemic. The second plague pandemic, also known as the Black Death, began in Central Asia in 1347 and then spread to Europe, Asia, and Africa. It killed an estimated 50 million people. The current (third) plague pandemic began in China and then spread worldwide along shipping routes in 1899–1900. *Y. pestis* is a gram-negative, nonmotile, facultatively anaerobic, non-spore-forming coccobacillus that is approximately 0.5 to 0.8 μm in diameter and 1 to 3 μm in length. Genomic sequencing shows that *Y. pestis* is a recently emerged clone of *Y. pseudotuberculosis*.

Epidemiology

Plague is a zoonosis for which urban and sylvatic rodents (e.g., rats, prairie dogs, and marmots) are the most important enzootic reservoirs. Additionally, domestic cats and dogs have been linked to human disease. Human plague occurs in North and South America, Asia, and Africa. Recent outbreaks reported to the World Health Organization (WHO) have occurred in the Democratic Republic of Congo (2005, 2006), China (2009), and Peru (2010). Plague is endemic in Madagascar, and between 2004 and 2009, 30% of all human cases worldwide were reported from this country. A new epidemic was identified August 1, 2017, and contained November 27, 2017. A total of 2417 cases (77% pneumonic) with a 9% case fatality ratio were reported. From 2000 to 2009, a total of 21,725 cases of plague with a 7.4% fatality rate were reported worldwide. Between 2010 and 2015 another 3248 cases of plague were reported to the WHO. In North America, most human cases occur in New Mexico, Arizona, California, Colorado, and Texas. Between 1900 and 2012, 1006 confirmed or probable cases have occurred in the U.S. with over 80% of these attributable to bubonic plague.

Modes of Transmission

Most human infections are transmitted from rodent to humans via the bite of an infected flea. Infection also can be acquired by contact with body fluids from infected animals, such as during field dressing of game or by inhalation of respiratory droplets from animals, particularly cats, or humans with pneumonic plague.

Bioterrorism Threat

Plague was used as an agent of biowarfare by the Japanese in World War II and was a focus of intensive research and development in the former Soviet Union during the Cold War. Primary pneumonic plague is the most likely form of exposure because of biowarfare or bioterrorism. Recent increases in terrorism worldwide have increased the focus of public health management groups to develop comprehensive statements regarding plague as a biological weapon.

Pathogenesis and Clinical Syndromes

Transdermal inoculation of bacilli from the bite of an infected flea ultimately leads to infection of the regional lymph nodes in which massive replication of bacteria creates the bubo (derived from the Greek *bubon* or "groin"), a swollen, erythematous, and painful lymph node in the groin, axilla, or cervical region.

Bacteremia and septicemia frequently develop and lead to secondary infection of other organs including the lungs, spleen, and central nervous system. Primary pneumonic plague is a rare natural occurrence and results from the inhalation of respiratory droplets containing *Y. pestis* bacilli from another case of pneumonic plague, usually in humans or in cats. Although plague in dogs is rare, human outbreaks have been traced to sick dogs with wildlife exposure. Secondary pneumonic plague results from seeding of the lungs by blood-borne bacteria in the setting of either bubonic or septicemic plague. Septicemic plague also begins with transdermal exposure but manifests as primary bacteremia/septicemia without the bubo. Less common manifestations include meningitis, pharyngitis, and gastroenteritis.

Bubonic plague is an acute febrile lymphadenitis that develops 2 to 8 days after inoculation. Inflamed lymph nodes are usually 1 to 6 cm in diameter and painful. Abrupt onset of fever is an almost universal finding and occurs simultaneously with, or up to 24 hours before, the appearance of the bubo. Headache, malaise, and chills are frequent, along with nausea, vomiting, and diarrhea. Most patients are tachycardic, hypotensive, and appear prostrate and lethargic with episodic restlessness. Leukocytosis with a left shift is typical. Complications include pneumonia, shock, disseminated intravascular coagulation, purpuric skin lesions, acral cyanosis, and gangrene. The differential diagnosis of bubonic plague includes tularemia and Group A β-hemolytic streptococcal adenitis with bacteremia.

Symptoms of septicemic plague are similar to those caused by other gram-negative bacteria, and are very similar to those of bubonic plague except that abdominal pain is more common in septicemic plague. Septicemic plague must be differentiated from fulminating septicemia caused by other gram-negative bacteria. Primary pneumonic plague has an abrupt onset of fever and influenza-like symptoms 1 to 5 days after inhalation exposure. Symptoms include shortness of breath, cough, chest pain, and bloody sputum with rapid progression to fulminating pneumonia and respiratory failure. Patients with secondary pneumonic infection show respiratory symptoms in addition to those attributed to the bubo or sepsis. Radiographic findings include patchy bronchopneumonia, multilobar consolidations, cavitations, and alveolar hemorrhage and are not pathognomonic of *Y. pestis*. Plague pneumonia must be differentiated from severe influenza, inhalation anthrax, and overwhelming community-acquired pneumonia.

Diagnosis

Plague is diagnosed by demonstrating *Y. pestis* in blood or body fluids such as a lymph node aspirate, sputum, or cerebrospinal fluid. A tentative diagnosis of bubonic plague can be made rapidly with fluid aspirated from a bubo showing gram-negative coccobacilli with bipolar staining. It is important to remember that automated diagnostic systems might misidentify *Y. pestis*. In an outbreak in Colorado, the misidentification of *Y. pestis* as *Pseudomonas luteola* delayed the recognition of the outbreak. Serology showing a fourfold rise in antibody titers to F1 antigen or a single titer of more than 1:128 is also diagnostic. Rapid tests using monoclonal antibodies to detect *Y. pestis* F1 antigen in bubo aspirates and sputum have been developed and field tested. The use of mass spectrometry as a more rapid and cost-effective diagnostic tool has also been studied.

Treatment

The aminoglycosides (gentamicin[1] and streptomycin), the fluoroquinolones (ciprofloxacin [Cipro] moxifloxacin [Avelox] and levofloxacin [Levaquin]) and doxycycline (Vibramycin) are the first-, second-, and third-line classes of antibiotics, respectively. Typical minimal inhibitory concentrations for 90% (MIC_{90}) of tested strains for the fluoroquinolones are less than 0.03 to 0.25 μg/mL compared with less than 1.0 μg/mL and less than 1.0 μg/

---

[1]Not FDA approved for this indication.

mL to 4.0 μg/mL for gentamicin and streptomycin, respectively, and less than 1.0 μg/mL for doxycycline. Streptomycin (15 mg/kg up to 1 g intramuscularly [IM] every 12 hours) and gentamicin (5 to 7 mg/kg/day intravenously [IV]/IM in one or two doses daily) are the drugs of choice for severe infection. Standard fluoroquinolone dosing includes ciprofloxacin 400 mg IV/500 mg orally every 12 hours; levofloxacin 500–750 mg IV/orally daily; and moxifloxacin 400 mg IV/orally daily. Doxycycline is administered starting with a 200 mg loading dose followed by 100 mg IV/orally every 12 hours. Chloramphenicol (25 mg/kg IV/orally every 6 hours) can be used in select circumstances. Antibiotic therapy should be continued for a total of 10 days; some experts will extend the duration of therapy to 14 days when a bacteriostatic agent like a tetracycline is used.

Prevention and Control

Standard infection control procedures should include a disposable surgical mask, latex gloves, devices to protect mucous membranes, and good hand washing. Hospitalized patients with known or suspected pneumonic plague should be isolated under respiratory droplet precautions for at least 48 hours after appropriate antibiotics are initiated. Patients without respiratory plague can be managed under standard precautions. Postexposure prophylaxis should be given to individuals with close contact (less than 2 meters) with an infectious case or who have had a potential respiratory exposure. The recommended adult antibiotics for prophylaxis are doxycycline or ciprofloxacin in the same doses used for treatment. Postexposure prophylaxis can be given orally and should be continued for 7 days following exposure. Currently, there is no licensed plague vaccine. An encapsulated *Y. pseudotuberculosis*, strain V674pF1[5], is an efficient live oral vaccine against pneumonic plague in mice. Recently, flea resistance to insecticides such as DDT and Deltamethrin in Madagascar has prompted an immediate need for alternative insecticides to prevent future plague outbreaks.

---

[5] Investigational drug in the United States.

References

Andrianaivoarimanana V, et al: Understanding the persistence of plague foci in Madagascar, *PLoS Negl Trop Dis.* 7(11):e2382, 2013.

Boulanger LL, Ettestad P, Fogarty JD, et al: Gentamicin and tetracyclines for the treatment of human plague: review of 75 cases in New Mexico, 1985–1999, *Clin Infect Dis* 38:663–669, 2004.

Boyer S, et al: Xenopsylla cheopis (Siphonaptera: Pulicidae) susceptibility to deltamethrin in Madagascar, *PLoS One* 9(11), 2014. e111998.

Butler T: A clinical study of bubonic plague. Observations of the 1970 Vietnam epidemic with emphasis on coagulation studies, skin histology and electrocardiograms, *Am J Med* 53:268–276, 1972.

Butler T: Plague gives surprises in the first decade of the 21st century in the United States and worldwide, *Am J Trop Med Hyg* 89(4):788–793, 2013.

CDC. Maps and Statistics. http://www.cdc.gov/plague/maps/index.html.

Cler DJ, Vernaleo JR, Lombardi LJ, et al: Plague pneumonia disease caused by Yersinia pestis, *Semin Respir Infect* 12:12–23, 1997.

Derbise A, Cerdà Marín A, et al: An encapsulated Yersinia pseudotuberculosis is a highly efficient vaccine against pneumonic plague, e1528 *PLoS Negl Trop Dis* 6(2), 2012.

Gage KL, Dennis DT, Orloski KA, et al: Cases of cat-associated human plague in the Western US, 1977–1998, *Clin Infect Dis* 30:893–900, 2000.

Inglesby TV, Dennis DT, Henderson DA, et al: Plague as a biological weapon: Medical and public health management. Working Group on Civilian Biodefense, *JAMA* 283:2281–2290, 2000.

Perry RD, Fetherston JD: Yersinia pestis—etiologic agent of plague, *Clin Microbiol Rev* 10:35–66, 1997.

Prentice MB, Rahalison L: Plague, *Lancet* 369:1196–1207, 2007.

Runfola JK, et al: Outbreak of human pneumonic plague with dog-to-human and possible human-to-human transmission, *MMWR Morb Mortal Wkly Rep* 64(16):429–434, 2015.

Wang H, et al: A dog-associated primary pneumonic plague in Qinghai Province, China, *Clin Infect Dis* 52(2):185–190, 2011.

Wong JD, Barash JR, Sandfort RF, Janda JM: Susceptibilities of Yersinia pestis strains to 12 antimicrobial agents, *Antimicrob Agents Chemother* 44:1995–1996, 2000.

World Health Organization. Plague Outbreaks Situation Report.

WHO external Situation report 14 - 04 December 2017

CLOSTRIDIUM DIFFICILE COLITIS

Method of
Jeffery D. Semel, MD

CURRENT DIAGNOSIS

- *Clostridium difficile* (renamed *Clostridioides difficile*) infection is diagnosed by a combination of clinical and laboratory findings.
- Diagnosis requires a positive test for the presence of *C difficile* toxins.
- GDH, or glutamate dehydrogenase, produced by *C difficile*, can be detected in stool. However, it is not specific and can be produced by non-toxigenic *C. difficile*.
- Enzyme immunoassay testing for toxin A and or B has a variable sensitivity and specificity and a turnaround time of about 24 hours and correlates well with disease activity.
- Polymerase chain reaction testing has a high sensitivity and specificity and a turnaround time of less than 4 hours; correlates less with disease activity, thus identifying patients with colonization as well as active infection. Increasingly, combination testing is being employed to improve diagnostic accuracy.
- Laboratory testing for *C difficile* toxins should only be performed on patients with ≥3 unformed stools per 24 hours, who are not on laxatives and is not useful as a test of cure.
- Pathologic findings can help to confirm diagnosis.

CURRENT THERAPY

- If possible, the clinician should first consider discontinuing concurrent antibacterial therapy.
- Treatment should be initiated only after a positive test result for *C difficile* toxin unless the patient is at high risk for *C difficile* infection or is severely ill, in which case empirical therapy is justified.
- Treatment recommendations depend on the severity of the disease and whether the patient has a first-time diagnosis or recurrence.
- Clinical parameters that guide treatment include increasing age, leukocytosis, elevation of serum creatinine, and presence of hypotension, shock, ileus, or megacolon.
- Oral vancomycin (Vancocin) or fidaxomicin (Dificid), are preferred for initial therapy. Metronidazole (Flagyl)[1] oral, can be used for non-severe disease if these are not available.
- Intravenous metronidazole and or rectal vancomycin (enema)[1],[6] can be added for severe disease.
- FMT (fecal microbiota therapy) is a safe and effective option for recurrent disease.

---

[1]Not FDA approved for this indication.
[6]May be compounded by pharmacists.

Pseudomembranous colitis is an inflammatory disease of the colon that is almost always associated with the toxin-producing bacteria *Clostridium difficile*. In very rare cases, other organisms can be responsible. In this article I discuss *C difficile* as an important cause of pseudomembranous colitis.

Epidemiology and Risk Factors

C difficile is the most common infectious cause of health care–associated diarrhea. Studies in US hospitals showed that mortality rates related to *C difficile* infection nearly quadrupled from 1999 through 2004. An active population and laboratory based study done by the US Centers for Disease Control and Prevention in 2011 suggested that 453,000 new cases occur in the United States annually; with a 30-day mortality rate of 6.4%. Higher rates of infection were found in whites, females, and those >65 years of age. A Canadian study in 2011 prospectively followed up 5422 hospitalized patients and showed that 7.4% had asymptomatic colonization only (60% of these were positive at the time of admission); 2.8% developed *C difficile* infection during hospitalization. Another study by the CDC found decreased hospital-associated infection rates in US hospitals between 2011 and 2015 but no change in the rate of *C. difficile* infections. Colonization of asymptomatic hospitalized patients with *C difficile* ranges from 0%–22% and is higher in residents of long-term care facilities.

Additional risk factors for the development of *C difficile* infection include antimicrobial or chemotherapeutic drug exposure, severe underlying illness, prior hospitalization (acute or long-term care), use of feeding tubes, recent gastrointestinal surgery, and gastric acid suppression. Exposure to antibiotics has been shown to lead to an alteration in the type and quantity of bacterial species found in the normal human intestinal microbiome. Most antibiotics have been associated with *C difficile* infection. Increased antimicrobial duration and dosage appear to be associated with higher risk of *C difficile* infection.

Epidemic strains have been described by pulsed-field gel electrophoresis (NAP1,4,7,11 etc.) that are associated with decreased regulatory gene function and increased toxin production. The risk and severity of infection are increased after exposure to the NAP1 strains. Failure of standard first-line therapy for *C difficile* infection may increase to 10% to 35% during infection with NAP strains.

C difficile infection occurs rarely without prior antibiotic exposure. Healthy peripartum women, children, and postsurgical patients rarely have *C difficile* infection develop after a single dose of an antibiotic. Newborns have a higher rate of colonization but generally a low rate of *C difficile* infection.

Infection is costly. It is estimated that each episode costs the US health care system $3,427– $16,307 per episode or $1.2 billion–$5.9 billion per year.

Microbiology and Pathophysiology

C difficile is a gram-positive, spore-forming, anaerobic rod. *C difficile* can exist as either a spore or vegetative form. The vegetative form is highly oxygen sensitive; slight exposure can kill the bacteria. The spore form is highly heat-stable and can survive harsh conditions such as the high acidity of the stomach. Spores have been shown to resist many commercial disinfectants. *C difficile* reproduces in intestinal crypts and releases exotoxins A and B, leading to severe inflammation. Toxin A (enterotoxin) attracts neutrophils and monocytes, and toxin B (cytotoxin) degrades colonic epithelial cells. Most strains of *C difficile* produce both toxin A and B; however, toxin production, and thus detection may fluctuate during infection. Toxins disrupt cell membranes and cause shallow ulcerations on the intestine mucosal surface. Ulcer formation leads to the release of proteins, mucus, and inflammation manifesting as a pseudomembrane. A pseudomembrane is virtually pathognomonic for *C difficile* infection.

Transmission occurs via the fecal–oral route, person to person, or via fomites. Following exposure to antibiotics, the normal gut flora is altered ("(dysbiosis"), allowing *C difficile* to become more dominant. Exposure to *C difficile* spores may result in no acquisition, asymptomatic colonization, mild diarrhea, or infection. Evidence showing colonization occurring during hospitalization as opposed to prior to hospitalization poses an increased risk for *C. difficile* infection, suggests that colonization in some patients induces immunity, and/or that more virulent strains are present in the hospital.

In addition, the host immune response to spore exposure is important in determining the clinical outcome. Approximately 60% of people have detectable levels of antibodies to toxin A and B. It is likely that prior exposure to *C difficile* spores or related clostridial species and subsequent colonization stimulates antibody production and immunity. Clostridium difficile has been found to be capable of creating a biofilm in vitro, which may impair the antibacterial activity of antibiotics such as metronidazole (Flagyl). Various studies are attempting to define the role of active or passive immunotherapy, including vaccination with nontoxigenic *C difficile*, to prevent *C difficile* infection.

Clinical Features

C difficile infection is diagnosed by a combination of clinical and laboratory findings. Diarrhea is defined as the passage of three or more unformed stools in a 24-hour period. Symptoms include fever, diarrhea, and cramplike abdominal pain. Patients can have nausea, vomiting, or hematochezia. In severe cases, abdominal tenderness and distention are present. Signs of septic shock can develop. The extent of leukocytosis frequently correlates with disease severity. Plain abdominal radiographs might show distended loops of bowel, ileus, or, in severe cases, toxic megacolon. Computed tomography (CT) image findings include colonic wall thickening and dilatation, mesenteric edema, and, rarely, perforation. Endoscopy can reveal pseudomembranes. However, sigmoidoscopy or colonoscopy may be complicated by perforation in severely ill patients and should be performed with caution.

Differential Diagnosis

The differential diagnosis includes bacterial causes such as *Shigella, Salmonella,* or *Campylobacter* species, protozoan infections such as *Entamoeba histolytica* or *Strongyloides stercoralis* (immunosuppressed patients), inflammatory disorders such as ulcerative colitis or Crohn's disease, drug toxicity (e.g., chemotherapeutic agents), and vascular disorders such as ischemic bowel disease.

Diagnosis

Various tests have been developed for the diagnosis of *C difficile* infection. Glutamate dehydrogenase (GDH) is produced by C difficile and can be detected in stool. It is very sensitive for C difficile but can be produced by non-toxigenic C. *difficile* and thus is non-specific.

Enzyme immunoassays (EIA) for toxin A and or B detect toxin production. The sensitivity is 63%–94% and specificity is 75%–100%. GDH and toxin assays correlate well with clinical disease activity.

Molecular tests such as polymerase chain reaction (PCR) can be performed in less than 4 hours. The sensitivity is approximately 93% and specificity is 97%. These tests target toxin genes and do not always correlate with clinical disease. Since the introduction of PCR, the number of cases diagnosed has increased further (though some may represent colonization). Thus positive *C difficile* testing must be correlated with clinical disease activity to determine if treatment is indicated. Increasingly, authors have recommended two-step testing using PCR and toxin EIA, or, GDH/ toxin EIA, followed by PCR.

Treatment

If possible, the clinician should first consider discontinuing concurrent antibacterial therapy, unless there is a compelling clinical indication to continue. Antimotility agents should be avoided because decreased gut motility can increase the potential for tissue toxin exposure and toxic megacolon. Treatment for *C difficile* infection should be initiated only after a positive *C difficile* test result unless the patient is at high risk for *C difficile* infection or is severely ill, in which case empirical therapy is reasonable even with negative test results.

Antibacterials used to treat *C difficile* infection can be administered orally, intravenously, or rectally. Oral therapies are preferred. Oral vancomycin (Vancocin) is not absorbed in the gastrointestinal tract and is eliminated in the feces. Fidaxomicin (Dificid), a macrocyclic antibiotic, has been shown to have equal efficacy to vancomycin but with a potentially lower rate of *C difficile* recurrence. Fidaxomicin is approved for patients 18 years or older. Oral metronidazole (Flagyl), a nitroimidazole antibiotic, is eliminated primarily in the urine, although 6% to 15% is eliminated in the feces, and may be less active as inflammation subsides.

The Society for Healthcare Epidemiology of America (SHEA) and the Infectious Diseases Society of America (IDSA) published treatment guidelines in 2018. Recommendations for the treatment of *C difficile* infection depend on the severity of the disease. Clinical parameters that correlate with severity include increasing age, leukocytosis, and elevation of the serum creatinine.

For all patients with a first episode of *C difficile* infection vancomycin 125 mg four times daily or fidaxomicin 200 mg twice daily, by mouth (PO) for 10 days is recommended. If these drugs are not available, metronidazole (Flagyl)[1] 500 mg three times daily by mouth can be used but should be avoided if the disease is severe.

A white blood cell count of at least 15,000 cells/μL or a serum creatinine at least 1.5 times the premorbid level suggests the possibility of severe infection.

Patients with an initial episode that is complicated by hypotension, shock, ileus, or megacolon should be treated with vancomycin 500 mg PO 4 times per day, plus metronidazole 500 mg IV[1] every 8 hours. If the patient has a complete ileus, the clinician may consider adding a rectal instillation of vancomycin[1,6] 500 mg every 6 hours.

Monitoring

The response to therapy should be monitored clinically. Reversal of hemodynamic instability, decreasing stool frequency, and a declining white blood cell count are objective measures of response. Stool tests for *C difficile* toxin are not valuable for monitoring disease elimination, because these tests can remain positive after improvement.

Complications and Recurrence

Another challenging problem in *C difficile* infection is recurrence. Recurrence is defined as another episode that occurs within eight weeks of the initial episode. Recurrence occurs in approximately 20% to 30% of cases following resolution of the initial episode. Continued use of antibacterials (other than treating agents), increased age, longer hospitalization, severe underlying disease, and inadequate antitoxin antibody response are risk factors for relapse. Even though treatment failure and relapse are common, resistance to metronidazole or vancomycin is uncommon.

For an initial recurrence, a tapered, pulsed dose regimen of vancomycin is often employed. This consists of vancomycin 125 mg PO 4 times per day for 2 weeks, followed by 125 mg PO 2 times per day for 1 week, followed by vancomycin 125 mg PO once daily for 1 week, followed by 125 mg PO once every 2 to 3 days for 2 to 8 weeks.

Fidaxomicin may be considered as an alternative to vancomycin for an initial recurrence.

Another option for recurrent *C difficile* infection is fecal reconstitution or fecal microbiota therapy (FMT). The goal is to reverse dysbiosis and restore normal colonic flora. Healthy donor stool is infused via colonoscopy, intraduodenal, or by frozen capsule. Numerous studies have shown the efficacy of FMT, although the exact place, timing and mode of installation continue to be under evaluation. Donor stool must be screened for infectious agents prior to installation. Additional promising options for prevention of recurrences include the addition of monoclonal antibodies directed against *C difficile* and the oral administration of non toxigenic *C difficile* strains. A monoclonal antibody, directed at toxin B. bezlotoxumab (Zinplava), is now available for prevention of recurrence in patients at high risk.

Probiotics[7] are live organisms that seek to restore the normal gastrointestinal microflora. Most studies have used *Lactobacillus* species or *Saccharomyces boulardii* in an effort to prevent, or treat *C difficile* infection. A recent Cochrane analysis has shown that the use of probiotics during antimicrobial administration may decrease the subsequent development of *C difficile* colitis. The optimal probiotic formula, dosing, and side effect profile remains to be determined. Probiotics have not shown benefit during active infection. Occasional cases of fungemia or bacteremia have been reported in immunocompromised patients and those with central venous catheters treated with probiotics. Probiotics should be avoided in these patients.

Total colectomy is often considered as a last measure for patients who remain critically ill despite standard therapy. The exact indications for surgery are not clear, although refractory shock, signs of peritonitis, megacolon, and multiorgan failure are most often cited. As expected, the mortality rate after total colectomy is high, ranging from 35% to 80%. Neal and colleagues reported that in a series of 42 patients, performance of a diverting loop ileostomy and intraoperative colonic lavage with polyethylene glycol, followed by postoperative antegrade vancomycin flushes, resulted in 19% mortality and 93% colon preservation.

Prevention

Given the current difficulties in controlling the spread of *C difficile*, prevention is critical. *C difficile* spores resist desiccation and can survive in the hospital environment for months. Environmental contamination is highest in and around the rooms of patients with *C difficile* infection. The risk of hospital-associated *C difficile* has been found to be increased for patients occupying the bed of a previous patient who received antibiotics. Items that have been found to harbor *C difficile* spores include clothing, blood pressure cuffs, telephones, toilets, doorknobs, oral and rectal thermometers, and other medical equipment. In addition, the hands of health care workers have been found to be a vehicle of transmission.

Current recommendations for prevention of transmission of *C difficile* include the following. Careful hand hygiene with soap and water is essential. Programs to monitor the compliance and technique of hand hygiene are recommended. Alcohol-based hand rubs, which are widely used, have been shown to be less effective at removing spores than conventional hand washing. Thus alcohol-based hand rubs should not be used for *C difficile* isolation when *C difficile* outbreaks are present. Barrier precautions with gowns and gloves should be used. Programs to ensure adequate and effective cleaning of health care facilities after use are recommended. Disposable electronic thermometers are recommended. Antimicrobial stewardship programs aimed at promoting the judicious use of antibacterial therapy have been found to be effective in reducing *C difficile* infection rates and should be used. In view of recent data that colonization at the time of admission increases the risk for *C difficile* infection, studies have been initiated to determine if contact isolation for *C difficile* colonized patients will be beneficial in decreasing transmission.

References

Agrawal M, Aroniadis OC, Brandt LJ, et al: The long-term efficacy and safety of fecal microbiota transplant for recurrent, severe, and complicated *Clostridium difficile* infection in 146 elderly individuals, *J Clin Gastroenterol* 50(5):403–407, 2016.

Feazel L, Malhotra A, Perencevich E, et al: Effect of antibiotic stewardship programmes on Clostridium difficile incidence: a systematic review and meta-analysis, *J Antimicrob Chemother.* 69:1748–1754, 2014.

Goldenberg JZ, Yap C, Lytvyn L, et al: Probiotics for the prevention of Clostridium difficile-associated diarrhea in adults and children, *Cochrane Database Syst Rev* 12:CD006095 2017 Dec 19, https://doi.org/10.1002/14651858.CD006095.pub4.

Hsu J, Abad C, Dinh M, et al: Prevention of endemic healthcare-associated *Clostridium difficile* infection: reviewing the evidence, *Am J Gastroenterol* 105:2327–2339, 2010.

Jiang ZD, Ajami NJ, Petrosino JF, et al: Randomised clinical trial: faecal microbiota transplantation for recurrent Clostridum difficile infection - fresh, or frozen, or lyophilised microbiota from a small pool of healthy donors delivered by colonoscopy, *Aliment Pharmacol Ther* 45(7):899–908, 2017 Apr. https://doi.org/10.1111/apt.13969. Epub 2017 Feb 21.

Kyne L, Warny M, Qamar A, et al: Asymptomatic carriage of *Clostridium difficile* and serum levels of IGG antibody against toxin A, *N Engl J Med* 342:390–397, 2000.

Kwon JH, Olsen MA, Dubberke ER: The morbidity, mortality, and costs associated with Clostridium difficile infection, *Infect Dis Clin N Am* 29:123–134, 2015.

Lessa E, Mu Y, Bamberg W, et al: Burden of *Clostridium difficile* infection in the United States, *N Engl J Med* 372:825–834, 2015.

Loo VG, Bourgalt A, Poirier L, et al: Host and pathogen factors for *Clostridium difficile* infection and colonization, *N Engl J Med* 365:1693–1703, 2011.

Magill SS, O'Leary SJ, Janelle DL, et al: Changes in prevalence of health - care associated infections in U.S. hospitals, *N Engl J Med* 379:1732–1744, 2018.

McDonald LC, Gerding DN, Johnson S, et al: Practice Guidelines for Clostridium difficile Infection in Adults and Children: 2017, *Clin Infect Dis* 2018 Feb 15. https://doi.org/10.1093/cid/cix1085 [Epub ahead of print].

Neal M, Alverdy JC, Hall DE, et al: Diverting loop ileostomy and colonic lavage: An alternative to total abdominal colectomy for treatment of severe, complicated *Clostridium difficile* associated disease, *Ann Surg* 254:423–427, 2011.

Semenyuk EG, Laning ML, Foley J, et al: Spore formation and toxin production in

---

[1] Not FDA approved for this indication.
[6] May be compounded by pharmacists.
[7] Available as a dietary supplement.

Clostridium difficile biofilms, *PLoS One* 9(1):e87757, 2014 Jan 30.

Shim JK, Johnson S, Samore MH, et al: Primary symptomless colonisation by *Clostridium difficile* and decreased risk of subsequent diarrhea, *Lancet* 351:633, 1998.

Truong C, Schroeder LF, Gaur R, et al: Clostridium difficile rates in asymptomatic and symptomatic hospitalized patients using nucleic acid testing, *Diagn Microbiol Infect Dis* 87(4):365–370, 2017 Apr https://doi.org/10.1016/j.diagmicrobio.2016.12.014. Epub 2017 Jan.

PSITTACOSIS

Method of
Christopher C. McGuigan, MB, ChB, MPH

CURRENT DIAGNOSIS

- The key to successful management of psittacosis is to consider this diagnosis, particularly in cases of community-acquired pneumonia (CAP), especially given a history of bird contact.
- The typical clinical pictures are of CAP, influenza-like illness, or fever of unknown origin. Psittacosis causes 1% of incident CAP cases. Onset is usually sudden with fever, chills and a prominent headache. Consider this diagnosis in a patient with CAP unresponsive to β-lactam antibiotics.
- Investigation will typically reveal a normal or slightly elevated white blood cell count with a left shift or toxic changes, increase in C-reactive protein (CRP) or erythrocyte sedimentation rate (ESR), mildly abnormal liver function tests, hyponatremia, and mild renal impairment. Chest x-ray may be more abnormal than examination alone would predict.
- Diagnosis can be confirmed with (ideally) paired serum samples: using either the complement fixation test (widely used but unable to differentiate between *Chamydophila* species), or the microimmunofuorescence test, which is specific for individual *Chamydophila* species. Either a single high titer or a fourfold rise in titer using samples collected at least 14 days apart are interpreted as positive. More recently, real-time polymerase chain reaction (rt-PCR) tests are used to detect specific DNA. These can provide a more rapid diagnosis, as well as subspecific genotype.

CURRENT THERAPY

- Therapy should commence when the diagnosis is suspected on clinical presentation and initial investigation.
- Tetracyclines are the drugs of choice; for example, doxycycline (Vibramycin) 100 mg bid for 10 to 14 days.
- Macrolides are suitable (but probably less effective) alternatives in those intolerant of tetracyclines (e.g., children and pregnant women).
- Notification to health authorities facilitates public health investigation and interventions to reduce transmission and control outbreaks.

Psittacosis is caused by infection with the bacterium *Chlamydophila psittaci* (formerly *Chlamydia psittaci*). It is twice as common in men than in women, and mainly affects adults typically aged 40 to 50 years. The main reservoir for psittacosis is birds, particularly psittacine birds (parrots, parakeets, budgerigars and cockatoos), but other bird species and mammals can be infected.

Risk Factors

The most common etiological factor is exposure to infected birds—especially a new, sick, or dead one—typically a pet or via occupational exposure (e.g., work as a veterinarian, zoo keeper, or poultry-worker). Most cases are sporadic, but outbreaks have occurred associated with pet shops, aviaries, and poultry-processing plants and with mowing lawns in areas with large numbers of psittacine birds. Person-to-person transmission is rare. Ingestion of poultry products is *not* a risk factor.

Pathophysiology

C psittaci infection is via the respiratory tract and is typically thought to be by inhalation of an aerosol of dried feces or other avian secretion. It then either travels via the blood to the liver and spleen (where it replicates, causing a secondary bacteremia) or directly infects respiratory epithelial cells.

Prevention

Prevention is aimed at controlling disease or colonization in susceptible host species: usually birds. This is facilitated by import restrictions including quarantine and treatment of suspected infections with tetracycline-impregnated feeds. Notification of health authorities is important for initiating public health investigations and interventions to reduce transmission and control of outbreaks.

Clinical Manifestations

The incubation period varies from 4 to 14 or more days. The typical presentation of psittacosis is of an influenza-like illness with sudden onset of fever, chills, and prominent headache, with or without rigors. A more gradual onset is also seen. A typically mild, dry cough usually starts later. There may also be diarrhea, pharyngitis, altered mental state, or shortness of breath. Chest examination is usually abnormal, but the findings are often minimal and less prominent than symptoms or x-ray findings would suggest. Pleural effusion is rare.

Patients might present with a fever of unknown origin without obvious respiratory involvement, or the disease can be misdiagnosed as meningitis because of prominent headache, sometimes with photophobia.

The white blood cell count is usually normal or slightly raised, but there is often a left shift or toxic changes. Increases in the C-reactive protein (CRP) and erythrocyte sedimentation rate (ESR) are common. Mildly abnormal liver function tests, hyponatraemia, and mild renal impairment are also common. The cerebrospinal fluid sometimes contains a few mononuclear cells but is otherwise normal. The chest x-ray usually shows more (nonspecific) abnormality than examination findings might predict. The most common finding is lobar consolidation, but bilateral consolidation and interstitial opacities are also common.

Confirmation of diagnosis is more commonly performed using serology. The complement fixation (CF) test is widely used, but cannot differentiate between *Chlamydophila* species. A fourfold rise in titer, using samples collected at least 14 days apart, or a single titer of 1:128 or higher, is interpreted as positive, but this test is not widely available. Culture of C *psittaci* is difficult and hazardous. Polymerase chain reaction (PCR) assays have been developed, but are not yet widely available for routine clinical use.

Diagnosis

Diagnosis is facilitated by eliciting a history of recent bird contact from a patient with a compatible clinical syndrome, most commonly an influenza-like presentation, community acquired pneumonia (CAP), or a fever of unknown origin. The diagnosis should be considered in a patient with CAP and prominent headache, splenomegaly, or failure to respond to β-lactam antibiotics.

Differential Diagnosis

Differential diagnosis of an atypical CAP, includes infection with *Legionella* species, *Mycoplasma pneumoniae*, or *Chlamydophila pneumoniae*.

Treatment

When the diagnosis is suspected on clinical presentation and initial investigations, empiric therapy should be commenced.

Tetracyclines are the drugs of choice, for example doxycycline (Vibramycin) 100 mg bid for 10 to 14 days. Tetracycline treatment usually leads to improvement in symptoms (including fever) within 24 to 48 hours. Macrolides are usually recommended for pregnant women, children, and other patients intolerant of tetracyclines. However, erythromycin (Erythrocin)[1] has been shown to fail in situations where a tetracycline was effective, and there are few clinical data on the efficacy of the other agents in this class. Some data suggest that quinolones may be effective. Tetracycline hydrochloride or doxycycline (4.4 mg/kg/d divided into two infusions) may be given intravenously for critically ill patients.

Monitoring

Symptomatic improvement usually occurs within 24 to 48 hours of starting a tetracycline; typically including reduction of fever.

Complications

The degree of illness varies from asymptomatic to life threatening. Given appropriate antimicrobial therapy, subsequent case-fatality is less than 1%. Elderly persons and pregnant women are susceptible to more severe illness. Neurologic consequences (e.g., meningo-encephalitis) are recognized but rare. Other less-common sequellae include hemoptysis, proteinuria, hepatosplenomegaly, and encephalitis. Cardiac manifestations include relative bradycardia and, rarely, myocarditis, culture-negative endocarditis, and pericarditis. Erythema nodosum and other skin manifestations have also been described. *C psittaci* has been demonstrated by PCR to be present in ocular adnexal lymphoma (OAL) in parts of Eurasia. Up to one half of such cases respond to antibiotic treatment. However, studies elsewhere suggest that this organism might not commonly play a role in OAL. Recovery with minimal residual deficit is normal.

References

Contini C, Seraceni S, Carradori S, et al: Identification of *Chlamydia trachomatis* in a patient with ocular lymphoma, *Am J Hematol* 84:597–599, 2009.
Grayston JT, Thom DH: The chlamydial pneumonias, *Curr Clin Top Infect Dis* 11:1–18, 1991.
Heddema ER, Beld MG, De Wever B, et al: Development of an internally controlled real-time PCR assay for detection of *Chlamydophila psittaci* in the LightCycler 2.0 system, *Clin Microbiol Infect* 12:571–575, 2006.
Hogerwerf L, DE Gier B, Baan B, VAN DER Hoek W: Chlamydia psittaci (psittacosis) as a cause of community-acquired pneumonia: a systematic review and meta-analysis. [Review], *Epidemiol Infect* 145(15):3096–3105, 2017.
Hughes P, Chidley K, Cowie J: Neurological complications in psittacosis: a case report and literature review, *Respir Med* 89:637–638, 1995.
National Association of State Public Health Veterinarians. Compendium of measures to control *Chlamydophila psittaci* infection among humans (psittacosis) and pet birds (avian chlamydiosis), 2010. Available at: http://www.nasphv.org/Documents/Psittacosis.pdf [accessed July 9, 2015].
Richards M. Psittacosis, Up to date 2006; Available at http://www.uptodate.com/physicians/pulmonology_toclist.asp [accessed 31.12.12; subscription required].
Williams J, Tallis G, Dalton C, et al: Community outbreak of psittacosis in a rural Australian town, *Lancet* 351:1697–1699, 1998.
Yung AP, Grayson ML: Psittacosis: a review of 135 cases, *Med J Aust* 148:228–233, 1988.

---

[1]Not FDA approved for this indication.

Q FEVER

Method of
Didier Raoult, MD, PhD

Q fever is a widespread zoonosis caused by *Coxiella burnetii*, a small, coccoid, strict intracellular gram-negative bacterium. It lives within the phagolysosome of its eukaryotic host cell at very low pH (4.5–4.8). It had previously been classified in the rickettsial family; however, recent phylogenic data based on study of the 16S rRNA gene sequence have shown that it belongs to *Legionellales* with the *Legionella* species and *Francisella tularensis*.

The bacterium has a sporelike life cycle, which explains its marked resistance to physicochemical agents. In cultures,

C. burnetii exhibits a phase variation (from virulent phase I to avirulent phase II) caused by a spontaneous chromosome deletion. The avirulent form paradoxically generates high antibody levels in patients, but only patients with chronic infection have high antiphase I immunoglobulin G (IgG) and IgA antibody titers.

The reservoir of *C. burnetii* is wide, and nearly all tested mammals, birds, and ticks can be infected. Outbreaks have also been reported in association with the birth products of mammals (including ungulates and pets), raw milk, slaughterhouses, and farm work. Laboratory outbreaks have been reported. The disease is prevalent everywhere in the world but in New Zealand and South Pacific Islands, but because its clinical spectrum is wide and nonspecific, the observed incidence is directly related to physician interest in Q fever. A recent outbreak has been observed in the Netherlands.

Clinical Features

Q fever is a reportable disease in the United States. In humans, infection is symptomatic in only 50% of patients. Most symptomatic patients experience a flulike syndrome lasting 2 to 7 days and consisting of severe headaches and cough; 5% to 10% of infected patients may be sick enough to be investigated. They initially have high fever and one or several of pneumonia, hepatitis, meningoencephalitis, rash, myocarditis, and pericarditis. Routine laboratory investigation commonly shows mildly elevated transaminase levels and mild thrombocytopenia.

In special hosts such as immunocompromised patients (specifically those with splenectomy), *C. burnetii* can cause endocarditis. In pregnant women it can lead to recurrent miscarriage, low-birth-weight offspring, and prematurity. *C. burnetii* could contribute to the evolution of lymphoma.

In patients with valvular heart disease and those with arterial aneurysms or a vascular prosthesis, it can cause chronic endocarditis or vascular infection in patients in the 2 years following primary infection. The clinical picture is that of a chronic blood culture–negative endocarditis; the modified Duke criteria are of diagnostic value in such cases. It is spontaneously fatal in most cases.

Diagnosis

Because Q fever is pleomorphic, the diagnosis is based mainly on comprehensive serum testing in patients with an unexplained infectious syndrome. Liver biopsy may be of diagnostic value, because the typical doughnut granuloma is quasispecific to acute Q fever. Valves obtained at surgery or autopsy can be used for culture, direct immunostaining, and polymerase chain reaction (PCR).

Three serologic techniques are used. Complement fixation lacks sensitivity, and one-third of patients with acute Q fever do not exhibit complement-fixing antibodies within 1 month after onset of the disease. However, a fourfold increase in antibodies to phase II antigen indicates acute Q fever, and antibody levels against phase I that are higher than 1:200 indicate persistent focalized Q fever. Indirect immunofluorescence assay is the reference method. A single titer of 1:200 for IgG antiphase II associated with a titer of 1:50 for IgM is diagnostic of acute infection. IgG antibody levels against phase I that are greater than 1:800 and IgA antibody levels greater than 1:50 are highly predictive of endocarditis or vascular infection. Enzyme-linked immunosorbent assay (ELISA) is useful for diagnosing acute infection in detecting IgM antiphase II.

PCR has recently been developed to detect *C. burnetii* DNA in the sera of patients with Q fever. Real-time PCR using multicopy gene *IS1111* is the more-sensitive technique. It is positive in the sera of patients with acute Q fever before IgG antibodies to *C. burnetii* become apparent. It is also positive in patients with untreated endocarditis. Contamination of PCR can occur, and many unconfirmed results are reported in the literature. Detection of patients at risk for endocarditis may be provided by systematic echocardiography in patients with acute Q fever specifically seeking for aortic bicuspidy and serologic follow-up at 3 and 6 months after acute infection. Antiphospholipid antibodies are relatively common during acute Q fever and predictive of endocarditis and deep vein thrombosis.

TABLE 1	Treatment	
Q FEVER	**RECOMMENDED TREATMENT**	**ALTERNATIVE TREATMENT**
Acute	Doxycycline (Vibramicyn) 100 mg PO q12h × 14 d	Ofloxacin (Floxin)[1] 200 mg PO q8h[3] × 14 d Cotrimoxazole (Bactrim)[1] 160/800 mg/PO q12h × 14 d
Endocarditis	Doxycycline 100 mg PO q12h *plus* hydroxychloroquine (Plaquenil)[1] 200 mg PO q8h[3] × 18–24 mo	Doxycycline 100 mg PO q12h *plus* ofloxacin[1] 200 mg PO q8h[3] for 3 y to lifetime
Acute in a patient with a valvular lesion	Same as chronic Q fever for 12 mo	
In pregnancy	Trimethoprim/ Sulfamethoxazole (Bactrim)[1] 160/800 mg PO q12h until term	

[1]Not FDA approved for this indication.
[3]Exceeds dosage recommended by the manufacturer.

Use of a positron emission tomography (PET) scanner may help in the diagnosis of endocarditis (and may reveal mycotic aneurisms), vascular infection, and joint infection.

Treatment

To be active against Q fever, an antibiotic compound has to enter the cell, be effective at an acidic pH (where *C. burnetii* multiplies), and have activity against *C. burnetii*. No antibiotic is bactericidal, but bactericidal activity can be achieved by the addition of hydroxychloroquine (Plaquenil)[1] to doxycycline (Vibramycin).

For acute Q fever, the reference treatment is doxycycline 100 mg orally twice daily for 2 to 3 weeks. Other compounds have been reported to be effective, such as trimethoprim-sulfamethoxazole (TMP-SMX) (Bactrim)[1], Rifampin (Rifadin)[1] 300 mg twice daily, and ofloxacin (Floxin)[1] 200 mg twice daily. In the case of Q fever in pregnant women, one double-strength TMP-SMX tablet (trimethoprim 160 mg, sulfamethoxazole 800 mg)[1] twice daily until delivery prevents fetal death (Table 1). Patients with acute Q fever and high antiphospholipid antibodies may be treated with hydroxychloroquine[1] until normalization.

Persistent focalized and acute endocarditis should be treated for 18 months to 2 years, and antibody levels should be monitored. Patients with prosthetic valves may be treated for 2 years. Two protocols have been evaluated: doxycycline 200 mg daily combined with ofloxacin[1] 400 mg daily for 4 years to lifetime, and doxycycline combined with hydroxychloroquine[1] for 1.5 to 2 years in an amount to achieve a 1 ± 0.20 µg/mL plasma concentration. Doxycycline serum levels greater than 4.5 µg/mL are associated with a more rapidly favorable outcome. This last regimen is apparently more efficacious in terms of relapse. However, regular ophthalmologic surveillance is critical to detect the accumulation of chloroquine in the retina. Both regimens expose the patient to a major risk of photosensitization.

The combination of doxycycline and hydroxychloroquine for 1 year has demonstrated efficacy in preventing endocarditis. Patients with high-level antiphospholipid antibodies may be treated by the same treatment until normalization of the antibody level.

[1]Not FDA approved for this indication.

Prevention

Prevention depends on avoiding exposure, particularly by pregnant women and patients with valvulopathy. No vaccine is currently available outside Australia.

References

Klee SR, et al: Highly sensitive real-time PCR for specific detection and quantification of Coxiella burnetii, *BMC Microbiol* 19:2, 2006.
Maurin M, Raoult D: Q fever, *Clin Microbiol Rev* 12:518–553, 1999.
Merhej V, Cammilleri S, Piquet P, et al: Relevance of the positron emission tomography in the diagnosis of vascular graft infection with *Coxiella burnetii*, *Comp Immunol Microbiol Infect Dis* 35(1):45–49, 2012.
Million M, Bardin N, Bessis S, et al: Thrombosis and antiphospholipid antibody syndrome during acute Q fever: a cross-sectional study, *Medicine (Baltimore)*. 96(29):e7578, 2017 Jul.
Million M, Roblot F, Carles D, et al: Reevaluation of the risk of fetal death and malformation after Q fever, *Clin Infect Dis* 59(2):256–260, 2014.
Million M, Thuny F, Richet H, Raoult D: Long-term outcome of Q fever endocarditis: a 26-year personal survey, *Lancet Infect Dis* 10:527–535, 2010.
Million M, Walter G, Thuny F, et al: Evolution from acute Q fever to endocarditis is associated with underlying valvulopathy and age and can be prevented by prolonged antibiotic treatment, *Clin Infect Dis* 57(6):836–844, 2013.
Raoult D: Chronic Q fever: expert opinion versus literature analysis and consensus, *J Infect* 65:102–108, 2012.
Rolain JM, Maurin M, Raoult D: Bacteriostatic and bactericidal activities of moxifloxacin against Coxiella burnetii, *Antimicrob Agents Chemother* 45:301–302, 2001.

RABIES

Method of
Alan C. Jackson, MD

CURRENT DIAGNOSIS

- A history of animal bite or exposure is often absent in North America.
- Pain, paresthesias, and pruritus are early neurologic symptoms of rabies, probably reflecting infection in local sensory ganglia.
- Autonomic features are common including hypersalivation, gooseflesh, cardiac arrhythmias, and priapism.
- Hydrophobia is a highly specific feature of rabies.
- Paralytic features may be prominent, and the clinical presentation can resemble that of Guillain-Barré syndrome.
- Saliva samples for reverse transcription polymerase chain reaction (RT-PCR) and a skin biopsy should be obtained to detect rabies virus antigen to make a laboratory diagnosis of rabies.

CURRENT THERAPY

- Details of an exposure determine whether postexposure rabies prophylaxis should be initiated.
- Wound cleansing is important after potential rabies exposure.
- Active immunization with a schedule of four doses of rabies vaccine (RabAvert or Imovax) at intervals is recommended. The four-dose series is a new Centers for Disease Control and Prevention (CDC) recommendation and is not yet reflected in the package insert, which calls for five doses.
- Passive immunization (if previously the patient was not immunized) consists of infiltrating human rabies immune globulin (HyperRAB, Imogam Rabies) into the wound, with the remainder of the 20 IU/kg dosage given intramuscularly.

Rabies is an acute infection of the nervous system caused by rabies virus, which is a member of the family Rhabdoviridae in the genus *Lyssavirus*. Other lyssaviruses have only very rarely caused rabies in locations outside of the Americas.

Pathogenesis

Rabies virus is usually transmitted by bites from rabid animals. Transmission has rarely occurred through an aerosol route (in a laboratory accident or bat cave containing millions of bats) or by transplantation of infected organs or tissues (e.g., corneas). The virus is in the saliva of the rabid animal and is inoculated into subcutaneous tissues or muscles via a bite.

During most of the long incubation period (lasting 20–90 days or longer), the virus is close to the site of inoculation. The virus binds to the nicotinic acetylcholine receptor at the postsynaptic neuromuscular junction and travels toward the central nervous system (CNS) in peripheral nerves by retrograde fast axonal transport. There is rapid dissemination throughout the CNS by fast axonal transport. Under natural conditions, degenerative neuronal changes are not prominent, and it is thought that the rabies virus induces neuronal dysfunction by mechanisms that are not well understood. In rabies vectors, the encephalitis is associated with behavioral changes that lead to transmission by biting. After the CNS infection is established, the virus spreads by autonomic and sensory nerves to multiple organs, including the salivary glands of rabies vectors in which the virus is secreted in saliva.

Clinical Features

In North America, where the bat is the most common rabies vector for human disease, a history of an animal bite is usually absent, and there may be no known contact with animals. The incubation period is usually between 20 and 90 days, but it occasionally lasts 1 year or longer. Prodromal features are nonspecific and include malaise, headache, and fever, and patients can also have anxiety or agitation. Approximately half of patients experience pain, paresthesias, or pruritus at the site of the wound, which has often healed, and these symptoms likely reflect infection and inflammation involving local sensory ganglia. Approximately 80% of patients with rabies have encephalitic rabies; approximately 20% have paralytic rabies.

In encephalitic rabies, there are characteristic periods of generalized arousal or hyperexcitability separated by lucid periods. Autonomic dysfunction is common and includes hypersalivation, gooseflesh, cardiac arrhythmias, and priapism. Hydrophobia is the most characteristic feature of rabies and occurs in 50% to 80% of patients; contractions of the diaphragm and other inspiratory muscles occur on swallowing. This can become a conditioned reflex, and even the sight or thought of water can precipitate the muscle contractions. Hydrophobia is thought to be caused by inhibition of inspiratory neurons near the nucleus ambiguus.

In paralytic rabies, prominent muscle weakness usually begins in the bitten extremity and progresses to quadriparesis; typically there is sphincter involvement. Patients have a longer clinical course than in encephalitic rabies. Paralytic rabies is often misdiagnosed as Guillain-Barré syndrome.

Coma subsequently develops in both clinical forms. With aggressive medical therapy, a variety of medical complications develop, and multiple organ failure is common. Survival is very rare and has usually occurred in the context of incomplete postexposure rabies prophylaxis that included administration of one or more doses of rabies vaccine.

Epidemiology

Worldwide about 60,000 human deaths per year are attributed to rabies. The impact is particularly significant in terms of years of life lost because children are commonly the victims. Most human rabies cases occur through transmission from dogs in developing countries with endemic dog rabies, particularly in Asia and Africa. In the United States and Canada, transmission of rabies virus occurs most commonly in human cases from insect-eating bats, and often there is no known history of a bat bite or exposure to bats. A bat bite might not be recognized. The rabies virus

variant responsible for most human cases is found in silver-haired bats and tricolored bats. These are small bats not often in contact with humans. Other rabies vectors in North American wildlife include skunks, raccoons, and foxes, but these species are rarely responsible for transmission to humans. This is likely because of effective postexposure rabies prophylaxis after recognized exposures.

Diagnosis

Most cases of rabies can be diagnosed clinically or the diagnosis will be strongly suspected, which is particularly important so that appropriate barrier nursing techniques can be initiated to prevent exposures of many health care workers. Some patients are candidates for an aggressive therapeutic approach. A serum-neutralizing titer can be useful for diagnosis in a previously unimmunized person, but a positive titer might not develop until the second week of clinical illness or later, and the result of the test might not be readily available. Detection of rabies virus antigen in a skin biopsy obtained from the nape of the neck using a fluorescent antibody technique is a useful diagnostic test. Detection of rabies virus ribonucleic acid (RNA) in saliva or in skin biopsies using RT-PCR amplification is an important recent advance for rapid rabies diagnosis. Rabies virus antigen can be detected in brain tissue obtained by brain biopsy or postmortem. Negative antemortem diagnostic laboratory tests do not exclude rabies and the tests may need to be repeated on subsequent samples.

Prevention

After a rabies exposure is recognized, rabies can be prevented with initiation of appropriate steps, including wound cleansing and active and passive immunization. After a human is bitten by a dog, cat, or ferret, the animal should be captured, confined, and observed for a period of at least 10 days; initiation of postexposure rabies prophylaxis is not necessary if the animal remains healthy. The animal should also be examined by a veterinarian prior to its release. If the animal is a stray, unwanted, shows signs of rabies, or develops signs of rabies during the observation period, the animal should be killed immediately, and its head should be transported under refrigeration for a laboratory examination. The brain should be examined via an antigen-detection method using the fluorescent antibody technique and viral isolation using cell culture or mouse inoculation.

The incubation period for animals other than dogs, cats, and ferrets is uncertain; these animals should be killed immediately after an exposure, and the head should be submitted for examination. If the result is negative, one may safely conclude that the animal's saliva did not contain rabies virus; if immunization has been initiated, it should be discontinued. If an animal escapes after an exposure, it should be considered rabid unless information from public health officials indicates this is unlikely, and rabies prophylaxis should be initiated. The physical presence of a bat might warrant postexposure prophylaxis when a person (such as a small child or sleeping adult) is unable to reliably report contact that could have resulted in a bite.

Local wound care should be given as soon as possible after all exposures, even if immunization is delayed, pending the results of an observation period. All bite wounds and scratches should be washed thoroughly with soap and water. Devitalized tissues should be débrided.

Purified chick embryo cell culture vaccine (RabAvert) and human diploid cell vaccine (Imovax) are licensed rabies vaccines in the United States and Canada. Other vaccines grown in either primary cell lines (hamster or dog kidney) or continuous cell lines (Vero cells) are also satisfactory and available in other countries. A regimen of four 1-mL doses of rabies vaccine should be given IM in the deltoid area (anterolateral aspect of the thigh is also acceptable in children). The four-dose series is a recent CDC recommendation and is an update from the five doses recommended in the current package insert. Ideally, the first dose should be given as soon as possible after exposure, but failing that, it should be given regardless of the length of a delay. Three additional doses should be given on days 3, 7, and 14. Pregnancy is not a contraindication for immunization. Live vaccines should not be given for 1 month after rabies immunization.

Local and mild systemic reactions are common. Systemic allergic reactions are uncommon, and anaphylactic reactions may be treated with epinephrine and antihistamines. Corticosteroids can interfere with the development of active immunity. Immunosuppressive medications should not be administered during postexposure therapy unless they are essential. The risk of developing rabies should be carefully considered before deciding to discontinue vaccination because of an adverse reaction. A serum-neutralizing antibody determination is necessary only after immunization of immunocompromised patients. Less-expensive vaccines derived from neural tissues are still used in some developing countries; these vaccines are associated with serious neuroparalytic complications.

Human rabies immune globulin (Imogam Rabies or Hyper-RAB) should also be administered as passive immunization for protection before the development of immunity from the vaccine. It should be given at the same time as the first dose of vaccine and no later than 7 days after the first dose. Rabies vaccine and human rabies immune globulin should never be administered at the same site or in the same syringe. The recommended dose of human rabies immune globulin is 20 IU/kg; larger doses should not be given because they can suppress active immunity from the vaccine. After wounds are washed, they should be infiltrated with human rabies immune globulin (if anatomically feasible), and the remainder of the dose should be given IM in the gluteal area. If the exposure involves a mucous membrane, the entire dose should be administered IM. With multiple or large wounds, the human rabies immune globulin might need to be diluted for adequate infiltration of all of the wounds. Adverse effects of human rabies immune globulin include local pain and low-grade fever.

After an exposure, a previously immunized patient should receive two 1-mL doses of rabies vaccine on days 0 and 3, but the patient should not receive human rabies immune globulin.

Management of Human Rabies

Only 25 people have survived rabies, and 24 received rabies vaccine prior to the onset of their disease. The possibilities for an aggressive approach were reviewed (see Jackson et al., 2003). There was one survivor in Wisconsin in 2004 who did not receive rabies vaccine. It is now doubtful whether the therapy she received played a significant role in her favorable outcome because a similar approach has failed in many cases (see Jackson, 2013), and there are concerns about its scientific rationale (see Zeiler and Jackson, 2016). Palliation is an important alternative approach and may be appropriate for many patients in whom rabies develops (see Jackson, 2019).

References

Fooks AR, Banyard AC, Horton DL, et al: Current status of rabies and prospects for elimination, *Lancet* 384:1389–1399, 2014.
Jackson AC: Human disease. In Jackson AC, editor: *Rabies: scientific basis of the disease and its management*, 3rd ed., Oxford, UK, 2013, Elsevier Academic Press, pp 269–298.
Jackson AC: Human rabies: a 2016 update, *Curr Infect Dis Rep* 18:38, 2016.
Jackson AC: Current and future approaches to the therapy of human rabies, *Antiviral Res* 99:61–67, 2013.
Jackson AC, Warrell MJ, Rupprecht CE, et al: Management of rabies in humans, *Clin Infect Dis* 36:60–63, 2003.
Jackson AC: *Rabies: scientific basis of the disease and its management*, 3rd ed., Oxford, UK, 2013, Elsevier Academic Press.
Jackson AC: Treatment of rabies. In: Hirsch MS, Edwards MS, Mitty J, eds. UpToDate. Waltham, MA: Wolters Kluwer, 2019.
Manning SE, Rupprecht CE, Fishbein D, et al: Human rabies prevention—United States, 2008: Recommendations of the Advisory Committee on Immunization Practices, *MMWR Recomm Rep* 57(RR-3):1–28, 2008.
World Health Organization: *WHO expert consultation on rabies. Third report*, WHO Technical Report Series 1012, Geneva, 2018, WHO.
Zeiler FA, Jackson AC: Critical appraisal of the Milwaukee protocol for rabies: this failed approach should be abandoned, *Can J Neurol Sci* 43:44–51, 2016.

RAT-BITE FEVER

Method of
Jatin M. Vyas, MD, PhD

CURRENT DIAGNOSIS

- Exposure to rats is the major risk factor. Transmission can occur with simple contact with infected animals or excreta.
- A maculopapular rash and septic arthritis after initial symptoms of fever or sepsis should raise the suspicion of rat-bite fever.
- Clinicians must maintain a high index of suspicion for this diagnosis.
- Notify microbiology laboratory of clinical suspicion (slow growth, 5%–10% CO_2 microaerophilic conditions, 20% normal rabbit serum media supplementation, and avoidance of sodium polyanethol sulfonate when collecting blood cultures from the patient).

CURRENT THERAPY

Bite Site
- Clean and disinfect the bite site.
- Administer tetanus toxoid (tetanus-diphtheria toxoids, Td), if indicated.
- Postexposure rabies prophylaxis (Imovax Rabies) for animal bites should be considered in consultation with local public health authorities, though there are no reports of rat-to-human transmission of the rabies virus.

Established and Suspected Cases
- Give intravenous penicillin G at a dose of 1.2 million U/day for 5 to 7 days, followed by oral penicillin (PenVK)[1] or ampicillin (Omnipen)[1] 500 mg qid for an additional 7 days.
- For penicillin-allergic patients, consider doxycycline (Vibramycin)[1] 100 mg IV/PO twice daily or tetracycline (Achromycin)[1] 500 mg PO four times daily.
- *S. moniliformis* can be resistant to gentamicin (Garamycin),[1] tobramycin (Nebcin),[1] ciprofloxacin (Cipro),[1] and levofloxacin (Levaquin).[1]

[1]Not FDA approved for this indication.

Rat-bite fever (RBF) is a systemic, febrile disease caused by infection with *Streptobacillus moniliformis* or *Spirillum minus*. As the name implies, this infection is transmitted by a rat bite. However, the bacteria can also be transmitted by simple contact with infected rats or even through ingestion of food contaminated with rat excreta. Diagnosis can be difficult, and a high degree of suspicion is necessary to make a correct diagnosis. Recognition and early treatment are crucial, because case fatality is as high as 25% in untreated cases.

Epidemiology

S moniliformis is part of the normal respiratory flora of the rat. From 50% to 100% of healthy wild, laboratory, and pet rats harbor *S moniliformis* in the nasopharynx. *S moniliformis* is also excreted in the urine. *S minus* causes rat-bite fever mostly in Asia, but this organism is found worldwide. *S minus* has been demonstrated in rat conjunctival secretions and blood. Thus rat-bite fever can be transmitted not only from a bite but also through scratches, handling of dead rats, handling litter material, or by contamination of rat excreta.

Although the rat is the natural reservoir and major vector of the disease, *S moniliformis* has also been found in other rodents such as mice, squirrels, gerbils, and weasels. No precise data are available on the true incidence of rat-bite fever because it is not a reportable disease. It appears to be unusual in Western countries, a rarity that might reflect failed diagnosis, empiric treatment of infected bites and scratches caused by animals, or spontaneous recovery.

Risk Factors

The major risk factor is exposure to rats, either as an occupational hazard for persons such as laboratory workers, veterinarians, or pet shop employees, or for persons who have rats for pets or feed rats to snakes, especially children. Classically, homelessness and lower socioeconomic status were described as major factors, but most cases reported in the last few years have involved pet rats. Thirty percent of patients with rat-bite fever do not report any exposure to rats or other rodents. Therefore the lack of documented exposure does not exclude this diagnosis.

Pathophysiology

Very little is known about the pathophysiology of *S moniliformis* infections. Presumably, the failure of local control by dendritic cells, tissue macrophages, neutrophils, and other components of the innate immune system results in deeper infection, leading to bacteremia. Studies using histologic analysis have revealed intravascular thrombosis near the port of entry.

Prevention

The role of prophylactic antibiotics is unknown, but some authors recommend the use of oral penicillin V (PenVK)[1] after documented exposure to rats and a break in the skin. Penicillin V should be given for 3 days at a dose of 2 g per day for adults. Primary prevention should be encouraged for patients with occupational risk by using protective gloves to handle animals or cages.

Clinical Manifestations

Rat-bite fever is a systemic febrile disease. Classically, following a rat bite and a short incubation of 2 to 10 days, systemic dissemination of the organism is associated with an abrupt onset with intermittent relapsing fever, rigors, myalgias, arthralgias, headache, sore throat, malaise, and vomiting. These symptoms are followed within the first week by the development of a maculopapular rash in 75% of patients. The rash can be pustular, purpuric, or petechial, and it typically involves the extremities, in particular the palms and soles. The bite site typically heals promptly, with minimal inflammation and no significant regional lymphadenopathy.

Following the rash, approximately 50% of infected patients develop an asymmetric migrating polyarthritis, which appears to be exceedingly painful and affects large and middle-sized joints. Joint effusion appears more common in adults. Infection can occur in any tissue. Although most cases of rat-bite fever resolve spontaneously, there have been reports of complications. These include meningitis, endocarditis (including prosthetic valve endocarditis), myocarditis, pericarditis, pneumonia, brain abscess, septic arthritis, DIC (disseminated intravascular coagulation), and infarcts of the spleen and kidneys. The mortality rate in untreated cases is around 10% to 15%, and it rises to more than 50% in the rare cases with cardiac involvement.

Two closely related variants have been described. In Haverhill fever, the organism is transmitted by ingestion of contaminated food. Haverhill fever tends to occur in epidemics and also causes rashes and arthritis, but upper respiratory tract symptoms and vomiting appear more prominent. It is important to note that these patients do not provide a history of exposure to rodents. Sodoku is a rat-bite fever caused by *S minus*; it is common in Japan. The course is more subacute, arthritic symptoms are rare, and if the bite initially heals, it then ulcerates and is associated with regional lymphadenopathy and a distinctive rash. *S minus* cannot be grown using synthetic media, and thus microbiologic diagnosis rests on visualization of these organisms in infected tissues.

Figure 1 Gram stain of *Streptobacillus moniliformis*. Gram stain of growth from anaerobic bottle, ×100 magnification [microphotography]. Reprinted with permission from Partners' Infectious Disease Images; accessed on August 11, 2016, from http://www.idimages.org/images/detail /?imageid=373.

Diagnosis

Diagnosis is difficult and requires a high clinical index of suspicion. The initial symptoms of rat-bite fever are nonspecific, triggering a broad differential diagnosis. Additionally, the fastidious nature of this organism makes isolation from blood cultures difficult. Clinicians should ask about rodent exposure when compatible symptoms are seen in patients. Rat-bite fever should not be ruled out in the absence of bite history, because transmission can occur without a bite, and pet owners or laboratory workers can minimize the significance of the bite, especially in the absence of a local reaction.

No reliable serologic test is available, and the definitive diagnosis requires isolation of *S moniliformis* from the wound, blood, or synovial fluid in patients with septic arthritis. The microbiology laboratory should be specifically notified of any clinical suspicion to enhance the chances of recovering the pathogen.

S moniliformis is a highly pleomorphic, nonencapsulated, nonmotile, gram-negative rod, which can stain positively on Gram stain (Figure 1). It is often dismissed as proteinaceous debris because of its numerous bulbous swellings with occasional clumping (*moniliformis*="necklace-like"). It grows slowly and requires a microaerophilic environment with 5% to 10% CO_2 or anaerobic conditions and media supplementation with 20% normal rabbit serum. Cultures can take up to 7 days to turn positive. Some experts recommend holding blood cultures for 21 days to permit sufficient time to grow this organism. *S moniliformis* is also inhibited by sodium polyanethol sulfonate, a common adjunct in most commercial blood culture media at a concentration as low as 0.0125%. *S moniliformis* has been identified using polymerase chain reaction amplification and 16S ribosomal ribonucleic acid (rRNA) sequencing, which shows great promise though it is available at reference laboratories. Fatty acid profiles obtained by gasliquid chromatography can also be used for identification.

S minus, the other etiologic agent of rat-bite fever, is a short, thick, gram-negative, tightly coiled spiral rod that measures 0.2 to 0.5 µm and has two to six helical turns.

Differential Diagnosis

Differential diagnosis for fever, rash, and polyarthritis is broad. Malaria, typhoid fever, and neoplastic disease can cause relapsing fevers, and the presence of a rash and polyarthritis might suggest viral and rickettsial diseases including Rocky Mountain spotted fever. An asymmetric oligoarthritis suggests disseminated gonococcal and meningococcal diseases in the context of cutaneous lesions on the palms and soles. Lyme disease, leptospirosis, or secondary syphilis can have a similar clinical presentation. Finally, when classic infectious symptoms such as fever or rash

---

[1]Not FDA approved for this indication.

are missing, any causes of polyarthritis, from crystal-induced arthropathies to rheumatoid arthritis, should be considered.

Treatment

All established cases of rat-bite fever should be treated with antibiotics because of the associated mortality and potential for complications. Intravenous penicillin G at a dose of 1.2 million units per day should be initiated as soon as the clinical diagnosis is made. Empiric therapy is necessary and should not be delayed for laboratory confirmation of this bacterial infection. The intravenous treatment should continue for 5 to 7 days. After treatment with IV penicillin and suitable clinical response, therapy should be continued with oral penicillin (PenVK)[1] or ampicillin (Omnipen)[1] at a dose of 500 mg qid for an additional 7 days. For patients allergic to penicillin, intravenous doxycycline (Vibramycin)[1] at a dose of 100 mg every 12 hours or oral tetracycline (Achromycin)[1] at a dose of 500 mg four times a day can be used.

Streptomycin[1] and cephalosporins including cefotamxine (Claforan)[1] have been reported to be potentially useful. Other antibiotics including azithromycin (Zithromax),[1] erythromycin,[1] carbapenems,[1] aztreonam (Azactam),[1] clindamycin (Cleocin),[1] vancomycin (Vancocin),[1] and nitrofurantoin (Macrodantin)[1] have shown efficacy in vitro, but they lack good clinical correlation to recommend them for routine use. Erythromycin has been associated with treatment failures. Trimethoprim-sulfamethoxazole (Bactrim),[1] polymyxin B,[1] gentamicin (Garamycin),[1] tobramycin (Nebcin),[1] ciprofloxacin (Cipro),[1] and levofloxacin (Levaquin)[1] should not be used because in vitro resistance has been demonstrated.

Typically, the bite site heals promptly. It should be cleaned and disinfected, as is typical for management of other wounds. Tetanus prophylaxis (tetanus-diphtheria toxoids, Td) administration is indicated as required by the patient's immunization record. Rabies prophylaxis (Imovax Rabies) is usually not required for rodent bite, but consultation with local public health authorities is encouraged. There are no reports of transmission of the rabies virus from rats to humans.

References

Abusalameh M, Mahankali-Rao P, Earl S: Discitis caused by rat bite fever in a rheumatoid arthritis patient on tocilizumab-first ever case, *Rheumatology (Oxford)* 57(6):1118–1120, 2018.

Adam JK, et al: Notes from the field: fatal rat-bite Fever in a child - San Diego County, California, 2013, *MMWR Morb Mortal Wkly Rep* 63(50):1210–1211, 2014.

Chen PL, Lee NY, Yan JJ, et al: Prosthetic valve endocarditis caused by *Streptobacillus moniliformis*: A case of rat bite fever, *J Clin Microbiol* 45:3125–3126, 2007.

Crews JD, Palazzi DL, Starke JR: A teenager with fever, rash, and arthralgia. *Streptobacillus moniliformis* infection, *JAMA Pediatr* 168(12):1165–1166, 2014.

Elliott SP: Rat bite fever and *Streptobacillus moniliformis*, *Clin Microbiol Rev* 20:13–22, 2007.

Fenn DW, et al: An unusual tale of rat-bite fever endocarditis, *BMJ Case Rep.* 2014: 2014.

Gaastra W, Boot R, Ho HT, Lipman LJ: Rat bite fever, *Vet Microbiol* 133:211–228, 2009.

Graves MH, Janda JM: Rat-bite fever (*Streptobacillus moniliformis*): A potential emerging disease, *Int J Infect Dis* 5:151–155, 2001.

Holroyd KJ, Reiner AP, Dick JD: *Streptobacillus moniliformis* polyarthritis mimicking rheumatoid arthritis: An urban case of rat bite fever, *Am J Med* 85:711–714, 1988.

King HY. Rat Bite Fever. UpToDate. http://www.uptodate.com/contents/rat-bitefever; [accessed April 21, 2018].

Lambe DW Jr., McPhedran AM, Mertz JA, Stewart P: *Streptobacillus moniliformis* isolated from a case of Haverhill fever: Biochemical characterization and inhibitory effect of sodium polyanethol sulfonate, *Am J Clin Pathol* 60:854–860, 1973.

Miura Y, Nei T, Saito R, Sato A, Sonobe K, Takahashi K: Streptobacillus moniliformis bacteremia in a rheumatoid arthritis patient without a rat bite: a case report, *BMC Res Notes* 8(1):694, 2005 Nov 19, https://doi.org/10.1186/s13104-015-1642-6.

Schachter ME, Wilcox L, Rau N, et al: Rat-bite fever, Canada, *Emerg Infect Dis* 12:1301–1302, 2006.

Stehle P, Dubuis O, So A, Dudler J: Rat bite fever without fever, *Ann Rheum Dis* 62:894–896, 2003.

Torres-Miranda D, Moshgriz M, Siegel M: Streptobacillus moniliformis mitral valve endocarditis and septic arthritis: the challenges of diagnosing rat-bite fever endocarditis, *Infect Dis Rep* 10(2):7731, 2018.

Washburn RG: Streptobacillus moniliformis (rat–bite fever). In Mandell GL, Bennett JE, Dolin R, editors: *Principles and Practice of Infectious Diseases, vol 2*, 6th ed, Philadelphia, 2005, Elsevier, pp 2708–2710.

[1]Not FDA approved for this indication.

RELAPSING FEVER

Method of
Diego Cadavid, MD

CURRENT DIAGNOSIS

- There are two forms of relapsing fever: epidemic and endemic.
- Epidemic relapsing fever is transmitted from person to person by the body louse *Pediculus humanus*.
- Endemic relapsing fever is transmitted from rodent reservoirs to humans exposed to endemic areas by soft-bodied ticks of the genus *Ornithodoros*.
- The hallmark of relapsing fever is two or more febrile episodes separated by periods of relative well-being.
- The diagnosis is confirmed by visualization of the etiologic spirochetes in thin peripheral blood smears prepared at times of febrile peaks by phase-contrast or darkfield microscopy or light microscopy after Wright or Giemsa staining.

CURRENT THERAPY

- The antibiotic of choice for treatment of relapsing fever is doxycycline except in children or pregnant women. In children <8 years of age, erythromycin[1] or oral penicillin is used instead of tetracycline (Table 3).
- Relapsing fever, if severe or complicated with neuroborreliosis, requires treatment with the intravenous antibiotics ceftriaxone or penicillin G (Table 3).
- The louse-borne epidemic form is treated with a single dose, whereas the endemic tick-borne form is treated with multiple doses for at least 1 week (Table 3).
- Antibiotic treatment of relapsing fever results in the Jarisch-Herxheimer reaction (JHR) in as many as 60% of cases, more often in the epidemic than in the endemic forms. It is characterized by the sudden onset of tachycardia, hypotension, chills, rigors, diaphoresis, and high fever. To reduce the risk of JHR, antibiotics should be started between but not at times of febrile peaks.

[1]Not FDA approved for this indication.

Relapsing fever is one of several diseases caused by spirochetes. Other human spirochetal diseases are syphilis, Lyme disease, and leptospirosis. Notable features of spirochetes are wavy and helical shapes, length-to-diameter ratios of as much as 100 to 1, and flagella that lie between the inner and outer cell membranes. The spirochetes that cause relapsing fever are in the genus *Borrelia*. Other *Borrelia* species cause Lyme disease, avian spirochetosis, and epidemic bovine abortion. Table 1 shows the main *Borrelia* species of relapsing fever, their vectors, and an estimate of their geographic ranges. In the United States, relapsing fever was considered a disease endemic only in the West. However, the recent finding of relapsing fever–like *Borrelia* in ticks and dogs in the eastern United States suggests that the risk of relapsing fever may extend into the East.

Epidemiology

There are two forms of relapsing fever: epidemic transmitted to humans by the body louse *Pediculus humanus* (louse-borne relapsing fever [LBRF]) and endemic transmitted to humans by soft-bodied ticks of the genus *Ornithodoros* (tick-borne relapsing fever [TBRF]). In LBRF, itching caused by skin infestation with lice leads to scratching, which may result in crushing of lice and release of infected hemolymph into areas of skin abrasion. Louse

TABLE 1	Relapsing Fever *Borrelia* Species Pathogenic to Humans		
RELAPSING FEVER	**BORRELIA SPECIES**	**ARTHROPOD VECTOR**	**DISTRIBUTION OF DISEASE**
Endemic	*Borrelia hermsii*	*Ornithodoros hermsi*	Western North America
	Borrelia turicatae	*Ornithodoros turicata*	Southwestern North America and northern Mexico
	Borrelia venezuelensis	*Ornithodoros rudis*	Central America and northern South America
	Borrelia hispanica	*Ornithodoros marocanus*	Iberian peninsula and northwestern Africa
	Borrelia crocidurae	*Ornithodoros erraticus*	North and East Africa, Middle East, southern Europe
	Borrelia duttoni	*Ornithodoros moubata*	Sub-Saharan Africa
	Borrelia persica	*Ornithodoros tholozani*	Middle East, Greece, Central Asia
	Borrelia uzbekistan *Borrelia miyamotoi*	*Ornithodoros pappilipes* *Ixodes* spp.	Tajikistan, Uzbekistan Asia, Europe, North America
Epidemic	*Borrelia recurrentis*	*Pediculus humanus*	Worldwide (recently only in East Africa including immigrants to Europe)

infestation is associated with cold weather and a lack of hygiene. Migrant workers and soldiers at war are particularly susceptible to this infection. Historically, massive outbreaks of LBRF occurred in Eurasia, Africa, and Latin America, but currently the disease is found only in Ethiopia and neighboring countries. However, immigrants can spread LBRF to other parts of the world.

The main risk factor for TBRF is exposure to endemic areas (Table 1). The risk of infection increases with outdoor activities in areas where rodents nest, like entering caves or sleeping in rustic cabins. *Ornithodoros* ticks are soft-bodied and feed for short periods of time (minutes), usually at night. They can live many years between blood meals and may transmit spirochetes to their offspring transovarially. Infection is produced by regurgitation of infected tick saliva into the skin wound during tick feeding. There are several natural vertebrate reservoirs for TBRF, but most common are rodents (deer mice, chipmunks, squirrels, and rats). In contrast, the body louse *Pediculus humanus* is a strict human parasite, living and multiplying in clothing. Hard-tick-borne relapsing fever (HTBRF) is an emerging infectious disease throughout the temperate zone caused by *Borrelia miyamotoi*. *Borrelia miyamotoi* is a spirochete closely related to the bacteria that cause TBRF. It is more distantly related to the bacteria that cause Lyme disease. First identified in 1995 in ticks from Japan, *B miyamotoi* has since been detected in two species of North American ticks, the black-legged or "deer" tick (*Ixodes scapularis*) and the western black-legged tick (*Ixodes pacificus*). These ticks are already known to transmit Lyme disease, anaplasmosis, and babesiosis.

Clinical Diagnosis

Relapsing fever should be suspected in any patient presenting with two or more episodes of high fever and constitutional symptoms spaced by periods of relative well-being. The index of suspicion increases if the patient has been exposed to endemic areas for TBRF or to countries where LBRF still occurs (Table 1). Whereas LBRF is usually associated with a single febrile relapse, TBRF usually has multiple relapses (up to 13). Only about 10% of cases of HTBRF have febrile relapses. In LBRF the second episode of fever is typically milder than the first; in TBRF the multiple febrile periods are usually of equal severity. The febrile periods last from 1 to 3 days, and the intervals between fevers last from 3 to 10 days. During the febrile periods, numerous spirochetes are circulating in the blood. This is called *spirochetemia* and is sometimes unexpectedly detected during routine blood smear examinations. Between fevers, spirochetemia is not observed because the numbers are low. The fever pattern and recurrent spirochetemia are

TABLE 2	Frequent Clinical Manifestations of Tick-Borne Relapsing Fever
SIGN OR SYMPTOM	**FREQUENCY (%)**
Headache	94
Myalgia	92
Chills	88
Nausea	76
Arthralgia	73
Vomiting	71
Abdominal pain	44
Confusion	38
Dry cough	27
Ocular pain	26
Diarrhea	25
Dizziness	25
Photophobia	25
Neck pain	24
Rash	18
Dysuria	13
Jaundice	10
Hepatomegaly	10
Splenomegaly	6

the consequences of antigenic variation of abundant outer membrane lipoproteins of relapsing fever *Borrelia* species that are the target for serotype-specific antibodies.

The mean latency between exposure to ticks in the endemic form or to lice in the epidemic form and onset of symptoms is 6 days (range, 3–18 days). Because *Ornithodoros* ticks feed briefly and painlessly at night, patients with TBRF may not be able to recall having been bitten by a tick. The clinical manifestations of TBRF and LBRF are similar, although some differences do exist. Table 2 lists the frequency of the most common manifestations of TBRF.

The usual initial presentation is sudden onset of chills followed by high fever, tachycardia, severe headache, vomiting, myalgia and arthralgia, and often delirium. In the early stages, a reddish rash may be seen over the trunk, arms, or legs. The fever remains high for 3 to 5 days, and then it clears abruptly. After an asymptomatic period of 7 to 10 days, the fever and other constitutional symptoms can reappear suddenly. The febrile episodes gradually become less severe, and the person eventually recovers completely. As the disease progresses, fever, jaundice, hepatosplenomegaly, cardiac arrhythmias, and cardiac failure may occur, especially with LBRF. Jaundice is more common at times of relapses. Patients with LBRF are more likely to develop petechiae on the trunk, extremities, and mucous membranes; epistaxis; and blood-tinged sputum. Rupture of the spleen may rarely occur. Multiple neurologic complications can occur as a result of disseminated intravascular coagulation in LBRF and as a result of infection of the meninges and cranial and spinal nerve roots by spirochetes in TBRF. The most common neurologic complications of TBRF are aseptic meningitis and facial palsy. Relapsing fever in pregnant women can cause abortion, premature birth, and neonatal death. Sometimes patients can have nonfebrile relapses, consisting of periods of severe headache, backache, weakness, and other constitutional symptoms without fever that occur at the time of expected relapses. Delirium may persist for weeks after the fever resolves, and, rarely, symptoms may be protracted.

Relapsing fever may be confused with many diseases that are relapsing or cause high fevers. These include typhoid fever, yellow fever, dengue, African hemorrhagic fevers, African trypanosomiasis, brucellosis, malaria, leptospirosis, rat-bite fever, intermittent cholangitis, cat-scratch disease, and echovirus 9 infection, among others. Relapsing fever *Borrelia* spp. have antigens that are cross reactive with Lyme disease *Borrelia* spp. and inasmuch as the endemic areas of relapsing fever and Lyme disease overlap to some extent, confusion between the two infections can be expected. In fact, the same species of ticks can transmit HTBRF and Lyme disease, although erythema migrans rash is rare in the former and common in the latter.

Laboratory Diagnosis

Although the pattern of recurring fever is the clue to diagnosing relapsing fever, confirmation of the diagnosis requires demonstration of spirochetes in peripheral blood taken during an episode of fever. The comparatively large number of spirochetes in the blood during relapsing fever provides the opportunity for the simplest method for laboratory diagnosis of the infection, light microscopy of Wright- or Giemsa-stained thin blood smears or darkfield or phase-contrast microscopy of a wet mount of plasma. The blood should be obtained during or just before peaks of body temperature. Between fever peaks, spirochetes often can be demonstrated by inoculation of blood or cerebrospinal fluid (CSF) into special culture medium (BSK-H with 6% rabbit serum available from Sigma) or experimental animals. Enrichment for spirochetes is achieved by using the platelet-rich fraction of plasma or the buffy coat of sedimented blood. In the United States the most common causes of relapsing fever are *Borrelia hermsii* and *Borrelia turicatae*; both grow in BSK-H medium and in young mice or rats. Whereas direct visual detection of organisms in the blood is the most common method for laboratory confirmation of relapsing fever, immunoassays for antibodies are the most common means of laboratory confirmation for Lyme disease. Although serologic assays have been developed for the agents of relapsing fever, these are not widely available and of dubious utility. The antigenic variation displayed by the relapsing fever species means there are hundreds of different "serotypes." If a different serotype or species is used for preparing the antigen, only antibodies to conserved antigens may be detected. For this reason, a standardized enzyme-linked immunosorbent assay (ELISA) with Lyme disease *Borrelia* as antigen may be the best available serologic assay for relapsing fever. ELISA for *Borrelia burgdorferi* antibodies is routinely done across the United States and Europe. If a positive result for IgM or IgG antibodies

| **TABLE 3** | Treatment Options for Tick-Borne Relapsing Fever* |

Adults

Nonsevere forms

   1. Doxycycline (Doryx oral), 100 mg PO bid for 1–2 wk†

   2. Tetracycline (Sumycin), 500 mg PO qid for 1–2 wk

   3. Erythromycin (Erythrocin),[1] 500 mg PO tid for 1–2 wk

Severe forms

   1. Ceftriaxone (Rocephin),[1] 2 g IV qd for 1–2 wk

   2. Penicillin G parenteral aqueous (Pfizerpen),[1] 4 million U IV q4h for 1–2 wk

Children (≤8 y)

Nonsevere forms

   1. Erythromycin suspension oral (EryPed),[1] 30–50 mg/kg/d divided tid for 1–2 wk

   2. Azithromycin oral suspension (Zithromax),[1] 20 mg/kg on the first day followed by 10 mg/kg/d for 4 more days

   3. Penicillin V (Pen-Vee K),[1] 25–50 mg/kg/d divided qid for 1–2 wk

   4. Amoxicillin (Amoxil),[1] 50 mg/kg/d divided tid for 1–2 wk

Severe forms

   1. Ceftriaxone (Rocephin),[1] 75–100 mg/kg/d IV for 1–2 wk

   2. Penicillin G parenteral aqueous (Pfizerpen),[1] 300,000 U/kg/d given IV in divided doses q4h for 1–2 wk

Abbreviations: IV = intravenous; PO = orally.
[1]Not FDA approved for this indication.
*The same oral agents are used for treatment of louse-borne (epidemic) relapsing fever but given as a single dose.
†In general, treatment for 1 wk is recommended in early/milder cases and for up to 2 wk for more severe cases.

is obtained, the Western blot for antibodies to *B burgdorferi* antigens would be expected to discriminate current or past Lyme disease from relapsing fever, as well as from syphilis, another cause of false-positive Lyme disease ELISA results. Other frequent laboratory abnormalities can occur in relapsing fever but are not diagnostic. These include elevated white blood cell count with increased neutrophils, thrombocytopenia, increased serum bilirubin, proteinuria, microhematuria, prolongation of the prothrombin time (PT) and partial thromboplastin time (PTT), and elevation of fibrin degradation products.

Treatment

Relapsing fever *Borrelias* are very sensitive to several antibiotics, and antimicrobial resistance is rare. Table 3 summarizes the treatment options for adults and children younger than 8 years. Children older than 8 years can be treated with the same antibiotics as adults, but the doses should be adjusted by weight. Before antibiotics are given, the possibility of causing the Jarisch-Herxheimer reaction (JHR) should be considered (see later). The tetracycline antibiotics are most commonly used for treatment of LBRF and TBRF. The first antibiotic of choice in adults and children older than 8 years is doxycycline (Doryx). In general, shorter treatments are needed for LBRF than for TBRF. Single-dose therapy is usually recommended for LBRF. In contrast, in TBRF even multiple doses of tetracyclines for up to 10 days may fail to prevent relapses, and retreatment can be required. *B. miyamotoi* is susceptible in vitro to doxycycline, azithromycin, and ceftriaxone. Physicians have successfully treated patients infected with *B miyamotoi* with a 2 to 4-week course of doxycycline.

Alternative oral antibiotics to the tetracyclines are erythromycin (E-Mycin)[1], azithromycin (Zithromax)[1], amoxicillin (Amoxil)[1], penicillin[1], and chloramphenicol (Chloromycetin).[1] However, oral chloramphenicol is not available in the United States. Erythromycin, azithromycin, and penicillin do not appear as effective as the tetracyclines; however, they are recommended for children younger than 8 years and for pregnant women. Amoxicillin is another alternative for young children with early Lyme disease; however, it is ineffective for human granulocytic ehrlichiosis, which sometimes occurs as a co-infection with Lyme disease. *Borrelia miyamotoi* may be resistant to amoxacillin.

Although treatment with antibiotics is usually given orally, they may need to be given intravenously if severe vomiting makes swallowing impractical. If there are symptoms and signs of meningitis or encephalitis without clinical or radiologic signs of increased intracranial pressure, the CSF should be examined to rule out central nervous system (CNS) infection. The finding of elevation of CSF cells and protein demands the use of parenteral antibiotics, such as penicillin G[1] or ceftriaxone (Rocephin).[1] Optimally, antibiotic treatment should be started during afebrile periods when the spirochetemia is low. Starting therapy near the peak of a febrile period may induce JHR, in which high fever and a rise and subsequent fall in blood pressure, sometimes to dangerously low levels, may occur. Dehydration should be treated with fluids given intravenously. Severe headache can be treated with pain relievers such as codeine, and nausea or vomiting can be treated with prochlorperazine (Compazine).

Jarisch-Herxheimer Reaction

Antibiotic treatment of relapsing fever causes JHR in as many as 60% of cases. JHR is more common in LBRF than in TBRF. It can also occur in HTBRF. It is characterized by the sudden onset of tachycardia, hypotension, chills, rigors, diaphoresis, and high fever. Patients with JHR have said that they felt as if they were going to die. JHR is caused by the rapid killing of circulating spirochetes 1 to 4 hours after the first dose of antibiotic, which results in the release of large amounts of *Borrelia* lipoproteins in the circulation followed by massive release of tumor necrosis factor and other cytokines. If possible, patients with JHR should be transferred to an intensive care unit for close monitoring and treatment. Over several hours, the temperature declines and the patient feels better. Large amounts of intravenous fluids (0.9% sodium chloride solution) may be required to treat hypotension. Steroids and nonsteroidal antiinflammatory agents have no effect on the frequency or severity of the JHR. One study found that pretreatment with anti-TNF-alpha monoclonal antibody (Humira)[1] suppressed JHR after penicillin treatment for LBRF and reduced the associated increases in plasma cytokines. Death can occur as a result of JHR secondary to cardiovascular collapse in up to 5% of patients with treated LBRF and much less frequently in TBRF.

Outcome

Complete recovery occurs in 95% or more of adequately treated patients. The prognosis for untreated cases or if treatment is delayed varies. A mortality rate as high as 40% is reported in untreated epidemics of LBRF. Relapsing fever also has a high mortality rate in neonates. Some neurologic sequelae can occur in patients with TBRF complicated with neuroborreliosis.

Prevention

Prevention of TBRF involves avoidance of rodent- and tick-infested dwellings such as animal burrows, caves, and abandoned cabins. Wearing clothing that protects skin from tick access (e.g., long pants and long-sleeved shirts) is also helpful. Repellents and acaricides provide additional protection. Diethyltoluamide (DEET) repels ticks when applied to clothing or skin, but it must be used with caution. It loses its effectiveness within 1 to several hours when applied to skin and must be reapplied; it is absorbed through

the skin and may cause CNS toxicity if used excessively. Picaridin (KBR 3023), which has been used as an insect repellent for years in Europe and Australia, is now available in the United States in 7% solution as Cutter Advanced Repellent (Spectrum Brands). The US Centers for Disease Control and Prevention (CDC) is recommending it as an alternative to DEET. Permethrin Insect Repellent, an acaricide, is more effective than DEET but should not be applied directly to skin. When applied to clothing, it provides good protection for 1 day or more. In LBRF, prevention can be achieved by promoting personal hygiene and by dusting undergarments and the inside of clothing with malathion[1] powder[2] or lindane[1] powder[2] when available. Widespread antibiotic use may be necessary to control epidemics of LBRF, using one or two doses of 100 mg doxycycline[1] given within 1 week of exposure.

References

Barbour AG, Hayes SF: Biology of *Borrelia* species, *Microbiol Rev* 50:381–400, 1986.
Bryceson AD, Parry EH, Perine PL, et al: Louse-borne relapsing fever, *Q J Med* 39:129–170, 1970.
Cadavid D, Barbour AG: Neuroborreliosis during relapsing fever: Review of the clinical manifestations, pathology, and treatment of infections in humans and experimental animals, *Clin Infect Dis* 26:151–164, 1998.
Fekade D, Knox K, Hussein K, et al: Prevention of Jarisch-Herxheimer reactions by treatment with antibodies against tumor necrosis factor alpha, *N Engl J Med* 335:311–315, 1996.
Kazragis RJ, Dever LL, Jorgensen JH, Barbour AG: In vivo activities of ceftriaxone and vancomycin against *Borrelia* spp. in the mouse brain and other sites, *Antimicrob Agents Chemother* 40:2632–2636, 1996.
Melkert PW: Fatal Jarisch-Herxheimer reaction in a case of relapsing fever misdiagnosed as lobar pneumonia, *Trop Geogr Med* 39:92–93, 1987.
Southern P, Sanford J: Relapsing fever, *Medicine* 48:129–149, 1969.
Taft W, Pike J: Relapsing fever. Report of a sporadic outbreak including treatment with penicillin, *JAMA* 129:1002–1005, 1945.

---

[1] Not FDA approved for this indication.
[2] Not available in the United States

RUBELLA AND CONGENITAL RUBELLA

Method of
Dee Ann Bragg, MD

CURRENT DIAGNOSIS

- Given its clinical overlap with other viral syndromes, suspected rubella infection must be confirmed with laboratory testing.
- Rubella serology or viral polymerase chain reaction (PCR) testing are available options for confirming a suspected diagnosis.

CURRENT THERAPY

- Rubella infection is largely self-limited with no specific treatment indicated.
- Infection during pregnancy should prompt further evaluation and counseling regarding risks and potential outcomes.
- Treatment of children with congenital rubella syndrome requires a multidisciplinary effort based on individual manifestations.
- Vaccination is essential in reducing the risk of rubella and congenital rubella syndrome.

Rubella typically presents in children and adults as a mild viral illness, but is one of the TORCH infections (toxoplasmosis, other, rubella, cytomegalovirus, herpes) known to cause congenital anomalies. Although vaccination efforts have led to the successful

---

[1] Not FDA approved for this indication.

eradication of rubella in the United States, it remains a significant cause of morbidity and death worldwide. Its name is derived from Latin and means "little red." Initially considered a variant of measles or scarlet fever, rubella was first described as its own entity in the German medical literature in 1814. Thus it is still often referred to as "German measles" in common nomenclature.

Pathophysiology and Virology

Rubella virus, a single-stranded RNA virus and the only member of the Rubivirus genus, is part of the Togaviridae family and is the causative agent of rubella infection. There are 13 recognized genotypes of rubella, each with minor differences in nucleotide sequencing and gene expression. Rubella typically presents as a mild and self-limited illness. During pregnancy, however, it can infect the placenta and disrupt organogenesis by creating systemic inflammation and inhibiting actin assembly. Outcomes of antenatal infection are variable but can include miscarriage, fetal death, and congenital rubella syndrome (CRS).

Multiple factors are involved in the pathogenesis of CRS. Rubella infection can cause necrosis of the chorionic epithelial and endothelial cells. These cells then enter fetal circulation and can incite thrombotic or ischemic lesions in the eyes, ears, brain, and heart. The virus also appears to trigger an immune-modulated upregulation of interferon and cytokines, which can alter the normal development and differentiation of fetal cells.

Epidemiology

Although rubella is less contagious than other viruses such as influenza or measles, large epidemics are associated with significant morbidity from complications including encephalitis, fetal loss, deafness, and blindness. Norman Gregg, an Australian ophthalmologist, was the first to recognize the teratogenic potential of rubella when in 1941 he noted an unusually high incidence of congenital cataracts after an area outbreak.

Rubella was successfully eradicated from the United States in 2004 due to widespread vaccination efforts, and most sporadic cases since that time have been documented in foreign-born young adults. In endemic areas, annual springtime outbreaks are common. However, sporadic cases can occur year-round in temperate climates. Outbreaks typically affect early school–aged children, and the mean age for an infected host is 5 to 9 years. Because lifelong immunity develops after natural infection, large cyclical epidemics tend to occur every 3 to 8 years as population immunity wanes.

Humans are the only known host of rubella infection, and the virus is transmitted from person to person through respiratory droplets. After transmission, rubella virus replicates in the respiratory mucosa and cervical lymph nodes before entering systemic circulation and spreading to target organs.

Clinical Manifestations

Acquired Rubella

After an incubation period of about 14 days (range, 12–23), a variety of clinical symptoms can appear. These are generally mild, and about 50% of cases are asymptomatic. In children, a skin rash is typically the initial manifestation of rubella. The rash usually appears on the face and then progresses downward from the head to the feet. It lasts about 3 days and is characteristically maculopapular, presenting with small pink non-coalescing papules that are occasionally pruritic. Bathing or showering in hot water tends to make the rash more evident.

Adults more often have a prodromal period of low-grade fever, malaise, and adenopathy lasting 1 to 5 days before the onset of skin findings. Lymphadenopathy may begin up to a week before the rash and can last for several weeks. The postauricular nodes are particularly commonly involved, and posterior cervical or suboccipital nodes may also be affected.

Sequelae

Polyarthritis and polyarthralgia are the most common complications of rubella, particularly in adult women, in whom they are seen up to 70% of the time. They appear with such frequency that they are often considered intrinsic to the virus itself rather than complications. Joint symptoms typically present around the same time or just after the onset of the rash. They usually last 3 to 4 days but can remain for up to 1 month. The most commonly affected joints are fingers, wrists, and knees. Chronic arthritis is rarely observed.

Other complications are uncommon but can carry a high degree of morbidity and death. Hemorrhagic events are more likely in children than adults and occur in about 1 in 3000 cases. They manifest as a result of vascular damage or thrombocytopenia. Skin purpura is the most common presentation, but gastrointestinal, cerebral, or intrarenal hemorrhage can occur. Encephalitis occurs in about 1 in 6000 cases, more commonly in adults than children. Rare complications include orchitis, neuritis, progressive panencephalitis, and Guillain-Barré syndrome.

Congenital Rubella Syndrome (CRS)

CRS can present transiently with low birth weight, thrombocytopenic purpura, or hemolytic anemia. However, permanent defects are the hallmark of CRS because it classically involves a triad of cataracts, cardiac anomalies, and sensorineural deafness. Of these, hearing loss is the most common and sometimes the only complication observed. Cardiac abnormalities can include patent ductus arteriosus, ventricular septal defect, pulmonary artery hypoplasia, and coarctation of the aorta. Other ocular defects such as glaucoma, retinopathy, and microphthalmia can also occur. Additional manifestations can include microcephaly, intellectual disability, psychomotor retardation, and delayed speech.

Notably, it can take 2 to 4 years for certain neurologic, endocrine, or cardiac abnormalities associated with CRS to manifest. Diabetes mellitus, thyroid disease, autism, and progressive panencephalopathy can all occur as late effects of CRS.

The risk of CRS and its associated congenital defects is greatest when infection occurs in the first trimester. Up to 85% of infants born under these conditions are found to be affected, whereas defects are rare when infection occurs after 20 weeks' gestation.

Diagnosis

Given its nonspecific nature and similarity to other viral infections, clinical diagnosis of rubella is challenging and largely unreliable. Suspected infection should be confirmed by 1 of 3 diagnostic methods: (1) rubella immunoglobulin M (IgM) serology, (2) a demonstrated rise in rubella virus immunoglobulin G (IgG) between acute and convalescent phases, or (3) detection of rubella virus by PCR.

Among the existing options for laboratory diagnosis, rubella IgM is the most accessible and widely used. However, collection timing is important to consider. Rubella IgM will only be detectable in about 50% of cases on the day of rash appearance but will be present in nearly all cases by 7 to 10 days after the rash. It will then remain positive for 4 to 12 weeks. Importantly, serum IgM testing is most sensitive and specific in the setting of local outbreaks. False-positive results occur more frequently in sporadic cases, and in those instances, additional means of analysis should be performed to confirm diagnosis.

Rubella IgG testing can be used to diagnose acute rubella infection under two circumstances: either (1) a negative rubella IgG during acute infection followed by a positive IgG in the convalescent phase, or (2) a fourfold increase in IgG titer over 10 to 14 days. IgG avidity testing may also be useful. This measures the strength of antigen-antibody binding, which is typically weaker in acute infection and increases over time. Therefore a low avidity index would indicate a more recent infection.

Viral isolation of rubella by PCR is quite valuable for diagnostic confirmation and can be performed on samples obtained from throat or nasopharyngeal swabs. These tests are not as widely available in postvaccination settings and may need to be performed in conjunction with local health departments or national epidemiology centers.

Diagnosis of CRS in infants can similarly be confirmed by one of three methods: (1) rubella IgM detection in serum or cord blood, (2) persistence of rubella IgG >6 months of age (past the time frame of passive maternal immunity), or (3) PCR isolation of rubella virus from respiratory or urinary samples. Because both rubella virus and IgM remain positive for several months in patients with CRS, the time frame for testing is less crucial than in cases of postnatal infection.

Treatment

There is no specific treatment for rubella and, because acquired cases are generally mild and self-limiting, basic supportive care is recommended. Detection of rubella infection in pregnancies before 18 weeks' gestation should prompt further investigation including maternal-fetal medicine referral, detailed ultrasound examination, support for adverse outcomes including neonatal hospice services, and follow-up examination and screening of the newborn. Maternal infections after 18 weeks can be followed with routine ultrasound monitoring along with newborn evaluation and testing.

Prevention

Rubella Vaccine

The first rubella vaccines became available in 1969, and a number of strains have been developed since that time. Of these, the RA 27/3 vaccine has been the most enduring, and all other strains were discontinued at the time of its introduction in 1979. The RA 27/3 rubella vaccine is a live attenuated virus that is administered in conjunction with measles and mumps as MMR, or with measles, mumps, and varicella as MMRV (ProQuad). Single-antigen rubella vaccine is not available in the United States.

Vaccination against rubella is safe and effective. Adverse events such as fever and rash are mild and are generally attributable to the measles and mumps portions of the vaccines. After a single dose, more than 95% of those vaccinated have serologic confirmation of rubella immunity, with evidence of lifelong immunity in the vast majority of responders. MMR or MMRV is recommended for all children at 12 months of age, followed by a second dose between 4 and 6 years of age. The second dose is generally indicated to stimulate measles and mumps immunity in those who did not respond to the first vaccine. MMR and MMRV are contraindicated in immunosuppression, pregnancy, and in patients with a history of anaphylaxis to neomycin or other vaccine components.

Preconception Counseling and Prenatal Care

Rubella immunity, defined as serum rubella IgG of 10 IU/mL or greater, should be documented in all women attempting to conceive. MMR vaccine should be given in cases of nonimmunity, and although it is recommended at least 4 weeks before conception, inadvertent vaccination after that time is unlikely to be associated with adverse events. Rubella IgG should likewise be checked in all pregnant females as part of routine obstetric care, and MMR should be administered postpartum to nonimmune women.

Eradication and Future Goals

Despite widely available effective vaccines and evidence of sustained eradication in the Western Hemisphere, there are still approximately 100,000 cases of CRS annually worldwide. Although some African and Asian nations have introduced routine rubella vaccination, public health efforts have been inconsistent in many developing countries. Dedicated personnel and funding will likely be necessary to decrease rubella and its complications on a global scale.

References

Baltimore RS, Nimkin K, Sparger K, et al: Case 4-2018: a newborn with thrombocytopenia, cataracts, and hepatosplenomegaly, *N Engl J Med* 378:564–572, 2018.
Bouthry E, Picone O, Hamdi G, et al: Rubella and pregnancy: diagnosis, management and outcomes, *Prenat Diagn* 34:1246–1253, 2014.
Centers for Disease Control and Prevention: *Epidemiology and Prevention of Vaccine-Preventable Diseases, 13th Edition.* Hamborsky J, Kroger A, Wolfe S, eds. Washington, DC: Public Health Foundation, pp 325–340, 2015.
Lambert N, Strebel P, Orenstein W, et al: *Rubella, Lancet* 385(9984):2297–2307, 2015.
Papania M, Wallace G, Rota P, et al: Elimination of endemic measles, rubella, and congenital rubella syndrome from the western hemisphere: the US experience, *JAMA Pediatr* 168:148–155, 2014.
Tipples G: Rubella diagnostic issues in Canada, *J Infect Dis* 204(Suppl 2):S659–S663, 2011.

SALMONELLOSIS

Method of
Arvid E. Underman, MD

CURRENT DIAGNOSIS

- More than 95% of nontyphoid salmonellosis presents as uncomplicated acute gastroenteritis.
- The clinical presentation of different causes of gastroenteritis and diarrhea overlaps significantly.
- The physician should be familiar with groups of patients at risk for complicated salmonellosis.
- Specific diagnosis requires culture of the stool or blood.
- Focal complications are always suspect in high-risk patients who are blood culture positive for nontyphoid *Salmonellae* (e.g., aortitis or mycotic aneurysm in patients older than age 60 years with atherosclerosis).

CURRENT THERAPY

- Fluid and electrolyte replacement is of paramount importance.
- The physician should avoid routine empiric antibiotic in acute uncomplicated patients.
- The physician should avoid antimotility agents for diarrhea presenting with fever or with mucus and blood present.
- More than 95% of patients with nontyphoid salmonellosis *will get better* on their own.
- Fluoroquinolone antibiotics should be reserved for when they are truly indicated clinically.
- Increasing resistance mandates sensitivity testing (including tests for ESBL) to guide therapy of bacteremia and its complications.
- Do not prescribe *prophylactic* antibiotics to prevent diarrhea in travelers.
- Stress personal hygiene and prudent food choice with proper preparation.

Abbreviation: ESBL = extended spectrum beta lactamases.

Salmonellosis refers to a group of infections caused by members of the genus *Salmonella*. This genus is named after Salmon, a pathologist who first isolated the organism, later designated as *Salmonella choleraesuis*, from the intestine of pigs with diarrhea. *Salmonellae* are widely distributed throughout nature and are adapted to a myriad of warm and cold-blooded hosts. In humans there are four main clinical presentations:
1. Acute gastroenteritis
2. Bacteremia
3. Focal extraintestinal infection
4. Chronic carriage (Table 1)

Microbiology

Salmonellae are motile, gram-negative, nonspore-forming bacilli that are differentiated from other *Enterobacteriaceae* by inability to ferment lactose and sucrose while producing acid, hydrogen sulfide, and gas (except *Salmonella typhi*). Members of the genus were more accurately classified into serotypes using the Kauffman-White schema, which differentiated and grouped them serologically dependent on their lipopolysaccharide somatic (O) and flagellar (H) antigens.

More recently, DNA analysis has divided the genus into two species. Initially the first of the two species was named *Salmonella choleraesuis* and was divided into six subspecies, each of which was then divided into more than 2400 serotypes (serovars) by Kauffman-White methodology. The second species, *Salmonella bongori*, is inconsequential. Serotypes were named historically from the host or the geographic locale of the first isolate, such as *Salmonella typhimurium* or *Salmonella dublin*. However, under the new DNA division, *choleraesuis* was both a species and a serotype. To avoid confusion the name *Salmonella enterica* has been widely adopted. The first of the six subspecies (Group I) is also named *enterica*. It contains the more than 1400 serotypes that occur in warm-blooded animals. Using nomenclature employed by the United States Centers for Disease Control (CDC) and the World Health Organization (WHO), the species and subspecies name is understood and the serotype is capitalized. Thus, the formal *S. enterica* subspecies *enterica* serotype *typhimurium* becomes simply *S. Typhimurium*, which except for the capital *T* is where we started!

Epidemiology

In the last 25 years, the incidence of nontyphoid salmonellosis has increased two- to threefold, with approximately 1.5 million cases occurring annually in the United States. This is an underestimate because most cases are sporadic (endemic) and go unreported. Children younger than 5 years of age have the highest incidence of gastroenteritis and constitute the greatest number of cases.

Animals are the source of nontyphoid salmonella infection in humans. Infection occurs from food of animal origin such as meat, poultry, eggs, and dairy products. Contamination may occur during the production, slaughter, processing, or distribution of these products. Outbreaks have been associated with eggs, ice cream, and processed meats. Increasingly there have been outbreaks associated with raw vegetables (e.g., scallions) that are crosscontaminated during growth and distribution. Restaurant or home outbreaks occur in the context of improper preparation, cooking, and refrigeration. Most of the outbreaks can be attributed to centralized mass production and preparation of food along with globalization of the food trade. Novel sources of human salmonella include pet turtles, lizards, iguanas, African hedgehogs, rattlesnakes, and even marijuana contaminated by manure.

Emergence of antibiotic resistant species is a formidable problem. It is believed that resistance is driven worldwide by improper antibiotics use. However, in developed countries it is attributable to widespread use in animal feeds. Large numbers of transferable-resistance plasmids have been described. Resistance rates of more than 50% to ampicillin, chloramphenicol (Chloromycetin), and trimethoprim-sulfamethoxazole (TMP-SMZ) (Bactrim) occur in parts of Asia, Africa, and Latin America. One strain of *S. Typhimurium* (DT104) is resistant to five antimicrobials; the three mentioned previously plus tetracycline and streptomycin. This organism has spread widely in livestock throughout the United States, Canada, the United Kingdom, Europe, and the Middle East. Likewise, resistance to third-generation cephalosporins is increasing and is mediated by plasmids producing both regular and extended-spectrum beta-lactamases (ESBLs). Even more disturbing is fluoroquinolone resistance caused by mutated DNA gyrase, topoisomerase IV, or efflux pumps. The latter literally expel the quinolone from the bacterium before it can act on its target. Fluoroquinolone resistance is most pronounced in Southeast Asia, Europe, and the Middle East.

Pathogenesis

Human infection usually requires 10^6 organisms. Fewer organisms may cause disease in patients who have hypochlorhydria or achlorhydria, have impaired cellular immunity, are at the extremes of age, or are taking certain drugs (Table 2). *Salmonellae* predominately infect the terminal ileum and proximal colon through attachment. Initially, host response is by neutrophils followed by lymphocytes and macrophages. Strains vary genetically in their virulence and invasiveness. The organisms can survive intracellularly, thus avoiding antibiotic agents that lack intracellular penetration. Bacteria that are not contained regionally in the gut or lymph nodes may enter the blood. There are many predisposing factors associated with this and subsequent focal complications (see Table 2).

Clinical Presentation

Gastoenteritis

Acute gastroenteritis is by far the most common clinical presentation of salmonellosis. It should be emphasized that there is

---

TABLE 1 Clinical Presentations of Salmonellosis

Acute gastroenteritis (90%–95% of cases)

Bacteremia (< 5% of cases)
• Transient during acute gastroenteritis
• Enteric fever (nontyphoid)
• Persistent or recurrent (especially HIV)

Focal complications following bacteremia
• Bronchopneumonia, empyema, chest wall abscess
• Aortitis with mycotic aneurysm
• Prosthetic graft or valve infection
• Endocarditis, endarteritis
• Osteomyelitis (especially with sickle cell anemia)
• Septic arthritis
• Soft tissue abscess
• Hepatic or splenic abscess
• Meningitis or brain abscess
• Suppurative urogenital disease

Carriage (asymptomatic)
• Convalescent excretors (<2 mo)
• Convalescent carriers (2–12 mo)
• Chronic carriers (>12 mo)

TABLE 2 Predisposing Factors for Salmonellosis

Gastrointestinal
• Achlorhydria
• Gastric surgery
• Inflammatory bowel disease

Immune or structural compromise
• Age (<6 mo, >60 y)
• Lymphoma
• Splenectomy
• Cirrhosis with portal hypertension
• Diabetes mellitus
• Chronic uremia
• Hemolytic anemia (iron overload)
• Sickle cell (bone infarct, autosplenectomy)
• Systemic lupus
• Atheromata, aortic aneurysm

Infections
• HIV/AIDS (decreased T-cells)
• Malaria
• Bartonellosis
• Schistosomiasis

Drugs
• H_2-blockers, H^+ proton pump inhibitors
• Antibiotic administration
• Antimotility agents
• Chemotherapy
• Corticosteroids
• Transplant antirejection agents

considerable overlap in its presentation with other infectious intestinal pathogens such as *Campylobacter* species. Given this, the incubation ranges from 6 to 96 hours but most commonly occurs between 12 and 48 hours. Initial symptoms include nausea and vomiting, followed by headaches, myalgias, malaise, chills, low-grade fever, abdominal cramps, and diarrhea. High temperatures (40°C [104°F]) should alert the clinician to invasive disease. Stools may be merely loose or profuse and watery. On direct examination, they may or may not contain polymorphonuclear leukocytes or occult blood. The presence of mucus or gross blood in the absence of hemorrhoids or fissures should alert the clinician to organisms causing dysentery such as *Shigella* species. The white blood cell count is most often normal or slightly elevated, with a left shift containing 10 to 15 bands. Low white blood cell counts with greater numbers of bands should alert the clinician to possible bacteremia or enteric fever. The diagnosis can be confirmed only by stool or blood culture. Serum serology examinations are not helpful. Most healthy adults have a self-limited, uncomplicated course, with resolution of symptoms without treatment within 48 to 72 hours.

Treatment

Fluid and Electrolyte Replacement

The sine qua non in the treatment of diarrhea is fluid and electrolyte replacement. In most cases increased oral intake of bland juices coupled with clear broth and temporary elimination of lactose-containing foods will suffice. Commercial electrolyte solutions (Pedialyte) may be useful. Although not readily available in the United States, rehydration salts are widely employed in many developing countries. WHO distributes packets containing its recommended formula of 90 mmol sodium, 20 mmol potassium, 80 mmol chloride, 30 mmol bicarbonate, along with 111 mmol glucose to dissolve in 1 L sterile or boiled water. This mixture should be consumed at a rate sufficient to compensate for diarrheal losses while maintaining an adequate output of dilute-appearing urine. Within 24 to 48 hours, the diet can be supplemented with bland, soft foods given in small, frequent feedings. If the patient has profuse vomiting or severe dehydration as determined by orthostatic changes in blood pressure, parenteral rehydration should be used. Frequently, this can be accomplished as an outpatient in an infusion room or with a home agency rather than through admission to hospital. When there is persistent emesis, profuse diarrhea, systemic toxicity, or abnormalities in serum electrolytes, parenteral rehydration in hospital is prudent.

Antimotility and Antinausea Agents

The use of agents such as atropine-diphenoxylate (Lomotil) or loperamide (Imodium) should be discouraged. Although they may result in symptomatic improvement in cramps and diarrhea, they can increase complications and even predispose to bacteremia. In general, if the patient has a fever and the diarrhea contains blood or mucus, their use should be eschewed. Most pediatricians feel they should never be used in children younger than 5 years of age. An alternative is bismuth subsalicylate (Pepto-Bismol). The adult dose is 1 ounce (2 tablespoons) or 2 tablets (262.5 mg) every 30 minutes for 8 hours. The pediatric dose is 1.1 mL/kg at 4-hour intervals for up to 5 days. Although nausea and vomiting are occasional presenting symptoms with enterocolitis, they rarely persist. Prochlorperazine (Compazine) or trimethobenzamide (Tigan) may be helpful. Both are available in oral, suppository, or parenteral form, even though injectable prochlorperazine (Compazine) has been in short supply. Suppositories usually stimulate further diarrhea. Vomiting may preclude oral administration. A singular muscular injection of prochlorperazine (Compazine) 5 to 10 mg, is often all that is needed. This may be repeated every 4 to 6 hours as needed. Promethazine hydrochloride (Phenergan) is more frequently used in children and may be used orally (0.5 mg/pound or 1 mg/kg every 6 hours) or intramuscularly in the same doses. A 5-HT$_3$ receptor antagonist such as ondansetron (Zofran)[1] is expensive and inefficacious.

Antibiotics

The routine empiric use of antibiotics, especially fluoroquinolones, for any and all cases of diarrhea is not only unjustifiable but should be decried. Certainly antibiotics are not needed in the treatment of uncomplicated *Salmonella* gastroenteritis in otherwise healthy children or adults. Studies have shown that they neither shorten the course nor improve symptoms. No doubt some of this usage is patient driven. However, overuse is contributing to the emergence of resistance, and may increase risk of symptomatic and bacteriologic relapse. Indeed, antibiotic use may actually prolong the convalescent excretion or contribute to chronic carriage of the organism. Postponing antibiotic therapy until the return of a stool culture often provides the physician with a way to avert the frequent demand for antibiotic therapy. Often patients are better by the time results become available. Nevertheless, high-risk patients, as previously identified (see Table 2), should receive treatment to prevent potential complications from bacteremia. Additionally, if patients are sick enough to require hospitalization, antibiotic therapy should be considered.

Appropriate antibiotic therapy should be guided by susceptibility testing. Initially, TMP-SMZ (cotrimoxazole, Bactrim, or Septra)[1] may be administered to the nonsulfonamide-sensitive patient. The dose is 5 to 8 mg/kg trimethoprim every 12 hours for children or 1 double-strength tablet (160 mg trimethoprim/800 mg sulfamethoxazole) every 12 hours for adults. Although widely used, trimethoprim-sulfamethoxazole has not yet received FDA approval. If the organism is susceptible, ampicillin, 50 mg/kg orally to 100 mg/kg/day intravenously, each in four divided doses for children, or 2 to 4 g/day in four divided doses for adults, may be administered. Amoxicillin (Amoxil)[1] in equivalent oral dosage may be substituted. The duration of therapy is generally 5 days.

Newer fluoroquinolone antibiotics, such as ciprofloxacin,[1] ofloxacin,[1] and norfloxacin,[1] are among the most effective agents, with excellent oral bioavailability and intracellular concentration. They are contraindicated in prepubertal children and pregnant women. Adult doses are ciprofloxacin (Cipro), 500 mg twice daily; ofloxacin (Floxin), 400 mg twice daily; or norfloxacin (Noroxin), 400 mg twice daily. It must be emphasized that the trend in the United States to use these agents empirically for all suspected bacterial diarrhea should be vigorously resisted by the thoughtful clinician.

Bacteremia and Focal Infection

Bacteremia in acute uncomplicated *Salmonella* gastroenteritis is infrequent. Therefore, blood cultures are not routinely necessary except for patients who are in high-risk categories. Shaking chills or high fever (40°C [104°F]) should alert the clinician to possible bacteremia. Focal suppurative infection following bacteremia is also infrequent but may occur at any site. Thus, *Salmonella* has been associated with bronchopneumonia, soft tissue infection, aortic mycotic aneurysms, endocarditis, septic arthritis, splenic or hepatic abscesses, meningitis, and osteomyelitis. The clinician should suspect an endovascular mycotic aneurysm in all blood culture–positive patients older than 50 years of age. *Salmonella* should always be suspected in individuals with sickle cell disease in whom bone and joint infection is the most frequent cause of extraintestinal infection. Meningitis occurs primarily in infants younger than 5 months of age. The diagnosis of a *Salmonella* bacteremia in HIV patients will almost always be accompanied by recurrent episodes.

Treatment

Antibiotics

Bacteremia and localized suppurative infection require antibiotic therapy. The choice of effective treatment is less predictable with the emergence of resistance. Therapy must be altered according to the results of susceptibility testing. Therefore the recovery of the organism is extremely important, and adequate cultures of blood or infected material must be obtained before initiation of therapy.

Parenteral ampicillin, 100 to 200 mg/kg/day divided into four doses, or TMP/SMZ,[1] 8 to 10 mg/kg of trimethoprim per day

---

[1] Not FDA approved for this indication.

[1] Not FDA approved for this indication.

in three divided doses, may be used. In the case of resistance or allergy to the foregoing, third-generation cephalosporins such as cefotaxime (Claforan) or ceftriaxone (Rocephin) have reasonable activity, but intracellular concentrations are not optimal. Cefotaxime, 1 to 2 grams every 6 to 8 hours for adults, or 100 to 200 mg/kg/day in three or four divided doses for children, has been found effective in bacteremia, osteomyelitis, septic arthritis, and a variety of other focal *Salmonella* infections. The use of chloramphenicol (Chloromycetin) is not recommended, but a preparation of it in oil (Typhomycine)[2] is in use in developing countries. Ciprofloxacin (Cipro)[1] 7.5 mg/kg intravenously twice daily is becoming a favored agent; not only is it effective, but oral bioequivalence facilitates the change to 500 to 750 mg by mouth twice daily. If fluoroquinolone resistance is encountered, imipenem (Primaxin)[1] may be tried. Efficacy data for it or other agents such as azithromycin (Zithromax)[1] are scant.

Surgery

Focal infection often requires surgery. Often this is as simple as the drainage of localized suppuration or lavage of a septic joint. However, in the case of infected aortic aneurysms, extensive resection and vascular reconstruction are required. Infected prosthetic grafts must be removed in nearly all cases, with courses of antibiotics before and after surgery.

The duration of therapy for simple bacteremia is 10 to 14 days. Septic arthritis is usually treated for 4 weeks whereas osteomyelitis and endovascular infections require 6 weeks. Oral fluoroquinolones such as ciprofloxacin (Cipro), 500 mg twice daily, may be helpful in treating osteomyelitis. TMP-SMZ (Bactrim)[1] can also be used in this manner. Both have adequate blood levels after oral administration. I have had to use continuous prophylaxis of either TMP-SMZ or ciprofloxacin in several HIV patients to prevent recurrent bacteremia. Because prophylactic TMP-SMZ is used chronically for *Pneumocystis*, it may be preferred.

Enteric Fever

The clinical picture of nontyphoid *Salmonella* enteric fever is indistinguishable from that of typhoid fever, which is discussed elsewhere in this publication. However, the following discussion also applies to enteric fever caused by nontyphoid *Salmonellae*.

Treatment

The adjunct and antibiotic therapy of nontyphoid enteric fever parallels that of the treatment of typhoid. Antibiotics should be adjusted and altered once the results of susceptibility testing are available. Acceptable regimens include ampicillin, amoxicillin,[1] and TMP-SMZ (Bactrim),[1] along with third-generation cephalosporins and fluoroquinolone antibiotics. My preference was cefotaxime (Claforan)[1] in the same doses as for bacteremic salmonellosis. The duration is 10 to 14 days. Relapse rates are low, and relapse is seen within 2 to 6 weeks. Relapse requires an equivalent course of therapy in both dose and duration. Currently, I prefer ciprofloxacin (Cipro)[1] intravenously 7.5 mg/kg every 12 hours continued until the patient is afebrile and clinically able to start taking it orally. Comparative studies are ongoing, using both third-generation cephalosporins, such as ceftriaxone (Rocephin)[1] or cefixime (Suprax),[1] and oral fluoroquinolones in short-course therapy of typhoid as well as nontyphoid enteric fever. Although these show some promise, they are currently not the standard of practice in the United States. Nevertheless, a strong case can be made for oral fluoroquinolones use, with obvious cost saving. Otherwise healthy young adults may be treated orally as outpatients. This advantage, if for no other reason, should prevent the physician from prescribing quinolones for uncomplicated gastroenteritis or other self-limited diarrheas of bacterial origin.

Adjunctive measures are of importance, including attention to fluid and electrolyte balance and nutrition. As in typhoid, the routine use of corticosteroids is controversial. Use in patients who are steroid dependent or believed to be hypoadrenal is indicated. In those who are delirious, obtunded, comatose, or in shock it may be warranted, but there are little supportive data. It has been my overall impression that nontyphoid enteric fever is somewhat milder than typhoid itself, and complications such as gastrointestinal bleeding or ileal perforation are exceedingly rare.

Carrier State

Asymptomatic excretion of organisms invariably occurs following clinical *Salmonella* gastroenteritis. It exceeds 8 weeks in 5% to 10% of patients. Chronic carriage, either in the stool or urine, is defined as excretion of the organism for more than 1 year. Its incidence is stated to be 1% in adults and 5% in children younger than 5 years of age. This is somewhat less than that seen with *S. typhi*. Convalescent excreters need only maintain strict personal hygiene to prevent transmission of the organism. Those involved in food preparation or in child care and health care should be kept off work until three successive cultures are negative at intervals required by the public health department. It goes without saying that all positive cases of salmonellosis are reportable by law to local public health authorities.

Recently, oral quinolones have been used (ciprofloxacin [Cipro],[1] 500 to 750 mg twice daily for 5 to 14 days) to curtail institutional outbreaks, as in nursing homes or psychiatric facilities. Although this may be expeditious, eliminating or preventing the source of the outbreak in a prospective fashion is preferable. In the case of food handlers and health care or child care workers, some feel that quinolone therapy eliminates the problem of convalescent excretion, hence individuals may return to work without delay. The data are debatable and the successive negative stool requirement will not be obviated.

The management of the chronic carriage of nontyphoidal salmonellosis is the same as that of *S. typhi*, which is discussed in detail elsewhere. A 4- to 6-week course of oral antibiotics may be tried when no evidence of gallbladder disease exists. However, if chronic cholecystitis and/or cholelithiasis are present, cholecystectomy is almost always necessary. Despite cholecystectomy, a certain number of individuals will continue to excrete organisms thought to be of hepatobiliary origin. Chronic carriage is seen, albeit rarely, in the United States with either *Schistosoma mansoni* or *Schistosoma haematobium*. When these parasites are treated, subsequent therapy of the *Salmonella* results in termination of the stool or urinary carrier state.

Prevention

Prevention of salmonellosis has both personal and public health dimensions. Food and leftovers should be rapidly refrigerated. I recommend separate plastic (not wood) cutting boards for meats and vegetables and washing them after each use. Spillage of raw animal juices should be immediately cleaned. All preparation surfaces should be washed and dried after each meal. Detergent rather than antibacterial cleaners should be used; bleach is beautiful.

Public health surveillance is essential via regular inspection of restaurants, food retailers, and industrial food processors. National efforts to coordinate and computerize surveillance systems such as FoodNet should be expanded and fully funded so as to guarantee our food supply. Preservation technologies, including irradiation, need study.

Finally, the practicing physician should take the time to reiterate to patients with HIV or malignancies or other immune-compromised patients (see Table 2) how they can avoid food-borne pathogens.

References

Brenner FW, Villar RG, Angulo FJ, et al: Salmonella nomenclature, *J Clin Microbiol* 38:2465, 2000.
Fierer J, Swancutt M: Non-typhoid *Salmonella*: A review. In Remington JS, Swartz MN, editors: *Current Clinical Topics in Infectious Diseases 20*, Boston, 2000, Blackwell Science, pp 134–157.

---

[1] Not FDA approved for this indication.
[2] Not available in the United States.

---

[1] Not FDA approved for this indication.

Herikstad H, Hayes P, Mokhtar M, et al: Emerging quinolone-resistant Salmonella in the United States, *Emerg Infect Dis* 3:371–372, 1997.

Molbak K: Human health consequences of antimicrobial drug resistant *Salmonella* and other foodborne pathogens, *Clin Infect Dis* 41:1613–1620, 2005.

Sirinivan S, Garner P: Antibiotics for treating Salmonella gut infections, *Cochrane Database Sys Rev* 93, 2000, CD001167.

Su LH, Chiu CH, Chu CS, et al: Antimicrobial resistance in nontyphoid *Salmonella*: A global challenge, *Clin Infect Dis* 39:546–551, 2004.

Voetsch AC, Van Gilder TJ, Angulo FJ, et al: FoodNet estimate of the burden of illness caused by nontyphoidal Salmonella infections in the United States, *Clin Infect Dis* 38(Suppl. 3):S127–S134, 2004.

SEVERE SEPSIS

Method of
Jerome Larkin, MD; and Marisa Holubar, MD

CURRENT DIAGNOSIS

Systemic Inflammatory Response Syndrome (SIRS)
- Diagnosis is based on the presence of two or more of the following:
  - Temperature >38°C or <36°C
  - Pulse >90 beats/min
  - Respirations >20 breaths/min or arterial partial pressure of carbon dioxide ($Paco_2$) <32 mm Hg
  - White blood cell count >12,000 or <4000 cells/mm³ or >10% bands

Sepsis
- Diagnosis is based on a finding of SIRS plus proven or suspected infection as the cause.

Severe Sepsis
- Diagnosis is based on a finding of sepsis plus organ dysfunction of one or more major systems (typically kidney, lung, or heart; less often, central nervous system).

Septic Shock
- Diagnosis is based on a finding of severe sepsis plus persistent hypotension despite aggressive fluid resuscitation (i.e., vasopressors are required to maintain mean arterial pressure >65 mm Hg).

Supportive Laboratory Findings
- Hyperglycemia
- Lactic acidosis
- Hyperbilirubinemia
- Acute renal failure
- Thrombocytopenia
- Coagulopathy
- Leukocytosis or leukopenia
- Elevated erythrocyte sedimentation rate or C-reactive protein

Supportive Physical Findings
- Decreased capillary refill or mottling of skin
- Mental status changes or obtundation
- Tachypnea or respiratory failure
- Tachycardia
- Anuria or oliguria
- Edema

CURRENT THERAPY

Initial 6 Hours
- Initiate fluid resuscitation with crystalloid or colloid to achieve central venous pressure of 12 mm Hg (or 15 mm Hg if intubated).

- Add dopamine (Intropin) or norepinephrine (Levophed) for persistent hypotension (mean arterial pressure <65 mm Hg).
- Obtain blood, urine, and other appropriate cultures (cerebrospinal fluid, abscess drainage, catheter tip, tissue, sputum).
- Administer empiric antimicrobial therapy.
- Perform appropriate imaging studies with urgent source control as indicated and allowed by clinical status; remove potentially infected foreign bodies.
- All interventions should be undertaken simultaneously and initiated within 1 hour after making a presumptive diagnosis of sepsis.

Subsequent Interventions
- Maintain glycemic control with a target blood glucose level of less than 150 mg/dL.
- Use unfractionated or low-molecular-weight heparin for prophylaxis against deep venous thrombosis.
- Use a histamine 2 (H_2) blocker or proton pump inhibitor for gastric ulcer prophylaxis.
- Initiate therapy with dobutamine (Dobutrex) for low cardiac output in the face of adequate filling pressures.
- Consider therapy with activated protein C (drotrecogin alfa [Xigris]) for patients with an Acute Physiology and Chronic Health Evaluation (APACHE) II score of 25 or greater.
- Consider therapy with hydrocortisone (Solu-Cortef)[1] for patients with continued hypotension despite adequate fluid resuscitation and vasopressors.
- Achieve adequate sedation.

[1]Not FDA approved for this indication.

Epidemiology

Sepsis is the tenth most common cause of death in the United States. The incidence is highest during the winter, most likely reflecting increased respiratory viral infections that precede the development of community-acquired pneumonia, which is itself a medical condition with increased risk of developing severe sepsis.

A remarkable aspect of sepsis, severe sepsis, and septic shock is the relatively small number of associated pathogens out of the more than 1000 microorganisms known to cause human disease. *Staphylococcus aureus*, streptococci, enterococci, and gram-negative rods are the most commonly isolated species. *Escherichia coli, Klebsiella, Pseudomonas, Serratia, Acinetobacter, Enterobacter, Citrobacter,* and *Neisseria meningitidis* (a gram-negative coccus) constitute the most common gram-negative pathogens. This relative paucity of etiologic bacterial pathogens has implications for empiric antimicrobial therapy. The emergence of resistant organisms, particularly methicillin-resistant *S. aureus* (MRSA) and gram-negative bacteria harboring extended-spectrum β-lactamases, increases the risk of antibiotic failure and attendant mortality. Fungal pathogens, particularly non-candidal species, continue to increase in incidence. This is most likely the result of better empiric management of gram-negative and candidal sepsis in patients with hematologic malignancies.

Although sepsis is most typically a disease of the elderly, the immune suppressed, and those with chronic medical problems, otherwise young and healthy individuals can also be stricken with no clear cause or known risk factor, such as in meningococcemia, toxic shock syndrome, and necrotizing fasciitis.

Definitions

The term *sepsis* derives from a Greek word that generally implies putrefaction. It also has a colloquial meaning, understood by most laypeople to mean a serious, potentially overwhelming infection. Historically, it has been intuitively understood by physicians to mean an infection, once localized, that has now disseminated and is life threatening. Bacteremia is implied if not always proven. Sepsis was usually fatal in the preantibiotic era, and its morbidity and mortality remain substantial.

In 2001, a consensus conference, sponsored by the American College of Chest Physicians and the Society of Critical Care Medicine and involving the European Society of Intensive Care Medicine, the Surgical Infection Society, and the American Thoracic Society, was convened to arrive at a specific definition of sepsis. They defined systemic inflammatory response syndrome (SIRS) as a state of immune activation characterized by the findings of fever with tachycardia, tachypnea, and/or leukocytosis or leukopenia. Although sensitive, this definition is so overly broad as to be rather unhelpful to an experienced clinician who would not need to resort to such terms to understand that a patient is seriously ill. Nonetheless, it provides a useful construct in beginning to arrive at a specific definition of sepsis. Both infectious and noninfectious processes—severe burns and pancreatitis being the most notable examples of the latter—can cause SIRS.

Sepsis is defined as the finding of SIRS in the presence of known or suspected invasion by a microbe into a normally sterile body site. Severe sepsis is sepsis that has become more generalized. The cardinal finding is organ dysfunction that is unrelated to the primary site of infection. Other typical findings include hyperglycemia, thrombocytopenia, hyperbilirubinemia, acidosis, coagulopathy, edema, oliguria, hypotension, ileus, hypoxia, and poor perfusion. Heart, kidney, and respiratory failure are the most common forms of organ dysfunction. Altered sensorium is also common. Septic shock refers to the presence of hypotension with systolic blood pressure lower than 90 mm Hg or mean arterial pressure lower than 60 mm Hg despite adequate fluid resuscitation. These terms (sepsis, severe sepsis, and septic shock) are all part of a continuum, implying a progressively graver degree of illness with associated increasing mortality. No single symptom, physical finding, organ dysfunction, or laboratory abnormality serves to make or exclude the diagnosis, although isolation of a microorganism in the setting of such findings is highly suggestive. Increasing numbers of physical findings and other abnormalities correlate with an increasing likelihood of the diagnosis of sepsis.

Pathophysiology

Infection of the immunocompetent host by a microorganism typically leads to immune activation. This serves to isolate the site and source of infection. Local tissue is often damaged, but eventually the infection is cleared, and repair and regeneration occur. This process is highly regulated, with a number of different cell types and mediators involved, all in delicate balance between proinflammatory and antiinflammatory effects. The patient may have few or no symptoms, or there may be systemic evidence of infection (i.e., SIRS). Sepsis is the failure of localization such that the process becomes generalized and leads to tissue destruction remote from the site of infection. Why the immune system enters this state of dysregulation remains unknown, although an enormous amount of research over the past 4 decades has elucidated many of the pathways and mediators involved. Tumor necrosis factor, platelet-activating factor, interleukins, eicosanoids, interferons, and nitric oxide are among the biologically active molecules characterized to date. Particular microbes also contribute to this process through the elaboration of toxins (typically by gram-positive organisms) and endotoxins (gram-negative–derived lipopolysaccharide). These events lead to tissue destruction as a result of ischemic insult, direct cytotoxicity, and accelerated apoptosis. The characterization of inflammatory mediators has led to attempts to modify the immune response through the use of novel therapies such as monoclonal antibodies directed against tumor necrosis factor. To date such attempts have not met with success, and investigation continues.

Diagnosis

The diagnosis of sepsis ultimately relies on the clinical suspicion of infection in the setting of SIRS. A constellation of other supportive evidence establishes a greater or lesser likelihood of the presence of sepsis (see the Current Diagnosis box). It is rare that specific microbiologic evidence for infection is available in a manner timely enough to determine that sepsis is present or to help guide the initial, typically urgent, therapy. When it is available, it usually is a Gram stain or other type of specialized microbiology stain that confirms the presence of a potential pathogen in a site where none should be (e.g., gram-positive cocci in cerebrospinal fluid). Early therapy therefore relies on aggressive resuscitative measures and the administration of empiric antibiotics.

Treatment

Early Goal-Directed Resuscitation: The First 6 Hours

Initial treatment of sepsis should focus on correction of hemodynamic parameters, early administration of antibiotics, and source control of potential sites of infection. The 2008 guidelines from the Surviving Sepsis Campaign, an international initiative to improve sepsis outcomes, emphasized the importance of aggressive fluid resuscitation. Therapy should be implemented according to a protocol directed at achieving the following specific goals:

- Central venous pressure 8 to 12 mm Hg, or 12 to 15 mm Hg in those who are mechanically ventilated or have decreased left ventricular compliance
- Central venous or mixed venous oxygen saturation 70% or greater
- Mean arterial pressure (MAP) 65 mm Hg or greater
- Urine output 0.5 mL/kg/hr or greater

Administration of fluid boluses of 1000 mL or more of crystalloids or 300 to 500 mL of colloids over 30 minutes should begin as soon as hypoperfusion is recognized. There is no evidence that one type of fluid is superior to the other, although crystalloid is substantially cheaper. In cases of profound intravascular volume depletion, more rapid and more frequent fluid administration may be needed. Hemodynamic improvement (decreased heart rate, increased blood pressure, increased urine output) and the goal of optimizing central venous pressure should direct the need for continued infusion of fluid while avoiding the development of volume overload and pulmonary edema. Transfusion of packed red blood cells should be considered if anemia is present, with a goal of achieving a hemoglobin level of 7.0 to 9.0 g/dL. If tissue hypoperfusion or hypoxia persists (central mixed venus oxygen saturation <70%) despite achieving a central venous pressure of 12 mm Hg, therapy with dopamine (Intropin) or norepinephrine (Levophed) should be initiated with a goal of achieving a MAP of 65 mm Hg. There is no role for the use of low-dose dopamine for renal protection. An arterial line for more precise and continuous measurement of blood pressure should be inserted as soon as possible after the initiation of vasopressor therapy. Ideally, vasopressors should not be introduced to increase MAP until after the fluid deficit has been corrected. However, in cases of severe shock, vasopressor therapy may be needed early in the resuscitation effort to improve perfusion to the peripheral vascular beds. If there is no response to dopamine and norepinephrine, the patient should be treated with epinephrine (Adrenalin).[1]

Appropriate antibiotics should be administered within 1 hour after diagnosis of severe sepsis or septic shock, because mortality increases in a linear fashion with each hour of delay. All efforts should be made to obtain appropriate cultures, in particular at least two sets of blood cultures. At least one of these should be peripheral, with the second from any long-term (>48 hours) vascular device. Cultures of urine, sputum, wounds, abscesses, and cerebrospinal fluid should also be obtained as appropriate and before the administration of antibiotics, assuming that such specimens can be obtained during the first hour. Specific antibiotic choices are discussed later.

Source Control

A survey for potential sources of infection should be performed, and early resuscitation efforts should occur concomitantly. Elimination of the source of infection is critical to reversing septic shock. Conditions that require emergent intervention, such as necrotizing fasciitis, cholangitis, and intestinal infarction, should be ruled

---

[1] Not FDA approved for this indication.

out within the first 6 hours after presentation. Potentially infected indwelling devices should be removed as soon as possible. Necrotic tissue should be débrided and abscesses drained if either condition is detected. Practitioners must consider the risks and benefits of the specific invasive procedures and the timing of such interventions for each patient individually. Every effort should be made to limit the invasiveness of necessary procedures, to avoid further stress in patients with an already hemodynamically fragile state. Imaging studies such as computed tomography of the head, chest, abdomen, and pelvis are necessary to identify or rule out potential sources of infection. An exception to the mandate to drain or débride infected collections is the presence of infected pancreatic necrosis, in which case surgical intervention should be delayed.

Other Interventions

After hemodynamic parameters have been stabilized with fluid and vasopressors, cultures have been obtained, antibiotics have been administered, and initial source control of infected foci has been achieved, other interventions may be appropriate. Many of these are typical components of good critical care.

Cardiac Dysfunction. Patients who have adequate left ventricular filling pressures (as determined by a central venous pressure ≥12 mm Hg) but low cardiac output may benefit from therapy with dobutamine (Dobutrex) to increase cardiac output and improve tissue perfusion.

Corticosteroid Therapy. Activation of the hypothalamic-pituitary axis and the consequent increase in serum cortisol levels are vital aspects of the body's acute stress response to shock. Recent data suggest that critical illness–related corticosteroid insufficiency is more prevalent in septic shock than previously thought, with rates as high as 60%. Therapy with corticosteroids is indicated only for those patients who have continued hypotension in the face of adequate fluid resuscitation and vasopressor support. Hydrocortisone (Solu-Cortef)[1] should be administered intravenously 200–300 mg/day for 7 days, either divided every 6 hours or as a continuous infusion. Dexamethasone (Decadron)[1] should not be used unless hydrocortisone is not available. Because of the unclear long-term benefits and the known immunosuppressive side effects of corticosteroids, patients should be weaned from hydrocortisone as soon as vasopressors are no longer necessary. If another form of corticosteroid other than hydrocortisone is used, then fludrocortisone (Florinef)[1] at a dose of 50 mcg/day should be added for mineralocorticoid effect.

Activated Protein C. Patients who are at increased risk of death with Acute Physiology and Chronic Health Evaluation (APACHE) II scores (https://www.mdcalc.com/apache-ii-score) of 25 or higher and those with multiple organ dysfunction may benefit from infusion of activated protein C (drotrecogin alfa [Xigris]). This drug has numerous contraindications, including current active bleeding, recent (within 3 months) hemorrhagic stroke, recent (within 2 months) severe head trauma or intracranial or intraspinal surgery, trauma with a risk of life-threatening bleeding, presence of an epidural catheter, and intracranial neoplasm or mass lesion or evidence of herniation. It is not recommended for use in children. It is given as a 96-hour continuous infusion.

Glycemic Control. Maintenance of the blood glucose concentration lower than 150 mg/dL is associated with decreased mortality and length of stay in the intensive care unit. Control should be achieved with intravenous insulin, paying close attention to serum glucose levels every 1 to 2 hours until stable, with adjustments made on the basis of a validated protocol. Patients receiving intravenous insulin should simultaneously receive some form of glucose as a calorie source to minimize the risk of hypoglycemia.

Sedation and Paralytics. Sedation and treatment of pain should be aggressively managed according to validated protocols. Daily interruption of sedation allows for more accurate titration of drug and decreases the total time of mechanical ventilation. Paralytics should be avoided or used only briefly if required.

Anticoagulation. Patients should receive prophylaxis for deep venous thrombosis with either low-molecular-weight heparin or unfractionated heparin unless contraindicated by severe thrombocytopenia, recent intracranial bleeding, or coagulopathy. Those patients who cannot receive heparin should receive prophylaxis with graduated compression stockings or intermittent compression devices. Patients who are at especially high risk for deep venous thrombosis (e.g., prior history of clot, orthopaedic surgery, trauma) should receive both pharmacologic and mechanical prophylaxis. Low-molecular-weight heparin is preferred to unfractionated heparin in high-risk patients.

Ulcer Prophylaxis. Patients should receive prophylaxis with a proton pump inhibitor or a histamine 2 (H_2) blocker to prevent upper gastrointestinal bleeding.

Bicarbonate Therapy. There is no role for the administration of bicarbonate to correct acidosis or improve hemodynamic status.

Antibiotics

Antibiotic choices should take into account the most likely pathogens for the suspected site or process. In general, initial empiric therapy (Table 1) should be broad, with an intention to narrow therapy once a microorganism has been isolated or a more precise clinical diagnosis has been made. Such a reevaluation should take place approximately 72 hours after the initiation of therapy. Numerous studies have documented the mortality associated with initial therapy that did not include agents active against the pathogen eventually isolated. In general, drugs from the β-lactam and related classes of antibiotics should be preferred for at least a part of most empiric regimens.

Special considerations include patients with neutropenia and fever, who should always be treated with at least one agent active against *Pseudomonas*. Some debate continues regarding the use of two anti-pseudomonal drugs as part of the initial antibiotic regimen. Given the possibility of resistance on the part of this pathogen, it would seem reasonable to use two drugs initially, until *Pseudomonas* has been isolated (if present) and its susceptibilities are known, allowing coverage to be narrowed. The Surviving Sepsis Campaign guidelines advocate this approach. There is no benefit in treating with two drugs known to be active in an attempt to achieve a supposed synergy.

Patients with hematologic malignancies are at increased risk for sepsis from fungal organisms. Severe sepsis or septic shock in such patients warrants empiric treatment with an echinocandin, a broad-spectrum azole such as voriconazole (Vfend) or posaconazole (Noxafil), or amphotericin (Fungizone).

MRSA continues to increase in incidence nationally and is now common as a community-acquired pathogen. It is also to be suspected as a cause of postinfluenza bacterial pneumonia. Empiric treatment with an antibiotic active against this bacterium, such as vancomycin (Vancocin), linezolid (Zyvox), or daptomycin (Cubicin), should be strongly considered in septic patients in communities where the rate of MRSA in bloodstream infections exceeds 10%. This pathogen should always be considered in a patient with a long-term intravenous catheter, prosthetic device, or other indwelling foreign body. Although vancomycin-resistant *S. aureus* is extremely rare, caution should be taken when using daptomycin and linezolid as empiric therapy, because resistance has been reported.

Prior administration of antibiotics and the attendant risk of infection by a pathogen resistant to the previous therapy should be considered in arriving at a course of empiric therapy. A typical scenario is a patient who presents with a catheter-related bloodstream infection while taking vancomycin. One would expect a gram-negative bacterium, a fungal organism, or, potentially, a vancomycin-resistant enterococcus as the pathogen. Recent hospitalization or residence in a nursing home places patients at risk for colonization and subsequent infection with resistant gram-negative rods.

Prognosis and Limits of Care

Patients who present with severe sepsis or septic shock often have substantial prior medical morbidity, decreasing their chances of

TABLE 1	Empiric Antibiotic Choices for Severe Sepsis*		
SOURCE	**ANTIBIOTIC AND DOSE**	**COMMENTS**
Community-acquired pneumonia	Ceftriaxone (Rocephin) 2 g q24h *plus* azithromycin (Zithromax) 500 mg q24h	Should include atypical coverage; alternative is moxifloxacin (Avelox)
Health care–associated pneumonia	Piperacillin/tazobactam (Zosyn) 4.5 g q6h *or* meropenem (Merrem)[1] 2 g q8h[3] *plus* vancomycin (Vancocin)[1] 1 g q12h	Should cover for *Pseudomonas* and other resistant gram-negative rods
Neutropenia/fever	Piperacillin/tazobactam[1] 4.5 g q6h *or* meropenem[1] 2 g q8h[3]	Consider empiric fungal coverage for prolonged neutropenia
Abdominal sepsis	Ampicillin/sulbactam (Unasyn) 3 g q6h *or* piperacillin/ tazobactam 4.5 g q6h	Consider coverage for yeast, MRSA
Urosepsis	Ampicillin/sulbactam[1] 3 g q6h *or* piperacillin/tazobactam[1] 4.5 g q6h	Obtain imaging and decompression as appropriate
Foreign body/vascular catheter–related sepsis	Piperacillin/tazobactam[1] 4.5 g q6h *or* meropenem[1] 2 g q8h[3] *plus* vancomycin 1 g q12h	Vascular catheters or other foreign bodies should be removed urgently
Meningitis	Ceftriaxone 2 g q12h *plus* vancomycin[1] 750 mg q8h *plus* rifampin (Rifadin)[1] 600 mg q24h	Consider steroid therapy before or simultaneously with administration of antibiotics
Soft-tissue infection	Cefazolin (Ancef) 2 g q8h *plus* vancomycin 1 g q12h	Image for abscess with débridement as appropriate
Necrotizing fasciitis	Ampicillin/sulbactam 3 g q6h *plus* vancomycin 1 g q12h *plus* clindamycin (Cleocin) 900 mg q8h	Obtain urgent surgical consultation
Unknown	Piperacillin/tazobactam 4.5 g q6h *or* meropenem 2 g q8h[3] *plus* vancomycin 1 g q12h *plus* tobramycin (Tobrex) 7 mg/kg q24h	Obtain appropriate imaging studies, especially of abdomen, pelvis, central nervous system

[1]Not FDA approved for this indication.
[3]Exceeds dosage recommended by the manufacturer.
*In all cases, prior antimicrobial therapy, kidney and liver dysfunction, and the probable source of sepsis should be carefully considered. Always consider coverage for methicillin-resistant *Staphylococcus aureus* (MRSA) in areas where incidence in bloodstream isolates is >10%.

survival. The overall mortality rate remains between 20% and 40%. Patients often have expressed wishes regarding limits of care to family members or others close to them before becoming ill. It is always appropriate to discuss goals of therapy, possible and probable outcomes, and plans for further evaluation and treatment with patients (if possible) and their proxies in all instances. Decisions to proceed with or limit care should be made within the context of a patient's expressed or expected wishes and should take into account unfolding clinical data and circumstances. Time spent in this endeavor can substantially decrease the amount of futile care rendered to a patient and lead to care that more truly reflects the patient's wishes regarding life-prolonging measures. The stress and anxiety experienced by family members may also be reduced.

Substantial progress has been made in the past 3 decades in decreasing the mortality associated with severe sepsis and septic shock. Nevertheless, the mortality rate remains unacceptably high, and the overall incidence and severity of disease appear to be increasing, by as much as 1.5% annually by some estimates. The risk of death for an individual patient appears to stabilize approximately 6 months after the original illness. Many patients who do survive remain with the same risk factors (e.g., diabetes, vascular disease, prosthetic devices, immunosuppression) that contributed to their infection and therefore are at risk for recurrence. Moreover, certain organisms, such as MRSA, resistant gram-negative rods, and fungi, remain difficult to treat, and success rates are relatively low despite aggressive, timely, and prolonged therapy.

There is some cause for optimism. The Surviving Sepsis Campaign has now entered phase III. This is a program in which a core set of recommendations, described in the guidelines, is being implemented with opportunities to measure outcomes, assess physician behavior, and provide feedback to improve survival through evidence-based interventions. This effort involves more than 12,000 patients in 239 hospitals in 17 countries and will undoubtedly change the future course of this lethal disease.

References

Bone RC: Immunologic dissonance: A continuing evolution in our understanding of the systemic inflammatory response syndrome (SIRS) and the multiple organ dysfunction syndrome (MODS), *Ann Intern Med* 125:680–687, 1996.

Delinger RP, Levy MM, Carlet JM, et al: Surviving Sepsis Campaign: Internatonal guidelines for management of severe sepsis and septic shock—2008, *Crit Care Med* 36:296–327, 2008.

Dombrovskiy VY, Martin AA, Sunderram J, Paz HL: Rapid increase in hospitalization and mortality rates for severe sepsis in the United States: A trend analysis from 1993 to 2003, *Crit Care Med* 35:1244–1250, 2007.

Ibrahim EH, Sherman G, Ward S, et al: The influence of inadequate antimicrobial treatment of bloodstream infections on patient outcomes in the ICU setting, *Chest* 118:146–155, 2000.

Jimenez MF, Marshall JC: Source control in the management of sepsis, *Intensive Care Med* 27(Suppl. 1):S49–62, 2001.

Kumar A, Roberts D, Wood KE, et al: Duration of hypotension before initiation of effective antimicrobial therapy is the critical determinant of survival in human septic shock, *Crit Care Med* 34:1589–1596, 2006.

Leibovici L, Shraga I, Drucker M, et al: The benefit of appropriate empirical antibiotic treatment in patients with bloodstream infection, *J Intern Med* 244:379–386, 1998.

Levy MM, Fink MP, Marshall JC, et al: 2001 SCCM/ESICM/ACCP/ATS/SIS International Sepsis Definitions Conference, *Intensive Care Med* 29:530–538, 2003.

Martin GS, Mannino DM, Easton S, et al: The epidemiology of sepsis in the United States from 1979 through 2000, *N Engl J Med* 348:1546–1554, 2003.

McDonald JR, Friedman ND, Stout JE, et al: Risk factors for ineffective therapy in patients with bloodstream infection, *Arch Intern Med* 165:308–313, 2005.

Miller PJ, Wenzel RP: Etiologic organisms as independent predictors of death and morbidity associated with bloodstream infection, *J Infect Dis* 156:471–477, 1987.

Sasse KC, Nauenberg E, Long A, et al: Long-term survival after intensive care unit admission with sepsis, *Crit Care Med* 23:1040–1047, 1995.

SMALLPOX

Method of
Raul Davaro, MD

Smallpox, a disease unique to humans, is one of the oldest recorded infections affecting humankind. In endemic forms and in epidemic waves, smallpox killed and disfigured millions of people throughout history. This viral infection, spread by respiratory droplets, continued to have worldwide distribution at the beginning of the 20th century. Because smallpox confers immunity in the survivors of an attack, its persistence depends on contact of nonimmune persons with infected persons in the initial 2 weeks of acquiring the infection.

Centuries ago, physicians realized that inoculating smallpox matter into nonimmune persons conferred partial or total immunity against smallpox. This practice was known in India and China as *variolation*. Variolation was introduced in England in 1721 by the wife of Ambassador Montagu, Lady Montagu, who herself was disfigured by smallpox. The practice spread rapidly in England despite skepticism from the scientific community and resistance from the Church. Variolation was risky and sometimes fatal. In 1783 Octavius, the son of King George III, died as a result of complications from variolation. Benjamin Franklin was an ardent supporter of variolation in the American colonies.

In 1778, Edward Jenner, an English physician, reported that milkmaids infected with cowpox were immune to smallpox during epidemics. In 1796 he decided to test his hypothesis by injecting cowpox material into James Phipps. Phipps developed no signs or symptoms of smallpox 2 months after the inoculation, when he had variolation. This experiment was the birth of vaccination (Latin *vacca*, "cow") against smallpox. With the support of King George IV, vaccination was implemented in England, and variolation was slowly abandoned and finally declared illegal in 1840. Vaccination was introduced in the United States in 1800 by Dr. Benjamin Waterhouse, a Harvard physician, and supported by President Thomas Jefferson, who immunized members of his household. The last-documented natural case of smallpox in the United States was documented in 1947.

The World Health Organization (WHO) designed an Intensified Eradication Program based on a ring vaccination strategy that began in 1966 and eradicated smallpox from humans in an unprecedented effort in less than 10 years. The last natural case was documented in Somalia in 1977. Routine immunization against smallpox ceased in the United States in 1972 and worldwide in 1980. It was thought that without a human reservoir, reemergence of this infection would not occur.

Smallpox virus stocks are still available in the United States at the CDC in Atlanta, Georgia, and in Russia at the State Center for Virology and Biotechnology in Novosibirk, Siberia. These stocks are maintained under strict bio-containment measures. In the aftermath of the terrorist attacks on September 11, 2001 and the deliberate distribution of *Bacillus anthracis* afterwards, President Bush announced plans to immunize health care workers and first responders against smallpox by 2003. Although the plan fell short of it goals, 40,000 first responders and health care workers were vaccinated by the end of 2003.

The Agent
Smallpox is a single, linear double-stranded DNA virus that belongs to the *Orthopoxvirus* genus, family Poxviridae. The poxviruses replicate in cell cytoplasm. They are brick-shaped and measure about 300 by 250 by 200 nm.

Epidemiology
The natural reservoir of smallpox is the patient suffering from the disease. Smallpox spreads from person to person through droplet nuclei or fine-particle aerosols released from the pharynx of infected persons. Smallpox can also be transmitted by fomites such as clothing and bedding. Smallpox patients are not infectious until the third day of the clinical disease, typically 1 day before the skin eruption. The secondary attack rate of smallpox is 37% to 88% among unvaccinated contacts, depending on many variables.

Clinical Presentation
Smallpox occurs as either variola major or variola minor (Alastrim). Variola major had a mortality rate of 30% compared with 1% for variola minor.

After an incubation period of 10 to 14 days, the illness begins with intense prostration and high fever lasting 4 to 6 days (Figure 1). Headache, photophobia, and vomiting are noted. During the prodrome phase most patients are bedridden. Around the fourth day the fever breaks and the patient feels better.

The eruptive phase is signaled by an enanthem involving the buccal mucosa and pharynx and a centrifugal exanthem that begins on the face and forearms. The initial rash is macular and turns pustular in 1 to 2 days. Within 2 days the papules evolve into vesicles that become cloudy and pustular. Most patients exhibit lesions on their soles and palms. A typical feature of variola is that the exanthem everywhere is in the same state of evolution, unlike the exanthem of chickenpox, in which lesions exhibit all stages of evolution. At the end of day 8 to 10 the skin rash crusts and dries; it takes 3 to 4 weeks from the onset of the disease for all the scabs to fall off. The period of contagiousness ends when the last scab falls off. Scarring and pitting of the skin are common sequelae.

Patients with hemorrhagic disease develop severe prostration, high fever, abdominal pain, petechiae, and extensive cutaneous ecchymoses. In the malignant or flat form, the lesions fail to progress to the pustular stage. In the hemorrhagic and the malignant forms, death invariably occurs within 1 week.

History of smallpox vaccination modifies the course of the disease. Vaccinated persons who contract smallpox have fewer skin lesions and an accelerated clinical course.

Complications
Bacterial infections of the skin and other organs are common. Ocular involvement may result in blindness. Encephalitis (one in 500 cases of variola major) is a devastating complication.

Differential Diagnosis (Figure 2)
Many rashes can be confused with smallpox, especially at the outset of the eruption, when the rash is maculopapular. Herpes zoster, chickenpox, herpes simplex, impetigo, scabies, erythema multiforme, and syphilis are some of the conditions that can be confused with smallpox (Box 1). When smallpox was endemic, chickenpox was the most common condition confused with smallpox. The most useful clinical points of smallpox are the following:
- Centrifugal distribution of the lesions
- All the lesions in the same stage of development
- Progression of the rash from the face to the arms, trunk and legs
- A severe prodrome phase that lasts 4 days
- In an epidemic, known contact with an active case

Diagnosis
The identification of a suspected case of smallpox should be treated as an international health emergency. Clinical samples may be collected from vesicular or pustular fluid, blood, tonsillar swabs, and skin biopsy and must be transported to a Biosafety level 4 facility for processing and testing with real-time polymerase chain reaction (PCR) assays to detect virus DNA.

Lesions of varicella zoster virus (chickenpox, herpes zoster) demonstrate multinucleated giant cells on Tzanck smears; lesions of smallpox do not. Serology or electronic microscopy are not recommended for the diagnosis of smallpox because these modalities cannot distinguish among different Orthopoxviruses.

Treatment
A suspected case of smallpox should be placed in a negative-pressure room with strict respiratory and contact isolation precautions. Ideally to minimize the risk of contagion in health care personnel, patient with smallpox should be assisted by providers documented to have been immunized against this condition. Patients with smallpox require careful care of their eyes to avoid complications and this is accomplished with daily eye rinsing. Patients must receive

Figure 1 Clinical manifestations and pathogenesis of smallpox and the immune response. **A,** The initial phases of infection and the clinical manifestations include temperature spikes and progressive skin lesions (photographs of lesions courtesy of Dr. David Heymann, World Health Organization). **B,** The pathogenesis of the infection. The photographs on the *right* show the characteristic features of the vesicles caused by smallpox (H&E, ×90). **C,** The immune response to smallpox and the period of infectiousness.
Abbreviations: CF = complement fixation; HI = hemagglutination inhibition.
(Reprinted with permission from Breman JG, Henderson DA. Diagnosis and management of smallpox. N Eng J Med 2002;346:1300–1308.)

```
                    ┌──────────────────────┐
                    │  Patient with acute, │
                    │ generalized vesicular│
                    │ or pustular rash     │
                    │     illness          │
                    └──────────────────────┘
                               │
                    ┌──────────────────────┐
                    │ Institute airborne and│
                    │ contact precautions; │
                    │ alert infection control│
                    │    on admission      │
                    └──────────────────────┘
```

Low risk of smallpox

Moderate risk of smallpox

High risk of smallpox

History and examination highly suggestive of varicella

Diagnosis uncertain

Infectious disease or dermatologic consultation, or both; varicella +/– other laboratory testing as indicated

Infectious disease or dermatologic consultation, or both; alert public-health agency immediately

Varicella testing optional

Test for varicella and other disorders as indicated

Non-smallpox diagnosis confirmed: report results to infection control

No diagnosis made; ensure adequacy of specimen: infectious disease or dermatologic consultant reevaluates patient

Public health agency advises on management and collection of samples

Cannot rule out smallpox: classify as high risk

Variola testing at approved laboratory

Not smallpox: further testing

Smallpox

■ High risk of smallpox: report immediately
□ Moderate risk of smallpox: urgent evaluation
▨ Low risk of smallpox: manage as clinically indicated

Figure 2 Algorithm for assessing patients for smallpox. Reprinted with permission from Moore ZS, Seward JF, Lane JM: Smallpox. Lancet 2006;367:425–435.

adequate nutrition and hydration. Skin and soft issue infections must be treated with an antistaphylococcal β-lactams, and initially pending results of cultures, with an antimicrobial with activity against methicillin-resistant Staphylococcus aureus. There is no antiviral drug with demonstrated activity against smallpox.

Vaccines and Vaccination

Sanofi's U.S.-licensed ACAM2000, a second-generation vaccine, was made from cell culture-derived vaccinia virus found in Dryvax, a first-generation vaccine that is no longer produced. ACAM2000 is indicated for active immunization of people who are determined to be at high risk for smallpox. A two-pronged stainless steel (or bifurcated) needle is dipped into the vaccine solution and the skin is pricked several times in the upper arm with a droplet of the vaccine. The virus begins growing at the injection site causing a localized infection or "pock" to form. A red, itchy sore spot at the site of the vaccination within 3-4 days is an indicator that the vaccination was successful; that is, there is "a take." A blister develops at the vaccination site and then dries up forming a scab that falls off in the third week, leaving a small scar. If no evidence of vaccine take is apparent after 7 days, the person can be vaccinated again.

The vaccine causes local and systemic symptoms. There is an eruption at the injection site with redness and pain, systemic symptoms such as fever, and headaches. Swelling and tenderness of regional lymph nodes begin 3 to 10 days after vaccination and can last up to a month.

Complications

Adverse events of vaccinia have been reviewed extensively and include postvaccinial encephalitis, progressive vaccinia, eczema vaccinatum, and generalized vaccinia (Table 1). The most common complication is inadvertent autoinoculation causing self-limited satellite lesions. Generalized vaccinia results from viremia and may be life threatening in immunocompromised patients. Progressive vaccinia is characterized by necrosis at the inoculation site and distal sites such as bones and internal organs. Progressive vaccinia is often a fatal complication. Myopericarditis was observed with the use of adult vaccines in the United States in 2002 (Table 1).

Contraindications to Vaccination

Persons who are immune compromised or who have severe eczema or who are pregnant should not receive Post-exposure vaccination against smallpox. However, in the event of exposure to a patient with smallpox, no absolute contraindication is applicable.

Control of Outbreaks

As soon as a diagnosis of smallpox is considered, suspected persons should be isolated and close contacts should be immunized. Post-exposure vaccination within the first 4 days can greatly mitigate subsequent illness. Contact isolation and ring vaccination are the strategies of choice to contain an outbreak of smallpox.

Use in Warfare

During the 15th century, variola-laden clothing and blankets were distributed by Europeans among Native Americans to spread smallpox in the local population. British soldiers used variola- contaminated blankets among the natives supporting the French during the French and Indian wars. The use of infectious agents in warfare is not new, and the potential use of smallpox as a weapon increased when routine immunization against smallpox ceased and worldwide immunity waned.

Because natural smallpox has been eradicated, the only possibility of a smallpox outbreak is the deliberate release of smallpox in a population by a nation or a terrorist group to inflict casualties in a civilian population. Preemptive vaccination of first responders and ring immunization of those exposed are the means available to avoid massive propagation of smallpox.

BOX 1	Conditions that Might Be Confused with Smallpox

Maculopapular Stage
Measles
Rubella
Drug eruptions
Secondary syphilis
Erythema multiforme
Scabies, insect bites
Acne
Scarlet fever

Vesicular/Pustular Stage
Chickenpox
Disseminated herpes zoster
Disseminated herpes simplex virus
Drug eruptions
Contact dermatitis
Erythema multiforme (including Stevens-Johnson syndrome)
Enteroviral infections
Secondary syphilis
Acne
Generalized vaccinia
Monkeypox
Impetigo
Scabies, insect bites
Disseminated molluscum contagiosum

TABLE 1	Rates of Complications from Vaccinia, According to Vaccination Status and Age*

COMPLICATIONS	PRIMARY VACCINATION (*N* = 650,000)				REVACCINATION (*N* = 996,000)			
	0–4 YR	5–19 YR	>20 YR	ALL AGES	1–4 YR†	5–19 YR	>20 YR	ALL AGES
Accidental infection	564	371	606	529	198	48	25	42
Generalized vaccinia	263	140	212	242	0	10	9	9
Erythema multiforme	299	87	30	165	73	2	9	10
Eczema vaccinatum	39	35	30	39	0	2	5	3
Postvaccinal encephalitis	15	9	0	12	0	0	5	2
Progressive vaccinia	3	0	0	2	0	0	7	3
Other	222	214	6636	266	18	24	55	39

*Data are from a 1968 survey of 10 states. No deaths occurred.
Reprinted with permission from Breman JG, Henderson DA: Diagnosis and management of smallpox. N Engl J Med 2002;346:1300–1308.
†No children younger than 1 year were revaccinated.

References

Behbehani A: The smallpox story: Life and death of an old disease, *Microbiol Rev* 47:455–509, 1983.

Breman JG, Henderson DA: Diagnosis and management of smallpox, *N Engl J Med* 346:1300–1308, 2002.

Bronze MS, Huycke MM, Machado LJ, et al: Viral agents as biological weapons and agents of bioterrorism, *Am J Med Sci* 323:316–325, 2002.

Centers for Disease Control and Prevention. Smallpox vaccination. Information for Health Care professionals. Available at http://www.bt.cdc.gov/agent/smallpox/vaccination/ [accessed 05.05.15].

Cleri DJ, Porwancher RB, Ricketti AJ, et al: Smallpox as a bioterrorist weapon: Myth or menace? *Infectious Dis Clin North Am* 20:329–358, 2006.

Kempe HC: Variola. In Beeson PB, McDermott W, editors: *Textbook of Medicine*, 12th ed., Philadelphia, 1967, WB Saunders, pp 44–46.

Lofquist J, Weimert NA, Hayney MS: Smallpox: A review of clinical disease and vaccination, *Am J Health Syst Pharm* 60:749–758, 2003.

Moore ZS, Seward JF, Lane JM: Smallpox, *Lancet* 367:425–435, 2006.

Weiss MM, Weiss PD, Mathisen G, et al: Rethinking smallpox, *Clin Infect Dis* 29:1668–1673, 2004.

Whitley RJ: Smallpox: A potential agent of bioterrorism, *Antiviral Res* 57:7–12, 2003.

TETANUS

Method of
Dilip R. Karnad, MD

Tetanus is a potentially fatal illness caused by the neurotoxin produced by the spore-bearing anaerobic bacterium *Clostridium tetani*. As the causative organism and its spores are ubiquitous, nonimmune individuals in any part of the world may get tetanus unless they are protected by the highly effective vaccine.

Epidemiology

As a result of effective universal immunization, tetanus is rare in the developed world. Twenty to 40 cases of tetanus occur annually in the United States and 12 to 15 cases per year have been reported from the United Kingdom in the last 10 years. Although progressively declining in the developing world due to improved immunization coverage, according to WHO figures, more than 500 cases were reported in 2012 from each of these nations: Angola, Bangladesh, Congo, India, and Uganda. While tetanus may affect individuals of all ages, a significant number of cases in developed countries are elderly people who did not receive a primary immunization or lacked the booster dosage needed to maintain protective immunity. In developing countries, most cases are neonates (*tetanus neonatorum*), children who are born to nonimmunized mothers and thus lack transplacentally acquired passive immunity. Infection of the umbilical stump due to poor hygiene results in severe tetanus that has mortality in excess of 60%.

The infection is caused by the gram-positive, spore-bearing bacterium *C. tetani*, the spores of which exist in the soil, in animal feces, and even in the human gastrointestinal tract. Spores remain dormant and viable for several months and are destroyed by autoclaving at 1 atmosphere pressure at 120°C for 15 minutes. When inoculated into human or animal tissues, they transform into motile bacilli in an anaerobic environment that produce a potent exotoxin, tetanospasmin, which produces the manifestations of tetanus. It must be emphasized that tetanus is not transmitted from human to human, and patients do not require isolation.

Risk Factors

Elderly individuals are at increased risk, as they may not have received adequate immunization or may have waning immunity. Other predisposed groups include immigrants from countries with an unreliable immunization program, immunosuppressed individuals (with HIV infection or receiving immunosuppressive drugs), and intravenous drug addicts. Local factors include wounds with crushed, devitalized tissue or contaminated by dirt or rust, such as open fractures, punctures, and abscesses. However, even scratches, chronic ulcers, or tattooing may cause tetanus. In developing countries, unsafe practices related to termination of pregnancy may cause maternal tetanus; newborn babies born outside of medical facilities are at risk of neonatal tetanus.

Pathophysiology

Tetanospasmin is a highly toxic protein released by *C. tetani*. It is absorbed into the circulation and reaches the ends of motor axons all over the body, from where it is transported proximally along the axonal cytoplasm to motor nuclei in the brainstem and spinal cord at a rate of 3 to 13 mm/hour. A fragment of the toxin then binds inhibitory interneurons that produce gamma-amino butyric acid (GABA) and glycine and inactivates synaptobrevin, a protein that is essential for the release of these neurotransmitters from presynaptic vesicles.

The loss of normal inhibition at motor and autonomic neurons results in spontaneous discharge of nerve impulses as well as exaggerated responses to stimuli manifesting as tonic muscle contraction with superadded intermittent muscle spasms. As tetanospasmin reaches the motor nuclei of the shortest motor axons first, muscles innervated by motor cranial nerves are affected first, followed by trunk muscles, and finally the extremities. Autonomic overactivity results in severe tachycardia, swings in blood pressure, profuse sweating, and (rarely) ileus. An exaggerated startle-like response to stimuli with motor and autonomic components is also typical. Generalized spasms may mimic tonic seizures.

Clinical Manifestations

An attempt should be made to locate the predisposing wound, such as cuts, abrasions, burns, puncture wounds, and other skin lesions. Uncommon causes include needle-sticks in intravenous drug abusers, ulcerated malignant tumors, and chronic middle-ear infection in children (otogenic tetanus). In up to 30% of patients, no site of infection is discovered. The incubation period is the interval between the injury and the onset of symptoms and can range from a few days to a few months (usually 3–21 days). A short incubation period (<7 days) suggests the likelihood of developing severe tetanus; however, a long incubation period does not necessarily indicate a milder disease. The period of onset (the interval between the first symptom and first paroxysmal muscle spasm) is a better predictor of severity: early elective tracheal intubation and mechanical ventilation are usually required if the interval is <48 hours.

Generalized Tetanus

Initial symptoms include an inability to open the mouth (lockjaw or trismus), difficulty in chewing and swallowing, and stiffness of neck muscles. The contraction of facial muscles produces the characteristic sneering smile (*risus sardonicus*) (Figure 1). In severe cases, intermittent spasms are provoked by attempts to speak or swallow. Pooled saliva from hypersalivation and dysphagia may trigger cough and laryngeal spasms; if prolonged, these may prove fatal. Rigidity of paraspinal muscles follows, and hyperextension of the spine results in opisthotonus (Figure 2). Finally, proximal muscles of the extremity are also affected. Deep tendon reflexes are always exaggerated and ankle clonus is common. Tonic muscle spasms may affect head and neck muscles and laryngeal muscles, or may be generalized. Paroxysmal spasms occur spontaneously or in response to loud noise, bright lights, or attempts to speak or swallow. Prolonged spasms may compromise breathing.

The Ablett classification is commonly used to grade the severity of tetanus. Grade I (mild) tetanus is characterized by moderate trismus and general spasticity without spasms, dysphagia, or respiratory distress. Grade II (moderate) tetanus has severe trismus, intermittent short spasms, mild tachypnea, and dysphagia. Grade III (severe) tetanus is associated with severe rigidity, prolonged spasms, severe dysphagia, tachypnea, apneic spells, and tachycardia. The presence of additional violent autonomic disturbances with persistent or intermittent episodes of severe hypertension and tachycardia alternating with hypotension and bradycardia is classified as Grade IV (very severe) tetanus. Cardiac arrhythmias, peripheral vasoconstriction, and sudden asystole may also occur in very severe tetanus.

Figure 1 Typical facial expression with the sneering smile *(risus sardonicus)*, wrinkled forehead, narrow palpebral fissures, and "crow's feet" at the lateral palpebral margins from the tonic contraction of muscles of facial expression in moderate tetanus.

Figure 2 Spasm of paraspinal muscles, producing the hyperextended opisthotonic posture in severe tetanus.

Figure 3 Cephalic tetanus: This 6-year-old child developed mild tetanus 3 weeks after a wound on his right cheek was sutured. He had cephalic tetanus characterized by partial paralysis of the right facial nerve along with overactivity of the unaffected nerve fibers. **A,** Note the overactivity of the facial muscles with a narrow palpebral and prominent nasolabial fold on the same side as the injury. On asking him to shut his eyes tight **(B),** weakness of the orbicularis oculi and other facial muscles on the right side become manifest.

Despite the use of antitetanus immune globulin (HyperTET) to neutralize circulating tetanus toxin, the disease may progress for up to 2 weeks as more intraaxonal toxin continues to reach the central nervous system. Manifestations persist for another 2 to 3 weeks before gradually subsiding. During this period, an apparently stable patient is at risk of developing sudden asphyxia due to severe generalized or laryngeal spasms. Patients may develop fever, rhabodomyolysis, and hyperthermia due to excessive muscular activity.

Cephalic Tetanus
Following injuries to the head or face, in some patients, the toxin reaches the local motor nuclei earlier and produces a combination of partial paralysis and overactivity—more severely affected motor neurons stop functioning while the remaining fibers are overactive and cause muscle spasm (Figure 3).

Localized Tetanus
In this rare form of tetanus, manifestations are restricted to muscles in the region of the wound. These patients have a good prognosis.

Diagnosis
C. tetani can be isolated from the wound in <30% of cases, and microbiological and other laboratory tests do not help in confirming the diagnosis. The diagnosis is entirely clinical. In an individual with a predisposing injury, the presence of trismus, rigidity of neck, abdominal and paraspinal muscles, and severe hyperreflexia are suggestive. The spatula test is a useful bedside test: A spatula (tongue depressor) is inserted into the mouth to touch the posterior pharyngeal wall. Normally, a gag reflex is activated in an attempt to expel the spatula. In tetanus, severe spasms of the masseters results in the patient biting on the spatula, making it difficult to withdraw—a positive test. In one study, the spatula

test was positive in 94% of patients with tetanus and in none without tetanus. The electromyogram shows the continuous discharge of motor units in moderate tetanus and the absence of the normal silent period.

Differential Diagnosis
While the diagnosis of tetanus is easy in severe tetanus, it may be mistaken for other conditions in its initial stages (Table 1). The spatula test is negative in other conditions causing trismus. Abdominal muscles usually relax after adequate sedation. As in spasticity due to cord compression, deep reflexes are exaggerated; however, the plantar response, which is extensor in spinal cord disorders, is always flexor with tetanus. Unlike seizures or other intracranial diseases, the patient with tetanus is always fully alert and awake.

Treatment
In patients with life-threatening spasms, prompt, adequate sedation is the first step in management. Patients must be observed in an intensive care unit because the disease may rapidly worsen. They should be nursed in a quiet, dimly lit room in order to keep external stimuli to a minimum—this is difficult in modern intensive care units.

Neutralization of Toxin
Although unsupported by randomized studies, human tetanus immune globulin (HyperTET) (3000–6000 units) is administered intramuscularly to neutralize the circulating toxin. This does not bind to the toxin that has already entered neurons. There is insufficient evidence favoring intrathecal administration[1] of tetanus

---

[1] Not FDA approved for this indication.

TABLE 1	Conditions that Mimic Clinical Manifestations of Tetanus
CLINICAL FEATURE	**DIFFERENTIAL DIAGNOSIS**
Trismus	Acute tonsillar abscess, temporomandibular joint disease, extraptramidal reaction to drugs, dental pathology
Neck stiffness	Cervical spine disease; extrapyramidal reaction to drugs such as antipsychotics, antiemetics, or metoclopramide; meningitis; subarachnoid hemorrhage
Abdominal rigidity	Acute abdomen
Dysphagia	Myasthenia gravis, acute bulbar paralysis, rabies
Muscle spasms	Seizures, spasticity due to spinal cord disease, stiff man syndrome

immune globulin over the usual intramuscular route, although one randomized study showed a shortening of the course of tetanus. Equine antiserum[2] (10,000–20,000 units) may be administered after skin testing for hypersensitivity. Though rarely used today due to the risk of anaphylaxis or serum sickness, it has the advantage of being administered intravenously.

Control of Clostridial Infection

Benzylpenicillin (Penicillin G) in a dose of 10 to 12 million units per day is given intravenously for 10 days. In one study, metronidazole (Flagyl) (500 mg every 6 hour for 10 days) was superior to procaine penicillin (Wycillin),[1] presumably because procaine and penicillin are GABA antagonists and may worsen manifestations of tetanus. However, a more recent study showed that a single intramuscular injection of 1.2 million units of benzathine penicillin (Bicillin LA)[1] was as effective as benzylpenicillin or metronidazole. Fortunately, resistance to these antibiotics has not been reported. Debridement of the infected wound and abscess drainage should be performed after spasms have been adequately controlled.

Control of Muscle Spasms

Benzodiazepines (diazepam [Valium] or lorazepam [Ativan][1]) are the preferred drugs and act by enhancing the effect of GABA on its receptor on the postsynaptic membrane, thus potentially antagonizing the effect of tetanospasmin. However, as very little GABA is released in tetanus, large doses (up to 1000 mg/day[3]) of diazepam may be required to achieve adequate sedation and muscle relaxation. Diazepam may be administered intravenously (10–30 mg in 5 mg boluses every 5 minutes)[3] or through a nasogastric tube (10–40 mg every 1 to 2 hours).[3] Barbiturates and chlorpromazine (Thorazine)[1] are alternative agents. Other sedative hypnotic agents such as midazolam (Versed)[1] and propofol (Diprivan)[1] have also been used with good effect. In mild to moderate tetanus, drug doses can be titrated to achieve moderate sedation and control rigidity and spasms without causing respiratory depression. In severe cases, however, spasms may not be controlled despite large doses, increasing the risk of severe central nervous system (CNS) depression. In these patients, heavy sedation combined with neuromuscular blockade and mechanical ventilation is required. In about 10% of cases, benzodiazepines may produce paradoxical excitation instead of sedation; increasing doses make the patient more wakeful, agitated, and delirious, with increased spasms. Discontinuation of diazepam and the use of barbiturates and chlorpromazine may prevent the need for paralysis and mechanical ventilation. Pancuronium (Pavulon),[1] vecuronium (Norcuron),[1] and rocuronium (Zemuron)[1] are often used for neuromuscular blockade. Atracurium (Tracrium)[1] could also be used but may have unfavorable cardiovascular effects. Intravenous and intrathecal baclofen (Lioresal Intrathecal)[1] have been used in some case.

Airway Management

Tracheostomy or endotracheal intubation is required in moderate and severe tetanus to prevent respiratory failure due to laryngeal spasm and aspiration of oropharyngeal secretions. In most developing countries, elective tracheostomy is performed early in severe tetanus. In countries with superior intensive care facilities, heavy sedation, neuromuscular blockade, endotracheal intubation, and mechanical ventilation are preferred, with tracheostomy being reserved for those who need prolonged ventilation.

Control of Autonomic Disturbances

With good intensive care, mortality due to respiratory failure has been drastically reduced. Autonomic dysfunction is now the major challenge in patients with severe tetanus; it is common even in sedated and paralyzed patients. Various measures to control autonomic fluctuations include intravenous fluid loading, oral and parenteral beta-blockers, alpha-blockers, centrally acting sympatholytics such as clonidine (Catapres)[1] or dexmedetomidine (Precedex),[1] and epidural or spinal bupivacaine (Marcaine).[1] More recently, infusion of dexmedetomidine has been used by some authors. Many patients may develop sudden asystole, possibly due to sudden parasympathetic discharge, catecholamine-induced myocardial damage, or sudden loss of sympathetic drive. Consequently, the use of long-acting antiadrenergic drugs should be avoided. Increasing the level of sedation itself is also effective, to a significant extent.

The agent most frequently used for autonomic dysfunction is intravenous magnesium sulfate.[1] A randomized controlled trial in Vietnamese patients showed that magnesium sulfate did not decrease mortality, ICU stay, or the need for mechanical ventilation but did reduce the dose of sedatives and neuromuscular blocking drugs required. This study used a loading dose of 40 mg/kg over 30 minutes, followed by intravenous infusion of 2 g/hour in patients >45 kg and 1 to 5 g/hour in patients ≤45 kg. Infusion was titrated to maintain serum magnesium levels between 2 and 4 mmol/L.

Other Measures

Continuous muscle hyperactivity and spasms greatly increase caloric requirements. Most patients require nasogastric tube feeding because of trismus and dysphagia. A catabolic state similar to sepsis may develop in very severe tetanus. Consequently, patients lose up to 15% of their body weight during the illness. Good nursing care is essential to prevent pressure sores, deep vein thrombosis, stress ulcers, and aspiration pneumonia. Urinary catheterization is required in most patients as urinary retention is common and distension of the urinary bladder may provoke spasms and autonomic overactivity. All patients should be started on a primary immunization schedule against tetanus.

Complications

Respiratory failure may occur due to laryngeal obstruction, prolonged spasm of respiratory muscles, aspiration pneumonia, or sedative drugs. Severe spasms may result in tongue-bite, compression fractures of midthoracic vertebrae, rhabdomyolysis, myoglobinuria, and renal failure. Rarely, patients may develop acute respiratory distress syndrome (ARDS) either due to tetanus itself or as a result of secondary bacterial sepsis. Cardiac arrhythmias and sudden asystole are common in patients with autonomic dysfunction. Acute myocardial infarction may occur in elderly patients with underlying coronary artery disease due to sympathetic overactivity. Deep vein thrombosis and pressure

---

[2] Not available in the United States.
[3] Exceeds dosage recommended by the manufacturer.

[1] Not FDA approved for this indication.

sores are preventable complications. The overall mortality ranges from 40% to 60% in countries with inadequate health care facilities. With good intensive care, mortality as low as 10% is reported in some series. Mortality is higher in neonates, the elderly, and patients with a short incubation period and period of onset.

Prevention

Adsorbed tetanus toxoid (Tt), derived from formaldehyde-treated tetanus toxin, is extremely effective in inducing active immunity. It is available as a single-antigen preparation or in combination with diphtheria toxoid as pediatric diphtheria-tetanus toxoid (DT) or adult tetanus-diphtheria (Td), and with both diphtheria toxoid and acellular pertussis vaccine as DTaP (Infanrix, Tripedia) or Tdap (Adacel, Boostrix) (lower-case alphabets indicate lower doses of antigens). Pediatric vaccines (DT and DTaP) contain identical amounts of tetanus toxoid as adult vaccines, but three to four times as much diphtheria toxoid. The usual schedule for primary immunization in children <7 years consists of four doses of DTaP or DT at age 2, 4, 6, and 15 to 18 months. A booster dose is recommended at 4 to 6 years of age. In individuals aged 7 years or older, three doses of the adult formulation are administered; the second dose is given 4 to 8 weeks after the first, and the third dose after another 4 to 6 months. Further booster doses are needed every 10 years to maintain antibody titers above the protective level of 0.1 IU/mL.

After administration of Tt to individuals with wounds, protective titers of antibody are achieved after at least 2 weeks. Consequently, passive immunization with 250 units of human tetanus immune globulin (HyperTET) or 1500 units of equine antitetanus serum[2] administered intramuscularly is needed to confer protection during these initial few weeks. This is especially required in individuals with tetanus-prone wounds who have not received at least three doses of tetanus toxoid in the past. Previously unimmunized individuals with clean, minor, nontetanus prone wounds do not need any passive immunization, but should receive active immunization. Passive immunization is not necessary in those who have received three or more doses of the toxoid. These individuals should receive a dose of Tt (or Td) if more than 10 years have elapsed since the last booster dose and they have nontetanus prone wounds or if >5 years have elapsed after the booster dose and they have a tetanus-prone wound. In countries where neonatal tetanus is common, primary immunization of women during pregnancy has been advocated as a public health program to prevent neonatal tetanus.

References

Apte NM, Karnad DR: The spatula test: A simple bedside test to diagnose tetanus, *Am J Trop Med Hyg* 53:386–387, 1995.
Centers for Disease Control and Prevention: In Atkinson W, Wolfe S, Hamborsky J, editors: *Epidemiology and Prevention of Vaccine-Preventable Diseases*, ed 12th, Washington, DC, 2011, Department of Health and Human Services, Centers for Disease Control and Prevention, pp 291–299.
Farrar JJ, Yen LM, Cook T, et al: Tetanus, *J Neurol Neurosurg Psychiatry* 69:292–301, 2000.
Gibson K, Uwineza JB, Kiviri W, Parlow J: Tetanus in developing countries: A case series and review, *Can J Anaesth* 56:307–315, 2009.
Lisboa T, Ho YL, Filho GTH, et al: Guidelines for the management of accidental tetanus in adult patients, *Rev Bras Ter Intensiva* 23:394–409, 2011.
Rodrigo C, Samarakoon L, Fernando SD, Rajapakse S: A meta-analysis of magnesium for tetanus, *Anaesthesia* 67:1370–1374, 2012.
Roper MH, Vandelaer JH, Gasse FL: Maternal and neonatal tetanus, *Lancet* 370:1947–1959, 2007.
Thwaites CL, Yen LM, Loan HT, et al: Magnesium sulphate for treatment of severe tetanus: A randomized controlled trial, *Lancet* 368:1436–1443, 2006.
Trujillo MH, Castillo A, Espana J, et al: Impact of intensive care management on the prognosis of tetanus. Analysis of 641 cases, *Chest* 92:63–65, 1987.

---

[2]Not available in the United States.

TICKBORNE RICKETTSIAL DISEASES (ROCKY MOUNTAIN SPOTTED FEVER AND OTHER SPOTTED FEVER GROUP RICKETTSIOSES, EHRLICHIOSES, AND ANAPLASMOSIS)

Method of
Robert Wittler, MD

CURRENT DIAGNOSIS

- Early diagnosis of Rocky Mountain spotted fever (RMSF) and other tickborne rickettsial diseases is made clinically. RMSF should be considered in the setting of fever, headache, rash, and a history of possible tick exposure. The rash is not always present and typically occurs 2 to 4 days after the onset of fever.
- Diagnostic laboratory tests for rickettsial diseases, particularly RMSF, are usually not helpful in making a timely diagnosis during the initial states of illness.
- Tickborne rickettsial diseases can be confirmed by polymerase chain reaction (PCR) during the acute stage if readily available (whole blood for ehrlichiosis and anaplasmosis and skin biopsy or whole blood for RMSF) or at later stages by subsequently demonstrating a fourfold increase between acute and convalescent (ideally 2 to 4 weeks apart) serum immunoglobulin G (IgG) indirect immunofluorescence antibody titers. PCR of whole blood for RMSF has low sensitivity, although sensitivity increases in patients with severe disease.
- Typical findings of ehrlichiosis and anaplasmosis include fever, headache, malaise, leukopenia, thrombocytopenia, and elevated serum transaminases. Rash is often not present.

CURRENT THERAPY

- Treatment of choice for all tickborne rickettsial diseases in patients of all ages (including children less than 8 years of age) is doxycycline (Vibramycin).
- The dose for doxycycline is 100 mg twice daily (intravenously [IV] or orally depending on severity of illness) for adults. For children weighing <45 kg,[1] the recommended dose is 2.2 mg/kg/dose IV or orally twice daily.
- Delay in recognition and appropriate treatment is the most important factor associated with death from RMSF. Empiric treatment within 5 days of the onset of symptoms with doxycycline is the best way to prevent morbidity and death. Treatment decisions should never be delayed while awaiting laboratory confirmation, nor should treatment be discontinued solely on the basis of a negative test result with an acute-phase specimen.
- Although optimal duration of therapy has not been well studied, a common treatment course for RMSF and ehrlichiosis is at least 3 days after the patient defervesces (typically the minimum total course is 5–7 days) or longer for severe illness. Anaplasmosis should be treated for 10 days to provide appropriate therapy for possible coinfection with *Borrelia burgdorferi*.
- Historically chloramphenicol has been recommended for the treatment of RMSF during pregnancy based on adverse effects of older tetracycline drugs (but not specifically doxycycline). Although there is limited evidence, doxycycline has not been associated with teratogenicity or maternal hepatic toxicity during pregnancy, and doxycycline has been used successfully to treat tickborne rickettsial disease in several pregnant women without adverse effects.
- Chloramphenicol is not an alternative treatment for human monocytic ehrlichiosis (HME) or HGA. Chloramphenicol treatment of RMSF has been associated with a greater risk of death compared with doxycycline treatment.

Tickborne rickettsial diseases in humans often share clinical features but are epidemiologically and etiologically distinct. In the United States included diseases are (1) Rocky Mountain spotted fever (RMSF) caused by *Rickettsia rickettsii*; (2) other spotted fever group (SFG) rickettsioses, caused by *Rickettsia parkeri* and *Rickettsia* species 364D; (3) *Ehrlichia chaffeensis* ehrlichiosis, also called human monocytic ehrlichiosis (HME); (4) other ehrlichioses, caused by *Ehrlichia ewingii* and *Ehrlichia muris*-like agent; and (5) anaplasmosis, caused by *Anaplasma phagocytophilum*, also called human granulocytic anaplasmosis (HGA). The reported incidence of tickborne rickettsial diseases has increased in the United States. Tickborne rickettsial diseases, especially RMSF, continue to cause severe illness and death in otherwise healthy adults and children, despite the availability of effective antibiotic therapy. SFG rickettsioses (including RMSF), ehrlichioses, and anaplasmosis are nationally notifiable diseases in the United States. Providers report potential cases to state or local health departments. In 2010, the reporting category of RMSF was changed to spotted fever rickettsiosis, as serology does not readily distinguish RMSF from other SFG rickettsioses.

Epidemiology

Tickborne rickettsial pathogens are maintained in natural cycles involving domestic or wild vertebrates and ticks. The epidemiology of each disease reflects the geographic distribution and seasonal activities of the tick vectors and the natural vertebrate hosts, as well as the human activities resulting in tick exposure. Although cases have been reported in every month, most cases occur during April to September, coincident with peak levels of tick host-seeking activity.

RMSF is the rickettsiosis in the United States that is associated with the highest rates of severe and fatal outcomes. The case-fatality rate in the preantibiotic era was ~25%. Current case-fatality rates are estimated at 5% to 10%. From 2008–2012, the estimated average annual incidence from passive surveillance of SFG rickettsioses was 8.9 cases per million persons. Reported annual incidence has increased during the past two decades. The highest incidence occurs in persons aged 60 to 69 years, and the highest case-fatality rate is among children aged <10 years. Additional epidemiologic risk factors for fatal RMSF include age ≥40 years, alcohol abuse, and glucose-6-phosphate dehydrogenase deficiency. From 2008 to 2012, 63% of reported SFG rickettsiosis cases came from Arkansas, Missouri, North Carolina, Oklahoma, and Tennessee. SFG rickettsiosis has been reported from all the contiguous 48 states and the District of Columbia.

In the United States, the tick species most frequently associated with transmission of *R rickettsii* is the American dog tick, *Dermacentor variabilis*, which is found primarily in the eastern, central, and Pacific Coast regions. The Rocky Mountain wood tick, *Dermacentor andersoni*, is associated with transmission in the western United States. Larval and nymphal stages of most *Dermacentor* spp ticks usually do not bite humans. Adult *D variabilis* and *D andersoni* ticks bite humans, but the principal hosts are deer, dogs, and livestock.

The brown dog tick, *Rhipicephalus sanguineus*, which is located throughout the United States, is an important vector in parts of Arizona and along the United States–Mexico border. All stages (larvae, nymphs, and adults) of *Rh sanguineus* bite humans and can transmit *R rickettsia*. Domestic dogs are the preferred host. On Arizona tribal lands, the warm climate and proximity of ticks to domiciles (tick-infested dogs) provide a suitable environment for *Rh sanguineus* to remain active year-round, resulting in cases of RMSF in Arizona every month of the year.

Rickettsia parkeri is transmitted by the Gulf Coast tick, *Amblyomma maculatum*. *R parkeri* rickettsiosis cases have not been documented in children, and no fatal cases have been reported. The first confirmed case of Rickettsia species 364D was in 2010 and likely transmitted by the Pacific Coast tick, *Dermacentor occidentalis*. All reported cases have been from California.

The average annual incidence of ehrlichiosis from 2008 to 2012 was 3.2 cases per million persons, with the most common cause being *E chaffeensis*. The highest incidence is in persons aged 60 to 69 years. The case fatality rate is ~3% and is highest among children aged <10 years, adults aged ≥70 years, and immunosuppressed persons. *E chaffeensis* is transmitted to humans by the lone star tick, *Amblyomma americanum*, which is the most commonly encountered tick in the southeastern United States, with a range that extends into areas of the Midwest and New England. Arkansas, Delaware, Missouri, Oklahoma, Tennessee, and Virginia have the highest reported incidence. The white-tailed deer is an important natural reservoir for *E chaffeensis*, and most cases occur during May to August.

The principal vector for *E ewingii* ehrlichiosis is also *A americanum*. Cases have primarily been reported from Missouri. No fatal cases of *E ewingii* ehrlichiosis have been reported. *Ehrlichia muris*–like agent (EML) has recently been recognized as a human pathogen. Reported cases have been from Minnesota and Wisconsin. The blacklegged tick, *Ixodes scapularis*, is an efficient vector for EML in experimental studies. EML agent DNA has been detected in *I scapularis* collected in Minnesota and Wisconsin but has not been detected in *I scapularis* from other states.

The incidence of human anaplasmosis during 2008–2012 was 6.3 cases per million persons. Incidence is highest in the northeastern and upper midwestern states, and the geographic range seems to be expanding. The case fatality rate is <1%. *I scapularis* is the vector for *Anaplasma phagocytophilum* in the northeastern and midwestern United States, whereas the western blacklegged tick, *Ixodes pacificus*, is the principal vector along the West Coast. The seasonality is bimodal, with the first peak June–July and a smaller peak in October, corresponding to the emergence of the adult stage of *I scapularis*. *I scapularis* also transits *Borrelia burgdorferi* (Lyme disease), *Babesia microti* (babesiosis), *Borrelia miyamotoi* (tickborne relapsing fever), and deer tick virus (a cause of tickborne encephalitis). Simultaneous infections with *A phagocytophilum* and *B burgdorferi* or *B microti* have occurred.

Pathophysiology

The agents causing RMSF, ehrlichiosis, and anaplasmosis are all obligate intracellular pathogens, but the target host cells they infect and subsequent pathology vary by organism.

R rickettsii is transmitted from the tick to humans via a painless bite, which often goes unrecognized. The organism resides in the salivary gland of the tick and is passed during acquisition of a blood meal. *R rickettsii* can be transmitted as early as 10 to 24 hours after tick attachment. When transmitted to a human host, *R rickettsia* localize and multiply in vascular endothelial cells, and, less commonly, underlying smooth muscle cells of small and medium vessels, resulting in vasculitis. The vasculitis is the underlying mechanism for most of the clinical features and laboratory abnormalities of RMSF. Injury to the vascular endothelium results in increased capillary permeability, microhemorrhage, and platelet consumption. Late-stage complications of pulmonary edema (acute respiratory distress syndrome) and cerebral edema are consequences of the microvascular leakage.

E chaffeensis predominantly infects monocytes and tissue macrophages and replicates in cytoplasmic vacuoles called morulae. Unlike RMSF, direct vasculitis and endothelial injury are rare in human monocytic ehrlichiosis. Frequent pathologic findings include granuloma formation, myeloid hyperplasia, and megakaryocytosis in the bone marrow. The severe pathology and multiorgan involvement in severe and fatal HME in immunocompetent patients is believed to be due to dysregulation of the host immune response that leads to tissue damage and eventually multiorgan failure. *E ewingii* has a predilection for neutrophils, and morulae can be observed in granulocytes of the blood, cerebrospinal fluid (CSF), and bone marrow.

A phagocytophilum is found predominantly in neutrophils in the peripheral blood and tissues from infected individuals. *A phagocytophilum* has the unique ability to selectively survive and multiply within cytoplasmic vacuoles (morulae) of polymorphonuclear cells by delaying their apoptosis. Infection with *A phagocytophilum* induces a systemic inflammatory response, which is believed to be the mechanism for tissue damage. Pathologic findings with human granulocytic anaplasmosis include normocellular or hypercellular bone marrow, erythrophagocytosis, hepatic apoptosis, focal splenic necrosis, and mild interstitial pneumonitis and pulmonary hemorrhage.

Clinical Manifestations

A detailed history should include information about known tick bites or activities that might be associated with tick exposure. Unrecognized tick bites are common. A history of a tick bite within 14 days of illness onset is reported in only 50% to 60% of RMSF cases and 68% of ehrlichiosis cases. Absence of a tick bite should never dissuade providers from considering tickborne rickettsial disease in the appropriate clinical context. Contact with pets, especially dogs, and a history of tick attachment or recent tick removal from pets can be useful in assessing human tick exposure.

Tickborne rickettsial diseases commonly have nonspecific clinical signs and symptoms early in the course of disease. Although there is overlap in the clinical presentations of tickborne rickettsial diseases, the frequency of certain associated signs and symptoms (e.g., rash and other cutaneous findings) and typical laboratory findings differ by pathogen and assist providers in developing a differential diagnosis, beginning appropriate antibacterial treatment, and ordering confirmatory diagnostic tests.

Symptoms of RMSF typically begin 3 to 12 days after the bite of an infected tick or 4 to 8 days after discovery of an attached tick. The incubation period is generally shorter (≤5 days) in patients who develop severe disease. Initial symptoms are often nonspecific and include the sudden onset of fever, chills, malaise, and myalgia. Clinical suspicion for RMSF should be maintained in cases of nonspecific febrile illness and sepsis of unclear cause, particularly during the spring and summer months.

The classic triad of fever, rash, and reported tick bite is present in only a minority of RMSF patients during the initial presentation to health care; therefore it is crucial not to wait for development of this triad before considering a diagnosis of RMSF and beginning treatment. A rash typically occurs 2 to 4 days after the onset of fever; however, many patients initially seek medical care before the rash. In one large series of patients with RMSF, 88% of patients had a rash, but only 49% had a rash in the first 3 days. Children more frequently have rash (97%) and develop the rash earlier. The rash typically begins as small, blanching macules on the ankles, wrists, or forearms that then spreads to the palms, soles, arms, legs, and trunk, usually sparing the face. The generalized petechial rash appears later (day 5 or 6) and is indicative of advanced disease. An inoculation eschar is rarely present with RMSF. In addition to rash, the most frequent clinical findings at any point in the illness are fever (99%), headache (91%), and myalgia (82%).

The total white blood cell count is typically normal or mildly increased with RMSF, and increased numbers of immature neutrophils are often present. Thrombocytopenia, slight elevations of AST or ALT, and hyponatremia might be present, particularly as the disease advances. Laboratory values cannot be relied on to guide early treatment decisions because they are often within or slightly deviated from normal reference values early in the course. When CSF is obtained, a lymphocytic (less commonly neutrophilic) pleocytosis can be present, along with a moderately elevated CSF protein. CSF glucose is generally normal.

R parkeri rickettsiosis is a milder illness compared with RMSF; no severe manifestations or death has been reported. Symptoms develop a median of 5 days (range, 2–10 days) after the bite of an infected tick. The first manifestation in nearly all patients is an inoculation eschar, which generally is nonpruritic, nontender or mildly tender, and surrounded by an indurated, erythematous halo and occasionally a few petechiae. Shortly after the onset of fever (0.5–4 days later), a nonpruritic maculopapular or vesicopustular rash develops in 90% of patients. The rash primarily involves the extremities and trunk and in ~half of patients involves the palms and soles. Headache (86%) and myalgia (76%) are common. Laboratory findings include modest elevation of hepatic transaminases (78%), mild leukopenia (50%), and thrombocytopenia (40%).

Few patients with *Rickettsia* species 364D have been reported, so the full clinical spectrum has yet to be described. It does appear to be relatively mild and characterized by an eschar or ulcerative skin lesion with regional lymphadenopathy. Fever, headache, and myalgia occur, but rash has not been a notable feature.

Symptoms of *E chaffeensis* ehrlichiosis typically occur a median of 9 days (range, 5–15 days) after an infected tick bite. Fever (96%), headache (72%), malaise (77%), and myalgia (58%) are common. Abdominal pain, vomiting, and diarrhea can occur, particularly in children. Rash (maculopapular, petechial, or diffuse erythema) occurs in approximately one-third of patients and is more frequent in children. The rash occurs a median of 5 days after illness onset and can involve the palms and soles. Neurologic manifestations are present in ~20% of patients. Characteristic laboratory findings in the first week include leukopenia, thrombocytopenia, and elevated levels of hepatic transaminases. *Ehrlichia ewingii* and *Ehrlichia muris*-like agent ehrlichiosis have similar clinical and laboratory features as *E chaffeensis* ehrlichiosis, although rash and gastrointestinal symptoms are less common.

Symptoms of human granulocytic anaplasmosis typically occur 5 to 14 days after an infected tick bite. Fever (92%–100%), headache (82%), malaise (97%), and myalgia (77%) are common. Rash is present in <10% of patients, and central nervous system involvement is rare. Laboratory findings are similar to ehrlichiosis.

Diagnosis

Early diagnosis and initiation of treatment of tickborne rickettsial diseases is based on clinical and epidemiologic findings, as rapid confirmatory assays are often not available or reliable to guide treatment decisions early in the clinical course. Confirmatory diagnostic tests are serologic assays, nucleic acid detection, immunostaining of biopsy tissue, blood-smear microscopy, and culture.

Assays using paired acute and convalescent sera (ideally collected 2–4 weeks apart) are the standard for serologic confirmation. Assays are insensitive during the first week of rickettsial infection. After 7 days of illness, the sensitivity increases. Assays are highly sensitive 2 to 3 weeks after illness onset. Early therapy with doxycycline may diminish or delay the development of antibodies in RMSF.

A diagnosis of tickborne rickettsial diseases is confirmed with a ≥fourfold increase in antibody titer in patients with a clinically compatible acute illness. A single IgG antibody reciprocal titer ≥64 is supportive of, but not confirmatory for, the diagnosis. In the United States, *R rickettsia*–reactive IgG antibody reciprocal titers ≥64 can be found in 5% to 10% of the population who do not acutely have RMSF. Some laboratories also perform assays for IgM antibodies. However, because of the lower specificity of IgM compared with IgG assays, IgM titers should not be used as a stand-alone method for diagnosis.

PCR amplification of DNA from whole blood specimens collected during the acute stage of illness is particularly useful for confirming *E chaffeensis*, *A phagocytophilum*, *E ewingii*, and EML agent infections due to the tropism of those organisms for circulating cells. PCR detection of *R rickettsia* in whole blood is less sensitive, as low numbers of rickettsiae typically circulate in the blood in the absence of advanced disease. Tissue specimens such as a skin biopsy are a more useful source of SFG rickettsial DNA compared with blood samples. Doxycycline treatment decreases the sensitivity of PCR. Obtaining blood before treatment is recommended to decrease false-negative results.

Immunostaining of a skin punch biopsy is useful for diagnosing RMSF with 100% specificity and 70% sensitivity. Microscopic examination of blood smears or buffy-coat preparations during the first week of illness may reveal leukocyte morulae in patients infected with *E chaffeensis* or anaplasmosis, although it is relatively insensitive, and accuracy is dependent on having experienced microscopists. Culture is the reference standard for microbiologic diagnosis, but the agents that cause tickborne rickettsial diseases require cell culture techniques that are not widely available.

Differential Diagnosis

The differential diagnosis of fever and rash is broad, and during the early stages of illness tickborne rickettsial diseases can be indistinguishable from many viral exanthams, particularly in children. In addition to viral infections, conditions that should be considered include meningococcemia, Kawasaki disease, secondary syphilis, disseminated gonococcal infection, bacterial endocarditis, scarlet fever, leptospirosis, typhoid, drug eruptions, Stevens-Johnson syndrome, toxic shock syndrome, and thrombotic thrombocytopenic purpura.

Treatment

Doxycycline is the drug of choice for treatment of all tickborne rickettsial diseases in patients of all ages and should be initiated immediately in persons with signs and symptoms suggestive of rickettsial disease. Treatment decisions should never be delayed awaiting laboratory confirmation. Multiple studies have noted a delay in appropriate treatment of tickborne rickettsial diseases, particularly after the fifth day of illness for RMSF, to be a significant potentially preventable risk factor for severe disease, increased mortality rates, and long-term sequelae. Because of the nonspecific signs and symptoms of tickborne rickettsial diseases, concomitant empiric treatment for other conditions in the differential diagnosis should be administered (e.g., treatment with ceftriaxone for meningococcemia).

The recommended dose of doxycycline is 100 mg twice daily (IV or oral) for adults and 2.2 mg/kg twice daily (IV or oral) for children weighing <45 kg.[1] Oral therapy is appropriate for patients with early-stage disease who can be treated as outpatients. The recommended duration of therapy for RMSF and ehrlichiosis is at least 3 days after fever resolves and until evidence of clinical improvement is noted; typically, the minimum total course is 5 to 7 days. Severe or complicated disease could require a longer course. HGA should be treated for 10 days to provide appropriate therapy for possible coinfection with Lyme disease.

The use of doxycycline to treat children with suspected tickborne rickettsial disease should no longer be a subject of controversy. The American Academy of Pediatrics and CDC recommend doxycycline as the treatment of choice for children of all ages with suspected tickborne rickettsial disease. Doxycycline used at the recommended dose and duration for RMSF in children aged <8 years, even after multiple courses, has not resulted in tooth staining or enamel hypoplasia.

Chloramphenicol in the past was used as an alternative drug for treating RMSF. However, chloramphenicol has been associated with a higher risk of death compared to patients treated with a tetracycline; in vitro evidence indicates that chloramphenicol is not effective treatment for ehrlichiosis or anaplasmosis. Chloramphenicol is no longer available in the oral form in the United States, and the IV form is not readily available at all institutions.

Chloramphenicol has been recommended for the treatment of RMSF during pregnancy based on adverse effects of older tetracycline drugs (but not specifically doxycycline). Although there is limited evidence, doxycycline has not been associated with teratogenicity or maternal hepatic toxicity during pregnancy, and doxycycline has been used successfully to treat tickborne rickettsial diseases in several pregnant women without adverse effects.

Rifamycins demonstrate in vitro activity against *E chaffeensis* and *A phagocytophilum*. Case reports document favorable outcomes in small numbers of pregnant women treated with rifampin for anaplasmosis. Rifampin[1] could be an alternative for treatment of confirmed mild anaplasmosis (RMSF ruled out) during pregnancy or documented allergy to tetracycline-class drugs. Rifampin is not acceptable treatment for RMSF or potential coinfection with *B burgdorferi*.

Treatment of symptom-free persons seropositive for tickborne rickettsial disease is not recommended, regardless of past treatment, because antibodies can persist for months to years after infection.

Monitoring and Complications

Fever with tickborne rickettsial diseases typically subsides within 24 to 48 hours when treated with doxycycline in the first 4 to 5 days of illness. Lack of a clinical response within 48 hours of early treatment with doxycycline could indicate the illness is not a tickborne rickettsial disease, and alternative diagnoses or coinfection should be considered. Severely ill patients may require >48 hours of treatment before clinical improvement is noted. Patients with mild disease treated on an outpatient basis need close follow-up to ensure they are responding appropriately.

Patients with evidence of organ dysfunction, severe thrombocytopenia, mental status changes, or the need for supportive therapy should be hospitalized. Other considerations for hospitalization include the likelihood and ability to take oral medication and existing comorbid conditions, including the patient's immune status. Infection with RMSF and to a somewhat lesser extent HME are most likely to have a severe disease or death. Severe, late-stage manifestations of RMSF include meningoencephalitis, acute respiratory distress syndrome (ARDS), acute renal failure, arrhythmia, and seizures. Severe manifestations of HME include ARDS, shock-like syndromes, renal failure, hepatic failure, coagulopathies, and hemorrhagic complications.

Severe or life-threatening manifestations are less frequent with anaplasmosis than with RMSF or HME. Predictors of a more severe course of anaplasmosis include advanced age, immunosuppression, comorbid medical conditions, and delay in diagnosis and treatment. Confirmed *A phagocytophilum* coinfection has been reported in <10% of patients with Lyme disease. Response to treatment can provide clues to possible coinfection with Lyme disease or babesiosis. If the clinical response to treatment with doxycycline is delayed, coinfection or an alternate infection should be considered. Conversely, if Lyme disease is treated with a beta-lactam antibiotic in a patient with unrecognized *A phagocytophilum* infection symptoms could persist.

Prevention

The best prevention for all the tickborne rickettsial diseases is to avoid tick bites, perform regular tick checks on humans and pets, and promptly remove attached ticks. Longer periods of tick attachment increase the probability of transmission of tickborne diseases. Repellents and protective clothing can reduce the risk for tick bites. Products containing 20% to 30% N,N-Diethyl-meta-toluamide (DEET) effectively repel ticks and can be applied directly to the skin. DEET is not recommended for use on infants younger than 2 months. Permethrin-treated or -impregnated clothing can significantly reduce tick bites. Prophylactic treatment is not recommended in persons who have had recent tick bites and are well.

References

Biggs HM, Behravesh CB, Bradley KK, et al: Diagnosis and management of tickborne rickettsial diseases: Rocky Mountain spotted fever and other spotted fever group rickettsioses, ehrlichioses, and anaplasmosis—United States, *MMWR Recomm Rep* 65:1–44, 2016.

---

[1]Not FDA approved for this indication.

[1]Not FDA approved for this indication.

Buckingham SC, Marshall GS, Schutze GE, et al: Clinical and laboratory features, hospital course, and outcome of Rocky Mountain spotted fever in children, *J Pediatr* 150:180–184, 2007.

Cross R, Ling C, Day NPJ, McGready R, Paris DH: Revisiting doxycycline in pregnancy and early childhood—time to rebuild its reputation? *Expert Opin Drug Saf* 15:367–382, 2016.

Dahlgren FS, Holman RC, Paddock CD, Callinan LS, McQuiston JH: Fatal Rocky Mountain spotted fever in the United States, 1999–2007, *Am J Trop Med Hyg* 86:713–719, 2012.

Hamburg BJ, Storch GA, Micek ST, Kollef MH: The importance of early treatment with doxycycline in human ehrlichiosis, *Medicine (Baltimore)* 87:53–60, 2008.

Helmick CG, Bernard KW, D'Angelo LJ: Rocky Mountain spotted fever: clinical, laboratory, and epidemiological features of 262 cases, *J Infect Dis* 150:480–488, 1984.

Ismail N, McBride JW: Tick-borne emerging infections: ehrlichiosis and anaplasmosis, *Clin Lab Med* 37:317–340, 2017.

Kirkland KB, Wilkinson WE, Sexton DJ: Therapeutic delay and mortality in cases of Rocky Mountain spotted fever, *Clin Infect Dis* 20:1118–1121, 1995.

Marshall GS, Stout GG, Jacobs RF, et al: Antibodies reactive to Rickettsia rickettsii among children living in the southeast and south central regions of the United States, *Arch Pediatr Adoles Med* 157:443–448, 2003.

TOXIC SHOCK SYNDROME

Method of
Julius Larioza, MD; and Richard B. Brown, MD

KEY DIAGNOSTIC AND THERAPEUTIC POINTS

- Toxic shock syndrome (TSS) secondary to *Staphylococcus aureus* and *Streptococcus pyogenes* (Group A Streptococcus [GAS]) is an acute-onset illness causing systemic symptoms of fever, hypotension, and desquamative rash with the potential for high morbidity and rapid mortality. Clostridium species TSS may lack fever and rash but is often fatal.

- TSS secondary to staphylococcus and streptococcus is associated with elaboration of bacterial toxins, with a resultant vigorous cytokine cascade leading to multiorgan failure. Clostridium species toxins have a direct cellular effect on vascular endothelium.

- Diagnosis of TSS is based on fulfillment of criteria that involve identification of a constellation of clinical and laboratory data.

- A strong suspicion, early recognition, and aggressive management may decrease overall mortality and morbidity. Treatment consists of strategies to control the source of infection, decrease toxin production, and provide appropriate antibiotic therapy, surgical intervention, and clinical support with close monitoring of end-organ function. Three major causes of TSS have been identified. Those caused by toxin-producing strains of *Staphylococcus aureus* and *Streptococcus pyogenes* produce an acute, desquamative febrile illness. Clostridium species (*Clostridium sordellii, Clostridium perfringens*) TSS lacks the febrile illness or rash but may rapidly lead to multiorgan system failure with substantial morbidity and mortality.

Epidemiology

Staphylococcal toxic shock syndrome (TSS) was first reported in 1978 in previously healthy children with *Staphylococcus aureus* infection. Estimated incidence peaked in the early 1980s, with between 6.2 and 12.3 cases per 100,000 population. Ninety percent of cases were associated with tampon use in healthy, young menstruating women. With a decrease in tampon absorbency, changes in tampon composition and usage patterns, standardized labeling, and greater awareness among women and physicians, incidence fell to about 1 case per 100,000 population in the United States. By 1986 rates of menstrual and nonmenstrual TSS cases were 1 and 0.3 per 100,000, respectively. Menstrual TSS declined from 91% of all TSS cases (1979–1980) to 59% (1987–1996). Of nonmenstrual causes, almost 20% were reported following surgery, 11.5% were postpartum or postabortion, and 23% were associated with nonsurgical cutaneous lesions. Incidence of postoperative cases of TSS following all types of surgery was estimated to be 3 per 100,000 population and was

higher following ear, nose, and throat surgery, likely related to nasal packing. The latest population-based report of incidence between 2000 and 2006 in Minneapolis–St. Paul showed menstrual cases at 0.69 and nonmenstrual cases at 0.32 per 100,000 population. The crude mortality rate from staphylococcal TSS is 5% to 8%, with acute respiratory distress syndrome being a major cause of death.

The incidence of streptococcal TSS corresponds to that of invasive group A streptococcal (GAS) disease. In the United States approximately 10,000 cases of invasive GAS occur each year, with an annual incidence of 3 to 3.5 cases per 100,000 population. TSS complicates 10% to 15% of cases. The crude mortality rate is significantly higher than with staphylococcal TSS and reaches 30% to 80% in adults and 5% to 10% in children.

The current passive surveillance system for TSS is limited given the complexity of the clinical diagnosis and lack of a single test. Because studies related to incidence of both staphylococcal and streptococcal TSS use the Centers for Disease Control and Prevention (CDC) case definition that identifies the most severe cases, they may underestimate the total TSS disease burden.

Clostridium species are uncommon causes of TSS but have been reported to cause fatal disease after medical or spontaneous abortion. These organisms are found in the vaginal tract of pregnant women and likely ascend to cause disease after abortion with or without cervical instrumentation. There are no available incidence data for clostridium species TSS, but it has been reported in case series and is associated with a case fatality rate of at least 70%.

Risk Factors

In patients with staphylococcal TSS, previous antibiotic treatment and hospital exposure may predispose to colonization with toxigenic strains of *Staphylococcus aureus*. Primary staphylococcal infections such as pneumonia, postsurgical state, disruption of skin or mucous membranes, abscesses or burns, and foreign body placement have also been noted as risk factors. The absence of protective antitoxin antibodies may be a predisposing factor.

A major risk factor for streptococcal TSS is extremes of age. This is more common in persons ≥65 years old, followed by those <2 years old. Higher incidence was also observed in persons with underlying chronic illnesses, in pregnancy as well as childbirth, after varicella infection, and with use of nonsteroidal antiinflammatory drugs. Any disease or injury compromising the mucosal surface or skin barrier may predispose a patient to streptococcal TSS. Transfer of the disease from one individual to another may also occur, as clusters of GAS infections have been described in nursing homes and among health-care workers and family members.

Main risk factors of clostridium species TSS are pregnancy, abortion, injection drug use, recent trauma, or (less commonly) cadaveric musculoskeletal graft surgery.

Pathophysiology

The hypothesis for the development of TSS is that infection with *Staphylococcus aureus* or *Streptococcus pyogenes* results in the production of toxins that act as superantigens. Staphylococcal TSS is normally associated with TSST-1, staphylococcal enterotoxin (SE) serotype B (SEB) or serotype C (SEC). Most cases of streptococcal TSS have been associated with streptococcal pyrogenic exotoxin (SPE) serotypes A (SPE A) and C (SPE C). These proteins share the ability to trigger excessive T-cell activation. Whereas conventional antigens stimulate on the order of 1 in 10,000 T cells, superantigens may stimulate over 20% of all T cells. This large expansion of T cells is believed to be responsible for severe clinical consequences such as capillary leakage leading to hypotension, shock, multiorgan failure, and death.

Clostridium sordellii and *C. perfringens* secrete lethal and hemorrhagic toxins. Unlike staphylococcal or streptococcal TSS, these toxins do not act as superantigens. Rather, they are large molecular weight proteins that have glycosyl transferase activity, modifying members of the Rho GTPase superfamily to disrupt crucial cell processes that particularly affect vascular endothelial cells. These culminate in vascular leak and are suggested to be the main virulence factors that lead to rapid progression to shock and death.

Clinical Manifestations

Staphylococcal TSS typically presents abruptly with an influenza-like prodrome consisting of fever, gastrointestinal upset, and myalgia, followed commonly by confusion, lethargy, and agitation. Symptoms of hypovolemia are common. If present, a focus of infection is more likely to be superficial, may complicate burns or a surgical wound, or may result from a foreign body. Desquamation is a characteristic late feature. Blood cultures are positive in <5% of cases. After the onset of symptoms, progression is rapid and multiorgan failure can present in 8 to 12 hours.

Streptococcal TSS more commonly arises from deep-seated, invasive, soft-tissue infections such as necrotizing fasciitis and myositis. An influenza-like illness is also common in the early stage with fever, sore throat, swollen lymph nodes, and gastrointestinal upset. Local pain may be severe and is one of the most common reasons for seeking medical attention. Patients with a defined entry site may have early and visible signs of inflammation. In the absence of a definite portal of entry, clinical evidence of a deep infection becomes more obvious as the illness progresses. The initiating injury may be blunt trauma, muscle strain, and hematoma or joint effusion and may seem trivial. Like staphylococcal TSS, hypotension and organ dysfunction are rapidly progressive but unlike it, most (60%) patients with streptococcal TSS have positive blood cultures. Bacteremia alone, however, is not sufficient to explain the complications and increased mortality associated with streptococcal TSS.

Clostridium species toxic shock was suggested in previously healthy women with recent mifepristone (Mifeprex) and misoprostol (Cytotec) pregnancy termination. Women were noted to have nonspecific complaints of sudden onset of weakness, nausea, vomiting, diarrhea, and abdominal pain. A rapid sequence of progressive hypotension and local and spreading edema was associated with severe hemoconcentration and marked leukemoid reaction. The syndrome was described with the identification of Clostridium sordellii or C. perfringens and exclusion of a staphylococcal cause of the rapidly progressive shock. Absence of fever, presence of refractory tachycardia, local edema at the infected site, and subsequent pleural and peritoneal effusions are seen.

Diagnosis

The diagnostic criteria for TSS are based on the clinical case definitions updated by the CDC in 2010 and 2011 for streptococcal TSS and staphylococcal TSS, respectively. They are presented in Table 1.

Additional laboratory abnormalities include an increase in bands, anemia, hypocalcemia, and hypoproteinemia. Cultures from sites of infection are usually positive and should be sought.

In clostridium species TSS, case definition is incomplete. The clinical manifestations as described should be confirmed by additional laboratory tests such as anaerobic culture of the cervix, histopathologic, immunohistochemical, and molecular studies of surgical or autopsy tissue to confirm necrotizing endometritis, and presence of clostridium species.

Differential Diagnoses

TSS can be confused with acute pyelonephritis, acute rheumatic fever, acute viral syndrome such as measles, Legionnaire disease, leptospirosis, Lyme disease, pelvic inflammatory disease, osteomyelitis, scarlet fever, typhus, meningococcemia, Rocky Mountain spotted fever, ehrlichiosis, and gram-negative sepsis. Noninfectious illnesses that lead to septic shock, severe drug reactions, Kawasaki disease (in children), flares of autoimmune illnesses such as systemic lupus erythematosus, tumors, and hemolytic uremic syndrome may also mimic the syndrome.

Therapy

Poor outcome is due in part to the nonspecific features at presentation leading to missed or delayed diagnosis and underestimation of the aggressive nature of the infection delaying treatment. Highest probability for successful outcome lies with early identification and a therapeutic strategy that involves hemodynamic stabilization and specific antibiotics to eradicate the bacteria and control toxin synthesis. Vigorous attempts at source control are mandatory. Timely management of hypovolemic shock is critical. Microbial

TABLE 1 Diagnostic Criteria for Toxic Shock Syndrome (TSS)	
CASE DEFINITION	
STAPHYLOCOCCAL TSS (2011)	**STREPTOCOCCAL TSS (2010)**
Clinical Manifestation	**Clinical Manifestation**

Fever: temperature ≥102° F
Rash: diffuse macular erythroderma
Desquamation: 1–2 weeks after onset of rash
Hypotension: systolic blood pressure ≤90 mm Hg for adults or <5th percentile by age for children <16 years old
Multisystem involvement (three or more of the following organ systems):
  Gastrointestinal: vomiting or diarrhea at onset of illness
  Muscular: severe myalgia or creatinine phosphokinase level at least twice the upper limit of normal
  Mucous membrane: vaginal, oropharyngeal, or conjunctival hyperemia
  Renal: blood urea nitrogen or creatinine at least twice the upper limit of normal or urinary sediment with pyuria (≥5 leukocytes per high-power field) in the absence of urinary tract infection
  Hepatic: total bilirubin, alanine aminotransferase enzyme (ALT), or aspirate aminotransferase (AST) enzyme levels at least twice the upper limit of normal
  Hematologic: platelets <100,000/mm³
  Central nervous system: disorientation or alterations in consciousness without focal neurologic signs when fever and hypotension are absent
	Hypotension
	Multisystem involvement (two or more of the following organ systems):
	  Renal: creatinine ≥2 mg/dL for adults or greater than twofold the upper limit of normal for age. In patients with preexisting renal disease, a greater than twofold elevation over baseline level
	  Coagulopathy: platelets <100,000/mm³ or disseminated intravascular coagulation, defined by prolonged clotting times, low fibrinogen level, and presence of fibrin degradation products
	  Hepatic: ALT, AST, or total bilirubin levels more than twice the upper limit of normal for the patient's age. In a patient with preexisting liver disease, a greater than twofold increase over the baseline level
	  Acute respiratory distress syndrome: defined by acute onset of diffuse pulmonary infiltrated and hypoxemia in the absence of cardiac failure or by evidence of diffuse capillary leak manifested by acute onset of generalized edema, or pleural or peritoneal effusions with hypoalbuminemia
	A generalized erythematous macular rash that may desquamate
	Soft-tissue necrosis, including necrotizing fasciitis or myositis, or gangrene

Laboratory Criteria	**Laboratory Criteria**
Negative results on the following tests, if obtained: Blood or cerebrospinal fluid (CSF) cultures (blood cultures may be positive for Staphylococcus aureus) Negative serologies for Rocky Mountain spotted fever, leptospirosis, or measles	Isolation of group A Streptococcus
Case Classification	**Case Classification**
Probable: meets the laboratory criteria and with four of the five clinical findings shown above present Confirmed: meets the laboratory criteria and with all five of the clinical findings above present including desquamation, unless the patient dies before desquamation occurs	Probable: meets the clinical case definition in the absence of another identified etiology for the illness and with isolation of group A Streptococcus from a nonsterile site Confirmed: meets the clinical case definition and with isolation of group A Streptococcus from a normally sterile site (e.g., blood or CSF or, less commonly, joint, pleural, or pericardial fluid)

documentation is rarely available at the onset of management; thus early antimicrobial therapy should be broad. At present the best empiric choices for serious gram-positive infections include vancomycin (Vancocin), linezolid (Zyvox), daptomycin (Cubicin), and tigecycline (Tygacil). The dosing schedule is summarized in

Table 2. Antimicrobial coverage may then be narrowed as the clinical picture and culture results become available to the clinician.

Semisynthetic penicillins and cephalosporins increase TSST-1 in culture, probably by lysis or increased cell membrane permeability. In the setting of increasing incidence of methicillin-resistant *Staphylococcus aureus*, these drugs should be avoided as empiric therapy. There is no obvious direct effect of vancomycin on toxin production while clindamycin has been shown to reduce TSST-1 by 90%. Thus, use of clindamycin in combination with a second agent such as vancomycin results in a potentially beneficial effect by decreasing the synthesis of TSST-1.

For streptococcal TSS, clindamycin is more effective because its antimicrobial activity is not affected by the inoculum size or dependent on penicillin-binding proteins; because it acts by inhibiting protein synthesis, it also inhibits the synthesis of antiphagocyte M protein and bacterial toxins (SPEs), subsequently reducing the superantigenicity of SPEs. It has a longer postantibiotic effect than β-lactams. Thus clindamycin is recommended although not as empiric monotherapy because up to 20% of GAS are resistant to it. Linezolid also has the ability to suppress toxin synthesis and may be an alternative as monotherapy or in combination with vancomycin.

Antimicrobial therapy should be continued for at least 10 to 14 days to eradicate the organism and prevent recurrences. The total duration should be based on the usual duration established for the underlying focus of infection.

TABLE 2	Empiric Antibiotics for Gram-Positive Infections	
AGENT	**DOSE (ADJUST FOR RENAL DYSFUNCTION)**
Vancomycin* (Vancocin)	15–20 mg/kg q12h (up to 4 g daily)[3]
Tigecycline (Tygacil)	Start with 100 mg×1, then 50 mg q12h
Daptomycin* (Cubicin)	6–8 mg/kg q24h[3]
Clindamycin (Cleocin)	900 mg q8h
Linezolid (Zyvox)	600 mg q12h

[3]Exceeds dosage recommended by the manufacturer.
*Requires renal adjustment.

A thorough and continuous search for possible sites of infection is key to eliminate any preformed toxin and to prevent further synthesis of toxins. Removal of suspect foreign bodies especially tampons is mandatory. Surgical wounds should be considered as possible reservoirs of infection, even if no superficial signs of local infection or purulent discharge are present. Infected wounds should be inspected, any packing should be removed, and abscesses should be drained and irrigated. Culture specimens from all possible sites should be obtained. Patients suspected of having necrotizing fasciitis should have urgent surgical intervention for fasciotomy and debridement.

With clostridium species, the presence of an anaerobic environment enhances growth and toxin production. Thus drainage and aggressive removal of necrotic tissue is important. Older literature suggests that total hysterectomy is often required. Antimicrobial agents with anaerobic coverage should be foremost for gram-positive infection. Inhibitors of protein synthesis such as clindamycin, linezolid, and fluoroquinolones may be of additional benefit.

Intravenous immunoglobulin (IVIG)[1] may be of value when given in addition to appropriate antimicrobial therapy. The neutralizing and protective activity against the superantigenic toxins has been reviewed but results appear variable. There are no current guidelines for the use of IVIG, but it may be used for TSS resulting from an infection refractory to several hours of aggressive therapy.

Monitoring

Control and monitoring of shock and individual organ dysfunction are best achieved in the setting of the intensive-care unit. There, active fluid resuscitation, early use of vasopressors or inotropes, or both, and mechanical ventilation if required are done. Appropriate management of associated problems such as renal failure and adult respiratory distress syndrome must be addressed. Monitoring of hemodynamic status and constant surveillance by repeated clinical examination and laboratory investigation searching for evidence of increasing burden of toxin production and subsequent clearance of the source of infections provide the highest chances of survival and equally prevention of further comorbidities related to irreversible organ system damage. Table 3 summarizes the characteristics of TSS by organism.

[1] Not FDA approved for this indication.

TABLE 3	Summary of Toxic Shock Syndrome by Organism		
CHARACTERISTIC	**STAPHYLOCOCCUS AUREUS**	**STREPTOCOCCUS PYOGENES**	**CLOSTRIDIUM SORDELLII, C. PERFRINGENS**
Fatality rate (%)	5–8	30–80	≥70
Major risk factors	Tampon use Skin and soft tissue infection Foreign body	Mucosal or skin barrier compromise Extremes of age	Cervical or intrauterine manipulation Pregnancy and/or termination
Pathophysiology	Toxins produced (TSST-1, SEB, SEC) act as superantigens	Toxins produced (SPE A, SPE C) act as superantigens	Toxins produced (lethal, hemorrhagic) act directly on vascular endothelium
Clinical manifestation	Flulike illness Fever Gastrointestinal (GI) upset Myalgia Desquamate late Superficial infection	Flulike illness Fever Sore throat, cervical lymphadenopathy GI upset Severe myalgia Desquamate early Deeper infection	Absent fever Absent rash GI upset Edema Abdominal pain Intrauterine manipulation Pleural and peritoneal effusion
Laboratory findings White blood cell count Red blood cell count Platelets Creatine phosphokinase Calcium TP	↑ ↓ ↓ ↑ ↓ ↓	↑ ↓ ↓ ↑↑ ↓	↑↑ ↓ / ↑↑ ↓ ↑↑

Continued

TABLE 3 Summary of Toxic Shock Syndrome by Organism—cont'd

CHARACTERISTIC	STAPHYLOCOCCUS AUREUS	STREPTOCOCCUS PYO-GENES	CLOSTRIDIUM SORDELLII, C. PER-FRINGENS
Empiric therapy	Vancomycin Daptomycin Tigecycline + clindamycin + linezolid + rifampin[1] (never as monotherapy) β-Lactamase inhibitor (if no methicillin-resistant *Staphylococcus aureus*)	β-Lactams Vancomycin Daptomycin Tigecycline + clindamycin + linezolid	Gram-positive antimicrobial with anaerobic coverage (carbapenem, piperacillin-tazobactam [Zosyn], tigecycline, moxifloxacin [Avelox]) + clindamycin + linezolid
Surgical intervention	±	+	++

[1]Not FDA approved for this indication.

Abbreviations: SEB=staphylococcal enterotoxin serotype B; SEC=staphylococcal enterotoxin serotype C; SPE A=streptococcal pyrogenic exotoxin serotype A; SPE C=streptococcal pyrogenic exotoxin serotype C.

Complications

Besides the obvious mortality, long-term morbidity was observed in up to 90% of TSS cases, with 20% experiencing recurrent episodes, 50% having long-term memory loss and abnormal electrocardiographic findings, and 23% having recurrent syncope or cardiomyopathy.

References

Andrews M, Parent EM, Barry M, Parsonnet J: Recurrent nonmenstrual toxic shock syndrome: clinical manifestations, diagnosis, and treatment, *Clin Infect Dis* 32:1470–1479, 2001.

Annane D, Clair B, Salomon J: Managing toxic shock syndrome with antibiotics, *Expert Opin Pharmacother* 5:1701–1710, 2005.

Aranoff DM, Ballard JD: Clostridium sordellii toxic shock syndrome, *Lancet Infect Dis* 9:725–726, 2009.

Centers for Disease Control and Prevention: Toxic Shock Syndrome, *Case definition*, 2011. https://wwwn.cdc.gov/nndss/conditions/streptococcal-toxic-shock-syndrome/case-definition/2010 . [Accessed August 11, 2016].

Centers for Disease Control and Prevention: Streptococcal Toxic Shock Syndrome. Case definition, 2010. https://wwwn.cdc.gov/nndss/conditions/toxic-shocksyn-drome-other-than-streptococcal/case-definition/2011. [Accessed August 11, 2016].

Cohen AL, Bhatnagar J, Reagan S, et al: Toxic shock associated with *Clostridium sordellii* and *Clostridium perfringens* after medical and spontaneous abortion, *Obstet Gynecol* 110:1027–1033, 2007.

Devries AS, Lesher L, Schlievert PM, et al: Staphylococcal toxic shock syndrome 2000–2006: epidemiology, clinical features, and molecular characteristics, *PLoS One* 6(8):e22997, 2011. https://doi.org/10.1371/journal.pone.0022997. [accessed 01.12.11].

Herzer CM: Toxic shock syndrome: broadening the differential diagnosis, *J Am Board Fam Pract* 14:131–136, 2001.

Lappin E, Ferguson AJ: Gram-positive toxic shock syndromes, *Lancet Infect Dis* 9:281–290, 2009.

McCormick JK, Yarwood JM, Schlievert PM: Toxic shock syndrome and bacterial superantigens: an update, *Annu Rev Microbiol* 55:77–104, 2001.

Stevens DL: Streptococcal toxic-shock syndrome: spectrum of disease, pathogenesis, and new concepts in treatment, *Emerg Infect Dis* 1:69–78, 1995.

Stevens DL, Wallace RJ, Hamilton SM, Bryant AE: Successful treatment of staphylococcal toxic shock syndrome with linezolid: a case report and in vitro eradication of the production of toxin shock syndrome staphylococcal toxin type 1 in the presence of antibiotics, *Clin Infect Dis* 42:729–730, 2006.

TOXOPLASMOSIS

Method of
Carlo Contini, MD

CURRENT DIAGNOSIS

- The diagnosis of *Toxoplasma gondii* infection mostly relies on serologic detection of specific IgM and IgG antibodies.
- Specific IgM antibodies with low IgG (IgG-avidity testing) are consistent with recent infection in immunocompetent persons. Positive IgG antibodies in the absence of IgM in healthy persons indicate past infection and resistance to reinfection.
- Amniocentesis and polymerase chain reaction (PCR)–based analysis on amniotic fluid (AF) [past 18 weeks' gestation] are useful to establish a certain or presumed seroconversion in pregnancy and to determine whether the infection was transmitted to the offspring.
- IgM, IgA, or both at birth indicate probable congenital infection.
- Serologic testing is not useful for the diagnosis of TE in AIDS patients, who should instead undergo computed tomography (CT) or magnetic resonance imaging (MRI), cerebrospinal fluid (CSF)–*T-gondii* DNA PCR testing, or demonstration of tachyzoites by histology.
- Serologic screening is helpful in identifying transplant patients at risk, especially seronegative recipients with seropositive donors, and can help in establishing the diagnosis by showing seroconversion. Serologic follow-up combined with PCR after allogeneic hematopoietic stem cell transplantation (HSCT) is recommended in all patients at risk for toxoplasmosis.

CURRENT THERAPY

- All immunocompetent patients, as well as nonpregnant women with acute toxoplasmosis presenting with lymphadenitis and fever, generally do not require specific antimicrobial treatment because the infection is self-limited and usually subclinical.
- Pyrimethamine (Daraprim) plus sulfadiazine[1] plus folinic acid (Leucovorin)[1] is the standard and preferred regimen against toxoplasmosis. It is recommended for acute *T gondii* infection in immunocompetent adults with acute illness; pregnant women who acquire the infection after 18 weeks' gestation or in whom fetal infection is documented (positive PCR-AF); and immunosuppressed patients, including AIDS patients. Patients who do not tolerate the standard regimen should be given alternative drugs such as clarithromycin (Biaxin),[1] azithromycin (Zithromax),[1] atovaquone (Mepron),[1] and dapsone.[1]
- Trimethoprim-sulfamethoxazole (TMP-SMX, Bactrim)[1] has been shown to have efficacy similar to pyrimethamine-sulfadiazine and may be used as an alternative if patients do not have sulfa allergy and pyrimethamine is not tolerated or is not available.
- Oral spiramycin (Rovamycine)[2] is the drug most often used in the prenatal therapy of congenital toxoplasmosis (before 18 weeks of gestation) because of high concentration in placenta without crossing it and of its relative lack of toxicity compared with the teratogenic effects of pyrimethamine.

Toxoplasma gondii is a ubiquitous protozoan parasite that is extremely widespread and of great medical importance, infecting all mammalian cells and responsible for human and veterinary diseases. It was initially described in Tunis by Nicolle and Manceaux (1908) in the tissues of the rodent gundi (*Ctenodoactylus gundi*) and later in Brazil by the microbiologist Alfonso Splendore (1908) in the rabbit. Its identification was rapidly followed by the recognition that it was a human pathogen. In this regard, the Italian bacteriologist Castellani (1914) was probably the first to describe a *T gondii*–like parasite in smears of blood and spleen from a 14-year-old Singhalese boy who died of a disease characterized by severe anemia, fever, and splenomegaly. However, it was not until the 1960s and 1970s that the parasite was identified as a coccidian and the cat recognized as the definite host.

Toxoplasma belongs to the phylum *Apicomplexa*, which contains many other protozoan pathogens of human and veterinary importance, such as *Plasmodium* spp. (malaria), *Cryptosporidium* spp (cryptosporidiosis), and *Eimeria* spp (poultry coccidiosis).

Disease can occur through acute infection after recent contact with *T gondii* cysts or oocysts or through endogenous reactivation. Primary infection is usually subclinical, but in some patients cervical or occipital lymphadenopathy or ocular disease is present. Infection acquired during pregnancy can cause severe damage to the fetus if *Toxoplasma* crosses the placental barrier, and it causes abortion or congenital birth defects if the mother becomes infected for the first time shortly before or during pregnancy.

In patients with AIDS and others who are immunocompromised, reactivation of latent disease can cause life-threatening encephalitis. Ocular infection by *Toxoplasma* is a major cause of retinochoroiditis in several geographic areas in both immunocompetent and immunocompromised persons. Due to the heterogeneous parasitologic outcomes and limited immunological data, the role of aging in toxoplasmosis evolution remains poorly understood.

Epidemiology and Risk Factors

Toxoplasmosis is a cosmopolitan zoonotic disease that has important implications for public health because it affects one-third of the world's population. It is also a significant veterinary pathogen that can infect many species of warm-blooded animals. *T gondii* is one of the world's most successful parasites, in part because of its ability to infect and persist in most warm-blooded animals. In general, the prevalence in animals is much higher than that in humans. In China, among the major animals monitored, pigs were the most frequently infected by *T gondii*, reaching 70% in some areas and farms. This high *T gondii* prevalence increases the risks of human infection through meat consumption, because pork is the main meat Chinese people consume. Among other meat-producing animals, sheep and chickens have also high *T gondii* infection rates, and economic losses caused by abortions and other diseases from sheep toxoplasmosis are predicted to be huge in the forthcoming decades.

In humans, the incidence of positive serology for *Toxoplasma* varies greatly around the world and is influenced by different cultures. In Colombia, approximately half of the women of child-bearing age have *T gondii* antibodies, and the clinical disease in congenitally infected children is more severe than in Europe. In humans, seroprevalence of *T gondii* infection rises with age; does not vary greatly between sexes; and is lower in cold regions, hot and arid areas, and at high elevations. Prevalence rates, which range worldwide from <10% to >60%, are thought to depend on food production and harvesting practices, water treatment, environment, climate, and exposure to soil or sand. In the United States, the seroprevalence of *T gondii* appears to be declining. Seroprevalence in Europe is high, up to 54% in southern European countries; it decreases with increasing latitude to 5% and 10% in northern Sweden and Norway, respectively. As is the case of most other protozoa, the prevalence of Toxoplasma is higher in Africa, South America, and in developing areas of the world. In Brazil, there is a higher prevalence of *T gondii* infection among male patients (79.0%) than among female patients (63.4%), according to data obtained from a blood bank.

The sexual cycle of *T gondii* occurs in felines. The estimated seroprevalence for *T gondii* in domestic cats (*Felis catus*), worldwide, is 30% to 40%. Most feline infections occur postnatally through ingestion of infected tissue cysts or rarely oocysts, although congenital infections occur. Tens of millions of unsporulated oocysts may be released in the feces of a single cat in a day, depending on the stage of *T gondii* ingested. These sporulate in 1 to 21 days and are highly infectious to the parasite's intermediate hosts (asexual cycle), which include almost any warm-blooded animal, such as birds, humans, and sea otters.

Sporulated oocysts are very resistant to environmental conditions and to disinfectants; however, they are killed within 1 to 2 minutes by heating to 55°C to 60°C, and the risk of infection is reduced by deep-freezing meat (–12°C or lower) before cooking.

Feline infections are typically subclinical. Common symptoms of *T gondii* infection in cats can include fever, ocular inflammation, anorexia, lethargy, abdominal discomfort, and neurologic abnormalities. Occasionally, pneumonia, liver damage, and loss of vision develop. Why only some cats show symptoms is not known.

Identification of locally prevalent risk factors is critical for health education, and it is generally important for policy. The most important recognized factors influencing the risk of *T gondii* infection are having a cat or a dog, doing household work, having a lower education level, having poor hygiene habits, eating raw vegetables, and working in contact with soil.

Most people are infected inadvertently, and thus the specific route of transmission usually cannot be established. Contact with this obligate intracellular protozoan can occur through the ingestion of oocysts containing sporozoites or cysts containing bradyzoites in contaminated food or water. The major risk factors for *T gondii* exposure are directly related to exposure to cats and more specifically to cat feces, which represent the source of ingestion of sporozoites from the environment. Because cats are the primary host for *T gondii*, cats in the house or stray cats in and around the house or property are considered a primary risk factor for acquiring this parasite during pregnancy. Moreover, any job or activity that puts a pregnant woman in direct contact with soil, sand, or materials such as fruit, vegetables, or drinking water that could have been contaminated by cat feces puts her at risk for being infected. In this setting, rain and surface water can transport infectious oocysts into drinking water supplies and irrigation waters. Coprophagous insects that can contaminate food and fertilizer also contribute to the spread of oocysts. Climate plays an indirect role in allowing better (in the case of moist and hot climate) or worse (in the case of dry and cold climate) survival of oocysts in the environment.

Consumption of undercooked meat of secondary hosts such as pigs and sheep is also a major route of transmission of the disease to humans. The ingestion of undercooked or raw meat during pregnancy is also an important risk factor, because the tissue can contain *T gondii* cysts that, unless destroyed by cooking or by food-preparation practices, could infect a pregnant woman. Heating at 60°C to 100°C for 10 minutes, freezing at either –10°C for 3 days or –20°C for 2 days, or irradiation at doses of 75 to 100 kilo rad is sufficient to kill tissue cysts. Tissue cysts are also killed by gamma irradiation at a dose of 1.0 kGy, but irradiation of meat has not been approved in the European Union (EU). Neither cooking in a microwave oven nor chilling at 5°C for 5 days is sufficient to kill tissue cysts.

The risk of infection rises also in women who taste meat when preparing meals or who eat raw or undercooked beef, lamb, or other meats, but not pork. Eating raw horsemeat imported from non-EU countries can expose consumers to high inocula of highly virulent atypical *T gondii* strains, which can cause a life-threatening primary infection or severe congenital toxoplasmosis with atypical outcome. Transmission during breast-feeding or direct human-to-human transmission other than from mother to fetus (discussed later in the chapter) has not been recorded. Drinking unpasteurized milk and consuming milk products also correlates with increased risk of infections. Although oral transmission is considered the main route of infection, it does not explain the common occurrence of toxoplasmosis in a variety of hosts, such as herbivorous animals, birds, and wild rodents. In this regard, *T gondii* infection has been discovered in particular ticks (i.e., *Haemaphysalis longicornis*) that could serve as a reservoir for secondary toxoplasmosis transmission to other common hosts, if ingested. Other routes are transplacental infection of the fetus, transfusion of white blood cells, and organ transplantation from a seropositive donor to a seronegative recipient.

It is not uncommon for health care professionals, laboratory workers, pet lovers (especially cat owners), butchers, cooks (those handling raw meat), veterinarians, and farmers to acquire acute toxoplasmosis.

Finally, an interesting hypothesis suggested that toxoplasmosis may be transmitted from infected men to noninfected women during unprotected sexual intercourse, resulting in the most dangerous form of disease, the congenital toxoplasmosis. *T gondii* tachyzoites in fact, are present in the seminal fluid and tissue of the testes of various animals including humans.

Dogs can also have a role in the transmission of toxoplasmosis as a mechanical vector by rolling in foul-smelling substances and by ingesting fecal material. Unlike in cats, *T gondii* does not replicate in the dog's gut and no cysts are shed. In areas where dogs and cats are plentiful, immunocompromised persons and pregnant women should be warned of the possibility of acquiring *T gondii* from dogs, as well as from soil contaminated by cats. People should be encouraged to wash their hands after contact with soil, dogs, or cats, as well as before eating.

Pathophysiology

Disease can occur through acute infection after recent contact with *T gondii* cysts or oocysts or through endogenous reactivation. After ingestion, the sporozoites or bradyzoites invade the intestinal epithelium and differentiate to tachyzoites, which disseminate in the blood and replicate within the new host. The parasite translocation into the blood stream may be a possible consequence of localized intestinal inflammation and enteropathy generated by the parasite, which collectively results in impaired integrity of the intestinal mucosa and gut–blood barrier. Transport of the parasite via the bloodstream can occur intracellularly within dendritic cells or monocytes or as a free tachyzoite. Certain Toxoplasma surface antigens aid in the interaction between the tachyzoite and the host cell. One is the perforin-like protein 1 (PLP-1) forming pores in the host cell membrane after binding, as well as playing a role in egress. The success of *Toxoplasma* as a widespread pathogen is due to the effortlessness with which it can be transmitted among the intermediate hosts. Once inside a host, the parasite develops powerful tools to modulate its host cell and to develop into a chronic infection, undergoing bradyzoite development that can evade the host's immune system as well as, in contrast with acute toxoplasmosis, all known antitoxoplasmic drugs.

Host protection from *T gondii* results from a complex cell-mediated immune response involving inflammatory cells, lymphocytes and macrophages, and cytokines. Inoculum size, parasite virulence (strain), genetic background, time of infection (congenital versus postnatal contamination), and sex also contribute to affect the course of infection in human beings and animal models of toxoplasmosis. In particular, the *T gondii* genotype affects its replication rate, migration, and tendency to differentiate to bradyzoites, virulence, and epidemiologic pattern of occurrence. Type II genotypes (most strains isolated from AIDS patients and newborns with congenital disease) and type III genotypes (mostly isolated from animals) are generally less virulent and more cystogenic compared with type I genotypes (also found in congenital disease). Ocular toxoplasmosis in humans is associated with type I but not type II or III genotypes.

Other than the three major Toxoplasma clonal lineages designated as types I, II and III, which are only predominant in Europe and North America (mostly type 2 strain), there are highly polymorphic strains referred to as atypical in South America and Africa, termed Africa 1, 2, and 3.

Genetic background also plays a significant role in increased susceptibility to *T gondii* in humans; HLA-DQ3 appears to be a genetic marker associated with susceptibility to development of TE in patients with AIDS. The mechanisms by which *T gondii* invades host cells and forms an intracellular niche have been extensively reviewed, and several aspects of this process are directly relevant to immunity and pathogenesis. During invasion, three successive waves of proteins are secreted from parasite organelles, (the micronemes, dense granules, and rhoptries) into the host cell. Rhoptry proteins are the major virulence factors of *T gondii* and are located in different parts of the host cells. Blocking the cell intrinsic defense mechanisms of the host lets *T gondii* invade, parasitize, and proliferate in the host successfully. These proteins can alter host cell function and inhibit the immune response directed toward the parasite.

During infection in the intermediate host, *T gondii* undergoes stage conversion between the rapidly dividing tachyzoite that is responsible for acute toxoplasmosis and the slowly replicating, encysted bradyzoite stage. This process of tachyzoite-bradyzoite interconversion is central to the pathogenesis and longevity of infection. In normal conditions, the tachyzoite stage is thwarted by the prompt and efficient interferon-γ-dependent cell-mediated immune response, which eventually kills off the majority of the disseminating tachyzoites before eventually entering the persistent form, the bradyzoite. Bradyzoites are encysted within various tissues, most notably the brain but also muscle, eye, and lung, and are infectious to another intermediate host or the cat if eaten. Cell-mediated immune mechanisms thus play a major role in the control of *T gondii* infection because the parasite is exclusively localized intracellularly.

After infection, *T gondii* evokes a powerful and persistent T-helper-1 (Th1) response (dendritic cell activated) together with neutrophils, inflammatory monocytes, and macrophages. The response is characterized by production of proinflammatory cytokines, including interleukin (IL)-12, INF-α and tumor necrosis factor (TNF)-α, which, together with other immunologic mechanisms, protect the host against rapid replication of tachyzoites and subsequent pathologic changes. The outcome of toxoplasmic infection depends on a balance between proinflammatory (IL-12, TNF-α) and downregulatory (IL-10, IL-27) cytokines that suppress parasite proliferation and control the inflammatory response, respectively.

Clinical Presentation in the Immunocompetent

Acute acquired toxoplasmosis has traditionally been considered an oligosymptomatic and self-limited infection in previously healthy patients. The typical clinical presentation of acute *T gondii* infection is a short flulike or mononucleosis-like illness that includes prolonged fever, headache, persistent enlarged but firm lymph nodes (rarely painful but initially tender) unattached to the overlying skin, and, occasionally, myalgia and gastrointestinal symptoms that rarely need treatment. Other infectious or non-infectious diseases cause similar symptoms and should always be included in the differential diagnosis: mononucleosis, cat scratch disease, tuberculosis, primary HIV infection, sarcoidosis, metastatic cancer, and lymphoma. In these cases, serologic testing is the initial and primary method of diagnosis.

Lymph node biopsy should be reserved for when *Toxoplasma* serology is uncertain and all other infectious serologic investigations are negative. Hepatomegaly and hepatitis with a moderate increase in liver enzyme levels (a 5- to 10-fold elevation) are common. Lymphocytosis and atypical lymphocytes are other laboratory hallmarks of toxoplasmosis. The spleen appears to be involved early in toxoplasmosis, but palpable splenomegaly is uncommon.

Pneumonia as well as myocarditis, polymyositis, or encephalitis are rarely described in immunocompetent hosts.

Although malaria and dengue are the most common causes of fever in travelers, toxoplasmosis should be considered in the differential diagnosis of fever, particularly in travelers with nonspecific symptoms such as fatigue, fever, headache and lymphadenopathy.

Latent toxoplasmosis is characterized by the lifelong presence of cysts of the parasite in different host tissues, including the nervous system, and by the presence of anamnestic *T gondii* immunoglobulin (Ig) G antibodies in the serum. Long considered asymptomatic, latent toxoplasmosis might increase the risk of schizophrenia and Parkinson's disease; influence human personality and behavior; impair psychomotor performance and increase the risk of suicide (suicide rates have been shown higher in countries with greater *T gondii* prevalence, regardless of national wealth or gross domestic product), traffic accidents, and the probability of the birth of male offspring. Recent studies have also hypothesized that *T gondii* is a risk factor for increasing aggressiveness as well as a murder behavior in women.

Higher rates of *T gondii* seropositivity have been reported for several psychiatric conditions affecting neurotransmitters, especially dopamine, that are implicated in the emergence of psychosis and behavioral Toxoplasma-induced abnormalities and in inducing brain inflammation by the direct stimulation of inflammatory cytokines in the central nervous system. Also, there is increasing evidence for a prominent role of immune dysregulation in psychosis and bipolar disorders. Accumulating evidence suggests that a permeabilized gut–blood barrier is present in psychiatric disorders, as demonstrated through studies of microbial translocation and microbiome sequencing that seem to indicate an actively dysbiotic environment in subsets of individuals with psychiatric disorders. RhD phenotype seems to play an important role in the strength and direction of association between latent toxoplasmosis and personality and intelligence.

Toxoplasmosis should also be regarded as an epilepsy risk factor. Epileptogenic mechanisms are probably multifactorial (direct lodgment of parasite, direct modulation of neuronal functions, abnormalities in GABA, role of calcium, etc.), etc. Recently, it was suggested that chronic latent neuroinflammation caused by the parasite may be responsible for the development of several neurodegenerative diseases manifesting with the loss of smell. Olfactory dysfunction reported in Alzheimer's disease, multiple sclerosis, and schizophrenia was frequently associated with the significantly increased serum anti-*T gondii* immunoglobulin G antibody levels.

In addition to above-mentioned manifestation, several recent studies performed in human and animal models have demonstrated that latent or acute toxoplasmosis is associated with reproductive organs disorders, infertility, sperm abnormalities, behavioral changes, and neurological disorders in pregnant women and other people.

A meta-analysis also suggested chronic toxoplasmosis as a possible risk factor for type 2 diabetes mellitus. However, more accurate studies are needed to better understand this association.

A very important aspect that has emerged in recent years concerns the possible occurrence of toxoplasmosis in patient receiving biotherapies, particularly anti-TNF-α agents for the treatment of rheumatologic diseases and other conditions that need biotechnological drugs. *Toxoplasma* serology should be performed in patients before treatment with TNF-α antagonists is initiated, and patients should be advised to avoid situations that increase risk of exposure to *Toxoplasma*.

Clinical Presentation in Immunocompromised Patients

The presence of latent bradyzoite cysts, along with the ability of bradyzoites to reconvert into the active and rapidly growing tachyzoites that can result in often fatal injury, explains the high incidence of acute toxoplasmosis often observed in immunocompromised persons. In immunocompromised hosts and in patients with AIDS, the central nervous system (CNS) is the site most typically affected by infection, and toxoplasmic encephalitis (TE) is the most common manifestation, which typically consists of single or multiple brain lesions. In individuals with AIDS and a CD4 T-cell count <100 cells/μL, the incidence of TE is 28% in seropositive patients not taking prophylaxis. Ocular and pulmonary diseases are the most common extracerebral sites of infection. For *Toxoplasma*, various mechanisms have been proposed for CNS entry, including the so-called "Trojan horse" mechanism, whereby an infected immune cell crosses the BBB, bringing the intracellular parasite with it. TE is also the third most common condition associated with AIDS in Brazil, still accounting for high mortality and morbidity rates despite free access to antiretroviral therapy (ART). However, as in transplant patients or those with malignant hemolymphopathies or solid tumors, other organs such as the lungs or eyes may be involved. Most of these cases result from reactivation of latent infection, although reinfection with a different *T gondii* strain in the transplanted organs can also occur. Although the mortality rate of pulmonary toxoplasmosis was high before the advent of ART, patients with AIDS and recipients of bone marrow transplants are also at risk for development of pulmonary toxoplasmosis, especially patients with very low CD4 cell counts. The clinical manifestations are nonspecific and are similar to those of *Pneumocystis jirovecii*.

In immunocompromised patients with suspected pulmonary toxoplasmosis, conventional staining is the most appropriate method to diagnose for experienced microbiology laboratories, whereas *T gondii*–specific PCR may be useful for laboratories with less experience in parasitology.

The predictive value of elevated blood levels of lactate dehydrogenase is of uncertain value. Patients with TE typically present with headache, confusion, altered mental status, and motor weakness. Focal neurologic deficits or seizures, weakness, sensory abnormalities, cerebellar signs, and neuropsychiatric manifestations are also common. Fever is usually, but not reliably, present. Accompanying nausea or vomiting usually indicates elevated intracranial pressure. Computed tomography (CT) scan or magnetic resonance imaging (MRI) of the brain typically shows multiple contrast-enhancing lesions, often with associated edema. These should be distinguished from other infectious or noninfectious CNS diseases in the course of AIDS.

In immunocompromised patients, the infection can disseminate rapidly and manifests with nonspecific symptoms such as fever and malaise. It can affect a number of organs, including the brain, cerebellum (an uncommon presentation), eye, liver, and lungs, as well as skeletal muscle, bone marrow, bladder, and spinal cord. Cardiac toxoplasmosis can occur during the course of multivisceral dissemination. However, in patients with AIDS, it is usually asymptomatic and found only at autopsy, typically in the setting of widely disseminated infection. Acquired toxoplasmosis with cutaneous involvement can also occur in the pediatric population, particularly in immunocompromised patients after stem cell transplantation. Early diagnosis and treatment of this life-threatening opportunistic infection may improve patient outcomes.

Toxoplasmosis of the Eye

Ocular toxoplasmosis is the major cause of visual impairment in high *T gondii* endemic regions of the United States and Europe, where it accounts for 30% to 50% of the infectious posterior uveitis. Toxoplasmosis can affect the retina and the underlying choroid, causing retinochoroiditis, the most common manifestation of ocular toxoplasmosis, which consists in an acute focal-necrotizing retinochoroiditis often adjacent to an old chorioretinal scar. Although the inner retina is the primary site of infection, vitreous, choroid, and sometimes sclera are secondarily affected. Many lesions are self-limiting and heal, forming characteristic unilateral or bilateral pigmented scars in the retina, where Toxoplasma cysts are found. Ocular lesions can recur in adolescence and adulthood, even after treatment in infancy. The severity of the disease is mainly a function of the parasite genotype and the host's immune status. Diagnosis in immunocompetent patients is based on the findings of typical ocular manifestations, including eye pain and decreased visual acuity, and may be confirmed by biologic tools applied to intraocular samples for antibody detection (local synthesis of specific antibodies), although PCR is becoming more widely available for direct identification of the parasite DNA in the vitreous and aqueous humor, especially with new methods of detection that can improve its sensitivity. When the clinical symptoms first manifest in immunocompetent patients, the intraocular inflammatory response may reduce the parasitic burden in the aqueous humor and vitreous, thus decreasing the amount of target DNA for PCR amplification. Secretory IgA antibodies in tears have been suggested as a reliable marker of acute ocular toxoplasmosis. Symptoms and signs in immunocompromised patients do not distinguish ocular toxoplasmosis from other ocular infections in HIV, including tuberculosis, P jirovecii pneumonia, and CMV retinitis. Toxoplasmic chorioretinitis appears as raised yellow-white, cottony lesions in a nonvascular distribution, unlike the perivascular exudates of CMV retinitis. Vitreal inflammation is usually present, in contrast to ocular toxoplasmosis in immunocompetent patients. Up to 63% of AIDS patients with Toxoplasma chorioretinitis have concurrent CNS lesions.

Maternal Infection and Congenital Toxoplasmosis

Infection with T gondii is particularly dangerous for pregnant women because it can lead to the transplacental passage of the parasite from the circulation of the primarily infected mother. Successful pregnancy involves an elegant equilibrium in organizing the immune system at the fetal-maternal and uteri milieu resulting in tolerance (TH2) of the fetus and defense (TH1) against the pathogenic agents. The placenta also plays an important role in trans-placental transmission, as it is a natural barrier to protection of the fetus against infectious agents and also a target tissue for parasite multiplication. In fact, the placental barrier is more efficient to inhibit the tachyzoites transmission at the beginning of gestation, but becomes more permeable at the end of pregnancy.

As tachyzoites bypass the placental blood barrier and invade the fetal organs, they propagate and compromise the embryonic developmental process.

During pregnancy, the prevalence of toxoplasmosis increases throughout the second and third quarter of gestation; simultaneously, progesterone and 17β-estradiol also increase and can aggravate or reduce parasite reproduction. Infection of the placenta is a prerequisite for congenital transmission. More than 60% of infected pregnant women do not experience any symptoms or signs, and the clinical features, when present, are the same as in other immunocompetent persons.

Currently, congenital toxoplasmosis is the second most common intrauterine infection and remains a public health problem throughout the world. The global annual incidence of congenital toxoplasmosis has been estimated to be 190,100 cases (95% credible interval, CI: 179,300–206,300). This is equivalent to a burden of 1.20 million DALYs (95% CI: 0.76–1.90). High burdens are seen in South America and in some Middle Eastern and low-income countries. The risk of transmission of T gondii to the fetus ranges from 0.6 to 1.7 per 1000 pregnant women.

According to Massachusetts Department of Health (United States), about 1 case of congenital toxoplasmosis occurs for every 10,000 live births. Moreover, from 4,000,000 live births each year in the United States, 400 have acquired congenital toxoplasmosis. This rate is markedly higher for other developing countries. In France, about 300 cases are reported each year to the National Reference Center. The frequency of transmission and severity of disease are inversely related.

The development of possible consequences depends on many factors, including the degree of parasitemia in the mother, the maturity of the placenta, the age of the fetus, and immunologic maturity. Early maternal infection (first trimester) can cause severe congenital toxoplasmosis and can result in death of the fetus in utero and spontaneous abortion. Clinical manifestations of congenital toxoplasmosis observed in infancy are numerous and include jaundice, rash, hepatosplenomegaly, anemia, thrombocytopenia, hydrocephalus, microcephalus, intracranial calcifications, convulsions, psychomotor and mental retardation, chorioretinitis, microphthalmia, blindness, strabismus, visual and auditory inflammatory disorders, cardiovascular abnormalities, and pains. All these signs and symptoms are included in the general workup of suspected congenital TORCH infections: toxoplasmosis, other (syphilis, varicella-zoster, parvovirus B19, HIV infection, listeriosis, hepatitis B, Zika virus), rubella, cytomegalovirus, and herpes. The classic triad of bilateral chorioretinitis, hydrocephalus, and cerebral calcifications is exceptional.

Fetal infection at the second trimester results in milder complications, which include splenomegaly, hepatomegaly, cerebral calcifications, pneumonitis, anemia, epilepsy, thrombocytopenia- induced petechiae, rash, and retinochoroiditis. When maternal infection occurs during the third trimester, most of neonates (more than 80%) are asymptomatic; however, retinochoroiditis and neurologic deficits in newborn who may be at high risk for seizures, mental retardation, or delay in growth, as well as in early adulthood, might be developed if these newborns are not treated appropriately in early age. In multiparous women, the risk of infections has been shown twice as high as in nulliparas.

The clinical course of the disease in a child with congenital toxoplasmosis is not influenced by whether the mother showed any clinical symptoms of the disease or was entirely asymptomatic. Infants born to women infected simultaneously with HIV and T gondii should be evaluated for congenital toxoplasmosis, considering the increased risk of reactivation of parasitemia and disease in these mothers.

Diagnosis in the Immunocompetent

In immunocompetent persons, confirmation of acute infection can exclude other potentially more serious etiologies. In other clinical settings where Toxoplasma infection can result in severe sequelae, the interpretation of laboratory findings poses significant challenges. The parasite can in fact be present in acute, chronic, latent, or reactivated form. Thus, discrimination of these forms is often crucial in understanding clinical relevance. A schematic diagnostic pathway that can be followed for the diagnosis of toxoplasmosis is shown in Figure 1. Methodical serologic screening for T gondii IgG and IgM antibodies in adult symptomatic immunocompetent persons, in pregnant women as early in gestation as possible (preferably in first trimester), and in seronegative women each month or trimester thereafter is optimal. Such screening allows detection of seroconversion and early initiation of treatment.

The laboratory tests used most commonly for initial investigation are serologic, targeting detection of IgG, IgM, and IgA specific for T gondii by available commercial kit. In addition to confirming infection, these tests can aid in determining prognosis, influence management, and assist in monitoring response to treatment. Typically, acute-phase IgM appears first about 1 to 2 weeks after infection, closely followed by IgA and IgE. Generally, IgM peaks at about 2 months. The time at which immunoglobulins can no longer be detected is highly variable depending on the test employed, usually about 6 to 9 months. In a small minority of cases IgM can persist at high levels for up to 18 months or for years, leading to an inaccurate assessment of when the exposure occurred. This circumstance can be problematic because congenital toxoplasmosis can occur if the mother was infected during her pregnancy, and it is thus important to ascertain in which trimester of pregnancy the infection occurred. IgA antibodies are considered to be a marker of acute toxoplasmosis as their kinetics are faster than those of IgM antibodies; however, they can also persist for more than a year, and their detection, together with IgM detection, strongly suggests neonatal infection. IgE serology is highly specific in pregnant women but has low sensitivity, remaining detectable for less than 4 months after infection; moreover, it is not useful in samples from newborns.

To date, an IgM test is still used by most laboratories to determine if a patient has been infected recently or in the distant past, but confirmatory testing (double sandwich or capture IgM-ELISA [enzyme-linked immunosorbent assay] kits and the immunosorbent agglutination assay [IgM-ISAGA]) should always be performed owing to the difficulties in interpreting a positive IgM test result for the relatively high incidence of false-positive results (due to the rheumatoid factor and antinuclear antibodies in some IgM-IFA tests). Thus, a positive IgM test result in a single serum sample can be interpreted as a true-positive result in the setting of a recently acquired infection, a true-positive result in the setting of an infection acquired in the distant past, or a false-positive result. IgM levels decline more rapidly than IgG antibodies, which typically reach maximal levels at about 4 months, then decline to a lower level over the next 12 to 24 months but persist for decades. Elevated IgG levels confirm if a patient has been exposed to the parasite, but they do not differentiate between a recent or past exposure, because IgG persists at a low level throughout the life of the patient. The absence of IgG antibodies in early pregnancy indicates that women are at risk for acquiring toxoplasmosis.

The most commonly used tests for the measurement of IgG antibody are the Sabin-Feldman dye test (still considered the gold standard diagnostic test; it measures primarily IgG antibodies to *T gondii*, but it requires viable *Toxoplasma* organisms), the ELISA, the IFA, and the modified direct agglutination test. Other immunological methods, including chemiluminescence assays (CLIA), enzyme-linked fluorescence assay (ELFA), and immunochromatographic test (ICT), have been developed to improve the ability of diagnosis of *T gondii* infection.

Depending on the method used, the avidity tests currently available (serum IgG avidity test and immunosorbent agglutination

All Persons With Suspected Toxoplasmosis, Including Pregnant Women: First Visit

First-level T. gondii Diagnostic Test

Detection of serum anti–T. gondii IgM and IgG in first trimester
- If IgM and IgG negative: absence of specific immunity; mother prophylaxis, monthly serologic control*
- If only IgG is detected: infection likely took place 6–12 months before or before pregnancy; immunity
- If only IgM is detected: initial phase seroconversion of false IgM positivity[†]
- If IgM and IgG are detected: possible recent infection; consider a more thorough workup (reference laboratory) to try to determine the time of infection in the mother[‡]

↓

Second-level Diagnostic Test

IgG avidity assay
- If negative (high avidity): infection occurred 3–5 months before testing
- If positive (low avidity): probable recent *T. gondii* infection; repeat serology 3 weeks after the first sample; start spiramycin, ecographic surveillance
Try to establish a certain or presumed seroconversion in pregnancy and to determine whether the infection was transmitted to the product of conception.

↓

Third-level Diagnostic Tests (further maternal and fetal assessment)

In the mother

Detection of T. gondii-specific DNA by PCR-AF at 18 weeks of gestation[§]
- If positive: the fetus has been infected; consider starting treatment and monthly fetal ultrasound examination to detect abnormalities; start pyrimethamine-sulfadiazine[‖]
- If negative: fetus unaffected; *T. gondii* has not crossed the placental barrier; continue spiramycin[¶]
- Parasite isolation on tissue culture: mouse inoculation[**]

In the newborn

Detection of serum anti-T. gondii IgM and IgA[††]
- If IgM and/or IgA are present at birth: probable connatal infection
- If IgM and/or IgA are not present at birth: monthly control

Western blot assay of serum IgG and IgM from mother-baby pairs[‡‡]
- If positive: confirmation of early postnatal diagnosis; therapy and serological control[§§]
- If negative: monthly control for the first 3 months

Figure 1 A schematic diagnostic pathway for the diagnosis of toxoplasmosis. *No treatment is required. [†]Repeat the tests weekly to detect the appearance of IgG antibodies to confirm the seroconversion. [‡]Given that IgM may persist for several months, try to date the beginning of infection through education and counseling to guide the prenatal diagnosis of the patient. [§]PCR sensitivity is significantly higher for infections occurred between the 17th and 21st week of gestation. [‖]If ecographic abnormalities, consider abortion. [¶]A negative PCR cannot completely rule out congenital infection; consider follow-up through ultrasounds and continue prophylaxis with spiramycin (Rovamycine) until delivery and neonatal testing. [**]For confirmation of PCR results; however, they are complex, expensive, and relatively insensitive. [††]Limitations because IgA antibodies may persist for several months and are not always produced. [‡‡]This test is not widely used mainly because of its technical complexity and high price. [§§]Administer pyrimethamine (Daraprim)-sulfadiazine therapy and serologic controls after cessation of therapy and every 6 months for the first 2 years.

assays (ISAGA) are helpful primarily to rule out that a patient's infection occurred within the prior 4 to 5 months and that the fetus is not at risk for congenital toxoplasmosis. The avidity test that shows low IgG values in a recent *T gondii* infection is most important when only a single serum sample is available at the time when critical decisions must be made. A major problem with this test is that the maturation of the IgG response after a primary *Toxoplasma* infection varies considerably among patients; in fact, low-avidity results can persist for as long as 1 year, and substantial numbers of patients have borderline or equivocal results. These equivocal cases require that in addition to a more careful interpretation of all laboratory test results in conjunction with other clinical findings, other serologic methods should then be undertaken in serology reference laboratories. Recently, a growing number of studies have demonstrated the potential advantages of chimeric or synthetic peptide antigens (EC2 (containing MIC1 and MIC2 antigenic regions) and EC3 (containing M2AP, GRA3 and GRA7 antigenic regions) for the serological diagnosis of toxoplasmosis.

The employment of polymerase chain reaction (PCR) to identify *T gondii* DNA in amniotic fluid (AF) obtained by amniocentesis at 18 weeks and later represents a milestone in the early diagnosis of intrauterine *T gondii* infection, thereby avoiding the use of more invasive procedures on the fetus. Sensitivity and specificity of PCR may even increase when performed on AF samples obtained from the sixteenth week of pregnancy onward. The specificity and positive predictive value of PCR on AF samples is close to 100%, although different protocols influence its sensitivity and specificity. PCR is generally carried out with various gene targets, of which the most widely used is the 35-fold repetitive gene *B1*. Following it, several multicopy targeting genes including 18S rRNA-, P30-, B1-genes, 529-bp repeat fragment or the AF146527 element have been used for the detection of *T gondii* in different biologic samples. In particular, PCR with the 529-bp RE gene is 10–100 times more sensitive than the B1 gene.

Results of studies indicated that loop-mediated isothermal amplification (LAMP) and real-time-PCR using AF and CSF are more sensitive and specific methods in congenital infection and immunocompromised patients, respectively, and could be used for early diagnosis of infection and also in follow-up after treatment. Moreover, LAMP on cord blood or whole blood is highly sensitive, specific, and easy to perform, as it doesn't require expensive equipment.

However, a definitive correlation between the number of *Toxoplasma* organisms in AF and the severity of congenital infection has not yet been demonstrated. PCR should be considered for pregnant women (without a contraindication for the procedure) with positive diagnostic serology or highly suggestive of an infection because of ultrasonographic abnormalities in the fetus acquired during gestation or shortly before conception. If the PCR-AF test result is negative, the fetus should be unaffected, presumably because *T gondii* has not yet crossed the placental barrier even if it is theoretically possible that fetal infection can occur later in pregnancy from a placenta that was infected earlier in gestation. Samples obtained by cordocentesis, funipuncture, or periumbilical fetal blood sampling should not be used, because fetal risk of contamination with maternal blood is higher than with amniocentesis, and cordocentesis is less sensitive.

In the newborn, diagnosis of infection is based on detection of serum anti-*Toxoplasma* IgM and IgA antibodies that do not cross the placenta, unlike maternal IgG antibodies. Better results are obtained if the ISAGA method is used. Maternal IgG antibodies present in the newborn can reflect either past or recent infection in the mother and require serologic follow-up of the newborn for the 1st year of life until the complete disappearance of these antibodies. A negative *T gondii*–specific IgG test result at 1 year of age essentially rules out congenital toxoplasmosis. Detection of IgG in oral fluid appears to be a promising tool for monitoring infants with suspected congenital toxoplasmosis.

Detection of specific IgA antibodies appears to be more sensitive than detection of IgM antibodies for establishing infection in the newborn, because these antibodies may be present when there is no *T gondii*–specific IgM, and the converse can also occur. However, transmission of maternal IgM or IgA antibodies can occur during the birth process. Because of the relatively brief half-life of IgM and IgA, positive tests for these antibodies usually must be confirmed by repeat testing at 2 to 4 days of life in the case of IgM antibodies and at 10 days of life for IgA antibodies.

Evaluation of infants with suspected congenital toxoplasmosis should always include ophthalmologic examination, electroencephalogram, hearing test, blood tests, non-contrast CT scanning or ultrasound of the brain, and examination of CSF. Although CT scanning is the first-line diagnostic method used in the United States to detect CNS abnormalities caused by toxoplasmosis, ultrasound can be used as an alternative diagnostic method to avoid the effects of radiation in the neonatal period. Ultrasound is recommended for women with suspected or diagnosed acute infection acquired during or shortly before gestation. This technique can reveal fetal abnormalities, including hydrocephalus, brain or hepatic calcifications, splenomegaly, and ascites. Because most infants do not show signs of toxoplasmosis at birth, a negative ultrasound does not rule out the possibility of infection and might need to be followed by a CT scan for confirmation, because ultrasound results can vary depending on the examiner and technology used. Newborns thus need a thorough examination after birth and follow-up blood tests during the first year of life.

Diagnosis in the Immunocompromised

In immunocompromised persons and AIDS patients with TE, indirect serologic methods widely used in immunocompetent patients are unreliable because they fail to produce significant titers of specific antibodies. Although incidence of TE among HIV-infected persons directly correlates with the prevalence of anti–*T gondii* antibodies, the absence of IgG antibody makes a diagnosis of toxoplasmosis unlikely, but not impossible. Anti-*Toxoplasma* IgM antibodies are usually absent. CSF findings are normal or show nonspecific alterations such as lymphocytic pleocytosis and discrete CSF hyperproteinorrachia.

In clinical practice, the diagnosis of TE is presumptive and mainly based on clinical presentation, imaging, and laboratory test results. Imaging includes CT or MRI, preferably with gadolinium contrast, and shows isodense or hypodense single or multiple lesions with a mass effect, taking up the contrast dye in a ringlike or nodular manner in more than 90% of cases. However, as neither CT nor MRI can reliably distinguish CNS infections, such as toxoplasmosis, from lymphoma in HIV-1–positive patients, the use of FDG-PET has been shown to offer better sensitivity to noninvasively differentiate cerebral toxoplasmosis and other infectious diseases from primary CNS lymphoma. Laboratory results include the presence of serum-specific *T gondii* IgG antibodies. Diagnosis is also made from an objective response, on the basis of clinical and radiographic improvement, to specific anti–*T gondii* therapy in the absence of a likely alternative diagnosis. In general, the occurrence of low CD4+ T-cell count (less than 150–200/mm³) and the presence of *T gondii* IgG antibody is habitually accepted as being a good predictor of TE reactivation, although less than 6% of TE patients show negative tests. If the suspected diagnosis of toxoplasmosis is correct, clinical or radiographic improvement should become evident by more than 50% within 7 to 14 days. If symptoms persist, a brain biopsy should be performed. This should be considered in immunocompromised patients with presumed CNS toxoplasmosis with a single MRI lesion, absence of IgG antibodies, or an unsatisfactory clinical response to specific anti–*T gondii* treatment.

Diagnosis of TE is crucial because other brain diseases—such as CNS lymphoma, bacterial abscess, progressive multifocal leukoencephalopathy, viral or fungal encephalitis, neurotuberculosis, cytomegalovirus encephalitis, and focal lesions caused by fungi (*Cryptococcus neoformans*, *Aspergillus* spp., and *Nocardia* spp.)—could share similar clinical and CT scan signs. In general, no imaging technique is completely specific. Thallium single-photon emission computed tomography (SPECT) and positron emission tomography (PET) can be useful in distinguishing toxoplasmosis or other infections from CNS lymphoma. CNS lymphoma has greater thallium uptake on SPECT and greater glucose and methionine metabolism on PET than neurotoxoplasmosis or other infections.

Definitive diagnosis of TE is made by pathologic examination of brain tissue obtained by open or stereotactic CT-guided brain biopsy, although there is morbidity and even death associated with the biopsy procedure. Tachyzoites are demonstrated on hematoxylin and eosin stains or immunoperoxidase staining, which can increase diagnostic sensitivity, or by Giemsa on cytocentrifuged CSF samples. Toxoplasma organisms must be distinguished from other intracellular organisms such as *Histoplasma*, *Trypanosoma cruzi*, and *Leishmania*.

Since the turn of the twenty-first century, molecular techniques have allowed significant improvement and have been shown to be an important diagnostic tool in laboratory diagnosis of TE. Their use is principally appropriate for immunocompromised patients because these techniques are not affected by the immunologic status of the host. PCR-based assays, in particular, have been shown to be rapid, sensitive, and specific enough to be used as a front-line test for detecting CSF *T gondii* DNA in most patients with CNS infection, thus avoiding invasive and expensive brain biopsy procedures. However, results usually are negative once specific anti-*Toxoplasma* therapy has been started. Moreover, parasite levels in blood and CSF may be very poor in some patients and cause difficulties in interpreting the PCR product. For this reason, a number of quantitative real-time PCRs with specific *T gondii* genome sequence have been developed in the last decade and used in patients with AIDS and CNS damage with different rates of sensitivity and specificity. In this setting, the recent sensitive and specific real-time PCR technique targeting the 529-bp repeat fragment of the *AF146527* element repeated 300 times in the genome of *T gondii* has been demonstrated to exactly quantify the parasite load, allowing correlation with clinical symptoms and impact of treatment. Moreover, the use of real-time PCR with primers targeting the genes SAG4 and MAG1 (located in the bradyzoites) and SAG1 (located in tachyzoites) has shown to be useful to identify relapses of TE in patients in whom the use of PCR with B1 gene failed to detect DNA, in AIDS patients and other immunocompromised patients especially, when prophylaxis or treatment has been started.

Diagnosis of TE in AIDS patients can also be supported by demonstration of intrathecal antibody production based on detection of oligoclonal bands in CSF with antibody-specific index (ASI) and affinity-mediated immunoblot (AMI) techniques. This approach has also been shown to discriminate TE from other opportunistic CNS infections in AIDS.

In non-AIDS–immunocompromised patients, regular PCR follow-up of allogeneic hematopoietic stem-cell transplant (allo-HSCT) patients could guide preemptive treatment and improve outcome.

Treatment

An ideal treatment for toxoplasmosis should achieve therapeutic, systemic brain and eye concentrations to be effective in the organs where the majority of disease occurs and should be active against both the acute replicating tachyzoite and latent bradyzoite stages of the parasite. However, current treatments are only capable of suppressing the rapidly dividing tachyzoyte stage of the organism. The main goal of treatment is to interrupt the replication of the parasite and prevent further damage to the organs involved. Nonpregnant immunocompetent patients with acute toxoplasmosis plus lymphadenitis generally do not require antimicrobial therapy because the infection is self-limiting and usually subclinical. Chronic lymphadenopathy accompanied by fever and marked weakness can be cured with specific therapy. Patients whose *T gondii* infection occurred during laboratory accidents or blood transfusions need specific treatment. Pregnant women must be treated to reduce the risk and severity of congenital infection. Immunocompromised patients, including patients with AIDS and

transplant recipients, should always be treated with antitoxoplasmic agents. For eye disease, treatment usually includes anti-*Toxoplasma* agents plus systemic corticosteroids. The most important treatment and prophylactic regimens for the therapy of toxoplasmosis are shown in Tables 1 and 2.

The folate synthesis pathway being the best-known therapeutic target against Toxoplasma, the main enzymes targeted by pharmaceuticals are the dihydropteroate synthase and dihydrofolate reductase. Since the dihydropteroate enzyme is not found in mammalian cells, it provides a specific target against Toxoplasma. The standard pyrimethamine (Daraprim) and trimethoprim (Trimpex)[1] are the most widely used dihydrofolate reductase inhibitors. Pyrimethamine, however, is more effective then trimethoprim and is usually administered in conjunction with a dihydropteroate synthase inhibitor (sulfonamide compounds such as sulfadiazine and sulfamethoxazole).

First-line therapy for acquired toxoplasmosis in both immunocompetent and immunodeficient patients consists of the synergistic combination of pyrimethamine and sulfadiazine. Pyrimethamine plus sulfadiazine[1] plus folinic acid (Leucovorin)[1] to prevent hematologic toxicity is the preferred regimen. Azithromycin (Zithromax)[1] or atovaquone (Mepron)[1] may be used as alternate therapy in combination with pyrimethamine or sulfonamides for the treatment and prophylaxis of toxoplasmosis when first-line line therapy is contraindicated. Both compounds have been shown to be partially effective against tissue cysts in experimental studies. More recently, however, the search for new and efficient pharmacologic treatments directed against proliferating tachyzoites or the tissue cyst of Toxoplasma is under intense and frequent evaluation.

Treatment During Pregnancy

Management of maternal and fetal infection of *T gondii* varies considerably between different countries and even centers in the same country. According to the European Multicentre Study on Congenital Toxoplasmosis (EMSCOT) data, which suffer from the lack of a large-scale controlled clinical trial, treatment for the fetus should be started immediately (within 3 weeks of infection) after diagnosis of recently acquired maternal infection. This has been shown to significantly reduce sequelae and to have a beneficial effect when therapy is begun soon after birth. Later treatment has been shown to have no effect.

The macrolide antibiotic spiramycin (Rovamycine)[2] is prescribed immediately after diagnosis of maternal infection in most centers in Europe and the United States, and there has been no evidence that this drug is teratogenic. Spiramycin does not cross the placenta but is concentrated in the placenta and protects the fetus from contact with the parasite. It has been estimated to reduce the incidence of vertical transmission of *T gondii* by about 60%. It is used 1 g every 8 hours in many EU countries, especially France, and in Asia and South America and does not seem to have any fetal effects, although a small percentage of women have developed gastrointestinal side effects.

Spiramycin should be continued as prophylaxis until delivery, along with periodic ultrasound examination, because the placenta could have been infected earlier in gestation.

In the case of positive PCR-AF at or immediately after 18 weeks' gestation, or with high probability of fetal infection acquired late in the second trimester (after 18 weeks) or during the third trimester of gestation (because of ultrasound abnormalities), and in women who cannot undergo amniocentesis, the spiramycin regimen should be replaced with the drug combination of sulfadiazine[1] and pyrimethamine plus folinic acid (Leucovorin).[1] This treatment strategy varies in some U.S. and European centers. Folinic acid prevents the toxicity of pyrimethamine without activity against Toxoplasma. This combination therapy is used only after confirmed or strongly suspected fetal infection and is never administered in the first trimester of pregnancy due to

---

[1]Not FDA approved for this indication.
[2]Not commercially available in the United States.

| TABLE 1 | Treatment Regimens for Toxoplasmosis | | | |

PATIENTS	DRUG OF CHOICE	RECOMMENDED DOSAGE	LENGTH OF ADMINIS-TRATION	ADVERSE EFFECTS
Acute infection in *T gondii* seropositive pregnant patients with undocumented fetal infection	Spiramycin (Rovamycine)[2]	1000 mg PO q8h (without food)	Throughout pregnancy or until fetal infection is documented	Mild GI disturbances, possible skin eruptions
Acute infection in a pregnant patient with documented fetal infection (positive PCR-AF)	Pyrimethamine (Daraprim)* *plus*	Loading dose, 50 mg PO q12h × 2 d, then 50 mg PO daily	Throughout pregnancy; avoid before 18th wk of gestation because of high risk of teratogenesis	Pyrimethamine is a potential teratogen (kidney and heart malformation) and should be used only after the first trimester Sulfadiazine can cause crystal-induced nephropathy‡
	Sulfadiazine[1] *plus*	Loading dose 75 mg/kg PO, then 50 mg/kg q12h (max 4 g daily) 10–20 mg PO daily	Throughout pregnancy; do not administer before 18th wk of gestation†	
	Folinic acid (Leucovorin)[1]		During and for 1 wk after pyrimethamine use	Complete regimen: rash, fever and dose-dependent myelosuppression; weekly monitoring of blood cell counts
Congenital infection in the infant	Pyrimethamine *plus*	Loading dose 2 mg/kg PO daily × 2 d; then 1 mg/kg PO daily × 2–6 mo; then 1 mg/kg tiw	1 y	Same as above
	Sulfadiazine[1] *plus*	50 mg/kg PO q12h	1 y	
	Folinic acid[1]	10 mg/kg PO tiw	During and for 1 wk after pyrimethamine use	
Acute *T gondii* infection in adult immunocompetent patients and in pregnant patients infected > 6 mo before conception	Treatment not recommended or, if acutely ill: Pyrimethamine *plus*	Loading dose 200 mg PO daily in 2 divided doses, then 0.5–1 mg/kg/d (max 50 mg/d; 75 mg (if >60 kg)	4–6 wk, or 1–2 wk after resolution of symptoms	Same as above
	Sulfadiazine[1] *plus*	1000–1500 mg PO q6h	During and 1 wk after pyrimethamine use	
	Folinic acid[1]	5–20 mg PO tiw		
Chorioretinitis in immunocompetent patients	Pyrimethamine§,[1] *plus*	200 mg loading dose, then 50–75 mg PO daily	1–2 wk after resolution of symptoms	
	Sulfadiazine§,[1] *plus*	1000–1500 mg PO q6h	1–2 wk after resolution of symptoms	
	Folinic acid[1] *plus*	5–20 mg PO tiw	During and for 1 wk after pyrimethamine use	
	Prednisone	1 mg/kg daily in 2 divided doses	Until resolution of signs and symptoms	
Alternatives				
	TMP-SMX (Bactrim)[1] *or*	160–800 mg q12h	6 wk	Skin rash, fever, leukopenia, thrombocytopenia, hepatotoxicity; also available as an IV formulation Not reported
	Azithromycin (Zithromax)[1] alone or associated with pyrimethamine *or*	500 mg/d	5 wk	
	Intravitreal clindamycin (Cleocin)[1]-dexamethasone (Decadron)	One injection 1–400 mcg	Not reported	Not reported

TABLE 1 Treatment Regimens for Toxoplasmosis—cont'd

PATIENTS	DRUG OF CHOICE	RECOMMENDED DOSAGE	LENGTH OF ADMINIS-TRATION	ADVERSE EFFECTS
For untreatable cases only				
	Photocoagulation	Not usually done	Not reported	Not reported
Immunocompro-mised patients and patients with TE‖	Pyrimethamine *plus*	Loading dose 200 mg PO, then 50–75 mg PO daily	At least 4–6 wk after signs and symptoms resolve	Same as above
	Folinic acid[1] *plus either*	10–20 mg PO or IV or IM daily (max 50 mg daily)		
	Sulfadiazine *or*	1000–1500 mg PO q6h	During and for 1 wk after pyrimethamine use	Rash, fever, diarrhea, hepatotoxicity
	Clindamycin[1,¶] *plus*	600 mg PO or IV q6h (max 1200 mg q6h)	At least 4–6 wk after signs and symptoms resolve	Fever, rash, diarrhea, hepatotoxicity
	Prednisone	1 mg/kg daily in 2 divided doses	Until improvement of edema or mass effect related to focal lesion	
	Alternatives TMP-SMX[1] alone *or*	5 mg/kg TMP PO or IV q12h (max 15–20 mg/kg/d)	Same as above	Same as above
	Pyrimethamine *plus* folinic acid[1] *plus one of the following:*	Same as above pyrimethamine and folinic acid doses 500 mg PO q12h	Same as above	Same as above
	Clarithromycin (Biaxin)[1]	750 mg PO q6h	At least 4–8 wk after resolution of signs and symptoms	
	Atovaquone (Mepron)[1]	1200–1500 mg PO daily	Not reported	Atovaquone can increase LFTs and skin rash Take with a meal to enhance absorption
	Azithromycin[1]	100 mg PO daily	Not reported	
	Dapsone[1]	750 mg PO q6h	Not reported	
	Atovaquone (Mepron)[1] alone or with sulfadiazine	1000–1500 mg PO q6h	Not reported	
Acute infection in patients with *T gondii* and HIV infection**	Spiramycin[2] (as for immunocompetent pregnant women)	1,000 mg PO q8h (without food)	Throughout pregnancy or until fetal infection is documented	

[1]Not FDA approved for this indication.
[2]Not commercially available in the United States.
*Take with food to minimize gastrointestinal adverse effects.
†This might change in some European countries.
‡Should be taken on an empty stomach with adequate water.
§Take both for 3 weeks followed by 1 week off; repeat for 3 or 4 cycles.
‖After initial phase of therapy, maintenance therapy must be continued as long as the patient remains immunocompromised.
¶Clindamycin can be used instead of sulfadiazine in patients intolerant to sulfonamides.
**Amniocentesis should be avoided because of the risk of transmitting HIV infection to the fetus.
Abbreviations: GI, gastrointestinal; LFT, liver function test; PCR-AF, polymerase chain reaction testing of amniotic fluid; TMP-SMX, trimethoprim-sulfamethoxazole.

its teratogenic and hematological adverse effects, in addition to symptoms of nausea in the mother.

Throughout the pregnancy, therapy with pyrimethamine in conjunction with folinic acid should be continued to prevent hematologic toxicities, along with monitoring of blood cell counts and rigorous periodic ultrasound examination. Because spiramycin does not readily cross the placenta, it is not reliable for the treatment of infection in the fetus. In the absence of clinical and laboratory signs suggestive of congenital toxoplasmosis, therapy is not indicated in infants, but it is necessary to inform the specialist and to plan, with the specialist, periodic clinical and serologic controls. In symptomatic infants, the combination of pyrimethamine plus sulfadiazine plus leucovorin is recommended. The duration of this treatment is not specifically defined, but it must be continued for up to a year, possibly alternating cycles of antifolate for 4 weeks with spiramycin cycles of equal duration.

Ocular Toxoplasmosis

In immunocompetent patients, *Toxoplasma*-related chorioretinitis is usually a self-limited infection and generally may resolve spontaneously in a period of 4 to 8 weeks. However, treatment is recommended for lesions within the vascular arcades, adjacent to the optic disk, or larger than 2 optic disk diameters to reduce the chance of vision loss. In general, pyrimethamine, sulfadiazine[1] plus folinic acid[1], and corticosteroids form the most common drug combination currently used to treat ocular toxoplasmosis. Patients may also be treated with TMP-SMX,[1] which appears to be a safe and effective substitute for pyrimethamine, sulfadiazine, and folinic acid, or with azithromycin[1] or intravitreal clindamycin (Cleocin)[1] and prednisone for 4 to 6 weeks. Pyrimethamine plus azithromycin is another drug combination that is similar to the standard treatment and can be considered an acceptable alternative treatment for sight-threatening ocular toxoplasmosis. *Toxoplasma* retinochoroiditis in immunocompromised patients requires immediate treatment. Atypical presentations also warrant treatment.

Recurrent toxoplasmic retinochoroiditis, probably related to the rupture of the dormant retinal cyst or *Toxoplasma* circulating in peripheral blood, remains a major health crisis and can be associated with severe morbidity if the disease extends to structures critical for vision, including the macula and optic

TABLE 2 Prophylaxis Regimens for Toxoplasmosis

PATIENTS WHO SHOULD RECEIVE PROPHYLAXIS	DRUG OF CHOICE*	RECOMMENDED DOSAGE	LENGTH OF ADMINISTRATION
Primary prophylaxis for immunocompromised patients, including advanced pregnant HIV-positive women (CD4+ count < 100 cells/mm³ and *T gondii* IgG positive)	First choice: TMP-SMX (Bactrim)[1] *Alternatives* Pyrimethamine (Daraprim)[1] *plus* Dapsone[1] *plus* Folinic acid[1] *or* Pyrimethamine-sulfadoxine (Fansidar)[1] *plus* Folinic acid[1] *or* Atovaquone (Mepron)[1]	1 DS tab 160–800 mg PO daily 50–75 mg/wk 50 mg/d 25 mg/wk 1 tab twice weekly 25 mg/wk 1,500 mg PO daily	For life or until immunoreconstitution has occurred[†] Same as above Same as above Same as above
Secondary prophylaxis for immunocompromised patients after primary or induction treatment	Same regimen used in the acute phase: TMP-SMX[1]	Half doses of those used in the acute phase 2.5 mg/kg TMP PO or IV q12h, max 15–20 mg/kg/d	For life or until immunoreconstitution has occurred[†]
Prophylaxis in adults receiving heart, lung, or liver transplant, especially in the case of a seropositive donor (D +) and seronegative recipient (R −)[‡]	First choice: TMP-SMX[1] *Alternative* Pyrimethamine[1] *plus* Folinic acid[1]	80 mg TMP/400 mg SMX (1 tab single-strength Bactrim) twice daily 50–75 mg PO daily 5–10 mg PO daily	For 6 wk after transplant Same as above During and for 1 wk after pyrimethamine use
Prophylaxis in adults receiving bone marrow and allogeneic stem cell transplants[§] Prophylaxis for accidental laboratory exposure and blood transfusions	First choice: TMP-SMX[1] *Alternatives*[¶]: Pyrimethamine[1] *plus* Clindamycin (Cleocin)[1] *plus* Folinic acid[1] Pyrimethamine[1] *plus* Sulfadiazine[1] *plus* Folinic acid[1]	Same as above[‖] Not standardized Same as for acute infection**	For more than 6 mo Not reported 2 wk

[1]Not FDA approved for this indication.

*For side effects, see Table 1.

[†]In patients with AIDS, primary and secondary prophylaxis are generally discontinued when the patient's CD4+ cell count has returned to more than 200 cells/μL and HIV PCR peripheral blood viral load has been reasonably controlled for at least 6 months following ART.

[‡]Preemptive antiparasite treatment should be considered for all symptomatic, seropositive, immunocompromised patients in whom toxoplasmosis is suspected.

[§]There are no clear recommendation for anti–*T gondii* prophylaxis in allogeneic stem cell transplantation, because the optimal regimen has not yet been determined.

[‖]Not specifically codified.

[¶]Alternative regimen in sulfonamide-allergic patients.

**Presumptive therapy should be given with the same dosages as for acute infection and monitored serologically for several months after the exposure or until seroconversion is noted; that is, testing immediately after the exposure, weekly for at least 1 month, and at least monthly thereafter. Seroconversion can occur despite presumptive therapy. Although presumptive therapy typically prevents disease or at least substantial morbidity, it does not necessarily prevent infection.

Abbreviations: ART, highly active retroviral therapy; PCR, polymerase chain reaction; TMP-SMX, trimethoprim-sulfamethoxazole.

disk. Severe morbidity can also occur if there is damage to the eye from inflammation or if there are complications such as retinal detachment or neovascularization. In patients with frequent recurrences, the rate of recurrent toxoplasmic retinochoroiditis can be significantly reduced by long-term intermittent treatment with TMP-SMX 160 mg/800 mg (Bactrim DS)[1], with one tablet administered three times a week as a prophylactic regimen. Intravitreal clindamycin[1] injection and possibly steroids may be an acceptable alternative to the classic treatment in ocular toxoplasmosis. It can offer the patient more convenience, a safer systemic side effect profile, greater availability, and fewer follow-up visits and hematologic evaluations. Although research has identified wide variation in practices regarding the use of corticosteroids, a recent Cochrane review did not identify evidence from randomized controlled trials for the role of corticosteroids in the management of ocular toxoplasmosis. The question of foremost importance, however, is whether they should be used as adjunct therapy (that is, in addition) to antiparasitic agents. There is no evidence to support that one antibiotic regimen is superior to another, so choice needs to be informed by the safety profile. Intravitreous clindamycin with dexamethasone[1] seems to be as effective as systemic treatments. There is currently level I evidence that intermittent trimethoprim-sulfamethoxazole prevents recurrence of the disease.

Toxoplasmosis in Immunosuppressed Patients

With the advent of the ART, the natural course of HIV infection has markedly changed, and opportunistic infections including toxoplasmosis have declined and changed in presentation, outcome, and incidence. However, TE is a major cause of morbidity and mortality, especially in resource-poor settings, and it is a common neurologic complication in some countries despite the availability of ART and effective prophylaxis. The initial therapy of choice in TE patients consists of the combination of pyrimethamine, which is able to penetrate the brain parenchyma efficiently even in the absence of inflammation, plus sulfadiazine or clindamycin[1] plus folinic acid.[1]

Adjunctive corticosteroids should be administered when clinically indicated only for treatment of a mass effect associated with focal lesions or associated edema and for a short time because of their potential immunosuppressive effects. Patients receiving corticosteroids should be closely monitored for the development of other effects, including CMV retinitis and tuberculosis. Anticonvulsants should be administered to patients with a history of seizures, but should not be administered prophylactically to all patients. Drug interactions between anticonvulsants and antiretroviral agents should be carefully evaluated, and doses should be adjusted according to established guidelines. The preferred alternative regimen for patients unable to tolerate or who fail to respond to first-line therapy is pyrimethamine plus clindamycin[1] plus leucovorin.[1]

Common clindamycin toxicities include fever, rash, nausea, diarrhea (including pseudomembranous colitis or diarrhea related to *Clostridium difficile* toxin), and hepatotoxicity. Other alternative regimens shown in Table 1 are active in the treatment of TE and may be used in sulfa-intolerant patients or those who have not responded to treatment, although their relative efficacy compared with the previous regimens is unknown.

The combination of atovaquone (Mepron)[1] with either pyrimethamine or sulfadiazine has demonstrated utility for the treatment of acute TE in patients with a Karnofsky Performance Status Score greater than 30, which combines the ability to work, to undertake normal activities without external assistance, and to take care of personal needs. Acute therapy should be continued for at least 6 weeks, if there is clinical and radiologic improvement. This should be followed by maintenance therapy (lifelong secondary prophylaxis), usually with the same regimen that was used in the acute phase but at half doses (see Table 2).

Recent findings indicate that daily pyrimethamine-based maintenance therapy is likely more efficacious in preventing TE relapse compared with intermittent therapy. Moreover, the likelihood of relapse associated with pyrimethamine-based therapy in patients with HIV and TE decreased after the introduction of HAART to approximately 11%. Relapse may thus affect a patient's disease severity and prognosis, increase utilization of health care resources, and result in additional health care expenditure. Currently, maintenance treatment should be continued for the life of the patient or until underlying immunosuppression has ceased (immune reconstitution resulting from ART). Adult and adolescent patients appear to be at low risk for recurrence of TE when they have successfully completed initial therapy, remain asymptomatic with respect to signs and symptoms, and have a sustained (i.e., more than 6 months) increase in their CD4+ T-lymphocyte counts to greater than 200 cells/μL on ART. AIDS patients with CD4+ T-cell counts less than 100/μL and IgG *Toxoplasma* antibody should receive primary prophylaxis for toxoplasmosis. Fortunately, the same daily regimen of one double-strength tablet of TMP/SMX (Bactrim DS) used for *Pneumocystis jirovecii* prophylaxis provides adequate primary protection against toxoplasmosis. Secondary prophylaxis for toxoplasmosis may be discontinued in the setting of effective ART and when CD4+ T-cell counts increase to more than 200/μL for 6 months.

Prophylaxis and treatment measures of disease in bone marrow transplant recipients as well as in those receiving organ transplantation are shown in Table 2. Universal prophylaxis with TMP/SMX in allo pre-hematopoietic cell transplant seropositive recipients (HCTSP) should be implemented by all transplant programs. Preemptive treatment with routine blood PCR monitoring is an option if prophylaxis cannot be used.

T *gondii* Infection During Pregnancy in HIV-Positive Women

Immunocompromised women with chronic infection do rarely transmit the parasite to the fetus, resulting in congenital infection. This includes women with AIDS, as well as those on immunosuppressive treatment. Vertical transmission occurs in up to 4% of cases, particularly when the CD4+ count is less than 100/mm³. The risk of transmission is low when the CD4+ count is greater than 200/mm³ (see Table 2).

Consideration should be given to screening all immunosuppressed women for evidence of maternal T *gondii* serologic status to establish an early diagnosis of reactivation. Seropositive women with low CD4 counts should receive TMP-SMX (Bactrim)[1] to prevent reactivation of *Toxoplasma*. Because of reports of congenital toxoplasmosis in mildly or moderately immunosuppressed women, it is recommended that immunocompromised women not infected with HIV and women who are infected with HIV and who have CD4 counts less than 200/mm³ be treated with spiramycin (Rovamycine)[2] for the duration of the pregnancy. A nonpregnant woman who has been diagnosed with an acute T *gondii* infection should be counseled to wait 6 months before attempting to become pregnant. Each case should be considered separately in consultation with an expert.

Detailed ultrasound examination of the fetus specifically evaluating for hydrocephalus, cerebral calcifications, and growth restriction should be done for HIV-1-infected women with suspected primary or symptomatic reactivation of T *gondii* during pregnancy.

Prevention
Strategies for the primary prevention of toxoplasmosis in pregnant women and in immunosuppressed patients with negative serology are shown in Box 1.

Screening
Secondary prevention by serologic monitoring of seronegative pregnant women should be closely connected with detailed primary prevention. Routine toxoplasmosis screening programs for pregnant women have been established in France, Austria, and Brazil. In France, guidelines recommend that nonimmune pregnant women be tested monthly throughout pregnancy to detect seroconversion to *Toxoplasma* infection. In the United States, routine serologic screening is not performed. In Italy, serologic screening is recommended to prevent congenital toxoplasmosis as part of the antenatal care protocol (TORCH). Serologic screening of women should begin before conception, with follow-up monthly tests during pregnancy to detect seroconversion. This is the basis for the French screening program and the Austrian Toxoplasmosis Prevention Program, which recommend routine serologic testing. Treatment is recommended if one of the tests suggests definite or probable primary maternal infection.

Vaccine
Vaccination is one of the most efficient strategies to prevent and control the spread of toxoplasmosis by immunization of humans and animals (the source of infection). To date, there is much debate about whether a human vaccine is feasible. Costs, target population, method for testing the vaccine, and risks associated with the vaccine are important factors affecting development of the vaccine. Much of the work has been focused on SAG1, a surface antigen expressed on tachyzoites, in attempts to induce protective immune response when introduced to the host with various adjuvants. SAG1 is primarily involved in adhesion, signal transduction, invasion, material transport and host immune responses. Thus, this protein may be crucial for both the diagnosis of T *gondii* infection and the ability to immunize against this parasite.

---

[1]Not FDA approved for this indication.

---

[1]Not FDA approved for this indication.
[2]Not commercially available in the United States.

BOX 1 Strategies for the Primary Prevention of Toxoplasmosis in Pregnant Women and in Immunosuppressed Patients With Negative Serology

- Check immunity to toxoplasmosis. If the patient has no protection (absence of anti-*Toxoplasma* IgG), take direct or indirect prophylactic measures against cats, food, and water.
- Universal prophylaxis with TMP/SMX[1] in all pre-HCTSP patients should be implemented by all transplant programs. Preemptive treatment with routine blood PCR monitoring is an option if prophylaxis cannot be used.
- Avoid contact with food (including unwashed fruit or vegetables) or water potentially contaminated with cat feces. Wash before consuming.
- Avoid any job or activity that requires contact with dirt, soil, or other material potentially contaminated with cat feces (e.g., gardening or handling cat litter). Wear gloves when gardening or handling cat litter.
- Keep cats inside. Do not adopt or handle stray cats. Do not feed cats raw or undercooked meat but only canned or dried commercial food or well-cooked food. Do not obtain a new kitten or cat during pregnancy.
- Disinfect the cat litter box with near-boiling water for 5 minutes before handling.
- Wash hands thoroughly after contact with raw meat.
- Kitchen surfaces and utensils that have come in contact with raw meat should be washed.
- Avoid ingesting raw or dried meat, raw eggs, or unpasteurized milk.
- Avoid eating raw oysters, clams, or mussels.
- Protect foods from flies, cockroaches, and other insects.
- Avoid touching the eyes or face or any mucous membrane during or immediately after preparing food.
- Cook meat thoroughly. Pork, lamb, beef, veal, and poultry should be cooked until the meat reaches 80°C in the center.
- Refrain from skinning animals.
- Avoid children's sandboxes.
- Avoid contact with stray dogs (xenosmophilia); if this is not possible, wash your hands after contact.

[1]Not FDA approved for this indication.

In general, a simpler route to prevent human disease would be to vaccinate animals (cats and intermediate hosts) that are responsible for transmission to humans, as demonstrated using a live attenuated vaccine developed for the prevention of chronic infection in sheep. However, it cannot be used in humans because of the risk of reversion to a pathogenic form. Vaccine development to prevent feline oocyst shedding is ongoing, mostly involving live vaccines. More recently, *T gondii* dense granule proteins including GRA-6, a secretory vesicular organelle that produces proteins that participate in the modification of the parasitophorous vacuole, have been shown to be suitable as possible DNA vaccines for immunity against toxoplasmosis. Recombinant rhoptry effector protein 54 (ROP54) plasmid has demonstrated to provide partial protection against acute and chronic toxoplasmosis. Finally, aspartic protease 1 (Asp 1) has also shown to play an essential role in the *T gondii* lifecycle, thus being a potential vaccine candidate against toxoplasmosis.

In summary, the immune evasive nature and complex life cycle of *T gondii* has made the design of immunotherapeutics aimed at providing complete protection, a discouraging challenge. Generally, vaccine studies thus far have shown that multi-antigenic formulations confer better protection than single-subunit vaccines.

References

Alaa Tareq Shakir Al-Hassnawi: Toxoplasma gondii may be an advisor for aggressiveness: seroprevalence of toxoplasmosis in murderer women in Iraq, *American Journal of Biology and Life Sciences* 2(6):187–190, 2014.

Boothroyd JC: Toxoplasma gondii: 25 years and 25 major advances for the field, *Int J Parasitol* 39:935–946, 2009.

Connolly MP, Haitsma G, Hernández AV, Vidal JE: Systematic review and meta-analysis of secondary prophylaxis for prevention of HIV-related toxoplasmic encephalitis relapse using trimethoprim-sulfamethoxazole, *Pathog Glob Health*. 111(6):327–331, 2017 Sep, https://doi.org/10.1080/20477724.2017.1377974.

Contini C: Clinical and diagnostic management of toxoplasmosis in the immunocompromised patient, *Parasitologia* 50:45–50, 2008.

Contini C, Seraceni S, Cultrera R, et al: Evaluation of a real-time PCR-based assay using the lightcycler system for detection of Toxoplasma gondii bradyzoite genes in blood specimens from patients with toxoplasmic retinochoroiditis, *Int J Parasitol* 35:275–283, 2005. Epub 2005 Jan 18.

Del Grande C, Contini C, Schiavi E, et al: Bipolar disorder with psychotic features and ocular toxoplasmosis: a possible pathogenetic role of the parasite? *J Nerv Ment Dis* 205(3):192–195, 2017.

Derouin F, Pelloux H: ESCMID study group on clinical parasitology: prevention of toxoplasmosis in transplant patients, *Clin Microbiol Infect* 14:1089–1101, 2008.

Dupont CD, Christian DA, Hunter CA: Immune response and immunopathology during toxoplasmosis, *Semin Immunopathol* 34:793–813, 2012. Epub 2012 Sep 7.

Elmore SA, Jones JL, Conrad PA, et al: Toxoplasma gondii: epidemiology, feline clinical aspects, and prevention, *Trends Parasitol* 26:190–196, 2010.

Flegr J, Preiss M, Klose J: Toxoplasmosis-associated difference in intelligence and personality in men depends on their Rhesus blood group but not ABO blood group, *PLoS One* 8, 2013. e61272.

Homan W, Vercammen M, De Braekeleer J, Verschueren H: Identification of a 200- to 300-fold repetitive 529 bp DNA fragment in Toxoplasma gondii, and its use for diagnostic and quantitative PCR, *Int J Parasitol*. 30:69–75, 2000.

Jasper S, Vedula SS, John SS, et al: Corticosteroids for ocular toxoplasmosis, *Cochrane Database Syst Rev* 30(4), 2013. CD007417.

Maenz M, Schlüter D, Liesenfeld O, et al: Ocular toxoplasmosis past, present and new aspects of an old disease, *Prog Retin Eye Res* 39:77–106, 2014.

Montoya JG, Liesenfeld O: Toxoplasmosis, *Lancet* 363:1965–1976, 2004.

Ngoungou EB, Bhalla D, Nzoghe A, Darde ML, Preux PM: Toxoplasmosis and epilepsy—systematic review and meta analysis, *PLoS Negl Trop Dis* 9(2), 2015. e0003525.

Petersen E: Toxoplasmosis, *Semin Fetal Neonatal Med* 12:214–223, 2007.

Peyron F, Mc Leod R, Ajzenberg D, et al: Congenital toxoplasmosis in France and the United States: one parasite, two diverging approaches, *PLoS Negl Trop Dis* 11(2), 2017. e0005222.

Remington JS, McLeod R, Thulliez P, et al: Toxoplasmosis. In Remington JS, Klein J, Wilson CB, Baker MD, editors: *Infectious Disease of the Fetus and Newborn Infant*, 6th ed., Philadelphia, 2006, Saunders, pp 946–1091.

Sathekge M, Maes A, Van de Wiele C: FDG-PET imaging in HIV infection and tuberculosis, *Semin Nucl Med* 43(5):349–366, 2013.

Shiadeh MN, Niyyati M, Fallahi S, et al: Human parasitic protozoan infection to infertility: a systematic review, *Parasitol Res* 115:469–477, 2016.

Sullivan Jr WJ, Jeffers V: Mechanisms of Toxoplasma gondii persistence and latency, *FEMS Microbiol Rev* 36:717–733, 2012.

Villard O, Cimon B, L'Ollivier C, et al: Serological diagnosis of Toxoplasma gondii infection, *recommendations from the French National Reference Center for Toxoplasmosis, Diagn Microbiol Infect Dis* 84:22–33, 2016.

TYPHOID FEVER

Method of
Tamilarasu Kadhiravan, MD

CURRENT DIAGNOSIS

- Typhoid fever typically manifests as an undifferentiated acute febrile illness.
- Soft splenomegaly, normal or low white blood cell count, and elevated liver enzymes are subtle diagnostic pointers.
- Blood culture, drawn before antibiotic administration, is the most useful investigation.
- Consider presumptive treatment in appropriate epidemiologic settings.

CURRENT THERAPY

- Intermediate susceptibility and resistance to fluoroquinolones are widespread among *Salmonella enterica* Typhi.
- High-dose fluoroquinolones are suboptimal for treating such infections.

- Azithromycin (Zithromax)[1] is the preferred drug for uncomplicated typhoid fever.
- Ceftriaxone (Rocephin)[1] is preferred for treating hospitalized and seriously ill patients.
- Extensively drug-resistant (XDR) typhoid fever, which is resistant to ceftriaxone and fluoroquinolones, is an emerging threat.

[1]Not FDA approved for this indication.

Typhoid fever is a bacteremic infection caused by the gram-negative bacillus *Salmonella enterica* serovar Typhi. *S enterica* Paratyphi also causes an illness clinically indistinguishable from typhoid fever. Humans are the only known host of *S enterica* Typhi, and it is transmitted by ingestion of contaminated food or water. Improvement in sanitation and hygiene led to the elimination of typhoid fever from the developed world long before the advent of antibiotics. On the other hand, in parts of the world lacking sanitation, it continues to be an important cause of febrile illness despite the availability of effective antibiotics.

Epidemiology
Typhoid fever is endemic in the developing world, especially the South and South East Asian countries of India, Nepal, Pakistan, Bangladesh, Vietnam, and Indonesia. Annual incidence in endemic settings is typically more than 100 cases per 100,000 population, and it predominantly affects children and young adults. Apart from sick persons with typhoid fever, convalescent carriers and asymptomatically infected food handlers (long-term carriers) are the sources of infection. Potential vehicles of infection include food or water consumed from roadside eateries, ice cubes and ice cream made from contaminated water, and raw vegetables and fruits. In contrast, most cases of typhoid fever in developed countries are imported by travel, especially to the Indian subcontinent.

Pathogenesis and Clinical Features
Following ingestion, the bacilli invade and multiply in the small-intestinal lymphoid tissue before entering the bloodstream. This primary bacteremia leads to widespread seeding of the reticuloendothelial system and intestinal lymphoid tissue, where the infection is amplified and spills over into the circulation. Onset of symptoms usually coincides with this secondary bacteremia. Interestingly, unlike other gram-negative bacteremic infections, septic shock develops relatively late in the course of illness, and the infection can be eminently cured by oral antibiotic therapy. Nonetheless, it should be emphasized that any delay in initiating antibiotic therapy increases the risk of complications (Box 1).

During the first week, temperature gradually increases in a stepladder fashion. Localizing symptoms are usually minimal. Anorexia, lassitude, and malaise are often marked. Headache and vomiting are common; however, a supple neck helps rule out meningitis. Abdominal symptoms such as constipation, loose stools, and abdominal pain are not infrequent, but they are nonspecific and often overlooked. Soft, tender enlargement of liver or spleen is seen in about half the patients. Rose spots and relative bradycardia, though classic, are rare. When the infection goes untreated, hypertrophied lymphoid tissue of the Peyer's patches can ulcerate toward the end of the second week, resulting in torrential gastrointestinal bleeding, small intestinal perforation, and secondary bacterial peritonitis. Patients with severe illness can present with a muttering delirium described as *coma vigil*. Untreated typhoid fever often resolves spontaneously in about 4 to 6 weeks. However, the risk of death is high (>10%), and relapses are frequent. Many patients excrete *S enterica* Typhi in feces and urine during convalescence (convalescent carriers), and some of them continue to excrete beyond 1 year (long-term carriers).

Current Pattern of Antimicrobial Susceptibility
Since 1990, a sea change has occurred in the antimicrobial susceptibility of *S enterica* Typhi in endemic countries and elsewhere.

Unregulated use of fluoroquinolones initially led to the emergence of *S enterica* Typhi strains with decreased susceptibility. These strains had a subthreshold increase in minimal inhibitory concentration (MIC) that was not detected by conventional disk-diffusion testing. Hence, resistance to nalidixic acid (NegGram)[2] (a quinolone) was often used as a surrogate marker for such strains. Currently, determination of MIC is recommended to identify fluoroquinolone susceptibility. Most infections in endemic countries are now caused by *S. enterica* Typhi with intermediate susceptibility or resistance to fluoroquinolones. Not surprisingly, this change is reflected in far-away geographic locales such as the United States and the United Kingdom. Of late, sporadic instances of resistance to azithromycin and third-generation cephalosporins have been reported. Notably, an ongoing outbreak of extensively drug-resistant (XDR) *S. enterica* Typhi with extended-spectrum β-lactamase–mediated resistance to third-generation cephalosporins has been reported in the Sindh province of Pakistan. A few travel-associated XDR-typhoid cases have been reported from the United States, United Kingdom, and Canada.

Diagnosis
Clinical features are nonspecific, and laboratory testing is essential to confirm a diagnosis of typhoid fever. A soft splenomegaly, absence of leukocytosis, mild leukopenia, and modest elevation of transaminases are subtle pointers to a diagnosis of typhoid fever. Blood culture drawn early in the illness before initiation of antibiotics is often fruitful and is the gold standard for the diagnosis of typhoid fever. The time-honored Widal test, which detects agglutinating antibodies to somatic and flagellar antigens of *S enterica* Typhi, adds little to decision making. Initial enthusiasm about rapid serologic tests such as Typhidot and Tubex TF has not been confirmed in community-based studies. None of these tests are sensitive enough to rule out typhoid. In a patient who has nonlocalizing acute febrile illness lasting more than 5 to 7 days in a suggestive epidemiologic setting (residence in or travel to endemic area; outbreaks), it is prudent to treat presumptively for typhoid fever, after reasonably ruling out competing diagnoses such as malaria, dengue, leptospirosis, and rickettsial infection.

Treatment
Fluoroquinolones (ciprofloxacin [Cipro] or ofloxacin [Floxin][1] 7.5 mg/kg twice a day for 5–7 days) were unparalleled in efficacy

[1] Not FDA approved for this indication.
[2] Not available in the United States.

TABLE 1 Outcomes of Alternative Treatments for Nalidixic Acid–Resistant *S enterica* Typhi (NARST) Infection Evaluated in Randomized, Controlled Trials

DRUG	DOSAGE	FEVER CLEARANCE TIME (MEDIAN OR MEAN)	RATE OF TREATMENT FAILURE	RELAPSE RATE	COMMENTS
High-dose ofloxacin (Floxin)[1]	10 mg/kg[3] bid × 7 d	8.2 d	36%	<1%; insufficient data	Not recommended
Gatifloxacin (Tequin)[2]	10 mg/kg qd × 7 d	4.4 d	9%	3%	Serious concerns about dysglycemia; resistance emerging in Nepal
Azithromycin (Zithromax)[1]	10–20[3] mg/kg qd × 7 d	4.4 d	9%	<1%; insufficient data	Effective in XDR-typhoid. Unproven in complicated typhoid fever
Cefixime (Suprax)[1]	10 mg/kg[3] bid × 7 d	5.8 d	27%	9%	High cost; not recommended
Ceftriaxone (Rocephin)[1]	60 mg/kg qd × 7 d	2.8 d	7%	7%	Experts suggest treatment for 10–14 d

Data from Arjyal A, Basnyat B, Nhan HT, et al: Gatifloxacin versus ceftriaxone for uncomplicated enteric fever in Nepal: an open-label, two-centre, randomised controlled trial. Lancet Infect Dis 2016;16:535. Dolecek C, Tran TP, Nguyen NR, et al: A multi-center randomised controlled trial of gatifloxacin versus azithromycin for the treatment of uncomplicated typhoid fever in children and adults in Vietnam. PLoS One 2008;3:e2188; Pandit A, Arjyal A, Day JN, et al: An open randomized comparison of gatifloxacin versus cefixime for the treatment of uncomplicated enteric fever. PLoS One 2007;2:e542; and Parry CM, Ho VA, Phuong le T, et al: Randomized controlled comparison of ofloxacin, azithromycin, and an ofloxacin-azithromycin combination for treatment of multidrug-resistant and nalidixic acid-resistant typhoid fever. Antimicrob Agents Chemother 2007;51:819.

[1]Not FDA approved for this indication.
[2]Not available in the United States.
[3]Exceeds dosage recommended by the manufacturer.

for treating fully susceptible *S enterica* Typhi strains. However, their use was associated with frequent treatment failures, prolonged defervescence, and higher rates of complications in nalidixic acid-resistant *S. enterica* Typhi (NARST) infections. Given the widespread emergence of reduced susceptibility, fluoroquinolones are no longer considered the drug of choice. Several alternatives have been evaluated in randomized, controlled trials for treating uncomplicated typhoid fever caused by NARST (Table 1). Ease of oral administration, proven efficacy, and safety (under FDA review) make azithromycin (Zithromax)[1] a good first choice for uncomplicated typhoid fever. In hospitalized seriously ill patients and treatment failures, parenteral ceftriaxone (Rocephin)[1] is preferred. Usually, it takes about 4 to 7 days for defervescence after the initiation of antibiotics. Recently, combining oral azithromycin (500 mg qd) with ceftriaxone (2 g qd) for inpatient or cefixime (Suprax)[1] (400 mg qd) for outpatient treatment was found to shorten the fever clearance time by about 7 hours, and fewer patients had persistent bacteremia on Day 3 (17% vs 4%). This clinical trial had certain limitations, and I do not recommend using a combination of antibiotics to treat typhoid fever. Despite in vitro susceptibility, aminoglycosides and first- and second-generation cephalosporins are not effective clinically for treating typhoid fever. Antipyretics should be used for symptom relief; ibuprofen (Motrin; 10 mg/kg every 6 hours) is superior to acetaminophen (Tylenol; 12 mg/kg every 6 hours). However, ibuprofen should be avoided when dengue fever is a possibility. A soft, low-residue diet is traditionally advised to prevent intestinal perforation. Such a practice, however, is not founded on scientific evidence. Treatment of *S enterica* Paratyphi infection is identical to that of *S enterica* Typhi infection.

Prevention

Sustained improvement in sanitation and access to safe drinking water are essential to control typhoid fever in endemic areas. Avoiding potentially contaminated food and beverages and being vaccinated before travel decrease the risk of typhoid fever among travelers (see the article on travel medicine). Mass administration of the Vi polysaccharide vaccine (Typhim Vi, Typherix [outside United States]) has been found to confer herd immunity and is a potential tool for the control of typhoid fever in endemic settings.

References

Arjyal A, Basnyat B, Nhan HT, et al: Gatifloxacin versus uncomplicated enteric fever in Nepal: an open- label, two-centre, randomised controlled trial, *Lancet Infect Dis* 16:535, 2016.
Chatham-Stephens K, Medalla F, Hughes M, et al: Emergence of extensively drug-resistant *Salmonella* Typhi infections among travelers to or from Pakistan - United States, 2016-2018, *MMWR Morb Mortal Wkly Rep* 68:11, 2019.
Dolecek C, Tran TP, Nguyen NR, et al: A multi-center randomised controlled trial of gatifloxacin versus azithromycin for the treatment of uncomplicated typhoid fever in children and adults in Vietnam, *PLoS ONE* 3, 2008:e2188.
Effa EE, Bukirwa H: Azithromycin for treating uncomplicated typhoid and paratyphoid fever (enteric fever), *Cochrane Database Syst Rev*(4), 2008:CD006083.
Karki S, Shakya P, Cheng AC, et al: Trends of etiology and drug resistance in enteric fever in the last two decades in Nepal: a systematic review and meta-analysis, *Clin Infect Dis* 57, 2013:e167.
Pandit A, Arjyal A, Day JN, et al: An open randomized comparison of gatifloxacin versus cefixime for the treatment of uncomplicated enteric fever, *PLoS ONE* 2, 2007:e542.
Parry CM, Ho VA, Phuong le T, et al: Randomized controlled comparison of ofloxacin, azithromycin, and an ofloxacin- azithromycin combination for treatment of multidrug-resistant and nalidixic acid resistant typhoid fever, *Antimicrob Agents Chemother* 51:819, 2007.
Vinh H, Parry CM, Hanh VT, et al: Double blind comparison of ibuprofen and paracetamol for adjunctive treatment of uncomplicated typhoid fever, *Pediatr Infect Dis J* 23:226, 2004.
Wijedoru L, Mallett S, Parry CM: Rapid diagnostic tests for typhoid and paratyphoid (enteric) fever, *Cochrane Database Syst Rev* (5), 2017.CD008892.
Zmora N, Shrestha S, Neuberger A, et al: Open label comparative trial of mono versus dual antibiotic therapy for typhoid fever in adults, *PLoS Negl Trop Dis* 12:e0006380, 2018.

VARICELLA (CHICKENPOX)

Method of
Cassie Scripter, MD

CURRENT DIAGNOSIS

- Clinical diagnosis is marked by a characteristic pruritic rash. The rash starts with erythematous macules progressing to papules and then vesicles ("dewdrop on a rose petal" appearance) that then crust. All stages of the rash are present simultaneously.
- Polymerase chain reaction can aide in the diagnosis. Specimens are collected by unroofing a vesicle and swabbing the base or collecting the crust from a lesion.

CURRENT TREATMENT

- Supportive care is recommended for immunocompetent individuals 1 to 12 years of age.
- Aspirin should not be used because of the risk of Reye's syndrome.
- Antiviral treatment with acyclovir (Zovirax) or valacyclovir (Valtrex) for individuals <1 year, >12 years, and immunocompromised individuals. Acyclovir is available in liquid suspension.
- Post-exposure prophylaxis with varicella immunization is recommended for children and adults without evidence of immunity.

Varicella (chickenpox) is an acute, self-limited primary infection of childhood caused by the varicella zoster virus (VZV), a herpesvirus. Transmission occurs by respiratory secretions or direct contact with skin lesions.

Epidemiology

In temperate climates varicella previously infected >90% of individuals before adolescence with epidemics every 2 to 5 years in late winter to early spring. Varicella was less common in tropical climates but more frequently affected young adults. In the early 1990s, an average of 4 million cases occurred in the United States annually, resulting in up to 150 annual deaths. A one-dose varicella immunization (Varivax) was introduced in 1995, and by 2005 the overall incidence of varicella and its associated complications had decreased by up to 90%. In the early 2000s, there were several outbreaks of mild varicella among immunized children, which led to the Centers for Disease Control and Prevention (CDC) 2006 recommendation of a routine second dose of varicella immunization for US children. The incidence has continued to decline since, although nearly 9000 cases of varicella and 3 deaths were reported in the United States in 2016.

Risk Factors and Prevention

There are no risk factors for varicella infection other than exposure to the virus. Complications are more likely in adults, infants <1 year of age, and immunocompromised individuals.

The CDC recommends a two-dose live, attenuated varicella immunization (Varivax). The first dose is administered between 12 and 15 months of age and the second between 4 and 6 years. The second dose may be given before 4 years of age if 3 months have elapsed since the first dose. A two-dose immunization regimen is recommended for all persons 13 years and older without evidence of immunity to varicella. The two doses should be separated by at least 4 weeks. Evidence of immunity requires documentation of age-appropriate immunization, laboratory evidence of immunity or confirmation of disease, verification of history or diagnosis by a healthcare provider, or birth in the United States before 1980, although birth in the United States before 1980 is not considered a sufficient criteria for healthcare personnel or pregnant women.

Pathophysiology

VZV enters the mucosa of the nasopharynx and conjunctivae through aerosolized droplets or direct contact with lesions. The virus replicates in regional lymph nodes before disseminating and replicating in the liver and spleen. After 14 to 16 days (range 10-21 days), VZV-infected cells spread to the nasopharyngeal surface and the skin, resulting in skin lesions. During the primary infection and after immunization, VZV can infect neurons and become latent in the dorsal root and other ganglia, including those of the cranial and autonomic systems. Reactivation of latent VZV causes herpes zoster (shingles).

Clinical Manifestations

Primary infection in non-immunized individuals begins with a mild prodrome of fever, malaise, headache, pharyngitis, and anorexia followed by the development of pruritic cutaneous lesions. The 1- to 4-mm lesions present on the head, scalp, trunk, and extremities. Lesions begin as erythematous macules, progress to papules, and then become vesicles that crust after 1 to 2 days. Crusts fall off within 1 to 2 weeks. The vesicular lesions on an erythematous base are described as having a "dewdrop on a rose petal" appearance (Figure 1). New lesions develop in successive crops for 3 to 5 days (range 1-7), with lesions in various stages of development simultaneously present (Figure 2). The median number of lesions is 200 to 400 in 2 to 4 successive crops. Patients are contagious from 1 to 2 days before the onset of the rash until all lesions have crusted over. The vesicular phase is the most contagious period. Lesions can occur on mucous membranes in the oropharynx, respiratory tract, conjunctiva, cornea, and vagina.

Breakthrough varicella is defined as a VZV infection more than 42 days after immunization and is due to incomplete immunity to the VZV virus. The course is mild, short-lasting, and has fewer skin lesions (<50) than primary infection. The rash is more likely to be macular than vesicular and may not follow the characteristic progression described above, making it more difficult to make a diagnosis on clinical presentation alone.

Diagnosis

Traditionally the diagnosis was based on the characteristic rash and clinical features. As more cases now occur in immunized individuals, atypical rashes present a diagnostic challenge. Infections in the immunocompromised may be severe, atypical, and difficult to diagnose based on clinical criteria. Polymerase chain reaction is recommended to confirm varicella infection if the diagnosis is unclear. Specimens are collected by unroofing a vesicle and swabbing the base of the lesion or by collecting the crust from a lesion. Specimens may be obtained from vesicular fluid or cerebrospinal fluid, blood, saliva, throat swabs, or biopsy tissue. Compared with polymerase chain reaction technology, testing for immunoglobulin M antibody using commercial kits is not recommended because of low sensitivity.

Differential Diagnosis

History and physical examination, particularly the characteristics of the rash, are key in differentiating varicella from other conditions. Smallpox was previously the most serious consideration in the differential diagnosis for varicella. Since its eradication via natural transmission, bioterrorism and laboratory exposure are the most likely sources of smallpox transmission. Smallpox has more prominent constitutional symptoms with lesions in the same stage of development. Zoster rashes appear in a dermatomal distribution. Other considerations include impetigo, diffuse herpes simplex virus, hand-foot-mouth disease, guttate psoriasis, allergic reaction (Stevens-Johnson syndrome), and viral exanthema (coxsackie virus, enterovirus).

Treatment

Patient age, immune status, and duration since rash eruption are key in management decisions. Symptomatic treatment is recommended in healthy children younger than 13 years because of the self-limited nature of the disease. Aspirin is not recommended because of the risk of Reye syndrome.

Oral antiviral therapy is indicated for immunocompetent individuals older than 12 years, individuals receiving long-term salicylate therapy or short, intermittent, or aerosolized courses of corticosteroids, and those with chronic dermatologic or pulmonary disease. Antivirals are most effective if administered within 48 hours of rash eruption. They decrease the duration of fever and rash, as well as the risk of severe and fatal disease. Valacyclovir (Valtrex) is preferred because of increased bioavailability. The oral dose of valacyclovir is 20 mg/kg up to 1000 mg three

Figure 1 **A,** "Dewdrop on a rose petal"; a thick-walled vesicle with clear fluid forms on a red base. **B,** The vesicle becomes cloudy and depressed in the center (umbilicated); the border is irregular (scalloped). **C,** A crust forms in the center and eventually replaces the remaining portion of the vesicle at the periphery.

Figure 2 The disease starts with lesions on the trunk and then spreads to the face and extremities.

times daily for 5 days. Dosing for acyclovir (Zovirax) (>40 kg) is 800 mg five times daily[3] for 5 days. Acyclovir is available in liquid suspension (200 mg/5 mL) and is dosed 20 mg/kg every 6 hours for 5 days in individuals older than 2 years old and less than 40 kg. The maximum daily dose is 3200 mg. Foscarnet (Foscavir)[1] is not considered first-line therapy due to potential nephrotoxicity and other adverse effects.

Infants and immunocompromised patients are treated with intravenous acyclovir at 10 to 15 mg/kg every 8 hours for 7 to 10 days. Dosing adjustment for renal impairment is recommended because intravenous antivirals can be nephrotoxic. A switch from intravenous to oral antivirals should be considered when patients have been fever free and without new lesions for 24 hours.

Pregnant women with varicella are at high risk of pulmonary complications, and antiviral treatment is recommended for any pregnant woman with pulmonary involvement. Acyclovir is a category B drug.

Post-exposure Prophylaxis

Post-exposure prophylaxis with varicella immunization[1] is effective in preventing illness or decreasing the severity of illness if administered to children up to 3 days, and possibly 5 days, after exposure. Although studies have only been conducted on children, one-dose varicella vaccination is recommended for both children and adults who have no evidence of immunity after exposure to varicella. During an outbreak, individuals who received only one dose of vaccine should receive a second dose if the appropriate time interval has lapsed. Varicella zoster immune globulin (VariZig) is available for post-exposure prophylaxis for individuals without evidence of immunity who are at greatest risk of severe disease and related complications or for those who have a contraindication to the varicella vaccine.

Complications

Varicella is typically self-limited in immunocompetent patients, but complications can occur. Secondary skin and soft tissue infections with *Staphylococcus aureus* or *Streptococcus pyogenes* are the most common complications. Other complications include pneumonia, subclinical hepatitis, encephalitis, and ataxia. Invasive infection occurs more commonly in infants younger than 1 year, adolescents, adults, immunocompromised patients, and newborns whose mothers develop a rash within 5 days before and 2 days after delivery. Congenital malformations, especially involving the central nervous system, are more likely to occur if the mother is infected during the first two trimesters. Disseminated varicella may result if infection occurs during the third trimester.

Varicella zoster virus lies dormant in the dorsal root ganglia and may activate causing herpes zoster. The incidence of shingles is approximately 10 cases per 1000 US population in those aged 60 years and older. Shingles most commonly presents as a unilateral maculopapular rash that becomes vesicular. The characteristic dermatomal distribution of the rash and any preceding pain and paresthesia are usually diagnostic. Postherpetic neuralgia, persistent pain in the area after resolution of the rash, is the most common complication of zoster and can last a few days to years. Immunocompromised hosts are more likely to experience severe complications. Two shingles vaccines are currently available in the United States, Zostavax and Shingrix. The CDC recommends two doses of Shingrix 2 to 6 months apart for those 50 years and older, even in those who have previously received Zostavax. If patients have already received Zostavax, 2 months should be allowed before administering Shingrix. Current data show 90% effectiveness in preventing shingles and postherpetic neuralgia with two doses of Shingrix. Individuals who have had shingles should receive the Shingrix series after acute symptoms of zoster have subsided.

References

American Academy of Pediatrics: Varicella-zoster infections. In Kimberlin D, Brady M, Jackson M, Long S (editors): Red Book: 2015 Report of the Committee on Infectious Diseases, 30th ed., American Academy of Pediatrics, Elk Grove Village, IL 2015, pp 846–860, 919, 925.

Centers for Disease Control and Prevention: Epidemiology and prevention of vaccine-preventable diseases. Varicella. In: Hamborsky J, Kroger A, Wolfe S, eds. 13th ed. Washington, DC, Public Health Foundation, 2015.

Centers for Disease Control and Prevention. National Notifiable Infectious Diseases and Conditions: United States. https://wonder.cdc.gov/nndss/static/2016/annual/2016-table2o.html. [Accessed April 20, 2018].

Dooling KL, Guo A, Patel M, et al: Recommendations of the Advisory Committee on Immunization Practices for Use of Herpes Zoster Vaccines, *MMWR Morb Mortal Wkly Rep* 67:103–108, 2018.

Gershon A: Is chickenpox so bad, what do we know about immunity to varicella zoster virus, and what does it tell us about the future? *J Infect.* 74(suppl1):S27–S33, 2017.

Lopez AS, Zhang J, Marin M: Epidemiology of varicella during the 2-dose varicella vaccination program—United States, 2005–2014, *MMWR Morb Mortal Wkly Rep* 65:902–905, 2016.

Marin M, Guris D, Chaves S, et al: Prevention of varicella: recommendations of the Advisory Committee on Immunization Practices (ACIP), *MMWR Recomm Rep* 56:1–40, 2007.

Marin M, Marti M, Kambhampati A, et al: Global varicella vaccine effectiveness: a meta-analysis, *Pediatrics* 137(3):e20153741, 2016.

Mueller NH, Gilden DH, Cohrs RJ, et al: Varicella zoster virus infection: clinical features, molecular pathogenesis of disease, and latency, *Neurol Clin* 26:675–697, 2008.

Su J, Leroy Z, Lewis P: Safety of a second-dose single antigen varicella vaccine, *Pediatrics* 139(3):e20162536, 2017.

[1] Not FDA approved for this indication.
[3] Exceeds dosage recommended by the manufacturer.

YELLOW FEVER

Method of
Lucius M. Lampton, MD

CURRENT DIAGNOSIS

- Yellow fever is a historically important mosquito-borne Flavivirus with high morbidity and mortality.
- Travel to yellow fever–endemic areas in Sub-Saharan Africa and tropical Central and South America is the essential risk factor.
- Symptoms may include abrupt onset of fever, relative bradycardia, headache, and, if severe, jaundice, hemorrhage, and multiorgan failure.
- Diagnosis is with viral culture and serologic tests.
- Although infectious disease experts consider it improbable that yellow fever outbreaks will return to the continental United States, this reemerging disease is threatening to become more prevalent and deadly in tropical South America and Africa. Travel-related cases should be anticipated in the United States and its territories, as well as the possibility of brief episodes of local dissemination in areas bordering the Gulf of Mexico, where the vector, the *Aedes aegypti* mosquito, can be found.

CURRENT THERAPY

- Prevention is key and accomplished by vaccination and mosquito avoidance and control.
- Supportive care is the only treatment.

Epidemiology

Yellow fever is one of the great epidemic diseases of tropical Africa and the Americas. It receives its appellation "yellow" from the symptom of jaundice, which appears in severe disease, and it is caused by an RNA virus, specifically a Flavivirus (a family name derived from yellow fever, with *flavus* Latin for yellow), that is held in natural reservoirs by forest monkeys and spread to people via mosquitoes. The disease, termed an acute hemorrhagic fever, infects humans, all species of monkeys, and certain other small mammals and is transmitted among its hosts by several species of mosquitoes.

There are three types of yellow fever infection: urban, jungle, and intermediate. In urban or classical yellow fever, human-to-human spread occurs by the bite of the *A. aegypti* mosquito, which breeds in urban unpolluted water and bites principally in the daytime. Reinvasion of this mosquito in Central and South America has occurred beginning in the 1970s owing to increases in breeding sites resulting from urbanization and the collapse of vector control efforts. In jungle or sylvatic yellow fever, which was first recognized in 1933, the disease is perpetuated by enzootic infection of mammalians, usually monkeys, disseminated by several different mosquitoes: in South America via the *Haemagogus* and *Sabethes* spp.; in East Africa via *Ae. africanus*; and in West Africa via a variety of species of *Aedes*. Human infection arises by jungle exposure to these mosquitoes. In intermediate or savannah yellow fever, which commonly occurs in Africa, the virus disseminates from mosquitoes to humans residing or working in areas bordering jungles. This cycle also involves spread of the virus from monkey to human or from human to human via the bite of a mosquito.

Yellow fever, also termed Yellow Jack, the Saffron Scourge, fievre jaune, Bronze John, and Black Vomit (the Spanish name is vómito negro), is the deadliest arthropod virus ever to emerge in the Americas. Both the molecular taxonomic research of viral strains and the annals of history reveal an African origin. Most authorities assert it was introduced to the new world by *A. aegypti*–infested slave ships voyaging from West Africa, with its first recognition in the Americas occurring in Yucatan, Mexico, in 1648 (although research suggests the disease was present in the Americas as early as 1498). Over the next two and a half centuries, yellow fever erupted with regularity in American and European port cities, with hundreds of thousands of deaths, earning the virus deserved recognition as one of the worst plagues the world had ever seen. Two of the most significant North American epidemics occurred in Philadelphia in 1793 and in the Mississippi Valley in 1878. American epidemics were the result of the introduction of the mosquito vector and infected humans along routes of trade, especially sea and river ports and rail lines, with particular virulence associated with the Gulf region where *A. aegypti* resided. Early attempts at control focused on quarantine and sanitary measures. The devastation associated with American epidemics was an important impetus in the nation's early public health and sanitation movements for the creation of city, state, and national boards of health.

Although two 19th-century physicians, Josiah Nott and Carlos Juan Finlay, suggested the mosquito was the infectious agent for yellow fever, it was not until 1900 that the work of the US Army Commission in Cuba under Major Walter Reed established that the vector of the urban form of this disease was the *A. aegypti* mosquito, with its viral cause not established until after 1928. Max Theiler developed an attenuated vaccine strain in 1937, which was recognized with a Nobel Prize. In what is acknowledged as one of the most successful campaigns in history against infectious disease, mosquito eradication and control efforts and this vaccine effectively controlled and eliminated urban yellow fever in the Americas and the West Indies, with the last large outbreak occurring in the continental United States in New Orleans in 1905. However, the disease persisted in its jungle form in forest areas in Africa and South America. Vaccine administration remains incomplete in endemic areas, and outbreaks periodically recur. As well, mosquito eradication efforts in both the Americas and Africa have recently slackened, with the resulting resurgence of *A. aegypti* into nearly all of the tropical American countries, placing this region at extraordinary risk for urban outbreaks. Also, while only travel-related cases have been documented in Asia, theoretic anthroponotic dissemination could also take place there in the many areas where the urban vector resides.

Official statistics suggest the incidence of yellow fever fluctuates, with 90% of the 200,000 annual cases reported in Africa. However, authorities warn that these statistics considerably underestimate (owing to underreporting) the true magnitude of epidemics, which field studies estimate as 50 times greater. A frightening prospect associated with failing mosquito control in urban habitats is the potential reemergence of yellow fever similar to the recent rapid resurgence of dengue, which is also transmitted by the vector *A. aegypti*. Experts contend that one of the most profound mysteries of tropical medicine is that this dangerous virus has not emerged more frequently where a susceptible, unimmunized human population and the vector density coexist. However, since the 1980s, a resurgence of yellow fever has been seen across South America and Africa, which augurs potential risk for the United States. While yellow fever outbreaks remain unlikely in the Unites States, travel-related cases should be expected, as well as the possibility of brief urban cycle transmission in the American Southeast.

The 2015–2019 outbreaks in Brazil and Africa portend ominously that yellow fever appears to be moving from its typical rural setting toward urban areas. A large urban outbreak in Angola, which began in December 2015 and subsequently spread to the Democratic Republic of the Congo, resulted in 962 confirmed cases and 393 deaths and included multiple travel-related cases appearing in nonendemic areas internationally such as China. The outbreak in Brazil was first recognized in December 2016, with more than 2246 confirmed cases and 762 deaths noted as of April 18, 2019, including two dozen travel-related cases. This upsurge of human cases, which is the highest observed in the Americas for decades, reflects the spread into densely populated metropolitan areas, such as Rio de Janeiro and Sao Paulo, which in the past were not considered at risk for transmission. This outbreak has impacted not only Brazil but six other American countries: Bolivia, Colombia, Ecuador, French Guiana, Peru, and Suriname. In the current outbreak, all human cases have been linked only to *Haemagogus* and *Sabethes* mosquitoes.

In response to yellow fever's reemergence in Africa, the World Health Organization (WHO) launched the Yellow Fever Initiative in 2006, vaccinating in mass campaigns more than 105 million people in West Africa and attempting to secure a global vaccine supply. In 2017, the Eliminate Yellow Fever Epidemics (EYE) strategy was initiated with more than 50 partners supporting 40 at-risk countries in the Americas and Africa to prevent, detect, and contain global outbreaks. By 2026, it is projected that 1.38 billion people will be vaccinated against the disease. In March 2018, Brazil's health minister announced that all of the country's 78 million people will be targeted in a large-scale vaccination campaign.

Yellow fever remains the most dangerous arbovirus ever to inhabit the Western Hemisphere. Despite ongoing vaccination and mosquito control efforts in endemic areas, sylvatic and intermediate transmission cycles persist and appear to be expanding toward urban spread. Public health leaders encourage clinicians to utilize heightened suspicion and awareness for the virus, especially among travelers to tropical areas. Recent yellow fever outbreaks underscore boldly the potential threat this disease poses for the international community.

Risk Factors

Travel to yellow fever–endemic areas in Sub-Saharan Africa and tropical Central and South America, between the 15th parallel north and the 15th parallel south, is the essential risk factor.

Pathophysiology

Yellow fever virus has three types or cycles of transmission: urban, jungle (sylvatic), and intermediate (savannah). In urban yellow fever, the virus is spread by the bite of an *A. aegypti* mosquito infected about 2 weeks previously by feeding on a person with viremia. In jungle (sylvatic) yellow fever, the virus is transmitted by various forest canopy mosquitoes that acquire it from wild primates and then disseminate it to humans who are visiting or working in the jungle. Incidence of the disease is highest during months of peak temperature, rainfall, and humidity in South America and during the late rainy and early dry seasons in Africa. In the intermediate (savannah) cycle, which is most common in Africa, transmission of the virus to humans results from humans living or working in jungle border areas, with the virus spread from monkey to human or from human to human by mosquitoes. Humans infected with the virus are infectious to mosquitoes (what is termed being "viremic") shortly before the onset of illness and up to 5 days after onset. Yellow fever is not transmissible by contact, only via a vector's bite.

Prevention

Yellow fever is a mosquito-borne infection that can be prevented by mosquito avoidance and vaccination. Recovery from yellow fever imparts lifelong immunity against the virus.

Mosquito control is an essential component of any strategy to prevent the spread of yellow fever. Before the development of the vaccine and after the mosquito was proven as the vector, eliminating mosquito-breeding sites and decreasing exposure to *A. aegypti* mosquitoes proved successful in ending yellow fever outbreaks in North America and also in the building of the Panama Canal. Today, it remains critical not only to reduce the number of mosquitoes through larvicides and insecticides but also to limit mosquito bites through the use of house screening, mosquito netting, the wearing of protective attire, and the use of insect repellants such as diethyltoluamide (DEET). During jungle outbreaks, mosquito elimination is impractical and evacuation is essential until individuals are immunized and mosquitoes controlled. To prevent further mosquito transmission during outbreaks, infected patients should be isolated in well-screened rooms sprayed with insecticides.

Immunization is the most effective and reliable way to prevent yellow fever in areas in which it is endemic. Live attenuated yellow fever virus vaccine (17D strain) (YF-VAX) should be given (0.5 mL subcutaneously every 10 years) at least 10 days before travel to endemic areas in Africa and Central and South America. A single dose of vaccine gives greater than or equal to 99% protection and confers lifelong immunity. (Although required by some countries, a booster dose of the vaccine is not medically needed.) Although infection is uncommon in most of the endemic areas, vaccination is legally required for entry into many of these countries. The typically well-tolerated vaccine is contraindicated in pregnant women, in individuals with concurrent febrile illness or compromised immunity, and in infants younger than 6 months. If infants aged 6 to 8 months cannot avoid travel to a high-risk location, parents should discuss immunization with their physician, since the vaccine is usually not offered until the age of 9 months. In the United States, the vaccine is given only at US Public Health Service-authorized Yellow Fever Vaccination Centers. The International Certificate of Vaccination is valid for 10 years from 10 days after immunization or immediately after reimmunization.

After the 2016 outbreaks depleted global vaccine supplies, experts suggested as a dose-sparing strategy the utilization of a fractional dose of the vaccine among children 2 years of age or older and among nonpregnant adults.[3] In an observational study, a one-fifth dose of the vaccine induced seroconversion in 98% of recipients. In the 2018 and 2019 outbreaks, mass vaccination campaigns have utilized primarily fractional dosing.

Clinical Manifestations

Yellow fever is characterized by the swift onset of fever, rigors, myalgias, headache, nausea, and vomiting. With an incubation period lasting 3 to 6 days, the illness is typically biphasic, with a two-stage course during which the pulse slows and kidney involvement occurs along with bleeding disorders. Between 5% and 50% of the cases are so mild they are inapparent. In those cases recognized, the pulse is usually rapid initially but by the second day becomes slow for the degree of fever (Faget sign). A tendency to bleed may be seen early in the disease. Often, the face is flushed, with facial edema and conjunctival injection. Restlessness, irritability, and leukopenia are also common. In most cases, this initial period of mild infection resolves after 1 to 3 days, occasionally longer, and the illness concludes with rapid recovery and no sequelae. However, approximately 15% of those infected progress further into the moderate to severe phases. In these cases, the falling fever and remission of symptoms 2 to 5 days after onset are only transitory, and a deadly phase soon begins with renewal of malignant symptoms. This stage of the illness, called intoxication, is marked by the fever returning, and although the pulse remains slow, the blood pressure drops, with resultant renal failure. The flushed face is replaced by a dusky pallor, with swollen, bleeding gums and a pronounced hemorrhagic tendency with telltale black vomit (one of the disease's monikers and classic symptoms) and melena. The skin and eyes may appear yellow (jaundice), the symptom that gave rise to the disease's popular name. (However, this jaundice is generally a symptom of convalescence more than acute disease.) Liver and renal failure (which may progress to acute tubular necrosis) and epigastric tenderness with hematemesis and gastrointestinal hemorrhage often occur. There may be oliguria, albuminuria, disseminated intravascular coagulopathy, backache, dizziness, ecchymoses, myocarditis, agitated delirium, intractable hiccups, seizures, coma, and multiple organ failure. During recovery, bacterial superinfections, particularly pneumonia, may occur.

---

[3] Exceeds dosage recommended by the manufacturer.

In terminal cases, death usually transpires within 7 days of onset and is rare beyond 10 days of illness. In patients with intoxication (malignant yellow fever), a 20% to 60% mortality may be seen, with survival depending on the quality of supportive management. At autopsy, the kidneys, liver, heart, and spleen appear to be the organs most impacted by the disease.

Diagnosis

Yellow fever is suspected in patients in endemic areas or returning from them if they develop classic clinical features such as sudden fever with relative bradycardia and jaundice. Mild infection often escapes recognition by the patient or clinician. Complete blood count, urinalysis, liver function tests, coagulation studies, viral blood cultures, and serologic tests should be done. Leukopenia with relative neutropenia is common, as are thrombocytopenia, prolonged clotting, and increased prothrombin time. Bilirubin and aminotransferase levels may be elevated acutely and for several months. Albuminuria, which occurs in 90% of patients, may reach 20 g/L. This finding helps differentiate yellow fever from viral hepatitis. In malignant yellow fever, hypoglycemia and hyperkalemia may occur terminally.

Diagnosis is confirmed by viral culture, serology, the identification of viral antigens and virus-specific immunoglobulin M (IgM) and neutralizing antibodies in serum by several rapid diagnostic methods, or detecting characteristic midzonal hepatocyte necrosis at autopsy. Suspected or confirmed cases must be quarantined and health departments notified. Needle biopsy of the liver during illness is contraindicated because of high risk of hemorrhage.

Differential Diagnosis

Mild yellow fever appears clinically like a broad expanse of other infections presenting with similar symptoms, including dengue, viral hepatitis, malaria, typhus, Q fever, typhoid, Rift Valley fever, leptospirosis, drug-induced syndromes, and toxic causes. Yellow fever may be distinguished from malaria by the findings of conjunctival suffusion or relative bradycardia. The other viral hemorrhagic fevers, which include dengue, Lassa fever, Marburg disease, Ebola, Crimean-Congo hemorrhagic fever, and Bolivian and Argentine hemorrhagic fevers, usually present without jaundice. As well, albuminuria is a reliable hallmark of yellow fever that allows its differentiation from other causes of viral hepatitis.

Treatment

Since no antiviral therapy is currently available, treatment is supportive, focused on aggressive symptom management designed to correct the acid-base imbalance and electrolyte abnormalities caused by emesis, heart failure, and renal derangements. Placement in an intensive care unit is recommended. Transfusions of blood, fresh-frozen plasma, and vitamin K[1] may be utilized with hemorrhagic symptoms. As well, a proton pump inhibitor, H2 blocker, and sucralfate (Carafate)[1] can be helpful as prophylaxis for gastrointestinal bleeding and should be considered in all hospitalized patients. Antipyretics, oxygen, vasopressors, and IV hydration may also be helpful. Avoidance of sedatives and drugs metabolized hepatically is prudent, and medication dosing should be adjusted in the face of declining renal function. Antibiotic therapy for secondary bacterial sepsis is often necessary during the recovery period. Owing to the increased risk of bleeding, avoidance of aspirin and other nonsteroidal antiinflammatory drugs, such as naproxen and ibuprofen, is recommended.

Complications

The majority of those infected with yellow fever will be asymptomatic or experience only mild disease with total recovery. The mortality rates in tropical America range from 45% to 75%, compared with less than 30% in Africa. This difference suggests genetic factors play a role in the course of the illness, as well as the viral strain. The convalescence of a yellow fever patient is usually prolonged and varies from patient to patient. Although uncommon, late death (weeks after the acute illness) can occur as a result of cardiac complications or renal failure. Profound asthenia and fatigue usually last for 1 to 2 weeks, but in some cases can last many months. Jaundice and the elevation of liver enzymes have been known to last an extended period (several months) during convalescence. Survival of an attack imparts life-long immunity against subsequent infection.

References

A global strategy to Eliminate Yellow fever Epidemics 2017–2026, Geneva: World Health Organization;

Ahuka-Mundeke S, Casey RM, et al: Immunogenicity of fractional-dose vaccine during a yellow fever outbreak—preliminary report, N Engl J Med 2018.

Bennett JE, Dolin R, Blaser M: Mandell, Douglas, and Bennett's Principles and Practice of Infectious Diseases, 8th ed., Philadelphia, 2015, Elsevier Saunders2015.

Centers for Disease Control and Prevention. Yellow fever. Available at: https://www.cdc.gov/yellowfever/index.html [accessed June 1, 2019].

Fauci AS, Paules CI: Yellow fever—once again on the radar screen in the Americas, N Engl J Med 376:1397–1399, 2017.

Hamer DH, Angelo K, Caumes E, et al: Fatal yellow fever in travelers to Brazil, 2018, MMWR Morb Mortal Wkly Rep 67:340–341, 2018.

Kimberlin DW, editor: In Red Book: 2015 Report of the Committee on Infectious Diseases, 13th ed., Elk Grove Village, IL, 2015, American Academy of Pediatrics.

Knipe DM, Howley P: Fields Virology, 5th ed., Philadelphia, 2007, Lippincott Williams and Wilkins2007.

Moritz UG Kraemer, et al: Spread of yellow fever virus outbreak in Angola and the Democratic Republic of the Congo 2015–16: a modelling study, The Lancet Infectious Diseases 17(3):330–338, 2017.

National Notifiable Diseases Surveillance System (NNDSS): Yellow Fever Case Definition 2019. Available at: https://wwwn.cdc.gov/nndss/conditions/yellow-fever/case-definition/2019/ [accessed June 1, 2019].

Wilder-Smith A, Monath TP: Responding to the threat of urban yellow fever outbreaks, The Lancet Infectious Diseases 17(3):248–250, 2017.

World Health Organization. Yellow fever factsheet. Available at: http://www.who.int/mediacentre/factsheets/fs100/en/ [accessed June 2, 2019].

WHOOPING COUGH (PERTUSSIS)

Method of
Deon Regis, MD

CURRENT DIAGNOSIS

- Primarily a toxin-mediated disease
- Incubation period 7 to 10 days (range 4 to 21 days)
- Insidious onset, similar to the common cold with nonspecific cough
- Catarrhal stage: 1 to 2 weeks
- Paroxysmal cough stage: 1 to 6 weeks
- Convalescence: weeks to months
- Nasopharyngeal culture—gold standard

CURRENT TREATMENT

- Vaccination is key for prevention.
- Early treatment eradicates the organism from secretions, decreasing transmission, and may shorten the course of the illness.
- Macrolides are the treatment of choice, specifically azithromycin (Zithromax).[1]

[1]Not FDA approved for this indication.

Pertussis, or whooping cough, is an acute infectious disease caused by the bacterium *Bordetella pertussis*. Outbreaks of pertussis were first described in the 16th century, and the organism was first isolated in 1906.

[1]Not FDA approved for this indication.

In the 20th century, pertussis was one of the most common childhood diseases and a major cause of childhood mortality in the United States. In 1932, an outbreak of whooping cough hit Atlanta, Georgia, and a pediatrician by the name of Leila Denmark began her study of the disease. In partnership with Emory University and Eli Lilly & Company, she developed the first pertussis vaccine. Before the availability of the pertussis vaccine in the 1940s, more than 200,000 cases of pertussis were reported annually. Since widespread use of the vaccine began, incidence has decreased more than 80% compared with the pre-vaccine era.

Epidemiology

Worldwide, it is estimated that there are about 16 million pertussis (whooping cough) cases and about 195,000 pertussis deaths in children per year. Despite generally high coverage with childhood pertussis vaccines, pertussis is one of the leading causes of vaccine-preventable deaths worldwide. Most deaths occur in infants who are either unvaccinated or incompletely vaccinated. The World Health Organization (WHO) estimates that in 2008, global vaccination against pertussis prevented approximately 687,000 deaths. The year 2012 was the peak year in which there were more than 48,000 reported cases in the United States, which drew the attention of the public health community.

Transmission

Pertussis is a human disease. There is no animal, insect source, or vector. Adolescents and adults are an important reservoir for *B. pertussis* and are often the source of infection for infants.

Transmission most commonly occurs by the respiratory route through aerosolized respiratory droplets or by direct contact with airborne droplets of respiratory secretions. Transmission occurs less frequently by contact with freshly contaminated articles of an infected person as the bacteria cannot not survive long outside of the reservoir. Pertussis is highly communicable. Persons with pertussis are most infectious during the catarrhal period and the first 2 weeks after cough onset.

Microbiology

B. pertussis is a small, aerobic, gram-negative rod. *B. pertussis* produces multiple antigenic and biologically active products, including pertussis toxin (PT), filamentous hemagglutinin (FHA), agglutinogens, adenylate cyclase, pertactin, and tracheal cytotoxin. These products are responsible for the clinical features of pertussis disease, and an immune response to one or more produces immunity following infection.

Pathogenesis

Pertussis is primarily a toxin-mediated disease. The bacteria attach to the cilia of the respiratory epithelial cells, causing inflammation, and produce toxins that paralyze the cilia, which interferes with the clearing of pulmonary secretions.

The steps in pathogenesis are:
- Exposure/inoculation
- Tissue tropism/attachment
- Proliferation and production of virulence factors
- Evasion/modulation of host defenses
- Local and systemic cell and tissue dysfunction/damage
- Clearance and resolution of symptoms or chronic infection or death

Pertussis Toxin*

PT is important as its effects include induction of lymphocytosis, alteration in insulin secretion, and enhancement of sensitivity to histamine and other mediators.

Filamentous Hemagglutinin*

This large surface protein can participate in the interaction of *B. pertussis* with host cells and exerts immunomodulatory effects; thus it is appropriately classified as an adhesion.

Pertactin*

Pertactin (PRN) can contribute to bacterium–host cell interaction as an adhesion and was found to have a role in host defense against neutrophils.

Fimbriae*

These surface appendages, similar to those in other bacteria, function as adhesins and make up several of the agglutinogens, which are used for *Bordetella* serotyping.

Adenylate Cyclase Toxin

This toxin increases cyclic adenosine monophosphate (cAMP) levels, resulting in inhibition of phagocyte function and activation of apoptosis in some cell types. Adenylate cyclase toxin is a critical virulence factor.

Tracheal Cytotoxin

The cytotoxin kills respiratory epithelial cells by a mechanism involving intracellular interleukin-1 and nitric oxide.

Clinical Features

The whole clinical course of the illness can typically last from 30 to 90 days and is divided into three stages. The incubation period of pertussis is commonly 7 to 10 days but can range anywhere from 4 to 21 days.

The first stage, the catarrhal stage, is similar to the symptoms of the common cold, which makes early diagnosis difficult. It is characterized by sneezing, low-grade fever, rhinitis, and a mild, occasional cough. This cough gradually becomes more severe over 1 to 2 weeks, which transitions to the second, or paroxysmal, stage.

It is during the paroxysmal stage that the diagnosis of pertussis is usually suspected. Typically the patient has severe paroxysms. Due to the length and force of the paroxysm, a long deep inspiratory effort is usually accompanied by a distinguishing high-pitched "whoop." Children and young infants usually appear very ill and distressed during these occurrences. Post-tussive vomiting and exhaustion commonly follow the episode. There have also been reported rib fractures due to the force of the cough. Between attacks, the patient may not appear ill.

During the first 1 or 2 weeks of this stage, the attacks increase in frequency and severity, remain at the same level for 2 to 3 weeks, and then gradually decrease. The paroxysmal stage usually lasts 1 to 6 weeks but may persist for up to 10 weeks.

In the convalescent stage, recovery is gradual. The cough becomes less paroxysmal and disappears in 2 to 3 weeks. However, paroxysms often recur with subsequent respiratory infections for many months.

Complications

The most common complication and the cause of most pertussis-related deaths is secondary bacterial pneumonia. Young infants are at highest risk for acquiring pertussis-associated complications. Neurologic complications such as seizures and encephalopathy may occur as a result of hypoxia or possibly from the toxin itself. Neurologic complications of pertussis are more common among infants. Other less serious complications of pertussis include otitis media, anorexia, and dehydration. Complications resulting from pressure effects of severe paroxysms include pneumothorax, epistaxis, subdural hematomas, hernias, and rectal prolapse.

In 2008 through 2011, a total of 72 deaths from pertussis were reported to the Centers for Disease Control and Prevention (CDC). Children 3 months of age or younger accounted for 60 (83%) of these deaths.

Prognosis

Most healthy older children and adults fully recover, but those with comorbid conditions have a higher risk of morbidity and mortality.

Infection in newborns is particularly severe. Pertussis is fatal in an estimated 1.6% of hospitalized U.S. infants younger than 1 year of age. First-year infants are also more likely to develop complications, such as pneumonia (20%), encephalopathy (0.3%), seizures (1%), failure to thrive, and death (1%).

Diagnosis

The diagnosis of pertussis is based on a characteristic clinical history (cough for more than 2 weeks with whoop, paroxysms, or posttussive vomiting), as well as a variety of laboratory tests (culture, polymerase chain reaction [PCR], and serology).

An elevated white blood cell count with a lymphocytosis is usually present in classical disease of infants. However, lymphocytosis is not absolute. Chest radiographs may show peribronchial consolidation, interstitial edema, or variable atelectasis, all of which are non-specific.

Culture is considered the gold standard laboratory test and is the most specific of the laboratory tests for pertussis. However, *B. pertussis* is difficult to culture. As with any sample, the yield of culture can be affected by specimen collection, transportation, and isolation techniques. Specimens should be obtained from the posterior nasopharynx, not the throat. Successful culture rates are highest during the first 2 weeks of illness (catarrhal and early paroxysmal stages). Since adolescents and adults have often been coughing for several weeks before they seek medical attention, it is often too late for culture to be useful.

PCR is a rapid test and has excellent sensitivity. PCR tests vary in specificity, so obtaining culture confirmation of pertussis for at least one suspicious case is recommended any time there is suspicion of a pertussis outbreak. Results should be interpreted along with the clinical symptoms and epidemiologic information.

All positive test results should be reported to the local health department.

Treatment

Early treatment of pertussis is very important. The earlier a person, especially an infant, starts treatment the better. If treatment for pertussis is started early in the course of illness, during the first 1 to 2 weeks before coughing paroxysms occur, symptoms may be lessened. *Clinicians should strongly consider treating prior to receiving test results if clinical history is strongly suggestive or the patient is at risk for severe or complicated disease (e.g., infants).*

If the patient is diagnosed late, antibiotics will likely not alter the course of the illness, but they will help to eradicate the organism from secretions, thereby decreasing communicability. Recommended first-line antibiotics are macrolides. Options are as follows:

- Azithromycin (Zithromax)[1]
- Erythromycin (Ery-Tab)[1]
- Fluoroquinolones[1]
- Trimethoprim-sulfamethoxazole (least effective)[1]

Postexposure Antimicrobial Prophylaxis

The CDC supports targeting postexposure antibiotic use to persons at high risk of developing severe pertussis and to persons who will have close contact with those at high risk of developing severe pertussis.

Prevention

The primary method of prevention for pertussis is vaccination. Refer to the CDC recommended immunization schedule for details. There is insufficient evidence to determine the effectiveness of antibiotics in those who have been exposed but are without symptoms. Preventive antibiotics, however, are still frequently used in those who have been exposed and are at high risk of severe disease (such as infants).

References

Altunaiji S, Kukuruzovic R, Curtis N, Massie J: Antibiotics for whooping cough (pertussis), *Cochrane Database Syst Rev*(3):CD004404, 2007.
Atkinson W: Pertussis epidemiology and prevention of vaccine-preventable diseases. In ed 12th, Washington DC, 2012, Public Health Foundation, pp 215–230.

Black RE, Cousens S, Johnson HL, et al, for the Child Health Epidemiology Reference Group of WHO and UNICEF: Global, regional, and national causes of child mortality in 2008: A systematic analysis, *Lancet* 375:1969–1987, 2010.
Centers for Disease Control and Prevention: *International Bordetella Pertussis Assay Standardization and Harmonization Meeting Report*, Atlanta, GA, 2007, Centers for Disease Control and Prevention. July 19–20.
Centers for Disease Control and Prevention. Pertussis (whooping cough) causes & transmission. September 4, 2014. Available at http://www.cdc.gov (accessed February 12, 2015).
Centers for Disease Control and Prevention. Pertussis (whooping cough) complications. August 28, 2013. Available at http://www.cdc.gov (accessed February 12, 2015).
Centers for Disease Control and Prevention. Pertussis (whooping cough) fast facts. February 13, 2014. Available at http://www.cdc.gov (accessed February 12, 2015).
Centers for Disease Control and Prevention. Pertussis (whooping cough) prevention. October 10, 2014. Available at http://www.cdc.gov (accessed February 13, 2015).
Centers for Disease Control and Prevention. Pertussis | whooping cough | surveillance | cases by year | CDC. Available at http://www.cdc.gov (accessed April 10, 2017).
Centers for Disease Control and Prevention. Pertussis (whooping cough) treatment. August 28, 2013. Available at http://www.cdc.gov (accessed February 13, 2015).
Centers for Disease Control and Prevention. Pertussis | whooping cough | vaccination | CDC. Available at http://www.cdc.gov (accessed May 27, 2017).
Centers for Disease Control and Prevention: Updated recommendations for use of tetanus toxoid, reduced diphtheria toxoid, and acellular pertussis vaccine (Tdap) in pregnant women — Advisory Committee on Immunization Practices (ACIP), *MMWR* 62(7):131–135, 2012.
Crowcroft NS, Stein C, Duclos P, et al: How best to estimate the global burden of pertussis, *Lancet Infect Dis* 3:413–418, 2003.
Edwards KM, Decker MD: Pertussis vaccines. In Plotkin SA, Orenstein WA, Offit PA, editors: *Vaccines*, ed 6, Philadelphia, 2013, Saunders.
Falleiros Arlant LH, de Colsa A, Flores D, et al: Pertussis in Latin America: Epidemiology and control strategies, *Expert Rev Anti Infect Ther* 12:1265–1275, 2014.
GBD 2015 Disease and Injury Incidence and Prevalence, Collaborators: Global, regional, and national incidence, prevalence, and years lived with disability for 310 diseases and injuries, 1990-2015: A systematic analysis for the Global Burden of Disease Study 2015, *Lancet* 388(10053):1545–1602, 2016.
Gregory DS: Pertussis: A disease affecting all ages, *Am Fam Physician* 74(3):420–426, 2006.
van Amersfoorth SCM, Schouls LM, van der Heide HGJ, et al: Analysis of *Bordetella pertussis* populations in European countries with different vaccination policies, *J Clin Microbiol* 43:2837–2843, 2005.
Wang K, Bettiol S, Thompson MJ, et al: Symptomatic treatment of the cough in whooping cough, *Cochrane Database Syst Rev*(9):CD003257, 2014.
Wendelboe AM, Van Rie A, Salmaso S, Englund JA: Duration of immunity against pertussis after natural infection or vaccination, *Pediatr Infect Dis J* 24(5 Suppl):S58–S61, 2005.
World Health Organization. Pertussis. (accessed March 23, 2016).

ZIKA VIRUS DISEASE

Method of
Scott Kellermann, MD, MPH and Rick D. Kellerman, MD

Zika virus is a mosquito-borne flavivirus. In 1947, researchers at the East African Research Institute in Entebbe, Uganda, were studying yellow fever and placed a caged rhesus macaque in the nearby Zika Forest. The monkey developed a fever and from its serum was isolated a transmissible agent that was first described as Zika virus in 1952. Initially, Zika virus, borne by arboreal mosquitoes such as *Aedes africanus,* infected wild primates and rarely infected humans, even in highly enzootic areas. From its discovery until 2007, there were only 14 confirmed human cases of Zika virus infection, the vertebrate life cycle primarily involving monkey-mosquito-monkey, with rare spread to humans. Prior to 2007, the virus circulated silently in West Africa. Although endemic in many African and Asian countries, reports of outbreaks on these continents is rare. In 2007, an outbreak was identified in the Yap Islands. In 2013-2014, an outbreak affecting an estimated 30,000 people occurred in French Polynesia. Other isolated outbreaks followed. In 2015-2016, a major outbreak occurred in Brazil and other South American, Central American, and Caribbean countries. The first locally transmitted cases on the United States mainland were reported in 2016. The Zika virus appears to have mutated in character while expanding its geographical range, transforming from a localized endemic, mosquito-borne infection producing only a mild illness to a disease causing explosive outbreaks linked with neurological disorders including Guillain-Barré syndrome and microcephaly. Estimates are that, between October 2015 and January 2016,

---

[1] Not FDA approved for this indication.

approximately 1.5 million Brazilians were infected by Zika with 3,500 cases of microcephaly reported and with the three poorest states of Paraiba, Pernambuco, and Bahia having the highest incidence. The strain of Zika virus most closely related to the one that emerged in Brazil was originally isolated from patient samples in French Polynesia. In all probability, Zika virus arrived in Brazil in 2014 during the Confederation Cup, when Tahiti's soccer team and its supporters visited a variety of Brazilian venues.

In November 2016, the World Health Organization declared that "The Zika virus and associated consequences remain a significant enduring public health challenge requiring intense action but no longer represent a public health emergency of international concern."

Zika virus cases in the Americas have dramatically decreased since August 2017. In 2018, no local mosquito-borne transmission of Zika virus was reported on the mainland of the United States.

Epidemiology

Zika virus is transmitted by the daytime-active Aedes mosquitoes, such as A. aegypti and A. albopictus. With the exception of West Nile virus, which is predominantly spread by culex-species mosquitoes, the arboviruses reaching the Western Hemisphere have all been transmitted by Aedes mosquitoes. Millennia ago, North African villagers began storing water in their dwellings, giving arboreal A. aegypti a ready medium for depositing their eggs—domestic water-containing vessels. The hatched mosquitoes then fed on humans, evolving into an entirely new maintenance cycle of human–A. aegypti–human transmission. Now, thousands of years later, the worst effects of this evolutionary cascade have been seen in the repeated emergence of arboviruses in human ecosystems.

The distribution of A. aegypti is more extensive now than ever recorded, extending across all continents including North America.

Another significant Zika virus vector is Aedes albopictus, commonly known as the Asian tiger mosquito, named for its white striped legs. A. albopictus is of medical importance due to its aggressive daytime human-biting behavior and ability to vector many viruses, including dengue, La Crosse, and West Nile. Figure 1 shows the estimated range of the Aedes aegypti and Aedes albopictus mosquitoes in the United States (Table 1).

Most significantly, pregnant mothers may vertically transmit the virus to the developing fetus, potentially resulting in microcephaly. Zika virus has been isolated in semen and vaginal secretions. Male to female as well as female to male sexual transmission of the Zika virus has been reported. Blood transfusions have been a source of transmission outside of the United States. The blood supply in the United States is tested for Zika virus. Although Zika virus has been detected in breast milk, there are no reports of infants being infected with Zika virus through breastfeeding.

Zika has followed a pattern of dispersion analogous to chikungunya, spreading pandemically from west to east. Both viruses now encircle the globe. It appears that both viruses migrated from East Africa to Asia. There is a similar striking movement of Zika and chikungunya from Asia into the Pacific Islands and then to the Americas. Analogous ecological factors might be responsible for their similar spread and may be a key to understanding effective prevention strategies.

Risk Factors

The risk of Zika virus infection for pregnant women is pronounced because of the potential link to microcephaly of the infant. The risk is greatest if the infection is obtained early in pregnancy. There is no evidence that pregnant women are more susceptible to Zika virus infection or that the disease is more severe during pregnancy. Although the transmission of Zika virus is most common due to the bite of an infected mosquito, transmission has also been documented through sexual contact, blood transfusion, laboratory exposure, and both intrauterine and intrapartum transmission. The CDC reports that although

Zika virus has been found in breast milk and possible Zika virus infections have been identified in breastfeeding babies, Zika virus transmission through breast milk has not been confirmed. Based on what is known about similar arbovirus infections, once a person has been infected and developed antibodies to Zika virus, he or she is likely to be protected from a future Zika infection. Based on currently available evidence, once the virus has cleared from the blood of a Zika-infected woman, she is not felt to be at future risk for having a child with a Zika-related birth defect.

Pathophysiology

The Zika virus is a member of the Flaviviridae virus family, which includes dengue, yellow fever, West Nile, and Japanese encephalitis viruses. Zika is a single-stranded, positive-sense RNA virus that has been fully sequenced. It is one of many arthropod-borne arboviruses. Monkeys are the common vertebrate host of the virus. Arboviruses oftentimes have complex natural transmission cycles involving mammals, birds, and blood-feeding arthropod vectors.

Until recently, only a few arboviruses have caused clinically significant human diseases. These include mosquito-borne alphaviruses such as chikungunya and flaviviruses such as dengue and West Nile. The most historically important of these is the yellow-fever virus, the first recognized viral cause of deadly epidemic hemorrhagic fever.

Prevention

Population-based mosquito control measures are recommended to prevent the spread of Zika virus. Although yellow fever has historically been prevented entirely by aggressive mosquito control, in the modern era vector control has been problematic because of the expense, logistics, public resistance, the development of resistance to the pesticides used and their collateral adverse effects on humans. Although a chemical war against the vector may provide short-term control, programs for improving urban infrastructure and environmental sanitation with a stable supply of potable water would offer more durable results. Among the best preventive measures against Zika virus are house screens, air conditioning, and removal of yard and household debris and containers that provide mosquito-breeding sites, luxuries often unavailable to impoverished residents of crowded urban locales where such epidemics take their greatest toll. Releasing mosquitoes that are sterile or genetically modified to die before they can reproduce is being investigated. Researchers funded by the Bill and Melinda Gates Foundation have proposed infecting mosquitoes with the Wolbachia bacteria, which seem to inhibit the transmission of dengue and other viruses by the mosquito.

Because of the association between Zika virus infection and microcephaly in fetuses, the United States Centers for Disease Control and Prevention (CDC) should be consulted for travel guidelines when pregnant women or women considering pregnancy are traveling to affected countries. In some cases, travel may need to be postponed. Pregnant women and those considering pregnancy should reference the CDC website at https://wwwnc.cdc.gov/travel/page/zika-information. Women who are considering becoming pregnant should consult with their physicians for preconception counseling.

The CDC recommends that women who have had Zika virus exposure through travel or sexual contact and do not have ongoing risks for exposure should wait at least 8 weeks from date of diagnosis, symptom onset (if symptomatic), or last possible exposure before attempting to conceive. During this waiting period, either abstinence should be practiced or barrier contraception with condoms should be used. The 8-week waiting period may decrease the risk of maternal-fetal transmission of the Zika virus.

Zika virus typically remains in the semen for longer periods of time than other body fluids. Accordingly, the CDC recommends waiting at least 3 months from date of diagnosis, symptom onset (if symptomatic), or after the last possible exposure before attempting conception with their partner. During this waiting period, either abstinence should be practiced or barrier

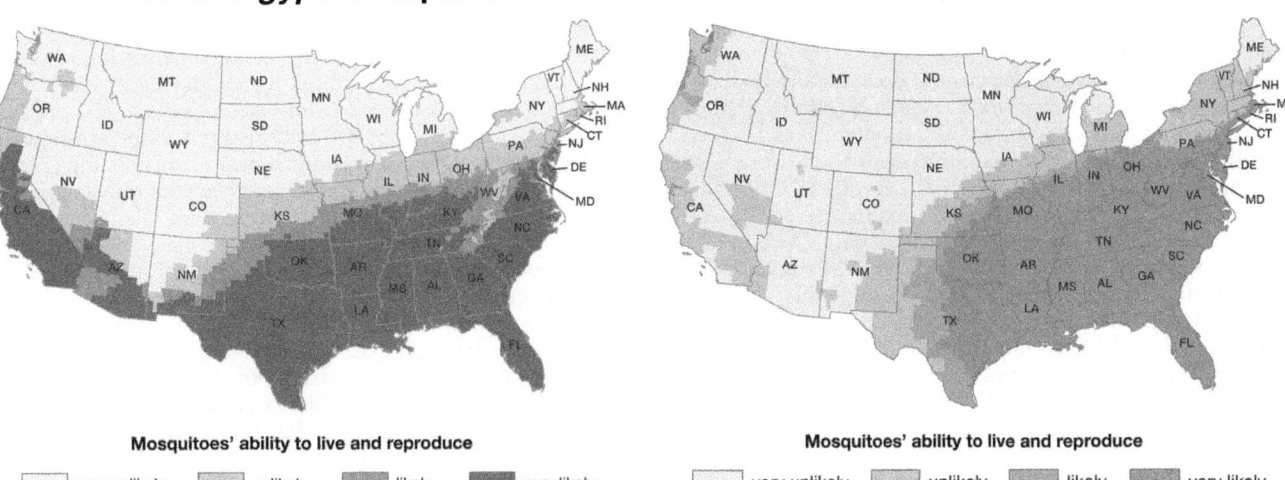

Figure 1 Range of Zika-transmitting mosquitoes in the United States. (Source: https://www.cdc.gov/zika/pdfs/Zika-mosquito-maps.pdf.)

TABLE 1	Prevention of Mosquito Bites

- Remove yard debris (e.g., old tires) and containers that collect water and may provide mosquito breeding sites.
- Wear long-sleeved shirts, long pants, and socks. Tuck pants into socks.
- Apply permethrin to outer clothing.
- Use window screens.
- Use mosquito netting at night if sleeping quarters are not screened.
- Use mosquito netting when children less than 2 months of age—before they can use mosquito repellants—must go outside.
- Apply mosquito repellents directly to exposed skin. When applying mosquito repellants to the face, spray it on the hands, then rub it in. Avoid the eyes and mouth.
- Do not allow young children to apply mosquito repellants themselves. Children who rub mosquito repellant into their own skin are prone to putting their hands into their mouths or touching their eyes.
- Adults should apply mosquito repellant on children by putting the repellant on their own hands and rubbing it into the child's skin.
- To limit the total amount of mosquito repellant that might be absorbed, do not apply to skin under clothing or on skin that is broken (i.e., cuts, rashes).
- Do not use mosquito repellants near food. Wash hands before eating or drinking.
- Wash off mosquito repellant from the skin when it is no longer needed.
- At the end of the day, wash treated skin with soap and water.

contraception with condoms should be used. The recommendation to wait at least 3 months for asymptomatic men is based on the length of time the Zika virus RNA has been detected in semen. The median and 95 percentile for the time until the loss of Zika RNA detection are 42 days and 120 days, respectively, for semen compared to 15 days and 41 days, respectively, for serum and 11 days and 34 days, respectively, for urine. The longest duration of detection of Zika RNA in semen is 370 days, although shedding of infectious Zika virus is believed to be limited to the first few weeks after the onset of illness. There is a lack of evidence that the risk of sexual transmission differs in symptomatic and asymptomatic men.

Between 2015 and July 2018, 52 cases of confirmed sexual transmission of Zika virus infection had been reported in the United States. Documented reports of sexual transmission have primarily involved transmission from a man to a woman; however, transmission has also been documented from a man to another man and from a woman to a man. The longest period from symptom onset in the index case to potential sexual transmission to a partner was between 32-41 days; most reports are of much shorter intervals.

Recommendations for men with possible Zika virus exposure whose partners are pregnant are advised to consistently and correctly use condoms during sex or abstain from sex for the duration of the pregnancy. Despite limited generalizabilty to humans, preliminary data from animal studies suggest that sexual transmission of Zika virus during pregnancy might pose a higher risk to the fetus than mosquito-borne transmission.

Pregnant women and men and women who are considering parenthood and who have visited or are considering traveling to areas at risk should consult their physician and reference the CDC website for travel alerts and pregnancy counseling recommendations.

Avoiding mosquito bites is important for disease control. There are hundreds of insect repellants sold in the United States. These insect repellants have different ingredients, different concentrations of ingredients, and different combinations of ingredients. Furthermore, different species of mosquitoes may be differentially repelled by different repellants. Though research is limited, the *Aedes aegypti* and *Aedes albopictus* mosquitoes seem to be most effectively repelled by products that contain at least 25% DEET (N,N-diethyl-m-toluamide), 30% Oil of Lemon Eucalyptus, or 20% picaridin. When applied appropriately, these ingredients may repel mosquitoes for approximately 7 hours and seem to be safe when used during pregnancy. Products with lower concentrations of DEET, Oil of Lemon Eucalyptus, and picaridin are much less effective. Products containing IR3535, 2-undecanone, and products made from natural plant oils such as citronella, lemongrass oil, cedar oil, rosemary oil, cinnamon oil, and geraniol seem to be ineffective against Zika-transmitting mosquitoes. Insect repellents can be used with sunscreen, but the sunscreen should be applied first.

Additional protection from mosquito bites can be achieved by treating outer clothing with permethrin. Permethrin, a derivative of *Chrysanthemum cinerariifolium*, is an insect repellent and insecticide. Though it is poorly absorbed and rapidly inactivated permethrin should not be applied directly to the skin and it should not be used on underclothing. The Environmental Protection Agency (EPA) recommends that clothes treated with permethrin should be washed separately from clothes that are not treated. If washed together, underclothing may absorb permethrin into the fabric which may increase the risk of absorption through the skin. Permethrin-treated clothing will retain repellent activity through multiple washes. The EPA indicates there is no evidence that exposure to permethrin results in adverse effects for pregnant or nursing mothers or adverse developmental effects in their children. Permethrin is listed as pregnancy category B. It can be used on the outer clothing of children older than 2 months of age.

At present no Zika vaccines are available, although Phase 1 and Phase 2 studies are underway.

Clinical Manifestations

The incubation period for Zika virus is estimated to be 3 to 12 days. Serosurvey results from the Yap Islands indicate that only 19% of persons who were infected had symptoms that were attributable to Zika virus. Common symptoms were macular or papular rash (90% of patients), fever (65%), arthritis or arthralgia (65%), nonpurulent conjunctivitis (55%), myalgia (48%), headache (45%), retro-orbital pain (39%), edema (19%), and vomiting (10%). The rash is generally maculopapular and pruritic. Fever, when present, is generally short-term and low-grade. Rarely, immune thrombocytopenia purpura has been linked to Zika. In more than 60 years of observation, severe disease requiring hospitalization is uncommon and case fatality is low.

Diagnosis

In a "pure" Zika epidemic, a diagnosis can be ascertained on clinical grounds. However, dengue and chikungunya have similar clinical presentations and have been epidemic in the Americas, confounding the clinical diagnosis.

The CDC website should be consulted for Zika virus testing recommendations for women who are symptomatic or asymptomatic during pregnancy. Instructions for testing can be found at https://www.cdc.gov/zika/hc-providers/types-of-tests.html.

Cross-reaction with related flaviviruses (e.g., dengue and yellow-fever viruses) is common, complicating the immunologic interpretation of infection. Physicians who deliver an infant suspected of suffering the effects of maternal Zika virus infection should consult the CDC to discuss blood, placental, and umbilical cord sampling. Zika virus infection is a nationally notifiable disease.

Differential Diagnosis

Differential diagnosis encompasses a wide variety of other viral diseases such as dengue, chikungunya, Mayaro virus disease, Ross River fever, Barmah Forest disease, o'nyong-nyong disease, and Sindbis fever. In addition, the CDC lists group A streptococcus, leptospirosis, malaria, rickettsia, rubella, measles, parvovirus, enterovirus, and adenovirus in the differential diagnosis.

Treatment

At present, there is no treatment or vaccine for Zika virus disease. Because symptoms are usually absent or mild, most acutely infected patients do not access the medical system and treat themselves symptomatically. Antiviral medication is ineffective. The mainstays of management are bed rest and supportive care. When multiple arboviruses are co-circulating, testing for a specific viral diagnosis, if available, can be important in anticipating, preventing, and managing complications.

Although the Zika virus has not been associated with hemorrhagic fever, it is probably best to avoid aspirin and nonsteroidal antiinflammatory medications due to their association with hemorrhagic fever syndromes and death when taken for the treatment of similar viruses. The use of aspirin should be avoided in children due to the risk of Reye syndrome. Guidelines for pregnant women during a Zika virus outbreak can be accessed at the CDC website: https://www.cdc.gov/pregnancy/zika/women-and-their-partners.html.

Because of the rapidly evolving knowledge about the Zika virus, clinicians are encouraged to freely consult the CDC and WHO websites for clinical guidance.

Monitoring

Pregnant women should be asked about their travel history. Currently the WHO recommends anomaly ultrasound investigations at 18 to 20 weeks' gestation to identify, monitor, or exclude fetal brain abnormalities, particularly microcephaly, for all pregnant women living in areas with ongoing Zika virus transmission.

International monitoring of Zika virus infection is important. Each year, nearly 10 million international travelers depart from Brazilian airports favorable to year-round transmission of the Zika virus, and over one-quarter of these travelers are headed to the United States. In the United States, during 2017, 424 symptomatic Zika virus disease cases were reported, 414 occurred in travelers returning from affected areas, 4 cases presumed were contracted through local mosquito-borne transmission (Florida-2, Texas-2) and 6 cases acquired through sexual transmission.

In 2017, 452 symptomatic Zika virus disease cases were reported in the United States excluding congenitally acquired disease. Four hundred thirty seven cases were in travelers returning from affected areas, 7 cases were presumably acquired through local mosquito-borne transmission (Florida -2; Texas -5), 7 cases were acquired through sexual contact, and one was acquired through laboratory transmission. In 2018, although statistical counts are not complete, 72 Zika virus disease cases were reported in the United States, all in travelers returning from affected areas.

Complications

The major complication of Zika virus disease is the potential risk of microcephaly as a result of vertical transmission. Amniocentesis has been used to detect the presence of Zika virus in amniotic fluid of women who had ultrasound confirmation of microcephalic fetuses. The virus has been isolated in the brains of newborns and miscarried fetuses. It is unclear whether there may be contributory factors to the development of microcephaly such as nutritional and environmental factors or concomitant infection with other micro-organisms. Other fetal findings have included intracranial calcifications, orbital calcifications, and microphthalmia. It does not appear that the proportion of birth defects differs among mothers who experience symptoms versus those who are asymptomatic.

Microcephaly, other brain abnormalities, and eye anomalies can result from infection during any trimester. A study of pregnancy outcomes in French Territories demonstrated that neurological birth defects occurred in 12.7%, 3.6%, and 5.3% of babies when Zika infection occurred during the first, second, and third trimester, respectively. In a study of pregnancy outcomes in US territories, among pregnancies with confirmed Zika virus infection in the first, second, and third trimesters, the percentages of fetuses or infants with possible Zika-association birth defects was 8%, 5%, and 4%, respectively. According to data in the US Zika Pregnancy and Infant Registry, 5% of pregnancies with suspected Zika virus infection and 10% of pregnancies with laboratory-confirmed Zika infection result in a fetus or newborn with a birth defect, while 15% had a birth defect if the infection occurred in the first trimester. The microcephaly may be subtle. Children may have a craniofacial disproportion and abnormal cranial shape. The fontanelles may be closed or very small and the sutures may be uneven or overlapping. In addition to microcephaly, a phenotypic spectrum has been identified in congenital Zika syndrome. Neurologically, there may be changes in motor activity, severe muscle hypertonia, feeding difficulties, and excessive and inconsolable crying. Musculoskeletal problems include joint immobility, hand and finger contractures, feet contractures and malposition, deep and multiple dimples over joints, abnormal palmar creases and generalized arthrogryposis. Skin on the scalp and other areas of the body may be redundant. Brain imaging may show calcifications, abnormal gyral patterns, enlarged ventricles, and marked decreases in the volume of gray and white matter. The corpus callosum may be thin or absent. The brainstem and cerebellum may be underdeveloped. Seizures, especially in infants between 3 and 6 months of age, may develop and children may exhibit visual problems, hearing loss, and impaired growth. Children exposed to Zika virus in utero who do not have overt signs of Zika virus-associated clinical manifestations or abnormal neuroimaging may have a higher risk of neurodevelopmental delay. The viruses' strong affinity for neural cells may cause neurologic damage that only becomes apparent as children age. Although the full range of birth defects and disabilities associated with Zika virus disease remains to be fully delineated, neural tube defects do not seem to be associated. It is unclear whether infants and children who contract Zika in infancy or early childhood may develop neurologic complications.

Retrospective data from the French Polynesia Zika virus outbreak from October 2013 to April 2014 indicate a close association with Guillain-Barré syndrome. Of the 42 patients diagnosed with Guillain-Barré syndrome, 41 (98%) had anti-Zika virus IgM or IgG, and all (100%) had neutralizing antibodies against Zika virus compared with 54 (56%) of 98 in the control group.

Much still needs to be learned about Zika virus and its geographic spread, transmission, teratogenicity, and long-term complications, including the potential for late onset symptoms in adulthood in previously asymptomatic individuals. A larger issue still to be elucidated in the emergence of Zika and other novel infectious diseases is the role played by urban crowding, ease of international travel, and human encroachments into complex ecosystems.

References

Byrne S: Consumer reports, Mosquito repellents that best protect against Zika. April 16, 2016. http://www.consumerreports.org/insect-repellents/mosquito-repellents-that-best-protect-against-zika/.

Centers for Disease Control and Prevention. Zika virus. Available at https://www.cdc.gov/zika/index.html (accessed June 15, 2019).

del Campo M, Feitosa IM, Ribeiro EM, et al: The phenotypic spectrum of congenital Zika syndrome, *Am J Med Genet* 173:841–857, 2017.

Duffy MR, Chen TH, Hancock WT, et al: Zika virus outbreak on Yap Island, Federated States of Micronesia, *N Engl J Med* 360:2536–2543, 2009.

Environmental Protection Agency: Repellent-treated clothing. https://www.epa.gov/insect-repellents/repellent-treated-clothing#.

Faria NR, Azevedo Rdo S, Kraemer MU: Zika virus in the Americas: Early epidemiological and genetic findings, *Science* 352:345–349, 2016.

Fauci AS, Morens DM: Zika virus in the Americas—yet another arbovirus threat, *N Engl J Med* 374:601–604, 2016.

Honein MA: Recognizing the global impact of Zika virus infection during pregnancy, *N Engl J Med* 378:1055–1056, 2018.

Hoen B, Schaub B, Funk AL, et al: Pregnancy outcomes after ZIKV infection in French territories in the Americas, *N Engl J Med* 378:985–994, 2018.

Kleber de Oliveira W, Cortez-Escalante J, De Oliveira WT, et al: Increase in reported prevalence of microcephaly in infants born to women living in areas with confirmed Zika virus transmission during the first trimester of pregnancy—Brazil, *MMWR Morb Mortal Wkly Rep* 65:242–247, 2016.

Lucey DR, Gostin LO: The emerging Zika pandemic: enhancing preparedness, *JAMA* 315:865–866, 2016.

Lupi E: The efficacy of repellents against Aedes, Anopheles, Culex and Ixodes spp.—a literature review, *Travel Med Infect Dis* 11(6):374–411, 2013.

Musso D: Zika virus transmission from French Polynesia to Brazil (letter to the editor), *Emerg Infect Dis* 21:1887, 2015.

Paz-Bailey G, Rosenberg ES, Doyle K: Persistence of Zika Virus in Body Fluids – Final Report, *NEJM* 379:1234–1243, 2018.

Peterson LR, Jamieson DJ, Powers AM, Honein MA: Zika virus, *N Engl J Med* 374:1552–1563, 2016.

Reynolds MR, Jones AM, Petersen EE, et al: Vital signs: update on Zika virus–associated birth defects and evaluation of all U.S. infants with congenital Zika virus exposure – U.S. Zika Pregnancy Registry, 2016, *MMWR* 66:366–373, 2017.

Rodriguez SD, et al: The efficacy of some commercially available insect repellents for Aedes aegypti (Diptera: Culicidae) and Aedes albopictus (Diptera: Culicidae), *J Insect Sci* 15(1):140, 2015.

Shapiro-Mendoza CK, Rice ME, Galang RR, et al: Pregnancy Outcomes After Maternal Zika Virus Infection During Pregnancy – U.S. Territories, January 1, 2016–April 25, 2017, *MMWR* 66:615–621, 2017.

World Health Organization. Zika virus. Available at https://www.who.int/news-room/fact-sheets/detail/zika-virus (accessed June 15, 2019).

Nervous System

ACUTE FACIAL PARALYSIS

Method of
Steven L. Meyers, MD

CURRENT DIAGNOSIS

- Typical cases of acute facial paralysis are diagnosed based on examination and do not require additional evaluation.
- All patients with acute facial paralysis should have a complete neurologic and head and neck examinations.
- The presence of atypical features such as a slowly progressive course, failure to improve, recurrent attacks, or other neurologic findings should prompt additional evaluation with computed tomography (CT) or magnetic resonance imaging (MRI) of the head and a specialist consultation.

CURRENT THERAPY

- Steroid therapy, such as prednisone[1] 60–80 mg daily for 7 days, initiated within 3 days of onset of the facial paralysis, increases the chances of recovery
- The use of antiviral therapy remains controversial without strong evidence of benefit, but valacyclovir (Valtrex)[1] 1000 mg three times daily for 7 days may be beneficial in patients with severe paralysis.
- Eye care with artificial tears, ophthalmic ointments at night, and eye protection should be used in patients with severe facial paralysis.

[1]Not FDA approved for this indication.

Acute facial nerve paralysis, or Bell's palsy, is a common disorder manifesting with the acute to subacute onset of unilateral paralysis of the muscles of facial expression. The Scottish physician Sir Charles Bell described cases of facial paralysis due to trauma in the 1800s, and the idiopathic condition carries his name today. However, there are many possible causes of facial paralysis, and each patient requires a careful history and complete neurologic examination to exclude these possibilities.

Epidemiology and Risk Factors
The annual incidence rate is between 13 and 34 cases per 100,000 population. All age ranges can be affected, but persons between the ages of 15 and 40 years are most commonly affected. Diabetics, pregnant women in the third trimester, and women in the immediate postpartum period are at increased risk. There is no gender, race, or geographic predilection.

Pathophysiology
The seventh cranial, or facial, nerve arises from the pontomedullary junction and runs in close proximity to the eighth cranial nerve to the internal auditory meatus. The nerve then runs through the bony fallopian canal before exiting the skull at the stylomastoid foramen. The labyrinthine portion of the fallopian canal is very narrow, and it is postulated that swelling of the nerve results in compression in this region.

Three branches arise from the facial nerve within the fallopian canal. The greater petrosal nerve arises from the geniculate ganglion, passes to the pterygopalatine ganglion, and eventually supplies innervation to the lacrimal and palatine glands. The second branch is the nerve to the stapedius muscle in the middle ear. The final branch is the chorda tympani, which supplies taste sensation from the anterior two thirds of the tongue.

The pathophysiology of Bell's palsy is uncertain, but a viral cause is the most commonly accepted hypothesis. Many different viruses have been associated with facial paralysis, with herpes simplex virus (HSV) having the strongest evidence. HSV-1 DNA has been detected by polymerase chain reaction assay in endoneural fluid in patients with Bell's palsy undergoing facial nerve decompression.

Herpes zoster is another virus associated with facial nerve paralysis. Herpes zoster oticus (Ramsey Hunt syndrome) is diagnosed when vesicles are seen in the external auditory canal or on the auricle. Other viruses implicated include cytomegalovirus, Epstein–Barr virus, adenovirus, rubella, mumps, influenza B, and coxsackievirus.

The histopathology of the facial nerve supports an inflammatory etiology with findings similar to those seen in herpes zoster infection. The perineurium is edematous, with diffuse infiltration of inflammatory cells between nerve bundles and surrounding the intraneural vessels.

Clinical Manifestations
The clinical presentation of Bell's palsy is typically dramatic and very stereotypical. Pain behind the ear in the region of the mastoid can precede the onset of weakness by hours to days. Weakness of the muscles of facial expression on one side progresses over a period up to 48 hours. Progression over more prolonged periods raises the possibility of a neoplasm affecting the nerve. The degree of weakness can range from quite subtle to complete paralysis of all muscles of facial expression. Typical features include inability to close the eye, sagging of the eyelid, loss of the nasolabial fold, and inability to wrinkle the forehead muscles. Sparing of the forehead muscles suggests a central or upper motor neuron lesion because these muscles receive bilateral innervation. Additional symptoms that may be reported include hyperacusis caused by paralysis of the stapedius muscle, loss of taste in the anterior tongue due to involvement of the chorda tympani, and decreased tearing due to dysfunction of the parasympathetic innervation of the lacrimal gland. However, most patients actually report increased tearing from the affected eye owing to diminished blinking.

Diagnosis and Differential Diagnosis
There is no specific diagnostic test for Bell's palsy. The diagnosis is based on a typical history and examination. Atypical features mandate a search for other causes. A slowly progressive course, parotid gland mass, or involvement in selected branches of the facial nerve can suggest neoplastic compression. Vesicles over the ear or internal auditory canal suggests herpes zoster infection. Patients should be asked about preceding fevers, rashes, and arthralgias, which can prompt evaluation for Lyme disease. However, in the absence of

BOX 1 Differential Diagnosis of Acute Facial Nerve Paralysis

Idiopathic
Idiopathic cases account for 65%

Infectious
Common
• Herpes zoster
• Herpes simplex
• Borreliosis
Uncommon
• Lyme disease
• Epstein-Barr virus
• Human immunodeficiency virus
• Tuberculosis
Rare
• Acute otitis media
• Chronic otitis media

Trauma
Temporal bone fractures
Penetration wounds

Neoplasm
Parotid
Metastases
Schwannoma
Cholesteatoma

Metabolic and Toxic
Diabetes
Thyroid disease
Alcoholism
Carbon monoxide poisoning (rare)

Other
Sarcoidosis
Multiple sclerosis
Sjögren syndrome

these features, routine serologic testing is not recommended. Sarcoid is a rare cause of usually bilateral facial paralysis. The onset of facial paralysis in the setting of head injury, particularly in the presence of ipsilateral hearing loss, should prompt imaging of the skull base to rule out a temporal bone fracture (Box 1).

Treatment

Treatment of Bell's palsy can be divided into three categories: general medical therapy, specific medical therapy, and surgical therapy. General medical care includes proper eye care. Reduced blinking and inability to completely close the eye increases the risk of corneal abrasion and ulceration. Artificial tears and ophthalmic ointments can prevent these complications. Patients should be instructed to use proper eye protection to prevent injuries. Facial muscle massage and facial nerve stimulation have no evidence to support their use.

Medical Therapy

Specific medical therapy includes glucocorticoid and antiviral medications. Glucocorticoid therapy has been demonstrated to be effective in both meta-analyses and randomized trials. The two largest trials of glucocorticoid and antiviral therapy demonstrated benefit for steroids but no benefit for antiviral therapy when used either alone or in combination with steroids. Treatment in these trials was begun within 72 hours of onset of paralysis and consisted of relatively high–dose prednisolone (Millipred)[1] 50 to 60 mg daily for 10 days. Antiviral therapy evaluated included acyclovir (Zovirax)[1] 400 mg five times daily for 10 days and

valacyclovir (Valtrex)[1] 1000 mg three times daily for 7 days, neither of which showed benefit.

Smaller, lower-quality studies have suggested a benefit of combining antiviral therapy with glucocorticoids, particularly in patients with more severe baseline dysfunction.

Surgical Therapy

Surgical decompression of the facial nerve is not recommended. A 2011 Cochrane review and a 2001 review by the American Academy of Neurology both found no good evidence supporting this treatment modality. Only two small randomized studies showed no differences in outcome between surgical and medical therapy.

Monitoring and Complications

The overall prognosis of Bell's palsy is favorable. In one study of untreated patients, 85% showed signs of recovery within 3 weeks. Ultimately, 71% experienced complete recovery and an additional 13% were felt to have only slight residual weakness. The degree of weakness at onset is an important prognostic indicator: 94% of patients with incomplete paralysis experienced complete recovery. The absence of any improvement, no matter how small, at 3 to 4 months should raise concern regarding the diagnosis and lead to a search for alternative etiologies.

Motor nerve conduction studies, or electroneurography, can be used to help predict prognosis in selected patients. Patients with incomplete lesions that have an excellent prognosis do not require further evaluation. Motor nerve conduction studies involve stimulating the facial nerve electrically and recording muscle responses with surface electrodes over appropriate muscles. The amplitude of the evoked muscle response on the affected side at 10 days can be compared with the unaffected side, giving an estimate of the degree of axonal loss. A 90% drop in amplitude predicts less than complete recovery, and loss greater than 98% predicts significant residual weakness and synkinesis.

In severe cases of facial paralysis, attention to good eye care as previously discussed is important to prevent eye damage and vision loss.

During recovery from severe nerve injury, axonal regrowth may be misdirected, resulting in synkinesis. Voluntary activation of one muscle group can cause activation of other muscles. Attempts at blinking can result in twitching of the mouth, or smiling can cause involuntary blinking. Misdirection of autonomic fibers can result in the syndrome of "crocodile tears," involuntary lacrimation while eating.

Recurrent attacks of facial paralysis on the ipsilateral or contralateral side occur in up to 15% of patients even after many years. Additional recurrences are quite rare, being reported at a rate between 1% and 3%.

References

Engstrom M, Berg T, Stjernquist-Desatnik A, et al: Prednisolone and valaciclovir in Bell's palsy: A randomised, double-blind, placebo-controlled, multicentre trial, *Lancet Neurol* 7:993–1000, 2008.
Gilden DH: Bell's palsy, *N Engl J Med* 351:1323–1331, 2004.
Grogan PM, Gronseth GS: Practice parameter: Steroids, acyclovir, and surgery for Bell's palsy (an evidence based review): Report of the Quality Standards Subcommittee of the American Academy of Neurology, *Neurology* 56:830–836, 2001.
Madhok VB, Gagyor I, Somasundara D, et al. Corticosteroids for Bell's palsy (idiopathic facial paralysis), *Cochrane Database Syst Rev*, 2016, Issue 7, Art. No.: CD001942. https://10.1002/14651858.CD001942.pub5.
Peitersen E: The natural history of Bell's palsy, *Am J Otol* 4:107–111, 1982.
Ronthal M: Bell's palsy: Pathogenesis, clinical features, and diagnosis in adults, *Up to Date*, December 22, 2011. Available at http://www.uptodate.com/contents/bells-palsy-pathogenesis-clinical-features-and-diagnosis-in-adults?source=search_result&search=bell%27s+palsy&selectedTitle=2~26 [accessed 27.08.14].
Ronthal M: Bell's palsy: Prognosis and treatment in adults, *Up to Date*, May 10, 2012. Available at http://www.uptodate.com/contents/bells-palsy-prognosis-and-treatment-in-adults?source=search_result&search=bell%27s+palsy&selectedTitle=1~26 [accessed 27.08.14].
Sullivan FM, Swan IR, Donnan PT, et al: Early treatment with prednisolone or acyclovir in Bell's palsy, *N Engl J Med* 357:1598–1607, 2007.
Yeo SG, Lee YC, Park DC, Cha CI: Acyclovir plus steroid vs steroid alone in the treatment of Bell's palsy, *Am J Otolaryngol* 29:163–166, 2008.
Zandian A, Osiro S, Hudson R, et al: The neurologist's dilemma: A comprehensive clinical review of Bell's palsy, with emphasis on current management trends, *Med Sci Monit* 20:83–90, 2014. https://10.12659/MSM.889876.

[1]Not FDA approved for this indication.

ALZHEIMER'S DISEASE

Method of
Philip D. Sloane, MD, MPH; and Daniel I. Kaufer, MD

CURRENT DIAGNOSIS

- Routine screening for cognitive impairment is controversial but may be beneficial for early diagnosis and identifying treatable causes.
- Combining the Mini-Cog screening test with screening questions on the informant-based AD8 provides a rapid, sensitive, validated screening assessment.
- A comprehensive dementia evaluation includes a battery of cognitive tests, a laboratory panel for treatable causes, a neurologic examination, a brain MRI, and other testing (e.g., depression screen), as indicated.
- The diagnosis of Alzheimer's disease (AD) continues to rest on having a presentation and course of dementia that is consistent with the disease, and ruling out other identifiable etiologies.
- AD often coexists with cerebrovascular disease; atypical and non-AD dementias generally merit a consultation with a neurology or geriatric specialist.

CURRENT THERAPY

- Patient and family education and support are the cornerstones of effective care.
- Preventive measures with the strongest supporting evidence include hypertension control; head injury prevention; physical, cognitive, and social activity; and a Mediterranean diet.
- "Review medications and reduce anticholinergic burden to the extent feasible".
- Cholinesterase inhibitors and memantine (Namenda) alone or jointly have a modest effect on improving or slowing cognitive decline.
- The primary approach to managing behavioral symptoms is person-centered care using dementia-focused communication skills.
- First-line drug agents that may help control behavioral symptoms include cholinesterase inhibitors and mood stabilizers; anticonvulsants and antipsychotics may be helpful for moderate to severe agitation.

Alzheimer's disease (AD) and related disorders of cognitive function are a common and growing issue for all clinicians who provide care to older adults. In discussing this condition, several related but distinctly different terms are used:

- *Cognitive impairment* refers to the presence of one or more measurable deficits in cerebral function when compared with normal persons of the same age.
- *Neurocognitive disorder* generally refers to a clinical syndrome involving cognitive decline from a previous level of functioning, most commonly associated with Alzheimer's disease. Each neurocognitive disorder is divided into mild and major forms, with the latter distinguished by clinically significant functional disability due to compromise in multiple domains. Within this new DSM-V framework, mild cognitive impairment is now referred to as mild neurocognitive disorder, and dementia is now referred to as major neurocognitive disorder.
- *AD* is the most common cause of dementia; it has a characteristic pathophysiology and clinical presentation.

Lack of a simple, reliable diagnostic test makes it difficult to know with certainty how many persons in the United States currently have AD, but estimates place the number between 5 million and 8 million. Onset can occur when people are in their 40s or 50s, but it is largely a disease of older persons, with the prevalence approximately doubling every 5 years after age 65. By age 85 to 90, up to 50% of individuals will meet criteria for dementia, often with mixed features of AD and cerebrovascular disease.

Risk Factors

Numerous risk factors have been associated with AD (Table 1); however, the strongest ones—age and a positive family history—cannot be modified. Of the modifiable risk factors, current emphasis is being placed on reduction of risk factors for atherosclerotic disease (especially hypertension) and traumatic brain injury, particularly sports-related concussions.

AD is associated with the pathological hallmarks of extracellular amyloid plaques and intracellular neurofibrillary tangles that are composed of hyper-phosphorylated tau protein. How these two protein markers of AD lead to the gradual loss of neuronal cell connections and eventually cell death remains poorly understood. New brain-imaging techniques have shown that amyloid deposits may begin decades before the onset of clinical signs, whereas the presence of neurofibrillary tangles composed of abnormal tau protein is much more strongly correlated with disease severity. Genetic mutations that cause AD and the strongest known AD genetic risk factor, the epsilon 4 allele of the apolipoprotein E locus, have led to a primary focus on abnormal amyloid protein processing, but amyloid-based therapeutics to date have been ineffective.

Despite intensive research efforts, the precise mechanisms and interrelationships between extracellular amyloid plaque and intracellular neurofibrillary tangle deposition remains elusive.

Prevention

With the disappointing lack of progress in developing safe, effective new medications to treat AD, increased emphasis is being placed on prevention through (a) modification of vascular risk factors, prevention of neural injury, and buildup of neuronal reserves (see Table 1). Among the preventive measures that can be recommended to persons with a family history of AD or other risk factors for the disease include:

- Control of hypertension, with the goal of a blood pressure of 130 to 140 or 80 to 90. Lower blood pressures are not generally advocated, especially in older persons, because of concern that more aggressive blood pressure reduction in persons with existing vascular disease may reduce cerebral perfusion, leading to ischemic damage.
- Reduction in other cardiovascular risk factors by not smoking and by treating hyperlipidemia and diabetes.
- Avoidance of and/or treatment of anything else that causes injury to brain cells, including head trauma, alcoholism, and obstructive sleep apnea.
- Maintenance of good general health by engaging in regular physical activity, being socially active, and adhering to healthy dietary principles, such as the Mediterranean diet.
- Avoidance when possible of medications that have anticholinergic side effects, depleting acetyl-choline and increasing the risk of memory loss.
- Promotion of brain use and activity through such activities as learning a language and doing puzzles.
- Failure to treat mid-life hearing loss and depression are other factors that have recently been identified as being associated with a greater relative risk of dementia.

Clinical Features

Diagnostic criteria for *dementia* include a chronic, progressive disease characterized by (a) memory impairment; (b) impairment of one or more other aspects of neurologic function, such as executive function, visuospatial function, aphasia, apraxia, and/or agnosia; and (c) significant reduction in social or occupational function from the person's previous level of performance, which is not explained by another psychiatric or neurologic disorder. Diagnostic criteria for *AD* include meeting all criteria for

TABLE 1 Major Risk Factors for Alzheimer's Disease and Evidence of Ability to Modify Risk

RISK FACTOR	DIRECTION OF EFFECT	MODIFIABLE?/ STRATEGY	EVIDENCE OF RISK REDUCTION*
Older age	↑	No	–
Family history of Alzheimer's	↑	No	–
Head injury history	↑	Yes/head protection in sports	B
Hypertension	↑	Yes/treat to ≤ 140/90	A
Other cardiovascular risk factors	↑	Yes/risk factor reduction	C
Apolipoprotein E4 allele	↑	No	–
Physical activity	↓	Yes/aerobic and strength training	B
Mediterranean diet	↓	Yes/diet modification	B
Diabetes	↑	Yes/treatment to reduce HbA1c	C
Moderate alcohol use	↓	Yes/encourage limited use	C
Heavy alcohol use	↑	Yes/successful alcoholism treatment	C
Cognitive and social activity	↓	Yes/brain health activities	B

*A = consistent, good-quality patient-oriented evidence; B = inconsistent or limited-quality patient-oriented evidence; C = consensus, disease-oriented evidence, usual practice, expert opinion. For information about the SORT evidence rating system, see http://www.aafp.org/afpsort.xml.

dementia and ruling out delirium and the other dementias (see next section). Over time, these criteria may change: In 2011 the Alzheimer's Association and the National Institute on Aging defined AD to include a preclinical stage and mild cognitive impairment (MCI); however, at present, these definitions are for research purposes only.

The cardinal feature of AD is short-term memory loss or difficulty learning new information, which is often accompanied by a lack of awareness or concern of the memory problem. Word-finding difficulties, loss of time orientation, getting lost or misplacing things, and impaired judgment and planning are other common features. On average, the person with AD lives 6 to 10 years after the diagnosis and progresses through several stages. Over time, progressive cognitive disturbances become more pervasive, leading to impairment in instrumental activities of daily living (IADLs) and later even basic activities of daily living (ADLs). Ultimately, if the person does not die from some other cause, they will progress to being unable to express themself verbally and will be relatively immobile, with contractures, swallowing problems, cachexia, weight loss, and eventually death.

Differential Diagnosis

The most important considerations in the differential diagnosis of AD are the following:
- Vascular dementia (VaD). There are two general types: (a) cortical—resulting from multiple infarcts in the cerebral cortex; and (b) subcortical—resulting from small-vessel disease with multiple lacunar infarcts. Presentation is highly variable; however, memory deficits are typically less prominent than in AD.
- Frontotemporal dementia (FTD). This diagnosis is relatively uncommon but accounts for up to half of all cases before age 65. The clinical presentation is highly variable, depending on the lateral distribution of pathological changes. Language disturbances involving expression or comprehension or prominent changes in behavior and personality (e.g., apathy, disinhibition, repetitive motor behaviors, loss of empathy) are the two main clinical subtypes (left and right side predominant, respectively). Clinical diagnosis can be aided by MRI brain imaging showing severe focal atrophy in the frontal and/or temporal lobes, which may not always be appreciated on radiology reports.
- Lewy body dementia (LBD) is an umbrella term for dementia with Lewy bodies (DLB) and Parkinson's disease dementia (PDD). DLB is used to describe the syndrome when cognitive

symptoms predominate in conjunction with parkinsonian motor signs (bradykinesia, rigidity, and tremor), prominent visual hallucinations, and sleep-wake disturbances (e.g., fluctuating arousal, daytime somnolence, acting out dreams). PDD refers to late-occurring dementia in a patient with Parkinson's disease, often with other clinical features associated with DLB, though lacking formal diagnostic criteria.
- Rare but distinctive forms of dementia. These include progressive supranuclear palsy, corticobasal degeneration, normal-pressure hydrocephalus, Creutzfeldt-Jakob disease, post-anoxic dementia, post-traumatic brain injury, chronic subdural hematoma(s), and Huntington's disease.
- MCI. This is a condition in which the person is able to carry out his or her normal activities but has deficits in certain areas of higher function such as short-term memory, judgment, and planning. There are two kinds of MCI: *amnestic*, which is characterized by isolated short-term memory loss; and *non-amnestic*, in which one or more other cognitive domains are affected. Amnestic MCI is particularly likely to progress to AD and in such cases reflects a prodromal stage of the disease.
- Delirium. In contrast to the dementias, delirium tends to be subacute or acute in onset and to be completely or partially reversible. Key characteristics include fluctuating consciousness, confusion, and hallucinations or delusions. The cause is usually identifiable and is most often because of medication, stress (such as infection or surgery), or a metabolic disturbance. Delirium often occurs in patients with dementia, reflecting increased vulnerability of a compromised brain to toxic, metabolic, or infectious insults.
- Depression. Decades ago, depression was at times mistaken for dementia and termed "pseudo-dementia," because people with depression often say "I don't know" in response to cognitive status questions. Improved interviewing techniques and routine use of depression screening tests as part of a dementia evaluation have largely eliminated this confusion. However, depression remains an important consideration in the dementia evaluation because it frequently coexists with dementia, particularly in early stages of the illness.

Screening for Cognitive Impairment

Whether to screen for AD is highly controversial. Advantages of early diagnosis include offering earlier treatment and research participation, allowing the person an opportunity to make life-planning decisions at a point where his or her residual cognitive function is at its best, helping family understand what is happening and learn how best to provide support, providing guidance to patient and family about managing finances wisely and avoiding scams, and providing time for decision making about such things as durable power of attorney and advance-care planning. Medicare currently requires cognitive screening as part of the annual Medicare wellness visit; in addition, we recommend screening anyone age 75 and older and anyone for whom a memory lapse or vagueness noted in an interview or an error in judgment (e.g., causing an auto accident) raises suspicion of cognitive impairment.

Primary care physicians can conduct expedient, reliable screening for dementia by employing the Mini-Cog (patient) and the AD8 (informant). Each can be administered simultaneously by a nurse or medical assistant in about 3 minutes.

- The *Mini-Cog* consists of asking the person to remember three items; to draw a clock face, putting in the numbers and placing the hands at "10 after 11"; and then to recall the three items. A positive screen occurs if the person cannot recall any of the items (regardless of the clock drawing), or if they recall one to two items and the clock is drawn incorrectly.
- The *AD8* requires the person being screened to be accompanied by a spouse, child, or other person who knows him or her well. It inquires about whether the person has had a change over the past several years in eight areas: judgment, interest in hobbies/activities, repeating things, learning, orientation, financial management, remembering appointments, and other memory. A change in two or more items is a positive screen.

Downloadable, printable copies of both instruments with instructions are available at https://carolinamemorycarenet.com/.

Diagnostic Evaluation
There are five general steps in a diagnostic evaluation for AD: (1) history; (2) cognitive assessment; (3) physical examination, with a focus on the neurologic evaluation; (4) laboratory testing; and (5) establishment of a working diagnosis (including consideration of and attempts to rule out other depression, delirium, and non-Alzheimer's dementias). Each of these is discussed below.

History
Patients suspected of having AD typically present either because a family member reports changes in their behavior and function or because of a positive screening evaluation. Judgment and decision-making can be impaired early in the disease, which may lead to an incident that draws attention to the problem. Examples include auto accidents, uncharacteristic purchases or donations, problems managing a household budget, or being victimized by a scam. Increased awareness of early warning signs and following the Medicare requirement for cognitive screening should help identify a higher proportion of patients with mild, as opposed to major, neurocognitive disorder.

An individual who presents with memory or other cognitive difficulties may not be able to provide a reliable history. The primary or at least collateral source of historical information about functional change needs to be a family member close to the individual. Such a history typically includes gradual functional decline in multiple domains including short-term memory (repeating oneself), getting lost while driving, having trouble managing a checkbook, saying things that the person normally wouldn't have said, and difficulty making decisions.

An important element of the history should be questions aimed at identifying other potential causes of cognitive impairment, such as alcoholism, illicit drug use, and prescription medications.

In addition, inquiry about a person's psychiatric history should be undertaken as well as screening for anxiety and depression. A formal screening tool, such as the Geriatric Depression Scale or the Patient Health Questionnaire nine-item depression screen (PHQ-9), is recommended.

Cognitive Status Examination
The cognitive status examination should include a standardized cognitive test, both for comparison with other patients and to provide a numerical result that can be followed over time. We recommend either the St. Louis University Mental Status Examination (SLUMS) or the Montreal Cognitive Assessment examination (MoCA), both of which cover a wide range of cognitive domains, are more sensitive to detecting cognitive impairment compared to older tests (e.g., Mini-Mental State Examination), have been validated in many populations, and are freely available in the public domain (i.e., available for download from the Internet).

The standardized examination should be supplemented by several other components to help round out the evaluation, identify behavioral issues, and screen for non-Alzheimer's dementias. Supplementary examination components that are useful include

- Verbal fluency testing—naming as many objects, such as animals, as they can in 1 minute (category fluency) and as many words beginning with a single letter such as "F" as they can in 1 minute (letter fluency). These not only tap into early loss cognitive areas but also help differentiate between AD (where category fluency tends to be more impaired) and other dementias, where impairment is similar (e.g., VaD) or letter fluency tends to be more impaired (e.g., FTD and LBD).
- Trail-Making Test B:—this is a timed paper-and-pencil test; it is a particularly sensitive test for early cognitive changes in non-memory domains (visuospatial and executive).
- Psychological and behavioral symptom evaluation—this is best obtained from a family member using a questionnaire tool such as the Neuropsychiatric Inventory (NPI).

Physical Examination
After evaluating cardiovascular and pulmonary status, the physical examination should focus on neurologic function, looking for signs that suggest a diagnosis other than AD. In particular, the examination should look for asymmetry in strength and/or motor function (suggesting one or more prior strokes), tremor and bradykinesia (suggesting parkinsonism), abnormalities of eye movement, especially inability to gaze downward (suggesting progressive supranuclear palsy), and peripheral neuropathy (suggesting the possibility of vitamin B12 deficiency, hypothyroidism, alcoholism, or neurosyphilis [although diabetes is more often the cause]).

Laboratory Testing and Neuroimaging
If the cognitive status examination confirms dysfunction, then a laboratory battery should be conducted largely to help identify remediable causes of cognitive impairment. Basic testing should include a complete blood count, blood glucose, electrolytes, renal function (BUN/creatinine), thyroid function, liver function tests, vitamin B12 level, and, if appropriate, a serologic test for syphilis.

Although research advances in brain imaging offer promise for more early and definitive diagnosis, a routine brain MRI remains the standard of clinical practice. It can identify cerebrovascular disease as discrete old infarcts (usually cortical) or as greater-than-normal deep white-matter changes (leukoariosis, suggesting subcortical vascular disease). The MRI is also useful in ruling out tumor or normal pressure hydrocephalus and in identifying focal cortical atrophy consistent with FTD.

Recently, positive emission tomography (PET) scanning for brain amyloid (florbetapir F 18 or Amyvid) has become commercially available, but is currently reimbursed by Medicare only if done as part of a research protocol. A large multicenter study is currently underway to evaluate the potential impact of amyloid brain PET imaging on clinical care for AD patients. Future therapeutic advances in MCI and early AD will likely usher in the selective, if not routine use of amyloid brain imaging in clinical care. At present, however, the only clinical indication for routine metabolic brain PET reimbursed by Medicare is to distinguish FTD from AD.

TABLE 2	Differential Diagnosis of Alzheimer's Disease		
DIAGNOSIS	**TYPICAL PRESENTING HISTORY**	**KEY EXAMINATION FINDINGS**	**BRAIN IMAGING/LAB FINDINGS**
Alzheimer's disease (AD)	Progressive, gradual onset; behavioral symptoms variable		
Mild	Short-term memory loss; IADL and judgment problems	Mild praxis or gait difficulty may be present	Normal CT or medial temporal atrophy; + amyloid brain PET scan
Moderate	ADL impairment; prominent memory deficits and confusion	May have frontal release signs	Medial temporal and parietal lobe atrophy; + amyloid PET scan
Mild cognitive impairment (MCI)	Impaired short-term memory without functional impairment	Mild praxis or gait difficulty may be present	Variable medial temporal atrophy (nonspecific)
Vascular dementia (VaD)	Stepwise progression; stroke history and/or vascular risk factors; gait problems early	Abnormal neurologic examination with lateralizing findings (may be subtle)	MRI shows cortical and/or subcortical infarcts, leukoariosis
Frontotemporal dementia (FTD)	Behavioral, personality, language changes; apathy	Variable, gait apraxia, frontal release signs	Marked atrophy in frontal and/or temporal lobes
Lewy body dementia (LBD)	Fluctuating attention, visual hallucinations, gait/motor/sleep disturbance (act out dreams)	Limb rigidity, bradykinesia, may see intention tremor and gait disturbance	MRI nondiagnostic
Parkinson's dementia	History of Parkinson's disease, later-onset cognitive dysfunction	Limb rigidity, bradykinesia, resting tremor, gait disturbance	MRI nondiagnostic
Delirium	Acute onset; identifiable pharmacologic, metabolic, toxic, or infectious cause	Fluctuating attention, fidgety, agitated, tremulous, or apathetic; may be obtundant	Diffuse EEG slowing, evidence of drug or metabolic toxicity, infection

Establishment of a Working Diagnosis

Because no gold-standard clinical test exists for diagnosing AD, the evaluation usually results in a working diagnosis. If the evaluation raises suspicions that a non-AD dementia may be involved (Table 2), then consultation with a specialist in neurology or geriatric medicine is advised. General principles of management apply to all dementias; however, different dementias respond differently to certain medications discussed later in this chapter, and so consultation may help direct appropriate therapeutic interventions in addition to clarifying the diagnosis.

Treatment

In managing AD, the physician needs to treat at least two individuals: the person with the disease and the person (or persons) who serves as the primary caregiver. A common thread in this dualistic approach is to promote safety and quality of life for all involved. While cognitive function is the key to diagnosis, behavioral symptoms are often the most important to address in the context of management and burden of care. Table 3 reviews the main therapeutic targets and interventions.

Counseling and Caregiver Support

The patient and caregiver should be counseled about the disease course, about increased safety risks from such things as operating machinery and driving a motor vehicle, about the desirability of establishing a durable power of attorney for health care decisions, and about the value of having conversations early on about desires for end-of-life care, including completion of advance directives. As the disease progresses, regular meetings with the patient and family are important so as to anticipate and address key decision points.

TABLE 3	Alzheimer's Disease Management Strategies		
OUTCOME TO BE AFFECTED	**INTERVENTION**	**COMMENTS**	**LEVEL OF EVIDENCE***
Cognitive symptoms (memory, judgment, etc.)	Cholinesterase inhibitors (donepezil [Aricept], rivastigmine [Exelon], galantamine [Razadyne], memantine [Namenda]) Medical food: Caprylidene (Axona) Cognitive training Physical activity and adequate rest	Effective for mild, moderate, and severe dementia. Effect equal to slowing decline by 6 months Modest benefits in apo E4 negative subjects only Improved ability specific to the abilities trained Improved alertness and physical function; reduced depression	A B/C B B
Behavioral symptoms (agitation, resistance to care, physical violence)	Mediterranean or modified Mediterranean (MIND) diet Individualized, person-centered ADL care Cognitive enhancers (e.g., donepezil, memantine) Antipsychotic drugs Anticonvulsants	Reduced risk of onset of Alzheimer's disease Reduced agitation; improved quality of life Effects modest but fewer adverse effects than other medications Only a minority of patients clearly benefit; high adverse effect profile; "black box" warning on atypical antipsychotics for increasing cardiovascular disease but typical antipsychotics also have adverse effects Carbamazepine (Tegretol)[1] reduces agitation, anxiety, and restlessness; ataxia and hematologic toxicity occur	B A A A B

Continued

TABLE 3 Alzheimer's Disease Management Strategies—cont'd

OUTCOME TO BE AFFECTED	INTERVENTION	COMMENTS	LEVEL OF EVIDENCE*
Caregiver stress, burden, and depression	Education, group programs, respite services	Early disease—education and group activities for caregiver and person with dementia; respite Moderate/advanced disease—caregiver support group; respite	A
Depression in persons with dementia	Selective seratonin reuptake inhibitors (SSRIs) (sertraline [Zoloft], citralopram [Celexa]) Physical activity/exercise	Mild to moderate effects on mood; no effect on agitation, aggression Formal program of caregiver education and exercise for the person with dementia; improved depression	A B
Quality of life; well-being	Pleasant sensory stimulation		A

*A = consistent, good-quality patient-oriented evidence; B = inconsistent or limited-quality patient-oriented evidence; C = consensus, disease-oriented evidence, usual practice, expert opinion. For information about the SORT evidence rating system, see http://www.aafp.org/afpsort.xml.
[1]Not FDA approved for this indication.

AD leads to progressive dependency; maintaining the health and well-being of the caregiver(s) is a critical component of care. Make sure the caregiver has a physician and is under treatment for any medical problems he or she may have. In addition, the caregiver should be advised about community resources that can provide assistance, such as the local chapter of the Alzheimer's Association, programs for persons with early-stage dementia, support programs for caregivers, local adult day care centers, and respite programs. In addition, because the majority of persons with AD spend their final days in a nursing home or assisted living community, health care providers should be prepared to provide support for that decision when appropriate.

Management of Cognitive Symptoms
The lack of novel therapeutic approaches during the past 10 years, in spite of very active research, has been a major disappointment. The cholinesterase inhibitors and memantine (Namenda) remain mainstays of treatment. Key points in using these drugs include the following (see Table 4):
- There is no demonstrated value to withholding drugs for later, when the patient gets worse.
- The overall benefit of treatment may be difficult to assess clinically; "real-world" changes noted by caregivers may be more important than cognitive test scores.
- Side effects are largely gastrointestinal (pain, bloating, nausea). Treatment should involve reducing the dose or switching to another agent. Donepezil (Aricept), while generally given at bedtime, may cause leg cramps, insomnia, or vivid bizarre dreams that often abate by switching to morning dosing.

- Studies indicate that combining a cholinesterase inhibitor with memantine (Namenda) produces a modest additive benefit.
- Long-term treatment effects involve symptom reduction and are not cumulative; if the efficacy of one or more drug treatments is in question, it is reasonable to pursue a sequential trial taper and withdrawal (resuming the previous dose or medication if acute decline is noted by informants).
- Ensuring adequate sleep, activity, and nutrition is important for optimizing the patient's functional abilities.

Management of Behavioral Symptoms
A wide variety of behavioral symptoms can develop. Among the more common are (a) early in the disease—repetitive questions, wandering, and refusing assistance; (b) in the mid-stage of the disease—resistance to care, agitation or pacing, verbal and physical agitation and aggression, and antisocial behaviors such as inappropriate sexual remarks; (c) late in the disease—resistance to care and repetitive vocalizations such as moaning and screaming.

The key to managing most behavioral symptoms rests on nonpharmacologic approaches involving good adaptive dementia communication skills. Key elements include making eye contact before speaking; using simple language; speaking slowly, clearly, and in a low-pitched voice; communicating empathy through such actions as smiling and giving a hug; asking only one question at a time and allowing the patient adequate time to respond; breaking instructions down into small steps and presenting one at a time; and backing off and trying later if the person becomes agitated or refuses. If the person doesn't seem to understand a statement, repeat the statement using the same wording; if this does not work,

TABLE 4 Drug Therapy for Cognitive Symptoms in Alzheimer's Disease

	DONEPEZIL (ARICEPT™)	RIVASTIGMINE (EXELON™ TRANSDERMAL PATCH)*	GALANTAMINE (RAZADYNE™)	MEMANTINE (NAMENDA™)
Mechanism	Cholinesterase-inhibitor	Cholinesterase-inhibitor	Cholinesterase-inhibitor	NMDA antagonist
Doses	5, 10 mg (qd) SR: 23 mg	4.6, 9.5, 13.3 mg qd	4, 8, 12 mg (bid) ER: 8, 16, 24 mg	5, 10 mg (bid) XR: 7, 14, 21, 28 mg
Target dose	5–10 mg/d; 23 mg SR for moderate - severe	4.6–13.3 mg/d	16–24 mg/d	10–20 mg/d 28 mg/d*
Half-life	70 h	> 24 h	6–8 h	60–80 h
Metabolism	Hepatic	Nonhepatic	Hepatic	Nonhepatic
Protein-binding	96%	40%	19%	45%
Most common adverse effects	Nausea (13%) Diarrhea (10%) Insomnia (8%)	Nausea (12%) Vomiting (10%) Diarrhea (6%)	Nausea (12%) Vomiting (9%) Anorexia (6%)	Headaches (3%) Dizziness (2%) Constipation (2%)

SR: sustained release (qd).
*Transdermal patch (oral dosing with high incidence of GI side effects not listed). ER: extended release (qd). XR: extended-release (qd).

rephrase and allow time for processing. When a specific problem develops, such as resistance to care or unwanted exiting, caregivers should use a structured problem-solving approach that defines the symptom, tries to identify reasons (including emotions and delusions) behind the symptom, and develops a management strategy to try and evaluate, using a quality improvement approach.

At times, however, families or facility caregivers report aggressive, frightening, or socially unacceptable behaviors that do not remit even in spite of excellent personalized psychosocial care. In these situations, medical providers are often asked for a prescription. Sometimes all that is needed is time, as aberrant behaviors tend to moderate over time. If a medication is needed, the first step should be a cholinesterase inhibitor, which has been shown to have potential benefits on apathy, delusions, and purposeless motor behaviors. If that is unsuccessful, then an antipsychotic or anticonvulsant should be considered, starting at a low dose and increasing until improvement is seen or intolerable side effects occur. Patients who demonstrate, or later develop, prominent behavioral features (e.g., visual hallucinations, disinhibition) should be referred to an appropriate specialist in neurology, geriatrics, or psychiatry. Caution is particularly warranted in managing psychotic symptoms in patients with Lewy body dementias, including Parkinson's disease with dementia. Eliminating anticholinergic or reducing dopaminergic medications should be the first line of treatment.

Monitoring

Patients and caregivers should be reevaluated every 3 to 6 months. If the person with AD resists going to the doctor (a common feature early in the disease), then some of these check-in evaluations can be handled by telephone. Indeed, telephone consultation is highly valued by caregivers, for whom a trip to the doctor can be costly and disruptive. To help provide readily available consultation, primary care practices are encouraged to designate a nurse, nurse practitioner, or physician assistant to focus on dementia treatment and care. This focus would include coordinating dementia screening in the practice, knowing each of the patients and families with dementia, coordinating a support group (if the practice chooses to have one), and responding to questions from caregivers.

References

Boustani M, Campbell N, Munger S, Maidment I, Fox C: Impact of anticholinergics on the aging brain: a review and practical application, *Aging Health* 4(3):311–320, 2008.

Jack CR Jr. Albert MS, Knopman DS, et al: Introduction to the recommendations from the National Institute on Aging—Alzheimer's Association workgroups on diagnostic guidelines for Alzheimer's disease, *Alzheimers Dement* 7:257–262, 2011.

Galvin JE, Sadowski CH: Practical guidelines for the recognition and diagnosis of dementia, *J Am Board Fam Med* 25:367–382, 2012.

Livingston G, Sommerlad A, Orgeta V, et al: Dementia prevention, intervention, and care, *Lancet* 379:2673–2734, 2017.

Odenheimer G, Borson S, Sanders AE, et al: Quality improvement in neurology: dementia management quality measures, *Neurology* 81:1545–1549, 2013.

BRAIN TUMORS

Method of
Ryan Merrell, MD

CURRENT DIAGNOSIS

- Subacute to chronic onset of generalized and/or focal neurologic symptoms should alert the physician to order neuroimaging to investigate the possibility of a brain tumor.
- Magnetic resonance imaging (MRI) is preferable to computed tomography (CT) for imaging tumors.
- A biopsy or resection is necessary to diagnose a primary brain tumor or a metastatic tumor of unknown primary origin. The diagnostic yield is increased with a resection.
- Neuroimaging suggestive of meningioma does not require a tissue diagnosis and in many cases can be followed closely with serial neuroimaging.

- If a primary central nervous system (CNS) lymphoma is suspected, corticosteroids should not be given unless absolutely necessary in order not to confound the biopsy diagnosis.

CURRENT THERAPY

- Surgical resection is preferred for patients with most types of brain tumors as long as the resection does not leave the patient with permanent neurologic deficits.
- Whole-brain radiotherapy and stereotactic radiosurgery are the primary treatment modalities for patients with metastatic brain tumors.
- Surgical resection is preferred for patients with large or symptomatic meningiomas that are surgically accessible and in patients who can tolerate surgery.
- Patients with gliomas are treated with fractionated radiotherapy alone or in combination with chemotherapy.
- Patients with primary central nervous system (CNS) lymphoma are treated with high-dose methotrexate[1] alone or in combination with other chemotherapy drugs.

[1]Not US Food and Drug Administration (FDA) approved for this indication.

Brain tumors are categorized as metastatic or primary. The incidence and prevalence of metastatic tumors outweigh those of primary tumors up to 10:1. Lung and breast carcinoma make up the majority of metastatic tumors, largely because of their increased prevalence in the population compared with other tumors. Melanoma is a less prevalent malignancy but has a high propensity to metastasize to the brain. Meningioma is usually a benign tumor that is found most often in the fourth through sixth decade, with a female-to-male ratio of 2:1. Gliomas are primary brain tumors that are categorized as high-grade gliomas or low-grade gliomas. High-grade gliomas usually affect patients in the fifth and sixth decades and older, whereas low-grade gliomas usually affect patients in the third and fourth decades. Primary central nervous system (CNS) lymphoma is a rare tumor that usually affects patients in the sixth decade and older.

There are very few identifiable risk factors for brain tumors. The histology of the primary neoplasm confers the risk of brain metastases because lung cancer, breast cancer, and melanoma are more likely to metastasize to the brain, whereas colorectal, ovarian, and prostate cancers are less likely to metastasize to the brain. Past exposure to ionizing radiation and a family history of a genetic cancer syndrome are the only known risk factors for primary tumors. Despite much press, cell phone use has not been irrefutably shown to be a risk factor for brain tumors. Immunocompromise such as human immunodeficiency virus (HIV) infection is a well-known risk factor for primary CNS lymphoma.

Presentation

Brain tumors manifest with the subacute or chronic onset of generalized symptoms such as confusion, headaches, seizures, and nausea or focal symptoms and signs such as visual field deficit, loss of language, unilateral weakness, sensory neglect, or difficulty walking. There are no symptoms or signs specific to any brain tumor because the anatomic location of the tumor in the brain dictates the presentation. These symptoms and signs should prompt neuroimaging with magnetic resonance imaging (MRI). MRI has largely replaced computed tomography (CT) for evaluating brain tumors, although CT serves as a quick screening modality and must be used in patients who have contraindications to MRI.

Evaluation

Radiographic features on MRI can predict the type of tumor but cannot accurately confirm the pathology. A tissue diagnosis through a biopsy or surgical resection is necessary to confirm the pathology, except in patients with metastatic tumors with a known primary tumor. The differential diagnosis of mass lesions in the brain includes abscess, demyelinating lesion, inflammatory disease, and other infections such as toxoplasmosis and cysticercosis.

A biopsy or surgical resection provides the definitive diagnosis of the tumor. For most tumors, a resection is preferred when safely possible, because the greater amount of tissue obtained avoids the sampling error that can occur with a biopsy. In addition, maximal surgical debulking can provide significant relief of symptoms. The goal of surgery for all brain tumors is to provide a maximal resection while leaving the patient free of permanent neurologic deficits.

Classification

Metastatic brain tumors are classified according to the cell of origin. Primary brain tumors are classified according to the World Health Organization (WHO) classification system. Additional molecular classification that can provide prognostic and therapeutic information is often obtained on select primary brain tumors. Oligodendroglioma is a primary brain tumor that has well-characterized chromosomal deletions on the short arm of chromosome 1 and the long arm of chromosome 19 (1p/19q codeletion) that have been shown to predict improved survival and increased sensitivity to treatment. Similarly, O-6-methylguanine-DNA-methyltransferase (MGMT) promoter methylation is a marker that predicts improved survival and may predict improved response to treatment in high-grade glioma.

Metastatic Tumors

Metastatic brain tumors are the most common brain tumors, with as many as 170,000 new cases diagnosed in the United States each year. Metastatic tumors can occur with or without evidence of a primary neoplasm. Findings on brain MRI suspicious for a metastatic tumor should prompt an investigation for a primary malignancy with body imaging (Figure 1). The discovery of a systemic mass that can be biopsied might avoid a brain biopsy or resection in select patients. Occasionally, after an extensive evaluation, no evidence of a primary tumor is found. Approximately 50% of patients have a single metastasis, and the rest have multiple tumors. In general, prognosis is poor, but some patients with less-aggressive primary tumors (melanoma, breast, non–small cell lung carcinoma [NSCLC]) can achieve long-term survival. This is particularly true for tumors with targetable mutations such as *BRAF* in melanoma and *EGFR* and *ALK* in NSCLC. In addition, immunotherapy has had significant impact on melanoma and other tumors. Clinical trials are evaluating whether treatment with targeted drugs can allow delaying radiotherapy in select patients.

Tumors can metastasize to the nervous system through infiltration of the cerebrospinal fluid (CSF), a process termed *leptomeningeal carcinomatosis* or *carcinomatous meningitis*. Symptoms suggesting leptomeningeal carcinomatosis include altered mental status, headaches, loss of vision, double vision, slurred speech, difficulty swallowing, and lower extremity pain and weakness. Brain MRI can show enhancement of the meninges, and CSF from lumbar puncture shows low glucose and elevated protein with malignant cells. A lumbar puncture is not necessary to confirm the diagnosis in a patient with a known primary malignancy and characteristic clinical presentation and MRI findings. The prognosis is poor, on the order of several months. Patients with lymphoma and breast cancer might realize longer survival.

Several factors determine the approach to treatment of metastatic tumors. The age, comorbidities, functional status, degree of neurologic impairment, and extent of the systemic disease determine whether surgery is indicated. Solitary metastases and large symptomatic tumors in patients with multiple tumors are generally resected in patients who are good surgical candidates. Whether a patient undergoes surgical resection or not, radiotherapy is the mainstay of treatment for metastatic tumors.

Figure 1 Contrast-enhanced magnetic resonance image shows a homogeneously enhancing mass with surrounding edema at the gray-white junction, suggesting a metastatic tumor.

The two approaches to radiotherapy are whole-brain radiotherapy and stereotactic radiosurgery. In whole-brain radiotherapy, a dose of radiation is fractionated into several treatment sessions and given to the entire brain. In stereotactic radiosurgery, a high dose of radiation is given only to areas of brain involved with tumor and often in one treatment session. The effectiveness of whole-brain radiotherapy versus stereotactic radiosurgery has not been established in large randomized trials. Whole-brain radiotherapy is more suited for patients with multiple metastases or large tumors (>3 cm in diameter). Stereotactic radiosurgery is indicated for patients with fewer than four metastases, for smaller-volume tumors (<3 cm in diameter), and for radioresistant tumors such as melanoma. Whole-brain radiotherapy has the advantage of treating the visible and undetectable tumors, but it carries a risk of delayed neurotoxicity that often manifests as cognitive impairment. Recent studies have shown that this cognitive toxicity can be lessened through whole-brain radiation with hippocampal sparing and addition of the drug memantine during radiation. Stereotactic radiosurgery has the advantage of local control by treating the visible tumors and carries less risk of delayed neurotoxicity. Stereotactic radiosurgery can be repeated if new tumors develop in areas of brain not previously radiated. The disadvantage of stereotactic radiosurgery is the potential for new tumors to develop in areas of brain not treated.

Treatment of leptomeningeal carcinomatosis involves chemotherapy or radiotherapy. Chemotherapy is often administered directly into the spinal fluid (intrathecal), usually through a ventricular (Omaya) reservoir. Alternatively, chemotherapy can be given systemically. Common chemotherapeutic agents include methotrexate (Methotrexate PF)[1], cytarabine (Cytarabine PF)[1], and thiotepa[1]. Radiotherapy is usually only used as a salvage treatment after chemotherapy failure.

Meningiomas

Meningiomas are the most common primary brain tumor, accounting for more than 32% of all tumors. Meningiomas arise from the arachnoid cap cells. They are often discovered incidentally when a patient undergoes neuroimaging for symptoms that

---

[1] Not FDA approved for this indication.

Figure 2 Contrast-enhanced magnetic resonance image shows a homogeneously enhancing mass arising from the dura, with the typical appearance of a meningioma.

are unrelated to the meningioma. The radiographic appearance of meningiomas is one of the most specific of all brain tumors and allows a confident diagnosis without the need for a confirmatory biopsy (Figure 2). The most common radiographic mimicker is a metastatic tumor to the meninges, but usually a patient in this circumstance has a known history of malignancy. Small meningiomas may be followed with serial imaging. Meningiomas that correlate with neurologic deficits or tumors that have grown significantly over time should be treated.

Surgical resection is the preferred treatment if it can be safely accomplished, but it should be avoided in the elderly. Meningiomas are graded WHO I to III; 90% are grade I (benign), and grade III (anaplastic) are the most aggressive and likely to recur. Complete resection is curative in most cases, but some meningiomas recur. If recurrent tumors are large or symptomatic, surgery is the preferred treatment if possible. Radiotherapy, either fractionated or stereotactic radiosurgery, can be used postoperatively to treat residual tumor or to treat tumors that cannot be resected. Meningiomas have an intermediate response to radiotherapy, and grade III tumors often show minimal response.

There is no defined chemotherapy for meningiomas, although several drugs are being actively investigated.

Gliomas

Gliomas consist of astrocytomas, oligodendrogliomas, and ependymomas, in decreasing order of prevalence. It was once thought that these tumors derived from mutations of normal glial cells, but it is increasingly recognized that gliomas derive from brain tumor progenitor cells. Glioblastoma is the most malignant glioma and accounts for 60% to 70% of all gliomas. Gliomas are classified by the glial cells from which they originate and the histologic features that give them a grade according to the WHO classification (Table 1). Grade III and IV tumors are high-grade gliomas, and grade II tumors are low-grade gliomas. Grade I glioma (pilocytic astrocytoma) is rarely seen in adults. A maximal surgical resection that leaves the patient with minimal neurologic deficits is the preferred initial treatment for all grades of gliomas.

TABLE 1 World Health Organization Classification of Common Gliomas in Adults

SUBTYPE	WORLD HEALTH ORGANIZATION GRADE
Low-Grade Gliomas	
Astrocytoma	II
Oligodendroglioma	II
Oligoastrocytoma	II
High-Grade Gliomas	
Anaplastic astrocytoma	III
Anaplastic oligodendroglioma	III
Anaplastic oligoastrocytoma	III
Anaplastic ependymoma	III
Glioblastoma	IV

Figure 3 Contrast-enhanced magnetic resonance image shows a ring-enhancing mass with surrounding edema with the typical appearance of glioblastoma.

High-Grade Gliomas

Most high-grade gliomas are glioblastoma or anaplastic astrocytoma (WHO grade III); anaplastic oligodendroglioma and anaplastic ependymoma are less common. The brain MRI often shows a ring-enhancing mass centered in the white matter surrounded by edema and causing mass effect (Figure 3). A maximal surgical resection that leaves the patient without permanent neurologic deficits is the goal in high-grade glioma. A maximal resection, younger age, and good performance status are favorable prognostic factors. Methylation of the MGMT promoter correlates with improved survival. High-grade gliomas are aggressive, incurable tumors; the median survival for glioblastoma is 14 to

TABLE 2	Common Chemotherapy for Gliomas	
GENERIC NAME	**TRADE NAME**	**DOSE**
Temozolomide	Temodar	75 mg/m² daily during radiotherapy, 150–200 mg/m² after radiotherapy on 5 days per 28 days schedule 50 mg/m² daily or 75 mg/m² 3 weeks on, 1 week off, for recurrent high-grade glioma
Bevacizumab	Avastin	10 mg/kg every 2 weeks

18 months and for anaplastic astrocytoma is 2 to 2.5 years. The isocitrate dehydrogenase I (IDH 1) mutation is less commonly seen in high-grade gliomas and correlates with improved survival.

Treatment of high-grade glioma is based on the histology of the tumor. The standard treatment of glioblastoma consists of fractionated radiotherapy given over 6 weeks with temozolomide (Temodar), an oral chemotherapeutic drug. Temozolomide is given 1 month after the completion of radiotherapy until tumor progression, which occurs on average around 7 months after the original diagnosis for glioblastoma (Table 2). There is no consensus on treatment of anaplastic gliomas, and two clinical trials are ongoing (CATNON and CODEL). Patients with anaplastic astrocytoma are usually treated with 6 weeks of radiotherapy alone followed by adjuvant temozlomide. Patients with glioblastoma and anaplastic astrocytoma are usually treated with 6 months of temozolomide, although some practitioners will treat up to 12 months. Tumor treating fields (TTFs) is a cap-like device worn on a shaved scalp. TTFs deliver radiofrequency pulses to the tumor. Based on the results of a large randomized clinical trial, TTFs were approved to add on to the standard therapy of radiation with temozolomide for newly diagnosed glioblastoma.

Careful consideration should be given to neuroimaging findings suggesting tumor progression within the first 6 months after radiotherapy because these changes can reflect radiation necrosis (pseudoprogression) rather than true tumor progression.

In the setting of tumor progression, salvage chemotherapy is the mainstay of treatment. Bevacizumab (Avastin), a drug that inhibits blood vessel formation around tumors, is the most common drug that is given at tumor recurrence. Temozolomide given in low doses daily is another approach for recurrent high-grade glioma. TTF can also be used in the recurrent setting if not used at initial diagnosis. Experimental chemotherapy through a clinical trial is a common option used in recurrent high-grade glioma. Occasionally, surgical resection is indicated to improve symptoms, but it has not been shown to improve survival. Likewise, focused radiation such as stereotactic radiosurgery has not been shown to affect survival.

Anaplastic oligodendroglioma is usually treated with radiation followed by chemotherapy, either PCV (procarbazine [Matulane][1], 1-(2-chloroethyl-3-cyclohexyl)-1-nitrosurea [CCNU; Lomustine], and vincristine[1]) or temozolomide, whereas anaplastic ependymoma is usually treated with radiotherapy alone. Anaplastic oligodendrogliomas with chromosomal 1p/19q co-deletions carry better prognosis and response to treatment.

Low-Grade Gliomas

Despite being lower-grade tumors, low-grade gliomas are not benign. The natural history is that patients with low-grade gliomas ultimately progress to high-grade glioma. Low-grade gliomas account for approximately 15% of all primary brain tumors. Low-grade gliomas are more likely to manifest with seizures than high-grade gliomas. The brain MRI often shows a nonenhancing mass with involvement of white matter and sometimes abutting the cerebral cortex (Figure 4). As in high-grade gliomas, a maximal surgical resection confers a survival advantage in low-grade gliomas. Prognosis varies considerably by tumor histology: Patients with astrocytoma live 5 to 10 years after diagnosis, whereas patients

---

[1] Not FDA approved for this indication.

Figure 4 Fluid-attenuated inversion recovery magnetic resonance image shows a nonenhancing tumor abutting the cerebral cortex with the typical appearance of a low-grade glioma. The tumor proved to be a grade II oligodendroglioma.

with oligodendroglioma live 10 to 15 years after diagnosis. The IDH 1 mutation correlates with improved survival. This mutation is seen in the majority of patients with low-grade glioma.

The results of a recent randomized clinical trial revealed superior progression free survival and overall survival in patients with low-grade gliomas treated with radiation followed by adjuvant PCV.

In the absence of a head-to-head clinical trial of PCV with temozolomide, many clinicians would use temozolomide in place of PCV because temozolomide is better tolerated. Therefore radiation followed by PCV or temozolomide has become the standard of care for all patients with low-grade gliomas. It is still a common practice to take a watch-and-wait approach in select patients with newly diagnosed low-grade glioma who have had a gross total resection. Clinical trials evaluating IDH inhibitors are ongoing. When patients with low-grade gliomas have findings on neuroimaging that suggest progressive tumor, a surgical resection or biopsy is often conducted to alleviate symptoms and to establish the grade of the tumor. Patients with low-grade gliomas that progress to high-grade glioma are treated similarly to patients with de novo high-grade glioma but with consideration to previous treatments.

Primary Central Nervous System Lymphoma

Primary CNS lymphoma is a rare non-Hodgkin lymphoma that affects the brain, eyes, meninges, and spinal cord, and accounts for approximately 5% of all brain tumors. This tumor is associated with the immunocompromised state, but it has a significant incidence in the immunocompetent. The characteristic radiographic appearance suggests but does not confirm the diagnosis (Figure 5). If primary CNS lymphoma is suspected, corticosteroids should not be given unless they are necessary to reduce increased intracranial pressure. This is because corticosteroids are directly cytotoxic to lymphoma cells, which can confound the tissue diagnosis. Occasionally, the diagnosis can be obtained through CSF testing, but a brain biopsy is often necessary.

Surgical resection has no role in treating this tumor because lymphoma is sensitive to chemotherapy and radiotherapy. The exception is in large tumors causing significant mass effect. Staging tests are necessary to rule out a systemic lymphoma that has metastasized to the CNS. Despite being incurable, primary CNS

Figure 5 Contrast-enhanced magnetic resonance image shows a homogenously enhancing mass near the surface of the ventricle, suggesting primary central nervous system lymphoma.

lymphoma is a more treatable tumor, and many patients live 5 years or longer after diagnosis.

Primary CNS lymphoma is treated with intravenous or intrathecal chemotherapy with or without radiotherapy. Methotrexate[1] is the principal drug used either alone or in combination with other chemotherapy drugs. High doses of methotrexate (3.5–8 g/m²)[3] must be used to overcome the blood-brain barrier. Owing to the potential for renal toxicity, high-dose methotrexate must be given in a setting where kidney function can be carefully monitored (usually the inpatient setting).

Radiotherapy was previously used as an initial treatment, but it is associated with profound cognitive impairment, especially in patients older than 60 years. However, more recent approaches have used lower doses of radiotherapy combined with chemotherapy with less neurotoxicity reported. Opinion is divided about the use of radiotherapy. Chemotherapy can also be used as a salvage treatment. Besides methotrexate, other commonly used chemotherapy drugs include cytarabine[1], etoposide (Toposar)[1], rituximab (Rituxan)[1], procarbazine (Matulane)[1], and temozolomide (Temodar)[1]. In younger patients, an increasingly used treatment at the time of relapse is high-dose chemotherapy with autologous stem cell transplantation. This approach is increasingly being investigated in the newly diagnosed setting. Newer drugs that are being used for salvage therapy include lenalidomide (Revlimid)[1] and ibrutinib (Imbruvica)[1].

---

[1] Not FDA approved for this indication.

[3] Exceeds dosage recommended by the manufacturer.

References

Ellis TL, Neal MT, Chan MD: The role of surgery, radiosurgery, and whole brain radiation therapy in the management of patients with metastatic brain tumors, *Int J Surg Oncol* 952345, 2012, 2012.

Gerstner ER, Batchelor TT: Primary central nervous system lymphoma, *Arch Neurol* 67:291–297, 2010.

Norden AD, Drappatz J, Wen PY: Advances in meningioma therapy, *Curr Neurol Neurosci Rep* 9:231–240, 2009.

Sanai N, Chang S, Berger MS: Low-grade gliomas in adults, *J Neurosurg* 115:948–965, 2011.

Wen PY, Kesari S: Malignant gliomas in adults, *N Engl J Med* 359:492–507, 2008.

GILLES DE LA TOURETTE SYNDROME

Method of
Steve W. Wu, MD; and Donald L. Gilbert, MD, MS

CURRENT DIAGNOSIS

- Multiple motor and one or more vocal tics have been present for some time during the illness, although not necessarily concurrently.
- The tics may wax and wane in frequency but have persisted for more than 1 year since first tic onset.
- Onset occurs before age 18 years.
- The disturbance is not caused by the direct physiologic effects of a substance or a general medical condition.

Gilles de la Tourette syndrome, or Tourette syndrome, was named after French neurologist Georges Gilles de la Tourette, who in 1885 described a series of nine patients with chronic tics. Tourette syndrome is a neuropsychiatric illness that begins in childhood. It is characterized by multiple motor and vocal tics that last for longer than 1 year (see Current Diagnosis box). The prevalence of Tourette syndrome varies greatly among epidemiologic studies, ranging from 0.1% to 3.8%. The prevalence of tic disorders is even higher, especially in children requiring special education.

Simple motor tics are sudden, brief, patterned movements such as eye blinking, facial grimace, head jerk, or shoulder shrug. Complex motor tics can involve a series of simple tics or a seemingly purposeful action, such as jumping, touching, or copropraxia (i.e., performing obscene gestures). Simple vocal tics consist of sounds such as throat clearing, sniffing, and coughing. Patients with complex vocal tics may exhibit echolalia (i.e., repeating others' words), palilalia (i.e., repeating their own words), or coprolalia (i.e., utterance of foul language).

Older children and adolescents often describe a premonitory urge before their tics. Tics can usually be transiently suppressed and are often diminished during focused mental or physical activities. Unlike myoclonus or chorea, tics usually do not affect activities of daily living or occupational or recreational activities. After the brief suppression, the release of the tic often brings relief to the patient. Tic severity commonly worsens during times of emotional stress. Fatigue or illness may also increase tics. Parents often notice more tics when the child is bored or unoccupied with an activity. Tics can occur during light sleep and rapid eye movement (REM) sleep.

Clinical Course

The onset of tics can occur after children are 3 years old, but they usually begin in children 6 to 7 years old. Children often present with motor tics first, followed by the development of vocal tics. Tics often wax and wane in the course of Tourette syndrome. During the early school years, tics often can go unnoticed or be mislabeled as a habit. If tics are noticed by fellow students, bullying is typically not an issue at this age. However, when parents notice the tics, they are often distressed and frequently tell their children to stop the movements.

Tic severity usually increases in the later elementary school years and into adolescence. This is the time when social interference such as bullying begins to occur. By late adolescence and early adulthood, most patients with Tourette syndrome have minimal tics, and some may "outgrow" tics. Because of this pattern, most individuals presenting for medical attention for tics are children.

Patients with Tourette syndrome frequently present with comorbid attention-deficit/hyperactivity disorder (ADHD) and obsessive-compulsive disorder (OCD). They also tend to have more sleep problems, anxiety, and mood disorders.

BOX 1 — Therapeutic Approach for Tourette Syndrome

- Educate the patient and family about tics and how tics often diminish spontaneously. Long-term reductions in tics may occur in the late teens, irrespective of pharmacologic therapy.
- Rank the tics, attention-deficit/hyperactivity disorder (ADHD), obsessive-compulsive disorder (OCD), anxiety, mood problems, learning problems, and behavior problems in order of the patient's or the family's perception of severity.
- Consider nonpharmacologic and pharmacologic treatment for each symptom in the order of perceived severity or impairment.
- Provide information to educate teachers and classmates to reduce social impairment.
- If the patient has learning problems, encourage formal assessment through the school or a psychologist. These children may qualify for modified educational methods.
- If ADHD is the most concerning problem, consider treating with clonidine (Kapvay), guanfacine (Intuniv), atomoxetine (Strattera), or methylphenidate (Ritalin). Stimulants are *not* absolutely contraindicated in patients with Tourette syndrome. However, if symptoms of OCD, anxiety, or pervasive developmental disorder are present, ticcing or compulsions may escalate on stimulants. If a patient has done well for months to years on stimulants for ADHD before an exacerbation of tics, it usually is not necessary to discontinue stimulants.
- If behavior problems are the most concerning problem or if a first-degree family member has a bipolar or psychotic disorder, refer the patient to a psychologist or psychiatrist.
- Anxious parents often worsen tic severity. If the family's anxiety is excessive, refer family members to a psychologist.
- If OCD or generalized anxiety disorder is the most severe problem, treatment with a selective serotonin reuptake inhibitor may be considered.
- Do not begin treatment with more than one central nervous system drug simultaneously. Start one, wait 2 to 4 weeks, and then reassess all symptoms before starting the next medication.
- Monitor the benefits and side effects at regular intervals.
- Maintain stable dosing during the school year; consider tapering medications in the summer.
- Consider weaning tic-suppressing medications in the middle to late teen years if tics wane.

Diagnosis and Differential Diagnosis

Diagnosis of tic disorders depends on correctly recognizing that the abnormal movements are tics by means of a careful history and thorough physical examination. Laboratory and imaging studies are rarely needed.

Tics may resemble other abnormal movements, such as stereotypy, chorea, ballism, dystonia, and myoclonus. *Stereotypies* are repetitive, simple movements that are suppressible and that usually occur when a child is excited. Stereotypies usually start when the child is younger than 3 years. *Chorea* consists of a sequence of random, continual, involuntary, nonpurposeful, nonrhythmic movements. Choreic movements often flow from one body part to another. *Ballism* is a large-amplitude choreic movement affecting the proximal limb. *Myoclonus* is an involuntary, sudden, shocklike movement. Chorea, ballism, and myoclonus cannot be volitionally suppressed. *Dystonia* is produced by co-contraction of agonist and antagonist muscles, leading to abnormal postures, and its twisting movements typically are slower than tics.

Vocal tics may sometimes lead to the misdiagnosis of asthma, chronic cough, or allergic rhinitis. Other primary tic disorders include Provisional Tic Disorder, Persistent (Chronic) Motor or Vocal Tic Disorder, Other Specified Tic Disorder and Unspecified Tic Disorder (DSM-5).

Tics are nonspecific and may occur in drug-induced movement disorders, after head trauma, and in a variety of neurodevelopmental and neurodegenerative disorders. Complex or atypical cases with multiple comorbidities or multiple abnormalities identified on a general or neurologic examination should be referred for specialist consultation.

A controversial diagnosis in which tics or OCD may occur is called pediatric autoimmune neuropsychiatric disorders associated with streptococcal infections (PANDAS). Criteria for this diagnosis classically include abrupt appearance in prepubertal children of tics or OCD on two or more occasions after documented group A β-hemolytic streptococcal (GABHS) infections. The paradigm for this diagnosis is rheumatic (Sydenham's) chorea; however, PANDAS has no arthritis, carditis, or nephritis and is not thought to be a rheumatic disease. As a result of recent epidemiological studies, tics are no longer considered a primary symptom of PANDAS. The following interventions are not routinely recommended: diagnostic throat cultures and antistreptococcal antibody tests; therapeutic or preventive antibiotics; and immune-modulating therapies such as steroids, intravenous immunoglobulins, or plasmapheresis. Specialty consultation should be considered.

Treatment

There are many factors to consider when treating a patient with Tourette syndrome, including the presence of common symptoms such as inattentiveness, hyperactivity, obsessive or compulsive behaviors, depression, and anxiety (Box 1). When deciding to treat the patient, it is important to prioritize all the neuropsychiatric symptoms and provide accurate educational information. Tics may not always need to be treated medically, and if treatment is needed, tics may not be the first symptom to manage. Daily tic-suppressing medication is considered when there is functional interference, social interference, pain, or classroom or occupational disruption.

The first step in treating Tourette syndrome is educating the patient, parents, and other adult caregivers. Parents, teachers, and other adult caregivers are discouraged from telling the child to stop ticcing because this produces emotional anxiety that may worsen the tics. Educational materials for teachers often promote a conducive environment for the child at school. The patient is encouraged to openly talk about his or her disorder to classmates to promote understanding and minimize bullying. Newer cognitive-behavioral treatments for tic suppression appear to be helpful for children and adolescents, and they should be considered.

Clinical trials enrolling patients with Tourette syndrome are usually small and show small effect sizes. Most commonly used tic-suppressing medications belong to two classes: α_2-adrenergic agonists and dopamine receptor blocking agents (Table 1). Other agents may show modest benefit. Because Tourette syndrome is a chronic, nonfatal disorder, it is prudent to start treatment with medications that carry the least side effects. For this reason, α_2-adrenergic agonists are usually the first-line treatment. Although it is unclear what the second-line agents should be, it is reasonable in many cases to restrict dopamine receptor blocking agents to the most severe cases.

α_2-Adrenergic Agonists

Clonidine (Catapres)[1] and guanfacine (Tenex)[1] are α_2-adrenergic agonists often used to treat tics. Several randomized trials have shown that these agents reduce tic and ADHD symptoms. The main side effects are sedation and lightheadedness due to mild hypotension. Sedation is more common with clonidine. The clonidine patch (Catapres-TTS)[1] may produce less peak sedation, but it commonly produces local skin irritation.

---

[1]Not FDA approved for this indication.

| **TABLE 1** | Therapy for Tics in Tourette Syndrome | | | |
MEDICATION	STARTING DOSE	TITRATION	GOAL DOSE
Clonidine (Kapvay)[1]	0.05 mg qhs	0.05 mg every 3–7 d	0.05–0.1 mg tid
Clonidine patch (Catapres-TTS)[1]	Catapres TTS-1 weekly*	Weekly as needed	Catapres TTS-1, TTS-2, or TTS-3 weekly*
Guanfacine (Intuniv)[1]	0.5 mg qhs	0.5 mg every 3–7 d	1–4 mg divided bid
Baclofen (Lioresal)[1]	10 mg qhs	10 mg every 3–7 d	40–90 mg/d divided bid/tid
Clonazepam (Klonopin)[1]	0.5 mg qhs	0.5 mg every wk	1–2 mg bid
Topiramate (Topamax)[1]	25 mg qhs	25–50 mg weekly	50–100 mg bid
Pimozide (Orap)	1 mg qhs	1 mg every 3–5 d	1–4 mg/d divided daily or bid
Haloperidol (Haldol)	0.25–0.5 mg qhs	0.25–0.5 mg every 5–7 d	1–4 mg/d divided daily or bid
Fluphenazine (Prolixin)[1]	0.5 mg qhs	0.5 mg every 3–5 d	1–4 mg/d divided daily or bid
Risperidone (Risperdal)[1]	0.5 mg qhs	0.5 mg every 3–5 d	1–4 mg/d divided daily or bid
Ziprasidone (Geodon)[1]	20 mg qhs	20 mg every wk	20–80 mg/d divided daily or bid
Aripiprazole (Abilify)	1 mg qhs	1 mg every wk	1–20 mg daily or divided bid
Botulinum toxin type A (Botox)[1]	Not applicable	Not applicable	30–300 units in one or more focal sites, injected once every 3 mo

[1]Not FDA approved for this indication.

*The system areas are 3.5 cm^2 (Catapres TTS-1), 7.0 cm^2 (Catapres TTS-2), and 10.5 cm^2 (Catapres TTS-3), and the amount of drug released is directly proportional to the area.

Dopamine Receptor Blocking Agents

Typical and atypical neuroleptics are dopamine receptor blocking agents that can be used to treat tics. Neuroleptics such as pimozide (Orap) and haloperidol (Haldol) can be very effective in tic suppression, but they can cause acute akathisia, dystonic reactions, cognitive blunting, acute anxiety with somatizations and school refusal, sedation, weight gain, metabolic syndrome, and QT prolongation. Monitoring for tardive dyskinesia is also important. Some experts recommend baseline electrocardiograms, particularly for individuals with personal or family history of cardiac arrhythmias. Weight gain and metabolic syndrome should be considered when starting neuroleptics, particularly risperidone (Risperdal)[1] and aripiprazole (Abilify).[1] Some experts recommend obtaining baseline values for weight, blood pressure, fasting glucose, and lipid profile, with follow-up monitoring every 3 months to detect drug-induced metabolic syndrome. Diet modification, routine exercise, or medical therapy may be needed.

Other Tic-Suppressing Medications

Several small, controlled studies show benefit for topiramate (Topamax),[1] dopamine agonists,[1] baclofen (Lioresal)[1], benzodiazepines,[1] and botulinum toxin type A (Botox)[1] injections for focal, strong tics. Tetrabenazine (Xenazine)[1] has been reported to reduce tics.

Behavioral Therapy

Recent clinical trials show that Comprehensive Behavioral Intervention for Tics, in which the patient learns to increase self-awareness of tics and premonitory urges and to perform antagonistic movements, reduces tics.

Treatment of Comorbid Conditions

ADHD and OCD are common comorbid conditions in Tourette syndrome. These comorbid symptoms are often more debilitating than the tics. Concern about stimulant therapy worsening tics was addressed by the Tourette Syndrome Study Group in the landmark Treatment of ADHD in Children with Tics (TACT) study. In this study, children treated with methylphenidate (Ritalin) had, on average, reduced tic severity, contrary to the widely held belief that stimulants exacerbate tics.

Medical treatment options for ADHD include psychostimulants, α_2=adrenergic agonists guanfacine (Intuniv) and clonidine (Kapvay), and the selective norepinephrine reuptake inhibitor atomoxetine (Strattera). OCD management includes cognitive-behavioral therapy, clomipramine (Anafranil), and any of the selective serotonin reuptake inhibitors.

Summary

Tourette syndrome is a complex neuropsychiatric illness with many potential symptoms that may need medical and nonmedical therapies. Cooperation among the primary care physician, neurologist, psychiatrist, and psychologist is imperative for the comprehensive care of severely affected patients. If a patient has mild tics and few or no comorbid symptoms, medical therapy may not be needed. However, if the tics are severe in the presence of many neuropsychiatric symptoms, it is reasonable to refer patients to specialists.

References

Bloch MH, Panza KE, Landeros-Weisenberger A, Leckman JF: Meta-analysis: treatment of attention-deficit/hyperactivity disorder in children with comorbid tic disorders, *J Am Acad Child Adolesc Psychiatry* 48:884–893, 2009.

Gilbert DL, Jankovic J: Pharmacological treatment of tourette syndorme, *Journal of Obsessive-Compulsive and Related Disorders* 3:407–414, 2014.

Leckman JF, King RA, Gilbert DL, et al: Streptococcal upper respiratory tract infections and exacerbations of tic and obsessive-compulsive symptoms: a prospective longitudinal study, *J Am Acad Child Adolesc Psychiatry* 50:108–118, 2011. e3.

Piacentini J, Woods DW, Scahill L, et al: Behavior therapy for children with Tourette disorder: a randomized controlled trial, *JAMA* 303:1929–1937, 2010.

Zinner SH, Mink JW: Movement disorders I: tics and stereotypies, *Pediatr Rev* 31:223–233, 2010.

SPORTS-RELATED HEAD INJURIES

Method of
Brandon Hockenberry, MD; Margaret Pusateri, MD; and Christopher McGrew, MD

CURRENT DIAGNOSIS

- Initial evaluation of any sports-related head injury should follow standard emergency medicine procedures.
- Presence of any "red flag" symptoms is concerning for a more serious head injury (skull fracture and intracranial hemorrhage) and requires emergency evaluation.
- If advanced imaging is indicated, a noncontrast computed tomography (CT) scan of the head is the initial study of choice.
- If no "red flag" symptoms are present, one of several validated neuropsychological tests should be administered to evaluate cognitive function (e.g., Sports Concussion Assessment Tool, version 5 [SCAT 5]; https://bjsm.bmj.com/content/bjsports/early/2017/04/26/bjsports-2017-097506SCAT5.full.pdf).
- Ultimately, concussion is still a clinical diagnosis.
- Advanced neuroimaging, fluid biomarkers, genetic testing, helmet sensors, and video surveillance have all been purported as possible prognostic indicators but require further validation.

CURRENT THERAPY

- Blood pressure control is critical for patients with an intracranial hemorrhage.
- Small intracranial hemorrhages without midline shift or significant symptoms may be monitored, but surgical decompression is otherwise required.
- For patients requiring sedation, propofol (Diprivan)[1] is often preferred due to its short half-life, making it easier to monitor neurologic status.
- Mannitol can also be used to help lower intracranial pressure.
- For posttraumatic seizures, phenytoin (Dilantin)[1] is the preferred medication.
- If there is any concern for concussion, the athlete should immediately be removed from play.
- An athlete should never be allowed to return to play on the same day as the injury.
- After an initial rest period of 24 to 48 hours, an athlete should begin progressing through return-to-play and "return-to-learn" protocols (https://www.cdc.gov/headsup/providers/return_to_activities.html).
- In the first 24 hours after injury, acetaminophen is the treatment of choice for associated headaches; nonsteroidal antiinflammatory drugs (NSAIDs) and aspirin can worsen an undiagnosed intracranial hemorrhage.
- If headaches persist greater than 3 to 5 days, medications that do not have a risk for rebound headaches (e.g., tricyclic antidepressants) can be used.
- Good sleep hygiene is important for recovery. If insomnia persists more than 2 to 3 days after injury, medications can be considered.
- Typical recovery time is up to 2 weeks in adults and 4 weeks in children.
- Access to a multidisciplinary team including physical therapists, neurologists, and psychiatric providers is beneficial for athletes with complicated or prolonged recoveries.
- If an athlete has a history of a learning disability, depression, anxiety, or chronic headaches, recovery can be complicated by an exacerbation of their underlying disease.

---

[1]Not FDA approved for this indication.

Introduction and Epidemiology

Sports-related head injuries include a heterogenous group of insults to the brain caused by either direct impact to the head or by an impact to the body associated with energy transfer into the head.

In the United States, sports are one of the leading causes of head injuries. Specifically between the ages of 15 and 24 years, athletic activities are the second-leading cause of head injuries, and only motor vehicle accidents have a higher incidence. Athletic and recreational activities vary widely in terms of biomechanics and kinetics, resulting in a wide range of associated risks. Many sports are limited by the speed at which an athlete can run (rugby or soccer), but others allow athletes to compete at much higher speeds, some nearly equivalent to motor vehicles (cycling or skiing). These sports potentially put athletes at a higher risk of more severe head injuries.

Sports- and recreation-related traumatic brain injuries (SRR-TBIs) are monitored by the National Electronic Injury Surveillance System-All Injury Program (NEISS-AIP). According to the NEISS-AIP, there were more than 3.4 million visits to emergency departments (EDs) across the United States for SRR-TBIs between 2001 and 2012, or approximately 340,000 per year.

Concussions are by far the most common head injury associated with athletic activity. It is estimated that there are 1.7 to 3.0 million concussions per year related to sports and recreational activities. The overall rate is 2.5 concussions per 10,000 athletic events, and concussions make up 5% to 18% of reported injuries in the National Collegiate Athletic Association. It is estimated that 50% of concussions go unreported or undiagnosed. The most common severe head injury is a subdural hematoma, which accounts for greater than 90% of all sport-related catastrophic head injuries. These are most often seen in American football, cheerleading, and skiing/snowboarding and occur in less than 1 per 100,000 athletic events. Fatalities from sports-related head injuries are very rare; however, subdural hematoma is a serious injury. In one study, it was reported that American football players with subdural hematoma had a fatality rate of 8.5% and a 48% rate of suffering permanent neurologic deficits.

Risk Factors

Every athlete is potentially at some risk for a head injury during activity. Many factors contribute to relative risk, with the type of activity being the largest contributing factor. In younger years, males sustain the most head injuries playing football or wrestling, whereas bicycling and basketball take over top spots after high school and college years. In females, bicycling and horseback riding contribute the most head injuries. It should be noted that some activities have higher incidence rates of head injuries than the aforementioned activities (men's/women's ice hockey) but are not as commonly played and therefore do not contribute to the sheer volume of injuries that other activities do. With respect to concussion specifically, men's ice hockey and football have the highest incidence rates (5.5 to 6.5 concussions per 10,000 athletic events) in the high school and college populations. On the women's side, soccer and lacrosse have the highest rates (3 to 3.5 concussions per 10,000 athletic events).

Children and teens are at increased risk for head injuries because of their immature development and increased participation in activities that have higher risk for head trauma. Overall, 70% of all SRR-TBIs are in the age group of 0 to 19 years. In the young athlete, a larger head-to-neck ratio, smaller amount of neck/shoulder musculature, and thinner cranial bones all contribute to an increased chance that a blow to the head will cause a head injury. The active elderly have better balance, fewer falls, and fewer TBIs than their more chronically ill counterparts. Therefore increased age is not an independent risk factor for SRR-TBIs.

At the high school and college level, men have more concussions than do women in sheer numbers but a lower incidence rate overall. Females may have greater risk because of decreased neck musculature compared with males. Female sex

TABLE 1	Red Flag Symptoms
Persistent vomiting	
Seizure	
Severe "worst headache of my life"	
Focal neurologic deficit	
Blurred vision	
Slurred speech	
Significant drowsiness/poor awakening	
Poor orientation to person/place/time	
Declining mental status	

The presence of any of these symptoms should prompt consideration of emergency department evaluation and head imaging. If no red flags are present, the clinician may be able to send the athlete home safely and follow up in the office the next day.

TABLE 2	Memory Assessment: Maddocks Questions
What venue are we at today?	
What half is it now?	
Who scored last in the game?	
What team did you play last week?	
Did your team win the last game?	
Note: Can be adapted to specific sports as necessary.	

These questions help make diagnosis of concussion. No official score cutoff is diagnostic; however, inability to answer them all correctly should raise suspicion for concussion or more severe head injury. Questions can be changed slightly if they are not relevant to a sport, such as swimming.

TABLE 3	Glasgow Coma Scale		
Best Eye Response (E)	**Best Verbal Response (V)**	**Best Motor Response (M)**
Eye opening spontaneously—4	Oriented—5	Obeys commands—6
Eye opening to voice—3	Confused—4	Localizes to pain—5
Eye opening to pain—2	Inappropriate words—3	Flexion/withdrawal from pain—4
No eye opening—1	Incomprehensible sounds—2	Abnormal flexion to pain—3
	No verbal response—1	Abnormal extension to pain—2
		No motor response—1

Used to rate severity of head injury. Scores in each category are added for a total of 15 points. Athletes with concussion typically have a Glasgow Coma Scale score of 14 (losing 1 point in the verbal response category) or 15. Scores less than 14 should prompt a visit to the emergency department for head imaging.

has been associated more commonly with abnormal imaging, surgical intervention, complication, and death. A history of previous concussion increases risk for future concussions compared with nonconcussed athletes, and the greatest risk for repeat concussion is during the 10-day period after the most recent concussion.

Pathophysiology

The pathophysiology of SRR-TBIs and sports-related concussion (SRC) is multifactorial. Several mechanisms have been identified. Biomechanically, a combination of acceleration, deceleration, rotational, and translational forces directly applied or transmitted to the head affect change at the level of individual cells. Metabolic derangements, neurotransmitter dysfunction, changes in cerebral blood flood, neuroinflammation, microstructural damage, and diffuse axonal injury have all been implicated as potential pathways. Helmet-based measurement studies have attempted to quantify head impacts, providing information on force, frequency, and location. However, results vary widely among athletes diagnosed with concussions. In addition, the accuracy of the data detected by helmet sensors and video surveillance systems has been called into question; it does not necessarily reflect the impact to the brain itself, and there is no evidence to support the use of such systems to attempt to diagnose SRC.

Assessment and Diagnosis of Sports-Related Head Injury

The initial assessment of any sports-related head injury should follow standard emergency medicine procedures. Assessment of the "ABCs" (airway, breathing, and circulation) and evaluation for concomitant cervical spine injury should be the first step in management. The presence of any "red flag" symptoms (Table 1) should raise concerns for a serious head injury, such as an intracranial hemorrhage or skull fracture, and requires immediate evaluation in the ED, likely advanced head or neck imaging, and possible specialist consultation. The appropriate emergency action plan should be initiated and the athlete stabilized and transported to the designated medical facility.

Once in the ED, the decision whether to obtain images needs to be made. Some assessment tools have been developed such as the Pediatric Emergency Care Applied Research Network (PECARN; https://www.mdcalc.com/pecarn-pediatric-head-injury-trauma-algorithm) and Canadian CT Head Injury algorithms. Glasgow Coma Scale score less than 14, palpable skull fracture, or presence of red flag symptoms would all be reasons to image acutely. The imaging test of choice after head injury is noncontrast head CT. A noncontrast CT will show fractures, intracranial hemorrhage, midline shifts, and signs of edema. CT with angiography will show decreased blood flow into cerebral vessels because of increased intracranial pressure. However, if increased intracranial

pressure due to malignant brain edema or expanding hematoma is suspected, more invasive intracranial pressure monitoring is a more accurate measure and will be more useful to management (see Table 1).

If no "red flag" symptoms are present and the athlete does not require emergency medical treatment, he or she should be removed from the field of play if there is any suspicion for possible SRC. Several brief neuropsychological tests have been developed to evaluate cognitive function. Examples of practical and validated tests include the Sports Concussion Assessment Tool version 5 (SCAT 5) and the Standardized Assessment of Concussion (SAC). The SCAT 5 is broken down into six steps: immediate or on-field assessment, symptom evaluation, cognitive screening, neurologic screening, delayed recall, and decision. In addition to an assessment of the aforementioned "red flag" symptoms, the immediate or on-field assessment section of the SCAT 5 also includes a review of observable signs (e.g., lying motionless on playing field, facial injury after head trauma, and blank or vacant look), a memory assessment using the Maddocks Questions (Table 2), a measure of the Glasgow Coma Scale (Table 3), and a cervical spine assessment. It has been found that standard orientation questions (name, location, and year) are not reliable in the immediate assessment of SRC. The Maddocks Questions, which focus on sport-specific memory assessment, provide better information to help the examiner determine whether there is a concern for an SRC. Once the initial assessment is complete, if there is any concern for an SRC, the athlete should be removed from the sporting environment and not allowed to return to play on the day of injury.

Diagnosis of SRC remains a clinical diagnosis. Over the past two decades, multiple investigations have focused on the use of advanced neuroimaging (e.g., functional magnetic resonance imaging [f-MRI] and electroencephalogram [EEG]) and body fluid analysis (blood, saliva, and cerebrospinal fluid) as potential tools to aid in the diagnosis of SRCs. (In addition, these modalities have also been explored as potential prognostic indicators, attempting to predict clinical recovery or assess the cumulative risk of repetitive trauma.) At this time, advanced neuroimaging, fluid biomarkers, and genetic testing are important research tools but require further validation to determine their ultimate clinical utility in evaluation and diagnosis of SRC.

Clinical Manifestations

Clinical manifestations after an SRR-TBI and SRC can be varied. The brain itself is a complex organ. Depending on which area is injured, different symptoms may present. With regard to the more serious diseases, such as intracranial hemorrhages or diffuse axonal injury, the athlete is often critically injured, again demonstrating "red flag" symptoms and signs of increased intracranial pressure. However, SRC is an evolving injury within the acute phase and can often have an initially subtle presentation. Signs and symptoms rapidly change, especially over the first 24 to 48 hours. Classically, symptoms fall into one of four categories: physical (headache, nausea, and dizziness), cognitive (difficulty concentrating and slowed reaction times), emotional (anxiety and irritability), and sleep disturbances (insomnia and hypersomnia). As part of the SCAT 5 and other concussion assessment tools, an in-depth symptom checklist is used to evaluate SRCs both initially and during follow-up. For example, Table 4 outlines the SCAT 5's symptom checklist. It is important to note that there are no specific scoring guidelines that are diagnostic of concussion. The scores are most commonly used to monitor an athlete's recovery, tracking improvement or decline over time. Of note, higher scores at the time of initial injury are associated with longer recoveries.

Treatment

Presence of red flag symptoms listed in Table 1 or a Glasgow Coma Scale of less than 14 should raise suspicion for a more severe SSR-TBI, such as a skull fracture or intracranial hemorrhage, rather than a typical concussion. If an athlete sustains an SSR-TBI other than concussion, they should be evaluated in the ED. In the event of an intracranial hemorrhage of any kind, the largest concern is increasing intracranial pressure. Strict blood pressure control is incredibly important because an increased blood pressure will increase the pressure in the bleeding vessel and thus the rate and severity of the bleed. Intracranial hemorrhages may be monitored if the bleed is small and not causing a midline shift or significant symptoms. However, definitive treatment with surgical decompression is preferred for subdural and epidural hemorrhages. Most patients will require intubation, sedation, and intracranial pressure monitoring. For sedation, propofol (Diprivan)[1] is the preferred agent at many institutions because it has a short half-life and makes it easier to monitor the patient's neurologic status. In the presence of malignant brain edema, mannitol (Osmitrol) can be added to decrease intracranial pressure when strict blood pressure and pain control has failed. For a TBI causing posttraumatic seizure, phenytoin (Dilantin)[1] remains the preferred medication, although many institutions will use older antiepileptic drugs such as valproate (Depakote)[1] or carbamazepine (Tegretol)[1] as treatments of choice.

Current recommendation for management of SRC is to remove the athlete from athletic activity and not allow to return the same day. The athlete should avoid physical exertion and mental activities that make symptoms worse. After an initial rest period of 24 to 48 hours, the patient should begin progressing both physical (noncontact) and mental activities. The athlete should return to normal activities of daily living as much as is tolerated without symptom exacerbation. The newest consensus statement on concussion in sport outlines not only a return-to-play protocol but also a "return-to-learn" protocol. These are outlined in Tables 5 and 6.

[1]Not FDA approved for this indication.

TABLE 4	SCAT 5 Symptoms Checklist
SYMPTOM	**SEVERITY**
Headache	0 1 2 3 4 5 6
"Pressure in head"	0 1 2 3 4 5 6
Neck pain	0 1 2 3 4 5 6
Nausea or vomiting	0 1 2 3 4 5 6
Dizziness	0 1 2 3 4 5 6
Blurred vision	0 1 2 3 4 5 6
Balance problems	0 1 2 3 4 5 6
Sensitivity to light	0 1 2 3 4 5 6
Sensitivity to noise	0 1 2 3 4 5 6
Feeling slowed down	0 1 2 3 4 5 6
Feeling like "in a fog"	0 1 2 3 4 5 6
"Don't feel right"	0 1 2 3 4 5 6
Difficulty concentrating	0 1 2 3 4 5 6
Difficulty remembering	0 1 2 3 4 5 6
Fatigue or low energy	0 1 2 3 4 5 6
Confusion	0 1 2 3 4 5 6
Drowsiness	0 1 2 3 4 5 6
More emotional	0 1 2 3 4 5 6
Irritability	0 1 2 3 4 5 6
Sadness	0 1 2 3 4 5 6
Nervous or anxious	0 1 2 3 4 5 6
Trouble falling asleep (if applicable)	0 1 2 3 4 5 6
Total number of symptoms	Of 22
Symptom severity score	Of 132

There is no score cutoff that is diagnostic of concussion; it is simply used to monitor a patient's improvement or decline over time. Higher scores at time of injury are associated with longer recovery times.
SCAT 5, Sports Concussion Assessment Tool version 5.

Children and adolescents should not return to sport until they have fully returned to school. It is important to note that there is no evidence to suggest that any medications or nutritional supplements will improve rate of recovery from concussion. Medications in concussion treatment are primarily used for symptomatic relief.

Monitoring Concussions

After concussion diagnosis, the clinically stable athlete can be sent home if a responsible adult is available. Sleep is encouraged, and the athlete does not need to be awakened for evaluation. The athlete should be followed up in a qualified healthcare provider's office within 24 to 48 hours for reevaluation. Follow-up examination should include a symptom severity checklist (see Table 4), history, and neurologic examination at a minimum. Completing a full SCAT 5 evaluation is unnecessary if the athlete had one done at time of injury and still has symptoms. Advanced neuroimaging with MRI is not needed to monitor a concussion and by definition should be normal.

As the athlete returns to play, close supervision under a qualified healthcare provider such as a certified athletic trainer or physical therapist is ideal but not always possible. When an athlete has progressed through the return-to-play protocol (see Table 5), follow-up with an appropriate qualified healthcare provider should be made to obtain full medical clearance to return to full contact activity.

TABLE 5 Graduated Return to Play Protocol as Outlined by the Consensus Statement on Concussion in Sport

STAGE	AIM	ACTIVITY	GOAL OF EACH STEP
1	Symptom-limited activity	Daily activities that do not provoke symptoms	Gradual reintroduction of work/school activities
2	Light aerobic exercise	Walking or stationary cycling at slow to medium pace; no resistance training	Increase heart rate
3	Sport-specific exercise	Running or skating drills; no head impact activities	Add movement
4	Noncontact training drills	Harder training drills, e.g., passing drills; may start progressive resistance training	Exercise, coordination, and increase thinking
5	Full-contact practice	After medical clearance, participate in normal training activities	Restore confidence and assess functional skills by coaching staff
6	Return to sport	Normal game play	

Start step 1 after initial 24 to 48-hour period of rest. Each step should take a minimum 24 hours to progress through.

TABLE 6 Example of a Graduated "Return-to-Learn" Protocol as Outlined by the Consensus Statement on Concussion in Sport

STAGE	AIM	ACTIVITY	GOAL OF EACH STEP
1	Daily activities that do not give the child symptoms	Typical activities of the child during the day as long as they do not increase symptoms (e.g., reading, texting, screen time). Start with 5–15 min at a time and build up	Gradual return to typical activities
2	School activities	Homework, reading, or other cognitive activities outside of the classroom	Increase tolerance to cognitive work
3	Return to school part time	Gradual introduction of schoolwork. May need to start with a partial school day or increased breaks during the day	Increase academic activities
4	Return to school full time	Gradually progress school activities until a full day can be tolerated	Return to full academic activities and catch up on missed work

Unlike the return-to-sport protocol, there is not a minimum required time for each stage. Some children may be able to tolerate a full school day immediately after injury without difficulty, depending on symptom severity.

Management of Concussion Complications

Headaches are one of the most common symptoms of a concussion and often the symptom that bothers the athlete the most. In the acute period after the injury, medications have some potential to mask important symptoms. For the first 1 to 2 hours after the injury, it is important to be able to accurately monitor the patient for changing clinical picture, which could suggest that the head injury is not a concussion but rather an evolving epidural or subdural hematoma. For the first 24 hours, nonsteroidal antiinflammatory drugs (NSAIDs) and aspirin should be avoided because they can thin the blood and potentially make an undiagnosed hematoma become a more significant bleed. Acetaminophen (Tylenol) is the preferred medication for headache in the first 24 hours. After the first day, it is safe to switch to ibuprofen (Motrin), which may have more benefit. If headaches are not improving after 3 to 5 days, it is advisable to switch to another medication that does not have the risk of creating rebound headaches. Tricyclic antidepressants are a good choice and work very well. Nortriptyline (Pamelor)[1] at a low dose (25 mg/day) is generally well tolerated in children as well as adults and may be stopped abruptly without withdrawal symptoms once the athlete is feeling well and ready to progress back to activities.

Sleep disturbances in athletes with concussion are also very common. Many will not sleep well the first night after injury and want to nap during the days. Other athletes may sleep much more than usual after initial injury. Although there are no clear studies proving the optimal amount of sleep, current trends are to try to return the athlete to normal sleep cycles and daily living as much as possible. Emphasizing sleep hygiene in the first few days is standard. If insomnia persists after 2 to 3 days, consider medications. Melatonin[7] is over the counter, has very few side effects, and is generally well tolerated. The next step would be amitriptyline (Elavil)[1] at a low dose (10 to 25 mg/day). This can be especially effective if the athlete has both headaches and poor sleep because it is more sedating than nortriptyline.

A concussion is expected to last no more than 14 days in an adult and less than 4 weeks in the pediatric population. Each individual physician will have a different comfort level treating concussion; however, it is reasonable to consider a referral to a specialty physician once an athlete has passed the normal expected recovery time and is not categorized as a "prolonged concussion." Each city or region will have a different culture about who takes care of the prolonged concussions. Neurologists, sports medicine physicians, and physical medicine and rehabilitation physicians are all well equipped to take care of these athletes. Physical therapists, particularly those who specialize in vestibular rehabilitation, can be very helpful in patients with continued balance problems, concentration difficulties, and other visual symptoms. Last, neuropsychologists can be incredibly helpful in difficult cases. Some athletes have complicated clinical histories prior to the injury. Attention-deficit/hyperactivity disorder, depression, anxiety, and chronic headaches can all make the clinical picture very confusing when the athlete is having symptoms such as concentration difficulties, mood swings, insomnia, or headaches that are not improving as expected. It is important to remember that many athletes would not rate their symptom severity score as all zeros at baseline, so expecting them to achieve this goal post injury is impractical. When this scenario is suspected, referral for neuropsychiatric testing can help divide out which symptoms may be concussion related and which could be more chronic in nature.

---

[1]Not FDA approved for this indication.

[7]Available as a dietary supplement.

Prevention

Helmets have been shown to reduce sports-related skull fractures and intracranial hemorrhages but have not been shown to decrease rates of concussion. Mouth guard use decreases the rate of dental injuries and lip lacerations but has not been definitively proven to decrease the rate of concussion or other brain injuries. Sport-specific rule changes have resulted in reduced rates of head injury. The most prominent and well-studied example is that of youth ice hockey. Introduction of the 2013 Canadian national body checking policy change disallowing body checking in Pee Wee hockey players below the age of 13 years resulted in a 50% relative reduction in injury rate and a 64% reduction in concussion rate in 11-year-old and 12-year-old hockey players in Alberta. Reduction of contact practices in certain team sports such as American football reduces exposure to head injury as well. Finally, epidemiologic evidence demonstrated that the most likely period for repeat sports-related concussion is in the first 10 days after the most recent concussion, so disallowing contact activity during this interval has potential to reduce repeat concussions.

References

Black AM, Hagel BE, Palacios-Derflingher L, et al: The risk of injury associated with body checking among Pee Wee ice hockey players: an evaluation of Hockey Canada's national body checking policy change, *Br J Sports Med* 51:1767–1772, 2017.

Coronado VG, Haileyesus T, Cheng TA, et al: Trends in sports-and recreation-related traumatic brain injuries treated in US emergency departments: The National Electronic Injury Surveillance System-All Injury Program (NEISS-AIP), 2001–2012, *J Head Trauma Rehabil* 30:185–197, 2015.

Gessel LM, Fields SK, Collins CL, et al: Concussions among United States high school and collegiate athletes, *J Athl Train* 42:495–503, 2007.

Harmon KG, Clugston JR, Dec K, et al: American Medical Society for Sports Medicine position statement on concussion in sport, *Br J Sports Med* 53:213–225, 2019.

Kerr ZY, Roos KG, Djoko A, et al: Epidemiologic measures for quantifying the incidence of concussion in National Collegiate Athletic Association sports, *J Athl Train* 52:167–174, 2017.

McCrory P, Meeuwisse W, Dvorak J, et al: Consensus statement on concussion in sport—the 5th international conference on concussion in sport held in Berlin, October 2016, *Br J Sports Med* 51:838–847, 2017.

Munivenkatappa A, Agrawal A, Shukla DP, et al: Traumatic brain injury: Does gender influence outcomes? *Int J Crit Illn Inj Sci* 6(2):70–73, 2016.

Nagahiro S, Mizobuchi Y: Current topics in sports-related head injuries: a review, *Neurol Med Chir (Tokyo)* 54:878–886, 2014.

Steenerson K, Starling AJ: Pathophysiology of sports-related concussion, *Neurol Clin* 35:403–408, 2017.

INTRACEREBRAL HEMORRHAGE

Method of
Joshua N. Goldstein, MD, PhD

CURRENT DIAGNOSIS

- Obtain a thorough history, including time of symptom onset
- Imaging of the cerebral vessels should be performed in patients younger than 55 years and should be strongly considered in all patients in whom underlying aneurysm or arteriovenous malformation is suspected.
- Obtain contrast-enhanced neuroimaging if underlying cerebral mass or tumor is suspected.

CURRENT THERAPY

- Maintain airway, breathing, and circulation; stabilize the neck if fracture is considered.
- Detect and emergently correct coagulopathy.
- Arrange emergent neurosurgical consultation for cerebellar hemorrhage and intraventricular hemorrhage.

Epidemiology

Intracerebral hemorrhage (ICH) is most often the acute manifestation of a chronic, progressive disorder of the blood vessels of the brain. With an estimated incidence rate of between 35 and 45 cases per 100,000 population in Europe and North America, ICH generally accounts for between 10% and 15% of acute strokes on those continents. The incidence is higher in East Asia, with estimates that ICH accounts for as many as 30% to 40% of acute stroke cases in those countries. Hospital-based series consistently suggest that mortality from ICH ranges between 35% and 65% and substantial permanent disability occurs in at least 50% of survivors.

Risk Factors

Risk factors for primary ICH include chronic conditions, chronic exposures, and acute physiologic derangements. Secondary ICH refers to hemorrhage that develops in the setting of vascular malformations, including saccular aneurysms, brain tumor, cerebral venous thrombosis, or hemorrhagic conversion of an ischemic infarct. Among patients older than 55 years, who account for the majority of cases, chronic hypertension, cerebral amyloid angiopathy, and chronic use of antithrombotic medication are the leading risk factors for primary ICH. History of a prior stroke, chronic alcohol use, and family history of ICH also contribute, and patients with severe coagulopathy, cocaine abuse, and liver disease are also at higher risk for ICH. Accumulating data suggest that aggressive lowering of serum cholesterol or chronic use of statin therapy can increase risk for ICH in the elderly. Although chronic hypertension has long been identified as contributing to the largest proportion of ICH cases, recent population-based studies demonstrate a substantial fall in hypertension-associated ICH. In parallel, however, the aging of the population has led to the broader use of antithrombotic medications as well as increases in the prevalence of amyloid angiopathy. The result is that ICH incidence rates overall have not fallen.

Pathophysiology

ICH arises when a blood vessel within the brain ruptures and blood leaks out to form a hematoma. Because the skull is fixed in volume and is completely filled by brain, blood, and CSF, any accumulation of blood within the brain must necessarily compress, distort, and disrupt surrounding brain structures. The result is that the damage caused by ICH is due to mass effect of the hematoma as well as the toxic effects of the blood itself. The volume of blood that leaks out is thus the most potent predictor of outcome from ICH. In addition, extravasated blood can enter the CSF drainage system, leading to hydrocephalus, another predictor of poor outcome.

Bleeding in ICH often occurs over hours, a phenomenon that can be documented with serial head computed tomography (CT) scans. The volume of ICH can be compared between a CT scan obtained at the time of presentation to the emergency department and one obtained several hours later. The shorter the time interval between symptom onset and presentation to the emergency department, the more likely the patient is to have ongoing bleeding and hematoma expansion after the initial CT scan.

Location of the ICH within the brain can be a clue to the underlying vessel abnormality responsible for the rupture. Among patients 55 years and older, hemorrhage in lobar locations, the junction of the cortical gray matter and underlying white matter, is most commonly a manifestation of underlying cerebral amyloid angiopathy, although other underlying conditions such as chronic hypertension and an underlying vascular malformation may instead be responsible. By contrast, hemorrhages centered in the deep gray structures of the basal ganglia, thalamus, and the brain stem arise most often as a complication of chronic hypertension, with amyloid angiopathy playing no role. Hemorrhages in the cerebellum can arise from any of these conditions.

ICH in the setting of chronic antithrombotic therapy is increasing in incidence as use of anticoagulants becomes increasingly widespread. Although it is likely that excessive doses of antithrombotic medication can cause ICH, the majority of cases in patients receiving antithrombotic medication occur in the absence of an overdose. This suggests that the majority of cases of antithrombotic-associated ICH arise in patients with an underlying disorder of the cerebral vessels such as cerebral amyloid angiopathy or hypertensive vasculopathy.

Recurrent ICH is common among survivors of ICH. In particular, patients 55 years and older who survive a lobar hemorrhage have a risk of recurrent lobar ICH in the range of 10% per year. The explanation for this is likely the inexorable progression of the underlying blood vessel disease, amyloid angiopathy. On the other hand, whereas survivors of ICH in the nonlobar regions are also at high risk for recurrent ICH, adequate control of hypertension following the initial ICH appears to substantially reduce that risk, suggesting that hypertension-related disease of the cerebral blood vessels can be arrested.

Prevention

Adequate control of chronic hypertension reduces the incidence of ICH in addition to reducing the incidence of a broad range of other cardiovascular conditions. Although no specific therapies have been shown to be effective in preventing ICH in patients with cerebral amyloid angiopathy, recognition of this condition might become useful in selecting patients for long-term antithrombotic use. Chronic statin therapy can increase risk of ICH, but more studies are required to inform the decision to withhold statins from patients at high risk for ICH.

Clinical Manifestations

Symptomatic ICH manifests with an acute stroke syndrome such as the sudden development of impaired consciousness, language difficulty, disorientation, or weakness. Nausea and vomiting can be prominent, particularly in patients with cerebellar hemorrhages as well as those who rapidly develop substantial mass effect or hydrocephalus. Headache and seizure at the onset of symptoms are more common in ICH than in ischemic stroke.

Small asymptomatic ICH also occurs in the setting of diseases like chronic hypertension and cerebral amyloid angiopathy. These hemorrhages, usually only detectable on magnetic resonance imaging (MRI) of the brain that includes susceptibility-weighted sequences sensitive to the permanent hemosiderin deposits left by all hemorrhages, are increasingly recognized as contributing to age-related deterioration in cognition, memory, and gait.

Diagnosis

ICH is a medical emergency. Rapid diagnosis and urgent critical care management (airway, breathing, circulation) are essential, particularly because ICH patients can deteriorate rapidly within hours of presentation. Noncontrast CT scan of the brain is the gold standard for confirming acute ICH, and all patients with suspected acute stroke or ICH should undergo an emergent noncontrast CT scan. In centers where emergent MRI is available, it can be substituted for noncontrast CT only if susceptibility-weighted sequences are performed. Angiographic imaging in the form of traditional catheter-based angiography or CT angiography should be performed in any patient younger than 55 years or in patients in whom underlying vascular malformation or ruptured saccular aneurysm is suspected. The history and laboratory evaluation, summarized in Box 1, should be focused on identifying possible contributing causes as well as targets for treatment.

Differential Diagnosis

Emergent neuroimaging can confirm the presence of ICH (Box 2). For patients in whom the history is not obtainable, or who have associated trauma, it is sometimes difficult to distinguish traumatic from nontraumatic ICH. It is therefore essential to examine head imaging for skull fractures and the presence of subdural or subarachnoid hemorrhage, which might be traumatic in origin.

Treatment

After the focused evaluation (see Box 1) is completed, emergency care is devoted to preventing neurologic deterioration (Box 3). Blood pressure elevation is common in ICH; clinical trials suggest that reducing systolic blood pressure below 140 is safe but does

---

BOX 1   Focused Evaluation of Intracerebral Hemorrhage

Assess airway, breathing, circulation

History
Time of symptom onset (or when last seen well)
Recent trauma or surgery
Headache
Seizures
Alcohol or drug abuse
History of hypertension
Prior stroke
Liver disease
Cancer
Coagulopathy
Medications, including antithrombotics

Physical Examination
General physical examination
Glasgow Coma Scale
NIH stroke scale

Neuroimaging
Computed tomography, magnetic resonance imaging
CT angiography for patients younger than 55 years or in whom an underlying vascular lesion is suspected
Venography if venous sinus thrombosis is suspected
Cervical spine imaging if trauma is suspected

Laboratory
Electrolytes
Complete blood count
Coagulation panel
Toxicology screen
Electrocardiogram

Abbreviation: NIH = National Institutes of Health.

BOX 2   Differential Diagnosis of Intracerebral Hemorrhage

Primary Intracerebral Hemorrhage
Cerebral small-vessel disease
Cerebral amyloid angiopathy
Hypertensive vasculopathy

Secondary Intracerebral Hemorrhage
Vascular malformations
Cerebral venous thrombosis
Hemorrhagic conversion of an ischemic infarct
Moya moya disease
Cerebral vasculitis
Bacterial endocarditis
Brain tumor
Trauma

---

not clearly improve outcomes. Many clinicians lower systolic blood pressure below 160.

Because ICH is a devastating condition that most commonly affects the elderly, physicians and families are often confronted with the question of whether their patient or loved one would choose to survive the event. Accurate prediction of prognosis is essential to guide such decision-making. The most commonly used tool to risk stratify patients for mortality is the ICH score (Table 1). A tool to predict the likelihood of functional recovery among survivors is the FUNC score (Table 2). Tools such as the FUNC score calculator (http://www.massgeneral.org/stopstroke/funcCalculator.aspx) can be useful in guiding decisions about aggressiveness of care, but their precision remains to be proved. Clinicians are advised to provide care according to the principles outlined in this chapter for all patients at the outset, and to defer decisions to limit aggressiveness of care for the first 24 hours.

BOX 3 | Targeted Therapy to Prevent Deterioration in Acute Intracerebral Hemorrhage

Neck stabilization in any patient at risk for cervical spine injury

Anticoagulant-associated ICH: In those on vitamin K antagonists, correct prothrombin time as rapidly as possible using intravenous vitamin K and prothrombin complex concentrate. Dabigatran (Pradaxa) can be reversed with idarucizumab (Praxbind). Rivaroxaban (Xarelto) and apixaban (Eliquis) can be reversed with andexanet (Andexxa), although many centers use prothrombin complex concentrates.

Severe thrombocytopenia or coagulation factor deficiency: Platelet and/or factor replacement. Platelet transfusion should not be given simply to treat those taking oral antiplatelet agents, as it worsens outcomes.

Blood pressure: Reduce systolic BP to less than 180 mm Hg for patients whose systolic BP is >220 mm Hg.

Avoid hypoglycemia.

Maintain euthermia.

Anticonvulsant medication: Only in patients who have had a seizure.

External ventricular drainage catheters: Consider for any patient with hydrocephalus or intraventricular hemorrhage.

Emergent surgical clot removal: Indicated for cerebellar hemorrhage with brain stem compression or neurologic deterioration.

Prevention of deep venous thrombosis: Intermittent pneumatic compression device and elastic stockings. Low-dose heparin should be started once serial CT scans confirm that bleeding has stopped and there is no longer any ICH expansion occurring.

Rehabilitation: Multidisciplinary rehabilitation should be offered to all ICH patients.

Abbreviations: BP = blood pressure; CT = computed tomography; ICH = intracerebral hemorrhage.

TABLE 2 | FUNC Score

COMPONENT	FUNC SCORE POINTS
ICH Volume (cm³)	
<30	0
30–59	2
≥60	3
Age (y)	
<70	0
70–79	1
≥80	2
ICH Location	
Lobar	0
Deep	1
Infratentorial	2
Glasgow Coma Scale Score	
≥8	0
<8	2
Pre-ICH Cognitive Impairment	
No	0
Yes	1
Total FUNC score	0–10

Abbreviation: ICH = intracerebral hemorrhage.

Monitoring

Initial monitoring of the ICH patient is best provided by an intensive care unit with neurointensive care specialists available. Because subclinical seizures are common in ICH patients, EEG monitoring should be considered in any patient who has had a seizure or whose level of consciousness is altered. Invasive monitoring of intracranial pressure should be considered in patients with evidence of shift of the intracranial contents on neuroimaging.

Complications

Prevention of ICH, particularly recurrent ICH, is increasingly recognized as a priority in making decisions about whether or not to offer chronic anticoagulation to elderly patients with atrial fibrillation, prosthetic heart valves, and other conditions accompanied by high risk of thromboembolic ischemic stroke. Given the established benefit of antithrombotic therapy for preventing ischemic stroke, decision-analysis models suggest that only patients at very high risk for ICH might benefit from antiplatelet therapy rather than anticoagulation, or even neither therapy. Factors that must be considered include the patient's risk for recurrent ICH, risk for thromboembolic stroke, expected outcomes from each should they occur, and the patient's preferences.

TABLE 1 | ICH Score

COMPONENT	ICH SCORE POINTS
Glasgow Coma Score	
3-4	2
5-12	1
13-15	0
Age (y)	
<80	0
≥80	1
ICH Volume	
<30	0
>=30	1
Intraventricular Hemorrhage	
No	0
Yes	1
Infratentorial location	
No	0
Yes	1
Total ICH score	0–6

References

Eckman MH, Rosand J, Knudsen KA, et al: Can patients be anticoagulated after intracerebral hemorrhage? A decision analysis, *Stroke* 34:1710–1716, 2003.

Eckman MH, Wong LK, Soo YO, et al: Patient-specific decision-making for warfarin therapy in nonvalvular atrial fibrillation: how will screening with genetics and imaging help? *Stroke* 39:3308–3315, 2008.

Kothari RU, Brott T, Broderick JP, et al: The ABCs of measuring intracerebral hemorrhage volumes, *Stroke* 27:1304–1305, 1996.

Hemphill, et al: Guidelines for the management of spontaneous intracerebral hemorrhage, *Stroke* 2015.

Hemphill 3rd JC, Farrant M, Neill TA Jr, Prospective validation of the ICH Score for 12-month functional outcome, *Neurology* 73(14):1088–1094, 2009 Oct 6.

Qureshi AI, et al: Intensive Blood-Pressure Lowering in patients with acute cerebral hemorrhage, *NEJM* 375(11):1033–1043, 2016 Sep 15.

Steiner T, et al: Fresh frozen plasma versus prothrombin complex concentrate in patients with intracranial haemorrhage related to vitamin K antagonists (INCH): a randomised trial, *Lancet Neurol* 15(6):566–573, 2016 May.

ISCHEMIC CEREBROVASCULAR DISEASE

Method of
Alvaro Cervera, MD, PhD; and Geoffrey A. Donnan, MD

Treatment of ischemic stroke has improved significantly in the past few years, and mortality and disability rates owing to this condition have decreased. The management of patients in stroke units and the demonstration of the efficacy of thrombolysis and thrombectomy have been crucial in this achievement. Control of vascular risk factors has decreased the number and severity of events. However, recent studies have found an increased incidence of ischemic stroke in the young. Improved management has included high-quality rehabilitation, which has to start early to improve the recovery (i.e., functional independence) of stroke survivors. The multidisciplinary management of stroke can be improved with specific educational programs aimed at increasing awareness of stroke in the general population and among professionals. The concept of *time is brain* has great value in emphasizing that stroke is an emergency. Because the window for the available time-dependent treatments is very narrow, avoiding delay is the major goal in the prehospital phase of acute stroke care. Therefore it is important to transport all stroke patients as soon as possible to the closest hospital with a stroke unit. In rural or remote areas with no stroke unit facilities, telemedicine has proven to be a valid alternative.

Prevention

Lifestyle modification can be a major contributor to reducing the risk of ischemic stroke. Strategies to achieve this protection include avoiding smoking and excessive alcohol consumption, keeping a low/normal body mass index, practicing regular exercise, and having a diet low in salt and saturated fat, high in fruits and vegetables, and rich in fiber. In addition, Mediterranean diet supplemented with nuts is associated with a decreased risk of vascular events. There is no need to add vitamin supplements to the diet because they have no impact in stroke prevention.

Regular assessment of vascular risk factors (e.g., hypertension, diabetes, and hypercholesterolemia) is important because their control can reduce significantly the incidence of vascular events. In the case of blood pressure, this can be done with diet and pharmacologic therapy, aiming at normal levels of 120/80 mm Hg. After an ischemic stroke, blood pressure should be lowered even in patients with normal blood pressure. Diabetes should be managed with lifestyle modification and pharmacologic therapy as required, and blood pressure needs to be more tightly controlled in these patients (<130/80 mm Hg). The best antihypertensive treatments for diabetics are angiotensin-converting enzyme inhibitors or angiotensin receptor antagonists. Hypercholesterolemia should be managed with lifestyle modification and a statin. After a noncardioembolic ischemic stroke, statins are beneficial in all patients for secondary prevention.

Postmenopausal hormone replacement therapy should be avoided for the primary or secondary prevention of stroke because it can increase the risk of new vascular events. Other strategies to prevent stroke include the treatment of obstructive sleep apnea with continuous positive airway pressure breathing.

Antithrombotic Therapy

Low-dose aspirin can be used for the primary prevention of stroke in women or of myocardial infarction in men. Nevertheless, its effect is very small, and it cannot be recommended on a population-wide basis. Aspirin is beneficial for the prevention of stroke in patients with asymptomatic carotid stenosis.

In patients with atrial fibrillation, the CHA2DS2-VASc scale (Table 1) is used to decide whether to use anticoagulation. If the score (https://www.mdcalc.com/chads2-score-atrial-fibrillation-stroke-ris) is 2 or more, treatment with oral anticoagulants is indicated. With a score of 1, the decision should be made according to the presence of risk factors, risk of bleeding, and patient choice. If the score is 0, there is no need to start antithrombotic treatment, neither antiplatelets nor anticoagulants. All patients with stroke or transient ischemic attack (TIA) should be anticoagulated, unless strictly contraindicated. Patients with valvular atrial fibrillation require anticoagulation with warfarin, aiming at an international normalized ratio (INR) of 2.0 to 3.0. Patients with prosthetic heart valves should also receive warfarin, and the target INR depends on the prosthesis type. In nonvalvular atrial fibrillation, the treatment options include warfarin (INR 2.0 to 3.0) or one of the new direct oral anticoagulants (dabigatran [Pradaxa], apixaban [Eliquis], rivaroxaban [Xarelto], and edoxaban [Savaysa]). The newer agents are associated with a decreased risk of intracranial hemorrhage when compared with warfarin. Dabigatran (150 mg twice daily) and apixaban (5 mg twice daily) have shown to be superior to warfarin in stroke prevention. The dose of the direct oral anticoagulants needs to be adjusted depending on age, renal function, or weight.

After an ischemic stroke, all patients should receive antithrombotic therapy. Antiplatelet agents are the first choice unless anticoagulation is required. The most effective regimen is clopidogrel (Plavix) or aspirin plus dipyridamole (Aggrenox). However, low-dose aspirin is a reasonable alternative. During the first 3 weeks after a minor stroke or TIA, the combination of aspirin plus clopidogrel can be more effective in reducing ischemic events than clopidogrel alone, although the evidence is scarce. However, dual antiplatelet treatment is not recommended in the long term, except if there is an association with unstable angina or non–Q wave myocardial infarction or if there has been a recent stenting. Anticoagulation is usually indicated for secondary prevention if the stroke cause is cardioembolic and in specific situations such as aortic arch atheroma or fusiform aneurysms of the basilar artery. However, level 1 evidence is lacking for these approaches.

Management of Carotid Stenosis

In patients with asymptomatic carotid stenosis (≥60%), surgery is indicated only if the risk of stroke is high. Endarterectomy is the treatment of choice if the stenosis is symptomatic (i.e., has been associated with an ipsilateral stroke or TIA) and severe (70% to 99%). Surgery should be performed in centers with a perioperative complication rate of less than 6% and as soon as possible after the last ischemic event.

Endarterectomy may be indicated for certain patients with moderate stenosis (50% to 69%), although it should be performed only in centers with a perioperative complication rate of less than 3% to be effective. In cases of symptomatic carotid lesions, angioplasty plus stenting is a reasonable alternative, mainly in patients younger than 70 years old. If stenting is performed, a combination of clopidogrel and aspirin is required immediately before the procedure and for at least 1 month to prevent stent thrombosis.

In patients with intracranial atheromatosis and stroke recurrences, intensive medical treatment is the preferred option. Angioplasty and stenting are not recommended.

TABLE 1 Prevention of Stroke in Patients With Atrial Fibrillation

CHA2DS2-VAS SCALE	
RISK FACTOR	**SCORE**
Congestive heart failure	1
Hypertension	1
Age ≥75	2
Age 65–74	1
Diabetes mellitus	1
Stroke or transient ischemic attack	2
Vascular disease	1
Female sex	1

BOX 1 — Treatment of Acute Ischemic Stroke: Intravenous Administration of Tissue Plasminogen Activator

- Infuse 0.9 mg/kg (maximum dose 90 mg) of tissue plasminogen activator (tPA [Activase]) over 60 min, with 10% of the dose given as a bolus over 1 min.
- Admit the patient to a stroke unit for monitoring. Perform neurologic assessment and blood pressure measurement every 15 min during the infusion, every 30 min thereafter for the next 6 h, and then hourly until 24 h after treatment. Administer antihypertensive medications to maintain systolic blood pressure ≤180 mm Hg and diastolic ≤105 mm Hg.
- If intracranial hemorrhage is suspected, discontinue the infusion and obtain an emergency computed tomography scan.
- Obtain a follow-up computed tomography scan at 24 h before starting anticoagulants or antiplatelet agents.

Management of Patent Foramen Ovale

The presence of a patent foramen ovale (PFO) is associated with cryptogenic stroke in the young. There is evidence that in selected patients with stroke or TIA (younger than 60 years of age, nonlacunar stroke, and exclusion of other causes of stroke) the percutaneous transcatheter closure of the PFO is associated with a significant reduction of new vascular events, although with more frequent atrial fibrillation postprocedure, usually transient. Otherwise, there is no evidence indicating that anticoagulation is more effective than antiplatelets for stroke prevention in patients with PFO.

Management of Acute Ischemic Stroke

All stroke patients should be treated in a stroke unit, because this is associated with a reduction of death, dependency, and the need for institutional care. This effect is present in all stroke patients, irrespective of gender, age, stroke subtype, and stroke severity. Patients with stroke should have a careful clinical assessment, including a neurologic examination. The use of a stroke rating scale, such as the National Institutes of Health Stroke Scale (NIHSS), provides important information about the severity of stroke.

Urgent cranial computed tomography (CT) is mandatory after an ischemic stroke before starting any therapy. Alternatively, magnetic resonance imaging (MRI) or CT perfusion (CTP) can be performed and provide additional information about the selection of patients for mechanical thrombectomy within 6 to 24 hours from symptom onset. However, there is not enough evidence to recommend its routine use in the acute stroke setting.

For the detection and early management of the medical complications of stroke, neurologic status, pulse, blood pressure, temperature, and oxygen saturation should be monitored. Similarly, serum glucose levels need to be monitored and hyperglycemia treated with insulin accordingly. Normal saline is recommended for fluid replacement during the first 24 hours after stroke. If the patient has a fever, treatment with paracetamol (acetaminophen) may be used while sources of infection are being sought. Reducing blood pressure is recommended only in patients with extremely high blood pressure or when indicated by other medical conditions. Blood pressure should be lowered gradually, avoiding abrupt changes.

Thrombolysis

All patients with an ischemic stroke within 4.5 hours of onset should receive thrombolytic treatment with intravenous tissue plasminogen activator (tPA [Activase]) unless contraindicated, because it is effective in improving stroke outcome (Box 1). It is very important to start treatment as soon as possible, because pooled analysis has demonstrated that earlier treatment results in a better outcome. Thrombolysis with tPA is effective in all different population subgroups, including the very elderly, even with significant comorbidities.

BOX 2 — Reperfusion Therapies in Acute Ischemic Stroke

- Symptom onset between 0 and 4.5 h:
  - No contraindications for thrombolysis.
    - Perform CT scan.
    - Administer IV tPA (Activase)
    - Perform multimodal imaging (this could be done before if it does not delay treatment with IV tPA
    - Mechanical thrombectomy (MT): if occlusion of intracranial internal carotid artery or middle cerebral artery (segment 1, M1), NIHSS score ≥6, no premorbid disability (mRS 0–1), and ASPECTS of ≥6. Groin puncture within 6 h of symptom onset.
- Contraindications for thrombolysis (or symptom onset within 4.5–6 h):
  - Perform multimodal imaging
  - Proceed to MT: if occlusion of intracranial internal carotid artery or middle cerebral artery (M1), NIHSS score ≥6, no premorbid disability (mRS 0-1) and ASPECTS of ≥6. Groin puncture within 6 hours of symptom onset.
- Symptom onset between 6 and 24 h:
  - Perform multimodal imaging
  - If occlusion of the intracranial internal carotid artery, middle cerebral artery (M1), or both.
    - Proceed to MT if significant penumbra according to DAWN or DEFUSE 3 trial (this is variable depending on age, NIHSS, and size of infarct core)
    - Otherwise, standard medical management.
- Other circumstances:
  - MT could be a reasonable option in selected cases with distal occlusion of the middle cerebral artery (M2 or M3).
  - MT is a reasonable therapeutic option for selected patients with occlusion of the anterior cerebral arteries, vertebral arteries, basilar artery, or posterior cerebral arteries.
  - Selected patients could benefit from MT even with premorbid conditions (mRS >1), ASPECTS <6, or NIHSS score <6.

ASPECTS, Alberta stroke program early CT score; *CT,* computed tomography; *IV,* intravenous, *mRS,* modified Rankin Scale; *NIHSS,* National Institutes of Health Stroke Scale; *tPA,* tissue plasminogen activator.

Endovascular Thrombectomy

Mechanical thrombectomy using stent retrievers in addition to thrombolysis is more effective in improving outcome than thrombolysis alone in anterior circulation strokes and a large artery occlusion, with a time window of up to 6 hours. This treatment is also effective when there are contraindications for intravenous thrombolysis. In a recent meta-analysis of five major trials (MR CLEAN, ESCAPE, REVASCAT, SWIFT PRIME, and EXTEND IA), endovascular thrombectomy led to significantly reduced disability at 90 days compared with control (odds ratio 2.49), with a number needed to treat of 2.6. All subgroups of patients benefit from this effect. Therefore health authorities have to implement access to thrombectomy within a reasonable time range in a network including stroke centers.

There is recent published evidence indicating that therapeutic window could be extended significantly when using multimodal imaging to select patients who have marked penumbra. Thus the DAWN trial showed that patients with ischemic penumbra could benefit from thrombectomy up to 24 hours since symptom onset, in comparison with standard care. This result was replicated by the DEFUSE 3 trial, although including patients up to 16 hours from onset. In Box 2, there is a simplified algorithm for the use of reperfusion therapies in acute ischemic stroke.

Antithrombotic Drugs

All ischemic stroke patients should receive a low dose of aspirin daily. This can be started as soon as possible in patients who have not received reperfusion therapies, always within 48 hours after onset. However, in patients that received thrombolysis, aspirin should be delayed for 24 hours. The use of other antiplatelet agents during the acute phase of stroke cannot be recommended based on available evidence. Similarly, early administration of unfractionated heparin, low-molecular-weight heparin, or heparinoids is not indicated in patients with acute ischemic stroke.

Treatment of Stroke Complications

Brain edema develops between the second and fifth day after stroke onset and is the cause of early deterioration and death. In the case of a malignant infarction of the middle cerebral artery, the mortality rate is 80%. In patients younger than 60 years with this pattern of cerebral infarction, hemicraniectomy has been effective in reducing mortality and severe disability, as shown in the pooled analysis of the DECIMAL, DESTINY, and HAMLET trials. Decompressive hemicraniectomy is also effective in reducing mortality in patients older than 60 years, although the rates of severe disability are very high. Surgery needs to be performed within 48 hours after symptom onset. Surgical decompression is also indicated in the case of large cerebellar infarctions that compress the brainstem.

Stroke-associated infections require appropriate antibiotics, but prophylactic administration is discouraged. Venous thromboembolism is a frequent complication after stroke, but its incidence can be reduced with appropriate hydration and graded compression stockings. If the risk of deep venous thrombosis or pulmonary embolism is high, the use of subcutaneous heparin or low-molecular-weight heparin is beneficial. Early mobilization is an effective way of preventing complications such as aspiration pneumonia or pressure ulcers. Anticonvulsants are administered only to prevent recurrent seizures but are not used prophylactically.

In case of urinary incontinence, specialist assessment and management are recommended. Dysphagia is common after stroke and is associated with a higher incidence of medical complications and increased mortality. Malnutrition also predicts a poor functional outcome and increased mortality, and it is important to assess the swallowing capacity and the nutritional status of the patient.

Rehabilitation should be started after admission to the stroke unit. The optimal timing of first mobilization is unclear, but mobilization within the first few days appears to be well tolerated. However, very early mobilization can be associated with a worse outcome, as shown in the AVERT trial. An early, lower-dose out-of-bed activity regimen is preferable to very early, frequent, higher-dose intervention. It is important to assess cognitive deficits and depression during the patient's hospital stay, because this may require specific intervention, although evidence about the type is lacking.

References

Albers GW, Marks MP, Kemp S, et al: DEFUSE 3 Investigators. Thrombectomy for stroke at 6 to 16 hours with selection by perfusion imaging, *N Engl J Med* 378(8):708–718, 2018 Feb 22.

AVERT Trial Collaboration Group, Bernhardt J, Langhorne P, et al: Efficacy and safety of very early mobilisation within 24h of stroke onset (AVERT): A randomised controlled trial, *Lancet* 386(9988):46–55, 2015.

European Stroke Organisation (ESO): Executive Committee, ESO Writing Committee: Guidelines for management of ischaemic stroke and transient ischaemic attack 2008, *Cerebrovasc Dis* 25:457–507, 2008.

Goyal M, Menon BK, van Zwam WH, et al: Endovascular thrombectomy after large-vessel ischaemic stroke: A meta-analysis of individual patient data from five randomised trials, *Lancet* 387(10029):1723–1731, 2016.

Hacke W, Kaste M, Bluhmki E, et al: Thrombolysis with alteplase 3 to 4.5 hours after acute ischemic stroke, *N Engl J Med* 359:1317–1329, 2008.

Kent DM, Thaler DE: Stroke prevention—Insights from incoherence, *N Engl J Med* 359:1287–1289, 2008.

Nogueira RG, Jadhav AP, Haussen DC, et al: DAWN Trial Investigators. Thrombectomy 6 to 24 hours after stroke with a mismatch between deficit and infarct, *N Engl J Med* 378(1):11–21, 2018 Jan 4.

Powers WJ, Rabinstein AA, Ackerson T, et al: American Heart Association Stroke Council. 2018 Guidelines for the Early Management of Patients With Acute Ischemic Stroke: A Guideline for Healthcare Professionals From the American Heart Association/American Stroke Association, *Stroke* 49(3):e46–e110, 2018 Mar.

Vahedi K, Hofmeijer J, Juettler E, et al: Early decompressive surgery in malignant infarction of the middle cerebral artery: A pooled analysis of three randomised controlled trials, *Lancet Neurol* 6:215–222, 2007.

MIGRAINE HEADACHE

Method of
Anne Walling, MB, ChB

CURRENT DIAGNOSIS

- Recurrent headaches accompanied by nausea/vomiting and/or photophobia and phonophobia.
- Each episode lasts 4–72 h and often ends with sleep.
- The headache has at least two of the classical features: unilateral, pulsating, moderate-to-severe intensity, and/or aggravated by movement.
- Five similar episodes must occur for diagnosis.
- No other condition better accounts for symptoms.

CURRENT THERAPY

Acute Migraine Episodes
- Acetaminophen
- Nonsteroidal antiinflammatory drugs (NSAIDs)
- Triptans
- Ergots
- Antiemetics
- Isometheptene-containing products
- Combination medications

Prophylaxis
- β-Blockers
- Tricyclic antidepressants
- Anticonvulsants

Definition

Migraines are episodic headaches accompanied by nausea and/or photophobia plus phonophobia. The headache must last 4 to 72 hours and have at least two of the defining features (i.e., unilateral, pulsating, moderate-to-severe intensity, and/or aggravated by movement). Five attacks and the exclusion of other conditions are required for diagnosis. Patients with migraine may also suffer from other types of headaches (e.g., tension-type headache).

Epidemiology

About 45 million US adults (18% to 23% of women, 6% to 9% of men) report migraine. Onset is usually between ages 12 and 30. Prevalence peaks in young adults. Migraine is diagnosed in about 30% of family medicine headache patients. A positive migraine diagnosis by a family physician is over 95% accurate, but cases may be misdiagnosed, especially as a tension or sinus headache.

Risk Factors

Besides age and female sex, the biggest risk factor is family history.

Pathophysiology

Migraine results from complex interactions among multiple genetic and environmental factors. The primary neuronal process may be a depolarizing wave (Leão's cortical spreading depression) activating the trigeminal nerve afferents and causing vasoactive neuropeptide release, local inflammation, vascular instability, and blood-brain barrier changes. The type and location of symptoms depend on which parts of the trigeminovascular system are activated. This system innervates pain-sensitive blood vessels and meninges and connects with various areas of the brain, including the thalamus and sensory cortex. Biochemically, serotonin, calcitonin gene-related peptide (CGRP), and other substances are implicated in migraine.

The role of right–left cardiac shunts, especially patent foramen ovale, has not been validated.

TABLE 1	Medications for Migraine Prophylaxis			
	β-BLOCKERS	ANTIEPILEPTICS	ANTIDEPRESSANTS	OTHERS
Level A: Established efficacy	Metoprolol (Lopressor)[1] 100–200 mg/day Propranolol (Inderal) 40–240 mg/day Timolol (Blocadren) 10–15 mg bid	Divalproex sodium (Depakote ER) 750–1500 mg/day[2] Sodium valproate (Depakene)[1] 800–1500 mg/day[2] Topiramate (Topamax) 25–100 mg/day		Frovatriptan (Frova)[1] 2.5 mg daily or bid* (menstrual migraine) Onabotulinumtoxin A 155 units (chronic migraine)
Level B: Probably effective	Atenolol (Tenormin)[1] 50–200 mg/day Nadolol (Corgard)[1] 20–160 mg/day		Amitriptyline (Elavil)[1] 50–150 mg/day Venlafaxine (Effexor)[1] 75–150 mg/day	Fenoprofen (Nalfon)[1] 1800 mg/day Ibuprofen (Motrin)[1,†] Ketoprofen (Orudis)[1] 150 mg/day Naproxen (Naprosyn)[1,†] Naproxen sodium (Anaprox)[1] 1100 mg/day Naratriptan (Amerge)[1] 1 mg bid ×5 days premenses Naproxen sodium (Anaprox DS)[1] 550 mg bid Riboflavin[3] 400 mg bid Magnesium 600 mg Trimagnesium dicitrate[3] Feverfew[3] 50–300 mg bid (2.08–18.75 MIG-99 preparation) Zolmitriptan (Zomig)[1] 2.5 mg bid or tid*
Level C: Possibly effective	Nebivolol (Bystolic)[1] 5 mg/day Pindolol (Visken)[1,†]	Carbamazepine (Tegretol)[1] 600 mg/d		Cyproheptadine (Periactin)[1,†] Lisinopril (Prinivil)[1,†] Candesartan (Atacand)[1,†] Clonidine (Catapres)[1] 0.075–0.15 mg/day Guanfacine (Intuniv)[1] 1 mg/day

Emerging Injectable Agents

Erenumab (Aimovig) 70 or 140 mg SC monthly
Fremanezumab (Ajovy) 225 mg monthly or 675 mg SC quarterly
Galcanezumab (Emgality) 240 mg loading dose then 120 mg SC monthly

[1]Not FDA approved for this indication.
[2]Exceeds dosage recommended by the manufacturer.
[3]Available as dietary supplement.
*Short-term use only.
†Dosage not established.
Source: American Headache Society. The American Headache Society position statement on integrating new migraine treatments into clinical practice. *Headache.* 2019;59:1–18; Dosages from Becker WJ, Gawel M, Mackie G, et al. Migraine treatment. *Can J Neurol Sci.* 2007;34:S10–S19; Evers S, Afra J, Frese A, et al. EFNS guideline on the drug treatment of migraine: Revised report of an EFNS task force. *Eur J Neuro.* 2009;16:968–981; Ramadan NM, Silberstein SD, Freitag F, et al. Evidence-based guidelines for migraine headache in the primary care setting: Pharmacological management for prevention of migraine. *U.S. Headache Consortium.* 2000. Available at https://www.aan.com/Guidelines/home/ByTopic?topicId=16.

Prevention

The vulnerability to migraine cannot be eliminated, but patients can be assisted to reduce the number of attacks and minimize the negative impact of migraine through managing triggers and use of prophylaxis.

Triggers

Some who experience migraine have specific precipitants for an attack. These triggers may be identified by use of a headache diary. The strongest evidence implicates stress, menstruation, missed meals, weather changes, and sleep disturbances as migraine triggers. Migraines may be associated with stress or its relief (weekend migraine). Avoiding or minimizing triggers may reduce the likelihood of a migraine.

Prophylactic Medications

Guidelines recommend discussing prophylaxis with patients who meet the following criteria:

- severe and/or frequent symptoms (>4 days per month) that disrupt daily activities despite adequate acute treatment.
- poor efficacy, medication overuse, or inability to use standard treatments for acute attacks (e.g., because of adverse effects, contraindications, cost).

- specific rare migraine syndromes associated with dangerous neurologic complications (e.g., basilar migraine, prolonged aura, hemiplegic migraine).

Successful prophylaxis depends on balancing potential benefits against adverse effects and the demands of adherence to long-term medications. Selection of a prophylactic medication depends on patient factors (e.g., personal preferences, comorbidities such as hypertension and depression) and medication issues (including efficacy, cost, pharmacokinetics, adverse effects, and medication interactions).

Prophylactic medication should be started at a low dose and gradually increased until benefit is demonstrated, or adverse effects outweigh benefits. Individual patients show enormous variation in the effective dose of prophylactic medication. An adequate trial of prophylaxis requires several months. A patient may have poor outcomes from one agent but good response to one from a different class. A headache diary is useful to monitor symptoms and adverse effects. Therapy should be reevaluated every 3 to 6 months.

The most recent evidence-based recommendations for pharmacologic migraine prophylaxis based on efficacy and potential adverse effects are summarized in Table 1. For herbal and complementary treatments, level A evidence was established

Migraine Headache

TABLE 2	Diagnostic Probability of Symptoms for Migraine (POUND Mnemonic)

Character of headache described as **P**ulsing or throbbing
Duration average **O**ne day (4–72 h)
Location **U**nilateral
Associated symptoms include **N**ausea or vomiting
Severity ranked as **D**isabling
Probability of migraine in a primary care patient is 92% with 4 POUND symptoms, 64% with 3, and 17% with 0–2.

From Ebell MH. Diagnosis of migraine headache. *Am Fam Physician.* 2006;74(12):2087–2088.

TABLE 3	"Red Flag" Findings Associated With Increased Risk of Underlying Pathology in Headache

Acute onset. "Thunderclap" headache (maximum severity reached within 1 min of onset) or "the worst headache ever"
New onset or change in established headache pattern after 50 years of age
History, signs or symptoms (e.g., fever, hypertension, myalgia, weight loss) of systemic disorders, including cancer, human immunodeficiency virus
Neurologic symptoms, seizures, or abnormal neurologic examination
Occipitonuchal location of headache
Persistent headache after Valsalva maneuver or exertion
Progressively increasing headache frequency and/or severity

Notes: In the emergency department setting, patients over 50 years of age with acute onset and neurologic signs had 98.6% specificity for serious intracranial pathology.
Adapted from Silberstein SD. Practice parameter: evidence-based guidelines for migraine headache (an evidence-based review): report of the Quality Standards Subcommittee of the American Academy of Neurology, *Neurology.* 2000;55:754–762; and Detsky ME, McDonald DR, Baerlocher MO, et al. Does this patient with headache have a migraine or need neuroimaging? *JAMA.* 2006;296(10):1274–1283.

for petasites (butterbur extract) 50 to 75 mg twice daily but was withdrawn due to concerns about hepatotoxicity, carcinogenesis, and poorly standardized manufacture. Magnesium (400 to 600 mg)[1], feverfew[7] (as MIG-99 extract, 6.25 mg, three times daily), and riboflavin (400 mg) were classified as level B and coenzyme Q10 (100 mg three times daily) was classified as level C.

Onabotulinumtoxin A (Botox) is approved for the prevention of chronic but not episodic migraine.

Newly-developed injectable monoclonal antibodies erenumab (Aimovig), fremanezumab (Ajovy), and galcanezumab (Emgality) are approved for the prevention of both episodic and chronic migraine, but the current indications for initiating these therapies stress their use *only* in patients with frequent migraine and confirmed failure of alternative treatments. Similarly, the criteria for continuation require documented reduction by at least 50% in monthly headache days plus achievement of specified reductions in at least one migraine-specific impact scale, such as the Migraine Disability Scale (MIDAS), Migraine Physical Function Impact Diary (MPFID), or Headache Impact Test (HIT-6). Other new agents targeting the CGRP receptor or ligand are anticipated to become available in the near future.

Nonpharmacologic Therapies

Behavioral therapies to prevent migraine attacks may be preferred by some patients and can be combined with medication, education, and lifestyle modifications for a potentially greater benefit. Relaxation training, biofeedback therapy, and cognitive-behavioral therapy (CBT) have grade A evidence for migraine prevention. These therapies are especially recommended for patients with contraindications or poor response to pharmacotherapy as well as for those who have a history or high risk for medication overuse or show significant stress or poor coping skills.

Two forms of neuromodulation, singe-pulse transcranial magnetic stimulation and electrical trigeminal nerve stimulation, have recently been cleared by the FDA for migraine prophylaxis.

Clinical Manifestations

Prodrome: About 60% of migraine sufferers experience 1 to 2 days of symptoms, such as yawning, intense hunger, mild euphoria, or depression/irritability, before an attack.

Aura

About 25% of migraine sufferers report consistent, specific neurologic changes about 5 to 60 minutes before the onset of headache. Common aura symptoms include visual (flashing lights, zigzag lines, scotoma), sensory (paresthesia, numbness), or speech disturbances.

Symptoms

Migraine combines a specific type of headache (unilateral, throbbing, moderate-to-severe, worse with activity) with other diagnostic symptoms (nausea/vomiting and/or photophobia/phonophobia). Many patients also experience vertigo, allodynia, and

fatigue. Additional symptoms may be prominent in migraine subtypes such as basilar or ophthalmoplegic migraine. Patients vary enormously in the symptom pattern as well as in the frequency, intensity, and impact of attacks. Some have infrequent episodes with mild symptoms, whereas others are incapacitated by recurrent, severe attacks.

Duration and Complications

Classically, migraine patients lie still in a dark room until sleep resolves symptoms. Afterward, some patients feel refreshed, while others are tired, and a few experience localized skull tenderness or headache on movement.

Status migrainosus is a debilitating migraine episode lasting more than 72 hours. The patient may be dehydrated, exhausted, and/or suffering adverse medication effects. Very rarely, migraine subtypes (basilar, ophthalmoplegic, hemiplegic) are complicated by seizure or cerebral infarction. Chronic migraine (defined as symptoms on more than 15 days per month) requires investigation, especially for medication overuse headache (MOH) or serious secondary causes of headache. With inappropriate therapy, episodic migraine can become complicated by superimposed MOH, resulting in chronic headaches that cause significant disability.

Diagnosis

Migraine diagnosis depends on history. Identifying classic symptoms has a high probability of accurate diagnosis (Table 2). The headache pattern should distinguish migraine from other primary headaches (e.g., tension, cluster). The clinical history and examination target identifying conditions that could cause secondary headache. Neurologic examination must be documented, because change over time is crucial in detecting the rare cases of intracranial pathology that present with migraine-type symptoms.

Diagnostic imaging is not indicated in migraine patients with normal neurologic examination. Guidelines recommended imaging only for atypical symptoms or "red flag" indications of serious pathology. There is limited evidence that neuroimaging benefits patients who are excessively anxious about the cause of their headaches (Table 3). Other testing (e.g., complete blood count, sedimentation rate, analysis of cerebrospinal fluid) are selected to identify specific potential causes of symptoms in individual patients. Guidelines stress that testing should be done only if results are likely to change management.

Differential Diagnosis

Other recurrent headaches, especially tension or cluster, can usually be distinguished by the combination of features (unilaterality, nausea, photo/phonophobia) and pattern (frequency and duration of episodes).

---

[1] Not FDA approved for this indication.
[7] Available as dietary supplement.

TABLE 4 Medications for Treatment of Acute Migraine

	MEDICATION (INITIAL ORAL DOSE mg)	LEVEL OF EVIDENCE
First Line	Aspirin (250 mg), acetaminophen (250 mg), caffeine (65 mg) (Excedrin Migraine)	A A A†
	Nonsteroidal antiinflammatory drugs:	A
	Naproxen (Naprosyn) (250–500 mg)	A
	Ibuprofen (Motrin) (200–800 mg)	A
	Aspirin*	A
	Triptans:	A
	Almotriptan (Axert) (6.25–12.5 mg) tab	A
	Eletriptan (Relpax) (20–40 mg) tab	A
	Frovatriptan (Frova) (2.5 mg) tab	A
	Naratriptan (Amerge) (1–2.5 mg) tab	
	Rizatriptan (Maxalt) (5–10 mg) tab (also oral disintegrating tab)	
	Sumatriptan (Imitrex) (25–100 mg) tab (also nasal spray [5–20 mg], subcutaneous injection [6 mg])	
	Zolmitriptan (Zomig) (2.5, 5 mg) tab (also oral disintegrating tab, nasal spray [2.5, 5 mg])	
Other Agents	Ergots:	B
	Dihydroergotamine nasal spray (Migranal [1 spray each nostril])	B
	Dihydroergotamine IV (D.H.E. 45) IV (0.5–1 mg), IM (0.5–1 mg), SC (1 mg)	B
	Ergotamine (Ergomar) (2 mg) tab	B
	Ergotamine (2 mg) plus caffeine (200 mg) tab (Cafergot)	
	Antiemetics:	
	Prochlorperazine (Compazine)¹ IV (10 mg), PR (25 mg)	
	Metoclopramide (Reglan)¹ (10 mg) oral, IM, IV	
	Isometheptene-containing product:	
	Acetaminophen 325 mg + dichloralphenazone 100 mg + isometheptene 65 mg (Midrin)	

¹Not FDA approved for this indication.
*Doses less than 1000 mg in combination with antiemetics and other agents in studies.
†Not included in U.S. Headache Consortium Guidelines, 2000.
IM, Intramuscular; *IV*, intravenous; *PR*, per rectum; *SC*, subcutaneous.

Intracranial pathology (including acute or chronic bleeding, infection, or space-occupying lesions) can cause headache resembling migraine. This can also occur with head and neck conditions such as temporal arteritis, sinusitis, temporomandibular joint syndrome, and various neuralgias as well as systemic conditions including carbon monoxide poisoning, sudden rise in blood pressure, or the adverse effects of medications. Diagnosis depends on recognizing that the clinical picture is not completely congruent with migraine, and also on identifying risk factors, symptoms, and signs, along with positive targeted testing for the underlying condition. Medication overuse should be suspected in patients with frequent migraine episodes.

Treatment

Treatment goals for acute migraine are rapid symptom control, minimizing adverse effects, preventing recurrence, and optimizing function. Self-management and efficient use of resources are priorities. Individual patients vary enormously in response to specific medications and in the effective dose. Patients who do not respond to an appropriate dose of one medication may have good outcomes from another agent in the same class or one from a different class. Medications should be taken in adequate dosage as early as possible during a migraine attack. Non-oral formats or adjunct medications (antiemetics) may be necessary because of vomiting or poor medication absorption due to gastric stasis.

Many medications have antimigraine activity (Table 4). Considerations in selecting an agent include patient comorbidities (e.g., hypertension or depression) and the medication's potential adverse effects. Cost may be a significant concern.

Of first-line therapies, NSAIDs or combination analgesics with caffeine are recommended for mild-to-moderate attacks or more severe attacks that have previously responded to these agents. Evidence also supports intramuscular ketorolac (Toradol) as a useful strategy for vomiting patients.

Triptans are recommended for moderate-to-severe migraine and for mild-to-severe attacks that have not responded adequately to other first-line therapies. Individual triptans have comparable efficacy and tolerability but differ in speed of onset and duration of action. This allows for the selection of an agent with pharmacokinetics that correspond to the patient's migraine symptom pattern. The most effective agent and dose for each patient can only be established by experience. Triptans may be combined synergistically with NSAIDs. Potential triptan adverse effects include vasoconstriction and serotonin syndrome.

Ergotamines are effective in migraine but limited by adverse effects, especially vasoconstriction. They are less effective than triptans but may have good results in some patients. Nasal spray is useful if the patient cannot take oral medications. In emergency room studies, parenteral dihydroergotamine (D.H.E. 45) combined with antiemetics has been as effective as opiates. Opiates are rarely appropriate for migraine. Studies show that other agents are more effective with fewer adverse effects and no risk of addiction or exploitation.

Emerging acute treatments such as CGRP receptor antagonists and selective serotonin receptor agonists are currently recommended for acute migraine treatment only in patients who have failed appropriate treatment with at least two oral triptans. Access may be limited by cost and insurance considerations. Guidelines published in 2019 recommend IV magnesium, single-pulse transcranial magnetic stimulation, noninvasive vagus nerve stimulation, or electrical trigeminal nerve stimulation when drug treatment is ineffective, intolerable, contradicted, or declined by patients with acute migraine.

Chronic Migraine

Each year, an estimated 3% of migraine sufferers progress to chronic migraine, defined as at least 3 months of headache on 15 or more days per month with headaches fulfilling criteria for migraine on at least 8 days per month. Other causes of symptoms must be excluded for diagnosis of chronic migraine. Approximately half of patients diagnosed with chronic migraine actually suffer from MOH. Persistent changes in brain structure and function occur in chronic migraine, resulting in central sensitization, intractable symptoms, and vulnerability to psychiatric comorbidities. Treatment requires lifestyle modification, consideration of non-pharmacological therapies, management of symptoms, and prophylactic therapy. Topiramate (Topamax) and other prophylactic therapies may reduce the frequency and impact of recurrent migraine headaches in patients with chronic migraine.

Monitoring

Regular monitoring can allow for the adjustment of medication for maximum efficacy and minimal adverse effects, promote healthy lifestyles, and aid in screening for migraine comorbidities, especially depression. Development of MOH in addition to migraine is a major concern. By definition, MOH is a new or significantly worse headache occurring on 15 or more days per month in a patient with a pre-existing primary headache (including migraine) that develops as a consequence of regular overuse of headache medication for more than 3 months and usually resolves after the overuse is stopped. "Overuse" is defined as 15 or more days per month for non-opioid analgesics (including aspirin, NSAIDs, and acetaminophen), and 10 or more days per month for triptans, ergotamines, opioids, and combination-analgesics. Individuals can develop MOH at much lower levels of regular medication use. Physicians should ensure that patients are aware of the risk of MOH and limit medication use well below these levels.

References

American Headache Society: The American Headache Society position statement on integrating new migraine treatments into clinical practice, *Headache* 59:1–18, 2019.

Aurora SK, Brin MF: Chronic migraine: an update on physiology, imaging, and the mechanism of action of two available pharmacologic therapies, *Headache* 20 57:109–125, 2017.

Burch RC, Loder S, Loder E, Smitherman TA: The prevalence and burden of migraine and severe headache in the United States: updated statistics from government health surveillance studies [published correction appears in *Headache*, 55(2):356, 2015] *Headache* 55(1):21–34, 2015.

Detsky ME, McDonald DR, Baerlocher MO, et al: Does this patient with headache have a migraine or need neuroimaging? *JAMA* 296(10):1274–1283, 2006.

Headache Classification Committee of the International Headache Society (IHS): Classification and diagnostic criteria of headache disorders, 3rd edition. *Cephalalgia* 38(1):1–211, 2018.

Loder E, Burch R, Rizzoli P: The 2012 AHS/AAN Guidelines for prevention of episodic migraine: a summary and comparison with other recent clinical practice guidelines, *Headache* 52:930–945, 2012.

Marmura MJ, Silberstein SD, Schwedt TJ: The acute treatment of migraine in adults: the American Headache Society evidence assessment of migraine pharmacotherapies, *Headache* 55:3–20, 2015.

Mayans L, Walling A. acute migraine headache: treatment strategies. *Am Fam Physician* 97(4):243–251, 2018.

Silberstein SD: Practice parameter: Evidence-based guidelines for migraine headache (an evidence-based review): Report of the Quality Standards Subcommittee of the American Academy of Neurology, *Neurology* 55:754–762, 2000.

MULTIPLE SCLEROSIS

Method of
B. Mark Keegan, MD

CURRENT DIAGNOSIS

- Multiple sclerosis (MS) is an autoimmune demyelinating disease of the central nervous system (CNS)
- Diagnosis is secured from having repeated CNS demyelinating attacks or new CNS demyelinating lesions on magnetic resonance imaging (MRI) or progressive neurologic dysfunction consistent with MS with no better alternative explanation.
- Presence of cerebrospinal fluid (CSF)-specific oligoclonal bands, characteristic of MS, aids in the diagnosis.

CURRENT THERAPY

- Acute attacks of multiple sclerosis (MS) are treated with high-dose corticosteroids and, in severe cases, plasma exchange.
- Therapy is directed at relapsing-remitting disease with one of the following type 1 interferon β medications: glatiramer acetate, fingolimod (Gilenya), teriflunomide (Aubagio), dimethyl fumarate (Tecfidera), and natalizumab (Tysabri). Therapy for primary progressive MS (progressive disease from onset without prior relapse) is ocrelizumab (Ocrevus).
- Novel MS medications, including further oral medications, and infusion-based monoclonal antibodies are currently under scientific evaluation.

Multiple sclerosis (MS) is an autoimmune inflammatory demyelinating disease of the central nervous system (CNS) that affects approximately one million people in the United States alone.

Risk Factors

Women are at least twice as likely to develop MS as are men. Other known risk factors for the development of MS include ethnicity, genetic background, and socioeconomic and environmental exposures. People of European ethnicity, particularly those born and reared in extreme northern or southern latitudes, are particularly susceptible to MS, although recent data suggests

African Americans are often less likely to be diagnosed with MS and may have a more severe clinical course. Genetic susceptibility is associated with the major histocompatibility allele HLA-DRB1, as well as with interleukin-2 and interleukin-7 receptors. Low serum vitamin D levels are associated with an increased risk of development of MS and may influence the severity of its clinical course. There are intriguing, but as yet unproven, associations with infection with Epstein-Barr virus (infectious mononucleosis), particularly if this is contracted later in adolescence. Exposure to Epstein-Barr virus may be necessary but insufficient for developing MS. Comorbid chronic vascular diseases and mood disorders complicate and worsen the MS disease course. Cigarette smoking is associated with an increased risk for the development of MS and is likely associated with an increased severity and clinical course of MS, including that of cognitive impairment.

Pathophysiology

The etiology and pathophysiology of MS as a whole remains uncertain. However, most evidence supports an inflammatory demyelinating disease induced by uncertain environmental factors in a genetically susceptible host. Animal studies, including experimental allergic encephalomyelitis and Theiler murine encephalomyelitis virus, also point to an autoimmune inflammatory demyelinating etiology, possibly associated with viral infection. Studies that suggested chronic cerebrospinal vascular insufficiency has an important association with MS have been refuted.

Pathophysiology likely varies among individual patients with MS. Four distinct pathologies in active demyelinating MS lesions have been described. Pattern 1 displays marked macrophage infiltration without humoral abnormalities. Pattern 2 shows distinct humoral abnormalities with complement activation and immunoglobulin (Ig) deposition. Pattern 3 involves primary oligodendrocyte degeneration and early loss of myelin-associated glycoprotein. Pattern 4 reveals oligodendrocyte dystrophy in periplaque white matter. Early studies suggest there could be a therapeutic advantage with different therapies for different types of demyelinating disease.

Prevention

Currently, there is no known way to prevent the development of MS. Patients with a single clinical attack of demyelination and abnormal magnetic resonance imaging (MRI) (a "high-risk," clinically isolated syndrome) have a delayed onset to MS diagnosis with immunomodulatory therapy; however, there is no evidence to support that this prevents the eventual development of MS.

Clinical Manifestations

The clinical course of MS is varied. Approximately 85% of patients present with a relapsing-remitting course. This entails an acute impairment within the CNS, depending on the area of inflammation. A demyelinating cause of a focal neurologic symptom is suggested by an onset over hours to days, with a plateau of impairment over a few weeks. Symptoms then improve, either spontaneously or with the use of corticosteroids, over a number of days to weeks or longer. Following this, however, symptoms might not completely resolve. Inflammation within the optic nerve (optic neuritis) is heralded by painful, unilateral, central monocular visual deficit (central scotoma). Symptoms of brain stem dysfunction include binocular diplopia, sensory deficits unilaterally on the face and contralaterally on the arm and leg, significant dysarthria, and vertigo. Cerebellar dysfunction is seen with pure ataxia that is typically unilateral. Spinal cord inflammation is indicated by a distinctive, usually gradually rising sensory level of deficit that is commonly accompanied by bowel and bladder impairment and paraparesis or quadriparesis, depending on a thoracic versus cervical level of the lesion.

Progressive forms of MS include secondary progressive MS and primary progressive MS. These are heralded by a slow (months to years) but steady and insidious, progressive neurologic deficit, usually a progressive myelopathy of upper motor neuron gait disorder with spasticity, neurogenic bladder and bowel impairment,

Figure 1 Magnetic resonance image showing brain T_1 gadolinium-enhancing lesions (A) and T_2 thoracic spine (B) typical of multiple sclerosis.

and progressive weakness. Occasionally, patients with progressive MS have insidious cerebellar ataxia or dementia in isolation or in association with the myelopathy. Secondary progressive MS is diagnosed when a patient has had a prior history of at least one clinical attack (relapse) with improvement in the past. Primary progressive MS is diagnosed with progressive CNS disease consistent with MS and typical MRI brain or spinal lesions from onset without any prior relapse, often with cerebrospinal fluid (CSF) or visual evoked potential abnormalities that support the diagnosis.

Diagnosis

The diagnosis of MS is formalized by the continually revised McDonald criteria. This entails having two or more clinical attacks (relapses) in the accompaniment of two or more objective lesions seen on clinical examination or with evidence for dissemination in space and time diagnosed by further development of new MRI lesions. Additionally, patients with a single clinical attack who have both the presence of MRI gadolinium enhancing lesions (indicative of acute MS lesions) and nongadolinium enhancing lesions (indicative of prior MS lesions) are diagnosed with relapsing-remitting MS. Progressive MS is diagnosed when there is progressive CNS disease characteristic of MS for at least 1 year and abnormal brain or spinal cord MRI scan with or without CSF-specific oligoclonal bands (Figure 1). Occasionally, visual-evoked potentials and somatosensory-evoked potentials are used to further document the dissemination of MS within the CNS. Serologic investigations are done primarily to rule out MS mimickers depending on and directed by any accompanying systemic symptoms and the clinical setting in individual patients. These may include antinuclear antibodies (ANA for lupus), erythrocyte sedimentation rate, anticardiolipin antibodies, vitamin B_{12}, Lyme serology, and chest imaging for CNS sarcoidosis.

Differential Diagnosis

Other CNS demyelinating diseases can mimic relapsing or progressive MS. Acute disseminated encephalomyelitis (ADEM) is an acute, typically monophasic, and postinfectious CNS inflammatory demyelinating disease. It may be severe; however, if recurrent episodes occur separated by at least 3 months, a diagnosis of relapsing-remitting MS is by far more likely.

Neuromyelitis optica is an autoimmune disease with severe acute attacks but is relatively restricted to the optic nerves and spinal cord. Other brainstem and deep cerebral structures, such as the area postrema, cerebral white matter, and hypothalamus, can also be affected by neuromyelitis optica. Brain MRI scan is usually not consistent with MS, at least early on in the disease, and a specific autoantibody (neuromyelitis optica IgG) directed against the aquaporin 4 water channel is found in most cases.

Clinical syndromes of CNS demyelination with inflammatory myelopathies, inflammatory optic neuritis, and ADEM with serologic presence of antibodies to myelin oligodendroglial protein (MOG-Ab) are increasingly recognized.

Optic neuritis may further be mimicked by acute ischemic optic neuropathy. This condition is typically painless, occurs suddenly, and occurs in patients with advanced age and preexisting vascular risk factors.

Progressive myelopathies that mimic primary progressive MS or secondary progressive MS include a compressive myelopathy from cervical spondylosis, disk disease, or neoplastic infiltration; nutritional deficiencies (such as vitamin B_{12} or copper deficiencies); paraneoplastic disease (e.g., CRMP-5 auto-antibodies); or a vascular progressive cause due to dural arteriovenous fistula.

Treatment

Acute demyelinating MS attacks (relapses) may be treated with high doses of corticosteroids. These may be given orally or intravenously; however, high doses of corticosteroids are necessary and superior to low doses. For example, a typical regimen is intravenous methylprednisolone (Solu-Medrol) 1000 mg once daily for 3 to 5 days without oral corticosteroid tapering doses. The oral equivalent to this intravenous regimen is prednisone 1000 to 1250 mg orally once daily for 5 days with no oral corticosteroid taper afterward. Gastrointestinal intolerance occurs in some patients, and concomitant use of stomach-protecting agents such proton pump inhibitors may be recommended. Typical acute corticosteroid side effects include insomnia, irritability, and increased appetite as well as an extremely rare association with avascular hip necrosis. Chronic corticosteroid side effects such as diabetes mellitus, cataracts, and weight gain and cushingoid habitus are more associated with chronic corticosteroid use and not short courses of steroids.

Generally, only MS attacks that are associated with functional impairment (vision loss, diplopia, motor weakness, or ataxia) are treated because clinical recovery is hastened, but final clinical recovery is not found to be altered by this therapy. Rarely, patients have very severe acute attacks of MS or other demyelinating disease that does not improve with the use of high-dose corticosteroids. In these rare patients, the use of plasma exchange (seven exchanges over approximately 14 days) is recommended. Approximately 45% of patients experience functional recovery within 1 month following plasma exchange. Side effects of plasma exchange therapy include paresthesias related to hypocalcemia, anemia, thrombocytopenia, or complications of central venous access that is required for many patients. Intravenous immunoglobulin (Gammagard)[1] has not yet been shown to improve severe clinical attacks of demyelinating disease.

Chronic parenteral therapy for relapsing–remitting MS includes the use of type 1 β interferons (IFN-β1), glatiramer acetate (Copaxone), natalizumab (Tysabri), alemtuzumab (Lemtrada), or ocrelizumab (Ocrevus) (Table 1). Patients with relapsing-remitting MS may be treated with traditional injectable therapies with preparations of IFN-β1, or glatiramer acetate. Alternatively, oral therapies with fingolimod (Gilenya), siponimod (Mayzent), teriflunomide (Aubagio), and dimethyl fumarate (Tecfidera) are increasingly used as first-line therapies. Cladribine (Mavenclad) is an oral medication for treatment resistant disease as a second line therapy. Ocrelizumab is approved for the treatment of primary progressive MS course as well, and siponimod is approved for secondary progressive MS with active inflammatory disease. The side-effect profile is well known for traditional injectable agents such as interferons and glatiramer acetate (see Table 1), and they have been safely used for many years. The safety profile for oral therapies seems satisfactory, but their long-term side-effect profile is still being assessed. For fingolimod, first dose monitoring for 6 hours is required to assess heart rate and rhythm, and occasional patients have developed progressive multifocal leukoencephalopathy (PML). Teriflunomide may be associated with liver disease and teratogenicity. Dimethyl fumarate is associated with flushing, gastrointestinal discomfort, and rare patients have developed PML on dimethyl fumarate. Highly active MS therapy may be indicated with natalizumab, alemtuzumab, or ocrelizumab if first-line medications are intolerable, if therapeutic response is suboptimal (continued MS attacks or marked ongoing and new inflammatory disease on MRI despite therapy), or when a concerning clinical onset (severe attack with multiple lesions and incomplete recovery) occurs. The goal of chronic immunomodulatory therapy for MS is a reduction in clinical attacks of MS (somewhere between 30% and 60%, depending on the agent) and reduction in new inflammatory MRI lesions (somewhere between 40% and 90%, depending on the agent). Patients and healthcare professionals should realize that the medications are not a cure or for symptomatic benefit (making people feel better) but specifically for reduction in relapse-related disease.

Natalizumab is clearly associated with the development of PML, a severely impairing and often fatal opportunistic brain infection caused by reactivation of dormant JC virus. In North America, natalizumab is only available through the TOUCH (Tysabri outreach: unified commitment to health) prescribing program. Risk factors for PML in natalizumab-treated patients include the presence and index value of JC virus serum antibody (JCV-AbAB), duration of therapy of at least 2 years, and a history of prior immunosuppressive medication therapy (e.g., methotrexate and azathioprine [Imuran]). Seropositivity of MS patients for JC virus antibody is over 55%. The seroconversion rate from JC virus Ab negativity to positivity is approximately 2% to 5% per year, and false-negative results are rare (<3%). Currently, no cases of PML have been found in patients persistently seronegative for JCV antibodies. Risk prevalence estimation after 2 years of treatment in JCV Ab–positive patients range from 1:250 for those without a history of immunosuppression to 1:90 in those with a history of prior immunosuppressive therapy. Mitoxantrone (Novantrone) is a chemotherapy agent that is approved for secondary progressive MS but given its severe side effect profile (acute and delayed cardiotoxicity, cases of acute myelogenous leukemia), it is rarely used today. Siponimod (Mayzent) is a selected

sphingosine 1 phosphate agonist approved for relapsing forms of MS as well as secondary progressive MS with active disease.

Alemtuzumab (Lemtrada) is a monoclonal antibody (anti-CD52; T and B cells) for relapsing-remitting MS with major safety precautions that include the development of the following: autoimmune thyroid disease, immune thrombocytopenia, and, rarely, antiglomerular basement membrane disease. Daclizumab (Zinbryta) (anti-CD25, IL2 receptor) was voluntarily withdrawn from the market worldwide because of case reports of an association with presumably immune-mediated encephalitis. Ocrelizumab (anti-CD20 B cells; humanized form) is approved for relapsing-remitting MS and is the only therapy approved for primary progressive MS.

Autologous bone marrow transplantation with stem cell delivery for recovery is under evaluation to determine which cases may respond favorably to it and whether it is equivalent or not to highly active MS therapies.

Monitoring

Most, if not all, MS patients should be followed by a neurologist at least occasionally. Recommendations for clinical assessment range from 6 to 18 months, depending on clinical activity of relapses and disability. The ideal scheduling of repeat brain MRI scans is controversial and varies depending on MS clinical activity, but general recommendations are every 1 to 2 years.

Complications

MS is one of the main causes of impairment at a young age and trails only acute trauma. Often, patients need gait assistance when impairment becomes more severe. This includes the use of a single gait aid, such as a cane or walking stick, or an ankle-foot orthosis for symptomatic foot drop.

Patients often experience symptoms of neurogenic bladder dysfunction. This includes symptoms of urgency and urge-related incontinence. Bladder stimulants such as caffeine need to be avoided. Patients with this symptom should be investigated for completeness of bladder emptying. If there is severe impairment in bladder emptying, urinary catheterization is often recommended. If bladder emptying is complete or only mildly impaired (<100 mL postvoid residual), the use of medications such as oxybutynin (Ditropan) or tolterodine (Detrol) may be recommended for urge-related symptoms; however, ongoing monitoring of bladder emptying is recommended. Some patients require formal urodynamic evaluation for complex bladder symptoms.

Fatigue is a common MS-related symptom. A complete sleep history to ensure appropriate sleep hygiene is imperative. This includes initiating sleep promptly, maintaining sleep throughout the night, and awakening feeling refreshed. Encouragement of a formal exercise program to facilitate restful sleep and daytime vigor is important. Obstructive sleep apnea, restless legs syndrome, and other parasomnias need to be ruled out as additional contributing factors to fatigue. If sleep hygiene is entirely normal and late afternoon fatigue remains a problem, pharmacologic therapy for MS-related fatigue can proceed. Pharmacologic recommendations are limited but include amantadine hydrochloride (Symmetrel) 100 mg by mouth twice daily. Modafinil (Provigil)[1] has been shown in some studies to have an effect on MS-related fatigue at a dose of 200 mg by mouth once daily.

Spasticity associated with upper motor neuron weakness in the lower extremities may be treated with an active daily exercise program directed by physical therapists and physiatrists. Judicious use of baclofen (Lioresal) is helpful (starting at 10 mg once to three times by mouth daily with no more than a maximum of 80 mg/day). Baclofen side effects include drowsiness and liver enzyme elevations. Some patients with significant lower extremity weakness are assisted in their gait by the leg support provided by spasticity, and if spasticity is reduced pharmacologically, this can in fact worsen their gait. Alternatives to baclofen include tizanidine (Zanaflex) and clonidine (Catapres).[1]

MS is a common CNS inflammatory demyelinating disease with heterogenous presentation and prognosis. Relapsing-remitting or

---

[1]Not FDA approved for this indication.

TABLE 1 Approved Immunomodulatory Therapy for Relapsing-Remitting Multiple Sclerosis

MEDICATION	DOSING	SIDE EFFECTS	MONITORING	ADDITIONAL INFORMATION
Interferon β1a (Avonex)	30 µg IM injection 1×/week	Flu-like symptoms (fever, chills, arthralgias, myalgias, and headaches), elevated liver function tests, anemia, leukopenia, thrombocytopenia, depression Localized injection-site rejections	CBC with differential, AST, ALT, ALP, and total bilirubin level every 3 months while on therapy Thyroid function cascade upon initiation of therapy	Premedication with acetaminophen can ameliorate any postinjection flu-like symptoms Ibuprofen and naproxen Pregnancy category C medication
Interferon β1a (Rebif)	22 µg or 44 µg SC injection 3×/week	Flu-like symptoms (fever, chills, arthralgias, myalgias, and headaches), elevated liver function tests, anemia, leukopenia, thrombocytopenia, depression Localized injection-site rejections	CBC with differential, AST, ALT, ALP, and total bilirubin level every 3 months while on therapy Thyroid function cascade on initiation of therapy	Premedication with acetaminophen can ameliorate any postinjection flu-like symptoms Ibuprofen and naproxen Pregnancy category C medication
Peginterferon β1a (Plegridy)	125 µg SC every 14 days	Flu-like symptoms (fever, chills, arthralgias, myalgias, and headaches), elevated liver function tests, anemia, leukopenia, thrombocytopenia, and depression Localized injection-site rejections	CBC with differential, AST, ALT, ALP, and total bilirubin level every 3 months while on therapy Thyroid function cascade upon initiation of therapy	Premedication with acetaminophen may ameliorate any postinjection flu-like symptoms Ibuprofen and naproxen Pregnancy category C medication
Interferon β1b (Betaseron, Extavia)	250 µg SC injection every other day	Flu-like symptoms (fever, chills, arthralgias, myalgias, and headaches), elevated liver function tests, anemia, leukopenia, thrombocytopenia, depression Localized injection-site rejections	CBC with differential, AST, ALT, ALP, and total bilirubin level every 3 months while on therapy Thyroid function cascade on initiation of therapy	Premedication with acetaminophen can ameliorate any postinjection flu-like symptoms Ibuprofen and naproxen Pregnancy category C medication
Glatiramer acetate (Copaxone)	20 mg SC injection daily or 40 mg SC injection 3×/week	Injection-site reactions (erythema, edema, pruritus, pain), transient chest pain, palpitations, facial flushing, anxiety, shortness of breath	None	Pregnancy category B medication
Fingolimod hydrochloride (Gilenya)	0.5 mg by mouth once daily	Headache, flu, diarrhea, back pain, liver enzyme elevations, and cough New FDA labeling required; investigating unexplained deaths occurring during treatment with fingolimod	Ophthalmologist review before therapy and in 3–4 months for macular edema, repeated annually in those with diabetes mellitus or uveitis. Serology for VZV-IgG to determine immunity CBC with differential, AST, ALT, ALP, and total bilirubin level, ECG ECG before first dose and after 6-h monitoring; first dose must be monitored for 6 h for heart-rate reduction and blood-pressure changes; 6-h monitoring following oral dose must be repeated for patients who discontinue therapy for 14 or more consecutive days. For VZV nonimmune patients, vaccination (2 doses at least 1 month apart) before starting treatment is needed, and treatment may commence 1 month after the second VZV vaccination	Should not be used in patients with recent MI, unstable angina, stroke, TIA, 2nd- or 3rd-degree AV block, CHF, SSS without cardiac pacing, or QTc >500 ms, or with Class Ia or III antiarrhythmic drugs Overnight continuous ECG monitoring recommended for those with: preexisting cardiac or cerebrovascular disease; recurrent syncope; severe, untreated obstructive sleep apnea; use of β-blockers; or prolonged QTc Occasional PML Pregnancy category C medication

Continued

TABLE 1   Approved Immunomodulatory Therapy for Relapsing-Remitting Multiple Sclerosis—cont'd

MEDICATION	DOSING	SIDE EFFECTS	MONITORING	ADDITIONAL INFORMATION
Siponimod (Mayzent)	The recommended maintenance dosage for most is 2 mg PO once daily The recommended maintenance dosage in patients with a CYP2C9*1/*3 or *2/*3 genotype is 1 mg PO once daily	Herpes infections, upper respiratory infections, fungal skin infections. Macular edema Severe exacerbation of MS rarely reported after discontinuation of a S1P receptor modulator (fingolimod)	CYP2C9 genotype determination, CBC, fundus evaluation (OCT), electrocardiogram recent (i.e., within last 6 months), liver transaminase and bilirubin levels • First-dose monitoring is recommended for patients with sinus bradycardia, first- or second-degree (Mobitz type I) atrioventricular (AV) block, or a history of myocardial infarction or heart failure	Concomitant use of siponimod and moderate or strong CYP3A4 inducers (e.g., modafinil [Provigil], efavirenz [Sustiva]) is not recommended for patients with CYP2C9*1/*3 and*2/*3 genotype
Teriflunomide (Aubagio)	7 mg or 14 mg PO once daily	Diarrhea, abnormal liver tests, nausea, influenza, alopecia, potential for hepatotoxicity, may cause significant birth defects if used during pregnancy (pregnancy category X), peripheral neuropathy, transient acute renal failure, and hyperkalemia	CBC monthly for the first 6 months Liver enzymes Tuberculin skin test Pregnancy test (women of childbearing potential)	Prolonged half-life; recommend removal by activated charcoal or cholestyramine when required Pregnancy category X medication
Dimethyl fumarate (Tecfidera)	120 mg PO twice daily for 7 days, then 240 mg PO twice daily	Flushing, abdominal pain, nausea, diarrhea	CBC Consider serum JCV Ab serology	CBC annually PML rare
Ocrelizumab (Ocrevus)	600 mg³ IV X 2 q 2 weeks then 600 mg IV q 24 weeks	Infusion reactions (~34%) Infections respiratory tract, herpes infections Possible increased risk of cancer including breast cancer	CBC, Rule out hepatitis B virus before first dose	Approved for RRMS and PPMS PMS Do not administer if signs of infection delay until infection resolves. Administer vaccines >6 weeks before ocrelizumab infusions Live and live-attenuated vaccines not recommended until B-cell counts recover after discontinuation
Natalizumab (Tysabri)	300 mg IV once every 28 days	Urticaria and anaphylaxis, headache, arthralgias, nausea, fatigue, depression, and infections (urinary tract, pneumonia, herpes simplex or reactivation)	Before treatment: JCV Ab serologic study, head MRI with or without gadolinium, CBC with differential, AST, ALT, ALP, and total bilirubin and pregnancy test if applicable. Every 6 months: JCV Ab serology if seronegative (no need to repeat if JCV Ab is seropositive); head MRI with and without gadolinium every 6 months while on therapy; if PML is suspected, discontinue therapy immediately; PLEX to remove drug, MRI head with and without gadolinium with diffusion-weighted imaging; CSF for JCV PCR	Monotherapy approved Risk of PML may be greater in patients with prolonged therapy and those previously treated with immunosuppressive medications Prescribing professional requires TOUCH enrollment Pregnancy category C medication

Continued

TABLE 1 Approved Immunomodulatory Therapy for Relapsing-Remitting Multiple Sclerosis—cont'd

MEDICATION	DOSING	SIDE EFFECTS	MONITORING	ADDITIONAL INFORMATION
Alemtuzumab (Lemtrada)	IV infusion over 4 h × 2 treatment course. First Course: 12 mg/day on 5 consecutive days Second course: 12 mg/day on 3 consecutive days 12 months after the first treatment course	Infusion reactions with anaphylaxis Autoimmune thyroid disorders, immune thrombocytopenia, antiglomerular basement membrane disease Malignancies, including thyroid cancer, melanoma, and lymphoproliferative disorders	CBC with differential, monthly for 48 months after last dose Creatinine, urinalysis with urine cell counts periodically for 48 months after last dose Baseline and yearly skin examinations	Premedicate with high dose corticosteroids, check VZV status and vaccinate those VZV antibody negative
Cladribine (Mavenclad)	2 treatment courses (1.75 mg/kg per treatment course) One treatment course per year for a total of 2 years Each treatment course is divided into 2 treatment weeks: one at the beginning of the first month and one at the beginning of the second month of the respective treatment year. Each treatment week consists of 4 or 5 days on which a patient receives 10 mg or 20 mg (one or two tablets) as a single daily dose, depending on body weight	Contraindicated in patients with current malignancy, pregnant women, and women and men of reproductive potential who do not plan to use effective contraception during cladribine dosing and for 6 months after the last dose in each treatment course, HIV infection, active chronic infections (e.g., hepatitis or tuberculosis), women intending to breastfeed on a cladribine treatment day and for 10 days after the last dose	Follow standard cancer screening guidelines CBC 2 and 6 months after the start of each treatment course Monitor CBC annually thereafter If the lymphocyte count at month 2 is below 200 cells/µL, monitor monthly until month 6 Hold cladribine therapy if the lymphocyte count is below 200 cells/µL	If VZV-IgG is negative, vaccinate with recombinant zoster vaccine (Shingrix) prior to initiating cladribine Administer live-attenuated or live vaccines at least 4–6 weeks prior to starting cladribine Avoid vaccination with live-attenuated or live vaccines during and after cladribine treatment while the patient's white blood cell counts are not within normal limits

Ab, Antibody; *ALP,* alkaline phosphatase; *ALT,* alanine aminotransferase; *AST,* aspartate aminotransferase; *AV,* atrioventricular; *CBC,* complete blood count; *CHF,* congestive heart failure; *CSF,* cerebrospinal fluid; *ECG,* electrocardiogram; *FDA,* US Food and Drug Administration; *HIV,* human immunodeficiency virus; *JCV,* JC virus; *MI,* myocardial infarction; *MRI,* magnetic resonance imaging; *PCR,* polymerase chain reaction; *PLEX,* plasma exchange; *PML,* progressive multifocal leukoencephalopathy; *SSS,* sick sinus syndrome; *TIA,* transient ischemic attack; *TOUCH,* Tysabri Outreach: Unified Commitment to Health; *VZV-IgG,* varicella zoster virus immunoglobulin G.

attack-related MS is treated with corticosteroids to hasten resolution of acute relapses and with chronic immunomodulatory medications such as IFN-β, glatiramer acetate, fingolimod, siponimod, cladribine, teriflunomide, dimethyl fumarate, alemtuzumab, and natalizumab to reduce the number of future clinical attacks and new MRI lesions. Ocrelizumab is the only medication approved for primary progressive MS. Symptomatic care is important in those patients, including the treatment of gait disorder, spasticity, neurogenic bladder dysfunction, and fatigue.

---

[1]Not FDA approved for this indication.

References

Diagnosis of multiple sclerosis: 2017 revisions of the McDonald criteria. Thompson AJ, Banwell BL, Barkhof F, Carroll WM, Coetzee T, Comi G, Correale J, Fazekas F, Filippi M, Freedman MS, Fujihara K, Galetta SL, Hartung HP, Kappos L, Lublin FD, Marrie RA16, Miller AE15, Miller DH17, Montalban X18, Mowry EM19, Sorensen PS20, Tintoré M21, Traboulsee AL22, Trojano M23, Uitdehaag BMJ24, Vukusic S25, Waubant E26, Weinshenker BG27, Reingold SC28, Cohen JA29. Lancet Neurol. 2018 Feb;17(2):162-173. https://doi.org/10.1016/S1474-4422(17)30470-2. Epub 2017 Dec 21

Ho PR, Koendgen H, Campbell N, Haddock B, Richman S, Chang I: Risk of natalizumab-associated progressive multifocal leukoencephalopathy in patients with multiple sclerosis: a retrospective analysis of data from four clinical studies, *Lancet Neurol* 16:925–933, 2017.

Incidence of multiple sclerosis in multiple racial and ethnic groups Annette Langer-Gould, Sonu M. Brara, Brandon E. Beaber, Jian L. Zhang Neurology May 2013, 80 (19) 1734-1739. https://doi.org/10.1212/WNL.0b013e3182918cc2.

Lublin FD, Reingold SC, Cohen JA, et al: Defining the clinical course of multiple sclerosis: the 2013 revisions, *Neurology* 83:278–286, 2014.

Montalban X, Belachew S, Wolinsky JS: Ocrelizumab in primary progressive and relapsing multiple sclerosis, *N Engl J Med* 376:1694, 2017.

Prevalence of extracranial venous narrowing on catheter venography in people with multiple sclerosis, their siblings, and unrelated healthy controls: a blinded, case-control study Anthony L Traboulsee, Katherine B Knox, Lindsay Machan, Yinshan Zhao, Irene Yee, Alexander Rauscher, Darren Klass, Peter Szkup, Robert Otani, David Kopriva, Shanti Lala, David K Li, Dessa SadovnickLancet 2014;383:138–145 Published Online October 9, 2013. https://doi.org/10.1016/S0140-6736(13)61747-X.

Reich DS, Lucchinetti CF, Calabresi PA: Multiple sclerosis, *N Engl J Med* 378:169–180, 2018.

Thompson AJ, Banwell BL, Barkhof F, et al: Diagnosis of multiple sclerosis: 2017 revisions of the McDonald criteria, *Lancet Neurol* 17:162–173, 2018.

The prevalence of MS in the United States Mitchell T. Wallin, William J. Culpepper, Jonathan D. Campbell, Lorene M. Nelson, Annette Langer-Gould, Ruth Ann Marrie, Gary R. Cutter, Wendy E. Kaye, Laurie Wagner, Helen Tremlett, Stephen L. Buka, Piyameth Dilokthornsakul, Barbara Topol, Lie H. Chen, Nicholas G. LaRocca Neurology Mar 2019, 92 (10) e1029-e1040. https://doi.org/10.1212/WNL.0000000000007035.

Wingerchuk DM, Banwell B, Bennett JL, et al: International consensus diagnostic criteria for neuromyelitis optica spectrum disorders, *Neurology* 85:177–189, 2015.

MYASTHENIA GRAVIS

Method of
Taylor B. Harrison, MD and William P. Roche, MD

CURRENT DIAGNOSIS

- Myasthenia gravis (MG) is an autoimmune disorder that affects the neuromuscular junction, resulting in fatigable skeletal muscle weakness.
- Diagnosis may be based on clinical history and exam in combination with identification of autoantibodies (Ach-R Abs) or abnormalities on electrodiagnostic testing.
- Myasthenic crisis, defined by respiratory failure, can stem from respiratory or oropharyngeal weakness. It may develop abruptly and typically occurs in the setting of illness, change in medications, or early in the disease course.

CURRENT THERAPY

- Mild symptoms can respond well to anticholinesterase inhibitors such as pyridostigmine (Mestinon).
- A wide range of medications may be used to treat MG, including steroids, nonsteroidal immunosuppressants, as well as intravenous immunoglobulin[1] and plasmapheresis. Thymectomy may be considered in patients with acetylcholine receptor antibodies.
- It is important to recognize that certain medications may worsen MG.
- Myasthenic crisis is a medical emergency, and patients should be treated in the intensive care unit with close respiratory monitoring and possibly intubation. Intravenous immunoglobulin[1] and plasmapheresis are treatment options for myasthenic crisis.

[1]Not FDA approved for this indication.

Epidemiology

Myasthenia gravis (MG) is the most common acquired disorder of neuromuscular transmission, with an incidence of 8 to 10 per million annually. The prevalence is 150 to 250 per million, reflecting the disease's low mortality rate. An estimated 700,000 people are living with MG worldwide, with between 36,000 to 60,000 living in the United States.

There exists a bimodal age distribution with two peaks of incidence: the first peak in the second to third decades of life, and a second peak in the seventh to eighth decades. Women predominate in early-onset MG (defined by onset <50 years of age) whereas men predominate with late-onset disease (>50 years of age).

Risk Factors

MG is associated with thymoma: approximately one-third of patients with thymoma will develop myasthenia, and 10% of myasthenic patients have a thymoma. Certain HLA subtypes, which are known to predispose to autoimmune disorders in general, also increase the risk of MG. Other autoimmune disorders are present in about 15% of myasthenic patients, most commonly thyroiditis, followed by systemic lupus erythematosus and rheumatoid arthritis. A small percentage of patients may have a myasthenia-myositis overlap syndrome (Tables 1 and 2).

Pathophysiology

To understand the pathophysiology, a review of normal physiology is needed. In normal muscle contraction, an action potential (AP) travels down a motor nerve to the presynaptic axon terminal. At the axon terminal, the AP triggers voltage-gated calcium channels to open, causing calcium influx. Calcium influx causes synaptic vesicles containing acetylcholine to fuse with the cell membrane, resulting in exocytosis of acetylcholine into the synaptic cleft. Acetylcholine diffuses across the synaptic cleft and binds with nicotinic acetylcholine receptors (AchRs) on the cell membrane of the muscle fiber. The AchRs are ligand-gated ion channels that, once opened, allow cation influx, generating an end plate potential (EPP). When the EPP reaches a threshold value, it triggers voltage-gated sodium channels in the postsynaptic membrane to open, resulting in further cation influx and membrane depolarization, resulting in a muscle fiber AP and muscle fiber contraction. Excess acetylcholine is then broken down by the enzyme acetylcholinesterase (AchE) in the synaptic cleft.

The safety factor is an important concept in understanding the muscle fatigability of MG. The safety factor is the ratio of postsynaptic EPP generated by a quantity of acetylcholine to the threshold required to generate an all-or-none muscle fiber AP and thus muscle fiber contraction. In the healthy state, more acetylcholine is released than is needed to generate a muscle fiber AP.

TABLE 1 Medications That May Exacerbate or Precipitate MG

Black box warnings:

Telithromycin (Ketek)[2]

Fluoroquinolones (ciprofloxacin [Cipro], moxifloxacin [Avelox], levofloxacin [Levaquin])

Drugs to avoid:

D-penicillamine (Cuprimine)

Checkpoint inhibitors (ipilimumab [Yervoy], pembrolizumab [Keytruda], nivolumab [Opdivo])

Quinine

IV Magnesium

Use only with caution:

Macrolidess (erythromycin, azithromycin [Zithromax], clarithromycin [Biaxin])

Aminoglycosides (gentamycin [Garamycin], neomycin, tobramycin)

Procainamide (Pronestyl)

Desferrioxamine (Desferal)

Beta blockers (propranolol, metoprolol [Lopressor], carvedilol [Coreg])

Statins (atorvastatin [Lipitor], pravastatin [Pravachol], rosuvastatin [Crestor], simvastatin [Zocor])

[2]Not available in the United States.

TABLE 2 Suggested Medication Monitoring

MEDICATION	SUGGESTED MONITORING
Azathioprine (Imuran)	CBC, LFTs weekly for the first month then monthly to every 3 months
Cyclosporine (Sandimmune)	Monthly CBC, LFTs, renal function monthly for 3 months then quarterly Periodic trough level Blood pressure checks
Cyclophosphamide (Cytoxan)	CBC (attention to neutrophil count), electrolytes and renal function, LFTs, UA every 2–4 weeks
Eculizumab (Soliris)	CBC, renal function, LFTs
IVIG (Gammagard)	Renal function monthly, with repeated dosing maybe every 3 months
Methotrexate (Trexall)	CBC, LFTs monthly initially, then at stable dose at least every 3 months
Mycophenolate mofetil	CBC every 2 weeks for first month, then monthly to quarterly
Plasma exchange	Blood pressure and serum calcium
Prednisone	Weight and blood pressure Periodic potassium and HgbA1c Bone density test Periodic eye exam
Rituximab (Rituxan)	CD 20 counts may be considered but varies among providers

CBC, Complete blood count.

In myasthenia the safety factor is lower, and sufficient acetylcholine may not be released to generate successive APs with repeated contractions. Exercise will result in insufficient neuromuscular transmission over time because of this reduction in safety factor, and as muscle fibers fail to reach threshold to generate an AP, fatigable weakness ensues.

MG is caused by antibodies targeting antigens of the postsynaptic membrane of the neuromuscular junction. In myasthenia gravis, the normal action of acetylcholine at the postsynaptic muscle cell membrane is disrupted by one of several antibody-mediated mechanisms. Most commonly, antibodies are formed against the AchR itself. These AchR antibodies interrupt normal transmission by cross-linking the receptors causing increased turnover or complement-mediated degradation or by inducing conformational changes in the channel, keeping acetylcholine from activating the channel. Other antibodies have been found to cause MG, including antibodies against muscle-specific kinase (MUSK), lipoprotein-related protein 4 (LRP4), or agrin. The postsynaptic cell membrane is folded into secondary synaptic folds, increasing the surface area of the cell membrane, and AchRs are organized in clusters at the peaks of these folds (adjacent to the nerve axon terminal). MUSK, LRP4, and agrin are proteins that participate in AchR clustering on these peaks. Antibody-mediated disruption of the function of these proteins causes reduced AchR concentration on the postsynaptic membrane with reduced safety factor, resulting in a myasthenia phenotype.

Some patients do not have antibodies that are detectable by current serologic testing. These patients are presumed to have antibodies against components of the postsynaptic membrane that have not yet been identified.

Prevention

Although there is no recognized prevention for developing myasthenia, exacerbations (myasthenic crises) are preventable by avoiding certain drugs. In particular, beta blockers, some antibiotics (aminoglycosides, fluoroquinolones, and macrolides), and chelating agents (penicillamine [Cuprimine]) should be avoided in myasthenic patients (see Box 1). Statins should be used cautiously and only at the lowest effective dose.

Clinical Manifestations

Patients with MG will present with weakness of the extraocular, bulbar, axial, or limb muscles. The most characteristic feature of the weakness seen in myasthenia is fatigability; that is, the tendency of a muscle to get weaker with repeated use. Thus, when thinking about weakness from MG, it is important to get a sense of whether the patient's symptoms are exacerbated by exercise, or demonstrate a diurnal fluctuation (with the most typical pattern being weakness that is worse at the end of the day).

Ocular symptoms (ptosis and diplopia) are the first symptoms of myasthenia in approximately 60% of patients, and in 15% to 20% of all myasthenic patients, weakness remains limited to the eye muscles (so-called "ocular myasthenia"). Patients will complain of a drooping eyelid or binocular double vision (that improves with closing one eye) that frequently fluctuates throughout the day or with activity. On physical examination, these patients have ptosis or limitations in extraocular movements that are triggered or exaggerated by sustained upgaze for 60 seconds (so-called "upgaze paresis"). The extraocular manifestations are rarely symmetric, and the ptosis is very often more significant on one side.

Weakness of the limbs tends to be symmetric and usually affects proximal more than distal muscles. Patients will frequently complain of reduced ability to perform repetitive actions of the proximal muscles, such as lifting an arm to comb hair or climbing stairs. On physical examination, fatigability can be demonstrated by having the patient activate the deltoids (arm abduction) or iliopsoas (hip flexion) either against gravity for 2 minutes or against examiner resistance for 5 repetitions of 5 seconds each. Typically, myasthenic patients with weakness of these muscle groups will have a significant decrement in strength between the first repetition and the last. Similar maneuvers can be performed using whichever muscle groups are affected, according to the patient's complaints.

Bulbar weakness manifests as difficulty with speech (dysarthria) or swallowing (dysphagia). These symptoms may also be fatigable; for example, patients may notice more difficulty enunciating toward the end of the day or at the end of a speech, or more trouble swallowing toward the end of a meal or when eating chewy foods such as steak. If shortness of breath is present, it typically improves moving from a supine to sitting position, which helps with diaphragm excursion. Strength of sniff and cough can be easily assessed at the bedside, and weakness of neck flexion may indicate risk for diaphragmatic weakness.

Sensation is not affected in MG. If a patient has sensory loss, static weakness that does not fluctuate with exercise, or other neurologic symptoms aside from weakness, this should prompt the examiner to consider an alternate diagnosis. Deep tendon reflexes are normal in myasthenia gravis.

Diagnosis

It is important to understand the proper diagnostic algorithm for MG, which is based on the combination of clinical history, examination findings, presence of autoantibodies, and results of electrodiagnostic testing. In the setting of a good clinical history and positive examination findings, the presence of pathologic autoantibodies is likely sufficient to confirm the diagnosis. When the clinical history or examination is suggestive but autoantibodies are not present, electrodiagnostic testing is important to confirm a suspected diagnosis, particularly if immunosuppressive or interventional therapies are considered.

Bedside tests to support a diagnosis include the ice pack test and edrophonium. Placement of ice over a ptotic eyelid may lead to clinical improvement, as cool temperature slows down the breakdown of Ach in the synapse due to slowed action of AchE. Edrophonium (Enlon, previously marketed as Tensilon) is a short-acting AchE inhibitor may be used to help confirm a clinical diagnosis. It is best used if the patient has ptosis or extraocular paresis because there is less subjectivity in assessing improvement. Edrophonium is given intravenously (IV) with 0.1 mL of a 10 mg/mL solution administered initially as a test to assess tolerance, and if no unwanted effects are noted, the remainder of the drug is injected and the patient is observed for a clinical response. If a cholinergic reaction occurs, which may include bradycardia or hypotension, then administer 0.5 mg atropine IV.

Laboratory evolution of autoantibodies is standard of care in patients with suspected MG. In generalized MG, Ach-R Abs are generally present in up to 85% of affected individuals with generalized MG. Ach-R Abs may include blocking, binding, as well as modulating antibodies. Of those patients with generalized MG who are seronegative for Ach-R Ab, approximately 30% to 40% are seropositive for MUSK antibodies. In ocular MG, where symptoms are limited to ptosis or binocular diplopia, only about 15% are seropositive for autoantibodies, and if present, those autoantibodies are Ach-R ab. The vast majority are seronegative and require further evaluation for confirmation of the diagnosis.

Electrodiagnostic testing for a disorder of neuromuscular transmission includes slow repetitive nerve stimulation (RNS). A stimulator is used to depolarize a motor nerve (resulting in an all-or-none nerve AP) and generate a muscle twitch recorded as a compound motor action potential (CMAP). A train of stimuli (between 4 to 6) are performed at a rate of 3 to 5 per second. In MG the dysfunction at the postsynaptic muscle membrane results in some muscle fibers not achieving depolarization sufficient to cause an all-or-none muscle fiber AP, and the size of the overall CMAP (from multiple muscle fibers) is reduced. The threshold for abnormality is a CMAP decrement of >10%, generally between the first and fourth stimuli. If a baseline study at rest is normal, the patient is asked to exercise the muscle for 1 minute, and the study is repeated at 1-minute intervals to assess for the development of decrement. It should be noted that the sensitivity of RNS is increased with the presence of fatigable weakness

on examination, because the clinical correlate of a decrement is weakness. Aside from distal hand muscles, trapezius or facial muscles such as nasalis can be studied.

Single fiber electromyography looks for "jitter" or loss of synchronization of individual muscle fibers innervated by a single anterior horn cell in the spinal cord. This is the most sensitive electrodiagnostic test for MG.

Differential Diagnosis

The differential diagnosis for diplopia and ptosis includes cranial nerve palsies: oculomotor (cranial nerve III), trochlear (cranial nerve IV), and abducens (cranial nerve VI). Horner's syndrome may also cause ptosis due to weakness in Mueller's muscle, although other signs such as anisocoria (unequal pupils) that is worsened in the dark is present. Thyroid eye disease may cause any of these symptoms as well. The differential diagnosis for appendicular weakness without sensory loss includes myopathy, pure motor neuropathy, anterior horn cell disease, or a central nervous system pathology involving the motor pathways. These causes of weakness result in static rather than fluctuating weakness.

The main differential diagnosis for fatigable weakness as seen in MG is the Lambert-Eaton myasthenic syndrome (LEMS). LEMS is caused by antibodies against voltage-gated calcium channels on the presynaptic neuromuscular junction and may be paraneoplastic (small cell carcinoma of the lung) or autoimmune. MG and LEMS can be differentiated by the presence of postexercise facilitation of reflexes (after 10 seconds of sustained exercise), as well as antibody and electrodiagnostic testing.

Therapy

Overall, the treatment goal is to achieve freedom from symptoms or functional limitations, recognizing that patients may still have some weakness of some muscles (this is known as minimal manifestation status). Mainstays of treatment include anticholinesterase inhibitors, as well as oral steroids, and a variety of immunosuppressants, as well as intravenous immunoglobulin (IVIG),[1] and plasmapheresis may be used. Broadly, medical therapy can be classified as symptomatic or disease-modifying, the latter with an immunomodulatory effect targeting the underlying disease pathophysiology.

It should be noted that there exists wide variation in therapeutic approaches, and there are limited head-to-head data comparing individual medications. Current treatments, as well as advances in clinical care, have significantly improved the mortality rate of MG and outcomes of myasthenic crisis.

Symptomatic Therapy

Pyridostigmine (Mestinon) is an AchE inhibitor that increases the amount of acetylcholine in the synaptic cleft by slowing its breakdown by AchE and should be considered as initial therapy. Onset of action is typically within 30 minutes, with benefit generally lasting 3 to 4 hours. As such it is initially dosed 60 mg 3 times daily by mouth and may be increased to 120 mg every 3 to 4 hours while awake, with the total dose typically not exceeding 480 mg/d. It does not penetrate the central nervous system, and most side effects are gastrointestinal. Side effects may include nausea, vomiting, abdominal cramping, diarrhea, sweating, blurred vision, or muscle twitching and cramps. Anticholinergic agents such as glycopyrrolate (Robinul)[1] 1 mg or hyoscyamine sulfate (Levsin)[1] 0.125 mg with each pyridostigmine dose can usually treat these muscarinic side effects effectively. Data suggest that MUSK Ab–positive patients may have a lesser response to acetylcholinersterase therapy when compared with ACH-R–seropositive patients. In the setting of ocular myasthenia, there appears to be more of response in ptosis when compared with diplopia.

Corticosteroids

Corticosteroids, typically prednisone,[1] are a mainstay of immunotherapy and used when pyridostigmine alone does not achieve an adequate treatment response. Two general approaches exist,

---

[1] Not FDA approved for this indication.

using either a low-dose or high-dose regimen. Decisions may be dictated by the severity of weakness, presence of significant bulbar dysfunction, or comorbid conditions (such as diabetes). A "low-dose" approach is used with milder disease and includes initiation of 10 to 20 mg daily, and increasing by 5 mg orally weekly to a lower target dose (generally 40–60 mg/d). Oral high-dose (1 mg/kg/d) steroid therapy may be used with moderate-severe weakness and generally has a latency of 2 to 4 weeks before onset of benefit with maximal benefit in 5 to 6 months. It is important to recognize that early clinical deterioration is possible (reported up to 50%) approximately 7 to 10 days after treatment initiation, generally when steroids are dosed at 1 mg/kg/d or higher. In those patients for whom high-dose therapy is introduced, concomitant treatment with either IVIG or plasma exchange (PLEX), discussed herein, may provide protection against early clinical deterioration.

For a patient who has achieved the treatment goal of minimal manifestation on a particular dose of steroids, it is important to consider weaning the dose to reduce side effects. A common approach is a slow taper decreasing 5 mg/d per month on alternate days, with a slower taper once a total dose of 10 mg daily is achieved. Many patients can be maintained on low doses of steroids.

Some patients have an inadequate response to steroids or intolerable side effects or are unable to taper because of recurrence of symptoms. These patients are typically treated with alternative, steroid-sparing, immunomodulatory therapies. Some patients with comorbidities that limit steroid dosing are started on steroids and nonsteroidal immunosuppressant medications concurrently.

Thymectomy
Thymectomy is considered standard of care for those with thymoma, which is present in approximately 15% of patients with generalized MG. A recent study supports thymectomy in Ach-R Ab–positive patients with at least moderately severe disease. Thymectomy patients demonstrated improved outcomes compared with placebo, required less steroids, fewer required steroid-sparing immunosuppressants, and experienced fewer hospitalizations. Thymectomy is controversial for mild symptoms, purely ocular disease, older age (>60 years), and there exist various surgical approaches. It is considered standard of care to pretreat with IVIG or PLEX before surgery if patients are symptomatic.

Other Immunomodulatory Therapies
Azathioprine (Imuran)[1] is a purine analogue that inhibits nucleic acid synthesis, as well as T- and B-cell proliferation. It is a commonly used steroid-sparing immunosuppressant that is considered first-line and has shown efficacy in a randomized clinical trial. Azathioprine allows reduced steroid dose, reduces relapse rate, and prolongs duration of remission. Treatment is generally started at 50 mg daily, increasing by 50 mg every 1 to 2 weeks to approximately 150 to 200 daily (2–3 mg/kg/d), generally in split doses. Onset of action is estimated at 4 to 8 months, and therapy requires regular blood count and liver function monitoring. Side effects include a flulike illness at initiation (reported in up to 10% to 20%, requires cessation), leukopenia, and transaminitis. Thiopurine methyltransferase enzyme testing can be performed, if available, before starting to identify patients at high risk of bone marrow suppression (although monitoring of blood counts is favored by many practitioners).

Intravenous immunoglobulin (IVIG, Gammagard)[1] has been shown to improve weakness in MG. Its mechanism of action is unclear although presumed to stem from neutralizing circulating pathogenic autoantibodies. A dose of 2 g/kg spread over 5 days is a common algorithm for initial treatment, although in patients who previously tolerated it, IVIG could be given as 1 g/kg/d over 2 days. Onset of action is typically within the first week, and benefit may be sustained for 3 to 4 weeks after treatment. Side effects include headache (sometimes severe and related to aseptic meningitis), thrombosis because of increased serum viscosity, and renal failure. Avoidance of sucrose-containing products may decrease risk of renal failure. Slowed infusion rates may help avoid decompensation of heart failure. Patients on maintenance dosing may receive IVIG 1 g/kg every 3 to 4 weeks.

Mycophenolate mofetil (Cellcept)[1] inhibits guanosine nucleotide synthesis that is needed for B and T lymphocytes. Although there have been two negative randomized clinical trials, there are several retrospective reports supporting efficacy and consensus expert opinion is that it remains a treatment option. It is started at 500 mg twice daily and titrated to 1000 to 1500 mg twice daily. Side effects include nausea, vomiting, diarrhea, and leukopenia. It has teratogenic potential and should not be used in pregnancy.

Cyclosporine (Sandimmune)[1] is a calcineurin inhibitor that has suppressed inflammatory cytokines and has multiple effects on T-cell function. It is initiated at approximately 3 mg/kg daily as a twice-daily split dose and may be titrated up to 5 mg/kg/d with a target trough level <300 ng/mL. Onset of action is approximately 2 to 3 months. Side effects include hirsutism, hypertension, clinically significant nephrotoxicity, and increased cancer risk (including dermatologic cancers). Cyclosporine level may be affected by multiple drug interactions, and concomitant medications should be reviewed.

Methotrexate (Trexall)[1] is a folate antimetabolite that may be dosed orally or subcutaneously. A typical oral dose is initiated at 10 mg weekly and titrated to 15 to 25 mg orally once a week. It is recommended that the patient take folate[1] supplementation of approximately at least 1 mg daily. Side effects include stomatitis (folate supplementation may help prevent this), bone marrow suppression, as well as interstitial lung disease (rare). It is important to note that methotrexate is a known teratogen and should be avoided in women of childbearing potential.

Plasmapheresis or PLEX removes plasma from the circulation and replaces it, typically with albumin, with the net effect of removing pathologic autoantibodies and inflammatory cytokines. Typically five exchanges are performed over a period of 1 to 2 weeks, and benefit is typically observed by the third exchange. PLEX requires placement of a vascath or (if to be used as a maintenance therapy) a permacath. When used as a maintenance therapy, 1 to 2 exchanges are typically performed, at variable intervals, as frequently as weekly. There is a risk of deep venous thrombosis or line infection. Hypotension may occur because of citrate-induced hypovolemia, and it may be associated with hypocalcemia. ACE inhibitors need to be held 24 hours because of bradykinin-related vasodilation.

Rituximab (Rituxan)[1] is a CD20 antibody that has been evaluated in a randomized controlled trial, the results of which are pending. There exists retrospective data to support efficacy, particularly in MUSK Ab patients who have failed initial therapy. It is dosed 325 mg/m[2] weekly for 4 weeks, although it can also be dosed 1 g/m[2] with a second dose 2 weeks later. Dosing may be repeated at 6-month intervals. Side effects include infusion-related symptoms including pruritis, headache, hypotension, nausea, and chills. Rituximab may additionally result in leukopenia, anemia, or thrombocytopenia. Infusion-related symptoms can be pretreated with acetaminophen and diphenhydramine.

Eculizumab (Soliris) is a complement inhibitor that was recently FDA approved for AchR Ab generalized myasthenia gravis. It is dosed at 900 mg weekly for 4 weeks, followed by 1200 mg for the fifth week and thereafter 1200 mg every 2 weeks. Generally only mild infusion reactions are reported, typically managed by pretreatment acetaminophen and diphenhydramine, although there is risk for severe meningococcal infection. Meningococcal immunization is recommended before treatment initiation.

Cyclophosphamide (Cytoxan)[1] is typically reserved for treatment-refractory patients. It may be administered orally with a daily dose ranging from 1.5 to 5 mg daily. Potential side effects of oral cyclophosphamide include cystitis as well as bladder

---

[1]Not FDA approved for this indication.

[1]Not FDA approved for this indication.

cancer, leading many treating physicians to use IV pulse dosing. A common approach for pulse dosing is 1 gm/m² monthly for 6 months (less toxic). Onset of action with pulse dosing is relatively quick, generally about 1 month.

Treatment Considerations in Pregnancy

Pregnancy and postpartum status have been reported to be triggers for worsening of myasthenia. Ideally, prepregnancy planning allows for optimization of clinical status to improve pregnancy outcomes. These patients require expert multidisciplinary care through the postpartum period. In pregnancy the treatment of choice is pyridostigmine, with steroids being the immunosuppressant of choice. Azathioprine[1] and cyclosporine[1] are relatively safe in expectant mothers who are not satisfactorily controlled or cannot tolerate corticosteroids. IVIG[1] and PLEX may also be treatment options.

Transient neonatal myasthenia may affect the newborn infant. This is difficult to predict and requires close attention for signs after delivery. Neonatal critical care support should be readily available for these infants.

Monitoring

After a diagnosis of MG is confirmed, additional testing or monitoring is indicated. The frequency of clinical assessment should be dictated by the severity and nature of the patient's symptoms, as well as the impact of the disease on function. Patients with MG should be managed in concert with a neurologist. Refractory MG is defined by symptoms that affect function and are unchanged or worse after corticosteroids and at least two other immunosuppressive agents used in adequate doses for adequate duration. Patients meeting criteria for refractory MG should be referred to a physician or medical center with expertise in MG.

Computed tomography of the chest should be performed to screen for thymoma. Assessment of thyroid function is important. If immunomodulatory medications are used for disease control, TB screening should be performed.

Pulmonary and swallowing dysfunction may be encountered. Pulmonary function testing should be performed for patients with symptomatic generalized MG, particularly if there are complaints of dyspnea. Speech therapy referral for a swallow evaluation should be performed if there is concern for dysphagia.

Periodic laboratory monitoring is required with use of immunomodulatory medications, which may vary depending on the specific medication used. Suggested tests and monitoring algorithms are detailed in Box 2.

Complications

The most severe complication of MG is myasthenic crisis, which is defined by worsening of weakness requiring intubation or noninvasive ventilation. Myasthenic crisis may be seen in up to 20% of patients at some point in disease course. Myasthenic crisis is most commonly encountered in the setting of concomitant illness, change in medications, or early in the disease course because maximum weakness occurs in the first year of the disease in 66% of patients. Respiratory failure can result from respiratory muscle weakness, oropharyngeal weakness, or a combination of both. It is important to recognize that new respiratory or swallowing complaints can quickly escalate, and patients with these complaints should be quickly assessed. One can assess diaphragm strength by the force of a strong sniff or cough; patients should be able to count to 20 after a deep breath. Staccato speech or dyspnea that precludes speaking in full sentences is of high concern for myasthenic crisis. Spirometry with forced vital capacity <2 L or negative inspiratory force of <40 cm H₂O should be sent to the hospital for further evaluation. Assessment of swallowing function by speech therapy and possible modified barium swallow should be considered in the context of dysphagia for solids and liquids.

IVIG and PLEX have comparable outcomes for the treatment of patients with moderate-to-severe weakness. The response to

---

[1] Not FDA approved for this indication.

PLEX may be more predictable than IVIG in severe MG exacerbations, and retrospective data suggests PLEX may be more effective than IVIG in myasthenic crisis. PLEX, however, may be associated with more complications, as well as longer hospital stay and associated hospital costs.

References

Farmakidis C, Pasnoor M, Dimachkie M, Baron R: Treatment of myasthenia gravis, *Neurol Clin* 36:311–337, 2018.
Gilhus NE, Verschuuren JJ: Myasthenia gravis: subgroup classification and therapeutic strategies, *Lancet Neurol* 14:1023–1036, 2015.
Gilhus NE: Myasthenia gravis, *N Engl J Med* 375:2570–2581, 2016.
Myasthenia Gravis Foundation of America. Myasthenia Gravis: A Manual for the Healthcare Provider. Available at http://myasthenia.org/. [accessed April 1, 2018].
Sanders DB, Wilfe GI, Benatar M, et al: International consensus guidance for management of myasthenia gravis, *Neurology* 87:419–425, 2016.
Wilfe GI, Kaminski HJ, Aban IN, et al: Randomized trial of thymectomy in myasthenia gravis, *N Engl J Med* 375:511–522, 2016.

NEUROFIBROMATOSIS (TYPE 1)

Method of
Jason E. Marker, MD, MPA

CURRENT DIAGNOSIS

- Neurofibromatosis Type 1 (NF1) can be diagnosed by physicians based on well-defined diagnostic criteria that can be met with a careful history and physical exam.
- Additional testing may be needed in some cases (including genetic testing) to confirm the diagnosis or to provide information that will be important for both short- and long-term management.
- NF1 has important genetic underpinnings, can have extremely variable expression within families and will evolve in its need for medical intervention throughout the lifetime of the patient.

CURRENT THERAPY

- There is no treatment for NF1. However, there are many therapies for both the common and uncommon manifestations and complications of the condition.
- Many therapies are similar to those used for non-NF1 patients with the same symptoms. However, there are some manifestations where unique therapies are needed, and physicians need to know the difference between these.
- Proper monitoring of the patient aids in the identification of treatable symptoms and allows opportunities for anticipatory guidance and counseling.
- There are several emerging therapies related to the heritability of NF1 that are important for patients of childbearing age to be aware of.

Introduction and Epidemiology

Neurofibromatosis encompasses three distinct genetic entities: NF1, neurofibromatosis type 2 (NF2), and schwannomatosis. Because NF1 is so much more common (incidence of 1:1900 to 1:3000 livebirths) than NF2 (incidence of 1:25,000 to 1:33,000 livebirths) and schwannomatosis (incidence of 1:40,000 to 1:1.7M livebirths), when the word "neurofibromatosis" is used (or the older name, "Von Recklinghausen Disease), it is generally referring to NF1. NF1 is the primary topic of this chapter.

NF1 is an autosomal dominant genetic disorder and is progressive in that its clinical manifestations evolve over the lifespan. About half of the cases of NF1 are familial and the remainder are the result of new, spontaneous mutations. Life expectancy is reduced by 5 to 15 years and is related to the severity of the clinical manifestations, the emergence of malignant tumors, and excess hypertensive and vascular disease risk. There is no predilection based on race, ethnic origin, or country of birth.

Risk Factors

NF1 is an autosomal dominant condition and affects 50% of the offspring of parents where one parent is affected, making family history the primary predictable risk factor. Advanced paternal age increases the likelihood of a de novo mutation. Eighty percent of newly occurring mutations are believed to come from the paternally derived chromosome.

Pathophysiology

NF1 is the result of mutations in the *NF1* gene (chromosome 17q11.2) that codes for the protein Neurofibromin. Neurofibromin is a protein in the GTPase-activating family that stimulates the Ras pathway for tumor suppression. Loss of neurofibromin results in "de-suppression" of tumor growth within susceptible tissues. Although genetic penetrance in NF1 is complete, NF1 is highly variable in its expression (even within families). This is because germline mutations must be coupled with somatic mutations in order for symptoms to manifest clinically.

Several thousand distinct *NF1* mutations have been identified. Many small mutations have demonstrated no genotype-phenotype correlation, while some individuals (1% to 5% of NF1 patients) will have complete loss of the 1.4 to 1.5Mb of the *NF1* gene and are quite severely affected. Due to the large size of this gene, mutations in the *NF1* gene occur more often than in any other human gene.

Somatic and germline (rare) mosaicism occurs and can result in phenotypically unaffected offspring who could later transmit the mutated gene to their own children.

Prevention

There is no specific prevention for any of the clinical manifestations of NF1. Due to its variable expression, some individuals will simply be more or less affected. To the extent that having a diagnosis of NF1 *could* cause academic challenges, interpersonal hardships and social isolation, robust anticipatory guidance throughout the lifespan can help these individuals develop proper support systems and personal resilience, preventing some of the morbidity of the disease.

Affected individuals of child-bearing age now have the option of genetic testing of fertilized eggs to select unaffected eggs for implantation. This is an emerging prevention strategy.

Clinical Manifestations

There are a number of clinical manifestations of NF1. Because of the variability of expression of the *NF1* gene, these manifestations may be variably present in any affected individual. The following section on diagnosis will discuss how these clinical manifestations fit into the diagnostic criteria for NF1.

Café-au-lait spots are flat, irregularly shaped, uniformly hyperpigmented macules that appear during the first year of life and then increase in number through childhood. These macules are present in 95% of adults with NF1 but tend to fade and become more indistinct later in life. Among the general population of individuals who do not have NF1, 15% will have one to three café-au-lait macules.

Freckling (primarily in areas of skin apposition like the axillae and inguinal folds) is distinct from café-au-lait macules as the freckles are smaller, more clustered, and generally appear later in childhood than the café-au-lait macules.

Lisch nodules are tan-colored hamartomas of the iris. Lisch nodules do not affect vision and may be seen with simple ophthalmoscopy (although the use of a slit lamp will help identify small nodules and distinguish them from iris nevi). These nodules are seen in up to 90% of adults with NF1, but fewer than 10% of children under 6 years old.

Neurofibromas present as several types of lesions with variable characteristics, risk of pathology, and symptomatology.

Cutaneous peripheral neurofibromas are benign peripheral nerve sheath tumors that are generally soft, mobile, and fleshy. They may be dermal or epidermal on a broad or pedunculated base. These neurofibromas are nontender, are usually more common on the trunk and can number from a few to thousands. Cutaneous peripheral neurofibromas do not degenerate into malignant peripheral nerve sheath tumors (MPNSTs). **Plexiform peripheral neurofibromas** can be superficial or deep inside the body. They tend to be more diffuse and involve plaques and tangles of abnormal tissues that can grow into a complex mass. On whole-body scanning, 50% of patients with NF1 will have at least one plexiform neurofibroma. Large plexiform neurofibromas can create symptoms by compressing nearby structures and, unlike cutaneous neurofibromas, they have the capacity to degenerate into MPNSTs. **Nodular neurofibromas** are firm and rubbery. Unlike the cutaneous neurofibromas, they are sometimes tender, often deeper and usually less mobile. They are not as invasive as the plexiform neurofibromas but can undergo degeneration into MPNSTs.

Optic pathway gliomas (OPGs) occur in 15% of children younger than 6 (but rarely in older individuals) and can grow anywhere along the optic tracts. Most individuals are asymptomatic, but advanced tumors can affect vision or even upset the normal function of the hypothalamus with growth rate variations and premature or delayed puberty.

Orthopedic abnormalities are primarily long-bone dysplasias and pseudoarthroses. Anterolateral bowing of the tibia (usually unilateral) in infants and young children can easily go undetected until a pathologic fracture develops at the onset of ambulation. One half of fractures occur during the toddler years. Long-bone pseudoarthrosis has a male predisposition (1.7:1) and NF1 accounts for 50% to 70% of all long-bone pseudoarthroses. Other orthopedic findings in NF1 patients may include short stature (13% have a height less than 2 standard deviations below the mean), scoliosis (10% to 15% of NF1 patients are affected), sphenoid wing dysplasia (leading to facial asymmetry), osteoporosis, and macrocephaly.

Neurologic abnormalities encompass cognitive defects and learning disabilities as well as the risk of seizures. Although profound intellectual disability is rare (the likelihood of having an IQ <70 is similar to the general population), 81% of NF patients will have some impairment in one or more areas of cognitive functioning. While less than half of NF1 patients have a specific learning disability, more than half will have some amount of neuropsychological impairment, including speech articulation problems, AD/HD, or impairment of executive functioning. Seizures occur twice as often in patients with NF1 (prevalence 4% to 6%) as in the general population and can be of any type and occur at any age.

Other manifestations of concern: Rarely, other **central nervous system (CNS) neoplasms** develop. CNS astrocytomas usually arise during childhood and, when not an incidental finding on a scan being done for another purpose, may present with symptoms of increased intracranial pressure. Rare brainstem gliomas are usually symptomatic at presentation. **Malignant peripheral nerve sheath tumors** are highly malignant tumors that can arise from a pre-existing plexiform or nodular neurofibromas. The lifetime risk of developing an MPNST in a patient with NF1 is 5% to 13% and most commonly occurs in teenagers and young adults. MPNSTs are usually diagnosed when a plexiform or nodular neurofibroma goes through a period of pain, change in consistency, and rapid growth. **Hypertension**, including hypertension as early as childhood, is common among NF1 patients. Although rare, renal neurovascular lesions can be the cause, and NF1 patients with hypertension should be evaluated for renal artery stenosis.

Diagnosis

The diagnosis of NF1 can be made reliably by a primary care team, but a multidisciplinary team of sub-specialists is often involved in the long-term care of these individuals, including during the diagnostic phase. A comprehensive history (including a detailed family history) and examination should be undertaken. Additional testing or referral, as indicated by the initial evaluation, should be pursued to clarify the diagnosis, seek findings amenable to treatment, and facilitate proper anticipatory guidance and patient/family education.

The US National Institutes of Health (NIH) Consensus Conference in 1997 set forth the following diagnostic criteria for NF1:

At least two of the following clinical features must be present to make the diagnosis of NF1:

- Six or more café-au-lait macules greater than 5 mm (prepubertal) or greater than 15 mm (postpubertal) in longest diameter
- Two or more neurofibromas of any type (or a single plexiform neurofibroma)
- Freckling in the axillary or inguinal regions
- Optic glioma
- Two or more Lisch nodules
- A distinctive bony lesion (sphenoid dysplasia or a long-bone dysplasia with or without pseudoarthrosis)
- A first-degree relative with NF1 based on the previous criteria

These NIH criteria are both sensitive and specific, and are met by 97% of NF1 patients by the age of 8 years (100% by the age of 20 years). Nearly half of individuals with a new sporadic mutation fail to meet these criteria by the age of 1 year. Therefore, in an infant with one clinical feature, close observation is needed to determine if other criteria will be met. If, by the age of 4 years, only one criterion is met, referral for a genetic diagnosis may be warranted.

Other specific testing may be needed to make the diagnosis, to determine the extent of involvement of the disorder, or to decide on treatment. These include the following:

- Dermatologic evaluation: If the identification of café-au-lait spots, whether café-au-lait spots meet diagnostic criteria, or the identification of criteria-meeting freckling is in question, referral to Dermatology may be needed. Likewise, the spectrum of neurofibromas is broad and a dermatologist may be needed to properly identify these lesions.
- Lisch nodules: Although occasionally seen with the naked eye or through an office ophthalmoscope, formal ophthalmologic consultation is recommended to look for small Lisch nodules and to assess for optic disk findings suggestive of OPGs or increased intracranial pressure.
- Optic pathway gliomas: Ophthalmologic evaluation is recommended as noted above. Brain MRI imaging is not recommended for asymptomatic patients with normal ophthalmologic evaluations.
- Orthopedic abnormalities: Plain radiographs of long bones or CT imaging of craniofacial bones may be needed to identify the diagnostic findings in these areas.
- Neurologic abnormalities: Because new focal seizures could be the result of a new intracranial neoplasm, neuroimaging is warranted with any new seizure activity.
- Other manifestations of concern: MPNSTs are best differentiated from benign plexiform or nodular neurofibromas by positron emission tomography (PET) scan. Evaluating for renal artery stenosis in individuals with new onset hypertension (including children) is indicated.
- Genetic counseling and testing: Genetic testing is usually reserved for cases where the diagnosis remains in question following a thorough history, examination, and nongenetic testing. Additionally, genetic testing may be indicated for family members of the affected individual. Knowing that expression is extremely variable, preconception, embryonic preimplantation, or prenatal (amniocentesis or chorionic villi sampling) testing for individuals in families with NF1 should be considered.

Differential Diagnosis

Because of the well-established diagnostic criteria and availability of genetic testing, the differential diagnosis of NF1 is limited. As noted at the outset, NF2 and schwannomatosis are lumped together with NF1 under the general diagnosis of Neurofibromatosis. Schwannomatosis is a complex regional pain syndrome

with some common underlying pathophysiology but no overlapping symptoms and unrelated genetics. NF2 will be discussed briefly in the discussion below.

Legius syndrome includes café-au-lait macules, axillary freckling, and macrocephaly. It does *not* include neurofibromas or CNS tumors, however. Like NF1, Legius syndrome is an autosomal dominant disorder for loss of a tumor suppressor protein, but it affects an entirely different gene.

Constitutional mismatch repair-deficiency syndrome (CMMR-D) is a rare autosomal recessive condition that results in café-au-lait macules (and occasionally axillary freckling and Lisch nodules). Unlike in NF1, individuals with CMMR-D are at risk for hematologic malignancies in infancy and childhood, brain tumors (primarily glioblastomas) in mid-childhood, and colorectal cancer in adolescence and young adulthood. Rhabdomyosarcomas and optic pathway gliomas may occur rarely in CMMR-D.

NF2 is caused by the *NF2* gene on chromosome 22, which encodes for the tumor suppressor protein merlin (or schwannomin), which is a functionally different protein than that produced by *NF1*. Key differences between NF1 and NF2 include the following points about NF2:

- Few or nonexistent café-au-lait macules
- No Lisch nodules
- No risk of MPNSTs
- Spinal root tumors are schwannomas in NF2 (neurofibromas in NF1)
- No cognitive impairment
- High prevalence of bilateral acoustic schwannomas and resulting hearing loss in 90% to 95% of patients by the age of 30 years.
- 60% to 80% have cataracts
- Presence of meningiomas

Noonan syndrome is characterized by short stature and may include café-au-lait macules that may meet the size and number criteria for NF1. Sometimes, the facial features of Noonan syndrome can overlap with the appearance of NF1. However, the webbed neck of Noonan syndrome and the association with pulmonic stenosis are not part of NF1. Although the Ras signaling pathway is involved in Noonan syndrome, the underlying genetics are entirely different.

Surveillance and Therapy

There is no treatment for NF1, and there are no therapeutic agents approved for the problems encountered that are specific to these patients because of their NF1 diagnosis. There are many ongoing, NF-specific clinical trials for the problems that are commonly encountered by individuals with NF1.

The following areas of surveillance should be undertaken. Where research or expert opinion suggests a proper frequency, it is listed, although shared decision making with the patient/family as well as communication with your medical colleagues will be required to develop appropriate timelines. Therapeutic options are listed below for many of the common issues NF1 patients face, while the management of less common complications is outlined in the next section.

- Yearly examination of the skin for new neurofibromas and any signs of change within an existing neurofibroma should be done. Especially when nodular or plexiform neurofibromas exist (those at risk of malignant transformation), any history of rapid change or new pain should be evaluated thoroughly. A PET scan can distinguish between benign and malignant lesions. Referral to surgical and/or dermatologic colleagues should be made regarding these nodular or plexiform neurofibromas (for biopsy and management decisions) and should be strongly considered for all but the most clear and superficial cutaneous neurofibromas.
- Cutaneous neurofibromas that develop pruritus are often not responsive to antihistamines, although the itching is often improved by the use of gabapentin (Neurontin)[1].

---

[1]Not FDA approved for this indication.

- Yearly blood pressure measurement, even in children and young adults, should be done. Once the diagnosis of essential hypertension is made following testing that excludes the diagnosis of renal artery stenosis, blood pressure should be controlled following standard blood pressure goals and treatment algorithms. Hypertension that becomes hard to control may prompt an evaluation for pheochromocytoma, a rare finding in NF1.
- Growth tracking of weight, height, and head circumference should be done through childhood and adolescence in the usual manner. Additionally, any signs of premature or delayed puberty should be evaluated further. Growth and pubertal abnormalities should prompt an age-appropriate endocrinology referral for additional testing (serum, urine, and/or neuroimaging) and treatments based on these results.
- Neurodevelopmental and academic assessment should be undertaken, involving family members and school personnel when appropriate. Individuals who develop neuropsychiatric and academic problems should undergo formal neurodiagnostic testing, and any identified diagnoses should be treated. These treatments are no different than those used for non-NF1 individuals who carry the same neuropsychiatric diagnosis. Neuroimaging is not indicated in the evaluation of neuropsychiatric conditions unless neurologic deficits exist.
- NF1 patients who develop seizures are treated with the usual seizure management algorithms following neuroimaging to look for new intracranial pathologies. An electro-encephalogram (EEG) is not indicated for asymptomatic individuals.
- Evaluation for skeletal changes including scoliosis, facial asymmetry, or long bone abnormalities should be performed yearly during childhood and adolescence, and then at the typical wellness visits into young adulthood (with prompting in these older ages to report any changes that are noticed between visits). Any abnormalities that are encountered should prompt additional imaging and referral to subspecialty care.
- Women with NF1 develop osteoporosis at an earlier age than their non-NF1 peers and should undergo earlier screening in accordance with this fact and with other standard risk factors they may have. When diagnosed, this osteoporosis is treated like it would be for any other patient.
- For unclear reasons, women with NF1 have an increased risk of breast cancer, especially women under the age of 40 (at the age of 70, the risk approximates that of the general population). These are usually invasive ductal carcinomas (the most common type overall) and are managed in the usual way, although these patients need both earlier education about, and screening for, breast cancer.
- Formal ophthalmologic evaluation for visual screening, slit lamp and intraocular examination should take place yearly at least through adolescence, usually in the context of a comprehensive examination. Lisch nodules are nonpathologic and no treatment is needed, but any signs of elevated intracranial pressure or optic disc pathology warrant further testing and management. The optimal frequency of MRI surveillance of an optic pathway glioma is unknown but should be based on symptomatology, size, and rate of progression.
- Brain MRI is not recommended as a routine screening test. It may be a part of the initial diagnostic work-up but should not need to be repeated for asymptomatic patients who are otherwise receiving comprehensive surveillance. Of note, "NF-associated bright spots" may be seen on MRI imaging, and the data are inconclusive on the relationship between these spots and any pathologic process. These spots often resolve spontaneously by late childhood.
- Whole body MRI screening or MRI of nonbrain areas of potential concern (such as visible but stable and asymptomatic plexiform or nodular neurofibromas) is not recommended by most authorities. Likewise, screening PET scanning is not recommended.

Management of Complications

The section above outlines the surveillance of and treatment for most of the common concerns for patients with NF1. Rarely, more significant complications present themselves. These are listed below along with their management plan.

- Symptomatic cutaneous neurofibromas that are cosmetically unacceptable, painful, itchy, or disfiguring will sometimes need to be managed. Once it is clear that the lesions in question are truly simple cutaneous neurofibromas, they may be removed in any manner, including by excision, cryotherapy, laser, or electrodessication.
- Symptomatic plexiform neurofibromas that have not degenerated into MPNSTs that are deemed in need of management or removal should be managed by a multidisciplinary team of surgeons and oncologists who are familiar with this type of tumor. These invasive tumors require nonstandard operative approaches and consideration of emerging chemotherapeutic agents.
- MPNSTs are often due to a co-mutated *SUZ12* gene (which lies contiguous to *NF1*). Individuals with large or complete deletions of the *NF1* gene (those who are generally more severely affected) are at an increased risk of this complication. MPNSTs are usually managed by surgeons and oncologists familiar with NF1 and often involve surgical excision with adjunctive radiation and possibly emerging chemotherapeutic agents.
- Optic pathway gliomas are most commonly found to be low-grade pilocystic astrocytomas. As such, they are often sensitive to the standard oncologic treatments for that type of tumor—but when to observe and when to proceed to treatment is controversial.
- Because the bony architecture of pathologic skeletal lesions is inherently abnormal in these patients, the risk of complications from corrective treatments is higher than in non-NF1 patients. Your local orthopedic colleagues need to be aware of this and obtain tertiary care back-up when needed. Amputation is often the best long-term plan for long bone lesions.
- Refractory hypertension in the absence of renal artery stenosis that is ultimately found to be the result of pheochromocytoma should be managed by a multidisciplinary team experienced in the management of this diagnosis. It is managed in the same manner as non-NF1 patients with a pheochromocytoma.
- Short stature is often correctible with growth hormone therapy. However, this treatment is not often used because it compounds the inherent protumorgenic nature of NF1. In extreme cases of short stature when growth hormone is used, clinicians need to be alert to the evolution and potential malignant degeneration of new or existing tumors.
- NF1 patients are at a high risk of psychosocial issues arising from the symptoms they may experience from their NF1, its lack of treatability, and its genetic underpinnings. These symptoms may affect relationship building and reproductive decisions. Extra professional support may be needed, particularly during adolescence.

Although pregnancy is not a "complication" of NF1, its management can certainly be complicated by the diagnosis. Pregnant NF1 patients have increased morbidity (but not mortality) due to hypertensive and vascular complications. These complications should be anticipated and managed by an appropriately trained medical team. Genetic counseling should be recommended, ideally prior to conception, and steps taken to ensure proper evaluation and surveillance for the newborn.

References

Defendi GL: Genetics of neurofibromatosis type 1 and type 2. Available at https://emedicine.medscape.com/article/950151-overview. [Accessed 15 November 2018].

Evans DG: Neurofibromatosis type 2. Available at https://www.uptodate.com/contents/neurofibromatosis-type-2. [Accessed 15 November 2018].

Ferner RE, Huson SM, et al: Guidelines for the diagnosis and management of individuals with neurofibromatosis 1, *J Med Genet* 44:81–88, 2007.

Hart L: Primary care of patients with neurofibromatosis 1, *The Nurse Practitioner* 30(6), 2005.

Hersh JH: Committee on Genetics of the American Academy of Pediatrics: Health Supervision of Children with Neurofibromatosis, *Pediatrics* 121:633–645, 2008.

Human Genetics Society of Australia: *Choosing Wisely Australia: 5 Things Clinicians and Consumers Should Question*, October 2016. Available at http://www.choosingwisely.org.au/getmedia/bbc1ca07-7340-49ca-9e85-ad4c1a7bc197/GESA_Choosing_Wisely_Recommendations.pdf.aspx. [Accessed 15 November 2018].

Korf BR: Neurofibromatosis type 1 (NF1): Management and prognosis. Available at https://www.uptodate.com/contents/neurofibromatosis-type-1-nf1-management-and-prognosis. [Accessed 15 November 2018].

Korf BR: Neurofibromatosis type 1 (NF1): Pathogenesis, clinical features, and diagnosis. Available at https://www.uptodate.com/contents/neurofibromatosis-type-1-nf1-pathogenesis-clinical-features-and-diagnosis. [Accessed 15 November 2018].

Stewart DR, Korf BR, et al: Care of adults with neurofibromatosis type 1: a clinical practice resource of the American College of Medical Genetics and Genomics (ACMG), *Genet Med* 20(7):671–682, 2018 Jul.

Tonsgard JH: Clinical manifestations and management of neurofibromatosis type 1, *Seminars in Pediatric Neurology*, Elsevier 13:2–7, 2006.

Williams VC, Lucas J, et al: Neurofibromatosis type 1 revisited, *Pediatrics* 123:124–133, 2009.

OPTIC NEURITIS

Method of
Heather E. Moss, MD, PhD

CURRENT DIAGNOSIS

- Vision is impaired, including visual acuity, visual field, and/or color perception.
- Patients typically have eye pain that is worse with eye movement.
- There is a relative afferent papillary defect if only one eye is affected.
- The anterior optic nerve has a normal appearance in two-thirds of affected patients.

CURRENT THERAPY

- Consider IV methylprednisolone (Solu-Medrol, 1 g/day IV for 3 days) followed by oral steroids (1 mg/kg per day for 11 days).
- Avoid low-dose oral steroid monotherapy, as this is associated with a higher relapse rate.
- If brain MRI or blood testing suggest a high-risk, clinically isolated syndrome, consider disease-modifying therapy to delay progression to Multiple Sclerosis (MS) or Neuro-myelitis optica (NMO).
- If the clinical features suggest NMO spectrum optic neuritis, consider IV methylprednisolone and plasma exchange therapy.
- If the patient's history and testing suggest MS or NMO, consider treatment for these conditions.

Epidemiology

The incidence of optic neuritis is approximately 1 to 5 in 100,000. Though it typically affects women in their fourth decade of life, 1 in 4 patients are male, and patients have been reported ranging from the first to seventh decades of life. Optic neuritis occurs worldwide in persons of various ethnicities.

Optic neuritis can be classified as a clinically isolated syndrome or in association with a disease such as multiple sclerosis (MS) or neuromyelitis optica (NMO). NMO is clinically distinguished by more frequent involvement of the optic nerves and spinal cord and less involvement of the brain than MS and by distinct pathophysiology. A recently identified distinct classification is anti-myelin oligodentrocyte glycoprotein (MOG) associated optic neuritis. Approximately half of patients with optic neuritis as a clinically isolated syndrome develop MS. A small percentage develop NMO.

Risk Factors

A diagnosis of a disease associated with optic neuritis, such as MS or NMO, increases the risk of developing optic neuritis. In one study, more than 70% of patients with MS and 100% of patients with NMO had unilateral optic neuritis at some point.

Pathophysiology

Most optic neuritis occurs as a result of inflammation causing demyelination of the ganglion cell axons that compose the optic nerve. This is thought to be an immune-mediated process.

Prevention

Disease-modifying therapies have been shown to reduce risk of neurologic relapses in patients with MS or NMO. These therapies presumably also decrease the risk of MS- or NMO-associated optic neuritis because optic neuritis is a common relapse syndrome in these conditions.

Clinical Manifestations

A typical optic neuritis patient experiences acute or subacute loss of vision characterized by decreased visual acuity, visual field loss, and/or color vision loss, accompanied or preceded by pain in the affected eye that is worse with eye movements. However, 8% of patients do not have pain. Other symptoms include positive visual phenomena in 30% of patients. Other signs include a relative afferent papillary defect in cases where one eye is affected and a mildly swollen optic nerve head in approximately one-third of patients. Optic neuritis in NMO is more likely to have bilateral involvement and severe visual impairment. The spectrum of anti-MOG associated optic neuritis is being defined with initial case series describing a higher prevalence of optic nerve head swelling than MS or NMO associated optic neuritis.

The natural history of clinically isolated optic neuritis includes resolution of pain 3 to 5 days after onset and nadir of vision 7 to 14 days after onset. Spontaneous improvement in vision is typically evident within 3 weeks, and almost 70% of affected patients recover 20/20 visual acuity even in the absence of treatment. Optic neuritis associated with NMO tends to have less spontaneous recovery of vision and early recognition is important due to benefits of early treatment.

Diagnosis

The diagnosis is based on the clinical presentation. Where there is uncertainty, magnetic resonance imaging (MRI) of the orbits, including fat-saturated sequences (T2 and T1 with and without gadolinium contrast), can help visualize inflammation in the retrobulbar optic nerve. Changes on MRI involving the chiasm or more than 50% of the optic nerve are suggestive of NMO spectrum optic neuritis. Anti-MOG optic neuritis may have distinct imaging features.

Optic neuritis is often associated with other demyelinating syndromes, most commonly MS. Therefore it is important to screen for historical and current neurologic impairment through history and examination. MRI and/or and cerebrospinal fluid analysis documenting evidence of dissemination in time and space is diagnostic of MS in patients with clinically isolated optic neuritis. In addition, for patients not meeting criteria for MS at time of presentation with clinically isolated optic neuritis, MRI of the brain has been shown to be an important prognostic indicator for development of MS. MRI of the brain showing 0, 1, or more than 3 lesions typical for MS is associated, respectively, with a 25%, 60%, and 78% risk of progression to clinically definite MS.

Less commonly, optic neuritis is associated with other demyelinating syndromes such as NMO. This should be considered in patients with severe vision loss, bilateral involvement, or history of prior optic neuritis or transverse myelitis. A serum antibody (anti-aquaporin 4 or NMO antibody) has been identified as a pathologic agent in this disorder. Testing for this is commercially available with a published sensitivity and specificity of 63% and

99%, respectively. Positive testing for anti-AqP4-IgG in a patient with optic neuritis is diagnostic of NMO per published consensus criteria. A serum antibody (MOG-IgG) is commercially available and aids in the identification of Anti-MOG associated optic neuritis.

Differential Diagnosis

Other diagnostic considerations in a patient with unilateral painful vision loss without explanatory pathology evident on ophthalmic examination include other optic neuropathies such as those due to sarcoidosis, lupus, vasculitis, neoplastic, vascular, and infectious causes. Atypical features for optic neuritis such as systemic symptoms, history of cancer, pain that persists beyond 2 weeks, progressive vision loss beyond 14 days, no spontaneous improvement in vision, retinal hemorrhages, cotton-wool spots, or macular exudates should prompt diagnostic evaluation for etiologies other than optic neuritis.

Treatment and Monitoring

The Optic Neuritis Treatment Trial (ONTT) was a randomized trial comparing placebo, oral prednisone, and IV methylprednisolone (1 g/day IV for 3 days) followed by oral prednisone (1 mg/kg per day for 11 days) for acute optic neuritis. IV steroids hastened recovery of vision without affecting final visual outcome compared with placebo treatment. Treatment with low-dose oral prednisone alone (1 mg/kg/day for 14 days) was associated with an increased risk of relapse compared with placebo treatment. The 15-year follow-up results, published in 2008, demonstrated persistence of visual recovery. Studies have demonstrated noninferiority of high-dose oral steroids (1250 mg prednisone/day for 3 days) to IV methylprednisolone with regards to vision recover following acute optic neuritis.

Many clinicians offer IV or high-dose oral steroid treatment to hasten visual recovery. Monotherapy with low-dose oral prednisone should be avoided. Regardless of the decision to treat or not with steroids, all patients should be monitored closely. Continued progression of vision loss, failure to spontaneously recover vision, or persistent pain should prompt additional diagnostic workup as well as consideration for additional IV steroid therapy for atypical optic neuritis. If this is not effective, plasma exchange has been reported as an effective acute therapy for atypical optic neuritis including NMO-spectrum optic neuritis.

In patients with acute optic neuritis and NMO or acute optic neuritis on the NMO-spectrum, treatment with plasma exchange or rituxamab (Rituxan)[1] should be considered to improve functional visual outcome.

In patients with a clinically isolated syndrome, consideration should be given to institution of disease-modifying therapy for MS based on the type and number of lesions on brain MRI and oligoclonal bands in cerebrospinal fluid. Several clinical trials have shown an association between early treatment with MS therapies and decreased incidence of progression to clinically definite MS in patients with a recent clinically isolated syndrome and clinically silent lesions on brain MRI.

In patients who meet diagnostic criteria for either MS or NMO, consideration should be given to treating the underlying disease.

Complications

Though more than 70% of patients with optic neuritis recover objectively normal visual acuity, many have residual subjective visual disturbances. These often worsen or recur in heat, which is known as Uhtoff's phenomenon.

Complications of steroid therapy include insomnia, agitation, and stomach irritation. Long-term side effects of steroid treatment for this condition are rare owing to the brief period of treatment. Complications of disease-modifying therapies for MS and NMO are reviewed elsewhere.

[1]Not FDA approved for this indication.

References

Beck RQ, Cleary PA, Anderson MM, et al: A randomized, controlled trial of corticosteroids in the treatment of acute optic neuritis, *The Neuritis Study Group, N Engl J Med* 326:581–588, 1992.

Biotti D, Bonneville F, Tournaire E, et al: Optic neuritis in patients with anti-MOG antibodies spectrum disorder: MRI and clinical features from a large multicentric cohort in France, *J Neurol.* 264:2173–2175, 2017.

Bonnan M, Valentino R, Debeugny S, et al: Short delay to initiate plasma exchange is the strongest predictor of outcome in severe attacks of NMO spectrum disorders, *J Neurol Neurosurg Psychiatry.* 89:346–351, 2018.

Hickman SJ, Ko M, Chaudhry F, et al: Optic neuritis: an update on typical and atypical optic neuritis, *Neuro-ophthalmology* 32:237–248, 2008.

Merle H, Olindo S, Bonnan M, et al: Natural history of the visual impairment of relapsing neuromyelitis optica, *Ophthalmology* 114:810–815, 2007.

Morrow SA: Fraser JA, Day C et al: *Effect of treating acute optic neuritis with bioequivalent oral vs. intravenous corticosteroids: a randomized clinical trial. JAMA Neurol.* Epub ahead of print March 5, 2018.

Moss HE: Visual consequence of medications for multiple sclerosis: the good, the bad, the ugly and the unknown, *Eye Brain.* 29:13–21, 2017.

Optic Neuritis Study Group: The clinical profile of optic neuritis: experience of the optic neuritis treatment trial, *Arch Ophthalmol* 109:1673–1678, 1991.

Optic Neuritis Study Group: Multiple sclerosis risk after optic neuritis: final optic neuritis treatment trial follow-up, *Arch Neurol* 65:727–732, 2008.

Optic Neuritis Study Group: Visual function 15 years after optic neuritis, *Ophthalmology* 115:1079–1082, 2008.

Roesner S, Appel R, Gbadamosi J, et al: Treatment of steroid-unresponsive optic neuritis with plasma exchange, *Acta Neurol Scand* 126(2):103–108, 2012.

Thompson AJ, Banwell BL, Carroll WM, et al: Diagnosis of multiple sclerosis: 2017 revisions of the McDonald criteria, *Lancet Neurol.* 17:162–173, 2018.

Vodopivec I, Matiello M, Prasad S: Treatment of neuromyelitis optica, *Curr Opin Ophthalmol* 26(6):476–483, 2015.

Winferchuk DM, Banwell B, Bennett JL, et al: International consensus diagnostic criteria for neuromyelitis optica spectrum disorders, *Neurology* 85:177–189, 2015.

PARKINSON DISEASE

Method of
Jessica Tate, MD

CURRENT DIAGNOSIS

- Clinical diagnosis based on four cardinal features:
  - Bradykinesia
  - Rigidity
  - Resting tremor
  - Postural instability
- Supportive features: asymmetric onset, response to dopaminergic medication, and presence of nonmotor features such as REM behavior disorder and anosmia.
- Single-photon emission tomography or olfactory testing may aid diagnosis in specific circumstances.

CURRENT THERAPY

- Initial symptomatic treatment with monoamine oxidase-B (MAO-B) inhibitor, dopamine agonist, or carbidopa/levodopa.
  - Carbidopa/levodopa (Sinemet) first line for patients >70; should be initiated in younger patients when severity of motor symptoms warrants it, rather than strict levodopa-sparing approach.
  - Anticholinergic can be used as first-line treatment in younger patients with predominant tremor.
- MAO-B inhibitor, dopamine agonist, or catechol-O-methyltransferase (COMT) inhibitor can be added to levodopa to reduce on-off fluctuations.
- Amantadine (Symmetrel) can reduce levodopa-induced dyskinesias.
- Deep brain stimulation (DBS) is effective for patients with medication-refractory tremor.
- DBS or carbidopa/levodopa enteral suspension (Duopa) is more effective than oral medication alone for patients with severe motor fluctuations.
- Exercise is crucial at all stages and may have neuroprotective benefits.

Epidemiology

Parkinson disease (PD) affects roughly 1% of the population over the age of 60 years and is projected to affect approximately 1 million people in the United States by 2020. Updated epidemiologic studies are currently under way. PD is more common in men than women and is suggested to be more common in whites than other racial groups, although this may relate to disparities in healthcare. The average age of onset is in the seventh decade of life, but onset is before age 40 in 3% to 5% of cases. Ninety percent of cases are considered sporadic or idiopathic, whereas approximately 10% are inherited.

Risk Factors

Age is the most significant risk factor. Other proposed risk factors include exposure to pesticides, herbicides, solvents, and well water. Cigarette smoking, coffee consumption, regular exercise, and elevated uric acid levels may be protective. Risk of PD is doubled in first-degree relatives of those affected.

Pathophysiology

The formation of Lewy bodies, intracellular accumulations of the protein α-synuclein, is central to the pathogenesis of PD. This leads to degeneration of dopamine-producing neurons in the substantia nigra pars compacta, setting off a chain of altered signaling in the basal ganglia and ultimately reduced activation of the motor cortex. However, Lewy body deposition and neurodegeneration also occurs in other brain regions, perhaps well before the degeneration of the substantia nigra. This may explain the myriad nonmotor manifestations of PD, such as early loss of smell and REM behavior disorder, which are under consideration as prodromal symptoms of PD.

Unfortunately, the pathophysiological process that leads to Lewy body formation is not well understood at this time, and several different mechanisms have been proposed. PD is likely caused by a combination of genetic predisposition and environmental factors, which may differ from one individual to another depending on the specific gene or genes responsible. Early disease-modifying interventions, when they become available, are likely to target specific genetic subtypes, and thus genetic testing will likely play a more crucial role in the future diagnosis and treatment of PD.

Clinical Manifestations

The hallmark signs and symptoms of PD are bradykinesia (slow, small-amplitude movement or lack of movement), muscle rigidity (increased resistance to passive movement of the joints that is not velocity-dependent), and resting tremor. Although tremor is a common presenting symptom in PD, some patients with PD *never* develop tremor. The other hallmark symptoms of gait dysfunction and postural instability (loss of postural reflexes crucial to maintaining balance) are uncommon in the early stages of PD but occur later in the disease course.

Loss of dexterity with fine motor tasks, micrographia (small handwriting), hypophonia (soft speech), masked facies (diminished facial expression and reduced blinking), shortened strides, and decreased arm swing while walking are all potential manifestations of bradykinesia.

Rigidity can lead to complaints of stiffness, aching, or cramping. This symptom can lead a patient to explore musculoskeletal causes, such as seeking out a specialist in sports medicine, before realizing it has a neurologic basis. Many physicians believe "cogwheeling" to be specific to a diagnosis of PD. However, cogwheeling typically will not be evident in PD patients without tremor. In addition, patients with essential tremor can exhibit cogwheeling without underlying rigidity.

Parkinsonian tremor most classically starts in one hand, although it can be seen in the jaw and lower extremity as well. It has a slow frequency (4 to 6 Hz) and is visualized with the affected body part at rest. It is often enhanced by distraction (conversation, having the patient perform calculations or name the months backward) and can be temporarily alleviated by concentration or repositioning. When a patient with PD tremor extends an affected upper extremity, the tremor may reappear after a delay. This is referred to as "reemergent rest tremor" and differs from essential tremor, which is typically present immediately on extending the arms.

Early gait changes can include bent posture and shuffling or dragging of the feet, often initially on one side of the body. Later gait changes can include freezing (hesitancy and difficulty initiating a stride with a sensation of feeling stuck to the floor) and festination (a series of small, rapid steps with a sensation of being propelled forward and unable to stop). Postural instability is assessed with the "pull test," in which the examiner stands behind the patient and tugs back firmly on his or her shoulders. An abnormal response is defined by taking two or more steps backward or, in severe cases, by complete lack of response, leading to the examiner catching the patient as he or she falls back.

Diagnosis

The diagnosis of PD is still made clinically in most cases, with a detailed history and neurologic examination. Often, the United Kingdom Parkinson's Disease Society Brain Bank Criteria is used, which requires the presence of bradykinesia along with at least one other cardinal feature as described above. When patients are seen by a movement disorders specialist (a neurologist with additional subspecialty training in PD and related conditions), these clinical features are often objectively scored and tracked over time using a validated measure such as the Unified Parkinson's Disease Rating Scale. Additional supportive diagnostic criteria are also required, which can include unilateral onset, persistent asymmetry, progression with time, and response to levodopa. Patients also should be questioned about the presence of specific nonmotor symptoms suggestive of PD. These can include loss of smell or presence of REM sleep behavior disorder, which can precede onset of motor symptoms by years or even decades, and autonomic symptoms such as constipation, urinary frequency and urgency, sexual dysfunction, or drooling. These are discussed further in Table 1.

Differential Diagnosis

The differential diagnosis for PD varies somewhat depending on age of onset. In young patients, secondary Parkinsonism should be excluded with testing for Wilson disease. Dopa-responsive dystonia (DRD) can also mimic PD in younger patients. Drug-induced Parkinsonism, usually secondary to dopamine-blocking agents such as atypical antipsychotics or antiemetics, can occur at any age. In older patients, vascular Parkinsonism can resemble idiopathic PD but is secondary to accumulation of significant chronic microvascular ischemic changes, often in the periventricular brain regions, or an accumulation of acute cerebral infarcts over time. These findings can be easily visualized on a noncontrast magnetic resonance imaging (MRI) scan of the brain. An MRI scan can also reveal disproportionate enlargement of the ventricles that may raise suspicion for normal pressure hydrocephalus, a poorly understood and somewhat controversial condition that can lead to a shuffling gait or freezing of gait resembling PD. Atypical Parkinsonism syndromes include progressive supranuclear palsy (PSP), multiple systems atrophy (cerebellar and Parkinsonian types), corticobasal degeneration, and Lewy body dementia. These conditions can be very difficult to differentiate from idiopathic PD early in their course. Red flags include symmetric onset, lack of response (distinguished from intolerance) to an appropriate dose of levodopa, and early onset of symptoms typically seen in advanced stages of PD such as gait freezing, postural instability, severe autonomic dysfunction such as symptomatic orthostatic hypotension, or hallucinations.

In specific situations, particularly those in which DRD, vascular Parkinsonism, or drug-induced Parkinsonism are suspected, a [123I]FP-CIT single-photon emission tomography scan—known as a DaTscan—can be used to provide supportive information. This scan is designed to detect reduced presynaptic dopamine activity in the caudate and putamen. Uptake is expected to be normal in essential tremor, DRD, drug-induced Parkinsonism, and most cases of vascular Parkinsonism, whereas it is reduced in neurodegenerative

SYMPTOMS	MANAGEMENT SUGGESTIONS	CONSIDERATIONS
Mood disorders Depression Anxiety disorders	If periodic, optimize PD treatment to minimize on-off fluctuations If more static, typical individualized treatment options including selective serotonin reuptake inhibitors (SSRIs), serotonin and norepinephrine reuptake inhibitors (SNRIs), tricyclic antidepressants (TCAs), counseling, psychotherapy, transcranial magnetic stimulation, etc.	Multiple antidepressants shown to be safe in combination with MAO-B inhibitors, but be aware of rare risk of serotonin syndrome
Sleep disturbances REM sleep behavior disorder (REM-BD) Insomnia Restless leg syndrome (RLS)	For REM-BD, melatonin[7] or clonazepam (Klonopin)[1] at bedtime For insomnia, sleep hygiene counseling, screening for sleep apnea with referral for sleep study if warranted, management of nocturia, treatment of nocturnal stiffness or cramping, etc. For RLS, iron supplementation if ferritin <75, dopamine agonists, gabapentin (Neurontin)[1]	Avoidance of sedative hypnotics due to high risk of adverse effects
Psychosis Illusions Hallucinations Delusions	Lower PD medication dosages *if* possible; discontinuation of other potential offending medications Acetylcholinesterase inhibitors, quetiapine (Seroquel)[1] or clozapine (Clozaril)[1], pimavanserin (Nuplazid)	If acute, requires full medical/neurologic evaluation for infection and other possible causes
Constipation	Hydration, exercise, removal of offending medications if possible PEG 3350 (Miralax)	
Urinary dysfunction	Mirabegron (Myrbetriq) may be helpful for patients without benign prostatic hypertrophy	Urodynamic testing recommended, since multiple factors may be at play (such as BPH) Caution regarding anticholinergics; possible delirium
Orthostatic hypotension	Abdominal binder or compression stockings Midodrine (Proamatine) fludrocortisone (Florinef)[1], or droxidopa (norepinephrine precursor) (Northera)	Extra caution in the hour following levodopa doses Must balance with supine hypertension, which may improve by raising head of bed 30 degrees or a nighttime antihypertensive
Fatigue	Exercise, treatment of depression or sleep disorders if present Avoiding under-medication of PD symptoms Selegiline (Eldepryl), amantadine (Symmetrel) Stimulants such as methylphenidate (Ritalin)[1] (rarely, in extreme cases)	
Drooling	Hard candy or gum Rimabotulinum toxin B (Myobloc)[1] injections in salivary glands Sublingual atropine[1]	
Weight loss	Monitoring, nutritional supplementation, referral to nutritionist	Associated with negative outcomes in PD including dementia and earlier death; unclear if causal

[1]Not FDA approved for this indication.
[7]Available as a dietary supplement.
MAO-B, Monoamine oxidase type B; *PD*, Parkinson disease.

Parkinsonism. A major limitation of the DaTscan is its inability to differentiate between PD and atypical Parkinsonism such as PSP.

Treatment

Exercise is believed to have neuroprotective benefits and should be strongly encouraged in all stages of PD. Most emphasis has been on cardiovascular forms of exercise, but strength and balance training are likely to be beneficial in this population as well. There are multiple Parkinson's-specific exercise programs appearing nationwide, including stationary cycling, noncombat boxing, and dance.

Symptomatic medication is often initiated either when tremor becomes bothersome, or when motor disability is affecting day-to-day activities. A sizable minority of patients with PD may have medication-refractory tremor, an important point to keep in mind because a patient with isolated tremor and lack of improvement with dopaminergics should not necessarily be considered a nonresponder. Dopaminergics may still be useful to those patients in the future for symptoms such as bradykinesia and rigidity.

For early-stage PD, there are three classes of drugs that are frequently used: monoamine oxidase (MAO)-B inhibitors, dopamine agonists, and levodopa. Levodopa may be chosen as initial therapy in a patient 70 years of age or older because of the

lower potential for side effects. In younger patients, it is common to start with an MAO-B inhibitor or dopamine agonist and escalate to levodopa if either of those are poorly tolerated or ineffective. Although a levodopa-sparing strategy has been commonly adopted by clinicians, evidence suggests that earlier initiation of levodopa is associated with better long-term outcomes for patients. Regardless of the patient's age, levodopa should be started when the patient is experiencing disabling symptoms that have not responded to other medication choices. Especially for patients on levodopa, it is best practice to treat with the lowest effective dose to help reduce the risk of dyskinesias. This symptom will be discussed in further detail in the next section. Typical dosages and side effects to consider can be found in Table 2.

Patients with moderate to advanced PD have typically reached a degree of symptom severity that necessitates levodopa. Eventually, they will begin to develop medication fluctuations. These include wearing-off of symptomatic benefits before the next dose, erratic failures of dosages to take effect, and dyskinesias. Dyskinesias are rocking, writhing, or twisting movements that can affect any region of the body. They most commonly occur at the peak of a levodopa dose but, for some patients, can occur at the end of a dose or in a diphasic manner. The pathophysiology behind dyskinesias is not fully understood,

TABLE 2	Medication Choices in Early Parkinson Disease.			
DRUG CLASS	**MEDICATION NAMES**	**TYPICAL DOSE RANGE**	**SIDE EFFECTS TO CONSIDER**	**COMMENTS**
MAO-B Inhibitors				
	Selegiline (Eldepryl)	5 mg daily to 5 mg BID	Insomnia, confusion, hallucinations	Controversy re: neuroprotective benefits Potential medication interactions (serotonin syndrome)
	Rasagiline (Azilect)	0.5–1 mg daily		
Anticholinergics				
	Benztropine (Cogentin)	0.5 mg daily to 1 mg TID	Dry mouth, cognitive impairment, hallucinations, urinary retention, blurred vision	Useful for tremor, high risk in elderly
	Trihexyphenidyl (Artane)	1 mg daily to 3 mg BID		
Dopamine Agonists				
	Pramipexole (Mirapex)	IR 0.125–1.5 mg TID ER: 0.375–4.5 mg daily	Nausea, leg edema, weight gain, daytime sleepiness, impulse control disorders, hallucinations Patch: skin irritation	Less favorable side effect efficacy profile than levodopa
	Ropinirole (Requip)	IR 0.25–8 mg TID XL: 2–24 mg daily		
	Rotigotine (Neupro)	Transdermal 2–8 mg/24 h		
Oral Levodopa Preparations	Carbidopa/levodopa (Sinemet) C/L controlled release (Sinemet CR)	25/100 mg BID-TID to 50/200 mg BID-TID	Nausea, daytime sleepiness, orthostatic hypotension, hallucinations	Dyskinesias are a long-term complication of therapy

BID, Two times daily; *C/L,* carbidopa/levodopa; *ER,* extended release; *MAO-B,* monoamine oxidase type B; *PD,* Parkinson disease; *TID,* three times daily.

but they are believed to be a function of both disease stage and dosage of levodopa. If dyskinesias are not bothersome to the patient, they do not require treatment. If they are bothersome, dosage reduction can be considered but is not always possible due to worsening of motor symptoms. The addition of amantadine (Symmetrel) can be helpful. For early wearing-off, dosing—particularly frequency—of levodopa can be modified, or adjunctive medication can be used such as an MAO-B inhibitor, a dopamine agonist, or entacapone (Comtan). Patients should also be counseled about the potential effect of protein on levodopa absorption and encouraged to space their doses 30 to 60 minutes from meals. For dose failures or abrupt wearing-off, apomorphine (APOKYN) injections can be used to provide rapid onset of symptom relief. Typical dosages and side effects of drugs used for advanced PD are summarized in Table 3. When medication fluctuations are severe, the patient may be considered for an advanced treatment option such as DBS or carbidopa-levodopa enteral suspension (Duopa). The ideal candidate for DBS has idiopathic PD, does not have dementia, and is typically receiving less-than-ideal benefit from medications for one of two reasons. In the first circumstance, levodopa is providing definite symptom reduction, but medication fluctuations have become a significant problem. In the second circumstance, the patient has medication-refractory tremor with or without additional troublesome motor symptoms. The enteral suspension, delivered continuously to the small intestine via a percutaneous endoscopic transgastric jejunostomy (PEG-J) tube and pump, is for patients experiencing significant motor fluctuations with oral medications.

Monitoring

Swallowing function should be monitored periodically, typically with a modified barium swallow, and modifications in diet and swallowing technique may reduce aspiration risk. A cognitive screening tool such as the Montreal Cognitive Assessment

should be administered yearly. Supportive treatment strategies should be used on an ongoing basis, including speech/swallow therapy, physical therapy, and occupational therapy. Therapists with specific training in neurologic disorders should be used when possible. PD-specific programs such as the Lee Silverman Voice Therapy Loud (speech therapy) and Big (physical therapy) programs are particularly helpful.

Complications and Nonmotor Symptoms

Nonmotor symptoms of PD can be more disabling in some cases than the more well-known motor symptoms. These are summarized in Table 1. Depression and anxiety, in particular, affect high numbers of patients with PD. Psychosis is not an inevitable occurrence but affects approximately 50% of patients, usually in more advanced stages of the disease. When PD psychosis is causing fear or agitation, it should be treated with an escalating strategy. Typically, acetylcholinesterase inhibitors will be introduced first, followed by either low-dose quetiapine (Seroquel)[1] or pimavanserin (Nuplazid) if symptoms are not stabilized. Pimavanserin is the only drug approved by the Food and Drug Administration for Parkinson's psychosis. Atypical antipsychotics have been associated with an increased risk of death in the elderly, and deaths have also been reported in patients receiving pimavanserin, although causality is not necessarily clear. Risks and benefits must be carefully weighed, but currently these medications may be the only option for a patient experiencing severe psychosis.

The gradual progression of PD is inevitable but highly variable in speed and severity from one individual to another. This is likely dependent on age of onset, other comorbid health conditions, access to expert care, and level of physical activity among other factors. Abrupt worsening of any symptoms of PD should prompt a workup for provoking medical conditions, such as

---

[1] Not FDA approved for this indication.

TABLE 3 Medication Choices in Advanced Parkinson Disease.

DRUG CLASS	MEDICATION NAMES	TYPICAL DOSE RANGE	SIDE EFFECTS TO CONSIDER	COMMENTS
MAO-B Inhibitors				
	Selegiline (Eldepryl)	5 mg daily to 5 mg BID	Insomnia, confusion, hallucinations	Adjunct to levodopa
	Rasagiline (Azilect)	0.5–1 mg daily		
	Safinamide (Xadago)	50–100 mg daily		
Dopamine Agonists				
	Pramipexole (Mirapex)	IR 0.125–1.5 mg TID ER: 0.375–4.5 mg daily	Nausea, leg edema, weight gain, daytime sleepiness, impulse control disorders, hallucinations	Adjunct to levodopa
	Ropinirole (Requip)	IR 0.25–8 mg TID XL: 2–24 mg daily		
	Rotigotine (Neupro)	Transdermal 2–8 mg/24 h	Skin irritation	
	Apomorphine (APOKYN)	Subcutaneous 0.2 mL (2 mg) to 0.6 mL (6 mg)	Orthostatic hypotension	Rapid onset within 10 min, used as rescue medication
COMT Inhibitor	Entacapone (Comtan)	200 mg with each dose of levodopa, up to 8 times daily	Orange urine, diarrhea	Used to prolong levodopa effects Can worsen dyskinesias
Levodopa Preparations				
	C/L (Sinemet) C/L controlled release (Sinemet CR)	Variable—total of 1200–2500 mg levodopa/d	Nausea, daytime sleepiness, orthostatic hypotension, hallucinations	Escalating dosage and frequency in advanced PD to combat wearing-off, must be balanced with side effects
	C/L ER capsules (Rytary)	23.75 mg/95 mg TID—variable		
	C/L/entacapone (Stalevo)	25/100/200 mg TID to 50/200/200 mg 6 times/d	Orange urine, diarrhea	
	Levodopa inhalation powder (Inbrija)	84 mg 1–5 times daily	Cough, upper respiratory infection, nausea, discolored sputum	Used as rescue medication for off periods Contraindicated in patients with lung disease
NMDA Antagonist				
	Amantadine (Symmetrel)	50 mg daily to 100 mg TID	Livedo reticularis, leg edema, insomnia, dry mouth, confusion, hallucinations, myoclonus	Reduces dyskinesias Can also be used for mild, early PD symptoms but now less commonly
	Amantadine ER (Gocovri)	137–274 mg nightly		FDA-approved for PD dyskinesia May reduce off time as well
	Amantadine ER (Osmolex ER)	129–322 mg		

C/L, Carbidopa/levodopa; COMT, catechol-O-methyltransferase; ER, extended release; MAO-B, monoamine oxidase type B; NMDA, N-methyl-D-aspartate PD, Parkinson disease; TID, three times daily.

occult urinary tract infection. PD does not directly lead to death, but death can occur in the setting of dysphagia leading to failure to thrive or aspiration pneumonia, or from serious injuries incurred from falls.

References

Bloem BR, de Vries NM, Ebersbach G: Nonpharmacological treatments for patients with Parkinson's disease, *Mov Disord* 30;1504–1520, 2015.

Cumming K, Macleod AD: Early weight loss in parkinsonism predicts poor outcomes: evidence from an incident cohort study, *Neurology* 89:2254–2261, 2017.

de Lau LM, Breteler MM: Epidemiology of Parkinson's disease, *Lancet Neurol* 5:525–535, 2006.

Fahn S, Elton R: Members of the UPDRS Development Committee. In Fahn S, Marsden CD, Calne DB, Goldstein M, editors: *Recent Developments in Parkinson's Disease*, Vol 2. Florham Park, NJ, 1987, Macmillan Health Care Information, pp 15, 3–163, 293–304.

Fox SH, Katzenschlager R, Lim SY, et al: Evidence based medicine publications. International Parkinson and Movement Disorder Society. Available at www.movementdisorders.org/MDS/resources/publications-reviews/EBM-Reviews1.htm. Accessed 15 April 2018.

Gibb WR, Lees AJ: The relevance of the Lewy body to the pathogenesis of idiopathic Parkinson's disease, *J Neurol Neurosurg Psychiatr* 51:745–752, 1988.

Gray R, Ives N, Rick C, et al: Long-term effectiveness of dopamine agonist and monoamine oxidase B inhibitors compared with levodopa as initial treatment for Parkinson's disease (PD MED): a large, open-label, pragmatic randomized trial, *Lancet* 384(9949):1196–1205, 2014.

Jankovic J, Schwartz KS, Ondo W: Re-emergent tremor of Parkinson's disease, *J Neurol Neurosurg Psychiatr* 67:646–650, 1999.

Shrag A, Schott JM: Epidemiological, clinical, and genetic characteristics of early-onset parkinsonism, *Lancet Neurol* 5:355–363, 2006.

REHABILITATION OF THE STROKE PATIENT

Method of
Marlís González-Fernández, MD, PhD; and Dorianne Feldman, MD, MSPT

CURRENT THERAPY

- Stroke rehabilitation improves functional outcomes.
- A comprehensive rehabilitation team composed of physicians, nurses, therapists, and community reintegration professionals can achieve the best outcomes.
- Early evaluation of family support and the home environment is critical to prevent unnecessary institutionalization.
- Evaluation and management of modifiable stroke risk factors, such as smoking, hypertension, and diabetes, are imperative during stroke rehabilitation to prevent stroke recurrence.
- Rehabilitation of the stroke patient can be hindered by conditions such as pneumonia (usually caused by aspiration), deep venous thrombosis, urinary tract infections, shoulder pain, depression, and spasticity. Early identification and treatment of these conditions are necessary to maximize functional outcomes.

According to the National Center for Health Statistics, 5.6 million Americans live with the disability caused by a previous stroke. Stroke is the leading cause of permanent disability in adults. Conservative estimates suggest that about 45% of stroke patients have moderate to severe disabilities requiring rehabilitation.

The goals of stroke rehabilitation are to maintain and optimize medical management, to maximize functional recovery, to minimize disability, and to improve quality of life and participation in society. The rehabilitative approach endeavors to provide patient-centered care that is organized, comprehensive, and specific to the needs of the stroke patient. The concerted efforts of the patient, family, and rehabilitation team are essential for achieving these goals. Recovery after stroke can be a long and challenging process for the patient and the family. Although functional gains occur most rapidly in the first year after a stroke, additional motor recovery is possible beyond 1 year when patients are involved in targeted rehabilitation programs.

The rehabilitation team is composed of rehabilitation physicians (physiatrists), other physicians such as neurologists and neurosurgeons, rehabilitation nurses, occupational therapists, physical therapists, speech and language pathologists, rehabilitation neuropsychologists, social workers, case managers, nutritionists, vocational counselors, and pharmacists. A goal of the acute inpatient rehabilitation team is discharging the patient to the least restrictive environment, ideally home. To accomplish this goal, it is critical to evaluate family support and the home environment.

Rehabilitation should start as part of the acute stroke inpatient stay. The decision-making process to determine the appropriate rehabilitation setting after discharge is described in Figure 1. Speech-language pathologists, physical therapists, and occupational therapists evaluate deficits in cognition, communication, deglutition, mobility, and activities of daily living. The severity of deficits in these major areas and the ability of the patient to tolerate therapy determine the appropriate rehabilitation setting.

Stroke patients with mild deficits are able to return home with home or outpatient therapy services. Patients with moderate to severe strokes benefit from more intensive therapy in an institutional setting. Comprehensive inpatient rehabilitation is suitable for patients with moderate to severe deficits who can tolerate intensive rehabilitation (3 h/day for 5 days each week or 15 hours of therapy over a 7 day period). If the severity of deficits or medical comorbidities limits the ability of the patient to participate in intensive therapy, alternate settings can be considered.

During the inpatient rehabilitation stage, medical management focuses on secondary stroke prevention: diet; exercise; smoking cessation; and reducing complications, including optimizing blood pressure control while maintaining cerebral perfusion, preventing and treating lipid disorders, and managing post-stroke pain, depression, and abnormal muscle tone. During this stage, much of the rehabilitation effort is directed toward educating stroke survivors about complications and the importance of adherence to medical recommendations.

Medical complications, such as deep venous thrombosis and related thromboembolism, pneumonia (usually related to aspiration), skin breakdown, and urinary infections, can hinder a

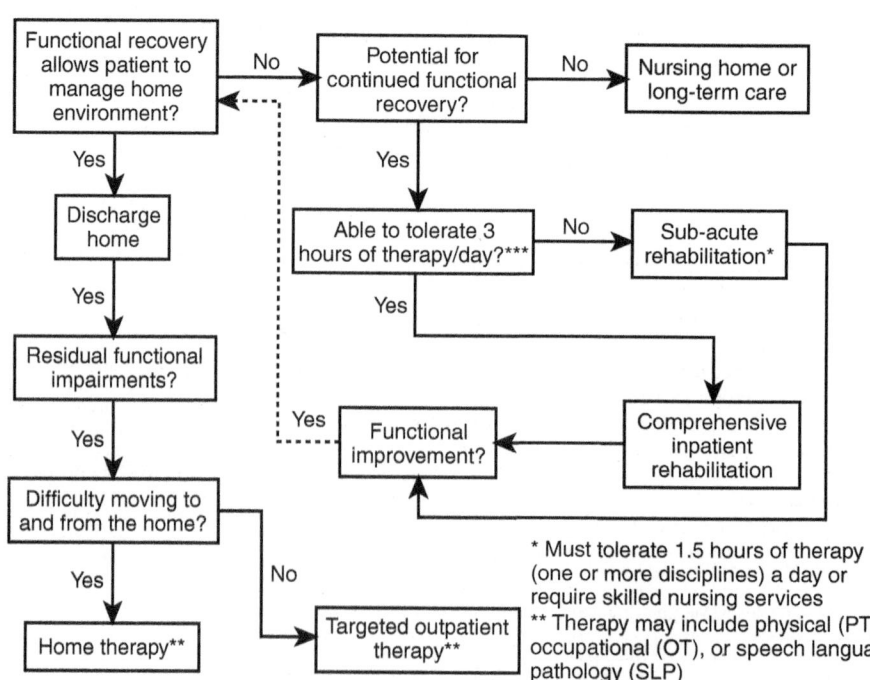

Figure 1 Determination of rehabilitation needs of patients being discharged after an acute stroke.

patient's recovery. Early identification of these complications is necessary to maintain progress in the rehabilitation effort. Other complications, such as seizures and cardiac decompensation, are possible and should be monitored.

Stroke often causes significant impairment and activity limitations. Deficits in strength, swallowing, vision, balance, muscle tone, communication, comprehension, cognition, attention, sensory perception, and bladder function are common and can cause difficulty completing activities of daily living, walking, transferring to and from different surfaces, and getting in and out of the bed. Post-stroke depression, fatigue, and pain are common and should be addressed to maximize participation in rehabilitative efforts.

Transition to the chronic phase begins after the patient is medically stable and inpatient therapy goals are met. Outpatient therapy services are initiated in conjunction with physiatric, primary care, and neurologic follow-up.

Hemiparesis

Hemiparesis, or one-sided weakness, is one of the most frequent complications after stroke. Recovery of motor function varies. Often, it is limited by muscle atrophy, co-contraction of agonists and antagonists, and abnormal tone. Usually, motor recovery is preceded by the development of patterned muscle movements, or synergies. Synergies occur when select muscles contract in a predictable manner. In the paretic upper extremity, a flexion synergy pattern (i.e., humeral adduction, internal rotation, elbow flexion, forearm pronation, and wrist and finger flexion) is common. In the lower extremity, extension synergies (i.e., hip internal rotation, adduction, extension, knee extension, and ankle extension and inversion) predominate. These patterns can be regarded as functional and nonfunctional. For instance, extension synergy patterns of the lower limb can augment rehabilitation because this position fosters early ambulatory therapy. Conversely, flexion synergy patterns in the upper extremity can significantly impair arm function.

Rehabilitation of the patient with hemiparesis should concentrate on maintaining range of motion and improving strength and posturing. Exercise programs should incorporate functional use of the hemiparetic limb and weight bearing to promote limb recognition, better alignment, muscle elongation, and muscle tone reduction.

Hemiparesis can lead to contracture, particularly when profound weakness is present, and contracture occurs most commonly in the wrist and ankle. Resting hand splints and solid ankle-foot orthoses can be used to maintain the limb in a neutral position. These devices can be used to prevent loss of motion, control muscle tone, and aid in positioning, particularly when wheelchairs are necessary.

Functional electrical stimulation (FES) has gained increasing interest as a means of enhancing functional movement and strength. Muscle contraction is induced with electrical stimulation. Many products on the market incorporate FES technology for the treatment of footdrop and hand weakness.

Preservation of scapulohumeral positioning is a critical component of rehabilitation. With shoulder weakness, the scapula becomes downwardly rotated, causing the glenoid fossa to move vertically and resulting in humeral subluxation. Traditionally, shoulder slings have been prescribed for the hemiplegic shoulder, but their effectiveness in preventing subluxation is questionable.

FES has been used to augment motor return in the hemiplegic shoulder and prevent subluxation. Despite advances in the treatment of the hemiplegic shoulder, it is still unclear which therapeutic interventions should constitute the standard of care.

Constraint-induced therapy (CIT), a therapeutic approach in which the nonparetic limb is restrained, can improve functional movement of the paretic upper extremity in patients with residual hand and wrist movement, even in patients more than 1 year after a stroke. More recently, CIT concepts have been applied to the treatment of aphasia. By limiting the use of nonverbal communication and stimulating verbal output, participants were able to improve language performance and communication.

Weight-supported treadmill training has been proposed to enhance gait training after a stroke. Although a recent clinical trial showed no clear benefit from weight-supported treadmill training on improving gait speed, walking ability, or balance, some advocate for continued research on the effects of this training on overall health, including maintaining bone mass and decreasing insulin resistance.

Dysphagia

Dysphagia after stroke occurs acutely in approximately 50% of stroke patients. Identifying dysphagia in this population is essential for preventing associated morbidity and mortality. Stroke patients with dysphagia are at risk for dehydration, malnutrition, and aspiration pneumonia. As allowed by their overall clinical status and consciousness level, stroke patients should be evaluated as early as possible during their acute hospital stay. Trained clinicians (most commonly speech-language pathologists) should evaluate the patient to make recommendations regarding further dysphagia evaluation or testing and the need for diet modifications or dysphagia rehabilitation.

Hemiplegic Shoulder Pain

Stroke survivors with residual hemiparesis or weakness are at risk for pain syndromes (particularly in the upper extremity), which can significantly limit rehabilitation efforts. These pain syndromes are usually multifactorial. In the rehabilitation setting, prevention of shoulder pain is key, and interventions should focus on proper positioning, handling, and transfer techniques.

In severe cases, shoulder pain can be accompanied by hand swelling, tenderness, skin changes, erythema, hyperhidrosis, and allodynia. When this occurs, it is referred to as *shoulder-hand syndrome*, a subtype of complex regional pain syndrome (CRPS). Although the mechanism and cause are unclear, it has been suggested that this process is the result of an overreaction to a neurologic insult and may be inflammatory in nature. In some cases, the pain is severe, resulting in decreased and guarded movements of the limb that limit functional use. Shoulder pathology such as rotator cuff strains or tears, bicipital tendonitis, subacromial and subdeltoid bursitis, and glenohumeral subluxation or dislocation contribute to poststroke shoulder pain and should be treated.

Nonpharmacologic treatment focuses on desensitization techniques, gentle range-of-motion exercises, and physical modalities (e.g., heat, cold, transcutaneous electrical nerve stimulation [TENS], FES). Pharmacologic management includes medications typically used for neuropathic pain syndromes, such as anticonvulsants, tricyclic antidepressants (TCAs), nonsteroidal anti-inflammatory drugs, topical agents (e.g., lidocaine [Xylocaine],[1] clonidine [Catapres-TTS],[1] capsaicin [Zostrix][1]), and injections of steroid or local anesthetics. Antispasmodic medications have been used. When pain relief is not achieved with conservative treatment, sympathetic blocks can be considered. Sympathectomies and spinal cord stimulators can be considered as last resorts.

Spasticity

Spasticity after stroke can significantly impact rehabilitation. The classic upper extremity flexor synergy pattern (i.e., adducted shoulder with flexed elbow, wrist, and fingers) can markedly interfere with the function of the affected arm. Conversely, the classic lower extremity extensor synergy pattern (i.e., extended hip and knee and ankle plantar flexion) can be advantageous for ambulation if plantar flexion can be controlled by physical or pharmacologic agents. If untreated, these patterns can lead to abnormal positioning and contracture.

Treatment of spasticity after stroke should address positioning and exacerbating factors. Splinting or bracing, appropriate wheelchair sitting position, and physical therapy techniques are important to prevent contracture and promote motor recovery. Painful or noxious stimuli can exacerbate spasticity. Shoulder pain, pressure sores, deep venous thrombosis, bladder distention,

---

[1] Not FDA approved for this indication.

and constipation are examples of stimuli that can exacerbate spasticity. Pharmacologic treatment should take into account the presence of these triggers because spasticity is likely to improve after the stimuli are resolved or relieved.

Pharmacologic treatment of post-stroke spasticity presents some challenges. Effective antispasticity agents such as baclofen (Lioresal) or tizanidine (Zanaflex) can cause somnolence or weaken unaffected muscles, which can significantly affect rehabilitation. Localized treatments such as botulinum toxins (Botox, Dysport, Myobloc, Xeomin)[1] injections or phenol blocks[1] can be useful, because treatment can be directed toward muscles that are affecting functional use of the limbs. Surgical interventions can be used for patients with severe spasticity limiting functional positioning or for those with the potential for functional grip if tendon lengthening or transfer can be considered.

Cognitive Dysfunction

Stroke patients can experience many cognitive deficits, including visuospatial neglect, cognitive-linguistic deficits, apraxia, memory loss, and attention deficits. Cognitive rehabilitation should concentrate on treatment of the specific deficits of the patient. Visuospatial rehabilitation (including scanning training) is recommended for deficits associated with visual neglect after right stroke. Cognitive-linguistic therapies are recommended for left hemispheric stroke patients with language deficits. Treatment of apraxia should include specific gestural and strategy training.

The use of medications that may impair cognitive function should be limited. Medications that are commonly considered during a stay in a rehabilitative facility that may have a significant impact on cognition and rehabilitation are highlighted in Table 1.

Depression and Neuropharmacology

Depression can be seen in up to one half of all stroke patients. It has been associated with poor functional outcomes and more severe impairments. Vegetative symptoms can have a significant impact on rehabilitative efforts because participation in therapy is critical.

Psychoactive drugs can be beneficial and should be considered. Selective serotonin reuptake inhibitors (SSRIs) are recommended in this population because of a better side effect profile and because of the undesirable anticholinergic side effects of TCAs. In cases unresponsive to treatment with SSRIs, nortriptyline (Pamelor) may be helpful. In the rehabilitation setting when rapid short-term improvement in symptoms is necessary to increase participation in therapy, the use of psychostimulants (e.g., methylphenidate [Ritalin][1]) may be indicated. Table 1 shows the neuropharmacologic agents commonly used during

---

[1] Not FDA approved for this indication.

stoke rehabilitation. Psychotherapy has been associated with modest improvement in post-stroke depression and is considered to be part of a multidisciplinary approach. Research has demonstrated the benefit of the antidepressant fluoxetine (Prozac)[1] on motor recovery; administration of the drug for 3 months as an adjunct to physical therapy improved motor functioning in poststroke patients.

Bladder Dysfunction

Bladder dysfunction after stroke depends on the stroke's location. During the rehabilitation phase, the most common problem is urinary incontinence and urgency associated with uninhibited bladder contraction. Ultrasound bladder scans (usually every 4 hours and after voiding) should be ordered to detect bladder distention and urinary retention. It is standard practice to intervene when bladder volumes are greater than 500 mL. If volumes exceed this cutoff point, intermittent catheterization should be started. Intermittent catheterization is preferable to indwelling catheters because the risk of urinary tract infection is higher with the latter. Bladder scans are usually discontinued when post-voiding residual volumes at 3- to 4-hour intervals are low (<150 mL) for a period of 24 to 48 hours.

Mobility and Use of Adaptive Equipment

Activity limitations vary among stroke survivors and can include difficulties with bed mobility, wheelchair propulsion, transfers, gait, stairs, and the basic activities of daily living. The goal of physical therapy and occupational therapy is to maximize functional independence. Addressing mobility limitations is fundamental in stroke rehabilitation because it is related to long-term care needs and independence.

Transfer training comprises learning how to maneuver from one surface or height to another. Ideally, patients should learn to roll and transfer toward the involved and uninvolved sides; however, early mobility efforts are directed to the uninvolved side to minimize the risk of injury.

Gait deviations are common after stroke and interfere with safety and efficiency of locomotion. If an assistive device is needed, the goal of physical therapy is to progress to the least restrictive device possible. Hemiwalkers and wide-based quad canes provide the most stability. An ankle-foot orthosis may be indicated for patients with decreased ankle control and footdrop. Instruction in ascending or descending stairs depends on assistive device requirements. With weakness, stairs are ascended by initiating movement with the uninvolved or stronger lower extremity. This process is reversed when descending.

---

[1] Not FDA approved for this indication.

TABLE 1	Neuropharmacologic Agents Commonly Used During Stroke Rehabilitation		
DRUG CLASS	**DRUG NAME**	**INDICATION**	**POTENTIAL PROBLEMS**
Benzodiazepines	Diazepam (Valium)	Agitation,[1] spasticity	Sedation, confusion, sundowning
	Lorazepam (Ativan)	Agitation,[1] seizures	Sedation, paradoxical reactions, confusion, sundowning
Tricyclic antidepressants (TCAs)	Nortriptyline (Pamelor) Amitriptyline (Elavil)	Depression, neuropathic pain,[1] central pain[1]	Anticholinergic effects, sedation
Selective serotonin reuptake inhibitors (SSRIs)	Sertraline (Zoloft) Escitalopram (Lexapro) Citalopram (Celexa)	Depression, stimulation[1]	Long titration period, suicidal ideations, serotonin syndrome, syndrome of inappropriate antidiuretic hormone (SIADH), somnolence, seizures
	Fluoxetine (Prozac)	Depression motor recovery[1]	As above for other SSRIs
Stimulants	Modafinil (Provigil) Methylphenidate (Ritalin)	Drowsiness,[1] decreased alertness,[1] impaired concentration,[1] diminished attention[1]	Arrhythmia, seizures, hepatotoxicity, blood pressure changes

[1] Not FDA approved for this indication.

For some stroke survivors, functional ambulation is not a realistic goal. In these cases, the wheelchair becomes the primary means of locomotion. Wheelchair prescription requires considerable skill and training and must take into account posturing, body habitus, cognition, physical fitness level, and the home environment. An appropriate wheelchair prescription is required to maximize mobility and prevent complications such as shoulder pain. Physical and occupational therapists should evaluate the patient before providing wheelchair recommendations to vendors. Hemi wheelchairs (i.e., wheelchairs situated closer to the ground) and one-arm drive wheelchairs allow hemiplegic patients to use the uninvolved side for wheelchair propulsion. Lap boards with arm supports can be added to improve hemiparetic arm posturing and sitting symmetry.

For some stroke survivors, the ability to return to driving is considered one of the most important long-term rehabilitation goals. Formal driving rehabilitation programs are available to evaluate and improve driver safety. Driver rehabilitation specialists perform vision, cognitive, and perceptual examinations. Perception tests assess reaction times to visual and auditory stimuli. Values for vision and reaction times are standardized and state-dependent. Specialists should also perform a behind-the-wheel assessment, beginning in a parking lot and progressing to the negotiation of more complex traffic situations. Many modifications can increase independence and assist with a return to driving, including a spinner knob, which can be attached to the steering wheel to allow one-arm control; hand controls for acceleration and braking; left foot pedals to compensate for right foot impairment; and wheelchair lifts.

Adaptive equipment, including bracing, shoe modification, and other tools, increases independence through completion of activities of daily living (e.g., long-handled sponge, reacher, shoe horn, mirror, sock aids) and is extremely beneficial for those with moderate to severe strokes, particularly if hemiparesis is dense (Figure 2). Silverware, pens, and other utensils can be modified for easier maneuverability. Multipodus boots can be used to prevent plantar flexion contracture development in the hemiparetic limb.

Falls

Falls are common after moderate to severe strokes. In rehabilitation settings, fall prevention usually requires a multimodal approach. Strategies include use of bed-chair alarms, placing those at risk close to the nursing station, wearing skid socks, limiting or refraining from polypharmacy, eliminating slick or irregular floors, and in some cases, providing a sitter for closer monitoring. Physical and occupational therapists must include general safety and fall recovery as part of the treatment plan.

Visual Impairment

Depending on the location of the stroke, the visual system may be involved. One of the most debilitating visual impairments is visuospatial neglect, a complication of right hemisphere strokes. Left-sided stimuli are not attended to or recognized, and affected individuals must learn to deal with this deficit. Other complications include gaze weakness or paralysis, diplopia, visual field loss, ptosis, tracking disorders, decreased visual acuity, and cortical blindness.

Screening for primary visual skills, including visual acuity, visual fields, and visual tracking, should be done by physiatrists, neurologists, and occupational therapists. If problems are identified, patients should be referred to neuro-ophthalmologists and low-vision rehabilitation programs. Visual acuity problems often can be addressed by incorporating the use of glasses into the therapy session or by changing the prescription. Eye movement disorders and visual field deficits usually lessen as time elapses and may respond to treatment with prisms, head positioning, and unilateral eye occlusion with tape or a patch technique. Prism therapy has also shown promise in treating hemispatial neglect. Those with continued visual field impairment should be taught eye movement techniques to expand the visual area.

Brain-Based Therapies: Noninvasive Brain Stimulation

Repetitive transcranial magnetic stimulation (rTMS) applies a brief magnetic field to the scalp with enough intensity to penetrate the skull and induce neuronal activation. Some promising results have been seen when rTMS is used after stroke. A second modality, transcranial direct current stimulation (tDCS), applies low-voltage electrical current to stimulate or modify neuronal activity in the brain cortex. The stimulation is applied to discrete areas of the head to target affected areas. Although the side-effect profile of these techniques is positive, more research is necessary to determine best candidates for treatment and optimal treatment protocols.

Robotics

The aim of robotic technology is to use an adjustable, programmable device to augment mobility in a task-specific manner. Robots can serve in an assistive (perform desired function) or therapeutic capacity (enhance gait or upper extremity function) and are suitable for this purpose as they not only enable more intensive therapy than conventional modes but also incorporate a greater degree of activity repetition. Present recommendations are for use as an adjunct to traditional rehabilitation interventions.

Figure 2 Adaptive equipment commonly used during stroke rehabilitation. The tapered front scoop dish (**A**) has nonskid feet to keep the plate from sliding. The curved edge simplifies scooping food. The dish is especially suited for individuals who have limited flexibility, have decreased motor coordination, or feed using one hand, such as a hemiparetic stroke patient. The reacher (**B**) is used to get items from the floor. The long-handled dressing aid (**C**) is used to reach clothes on the floor or to bring clothes up the paretic side. The long-handled shoe horn (**D**) aids with slipping into shoes. The long-handle sponge (**E**) is used for reaching the involved side while bathing or when the shoulder range of motion does not allow reaching. The leg lifter (**F**) and the sound upper limb can be used to assist in moving the paretic lower limb. Adapted feeding utensils (**G**) are used for patients with grip weakness or difficulties with upper limb range of motion; *left to right*: bent-handle spoon, no-grip fork, rocker bottom knife, and thick-handle spoon. No-tie laces (**H**) are elastic shoelaces that do not require tying. When using the sock-donning aid (**I**), the sock slides onto the plastic portion of the device, and the strap is used to pull the sock with the device on the foot.

Conclusions

Stroke rehabilitation requires the concerted efforts of the patient, family, and medical professionals. A multidisciplinary team with training to address the particular impairments and functional limitations of the stroke patient is critical. The physician's efforts should focus on preventing complications and treating stroke sequelae with the primary goal of improving overall function and participation in society.

References

Barrett AM, Oh-Park M, Chen P, et al: Neurorehabilitation: Five new things, *Neurol Clin Pract* 3:484, 2013.

Bhakta BB: Management of spasticity in stroke, *Br Med Bull* 56:476, 2000.

Cicerone KD, Dahlberg C, Malec JF, et al: Evidence-based cognitive rehabilitation: Updated review of the literature from 1998 through 2002, *Arch Phys Med Rehabil* 86:1681, 2005.

Chang WH, Kim YH: Robot-assisted therapy in stroke rehabilitation, *J Stroke* 15:174, 2013a.

Chollet F, Tardy J, Albucher JF, et al: Fluoxetine for motor recovery after acute ischaemic stroke (FLAME): A randomised placebo-controlled trial, *Lancet Neurol* 10:123, 2011.

Hackett ML, Anderson CS, House A, et al: Interventions for treating depression after stroke, *Cochrane Database Syst Rev*: CD003437, 2008.

Jones SA, Shinton RA: Improving outcome in stroke patients with visual problems, *Age Ageing* 35:560, 2006.

Kelly-Hayes M, Beiser A, Kase CS, et al: The influence of gender and age on disability following ischemic stroke: The Framingham Study, *J Stroke Cerebrovasc Dis* 12:119, 2003.

Lannin NA, Cusick A, McCluskey A, et al: Effects of splinting on wrist contracture after stroke: A randomized controlled trial, *Stroke* 38:111, 2007.

Legg L, Drummond A, Leonardi-Bee J, et al: Occupational therapy for patients with problems in personal activities of daily living after stroke: Systematic review of randomised trials, *BMJ* 335:922, 2007.

Pertoldi S, Di Benedetto P: Shoulder-hand syndrome after stroke. A complex regional pain syndrome, *Eura Medicophys* 41:283, 2005.

Poole D, Chaudry F, Jay WM: Stroke and driving, *Top Stroke Rehabil* 15:37, 2008.

Starkstein SE, Mizrahi R, Power BD: Antidepressant therapy in post-stroke depression, *Expert Opin Pharmacother* 9:1291, 2008.

Stein J: Stroke. In Frontera WR, Silver JK, editors: *Essentials of Physical Medicine and Rehabilitation*, Philadelphia, 2002, Saunders, p. 778–783.

Stein J, Harvey RL, Macko RF, et al: *Stroke Recovery & Rehabilitation*, New York, 2009, Demos Medical Publishing2009.

Umphred DA: *Neurological Rehabilitation*, St Louis, 1995, Mosby Elsevier Health Science1995.

van Wijk I, Algra A, van de Port IG, et al: Change in mobility activity in the second year after stroke in a rehabilitation population: Who is at risk for decline? *Arch Phys Med Rehabil* 87:45, 2006.

Wolf SL, Winstein CJ, Miller JP, et al: Effect of constraint-induced movement therapy on upper extremity function 3 to 9 months after stroke: The EXCITE randomized clinical trial, *JAMA* 296:2095, 2006.

Chang WH, Kim YH: Robot-assisted therapy in stroke rehabilitation, *J Stroke* 15:174, 2013b.

SEIZURES AND EPILEPSY IN ADOLESCENTS AND ADULTS

Method of
Jose A. Padin-Rosado, MD

CURRENT DIAGNOSIS

- Obtain a thorough clinical history, including a detailed description of the paroxysmal events from the patient and from witness accounts.
- Perform a thorough physical and neurologic examination.
- Perform laboratory tests, including electrolytes, blood glucose, liver function, and toxicology.
- Obtain a lumbar puncture if signs of infection are present.
- Neuroimaging is strongly recommended. Magnetic resonance imaging (MRI) is the preferred test due to higher resolution. Head computed tomography (CT) is acceptable in the acute setting to rule out hemorrhage.
- Routine electroencephalography (EEG) with sleep deprivation and activation procedures should be performed as close to the time of occurrence of the paroxysmal event to increase the diagnostic yield.

CURRENT THERAPY

- Choose the right medication for the type of epilepsy and epilepsy syndrome.
- Consider the side-effect profile, cost, and drug-dosing schedule, and adapt to the unique patient characteristics, taking into consideration the patient comorbidities.
- Aim for monotherapy whenever possible.
- Start low and increase slowly when initiating antiepileptic drug (AED) therapy to minimize side effects and increase compliance.
- An adequate AED trial with titration of the medication until clinical effectiveness or side effects occur is recommended.
- When switching from one drug to another, consider overlapping medications to provide protection until the first drug is discontinued.
- If the two AEDs fail, the patient should be referred to an epilepsy center for evaluation.
- If the patient is seizure free after 2 years of treatment, consider withdrawing AEDs for epilepsies of unknown etiology or epilepsy syndromes known to resolve.

Epilepsy is a disease characterized by an enduring predisposition to generate seizures and by the neurobiologic, cognitive, psychological, and social consequences of this condition. Epilepsy is commonly defined as having two or more unprovoked seizures greater than 24 hours apart. However, as per the new classification proposed by the International League Against Epilepsy (ILAE), a single seizure can be classified as epilepsy if risk of seizure recurrence is high (see "Classification" section).

A seizure is defined as transient signs or symptoms caused by abnormal excessive synchronous activity of brain neurons. Seizures can be classified as either acute symptomatic (provoked) or unprovoked. Acute symptomatic seizures are associated with a transient systemic or brain insult and will usually not require treatment with antiepileptic drugs (AEDs) because of the transient nature of the precipitant and the associated low risk for development of epilepsy. Unprovoked seizures, on the other hand, may represent the beginning of epilepsy.

Epidemiology

Epilepsy is one of the most common neurologic conditions, affecting more than 50 million people worldwide. The prevalence of epilepsy (number of people with active epilepsy) is approximately 1% in the United States, with 3.4 million people (3 million adults and 470,000 children) suffering from the disease. The incidence of epilepsy (number of new cases of epilepsy) is around 150,000 each year or 55 per 100,000 population. The incidence is highest in infants younger than age 1 year and in people older than age 65 years. Men have a slightly higher risk of developing epilepsy than women. African Americans and disadvantaged populations are affected at a higher rate than Caucasians. The lifetime risk of developing a seizure is around 9% to 10%.

Classification
Definition of Epilepsy

In 2014, the ILAE published a practical definition of epilepsy. The new definition classifies epilepsy as a disease of the brain characterized by any of the following criteria: at least two unprovoked or reflex seizures occurring 24 hours apart, one unprovoked or reflex seizure and a probability of recurrent seizures similar to the general recurrence risk (60%) after two unprovoked seizures, occurring over the next 10 years or a diagnosis of an epilepsy syndrome.

In 2017, the ILAE released a major revision of both the classification of the epilepsies and epilepsy syndromes and the classification of seizure types. The classification of the epilepsies and epilepsy syndromes has three levels: (1) classification of the

ILAE 2017 Classification of Seizure Types Expanded Version[1]

Focal Onset	Generalized Onset	Unknown Onset

Focal Onset

Aware | Impaired Awareness

Motor Onset
- automatisms
- atonic[2]
- clonic
- epileptic spasms[2]
- hyperkinetic
- myoclonic
- tonic

Non-Motor Onset
- autonomic
- behavior arrest
- cognitive
- emotional
- sensory

Focal to bilateral tonic-clonic

Generalized Onset

Motor
- tonic-clonic
- clonic
- tonic
- myoclonic
- myoclonic-tonic-clonic
- myoclonic-atonic
- atonic
- epileptic spasms[2]

Non-Motor (absence)
- typical
- atypical
- myoclonic
- eyelid myoclonia

Unknown Onset

Motor
- tonic-clonic
- epileptic spasms

Non-Motor
- behavior arrest

Unclassified[3]

1 Definitions, other seizure types and descriptors are listed in the accompanying paper and glossary of terms.

2 These could be focal or generalized, with or without alteration of awareness.

3 Due to inadequate information or inability to place in other categories.

Figure 1 Classification of seizure types. (From Fisher RS, Cross JH, French JA, et al. Operational classification of seizure types by the International League Against Epilepsy: Position paper of the ILAE Commission for Classification and Terminology. *Epilepsia*. 2017;58:522–530. Wylie Journal: Figure 2, page 525.)

seizure type, (2) classification of the epilepsy type, and (3) diagnosis of an epilepsy syndrome whenever possible. The cause and associated comorbidities are considered at each diagnostic step because these carry treatment implications.

The first step is to classify the type of seizure (Figure 1 and Box 1). It assumes that the patient has been diagnosed with an epileptic seizure and then organizes the seizures by where they originate in the brain into either focal onset seizures, formerly known as partial-onset seizure (emanating from networks in one lobe or hemisphere), generalized-onset seizure (seizures engaging bilateral neural networks), and unknown-onset seizures. The term *secondary generalized seizure* is replaced by focal to bilateral tonic-clonic seizure, and it is placed in a special category. Then focal-onset seizures can be optionally classified into seizures with preserved awareness as focal aware seizures (formerly known as simple partial seizures) and seizures with impaired awareness as focal impaired awareness seizures (formerly known as complex partial seizures). Focal-onset seizures, generalized-onset seizures, and unknown-onset seizures can be optionally and further subdivided into whether they have associated motor symptoms or other nonmotor symptoms. In some settings, classification into seizure type will be the only attainable level possible for diagnosis because there may be no access to EEG, video, and imaging studies or too little information available to make a higher level of diagnosis.

The second step is to classify the type of epilepsy (Figure 2). This step in the classification assumes that the patient fulfills the diagnosis of epilepsy (ILAE 2014 definition of epilepsy—as discussed earlier) and classifies the epilepsies into focal (focal clinical features and EEG with focal epileptiform abnormalities), generalized (bilateral clinical features and EEG with generalized epileptiform abnormalities), combined generalized and focal (features of both on clinical evaluation and on EEG), and unknown type (either no clinical information available and normal or no EEG available).

The third step is the diagnosis of an epilepsy syndrome whenever possible. A syndrome refers to a cluster of features such as seizure type, EEG findings, and imaging features that tend to occur together and may give information regarding treatment implications and prognosis. Within the generalized epilepsies, a well-known subgroup, known as the idiopathic primary generalized epilepsies, exists and includes four distinct syndromes: childhood absence epilepsy, juvenile absence epilepsy, juvenile myoclonic epilepsy, and generalized tonic-clonic seizures.

BOX 1 Changes in Seizure Type Classification from 1981 to 2017

- Change of "partial" to "focal."
- Certain seizure types can be either of focal, generalized, or unknown onset.
- Seizures of unknown onset may have features that can still be classified.
- Awareness is used as a classifier of focal onset seizures.
- The terms *dyscognitive, simple partial, complex partial, psychic,* and *secondary generalized* were eliminated.
- New focal seizure types include automatisms, autonomic, behavioral arrest, cognitive, emotional, hyperkinetic, sensory, and focal to bilateral tonic-clonic seizures. Atonic, clonic, epileptic spasms, myoclonic, and tonic seizures can be either focal or generalized.
- New generalized seizure types include absence with eyelid myoclonia, myoclonic absence, myoclonic tonic-clonic, myoclonic atonic, and epileptic spasms.

From Fisher RS, Cross JH, French JA, et al. Operational classification of seizure types by the International League Against Epilepsy: Position paper of the ILAE Commission for Classification and Terminology. *Epilepsia*. 2017;58:522–530.

From the moment the patient is diagnosed with having an epileptic seizure, a cause should be sought. Etiologies include structural etiology (structural abnormality seen on brain MRI that is strongly associated with the development of seizures), for example, temporal lobe seizures from mesiotemporal sclerosis; genetic etiology (epilepsies with a presumed genetic mutation), for example, benign familial neonatal epilepsy with mutation in *KNCQ2* or *KNCQ3* (potassium channels); infectious etiology, for example neurocysticercosis; metabolic etiology, for example, porphyria and pyridoxine-dependent seizures; immune etiology, for example, anti-N-methyl-D-aspartate (NMDA) receptor encephalitis and anti-LG1 encephalitis and unknown etiology.

Comorbidities should be considered for every patient with epilepsy at each stage of classification just like etiology. Comorbidities include learning, psychological, and behavioral problems. The term *benign* is replaced by self-limiting (likely spontaneous

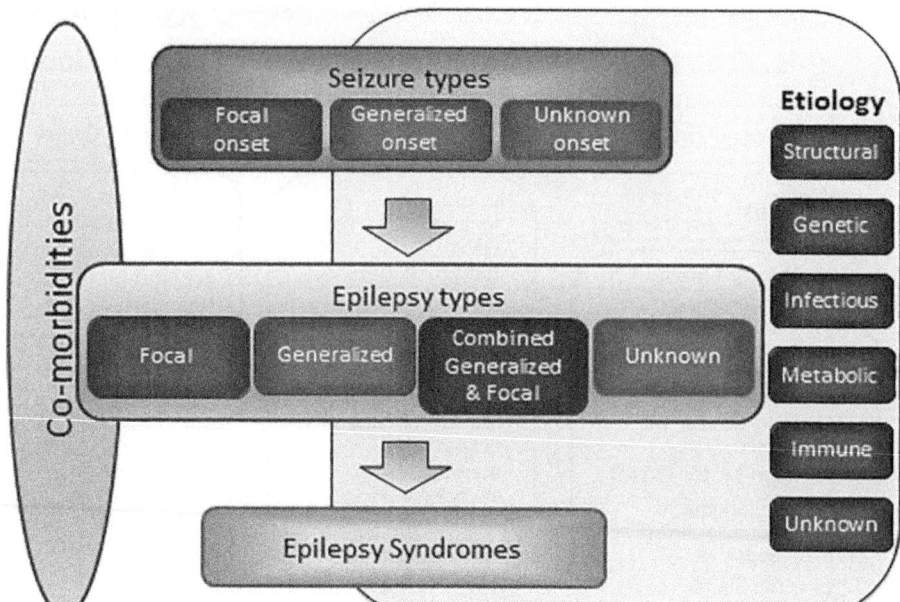

Figure 2 Classification of the epilepsies. (From Scheffer IE, Berkovic S, Capovilla G, et al. ILAE classification of the epilepsies: position paper of the ILAE Commission for Classification and Terminology. *Epilepsia*. 2017;58:512–521. Wylie Journal: Figure 1, page 515.)

resolution of a syndrome) and pharmacoresponsive (the epilepsy syndrome will be controlled with appropriate AED treatment). This new classification is aimed at providing tools for improved diagnosis and understanding of etiology and targeted therapies to the patient's disease.

Diagnosis

The diagnosis of a seizure and epilepsy is largely a clinical one and is highly dependent on the history and physical examination. The clinical history should be obtained from the patient and from a witness. After the aforementioned is obtained, the information is analyzed to determine whether indeed the paroxysmal event in question represents a true seizure or a seizure mimicker. If the event of concern represents a seizure, then it is further classified into focal or generalized and into acute symptomatic, a transient phenomenon with lower seizure recurrence, or unprovoked, which confers a higher risk for seizure recurrence and development of epilepsy.

The clinical history is aimed at obtaining a clear description of the prodromal or premonitory state, the pre-ictal state, the ictal state, and the postictal state. The prodromal state occurs hours to days prior to the ictus and is most commonly seen in generalized seizures but may also occur in focal onset seizures and consists of behavioral changes, mood swings, fatigue, and changes in sleep patterns. Regarding the pre-ictal period, the patient should be questioned about the presence of warning signs immediately before the seizure onset, also known as auras. An aura is a simple partial seizure or seizure without impaired awareness. An aura points to a focal seizure onset and according to the description of the aura, we can potentially determine the lobe of onset. For example, a rising gastric sensation and a sensation of déjà vu points to seizure onset in the temporal lobe and visual hallucinations point to the occipital lobe.

Then ask what happened during the event (ictal period). Issues to consider include the level of awareness, the presence of ability to speak, the presence of automatisms (lip-smacking, ipsilateral hand automatisms, and contralateral dystonia points to ipsilateral temporal lobe seizures), other behavior, and the duration of the event (true seizures usually last less than 2 minutes whereas nonepileptic events are usually of longer duration).

Next, focus on what happened after the event (postictal period): whether there is any confusion or fatigue, how long it takes the patient to come back to baseline, presence of tongue bites and muscle aches, and urinary incontinence (commonly seen with true seizures). Also, ask for triggers including sleep deprivation, stress, drug intake, and alcohol withdrawal.

Other information to obtain includes the presence of diurnal variations; for example, frontal lobe seizures usually occur at nighttime, and generalized tonic-clonic and myoclonic seizures occur mostly during the morning. If more than one seizure occurs, then ask for maximum seizure-free period, seizure frequency to assess for severity of disease and response to treatment, number of visits to the hospital or the emergency department to assess for seizure severity, as well as the presence of falls or injuries during seizures to assess for risks and degree of seizure control.

Medical history should include questions on patient's prenatal history and development to assess for remote symptomatic causes of seizures, history of febrile seizures, history of central nervous system (CNS) lesions (tumors, stroke) and infections, history of brain trauma specifically with associated penetrating injuries with intraparenchymal blood, skull fractures, and prolonged loss of consciousness, and family history of epilepsy.

Social history should include questions on level of education and employment. Patients with a higher level of education usually will have a better understanding of their diagnosis and prognosis. Employment is important, because patients at higher risk for development of subsequent seizures after a first seizure have a higher risk of injury if they work in a high-risk job (e.g., in construction handling heavy machinery). Patients with altered awareness during a seizure should not be driving. Clinicians should be familiar with the specific state laws regarding driving in patients with seizures and epilepsy. Use of drugs and alcohol are risk factors for the development of a first provoked seizure, and some illegal drugs may exacerbate or cause seizures. Patients should be discouraged from using illegal drugs and from the excessive intake of alcohol. Review of current medications or newly started medications should be performed to determine whether any can precipitate seizures (e.g., tramadol, bupropion).

After the medical history is obtained, a thorough physical and neurologic examination should be performed. The clinician should look for skin abnormalities such as neurocutaneous manifestations of diseases (tuberous sclerosis and neurofibromatosis). Test for muscle strength to rule out subtle weakness or postictal Todd paralysis; look for lateral tongue/cheek bites, which are commonly seen in true epileptic seizures; also look for bruises, scrapes from falls, burns, and muscle and back pain commonly seen in compression fractures caused by convulsive seizures.

The evaluation of a new-onset seizure should be aimed at determining whether the seizure represents an acute symptomatic seizure, usually a transient phenomenon or an unprovoked seizure.

If the history and examination points to a probable acute symptomatic seizure, then life-threatening conditions should be ruled out (hemorrhage, CNS infection, neoplasms) as soon as possible. Basic laboratory tests should be ordered including complete blood count, electrolytes (sodium), blood glucose, liver function tests, and toxicology to rule out drug use. If signs of CNS infection are present (fever, nuchal rigidity), consider performing a lumbar puncture. Emergency neuroimaging (usually head CT [HCT] in acute setting) should also be performed. If the patient continues to be altered or confused or to have focal deficits not explained by neuroimaging or is not at baseline 30 to 60 minutes after a seizure, emergency EEG or continuous video EEG monitoring should be performed to look for subclinical seizures. If there is evidence of provoking factors (sleep deprivation, alcohol or drug use), normal neuroimaging and the patient is back to baseline, then the EEG can be delayed and performed in the outpatient setting. The EEG is important, because some patients with symptomatic seizures can also have epileptiform abnormalities perhaps requiring AED treatment (alcohol withdrawal seizure with focal interictal epileptiform discharges [IEDs] coming from area of encephalomalacia due to falls).

Unprovoked seizures are classified into seizures of unknown etiology and seizures with a preexistent brain lesion (remote symptomatic). If the initial workup points to a probable unprovoked seizure, an MRI with epilepsy protocol (3 Tesla MRI with 1- to 3-mm slices and coronal fluid-attenuated inversion recovery sequences) interpreted by a neuroradiologist should be performed to rule out subtle lesions such as cortical dysplasias and mesiotemporal sclerosis, which confer higher risk of development of epilepsy. Also, the EEG is of paramount importance to stratify patients at risk for recurrent seizures. The EEG should be performed with sleep deprivation and with activating procedures and as close as possible to the seizure (within 24 hours) to increase the yield of detecting interictal epileptiform abnormalities. There is a 51% chance of recording epileptiform abnormalities if EEG is performed 24 hours after a seizure.

Differential Diagnosis

The diagnosis of a seizure or epilepsy can be challenging. There are many paroxysmal conditions, both psychiatric and organic, that may mimic seizures. Of all the seizure mimickers, psychogenic nonepileptic attacks (also known as psychogenic nonepileptic seizures) are the condition most commonly misdiagnosed as epilepsy. The estimated prevalence of psychogenic nonepileptic attacks is 2 to 33 per 100,000 and most patients are younger females. The clinical history and physical examination usually point to the diagnosis of psychogenic nonepileptic attacks. Red flags include poor control on multiple AEDs with a series of normal EEGs, psychiatric history, unusual triggers such as pain and getting upset, diagnosis of chronic pain syndrome and fibromyalgia, seizures in the outpatient clinics or at doctor's visit (presence of an audience), and a never-ending list of symptoms on review of systems. Some of these patients also have history of sexual, emotional, or physical abuse. The physical examination may reveal give-way weakness and histrionic behavior. The "gold standard" for the diagnosis of psychogenic nonepileptic events is continuous video EEG monitoring. The combination of atypical semiology and lack of EEG findings during the paroxysm allows for a definitive diagnosis. Common behaviors seen during a nonepileptic paroxysmal event include position of convenience, ictal eye closure, retained awareness with bilateral motor features resembling a convulsive event, opisthotonic posturing (arched back), pelvic thrusting, crying/weeping, ictal stuttering, baby talk, side-to-side head movements, pseudo-sleep, irregular out-of-phase motor activity (like a fish out of water), gradual onset and termination, prolonged attacks, and stop-and-go phenomena.

Syncope is the second most common paroxysmal event misdiagnosed as seizures. Syncope represents a transient lack of blood flow to the brain. Some features are helpful in differentiating syncope from true seizures, and these include prodromal symptoms of general malaise, sweating, dizziness, nausea, palpitations and chest pain, and loss of consciousness with rapid recovery after hitting the ground due to rapid brain reperfusion. The challenging part is the fact that many syncopal events show "convulsive-like" behavior such as clonic phenomena, making the diagnosis more challenging. Syncopal attacks are usually shorter than typical convulsive seizures and recovery is faster with no postictal state and usually no tongue-bites or urinary incontinence, a feature commonly seen in true convulsive seizures. The most common type of syncope is vasovagal and is precipitated by some situations such as pain and sight of blood. The other type is reflex syncope due to micturition, cough, Valsalva maneuver, and defecation. The EEG shows a typical progression of generalized slowing followed by suppression without any associated ictal features. Cardiac mechanisms should be explored because some could be life-threatening (e.g., Brugada syndrome or other arrhythmias) and require immediate intervention.

Migraines, especially complicated migraines, and migraine auras cause positive focal symptoms such as visual auras, sensorimotor phenomena, and weakness, which could potentially mimic partial seizures. The course, however, for migraines is in the range of minutes and of seizures in the range of seconds. A complicated migraine may be misdiagnosed as Todd paralysis. Patients with migraines do have history of headaches and retained awareness during the attack; these two features favor the diagnosis of migraine headaches.

Transient ischemic attacks or TIAs should not be misdiagnosed as seizures because this entity has marked focal negative phenomena (weakness, numbness, aphasia), whereas seizures present mostly positive phenomena (movement, automatisms, jerking). Positive symptoms rarely occur during TIAs (limb-shaking TIA).

Other conditions that may mimic seizures include hypoglycemia, panic attacks, paroxysmal movement disorders, nonepileptic myoclonus, sleep disorders, parasomnias, cataplexy, and hypnic jerks. It important, therefore, to obtain a detailed history, followed by continuous video-EEG monitoring to try to capture these events for final diagnostic purposes, because it is not uncommon to misdiagnose and mislabel these conditions as epilepsy.

Treatment

Treatment should be initiated only if the potential benefit from treatment exceeds the potential for harm. In general, if the patient has an acute symptomatic seizure, treatment with AEDs is usually not necessary because these seizures are caused by a transient and reversible precipitating factor. In these cases, it is best to treat the provoking factor (discontinue an offending drug or treating electrolyte abnormality) or allow adequate time for the acute provoking etiology to resolve.

If an acute symptomatic cause cannot be found, then it is possible that the patient's seizure represents the first unprovoked seizure of an underlying epileptic disorder. About 150,000 adults will have an unprovoked first seizure. Unprovoked seizures are classified into remote symptomatic seizures (preexistent brain lesion) or seizures of unknown etiology. The rate of seizure recurrence after an unprovoked single seizure ranges from 31% to 56% over 2 to 5 years, and most patients will experience a recurrence in the first year. Seizure recurrence rates are significantly higher if there is a prior brain insult (twofold increase), if the EEG shows epileptiform abnormalities, if there is an abnormality on neuroimaging, and if the seizure occurs out of sleep (nocturnal seizure). If any of the aforementioned factors are present, then AED treatment may be warranted. If AED treatment is recommended, then patients should be advised that the risk of side effects will range between 7% and 31%, and these are mild and reversible. Patients should be informed that immediate AED therapy will reduce the risk of seizure recurrence in the first 2 years after the seizure but will not improve the long-term (>3 years) chance of attaining seizure remission. Also, a single seizure can potentially be treated if the consequences of a recurrent seizure will significantly impact quality of life such as driving, work, or general safety. If two or more unprovoked seizures separated by 24 hours occur or if seizure recurrence risk is equal to 60% or more after a single event, then epilepsy is diagnosed, and AED treatment is strongly recommended.

The goal of therapy is complete seizure freedom with no side effects. Around 50% to 60% of patients become seizure free on a single drug. Unfortunately, this is not possible in 30% to 40% of patients, necessitating referral to epilepsy centers for evaluation to rule out seizure imitators, evaluate for the presence of possible surgically remediable syndromes, and to try other options including diets and/or devices (vagal nerve stimulator, responsive nerve stimulator [RNS]).

When starting AED treatment, always choose the medication that is effective for the seizure type or epilepsy syndrome. Of all the available AEDs, there are five that have a "broad spectrum" of action (work for both focal and generalized seizures): valproate (Depakote), lamotrigine (Lamictal), levetiracetam (Keppra), topiramate (Topamax), and zonisamide (Zonegran)[1]. Consider a broad-spectrum AED if the type of seizure is unknown. All the available AEDs are effective against focal seizures except ethosuximide (Zarontin); this medication is only effective in the treatment of typical absence epilepsy.

Next, consider the side-effect profile, cost, and drug dosing schedule, and adapt to the unique patient characteristics, taking into consideration the patient comorbidities (Tables 1 and 2). For example, drugs with a once-a-day schedule are optimal for patients with history of prior poor compliance and for the elderly; in patients taking multiple drugs for other comorbidities, administration of liver enzyme inducers (phenytoin) should be avoided. If the patient suffers from obesity, topiramate should be considered. In patients with migraine, either valproate or topiramate should be considered because these drugs are also effective for migraine prophylaxis.

Aim for monotherapy whenever possible to decrease side effects and drug interactions. Begin titration with a low dose and increase slowly to maximize compliance and decrease side effects. If mild side effects occur, reassure the patient, because most are usually transient.

Increase AED dose until seizure freedom is achieved or until side effects occur. If side effects occur, decrease dose to the maximum tolerated dose. When switching from one AED to another, always overlap the medications. For example, if a new medication is added, consider titrating to effective dose before decreasing the failed medication. This approach provides some protection against breakthrough seizures during medication transitions.

If polytherapy is needed, consider AEDs with different mechanism of actions (rational polytherapy); for example, a sodium channel blocker with a GABA enhancer or synergistic mechanisms (e.g., valproate and lamotrigine). Consider medications with parenteral formulations and a rapid time to therapeutic onset for rapid control of seizures if you want to discharge the patient from the ED with an adequate therapeutic dose. Drug levels should be obtained when compliance is an issue. Medication drug levels are a guide and not a goal. Always follow the patient's clinical response to AEDs.

In general, it is reasonable to consider AED discontinuation in patients who have been seizure free for 2 years. The reported relapse rates after stopping AEDs is around 41% or less. Factors associated with higher relapse include symptomatic epilepsy, age of onset between 10 and 12 years, cognitive delay, abnormal neurologic examination, juvenile myoclonic epilepsy, symptomatic partial epilepsy, abnormal EEG, family history of seizures or epilepsy, poor initial response to drug, and more than 1 drug before discontinuation. If epileptiform abnormalities are seen and there is worsening of the EEG (increased EEG abnormalities) during discontinuation, then relapse rates are higher. Therefore, consider performing EEG before and after AED discontinuation.

Characteristics of Specific Antiepileptic Drugs
Phenytoin
Phenytoin (Dilantin) is one of the most used antiepileptic medications. It is effective in the treatment of focal seizures and generalized seizures, prophylaxis after neurosurgical procedures, and status epilepticus that do not respond to benzodiazepines. It can exacerbate absence seizures and myoclonus. Phenytoin exerts its antiepileptic effect by blocking sodium channels, thereby preventing posttetanic potentiation. It is metabolized by the cytochrome P-450 enzyme in the liver and follows zero order or nonlinear kinetics, and therefore very steep elevations in blood levels can occur with minimal dose increases when the blood level is close to 20 µg/mL. Idiosyncratic reactions include blood dyscrasias and hepatitis, but these are rare. Common cumulative side effects include gum hyperplasia, coarsening of facial features, hirsutism, ataxia caused by cerebellar degeneration, nystagmus, drowsiness, lethargy, rash, headaches, nausea, vomiting, bone marrow hypoplasia, vitamin K and folate deficiency, and osteoporosis. Phenytoin is a strong inducer of hepatic enzymes, and it alters the metabolism of other drugs.

Fosphenytoin sodium (Cerebyx) is a prodrug, with phenytoin as its active metabolite. This medication is intended for parenteral administration; it is better tolerated than parenteral phenytoin because it is an aqueous solution with a neutral pH and can be administered three times as fast as phenytoin (150 mg/min vs. 50 mg/min). It has fewer cardiovascular side effects, including less hypotension, because, unlike phenytoin, it is not mixed with polyethylene glycol and it won't cause vein irritation or purple glove syndrome because of its neutral pH.

Carbamazepine
Carbamazepine (Tegretol) is one of the most used AEDs in the world. It has been used in the United States since 1974 for the treatment of focal epilepsies and generalized tonic-clonic seizures. It is highly effective and usually well tolerated. Carbamazepine, like phenytoin, blocks sodium channels. This medication is metabolized in the liver, and the major metabolic pathway is epoxidation to CBZ 10-11-epoxide. This epoxide confers most of the toxicity associated with this drug. It undergoes autoinduction and therefore induces its own metabolism in the first 3 to 5 weeks, and it takes longer to reach steady-state blood levels. Usually the extended-release formulations (Carbatrol and Tegretol XR) are better tolerated than the immediate-release formulations. Idiosyncratic side effects are rare and include aplastic anemia, agranulocytosis, hyponatremia, thrombocytopenia, hepatitis, and Stevens-Johnson syndrome. White blood cell counts may drop mildly and do not require intervention unless the level drops below 3000 per mm[3]. Dose-related side effects include diplopia, dizziness, nausea, and ataxia.

Phenobarbital
Phenobarbital (Luminal) is the most commonly used AED of the 20th century. It is inexpensive and long acting, but due to the poor side-effect profile, it has fallen out of favor for newer AEDs. It is used for the treatment of focal-onset, generalized seizures and neonatal seizures.[1] It is a barbiturate and acts on the GABA-A barbiturate binding site and therefore prolongs the duration of calcium channel opening stabilizing neuronal membranes. It has a very long half-life (70 to 120 hours) in adults and therefore is suitable for once-a-day administration. It is a powerful inducer of microsomal liver enzymes. Side effects include cognitive problems, sedation, psychomotor slowing, depression, coarsening of facial features, osteopenia, folic acid deficiency, Dupuytren contractures, megaloblastic anemia, and hepatitis (autoimmune reaction). Withdrawal of this medication should be performed very slowly because of the high risk of withdrawal seizures.

Primidone (Mysoline) is metabolized to phenobarbital (main active metabolite) and phenylethylmalonamide. It is a second-line agent used for the treatment of focal seizures and secondary generalized seizures, and the side-effect profile is similar to phenobarbital.

---

[1] Not FDA approved for this indication.

[1] Not FDA approved for this indication.

TABLE 1 Dosage and Side-Effect Profile of Commonly Prescribed Antiepileptic Drugs

DRUG	HALF-LIFE	INITIAL DOSAGE	MAINTENANCE DOSAGE	INCREMENT	DOSING SCHEDULE	ADVERSE EFFECTS
Carbamazepine (Tegretol)	12–17 h	200 mg BID	600–1800 mg[3]	200 mg q wk	TID–QID	Hyponatremia, leukopenia, rare aplastic anemia, and hepatitis
Gabapentin (Neurontin)	5–7 h	300 mg QD	1200–3600 mg	300 mg q3–7 d	TID	60% removed by hemodialysis, prolonged half-life to 51 h with hemodialysis Dosed 300 mg after hemodialysis
Lacosamide (Vimpat)	13 h	50 mg QD	300–600 mg[3]	100 mg q wk	BID	Extra 50% of dose after each hemodialysis Can prolong PR interval at high doses
Lamotrigine (Lamictal)	25 h alone; 60 h with VPA	6.25–12.5 mg QD to QOD	400 mg alone 100 mg with VPA	12.5–25 mg	BID q2 wk	Life-threatening rash, especially with rapid titration and VPA Titration and maintenance doses vary based on other AEDs
Levetiracetam (Keppra)	7 h	500 mg QD	2000–4000 mg[3]	500 mg q wk	BID	Decrease dose in chronic renal insufficiency, severe hepatic disease
Oxcarbazepine (Trileptal)	9–11 h	300 mg QD	900–2400 mg	300 mg q wk	BID	Hyponatremia Fewer side effects than carbamazepine
Phenobarbital	80–100 h	30–60 mg QD	60–120 mg	30 mg q1–2 wk	QD–BID	Sedation, Dupuytren contractures, rebound seizures with rapid tapering
Phenytoin (Dilantin)	22 h	200 mg QD	200–300 mg	100 mg q wk	QD–BID	Gum hypertrophy, hirsutism, cerebellar ataxia or atrophy, peripheral neuropathy, rare hypersensitivity, hepatitis
Pregabalin (Lyrica)	6 h	50 mg QD	150–600 mg	50 mg q3–7 d	BID–TID	Weight gain
Topiramate (Topamax)	21 h	25 mg QD	200–400 mg	25 mg q1–2 wk	BID	Cognitive impairment at >400 mg/d, rare kidney stones, glaucoma, oligohidrosis
Valproic acid (Depakene)	9–16 h	250 mg QD	750–3000 mg	250 mg q3–7 d	TID–QID	Tremor, weight gain, alopecia, thrombocytopenia Rare hepatitis and pancreatitis Risk of teratogenesis and neural tube defects
Zonisamide (Zonegran)	63 h	100 mg QD	200–400 mg	100 mg q2 wk	BID	Kidney stones, oligohidrosis, rare blood dyscrasias

[3]Exceeds dosage recommended by the manufacturer.
AED, Antiepileptic drug; *BID,* 2 times daily; *q,* every; *QD,* every day; *QID,* 4 times daily; *QOD,* every other day; *TID,* 3 times daily; *VPA,* valproic acid.

735

Valproic Acid

Valproic acid (Depakene) and its sodium salt divalproex (Depakote) are "broad-spectrum" medications and the drugs of choice for the treatment of primary generalized epilepsies such as juvenile myoclonic epilepsy, absence epilepsy, photosensitive epilepsy, Lennox-Gastaut Syndrome (LGS), and second-line in epileptic spasms; it is also approved for the treatment of focal-onset epilepsies, although higher doses are needed to treat focal epilepsy. A parenteral form (Depacon) is available for the treatment of status epilepticus. It works by enhancing GABA function; it may increase GABA by stimulation of glutamate decarboxylase (GAD) and by selective modulation of voltage-gated sodium channels. Divalproex sodium (Depakote) is a powerful inhibitor of both oxidation and glucuronidation. Common side effects include dyspepsia, thinning and curling of hair, weight gain, tremor, rashes, bone marrow suppression, polycystic ovarian syndrome, amenorrhea with anovulatory cycles, thrombocytopenia, hepatitis and pancreatitis which could be life threatening, hyperammonemia, and sedation. Valproic acid should not be given to women of childbearing potential because of the high risk of fetal defects (10%), specifically neural tube defects. Decreased IQ scores have been noted in children whose mothers were treated with valproate during pregnancy.

Ethosuximide

The ethosuximide (Zarontin) mechanism of action is blockade of T-type calcium channels, and it is indicated in the treatment of typical absence epilepsy. This medication will not work to control any other seizure types. Common side effects are minimal and include dyspepsia, nausea, loss of appetite, and tiredness.

Felbamate

Felbamate (Felbatol) is effective in the treatment of multiple seizure types, but because of the occurrence of aplastic anemia and hepatic failure, it was briefly withdrawn from the US market in 1994. It is now available only for patients with intractable seizures in whom other medications have failed and when benefits

TABLE 2 Choice of Antiepileptic Drug in Special Situations

SPECIAL SITUATION	DRUG OF CHOICE	COMMENTS
Partial seizures	Carbamazepine, lamotrigine, levetiracetam, oxcarbazepine, topiramate, gabapentin	
Refractory partial seizures	Lacosamide, pregabalin, zonisamide	Second-line treatment
Generalized epilepsies	Lamotrigine, topiramate, valproic acid,[1] zonisamide[1]	Avoid valproic acid in women
Absence seizures	Ethosuximide, lamotrigine,[1] valproic acid, topiramate[1]	Ethosuximide is the choice for only pure absence seizures and is insufficient in other associated generalized tonic-clonic or myoclonic seizures
Juvenile myoclonic epilepsy	Valproic acid,[1] topiramate,[1] lamotrigine,[1] zonisamide,[1] levetiracetam	Avoid valproic acid in women
Myoclonic seizures	Clonazepam, valproic acid,[1] levetiracetam	Lamotrigine occasionally exacerbates myoclonic seizures
Women of childbearing potential	Lamotrigine, topiramate, levetiracetam, oxcarbazepine	Avoid enzyme-inducing agents that alter steroid hormones and OCP levels; use OCPs with ≥50 μg of estrogen; OCPs increase the elimination of lamotrigine Significant increased risk of teratogenicity with valproic acid
Elderly patients	Lamotrigine, gabapentin, levetiracetam, topiramate	Avoid polypharmacy and highly protein-bound AEDs and AEDs with high drug-drug interactions
Depression	Lamotrigine,[1] topiramate[1]	
Bipolar disorder	Valproic acid,[1] carbamazepine, lamotrigine, topiramate[1]	
Migraine	Valproic acid, topiramate	Consider the choice according to sex, side-effect profile, and seizure type
Chronic pain	Pregabalin,[1] gabapentin[1]	
Neuropathic pain	Carbamazepine,[1] gabapentin,[1] pregabalin	

[1]Not FDA approved for this indication.
AED, Antiepileptic drug; *OCP*, oral contraceptive pill.

outweigh the risks. Its mechanism of action is blockade of NMDA receptors, modulation of sodium channels, and blockade of calcium channels. The risk for hepatic failure is 14 of 110,000 patients and increases with polytherapy.

Gabapentin
Gabapentin (Neurontin) is similar to the structure of GABA but has no effect on the GABA receptor. It enhances GAD, thereby increasing levels of GABA. This medication has no drug interactions. It is excreted entirely unchanged in kidneys. Gabapentin is used for the treatment of focal seizures with or without secondary generalization. It is ineffective in myoclonus and primary generalized seizures, and it is ineffective at lower doses. Dose should be adjusted in patients with renal disease according to creatinine clearance.

Pregabalin
Pregabalin (Lyrica) is an analogue of GABA but, like gabapentin (Neurontin), has no effect on the GABA receptor. It has no drug interactions, and it is usually well tolerated. It must be dose-adjusted in patients with renal failure, and it is 50% removed after hemodialysis. It is used as an adjunct in adult patients with focal epilepsies. Common side effects include dizziness, drowsiness, weight gain, dry mouth, and edema.

Lamotrigine
Lamotrigine (Lamictal) works by sodium channel blockade and inhibits release of glutamate. It is "broad spectrum," and it is used for adjunctive treatment of focal-onset seizures with or without secondary generalization, crossover to monotherapy, and in LGS. It is also effective in atypical absence[1], tonic/atonic seizures, and in myoclonic seizures, although it may cause exacerbations

[1]Not FDA approved for this indication.

in some patients with juvenile myoclonic epilepsy. It is one of the preferred drugs to treat elderly patients and pregnant women because of the good safety and pharmacokinetic profile. Lamotrigine levels should be closely watched and will increase significantly with coadministration of valproate; these two medications cause a synergistic therapeutic effect but could also increase adverse reactions (rash). It could cause a rash (5%) if the drug is titrated too quickly; this rash could progress into a life-threatening condition (Stevens-Johnson syndrome [0.1%]) and is more common in children with concomitant valproate use. If rash occurs, the medication should be stopped immediately. Other common side effects include tremor, insomnia, headaches, ataxia, and somnolence. Pregnancy increases lamotrigine clearance by 50%, necessitating dose adjustments; therefore, lamotrigine levels should be monitored before, during, and after pregnancy, and doses should be adjusted accordingly.

Levetiracetam
Levetiracetam (Keppra) is one of the most widely used AEDs because of its good pharmacokinetics, favorable side-effect profile, and multiple formulations, including parenteral and liquid (ease of administration). It is a "broad-spectrum" drug. It has a unique mechanism of action (binds to synaptic vesicle protein 2A-SV2A). It does not induce liver enzymes and therefore does not affect the metabolism of other drugs and does not bind to proteins in plasma. This medication needs to be dose-adjusted in patients with renal disease and after hemodialysis (add an extra 500 mg). It is one of the only AEDs that decreases the interictal epileptic burden, the other one being Depakote. It is approved as adjunctive treatment of primary generalized tonic-clonic seizures in adults and children 6 years of age and older with idiopathic generalized epilepsy, adjunctive treatment of focal onset seizures in adults and children 4 years of age and older, and adjunctive treatment of myoclonic seizures in adults and adolescents 12

years or older with juvenile myoclonic epilepsy. It is also used off-label for prophylaxis in patients after traumatic brain injury and in status epilepticus. Common adverse effects include behavioral changes (avoid in patients with psychiatric conditions), somnolence, asthenia, headache, dizziness, and flu-like symptoms. It does not have any serious idiosyncratic reactions and is safe for the elderly and probably safe to take during pregnancy. Consider obtaining levels during pregnancy, because clearance is increased during pregnancy, necessitating dose adjustments.

Brivaracetam

Brivaracetam (Briviact) is a chemical analog of levetiracetam, with a similar mechanism of action but a higher affinity (20-fold) for the SV2A receptor. It exhibits linear kinetics with a good side-effect profile such as levetiracetam. It is indicated as adjunct treatment of focal-onset seizures with or without secondary generalization in adults and children aged 16 years and older. It does not have added therapeutic benefit if coadministered with levetiracetam. It may increase serum concentrations of carbamazepine epoxide and phenytoin.

Oxcarbazepine

Oxcarbazepine (Trileptal) is an analogue of carbamazepine but without the toxic epoxide. Thus, it is better tolerated than carbamazepine (Tegretol). It is metabolized to 10 monohydroxy metabolite (MHD), which confers its pharmacologic effect. It is used as monotherapy or adjunctive therapy in focal epilepsies in adults and as monotherapy in the treatment of focal epilepsies in children 4 years and older and as adjunctive in children 2 years and older. It may exacerbate myoclonic seizures and absence seizures. It interacts with oral contraceptives (OCPs), thereby reducing its efficacy. Hyponatremia is rare in children but may be higher in elderly populations. Other side effects include dizziness, fatigue, and headache, and these are dose dependent. Patient who develop rash with carbamazepine (Tegretol) may develop rash if treated with oxcarbazepine (Trileptal) because of cross-reactivity.

Tiagabine

Tiagabine (Gabitril) works by reversible inhibition of the GABA-transporter-1, thereby increasing the availability of GABA in the synaptic cleft. It is approved as an add-on medication in the treatment of refractory focal-onset seizures. It can worsen absence seizures and cause status epilepticus in patients with primary generalized epilepsy. Common side effects include tremor, nervousness, dizziness, abdominal pain, diarrhea, and emotional lability.

Topiramate

Topiramate (Topamax) is a broad-spectrum AED with multiple mechanisms of action. It works by inhibiting sodium conductance and weakly carbonic anhydrase, blocks the alpha-amino-3-hydroxy-5-methyl-4-isoxazole propionic acid (AMPA) glutamate receptor, and enhances GABA. It is approved for the treatment of focal-onset seizures or primary generalized epilepsy as add-on and in the treatment of LGS. Enzyme inducers (e.g., phenytoin) decrease levels of topiramate by 50%. This medication will need dose adjustments in patients with renal failure. Topiramate (Topamax) reduces the levels of OCPs, thereby decreasing its effectiveness. Common side effects include word finding difficulties, weight loss (decreased appetite), paresthesias in fingers and mouth, kidney stones, and anhidrosis due to the carbonic-anhydrase effect of this drug, acute myopia in close-angle glaucoma, ataxia, and tiredness. Usually doses >400 mg are poorly tolerated.

Zonisamide

Zonisamide (Zonegran) is a "broad-spectrum" AED used in the treatment of focal epilepsy with or without secondary generalization. It is also effective in the treatment of myoclonus (juvenile myoclonic epilepsy [JME])[1] and absence seizures (T-type calcium channel blockade). This AED has a structure similar to the sulfonamides; therefore, it is contraindicated in patients with allergies to these antibiotics. It has a long-half life (>60 hours); therefore, it can be taken once a day, which increases compliance. The major mechanism of action is by the blockade of sodium channels. It also works on T-type calcium channels and weak inhibition of carbonic anhydrase. Enzyme inducers and valproate (Depakote) decrease half-life. The most common adverse reactions include anorexia with associated weight loss, headache, mental slowing, confusion, ataxia, dizziness, kidney stones (1%), oligohidrosis, and paresthesias (carbonic anhydrase inhibition).

Vigabatrin

Vigabatrin (Sabril) is a structural analogue of GABA and binds irreversibly to the GABA-T (GABA transaminase), thereby increasing GABA concentrations in the brain. It is indicated for treatment of epileptic spasms in tuberous sclerosis and in refractory focal-onset epilepsies. It may exacerbate absence seizures and myoclonic seizures and, like tiagabine, may cause generalized spike-and-wave status epilepticus in patients with absence seizures or primary generalized epilepsy. This AED causes visual field defects (nasal constriction and concentric constriction with preserved central vision), and these may be irreversible. Other side effects include fatigue, dizziness, headache, tremor, and double vision.

Rufinamide

Rufinamide's (BANZEL) mechanism of action is probable modulation of sodium channels (prolongation of inactive state of the channel). It is indicated as adjunctive treatment of seizures associated with LGS in both children and adults.

Lacosamide

Lacosamide (Vimpat) has a novel mechanism of action by enhancing the slow inactivation of voltage-gated sodium channels. It is approved for the adjunctive treatment and conversion to monotherapy and monotherapy treatment of focal onset epilepsies. It is also used off-label for the treatment of status epilepticus in the intensive care unit because of availability of IV formulation. This medication does not have significant drug interactions.

Clobazam

Clobazam (Onfi) is a benzodiazepine with a 1,5 substitution instead of the common 1,4 substitution; therefore, it has less anxiolytic and sedative effects. It works by binding to the GABA-A receptor. It is approved for the adjunctive treatment of LGS. It may also be effective in the treatment of primary or focal seizures with secondary generalized seizures[1], as well as catamenial epilepsy. It has no significant clinical interactions. Side effects include sedation, dizziness, ataxia, and weakness. No idiosyncratic reactions have been identified.

Perampanel

Perampanel (Fycompa) is a noncompetitive AMPA receptor antagonist and is indicated in the adjunctive treatment of focal-onset seizures with or without secondary generalization and in primary generalized seizures in adults and adolescents 12 years of age and over. The recommended dose is 8 to 12 mg/d for focal seizures and 8 mg/d for primary generalized seizures. This medication has a black box warning because of severe psychiatric and behavioral reactions (aggressiveness, suicidality, homicidal threats and ideations, and irritability). Common adverse effects include somnolence, headache, dizziness, and fatigue.

Eslicarbazepine

Eslicarbazepine (Aptiom) is a prodrug to s-licarbazepine with a mechanism of action similar to oxcarbazepine (Trileptal) sodium channel blockade. It is approved as monotherapy or adjunct therapy for the treatment of focal-onset seizures. Common adverse effects include dizziness, nausea, diplopia, and headache.

---

[1] Not FDA approved for this indication.

[1] Not FDA approved for this indication.

Cannabidiol

Cannabidiol (EPIDIOLEX) is the first prescription pharmaceutical formulation of purified CBD oil approved by the FDA on June 25, 2018, for the treatment of seizures associated with Lennox Gastaut and Dravet syndrome in patients two years of age or older.

The most common side effects of this drug include increase in liver enzymes especially when used in conjunction with valproate or valproate and clobazam, decreased appetite, diarrhea, rash, tiredness, rash, sleepiness, and infections.

Special Populations

Women

Epilepsy is one of the most common conditions occurring in women of reproductive age (1.1 million). Women of reproductive age and with epilepsy and taking AEDs should be counseled on the possibility of teratogenicity from AED therapy and the potential interaction with contraception. Some AEDs (enzyme inducers) affect OCPs, leading to decreased effectiveness and unwanted pregnancies. These AEDs are phenobarbital, phenytoin, carbamazepine, oxcarbazepine, eslicarbazepine, felbamate, topiramate (at higher doses >200 mg/d), lamotrigine (doses >300 mg/d), primidone, rufinamide, and clobazam. OCPs can reduce the levels of lamotrigine, leading to breakthrough seizures. In patients taking these AEDs, a second barrier method versus changing to a nonenzyme-inducing AED is recommended. Seizures during pregnancy will remain the same or decrease, but around 15% to 30% will have an increase in seizure frequency. Most (84% to 92%) women with epilepsy who were seizure free 9 months before pregnancy will remain free of seizures during the pregnancy. Blood levels of lamotrigine, phenytoin, and, to a lesser extent, carbamazepine, and possibly levetiracetam and the active oxcarbazepine metabolite (MHD), will decrease during pregnancy because of increased clearance, and therefore these AED levels should be monitored, and medication dosages adjusted as needed. The risk from seizures to the fetus (especially convulsive seizures) is higher than the risk to the fetus from AEDs. More than 90% of female patients with epilepsy will deliver a normal baby. The rates of congenital malformations in women with epilepsy taking AEDs is around 4% to 6% (double that of general population) but remain low. Risk of malformations increases with polytherapy and with higher dose of AEDs. Valproate/valproic acid is the AED that carries the highest teratogenicity (6% to 10%), mostly associated with neural tube defects. It also produces long-term cognitive problems, with a reduction in children's IQs when mothers take valproate (Depakote) during pregnancy. Therefore, valproic acid is contraindicated and should not be used as a first-line treatment in women of childbearing potential. Women with epilepsy and of childbearing potential should be supplemented with folic acid at a dose of 0.4 mg/d to decrease the risk of congenital malformations if they become pregnant. Breastfeeding is an important concern in the postpartum period in women taking AEDs. Even though some AEDs (e.g., primidone and levetiracetam) transfer into breast milk, breastfeeding is encouraged. The baby should be monitored for increased sedation if mothers are on those two AEDs.

Elderly Patient

The current world population is aging, and the risk for epilepsy increases dramatically after the age of 65. The recognition of seizures in this group may be more complicated because the presentation may be atypical. Also, many other conditions may mimic seizures in the elderly, making diagnosis a challenging proposition. The most common seizure type in the elderly is complex partial seizures and present with confusion, staring, change in mental status, and unresponsiveness. The most common cause of epilepsy in this group is cerebrovascular disease. Other conditions that may cause epilepsy include neurodegenerative conditions (Alzheimer disease), head trauma, and brain tumors. When treating elderly patients, pharmacokinetic and pharmacodynamic properties of medications should be considered. Older people have reductions in protein binding, renal elimination, and hepatic metabolism, thereby conferring a higher risk for idiosyncratic reactions and altered kinetics. Gabapentin, lamotrigine, levetiracetam, pregabalin, and oxcarbazepine are usually well tolerated and recommended as first-line treatment in this patient population. AEDs with hepatic enzyme-inducing mechanisms are not recommended in elderly patients because of the potential for interactions with other drugs. Fortunately, seizures in this population are easy to control, and monotherapy is usually effective.

Drug Resistant Epilepsy

Drug resistant or intractable epilepsy (DRE) is defined as the failure of adequate trials of two tolerated, appropriately chosen and used AEDs as monotherapy or polytherapy to achieve sustained seizure freedom. DRE affects one third of patients living with epilepsy.

These patients should be referred to an epilepsy center for further management, including evaluation by an epileptologist who will perform a detailed clinical and physical examination and will order further diagnostic tests including video EEG monitoring to record the patient's events for final diagnostic purposes and for evaluation for possible epilepsy surgery. Surgical resection of the epilepsy focus is the only available treatment to cure epilepsy. Seizure freedom rates after temporal lobectomy for mesiotemporal sclerosis is in the range of 70% to 90% and of 40% to 70% in neocortical resections. In patients who are not suitable candidates for epilepsy surgery, dietary treatment or neurostimulation is recommended. Dietary options include the ketogenic diet, the modified Atkin's diet, and the low glycemic index diet.

These diets can be used as an add-on therapy in combination with AEDs and devices (vagus nerve stimulator [VNS]). These diets have a similar seizure reduction rates (around 50%) in half of patients. The low glycemic index diet is better tolerated and less restrictive than the modified Atkin's diet and the classic ketogenic diet.

Devices approved for the treatment of pharmacoresistant epilepsy in the United States include the VNS, the RNS, and Deep Brain Stimulation (DBS). The VNS works by delivering an intermittent mild current to the left vagus nerve. The mechanism of action is unknown but believed to include alterations in the reticular activating system, the central autonomic network, the limbic system, and the diffuse noradrenergic projection system. With long-term use, this device provides >50% seizure reduction in about 50% to 60% of patients, with around 8% becoming seizure free after 2 years. The new AspireSR generator combines traditional VNS therapy with seizure detection technology via changes in cardiac rhythms.

Responsive neurostimulation or RNS therapy (Neuropace) was approved by the Food and Drug Administration in 2013 for the treatment of refractory focal-onset seizures. This device continuously monitors and detects abnormal electrical activity that can lead to a seizure and then delivers electrical stimulation to the area of seizure generation to try to abort the seizure. It has two leads, and either subdural or depth electrodes or a combination of both can be used and placed close or over the epileptogenic zone. These leads are connected to the generator that seats on the skull. Treatment with the RNS system is recommended in patients who are not amenable to surgery and have multifocal epilepsy with no more than two discrete seizure onset zones. The median seizure reduction at 5 years was >65%, with 15% of patients achieving seizure freedom.

DBS was approved by the FDA in 2018 as adjunctive for the treatment of patients with drug-resistant focal onset epilepsy who are 18 years of age and older. This device is particularly useful if the seizure focus is difficult to localize to one or two brain regions. Leads are placed in the anterior nucleus of the thalamus for delivery of electrical stimulation. According to the SANTE (Stimulation of the Anterior Nuclei of the Thalamus for Epilepsy) trial with 110 patients randomized to receive active stimulation versus sham stimulation, at the end of five years a median reduction in seizures of 69% from baseline was observed and seizure severity and quality of life improved significantly.

References

Ahmed NS, Spencer SS: An approach to the evaluation of a patient for seizures and epilepsy, *Wisc Med J* 103(1):49–55, 2004.

Benbadis S: The differential diagnosis of epilepsy: a critical review, *Epilepsy Behav* 15:15–21, 2009.

Britton JW: Antiepileptic drug therapy: when to start, when to stop, *Continuum Lifelong Learning Neurol* 16:105–120, 2010.

Fisher RS, Acevedo C, Arzimanoglou, et al: ILAE official report: a practical clinical definition of epilepsy, *Epilepsia* 55:475–482, 2014.

Fisher RS, Cross JH, French JA, et al: Operational classification of seizure types by the International League Against Epilepsy: Position Paper of the ILAE Commission for Classification and Terminology, *Epilepsia* 58:522–530, 2017.

Gavvala JR, Schuele SU: New-onset seizure in adults and adolescent: a review, *JAMA* 36:2657–2668, 2016.

Harden CL, Meador KJ, Pennell PB, et al: Management issues for women with epilepsy—focus on pregnancy (an evidence-based review): II. Teratogenesis and perinatal outcomes: Report of the Quality Standards Subcommittee and Therapeutics and Technology Subcommittee of the American Academy of Neurology and the American Epilepsy Society, *Epilepsia* 50:1237–1246, 2009.

Harden CL, Pennell PB, Koppel BS, et al: Management issues for women with epilepsy—focus on pregnancy (an evidence-based review): III. Vitamin K, folic acid, blood levels, and breast-feeding: Report of the Quality Standards Subcommittee and Therapeutics and Technology Assessment Subcommittee of the American Academy of Neurology and the American Epilepsy Society, *Epilepsia* 50:1247–1255, 2009.

Hesdorffer DC, Logroscino G, Benn EKT, et al: Estimating risk for developing epilepsy: a population-based study in Rochester, Minnesota, *Neurology* 76:23–27, 2011.

Krumholz A, Wiebe S, Gronseth G, et al: Practice parameter: evaluating an apparent unprovoked first seizure in adults (an evidence-based review): Report of the Quality Standards Subcommittee of the American Academy of Neurology and the American Epilepsy Society, *Neurology* 69:1996–2007, 2007.

Kwan P, Arzimanoglou A, Berg AT, et al: Definition of drug resistant epilepsy: concensus proposal by the ad hoc Task Force of the ILAE Commission of Therapeutic Strategies, *Epilepsia* 51(6):1069–1077, 2010.

Kwan P, Brodie MJ: Early identification of refractory epilepsy, *N Engl J Med* 342(5):314–319, 2000.

Kwan P, Brodie MJ: Effectiveness of first antiepileptic drug, *Epilepsia* 42(10):1255–1260, 2001.

Ochoa JG: Antiepileptic Drugs. Available at https://emedicine.medscape.com/article/1187334-overview. Accessed 22 March 2018.

Salanova V, et al: Long-term efficacy and safety of thalamic stimulation for drug resistant partial epilepsy, *Neurology* 84(10):1017–1025, 2015.

Scheffer IE, Berkovic S, Capovilla G, et al: ILAE classification of the epilepsies: Position Paper of the ILAE Commission for Classification and Terminology, *Epilepsia* 58:512–521, 2017.

SLEEP DISORDERS

Method of
Meghna P. Mansukhani, MD; Bhanu Prakash Kolla, MD, MRCPsych; Erik Kent St. Louis, MD, MS; and Timothy I. Morgenthaler, MD

Sleep is a universal biological imperative for all mammals. Sleep deprivation and sleep disorders are frequent and underappreciated determinants of health status. Sleep is essential for survival, and sleep loss and sleep disorders are associated with major health problems, including cardiovascular, metabolic, neuropsychiatric, and neoplastic disorders, as well as neurobehavioral-associated accidents and risks. Healthy sleep must be regarded along with nutrition and exercise as key pillars for good health.

Recent evidence has suggested that a chief purpose of sleep may be to maintain cerebral metabolic homeostasis, clearing waste products that accumulate during wakefulness such as beta-amyloid, a protein known to abnormally accumulate in Alzheimer's disease. Insufficient sleep quantity appears to be associated with a variety of health problems and may contribute to mortality and dementia risk. Total sleep deprivation, as well as selective deprivation of nonrapid eye movement (NREM) or rapid eye movement (REM) sleep, may be lethal in laboratory animals. Adequate sleep quality is similarly necessary to ensure optimal daytime functioning because basic vigilance, attention and cognitive performance, and overall quality of life are each substantially eroded by disordered sleep, and insufficient sleep and sleep-disordered breathing (SDB) pose significant health hazards. Unfortunately, insufficient sleep quantity and quality is a widespread public health crisis in children and adults worldwide in the developed world, and primary sleep disorders are a highly prevalent cause of morbidity, an important contributor to mortality,

and a public health hazard that raises risk for motor vehicle collisions and catastrophic occupational injuries and accidents.

The clinical specialty of sleep medicine initially emerged during the 1970s and 1980s, surrounding growing clinical application of diagnostic polysomnography (PSG). While the main diagnostic use remains evaluation and initial treatment for SDB, PSG and related techniques have tremendous utility for the evaluation of selected patients with nocturnal events, periodic limb movement disorder (PLMD), narcolepsy and related primary central nervous system (CNS) hypersomnias.

In this chapter, we review the classification of common sleep disorders, a practical bedside approach toward interviewing and examining patients with sleep problems, advantages and limitations of diagnostic implements within the sleep laboratory, and summarize diagnostic and therapeutic approaches to common sleep disorders.

The International Classification of Sleep Disorders

The International Classification of Sleep Disorders (ICSD) provides a common nomenclature and taxonomy for disorders of sleep for clinicians and researchers alike. The most current ICSD, ICSD-3, divides sleep disorders into six distinct categories. The ICSD-3 nomenclature is shown in Box 1, and the most common sleep complaints and disorders are presented and discussed in detail throughout this chapter.

Clinical Approach to the Sleep Medicine Patient: The Interview and Examination

The three most common clinical presenting sleep-related complaints are hypersomnia, insomnia, and unusual behaviors or events at night (parasomnias). Hypersomnia, which is excessive sleepiness during waking hours, is often multifactorial and may be related to insufficient sleep quantity, quality, or timing; SDB; sedating medications; or certain medical, psychiatric, or neurologic conditions. Insomnia may be regarded as a problem in initiating or maintaining sleep under conditions that are normally conducive to sleep. Parasomnias are unusual behaviors that are often dangerous to the patient or bed partner during sleep.

Insomnia is a subjective complaint. To some patients it is not at all bothersome to require 20 to 30 minutes to fall asleep, while to others it seems very wrong. While insomnia is fundamentally a subjective symptom, the manifestations follow common patterns. Sleep latency, the time taken to fall asleep, varies significantly, but initial sleep latency longer than 30 minutes may be considered prolonged, once proper sleep-conductive conditions have been established (lights off, dark and quiet sleep environment without distracting stimuli). There is also significant variation in what degree of subjective sleep disruption reflects sleep-maintenance insomnia, as normal individuals may briefly awaken as often as 10 to 15 times each hour, with most such arousals being below the threshold of conscious awareness. Multiple nocturnal awakenings that are disturbing to the patient, especially when there is difficulty reinitiating sleep and prolonged wake after sleep-onset time, may be regarded as sleep-maintenance insomnia. Patients admitting to insomnia should be asked to estimate what amount of their problem is ascribable to an active mind or worries, restless legs, or body pain. Disturbing influences in the sleep environment such as the ambient light, temperature, and noise conditions in the bedroom should be sought. A precise diagnosis is not possible without detailed knowledge of sleep and wake behavior over the entire circadian cycle during a more protracted time, such as 1 to 2 weeks. A sleep diary can be very helpful in gaining needed insights for diagnosis. Increasingly, helpful information about timing and duration of sleep may be logged in applications for personal mobile computing devices.

The patient and physician may at times have difficulty differentiating between hypersomnia and complaints of fatigue (a sense of lacking enough energy to carry out usual daily activities, without the tendency toward dozing or nodding off inadvertently). A quick, incisive bedside test that helps distinguish between

Insomnia
- Chronic insomnia disorder
- Short-term insomnia disorder
- Other insomnia disorder
  Isolated symptoms and normal variants
- Excessive time in bed
- Short sleeper

Sleep-Related Breathing Disorders

The continuum of obstructive sleep-disordered breathing: snoring, Upper-airway resistance syndrome, and obstructive sleep apnea (OSA)

Obstructive sleep apnea (OSA) disorders
- OSA, adult
- OSA, pediatric

Central sleep apnea syndromes
- Central sleep apnea with Cheyne-Stokes breathing
- Central apnea due to medical disorder without Cheyne-Stokes breathing
- Central sleep apnea due to high altitude periodic breathing
- Central sleep apnea due to a medication or substance
- Primary central sleep apnea
- Primary central sleep apnea of infancy
- Primary central sleep apnea of prematurity
- Treatment-emergent central sleep apnea

Sleep-related hypoventilation disorders
- Obesity hypoventilation syndrome
- Congenital central alveolar hypoventilation syndrome
- Late-onset central hypoventilation with hypothalamic dysfunction
- Idiopathic central alveolar hypoventilation
- Sleep-related hypoventilation due to a medication or substance
- Sleep-related hypoventilation due to a medical disorder
- Sleep-related hypoxemia disorder
  Isolated symptoms and normal variants
- Snoring
- Catathrenia

Central Disorders of Hypersomnolence
- Narcolepsy Type I
- Narcolepsy Type II
- Idiopathic hypersomnia
- Kleine-Levin syndrome
- Hypersomnia due to a medical disorder
- Hypersomnia due to a medication or substance
- Hypersomnia associated with a psychiatric disorder
- Insufficient sleep syndrome
  Isolated symptoms and normal variants
- Long sleeper

Circadian Rhythm Sleep-Wake Disorders
- Delayed sleep-wake phase disorder
- Advanced sleep-wake phase disorder
- Irregular sleep-wake rhythm disorder
- Non-24-hour sleep-wake rhythm disorder
- Shift work disorder
- Jet lag disorder
- Circadian rhythm sleep-wake disorder not otherwise specified

Parasomnias

NREM-related parasomnias
- Disorders of arousal (from NREM sleep)
- Confusional arousals
- Sleepwalking
- Sleep terrors
- Sleep-related eating disorder

REM-related parasomnias
- REM sleep behavior disorder
- Recurrent isolated sleep paralysis
- Nightmare disorder

Other parasomnias
- Exploding head syndrome
- Sleep-related hallucinations
- Sleep enuresis
- Parasomnia due to a medical disorder
- Parasomnia due to a medication or substance
- Parasomnia, unspecified
  Isolated symptoms and normal variants
- Sleep talking

Sleep-Related Movement Disorders
- Restless legs syndrome
- Periodic limb movement disorder
- Sleep-related leg cramps
- Sleep-related bruxism
- Sleep-related rhythmic movement disorder
- Benign sleep myoclonus of infancy
- Propriospinal myoclonus at sleep onset
- Sleep-related movement disorder due to a medical disorder
- Sleep-related movement disorder due to a medication or substance
- Sleep-related movement disorder, unspecified

Isolated symptoms and normal variants
- Excessive fragmentary myoclonus
- Hypnagogic foot tremor and alternating leg muscle activation
- Sleep starts (hypnic jerks)

Other Sleep Disorders
- Fatal familial insomnia
- Sleep-related epilepsy
- Sleep-related headaches
- Sleep-related laryngospasm
- Sleep-related gastroesophageal reflux
- Sleep-related myocardial ischemia

Abbreviations: CNS = central nervous system; NREM = non–rapid eye movement [sleep]; REM = rapid eye movement [sleep].

hypersomnia and fatigue is the Epworth Sleepiness Scale (ESS), a short questionnaire asking the patient his or her likelihood of dozing inadvertently during usual permissive daytime sedentary settings including reading, watching television, or traveling in a car. An online version is available at http://www.stanford.edu/~dement/epworth.html. Scores over 10 are considered abnormal and indicative of a possible underlying primary sleep disorder and suggest the need for further evaluation. Complaints of hypersomnia must be placed into the context of the sleep history with particular emphasis on the quantity, timing, and quality of sleep.

Patients may also present with complaints of disturbing or unusual activities during sleep (parasomnias). Key diagnostic points in determining the diagnosis for parasomnias include their onset, duration, frequency, time of night, stereotypy, injuries sustained, and whether there is any further behavioral change following the parasomnia episode.

Collateral history obtained from a bed partner may be particularly instructive. Patients should be asked whether they are reported to snore, whether the snoring is intermittent or constant, and if the snoring volume is related to sleeping in a supine position. Disruptive snoring loud enough to be heard outside a closed bedroom door, or witnessed stop-breathing episodes indicating apneas or self-awareness of arousals related to a snort or gasp, are particularly suggestive symptoms of obstructive sleep apnea

(OSA). Symptoms such as morning dry mouth and sore throat, frequent morning headaches, or heartburn may indicate a higher likelihood of significant SDB. Patients should be asked about awareness of restless legs symptoms or movements during sleep, and whether they have been told of peculiar sleep-related behaviors or evidence of acting out their dreams, yelling or thrashing in sleep, or exhibiting sleep walking or other amnestic behaviors during sleep.

In addition to a detailed sleep history, taking a thorough general medical history is important because sleep disorders are frequently tightly linked to other diseases. OSA is closely associated with hypertension, coronary artery disease, cerebrovascular disease, atrial fibrillation, obesity, and the metabolic syndrome. Congestive heart failure, even when well compensated, is frequently associated with central sleep apnea syndrome. Restless legs syndrome and periodic limb movements in sleep (PLMS) are more common in patients with systemic iron deficiency or renal impairment, or in those with spinal cord or peripheral nerve pathologies. Hypoventilation is more prevalent in patients with neuromuscular disease; advanced obstructive lung disease; kyphosis; and in traumatic, vascular, neoplastic, or degenerative disorders that affect the medullary centers of the brain. Various genetic syndromes such as trisomy-21 produce craniofacial abnormalities predisposing to OSA due to anatomic narrowing of the upper airway.

Physical examination in sleep medicine focuses on signs indicating predisposition or associated sequelae of SDB. Careful inspection of the oropharynx and nares is particularly important because significant oropharyngeal narrowing is the chief anatomic substrate for obstructive SDB, while nasal septal deviation or other nasal obstruction, in addition to a thickened neck and overweight body habitus, may also contribute toward sleep apnea. Careful inspection for signs of neuromuscular disease, such as weakness of cervical flexor or extensor muscles, fasciculations or thoracoabdominal paradox, may help detect the underlying cause for sleep-related hypoventilation. Elevated blood pressure, a cardiac gallop, wet rales, and peripheral edema may be present as signs of systemic hypertension, heart failure, or cor pulmonale associated with untreated SDB.

Diagnostic Tools in the Sleep Laboratory
Polysomnography
Laboratory polysomnography (PSG) is the "gold standard" for formal assessment of suspected SDB, hypersomnia, or parasomnias. PSG is a diagnostic test most often performed in a sleep laboratory; attended by trained technicians; and combining evaluation of sleep, breathing, and movement. During PSG, several polygraphic physiologic variables are analyzed, including electroencephalography (EEG) as well as chin electromyography (EMG) to allow determination of sleep staging, limb EMG leads to analyze periodic leg movements that may disrupt sleep, oronasal airflow measured by a thermistor and nasal pressure sensors, electrocardiography, and respiratory effort measured by inductance plethysmography or piezocrystal monitors. Body position is also analyzed to delineate effects of sleeping position on breathing.

Each 30-second epoch of the PSG is subsequently scored by a sleep technologist as either wake, NREM sleep (N1 or N2 light NREM, or N3 slow wave sleep), or REM sleep according to well-defined guidelines. Sleep architecture, or the composition of sleep by different stages, varies greatly by age, but in middle-aged adults is approximately 60% to 75% N1-N2, 10% to 20% N3, and 15% to 25% REM sleep. Children usually have higher, and elderly individuals have lower, percentages of N3 and REM. Arousals from sleep and their mechanisms, whether due to breathing, movement, or spontaneous causes, are determined. Accordingly, a precise determination of the duration of a patient's total sleep time, sleep efficiency (total time spent asleep divided by time in bed), and disrupting influences on sleep, such as abnormal respiration or movement, may be determined. The effects of confounding medications and medical disorders on sleep architecture, such as selective-serotonin reuptake inhibitors (SSRI) that suppress and delay REM sleep, or benzodiazepines that reduce the N3 and REM amounts and increase sleep stage

shifting leading to heightened light NREM N1 and N2, must also be considered.

Attended PSG is advantageous because it allows precise measurement of sleep and relevant cardiorespiratory and neurologic behaviors and allows intervention with therapeutic positive airway pressure (PAP) trials if indicated. Disadvantages of PSG include patient inconvenience, a foreign sleep environment, and expenses due to highly trained personnel and technology. For those patients whose disease severity is difficult to predict, or who may have other complicating medical illnesses that would render interpretation of an out-of-center cardiopulmonary sleep test inaccurate (such as those with significant cardiopulmonary or neurologic diseases), or those who may require noncontinuous PAP modalities, or for those with parasomnia symptoms, attended PSG and treatment design is needed. Split-night PSG remains a cost-effective strategy for many patients.

PSG is currently the only way to actually measure sleep; although the sleep state is currently defined by the variables measured in PSG (EEG, EMG, and EOG), the science of sleep medicine may develop other ways of characterizing the sleep state that are more convenient, precise, and correlate even better with health and disease.

Home Sleep Apnea Testing
PSG is comprehensive, but for patients with characteristic clinical presentations for OSA syndrome, it is often possible to arrive at a diagnosis using a significantly reduced number of recording channels that may be conducted in the home setting. A recent systematic review concluded that many commercially available home monitoring devices do not perform well in sensitivity or specificity. The best out-of-center testing devices use similar measures as PSG but exclude EEG, EMG, or EOG channels needed to score sleep. Thus, these devices typically measure at a minimum airflow using thermistors and nasal pressure transducers, breathing effort using respiratory impedance plethysmography, oxygen saturation using pulse oximetry, and snoring. Using these signals, the frequency of apneas and hypopneas per hour of recording, called the respiratory event index (REI), may be determined. Some testing devices add markers for sleep, such as actigraphy (see below), position sensors, or pattern recognition of pulse or autonomic variability to estimate sleep time (called peripheral arterial tonometry). Home sleep apnea testing (HSAT) devices are thus far only considered for evaluation of OSA syndrome and are not suitable for diagnostic evaluation of other sleep disorders. Because of limited sensitivity, they are best employed when there is a high pretest probability that the patient has at least moderately severe OSA syndrome. Patients appropriate for HSAT would be those who satisfy three criteria: have a high likelihood of having at least moderately severe OSA, will be good candidates for either autotitrating continuous PAP (CPAP) or an oral appliance, and do not have underlying diseases that either will obscure HSAT or who may have other disorders that require PSG for diagnosis. Because of the poor sensitivity of HSAT, a negative result should be cause for PSG: the patient should have had a high pretest probability for having at least moderately severe OSA.

For medically uncomplicated patients fitting the above criteria, using HSAT followed by APAP most often leads to similar results as attended PSG with CPAP therapy based upon in-lab titration of pressure. This strategy is increasingly being used, largely owing to reduced costs. These good results depend, however, upon expert PAP mask fitting and follow-up. It is best to remember that treatment is chronic and requires ongoing follow-up. More is written about this in the section on OSA below.

Multiple Sleep Latency and Maintenance of Wakefulness Testing
The multiple sleep-latency test (MSLT) provides an objective measure of sleepiness compared with normal individuals lacking primary sleep disorders. The chief clinical indication for MSLT is for evaluation of narcolepsy and related primary CNS hypersomnias such as idiopathic hypersomnia and Kleine-Levin syndrome.

A MSLT is carried out during the daytime in a sleep laboratory following nocturnal PSG, with four or five nap opportunities at standard times and intervals, usually at 9:00 and 11:00 AM and 1:00, 3:00, and 5:00 PM. Careful inspection of each nap is subsequently performed to determine the timing of sleep onset relative to commencement of each nap, and whether REM sleep occurs during each nap. A mean sleep latency is then calculated from the average initial sleep latency from each nap. Mean sleep latencies shorter than 8 minutes are considered abnormal and indicative of pathologic excessive daytime sleepiness. Whether or not a sleep-onset REM period (a SOREM, i.e., reaching REM sleep within 15 minutes of sleep onset during a nap) is captured is also considered and tabulated. More than one SOREM is abnormal and is consistent with the diagnosis of narcolepsy.

There are several considerations prior to performing and interpreting a valid MSLT. Patients should be instructed to sleep well for at least 2 weeks preceding the study, to allow at least 6 to 7 hours per night (and when possible, extending time in bed to 8-9 hours), and many sleep specialists document the quantity of sleep before the test with actigraphy monitoring or a sleep diary to ensure adherence to this recommendation and exclude the contaminating influence of insufficient sleep quantity. If it is safe and practically possible to do so, patients should be instructed to taper or discontinue sedative, stimulant, or REM suppressant medications (i.e., opiate analgesics, antidepressants, or other psychotropic or CNS active drugs) with the oversight and permission of other relevant treating primary care, psychiatry, and pain physicians at least 2 weeks prior to MSLT, and certain psychotropic drugs such as fluoxetine (Prozac) with a long elimination half-life should be discontinued for at least a month prior to MSLT to avoid decrease in MSLT sensitivity for delay of REM latency. Patients should undergo a full-night diagnostic PSG the night before a MSLT study to ensure that there is not another primary sleep disorder, such as SDB or PLMD, that could provide an alternative reason for significant sleepiness and to ensure that sufficient sleep quantity of 6 hours or more is obtained.

While the MSLT is designed to assess sleepiness, the maintenance of wakefulness test (MWT) is used to assess the ability to remain awake. The MWT is most useful when an objective measure of the effectiveness of treatment for disorders causing hypersomnolence is needed. The patient is seated in a dim room in a comfortable, semi-reclined position and asked to remain alert but passive for four 40-minute periods that are 2 hours apart. EEG, EOG, and chin EMG are measured, and the signals are analyzed to detect any epochs of unequivocal sleep during each 40-minute period. Normal patients have a mean time to epochs of unequivocal sleep of 30.4 minutes; however, the data is not normally distributed, and 42% of all patients remain awake for the entire 40 minutes on all four opportunities. Since simulated and actual driving performance is compromised with sleep times of 19 minutes or less on MWT, this is a reasonable threshold for the distinction of clinically significant daytime sleepiness, and driving or other safety sensitive tasks should be curtailed when sleep latencies are 19 minutes or shorter.

Actigraphy Monitoring

Wrist actigraphy monitoring is utilized to provide a rigorous estimation of sleep quantity and its circadian pattern. The actigraphy monitor may be worn like a wristwatch and contains an accelerometer that detects movements, which are recorded over time periods lasting up to weeks. The magnitude and pattern of movements may be analyzed and modeled to infer the sleep-wake pattern and provides a graphic representation of the patient's sleep schedule. The test is used in the evaluation of suspected circadian rhythm disorders, to assess response to treatment of insomnia, and for investigating patients with hypersomnia prior to PSG and MSLT to more accurately document the adequacy of sleep prior to the assessment for sleepiness. Recent applications utilizing the accelerometer in smartphones and wrist-worn fitness devices show promise, but most have not been validated as diagnostic tools.

Diagnostic and Therapeutic Approach to Common Sleep Disorders

Insomnia

The insomnia disorders all share three basic components: repeated complaints of insomnia, which may involve difficulties falling asleep, staying asleep, poor sleep quality, or waking undesirably early; an adequate time and opportunity for sleep; and a complaint of resultant daytime impairment. Insomnia is the most common of sleep complaints: nearly 45% of people were affected intermittently within the past year in some large studies, and up to 15% suffer chronic insomnia disorders. Risks for insomnia include female sex, older age, and a psychiatric or medical comorbidity. Chronic insomnia should be distinguished from short-term insomnia, which may occur in anyone occasionally (e.g., the night before an important job interview, or during increased stress). Per the ICSD-3, the sleep disturbance and associated daytime symptoms have to occur at least three times a week for at least three months to meet criteria for chronic insomnia disorder (see Box 1). Insomnia may begin in childhood, continue throughout a patient's lifetime, and appear as a manifestation of neurologic hyperarousal, with demonstrable increases in cerebral metabolism via functional MRI and increases in beta and theta EEG activity as well as generalized increased metabolism and stress hormone production compared with normals in either wake or sleep states. To a lesser extent, these same markers for hyperarousability are seen in other causes of primary insomnia (see Box 1).

In the past, insomnia was classified into primary and secondary, with secondary insomnia being far more common. Secondary insomnia was thought to be a result or accompaniment of an underlying illness. This may be incorrect. For example, it has previously been thought that treatment of secondary insomnia ought to focus on treatment of the underlying disorder. Newer evidence indicates that this approach may be suboptimal for the following reasons: secondary insomnia does not reliably improve when the underlying disorder does; secondary insomnia in general responds to treatment directed at insomnia; and in some cases, the underlying disorder, such as depression, responds better to treatment when the insomnia is addressed directly and concurrently. Furthermore, in several illnesses, such as depression, insomnia may predate the depression by months, and insomnia is a risk factor for future development of many psychiatric illnesses. In addition, primary insomnia was further divided into subtypes of idiopathic insomnia, psychophysiologic (learned) insomnia and paradoxical insomnia (sleep state misperception). Secondary insomnia was also divided into various subtypes such as inadequate sleep hygiene, insomnia due to medical condition, mental disorder, drug or substance. However, it is rare to encounter patients who fit under one of these subtypes exclusively. Most patients with insomnia, primary and secondary, tend to have some diagnostic criteria listed under many of these subtypes. Thus, in the current ICSD-3 insomnia is no longer classified into primary and secondary insomnia and no distinction is made between various etiologic subtypes of primary and secondary insomnia.

Chronic insomnia may be preceded in predisposed individuals by precipitating factors such as illness or stress and may be propagated by behavioral or maladaptive cognitive factors. Some individuals do not appear to require precipitating or propagating factors to develop chronic insomnia and have underlying redisposition toward insomnia. They are prototypic for an underlying predisposition toward insomnia. These individuals manifest insomnia from infancy and persist despite optimization of sleep hygiene and habit. However, in most cases of insomnia, precipitating and/or propagating influences may be found through careful interview and help establish a secure diagnosis.

In these individuals, identifiable precipitating causes that may be traumatic, stressful periods or struggles, medical illness, drugs, or toxins. However, even when the cause is removed, a conditioned response built upon associated and at times maladaptive sleep-related behaviors ensues. Instead of beginning to relax for sleep under permissive circumstances, the affected patient experiences

TABLE 1	Therapeutic Tools for Treating Insomnia	
THERAPY TYPE	**SPECIFIC THERAPIES/COMPONENTS**	**GOALS**
Education/sleep hygiene	Improve knowledge about behaviors that foster or hinder healthy sleep	Improve opportunity and environment for sleep
Behavioral therapies	Stimulus control • Unmodified extinction • Graduated extinction • Positive routines/faded bedtime with response cost • Scheduled awakeningsSleep restriction	Dissociate anxiety or conditioned autonomic response from the process or location of going to sleep
	Relaxation training • Progressive muscle relaxation • Passive relaxation • Autogenic training-biofeedback • Imagery training • Meditation • HypnosisParadoxical intention	Increase pressure for sleep by decreasing the time allotted for sleep, increasing the probability of successful sleep attempts Reduce physiologic and/or cognitive arousal that hinders or disrupts sleep
		Reduce performance anxiety that confounds ability to successfully go to sleep
Cognitive therapies	Cognitive restructuring Decatastrophizing Reappraisal Attention shifting	Decrease unrealistic expectations about sleep, misconceptions, or misattributions regarding causes of insomnia, consequences of insomnia, ability to control sleep; produce a more appropriate and adaptive mind-set
Pharmacologic therapies	Hypnotics Sedating antidepressants Herbal supplements	Enhance sleepiness at appropriate times or to enhance convenience of sleep time and/or duration

paradoxical arousal as they approach their sleep conditions. The patient under the influence of the precipitating cause may have spent many hours worrying, uncomfortable, clock-watching, or otherwise raising their anxiety levels. Propagating factors include these same behaviors that help maintain sleeplessness once it has begun and may additionally include irregular sleep schedules and the use of drugs. Abuse of alcohol may contribute or be secondary to the sleep disturbance.

Effective treatment strategies for insomnia focus on removing any residual precipitating influences and mitigating or eliminating propagating influences. The main therapies for insomnia are sleep hygiene, behavioral therapies, cognitive therapies, and pharmacologic therapies. Patients often respond best to combined modalities. There is high-level evidence that combined cognitive/behavior therapies (CBT) are at least as effective as pharmacologic therapy for most patients with insomnia. CBT also appears to have enhanced rates of insomnia remission, so these approaches ought generally to be employed first. The addition of hypnotics to CBT has resulted in more rapid remission in some, but not all, studies. Growing recognition of the adverse effect profile of sedative-hypnotic drugs, particularly zolpidem (Ambien), which has been associated with heightened risks of falls and sleep walking, sleep eating, and related amnestic behaviors, has also encouraged a shift toward an earlier application of behavioral approaches to coping with insomnia.

In childhood, the most common causes of insomnia are behavioral. Insomnia may occur when parents fail to establish and enforce an appropriate nightly bedtime, so that their child may subsequently stall and refuse to go to bed in a timely fashion. In other cases, insomnia may occur when a child cannot fall asleep until a usual condition is present, such as being held, rocked, or fed. Appropriate advice and treatments include strict limit-setting for bedtime resistance; maintaining regular sleep schedules with avoidance of napping during the daytimes; and curtailing disrupting influences, such as television watching, gaming, and computer use. Suggesting a nightly cell phone or personal device (i.e., iPod, iPad, or Wii U) check-in procedure is especially helpful in teenage children, and caffeinated soda and excessively stimulating activities should be avoided during the evenings. Selected children benefit

from incentives such as a patient-parent contract that offers privileges for slightly later bedtimes on weekends after the child adheres regularly to a specified sleep schedule during school nights.

Four considerations for restoring normal sleep hygiene to discuss with all insomnia patients in the office include these three central concepts:
- Maintain a regular sleep schedule. Go to bed and arise at the same time each day. Ideally, the schedule should match the patient's biologic clock, with nocturnal sleep and bedtime/rise time matching their tendency for sleepiness and alertness (sleep education/hygiene).
- Avoid lying sleepless in bed. After 20 to 30 sleepless minutes spent trying to fall asleep, the patient should be instructed to leave the bedroom to pursue a quietly distracting activity, such as reading mundane material or watching a boring television program, and waiting until he or she feels sleepy enough to return to bed. Patients should explicitly avoid reading in bed, listening to the radio in bed, or watching television in bed if they are having difficulty initiating or maintaining sleep. This is a practical form of stimulus control (Table 1).
- Avoidance of clock-watching behavior. Patients should be instructed to remove clocks from their bedrooms or hide the clock face so as to make the insomnia period timeless and of uncertain duration. Falling asleep should not be a race against time, and repetitive checking of the time only serves to reinforce anxiety and further activate the mind (see stimulus control, Table 1). For the same reason, when watching television, discourage patients from watching news shows with scrolling tickertape newsflashes with clock time shown.
- Schedule thinking time earlier in the evening, well in advance of the sleep period. Patients who worry, plan, or think out their problems in bed should be encouraged to schedule a time earlier in the evening, well in advance of their normal bedtime, to attempt to work out these concerns prior to carrying them into bed. This "constructive worry" or "worry time" represents a practical form of cognitive and stimulus control therapy.

There are numerous other associated issues and behaviors that may be useful for application in selected patients, such as cutting down overall time in bed (sleep restriction), establishing a regular and relaxing bedtime routine (such as by taking a relaxing bath, listening to soothing music, or having a light snack before bed), avoiding daytime naps, avoiding caffeinated beverages after noontime, and establishing a regular morning exercise routine and avoiding evening exercise. It is important for the physician to avoid overloading the patient with too many considerations and tasks at once, however, as the burden of implementing these suggestions then becomes tantamount to too many obtrusive "swing thoughts" during a golf swing. One or two concepts to start with are sufficient, and once mastered and implemented, the patient can gradually phase in other ideas over time. Relaxation training and cognitive behavioral therapy can be very helpful in selected receptive patients who have failed the above typical self-help measures, and as a last resort, periodic or even scheduled chronic pharmacotherapy can also be implemented.

There are now several highly effective and tolerable hypnotic medications available for short-term, intermittent, and chronic use. The class of nonbenzodiazepine receptor agonists (the so-called "Z" drugs, or zolpidem [Ambien], zaleplon [Sonata], and eszopiclone [Lunesta]) are preferred by most sleep specialists but some of them remain costlier than the older generation choices, including the benzodiazepines—which have adverse effects on sleep architecture—as well as diphenhydramine (Benadryl) and trazodone (Desyrel),[1] which each have less specific sleep-promoting effects and more adverse effects and potential for drug-drug interactions, especially in elderly patients. The clinical pharmacology of the most commonly prescribed and most useful hypnotic medications are summarized in Table 2. A concern with each of these may be the potential for habituation of efficacy; fall risk; and the potential to cause sleepwalking, sleep eating, or other amnestic behaviors during sleep. If these adverse effects result, the hypnotic drug should be promptly discontinued with a shift toward the use of cognitive behavioral therapy strategies. In women, zolpidem should be used with particular caution given the slower metabolism of the drug, thereby promoting vulnerabilities to carryover sedation and unpleasant "hangover" type feelings or driving safety risks during the commute the next morning. Pharmacologic therapy of insomnia may be bolstered by the advent of suvorexant (Belsomra), a novel hypocretin antagonist that has a wake-suppressing rather than sleep-promoting mechanism of action. However, it should be noted that the higher doses that were primarily studied were determined as overly sedating and unsafe by the FDA and only the lower doses were approved. Further clinical experience will likely be necessary to establish the role of this medication as a treatment for insomnia.

Sleep-Disordered Breathing

Breathing during sleep is carefully regulated to maintain homeostasis of oxygen, carbon dioxide, and blood pH. The mechanisms and homeostatic set points for ventilation vary systematically between wake, non-REM sleep, and REM sleep. In wake, the resulting ventilatory pattern is governed by careful integration of classic feedback systems designed to keep blood pH at approximately 7.40, arterial $Paco_2$ at approximately 38 to 45 mm Hg, and Pao_2 greater than approximately 60 mm Hg with cortical influences that govern functions such as speaking, laughing, eating, singing, and other voluntary activities. During non-REM sleep, ventilation is considerably more rhythmic and is governed almost exclusively by the chemoresponsive feedback systems indicated above; during REM sleep, the chemoresponsive feedback system is further influenced by additional input from REM-influenced neurons, resulting in a less rhythmic and less-carefully regulated metabolic milieu.

Significant deviation from these norms is termed "sleep-disordered breathing" (SDB), and is marked by several distinct event types. Apneas are total or near-total cessations of airflow. Hypopneas are significant declines in tidal volume sufficient to result in significant reduction in oxygenation. Excess effort for

breathing may result in arousals from and disturbance of sleep, and are termed respiratory effort-related arousals (RERAs). These types of events are often related as a rate, either as the apnea-hypopnea index (AHI; apneas+hypopneas per hour of sleep), the respiratory disturbance index (apneas+hypopneas+RERAs per hour of sleep), or the REI (apneas+hypopneas per hour of recording when sleep is not measured directly). In addition to these types of SDB, the general baseline minute ventilation may fall to the point where sustained hypoventilation takes place during sleep, termed sleep-related alveolar hypoventilation.

Obstructive SDB: Snoring and OSA

The dynamic upper-airway obstruction, which occurs as a result of sleep in some persons, leads to a continuum of SDB varying from mild snoring to hypopneas to obstructive apneas. The likelihood and extent of upper-airway collapse is determined by the neural input into the dilating upper-airway muscles, influence of sleep state, and upper-airway anatomy. Obstructive events are more likely to occur in REM sleep when muscle tone is lowest, during transitions from lighter non-REM sleep to deep non-REM sleep when sleep is unstable, or when muscle tone is decreased by substances such as alcohol or drugs. The single biggest risk factor for snoring or OSA is obesity, wherein fatty deposition reduces upper-airway dimension, humoral factors reduce net dilating forces of the muscles, and the mechanical effects of obesity reduce lung volumes and the stabilizing effect of tracheal traction on the upper airway. Beyond obesity, many but not all patients have a predisposing anatomy of a narrowed oropharynx, such as a low-lying palate or redundant soft palate tissue, a thickened tongue base, or a narrow hypopharynx, although nasal anatomy with septal deviation or chronic congestion may also aggravate the problem.

Snoring without other symptoms, signs, or polysomnographic evidence of upper-airway obstructions such as hypersomnia, frequent associated arousals, or significant airflow limitation is termed primary snoring. While snoring may be a socially objectionable symptom or disruptive to the patient's sleep partner, snoring in isolation is otherwise not considered to be abnormal and such patients may be reassured if their bed partners are not bothered by their snoring. If treatment is desired, options include relieving nasal obstruction if present, commercially available lubricant throat sprays, mandibular positioning devices, and nasal or upper-airway surgical approaches such as nasal septal repair or uvulopalatopharyngoplasty (UPPP, or UP3 procedure). An otorhinolaryngology consultation may be helpful in determining which surgical approaches may be most beneficial for the individual.

OSA is an extremely common public health problem present in at least 2% to 4% of the general population and has been linked to development of hypertension and is a risk factor for incidental development of stroke, coronary artery disease, congestive heart failure, and atrial fibrillation. OSA has been shown to be associated with a wide variety of endothelial and metabolic abnormalities that favor vascular disease, and when patients with moderate to severe OSA are compared to normals or treated OSA patients, they appear to have a higher mortality and cardiovascular event frequency. Thus, the two main reasons to detect and treat OSA are to improve symptoms and to decrease cardiovascular risks. There are good data to show that treatment of OSA improves symptoms and quality of life. Data regarding the reversal of cardiovascular risk are not as firm, but most experts agree that at least moderate and severe OSA ought to be treated, regardless of symptom severity.

OSA severity is rated by the polysomnographic AHI, the hourly rate of apneas and hypopneas averaged over the total sleep time, or, in the case of HSAT, by the REI. An AHI of 4 per hour or less is considered normal. Mild OSA is diagnosed with an AHI of 5 to 14 per hour, moderate OSA with AHI of 15 to 29 per hour, and severe OSA with AHI being 30 per hour or higher. In most laboratories, correlation of the AHI with specific sleep stages and body positions is usually performed to determine whether

---

[1]Not FDA approved for this indication.

TABLE 2 Clinical Pharmacology of Hypnotic Medications

	MECHANISM OF ACTION	DOSAGE (MG)	DURATION OF ACTION ($T^{1/2}$)	TYPICAL ADVERSE EFFECTS	INTERACTIONS
Older Hypnotics					
Diphenhydramine (Benadryl)	H1	25–50	Intermediate (2.4–9.3 h)	Dry mouth, constipation, urinary retention	Nonsignificant
Trazodone (Desyrel)[1]	SRI	50–150	Short (3–6 h)	Dry mouth, dizziness, rash	CYP substrate; several others
Triazolam (Halcion)	BRA	0.125–0.5	Short (1.5–5.5 h)	Tolerance	CYP induction
Temazepam (Restoril)	BRA	7.5–30	Intermediate (8–18 h)	Tolerance	Nonsignificant
Melatonin[2]	MT1–MT2	1–3	Ultra-short (35–50 min)	Hangover type effect	None
Newer Hypnotics					
Zolpidem (Ambien)	NBRA	5, 10	Short (2–2.6 h)	Amnestic behavior	Numerous
Zaleplon (Sonata)	NBRA	5, 10	Short (1 h)	Headache, amnestic behavior	Several
Eszopiclone (Lunesta)	NBRA	1–3	Intermediate (6 h)	Headache, amnestic behavior, rash possible	Nonsignificant
Ramelteon (Rozerem)	MT1-MT2	8, 16[3]	Short (1–2.6 h)	Hyperprolacti nemia	Ketoconazole (Nizoral), rifampin
Doxepin (Silenor)	H1	3,6	Intermediate (12-15 h)	Dizziness, tachycardia	Nonsignificant
Suvorexant (Belsomra)	Orexin antagonist	10-20	Intermediate (12 h)	Headache, dizziness, abnormal dreams	CYP3A4 inducer

Abbreviations: $t^{1/2}$=half-life of drug; h=hours; H1=antihistaminergic H1 receptor blocker; SRI=serotonin reuptake inhibitor; BRA=benzodiazepine receptor agonist; CYP substrate=metabolized by cytochrome metabolism, susceptible to enzyme inhibition and elevated serum levels by multiple drugs; CYP induction=cytochrome enzyme inducer, may cause multiple potential drug-drug interactions via this mechanism; NBRA=nonbenzodiazepine benzodiazepine receptor agonist; MT1/MT2=melatonin type 1 and type 2 receptor agonist.

[1]Not FDA approved for this indication.
[2]Available as dietary supplement.
[3]Exceeds dosage recommended by the manufacturer.

positional therapy may be offered, as many patients have OSA only during the supine sleep position (position-dependent OSA), and some manifest OSA only during REM sleep in the supine position.

A form of OSA called the upper-airway resistance syndrome is defined by a clinical complaint of hypersomnia, often accompanied by snoring but without an abnormally high frequency of overt apneas or hypopneas resulting in significant decline in oxygen saturation. PSG confirms repetitive arousals related to the increased respiratory effort (respiratory effort-related arousals, or RERAs, during PSG) required to overcome upper-airway obstruction. Because of the similar pathogenesis and treatment response to relieve upper-airway obstruction, this is considered a variant of OSA.

Therapeutic options for snoring and sleep apnea include reducing nasal congestion or obstruction, positional therapy, nasal continuous positive airway pressure, oral appliances, the nasal expiratory positive airway pressure device, oral pressure therapy (OPT), or surgical management (Table 3). Patients with OSA have higher morbidity from vascular events and higher motor vehicle accident rates. Assessment and appropriate counseling for weight loss, cardiovascular risk factors, and driving while untreated (or extreme caution) should be part of a treatment plan.

Weight loss. Weight loss may reduce soft tissue in the neck, making the oropharynx less compressible. The improvement in lung volumes accompanied by weight loss also favor enhancement of longitudinal traction on the upper airway, the so-called "tracheal tug." About 30% to 40% of patients who are able to achieve substantial weight loss may become cured of their OSA. Careful follow-up is needed because many remissions are not permanent. Alcohol and other substances that reduce upper-airway tone or cause sedation or reduced responsiveness worsen OSA and should be prudently avoided.

Positional therapy. Among the lifestyle or behavioral changes, positional therapy involves employing one or more simple strategies to enforce sleep only in nonsupine body positions, usually on the side. One method is the "tennis ball in T-shirt" approach. The patient wears a snug-fitting T-shirt with a pocket sewn onto the back between the shoulder blades with two or three tennis or wiffle balls inserted into it to discourage the patient from turning onto the back during sleep. Other options include similar commercially marketed shirts or vests (the FDA-approved ZZoma sleep apnea pillow, the "snoring backpack," and similar strategies) and body pillows propped or wedged behind the patient or hugged by the patient. A correctional device for positional sleep apnea is also approved in the European Union. Unfortunately, shoulder or hip pain often limits the application of positional therapy, especially in elderly persons, and long-term adherence or compliance remains poor, with only about one-third of patients able to perpetuate positional therapy strategies in long-term follow-up. Patients with position-dependent OSA should be counseled to be cautious for development of severe OSA problems during any future anticipated prolonged periods of supine sleep, such as postoperative recovery periods following surgery or following a major injury.

Positive airway pressure. The mainstay of treatment for OSA for the majority of patients remains positive airway therapy (PAP). The main components of PAP appliances are the blower unit, which delivers calibrated pressures to hold open the airway; tubing to conduct the pressurized air to the patient; an interface such as a nasal or oronasal mask; and a harness to hold the mask firmly to the patient's face during use. Of the PAP therapies, continuous positive airway pressure (CPAP), which delivers a continuous set pressure between 5 and 20 cm H_2O, is usually first tried in the setting of PSG; in many sleep centers, the practice of performing split-night PSG (an initial diagnostic phase followed by a treatment phase of CPAP titration toward an optimal pressure for the individual patient) allows diagnosis and treatment prescription to occur in an efficient manner. If an optimal pressure cannot be determined by laboratory titration or data is not available to

TABLE 3 Treatment of Sleep-Related Breathing Disorders

SLEEP-RELATED BREATHING DISORDER	TREATMENT MODALITY		GOAL
OSA syndrome	Lifestyle/behavior modification	• Weight loss	Reduced weight may result in improvement airway patency
		• Alcohol avoidance	Alcohol worsens OSA; avoidance of exacerbating factor is encouraged
	Positive airway pressure	• Positional therapy	Enhance airway patency by nonsupine sleeping
		• Continuous positive airway pressure (CPAP)	Counteract collapsing forces in upper airway; "stent" open the upper airway
		• Bilevel positive airway pressure (BPAP)	End expiratory pressure stents open airway; inspiratory pressure enhances minute ventilation or decreases hypopneas
	Upper airway stimulation	Inspire™	Stimulation to upper airway muscles during sleep resulting in increased airway patency
		• Autotitrating positive airway pressure (APAP)	Uses feedback algorithms to adjust pressure in response to airway conditions in order to provide airway patency with minimal mean pressure
	Oral appliances	• Mandibular positioning devices • Tongue retention devices	Enhance airway patency by stabilizing lateral pharyngeal walls and enhancing AP airway dimensions at the velopharyngeal level
	Surgical modification of the upper airway	• Palatal surgeries (uvulopalatopharyngo plasty, others)	Enhance airway patency by reconfiguring soft tissues and/or skeletal structures
		• Maxillo-mandibular advancement	Enhance airway patency by reconfiguring soft tissues and skeletal structures
Central sleep apnea syndromes	Correct underlying disorders (treat heart failure, etc.)	• Various	Reduce stimuli to ventilatory hyperresponsiveness
	Gases	• Oxygen	Reduce responsiveness to variation in CO_2
	Positive airway pressure	• CPAP	Reduce stimulation to ventilate by decreasing lung water, improving V/Q matching, reducing airway resistance
		• Noninvasive positive pressure ventilation (NIPPV), also referred to as BPAP-ST (Avoid in heart failure patients with ejection fraction<45%)	Provide ventilatory assistance in order to avoid hypercapnia/hypoxemia associated with central apneas or hypopneas, thus reducing hyperventilatory feedback
		• Adaptive servoventilation (Avoid in heart failure patients with ejection fraction<45%)	Provide ventilatory assistance in proportion to needs, reducing or eliminating variability in ventilation and ventilatory drive; avoid hypercapnia/hypoxemia associated with central apneas or hypopneas, thus reducing hyperventilatory feedback.
Hypoventilation syndromes	Positive airway pressure	• Noninvasive positive pressure ventilation (NIPPV), also referred to as BPAP-ST	Provide ventilatory assistance in order to avoid hypercapnia/hypoxemia associated with central apneas or hypopneas
		• Tracheostomy with mechanical ventilation	Provide ventilatory assistance in order to avoid hypercapnia/hypoxemia associated with central apneas or hypopneas, protect or control airway

guide prescription of a specific pressure for a patient, application of an autotitrating PAP device may be considered, offering flexibility for delivering a relatively wide range of self-adjusting treatment pressures as the patient changes sleep position and enters different sleep stages through the night with accordingly varying apnea severity. Autotitrating PAP has been found to be efficacious in most patients diagnosed with OSA by HSAT. However, close clinical follow-up is needed in all patients who have recently started PAP.

PAP is typically delivered through an interface chosen as most comfortable by the patient, either a nasal mask, nasal pillows, or an oronasal. Nasal pillows, a type of cannula that provides a tight seal within the nares, and a newer tube-like frame that sits in front of and not within the nares are most effective at lower treatment pressures; they may be favored by many patients with claustrophobia but may dislodge at higher pressures or with frequent nocturnal movement. Nasal masks of various types are used in many patients, but if mouth breathing and consequent leak are a problem, a chin strap may be added, or an oronasal face mask may be substituted. Many newer PAP machines offer the feature

of pressure relief during exhalation, which may enhance patient tolerability at higher level PAP pressures by "giving way" as the patient expires. Bilevel positive airway pressure (BPAP) may also be employed at higher treatment pressures if CPAP is not well tolerated. Setting a pressure delta ≥4 cm between the inspired and expired pressure may also add a degree of positive pressure ventilation for patients with concurrent sleep-related hypoventilation from an intrinsic pulmonary disease or neuromuscular respiratory muscle weakness.

Oral appliances. Oral appliances may be fitted by a dental sleep specialist. They provide a means of advancing the mandible that pull the tongue base forward slightly, opening the oropharyngeal airway to some degree and obviating some apnea and hypopnea events. The device is most effective for mild to moderate severity and supine position-dependent OSA and generally less predictably effective for most cases of severe OSA. However, the use of oral appliances is increasing due to greater availability of competent dental professionals working with the devices, awareness that for some patients adherence is better with OAs than PAP, and improvements in appliance design that allow enhanced efficacy in some instances. Because oral appliances are less reliably effective in controlling SDB, repeat testing—either with out-of-center sleep testing or PSG after maximal adjustment—is needed to confirm efficacy.

Nasal valve appliances. An expiratory nasal resistance valve appliance (Provent) was approved by the FDA for treatment of OSA. The device may be an alternative for some patients with OSA who fail to tolerate CPAP therapy. The device is a small, disposable oval appliance that is affixed over each of the patient's nares by self-adhesive with an airflow port that offers resistance to expiratory airflow, thereby producing expiratory positive airway pressure and preserving nasal and oropharyngeal airway patency with minimal impedance to inspiratory airflow. The device was proven to significantly reduce polysomnographic AHI and subjective sleepiness on the ESS in a sham-controlled randomized trial. Because they are disposable, a new device must be affixed each night. Appropriate patient characteristics and long-term results are not yet clear, but these may be considered in patients who do not prefer CPAP or oral appliances and are agreeable to follow-up to ensure efficacy.

Oral pressure therapy. A newer option for treatment of mild to moderate OSA is OPT (Winx), which combines an oral appliance with negative intraoral pressure to help keep the tongue and soft palate in a more anterior position, enlarging the retrolingual and retropalatal space. There is as yet limited experience with the device; however, this may be an option for some patients who are averse to or intolerant of other therapies.

Surgery. Surgical modifications of the upper airway are principally of two basic approaches, palatal approaches, tongue-based procedures (genioglossus advancement, hyoid myotomy and suspension, lingualplasty), or maxillomandibular advancement (MMA). Palatal approaches such as UPPP, or "UP3" performed by otorhinolaryngologists are effective for relief of snoring but mostly ineffective for treatment of OSA, especially if severity is moderate or greater in degree. MMA appears to be quite effective in mild to moderate OSA and can even be applied with good effect even in selected severe OSA cases; however, morbidity from perioperative pain is considerable and long-term outcomes remain unclear. A hypoglossal nerve stimulation implant (Inspire) is a novel surgical treatment for PAP-intolerant patients. A recently published randomized controlled trial demonstrated efficacy and reasonable tolerability; however, this device was only recently FDA approved and there is limited clinical experience with it, thus, its future role and scope of use in OSA management remains to be determined.

Central Sleep Apnea Syndrome

Central sleep apnea syndrome results from an unstable ventilatory drive during sleep, resulting in periods of insufficient ventilation and compromise of gas exchange despite a patent oropharyngeal airway. Clinically, patients may share similar symptoms with those with OSA, including snoring, except patients with central sleep apnea more frequently complain of insomnia than hypersomnia. Central sleep apnea has a heterogeneous pathophysiology and may be idiopathic or due to high-altitude-induced periodic breathing, due to Cheyne-Stokes breathing, or narcotic-induced. Neurologic causes—such as brainstem infarction or neurodegenerative disorders, including multiple system atrophy—may also cause central apnea. In heart failure, the presence of central sleep apnea syndrome or Cheyne-Stokes breathing imparts a poor prognosis. A high-quality clinical trial showed that on average, CPAP did not reduce mortality. However, central sleep apnea is often at least partially resistant to treatment with conventional nasal CPAP therapy, and while CPAP may effect improved mean oxygenation, frequent arousals that fragment sleep often continue. However, a recent large multicenter randomized control trial, the SERVE-HF study, showed elevated all-cause and cardiovascular mortality risk in patients with central sleep apnea and symptomatic heart failure with an estimated ejection fraction of ≤45% who were randomized to ASV. Therefore, use of ASV in this patient population is not advised at the current time.

Treatment-Emergent Central Sleep Apnea Syndrome

Treatment-emergent central sleep apnea syndrome is a subtype of central sleep apnea wherein patients have significant obstructive/anatomical problems with ventilation, but also have unstable ventilatory patterns noted in patients with central sleep apnea syndromes. These patients have a clinical and PSG presentation of OSA, but once the upper airway is opened with CPAP, they experience frequent central apneic events that may or may not later resolve with continued exposure to PAP in the home setting. Some patients clearly continue to manifest frequent central sleep apneic events more than five times per hour, leading to the suboptimal outcomes of persisting clinical complaints of hypersomnia and medical risk. Treatment-emergent central sleep apnea syndrome may occur in as many as 4% to 15% of those with OSA. There is emerging evidence that alternative modes of PAP—particularly ASV—may be superior to conventional CPAP for treatment of treatment-emergent central sleep apnea syndrome. A randomized controlled trial recently showed that ASV more reliably relieves SDB, while CPAP fails to control SDB in up to one-third of cases. However, there is also evidence to suggest that treatment-emergent central sleep apnea resolves over time in a substantial number of patients who continue to remain on CPAP therapy.

Sleep-Related Hypoventilation

The causes of hypoventilation during sleep include primary pulmonary parenchymal disorders, neuromuscular conditions affecting bellows musculature, or restrictive physiology of the chest wall accompanying kyphoscoliotic disorders or morbid obesity. While each of these disorders may also ultimately cause daytime hypoventilation, sleep recumbency, especially supine sleep positioning, and REM sleep stage (which leads to relative paralysis of the chest wall and sole dependency on diaphragmatic excursion to drive respiratory effort) often lead to exclusive or initial sleep-related hypoventilation with subsequent medical risk consequent to suboptimal nocturnal oxygenation. Failure to treat significant nocturnal hypoventilation may result in the development of sequelae of hypoxemia such as polycythemia, pulmonary hypertension, and right heart failure, or of hypercapnic respiratory failure. Treatment most often involves use of NIPPV (see Table 4). A newer modality of positive pressure ventilation, volume-assured pressure support ventilation (AVAPS™), consists of a short delivery of a provider-set tidal volume, which, when coupled with a set backup respiratory rate, assures delivery of a minimum minute ventilation, even when changes in the patient's muscular strength or ventilatory load change. These therapies are best titrated in the context of a supervised overnight laboratory polysomnogram under the direction of a sleep or pulmonary medicine specialist. One must be careful not to resort to the potentially dangerous solution of added oxygen therapy alone in severe COPD or neuromuscular etiologies of sleep-related hypoventilation, because as ventilation fails and hypercapnea results, the hypoxic drive to breathe may become the chief factor leading to continued ventilatory effort and oxygen in this context may precipitate acute respiratory failure in some individuals. A morning arterial blood gas on room air following PSG is indicated to assess for potential hypercapnia and assess the impact of ventilatory support. In the context of severe hypercapnia (i.e., PCO_2 of 55 or greater), serial arterial blood gases to monitor the effects of ventilatory support, oxygenation, and accumulating hypercapnia may help determine whether nocturnal mechanical ventilatory support is indicated.

Narcolepsy and Central Disorders of Hypersomnolence

Narcolepsy is the prototypical central disorder of hypersomnolence. Narcolepsy is categorized further as Narcolepsy Type I (previously called narcolepsy with cataplexy) and Narcolepsy Type II (previously called narcolepsy without cataplexy). Cataplexy is a distinctive and highly specific symptom characterized by emotionally provoked muscle atonia intruding into wakefulness that is seen in a minority of patients overall and may precede but more often follows onset of the main symptom of hypersomnia.

TABLE 4 Clinical Pharmacology of Stimulant and Wake-Promoting Medications

	MECHANISM OF ACTION	DOSAGE (MG)	DURATION OF ACTION ($T\frac{1}{2}$)	TYPICAL ADVERSE EFFECTS	INTERACTIONS
Modafinil (Provigil)	Unknown	100–600[3]	Intermediate (15 h)	Tremor, jitteriness, palpitations, hypertension	Oral contraceptives
Armodafinil (Nuvigil)	Unknown	150–450[3]	Intermediate (15 h)	Tremor, jitteriness, palpitations, hypertension	Oral contraceptives
Methylphenidate (Ritalin)	DNRI	15–100[3]	Short (2–4 h)	Tremor, jitteriness, palpitations, hypertension	Nonsignificant
Methylphenidate SR (Concerta)[1]	DNRI	18–72	Intermediate (3.5 h)	Tremor, jitteriness, palpitations, hypertension	Nonsignificant
Amphetamine/ dextroamphetamine (Adderall)	DNRI	15–100[3]	Intermediate (10–13 h)	Tremor, jitteriness, palpitations, hypertension, QTc prolongation	Beware MAOIs, SSRIs, SNRIs, TCAs, bupropion (Wellbutrin)
Dextroamphetamine (Dexedrine)	DNRI	15–100[3]	Long (10–28 h)	Tremor, jitteriness, palpitations, hypertension, QTc prolongation	Beware MAOIs, SSRIs, SNRIs, TCAs, bupropion
Lisdexamfetamine (Vyvanse)[1]	DNRI	20–100[3]	Short (<1 h as prodrug) (10–28 h as dextroamphetamine)	Tremor, jitteriness, palpitations, hypertension, QTc prolongation	Beware MAOIs, SSRIs, SNRIs, TCAs, bupropion
Methamphetamine (Desoxyn)[1]	DNRI	15–100[3]	Intermediate (9–15 h)	Tremor, jitteriness, palpitations, hypertension, QTc prolongation	Beware MAOIs, SSRIs, SNRIs, TCAs, bupropion

[1]Not FDA approved for this indication.
[3]Exceeds dosage recommended by the manufacturer.
Abbreviations: $t\frac{1}{2}$=half-life of drug; h=hours; DNRI=dopamine and norepinephrine monoamine reuptake inhibitor; QTc=corrected QT interval; MAOI=monoamine oxidase inhibitor; SSRI=serotonin selective reuptake inhibitor; SNRI=selective norepinephrine reuptake inhibitor; TCA=tricyclic antidepressant (the potential interaction with all these agents is largely theoretical concern for potentiation of serotonin syndrome).

In the absence of cataplexy, a diagnosis of Narcolepsy Type I may also be made if cerebrospinal fluid (CSF) hypocretin-1 concentration, measured by immunoreactivity, is <110 pg/mL or <1/3 of mean values obtained in normal subjects with the same standardized assay. In Narcolepsy Type II, there is no cataplexy, and the CSF hypocretin level does not meet the above criteria or has not been measured. In addition to sleepiness and cataplexy, the full clinical pentad of narcolepsy also includes symptoms of sleep paralysis (the inability to move the body upon awakening), hypnogogic hallucinations (the intrusion of dream imagery and mentation into conscious awareness following awakening), and sleep-maintenance insomnia (with frequent nocturnal arousals and difficulty maintaining sleep). However, narcolepsy is most frequently monosymptomatic, with the sole symptom being pervasive, enduring sleepiness and decreased vigilance with a tendency toward dozing off inadvertently in permissive settings and the overwhelming desire to nap during the daytime, especially in the afternoons. Naps are most often highly refreshing; scheduled naps can be utilized to therapeutic advantage or indeed, in rare patients, as the sole treatment for those bent on avoiding stimulant pharmacotherapy. Narcolepsy is relatively uncommon, affecting approximately 1:2000 of the general population. While the etiology of narcolepsy remains unknown, most experts continue to favor a long hypothesized autoimmune cause. Major advances in the understanding of the neurobiology of narcolepsy over the past two decades have included the clear linkage of the HLA DQB1*0602 haplotype in up to 90% patients having narcolepsy with cataplexy, discovery of wake-promoting hypocretin/ orexin peptides produced by the perifornical posterolateral hypothalamus, and low to unmeasurable CSF hypocretin in nearly 90% of narcolepsy with cataplexy patients. Within the last few years, epidemic narcolepsy-cataplexy following H1N1 vaccination in Europe and Asia also provided further support for the autoimmune hypothesis of narcolepsy. Unfortunately, these tantalizing discoveries have not yet yielded clear insight into pathogenic mechanisms nor more specific therapies for patients, and the mainstay of treatment for the condition remains the use of older stimulant and wake-promoting medications, or prescribed therapeutic napping, as naps are most often highly refreshing and restorative in narcolepsy patients. Supportive laboratory evidence for narcolepsy includes a relatively normal polysomnogram to exclude other causes of hypersomnia such as OSA or PLMD, followed by a confirmatory MSLT, which demonstrates mean sleep latency shorter than 8 minutes and two or more sleep-onset REM periods during four or five nap opportunities.

Idiopathic hypersomnia is a closely related condition often difficult to distinguish from narcolepsy without cataplexy, although a few nuanced clinical features tend to distinguish it from narcolepsy, chiefly a characteristically reported unrefreshing nocturnal sleep and nap quality. Idiopathic hypersomnia has previously been further subclassified as variants with or without prolonged sleep period, although these phenotypes are overlapping and current diagnostic standards have eliminated this distinction. Other similar enigmatic and poorly understood primary CNS hypersomnias include posttraumatic hypersomnia when there is a history of temporally related antecedent substantial head injury, and recurrent hypersomnia, also known as the Kleine-Levin syndrome, which in addition to hypersomnia includes other neuropsychiatric sequelae such as cognitive and behavioral changes like hypersexuality and hyperphagia. Hypersomnia is also commonly associated with as many as 50% of those with myotonic dystrophy type 1.

The mainstay of treatment for each of these conditions is stimulant and wake-promoting agent therapy, with the goal of improved vigilance and psychomotor functioning. Stimulants and wake-promoting agents range in intensity from lower to higher intensity and efficacy/tolerability options, from modafinil (Provigil) and armodafinil (Nuvigil) on the milder end of the spectrum—although selected narcolepsy patients respond quite well to these drugs—to methylphenidate (Ritalin), and to the amphetamine/dextroamphetamine (Adderall). Relevant clinical pharmacology of the stimulant medications commonly used in clinical practice are summarized in Table 4. Pitolisant (Wakix), a selective

H3 subtype histamine inverse agonist/antagonist proven effective as a wake promoting agent for narcolepsy, recently received European Medicines Agency marketing authorization but is currently unavailable in the United States. Patients with uncontrolled hypersomnias should be cautioned against driving, operating dangerous machinery, or engaging in other similarly dangerous activities or hobbies while they are drowsy, as they may be prone to sudden and unpredictable sleep attacks. Sodium oxybate (gamma hydroxy butyrate) is an FDA approved tightly controlled substance for the treatment of sleepiness and cataplexy in patients with narcolepsy. Sodium oxybate (Xyrem) is usually given in two divided doses, before bedtime and in the middle of the night; it can be dangerous in the setting of uncontrolled OSA or respiratory conditions and central nervous system depressants. Other REM suppressing medications such as tricyclic antidepressants, SSRIs and SNRIs are also used in the treatment of cataplexy.

Circadian Rhythm Sleep Wake Disorders

Circadian rhythm sleep disorders result in misalignment of the timing of the sleep period relative to the desired bed and rise times, resulting in concurrent insomnia and hypersomnia symptoms despite normal total sleep time. The most common circadian rhythm disturbances are actually exogenous influences on the patient and his/her circadian axis, which in these cases is functioning normally but is unable to adjust rapidly enough to the required new temporal milieu. These exogenous disorders include jet lag disorder and shift work disorder, resulting either from imposed transmeridian travel or alternating work shifts, respectively, that disturb the patient's environmental entraining cues and homeostatic drives for sleep and wakefulness, thereby resulting in misalignment of the patient's endogenous biological sleep drive and typical sleep schedule to the clock time and environment to which they must rapidly adapt.

Jet lag disorder results when an individual crosses across several transmeridian time zones in a single day. Crossing one or two time zones is usually not too difficult for the traveler to accommodate, but crossing three time zones typically causes symptoms of jet lag. Flying eastward is generally much more difficult than flying westward, as patients more easily accommodate phase delay then phase advancing, or "loss" of time. Treatments for jet lag syndrome usually involve efforts to rapidly reentrain the patient to the new environment, and protocols for advance preparation including setting back (for eastward travel) or setting ahead (for planned westward travel) one's daily routine 2 to 3 weeks prior to the trip so that the traveler is already partially reset in his or her circadian routine before departing. Also critical is attempting to rapidly adapt to the new time zone, such as by seeking regular sunlight exposure during the daytime and avoiding light exposure in the evening. Brief use of a hypnotic medication and regular daily doses of melatonin[7] 0.5 to 5.0 mg at bedtime for the first few nights after arrival can help reset the sleep schedule in the new time zone.

Shift-work sleep disorder results from workers who must constantly and regularly alter or rotate their work schedules between different shifts (so-called "swing shifts") or workers who must accommodate a regularly scheduled second or third shift (i.e., shifts other than a day shift). Shift workers often have difficulty adapting and shifting their sleep-wake schedules and develop symptoms of insomnia or hypersomnia. Shift workers must be educated to prioritize regularly obtaining a sufficient quantity of sleep, regardless of their work circumstances. Swing shift workers should also be counseled to avoid working more than five night shifts in a row, as night shift work frequently leads to a greater degree of sleep deprivation over time. Shift workers should also be counseled to avoid rotating swing shifts whenever possible, to strictly avoid scheduling overtime duty, and to avoid long commutes (and to exercise special caution to avoid drowsy driving). Judicious use of caffeinated beverages, or prescribed stimulant therapy with modafinil may be helpful for enhancing vigilance in some patients, but should be used with caution as they might interfere with sleep initiation.

[7]Available as a dietary supplement.

The two most common endogenous circadian disorders are delayed sleep-wake phase disorder (DSWPD) and advanced sleep-wake phase disorder (ASWPD), disorders that are most prevalent in opposite extremes of life. DSWPD is seen most often in adolescents and young adults who are biological night owls in their circadian preference, preferring a delayed bedtime and rise time (i.e., bedtimes well past midnight and subsequent arising times in the late morning or early afternoon). DSWPD patients have an extreme and enduring form of this tendency, however, resulting in persisting misalignment of the patient to societal norms. Adolescent and young adult patients present with profound intractable initial insomnia due to their inability to fall asleep at a conventional bedtime as required for school or most daytime occupations, and profound daytime hypersomnia due to their inability to arise and function in the morning hours. Diagnosis is easily recognized by clinical history and sleep diaries, with or without adjunctive actigraphy to objectively verify the pattern of consistent delayed sleep-phase periods. Contrarily, ASWPD is more common in elderly individuals who are biological larks (i.e., preferring an early bedtime and early rise time by nature). However, the ASWPD elderly are unable to stay awake for desired evening activities (often even unable to go out to dinner with friends), and awaken undesirably early in the morning with a consequent inability to fall back asleep in early morning hours. The presentation can mimic depression, whose hallmark biological sign is often noted to be an early morning awakening; care should be taken to carefully distinguish between these two diagnoses. Treatment of each is difficult; options include specifically timed bright light therapy, with or without light restriction, and timed administration of low dose melatonin. The time of administration differs for the two disorders, and is determined by the patient's own endogenous dim light melatonin onset and arise time, and the phase response curve for light and melatonin administration. Bright light therapy is administered at approximately 2500 lx intensity for at least 30 minutes. The timing of bright light administration is first thing in the morning after arising in DSWPD, where a phase-advancing influence is desired; for ASWPD patients, bright light is prescribed in the late afternoon and early evening hours where it will have a phase-delaying effect. Weeks to a few months of regular therapy are necessary to achieve effect. Adherence is difficult and compliance unable to be verified. Specifically timed melatonin usually given at very low doses for this indication (contrary to its use in higher supraphysiologic doses as a hypnotic agent by many patients in other contexts of insomnia, or its high-dose use in REM sleep behavior disorder [RBD]) may also be administered, but its dose and timing are complicated; it must be given in accordance with the circadian phase response curve to have optimal effects and to avoid complicating the problem. For most patients with DSWPD, immediate release melatonin 0.5 mg should be administered at approximately 1 hour before desired bedtime; in ASWPD, melatonin would instead be given prior to the time point of 8 hours following the patient's usual rise time (so as to have a phase-delaying effect). Adjunctive light restriction is recommended in the late afternoon and evenings for DSWPD to avoid precipitating additional phase delays—such as the avoidance of working with luminescent computer screens or viewing video media from close distance in the late evenings—and some experts advocate the use of commercially available blue light restricting glasses as biologically reasonable, as blue light stimuli in evening hours may exacerbate phase delay and confound other recommended treatment effects. However, the efficacy of blue light restriction currently lacks explicit evidence from large clinical trials. As a last resort, the measure of chronotherapy, a progressive delay of bedtime every few days, is prescribed, with the bed and rise times being progressively and successively delayed until the desired bed and rise times are achieved. Attempts to then entrain the patient on this schedule with the aforementioned measures are again attempted with scheduled bright light and prescribed timed melatonin dosing. This is a lengthier process for DSWPD patients and necessitates work restriction during the approximate 2-week time frame necessary to achieve a turnaround of the desired patient's sleep/wake schedule.

Parasomnias and Other Nocturnal Events

Parasomnias are nocturnal events that disrupt sleep but usually do not appreciably disturb sleep quality. As such, nocturnal events do not typically present with symptoms of insomnia or hypersomnia unless there are other comorbid primary sleep disorders such as OSA, which is a frequent comorbidity presenting along with the parasomnias, especially in adult patients.

Parasomnias may arise from either NREM or REM sleep. The NREM parasomnias are essentially all variations on the theme of disorders of arousal, where the behavioral sleep state lingers into awakening, leaving arousal from sleep incomplete. Consequent clinical manifestations are surprisingly heterogeneous and often age related, with specific syndromes such as sleep terrors (also called night terrors) in children, sleep walking and confusional arousals seen in children and adults, and sleep-related eating behavior seen almost exclusively in adults, especially those receiving zolpidem or other newer prescribed hypnotics. NREM disorders of arousal are especially common in children in the first decade of life and are regarded as a relatively normal variant (and perhaps in some cases simply representing an exaggerated manifestation of the physiological difficulty in arousing from the characteristically deeper N3 NREM sleep inherent in the developing brain). As such, pediatric parasomnias are frequently outgrown; however, in some patients, they do endure throughout life. In adult patients who present with newly evolved nocturnal events proven to be NREM disorders of arousal, one should be highly suspicious of comorbid primary sleep disorders that provoke arousing events, such as SDB or PLMD.

REM parasomnias include nightmares and RBD. Nightmares are undesirable, disturbing dreams that lead to sudden arousal from sleep with heightened autonomic sequelae of sweating, hypervigilance, tachycardia, and tachypnea. Nightmares and vivid dreaming are present in between 10% and 50% of normal young children and in about 50% of adults, but become abnormally disturbing in content or frequency much less frequently, and the true prevalence of nightmare disorder remains unknown. Patients who present with a chief complaint of frequent nightmares should be reassured as to their biological nature and receive a detailed physical and neurologic history and examination to exclude potential provoking comorbid causes such as a recent medication change in type or dosage, mood or anxiety disorder, or primary sleep disorder such as SDB. If no certain readily reversible triggering cause may be identified, referral for consideration of hypnosis, behavior treatment in the form of imagery rehearsal therapy, or pharmacotherapy with clonazepam (Klonopin)[1] may be helpful in some cases. Nightmares that involve flashbacks of previous traumatic events, most often also with similar daytime flashbacks, suggest the alternative diagnosis of posttraumatic stress disorder (PTSD) and the need for psychiatric evaluation. Recent evidence has suggested that alpha-blocking medications such as prazosin (Minipress)[1] or terazosin (Hytrin)[1] may be helpful in suppressing nightmares associated with PTSD.

RBD is characterized by potentially injurious dream enactment behaviors that mirror frightening dream content (characteristically involving fighting off attackers or defending oneself against assailants). In RBD, bed partners will describe objective witnessed dream enactment manifested by violent limb thrashing movements such as punching or kicking and screaming or shouting vocalization during sleep. While RBD patients rarely leave the bed and sleepwalk, falls or other injurious behavior to self or the bed partner are frequent. Importantly, RBD is strongly associated with future development of neurodegenerative disorders. Elderly patients newly diagnosed with RBD harbor up to an 91.9% risk of developing Parkinsonism within 15–25 years of symptom onset, with a shorter-term risk of 30% to 50%, so that all patients with RBD require serial neurologic examinations and follow-up. RBD in young adults may, however, be caused by antidepressant medications, especially the SSRIs, and removal of the offending drug may lead to resolution of dream enactment in some cases. Diagnosis of RBD is by clinical history as well as confirmatory evidence for increased REM sleep muscle tone evident on polysomnographic electromyogram (EMG) leads in the chin and limbs (known as REM sleep without atonia). Treatment options include melatonin, initially at doses of 3 to 6 mg and gradually titrating toward 12 mg nightly as needed to suppress witnessed injurious behaviors, or clonazepam (Klonopin)[1] 0.5 to 1.0 mg increased to 2 to 3 mg nightly. Great care should be taken to first exclude comorbid OSA prior to use of clonazepam, a potential respiratory and upper-airway suppressant.

Nocturnal epilepsies or psychogenic nonepileptic spells may also arise from sleep or apparent sleep and are additional diagnostic considerations in the differential diagnosis of parasomnias. A high degree of stereotypy (one attack being essentially identical to the next) with multiple attacks within a single night are features suggestive of organic partial extratemporal (frontal lobe) epilepsy, even in the absence of EEG changes between or during an episode. In children, benign rolandic epilepsy may lead to stereotyped episodes of facial twitching and drooling, with or without secondary generalized tonic clonic seizures. Children or adults with autosomal dominant nocturnal frontal lobe epilepsy (ADNFLE) may present with bizarre brief motor behavior (typically of 10- to 60-second duration) without postictal sleepiness. ADNFLE has recently been mapped in several kindreds as a channelopathy, producing a defect of the neuronal nicotinic acetylcholine receptor. Psychogenic nonepileptic spells are instead characterized by nonstereotypic and often prolonged attacks that arise from a behavior state of apparent sleep that is instead confirmed during video-EEG PSG to represent normal waking EEG background. Distinguishing features for the differential diagnosis of nocturnal events are shown in Table 5.

Sleep-Related Movement Disorders

Sleep-related movement disorders include restless legs syndrome (RLS), periodic limb movement disorder (PLMD), leg cramps, bruxism, rhythmic movement disorder, and others.

RLS and PLMS

Diagnosis of RLS is based completely on a clinical history and typically requires four central elements of the described symptoms: an uncomfortable urge to move the legs, with or without uncomfortable leg sensations; temporary relief by movement; symptoms occurring solely or predominantly at rest; and nocturnal worsening of symptoms. About 50% of patients with RLS will carry a positive family history of the disorder, but positive family history is not necessary for the diagnosis. The nature of the symptoms as described by the patient may be quite variable with regard to the symptom quality, location or distribution, temporal occurrence, frequency, and severity. RLS symptoms are usually described as uncomfortable, although not really painful, with a sense of a creepy-crawly or prickling discomfort, often below the knees and centered about the shins or calves, but sometimes more proximally in the thighs, or even isolated to the feet and ankles. Symptoms may occur in the arms as well, especially proximally near the shoulders. Augmentation is common, occurring in about 50% of patients treated with dopaminergic drugs and involves a worsening of the symptoms: symptom onset occurs earlier during the day, becomes more intense, and spreads up to the arms. RLS has been linked to deficient iron stores and dopaminergic neurotransmission in the brain and is more common in patients with parkinsonism, multiple sclerosis, epilepsy, and in those with chronic renal insufficiency.

While periodic limb movements of sleep (PLMS) are seen in 80% to 90% of RLS patients, PLMS are not necessary for the diagnosis of RLS. Furthermore, PLMS are also extremely frequent in the general population, seen in 5% to 15% of younger adults and as many as 45% of elderly individuals. PLMD is diagnosed when PLMS is thought to cause daytime hypersomnia in the absence of other sleep disorders.

Nonpharmacologic treatments including warm or cool baths, massage, stretching, or even the application of spontaneous compression devices have been reported to be effective anecdotally and

---

[1]Not FDA approved for this indication.

TABLE 5 Distinguishing Features of Nocturnal Events

	PREMONITORY SYMPTOMS	BEHAVIORAL CHARACTERISTICS	DURATION	FREQUENCY	EEG/PSG FINDINGS
NREM Parasomnias					
Night terrors	None	Inconsolable screaming	Minutes	1 or less nightly	Arousal from N2-N3
Confusional arousals	None	Confused, amnestic	Seconds to minutes	1 or less nightly	Arousal from N3>N2
Sleepwalking	None	Ambulation, amnesia	Minutes	1 or less nightly	Arousal from N3 » N2
REM Parasomnias					
Nightmares	Dream recall	Arousal, frightened, palpitations	Seconds	Generally 1/nightly	Arousal from REM
RBD	Variable dream recall	Thrashing, complex motor behavior	Seconds to minutes	>1/night, second>first half	REM sleep without atonia
Epilepsies					
BECTS	Facial twitching, hypersalivation	Focal motor or GTC, postictal	Seconds to minutes	>1/night	Arousal from NREM, IEDs EEG pattern
ADNFLE	Bizarre stereotyped motor behavior	Focal motor, bizarre motor	Seconds, < 1 min	1 or multiple attacks/night	Arousal from N2
TLE	Aura variable	CPS, postictal	1–2 min	1 or multiple attacks/night	Arousal from N2
Psychogenic spells	Variable	Variable	often>5 min	1 or multiple attacks/night	Normal awake EEG

Abbreviations: NREM=nonrapid eye movement sleep; N2=stage 2 NREM sleep; N3=stage 3 NREM sleep; REM=rapid eye movement sleep; IEDs=interictal epileptiform discharges; EEG=electroencephalogram; PSG=polysomnogram; BECTs=benign epilepsy of childhood with centro-temporal spikes; ADNFLE=autosomal dominant nocturnal frontal lobe epilepsy; TLE=temporal lobe epilepsy; RBD=REM sleep behavior disorder.

TABLE 6 Clinical Pharmacology of Treatments for Restless Leg Syndrome

	MECHANISM OF ACTION	DOSAGE	TYPICAL ADVERSE EFFECTS	INTERACTIONS
Iron Replacement				
Ferrous sulfate1	Fe	324 mg, 1 tab every alternate day	Nausea, constipation	None
Ferrous fumarate+vit C1	Fe	200/125 mg, 1 tab every alternate day	Nausea, constipation	None
Carbidopa-Levodopa (Sinemet)1	DA	25/100 1–2 prn	Nausea, dizziness, ICD	None
Pramipexole (Mirapex)	DA	0.125–1.0 mg^2 qhs	Nausea, dizziness, ICD	None
Ropinirole (Requip)	DA	1–6 mg^2 qhs	Nausea, dizziness, ICD	None
Rotigotine (Neupro Transdermal Patch)	DA	1–3 mg qam	Nausea, dizziness, ICD	None
Gabapentin (Neurontin)1	Unknown	300–1200^2 mg qhs	Nausea, dizziness, pedal edema, weight gain	None
Gabapentin Enacarbil (Horizant)	Unknown	600 mg	Nausea, dizziness, pedal edema, weight gain	None
Pregabalin (Lyrica)1	Unknown	100–600 mg qhs	Nausea, dizziness, pedal edema, weight gain	None
Tramadol (Ultram)1	MRA	50 mg	Nausea, dizziness	None
Codeine	MRA[1]	400 mg qhs 30–60 mg	Nausea, dizziness	None
Oxycodone1	MRA	5–15 mg	Nausea, dizziness	None

[1]Not FDA approved for this indication.
[2]Exceeds dosage recommended by the manufacturer.
Abbreviations: mg=milligrams; Fe=iron replacement; DA=dopamine agonist; MOR=mu opiate receptor agonist.

in small case series, but an evidence base for these measures remains poor, and most patients seeking medical care for the symptom have severe enough symptoms to merit pharmacologic treatment.

Iron and pharmacologic treatments for RLS are outlined in Table 6. Iron deficiency, or even low normal body iron stores, may worsen or precipitate symptoms. Measuring a serum ferritin should be considered early in all RLS patients, with iron replacement therapy begun if serum ferritin values are less than 50 mcg/L. Iron therapy can be constipating or cause GI distress, and the formulation of iron with added vitamin C (Ferrex 150 Plus, Vitelle Irospan) is often better tolerated by those who cannot stomach ferrous sulfate.

Carbidopa-levedopa (Sinemet)[1] may be used for patients with only intermittently disturbing symptoms, but chronic nightly use of carbidopa-levodopa, especially above a dosage of 200 mg daily, may raise the risk of augmentation. For nightly use, the newer dopaminergic agonist medications pramipexole (Mirapex) or ropinirole (Requip) remain a mainstay of treatment. Pramipexole may be initiated at 0.125 to 0.25 mg nightly and titrated every few days to the 0.375 to 0.50 mg range or beyond if needed for symptom control. Doses beyond 1.0 mg[3] are typically not additionally effective and appear to raise augmentation risk. Ropinirole may be initiated at 0.5 to 1.0 mg with gradual upward titration to the 4 to 6 mg[3] range as needed and tolerated. Generally, dosing 1 hour prior to bedtime is sufficient, but if earlier evening or late afternoon symptoms emerge, cautious application of divided doses may be utilized, and some experts advice at least a low morning dosage administered daily to achieve a more chronic steady state of dopamine administration since this may be a sensible strategy to minimize augmentation risk. For either initial first-line therapy, or particularly when patients are beginning to experience earlier symptom onset during the day and may have failed the other short-acting dopaminergic drugs pramipexole and ropinirole, a rotigotine (Neupro) patch has been an advent in RLS management and often may be substituted for those other agents to provide more day-long symptom relief and reduce a growing augmentation tendency. Rotigotine offers several other advantages, as its transdermal delivery system provides continuous day-long release of medication that may minimize peak/trough serum concentration variation and minimize the occurrence of other potential adverse effects. Rotigotine also appears to result in augmentation less frequently than other dopaminergic drugs. All patients receiving dopaminergic agents should be counseled upfront about the approximate 15% idiosyncratic risk of impulse control disorder symptoms (such as pathologic gambling, shopping, or hoarding/punding behaviors), and be forewarned that should such problems result, the medication must be withdrawn and another nondopaminergic drug substituted for symptom control. Typical dose-related adverse effects are also described further in Table 6.

Gabapentin (Neurontin) is increasingly becoming an alternative first-line medication for RLS, dosed 300 to 1200[2] mg every night at bedtime as needed and tolerated. Gabapentin may be the agent of choice in patients with comorbid anxiety, pain and insomnia or in patients who are intolerant, resistant to, or have developed augmentation with dopamine agonist medications. On the other hand a dopamine agonist is still generally the first choice for pharmacologic treatment of RLS in severe cases and may be preferred over gabapentin in patients with comorbid depression, obesity, metabolic syndrome, OSA and history of falls. Gabapentin enacarbil (Horizant) is a prodrug of gabapentin that is better absorbed and carries an indication for RLS, but generic gabapentin is also frequently effective and well tolerated, and there has been no head-to-head trial showing superiority of the more expensive prodrug gabapentin encarbil over that of gabapentin. Other alternatives include clonazepam[1] and tramadol (Ultram).[1] For patients unresponsive to these measures, opiate treatment with oxycodone (Roxicodone)[1] 5 to 15 mg at bedtime, hydromorphone (Dilaudid),[1] or methadone (Dolophine)[1] are often effective. A large randomized trial showed that the combination oxycodone-naloxone (Targiniq ER)[1] resulted in substantial improvements in RLS symptoms in patients who had previously shown inadequate response to dopamine agonists. Small case series suggest other alternatives for refractory RLS such as carbamazepine (Tegretol),[1] oxcarbazepine (Trileptal),[1] and lamotrigine (Lamictal).[1] The impact of comorbid OSA should also be considered, as optimization of treatment for SDB may improve both subjective RLS symptoms as well as PLMD frequency in many patients.

Sleep-Related Leg Cramps

Sleep-related leg cramps are a common and enigmatic problem affecting 7% to 10% of children and up to 70% of elderly adults. Unfortunately, despite their extremely common occurrence and impact on the quality of life of cramp sufferers, little is known about the pathophysiology or treatment of this condition. Cramps are painful, involuntary sustained muscle contractions, lasting 2 to 10 minutes and affecting the unilateral or bilateral calves, thighs, or feet, with residual tenderness of the affected muscle lasting up to an hour or longer. The clinical approach to sleep-related leg cramps is to first determine whether they are also present during daytime in addition to sleep. If daytime cramping is prominent, exclusion of a precipitating neuromuscular disorder is paramount, including amyotrophic lateral sclerosis, peripheral neuropathy, myositis, or cramp-fasciculation syndrome. In elderly men, peripheral vascular disease and other systemic medical comorbidities are also common. (The reader is referred to the chapter on neuromuscular disorders for further advice on the diagnosis of these conditions.) A neurologic examination should be conducted on all cramp sufferers, and those having sensorimotor findings, fasciculations, or pathologic reflex findings should be referred for EMG, serum creatinine kinase, or additional blood and urine tests for exclusion of symptomatic causes of neuropathy as appropriate. While additional testing for electrolyte abnormalities such as hypomagnesemia, hypocalcemia, hyponatremia, and hypokalemia can be considered, they are of extremely low yield. When examination findings are normal and cramps are isolated to the sleep state, further diagnostic work-up can usually be avoided. Symptomatic treatment measures for sleep-related leg cramps include tonic water with lemon and advising adequate hydration and nightly stretching of the calves and thighs. Prescription quinine (Qualaquin)[1] carries a FDA black box warning for leg cramp treatment and is essentially no longer used for this indication. For refractory frequent cramp sufferers, a sodium-channel blocking anticonvulsant such as carbamazepine[1], oxcarbazepine[1], or lamotrigine[1] may also be considered.

Sleep-Related Bruxism

Sleep-related bruxism, rhythmic grinding of the teeth during sleep, may lead to significant tooth wear and dental or jaw pain. The condition is usually idiopathic, although it may be associated with psychiatric conditions such as mood or anxiety disorders, especially if it is also present during daytime. Treatment usually involves dental referral for consideration of a fitted mouth guard, although in extreme cases pharmacotherapy with clonazepam[1] or consideration of botulinum toxin (Botox)[1] may be necessary.

Other Sleep-Related Movement Disorders

Sleep-related rhythmic movement disorder usually occurs in patients with psychomotor maldevelopment and involves repetitive head and neck or axial body movements. This behavior is not strictly voluntary and often persists during PSG into deep drowsiness or light NREM sleep, so behavioral treatments alone are often ineffective. Head banging behavior, sometimes into the headboard of the bed, can be injurious at times: a protective helmet or treatment with clonazepam[1] is advisable in some cases. Most other movement disorders, such as organic tremors, myoclonus, or dyskinesias generated by the basal ganglia, are suppressed during sleep but may reemerge during drowsiness or nocturnal awakenings.

Propriospinal myoclonus at sleep onset is characterized by myoclonic jerks having their primary and earliest onset in abdominal and axial muscles prior to spreading to the limbs and may be associated with thoracic spinal cord pathology. Spinal imaging with MRI is advised. Treatment with clonazepam[1] is usual for this uncommon diagnosis, although it is unfortunately often ineffective, and many cases of propriospinal myoclonus are instead found to represent a functional movement disorder.

---

[1]Not FDA approved for this indication.
[2]Not available in the United States.
[3]Exceeds dosage recommended by the manufacturer.

---

[1]Not FDA approved for this indication.

Isolated Symptoms and Normal Variants

These conditions are felt largely to represent either normal variants or otherwise largely benign disorders. The definition of long and short sleepers are somewhat arbitrary, but may be considered as greater than 10 hours or shorter than 5 hours of habitual sleep. Short or long sleep time are each assumed to be variants of normal behavior in the absence of hypersomnia or nighttime symptoms of insomnia.

Sleep talking, or somniloquy, in isolation is rarely of concern. History is often lifelong in such patients. When sleep talking is newly evolved in an elderly individual or a younger patient receiving antidepressant therapy, RBD should be considered in the differential diagnosis, and the patient should be questioned about other potential evidence for dream enactment behavior. A careful medication history and neurologic examination alone will usually dictate whether further evaluation with PSG may be indicated, but in most cases isolated sleep talking is not a cause for concern.

Sleep starts, hypnic jerks or physiologic myoclonus are near universal in their occurrence and often associated with recent excessive caffeine intake or emotional or physical stress. A history of occurrence of jerks limited to the arms, legs, or axial musculature causing arousal within the first 5 to 10 minutes of sleep, and lacking later recurrence during the night, is typical. Reassurance and avoidance of precipitating factors is advised; however, if hypnic jerks are excessive or recur later in the night, PSG is occasionally necessary to distinguish this benign diagnosis from PLMD or propriospinal myoclonus. Propriospinal myoclonus at sleep onset is characterized by myoclonic jerks having their primary and earliest onset in abdominal and axial muscles prior to spreading to the limbs and may be associated with thoracic spinal cord pathology. Spinal imaging with MRI is advised. Treatment with clonazepam[1] is usual for this uncommon diagnosis.

Other Sleep Disorders

Undesirable influences in the patient's sleep environment can serve to regularly distract or disturb him or her from initiating or maintaining sleep. Typical influences include a bed partner who snores loudly or who causes bed motion due to restless or disturbed sleep; pets who sleep in bed with the patient and cause awakening; environmental noise from neighborhood dogs, car alarms, or neighboring freeway or train way; too much outdoor ambient light; or undesirable household ambient temperature. There is considerable overlap in this category of environmental sleep disturbance with inadequate sleep hygiene, as activating stimuli in the environment may lead the patient toward chronic insomnia and adapting undesirable sleep-related behaviors that serve to further disrupt restful sleep.

Sleep-Related Medical and Neurologic Disorders

Fatal familial insomnia is an exceedingly rare, autosomal dominant variant form of familial Creutzfeldt-Jakob disease, a prion disorder that leads to progressive insomnia and progressive cognitive impairment, with death inevitably occurring within 3 years of onset. Aggregate prion protein accumulates in the thalamus and other brain regions, and relentlessly progressive insomnia, panic disorder, hallucinosis, and dementia ensue. Unfortunately, no treatments are currently known for this rare disorder.

Conclusions

Sleep disorders are common and result in significant patient morbidity, daytime dysfunction, and impaired quality of life. Untreated sleep disordered breathing (SDB) may also raise the risk for hypertension, vascular events, and mortality. The most common presenting symptoms of sleep disorders include insomnia, characterized by difficulty initiating and maintaining sleep with poor sleep quality, and hypersomnia, the symptom of excessive daytime sleepiness. Evaluation begins with a detailed history and physical examination, which in select cases may require support and clarification by polysomnography and multiple sleep-latency testing. Fortunately, effective therapies are available for the majority of sleep disorders. Insomnia typically requires behavioral or pharmacologic interventions, while SDB may be effectively treated in most cases with positive airway pressure (PAP) therapy. Primary CNS hypersomnias including narcolepsy require stimulant management in most cases, while most parasomnias benefit from clonazepam.[1] Circadian sleep disorders may require timed light and melatonin therapies. Patients having RLS and PLMD should be evaluated for iron deficiency and may enjoy symptom control through dopaminergic or other alternative symptomatic treatments. The majority of patients with sleep disorders benefit from a careful clinical evaluation and appropriately selected therapies.

---

[1]Not FDA approved for this indication.

References

American Academy of Sleep Medicine: *International Classification of Sleep Disorders: Diagnostic and Coding Manual*, ed 3, Darien, IL, 2014, American Academy of Sleep Medicine2014.

Auger RR, Burgess HJ, Emens JS, et al: Clinical practice guideline for the treatment of intrinsic circadian rhythm sleep-wake disorders: Advanced Sleep-Wake Phase Disorder (ASWPD), Delayed Sleep-Wake Phase Disorder (DSWPD), Non-24-Hour Sleep-Wake Rhythm Disorder (N24SWD), and Irregular Sleep-Wake Rhythm Disorder (ISWRD). An update for 2015. An American Academy of Sleep Medicine Clinical Practice Guideline, *J Clin Sleep Med* 11:1119–1236, 2015.

Chesson AL, Anderson WL, Pancer JP, Wise M: Practice parameters for the indications for polysomnography and related procedures: An update for 2005, *Sleep* 28:499–521, 2005.

Collop NA, Tracy SL, Kapur V, et al: Obstructive sleep apnea devices for out-of-center (OOC) testing: Technology evaluation, *J Clin Sleep Med* 7:531–548, 2011.

Johns MW: A new method for measuring daytime sleepiness: The Epworth sleepiness scale, *Sleep* 14:540–545, 1991, Also available online in a patient fillable version at http://www.stanford.edu/~dement/epworth.html.

Kushida CA, Littner MR, Morgenthaler T, et al: Indications for positive airway pressure treatment of adult obstructive sleep apnea patients: A consensus statement, *Chest* 115:863–866, 1999.

Luyster FS, Strollo Jr PJ, Zee PC, et al: Sleep: A health imperative, *Sleep* 35:727–734, 2012.

Morgenthaler TI, Lee-Chiong T, Alessi C, et al: Standards of Practice Committee of the American Academy of Sleep Medicine. Practice parameters for the clinical evaluation and treatment of circadian rhythm sleep disorders, *Sleep* 30:1445–1459, 2007.

Schutte-Rodin S, Broch L, Buysse D, et al: Clinical guideline for the evaluation and management of chronic insomnia in adults, *J Clin Sleep Med* 4:487–504, 2008.

Silber MH, Becker PM, Earley C, et al: Willis-Ekbom Disease Foundation revised consensus statement on the management of restless legs syndrome, *Mayo Clin Proc* 88:977–986, 2013.

St. Louis EK: Key sleep neurologic disorders: Narcolepsy, restless legs syndrome/Willis-Ekbom disease, and REM sleep behavior disorder, *Neurol Clin Pract* 4:16–25, 2014.

Wise MS, Arand DL, Auger RR, et al: American Academy of Sleep Medicine. Treatment of narcolepsy and other hypersomnias of central origin, *Sleep* 30:1712–1727, 2007.

TARGETED TEMPERATURE MANAGEMENT (THERAPEUTIC HYPOTHERMIA)

Scott Leikin, DO, Jennifer Wang, DO, and Adel Bassily-Marcus, MD

 CURRENT THERAPY

- Targeted temperature management (therapeutic hypothermia) should be considered following resuscitation from cardiac arrest to reduce the risk of anoxic brain injury.
- There does not appear to be a benefit to cooling to a temperature of 33°C when compared to cooling to a temperature of 36°C (97°F).
- There is a paradigm shift of therapeutic hypothermia to preventing fever and instituting a targeted temperature.
- Cooling pads are the most commonly used method to induce hypothermia.

---

[1]Not FDA approved for this indication.

Introduction

Inducing patients to a targeted temperature to reduce anoxic brain injury post cardiac arrest has now become the standard of care at medical institutions around the world. Although the theory has multiple applications for multiple conditions, post cardiac arrest is the most common and studied indication and the focus of this chapter. Although each institution has their own protocol, there are common tenets that are included in each institution's protocols. Current nomenclature is Targeted Temperature Management (TTM) as the theories on ideal temperature for the post cardiac arrest patient have evolved from therapeutic hypothermia. The evolution of TTM is important to understand, as the current theory is fever prevention is where the benefit is and fever is what is associated with poor neurologic outcomes in the post cardiac arrest time period.

The first multicenter, randomized control study on post cardiac arrest care was conducted in Europe and published in the New England Journal of Medicine (NEJM) in 2002. A total of 3551 patients were deemed eligible, but only 275 were included. In the study, 137 were assigned to hypothermia (32 to 34°C as measured by bladder temperature for 24 hours) and 138 to normothermia. To qualify in the study, subjects must have had a witnessed cardiac arrest, with an initial rhythm of ventricular fibrillation (VF) with return of spontaneous circulation (ROSC). The results showed a favorable neurologic outcome in 75/136 patients (55%) in the hypothermia group compared to 54/137 patients (39%) in the normothermia group at 6 months as measured by the Pittsburgh cerebral-performance category. The mortality difference at 6 months was 41% in the hypothermia group and 55% in the normothermia group. This validated the utilization of mild therapeutic hypothermia to improve neurologic outcomes and decrease mortality for witnessed VF cardiac arrest.

In 2002, a NEJM study described survival with good neurologic outcome to hospital discharge in patients who were unconscious after ROSC in out-of-hospital cardiac arrest. In the study, 77 patients were assigned to normothermia or moderate hypothermia (core body temperature of 33°C within 2 hours of ROSC for 12 total hours). Usually, out-of-hospital cardiac arrests have survival rates of only 5% to 35%. The investigators found 21/43 (49%) patients in the hypothermia group survived and had a favorable neurologic outcome compared to 9/34 (26%) in the normothermia group with (P = .046). The authors concluded that moderate hypothermia improved outcomes in patients with coma after ROSC in out-of-hospital cardiac arrest patients.

In 2010, the American Heart Association (AHA) released a class I recommendation for post VF/VT TTM. Pulseless electrical activity/asystole was given a IIb recommendation. TTM is generally defined as a core temperature of 33 to 36°C. Since this recommendation, TTM has been adopted as common practice post cardiac arrest in comatose adult patients.

In May 2011, the Society of Critical Care Medicine published "Targeted temperature management in critical care: A report and recommendations from five professional societies" and determined that TTM with a core body temperature goal of 32 to 34°C be used for post out-of-hospital VF/VT arrest.

In December 2013, the NEJM published a study titled "Targeted Temperature Management at 33°C versus 36°C after Cardiac Arrest." This international multicenter study aimed to determine the optimal temperature associated with improved neurologic outcomes for out-of-hospital cardiac arrest patients. They found no significant 180-day neurologic outcome or mortality difference between the patients in the 33°C arm and the patients in the 36°C arm. There were no adverse effects or benefits to patients cooled to 33°C. The authors concluded that in patients who were unconscious after ROSC was obtained in out-of-hospital cardiac arrest, a temperature of 33°C did not confer a benefit compared to a temperature of 36°C. This shifted the paradigm of therapeutic hypothermia to preventing fever and instituting a targeted temperature.

The International Liaison Committee on Resuscitation and the AHA Emergency Cardiovascular Care Committee and the Council on Cardiopulmonary, Critical Care and Perioperative and Resuscitation reviewed 5045 studies, of which 6 were RCTs and 5 were observational. They recommended: target core temperatures between 32 and 36°C for at least 24 hours and against using pre-hospital cooling with cooled intravenous fluids.

The theoretical benefits of TTM are that it can reduce brain oxygen usage by 6% for every 1°C reduction while also preventing inflammation and cerebral edema. TTM is currently being studied for encephalopathy, bacterial meningitis, cardiogenic shock, traumatic brain injury, and organ donation.

Initiation

With few absolute contraindications, TTM should be considered in all patients who achieved ROSC post cardiac arrest regardless of the underlying rhythm during the cardiac arrest. Many post cardiac arrest patients with ROSC will go to the cardiac catheterization lab for an angiogram and this should not delay the initiation of TTM. Determining the etiology for the cardiac arrest is still extremely important and should not have a bearing on the initiation of TTM. The patient populations in whom TTM is considered a relative contraindication include intracranial hemorrhage, exsanguination, hypotension refractory to multiple vasopressors, severe sepsis, and pregnancy. At our tertiary care academic medical center, the only absolute contraindications are cryoglobulinemia, traumatic injury leading to cardiac arrest, and family refusal or advanced directives that preclude the use of TTM.

Eligibility requires a comatose patient; the patient should not be able to follow commands or respond to noxious stimuli. This is equivalent to a Richmond Agitation Sedation Score of −4 or −5 or Glasgow Coma Scale <8. The patient must have a sustained cardiac rhythm that results in adequate brain perfusion.

The most studied rhythms in cardiac arrest which benefited from TTM were VT or VF. It is uncertain whether pulseless electrical activity and a "nonshockable rhythm" would benefit from TTM but we would advocate that any patient regardless of the underlying rhythm have TTM utilized if ROSC is obtained. This is in line with the 2015 AHA guidelines on post cardiac arrest care and emergency cardiovascular care. The guideline committee came to this conclusion because cohorts who did not receive TTM had such significant neurologic morbidity that the benefits were considered to outweigh the risks. Significant head trauma should be ruled out in patients who present to an emergency department with a noncontrast head computed tomography (CT) scan. Ideally, TTM should be initiated as soon as ROSC is obtained but it is acceptable to initiate it within the first 6 hours, and even up to 12 hours post arrest. We strongly advocate initiating the process as soon as feasible. We would also recommend that pacer pads be applied to the patient's skin and kept in place. The target core temperature should be maintained at the desired temperature for 24 hours. Based on a review of the literature, initiating a core temperature between 32 and 36°C for these patients with external cooling pads is the target.

The most commonly used method to induce hypothermia is with external cooling pads. Once the process is started, the time to target temperature should be within 2 hours. Other less commonly used options include ice bags at the groin, chest, axilla, and neck, and infusing cold saline. Cooled intravenous saline will reduce core temperature by 1°C every 30 minutes. The 2015 AHA guidelines recommend against cooling patients in the prehospital setting with intravenous cooled saline, as survival and neurologic recovery were not shown to be improved in various trials. Urinary catheters with temperature probes are often used to measure core temperature. Other acceptable methods of temperature measurement include esophageal, rectal, central, tympanic, or nasal probes. Axillary and oral temperature measurements are not reliable in measuring core temperature. Potential complications of cooling include electrolyte abnormalities, hyperglycemia, coagulopathy, and arrhythmias.

Maintenance

In TTM, the targeted core temperature should be maintained within 0.5°C for 24 hours. Shivering should be avoided as it creates heat, thereby increasing oxygen demand. Bedside Shivering Assessment Scale (BSAS) should be utilized to help guide therapy for shivering. For sedation purposes, our recommended first-line treatment is propofol (Diprivan) 15 to 20 µg/kg/min. Midazolam (Versed) 1 to 2 mg/h is an alternative. Fentanyl 25 µg/h infusion can be used if adequate sedation is not achieved.

The BSAS treatment algorithm should be utilized to eliminate shivering. In the BSAS, neuromuscular blockade with an agent such as cisatracurium (Nimbex) 0.15 mg/kg IV bolus followed by an infusion of 1 µg/kg/min can be used, although this protocol may mask seizures. The lowest dose that eliminates shivering using agents with a short half life is recommended because hypothermia slows medication metabolism and elimination.

TTM may worsen or cause hemodynamic derangements and arrhythmias, such as hypotension and bradycardia, that are common post cardiac arrest. Maintenance of a mean arterial pressure (MAP) of 80 to 100 mm Hg will help ensure adequate brain perfusion.

TTM patients are mechanically ventilated, and some institutions use esophageal probes to track body temperature, although this is less common, as it is invasive. Oxygen saturation should be maintained at 94% to 96% to avoid hypoxia or hyperoxygenation. Hyperglycemia is common with TTM, so serum glucose should be checked at set intervals, with a goal <180 mg/dL. If serum glucose is persistently >200 mg/dL despite treatment, an insulin drip should be considered. Electrolyte abnormalities, especially hypokalemia, are common during TTM. Therefore, the serum potassium level should be checked every 4 to 6 hours and replenished if lower than 3.5 meq/L. Rewarming may increase potassium levels.

It has been reported in the literature that up to 66% of TTM patients will develop an infection. Fever and leukocytosis may be present in the absence of infection and are not reliable indicators of infection. A comprehensive plan needs to be developed for every patient when signs of infection are potentially present. Even if a high percentage of patients develop an infection, this has not been shown to affect mortality.

Rewarming

Rewarming should occur 24 hours after achieving the targeted temperature. Rewarming should not occur at a rate that is faster than 0.2°C/h until the patient reaches 37°C; this will likely take between 6 to 12 hours. Once at 37°C, this temperature should be maintained for 48 to 72 hours, as rebound hyperthermia is associated with poor neurologic outcomes. Electrolyte abnormalities such as hyperkalemia, hypoglycemia, and hypotension may occur. Blood pressure should be carefully monitored during the rewarming period.

Post-Therapeutic Hypothermia/Prognosis

The AHA recommends 72 hours before prognosticating neurologic recovery. Presence of at least two of the following: incomplete brain stem reflexes, presence of myoclonus, unreactive electroencephalography (EEG), and absent cortical somatosensory-evoked potentials suggest poor neurologic outcome. A full neurologic examination should be done daily. Involving neurology or neurocritical care is advised to help prognosticate neurologic recovery in post cardiac arrest TTM patients.

References

Badjatia N, Strongilis E, Gordon E: Metabolic impact of shivering during therapeutic temperature modulation the bedside shivering assessment scale, *Stroke* 39(12):3242–3247, 2008, Available at: https://doi.org/10.1161/STROKEAHA.108.523654.

Bernard, Gray, Buist: Treatment of comatose survivors of out-of-hospital cardiac arrest with induced hypothermia. *New England Journal of Medicine*, 346: 557–563, 2002, https://doi.org/10.1056/NEJMoa003289.

Callaway Clifton W, et al: American heart association guidelines update for cardiopulmonary resuscitation and emergency cardiovascular care, *Circulation* 132(18):S315–S367, 2015, Available at: https://doi.org/10.1161/CIR.0000000000000252, 3 Nov. 2015.

Donnino MW, Anderson LW, Berg KM, Reynolds JC: Temperature management after cardiac arrest an advisory statement by the advanced life support task force of the international liaison committee on resuscitation and the american heart association emergency cardiovascular care committee and the council on cardiopulmonary, critical care, perioperative and resuscitation, *Circulation* 132(25):2448–2456, 2015. Available at: https://doi.org/10.1161/CIR.0000000000000313.

Friedman OA: *Critical care: targeted temperature management after cardiac arrest*, In JM Orpopello, V Kvetan, SM Pastores. Eds. New York, NY: McGraw Hill, Lange, 2017.

Moler MD, Silverstein FS, Hulubkov R, et al: Therapeutic hypothermia after out-of-hospital cardiac arrest in children, *New Eng Journal of Medicine*, 372: 1898–1908, 2015, Available at: https://doi.org/10.1056/NEJMoa1411480.

Nielson MD, PhD, Wetterslev N, MD, PhD, J, & Cronberg, MD, PhD, T: Targeted temperature management at 33°c versus 36°c after cardiac arrest. *New England Journal of Medicine* 369:2197–2206, 2013, Available at: https://doi.org10.1056/NEJMoa1310519.

Nunnally M, Jaeschke R, Bellingan G: Targeted temperature management in critical care: a report and recommendations from five professional societies, *Critical Care Medicine* 39(5):1113–1125, 2011, Available at: https://doi.org/10.1097/CCM.0b013e318206bab2.

T.: Mild therapeutic hypothermia to improve the neurologic outcome after cardiac arrest, *New England Journal of Medicine* 346:549–556, 2002, Available at: https://doi.org/10.1056/NEJMoa012689.

Scirica BM: Therapeutic hypothermia after cardiac arrest, *Circulation, Clinician update* 127(2):244–250, 2013, https://doi.org/10.1161/CIRCULATIONAHA.111.076851.

Yunen JR, Tolentino R: *Critical care: chapter: controversies in therapeutic hypothermia*, In JM Oropello, V. Kvetan, SM Pastores. Eds.). New York, NY: McGraw Hill Lange, 2017.

TRIGEMINAL NEURALGIA

Method of
Karlynn Sievers, MD; and Hugh Silk, MD, MPH

CURRENT DIAGNOSIS

International Headache Society Diagnostic criteria (classical):
A. At least three attacks of unilateral facial pain fulfilling criteria B and C
B. Occurring in one or more divisions of the trigeminal nerve, with no radiation beyond the trigeminal distribution
C. Pain has at least three of the following four characteristics:
   1. Recurring in paroxysmal attacks lasting from a fraction of a second to 2 minutes
   2. Severe intensity
   3. Electric shock-like, shooting, stabbing, or sharp in quality
   4. Precipitated by innocuous stimuli to the affected side of the face
D. No clinically evident neurologic deficit
E. Not better accounted for by another diagnosis.
International Headache Society Diagnostic criteria (secondary)
Same as above, except E. Secondary trigeminal neuralgia is secondary to another disease process.

CURRENT THERAPY

- Medications
  - Carbamazepine: start 100 mg two times daily, and increase by 200 mg/day to max 1200 mg/day (number needed to treat = 2)
  - Alternative treatments are available but have not been proven to be as effective (see Table 1)
  - For patients with refractory or severe symptoms, surgical treatment (e.g., microvascular decompression, radiosurgery, alternative invasive procedures) can be helpful for some.

TABLE 1	Treatment Options for TN, With Evidence of Effectiveness	
	TREATMENT TYPE	EVIDENCE OF EFFECTIVENESS
Medical therapy		
	Carbamazepine (Tegretol)	Likely to be beneficial (gold standard)
	Oxcarbazepine (Trileptal)[1]	Likely to be beneficial*
	Baclofen (Lioresal)[1]	Likely to be beneficial,* particularly in patients with TN caused by MS
	Gabapentin (Neurontin)[1]	Unknown effectiveness
	Lamotrigine (Lamictal)[1]	Unknown effectiveness
Surgical therapy		
	Microvascular decompression	Trade-off between benefits and harms*
	Stereotactic radiosurgery	Trade-off between benefits and harms*
	Percutaneous destructive radiosurgical techniques	Trade-off between benefits and harms*

Abbreviations: TN = trigeminal neuralgia; MS = multiple sclerosis.
*Based on observational studies and/or consensus.
[1]Not FDA approved for this indication.

Epidemiology

The incidence of trigeminal neuralgia is estimated to be 5.9/100,000 women and 3.4/100,000 men. The peak incidence is in patients age 60 to 70 years. It has also been called "tic douloureux" because of facial spasms that often accompany the disorder.

Risk factors

Increasing age is a risk factor. It is rarely diagnosed in patients younger than 40 years of age. Other risk factors include multiple sclerosis (the incidence of trigeminal neuralgia in this population is 1% to 2%), stroke, and hypertension (especially in women). There is no racial predominance.

Pathophysiology

It is currently hypothesized that trigeminal neuralgia results from demyelination of the fifth cranial nerve, leading to electrical transmission of nerve impulses that are not mediated by neurotransmitters and that generate pain. Demyelination is most commonly caused by aberrant or tortuous blood vessels that cause nerve compression but can also be attributed to sources such as multiple sclerosis or amyloid deposition.

The most commonly used classification system for trigeminal neuralgia has four categories: classical, symptomatic, secondary, and idiopathic. With classical trigeminal neuralgia, there is no underlying cause for the demyelination other than vascular compression, as described previously. With secondary trigeminal neuralgia, an alternate cause such as multiple sclerosis or tumor is responsible for the demyelination. Symptomatic trigeminal neuralgia is caused by herpes, trauma, or another disorder. A fourth category would include idiopathic trigeminal neuralgia, where there are no radiologic findings that account for the patient's symptoms.

Prevention

There is no known method of prevention for trigeminal neuralgia.

Clinical manifestations

Trigeminal neuralgia is a clinical diagnosis made on the basis of recurrent attacks of unilateral facial pain. Pain is intense, and is usually described as sharp, shock-like, or stabbing. Any of the branches of the trigeminal nerve can be affected, but the maxillary branch is the most common, and the ophthalmic branch the least common. The pain lasts for seconds, and most patients are asymptomatic between attacks (though some patients will have a mild, dull, persistent ache in the area of the affected nerve). Attacks can recur infrequently or hundreds of times per day.

Often, patients have trigger zones that will set off paroxysms of pain with minimal stimulation. Activities such as chewing, teeth brushing, or touching a trigger area can set off attacks; sometimes even minimal stimulation such as a light breeze can trigger episodes. Not all patients have trigger zones; however, the presence of these is nearly pathognomonic for trigeminal neuralgia.

Diagnosis

Diagnosis is clinical, based on the commonly described symptoms listed above. Diagnosis of trigeminal neuralgia should be considered in all patients who describe unilateral intense paroxysmal facial pain on three or more occasions. Careful examination of the head and neck and thorough neurologic examination should be performed in all patients. Exam findings are typically normal in patients with trigeminal neuralgia, and so exam abnormalities should prompt reconsideration of the diagnosis. Sensory abnormalities (including vision or hearing loss), facial muscle weakness, or loss of corneal reflex are not associated with trigeminal neuralgia and warrant further workup.

Laboratory studies are typically not helpful in making the diagnosis. Temporal mandibular joint or dental radiographs may be helpful to rule out other pathology for those who present with mid or lower face symptoms. MRI (with and without contrast) of the brain can be helpful in distinguishing between classical and symptomatic trigeminal neuralgia and should be considered in all patients with new onset of symptoms. There is some early evidence that structural MRI techniques can help identify changes associated with trigeminal neuralgia and help predict those that will respond well to surgical intervention, but more research is needed in this area.

Differential Diagnosis

Differential diagnosis includes other types of headaches (migraine, cluster headache, paroxysmal hemicrania), dental sources (cracked teeth, caries, dental abscess), infectious causes (sinusitis, otitis media, postherpetic neuralgia), nervous system pathology (intracranial tumors, multiple sclerosis), temporomandibular joint syndrome, and giant cell arteritis. Many of these other diagnoses will have specific exam findings.

Treatment

Medical treatment should be initiated for all new cases of trigeminal neuralgia. Carbamazepine (Tegretol) has been shown in multiple randomized control trials to reduce pain in trigeminal neuralgia and is considered the gold standard for medical treatment. The number needed to treat is 2. Dosing starts at 100 mg two times daily and increases gradually in increments of 200 mg daily to a maximum dose of 1200 mg daily. Carbamazepine can have side effects such as drowsiness, dizziness, hepatotoxicity, pancreatitis, blood dyscrasias, and ataxia. Consensus opinion is that it has a greater than 50% failure rate for long-term (5 to 10 years) pain control. Oxcarbazepine (Trileptal)[1] has equal efficacy in some studies to carbamazepine. For both medications, consider testing for HLA-B*15:02 allele in at-risk patients (e.g., Asian ancestry) to avoid Stevens-Johnson reaction. Pimozide (Orap)[1] has been promoted as equal to carbamazepine; however, the studies are of low quality with no adverse effect comparison. Tizanidine (Zanaflex)[1] has been shown to be as effective as carbamazepine but also with low-quality studies, and pimozide can have serious side effects. Lamotrigine (Lamictal)[1] can be used in patients who do not tolerate carbamazepine or as an adjunct to those without full benefit from carbamazepine, but the dose must be titrated slowly, so it is not as effective in acute pain control. Baclofen (Lioresal)[1] and gabapentin (Neurontin)[1] may be useful

---

[1]Not FDA approved for this indication.

in patients with multiple sclerosis who also have trigeminal neuralgia, but evidence is lacking regarding their effectiveness in classical trigeminal neuralgia.

Recent studies have shown some weak data that botulinum toxin A (Botox)[1] to be an effective treatment in reducing both pain intensity and frequency of paroxysms in trigeminal neuralgia; adverse events include facial asymmetry and edema or hematoma at the injection site. Alcohol injections[1] and cryotherapy have also been used for trigeminal neuralgia pain.

For patients with refractory or severe symptoms, surgical treatment can be helpful for some. Microvascular decompression and radiosurgery are both common techniques for treatment of trigeminal neuralgia, with microvascular decompression generally considered to be first-line surgical intervention. Other surgical techniques can include radiofrequency thermocoagulation, glycerol rhyzolysis, stereotactic radiosurgery, balloon compression, peripheral nerve section, partial sensory root section, and gamma-knife radiosurgery. Studies have noted sensory side effects, and most evidence for neurosurgical approaches comes from observational studies. Treatment for secondary trigeminal neuralgia typically includes treating the underlying cause.

Monitoring
Although there is no standard protocol for monitoring patients with trigeminal neuralgia, the condition is extremely painful, and there have been incidents reported of patients accidentally overdosing on medications or taking their own lives. Therefore it is recommended that patients are monitored at regular intervals to ensure their pain is controlled and to monitor for side effects from treatment.

Management of Complications
The disease can have relapses and remissions. Medications or alternative treatments should be reinstituted as needed. Tests should be run as needed based on side effect symptoms, and treatments stopped and others considered based on efficacy and patient tolerance.

References
Gubian A, Rosahl SK. Meta-analysis on safety and efficacy of microsurgical and radiosurgical treatment of trigeminal neuralgia, World Neurosurg 103:757–767, 2017.
International Headache Society. International Classification of Headache Disorders (3rd edition – beta version). Available at http://www.ihs-headache.org/ichd-guidelines/ihs-guidelines.
Khan M, Nishi SE, Hassan SN, et al: Trigeminal neuralgia, glossopharyngeal neuralgia, and mysfascial pain dysfunction syndrome: an update, Pain Res Manag 7438326, 2017. https://doi.org/10.1155/2017/7438326. Epub 2017 Jul 30.
Krafft R: Trigeminal neuralgia, Am Fam Physician 77:1291–1296, 2008.
Wiffen PJ, Derry S, Moore RA, et al: Carbamazepine for acute and chronic pain. In: The Cochrane Library, Issue 8 2013, Chichester, UK: John Wiley & Sons, Ltd. Search date 2010.
Zakrzewska JM, Linskey ME: Trigeminal neuralgia, Am Fam Physician 94(2):133–135, 2016.
Zakrzewska JM, Linskey ME: Trigeminal neuralgia, BMJ 350:h1238, 2015.
Zhang J, Yang M, Zhou M, He L, Chen N, Zakrzewska JM: Non-antiepileptic drugs for trigeminal neuralgia, Cochrane Database Syst Rev (12), 2013.

VIRAL MENINGITIS

Method of
Joanna Thomson, MD, MPH; and Samir S. Shah, MD, MSCE

CURRENT DIAGNOSIS

- Typical presentation includes fever, headache, and neck stiffness or pain. Constitutional symptoms include mild lethargy, myalgias, nausea, and vomiting.
- Neonates often present with nonspecific signs and symptoms including lethargy, irritability, and poor feeding.
- Cerebrospinal fluid (CSF) profile should be performed. Results show elevated white blood cell count (often but not always with mononuclear cell predominance), normal to slightly elevated protein, normal glucose, normal to slightly elevated opening pressure, and negative bacterial Gram stain and culture.
- Diagnostic polymerase chain reaction (PCR) and serologic studies can identify the etiologic agent.
- Consider neuroimaging before lumbar puncture if there is concern for increased intracranial pressure or if encephalitis is possible.

CURRENT THERAPY

- Symptomatic and supportive management includes analgesia, antipyretics, antiemetics, and intravenous fluids.
- Hospitalization is recommended for infants (younger than 1 year), elderly patients (older than 65 years), and immunocompromised patients, as well as for patients presenting with altered mental status, seizures, focal neurologic signs, or the absence of classic viral CSF findings.
- Few medications, with the exception of acyclovir (Zovirax) for HSV, effectively treat viral meningitis.

Epidemiology
The true epidemiology of viral meningitis is unknown because it is not a reportable disease. However, the Centers for Disease Control and Prevention (CDC) estimate 25,000 to 50,000 hospitalizations per year. There is also yearly variation in disease burden. Causes of viral meningitis vary by age group, immune status, season, and geography. There is increased incidence in summer and early fall owing to the high prevalence of enteroviruses and arthropod-borne viruses (arboviruses). Common etiologic agents include enteroviruses, herpes simplex virus (HSV), arboviruses, lymphocytic choriomeningitis virus (LCMV), cytomegalovirus (CMV), varicella zoster virus (VZV), and Epstein–Barr virus (EBV). See Table 1 for features of the common and some less-common viral agents that cause meningitis.

Pathophysiology
Viral infection begins at the mucosal surface of the respiratory tract or gastrointestinal tract, with viral replication occurring in regional lymph nodes. A secondary viremia then occurs that provides access to the central nervous system (CNS). Symptoms of viral meningitis are due to either an immune response to the virus within the CNS (e.g., enterovirus) or direct viral invasion of neural tissue (e.g., HSV1/2).

Prevention
To prevent spread of viral agents responsible for meningitis, hand-washing and other infection-control measures are most important. The infection-control precautions necessary during patient contact depend on mode of transmission of the virus (see Table 1). Vaccines are available for some of the viruses that are known to cause meningitis, including polio (an enterovirus), mumps, measles, and varicella.

Clinical Manifestations
Viral meningitis can be difficult to distinguish from bacterial meningitis. Fever, headache, and neck stiffness and pain are the usual presenting complaints. Headache can be localized to the frontal or retro-orbital areas and may be associated with photophobia. Although neck stiffness and pain are usually present, neck rigidity (positive Kerning's sign or positive Brudzinski's sign) is not always present on examination. Constitutional symptoms can include lethargy, myalgias, and nausea or vomiting. There is often

a history of concomitant viral respiratory or gastrointestinal illness at the time of presentation. Seizures can occur with viral causes of meningitis, especially HSV, but should prompt consideration of other diagnostic possibilities.

In contrast to children and adults, neonates often present with nonspecific findings such as lethargy, irritability, and poor feeding. See Table 1 for clinical manifestations associated with specific etiologic agents.

Viral meningitis can also manifest with signs of encephalitis, in which case the encompassing diagnosis is meningoencephalitis. Encephalitis or meningoencephalitis are likely if any of the following are present: altered mental status, seizures, focal neurologic deficits (including aphasia, anosmia, ataxia, cranial nerve deficits, motor weakness, or involuntary movements), or behavioral changes.

Diagnosis

Diagnosis of viral meningitis requires lumbar puncture for CSF studies including cell count, protein, glucose, Gram stain and culture, and specific viral studies. Although a lymphocytic pleocytosis is associated with viral infections, most viral CNS infections initially have a neutrophilic pleocytosis. However, neutrophilic pleocytosis is also associated with bacterial meningitis. In viral meningitis, though CSF protein is normal to slightly elevated, CSF glucose is normal, and no organisms are identified on CSF bacterial Gram stain or culture compared with elevated CSF protein, low CSF glucose, and positive CSF bacterial culture in bacterial meningitis.

Studies to identify a specific virus as the etiologic agent are recommended for patients with severe illness or a complicated course. Viral cultures of CSF are not generally useful given their poor sensitivity, and serologic viral studies require both acute and convalescent titers to demonstrate antibody response to the suspected viral antigen. CSF PCR studies that detect viral DNA or RNA are more sensitive than viral culture and provide more rapid results than serologic viral studies (see Table 1). Multiplex PCR techniques allow for testing of multiple viruses and bacteria with a single CSF sample and a single test. Where available, multiplex PCR may result in considerable savings in time and effort, while improving diagnostic capacity. In some cases, it is useful to perform viral PCR studies on blood (HSV, EBV, CMV, and human herpesvirus [HHV]6), urine (CMV), stool (enterovirus), and skin vesicles (HSV) to further support the diagnosis. However, a positive PCR study from blood, urine, stool, or skin does not provide direct evidence of CNS infection by the same virus. For example, enterovirus isolated from the stool can represent asymptomatic infection or prior infection but may also be isolated from the stool at the same time as concomitant enteroviral meningitis.

Most other testing is not helpful, but further testing (including complete blood count, renal profile, liver function, pancreatic enzymes, and HIV studies) should be guided by the patient's presentation and clinical status.

Neuroimaging (computed tomography [CT] or magnetic resonance imaging [MRI]) should be obtained before lumbar puncture if there is concern for increased intracranial pressure. It is also recommended if symptoms of encephalitis are present (including altered consciousness, seizures, focal neurologic deficits, behavioral changes) to exclude other CNS disease.

Differential Diagnosis

The major item on the differential diagnosis for viral meningitis is bacterial meningitis. The bacterial meningitis score, validated in children 29 days to 19 years, is a clinical prediction rule that identifies patients as at very low risk (0.1%) for bacterial meningitis if they lack all of the following: positive CSF Gram stain, CSF absolute neutrophil count (ANC) of at least 1000 cells/μL, CSF protein of at least 80 mg/dL, peripheral blood ANC of at least 10,000 cells/μL, and a history of seizure before or at the time of presentation. While C-reactive protein (CRP) is not generally useful because it can be high in viral meningitis and low in the initial stages of bacterial disease, elevated serum procalcitonin levels (>0.5 μg/mL in children and >0.2 μg/mL in adults) are more sensitive and specific for distinguishing viral from bacterial meningitis.

Other diagnoses to consider include parameningeal infections (i.e., subdural or epidural empyema, brain abscess), meningitis due to fungi, mycobacteria, rickettsia, mycoplasma, parasites, and other CNS infectious or inflammatory processes including malignancy, drug exposure, rheumatologic disease (e.g., systemic lupus erythematosus), or autoimmune (e.g., anti-NMDA receptor encephalitis).

Treatment

Symptomatic care remains the mainstay of therapy for viral meningitis. Therapy should be directed at pain and fever control (e.g., ibuprofen [Motrin], acetaminophen [Tylenol], ketorolac [Toradol]), management of nausea and vomiting (e.g., ondansetron [Zofran]), and intravenous fluids. Hospitalization is recommended for patients younger than 1 year, the elderly, and the immunocompromised. Patients who present with altered mental status, seizures, focal neurologic signs, or a CSF profile that does not have the classic viral profile should also be hospitalized for clinical management and for antibiotic treatment until bacterial meningitis can be excluded. Advanced care including management of respiratory failure, cardiovascular instability, seizures, disturbed fluid and electrolyte balance, and cerebral edema may be necessary.

Empiric antibiotic coverage may be considered while awaiting CSF culture results in the young, elderly, and immunocompromised, especially if there is suspicion of bacterial meningitis or partially treated bacterial meningitis.

Acyclovir (Zovirax) should be initiated in cases of suspected HSV while waiting PCR confirmation. Dosing of acyclovir is age and weight dependent: 20 mg/kg per dose IV every 8 hours for patients younger than 12 years; 10 mg/kg per dose IV every 8 hours for patients older than 12 years.

In the immunocompromised patient, HHV6 may be treated with foscarnet (Foscavir)[1] or ganciclovir (Cytovene)[1], and CMV may be treated with ganciclovir, valganciclovir (Valcyte), foscarnet, or cidofovir (Vistide). Case reports suggest benefit of such antiviral therapies in the immunocompromised, but no controlled trials have been performed.

Complications

The prognosis of viral meningitis depends on cause and severity of illness as well as age. Non-HSV viral meningitis has low mortality rates in adults and children alike. Mortality and morbidity are associated with other organ system involvement, including meningoencephalitis. Although up to 10% of infants hospitalized with non-HSV viral meningitis experience seizures, altered mental status, or increased intracranial pressure during the acute illness, studies have shown no evidence of long-term neurodevelopmental delay. Most adults recover fully within a week without long-term sequelae. Persistent neurologic sequelae (including headaches, incoordination, concentration difficulties, muscle weakness, and focal neurologic deficits) occur more often in patients with meningoencephalitis.

HSV is associated with high rates of morbidity and mortality. Neonatal isolated CNS HSV has a 4% mortality rate even with acyclovir treatment; mortality is 50% without acyclovir treatment. Unfortunately, acute treatment does not affect morbidity, as 70% of infants with neonatal CNS HSV infection will suffer from neurodevelopmental impairments. Recent studies have demonstrated improved outcomes in these infants with long-term oral acyclovir suppression therapy. Outside of the neonatal period, CNS HSV infection has a 28% mortality rate with antiviral treatment (70% mortality rate without treatment). Long-term neurologic sequelae occur in two-thirds of survivors who received antiviral therapy, compared with virtually all of those who did not receive treatment.

---

[1] Not FDA approved for this indication.

TABLE 1 Clinical and Laboratory Characteristics of Viral Meningitis

VIRUS	TRANSMISSION	KEY CLINICAL FEATURES	DIAGNOSIS	COMMENTS
Enterovirus	Fecal-oral	May have rash on exam (e.g., Coxsackie, hand–foot–mouth) Patients with impaired humoral immunity or those <2 wk old can present with a sepsis-like syndrome with multiorgan dysfunction, DIC, cardiovascular collapse	CSF enterovirus PCR	More prevalent in summer and fall
Herpes simplex viruses 1 and 2	Vertical transmission during birth (HSV2), horizontal transmission via contact (HSV1 or HSV2)	10%–30% of adults have symptoms of meningitis with primary HSV2 infection; look for genital vesicular lesions on exam Mollarets meningitis: >3 episodes of fever and meningismus lasting 2–5 d, with spontaneous resolution; episodes may be months to years apart often due to chronic HSV2 CNS infection	CSF HSV1/HSV2 PCR	Meningitis is uncommon with nonprimary HSV2 infection
Arboviruses	Subcutaneous inoculation via mosquito or tick Prevention: Minimize tick and mosquito exposure with personal protection measures including insect repellents and covering exposed skin	Zika virus associated with Guillan-Barré syndrome and in newborn infants microcephaly; sexual transmission is possible	CSF arboviral PCR Zika RT-PCR (performed at CDC Arbovirus laboratory on CSF or serum within first 5–7 days of symptoms); Zika IgM cross reacts with other flaviviruses (e.g., Dengue)	More prevalent in summer and fall Geographic distribution within the United States: Eastern equine encephalitis: Eastern U.S. Western equine encephalitis: Western U.S. St. Louis encephalitis: Across the U.S. (majority of cases in Central and Eastern U.S.) West Nile virus: Across the U.S. California encephalitis (LaCrosse): Midwestern, mid-Atlantic, and Southeastern U.S. Zika virus: Small epidemics have been reported in Southeastern U.S. and Gulf Coast states
Lymphocytic choriomeningitis virus	Virus is present in rodent secretions, feces, and urine Ingestion of contaminated food, exposure of open wounds, or inhalation of aerosolized virus Lab workers, pet owners, and those living in impoverished conditions are highest risk for illness	Accompanied by a flulike illness	Serum LCMV titers (acute and convalescent) CSF findings: May have decreased glucose and WBC count >1000/mL	More prevalent in winter and spring
Cytomegalovirus	Exposure to infected body fluids (e.g., saliva, blood)		CSF CMV PCR	Reactivation of prior infection typically only occurs in the immunosuppressed
Epstein–Barr virus	Exposure to infected body fluids (e.g., saliva, blood)	Alice in Wonderland syndrome: altered body image and distortion of visual perception	CSF EBV PCR	Most common neurologic complication with primary infection
HIV	Exposure to contaminated blood or other body fluids (e.g., transfusion, sexual contact, percutaneous blood exposure)	During primary infection, a subset have meningitis or meningoencephalitis May expect thrush and cervical lymphadenopathy	HIV studies	Treatment with HAART
Human herpesvirus 6	Respiratory	Roseola: febrile illness followed by viral exanthem	CSF HHV6 PCR	HHV6 has been demonstrated in the CSF of asymptomatic persons Immunosuppressed persons at risk for symptomatic infection and reactivation

VIRUS	TRANSMISSION	KEY CLINICAL FEATURES	DIAGNOSIS	COMMENTS
Varicella	Respiratory	Typical vesicular skin lesions of chickenpox on exam CSF pleocytosis has also been demonstrated with reactivation; can also occur in the absence of cutaneous findings of herpes zoster ("zoster sine herpete")	CSF VZV PCR	Rarely diagnosed during acute chickenpox infection; usually a postinfectious complication Other neurologic sequelae of varicella infection are more common than aseptic meningitis; most common is cerebellar ataxia
Mumps	Respiratory	Parotitis on exam is the most prominent sign of infection Aseptic meningitis can precede or follow clinical exam findings CSF profile can demonstrate an unusually high protein with a mild pleocytosis and normal glucose	Serum titers	More common in winter and spring
Measles	Respiratory	CSF pleocytosis in ≤30% of patients with measles; patients are usually without clinical meningitis	Serum titers	In the United States, most cases are imported (e.g., occur in returning travelers)
Influenza	Respiratory	Aseptic meningitis is a less common neurologic complication of influenza infection (encephalopathy is more common)	CSF influenza PCR	More prevalent in winter Increased risk of neurologic complication in young patients and in those with pre-existing medical disease

Abbreviations: CMV = cytomegalovirus; CNS = central nervous system; CSF = cerebrospinal fluid; DIC = disseminated intravascular coagulopathy; HHV = human herpesvirus; HSV = herpes simplex virus; LCMV = lymphocytic choriomeningitis virus; PCR = polymerase chain reaction; VZV = varicella zoster virus; WBC = white blood cell.

References

Centers for Disease Control and Prevention. Zika Virus. http://www.cdc.gov/zika/index.html. Accessed February 12, 2016.

Dubos F, Korczowski B, Aygun DA, et al.: Serum procalcitonin level and other biological markers to distinguish between bacterial and aseptic meningitis in children: a European multicenter case cohort study, *Arch Pediatr Adolesc Med* 162:1157–1163, 2008.

Hawkes MT, Vaudry W: Nonpolio enterovirus infection in the neonate and young infant, *Paediatr Child Health* 10:383–388, 2005.

James SH, Kimberlin DW, Whitley RJ: Antiviral therapy for herpesvirus central nervous system infections: neonatal herpes simplex virus infection, herpes simplex encephalitis, and congenital cytomegalovirus infection, *Antiviral Res* 83:207–213, 2009.

Khetsuriani N, Quiroz ES, Holman RC, Anderson LJ: Viral meningitis associated hospitalizations in the United States, 1988–1999, *Neuroepidemiology* 22:345–352, 2003.

Kimberlin DW, Lin CY, Jacobs RF, et al.: Safety and efficacy of high-dose intravenous acyclovir in the management of neonatal herpes simplex virus infections, *Pediatrics* 108:230–238, 2001.

Kimberlin DW, Whitley RJ, Wan W, et al.: Oral acyclovir suppression and neurodevelopment after neonatal herpes, *N Engl J Med* 365:1284–1292, 2011.

Nigrovic LE, Fine AM, Monuteaux MC, et al.: Trends in the management of viral meningitis at United States children's hospitals, *Pediatrics* 131:670–676, 2013. [PMID: 23530164].

Nigrovic LE, Kuppermann N, Macias CG, et al.: Clinical prediction rule for identifying children with cerebrospinal fluid pleocytosis at very low risk of bacterial meningitis, *JAMA* 297:52–60, 2007.

Rorabaugh ML, Berlin LE, Heldrich F, et al.: Aseptic meningitis in infants younger than 2 years of age: acute illness and neurologic complications, *Pediatrics* 92:206–211, 1993.

Rotbart HA: Viral meningitis, *Semin Neurol* 20:277–292, 2000.

Sakushima K, Hayashino Y, Kawaguchi T, et al.: Diagnostic accuracy of cerebrospinal fluid lactate for differentiating bacterial meningitis from aseptic meningitis: a meta-analysis, *J Infect* 62:255–262, 2011.

Viallon A, Zeni F, Lambert C, et al.: High sensitivity and specificity of serum procalcitonin levels in adults with bacterial meningitis, *Clin Infect Dis* 28:1313–1316, 1999.

10 Psychiatric Disorders

ALCOHOL USE DISORDERS

Method of
Richard N. Rosenthal, MD

CURRENT DIAGNOSIS

Risky or Hazardous Drinking (Need Further Evaluation)
- Men who drink more than four standard drinks per day or 14 standard drinks per week.
- Women and those older than 65 years who drink more than three standard drinks per day or more than seven standard drinks per week.
- Drinking concurrent with any medical condition where alcohol is contraindicated.

Alcohol Use Disorder
- Repeated failure to fulfill obligations at home, school, or work.
- Increased risk of physical harm.
- Drinking despite causing social or interpersonal problems.
- Episodes of alcohol craving or strong urges.
- Cannot cut down or stop.
- Decreased time spent in other usual activities.
- Drinking despite physical or psychological consequences.
- Drinking more than intended.
- Physical tolerance.
- Preoccupied with drinking.
- Withdrawal episodes.

CURRENT THERAPY

All At-Risk Patients
- Assess: Screen patients with standard instruments and compute average standard drinks per week.
- Advise: Give feedback, express concern, present findings and conclusions, and recommend specific behavioral changes.
- Agree: Determine the patient's readiness to change, encourage reflection, listen empathically, elicit patient concerns, avoid arguing, express optimism, set a specific reduction or abstinence goal.
- Assist: Formulate concrete implementation plan, including avoiding high-risk situations, recording alcohol intake, and eliciting family and community support for patient goals.
- Arrange: Set up follow-up visits and refer patients meeting dependence criteria for specialty treatment.

Additionally for Alcohol-Dependent Patients
- Offer or arrange for detoxification if indicated.
- Offer or arrange for specialty alcoholism treatment and/or mutual help groups.
- Offer pharmacotherapy to support maintenance of abstinence: naltrexone (ReVia, Vivitrol), acamprosate (Campral), or disulfiram (Antabuse).
- Offer medication management support during follow-up visits.

Epidemiology

Alcohol use disorders are among the most prevalent mental disorders in the population, occurring at frequencies that rival those of mood and anxiety disorders. In any year, almost 8.5% of the US population older than 18 years meets criteria for a formal alcohol use disorder (alcohol abuse or dependence), and almost 4% meets criteria for alcohol dependence.

Economic and Medical Sequelae

Alcohol use disorders are important to identify and treat for several reasons. The first is the direct negative impact of chronic heavy alcohol exposure on cognitive, physical, social, and vocational functioning. The second is the well-described long-term medical sequelae of alcohol dependence such as hepatic cirrhosis, pancreatitis, and dementia. Chronic heavy drinking, even in the absence of a formal diagnosis of alcohol dependence, is associated with an increased risk of diabetes mellitus, hypertension, gastrointestinal bleeding, hemorrhagic stroke, and several forms of carcinoma. The third reason for identification and treatment is the public impact of alcohol use disorders, which covers associated traumatic injuries from motor vehicle and job-related accidents, alcohol-related crime, and their associated economic costs. More than $180 billion is lost to the US economy each year as a result of alcohol-related crime, injury, healthcare costs, and lost productivity in the workplace.

Screening
Screening Rationale
Screening for alcohol problems arrays patients on a continuum from abstinence to dependence and is a highly efficient way to identify patients who are at acute risk for the effects of alcohol abuse and dependence as well as those who do not currently meet formal alcohol-related diagnoses but who are at risk for long-term medical and social consequences of heavy alcohol exposure (Box 1). The US Preventative Services Task Force (USPSTF) found that screening could accurately identify patients whose levels or patterns of alcohol consumption do not meet criteria for alcohol dependence but that place them at risk for increased morbidity and mortality. The USPSTF also found good evidence that brief interventions that consist of behavioral counseling and follow-up can reduce alcohol consumption for 6 to 12 months or longer and that the benefits outweigh any potential harms. Thus, it is recommended that alcohol screening and brief interventions be performed in primary care settings to reduce alcohol problems for adults, including pregnant women.

Brief Screening
Every patient should be asked about alcohol use. Because drinking is normative in the United States, if drinking is denied, it is useful to determine if the patient used to drink but has stopped because of a past problem. After determining if a patient currently uses any alcohol, the simplest strategy is to ask about the number of heavy drinking days in the past year, where heavy drinking is defined as more than five drinks for men and more than four drinks for women in one day. If that threshold is reached (0 = negative screen; >0 = positive screen), which corresponds to at-risk or hazardous drinking, then further evaluation of alcohol-related problems is indicated through the use of screening instruments,

---

BOX 1 Current Risk Terms

Abstinence
- No alcohol use.

Moderate Drinking
- Men: No more than 2 standard drinks per drinking day.
- Women: No more than 1 standard drink per drinking day.
- Elderly persons (>65 years): No more than 1 standard drink per drinking day.

Risky or Hazardous Drinking
- Men
  - More than 4 standard drinks per drinking day.
  - More than 14 standard drinks per week.
- Women
  - More than 3 standard drinks per drinking day.
  - More than 7 standard drinks per week.
- Elderly persons (>65 years):
  - More than 3 standard drinks per drinking day.
  - More than 7 standard drinks per week.

BOX 2 Standard Drinks

Each equivalent drink contains about 14 g of pure alcohol:
- 12 oz of beer or wine cooler
- 8–9 oz of malt liquor
- 5 oz of wine
- 3–4 oz of fortified wine (e.g., port)
- 1½ oz of 80-proof distilled spirits (or 1 jigger of liquor before mixing)

---

such as the three-item AUDIT-C, in the following. A standard drink is the same amount of alcohol contained in different volumes of alcoholic beverages (Box 2).

The Alcohol Use Disorders Identification Test (AUDIT) (Table 1) is a 10-item screen developed by the World Health Organization. Given its length, the AUDIT can be used as a self-report screener that patients can fill out in the waiting area before seeing the clinician. The minimum score is 0 and the maximum score is 40. A score of 8 or more for men or 4 or more for women, adolescents, and persons older than 65 years, like a positive endorsement of any heavy drinking days, indicates the need for further evaluation of alcohol use and an increased risk of an alcohol use disorder. For brevity, the AUDIT-C, a truncated version of the AUDIT consisting of the first three AUDIT questions focused on alcohol consumption, can be used as a part of a waiting-room health history form. A score of 6 or more for men or 4 or more for women on the AUDIT-C indicates a need for further evaluation.

Asking about alcohol consumption during a routine clinical interview is best bundled with other questions about lifestyle and health, such as diet, smoking, and exercise. In addition to giving the patient a pre-examination questionnaire to fill out such as the AUDIT, another screening strategy is to ask the CAGE questions (Box 3) during the clinical examination. A positive answer to any of these questions also indicates the need for further evaluation of alcohol use. Two or more CAGE questions answered affirmatively identifies a patient at high risk for alcohol dependence. Because the CAGE screens for consequences, it is not as sensitive for risky drinking.

There are other question sets that are more sensitive than the CAGE in specific demographic subsets, and these can also be easily asked during a routine history. The five-item TWEAK questionnaire (Table 2) may be a more optimal screening questionnaire for identifying women (including pregnant women) with risky drinking or alcohol use disorders in racially mixed populations. The CRAFFT (Box 4) is a six-item question set that has high sensitivity in screening adolescents for alcohol and other substance-abuse problems. For patients older than 65 years, the Short Michigan Alcoholism Screening Test—Geriatric (S-MAST-G) (Box 5) is useful in identifying those at risk for alcohol problems, because these patients might not need the same volumes of alcohol intake as others to develop alcohol-related problems. To complete the initial screening, one should compute the average number of drinks per week by multiplying the days per week on average that the patient drinks by the number of drinks consumed on a typical drinking day.

Laboratory testing for elevations of alanine aminotransferase (ALT), aspartate aminotransferase (AST), γ-glutamyltransferase (GGT), or carbohydrate-deficient transferrin (CDT) have no incremental sensitivity over those of validated screening instruments, and they may be better suited to monitoring patients already in treatment for alcohol use disorders. The patient must still be asked about quantity and frequency of alcohol use. However, laboratory testing can provide indicators of covert heavy drinking (e.g., elevated GGT and CDT) when the patient does not reveal the extent of alcohol intake. CDT, which is perturbed less than other indices by nonalcoholic liver disease, may be a more specific and sensitive indicator of heavy drinking.

Diagnosis

Screening can identify those who are at risk for the sequelae of risky or hazardous drinking and who might benefit from a brief intervention conducted in the primary care office, but only a diagnostic evaluation can confirm the clinician's suspicion that the patient's use of alcohol meets syndromal criteria and warrants specific medical and psychosocial treatment beyond the brief intervention. According to *Diagnostic and Statistical Manual of Mental Disorders*, fifth edition (DSM-5) criteria (Table 3), the patient has a diagnosis of an alcohol use disorder if he or she has two or more of the following criteria over a 12-month period related to alcohol use: physical tolerance; symptoms of withdrawal; repeatedly drinking more than intended; unsuccessful reduction or quit attempts; repeated episodes of failure to fulfill obligations at home, school, or work; episodes of increased risk of physical harm; recurrent problems with significant others; increased time drinking or recovering from drinking; reduced time in other pleasurable or important activities; and continued drinking despite physical or psychological problems. With DSM-5, the term *alcohol dependence* describes the symptoms of physical tolerance and withdrawal, not the use disorder syndrome. Severity is defined as: Mild, 2 to 3 symptoms; Moderate, 4 to 5 symptoms; and Severe, 6 or more symptoms.

Rates of co-occurring mood and anxiety disorders are especially high among those with alcohol use disorders. Untreated mood and anxiety disorders tend to have a negative impact on alcoholism recovery. Among treatment-seeking patients in the National Epidemiologic Survey on Alcohol and Related Conditions (NESARC) sample with a current alcohol use disorder, 40% had at least one current independent mood disorder, and more than one-third had at least one current independent anxiety disorder. Heavy alcohol intake can also induce symptoms of mood and other mental disorders. To differentiate alcohol-induced symptoms from independent disorders, it is optimal to reassess symptoms of a mental disorder several weeks after cessation or significant reduction of alcohol intake.

Brief Intervention

Intention

Although risky or hazardous drinking is not a formal diagnosis, it describes a group with a higher likelihood to develop alcohol problems with risk for accidents, injuries, and social and health problems compared with the general population (see Box 1). Thus, even without a formal diagnosis, it is beneficial to help the patient with risky drinking to change his or her drinking behavior. Several well-described short interchanges between the clinician and the patient, organized under the rubric of *brief interventions*,

TABLE 1 Alcohol Use Disorders Identification Test (AUDIT)

QUESTIONS	SCORING				
	0	**1**	**2**	**3**	**4**
Consumption (AUDIT-C)					
How often do you have a drink containing alcohol?	Never	Monthly or less	2–4 times a month	2–3 times a week	4 or more times a week
How many drinks containing alcohol do you have on a typical day when you are drinking?	1 or 2	3 or 4	5 or 6	7–9	10 or more
How often do you have five or more drinks on one occasion?	Never	Less than monthly	Monthly	Weekly	Daily or almost daily
Personal Consequences					
How often during the last year have you found that you were not able to stop drinking once you had started?	Never	Less than monthly	Monthly	Weekly	Daily or almost daily
How often during the last year have you failed to do what was normally expected of you because of drinking?	Never	Less than monthly	Monthly	Weekly	Daily or almost daily
How often during the last year have you needed a first drink in the morning to get yourself going after a heavy drinking session?	Never	Less than monthly	Monthly	Weekly	Daily or almost daily
How often during the last year have you had a feeling of guilt or remorse after drinking?	Never	Less than monthly	Monthly	Weekly	Daily or almost daily
How often during the last year have you been unable to remember what happened the night before because of your drinking?	Never	Less than monthly	Monthly	Weekly	Daily or almost daily
Social Consequences					
Have you or someone else been injured because of your drinking?	No		Yes, but not in the last year		Yes, during the last year
Has a relative, friend, doctor, or other healthcare worker been concerned about your drinking or suggested you cut down?	No		Yes, but not in the last year		Yes, during the last year
Scoring and Interpretation					
Add all scores to obtain a total: >8 points for men or >4 points for women indicates a high risk of alcohol use disorder.					
AUDIT-C (first three AUDIT questions): >6 points for men or >4 points for women indicates a need for further evaluation.					

BOX 3 CAGE Questionnaire

- Have you ever felt that you should *Cut down* on your drinking?
- Have people *Annoyed* you by criticizing your drinking?
- Have you ever felt bad or *Guilty* about your drinking?
- Have you ever taken a drink *(Eye opener)* first thing in the morning to steady your nerves or to get rid of a hangover?
One yes response indicates need for further assessment. Two yes responses indicate risk of an alcohol use disorder.

TABLE 2 TWEAK Questionnaire

FEATURE	QUESTION	ANSWER	SCORE
Tolerance	How many drinks does it take before you begin to feel the first effects of alcohol?	≥3	2
Worry	Have your friends or relatives worried or complained about your drinking in the past year?	Yes	2
Eye-opener	Do you sometimes take a drink in the morning when you first get up?	Yes	1
Amnesia	Are there times when you drink and afterward you can't remember what you said or did?	Yes	1
Kut	Do you sometimes feel the need to cut down on your drinking?	Yes	1
Scoring and interpretation: Two or more points indicate a possible alcohol problem.			

have been validated in randomized trials as decreasing alcohol intake in those who drink too much but do not have a diagnosis of alcohol dependence. Brief intervention has been demonstrated to reduce weekly alcohol use, frequency of binging, liver enzymes associated with heavy drinking, blood pressure, emergency department visits, hospital days, and psychosocial problems, typically for 6 to 12 months, and to reduce drinking and hospital days at up to 4 years in one study. Because most at-risk patients seen in primary care settings are subsyndromal for alcohol use disorders, the typical clinical interaction related to alcohol will be that of screening and then a brief intervention for positive cases. The two are typically referred to together under the acronym SBI (screening and brief intervention).

The basic intention of a brief intervention is to educate the patient about the risks of heavy alcohol use in such a way as to motivate him or her to reduce weekly alcohol consumption. The standard initial brief intervention takes about 15 minutes and

consists of feedback, advice, and goal setting. It can be performed wholly in the primary care setting by the physician or other members of the health delivery team. Including alcohol screening, the USPSTF suggests five **A**'s to conducting SBI: *assess* the patient's alcohol consumption with a screening tool and clinical evaluation

BOX 4 CRAFFT Questionnaire

- Have you ever ridden in a **C**ar driven by someone (including yourself) who was high or had been using alcohol or drugs?
- Do you ever use alcohol or drugs to **R**elax, feel better about yourself, or fit in?
- Do you ever use alcohol or drugs while you are **A**lone?
- Do you ever **F**orget things you did while using alcohol or drugs?
- Do your **F**amily or Friends ever tell you that you should cut down on your drinking or drug use?
- Have you ever gotten into **T**rouble while you were using alcohol or drugs?

One yes response indicates need for further assessment. Two yes responses indicate risk of alcohol use disorder.

BOX 5 S-MAST-G Questionnaire

- When talking with others, do you ever underestimate how much you actually drink?
- After a few drinks, have you sometimes not eaten or been able to skip meals because you didn't feel hungry?
- Does having a few drinks help decrease your shakiness or tremors?
- Does alcohol sometimes make it hard for you to remember parts of the day or night?
- Do you usually take a drink to relax or calm your nerves?
- Do you drink to take your mind off your problems?
- Have you ever increased your drinking after experiencing a loss in your life?
- Has a doctor or nurse ever said that he or she was worried or concerned about your drinking?
- Have you ever made rules to manage your drinking?
- When you feel lonely, does having a drink help?

Two or more yes responses indicate a probable alcohol problem.

S-MAST-G, Short Michigan Alcoholism Screening Test—Geriatric.

TABLE 3 Diagnosis of Alcohol Use Problems

CRITERIA	TYPICAL SYMPTOMS AND HISTORY
Alcohol Use Disorder (≥2 in the last 12 months)	
Alcohol has caused or contributed to repeated:	
Failure to fulfill obligations at home, school, or work	Hangovers at work, truancy at school, missing appointments
Episodes of increased risk of physical harm	Driving, swimming, or operating machinery under the influence of alcohol
Craving, or a strong desire or urge to use alcohol	Inability to refrain from drinking due to strong impulses
Problems with significant others	Spousal strife, physical fights
Development of physical tolerance	Drinks more for the same effect
Episodes of withdrawal syndrome (see below)	Morning shakes, nausea, anxiety
Drinking more than intended repeatedly	Binging episodes
Unsuccessful efforts to cut down or stop drinking	Failed New Year's resolution
Increased time planning for drinking, or recovering from drinking	Instead of being with kids, spends weekend mornings sleeping in
Reduced time in other pleasurable or important activities	Stopped socializing with friends, withdrew from hobby group
Drinking persists despite physical or psychological problems	Developed depressed mood, but kept on drinking
Alcohol Withdrawal (≥2 within h to days after lowered blood alcohol levels)	
Autonomic hyperactivity	Heart rate ≥ 100 bpm, diaphoresis
Hand tremor	Hands shake when extended
Insomnia	Difficulty falling asleep
Nausea or vomiting	Feels queasy
Anxiety	Spontaneous report of fear
Psychomotor agitation	Inability to keep still, pacing
Hallucinations or illusions	Reports visual disturbances
Seizures	Tonic-clonic movements

as indicated; *advise* reduction of alcohol consumption to appropriate levels, including abstinence if indicated; *agree* on individual goals for reducing alcohol use, including abstinence if indicated; *assist* patients in obtaining the motivation, skills, or supports needed to institute changes in drinking; and *arrange* for follow-up support, including specialty treatment referral for dependent patients. The most effective interventions are multicontact ones that provide ongoing assistance and follow-up.

Procedure

Assess

Screen patients with the AUDIT or with the CAGE, TWEAK, CRAFFT, or S-MAST-G questionnaires as appropriate, and compute average drinks per week.

Advise

Give feedback in the form of expression of concern, direct conclusions, and recommendations. Present medical findings, such as elevated liver enzymes, to back up conclusive statements such as "I'm concerned that your alcohol intake exceeds safe limits." Show the patient information comparing use with population norms and the associated health risks. Educate the patient about how alcohol can lead to medical, psychosocial, and legal consequences. Where possible, link the patient's current symptoms to alcohol use. Recommend appropriate and specific changes in behavior, such as "I strongly recommend you cut down your drinking," or in the case in which any drinking places the patient at high risk, "I strongly suggest you quit drinking."

Agree

Determine the patient's readiness to change drinking behavior, such as asking, "Do you think that cutting down on your drinking is something you are willing to talk about?" If the patient is ambivalent, avoid labeling the patient's behavior with a diagnosis at this stage, which can increase resistance to change, but encourage the patient to reflect on the positive reasons for drinking and the negative consequences of drinking. Offer concerns that continued drinking at the same level will impede the patient's achievement of goals such as decreased gastric distress or improved sleep patterns.

Empathic listening is generally more effective than a confrontational approach, and it is useful to express optimism about the patient's capacity to change. Elicit what the patient's concerns are about cutting down or quitting. Avoid arguing or challenging when the patient is unready to change, but schedule a follow-up visit to continue the dialogue and reassess drinking behavior. Restate your commitment to help when the patient is ready and that you remain open to questions.

When the patient concurs that a change in drinking would be beneficial, agree on a specific goal to cut down to particular daily and weekly limits for low-risk drinking or to stop drinking, if indicated, for a specific period of time. The agreement should be recorded and a copy given to the patient both as a reminder and motivator for behavioral change.

Assist

Work with the patient to formulate concrete steps to implement the drinking reduction plan. These steps include how to avoid high-risk drinking situations, how to keep a record of alcohol intake, and who can support the patient in meeting his or her goals. Provide resources in the form of patient educational materials, examples of which can be downloaded from the National Institute of Alcohol Abuse and Alcoholism (NIAAA) website (www.niaaa.nih.gov).

Arrange

Set up follow-up support and counseling visits or refer patients meeting dependence criteria for specialty treatment. Advise the patient to seek immediate medical treatment if withdrawal symptoms occur.

Treatment

Detoxification

Put simply, detoxification is medical stabilization that offers an opportunity to engage patients in alcoholism treatment, but it is not in itself treatment for alcohol dependence. Patients who drink more than 250 g of alcohol daily are likely to experience physiologic withdrawal symptoms on cessation of drinking, but volume is not the only predictor of withdrawal severity. Although often mild, untreated alcohol withdrawal can result in seizures or delirium tremens (DTs), with increased risk of mortality.

Assessment

The Clinical Institute Withdrawal Assessment for Alcohol Scale, Revised (CIWA-Ar) is a public domain scale that scores 10 signs and symptoms of withdrawal by severity ranging from not present to severe (Box 6). A score of less than 8 indicates mild withdrawal, characterized by increased autonomic activity with low-grade anxiety, diaphoresis, agitation, nausea, and elevated blood pressure, temperature, and heart rate. Scores of 8 to 15 indicate moderate withdrawal, and scores of 15 or more indicate more severe withdrawal states. In severe withdrawal, in the context of autonomic hyperarousal, the patient can become disoriented and have a clouded sensorium—the hallmarks of delirium.

Prior history of severe withdrawal, such as DTs, is a reasonable predictor of similar future responses to alcohol withdrawal. Risk for withdrawal delirium is increased if the patient has a heart rate of greater than 120 bpm before treatment, a current infectious disease, withdrawal symptoms in the context of a blood alcohol concentration greater than 100 mg/dL, a prior history of either delirium or seizures, or a high CIWA-Ar score, indicating severe autonomic hyperactivity. Patients who have severe withdrawal symptoms, who are at high risk for seizures, or who have a medical condition likely to be exacerbated by withdrawal, such as type 1 diabetes or coronary artery disease, should have medically supervised inpatient detoxification.

Pharmacologic Therapy

Alcohol withdrawal is best treated with sedative hypnotic medications that are cross-tolerant with alcohol, such as benzodiazepines. Longer-acting benzodiazepines such as diazepam (Valium) and chlordiazepoxide (Librium) are easier to titrate against withdrawal symptoms and give a gradual offset in plasma concentration, but shorter-acting benzodiazepines such as lorazepam (Ativan)[1] are less likely to oversedate the patient. Rapid-onset benzodiazepines have a higher abuse liability and are generally best avoided. However, patients with severe hepatic impairment (elevated total bilirubin) are best treated with benzodiazepines that are not oxidized by the liver, such as oxazepam (Serax) or lorazepam.

Typical dosing is chlordiazepoxide 50 to 100 mg, diazepam 10 to 20 mg, oxazepam 20 to 40[3] mg, or lorazepam 2 to 4 mg. The typical front-loading style of dosing is to administer medication at the higher end of the dose range every 1 to 2 hours so that the CIWA-Ar score is less than 8 for 24 hours.

With long-acting medications, once symptoms subside, there is often no need to taper doses. The short-acting benzodiazepines and long-acting benzodiazepines given to patients at high-risk for seizures or DTs are best given on a fixed-dose regimen of four times daily for the first 24 hours, with the patient reassessed 1 to 2 hours after each dose, and additional medication given as needed. On days 2 and 3, 50% of the dose can be given four times daily.

Long-acting barbiturates, such as phenobarbital, can be also used on a fixed-dose regimen of 60 mg every 4 to 6 hours, with a loading dose of 120 mg orally or intramuscularly every hour for acute withdrawal symptoms (e.g., pulse >110 bpm) or a CIWA-Ar score of 10 or more.

Anticonvulsants such as carbamazepine (Tegretol), valproate (Depakote), or gabapentin (Neurontin) have also been used effectively in uncomplicated withdrawal, but they are unproved in preventing withdrawal-related seizures and in treating DTs.

Although phenothiazines and haloperidol (Haldol) are somewhat effective compared with benzodiazepines in reducing withdrawal symptoms such as agitation, they are not as protective against seizures or delirium and thus are not recommended.

Thiamine (vitamin B_1) supplementation of 100 mg/day for 3 days can counteract the thiamine deficiencies that are common in alcoholic patients.

Psychosocial Interventions for Alcohol Use Disorder

In addition to brief interventions for risky alcohol use, the most opportune and practical psychosocial intervention that the primary care office can provide is clinical behavioral support for pharmacotherapy for alcohol dependence. Simply put, medication management support consists initially of feedback to the patient of screening and medical evaluation results and the negative health effects of continued heavy drinking, as in a brief intervention. The patient is then given the basis for the diagnosis of alcohol dependence, the rationale for abstinence, and recommendation for pharmacotherapy. The patient is given information about medication and the appropriate prescriptions and is encouraged to seek community support for sobriety in mutual help groups such as Alcoholics Anonymous or to follow a plan such as Rational Recovery. Follow-up visits consist of assessment of medication side effects, patient adherence to the medication regimen, assessment of abstinence or quantity and pattern of alcohol intake, and assessment of overall functioning. Problems with medication adherence are identified and addressed.

There are evidence-based psychosocial interventions that are typically performed in the context of specialty programs for alcohol dependence, but they can be offered by clinical personnel in the context of the physician's office. Cognitive behavior therapy, network therapy, behavioral family therapy, and motivational interviewing are effective approaches for the treatment of alcohol dependence. Motivational interviewing is especially adaptable for use in primary care settings in that it is an approach to interacting with the alcohol-dependent patient that can be learned quickly and executed by any staff with clinical contact. A motivational enhancement manual can be accessed at the NIAAA website (http://www.niaaa.nih.gov/).

Medication Management of Alcohol Dependence

There are currently four US Food and Drug Administration (FDA)-approved medications for the treatment of alcohol dependence. Any of these medications can and should be given concurrently with other interventions such as psychosocial treatment or mutual help groups.

Disulfiram (Antabuse) works by inhibiting the metabolism of ethyl alcohol, causing a buildup of acetaldehyde, a noxious

BOX 6 Clinical Institute Withdrawal Assessment for Alcohol Scale, Revised (CIWA-Ar)

Patient:_____ Date:_____ Time:_____ (24-hour clock, midnight = 00:00)

Pulse or heart rate, taken for 1 minute:_____ Blood pressure:_____ mm Hg

Nausea and Vomiting—Ask, "Do you feel sick to your stomach? Have you vomited?" Observation:
0 no nausea and no vomiting
1 mild nausea with no vomiting
2
3
4 intermittent nausea with dry heaves
5
6
7 constant nausea, frequent dry heaves, and vomiting

Tremor—Arms extended and fingers spread apart. Observation:
0 no tremor
1 not visible, but can be felt fingertip to fingertip
2
3
4 moderate, with patient's arms extended
5
6
7 severe, even with arms not extended

Paroxysmal Sweats—Observation:
0 no sweat visible
1 barely perceptible sweating, palms moist
2
3
4 beads of sweat obvious on forehead
5
6
7 drenching sweats

Anxiety—Ask, "Do you feel nervous?" Observation:
0 no anxiety, at ease
1 mild anxious
2
3
4 moderately anxious, or guarded, so anxiety is inferred
5
6
7 equivalent to acute panic states as seen in severe delirium or acute schizophrenic reactions

Agitation—Observation:
0 normal activity
1 somewhat more than normal activity
2
3
4 moderately fidgety and restless
5
6
7 paces back and forth during most of the interview or constantly thrashes about

Tactile Disturbances—Ask, "Have you any itching, pins and needles sensations, any burning, any numbness, or do you feel bugs crawling on or under your skin?" Observation:
0 none
1 very mild itching, pins and needles, burning, or numbness
2 mild itching, pins and needles, burning, or numbness
3 moderate itching, pins and needles, burning, or numbness
4 moderately severe hallucinations
5 severe hallucinations
6 extremely severe hallucinations
7 continuous hallucinations

Auditory Disturbances—Ask, "Are you more aware of sounds around you? Are they harsh? Do they frighten you? Are you hearing anything that is disturbing to you? Are you hearing things you know are not there?" Observation:
0 not present
1 very mild harshness or ability to frighten
2 mild harshness or ability to frighten
3 moderate harshness or ability to frighten
4 moderately severe hallucinations
5 severe hallucinations
6 extremely severe hallucinations
7 continuous hallucinations

Visual Disturbances—Ask, "Does the light appear to be too bright? Is its color different? Does it hurt your eyes? Are you seeing anything that is disturbing to you? Are you seeing things you know are not there?" Observation:
0 not present
1 very mild sensitivity
2 mild sensitivity
3 moderate sensitivity
4 moderately severe hallucinations
5 severe hallucinations
6 extremely severe hallucinations
7 continuous hallucinations

Headache, Fullness in Head—Ask, "Does your head feel different? Does it feel like there is a band around your head?" Do not rate for dizziness or lightheadedness. Otherwise, rate severity:
0 not present
1 very mild
2 mild
3 moderate
4 moderately severe
5 severe
6 very severe
7 extremely severe

Orientation and Clouding of Sensorium—Ask, "What day is this? Where are you? Who am I?"
0 oriented and can do serial additions
1 cannot do serial additions or is uncertain about date
2 disoriented for date by no more than 2 calendar days
3 disoriented for date by more than 2 calendar days
4 disoriented for place or person

Total CIWA-Ar Score_____
Rater's Initials_____
Maximum Possible Score: 67

The CIWA-Ar *is not* copyright and may be reproduced freely. This assessment for monitoring withdrawal symptoms requires approximately 5 min to administer.

From Sullivan JT, Sykora K, Schneiderman J, et al. Assessment of alcohol withdrawal: The revised Clinical Institute Withdrawal Assessment for Alcohol scale (CIWA-Ar). *Br J Addiction.* 1989;84:1353–1357.

substance, which causes a strong stereotypic aversive response (flushing, diaphoresis, nausea, tachycardia) in the patient. Standard dosing is 250 mg/day (range, 125 to 500 mg). The major clinical concern with disulfiram is patient noncompliance with the medication regimen. Thus, it is most likely to be effective when there is a concrete method for supporting compliance in place, such as directly observed therapy by a spouse or in a clinic.

More recently, the opioid antagonist naltrexone (ReVia) was approved for the treatment of alcohol dependence. It is dosed at 50 mg orally once daily. Naltrexone reduces days of heavy drinking and can reduce alcohol craving. Naltrexone in a long-acting intramuscular formulation (Vivitrol) allows once-monthly dosing (380 mg) and reduces the risk of noncompliance. It reduces heavy drinking overall and helps maintain abstinence in those who are abstinent at initial drug administration. Both oral and intramuscular (IM) naltrexone formulations carry FDA black-box warnings related to findings of reversible elevations of liver enzymes at three to six times the standard dosage; however, naltrexone is safe at the recommended dose.

Acamprosate (Campral) is a taurine analogue that has been demonstrated to reduce relapse to any drinking as well as reducing heavy drinking in nonabstinent patients. It is dosed as two 333-mg tablets three times a day to patients who have ceased alcohol intake. It is excreted unchanged through the kidneys and has no interactions with other medications. The side effects are benign, and the most frequent is loose stools, which are mild to moderate and self-limited.

Topiramate (Topamax)[1] titrated over 5 weeks between 50 and 300 mg daily appears to reduce heavy drinking and days of any drinking over the short term (12 weeks) in alcohol-dependent patients who have not established abstinence prior to treatment. Common side effects include paresthesias, taste perversion, decreased appetite, and difficulty concentrating.

---

[1] Not FDA approved for this indication.

References

American Psychiatric Association: In *American Psychiatric Association: Diagnostic and statistical manual of mental disorders, 5th ed. (DSM-5)*, Washington, DC, 2013, American Psychiatric Publishing (DSM-5).

Bertholet N, Daeppen J-B, Wietlisbach V, et al: Reduction of alcohol consumption by brief alcohol intervention in primary care systematic review and meta-analysis, *Arch Intern Med* 165:986–995, 2005.

Bradley KA, Boyd-Wickizer J, Powell SH, Burman ML: Alcohol screening questionnaires in women: a critical review, *JAMA* 280:166–171, 1998.

Fleming MF, Mundt MP, French MT, et al: Brief physician advice for problem drinkers: long-term efficacy and cost-benefit analysis, *Alcohol Clin Exp Res* 26:36–43, 2002.

Grant BF, Stinson FS, Dawson DA, et al: Prevalence and co-occurrence of substance use disorders and independent mood and anxiety disorders: results from the National Epidemiologic Survey on Alcohol and Related Conditions, *Arch Gen Psychiatry* 61:807–816, 2004.

Johnson BA, Rosenthal N, Capece JA, et al: Topiramate for treating alcohol dependence: a randomized controlled trial, *JAMA* 298:1641–1651, 2007.

Knight JR, Sherritt L, Shrier LA, et al: Validity of the CRAFFT substance abuse screening test among adolescent clinic patients, *Arch Pediatr Adolesc Med* 156(6):607–614, 2002.

Kranzler HR, Knapp CM, Ciraulo DA: Alcohol. In Kranzler HR, Ciraulo DA, Zindel LR, editors: *Clinical Manual of Addiction Psychopharmacology*, Washington, DC, 2014, American Psychiatric Publishing, pp 1–69.

Maisto SA, Saitz R: Alcohol use disorders: Screening and diagnosis, *Am J Addict* 12(Suppl. 1):S12–S25, 2003.

McCaul ME, Petry NM: The role of psychosocial treatments in pharmacotherapy for alcoholism, *Am J Addict* 12(Suppl. 1):S41–S52, 2003.

McNeely J, Cleland CM, Strauss SM, et al: Validation of self-administered single-item screening questions (SISQs) for unhealthy alcohol and drug use in primary care patients, *J Gen Intern Med* 30:1757–1764, 2015.

National Institute on Alcohol Abuse and Alcoholism: *Helping patients who drink too much: a clinician's guide*, Rockville, MD, 2005, National Institute on Alcohol Abuse and Alcoholism, Available at http://pubs.niaaa.nih.gov/publications/Practitioner/CliniciansGuide2005/guide.pdf. Accessed 20 July 2014.

Saitz R: Unhealthy alcohol use, *N Engl J Med* 352:596–607, 2005.

Saunders JB, Aasland OG, Babor TF, et al: Development of the Alcohol Use Disorders Screening Test (AUDIT) WHO collaborative project on early detection of persons with harmful alcohol consumption, *Addiction* 88:791–804, 1993.

Sullivan JT, Sykora K, Schneiderman J, et al: Assessment of alcohol withdrawal: the revised Clinical Institute Withdrawal Assessment for Alcohol scale (CIWA-Ar), *Br J Addict* 84:1353–1357, 1989.

U.S. Preventive Services Task Force: Screening and behavioral counseling interventions in primary care to reduce alcohol misuse: recommendation statement, *Ann Intern Med* 140:554–556, 2004.

AUTISM

Method of
Rachel Brown, MBBS

CURRENT DIAGNOSIS

- Autism spectrum disorder (ASD) is characterized by the presence of persistent deficits in social communication and social interaction as well as by restricted, repetitive patterns of behavior, interests, or activities
- Symptoms must be present in the early developmental period, cause clinically significant impairment in important areas of functioning, and not be better explained by intellectual disability or global developmental delay.
- ASD may co-occur with intellectual disability, language impairment, with another medical, genetic, environmental, neurodevelopmental, mental or behavioral disorder, or with catatonia.
- Patients with ASD require different levels of support.

CURRENT TREATMENT

- Early identification and intensive intervention is associated with improved outcomes.
- Intervention should start in early childhood and may need to be lifelong. It should focus on improving functional independence through structured education, supported employment and daily living, therapy focused on social skills and communication, and behavioral therapy, especially applied behavioral analysis (ABA).
- Ongoing surveillance and the management of co-occurring medical (sleep, constipation, etc.) and psychiatric (ADHD, anxiety, etc.) conditions is important.
- No biomedical agent reliably improves the core symptoms.
- Stimulants, guanfacine (Intuniv), and atomoxetine (Strattera) have shown benefit for co-occurring ADHD. Treatment of anxiety and depression should follow practice guidelines for those conditions. Antipsychotic agents, such as risperidone (Risperdal) and aripiprazole (Abilify), reduce symptomatic challenging behaviors. However, potential adverse effects include weight gain, sedation, and extrapyramidal symptoms.

Epidemiology

Older epidemiologic studies suggested that autism spectrum disorder (ASD) was a rare disorder, with a prevalence of only 4 in every 10,000 population. With time, estimates of prevalence have steadily increased, and current estimates are 0.6% to 0.7%, with some as high as 1% to 2%. The reasons for the increase are not completely known. Improved awareness of the disorder, especially in those less severely affected, and broader diagnostic criteria have played a significant role. However, a real increase in prevalence remains a possibility. Approximately 45% of individuals with ASD also have intellectual disability.

Studies have consistently shown that males with ASD outnumber females by a factor of at least 2–3 to 1. Older studies placed the male predominance even higher, and there is a suggestion that females have been historically under-recognized. Girls are diagnosed somewhat later in life, and studies suggest that more concurrent behavioral or cognitive problems need to be present in girls for the disorder to be recognized. Around a third of individuals with ASD have a pattern of regression (loss of previously acquired skill) occurring in the second year of life.

Risk Factors, Etiology, and Pathophysiology

The theory that ASD is the consequence of maternal mistreatment has been disproven, and there is no evidence that ASD is caused by vaccination. Both genetic and environmental factors probably play a role. Studies have consistently shown a familial pattern for ASD. Twin studies demonstrate a much higher concordance for monozygotic twins (between 80% and 90%), compared to dizygotic and other siblings, where the risk ranges from around 7% to as high as 20%. The data is somewhat complicated because of the recognition of a so-called "broader autism phenotype" that includes milder but qualitatively similar features to the defining features of autism. Some conditions with known genetic etiology are associated with high rates of ASD. Those include fragile X, Rett, tuberose sclerosis, Down, Angelman, and a variety of others. For the majority of patients with ASD, however, specific syndromes are not present, and the search for a single "autism gene" has been fruitless. Instead, a wide variety of genes are probably associated with ASD susceptibility. Many of the genes are related to transcriptional control, chromatin remodeling, protein synthesis and cellular metabolism, and synapse development and function. Although the estimated heritability of ASD is relatively high, environmental factors also play a part. Recognized risk factors include older maternal and paternal age, gestational hypertension and diabetes, prematurity, and maternal immune activation. Studies of the neurobiology of autism suggest that autism is associated with atypical neural connectivity, and is a problem of neural networks, rather than a structurally discrete abnormality. One commonly reported feature is generalized brain overgrowth in the first 2 years of life, manifested by a larger than average head circumference in a portion of patients with ASD. Studies have also shown some consistent neurologic abnormalities of both white and grey matter in a variety of brain regions, as well as evidence of cortical dysgenesis. Alterations in serotonin and γ-aminobutyric-acid (GABA) systems, as well as oxytocin, vasopressin, and androgens/estrogens are under active investigation. Information about the genetics and neurobiology of this condition are rapidly evolving. It is likely that, in time, ASD may be subclassified into a number of related conditions, each of which may be diagnosed and treated differently, according to the underlying etiology.

Clinical Manifestations

For the diagnosis of ASD to be made, patients must have both persistent deficits in social communication and interaction as well as repetitive, restrictive behaviors emerging in early childhood (Table 1). Human beings, including children and young babies, are inherently social and interaction seeking. However, in patients with ASD, social approach and interaction is either absent or qualitatively abnormal. In some patients, the onset of abnormality is present from the beginning, while in others there is a period of normal development followed by loss of skills, most commonly in the second year of life. There is a failure of normal back-and-forth conversation and a reduction or absence of normal sharing of interests, affect, and emotion. Normal nonverbal communicative behavior is also abnormal and/or poorly integrated with verbal communication. That means that facial expression may be flat, eye contact disconnected from gestures, such as pointing for shared enjoyment, and from language, including the requesting of preferred objects. Typical gestures, such as waving bye-bye, playing pat-a-cake, and head shaking may be absent or delayed. Children with ASD have difficulties adjusting to social situations and are either disinterested in peers or experience significant difficulty in making friends and sharing interests, including shared imaginative play. Repetitive, restrictive behaviors typically described include motor abnormalities, sometimes known as "stimming," such as spinning and hand flapping, interests focused on a limited number of play items that are not used for imaginative play, resistance to change

TABLE 1	Examples of Typical Symptoms in Autism Spectrum Disorder
Social impairment	Lack of or abnormalities in eye contact
	Lack of interest in peers
	Lack of empathy for others
	Diminished facial expression
	Diminished/absent pointing to share enjoyment
	Abnormal requesting of items, e.g., use of another's hand as a tool
	Failure to respond to name
	Poorly developed/absent friendships
	Difficulties modulating social interactions
Communication	Complete lack of language
	Absence of babbling
	Use of stereotyped phrases
	Idiosyncratic use of language
	Pronoun reversal
	Echolalia
	"Scripting" (e.g. repeating of movie scripts, etc.)
	Failure to use language for social interaction; unusual prosody
	Inability to have a back and forth conversation
Repetitive, restricted behaviors	Hand flapping, toe walking, spinning, etc., also known as "stimming"
	Excessive attachment to inanimate objects
	Abnormal response to pain, noise, textures, etc.
	Difficulty with transitions between activities
	Difficulty with changes in routine

and transition, and sensory sensitivity, such as overreaction to loud noises, food textures, and pain. Onset of symptoms must be in "early childhood." Delay in diagnosis may be seen, especially in those with higher intellectual ability, more verbal facility, and in girls. Patients who are not diagnosed in early childhood nonetheless present with deficits in communication and interaction, including social isolation, difficulties in making friends, and focused interests/activities.

Diagnosis

The diagnosis is based on clinical symptoms consistent with the *Diagnostic and Statistical Manual of Mental Disorders*, fifth edition (DSM-5). Symptoms must be present in the early developmental period and cause clinically significant impairment in social, occupational, or other important areas of functioning. ASD may occur with or without accompanying intellectual impairment and language impairment. ASD may be associated with a known genetic or medical condition, with another neurodevelopmental or behavior disorder, and with catatonia. Full evaluation should include a detailed history of presenting symptoms and early development, and observation of the child in a setting where social interaction is required. Although there is no psychological "test" for ASD, validated, structured observation tools may be employed as a component of a detailed diagnostic evaluation. Of these, the most commonly seen is the Autism Development Observation Scale (ADOS), available in multiple versions appropriate for different age groups, and including a version for diagnosis in adults. It is important for practitioners to be aware of local regulations. In some states, access to resources (e.g. early childhood intervention, respite care, applied behavioral analysis, etc.) may only be triggered after specific evaluation requirements are met; those may include assessment by certain kinds of professionals, evaluation in approved settings, or the use of specific tools.

There is a difference between a clinical diagnosis of ASD and a determination that a child is eligible for autism-related educational services. Children with a clinical diagnosis may not necessarily be eligible for special educational services. The latter are determined by assessment for educational need and may be delivered through an Individualized Education Plan (IEP). Families may benefit from advocacy in accessing educational services for social and behavioral difficulties, even when their child is doing well academically. On the other hand, not every child deemed eligible for educational services for autism will have received a formal clinical diagnosis. The latter is important when a child transfers to adult services, when a clinical diagnosis may be necessary to determine eligibility for disability, guardianship, vocational education, or sheltered workshops and group homes.

Differential Diagnosis

DSM-V states that disturbances in development and behavior must not be better explained by intellectual disability or global developmental delay. The latter are the most common differentials. Many individuals with ASD also have intellectual disability. However, to make comorbid diagnoses of ASD and intellectual disability, social communication should be below the general developmental level, and significant repetitive, restrictive activities must be present. Additional differential diagnoses include communication disorders, of which social (pragmatic) communication disorder is the most difficult to distinguish. Language delay is no longer required for the diagnosis of ASD but is very common. Social (pragmatic) language disorder is diagnosed in patients who have deficits in communication but do not have the characteristic repetitive behaviors seen in patients with ASD. Specific sensory deficits in hearing and vision must be excluded. Finally, studies of individuals who have suffered extraordinary and extreme early childhood neglect show that some of these children later demonstrate a pattern of "pseudo-autism."

Screening, Clinical Assessment, Intervention, and Monitoring

Because of the increasing evidence that early intervention for children with ASD may be critical to long term outcomes, routine early screening for ASD is essential. Primary care physicians should follow recommendations for the developmental screening of babies and young children, which include specific screening for ASD at 18 and 24 months. A positive screen should result in a referral for a comprehensive evaluation from a qualified specialist, such as a behavioral pediatrician, child and adolescent psychiatrist, or pediatric neurologist. The comprehensive evaluation will likely be multidisciplinary, and may include evaluations by psychology, speech and language therapy, and occupational therapy. Critical elements include a detailed birth, developmental and medical history, and family medical and psychiatric history, and may include structured interviews of the parent(s). Careful observation of the child is essential and is often supplemented by structured clinical observation. Assessments of adaptive skills should be included, along with intellectual ability and academic and work-related performance where appropriate. Primary care physicians may contribute by completing a full medical examination, including measurement of head circumference, screening for vision and hearing anomalies, careful review for dysmorphology, and assessment for seizure disorder, which is present in 20% of patients with ASD. Children with suspected genetic syndromes should be referred for expert evaluation and follow-up, as should those with suspected specific sensory impairments and seizure disorders. Recommended blood work for children with ASD includes comprehensive blood count, lead level and chromosomal microarray with Fragile X.

There may be a significant delay before the results of a full evaluation become available. However, a child with a significant delay in development should be referred promptly to early intervention, whether or not the diagnosis of ASD has been confirmed. Every state has an early intervention program for children from birth to 3 years, and older preschool-age school children may be eligible for early childhood special education. Additional referrals for occupational, physical, and speech therapy may also be made, as well as for other enrichment programs, such as Headstart.

As in the management of any other complex medical condition in a child, support for parents and families, and coordination of services is a critical role for primary care. Parent-parent resources may be helpful, both local and internet-based. Although there will be geographic variation in the availability of specific programming, the cornerstone of intervention throughout life should be an individualized program designed to optimize a particular patient's strengths and address deficits, with interventions targeted at maximizing function and quality of life.

Behavioral approaches supplemented by other therapies and interventions supporting social engagement are recommended for children with ASD diagnoses. Programs focus on the development of language and social skills, and reductions in disability and comorbidity, particularly the impairments associated with behavioral disinhibition and aggression. Early intensive behavioral intervention should include applied behavioral analysis, which focuses on the building of discrete skills as well as on diminishing problematic behavioral patterns. Interventions may be delivered through comprehensive programs such as the Early Start Denver Model or TEACCH (Treatment and Education of Autistic and related Communication Handicapped Children), or via a combination of behavioral and educational services and therapy interventions. Programming typically involves parents in the delivery of interventions designed to enhance emotional engagement and communication. Communication is facilitated where necessary through visual scheduling (Picture Enhanced Communication Systems [PECS]), technology enhanced communication, and the use of sign language. Many children with ASD benefit from ongoing special educational interventions, which should target behavioral and social skills training as well as academic interventions. Vocational intervention is recommended for older children, adolescents, and adults. The transition to adult services may be challenging both for patient and family. Planning should start in early adolescence and, besides the transition of medical services if needed, should include careful consideration and planning for appropriate independence and support, including safe driving, options for further education and employment, and the need for possible ongoing guardianship by parents or other relatives. Unemployment is, sadly, very common in adults with ASD, who may become very isolated. Supports should be designed to facilitate their fullest possible engagement with their community, while protecting them, where necessary, from exploitation and abuse.

Patients with ASD may respond in unusual ways to common medical conditions, especially those that are painful and uncomfortable such as dental pain, headache, sinus pain, menstrual cramps, etc. This may be because of unusual response to physical symptoms, because of difficulty in communication, or both. Routine preventive medical and dental visits should be encouraged from early childhood onward. New onset and exacerbations of agitation, irritability, or self-injury in a patient with limited ability to communicate should always prompt a search for a physical cause, including a thorough physical examination.

Certain medical conditions (sleep disturbance; gastrointestinal problems, especially constipation; and seizure disorders) are particularly common in individuals with ASD and are associated with increased likelihood of irritability and behavioral disturbance. Routine surveillance should include attention to these conditions as well as appropriate management and referral. Seizure onset may be in later childhood or adolescence, and poorly controlled seizures are associated with both educational and behavioral deterioration. Some individuals with ASD have very limited dietary intake. Careful enquiry may be followed by blood work if indicated, including blood count, ferritin, vitamin D, and zinc. Referral may be made to a dietician, to behavioral therapy for mealtime related behaviors and/or to occupational therapy if the eating problems are related to problems with texture or swallowing. Many children with ASD have constipation and other gastrointestinal issues such as reflux, diarrhea, and inflammatory bowel disease. These conditions should be monitored and managed aggressively. Finally, sleep difficulties may be prominent,

TABLE 2 — Psychopharmacology in Patients With Autism Spectrum Disorder

MEDICATION	TARGET	EVIDENCE FOR EFFECTIVENESS	RELATED CONSIDERATIONS
Atypical antipsychotics—risperidone (Risperdal) and aripiprazole (Abilify)	Agitation, aggression, irritability in patients with ASD	Moderate to high, however, side effects may limit utility	Practice guidelines for monitoring; weight gain (for which metformin may be helpful), sedation, extrapyramidal symptoms, and elevated prolactin
SSRI's—citalopram (Celexa)[1], escitalopram (Lexapro), fluoxetine (Prozac)[1], sertraline (Zoloft)[1] and others	Anxiety and mood disorders	Little data for patients with ASD and co-occurring anxiety/depression. Not effective for core ASD symptoms	Common side effects include gastro-intestinal symptoms and increased irritability
Stimulants (methylphenidate [Ritalin], dextroamphetamine [Dexedrine])	ADHD	Well established for ADHD in patients without ASD; moderate evidence for ADHD in patients with ASD	Probably effective in a lower percentage of ASD patients than in uncomplicated ADHD. Side effects include irritability, decreased appetite, insomnia, weight loss, and headache
Melatonin[7]	Sleep disturbance	Some support	Use as an adjunct to CBT for sleep

[1]Not FDA approved for this indication.
[7]Available as dietary supplement.
ADHD, Attention deficit hyperactivity disorder; *ASD*, autism spectrum disorder.

especially in many young children with ASD. Nonpharmacologic approaches (psychoeducation and cognitive-behavioral therapy [CBT]) should be implemented first; these typically include education about the nature and function of sleep and the implementation of good sleep hygiene and bedtime routines. There is some evidence that the use of melatonin as a supplement to sleep-focused CBT may be helpful.

Co-occurring psychiatric disorders are not uncommon in individuals with ASD. Historically, the diagnosis of attention deficit hyperactivity disorder (ADHD) was not possible in patients with ASD, but this changed with the DSM-5. There is suggestive evidence that stimulants, α-2 agonists and atomoxetine (Strattera) are helpful for ADHD, though potentially in a lower percentage of patients and with a higher frequency of side effects compared to the non-ASD population. Anxiety, particularly social anxiety, and generalized anxiety disorders, may present in older children, adolescents, and adults, along with depression and other mood symptoms. CBT is an established treatment in ASD patients without intellectual disability who present with anxiety. There are less data to support the use of CBT in ASD patients who have an intellectual disability and in those who experience mood symptoms rather than anxiety.

Pharmacotherapy

There are currently no pharmacologic interventions available that address the underlying core deficits of autism, though studies targeting the cholinergic, glutaminergic, and oxytocin systems are under way. Psychotropic medication interventions may be used for co-occurring psychiatric conditions, where those are present. Stimulant medications, guanfacine (Intuniv), and atomoxetine may be used for ADHD in patients with ASD. Some supporting data shows efficacy, but in a smaller percentage of ASD than non-ASD patients and with a higher side effect burden. Psychopharmacologic intervention for anxiety and depression should follow clinical guidelines for patients without ASD, including the use of selective serotonin reuptake inhibitors (SSRIs), with awareness that side effects, especially irritability, may be more common (Table 2). Antipsychotic medications have been shown to be effective for symptomatic relief of aggressive, agitated behaviors in adolescents with ASD; however, studies are relatively short term, and the side effects of this group of medications limit their utility. Practice guidelines include specific monitoring for weight gain and associated metabolic abnormalities.

TABLE 3 — Educational Resources for Patients and their Families

1. Autism Speaks: www.autismspeaks.org
2. The American Academy of Pediatrics official parenting website https://www.healthychildren.org/English/Pages/default.aspx
3. The American Academy of Child and Adolescent Psychiatry: Facts for Families and Medication Guide for Treating Autism Spectrum Disorders: www.aacap.org/AACAP/Families_and_Youth/Home
4. Missouri Family to Family Lifecourse: https://www.lifecoursetools.com/
5. The MIND Institute Autism Distance Education Parent Training: https://health.ucdavis.edu/mindinstitute/centers/cedd/adept.html
6. Centers for Disease Prevention: Learn the Signs. Act Early: https://www.cdc.gov/ncbddd/actearly/milestones/index.html

Patients with ASD have been the target of many complementary and alternative interventions (e.g., high dose vitamin regimes, dietary modification such as gluten-casein free diets, omega-3 fatty acids, secretin, chelation, hyperbaric oxygen, antifungal regimes, etc.), none of which have proven efficacy and some of which are frankly dangerous. Patients and their families may need support and guidance in resisting inaccurate, nonscientific claims made by organizations marketing unproven interventions (Table 3).

References

Ameis SH, Kassee C, Corbett-Dick P, et al: Systematic review and guide to management of core and psychiatric symptoms in youth with autism, *Acta Psychiatr Scand* 138(5):379–400, 2018.

American Academy of Child and Adolescent Psychiatry: *Practice Parameter for the Assessment and Treatment of Children and Adolescents with Autism Spectrum Disorder*, Available at: https://www.aacap.org/app_themes/aacap/docs/practice_parameters/autism.pdf 2013

American Academy of Pediatrics Screening Recommendations: Available at: https://www.aap.org/en-us/advocacy-and-policy/aap-health-initiatives/Screening/Pages/Screening-Recommendations.asp

American Psychiatric Association, DSM-5 Task Force: *Diagnostic and Statistical Manual of Mental Disorders: DSM-5*, ed 5, Washington, DC, 2013, American Psychiatric Association.

Lai M-C, Lombardo MV, Baron-Cohen S: Autism, *The Lancet* 383:896–910, 2014.

Sahin M, Sur M: Genes, circuits and precision therapies for autism and related neurodevelopmental disorders, *Science* 350(6263), 2015.

Santosh PJ, Bell L, Fiori F, et al: Pediatric antipsychotic use and outcomes monitoring, *J Child Adolesc Psychopharmacol* 27(6):546–554, 2017.

DELIRIUM

Method of
Kari R. Clouse, MD

CURRENT DIAGNOSIS

- Delirium is an acute, fluctuating syndrome of altered attention, awareness, and cognition.
- Hypoactive delirium presents with at least four of the following behaviors: unawareness, decreased alertness, reduced or delayed speech, lethargy, slowed movements, staring, apathy, diminished appetite, or new incontinence.
- Hyperactive delirium is distinguished by at least three of the following behaviors: hypervigilance, restlessness, fast or loud speech, irritability, combativeness, impatience, swearing, singing, laughing, uncooperativeness, euphoria, anger, wandering, easy startling, fast motor responses, distractibility, tangentiality, nightmares, or persistent thoughts.
- Mixed delirium is distinguished by a combination of hypoactive and hyperactive behaviors.
- The Diagnostic and Statistical Manual of Mental Disorders, Fifth Edition, offers diagnostic criteria for delirium (see the diagnosis section).

CURRENT THERAPY

- Prevention is best achieved by assessing predisposing and precipitating risk factors.
- Treatment should be targeted at reversing underlying causes and implementing nonpharmacologic interventions.
- Pharmacologic therapies should be reserved for severely agitated patients, psychotic individuals, or those who threaten substantial harm to self or others.

Epidemiology

Delirium is a common medical condition seen in various care settings. Although rates vary by location, delirium prevalence in long-term care facilities has been reported up to 60% and as high as 80% in intensive care units (ICUs). Patients who suffer from delirium have longer hospital stays, higher costs of care, greater risk of long-term cognitive impairment, and increased mortality rates.

Risk Factors

Once viewed as a reversible process caused by a single underlying cause, delirium is now believed to be multifactorial. Several risk factors have been identified and can be divided into predisposing and precipitating factors as noted in Table 1. A complex relationship exists between predisposing factors and exposures to precipitating events. A vulnerable patient may only require a small triggering incident whereas a healthy patient may be subject to multiple noxious insults, but both could result in delirium.

Pathophysiology

Delirium is a complex, multifactorial neurobehavioral syndrome and the exact pathophysiology is difficult to elucidate. Recent evidence suggests that several different sets of interacting biologic factors instigate the disruption of large-scale neuronal networks in the brain, leading to acute cognitive dysfunction. Ultimately, multiple insults can result in neuronal cell apoptosis and decreased synaptic plasticity. Contributing biologic factors may include neuroinflammatory processes, neurotransmitter disruption, and circadian rhythm dysregulation. For example, insults such as severe infection, surgery, and trauma are known to increase inflammatory cytokines and endotoxins. The inflammatory process is

TABLE 1	Risk Factors for Delirium
PREDISPOSING FACTORS	**PRECIPITATING FACTORS**
Cognitive impairment	Environmental triggers
Dementia	Sleep deprivation
Depression	Physical restraints
Medical comorbidities	Foley catheter
Sensory loss	Arterial catheter
Chronic medical conditions	Gastric tube
Persistent pain	Multiple IV infusions
Pressure ulcers	Lack of visitors
Urinary incontinence	Length of stay in ICU
Malnutrition	Medical insults
Alcohol abuse	Medications
Terminal illness	Infection
Geriatric factors	Hypoxia
Dehydration	Ischemia
Age >65 years	Severe illness
Elder abuse	Uncontrolled pain
Frequent falls	Surgery
Functional dependence	
Polypharmacy	

thought to degrade the blood-brain barrier, activate microglia, cause endothelial dysfunction, alter cerebral blood flow causing hypoperfusion, and change neurotransmitter levels. Alteration of neurotransmitter levels, such as excess dopamine, depletion of acetylcholine, or melatonin deficiency are likely involved in the development of delirium. However, treatments targeted at correcting these imbalances have mixed outcomes, further accentuating the complexity of the illness. Moreover, predisposing factors such as cognitive dysfunction, advanced age, and chronic medical conditions affect the magnitude of neuronal resiliency needed to withstand precipitating events.

Prevention

Delirium is considered to be preventable 30% to 40% of the time. To minimize the possibility of delirium, modifiable variables should be assessed and eliminated. Resources available to help prevent, assess, and manage delirium can be found on the ICU Delirium and Cognitive Impairment Study Group website (http://www.icudelirium.org). The delirium prevention mnemonic "ABCDEF" outlines a bundle of measures beneficial in the prevention and management of delirium in the ICU.

*A*ssess for and manage pain
*B*oth spontaneous awakening and breathing trials (SAT, SBT)
*C*hoice of sedation and analgesia
*D*elirium monitoring and management
*E*arly mobility
*F*amily or companion involvement

Clinical Manifestations

Delirium presents as an acute, fluctuating syndrome of confusion, altered attention, reduced perceptual awareness of surroundings, disorganized thinking, and cognitive impairment. Three subtypes of delirium have been identified:

- Hypoactive (at least four of the following): unawareness, decreased alertness, reduced or delayed speech, lethargy, slowed movements, staring, apathy, diminished appetite, or new incontinence.

- Hyperactive (at least three of the following): hypervigilance, restlessness, fast or loud speech, irritability, combativeness, impatience, swearing, singing, laughing, uncooperativeness, euphoria, anger, wandering, easy startling, fast motor responses, distractibility, tangentiality, nightmares, or persistent thoughts.
- Mixed (combination of hypoactive and hyperactive behaviors).

Diagnosis

Unfortunately, lack of recognition by health-care professionals is a significant issue and the diagnosis of delirium is commonly missed. The key to early identification is having a high clinical suspicion of the syndrome. According to the *Diagnostic and Statistical Manual of Mental Disorders*, Fifth Edition, the following five criteria must be fulfilled to accurately diagnosis delirium.

1. A disturbance in attention (i.e., reduced ability to direct, focus, sustain, and shift attention) and awareness (reduced orientation to the environment) exists;
2. An additional disturbance in cognition (e.g., memory deficit, disorientation, language, visuospatial ability, or perception) exists;
3. The disturbance develops over a short period of time (usually hours to a few days), represents a change from baseline attention and awareness, and tends to fluctuate in severity during the course of a day;
4. The disturbances in criteria 1 and 2 are not explained by another preexisting, established, or evolving neurocognitive disorder and do not occur in the context of a severely reduced level of arousal such as coma;
5. There is evidence from the history, physical examination, or laboratory findings that the disturbance is a direct physiologic consequence of another medical condition, substance intoxication or withdrawal (i.e., due to a drug of abuse or to a medication), exposure to a toxin, or is due to multiple etiologies.

Several assessment tools exist to identify this complex syndrome. One of the most effective and commonly used is the Confusion Assessment Method (CAM). When performed by a trained individual, this instrument is reported to have 94% to 100% sensitivity and 90% to 95% specificity in detecting delirium. It can also be used as an indicator of severity. For efficiency, a shortened version of this test, CAM-Short (CAM-S) also exists, but lacks the ability to characterize severity. Several other evaluation methods are available and can be found on the Hospital Elder Life Program website (http://www.hospitalelderlifeprogram.org/delirium-instruments). A basic laboratory and imaging workup is routinely indicated. For most patients this includes a complete blood count, complete metabolic panel, urinalysis, chest radiograph, and electrocardiogram. Individual scenarios may warrant additional diagnostic investigation such as a computerized tomography scan, electroencephalogram, lumbar puncture, or supplementary laboratory tests.

Differential Diagnosis

Several clinical scenarios can mimic delirium. This contributes to the underdiagnosed nature of this syndrome. Multiple mnemonics have been created to aid in identification of underlying clinical conditions that might cause or contribute to delirium. One helpful mnemonic is "I WATCH DEATH."

Infection	Urinary tract infection, pneumonia, sepsis, human immunodeficiency virus, syphilis, abscess
Withdrawal	Alcohol, barbiturates, sedative-hypnotics
Acute metabolic	Acidosis, alkalosis, electrolyte disturbance, hepatic/renal failure, dehydration
Trauma	Head injury, postoperative state, hyper/hypothermia, burns
CNS pathology	Cerebrovascular accident, tumors, metastasis, seizures, hemorrhage, encephalitis, meningitis, vasculitis
Hypoxia	Anemia, cardio/pulmonary failure, hypotension
Deficiencies	Thiamine, B_{12}, niacin, folate
Endocrinopathies	Hyper/hypothyroid, hyper/hypoglycemia, adrenal dysfunction, parathyroid disorders
Acute vascular	Hypertensive emergency, subarachnoid hemorrhage, sagittal vein thrombosis
Toxins/drugs	Medications, alcohol, illicit drugs, synthetic cannabinoids, pesticides, industrial poisons, carbon monoxide, cyanide, solvents, synthetic cathinones
Heavy metals	Lead, mercury, manganese

Additional memory aids can be located on the ICU Delirium and Cognitive Impairment Study Group website (http://www.icudelirium.org).

Treatment

The treatment of delirium consists of both nonpharmacologic and pharmacologic therapies and should be centered on the patient's medical condition, risk factors, and environmental insults. For initial symptom management, nonpharmacologic tactics are the first-line strategy. The most widely disseminated approach is the Hospital Elder Life Program, a multicomponent hospital intervention strategy involving health-care professionals, families, caregivers, and patients. The program has proven effectiveness and demonstrated reductions in the cost of care (http://www.hospitalelderlifeprogram.org). *Pharmacologic therapies should be reserved for severely agitated patients, psychotic individuals, or those who threaten substantial harm to self or others.* Low starting doses should be used. Currently, there are no antipsychotic medications that are Food and Drug Administration–approved for prevention or treatment of delirium. Clinical trials are currently evaluating the effectiveness of dexmedetomidine, a sedative α_2-agonist, in ICU patients requiring sedation for agitated delirium. Types of management are outlined in Tables 2 and 3.

Monitoring

Once identified, regular monitoring of delirium can focus treatment targets. Multiple screening tools are available and can be found at the Hospital Elder Life Program website. Situations that warrant a significant and prompt reevaluation include a dramatic vital change, new focal neurologic deficits, respiratory distress, escalating behaviors, or danger to self or others.

TABLE 2	**Nonpharmacologic Management of Delirium**

Target and address underlying causes first
Medication review and appropriate management
Nutritional and fluid replacement
Sleep enhancement through proper sleep hygiene, relaxation, and creation of quiet, soothing, warm environment
Adequate pain control, preferably nonopioid
Cognitive orientation by family or companion involvement, consistent medical staff, clocks, and calendars
Early and continued mobilization
Improved exposure to daylight to promote circadian rhythm
Sensory enhancement with glasses, hearing aids, or other adaptive equipment
Daily cognitive assessment with standardized tool

TABLE 3	**Pharmacologic Management of Delirium**

Typical Antipsychotics[1]

Haloperidol (Haldol) 0.5–2.0 mg bid orally every 4 hours or intramuscularly every 30–60 minutes prn; maximum dose 20 mg in 24 hours
Most commonly used agent

Atypical Antipsychotics[1]

Quetiapine (Seroquel) 25–200 mg orally bid
Risperidone (Risperdal) 0.25–2 mg orally divided once daily to bid
Olanzapine (Zyprexa) 2.5–10 mg orally once daily
Ziprasidone (Geodon) 20–80 mg orally bid
Aripiprazole (Abilify) 10–30 mg orally once daily

Benzodiazepines[1]

Lorazepam (Ativan) 0.5–1.0 mg orally every 4 hours prn
Reserve for alcohol withdrawal
Can worsen delirium caused by other factors

[1]There are no antipsychotic medications and benzodiazepines that are FDA approved for prevention or treatment of delirium.

Complications

Long-term complications of delirium are significant. Patients with delirium can experience postoperative setbacks, prolonged hospitalization, loss of functional independence, posttraumatic stress disorder, and permanently reduced cognitive function. These individuals are at high risk for readmission, particularly if over the age of 75. Medications used to treat delirium can result in many adverse effects such as extrapyramidal symptoms, cardiac conduction abnormalities, hypotension, somnolence, and anticholinergic effects. Finally, delirium is associated with increased mortality, with rates ranging from 14.5% to 37%.

References

American Psychiatric Association: *Desk Reference to the Diagnostic Criteria from DSM-5*, Arlington, VA, 2013, American Psychiatric Association.
Hospital Elder Life Program (HELP) for Prevention of Delirium. Available at http://www.hospitalelderlifeprogram.org. Accessed March 10, 2016.
ICU Delirium and Cognitive Impairment Study Group. Available at http://www.icudelirium.org. Accessed June 3, 2017.
Inouye SK, Robinson T, et al: Postoperative delirium in older adults: best practice statement from the American Geriatrics Society, *J Am Coll Surg* 220(2):136–148. e1, 2015.
Inouye SK, Westendorp RG, Saczynski JS: Delirium in elderly people, *The Lancet* 383(9920):911–922, 2014.
Jackson P, Khan A: Delirium in critically ill patients, *Crit Care Clin* 31(3):589–603, 2015.
Kalish VB, Gillham JE, Unwin BK: Delirium in older persons: Evaluation and management, *Am Fam Physician* 90(3):150–158, 2014.
Lawlor PG, Bush SH: Delirium diagnosis, screening and management, *Curr Opin in Support and Palliat Care* 8(3):286–295, 2014.
Meagher DJ, McLoughlin L, Leonard M, et al: What do we really know about the treatment of delirium with antipsychotics? Ten key issues for delirium pharmacotherapy, *Am J Geriatr Psychiatry* 21:1223–1238, 2013.
Pendlebury ST, Lovett NG, Smith SC, et al: Observational, longitudinal study of delirium in consecutive unselected acute medical admissions: age-specific rates and associated factors, mortality and re-admission, *BMJ Open*, 2015. Available at http:/bmjopen.bmj.com. Accessed February 16, 2015.

DRUG ABUSE

Method of
William M. Greene, MD; and Mark S. Gold, MD

CURRENT DIAGNOSIS

- Screen for substance use in all primary care and emergency settings.
- The clinical interview remains the mainstay of diagnosis.
- Clinicians should have a low threshold for ordering a urine drug test.
- Collateral information should be obtained from family or other sources.
- DSM-5 offers current diagnostic criteria for substance use disorders (see Box 1).

CURRENT THERAPY

- Effective pharmacologic and psychosocial treatments exist.
- Formal detoxification is indicated for dangerous withdrawal states or in patients with serious medical comorbidity.
- Pharmacologic relapse prevention treatment options are substance-specific, and particularly useful options exist for nicotine and opioids.
- Psychosocial treatments remain the mainstay of substance treatment, and these range along a continuum of intensity from outpatient counseling to long-term residential treatment.
- Patients should be referred to self-help groups (e.g., Narcotics Anonymous) to complement other therapies.
- Indefinite remission is an attainable goal for many—a relapse does not constitute total failure but gives opportunity to reevaluate the treatment approach.

Epidemiology

Widespread pathologic use of intoxicating substances, both legal and illegal, remains one of the greatest public health concerns facing our nation. According to the 2010 National Survey on Drug Use and Health, 22.6 million Americans (8.9% of the population) aged 12 years and older used an illicit drug within the past month. By order of frequency, these include marijuana, nonmedical use of prescription drugs, cocaine, hallucinogens, inhalants, and heroin. In addition, 69.6 million Americans (27.4%) aged 12 years and older used tobacco within the past month, mostly in the form of cigarettes. Each year in the United States, approximately 443,000 people die of an illness attributable to cigarette smoking, making this the foremost cause of preventable death. The estimated annual economic cost of drug abuse is over $600 billion in the United States alone: $185 billion for illicit drugs, $235 billion for alcohol, and $193 billion for tobacco. These costs include only direct health-related, crime-related, and lost-productivity costs, thus underestimating the full impact of drug abuse on society.

From 2002 to 2010, the rate of past-month cigarette use among 12- to 17-year-olds has steadily dropped from 13.0% to 8.3%. The 2010 Monitoring the Future survey data confirm that cigarette smoking has continued to fall to the lowest rate in the survey's history (i.e., past month use among 12th graders is now at 19%). Since 2000, overall rates of illicit drug use have slowly dropped, but use of marijuana has recently slowed its rate of decline and initiation of illicit prescription drugs is now on the rise. In 2006, new users of illicit prescription drugs caught up with new users of marijuana for the first time; however, since then, first-time use of marijuana has regained its ascendancy, with 2.4 million first-time users estimated in 2010. As of 2010, 48.2% of 12th graders still report having used an illicit drug at some point in their life. Despite advances in our understanding and treatment of substance use disorders, drug abuse remains an epidemic, especially in the areas of drugged driving and drug use (including tobacco) in pregnancy.

Diagnosis

With the publication of the DSM-5 in 2013, the diagnostic categories of substance abuse and substance dependence have been entirely eliminated. In the interest of consistency and clarity, and based on large population data, these have been replaced with a new diagnostic entity: "substance use disorder" (Box 1). It is no longer necessary for the clinician to decide between two different diagnoses. Those familiar with DSM-IV terminology will find the new criteria quite familiar, as they essentially represent a combination of the old abuse and dependence criteria, with two notable exceptions: one, legal problems has been eliminated; and two, a craving criterion has been added. When diagnosing a substance use disorder, the specific substance for which criteria are met must be listed. In addition, it is also important to document the severity of the disorder based on the number of symptoms present. Examples of specific diagnoses using the new nomenclature would be "alcohol use disorder, moderate" or "alprazolam use disorder, severe." This simpler, evidence-based, diagnostic schema should eliminate some of the confusion previously surrounding the term "dependence," which was often mistaken to be synonymous with "physiological dependence." It has long been understood, in the context of certain prescribed drugs, that the presence of tolerance and withdrawal is not pathological in nature; rather, these represent an expected state of neuroadaptation. This fact is reflected in the new criteria for opioid use disorder; stimulant use disorder; and sedative, hypnotic, or anxiolytic use disorder. For these three categories, the tolerance and withdrawal criteria are not considered to be met if present when the substance is taken solely under appropriate medical supervision. It should be noted this exception does not apply to cannabis, even if it is "prescribed."

Despite the importance and usefulness of the DSM-5, many patients (and clinicians) may still be left wondering if the problem at hand would appropriately be characterized as "addiction." In a 2011 public policy statement, the American Society

BOX 1 DSM-5 Diagnostic Criteria for "Substance Use Disorder"

A problematic pattern of use leading to clinically significant impairment or distress as manifested by two or more of the following in a 12-month period:

1. Often taken in larger amounts or longer period than intended.
2. Persistent desire or unsuccessful efforts to cut down or control use.
3. Great deal of time spent in activities necessary to obtain, use, or recover from effects.
4. Craving, or strong desire or urge to use.
5. Recurrent use resulting in failure to fulfill major role obligations at work, school, or home.
6. Continued use despite having persistent/recurrent social or interpersonal problems caused or exacerbated by the substance.
7. Important social, occupational, or recreational activities are given up or reduced because of use.
8. Recurrent use in situations in which it is physically hazardous.
9. Continued use despite knowledge of having a persistent/recurrent physical or psychological problem likely to have been caused or exacerbated by the substance.
10. Tolerance (needing increased amounts for desired effect, or diminished effect with same amount).
11. Withdrawal (manifested by characteristic syndrome or taking more to relieve/avoid withdrawal).

Specify current severity:

Mild: Two to three criteria are met

Moderate: Four to five criteria are met

Severe: Six or more criteria are met

---

of Addiction Medicine offered the following short definition of addiction, which has been well received: *"Addiction is a primary, chronic disease of brain reward, motivation, memory and related circuitry. Dysfunction in these circuits leads to characteristic biological, psychological, social and spiritual manifestations. This is reflected in an individual pathologically pursuing reward and/or relief by substance use and other behaviors. Addiction is characterized by inability to consistently abstain, impairment in behavioral control, craving, diminished recognition of significant problems with one's behaviors and interpersonal relationships, and a dysfunctional emotional response. Like other chronic diseases, addiction often involves cycles of relapse and remission. Without treatment or engagement in recovery activities, addiction is progressive and can result in disability or premature death."*

Tobacco and Nicotine

Nicotine is the main addictive component in tobacco, which is administered via smoking (e.g., cigarettes, cigars, pipes, bidis, hookah) or in smokeless formulations (e.g., dip, snuff, snus, chew). However, smoking tobacco is clearly not equivalent to taking nicotine. Cigarette smoking causes nicotine, brain monoamine oxidase (MAO), and other effects in the smoker, some resulting from the smoke and others resulting from the nicotine.

Following administration, nicotine rapidly binds to nicotinic acetylcholine receptors in the central nervous system (CNS), where it acts as a mild psychostimulant and mood modulator in a nonimpairing yet profoundly addictive manner. When the user is tired, smoking has a stimulating effect. When the user is anxious or stressed, smoking exerts a calming effect. Smoking is like an injection without the needle, and given its short half-life, repeated self-administration serves to effectively relieve unpleasant withdrawal symptoms from the nicotine itself. Repeated use quickly leads to both physiologic and psychological dependence.

As with other drugs of abuse, cue-induced cravings play an important role in maintaining the addiction. For example, the smell of the smoke, the sound of a lighter, and the feel of a cigarette on the lips all contribute to an overall process addiction beyond just addiction to the nicotine itself. Tobacco use is also strongly associated with alcohol use, with which it has synergistic toxic effects.

Toxicities from tobacco use are well described and include severe pulmonary disease, cardiovascular disease, and carcinomas of the upper aerodigestive tract and bladder. Even second-hand smoke, previously considered harmless, is now correctly regarded as a serious health risk to the nonsmoker and a "drug" itself. Cigarette smoke contains more than nicotine (up to 4700 components, all of which affect the smoker). Additionally, secondhand tobacco exposure in utero can cause addiction and lead to serious health-related consequences.

Although quitting remains difficult for even the most motivated tobacco users, effective treatments for nicotine dependence now exist. Clinical trials indicate a combination of counseling and medications offers the best chance for success and should be offered to patients who are willing to make a quit attempt. A wide range of FDA-approved nicotine replacement therapies are readily available and have similar rates of efficacy (Table 1). Patches (Nicoderm CQ), gums (Nicorette), and lozenges (Commit) are available over the counter, but the nasal spray (Nicotrol NS) and inhaler (Nicotrol Inhaler) are available by prescription only. Recently, "electronic cigarettes" have gained in popularity, but unlike other nicotine products, they are not regulated as a drug by the FDA.

Non-nicotine prescription medications with proven efficacy are available. Bupropion HCl (Wellbutrin) is an antidepressant that was serendipitously noted to dramatically reduce nicotine cravings in some patients, and it is now widely used for this purpose (as Zyban). Varenicline (Chantix) was specifically developed to treat nicotine dependence and represents a considerable advancement, with improved smoking cessation rates. It acts as a partial agonist at the nicotine receptor and effectively serves to satisfy cravings while simultaneously blocking the effects of exogenously administered nicotine. Although probably the most effective agent, varenicline carries significant risk of psychiatric side effects. The "nicotine vaccine" (NicVAX),[1] a novel approach, is currently in phase III clinical trials, and appears promising.

Nicotine replacement, bupropion, and varenicline are all considered first-line pharmacotherapy. Bupropion, but not varenicline, may also be used in combination with nicotine replacement therapies. All pharmacotherapy options are enhanced with coadministration of counseling or behavioral therapies. Helpful resources for patients interested in quitting include www.smokefree.gov (a government website dedicated to helping people quit smoking), 1-800-QUIT-NOW (a free phone-based services with coaches and educational materials) and a variety of resources available through the American Cancer Society and American Heart Association.

Cannabis

Cannabis (marijuana, pot, weed, grass, ganja, hash) remains the most-used illicit drug in the world. In Americans older than 12 years, 45% have used cannabis at least once, and 7.4% have used it in the past month. Cannabis is readily harvested from *Cannabis sativa*, and typically it is smoked, although it may also be ingested or vaporized. Despite a recent trend advocating legitimate medicinal use, it is still listed in Schedule I by the Drug Enforcement Agency (DEA), with high potential for abuse and no currently accepted medical use. Delta-9-tetrahydrocannabinol (THC) is the active ingredient, which exerts its desired psychoactive effects at CB_1 receptors diffusely throughout the CNS. Marijuana's THC concentration has been steadily increasing as a result of selective plant breeding. Annual analysis of DEA seizures indicates average THC concentrations increased from

---

[1] Not FDA approved for this indication.

				TABLE 1 Pharmacotherapy for Nicotine Dependence				

DRUG	MECHANISM OF ACTION	DOSAGE	INSTRUCTIONS	COMMENTS
Nicotine patch (Nicoderm CQ)	NRT	7 mg, 14 mg, 21 mg	1 patch daily	Tapering doses recommended to discontinue
Nicotine gum (Nicorette)	NRT	2 mg, 4 mg	Chew slightly then "park" on oral mucosa	Tapering doses recommended to discontinue
Nicotine lozenge (Commit)	NRT	2 mg, 4 mg	Absorbed through oral mucosa; minimize swallowing	Tapering doses recommended to discontinue
Nicotine inhaler (Nicotrol Inhaler)	NRT	4 mg/cartridge	6–16 cartridges/day	By prescription only; tedious administration
Nicotine nasal spray (Nicotrol NS)	NRT	0.5 mg/spray	1–2 sprays each nostril q1h; max 80 sprays/day	By prescription only
Bupropion HCl (Wellbutrin,[1] Zyban)	Inhibits reuptake of NE and DA	150 mg SR tab, 300 mg XL tab	300 mg PO (divided qd [XL tab]-bid [SR tab]) daily × 7–12 wk	Helps with comorbid depression; can help prevent weight gain
Varenicline (Chantix)	Partial agonist at $\alpha_4\beta_2$ nicotinic acetylcholine receptor	0.5 mg, 1 mg	0.5 mg PO qd × 3 d, then 0.5 mg PO bid × 4 d, then 1 mg PO bid × 11 wk	May smoke during 1st wk; may continue additional 12 wk
Nicotine vaccine (NicVAX)	Antibody sequestration of nicotine	n/a	n/a	In clinical trials

Abbreviations: DA = dopamine; max = maximum; n/a = not applicable; NE = norepinephrine; NRT = nicotine replacement therapy; SR = sustained release; XL = extended release.
[1]Not FDA approved for this indication.

approximately 1% in 1975 to approximately 10% in 2008. To what extent this makes the drug more dangerous or more addictive remains unclear.

Acute psychoactive effects of cannabis include euphoria, relaxation, heightened sensations, increased appetite, distorted sense of time, slowed reaction time, illusions and hallucinations, paranoia, and anxiety. Acute somatic effects include conjunctival injection, xerostomia, increased heart rate and blood pressure, muscle relaxation, and reduced intraocular pressure. There is no known risk of dangerous overdose, and withdrawal symptoms are generally mild but include irritability, cravings, diminished appetite, and insomnia. Cannabis is now recognized as unequivocally addictive. Abusers of this drug rapidly develop tolerance and commonly demonstrate loss of control and continued use despite negative consequences—the hallmarks of addiction. It is estimated that 1 million Americans sought treatment for cannabis as their primary drug of choice in 2010.

Not surprisingly, with more than 400 chemicals identified in its smoke, cannabis is dangerous with respect to long-term health. Chronic cannabis use is associated with lung cancer, chronic obstructive pulmonary disease, cardiovascular disease, impaired immunity, persistent disruption of memory and attention, and various psychiatric disorders, most commonly anxiety disorders and depressive disorders. There is a growing body of evidence that cannabis abuse can lead to lasting psychosis (i.e., schizophrenia) in predisposed persons.

Currently, treatment of cannabis dependence remains entirely psychosocial. Various existing drugs (including fluoxetine [Prozac],[2] lithium, buspirone [Buspar][2]) have been investigated. However, well-controlled clinical trials to support their use are lacking. Preliminary data suggest that dronabinol (Marinol) may be of some utility in relieving cravings and withdrawal symptoms without causing intoxication. Rimonabant (Acomplia),[3] a CB_1 antagonist previously prescribed for weight loss in Europe, showed promise but has failed to achieve FDA approval because of psychiatric side effects.

[2]Not available in the United States.
[3]Exceeds dosage recommended by the manufacturer.

Cocaine, Methamphetamine, and Other Stimulants

As a class, cocaine and other stimulants work primarily by enhancing dopamine transmission in a dose-dependent fashion, either directly (amphetamines) or by blocking reuptake (cocaine). Cocaine and a variety of amphetamines (e.g., amphetamine/dextroamphetamine [Adderall], dextroamphetamine [Dexedrine], methamphetamine [Desoxyn], methylphenidate [Methylin, Ritalin]) are available for legitimate medical use as Schedule II drugs. Cocaine (in solution) is still used as a topical anesthetic, and amphetamine derivatives are used to treat attention-deficit/hyperactivity disorder (ADHD), narcolepsy (amphetamine and methylphenidate), and obesity (methamphetamine only). Any of these agents may be abused and carry significant potential for addiction. Even newer "safer" agents such as modafinil (Provigil) and armodafinil (Nuvigil) are associated with abuse and dependency, albeit less commonly than with traditional stimulants.

Prescription stimulant abuse can involve using excessive doses to achieve a euphoric high, or via nonmedical use or diversion of prescriptions (e.g., students sharing medication to facilitate studying). When taken at prescribed doses for an appropriate condition, even methamphetamine is generally safe and effective. In contrast, when it is synthesized in clandestine laboratories and smoked or injected in extreme quantities, methamphetamine (crystal meth, ice, crank, speed) is alarmingly dangerous. No other commonly abused drug is so strongly associated with permanent brain damage, resembling that seen in traumatic brain injury victims. As ADHD becomes more recognized and treated, physicians must be aware of the potential for abuse of their well-intentioned prescriptions. To this end, several recent pharmacologic developments have introduced improved options for treatment. Time-released formulations of methylphenidate (e.g., Concerta) and amphetamine/dextroamphetamine (Adderall XR) are considered to have less abuse potential than the short-acting formulations. Better still, the formulation of lisdexamfetamine (Vyvanse) includes the amino acid lysine coupled with the amphetamine molecule, consequently acting as a prodrug with the least abuse potential of all ADHD stimulants.

Cocaine and other stimulants induce sympathomimetic effects including tachycardia, hypertension, mydriasis, and diaphoresis. These drugs are commonly associated with seizures, myocardial infarction, hemorrhagic strokes, dyskinesias and dystonias, and psychosis when taken at the doses typically used to achieve euphoria. Withdrawal is generally experienced as a crash and includes fatigue, depressed mood, increased appetite, and cravings. Considered nonaddictive until about 1980, cocaine is now widely recognized as one of the most addictive drugs, particularly in the base form (crack or freebase). MDMA (methylenedioxymethylamphetamine), or ecstasy, shares the pharmacodynamic properties of the stimulants, combined with serotoninergic effects of the hallucinogens.

Currently, no medication has demonstrated efficacy in treating cocaine or stimulant dependence. Pharmacologic treatment remains symptomatic during the acute withdrawal phase. Stimulant-induced psychosis and mania respond well to traditional psychotropics when warranted; however, to date, no medications have reliably demonstrated efficacy in preventing relapse. A "cocaine vaccine,"[2] which enlists the immune system to develop antibodies rendering cocaine useless, is currently in phase II clinical trials and holds promise for the future. In the meantime, traditional psychosocial treatments remain the mainstay of clinical care.

Opioids

Opioids are categorized as endogenous (endorphins, enkephalins, dynorphins), opium alkaloids (morphine, codeine), semisynthetic (heroin, oxycodone [Roxicodone, OxyContin]), or synthetic (methadone [Dolophine], fentanyl [Sublimaze, Duragesic]). The last three categories have a wide range of clinical uses including analgesia, anesthesia, antidiarrhea, cough suppression, and detoxification and maintenance therapy.

Opioids exert their clinical effect at mu, delta, and kappa opioid receptors. The effect on mu receptors is considered the most important, with its activation directly linked to both analgesic and euphoric effects. Most humans subjectively experience opioids with a neutral to aversive response. However, when used in sufficient quantities by genetically vulnerable persons, some users experience energy, relief of emotional pain, and a euphoria many describe as a "total body orgasm." Intoxication manifests with miosis, impaired consciousness, slurred speech, bradycardia, and depressed respiration. Overdose is potentially fatal via respiratory depression, but it is quite amenable to treatment with repeated doses of intravenous naloxone (Narcan). The withdrawal syndrome is characterized by a constellation of miserable but not life-threatening symptoms including mydriasis, piloerection, muscle cramps, diaphoresis, vomiting, lacrimation, rhinorrhea, chills, insomnia, cravings, and autonomic hyperactivity.

Since pain was recognized as "the fifth vital sign" in the 1990s, concurrent with heavy marketing campaigns from pharmaceutical companies, the United States has experienced a veritable explosion of widespread opioid prescribing for nonmalignant pain. An entire industry of pain management has developed, with the unfortunate side effect of having a sizable proportion of its output being used nonmedically. It is important for prescribers to recognize that the abuse potential of prescription opioids matches, or in some cases even exceeds, that of heroin. Today, oxycodone has a street value of approximately $1.00 per milligram.

The most common method of abuse involves simply taking more than prescribed, usually by the appropriate route of administration. Alternatively, opioid abusers commonly take their medications via nasal insufflation or inject them intravenously. The time-release property of certain medications, such as oxycodone (OxyContin), is easily circumvented by crushing the pills, which greatly enhances the euphoric effect. Even transdermal fentanyl patches (Duragesic) are abused via any number of methods, such as applying heat to a worn patch, employing complex extraction techniques described on the Internet, or simply sucking on the patch itself (a common finding by the coroner). Once the prescription is finished early, the user must either supplement the supply or face the unpleasant effects of withdrawal.

There is no shortage of easy methods to obtain opiates illegally. These include seeing multiple prescribers (doctor shopping), purchasing online at foreign "pharmacies," and general trade or purchase on the black market. Also alarming is the growing problem of diversion from hospitals and pharmacies by health care professionals, who are not immune to the disease of addiction. Many states are implementing controlled substance databases aimed to curb the problem of abuse of opioids and other prescription drugs.

Acute detoxification from opioids is achieved via one of two basic strategies: symptomatic treatment with unrelated medications, or substitution with a cross tolerant (opioid) drug with less abuse potential (Table 2). The first strategy may employ the use of clonidine (Catapres),[2] an α2-adrenergic agonist, to help with the autonomic component of withdrawal. This is commonly done in combination with other symptomatic treatments on an as-needed basis, such as diazepam (Valium) for anxiety, loperamide (Imodium) for diarrhea, and promethazine (Phenergan)[2] or ondansetron (Zofran)[2] for nausea.

The second strategy typically involves either methadone or buprenorphine (Subutex). Methadone, a pure mu agonist with a half-life of about 36 hours, is usually started in the 20- to 30-mg range and titrated cautiously by 10 mg every 4 to 7 days. Maintenance therapy with methadone occurs only in highly regulated methadone clinic settings. Buprenorphine, a partial agonist at the mu receptor (and kappa antagonist) is administered sublingually and has a half-life similar to that of methadone. It was approved in 2002 for office-based treatment of opioid addiction, making pharmacotherapy much more widely available. Caution should be used to not administer buprenorphine too soon (before onset of withdrawal syndrome), or acute withdrawal can actually be precipitated. Buprenorphine is available either alone or in combination with naloxone (Suboxone). Here, the role of naloxone is solely to deter intravenous abuse, because naloxone is inactive when taken sublingually as prescribed.

Buprenorphine and methadone are useful in managing acute withdrawal as well as long-term (months to years) maintenance therapy for preventing relapse to heroin or the opioid of choice. As maintenance therapy, these agents serve to block euphoria, satisfy cravings, and reduce illicit use, with consequent verifiable harm reduction. Buprenorphine, with a built-in ceiling effect because of its unique pharmacology, is much safer than methadone, which is often fatal in overdose. Increasingly, buprenorphine is being used as an analgesic as well (Butrans), and it may be an ideal choice in patients with comorbid pain and addiction who have demonstrated an inability to safely use other opioids.

Also approved for prevention of opioid relapse is naltrexone, an opioid antagonist, which is available in oral (ReVia) and intramuscular depot formulations (Vivitrol).

Sedative-Hypnotics

This class of drugs includes a wide array of compounds (benzodiazepines, barbiturates, and various related compounds) (Table 3), most of which have at least some potential for abuse. Overall, these medications do much more good than harm, and are useful in treating anxiety disorders, insomnia, seizures, and muscle spasms. They are also important in managing withdrawal states and as a component of surgical anesthesia. These drugs act as CNS depressants, and their primary mechanism of action is to enhance inhibitory GABA neurotransmission. The risk of toxicity is by respiratory depression, which is magnified by concomitant use of opioids or other CNS depressants, such as alcohol.

Sedative-hypnotic intoxication and withdrawal states closely resemble those of alcohol, except for a more protracted time course of withdrawal. Anxiety, restlessness, insomnia, tremor, nystagmus, tachycardia, and hypertension usually appear 2 to 12

---

[2]Not available in the United States.

[2]Not available in the United States.

| TABLE 2 | Useful Medications in Treating Opioid Use Disorders |

DRUG	UTILITY	FORMS	ADMINISTRATION	NOTES
Naloxone (Narcan)	Overdose; additive to prevent abuse[1]	SC, IM, IV	0.4–2 mg q2–3 min prn	$T_{1/2}$ = 1 h, wears off quickly
Naltrexone (ReVia, Vivitrol)	Prevention of relapse	PO, IM	ReVia: 50–100 mg PO daily; Vivitrol: 380 mg IM q4wk	Potential for hepatotoxicity; precipitates withdrawal; useful for ETOH as well
Clonidine (Catapres, Catapres-TTS patch)[1]	Withdrawal	PO, transdermal	0.1–0.2 mg PO tid prn; 0.1–0.3 mg/24 h transdermal via weekly patch	Monitor for hypotension
Methadone (Dolophine)	Withdrawal; maintenance	PO	Start 20–30 mg PO qd Target 80–120 mg PO qd	Restricted to methadone clinics
Buprenorphine (Subutex, Suboxone [with naloxone], Buprenex injection[1])	Withdrawal; maintenance	SL IM, IV	Start 2–4 mg SL qd-bid Target 4–32 mg SL daily divided qd-tid	Requires special DEA certification

Abbreviations: DEA = Drug Enforcement Administration; ETOH = ethanol.
[1]Not FDA approved for this indication.

| TABLE 3 | Common Sedative-Hypnotics, Equivalent Dose Conversions |

GENERIC NAME	TRADE NAME	DOSE (MG)
Benzodiazepines		
Diazepam	Valium	10
Alprazolam	Xanax, Niravam	0.5–1
Lorazepam	Ativan	2
Clonazepam	Klonopin	1–2
Chlordiazepoxide	Librium	25
Clorazepate	Tranxene	7.5
Oxazepam	Serax	10–15
Temazepam	Restoril	15
Triazolam	Halcion	0.25
Flurazepam	Dalmane	15
Barbiturates		
Phenobarbital	n/a	30
Pentobarbital	Nembutal	100
Secobarbital	Seconal	100
Butalbital (with caffeine and aspirin or acetaminophen)	Fiorinal, Fioricet	100
Amobarbital	Amytal	100
Related Compounds		
Carisoprodol	Soma	700
Meprobamate	Miltown, Equanil	1200
Chloral hydrate	Noctec	500
Methaqualone[1]	Quaalude	300
Ethchlorvynol[1]	Placidyl	500
Zolpidem	Ambien	20
Zaleplon	Sonata	20
Eszopiclone	Lunesta	3

n/a, not applicable.
[1]Not FDA approved for this indication.

hours after the last dose, and symptoms gradually resolve over 1 to 2 weeks. Withdrawal seizures, psychosis, and delirium are fairly common. Detoxification is best accomplished on an inpatient basis and typically involves tapering doses of a long-acting benzodiazepine (e.g., clonazepam [Klonopin], diazepam, clorazepate [Tranxene]) at a rate of about 10% of initial daily requirement per day. Acute sedative overdose is managed primarily with supportive care and airway management. Flumazenil (Romazicon) 0.2 to 0.5 mg/min IV may be used with caution for acute overdose of benzodiazepines because it can precipitate severe acute withdrawal symptoms.

Since their introduction in the 1960s, benzodiazepines have largely replaced barbiturates, given their enhanced safety profile. However, barbiturates still in common use include phenobarbital and butalbital. Phenobarbital, used mainly for treating seizures, is considered to have low potential for abuse. Butalbital, compounded with caffeine plus acetaminophen or aspirin (Fioricet, Fiorinal), has moderate abuse potential, typically in combination with other drugs. Carisoprodol (Soma), although not a barbiturate, is metabolized into meprobamate, a barbiturate-like drug. Commonly taken in combination with opioids and other sedatives, carisoprodol is highly abused.

Alprazolam (Xanax) stands out among its peers as the single most abused, most addictive, and yet currently most prescribed sedative-hypnotic. Its rapid onset (T_{max} 1–2 h) and relatively short half-life (6–14 h) contribute to its abuse liability and propensity for withdrawal seizures. Diazepam, historically the most prescribed sedative, also has relatively rapid onset and significant abuse potential, but its long half-life makes it an ideal agent for use in treating withdrawal from other sedatives. Flunitrazepam (Rohypnol, "roofies") is a benzodiazepine that causes anterograde amnesia and is now illegal in the United States because of its use in drug-facilitated sexual assaults.

γ-Hydroxybutyric acid (GHB) and baclofen (Lioresal) also act as GABAergic CNS depressants, with intoxication and withdrawal states consistent with the class. Oddly, GHB is considered a Schedule I drug with high abuse potential and no accepted medical use, but marketed as sodium oxybate (Xyrem), GHB is available as a Schedule III drug (with special restrictions) when used to treat narcolepsy. Baclofen, on the other hand, appears to have rather low abuse potential and may actually play a role in the treatment of alcoholism.[1]

Relatively new drugs such as zolpidem (Ambien), zaleplon (Sonata), and eszopiclone (Lunesta) are benzodiazepine-like drugs with CNS depressant activity, approved for short-term

[1]Not FDA approved for this indication.

treatment of insomnia, and have at least some potential for abuse and dependence. Clonazepam is generally considered to have the lowest potential for euphoria and abuse and is the agent of choice if a benzodiazepine must be given to patients with a relative contraindication, such as a history of any drug abuse or dependence.

Conclusion

Despite intensive supply-reduction strategies, improved primary prevention efforts, and the many recent pharmacotherapy advances, drug abuse remains largely unchanged in its overall scale, with the exceptions of increasing use, abuse, and dependence of both marijuana and prescription opioids. Another notable exception is the significant reduction in tobacco use since the turn of the century. It is estimated that 25% of patients seen in office settings and 50% of those seen in emergency department settings have active problems related to substance abuse. All patients in primary care settings must be screened for tobacco, alcohol, and illicit drug abuse. Patients should be asked directly about substance use at the initial point of contact (e.g., emergency departments, primary care offices), and clinicians should maintain a healthy degree of skepticism toward patients' responses, remembering that most patients minimize substance use. When any suspicion exists, urine drug screens should be readily utilized without hesitation or fear of communicating mistrust. A variety of affordable quick screen kits are available, which can be sent out for laboratory confirmation of positive results if necessary.

Physicians and other health care professionals are in a unique position to intervene with drug abuse at the individual level, because it is encountered commonly in clinical practice. The problem must first be identified, and depending on the skill set of the primary provider, patients should be treated or referred to an appropriate treatment provider. There is an initiative to incorporate formal SBIRT (screening, brief intervention, and referral to treatment) into routine clinical practice. Current procedural terminology (CPT) codes and a reimbursement schedule for screening and brief intervention may be located online at https://www.samhsa.gov/sbirt/coding-reimbursement. Screening may involve the written or verbal assessment of substance use to determine whether the patient exhibits problematic levels of use. The brief intervention aspect of SBIRT targets those with milder substance use problems and provides effective strategies for intervention before the need for more extensive or specialized treatment arises. Referral to specialized treatment is recommended for patients with moderate-to-severe substance use disorders. Data suggest this approach is successful in modifying problematic substance-use behavior. In addition to formal treatment, physician referral to local 12-step recovery meetings (Alcoholics Anonymous, Narcotics Anonymous) has proved beneficial. Local chapters provide physicians with names and telephone numbers of members willing to welcome newcomers (www.aa.org).

Physicians are usually well equipped to treat the sequelae of drug abuse, but they often forget that addiction is a treatable disease entity itself. Treatment ranges in intensity along a continuum including medically managed inpatient detoxification, partial hospitalization, intensive outpatient treatment, and outpatient care. The American Society of Addiction Medicine provides patient placement criteria that dictate the appropriate level of treatment based on a multidimensional assessment. Health care professionals should be familiar with the treatment centers in their area, which can place the patient in the appropriate level of care.

It is important to remember that relapse is a characteristic of addiction and does not equate to treatment failure, but rather indicates a need for an adjustment in the treatment level or monitoring. Other chronic diseases, such as diabetes or hypertension, necessitate the ongoing monitoring and adjustment of treatment interventions as needed, and so is the case with addiction. Recently published data on the treatment and monitoring of recovering physicians (a subgroup of addicts that boasts a 5-year success rate greater than 78%) teaches us the lesson that adequate initial treatment coupled with ongoing monitoring is critical. Sustained recovery from substance use disorders is attainable and is characterized by voluntary sobriety, improved personal health, and improved citizenship.

References

American Psychiatric Association: *Diagnostic and Statistical Manual of Mental Disorders*, 5th ed., Washington, DC, 2013, American Psychiatric Publishing.

American Society of Addiction Medicine: Public policy statement: Definition of addiction. August 15, Available at http://www.asam.org/docs/publicy-policy-statements/1definition_of_addiction_long_4-11.pdf, 2011.

Bailey JA, Hurley RW, Gold MS: Crossroads of pain and addiction, *Pain Med* 11:1803–1818, 2010.

Centers for Disease Control, Prevention: Annual smoking-attributable mortality, years of potential life lost, and productivity losses—United States, 1997–2001, *MMWR Morb Mortal Wkly Rep* 54:625–628, 2005.

DuPont RL, McLellan AT, White WL, et al: Setting the standard for recovery: physicians health programs, *J Subst Abuse Treat* 36:159–171, 2009.

Fowler JS, Volkow ND, Wang GJ, et al: Neuropharmacological actions of cigarette smoke: brain monoamine oxidase B (MAO B) inhibition, *J Addict Dis* 17:23–24, 1998.

Gold MS, Kobeissy FH, Wang KK, et al: Methamphetamine- and trauma-induced brain injuries: comparative cellular and molecular neurobiological substrates, *Biol Psychiatry* 66:118–127, 2009.

Haney M, Hart CL, Foltin RW: Effects of baclofen on cocaine self-administration: opioid- and nonopioid-dependent volunteers, *Neuropharmacology* 31:1814–1821, 2006.

Johnston LD, O'Malley PM, Bachman JG, et al: *Monitoring the Future: National Results on Adolescent Drug Use: Overview of Key Findings, 2010*, Ann Arbor, 2011, Institute for Social Research, The University of Michigan.

Office of National Drug Control Policy: *The Economic Costs of Drug Abuse in the United States: 1992–2002*, Washington, DC, 2004, Executive Office of the President. [Publication No. 207303].

Small E, Shah HP, Davenport JJ, et al: Tobacco smoke exposure induces nicotine dependence in rats, *Psychopharmacology (Berl)* 208:143–158, 2010.

EATING DISORDERS

Method of
Sarah Forsberg, PsyD and James Lock, MD, PhD

Bulimia Nervosa

CURRENT DIAGNOSIS

- Binge eating episodes occur at least once per week for 3 months (eating objectively large quantities of food accompanied by a loss of control while eating).
- Compensatory purging episodes occur at least once per week for a period of 3 months (e.g., self-induced vomiting, laxatives, diuretics, excessive and driven exercise, enemas).
- Shape and weight are overvalued in self-worth and self-esteem.
- Weight is at or above expected range given age, height, and historical growth curves.

CURRENT TREATMENT

- Cognitive behavioral therapy (CBT) is the most evidence-based treatment for bulimia nervosa (BN).
- Interpersonal psychotherapy (IPT) is an appropriate alternative.
- Family-based treatment (FBT) is useful for adolescents with BN.
- Antidepressant treatment (selective serotonin reuptake inhibitors [SSRIs]) may be useful in augmenting psychotherapy, or as an alternative in the event that psychotherapy is not effective, is refused, or is unavailable. It is not as effective as CBT and thus not a front-line approach.

Diagnosis

To diagnose bulimia nervosa (BN), an individual must engage in recurrent binge episodes with compensatory behaviors (e.g., self-induced vomiting, diuretic or laxative use, excessive exercise).

A binge is a discrete episode of eating a quantity of food that is more than the average person would eat in the same setting. While binging, there is a loss of control or sense of being unable to stop eating. A disproportionate emphasis on weight and shape in one's self-evaluation is also required in diagnosing BN. DSM-5 criteria require that these episodes occur at a minimum of once weekly for 3 months. Unlike individuals with anorexia nervosa (AN), who may binge and purge, individuals with BN are within range of or above the median BMI.

Significant health consequences may accompany BN. Laboratory studies often reveal electrolyte abnormalities, which can lead to cardiac arrhythmias and cardiac arrest in severe cases. Physical examination may detect enamel decay and parotid gland enlargement because of recurrent vomiting. When ipecac[1] is used to induce vomiting, severe cardiac and skeletal myopathies may develop. Laxative abuse is associated with metabolic acidosis and elevated serum amylase levels. BN has an elevated risk for mortality (crude mortality of 3.9%-6% in an inpatient sample), with many dying by suicide. Most common comorbid psychiatric diagnoses are mood, anxiety, personality disorders (specifically borderline personality), and substance use disorders.

Epidemiology

BN behaviors typically first occur in middle adolescence (ages 14–16), with onset of full syndrome BN in later adolescence and early adulthood (ages 17–24). The lifetime prevalence estimate of DSM-5 BN ranges from 4%-6.7%, and while less is known about males, at minimum they are estimated to account for between 10% to 25% of all cases. Symptoms may persist for a number of years, with intermittent periods of remission. A review of existing treatment studies suggests that approximately 45% of patients fully recover, with 27% improving considerably and the remaining 23% exhibiting a chronic course.

Etiology

BN can be explained by a confluence of biological, sociocultural, psychological, and familial factors. From a biological standpoint, BN clusters in families; in twin studies, about half of the variance in heritability can be explained by genetic factors. Serotonin levels may be reduced, and imaging studies show abnormal serotonergic circuitry in the orbital-frontal cortex. Internalization of cultural ideals of beauty may present as a focus on thinness for women, where for males there is often pressure to be muscular with low body fat. Participation in sports where weight and appearance are tied to performance (e.g., gymnastics, wrestling) may increase risk. Early puberty and childhood obesity are common precipitants, as are experiences with peer weight-related teasing. Personality characteristics of individuals with BN may include perfectionism, impulsivity, and instability in interpersonal relationships. Childhood sexual and physical abuse increases the risk for BN.

Treatment

Given the significant physical, social, and emotional consequences associated with BN, effective treatment requires addressing wide-ranging difficulties. Over 70 randomized controlled treatment trials (RCTs) exist for adults with BN, yet only four focus on adolescents. Most studies have examined behavioral therapies, medications, or a combination thereof. CBT is established as the treatment of choice for adults with BN and has been subjected to a large number of RCTs. The underlying assumption of CBT is that bulimic behaviors are maintained by dysfunctional attitudes about shape, weight, and physical appearance, which thereby lead to an overemphasis of these aspects in self-evaluation. Excessive dieting typically ensues, resulting in physiologic and psychologic deprivation that increases vulnerability to binge eating. Feelings of guilt and fear about weight gain are mitigated through engaging in purging behaviors. CBT targets this cycle through the use of self-monitoring to increase an awareness of patterns in behaviors, thoughts and emotions that maintain BN.

CBT is found to be more effective than no treatment, pill placebo, nondirective supportive psychotherapy, nutritional counseling, stress management, and antidepressant medication therapy. Response to CBT is good, with approximately 50% recovered and 20% with significant reductions in symptoms at the end of treatment. CBT is acceptable and feasible with adolescents, however a more recent RCT had a 20% rate of abstinence, compared to previous rates of 56% in a case series and 36% in a guided self-help (GSH) version at the end of treatment. When compared to an alternative intervention, interpersonal psychotherapy (IPT), CBT demonstrates a greater probability of remission and reduction in symptoms at the end of treatment. However, these initial differences appear to diminish at a 1-year follow-up, suggesting that, while less efficient, IPT is a viable alternative. IPT was adapted for BN to target interpersonal factors thought to contribute to the development and maintenance of the disorder. IPT has yet to be studied with adolescents.

More recently, CBT has been expanded to address other maintaining features of eating disorders more broadly (e.g., interpersonal difficulties, clinical perfectionism, low self-esteem, and mood intolerance). Enhanced CBT (CBT-E) addresses these features and is delivered in a focused or broad (addressing aforementioned maintaining features) format. For individuals with more complex psychopathology, the broad version may be more effective. Further, a novel treatment, integrative cognitive affective therapy for BN (ICAT-BN), may be preferable to CBT-E for individuals with greater affective lability and stimulus seeking.

Other interventions show promise in the treatment of BN and require further examination. For adolescents, FBT may be helpful, demonstrating higher rates of binge/purge abstinence (40%) than supportive psychotherapy in one study, and than CBT (FBT: 39% vs. CBT: 20%) in another. Derived from FBT for AN, parents are supported to directly change dysfunctional eating behaviors. For adults, dialectical behavior therapy (DBT) has been shown to significantly decrease binge/purge episodes when delivered in an individual format. Similar effects were found when an appetite-awareness component was added to standard DBT.

Antidepressants (SSRIs) are the most studied medication treatment for BN. Fluoxetine (Prozac) demonstrates greater reductions in binge eating, purging, and eating-related cognitions than placebo when prescribed at higher doses (60 mg/day). A small pilot study of fluoxetine with adolescents suggests it is acceptable and may decrease BN symptoms. Antidepressants alone are not as effective as when combined with CBT, or as CBT alone.

Binge Eating Disorder

 CURRENT DIAGNOSIS

- Recurrent episodes of binge eating, defined as eating an objectively large amount of food in a discrete period of time with an experience of loss of control.
- Binge eating is associated with at least three of the following: eating rapidly; eating until uncomfortably full; eating outside of physical hunger; eating alone because of embarrassment; and subsequent feelings of disgust, depression, or guilt.
- There is marked distress associated with binge eating.
- These episodes occur at least once per week over 3 months.
- There is no associated compensatory behavior (e.g., purging), and binging does not occur in the context of another eating disorder diagnosis (anorexia or bulimia nervosa [BN]).

---

[1]Not FDA approved for this indication.

CURRENT TREATMENT

- CBT and IPT have good evidence of efficacy among adults.
- GSH CBT may be effective for those with less psychopathology.
- DBT requires further study to determine if good outcomes are sustained over time.
- There is no evidence-based treatment for young patients with binge eating disorder (BED)-pharmacologic treatments should be considered as an adjunct to psychotherapy.

Diagnosis

Binge episodes are characterized by eating quantities that are larger than others would eat in a similar setting and are accompanied by a feeling of being out of control. Individuals with BED do not engage in compensatory behaviors (e.g., self-induced vomiting, excessive exercise) as in BN. DSM-5 criteria require that the episodes occur at a minimum frequency of once per week over a 3-month period. Binge eating (BE) is commonly associated with feelings of guilt and embarrassment and may result in attempts to hide eating. Further, during binge episodes, eating is often rapid and results in feeling uncomfortably full. Most individuals with BED have at least one comorbid psychiatric diagnoses (79% of respondents in one study).

Epidemiology

Lifetime prevalence of BE among adult females was 3% and 3.6% in two separate studies, and 2.1% in males. It occurs at equal rates across ethnic and racial groups. BE most typically onsets in later adolescence or early adulthood, although it does occur in children and is often associated with overweight and obesity as well as psychological symptoms. Among adolescents with obesity, an estimated 1% meet the criteria for BED and up to 26% experience BE/loss of control eating. In BED, obesity often predates dieting and subsequent BE, with women having an earlier onset of both dieting and BE. Remission rates in BED are higher than in other eating disorders, although duration and severity is similar to BN.

Etiology

The etiology of BED is unknown. Restrictive dieting, body image dissatisfaction, pressure to be thin, low self-esteem, depressive symptoms, and limited social support increase the risk for the onset of adolescent BE. Increased rates of BE in families suggests there may be a genetic link. Potential medical causes for BE include CNS tumors, Kleine-Levin syndrome, Kluver-Bucy syndrome, Prader-Willi syndrome, and gastrointestinal pathology, and these causes should be ruled out during assessment. Comorbid psychiatric disorders are common among adults with BED, including mood disorders, anxiety disorders, and, at lesser frequency, substance use disorders and personality disorders. There are high rates of obesity among individuals with BED; however, psychiatric symptoms are linked to the severity of BE rather than obese status.

Treatment

Treatment for adults with BED has received considerable attention in RCTs compared to other eating disorder diagnoses. Most treatments target reduction in BE, psychological symptoms, and weight loss for those who are overweight. CBT has been applied in multiple formats (group, GSH, CD-ROM delivered, and in combination with medication) and appears to have the highest rates of abstinence. Individual CBT outperformed group CBT in one trial, and a GSH version was more effective in reducing BE than behavioral weight-loss (BWL). CBT targets underlying dysfunctional attitudes and behaviors that maintain BE. An alternative treatment, IPT, is a time-limited psychodynamic therapy targeting interpersonal difficulties that underlie the disorder. IPT is helpful in reducing the frequency of BE. IPT, CBT, and motivational interviewing (MI) all lead to improvements in cognitive restraint, disinhibition, and shape and weight concerns thought to maintain BE.

Dialectical behavior therapy (DBT) is another treatment adapted for BED with the aim of targeting affected regulation difficulties formulated to be a maintaining mechanism of BE. Women in a small trial comparing group DBT to a waitlisted group had significantly greater decreases in BE and related eating disorder thoughts and behaviors, with over half abstinent from BE at follow-up. However, when compared to supportive psychotherapy, the rate of abstinence, while achieved more quickly in the DBT group, did not differ between the groups at follow-up. Pilot data suggest comprehensive DBT (individual, group, and skills coaching) may be effective.

Pharmacologic treatments targeting BE and weight loss have been tested alone and in combination with psychotherapy. There may be improvement in weight loss with addition of pharmacotherapy. The combination of CBT with topiramate (Topamax)[1] resulted in greater weight loss and better psychosocial outcomes than CBT with fluoxetine.[1] A high dose of the SSRI escitalopram (Lexapro)[1], anticonvulsants topiramate and zonisamide (Zonegran)[1], lisdexamfetamine (Vyvanse) at a dose of 50 mg or 70 mg, and the selective norepinephrine reuptake inhibitor atomoxetine (Strattera)[1] were each associated with significantly decreased binge eating and weight in separate placebo-controlled trials.

Anorexia Nervosa

CURRENT DIAGNOSIS

- Persistent restriction of energy (caloric) intake relative to requirements, leading to significantly low weight (e.g., accounting for age, sex, developmental trajectory, and physical health).
- Fear of becoming fat or ongoing behavior interferes with weight gain.
- Disturbance in the perception of shape, weight, overvaluation of weight, and shape in self-evaluation, or lack of acknowledgment of seriousness of low weight.
- Either meets criteria for restricting type—with absence of binge or purge behaviors, or binge eating/purging type.

CURRENT TREATMENT

- Family-based treatment (FBT) for adolescents with AN is the most evidence-based approach.
- Adolescent-focused therapy (AFT) may be a helpful alternative.
- There are no first-line treatments for adults with AN.
- CBT may prevent relapse in weight-restored individuals.

Diagnosis

AN is characterized by dietary restriction that is severe enough to lead to seriously low weight, fear of weight gain, and difficulty or inability to accurately perceive shape or weight. Secondary amenorrhea is no longer required for a diagnosis of AN in DSM-5. Individuals may be classified as AN-restricting type or AN-binge/purge subtype. The definition of low weight is less than "minimally normal" among adults or "minimally expected" among children and adolescents. Growth charts normed by age

---

[1]Not FDA approved for this indication.

and gender are necessary to calculate expected BMI for individuals under 18 and growth curves may help detect deviations from an individual's growth trajectory. A BMI at or below the 10th percentile is a benchmark reflecting malnourishment associated with AN, and BMI below 18.5 kg/m^2 may be used as guidelines. When an individual meets all criteria for AN, but despite significant weight loss weighs within or above the median BMI range, atypical AN may be diagnosed.

A wide variety of medical and psychiatric symptoms accompany AN. Potentially life-threatening medical conditions may develop as a result of semistarvation. Vital sign abnormalities (bradycardia, orthostasis, hypothermia) and amenorrhea are common consequences of malnutrition. Bone loss resulting in osteopenia and, in more severe cases, osteoporosis may occur. Abnormal laboratory findings may occur in some patients with AN who use laxatives, diuretics, and diet pills and who engage in self-induced vomiting.

The lifetime rate of comorbid psychiatric diagnoses among adolescents with AN is approximately 55%. Most commonly, these comorbidities include anxiety disorders (social anxiety, separation anxiety, generalized anxiety and obsessive compulsive disorder [OCD]), depression, and substance abuse. There is significant overlap in OCD symptoms and AN, thus careful consideration must be given to the content of obsessions and compulsions in diagnosis. In AN, obsessional preoccupations are related to eating, food, weight, and shape, and compulsions may appear as calorie counting, excessive exercise routines, and mealtime rituals. Depressive symptoms such as dysphoric thought, low energy, difficulty concentrating, and low self-esteem also manifest in AN and may not indicate a separate depressive disorder.

Epidemiology

Peak age of onset for AN is between 14 and 18 years. Lifetime prevalence of females with a DSM-5 diagnosis of AN in the United States is estimated to be between .8% and 3.6%, based on method of data collection. The incidence of AN among males is less studied, but recent estimates suggest that 1 out of every 4 cases are male. Little is known about the prevalence of AN across racial and ethnic groups. A recent study did not reflect significantly higher rates of AN among non-Hispanic white adolescents as compared to Hispanic and non-Hispanic black peers; however, other evidence suggests that it is less common among persons of African origin.

AN has the highest mortality rate of any psychiatric illness, with reports as high as 5% per decade. Rates of chronicity obtained from long-term adult follow-up studies (AN diagnosis persisting greater than 5 years) are estimated between 7% and 15%. Death occurs most commonly secondary to medical complications of starvation or suicide. Prognosis for adolescents with short duration (less than 3 years) is better than adults.

Etiology

The causal mechanisms of AN are multiply determined through the interface of biological/genetic, psychological, and sociocultural factors. Heritability estimates from twin studies range from 48% to 74%, and family aggregation studies report that AN occurs at about five times the expected rate in affected families. The interactional effect between genes and developmental processes is reflected in studies demonstrating greater heritability among 17-year-old twins as compared to 11-year-old twins. Hormonal changes during adolescence could mediate gene expression during puberty, explaining this difference.

Perfectionistic and avoidant personality features are associated with AN, and are likely heritable. Neurocognitive features including cognitive rigidity and an overly detailed style of information processing are common and may represent an endophenotype as those who are recovered as well as unaffected siblings who demonstrate similar cognitive styles. Common developmental

challenges associated with adolescence may also precipitate or emerge as a consequence of AN—these include navigating issues of autonomy, self-efficacy, and intimacy. Sociocultural factors including exposure to a Westernized "thin ideal" of beauty for females and an overly muscular ideal for males may be internalized, thereby triggering extreme dieting or exercise. Further, activities where weight or appearance is intertwined with performance may also elevate risk (e.g., gymnastics, ballet, wrestling, figure skating).

Treatment

Given the severity of psychological, social, and health consequences of AN, both close medical monitoring and psychotherapy are the standard of care. In severe cases, inpatient medical monitoring may be required, and standard criteria for hospitalization are available for physicians. Findings from RCTs among adults are inconclusive because of dropout rates as high as 50%. Medication trials of antidepressants (serotonin reuptake inhibitors and tricyclics) have high dropout rates and little to no improvement in weight or eating disorder behaviors. Therefore, these should not be used independent of psychotherapy. A recent trial demonstrated an average of 1 lb per month greater weight gain for those taking olanzapine (Zyprexa)[1] than not; however, potential risks, including tardive dyskinesia and metabolic side effects, need be considered. CBT may help prevent relapse for individuals who are already weight-restored. For underweight individuals, findings are mixed, and nonspecific therapies such as nonspecific supportive clinical management (NSCM) showed better outcomes compared to IPT and CBT at end of treatment. However, improvements in NSCM appear to decline over time, and IPT may catch up to CBT.

Recent treatment studies have focused on improving retention. For example, an enhanced version of outpatient CBT (CBT-E), which employs motivational enhancement strategies, retained 64% of the original sample, improving on previous trends in attrition. Individuals completing treatment had clinically significant improvements in weight and eating disorder psychopathology. When CBT-E was compared to focal psychodynamic therapy and treatment as usual (TAU) in the community, weight gain and improvements in eating disorder symptoms were more rapid. However, focal psychodynamic treatment had the highest rates of recovery at follow-up (35%), though these were only significantly higher than the TAU group.

FBT, otherwise known as Maudsley family therapy, has been studied in seven RCTs with superior outcome to other individual therapies. This outpatient treatment empowers parents to disrupt self-starvation and other behaviors that maintain AN. In the initial phase of treatment, parents take full control over managing eating-related behaviors. FBT demonstrates rates of remission ranging from 49% (full remission in weight and eating disorder thoughts and behaviors) to 89% for partial remission. Rates of relapse are about 10% and there is minimal dropout, suggesting it is acceptable to families. FBT delivered in a parent-focused format may be just as effective, and preferable to conjoint FBT for families with high levels of expressed emotion.

Adolescent Focused Therapy (AFT) may be an alternative approach for individuals whose family members are unable to participate. The focus in AFT is on helping an adolescent move toward healthy individuation and increased self-efficacy. AN is conceptualized as an ineffective strategy that the adolescent has adopted in managing common developmental challenges. In AFT, adolescents learn new skills to support eating and weight gain and parents are involved in separated collateral sessions. CBT has also been studied in adolescents; when compared to TAU and hospitalization, it appeared to be the most cost-effective approach.

---

[1]Not FDA approved for this indication.

Avoidant-Restrictive Food Intake Disorder

CURRENT DIAGNOSIS

- Disturbance in eating/feeding resulting in persistent failure to meet nutritional and/or energy needs.
- The disorder must result in one of the following consequences: significant weight loss or faltering growth; significant nutritional deficiency; dependence on nutritional supplements or enteral feeding; and interference with psychosocial functioning.
- The eating/feeding disturbance is not better explained by another medical or psychiatric condition or by cultural or religious practices.

CURRENT TREATMENT

- There are no established treatments for this new diagnosis.
- CBT or family interventions that employ behavioral strategies are being explored as potential treatment options.

Diagnosis

Avoidant-restrictive food intake disorder (ARFID) is a new diagnosis included in the DSM-5, which reflects the recognition of "food neophobia" or extreme picky eating as challenges. Individuals with ARFID can be of any age and exhibit clinically significant feeding/eating difficulties, which result in failure to meet energy (caloric) or nutritional needs. In response, individuals have low weight or failure to meet expectations for growth, significant nutritional deficiency, a need for enteral feeding or oral nutritional supplementation, or impairment in psychosocial functioning. Although there may be failure to thrive or to make expected weight gain/weight loss, it is distinguished from AN by the absence of body image disturbance. Low weight can be determined through clinical judgment and examination of developmental trajectory using growth charts. Nutritional deficiency may be assessed through dietary history as well as physical examination. Related medical consequences may follow those seen in malnourished individuals with AN (e.g., bradycardia, anemia, hypothermia), and can be life threatening. Individuals with ARFID treated in an inpatient setting are more likely to require nasogastric feeding than those with AN. If limited food intake is better explained by cultural or religious practice, an eating disorder in which there is disturbance in experience of shape/weight, or current physiologic or psychiatric conditions that explain the symptoms, ARFID is not diagnosed. Further, in the event of a coexisting medical diagnosis, food refusal is serious enough to warrant separate clinical attention. Thorough assessment should include examination of feeding, and eating history, psychiatric symptoms, development, and underlying medical causes must be ruled out before making a diagnosis.

Individuals with ARFID often exhibit selective eating, food neophobia, and hypersensitivity to sensory features of food (texture, taste, temperature, appearance). Similar clinical presentations may have varying etiology, requiring individualized treatment plans. In some, development of food avoidance can be traced to a specific aversive event, trauma, or related gastrointestinal problem, or may arise out of a choking, swallowing, or vomiting phobia. Individuals may also have a lack of drive or interest in eating or heightened textural sensitivity, which is common in autism spectrum disorders.

Epidemiology

No data exist on prevalence, course, and outcome of this disorder. Surveillance studies are underway in the UK and Canada for related "food avoidance emotional disorder," with overlap in clinical features. In pediatric inpatient ED programs, rates of ARFID are reported to be between 5% and 14% comprised of a higher proportion of males than other ED diagnoses. ARFID appears to arise most commonly in infancy and early childhood, but can occur at any age and last into adulthood. Preliminary data suggest ARFID occurs at equal rates in males and females. There is no evidence to guide for whom clinical intervention is warranted versus those whose symptoms resolve over time.

Treatment

There are no systematically studied treatments to date for ARFID; however, behavioral interventions with contingency management have been successfully utilized among children who have food neophobia in the context of a developmental disability. Given limited data, individualized treatment plans are best derived through assessment of medical history, temperament, psychiatric symptoms, and development. Food avoidance may be treated through use of behavioral strategies (e.g., shaping, chaining, contingency management, extinction) that systematically desensitize individuals to a wider range of foods. Related anxiety management techniques (relaxation training, visualization for mastery) and cognitive strategies derived from CBT may address maintaining psychiatric features. CBT was successfully applied in a case study of young adults with food neophobia. In most severe cases of malnutrition, hospitalization for medical stabilization purposes may be needed before outpatient therapy.

References

Bulik CM, Berkman ND, Brownley KA, et al: Anorexia nervosa treatment: a systematic review of randomized controlled trials, *Int J Eat Disord* 40:310–320, 2007.
Call C, Walsh B, Attia E: From DSM-IV to DSM-5: changes to eating disorder diagnoses, *Curr Opin Psychiatry* 26:532–536, 2013.
Hay P: A systematic review of evidence for psychological treatments in eating disorders: 2005-2012, *Int J Eat Disord* 46:462–469, 2013.
Kreipe R, Palomski A: Beyond picky eating: avoidant/restrictive food intake disorder, *Curr Psychiatry Rep* 14:421–431, 2012.
Le Grange D, Lock J, editors: *Eating Disorders in Children and Adolescents: A Clinical Handbook*, New York, 2011, The Guilford Press.
Peat C, Brownley K, Berkman N, et al: Binge eating disorder: evidence-based treatments, *Curr Psychiatry* 11:32–39, 2013.
Shapiro J, Berkman N, Brownley K, et al: Bulimia nervosa treatment: a systematic review of randomized controlled trials, *Int J Eat Disord* 40:321–336, 2007.
Smink F, van Hoeken D, Hoek H: Epidemiology of eating disorders: incidence, prevalence and mortality rates, *Curr Psychiatry Rep* 14:406–414, 2012.
Steinhausen H, Weber S: The outcome of bulimia nervosa: findings from one-quarter century of research, *Am J Psychiatry* 166:1331–1341, 2009.

GENERALIZED ANXIETY DISORDER

Method of
Natalie C. Dattilo, PhD; and Andrew W. Goddard, MD

CURRENT DIAGNOSIS

- Generalized anxiety disorder (GAD) is the most common psychiatric disorder seen in the primary care setting.
- GAD is characterized by feelings of dread, negative anticipation, and worry that are difficult to control and may include hypervigilance, excessive reassurance seeking, and behavioral avoidance of anxiety-provoking situations.
- Symptoms of GAD most often include agitation, irritability, restlessness, muscle aches or tension, dizziness, fatigue, racing heart, dry mouth, nausea, decreased sexual desire, sleep or appetite disturbances, and an inability to relax.
- A thorough medical examination and laboratory work may be indicated to rule out underlying physiologic causes, adverse reaction to medication, caffeine or substance use, and drug or alcohol withdrawal.
- Symptoms that are persistent, disruptive, or distressing warrant treatment.

- The Generalized Anxiety Disorder – 7 (GAD-7) is a screening instrument used to assess symptoms of GAD in primary care settings. Scores of 5, 10, and 15 are taken as the cut-off points for mild, moderate, and severe anxiety, respectively. When used as a screening tool, further evaluation is recommended when the score is 10 or greater.

CURRENT THERAPY

- Effective treatments for GAD include serotonergic antidepressants, certain forms of psychotherapy, or a combination of both.
- Educate the patient and family members about treatment options as well as realistic treatment expectations.
- Depending on the patient's preference, treatment may include a selective serotonin reuptake inhibitor (SSRI) or a serotonin norepinephrine reuptake inhibitor (SNRI), starting at low doses with careful titration so as not to exacerbate anxiety symptoms.
- Treatment may also include a trial of cognitive-behavioral therapy (CBT) monotherapy or in combination with medication management.
- Refer to or consult with a psychiatrist for patients with severe or particularly complex cases or for patients with a less-than-expected response to treatment.
- Refer to a CBT specialist for patients with a preference for behavioral, skills-based, or nonmedication therapy or for whom pharmacotherapy may be contraindicated.

Epidemiology

Anxiety disorders are among the most prevalent psychiatric disorders in the world. In the United States, it is estimated that an anxiety disorder is diagnosed in approximately 16 million adults each year and approximately 30 million meet criteria for an anxiety disorder over the course of their lifetimes. Second to depression, anxiety disorders are the most common mental health problem seen by physicians in the general medical setting. In fact, patients with anxiety are more likely to present initially to a generalist physician office than to a mental health care provider.

Anxiety disorders tend to be chronic and disabling and impose a high individual and societal burden. It has been estimated that the United States spends approximately $40 billion to $60 billion per year for costs associated with anxiety disorders. These include not only direct costs associated with treatment but also indirect costs associated with lost productivity. Thus early detection and treatment is critically important.

Risk Factors

Risk factors associated with anxiety disorders include personal or family history of anxiety; recent increase in stressful life events; lack or perceived lack of social support; ineffective emotional coping strategies; being female; experiencing childhood adversity, including trauma or witnessing a traumatic event; having a chronic health condition or serious illness; having an acute or chronic pain condition; and substance abuse. Having a genetic predisposition to developing an anxiety disorder is likely, although environmental stressors clearly play a role. Research has also shown that patients suffering from anxiety are generally more sensitive to physiologic changes than nonanxious patients. This heightened sensitivity leads to diminished autonomic flexibility, which may be the result of faulty central information processing in anxiety-prone persons.

Pathophysiology

Current evidence suggests that anxiety symptoms are likely caused by dysregulation in the central nervous system fear circuit.

Physical and emotional manifestations of this dysregulation can result in a state of hyperarousal. Several neurotransmitter systems have been implicated in the development of this state.

The most commonly considered are the serotoninergic and noradrenergic neurotransmitter systems. Very simply, it is believed that an underactivation of the serotoninergic system and an overactivation of the noradrenergic system are involved, resulting in dysregulation of physiologic arousal and the emotional experience of this arousal. Disruption of the γ-aminobutyric acid (GABA) system has also been implicated because of the response of many of the anxiety-spectrum disorders to treatment with benzodiazepines.

There has also been some interest in the role of corticosteroid regulation and its relation to symptoms of fear and anxiety. Corticosteroids might increase or decrease the activity of certain neural pathways, affecting not only behavior under stress but also the brain's processing of fear-inducing stimuli. The stress response is hardwired into the brain and is most often triggered when survival of the organism is threatened. The stress response, however, can be triggered not only by a physical challenge or threat but also by the mere anticipation (or fear) of threat. As a result, when humans chronically and erroneously believe that a threatening event is about to occur, they begin to experience the physical and psychological symptoms of anxiety and panic.

Finally, a subcortical neural structure, the amygdala, serves an important role in coordinating the cognitive, affective, neuroendocrine, cardiovascular, respiratory, and musculoskeletal components of fear and anxiety responses (fear expression). It is central to registering the emotional significance of stressful stimuli and creating emotional memories. The amygdala receives input from neurons in the sensory cortex. When activated, the amygdala stimulates regions of the midbrain and brainstem, causing autonomic hyperactivity, which can be correlated with the physical symptoms of anxiety.

Prevention

No biological markers are specific enough yet to detect anxiety early, and there is no available evidence to suggest that current medications prove efficacious in preventing these disorders. Therefore, it is important to screen for specific risk factors, such as family history and substance abuse. If a person is anxiety prone, he or she should first be encouraged to adopt healthy lifestyle habits. Exercise has been shown to relieve tension, anxiety, and stress. Patients should avoid stimulants such as caffeine and nicotine, which can exacerbate symptoms. Reducing alcohol intake should be encouraged as well. Educating patients on healthy sleep habits can prevent conditioned (or secondary) insomnia issues. It is also recommended that anxiety-prone persons reduce subjective levels of stress by practicing effective methods of relaxation and other stress management activities, like meditation, yoga, social connection, gratitude journaling, and pleasant event scheduling.

Clinical Manifestations

GAD is characterized by subjective feelings of worry, dread, or anticipation of negative events and can include hypervigilance and avoidance of anxiety-producing situations. Physical symptoms can include jitteriness or shakiness, trembling, muscle aches and tension, sweating, cold or clammy hands, dizziness, or vertigo; fatigue; racing or pounding heart; hyperventilation; sensation of a lump in the throat, choking sensation, or dry mouth; numbness and tingling in the hands, feet, or other body parts; upset stomach, nausea, vomiting, or diarrhea; decreased sexual desire; and sleep and appetite disturbances.

Psychological symptoms include, most predominantly, unrealistic or excessive worry and apprehension, hypervigilance or an inability to relax, distractibility, indecisiveness, and insecurity. Patients often express feelings of impatience, agitation, irritability, and fear. They may ask multiple questions repeatedly in an attempt to quell the anxiety through excessive information or reassurance seeking. In GAD, the worries a patient may express tend to be nonspecific and all-encompassing. They tend to be "worst-case scenario" and "what if?" thinkers. Some patients also exhibit specific phobias such as fear of being far from home or fear of social contact. Patients with GAD may report difficulty falling asleep because they "can't turn their mind off" at night. If a patient reports these symptoms or displays one of several behavioral manifestations of GAD leading to significant distress and/or impairment of function, the condition is unlikely to remit on its own and treatment is warranted.

Diagnosis

A diagnosis of GAD is made when a patient meets the specific diagnostic criteria outlined in the *Diagnostic and Statistical Manual of Mental Disorders, Fifth Edition* (DSM-5). Persons with GAD experience uncontrollable, excessive anxiety and worry involving several areas of functioning on most days for at least 6 months. The anxiety must be associated with at least three of the following symptoms: restlessness, fatigue, impaired concentration, irritability, muscle tension, or sleep problems. Patients tend to express chronic excessive nervousness, exaggerated worry, tension, and irritability that appear to have no cause or are more intense than the situation warrants. Physical signs such as headaches, trembling, twitching, or sweating often develop, which lead to further worries. GAD symptoms tend to wax and wane over time, with short-term exacerbations of acute anxiety in response to stress. Symptoms show substantial overlap with those of other medical and psychological disorders, particularly major depressive disorder, substance abuse disorders, and other anxiety disorders, which tends to complicate diagnosis.

Differential Diagnosis

It is important to perform a thorough medical workup when initially assessing the patient with anxiety symptoms. The differential diagnosis can include several organic causes, such as endocrine dysfunction, intoxication or withdrawal, hypoxia, metabolic abnormalities, and neurologic disorders. It is also important to rule out other comorbid psychiatric disorders. Severe depression, bipolar disorder, prodromal schizophrenia, delusional disorder, and adjustment disorder can often be accompanied by severe anxiety. Many organic causes can be ruled out by a thorough history and basic laboratory work, including thyroid-stimulating hormone, urine toxicology, electrocardiogram, complete blood count, and metabolic panel. The most common medical conditions associated with anxiety are presented in Box 1.

The list of drugs suspected of causing anxiety is extensive. Drugs commonly associated with anxiety include stimulants such as amphetamine, cocaine, methamphetamine, and caffeine. Drugs such as lysergic acid diethylamide (LSD) and 3,4-methylenedioxymethamphetamine (MDMA, or "ecstasy") can also cause acute and chronic anxiety. Prescription medications to consider include sympathomimetics, antihypertensives, and nonsteroidal antiinflammatory drugs (NSAIDs).

Treatment and Monitoring

Current practice guidelines indicate that the treatment of an anxiety disorder begins with education. Many people are confused, scared, or frustrated by the symptoms and behavior and are reassured to know they are not alone and that there are effective interventions. The patient should receive an appropriate medical workup, such as a physical examination, and studies (e.g., electrocardiogram, thyroid-stimulating hormone) when indicated. After ruling out a medical condition, developing a good working alliance with the patient provides a basis for ongoing disease management and prevents unnecessary utilization or overutilization of the medical system, as well as potential exacerbation of symptoms.

A combination of psychotherapy and medication management is recommended as first-line treatment for GAD. CBT has the strongest empirical support to date for the treatment of anxiety. Mindfulness-based stress reduction (MBSR) has an emerging evidence base as an effective alternative or complementary behavioral treatment program for anxiety. Both offer a skills-based approach to treatment. In CBT, the therapist and patient

---

| **BOX 1** | Medical Conditions Often Associated With Anxiety Symptoms |

Cardiopulmonary
Angina
Mitral valve prolapse
Pulmonary embolism
Chronic obstructive pulmonary disease (COPD)
Asthma

Endocrine
Hyperthyroidism
Pheochromocytoma
Cushing syndrome
Menopause

Gastrointestinal
Gastroesophageal reflux
Irritable bowel syndrome (IBS)
Gastritis

Neurologic
Dementia
Substance intoxication or withdrawal
Seizure disorder
Migraine

---

work collaboratively and in an active and problem-solving manner. It is structured and generally short term with an emphasis on reducing symptoms and preventing "flare-ups" by monitoring and changing unhelpful or inaccurate thinking patterns that result in feelings of anxiety and worry. Another critical component of CBT for GAD is learning and applying behavioral relaxation techniques (e.g., diaphragmatic breathing, guided imagery, progressive muscle relaxation) and distress tolerance skills (e.g., mindfulness, acceptance). Volumes of evidence support the efficacy of CBT interventions for GAD, but success requires commitment to treatment on the part of the patient. Its efficacy is also contingent upon the ability of the therapist and the length of time in treatment. Studies show that when compared with patients undergoing monotherapy, patients treated with a combination of CBT and medication experience nearly twice the remission rate.

SSRIs have been shown to be the best-tolerated class of medication, and response rates are significantly higher than placebo for GAD. SSRI medications includes fluoxetine (Prozac),[1] fluvoxamine (Luvox),[1] citalopram (Celexa),[1] escitalopram (Lexapro), paroxetine (Paxil), and sertraline (Zoloft).[1] Some improvement in symptoms should be noted within 3 or 4 weeks, and the dose should be increased if no improvement is seen. In treating any anxiety disorder, SSRIs should be started at low doses and gradually titrated up to therapeutic levels to avoid an initial exacerbation of anxiety. Pharmacotherapy options for the treatment of GAD are presented in Table 1.

Benzodiazepines, which have been commonly used in the past to treat anxiety disorders, are not recommended except in cases of extreme impairment of function and only for very short-term use. The tolerability and lack of addiction potential make the SSRIs more desirable for long-term management, but the delay in response makes short-term symptom relief with a benzodiazepine desirable for those with the greatest impairment. Because of the risk for rebound anxiety when withdrawing from benzodiazepines with short half-lives, such as alprazolam (Xanax), many prefer the longer-acting benzodiazepines, such as clonazepam (Klonopin).[1] However, the addiction potential and the potential for abuse with either drug make this the treatment option of last resort.

---

[1] Not US Food and Drug Administration (FDA) approved for this indication.
[1] Not FDA approved for this indication.

TABLE 1	Pharmacotherapy for the Treatment of Generalized Anxiety Disorder		
DRUG	**STARTING DOSE**	**TARGET DOSE**	
Selective Serotonin Reuptake Inhibitors			
Paroxetine (Paxil)*	10 mg qd	10–60 mg qd	
Escitalopram (Lexapro)*	5–10 mg qd	10–20 mg qd	
Sertraline (Zoloft)	12.5–25 mg qd	50–200 mg qd	
Fluoxetine (Prozac)	10 mg qd	20–40 mg qd	
Serotonin-Norepinephrine Reuptake Inhibitors			
Venlafaxine (Effexor XR)*	37.5 mg qAM	150–300 mg qAM†	
Duloxetine (Cymbalta)*	30 mg qd	60–90 mg qd	
Other			
Buspirone (BuSpar)	5 mg bid–tid	10 mg tid	

*U.S. Food and Drug Administration indication for generalized anxiety disorder.
†Exceeds dosage recommended by the manufacturer.

TABLE 2	Helpful Resources for Family Members and Patients With Anxiety Disorders
ORGANIZATION	**WEBSITE**
American Family Physician	www.familydoctor.org/condition/generalized-anxiety-disorder
American Psychiatric Association	www.psychiatry.org/patients-families/anxiety-disorders
American Psychological Association	www.apa.org/topics/anxiety
Anxiety Disorders Association of America	www.adaa.org
Association for Behavioral and Cognitive Therapies	www.abct.org
Mental Health America	www.mentalhealthamerica.net/conditions/anxiety-disorders
National Institute of Mental Health	www.nimh.nih.gov/index.shtml

If the patient does not respond to the combination of CBT and medication, a reevaluation of symptoms might reveal a comorbid disorder missed on the first examination. Comorbid psychiatric disorders significantly lower the likelihood of recovery from anxiety and increase recurrence rates. Some clinicians try switching to a different SSRI before considering the next step in treatment; however, a referral to a psychiatrist or integrated care consultant for further evaluation and management may be necessary. Treatment-refractory anxiety can be extremely frustrating for the patient, the patient's family, and the treating physician. If benzodiazepine treatment was initiated, this frustration can and does often lead to an increased dependence on the medication and a requirement of increasingly higher doses to achieve the same effect. For long-term gains, therapy in addition to medication treatment should be recommended.

Education is critical to reassure the patient that effective treatment is available, but that patience may be necessary until the right combination of modalities is found. Although all anxiety disorders display a significant amount of chronicity, most patients have an improved outcome with appropriate treatment. Response rates improve when comorbidity is low. Patients with an earlier onset of symptoms (childhood or adolescence) can generally expect a more chronic course and their anxiety symptoms may be more difficult to treat. Patients rarely have a spontaneous remission of symptoms, but most can continue to function despite the symptoms. Nevertheless, time to resolution of symptoms is shortened and overall functioning typically improves with treatment.

Pharmacotherapy often helps to prevent relapse, and rates are improved when effective treatment is continued for 12 months. When considering termination of pharmacologic treatment, the risk for relapse in GAD should be discussed with the patient. When discontinuing the SSRIs, a slow taper is recommended, with close monitoring for withdrawal symptoms (e.g., headache, gastrointestinal upset, restlessness, and other flulike symptoms). Also monitor for rebound anxiety symptoms. If relapse occurs, reinstituting treatment is indicated, and many patients opt for indefinite treatment to maintain remission of symptoms. Lifelong management with pharmacotherapy or psychotherapy, or both, is not unusual for many patients. For many, a maximum reduction of symptoms, rather than a full remission, is an acceptable outcome.

Complications

Untreated anxiety disorders can lead to, or worsen, other mental and physical health conditions, including bruxism (teeth grinding), cognitive impairment, depression, gastrointestinal disorders, headache, insomnia, heart disease, substance abuse, and significantly impaired quality of life.

Conclusion

Anxiety disorders are highly prevalent in the United States. GAD is one of the most common psychiatric conditions seen in primary care, second only to major depression. This condition can be disabling and costly to the patient and to the health care system. Despite the prevalence of anxiety disorders, patients often remain undiagnosed and untreated, and patients with unrecognized anxiety disorders tend to be higher utilizers of general medical care. Patients with anxiety disorders can present with multiple somatic complaints and comorbid disorders, causing great effort and expense in identifying the cause of unexplained symptoms. Once an anxiety disorder is identified, patients may be treated using well-tested and efficacious pharmacologic and psychotherapeutic treatments. Helpful resources for patients and families are listed in Table 2.

References

American Psychiatric Association: *Diagnostic and Statistical Manual of Mental Disorders*, ed 5, Washington, DC, 2013, American Psychiatric Association.

American Psychiatric Association: *Practice Guideline for the Treatment of Patients with Panic Disorder*, ed 2, Washington, DC, 2009, American Psychiatric Association.

Campbell-Sills L, Stein MB: *Guideline Watch: Practice Guidelines for the Treatment of Patients With Panic Disorder*, Arlington, VA, 2006, American Psychiatric Association.

Davidson JRT, Feltner DE, Dugar A: Management of generalized anxiety disorder in primary care: Identifying the challenges and unmet needs, *Prim Care Companion J Clin Psychiatry* 12: 2010.

Gabbard GO: *Gabbard's Treatment of Psychiatric Disorders*. ed 3, Washington, DC, 2001, American Psychiatric Publishing.

Goddard AW, Coplan JD, Shekhar A, et al: Principles of the pharmacotherapy of anxiety disorders. In Charney DS, Nestler EJ, editors: *The Neurobiology of Mental Illness*, ed 2nd, New York, 2004, Oxford University Press, pp 661–682.

Kessler RC, Berglund P, Demler O, et al: Lifetime prevalence and age-of-onset distributions of DSM-IV disorders in the National Comorbidity Survey Replication, *Arch Gen Psychiatry* 62:593–602, 2005.

Kroenke K, Spitzer RL, Williams JBW, et al: Anxiety disorders in primary care: Prevalence, impairment, comorbidity, and detection, *Ann Intern Med* 146:317–325, 2007.

Lépine JP: The epidemiology of anxiety disorders: Prevalence and societal costs, *J Clin Psychiatry* 63(Suppl. 14):4–8, 2002.

Sadock BJ, Sadock VA: *Kaplan and Sadock's Synopsis of Psychiatry: Behavioral Sciences/Clinical Psychiatry*, ed 10, Philadelphia, 2007, Lippincott Williams & Wilkins.

Spitzer RL, Kroenke K, Williams JBW, Lowe B: A brief measure for assessing generalized anxiety disorder, *Arch Intern Med* 166:1092–1097, 2006.

Stein MB: Attending to anxiety disorders in primary care, *J Clin Psychiatry* 64(Suppl. 15):35–39, 2003.

DEPRESSIVE, BIPOLAR, AND RELATED MOOD DISORDERS

Method of
Andrei Novac, MD

CURRENT DIAGNOSIS

- Clinical evaluation of mood disorders starts with a thorough psychosocial and medical history.
- Identify symptoms and patterns of the appearance of mood changes.
- Differentiate between unipolar and bipolar symptom patterns.
- Use collateral history, if possible.
- For recent-onset disorder, rule out new medical disorders. Always check thyroid function.

CURRENT THERAPY

- Any underlying medical conditions must be treated simultaneously.
- The mainstay of treatment for all mood disorders remains the combination of pharmacology and psychotherapy.
- Monitor frequently for suicidality.
- Allow at least 2 to 4 weeks for response before a medication switch.
- Switch medication early in cases of intense side effects.
- Monitor for hypomanic switch on medications in undiagnosed bipolarity.

Introduction

Unipolar and bipolar mood disorders are part of a large group of psychiatric conditions referred to as mood or affective disorders. They are among the medical conditions that are most commonly encountered in everyday clinical practice. While current psychiatric texts classify mood disorders in two broad categories (unipolar and bipolar), the clinician has to keep in mind that many mood disorders are mixed and manifest in many co-morbid and atypical forms. Thus, mood disorders and related mood dysregulation encompass a broad range of human experiences: (1) psychiatric disorders, well defined and described in medical texts; (2) a variety of mood syndromes, often comorbid and less well classified and often undiagnosed, which coexist with medical and other psychiatric disorders alike; and (3) mood dysregulation, an aggregate of dispositional traits, at times transient in nature, that are outside clear-cut psychiatric diagnosis but are often related to disturbances of personality. They all deserve particular attention because they can gravely impact the level of functioning, compliance, treatment outcome, and quality of life.

Mood Disorders*

Both the *Diagnostic and Statistical Manual of Mental Disorders*, Fifth Edition (DSM-5), and the ICD-10-CM classify mood disorders into similar types. These include major depressive disorders (unipolar, single episodes, and recurrent), persistent depressive disorder (dysthymia), bipolar I disorder, bipolar II disorder, cyclothymic disorder, and mood disorder due to medical conditions, substance-induced mood disorders, and the "unspecified" unipolar and bipolar disorders. In addition, the DSM-5 has included new clinical entries, such as disruptive mood dysregulation disorder (DMDD), persistent depressive disorder (dysthymia) with

*In this chapter, no DSM-5 or ICD-10-CM diagnostic codes are included. The clinician is advised to consult the DSM-5 for specific diagnostic codes.

intermittent major depressive disorders, and premenstrual dysphoric disorder. The previously entitled "not otherwise specified" syndromes are now called "unspecified mood disorders." New to the DSM-5 are the following *specifiers* that apply to *both* bipolar and unipolar disorders: (1) with anxious distress (a mixture of mood disorder and anxiety disorder), (2) with mixed features, (3) with melancholic features, (4) with atypical features, (5) with psychotic features, (6) with catatonia, (7) with peripartum onset, and (8) with seasonal pattern.

Epidemiology for Unipolar and Bipolar Disorders

Most recent data regarding prevalence comes from the National Comorbidity Survey, which has exposed in detail the rates of subtypes of mood disorders: unipolar, bipolar, and the subthreshold disorders. The lifetime prevalence of any mood disorder was found to be 21.4% (female 24.9%, male 17.5%), with major depression occurring at a lifetime prevalence of 16.9% (female 20.2%, male 13.2%) and 12-month prevalence of 6.8%. Persistent depressive disorder (dysthymia) occurs at a lifetime prevalence of 2.5% (female 3.1%, male 1.8%) and 12-month prevalence of 1.5%. The DSM-5 specifies the prevalence for dysthymia as being approximately 0.5% and for the chronic form of major depressive disorder as 1.5%. Bipolar disorders present with a lifetime prevalence of 4.4% (female 4.5%, male 4.3%). If broken down, bipolar I disorder occurs at a lifetime prevalence of 1.0%, and 0.6% of new cases over 12 months. Bipolar II disorder occurs at a prevalence of 1.1% and 0.8%, respectively. Subthreshold bipolar disorder is twice as common at 2.4% lifetime and 1.4% new cases over 12 months.

Risk Factors Common to Unipolar and Bipolar Disorders

For unipolar major depressive disorders, risk factors include gender (women at greater risk), age (18 to 44 years of age at greater risk), marital status (separated and divorced at greater risk), family history (relatives with depression), early parental death, life events (negative stressful events, chronic exposure to stress), low confidence, and urban environments. For bipolar disorder, risk factors are similar. In addition, for bipolar disorder, higher rather than lower socioeconomic status and suburban environments have been cited as risk factors.

Individuals with anxiety disorder, chronic exposure to stress and trauma, substance abuse, psychotic disorders, and chronic medical conditions are all known to be at risk for mood disorders.

Additionally, results from the World Health Organization (WHO) World Mental Health Surveys revealed that 22.9% of adult mood disorders and 31% of anxiety disorders are attributed to childhood adversity. Certain types of adversity, such as frequent childhood bullying, result in a high risk of poor social health and economic outcomes with an increase of suicidality, depression, anxiety disorders, and alcohol dependency, nearly four decades after exposure. In addition, psychiatric symptoms that are present in childhood constitute a risk factor for adult psychopathology, including mood disorders. Anxiety/depression, labile affect, and manic symptoms are all predictors for future onset of bipolar spectrum disorder. Acute and transient psychotic disorder resulted in 28% onset of affective disorder, but only 15% schizophrenia at 1-year follow-up. Finally, a more recently identified risk factor for mood disorders constitutes a gene environment interaction that results in methyltetrahydrofolate reductase (MTHFR) deficiency, and inadequate homocysteine metabolism, a risk factor for depressive disorders. MTHFR activity can be evidenced by readily available genetic testing (i.e., GeneSight). More recently, studies have pointed to the relationship between severity of depression and abnormalities in immune response. Depression has been associated with high levels of C-reactive protein and low levels of fractional exhaled nitric oxide.

Unipolar Depressive Disorder

The DSM-5 reclassifies unipolar depression into: DMDD; Major Depression; Persistent Depressive Disorder (Dysthymia); Pre-Menstrual Dysphoric Disorder; Substance/Medication Induced;

Depressive Disorders due to Another Medical Condition; Other Specified Depressive Disorders; and Unspecified Depressive Disorders.

Below, we are first presenting Major Depression as the prototype of most of depression encountered in clinical practice.

Major Depression

The mainstay of major depressive disorder is a major depressive episode. The DSM-5 provides criteria according to a threshold of symptoms, yet all mood disorders have to be understood as lying on a continuum. Therefore, even individuals who do not meet all criteria have to be carefully followed, and in many cases preventive treatment is warranted.

At least five or more of the following symptoms during the same 2-week period are required: (1) depressed mood most of the day, nearly every day (sadness, feelings of emptiness, and tearfulness); (2) marked diminished interest or pleasure in almost all activities; (3) significant weight loss or weight gain or fluctuations in appetite; (4) insomnia or hypersomnia; (5) psychomotor retardation or agitation nearly every day; (6) fatigue or loss of energy; (7) feelings of worthlessness and/or inappropriate guilt; (8) inability to concentrate, think, and make decisions; and (9) recurrent thoughts of death and/or suicidal ideations. These symptoms (1) cause significant distress or impairment in social, occupational, and/or personal functions and (2) are not due to a general medical condition. In the DSM-5, contrary to previous classifications, bereavement and depression are not mutually exclusive. In fact, bereaved individuals can also develop major depression, which would warrant additional medical treatment (see Table 1). The following are some forms of manifestations:

- Major depressive disorder, single episode: Episodes may occur only one time in life or may occur again years later, usually triggered by major stressful events.
- Major depressive disorder, recurrent type: Episodes reoccur at shorter intervals. Often the distance between episodes shortens with advancement in age. The first few episodes are more likely to be triggered by stressful life events, while in time the condition becomes self-maintained and self-triggered.
- Depressive disorder with catatonic features (motoric immobility, catalepsy, stupor, extreme opposition, posturing, and echolalia).
- Major depression occurring after giving birth may predict further depressive episodes years later. Postpartum depression has also been associated with bipolar disorder.

Depressive disorder can also take a chronic course. Some patients present with *melancholic features* (profound loss of pleasure, depression worse in the morning, early morning awakening, severe psychomotor retardation, severe anorexia, and weight loss). Melancholia may be a predictor of relatively good response to medications. *Atypical depression* features are characterized by inverted functional shift (weight gain and increased appetite, craving for sweets, hypersomnia, leaden paralysis, and long-standing interpersonal rejection sensitivity). Table 2 presents the subtypes (specifiers) of mood disorders according to the DSM-5. These subtypes are encountered both in unipolar and in bipolar mood disorders. Under these new DSM-5 classifications, conditions such as catatonia, seasonal affective disorders (SAD), and atypical depression may occur both in individuals with unipolar disorder and in individuals with bipolar disorders.

Major depression *with psychosis* is more often encountered in inpatient settings. However, early prodromal symptoms, which start with suspicion, paranoid features, or transient perceptive abnormalities, are relatively common. As most of the time, patients with prodromal psychotic features do not volunteer such symptoms, clinicians need to ask, specifically, about the presence of suspicions, "unusual perceptions," which carry a significant, severe prognosis. Such clinical features of psychosis may complicate the treatment regimen. Antidepressive medications alone may sometimes be insufficient or exacerbate some of the psychotic features. In such cases, the addition of antipsychotic medications, frequent

monitoring, and psychiatric consultation is necessary. *Seasonal Affective Disorder* is a recurrent type of depression, often combined with bipolar features. Most patients develop major depression of different degrees, between October and February-March, in the northern hemisphere. Clinicians need to specifically inquire about this pattern of occurrence. Curiously, many patients with this subtype of depression have limited awareness of their seasonal pattern. Specific modalities that have emerged in recent years for SAD include light therapy and social rhythm therapy.

Persistent Depressive Disorder (Dysthymia)

Persistent depressive disorder, the new designation for dysthymic disorder, is a chronic form of depression in which the depressed mood has persisted for at least 2 years (in children for at least 1 year), as manifested by at least two of the following symptoms: (1) poor appetite or overeating, (2) insomnia or hypersomnia, (3) low energy or fatigue, (4) low self-esteem, (5) poor concentration or difficulty making decisions, and (6) feelings of hopelessness. These manifestations are distinct from any major depressive episode, there have been no manic symptoms, and there is significant distress or impairment in social, occupational, or personal functioning. Dysthymia can occur in any age and can co-occur with major depressive disorder.

The following clinical forms have been identified: (1) with pure dysthymic syndrome: no full criteria of major depression have been met in the past 2 years; (2) with persistent major depressive episode: full criteria of a major depressive episode have been present in the past 2 years; (3) with intermittent major depressive episodes, with current episode: full criteria for major depressive episodes are currently met but there have been periods of at least 8 weeks in the last 2 years when major depression criteria have not been met; and (4) with intermittent major depressive episodes, without current episode: no current major depression is identified (only symptoms of dysthymia) but there has been one or more major depressive episode(s) in the past 2 years. Persistent depressive disorder may also qualify for any of the specifiers described in Table 2. (Note: Table 2 specifiers can apply to any of the unipolar and bipolar forms of mood disorders.) The term "minor depression" to distinguish from "major depression" has also been used in earlier contributions. Minor depression refers to two to four symptoms of depression lasting for more than 2 weeks but less than 2 years. This clinical variant falls within the spectrum of persistent depressive disorder (dysthymia). Major depression and persistent depressive disorder (dysthymia) can co-exist. More often, an individual suffering from dysthymia develops major depression as a complication. An earlier literature refers to these complications as "double depression." Such patients necessitate long-term maintenance treatment beyond the acute major depressive episode.

Disruptive Mood Dysregulation Disorder

This condition occurs in childhood or adolescence between the ages of 6 and 18. It is characterized by (1) severe recurrent temper outbursts manifested verbally (verbal rages) and/or behaviorally (physical aggression toward people or property) that are grossly out of proportion in intensity or duration to the situation or provocation; (2) temper outbursts that are inconsistent with developmental level; (3) temper outbursts that occur on average three or more times per week; (4) a mood between temper outbursts that is persistently irritable or angry most of the day, nearly every day, and is observable by others; (5) the previous criteria, which have been present for 12 or more months (with no lapse in symptoms for a duration of 3 or more months); and (6) an age of onset that is before 10 years. Diagnosis should not be made before the age of 6 years or after 18 years.

DMDD was introduced into the DSM-5 for a subgroup of children with mood dysregulation and as an alternative to the diagnosis of childhood bipolar disorder. Some of these patients do move on to develop bipolar disorder. There is a significant overlap between DMDD and the onset of bipolar disorder. In one study of children in psychiatric hospitals, 30.5% met criteria for DMDD by parent report and 15.9% by inpatient unit

TABLE 1	Guidelines to the Differential Diagnoses			
DIAGNOSIS	**SIMILARITIES**	**DIFFERENTIATING DETAILS**	**CLINICAL CLUES**	**TREATMENT RESPONSE**
Major depression (MDD) versus persistent depressive disorder (dysthymia) (PDD)	Depressed mood; depressive cognition (pessimism); and vegetative symptoms (physical)	MDD: Acute or subacute onset; possible recent life stressors; and often more numerous symptoms PDD: May overlap with MDD; chronic, fluctuating course	MDD: Usually a marked drop in functionality PDD: Significant chronic impairment; often symptoms are ego-syntonic; and "personality disorder" flavor	MDD: Antidepressants and/or initial antianxiety medications; consider psychotherapy PDD: Cognitive-behavioral psychotherapy; antidepressants (often long term); sometimes enhancement pharmacology
Mixed mania versus agitated depression	Psychomotor agitation; dysphoria; and mood swings	Mixed mania: Labile affect; often rapid switch with brief euphoric states	Mixed mania: Personal and family history	Mixed mania: Mood stabilizers; caution regarding antidepressants: can cause worsening
		Agitated depression: No euphoric states; severe anxiety, including sympathetic symptoms	Agitated depression: Anxiety symptoms, often subtle, precede depressive symptoms	Agitated depression: Antidepressants and sedating mood stabilizers; avoid long-term tranquilizers
Mania versus cyclothymia	Intermittent states of high energy and euphoria with or without recurrent depression	Mania: Distinct states of high energy; depression is sometimes unnoticed	Mania: More often severe insomnia without fatigue; severity of mania and insomnia directly related	Mania: Mood stabilizers; caution about antidepressants; and atypical antipsychotics if needed
		Cyclothymia: Distinct cycling from depression to hypomania	Cyclothymia: May take unpredictable forms; fluctuation of mood and sleep	Cyclothymia: Same as above, according to clinical judgment
Substance abuse disorder versus cyclothymia	Intermittent use of stimulant abuse may mimic cycling mood disorder; may coexist	Substance abuse: Substance abuse tends to escalate	Substance abuse: Look for specific syndromes; drug screen	Substance abuse: Rehabilitation; treat underlying psychiatric symptoms
		Cyclothymia: Cyclothymia may remain constant for years (even lifelong)	Cyclothymia: Negative drug screens; no withdrawals; and no drug culture history	Cyclothymia: Mood stabilizers and/or antidepressants and/or atypical antipsychotics
Personality disorder versus mood disorder	More often overlap; requires concomitant treatment	Personality disorder: Long-term pervasive history since adolescence	Personality disorder: Borderline personality disorder includes mood lability/depressive episodes; often narcissistic personality includes grandiose/hypomanic states	Personality disorder: Acute decompensation; long-term psychotherapy; mood stabilizers; and atypical antipsychotics
		Mood disorder: More often episodic	Mood disorder: More often symptoms are egodystonic	Mood disorder: See treatment of mood disorders
Bereavement versus MDD	May overlap; attention to recent major loss; sometimes similar picture; bereavement and MDD may co-occur	Bereavement: Tends to improve over time	Bereavement: Preoccupation with loss persists	Bereavement: Social support; grief counseling; psychotherapy; and if MDD present, treat as MDD
		MDD: Tends to worsen over time	MDD: Duration of average major depressive episode is 9 months	MDD: See treatment of MDD
Terminal illness–related mood (TIRM) changes versus MDD	May overlap; attention to symptom patterns	MDD has better response to medications	Fear of and preoccupation with death often progress with progression of medical condition	Both warrant trial with antidepressants, recommended prior to any end-of-life decisions
		TIRM dominated by sadness and grief		Experimental only: Treatment with entheogen-enhanced psychotherapy (psilocybin, lysergic acid diethylamide (LSD), methylenedioxymethamphetamine (MDMA))*

TABLE 1   Guidelines to the Differential Diagnoses—cont'd

DIAGNOSIS	SIMILARITIES	DIFFERENTIATING DETAILS	CLINICAL CLUES	TREATMENT RESPONSE
Primary mood disorder versus mood disorder arising from medical condition	Clinical picture may be identical	Primary mood disorder: May be triggered by external stressful events	Neurologic, endocrine, infectious, systemic, and blood disorders†	Treat both primary medical condition and mood disorder; treatment same as for primary mood disorder
		Medical condition: Often onset is insidious; sometimes precedes medical condition		

*Not yet approved for use in the United States.

†Medical conditions complicated by mood disorders: Addison disease, AIDS, anemia, brain tumors, chronic pain, complex partial seizures, Cushing disease, cerebrovascular accident, dementia, diabetes mellitus, encephalitis, head trauma, hepatitis, hyperparathyroidism, hyperthyroidism, hypopituitarism, hypothyroidism, infectious mononucleosis, influenza, lupus erythematosus disseminatus, meningitis, multiple sclerosis, pneumonia, porphyria, rheumatoid arthritis, scleroderma, sleep apnea, toxoplasmosis, and others.

TABLE 2   Subtypes of Mood Disorders (Specifiers) Common to Both Unipolar and Bipolar Mood Disorders

SUBTYPE WITH	PRESENTATION	FEATURES
Anxious distress (with elements of mood disorder and anxiety disorder) 74.6% of MDD	During the majority of days of depressive, manic, or hypomanic episode	Feeling keyed up or tense, feeling restless, unable to concentrate, fear that something awful may happen, etc.
Mixed features 15.5% of MDD	Meets criteria for either mania, hypomania, or depression	With mixed symptoms (if manic, there is associated dysphoria and depression), observable by others
Melancholic features	During the most severe period	Severe anhedonia, worse in the morning, early-morning awakening, psychomotor retardation or agitation, and weight loss or gain
Typical features	During majority of days of a major depressive episode	Inverted functional shift (hypersomnia, hyperphasia, and weight gain), leaden paralysis, and long-standing pattern of interpersonal rejection sensitivity
Psychotic features	The presence of delusions and/or hallucinations	Mood-congruent psychosis (delusions/hallucinations include themes consistent with the type of mood [manic or depressed]) Mood-incongruent psychosis
Catatonia	The presence of catatonia	Catatonic features are present during most of depressive or manic episodes
Peripartum onset	Mania, hypomania, major depression in bipolar I or II disorders	During pregnancy or in the 4 weeks following delivery
Seasonal pattern	At least one type of episode (mania, hypomania, or depression) within a seasonal pattern	Temporal relationship between an episode and a particular time of the year (fall or winter, in bipolar I or II)

observation. In clinical practice, young children may present with symptoms of Attention-Deficit Disorder, Hyperactive Type, and comorbid DMDD. Such patients often require careful assessment, complex pharmacologic treatment, and monitoring for possible worsening of bipolar symptoms.

Premenstrual Dysphoric Disorder

- The condition is characterized by the majority of menstrual cycles that include five symptoms. The following symptoms occur in the final week before the onset of menses and begin to improve within a few days after the onset of menses.
- One or more of the following symptoms must be present: (1) marked affective lability (mood swings, feeling suddenly sad or tearful, increased sensitivity to rejection); (2) marked irritability or anger or increased interpersonal conflict; (3) marked depressed mood, feelings of hopelessness, or self-deprecating thoughts; (4) marked anxiety, tension, and/or feelings of being keyed up or on edge.

One or more of the following symptoms must be present to reach a total of five symptoms: decreased interest in usual activities; subjective difficulty in concentration; lethargy; easily fatigued; marked changes in appetite, overeating, or specific food cravings; hypersomnia or insomnia; a sense of being overwhelmed or out of control; physical symptoms such as breast tenderness or swelling, joint or muscle pain, or bloating or weight gain.

TABLE 3	Examples of Medications Known to Trigger Depression as a Side-Effect
CLASS	**EXAMPLES**
Antihypertensives	Clonidine, reserpine, β-blockers
Cardiovascular	Digitalis
Steroids	Prednisone and dexamethasone (Decadron)
Antiarthritic	Indomethacin (Indocin)
Hormonal substitutes	Estrogen, progesterone, testosterone, anabolic steroids, and birth-control pills
Cancer medications	Most chemotherapy combinations, i.e., cycloserine (Seromycin), tamoxifen (Nolvadex), vinblastine (Velban), and vincristine (Vincasar)
Tranquilizers and hypnotics	Diazepam (Valium), triazolam (Halcion), and zolpidem (Ambien)
Analgesics	Codeine, propoxyphene[2], and potentially all opiates
Anti-Parkinson's medication	Levodopa (L-Dopa) and bromocriptine (Parlodel)
Other	Anti-HIV; Medications used in the treatment of hepatitis C

[2]Not available in the United States.

Substance/Medication-Induced Depressive Disorder

This diagnosis is used when persistent disturbance in mood predominates the clinical picture and is characterized by depression and diminished interest or pleasure in activities. These symptoms occur during or soon after substance intoxication or withdrawal or after exposure to a medication. The substance in question has to be known to cause symptoms of depression. Many substances that are abused (illicit and prescription) can cause depression. A 2018 study by Qato, et al., which included 26,000 patients, found that more than one-third of American adults could be experiencing depression due to their prescription medication. Table 1 lists principle groups of medications to be considered when assessing patients with depression.

Depressive Disorder Due to Another Medical Condition

This diagnosis is used when a depressive disorder is triggered by a medical condition (diagnosed by physical examination and laboratory findings) known to cause symptoms of depression. These may include disorders of the central nervous system (CNS), systemic disorders (lupus and cancer), and so forth. Additionally, depression can aggravate many medical conditions, including chronic pain, multiple sclerosis, and cardiovascular disease.

Other Specified Depressive Disorders

These are depressions that do not fully meet the criteria of the previously described conditions. However, they may appear in one of the following forms:

- Recurrent brief depression (symptoms of depression lasting from 2 to 13 days at least once per month) not associated with menstrual cycles
- Short-duration depressive episode (lasting from 4 to 13 days), with at least four symptoms of major depressive episode associated with clinical distress and impaired functioning that persist but never meet criteria of major depression
- Depressive episode with insufficient symptoms (at least one of the symptoms of major depression associated with distress

and impairment persisting for at least 2 weeks with no prior history of major depression)

These "other specified depressive disorders" are helpful to clinicians in refining the description of a clinical pattern exhibited by a particular patient.

Unspecified Depressive Disorder

Finally, the previously used designation of "not otherwise specified" now reads "unspecified depressive disorder" (when none of the criteria are fully met, yet the patient is suffering from a mood disorder).

Bipolar Mood Disorders
Manic Episode

A manic episode is characterized by a period of at least 1 week with abnormal and persistently elevated, expansive, or irritable mood. At least three of the following should also be present: (1) inflated self-esteem or grandiosity, (2) decreased need for sleep (yet still feeling rested), (3) more talkative than usual or inability to stop talking, (4) flight of ideas or racing thoughts, (5) distractibility, (6) increase in goal-oriented activities (socially, sexually) or psychomotor agitation, and (7) excessive involvement in pleasurable activities with little regard for consequences (e.g., sexual indiscretions and unwise investments). These symptoms (1) result in marked impairment in most areas of life and (2) are not due to substance abuse or general medical conditions.

Hypomania

A hypomanic episode is similar to, but less intense than, a manic episode. At least three symptoms from the same symptom cluster (inflated self-esteem, decreased need for sleep, excessive talking, racing thoughts, hyperactivity, and increased involvement in pleasurable activities) are required, but the condition is not severe enough to cause marked impairment in social, occupational, and personal functioning, and it does not necessitate hospitalization. However, functional impairment is noticeable over time.

"Bipolar I" disorder requires only one full manic episode for the diagnosis. Usually, individuals with bipolar I disorder also have both manic and depressive episodes, but the depressions can range from severe and disabling to very brief and unnoticed. Therefore, a history of a depressive episode is not required for the diagnosis.

"Bipolar II" disorder is characterized by long periods of hypomania, with occasional major depressive episodes. Such individuals are usually not hospitalized for their hypomania and tend to function relatively well between depressive episodes. Hypomanic states are episodic and exhibit an unequivocal change in functioning that is uncharacteristic for the individual when not symptomatic. These changes are observable by others. Depressions tend to be severe and disabling. Bipolar II disorders do not include full manic episodes.

Mixed States and Rapid Cycling

The particular specifiers for bipolar disorder are mixed states and rapid cycling. *Mixed states* refer to manic or hypomanic episodes with at least three of the following depressive symptoms: prominent dysphoria or depressed mood, diminished interest in activities, psychomotor retardation, fatigue or loss of energy, feelings of worthlessness, and recurrent thoughts of death. Often there is a rapid alternation between mania and depression (rapid cycling). Contingent upon severity, mixed states are usually accompanied by severe impairment. *Rapid cycling* refers to bipolar disorder that includes at least four episodes of illness per year. In addition, bipolar disorders may include any of the specifiers described in Table 2.

Cyclothymic Disorder

Cyclothymic disorder is a cycling mood disorder lasting for 2 years or more and is characterized by numerous periods with hypomanic symptoms and depressive symptoms that do not

TABLE 4 Other Specified and Unspecified Bipolar Disorders

SUBTYPE	PRESENTATION	FEATURE
Substance/medication-induced bipolar and related disorder	Persistent disturbance of mood characterized by mania, hypomania, with or without depressed mood, which occurs soon after substance intoxication or withdrawal or after administration of a medication	• Substance involved is capable of producing described mood symptoms • Does not occur in the course of delirium • There is significant stress or impairment
Bipolar and related disorder due to another medical condition	• Persistent period of abnormally elevated expansive or irritable mood • Evidence from history, physical examination, and laboratory findings that disturbance is a direct pathophysiologic consequence of another medical condition	• With manic features • With manic or hypomanic-like episode • With mixed features (depression is also present)
Other specified bipolar and related disorder	Symptoms of bipolar disorder, but do not meet full criteria	• Short-duration hypomanic episodes (2–3 days) and major depressive episodes • Hypomanic episodes with insufficient symptoms and major depressive episodes • Hypomanic episode without prior major depressive episode • Short-duration cyclothymia (<24 months)
Unspecified bipolar and related disorders	Patients with bipolar symptoms and clinical distress and impairment; however, the clinician chooses not to specify the reason that the criteria are not met	

meet criteria for bipolar disorder or major depression. During a 2-year period (1 year in children and adolescents), hypomanic and depressive periods have been present for at least half the time, and the individual has not been without symptoms for more than 2 months at a time. Criteria for major depression, mania, or hypomanic episodes have never been met. However, in the long run, some patients may develop symptoms of bipolar affective disorder. These symptoms should not be attributable to the effect of a substance (drug abuse and medication) or another medical condition (hyperthyroidism, Cushing disease, etc.). The condition is significantly impairing and includes psychological distress. Cyclothymia has the specifier (subtype) "cyclothymia with anxious distress." This condition consists of cyclothymia and features of anxious distress as outlined in Table 2. A variety of subclinical forms of *subthreshold cyclothymia* may be encountered in clinical practice. Such patients tend to develop overt symptoms of cyclothymia, or even bipolar disorder, when exposed to a variety of psychosocial stressors, substance abuse, and/or a variety of medications. Finally, Table 4 presents subtypes of bipolar disorder currently listed in the DSM-5 as "other specified bipolar and related disorders" and "unspecified bipolar and related disorder."

Specifiers for Bipolar and Related Disorders
Please refer to Table 2 for specifiers of depressive disorders that apply to bipolar disorders as well.

Diagnosis. When faced with symptoms of mood disorder, a clinician has to decide whether these are transient manifestations related to life circumstances or symptoms of treatable psychopathology. The clinical evaluation of patients with mood disorders starts with a thorough history of the present illness. A thorough medical history is paramount given the numerous medical disorders that present with depression or mania. Mood disorders are, in general, recurrent conditions. Past history will provide not only a suspicion toward a diagnosis but also clues toward clinical manifestations, which, in the cases of depression and mania, are often similar to previous episodes. An early history of childhood behavioral problems can constitute a precursor of mood disorders. The Mental Status Examination provides further clues to the diagnosis. For depressive states, patients often exhibit psychomotor retardation; slow speech; constricted affect; and slow, observable mental activity. For mania and hypomania, the opposite can be observed. Patients

show increased psychomotor activity, pressured speech, full or labile affect, and elevated mood. Often, they will appear unrealistically optimistic. In general, the diagnosis of mood disorder is aided significantly by obtaining a collateral history from friends or family members. The value of the Mental Status Examination is enhanced if the clinician knows the patient from before the mood disorder episode. A variety of psychological tests and depression rating scales exist, including the Beck Depression Inventory, the Hamilton Depression Rating Scale, and the Profile of Mood States (POMS) Depression Scale. While extremely useful in quantifying symptoms of depression, psychological testing is time-consuming and not necessary for the initial diagnosis of a mood disorder.

A thorough account of all symptoms present in a patient can point to treatment choice and outcome. Depression symptoms can be classified into at least three major groups:
- Emotional symptoms: sadness, dysphoria, emotional numbness
- Physical symptoms: low energy, sluggishness with difficulties in initiating activities, difficulties concentrating, and sleep and appetite problems
- Cognitive (mental) symptoms: pessimism, loss of enthusiasm, hopelessness, and thoughts of death

Not all three groups of symptoms are present from the beginning. In many individuals, the presence of cognitive symptoms may be a sign of chronicity. At other times, it may have been a premorbid feature or a constant presence between episodes. Cognitive symptoms tend to respond both to medication and to psychotherapy (cognitive-behavioral techniques), and their monitoring is paramount to suicide prevention. If a mood disorder is secondary to a medical condition, the diagnosis will be made both by monitoring for mood symptoms and by pathognomonic medical findings.

Differential Diagnosis
Given the multitude of clinical manifestations, a differential diagnosis both between subtypes of mood disorders and between mood and other psychiatric disorders is necessary. Table 1 presents comparisons and differences between subtypes of mood disorders and guidelines to the differential diagnoses.

Given the frequent overlap of anxiety and mood disorders, it is useful to inquire about the presence of anxiety disorder in a systematic manner. Anxiety disorder symptoms can also be classified into at least three major groups:

- Emotional symptoms: anxiety and/or fear, either fluctuating or in the form of attacks
- Physical symptoms: palpitations, tachycardia, diaphoresis, sweaty palms, sensation of a knot in the throat, muscle tension, shortness of breath, gastrointestinal symptoms, insomnia, and so forth
- Cognitive symptoms: (1) intrusive thoughts (such as "What if...," "I should have...," other specific exaggerated worries), (2) racing thoughts, (3) ruminative thoughts, and so forth

Because of the long-term, chronic, egosyntonic nature of these symptoms, they are often not readily volunteered by the patient unless specifically asked about. Between mood disorders and anxiety disorders, there is a comorbidity of more than 50%, with generalized anxiety, panic disorders, and posttraumatic stress disorders constituting both a risk factor for and a possible complication of mood disorders. Please note that the DSM-5 allows for a specifier "with anxious distress" that can be applied to both unipolar and bipolar mood disorders. Depending on the primary diagnosis, the clinician may choose between adding this specifier or the comorbid separate diagnosis of "anxiety disorder" in addition to mood disorder.

Treatment

Currently, psychopharmacology and psychotherapy are the mainstay of care for mood disorders. As we will see below, a variety of novel treatments (transcranial magnetic stimulation [TMS], ketamine, entheogens) have recently emerged. An accurate initial diagnosis directs the first choice of treatment. Close monitoring of treatment with frequent visits usually predicts better outcome. In general, response is considered to be a 50% reduction of symptoms, while remission refers usually to the absence or only minimal symptoms for 6 months or more. By Tohen and colleagues' opinion, relapse is considered a return of symptoms within 6 months, while recurrence is after 6 months of remission.

Among risk factors for severity, treatment resistance has been a major clinical challenge. Four predictors have been recently identified. They include symptom severity (3.3-fold increase in likelihood for treatment resistance); suicidal risk (a 1.74-fold increase in treatment resistance); comorbid disorder (1.68-fold increase risk); and lifetime number of major depressive episodes (15% increase in treatment resistance per prior episode).

Treatment of Unipolar Depression (Major Depression and Dysthymia)

Given the fact that many depressive disorders occur along a spectrum, the treatment of major depression and dysthymia will be covered together.[†] In addition, a more recent study confirms the fact that comorbidity features, with anxiety, are significant: the anxious/distressed specifier occurs in 74.6% of cases and mixed-features specifier in 15.5% of major depressive disorder patients.

Psychopharmacology

First, a thorough medical workup should be performed in any new case of mood disorder. The National Institutes of Health (NIH)-sponsored STAR*D study (Sequenced Treatment Alternatives to Relieve Depression) recommends the initial choice of a selective serotonin reuptake inhibitor (SSRI) (citalopram [Celexa]). In the study, nonresponders were then switched to sertraline (Zoloft)

and/or venlafaxine XR (Effexor XR). In clinical practice, other factors have to be weighed when choosing the first antidepressant. *Prior response history* (italics added) to a specific antidepressant or to an overall treatment modality should take precedence in the first choice of treatment. If such a history is unavailable, any family history of response to a specific treatment should be considered. Response to treatment seems to be similar among blood relatives. Table 5 includes a list of the more common medications used in clinical practice for the treatment of unipolar and bipolar disorder. Given the possibility of manic switch with antidepressants, it is recommended that in bipolar depression, mood stabilizers be started concomitantly with antidepressants.

Although myriad side effects are known to exist for each medication, all SSRIs and serotonin norepinephrine reuptake inhibitors (SNRIs) are generally well tolerated. Any trial of medications should be continued for 4 to 6 weeks before failure is declared. However, clinical judgment in assessing each circumstance, especially regarding suicide risk, is crucial. Often in the initial phase of response, the physical symptom of low energy remits first while cognitive symptoms of depression (persistent thoughts of death) persist. The coexistence of higher energy and thoughts of death may constitute a temporary suicide risk in the initial phase of antidepressant treatment. Currently, biological markers for the prediction of treatment response and side effects are being considered. Psychiatric EEG Evaluation Registry (PEER), by using quantitative EEG technology, compares variations of normal awake EEG readings with a large database of medication responders. Results are available for antidepressants, mood stabilizers, stimulants, second-generation antipsychotics, and so forth. The validity of PEER has been supported by a wealth of published literature; however, more recently the usefulness of PEER has been disputed. The AmpliChip CYP450 Test is a method that predicts side effects by measuring the activity of genes that control the P450 hepatic enzyme system and, implicitly, the ability to metabolize a specific drug. Both methods are promising, but high cost and questions about large individual variability of response, have had so far prevented general use.

Given the risk of suicide, close monitoring during the treatment of major depression is required. The choice of medication and adjustment has to be tailored according to the most dominant initial presentation. For patients with severe insomnia, an SSRI is indicated. If the initial choice (e.g., citalopram [Celexa], escitalopram [Lexapro], or sertraline [Zoloft]) shows little impact in improving sleep, the temporary addition of a sleep aid is a reasonable choice. Alternatively, some clinicians prefer to avoid hypnotics, which may allow close monitoring of the natural improvement in sleep during the first 2 weeks of SSRI treatment. This in turn may predict a good response. In geriatric patients, long-term SSRI treatment has been found to delay progression from mild cognitive impairment to dementia. For many years, in patients with hypersomnia and hyperphagia—a variant known as "atypical depression"—the first choice was a monoamine oxidase inhibitor (MAOI). Currently, for atypical depression, clinicians prefer as a first choice a norepinephrine/serotonin reuptake inhibitor (venlafaxine [Effexor], desvenlafaxine [Pristiq]), or a norepinephrine/dopamine active medication (bupropion [Wellbutrin]). Response to medications is often difficult to predict. Again, early in treatment, a thorough medical workup, which should always include a thyroid panel, should be the norm. Sometimes, switches to other classes of antidepressants (dopamine enhancers, tricyclics) are necessary before a result is obtained. Pharmacologic augmentation with mood stabilizers, neuroleptics, and thyroid hormone has been used in cases of treatment-resistant depression. In cases where severe anxiety, insomnia, and poor appetite dominate the picture, the early addition of a second-generation neuroleptic (olanzapine [Zyprexa][1], quetiapine [Seroquel XR], risperidone [Risperdal][1], aripiprazole [Abilify], and, more recently, cariprazine [Vraylar][1]) is recommended (see Table 5). Medication

---

[†] The newly introduced DSM-5 diagnosis of disruptive mood dysregulation disorder is a condition of childhood and adolescence. Prior to the publication of the DSM-5, many of these patients were diagnosed as bipolar. Many clinicians prefer to initiate treatment with psychotherapy, which includes addressing a variety of family issues before initiating psychopharmacologic intervention. Premenstrual dysphoric disorder, also newly introduced in the DSM-5, is treated, depending on the intensity of symptoms, by using protocols similar to those utilized in the treatment of dysthymic and/or cyclothymic disorders.

*For specifiers and diagnostic codes, please see the DSM-5 and/or ICD-10-CM.

---

[1] Not FDA approved for this indication.

TABLE 5 Medications Used for the Treatment of Unipolar and Bipolar Depression

MEDICATION GROUP	MEDICATION	USUAL DAILY DOSE	CAUTIONS
SSRI	Fluoxetine (Prozac) Sertraline (Zoloft) Paroxetine (Paxil) Citalopram (Celexa) Escitalopram (Lexapro) Fluvoxamine (Luvox)*	10–80 mg 25–200 mg 5–60 mg 10–40 mg 5–20 mg 50–300 mg	All can cause sedation, agitation, insomnia, GI side effects, and sexual dysfunction
SSRIs with combined action	Vilazodone (Viibryd) Functions of SSRI and a 5-HT$_{1A}$ receptor agonist Vortioxetine (Brintellix) Functions of SSRI and multiple serotonin receptor agonists and antagonists	10–40 mg 5–20 mg	Same as above
Serotonin-norepinephrine reuptake inhibitor (SNRI)	Venlafaxine XR (Effexor XR) Desvenlafaxine (Pristiq) Levomilnacipran ER (Fetzima)	37.5–225 mg 50–100 mg 40–120 mg	Insomnia, sedation, possible HTN Mydriasis, and urinary hesitation
Dopamine/norepinephrine agonist	Bupropion SR, XL (Wellbutrin SR, XL)	100–450 mg	Agitation, GI side effects, and possible HTN
Stimulants (usually used to enhance effects of other antidepressants)	Methylphenidate (Ritalin)* Dextroamphetamine (Dexedrine)* Amphetamine/dextroamphetamine mixed (Adderall)*	10–60 mg 5–60 mg 5–60 mg	Agitation, insomnia, psychosis, HTN, and seizures
Second-generation neuroleptics	Olanzapine (Zyprexa)* Quetiapine (Seroquel) Aripiprazole (Abilify) Risperidone (Risperdal)* Lurasidone (Latuda) mainly for bipolar disorder Cariprazine (Vraylar)*	2.5–20 mg (in unipolar depression, olanzapine 5 mg, plus fluoxetine 20 mg [Symbyax]) 50–300 mg (up to 800 mg in bipolar disorder) 2–30 mg 0.5–6 mg 20–120 mg/day 1.5–6 mg/day	Metabolic syndrome, sedation Oversedation, metabolic syndrome, and cardiovascular complications in elderly Oversedation, metabolic syndrome, and hyperprolactinemia Somnolence or agitation from akathisia and extrapyramidal symptoms
Tricyclic antidepressants	Amitriptyline (Elavil) Imipramine (Tofranil) Doxepin (Sinequan) Desipramine (Norpramin) Nortriptyline (Pamelor) Maprotiline (Ludiomil) Protriptyline (Vivactil)	50–300 mg 50–300 mg 50–300 mg 50–300 mg 20–200 mg† 100–225 mg 20–60 mg	All can cause anticholinergic effects and sedation; occasional agitation and weight gain
Mixed action (presynaptic and postsynaptic, multiple neurotransmitter action)	Mirtazapine (Remeron) Trazodone (Desyrel) Clomipramine (Anafranil)*	15–30 mg 150–600 mg 50–300 mg†	Sedation, weight gain
MAOI (dietary restrictions are obligatory)	Phenelzine (Nardil) Tranylcypromine (Parnate)	15–90 mg 30–60 mg	Hypertensive crisis, occasional sedation/activation
Mood stabilizers	Lithium carbonate/citrate/ER* Valproate (valproic acid, Depakote ER)* Lamotrigine (Lamictal)/XR* Carbamazepine (Tegretol)*	600–1800 mg (attaining blood level from 0.6 to 1.2 mEq/L) 250–1500 mg (attaining blood level from 50 to 100 mcg/mL) 50–400 mg 200–1000 mg (attaining blood level from 5 to 12 mdg/mL)	Signs of toxicity: tremor, nausea, vomiting, and staggering gait; monitor kidney and thyroid function Oversedation, GI side effects, may affect blood levels of other medications, and weight gain A variety of severe skin rashes, Stevens-Johnson syndrome Monitor blood count for aplastic anemia/agranulocytosis, possible Stevens-Johnson syndrome, and sedation

*Not U.S. Food and Drug Administration approved for this indication.
†Exceeds dosage recommended by the manufacturer.
ER, Extended release; GI, gastrointestinal; HTN, hypertension; MAOI, monoamine oxidase inhibitor; SSRI, selective serotonin reuptake inhibitor.

resistance (after several failed trials) dictates the reassessment of diagnosis to further rule out psychiatric and medical comorbidity. For medication-resistant mood disorders, Table 6 presents a list of further biological treatments. Some of these treatments are promising but have yet to be included as routine choices in some of the most difficult-to-treat patients.

Psychotherapy

For mood disorders, cognitive-behavioral, interpersonal and more recently, mindfulness-focused psychotherapy have been considered therapies of choice. Cognitive-behavioral and mindfulness directly address the negative, pessimistic bias of the depressive thinking, which is a maintenance factor of depressed mood. The

TABLE 6	Biological Treatments for Medication-Resistant Mood Disorders	
TYPE OF INTERVENTION	REPORTED RESPONSE	CURRENT AVAILABILITY
Electroconvulsive therapy (ECT)	50.9%–53.2% remission rate	Common
Transcranial magnetic stimulation (TMS)	41.5%–56.4% response rate, 26.5%–28.7% remission rate	Accepted by several insurance plans
Vagal nerve stimulation (VNS)	53% response rate, 33% remission after 1 year	Rare (neurosurgical)
Deep brain stimulation (DBS)	29% response rate at 1 year	Rare (neurosurgical)
Ketamine (Ketalar) infusion[1]	79% response rate	Very rare (only in selective institutions)
Anterior cingulotomy	33.3% response rate, after 30 months	Very rare (only in selective institutions, neurosurgical)

[1]Not FDA approved for this indication.

latter addresses social and interpersonal functioning by enhancing coping abilities. Their popularity has been increasing; however, they require special training and supervision. In clinical practice, though, the most readily available therapies remain supportive and insight-oriented psychotherapy. They too complement the effect of pharmacology. Brain imaging studies have revealed that the activity of the subgenual anterior cingulate cortex (Brodmann area 25) predicts the outcome of response to cognitive-behavioral psychotherapy in depression. As a general rule, therapies should have specific goals that need to be discussed with patients at the onset of treatment. This needs to be part of an overall "informed consent" approach to treatment. Given the availability of a variety of clinicians with different levels of expertise that provide psychotherapy, it is important to monitor results and coordinate care. If "split" treatment (pharmacology and psychotherapy provided by different clinicians) is chosen, communication between parties of the treatment team remains a crucial requirement for rapid response and recovery. Other therapeutic measures, such as an increase in physical activity, normalization of sleep, and improvement of social support, are particularly important in promoting recovery.

Neurostimulation
TMS was approved by the FDA in 2008. Over the past 2 years, the majority of insurance plans and Medicare have approved TMS treatment for major depression. It is the treatment modality approved by the FDA that has made the greatest strides in providing neuromodulation treatment for patients with major depressive disorder in over 1000 centers nationwide. Table 6 includes other neuromodulation treatments, which need to be considered when TMS remains ineffective.

Treatment of Bipolar Disorders (Bipolar Type I, Type II, Mixed Type, and Cyclothymia)
The treatment of bipolar disorder has been well refined over the years by a large body of literature. For acute mania, treatment with mood stabilizers and/or antipsychotics has remained the main approach for the past several decades. Severe forms of mania and psychosis usually require hospitalization. Table 7 indicates intervention options for different phases of bipolar disorder.

As indicated in the table, some of the medication choices overlap between different clinical presentations. For chronic forms of bipolarity, such as mixed bipolar and cyclothymic disorder, a variety of new approaches has been developed, including social rhythm therapy. The latter includes monitoring and optimization of social interactions, sleep, and circadian rhythms that seem to benefit bipolar patients. Chronic bipolarity, with its significant impairment and suicide risk, remains a major problem, often requiring multidisciplinary consultations and referral to a tertiary institution. In treatment-resistant cases, employment of electroconvulsive therapy and other novel biological approaches can be lifesaving. Even with partial treatment response, maintenance is paramount. Lifelong maintenance treatment is likely to prevent suicide and further functional deterioration. More recently, suicide prevention both

TABLE 7	Intervention Options for Phases of Bipolar Disorder
PHASE OF DISORDER	INTERVENTIONS
Acute	Hospitalization if necessary Antipsychotics, tranquilization, and start mood stabilizers
Subacute	Antipsychotics/neuroleptics, mood stabilizers If already medicated, adjust dose
Rapid cycling/mixed	As in acute phase; check thyroid; and medical workup Rule out substance abuse May require treatment indefinitely
Cyclothymia	Mood stabilizers, long term, with or without antidepressants based on history Close initial monitoring May need treatment indefinitely

in chronic mood disorders and in personality disorders has been reported with maintenance treatment of lithium carbonate and clozapine (Clozaril)[1]. Among bipolar patients, chronic depression is one of the most treatment-resistant conditions in psychiatry. In any patient with treatment-resistant, undiagnosed bipolar depression, the addition of mood stabilizers may result in the conversion of a treatment nonresponder to a responder. In addition, the value of treatment with lithium carbonate has been recently reiterated in a Finnish study. Lithium carbonate, besides an effective antimanic treatment, can prevent re-hospitalization for bipolar disorder. One 2018 study revealed a significant response when 7000-lux bright white light was administered daily for 4 to 6 weeks, in conjunction with mood stabilizers. The response rate was 68.2% compared to 22.2% in the placebo group. Among the treatment cases, no mood polarity switches occurred. This improvement occurs even in patients who are not diagnosed with SAD. Further replication of these findings may reveal bright light to be a new modality of treatment for bipolar depression, which is readily available and free of significant side effects.

Mood Dysregulation
Mood dysregulation is a broad phenomenon encountered both in clinical and in nonclinical settings. For clinicians, a variety of difficult-to-classify syndromes remain relevant (referred to here as "mood syndrome variants"). These mood syndrome variants present anecdotal but clinically pertinent manifestations collected from the medical literature of the past century. Psychiatric and medical disorders often coexist with different degrees of mood dysregulation. A more detailed description of each clinical entity

[1]Not FDA approved for this indication.

TABLE 8 Examples of Mood Syndrome Variants With Different Degrees of Mood Dysregulation as Encountered in the Literature Over the Past Century

I MSV WITH MANIFESTATIONS OF OTHER PSYCHIATRIC DISORDERS	II MSV WITH UNUSUAL SYMPTOMS (MASKED DEPRESSION)	III MSV AS PART OF OTHER CONDITIONS
Atypical depression	Mood dysregulation and thrill-seeking behavior (gambling, racing, substance abuse, hypersexuality)	Postpartum depression
Subaffective dysthymia		Depression secondary to chronic pain
Hysteroid dysphoria	Reactive overeating	Substance- and medication-induced mood dysregulation*
Pseudodementia	Isolated sleep disturbance and mood dysregulation	
Pseudoborderline		"Organic" mood disorders (due to central nervous system disorders)
Somatic depression	Atypical facial pain	
Underground depression	Dysphagia	Vicarious traumatization†
Neurasthenia	Monosymptomatic hypochondriasis	
Mood syndrome as part of personality disorders	Monosymptomatic delusions	
Mood syndromes and depression in schizophrenia		

*Medications more often associated with depression are, among others, reserpine, α-methyldopa (Aldomet), some α- and β-blockers, sedative hypnotics, cimetidine (Tagamet), indomethacin (Indocin), anticancer medications, oral contraceptives, and corticosteroids.
†It has been described as a form of secondary trauma in mental health professionals who treat victims of trauma.
MSV, Mood Syndrome Variant.
Novac and Djenderedjian, unpublished data.

in Table 8 is beyond the scope of this chapter. As seen from the table, different forms of mood dysregulation can occur both within and outside DSM diagnoses. For instance, atypical depression has been included in the DSM, whereas other syndromes, such as neurasthenia, remain unclassified. When encountered, any of the listed syndromes should raise suspicion of an underlying mood disorder. A diagnosis of "unspecified depressive disorder" (F32.9) can be made, and the entire mood disorder treatment armamentarium should be considered.

Clinical Course and Prognosis of Mood Disorders

Given the heterogeneity of mood disorders, there is great variation in clinical outcome. Clinical course and outcome depend on whether treatment is available, whether an individual is sensitive or resistant to the treatment, and the degree of compliance. Many individuals with mild and subsyndromal disorders remain undiagnosed, whereas others with severe forms of mood disorders refuse treatment. As a general rule, most untreated mood disorders tend to become chronic. Episodic disorders, such as bipolar I and II and depression, recurrent type, may show more frequent recurrences with advancement in age. Other patients with hyposymptomatic presentations and infrequent episodes may show long-term remissions. Such remissions are favored by stable, low-stress lifestyles. Dyslipidemia, hypertension, type 2 diabetes, coronary vascular disease, and stroke are among the numerous medical complications of chronic mood disorders. Some of these complications are direct side effects of long-term use of psychotropic medications, in particular second-generation antipsychotics. They all contribute to shortened life expectancy of individuals with mood disorders. Table 9 demonstrates the severe impact on life expectancy of bipolar disorder. Mortality comes from suicide, cardiovascular disease, and respiratory disorders. However, treatment can at least partially reverse these trends.

Prevention

Primary prevention of mood disorders requires a concerted effort to educate the public and policymakers for funding of prevention. Depression Awareness Week and other community efforts enhance awareness and decrease stigma. Primary prevention may also include the promotion of general health and healthy work environments and addressing of major social problems, including the avoidance of early trauma and family problems, as well as prevention of excessive stress and trauma in adults. These are all known to be associated with mental illness. Populations at risk need to be identified in primary care settings. Secondary prevention requires the availability of mental health services, including early detection, education about the need for adequate treatment, and continuity of care to prevent impairment. Tertiary prevention would include the continuation of treatment to prevent

TABLE 9 Causes of Mortality in Patients With Bipolar Disease: Index Group Compared to the General Population

CAUSE OF DEATH	OBSERVED DEATHS (% STUDY GROUP)	EXPECTED DEATHS (% REGISTRAR GENERAL'S* FIGURES)	MORTALITY RATIO (ACTUAL STUDY)
Suicide	15.7	0.67	23.4
Cardiovascular system	42.1	14	3.0
Respiratory system	33.3	1.08	30.8

*Edinburgh Registrar General's Office.
Data from Sharma R, Markar HR. Mortality in affective disorder. *J Affect Disord.* 1994;31:91–96.

comorbidity of other psychiatric disorders and catastrophic complications, including suicide. Finally, in the case of mood disorders, quaternary prevention would include long-term follow-up, monitoring of recurrences, and medical comorbidity (accidents, cardiovascular, respiratory, and other medical conditions) to avoid overburdening the health system.

The high medical comorbidity rate recently found among patients with mood disorders varies by medical diagnosis and socioeconomic background. Chronic pain, neurologic conditions, gastrointestinal disorders, cardiovascular disorders, and metabolic syndrome are the most common medical conditions associated with mood disorders. Except for thyroid disorders, the seriousness of the comorbid condition seems to be even higher among patients of lower socioeconomic background. This poses a significant medical and socioeconomic burden of untreated mood disorders.

References

Amare AT, Schubert KO, Klingler-Hoffman M, et al: The genetic overlap between mood disorders and cardiometabolic diseases: A systematic review of genome wide and candidate gene studies, *Transl Psychiatry* 7, 2017. Available at: https://doi.org/ 10.1038/tp.2016.261.

American Psychiatric Association: *Diagnostic and Statistical Manual of Mental Disorders (DSM-5)*, ed 5, Washington, DC, 2013, American Psychiatric Publishing.

Bartels C, Wagner M, Wolfsgruber S, et al: Impact of SSRI therapy on risk of conversion from mild cognitive impairment to Alzheimer dementia in individuals with previous depression, *Am J Psychiatry* 175:232, 2018.

Binzer S. Multiple Sclerosis. Presented at European Committee for Treatment and Research in Multiple Sclerosis. Abstract 99: 2018; 24(Suppl 2) p. 41.

Cepeda MS, Stang P, Makadia R: Depression is associated with high levels of C-reactive protein and low levels of fractional exhaled nitric oxide: Results from the 2007-2012 National Health and Nutrition Examination Surveys, *J Clin Psychiatry* 77(12), 2016 December.

Connolly KR, Thase ME: If at first you don't succeed: A review of the evidence for antidepressant augmentation, combination and switching strategies, *Drugs* 71:43–64, 2011. Available at: https://doi.org/10.2165/11587620-000000000-00000.

Dobson KS, Dozois DJA, editors: *Risk Factors in Depression*, San Diego, CA, 2008, Academic Press (Elsevier).

Fogel J, Eaton WW, Ford DE: Minor depression as a predictor of the first onset of major depressive disorder over a 15-year follow-up, *Acta Psychiatr Scand* 113(1):36–43, 2006.

Frank E, Kupfer DJ, Thase ME, et al: Two-year outcomes for interpersonal and social rhythm therapy in individuals with bipolar I disorder, *Arch Gen Psychiatry* 62:996, 2005.

Griffiths R, Johnson M, Carducci M, et al: Psilocybin produces substantial and sustained decreases in depression and anxiety in patients with life-threatening cancer: A randomized double-blind trial, *J Psychopharmacol* 30(12):1181–1197, 2016.

Hasin DS, Sarvet AL, Meyers JL, et al: Epidemiology of adult *DSM-5* major depressive disorder and its specifiers in the United States, *JAMA Psychiatry* 75(4):336–346, 2018. Available at: https://doi.org/10.1001/jamapsychiatry.2017.4602.

Iosifescu DV, Neborsky RJ, Valuck RJ: The use of the Psychiatric Electroencephalography Evaluation Registry (PEER) to personalize pharmacotherapy, *Neuropsychiatric Dis Treat* 12:2131–2142, 2016. Available at: https://doi.org/10.2147/NDT.S113712.

Janicakk PG. What's new in transcranial magnetic stimulation: Recent developments have enhanced the benefits of this treatment. *Current Psychiatry* 18(3):11-16.

Lahteenvulo M, Tanskanen A, Taipale H, et al: Real-world effectiveness of pharmacologic treatments for the prevention of rehospitalization in a Finnish nationwide cohort of patients with bipolar disorder, *JAMA Psychiatry* 75:347–355, 2018.

Lamers F, van Oppen P, Comijs HC, et al: Comorbidity patterns of anxiety and depressive disorders in a large cohort study: The Netherlands Study of Depression and Anxiety (NESDA), *J Clin Psychiatry* 72:341–348, 2011. Available at: https://doi.org/10.4088/JCP.10m06176blu.

Laursen TM, Musliner KL, Benros ME, et al: Mortality and life expectancy in persons with severe unipolar depression, *J Affect Disord* 193:203–207, 2016.

Merikangas KR, Akiskal HS, Angst J, et al: Lifetime and 12-month prevalence of bipolar spectrum disorder in the national comorbidity survey replication, *Arch Gen Psychiatry* 64:543–552, 2007. Available at: https://doi.org/10.1001/archpsyc.64.5.543.

Metcalf CA, Gold AK, Davis BJ, Sylvia LG, Battle CL: Mindfulness as an intervention for depression, *Psychiatric Annals* 49(1): 2019.

National Comorbidity Survey-Replication: *Appendix Tables: Table 1 and 2*, 2011. Available at: http://www.hcp.med.harvard.edu/ncs/publications.php. Accessed 13 August 2013.

Qato DM, Ozenberger K, Olfson M: Prevalence of prescription medications with depression as a potential adverse effect among adults in the United States, *JAMA* 319(22):2289–2298, 2018. Available at: https://doi.org/10.1001/jama.2018.6741.

Sachs GS, Dupuy JM, Wittmann CW: The pharmacologic treatment of bipolar disorder, *J Clin Psychiatry* 72:704–715, 2011.

Sharma R, Markar HR: Mortality in affective disorder, *J Affect Disord* 31:91–96, 1994.

Siegle GJ, Thompson WK, Collier A, et al: Toward clinically useful neuroimaging in depression treatment: Prognostic utility of subgenual cingulate activity for determining depression outcome in cognitive therapy across studies, scanners, and patient characteristics, *Arch Gen Psychiatry* 69:913–924, 2012. Available at: https://doi.org/10.1001/ archgenpsychiatry.2012.65.

Sit DK, McGowan J, Wiltrout C, et al: Adjunctive bright light therapy for bipolar depression: A randomized double-blind placebo-controlled trial, *Am J Psychiatry* 175:131–139, 2018. Available at: https://doi.org/10.1176/appi.ajp.2017.16101200.

Smith D, Court H, McLean G, et al: Depression and multimorbidity in psychiatry and primary care, *J Clin Psychiatry* 75(11):1202–1208, 2014.

Tohen M, Frank E, Bowden CL, et al: The International Society for Bipolar Disorders (ISBD) Task Force report on the nomenclature of course and outcome in bipolar disorders, *Bipolar Disord* 11:453–473, 2009.

Weissman M: The psychological treatment of depression, *Arch Gen Psychiatry* 36:1261–1269, 1979.

OBSESSIVE-COMPULSIVE DISORDER

Method of
Rachna Kalia, MD; and Anne Walling, MB, ChB

CURRENT DIAGNOSIS

- Obsessive-compulsive disorder (OCD) is characterized by obsessions (recurrent, persistent, and intrusive unwelcome thoughts, urges, or images) and compulsions (repetitive behaviors or activities that the patient feels forced to perform in response to an obsession).

- Obsessions and compulsions are unwelcome and time-consuming, impair functioning, and usually cause significant anxiety or distress.
- The obsessions or compulsions are not attributable to any toxin, medication, or another medical condition.
- Patients may be unwilling to reveal symptoms of OCD or may lack insight into abnormal thoughts or behaviors.
- Patients with OCD may present with symptoms of depression, another comorbid psychiatric condition, or physical sequelae such as skin damage, fatigue, or insomnia.

CURRENT TREATMENT

- Selective serotonin reuptake inhibitors (SSRIs) and exposure and response prevention (ERP) behavioral therapy are first-line treatments for OCD with good evidence of effectiveness.
- SSRIs, clomipramine (Anafranil), serotonin-norepinephrine reuptake inhibitors (SNRIs), and monoamine oxidase inhibitors (MAOIs) have demonstrated efficacy in the treatment of OCD.
- Effective SSRI therapy often requires high dosages and 8 to 12 weeks of treatment. Long-term adherence is essential. If a patient fails an adequate trial of SSRI monotherapy, a trial of another SSRI is recommended.
- Evidence-based augmentation strategies for treatment-resistant cases include low-dose antipsychotics.
- Comorbid conditions, including depression with suicidal ideation, must be identified and addressed.

Epidemiology

Clinically significant OCD has an estimated lifetime prevalence in US adults of 1.9% to 3.0%. About 2.0% of adults report symptoms that meet criteria for the diagnosis within the prior year. Many more individuals suffer from OCD symptoms that do not reach diagnostic thresholds. Approximately 90% of patients with OCD suffer from at least one additional psychiatric condition, mainly anxiety (75.8%), mood disorders (63.3%), impulse control (55.9%), and substance use disorders (38.6%). Patients report that OCD persists for a mean of 8.9 years. The duration, high morbidity, and significant role impairment place heavy demands on patients and families. The World Health Organization (WHO) ranks OCD as one of the 10 most disabling medical conditions worldwide.

The mean age of onset of OCD is 19.5 years, and new cases are rarely diagnosed after age 35. The majority of childhood and adolescent cases are in males. Nearly a quarter of males report onset before 10 years of age. The onset in females tends to be in adolescence and early adulthood. In adults, the prevalence is approximately equal in men and women. No strong evidence supports racial or ethnic difference in the prevalence of OCD.

Risk Factors, Etiology, and Pathophysiology

Several studies confirm a familial pattern for OCD, especially in childhood-onset forms. Twin studies implicate both genetic and environmental factors. Multiple genes have been implicated, notably areas on chromosomes 9 and 15. Current theory focuses on dysregulation in a network of genes influencing the glutamatergic, serotonergic, and dopaminergic systems, and possibly other parts of the brain, as underlying the development of OCD. The heritability of OCD is estimated to be approximately 40% with the remaining variation attributed to adverse environmental factors. Suggested environmental triggers for OCD include perinatal events, psychosocial stress, trauma, and inflammatory processes, especially streptococcal infection. Neuroimaging and neuropsychiatric studies indicate OCD-related changes in the

TABLE 1	Examples of Common Obsessions and Compulsions

OBSESSIONS	COMPULSIONS
Contamination or infection ("germophobia")	Avoidance of people or situations perceived as dirty, infectious, or corrupting; excessive cleaning or use of protective materials (surgical gloves, masks, sanitizer)
Control: Fear of losing control of speech or actions in public; making inappropriate comments; doing shameful or hurtful activities in public; inviting ridicule or negative reactions from others	Avoidance of others and public places; guarded behavior and curtailed speech to minimize contact with others
Religious, especially unworthiness, sinfulness, guilt	Praying, ritualizing acts of penance, seeking forgiveness (expression depends on religious belief/tradition of patient)
Sexual: concerns about acting inappropriately or being deviant	Avoidance of sexual situations, materials
Symmetry, correctness, precision	Arranging, ordering, scheduling, checking; "correcting" work of others
Violence; fear of harming others or becoming dangerous	Vigilance, attention to violent incidents, requiring reassurance

TABLE 2	Examples of Screening Questions for Obsessive-Compulsive Disorder

Do you check things repeatedly or wash your hands over and over?
Do you have unpleasant or unusual thoughts that you can't seem to get rid of?
Do you need things symmetrically arranged or always in a certain order?
Do you have trouble discarding things, so that your house is quite cluttered?

cortico–striato–thalamo–cortical (CSTC) circuit, known to be critical in evaluating and taking steps to neutralize perceived threats.

Obsessive-compulsive disorder has several subtypes. Some of the childhood-onset forms are comorbid with Tourette's and other chronic tic syndromes. In adults, the common associations with schizophrenia or schizoaffective disorder, bipolar disorder, and eating disorders could indicate that the conditions have overlapping etiologies or that one condition is a risk factor for the other. Clinicians should have an increased awareness of the possibility of OCD in adolescent and young adult patients presenting with a range of psychiatric conditions.

Clinical Manifestations

The core features of OCD are obsessions and compulsions (Table 1). Most patients have both. Obsessions are recurrent, persistent, and intrusive thoughts, urges, or images that are unwelcome and usually cause significant anxiety or distress. Patients attempt to ignore obsessions or to suppress or neutralize them by imposing other thoughts or performing specific activities. Compulsions are repetitive behaviors (e.g., handwashing, organizing, or checking) or activities (e.g., praying, counting, or repeating words silently) that the patient feels forced to perform in response to an obsession. Compulsions are characterized by rigid rules and inflexible behaviors but are not connected in a realistic way with what they are designed to neutralize or prevent and are clearly excessive responses to the intrusive thoughts, urges, or images.

Children may be unable to articulate symptoms and adults may be unwilling to disclose experiences that they recognize as abnormal. Individuals with OCD tend to be secretive about their symptoms, because most of them retain insight into the abnormal nature of their fears or behaviors. The estimated 14% to 30% of patients who have poor insight often have more severe and intractable symptoms. By the time patients present to medical attention, OCD is usually impacting function in society and/or eliciting concern from others about the patient's symptoms. The reported average time from onset of symptoms to diagnosis is 11 years. Other psychiatric conditions are commonly comorbid with

OCD, and many patients present or are misdiagnosed as suffering primarily from depression or anxiety. Physical symptoms such as skin damage ("intractable dermatitis") from recurrent handwashing or scratching may be the presenting feature of OCD.

Without intervention, OCD is usually a chronic relapsing condition with adult rates of spontaneous remission estimated at about 20%. Remission in treated patients is associated with shorter duration of symptoms, emphasizing the need for prompt recognition and effective therapy. The risk of suicide is high in patients with OCD, particularly those with depression, posttraumatic stress disorder, or impulse control disorders. One large study reported that 20% made suicidal plans and 11% attempted suicide.

Diagnosis

The diagnosis is based on clinical symptoms consistent with *Diagnostic and Statistical Manual of Mental Disorders,* Fifth Edition (DSM-5) criteria for obsessions and compulsions (see Table 1). The obsessions and compulsions must be time-consuming, often regarded as requiring more than 1 hour per day, or cause clinically significant distress or impairment in social, occupational, or other important areas of functioning. Simple screening questions have been suggested (Table 2). Several more-detailed inventories are available to document symptoms and their impact, but these are of limited use in diagnosis in a primary care setting.

A diagnosis of OCD also requires eliminating other potential causes of symptoms, as described next.

Differential Diagnosis

Identifying underlying OCD may be challenging in patients presenting with depression, anxiety, or another comorbidity. Some key features help in distinguishing OCD from these conditions (Table 3).

Insight distinguishes OCD from delusions and other features of schizophrenia. An important distinction is between OCD and obsessive-compulsive personality disorder (OCPD). In OCPD, behavior is ego-syntonic, that is, driven by desire or pleasure seeking rather than fear. Clinical OCD also needs to be distinguished from normal individuals who are meticulous and have rigid, inflexible thought processes or from individuals who describe compulsive behaviors such as eating or gambling that are or were pleasurable.

Obsessive-compulsive symptoms can occur in several neurologic conditions such as brain trauma, stroke, encephalitis, temporal lobe epilepsy, Prader-Willi syndrome, Huntington disease, Parkinson disease, carbon monoxide poisoning, or manganese poisoning, but these can usually be identified by the predominant other symptoms.

Treatment and Monitoring

Obsessive-compulsive disorder is a chronic condition with low frequency of spontaneous improvement but high probability of response to therapy if adherence and social support are maintained and comorbidities addressed. Short-term and long-term treatment goals should be established with each patient and those in his or her support system. Goals should focus on management of symptoms to optimize function and quality of life rather than complete resolution of symptoms. Adherence is critical to prognosis. Close follow-up must be secured, especially early in treatment. Given the secretive nature of the illness, the initial presentation may be

TABLE 3 Key Features That Help with Differential Diagnosis

ALTERNATIVE DIAGNOSIS	SYMPTOMS TYPICAL OF OBSESSIVE-COMPULSIVE DISORDER (OCD)	SYMPTOMS TYPICAL OF ALTERNATIVE DIAGNOSIS
Depressive disorders	Focus and content of obsessions is usually broader	Content of depressive ruminations is self-criticism, failures, guilt, regret, or pessimism
Generalized anxiety disorder	Obsessions may not be reality based. Rituals may be present	Worries focus on real-life problems, generally more vague. Usually no rituals
Posttraumatic stress disorder	Intrusive thoughts are anticipation of future events	Intrusive thoughts are replay of actual events
Schizophrenia, mania	Content is related to OCD. Insight usually present	Content is related to persecution, grandiosity, ideas of reference. Insight usually absent
Hypochondriasis	Insight usually present. Origin is external based	Insight usually absent. Origin is misinterpretation of physical signs and symptoms

the only chance to engage these patients in treatment, and must not be missed. Providing patients and families with educational information and access to community resources can help with adherence and social stabilization. Education for patients and others regarding what to expect from pharmacotherapy, including potential adverse effects and the lag period before benefit, can help ease anxiety and improve adherence and prognosis.

Once the diagnosis of OCD has been confirmed, the appropriate setting and strategy for treatment must be decided. The spectrum of treatment settings includes outpatient, adult partial-day programs, residential facilities, and inpatient psychiatric hospitalization. Factors such as suicide assessment, severity of illness, treatment cost, insurance coverage, and social support availability need to be explored to determine the optimal treatment environment.

Both pharmacotherapy and psychotherapy are recommended first-line treatment either alone or in combination (Figure 1). Combined therapy may be more effective than pharmacotherapy alone but has not been shown to be superior to behavioral therapy. Combination therapy may be most useful in patients with a coexisting psychiatric condition for which SSRIs are effective, those with poor response to initial monotherapy, or those who wish to discontinue medication as soon as possible. Practice guidelines recommend use of an approved symptom rating scale to monitor response to therapy, such as the 10-item Yale-Brown Obsessive Compulsive Scale (Y-BOCS).

Pharmacotherapy

SSRIs are first-line treatment agents for OCD (Table 4). Fluoxetine (Prozac), clomipramine (Anafranil), fluvoxamine (Luvox), paroxetine (Paxil), and sertraline (Zoloft) are approved by the U.S. Food and Drug Administration (FDA) and appear to be equally effective. Medication selection depends on factors including adverse effect profile, cost, concomitant medications, comorbid medical conditions, previous experience with the medication, and patient preference. The selected medication should be initiated at low dose and slowly titrated to effective levels. The optimal response may require a dose exceeding the manufacturer's recommended maximum dose. The "start low, go slow" strategy minimizes adverse effects, especially

in older patients, and improves adherence. Common adverse effects include gastrointestinal upset, agitation, insomnia, fatigue, and sexual side effects. Many adverse effects are transitory. Serotonin syndrome is a serious potential risk at high doses. Patients with OCD are at risk of suicide and self-harm, but studies do not indicate increased risk in those treated with SSRIs, including adolescents.

Most patients will not experience substantial improvement for 4 to 6 weeks, and many require 10 to 12 weeks of treatment at optimal dosage. Although full remission of symptoms is reported in only about 10% of patients treated with SSRIs, 40% to 65% improve. The mean improvement in symptoms is 20% to 40%. Effective therapy should be maintained for at least a year and possibly indefinitely. If medication is discontinued, gradual tapering is recommended. Relapse rates in patients who discontinue medication after 2 years of treatment are 25% to 40% and up to 80% after shorter periods of treatment.

If response continues to be inadequate and adherence is confirmed, options include changing the primary agent to clomipramine, venlafaxine (Effexor),[1] or mirtazapine (Remeron),[1] or augmentation with a second-generation antipsychotic agent. Referral to a psychiatric provider with expertise in OCD therapy may be the best option for treatment-resistant cases.

A patient may respond well to a different SSRI, but a full trial of several weeks at adequate dose is necessary before changing medication. Clomipramine is as effective as SSRIs but carries safety concerns. It is strongly serotonergic and anticholinergic and may increase risk of seizure or cardiac arrhythmia. Addition of risperidone (Risperdal)[1] and possibly aripiprazole (Abilify)[1] may benefit some treatment-resistant patients. The efficacy of quetiapine (Seroquel)[1] and olanzapine (Zyprexa)[1] is unclear. All antipsychotic agents require careful monitoring for adverse effects. Medications sometimes used for OCD but with only limited evidence of efficacy include topiramate (Topamax),[1] ondansetron (Zofran),[1] pindolol,[1] buspirone,[1] memantine (Namenda),[1] pregabalin (Lyrica),[1] N-acetylcysteine (Acetadote),[1] naltrexone (Vivitrol),[1] and riluzole (Rilutek).[1]

Psychological Therapy

The strongest evidence for effective behavioral treatment of OCD supports exposure and response prevention (ERP), a form of cognitive-behavioral therapy (CBT) in which patients learn alternative responses to anxiety-provoking stimuli or situations. Weekly or twice-weekly sessions for a total of 20 to 30 hours are recommended followed by monthly "booster" sessions for 3 to 6 months. Studies report considerable reduction in symptoms in up to 80% of patients with improvement maintained for up to 5 years. Remote-delivery formats of ERP using the telephone, a computer, or the Internet may provide effective and more accessible alternatives to traditional therapist consultation. ERP therapy not only is first-line treatment for OCD but also has strong evidence of effectiveness as an augmentation strategy to pharmacotherapy.

Cognitive therapy focusing on recognizing and changing interpretation of unrealistic thoughts is also associated with improvement in 60% to 80% of patients with OCD and is a good alternative for those unwilling to undertake ERP.

Other Treatment Options

Deep brain stimulation at the ventral capsule/striatum was approved by the FDA in 2009 for refractory OCD. Good results are reported in about half of patients treated in small trials compared with sham stimulation. Neurosurgical procedures may be recommended for selected patients with intractable OCD. Robust trials of ERP, two or more treatments with different SSRIs, a course of clomipramine, and at least three trials of augmentation therapy are recommended before considering neurosurgical approaches. These include ablative surgeries such as anterior cingulotomy, anterior capsulotomy, subcaudate tractotomy, and limbic leucotomy. These last-resort invasive procedures have had mixed success and carry risk of serious adverse effects. The

---

[1]Not FDA approved for this indication.

Figure 1 Treatment algorithm for obsessive-compulsive disorder.

TABLE 4	Dosing of Selective Serotonin Reuptake Inhibitors (SSRIs) to Treat Obsessive-Compulsive Disorder

	DOSAGE (MG/DAY)		
SSRI	**STARTING**	**TARGET**	**USUAL MAXIMAL**
Citalopram (Celexa)*	20	40	40
Escitalopram (Lexapro)*	10	20	40†
Fluoxetine (Prozac)	20	40–60	80
Fluvoxamine (Luvox)	50	200	300
Paroxetine (Paxil)	20	40–60	60
Sertraline (Zoloft)	50	200	200

*Not U.S. Food and Drug Administration approved for this indication.
†Exceeds dosage recommended by the manufacturer.

TABLE 5	List of Educational Resources for Patients and Their Families

1. Obsessive-Compulsive Foundation: http://www.ocfoundation.org.
2. Obsessive-Compulsive Information Center: http://www.miminc.org/aboutocic.html.
3. Baer L. Getting Control: Overcoming Your Obsessions and Compulsions. New York: Plume Books; 2000.
4. Gravitz HL. Obsessive Compulsive Disorder: New Help for the Family. Santa Barbara, CA: Healing Visions Press; 1998.
5. Steketee GS. Overcoming Obsessive-Compulsive Disorder: Client Manual. Oakland, CA: New Harbinger Publications; 1999.
6. Van Noppen B, Pato M, Rasmussen S. Learning to Live with OCD. New Haven, CT: Obsessive Compulsive Foundation; 2003.

American Psychiatric Association (APA) warns that they should be performed only at specialist centers.

Table 5 provides a list of educational resources for patients and their families.

References

American Psychiatric Association, DSM-5 Task Force: *Diagnostic and Statistical Manual of Mental Disorders: DSM-5*, ed 5, Washington, DC, 2013, American Psychiatric Association.

Fenske JN, Petersen K: Obsessive-compulsive disorder: Diagnosis and management, *Am Fam Physician* 92:896–903, 2015.

Goodman WK, Alterman RL: Deep brain stimulation for intractable psychiatric disorders, *Ann Rev Med* 63:511–524, 2012.

Goodman WK, Grice DE, Lapidus KAB, Coffey BJ: Obsessive-compulsive disorder, *Psychiatr Clim N Am* 27:257–267, 2014.

Grant JE: Clinical practice: Obsessive–compulsive disorder, *N Engl J Med* 371:646–653, 2014.

Komossa K, Depping AM, Meyer M, et al: Second-generation antipsychotics for obsessive-compulsive disorder, *Cochrane Database Syst Rev*: CD008141, 2010.

Koran LM, Simpson HB. Guideline watch (March 2013): Practice guideline for the treatment of patients with obsessive-compulsive disorder. Available at: http://psychiatryonline.org/pb/assets/raw/sitewide/practice_guidelines/guidelines/ocd-watch.pdf [accessed February 2017].

Pauls DL, Abramovitch A, Rauch SL, Geller DA: Obsessive-compulsive disorder: An integrative genetic and neurobiological perspective, *Nat Rev Neurosci* 15(6):410–424, 2014.

Ponniah K, Magiati I, Hollon SD: An update on the efficacy of psychological therapies in the treatment of obsessive compulsive disorder in adults, *J Obsessive Compuls Relat Disord* 2:207–218, 2013.

Romanelli RJ, Wu FM, Gamba R, et al: Behavioral therapy and serotonin reuptake inhibitor pharmacotherapy in the treatment of obsessive-compulsive disorder: A systematic review and meta-analysis of head-to-head randomized controlled trials, *Depress Anxiety* 31:641–652, 2014.

Ruscio AM, Stein DJ, Chiu WT, Kessler RC: The epidemiology of obsessive-compulsive disorder in the National Comorbidity Survey Replication, *Mol Psychiatry* 15:53–63, 2010.

Veale D, Miles S, Smallcombe N, et al: Atypical antipsychotic augmentation in SSRI treatment refractory obsessive-compulsive disorder: A systematic review and meta-analysis, *BMC Psychiatry* 14:317–330, 2014, https://doi.org/10.1186/s12888-014-0317-5.

PANIC DISORDER

Method of
Cheryl Wehler, MD

CURRENT DIAGNOSIS

- Panic disorder (PD) is characterized by the presence of multiple untriggered panic attacks.
- These unexpected panic attacks are associated with significant anticipatory anxiety and/or changes in behavior to minimize the consequences or avoid another panic attack.
  - Patients worry about being negatively judged due to visible panic symptoms.
  - Patients worry about dying or "going crazy."
- The panic attacks are not attributable to another medical condition or to the effects of a substance (medication or drug of abuse).
- The panic attacks are not better explained by another mental disorder.
- Patients frequently present with concern about somatic symptoms (e.g., fear of heart attack because of shortness of breath and chest discomfort).
- Assess patients for suicidality, as suicide risk increases with panic attacks or recent diagnosis of panic disorder.

CURRENT THERAPY

- Pharmacology and psychotherapy are effective treatments for PD.
- Selective serotonin reuptake inhibitors (SSRIs), serotonin norepinephrine reuptake inhibitors (SNRIs), tricyclic antidepressants (TCAs), and benzodiazepines have demonstrated efficacy for the treatment of PD.
- The favorable safety profile of SSRIs and SNRIs make them first-line monotherapy agents.
- Although TCAs are effective, their side effects and greater toxicity in overdose limit their clinical utility.
- Monoamine oxidase inhibitors (MAOIs) also appear effective but are reserved for patients who are nonresponders to multiple first-line treatments because of their safety profile limitations.
- Benzodiazepines are not first-line monotherapy but are useful adjuncts to antidepressants if residual anxiety requires additional treatment.
- Although the more rapid response of benzodiazepines (compared with SSRIs/SNRIs) make them attractive, the inevitable physiological dependence make them less so.
- Patients with PD can be sensitive to medication side effects; therefore the adage "start low and go slow" is applicable to dosing.
- Cognitive behavioral therapy (CBT) or CBT with medications are first-line treatments for children and adults with PD.

Epidemiology

The 12-month prevalence estimate for panic disorder (PD) in the general population of the United States and Europe is approximately 2% to 3% in adults and adolescents. Non-Latino Caucasians and Native Americans have significantly higher rates than Latinos, African Americans, and Asian Americans. Adolescent and adult females are approximately twice as likely as males to be affected (although the clinical features of PD do not differ between males and females). The prevalence is highest in adult females. Prevalence rates decline in older individuals. The overall prevalence of PD is low in children (<14 years). PD is associated with the highest number of medical visits among all anxiety disorders.

Risk Factors

Risks factors for PD include a disposition to negativity, experience of childhood physical and sexual abuse, and family history, indicating genetic vulnerability. Respiratory disorders such as asthma are associated with panic disorder. Smoking is a risk factor for panic attacks and PD. PD is associated with social and occupational/physical disability and high economic cost. PD may be comorbid with a variety of other psychiatric diagnoses, such as depression, bipolar affective disorder, and other anxiety disorders.

Diagnosis

PD is defined by the *Diagnostic and Statistical Manual of Mental Disorders,* fifth edition (DSM-V) as recurrent unexpected panic attacks followed by at least 1 month of anticipatory anxiety about having another attack, and a significant change in behavior to avoid another panic attack. A panic attack, the core feature of panic disorder, is an abrupt surge of intense fear/anxiety with concurrent physical and cognitive symptoms (Box 1). To be diagnosed as having PD, a patient must have more than one panic attack that is not the result of an obvious trigger or cue. The best example might be a nocturnal panic attack in which the individual is waking from sleep, with no external cues, in a state of intense fear (panic) and experiencing physical and cognitive symptoms. Expected panic attacks, that is, those for which there is an obvious cue or trigger, also occur in patients with PD. In the United States and Europe, approximately half of individuals with PD experience expected panic attacks as well as unexpected panic attacks. The presence of expected panic attacks does not rule out the diagnosis but is insufficient to make the diagnosis of this disorder.

A thorough diagnostic evaluation, including a complete history and thorough physical examination, is necessary to rule out medical or substance-induced panic attacks and establish the diagnosis of PD. Atypical symptoms or features of a panic attack may be suggestive of a medical illness or pharmacologic substance as the precipitant. A workup that includes laboratory tests such as complete blood cell count, complete chemistry panel (including calcium level), thyroid-stimulating hormone (TSH) level, and urine drug screen may be helpful in determining a medical or substance-related cause. These tests may be followed by a chest radiograph, an electrocardiogram, and cardiac enzymes, as warranted. If the clinical examination or history is suggestive, a Holter monitor, EEG, CT scan, or urine catecholamine assay may be performed.

Clinical Manifestations

In the United States, the median age of onset for PD is 20 to 24 years. PD is rare in childhood but occurs in adolescents; their symptoms are similar to those in adults. Onset after age 45 is unusual. If untreated, the usual course is chronic, and attacks may wax and wane. Some individuals have a chronic course complicated by frequent attacks whereas others have rare episodic symptoms. A minority of individuals have full remission. Caffeine and several other substances can provoke a panic attack.

The severity and frequency of panic attacks vary widely. Individuals who have infrequent panic attacks resemble individuals with more frequent panic attacks with regard to symptoms, demographics, and family history. To be diagnosed with PD, an individual must have more than one full-symptom attack with more than four of the symptoms listed in Box 1. Individuals may, however, have limited-symptom attacks with fewer than four symptoms.

There are three symptomatic facets of PD: acute panic, anticipatory anxiety, and phobic avoidance. Phobic avoidance often includes restricting daily activities to minimize or avoid panic attacks. Panic disorder is associated with other psychopathology, such as other anxiety disorders, particularly agoraphobia.

BOX 1 DSM-5 Criteria for Panic Disorder

- Recurrent unexpected panic attacks. A panic attack is an abrupt surge of intense fear or intense discomfort that reaches a peak within minutes, and during which time four (or more) of the following symptoms occur:
  Note: The abrupt surge can occur from a calm state or an anxious state.
  - Palpitations, pounding heart, or accelerated heart rate
  - Sweating
  - Trembling or shaking
  - Sensations of shortness of breath or smothering
  - Feelings of choking
  - Chest pain or discomfort
  - Nausea or abdominal distress
  - Feeling dizzy, light-headed, faint, or unsteady
  - Chills or heat sensations
  - Parenthesis (numbness or tingling sensations)
  - Depersonalization (being detached from oneself) or derealization (feelings of unreality)
  - Fear of "going crazy" or losing control
  - Fear of dying
  Note: Culture-specific symptoms (e.g., tinnitus, neck soreness, headache, uncontrollable screaming or crying) may be seen. Such symptoms should not count as one of the four required symptoms [to diagnose PD].
- At least one of the attacks has been followed by 1 month (or more) of one or both of the following:
  - Persistent concern or worry about additional panic attacks or their consequences (e.g., losing control, having a heart attack, "going crazy")
  - A significant maladaptive change in behavior related to the attacks (e.g., behaviors designed to avoid having panic attacks, such as avoidance of exercise or unfamiliar situations)
- The disturbance is not attributable to the physiological effects of a substance (e.g., a drug of abuse, a medication) or another medical condition (e.g., hyperthyroidism, cardiopulmonary disorders)
- The disturbance is not better explained by another mental disorder (e.g., the panic attacks do not occur only in response to feared social situations, as in social anxiety disorder; in response to circumscribed phobic objects or situations, as in specific phobia; in response to obsessions, as in obsessive-compulsive disorder; in response to reminders of traumatic events, as in posttraumatic stress disorder; or in response to separation from attachment figures, as in separation anxiety disorder)

Although medical illness can precipitate a panic attack, individuals with anxiety, particularly PD, may be hypervigilant and misinterpret mild physical symptoms as harbingers of a catastrophic or fatal illness. Individuals with PD often report feelings of anxiety that are associated with health or mental health concerns.

Panic attacks often contribute to the presentation of other psychiatric illnesses, such as other anxiety disorders and major depression. A thorough history that documents the onset of symptoms, possible triggers, and context of symptoms is critical to establishing the diagnosis of PD. In addition to the history of the present illness and current symptoms, a psychiatric review of symptoms, past psychiatric history, general medical history and current medications, substance use history, family history, and mental status exam are valuable in constructing a psychiatric differential diagnosis and then a final working diagnosis. For instance, an individual with a history of a past trauma presenting with flashbacks, nightmares, and triggered panic attacks may have posttraumatic stress disorder (versus panic disorder).

TABLE 1 Differential Diagnosis of Panic Attacks

SYSTEM	POSSIBLE DIAGNOSES
Psychiatric	Mood disorder (panic attacks associated with depression or bipolar disorder) Anxiety disorders (panic attacks associated with social anxiety, specific phobia, posttraumatic stress disorder, generalized anxiety disorder, obsessive compulsive disorder) Agoraphobia Psychotic disorder (panic attacks associated with psychosis) Somatoform disorder Factitious disorder
Cardiac	Myocardial infarction Angina SVT or other arrhythmia Mitral valve prolapse Labile hypertension
Respiratory	Asthma COPD Pulmonary embolus
Neurologic	Seizure disorder Vestibular dysfunction
Endocrine	Thyroid disorder Hypoglycemia Adrenal dysfunction Hyperparathyroidism Pheochromocytoma
Substance Use	Excess caffeine Psychostimulants
Substance Withdrawal	Caffeine Nicotine Alcohol or sedative Opioid

Suicidal behavior in individuals with anxiety disorders has long been attributed to co-occurring risk factors, such as depression. New research suggests that an anxiety disorder is associated with suicidal ideation and suicide attempts beyond the effects of co-occurring mental disorders. Panic attacks and a recent diagnosis of PD are associated with a higher rate of suicide attempts and suicidal ideation.

Differential Diagnosis

The differential diagnosis of PD is wide ranging (Table 1). PD is not diagnosed if panic attacks are the direct physiological consequence of another medical condition or substance. Medical conditions that can cause panic attacks include cardiopulmonary conditions such as arrhythmias and asthma or chronic obstructive pulmonary disease (COPD). Endocrine and neurologic disorders such as hyperthyroidism, pheochromocytoma, vestibular dysfunction, and seizures may also cause panic attacks. In addition, central nervous system (CNS) stimulants and withdrawal from CNS depressants may precipitate a panic attack. On the other hand, a panic attack may mimic a wide variety of medical disorders.

Treatment

PD is a common mental disorder. It is associated with social and occupational/physical disability and high economic cost. When symptoms cause significant distress or interfere with functioning, treatment is warranted. Regardless of the modality chosen, the goal of treatment is a reduction in the frequency and severity of

TABLE 2 Pharmacologic Treatments of Panic Disorder

MEDICATION (TRADE NAME)	INITIAL DOSE (MG/DAY)	DOSE RANGE (MG/DAY)
SSRIs		
Citalopram (Celexa)[1]	10–20	20–40
Escitalopram (Lexapro)[1]	5–10	10–20
Fluoxetine (Prozac)	10–20	20–80
Fluvoxamine (Luvox)[1]	50	100–300[†]
Fluvoxamine CR (Luvox CR)[1]	100	100–300
Paroxetine (Paxil)	10–20	20–60
Paroxetine CR (Paxil CR)	12.5–25	25–75
Sertraline (Zoloft)	25	50–200
SNRIs		
Duloxetine (Cymbalta)[1]	30	60–120
Venlafaxine (Effexor)[1]	25–50	150–225
Venlafaxine ER (Effexor ER)	37.5	75–225
TCAs		
Desipramine (Norpramin)	25–50	100–200
Clomipramine (Anafranil)[1]	25	50–150
Imipramine (Tofranil)[1]	25	50–150
Nortriptyline (Pamelor)[1]	10–25	75–150
MAOIs		
Phenelzine* (Nardil)[1]	45[†]	45-75[§]
Benzodiazepines		
Alprazolam (Xanax)	0.25–0.5 tid	5–6
Alprazolam XR (Xanax XR)	0.5–1	3–6
Lorazepam (Ativan)[1]	0.25 tid	2–8[‡]
Clonazepam (Klonopin)	0.25 bid	0.5–2[†]

[1]Not FDA approved for this indication.
*Dietary restrictions required (low-tyramine diet); 2-week washout required before initiation and after termination of monoamine oxidase inhibitor (MAOI) trial.
[†]Divided doses may be given.
[‡]Total daily dosage divided across 2–4 doses/day.
[§]Usually administered tid.

panic attacks as well as the resultant anticipatory anxiety and avoidance behaviors.

Research has confirmed the efficacy of multiple psychosocial and pharmacologic interventions in treating PD. Choice of treatment depends on multiple factors, including patient preference; risks and benefits for an individual patient; cost; past treatment history; and co-occurring medical, psychiatric, or substance abuse issues.

Selective serotonin reuptake inhibitors (SSRIs), serotonin norepinephrine reuptake inhibitors (SNRIs), tricyclic antidepressants (TCAs), and benzodiazepines have demonstrated efficacy for the treatment of PD. The favorable safety profile of SSRIs and SNRIs makes them first-line monotherapy agents. Although TCAs are effective, their side effects and toxicity in overdose limit their clinical utility. Monoamine oxidase inhibitors (MAOIs) also appear effective but are reserved for patients who are nonresponders to multiple first-line treatments because of their safety profile. Benzodiazepines are not first-line monotherapy but are useful adjuncts to antidepressants if residual anxiety requires additional treatment (Table 2).

An important consideration when using psychopharmacologic treatments in PD is the side-effect profile of a particular agent. Because patients with PD can be acutely sensitive to medication side effects, it is prudent to start medications at low doses and gradually increase them to therapeutic doses as tolerated. An effective dose is patient dependent—the goal is to prevent (versus respond to) panic attacks. If a decision is made to discontinue a SSRI, SNRI, or TCA, the medication should be gradually tapered when feasible.

Cognitive behavioral therapy (CBT) and CBT with medications are first-line treatments for children and adults with PD. CBT presents the most evidence of efficacy from random control trials. CBT for panic disorder generally includes psychoeducation, episode monitoring and response, self-awareness of anxious automatic thoughts and beliefs, controlled exposure to fear cues, modification of anxiety-reducing behaviors, and prevention of relapse. Psychosocial interventions, such as CBT, may enhance long-term outcomes by reducing the likelihood of relapse.

References

American Psychiatric Association: *Diagnostic and Statistical Manual of Mental Disorders*, ed 5, Arlington, VA, 2013, American Psychiatric Association.
American Psychiatric Association: *Practice Guideline for the Treatment of Patients with Panic Disorder*, ed 2, Arlington, VA, 2010, American Psychiatric Association.
Craske MG, Kircanski K, Epstein A, et al: Panic disorder: A review of DSM-IV panic disorder and proposals for DSM-V, *Depress Anxiety* 27:93–112, 2010.
Thibodeau MA, Welch PG, Sareen J, Asmundson GJG: Anxiety disorders are independently associated with suicide ideation and attempts: Propensity score matching in two epidemiological samples, *Depress Anxiety* 30:947–954, 2013.
Locke AB, Kirst N, Shultz CG: Diagnosis and management of generalized anxiety disorder and panic disorder in adults, *Am Fam Physician* 91(9):617–624, 2015.
Marchesi C: Pharmacological management of panic disorder, *Neuropsychiatr Dis Treat* 4:93–106, 2008.
Milrod B, Chambless DL, Gallop R, et al: Psychotherapies for panic disorder: a tale of two sites, *J Clin Psychiatry* 9, 2015, Jun (Epub ahead of print).
Stahl SM: *Stahl's Essential Psychopharmocology: The Prescriber's Guide*, ed 5, New York, 2014, Cambridge University Press.
Andrisano C, Chiesa A, Serretti A: Newer antidepressants and panic disorder: A meta-analysis, *Int Clin Psychopharmacol* 28:33–45, 2013.

POSTTRAUMATIC STRESS DISORDER

Method of
Natalie C. Dattilo, PhD

CURRENT DIAGNOSIS

- Posttraumatic stress disorder (PTSD) is quickly becoming one of the most common psychiatric disorders seen in the primary care setting.
- PTSD is diagnosed after a person experiences symptoms for at least 1 month following a traumatic event. However, symptoms may not appear until several months or even years later and can persist as a chronic condition.
- The disorder is characterized by three main types of symptoms: (1) reexperiencing the trauma through distressing recollections, (2) emotional numbness and behavioral avoidance, and (3) increased arousal such as feeling jumpy and easily angered.
- A thorough medical examination and laboratory workup may be indicated to rule out contributing physiologic factors and comorbidities, substance use or misuse, and drug or alcohol withdrawal.
- Symptoms that are persistent, disruptive, or distressing warrant treatment.
- The PTSD Checklist-5 (PCL-5) is a 20-item self-report measure that assesses the 20 *Diagnostic and Statistical Manual of Mental Disorders,* Fifth Edition (DSM-5) symptoms of PTSD. The gold standard for diagnosing PTSD is a structured clinical interview such as the Clinician-Administered PTSD Scale (CAPS-5). When necessary, the PCL-5 can be scored to provide a provisional PTSD diagnosis.

CURRENT THERAPY

- Effective treatments for PTSD include serotonergic antidepressants, certain forms of trauma-based psychotherapy, or a combination of both.
- Educating the patient and family members about treatment options and setting realistic treatment expectations are critical.
- Depending on the patient's preference, treatment may include a selective serotonin reuptake inhibitor (SSRI) starting at low doses with careful titration so as not to exacerbate anxiety or agitation.
- Treatment may also include a trial of cognitive-behavioral therapy, cognitive processing therapy, or prolonged exposure therapy to boost response rates and prevent relapse.
- Refer to or consult with a psychiatrist for patients with severe or particularly complex cases or for patients with a less-than-expected response to treatment.
- Refer to a cognitive-behavioral therapy specialist for patients with a preference for behavioral, skills-based, or nonmedication therapy or for whom pharmacotherapy may be contraindicated.

Epidemiology

In the United States, it is estimated that PTSD is diagnosed in approximately 10.5 million adults (3.5%) each year, and approximately 20.4 million (6.8%) will meet criteria over the course of their lifetimes. The lifetime prevalence of PTSD among men is 3.6% and among women is 9.7%. The 12-month prevalence is 1.8% among men and 5.2% among women. As with depression and anxiety disorders, patients with PTSD are more likely to present initially to a general practitioner's office than to a mental health care provider.

Owing, in part, to increased public awareness, PTSD is quickly becoming one of the most frequently seen clinical problems in primary care. Symptoms frequently overlap with other complaints, such as insomnia, irritability, or pain. Most behavioral symptoms of PTSD are a result of anxiety and hypervigilance, and the clinical presentation shares many phenotypic similarities with other anxiety disorders, such as panic disorder (PD) and generalized anxiety disorder (GAD).

Risk Factors

Risk factors associated with PTSD include exposure to trauma, being female, having lower levels of education and income, being divorced or widowed, having a history of behavioral or psychological problems, family history of behavioral or psychological problems including substance abuse, recent increase in stressful life events, lack or perceived lack of social support, ineffective emotional coping strategies, experiencing childhood adversity or trauma, having a chronic health condition or serious illness, having an acute or chronic pain condition, and substance abuse. Although a genetic predisposition to developing PTSD is likely, environmental stress and early trauma clearly play a role.

Pathophysiology

Our current understanding of PTSD is incomplete; however, several neurobiologic systems have been implicated in the pathophysiology and vulnerability toward developing PTSD after trauma exposure. As in other anxiety disorders, PTSD symptoms are believed to be due to dysregulation of neuronal activity within the central nervous system (CNS), in particular the fear circuit. This dysregulation causes a state of hyperarousal, which gives rise to the physical and emotional manifestations of the condition. Several neurotransmitter systems have been implicated in the genesis of this hyperaroused state. Overstimulation of the CNS and the autonomic sympathetic activity it generates affect the prefrontal cortex and the limbic system (e.g., amygdala, hypothalamus), both of which play an important role in our ability to discern stimuli as aversive or threatening and regulate our stress response.

The two most commonly implicated neurotransmitter systems to date include the serotoninergic and noradrenergic neurotransmitter systems. Very simply, it is believed that an underactivation of the serotoninergic system and an overactivation of the noradrenergic system are involved. These systems interact with other neuronal circuits in various regions of the brain, including the locus ceruleus (LC) and the limbic structures, resulting in a dysregulation of physiologic arousal and the emotional interpretation of this arousal, respectively. Disruption of the γ-aminobutyric acid (GABA) system has also been implicated because of the response of many of the anxiety-spectrum disorders to treatment with benzodiazepines.

There has also been some interest in the role of corticosteroid regulation and its relation to symptoms of fear and anxiety. Corticosteroids might increase or decrease the activity of certain neural pathways, affecting not only an individual's behavior under stress but also how the brain perceives and processes threatening stimuli. The stress response is hardwired into the brain and is most often triggered when survival of the organism is threatened. The stress response, however, can be triggered not only by a physical challenge or threat but also by the mere anticipation (or fear) of threat. As a result, when humans chronically and erroneously believe that a threatening event is about to occur, they begin to experience the physical and psychological symptoms of anxiety and panic.

The hypothalamic–pituitary–adrenal (HPA) axis is another neurocircuit implicated in the initiation of a stress response. The HPA axis assists with the adaptation to stress and the maintenance of homeostasis after challenge. It connects the CNS and the endocrine system, and a dysfunctional HPA axis is associated with numerous psychosomatic and psychiatric disorders. Corticotropin-releasing factor (CRF) is a molecule produced by cells in the hypothalamus in response to physical or psychological stress. Increased levels of CRF in the hypothalamus in response to stress results in the activation of the HPA axis and increased release of cortisol. It is believed that high CRF levels at the time of trauma may facilitate encoding of traumatic memory and enduring anxiety effects. Patients with PTSD exhibit increased cerebrospinal fluid levels of CRF and other abnormalities in the HPA axis system.

Finally, a subcortical neural structure, the amygdala, serves an important role in coordinating the cognitive, affective, neuroendocrine, cardiovascular, respiratory, and musculoskeletal components of fear and anxiety responses. It is central to registering the emotional significance of stressful stimuli and creating emotional memories. The amygdala receives input from neurons in the sensory cortex. When activated, the amygdala stimulates regions of the midbrain and brainstem, causing autonomic hyperactivity, which can be correlated with the physical symptoms of anxiety.

Prevention

No biological markers are specific enough yet to detect which individuals are more likely to develop PTSD after experiencing a trauma, and there is no available evidence to suggest that current medications prove efficacious in preventing this disorder. Therefore it is important to screen for specific risk factors, such as exposure to trauma (either recent or remote), family history of mental health issues, recent increase in stressful life events, or substance abuse. If a person is found to be at risk, but not symptomatic, he or she should first be encouraged to adopt healthy lifestyle habits. Aerobic exercise and other forms of physical activity have been shown to relieve stress and anxiety and improve mood relatively quickly. These patients should also be encouraged to avoid stimulants such as caffeine and nicotine, which can exacerbate symptoms and contribute to insomnia. It is also highly recommended that anxiety-prone persons manage stress by learning effective methods of behavioral relaxation, applied meditation, and other healthy stress reduction techniques.

Clinical Manifestations

PTSD can manifest in many ways. Behavioral signs may include increased alcohol consumption, change in communication, change in sexual functioning, emotional outbursts, inability to rest or relax, change in appetite, pacing, suspiciousness, self-destructive behavior, or social isolation. Cognitive signs may include changes in alertness, confusion, hypervigilance, memory problems, poor attention and concentration, poor decision making or problem solving, and suicidal ideation. Emotional signs may include agitation, anxiety, apprehension, depression, fear, feeling overwhelmed, grief, guilt, irritability, and loss of emotional control. Sleep is also affected for individuals suffering from PTSD, and they will often report insomnia or nightmares. Other common features include a sense of emotional detachment from others and unwanted or intrusive thoughts; however, these can be difficult for clinicians to identify and patients rarely self-report. Physical symptoms can include chills, difficulty breathing, dizziness, elevated blood pressure, fainting, fatigue, grinding teeth, headaches, muscle tremors, nausea, pain, profuse sweating, rapid heart rate, twitches, and weakness. These symptoms cause significant distress and impairment of function.

Diagnosis

A diagnosis of PTSD is made when the patient meets specific diagnostic criteria as outlined in the DSM-5. In previous versions of the DSM, PTSD was categorized as an anxiety disorder. The diagnosis of PTSD now falls under its own category of mental disorders, called "Trauma and Stressor-Related Disorders," owing to the myriad ways it can present clinically.

PTSD may develop after a person experiences, witnesses, or confronts a physically or psychologically traumatic event. The event may involve actual or threatened death, serious or life-threatening injury or threat of severe injury, or sexual violence or threat of sexual violence. An individual may directly experience the traumatic event; witness, in person, the traumatic event; or learn that the traumatic event occurred to a close family member or close friend. An individual may also develop PTSD after experiencing repeated or extreme exposure to aversive details of the traumatic events. Examples may be first responders collecting human remains or police officers repeatedly exposed to details of child abuse. Note: This does not apply to exposure through electronic media, television, movies, or pictures, unless exposure is work related.

The disorder is characterized by three main types of symptoms: (1) reexperiencing the trauma through distressing recollections, (2) emotional numbness and behavioral avoidance, and (3) increased arousal such as feeling jumpy and easily angered.

A diagnosis of PTSD can be made in adults, adolescents, and children over the age of 6 when one or more of the following reexperiencing symptoms are present:

- Spontaneous or cued recurrent, involuntary, and intrusive distressing memories of the traumatic events (Note: In children repetitive play may occur in which themes or aspects of the traumatic events are expressed.)
- Recurrent distressing dreams in which the content or affect (i.e., feeling) of the dream is related to the events (Note: In children there may be frightening dreams without recognizable content.)
- Flashbacks or other dissociative reactions in which the individual feels or acts as if the traumatic event is recurring (Note: In children trauma-specific reenactment may occur in play.)
- Intense or prolonged psychological distress at exposure to internal or external cues that symbolize or resemble an aspect of the traumatic events
- Physiologic reactions to reminders of the traumatic events

A diagnosis of PTSD can be made in adults, adolescents, and children over the age of 6 when two or more of the following emotional numbness or behavioral avoidance symptoms are also present:

- Inability to remember an important aspect of the traumatic events (not due to head injury, alcohol, or drugs)
- Persistent and exaggerated negative beliefs or expectations about oneself, others, or the world (e.g., "I am bad," "No one can be trusted," "The world is completely dangerous")
- Persistent, distorted blame of self or others about the cause or consequences of the traumatic events
- Persistent fear, horror, anger, guilt, or shame
- Markedly diminished interest or participation in significant activities
- Feelings of detachment or estrangement from others
- Persistent inability to experience positive emotions

In addition to reexperiencing and avoidance, a diagnosis of PTSD can be made in adults, adolescents, and children over the age of 6 when two or more of the following marked changes in arousal and reactivity are also present:

- Irritable or aggressive behavior
- Reckless or self-destructive behavior
- Hypervigilance
- Exaggerated startle response
- Problems with concentration
- Difficulty falling or staying asleep or restless sleep

Finally, the diagnosis is made if the symptoms have been present for at least 1 month and cause clinically significant distress or impairment in functioning.

Differential Diagnosis

It is important to perform a thorough medical workup when initially assessing the patient with PTSD symptoms. Differential diagnoses can include several organic causes, such as endocrine dysfunction, intoxication or withdrawal, hypoxia, metabolic abnormalities, and neurologic disorders. It is also important to consider and rule out any cooccurring psychiatric disorders. Major depression with or without suicidality, bipolar disorder, panic disorder, delusional disorder, polysubstance dependence, and adjustment disorder can often accompany PTSD, in addition to relationship problems and difficulty at work or in social situations.

It is not uncommon for patients with PTSD to report chronic pain or present with "ill defined" or "medically unexplained" somatic symptoms such as headaches, dizziness, tinnitus, and blurry vision or medical issues including diabetes, obesity, and cardiovascular, respiratory, musculoskeletal, neurologic, or gastrointestinal problems. Frequently reported medical comorbidities with PTSD across various studies include cardiovascular disease, especially hypertension, and immune-mediated disorders. Because PTSD is associated with limbic dysfunction and alterations in the HPA axis, neuroendocrine and immune function can be significantly disrupted, and because of its impact on the CNS, pseudo-neurologic symptoms and disorders of sleep–wake regulation are also common.

It is also not uncommon for patients with PTSD to "self-medicate" or cope with their symptoms by drinking alcohol, smoking cigarettes, or using drugs, including cannabis and prescription pain medications or anxiolytics. Studies show that people with PTSD have more issues with drugs and alcohol both before and after being diagnosed with PTSD. In addition, having PTSD increases the risk that one will develop a drinking or drug problem, even in the absence of any prior drug or alcohol use.

Treatment and Monitoring

Current practice guidelines for the treatment of PTSD begin with education. Many people are confused, scared, or frustrated by the symptoms and behavior and are reassured to know they are not alone and that there are effective interventions. The patient should receive an appropriate medical workup, including a physical examination and studies (e.g., electrocardiogram, thyroid-stimulating hormone) when indicated. In addition to treating any cooccurring or underlying medical conditions, developing a good working alliance with the patient and family provides a basis for ongoing disease management and prevents unnecessary utilization or overutilization of the medical system, as well as potential exacerbation of symptoms.

A combination of psychotherapy and medication management is recommended as first-line treatment for PTSD. Psychological treatments with the most robust empirical support include trauma-focused psychotherapies utilizing exposure techniques, cognitive restructuring, relaxation/stress modulation training, and psychoeducation.

Cognitive-behavioral therapy (CBT) is the most effective non-medication treatment for PTSD. The two types of CBT recommended for PTSD are cognitive processing therapy (CPT) and prolonged exposure (PE). In CPT one examines what he or she is thinking and telling him- or herself about the trauma and decides whether those thoughts are accurate or inaccurate. It can be done individually or in a group. PE works through repeated exposure to thoughts, feelings, and situations the person has been avoiding and helps him or her learn that reminders of the trauma do not have to be avoided. PE is done individually with a therapist. Both CPT and PE offer a skills-based approach to treatment. The therapist and patient work collaboratively and in an active and problem-solving manner. The work structured and generally short term with an emphasis on reducing symptoms. Volumes of evidence support the efficacy of CBT interventions for PTSD, but success requires commitment to treatment on the part of the patient. Its efficacy is also contingent upon the ability of the therapist and the length of time in treatment. Studies show that when compared with patients undergoing monotherapy, patients treated with a combination of CBT and medication experience nearly twice the remission rate.

If combination therapy is initiated owing to symptom severity or patient preference, the SSRIs have been shown to be the best-tolerated class of medications, and response rates are significantly higher than placebo. This class of medication includes fluoxetine (Prozac),[1] fluvoxamine (Luvox), citalopram (Celexa), escitalopram (Lexapro), paroxetine (Paxil), and sertraline (Zoloft). Some improvement should be noted within 3 or 4 weeks, and the dose should be increased if no improvement is seen. In all cases, SSRIs should be started at low doses and gradually titrated up to therapeutic levels to avoid an initial exacerbation of anxiety or agitation. Pharmacotherapy and psychotherapy options for the treatment of PTSD are presented in Tables 1A and 1B.

Benzodiazepines, which have been commonly used in the past to treat anxiety symptoms, are not recommended except in cases of extreme impairment of function, for short-term use only, and only after a thorough substance abuse history has been obtained. The tolerability and lack of addiction potential make the SSRIs more desirable for long-term management, but the delay in response makes short-term symptom relief with a benzodiazepine desirable for those with the greatest impairment. Because of the risk for rebound anxiety when withdrawing from benzodiazepines with short half-lives, such as alprazolam (Xanax), many prefer the longer-acting benzodiazepines, such as clonazepam (Klonopin).[2] However, the addiction potential and the potential for abuse with either drug make this the treatment option of last resort.

If the patient does not respond to the combination of CBT and medication, a reevaluation of symptoms might reveal a comorbid disorder missed on first examination. Comorbid psychiatric disorders significantly lower the likelihood of recovery from PTSD and increase recurrence rates. Many clinicians try switching between SSRIs before considering the next step in treatment, but a referral to a psychiatrist for further evaluation and management may be necessary if this strategy does not work. Treatment-refractory anxiety can be extremely frustrating for both the patient and clinician. This can lead to increased dependence on benzodiazepines and an escalation of doses required for the same effect.

When approaching the start of therapy, the clinician should reassure the patient that effective treatment is available but that patience may be necessary until the right combination of modalities is found. Although PTSD, like all anxiety disorders, displays a significant amount of chronicity, most patients have an improved outcome with appropriate treatment. Response rates

---

[1] Not FDA approved for this indication.
[2] Not U.S. Food and Drug Administration (FDA) approved for this indication.

TABLE 1A	Pharmacotherapy for the Treatment of Posttraumatic Stress Disorder	
DRUG	**STARTING DOSE**	**TARGET DOSE**
Selective Serotonin Reuptake Inhibitors		
Paroxetine (Paxil)	10 mg qd	10–60 mg qd
Escitalopram (Lexapro)*	5–10 mg qd	10–20 mg qd
Sertraline (Zoloft)	12.5–25 mg qd	50–200 mg qd
Fluoxetine (Prozac)*	10 mg qd	20–40 mg qd

*Not US Food and Drug Administration approved for this indication.

TABLE 1B	Evidence-Based Psychotherapy for the Treatment of Posttraumatic Stress Disorder	
PSYCHOTHERAPY	**DESCRIPTION**	**FORMAT**
Trauma-Focused Cognitive-Behavioral Therapy (TF-CBT)		
Cognitive processing therapy (CPT)	Teaches you to reframe negative thoughts about trauma	Weekly individual or group meetings
Prolonged exposure (PE)	Teaches you to gain control by facing your fears	Weekly individual meetings

improve when comorbidity is low. Patients with an earlier onset of symptoms (childhood or adolescence) can generally expect a more chronic course and may be more difficult to treat. Occasionally, patients can have a spontaneous remission of symptoms and many can continue to function despite their symptoms. However, time to resolution of symptoms is shortened and overall functioning can improve with treatment.

Pharmacotherapy often helps to prevent relapse, and rates are improved when effective treatment is continued for 12 months. When considering termination of pharmacologic treatment, the risk for relapse in all the disorders should be discussed with the patient. When discontinuing the SSRIs, a slow taper is recommended, with close monitoring for withdrawal symptoms (e.g., headache, gastrointestinal upset, restlessness, and other flulike symptoms). Also monitor for rebound anxiety symptoms. If relapse occurs, reinstituting treatment is indicated, and many patients opt for indefinite treatment to maintain remission of symptoms. Lifelong management with pharmacotherapy or psychotherapy, or both, is not unusual for many patients. For many, a maximum reduction of symptoms, rather than a full remission, is an acceptable outcome.

Complications

Untreated anxiety disorders can lead to, or worsen, other mental and physical health conditions, including bruxism (teeth grinding), cognitive impairment, depression, gastrointestinal disorders, headache, insomnia, heart disease, substance abuse, and significantly impaired quality of life.

Conclusion

PTSD is a highly prevalent psychiatric condition that can be disabling and costly to the patient and to the health care system. Despite the prevalence of PTSD and other mental health disorders, a high percentage of patients often remain undiagnosed and untreated. These untreated patients also tend to be higher utilizers of general medical care. Patients with PTSD often present with multiple somatic complaints and comorbid disorders, causing great effort and expense in identifying the cause of unexplained symptoms. Once PTSD is identified, patients may be treated using well-tested and efficacious pharmacologic and psychotherapeutic treatments. Helpful resources for patients and families are listed in Table 2.

TABLE 2 Helpful Resources for Patients with Posttraumatic Stress Disorder

ORGANIZATION	WEBSITE
US Department of Veteran Affairs National Center for PTSD	https://www.ptsd.va.gov/index.asp
Anxiety and Depression Association of America (ADAA)	https://www.adaa.org/understanding-anxiety/posttraumatic-stress-disorder-ptsd
National Institute of Mental Health (NIMH)	https://www.nimh.nih.gov/health/topics/post-traumatic-stress-disorder-ptsd/index.shtml
American Academy of Family Physicians (AAFP)	http://www.aafp.org/afp/2000/0901/p1046.html

References

American Psychiatric Association: *Diagnostic and Statistical Manual of Mental Disorders*, ed 5, Washington, DC, 2013, American Psychiatric Association.

American Psychological Association: *Clinical Practice Guideline for the Treatment of Posttraumatic Stress Disorder (PTSD) in Adults*, Washington, DC, 2017, American Psychological Association.

Bailey C, Cordell E, Sobin S, Neumeister A: Recent progress in understanding the pathophysiology of posttraumatic stress disorder: Implications for targeted pharmacological treatment, *CNS Drugs* 27:221–232, 2013.

Gabbard GO: Treatment of Psychiatric Disorders, vols. 1–2. 3rd ed, Washington, DC, 2001, American Psychiatric Publishing.

Goddard AW, Coplan JD, Shekhar A, et al: Principles of the pharmacotherapy of anxiety disorders, In Charney DS, Nestler EJ, editors: *The Neurobiology of Mental Illness*, ed 2nd, New York, 2004, Oxford University Press, pp 661–682.

Gupta M: Review of somatic symptoms in post-traumatic stress disorder, *Int Rev Psychiatry* 25:86–99, 2013.

Kessler RC, Berglund P, Demler O, et al: Lifetime prevalence and age-of-onset distributions of DSM-IV disorders in the National Comorbidity Survey Replication, *Arch Gen Psychiatry* 62:593–602, 2005.

Kroenke K, Spitzer RL, Williams JBW, et al: Anxiety disorders in primary care: Prevalence, impairment, comorbidity, and detection, *Ann Intern Med* 146:317–325, 2007.

Lepine JP: The epidemiology of anxiety disorders: Prevalence and societal costs, *J Clin Psychiatry* 63(Suppl. 14):4–8, 2002.

National Comorbidity Survey: NCS-R appendix tables: Table 1. Lifetime prevalence of DSM-IV/WMH-CIDI disorders by sex and cohort. Table 2. Twelve-month prevalence of DSM-IV/WMH-CIDI disorders by sex and cohort. 2005. Available at: http://www.hcp.med.harvard.edu/ncs/publications.php.

Sadock B, Sadock V: *Kaplan and Sadock's Synopsis of Psychiatry: Behavioral Sciences/Clinical Psychiatry*, ed 10, Philadelphia, 2007, Lippincott Williams & Wilkins.

Stein M: Attending to anxiety disorders in primary care, *J Clin Psychiatry* 64:35–39, 2003.

SCHIZOPHRENIA

Method of
Brian J. Miller, MD, PhD, MPH; and Peter F. Buckley, MD

CURRENT DIAGNOSIS

- There are three primary symptom domains in schizophrenia:
  - Positive symptoms (i.e., hallucinations, delusions, disorganized thought, and abnormal psychomotor behavior)
  - Negative symptoms (i.e., restricted affect or avolition/asociality)
  - Cognitive symptoms (i.e., attention, language, memory, and processing speed)
- Symptoms last ≥ 1 month and there are continuous signs of illness for ≥ 6 months.
- There is significant impairment one or more major areas of functioning (work, interpersonal relations, or self-care).
- Rule out that psychosis is not due to a primary mood disorder, schizoaffective disorder, substance intoxication or withdrawal, or a general medical condition.

CURRENT THERAPY

- Antipsychotic medication, with monitoring for medication adherence and side effects.
- Adjunctive medications as needed, including antidepressants, mood stabilizers, benzodiazepines, beta-blockers, and anticholinergics.
- Aggressive monitoring for and management of medical comorbidities, substance use disorders, and suicidality, including collaboration with primary care physician.
- Psychosocial interventions.
- Involvement of family/support system in care.
- Long-term treatment, including outpatient medication management and therapy, with inpatient care for acute crisis intervention/illness exacerbation.

Schizophrenia is a complex, chronic, and often severe psychiatric disorder that is a leading cause of disability worldwide. Although the literal translation of the word schizophrenia is "split mind," patients with this disorder do not have a "split personality" or "multiple personality disorder" (known as dissociative identity disorder). Rather, schizophrenia is a psychotic disorder that interferes with a person's thinking, mood, behavior, and/or interpersonal relations. Schizophrenia often has devastating, lifelong consequences for affected individuals and their families and is associated with an increased risk of premature mortality, including deaths from suicide and cardiovascular disease. In this chapter, the epidemiology and diagnosis of schizophrenia are reviewed. We then discuss pharmacologic and psychosocial treatments for schizophrenia in the context of a chronic disease model. The risks of medical and substance use comorbidity and suicidality are also highlighted.

Epidemiology and Risk Factors

The etiology of schizophrenia is not known, but it is thought to involve interactions between genetic (or epigenetic) and environmental factors, including developmental problems that occur during gestation. The lifetime prevalence of schizophrenia is approximately 1% and is equal in men and women. The usual age of onset is in the late teens or early 20s to late 30s, although schizophrenia can have onset before age 10 (early onset) or after age 45 (late onset). The age of onset is usually younger for men than women.

Several lines of evidence support a genetic contribution to the risk of schizophrenia. There is a 40% lifetime risk of schizophrenia in a child of two parents with schizophrenia. Twin-twin concordance is 50% in monozygotic twins, and 12% in dizygotic twins. A recent genome-wide association study and meta-analysis found that schizophrenia is significantly associated with single nucleotide polymorphisms in the major histocompatibility complex region on chromosome 6p22.1 (which includes several immunity-related genes, particularly complement C4), although numerous other genes have been implicated. There are likely multiple candidate genes that increase the risk of schizophrenia, each with small effect size.

Replicated environmental risk factors for schizophrenia include season of birth (winter), advanced paternal age, prenatal stress throughout gestation (famine and acute maternal stress in the first trimester, prenatal infections with a myriad of different agents, loss of the father in the second or third trimester), obstetric complications (including gestational diabetes, low birth weight, asphyxia), severe childhood abuse, and cannabis use. It remains unclear whether some of these risk factors are causal to schizophrenia or represent early manifestations of disease.

Diagnosis

There are three primary symptom domains in schizophrenia: positive, negative, and cognitive symptoms. Positive symptoms are abnormalities of thought content, including hallucinations (abnormal sensory perceptions in the absence of external stimuli) and delusions (fixed, false beliefs), formal thought disorder (also called disorganized thinking), and abnormal psychomotor behavior (such as catatonia). Hallucinations are most commonly auditory but can occur in any sensory modality. Negative symptoms include impairments in emotional expression (blunted affect), motivation (avolition), social behavior (asociality), speech (alogia), and the ability to experience pleasure (anhedonia). Cognitive symptoms include impairments in attention, language, memory, processing speed, and executive function.

The most commonly used diagnostic criteria for schizophrenia are derived from the *Diagnostic and Statistical Manual of Mental Disorders*, Fifth Edition (DSM-5). These criteria include the presence of two or more characteristic symptoms—delusions, hallucinations, disorganized speech, grossly abnormal psychomotor behavior (such as catatonia), or negative symptoms (i.e., restricted affect or avolition/asociality)—for a significant portion of time during a 1-month period (or less if successfully treated), with continuous signs of the disturbance persisting for at least 6 months. At least one of these two characteristic symptoms should include delusions, hallucinations, or disorganized speech. During this period, there is significant impairment in one or more major areas of functioning, including work, interpersonal relations, or self-care. It must also be established that the disorder is not better accounted for by a primary mood disorder, schizoaffective disorder, substance intoxication or withdrawal, or other general medical condition. From these criteria, it is important to note that delusions and hallucinations, although common, are not required for the diagnosis. Furthermore, although cognitive symptoms are also not required for the diagnosis, they are a tremendous cause of illness-related disability. A diagnosis of schizophrenia is most definitively made by interviewing the patient, obtaining collateral history from family and/or friends, and completing a medical workup (physical examination, routine blood and urine tests). According to DSM-5 (released May 2013), the diagnostic criteria no longer identify subtypes of schizophrenia, primarily because of a lack of utility for clinicians. Also of note, the Psychoses Workgroup for DSM-5 considered the addition of "attenuated psychosis syndrome" (i.e., prodromal or high-risk psychosis) as a diagnostic category. Ultimately, attenuated psychosis syndrome is listed in DSM-5 among conditions that require further research before consideration as a formal disorder. Nevertheless, the early identification of individuals with prodromal or high-risk psychosis, investigation of risk factors and biomarkers that might predict conversion to fulminant psychotic disorder, and early interventions for individuals with prodromal or high-risk psychosis are areas receiving significant attention and effort in the field.

Treatment

At present there is no cure for schizophrenia. Although there is significant clinical heterogeneity within the disorder, schizophrenia is usually a chronic condition that requires long-term treatment. Comprehensive treatment involves outpatient medication management and psychotherapy, psychosocial interventions, involvement of the family/support system, inpatient care for acute crisis intervention/illness exacerbation, and collaboration with primary care physicians. Currently, there is a vigorous research effort for diagnostic, prognostic and theranostic biomarkers in schizophrenia, toward a more "personalized medicine" approach for patients.

Antipsychotic medications play an important role in the pharmacologic management of schizophrenia. So-called first-generation antipsychotics (FGAs) have been in clinical use since the introduction of chlorpromazine (Thorazine) in the 1950s. These agents block the dopamine D2 receptor, and common side effects include extrapyramidal side effects (EPS) (e.g., Parkinsonism, dystonia). The newer or "second-generation antipsychotics" (SGAs), in addition to D2 receptor blockade, are also serotonin 5-HT2 receptor antagonists. While the risk of EPS is lower for SGAs than FGAs, SGAs are associated with a heightened risk of weight gain and the metabolic syndrome. Table 1 provides a more detailed description of antipsychotic medications. The Texas Medication Algorithm Project (TMAP) currently recommends a trial of a single (non-clozapine) SGA for newly diagnosed patients with schizophrenia, or patients never before treated with an SGA. However, neither the TMAP nor the American Psychiatric Association (APA) guidelines for the treatment of schizophrenia preferentially endorse a particular antipsychotic. Clozapine (Clozaril) is primarily used for "treatment-refractory" schizophrenia, usually defined as a lack of/partial response to an adequate trial of monotherapy with two or three different antipsychotics.

Adjunctive medications may also play an important role in the pharmacologic treatment of some patients with schizophrenia. These include antidepressants for depression and anxiety, mood stabilizers for depression or mood elevation, benzodiazepines for anxiety or agitation, beta-blockers for akathisia, and anticholinergics for EPS.

Medication nonadherence is a major treatment issue in patients with schizophrenia at all phases of the illness. Reasons for nonadherence are complex and multifaceted but may include medication side effects, impaired insight into illness, psychopathology in all three symptom domains, lack of efficacy, and comorbid substance use. Over 70% of patients in the Clinical Antipsychotic Trials of Intervention Effectiveness (CATIE) Schizophrenia Trial discontinued medication within the first 18 months of treatment. Medication nonadherence leads to dramatically increased risk of illness relapse, hospitalization, and suicidal behavior and should be routinely assessed in clinical visits. The use of rapid-dissolving oral or long-acting injectable medications may improve adherence in some patients.

Psychosocial interventions are also a cornerstone of the comprehensive treatment of patients with schizophrenia, and when utilized in combination with medication, are more effective than antipsychotics alone. Psychotherapy, including cognitive-behavioral therapy, supportive therapy, and group therapy, promotes improved illness management and medication adherence. Involvement of the patient's family/support system in care, including family-based therapies and psychoeducation, has been shown to increase medication adherence and decrease illness relapse rates. Psychosocial rehabilitation, which may include assertive community treatment, social skills training, vocational rehabilitation, and cognitive remediation, can help maximize patients' psychosocial functioning. There is growing evidence that cognitive remediation therapy in combination with other psychosocial interventions, particularly vocational rehabilitation, can improve real-world functioning for patients with schizophrenia in a relatively short time period.

Although there is no "typical" patient with schizophrenia, the clinical course is often characterized by acute relapses of the illness with the inter-episode absence or attenuation of symptoms. Multiple factors increase a patient's risk of illness relapse, including medication nonadherence, psychosocial stressors, substance use, medical illnesses such as infections, and the natural history of the disorder itself. Hospitalization may be required for acute exacerbations of psychotic symptoms, including hallucinations, delusions, and impaired self-care. Hospitalization may also be required if a patient represents an acute danger to self or others.

The concept of the recovery model and recovery-oriented care is a movement that is currently transforming the delivery of mental health services. Integral to the recovery model are certified peer specialists (CPS). A CPS is a licensed professional who has progressed in their own recovery from mental illness and works to assist patients with schizophrenia and other mental illness in regaining control over their own lives and over their own recovery process. CPSs provide peer support services, serve as consumer advocates, are resources for psychoeducation, and offer the unique perspectives based on their individual experiences.

TABLE 1 Antipsychotic Medications

AGENT	MECHANISM OF ACTION*	TYPICAL DOSING	SIDE EFFECTS†	SIDE EFFECTS†	NOTES
First Generation					
Haloperidol (Haldol)	D$_2$-antagonist	1.5–15 mg/day	EPS/TD Akathisia	NMS Hyperprolactinemia	PO, IM, IV, and long-acting injection formulations
Loxapine (Adasuve)	D$_2$-antagonist	10 mg/day	Dysgeusia Sedation	Throat irritation	INH formulation; for treatment of acute agitation
Second Generation					
Aripiprazole (Abilify)	Partial D$_2$-agonist and 5-HT2A antagonist	10–30 mg/day	Weight gain (+) Dyslipidemia (+) Glucose dysregulation (+)	Headache EPS/TD Akathisia	PO, rapid-dissolving PO, IM, transdermal patch, and long-acting injection formulations
Asenapine (Saphris)	D$_2$-antagonist/5-HT$_2$ antagonist	10–20 mg/day	Weight gain (+) Dyslipidemia (+) Glucose dysregulation (+)	Sedation EPS/TD Akathisia	Rapid-dissolving PO formulation
Clozapine (Clozaril)	D$_2$-antagonist/5-HT$_2$ antagonist	300–900 mg/day	Weight gain (+++) Dyslipidemia (+++) Glucose dysregulation (++) Agranulocytosis Sedation	Orthostatic hypotension Seizures Myocarditis EPS/TD	PO and rapid-dissolving PO formulations
Iloperidone (Fanapt)	D$_2$-antagonist/5-HT$_2$ antagonist	12–24 mg/day	Weight gain (++) Dyslipidemia (+) Glucose dysregulation (+)	Dizziness Tachycardia Sedation EPS/TD	PO formulation
Lurasidone (Latuda)	D$_2$-antagonist/5-HT$_2$ antagonist	40–80 mg/day	Weight gain (+) Dyslipidemia (+) Glucose dysregulation (+)	Sedation Akathisia Nausea EPS/TD	PO formulation
Olanzapine (Zyprexa)	D$_2$-antagonist/5-HT$_2$ antagonist	5–30 mg/day	Weight gain (+++) Dyslipidemia (+++) Glucose dysregulation (++)	Sedation Dizziness Hyperprolactinemia EPS/TD	PO, rapid-dissolving PO, IM, and long-acting injection formulations
Paliperidone (Invega)	D$_2$-antagonist/5-HT$_2$ antagonist	6–12 mg/day	Weight gain (+) Dyslipidemia (+) Glucose dysregulation (+)	Tachycardia Headache EPS/TD	PO and long-acting injection formulations Active metabolite of Risperidone (Risperdal)
Quetiapine (Seroquel)	D$_2$-antagonist/5-HT$_2$ antagonist	200–800 mg/day	Weight gain (++) Dyslipidemia (+) Glucose dysregulation (+)	Sedation Headache Orthostatic hypotension EPS/TD	PO and extended-release PO formulations
Risperidone (Risperdal)	D$_2$-antagonist/5-HT$_2$ antagonist	2–6 mg/day	Weight gain (++) Dyslipidemia (+) Glucose dysregulation (+)	Sedation Hyperprolactinemia EPS/TD	PO, PO liquid, rapid-dissolving PO, and long-acting injection formulations
Ziprasidone (Geodon)	D$_2$-antagonist/5-HT$_2$ antagonist	80–160 mg/day	Weight gain (+) Dyslipidemia (+) Glucose dysregulation (+)	Sedation QTc prolongation EPS/TD	PO and IM formulations
Aripiprazole lauroxil (Aristada)	Partial D$_2$ agonist and 5-HT2A antagonist	441 mg/month or 882 mg/4–6 weeks	Weight gain (+) Dyslipidemia (+) Glucose dysregulation (+)	Headache EPS/TD Akathisia	Long-acting injection formulation
Brexpiprazole (Rexulti)	Partial D2 and 5-HT1A agonist and 5-HT2 antagonist	1–4 mg/day	Weight gain (+) Dyslipidemia (+) Glucose dysregulation (+)	Increased triglycerides EPS/TD Akathisia	PO formulation
Cariprazine (Vraylar)	Partial D2 and D3 agonist	1.5–6 mg/day	Weight gain (+) Dyslipidemia (+) Glucose dysregulation (+)	Headache EPS/TD Akathisia	PO formulation

Abbreviations: D$_2$ = dopamine D$_2$ receptor; +++, severe risk; EPS = extrapyramidal side effects; 5-HT$_2$ = serotonin 5-HT$_2$ receptor; ++ = moderate risk; TD = tardive dyskinesia; + = mild or low risk; NMS = neuroleptic malignant syndrome.
*All first-generation and second-generation antipsychotics have an FDA black box warning for an "association with an increased risk of mortality in elderly patients treated for dementia-related psychosis." All second-generation agents are D$_2$ and 5-HT$_2$ antagonists; however, many act on multiple receptors, including alpha-adrenergic, beta-adrenergic, histaminergic, muscarinic cholinergic, and D$_1$, and 5-HT$_1$ receptors.
†EPS and TD are possible side effects with all antipsychotics, but they occur less frequently with second-generation than first-generation drugs.

TABLE 2	Monitoring Second-Generation Antipsychotic (Excluding Clozapine)								
	BASELINE	4 WEEKS	8 WEEKS	12 WEEKS	QUARTERLY	ANNUALLY	IF SYMPTOMS ARISE	EVERY 5 YEARS	OTHER
Personal/family history*	X					X			
Pregnancy test†	X						X		
Weight/BMI	X	X	X	X	X				
Waist circumference	X					X			
Blood pressure	X			X		X			
Fasting glucose/HgbA1C	X			X		X			
Fasting lipid panel	X			X				X	
EKG‡	X						X		
Prolactin	X						X		
CBC with differential§									X

More frequent assessments may be warranted based on clinical status.
*Including obesity, diabetes, hypertension, and dyslipidemia.
†In all women of childbearing age.
‡For patients taking Ziprasidone (Geodon), which may prolong the QTc interval, and Clozapine (Clozaril).
§For patients taking Clozapine (Clozaril). CBC with differential required at baseline, then weekly for 6 months, then every other week for 6 months, then monthly thereafter.
    Baseline absolute neutrophil count (ANC) must be ≥ 1500/mm³ (or ≥1000/mm³ in patients with benign ethnic neutropenia) due to risk of agranulocytosis.

Comorbidity

Schizophrenia is associated with an increased risk of premature mortality, and cardiovascular disease is a leading cause of death in this patient population. Multiple factors contribute to this risk, including a high prevalence of smoking, poor health habits, poor health care, medication side effects, and (perhaps) the pathophysiology of the disorder itself. SGAs as a class are associated with weight gain and an increased risk of metabolic syndrome. Over 40% of the 1460 patients in the CATIE Schizophrenia Trial met the criteria for metabolic syndrome at baseline. Recommendations for monitoring of patients on SGAs, based on a consensus statement from the American Diabetes Association and the APA, are described in Table 2. Primary care physicians play an important collaborative role with psychiatrists in the detection and management of metabolic disturbances in patients with schizophrenia, in order to minimize the cardiovascular risks associated with these comorbidities.

Patients with schizophrenia are also at an increased risk of suicide, which is also a leading cause of premature mortality. The prevalence of completed suicide in patients with schizophrenia is about 10%, and suicide attempts occur with even greater frequency. Clinicians should routine assess patients for suicidal ideation and, if present, explore risk factors for completed suicide, which include a suicidal plan and intent, previous suicide attempts, a family history of suicide, age, sex, access to lethal means, social isolation, and comorbid substance use. Medications, psychotherapy, and/or hospitalization may be required.

Comorbid substance use disorders predominate in patients with schizophrenia, with an estimated prevalence of 40% to 50%. Common substances of abuse include alcohol, marijuana, and cocaine. Patients with schizophrenia and comorbid substance use are at increased risk of medication nonadherence, illness relapse, hospitalization, suicidal and violent behavior, and an overall poor response to treatment. Furthermore, up to 70% to 90% of patients with schizophrenia are tobacco users, which contribute to the increased risk of medical comorbidity. Clinicians are encouraged to routinely screen for and address substance use in their treatment plans.

Conclusions

Schizophrenia is a complex, heterogeneous, and chronic psychiatric disorder. Comprehensive treatment usually involves long-term medication management and therapy, education for patients and their families, and psychosocial interventions. Primary care physicians play an important collaborative role in the detection and management of medical comorbidities, substance use disorders, and suicidality. Physicians, patients, and families are encouraged to become involved in the National Alliance on Mental Illness (NAMI; www.nami.org), which is a tremendous resource for help, support, education, and advocacy for patients with schizophrenia and other mental illness.

References

American Diabetes Association, American Psychiatric Association, American Association of Clinical Endocrinologists, et al: Consensus development conference on antipsychotic drugs and obesity and diabetes, J Clin Psychiatry 65:267, 2004.
American Psychiatric Association: Practice guideline for the treatment of patients with schizophrenia, 2nd ed., Am J Psychiatry 161(Suppl):1717, 2004.
Buchanan RW, Carpenter WT: Schizophrenia and other psychotic disorders. In Sadock BJ, Sadock VA, editors. Kaplan and Sadock's Comprehensive Textbook of Psychiatry, 8th ed, Philadelphia, 2005, Lippincott Williams and Wilkins, pp 1329–1345.
Buckley PF, Miller BJ, Lehrer DS, et al: Psychiatric comorbidities and schizophrenia, Schizophr Bull 35:383, 2009.
Fusar-Poli P, Tantardini M, De Simone S, et al: Deconstructing vulnerability for psychosis: meta-analysis of environmental risk factors for psychosis in subjects at ultra high-risk, Eur Psychiatry 40:65–75, 2017.
Laursen TM, Munk-Olsen T, Vestergaard M: Life expectancy and cardiovascular mortality in persons with schizophrenia, Curr Opin Psychiatry 25:83, 2012.
Leucht S, Corves C, Arbter D, et al: Second-generation versus first-generation antipsychotic drugs for schizophrenia: a meta-analysis, Lancet 373:31, 2009.
Lieberman JA, Stroup TS, McEvoy JP, et al: Effectiveness of antipsychotic drugs in patients with chronic schizophrenia, N Engl J Med 353:1209, 2005.
McEvoy JP, Meyer JP, Goff DC, et al: Prevalence of the metabolic syndrome in patients with schizophrenia: baseline results from the clinical antipsychotic trials of intervention effectiveness (CATIE), Schizophr Res 80:19, 2005.
Messias EL, Chen CY, Eaton WW: Epidemiology of schizophrenia: review of findings and myths, Psychiatr Clin North Am 30:323, 2007.
Nelson B, Amminger GP, Yuen HP, et al: Staged treatment in early psychosis: a sequential multiple assignment randomised trial of interventions for ultra high risk of psychosis patients, Early Interv Psychiatry, 2017, https://doi.org/10.1111/eip.12459.
Rodrigues-Amorim D, Rivera-Baltanás T, López M, et al: Schizophrenia: a review of potential biomarkers, J Psychiatr Res 93:37–49, 2017.
Shi J, Levinson DF, Duan J, et al: Common variants on chromosome 6p22.1 are associated with schizophrenia, Nature 460:753, 2009.
Torrey EF: Surviving Schizophrenia, 7th ed., New York, 2019, Harper Perennial.

Schizophrenia

11 Respiratory System

BRONCHITIS AND VIRAL RESPIRATORY INFECTIONS

Method of
Tomoko Sairenji, MD

CURRENT DIAGNOSIS

- Most cases of acute bronchitis are caused by viruses and diagnosed clinically.
- Predominant symptom is acute cough, with or without sputum.
- Other diseases such as asthma, pneumonia, chronic obstructive pulmonary disease exacerbation, and heart failure should be ruled out.

CURRENT THERAPY

- Antibiotics are not recommended for most cases of acute bronchitis.
- Dextromethorphan, guaifenesin, and honey may be considered to relieve cough symptoms.
- Patient education: Cough can last 3 weeks or more.

Epidemiology

Acute cough is the most common reason for ambulatory care visits. Acute bronchitis, which is characterized by an acute cough, is most commonly caused by viruses such as rhinovirus, enterovirus, influenza A and B, parainfluenza, coronavirus, coxsackie, and respiratory syncytial virus. Bacterial causes such as *Mycoplasma pneumoniae*, *Chlamydia pneumoniae*, and *Bordetella pertussis* are much less common.

Pathophysiology

Acute bronchitis is caused by an acute inflammatory process in the mucosa of the trachea and bronchi with resultant injury to epithelium of the mucosa.

Clinical Manifestations

Cough is the primary symptom of acute bronchitis, but it can cause other symptoms such as nasal congestion, wheezing, dyspnea, fever, and nonspecific constitutional symptoms.

Diagnosis

Acute bronchitis is diagnosed clinically, characterized by an acute cough with or without sputum production. It is often a diagnosis of exclusion, in which other diseases such as asthma, pneumonia, chronic obstructive pulmonary disease exacerbation, and heart failure are ruled out. Initially, manifestations of acute bronchitis can be identical to the common cold and difficult to distinguish. Fever is less common in bronchitis after the first few days, and patients may have a mildly ill appearance. On auscultation, there may be wheezing or rhonchi that improve with coughing. A patient with

a high temperature, otherwise abnormal vital signs, and a more toxic appearance should raise concern for pneumonia or influenza.

Laboratory testing is usually not necessary for the typical patient in the outpatient setting, but testing for influenza and pertussis can be done when there is greater suspicion for these diseases.

Imaging such as chest x-rays are not necessary in most cases for patients who have normal vital signs, no bloody sputum, and have a normal lung examination result, because there are typically no findings in acute bronchitis. However, it is recommended in those older than 75 years of age, because pneumonia does not always mount a fever or cause tachycardia.

Differential Diagnosis
Common Cold/Upper Respiratory Infections (URI)

The common cold can be difficult to differentiate from acute bronchitis. On average, adults have 2 to 4, and young children as many as 6 to 10 episodes annually. It is most commonly caused by rhinoviruses but can also be caused by other respiratory viruses such as coronavirus, influenza, and respiratory syncytial virus and parainfluenza viruses. The symptomatic trajectory of the common cold is sore throat, malaise, and low-grade fever for 1 to 2 days, followed by nasal congestion, rhinorrhea, and cough. Cough can occur in 30% to 40% of cases, and fluid can accumulate in middle ear or sinus cavities. Symptoms generally are the worst on day 3 to 4 and start to improve by day 7. Symptoms that would warrant consideration for more serious disease are respiratory distress, difficulty swallowing, altered mental status, signs suggesting dehydration, stiff neck, rash, or sore throat for more than 5 days. Influenza (high fever with general myalgias), acute bacterial sinusitis (symptoms for more than 10 days without improvement, severe symptoms including fever ≥39°C, and purulent nasal discharge lasting more than 3 consecutive days), streptococcal pharyngitis (absence of cough with tender lymphadenopathy and tonsillar exudates), asthma exacerbations triggered by URI, and infectious mononucleosis (fatigue, fever, sore throat, and adenopathy more severe than typical URI) are other conditions on the differential. Testing is not warranted for the diagnosis of a common cold unless one of these diseases is suspected and needs to be ruled out.

Similar to acute bronchitis, antibiotics are strongly discouraged for the common cold because they provide no benefit in terms of reducing symptom severity or duration. If symptoms are severe, treatment focuses mostly on symptomatic management, of which most can be done using over-the-counter therapies. Rest as well as adequate hydration and nutrition are encouraged but not studied in trials. Acetaminophen and nonsteroidal antiinflammatory drugs can help with fever and discomfort. The combination of antihistamines and decongestants may be more beneficial than either component alone for nasal symptoms. When needed, dextromethorphan may provide symptom relief with cough suppression. Intranasal or inhaled cromolyn sodium[1] may help with rhinorrhea, throat pain, or cough. Various formulations of intranasal cromolyn sodium (NasalCrom) are available over the counter, and oral inhaled cromolyn sodium (Intal) is available by a

---

[1]Not FDA approved for this indication.

prescription. Regular use of vitamin C supplements[1,7] (at least 200 mg/d) may decrease duration of cold symptoms but is not effective if started after cold symptoms start. Oral zinc sulfate[1,7] may decrease URI symptom duration and severity, but it is not routinely recommended because of adverse effects (bad taste and nausea).

Croup

Croup affects children with a peak incidence between 6 and 36 months of age, annually affecting 3% of those in this age range. Parainfluenza virus types 1 to 3 constitute 75% of all cases, but infection with many different viruses can produce this illness. Although some cases of croup can be caused by bacteria, it does not change how it is managed.

Croup is diagnosed clinically. Initially, patients experience cold-like symptoms: low-grade fevers and coryza. Inspiratory stridor, hoarseness, and a barking cough are typical findings that follow, peaking between 24 to 48 hours after onset. These symptoms are caused by mucosal inflammatory swelling of the larynx, trachea, and bronchi. Symptoms are often worse at night and can be exacerbated by emotional distress. Most (85%) cases are considered mild, but nasal flaring and retractions, increased respiratory rate, hypoxia, and tachycardia are indicators of more severe croup. Routine radiologic imaging is not encouraged, because the steeple sign that is often associated with croup is actually nonspecific and can be seen in other causes of glottic and subglottic narrowing such as epiglottitis and bacterial tracheitis.

Management of croup is dependent on the severity of the disease. Administration of corticosteroids (single dose of dexamethasone [Decadron][1] 0.6 mg/kg) are recommended for croup of any severity because it reduces return visits and hospitalization rates. Oxygen should be given to children with hypoxia or respiratory distress. Nebulized epinephrine[1] (0.05 mL/kg of racemic epinephrine 2.25% [max dose = 0.5 mL] or 0.5 mL per kg of L-epinephrine 1:1,000 via nebulizer [max dose = 5 mL]) is recommended for moderate or severe croup. It takes effect by vasoconstriction of the upper airway mucosa, leading to decreased edema. It has a quick onset of action, but efficacy wanes after 1 to 2 hours, so monitoring patients beyond 2 hours is recommended.

Humidified air has been commonly used for croup, but it has not been shown to be effective in decreasing croup symptoms or hospital admissions in moderate croup.

Pertussis

Pertussis should be suspected when patients have a persistent cough of more than 2 weeks with a characteristic paroxysmal cough, whooping cough, and post-tussive emesis or recent pertussis exposure. Most pertussis is caused by B pertussis. The number of outbreaks and pertussis incidence has increased in recent years. In the early catarrhal stage (1–2 weeks), it is difficult to discern from a common cold. The cough becomes more frequent, and severe bouts characterize the following paroxysmal stage (1–6 weeks, maximum of 10 weeks). Paroxysms of cough can be debilitating and cause post-tussive emesis, weight loss, and other conditions related to severe cough, but there are few symptoms otherwise. After this stage, the cough gradually improves over the course of a few weeks.

Atypical presentations are not uncommon, because those who have acquired immunity can present with a lesser degree of paroxysm. Thus pertussis should be suspected if cough symptoms last more than 3 weeks. Infants may also have atypical presentation of cough without paraoxysmal whooping.

Diagnosis should be confirmed with either culture, polymerase chain reaction (both better for early stages), or serology (accurate in later stage). Efficacy of antibiotics is questionable because treatment does not improve symptoms. However, antibiotics (Azithromycin [Zithromax][1] is first line—Children: 10 mg/kg/d for 3 days, or 10 mg/kg on day 1, then 5 mg/kg/d on

days 2-5; Adults: 500 mg/d for 3 days, or 500 mg on day 1, then 250 mg/d on days 2–5) are still recommended because they eradicate B pertussis from the nasopharynx and may decrease transmission. Immunization is critical to prevent further outbreaks of pertussis.

Bronchiolitis

Bronchiolitis is the most common cause for infant hospitalization of infants. Respiratory syncytial virus is the most common cause of bronchiolitis. Bronchioles become plugged with detached epithelium and inflammatory cells. Onset of upper respiratory symptoms is often soon followed by rapid development of wheezing and labored breathing. Infants with bronchiolitis typically do not have a marked response to asthma treatment with bronchodilators and corticosteroids, despite similar presenting symptoms. Treatment primarily consists of supplemental oxygen and intravenous fluids as needed to prevent dehydration. Palivizumab (Synagis) is used to prevent hospitalization rate for high-risk infants, such as those with premature birth, chronic lung disease, and hemodynamically significant congenital heart disease.

Therapy (or Treatment)

Decreasing Antibiotic Use

Antibiotic use in the treatment of bronchitis is strongly discouraged in all major guidelines, but they are often prescribed regardless of the recommendations. The strongest predictor of whether a patient will receive antibiotics is whether the clinician perceives the patient desires them. Patient education such as setting the expectation that cough from acute bronchitis can last 3 weeks, that antibiotics would not effectively aid in shortening the duration of symptoms, and explaining the undesired consequences of inappropriate antibiotic use such as antibiotic resistance and adverse effects is important. One in five patients treated with antibiotics will experience side effects such as headache, nausea, skin rash, diarrhea, and vaginitis. Patients are more likely to respond to this sort of education if they feel their concerns have been heard and addressed. In some cases, using a delayed prescription strategy wherein patients would need to call for a prescription or agree to pick up antibiotics after a certain number of days may be effective in decreasing antibiotic use. Providing methods for symptomatic management is also important for patients who desire treatment.

Recommended Cough Treatment

Dextromethorphan, guaifenesin, and honey may be considered to relieve cough symptoms. Dextromethorphan (30 mg orally every 6 to 8 hours) is a central-acting antitussive that reduces the cough reflex. In placebo-controlled studies, it was shown to decrease coughs by 19% to 36% (8 to 10 fewer coughs per 30 minutes) compared with placebo. Guaifenesin ([immediate-release] 200 to 400 mg orally every 4 hours) is an expectorant that increases respiratory tract secretions, hence decreasing mucus thickness. Study results vary, but it has been shown to decrease cough frequency and severity compared with placebo. Honey (2.5–10 mL [0.5–2 teaspoons]) has been compared with dextromethorphan, diphenhydramine, and no treatment in children. It was found to be better than no treatment in its effectiveness in decreasing cough severity and frequency and improving sleep quality. Honey would be an option for children older than 1 year, because antitussive use is not recommended in small children.

Cough Treatments that are not Recommended

There is no evidence that centrally acting antitussive codeine[1] has any effect to decrease cough symptoms, and benzonatate (Tessalon Perles), a peripherally acting antitussive has only been shown to be effective in conjunction with guaifenesin. Unfortunately, many over-the-counter therapies do not significantly impact acute bronchitis symptoms. Clinical trials have shown that ibuprofen

---

[7]Available as a dietary supplement.
[1]Not FDA approved for this indication.

---

[1]Not FDA approved for this indication.

(Motrin)[1] and antihistamines are not effective in reducing symptoms of cough. The FDA warns against using cough medications that have antihistamines and antitussives because of the high risk for potential harm in children younger than 4 years of age. Use of beta-agonists is also not recommended, unless the patient presents with wheezing at the time of presentation.

References

Altunaiji S, Kukuruzovic R, Curtis N, et al: Antibiotics for whooping cough (pertussis), *Cochrane Database Syst Rev* (3):CD004404, 2007.

Barnett ML, Linder JA: Antibiotic prescribing for adults with acute bronchitis in the United States, 1996-2010, *JAMA* 311:2020–2022, 2014.

Ebell MH, Lundgren J, Youngpairoj S: How long does a cough last? Comparing patients' expectations with data from a systematic review of the literature, *Ann Fam Med* 11:5–13, 2013.

Kinkade S, Long N: Acute bronchitis, *Am Fam Physician* 94:560–565, 2016.

Oduwole O, Meremikwu MM, Oyo-Ita A, et al: Honey for acute cough in children, *Cochrane Database Syst Rev* Rev (12):CD007094, 2014.

Petrocheilou A, Tanou K, Kalampouka E, et al: Viral croup: diagnosis and a treatment algorithm, *Pediatr Pulmonol* 49:421–429, 2014.

Russell KF, Liang Y, O'Gorman K, et al: Glucocorticoids for croup, *Cochrane Database Syst Rev* Rev (1):CD001955, 2011

Smith D, McDermott A, Sullivan J: Croup: diagnosis and management, *Am Fam Physician* 97:575–580, 2018.

Smith SM, Fahey T, Smucny J, et al: Antibiotics for acute bronchitis, *Cochrane Database Syst Rev* Rev (3):CD000245, 2014

Smith SM, Schroeder K, Fahey T: Over-the-counter (OTC) medications for acute cough in children and adults in community settings, *Cochrane Database Syst Rev* Rev (11):CD001831,2014.

ACUTE RESPIRATORY FAILURE

Method of
Anthony J. Faugno III, MD; and Scott K. Epstein, MD

CURRENT DIAGNOSIS

- History and physical examination can give insight into the etiology of hypoxic and hypercapneic respiratory failure but may be insufficient to make a definitive diagnosis and guide therapy.
- An arterial blood gas is mandatory to define severity and whether hypoxic or hypercapneic (or both) respiratory failure is present.
- Additional diagnostic modalities, including chest radiograph, electrocardiogram, cardiac laboratory tests (troponin, brain natriuretic peptide), echocardiography, and selected use of a pulmonary artery catheter, can help identify a specific etiology.

CURRENT THERAPY

- Treatment of acute respiratory failure often begins with non-specific approaches such as oxygen and mechanical ventilation (noninvasive or invasive).
- The goal of mechanical ventilation is to improve gas exchange and rest the respiratory muscles while waiting for the beneficial effects of specific therapy aimed at the underlying cause (e.g., bronchodilators, antibiotics, and corticosteroids in acute exacerbations of chronic obstructive pulmonary disease [COPD]).
- Noninvasive ventilation avoids many complications associated with invasive ventilation and improves outcomes for patients with acute cardiogenic pulmonary edema and acute exacerbations of COPD.
- High-flow nasal cannula is emerging as the preferred therapy for hypoxic respiratory failure in patients with non-cardiogenic pulmonary edema who do not require urgent intubation.

- Invasive mechanical ventilation can be lifesaving but can cause clinical deterioration if not properly administered.
- Using low tidal volumes (6 mL/kg ideal body weight) can help avoid dangerous dynamic hyperinflation in acute exacerbations of COPD and further lung injury in acute lung injury (e.g., volutrauma, barotrauma).
- Once signs of improvement are evident, focus rapidly shifts to liberating the patient from the ventilator using spontaneous breathing trials to assess the need for ventilatory support followed by airway assessment to determine readiness for extubation.

The respiratory system serves many complex physiologic functions, the most important of which is gas exchange. Using the interface between the alveolar space and capillaries, O_2 is taken up and CO_2 is eliminated. Acute respiratory failure, a life-threatening entity, is present when this system fails, over the course of minutes to hours, resulting in hypoxemia (type I) or hypercapnia (type II), or both. Most patients with acute respiratory failure present with dyspnea, although the correlation with disease severity is poor. Indeed, dyspnea might seem mild in those with baseline chronic respiratory failure, and it might be absent in those with an underlying neurologic process (e.g., drug overdose). Other symptoms and signs such as cough, chest pain, orthopnea, fever, tachypnea, rales, and wheezing are insensitive and nonspecific.

This chapter outlines the general pathophysiology and therapeutic approach to acute respiratory failure by using the examples of three common entities: acute respiratory distress syndrome (ARDS), cardiogenic pulmonary edema (congestive heart failure [CHF]), and acute exacerbation of chronic obstructive pulmonary disease (AECOPD).

Definitions and Pathophysiology

Acute Hypoxic Respiratory Failure

Hypoxic respiratory failure is conventionally defined as an arterial oxygen tension (PaO_2) of less than 60 mm Hg. Because this definition ignores the inspired fraction of oxygen (FiO_2), some favor a PaO_2/FiO_2 ratio of less than 300. To account for the arterial CO_2 tension ($PaCO_2$), others favor an alveolar–arterial (A–a) O_2 gradient greater than 250 mm Hg, using the equation

$$A\text{–a } O_2 \text{ gradient} = PAO_2 - PaO_2$$
$$= (713 \times FiO_2) - (PaO_2 + PaCO_2/0.8)$$

where 713 is the barometric pressure (760) minus the water vapor pressure. A normal A–a O_2 is less than 10 mm Hg, but this threshold value increases with age. The determination of PaO_2 requires an invasive test, an arterial blood gas. Oxygenation can be continuously monitored noninvasively by pulse oximetry, which provides an estimate of arterial oxygen saturation (SaO_2). In general, an SaO_2 of 0.90 corresponds to a PaO_2 of 60 mm Hg, but the relation depends on temperature, pH, $PaCO_2$, and 2,3-diphosphoglycerate (2,3-DPG). Accuracy is adversely affected by low perfusion states, dark skin pigmentation, nail polish, dyshemoglobins (e.g., carboxyhemoglobin, methemoglobin), intravascular dyes, motion, and ambient light.

Clinicians tend to focus on PaO_2 and SaO_2, but the real parameter of interest is O_2 delivery (DO_2) to organs and tissues. DO_2 depends on cardiac output and O_2 carrying capacity of arterialized blood (CaO_2):

$$DO_2 = CO \times CaO_2$$

where

$$CaO_2 = k(Hb \times SaO_2) + 0.003\ PaO_2$$

where k is a constant. DO_2 decreases when cardiac output or hemoglobin is reduced despite a normal PaO_2 and SaO_2. The peripheral response to reduced DO_2 is an increased O_2 extraction ratio (O_2ER), allowing oxygen uptake ($\dot{V}CO_2$), an indicator of metabolic demand, to remain constant. Cellular and organ dysfunction occurs when DO_2 and O_2ER are outstripped by

TABLE 1 Pathophysiologic Mechanisms of Acute Hypoxic Respiratory Failure

MECHANISM	A–a O_2 GRADIENT	$PaCO_2$	RESPONSE TO 100% O_2	CAUSE
Diffusion abnormality	↑	↑ Normal	↑↑	Severe interstitial lung disease ARDS, pneumonia
Hypoventilation	Normal	↑	↑↑↑	Narcotic overdose, obesity hypoventilation syndrome, respiratory muscle weakness
↓ FiO_2	Normal	Usually ↓	↑↑↑	High altitude, smoke inhalation
↓ MvO_2	↑	Usually ↓	↑	ARDS, shock, CHF, PE
Shunt	↑	Usually ↓	None or ↑	ARDS, pneumonia, CHF, atelectasis, PE
$\dot{V}/\dot{Q}$ mismatch	↑	↑, Normal, ↓	↑↑↑	AECOPD, asthma, PE, ARDS, pneumonia

↑, Increased; ↓, decreased; *A–a O_2*, alveolar–arterial O_2; *AECOPD*, acute exacerbation of chronic obstructive pulmonary disease; *ARDS*, acute respiratory distress syndrome; *CHF*, cardiogenic pulmonary edema; *FiO₂*, fraction of inspired oxygen; *MvO₂*, mixed venous oxygen saturation; *PaCO₂*, partial pressure of arterial CO_2; *PE*, pulmonary embolism; $\dot{V}/\dot{Q}$, ventilation–perfusion ratio.

metabolic demand. The balance between DO_2 and demand can be estimated by examining the mixed venous O_2 saturation (MvO_2) using the rearranged Fick equation:

$$MvO_2 = SaO_2 - \left(\dot{V}O_2/CO \times Hb\right)$$

When MvO_2 falls below 65% to 75%, imbalance is present. When cellular injury is present, extraction capabilities are limited and cellular hypoxia occurs despite "adequate" DO_2. Under these circumstances, the MvO_2 can be paradoxically normal. These parameters can be determined using a pulmonary artery catheter. The data obtained may be useful in individual patients, but randomized, controlled trials show no benefit when the pulmonary artery catheter is used routinely to guide therapy.

The pathophysiologic mechanisms of type I respiratory failure are listed in Table 1. The most common mechanism is ventilation–perfusion ($\dot{V}/\dot{Q}$) mismatch, characterized by a widened A–a O_2 gradient, a dramatic increase in PaO_2 in response to supplemental O_2, and a variable $PaCO_2$. When areas of low ($\dot{V}/\dot{Q}$) predominate (e.g., reduced ventilation with normal perfusion), the $PaCO_2$ may be low as the patient hyperventilates in an effort (only partially effective) to increase the PaO_2. When areas of high ($\dot{V}/\dot{Q}$) predominate, much ventilation is wasted, and hypercapnia is also present. Areas of lung that are perfused but not ventilated characterize shunt. The resulting fall in PaO_2 depends on the percentage of cardiac output circulating through the shunt and the O_2 content of that blood. Supplemental O_2 has minimal or small effect on PaO_2 because the shunted blood is not exposed to the increased FiO_2. Therefore, treatment is aimed at decreasing shunt by improving ventilation to the affected area or reducing perfusion to that area. When shunt results from a unilateral process (e.g., pneumonia, atelectasis), placing the good lung in the dependent position decreases shunt perfusion, and oxygenation improves.

Acute Hypercapneic Respiratory Failure
Hypercapneic respiratory failure is defined as a $PaCO_2$ greater than 45 mm Hg. The equation used to determine $PaCO_2$ provides insight into the three basic mechanisms underlying hypercapnia:

$$PaCO_2 = k\left(\dot{V}CO_2\right)/V_E\left(1 - V_D/V_T\right)$$

where k is a constant, V_E is total minute ventilation (respiratory rate times tidal volume), and V_D/V_T is the dead space. Therefore, hypercapnia can result from increased CO_2 production $\dot{V}CO_2$, increased physiologic dead space (V_D/V_T), and decreased minute ventilation (Box 1). Increased $\dot{V}CO_2$ alone is usually insufficient to cause hypercapnia because the respiratory system responds by increasing minute ventilation to keep $PaCO_2$ normal (37 to 43 mm Hg). Conversely, with abnormalities of respiratory muscle function or respiratory drive, or with increased dead space (and diminished reserve), the respiratory response to increased $\dot{V}CO_2$ may be insufficient, and hypercapnia results.

BOX 1 Pathophysiologic Mechanisms of Hypercapnia

Increased Carbon Dioxide Production $\left(\dot{V}CO_2\right)$
Fever
Overfeeding
Seizure
Sepsis
Thyrotoxicosis

Decreased Ventilation (V_E)
Depressed respiratory drive
Phrenic nerve injury
Respiratory muscle weakness

Increased Dead Space (V_D/V_T)
Acute exacerbation of chronic obstructive pulmonary disease
Interstitial lung disease (e.g., pneumonia, interstitial fibrosis, etc.)
Pulmonary vascular disease

Treatment
Treatment of acute hypoxemic and hypercapneic respiratory failure combines nonspecific (e.g., supplemental O_2, mechanical ventilation) and specific therapy (Boxes 2 and 3).

Oxygen Therapy
In the hospital, 100% O_2 is supplied from a wall source with a regulator determining flow rate in liters per minute. The final delivered oxygen concentration (FiO_2) depends on this flow rate and the amount of room air breathed by the patient. The O_2 flow rate is almost never sufficient to meet all of the patient's ventilatory demands, so varying amounts of room air are entrained to meet these needs. The final inspired oxygen concentration depends on the relative fraction of each gas, total minute ventilation, and the pattern of breathing (including the inspiratory-to-expiratory ratio). O_2 may be administered using nasal prongs, a facial mask, or high-flow devices designed to deliver higher FiO_2 (Table 2). High-flow nasal cannula (HFNC) devices are more capable of meeting the inspiratory flow demands during respiratory distress (in excess of 40 L/min) and more reliably deliver the set FiO_2 because they can overcome the entrainment phenomenon. Other reported benefits of HFNC include reduction in respiratory rate and work of breathing and increased end expiratory lung volume. A modest amount of positive end expiratory pressure, approximately 0 to 5 cm H_2O, is supplied by HFNC when breathing with a closed mouth.

Regardless of oxygenation strategy it is important to titrate oxygen support to physiologic endpoints, generally a $SaO_2 > 92\%$. Recent clinical data suggest evidence of potential harm

BOX 2	Causes of and Treatments for Acute Hypoxemic Respiratory Failure

Acute Exacerbation of Chronic Obstructive Pulmonary Disease
Antibiotics
Bronchodilators
Systemic steroids

Acute Respiratory Distress Syndrome
Efforts to decrease lung water
Lung-protective mechanical ventilation
Treatment of specific etiology or removal of injurious trigger

Congestive Heart Failure
Afterload reduction
Diuretics
Inotropes

Lobar Collapse or Atelectasis
Bronchoscopy
Pulmonary toilet (airway suctioning to improve clearance of secretions)

Pneumonia
Antibiotics
Chest physiotherapy

Pneumothorax
Tube thoracostomy to drain pleural air and facilitate lung re-expansion

Pulmonary Embolism
Anticoagulation
Thrombolytic therapy

Status Asthmaticus
Bronchodilators
Systemic steroids

BOX 3	Causes of and Treatments for Acute Hypercapneic Respiratory Failure

Acute Exacerbation of Chronic Obstructive Pulmonary Disease
Antibiotics
Bronchodilators
Systemic steroids

Acute Respiratory Muscle Weakness (e.g., myasthenic crisis)
Acetylcholinesterase therapy

Drug Overdose
Flumazenil (Romazicon)
Naloxone (Narcan)
Other antidotes

Guillain-Barré Syndrome
Immunoglobulin
Plasmapheresis

Spinal Cord Injury
Intravenous methylprednisolone

Status Asthmaticus
Bronchodilators
Systemic steroids

Toxin (e.g., botulinum toxin)
Antitoxin

for supraphysiologic blood oxygen tensions, and that an upper limit of supplemental oxygenation should be observed in all patients. The goal here is likely a PaO_2 between 70 and 120 mm Hg with an upper threshold of 98% SaO_2, though this requires further prospective evaluation. In hypercapneic patients (e.g., with AECOPD), high-flow O_2 can lead to worsening hypercapnia and acute respiratory acidosis. The mechanisms are multifactorial: worsening $\dot{V}/\dot{Q}$ matching (increased dead space), decreased intracellular binding of CO_2, and minute ventilation inadequate for the amount of CO_2 produced. Therefore, the goal in these patients is to achieve a PaO_2 of 55 to 60 mm Hg (SaO_2 88% to 90%) with low-flow oxygen (~24% to 28% O_2). If this (often delicate) balance between maintaining tissue oxygenation and avoiding significant respiratory acidosis cannot be achieved, short-term mechanical ventilation may be required.

Mechanical Ventilation

Mechanical ventilation can be delivered noninvasively through a tight-fitting face mask or invasively via an endotracheal tube. The goals of mechanical ventilation are to correct severe arterial blood gas abnormalities, provide respiratory support while specific therapy is used, and unload and rest the respiratory muscles. The ventilator should be set to optimize patient–ventilator interaction and avoid dynamic hyperinflation and intrinsic positive end-expiratory pressure (PEEPi). PEEPi can worsen gas exchange, predispose to barotrauma, and cause hypotension.

Noninvasive Ventilation

Noninvasive ventilation is most commonly applied as continuous positive airway pressure (CPAP), when airway pressure is kept constant throughout the respiratory cycle, or by bilevel positive airway pressure (BiPAP), when inspiratory pressure support actively assists each inspiration. Noninvasive ventilation

offers numerous advantages over invasive ventilation, including increased comfort; maintenance of normal swallowing, speech, and cough; less need for sedation; and avoiding the trauma of intubation.

The effective application of noninvasive ventilation starts with carefully explaining the procedure to the patient, followed by selection of a proper-fitting face mask. The mask is placed close to the face to acclimate the patient to high inspiratory flow. The mask is then secured using straps (but not too tightly), and ventilator settings are adjusted to minimize leaks and ensure comfort. The patient is reassessed frequently. Failure to improve within 2 to 4 hours (e.g., reduction in dyspnea, respiratory rate, accessory muscle use, and hypercapnia) signals noninvasive ventilation failure and need for intubation.

Noninvasive ventilation improves outcome (avoids intubation, decreases length of stay, improves survival) in a number of conditions (Table 3). Although randomized, controlled trials show dramatic benefit in AECOPD, other studies show no or uncertain benefit in community-acquired pneumonia, ARDS, pulmonary fibrosis, and routinely after planned extubation. One mechanism for improved outcome is the reduction in infection (pneumonia, sepsis) seen with noninvasive ventilation compared with intubated patients. Noninvasive ventilation should not be used in the presence of respiratory arrest, shock, excessive secretions, inability to protect the airway, an agitated or uncooperative patient, and facial abnormalities that preclude proper application of the mask. Comparison of noninvasive ventilation to high-flow nasal cannula in ARDS suggests evidence of harm in patients with more severe hypoxemia. This phenomenon is hypothesized to be related to ventilator-induced lung injury where tidal volumes are less strictly regulated in noninvasive as compared to invasive ventilation.

Invasive Ventilation

Invasive mechanical ventilation is delivered via an endotracheal tube. The set parameters include FiO_2 and positive end-expiratory pressure (PEEP). For volume-assist control, the clinician chooses respiratory rate and tidal volume. For pressure support, the clinician chooses the inspiratory pressure level above PEEP, and the patient determines respiratory rate. The resulting tidal volume depends on inspiratory pressure level and patient factors including respiratory muscle strength and

TABLE 2 Short-Term Oxygen Delivery Systems

DELIVERY SYSTEM	O₂ FLOW RATE (L/MIN)	FiO₂ RANGE	COMMENTS
Basic Systems			
Nasal cannula (prongs)	1–6	0.22–0.40	Comfortable
			Facilitates communication and oral intake
			Humidification required at high flow rates
Simple masks	5–6	0.30–0.50	Mask acts as reservoir to increase FiO_2
			High flow combats CO_2 rebreathing
			Less comfortable
			Must be removed to facilitate communication and oral intake
			Easily displaced with movement
Reservoir Masks			
Nonrebreathing	4–10	0.60–1.00	One-way valve between the mask and the reservoir bag
			Inspired O_2 from wall source and reservoir bag
Partial rebreathing	5–10	0.35–0.90	Lacks one-way valve
Venturi masks	4–10	0.24–0.40	Uses Bernoulli principle (fixed amount of entrained room air added to O_2)
			Maximum delivered FiO_2 can be controlled
			Often used in COPD to avoid excessive FiO_2 and risk for hypercapnia
High-flow nasal cannula	10–60	0.21–1	Can overcome room air entrainment, set FiO_2 more accurate
			Generates modest amount of positive end expiratory pressure
			Reduces CO_2 rebreathing by anatomic dead space washout
			Reduction in work of breathing in select patients

COPD, Chronic obstructive pulmonary disease; *FiO₂*, fraction of inspired oxygen.

respiratory system mechanics. Initially the ventilator is set to meet most of the patient's minute ventilation, allowing respiratory muscle rest. Such full support should not be prolonged because diaphragmatic dysfunction can result. Most patients require sedation, but excessive sedation levels are associated with worse outcomes. Therefore, strategies to minimize continuous intravenous sedation using a sedation protocol or once-daily interruption of sedation are recommended.

Invasive mechanical ventilation, especially when prolonged, is associated with numerous complications including ventilator-associated pneumonia, sinusitis, airway injury, thromboembolism, and gastrointestinal bleeding. Therefore, once significant clinical improvement occurs, efforts should focus on rapidly removing the patient from the ventilator. This is achieved by daily screening for readiness (Box 4) followed by a 30- to 120-minute spontaneous breathing trial on minimal or no ventilator support. Patients tolerating the spontaneous breathing trial are extubated if they have a good cough, manageable respiratory secretions, and an adequate mental status to protect the airway. Approximately 25% of patients do not tolerate the spontaneous breathing trial; they should be returned to full ventilator support for 24 hours and undergo careful evaluation for reversible causes. The clinician should consider a more gradual approach to weaning these patients.

Specific Causes of Acute Respiratory Failure
Acute Exacerbation of Chronic Obstructive Pulmonary Disease

Patients with COPD can experience two or three exacerbations per year, especially if they are actively smoking. The best predictor of future exacerbations is a history of previous exacerbations. Other risk factors for exacerbation include serum eosinophilia, pulmonary hypertension and gastric reflux. Hospital mortality ranges from 2% to 11%, rising to 25% for those requiring critical care.

AECOPD is defined by increased sputum volume, purulence, and dyspnea. Physical examination is notable for tachypnea, use of accessory respiratory muscles, diminished breath sounds, prolonged expiratory phase with wheezing, thoraco-abdominal paradox (inward inspiratory abdominal motion), and Hoover sign (inward inspiratory motion of the lower rib cage). The latter two physical signs indicate the presence of dynamic hyperinflation and diaphragmatic dysfunction. AECOPD is further characterized by hypoxemia (resulting from $\dot{V}/\dot{Q}$ mismatch) and hypercapnia. Patients with more severe underlying disease might demonstrate evidence of acute and chronic respiratory acidosis.

Etiology and Diagnosis
Approximately 50% of AECOPDs result from bacterial infection (e.g., *Pneumococcus* species, *Haemophilus influenzae*, *Moraxella catarrhalis*, and *Pseudomonas* species). The remainder result from viral infection and air pollution. In many cases a cause cannot be identified, although there is increasing appreciation that acute myocardial infarction and pulmonary embolism may be present in up to 25%. Pulmonary embolism may be suggested by a $PaCO_2$ lower than baseline and the need for a higher than expected FiO_2 to maintain the SaO_2 at greater than 90%. Computed tomographic pulmonary arteriogram is recommended to make the diagnosis, because $\dot{V}/\dot{Q}$ scanning is nondiagnostic in nearly half of COPD patients, and false-positive high-probability scans occur.

Treatment
Treatment for AECOPD is based on high-quality evidence consisting of numerous randomized, controlled trials and well-performed meta-analyses. Bronchodilator therapy is essential. Nebulized combination therapy (albuterol and ipratropium [DuoNeb]) is effective, but it is not demonstrably superior to single-agent therapy delivered via a metered-dose inhaler. Theophylline should generally be avoided because toxicity outweighs

TABLE 3 Efficacy of Noninvasive Ventilation in Various Conditions

CONDITION	QUALITY OF EVIDENCE	COMMENT
AECOPD	Strong	↓ Need for intubation
		↓ Nosocomial pneumonia
		↑ Survival
Acute cardiogenic pulmonary edema	Strong	↓ Need for intubation
		↑ Survival
Facilitating weaning in select patients	Strong	↓ Duration of intubation
		Most effective in AECOPD
High risk for extubation failure	Strong	↓ Need for reintubation
Extubation failure in heterogeneous patient population	Moderate	Not effective, two RCTs
Routinely after extubation	Moderate	Not effective, single RCT
Extubation failure in AECOPD	Moderate	Single case-control study
Type I RF, diffuse infiltrates, not ICH	Moderate	↓ Need for intubation
		May ↓ survival, requires close monitoring
Hypoxemic respiratory in ICH with diffuse pulmonary infiltrates	Moderate	↓ Need for intubation
		↑ Survival
Postoperative respiratory failure	Moderate	↓ Need for intubation
		↓ Nosocomial pneumonia
		↑ Survival
Asthma	Weak	Uncertain effect on mortality
		Uncertain effect on intubation
		Benefit may be in ACOS
Obesity hypoventilation	No RCTs	Probably effective in ↓ need for intubation
Do not intubate patients	Observational studies	Most effective with CHF, COPD
Pulmonary fibrosis	Observational studies	Not effective

ACOS, Asthma COPD Overlap Syndrome; *AECOPD,* acute exacerbation of chronic obstructive pulmonary disease; *CHF,* cardiogenic pulmonary edema; *COPD,* chronic obstructive pulmonary disease; *FiO2,* fraction of inspired oxygen; *ICH,* immunocompromised host; *RCT,* randomized, controlled trial; *RF,* respiratory failure.

BOX 4 Screening Criteria to Assess Readiness to Undergo a Trial of Spontaneous Breathing

Required Criteria
$PaO_2/FiO_2 \geq 150$ *or* $SaO_2 \geq 90\%$ *or* $FiO_2 \leq 40\%$ *and* PEEP ≤5 cm H_2O
Absence of hypotension

Additional Criteria (optional criteria)
Weaning parameters*
- Negative inspiratory force <−20 to −25 cm H_2O
- Respiratory rate (f) ≤35 breaths/min
- Spontaneous tidal volume (V_T) >5 mL/kg
- f/V_T <105 breaths/L per min.

Absence of significant anemia (e.g., Hb ≥8–10 mg/dL)
Absence of fever (e.g., core temperature ≤38.5°C)
Adequate mental status: patient awake and alert or easily aroused.

---

*Recent studies indicate that these parameters are often unnecessary in deciding whether to initiate trials of spontaneous breathing.
Hb, Hemoglobin; *PEEP,* positive end-expiratory pressure.

---

benefits. Antibiotics improve outcome, especially in the presence of fever and increased sputum purulence and volume. Older agents, such as amoxicillin and tetracycline, appear to be less effective than newer macrolides and fluoroquinolones though local resistance patterns should drive antibiotic selection.

Corticosteroids enhance β-agonist activity and counteract the inflammatory state seen in AECOPD. Oral prednisone at a dose of 30 to 40 mg is recommended with a duration of 5 days being noninferior to longer courses. Intravenous therapy (methylprednisolone [Solu-Medrol] 125 mg every 6 hours for 72 hours followed by oral prednisone) should be used in the critically ill patient or when response to oral therapy is suboptimal. There is no role for mucolytic agents or chest physiotherapy during acute exacerbation. Continuation of beta blockers, previously thought to contribute to bronchoconstriction, may in fact be associated with decreased mortality and exacerbations because of impact on COPD comorbidities such as coronary artery disease.

Admission to the intensive care unit (ICU) is indicated for patients with hemodynamic instability, confusion, lethargy and coma, severe dyspnea unresponsive to emergency management, or severely abnormal gas exchange despite initial therapy (PaO_2 <40 mm Hg, $PaCO_2$ >60 mm Hg, pH <7.25). Randomized, controlled trials demonstrate that noninvasive ventilation decreases the risk for intubation and improves survival in AECOPD when there is severe dyspnea, hypoxemia, tachypnea, and significant respiratory acidosis ($PaCO_2$ >45 mm Hg and pH <7.35). Patients who fail noninvasive ventilation or who are not candidates require intubation and mechanical ventilation.

A major risk is the development of dynamic hyperinflation (PEEPi), which occurs when expiratory time is not sufficient to reach functional residual capacity. The resulting air trapping within the thorax can worsen gas exchange, predispose to barotrauma (e.g., pneumothorax), and cause hypotension. PEEPi is minimized by keeping delivered minute ventilation at 5 L/min or less; achieved by lowering tidal volume (e.g., 6 mL/kg ideal body weight) or respiratory rate (8 to 10 breaths/min), or by increasing inspiratory flow rate, allowing more time for expiration. PEEPi is suggested by an elevated plateau pressure or persistent expiratory flow at the time of the next ventilator breath. PEEPi can also increase work of breathing by increasing the patient's inspiratory effort to trigger the ventilator. When extrinsic PEEP is at or just below the PEEPi level, the patient triggers more easily and work of breathing is reduced. The approach to weaning and extubation in AECOPD is similar to that for other conditions, although the risk of failing a spontaneous breathing trial is increased.

Acute Respiratory Distress Syndrome
Etiology and Diagnosis
ARDS is the result of an acute process and is characterized by hypoxemia (PaO_2/FiO_2 <300) with bilateral diffuse alveolar infiltrates, and no evidence of cardiac etiology. Lung injury in this syndrome can result from both pulmonary and extrapulmonary etiologies. Pulmonary causes include pneumonia, gastric aspiration, near drowning, toxic gas inhalation, medication side effects, and lung contusion. Extrapulmonary causes include sepsis, pancreatitis, fat embolism, drug overdose, nonthoracic trauma, and massive transfusion. Conditions that can mimic the clinical findings of ARDS include CHF, diffuse alveolar hemorrhage (DAH), acute cryptogenic organizing pneumonia (COP), and acute eosinophilic pneumonia (AEP). These latter three entities can be diagnosed by bronchoscopy (DAH, AEP) or by open lung biopsy (COP), all of which are treated with high doses of corticosteroids.

Differentiating cardiogenic pulmonary edema from ARDS can be challenging, especially because these conditions can coexist. Physical findings of jugular venous distention and a positive third heart sound, abnormal electrocardiogram (ECG), elevated brain natriuretic peptide (BNP), and positive cardiac enzymes (troponin) point to a cardiac etiology. A chest radiograph showing cardiomegaly, vascular redistribution, widened vascular pedicle, perihilar alveolar infiltrates, and pleural effusions also suggests a cardiac cause. Bedside echocardiography can demonstrate reduced left ventricular function. A pulmonary artery catheter provides definitive evidence of an elevated pulmonary capillary wedge pressure and reduced cardiac output. That said, recent randomized, controlled trials demonstrate no improvement in survival with routine use of the pulmonary artery catheter in ARDS.

Treatment
The first principle of ARDS management is to prevent further lung injury by employing a lung protective ventilation strategy limiting the transpulmonary pressure, using the plateau pressure as a surrogate. In general this is accomplished by titrating the set tidal volume to 6 to 8 mL/kg of ideal body weight. Once this is achieved the tidal volume is titrated down to achieve a plateau pressure of 30 cm H_2O or less, with lower pressures being more protective. This plateau pressure is measured on the ventilator with an inspiratory hold, and approximates the alveolar pressure. Failing to accomplish this places the lungs at risk for further injury by creating significant shear stress with repeated opening of atelectatic areas (atelectrauma) and overdistending less affected areas (volutrauma, barotrauma). Using small tidal volumes often results in significant hypercapnia, which can have an independent protective effect (permissive hypercapnia). The application of PEEP recruits and opens atelectatic lung, thereby reducing harmful shear forces. The optimal level of PEEP remains uncertain; individual studies have tended to show no mortality

benefit of a high PEEP versus a low PEEP ventilatory strategy, however trends in mortality reduction and decreased salvage therapy are seen with a higher PEEP strategy in meta-analysis.

The severity of ARDS is generally subdivided by PaO_2/FiO_2 ratios indicating mild (300 to 200), moderate (200 to 100), and severe (<100) disease; these thresholds correspond to rising risk of mortality. A PaO_2/FiO_2 ratio of less than 150 suggests a higher mortality ARDS phenotype where therapy in addition to lung protective ventilation may provide benefit. Placing the patient in the prone position may reduce mortality. The routine use of neuromuscular blockade is controversial with the most recent trial indicating no mortality benefit. Inhaled pulmonary vasodilators, to optimize V/Q matching, do improve oxygenation but have no impact on mortality. The benefit of extracorporeal membrane oxygenation is yet unclear and is reserved for very severe, high-mortality disease to be used in expert centers. Numerous studies indicate that corticosteroids do not improve the outcome of acute lung injury (ALI)/ARDS in a heterogenous population, nor do antioxidants.

Cardiogenic Pulmonary Edema
Cardiogenic pulmonary edema occurs in patients with cardiomyopathy or acutely when ischemia is present. Diagnosis is suggested by jugular venous distension, a third heart sound, diffuse rales, abnormal ECG, and a chest radiograph showing cardiomegaly, diffuse alveolar infiltrates, and bilateral pleural effusion. A markedly elevated BNP or pro-BNP further suggests a cardiac etiology.

Therapy consists of oxygen, nitrates, diuretics, afterload reduction, and anti-ischemic therapy if the history or ECG is suggestive. Mechanical ventilation produces positive intrathoracic pressure, which improves cardiac function by decreasing both left ventricular preload and afterload, reversing hypoxemia, and decreasing work of breathing. In hemodynamically stable patients without active ischemia, CPAP at levels of 8 to 12 cm H_2O should be used. A meta-analysis of 15 randomized, controlled trials showed that noninvasive ventilation decreased the need for intubation and improved survival. CPAP and BiPAP appear to be equivalent, although many prefer BiPAP when hypercapnia is present.

Because cardiogenic pulmonary edema is rapidly reversible, intubated patients can often be extubated within 24 hours. That said, the transition from positive pressure ventilation to negative ventilation (e.g., T-piece or extubation) can precipitate pulmonary edema. These patients may benefit from lower peri-extubation respiratory support to anticipate postextubation pulmonary edema.

References

Acute Respiratory Distress Syndrome: The Berlin Definition, *JAMA* 307(23), 2012.

Acute Respiratory Distress Syndrome Network: Ventilation with lower tidal volumes as compared with traditional tidal volumes for acute lung injury and the acute respiratory distress syndrome, *N Engl J Med* 342:1301–1308, 2000.

Briel M, Meade M, Mercat A, et al: Higher vs lower positive end-expiratory pressure in patients with acute lung injury and acute respiratory distress syndrome: Systematic review and meta-analysis, *JAMA* 303(9):865, 2010.

Ely EW, Baker AM, Dunagan DP, et al: Effect on the duration of mechanical ventilation of identifying patients capable of breathing spontaneously, *N Engl J Med* 335:1864–1869, 1996.

Epstein SK: Complications in ventilator supported patients. In Tobin M, editor: *Principles and Practice of Mechanical Ventilation*, New York, 2006, McGraw Hill, pp 877–902.

Frat J-P, Thille AW, Mercat A, et al: High-flow oxygen through nasal cannula in acute hypoxemic respiratory failure, *N Engl J Med* 372(23):2185–2196, 2015.

Girardis M, Busani S, Damiani E, et al: Effect of conservative vs conventional oxygen therapy on mortality among patients in an intensive care unit: the oxygen-icu randomized clinical trial, *JAMA* 316(15):1583, 2016.

Kress JP, Pohlman AS, O'Connor MF, et al: Daily interruption of sedative infusions in critically ill patients undergoing mechanical ventilation, *N Engl J Med* 342:1471–1477, 2000.

Masip J, Peacock WF, Price S, et al: Indications and practical approach to non-invasive ventilation in acute heart failure, *European Heart Journal* 39(1):17–25, 2018.

Ouellette DR, Patel S, Girard TD, et al: Liberation from mechanical ventilation in critically ill adults: An official American College of Chest Physicians/American Thoracic Society Clinical Practice Guideline, *Chest* 151(1):166–180, 2017.

Rochwerg B, Brochard L, Elliott MW, et al: Official ERS/ATS clinical practice guidelines: noninvasive ventilation for acute respiratory failure, *Eur Respir J* 50(2):1602426, 2017.

Vogelmeier CF, Criner GJ, Martinez FJ, et al: Global strategy for the diagnosis, management, and prevention of chronic obstructive lung disease 2017 report. GOLD Executive Summary, *Am J Respir Crit Care Med* 195(5):557–582, 2017.

ASTHMA IN ADOLESCENTS AND ADULTS

Method of
Matthew A. Rank, MD; and Michael Schatz, MD, MS

CURRENT DIAGNOSIS

- Confirm the diagnosis by demonstrating an increase in forced expiratory volume in 1 second (FEV$_1$) by 12% or more after asthma therapy.
- Assess past severity by a history of exacerbations requiring oral corticosteroids, emergency department visits, hospitalization, or intubation.
- Identify environmental exposures, allergic sensitization, and comorbidities that may be aggravating asthma.
- Assess current *severity* in patients not taking long-term control medications and assess *control* in patients who are taking long-term control medications based on symptom frequency, nocturnal awakenings, rescue therapy use, activity limitation, spirometry, and recent exacerbation history.

CURRENT THERAPY

- Nonpharmacologic therapy includes asthma education (especially regarding inhaler technique, self-monitoring, self-management, and importance of adherence to medication), reduction in environmental triggers, addressing any relevant psychosocial issues, and allergen immunotherapy for select patients.
- Preferred step therapy for long-term asthma management is (in order): low-dose inhaled corticosteroids; medium-dose inhaled corticosteroids or low-dose inhaled corticosteroids plus long-acting β-agonists; medium-dose inhaled corticosteroids plus long-acting β-agonists; high-dose inhaled corticosteroids plus long-acting β-agonists; high-dose inhaled corticosteroids plus long-acting β-agonists plus long-acting muscarinic antagonists; asthma biologics; and oral prednisone.
- Asthma exacerbations should be treated with high-dose inhaled β-agonists and early use of systemic corticosteroids.

Asthma is an extremely common chronic medical condition that causes substantial morbidity among its sufferers. In addition to discomfort, asthma can cause sleep disruption, missed school and work, limitations of recreational activities, and acute episodes requiring emergency hospital care. Although the past 40 years have seen the introduction of increasingly effective and convenient medications, recent surveys continue to suggest that asthma remains suboptimally controlled in a substantial proportion of patients. The purpose of this article is to describe an approach to assessment and therapy that leads to optimal asthma control. It is based on the National Asthma Education and Prevention Program (NAEPP) Expert Panel Report 3: Guidelines for the Management of Asthma (https://www.nhlbi.nih.gov/health-topics/guidelines-for-diagnosis-management-of-asthma) but includes recommendations that stem from studies published since this guideline was released.

Diagnosis

The first step in evaluating a patient with asthma is to confirm the diagnosis. This is particularly important in patients with atypical symptoms or a poor response to asthma therapy. Asthma is confirmed by the demonstration of reversible airways obstruction, which most commonly is an increase in forced expiratory volume in 1 second (FEV$_1$) by 12% or more and at least 200 mL after an inhaled bronchodilator. For some patients, 2 to 4 weeks of chronic inhaled asthma therapy or 2 weeks of oral corticosteroid therapy is necessary to demonstrate reversibility. The latter is particularly important in adults with a history of smoking in whom chronic obstructive pulmonary disease (COPD) is a diagnostic consideration. In patients with normal pulmonary function, asthma can also be confirmed by means of methacholine (Provocholine) or exercise challenge. In addition, an elevated fractional exhaled nitric oxide (FENO >50 ppb) can be suggestive of a diagnosis of asthma.

Particularly important masqueraders of asthma include vocal cord dysfunction, panic attacks, hyperventilation, and cough due to postnasal drip, reflux, or angiotensin-converting enzyme (ACE) inhibitor therapy. All of these can also coexist with asthma, so their presence does not exclude asthma. Even when these conditions coexist with asthma, their diagnosis and appropriate therapy usually reduce the patient's respiratory symptoms.

Assessment

Assessment of asthmatic patients involves assessment of past severity, identification of aggravating factors, and definition of current status regarding treatment and clinical severity or control.

Past Severity

Asthma can be a mild, infrequent illness or a daily severe one. Certain severity markers identify patients who are more likely to experience severe exacerbations or to have symptoms that are more difficult to control and who thus require more careful surveillance. These include histories of asthma hospitalization, especially requiring intensive care or intubation, past requirement for oral corticosteroids, and exacerbation by aspirin or other NSAIDs. In patients with prior severe exacerbations, the rapidity of the onset of the exacerbation should be ascertained.

Aggravating Factors

Factors that appear to trigger asthma symptoms should be assessed because they may be targets for avoidance therapy. Certain aspects of the patient's environment that can contribute to asthma triggering should be specifically ascertained, including occupational exposures, age of the home, pets, carpeting, visible mold, passive smoke, and cockroach exposure. Patients with persistent asthma should have in vitro or skin tests to identify allergic sensitization to pollens, house dust mites, mold spores, animal dander, and cockroaches that can contribute to the maintenance of asthma inflammation or can trigger episodes. The presence of comorbidities that can aggravate asthma, including cigarette smoking, obesity, rhinitis, sinusitis, reflux, and COPD, should be identified and treated. Finally, psychosocial factors to assess include a history or symptoms of anxiety or depression, attitudes toward asthma and asthma therapy, adherence to therapy, and social support. These may be targets for therapy or may be necessary to understand to create an effective therapeutic plan and therapeutic alliance.

Current Status

Assessment of the current therapy the patient is actually taking is necessary for understanding the asthma's severity and to appropriately initiate or change therapy. It is particularly important to determine if the patient is taking long-term control medications, such as inhaled corticosteroids, long-acting β-agonists, leukotriene modifiers, or long-acting muscarinic antagonists. If the patient is not taking controllers, severity should be assessed, as described in Table 1, based on symptom frequency, nocturnal awakenings, rescue therapy use, activity limitation, spirometry, and exacerbation history. If the patient is already taking controllers, control should be assessed (Table 2). Normal FEV$_1$/FVC (forced vital capacity) by age is shown in Table 3.

Long-Term Management

The goals of long-term management are to achieve and maintain well-controlled asthma. Both nonpharmacologic and pharmacologic therapy must be considered.

TABLE 1	Classifying Asthma Severity and Initiating Treatment in Patients 12 Years and Older Not Currently Taking Long-Term Control Medications			
COMPONENTS OF SEVERITY	**CLASSIFICATION OF SEVERITY***			
	INTERMITTENT	**PERSISTENT**		
		MILD	**MODERATE**	**SEVERE**
Impairment				
Symptoms	≤2 days/week	>2 days/week but not daily	Daily	Throughout the day
Nighttime awakenings	≤2 times/month	3–4 times/month	>1 time/week but not nightly	Often 7 times/week
Short-acting β₂-agonist use for symptom control (not prevention of EIB)	≤2 days/week	>2 days/week but not daily, and not more than 1 time on any day	Daily	Several times per day
Interference with normal activity	None	Minor limitation	Some limitation	Extremely limited
Lung function†	Normal FEV₁ between exacerbations; FEV₁ >80% predicted	FEV₁ >80% predicted	FEV₁ >60% but <80% predicted	FEV₁ <60% predicted
	FEV₁/FVC normal	FEV₁/FVC normal	FEV₁/FVC reduced 5%	FEV₁/FVC reduced >5%
Risk				
Exacerbations requiring oral systemic corticosteroids	0–1/year‡	≥2/year‡ ──→ ←────────── Consider severity and interval since last exacerbation. ──────────→ Frequency and severity may fluctuate over time for patients in any severity category. Relative annual risk of exacerbation may be related to FEV₁.		
Recommended Steps for Initiating Treatment§				
Initiation Follow-up	Step 1 In 2–6 weeks, evaluate level of asthma control and adjust therapy accordingly.	Step 2	Step 3¶	Step 4 or 5¶

*Level of severity is determined by assessment of both impairment and risk. Assess impairment domain by patient's/caregiver's recall of previous 2–4 weeks and spirometry. Assign severity to the most severe category in which any feature occurs.

†See Table 3 for normal FEV₁/FVC.

‡At present, there are inadequate data to correlate frequencies of exacerbations with different levels of asthma severity. In general, more frequent and intense exacerbations (e.g., requiring urgent, unscheduled care, hospitalization, or ICU admission) indicate greater underlying disease severity. For treatment purposes, patients who had ≥2 exacerbations requiring oral systemic corticosteroids in the past year may be considered the same as patients who have persistent asthma, even in the absence of impairment levels consistent with persistent asthma.

§See Table 6 for treatment steps. The stepwise approach is meant to assist, not replace, the clinical decision making required to meet individual patient needs.

¶And consider short course of oral systemic corticosteroids.

EIB, Exercise-induced bronchospasm; FEV₁, forced expiratory volume in one second; FVC, forced vital capacity; ICU, intensive care unit.

Data from the National Asthma Education and Prevention Program (NAEPP) Expert Panel Report 3: Guidelines for the Management of Asthma.

Nonpharmacologic Therapy

The first tenet of nonpharmacologic therapy in the long-term management of asthma is education. Patients need to understand the inflammatory pathophysiology of asthma and the relationships among airway inflammation, bronchospasm, and symptoms. Patients should be informed that the cause of asthma is unknown and there is no cure, but that triggers can be identified and asthma can be controlled. They should receive education regarding self-assessment, either based on symptoms or peak flow monitoring, and regarding the recognition of early signs of an impending exacerbation.

The next step is to discuss and agree on the goals of therapy. The NAEPP has defined the following goals:

- Prevent chronic and troublesome daytime and nighttime symptoms.
- Maintain optimal pulmonary function for that patient.
- Maintain normal activity, including work, school, leisure activity, and exercise.
- Prevent recurrent exacerbations, especially those requiring urgent medical visits.
- Provide pharmacotherapy with minimal or no adverse effects.
- Achieve patient and family satisfaction with asthma care.

The physician should let the patient know that these are the expectations of optimal management and confirm that those are the patient's goals as well.

A very important component of nonpharmacologic therapy is reduction of relevant environmental triggers. Information should be given regarding environmental control of pollen, mite, mold, animal dander, and cockroach antigens (Box 1) that appear to be relevant based on the history and results of skin or in vitro specific IgE tests. Inhalant allergen immunotherapy should be considered for patients who have persistent asthma when there is clear evidence of a relationship between symptoms and exposure to an allergen to which the patient is sensitive.

Finally, psychosocial issues should be considered and addressed. For many patients, the education and therapeutic alliance described earlier adequately addresses psychosocial concerns. For other patients, poor past adherence requires identifying the barriers to adherence and finding solutions together. Resources for patients with poor social support should be identified. Clinically significant anxiety or depression that can make asthma harder to control should be treated.

Pharmacologic Step Therapy

The main principle of asthma pharmacologic step therapy is to add therapy in steps until control is achieved (step up) and decrease therapy in reverse steps (step down) to establish the lowest effective dose necessary to maintain control.

There are two types of asthma medications: quick-relief medications (Table 4) and long-term control medications (Table 5). Systemic corticosteroids can be used either short-term to treat an exacerbation (see Table 4) or as long-term maintenance therapy for patients with severe disease (see Table 5). The generally

TABLE 2 Assessing Asthma Control and Adjusting Therapy in Patients 12 Years and Older

COMPONENTS OF CONTROL	CLASSIFICATION OF CONTROL*		
	WELL CONTROLLED	NOT WELL CONTROLLED	VERY POORLY CONTROLLED
Impairment			
Symptoms	≤2 days/week	>2 days/week	Throughout the day
Nighttime awakenings	≤2 times/month	1–3 times/week	≥4 times/week
Short-acting β2-agonist use for symptom control (not prevention of EIB)	≤2 days/week	>2 days/week	Several times per day
Interference with normal activity	None	Some limitation	Extremely limited
FEV1 or peak flow	>80% predicted or personal best	60%–80% predicted or personal best	<60% predicted or personal best
Validated Questionnaires†			
ACQ	≤0.75‡	≥1.5	N/A
ACT	≥20	16–19	≤15
ATAQ	0	1–2	3–4
Risk			
Exacerbations requiring oral systemic corticosteroids	0–1/year	≥2/year§ ──────────────────────────→	
Progressive loss of lung function	Evaluation requires long-term follow-up care.		
Treatment-related adverse effects	Medication side effects can vary in intensity from none to very troublesome and worrisome. The level of intensity does not correlate to specific levels of control, but it should be considered in the overall assessment of risk.		
Recommended action for treatment¶	Maintain current step	Step up 1 step and reevaluate in 2–6 weeks	Consider short course of systemic oral corticosteroids
	Regular follow-up every 1–6 months to maintain control	For side effects, consider alternative treatment options	Step up 1–2 steps and reevaluate in 2 weeks
	Consider step down if well controlled for ≥3 months		For side effects, consider alternative treatment options

*The level of control is based on the most severe impairment or risk category. Assess impairment domain by patient's recall of previous 2–4 weeks and by spirometry or peak flow measures. Symptom assessment for longer periods should reflect a global assessment, such as inquiring whether the patient's asthma is better or worse since the last visit.
†Validated questionnaires for the impairment domain (the questionnaires do not assess the risk domain). Minimal important difference. 0.5 for the ACQ, 1.0 for the ATAQ, and 3.0 for the ACT.
‡ACQ values of 0.76–1.4 are indeterminate regarding well-controlled asthma.
§At present, there are inadequate data to correlate frequencies of exacerbations with different levels of asthma control. In general, more frequent and intense exacerbations (e.g., requiring urgent, unscheduled care, hospitalization, or ICU admission) indicate poorer disease control. For treatment purposes, patients who had ≥2 exacerbations requiring oral systemic corticosteroids in the past year may be considered the same as patients who have not-well-controlled asthma, even in the absence of impairment levels consistent with not-well-controlled asthma.
¶See Table 6 for treatment steps. The stepwise approach is meant to assist, not replace, the clinical decision making required to meet individual patient needs. Before a step up in therapy, review adherence, inhaler technique, environmental control, and comorbid conditions. If an alternative treatment option was used in a step, discontinue it and use the preferred treatment for that step.
ACQ, Asthma Control Questionnaire; ACT, Asthma Control Test; ATAQ, Asthma Therapy Assessment Questionnaire; EIB, exercise-induced bronchospasm; FEV1, forced expiratory volume in one second; N/A, not applicable.
Data from the National Asthma Education and Prevention Program (NAEPP) Expert Panel Report 3: Guidelines for the Management of Asthma.

TABLE 3 Normal FEV1/FVC by Age

AGE RANGE (YEAR)	NORMAL FEV1/FVC (%)
8–19	85
20–39	80
40–59	75
60–80	70

FEV1, Forced expiratory volume in one second; FVC, forced vital capacity.
Data from the National Asthma Education and Prevention Program (NAEPP) Expert Panel Report 3: Guidelines for the Management of Asthma.

recommended steps of pharmacologic therapy are shown in Table 6. Definitions of low-, medium-, and high-dose inhaled corticosteroids for each of the available preparations are given in Table 7. At each therapeutic step level, the NAEPP Expert Panel has indicated preferred medications, which generally identify medications with the best balance of efficacy and safety in clinical trials for patients at that level of severity. However, these recommendations are based on population data and must be tailored to individual patient needs, circumstances, and responsiveness to therapy.

All patients with asthma should have an action plan that describes their pharmacologic self-management. Aspects of pharmacologic self-management include the maintenance medication schedule, rescue therapy doses for increased symptoms, when and how to increase controller medication therapy, when and how to use prednisone, how to recognize a severe exacerbation, and when and how to seek urgent or emergency care. Controller medications should be increased with an upper respiratory infection or with symptoms requiring more than two doses of rescue therapy in 12 hours. Although doubling the dose of inhaled corticosteroids does not appear to generally be sufficient to provide clinical benefit under these circumstances, greater increases may be effective (e.g., fourfold increases). The increased dose of controller medications should be maintained at least until increased

BOX 1   Measures to Control Environmental Factors That Can Make Asthma Worse

Allergens

Reduce or eliminate exposure to the allergen(s) the patient is sensitive to:

Animal Dander

- Remove animal from house or, at a minimum, keep animal out of the patient's bedroom and keep the bedroom door closed.

Dust Mites

- Recommended
  - Encase mattress in a special dust-proof cover.
  - Encase pillow in a special dust-proof cover or wash it weekly in hot water.
  - Wash sheets and blankets on the patient's bed in hot water weekly. Water must be hotter than 130°F to kill the mites. Cooler water used with detergent and bleach can also be effective.
- Desirable
  - Reduce indoor humidity to 60% or less.
  - Remove carpets from the bedroom.
  - Avoid sleeping or lying on cloth-covered cushions or furniture.
  - Remove carpets that are laid on concrete.

Cockroaches

- Keep all food out of the bedroom.
- Keep food and garbage in closed containers.
- Use poison baits, powders, gels, or paste (e.g., boric acid). Traps can also be used.
- If a spray is used to kill cockroaches, stay out of the room until the odor goes away.

Pollens (From Trees, Grass, or Weeds) and Outdoor Molds

- Try to keep windows closed
- If possible, stay indoors, with windows closed, during periods of peak pollen exposure, which are usually during the midday and afternoon.

Indoor Mold

- Fix all leaks and eliminate water sources associated with mold growth.
- Clean moldy surfaces.
- Dehumidify basements if possible.

Tobacco smoke

- Advise patients and others in the home who smoke to stop smoking or to smoke outside the home.
- Discuss ways to reduce exposure to other sources of tobacco smoke, such as from daycare providers and the workplace.

Indoor and Outdoor Pollutants and Irritants

- If possible, do not use a wood-burning stove, kerosene heater, fireplace, unvented gas stove or heater.
- Try to stay away from strong odors and sprays, such as perfume, talcum powder, hair spray, paints, new carpet, or particle board.

Data from the National Asthma Education and Prevention Program (NAEPP) Expert Panel Report 3: Guidelines for the Management of Asthma.

symptoms resolve. Prednisone is usually needed for patients with incomplete or temporary responses to adequate doses of β-agonists (4 puffs with a spacer, waiting at least 1 minute between puffs), substantial interference with sleep every night, requirement for 12 or more puffs of β-agonist in a 24-hour period, or a peak flow less than 60% predicted. Home treatment of exacerbations is further discussed later.

For patients not on long-term control medications, assess severity and select the level of treatment that corresponds to the patient's level of severity (see Table 1). Persistent asthma is most effectively controlled with daily long-term control medications, specifically antiinflammatory therapy. For patients receiving long-term control medications, identify their current step of therapy, based on what they are actually taking (see Table 6), and their level of control (see Table 2). In general, step up one step for patients whose asthma is not well controlled. For patients with very poorly controlled asthma, consider increasing by two steps, a course of oral corticosteroids, or both. Before increasing pharmacologic therapy, consider adverse environmental exposures, poor adherence, poor inhaler technique, or comorbidities as targets for intervention. For patients with troublesome or debilitating side effects from asthma therapy, explore a change in therapy.

There are now five biologic medications approved for severe asthma not controlled by standard therapy (see Table 5). These biologic medications can be considered for patients with frequent and/or severe asthma exacerbations, poor asthma control, or frequent and/or chronic use of systemic corticosteroids.

Follow-up

Patients whose asthma is not controlled should be seen every 2 to 6 weeks (depending on their initial level of severity or control) until control is achieved. Once control is achieved, follow-up contact at 1- to 6-month intervals is recommended. These checkups should ensure continued control, identify other changes in the patient's status, and update the patient's action plan.

When well-controlled asthma has been maintained for at least 3 months, a step down in therapy can be considered to determine the minimum amount of medication required to maintain control or reduce the risk of side effects. Reduction in therapy should be gradual because asthma can deteriorate at a highly variable rate and intensity. Doses of inhaled corticosteroids may be reduced about 25% to 50% every 3 months to the lowest dose possible to maintain control. Many patients with persistent asthma relapse if inhaled corticosteroids are totally discontinued.

Patients should be encouraged to contact their asthma physician for signs of loss of asthma control, such as nocturnal symptoms, increasing β-agonist use, or activity limitation. Consultation with an asthma specialist is recommended if the patient has difficulties achieving or maintaining control of asthma, immunotherapy or an asthma biologic is being considered, the patient requires step 4 care or higher, or the patient has had an exacerbation requiring hospitalization.

Treatment of Exacerbations

Asthma exacerbations are acute or subacute episodes of progressively worsening shortness of breath, cough, wheezing, or chest tightness associated with decreases in expiratory airflow.

Home Management

Patients' action plans should direct their home therapy of asthma exacerbations according to the following recommendations.

Initial therapy should be with inhaled short-acting β-agonists (2 to 6 puffs by metered-dose inhaler [MDI] or nebulizer). This may be repeated in 20 minutes. With a good response (minimal or no symptoms and peak expiratory flow (PEF) ≥80% predicted or personal best), the patient may continue β-agonists every 3 to 4 hours for 24 to 48 hours. If repeated β-agonists are needed, a short course of oral corticosteroids should be considered.

With an incomplete response to initial therapy (persistent wheezing and dyspnea and PEF 50% to 79% predicted or personal best), oral corticosteroids should be added, β-agonists should be repeated, and the clinician should be contacted that day.

With a poor response (marked wheezing and dyspnea at rest, PEF <50% predicted or personal best), oral corticosteroids should be added, the β-agonist should be repeated immediately, and the patient should call the clinician and usually proceed to the emergency department. For signs of severe distress (e.g., difficulty talking in full sentences, diaphoresis, drowsiness, confusion, or cyanosis), 911 should be called. Patients with histories of rapid-onset severe exacerbations can consider carrying self-injectable

TABLE 4   Usual Dosages for Quick-Relief Medications for Patients 12 Years and Older

MEDICATION	DOSAGE FORM	ADULT DOSE	COMMENTS
Inhaled Short-Acting β₂-Agonists (SABA)			
Metered-Dose Inhaler		*Applies to all three SABAs*	
Albuterol HFA (Proventil, Ventolin, ProAir)	90 µg/puff, 200 puffs/canister	2 puffs 5 min before exercise	An increasing use or lack of expected effect indicates diminished control of asthma.
Albuterol RespiClick (ProAir)	90 µg/puff, 200 puffs/canister	*or* 2 puffs q4–6h prn	Not recommended for long-term daily treatment. Regular use exceeding 2 days/week for symptom control (not prevention of EIB) indicates the need for additional long-term control therapy.
Levalbuterol HFA (Xopenex)	45 µg/puff, 200 puffs/canister		Differences in potencies exist, but all products are essentially comparable on a per-puff basis. May double usual dose for mild exacerbations. For levalbuterol, should prime the inhaler by releasing 4 actuations prior to use. For HFA, periodically clean HFA activator, as drug may block/plug orifice. Nonselective agents (epinephrine [Primatene Mist], isoproterenol [Isopro Aerometer], metaproterenol [Alupent]) are not recommended due to their potential for excessive cardiac stimulation, especially in high doses.
Nebulizer Solutions			
Albuterol (Accuneb, Proventil)	0.63 mg/3 mL 1.25 mg/3 mL 2.5 mg/3 mL 5 mg/mL (0.5%)	1.25–5 mg in 3 mL saline q4–8h prn	May mix with budesonide (Pulmicort) inhalant suspension, cromolyn (Intal) or ipratropium (Atrovent) nebulizer solutions. May double the dose for severe exacerbation.
Levalbuterol (R-albuterol) (Xopenex)	0.31 mg/3 mL 0.63 mg/3 mL 1.25 mg/0.5 mL 1.25 mg/3 mL	0.63 mg–1.25 mg q8h prn	Compatible with budesonide (Pulmicort) inhalant suspension. The product is a sterile-filled, preservative-free, unit-dose vial.
Anticholinergics			
Metered-Dose Inhalers			
Ipratropium HFA (Atrovent)	17 µg/puff, 200 puffs/canister	2–3 puffs q6h	Multiple doses in the emergency department (not hospital) setting provide additive benefit to short-acting β-agonists. Treatment of choice for bronchospasm due to β-blocker. Does not block EIB. Reverses only cholinergically mediated bronchospasm; does not modify reaction to antigen. May be alternative for patients who do not tolerate short-acting β-agonist. Evidence is lacking for ipratropium producing added benefit to β₂ agonists in long-term control asthma therapy.
Ipratropium with albuterol (Combivent)[1]	18 µg/puff of ipratropium bromide and 90 µg/puff of albuterol, 200 puffs/canister	2–3 puffs q6h	
Nebulizer Solutions			
Ipratropium bromide	0.2 mg/mL (0.2%)	0.5 mg q6h	
Ipratropium bromide with albuterol (DuoNeb)[1]	0.5 mg/3 mL ipratropium bromide and 2.5 mg/3 mL albuterol	3 mL q4–6h	Contains EDTA to prevent discoloration of the solution. This additive does not induce bronchospasm.
Systemic Corticosteroid			
Methylprednisolone (Medrol) Prednisolone (Delta-Cortef, Prelone) Prednisone (Deltasone, Orasone)	2, 4, 6, 8, 16, 32 mg tab 5 mg tabs; 5 mg/5 mL, 15 mg/5 mL 1, 2.5, 5, 10, 20, 50 mg tabs; 5 mg/mL, 5 mg/5 mL	Short course (burst): 40–60 mg/day as single or 2 divided doses for 3–10 days	Short courses (bursts) are effective for establishing control when initiating therapy or during a period of gradual deterioration. Action may begin within an hour. The burst should be continued until symptoms resolve. This usually requires 3–10 days but can require longer. There is no evidence that tapering the dose following improvement prevents relapse in asthma exacerbations.
Dexamethasone (Decadron)	0.5, 0.75, 1, 1.5, 2, 4, and 6 mg tablets and 0.5 mg/5 mL and 1 mg/5 mL	0.6 mg/kg as a single dose	Can be considered as an alternative for children presenting to the ED with asthma
Repository Injection			
Methylprednisolone acetate (Depo-Medrol)	40 mg/mL 80 mg/mL	240 mg[3],* IM once	May be used in place of a short burst of oral steroids in patients who are vomiting or if adherence is a problem.

[1]Not FDA approved for this indication.
[3]Exceeds dosage recommended by the manufacturer.
*80–120 mg per package insert.
CFC, Chlorofluorocarbon; *EDTA*, edetic acid; *EIB*, exercise-induced bronchospasm; *HFA*, hydrofluoroalkane; *PEF*, peak expiratory flow; *tab*, tablet.
Data from the National Asthma Education and Prevention Program (NAEPP) Expert Panel Report 3: Guidelines for the Management of Asthma.

TABLE 5	Usual Dosages for Long-Term Control Medications for Patients 12 Years and Older			
MEDICATION	**DOSAGE FORM***	**ADULT DOSE**	**COMMENTS**

Systemic Corticosteroids

Methylprednisolone (Medrol)	2-, 4-, 8-, 16-, 32-mg tab	7.5–60 mg qd in a single dose in a.m. or qod as needed for control	For long-term treatment of severe persistent asthma, administer single dose in a.m. either daily or on alternate days (alternate-day therapy may produce less adrenal suppression).
Prednisolone (Delta-Cortef, Prelone)	5-mg tab 5 mg/5 mL, 15 mg/5 mL	Short-course (burst) to achieve control, 40–60 mg/day as single or 2 divided doses for 3–10 days	Short courses (bursts) are effective for establishing control when initiating therapy or during a period of gradual deterioration. There is no evidence that tapering the dose following improvement in symptom control and pulmonary function prevents relapse.
Prednisone (Deltasone, Orasone)	1, 2.5, 5, 10, 20, 50-mg tab/5 mg/mL, 5 mg/5 mL		

Inhaled Long-Acting β²-Agonists

| | | | Should not be used for relief of acute symptoms or exacerbations. Use only with ICS. |
| Salmeterol (Serevent) | DPI 50 μg/inhalation | 1 inhalation q12h | Decreased duration of protection against EIB may occur with regular use. |

Inhaled Combined Medications

Fluticasone and salmeterol (Advair and generic)	DPI 100 μg/50 μg, 250 μg/50 μg, 500 μg/50 μg	1 inhalation bid†	100/50 DPI or 45/21 HFA for patients not controlled on low-to-medium dose ICS.
	HFA 45 μg/21 μg 115 μg/21 μg 230 μg/21 μg	2 puffs bid†	250/50 DPI or 115/21 HFA for patients not controlled on medium-to-high dose ICS.
Fluticasone and salmeterol (AirDuo)	RespiClick 55 μg/14 μg 113 μg/14 μg 232 μg/14 μg	1 inhalation bid	
Budesonide and formoterol (Symbicort)	HFA MDI 80 μg/4.5 μg 160 μg/4.5 μg	2 inhalations bid†	80/4.5 for patients not controlled on low-to-medium dose ICS. 160/4.5 for patients not controlled on medium-to-high dose ICS.
Mometasone and formoterol (Dulera)	100 μg/5 μg 200 μg/5 μg	2 inhalations bid†	100/5 for patients not controlled on low-to-medium dose ICS. 200/5 for patients not controlled on medium-to-high dose ICS.
Fluticasone furoate/vilanterol trifenatate (Breo Ellipta)	100 μg/25 μg 200 μg/25 μg	1 inhalation daily	

Inhaled Long-acting Anticholinergic

| Tiotropium (Spiriva Respimat) | 1.25 μg or 2.5 μg / actuation | 2 puffs daily | May be as effective as LABA as add-on therapy to ICS. |

Leukotriene Modifiers

Leukotriene Receptor Antagonists

| Montelukast (Singulair) | 4 mg, or 5-mg chewable tab 10-mg tab | 10 mg qhs | Montelukast exhibits a flat dose-response curve. Doses > 10 mg do not produce a greater response in adults. |
| Zafirlukast (Accolate) | 10- or 20-mg tab | 40 mg/day (20-mg tab bid) | For zafirlukast: Administration with meals decreases bioavailability; take at least 1 h before or 2 h after meals. Zafirlukast is a microsomal p450 enzyme inhibitor that can inhibit the metabolism of warfarin. Doses of this drug should be monitored accordingly. Monitor for signs and symptoms of hepatic dysfunction. |

5-Lipoxygenase Inhibitor

| Zileuton (Zyflo) | 600-mg tab, immediate-release or extended-release tablets | 2400 mg daily (600 mg qid for immediate-release or 1200 mg bid for extended-release) | Monitor hepatic enzymes (ALT). Zileuton is a microsomal p450 enzyme inhibitor that can inhibit the metabolism of warfarin and theophylline. Doses of these drugs should be monitored accordingly. |

| TABLE 5 | Usual Dosages for Long-Term Control Medications for Patients 12 Years and Older—cont'd |||

MEDICATION	DOSAGE FORM*	ADULT DOSE	COMMENTS
Methylxanthines			
Theophylline (Slo-Phyllin, Theobid, Theo-Dur)	Liquids, sustained-release tab, cap	Starting dose 10 mg/kg/day up to 300 mg max Usual max 800 mg/day	Adjust dosage to achieve serum concentration of 5–15 µg/mL at steady-state (≥48 h on same dosage). Due to wide interpatient variability in theophylline metabolic clearance, routine serum theophylline level monitoring is essential. Patient should be told to discontinue if they experience symptoms of toxicity. Various factors (diet, food, febrile illness, age, smoking, and other medications) can affect serum concentration.
Asthma Biologics			
Omalizumab (Xolair)	Subcutaneous (SQ) injection 150 mg/1.2 mL following reconstitution with 1.4 mL sterile water for injection	150–375 mg SQ every 2–4 week, depending on body weight and pretreatment serum IgE level	For 6 years and older with moderate to severe allergic asthma not controlled by inhaled corticosteroids Monitor patient following injections; be prepared and equipped to identify and treat anaphylaxis that may occur. Do not administer more than 150 mg per injection site.
Benralizumab (Fasenra)	Solution 30 mg/1 mL	30 mg SQ every 4 weeks for first 3 doses, then every 8 weeks	For 12 years and older with severe eosinophilic asthma
Mepolizumab (Nucala)	Subcutaneous powder for solution: 100 mg	100 mg SQ every 4 weeks	For 12 years and older with severe eosinophilic asthma Monitor patient following injections; be prepared and equipped to identify and treat anaphylaxis that may occur.
Reslizumab (Cinqair)	Intravenous solution 10 mg/1 mL	3 mg/kg over 20–50 minutes every 4 weeks	For adults with severe eosinophilic asthma
Dupilumab (Dupixent)	Subcutaneous solution 300 mg/2 mL and 200 mg/1.14 mL	400 mg SQ loading followed by 200 mg every other week OR 600 mg SQ loading followed by 300 mg every other week	For 12 years and older with moderate to severe eosinophilic or corticosteroid-dependent asthma

*See Table 7 for estimated comparative daily dosages for inhaled corticosteroids.
†Dose depends on level of severity or control.
ALT, Alanine aminotransferase; amp, ampule; cap, capsule; DPI, dry powder inhaler; EIB, exercise-induced bronchospasm; HFA, hydrofluoroalkane; ICS, inhaled corticosteroid; LABA, long-acting β2-agonist; max, maximum; MDI, metered-dose inhaler; SABA, short-acting β2-agonist; tab, tablet.
Data from the National Asthma Education and Prevention Program (NAEPP) Expert Panel Report 3: Guidelines for the Management of Asthma.

| TABLE 6 | Stepwise Approach for Managing Asthma in Patients 12 Years and Older* ||

STEP	PREFERRED THERAPY	ALTERNATIVE THERAPY
1	Short-acting β-agonist prn	—
2	Low-dose ICS	LTRA, theophylline
3	Low-dose ICS *plus* LABA or Medium-dose ICS	Low-dose ICS *plus* LTRA *or* theophylline *or* zileuton (Zyflo) *or* tiotropium (Spiriva)[1]
4	Medium-dose ICS *plus* LABA	Medium-dose ICS *plus* LTRA *or* theophylline *or* zileuton (Zyflo) *or* tiotropium (Spiriva Respimat)
5	High-dose ICS *plus* LABA Consider omalizumab (Xolair) for patients who have allergies and benralizumab (Fasenra), mepolizumab (Nucala), reslizumab (Cinqair), or dupilumab (Dupixent) for patients who have eosinophilic asthma	Medium-dose ICS + LABA + tiotropium
6	High-dose ICS *plus* LABA *plus* oral corticosteroid† Consider omalizumab for patients who have allergies and benralizumab (Fasenra), mepolizumab (Nucala), reslizumab (Cinqair), or dupilumab (Dupixent) for patients who have eosinophilic asthma	—

[1]Not FDA approved for this indication.
*The stepwise approach is meant to assist, not replace, the clinical decision making required to meet individual patient needs.
†In step 6, before oral corticosteroids are introduced, a trial of high-dose ICS + LABA + either LTRA, theophylline, zileuton, or tiotropium may be considered, although this approach has not been studied in clinical trials.
ICS, Inhaled corticosteroid; LABA, long-acting β agonist; LTRA, leukotriene receptor antagonist.
Data updated from the National Asthma Education and Prevention Program (NAEPP) Expert Panel Report 3: Guidelines for the Management of Asthma.

| | | DAILY DOSE | | |
| TABLE 7 | Estimated Comparative Daily Dosages for Inhaled Corticosteroids for Patients 12 Years and Older | | | |
DRUG	DOSAGE FORM	LOW (µG)	MEDIUM (µG)	HIGH (µG)
Beclomethasone (QVAR RediHaler)	40 or 80 µg/puff	80–240	>240 to 480	>480
Budesonide DPI (Pulmicort)	90 or 180 µg/inhalation	180–540	>540 to 1080	>1080
Ciclesonide (Alvesco)	80 or 160 µg/actuation	160–320	>320 to 640	>640
Fluticasone-HFA (Flovent HFA)	MDI: 44, 110, 220 µg/puff	88–264	>264 to 440	>440
Fluticasone DPI (Flovent Diskus, ArmonAir RespiClick, Arnuity Ellipta)	DPI: 50, 100, and 250 µg/inhalation Flovent Diskus; 55, 113, and 232 µg/inhalation ArmonAir RespiClick; 100 and 200 µg/inhalation Arnuity Ellipta	100–300	>300 to 500	>500
Mometasone DPI (Asmanex)	110 or 220 µg/actuation	110–220	>220 to 440	>440

DPI, Dry powder inhaler; *HFA,* hydrofluoroalkane; *MDI,* metered-dose inhaler.
Data from the National Asthma Education and Prevention Program (NAEPP) Expert Panel Report 3: Guidelines for the Management of Asthma and *Ann Pharm.* 2009;43:519.

epinephrine (Adrenaclick, Auvi-Q, EpiPen)[1] at home to use at the onset of increased symptoms.

Emergency Department and Hospital Management

Assessment should rapidly determine the severity of the exacerbation based on intensity of symptoms, signs (heart rate, respiratory rate, use of accessory muscles, chest auscultation), peak flow (unless the patient is too dyspneic to perform), and pulse oximetry. Treatment should begin immediately following recognition of an exacerbation severe enough to cause dyspnea at rest, peak flow less than 70% predicted or personal best, or pulse oximetry oxygen saturation less than 95%. While treatment is being given, a brief, focused history and physical examination pertinent to the exacerbation can be obtained.

In patients with mild to moderate exacerbations (PEF >40% predicted), initial therapy is oxygen to achieve oxygen saturation greater than 93% and inhaled short-acting β-agonist by nebulizer or MDI (4 to 8 puffs) with holding chamber, which may be repeated up to three times in the first hour. Oral corticosteroids (prednisone 40 to 80 mg) are recommended if there is no immediate response to therapy or if the patient had been recently treated with oral corticosteroids.

In patients with severe exacerbations (PEF <40% predicted), initial therapy is oxygen as above, inhaled high-dose short-acting β-agonist (e.g., albuterol 5 mg) and ipratropium (0.5 mg) by nebulizer, and oral or intravenous corticosteroids (prednisone or methylprednisolone 80 mg). The albuterol may be repeated every 20 minutes or used continuously for 1 hour.

Repeated assessments of symptoms, signs, PEF, and oxygen saturation determine the responsiveness of the exacerbation to therapy. Such assessments should be made in patients presenting with severe exacerbations after the initial bronchodilator treatment and in all patients after three doses of bronchodilator therapy (60 to 90 minutes after initial treatment). In patients who are improving, short-acting β-agonists may be repeated every hour until a good response is achieved (no distress, PEF >70%). When this response is sustained at least 60 minutes after the last treatment, the patient may usually be discharged on a course of oral corticosteroids (generally prednisone 40 to 60 mg for 5 to 10 days), initiation or continuation of medium-dose inhaled corticosteroids, and arrangement for outpatient follow-up.

In patients who are not improving with the above therapy, adjunctive therapy, such as with intravenous magnesium sulfate[1] (2 g) or heliox, may be considered. Intubation and mechanical ventilation may be required for patients with respiratory failure in spite of treatment.

---

[1] Not FDA approved for this indication.

Summary

Asthma is a very common problem with the potential to cause substantial interference with quality of life. Although there is no cure for asthma, asthma can be well controlled in the majority of patients with proper management and an effective patient-physician relationship. We hope that the method described herein for assessing and managing asthma will help physicians help their patients achieve well-controlled asthma.

ATELECTASIS

Method of
Alykhan S. Nagji, MD; Joshua S. Jolissaint, MD; and Christine L. Lau, MD

CURRENT DIAGNOSIS

- Hypoxia
- Tachypnea
- Diminished breath sounds
- Wheezing
- Radiologic signs of atelectasis

CURRENT THERAPY

- Chest percussion or vibration
- Nasotracheal or bronchoscopic suctioning
- Incentive spirometry
- Positive-pressure ventilation
- Ambulation
- Postoperative pain control

Atelectasis refers to the collapse of alveoli that affects segmental or lobar regions of the lung or the entire lung and results in hypoventilation. However, recent studies have suggested that the alveoli are not collapsed but are filled with fluid and foam. These hypotheses are not mutually exclusive; collapsed alveoli and fluid- and foam-filled alveoli may be present concurrently in an atelectatic lung. Although atelectasis is considered a benign condition, early treatment, reversal, and prevention are essential to an overall improved outcome.

Etiology

Compression Atelectasis

Compression atelectasis occurs when the transmural pressure distending the alveolus is reduced to a level that allows the alveolus to collapse. To best illustrate this mechanism, consider the patient who has undergone induction of anesthesia. The diaphragm is relaxed and is displaced cephalad. In the supine position, the pleural pressures increase to the greatest extent in the dependent lung regions and can compress the adjacent lung tissue.

Surfactant Impairment

Surfactant serves to reduce the alveolar surface tension, thereby stabilizing the alveoli and preventing collapse. Reduction in surfactant occurs with certain types of anesthesia. Studies have shown that hyperinflation by means of increased tidal volume, sequential air inflations to the total lung capacity, or even a single cycle of increased tidal volume can increase the release of surfactant, aiding in recruitment and stabilization of alveoli.

Gas Resorption

One mechanism by which gas resorption results in atelectasis involves the patent airway. In regions of the lung with increased ventilation compared to perfusion, which produces a ventilation/perfusion (V/Q) mismatch, there is low alveolar oxygen tension. Increasing the fraction of inspired oxygen (FIO_2) initiates a cascade of events that increases alveolar oxygen tension (PAO_2) and decreases alveolar nitrogen tension (PAN_2), which results in loss of alveolar volume secondary to increased absorption of oxygen.

Another mechanism by which gas resorption leads to atelectasis occurs after complete airway occlusion. In such cases, gas is trapped distal to the obstruction. Gas uptake by the proximal blood flow continues without additional gas inflow. This causes the alveoli to collapse.

Pathophysiology

The trapping of air and hyperinflation of the alveoli are produced from the aforementioned mechanisms. The gases that are trapped are absorbed by the blood perfusing through that region of the lung, which eventually causes collapse of the alveoli. The atelectasis produces alveolar hypoxia and pulmonary vasoconstriction to prevent V/Q mismatching and to minimize arterial hypoxia. This vascular response is effective only if a large part of the lung is not collapsed; otherwise, intrapulmonary shunting occurs.

Clinical Presentation

The signs and symptoms of atelectasis are often nonspecific. The natural course of atelectasis may lead to fever, cough, tachypnea, wheezing, rhonchi, and chest pain. On physical examination, atelectasis may manifest as an area of localized reduced breath sounds with constant wheeze or reduced chest wall expansion or both.

Diagnosis

Chest radiographs aid in the diagnosis of atelectasis. They provide both direct and indirect signs that may indicate an atelectatic etiology for the patient's symptoms.

Direct signs include:
- Displaced pulmonary vessels
- Air bronchograms
- Displacement of intralobar fissures (most reliable sign)

Indirect signs include:
- Pulmonary opacification
- Diaphragmatic elevation
- Hyperexpansion of unaffected lung
- Tracheal, heart, and mediastinal shift toward atelectatic side
- Shift of the hilum toward the collapsed lobe
- Segmental ipsilateral rib approximation

Treatment

Treatment of atelectasis is geared toward the underlying cause. It is important to recognize respiratory distress and to intubate the patient if appropriate.

If the etiology is that of an obstructive atelectasis, chest percussion or vibration and nasotracheal or bronchoscopic suctioning may help in the clearing of secretions. With regard to lung re-expansion, incentive spirometry, continuous or intermittent positive-pressure ventilation, and early ambulation may be used.

Those patients who have a nonobstructive atelectasis caused by a pneumothorax or pleural effusion benefit from tube thoracostomy or thoracentesis. Additionally, appropriate pain management in the postoperative setting allows for proper ventilation.

References

Duggan M, Kavanagh BP: Pulmonary atelectasis: A pathogenic perioperative entity, *Anesthesiology* 102:838–854, 2005.
Duggan M, Kavanagh BP: Atelectasis in the perioperative patient, *Curr Opin Anaesthesiol* 20:37–42, 2007.
Hubmayr RD: Perspective on lung injury and recruitment: A skeptical look at the opening and collapse story, *Am J Respir Crit Care Med* 165:1647–1653, 2002.
Peroni DG, Boner AL: Atelectasis: Mechanisms, diagnosis and management, *Paediatr Respir Rev* 1:274–278, 2000.
Wagner PD, Laravuso RB, Uhl RR, West JB: Continuous distributions of ventilation-perfusion ratios in normal subjects breathing air and 100 per cent O_2, *J Clin Invest* 54:54–68, 1974.

BACTERIAL PNEUMONIA

Method of
Alison N. Huffstetler, MD; Arjun Muthusubramanian, MD, MPH; and Katharine C. DeGeorge, MD, MS

CURRENT DIAGNOSIS

- Diagnosis of community-acquired pneumonia requires symptoms plus radiographic findings consistent with pneumonia.
- Hospital-acquired pneumonia may be diagnosed in hospitalized patients who develop a pulmonary infection ≥48 hours after hospital admission in the absence of mechanical ventilation.
- Blood and sputum cultures are not necessary for all patients hospitalized with pneumonia.
- Biomarkers, such as procalcitonin and C-reactive protein, are not routinely recommended for the diagnosis of pneumonia.
- When determining the appropriate treatment setting, use a validated scoring system such as the pneumonia severity index (PSI) or CURB-65 to predict disease severity and risk of death.

CURRENT THERAPY

- Treat outpatients with uncomplicated bacterial pneumonia empirically with either a macrolide (azithromycin [Zithromax]) or doxycycline (Vibramycin).
- Patients hospitalized with pneumonia should be treated with a respiratory fluoroquinolone (levofloxacin [Levaquin] or moxifloxacin [Avelox]) or a select β-lactam (ceftriaxone [Rocephin] or ampicillin) PLUS a macrolide.
- Use broad-spectrum antibiotics to treat patients with hospital-acquired pneumonia; antibiotic selection should be based on local antibiograms, with consideration for coverage for *Pseudomonas aeruginosa* or methicillin-resistant *Staphylococcus aureus* (MRSA).
- Narrow antimicrobial therapy as soon as possible, based on culture results and sensitivities.
- Whenever MRSA is suspected, treatment with vancomycin (Vancocin) or linezolid (Zyvox) should be initiated; daptomycin (Cubicin)[1] should not be used to treat pulmonary MRSA infection.

[1]Not FDA approved for this indication.

Pneumonia is a leading cause of death in the United States and accounts for more than 400,000 emergency department (ED) visits annually. Pneumonia often presents with shortness of breath, fever, productive cough, with leukocytosis and radiographic findings of lobar infiltrate.

Diagnosis and treatment should be based on underlying characteristics of the patient and their risk factors. The most common cause of community-acquired pneumonia (CAP) is *Streptococcus pneumoniae*, whereas hospital-acquired pneumonia (HAP) is more frequently caused by gram-negative bacteria and places patients at a risk for multidrug-resistant organisms.

This chapter discusses diagnosis and treatment of community-acquired pneumonia (CAP) and HAP in adults. Although previous guidelines approached health care–associated pneumonia (HCAP) and HAP separately, these are now diagnosed and treated as a single disease process (HAP).

Epidemiology

Community-acquired pneumonia (CAP) affects approximately 5 to 6 people per 1000 persons per year, with seasonal variance resulting in higher incidence during winter. The associated morbidity and mortality rates are high; in 2015, 16.1 deaths per 100,000 people in the US population were attributed to pneumonia. Treating these patients comes at a cost of $10.6 to $17 billion in the United States annually. Men are affected more frequently than women, and African Americans more frequently than Caucasians. The very young and elderly (aged ≥65 years) are affected more often than younger adults. Despite our best efforts, advances in medical therapies have not significantly decreased the mortality rate associated with pneumonia since the advent of penicillin in 1928.

The incidence of HAP is approximately 1.6 to 3.6 cases per 1000 hospital admissions. HAP is a leading cause of hospital-acquired infections (HAI): 22% of HAIs are accounted for by HAP. HAP most frequently occurs in patients outside of the intensive care unit (ICU); however, those in the ICU and on mechanical ventilation are at high risk of ventilator-associated pneumonia (VAP). HAP is associated with complications including respiratory compromise, septic shock, acute renal failure, and empyema.

Etiology

Risk Factors

Predisposing factors for development of pneumonia include several prescription medications (angiotensin-converting enzyme inhibitors, antipsychotic medications, glucocorticoids, H_2 blockers, proton pump inhibitors, and sedatives), tobacco use, alcohol use, malnutrition, use of dentures at night, bronchial obstruction due to foreign body, altered mental status due to reversible causes, and pulmonary edema. Nonmodifiable risk factors include immotile cilia, cystic fibrosis, chronic obstructive pulmonary disease (COPD), Kartagener's syndrome, human immunodeficiency virus (HIV), lung cancer, and Young's syndrome.

Community-Acquired Pneumonia (CAP) Pathogens

Worldwide, *S pneumoniae* is the leading cause of pneumonia. In the United States, however, rates of streptococcal pneumonia have declined after implementation of the pneumococcal vaccine in both adults and children. "Typical" organisms that cause pneumonia in the United States include *Haemophilus influenza* (although less common after development of the *H influenza* vaccine in 1987), *S aureus*, group A streptococcus, *Moraxella catarrhalis*, anaerobes, and aerobic gram negative bacteria. "Atypical" organisms include *Mycoplasma pneumoniae*, *Legionella* spp, *Chlamydia pneumoniae*, and *Chlamydia psittaci*.

Existing pulmonary infection with influenza, RSV, human metapneumovirus, adenovirus, and rhinovirus increase the risk of developing a secondary bacterial pneumonia. Patients admitted to the ICU requiring invasive diagnostic testing frequently become infected with *S pneumoniae* but have a disproportionate incidence of *Legionella*, *S aureus*, *H influenza*, and enteric gram-negative bacilli (*Klebsiella pneumoniae*, *Pseudomonas aeruginosa*, *Acinetobacter* spp, *M catarrhalis*). Identification of the organism responsible for CAP is only established in approximately 40% of cases.

Specific patient risk factors should be considered to identify involved pathogens in CAP. Consider local trends and outbreaks for diagnosis of *Legionella*, *M pneumoniae*, and *C pneumoniae*. Alcoholism is frequently linked to anaerobic bacterial pneumonia, *K pneumoniae*, *Mycobacterium tuberculosis*, and *S pneumoniae*. Patients with high risk of aspiration also have higher rates of anaerobic oral flora underlying pneumonia. Patients with COPD frequently have pneumonia caused by *Chlamydophila pneumoniae*, *H influenza*, *Legionella* species, *M catarrhalis*, *P aeruginosa*, and *S pneumoniae*. Exposure to animals such as bats, birds, or farm animals increases risk of *Histoplasma capsulatum* and *Coxiella burnetii* (Q fever) infections. HIV is a risk factor for *H influenza*, *M tuberculosis*, and *S pneumoniae* in the early stages and a risk factor for *Pneumocystis jiroveci* in late stages with decreased CD4 count. Travel increases risk for *Blastomyces dermatitidis* and *Coccidioides* species. Severe infections that do not respond to initial therapy should raise concern for possible MRSA infection. When clinical management would be altered by confirmed diagnosis of microbial infection, effort should be made for more extensive diagnostic testing; Table 1 lists the conditions that should prompt more extensive testing to identify specific pathogen involvement and antibiotic sensitivities.

Hospital-Acquired Pneumonia

Acutely ill, hospitalized patients have a higher risk of aspirating, which accounts for many of the differences in involved pathogens in HAP as compared with CAP. Oropharyngeal colonization with microorganisms that are commonly found in hospitals may occur within 48 hours of admission. Aerobic gram-negative bacilli such as *Escherichia coli*, *K pneumonia*, *Enterobacter* spp, and *P aeruginosa* are more commonly identified in patients with HAP, but gram-positive cocci are also identified. HAP, distinct from CAP, places patients at higher risk for multidrug-resistant (MDR) pathogens. Prior intravenous (IV) antibiotic use is a strong risk factor for MDR HAP. MRSA is also more common in patients with HAP, primarily because of prior IV antibiotic use as well. MDR *P aeruginosa* is identified most frequently in patients who have received IV antibiotics, previously on mechanical ventilation, and with a history of COPD, cystic fibrosis, and bronchiectasis.

Diagnosis

Symptoms of pneumonia most often include fever, cough, shortness of breath, purulent sputum, and chest pain. Physical examination may demonstrate bronchial breath sounds and crackles, although breath sounds may also be entirely normal, especially in the elderly. Oxygen saturation is often reduced, and chest radiography may demonstrate lobar consolidation, pleural effusion, or cavitary lesions. Depending on the severity of illness, patients may be treated in the outpatient or inpatient acute care settings or may require intensive care for ventilatory or vasopressor support.

Community-Acquired Pneumonia (CAP)

Diagnosis of CAP requires the presence of symptoms (fever, cough, purulent sputum, pleuritis, and/or shortness of breath) plus chest radiographic findings consistent with pneumonia such as lobar consolidation, pleural effusion, or cavitary lesions. Blood oxygen saturation is frequently low and white blood cell counts may be elevated, often with a neutrophilic predominance. Presentation in the elderly may be more subtle, with atypical or absent symptoms, blunted febrile response, and lack of leukocytosis.

TABLE 1	Patient-Specific Indicators for More-Extensive Diagnostic Testing in CAP				
INDICATION	**BLOOD CULTURE**	**SPUTUM CULTURE**	**_LEGIONELLA_ UAT**	**PNEUMOCOCCAL UAT**	**OTHER**
Intensive care unit admission	X	X	X	X	X*
Active alcohol abuse	X	X	X	X	
Asplenia	X			X	
Cavitary infiltrates	X	X			X†
Chronic severe liver disease	X			X	
Failure of outpatient antibiotic therapy		X	X	X	
Leukopenia	X			X	
Pleural effusion	X	X	X	X	X‡
Positive _Legionella_ UAT result		X	NA		
Positive pneumococcal UAT result	X	X		NA	
Recent travel			X		X‡
Severe obstructive lung disease		X			

Abbreviations: CAP = community-acquired pneumonia; NA = not applicable; UAT = urinary antigen test.
*Endotracheal aspirate (intubated) or bronchoscopy or nonbronchoscopic bronchoalveolar lavage.
†Fungal and tuberculosis cultures.
‡Thoracentesis and pleural fluid cultures.

Patients diagnosed with bacterial pneumonia treated in the outpatient setting do not require specific microbial identification; neither noninvasive nor invasive testing is recommended for this population (including blood cultures, endotracheal aspirates, and urine antigen testing).

Expectorated sputum samples for gram stain and culture are optional for most patients with pneumonia but should be collected from those hospitalized requiring intensive care or with any of the risk factors listed in Table 1, ideally before treatment is initiated. Early gram staining can direct initial empiric therapy, especially with findings of less common pathogens. Sputum samples become lower yield as the time between treatment initiation and collection of the sample increases. Inadequate samples (<10 inflammatory cells per epithelial cell) should not be sent for gram stain or culture. Nebulized hypertonic saline may be used to induce sputum sample when necessary.

Blood cultures are optional for most patients with pneumonia but, similarly to sputum culture, should be obtained for those hospitalized requiring intensive care or with any factors listed in Table 1. In the general population of patients hospitalized with pneumonia, false-positive blood cultures are common and can increase the duration of hospital stay and potentially misinform treatment decisions. Additionally, false-positive blood cultures frequently lead to use of broad spectrum antibiotics, increasing microbial resistance patterns.

Biomarkers such as procalcitonin (PCT), soluble triggering receptor expressed on myeloid cells-1, and CRP are not routinely recommended for use in the diagnosis of pneumonia, although there is emerging evidence for their use in distinguishing bacterial pneumonia from other causes of pulmonary symptoms. These markers are better used in assessing response to treatment, discussed below in the treatment section.

Hospital-Acquired Pneumonia
The diagnosis of HAP can be made in hospitalized patients who develop pulmonary infection ≥48 hours after hospital admission. Criteria for HAP requires new or progressive findings on chest radiography, fever, leukopenia or leukocytosis, or altered mental status (for patients aged ≥70 years), and new or worsening clinical symptoms or signs consistent with bacterial pneumonia in the absence of mechanical ventilation. Similarly to CAP, sputum and blood cultures should be obtained only when clinically indicated

(Table 1), and biomarkers for diagnostic purposes are not routinely recommended.

Treatment Setting
Determination of appropriate treatment setting is important for both patient outcomes and health care costs. Inpatient care of pneumonia can be 25 times as costly as outpatient management and also increases risk of thromboembolic events and superinfection with drug-resistant or virulent organisms. However, inappropriate outpatient management of patients at higher risk of death can lead to potentially avoidable morbidity and death.

Several scoring systems have been developed to help predict short-term mortality and need for hospital or ICU admission in patients with bacterial pneumonia. The following clinical decision aids are the most commonly used:

Pneumonia Severity Index (PSI)
Commonly used, well-validated scoring system that evaluates 20 items with emphasis on the age of the patient. Higher PSI scores indicate higher risk of requiring ICU level care or short-term mortality. See Table 2 for details of PSI scoring. Patients classified as risk classes I and II should be managed as outpatients; those with risk class III should be treated in an observation unit or with short-stay hospitalization; risk classes IV and V should be admitted to the hospital.

CURB-65
Severity-of-illness score which incorporates <u>c</u>onfusion, <u>u</u>remia, <u>r</u>espiratory rate, low <u>b</u>lood pressure, and age ≥<u>65</u> years into a prognostic model to determine a patient's candidacy for outpatient therapy. A CURB-65 score of ≥2 is indicative of likely need for hospitalization, with consideration for ICU care for those with of scores 3 or greater. This shorter scoring system may be less cumbersome in a busy setting, but the effect on hospital admission rates and patient outcomes have been studied less extensively than the PSI score.

SMART-COP
Assists the physician in determining whether the patient requires ICU level care. The algorithm takes into account systolic blood pressure, multilobar chest x-ray findings of infiltrate, albumin,

TABLE 2	Pneumonia Severity Index	
RISK FACTORS		**POINTS**
Demographics		
Age, men		Age in years
Age, women		Age in years - 10
Nursing home resident		+10
Comorbid conditions		
Active neoplasm		+30
Liver disease		+20
History of CVA		+10
Chronic heart failure		+10
Chronic renal failure		+10
Physical examination		
Altered mental status		+20
Respiratory rate elevated >30		+20
Hypotension, SBP <90 mm Hg		+20
Temperature <95° or >40° C		+15
Tachycardia, pulse > 125 beats/min		+10
Laboratory and imaging findings		
Acidosis, arterial pH < 7.35		+30
Hyponatremia, Na <130 mmol/L		+20
BUN ≥ 30 mg/dL		+20
Glucose ≥ 250 mg/dL		+10
Hematocrit < 30%		+10
PaO_2 < 60 mm Hg		+10
Pleural effusion		+10
Total points		

Abbreviations: BUN= blood urea nitrogen; CVA= cerebrovascular disease; Na = sodium; PaO_2 = partial pressure of arterial oxygen; SBP = systolic blood pressure. Total points < 51 indicates low incidence of death from CAP. Patients with increased total points have higher risk of death; the greatest risk for those >130 total points with rate of death for adults diagnosed with CAP of 24.9%.

respiratory rate, tachycardia, confusion, oxygenation, and pH and stratifies patients into risk groups that estimate risk of requiring intensive respiratory or vasopressor support.

Patients with septic shock requiring vasopressor therapy in the setting of CAP should be admitted to the ICU. If there is clinical concern for impending airway compromise, the patient should be intubated and admitted to the intensive care unit. In several clinical studies, patients who were critically ill and were not initially admitted to the ICU had higher rates of morbidity and mortality.

Treatment

General recommendations for empiric treatment of both CAP and HAP are detailed in Table 3. Treatment of a nonsevere case of pneumonia in an outpatient should be empiric and include a macrolide (such as azithromycin [Zithromax]) or doxycycline (Vibramycin). Therapy for inpatients may rely on sputum cultures with targeted antibiotic regimens to reduce cost and complications of therapy. Common treatment regimens for CAP requiring hospitalization include a respiratory fluoroquinolone (such as moxifloxacin [Avelox]) or a beta-lactam (ceftriaxone [Rocephin]) plus a macrolide. Empiric treatment regimens for HAP should be broad and based on local antibiograms, with consideration for coverage for *P aeruginosa* or MRSA. Prevention of pneumonia is essential, and pneumococcal vaccines should be provided to children and adults over 65 years

of age and those with risk factors for developing pneumonia at a younger age. These antibiotics and supportive care (oxygen, IV fluids, and ventilatory or vasopressor support when necessary) are the mainstay of treatment for both community and hospital-acquired bacterial pneumonia. Antibiotic selection is guided by several factors:
- age
- severity of illness
- risk of infection by multidrug-resistant pathogen (see Table 4 for risk factors)
- setting (both timing and location) of pneumonia onset

Initiation of initial treatment should also be guided by geographic antibiograms, which should be available through local hospitals. The Centers for Disease Control and Prevention's Antibiotic Resistance Patient Safety Atlas provides similar information for the aggregate of hospital-acquired infections. Antibiotic therapy should be narrowed as soon as possible based on culture and subsequent sensitivity results, if culture was obtained.

PCT may be used as an indicator of response to therapy after diagnosis of CAP and HAP based on recent trial data. If procalcitonin measurements decrease to <0.1 μg/L, a provider may consider discontinuation of antibiotics.

In addition to antimicrobial therapy for those who require hospitalization, care should be taken to maintain appropriate oral hygiene and to maintain head of bed at 30° to 45° in efforts to minimize risk of aspiration. Serum glucose goal should be <180 mg/dL. A few additional considerations exist for patients who require an intensive care unit stay during hospitalization. These individuals should all receive dual antibiotic therapy, as noted in Table 3. For those who remain hypotensive despite adequate fluid resuscitation, consider screening for occult adrenal insufficiency. Those with hypoxemia or respiratory distress may receive a closely monitored trial of noninvasive ventilation followed by intubation as indicated. Low-tidal volume ventilation (6 mL/kg of ideal body weight) should be used.

Community-Acquired Pneumonia (CAP)

Patients with suspected CAP should first be risk stratified using one of the pneumonia severity scoring indices discussed above and in Table 2. If being admitted to the hospital, the first dose of empiric antibiotic (see Table 3) should be administered in the emergency department as soon as the diagnosis of pneumonia is made. Patients may be transitioned from intravenous to oral antibiotics when they are hemodynamically stable, able to tolerate oral medications, and are able to absorb these medications enterally. When possible, an oral antibiotic should be chosen from the same or similar antibiotic class as the intravenous antibiotic used. Observation of inpatients after transition to oral antibiotics is not necessary as long as the patient is clinically stable and has a safe disposition plan. The recommended duration of antibiotic therapy is at least 5 days, with discontinuation only after the patient has been afebrile for at least 48 to 72 hours and remains clinically stable. Concern for a coexisting extrapulmonary infection may affect antibiotic selection and extend duration of therapy.

Hospital-Acquired Pneumonia

All patients with suspected HAP should be treated with broad spectrum antibiotics (Table 3). Antibiotic choice should be governed by local antibiograms. As described in more detail in the diagnosis section, Table 1 details the circumstances that guide further diagnostic testing, including cultures and PCR testing. Also, as described in Table 3, if symptoms have a late onset or if risk factors for a multidrug resistant pathogen are present, then dual therapy is indicated. However, in selecting antimicrobial coverage, clinicians must weigh the benefit of initiating adequate coverage as soon as possible against the harms of uniform broad spectrum coverage, such as increased resistance rates, risk of *Clostridium difficile* infection, and adverse drug effects. Whenever MRSA is suspected, treatment with vancomycin (Vancocin) or linezolid (Zyvox) should be initiated; daptomycin (Cubicin)[1] should not be used to treat pulmonary MRSA infection.

---

[1]Not FDA approved for this indication.

TABLE 3 — Empiric Antibiotic Therapy for Pneumonia for Adults

TYPE OF PNEUMONIA	SETTING	ANTIMICROBIAL THERAPY
Community-acquired pneumonia		
	Outpatient, healthy patient	Macrolide (azithromycin [Zithromax] or clarithromycin [Biaxin]) OR
		Doxycycline (Vibramycin) OR
	Outpatient, patient with risk factors*	Respiratory fluoroquinolone[†] if failure with above therapy OR
		Macrolide PLUS β-lactam[‡]
	Inpatient, patient not in ICU	Respiratory fluoroquinolone[†] OR
		Select β-lactam (ceftriaxone [Rocephin], cefotaxime [Claforan], ertapenem [Invanz], or ampicillin) PLUS macrolide
	Inpatient, patient in ICU	Select β-lactam (ceftriaxone, cefotaxime, or ampicillin/sulbactam [Unasyn]) PLUS either a respiratory fluoroquinolone[†] or azithromycin
	Concern for *P. aeruginosa*	Antipseudomonal β-lactam[§] PLUS either ciprofloxacin (Cipro) or levofloxacin (Levaquin) OR
		Antipseudomonal β-lactam[§] PLUS aminoglycoside PLUS azithromycin
Aspiration pneumonia		
	Outpatient	Amoxicillin/clavulanate (Augmentin) OR clindamycin (Cleocin)
	Inpatient	β-Lactam/β-lactamase inhibitor (ampicillin/sulbactam [Unasyn],[1] piperacillin/tazobactam [Zosyn], ticarcillin/clavulanate [Timentin]) OR
		3rd or 4th generation cephalosporin PLUS either metronidazole (Flagyl) or clindamycin (Cleocin) OR
		fluoroquinolone PLUS either metronidazole or clindamycin OR
		Meropenem (Merrem),[1] ertapenem (Invanz), doripenem (Doribax),[1] or imipenem/cilastatin (Primaxin)
Hospital-acquired pneumonia		
	Early-onset AND No risk factors for MDR organisms	Ceftriaxone, cefotaxime, respiratory fluoroquinolone,[†] ampicillin/sulbactam, piperacillin/tazobactam, ticarcillin/clavulanate, or ertapenem
	Late-onset OR Risk factors for MDR organisms	Select β-lactam (cefepime, ceftazidime, imipenem, meropenem,[1] doripenem,[1] or piperacillin/tazobactam) PLUS one of ciprofloxacin, levofloxacin, or an aminoglycoside
MRSA suspected	Either community- or hospital-acquired	ADD vancomycin (Vancocin) or linezolid (Zyvox) to regimen

*Presence of comorbid conditions (chronic heart, lung, liver, or renal disease; diabetes mellitus; alcoholism; malignancies, asplenia, immunosuppression [iatrogenic or pathologic]), use of antimicrobials within the past 3 months, high-rate (>25%) of macrolide-resistant *S pneumoniae*
[†]Respiratory fluoroquinolones include levofloxacin (Levaquin), moxifloxacin (Avelox), or Gemifloxacin (Factive).
[‡]High-dose amoxicillin, amoxicillin/clavulanate (Augmentin), ceftriaxone (Rocephin), cefuroxime (Ceftin), cefpodoxime (Vantin)
[§]Antipseudomonal beta-lactams include piperacillin/tazobactam (Zosyn), cefepime (Maxipime), ceftazidime (Fortaz), imipenem/cilastatin (Primaxin), doripenem (Doribax),[1] and meropenem (Merrem).
[1]Not FDA approved for this indication.

TABLE 4 — Risk Factors for Multidrug Resistant Pathogens in Hospital-Acquired Pneumonia

Antimicrobial therapy in preceding 90 days

Current hospitalization greater than or equal to 5 days

High frequency of antibiotic resistance in the community or specific hospital unit

Presence of risk factors for health care–associated pneumonia

Hospitalization for 2 or more days in preceding 90 days

Residence in nursing home or extended-care facility

Home infusion therapy (including antibiotics)

Chronic dialysis in preceding 30 days

Home wound care

Family member with MDR pathogen

Immunosuppressive disease or therapy

MDR, multidrug-resistant.

Prevention

Immunization against influenza, *S pneumoniae,* and *H influenza* is the best protection against bacterial pneumonia in adults and children. Recommended vaccine schedules are described in Table 5. In general, everyone should receive an annual influenza vaccine and individuals should receive *H influenza* and pneumococcal immunization on a schedule based on age and risk factors. The pneumococcal vaccines have a 44%–75% efficacy against invasive disease from *S pneumoniae* for persons 65 years and older and have been shown to be cost effective in populations aged 50 years and older. A systematic review demonstrated that the influenza vaccine effectively reduces pneumonia, hospital admission, and death. Annual influenza immunization is recommended, as neuraminidase and hemagglutinin evolve rapidly, and new formulations targeting predicted strains are needed.

References

Centers for Disease Control and Prevention. FastStats—Pneumonia. https://www.cdc.gov/nchs/fastats/pneumonia.htm. Published 2017. Accessed March 10, 2018.
Centers for Disease Control and Prevention: *Immunization Schedules.* https://www.cdc.gov/vaccines/schedules/index.html.

TABLE 5 Recommended Vaccinations for the Prevention of Pneumonia

VACCINE	POPULATION	RECOMMENDATIONS
Influenza	All persons older than 6 months	Annually If first lifetime dose of influenza vaccine, 2nd dose should be given 4 weeks after 1st dose
Pneumococcal		
	All adults	Should receive 1 dose of PCV13 (Prevnar) and either 1, 2, or 3 doses of PPSV23 (Pneumovax 23). See below for guidance regarding the number and timing of vaccine doses.
	Immunocompetent adults 19–64 years who smoke tobacco or who have chronic heart disease (excluding hypertension), chronic lung disease, chronic liver disease, alcoholism, or diabetes mellitus	1 dose of PPSV23. At age 65 or older, they should receive 1 dose of PCV13 and 1 dose of PPSV23 at least 1 year after dose of PCV13 AND at least 5 years after previous dose of PPSV23.
	All immunocompetent adults 65 years and older	At 65 years or older they should receive 1 dose of PCV13, followed by PPSV23 at least 1 year after PCV13. If they received dose of PPSV23 before age 65, dose of PCV13 should be given at least 1 year after 1st dose of PPSV23 and dose of PPSV23 should be given at least 5 years after 1st dose of PPSV23.
	Adults 19 and older with immunocompromising conditions*	Administer 1 dose of PCV13 first and then dose of PPSV23 at least 8 weeks after dose of PCV13 and a second dose of PPSV23 5 years after 1st dose of PPSV23. At age 65 and older, administer one final dose of PPSV23 at least 5 years after previous dose of PPSV23 and at least 8 weeks after dose of PCV13.
	Adults 19 and older with cerebrospinal fluid leak or cochlear implant	Administer 1 dose of PCV13 first and then a dose of PPSV23 at least 8 weeks after the dose of PCV13. At age 65 and older, administer 1 final dose of PPSV23 at least 5 years after previous dose of PPSV23 and at least 8 weeks after dose of PCV13.
Haemophilus influenza type B	All children younger than 5 years old, unvaccinated older children and adults with certain medical conditions,* people who receive bone marrow transplant	Administer 1 dose of HiB at age 2, 4, 6 (per product) and 12–15 months with minimum of age 6 weeks. Children with 1 dose at age >15 months need no further doses. For high-risk conditions, children age 12-59 months who previously received 1 or no doses should receive 2 additional doses of HiB, 8 weeks apart. For children who received 2 doses before 12 months of age should receive 1 additional dose. Hib may be given to high-risk adults.

HiB, *Haemophilus influenza* type B; PCV, pneumococcal conjugate vaccine; PPSV23, 23-valent pneumococcal polysaccharide vaccine.
*B- or T-lymphocyte deficiency, complement deficiencies, phagocytic disorders (excluding chronic granulomatous disease), HIV infection, chronic renal failure, nephrotic syndrome, leukemia, lymphoma, Hodgkin disease, generalized malignancy, multiple myeloma, solid organ transplant, iatrogenic immunosuppression, anatomic, or functional asplenia.

Jones RN: Microbial etiologies of hospital-acquired bacterial pneumonia and ventilator-associated bacterial pneumonia, *Clin Infect Dis* 51(S1):S81–S87, 2010.

Kaysin A, Viera AJ: Community-acquired pneumonia in adults: diagnosis and management, *Am Fam Physician* 94:698–706, 2016.

Kalil AC, Metersky ML, Klompas M, et al: Management of adults with hospital-acquired and ventilator-associated pneumonia: 2016 Clinical Practice Guidelines by the Infectious Disease Society of America and the American Thoracic Society, *Clin Infect Dis* 63(5):61–111, 2016.

Mandell LA, Wunderink RG, Anzueto A, et al: Thoracic Society consensus guidelines on the management of community-acquired pneumonia in adults, *Clin Infect Dis* 44:S27–S72, 2007.

Musher DM, Thorner AR: Community-acquired pneumonia, *N Engl J Med* 371(17):1619–1628, 2014.

Wilson JW, Estes LL:(2012). *Mayo Clinic Antimicrobial Therapy: Quick Guide*, 2nd ed. 2012.

- Blastomycosis should be suspected in the appropriate clinical context in patients who have resided or traveled to an endemic area.
- Blastomycosis has a broad range of manifestations, mimicking other infectious (e.g., bacteria, mycobacteria) and neoplastic processes.
- Blastomycosis may be asymptomatic, or it can manifest with disease involving the lung, skin, bone and joints, genitourinary system, or central nervous system.
- Diagnosis requires microscopic examination and/or culture of clinical specimens. *Blastomyces* antigen detection is also useful. Serology has no diagnostic value.

BLASTOMYCOSIS

Method of
John M. Embil, MD; and Donald C. Vinh, MD

CURRENT DIAGNOSIS

- Blastomycosis is caused by the thermally dimorphic fungus *Blastomyces dermatitidis* and *gilchristi*.
- *Blastomyces* spp. are endemic to the United States (southeastern and south central states bordering Mississippi and Ohio rivers; upper Midwestern states bordering the Great Lakes) and to Canada (Manitoba and Ontario bordering the Great Lakes; Quebec adjacent to St. Lawrence River).

CURRENT THERAPY

- Treatment varies with the severity of disease.
- Long-term suppressive therapy may be required for those who are immunosuppressed.

Blastomyces dermatitidis, and the recently identified *B. gilchristii*, are the thermally dimorphic fungi that causes blastomycosis. These fungi exist in mycelial form in the environment but grow as yeast forms at body temperature. Although *Blastomyces* spp. are endemic to certain specific regions within North America, numerous cases have been reported from areas where they are not considered endemic. It is presumed that those patients acquired infection in the endemic areas and subsequently presented outside of these geographic locations. However, it is also possible that the natural reservoirs of the fungus are evolving. The clinical manifestations of blastomycosis can be diverse, and therefore this infection should be suspected within the appropriate clinical context in persons with a history of residence or travel to such endemic areas.

Epidemiology

Our knowledge of the exact geographic distribution of *B. dermatitidis*, and of the newer *B. gilchristii*, is limited by the fact that the fungus cannot be readily recovered from nature; thus, identification of the endemic area has been largely derived from outbreak investigations and small case series. Most epidemiologic studies have depended upon recovery of *B. dermatitidis* in culture from clinical specimens or histologic visualization to establish the diagnosis. In addition, the incidence and prevalence of blastomycosis has been difficult to establish because suitable serologic or skin-prick assays (demonstrating acceptable sensitivity and/or specificity) to confirm infection are lacking. The geographic niche of *Blastomyces* spp. may therefore be greater than is currently believed.

The currently known areas of endemnicity for *B. dermatitidis/gilchristii* are the south central and upper midwestern United States, including areas surrounding the Great Lakes. *B. dermatitidis* is also endemic in Wisconsin (1.3 cases per 100,000 population) and Mississippi (1.4 cases per 100,000 population), as well as parts of Missouri, Kentucky, Tennessee, Arkansas, and Alabama. In Canada, the major areas of endemicity include the province of Manitoba (0.62 cases per 100,000 population), the southern region of Québec (0.46–0.79 cases per 100,000 population), and the Kenora region of the province of Ontario (7.11 cases per 100,000 population). Although most cases of blastomycosis are concentrated in these regions, it should be remembered that persons can acquire infection with *Blastomyces* spp. in these areas but present at a later time to health care providers in locations where blastomycosis is not usually observed. Inquiring about residence or travel to these areas is important to help establish the diagnosis.

Risk factors for acquiring blastomycosis have been defined by case reports, case series, and a small number of case-control studies and have not been conclusively established. Exposure while in endemic regions to soil, decaying wood, or to dust clouds generated by soil disruption is important; however, specific outdoor occupations or activities have not been confirmed. The fungus may also be associated with exposure to river waterways.

Race may be a contributing factor to disease. In one study from Mississippi, African-American race and prior history of pneumonia were independent risk factors for blastomycosis; however, neither environmental nor socioeconomic risk factors were detected. These findings were in contrast to previously noted studies where race and gender were not identified as specific risk factors for acquisition of blastomycosis. One study in Canada noted an increased incidence among the aboriginal population of Manitoba. Thus, it remains unclear if certain ethnic groups are at increased risk for disease or simply reflect differences in exposure.

Immunosuppression may also be an important risk factor, particularly for the tendency to develop severe disease. Blastomycosis has been reported in pregnant women, persons with diabetes mellitus, organ transplant recipients, and persons infected with HIV.

Dogs and humans are the species most commonly affected by *B. dermatitidis*. Anecdotally, dogs can serve as a sentinel marker for human disease (i.e., dogs present with systemic infection before their owners), leading to early suspicion of human infections by astute veterinarians. In such cases, it is speculated that humans and their pet dogs have a simultaneous exposure to the same source of fungus and therefore develop synchronous infection. This hypothesis, however, remains to be confirmed, and in a more recent study, canine blastomycosis was not deemed to predict human disease among the human owners. Additional studies are required to establish the relationship between blastomycosis in humans and disease in their pet dogs.

The most common mode of transmission is presumed to be by inhalation of aerosolized conidia from the environment. There are, however, reports of cutaneous blastomycosis occuring after accidental cutaneous inoculation, for example in the laboratory setting during autopsy or after dog bites. The median incubation period, established by reviewing the results of point-source outbreaks, ranges from 30 to 45 days.

Pathophysiology

Following inhalation of conidia into the lungs, the fungus is phagocytosed by alveolar macrophages. The human body temperature allows the fungus to transform to the yeast phase. It is speculated that a process similar to infection with *Mycobacterium tuberculosis* then occurs. The fungus might spread to other organs via the bloodstream and lymphatics. The primary defense against *B. dermatitidis* is through a suppurative response initially with neutrophils, followed by influx of monocytes with establishment of cell mediated immunity, resulting in noncaseating granuloma. The patient with intact immunologic responses can contain the process without progression to clinical disease. Alternatively, the patient can develop a symptomatic pneumonia and then mount a suitable immunologic response and recover. Impaired immunity favors the development of progressive pulmonary disease with or without extrapulmonary manifestations. It has also been suggested that reactivation of disease can occur at pulmonary or extrapulmonary sites. The pathophysiology of *B. gilchristii* is thought to be similar to that of *B. dermatitidis*. A vaccine that protects humans against infection with *Blastomyces* spp. is unavailable.

Clinical Manifestations

After inhalation of the conidia, an initial infection can occur. Most primary infections (at least 50%) are asymptomatic or mild and usually go unrecognized, resolving spontaneously. In others, a symptomatic pneumonia can develop; recovery can occur either spontaneously or with therapy, without further progression. Some persons develop progressive pneumonia or extrapulmonary manifestations. The type of clinical manifestations (localized, extrapulmonary or disseminated disease) can have a seasonal variation: Persons with manifestations occurring early after exposure (1–6 months) developed localized pneumonia, whereas those who presented later after exposure (4–9 months) tended to have isolated extrapulmonary or disseminated disease. Blastomycosis has been termed "the great mimic," because its clinical manifestations are nonspecific and can be similar to those of many different clinical entities. The most common organ systems involved in blastomycosis, in descending order of frequency, include lung, skin, bone, genitourinary, and central nervous systems (CNS). Box 1 summarizes the key clinical manifestations of blastomycosis.

Blastomycosis in Special Populations

Children account for a small percentage of the cases of blastomycosis, ranging from 2% to 11%. Children demonstrate a similar spectrum of manifestations as in adults (excluding prostatic disease). The most common symptoms include cough, headache, chest pain, weight loss, fever, abdominal pain, and night sweats. It is postulated that children experience disseminated infection more frequently than do adults.

Although there are few published reports of blastomycosis in pregnancy, disease has been observed in pregnant women, with presumed subsequent intrauterine and perinatal transmission.

Blastomycosis has been reported in persons with advanced HIV and among those who have undergone solid organ transplants. In immunocompromised hosts, it appears that a significant percentage developed rapidly progressive pulmonary disease, leading to respiratory failure and death. For those who are immunocompromised, the reported mortality rate range is 30% to 40%, with death occurring within the first few weeks of disease onset.

Diagnosis

The most reliable technique for confirming the diagnosis of blastomycosis is recovery of the fungus in culture. Alternatively, direct observation of the pathogen by light microscopy or with calcofluor

| BOX 1 | Clinical Manifestations of Blastomycosis |

Lung

Acute Pneumonia

Acute pneumonia is clinically indistinguishable from bacterial pneumonia.

Patients may present with fevers, chills, dyspnea, and cough, which initially might not be productive but, with time, may be accompanied by sputum production.

Radiographic findings can also be difficult to discern from those due to a bacterial pneumonia.

The radiographic pattern of pulmonary blastomycosis includes the following:

- Lobar infiltrates that mimic bacterial pneumonias
- Cavitary lung lesions and miliary patterns, which can mimic tuberculosis
- Mass lesions that may be mistaken for neoplasms
- Cystic lesions that resemble abscesses

There is no definitive plain radiograph or computed tomographic scan findings characteristic of pulmonary blastomycosis.

The spectrum of clinical pulmonary disease ranges from spontaneous resolution to pneumonia, with or without the acute respiratory distress syndrome; the latter is accompanied by high (50%–89%) mortality rates.

Chronic Pneumonia

A nonresolving pneumonia is one of the hallmarks of pulmonary blastomycosis.

Chronic pneumonia may be associated with fever, chills, weight loss, sputum-producing cough, and hemoptysis.

There is no characteristic radiographic appearance to help establish the diagnosis.

Skin

Cutaneous lesions are the most common extrapulmonary manifestations of blastomycosis. Lesions usually result from dissemination of a primary pulmonary lesion or rarely from direct inoculation.

Lesions can have a number of different appearances, with verrucae (wartlike lesions) and ulcers being the most common

manifestations. The verrucous lesions have a heaped-up appearance with a raw excoriated center. These lesions can mimic squamous cell carcinomas. Cutaneous abscesses may be associated with these lesions.

Ulcerative lesions initially manifest as pustules that eventually erode, producing a bed of granulation tissue that is friable and bleeds when traumatized. Other skin lesions include subcutaneous nodules and isolated abscesses.

Bone and Joint

The most common manifestation of extrapulmonary blastomycosis, after cutaneous disease, is involvement of bones and joints.

Any bone may be involved, although the long bones and axial skeleton are the most commonly affected.

The radiographic findings are indistinguishable from bacterial osteomyelitis and arthritis.

Genitourinary Tract

In the genitourinary tract, the prostate has been reported to be commonly affected by blastomycosis.

Symptoms can mimic prostatitis, and patients can present with obstructive uropathy.

Central Nervous System

The CNS is infrequently affected by *B. dermatitidis*. Infection may occur in isolation or with concomitant non-CNS infection.

CNS blastomycosis can occur in immunocompromised patients (e.g., HIV, solid organ transplant), as well as in patients with little/no risk factors (e.g., diabetes mellitus alone; persons with no underlying co-morbidities).

Clinical manifestations depend on the area of involvement and range from focal neurologic findings (e.g., due to mass lesions in the brain parenchyma) to symptoms of meningitis due to involvement of the meninges.

Radiographically, the findings may be indistinguishable from bacterial processes. Other sites of involvement have been described but are infrequent compared to those summarized above.

white stain or in histopathologic examination of tissue establishes a presumptive diagnosis. *Blastomyces* spp. are characteristically observed as a thick-walled, broad-based budding yeast. Because colonization does not occur, identification of *B. dermatitidis/gilchristii* should never be considered a contaminant. Serologic assays are extremely variable in their sensitivity and specificity and do not play a role in confirming or excluding the diagnosis, thus limiting their value in therapeutic decision making. A reliable skin test is unavailable, but a urinary antigen detection assay exists that may aid in diagnosis and may be of benefit to follow the efficacy of treatment in established infections. Box 2 summarizes techniques for establishing the diagnosis of blastomycosis.

Treatment

The treatment recommendations for blastomycosis from the Infectious Diseases Society of America (IDSA) are summarized in Table 1. Amphotericin B deoxycholate (Fungizone) is the agent with which there is the greatest experience, particularly for the treatment of patients with severe blastomycosis or for those who have CNS involvement. Lipid preparations of amphotericin B (Abelect, Amphotec, AmBisome)[1] have been shown to be effective in animal models, although clinical trial data are unavailable for these agents in humans. Clinical experience suggests that the lipid formulations are as effective but less toxic than the deoxycholate preparation.

It is generally accepted that in patients with severe disease or CNS involvement, amphotericin B-based products should be used

to initiate therapy until the patient is stable, followed by step-down to an azole, specifically itraconazole (Sporanox), to complete the total duration of therapy. Patients on itraconazole should have serum levels of the antifungal drug measured after at least 2 weeks of therapy, targeting a level >1.0 mcg/mL and <10.0 mcg/mL. Ketoconazole (Nizoral), although once recommended as the agent of choice, is less effective and more toxic than itraconazole. Experience with fluconazole (Diflucan)[1] for the treatment of blastomycosis is limited, although *in vitro* studies have demonstrated that fluconazole is effective against *B. dermatitidis*. Fluconazole does, however, have excellent penetration into the CNS; therefore, fluconazole may be considered as an alternative treatment of CNS blastomycosis. There are also a number of reports of voriconazole (Vfend)[1] being used for the successful treatment of CNS blastomycosis, as well as in persons with refractory blastomycosis. A case series of patients with CNS blastomycosis suggested that voriconazole may be the most desirable azole for the management of CNS disease. Similarly, there are reports on the successful use of posaconazole (Noxafil)[1] and isavuconazole (Cresemba)[1] for blastomycosis. The echinocandins (caspofungin [Cancidas],[1] micafungin [Mycamine],[1] and anidulafungin [Eraxis][1]) have limited activity against *B. dermatitidis* and are not considered appropriate choices.

Box 2 summarizes the therapeutic options for treatment of various types of blastomycosis. Amphotericin B-based therapy is usually the treatment option of choice in persons who have severe disease. Whenever the patient is clinically stable, it is desirable to switch from

[1]Not FDA approved for this indication.

[1]Not FDA approved for this indication.

BOX 2 | Establishing the Diagnosis of Blastomycosis

Direct Examination

A wet preparation of respiratory secretions or a touch preparation of tissues examined under high magnification by light microscopy can reveal the characteristic thick-walled, broad-based budding yeast form. However, this method has a low diagnostic yield: 36% for a single specimen and 46% for multiple specimens.

Calcofluor white stains can help in identifying the pathogen but require fluorescence microscopy.

Histopathologic Examination

The fungus may be difficult to identify with hematoxylin and eosin stain.

If there is a high index of suspicion, the Gomori methenamine-silver stain should be used to optimize detection of thick-walled, broad-based budding yeast forms compatible with *B. dermatitidis*.

Culture

Diagnostic yield ranges from approximately 86% from sputum to 92% from specimens obtained by bronchoscopy.

Culture is the gold standard for diagnosis. However, the fungus can take several weeks to be isolated in culture.

Confirmation of identity traditionally requires demonstration of thermal-dimorphism (mycelial-to-yeast conversion), which can further delay diagnosis.

Isolation of *B. dermatitidis* should not be considered a contaminant.

Serology

Current serologic assays are neither sensitive nor specific, and they should not be used to establish or refute a diagnosis or in therapeutic decision making.

Nucleic Acid Detection

This method permits genetic-based identification of *B. dermatitidis* from culture of clinical specimens, rather than relying on thermal-dimorphism to confirm identity of the fungus, thus reducing the time required for its identification.

Antigen Detection

The only currently available antigen detection assay has its greatest sensitivity in urine, although antigens can be detected in serum and other body fluids.

Cross reaction with antigens from other fungi (e.g., *Histoplasma* spp.) can occur.

The greatest benefit of the antigen detection assay may be to follow efficacy of treatment in patients with established disease (antigen levels decrease with successful treatment or rise with recurrence).

Skin Testing

A commercially available standardized reagent for skin testing is not available.

Modified from Chapman SW, Bradsher RW, Campbell GD, et al: Practice guidelines for the management of patients with blastomycosis. Cin Infect Dis 2000;30:679–683; and Martynowicz MA, Prakash UBS: Pulmonary blastomycosis: An appraisal of diagnostic techniques. Chest 2002;121:768–773.

TABLE 1 | Treatment Suggestions for Infections Caused by *Blastomycosis dermatitidis*

MANIFESTATION	TREATMENT RECOMMENDATIONS		COMMENTS
	PRIMARY RECOMMENDATION	ALTERNATIVE RECOMMENDATION	
Pulmonary Infection			
Mild to moderate	Itraconazole (Sporanox) 200 mg PO tid × 3 days, then qd or bid × 6–12 mo	Fluconazole (Diflucan)[1] 400–800[3] mg/day or ketoconazole (Nizoral) 400–800 mg/kg × 6–12 mo	For Itraconazole, measure serum levels after at least 2 weeks, to ensure adequate drug exposure. Target level: >1.0 mcg/mL and <10.0 mcg/mL
Moderate to severe	Lipid formulation of amphotericin B (AmBisome, Abelect, Amphotec)[1] 3–5 mg/kg/day OR Amphotericin B deoxycholate (Fungizone) 0.7–1 mg/kg/d for 1–2 wk or until improvement, followed by itraconazole 200 mg PO tid × 3 days then 200 mg PO bid × 6–12 mo		Amphotericin B toxicity can be attenuated by minimizing the duration of therapy and switching to oral therapy when the patient is stable. For Itraconazole, measure serum levels after at least 2 weeks, to ensure adequate drug exposure. Target level: >1.0 mcg/mL and <10.0 mcg/mL
Disseminated Infection Not Involving the Central Nervous System			
Mild to moderate	Itraconazole 200 mg PO tid × 3 days then qd or bid × 6–12 mo		
Moderate to severe	Lipid formulation of amphotericin B 3–5 mg/kg/d OR Amphotericin B deoxycholate 0.7–1 mg/kg/d for 1–2 wk or until improvement, followed by Itraconazole 200 mg PO tid × 3 days then 200 mg PO bid to complete at least 12 mo		To minimize toxicity, switching to oral therapy once the patient is stable should be considered. Bone and joint infections are usually treated for at least 12 mo with itraconazole. For Itraconazole, measure serum levels after at least 2 weeks, to ensure adequate drug exposure. Target level: >1.0 mcg/mL and <10.0 mcg/mL

continued

| | TREATMENT RECOMMENDATIONS | | |
MANIFESTATION	PRIMARY RECOMMENDATION	ALTERNATIVE RECOMMENDATION	COMMENTS
Central Nervous System Involvement (with or without other manifestations)			
	Lipid preparations of amphotericin B[1] 5 mg/kg/d × 4–6 wk followed by an oral azole for ≥12 mo		It has been suggested that liposomal amphotericin B achieves higher CNS levels than other lipid formulations When switching to oral azole, options include fluconazole[1] 800 mg PO qd,[3] itraconazole 200 mg PO bid or tid,[3] or voriconazole (Vfend)[1] 200–400[3] mg PO bid Longer durations of therapy may be necessary in the immunocompromised host
Special Populations			
Immunocompromised	Lipid formulation of amphotericin B 3–5 mg/kg/d OR Amphotericin B deoxycholate 0.7–1 mg/kg/d for 1–2 wk or until improvement, followed by Itraconazole 200 mg PO tid × 3 days then 200 mg PO bid to complete at least 12 mo		Lifelong suppression with itraconazole 200 mg PO qd may be required for those in whom immunosuppression cannot be reversed
Pregnant patients	Lipid formulation of amphotericin B 3–5 mg/kg/d		No duration of lipid formulation amphotericin B treatment provided; continue until clinical cure During pregnancy, azoles should be avoided because of potential teratogenicity If the placenta or newborn demonstrates evidence of infection, give amphotericin B deoxycholate 1.0 mg/kg/d
Children: mild to moderate	Itraconazole[1] 10 mg/kg/d for 6–12 mo		Maximum dose of itraconazole should be 400 mg/d
Children: moderate to severe	Amphotericin B deoxycholate 0.7–10.0 mg/kg/d OR Lipid formulation amphotericin B 3–5 mg/kg/d × 1–2 wk followed by itraconazole 10 mg/kg/d × 12 mo		

Modified from Chapman SW, Bradsher RW, Campbell GD, et al: Practice guidelines for the management of patients with blastomycosis. Clin Infect Dis 2000;30:679; and Chapman SW, Dismukes WE, Proia LA, et al: Clinical practice guidelines for the management of blastomycosis: 2008 update by the Infectious Diseases Society of America. Clin Infect Dis 2008;46:1801–12.
[1]Not FDA approved for this indication.
[3]Exceeds dosage recommended by the manufacturer.

the potentially toxic amphotericin B to a less-toxic agent (usually an azole). It is important to note that amphotericin B in cumulative doses of 1.5 to 2.5 grams for persons with disseminated blastomycosis, with life-threatening disease, or in those who are immunocompromised or pregnant, can lead to cure without relapses.

In patients with overwhelming pulmonary disease, amphotericin B-based products are the therapeutic agents of choice. Although acute respiratory distress syndrome (ARDS) can complicate the management of these patients, data on the beneficial role of corticosteroids in the management of patients with overwhelming pulmonary disease or ARDS are limited to few case reports. For patients with less-severe pulmonary disease, an alternative to amphotericin B is a 6- to 12-month course of oral itraconazole. A similarly prolonged course of oral itraconazole is also appropriate for persons with bone and joint disease. The precise duration of therapy, however, is unknown and should be individualized. The same is true for cutaneous blastomycosis. For persons with CNS blastomycosis, an initial treatment course of 4 to 6 weeks with intravenous lipid formulation of amphotericin B should be followed with an oral azole to complete at least 12 months of therapy. For those who are immunocompromised, prolonged therapy is also necessary. Patients who are immunosuppressed and in whom the immunosuppression cannot be reversed can require lifelong suppressive itraconazole therapy at 200 mg per day. Additional details for the management of the various stages of blastomycosis should be sought from the most current version of the IDSA guidelines.

References

Bariola JR, Perry P, Pappas PG, et al: Blastomycosis of the central nervous system: a multicenter review of diagnosis and treatment in the modern era, *Clin Infect Dis* 50:797–804, 2010.

Bush JW, Wuerz T, Embil JM, Del Bigio MR, McDonald PJ, Krawitz S: Outcomes of persons with blastomycosis involving the central nervous system, *Diagn Microbiol Infect Dis* 76(2):175–181, 2013.

Chapman SW, Sullivan DC: Blastomyces dermatitidis. In Mandell GL, Bennett JE, Dolin R, editors: *Mandell, Douglas, and Bennett's Principles and Practice of Infectious Diseases*, 7th ed., Philadelphia, 2010, Elsevier, pp 3319–3332.

Chapman SW, Lin AC, Hendricks KA, et al: Endemic blastomycosis in Mississippi: Epidemiological and clinical studies, *Semin Respir Infect* 12:219–228, 1997.

Chapman SW, Dismukes WE, Proia LA, et al: Clinical practice guidelines for the management of blastomycosis: 2008 update by the Infectious Diseases Society of America, *Clin Infect Dis* 46:1801–1812, 2008.

Choptiany M, Wiebe L, Limerick B, et al: Risk factors for acquisition of endemic blastomycosis, *Can J Infect Dis Med Microbiol* 20:117–121, 2009.

Crampton TL, Light RB, Berg GM, et al: Epidemiology and clinical spectrum of blastomycosis diagnosed at Manitoba hospitals, *Clin Infect Dis* 34:1310–1316, 2002.

Litvinov IV, St-Germain G, Pelletier R, Paradis M, Sheppard DC: Endemic human blastomycosis in Quebec, Canada, 1988–2011, *Epidemiol Infect* 141(6):1143–1147, 2013.

Martynowicz MA, Prakash UBS: Pulmonary blastomycosis: An appraisal of diagnostic techniques, *Chest* 121:768–773, 2002.

Meyer KC, McManus EJ, Maki DG: Overwhelming pulmonary blastomycosis associated with the adult respiratory distress syndrome, *N Engl J Med* 329:1231–1236, 1993.

Oppenheimer M, Cheang M, Trepman E, et al: Orthopedic manifestations of blastomycosis, *South Med J* 100:570–578, 2007.

Pappas PG: Blastomycosis in the immunocompromised patient, *Semin Respir Infect* 12:243–251, 1997.

Ward BA, Parent AD, Raila F: Indications for the surgical management of central nervous system blastomycosis, *Surg Neurol* 43:379–388, 1995.

CHRONIC OBSTRUCTIVE PULMONARY DISEASE

Method of
Michael L. Corriveau, MD; and J. Barry Fagan, MD

CURRENT DIAGNOSIS

- Chronic obstructive pulmonary disease (COPD) is a treatable, though not curable, disease.
- Smoking is the most common risk factor for COPD worldwide.
- Eleven million Americans are diagnosed with COPD. An additional 11 million Americans have COPD but have not been diagnosed.
- Alpha 1 antitrypsin deficiency occurs in 1 in every 1500 to 3000 individuals of European ancestry and is treatable by alpha-1 antitrypsin augmentation.
- Dyspnea, cough, and sputum production are common presenting complaints.
- Exam may reveal use of accessory muscles of ventilation, increased AP diameter, diminished breath sounds, wheezing, rhonchi, or crackles.
- Spirometry is the cornerstone of the diagnosis of COPD. COPD is defined by a reduction in the forced expiratory volume in 1 second/forced vital capacity (FEV1/FVC).
- The severity of COPD is defined by the FEV1 percent of predicted; mild (stage 1) FEV1 >79%; moderate (stage 2) FEV1 50% to 79%; severe (stage 3) FEV1 30% to 49%; very severe (stage 4) FEV1 <30%.

CURRENT THERAPY

- Smoking cessation is the cornerstone of COPD management. Counselling and pharmacotherapy improve quit rates.
- Patients with COPD should receive both pneumococcal and influenza vaccines.
- Pulmonary rehabilitation improves activity capacity and quality of life and decreases dyspnea and hospitalization.
- Supplemental oxygen is used for resting, nocturnal, or exertional hypoxemia. Supplemental oxygen use prolongs life in those with resting hypoxemia (PaO2 < 89%).
- Pharmacotherapy can improve symptoms and decrease exacerbation rate.
- Proper inhaler technique is necessary for maximal benefit from inhaled medications.
- Short-acting beta agonists are appropriate for mild, intermittent symptoms.
- A long-acting beta agonist (LABA), long-acting antimuscarinic (LAMA), or both may be added in patients with more frequent or severe dyspnea.
- Inhaled corticosteroids can decrease exacerbation frequency.
- Attention should be paid to management of retained secretions.
- Noninvasive ventilation can decrease hypercapnia and dyspnea in patients with chronic hypercapnic respiratory failure.
- A selected group of patients with severe disease may benefit from endobronchial valve treatment or surgical interventions, such as lung volume reduction surgery or lung transplantation.
- Exacerbations of COPD in outpatients may be managed with increased frequency of short-acting bronchodilators, systemic corticosteroids, and antibiotics.
- Palliative care is appropriate for patients with severe, refractory symptoms.

Epidemiology

Over 11 million Americans have chronic obstructive pulmonary disease (COPD), but including those undiagnosed, the number may be as high as 24 million. Prevalence varies state by state, from as low as 4% in Wisconsin and South Dakota to 10.4% in Kentucky. The global incidence in 2010 was estimated to be 384 million, with a global prevalence of 11.7%. The medical cost of COPD was estimated to be $32 billion/year in 2010 with an additional loss of $3.9 billion from absenteeism. These combined costs are estimated to increase to $49 billion annually by 2020. COPD is the third leading cause of death in the United States, accounting for more than 480,000 deaths/year, and is the fourth leading cause of death worldwide. Although the death rate from COPD in men in the United States has been dropping, the death rate in women is stable to rising.

Risk Factors

Smoking is the leading risk factor for COPD in the United States and around the world. 15.1% of American adults over age 18 are smokers (16.7% of men and 13.6% of women), which is approximately 36.5 million people. Globally, some 8 million people use the burning of biomass fuels or coal as their main source of energy for both cooking and heating. This indoor pollution is a significant risk factor for COPD in non-smoking women and children in the Middle East, Africa, and Asia, and it is estimated to kill 2 million women and children each year. Occupational dusts and chemicals are additional risk factors. Alpha-1 antitrypsin (A1A) deficiency is an important genetic risk factor for COPD. A1A occurs in 1 in every 1500 to 3000 individuals of European ancestry, but is less common in Asian and black populations. The metalloproteinase 12 gene is associated with decline in lung function; the relationship between other genes and reduction in lung function is less well understood. It appears that women are more susceptible to the effects of cigarette smoke than men. Other factors possibly playing a role in COPD development include childhood respiratory infections, asthma, and low socioeconomic status.

Pathophysiology

COPD is an inflammatory lung disease, caused by an imbalance between pro-inflammatory cytokines, enzymes, and effector cells, and the pulmonary defense mechanisms. An increase is seen in the number of pro-inflammatory cells, including circulating neutrophils and CD8 T lymphocytes as well as the number of macrophages in bronchial mucosa. CD8+ cells have the potential to release tumor necrosis factor α, perforins, and granzymes, though the exact role of T lymphocytes in COPD remains unclear. Neutrophils produce proteases which have the potential to cause alveolar destruction, elastase destruction, and mucus hypersecretion. Macrophages produce proteases as well as a variety of inflammatory mediators. Cigarette smoke promotes the release of these pro-inflammatory mediators and also inactivates several antiproteases, causing an inflammation/antiinflammation imbalance. This imbalance causes a cycle of injury and repair which results in permanent damage to airways, lung parenchyma, and vasculature. The airways become narrowed by increased numbers of goblet cells, increased size of submucosal glands, mucosal thickening, collagen deposition, ciliary dysfunction (promoting retention of secretions within the airway), and destruction of alveolar walls and alveolar support. Loss of pulmonary vascular bed, vascular remodeling, and arterial vasoconstriction lead to hypoxemia from ventilation perfusion mismatch and pulmonary hypertension.

Airway obstruction results in air trapping, hyperinflation, and flattening of the diaphragms. As the diaphragms flatten, the patient requires the use of accessory muscles of ventilation to move air. Airway narrowing or collapse increases the resistance to airflow, increasing the work of breathing and resulting in dyspnea. Lung compliance is decreased at high lung volumes, so breathing at high lung volumes due to hyperinflation also results in dyspnea. Work of breathing is increased at rest in COPD and increases exponentially with activity. Dyspnea often leads to the vicious cycle of decreased activity, deconditioning, and progressive disability.

Diagnosis

Most patients with COPD present to their provider with complaints of dyspnea, cough, and sputum production, or decreased activity capacity. This presentation may be relatively late in the disease course. Many smokers accept their cough as a "smoker's cough." Non-smokers have a large ventilatory reserve; we breathe about 5 L/min, but our maximum ventilatory volume is approximately 180 L/min. Because of this, especially if the patient is sedentary, they may not notice dyspnea until there has been considerable loss of pulmonary function.

The diagnosis of COPD should be considered in all patients with dyspnea, cough, sputum production, or exposure to risk factors. A careful history should include questions regarding quantity and duration of smoking and exposure to passive smoking or other occupational or environmental exposures. The patient should be asked about activity capacity; activities resulting in dyspnea, cough, and mucus production; and ease or difficulty clearing secretions. The input from a family member or friend is valuable, in that the patient may have become desensitized to dyspnea. On observation, the patient may be found in the "tripod" position, resting arms on a surface elevating the clavicles, which places the accessory muscles of ventilation at better mechanical advantage. (This is why patients will often relate that they can walk further while using a shopping cart "tripoding" on the cart's handles.) Patients may be observed to be pursed lip breathing, exhaling through pursed lips, elevating the pressure in the airways, stenting them open and allowing a fuller expiration, decreasing air trapping and hyperinflation. Percussion may reveal evidence of hyperinflation. Auscultation may reveal wheezing or prolonged expiration resulting from airway obstruction, as well as rhonchi from retained secretions in the airways. Normal breath sounds originate in the terminal airways, and emphysematous destruction of these airways results in diminished breath sounds. Emphysema results in increased compliance of the lung, which raises the closing volume (the volume of air within the lung at which airways close). The closing volume may rise above functional residual capacity (the normal end-expiratory volume) causing inspiratory crackles.

Spirometry is the cornerstone of diagnosis of COPD. Airway obstruction is defined by an FEV1/FEC of <70%. Patients with airway obstruction may be able to exhale much of their vital capacity (VC), but because of airways narrowing, they cannot do it very quickly, resulting in the low ratio. The degree of obstruction is defined by the FEV1 percent of predicted value (Figure 1). It is recommended that an A1A be obtained in all patients diagnosed with COPD. It is important to note that A1A is an acute-phase reactant and can be elevated during an exacerbation of COPD; it is therefore best to obtain when the patient is clinically stable.

Differential Diagnosis

COPD may be confused with other obstructive airway diseases, most notably asthma. Asthma will most often present at a younger age, though it may be diagnosed during any decade of

SEVERITY	SPIROMETRY
Stage I: mild	FEV1/FVC <70% FEV1 ≥80%
Stage II: moderate	FEV1/FVC <70% 50% ≤FEV1 <80%
Stage III: severe	FEV1/FVC <70% 30% ≤FEV1 <50%
Stage IV: very severe	FEV1/FVC <70% FEV1 <30%

Abbreviations: FEV1 = forced expiratory volume in 1 second; FVC = forced vital capacity

Figure 1 Chronic obstructive pulmonary disease staging. *FEV1,* Forced expiratory volume in 1 second; *FVC,* forced vital capacity.

life. Asthmatics generally have more reversibility and less fixed obstruction, but overlap is seen. Both may have hyperinflation and reduction in forced expiratory flows on pulmonary function testing, but a reduction in diffusing capacity would be more characteristic of COPD. Exhaled NO will more often be elevated in asthma. Eosinophils are characteristically elevated in the sputum blood and BAL fluid in asthmatics, whereas neutrophils are more commonly elevated in patients with COPD. Considerable overlap occurs in each of these areas. There are a small percentage of patients where COPD and asthma cannot be differentiated; this is called the "overlap syndrome."

Treatment of Stable Chronic Obstructive Pulmonary Disease

The goals of treatment of COPD include improving quality of life, decreasing dyspnea, increasing activity capacity, preventing and treating complications and exacerbations, and prolonging life.

Smoking Cessation

Smoking cessation is the cornerstone of management of COPD. Stopping smoking, along with supplemental oxygen in patients with severe chronic hypoxemia, are the only two interventions which prolong life in patients with COPD. During each clinical interaction with a patient who smokes, it is appropriate to *ask* about their smoking status, *advise* all smokers to quit, *assess* the willingness of the patient to quit, *assist* the patient in quitting, and *arrange* a follow-up visit. Brief counselling alone can improve quit rate. In those patients who express a willingness to attempt to quit, adding pharmacotherapy to counselling is appropriate. Considerations for pharmacotherapy include nicotine replacement therapy, bupropion (Zyban), and varenicline (Chantix) (Figure 2). E-cigarettes are not currently recommended to assist with smoking cessation.

Pulmonary Rehabilitation

Pulmonary rehabilitation programs are widely available and can be defined as multidisciplinary programs, which seek to improve the quality of life for patients with COPD or other lung diseases. Programs vary in content, but will always include an exercise and an educational component, supervised by a respiratory therapist. They often meet 2 or 3 times weekly and last about 6 to 8 weeks. The educational component includes information on the disease state, medications used to manage COPD, energy-conserving techniques such as pacing activities, breathing techniques such as pursed-lip breathing, and what steps to take during an exacerbation. Programs may include nutritional advice, smoking cessation education, or psychosocial counselling. The exercise component is tailored to the individual patient and often includes treadmill or stationary bicycle exercise, light weights, arm ergometry, and stretching. Programs stress the importance of maintaining exercise following completion of the program and may offer a phase 3 component for continued exercise. Pulmonary rehabilitation has many proven benefits, including decreased dyspnea, improved quality of life, improved activity capacity, and decreased hospitalization. Pulmonary rehabilitation may be offered to any COPD patient with symptoms or high risk of exacerbation.

Vaccinations

Annual influenza vaccines are recommended for all patients with COPD. Polysaccharide pneumococcal vaccines (PPSV23) are recommended for all patients who smoke and/or have COPD with a repeat dose given 5 years after the first dose. At age 65, PCV13 is given, since it is more important for those that are immunocompromised, which happens with more advance age.

Medications

Commonly used medications for the treatment of stable COPD are listed in Figure 3. The beta-agonists stimulate beta 2 receptors on airway smooth muscle, causing muscle relaxation and bronchodilation. The short-acting beta-agonists have onset of action in 1 to 3 minutes and duration of action 4 to 6 hours. Because of their quick onset and short duration of action, they are used

Medication	Dosage and Administration
Nicotine Transdermal (NicoDerm CQ)	21 mg/24 hours, 14 mg/24 hours, 7 mg/24 hours If >10 cigarettes/D, then use 21 mg/D for 6 weeks, then 14 mg/D for 2 weeks, then 7 mg/D for 2 weeks, If <10 cigarettes/D, then use 14 mg/D for 6 weeks, then 7 mg/D for 2 weeks
Nicotine lozenges (Nicorette)	4 mg, 2 mg weeks 1–6, 1 lozenge every 1–2 hours, weeks 7–9 1 lozenge every 2–4 hours, weeks 10–12, 1 lozenge every 4–8 hours
Nicotine gum (Nicorelief, Thrive)	4 mg, 2 mg weeks 1–6, 1 gum every 1–2 hours, weeks 7–9 1 gum every 2–4 hours, weeks 10–12, 1 gum every 4–8 hours
Nicotine inhaler (Nicotrol)	10 mg/cartridge up to 12 weeks, 6–16 cartidges/day up to 12 weeks (if necessary), gradual reduction
Nicotine nasal spray (Nicotrol NS)	0.5 mg/spray each nostril, beginning 1–2/hour, maximum /hour, maximum 80 sprays/day up to 8 weeks, then taper up to 6 weeks
Bupropion hydrochloride SR (Zyban)	150 mg per day, first 3 days, then 150 mg bid
Varenicline (Chantix)	Day 1–3, 0.5 mg q day, day 4–7, 0.5 mg bid, day 8–end of treatment, 1 mg bid. Patients who quit at 12 weeks may be treated an additional 12 weeks.

Figure 2 Smoking cessation medications.

Medication	Dosage
Short-acting bronchodilators:	
Albuterol (multiple brands)	2 puffs q 4–6 hours, prn
Levalbuterol (Xopenex)	1–2 puffs q 4–6 hours prn
Ipratropium (Atrovent)	2 inhalations 4 times a day
Albuterol/ipratropium (Combivent Respimat)	1 inhalation 4 times a day
Long-acting beta agonists:	
Salmeterol (Serevent)	one inhalation twice daily
Indacaterol (Arcapta)	inhale contents of one capsule q day
Olodaterol (Striverdi)	2 puffs once a day, same time of day
Long-acting antimuscarinics:	
Tiotropium (Spiriva Handihaler,	2 inhalations of the powder contents of a single Spiriva capsule once daily
Spiriva Respimat)	2 inhalations once daily
Aclidinium (Tudorza)	1 inhalation twice daily
Combination medications:	
Umeclidinium/vilanterol (Anoro)	1 inhalation once daily
Budesonide/formoterol (Symbicort 160/4.5, 80/4.5)	2 puffs twice daily
Fluticasone/salmeterol (Advair Diskus 100/50, 250/50, 500/50)	1 inhalation twice daily
(Advair HFA 45/21, 115/21, 230/21)	2 puffs twice daily
Mometasone/formoterol (Dulera 100/5, 200/5)	2 inhalations twice daily
Olodaterol/tiotropium (Stiolto)	2 inhalations once daily
Fluticasone/vilanterol (Breo 100/25, 200/25)	1 inhalation once daily
Formoterol/glycopyrrolate (Bevespi)	2 inhalations twice daily
Fluticasone/umeclidinium/vilanterol (Trelegy)	1 inhalation once daily

(Advair Diskus 100/50, 250/50, 500/50[1]) (Advair HFA 45/21, 115/21, 230/21)

Figure 3 Commonly used inhaled medications for stable chronic obstructive pulmonary disease.

as "rescue" or prn medications. Some long-acting beta-agonists also have rapid onset of action, but the duration of action is 12 to 24 hours. Potential side effects of beta-agonists include tremor, tachycardia, and, uncommonly, hypokalemia.

The antimuscarinic bronchodilators bind to muscarinic receptors, which are found on smooth muscle and submucosal glands. Two of these receptors, the M1 and M3 receptor, facilitate acetylcholine transmission which results in bronchoconstriction. Potential side effects of the antimuscarinics include dry mouth and urinary hesitancy. The beta-agonists and antimuscarinics have additive effects on bronchial smooth muscle. Inhaled corticosteroids decrease airway inflammation and have been shown to decrease the frequency of exacerbation of COPD. Unlike asthma, inhaled corticosteroids are not used as sole maintenance therapy in COPD. Potential side-effects of the inhaled corticosteroids include a small increase in risk of pneumonia and oral candidiasis. There are now many varieties of inhaler devices. Instruction in the use of the devices and observation of proper technique is necessary to ensure maximal benefit.

In the 2019 Global Initiative for Chronic Obstructive Lung Disease (GOLD) guidelines (https://www.guidelines.co.uk/respiratory/gold-copd-2019-strategy/454454.article), medication recommendations are dictated by a classification system based on symptom score and exacerbation history. Patients are categorized as having either zero or one exacerbation, not requiring hospitalization, or two or more exacerbations, or at least one exacerbation requiring hospitalization. Symptom severity is based on a symptom scoring scale, such as the COPD Assessment Test (Figure 4). On the COPD Assessment Test, the patient is asked a series of 8 questions, grading severity as 0 to 5. The sum of the scores is used to categorize the patient in the GOLD classification grid.

Patients in group A are given a trial of short- or long-acting bronchodilator. The medication is continued if the patient is determined to have benefitted from the intervention. Group B patients should be started on a long-acting bronchodilator, either LABA or LAMA. If the patient has continued dyspnea, LAMA and LABA may be used together. For patients with severe dyspnea,

treatment may begin with both agents. Initial therapy for group C patients is a LAMA. For patients with persisting exacerbations adding a LABA is the primary choice. Adding an ICS would be a secondary choice. Recommended initial treatment for group D patients is a LABA/LAMA combination. Consideration could be given to initiating treatment with a LABA/ICS combination, in patients with prominent asthmatic symptoms or an eosinophil count ≥300 cells/microLiter. Patients with continuing exacerbations may be switched to a LABA/LAMA/ICS combination. In patients with persisting exacerbations on this treatment, the phosphodiesterase-4 inhibitor roflumilast (Daliresp) 500 mcg/day or prophylactic azithromycin (Zithromax)[1] 250 mg/day or 500 mg on Monday, Wednesday, and Friday have been shown to decrease the frequency of exacerbations.

Sustained release theophylline preparations have a mild bronchodilator effect and may be added to an otherwise maximized regimen, or used when cost considerations prohibit the use of long-acting bronchodilators.

Retained secretions may increase dyspnea and hypoxemia. Management may include use of guaifenesin[1] 200 to 400 mg orally every 4 hours as needed, not to exceed 2.4 g/day; potassium iodide (SSKI) 0.3 mL (300 mg) or 0.6 mL (600 mg) diluted in one glassful of water, fruit juice or milk 3 to 4 times daily, and positive expiratory pressure devices, such as the Acapella.

On follow-up visits, medications may be escalated or de-escalated based on symptoms or exacerbations.

Noninvasive Ventilation

Bi-level ventilation has been used in patients with chronic hypercapnic respiratory failure. Regular use of noninvasive ventilation in this population has shown improvement in walk distance, dyspnea, and hypercapnia by increasing minute ventilation and decreasing work of breathing. Medicare guidelines for prescribing require documented hypercapnia ($PaCO_2$ >51) and also require a nocturnal oximetry showing desaturation to SaO_2 <89% for at least 5 consecutive minutes during sleep. Initial settings are somewhat empiric, often beginning at IPAP 12 cm H_2O and EPAP 5 cm H_2O. These settings may be adjusted based on comfort and degree of hypercapnia.

Surgical Remedies

Lung volume reduction surgery is a consideration for patients with severe disease meeting certain criteria. The rationale is that removing the most diseased portions of lung in patients with emphysema will decrease hyperinflation, improve ventilation/perfusion matching, and decrease lung compliance. This elevates the diaphragms, placing them at better mechanical advantage, and stents open the airways. Selection criteria come from the National Emphysema Therapy Trial (NETT) and include patients with emphysema who are <75 years old, smoke-free for 6 months, on no more than 20 mg/day of prednisone with functional limitation good compliance, and severe dyspnea despite maximum medical therapy. Laboratory evaluation must demonstrate upper lobe predominant emphysema on chest CT, hyperinflation, low FEV1 (≤45% predicted; ≥15% predicted if age over 70), and post-rehabilitation 6-minute walk >140 m. Exclusionary criteria include morbid obesity, significant comorbidities, previous chest surgery or chest wall deformity which might interfere with the procedure, resting pulmonary hypertension, well-preserved exercise capacity, and significant pleural or interstitial disease.

Lung transplantation may be considered in patients < 65 years old (<60 years old for double lung transplant), with FEV1 <25% predicted and/or $PaCO_2$ >55 mm Hg and/or pulmonary hypertension, especially in patients with progressive disease requiring supplemental oxygen. Exclusionary criteria include other major organ dysfunction, recent malignancy, HIV-positive status, and hepatitis B or C.

I never cough	0 1 2 3 4 5	I cough all the time
I have no phlegm (mucus) in my chest at all	0 1 2 3 4 5	My chest is completely full of phlegm (mucus)
My chest does not feel tight at all	0 1 2 3 4 5	My chest feels very tight
When I walk up a hill or one flight of stairs I am not breathless	0 1 2 3 4 5	When I walk up a hill or one flight of stairs I am very breathless
I am not limited doing any activities at home	0 1 2 3 4 5	I am very limited doing activities at home
I am confident leaving my home despite my lung condition	0 1 2 3 4 5	I am not at all confident leaving my home because of my lung condition
I sleep soundly	0 1 2 3 4 5	I don't sleep soundly because of my lung condition
I have lots of energy	0 1 2 3 4 5	I have no energy at all

Figure 4 Chronic obstructive pulmonary disease assessment test.

---

[1] Not FDA approved for this indication.

An emerging therapy is endobronchial valve therapy, in which one-way valves are placed in some airways endoscopically to produce a nonsurgical lung volume reduction. This treatment has been shown to result in improved pulmonary function, exercise capacity, and quality of life in some patients with emphysema.

Supplemental Oxygen

The use of supplemental oxygen in patients with COPD is based on the fact that its use in severely hypoxemic patients helps prevent pulmonary hypertension, cor pulmonale, and premature death. Indications for continuous supplemental oxygen are resting PaO_2 ≤55 mm Hg or PaO_2 56 to 59 mm Hg with evidence of complication, such as pulmonary hypertension or polycythemia. Supplemental oxygen may be prescribed during activity for SaO_2 <89% during activity, and may be prescribed during sleep for patients with SaO_2 <89% for at least 5 minutes during sleep.

Treatment of Exacerbations of Chronic Obstructive Pulmonary Disease

COPD exacerbations are defined as an acute increase in symptoms requiring an adjustment in medication. They are defined as mild (requiring only bronchodilator adjustment), moderate (requiring antibiotics and/or oral corticosteroids), or severe (requiring hospitalization or emergency department management). Some factors which help to determine the need for hospitalization include severity of symptoms, failure to respond to initial management, increasing hypoxemia or hypercapnia, or mental status changes. Underlying comorbidities or lack of support at home may also contribute to the need for hospitalization. Exacerbations may be triggered by viral or bacterial infections or environmental factors.

An increase in frequency of use of as-needed short-acting beta agonists is initial management for exacerbations. Systemic corticosteroids improve pulmonary function measurement and shorten recovery time. Prednisone 40 mg/day for 5 days is effective and has been shown to have similar effect to intravenous steroid administration. The addition of an antibiotic course, 5 to 7 days, has been shown to improve outcomes in outpatients with either increased dyspnea or increased sputum production plus increased sputum purulence. Antibiotics have been shown to decrease mortality and the incidence of nosocomial infection in patients with exacerbation who require invasive or noninvasive mechanical ventilation.

References

Center for Disease Control and Prevention: Chronic Obstructive Pulmonary Disease, Available at https://www.cdc.gov/copd. Accessed 13 January 2017.
DeCamp M, Lipsom D, Krasna M: The evaluation and preparation of the patient for lung volume reduction surgery, *Proc Am Thorac Soc* 5:427, 2008.
Global Initiative for Chronic Obstructive Pulmonary Disease (GOLD): Global strategy for the diagnosis, management and prevention of COPD 2017, Available at http://www.goldcopd.org. Accessed 10 February 2017.
Hunninghake GM, Cho MH, Tesfaigzi Y, et al: MMP12, lung function and COPD in high risk populations, *N Engl J Med* 361:2599, 2009.
International guidelines for the selection of lung transplant candidates, *Am J Respir Crit Care Med* 158:335, 1998.
Klooster K, Hacken N, Hartman J, et al: Endobronchial valves for emphysema without interlobar collateral ventilation, *N Engl J Med* 373:2325, 2015.
MacNee W: Pathogenesis of chronic obstructive pulmonary disease, *Proc Am Thorac Soc* 2:258, 2005.
Quon BS, Gan WQ, Sin DD: Contemporary management of acute exacerbations of COPD: a systematic review and metaanalysis, *Chest* 133(3): 2008.
Silverman EK, Weiss ST, Drazen EM, et al: Gender-related differences in severe, early onset chronic obstructive pulmonary disease, *Am J Resp Crit Care Med* 162:2152, 2000.
Treating Tobacco Use and Dependence: Available at https://www.ahrq.gov/professionals/clinicians-providers/guidelines-recommendations/tobacco. Accessed February 19, 2017.
Woodhead M, Blasi F, Ewig S, et al: Guidelines for the management of adult lower respiratory tract infections, *Eur Respir J* 133(1): 2008.
World Health Organization: Chronic Respiratory Diseases. Available at: http://www.who.int/respiratory/copd. Accessed 3 January 2017.

COCCIDIOIDOMYCOSIS

Method of
Gregory M. Anstead, MD, PhD

CURRENT DIAGNOSIS

- Maintain a high index of suspicion in patients from endemic areas and travelers
- Diagnostic tests include:
  - Serologic detection of immunoglobulin M and immunoglobulin G antibodies by immunodiffusion, complement fixation, and enzyme immunoassay
  - Culture of sputum, exudates, cerebrospinal fluid, and tissue
  - Direct observation of *Coccidioides* spherules in histopathologic and cytologic specimens
  - Urine antigen enzyme immunoassay

CURRENT THERAPY

Pulmonary Infection

- No risk factors for dissemination; not severe disease—observe
- Risk factors; prolonged symptoms—fluconazole (Diflucan)[1] 400 mg/day or itraconazole (Sporanox)[1] 200 mg twice a day for 3 to 6 months
- Diffuse or severe pneumonia—amphotericin B (Fungizone) 1 mg/kg/day or lipid formulation of amphotericin (Abelcet, AmBisome)[1] 5 mg/kg/day; after improvement, switch to azole; treat for 1 year
- Chronic fibrocavitary disease—azole therapy for at least 1 year; resection in selected cases

Disseminated Disease

- Nonmeningeal, severe disease—amphotericin B 1 mg/kg/day or lipid formulation of amphotericin[1] 5 mg/kg/day; after improvement, switch to azole for 1 to 2 years; consider posaconazole (Noxafil)[1] suspension 200 mg four times daily or voriconazole (Vfend)[1] 400–600 mg/day daily in refractory cases
- Nonmeningeal, slowly progressive—azole therapy for 1 to 2 years; itraconazole[1] preferred for bony involvement; consider posaconazole[1] or voriconazole[1] (as above) in refractory cases
- Meningeal, central nervous system involvement—fluconazole[1] 800 to 2000 mg/day[3]; intrathecal amphotericin B[1] or voriconazole (Vfend)[1] 200 mg twice daily in refractory cases[1]; shunting for hydrocephalus; consider corticosteroids if vasculitis is present

[1]Not FDA approved for this indication.
[3]Exceeds dosage recommended by the manufacturer.

Coccidioidomycosis is caused by soil fungi of the genus *Coccidioides*, divided genetically into *Coccidioides immitis* (California isolates) and *Coccidioides posadasii* (isolates outside California). There are no distinct clinical differences between the two species. *Coccidioides* occurs only in the Western hemisphere, primarily in the southwestern United States (Arizona and parts of California, New Mexico, Utah, Nevada, and Texas) and in northern Mexico, areas characterized by arid to semiarid climates, hot summers, low altitude, alkaline soil, and sparse vegetation. Hyperendemic areas include the San Joaquin Valley of California and Pima, Pinal, and Maricopa Counties in Arizona. *Coccidioides* is also found in parts of Latin America (Guatemala, Honduras, Nicaragua, Argentina, Paraguay, Venezuela, and Colombia). Cases may be observed in nonendemic areas because of travel or reactivation of prior infection. In the United States, an estimated 150,000 cases of coccidioidomycosis occur annually, with the clinical presentation ranging from a self-limited respiratory infection to devastating disseminated disease. The incidence of coccidioidomycosis is increasing in the USA due to rising populations and the resulting construction in the endemic areas. Risk factors for increased severity of coccidioidomycosis include: receiving immunosuppressive medications (corticosteroids, transplant drugs, and tumor necrosis factor–alpha antagonists); pregnancy (esp. the third trimester); genetic factors (i.e., defects in the IL-12/interferon-γ axis and STAT3 pathways, certain ABO blood group and HLA types); and specific races/ethnicities (African Americans, Asian-Pacific Islanders, and Native Americans). Outbreaks may occur after dust storms, earthquakes, droughts, and activities causing soil disruption, such as construction and archeological digs. Persons with occupations involving exposure to soil are also at risk for acquiring coccidioidomycosis.

Coccidioides is dimorphic; in the soil, the organism exists in its mycelial form, which produces barrel-shaped arthroconidia. The usual means of infection is the inhalation of arthroconidia; uncommon routes include direct cutaneous inoculation and organ transplantation. Arthroconidia germinate to produce spherules filled with endospores, the characteristic tissue phase. Spherules rupture to release endospores, which form additional spherules. The spherules become surrounded by neutrophils and macrophages, which leads to granuloma formation. Both B and T lymphocytes are essential for host defense against this pathogen.

Clinical Manifestations

Coccidioidomycosis is asymptomatic in 60% of infected individuals. In the remaining 40% a self-limited, flu-like illness, with dry cough, pleuritic chest pain, myalgias, arthralgia, fever, sweats, anorexia, and weakness, develops 1 to 3 weeks after exposure. Primary infection may be accompanied by immune complex–mediated complications, including an erythematous macular rash, erythema multiforme, and erythema nodosum. Acute infection usually resolves without therapy, although symptoms may persist for weeks. In 5% of these patients, asymptomatic pulmonary residua persist, including pulmonary nodules and cavitation. Immunocompromised patients may develop chronic progressive pulmonary infection, with the evolution of thin-walled cavities that may rupture, leading to bronchopleural fistula and empyema formation.

Extrapulmonary disease develops in 1 of every 200 patients and can involve the skin, soft tissues, bones, joints, and meninges. The most common cutaneous lesions are verrucous papules, ulcers, or plaques. The spine is the most frequent site of osseous dissemination, although the typical lytic lesions may also occur in the skull, hands, feet, and tibia. Joint involvement is usually monoarticular and most commonly involves the ankle and knee. Fungemia may occur in immunocompromised patients and carries a poor prognosis.

In coccidioidal meningitis, the basilar meninges are usually affected. Cerebrospinal fluid findings include lymphocytic pleocytosis (often with eosinophilia), hypoglycorrhachia, and elevated protein levels. The mortality rate is greater than 90% at 1 year without therapy, and chronic infection is the rule. Hydrocephalus or hydrocephalus coexisting with brain infarction is associated with a higher mortality rate.

Coccidioidomycosis is a great imitator and has many diverse clinical presentations, including immune thrombocytopenia, ocular involvement, massive cervical lymphadenopathy, laryngeal and retropharyngeal abscesses, endocarditis, pericarditis, peritonitis, hepatitis, and lesions of the male and female genitals and urogenital tracts.

Diagnosis

Coccidioidomycosis may be diagnosed by direct observation of spherules in tissues or in wet mounts of sputa or exudates. The growth of *Coccidioides* in culture usually occurs in 3 to 5 days, with sporulation after 5 to 10 days. Definitive identification is made by DNA probe or exoantigen testing. Laboratory personnel should exercise extreme caution when handling cultures of *Coccidioides*.

Serologic methods are quite useful in establishing the diagnosis and for monitoring the course of the infection. Immunoglobulin M (IgM) antibodies are present soon after infection or relapse but then wane; quantification does not correlate with disease severity. The IgG antibody appears later and remains positive for months. Rising titers of IgG are associated with progressive disease, and declining titers are associated with resolution. The IgG antibodies are able to fix complement when combined with coccidioidal antigen, and can be detected by immunodiffusion for complement fixation (IDCF); titers of 1:16 or greater suggest disseminated disease. In the cerebrospinal fluid, a positive IDCF of any titer is considered diagnostic of meningitis and is much more sensitive than culture in making the diagnosis. An enzyme immunoassay is also available, but it is less specific. Recently, a specific urinary antigen test became available for the diagnosis of coccidioidomycosis; this assay has a sensitivity of 71% in moderate-to-severe disease, compared with 84% for culture, 29% for histopathologic examination, and 75% for serologic testing.

Treatment

In most patients, primary pulmonary infection resolves spontaneously without treatment. However, all patients require observation for at least 2 years to document resolution of infection and to identify any complications as soon as possible. For patients who have risk factors for disseminated disease (listed earlier), treatment is necessary. Other indications for treatment are severe disease (infiltrates involving both lungs or more than half of one lung; significant hilar or mediastinal lymphadenopathy; complement fixation titers >1:16) and highly symptomatic disease (weight loss >10%; night sweats present for >3 weeks; symptoms present for >2 months).

For diffuse or severe pneumonia, therapy with amphotericin B deoxycholate (Fungizone) 0.5 to 1.5 mg/kg/day, or a lipid formulation of amphotericin B (Abelcet or AmBisome)[1] 2 to 5 mg/kg/day should be given for several weeks, followed by an oral azole, such as itraconazole (Sporanox)[1] 200 mg twice daily or fluconazole (Diflucan)[1] 400 to 800 mg/day. The total duration of therapy should be at least 1 year; for immunosuppressed patients, oral azole therapy should be maintained as secondary prophylaxis. In HIV patients with CD4-positive T-cell counts greater than 250 cells/mm[3] who had focal pneumonias that responded to azoles, antifungals may be discontinued. Azole therapy may be used initially for less severe disease. During pregnancy, amphotericin B is the preferred drug, because of the teratogenicity of azoles.

An asymptomatic patient with a solitary nodule or pulmonary cavitation due to *C. immitis* does not require specific antifungal therapy or resection. However, the development of complications from the cavitation, such as hemoptysis or bacterial or fungal superinfection, necessitates initiation of azole therapy. Resection of the cavities is an alternative to antifungal therapy. Rupture of a cavity into the pleural space requires surgical intervention with closure by lobectomy with decortication, in addition to antifungal therapy. For chronic pneumonia, the initial treatment should be an oral azole for at least 1 year. If the disease persists, one may switch to another oral azole, increase the dose if fluconazole was initially selected, or switch to amphotericin B. Resection should be performed for patients with refractory focal lesions or severe hemoptysis.

The treatment of disseminated infection without central nervous system involvement is based on oral azole therapy, such as itraconazole[1] or fluconazole[1] (400 mg/day, or higher in case of fluconazole). If there is little or no improvement or if there is vertebral involvement, treatment with amphotericin B is recommended (dosage as for diffuse pneumonia). Concomitant surgical débridement or stabilization is also recommended. In patients with refractory coccidioidomycosis that has failed to respond to fluconazole, itraconazole, and amphotericin B and its lipid formulations, treatment with posaconazole (Noxafil)[1] suspension 200 mg four times daily with a fatty meal or voriconazole (Vfend)[1], at doses of 400–600 mg/day, has been successful. A posaconazole tablet with improved oral

---

[1] Not FDA approved for this indication.

bioavailability and an intravenous preparation are now available and likely these new forms of posaconazole are more efficacious. Clinical experience with voriconazole is limited.

For coccidioidal meningitis, lifetime treatment with azoles is indicated. Fluconazole[1], at doses of 800 mg/day or higher[3], is recommended. There have been a few reports of successful treatment of coccidioidal meningitis with voriconazole (Vfend)[1] 200 mg orally twice daily after a loading dose. Itraconazole is not recommended because of its irregular oral absorption. For patients with increased intracranial pressure at the time of meningitis diagnosis, repeated lumbar punctures are recommended. Obstructive hydrocephalus requires shunting. Intrathecal amphotericin B[1] is now strictly reserved for meningitis refractory to high-dose azoles or coccidioidal meningitis in the first trimester of pregnancy. In patients with CNS vasculitis with cerebrovascular accident due to coccidioidomycosis, those that received corticosteroids were less likely to develop additional infarcts compared to those who did not.

Reduction of immunosuppression is an important adjunct to antifungal therapy, including the initiation of antiretroviral therapy if the patient has HIV infection. In patients with AIDS and non-meningeal coccidioidomycosis, antifungal therapy can be discontinued when the CD4 count exceeds 250 cells/mm[3].

---

[1] Not FDA approved for this indication.
[3] Exceeds dosage recommended by the manufacturer.

References

Anstead GM, Corcoran G, Lewis J, et al: Refractory coccidioidomycosis treated with posaconazole, *Clin Infect Dis* 40:1770–1776, 2005.

Brown J, Benedict K, Park BJ, Thompson GR 3rd: Coccidioidomycosis: epidemiology, *Clin Epidemiol* 5:185–197, 2013.

Crum NF, Lederman ER, Stafford CM, et al: Coccidioidomycosis: a descriptive survey of a reemerging disease—clinical characteristics and emerging controversies, *Medicine (Baltimore)* 83:149–175, 2004.

Crum-Cianflone NF, Truett AA, Teneza-Mora N, et al: Unusual presentations of coccidioidomycosis: a case series and review of the literature, *Medicine (Baltimore)* 85:263–277, 2006.

Donovan FM, Zangeneh TT, Malo J, Galgiani JN: Top questions in the diagnosis and treatment of coccidioidomycosis, *Open Forum Infect Dis* 4:ofx197, 2017.

Freifeld A, Proia L, Andes D, et al: Voriconazole use for endemic fungal infections, *Antimicrob Agents Chemother* 53:1648–1651, 2009.

Gabe LM, Malo J, Knox KS: Diagnosis and management of coccidioidomycosis, *Clin Chest Med* 38:417–433, 2017.

Galgiani JN, Ampel NM, Blair JE, et al: 2016 Infectious Diseases Society of America (IDSA) clinical practice guideline for the treatment of coccidioidomycosis, *Clin Infect Dis* 63:e112–146, 2016.

Hartmann CA, Aye WT, Blair JE: Treatment considerations in pulmonary coccidioidomycosis, *Expert Rev Respir Med* 10:1079–1091, 2016.

Hector RF, Rutherford GW, Clarisse A, et al: The public health impact of coccidioidomycosis in Arizona and California, *Int J Environ Res Public Health* 8:1150–1173, 2011.

Johnson L, Gaab EM, Sanchez J, et al: Valley fever: danger lurking in a dust cloud, *Microbes Infect* 16:591–600, 2014.

Odio CD, Marciano BE, Galgiani JN, Holland SM: Risk factors for disseminated coccidioidomycosis, United States, *Emerg Infect Dis* 23(2), 2017.

Stockamp NW, Thompson GR 3rd: Coccidioidomycosis, *Infect Dis Clin North Am* 30:229–246, 2016.

Thompson GR 3rd, Blair JE, Wang S, et al: Adjunctive corticosteroid therapy in the treatment of coccidioidal meningitis, *Clin Infect Dis* 65:338–341, 2017.

Williams PL: Coccidioidal meningitis, *Ann N Y Acad Sci* 1111:377–384, 2007.

CYSTIC FIBROSIS

Method of
Hanna Phan, PharmD; and Cori L. Daines, MD

CURRENT DIAGNOSIS

- Cystic fibrosis (CF) is an autosomal recessive genetic disorder that causes dysfunction of the cystic fibrosis transmembrane conductance regulator (CFTR) on the apical surface of epithelial cells leading to inability to move adequate ions, specifically chloride, out of the cell.

- Basic defect leads to thick, dehydrated mucus in the respiratory tract manifesting as chronic cough and recurrent infections
- Diagnosis is made via a sweat chloride test using quantitative pilocarpine iontophoresis
- Close to 2000 mutations of CFTR are known, leading to a multitude of clinical phenotypes and severity of disease

CURRENT THERAPY

- A given patient's overall treatment regimen is often based on various factors including age, clinical presentation, organ systems involved, disease progression/severity, CFTR genotype, and comorbidities
- Primary treatment is augmented airway clearance with bronchodilators, mucolytics or mucus hydrators, and mechanical airway vibration
- Nutritional therapy consists of enzymes and vitamin replacement for those who are pancreatic insufficient

Epidemiology

Cystic fibrosis is an autosomal recessive, inherited multisystem disease caused by mutations of the cystic fibrosis transmembrane regulator (CFTR) on chromosome 7. There are currently close to 2000 mutations of CFTR known. Carriage of the gene is highest in individuals of Northern European decent, leading to an incidence of 1 in 3000 non-Hispanic Caucasians in the United States. Incidence is lower in Hispanic Caucasians and those of African descent. There are approximately 30,000 individuals with CF in the United States, 70,000 individuals worldwide, and approximately 1000 new diagnoses are made each year. Average life expectancy is increasing with new therapies but still varies among countries. In the United States and Canada, life expectancy is well beyond 40 years.

Pathophysiology

Cystic Fibrosis Transmembrane Regulator Genotypes—Genotype/Phenotype

CFTR is a protein in the adenosine triphosphate–binding cassette transporter family that has two transmembrane domains, two nucleotide-binding domains, and a regulatory domain. It shares structural elements with other membrane pumps. Mutations in the gene coding the CFTR fall broadly into six categories. The first category includes premature truncation mutations, leading to no full-length protein. The second category includes the Phe508del (i.e., F508del) mutation, which is the most common mutation, accounting for 75% of all mutations in the United States. The category II mutations are mutations that result in the cell degrading the CFTR prior to full maturation and function. Class III mutations result in a chloride channel at the cell surface that does not function or a "gating" mutation. Class IV mutations result in a chloride channel embedded at the cell surface that has decreased and ineffective chloride movement function, and class V mutations are promoter or splicing abnormalities resulting in reduced number of functional chloride channels at the cell surface. The newest class of mutations, class VI mutations, result in a chloride channel that is not stable on the cell surface and therefore, like class V mutations, insufficient quantities of chloride channel at the cell surface.

Understanding the genetics of any given individual with CF is vital in understanding the pathophysiology. Disease manifestation is directly related to the amount of chloride moved at the cell surface. Class I, II, and III mutations result in minimal chloride movement, less than 5% of normal, and result in "classic" or severe disease phenotype. Presence of one mutation in the class IV, V, or VI category results in greater chloride movement at the surface, typically 10% or more, and a "mild" or "nonclassic" phenotype. Approximately 15% of individuals with CF fall into this latter category and have some preserved chloride channel activity and milder disease phenotype.

Mechanism

CF affects all organs with epithelial cells expressing CFTR, which typically means cells lining a ductal system and the fluid outside that system are affected. In the lungs, the respiratory epithelium is lined with cells that express the CFTR. When the CFTR does not move appropriate amounts of chloride, chloride is trapped inside the cell, which leads to the epithelial sodium channel pumping additional sodium into the cell to balance. The resulting salt inside the cell creates an osmotic gradient across the cell surface and water enters the cell. The water first comes from the periciliary fluid layer, dehydrating the fluid around the cilia, making it difficult for them to beat. Secondly, water is removed from the outer mucus layer, also dehydrating it, making it thick and viscous. In the sinopulmonary tract, this inspissation of the mucus limits natural mucociliary clearance and leads to inflammation as well as an advantageous environment for bacterial colonization. Damage to the airways becomes irreversible and leads to loss of lung function.

A similar issue happens in other organs with any epithelial cell lining a ductal system. In the pancreas, for instance, epithelial cells line the ducts of the exocrine pancreas. The cells pull water from the normal pancreatic excretion, dehydrating it and clogging up the ducts. The enzymes then autodigest the exocrine pancreas rendering it nonfunctional. The same is true in the biliary ducts of the liver. In the sweat glands, salt and water are trapped in the ducts, making the sweat very salty and leading to the diagnostic test of the sweat chloride test.

Clinical Manifestations

Pulmonary

The normal tracheobronchial tree has poor mucocilliary clearance, as noted previously. People with CF have excessive cough, make mucus, and might wheeze. They have periodic episodes of exacerbation where there is an excessive mucus build up and bacterial infection. The thick mucus becomes a source of persistent infection with bacteria that are unable to be cleared. Often, the infections are caused by bacteria that are not present in the normal undamaged airway, especially *Staphylococcus aureus* and *Pseudomonas aeruginosa*. When the bacteria become active and the patient experiences an exacerbation, the cough and sputum production will worsen. Exacerbations in children are often triggered by viruses and typical childhood illnesses, and in adults, exacerbations may also be triggered by other environmental factors. With exacerbation, there may be shortness of breath, chest pain, wheezing, dyspnea on exertion or at rest, and fatigue. Other symptoms of a pulmonary exacerbation include weight loss, poor appetite, and fever. Over time, there is progressive loss of lung function owing to infections, mucus, and inflammation. Symptoms become more persistent and bothersome over time and exacerbations become more common.

Sinuses

The sinuses in CF have the same thick mucostasis that occurs in the lungs. The mucus impaction leads to chronic sinus congestion and obstruction, persistent infections, and persistent inflammation. Individuals with CF are more likely to develop polyps as well. Symptoms include nasal congestion or drainage, sinus headache, and inability to smell.

Pancreas

Poor growth occurs due to insufficient nutrient breakdown and absorption, with malabsorptive, greasy stools occurring owing

to this. Owing to malabsorption of fat, fat-soluble vitamins in the diet are also malabsorbed. Individuals with CF can develop significant deficiencies in vitamins A, D, E, and K. Generally, the endocrine pancreas that makes insulin is not initially affected in CF. Over time, individuals with CF often develop CF-related diabetes caused by global inflammation of the pancreas. More than 30% to 40% of adults will develop CF-related diabetes (CFRD).

Liver

In the liver, there is inspissation of the bile in the bile duct caused by excessive reabsorption of water from the bile. The resulting blockage of the bile ducts leads to hepatic inflammation. Generally, this is asymptomatic for the individual with CF and is found owing to checking laboratory levels of liver function tests. Occasionally, this bile blockage is severe and leads to chronic inflammation and biliary cirrhosis of the liver. A small percentage of individuals with CF, typically less than 5%, have fulminant liver failure with esophageal varices and splenomegaly and would need a liver transplant.

Intestines

Excessive reabsorption of fluid in the gut can lead to constipation and even small bowel obstruction. This can also occur when stools are malabsorptive. Some people with CF will have rectal prolapse caused by straining, with either malabsorptive or constipated stools. Other manifestations of CF in the intestines can be a result of medication side effects.

Sweat Gland

Excessive salt is trapped in the sweat leading to excessive salt loss in the sweat and electrolyte imbalance and dehydration.

Genitourinary

Males with CF generally all have congenital absence of the vas deferens, rendering them naturally infertile. Men still produce sperm but do not have the other structures. Women with CF may have decreased fertility owing to poor nutritional status but, typically, can have children.

Other

CF causes clubbing of the fingers, which is usually more prominent as lung disease progresses. CF-related arthropathies occur in a small percentage of individuals with CF, usually caused by inflammatory markers in circulation that deposit in the joints.

Diagnosis

Because CF is an insidiously progressive disease, it is important to make an early diagnosis and begin therapies as soon as possible. In the United States, the majority of diagnoses are made via newborn screening. Depending on the state, testing involves immunoreactive trypsinogen (IRT) levels with possible genetic panels of mutations. When the state reports a positive newborn screen, the care provider must order/obtain a sweat chloride test on the baby. Diagnoses are then based on results of the screens. The CF Foundation guidelines state that a positive sweat diagnosis of CF is greater than 30 mmol/L chloride, with 30 to 60 mmol/L chloride being the intermediate zone. Consensus remains that if a child has 2 mutations as well as symptoms and a sweat chloride, this is consistent with a diagnosis of CF. Children with symptoms and a sweat chloride greater than 60 mmol/L have CF as well. A secondary diagnosis of CF-related metabolic disorder (CRMS) designates those individuals whose diagnoses are unclear. Those with one mutation and an intermediate sweat (30 to 60 mmol/L) or those with 2 mutations and a negative sweat (<30 mmol/L) are followed prospectively for the development of symptoms and should have periodic sweat tests as well as periodic visits at the CF Center to evaluate for the evolution of symptoms.

As newborn screening has only been available for the last 10 to 20 years, children and adults who did not receive newborn screening are still being diagnosed the traditional way, which is the presence of symptoms and a positive sweat test. Here again, a positive sweat means a value of 60 mmol/L, while a value of 30 mmol/L or greater deserves further investigation, such as genetic testing. Sweat tests should be done at certified CF Centers where the testing methodology has been certified by the national Cystic Fibrosis Foundation. Traditional symptomatology per the CF Foundation is represented in the following:

- Very salty-tasting skin
- Persistent coughing, at times with phlegm
- Frequent lung infections, such as pneumonia or bronchitis
- Wheezing or shortness of breath
- Poor growth or poor weight gain in spite of a good appetite
- Frequent greasy, bulky stools or difficulty in bowel movements
- Nasal polyps
- Chronic sinus infections
- Clubbing or enlargement of the fingertips and toes
- Rectal prolapse
- Male infertility

If a diagnosis of CF is suspected owing to symptomatology, no matter what the age or status of newborn screening, a sweat test for definitive diagnosis should be performed.

Treatment
Pulmonary
Nonpharmacologic
Owing to the increased viscosity of the airway secretions and the subsequent obstruction and even mucus plugging in CF, there is a fundamental need for airway clearance or chest physiotherapy as part of chronic care. As a core component of therapy in the pulmonary management of CF, airway clearance or chest physiotherapy helps loosen this mucus, and help with expectoration should be done routinely two to three times per day as part of chronic management in all ages; increased frequency may be necessary during periods of pulmonary exacerbation. Manual physiotherapy or percussion and postural drainage is often the first type introduced into care. Other airway clearance techniques can be utilized, depending on age, access to devices, etc., such as autogenic drainage, active-cycle-of breathing, high frequency chest compression (e.g., vest) and/or oscillatory positive expiratory pressure (OPEP) devices, and exercise.

Pharmacological, Chronic Therapy
Selection of chronic medications used in the pulmonary management of CF is currently guided based on age and clinical need. This is based on current guidelines, US Food and Drug Administration approved indications for newer agents (e.g., CFTR modulators) as well as current evidence in cases of off-label medication use. Such pharmacotherapy consists of various medication classes, including bronchodilators, mucolytics, inhaled antibiotics, antiinflammatory agents, and CFTR modulators.

Inhaled medications are used in conjunction with chest physiotherapy to facilitate airway clearance, helping loosen mucus and expectoration as well as suppress bacterial growth of pathogens in the airways. The use of a short-acting β agonist, such as albuterol (Proventil, Ventolin)[1], in either meter dose inhaler or aerosolized or nebulizer form, facilitates mucocilliary clearance through bronchodilation paired with decreasing occurrence of bronchospasm from subsequent inhaled therapies such as hypertonic saline (sodium chloride 7% [HyperSal, PulmoSal]), dornase alfa (Pulmozyme), and antibiotics. Mucolytics are also fundamental in mucociliary clearance. Nebulized hypertonic saline, most commonly sodium chloride 7%, increases hydration of sputum through osmotic action, thinning sputum for airway clearance. Dornase alfa breaks down extracellular DNA in sputum, thereby decreasing its viscosity. This nebulized mucolytic is most commonly administered daily, usually following the use of nebulized hypertonic saline in sequence. The use of hypertonic saline and dornase alfa is recommended to help improve lung function

and reduce exacerbations. Inhaled corticosteroids with/without a long-acting β agonist are not used to treat CF itself, but in cases of concurrent asthma.

Some patients with CF may require the use of an inhaled antibiotic to help suppress bacterial burden in the airways and improve patient outcomes such as lung function and exacerbation frequency. Currently, the only FDA-approved inhaled antibiotics are tobramycin inhalation solution (Bethkis, Tobi), tobramycin inhalation powder (Tobi Podhaler), and aztreonam for inhalation solution (Cayston) for patients with CF with *Pseudomonas aeruginosa*. For those patients who newly acquire *P. aeruginosa*, it is recommended to use an inhaled antibiotic for treatment, with the preferred agent being tobramycin-inhaled solution, for 28 days, in an attempt to eradicate the pathogen. The use of an inhaled antibiotic to prevent acquisition of *P. aeruginosa* is not recommended. For patients with CF with persistent presence of *P. aeruginosa* from respiratory cultures, the chronic use of inhaled antibiotics, such as tobramycin or aztreonam, is recommended to improve lung function and reduce exacerbations. For chronic use, the cycling (i.e., on 28 days, off 28 days, etc.) of an inhaled antibiotic is common. The use of continuous inhaled antibiotic therapy, where two different inhaled antibiotics (e.g., tobramycin and aztreonam) are used rotationally, is not routine, but has been used by specialists in cases of multidrug resistant pathogens, advanced or severe lung disease, or in patients with frequent acute exacerbations.

Antiinflammatory agents, specifically, oral azithromycin and/or high-dose ibuprofen, are also noted in current guidelines. Azithromycin (Zithromax), a macrolide antibiotic, is not used in chronic CF for its antiinfective properties, but for its antiinflammatory and immunomodulary properties. For patients with CF with persistent presence of *P. aeruginosa* from respiratory cultures, the use of chronic azithromycin[1] is recommended to improve lung function and reduce exacerbations. The use in patients with CF who lack persistent presence of *P. aeruginosa* can be considered to help reduce frequency of exacerbations. Monitoring for presence of non-tuberculosis mycobacterium (NTM) in respiratory cultures and potential for drug interactions with azithromycin (e.g., medications that may prolong QT interval) is recommended with the use of chronic azithromycin. A less commonly used antiinflammatory agent used among CF centers is high-dose ibuprofen[1]. The therapeutic benefit of slowing the loss of lung function is greatest in children aged 6 to 17 years. This therapy requires therapeutic drug monitoring (i.e., pharmacokinetic assessment of serum ibuprofen levels) and dose adjustment. Subtherapeutic levels can have negative effects on lung function owing to increase in inflammatory mediators, and supratherapeutic levels increase the risk for toxicities (e.g., bleeding, nephrotoxicity). This therapy is less common in use owing to its potential for adverse effects, the need for laboratory monitoring, and the need for pharmacokinetic-based dosing. Routine, chronic use of systemic steroids such as prednisone is not recommended in the chronic management of CF.

CFTR modulators, a newer class of medications, are available for patients with CF with certain CF genotypes. The initial consideration for use and dosing of CFTR modulators is based on age, CF genotype, and concurrent therapy. There are three main types: potentiators, correctors, and amplifiers; however, the latter type is not currently available and is being developed and studied. Ivacaftor (Kalydeco) is a potentiator, increasing chloride movement through the CFTR protein channel. Ivacaftor is intended for patients with approved genotypes with gating and conducting mutations. Lumacaftor is a corrector, facilitating correct formation and stabilization of CFTR protein. Lumacaftor is combined with ivacaftor (Orkambi) for treatment and is intended for patients whose genotype is homozygous Phe-508del. Tezacaftor is also a corrector but is longer acting and has some differences compared to lumacaftor with regard to

---

[1]Not FDA approved for this indication.

[1]Not FDA approved for this indication.

drug interactions and side effects. Like lumacaftor, tezacaftor is combined with ivacaftor (Symdeko) for the chronic treatment of CF and is approved for patients whose genotype is homozygous Phe508del as well as a number of residual function mutations. All of the mentioned CFTR modulators have similar administration and monitoring considerations. Liver function tests aspartate aminotransferase (AST) and alanine aminotransferase (ALT) should be done prior to starting therapy, then every 3 months for the first year of therapy and annually thereafter. As noncongenital lens opacities or cataracts have been reported in pediatric patients, a baseline ophthalmologic exam is also recommended in those aged less than 18 years. Follow-up ophthalmologic exams are recommended but the frequency is not well defined. Doses should be taken with a fatty meal and with pancreatic enzymes (for those who require use of pancreatic enzymes as part of CF management). All the listed CFTR modulators are inducers and/or substrates of CYP3A4, so screening for and managing drug interactions are essential. Additionally, dosing modifications or discontinuation may be necessary for moderate or severe hepatic dysfunction.

Pharmacological, Acute Therapy

Many patients with CF, despite the use of chronic therapies, experience pulmonary exacerbations requiring treatment. In addition to increased frequency of airway clearance or chest physiotherapy, acute pulmonary exacerbations may require the use of systemic antimicrobials. Whenever possible, selection of systemic antimicrobial agents should be guided by patient-specific history of respiratory cultures as well as patient clinical response to past regimens.

When a systemic antimicrobial is required for outpatient management, an oral antibiotic is commonly used, with duration of most agents for 10 to 14 days. For example, if a given patient has history of *P. aeruginosa*, use of oral ciprofloxacin (Cipro)[1] or levofloxacin (Levaquin)[1] for 10 to 14 days may be appropriate. Patients who have inhaled antibiotics as part of their chronic regimen may continue treatment cycles during outpatient treatment for acute pulmonary exacerbation. Some CF centers may utilize home infusion services for intravenous antimicrobials; however, this requires additional logistic considerations including nursing support, infusion equipment, and laboratory monitoring. Additionally, factors related to adherence to airway clearance, social support system at home, and appropriateness of home intravenous access should be considered.

For inpatient management, the use of intravenous antibiotics is more common and the use of oral antibiotic(s) may also be part of the regimen. *P. aeruginosa* is often "double-covered" when it is possible, specifically when hospitalized and/or requiring intravenous antimicrobials. "Double-coverage" involves the use of two agents active against *P. aeruginosa* from two different antibiotic classes (e.g., beta lactam and aminoglycoside). The use of both inhaled and systemic (e.g., intravenous) antibiotics of the same class (e.g., aminoglycosides) simultaneously is not common. Another approach is starting intravenous antimicrobials in the inpatient setting, with transition and completion of the therapy course with home infusion services.

Nutrition/Gastrointestinal
Nonpharmacologic

Persons with CF often have greater dietary energy intake needs. Consistent, high-calorie dietary intake can be a challenge because of several physiologic factors, including loss of taste or smell caused by chronic sinusitis and chronic gastroesophageal reflux. Behavioral factors may affect nutritional intake, necessitating behavioral intervention by dietitians and/or psychologists. For patients of all ages with continued suboptimal growth, the use of enteral feeding modes may also be necessary. For patients who have chronic constipation or history of distal intestinal obstructive

syndrome (DIOS), appropriate hydration and increased fiber content in diet are recommended.

Infant formulas and breast milk do not provide adequate Na^+ for infants with CF. Owing to excessive loss of Na+ through insensible loss, infants are at risk of developing hyponatremic, hypochloremia dehydration. It is recommended that ⅛ teaspoon of table salt be provided from birth and increased with time to ¼ teaspoon by 6 months through 1 year of age, divided throughout the day by feedings. Additional supplementation may be necessary for children and adults living in high-temperature climates and/or involved in considerable physical activities (e.g., sports).

Pharmacological, Chronic Therapy

For patients who are pancreatic insufficient, the use of pancreatic enzyme replacement therapy (PERT) is needed. There are various brands of PERT that contain various amounts of lipase, protease, and amylase. Pancreatic enzymes should be taken at meal and snack times, as well as in coordination with enteral feeds (when applicable). Dosing of PERT is based on lipase component. Typical pancreatic enzyme initial dosing ranges from 500 to 1500 units of lipase per kilogram body weight per meal with a maximum of either 10,000 units of lipase per kilogram per day or 2500 units of lipase per kilogram per meal. Enzyme preparations come in a range of concentrations to accommodate all patient needs and minimize the number of capsules required. Given the number of medications a person with CF may require for chronic management, clinicians should be mindful about how many capsules are required per meal or snack when selecting a brand and strength of pancreatic enzyme. When maximal PERT dosing is reached and the individual continues to present with symptoms of malabsorption (e.g., steatorrhea), other etiologies should be investigated. Some clinicians may add an acid suppression agent (e.g., a proton pump inhibitor or H2 receptor antagonist) to help enhance the activity of pancreatic enzymes through decreasing duodenal acidity; however, the potential risks of long-term acid suppression (e.g., small intestinal bacterial overgrowth [SIBO]) should be considered. A proton pump inhibitor or H2 receptor antagonist may also be used to treat concurrent gastroesophageal reflux disease.

Supplementation of fat-soluble vitamins (i.e., A, D, E, K) should be provided via specially formulated multivitamins, available in various dosage forms with dosing based on age. Monitoring of vitamin levels are often done at least annually, with adjustments in supplementation of individual vitamins (e.g., vitamin D, cholecalciferol) based on adherence to current treatment, age, and level of deficiency.

For those who have chronic constipation or history of DIOS, chronic use of an osmotic laxative such as over-the-counter, polyethylene glycol 3350 (MiraLax)[1] may be helpful. Oral *N*-acetylcysteine (Mucomyst)[1] has also been used for the prevention of mucus accumulation in the gastrointestinal (GI) tract of some individuals with DIOS.

Pharmacological, Acute Therapy

Patients presenting with DIOS often require more aggressive treatment than that of chronic constipation related to CF. Treatment of DIOS may include laxatives at higher doses, use of electrolyte intestinal lavage solution (e.g., GoLYTELY)[1], or hyperosmolar enemas. Oral and/or rectal administration[1] of *N*-acetylcysteine solution has also been used for the treatment of mucus accumulation in the GI tract of some individuals with DIOS.

Monitoring

Monitoring of pulmonary symptoms should be done at each encounter. Spirometry to assess lung function is recommended as part of CF clinic visits to assess changes in forced expiratory volume in one second (FEV_1) relative to baseline. Additionally, routine respiratory cultures, including screening for acid-fast bacilli and fungal cultures to monitor for pathogens and susceptibilities

---

[1]Not FDA approved for this indication.

[1]Not FDA approved for this indication.

are recommended. Nutritional status (e.g., weight, height, weight for length, body mass index) should also be monitored regularly. Annual routine laboratory testing is also done through CF centers as well as screenings for complications (e.g., CFRD). Recommended monitoring for the various chronic therapies is discussed in the previous section.

Management of Other Complications

In addition to the general manifestation of CF (e.g., pulmonary, growth, and nutrition), complications may appear with age and disease progression. The following are examples and general management approaches. Referral to other specialists, such as endocrinology, gastroenterology, otorhinolaryngology, or transplant (if/when appropriate for advanced disease), may be necessary.

Sinusitis

Treatment of the acute exacerbations of sinusitis can include systemic (e.g., oral) antibiotics, which are also used in pulmonary exacerbations. The use of intranasal irrigations of antimicrobials (e.g., gentamicin)[1] may also be considered, although guidance defining and comparing intranasal irrigation agent selection, formulation, dosing, and monitoring are currently lacking.

Small Intestinal Bacterial Overgrowth

Treatment of SIBO in persons with CF is similar to that of those without CF, including use of oral antibiotics (e.g., rifaximin [Xifaxan][1]). Nonpharmacologic treatment may include dietary manipulation, such as reducing carbohydrate consumption, resulting in a high-fat, low-carbohydrate diet.

Cystic Fibrosis Related Diabetes

In addition to dietary modifications, when pharmacologic treatment is needed, insulin therapy includes a regimen consisting of long-acting insulin paired with carbohydrate counting and coverage with rapid-acting insulin. Acute pulmonary exacerbation or illness may complicate glucose control, especially if systemic corticosteroids are used as part of the management of severe, acute pulmonary exacerbations.

Hepatobiliary Disease

In addition to nutritional support, treatment with oral ursodeoxycholic acid or ursodiol (Actigall)[1] is currently recommended.

---

[1]Not FDA approved for this indication.

References

Borowitz D, Robinson KA, Rosenfeld M, et al: Cystic Fibrosis Foundation evidence-based guidelines for management of infants with cystic fibrosis, *J Pediatr* 155(6 Suppl):S73–S93, 2009 Dec.

Farrell PM, White TB, Ren CL, et al: Diagnosis of Cystic Fibrosis: Consensus Guidelines from the Cystic Fibrosis Foundation, *J Pediatr* 181S:S4–S15.e1, 2017 Feb. https://doi.org/10.1016/j.jpeds.2016.09.064.

Flume PA, Clancy JP, Retsch-Bogart GZ, et al: Continuous alternating inhaled antibiotics for chronic pseudomonal infection in cystic fibrosis, *J Cyst Fibros* 15(6):809–815, 2016 Nov.

Flume PA, Mogayzel Jr PJ, Robinson KA, et al: Clinical Practice Guidelines for Pulmonary Therapies Committee. Cystic fibrosis pulmonary guidelines: treatment of pulmonary exacerbations, *Am J Respir Crit Care Med* 180(9), 2009 Nov 1, 802-8.

Flume PA, Robinson KA, O'Sullivan BP, et al: Clinical Practice Guidelines for Pulmonary Therapies Committee. Cystic fibrosis pulmonary guidelines: airway clearance therapies, *Respir Care* 54(4), 2009 Apr, 522-37.

Lahiri T, Hempstead SE, Brady C, et al: Clinical practice guidelines from the Cystic Fibrosis Foundation for preschoolers with cystic fibrosis, *Pediatrics* 137(4), 2016 Apr.

LeGrys VA, Yankaskas JR, Quittell LM, Marshall BC, Mogayzel PJ: Cystic Fibrosis Foundation. Diagnostic sweat testing: The Cystic Fibrosis Foundation Guidelines, *J Pediatr* 151(1), 2007 Jul, 85-9.

Mogayzel Jr PJ, Naureckas ET, Robinson KA, et al: Cystic fibrosis pulmonary guidelines. Chronic medications for maintenance of lung health, *Am J Respir Crit Care Med* 187(7), 2013 Apr 1, 680-9.

Mogayzel Jr PJ, Naureckas ET, Robinson KA, et al: Cystic Fibrosis Foundation pulmonary guideline. pharmacologic approaches to prevention and eradication of initial Pseudomonas aeruginosa infection, *Ann Am Thorac Soc* 11(10), 2014 Dec, 1640-50.

Ren CL, Morgan RL, Oermann C, et al: Cystic Fibrosis Foundation Pulmonary Guidelines: Use of cystic fibrosis transmembrane conductance regulator modulator therapy in patients with cystic fibrosis, *Ann Am Thorac Soc* 15(3):271–280, 2018 Mar.

HISTOPLASMOSIS

Method of
David van Duin, MD, PhD

CURRENT DIAGNOSIS

- The most common symptomatic manifestation of histoplasmosis is acute pulmonary histoplasmosis, which is generally characterized by nonspecific symptoms including fevers, chills, malaise, a nonproductive cough, and chest pain.
- Other presentations of histoplasmosis include chronic pulmonary histoplasmosis, disseminated histoplasmosis in immunocompromised hosts, and extrapulmonary disease such as mediastinal histoplasmosis.
- A multimodality approach to diagnosis, which may include serology, histopathology, antigen testing, and culture, should be considered in the appropriate setting.

CURRENT THERAPY

- Oral itraconazole is the treatment of choice for most forms of histoplasmosis.
- Serum levels of itraconazole are unpredictable and should be monitored during treatment.
- Depending on localization and severity of disease, induction with amphotericin B formulations may be required.
- Careful monitoring of patients during and after treatment is recommended, because relapses are observed in a subset of patients.

Mycology and Pathogenesis

Histoplasma capsulatum var. *capsulatum* and *H. capsulatum* var. *duboisii* are the two varieties of *H. capsulatum* that cause human histoplasmosis. *H. capsulatum* var. *duboisii* is the causative agent of African histoplasmosis, which is characterized by skin, bone, lymph node, and subcutaneous tissue involvement. This chapter focuses solely on the manifestations and treatment of *H. capsulatum* var. *capsulatum*, hereafter referred to as *H. capsulatum*.

H. capsulatum is a thermally dimorphic fungal pathogen, which grows as a mold in the environment, and converts to a yeast at 37°C during infection. During mold growth, *H. capsulatum* forms macroconidia, which are 8 to 15 μm and have thick walls and protuberances, as well as microconidia, which are 2 to 4 μm and have a smooth surface.

Disruption of soil containing *H. capsulatum*, such as during a construction project, results in the aerosolization of microconidia, which are the infectious particles. Inhaled microconidia are phagocytized but are able to survive and convert to yeast phase inside pulmonary macrophages. The resulting dissemination through the reticuloendothelial system is usually quickly contained in immunocompetent hosts, but it can lead to severe disease in the absence of normal immunity. Microconidia can be carried for several miles by air currents. Therefore, persons who are not in the direct vicinity of the disrupted soil are also at risk for developing histoplasmosis.

In tissues, *H. capsulatum* is recognized as 2- to 4-μm oval yeast forms with narrow-based budding. *H. capsulatum* does not have a capsule; the name is derived from the erroneous interpretation by Samuel Darling of an apparent clearing surrounding these yeasts in tissues as a capsule.

Epidemiology

Histoplasmosis is most common in North and Central America, but cases occur worldwide, some in microfoci of infection.

Areas of high prevalence include the Mississippi and Ohio River valleys in the United States and Rio de Janeiro State in Brazil. *H. capsulatum* thrives in soil that is enriched with bird or bat guano, and it can be found in high quantities near bird roosts, chicken coops, abandoned old buildings, and bat-infested caves. Because *H. capsulatum* can enter a state of latency and reactivate years later, cases have been described in patients who have a remote history of living in or visiting endemic areas. A complete geographic history and a high index of suspicion are required for the correct diagnosis of such cases in nonendemic areas.

Clinical Manifestations

Most *H. capsulatum* infections are asymptomatic; it is estimated that less than 5% of infections lead to clinical symptoms. The occurrence and severity of a clinical syndrome are thought to be related to the immune status of the host, as well as the size of the infectious inoculum. The most common clinical scenario is acute pulmonary histoplasmosis, but a variety of other symptomatic histoplasmosis syndromes have been described. Also, a substantial number of cases come to clinical attention years after the initial infection during the course of a pulmonary nodule workup, when malignancy is suspected. Although they are asymptomatic, these cases can lead to anxiety, as well as the morbidity and health care costs associated with radiographic exposures and biopsy procedures.

Acute Pulmonary Histoplasmosis

Most commonly, acute pulmonary histoplasmosis is a self-limited flulike illness. Symptoms are generally nonspecific and include fevers, chills, malaise, a nonproductive cough, and chest pain. Chest radiographs can show diffuse infiltrates in one or more lobes, often with hilar lymphadenopathy. The differential diagnosis includes more common infections such as bacterial and viral pneumonias. Symptoms usually resolve without treatment in 2 to 3 weeks. However, more-severe cases do occur, even in seemingly immunocompetent hosts. In these cases, severe respiratory distress, prolonged symptoms, and even death can occur in the absence of adequate treatment. This highlights the importance of timely diagnosis and treatment when indicated.

Chronic Pulmonary Histoplasmosis

Some patients with acute pulmonary histoplasmosis fail to clear their infection and go on to develop a chronic pulmonary infection. A subset of these patients has chronic cavitary disease.

Chronic pulmonary histoplasmosis may be arbitrarily defined when the duration of symptoms from pulmonary histoplasmosis exceeds 6 weeks. The classic patient is a white middle-aged to elderly man with chronic obstructive pulmonary disease (COPD). Although these are clearly risk factors for the development of chronic disease, case series have illustrated that even never-smokers without preexisting lung disease are at risk for developing this complication.

A combination of systemic and pulmonary signs and symptoms is usually found in chronic pulmonary histoplasmosis. Fevers, night sweats, weight loss, lack of appetite, subjective loss of energy, and malaise are common systemic symptoms, and pulmonary symptoms include cough, sometimes with minimal hemoptysis, dyspnea, and sputum production. In patients with preexisting lung disease it may be difficult to distinguish these symptoms from baseline symptomatology. Radiology studies classically show cavitary disease without hilar lymphadenopathy. However, nodules, infiltrates, and lymphadenopathy are also seen, especially in nonsmoking women.

Untreated, this form of histoplasmosis can lead to death secondary to respiratory failure. With treatment, prognosis depends on coexisting pulmonary disease, and is generally favorable with regard to microbiological cure. However, relapses occur in up to 20% of cases even after prolonged treatment.

Disseminated Histoplasmosis

Most, if not all, episodes of histoplasmosis have a period of dissemination, during which infected macrophages spread throughout the body via the reticuloendothelial system. In the majority of cases this is a self-limited event, which is quickly contained upon activation of the immune system. However, about 1 in 2000 infections results in progressive disseminated disease. Almost invariably, these cases occur in immunocompromised hosts. Patients at risk for progressive disseminated disease include those with advanced HIV infection, solid organ transplant recipients, patients with hematologic malignancies, and those treated with immunomodulating agents, most notably corticosteroids or tumor necrosis factor α (TNF-α) inhibitors. Infants are also at risk.

Recognition of disseminated histoplasmosis can be challenging. Symptoms include fevers, malaise, anorexia, respiratory symptoms, and weight loss. Laboratory investigations often reveal elevated acute phase reactants, abnormal liver function tests, and pancytopenia. Hepatosplenomegaly and lymphadenopathy occur in about half of cases. Severe cases can be clinically indistinguishable from bacterial sepsis, and patients present with hypotension and multiorgan failure. A potential diagnostic clue to the diagnosis is the presence of mucosal ulcerations, which are generally painful and can occur anywhere in the oral, pharyngeal, or laryngeal mucosa. Various morphologies may be seen, ranging from superficial to verrucous. Adrenal involvement resulting in adrenal insufficiency can occur. These patients present with enlarged adrenals on imaging and clinical symptoms of Addison disease.

Although survival without antifungal therapy has been described, disseminated histoplasmosis is generally fatal if left untreated.

Mediastinal Manifestations of Histoplasmosis

Mediastinal disease can manifest itself as mediastinal fibrosis or granulomatous mediastinitis. Mediastinal fibrosis or fibrosing mediastinitis is an uncommon complication of pulmonary disease, in which extensive fibrotic tissue develops in the mediastinum in response to infection. Men between the ages of 20 and 40 years are at the highest risk for this complication. The fibrosis consists of mature collagen, rather than granulomatous tissue, which encases the structures of the mediastinum and can have a progressive course eventually leading to death. The prognosis depends on the extent of involvement of mediastinal structures. Bilateral disease in which the pulmonary veins are involved is especially associated with poor outcomes. No satisfactory treatment is available.

In contrast, granulomatous mediastinitis, also known as mediastinal granuloma, is characterized by a caseous inflammatory mass of mediastinal lymph nodes. Most patients remain asymptomatic, and cases are often recognized only as an incidental imaging finding. However, a subset of patients develops symptoms related to compromise of mediastinal structures. The prognosis is more benign; usually the process resolves and the involved lymph nodes calcify. The role of treatment in this entity remains unclear.

Central Nervous System Histoplasmosis

Central nervous system (CNS) involvement during *H. capsulatum* infection occurs infrequently. Like other extrapulmonary disease, CNS disease may be seen as a part of progressive disseminated histoplasmosis in about 5% to 10% of disseminated histoplasmosis cases. Additionally, isolated cases in which no other signs of dissemination are found have been reported. CNS histoplasmosis typically results in chronic lymphocytic meningitis, but parenchymal lesions can also be found. Symptoms are similar to those of other chronic infectious meningitides. The typical presentation is a combination of systemic symptoms including fevers, weight loss, and night sweats and localizing symptoms of headache, focal neurologic deficits, or behavioral changes. Treatment failures and relapses are common. Prognosis in the context of adequate treatment is dependent on the degree and the reversibility of immunosuppression.

Other Manifestations of Histoplasmosis

Involvement of all organ systems with *H. capsulatum* has been reported, either in the setting of clinical disseminated histoplasmosis or as an isolated extrapulmonary site of infection.

H. capsulatum as a cause of endovascular and cardiac infections is well established. In endocarditis cases, native and prosthetic valves may be involved. Pericarditis is found in around 5% of patients with pulmonary histoplasmosis, and it appears to represent an immunologic reaction. Consistent with this, symptoms usually resolve with nonsteroidal antiinflammatory drugs (NSAIDs) or corticosteroids. Bone, joint, and skin infections can also occur and can present diagnostic difficulty.

Urogenital involvement is often documented in autopsy series, but it infrequently results in clinical symptoms. Few cases of *H. capsulatum* causing symptomatic prostatitis, nephritis, epididymitis, vaginal and penile ulcers, and ovarian involvement have been reported. Similarly, although autopsy series report gastrointestinal involvement in disseminated histoplasmosis in up to 70% to 90% of cases, specific symptoms attributable to the gastrointestinal tract are much less common. Diarrhea, gastrointestinal bleeding, bowel perforation, or bowel obstruction can result from gastrointestinal histoplasmosis.

Diagnosis

Diagnosing histoplasmosis can be complicated, and the available specific diagnostic tests each have their limitations. If the diagnosis is suspected, using available modalities in combination is generally the right approach. Turn-around time can vary depending on circumstances, and in severe or disseminated cases, empiric therapy may be warranted. Obtaining tissue, when it is feasible to do so, is essential for a pathologic diagnosis.

Histopathology

One of the most useful modalities in reaching a diagnosis is histopathology. Necrotizing or non-necrotizing granulomas are often seen. An experienced pathologist can recognize the specific pattern of yeast forms, mostly inside but also outside of macrophages. The yeast forms are best visualized by a methamine silver stain, such as the Gomori-Grocott methenamine silver stain (GMS). Alternatively, periodic acid–Schiff (PAS) staining may be used. Confusion with other pathogens or, more commonly, staining artifacts can occur, and expert consultation is required in such cases. Obtaining tissue for histopathology is usually the real challenge, and a careful evaluation of the risk-to-benefit ratio for each individual patient needs to be made.

Cultures

Culture confirmation of histoplasmosis is desirable, but often the yield of cultures is limited. In addition, cultures may be subject to a substantial time delay of several weeks. In disseminated histoplasmosis, cultures are often positive from several sites, including blood and bone marrow. In acute pulmonary histoplasmosis, the yield of respiratory cultures is estimated to be between 9% and 40%, depending on the degree of lung involvement. In mild to moderate cases, cultures are rarely positive. In chronic cavitary lung disease, the yield of culture improves, probably as a reflection of the increased fungal burden in these patients, and cultures can grow *H. capsulatum* in as many as 85% of cases. A positive fungal culture, with microscopic characteristics suggesting *H. capsulatum*, should be confirmed by specific testing. This is usually accomplished by DNA probing.

Serology

Antibody testing can be helpful when used in conjunction with the clinical scenario and other specific testing. The presence of antibodies to *H. capsulatum* may be determined by complement fixation (CF) or immunodiffusion (ID). Immunodiffusion methods evaluate the presence of M and H precipitin bands. Mild acute infections may be characterized by presence of an M band in isolation. Presence of an H band generally indicates more severe or chronic infection and is usually found in combination with an M band. Complement fixation determines the level of antibodies directed against mycelial and yeast antigens separately. For diagnosis, a fourfold rise in either mycelial or yeast CF antibody titer is required.

The incidence of detectable antibodies in persons in endemic areas is much lower than the incidence of positive skin testing, which suggests that detectable antibodies probably wane after exposure to undetectable levels. Therefore, although an isolated antibody titer of 1:32 or greater is not diagnostic, it is very suggestive of histoplasmosis in a patient with a consistent clinical presentation. In addition, any positive titer should lead to additional work-up because a substantial number of patients with confirmed histoplasmosis have antibody titers that are in the low positive range. Antibodies take 2 to 6 weeks to appear, which limits their use in acute cases. Immunosuppressed states clearly diminish the sensitivity of serology, but positive serologies are found in around 50% of disseminated histoplasmosis in immunocompromised patients. Antibody testing may be particularly helpful in CNS histoplasmosis, where cerebrospinal fluid (CSF) cultures are often negative. The finding of detectable anti–*H. capsulatum* antibodies in the CSF is diagnostic in the right clinical setting.

Antigen Detection

A commercial assay is available to determine the presence of polysaccharide antigens shed by *H. capsulatum* in urine or serum. Previously, urine assays appeared to outperform serum assays, but the most recent generation of antigen assays seems to be equivalent in urine and serum. Measuring antigen shedding in bronchoalveolar lavage (BAL) fluid is a new and promising development. Preliminary data indicate that yields from BAL may be increased in pulmonary disease. In general, antigen detection assays are a valuable adjunct to diagnosis and should be obtained in any case in which histoplasmosis is suspected. Because direct shedding is measured, the yield of this test is not diminished in immunocompromised hosts. In limited disease with a minimal fungal burden, antigens are unlikely to be detected.

Treatment

In 2007, the Infectious Diseases Society of America (IDSA) published updated management guidelines for the treatment of histoplasmosis (Table 1). The IDSA emphasizes that all of its guidelines "cannot always account for individual variation among patients. They are not intended to supplant physician judgment with respect to particular patients or special clinical situations." Regarding acute pulmonary histoplasmosis, no evidence from clinical trials is available to guide treatment decisions, and the IDSA guidelines are relatively conservative, reserving treatment only for "moderately severe to severe" cases. No explicit definition of severity is provided. Also, when mild to moderate symptoms persist, treatment is not recommended until the patient has been symptomatic for more than 4 weeks. Here, careful clinical judgment is warranted. Although poor long-term outcomes are uncommon in these patients, symptom resolution upon antifungal treatment is the rule. Therefore, some experts treat even mild to moderate acute pulmonary disease with a symptom duration of less than 4 weeks, in contrast to IDSA guideline recommendations.

Recommended induction treatment for the first 1 to 2 weeks in moderately severe to severe acute pulmonary histoplasmosis is a lipid formulation of amphotericin B (AmBisome, Abelcet)[1] 3 to 5 mg/kg IV daily. During induction therapy, methylprednisolone (Solu-Medrol) may be used as needed for respiratory complications. After that, oral itraconazole (Sporanox) can be used (200 mg three times daily for 3 days and then 200 mg twice daily) for a total duration of treatment of 12 weeks. Oral itraconazole for 6 to 12 weeks is the treatment of choice when the decision is made to treat mild to moderate acute pulmonary histoplasmosis.

When itraconazole is used, careful instructions should be given to ensure optimal oral absorption. Using the solution results

---

[1] Not FDA approved for this indication.

TABLE 1 2007 IDSA Guidelines for Treating Histoplasmosis

CLINICAL MANIFESTATION	INDUCTION	DURATION	MAINTENANCE	TOTAL DURATION
Acute Pulmonary				
Mild to moderate <4 weeks	None			
Mild to moderate >4 weeks	None		Itra*	6–12 wk
Moderately severe to severe	AmB†	1–2 wk	Itra*	12 wk
Chronic Pulmonary				
	Itra*	3 day	Itra*	1–2 yr
Disseminated				
Mild to moderate	Itra*	3 day	Itra*	1 yr
Moderately severe to severe	AmB†	1–2 wk	Itra*	1 yr
Granulomatous mediastinitis	Itra*	3 day	Itra*	6–12 wk
CNS	AmB†	4–6 wk	Itra*	1 yr

Abbreviations: AmB = amphotericin B; CNS = central nervous system; ISDA = Infectious Diseases Society of America; Itra = itraconazole.
[1]Not FDA approved for this indication.
*Itraconazole (Sporanox) dosing for mild to moderate disease is 200 mg qd or bid; for all other indications a loading dose of 200 mg tid × 3 d is recommended followed by 200 mg qd or bid, guided by blood levels.
†Amphotericin B, in general liposomal (AmBisome)[1] or lipid formulations (Abelcet)[1] are preferred, but deoxycholate formulation of amphotericin B (Fungizone) may be used as an alternative in the treatment of acute pulmonary histoplasmosis. In CNS histoplasmosis, liposomal amphotericin B[1] is preferred.

generally in higher blood levels, but the unpleasant taste can be an issue for patients. To optimize absorption of the capsules, encourage patients to take them with a cola beverage. Because of substantial interpersonal variability in itraconazole metabolism, blood levels remain unpredictable. As a result, levels should be monitored on all patients whose treatment exceeds 2 weeks. In general, blood levels between 1.0 and 10.0 μg/mL are recommended, even though strong evidence for these cutoffs is lacking.

Chronic pulmonary histoplasmosis requires oral itraconazole therapy for 1 to 2 years. As noted earlier, relapses can occur even with prolonged therapy, and some patients require lifelong suppressive therapy. When an asymptomatic pulmonary nodule is found to be a histoplasmoma in the course of a malignancy workup, no treatment is generally indicated.

In disseminated histoplasmosis with moderately severe to severe symptoms, induction treatment with liposomal amphotericin B[1] (3 mg/kg IV daily) is recommended for the first 1 to 2 weeks. This is followed by oral itraconazole for a total of at least 1 year. When symptoms of disseminated histoplasmosis are mild to moderate, the induction phase can be omitted, and treatment with oral itraconazole for 1 year should suffice. The role of treatment in mediastinal complications of histoplasmosis depends on the etiology. If symptomatic and inflammatory findings predominate, as in granulomatous mediastinitis, treatment with oral itraconazole is warranted. In mediastinal fibrosis, antifungal treatment generally does not improve the prognosis. CNS histoplasmosis should be aggressively treated with liposomal amphotericin B (5 mg/kg daily intravenously) for 4 to 6 weeks, followed by oral itraconazole for at least 1 year.

References

Ashbee HR, Evans EG, Viviani MA, et al: Histoplasmosis in Europe: Report on an epidemiological survey from the European Confederation of Medical Mycology Working Group, *Med Mycol* 46(1):57–65, 2008.

Assi MA, Sandid MS, Baddour LM, et al: Systemic histoplasmosis: A 15-year retrospective institutional review of 111 patients, *Medicine (Baltimore)* 86(3):162–169, 2007.

Cuellar-Rodriguez J, Avery RK, Lard M, et al: Histoplasmosis in solid organ transplant recipients: 10 years of experience at a large transplant center in an endemic area, *Clin Infect Dis* 49(5):710–716, 2009.

Deepe Jr GS: Immune response to early and late *Histoplasma capsulatum* infections, *Curr Opin Microbiol* 3(4):359–362, 2000.

Gugnani HC: Histoplasmosis in Africa: A review, *Indian J Chest Dis Allied Sci* 42(4):271–277, 2000.

Hage CA, Bowyer S, Tarvin SE, et al: Recognition, diagnosis, and treatment of histoplasmosis complicating tumor necrosis factor blocker therapy, *Clin Infect Dis* 50(1):85–92, 2010.

Hage CA, Davis TE, Fuller D, et al: Diagnosis of histoplasmosis by antigen detection in bronchoalveolar fluid, *Chest* 137(3):623–628, 2010.

Hage CA, Wheat LJ, Loyd J, et al: Pulmonary histoplasmosis, *Semin Respir Crit Care Med* 29(2):151–165, 2008.

Kahi CJ, Wheat LJ, Allen SD, Sarosi GA: Gastrointestinal histoplasmosis, *Am J Gastroenterol* 100(1):220–231, 2005.

Kauffman CA: Histoplasmosis: A clinical and laboratory update, *Clin Microbiol Rev* 20(1):115–132, 2007.

Kauffman CA: Diagnosis of histoplasmosis in immunosuppressed patients, *Curr Opin Infect Dis* 21(4):421–425, 2008.

Kauffman CA: Histoplasmosis, *Clin Chest Med* 30(2):217–225, 2009.

Kennedy CC, Limper AH: Redefining the clinical spectrum of chronic pulmonary histoplasmosis: A retrospective case series of 46 patients, *Medicine (Baltimore)* 86(4):252–258, 2007.

Mata-Essayag S, Colella MT, Rosello A, et al: Histoplasmosis: A study of 158 cases in Venezuela, 2000-2005, *Medicine (Baltimore)* 87(4):193–202, 2008.

Nosanchuk JD, Gacser A: *Histoplasma capsulatum* at the host–pathogen interface, *Microbes Infect* 10(9):973–977, 2008.

Pasqualotto AC, Oliveira FM, Severo LC: *Histoplasma capsulatum* recovery from the urine and a short review of genitourinary histoplasmosis, *Mycopathologia* 167(6):315–323, 2009.

Thompson GR 3rd, Cadena J, Patterson TF: Overview of antifungal agents, *Clin Chest Med* 30(2):203–215, 2009.

Wheat LJ: Approach to the diagnosis of the endemic mycoses, *Clin Chest Med* 30(2):379–389, 2009.

Wheat LJ, Freifeld AG, Kleiman MB, et al: Clinical practice guidelines for the management of patients with histoplasmosis: 2007 update by the Infectious Diseases Society of America, *Clin Infect Dis* 45(7):807–825, 2007.

Wheat LJ, Kauffman CA: Histoplasmosis, *Infect Dis Clin North Am* 17(1):1–19, 2003 vii.

Wheat LJ, Musial CE, Jenny-Avital E: Diagnosis and management of central nervous system histoplasmosis, *Clin Infect Dis* 40(6):844–852, 2005.

HYPERSENSITIVITY PNEUMONITIS

Method of
David I. Bernstein, MD; and Haejin Kim, MD

CURRENT DIAGNOSIS

- Objective evidence of parenchymal and/or interstitial infiltrative disease by physical examination, spirometry, and radiography associated with exposure to a causative agent
- Improvement in symptoms, lung function, and radiographic abnormalities with avoidance of the causative agent

CURRENT THERAPY

- Avoidance of contact with the offending antigen is essential and is often curative if performed early in the course of the disease.
- Systemic corticosteroids are often required during the acute phase of hypersensitivity pneumonitis.

Hypersensitivity pneumonitis, also known as extrinsic allergic alveolitis, is an inflammatory disorder of the lungs that is mediated by immunologic hypersensitivity to a specific antigen, usually organic in nature. Although more than 200 causative antigens have been implicated, only a small number of individuals develop HP in response to exposure. Table 1 lists common causative agents in hypersensitivity pneumonitis. Comprehensive lists of causative agents are available.

Pathophysiology

Hypersensitivity pneumonitis is thought to involve primarily type IV (cell-mediated) hypersensitivity. Bronchoalveolar fluid obtained from patients with hypersensitivity pneumonitis shows a predominant CD8+ lymphocytosis supporting T cell–mediated

disease. Viruses are thought to play a role in the development of hypersensitivity pneumonitis through upregulation of costimulatory molecules on alveolar macrophages and dendritic cells, leading to increased activation of type 1 helper T cells. Adoptive transfer models in animals have shown that CD4+ T cells and cytotoxic T cells are the most important effector cells in experimental hypersensitivity pneumonitis, rather than cytokines, antibodies, or complement alone. Genetic susceptibility to this disorder could be associated with presence of specific MHC class II alleles.

Clinical Presentation and Diagnosis

The main clinical features for hypersensitivity pneumonitis are listed in Table 2. Hypersensitivity pneumonitis is most likely to be diagnosed if the history, physical findings, high-resolution chest CT, and pulmonary function tests indicate infiltrative and restrictive lung disease; exposure is documented to a recognized or new causative agent; and there is significant improvement in symptoms, lung function, and radiographic findings with avoidance of the offending cause. Antibody to the offending antigen may be demonstrated but is not required for diagnosis. These are the most widely accepted criteria, but evidence-based diagnostic guidelines have not been established. A careful home, environmental, and occupational history is essential to identify one or more causative antigens.

TABLE 1	Hypersensitivity Pneumonitis: Representative Sources and Causative Agents	
CONDITION OR PERSONS AT RISK	**SOURCE**	**CAUSATIVE ANTIGENS**
Dairy farmers	Hay, grains, silage	Thermophilic actinomycetes
Bird fancier's or pigeon breeder's disease	Avian droppings or feathers	Avian proteins
Humidifier lung	Contaminated water	Thermophilic actinomycetes or other microorganisms
Chemical workers	Polyurethane foam, varnishes, lacquers	Isocyanates
Machine workers	Metalworking fluid	*Pseudomonas fluorescens, Aspergillus niger, Staphylococcus capitis, Rhodococcus* spp., *Bacillus pumilus*
Familial hypersensitivity pneumonitis	Contaminated wood dust in walls	*Bacillus subtilis*
Hot tub lung	Mold on ceiling	*Cladosporium* spp., *Mycobacterium avium*

Modified from Richerson HB, Bernstein IL, Fink JN, et al: Guidelines for the clinical evaluation of hypersensitivity pneumonitis: Report of the subcommittee on hypersensitivity pneumonitis. J Allergy Clin Immunol 1989;84:839–844; and Hanak V, Golbin JM, Hartman TE, et al: High-resolution CT findings of parenchymal fibrosis correlate with prognosis in hypersensitivity pneumonitis. Chest 2008;134:133–138.

TABLE 2	Clinical Features of Hypersensitivity Pneumonitis		
FEATURE	**ACUTE**	**SUBACUTE**	**CHRONIC**
Exposure to antigen	Hours to days	Days to weeks	Months
Symptoms	Influenza-like illness ± cough/dyspnea	Cough and dyspnea with severe cyanosis	Increasing cough and exertional dyspnea; fatigue, weight loss
Physical findings	Fever; lungs normal or bibasilar crackles	Cyanosis; lungs normal or bibasilar crackles	Cyanosis; right-sided heart failure; lungs normal or bibasilar crackles
High-resolution computed tomography	Diffuse ground-glass infiltrates	Reticulation; small centrilobular nodules; air trapping on expiration	Honeycombing, traction bronchiectasis
Pulmonary function testing	↓ FEV$_1$ and FVC (restrictive pattern); ↓ TLC; ↓ PaO$_2$ on exercise challenge; ↓ D$_{LCO}$		
Other findings supportive of a diagnosis of HP	• Positive natural challenge or increase in signs and symptoms on reexposure • Positive precipitating antibodies to HP antigens or antigens cultured directly from the causative environment • Improvement with avoidance • Surgical lung biopsy: interstitial lymphocytic or plasma cell infiltrates and/or noncaseating granulomas; pulmonary fibrosis in advanced cases • BAL lymphocytosis with reduced CD4/CD8 ratio		

Abbreviations: BAL = bronchoalveolar lavage; D$_{LCO}$ = carbon monoxide diffusion in the lungs; FEV$_1$ = forced expiratory volume in 1 second; FVC = forced vital capacity; HP = hypersensitivity pneumonitis; PaO$_2$ = arterial partial pressure of oxygen; TLC = total lung capacity.
From Richerson HB, Bernstein IL, Fink JN, et al: Guidelines for the clinical evaluation of hypersensitivity pneumonitis: Report of the subcommittee on hypersensitivity pneumonitis. J Allergy Clin Immunol 1989;84:839–844; and Bernstein D, Lummus Z, Santilli G, et al: Machine operator's lung: A hypersensitivity pneumonitis disorder associated with exposure to metalworking fluid aerosols. Chest 2006;108:636–641.

Treatment

The primary treatment is cessation of exposure to the sources of offending antigens at home or in the workplace. Effective environmental control measures may include modification of work habits, improvement in ventilation, or change in manufacturing procedures. Systemic corticosteroids are often required and aid in recovery during the acute or subacute phases, but there are no long-term studies of their impact on disease progression or survival rates. Referral to a specialist in occupational lung diseases is recommended for proper diagnosis and identification of the sources of causative antigens.

References

Bernstein D, Lummus Z, Santilli G, et al: Machine operator's lung: A hypersensitivity pneumonitis disorder associated with exposure to metalworking fluid aerosols, Chest 108:636–641, 2006.

Girard M, Lacasse Y, Cormier Y: Hypersensitivity pneumonitis, Allergy 65:322–334, 2009.

Hanak V, Golbin JM, Hartman TE, et al: High-resolution CT findings of parenchymal fibrosis correlate with prognosis in hypersensitivity pneumonitis, Chest 134:133–138, 2008.

Jacobs RL, Andrews CP, Coalson JJ: Hypersensitivity pneumonitis: Beyond classic occupation disease: Changing concepts of diagnosis and management, Ann Allergy Asthma Immunol 95:115–128, 2005.

Lacasse Y, Assayag E, Cormier Y: Myths and controversies in hypersensitivity pneumonitis, Semin Respir Crit Care Med 29:631–642, 2008.

Nogueira R, Melo N, Novais E, et al: Hypersensitivity pneumonitis: Antigen diversity and disease implications, Pulmonology 25(2):97–108, 2019.

Richerson HB, Bernstein IL, Fink JN, et al: Guidelines for the clinical evaluation of hypersensitivity pneumonitis: Report of the subcommittee on hypersensitivity pneumonitis, J Allergy Clin Immunol 84:839–844, 1989.

Schuyler M, Gott K, French V: The role of MIP-1alpha in experimental hypersensitivity pneumonitis, Lung 182:135–149, 2004.

LEGIONELLOSIS (LEGIONNAIRES' DISEASE AND PONTIAC FEVER)

Method of
Julio A. Ramirez, MD

In the summer of 1976, an outbreak of approximately 182 cases of pneumonia occurred in persons attending the American Legion convention in Philadelphia. One year later, Dr. McDade reported the identification of *Legionella pneumophila*, the bacterium responsible for the infection. Today, the family of Legionellaceae is composed of more than 40 species, with some species having different serogroups. *L pneumophila* causes approximately 85% of all *Legionella* infections. *L pneumophila* serogroup 1 is the single most common member of the family causing clinical infections.

Epidemiology

Legionella is an intracellular organism that lives in natural water. In the aquatic environment, the bacteria live and multiply within freshwater amebae. The number of *Legionella* organisms in the water can increase significantly with appropriate local conditions such as warm temperature, lack of biocides, stagnant water, and presence of amebae and other nutrients. These special conditions can be present in artificial water systems such as cooling towers, whirlpools, decorative fountains, and respiratory therapy devices.

The susceptible host acquires the bacteria from water containing the organism. Infection can be acquired by inhaling aerosols containing *Legionella* organisms or by microaspiration of water contaminated with *Legionella*. The hospitalized patient with *Legionella* pneumonia does not require respiratory isolation because legionellosis is not transmitted from person to person.

Clinical Features

Once *Legionella* organisms reach the respiratory tract, based on the interactions of the organism with the host immune system, the patient can have four possible clinical outcomes: asymptomatic infection, Pontiac fever, Legionnaires' disease, or extrapulmonary disease involving the liver, heart, brain, or other organs. Pontiac fever is a nonpneumonic form of disease characterized by fever, headaches, myalgias, and malaise. The patient has an influenza-like illness, with resolution of disease in a few days without specific antimicrobial therapy. Patients with Legionnaires' disease present with community-acquired pneumonia associated with high fever, gastrointestinal complaints such as diarrhea, and central nervous system complaints such as headaches or mental status changes. Hospital-acquired pneumonia can occur if *Legionella* is present in the hospital water supply.

Diagnosis

The currently available laboratory tests for diagnosis of *Legionella* infections include the direct fluorescent antibody stain (DFA), culture, antigen detection in the urine, antibody detection in serum by indirect fluorescent antibody testing (IFA), and DNA amplification using the polymerase chain reaction (PCR). The DFA stain can detect all *L pneumophila* serogroups, but a large number of bacteria need to be present in sputum for a positive result. *Legionella* can be cultured from respiratory specimens on selective media composed of buffered charcoal–yeast extract agar. The urinary antigen detection has a specificity greater than 95%; the disadvantage is that the test detects only the antigen of *L pneumophila* serogroup 1. Clinical specimens that have been used to detect *Legionella* by PCR include throat swabs, sputum, tracheal suction, bronchoalveolar lavage fluid, pleural fluid, and lung tissue.

Treatment

In the pulmonary parenchyma, *Legionella* can infect and multiply inside alveolar macrophages, alveolar epithelial cells, and capillary endothelial cells. The poor clinical outcome with β-lactam antibiotics is due to their lack of penetration into cells. Antibiotics with good intracellular penetration that can be used as monotherapy for *Legionella* infections include macrolides, tetracyclines, and quinolones (Table 1). Rifampin (Rifadin)[1] is not used as monotherapy because resistance can rapidly emerge when it is used alone.

TABLE 1	Antibiotic Therapy for Legionella Infections	
	ORAL DOSE	**IV DOSE**
Macrolides		
Azithromycin (Zithromax)	500 mg qd	500 mg qd
Clarithromycin (Biaxin)[1]	500 mg bid	
Erythromycin (Ery-Tab)	500 mg q6h	1 g q6h
Quinolones		
Ciprofloxacin (Cipro)[1]	750 mg bid	400 mg bid
Levofloxacin (Levaquin)	750 mg qd	750 mg qd
Moxifloxacin (Avelox)[1]	400 mg qd	400 mg qd
Rifamycins		
Rifampin (Rifadin)[1]	300 mg bid	300 mg bid
Tetracyclines		
Doxycycline (Vibramycin)[1]	100 mg bid on day 1, then 100 mg qd	100 mg bid on day 1, then 100 mg qd
Omadacycline (Nuzyra)	450 mg qd on day 1 and 2[3], then 300 mg qd	100 mg bid on day 1, then 100 mg qd

[1]Not FDA approved for this indication.
[3]Exceeds dosage recommended by the manufacturer.

---

[1]Not FDA approved for this indication.

Therapy of the patient with severe disease is initiated with intravenous antibiotics. Once the patient reaches clinical stability, the intravenous therapy can be switched to oral therapy. Doses for the most common antibiotics for intravenous and oral therapy are depicted in Table 1. In the nonimmunocompromised patient, the recommended duration of therapy is 7 to 10 days. In immunocompromised patients, because they are at risk for relapsing infection, the recommended duration of therapy is 14 to 21 days.

Several antibiotics have demonstrated clinical efficacy in Legionnaires' disease. Data with several in vitro and animal studies comparing different anti-*Legionella* antibiotics indicate that erythromycin (Ery-Tab) is a weak anti-*Legionella* agent. If erythromycin is selected for therapy, it is important to add rifampin to the regimen to increase intracellular killing. From the family of macrolides, azithromycin (Zithromax) is the most active. The best bactericidal activity in the laboratory is achieved with quinolones. Retrospective observational studies indicate that patients treated with levofloxacin (Levaquin) have a shorter time to reach clinical stability and shorter duration of hospital stay. These antibiotics are considered primary anti-*Legionella* agents.

In clinical practice, I treat immunocompromised patients who have severe Legionnaires' disease with a combination of an intravenous quinolone plus an intravenous macrolide (e.g., levofloxacin plus azithromycin). This regimen is based only on the theoretical consideration that synergistic killing may be obtained using a quinolone to alter DNA synthesis and a macrolide to alter protein synthesis.

OBSTRUCTIVE SLEEP APNEA

Method of
Daniel P. Fox, MD; and Masayoshi Takashima, MD

CURRENT DIAGNOSIS

Symptoms
- Excessive daytime fatigue and somnolence
- Morning headaches
- Loud snoring and gasping for air
- Witnessed apneic episodes following loud snoring
- Frequent nocturia with no other underlying etiology
- Hypertension

Clinical Signs and Risk Factors
- Central obesity with body mass index (BMI) >30 kg/m²
- Large neck circumference (>17 inches in men, >16 inches in women)
- Being male or a postmenopausal woman
- Use of sedatives or alcohol before going to bed
- Family history of sleep apnea
- Craniofacial abnormalities: retrognathia, micrognathia, congenital malformations

CURRENT THERAPY

- Gold standard for treatment is positive airway pressure
- Weight loss, smoking cessation, avoidance of sedatives
- Improvement of sleep hygiene and sleep schedule
- Minimally invasive procedures (oral appliances, palatal stents, radiofrequency turbinate reductions) may be beneficial for a select patient population

- Surgical therapy is usually reserved for patients not tolerating or unable to use CPAP or BiPAP
- Initial procedures are focused on decreasing upper airway resistance to improve compliance with CPAP or BiPAP
- Identification of anatomic sites of obstruction is critical to successful surgical outcomes

Abbreviation: BiPAP = bilevel positive airway pressure; CPAP = continuous positive airway pressure.

Sleep-disordered breathing encompasses the spectrum from upper airway resistance syndrome to obstructive sleep apnea (OSA). OSA is characterized by episodes of partial or complete upper airway collapse leading to cessation or reduction of airflow. Such events lead to oxygen desaturation and sleep fragmentation, causing excessive daytime sleepiness, morning headaches, depression, memory loss, impaired alertness, decreased libido, and reduced cognitive function. Nighttime symptoms are often more telling, and obtaining a sleep history from a bed partner is exceptionally helpful. The most common symptoms include loud snoring, restless sleep, choking or gasping episodes, and awakenings during sleep. Nocturnal perspiration, nocturia, and symptoms of nocturnal gastroesophageal reflux are also commonly associated with severe OSA.

As the severity of OSA typically increases with age, nightly hypoventilation and activation of the sympathetic nervous system lead to pathophysiologic derangements, such as hypertension, ischemic heart disease, myocardial infarction, stroke, arrhythmia, and premature death. An apnea–hypopnea index (AHI) of greater than 5 has been shown to be associated with increased risk of cerebrovascular accident. An AHI greater than 20 is associated with increased mortality. Patients with oxygen desaturation below 90% have an elevated incidence of cardiac arrhythmias. These potentially severe consequences, along with a patient's decreased quality of life, substantiate the need for early recognition and treatment.

Definitions of terms related to sleep apnea are listed in Box 1.

BOX 1	Definitions of Sleep Medicine Terms

Apnea–hypopnea index (AHI): Sum of apneas and hypopneas per hour of sleep.

Obstructive apnea: Cessation of airflow for ≥10 seconds associated with ongoing ventilatory effort.

Obstructive hypopnea: 1. Decreased airflow by ≥30% which is ≥10 seconds and a ≥3% oxygen desaturation and or associated with an arousal. 2. Decreased airflow ≥30% which is ≥10 seconds which is associated with a ≥4% oxygen desaturation

Obstructive sleep apnea (OSA): AHI >5 events per hour of sleep, often associated with oxygen desaturation <90%. Mild OSA is defined by an AHI of 5 to 15. Moderate OSA is an AHI 15 to 30, and severe OSA is an AHI >30.

Obstructive sleep apnea syndrome: OSA in association with daytime symptoms of excessive sleepiness or other neurobehavioral symptoms.

Primary snoring: Snoring with an AHI <5 and no complaints of excessive daytime sleepiness.

Respiratory effort–related arousals: Sleep fragmentation that is caused by arousals from increasing respiratory effort but that does not meet criteria for an apnea or hypopnea. The event lasts longer than 10 seconds.

Respiratory disturbance index: Sum of apneas, hypopneas, and respiratory effort–related arousals per hour of sleep.

Upper airway resistance syndrome (UARS): Snoring in association with AHI <5, frequent arousals, and abnormally negative midesophageal pressure (less than –10 cm H₂O) or increased diaphragmatic electromyogram activity.

Epidemiology

Based on available population-based studies, the prevalence of OSA among adults between 30 and 60 years of age is estimated to be 6% for women and 13% for men. This represents relative increases over the last two decades of 14–55% amongst subgroups divided by age, gender, and BMI. OSA remains undiagnosed in 70% to 80% of patients because their symptoms are often vague, and OSA must be diagnosed with polysomnography.

Risk Factors

When controlling for gender and BMI, patients over age 50 have an increased prevalence of obstructive sleep apnea secondary to decreased muscle tone.

Obesity (body mass index [BMI] greater than $30\,kg/m^2$) is a risk factor for OSA. A 10% increase in weight is associated with a six-fold increase in risk for development of OSA, and a 10% weight loss is associated with 26% decrease in AHI. Patients undergoing bariatric surgery on average have post-surgical reductions in AHI of 29 events per hour. There is evidence of a potential link between OSA and insulin resistance.

Approximately 30% of hypertensive persons have OSA and up to 50% of OSA patients have hypertension. Resistant hypertension, which is defined as blood pressure >140/90 mmHg despite therapy with at least 3 different anti-hypertensive classes, is especially prevalent in the OSA population. It is estimated that 90% of male patients and 77% of female patients with resistant hypertension have OSA. A dose-effect relationship between OSA severity and severity of hypertension has been established. Mechanisms for hypertension center around hypoxemia and hypercapnia leading to increased oxidative stress, decreased nitric oxide secretion, and increased catecholamine, angiotensin II, aldosterone, renin, and endothelin-1 secretion.

Male patients are nearly twice as likely to have OSA as female patients. Estrogen and progesterone might have a protective role because population-based studies have demonstrated that post-menopausal women have a two- to threefold increased risk of OSA compared to premenopausal women.

African Americans and Asians are at greater risk for OSA than Caucasians. Being African American is an independent risk factor for severe sleep-disordered breathing, with an odds ratio of 2.55 compared with whites. Asians have a narrower cranial base, a higher Mallampati score, smaller thyromental distance, and steeper thyromental plane than whites, which might account for their increased risk.

Pathophysiology

Airway obstruction leading to OSA can occur anywhere along the pathway from the nostrils, soft palate, base of tongue, hypopharynx, and the epiglottis. The airway lacks skeletal structure and is vulnerable to influences such as muscle tone, fat deposition, and tissue redundancy.

Prevention

Lifestyle modification can prevent OSA. Patients should adopt a healthy and athletic lifestyle to develop good muscle tone and weight loss, avoid sedatives and alcohol at bedtime, establish regular sleeping patterns, avoid the supine sleeping position, and elevate the head when sleeping.

Diagnosis

Definitive diagnosis of OSA is made by polysomnography. Mild OSA is defined as an AHI of 5 to 15 per hour, moderate OSA is an AHI of 15 to 30 per hour, and severe OSA is an AHI greater than 30 per hour. Patients spend the night in a sleep laboratory during which multiple physiologic variables are continuously monitored. These include electroencephalogram (EEG), electrooculogram (EOG), electromyogram (EMG), oronasal airflow, chest wall effort, body position, snore volume, electrocardiogram (ECG), and oxyhemoglobin saturation. Laboratory testing also includes a complete accounting of sleep variables, monitoring of cardiac rhythm, and assessment of possible restless legs syndrome (RLS) or periodic limb movements (PLMs) during sleep. This information enables the clinician to determine the severity of the condition and identifies potentially relevant comorbidities.

A thorough diagnostic study requires at least 6 hours of sleep, allowing assessment of variability related to sleep stages. If there are sufficient apneas or hypopneas during the first half of the study (ideally 4 hours of diagnostic testing, with a minimum of 2 hours if an AHI >40 is confirmed), a split-night study may be performed, in which the second half of the night (minimum of 3 hours of sleep) is devoted to titration of continuous positive airway pressure (CPAP) therapy. If the criteria for a split-night sleep study are not achieved during the night, a second night for titration study is ordered. The split-night protocol is a cost-effective use of laboratory resources that is particularly well suited for patients with severe OSA.

According to the Institute for Clinical Systems Improvement (ICSI), polysomnography should be performed in patients with symptoms of OSA and one or more of the following: cardiovascular disease, hypertension, coronary artery disease, obesity, sleep complaint, type 2 diabetes mellitus, recurrent atrial fibrillation, and large neck circumference.

Treatment

Initially, patients should be counseled to avoid practices that can potentially worsen the severity of OSA. CNS depressants taken before sleep (alcohol, sleep medications, pain medications) can worsen upper airway collapse during sleep and should be discouraged. Weight loss and maintenance should always play a role in the treatment of these patients. Myofunctional Therapy, which is a series of isometric and isotonic exercises of the oral cavity and pharyngeal muscles, is designed to increase upper airway tone. Oral Pressure Therapy uses a mouthpiece to generate negative pressure to gently pull the palate forward, opening the retropalatal airway. End Positive Airway Pressure (EPAP) Therapy uses nasal appliances to increase expiratory resistance and prevent pharyngeal collapse.

In patients with positional OSA, defined as >2-fold difference in AHI between supine and non-supine positions, avoiding the supine position during sleep may suffice to normalize ventilation during sleep. There are several commercial devices worn around the neck or back that gently vibrate when a patient is supine. Nightly compliance rates are 75–96%.

Continuous Positive Airway Pressure Therapy

CPAP remains the therapeutic mainstay for primary treatment of OSA. It serves as a pneumatic stent for the upper airway and is effective in reducing the physiologic abnormalities measured on polysomnography. Additionally, CPAP is thought to augment lung volumes and elicit a reflex that increases tone in the upper airway musculature. Overall, it has been shown to reduce AHI, improve quality of life, and reduce cardiovascular risk.

There are many manufacturers of CPAP devices and many interfaces that help maximize comfort with treatment. Expiratory pressure release (EPR) is available through several CPAP manufacturers. EPR does not seem to compromise the effectiveness of CPAP therapy and improves the patient's sense of comfort with therapy, but it does not seem to systematically improve the level of adherence. Automatically-adjusting Positive Airway Pressure (APAP), is similar to CPAP but instead of delivering a constant pressure adjusts delivered pressure breath-to-breath.

Bi-level respiratory-assist devices deliver alternating levels of positive airway pressure and might be considered an alternative therapeutic option when standard CPAP is not tolerated or when oxygen saturation is not raised sufficiently with standard CPAP. In some cases of severe OSA (in particular among patients with

BOX 2 — Treatments for Obstructive Sleep Apnea

Nasal Obstruction
Septoplasty
Rhinoplasty or nasal valve surgery
Turbinate reduction
Adenoidectomy

Retropalatal Obstruction
Tonsillectomy
Uvulopalatopharyngoplasty
Z-palatoplasty
Lateral pharyngoplasty
Palatal stents
Radiofrequency soft palate surgery

Retrolingual Obstruction
Transoral robotic-assisted base of tongue reduction
Lingual tonsillectomy
Genioglossus advancement
Hyoid suspension
Tongue base suspension
Maxillomandibular advancement

underlying pulmonary conditions), supplemental oxygen can be used in conjunction with CPAP therapy.

The main disadvantage with positive airway pressure treatment is poor compliance. Multicenter trials show that CPAP adherence rates defined as at least 4 hours per night 70% of nights are between only 39-50% overall CPAP compliance. Treatment is effective as long as the patient uses the device for the entire night, every night. APAP, CPAP desensitization, and the use of integrated heated humidifiers helped improve adherence to therapy.

Oral Appliances

Oral appliances worn in the mouth during sleep can help maintain a patent airway, especially in patients with significant positional sleep apnea who sleep supine and experience airway collapse secondary to the tongue falling posteriorly. In general, there are two types of appliances, mandibular-advancement appliances and tongue-retaining devices. The mandibular-advancement appliances are currently used more often and have been more widely studied. They require viable dentition for retention and they are fitted to the maxillary and mandibular dentition to enable the protrusion of the mandible and therefore increase oropharyngeal patency. The most common side effect is drooling. Temporomandibular joint pain might limit the viability of this therapy, and chronic use of the appliance can result in a change of the dental occlusion. A dentist with expertise in sleep medicine should ideally implement and monitor this type of treatment.

Surgical Procedures

If patients are not tolerating CPAP and a significant upper airway anatomic obstruction is identified, surgery should be considered. A variety of procedures help stabilize the retropalatal region, and others are intended to stabilize the retrolingual airway (Box 2). Sleep surgery has been shown to be most effective when addressing multiple levels of obstruction. Procedures are often combined for maximum effectiveness, such as septoplasty, turbinate reduction, tonsillectomy, uvulopalatopharyngoplasty and genial tubercle advancement. With the advent of transoral robotic surgery, surgeons are now able to access the posterior oropharynx, base of tongue, and hypopharynx more easily, and procedures to address these areas are more common. A substantially more invasive procedure, the maxillomandiublar advancement, has been shown very effective in a number of case series. However, the only definitive surgical cure is tracheostomy, which completely bypasses the upper airway but is not without its comorbidities.

It is challenging to predict which patients are likely to have a successful surgical outcome. Much of this difficulty is associated with accurately identifying the site(s) of obstruction. The current gold standard is drug-induced sleep endoscopy (DISE), a procedure that examines the upper airway while the patient is in a drug-induced (propofol [Diprivan][1] or dexmedetomidine [Precedex]) sleep-resembling state. As the patient snores and obstructs, a flexible fiberoptic scope is passed through the nose to evaluate the upper airway for the site of obstruction.

Monitoring

The patient's response to therapy needs to be monitored. In the case of CPAP therapy, monitoring of CPAP adherence is critical, because subjective reports are inaccurate. Resolution of excessive sleepiness is the desired outcome for patients who are symptomatic at baseline. If excessive sleepiness remains problematic despite documentation of desirable CPAP adherence, treatment with modafinil (Provigil) 100 to 400 mg in the morning might be considered. Other potential conditions affecting sleep need to be monitored and, if necessary, treated. Often, other conditions such as poor sleep hygiene, restless legs syndrome, periodic limb movements, or psychophysiologic insomnia interfere with adequate response to therapy.

For patients who undergo surgery, retesting is indicated. The interval at which retesting should be done depends on the type of surgery that was performed. Retesting 3 months following the surgical intervention is adequate in most cases.

References

Al Lawati NM, Patel SR, Ayas NT: Epidemiology, risk factors, and consequences of obstructive sleep apnea and short sleep duration, *Prog Cardiovasc Dis* 51:285–293, 2009.

Ancoli-Israel S, Klauber MR, Stepnowsky C, et al: Sleep-disordered breathing in African-American elderly, *Am J Respir Crit Care Med* 52:1946–1949, 1995.

Ashrafian H, Toma T, Rowland SP, et al: Bariatric surgery or non-surgical weight loss for obstructive sleep apnoea? A systematic review and comparison of meta-analysis. *Obes Surg* 25(7):1239–1250, 2015.

Cai A, Wang L, Zhou Y. Hypertension and obstructive sleep apnea. Hypertens Res 2016;39:391–5.

Caples SM, Rowley JA, Prinsell JR, et al: Surgical modifications of the upper airway for obstructive sleep apnea in adults: a systematic review and meta-analysis, *Sleep* 33(10):1396–1407, 2010.

Dedhia RC, Strollo PJ, Soose RJ: Upper airway stimulation for obstructive sleep apnea: Past, present, and future, *Sleep* 38:899–906, 2015.

Fujita S, Conway W, Zorick F, Roth T: Surgical correction of anatomic abnormalities in obstructive sleep apnea syndrome; Uvulopalatopharyngoplasty, *Otolaryngol Head Neck Surg* 89(6):923–934, 1981.

Hsin-Ching L, Friedman M, Hsueh-Wen C, et al: The efficacy of multilevel surgery of the upper airway in adults with obstructive sleep apnea/hypopnea syndrome, *The Laryngoscope* 118:902–908, 2008.

Institute for Clinical Systems Improvement (ICSI): *Diagnosis and Treatment of Obstructive Sleep Apnea in Adults*, Bloomington, MN, 2008, Institute for Clinical Systems Improvement.

Levendowski DJ, Seagraves S, Popovic D, Westbrook PR: Assessment of a neck-based treatment and monitoring device for positional obstructive sleep apnea, *J Clin Sleep Med* 10:863–871, 2014.

Li KK, Powell NB, Kushida C, et al: A comparison of Asian and white patients with obstructive sleep apnea syndrome, *Laryngoscope* 109:1937–1940, 1999.

Peppard PE, Young T, Palta M, et al: Prospective study of the association between sleep-disordered breathing and hypertension, *N Engl J Med* 342:1378–1384, 2000.

Peppard PE, Young T, Palta M, et al: Longitudinal study of moderate weight change and sleep-disordered breathing, *JAMA* 284:3015–3021, 2000.

Punjabi NM: The epidemiology of adult obstructive sleep apnea, *Proc Am Thorac Soc* 5:136–143, 2008.

Quan SF, Howard BV, Iber C, et al: The Sleep Heart Health Study: Design, rationale, and methods, *Sleep* 20:1077–1085, 1997.

Sher AE, Schechtman KB, Piccirillo JF: The efficacy of surgical modifications of the upper airway in adults with obstructive sleep apnea syndrome, *Sleep* 19(2):156–177, 1996.

Vilaseca I, Morello A, Montserrat JM, et al: Usefulness of uvulopalatopharyngoplasty with genioglossus and hyoid advancement in the treatment of obstructive sleep apnea, *Arch Otolaryngol Head Neck Surg* 128:435–440, 2002.

---

[1] Not FDA approved for this indication.

PLEURAL EFFUSIONS AND EMPYEMA THORACIS

Method of
David J. Finley, MD; and Raja Flores, MD

Pleural effusions have multiple etiologies, making the diagnosis and management a common clinical issue. Though the amount of fluid produced varies significantly, an average 0.1 to 0.2 mL/kg is maintained within the pleural space. Production of fluid is matched with removal during normal physiologic states, but aberrations of this homeostasis with local or systemic diseases lead to the formation of an effusion. Symptoms are related to the volume of fluid and the etiology of the fluid accumulation, including both benign and malignant processes. Secondary infection of a pleural effusion, known as an empyema, is a significant complication necessitating aggressive treatment of both the underlying cause and the empyema itself.

Symptoms are variable and include dyspnea, shortness of breath, cough, and chest discomfort, though patients can be asymptomatic, even with very large effusions. Dullness to percussion and decreased breath sounds are often hallmarks of effusions, but these signs are also seen with lung masses and consolidative pneumonias. A clinical history, physical examination, and imaging studies are often needed in combination to diagnose an effusion.

Etiology

Many local and systemic illnesses are associated with the formation of a pleural effusion. Systemic symptoms can indicate the most common cause of the effusion, but diagnostic procedures are often necessary to delineate the etiology. Determination of an exudative or transudative effusion can point out possible disease that may be the cause (Box 1).

Fluid that is low in total protein is a transudative effusion, which is most commonly caused by decreased oncotic pressure or increased capillary hydrostatic pressure. Transudative effusions can also be caused by fluid traversing the diaphragm, as seen in patients with ascites.

Exudative effusions are high in total protein (pleural fluid-to-serum ratio >0.5) and often have an elevated cell count. Increased capillary permeability and decreased lymphatic clearance, usually due to a local or systemic inflammatory illness, produce exudative effusions. The causes are varied, but the most common causes are malignancy, infection, and pulmonary emboli.

Diagnosis

Imaging

Approximately 200 to 500 mL of pleural fluid is necessary before it can be visualized on a posteroanterior upright chest x-ray, usually as blunting of the costophrenic angle. A lateral chest x-ray is more sensitive, often discerning fluid with as little as 100 mL present; layering of the fluid confirms that it is free flowing. Loculations can be seen on x-ray but may be mistaken for lung or pleural masses. Large effusion can completely opacify the hemithorax where the effusion is located. Ultrasound is useful in defining the location and extent of an effusion and can also identify loculated effusions, pleural thickening, and masses. When used to help guide thoracentesis, it can increase diagnostic accuracy and yield and decrease complications.

Chest computed tomography (CT) has distinct advantages over x-ray and ultrasound, though its utility is significantly decreased when there is a large effusion. Imaging with CT after initial drainage of a large effusion is recommended to obtain the most information regarding the possible etiologies of the effusion and aid in operative planning for treatment of an empyema. It also delineates pleural masses and helps differentiate pleural disease from lung pathology (e.g., loculated effusion vs. lung abscess).

Thoracentesis

Often it is difficult to discern the cause of an effusion solely based on the patient's clinical presentation and image studies. Also, when concerned about a malignant process or an infected effusion, these studies do not give enough information to make a definitive diagnosis. Thoracentesis is the diagnostic procedure of choice, allowing drainage of the fluid to relieve symptoms for the patient and provide a specimen for evaluation. Ultrasound should be employed to help guide thoracentesis, especially if the effusion is small or loculated. Care must be taken when draining a large amount of fluid in one setting due to the risk of reexpansion pulmonary edema. If a patient becomes symptomatic during the procedure (persistent cough, significant pleuritic pain, or shortness of breath) no more fluid should be removed at that time. Coagulopathy is a contraindication to thoracentesis due to the risk of intrathoracic bleeding.

Pleural Fluid

The initial evaluation of pleural fluid is done at the bedside by determining the nature of the fluid: clear, cloudy, bloody, or milky. One should also evaluate the fluid for odor and cellularity. These simple steps can point the clinician toward the correct diagnosis. In addition to bedside evaluation, the fluid should be sent for the following laboratory studies: pH, glucose, lactate dehydrogenase (LDH), protein, cytology, Gram stain, and culture (including fungal and viral). Serum pH, protein, LDH and glucose should be sent at the same time.

Light's criteria are helpful in differentiating between an exudative and transudative effusion (Box 2). The sensitivity and specificity of Light's criteria is 82% to 90%.

Transudative effusions rarely need any further intervention, and the goal of treatment is directed at the underlying condition (see Box 1). For exudative effusions, the cause of the effusion dictates the treatment. Incorporating the clinical picture and radiographs with the pleural fluid chemistry studies, cytology, and

---

BOX 1 | **Etiologies of Transudative and Exudative Effusions**

Transudative
Congestive heart failure
Cirrhosis
Pulmonary emboli
Peritoneal dialysis
Renal disorders
Myxedema
Sarcoidosis

Exudative
Malignancy
Infection
Drugs (e.g., nitrofurantoin [Marcodantin, Macrobid], methotrexate [Trexall])
Chylothorax
Pulmonary emboli
Gastrointestinal diseases (e.g., pancreatitis)
Collagen vascular disease (e.g., rheumatoid arthritis)
Asbestos exposure
Trauma (e.g., hemothorax, chest surgery)
Postpericardiectomy or postmyocardial infarction syndrome
Pleuropericarditis

BOX 2 | **Light's Criteria for an Exudative Effusion**

Pleural fluid-to-serum ratio of protein >0.5
Pleural fluid-to-serum ration of LDH >0.6
Absolute pleural fluid LDH >2/3 of upper limit of normal serum levels

Abbreviation: LDH = lactate dehydrogenase.

cultures, the diagnosis is often obtained. Malignant effusions can have positive cytology, but they are more likely to have a pleural fluid glucose level less than 60 mg/dL and to be bloody. An elevated amylase level is seen in esophageal perforation, pancreatitis, and malignant effusions. Chylothorax can be definitively diagnosed if the triglyceride level is more than 110 mg/dL within the pleural fluid. Finally, pH, glucose, and cultures are useful in the treatment of patients with a presumed infected pleural effusion (empyema).

Up to 25% of patients will not have a definitive diagnosis based on the clinical scenario and pleural fluid evaluation. These patients can require further diagnostic testing, including repeat thoracentesis or evaluation of the chest cavity via video-assisted thoracoscopic surgery (VATS) with pleural biopsies.

Treatment

After initial evacuation of the effusion, treatment is directed at controlling the underlying disease that caused the effusion. Malignant effusions are best managed with pleurodesis, usually employing talc (Sterile Talc), if lung re-expansion can be obtained. This is best performed via VATS, which allows biopsies to be performed, confirming the diagnosis and visually confirming lung re-expansion. Though it can be done via tube thoracostomy at the bedside, VATS pleurodesis has been shown to reduce hospital stay and the risk of recurrence. If the lung cannot expand fully, then the fluid is often best managed with an indwelling long-term silicone-elastic catheter for palliation. In patients with benign disease, pleurodesis is rarely done because of the high complication and failure rates.

Infected Pleural Space and Empyema

A parapneumonic effusion (exudative effusion in the setting of pulmonary infection) is seen in 20% to 40% of patients admitted for pneumonia, of whom 10% to 20% will develop a complicated parapneumonic effusion or empyema (pus in the pleural space). Progression to empyema is most often due to delay in treatment and leads to longer hospital stays and increased morbidity and mortality. Other causes of infected effusions are trauma, thoracic surgical procedures, perforated esophagus, systemic infection, and transdiaphragmatic spread.

Parapneumonic effusions can be separated into three stages: exudative (stage I), fibropurulent (stage II), and organizational (stage III). Though thoracentesis is indicated in each stage, it is usually sufficient for stage I effusions when coupled with appropriate antibiotics. These effusions are free flowing, have negative cultures, and often do not reaccumulate.

Complicated parapneumonic, or stage II, effusions require drainage beyond the initial thoracentesis. The fluid is more viscous and has positive bacterial cultures, a low glucose level, and low pH. Progression to frank pus, or empyema, occurs in this stage, with the formation of loculations as fibrin deposition increases. Complete evacuation of the effusion is required, and initial tube thoracostomy is indicated. If the patient does not improve over the next 24 hours or the space is not completely drained (residual loculations), then surgery is recommended. Randomized, placebo-controlled trials showed no improved outcomes with the use of fibrinolytics as compared to standard tube thoracostomy drainage. The introduction of DNase (Pulmozyme)[1] may be of benefit, but data are insufficient to recommend this treatment. We strongly recommend early intervention with VATS, which has been shown to reduce hospital stay and offers definitive treatment as compared to tube thoracostomy with fibrinolytic therapy.

Delayed or inadequate treatment causes the patient to progress to the organizational stage. This is characterized by heavy fibrin deposit with the formation of a thick peel throughout the pleura with loculations, trapping, and retarding lung re-expansion. Classic CT findings include thickened pleura with multiple loculations and inability of the lung to expand after tube thoracostomy. Decortication, either via VATS or thoracotomy, is required to completely remove the peel off the parietal and visceral pleura.

---

[1]Not FDA approved for this indication.

Without obliteration of the empyema space it is very unlikely that the infection can be cleared. In these situations an open thoracostomy, or Eloesser flap, may be required to eradicate the infection.

References

Cameron R, Davies HR: Intra-pleural fibrinolytic therapy versus conservative management in the treatment of adult parapneumonic effusions and empyema, *Cochrane Database Syst Rev*(2), 2008. CD002312.

de Campos JR, Vargas FS, de Campos Werebe E, et al: Thoracoscopy talc poudrage: A 15-year experience, *Chest* 119:801–806, 2001.

Light R: Clinical practice. Pleural effusion, *N Engl J Med* 346:1971–1977, 2002.

Light RW: Parapneumonic effusions and empyema, *Proc Am Thorac Soc* 3:75–80, 2006.

Luh SP, Chen CY, Tzao CY: Malignant pleural effusion treatment outcomes: Pleurodesis via video-assisted thoracic surgery (VATS) versus tube thoracostomy, *Thorac Cardiovasc Surg* 54:332–336, 2006.

Luh SP, Hsu GJ, Cheng-Ren C: Complicated parapneumonic effusion and empyema: Pleural decortication and video-assisted thoracic surgery, *Curr Infect Dis Rep* 10:236–240, 2008.

Rahman NM, Chapman SJ, Davies RJ: Diagnosis and management of infectious pleural effusion, *Treat Respir Med* 5:295–304, 2006.

Tokuda Y, Matsushima D, Stein GH, et al: Intrapleural fibrinolytic agents for empyema and complicated parapneumonic effusions: A meta-analysis, *Chest* 129:783–790, 2006.

PNEUMOCONIOSIS: ASBESTOSIS AND SILICOSIS

Method of
David N. Weissman, MD

CURRENT DIAGNOSIS

- History of inhalation of mineral or metal dust
- Respiratory symptoms such as cough and dyspnea
- Spirometry and lung volumes show restriction or mixed obstruction/restriction in advanced disease
- Interstitial lung disease can usually be demonstrated by chest imaging. Biopsy is usually unnecessary in the setting of good exposure history and typical findings on chest imaging.
- No other likely cause of interstitial lung disease is present

CURRENT THERAPY

- Treatment is symptomatic and similar to that for other patients with chronic lung disease
- Give pneumococcal and influenza vaccinations.
- Provide empiric treatment with short- and long-acting inhaled bronchodilators and inhaled corticosteroids when they are found to provide symptomatic relief.
- Give supplemental oxygen therapy if pulmonary hypertension is present or to prevent pulmonary hypertension if O_2 saturation is less than 88% at rest, with exercise, or with sleep.
- Consider lung transplantation in the setting of end-stage lung disease.

The pneumoconioses are a group of interstitial fibrotic lung diseases predominantly associated with occupational exposures. They are caused by inhalation of mineral or metallic dust particles small enough to penetrate into the deep lung (respirable size range) (Table 1). These agents interact with pulmonary target cells, including alveolar macrophages and alveolar epithelial cells, to activate a cascade of inflammatory mediators including growth factors. Although exposure to these dusts can induce other types of respiratory disease as well, the final common pathway leading to pneumoconiosis is alveolar epithelial cell damage and interstitial fibrosis. This chapter focuses on silicosis and asbestosis, two common forms of pneumoconiosis.

TABLE 1 Representative Pneumoconioses

SOURCE	MAIN CLINICAL FEATURES	OCCUPATION	DUST
Crystalline silica	Silicosis, CODP, increased susceptibility to TB, lung cancer, autoimmune diseases	Mining, stone cutting, pottery, foundry work	Free crystalline silica (SiO_2)
Asbestiform fibers	Asbestosis, bronchogenic carcinoma, mesothelioma, various forms of benign pleural disease	Insulation, shipbuilding, construction, some mining (e.g., vermiculite mining in Libby, MT)	Various asbestiform fibers
Coal	Coal workers' pneumoconiosis, COPD	Coal mining	Coal mine dust
Hard metal	Hard metal lung disease (cobalt lung), asthma	Machinists, metal workers	Hard metal, composed primarily of tungsten carbide and cobalt

COPD, chronic obstructive pulmonary disease; *TB*, tuberculosis.

Asbestosis

Asbestos is composed of strong, heat-resistant fibers of hydrated magnesium silicate classified morphologically as serpentine (chrysotile) or amphibole (crocidolite [riebeckite asbestos], amosite [cummingtonite-grunerite asbestos], anthophyllite asbestos, actinolite asbestos, and tremolite asbestos). In addition, certain asbestiform fibers (winchite, richterite, erionite) can cause adverse health effects identical to those of asbestos. Fiber dimensions and persistence in tissues are key determinants of toxicity. There is a dose–response effect between the quantity of asbestos inhaled and the severity of fibrotic lung disease. Asbestos is also a carcinogen, and increasing exposure is associated with increased risk for lung cancer, mesothelioma, ovarian cancer, and laryngeal cancer.

Although asbestos is no longer mined in the United States, importation of asbestos-containing products continues. Exposures also continue to occur, especially in construction and renovation (due to reservoirs of asbestos that are still present in many older buildings), the heating trades (where asbestos is often encountered), and with exposure to older or imported asbestos-containing automotive friction products such as brake linings and clutch facings. Workers exposed to asbestos can carry it home on their clothing, resulting in exposure of family members. Living near geological formations prone to asbestos formation in California has been implicated as a risk factor for mesothelioma.

The Occupational Safety and Health Administration (OSHA) permissible exposure limit (PEL) for asbestos is 0.1 fiber per cc air. This limit was based in part on the limits of the analytical methodology used in exposure assessment. Exposure to the PEL every day over a 45-year working lifetime has been estimated to be associated with an increased risk of cancer (lung, mesothelioma, and gastrointestinal) of 336 cases per 100,000 exposed persons and an increased risk of asbestosis of 250 cases per 100,000 exposed persons.

Asbestosis causes symptoms of dyspnea and cough. Latency between initial exposure and disease onset is related to exposure intensity. In the United States, this period is generally about two or more decades. The disease can lead to chronic respiratory failure. Effects of smoking add to the severity of the disease and can cause obstructive findings in addition to the expected decreased lung volume and diffusion capacity associated with fibrotic lung diseases. Bibasilar inspiratory crackles on auscultation, finger clubbing, and bibasilar small, irregular parenchymal opacities on chest x-ray with extension to mid- and upper-zones with advancing disease are characteristic.

The International Labour Organization (ILO) has established a system for classification (grading) of radiographs for the presence of radiographic abnormalities in lung parenchyma and pleura that are associated with pneumoconiosis, as well as their severity. The ILO classification system is widely used in epidemiology, surveillance, administrative, and legal settings. The small opacity profusion grades of 0/1 and 1/0 are often considered as defining the boundary between normal and abnormal lung parenchyma.

High-resolution computed tomography (CT) is the most sensitive imaging method for suspected asbestosis. Findings associated with asbestos exposure include lower lobe or diffuse irregular opacities, bronchial wall thickening, rounded atelectasis, and pleural abnormalities such as pleural plaques and diffuse pleural thickening. The presence of pleural plaques on radiography (particularly bilateral calcified pleural plaques); or uncoated asbestos fibers or fibers coated with an iron-rich proteinaceous material (asbestos bodies) in sputum, bronchoalveolar lavage, or lung biopsy help differentiate asbestosis from idiopathic pulmonary fibrosis.

Criteria for Diagnosis

Diagnosis is supported by radiographic chest imaging or lung biopsy findings of interstitial lung disease compatible with asbestosis; documentation of exposure to asbestos by history, the presence of pleural plaques (bilateral pleural plaques are essentially pathognomonic for asbestos exposure), or the presence of asbestos bodies or an excessive burden of uncoated asbestos fibers in lung biopsy tissue or possibly via bronchoalveolar lavage or sputum; and no other likely explanation for the diffuse fibrotic lung disease.

Asbestos-Related Benign Pleural Disease

Pleural plaques are characteristic forms of localized parietal pleural thickening that are usually bilateral and asymmetrical, involve the lower lung fields or the diaphragm, and spare the costophrenic angles and apices. Pleural plaques are a marker for exposure to asbestos and are often associated with other asbestos-related conditions. Pleural plaques generally result in minimal reductions in forced vital capacity and do not degenerate into malignant lesions.

In contrast, diffuse visceral pleural thickening can result in adhesions between the visceral and parietal pleura with major decreases in forced vital capacity and respiratory insufficiency sufficient for consideration of decortication.

Benign pleural effusions can occur in the first decade after asbestos exposure and contain erythrocytes and a mixed inflammatory cell infiltrate of lymphocytes, neutrophils, and eosinophils. The thickened visceral pleura and adjacent atelectatic lung tissue can result in a pleural-based area of rounded atelectasis, simulating a lung mass on chest radiography. CT can reveal the comet sign, a pleural band connecting the apparent mass to an area of thickened pleura.

Lung Cancer and Malignant Mesothelioma

Exposure to all forms of asbestos increases the risk of lung cancer. The peak risk occurs at about 30 to 35 years after the onset of exposure. Tobacco smoking increases this risk in a supra-additive fashion, increasing risk to a level greater than for asbestos or smoking alone. In contrast, smoking does not further increase the asbestos-associated risk for malignant mesothelioma. Asbestos-associated malignant mesothelioma can also affect the peritoneum (and sometimes the pericardium), but when it affects the pleura, this disease manifests with dyspnea, chest pain, and bloody pleural effusion (most often unilateral). A latency period of 30 years or longer after initial exposure is common. Special immunochemical stains and electron microscopy of pleural fluid or pleural biopsies may be necessary to differentiate mesothelioma from adenocarcinoma. It is currently unclear when to screen asbestos-exposed individuals at increased risk for lung cancer with low-dose chest computed tomography.

Treatment

Treatment of asbestosis is symptomatic and similar to that for other patients with chronic lung disease (Box 1). Lung transplantation should be considered in the setting of end-stage lung disease. Treatment of benign pleural disease is also symptomatic; as already noted, decortication is an option for managing severe cases of diffuse visceral pleural thickening. Depending on extent of disease, mesothelioma may be treated with surgery, radiation, chemotherapy, or some combination of these. In general, prognosis is poor. Mesothelioma-associated malignant pleural effusion can require palliation through procedures such as pleurodesis, pleurectomy, and decortication. Asbestos-associated lung cancer is managed in the same fashion as lung cancer occurring without a history of exposure to asbestos.

Silicosis

Silicosis is a fibrosing interstitial lung disease resulting from the inhalation of crystalline silicon dioxide (silica) in dust of respirable size. The commonest form of crystalline silica is quartz, which is the main component of sand and is present in most rocks. Noncrystalline (amorphous) silica, like that in diatomaceous earth or glass, does not cause silicosis. However, heating amorphous silica, as occurs in foundries when molten metal is poured into clay castings, can convert amorphous silica into cristobalite, a hazardous form of crystalline silica. Mining, stone cutting, sandblasting, and foundry work are all examples of trades associated with exposure to respirable dust containing crystalline silica. The International Agency for Research on Cancer (IARC) has designated crystalline silica as a Group 1 human lung carcinogen.

In 2016, OSHA established a new PEL for respirable crystalline silica of 0.05 mg/m^3. It also established requirements for engineering and administrative controls, personal protective equipment, and medical surveillance including periodic chest radiography and spirometry obtained at least every 3 years. Reporting of silicosis cases to public health authorities is required in some states.

Radiographic Patterns of Silicosis

Three main radiographic patterns of silicosis have been described. Two are nodular interstitial patterns and one is an alveolar-filling pattern. The *simple* pattern is associated with nodules that are smaller than 10 mm and that are predominantly rounded and in the upper lung zones. *Progressive massive fibrosis* (PMF) is found in more advanced interstitial disease. It is associated with multiple coalescent larger nodules, upper lobe fibrosis, upward retraction of the hila, and compensatory hyperinflation of the lower lobes. The large upper-zone opacities can cavitate, sometimes in the setting of superimposed mycobacterial infection. Hilar adenopathy can occur in association with either pattern, sometimes with an egg-shell pattern of hilar node calcification. A third radiographic pattern is an alveolar-filling process. Overwhelming silica exposure over a short period can cause a pathologic response called *silicoproteinosis*, in which alveoli become flooded with proteinaceous fluid. The condition resembles idiopathic pulmonary alveolar proteinosis. The radiographic alveolar filling pattern favors the lower lung zones and is not associated with the changes of simple silicosis or PMF.

Silicosis Syndromes

Three syndromes of silicosis can be defined based on clinical course and radiographic pattern. Chronic silicosis develops slowly, usually 10 to 30 years after first exposure. It most often has the simple radiographic pattern, but it can be associated with PMF.

Accelerated silicosis develops more rapidly, within 10 years after first exposure. It is associated with higher intensity exposures and can be associated with either the simple or PMF radiographic

Patients
Stop further exposure to silica or asbestos.
  Stop smoking, avoid exposure to tobacco products.

Physicians
Provide early treatment of respiratory infections with antibiotics.
Give pneumococcal and influenza vaccinations.
Maintain a high index of suspicion and provide early evaluation of symptoms for lung, laryngeal, and ovarian cancers and mesothelioma in asbestos-exposed patients.
Maintain a high index of suspicion for pulmonary infection with *Mycobacterium tuberculosis,* nontuberculous mycobacteria, and fungi in silica-exposed patients.
Screen silica-exposed patients for latent tuberculosis infection. Treat latent infections with one of the currently-approved drug protocols.
Provide empiric treatment with short- and long-acting inhaled bronchodilators and inhaled corticosteroids when they are found to provide symptomatic relief.
Give supplemental oxygen therapy if pulmonary hypertension is present or to prevent pulmonary hypertension if O_2 saturation is less than 88% at rest, with exercise, or with sleep.
Consider lung transplantation in the setting of end-stage lung disease.

patterns. Accelerated silicosis is differentiated from chronic silicosis by its more rapid course. Patients with accelerated courses are at greater risk for developing PMF. The clinical presentations of chronic and accelerated silicosis are variable but include cough, dyspnea, and a variety of chest findings ranging from a normal chest examination to crackles, rhonchi, or wheezing. PMF is associated with more severe symptoms and respiratory impairment. Findings compatible with both restrictive and obstructive lung disease (decreased forced vital capacity [FVC], forced expiratory volume at 1 sec [FEV_1], FEV_1/FVC, diffusion capacity) can occur, potentially leading to cor pulmonale and respiratory failure.

Acute silicosis is associated with very intense exposures to silica, leading to symptoms within a few weeks to a few years after exposure. Intense exposure results in lung injury caused by flooding of alveoli with proteinaceous material, or silicoproteinosis. As already noted, the radiographic appearance is that of an alveolar-filling pattern favoring the lower lung zones. Patients present weeks to a few years after exposure with cough, weight loss, fatigue, and occasional pleuritic chest pain, crackles on auscultation, and progression to respiratory failure often complicated by mycobacterial infection.

Criteria for Diagnosis

The diagnosis of silicosis is predicated on a history of exposure to respirable crystalline silica, typical chest x-ray findings, and the lack of a more likely diagnosis. High-resolution CT detects changes of silicosis with greater sensitivity than chest radiography. Lung biopsy is seldom required for diagnosis in the setting of a good exposure history and typical findings on chest imaging.

Treatment

Treatment is symptomatic and similar to that for other patients with chronic lung disease (see Box 1). Experimental therapies such as oral corticosteroid therapy and whole-lung lavage have been reported, but clinical benefit is unclear. Lung transplantation should be considered for patients with end-stage lung disease.

All forms of silicosis, as well as substantial exposure to crystalline silica in the absence of silicosis, are associated with an increased risk of pulmonary tuberculosis and fungal infections. Patients should be evaluated for latent tuberculosis infection by tuberculin skin testing or with an interferon gamma release assay. A positive tuberculin skin test in a patient with a history of substantial silica exposure of at least 10 mm of induration should be considered evidence of tuberculosis infection, regardless of previous immunization with bacille Calmette-Guérin. If testing for latent tuberculosis infection is positive, an evaluation for active tuberculosis should be performed and active disease treated. If active tuberculosis is not present, treat for latent infection. As in other settings, treatment for active or latent infection should be provided using one of the drug treatment protocols recommended by the Centers for Disease Control and Prevention. Vaccination for influenza should be provided annually. In addition, adults with silicosis should be vaccinated with 13-valent pneumococcal conjugate vaccine (PCV13, Prevnar 13) and 23-valent pneumococcal polysaccharide vaccine (PPSV23, Pneumovax 23) according to current Centers for Disease Control and Prevention recommendations.

Disclaimer

The findings and conclusions in this report are those of the authors and do not necessarily represent the views of the National Institute for Occupational Safety and Health or the Centers for Disease Control and Prevention.

References

American Thoracic Society: Diagnosis and initial management of nonmalignant diseases related to asbestos, *Am J Respir Crit Care Med* 170(6):691–715, 2004.
CDC (Centers for Disease Control and Prevention). 2016. Recommended vaccines by age. Available at: https://www.cdc.gov/vaccines/vpd/vaccines-age.html, accessed 3/14/2017.
Department of Labor: Mine Safety and Health Administration: 30 CFR Parts 56, 57, and 71. Asbestos exposure limit; proposed rule, *Fed Reg* 70:43950–43989, 2005.
Leung CC, Yu IT, Chen W: Silicosis, *Lancet* 379(9830):2008–2018, 2012.
Miller A: Radiographic readings for asbestosis: misuse of science—validation of the ILO classification, *Am J Ind Med* 50:63–67, 2007.
Oksa P, Wolff H, Vehmas T, Pallasaho P, Frilander H, editors: *Asbestos, Asbestosis, and Cancer—Helsinki Criteria for Diagnosis and Attribution 2014*, Tampere, 2014, Juvenes Print.
Petsonk FL, Rose C, Cohen R: Coal mine dust lung disease. New lessons from old exposure, *Am J Respir Crit Care Med* 187(11):1178–1185, 2013.

LUNG ABSCESS

Method of
Dan Schuller, MD

CURRENT DIAGNOSIS

- Lung abscess is usually a complication of aspiration in patients with gingivitis or periodontal disease.
- Mixed aerobic-anaerobic copathogens are common, but sputum cultures are not reliable.
- Lung abscesses are rare in edentulous patients and should prompt evaluation for bronchial obstruction.
- CT scan of the chest is very useful in the diagnostic evaluation.

CURRENT THERAPY

- Prolonged antimicrobial therapy (6–8 weeks) and postural drainage are the cornerstones of therapy.
- Clindamycin (Cleocin) or alternative anaerobic coverage is required even if sputum cultures grow only aerobic bacteria (colonizers or copathogens).
- Percutaneous or bronchoscopic drainage is reserved for selected cases refractory to medical management or at a high risk for complications.
- Surgical resection is seldom needed because of the success of medical therapy.
- Evaluation and management of underlying predisposing conditions should not be neglected.

Definition and Classification

Lung abscess is defined as a focal area of necrosis of the lung parenchyma resulting from microbial infection and usually measuring more than 2 cm in diameter. Smaller or multiple areas of necrosis in contiguous areas are referred to as *necrotizing pneumonia*. Primary lung abscess (80%) is due to direct infection or aspiration. Secondary lung abscess (20%) is secondary to bronchial obstruction, immunodeficiency, pulmonary infarction, trauma, or complications from surgery. Lung abscesses can also be classified according to pathogen (e.g., mixed anaerobic, *Pseudomonas,* mycobacterial, fungal) or duration of symptoms (e.g., chronic with symptoms for more than a month before presentation). If symptoms are present for more than one month, the lung abscess is considered chronic.

Epidemiology and Risk Factors

Most lung abscesses result from aspiration of oral secretions in patients who harbor high bacterial concentrations in the gingival crevices. Periodontal disease, especially gingivitis, is a major predisposing condition, particularly in hosts impaired by altered sensorium due to alcoholism, anesthesia, coma, drug overdose, seizures, or stroke. Because edentulous persons rarely develop lung abscesses, other causes such as malignancy should be carefully sought. Patients with dysphagia, esophageal disease, poor airway protection, or weak cough and respiratory clearance mechanisms are also at risk for developing lung abscess.

Patients whose immune systems are compromised by malignancy, HIV infection, malnutrition, diabetes, chronic use of corticosteroids, or previous organ transplantation are more likely to be infected with aerobic bacteria, mycobacterial or fungal pathogens. These patients are more likely to have multiple abscesses, less response to treatment, and a worse prognosis.

In children, consider secondary causes including foreign body aspiration, congenital cystic adenomatoid malformation, pulmonary sequestration, cystic fibrosis, bronchiectasis, bronchogenic cyst, congenital immunodeficiency, or severe underlying neurologic abnormality.

Lemierre's disease or jugular vein suppurative thrombophlebitis, usually caused by *Fusobacterium necrophorum,* is a rare infection that begins in the pharynx as a tonsillar or peritonsillar abscess and spreads to involve the internal jugular vein, with septic emboli to the lung with secondary cavitations.

Pathophysiology

The understanding of lower airway microbiota in humans as well as the capacity of a microorganism to cause damage in a host has evolved. The development of a lung abscess usually starts when an insult (e.g., inoculum of highly contaminated oral secretions) overcomes the pulmonary mechanisms of defense and begins a process of pneumonitis in the dependent areas affected by aspiration. Depending on the microbiology and the intensity of the inflammatory response, the acute pneumonitis evolves to tissue necrosis after 7 to 14 days and subsequent cavitation. At first, the enclosing wall is poorly defined, but with time and progressive fibrosis it becomes more discrete. When a communication with the airway exists, the suppurative debris from the abscess can partially drain, leaving an air-containing cavity with a radiographic air-fluid level. Occasionally, abscesses rupture into the pleural cavity yielding an empyema or a bronchopleural fistula (Figure 1). Primary abscesses due to aspiration are much more common on the right side than the left and are most often single. The most common locations include the superior segments of the lower lobes and the posterior segment of the right upper lobe.

Clinical Manifestations

Most patients present with insidious symptoms that evolve over a period of weeks to months. Cough productive of copious amounts of putrid, foul-smelling sputum that occurs in paroxysms after changing position are characteristic. Fevers, chills, night sweats, chest pain, dyspnea, general malaise, and fatigue are common. Hemoptysis can vary from blood-streaked sputum to

Figure 1 Primary lung abscess in the right lower lobe with rupture into the pleural space causing an empyema.

life-threatening hemorrhage. Physical findings can include fever, tachycardia, periodontal disease, halitosis, signs of lung consolidation or pleural effusion, amphoric breath sounds, and occasionally clubbing of the fingers and toes can appear within a few weeks after the onset of an abscess.

Diagnosis

Lung abscess is easily diagnosed when there is a classic clinical presentation with indolent symptoms lasting more than 2 weeks in a host with predisposing risk factors and a chest radiograph revealing a cavitary infiltrate or an air-fluid level. However, numerous pathogens are associated with this syndrome, and attempts to establish microbiological diagnosis and exclude other conditions are warranted.

Computed tomography (CT) scans can be useful for better anatomic definition, to evaluate possible associated conditions such as malignancy, and to rule out pleural involvement. Distinguishing between a lung abscess and an empyema with an associated bronchopleural fistula leading to an air-fluid level can sometimes be challenging, but it is crucial because the management of these conditions is very different. Features that suggest empyema include a lenticular shape or a larger diameter of the air-fluid level on the lateral view of the chest film, an obtuse angle of the cavity with the chest wall, and a split pleural sign with contrast enhancement of the pleura.

Most lung abscesses are caused by anaerobic or mixed aerobic and anaerobic infections. Anaerobic bacteria include *Peptostreptococcus, Prevotella, Bacteroides* spp., and *Fusobacterium* spp. and are difficult to isolate owing to technical issues and contamination by upper airway flora. Other pathogens, including *Staphylococcus aureus, Klebsiella pneumonia, Pseudomonas, Burkholderia pseudomallei, Nocardia, Actinomyces,* and mycobacterial or fungal organisms, are more likely to occur in secondary lung abscesses. The bacteriology of lung abscesses may be different in other parts of the world.

Sputum Gram stains and culture should be performed in all patients but interpreted with caution because prior antimicrobial therapy can inhibit growth, and contaminant strains can be misleading. Even when there is abundant growth of a species of aerobic bacteria, treatment should still be directed at covering anaerobes.

In the absence of positive blood or pleural fluid cultures, microbiological confirmation of a lung abscess requires other invasive methods such as a transthoracic needle aspirates (TTNA) or bronchoscopy with bronchoalveolar lavage (BAL) or protected specimen brush (PSB). The best timing for bronchoscopy is controversial because early intervention has the highest diagnostic yield but at the risk of provoking spillage of a relatively contained abscess into additional lobes or the contralateral lung. In patients who are edentulous or in whom there is a high suspicion

for malignancy, the indication for bronchoscopic evaluation is almost universal but should be scheduled when the risk for clinical deterioration (e.g., spillage with resultant respiratory failure) has been minimized.

Differential Diagnosis

In addition to the multiple necrotizing infections or an empyema with a bronchopleural fistula (see earlier), there are many noninfectious diseases that can cause cavitary lung lesions and mimic a lung abscess. The differential diagnosis includes neoplasm (primary or metastatic), bullae or cyst with air-fluid level, bronchiectasis, necrotizing vasculitis, or pulmonary infarction. In patients with multiple cavitary lesions, consider septic emboli.

Treatment

Lung abscess is best treated with a prolonged course of adequate antimicrobials and postural drainage. Percutaneous or bronchoscopic drainage and surgery are considered only for selected patients whose disease is refractory to standard care.

Initial empiric antibiotic treatment for a typical community-acquired lung abscess should consist of intravenous clindamycin (Cleocin) 600 to 900 mg every 6 to 8 hours, which has been shown to be superior to penicillin. For patients with a nosocomial or health care–associated lung abscess, additional coverage for enteric gram-negative pathogens including *Pseudomonas aeruginosa* and *Staphylococcus aureus* is appropriate.

Alternative antimicrobial options include ampicillin–sulbactam (Unasyn)[1] 1.5 to 3.0 g IV every 6 hours, piperacillin–tazobactam (Zosyn)[1] 3.35 g IV every 6 hours, cefoxitin (Mefoxin) 2 to 3 g every 6 to 8 hours, or a combination of moxifloxacin (Avelox)[1] 400 mg IV daily and metronidazole (Flagyl) 500 mg IV every 6 to 8 hours. The use of metronidazole as single agent has been associated with a high therapeutic failure rate.

After defervescence and radiographic improvement, parenteral antibiotics can be switched to oral bioequivalent therapy for 6 to 8 weeks or longer depending on the course. Shorter antimicrobial courses are associated with a high rate of relapse. Most experts suggest continuing therapy until there is radiographic resolution or a small stable lesion.

Indications for percutaneous or bronchoscopic drainage include persistent sepsis after 5 to 7 days of antimicrobial therapy, abscesses larger than 4 cm that are under tension or enlarging, and need for mechanical ventilator support. Percutaneous drainage should only be considered when there is a reasonable abscess–pleura symphysis and no associated coagulopathy. Lung resection is rarely needed and is reserved for operable cases refractory to medical treatment.

Postural drainage and chest physiotherapy facilitate removal of pus, relieving symptoms and improving gas exchange. Surgical resection is required in less than 10% of patients whose disease is refractory to medical management.

Finally, evaluation and management of the predisposing conditions leading to aspiration should take place after the patient is stabilized. This can include swallowing assessment, dental work, or oral surgery.

Prognosis

Primary lung abscesses in nonimmunocompromised hosts have cure rates of 90% to 95% with antimicrobial therapy and postural drainage alone. However, in immunocompromised patients and those with bronchial obstruction due to cancer, the mortality has been reported between 20% and 75%.

---

[1]Not FDA approved for this indication.

References

Bartlett JG: Anaerobic bacterial pleuropulmonary infections, *Semin Respir Med* 13:159–164, 1992.
Bartlett JG: The role of anaerobic bacteria in lung abscess, *Clin Infect Dis* 40:923–925, 2005.
Egyud M, Suzuki K: Post-resection complications: abscesses, empyemas, bronchopleural fistulas, *J Thorac Dis* 10:S3408, 2018.

Gudiol F, Manresa F, Pallares R, et al: Clindamycin vs. penicillin for anaerobic lung infections, *Arch Intern Med* 150:2525–2529, 1990.

Hammer DL, Aranda CP, Galati V, Adams FV: Massive intrabronchial aspiration of contents of pulmonary abscess after fiberoptic bronchoscopy, *Chest* 7:306–307, 1978.

Herth F, Ernst A, Becker HD: Endoscopic drainage of lung abscesses. Technique and outcome, *Chest* 127:1378–1381, 2005.

Levinson ME, Mangura CT, Lorber B, et al: Clindamycin compared with penicillin for the treatment of anaerobic lung abscess, *Ann Intern Med* 98:466–471, 1983.

Mandell LA, Niederman MS: Aspiration pneumonia, *N Engl J Med* 380:651–663, 2019.

Mandell LA, Wunderink RG, Anzueto A, et al: Infectious Diseases Society of America/American Thoracic Society consensus guidelines on the management of community-acquired pneumonia in adults, *Clin Infect Dis* 44:S27–72, 2007.

Mueller PR, Berlin L: Complications of lung abscess aspiration and drainage, *AJR Am J Roentgenol* 178:1083–1086, 2002.

Wang JL, Chen KY, Fang CT, et al: Changing bacteriology of adult community-acquired lung abscess in Taiwan: *Klebsiella pneumonia* vs anaerobes, *Clin Infec Dis* 40:915, 2015.

LUNG CANCER

Method of
Erin A. Gillaspie, MD, MPH; Jennifer Lewis, MD, MPH; Leora Horn, MD, MSc

CURRENT DIAGNOSIS

- An improvement in lung cancer outcomes is achievable with use of low-dose computed tomography (CT) for lung cancer screening
- All eligible patients should be screened with an annual low-dose CT scan
- The accurate staging of lung cancer is crucial in helping to guide treatment recommendations
- Many patients have no symptoms at the time of diagnosis
- Tissue diagnosis can be achieved through image-guided endobronchial and surgical biopsies
- All smokers should be counselled on smoking cessation

CURRENT THERAPY

- Treatment recommendations are based on stage of cancer and fitness of patient to tolerate surgery
- Surgically resectable non–small cell lung cancer (NSCLC) is more commonly approached in a minimally invasive fashion
- Early stage NSCLC is most often treated with definitive surgery with or without chemotherapy
- Locally advanced NSCLC requires a multimodality treatment regimen often using a combination of radiation, surgery, and systemic therapy
- Forty percent of patients will have advanced stage of disease at diagnosis, and systemic therapy is the mainstay of treatment
- All patients with Stage IV disease should have molecular and PD-L1 testing to help guide therapy
- Routine disease monitoring is important both after curative-intent treatment and during treatment for incurable disease
- Small cell lung cancer (SCLC) is aggressive and the mainstay of treatment is systemic therapy combined with radiation in early stage disease or immunotherapy in advanced disease

Epidemiology

Lung cancer is the second most common cancer diagnosed and the leading cause of cancer-related mortality in the United States among both men and women. The incidence rate is decreasing, more rapidly among men compared to women largely due to the historical trends in tobacco use. Lung cancer is predominantly a disease of older individuals, aged 60 to 84. There is an approximately equal distribution in lung cancer incidence among African Americans and Caucasians as a whole. Among males and females, African American males and Caucasian females have the highest lung cancer incidence compared to their counterparts. Incidence and mortality rates among Hispanics and Native and Asian Americans are approximately 40% to 50% of that of Caucasians. A large majority (79%) of cases are diagnosed at regional or advanced stages, which limits treatments available and accounts for the relatively poor overall survival. The 5-year relative survival rate for all stages is 19%; 56% local, 30% regional, and 5% distant stages.

Epithelial lung cancers are divided into four major cell types: SCLC, adenocarcinoma, squamous cell carcinoma, and large cell carcinoma; the latter three types are collectively known as NSCLCs. All histologic types of lung cancer can develop in current and former smokers, although squamous and small cell carcinomas are most commonly associated with heavy tobacco use. It is important to distinguish between SCLC and NSCLC because these tumors have quite different natural histories and therapeutic approaches. In addition, the histologic and molecular subtype of NSCLC has become an important part of treatment planning because some chemotherapeutic agents perform quite differently in squamous cell cancers versus adenocarcinoma, and patients with adenocarcinoma are more likely to harbor tumor mutations that make them candidates for oral therapy.

Risk Factors

Tobacco use (cigarettes, cigars, and pipes) is by far the greatest risk factor for lung cancer, accounting for approximately 80% to 90% of lung cancer deaths. This risk increases as tobacco exposure increases in both quantity and duration. Environmental tobacco smoke (ETS) or second-hand smoke is also an established cause of lung cancer. Radon gas is the second most common risk factor. Prolonged exposure to low-level radon in homes might impart a risk of lung cancer equal or greater than that of ETS. Additional risk factors include asbestos, radiation, agent orange, chromium, cadmium, and arsenic. Individuals with occupations in rubber manufacturing, roofing, paving, and chimney sweeping are also felt to be at an increased risk for developing lung cancer. Finally, family history of lung cancer is a risk factor, but the exact genetic driver remains unclear. Notably, the incidence of lung cancer in never smokers is increasing for reasons that are also unclear.

Prevention

Smoking cessation is the cornerstone of lung cancer prevention. Stopping tobacco use before middle age avoids more than 90% of the lung cancer risk attributable to tobacco. Moreover, smoking cessation in individuals with an established diagnosis of lung cancer is associated with improved survival and decreased toxicities from therapy. The combination of smoking cessation counseling with medications leads to a higher likelihood of successful quit attempts. US Food and Drug Administration (FDA) approved medications include nicotine replacement therapy (nicotine patches [Nicoderm CQ], lozenges [Nicorette], gum [Nicorelief, Nicorette], spray [Nicotrol NS]), varenicline (Chantix), and bupropion (Zyban). Nicotine patches, which provide longer periods of nicotine replacement, should be used in combination with gum or lozenges to treat short-term cravings. The results of a multicenter, double-blinded, randomized controlled trial, the Evaluating Adverse Events in Global Smoking Cessation Study (EAGLES trial), compared varenicline, bupropion, nicotine patch, and placebo in more than 8000 smokers and found that the efficacy of each medication was higher than placebo. The results of this trial also demonstrated that there was no increase in neuropsychiatric symptoms in smokers exposed to varenicline, leading the FDA to remove the black box warning on varenicline. Physicians must understand that the individual must want to stop smoking and must be willing to work hard to achieve the goal of smoking abstinence to achieve success. Counseling using the 5 As remains the recommended five major steps in intervention (Table 1). A shortened version, the 3 As, is an alternative for busy clinicians and involves **asking** and recording smoking status, **advising** patient of health benefits, and **acting** on patient's response.

TABLE 1	The 5As of Smoking Cessation
THE 5AS OF SMOKING CESSATION COUNSELING	
Ask	Ask and record smoking status
Advise	Advise smokers on benefit of stopping in a personalized, appropriate manner
Assess	Assess motivation to quit
Assist	Assist in smokers' quit attempt
Arrange	Arrange follow up with cessation services

TABLE 2	Clinical Signs & Symptoms of Lung Cancer	
TUMOR LOCAL EFFECTS	**DISTANT METASTASIS EFFECTS**	**PARANEOPLASTIC SYNDROME**
Cough	Bone pain	Hypercalcemia
Dyspnea	Headache	SIADH
Hemoptysis	Nausea and vomiting	Lambert-Eaton syndrome
Chest pain	Seizure	Cerebellar ataxia
Hoarseness	Weight loss	Encephalitis
SVC syndrome	Fatigue	Cachexia/anorexia
Postobstructive pneumonia	Abdominal pain	Cushing syndrome
Pleural effusion	Spinal cord compression	
Pericardial effusion	Pathologic fracture	

SIADH, syndrome of inappropriate antidiuretic hormone secretion; *SVC,* superior vena cava

Early Detection

Clinicians have an important opportunity to improve lung cancer outcomes through early detection. Increasing evidence demonstrates a mortality benefit when screening high-risk individuals with low-dose computed tomography (LDCT). Lung cancer screening with LDCT is recommended by the US Preventive Services Task Force (USPSTF) for individuals aged 55 to 80, current smokers or former smokers who have quit within the past 15 years, and smokers who have at least a 30 pack-year history of smoking. Medicare covers LDCT screening for a similar group of high-risk individuals, differing only in the upper age limit (ages 55–77). These policy decisions were made following the results of the National Lung Screening Trial (NLST).

The NLST was a large, multicenter, randomized controlled trial performed in the US that compared annual chest x-ray (CXR) to LDCT in 53,454 patients who were considered high-risk for the development of lung cancer. This trial was terminated early when it met its primary endpoint of achieving a 20% relative reduction in lung cancer mortality favoring the LDCT arm. Nearly twice as many early stage 1A cancers were detected in the LDCT group compared with the CXR group (40% vs 21%). The overall rates of lung cancer death were 247 and 309 deaths per 100,000 person-years in the LDCT and CXR groups, respectively. Compared with the CXR group, the rate of death in the LDCT group from *any* cause was reduced by 6.7% (95% CI, 1.2–13.6; *P* = .02). A common critique of the NLST is the high false positive rate. However, across three rounds of screening in the LDCT arm, only 24.2% of screening exams were positive and went on to require additional imaging or biopsy. The interpretation of screening LDCT continues to improve through the use of the American College of Radiology's structured reporting system, Lung-RADs, which has further decreased the false positive rate.

More recently, the Danish-Belgium Lung Cancer Screening Trial (NELSON) found a 26% relative reduction in lung cancer mortality when screening high-risk individuals with LDCT compared with no screening, further supporting the role for annual LDCT scans in high-risk individuals as part of health maintenance.

Clinical Manifestations

The location of tumors and the manifestation of paraneoplastic syndromes determine the clinical presentation of most patients with lung cancer. Most patients with early stage disease are asymptomatic and their cancer is discovered incidentally on chest x-ray or CT scans (Table 2).

Peripheral tumors may invade the chest wall and generally will present with pain. Centrally located tumors may cause symptoms from direct invasion or compression of mediastinal structures. Symptoms may include cough, hemoptysis, wheezing, stridor, or even postobstructive pneumonias. Patients may present with diaphragmatic paralysis due to phrenic nerve invasion, superior vena cava (SVC) syndrome with facial edema, bluish discoloration of the upper chest, and shortness of breath. They can even have dysphagia from esophageal compression. Mediastinal lymph node involvement can cause disruption of the recurrent laryngeal nerve, leading to hoarseness. Tumors arising in the superior sulcus, so-called Pancoast tumors, can result in a lower brachial plexopathy and Horner syndrome. Pleural effusion may also be the presenting sign for lung cancer and can cause pain, dyspnea or cough. (see Table 2).

Symptoms from metastatic disease may be the first sign of malignancy. Frequent sites of metastasis include supraclavicular and cervical lymph nodes, bone, brain, liver, and adrenal glands. Brain metastases occur in 10% to 30% of patients. Estimates are limited by sample size and therefore reported commonly in a range. Symptoms include seizures, nausea and vomiting, headache, or focal neurologic dysfunction. Bony metastases present with pain, pathologic fracture, or spinal cord compression. Liver metastases can cause biliary obstruction and jaundice; however, this is not particularly common. Constitutional symptoms may include anorexia, weight loss, weakness, fever, and night sweats.

Lung cancers are notable for ectopic production of hormones leading to several paraneoplastic syndromes. These are most commonly described in SCLC; however, it can occur in rare cases of NSCLC as well. The most common paraneoplastic syndromes in NSCLC are tumor cachexia and hypercalcemia. Although the causes of tumor cachexia are not well characterized, hypercalcemia is mediated by the production of parathyroid hormone–related peptide (PTHrP). The peptide stimulates release of calcium from bones, resulting in an elevation in calcium in the blood and osteopenia. This syndrome is treated effectively with bisphosphonate therapy. Hypertrophic pulmonary arthropathy can occur with NSCLC or SCLC and is characterized by digital clubbing and periostitis of the long bones that are demonstrable on plain x-rays.

Paraneoplastic syndromes unique to SCLC include Lambert-Eaton myasthenic syndrome (LEMS), syndrome of inappropriate antidiuretic hormone (SIADH), and Cushing syndrome. A patient presenting with LEMS should always be ruled out for malignancy; 50% of patients who present with this syndrome have cancer, and in 95% of those cases, it is SCLC. Another paraneoplastic syndrome related to SCLC is SIADH. SIADH generally resolves within 1 to 4 weeks of initiating chemotherapy. During this period, serum sodium can usually be managed and maintained above 128 mEq/L via fluid restriction. Demeclocycline (Declomycin)[1] can be a useful adjunctive measure when fluid restriction alone is insufficient. Vasopressin receptor antagonists also have been used in the management of SIADH but are costly and have increased unique toxicities such as liver injury. Cushing syndrome due to ectopic production of adrenocorticotropic

---
[1] Not FDA approved for this indication.

TABLE 3	TMN Staging		
PRIMARY TUMOR (T)		**LYMPH NODES (N)**	
T0	No evidence of primary tumor	N0	No regional lymph nodes involved
Tis	Carcinoma in situ	N1	Ipsilateral lymph node peribronchial and/or ipsilateral hilar or intrapulmonary lymph nodes involved
T1	Tumor ≤ 3cm, surrounded by lung or visceral pleura without bronchoscopic evidence of invasion more proximal than lobar bronchus	N2	Ipsilateral mediastinal or subcarinal lymph nodes involved
T1a	Tumor ≤ 1cm	N3	Contralateral mediastinal or hilar lymph nodes or ipsilateral or contralateral scalene or supraclavicular lymph nodes involved
T1b	Tumor > 1cm but ≤ 2cm	Distant Metastasis (M)	
T1c	Tumor > 2cm but ≤ 3cm	M0	No distant metastases
T2	Tumor > 3cm but ≤ 5cm or with any of the following: involves main bronchus but does not involve carina, invades visceral pleura, associated with atelectasis or obstructive pneumonitis	M1	Distant metastases present
T2a	Tumor > 3cm but ≤ 4cm	M1a	Separate tumor nodule(s) in contralateral lobe; pleural or pericardial nodule(s) or malignant pleural or pericardial effusion
T2b	Tumor > 4cm but ≤ 5cm	M1b	Single extrathoracic metastasis
T3	Tumor > 5cm but ≤ 7cm or with any of the following: separate tumor nodule(s) in same lobe as primary or directly invades	M1c	Multiple extrathoracic metastases in one or more organs
T4	Tumors >7 cm in greatest dimension or any tumor that invades the mediastinum, diaphragm, heart, great vessels, recurrent laryngeal nerve, carina, trachea, esophagus, spine or separate tumor in a different lobe of the ipsilateral lung		

hormone (ACTH) by SCLC and pulmonary carcinoids results in electrolyte disturbances rather than classic changes in body habitus. Treatment with standard medications such as metyrapone[1] and ketoconazole (Nizoral)[1] is largely ineffective. Cerebellar degeneration may be associated with anti-Hu, anti-Yo or P/Q channel autoantibodies. Cutaneous manifestations such as dermatomyositis are rare. Thrombosis including Trousseaus syndrome, marantic endocarditis, and coagulopathies are also uncommon and are usually associated with a worse prognosis.

Diagnostic Techniques

Once lung cancer is suspected, tissue biopsy is required to make a definitive diagnosis. In patients with suspected metastatic disease, a biopsy of a distant site of disease is preferred for tissue confirmation because it provides additional staging information. Several methods can be considered depending on the location of the tumor, and the technique should be tailored to the location of the primary tumor and the presence of mediastinal nodal involvement or metastatic disease. Transbronchial biopsy can be performed for centrally located tumors, and the yield may be increased by using endobronchial ultrasound (EBUS) techniques. Mediastinal nodal involvement or direct extension into the mediastinum may be evaluated by bronchoscopy paired with endoscopic ultrasound (EUS) or surgically by mediastinoscopy.

For peripheral lesions, a CT-guided needle biopsy may be considered. The advent of navigational bronchoscopy has allowed interventional pulmonologists to sample nodules in the periphery of the lungs

with very high yield. If equivocal results are obtained, transthoracic biopsies using a minimally invasive approach (video-assisted thoracoscopic surgery [VATS] or robotic-assisted thoracoscopic surgery [RATS]) may be used as both diagnostic and therapeutic options. For patients presenting with a pleural or pericardial effusion, cytologic examination of pleural fluid can establish the diagnosis.

The tenets of biopsy are the same no matter the method chosen: there should be adequate tissue for diagnosis, histologic subtyping, and molecular testing. If sufficient tissue is not obtained to further classify the subtype of lung cancer, additional procedures to obtain sufficient tissue are often warranted, particularly in patients with advanced stage disease.

Staging

The accurate staging of lung cancer is crucial in helping to guide treatment recommendations (Tables 3 and 4). Staging makes use of imaging modalities combined with biopsy to help determine size, location, and histology of a lesion. A complete history and physical examination along with assessment of performance status is important in evaluating a patient's ability to tolerate therapy. (Figure 1)

Imaging

CT scanning is a standard part of the work-up for lung cancer and determining the candidacy for resection. Although excellent in delineating the extent of the primary lesion disease and some sites of metastatic disease, it is the least sensitive and specific modality for the identification of lymph node involvement or distant metastatic disease. CT scan of the chest should always be

---

[1] Not FDA approved for this indication.

TABLE 4	Staging Groups		
STAGE	T	N	M
Stage 0	Tis	N0	M0
Stage IA1	T1a	N0	M0
Stage IA2	T1b	N0	M0
Stage IA3	T1c	N0	M0
Stage IB	T2a	N0	M0
Stage IIA	T2b	N0	M0
Stage IIB	T1a to c	N1	M0
	T2a	N1	M0
	T2b	N1	M0
	T3	N0	M0
Stage IIIA	T1a to c	N2	M0
	T2a to b	N2	M0
	T3	N1	M0
	T4	N0	M0
	T4	N1	M0
Stage IIIB	T1a-c	N3	M0
	T2a to b	N3	M0
	T3	N2	M0
	T4	N2	M0
Stage IVA	Any	Any	M1a
	Any	Any	M1b
Stage IVB	Any	Any	M1c

obtained with extension through the adrenal glands, a common site of metastatic disease.

Positron emission tomography (PET) scans play an important role in both nodal and extrathoracic staging. PET scans attempt to identify sites of malignancy based on glucose metabolism by measuring the uptake of ^{18}F-fluorodeoxyglucose (FDG). Rapidly dividing cells will preferentially take up ^{18}F-FDG and appear as a "hot spot." Combined ^{18}F-FDG PET-CT imaging has been shown to improve the accuracy of staging in NSCLC compared with visual correlation of PET and CT on either study alone. A standardized uptake value (SUV) of >2.5 on PET is highly suspicious for malignancy. False negatives can be seen in diabetes, in lesions <8 mm, and in slow-growing tumors (e.g., carcinoid tumors or well-differentiated adenocarcinoma). Confirmation of PET scan abnormalities with tissue diagnosis remains important because this modality of imaging also carries the risk of false positive upstaging; particularly in regions where histoplasmosis is prevalent.

Mediastinoscopy was once considered the gold standard diagnostic technique for the assessment of mediastinal lymph nodes. Mediastinoscopy can evaluate level lymph node stations 2R, 4R, 2L, 4L, and 7, and can send whole lymph nodes for analysis. This has been replaced in many centers by endobronchial ultrasound (EBUS), which is less invasive and offers the ability to sample both N1 and N2 nodes. Review of available publications reveals a median sensitivity of 89% and a very low risk of complications. In addition, rapid onsite cytologic evaluation (ROSE) confirms adequacy of samplings at the time of procedure to enhance overall yield.

An MRI scan of the brain is mandatory in all patients with SCLC. In patients with NSCLC, an MRI scan of the brain should also be performed in patients with nodal involvement, stage IV disease, or any neurologic symptoms.

Assessing Treatment Candidacy

After establishing the stage of cancer, a meticulous evaluation should be performed prior to recommending therapy (see Figure 1). Work-up should include history and physical examination, blood work including a complete blood count, renal function and liver function tests, pulmonary function tests, nutritional assessments, and cardiac clearance in patients being selected for surgery. Assessment of a patient's performance status has important prognostic and therapeutic implications and should be noted in all patients.

In patients who are being considered for surgery, smokers should be counselled to stop immediately. In addition to helping to reduce the risk of perioperative pulmonary complications and death, it will also help to reduce the long-term consequences related to tobacco abuse.

Assessment of Cardiovascular Risk

Major cardiac-related adverse events occur in approximately 2% to 3% of patients after pulmonary resection. The thoracic revised cardiac risk index is a validated tool that can be used to help guide which patients should be sent for additional preoperative consultation. Patients who score more than 1.5 in the cardiac index, or those describing limited exercise capacity or recent diagnosis of active heart disease all warrant evaluation by a cardiologist.

Assessment of Pulmonary Function

Patients undergoing pulmonary resection commonly have several coexisting conditions and exposures that can affect pulmonary function. It is therefore essential to ensure adequate pulmonary reserve prior to proceeding with resection. Most surgeons will request a spirometry and measurement of diffusion capacity for carbon monoxide (DLCO) for all patients undergoing pulmonary resection. These are calculated as a percentage of the predicted value. The forced expiratory volume in 1 second (FEV1), measured during spirometry, determines the mechanical function of the lung, that is, the airflow limitations of medium to large airways. The DLCO value provides a gross estimate of the function at the alveolar-capillary membrane. The DLCO (the actual and predicted postoperative percentage) have been shown in various studies to be the most important predictors of perioperative complications and mortality.

A postoperative predicted FEV1 or DLCO of less than 60% should prompt additional testing such as a shuttle walk test or stair-climbing exercise. If the postoperative predicted DLCO is less than 30% to 40%, this denotes an increased risk and warrants a formal cardiopulmonary exercise test with measurement of maximal oxygen consumption. This quantitative assessment has established thresholds associated with surgical risk. A ventilation-perfusion scan may also be helpful in patients with heterogeneous, underlying lung disease.

Surgical Approach to Lung Cancer

The approach to surgery and extent of pulmonary resection is determined by the size and location of the tumor and experience of the surgeon.

Open Lobectomy

The majority of pulmonary resections continue to be performed in open fashion via thoracotomy and often involve dividing muscle and taking out a portion of a rib.

Surgery is performed with a special endotracheal tube (a double lumen tube) that allows the operative lung to be collapsed. After thoracotomy, the chest is inspected to rule out metastatic disease and confirm that the tumor is resectable.

Surgery begins with the removal of N1 and N2 lymph nodes, which are sent to pathology. A lobectomy is performed by isolating the arteries, vein, and bronchus associated with the lobe and dividing each along with the fissure that connects the upper, middle (right), and lower lobes. Once the lobectomy is completed, the remaining lung is reinflated to fill the pleural space and chest tubes are positioned to help drain fluid and air while the patient recovers.

Figure 1 Approach to diagnosis. *CBC*, complete blood count; *PS*, performance status.

Lung resections carry a significant risk of perioperative morbidity, with 37% of patients experiencing some form of postoperative complication; atrial arrhythmia and prolonged air leak are the most common. Other complications can include infection, bleeding, hypoxia, and death.

Video-Assisted Thoracoscopic Surgery (VATS) Lobectomy

A VATS lobectomy is conducted in similar fashion to an open lobectomy but utilizes 2 to 3 small ports in the chest, each measuring approximately 1 cm, and a slightly larger utility incision measuring 3 cm through which the specimen is removed. VATS differs from open surgery in both the length of incisions and the minimal muscular division and no rib spreading. A camera and special instruments have been designed to make the surgery possible. Comparison of outcomes shows that both open surgery and VATS provide equal cancer-specific outcomes. Both VATS and open surgery have similar patterns of postoperative complications, although VATS occur at a lesser rate. Additional benefits of VATS include earlier recovery, earlier discharge, less pain, less impact on pulmonary function, better quality of life, and increased delivery of adjuvant therapy.

Robotic Lobectomy

Robotic lobectomies were first performed in 2003, and the use of this technology has continued to increase with time. Much like VATS, robotic lobectomy is performed through small (8 mm) incisions.

This newer technology has several advantages over traditional thoracoscopic surgery in that it provides a three dimensional, high definition field and the instruments have 9 degrees of freedom and include the ability to staple and seal vessels.

Extent of Resection: Lobar vs. Sublobar Resection

Lobectomy has long been considered the standard of care and the optimal oncologic procedure for the management of resectable lung cancer. More limited resections (including segmentectomy or wedge resection) were thought to be associated with higher risk of recurrence and historically were reserved for patients with limited cardiopulmonary reserve.

The advent of CT screening for lung cancer and improvements in imaging technology have led to the identification earlier stage cancers (<2 cm), and partially solid lesions or completely ground glass lesions. This has prompted a renewed interest in the possibility of more limited

resection that preserves more pulmonary function and thereby a patient's ability to undergo subsequent resections if required.

The recommended extent of resection remains highly controversial. Investigators have not been able to definitively define the ideal tumor size or histology for a sublobar resection. Detractors argue that most evidence supporting sublobar resections comes from single-institution, retrospective analysis with pooled histology and surgical technique (wedge or segmentectomy), resulting in confounded results that may not be broadly disseminated.

Treatment: Non–Small Cell Lung Cancer

General treatment recommendations by stage are summarized in Figure 2.

Early Stage Lung Cancer

Surgery is considered the treatment of choice for stage I and II NSCLC (Table 3; Figure 2). Based on the eighth edition staging system, this includes tumors that are node negative and up to 7 cm in size, tumors that involve the chest wall, and pericardium or satellite nodules in the same lobe. Surgery is also performed for patients who have smaller tumors up to 5 cm or tumors involving the main bronchus and ipsilateral, hilar nodes.

Operative mortality rates for patients undergoing pulmonary resection are lower if the resection is performed by a high volume surgeon (>70 procedures per year), and surgeons who have had dedicated thoracic surgical training.

Comprehensive pathologic staging is just as important at the time of surgery as it is in the workup of a patient. Lymph nodes should be sampled from N2 stations (on the right side, stations 4R, 7, and 9R; on the left side, stations 5, 6, 7, and 9L) and N1 stations (stations 10 through 14) at the time of surgery. There is notably a 6% to 8% rate of occult N2 disease discovered at the time of final pathology for patients with T1 tumors and negative preoperative assessments.

There is currently no clear role for neoadjuvant chemotherapy in these patients; however, adjuvant chemotherapy is recommended for tumors that are determined on final pathology to be greater than 4 cm or in patients with lymph node involvement. The benefit of adjuvant chemotherapy was firmly established in 2008 by a landmark meta-analysis (the Lung Adjuvant Cisplatin Evaluation Study [LACE]) that demonstrated a 5.4% improvement in 5-year survival for patients treated with surgery followed by adjuvant chemotherapy compared to surgery alone.

```
                                    ┌─────────────────────┐
                                    │      Stage IA:      │
                                    │      Surgery        │
                                    └─────────────────────┘
                                    ┌─────────────────────┐
                                    │ Stage IB (≥4 cm) –IIIA: │
                                    │  Surgery + chemotherapy │
                                    └─────────────────────┘
                 ┌──────────────┐   ┌─────────────────────────┐
                 │ Non-small cell │  │ Stage IIIA/IIIB (N2 and N3) │
                 │ lung cancer*   │  │  Chemotherapy + radiation   │
                 └──────────────┘   │  followed by durvalumab     │
                                    └─────────────────────────┘
 ┌──────────┐                       ┌─────────────────────┐
 │ Determine │                      │      Stage IV:      │
 │ histology │                      │   Systemic therapy  │
 └──────────┘                       └─────────────────────┘
                                    ┌─────────────────────┐
                                    │ Limited stage disease: │
                                    │     Chemo + RT         │
                                    │   followed by PCI      │
                 ┌──────────────┐   └─────────────────────┘
                 │ Small cell   │   ┌─────────────────────────┐
                 │ lung cancer  │   │ Extensive stage disease:   │
                 └──────────────┘   │ Carboplatin + etoposide +  │
                                    │     atezolizumab           │
                                    └─────────────────────────┘
```

* For patients with stage IV NSCLC knowledge of histologic subtype,
PD-L1 and molecular testing are essential for selecting systemic therapy

Figure 2 General treatment algorithm for lung cancer.

The benefit was primarily confined to patients with stage II or IIIA disease, with only a modest benefit in patients with tumors less than 4 cm. In 2011, the NSCLC Collaborative Group compiled a postoperative chemotherapy meta-analysis and reported a similar survival benefit in patients with stage II disease. There is no role for adjuvant chemotherapy in patients with stage IA NSCLC.

The optimal platinum-based chemotherapy regimen remains a topic of debate. Although the aforementioned trials employed different platinum doublets, cisplatin (Platinol)[1] and vinorelbine (Navelbine) was one of the most common regimens adopted. The E1505 trial assessed the addition of bevacizumab (Avastin) to cisplatin-based chemotherapy. While this trial demonstrated no benefit in overall survival, a post hoc analysis compared the different platinum doublet regimens (pemetrexed [Alimta], gemcitabine [Gemzar], docetaxel [Taxotere], and vinorelbine) and found no difference in either overall or disease-free survival but noted cisplatin and pemetrexed was associated with improved tolerance and was preferred among physicians for patients with nonsquamous NSCLC.

If a decision is made to proceed with adjuvant chemotherapy, treatment should be started within 6 to 12 weeks after surgery, assuming the patient has fully recovered, and should be administered for no more than four cycles. Although a cisplatin-based chemotherapy is the preferred treatment regimen, carboplatin (Paraplatin)[1] can be substituted for cisplatin in patients who are unlikely to tolerate cisplatin for reasons such as reduced renal function, presence of neuropathy, or hearing impairment.

Postoperative radiation is usually reserved for patients in whom there is a concern for residual disease (i.e., patients with positive margins on final pathology) or in patients with N2 disease.

In patients with stage I and II disease who either refuse or are not suitable candidates for surgery, stereotactic body radiation therapy (SBRT) is a treatment option for patients with tumors

[1] Not FDA approved for this indication.

that are ≤5 cm. Treatment is typically administered in three to five fractions delivered over 1 to 2 weeks and is associated with a disease control rate of approximately 90% and 5-year survival rates of up to 60%. Cryoablation is another technique occasionally used to treat small, isolated tumors (i.e., ≤3 cm). However, very little data exist on long-term outcomes with this technique.

Locally Advanced Lung Cancer
The treatment of locally advanced lung cancer is complex and requires a multidisciplinary approach.

T3N1 Tumors
T3N1 is a relatively infrequent stage of lung cancer but surgery has a well-defined role as the primary treatment for these tumors. T3 lung cancers range in size from 5 to 7 cm or invade structures that can be routinely taken en bloc with the lung: the chest wall, pericardium, or a single phrenic nerve. Often, hilar nodal involvement is discovered at the time of resection. The surgical goal is an en bloc resection with microscopically negative margins.

Surgical resection should be followed by adjuvant chemotherapy as described previously. If a complete resection is not technically feasible then concurrent chemoradiation is recommended as described in the following section.

Stage IIIA Tumors
This is a heterogenous group that comprises patients with: (1) small tumors (T1–T2) with ipsilateral mediastinal lymph node involvement (N2), (2) large tumors (T3–T4) with ipsilateral lymph node involvement (N1), and (3) large tumors (T4) without any lymph node involvement (N0). We will discuss some of the nuances of this complex group in the subcategories below: N2 disease, T4 tumors, and superior sulcus tumors.

N2 Disease
The optimal management of N2 disease is perhaps the most challenging and controversial area in thoracic oncology. Tumor

characteristics and nodal burden of disease as well as performance status play an important role in determining who should be considered for surgery. Patients with clinical stage I or II disease who are found to have N2 positive nodes at the time of resection should be referred for adjuvant chemotherapy as described previously. In most cases, pathologic involvement of mediastinal lymph nodes is documented preoperatively, and a combined modality approach is recommended because these patients are at high risk for local and distance recurrence.

In patients who are deemed surgically resectable, the optimal combination and order of treatments remains debated. Some centers favor a neoadjuvant chemotherapy approach and others a neoadjuvant chemoradiotherapy (6000 cGY).

The Intergroup 0139 study sought to help define the roles of therapy for N2 disease. The trial found no definitive survival benefit with surgery after neoadjuvant chemoradiation therapy compared to definitive chemoradiation therapy alone. The study outcomes were confounded by a very high mortality rate in patients undergoing pneumonectomy that likely impacted this outcome. Subgroup analysis did show a trend toward survival benefit in patients undergoing lobectomy as a part of trimodality treatment.

More contemporary studies (mostly single institution) have demonstrated significantly higher median survival and freedom-from-recurrence compared with the INT0139 trial for trimodality therapy. Vyfhuis et al. achieved a median survival of 60 months with trimodality therapy compared with 20-month survival for bimodality (chemotherapy and radiation) in surgically resectable patients.

Concurrent chemoradiation therapy with cisplatin[1] and etoposide (Toposar)[1] is the preferred therapeutic combination, although carboplatin (Paraplatin)[1] and paclitaxel (Taxol) is often substituted for patients who cannot tolerate cisplatin-based chemotherapy for reasons stated previously.

A recent randomized, placebo-controlled, phase III trial demonstrated a significant improvement in progression-free and overall survival in patients treated with concurrent chemoradiation followed by one year of therapy with the immune checkpoint inhibitor durvalumab (Imfinzi) compared to placebo. This trial has established this as a new standard of care for patients with locally advanced, unresectable disease. There is no role for durvalumab in patients treated with trimodality therapy.

Esophagitis and pneumonitis are the two most common toxicities associated with concurrent chemoradiation.

T4 Tumors

T4 tumors are locally aggressive with invasion of critical mediastinal structures such as the pulmonary artery, heart, aorta, superior vena cava (SVC), trachea, esophagus, spine, or diaphragm. Surgery can be considered as part of a multimodal therapy plan in high volume centers with dedicated thoracic surgeons. Meticulous preoperative planning and in some cases multidisciplinary surgical approach is necessary to ensure complete resection.

Superior Sulcus Tumors

Superior sulcus tumors, also known as Pancoast tumors, arise from the apical segment of the right upper or left upper lobe. These tumors may invade any of the structures in the apex of the chest: brachial plexus, subclavian artery, subclavian vein, musculature, ribs, paravertebral sympathetic chain, or spinal nerve roots. Patients may present with shoulder pain, Horner syndrome, or neurologic complications of the upper extremity.

As with other locally advanced tumors, multidisciplinary approach is the mainstay of management of superior sulcus tumors. Complete staging is important to help determine resectability. MRI is often used in conjunction with other imaging modalities to better assess chest wall invasion and neurologic involvement.

Treatment with neoadjuvant chemoradiotherapy followed by surgery results in superior survival for patients with N0 or N1

disease. Surgery is generally completed 3 to 5 weeks after completion of chemoradiotherapy and involves an en bloc resection of the tumor, chest wall, and any other involved structures with subsequent reconstruction.

Patients with unresectable disease (medical inoperability, positive mediastinal nodes) should be offered concurrent chemoradiation followed by durvalumab consolidation as described previously.

Stage IIIB

Stage IIIB includes any tumors with contralateral mediastinal nodal involvement or large tumors (>5 cm) with ipsilateral mediastinal nodal involvement. These tumors are considered inoperable because surgery has not been shown to confer any survival benefit. These patients should be treated with concurrent chemoradiation therapy followed by durvalumab as described previously.

Stage IV

Approximately 40% of patients present with stage IV disease at the time of diagnosis. Moreover, a significant proportion of patients who present with early stage NSCLC will relapse despite initial curative-intent therapy. Systemic therapy depends on a patient's performance status, histology, and PD-L1 and molecular status. Of note, the early application of palliative care in conjunction with chemotherapy is associated with improved survival and a better quality of life.

Chemotherapy. Chemotherapy has been an important therapeutic option for decades in the treatment of patients with stage IV NSCLC. A landmark meta-analysis in 1995 established cisplatin-based regimens conferred a survival benefit in patients with stage IV disease.

Treatment recommendations have continued to evolve over the years. Histology of the NSCLC has come to be very important in treatment consideration; phase III trials have demonstrated cisplatin[1] and pemetrexed to be superior to cisplatin and gemcitabine (Gemzar) in patients with nonsquamous NSCLC, while cisplatin and gemcitabine was superior in patients with squamous cell histology. This survival difference is thought to be related to the differential expression of thymidylate synthase (TS), one of the targets of pemetrexed, between tumor subtypes. Importantly, bevacizumab (Avastin), a monoclonal antibody that targets VEGF, was also established as unsafe to administer in patients with squamous NSCLC and is FDA approved in combination with carboplatin and paclitaxel as a first-line option only in nonsquamous NSCLC patients.

Immunotherapy. Immune checkpoint inhibitors have increasingly become part of the first-line treatment paradigm in patients with metastatic NSCLC and no driver mutations. Checkpoint inhibitors exert anti-tumor effects by inhibiting negative T-cell regulators. Regardless of histology, all patients with advanced stage lung cancer should have PD-L1 testing prior to embarking on therapy. A randomized phase III trial demonstrated a superior response rate and progression-free and overall survival rate when pembrolizumab (Keytruda) was compared to platinum-based chemotherapy in patients with tumors that were PD-L1 ≥ 50% and EGFR and ALK wild type. More recently, combination therapy with platinum-pemetrexed and pembrolizumab in nonsquamous NSCLC and platinum-taxane (paclitaxel or nab-paclitaxel) and pembrolizumab in squamous cell lung cancer was found to be superior to chemotherapy alone in patients regardless of PD-L1 status. However, the additive benefit of chemotherapy to patients with tumors that are PD-L1 ≥ 50% to pembrolizumab alone remains unclear beyond small subset analyses from the aforementioned trials. Combination chemotherapy with carboplatin, paclitaxel, bevacizumab and atezolizumab (Tecentriq) has also been shown to be superior to carboplatin, paclitaxel, and bevacizumab in patients regardless of PD-L1 status and is also FDA approved as a first-line treatment option for nonsquamous

---

[1] Not FDA approved for this indication.

[1] Not FDA approved for this indication.

Figure 3 Algorithm for the treatment of metastatic NSCLC.

In the figure:

Metastatic NSCLC treatment algorithm

Squamous
- PD-L1 ≥50%: Pembrolizumab +/- carboplatin and taxane
- PD-L1 <50%: Carboplatin + taxane + pembrolizumab

Non-squamous*
- EGFR positive: Osimertinib, Erlotinib, Afatinib, Gefitinib, Dacomitinib
- ALK positive: Alectinib, Crizotinib, Ceritinib, Brigatinib **, Lorlatinib **
- BRAF positive (V600E): Dabrafenib + Trametinib, Vemurafenib
- ROS1 positive: Crizotinib, Ceritinib, Entrectinib
- NTRK positive: Larotrectinib
- PD-L1 ≥50%: Pembrolizumab +/- carboplatin and pemetrexed
- PD-L1 <50%: Carboplatin + pemetrexed + pembrolizumab

* All patients with nonsquamous NSCLC should undergo molecular testing. In patients with a driver mutation who are also PD-L1 positive, the driver mutation is more important and first-line therapy should be a TKI

** Not FDA approved in first-line therapy

NSCLC (Figure 3). Numerous other trials are currently ongoing evaluating the use of immunotherapy in NSCLC, both alone and in combination with other immunological agents, chemotherapy, targeted therapy, and radiotherapy.

Targeted Therapy. Driver mutations have been detected in 50% of nonsquamous NSCLC including *KRAS*, *EGFR*, *ALK*, *BRAF*, *HER2*, *ROS1*, *RET*, *PIK3CA*, *MET*, *NRAS*, *MEK1*, *AKT1*, *FGFR1*, *DDR2*, and *NTRK*. Targeted therapy is FDA approved for patients with *EGFR* mutations, *ALK* rearrangements, *ROS1* rearrangements, *NTRKI* rearrangements, and *BRAF* mutations. In addition, promising agents are in clinical trials for patients with *KRAS* mutations, *RET* rearrangements, and *MET* exon 14 skipping mutations. In patients who harbor a mutation and are also strongly PD-L1 positive, the presence of the mutation should drive selection of therapy (see Figure 3).

EGFR mutations have been reported in approximately 15% of North American patients with metastatic nonsquamous NSCLC, of which 90% are exon 19 deletions or exon 21 L858R point-mutations. First- and second-generation *EGFR* tyrosine kinase inhibitors (TKIs) erlotinib (Tarceva), gefitinib (Iressa), and afatinib (Gilotrif) are approved as first-line therapy based on clinical trials demonstrating superior response rates, progression-free survival, and overall survival compared with chemotherapy in treatment-naïve patients with *EGFR* mutation–positive NSCLC. Despite the observed survival benefits, a majority of patients eventually develop therapeutic resistance. Furthermore, approximately 50% of patients who develop acquired resistance to *EGFR* TKI therapy acquire a second site mutation occurring within exon 20 (i.e., T790M) Consequently, osimertinib (Tagrisso), a third-generation mutant-specific *EGFR* inhibitor that irreversibly binds to the kinase domain of *EGFR* was recently approved for patients with T790M mutations who have acquired resistance to first- and second-generation *EGFR* inhibitors. Osimirtinib was also demonstrated in the FLAURA trial to have improved PFS when compared to the first-generation inhibitors erlotinib and gefitinib in patients with treatment-naïve *EGFR* mutation positive NSCLC, establishing osimertinib as the preferred first-line option for this cohort of patients.

ALK-positive NSCLC accounts for approximately 3% to 7% of patients diagnosed with NSCLC. Crizotinib (Xalkori) was the initial *ALK* tyrosine kinase inhibitor (TKI) to gain accelerated approval by the FDA in 2011 after two open label, randomized phase III trials demonstrated improved progression-free survival

with crizotinib compared with chemotherapy in both the first- and second-line setting. Ceritinib (Zykadia) is also approved as a front-line therapy option, demonstrating superior progression-free survival compared to chemotherapy in patients with *ALK* positive NSCLC. More recently, alectinib (Alecensa) and brigatinib (Alunbrig) demonstrated superior progression-free survival and central nervous system control compared to crizotinib in patients with *ALK* positive NSCLC, with alectinib receiving FDA approval and considered the preferred option as front-line therapy for *ALK* positive NSCLC. Lorlatinib (Lorbrena) is also approved in patients who have progressed on a prior *ALK* inhibitor and is particularly effective in patients who develop G1202R as a mechanism of resistance to *ALK* inhibitor therapy.

ROS1 rearrangements occur in approximately 1% to 2% of NSCLC. Crizotinib is the preferred first-line therapy for patients with *ROS1* positive NSCLC. Ceritinib and lorlatinib have also been shown to be active in this cohort of patients.

BRAF mutations occur in approximately 2% to 3% of NSCLC patients, and more than 50% of these are V600E. Dabrafenib (Tafinlar) and vemurafenib (Zelboraf)[1] have demonstrated promising results in phase II trials. Dabrafenib in combination with the MEK inhibitor trametinib (Mekinist) had response rates of more than 60% and progression-free survival of 9 months, establishing this combination as the preferred treatment options for patients with *BRAF* V600E positive NSCLC.

NTRK rearrangements have been reported in 1% of patients with NSCLC. Recently larotrectinib (Vitrakvi) received FDA approval for *NTRK* positive tumors based on a phase II trial that enrolled patients with *NTRK* positive tumors regardless of tumor type.

Second-Line Therapy and Beyond
Second-line therapy for advanced NSCLC was almost never recommended until a seminal study in 2000 showed that docetaxel (Taxotere) improved survival compared to supportive care alone. Over a decade later, docetaxel and ramucirumab (Cyramza) received FDA approval after a phase III trial found the combination to impart a modest improvement in response rate, overall survival, and progression-free survival compared with docetaxel alone. More recently, nivolumab (Opdivo) and atezolizumab

[1] Not FDA approved for this indication.

(Tecentriq) received approval in patients who progress on platinum-based chemotherapy, while pembrolizumab (Keytruda) is also approved in patients with tumors that are PD-L1 ≥ 1%. It should be noted that a patient who progresses on a first-line TKI or pembrolizumab should be considered for a platinum-based doublet as their second-line therapy, not single agent docetaxel or docetaxel and ramucirumab.

Oligometastatic Disease. The concept of oligometastatic disease (single site metastatic disease) was first proposed in 1995. Studies at this time described patients with disease in the adrenal gland or brain as actually having a relatively favorable prognosis. For these lesions, the standard of care includes surgical resection of both the primary and metastasis or recurrence. Generally, for synchronous disease (primary tumor and metastatic disease identified at the same time), the metastatic site is treated first. If this is not able to be successfully addressed, there is no benefit to resecting the primary.

Treatment: Small Cell Lung Cancer
Small Cell Lung Cancer
Small cell lung cancer (SCLC), which accounts for 15% to 20% of new lung cancer cases, is an aggressive disease characterized by rapid growth and early widespread metastasis. The primary etiologic agent responsible for SCLC is tobacco smoke. The aggressive nature of SCLC is underscored by its high mutational burden, including loss of expression of the tumor suppressor genes *p53* in 70% to 80% and retinoblastoma in almost 100% of tumors. Although there is a shift in recommendations for the staging of small cell lung cancer, most patients are still diagnosed using the traditional staging system of limited stage disease (LD) and extensive stage disease (ED). At the time of diagnosis, approximately 30% of patients have limited-stage disease (LD-SCLC), defined as tumors confined to the hemithorax that can be encompassed in a tolerable radiation port, while about 70% of patients have extensive-stage disease (ED-SCLC), defined as the presence of overt metastatic disease by imaging or physical examination. Regardless of stage at diagnosis, the majority of patients relapse and develop chemotherapy-resistant disease, with a median survival of 12 to 20 months for patients with limited stage disease and 7 to 11 months for patients with extensive stage disease; only 6% to 12% of patients with LD-SCLC and 2% of patients with ED-SCLC live beyond 5 years. For decades, first-line therapy consisted of four to six cycles of platinum-based chemotherapy with either cisplatin[1] or carboplatin [1]plus either etoposide (Toposar) or irinotecan (Camptosar)[1] followed by observation. A recent phase III trial in patients with advanced stage disease demonstrated superior survival when atezolizumab (Tecentriq) was combined with carboplatin and etoposide for four cycles followed by maintenance atezolizumab compared to carboplatin and etoposide alone, making combination chemotherapy with a checkpoint inhibitor a new treatment option for patients with this disease. Although up to 80% of patients will respond to first-line chemotherapy, the majority will eventually relapse and topotecan (Hycamtin) is the only approved agent in the second line. Nivolumab (Opdivo) has also received FDA approval in the third line setting, but this was in patients who had not received a checkpoint inhibitor in the first-line setting.

Radiation therapy is also an important component in the therapeutic armamentarium for patients with SCLC. Patients with LD are generally treated with concurrent chemoradiation therapy with four cycles of chemotherapy and radiation added with either cycle one or two of therapy. For patients who are not candidates for concurrent chemoradiation therapy, sequential therapy can also be considered with radiation after chemotherapy. Prophylactic cranial irradiation (PCI) should be considered in patients who have responded well to initial therapy. In patients with ED, thoracic radiation can be considered although has not been shown to improve overall survival. Similarly, a large phase III trial in patients without brain metastases following chemotherapy

[1]Not FDA approved for this indication.

demonstrated no improvement in overall survival for patients treated with PCI compared to observation. Long-term toxicities, including deficits in cognition, have been reported after PCI, and for many patients observation with an MRI every 3 months has been adopted as standard of care.

Surgery has for many decades played a very limited role in the treatment of SCLC due to its propensity to metastasize. The pendulum is beginning to shift for early stage, node-negative SCLC. More contemporary studies have demonstrated that surgery may play a beneficial role in a select group of patients.

Invasive mediastinal staging should be performed for patients without evidence of metastatic disease. In node-negative patients with T1 and T2 tumors, a lobectomy followed by adjuvant chemotherapy should be offered to medically fit patients. The 5-year survival in this group of patients is 40% to 50%.

Monitoring
Routine disease monitoring is important both after curative treatment and during treatment for incurable disease.

Non–Small Cell Lung Cancer
The NCCN guidelines have clear recommendations for follow up of NSCLC and SCLC divided by stage, and these are summarized in the following.

After completion of curative therapy for Stages I and II, a history and physical examination along with a chest CT (+/-) contrast every 6 months for the first 2 to 3 years should be performed. If there are no findings that would require alternative monitoring, the patient can be transitioned to annual history, physical examination, and a low-dose, non-contrasted CT scan of the chest.

Patients with Stages I and II who were treated with radiation rather than surgery should be followed by a slightly more aggressive regimen. Patients should have a history and physical examination along with a chest CT (+/-) contrast every 3 to 6 months for the first 3 years, then every 6 months for the next 2 years. If there are no findings that would require alternative monitoring, the patient can be transitioned to annual history, physical examination, and a low-dose, non-contrasted CT scan of the chest.

Patients with Stages III and IV oligometastatic disease should likewise be followed with history and physical examination along with a chest CT (+/-) contrast every 3 to 6 months for the first 3 years, then every 6 months for the next 2 years. If there are no findings that would require alternative monitoring, the patient can be transitioned to annual history, physical examination, and a low-dose, non-contrasted CT scan of the chest.

Any residual or new radiographic abnormalities will require consideration of more frequent imaging. Please note that a PET-CT and brain MRI are not routinely indicated as part of surveillance; however, they should be tailored to each patient and their primary sites of disease.

Symptoms of shortness of breath, cough, wheezing, new bone pain, headache, or constitutional symptoms should prompt immediate evaluation with imaging to rule out disease recurrence, and the patient's primary oncologist should be contacted.

While patients are being treated with palliative system therapy, scans are routinely obtained every 6 to 8 weeks while on chemotherapy or every 8 to 9 weeks while on immunotherapy.

Small Cell Lung Cancer
SCLC has a distinct follow-up recommendation. Patients who were diagnosed and treated for limited stage disease should have follow-up with history and physical, CT scan of the chest/abdomen every 3 months for the first year and every 6 months for the subsequent 2 years. At that time, the patients may transition to annual examinations and imaging. MRI scans of the brain are essential as well and are recommended every 3 to 4 months for year 1 and every 6 months for year 2.

Patients with extensive stage will have more frequent follow-ups. A history and physical with CT scans of the chest/abdomen should occur every 2 months for the first year, every 3 to 4 months for years 2 and 3, every 6 months in years 4 and 5, and then annually. Monitoring of the brain is the same as for limited stage, with an MRI scan of the brain recommended every 3 to 4 months for year 1 and every 6 months for year 2.

Any patient, regardless of type of cancer, should have a survivorship plan created as part of their follow-up. These plans apply to survivors across the continuum of care. This comprehensive, individualized plan includes the aforementioned cancer-specific follow-up but also highlights important nutritional considerations, physical activity, and immunizations. Patients should be encouraged to continue routine screening for other malignancies and routine health maintenance. Ongoing smoking cessation should be encouraged.

Summary

The treatment of cancers is rapidly changing with the advent of immunotherapy, targeted therapy, localized radiation treatments, and minimally invasive surgical approaches. The intricacies of treatment, now more than ever before, demand a multidisciplinary approach to ensure that patients are provided with the best possible care to optimize both their quantity and quality of life.

References

Antonia SJ, Villegas A, Daniel D, et al: Durvalumab after chemoradiotherapy in stage iii non-small-cell lung cancer, *N Engl J Med* 377(20):1919–1929, 2017.

Gaissert HA, Ferenandez FG, Crabtree T, et al: The Society of Thoracic Surgeons General Thoracic Surgery Database: 2017 Update on Research, *Annals Thor Surg* 104(5):1450–1455, 2017.

Gandhi L, Rodrigues Abreu D, Gadgeel S, et al: (Keynote-189). Pembrolizubman plus chemotherapy in metastatic non-small cell lung cancer, *NEJM* 327:2078–2092, 2018.

Horn L, Mansfield AS, Szczęsna A, et al: IMpower133 Study Group: First-line atezolizumab plus chemotherapy in extensive-stage small-cell lung cancer, *N Engl J Med* 379(23):2220–2229, 2018.

Paz-Ares L, Luft A, Vincente D, et al: (Keynote-407). Pembrolizumab plus chemotherapy for squamous non-small cell lung cancer, *NEJM* 379:2040–2051, 2018.

Peters S, Camidge RC, Shaw AT, et al: Alectinib versus crizotinib in untreated alk-positive non–small-cell lung cancer, *N Engl J. Med* 377:829–838, 2017.

Reck M, Rodriguez-Abreu D, Robinson AG, et al: Pembrolizumab versus chemotherapy for PD-L1-positive non-small-cell lung cancer, *N Engl J Med* 375(19):1823–1833, 2016.

Soria JC, Ohe Y, Vansteenkiste J, et al: Osimertinib in untreated egfr-mutated advanced non-small-cell lung cancer, *N Engl J Med* 378:113–125, 2018.

Spyratos D, Zarogoulidis P, Porpodis K, et al: Preoperative evaluation for lung cancer resection, *J Thorac Dis* 6(suppl1):S162–166, 2014.

The National Lung Screening Trial Research Team: Reduced lung-cancer mortality with low-dose computed tomographic screening, *NEJM* 365:395–409, 2011.

SARCOIDOSIS

Method of
Marc A. Judson, MD

CURRENT DIAGNOSIS

- The diagnosis of sarcoidosis is one of exclusion.
- Tissue biopsy, confirming noncaseating granulomatous inflammation, is required in most cases.
- Efforts should be made to search for the least invasive biopsy site.

CURRENT THERAPY

- Many cases of sarcoidosis do not require treatment.
- All patients should be evaluated for possible pulmonary, eye, and cardiac disease.
- When therapy is indicated, corticosteroids are most commonly used.
- Topical corticosteroids should be given whenever possible.

Sarcoidosis is a multisystem granulomatous disease of unknown cause. The lung is most commonly affected, but any organ may be involved. The natural course of sarcoidosis is variable, ranging from an asymptomatic state to a progressive disease causing significant organ dysfunction that may be life-threatening. This variability in organ involvement and disease presentation often makes the diagnosis of sarcoidosis problematic.

Epidemiology

Sarcoidosis occurs worldwide and affects all races and ages. Although the disease has been thought to be most common between ages 20 and 40, analyses from large databases have revealed that the incidence and prevalence of the disease is greatest between ages 45 and 65. There is an earlier onset of disease in blacks and males. A large analysis from an American national health care database found an incidence of 17.8 per 100,000 in African Americans and 8.1 per 100,000 in American whites, a prevalence of 141 per 100,000 in African Americans and 50 per 100,000 in American whites. Incidence and prevalence rates were lower in American Hispanics than whites and lower still in American Asians. The highest prevalence of sarcoidosis is found in whites in Scandinavia and in persons of African descent in the United States. The relative risk for having sarcoidosis increases significantly if a family member has it as well. In the United States, nearly 20% of African Americans with sarcoidosis have an affected first-degree relative, compared with 5% in whites.

The clinical presentation and severity of sarcoidosis vary among racial and ethnic groups. The disease tends to be more severe in African Americans, whereas whites are more likely to be asymptomatic at presentation. Extrathoracic manifestations are more common in certain populations, such as ocular and cardiac sarcoidosis in Japanese populations, chronic uveitis in African Americans, and erythema nodosum in Europeans. There is increasing evidence that genetic polymorphisms affect the risks and manifestations of the disease. This is consistent with the current theory that sarcoidosis does not have a single cause but is the result of an abnormal host (granulomatous) response to one of many potential antigens in a genetically susceptible person.

Immunopathogenesis

The exact immunopathogenesis of sarcoidosis is unknown, but it is thought to be similar to that of other granulomatous diseases. That is, antigen-presenting cells (APCs), usually either macrophages or dendritic cells, process and present an antigen via a human leukocyte antigen (HLA) class II molecule to T lymphocytes and their receptors. These T lymphocytes are usually of the CD4 T-helper 1 (T_H1) class. The antigen involved in this reaction is unknown, and there may be many antigens that are each associated with a specific HLA class II molecule and T-cell receptor. This could explain the inability to determine one specific cause of sarcoidosis and the varied phenotypic expressions of the disease.

The interaction of APCs and T lymphocytes activates the APCs to produce tumor necrosis factor α (TNF-α) and other cytokines. A proliferation of CD4 T_H1 lymphocytes also ensues, which results in the secretion of interferon-γ (IFN-γ), interleukin (IL)-2, IL-12, and other cytokines. These cytokines activate and recruit monocytes and macrophages and transform them into giant cells, which are important building blocks of the granuloma. Recent evidence suggests that an additional factor leading to this series of immunologic events is persistence of antigen, possibly related to production of soluble AA amyloid fibrils, that prevents antigen degradation.

The typical sarcoidosis lesion is a noncaseating (non-necrotic) granuloma. The sarcoid granuloma consists of a compact core of macrophage-derived epithelioid and multinucleated giant cells surrounded by a perimeter of monocytes, lymphocytes, and fibroblasts. Granulomas can resolve spontaneously or with therapy; however, they can also persist and lead to persistent hyalinization and fibrosis. The development of such fibrosis can cause permanent organ damage and in large part determines the prognosis.

Clinical Features and Clinical Course

Pulmonary Sarcoidosis

Between 30% and 60% of patients with pulmonary sarcoidosis are asymptomatic, and the disease is detected incidentally on chest x-ray. Some patients present with nonspecific pulmonary symptoms, such as dyspnea, cough, wheezing, and chest pain. Respiratory failure from sarcoidosis is extremely rare at presentation. Unlike in many other interstitial lung diseases, crackles are rarely heard on chest auscultation. Abnormalities on the chest radiograph occur in more than 90% of patients with pulmonary sarcoidosis. Bilateral hilar adenopathy occurs in 50% to 85% at disease presentation, and 25% to 50% have parenchymal infiltrates. Sarcoid granulomas have a predilection for the bronchovascular bundles, subpleural locations, intralobular septa, and the airways.

A radiographic staging system was developed several decades ago (Table 1). Groups of patients with higher radiographic stages have more-severe pulmonary dysfunction, lower remission rates, and greater mortality. However, there is significant overlap among these groups, and predictions concerning individual patients based on stage are highly inaccurate. (See Figure 1.)

Advanced pulmonary stage IV (fibrocystic) sarcoidosis displays destruction of the lung architecture, with upward traction of the hila, lung distortion, upper-lobe volume loss, fibrocystic disease, honeycombed cysts, and decreased lung volumes. Aspergillomas can develop in these large cystic lesions and may be associated with life-threatening hemoptysis. Bronchiectasis from airway distortion also can occur and is an additional potential cause of hemoptysis.

The majority of patients with pulmonary sarcoidosis have a vital capacity of greater than 70% of predicted at diagnosis. Pulmonary function and the chest radiographic findings are often discordant. In pulmonary sarcoidosis patients with a normal lung parenchyma (stage I), the vital capacity, diffusing capacity, partial pressure of arterial oxygen (Pao_2) at rest, Pao_2 with exercise, and lung compliance are abnormal in 20% to 40% of cases. Patients with abnormal lung parenchyma have abnormal pulmonary function tests 50% to 70% of the time. Patients with stage IV fibrocystic sarcoidosis tend to have the most severe pulmonary dysfunction.

Sarcoidosis is an interstitial lung disease with a restrictive ventilatory defect often found on spirometry. It is underappreciated, however, that endobronchial involvement is common in sarcoidosis, and therefore airflow obstruction may be the major abnormality found on pulmonary function testing. Wheezing may be the prominent presenting symptom of sarcoidosis, and many cases of sarcoidosis are misdiagnosed as asthma. Airflow obstruction is also common in chronic pulmonary sarcoidosis, where it is caused by airway distortion from fibrosis. The cause of dyspnea in pulmonary sarcoidosis is multifactorial. It may be the result of abnormalities of gas exchange or lung mechanics, weakness of the respiratory muscles, obesity from corticosteroid therapy, pulmonary hypertension, or sarcoidosis involvement of the heart.

Only 3% to 5% of patients die of sarcoidosis. In the United States, 75% of these deaths are the result of pulmonary involvement. Death from pulmonary involvement is rarely acute but normally is an insidious process that develops over 5 to 25 years with the development of progressive pulmonary fibrosis. Several studies have suggested that pulmonary hypertension is a major risk factor for death from pulmonary sarcoidosis. Patients with aspergillomas are also at risk for death from episodes of life-threatening hemoptysis. Both pulmonary hypertension and aspergillosis are most commonly found in the sarcoidosis patients with stage IV fibrocystic disease. Other organs that result in fatalities from sarcoidosis are the heart and the central nervous system. In Japan, death from sarcoidosis is more commonly caused by cardiac than pulmonary involvement.

Extrapulmonary Sarcoidosis

The extrapulmonary manifestations of sarcoidosis can predominate in many patients. Extrapulmonary disease can affect the prognosis and treatment options for sarcoidosis.

The eyes and skin are the most common extrapulmonary organs involved with sarcoidosis. Ocular manifestations occur in 25% to 50% of patients; anterior uveitis is the most common manifestation. Symptoms of anterior uveitis include red eyes, painful eyes, and photophobia. However, in one-third of patients with anterior uveitis from sarcoidosis have no ocular symptoms. In addition, an intermediate or posterior uveitis can cause vision problems or can be asymptomatic. For these reasons, all patients with sarcoidosis should undergo an eye examination by an ophthalmologist. Other ocular manifestations of sarcoidosis include conjunctivitis, keratoconjunctivitis sicca (dry eyes), scleritis, and optic neuritis.

Skin lesions in sarcoidosis can be classified into two categories: specific lesions that demonstrate noncaseating granulomas on biopsy and nonspecific lesions that do not. The specific skin lesions are often papular and have a predilection for areas of previous scars and tattoos. Lupus pernio is a type of specific skin

| TABLE 1 | Chest Radiograph Stages of Sarcoidosis |

RADIOGRAPHIC STAGE	BILATERAL HILAR LYMPH NODE ENLARGEMENT	PARENCHYMAL DISEASE
I	Yes	No
II	Yes	Nonfibrotic
III	No	Nonfibrotic
IV	No or yes	Fibrotic

Adapted from Judson MA, Baughman RP: Sarcoidosis. In Baughman RP, du Bois RM, Lynch JP, Wells AU (eds): *Diffuse Lung Disease: A Practical Approach.* London, Arnold, 2004, p 109–29.

A   B

Figure 1 Skin lesions of sarcoidosis. *A,* Sarcoid lesions may occur at any site, and they may take nodular, papular, or plaque forms. Biopsy is often necessary for diagnosis. *B, Lupus pernio* is the term used to describe a dusky-purple infiltration of the skin of the nose, cheeks, or ears in chronic sarcoidosis. (From Forbes CD, Jackson WF: *Color Atlas and Text of Clinical Medicine,* 3rd ed. London, Mosby, 2003, with permission.)

lesion causing disfiguring lesions on the face, often with erythema and significant induration. These lesions have a predilection for the nose, cheeks, medial and lateral sides of the eyes, and lateral sides of the mouth. Lupus pernio lesions are relatively recalcitrant to therapy and often respond only partially to corticosteroids. The most common nonspecific skin lesion is erythema nodosum, which is often seen with an acute sarcoidosis presentation of fever, arthritis (especially in the ankles), pulmonary symptoms, and bilateral hilar adenopathy on chest radiograph. This syndrome is known as *Löfgren's syndrome* and tends to have a good long-term prognosis.

Cardiac and neurologic sarcoidosis can be life threatening and are therefore important to recognize. Cardiac involvement is detected clinically in 5% of sarcoidosis patients during life but in 25% at autopsy. Cardiac sarcoidosis can cause left ventricular dysfunction and cardiac arrhythmias, possibly resulting in sudden death. All patients with sarcoidosis should be screened for cardiac sarcoidosis. Such screenings should include an electrocardiogram as well as eliciting symptoms of left ventricular dysfunction (e.g., orthopnea, peripheral edema) and cardiac arrhythmia (e.g., palpitations, sensation of skipped heartbeats, syncope). Echocardiography and Holter monitoring have been recommended by some as appropriate additional screening tests. The diagnosis of cardiac sarcoidosis is problematic, because the disease is patchy and diagnosed less than 25% of the time by endomyocardial biopsy because of sampling error. Often the diagnosis is made noninvasively, if a typical clinical presentation is coupled with detection of abnormalities on echocardiography, gallium scanning, thallium scanning, cardiac magnetic resonance imaging (MRI), or positron emission tomography (PET).

Clinically apparent neurosarcoidosis occurs in less than 10% of sarcoidosis patients. Palsy of the seventh cranial nerve is the most common manifestation of neurosarcoidosis, and it often predates the diagnosis of the disease. Sarcoidosis can affect any part of the peripheral nervous system and central nervous system and can cause a cranial nerve palsy, mononeuropathy or polyneuropathy, aseptic meningitis, seizures, mass lesions in the brain and spinal cord, and encephalopathy.

Sarcoidosis causes clinically apparent peripheral lymphadenopathy in more than 10% of patients. The spleen may be involved in up to 50% of patients, but it is usually asymptomatic and rarely causes hypersplenism.

Bone involvement is occasional, usually occurring as small cysts or cortical defects found in the small bones of the hands and feet. An acute sarcoid arthritis often is present at disease onset and has a good prognosis. This is commonly found in the ankles of patients who present with Löfgren's syndrome. Chronic sarcoid arthritis is rare. It is usually a nondestructive arthropathy of the shoulders, wrists, knees, ankles, and small joints of the hands and feet.

Sarcoidosis of the sinuses is underappreciated. It can occur in the nasopharynx, hypopharynx, larynx, or any of the sinuses and is known as *sarcoidosis of the upper respiratory tract*. Sarcoidosis of the upper respiratory tract is often relatively recalcitrant to therapy.

Histologic evidence of hepatic sarcoidosis is present in 50% to 80% of sarcoidosis patients, although most of these patients are asymptomatic and have normal liver function tests. Hepatomegaly, abdominal pain, and pruritus are the most common symptoms associated with hepatic sarcoidosis but are present only in 15% to 25% of patients with hepatic involvement. Elevation of the serum alkaline phosphatase is the most common liver function test abnormality.

Hypercalcemia or hypercalciuria leading to nephrolithiasis and renal dysfunction can occur with sarcoidosis. These phenomena are the result of the enzyme 1α-hydroxylase in activated macrophages that convert 25-hydroxyvitamin D to 1,25-dihydroxyvitamin D, the active form of the vitamin. This results in increased gut absorption and increased renal excretion of calcium that can cause nephrolithiasis.

Sarcoidosis rarely involves the thyroid, kidney, breast, renal parenchyma, GU tract, and GI tract.

Patients can have constitutional symptoms such as fever, night sweats, weight loss, malaise, and fatigue at presentation. These symptoms occasionally are associated with hepatic sarcoid involvement but may be a sign of the systemic nature of the disease, presumably from cytokine release, rather than specific organ involvement. A small fiber neuropathy may occur with sarcoidosis and cause pain or autonomic dysfunction. Patients who present with Löfgren's syndrome or with asymptomatic bilateral hilar adenopathy on chest radiograph have a good prognosis. African Americans tend to have a worse prognosis than whites, with lower forced vital capacity and more new organ involvement within 2 years of diagnosis. Box 1 lists risk factors associated with a poor prognosis.

Diagnosis and Initial Workup

The diagnosis of sarcoidosis requires a compatible clinical picture, histologic demonstration of noncaseating granulomas, and exclusion of other diseases capable of producing a similar histologic and clinical picture. It is prudent to bear a healthy degree of skepticism in the diagnosis and evaluate the patient closely for additional clues supporting an alternative diagnosis. Mycobacterial and fungal diseases must always be considered as alternative causes of granulomatous inflammation. Therefore stains and cultures of tissue specimens for mycobacteria and fungi always should be obtained when the diagnosis of sarcoidosis is considered. Hypersensitivity pneumonitis, a granulomatous lung disease from inhalation of bioaerosols, is another disease that may mimic sarcoidosis. Bioaerosols from hot tubs and birds are the most common causes of hypersensitivity pneumonitis, and clinicians should specifically inquire about these two exposures in individuals who are being evaluated for sarcoidosis. Sarcoidosis is a systemic disease, so signs or symptoms of extrathoracic disease such as uveitis, skin lesions, or an elevated serum alkaline phosphatase concentration should be sought. Because of the varied clinical presentation of sarcoidosis, there is no single diagnostic algorithm.

It is prudent to select a biopsy site associated with less morbidity, such as the skin if a lesion is present. Transbronchial lung biopsy has a diagnostic yield of 40% to more than 90% in pulmonary sarcoidosis. Endobronchial biopsy has a 40% to 60% sensitivity and adds to the yield of transbronchial biopsy. Although granulomas are almost universally obtained via mediastinoscopy when mediastinal lymphadenopathy is present, transthoracic needle aspiration under ultrasound guidance (EBUS-TBNA) of mediastinal lymph nodes via bronchoscopy has a high yield for the diagnosis of sarcoidosis and has supplanted mediastinoscopy at many centers.

Bronchoalveolar lavage (BAL) with examination of lymphocyte populations has been used in the evaluation of possible pulmonary sarcoidosis. In sarcoidosis, there is an increased number of BAL lymphocytes, and these are predominantly CD4+. It has been proposed that an increase in BAL lymphocytes and a BAL

BOX 1	Factors Associated With a Poor Prognosis in Sarcoidosis

No symptoms at presentation
African-American race
Extrathoracic disease
Stage II to III versus stage I on chest x-ray
Age >40 years
Splenic involvement
Lupus pernio
Disease duration >2 years
Forced vital capacity <1.5 L
Stage IV chest x-ray or aspergilloma
Pulmonary hypertension

Data from Judson MA, Baughman RP: Sarcoidosis. In Baughman RP, du Bois RM, Lynch JP, Wells AU (eds): *Diffuse Lung Disease: A Practical Approach*. London, Arnold, 2004, p 109–29.

Clinical or Laboratory Findings That Strongly Support a Diagnosis of Sarcoidosis Without a Tissue Biopsy

Löfgren's syndrome
Heerfordt's syndrome (uveoparotid fever)
Asymptomatic bilateral hilar adenopathy on chest x-ray
^{67}Ga scan showing a lambda sign and a panda sign

CD4/CD8 ratio greater than 3.5 makes the diagnosis of sarcoidosis highly likely.

Although serum angiotensin-converting enzyme (ACE) often is elevated in active sarcoidosis, the specificity and sensitivity of this test are inadequate for it to be used diagnostically. Serum ACE may be used as supportive evidence for the diagnosis, and it also may be used in some instances to follow disease activity.

Gallium-67 (^{67}Ga) scanning is cumbersome because it takes several days to complete and is infrequently used as a diagnostic test. However, bilateral hilar uptake and right paratracheal uptake (lambda sign) coupled with lacrimal and parotid uptake (panda sign) with ^{67}Ga strongly suggest a diagnosis of sarcoidosis.

Gadolinium enhancement on MRI and fluorodeoxyglucose PET scanning have essentially replaced ^{67}Ga scanning for detecting sarcoidosis activity, because evidence suggests that they may be more sensitive in detecting sarcoidosis activity and they can be performed in one sitting. Somatostatin receptor scintigraphy may also be a useful technique to detect sarcoidosis activity.

Ideally, the diagnosis of sarcoidosis requires demonstration of noncaseating granulomas in at least one organ. However, certain clinical presentations are so specific for the diagnosis of sarcoidosis that the diagnosis may be accepted without tissue biopsy. Extreme caution must be used in these situations to ensure that there is no clinical information that would suggest an alternative diagnosis that should prompt a tissue biopsy. Clinical or laboratory findings that strongly support the diagnosis of sarcoidosis without a tissue biopsy are listed in Box 2.

Treatment

Therapy is not mandated for sarcoidosis because the disease can remit spontaneously. Therapy is indicated for potentially dangerous disease and for disease causing significant quality of life impairment. Potentially dangerous disease includes neurosarcoidosis, cardiac sarcoidosis, hypercalcemia that does not respond to dietary measures, ocular sarcoidosis that does not respond to topical (eyedrop) therapy, and other life- or organ-threatening disease. Therapy also should be considered when the disease is progressive. Relative indications for therapy include arthritis that fails to respond to nonsteroidal antiinflammatory drugs (NSAIDs); a systemic inflammatory response syndrome of fever, night sweats, fatigue, and arthralgias; and symptomatic hepatic disease. In general, treatment is discouraged for asymptomatic elevations of serum liver function tests, specific levels of ACE, or asymptomatic uptake on ^{67}Ga scan (with the possible exceptions of the heart or brain).

The decision to treat sarcoidosis can be problematic, because the disease has a variable prognosis that must be weighed against the potential side effects of therapy. It is often most prudent to monitor patients without therapy if they are asymptomatic or have only mild organ dysfunction. For pulmonary sarcoidosis, asymptomatic patients and those with mild disease that might spontaneously remit usually are not treated. For patients with clinical findings that predict spontaneous remission (e.g., erythema nodosum), the benefits of treatment often are offset by the toxicity of therapy. Often these patients can be managed with palliative therapy such as NSAIDs for arthralgias and fever and bronchodilators and inhaled corticosteroids for wheezing and cough.

It is recommended that patients with mild to moderate pulmonary sarcoidosis be observed for 2 to 6 months, if possible. Patients who improve will have avoided the toxicity of corticosteroids, and patients who deteriorate over this period should be considered for treatment. Patients with pulmonary dysfunction who neither improve nor deteriorate during the observation period may be given a corticosteroid trial, or they may be observed further. Patients with severe pulmonary dysfunction or pulmonary symptoms causing significant impairment should be treated.

Corticosteroids often are used to treat sarcoidosis, but the dose, duration of therapy, and method by which one can assess effectiveness have not been standardized. Topical corticosteroid therapy should be used whenever possible in an attempt to minimize systemic complications. This includes corticosteroid eye drops for anterior sarcoid uveitis and corticosteroid creams and injections for localized skin lesions. Pulmonary sarcoidosis usually is treated initially with 20 to 40 mg/day of prednisone or its equivalent. Higher doses may be required for neurosarcoidosis and cardiac sarcoidosis. The patient usually is evaluated within 2 to 12 weeks for a response. Patients failing to respond to therapy within 3 months are unlikely to respond to a more protracted course of therapy or a higher dose. Among the responders, the corticosteroid dose is tapered to 5 to 10 mg/day of a prednisone equivalent or an every-other-day regimen. Treatment is usually continued for at least 6 months.

The relapse rate after corticosteroid therapy is withdrawn may be as high as 70%, and therefore patients need to be followed closely as the corticosteroid dose is tapered and discontinued. In some patients, there may be recurrent relapses requiring long-term low-dose therapy. On occasion, the chronic prednisone dose needed to prevent relapse is less than 5 mg/day. Patients who relapse after corticosteroids have been withdrawn should be re-treated with corticosteroids. Alternative agents, such as corticosteroid-sparing agents, to control the disease in a patient on a chronic low dose of prednisone should be considered. On occasion, alternative agents may completely replace corticosteroid therapy. In general, corticosteroid-sparing agents should not be considered unless the patient requires more than 7.5 mg/day of prednisone to control the disease.

Methotrexate (Rheumatrex)[1] and hydroxychloroquine (Plaquenil)[1] are the most-studied alternative sarcoidosis medications. They are usually used as corticosteroid-sparing agents but at times can be used as replacement therapy. Methotrexate is most useful for pulmonary, skin, joint, and eye sarcoidosis. Hydroxychloroquine is often used for sarcoidosis of the skin, joints, and nerves and for hypercalcemia from sarcoidosis. Azathioprine (Imuran)[1] may be useful for sarcoid uveitis, but usually it is added to corticosteroid plus methotrexate in this instance. Minocycline (Minocin)[1] and doxycycline (Vibramycin)[1] may be useful for skin sarcoidosis. Cyclophosphamide (Cytoxan)[1] is used occasionally and seems to have a potential role in neurosarcoidosis. Leflunomide (Arava)[1] has also been shown to be useful in the treatment of pulmonary and extrapulmonary sarcoidosis. Monoclonal antibodies against TNF-α, such as infliximab (Remicade)[1] and adalimumab (Humira)[1], are useful agents in sarcoidosis patients with severe disease and/or who fail to respond to the aforementioned treatments.

Therapy should also be considered for the non-granulomatous aspects of the disease. Sarcoidosis-associated small fiber neuropathy may respond to medications for neuropathic pain, monoclonal antibodies against TNF-α, or intravenous immunoglobulin[1]. Sarcoidosis-associated fatigue may benefit from a physical training program, neurostimulants, or monoclonal antibodies against TNF-α.

---

[1]Not FDA approved for this indication.

References

Baughman RP, Culver DA, Judson MA: A concise review of pulmonary sarcoidosis, *Am J Respir Crit Care Med* 183:573–589, 2011.

Baughman RP, Field S, Costabel U: Sarcoidosis in America: analysis based on health care use, *Ann Am Thorac Soc* 13:244–252, 2016.

Baughman RP, Nunes H, Sweiss NJ, et al: Established and experimental medical therapy of pulmonary sarcoidosis, *Eur Respir J* 41(6):1424–1438, 2013.

Baughman RP, Teirstein AS, Judson MA, et al: Clinical characteristics of patients in a case control study of sarcoidosis, *Am J Respir Crit Care Med* 164:1885–1889, 2001.

Chen ES, Song Z, Willett MH, et al: Serum amyloid A regulates granulomatous inflammation in sarcoidosis through Toll- like receptor-2, *Am J Respir Crit Care Med* 181:360–373, 2010.

Hamzeh N, Steckman D, Sauer W, Judson MA: Pathophysiology and clinical management of cardiac sarcoidosis, *Nature Rev Cardiol* 12:278–288, 2015.

Hunninghake GW, Costabel U, Ando M, et al: ATS/ERS/WASOG statement on sarcoidosis, *Am J Respir Crit Care Med* 160:736–755, 1999.

Judson MA: The diagnosis of sarcoidosis, *Clinics Chest Med* 29:415–427, 2008.

Judson MA: The clinical features of sarcoidosis: a comphrensive review, *Clinic Rev Allerg Immunol* 49:63–78, 2015.

Judson MA, Costabel U, Drent M, et al: The WASOG Sarcoidosis Organ Assessment Investigators. The WASOG Sarcoidosis Organ Assessment Instrument: an update of a previous clinical tool, *Sarcoidosis Vasc Diff Lung Dis* 31:19–27, 2014.

Lower EE, Baughman RP: Prolonged use of methotrexate in refractory sarcoidosis, *Arch Intern Med* 155:846–851, 1995.

Tavee JO, Karwa K, Ahmed Z, et al: Sarcoidosis-associated small fiber neuropathy in a large cohort: Clinical aspects and response to IVIG and anti-TNF alpha treatment, *Respir Med* 126:135–138, 2017.

Tremblay A, Stather DR, MacEachern P, Khalil M, Field SK: A randomized controlled trial of standard vs endobronchial ultrasonography-guided transbronchial needle aspiration in patients with suspected sarcoidosis, *Chest* 136:340–346, 2009.

TUBERCULOSIS AND OTHER MYCOBACTERIAL DISEASES

Method of
Jotam Pasipanodya, MD; Ronald Hall II, PharmD, MSCS; and Tawanda Gumbo, MD

Mycobacterial diseases are some of the oldest documented infectious diseases in humans, and they still cause significant morbidity and mortality. *Mycobacterium tuberculosis* complex, *Mycobacterium avium* complex (MAC), and *Mycobacterium leprae* are slow-growing, acid-fast bacilli that belong to the family Mycobacteriaceae of the order Actinomycetales. This chapter deals with management of diseases caused by *M. tuberculosis*, MAC, and *M. leprae*. A summary of diseases caused by other, less common mycobacteria is presented in Table 1.

Recent evidence suggests that the mycobacteria causing tuberculosis (TB) might have co-evolved with humans. Clues attesting to the success of mycobacteria as human pathogens include the prolonged period of latency and the ability to cause extensive disease in only a narrow host range. DNA evidence suggests that the *M. tuberculosis* strains causing the current waves of TB epidemics most likely evolved from a common ancestor. *Mycobacterium canetti* and the other strains that form the *M. tuberculosis* complex (i.e., *Mycobacterium africanum*, *Mycobacterium microti*, and *Mycobacterium bovis* strains) also evolved from the ancestral strain through successive loss of DNA. This is contrary to the belief that the *M. tuberculosis* complex evolved from *M. bovis*.

Tuberculosis
Epidemiology
TB remains a global pandemic, with 9.3 million new cases and 1.4 million deaths reported worldwide in 2007. Approximately 1 of every 7 patients who has TB is co-infected with the human immunodeficiency virus (HIV). Whereas global TB incidence trends are stabilizing after reaching a peak in 2004, rates in countries with a low TB burden have been declining gradually. An explanation could be the similar plateau and declines in HIV prevalence observed in the year 2000. On the other hand, this could merely reflect the natural ebbs and increases inherent to epidemic cycles.

Global estimates show that one third of humankind has been infected with *M. tuberculosis*, the TB disease-causing bacillus. About 80% of global TB is accounted for by the 22 high-burden countries. The top five countries in rank order are India, China, Indonesia, Nigeria, and South Africa. TB program priorities and approaches to combating the disease differ among and within countries. These differences are based on the availability of resources and the prevalence of HIV within communities. For example, program goals in areas of low TB incidence, such as the United States, are aimed at TB elimination. Therefore, in the United States, treatment of latent TB is a priority. Reducing TB transmission through increased diagnosis of patients with active TB disease is the primary goal in high-incidence areas.

Natural History
Susceptibility to *M. tuberculosis* infection and the subsequent progression of that infection to active TB disease is influenced by the complex interaction of host, pathogen, and environmental factors. Between 20% and 30% of people exposed to a person with active TB become infected. Animal models, twin studies, segregation studies, and candidate gene analysis studies provide insight into the role of host genetic factors in susceptibility to TB.

The immune system contains the infection in more than 90% to 95% of persons infected. Protective immunity mediated by subsets of T lymphocytes produces soluble lymphokines that enable macrophages to kill intracellular bacilli. The bacilli are often not completely eradicated and remain dormant in macrophages or other cells, with the potential to reactivate to active disease when the immune system wanes. This is termed latent TB infection (LTBI). The lifetime risk of reactivation to active TB disease is 5% to 10%. This risk of reactivation increases with several factors, including development of the acquired immunodeficiency syndrome (AIDS), renal failure, immunomodulatory therapy, and poorly controlled diabetes mellitus.

In a small subgroup of patients, *M. tuberculosis* infection is not brought under control during primary infection and quickly progresses to disseminated disease. TB that follows such a course is called progressive primary TB. Primary TB is associated with a higher mortality rate, and death typically occurs within 2 years after infection. The risk of developing TB disease after being infected is higher in males from infancy to 6 years of age. Males older than 45 years of age are also at an increased risk compared to females of the same age.

Diagnosis of Active Tuberculosis
In immunocompetent persons, pulmonary involvement is the most common presentation, followed by isolated extrapulmonary disease. Involvement of only extrapulmonary sites is rare, and most immunocompromised patients present with both pulmonary and extrapulmonary involvement. The presenting signs and symptoms of active TB disease are site specific. However, constitutional symptoms such as fever, night sweats, and fatigue are common and gradually evolve over many weeks. Patients should be specifically asked about constitutional symptoms, because these symptoms raise the index of suspicion. Atypical presentations are common in patients who are immunosuppressed and can delay diagnosis.

Definitive diagnosis is made on the basis of a positive culture. Therefore, all patients with suspected TB must have the appropriate specimens collected for microscopic and, if appropriate, histologic examination. Mycobacterial culture and sensitivity testing should also be performed, if available. Acid-fast bacillus (AFB) staining and microscopy is limited by poor sensitivity (45% to 80% with culture-confirmed TB cases) and poor positive predictive value (50% to 80%) for TB in settings where nontuberculous mycobacteria are commonly isolated. TB culture results are available only after 2 to 6 weeks. Nucleic acid amplification (NAA) testing can also be used to confirm a TB diagnosis in 24 to 48 hours, even when the specimen sample is limited. NAA tests can detect the presence of *M. tuberculosis* in 50% to 80% of AFB-negative and culture-positive specimens. The CDC now recommends that evaluation of at least the first diagnostic specimen include NAA testing.

Serial radiologic images can be used to exclude active TB and assess clinical improvement.

TABLE 1	Species of Mycobacteria		
MICROBE	**RESERVOIR**	**CLINICAL MANIFESTATION**	
Always Pathogenic in Humans			
M. tuberculosis	Humans	Pulmonary and disseminated tuberculosis	
M. bovis	Cattle, humans	TB-like disease	
M. africanum	Humans, monkeys	Rarely, TB-like pulmonary disease	
M. leprae	Humans	Leprosy	
M. canetti	Humans, possibly others	Rarely, TB-like pulmonary disease	
Potentially Pathogenic in Humans			
M. avium complex	Soil, water, birds, swine, cattle, environment	Disseminated and pulmonary TB-like disease	
M. microti	Rodents, llamas, cats, ferrets, and possibly humans	Rarely, TB-like pulmonary disease	
M. kansasii	Water, cattle	TB-like disease	
Uncommon or Rarely Pathogenic in Humans			
M. flavescens	Humans, environment	TB-like disease	
M. genavense	Humans, birds	Blood-borne disease with AIDS	
M. haemophilum	Unknown	Skin, joint, bone, and pulmonary infections in immunocompromised individuals; lymphadenitis in children	
M. malmoense	Environment, possibly others	TB-like pulmonary disease in adults; lymphadenitis in children	
M. marinum	Fish, water	Skin infections	
M. scrofulaceum	Soil, water	Cervical lymphadenitis	
M. simiae	Monkeys, water	TB-like pulmonary disease and disseminated disease with AIDS	
M. szulgai	Water, environment	TB-like pulmonary disease	
M. ulcerans	Humans, environment	Skin infections (Buruli ulcer)	
M. xenopi	Water, birds	TB-like pulmonary disease	

M., Mycobacterium; TB, tuberculosis.
Adapted from Coberly JS, Chaisson RE. Tuberculosis. In: Nelson KE, Williams CM, eds. *Infectious Disease Epidemiology: Theory and Practice.* 2nd ed. Boston: Jones and Bartlett; 2007.

Principles of Treatment

The goal of anti-TB therapy is cure. A secondary objective is minimizing the transmission of *M. tuberculosis* to others by curing the patient. Treatment outcomes are best when patient-centered treatments and care are offered, regardless of whether the treatment facility is private or public. Patient management and supervision plans should be tailored to the patient's clinical and social circumstances. Directly observed therapy (DOT) is recommended by regulatory bodies to help ensure adherence to treatment and is regarded as central to current case management. However, the efficacy of DOT compared with self-administration has been questioned in recent studies. There are three types of anti-TB therapy: prophylaxis, definitive TB therapy for drug-susceptible infection, and therapy for drug-resistant TB.

Chemoprophylaxis

The confusing terms of preventive therapy and chemoprophylaxis are sometimes used to describe treatment of LTBI. Preventive therapy, in this context, does not actually prevent infection; rather, it prevents development of active TB in those already infected. Therefore, the better descriptive term, treatment of LTBI, is preferred. Treatment of minimal or LTBI prevents subsequent evolution to active disease. A series of double-blind, placebo-controlled clinical trials done in the 1950s and 1960s provided evidence demonstrating the effectiveness of treatment of LTBI. Priority is usually given to those patients with the highest risk for reactivation.

Treatment of LTBI, particularly when it is targeted toward persons with higher risks of reactivation, is one of the major strategies for elimination of TB in the United States. Targets include people who have been recently infected and those who were remotely infected but have concurrent disease that puts them at higher risk for developing reactivation disease. There are more than 11 million people with LTBI in the United States, each with a 5% to 10% lifetime risk of developing TB disease.

The Mantoux method of tuberculin skin testing is commonly used to diagnose LTBI as well as active disease. Use of tuberculin skin testing is hampered by low sensitivity in immunocompromised patients, low specificity in persons who have received the bacille Calmette-Guérin (BCG) vaccine, and the requirement to return to a trained person to have the test read after 48 to 72 hours. Results are interpreted based on the patient scenario (Box 1).

Recently, various blood-testing methods that are based on detection of the interferon-γ (IFN-γ) released by T lymphocytes in response to *M. tuberculosis*–specific antigens have become available as an alternative to skin testing. These tests may be more specific than the tuberculin skin test in BCG-vaccinated and immunocompromised populations. However, IFN-γ release assays do not differentiate LTBI from active TB disease. Currently available IFN-γ release assays are QuantiFERON, QuantiFERON-Gold, and ELISPOT. The CDC recommends these tests for LTBI screening of healthcare workers, recent immigrants, injection drug users, prison and jail inmates and workers, and contacts of

BOX 1 Interpretation of a Tuberculin Skin Test

Reaction ≥5 mm of Induration
HIV-positive persons
Recent contacts of TB case patients
Fibrotic changes on chest radiography consistent with prior TB
Organ transplant recipients and other immunosuppressed
 patients (receiving the equivalent of ≥15 mg/d of
 prednisone for 1 month or longer)*

Reaction ≥10 mm of Induration
Recent immigrants (i.e., ≤5 years) from high-prevalence
 countries
Injection drug users
Residents and employees† of the following high-risk
 congregate settings:
• Prisons and jails
• Nursing homes and other long-term facilities for the elderly
• Hospitals and other healthcare facilities
• Residential facilities for patients with AIDS
• Homeless shelters
• Mycobacteriology laboratory personnel
Persons with the following clinical conditions that place them
 at high risk:
• Silicosis
• Diabetes mellitus
• Chronic renal failure
• Certain hematologic disorders (e.g., leukemias, lymphomas)
• Other specific malignancies (e.g., carcinoma of the head,
 neck, or lung)
• Weight loss (>10% of ideal body weight)
• Gastrectomy and jejunoileal bypass
Children <4 years of age; infants, children, and adolescents
 exposed to adults at high risk

Reaction >15 mm of Induration
Persons with no risk factors for TB

---

*Risk of TB in patients treated with corticosteroids increases with higher dose and
 longer duration.
†For persons who are otherwise at low risk and are tested at the start of employment, a
 reaction of >15 mm induration is considered positive.
AIDS, Acquired immunodeficiency syndrome; *HIV*, human immunodeficiency syndrome;
TB, tuberculosis.
Adapted from Centers for Disease Control and Prevention: Screening for tuberculosis
 and tuberculosis infection in high-risk populations: Recommendations of the
 Advisory Council for the Elimination of Tuberculosis. *Morb Mortal Wkly Rep MMWR.*
 1995;44(No. RR-11):19–34.

TB cases within schools, workplaces, and the military. Prohibitive costs limit the use of these assays in resource-limited places.

Table 2 summarizes the regimens currently recommended by the American Thoracic Society (ATS), CDC, and Infectious Diseases Society of America (IDSA) for treatment of LTBI. Because of high rates of hospitalization and death from liver injury, the ATS and the CDC no longer recommend the 2-month regimen of daily or twice-weekly rifampin (Rifadin) plus pyrazinamide for LTBI. Directly observed 12-dose once-weekly regimen of isoniazid (INH; Nydrazid) and rifapentine (RPT; Priftin) is recommended as an option equal to the standard INH 9-month daily regimen for treating LTBI in otherwise healthy people 12 years of age and older who were recently in contact with infectious TB, or who had tuberculin skin test or blood test for TB infection conversions, or those with radiologic findings consistent with healed pulmonary TB. In recent large clinical trials of mostly adults without HIV, this regimen was associated with fewer serious adverse events, higher completion rates, and equal efficacy, as compared with isoniazid for 9 months. Rifampin or rifabutin (Mycobutin)[1] may be used to treat LTBI in HIV-infected persons exposed to TB

---

[1]Not FDA approved for this indication.

that is resistant to isoniazid (INH; Nydrazid) and susceptible to rifampin, with dose adjustments and diligence taken to prevent cytochrome P-450–derived drug interactions with antiretroviral agents.

Definitive Therapy

The decision to initiate therapy is made based on local epidemiologic information; the patient's clinical, pathologic, and radiologic data; and the results of microscopic and culture examination. Therapy may be started immediately if the index of suspicion is high or if the patient is gravely ill. However, in general, clinicians should still collect initial specimens for microscopic evaluation and culture before starting treatment. HIV testing and baseline liver function testing, serum creatinine levels, and platelet counts should be conducted as part of standard medical care for patients with suspected or documented TB disease.

Achieving microbiologic cure by killing all bacilli and preventing emergence of clinically significant drug-resistant mutants are the primary goals of definitive TB therapy. Therapy is prolonged despite sputum conversion and resolution of symptoms, because some organisms persist in some tissues. DOT is generally recommended to ensure compliance with prescribed medications.

The four ATS/CDC/IDSA-recommended regimens used for treating TB caused by drug-susceptible organisms are shown in Table 3. Each regimen has an initial phase of 2 months followed by a choice of several options for the continuation phase of 4 or 7 months. Treatment of previously untreated TB consists of 2 months of an initial phase of four drugs: isoniazid, rifampin, pyrazinamide, and ethambutol (Myambutol) or streptomycin (generally not used in the United States). The newer rifamycins are also first-line drugs used under certain circumstances. Rifabutin[1] is used if rifampin is contraindicated, as in patients taking certain antiretroviral drugs; rifapentine (Priftin) is used in the once-weekly continuation phase with isoniazid in selected patients (see Table 3). If the organisms are later demonstrated to be susceptible to isoniazid and rifampin, ethambutol is discontinued. The continuation phase is usually 4 months of daily or intermittent isoniazid and rifampin or rifapentine. The 7-month continuation phase is recommended only for those patients with cavitary TB caused by susceptible organisms that remains sputum positive after 2 months of DOT, patients whose initial treatment phase did not include pyrazinamide, and patients on weekly isoniazid and rifapentine whose sputum smear was still positive at the end of the intensive phase. There is evidence from many clinical trials done worldwide that demonstrates the efficacy of supervised intermittent therapy is similar to daily dosing in terms of various clinical outcomes. Routine follow-up to monitor adverse events and adherence to the treatment regimen should occur at least monthly.

Approximately 80% of patients who take the four-drug therapy for susceptible organisms are expected to convert from culture positive to negative after 2 months, and 90% to 95% after 3 months. Failure of treatment is defined by positive culture or, at times, positive smears after 4 months of supervised therapy. Relapse is defined by recurrent TB at any time after completion of treatment or apparent cure. Relapses most commonly occur during the first 6 to 12 months after the end of therapy. Treatment of initially susceptible disease can fail for many reasons, including extensive cavitary disease, drug resistance, malabsorption of drugs, laboratory error, and biologic variation in response. In any case, positive smears or cultures after 2 months of supervised therapy should be carefully evaluated to determine the cause. In addition, a full course of therapy is determined by the number of doses completed. Hence, a 6-month daily regimen (including both initiation and continuation phases) consists of at least 182 doses of isoniazid and rifampin and 56 doses of pyrazinamide (see Table 3). All missed doses should be taken. Patients interrupting

---

[1]Not FDA approved for this indication.

TABLE 2 CDC-Recommended Treatment for Latent Tuberculosis Infection

| DRUG | INTERVAL* | ORAL DOSE (MG/KG) | | MONITORING |
		CHILDREN	ADULTS	
Isoniazid (INH, Nydrazid)	Daily Twice weekly	10–20[3] 20–40	5 15	Monthly, LFTs[†] at baseline, repeat in selected patients if initial results are abnormal; hepatitis risk increases with age and alcohol consumption; pyridoxine[1] 10–25 mg/d may prevent peripheral neuropathy and CNS effects
Rifampin (Rifadin)	Daily Twice weekly	10–20 —	10 10	Weeks 2, 4, and 8 with pyrazinamide; contraindicated in patients receiving antiretroviral drugs; baseline LFTs[†] and CBC and platelets
Rifabutin (Mycobutin)[1]	Daily Twice weekly	— —	5 5	Weeks 2, 4, and 8; baseline LFTs[†] and CBC and platelets; use adjusted daily doses of rifabutin and monitor for decreased antiretroviral activity and rifabutin toxicity if PIs or NNRTIs are taken concurrently; contraindicated with saquinavir (Invirase) or delavirdine (Rescriptor)
Pyrazinamide[‡]	Daily Twice weekly	— —	15–20 50	Weeks 2, 4, and 8; LFTs[†] at baseline; avoid in first trimester of pregnancy
Rifapentine (Priftin)[§]	Weekly	—	10–14 kg: 300 mg 14.1–25 kg: 450 mg 25.1–32.0 kg: 600 mg 32.1–49.9 kg: 750 mg ≥50.0 kg: 900 mg	Monthly, LFTs[†] at baseline, repeat in selected patients if initial results are abnormal; hepatitis risk increases with age and alcohol consumption

CBC, Complete blood count; *CDC*, Centers for Disease Control and Prevention; *CNS*, central nervous system; *LFT*, liver function test; *NNRTI*, non-nucleoside reverse transcriptase inhibitor; *PI*, protease inhibitor.
[1]Not FDA approved for this indication.
[3]Exceeds dosage recommended by the manufacturer.
*All intermittent dosing should be given by directly observed therapy (DOT).
[†]LFTs include aspartate aminotransferase (AST), alanine aminotransferase (ALT), and serum albumin.
[‡]Used with either rifampin or rifabutin in combination therapy for 2–4 months.
[§]Rifapentine (RPT) is formulated as 150-mg tablets in blister packs that should be kept sealed until usage. Combined with INH.
Adapted from American Thoracic Society: Treatment of tuberculosis. *Am J Respir Crit Care Med.* 2003;167:603–662.

therapy by more than 14 days during the initial phase or more than 3 months during continuation phase should be restarted on therapy from the beginning.

Treatment of Tuberculosis in Resource-Poor Settings
Direct observation of patients taking therapy is just one of five elements of DOTS recommended by the World Health Organization and the International Union Against Tuberculosis and Lung Disease for TB treatment programs in resource-poor settings. The five elements of DOTS are:

- Government commitment to sustained TB control activities
- Case detection by sputum microscopy in symptomatic patients self-reporting to health centers
- Standardized treatment regimen of 6 to 9 months for at least all confirmed sputum smear-positive cases, with DOT for at least the intensive phase
- Regular, uninterrupted supply of essential anti-TB drugs
- Standardized recording and reporting system that allows for patient and program assessments

Smear microscopy for AFB is emphasized because of cost concerns and because access to culture facilities is limited in most countries. Three AFB stains that include early-morning sputum smears are recommended for a diagnosis. However, some recent data refute the need for three sputum samples by suggesting that no significant benefit is derived from the third smear when performed in high-burden countries. A new molecular diagnostic test called Xpert MTB/RIF assay detects *M. tuberculosis* complex within 2 hours with an assay sensitivity that is much higher than that of smear microscopy, and detects multidrug-resistant tuberculosis at the same time. In HIV infected patients, the test has a rate of case detection that is increased by 45%, as compared to smear microscopy.

Susceptibility testing is strongly recommended for patients who fail to convert to smear-negative status after 2 months of treatment. The prevalence of drug resistance in areas of high TB burden is unknown because of limited laboratory capacity.

Individualized TB care in resource-limited areas is difficult to implement because most decisions are made based solely on clinical judgment or limited radiologic findings. These challenges result in the use of standardized treatments that emphasize cost-effectiveness for utilitarian returns. This "one size fits all" approach is likely to worsen the financial and clinical outcomes of some patients.

Treatment of Tuberculosis in Special Circumstances
Multidrug-Resistant Tuberculosis
In resource-poor settings, where susceptibility testing facilities usually are not available, the surrogate terms "retreatment" and "chronic" are used to define various forms of drug-resistant strains. In the United States, about 1.1% of TB cases reported in 2007 had primary multidrug resistance, which is defined as resistance to at least isoniazid and rifampin in a patient with no previous history of TB treatment. Combination therapy including first- and second-line drugs is used to treat multidrug-resistant TB, and at least one of the drugs must be an injectable agent. Some of the second-line TB drugs are levofloxacin (Levaquin)[1], cycloserine (Seromycin), ethionamide (Trecator), *p*-aminosalicylic-acid (Paser), capreomycin (Capastat), kanamycin (Kantrex), and amikacin (Amikin).

Therapy takes several years to complete. Treatment failure, costs, and drug-related side effects are higher with the second-line drugs. Patients with suspected treatment failure should be managed at specialized facilities with necessary expertise where the full range of drug susceptibilities can be performed. As a general rule, single drugs should never be added to failing regimens because this leads to acquired resistance to each new drug. Drug resistance in mycobacteria occurs through random genetic mutations, with minimal lateral transfer of genetic material. Chances of detecting primary resistance are greater when the bacillary load is high, for example in patients with multiple cavitary disease.

[1]Not FDA approved for this indication.

TABLE 3 Drug Regimen for Culture-Positive Pulmonary Tuberculosis Caused by Drug-Susceptible Organisms

REGIMEN	DRUGS	INTERVAL AND MINIMUM DURATION*	DOSE (MAXIMUM DOSE IN 24 HOURS OR MAXIMUM DURATION)	
			CHILDREN	ADULTS
Initial Phase				
1	Isoniazid (INH, Nydrazid) Rifampin (Rifadin) Pyrazinamide Ethambutol (Myambutol)	Once daily on 7 doses/week for 56 doses (8 weeks), or Once daily on 5 doses/wk for 40 doses (8 weeks)	10–20 mg/kg/d[3] (300 mg) 10–20 mg/kg/d (600 mg) 15–30 mg/kg/d (2000 mg) 15–25 mg/kg/d	5 mg/kg/d (300 mg) 10 mg/kg/d (600 mg) 15–30 mg/kg/d (2000 mg) 15–25 mg/kg/d
2	Isoniazid Rifampin Pyrazinamide Ethambutol	Once daily on 7 doses/wk for 14 doses (2 weeks), then twice weekly for 12 doses (6 weeks), or Once daily on 5 doses/wk for 10 doses (2 weeks), then twice weekly for 12 doses (6 weeks)	20–40 mg/kg/d (900 mg) 10–20 mg/kg/d (600 mg) 50–70 mg/kg/d (4000 mg) 50 mg/kg/d[3]	15 mg/kg/d (900 mg) 10 mg/kg/d (900 mg)[3] 50–70 mg/kg/d (4000 mg) 50 mg/kg/d[3]
3	Isoniazid Rifampin Pyrazinamide Ethambutol	Three times weekly for 24 doses (8 weeks)	20–40 mg/kg/d (900 mg) 10–20 mg/kg/d (600 mg) 50–70 mg/kg/d (3000 mg) 50 mg/kg/d[3]	15 mg/kg/d (900 mg) 10 mg/kg/d (900 mg)[3] 50–70 mg/kg/d (3000 mg) 50 mg/kg/d[3]
4	Isoniazid Rifampin Ethambutol	Once daily on 7 doses/wk for 56 doses (8 weeks), or Once daily on 5 doses/wk for 40 doses (8 weeks)		
Continuation Phase[†]				
1a	Isoniazid Rifampin	Once daily on 7 doses/wk for 126 doses (18 weeks), or Once daily on 5 doses/wk for 90 doses (18 weeks)	182–130 doses (max. 26 weeks)	
1b[‡]	Isoniazid Rifampin	Twice weekly for 36 doses (18 weeks)	92–76 doses (max. 26 weeks)	
1c[§]	Isoniazid Rifapentine	Once weekly for 18 doses (18 weeks)	74–58 doses (max. 26 weeks)	
2a[‡]	Isoniazid Rifampin	Twice weekly for 36 doses (18 weeks)	62–58 doses (max. 26 weeks)	
2b[§]	Isoniazid Rifapentine (Priftin)	Once weekly for 18 doses (18 weeks)	44–40 doses (max. 26 weeks)	
3a	Isoniazid Rifampin	Three times weekly for 54 doses (18 weeks)	78 doses (max. 26 weeks)	
4a	Isoniazid Rifampin	Once daily on 7 doses/wk for 217 doses (31 weeks), or Once daily on 5 doses/wk for 155 doses (31 weeks)	273–195 doses (max. 39 weeks)	
4b	Isoniazid Rifampin	Twice weekly for 62 doses (31 weeks)	118–102 doses (max. 39 weeks)	

[3]Exceeds dosage recommended by the manufacturer.
*When directly observed therapy (DOT) is used, drugs may be given on 5 doses/wk, with the necessary number of doses adjusted accordingly; therapy administered on 5 doses/wk should always be given by DOT.
[†]Patients with cavitation on initial chest radiography and positive cultures at 2 months should receive a 7-month (31-week) regimen of either 217 (daily) or 62 (twice weekly) doses in the continuation phase.
[‡]Not recommended for HIV-infected patients with CD4+ T-cell count <100 cells/mm[3].
[§]Use only in HIV-negative patients who have negative smears at 2 months and no cavitation on chest radiography.
Adapted from the American Thoracic Society. Treatment of tuberculosis. *Am J Respir Crit Care Med.* 2003;167:603–662.

In addition, selective pressure can induce the emergence of drug-resistant mutants.

Extrapulmonary and Sputum-Negative Tuberculosis

TB can involve any organ or tissue in the body. Therefore, histologic examination or smear microscopy with AFB staining of specimens from appropriate sites is necessary to confirm extrapulmonary TB. The specimens may include cerebrospinal, pleural, pericardial, or ascitic fluids and lymph node tissue, bone, bone marrow, or brain biopsy specimens. The yield of bacilli in staining or culture from body fluids is usually very low (<50% for pericardial fluid). A diagnosis of extrapulmonary TB can also be made based on clinical and radiologic improvement on empiric therapy if it is not possible to obtain a specimen.

The same four drugs and dosing regimens used to treat pulmonary TB are also used for extrapulmonary disease. Use of adjunct corticosteroids in patients with pericardial or meningeal TB was associated with lower mortality in some prospective and retrospective studies. Bone and joint TB is treated for 6 to 9 months, and central nervous system TB (including meningitis) for 9 to

12 months. Duration of treatment for TB in all other sites is 6 months if pyrazinamide is given during the first 2 months; otherwise, the continuation phase is prolonged to 7 months. The ATS/CDC/IDSA guidelines also recommend intermittent therapy. Once-weekly administration of isoniazid and rifapentine should be avoided in the continuation phase, because data to support the efficacy of this regimen in patients with extrapulmonary TB is lacking. However, recent data report poor long-term outcomes despite adequate therapy in patients successfully treated for pericardial and meningeal TB. These and other studies question the wisdom of using the same drug exposures to target organisms in different physiologic spaces, given that drug penetration, and therefore drug concentrations, in these spaces differs.

A diagnosis of sputum-negative TB is made in patients for whom the clinical and radiologic findings strongly suggest TB but the culture and AFB smears are negative. In addition, there is clinical and/or radiologic improvements at the end of 2 months of therapy. A 2-month continuation phase of isoniazid and rifampin is used for these patients, rather than the 4 months used for sputum-positive patients.

Mycobacterium avium Complex Infection

In patients with advanced AIDS and other causes of severe cell-mediated immune deficiency, MAC causes disseminated infections. In others with ill-defined immunologic disorders, and in those who are immunocompetent, MAC causes chronic pulmonary disease. Therapy for these patients is long and complicated, with many adverse effects. The same regimens are used for all patients regardless of their HIV/AIDS status. Drug resistance is frequent.

Culture from blood or other sites (e.g., lymph node, bone marrow) is required to demonstrate invasive or disseminated disease. Bacteriologic diagnosis should be based on positive cultures or smears (or both) from sputum or bronchial wash specimens. If sputum specimens are used to diagnose pulmonary disease, at least three positive sputum smears are needed for diagnosis. Clinical and radiologic findings must also be consistent with MAC.

Combination therapy is used to prevent selection of drug-resistant mutants and to capitalize on the additive and synergistic effects of antimycobacterial drugs. Clarithromycin (Biaxin) or azithromycin (Zithromax) together with ethambutol is now the cornerstone of MAC therapy. Three- or four-drug combinations that included ethambutol, a rifamycin (rifampin[1] or rifabutin), clofazimine (Lamprene), isoniazid, or ciprofloxacin (Cipro) were shown to clear bacteremia better in some AIDS patients, especially those with a bacillary burden of greater than $2 \log_{10}$ colony-forming units per milliliter. However, adherence to therapy was poor because of toxicity. Two-way interactions between anti-retroviral medications (e.g., protease inhibitors, non-nucleoside reverse transcriptase inhibitors) and the rifamycins as well as clarithromycin and rifabutin can make patient management complicated. AIDS patients with CD4-positive T-cell counts lower than 50 cells/mm^3 should be offered prophylactic therapy to protect against disseminated MAC. Azithromycin has greater efficacy, has fewer drug interactions, and can be given once weekly. Resistance has been observed in 16% of patients treated with azithromycin and in 29% to 58% of those treated with clarithromycin. Resistance of MAC to rifamycin is rare.

Mycobacterium leprae

Leprosy is a legendary disease that has been stigmatized throughout many societies and eras of human history. The causative organism is M. leprae. The global incidence of this disease has been on the decline. Fewer than 200 cases are diagnosed each year in the United States, almost exclusively in immigrants. Most practitioners in the United States will not encounter patients with this disease.

The important clinical features of leprosy are skin lesions, nerve involvement, disfigurement of the face, and reversal reactions. Skin lesions are hypopigmented anesthetic macules and papules. Peripheral nerve enlargement can also occur, as can disfigurement of parts of the face (e.g., leonine faces). Leprosy has a spectrum of manifestations. Some patients have multibacillary leprosy associated with poor cell-mediated immunity. Others have paucibacillary leprosy resulting in a few skin patches with a robust cell-mediated immunity. Skin reactions encountered in paucibacillary leprosy due to delayed hypersensitivity to M. leprae antigens are called reversal reactions. These may also occur when massive numbers of bacilli are killed by chemotherapy.

Diagnosis is established on the basis of a compatible clinical picture and demonstration of M. leprae in smears or on histologic analysis of skin and nerve biopsy specimens. The lepromin skin test is nonreactive in multibacillary disease but reactive in paucibacillary disease. Unlike other mycobacteria, M. leprae has stringent growth requirements; it can only grow when injected into foot pads of some animals and does not grow on artificial laboratory media.

The aim of leprosy treatment is total cure. As with other slow-growing mycobacteria, multidrug therapy is administered. Therapy consists of rifampin, clofazimine (Lamprene), and dapsone. Recently, fluoroquinolones have been investigated for a role in the treatment of leprosy. In the United States, the therapy for paucibacillary leprosy is oral rifampin 600 mg/day and dapsone 100 mg/day for 6 months, followed by dapsone monotherapy for at least 3 years. The treatment of multibacillary leprosy is similar to that of paucibacillary leprosy, with dual therapy being continued for 3 years. Clofazimine is added for reverse reactions and if there is dapsone resistance. After 3 years of dual or even triple therapy, dapsone monotherapy is continued for 10 years. These regimens differ from those recommended by the World Health Organization, which are utilized elsewhere.

Mycobacteria Other Than Tuberculosis

Mycobacteria other than tuberculosis (MOTT) are mycobacterial species that may cause human disease but do not cause TB (see Table 1). The incidence of infection is reported to be about 2 in 100,000, but this may be an underestimate. The common mycobacteria identified in the United States are M. avium, Mycobacterium gordonae, Mycobacterium fortuitum, Mycobacterium kansasii, and Mycobacterium chelonae. MOTT infections are not contagious, but some produce signs and symptoms similar to those of TB, whereas others cause suppurative-like disease. MOTT primarily affect the lungs, and disease progression is slow. MOTT cause reportable disease.

Diagnosis is based on clinical presentation, radiologic findings, examination of histologic specimens, culture, and smear staining for microscopy of sputa or bronchial washings. The diagnostic criteria for MOTT in AIDS and non-AIDS patients are

- Chest radiographs showing infiltrates or nodular or cavitary disease or computed tomographic scans consistent with bronchiectasis or small nodules
- Three positive cultures with negative AFB smears or two positive cultures and one positive AFB smear from three sputum or bronchial washing specimens obtained within the previous 12 months
- Positive culture from bronchial wash with AFB smear or growth on solid media greater than 2+
- Transbronchial or lung biopsy consistent with mycobacterium histologic features and sputum or bronchial washings that are nondiagnostic of another disease.
- For mycobacteria other than tuberculosis such as M. abscessus/chelonae therapy is more with standard antibiotics like ceftriaxone. However, all these patients should be reported to specialist centers.

References

Agins BD, Berman DS, Spicehandler D, et al: Effect of combined therapy with ansamycin, clofazimine, ethambutol, and isoniazid for Mycobacterium avium infection in patients with AIDS, J Infect Dis 159:784–787, 1989.

American Thoracic Society: Centers for Disease Control and Prevention, Council of the Infectious Diseases Society of America. Diagnostic standards and classification of tuberculosis in adults and children, Am J Respir Crit Care Med 161:1376–1395, 2000.

---

[1]Not FDA approved for this indication.

Bach MC: Treating disseminated *Mycobacterium avium-intracellulare* infection, *Ann Intern Med* 110:169–170, 1989.

Bellamy R, Beyers N, McAdam KP, et al: Genetic susceptibility to tuberculosis in Africans: A genome-wide scan, *Proc Natl Acad Sci U S A* 97:8005–8009, 2000.

Blumberg HM, Burman WJ, Chaisson RE, et al: American Thoracic Society/Centers for Disease Control and Prevention/ Infectious Diseases Society of America: Treatment of tuberculosis, *Am J Respir Crit Care Med* 167:603–662, 2003.

Brosch R, Gordon SV, Marmiesse M, et al: A new evolutionary scenario for the *Mycobacterium tuberculosis* complex, *Proc Natl Acad Sci U S A* 99:3684–3689, 2002.

Cegielski JP, Devlin BH, Morris AJ, et al: Comparison of PCR, culture, and histopathology for diagnosis of tuberculous pericarditis, *J Clin Microbiol* 35:3254–3257, 1997.

Centers for Disease Control and Prevention: *Reported Tuberculosis in the United States, 2007*, Atlanta, 2007, U.S. Department of Health and Human Services, CDC.

Comstock GW: Frost revisited: The modern epidemiology of tuberculosis, *Am J Epidemiol* 101:363–382, 1975.

Comstock GW: Tuberculosis in twins: A re-analysis of the Prophit survey, *Am Rev Respir Dis* 117:621–624, 1978.

Comstock GW, Livesay VT, Woolpert SF: Evaluation of BCG vaccination among Puerto Rican children, *Am J Public Health* 64:283–291, 1974.

Dannenberg Jr AM: Delayed-type hypersensitivity and cell-mediated immunity in the pathogenesis of tuberculosis, *Immunol Today* 12:228–233, 1991.

Engel ME, Matchaba PT, Volmink J: Corticosteroids for tuberculous pleurisy, *Cochrane Database Syst Rev* (4), CD001876.

Guerra RL, Hooper NM, Baker JF, et al: Use of the amplified *Mycobacterium tuberculosis* direct test in a public health laboratory: Test performance and impact on clinical care, *Chest* 132:946–951, 2007.

Guerra RL, Hooper NM, Baker JF, et al: Cost-effectiveness of different strategies for amplified *Mycobacterium tuberculosis* direct testing for cases of pulmonary tuberculosis, *J Clin Microbiol* 46:3811–3812, 2008.

Gumbo T, Louie A, Deziel MR, et al: Concentration-dependent *Mycobacterium tuberculosis* killing and prevention of resistance by rifampin, *Antimicrob Agents Chemother* 51:3781–3788, 2007.

Gumbo T, Louie A, Liu W, et al: Isoniazid bactericidal activity and resistance emergence: Integrating pharmacodynamics and pharmacogenomics to predict efficacy in different ethnic populations, *Antimicrob Agents Chemother* 51:2329–2336, 2007.

Haas CJ, Zink A, Palfi G, et al: Detection of leprosy in ancient human skeletal remains by molecular identification of *Mycobacterium leprae*, *Am J Clin Pathol* 114:428–436, 2000.

Iseman MD: *A Clinician's Guide to Tuberculosis*, Philadelphia, 2000, Lippincott Williams & Wilkins.

Kallmann FJ, Reisner D: Twin studies on the significance of genetic factors in tuberculosis, *Am Rev Tuberculosis* 47:549–574, 1943.

Kramnik I, Demant P, Bloom BB: Susceptibility to tuberculosis as a complex genetic trait: Analysis using recombinant congenic strains of mice, *Novartis Found Symp* 217:120–131, 1998.

Kramnik I, Dietrich WF, Demant P, Bloom BR: Genetic control of resistance to experimental infection with virulent *Mycobacterium tuberculosis*, *Proc Natl Acad Sci U S A* 97:8560–8565, 2000.

Mabaera B, Lauritsen JM, Katamba A, et al: Sputum smear-positive tuberculosis: Empiric evidence challenges the need for confirmatory smears, *Int J Tuberc Lung Dis* 11:959–964, 2007.

Mabaera B, Lauritsen JM, Katamba A, et al: Making pragmatic sense of data in the tuberculosis laboratory register, *Int J Tuberc Lung Dis* 12:294–300, 2008.

Mayosi BM, Wiysonge CS, Ntsekhe M, et al: Clinical characteristics and initial management of patients with tuberculous pericarditis in the HIV era: The Investigation of the Management of Pericarditis in Africa (IMPI Africa) registry, *BMC Infect Dis* 6(2), 2006.

Mayosi BM, Wiysonge CS, Ntsekhe M, et al: Mortality in patients treated for tuberculous pericarditis in sub-Saharan Africa, *S Afr Med J* 98:36–40, 2008.

Moonan PK, Weis SE: Assessing the impact of targeted tuberculosis interventions, *Am J Respir Crit Care Med* 177:557–558, 2008.

Moore DF, Guzman JA, Mikhail LT: Reduction in turnaround time for laboratory diagnosis of pulmonary tuberculosis by routine use of a nucleic acid amplification test, *Diagn Microbiol Infect Dis* 52:247–254, 2005.

Nerlich AG, Haas CJ, Zink A, et al: Molecular evidence for tuberculosis in an ancient Egyptian mummy, *Lancet* 350:1404, 1997.

Nuermberger E, Grosset J: Pharmacokinetic and pharmacodynamic issues in the treatment of mycobacterial infections, *Eur J Clin Microbiol Infect Dis* 23:243–255, 2004.

Prasad K, Singh MB: Corticosteroids for managing tuberculous meningitis, *Cochrane Database Syst Rev* (1): CD002244.

Stein CM, Nshuti L, Chiunda AB, et al: Evidence for a major gene influence on tumor necrosis factor-alpha expression in tuberculosis: Path and segregation analysis, *Hum Hered* 60:109–118, 2005.

Stein CM, Zalwango S, Malone LL, et al: Genome scan of M. *tuberculosis* infection and disease in Ugandans, *PLoS ONE* 3:e4094, 2008.

Volmink J, Garner P: Directly observed therapy for treating tuberculosis, *Cochrane Database Syst Rev* (4): CD003343.

Weis SE, Miller TL, Hilsenrath PE, Moonan PK: Comprehensive cost description of tuberculosis care, *Int J Tuberc Lung Dis* 9:467–468, 2005.

World Health Organisation: Global leprosy situation, *Wkly Epidemiol Rec* 80:289–295, 2005.

World Health Organization: *Global Tuberculosis Control: Epidemiology, Strategy, Financing: WHO Report 2009*, Geneva, 2009, WHO.

Zink A, Haas CJ, Reischl U, et al: Molecular analysis of skeletal tuberculosis in an ancient Egyptian population, *J Med Microbiol* 50:355–366, 2001.

VENOUS THROMBOEMBOLISM

Method of
Moniba Nazeef, MD, and John P. Sheehan, MD

CURRENT DIAGNOSIS

- A good history is the most important diagnostic tool to assess risk factors including recent surgery, bedridden state, trauma, orthopedic procedure, or active cancer. Risk tools such as Wells model may be useful.
- Moderately high–sensitivity D-Dimer assays (>85% sensitivity) can be used to exclude venous thromboembolism (VTE) if there is low clinical probability but should be combined with imaging in all other cases.
- Venous compression ultrasonography (CUS) is a noninvasive, affordable, and widely available test for the diagnosis of deep vein thrombosis (DVT).

CURRENT THERAPY

- The choice of initial therapy is frequently guided by the clinical scenario. Initial therapy includes unfractionated heparin (UFH), low-molecular-weight heparin (LWMH), fondaparinux (Arixtra), or the direct oral anticoagulants (DOACs) rivaroxaban (Xarelto) or apixaban (Eliquis)
- The traditional heparin-warfarin regimen has been increasingly supplanted by the use of direct oral anticoagulants (DOAC).
- Standard treatment for a new episode of DVT or Pulmonary Embolism (PE) has traditionally been 3 to 6 months of therapeutic anticoagulation. The recommended duration of anticoagulation for VTE requires individualized analysis of the clinical presentation and patient specific factors that weigh both recurrence and bleeding risk.

Venous thromboembolism (VTE) is a significant health problem, with surveillance data suggesting that 60,000 to 100,000 people die of VTE each year in the United States. Approximately 50% to 60% of this disease burden is associated with a recent hospitalization, underscoring the importance of VTE prophylaxis. VTE is comprised of superficial vein thrombosis (SVT), deep venous thrombosis (DVT), and pulmonary embolism (PE). DVT typically starts in the deep veins of the lower extremities and progresses proximally. If untreated, a clot can break off and travel to the lungs where it is trapped in the pulmonary circulation, resulting in PE. DVT confined to the deep veins of the calf is termed *isolated distal DVT*, whereas involvement of the popliteal or more proximal veins is termed *proximal DVT*. SVT represents thrombosis in the superficial veins of the legs or arms and rarely progresses to DVT. The focus of this chapter is to understand the risk factors, diagnosis, treatment, and prevention of DVT and PE.

Pathophysiology/Risk Factors

Venous blood flow is maintained by a delicate homeostatic balance of prothrombotic and antithrombotic factors. Virchow's triad describes the major factors leading to VTE from a pathophysiologic standpoint: (1) intrinsic hypercoagulability, (2) endothelial damage, and (3) venous stasis. Most often, a combination of these factors leads to the development of VTE. Based on the presence or absence of typical clinical risk factors, VTE occurrences can be considered either provoked (e.g., post-surgical) or unprovoked (spontaneous). Furthermore, provoking risk factors may be transient/reversible (e.g., estrogen use) versus nontransient/irreversible (e.g., lower extremity paresis), which has implications for decisions regarding duration of anticoagulant therapy Table 1.

TABLE 1 Risk Factors for Venous Thromboembolism

Transient/Reversible

Surgery (esp. lower limb orthopedic surgery)
General anesthesia >30 min
Immobility due to surgical or medical condition
Oral contraceptives/hormone replacement therapy
Pregnancy, puerperium
Major trauma
Acute inflammation
Indwelling venous catheters
Heparin induced thrombocytopenia
Travel-associated thrombosis
Medications- including tamoxifen, L-asparaginase,
    immunomodulatory agents (lenalidomide), EPO

Permanent/Non-Reversible

Active cancer
Antiphospholipid Syndrome
Myeloproliferative neoplasms
Paroxysmal nocturnal hemoglobinura (PNH)
Lower extremity paresis from neurologic disease
Sickle Cell Disease
Nephrotic Syndrome
Active autoimmune conditions (SLE, IBD, ITP,TTP)
Chronic infection/inflammation
Morbid obesity (BMI > 40)

EPO, Erythropoietin; SLE, systemic lupus erythematosus; IBD, inflammatory bowel disease; ITP, immune thrombocytopenic purpura; TTP, thrombotic thrombocytopenic purpura.

Acquired Risk Factors

Certain clinical conditions shift the balance between procoagulant and anticoagulant factors to promote thrombosis. These conditions include surgery, pregnancy and puerperium, inflammation, active cancer, major trauma, specific medications, and a variety of conditions that lead to immobility. A more comprehensive list is provided in Table 1. Many of these clinical conditions cause multiple changes relevant to VTE risk. For example, surgical interventions may induce endothelial damage, immobilization leading to venous stasis, platelet activation, and trigger inflammatory responses that increase fibrinogen, factor VIII, and von Willebrand factor levels. Orthopedic procedures involving the lower limbs and abdominopelvic surgeries in cancer patients are especially high risk from a VTE standpoint. Active cancer is associated with 20% of all VTE and involves a variety of mechanisms leading to hypercoagulability, including increased tissue factor expression, venous obstruction, indwelling catheters, reduced mobility, and chemotherapy.

Pregnancy and the puerperium, oral contraceptives (OC), and hormone replacement therapy (HRT) are important VTE risk factors in women. OC and HRT are associated with a number of changes in hemostatic protein levels and platelet function that appear globally prothrombotic. Higher estrogen content is associated with increased thrombotic risk and is modulated by a combination with specific progestins. Additionally, there is a higher risk of VTE in OCP users with a positive family history, suggesting an underlying genetic predisposition.

A variety of conditions that involve prolonged immobilization enhance VTE risk. Cast immobilization of the lower extremity, paresis after neurologic events, multiple trauma, orthopedic surgeries, travel-associated immobility (>4–6 hours) or a bedridden state due to a variety of medical or surgical conditions result in stasis that promotes venous thrombosis. Many of these clinical situations are also associated with an inflammatory state that concomitantly increases intrinsic hypercoagulability of the blood. Venous wall injury may occur via a variety of mechanisms, including surgical interventions, indwelling intravenous catheters, trauma, and vasculitis.

Genetics of Venous Thromboembolism

Although acquired clinical risk factors are critical to assessing risk, the genetic contribution to VTE is also substantial, with heritability of VTE estimated at 40% to 47%. Like many complex phenotypes, VTE has a multigenic basis in which most individual alleles make relatively small contributions to overall risk. Factor V Leiden and the prothrombin G20210A polymorphism are examples of such alleles (2- to 4-fold relative risk). At least 17 genes have been identified that harbor VTE-associated variants. Importantly, family history remains an independent risk factor even after excluding known gene variants associated with thrombophilia, suggesting that unidentified genes also contribute to VTE risk. Deficiencies of the coagulation inhibitors antithrombin, protein C, and protein S are rare conditions with a more substantial effect on the relative risk of VTE (10- to 20-fold increase) but tend to be diagnosed erroneously in the setting of acute thrombosis. The multigenic basis of VTE has implications for thrombophilia testing that include: (1) identification of minor alleles (e.g., FV Leiden) is not helpful for prediction of VTE recurrence risk; (2) a careful family history is generally more valuable than a thrombophilia evaluation; and (3) the *absolute* risk for carriers of thrombophilic alleles is generally quite small and does not justify indefinite anticoagulation. A robust estimate of individual genetic risk requires systematic screening of all known VTE risk genes or whole genome/exome sequencing approaches that are not routinely available. Thus current thrombophilia testing rarely contributes to clinical decision making in patients with VTE. Testing should never be pursued for provoked events and is best limited to selected situations such as presentations at a young age (<30 years) or known thrombophilic traits occurring in the context of a family history of VTE. A thorough personal and family history is generally sufficient to determine the likelihood of an underlying inherited hypercoagulable state.

Epidemiology and Natural History

The exact incidence of VTE is unknown, but it is estimated that about 300,000 to 600,000 Americans are affected by VTE each year. VTE incidence appears ~30% higher in African Americans and ~70% lower in Asian and Native American populations relative to Caucasians. Importantly, the incidence of VTE increases with age, particularly after age 50. Whereas overall VTE is slightly more common in men, women have an increased incidence before age 40 based on the impact of pregnancy and contraceptives. In older age groups, the frequency of PE is increased relative to DVT. Finally, the incidence of VTE has been increasing steadily since the mid-1980s, which may, in large part, represent the increased use and enhanced sensitivity of computed tomography (CT) scans and magnetic resonance imaging (MRI).

The natural history of VTE is impacted by the underlying clinical risk factors, provoked versus unprovoked nature of the event, reversibility of risk factors, and location/nature of the thrombotic event. In general, untreated thrombi tend to extend proximally, break off, and embolize to the pulmonary circulation, where they may result in infarction and pulmonary hypertension. The risk of PE is increased for proximal versus distal involvement with DVT. More than 75% of VTE starts in the calf veins, and 20% to 30% of these cases progress to involve proximal veins in the leg or pelvis. Approximately 50% of patients with untreated symptomatic proximal DVT develop symptomatic PE, whereas the incidence of asymptomatic PE is even higher. Importantly, 10% of symptomatic PE is rapidly fatal, and 30% of patients with untreated symptomatic nonfatal PE will have a fatal recurrence. Thus recognition of PE is of the utmost clinical importance. Anticoagulant therapy inhibits thrombus growth and largely prevents interval recurrence, whereas endogenous thrombolysis may result in partial or complete resolution of the thrombus. Uncommonly, progressive thrombosis in the presence of anticoagulation may occur in high-risk situations such as metastatic malignancy or the antiphospholipid syndrome.

The risk of VTE recurrence after stopping anticoagulation varies significantly based on clinical presentation. About 20% to 40% of VTE episodes are unprovoked in nature, which is associated with a substantially higher recurrence rate. For unprovoked clots, recurrence rate is estimated to be ~10% in one year, ~30%

in 5 years, and approaches ~40% in 10 years. In contrast, the recurrence risk of VTE associated with surgery (a transient risk factor) is less than 3% per year. Recurrences tend to occur in a similar site to the initial event, which is particularly important in the case of PE, as 25% of pulmonary embolism presents as sudden death. In contrast, the risk of recurrent VTE is much smaller in isolated distal (calf) DVT compared with proximal DVT and PE.

Long-Term Complications of VTE
Postthrombotic Syndrome (PTS)
About 20% to 50% patients with DVT develop some degree of PTS within the subsequent 1–2 years. Chronic venous obstruction, inflammation, endofibrosis, and valvular dysfunction contribute to the chronic venous insufficiency of PTS. Risk factors for PTS include persistent DVT symptoms after one month, extensive or recurrent DVT, inadequate anticoagulation, and advanced age. Manifestations include chronic leg edema, pain, heaviness, erythema, and venous ulcers that may result in significant disability. PTS is largely non-reversible, emphasizing the importance of DVT prevention. Graduated compression stockings provide symptomatic relief by preventing pooling of blood in the lower extremities, but do not prevent PTS. In the 5% to 10% of patients with severe PTS, active supportive care and consultation with vascular surgery, dermatology, or vein specialists should be sought early to avoid development of debilitating venous ulcers.

Chronic Thromboembolic Pulmonary Hypertension (CTEPH)
CTEPH is a long-term complication of PE affecting 3% to 4% patients despite adequate anticoagulation. CTEPH is characterized by progressive pulmonary hypertension and right-side heart failure due to remodeling of pulmonary vasculature by thrombotic material. Patients with large central or extensive pulmonary emboli, hemodynamic compromise, and right heart dysfunction at diagnosis are at highest risk. Chronic progressive dyspnea with exertion is the most common symptom, and the clinician must have a high clinical suspicion based on patient's history of PE. An echocardiogram revealing elevated pulmonary arterial hypertension should trigger evaluation with a VQ scan. The presence of chronic mismatched segmental perfusion defects on the VQ scan is diagnostic of CTEPH. If anatomically feasible, treatment of choice is pulmonary endarterectomy, which can reverse the hemodynamic and functional abnormalities. Early recognition and referral to a specialized surgical treatment center are critical to patient outcomes. Lifelong anticoagulation is recommended for all patients with CTEPH.

Diagnosis of Deep Venous Thrombosis
The diagnosis of DVT proceeds via determination of clinical probability, D-dimer screening, and confirmatory imaging.

Clinical Features
Diagnosis begins with evaluation of the clinical scenario for VTE risk factors and suspicious physical exam findings. Suggestive features in the patient's recent history include recent surgery or bedridden state, trauma or orthopedic procedure, active cancer, and other typical risk factors (**Table 1**). Classic symptoms of DVT include limb swelling, pain, and erythema. On exam, unilateral calf swelling, pitting edema, dilated veins, and tenderness on palpation can be seen. The clinical probability becomes stronger when more of these findings are present. Risk stratification systems such as the Wells model (Table 2) use these clinical features to rapidly classify patients as high (~60% thrombosis), moderate (~25%), or low (~5%) risk for DVT. Differential diagnosis of DVT includes trauma, cellulitis, osteomyelitis, chronic venous insufficiency, arterial ischemia, ruptured Baker's cyst, hematoma, and superficial thrombophlebitis. Because neither history nor physical examination findings are specific for DVT, D-dimer screening and objective imaging must be pursued if sufficient clinical suspicion exists. A simplified algorithm for diagnosis of DVT is provided (Figure 1).

TABLE 2	Wells Model for Predicting Pretest Probability of Deep Vein Thrombosis	
CLINICAL VARIABLE		**POINTS**
Active cancer (treatment ongoing or within previous 6 months or palliative)		1
Recently bedridden >3 days or major surgery within 4 weeks		1
Pitting edema confined to the symptomatic leg		1
Dilated superficial veins (non-varicose)		1
Previous documented DVT		1
Paralysis, paresis, or recent plaster immobilization of the 1 lower extremities		1
Localized tenderness along the distribution of the deep 1 venous system		1
Calf swelling 3 cm greater than asymptomatic side measured 10 cm below tibial tuberosity		1
Pitting edema confined to the symptomatic leg		1
Alternative diagnosis at least as likely as DVT		-2

Clinical probability by interpretation of total score: >2 points, high; 1 or 2, moderate; <1, low.

D-Dimer Screening
D-dimer is a specific fibrin degradation product generated by plasmin cleavage of cross-linked fibrin clot, formed by thrombin and Factor XIII activity. D-dimer represents a useful screening tool based on excellent sensitivity and a high negative predictive value for VTE. However, D-dimer lacks specificity, as it is increased in a variety of conditions, including acute inflammation, recent surgery or trauma, pregnancy, DIC, advanced age, or cancer. The level of clinical suspicion also impacts interpretation of D-dimer results. Specific D-dimer assays vary in sensitivity and specificity, although qualitative testing has largely been replaced by enzyme-linked immunosorbent assay–based quantitative assays. More recently, highly sensitive assays (>95% sensitivity) using latex-enhanced immunoturbidimetric immunoassays provide rapid quantitation for use in the diagnosis of VTE. Point-of-care (POC) testing with specified cutoff values are also available. Thus the clinician should be familiar with the type of D-dimer testing available locally. Highly sensitive assays have a good negative predictive value to rule out VTE without further testing. Moderately high–sensitivity assays (>85% sensitivity) can be used to exclude VTE if there is low clinical probability but should be combined with imaging in all other cases. Qualitative or semiquantitative assays are generally not reliable for excluding thrombosis. Finally, if clinical suspicion for DVT or PE is high, a negative D-dimer should not be used to rule out VTE, and appropriate imaging should be pursued to confirm the diagnosis.

Imaging
Ultrasonography
Venous compression ultrasonography (CUS) is a noninvasive, affordable, and widely available test for the diagnosis of DVT. The deep veins are assessed by use of a compression probe with lack of compressibility in a venous segment indicative of thrombus. Duplex technology or color-coded Doppler scanning visualizes blood flow to allow accurate identification of deep veins. Lack of flow plus non-compressibility increases diagnostic accuracy and also facilitates diagnosis in veins that cannot be compressed (e.g., pelvic and subclavian veins). Venous ultrasonography has an excellent sensitivity and specificity (~94%) for diagnosis of proximal limb DVT. The common femoral, femoral, and trifurcation of calf veins are readily visualized. In most cases, a negative test is sufficient to rule out proximal VTE. Currently two methods for CUS are used: (1) the two point compression

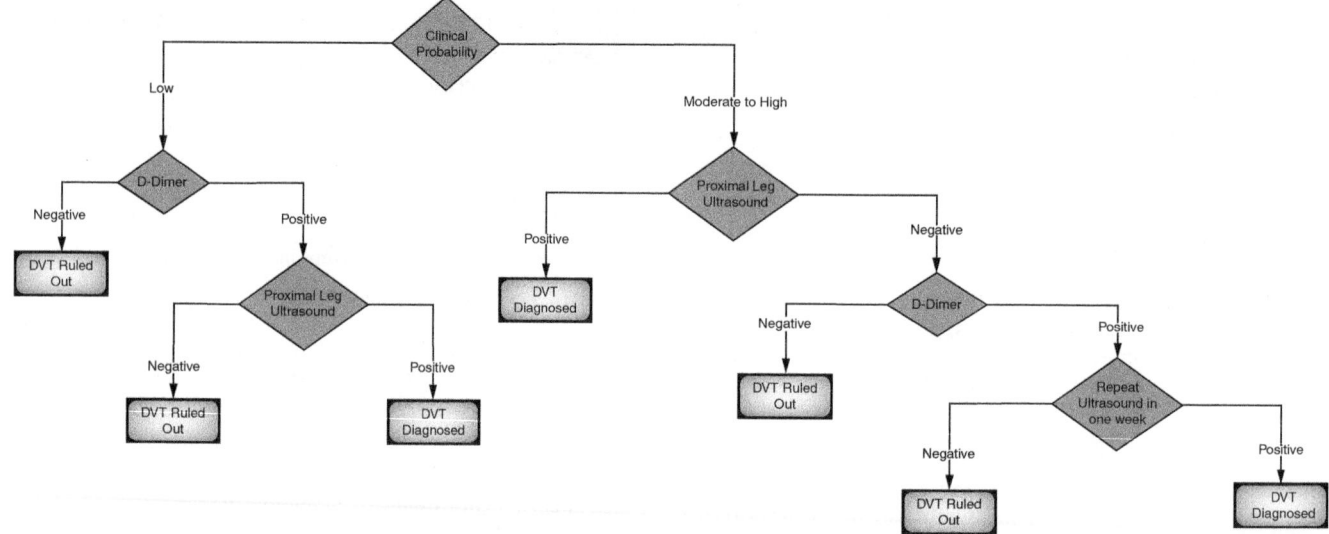

Figure 1 Suggested diagnostic algorithm for diagnosis of deep venous thrombosis (DVT).

technique, which only evaluates the proximal veins in the groin and popliteal fossa; and (2) whole-leg ultrasound scanning evaluating both proximal and distal veins. The sensitivity and specificity of CUS for calf vein DVT is significantly lower and highly operator dependent. Therefore many centers only perform the proximal vein assessment, which is reliable, reproducible, and efficient. If clinical suspicion remains high after a negative proximal vein ultrasound scan, repeat ultrasound scanning should be performed in about a week to assess for proximal extension in the deep venous system. If negative, no further testing is needed. A negative whole-leg CUS test result essentially rules out DVT and does not need follow-up testing. However, this approach is time consuming, may lead to increased diagnosis of calf vein thromboses, and potential overtreatment. The 3-month incidence of symptomatic proximal venous thrombosis in patients with a normal initial test are comparable at ~1% for both approaches. For upper extremities, compression ultrasonography is about 86% sensitive and specific.

Contrast Venography

Previously the gold standard for diagnosis of DVT, contrast venography is rarely used because it is invasive and requires contrast exposure. CT and MR venography have a sensitivity and specificity of >90% for DVT in lower extremities. However, these studies are also not widely used for diagnosis because of increased cost, radiation, and contrast exposure. CT and MR venography are useful to define anatomy in patients with multiple recurrent DVT (evaluation by CUS is problematic), an indeterminate abnormality on ultrasound scanning, or a thrombus diagnosed in the setting of very low clinical suspicion.

Diagnosis of PE

Similar to DVT, the diagnosis of PE requires determination of clinical probability, consideration of D-dimer testing, and confirmatory imaging.

Clinical Features

A patient presenting with risk factors for VTE and antecedent history of DVT should raise the suspicion for pulmonary embolism. The most common symptoms of PE are shortness of breath and chest pain. Pleuritic chest pain is typical, but PE may also present with substernal pressure or be confused with musculoskeletal pain. Other symptoms may include cough and hemoptysis. Clinical signs include tachypnea, tachycardia, and hypoxia. The findings of DVT in the lower extremities increase the probability of PE. The Well's model for PE provides a useful framework to estimate the pretest probability using these variables (Table 3).

TABLE 3	Wells Model for Predicting Pretest Probability of Pulmonary Embolism	
CLINICAL VARIABLE		**POINTS**
Clinical signs and symptoms of DVT (minimum leg swelling and pain with palpation of the deep veins		3
An alternative diagnosis is less likely than PE		3
Heart rate >100 beats/min		1.5
Immobilization or surgery in the previous 4 weeks		1.5
Previous DVT/PE		1.5
Hemoptysis		1
Active Cancer (treatment ongoing or within previous 6 months or palliative)		1

Clinical probability by interpretation of total score: >6 points, high; 4 to 6, moderate; <4, low.

Chest X-Ray, Electrocardiography, and Troponin

Chest x-ray should be performed in all suspected cases. The classical "Hampton's hump" or peripheral wedge-shaped opacity corresponding to a large pulmonary infarct is seldom appreciated and not very sensitive or specific. However, a chest x-ray is useful in assessing for other conditions such as pneumonia, pneumothorax, and pulmonary edema that can present in similar fashion. Electrocardiography (EKG) should be performed in anyone presenting with chest pain to rule out myocardial infarction. Evidence of right heart strain on EKG has predictive and prognostic value in assessment of pulmonary embolism. Similarly, a troponin level is usually obtained in evaluation for myocardial ischemia. An elevated troponin level in the absence of EKG evidence of ischemia can be suggestive of myocardial injury in the setting of massive or submassive PE.

Ventilation/Perfusion (V/Q) Scanning

V/Q scans have largely been replaced by computed tomography pulmonary angiography (CTPA). However, V/Q scans remain useful in selected patients with significant renal insufficiency (to avoid contrast dye) and young or pregnant females (to avoid radiation exposure). This technique uses inhaled and intravenous radioisotopes to evaluate ventilation and circulation in the pulmonary parenchyma and vasculature, respectively. A normal perfusion scan in the setting of a normal chest x-ray excludes PE. The addition of a ventilation scan increases specificity by accounting for other pulmonary disorders. A

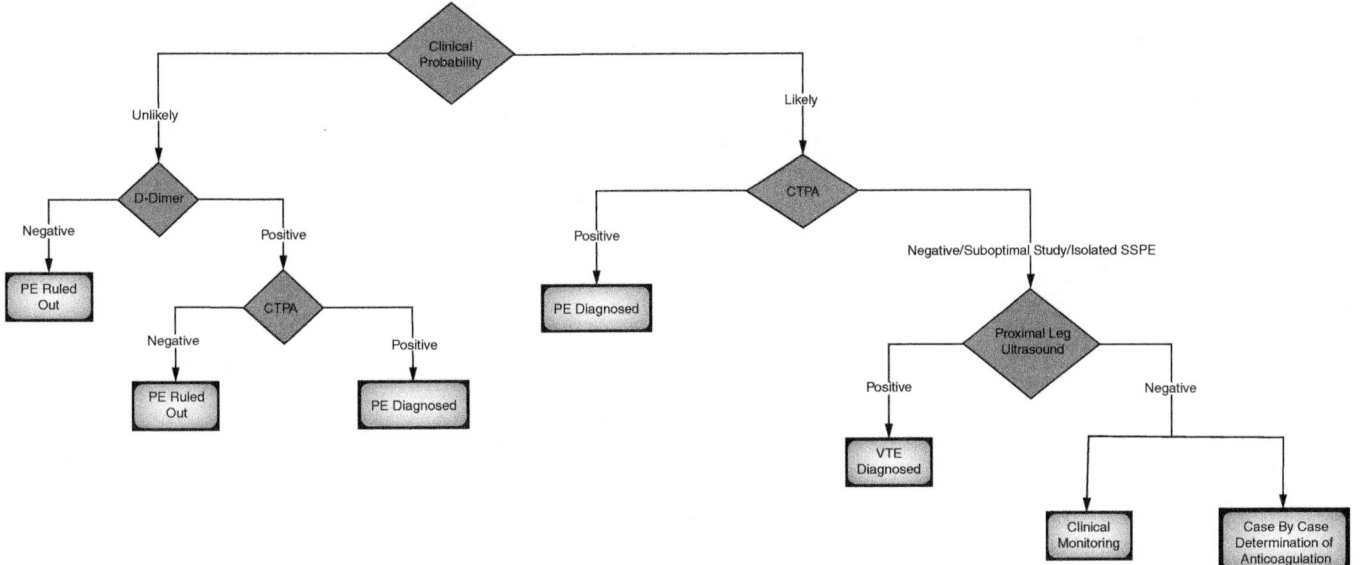

Figure 2 Suggested diagnostic algorithm for diagnosis of pulmonary embolism (PE). *CTPA*, computed tomography pulmonary angiography.

normal chest x-ray and ventilation scan in areas with multiple large perfusion defects that involve >75% of a segment (V/Q mismatch) is associated with >80% probability of PE and considered a high-probability V/Q scan. An intermediate-probability scan usually requires further diagnostic evaluation because it is considered nondiagnostic in most situations. Three-dimensional single-photon emission CT (SPECT) is now used by many centers in place of planar VQ scans. SPECT may be more accurate than planar VQ scanning, resulting in fewer nondiagnostic studies.

Computed Tomography Pulmonary Angiography
Computed tomography pulmonary angiography (CTPA) has become the modality of choice for diagnosis of PE. It is a relatively noninvasive procedure that can provide prompt diagnosis of PE. With recent advancements, the availability of thin-slice scans provides a detailed analysis of pulmonary vasculature that increases the sensitivity for detecting thrombi at the subsegmental and peripheral arterial level. In contrast to V/Q scanning, CTPA provides detailed visualization of the lung parenchyma, which can detect peripheral pulmonary infarctions and alternative diagnoses. When required, the CTPA examination can be extended to include the iliac veins, providing a detailed view with a single contrast exposure. CTPA has excellent sensitivity and specificity for diagnosis of lobar and segmental PE. Diagnostic accuracy is lower at the subsegmental level, and results should be interpreted in the context of clinical probability, proximal lower extremity ultrasound results, and D-dimer level. A simplified algorithmic approach to diagnosis of PE is provided (Figure 2). CTPA use is limited by costs, exposure to potentially nephrotoxic contrast dye, and chest radiation. It should be avoided in younger women because of the associated increased risk of breast cancer.

Pulmonary Angiography
Formerly the gold standard for the diagnosis of PE, pulmonary angiography is an invasive procedure that has been replaced by CTPA and is now very rarely performed.

Magnetic Resonance Angiography
Pulmonary contrast-enhanced magnetic resonance angiography (CE-MRA) is emerging as a useful alternative to CTPA in select patients such as younger females and those with severe iodinated contrast allergy. Currently, CE-MRA has limited availability and usefulness that is dependent on the expertise and experience of the available radiologists.

Diagnosis of Recurrent DVT
The diagnosis of recurrent DVT can be challenging, because signs and symptoms of PTS in the affected extremity can obscure the diagnosis. Clinical assessment of the probability for recurrent DVT is less well standardized than initial episodes; however, many predictive factors are expected to be shared. The clinician should assess for the presence of ongoing clinical risk factors, attempt to discern between chronic and acute signs and symptoms, and consider D-dimer testing. A negative D-dimer test can be used to exclude recurrent DVT, although the accuracy of this approach has not been well studied. If D-dimer testing is positive or has not been done, CUS is performed. The finding of non-compressibility of an ipsilateral femoral or popliteal vein segment, which was previously unaffected, can be considered diagnostic. For diagnosing recurrent DVT in a previously affected vein segment, an increase in thrombus diameter of at least 4 mm on serial CUS in combination with a D-dimer measurement can serve as helpful criteria. This diagnosis requires the expertise of an experienced radiologist with the previous ultrasound available for comparison. In practice, comparison with previous CUS is difficult, given the operator-dependent characteristics of the test. If comparison with the previous examination is equivocal or unavailable, CT or MR venography may be considered. An intraluminal filling defect suggests acute rather than remote thrombosis. Alternatively, a patient with initially equivocal CUS findings can undergo serial repeat examinations to detect DVT extension.

Treatment of Venous Thromboembolism
Anticoagulation Therapy for VTE
Patients with newly diagnosed VTE should be promptly initiated on therapeutic anticoagulation. In the absence of a severely symptomatic lower extremity, high thrombus burden pulmonary embolism with right ventricular dysfunction or significant cardiovascular comorbidity, management is predominantly outpatient. In the presence of PE, a simplified pulmonary embolism severity index (sPESI) is often used to assess appropriateness for outpatient therapy. The sPESI score includes the following factors (1 point each): age >80, history of cancer, chronic cardiopulmonary disease, pulse >110 beats/min, systolic blood pressure <100 mm Hg, arterial oxygen saturation <90%. Patients with a sPESI score ≥1 are considered "high risk" and should be considered for initial inpatient management.

Choice of Initial Anticoagulant Therapy
The choice of initial therapy is frequently guided by the clinical scenario. Initial therapy includes unfractionated heparin (UFH),

TABLE 4   Drugs for the Treatment of VTE

DRUG	DOSING	ELIMINATION	HALF-LIFE	MONITORING
UFH	80 units/kg IV bolus, then 18 units/kg/hour initial infusion rate	Complex, hepatic/renal metabolism	1–2 hours	APTT Anti-FXa activity
LMWH	Dalteparin (Fragmin): 200 U/kg SQ QD Enoxaparin (Lovenox): 1 mg/kg SQ QD[3]	Predominantly renal	3–5 hours	None required*
Fondaparinux (Arixtra)	5.0 mg SQ (<50 kg) 7.5 mg SQ (50–100 kg) 10 mg SQ (>100 kg)	Renal	17–21 hours	None required*
Warfarin (VKA) (Coumadin)	Initially 5 mg po QD, broad range (2.5–10 mg)	Extensive hepatic metabolism, Renal excretion for metabolites	Pharmacokinetics: 20–60 hrs, variable †Pharmacodynamics: 42–72 hours	PT/INR (2.0–3.0)
Dabigatran (Pradaxa)	Parenteral anticoagulant × 5-10 days, then dabigatran 150 mg po BID	>80% renal, 20% biliary Pro-drug	12–17 hours 14–17 hours (elderly)	None required
Rivaroxaban (Xarelto)	15 mg po BID × 21 days; then 20 mg po QD	66% renal, 33% biliary CYP450 substrate	5–9 hours 9–12 hours (elderly)	None required
Apixaban (Eliquis)	10 mg po BID × 7days, then 5 mg po BID	25% renal, 75% biliary CYP450 substrate	8–15 hours	None required
Edoxaban (Savaysa)	Parenteral anticoagulant × 5–10 days, then edoxaban 60 mg po QD (30 mg < 60 kg)	35% renal, 60% biliary	10–14 hours	None required
Betrixaban (Bevyxxa)‡	160 mg first dose, then 80 mg po QD for 35–42 days‡	11% renal 85% biliary	19–27 hours	None required

UFH, Unfractionated heparin; LMWH, low-molecular-weight heparin.
*Anti-FXa activity can be used in selected circumstances such as pregnancy and extremes of body weight (BW) (BW <45 kg or >100 kg).
†Pharmacodynamics of coagulation protein recovery most relevant to in vivo effect of VKA.
‡Betrixaban FDA approved for VTE prophylaxis only.
3Exceeds dosage recommended by the manufacturer.

low-molecular-weight heparin (LWMH), fondaparinux (Arixtra), or the direct oral anticoagulants rivaroxaban (Xarelto) or apixaban (Eliquis) (Table 4). Therapeutic UFH is administered intravenously (IV) and demonstrates complex pharmacokinetics (both hepatic and renal clearance) that requires laboratory monitoring of drug effect (aPTT or anti–factor Xa activity). Thus UFH therapy requires hospital admission and has largely been replaced by other options. UFH may still be appropriate for patients experiencing inpatient VTE events, especially if a need for invasive procedures is anticipated (half-life, 1–2 hours). The therapeutic target range for UFH is a 1.5- to 2.5-fold increase over the baseline aPTT or 0.3–0.7 U/mL anti–factor Xa activity. In contrast, LMWH is administered subcutaneously and primarily cleared by the kidneys, resulting in predictable pharmacokinetics. Subcutaneous administration facilitates outpatient treatment and predictable pharmacokinetics allow weight-based dosing without laboratory monitoring. Fondaparinux (synthetic pentasaccharide) is exclusively cleared by the kidneys with a long half-life (17–21 hours) that allows for once-daily, weight-adjusted subcutaneous dosing. Fondaparinux similarly does not require routine laboratory monitoring, but caution is warranted in patients with mild renal insufficiency where drug accumulation may increase bleeding risk. Heparin therapy (UFH, LWMH, or fondaparinux) for VTE is administered for a *minimum* of 5 days followed by transition to longer-term oral anticoagulation with an oral vitamin K antagonist (VKA) or a direct oral anticoagulant (DOAC). Alternatively, rivaroxaban or apixaban can be initiated immediately after VTE diagnosis and bypass the need for heparin therapy (see below).

Historically, vitamin K antagonists (VKA) are the primary oral anticoagulants for the long-term treatment of VTE. Warfarin (Coumadin) is the VKA used almost exclusively in the United States. Warfarin and other VKA inhibit vitamin K-dependent γ-carboxylation of the coagulation zymogens (proenzymes). This post-translational modification is required for both efficient protein secretion and function (membrane binding) of coagulation factors VII, IX, X, and II. Vitamin K is oxidized during γ-carboxylation of these coagulation factors, and warfarin inhibits enzymatic regeneration of the reduced form of vitamin K, creating a functional deficiency. This mechanism of action is the basis for (1) the reversibility of the warfarin by administration of the reduced form of vitamin K, (2) the reduction in warfarin effect by dietary vitamin K, and (3) the enhancement of the warfarin effect by many antibiotics, as bacterial flora are a major source of vitamin K. Warfarin also undergoes extensive metabolism by the liver, which provides multiple opportunities for drug interactions. Thus genetic variation in liver metabolism, variable dietary vitamin K intake, and numerous potential drug interactions generate substantial individual variation in warfarin dose requirements.

Warfarin (2.5- to 10-mg initial dose) is usually started the same day as heparin, overlapped with parenteral heparin therapy for a *minimum* of 5 days and discontinued once a therapeutic warfarin level is obtained on two consecutive days. The warfarin effect is monitored by the international normalized ratio (INR), which represents a prothrombin time (PT) that has been corrected for specific reagent sensitivity. The target INR for VTE treatment is 2.0 to 3.0. The pharmacodynamic effects of warfarin on the INR are primarily determined by the in vivo half-lives of the relevant coagulation factors. Thus the full effect of a warfarin dose change on the INR is usually not seen for 48 to 72 hours, correlating with the half-life of factors IX, X, and prothrombin (factor II). This delayed effect necessitates overlap with heparin therapy for at least 5 days, or longer if further warfarin dose titration is required to reach a therapeutic INR. Initial warfarin dosing should be conservative (2.5 mg daily) if enhanced sensitivity is expected, including patients that are elderly (>65 years old), low body weight (<45 kg), hypoalbuminemic (<2 g/dL), on antibiotic therapy or have poor oral intake.

TABLE 5	Reversal Agents		
DRUG	**REVERSAL AGENT**	**DOSING**	**COMMENTS**
Heparin	Protamine*	1–1.5 mg/100 U UFH IV	Hypersensitivity reactions, less effective vs. LMWH
Warfarin	4 factor PCC (Kcentra)	25–50 U/kg IV	Dose depends on INR, PCC favored over FFP
	FFP	2–4 liters	Volume overload, Transf rxn
	Vitamin K	1–10 mg oral or IV	Reversal takes 6–24 hours
Dabigatran	Idarucizumab (Praxbind)	2.5 g IV for 2 doses (within 15 min)	Drug specific monoclonal Fab fragment
Rivaroxaban Apixaban Edoxaban[1] Betrixaban[1]	Andexanet alfa (Andexxa)[1] 4 factor PCC[†]	800 mg IV bolus @ 30 mg/min, then 960 mg infusion @ 8 mg/min 50 U/kg IV	Reverses factor Xa active site inhibitors

*FDA approved for treatment of heparin overdose. Off-label uses: heparin neutralization (adults); intracranial hemorrhage associated with heparin or LMWH; LMWH overdose (adults).
[†]Evidence for reversal of factor Xa inhibitors by PCC is low quality.
[1]Not FDA approved for this indication.

The traditional heparin-warfarin regimen has been increasingly supplanted by the use of direct oral anticoagulants (DOAC). DOACs are orally available, low-molecular-weight compounds that directly inhibit the active site of either factor Xa (rivaroxaban [Xarelto], apixaban [Eliquis], edoxaban [Savaysa]), or thrombin (dabigatran [Pradaxa]). In general, these drugs possess predictable pharmacokinetics and relatively short half-lives, allowing fixed once- or twice-daily oral dosing without routine monitoring. Both rivaroxaban and apixaban are approved for initial use after the VTE diagnosis with a more intensive dose regimen that tapers to the standard maintenance dose after 21 days for rivaroxaban or 7 days for apixaban (Table 4). Edoxaban and dabigatran are approved for continued treatment of VTE at their standard maintenance dose after 5 to 10 days of a parenteral anticoagulant (usually LWMH). Differences in clearance mechanisms have implications for clinical usage. For instance, dabigatran is heavily dependent on renal clearance and can accumulate with increased bleeding risk in patients with significant renal insufficiency (CrCl <30 mL/min). In contrast, apixaban dosing is less affected by renal insufficiency but should not be used in patients with significant liver dysfunction or biliary stasis.

Comparison of Warfarin Versus DOACs
DOACs demonstrate equivalent efficacy to the traditional combination of LMWH and warfarin in the treatment of VTE. Advantages of the DOACs include rapid onset of action, predictable dose response, no monitoring requirement, elimination of parenteral therapy (rivaroxaban and apixaban), no significant diet interactions, limited drug interactions, and an overall safety signal equivalent to or better than warfarin. Meta-analysis of DOAC trials demonstrate that fatal bleeding, intracranial hemorrhage (ICH), and clinically relevant, non-major bleeding are reduced with DOACs compared to warfarin. The rate of GI bleeding was similar. Given the potentially life-changing nature of ICH, the lower rate with DOACs is particularly significant. Disadvantages of DOACs include cost, inability to monitor compliance with routine coagulation testing, the impact of renal function on drug clearance, and lack of widely available reversal agents. The relatively short half-lives of DOACs and recent development of reversal agents (Table 5) partially overcomes the reversibility advantage for warfarin. Largely based on safety profile and ease of use, recent guidelines provide a weak recommendation for DOACs over warfarin in patients without cancer.

Cancer-Associated Thrombosis
VTE associated with cancer accounts for ~20% of all cases and clearly is a heterogeneous patient population. Treatment of cancer-associated thrombosis is problematic in that patients are at increased risk for both VTE recurrence and bleeding complications. In addition to the multiple drug interactions that complicate VKA use in cancer patients, LMWH demonstrates significantly lower rates of recurrent VTE relative to VKA therapy. Thus LMWH for the first 6 months after the event has been the standard recommendation. The role of DOACs in cancer-associated thrombosis continues to evolve. Meta-analysis of subgroups from the large DOAC VTE trials demonstrates no difference in VTE recurrence or major bleeding compared with LMWH for primarily low-risk cancer patients. Subsequent comparison of edoxaban and dalteparin (Hokusai Trial) in a broader population of active cancer patients demonstrated a lower rate of VTE recurrence but higher rate of major bleeding. A randomized study comparing rivaroxaban to dalteparin (SELECT-D) demonstrated similar findings with reduced VTE rate and increased non-major bleeding in the DOAC arm. The increased bleeding was primarily observed in patients with upper GI or urothelial cancers in both studies. Ongoing studies will further address the role of DOACs in this setting. Duration of therapy is generally at least 6 months, but may be modified based on disease response, bleeding risk, and prognosis.

Special Considerations in the Acute Management of Venous Thromboembolism (VTE)
Although the vast majority of patients diagnosed with venous thromboembolism (VTE) should be promptly initiated on therapeutic anticoagulation, a limited number of acute presentations may require a modified approach. These presentations include the following:

Massive Pulmonary Embolism (PE)
With Hemodynamic Instability
Patients presenting with hemodynamically unstable PE (SBP < 90 mmHg for 15 minutes, requiring vasopressors or overt shock) are at high risk for right heart failure and death. The focus for these patients should be resuscitation (IV fluids, pressors, oxygenation, and airway control) and rapid confirmation of diagnosis (perfusion scan or CT pulmonary angiography). If highly unstable, then bedside ECHO may be used for a presumptive diagnosis based on right ventricular findings. Prompt thrombolytic therapy (tPA [Activase]100 mg IV) or consideration of emergency endovascular therapy should be pursued, with the former being more readily available.

Patients who present with worsening right heart failure, pre-resuscitation cardiopulmonary arrest, free-floating thrombus, or high thrombus burden in the absence of systemic hypotension may also be considered for thrombolytic therapy. Many institutions have a pulmonary embolism response team (PERT) to facilitate decision making and institution of therapy. However, for the majority of patients presenting with evidence of right ventricular dysfunction (by ECHO or CT) without systemic hypotension (i.e., "sub-massive" or intermediate risk PE), the use of thrombolytic therapy remains controversial. This controversy stems from both heterogeneity in patient selection for these trials and the inability to demonstrate long-term benefits over anticoagulation alone.

Broader use of thrombolytic therapy is primarily limited by the increased risk of major bleeding (9.2%) versus anticoagulation (3.4%), which includes a 1.5% incidence of intracranial bleeding. Contraindications include previous intracranial hemorrhage, known intracranial vascular lesion or malignancy, ischemic stroke within 3 months, suspected aortic dissection, active bleeding or bleeding diathesis, and closed head/facial trauma within 3 months. Relative contraindications include poorly controlled hypertension, recent surgery (14 days), and pregnancy. The use of combined modalities (catheter-based fibrinolysis, pharmaco-mechanical clot dissolution) and lower doses of tissue plasminogen activator (tPA 50 mg IV) may modulate the bleeding risk, but currently broader application of thrombolytic therapy remain controversial.

Extensive Proximal Vein Lower Extremity Thrombosis
Proximal iliac vein thrombosis is often highly symptomatic and may result in severe postthrombotic syndrome (PTS). Rarely, compromise of the arterial supply may occur, as described for phelgmasia alba dolens ("milk leg") and phlegmasia cerulea dolens. The former describes a swollen, white extremity with early compromise of arterial flow secondary to extensive DVT. The latter is an advanced stage characterized by severe swelling, cyanosis, and blue discoloration of the extremity—a precursor of venous gangrene. These entities are emergencies that require prompt anticoagulation, elevation, and consideration of endovascular intervention. The presence of bilateral proximal iliac vein thrombosis should prompt evaluation for IVC thrombus or agenesis, particularly in younger patients. Catheter-directed thrombolysis and endovascular approaches have been pursued in proximal iliofemoral venous thrombosis in an attempt to reduce the risk of severe PTS. Recent studies have been unable to demonstrate that the desired benefit in PTS reduction outweighs the increased risk of bleeding. Thus the routine use of thrombolytic therapy for proximal iliofemoral venous thrombosis cannot be recommended, and patient selection for this approach remains controversial.

Spontaneous Proximal Upper Extremity Thrombosis
The majority of upper extremity DVT is related to intravenous catheters, malignancy, or thrombophilia. Spontaneous upper extremity DVT in the absence of provocation is rare. This entity (Paget-Schroetter syndrome) tends to occur in a younger, often adolescent population with a recent history of exercise or strenuous activity usually involving the dominant upper extremity. This presentation in the absence of usual VTE risk factors should prompt an evaluation for venous thoracic outlet syndrome (TOS). Because of the younger age of these patients and significant disability associated with PTS in the upper extremity (particularly the dominant hand), the initial approach has included thrombolysis (within 14 days), anticoagulation, and evaluation for venous TOS. However, no rigorous comparison of these approaches or combinations of approaches has been undertaken. If evidence for venous TOS is demonstrated, first rib resection on the affected side is often recommended. In the absence of a predisposing anatomical abnormality, an underlying thrombophilic state or occult malignancy should be considered.

VTE Presenting With Paradoxical Embolism
The occurrence of arterial embolism, most commonly cryptogenic stroke, in the presence of DVT and a right-to-left shunt (i.e., patent foramen ovale or PFO) suggests the diagnosis of paradoxical embolus. Standard anticoagulation for VTE is recommended, followed by PFO closure when complete. If indefinite anticoagulation is planned, the additional benefit of PFO closure is unclear.

Acute Venous Thromboembolism With Contraindication to Anticoagulation
Occasional patients diagnosed with acute VTE will have an absolute contraindication to anticoagulation. Placement of a temporary IVC filter may be considered in these patients to provide short-term protection from PE. However, the vast majority of contraindications to anticoagulation are temporary and definitive anticoagulation therapy should be instituted as soon as feasible. IVC filter use is associated with increased risk of lower extremity DVT. Evaluation for IVC filter removal should be planned within 3 to 6 months, depending on the clinical scenario.

Isolated Subsegmental Pulmonary Embolism and Incidental VTE
The enhanced sensitivity of current CT scanners and extensive use of CT angiography has led to an increased diagnosis of isolated subsegmental PE. Treatment of isolated subsegmental PE (where proximal DVT has been excluded) is controversial as the natural history and benefit of anticoagulation is unclear. If an isolated subsegmental defect occurs in a clinical context that is high risk for recurrent VTE (e.g., malignancy), therapeutic anticoagulation is preferred. Alternatively, for an isolated subsegmental PE occurring in a patient that is otherwise low risk for VTE recurrence, clinical surveillance is preferred. Based on the frequency of diagnostic and staging CT scans in cancer patients, an incidental diagnosis of VTE is not an uncommon finding. Although outcome data are limited in this setting, incidental VTE appears to have similar effects on mortality and risk of VTE recurrence. Because the outcomes for incidental and symptomatic VTE in cancer patients appear similar, most cases of incidental VTE should be treated similar to symptomatic VTE.

Special Circumstances for Anticoagulant Monitoring
The predictable dose responses for LMWH, fondaparinux and the DOACs allow use without monitoring. However, select circumstances exist where monitoring may be desirable. LMWH is the preferred anticoagulant in pregnancy, but weight-based dosing may not be as accurate during pregnancy. Periodic confirmation of therapeutic target levels (0.5–1.2 U/mL anti–factor Xa activity) 4 hours after subcutaneous injection is often recommended. Likewise, the accuracy of weight-based LMWH dosing with a body weight <45 kg or >100 kg is not extensively validated. Confirmation of therapeutic peak levels in these individuals is recommended. Similarly, a need for DOAC drug levels may arise when assessing compliance, bleeding with potential drug-overdose, or for an emergent procedure. DOACs directed against factor Xa (rivaroxaban, apixaban, and edoxaban) are monitored with an anti–factor Xa activity assay using a drug-specific standard curve. Significant dabigatran drug effect is excluded with a normal thrombin time. Alternatively, dabigatran drug effect can be detected by prolongation of the APTT or more specialized coagulation tests. The INR is not sensitive to dabigatran.

Reversal Agents
Acute reversal of anticoagulation may be required for drug overdose with clinically significant bleeding or emergent procedures. If the situation is non-emergent, holding warfarin (4–5 days depending on INR) or DOACs (2–3 days depending on renal function) is preferable. If urgent reversal is required, specific agents exist for UFH, warfarin, and, more recently, DOACs (Table 5). Although UFH overdose may be reversed with dose-adjusted protamine, the short half-life of UFH and potential toxicity of protamine often mitigate against use. Protamine[1] is most commonly used to reverse high-dose UFH after cardiopulmonary bypass. LMWH overdose may also be treated with protamine, but significantly less effectively. Warfarin is fully reversed by administration of 4 factor prothrombin complex concentrate (PCC) or fresh frozen plasma (FFP). The 4-factor PCC dose is modified based on the INR and favored over FFP, which may be complicated by volume overload and transfusion reactions. Immediate reversal

---

[1]Not FDA approved for this indication.

Figure 3 Suggested algorithm for treatment of VTE. AC = anticoagulation. *Estrogen- related includes oral contraceptives, hormone replacement therapy, pregnancy and puerperium. **Indefinite anticoagulation includes reduced dose DOAC options after initial 3 months therapeutic AC.

with PCC or FFP should be followed with 5 to 10 vitamin K by the oral or IV route. Vitamin K takes 6 to 24 hours to act but is critical to maintaining anticoagulant reversal because the PCC or FFP effect will wane based on plasma half-life of the coagulation factors. Notably, high doses of vitamin K can result in relative warfarin resistance for the ensuing 1 to 2 weeks. Lower doses of vitamin K (1–2 mg) may be appropriate for less serious bleeding where early reinitiation of warfarin is anticipated. Highly specific agents for the reversal of DOACs are now available. Dabigatran is rapidly reversed by administration of idarucizumab (Praxbind), a humanized monoclonal Fab fragment that neutralizes the parent drug and major metabolites. DOACs targeting factor Xa (rivaroxaban, apixaban, edoxaban, betrixaban [Bevyxxa]) may be rapidly reversed with Andexanet alfa (Andexxa), a truncated, inactive form of recombinant factor Xa that acts as a decoy for small molecules targeting the factor Xa active site. Andexanet alfa is currently approved for patients treated with rivaroxaban and apixaban (ANNEXA-4). Given the relatively short half-lives of the DOACs and high costs of pharmacologic reversal, these agents should be reserved for truly emergent procedures or clinically significant anticoagulant-related bleeding.

Duration of Anticoagulation
Standard treatment for a new episode of DVT or PE has traditionally been 3 to 6 months of therapeutic anticoagulation. The recommended duration of anticoagulation for VTE requires individualized analysis of the clinical presentation and patient specific factors that weigh both recurrence and bleeding risk (Figure 3).

Clinical Presentation
Recurrence risk varies widely based on clinical presentation (see Natural History). The key distinction is between events that occur in the absence (unprovoked) versus the presence (provoked) of established VTE risk factors (Table 1). The majority of cases with clinical risk factors present may be categorized as transient/reversible (e.g., surgery, estrogen) or permanent/non-reversible (e.g., dense hemiplegia secondary to stroke). Surgery is a major transient risk factor for VTE with a low recurrence risk (3% at 5 years). Three months of anticoagulation is sufficient for this population, while shorter durations are associated with increased risk of recurrence. Estrogen-related events have a similarly low risk of recurrence if re-exposure is avoided. A second category of VTE events occurs in association with a nonsurgical transient risk factor (leg injury, significant medical illness, travel-associated) and demonstrates an intermediate recurrence risk (15% at 5 years).

This subgroup is substantially more heterogeneous than the surgical group, with a variety of triggering factors and broader recurrence risk estimates. VTE events associated with nonreversible clinical risk factors may require extended anticoagulation with periodic reassessment of risks and benefits. Unprovoked VTE demonstrates a high risk of recurrence (30% at 5 years) and, in many respects, behaves as a chronic disease. Finally, patients with an underlying malignancy represent ~20% of VTE cases but are usually excluded from natural history studies. Cancer-associated thrombosis demonstrates a 15% annualized recurrence risk with longer-term risk more difficult to estimate based on competing mortality from the underlying cancer. These patients have concomitant increased bleeding risk, complicating the risk–benefit analysis for anticoagulation.

Thrombus Site
Thrombus location significantly influences recurrence risk, with more proximal events demonstrating higher rates of recurrence. Patients with isolated distal or calf vein DVT are half as likely to have recurrent events compared to proximal DVT or PE. Patients presenting with proximal DVT have similar recurrence risk to patients with PE. However, patients initially presenting with PE are substantially more likely to have a PE recurrence relative to patients presenting with DVT only. This finding takes on particular importance when one considers the cause specific mortality rate associated with PE is greater than 10%. Thus patients presenting with unprovoked PE deserve particular attention with regard to consideration of indefinite anticoagulation.

Standard Versus Indefinite Anticoagulation
Clinical presentation categorizes patients with regard to recurrence risk, which is critical to the decision between standard (3 months) and indefinite anticoagulation (Figure 3). This decision is also influenced by bleeding risk and requires clinical judgment. As above, VTE associated with surgical or estrogen-related provoking factors and distal DVT (provoked or unprovoked) should be treated with therapeutic anticoagulation for 3 months. Conversely, most patients with unprovoked proximal DVT or PE should be considered for indefinite therapy based on their substantial recurrence risk, unless they also have high bleeding risk. There is little rationale for arbitrary extended periods of anticoagulation beyond the standard 3 to 6 months, unless awaiting resolution of a risk factor (e.g., extended immobilization). Prolongation of anticoagulation beyond 6 months in patients with unprovoked VTE delays but

clearly does not prevent recurrence. A number of strategies, including postanticoagulation D-dimer testing (3–5 weeks) and risk stratification models, have attempted to identify patients with unprovoked VTE for which anticoagulation may be safely stopped. Post-anticoagulation D-dimer testing is the most established strategy, further stratifying these patients into high (8.8%) and low (3.0%) first-year recurrence rates. Conversely, the presence of persistent or multiple antiphospholipid antibodies increases recurrence risk (1.8- to 4.5-fold) for patients presenting with unprovoked VTE. Alternative approaches to risk reduction in unprovoked VTE include indefinite anticoagulation with reduced intensity DOACs or daily ASA. ASA reduces recurrence risk by ~1/3 in unprovoked VTE but is inferior to reduced dose rivaroxaban and apixaban (EINSTEIN CHOICE, AMPLIFY-EXT).

VTE associated with nonsurgical risk factors is more problematic with regard to definitive assessment of recurrence risk. Patients who suffer VTE with minor provocations may have a recurrence rate that approaches unprovoked VTE. These patients should be treated for at least 3 months and reassessed. Clinical factors that may impact a decision for indefinite anticoagulation include underlying cardiopulmonary disease (decreased ability to tolerate recurrence), ongoing inflammation (inflammatory bowel disease, autoimmune disease, chronic infections), prolonged immobilization (stroke), and male sex. For patients with a prolonged but ultimately reversible risk factor (i.e., stroke immobility improving with physical therapy), prolongation of anticoagulation until resolution of the underlying risk factor is reasonable. Similarly, travel-associated thrombosis may be a recurring risk that requires an intermittent prophylaxis plan. Bleeding risk assessment is important to decisions regarding recommended duration of therapy. Major risk factors for bleeding on anticoagulation include: advanced age, previous bleeding history, cancer, renal or liver failure, previous stroke, diabetes mellitus, nonsteroidal inflammatory drugs or antiplatelet therapy, comorbidity and reduced functional capacity, recent surgery, frequent falls, and alcohol (Table 6). Additional risk assessment tools (e.g., HAS-BLED score) exist, primarily validated for warfarin therapy.

Clinical Decision Making

Particularly for clinical situations with modest evidence, shared decision making between physician and patient is desirable in determining the duration of anticoagulant therapy. Medical comorbidities affecting bleeding or fall risk in the elderly, patient anxiety about recurrent VTE events, and occupational/lifestyle risks for trauma may substantially impact anticoagulation decisions. Family history should be obtained with particular attention to first-degree relatives affected by VTE, including unprovoked events and age of presentation. Questions regarding the underlying cause for a VTE event often drive requests for thrombophilia evaluations. These requests generally fail to acknowledge the complex, multigenic basis for VTE and rarely contribute to clinical decision making (see "Genetics of Venous Thromboembolism"). The clinical presentation and family history are substantially more useful than identification of minor thrombophilia traits, which are poor predictors of VTE recurrence. Finally, when a decision is made to pursue indefinite anticoagulation, periodic reassessment of this decision is important. The risk-to-benefit ratio of anticoagulation may change as the patient's medical history evolves. The hematology consultant serves an important role in facilitating difficult anticoagulation decisions.

Prevention of Venous Thromboembolism

About 60% of VTE events are associated with recent hospitalization or surgery, and up to 70% of these cases are preventable. However, less than half of hospitalized patients receive appropriate prophylactic measures. Given the significant morbidity and mortality associated with VTE, primary prophylaxis strategies in high-risk situations are of great medical importance and may

TABLE 6 Risk Factors for Bleeding With Anticoagulant Therapy and Estimated Risk of Major Bleeding in Low-, Moderate-, and High-Risk Categories

Risk Factors

Age >65 y

Previous bleeding

Cancer

Metastatic cancer

Renal failure

Liver failure

Thrombocytopenia

Previous stroke

Diabetes

Anaemia

Antiplatelet therapy

Poor anticoagulant control

Comorbidity and reduced functional capacity

Recent surgery

Frequent falls

Alcohol abuse

Nonsteroidal antiinflammatory drug

Categorization of Risk of Bleeding

	ESTIMATED ABSOLUTE RISK OF MAJOR BLEEDING		
	LOW RISK (0 RISK FACTORS)	MODERATE RISK (1 RISK FACTOR)	HIGH RISK (≥2 RISK FACTORS)
Anticoagulation 0–3 mo			
Baseline risk (%)	0.6	1.2	4.8
Increased risk (%)	1.0	2.0	8.0
Total risk (%)	1.6	3.2	12.8
Anticoagulation after first 3 mo			
Baseline risk (%/y)	0.3	0.6	≥2.5
Increased risk (%/y)	0.5	1.0	≥4.0
Total risk (%/y)	0.8	1.6	≥6.5

Data from the 9th Edition of the Antithrombotic Guideline (AT9).

provide a cost savings. Risk stratification of patients based on surgery or medical illness, patient characteristics (previous VTE, active cancer, duration of immobility, etc.), and bleeding risk impact recommendations for pharmacologic and mechanical prophylaxis. Pharmacologic agents include LMWH, fondaparinux, low-dose UFH, VKA, and DOACs. The focus in this section is primarily on heparin and DOACs given the available evidence. Mechanical prophylaxis includes graduated compression stockings (GCS) that are >15mm Hg at the ankle or intermittent pneumatic compression devices (IPCs). IPCs enhance lower extremity deep vein blood flow and may increase fibrinolytic activity. These modalities can be used alone or in combination for patients with high bleeding risk who cannot use pharmacologic prophylaxis. IPCs are considered more effective than GCS alone, particularly after orthopedic surgery.

TABLE 7 | Risk Factor Stratification and Prophylaxis Options

RISK STRATIFICATION	RECOMMENDED PROPHYLAXIS	DURATION
Low Risk		
Same-day surgery Medical illness in a fully mobile patient	Early mobilization	-
Moderate Risk		
Most general surgery procedures	LMWH UFH IPC/GCS with or without pharmacologic prophylaxis as appropriate	5–14 days
Most acute medical illnesses	LMWH UFH Betrixaban^	Duration of inpatient stay Extended duration beyond hospitalization may be appropriate for very-high-risk patients in whom bleeding risk is low
High Risk		
Hip or knee replacement surgery	LMWH UFH Fondaparinux Rivaroxaban Apixaban Dabigatran* Adjusted dose Warfarin	At least 10–14 days Extended duration up to 4 weeks preferred ASA may be used subsequently for extended duration of therapy
General surgery with active cancer, previous VTE	LMWH** UFH Adjusted dose Warfarin	Extended duration (4 weeks) for abdominopelvic surgeries in cancer patients
Major Trauma, Spinal cord injury	IPC with or without GCS, use pharmacologic prophylaxis when appropriate	

Abbreviations: DVT: deep venous thrombosis; GC: graduated compression; IPC: intermittent pneumatic compression; LMWH: low-molecular-weight heparin; UFH: unfractionated heparin; VTE: venous thromboembolism.
^FDA approved for patients hospitalized for acute medical illness at high risk of VTE
*FDA approved for VTE prevention after hip replacement surgery
**Off-label use in cancer patients
^^Usually started postoperatively and adjusted to achieve an international normalized ratio of 2.0–3.0

General Surgery

For general surgery patients, well-established risk assessment tools such as the Caprini or Rogers scores stratify patients by VTE risk to identify those who would benefit from pharmacologic prophylaxis. In general, if the risk of VTE is moderate to high and bleeding risk is low, pharmacologic prophylaxis with LMWH or low-dose UFH should be given. If the bleeding risk is high, intermittent pneumatic compression with or without GCS should be used. Ideally, the minimal duration of prophylaxis is 5 to 10 days but varies widely based on duration of bed rest, inpatient stay, and comorbid conditions. In patients with active cancer undergoing abdominopelvic surgery, prophylaxis should be extended to 4 weeks after surgery.

Orthopedic Surgery

Orthopedic procedures are associated with high risk of VTE, especially those involving the lower extremities and pelvic region.

For patients undergoing total hip or total knee arthroplasty, pharmacologic prophylaxis using LMWH, UFH, DOACs, or adjusted-dose warfarin should be used if no contraindication exists. LMWH is quite effective and safe with the benefit of long-term experience with these agents. Low-dose DOACs have shown comparable efficacy to enoxaparin in this population with a similar low absolute risk of bleeding. Low-dose apixaban (2.5 mg twice daily), rivaroxaban (10 mg daily), and dabigatran (150 mg daily) appear safer than higher doses. Prophylaxis should continue at least 10 to 14 days, and prolongation up to a month should be considered for major orthopedic surgery. Low-dose aspirin has been shown to be effective for extended prophylaxis after initial acute phase of therapy (~5 days) with standard anticoagulant in patients undergoing total hip or knee arthroplasty; however, anticoagulants are generally favored for high-risk patients. IPCs should be used during the inpatient stay in addition to pharmacologic prophylaxis. If bleeding risk is high, IPCs should be used until pharmacologic agents can be safely administered. For arthroscopic procedures of the knee and other low-risk procedures, prophylaxis is generally not indicated unless other risk factors exist. A summary of available agents and recommendations for prophylaxis is provided (Table 7).

Acute Medical Illness

For hospitalized patients with medical illnesses, the risk of VTE is ~8 fold higher than the general population. Patients expected to be hospitalized with reduced mobility >3 days, a previous history of VTE, active infection or malignancy, recent surgery or trauma, heart failure or respiratory failure should be considered for prophylaxis. The Padua score is a prospectively validated risk assessment model that stratifies patients into groups with high (~11%) or low (0.3%) incidence of VTE. Current prophylaxis options for medical patients include LMWH, low-dose UFH, and fondaparinux. When bleeding risk is considered moderate to high, mechanical prophylaxis using IPCs or GCS should be used until it is safe to add anticoagulants. For low-risk patients admitted for short duration or remaining ambulatory, withholding prophylaxis may be appropriate. Clinical context and bleeding risk assessment should also impact these decisions.

Although pharmacologic prophylaxis is typically limited to the acute illness during the inpatient stay, analysis of population-based data suggests that ~75% of VTE events occur well after discharge, at a median of almost 3 weeks. Furthermore, increased compliance with inpatient prophylaxis over time has not resulted in the expected decrease in the rate of VTE. The effect of extended DOAC prophylaxis (35–42 days) has been examined in medical patients for apixaban, rivaroxaban, and betrixaban. Reduced-dose apixaban and rivaroxaban demonstrated similar VTE prevention to standard enoxaparin prophylaxis but increased bleeding events. Evaluation of betrixaban in a select patient group (elevated D-dimer and elderly) demonstrated modestly better VTE prevention relative to enoxaparin, with an increase in nonmajor but not major bleeding. Extended prophylaxis is an area of ongoing investigation with unresolved issues that include appropriate patient selection and discerning the impact of specific anticoagulants versus prophylaxis duration on outcomes.

References

Chatterjee S, Chakraborty A, Weinberg I, Kadakia M, Wilensky RL, Sardar P, et al: Thrombolysis for pulmonary embolism and risk of all-cause mortality, major bleeding, and intracranial hemorrhage: a meta-analysis, *JAMA* 311(23):2414–2421, 2014.

Connors JM: Thrombophilia testing and venous thrombosis, *N Engl J Med* 377:1177–1187, 2017.

Heit JA, Crusan DJ, Ashrani AA, Petterson TM, Bailey KR: Effect of a near-universal hospitalization-based prophylaxis regimen on annual number of venous thromboembolism events in the US, *Blood* 130:109–114, 2017.

Kearon C, Akl EA, Ornelas J, Blaivas A, Jimenez D, Bounameaux H, et al: Antithrombotic therapy for VTE disease: CHEST Guideline and Expert Panel Report, *Chest* 149:315–352, 2016.

Kearon C, Parpia S, Spencer FA, Baglin T, Stevens SM, Bauer KA, et al: Antiphospholipid antibodies and recurrent thrombosis after a first unprovoked venous thromboembolism, *Blood* 131:2151–2160, 2018.

Konstantinides SV, Vicaut E, Danays T, Becattini C, Bertoletti L, Beyer-Westendorf J, et al: Impact of thrombolytic therapy on the long-term outcome of intermediate-risk pulmonary embolism, *J Am Coll Cardiol* 69:1536–1544, 2017.

Raskob GE, van Es N, Verhamme P, Carrier M, Di Nisio M, Garcia D, et al: Edoxaban for the treatment of cancer-associated venous thromboembolism, *N Engl J Med* 378:615–624, 2018.

Vedantham S, Goldhaber SZ, Julian JA, Kahn SR, Jaff MR, Cohen DJ, et al: Pharmacomechanical catheter-directed thrombolysis for deep-vein thrombosis, *N Engl J Med* 377:2240–2252, 2017.

Weitz JI, Lensing AWA, Prins MH, Bauersachs R, Beyer-Westendorf J, Bounameaux H, et al: Rivaroxaban or aspirin for extended treatment of venous thromboembolism, *N Engl J Med* 376:1211–1222, 2017.

Zoller B, Ohlsson H, Sundquist J, Sundquist K: A sibling based design to quantify genetic and shared environmental effects of venous thromboembolism in Sweden, *Thromb Res* 149:82–87, 2017.

VIRAL AND MYCOPLASMAL PNEUMONIAS

Method of
Burke A. Cunha, MD; and Cheston B. Cunha, MD

CURRENT DIAGNOSIS

Influenza (human, avian, swine)

- Mild influenza A or B presents acutely with headache, fever, sore throat, plus/minus rhinorrhea.
- Severe influenza A presents with an acute onset (patients often able to name the hour the influenza began) and rapidly become bed bound.
- Headache, myalgias, and prostration may be severe.
- With swine influenza, gastrointestinal symptoms (e.g., nausea/vomiting or diarrhea) may be prominent.
- Auscultation of the lungs is quiet, disproportionate to the degree of respiratory distress. Influenza is an interstitial process and not alveolar, which explains the absence of rales.
- With severe influenza, patients rapidly become hypoxemic. Hypoxemia is accompanied by an A-a gradient >35, which indicates a interstitial oxygen diffusing defect.
- Severe tracheobronchitis is common and manifested by hemoptysis.
- Relative lymphopenia with monocytosis occurs early followed by thrombocytopenia and later leukopenia. Low titer elevations of cold agglutinins are not infrequent (≥1:18).
- Patients may have chest pain exacerbated by breathing mimicking pleuritic chest pain. This is the result of direct intracostal muscle involvement with the influenza virus, which results in myositis and pain on inspiration.
- The chest radiograph in early influenza, in mild to moderate cases, is normal or near normal, with minimal, if any, increase in interstitial markings. The chest radiograph in fulminant cases shows symmetrical bilateral patchy infiltrates without pleural effusion in 48 hours.
- Severe influenza A is accompanied by severe hypoxemia cyanosis, and may be followed by an early fatal outcome.
- Influenza pneumonia most often presents alone without bacterial superinfection, but bacterial infection may accompany (MSSA/CA-MRSA) or follow influenza (*S. pneumoniae* or *H. influenzae*).
- Purulent sputum with influenza indicates concurrent bacterial pneumonia usually caused by *S. aureus* (MSSA/MRSA). Bacterial pneumonia following influenza (after 1–2 weeks), is suggested by leukocytosis, focal or segmental pulmonary infiltrates, and purulent sputum; the pathogens are not *S. aureus*, but most commonly are *S. pneumoniae* or *H. influenzae*.
- A laboratory diagnosis may be made by multiplex PCR of respiratory secretions.

Mycoplasma pneumoniae

- In a patient with CAP and a dry nonproductive cough, without severe headache or myalgias, the most likely diagnosis is *M. pneumoniae*. *M. pneumoniae* CAP is commonly accompanied by nonexudative pharyngitis and/or loose stools or watery diarrhea.

- The temperature is usually less than 102°F (38.9°C) and is not accompanied by frank rigors or pleuritic chest pain.
- Relative bradycardia and elevations in the serum transaminases are not features of *M. pneumoniae* CAP.
- Respiratory viruses are often associated with mild elevations of cold agglutinins (≤1:16) but *M. pneumoniae* is the only pathogen causing CAP associated with highly elevated cold agglutinin titers (≥1:64). Elevated cold agglutinin titers occur in up to 75% of patients with *M. pneumoniae*, and occur early and transiently.
- In a patient with CAP, elevated cold agglutinin titers (>1:8) effectively rule out the typical pathogens, as well as *Legionella* species and *C. pneumoniae*.
- Elevated *M. pneumoniae* ELISA IgG titers indicate past exposure/infection and not current infection or co-infection with another pathogen.
- In the absence of an antecedent respiratory tract infection (e.g., nonexudative pharyngitis, otitis, etc., in the preceding 3 months), the presence of an increased *M. pneumoniae* ELISA IgM titer is diagnostic of acute infection.

CURRENT THERAPY

Viral Influenza

- The aim of therapy is to inhibit the influenza virus and prevent its attachment/spread to uninfected respiratory epithelial cells.
- The neuramidase inhibitors shorten the course of influenza by 1 to 2 days and have antiviral activity. These agents are active against both influenza A and B.
- Most strains of human and avian, but not swine flu strains, are resistant to amantadine (Symmetrel) or rimantadine (Flumadine).
- Amantadine and rimantadine may have an important therapeutic effect in severe influenza A by increasing distal airway dilation and increasing oxygen action.
- Peramivir (Rapivab) may be useful in those unable to take oral neuraminase inhibators.

Mycoplasma pneumoniae

- The agents active against *M. pneumoniae* are macrolides, tetracyclines, quinolones, and ketolides. β-Lactam antibiotics are not active against *M. pneumoniae* because the organisms do not contain a bacterial cell wall.
- Goals of therapy of *M. pneumoniae* CAP are to eradicate the infection, decrease the shedding of *Mycoplasma* in respiratory secretions posttherapy, and to prevent post-treatment asthma.
- Therapy is equally efficacious with macrolides, doxycycline (Vibramycin), or a respiratory quinolone intravenously, orally, or in combination for 1 to 2 weeks.
- The mode of administration is determined by the severity of the CAP and the setting. Outpatients are usually treated orally. Patients hospitalized with severe CAP are initially treated intravenously and then changed to an oral agent.
- Macrolide resistance to *M. pneumoniae* has been described in children and reported in adults.

Influenza pneumonia is the most important cause of viral pneumonia in adults. Influenza A is the predominant type of influenza found in adults, and influenza B is more common in children. Influenza A has the potential for severe disease, occurs seasonally, and is the predominant type involved in influenza pandemics. *Mycoplasma pneumoniae* community-acquired pneumonia (CAP) was first recognized decades ago as distinctive from bacterial and viral pneumonias. It was originally described by Eaton as "Eaton agent" pneumonia caused by a pleuropneumonia-like organism (PPLO), later shown to be caused by *M. pneumoniae*. *M. pneumoniae* is a common cause of pneumonia in all age groups, but the peak incidence of *M. pneumoniae* CAP is in young adults. *M. pneumoniae* CAP is a common cause of ambulatory CAP.

The term *atypical pneumonia* was first applied to viral pneumonias because the clinical laboratory and radiologic findings were different from those caused by typical bacterial pulmonary pathogens. In influenza pneumonia, the clinical findings are confined to the trachea, bronchi, lung parenchyma, and central nervous system. *M. pneumoniae* CAP is a systemic infection with a pulmonary component. Over the years, atypical pneumonia has come to refer to pneumonia caused by systemic nonviral/nonbacterial pathogen agents that have a pulmonary component. Viral pneumonias are no longer considered atypical pneumonias. Atypical pneumonias may be divided into nonzoonotic and zoonotic atypical CAPs. Nonzoonotic CAPs are most commonly caused by *M. pneumoniae*, *Chlamydia pneumoniae*, or *Legionella* species, whereas the three most common zoonotic atypical pneumonias are caused by *Chlamydia psittaci* (psittacosis), *Francisella tularensis* (tularemia), or *Coxiella burnetii* (Q fever). All of the atypical pneumonias are distinct clinical entities that may be differentiated on the basis of their characteristic pattern of extrapulmonary organ involvement. Although some viruses may occasionally have extrapulmonary manifestations (i.e., influenza, adenovirus with viral pneumonias), the primary clinical features are confined to the lungs. *M. pneumoniae* is a critical cause of nonzoonotic atypical CAP, particularly in the ambulatory setting. *M. pneumoniae* CAP may be severe in patients with impaired host defenses or those with severe, preexisting cardiopulmonary disease.

Influenza (Human, Avian, and Swine)

Viral influenza pneumonia affects children and adults. Influenza B is the primary type causing mild influenza in children and adults. Influenza A is primarily an infection of adults that may be mild to severe. Influenza A has the potential for pandemic spread (e.g., swine influenza [H_1N_1]).

Influenza occurs during the winter months, usually peaking in February. Influenza is spread by aerosolized droplet infection from person to person and via fomites. Influenza A is classified into subtypes based on hemagglutinin (H) and neuramidase (N) surface proteins. An important characteristic of influenza A virus is antigenic drift, which refers to minor changes in surface protein shift in the neuramidase or hemagglutinin receptors. With influenza A, these surface receptor proteins are important in cellular adherence of the influenza virus and spread of influenza from respiratory epithelial cells. The vaccine for the flu season most often includes the influenza hemagglutinin and neuramidase types seen at the end of the preceding year's season. Prevention of attachment and spread of the virus is helpful to controlling the spread of influenza; vaccine protection conferred by specific antibody response to influenza A is highly protective (approximately 80% in noncompromised hosts).

During the years when influenza B has been prevalent, vaccines for the subsequent year contain an influenza B component.

Clinical manifestations of influenza A in adults varies considerably from mild to fatal infection. Mild infection is usually manifested as an acute febrile illness characterized by headache and myalgias with dry unproductive cough and rhinorrhea. Mild influenza may be due to influenza A or B and usually resolves in a few days without complications in normal hosts who have good cardiopulmonary function.

Severe influenza A (human, avian, swine) occurs in normal healthy adults and may be fatal. The onset of severe influenza A (human, avian, swine) is sudden, and the patient often recalls the exact hour of onset. The patient is febrile with early/extreme prostration rendering the patient bedridden. Fever rapidly rises and may be accompanied by chills. Neck soreness, severe headache, and myalgias are typical. Sore throat, eye pain, conjunctival injection, and hemoptysis are frequently present. Chest pain worsened by deep inspiration is not truly pleuritic but rather reflects influenza A myositis of the intracostal muscles. Shortness of breath is

related to the degree of hypoxemia. Severe influenza A causes an oxygen diffusion defect as manifested by an increased A-a gradient (>35). Profound hypoxemia may be accompanied by cyanosis. Hypotension caused by hypoxemia and vascular collapse may follow. The course of fulminant viral influenza A is of short duration.

Physical findings are few in viral influenza (i.e., conjunctival suffusion). Auscultation reveals absolutely quiet lungs because the infectious process is interstitial and not alveolar. Routine blood tests are usually unremarkable except for leukopenia, relative lymphopenia, and thrombocytopenia. Atypical lymphocytes are not present, but low titers of cold agglutinins may be present. Cold agglutinins (if present) have low titers less than or equal to 1:18. In fatal cases, a pale bluelike hue of the skin may be noted, and there may be bleeding from multiple orifices preterminally. The chest radiograph in uncomplicated influenza A is unremarkable or may have minimal perihilar bilateral increased prominence of interstitial markings. In severe influenza A pneumonia, the chest radiograph shows bilateral symmetrical perihilar infiltrates without pleural effusions in <48 hours.

Patients may die from severe influenza A without superimposed bacterial pneumonia. Most deaths during the 1918–1919 pandemic were young military recruits who died early of influenza A pneumonia without bacterial pneumonia. Influenza may be complicated by bacterial pneumonia. Bacterial pneumonias complicating influenza may occur concurrently at presentation or may occur 1 to 2 weeks after an interval of improvement after the presentation of influenza. Influenza A presenting concurrently with bacterial pneumonia is caused by *Staphylococcus aureus*. In contrast to influenza alone, MSSA/CA-MRSA is manifested by an increase in fever, shaking chills, leukocytosis, purulent sputum, localized rales on auscultation, bacteremia, and focal/segmental infiltrates on chest radiograph that rapidly cavitate in less than 72 hours. Alternately, patients with influenza A may develop a secondary bacterial infection 1 to 2 weeks later. Secondary bacterial pneumonia is less severe and is usually caused by *Streptococcus pneumoniae* or *Haemophilus influenzae*.

Viral influenza-like illnesses (ILIs) most often present during the winter months or influenza season. For clinical and therapeutic purposes, it is important to differentiate influenza A from viral ILIs in hospitalized adults. Some clinical features may point to a specific ILI viral etiology, but a specific viral diagnosis can be made by viral respiratory PCR of nasopharyngeal swab specimens. The only viral ILI likely to mimic influenza A presenting with a fulminant severe viral CAP is MERS-CoA. The mimics of ILIs are presented (Table 1). The main non-viral mimic of influenza A in hospitalized adults is Legionnaire's disease (LD). LD may be different from influenza A and other viral ILIs by CXR findings and characteristic non-specific laboratory tests. With LD CAP, the CXR shows one or more non-focal infiltrates. Fever, usually > 102° F, is accompanied by relative bradycardia. With LD, the ESR is highly elevated > 90 mm/h, the ferritin is highly elevated > 2 xn, and the serum phosphorus is decreased early as is serum sodium. Although an elevated CPK and mild transaminitis often accompany LD, these findings are not uncommon in influenza A and some viral ILIs. There are few infections that may mimic the dry, productive cough of *Mycoplasma pneumoniae* CAP. Pertussis is most likely to mimic mycoplasma. Pertussis, unlike mycoplasma, is not accompanied by watery diarrhea. The distinguishing laboratory feature of mycoplasma CAP is elevated cold agglutinins not found with pertussis. The key non-specific laboratory finding in pertussis is marked lymphocytosis (Table 2).

Anti-Influenza Therapy

Therapy of viral influenza is directed at inhibiting viral replication and preventing further infection of respiratory epithelial cells. The neuramidase inhibitors zanamivir (Relenza), oseltamivir (Tamiflu), and peramivir (Rapivab) have anti-influenza A and B activity. Neuramidase inhibitors decrease the severity and duration of influenza symptoms by 1 to 2 days. Current flu strains are resistant to amantadine and rimantadine, but these drugs may still be useful to increase peripheral airway dilatation

TABLE 1	Mimics of Influenza A in Hospitalized Adults Presenting with Influenza-like illnesses (ILIs)	
INFLUENZA-LIKE ILLNESSES (ILIS)	**CHEST FILM FEATURES**	**CLINICAL CLUES**
MERS (MERS-CoA)	• Ill defined infiltrates (early) • Bilateral dense interstitial nodular infiltrates (late) • Severe cases often develop ARDS	• Recent travel to Middle East or contact with MERS case • Dry cough and sore throat • Hemoptysis (in some) • Diarrhea (common) • WBC count normal, thrombocytopenia • Elevated LDH
RSV	• Clear CXR (early) • Bilateral ill defined infiltrates on CXR (late) • Chest CT : GGO (non-specific)	• Antecedent/concurrent rhinorrhea • Hoarseness • Lymphocyte/monocyte ratio>2
HPIV-3	• Clear CXR (early) • Bilateral ill defined infiltrates on CXR (late)	• Hoarseness • Prolonged lymphocyte/monocyte ratio<2 • Monocytosis
EV-D86	• Clear CXR (early) • Bilateral ill defined infiltrates on CXR (late)	• Diarrhea (common) • Flaccid paralysis
Legionnaire's disease	• Rapidly progressive asymmetric ill defined infiltrates on CXR • Consolidation and small pleural effusions (common) • Cavitation (rare)	• High fevers (>102°F) • Highly elevated ESR (>90 mm/h) • Ferritin (>2 xn) • Leukocytosis with relative lymphopenia • Elevated CPK (in some) • Mild transient elevated transaminates common (early) • Microscopic hematuria (early)

Abbreviations: MERS=Middle East respiratory syndrome; RSV=respiratory syncytial virus; HPIV=human parainfluenza virus; EV=enterovirus; GGO=ground gloss opacity; CXR=chest x-ray; ARDS=acute respiratory distress syndrome.

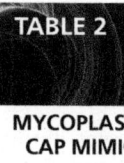

TABLE 2	Mimics of Mycoplasma pneumoniae in Community Acquired Pneumonia (CAP) Hospitalized Adults	
MYCOPLASMA CAP MIMICS	**CHEST FILM FEATURES**	**CLINICAL CLUES**
C. pneumoniae	• Ill defined lower lobe infiltrates (often ovoid) • No consolidation, cavitation or effusion	• No seasonal predisposition • Hoarseness • Protracted dry cough • Mycoplasma-like illness that doesn't respond to erythromycin • Wheezing (in some) • No diarrhea • No cold agglutinins • Rhinorrhea proceeds dry cough (1–2 weeks)
Pertussis	• Perihilar ill defined infiltrates ("shaggy heart" sign) • No consolidation, cavitation or effusions	• Protracted dry cough • Persistent cough (without typical "whoop" of children) • Afebrile or minimal fevers • Marked lymphocytes (>60%) • No cold agglutinins

and oxygenation, which may be of critical importance in severe influenza A with severe hypoxemia. Mild influenza A/B may be treated with neuramidase inhibitors. Mild cases of influenza A should be treated at the onset of the illness. For severe influenza A, neuramidase inhibitors provide optimal anti-influenza therapy (Table 3). For human and avian influenza (H_5N_1), these antiviral drugs may be ineffective, but are effective against swine influenza.

Mycoplasma pneumoniae
M. pneumoniae is a common cause of ambulatory CAP. It affects all age groups, and in normal hosts with intact cardiopulmonary function, *Mycoplasma* CAP is usually a mild, self-limiting infection. However, *M. pneumoniae* derives its importance from difficulty in diagnosis, the necessity for non–β-lactam therapy, and because of its effect on peripheral airways.

Mycoplasma CAP is one of the nonzoonotic causes of CAP (the others being *Legionella* and *Chlamydia pneumoniae*). *M. pneumoniae* is an atypical pneumonia that is a systemic infectious disease with a pulmonary component. It may be distinguished from other atypical pneumonias by its characteristic pattern of extrapulmonary organ involvement. *M. pneumoniae* CAP most closely resembles *C. pneumoniae* CAP clinically, but is very different from Legionnaires' disease in terms of its epidemiology, age distribution, pattern of extrapulmonary organ involvement, and severity.

Clinically, *M. pneumoniae* presents as a subacute febrile illness. Temperatures rarely exceed 102°F (38.9°C). Rigors are not a feature of *M. pneumoniae* CAP, but patients may complain of chilly sensations. Mild headache and/or myalgias are not uncommon. The most common presenting symptom in *Mycoplasma* CAP is the prolonged, nonproductive dry cough. Patients with *Mycoplasma* CAP often complain of or have mild nonexudative pharyngitis. Rhinorrhea and conjunctivitis are not features of *M. pneumoniae* CAP. Watery diarrhea is commonly present in *Mycoplasma* CAP, but abdominal pain is not a clinical finding. Other extrapulmonary manifestations are uncommon or rare (e.g., meningoencephalitis, pericarditis, hemolytic anemia, glomerular nephritis, Guillain-Barré syndrome, erythema multiforme). *M. pneumoniae* has a distinctive pattern of extrapulmonary organ involvement that does not include cardiac involvement (relative bradycardia) or hepatic involvement, including normal serum glutamate-oxaloacetate transaminase (SGOT) or serum glutamate-pyruvate transaminase (SGPT). The distinguishing laboratory feature of *M. pneumoniae* CAP is elevated cold agglutinin titers. Although a variety of infectious and noninfectious diseases are associated with cold agglutinin elevations, they are usually of low titer (i.e., <1:16). There are no pulmonary infections presenting as CAP that are associated with high elevations of cold agglutinin titers (i.e., ≥1:64). Although elevated cold agglutinins occur early in up to 75% of patients with *M. pneumoniae* CAP, they are still diagnostically important when present. In a patient with CAP and a

TABLE 3 **Adult Anti-Influenza Antivirals**

ANTIVIRAL	TREATMENT DOSE	PROPHYLACTIC DOSE
Mild Influenza A/B		
Zanamivir (Relenza)†	2 inhalations (5 mg per inhalation) q12h × 5 d	2 inhalations (5 mg per inhalation) q24h × 5 d
Influenza A		
Oseltamivir (Tamiflu)†	75 mg (PO) q12h × 5 d*	75 mg (PO) q24h × 7 d
Peramivir (Rapivab)	600 mg (IV) over 30 min × 1 d	None

*For avian (H5N1) influenza, 150 mg (PO) q12h may be effective.
†Currently most human and avian influenza strains are resistant.

cold agglutinin titer greater than or equal to 1:64, the diagnosis of *M. pneumoniae* CAP is very likely.

M. pneumoniae may be differentiated from the typical bacterial pneumonias because of the presence of extrapulmonary findings, including nonexudative pharyngitis, loose stools or watery diarrhea, erythema multiforme, and high cold agglutinin. Patients with typical bacterial CAP usually have a more acute onset of presentation, a productive cough, and temperatures that may exceed 102°F (38.9°C), often accompanied by chills. Patients with typical pneumonia often have pleuritic chest pain, which is not a feature of *M. pneumoniae* CAP. Among the atypical pneumonias, the zoonotic pneumonias (i.e., tularemia, psittacosis, Q fever) may be eliminated from consideration if there is a recent zoonotic contact history with the appropriate vector.

C. pneumoniae resembles closely *M. pneumoniae* CAP. *C. pneumoniae* may be distinguished by the absence of cold agglutinins and the presence of hoarseness, which is a feature of *C. pneumoniae* but not *M. pneumoniae* CAP. Loose stools or watery diarrhea are not usual features of *C. pneumoniae* CAP. The most common clinical problem is differentiating *Legionella* from *Mycoplasma* CAP; this may be done by appreciating the differences in the pattern of extrapulmonary organ involvement with each of these pathogens. *Legionella* may be clinically differentiated from *Mycoplasma* by acuteness of onset or severity, the presence of relative bradycardia, temperatures greater than 102°F (38.9°C), and the presence of abdominal pain. From a laboratory standpoint, highly elevated cold agglutinin titers argue strongly against the diagnosis of *Legionella* and point to *M. pneumoniae*. Nonspecific laboratory tests in a patient with CAP that suggest *Legionella* and argue against *M. pneumoniae* include otherwise unexplained hypophosphatemia, hyponatremia, microscopic hematuria, and increased creatinine. *Legionella* does not affect the upper respiratory tract as does *Mycoplasma* (e.g., nonexudative pharyngitis). Ear findings are not a feature of Legionnaires' disease but are common in *M. pneumoniae* CAP. The finding most likely to cause confusion between *M. pneumoniae* and *Legionella pneumophila* is the presence of loose stools or watery diarrhea, which is found in both.

M. pneumoniae may be cultured from the throat in viral culture media, but the diagnosis is usually made serologically. An elevated enzyme-linked immunosorbent assay (ELISA) or enzyme immuno-assay (EIA) IgM titer suggests acute or recent infection, but an elevated IgG titer indicates past exposure but not acute infection. Elevated IgG titers regardless of degree of elevation are not diagnostic of current infection with *M. pneumoniae* and only indicate previous antigenic exposure. *M. pneumoniae* ELISA IgM levels may take up to 3 months to decrease. Therefore, clinicians should take into account recent antecedent respiratory illness in order to properly interpret elevated IgM titers, including patients with nonexudative pharyngitis within 3 months prior to the presentation of CAP. The combination of an increased *M. pneumoniae* IgM titer and highly elevated cold agglutinin titers is virtually diagnostic of acute infection. Cold agglutinin titers are elevated transiently early and rapidly fall; the simultaneously elevated cold agglutinins and IgM titers of *M. pneumoniae* indicate active or current infection. In patients with CAP caused by another organism (e.g., *S. pneumoniae*), the presence of elevated *Mycoplasma* IgG titers does not indicate co-infection but only preexisting serologic exposure to *M. pneumoniae*.

Therapy

M. pneumoniae has a predilection for the respiratory epithelial cells and resides literally on their surface. Mycoplasmas have no definite cell wall like the typical pathogens causing CAP. Their position on the surface of the respiratory epithelium and their absence of a cell wall necessitates the therapeutic approach, which includes non–β-lactam antibiotics with the capacity to penetrate into the *Mycoplasma* organisms. Traditionally, macrolides and tetracyclines have been used successfully to treat *M. pneumoniae*. Both CAP tetracyclines and macrolides are effective against *Mycoplasma* because they interfere with intracellular protein synthesis at the ribosomal level. Tetracyclines penetrate intracellularly better than macrolides, with the exception of penetration into the alveolar macrophage, which is relevant in *Legionella*, but not *M. pneumoniae*, infections. Macrolides and tetracyclines are both active against *Mycoplasma*. Patients treated with macrolides or tetracyclines defervesce rapidly over 24 to 48 hours. Clinical defervescence manifests by an increased feeling of well-being and a decrease in fever. The dry cough persists during and after therapy regardless of the anti-*Mycoplasma* antimicrobial used.

There are important differences in the shedding rates of *Mycoplasma* from respiratory epithelial cells posttherapy when using tetracyclines instead of macrolides. Tetracycline therapy is associated with a more rapid decrease in shedding. Tetracyclines with better ability to penetrate intracellularly, such as doxycycline (Vibramycin), are the most rapid at decreasing *Mycoplasma* shedding, which is an important public health consideration. Mycoplasmas are transmitted by aerosolized droplet infection. Because patients with *Mycoplasma* have a prolonged cough, organisms not eliminated from respiratory epithelial cells may be aerosolized during coughing for weeks following the acute infection, spreading the infection to susceptible individuals via aerosolized droplets. The aim of therapy is to rapidly treat the patient's pneumonia and extrapulmonary sites of involvement. The secondary goal is to rapidly decrease shedding and aerosolization to prevent the spread of *Mycoplasma* to other individuals. An additional therapeutic goal is to decrease the incidence of post-*Mycoplasma* asthma seen in some patients. *M. pneumoniae* CAP may exacerbate preexisting asthma, but may also cause permanent post-CAP asthma in some individuals.

Until recently, doxycycline was the most active antimicrobial to use against *M. pneumoniae*. Currently, the "respiratory quinolones," levofloxacin (Levaquin) and moxifloxacin (Avelox), are highly active anti–*M. pneumoniae* antimicrobials. The respiratory quinolones and doxycycline penetrate cells efficiently and interfere with intracellular enzymes or protein synthesis of intracellular organisms. Respiratory quinolones and doxycycline are highly effective anti-*Mycoplasma* agents and rapidly decrease shedding of *M. pneumoniae* in respiratory secretions.

Therapy for *M. pneumoniae* is ordinarily 1 to 2 weeks. Patients who have impaired cardiopulmonary disease or compromised host may require 2 full weeks of therapy. In patients with borderline cardiopulmonary function, *M. pneumoniae* as with other relatively low virulence pathogens may present as severe CAP. Antimicrobial therapy for typical or atypical CAP should be directed against the presumed pathogen and not based on co-morbidities. Normal healthy hosts are treated with the same antimicrobial as patients hospitalized with severe CAP. Patients hospitalized with compromised cardiopulmonary function severe *Mycoplasma* CAP are most often initially treated intravenously

TABLE 4 Antibiotics Effective Against *M. pneumoniae*

ANTIBIOTIC	DOSE (ADULT)
Mild/Moderate CAP	
Doxycycline	100 mg (IV/PO) q12h
Erythromycin	500 mg (base, estolate, stearate) (PO) q6h
Erythromycin lactobionate	1 g (IV) q6h
Clarithromycin (Biaxin)	500 mg (PO) q12h
Azithromycin (Zithromax)	500 mg (IV) q24h × 2 doses, followed by 500 mg (PO) q24h
Severe CAP	
Levofloxacin (Levaquin)	500 mg (IV/PO) q24h, or 750 mg IV/PO q24h (may allow for shorter duration of therapy)
Moxifloxacin (Avelox)	400 mg (IV/PO) q24h

with doxycycline (Vibramycin), a macrolide, or a respiratory quinolone. Most patients with *M. pneumoniae* CAP present in the ambulatory setting, which permits therapy with oral doxycycline, macrolide, or a respiratory quinolone (Table 4).

References

Ali NJ, Sillis M, Andrews BE, et al: The clinical spectrum and diagnosis of *Mycoplasma pneumoniae* infection, *Q J Med* 58:241–251, 1986.
Cunha BA: Hepatic involvement in *Mycoplasma pneumoniae* community-acquired pneumonia, *J Clin Microbiol* 3:385–386, 2003.
Cunha BA: Influenza: Historical aspects of epidemics and pandemics, *Infect Dis Clin North Am* 18:141–155, 2004.
Cunha BA: The atypical pneumonia. Clinical diagnosis and importance, *Clin Microbiol Infect* 12:12–24, 2006.
Cunha BA: *Pneumonia Essentials*, 3rd ed., Sudbury, MA, 2010, Jones & Bartlett.
Cunha BA: *Antibiotic Essentials*, 14th ed., New Delhi: Jaypee Medical Publishers, 2015.
Cunha BA, Corbett M, Mickail N. Human parainfluenza virus type 3 (HPIV-3) viral community-acquired pneumonia (CAP) mimicking swine influenza (H1N1) during the swine flu pandemic. *Heart Lung* 2011;40:76–80.
Cunha BA, Pherez FM, Strollo S, Syed U, Laguerre M: Severe swine influenza A (H1N1) versus severe human seasonal influenza A (H3N2): clinical comparisons, *Heart Lung* 40:257–261, 2011.
Cunha BA, Raza M: During influenza season: all influenza-like illnesses are not due to influenza: dengue mimicking influenza. *J Emerg Med* 2015;48:e117–20.
Cunha CB, Opal SM. Middle East respiratory syndrome (MERS): a new zoonotic viral pneumonia, *Virulence* 5:650–654, 2014.
Cunha CB: The first atypical pneumonia: the history of the discovery of Mycoplasma pneumoniae, *Infect Dis Clin North Am* 24:1–5, 2010.
Debré R, Couvreur J: Influenza: Clinical features. In Debré R, Celers J, editors: *Clinical Virology: The Evaluation and Management of Human Viral Infections*, Philadelphia, 1970, WB Saunders, pp 507–515.
File TM: Tan JS: *Mycoplasma pneumoniae* pneumonia. In Marrie TJ, editor: *Community-Acquired Pneumonia*, New York, 2001, Kluwer Academic/Plenum Publishers, pp 487–500.
Foster N, Friedman N, Carl J, Piedimonte G: Enterovirus D68: a clinically important respiratory enterovirus, *Cleve Clin J Med* 82:26–31, 2015.
Hammerschlag MR: *Mycoplasma pneumoniae* infections, *Curr Opin Infect Dis* 14:181–186, 2001.
Hurt AC, Selleck P, Komadina N, et al: Susceptibility of highly pathogenic A(H5N1) avian influenza viruses to the neuraminidase inhibitors and adamantanes, *Antiviral Res* 73:228–231, 2007.
Louria DB, Blumenfield HL, Ellis JT: Studies on influenza in the pandemic of 1957–1958. II. Pulmonary complications of influenza, *J Clin Invest* 38:213–265, 1959.
Lu QB, Wo Y, Wang HY, Wei MT, Zhang L, Yang H, et al: Detection of enterovirus 68 as one of the commonest types of enterovirus found in patients with acute respiratory tract infection in China, *J Med Microbiol* 63:408–414, 2014.
Marrie TJ: Empiric treatment of ambulatory community-acquired pneumonia: Always include treatment for atypical agents, *Infect Dis Clin North Am* 18:829–841, 2004.
Murray HW, Masur H, Senterfit LS, Roberts RB: The protean manifestations of *Mycoplasma pneumoniae* infection in adults, *Am J Med* 58:229–242, 1975.
Nisar N, Guleria R, Kumar S, et al: Mycoplasma pneumoniae and its role in asthma, *Postgrad Med J* 83:100–104, 2007.
Yang Y, Guo F, Zhao W, Gu Q, Huang M, Cao Q, Shi Y, et al: Novel avian-origin influenza A (H7N9) in critically ill patients in China, *Crit Care Med* 43:339–345, 2015.

VIRAL RESPIRATORY INFECTIONS

Method of
Robert C. Welliver Sr., MD

CURRENT DIAGNOSIS

- Rapid diagnostic kits are available for many common respiratory viruses. These tests are used increasingly to establish that antibiotic therapy is not necessary in many patients with febrile respiratory illnesses or with lower respiratory tract infections.
- The presence of wheezing on physical examination virtually excludes bacterial infection from consideration in subjects with lower respiratory disease.

CURRENT THERAPY

- The management of most viral respiratory infections consists of rest, adequate caloric and fluid intake, and management of fever and malaise.
- Corticosteroids are essential in the management of croup.
- Specific antiviral therapy is available only for influenza virus infection, and beneficial effects have been more readily achieved in prevention rather than treatment.

Viral infections of the respiratory tract are among the most common infections in humans, and they account for significant morbidity at all ages. Infants and young children can sustain six to eight such infections annually, and adults have an average of nearly two such infections per year.

Rhinoviruses are the most commonly identified etiologic agents and cause illness year-round. Other common causative agents during winter months include influenza viruses and respiratory syncytial virus, and enteroviruses predominate in summer months. The parainfluenza viruses also commonly cause respiratory infection, particularly in autumn (type 1) and late spring or summer (type 3). Coronaviruses, metapneumoviruses, adenoviruses, and other agents are identified less often.

Although each of these agents can cause a common cold, some viral infections are associated with characteristic patterns of respiratory disease. Most of these viruses can also exacerbate asthma, cystic fibrosis, and chronic obstructive pulmonary disease (COPD).

Common Colds

Colds are the most common of the viral respiratory illnesses. Pharyngitis is usually the earliest sign of a cold, beginning a few days after infection has taken place. Nasal congestion and clear or slightly cloudy rhinorrhea usually follow within 24 to 48 hours. Cough occurs in approximately 30% to 40% of those infected, and fluid can accumulate in middle ear or sinus cavities that have become blocked as a result of mucosal swelling. Ear and sinus cavity infections occur when this fluid is trapped for a week or more. Treatment with antibiotics is ineffective before this time, and they are ineffective especially in the absence of other clinical signs of ear and sinus infections.

Colds are a frequent cause of missed school and work, and even of mild morbidity, but they are rarely serious in otherwise healthy persons. The most appropriate approach to treatment therefore entails rest, with adequate nutrition and hydration. Agents that inhibit the activity of cyclooxygenase probably represent the most effective form of pharmacologic intervention. These compounds include acetaminophen (Tylenol) and the nonsteroidal anti-inflammatory agents (NSAIDs) such as ibuprofen (Motrin). They are effective in reducing fever and, perhaps more importantly in most colds, reducing malaise, headache, and pharyngitis.

Nasal congestion and some rhinorrhea during colds are related to dilation of blood vessels in the nose and sinuses. Vasoconstrictors have therefore been used extensively to attempt to reverse these symptoms. Oral decongestants such as pseudoephedrine (Sudafed) have minimal effect on nasal congestion, and can result in systemic hypertension, anxiety, and difficulty sleeping. The propensity for these compounds to cause cardiac arrhythmias in the very young child has led to recommendations against their use in the first year or two of life. Nasal sprays containing vasoconstricting agents such as oxymetazoline (Afrin) can result in mild temporary relief of nasal obstruction. However, the use of these compounds for more than 3 or 4 days can result in rebound vasodilation and paradoxically increased rhinorrhea.

Numerous investigations have evaluated the role of antihistamines in colds. The release of histamine itself is not associated with fever, cough, or malaise, so effects on these symptoms would not be expected. Furthermore, nasal congestion and discharge may be more related to the release of kinins, and not histamine. Indeed, the administration of antihistamines in adults and, particularly, in children has not demonstrated strikingly positive results. As many as 40% of subjects treated with placebo report beneficial effects. Side effects of histamine use, primarily sedation and dry mouth, are commonly encountered.

Cough can be one of the most irritating symptoms during colds. Cough during colds is principally caused by secretions entering the airway (postnasal drip) and not by inflammation of the airway itself. Therefore, it is not surprising that cough suppressants, especially codeine, have little effect on cough induced by colds. Antihistamines have also been found to be ineffective in relief of cough during colds.

Influenza-Like Illness

The influenza syndrome is defined as the abrupt onset of fever, headache, and striking degrees of malaise and prostration, often with intense myalgia. Respiratory symptoms can occur concurrently, but they might not be prominent features. The principal cause is, of course, influenza virus, although infection with many other viruses can cause similar (although not as intense) symptoms. The illness is generally self-limited, and most symptoms resolve over 4 or 5 days. Lassitude can persist for up to 2 weeks.

Influenza virus infection and influenza-like illness are best treated symptomatically, relying on rest, adequate intake of fluids and calories, and appropriate analgesic therapy. Compounds referred to as *M2 inhibitors* such as amantadine (Symmetrel) and rimantadine (Flumadine) have been approved for therapy. Positive outcomes from therapy with these agents are observed only when therapy is instituted within 48 hours after the onset of symptoms, and benefits are not striking. In recent years, resistance to M2 inhibitors has been commonly observed among circulating epidemic strains of influenza virus.

More recently, inhibitors of the activity of influenza viral neuraminidase have been used in treatment and prevention of influenza virus infection in adults and children. The first such compound released, zanamivir (Relenza), was administered by inhalation but was unpopular because of its irritating effects on the airway. An oral compound, oseltamivir (TamiFlu), has been used to prevent and to treat influenza virus infection. As with M2 inhibitors, it is believed that treatment should be started within the first 48 hours of symptoms and that prophylaxis should be instituted within 48 hours of exposure. Treatment with oseltamivir shortens the duration of subsequent illness by only about 24 hours. Treatment can prevent some of the complications of influenza infection, including pneumonia. The drug may be more effective as a therapeutic agent, because it may be up to 90% effective in preventing culture-positive symptomatic influenza illness. The recommended dose for adults is 75 mg orally every 12 hours for 5 days. In children, the appropriate dose based on body weight is 30 mg twice daily for children weighing less than 15 kg, 45 mg twice daily for children weighing 15 to 23 kg, 60 mg twice

daily for children weighing 23 to 40 kg, and 75 mg twice daily for children weighing more than 40 kg. The principal side effect is nausea, which can be reduced by taking the drug with food.

A new type of antiviral (baloxavir marboxil [Xofluza]) was released for treatment of influenza infections in 2018. This drug acts by a different mechanism than previous antivirals used to treat influenza infections. The advantages are that it is given as a single dose for the entire course of treatment, and reduces the duration of influenza illness by approximately 24 hours. It does not seem more effective than oseltamivir in reducing influenza-related symptoms. The appropriate doses are 40 mg for individuals age 12 years or greater and weighing less than 40 kg (88 lbs.) to less than 80 kg (176 lbs), and 80 mg for individuals weighing greater than or equal to 80 kg (176 lbs.).

In 2009, a novel H1N1 strain of influenza caused a worldwide pandemic. At the time of this writing, both this epidemic H1N1 strain as well as the seasonal influenza A/H3N2 and type B strains continue to circulate in the world. The considerable majority of these epidemic and seasonal strains continue to show sensitivity to oseltamivir, while most are resistant to M2 inhibitors. All strains continue to show sensitvity to zanamivir.

Croup

Croup is defined by the occurrence of hoarseness or laryngitis, a deep, brassy or barking cough, and inspiratory stridor. Airway obstruction in croup is caused by constriction in the subglottic area, often noted on radiographs by a steeple-shaped narrowing of the air column in this region. Affected children are usually afebrile and nontoxic in appearance.

Parainfluenza virus type 1 is the primary cause of croup, although infection with many different viruses can produce this illness, and influenza virus can cause a particularly severe form of croup. Bacterial secondary infection occurs uncommonly, but it can result in fever and severe obstruction of the airway. Administration of dexamethasone (Decadron)[1] at 0.6 mg/kg either orally or intramuscularly markedly reduces the rate of hospitalization, admission to the intensive care unit, and intubation for croup.

Bronchiolitis

Bronchiolitis represents the most common cause for hospitalization of infants in developed countries. Infants present with a history of several days of upper respiratory symptoms, followed by the rapid onset of wheezing and labored breathing. Respiratory syncytial virus (RSV) is the most common cause and is the agent found in the most severe cases that result in respiratory failure. Contrasting with asthma, obstruction of the airway in bronchiolitis is a result of plugging of bronchioles with detached epithelium and inflammatory cells. Mucus plugging and constriction of smooth muscle are not prominent. Also in contrast with asthma is the absence of a sustained response to bronchodilators and corticosteroids among infants with bronchiolitis.

Therapy of bronchiolitis primarily consists of administration of supplemental oxygen and replacement of fluid deficits as needed. Ribavirin (Virazole)[1] is a compound with antiviral activity against RSV, but controlled studies have not demonstrated meaningful differences in outcomes between treated and untreated subjects. The compound is quite expensive and must be delivered via a special aerosol generator.

Palivizumab (Synagis), a preparation consisting of a monoclonal antibody against the fusion protein of RSV, has proved to be effective in reducing the rate of hospitalization for RSV infection by approximately 50% when given to high-risk infants. Infants who may be considered candidates for therapy include those with chronic lung disease, those born prematurely, and those with hemodynamically significant congenital heart disease. Doses of palivizumab (15 mg/kg) are given on a monthly basis throughout the local RSV season, usually November through March.

---

[1]Not FDA approved for this indication.

References

Akerlund A, Klint T, Olen L, Runderantz H: Nasal decongestant effect of oxymetazoline in the common cold: An objective dose-response study in 106 patients, *J Laryngol Otol* 103:743–746, 1989.

Buckingham SC, Jafri HS, Bush AN, et al: A randomized, double-blind, placebo-controlled trial of dexamethasone in severe respiratory syncytial virus (RSV) infection: Effects on RSV quantity and clinical outcome, *J Infect Dis* 185:1222–1228, 2002.

Curley FJ, Irwin RS, Pratter MR, et al: Cough and the common cold, *Am J Respir Crit Care Med* 138:305–311, 1988.

Flores G, Horwitz RI: Efficacy of β_2-agonists in bronchiolitis: A reappraisal and meta-analysis, *Pediatrics* 100:233–239, 1997.

Johnson DW, Jacobson S, Edney PC, et al: A comparison of nebulized budesonide, intramuscular dexamethasone, and placebo for moderately severe croup, *N Engl J Med* 339:498–503, 1998.

Muether PS, Gwaltney JM Jr, Jr.: Variant effect of first- and second-generation antihistamines as clues to their mechanism of action on the sneeze reflex in the common cold, *Clin Infect Dis* 33:1483–1488, 2001.

Randolph AG, Wang EL: Ribavirin for respiratory syncytial virus lower respiratory tract infection, *Arch Pediatr Adolesc Med* 150:942–947, 1996.

Tavorner D, Danz C, Economos D: The effects of oral pseudoephedrine on nasal patency in the common cold: A double-blind single-dose placebo-controlled trial, *Clin Otolaryngol* 24:47–51, 1999.

Treanor JJ, Hayden FG, Vrooman PS, et al: Efficacy and safety of the oral neuraminidase inhibitor oseltamivir in treating acute influenza: A randomized controlled trial. US Oral Neuraminnidase Study Group, *JAMA* 283:1016–1024, 2000.

Van Voris LP, Betts RF, Hayden FG, et al: Successful treatment of naturally occurring influenza A/USSR/77 H1N1, *JAMA* 245:1128–1131, 1981.

12 Rheumatology and the Musculoskeletal System

AXIAL SPONDYLOARTHRITIS

Method of
Atul Deodhar, MD; and Sonam Kiwalkar, MBBS

CURRENT DIAGNOSIS

- Axial spondyloarthritis (axSpA) is an umbrella term that includes ankylosing spondylitis (AS) and non-radiographic axial spondyloarthritis (nr-axSpA). Presence or absence of definitive sacroiliitis on radiographs differentiates AS (also called radiographic axSpA) from nr-axSpA. The latter is a condition with the same clinical features and similar disease burden as AS, except definitive radiographic features of sacroiliitis are lacking.
- In the absence of diagnostic criteria, the diagnosis of AS is made by the presence of definitive sacroiliitis on sacroiliac (SI) joint x-ray, plus either chronic (>3 months), inflammatory back pain, or restriction in spinal movements or chest expansion (Modified New York Criteria for Classification of AS).
- Because definitive sacroiliitis may take up to 10 years to appear on a radiograph from the start of chronic inflammatory back pain (the most common first symptom), early or mild disease can be missed.
- When AS is suspected with features of inflammatory back pain usually starting before age 45, along with other clinical features of spondyloarthritis (such as uveitis, psoriasis, enthesitis, asymmetric peripheral inflammatory arthritis, family history of spondyloarthritis, high C-reactive protein (CRP), inflammatory bowel disease, good response to nonsteroidal antiinflammatory drugs [NSAIDs]), but an x-ray of the SI joints is negative or uncertain for definitive sacroiliitis, MRI scan of the SI joints and/or HLA-B27 typing may help in making the diagnosis of axSpA.

CURRENT THERAPY

- Non-pharmacologic interventions include active physical therapy, self-directed physical exercise, patient education, and smoking cessation.
- NSAIDs are the first line of pharmacologic treatment.
- In those who are not adequately responding to NSAIDs, treatment with tumor necrosis factor-α inhibitors (TNFi) or interleukin-17 inhibitors (IL-17i) is recommended.
- Retrospective analysis in cohorts of patients with AS using long-term TNFi has shown reduced rate of new bone formation in the spine, though no pharmaceutical agents have shown "disease modifying" ability in prospective studies to date.
- Conventional synthetic anti-rheumatic drugs such as sulfasalazine or methotrexate[1] can be used to treat peripheral arthritis in axSpA patients, but they do not have efficacy in axial disease.

[1]Not FDA approved for this indication.

Definition and Spectrum of the Disease

Axial spondyloarthritis (axSpA) is an umbrella term that includes ankylosing spondylitis (AS) and non-radiographic axial spondyloarthritis (nr-axSpA). Presence or absence of definitive sacroiliitis on radiographs differentiates AS (also called radiographic axSpA) from nr-axSpA.

AxSpA is a chronic, immune-mediated inflammatory disorder involving the sacroiliac (SI) joints, the spine, and often the hips. In some, spinal bony fusion develops gradually over several years, and may lead to reduced spine and neck flexibility. The axial skeleton is always involved, and involvement of the peripheral joints occurs in approximately 30% of patients. Enthesitis is a common occurrence. Extra-articular manifestations include osteoporosis, psoriasis, acute anterior uveitis, and inflammatory bowel disease (IBD) (i.e., Crohn disease or ulcerative colitis).

Epidemiology

Based on the 2009–2010 National Health and Nutritional Examination Survey (NHANES), the estimated prevalence of axSpA in the US population is about 1.0%, of which 0.5% of patients reported to have AS. The prevalence of nr-axSpA is thus assumed to be the other 0.5%, as pelvic radiographs and SI MRI examinations were not carried out in this population-based study.

The prevalence of axSpA varies with the geographic region and, in general, depends on the prevalence of human leukocyte antigen (HLA)-B27. Prevalence of HLA-B27 is less than 1% in Japan, 3% in African Americans, 8% in Western Europe, 10% to 16% in Scandinavian countries, and more than 20% in some natives of Eastern Siberia and Alaska. AxSpA is thus rare in the Japanese and African American population. The prevalence of axSpA is about 0.5% in persons of European descent and 1.4% in Scandinavia, while it rises to 2% to 3% in Eastern Siberia and Alaska. The risk of axSpA is increased among those with an affected first-degree relative. The male to female ratio is 2:1 for the diagnosis of AS. In contrast patients with nr-axSpA show hardly any difference in its prevalence among males and females.

Pathogenesis

Genetics plays a major role in the pathogenesis of spondyloarthritis and HLA-B27 gene has a major association with AS. HLA-B27 is present in about 70% to 90% of patients with AS in most ethnic groups. The risk of disease in family members of patients with AS is 63% in monozygotic twins, 20% in dizygotic twins, 8.2% in first-degree relatives, 1% in second-degree relatives, and 0.7% in third-degree relatives. The overall contribution to AS heritability by HLA-B27 is estimated to be approximately 20%. Some other genes associated with AS such as endoplasmic reticulum aminopeptidases (ERAP-1 and ERAP-2) and interleukin-23 receptor (IL-23R) have been implicated to play a role in the pathogenesis.

Several hypotheses are put forth to explain the role of HLA-B27 in the pathogenesis of AS:

1. Arthritogenic peptide presentation: Certain antimicrobial peptides have molecular mimicry to self-peptides found in the joints, and it is hypothesized that HLA-B27 presents these to cytotoxic T cells. The activated T-cell lymphocytes then lead to autoreactivity, arthritis, and spondylitis.
2. HLA-B27 heavy chain homodimer: The heavy chains of HLA-B27 molecule can form homodimers when expressed on cell surface, resulting in recognition by natural killer cell receptors.

This can enhance the survival and proliferation of CD-4 T cells and increase IL-17 production in vivo.

3. HLA-B27 misfolding and unfolded protein response: HLA-B27 assembly takes place in the endoplasmic reticulum (ER) before it is expressed on the cell surface. The misfolded HLA-B27 molecules accumulate in the ER, leading to cellular stress secondary to unfolded protein response. This then activates the IL-23/IL-17 pathway of inflammation.

4. HLA-B27 shaping human gut microbiome: The human body contains a large community of commensals and symbiotic bacteria, fungi, and viruses, called microbiota. Microbiome refers to genomes of these microorganisms. The composition of the gut microbiome is influenced by genes and other environmental factors. It is postulated that HLA-B27 predisposes to AS by influencing gut microbiome. Studies have shown that microbiota composition of patients with AS differed from rheumatoid arthritis patients as well as healthy controls. Further, HLA-B27 positive healthy individuals had a different microbiome from HLA-B27 negative subjects.

In animal models of spondyloarthritis, HLA-B27 transgenic rats and mice when raised in a germ-free environment did not develop spondyloarthritis, but developed spondyloarthritis-like disease when housed in a typical laboratory environment, suggesting the role of microbes in the pathogenesis of spondyloarthritis. More than 60% of patients with AS have subclinical acute or chronic intestinal inflammation. This loss of architectural and functional integrity in the intestinal epithelium allows passage of microbial products into the submucosa and then in to systemic circulation. Innate and adaptive immune cells recognize these microbial products and produce proinflammatory cytokines. These microbial products and the immune cells travel from the gut to distant sites like peripheral joints and entheses causing inflammation.

Clinical Manifestations

The most common manifestations of axSpA include chronic inflammatory low back, hip, or buttock pain. The typical characteristics of inflammatory back pain include age of onset less than 40 years, insidious onset without any identifiable cause, improvement with exercise or activity and no improvement with rest, and pain in the second half of the night. Neck pain is rarely the presenting feature due to cervical spine involvement and, when present, is more commonly seen in women.

The limitation of spinal motion is initially the result of axial inflammation, and later is secondary to the ossification of ligamentous structures, bony fusion of apophyseal joints, and outer fibers of the annulus fibrosis of the intervertebral disks leading to development of syndesmophytes.

Hip involvement is seen in up to 40%. The typical symptoms are pain in the groin or radiation of pain to the medial thigh or the knee. Hip involvement is associated with significant functional impairment. Other peripheral joints such as the ankles, knees, shoulders and, to a lesser extent, the sternoclavicular joint, the temporomandibular joint, and small joints of the hands and feet may also be involved.

Enthesitis is a classic feature of axSpA. Enthesitis presents as pain, stiffness, and tenderness at the sites of insertions of ligaments, muscles, or tendons to a bone. Typical areas of enthesitis include the Achilles tendon, plantar fascia attachment to the calcaneum, costochondral junctions, and the paraspinal muscle attachment to the pelvic rim. Diffuse swelling of toes or fingers, called dactylitis ("sausage digits"), is occasionally seen in axSpA.

Extra-articular manifestations (EAMs) associated with axSpA include psoriasis, IBD, uveitis, and osteoporosis. A large epidemiological study found that 42% of axSpA patients had one or more EAMs; uveitis was present in 27%, IBD in 10%, and psoriasis in 11%. Uveitis seen in association with axSpA presents as eye discomfort during a prodromal phase, followed by an acute onset of eye redness, pain, photophobia, and miosis. The usual characteristics of uveitis associated with axSpA are acute in onset, unilateral, and involving the anterior part of the uvea. Even though overt IBD is seen in 10% of axSpA patients, more than 60% have subclinical mucosal inflammation in the gut.

Diagnosis

Within the United States, there is a significant delay of 10 to 14 years in the diagnosis of axSpA from symptom onset. There are many reasons for this, including the commonality of back pain in the general population, and rarity of axSpA as a cause of back pain. There are no specific physical findings or laboratory tests to diagnose axSpA, and the diagnosis is based on pattern recognition and clinical reasoning. Patients with back pain are generally seen by non-rheumatologists, who may not be familiar with features of inflammatory back pain and may not suspect axSpA. In the optimal clinical setting with a patient complaining of onset of chronic (more than 3 months) inflammatory back pain starting before age 45 years, the presence of other features of spondyloarthritis (as described above), a positive HLA B-27 test, and a plain x-ray of the SI joint showing sacroiliitis, the diagnosis of AS would be straightforward. Radiographic findings such as sclerosis; joint erosions; or widening, narrowing, or ankylosis of the SI joint suggest sacroiliitis.

During this early stage of disease (also known as nr-axSpA), MRI scan (without contrast) of the SI joints may show evidence of active inflammation, and may also show structural changes such as sclerosis, fatty metaplasia, or erosions that aid in making the diagnosis. The required sequence of MRI imaging, and the features that suggest a diagnosis of nr-axSpA, include:

1. T1 weighted sequence: Structural changes such as erosions and ankylosis can be seen. Fat metaplasia appears hyperintense.
2. Fat-suppressed T2 weighted (STIR) sequence: Osteitis, representing active inflammation and reported as bone marrow edema, appears hyperintense.

When the clinical suspicion of axSpA is high, but an x-ray of the SI joints is negative or inconclusive for sacroiliitis, the presence of the features noted above on MRI of the SI joints may help in confirming a diagnosis of nr-axSpA.

The changes of inflammation on short-TI inversion recovery (STIR) imaging (i.e., "osteitis") can be seen in professional athletes, military recruits, and even in normal individuals because of mechanical stress ("false positive MRI"). It is therefore important to emphasize that ruling out common causes of back pain, pattern recognition, and clinical reasoning is the key to diagnosis of axSpA.

Plain radiographs of the spine may show characteristic changes in AS. Romanus lesions or the "shiny corner sign" and squaring of the vertebral body are seen due to erosions at the attachments of the spinal ligaments at the vertebral corners in early disease. This is followed by ossification of the outer layer of annulus fibrosis leading to syndesmophyte formation on plain x-ray. In the late stages, ankylosis of the spine, also known as bamboo spine, may be seen in a small percentage of AS patients.

An elevated erythrocyte sedimentation rate (ESR) or C-reactive protein (CRP) is seen in only 30% to 40% of patients with active AS.

Differential Diagnosis

Chronic non-specific back pain is common in the general population (19% according to the NHANES study), hence mechanical causes of back pain should be considered first.

Diffuse idiopathic skeletal hyperostosis (DISH) is sometimes mistaken for "bamboo spine of AS." DISH is a non-inflammatory condition affecting the spine. It is more commonly seen in obese, diabetic males, often greater than the age of 50 years. Radiographically, DISH is characterized by calcification of the anterior longitudinal ligament involving at least four contiguous vertebral bodies, sometimes referred to as "flowing osteophytes." The flowing osteophytes are bulky and typically appear on the right side of the spine. SI joints are not involved in patients with DISH.

Osteitis condensans ilii (OCI) can be mistaken for sacroiliitis, but is usually an asymptomatic, benign disorder of multiparous women. OCI is characterized by radiographic findings of a triangular area of dense sclerosis on the lower and inferior part of iliac side of the SI joint. OCI is not associated with erosions or ankylosis of the SI joints.

Inflammatory back pain with sclerotic changes on SI joint x-ray can also be seen in conditions such as: (1) postpartum insufficiency fracture of the sacrum; (2) septic sacroiliitis from tuberculosis, brucellosis, fungi, and other infectious agents; and (3) rarely malignancies such as acute lymphoblastic leukemia.

Treatment

The goals of treatment of axSpA are to reduce symptoms, improve and maintain spinal flexibility and normal posture, reduce functional limitations, and decrease complications of the disease. The mainstay of treatment has been NSAIDs, exercise and physical therapy, and biologics such as tumor necrosis factor-α inhibitors (TNFi) and interleukin-17 inhibitors (IL-17i).

Treatment of axSpA can be divided into non-pharmacologic, pharmacologic, and surgical interventions.

Non-pharmacologic interventions: Non-pharmacologic interventions include active physical therapy (land or aquatic), self-directed physical exercise, patient education, and smoking cessation. These are recommended at all stages of the disease.

Pharmacologic interventions: Box 1 outlines pharmacologic interventions for the treatment of axSpA.

In clinical practice most of the treatment recommendations for nr-axSpA are extrapolated from studies based on AS. Recently, based on a 52-week placebo-controlled trial, Certolizumab pegol was approved by the FDA for the treatment of nr-axSpA in the US.

| BOX 1 | Pharmacologic Interventions for the Treatment of Ankylosing Spondylitis |

1. NSAIDs are used in full doses either continuously or on an "as required" basis depending on the severity of symptoms, comorbidities, and patient preferences. No particular NSAID is preferred over the other.
2. If patients continue to have symptoms despite a 4-week trial of full-dose NSAIDs, therapy is escalated to TNFi. Currently five TNFi agents are approved for the treatment of AS (and for nr-axSpA in certain countries):
   a. Soluble receptor of TNF—Etanercept 50 mg, SC injection once weekly.
   b. TNFi monoclonal antibodies –
      i. Adalimumab 40 mg SC every 2 weeks.
      ii. Golimumab 50 mg SC once a month or 2 mg/kg IV every 2 months.
      iii. Certolizumab pegol 200 mg SC twice a month or 400 mg SC once a month.
      iv. Infliximab 5 mg/kg intravenous infusion every 6 weeks.
   No TNFi is preferred over the other, except in patients with concomitant uveitis or IBD, monoclonal antibodies are preferred over soluble receptor TNFi.
3. If case of secondary failure of TNFi (failing after initial benefit), an alternative TNFi can be used. In case of primary failure of TNFi (no response), an IL-17i, secukinumab could be used, Secukinumab is given subcutaneously as 150 mg at weeks 0, 1, 2, 3, and 4, followed by 150 mg every 4 weeks.
4. Conventional synthetic DMARDs like sulfasalazine[1] up to 3 g/d and methotrexate up to 25 mg/wk are effective in treatment of peripheral joint involvement but not for axial disease in AS.
5. Local glucocorticoid injections for enthesitis or intra-articular injections for active peripheral arthritis can provide relief for flareups. However, injections of inflamed weight-bearing tendons such as the Achilles tendon is not recommended due to the risk of rupture. Systemic glucocorticoids do not have any benefit in AS, and should be avoided.

---

[1]not FDA approved for this indication.

AS, Ankylosing spondylitis; *DMARDs*, disease-modifying anti-rheumatic drugs; *IBD*, Inflammatory bowel disease; *IL-17i*, interleukin-17 inhibitors; NSAIDs, nonsteroidal antiinflammatory drugs; SC, subcutaneous; TNFi, tumor necrosis factor-α inhibitors.

Some of the side effects of TNFi and IL-17i include injection site reactions with subcutaneous preparations or infusion reactions with infliximab or golimumab. Use of biologics have been associated with increased risk of serious infections. These include bacterial infections, tuberculosis, and herpes zoster. Screening for latent tuberculosis should be performed before the initiation of these therapies because of the increased risk of reactivation of latent tuberculosis. Some of the other adverse effects of TNFi are development of demyelinating disease, worsening of heart failure, recurrence of lymphoma or malignant melanoma, and paradoxical development of psoriasis-like skin lesions. Some of the adverse events of IL-17i include leucopenia, candidiasis, and development or worsening of IBD.

Surgical interventions: Total hip arthroplasty should be considered in patients with refractory hip pain or functional decline in the presence of radiographic evidence of structural damage. Spinal corrective osteotomies are occasionally necessary for fixed kyphotic deformities seen in advanced AS, but should only be undertaken in centers of expertise.

Monitoring

Patients should be regularly monitored for disease activity, function impairment, and medication safety. The frequency of monitoring is individualized. Disease activity assessment can be done by:

1. Bath Ankylosing Spondylitis Disease Activity Index (BASDAI): This is a patient-administered questionnaire with 6 questions answered on a visual analogue scale of 0 to 10. A BASDAI score of ≥4 is indicative of an active disease. Clinically significant improvement is defined as an absolute change of ≥2.
2. Ankylosing Spondylitis Disease Activity Score (ASDAS): It incorporates 3 questions used in BASDAI, a patient global assessment of disease activity, and CRP. An ASDAS score of <1.3 is defined as inactive disease, 1.3 to 2.1 is low disease activity, 2.1 to 3.5 is high disease activity, and >3.5 is very high disease activity. A reduction of ≥1.1 in ASDAS is considered a significant improvement.

Structural damage due to axSpA can be measured by the modified Stoke Ankylosing Spondylitis Spine Score. This score correlates with disease activity as measured with ASDAS.

Functional impairment can be measured by the Bath Ankylosing Spondylitis Functional Index. It is a patient-administered questionnaire that includes 10 activities of daily living. The Bath Ankylosing Spondylitis Metrology Index (BASMI) is an index of spinal and hip mobility in patients with AS. It includes lateral lumbar flexion, tragus-to-wall distance, modified Schober test, maximal intermalleolar distance, and cervical rotation.

The ESR and CRP may be useful in monitoring disease activity. MRI of the SI joints or spine is expensive, and is not indicated to monitor disease activity of AS. Spine x-rays are not used for monitoring purposes in daily practice, though they could be used to counsel patients about life-style changes (such as stopping smoking), or to start biologic therapy.

Complications

The prevalence of osteoporosis is approximately 25% after 10 years of axSpA. Vertebral fractures are seen in about 10% of patients with AS. The lower cervical spine is the most commonly involved area, often accompanied by neurologic compromise. One should consider vertebral fractures in patients with neck and back pain that has changed in intensity or character from baseline. Another rare complication is the cauda equine syndrome from long-standing AS owing to the inflammation of the lumbosacral nerve roots caused by arachnoiditis. Cardiac manifestations including aortic valve insufficiency and conduction abnormalities. Pulmonary manifestations are rare and include chest expansion restriction from ossification of costovertebral joints and upper lobe predominant interstitial lung disease. Patients with AS can have IgA nephropathy, or in late stages, renal amyloidosis if the disease is left untreated. Cardiovascular disease is being recognized as a common comorbidity in patients with AS, and is linked to chronic inflammation. All patients with AS should be counseled about traditional risk factors of cardiovascular disease, and appropriate treatment instituted if necessary.

References

Bennett AN, McGonagle D, O'Connor P, et al: Severity of baseline magnetic resonance imaging-evident sacroiliitis and HLA-B27 status in early inflammatory back pain predict radiographically evident ankylosing spondylitis at eight years, *Arthritis Rheum* 58(11):3413–3418, 2008, Available at: https://doi.org/10.1002/art.24024.

Braun J, Sieper J: Ankylosing spondylitis, *Lancet (London, England)* 369(9570):1379–1390, 2007, Available at: https://doi.org/10.1016/S0140-6736(07)60635-7.

Brophy S, MacKay K, Al-Saidi A, Taylor G, Calin A: The natural history of ankylosing spondylitis as defined by radiological progression, *J Rheumatol* 29(6):1236–1243, 2002.

de Winter JJ, van Mens LJ, van der Heijde D, Landewé R, Baeten DL: Prevalence of peripheral and extra-articular disease in ankylosing spondylitis versus non-radiographic axial spondyloarthritis: A meta-analysis, *Arthritis Res Ther* 18(1), 2016, Available at: https://doi.org/10.1186/s13075-016-1093-z.

Deodhar A, Mease PJ, Reveille JD, et al: Frequency of axial spondyloarthritis diagnosis among patients seen by US rheumatologists for evaluation of chronic back pain, *Arthritis Rheumatol* 68(7):1669–1676, 2016, Available at: https://doi.org/10.1002/art.39612.

Reveille JD: Genetics of spondyloarthritis - Beyond the MHC, *Nat Rev Rheumatol* 8(5):296–304, 2012, Available at: https://doi.org/10.1038/nrrheum.2012.41.

Reveille JD, Witter JP, Weisman MH: Prevalence of axial spondylarthritis in the United States: Estimates from a cross-sectional Survey, *Arthritis Care Res* 64(6):905–910, 2012, Available at: https://doi.org/10.1002/acr.21621.

Rudwaleit M, Khan MA, Sieper J: Commentary: The challenge of diagnosis and classification in early ankylosing spondylitis: Do we need new criteria? *Arthritis Rheum* 52(4):1000–1008, 2005, Available at: https://doi.org/10.1002/art.20990.

Ward MM, Deodhar A, Akl EA, et al: American College of Rheumatology/Spondylitis Association of America/Spondyloarthritis Research and Treatment Network 2015 Recommendations for the Treatment of Ankylosing Spondylitis and Non-radiographic Axial Spondyloarthritis, *Arthritis Rheumatol*, 2016, Available at: https://doi.org/10.1002/art.39298.

Van Der Heijde D, Ramiro S, Landewé R, et al: 2016 update of the ASAS-EULAR management recommendations for axial spondyloarthritis, *Ann Rheum Dis*, 2017, Available at: https://doi.org/10.1136/annrheumdis-2016-210770.

BURSITIS AND TENDINOPATHY

Method of
Kyle Goerl, MD

CURRENT DIAGNOSIS

Tendinopathy
- Tendinitis is an inflammatory condition only present within the first weeks of a tendon injury.
- Tendinosis is a degenerative condition usually developing weeks after the initial injury.
- The diagnosis is typically made clinically with a thorough history and physical examination.
- Most tendinopathies occur secondary to overuse, and can be acute, chronic, or recurrent.
- Tendinopathies are usually characterized by pain, possible swelling, and dysfunction of the affected tendon.
- If the diagnosis is in question, magnetic resonance imaging and ultrasound are helpful diagnostic aides.

Bursitis
- Bursitis is an inflammatory reaction of a bursa.
- Bursitis is typically the result of overuse or trauma, but systemic illnesses can also cause bursitis.
- The olecranon, prepatellar, and trochanteric bursa are particularly susceptible to traumatic bursitis because of their location immediately under the skin with minimal subcutaneous fat for protection.
- Bursitis rarely occurs alone, so a search should be conducted for an associated condition such as tendinopathy or a tendon tear.

- Imaging studies demonstrate that lateral hip pain is usually tendinopathy, not "trochanteric bursitis," a term that should be reserved for image-proven bursitis.
- Septic bursitis usually only affects the olecranon and prepatellar bursa, and care must be taken to distinguish it from aseptic bursitis.
- Common pathogens in septic arthritis include *Staphylococcus aureus* and β-hemolytic *Streptococcus*.
- If the diagnosis of septic bursitis is in question, aspiration should be performed, and the aspirate sent for Gram stain, cell count and differential, culture and crystal analysis, and blood should be sent for culture, complete blood count, C-reactive protein, and erythrocyte sedimentation rate.

CURRENT THERAPY

Tendinopathy
- Given that tendonitis is an inflammatory condition, NSAIDs should be considered. Ice, activity modification, and rest are also effective.
- Tendinosis is not an inflammatory condition, so NSAIDs are not usually a part of the treatment regimen.
- Tendinosis responds well to physical therapy and, in particular, eccentric exercises. Deep tissue massage with tools is also an effective treatment modality.
- Steroid injections can be effective for short term pain relief, but not for long-term healing, and should not be a routine part of the treatment plan. Steroid injections can be considered if the patient is in too much pain to perform physical therapy.
- Injections of blood products such as whole blood and platelet-rich-plasma, prolotherapy and sclerotherapy have varying levels of evidence supporting their effectiveness, but are reasonable alternatives to surgery.
- When conservative measures fail, more invasive procedures such as tenotomy, tendon scraping, and open débridement should be considered, but are rarely needed.

Bursitis
- Early treatment should include NSAIDs, ice, activity modification, and rest.
- If an associated condition like tendinopathy is discovered, appropriate treatment should target that condition as well, and typically involves physical therapy.
- In the event of septic bursitis, antibiotic treatment should be initiated. Parenteral medication should be heavily considered, given the high failure rate of oral antibiotics.
- Surgery is rarely needed for bursitis.

Tendinopathy

Background

Tendon is a connective tissue used to attach muscle to bone. Normal tendon tissue is dense and has a highly regular and fibrillar pattern. Tendinopathy is the term used to describe a clinical syndrome typically resulting from overuse of a tendon. Traditionally the term tendonitis has been used to describe all tendon injuries, but the suffix "–itis" indicates the presence of inflammation, and inflammation is only present early on in the tendinopathy disease process. Inflammation may have resolved and inflammatory cells may no longer be present, but the patient may still have pain. At that point the disease process has changed from one of inflammation to a degenerative problem more appropriately termed tendinosis (Table 1).

Tendinopathies are characterized by pain, swelling, and impairment of functional activities of the affected region. They can be acute, chronic, or recurrent. The diagnosis is usually clinical based on history and physical examination. Typically, there is a history of repetitive motion, which can be anything from painting a wall to playing a sport like tennis. If this historical information is lacking, then a systemic medical condition should be considered.

With repetitive activities and inadequate recovery time tenocytes will begin producing inflammatory substances, and the load-bearing matrix of the tendon will begin to breakdown and become fibrotic. The collagen matrix becomes disorganized with fibers separating and healing in an erratic, disorganized manner. There is an increase in mucoid ground substance, hypercellularity, and pathologic vessel and sensory afferent nerve formation. The abnormal nerve formation likely contributes to the sensation of pain. This histopathological degenerative process is more appropriately called tendinosis. The degenerative mechanism appears to be multifactorial, with contributions from:

1. Classic inflammatory mediators like interleukins, prostaglandins, and substance P.
2. Altered load bearing on a tendon as in shoulder impingement.
3. Systemic influences such as aging.

Tendinopathy is occurring at higher rates in the developed world secondary to an increase in recreational sport participation. Lower extremity tendons, like the Achilles and patellar tendons, bear a large amount of tensile force (Table 2). Thirty percent of runners will suffer Achilles tendinopathy in their lifetime, with an odds ratio of 31:2 when compared with age matched controls, and repetitive exposure is a risk factor. One in 3 patients with Achilles tendinopathy do not participate in sports. With respect to patellar tendinopathy, jumping sports like volleyball and basketball are risk factors. Historically, most lateral hip pain was labeled "trochanteric bursitis." Research using imaging techniques, including magnetic resonance imaging (MRI) and ultrasound (), has concluded that lateral hip pain around the greater trochanter is more likely caused by tendon tears or tendinopathy of the gluteus medius and gluteus minimus muscle-tendon complex than inflammation of the trochanteric bursa. Rarely is there an actual bursitis present, so the diagnosis "trochanteric bursitis" should no longer be used regularly unless there is documented bursitis on an imaging study. This is important because the patient is more likely to benefit long-term from physical therapy (PT) as opposed to nonsteroidal antiinflammatory drugs (NSAIDs), or steroid injections, attributable to the underlying pathology being more likely tendon related than bursa related. Without an imaging study, the better

term for lateral hip pain at this time is greater trochanteric pain syndrome (GTPS).

Many upper extremity tendons, such as those of the wrist, are adapted to gliding through synovial sheaths. The most commonly affected tendons in the upper extremity are the rotator cuff, specifically the supraspinatus tendon, and the common extensor tendon (more precisely the extensor carpi radialis brevis) involved in lateral epicondylopathy, commonly known as *tennis elbow*. Despite names like tennis elbow and golfer's elbow, upper extremity tendinopathies (see Table 2) are more likely the result of repetitive motion from work or hobby related activities. When sports are a cause of upper extremity tendinopathy, they are typically sports requiring overhead motion like baseball, volleyball, and tennis. Up to 35% to 50% of adult tennis players will develop an elbow tendinopathy during their lifetime. A common cause of tendinopathy in the wrist is De Quervain tenosynovitis. De Quervain tenosynovitis affects the first dorsal compartment of the wrist containing the abductor pollicis longus and extensor pollicis brevis tendons. As the term "tenosynovitis" suggests, this condition results in irritation and swelling of not only the tendons themselves, but also of the synovial sheath encapsulating those tendons.

Some patients will develop tendinopathies without repetitive activity. Diseases of glucose metabolism and atherosclerosis are associated with a higher incidence of tendinopathy. Some common medications are also associated with tendinopathy including statins, fluoroquinolone antibiotics, and steroids, especially when steroids are injected intratendinously, which should be avoided.

Evaluation

On physical examination the affected tendon will sometimes appear swollen, and it is typically tender to palpation. The affected tendon-muscle complex may exhibit restricted flexibility, and stretching it or activating it against resistance may reproduce the patient's pain.

When the diagnosis of a tendinopathy is in question, imaging can be helpful. Radiographs of the affected area should be considered, to look for abnormalities such as large calcifications within tendons (Figure 1, A). When the diagnosis is in question or the patient has failed a course of physical therapy, advanced imaging should be considered. This is usually accomplished by either ultrasound or MRI. Ultrasound can reveal thickening or structural changes within the tendon consistent with degeneration and other abnormalities such as calcification. As tendinopathies are commonly associated with bursitis, bursal thickening consistent with bursitis may also be seen (Figures 1, B-C, 2, and 3). Similar findings may be demonstrated on MRI (Figure 4).

Determining which imaging modality to use can be challenging. MRI is considered the gold-standard for diagnosing tendinopathies and has the advantage of demonstrating an anatomic overview of the affected area, in addition to providing soft tissue contrast. However, in trained hands, the advantages of ultrasound include ease of use, point-of-care examination, dynamic evaluation of the tendon and muscles, better resolution than MRI, and guidance for injections and procedures.

Prevention

Prevention is always the best option. Tendons do not respond well to acute changes in routine or long periods of rest. This should be kept in mind by athletes during the off-season, someone taking on a new labor job on an assembly line, or a secretary with a new work space. These "potential patients" should be eased into their new routines, because all of these scenarios are classic setups for the development of a tendinopathy. Maintaining activity during the offseason and preparing one's self for changes in the workplace will help to mitigate the risk of tendinopathy development.

Treatment

Medications are rarely employed in the treatment of tendinosis because the patient usually does not present to the clinician's

TABLE 1	Tendinopathy Progression	
	TENDONITIS	**TENDINOSIS**
Pathology	Inflammatory	Degenerative
Timing	Days to weeks	Weeks to years
Imaging	Typically unnecessary	Radiographs initially Ultrasound or magnetic resonance imaging for persistent symptoms

TABLE 2	Common Tendinopathy Sites

Upper Extremity

- Rotator cuff (especially supraspinatus)
- Medial epicondyle
- Lateral epicondyle (especially extensor carpi radialis brevis)
- First dorsal compartment of the wrist (De Quervain)

Lower Extremity

- Gluteus medius and gluteus minimus
- Iliopsoas
- Patellar
- Achilles

Figure 1 A, AP of the patients shoulder demonstrating a calcific lesion near the humeral head. B, Long axis view; C, short axis view both by ultrasound of the same patient's supraspinatus tendon *(outline)* near its attachment at the humeral head. The humeral cortex shows as hyperechoic on the bottom of the tendon. The calcification is noted to be within the tendon near the attachment. Acoustic shadowing is noted underneath the calcification, which prevents viewing the entire calcific structure and the underlying humeral cortex. *Abbreviations:* CALC=calcification, SS=supraspinatus.

office until long after the disease process has begun. If the patient is caught early enough, for example within a week or two of the offending event (eg, lateral epicondylitis a week after painting a house), then the disease process is still likely an inflammatory one, and appropriately termed a tendonitis. In this case, NSAIDs are appropriate to try to stop the inflammatory process and ultimately try to prevent it from progressing to a degenerative process. Other effective treatments for tendonitis include activity modification, rest, and ice. However, if the patient has had pain for months, the process has likely progressed to tendinosis. The use of NSAIDs has been shown to negatively affect the repair mechanism involved in tendinosis, thus they should be used cautiously in this situation.

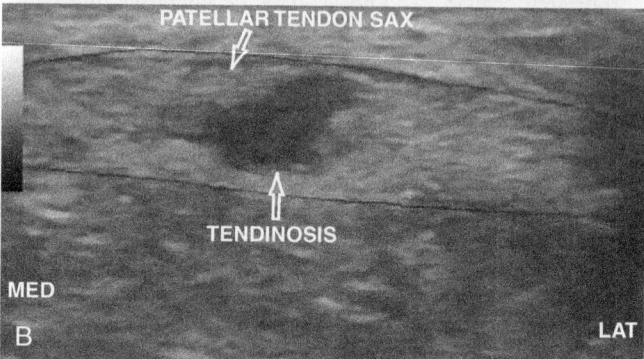

Figure 2 A, Long axis view; B, short axis view both by ultrasound of a patellar tendon *(outline)* demonstrating tendinosis as evidence by the hypoechoic heterogeneous region outline, which represents the degeneration and irregularity of tendinosis. *Abbreviations:* DIST=distal, HFP=Hoffa's fat pad, MED=medial, LAT=lateral, LAX=long axis, P=patella, PROX=proximal, SAX=short axis.

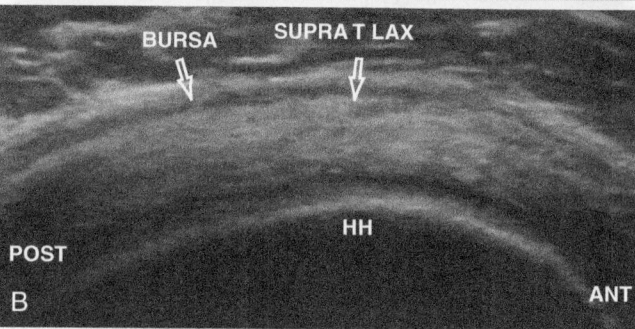

Figure 3 A, long axis view; B, short axis view both by ultrasound of a supraspinatus tendon with a subacromial-subdeltoid bursitis. The tendon is hyperechoic and fibrillar, which is in contrast to the overlying hypoechoic bursa. *Abbreviations:* ANT=anterior, GT=greater tuberosity, HH=humeral head, LAX=long axis, POST=posterior, SAX=short axis, SUPRA T=supraspinatus tendon.

Figure 4 MRI appearance of tendinopathy. Sagittal T1-weighted image of the knee in a professional basketball player demonstrates abnormal signal and increased size in the patellar tendon, consistent with severe tendinopathy *(arrow)*. The tendon is normally devoid of signal. (From Grainger RG, Allison DJ, Adam A, Dixon AK. Grainger and Allison's Diagnostic Radiology, 4th ed. Philadelphia: Churchill Livingstone; 2001.)

Expectations about healing tendinosis should be addressed early. To begin with, tendon healing takes significant time and effort on the part of the patient. Additionally, many of the treatment modalities used to heal tendons will produce a reasonable amount of pain in and of themselves. This is actually a good thing as it indicates the patient is working hard enough to heal and that the healing process is occurring. It is not uncommon to have minor setbacks during the rehabilitation process. There should be an overall trend from a state of disease to health, but the path to recovery is not typically linear. The initial management of tendinopathy should be rehabilitation through PT. The patient should be informed that the "work" of PT is not done at the therapist's office, but it is done at home on their own. Failing to adhere to the treatment program will almost ensure a lack of recovery.

The exercises performed in PT aim to reorganize the degenerative matrix, reduce tenocyte activity, improve tendon compliance, and provide analgesia. Specifically, eccentric exercises have proven to be an effective treatment. An eccentric exercise is one that strengthens the muscle-tendon complex while lengthening the complex. For example, if a patient is being treated for lateral epicondylosis, the eccentric exercise would be to move the wrist from extension to flexion against resistance, lengthening the common extensor tendon. Strengthening exercises also work to hypertrophy the muscle, which is commonly atrophied after long periods of abnormal use from compensatory movement by the patient to try to reduce pain. The time needed for the exercises to work well is 3 months, which correlates with the time needed to form new fibroblasts, the presumed mechanism by which eccentric exercises work.

PT exercises should be done bilaterally as there is a proven crossover effect for tendinopathies, whereby exercising the non-affected side actually improves the affected side. Adding static stretching to eccentric exercises has been shown to improve outcomes over eccentric exercises alone in patellar tendinopathy, and should be included in an effective rehabilitation program. Before releasing an athlete back to sports activity, the final components of an optimal rehabilitation program includes explosive concentric movements (e.g., weightlifting or box jumps), higher eccentric loading exercises (e.g., jumping from an elevated surface like a box and landing on the ground), and sports-specific movements like sprinting and cutting.

The other treatment modality commonly employed by a physical therapist in tendinosis is deep soft tissue massage with tools. These tools are used to scrape along the pathologic tendon, which promotes blood flow and inflammation leading to the breakdown of the degenerative tissue and ultimately healing of that tissue.

When these conservative measures fail, more aggressive treatment methods should be considered. It is important to point out that the following treatment options are supported by limited high quality evidence, but are nonetheless reasonable alternatives to a surgical procedure. Less invasive methods include extracorporeal shockwave therapy and low-intensity pulsed ultrasound. Glyceryl trinitrate patches are sometimes used to promote blood flow, and have been shown to provide some pain relief. Injections are common treatment modalities in tendinopathies. Steroid injections are commonly used, but usually provide short-term pain relief at best. There is evidence for long-term negative effects of steroids, so they should be used judiciously. A reasonable time to try a steroid injection is when the patient is experiencing so much pain that they are unable to perform therapy. Ultrasound guidance in the hands of a trained physician can help ensure that the injection is placed properly, and specifically not intratendinously. Other treatment options requiring a more trained physician, such as a sports medicine specialist, include prolotherapy, sclerotherapy, and biological blood product injections. Prolotherapy, the injection of hypertonic glucose, is thought to work by inducing a local inflammation-repair mechanism. In sclerotherapy, a sclerotic agent, typically polidocanol, is injected to degrade the tendinopathy pain generators, namely the abnormal vessels and sensory nerves within the tendinopathic tissue. Blood products, including whole blood and platelet-rich-plasma, are used with the intent to deliver a high concentration of growth factors to the tendinopathic tissue, where blood flow is typically low.

If the tendinopathy does not respond to these treatment options, then more invasive measures are typically considered. A tenotomy procedure uses a sharp object, typically a large bore needle, to repetitively fenestrate the degenerated portion of tendon tissue, as noted on ultrasound guidance, to cause bleeding, and stimulate tissue healing. There is a newer technique, whereby the outside of tendon is scraped with a needle or scalpel. The procedure is guided by increased color Doppler signal on ultrasound indicating high vascularity and presumed nerve formation. The recovery from these techniques is usually a minimum of 6 weeks, so they should be reserved for recalcitrant cases. Finally, an open procedure can be performed to remove macroscopically abnormal tissue through an incision in the tendon; unfortunately the recovery for this sort of a procedure is in the time frame of 4 to 12 months.

Bursitis
Background
Bursas are fluid filled sacs designed to reduce friction between various tissues including bones, skin, tendons, and muscles. Typically, there is little fluid within a bursa, but with irritation from overuse or trauma, the bursa may swell with fluid leading to pain and dysfunction. This is referred to as bursitis because of the inflammatory nature of the condition.

There are multiple locations in the body where bursitis more commonly occurs, including the shoulder, elbow, hip, and knee. Bursitis usually develops from either trauma or overuse, but systemic illnesses like rheumatoid arthritis, diabetes mellitus, gout or pseudogout, and immunosuppression may also lead to bursitis. Bursas that are more susceptible to traumatic bursitis include the prepatellar, olecranon, and trochanteric bursas; they are closer to the skin and have little subcutaneous fat over them, thus they are more likely to sustain a direct impact. Both the olecranon and prepatellar bursa are also at risk for chronic irritation and trauma. Olecranon bursitis is seen in patients who frequently rest on their elbows, as in desk workers and truck drivers. Prepatellar bursitis is seen in patients who kneel for work like carpet layers and house cleaners.

Septic bursitis is rare, and it most commonly affects the olecranon and prepatellar bursa. This occurs via direct inoculation from the traumatic event. The most common organisms isolated are *Staphylococcus aureus* followed by β-hemolytic *Streptococcus*, with about 10% being polymicrobial infections.

The other bursas in the body are more susceptible to overuse injuries. The bursas around the shoulder most commonly affected include the subacromial-subdeltoid bursa, and the scapulothoracic bursa. Athletes who perform overhead movements in sports like baseball, softball, tennis, volleyball, and swimming are at greater risk for irritating these bursas. Of course, athletes are not the only people at risk for bursitis. Manual laborers working with their arms, especially when flexed or abducted regularly can also develop bursitis around the shoulder.

The hip and pelvis have multiple bursas, but the more commonly affected include the bursas around the greater trochanter and iliopsoas. As stated in the tendinopathy section, lateral hip pain is rarely caused by "trochanteric bursitis," but there are bursa present under the gluteus maximus, gluteus medius, and gluteus minimus muscle-tendon complexes. Bursitis in this region is rarely found without an associated problem like gluteal tendinopathy, or iliotibial (IT) band syndrome. In fact, it is likely that one of these underlying problems led to the bursitis. There is also a bursa under the iliopsoas muscle as it crosses the iliopectineal eminence and anterior hip joint.

Rare causes of knee bursitis include irritation of the suprapatellar bursa, deep infrapatellar bursa, pes anserine bursa, semimembranosus bursa, and medial collateral ligament bursa (Voshell bursa). Bursitis at these locations is almost always from chronic overuse. In the ankle, the retrocalcaneal bursa may also be irritated from overuse.

Evaluation

Evaluation of a patient with suspected bursitis should always begin with a thorough history. Usually the clinician will discover a history of either trauma or overuse, but the patient should also be questioned about the presence of systemic illness. Physical exam of the affected region should include inspection for erythema and swelling. Warmth may be noted on palpation. Range of motion may be limited, but is not a consistent finding. Strength is rarely affected. The appearance of decreased strength may only reflect pain, not true weakness. True weakness would suggest an associated concern like tendinopathy or a tendon tear.

Patients with the presenting symptom of shoulder pain should be evaluated for rotator cuff tendinopathy and scapulothoracic dysfunction and winging, which predispose the athlete to impingement and bursitis. For patients complaining of hip pain, another symptom they may complain of is snapping. The patient should be questioned if the snap is reliably reproducible. If so, then have the patient demonstrate the snap. Snapping laterally is typically the gluteus maximus muscle or the iliotibial band snapping over the greater trochanter, and this is a risk factor for bursitis. If the snapping is anterior in the hip, it is likely the iliopsoas tendon snapping over the iliopectineal eminence or anterior femoral head, which can lead to iliopsoas bursitis.

For the olecranon and prepatellar bursas, special attention must be given to the fact that they are more likely to develop into a septic bursitis from a bacterial infection. If there is evidence of an abrasion in these particular areas, the physician needs to ensure there is not an associated infection. Erythema, progressive swelling, and painful range of motion may point towards the presence of an infection, but these symptoms are often present in aseptic bursitis as well, making the diagnosis difficult. Fever may be present, but its absence does not rule out infection. If there is any concern for infection, the bursa needs to be aspirated and fluid sent for cell count and differential, crystal analysis, gram stain, and culture before starting antibiotics. Blood should also be sent for a complete blood count, C-reactive protein, erythrocyte sedimentation rate, and cultures.

Imaging is not always necessary to diagnose bursitis. Swelling and erythema over a known bursa may be enough to make a diagnosis, but if the diagnosis is in question, then imaging typically begins with radiographs. Radiographs can evaluate for bony abnormalities that may suggest an underlying reason for bursitis. For example, spurring on the undersurface of the acromion can be a risk factor for subacromial-subdeltoid bursitis. Radiographs can also be used to rule out fracture or to evaluate for a foreign body, especially in the setting of olecranon or prepatellar bursitis.

Further evaluation is typically done with either MRI or ultrasound. MRI offers the advantage of global assessment of the affected region, in addition to allowing enhancement of soft tissues. In skilled hands, ultrasound is an effective tool to demonstrate bursitis throughout the body (see Figure 3). Ultrasound also has the distinct advantage of real-time imaging during a dynamic examination of the affected tissue. If aspiration or injection is needed, ultrasound can help guide the procedure. Both MRI and ultrasound modalities are useful in assessing for associated diagnoses like tendinopathy.

Treatment

Bursitis treatment usually begins with conservative measures like rest or activity modification, NSAIDs, compression, padded splinting, and ice. If the bursitis is acute, it is typically responsive to these basic treatments. As stated previously in this chapter, it is common to find associated problems with the bursitis. These include rotator cuff tendinopathy, gluteal tendinopathy, and iliotibial band syndrome. It is imperative that these issues be treated as well or the bursitis will likely reoccur. This typically requires a home exercise plan usually best directed by a physical therapist.

If these problems fail to respond to this conservative approach, including rehabilitation, then a steroid injection can be considered. There is reasonable evidence that doing the injection under ultrasound guidance will lead to better outcomes, especially for the subacromial-subdeltoid bursa, but blind injections are certainly reasonable if ultrasound is not available. Research reveals that steroid injections for greater trochanteric pain syndrome demonstrate clinically relevant relief at 3 months postinjection when compared with usual care, but that difference disappears by 12 months. This is a common finding with steroid injections. Thus, it is reasonable to consider a steroid injection for pain relief, especially if the patient is unable to participate in PT, but it is unlikely to "fix" the patient's problem long-term.

For olecranon and prepatellar bursitis, the clinician must first differentiate between septic and aseptic bursitis. If the bursa is infected, following aspiration and lab collection, antibiotics must be initiated. The decision about whether to use oral versus parenteral antibiotics and whether admission is warranted depends upon the severity of the infection and the reliability of the patient. Oral therapy should be used cautiously, as treatment failure has been seen in up to 39% to 50% of patients. The duration of antibiotic treatment is usually 10 to 14 days. Surgical intervention is rarely necessary, but should be considered in patients who fail to respond to incision and drainage and appropriate antibiotics, if there is suspicion of a foreign body, or there is an inability to adequately drain the bursa.

With aseptic bursitis of the prepatellar and olecranon bursas, the clinician should resist the urge to aspirate and inject with steroids. Aspiration and injection is a possible treatment option, but should only follow a failed conservative approach. The reason for this is that once drained, the bursa is likely to fill with fluid again quickly, and there is a risk for an iatrogenic infection. Steroids are also known to cause skin atrophy. A 6- to 8-week trial of the conservative approach is reasonable.

References

Ackermann PW, Renstrom P: Tendinopathy in sport, *Sports Health* 4:193–201, 2012.

Chang A, Miller TT: Imaging of tendons, *Sports Health* 1:293–300, 2009.

Long SS, Surrey DE, Nazarian LN: Sonography of greater trochanteric pain syndrome and the rarity of primary bursitis, *Am J Roentgenol* 201:1083–1086, 2013.

Reilly D, Kamineni S: Olecranon bursitis, *J Shoulder Elbow Surg* 25:158–167, 2016.

Scott A, Docking S, Vicenzino B, et al: Sports and exercise-related tendinopathies: a review of selected topical issues by participants of the second International Scientific Tendinopathy Symposium (ISTS) Vancouver 2012, *Br J Sports Med* 47:536–544, 2013.

Seroyer ST, Nho SJ, Bach BR, et al: Shoulder pain in the overhead throwing athlete, *Sports Health* 1:108–120, 2009.

Williams BS, Cohen SP: Greater trochanteric pain syndrome: a review of anatomy, diagnosis and treatment, *Anesth Analg* 108:1662–1670, 2009.

Wu T, Song HX, Dong Y, Li JH: Ultrasound-guided versus blind subacromial-subdeltoid bursa injection in adults with shoulder pain: A systematic review and meta-analysis, *Semin Arthritis Rheum* 45:374–378, 2015.

COMMON SPORTS INJURIES

Method of
Andrew S.T. Porter, DO

CURRENT DIAGNOSIS

- **Lateral Ankle Sprain**—Pain over lateral ankle ligament(s) with localized swelling. Often associated with laxity and pain with anterior drawer and/or talar tilt test. Obtain x-rays based on the Ottawa ankle and foot rules.
- **Medial Ankle Sprain**—Less common than lateral ankle sprain. Pain in the deltoid ligament with localized swelling. Obtain x-rays based on Ottawa ankle and foot rules.
- **High Ankle Sprain**—Syndesmotic injury. Pain with squeeze test and/or dorsiflexion with external rotation.
- **Osteochondral Ankle Injuries**—Most commonly seen in the talar dome. Associated with an ankle inversion injury and ankle pain. Often have a joint effusion and soft tissue swelling and can have mechanical symptoms (catching, locking, crepitus, and a feeling of giving way). Obtain x-rays initially and then magnetic resonance imaging (MRI) to grade degree of injury.
- **Anterior Cruciate Ligament (ACL) Injuries**—Most common after noncontact injuries. Physical examination reveals a diffuse knee effusion, positive Lachman, and/or anterior drawer test. Obtain x-rays then MRI for further evaluation.
- **Posterior Cruciate Ligament (PCL) Injuries**—Occur with varus/valgus stress with the knee in full extension. Physical examination reveals a positive posterior drawer and sag sign. Obtain x-rays then MRI for further evaluation.
- **Medial Collateral Ligament (MCL) Injuries**—Occur with valgus stress or twisting with or without contact. Physical examination reveals localized effusion and a positive valgus stress testing and tenderness to palpation along the MCL. Graded 1 to 3.
- **Osteochondral Knee Injuries**—Most commonly seen in the femoral condyle. Associated with a knee injury. Knee pain and, often, mechanical symptoms of the knee. Palpation of the femoral condyles with the knee in flexion reproduces pain. Obtain x-rays initially and then MRI to grade degree of injury.
- **Mallet Finger**—Disruption of the extensor mechanism insertion into the distal phalanx.
- **Jersey Finger**—Occurs after avulsion of the flexor digitorum profundus tendon from its insertion on the distal phalanx.
- **Proximal Interphalangeal (PIP) Joint Dorsal Dislocation**—Injury to the volar plate with or without an avulsion fracture.
- **Scaphoid Fracture**—Pain over the scaphoid with or without a fall on an outstretched hand injury is a scaphoid fracture until proven otherwise. Obtain wrist x-rays with a scaphoid view.

- **Tendinosis**—Repetitive chronic tendon injuries result in scarring, disorganization of fibers, degeneration, and are without an inflammatory component.
- **Stress Fractures**—Most often seen in active patients as a result of excessive stress on normal bone from overactivity or normal stress on a bone that is deficient (osteoporotic, poor nutrition, or in female athlete triad). History is positive for bone pain, and physical examination reveals tenderness to palpation in the affected bone and often a positive tuning fork test, hop test, and fulcrum test. Obtain x-rays first, then MRI or bone scan if needed.
- **Spondylolysis/Spondylolisthesis**—Most often seen in young athletes with insidious onset low back pain and history of repetitive extension. Positive stork test. X-rays initially, and if negative, may proceed with limited CT and SPECT scan or MRI.

CURRENT THERAPY

- **Lateral Ankle Sprain**—Treat with RICE (rest, ice, compression, elevation) and early rehab. Return to play (RTP) is generally 1 to 4 weeks and is based on functional progression. RTP with ankle brace.
- **Medial Ankle Sprain**—Treat with RICE and early rehab. RTP with ankle brace.
- **High Ankle Sprain**—Treat with RICE and boot for 1 to 3 weeks and then rehab. RTP takes a longer time compared with lateral ankle sprain.
- **Osteochondral Ankle Injuries**—Degree of injury is graded via MRI, and this guides treatment and RTP.
- **ACL Injuries**—ACL tears often need reconstruction that is individualized in active patients who require knee stability.
- **PCL Injuries**—Isolated PCL injuries often heal conservatively with protected weight bearing in an extension brace and knee rehab.
- **MCL Injuries**—Often heal conservatively with bilateral hinged knee brace and knee rehab. Generally, RTP in 2 to 6 weeks.
- **Osteochondral Knee Injuries**—Degree of injury is graded via MRI, and this guides treatment and RTP.
- **Mallet Finger**—Treat with continuous full-extension stack splinting of the distal interphalangeal joint for 6 weeks and then nighttime splinting and activity splinting for 6 weeks.
- **Jersey Finger**—Treatment is referral to orthopedic surgeon for surgical intervention.
- **PIP joint dorsal dislocation**—Reduce dislocation and obtain x-rays. Treat with progressive extension blocking splint with 30° to 40° of flexion and decrease by 10° per week.
- **Scaphoid Fracture**—If x-rays with scaphoid view are negative, place in a short-arm thumb spica cast and follow up in 2 weeks. If x-rays remain negative but pain persists, obtain a CT or MRI. Treat nondisplaced scaphoid fractures with short-arm thumb spica cast: proximal-third fractures 12 to 20 weeks, middle-third fractures 10 to 12 weeks, and distal-third fractures 4 to 6 weeks.
- **Tendinosis**—Treat by creating inflammation to facilitate healing.
- **Stress Fractures**—Treat with general treatment for stress fractures plus specific treatment based on stress fracture site.
- **Spondylolysis/Spondylolisthesis**—Treat with extension blocking brace, rest, rehabilitation with core strengthening and lower extremity flexibility, and gradual RTP.

Ankle Injuries

The ankle is the most common joint injured in athletes. Ankle sprains are common, as they represent 25% of all sports-related injuries. The Ottawa ankle and foot rules help in the decision to obtain x-rays (Box 1). In general, treatment will consist of RICE (rest, ice, compression, elevation), early mobilization, and rehab. Prevention of ankle injuries is important and consists of ankle braces, ankle taping, neuromuscular training program, and regular sport-specific warm-up exercises.

Lateral Ankle Sprain

The most common ankle sprain is a lateral inversion sprain that results from landing on an inverted foot with or without plantarflexion. The lateral ankle ligaments are the anterior talofibular ligament (ATFL), calcaneofibular ligament, and the posterior talofibular ligament. The ATFL is the most commonly sprained ligament. Lateral ankle sprains are most commonly treated with RICE initially, then early ambulation, range of motion, progression into strengthening, and then proprioception rehabilitation. Proprioception rehabilitation includes balancing on one leg and performing balancing exercises on a wobble board. For example, patients can balance on one leg when brushing their teeth. Athletes should return to play (RTP) with a lace-up/velcro ankle brace after injury with or without taping. This added stability will help prevent future ankle injuries and also decrease the severity of ankle injuries. Most athletes will RTP in a few days to 4 weeks; this return is based on pain, obtaining full active range of motion and full strength, and functional stability.

Medial Ankle Sprain

Medial ankle ligament sprains are rare, account for < 10% of ankle injuries, and are often accompanied with a lateral malleolar fracture or syndesmotic injury. The medial ankle ligament is the deltoid ligament and is injured via external rotation or eversion. These ankle sprains are treated similarly to lateral ankle sprains.

High Ankle Sprain

High ankle sprains, also known as syndesmotic ankle sprains, occur through forced external rotation of a dorsiflexed foot most commonly but also occur by forced internal rotation of a fixed plantar flexed foot. The syndesmotic ligaments connect and stabilize the distal tibia to the distal fibula. The syndesmotic ligaments are the anterior tibiofibular ligament, posterior tibiofibular ligament, transverse tibiofibular ligament, interosseous ligament, and the interosseous membrane. Palpate the fibular head for pain. Pain on palpation of the fibular head might indicate a maisonneuve fracture, a fracture of the proximal third of the fibula associated with syndesmotic disruption. A high ankle sprain has a longer healing time compared to a lateral ankle sprain. Often these need immobilization with a boot or cast for 1 to 4 weeks to help with healing before beginning rehab. RTP after a high ankle sprain depends on pain, achieving a full active range of motion, full strength, and functional stability. Incomplete healing of a high ankle sprain can result in distal tibia and fibula instability.

Osteochondral Ankle Injuries

Osteochondral injuries are injuries to the articular surface of a joint. These injuries range from small undisplaced depressions and cracks in the osteochondral surface to small pieces of articular cartilage and bone that break off of the articular surface and float within the joint. Osteochondral injuries occur most commonly on weight-bearing articular surfaces. In osteochondral injuries, osteonecrosis of subchondral bone occurs, resulting in separation of cartilage and subchondral bone from underlying, well-vascularized bone. The term *osteochondral lesion* (OCL) is favored over the previously used term *osteochondritis dessicans* because there might not be an inflammatory component of the injury. OCLs are often associated with repeated trauma or overuse in athletes. OCLs typically present with pain in the affected joint and can develop with a specific injury or over several months in highly active athletes. OCLs are more common in younger patients with open physes (growth plates) and are referred to as juvenile OCLs. Adult OCLs describe this condition in skeletally mature patients.

Osteochondral injuries are a cause for pain in up to 25% of ankle injuries and need to be considered when a patient presents with ankle pain. Acute osteochondral injuries in the ankle most commonly affect the talar dome (Figures 1–3) but can also be found in the distal tibia (Figure 4). OCLs are first evaluated by x-rays (see Figures 1 and 2) and then graded by magnetic resonance imaging (MRI) (Table 1). CT scan (see Figure 3) is sometimes utilized as well. Grade 1 to 3 juvenile OCLs and grade 1 to 2 adult OCLs are treated conservatively. Conservative treatment consists of no weight bearing (NWB) in a cast or boot for 6 to 10 weeks followed by partial weight bearing (PWB) to full weight bearing (FWB) over 2 to 6 weeks, followed with an ankle brace for 3 months, and ensuring adequate calcium and vitamin D intake to facilitate healing. Nonsteroidal antiinflammatory drugs (NSAIDs) should be avoided because they can slow bone healing, and OCLs are probably not an inflammatory process. For grade 4 juvenile OCLs, grade 3 and 4 adult OCLs, and those that have not clinically healed with conservative care operative treatment is required. Operative treatment options depend on OCL size and type and include removal of the OCL followed by transchondral drilling and microfracture to stimulate fibrocartilage formation, fixation of the OCL with an osteochondral allograft, osteochondral autograft transfer, and autologous chondrocyte implantation.

Knee injuries—The knee joint lacks intrinsic bone stability, so most stability is from the major knee ligaments.

Anterior Cruciate Ligament Injuries

The anterior cruciate ligament (ACL) is the key stabilizer of the knee and is one of two major intraarticular knee ligaments, the other being the posterior cruciate ligament (PCL). Most ACL tears occur from noncontact injuries. Women experience ACL tears up to nine times more often than men do. The main function of the ACL is to prevent excessive anterior tibial translation relative to the femur. Patients who sustain an injury to their ACL often describe hearing a pop, feeling instability in their knee, experiencing pain immediately after the injury, and develop an associated knee effusion. On-the-field evaluation is ideal in an ACL injury, as the hamstrings will often start to tighten up shortly after the injury, preventing anterior tibial translation. This will prevent an isolated test of the ACL and give the false impression that an ACL endpoint is present when in fact the ACL is completely torn. The anterior drawer (Figure 5) and Lachman test (Figure 6) are the main physical examination tests to evaluate the ACL. Obtain x-rays and then MRI if an ACL tear is suspected. The blood supply to the ACL is poor and is provided by the middle geniculate artery off of the popliteal artery. Because of the poor blood supply, ACL tears often need reconstruction if athletes want to return to a high level of activity and knee stability is needed. ACL reconstruction timing is important and often will occur 3 to 4 weeks after injury to allow for swelling to decrease, ROM and strength to improve,

Figure 1 X-rays of the left ankle, AP and mortise views, which demonstrate a grade 2 osteochondral lesion (OCL) along the medial talar dome.

Figure 2 X-ray of the left ankle, mortise view, which demonstrates a grade 4 OCL along the lateral talar dome.

Figure 3 CT scan without contrast. Sagittal image of ankle, which demonstrates a grade 4 OCL of the talar dome.

and inflammation to decrease. Also during this presurgical time, it is important to have patients perform pre-hab (presurgical rehabilitation), focusing on AROM and knee strengthening. A knee effusion will cause the quadriceps muscles to weaken and atrophy. Hamstring tendon autograft, patella tendon autograft, quadriceps tendon autograft, and allograft are all used for ACL reconstruction. Each graft has advantages and disadvantages and should be discussed with the orthopaedic surgeon before reconstruction and

individualized for each patient. Continuing to participate in high-level activity after an ACL tear if undiagnosed can lead to a knee dislocation and further intraarticular knee injury.

PCL Injuries

The PCL is the other major intraarticular knee ligament. Isolated PCL injuries are much less common than ACL injuries and make up only 3.5% of ligamentous knee injuries in sports, with the remaining 96.5% of PCL injuries associated with multiligamentous knee injuries. PCL injuries, unlike ACL injuries, are the result of external forces (e.g., a soccer player sliding into the goal post and tearing his or her PCL). The main function of the PCL is to resist posterior tibial translation. Posterior drawer testing (Figure 7) and a sag sign test (Figure 8) are the physical examination tests used to evaluate the PCL. Obtain x-rays then MRI if a PCL tear is suspected. The blood supply to the PCL is better than the blood supply to the ACL. Isolated PCL injuries (grades 1 and 2) are treated conservatively because surgical reconstruction has not been shown to be helpful. Conservative treatment consists

Figure 4 CT scan without contrast. Coronal image of ankle, which demonstrates a grade 1 OCL of the distal lateral tibia.

TABLE 1	Classification of Osteochondral Lesions	
STAGE	PLAIN X-RAY FINDINGS	MRI FINDINGS
1	Depressed osteochondral fragment	Articular cartilage thickening and low signal changes in subchondral bone
2	Osteochondral fragment attached by bone	Articular cartilage breached, no synovial fluid around fragment
3	Detached nondisplaced fragment	Articular cartilage breached, synovial fluid around fragment
4	Displaced fragment	Loose foreign body

Figure 5 Anterior drawer test for ACL laxity. Patient's knee is flexed 90°. Examiner applies anterior force to the tibia in relation to the patient's femur to evaluate for laxity.

Figure 6 Lachman test for ACL laxity. Patient's knee is flexed 20°–30°. Examiner grasps the distal femur and proximal tibia and applies anterior force to the tibia and posterior force to the femur to evaluate for ACL laxity.

Figure 7 Posterior drawer test for PCL laxity. Patient's knee is flexed 90°. Examiner applies posterior force to the tibia in relation to the patient's femur to evaluate for laxity.

Figure 8 Sag sign test for PCL laxity. Examiner views the tibia condyles from the lateral side to evaluate for a posterior sag (displacement) in the appearance that would indicate a PCL injury.

of protected weight bearing in an extension brace followed by quadriceps rehabilitation and ROM exercises. RTP is generally 4 to 6 weeks after a PCL injury. Surgical intervention is recommended for associated injuries to the ACL, medial collateral ligament (MCL), and posterior lateral corner (grade 3 PCL injury).

MCL Injuries

The MCL is an extraarticular ligament that resists knee valgus forces. An MCL sprain results from a valgus stress to a partially flexed knee. Athletes will present with localized pain and swelling along the medial aspect of the knee. Most MCL injuries are isolated ligament injuries, but more severe MCL injuries can involve tears of the medial meniscus and ACL, commonly referred to as the "terrible triad." The MCL is examined by palpation and valgus stress testing at 0° and 30° of knee flexion. MCL injuries are graded 1, 2, or 3 depending on severity of injury. A patient with a grade 1 MCL sprain has pain in the MCL but no valgus stress testing laxity. A grade 2 MCL sprain has valgus stress testing laxity but a solid endpoint. A grade 3 MCL sprain has no endpoint with valgus

Figure 9 X-ray of the bilateral knees, AP view, which demonstrates a grade 1 OCL along the right knee medial femoral condyle.

Figure 10 Magnetic resonance imaging (MRI) of the right knee, without contrast. Coronal T2 fat saturation image, which demonstrates a grade 4 OCL of the medial femoral condyle.

stress testing. Thankfully, the MCL has a rich vascular supply and can often heal conservatively. Treatment consists of RICE for the first 1 to 2 weeks and a bilateral hinged knee brace to facilitate healing. Weight bearing and ROM and strengthening exercises are started when they are tolerable. RTP after an MCL injury depends on the grade and generally takes 2 to 6 weeks.

Osteochondral Knee Injuries

Osteochondral injuries occur in the knee as well as in the ankle. Osteochondral injuries of the knee most commonly affect the lateral aspect of the medial femoral condyle but can be found anywhere along the medial or lateral femoral condyle, patella, or trochlea. History is significant for knee pain, with or without swelling and mechanical symptoms (catching, locking, crepitus, and feeling of giving way). On palpation, patients can have pain in the affected area with knee flexion with or without crepitus. Obtain x-rays initially (Figure 9) and then grade the OCL severity by MRI (Figure 10). CT scans are also utilized sometimes. Grade 1 to 3 juvenile knee OCLs and grade 1 to 2 adult knee OCLs are treated conservatively. Grade 4 juvenile OCLs, grade 3 to 4 adult OCLs and all OCLs that have failed conservative care are treated operatively.

Hand Injuries

Mallet Finger

A mallet finger occurs after forced flexion of an actively extended distal interphalangeal (DIP) joint, resulting in disruption of the extensor mechanism insertion into the distal phalanx. Patients with a mallet finger are unable to actively extend the DIP joint. This injury can be associated with an avulsion fracture (Figure 11). For acute injuries, general treatment consists of continuous extension splinting of the DIP joint (0° to 10° of hyperextension) for at least 6 weeks. The 6-week clock starts over if the DIP joint is allowed to flex at all during the initial 6 weeks of treatment or if, at the end of the 6 weeks, the mallet finger is not completely healed. After the initial 6 weeks, it is recommended to continue with nighttime splinting and activity splinting for another 6 weeks to ensure adequate healing and avoidance of surgery. To perform this splinting, a stack splint is well tolerated and is protective (Figure 12). Orthopaedic referral is indicated if the patient is unable to obtain full passive extension of the DIP joint or if the avulsion fracture involves over 30% of the joint space.

Jersey Finger

A jersey finger results from the avulsion of the flexor digitorum profundus tendon from its insertion on the distal phalanx. This commonly occurs in football and rugby players when the tip of their flexed finger is caught in a jersey and the DIP joint of the finger is then forcefully extended. After this injury occurs, the patient is unable to actively flex the DIP joint. Treatment is urgent referral to an orthopaedic surgeon for surgical intervention.

Proximal Interphalangeal Joint Dorsal Dislocation

Proximal interphalangeal (PIP) joint injuries are the most common joint injuries in sports. Most PIP dislocations are dorsal and

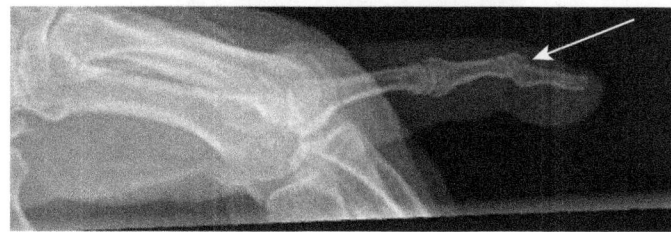

Figure 11 X-ray of the left hand, lateral view, which demonstrates a mallet finger of the fifth finger. Note the flexion of the DIP joint and avulsion fracture of the distal phalanx that involves about 30% of the joint space.

result from hyperextension with an axial load. Dislocations are described by the position of the distal fragment in relation to the proximal fragment. PIP dorsal dislocations cause injury to the volar plate with or without avulsion fracture. Pre-reduction x-rays are preferred if they can be obtained promptly (Figure 13). X-rays of the finger with at least one view being a true lateral view should be obtained to rule out fracture. However, many PIP dorsal dislocations occur on the playing field and it is reasonable to reduce these dislocations, buddy tape the affected finger, and allow the patient to RTP with x-rays obtained after the athletic competition. Reduction is usually uncomplicated and is performed urgently via hyperextending the joint, applying traction in plane with the finger, then flexing the joint. Post reduction films are a necessity (Figure 14). Stability testing of the collateral ligaments should be performed after the reduction. Full flexion and extension of the PIP joint will be possible if the joint is stable. A stable joint without a large avulsion fragment should be treated with a progressive extension blocking splint (Figures 15 and 16). Start with 30° to 40° of flexion and decrease by 10° per week over 3 to 4 weeks, then buddy tape the injured finger with activity PRN (8). Some PIP dorsal dislocations have a lateral component to them and these are treated similar to pure dorsal dislocations (see Figure 13). Orthopaedic surgeon referral is indicated if there is a large avulsion fracture or the joint is unstable.

Figure 12 Stack splint with Coban wrap added for stability that immobilizes the DIP joint at neutral to 5° of hyperextension.

Figure 14 X-ray of the left hand, lateral status postreduction view, which demonstrates a relocated proximal interphalangeal (PIP) joint. Note the avulsion fracture of the middle phalanx.

Figure 15 Dorsal extension blocking splint at 30°–40° of flexion at the PIP joint. Note that there is no pressure over the PIP joint volar plate and that flexion and extension at the DIP joint is possible.

Figure 13 X-ray of the left hand, oblique view, which demonstrates a proximal interphalangeal (PIP) joint dorsal and lateral dislocation.

Figure 16 Dorsal extension blocking splint at 30°–40° of flexion at the PIP joint. This figure illustrates the freedom of motion that is possible at the PIP joint (full flexion and limited extension) and the DIP joint (full flexion and extension).

Figure 17 Scaphoid view x-ray (AP view with ulnar deviation) is important to obtain in addition to your standard wrist views (AP, lateral, and oblique) when scaphoid fracture is suspected. This scaphoid fracture was not seen on the x-rays on the day of the injury. Patient continued to have wrist pain and then presented 10 weeks later, and x-rays were obtained demonstrating the scaphoid fracture.

Scaphoid Fracture

The scaphoid bone is the most common carpal bone that is fractured and is a common injury that is encountered in primary care. Interestingly, scaphoid fractures occur most commonly in young men. Scaphoid fractures occur less commonly in young children and the elderly because of the relative weakness of the distal radius compared with the scaphoid in these age groups. Often a scaphoid fracture is caused by a FOOSH (fall on an outstretched hand) injury. On physical examination, if the patient has pain over the scaphoid tubercle or in the anatomical snuffbox with or without a history of a FOOSH injury, the clinician needs to have a high index of suspicion for a scaphoid fracture when evaluating the wrist x-rays. Obtain the standard wrist

x-rays (AP, lateral, and oblique views) plus a dedicated scaphoid view (AP with ulnar deviation) and be aware that early imaging with x-rays is often unrevealing for a scaphoid fracture (Figure 17). If a fracture is not seen on x-rays, the clinician needs to have a high index of suspicion for a scaphoid fracture, place the patient in a short-arm thumb spica cast, and have the patient follow up in 2 weeks. If repeat x-rays remain negative and the patient continues to have scaphoid pain, proceed with an MRI of the wrist with T2 fat saturation views or a CT scan. If a scaphoid fracture is noted on imaging, the location of the scaphoid fracture will guide treatment. Because the blood supply to the scaphoid is distal to proximal, scaphoid fractures are harder to heal than other carpal fractures. Nondisplaced middle-third or proximal-third scaphoid fractures are treated with a long- or short-arm thumb spica cast with the wrist at 20° to 30° of extension and the thumb in slight extension and abduction for 10 to 20 weeks. Middle-third fractures should be immobilized for 10 to 12 weeks. Proximal-third fractures should be immobilized from 12 to 20 weeks. It is much easier to regain flexion in the wrist after casting than it is to regain extension. If the elbow is incorporated in the cast, it should be casted at 90° of flexion. A long-arm cast may decrease healing time, but it does not improve nonunion rates. A nondisplaced distal-third fracture should be treated in a short-arm thumb spica cast for 4 to 6 weeks. For displaced fractures or non-healing fractures, a referral to an orthopedic surgeon is recommended. Use acetaminophen for pain control and avoid nonsteroidal antiinflammatory drugs (NSAIDs) because NSAIDs can impair bone healing. Ensure adequate energy availability via diet and adequate calcium and vitamin D intake, and avoid tobacco exposure to help heal the fracture. Bone health and bone nutrition are a part of the big picture in fracture healing.

Overuse Injuries
Tendinosis

The paradigm and management of tendon overuse injuries is changing. The term *tendinitis* is generally used to refer to painful overuse tendon conditions and implies that inflammation is present. However, the most common pathology in chronic painful tendons is tendinosis. Tendinosis occurs after repetitive injuries to a tendon results in intertendinous scarring, disorganization of tendon fibers, and degeneration. Tendinosis does not have an inflammatory component. Early on in a tendon injury, there is inflammation resulting in tendinitis, but after about 6 weeks this generally evolves into tendinosis. Early activity modification and treatment of tendinitis with NSAIDs and rehabilitation may prevent the development of tendinosis. Tendinosis is a problematic condition that affects many active people, young and old. To address these more chronic tendon injuries, healing is facilitated by creating an inflammatory response. To create inflammation, treatments such as eccentric strengthening (Figure 18), deep soft tissue massage with tools (e.g., gua sha or Graston, or ASTYM) (Figure 19), nitroglycerin patches (Nitro-Dur),[1] and musculoskeletal ultrasound-guided percutaneous needle tenotomy (with or without injection of autologous blood, prolotherapy, or platelet-rich plasma) have all been utilized and have been shown to be effective (Table 2). It is important to avoid NSAIDs when trying to create inflammation because NSAIDs will prevent the inflammatory response. This concept of tendinosis diagnosis and treatment can be utilized for tendons throughout the body and is most commonly applied to the Achilles tendon, patella tendon, iliotibial (IT) band, piriformis, gluteus medius, hamstrings, biceps, common elbow flexor tendon, and common elbow extensor tendon.

Stress Fractures

Stress fractures occur when osteoclastic activity overwhelms osteoblastic activity. Bone injury unfolds over a continuum of time,

---

[1]Not FDA approved for this indication.

Figure 18 Eccentric exercises for Achilles tendinosis. (**A**) Patient begins with the injured leg straight and the ankle in flexion. The assistance of the uninjured leg was utilized to get in this starting position. (**B**) The ankle of the injured leg (right leg, in this case) is slowly lowered in a controlled fashion to full dorsiflexion to eccentrically strengthen (while lengthening the calf muscles) the right Achilles tendon. The left leg is then brought back down, and full plantarflexion in both ankles is performed, recruiting the uninjured leg to assist with getting back to position (**A**). (**C**) The eccentric exercise from (**B**) is repeated with the knee bent at 45°.

Figure 19 ASTYM® tools.

TABLE 3	Stress Fracture Physical Exam Tests
PHYSICAL EXAM TEST	**POSITIVE TEST**
Palpation	Pain over affected bone with palpation
Stork test (Figure 22)	Back extension with rotation while standing on one leg increases pain in the pars interarticularis region
Fulcrum test	Pain in fracture site while applying a bending force (e.g., over the exam table) to distal extremity while proximal extremity is kept relatively immobilized
Hop test	Hopping 10 times on affected leg reproduces pain at fracture site
Tuning fork test	Vibrating tuning fork over fracture site results in pain at site

TABLE 2	Treatment of Tendinosis
TREATMENT MODALITY	**DESCRIPTION**
Deep soft tissue massage with tools (gua sha, Graston, ASTYM) (Figure 19)	One to three times per week for 4–6 wk; most common with athletic trainer certified or physical therapist
Nitroglycerin patches (Nitro-Dur)[1]	0.1 mg/h patch, apply Q24 h to a different location on tendon for at least 6 wk
Eccentric strengthening (Figure 18)	3 sets of 15 exercises, twice daily, for 12 wk
Musculoskeletal ultrasound-guided percutaneous needle tenotomy with or without autologous blood injection, prolotherapy, or platelet-rich plasma	Referral to primary care sports medicine physician

[1]Not FDA approved for this indication.

starting with normal bone that progresses to stress reaction, then stress fracture, and finally fracture if the bone continues to be injured. This can occur as a result of excessive stress on normal bone from overactivity or normal stress on a bone that is deficient (osteoporotic, poor nutrition, or in female athlete triad). Stress fractures are common injuries in athletes and occur most often in the lower extremities. Running sports account for 69% of stress fractures. Stress fractures should be considered in someone who is active, presents with bone pain, and who performs repetitive activities with limited rest or with a recent increase in activity. Physical examination tests to perform in the area of interest are palpation, the tuning fork test, the fulcrum test, and the hop test (Table 3). If a stress fracture is suspected, x-rays should be obtained, keeping in mind that it takes 2 to 3 weeks for signs of stress fracture (i.e., periosteal reaction, callus formation, fracture line) to show up on an x-ray, and often stress fractures do not show up on x-rays. If x-rays are negative and a diagnosis is needed to help guide care and RTP, a bone scan or MRI with T2 fat saturation views (Figures 20 and 21) should be obtained. The bone scan and MRI are equally sensitive, but an MRI is more specific and avoids patient radiation exposure. An MRI is more expensive. Because a bone scan can stay positive for up to 18 months, clinical progress should not be monitored with a bone scan.

Figure 20 MRI of the right hip without contrast. Coronal T2 fat saturation image demonstrates a compression-sided femoral neck stress fracture (note surrounding bone edema in white).

Figure 21 MRI of the right hip without contrast. Axial T2 fat saturation image that demonstrates a compression sided femoral neck stress fracture (note edema in *white* and probable fracture line in *black* that measures up to 11 mm).

To prevent stress fractures, athletes should distribute loading forces on the bone with cross training and biomechanical adjustments (i.e., orthotics, proper shoes, stretches, strengthening, running mechanics), consume sufficient calories to maintain adequate energy availability, and ensure appropriate intake of calcium and vitamin D. A study by Lappe of female Navy recruits

TABLE 4	High-Risk Stress Fracture Initial Treatment
HIGH-RISK STRESS FRACTURE	**INITIAL TREATMENT (IF STABLE AND NONDISPLACED)**
Femoral neck (compression side) (Figures 20 and 21)	NWB for 6–8 wk then PWB to FWB over next 6–8 wk
Anterior tibia (tension side)	NWB for 6–8 wk then PWB to FWB over next 6–12 wk
Medial malleolus	Pneumatic lower leg boot for 6–8 wk
Navicular	NWB cast/boot for 6 wk then 6-wk RTP progression
Base of fifth metatarsal (Jones)	NWB cast/boot 6–8 wk
May consider surgery for quicker RTP	
Sesamoids	NWB cast/boot 6 wk

Abbreviations: NWB = non-weight bearing; PWB = partial weight bearing; FWB = full weight bearing.

TABLE 5	Low-Risk Stress Fracture Initial Treatment
LOW-RISK STRESS FRACTURE	**INITIAL TREATMENT**
Sacrum/pelvis	WBAT 7–12 wk
Femoral shaft	WBAT 6–8 wk
Posterior medial tibia (compression side)	WBAT boot 2–12 wk (longer time with cortical break) then transition to pneumatic tibial brace
Fibula	WBAT 1–4 wk
Metatarsal (2nd–5th)	Steel shank/walking boot 3–6 wk

Abbreviations: WBAT = weight bearing as tolerated.

showed reductions in stress fractures in those consuming 2000 mg of calcium[1] and 800 IU vitamin D[1] daily, either as a supplement or through consumption of dairy products. Tobacco should be avoided. Additionally, women of child bearing age should try to maintain regular menses by consuming adequate calories and avoiding a negative energy balance.

General treatment for stress fractures can be grouped into nutrition, medication, and biomechanical recommendations. Nutrition recommendations include optimizing energy availability in the diet, ensuring adequate calcium and vitamin D intake, and avoidance of tobacco exposure. Medication recommendations include using acetaminophen as needed for pain control and avoidance of NSAIDs. Biomechanical recommendations are to offload the affected bone and reduce activity to pain-free functioning and pain-free cross-training. Crutches may be needed to offload the injured area even more than a walking boot/cast or steal shank. The patient may require complete non-weight bearing (NWB) with the overall goal being to obtain pain-free ambulation during the initial treatment. Tables 4 and 5 outline recommended guidelines for protected weight bearing for specific stress fracture sites. Additional recommendations are to begin a rehabilitation program when tolerated and to stretch and strengthen supporting structures. Start a gradual increase in activity when the patient is pain-free.

Because of their propensity for delayed healing and nonunion, certain stress fractures are considered high risk, necessitate prompt treatment, and may ultimately require surgical fixation. Low-risk stress fractures have a lower incidence of delayed healing and nonunion. High-risk stress fractures that appear stable and

[1]Not FDA approved for this indication.

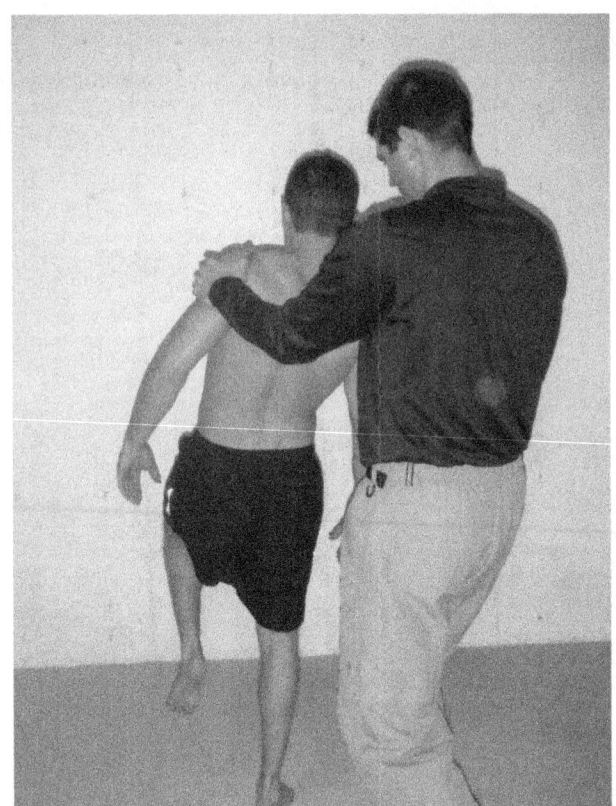

Figure 22 Stork test: To assess localized spondylolysis pain, a single leg hyperextension rotation test (stork test) is performed. The patient stands on one leg and hyperextends and rotates the spine. Reproduction of the patient's pain is suggestive of a spondylolysis.

Figure 23 Oblique view x-ray of the lumbar spine, which demonstrates a L3 and L4 spondylolysis.

Figure 24 SPECT scan lumbar spine, PA view, which demonstrates an acute bilateral L3 and L4 spondylolysis.

nondisplaced can be treated nonoperatively with close follow-up. Consider referral to an orthopaedic surgeon for failed conservative treatment. Biomechanical forces along the bone with activity are used to classify tibia and femur stress fractures. For example, during running, the tibia and femur have different forces exerted on different parts of the bone. The tibia compresses posteriorly, so there is more compression along the posterior tibia and more tension along the anterior aspect of the tibia. The femoral neck compresses inferiorly and medially with running, so there is more compression along the inferior medial aspect of the femoral neck and more tension along the superior lateral aspect of the femoral neck. These variable forces on different parts of the bone affect the potential for delayed healing and nonunion.

Spondylolysis and Spondylolisthesis

Spondylolysis is a nondisplaced stress fracture of the pars interarticularis. Spondylolisthesis occurs when there is bilateral spondylolysis with listhesis (slippage) of the vertebral body. Spondylolisthesis is graded 1 to 4 depending on how much slippage is present with each grade, accounting for 25% (i.e., grade 1 = 0–25%).

When a young athlete presents with low back pain, spondylolysis needs to be considered: this can be the cause of their pain up to 47% of the time. Spondylolysis is an overuse injury caused by repetitive hyperextension and/or rotation and has increased incidence in ballet dancers, gymnasts, divers, soccer players, and football linemen. L5 is the most common level for a spondylolysis. The history is significant for insidious onset of deep pain in the low back exacerbated by extension. Physical examination shows a positive Stork test (see Table 3), often with reproduction of pain on the side of weight bearing (Figure 22). If history and physical exam are suggestive of a pars interarticularis injury, x-rays of the lumbar spine, including oblique views, should be obtained. Oblique view x-rays provide the best view to identify a spondylolysis even though they only demonstrate spondylolysis about 30% of the time when it is present (Figure 23). If x-rays are negative, proceed with MRI or with SPECT scan. If the SPECT scan is positive (Figure 24), then proceed with limited CT scan (Figures 25 and 26). If radiation exposure is a concern, or if high-definition MRI is readily accessible, thinly sliced stacked axial cuts with T2 fat saturation views in all planes using a high-definition MRI is the test of choice (Figure 27). A spectrum of recommended treatments and conservative approaches that allow for a prompt and safe RTP are reasonable. For acute spondylolysis, the recommended treatment consists of a warm

Figure 25 CT scan without contrast. Axial image at L3 shows bilateral pars interarticularis fractures that appear acute with jagged and nonsclerotic fracture edges.

Figure 26 CT scan without contrast. Axial image at L4 shows bilateral pars interarticularis fractures. Right L4 pars fracture appears more chronic in appearance, with sclerotic fracture edges on the lateral aspect. Left L4 pars fracture appears more acute, with more jagged-appearing edges.

Figure 27 MRI lumbar spine without contrast. Axial T2 fat saturation image at L5 that demonstrates a right L5 spondylolysis signified by right pars interarticularis bone edema in white at L5.

Figure 28 Lateral view x-ray of the lumbar spine, which demonstrates a grade 1 L5 spondylolisthesis.

and form-extension-blocking back brace worn all day except for showering and bathing (23–24 hours per day) for the first month of treatment in conjunction with rest from activity. During the second month, use of the brace during the day with rehabilitation is suggested. Rehabilitation consists of core strengthening and lower extremity flexibility. The third month consists of a gradual return to activity, continuing core strengthening and flexibility, and wearing the brace with activity. When treating spondylolysis, a healed pars interarticularis injury is defined as pain-free activity that may include bony union of the pars interarticularis stress fracture or fibrous nonbony union. Generally, the patient should wear the brace for at least 1 year with activity and sometimes

longer depending on the severity of injury. Utilize acetaminophen for pain, avoid NSAIDs, ensure adequate energy availability, maximize calcium and vitamin D intake, and avoid tobacco exposure to facilitate bone healing.

The general goal for spondylolisthesis treatment is to prevent further slippage; treatment is similar to that for spondylolysis. Surgical referral is indicated for grade 2, 3, or 4 spondylolisthesis (Figure 28).

References

Almekinders LC: Anti-inflammatory treatment of muscular injuries in sports, *Sports Med* 15:139–145, 1993.

Bachmann LM, Kolb E, Koller M, et al: Accuracy of Ottawa ankle rules to exclude fractures of the ankle and mid-foot: systematic review, *Br Med J* 326:417–424, 2003.

Beynnon BD, Johnson RJ, Brown L: Knee. In DeLee JC, Drez D, Miller MD, editors: *DeLee & Drez's Orthopaedic Sports Medicine Principles & Practice*, 3rd ed., Philadelphia, 2009, Elsevier, pp 1579–1847.

Gellman H, Caputo RJ, Carter V, et al: Comparison of short and long thumb-spica casts for non-displaced fractures of the carpal scaphoid, *J Bone Joint Surg Am* 71:354–357, 1989.

Haskell A, Mann RA: Foot and ankle. In DeLee JC, Drez D, Miller MD, editors: *DeLee & Drez's Orthopaedic Sports Medicine Principles & Practice*, 3rd ed. Philadelphia, 2009, Elsevier, pp 1865–2205.

Kaeding C, Best TM: Tendinosis: Pathophysiology and nonoperative treatment, *Sports Health* 1:284–292, 2009.

Lappe J, Cullen D, Haynatzki G, et al: Calcium and vitamin D supplementation decreases incidence of stress fractures in female navy recruits, *J Bone Miner Res* 23:741–749, 2008.

Leggit JG, Meko CJ: Acute finger injuries: part I. Tendons and ligaments, *Am Fam Physician* 73:810–816, 2006.

Liem BC, Truswell HJ, Harrast MA: Rehabilitation and return to running after lower limb stress fractures, *Curr Sports Med Rep* 12:200–207, 2013.

Purcell L, Micheli L: Low back pain in young athletes, *Sports Health* 1:212–222, 2009.

Simon AM, Manigrasso MB, O'Connor JP: Cyclo-oxygenase 2 function is essential for bone fracture healing, *J Bone Miner Res* 17:963, 2002.

Tiemstra JD: Update on acute ankle sprains, *Am Fam Physician* 85:1170–1176, 2012.

CONNECTIVE TISSUE DISORDERS

Method of
Molly A. Hinshaw, MD; and Susan Lawrence-Hylland, MD

CURRENT DIAGNOSIS

Lupus Erythematosus

- The erythematous-violaceous and variably pruritic, tender, or scaly eruption is photosensitive.
- Mild to moderate systemic involvement may include arthritis and pleurisy.
- Severe systemic involvement may include nephritis, cerebritis, vasculitis, and severe cytopenias.
- Associated findings include antiphospholipid antibodies associated with thromboembolism or stroke, Raynaud's phenomenon, and sicca symptoms.

Dermatomyositis and Polymyositis

- Photosensitive, violaceous-erythematous, poikilodermatous, and variably scaly patches occur around eyes, on extensor extremities (especially over joints), upper back, scalp, and dystrophic nail folds with prominent telangiectasias.
- Patients may have or develop myositis or pulmonary involvement.
- Age-appropriate cancer screening is required for adults.

Scleroderma

- Patients have firm, variably pruritic, and indurated plaques.
- Localized scleroderma (i.e., morphea or asymmetric sclerotic plaques) may be seen.
- Limited systemic sclerosis is characterized by symmetric sclerosis of distal extremities, and patients may have systemic disease.
- Diffuse systemic sclerosis is characterized by symmetric sclerosis of the trunk and proximal extremities, and patients may have systemic disease.
- Sclerodactyly (i.e., thickening of skin of digits) may occur in patients with systemic sclerosis.
- Pulmonary, cardiac, and gastrointestinal screening should be done for patients with systemic sclerosis.
- Patients with systemic sclerosis should be evaluated and monitored for renal crisis.
- Raynaud's phenomenon may develop in patients with systemic sclerosis.

CURRENT THERAPY

Lupus Erythematosus

- Patients should be counseled on photoprotection measures.
- Localized cutaneous disease is treated with medium- to high-potency topical corticosteroids, and intralesional triamcinolone acetonide 10 mg/mL (Kenalog-10) is added if needed.
- Mild to moderate systemic involvement is treated with low- to medium-potency prednisone 5 to 20 mg/day and with antimalarials.
- Severe disease is treated with prednisone 1 mg/kg/day with a taper based on clinical response. Steroid-sparing agents include azathioprine (Imuran),[1] mycophenolate mofetil (CellCept),[1] methotrexate (Rheumatrex),[1] and cyclophosphamide (Cytoxan).[1]
- Thromboembolism or stroke is treated by anticoagulation with warfarin (Coumadin), aspirin, or heparin.
- Sicca syndrome is treated with frequent water intake, saliva replacement, artificial tears, routine dental care, and pilocarpine (Salagen).

Dermatomyositis and Polymyositis

- Patients should be counseled on photoprotection measures.
- Medium-potency topical corticosteroids and calcineurin inhibitors are used for cutaneous disease.
- Prednisone 1 mg/kg/day is first-line therapy for muscle or pulmonary disease.
- Methotrexate[1] 10 to 25 mg/week is a steroid-sparing agent used for muscle involvement.
- Hydroxychloroquine (Plaquenil)[1] 200 mg/day is used for persistent skin involvement.

Scleroderma

- For localized scleroderma, UVA[1] 20 to 60 J/cm² or psoralen plus UVA (PUVA) is used to resolve established lesions; high-potency corticosteroids and calcipotriene (Dovonex)[1] may help to reduce pruritus and inflammation in new lesions; and systemic prednisone[1] or methotrexate[1] may be used for rapidly progressive new lesions.
- Treatment of systemic sclerosis is primarily aimed at limiting complications.
- Physical therapy is used for contractures.
- Systemic sclerosis is treated with cyclophosphamide (Cytoxan),[1] mycophenolate mofetil (CellCept),[1] methotrexate[1] 10 to 25 mg/week, and photopheresis.
- Renal crisis is treated with captopril (Capoten)[1] 6.25 mg three to six times/day and titrated to effect.
- Raynaud's is treated with warming techniques, calcium channel blockers, antiadrenergic agents, antiplatelet drugs, and topical vasodilators.

[1]Not FDA approved for this indication.

Lupus Erythematosus

Lupus erythematosus is an autoimmune connective tissue disease that may localize to the skin or involve several organ systems. A complete review of systems with evaluation of positive findings is necessary to thoroughly assess patients for signs of systemic lupus as defined by the American Rheumatism Association. Cutaneous lupus erythematosus manifests in chronic, subacute, and acute forms. A punch biopsy from within an erythematous lupus lesion is useful for confirming the diagnosis.

Clinical Features

Discoid lupus and tumid lupus are the two forms of chronic cutaneous lupus erythematosus. Discoid lupus lesions are tender or pruritic, erythematous to violaceous, scaly plaques that typically occur on sun-exposed skin. The lesions resolve with scarring, and when the lesions affect the scalp, they cause scarring alopecia. Tumid lupus manifests as pruritic, erythematous to violaceous, nonscaly plaques that typically preferentially affect the face and trunk.

The lesions of subacute cutaneous lupus erythematosus occur as erythematous to violaceous, scaly macules and as annular or polycyclic patches. These lesions are commonly located on sun-exposed skin and heal without scarring.

Acute cutaneous lupus erythematosus is exemplified by malar erythema (i.e., butterfly rash) and by poikiloderma (i.e., hyperpigmentation, telangiectasias, and epidermal atrophy). It is a manifestation of systemic lupus erythematosus (SLE). Cutaneous lesions may be widespread. In addition to the American Rheumatism Association criteria, patients with SLE may also develop Raynaud's phenomenon, hypercoagulability, and overlap syndromes with Sjögren's disease, dermatomyositis, and other conditions.

Hydrochlorothiazide (HydroDIURIL), terbinafine (Lamisil), minocycline (Minocin), procainamide (Pronestyl), hydralazine (Apresoline), and isoniazid (Nydrazid) are a few of the pharmaceutical agents that cause drug-induced lupus. This disease manifests with synovitis, photosensitivity, and positive serology results, and it may have cutaneous lesions that do not necessarily abate with cessation of the medication.

Management
Prevention
All patients with lupus erythematosus should be counseled on photoprotection, including protecting skin from sunlight and avoiding sun exposure during peak hours (i.e., between 10 AM and 2 PM). Ultraviolet A and B wavelengths may cause lupus to flare. Broad-spectrum sunscreen with an SPF of 30 or higher and that contains titanium, zinc, Mexoryl (L'Oreal), or Helioplex (Neutrogena) should be used whenever patients are outdoors. Photoprotective clothing, available from multiple vendors, is useful for limiting sun exposure.

Patients with lupus are relatively immunosuppressed by their disease. Vaccinations should be kept up to date, although there is a debate about the necessity and safety of vaccination against meningococcal disease (*Neisseria meningitidis*) (Menactra, Menomune), varicella-zoster virus (Zostavax), and *Streptococcus* (Pneumovax).

Treatment of Cutaneous Lupus Erythematosus
Medium-potency topical corticosteroids should be used for lupus localized to the skin, and they are used as adjunct treatment for patients with systemic lupus. Use of triamcinolone 0.1% cream (Flutex) for lesions on the head and neck until symptoms subside or up to 2 weeks continuously is an appropriate starting strength. Ointment-based vehicles are useful for lesions on the trunk and extremities. They are also the vehicles of choice on the scalp of patients of African American descent. Foam or liquid- or lotion-based corticosteroids work well in the scalp of other ethnic groups and can be used on the trunk and extremities. If lesions persist, the corticosteroid can be occluded, or intralesional injections with triamcinolone can be repeated monthly as needed. Intralesional triamcinolone acetonide at concentrations of 5 mg/mL (Kenalog) can be injected into lesions on the face or neck and doses of 10 to 20 mg/mL (Kenalog-10, Kenalog) into lesions on the trunk or extremities. Intralesional corticosteroids may cause mild discomfort, atrophy of the skin or subcutis, or stretch marks. Topical calcineurin inhibitors such as pimecrolimus (Elidel)[1] or tacrolimus (Protopic)[1] may be used for maintenance treatment but are not recommended for new or active lesions because they do not work quickly. Recurrent or refractory cutaneous lesions require systemic treatment.

Treatment of Systemic Lupus Erythematosus
Antimalarials, including hydroxychloroquine (Plaquenil),[1] are disease-modifying agents that limit the progression of lupus. Hydroxychloroquine, chloroquine (Aralen),[1] and quinacrine[2] (at compounding pharmacies) raise the pH of inflammatory cells, inhibiting inflammatory pathways that cause end-organ damage in patients with SLE.

Hydroxychloroquine is typically used first at 200 mg daily for 2 weeks and then increased to 400 mg daily. Patients need laboratory monitoring and a baseline and then yearly eye examination because the medication may be deposited in the retina over time. Hydroxychloroquine exerts its effects within 2 to 3 months of beginning treatment. Its effects are diminished in smokers.

Depending on end-organ involvement in SLE, immunosuppression with systemic corticosteroids such as prednisone at doses of 1 mg/kg/day is appropriate. Steroid-sparing drugs such as methotrexate (Rheumatrex),[1] acitretin (Soriatane),[1] or mycophenolate mofetil (CellCept)[1] are added. After signs of inflammation subside, prednisone is tapered.

Treatment of Musculoskeletal Manifestations
Arthralgia is a common complaint that can usually be managed with acetaminophen or nonsteroidal antiinflammatory drugs (NSAIDs). For true arthritis unresponsive to the previously described measures, hydroxychloroquine[1] 200 mg twice daily can be added. After that, treatments similar to those used for rheumatoid arthritis can be added, although the antitumor necrosis factor agents usually are avoided in lupus. Methotrexate[1] 7.5 to 25 mg PO once weekly may be used along with folic acid[1] 1 mg daily to help limit side effects. Routine toxicity monitoring includes frequent complete blood cell counts and liver tests. Azathioprine (Imuran)[1] 0.5 to 2 mg/kg can be used with frequent monitoring of complete blood cell counts and liver tests. A sample for testing the thiopurine methyltransferase activity level should be drawn before initiating therapy because a genetic deficiency can lead to severe pancytopenia. Leflunomide (Arava)[1] 10 to 20 mg PO once daily can be used with frequent blood cell counts and liver tests. Low-dose glucocorticoids (prednisone 5–10 mg/day) may be used as a bridge to steroid-sparing therapy and to treat intermittent flares.

Treatment of Hematologic Manifestations
Autoimmune cytopenias are common and are often a defining feature of SLE. Lymphopenia (absolute lymphocyte count <1500 cells/microliter) does not require therapy. Hemolytic anemia in SLE is the result of antierythrocyte antibodies that activate complement, and it is treated with prednisone at a dose based on clinical severity. Typically, 1 mg/kg/day, or approximately 60 mg, is used for 4 to 6 weeks, with gradual tapering as long as the response is maintained. For severe hemolytic anemia, pulse methylprednisolone (Solu-Medrol) 1 g IV for 3 consecutive days can be tried, followed by the previously described standard dosing. For patients who do not respond to glucocorticoids or are unable to taper prednisone to low doses, other treatments can be used. They may include azathioprine[1] 1.5 to 2.5 mg/kg/day, mycophenolate mofetil[1] 1000 to 2000 mg/day in divided doses, danazol (Danocrine)[1] 300 to 600 mg/day in divided doses, intravenous immunoglobulin,[1] or rituximab (Rituxan)[1] 375 mg/m² weekly for four doses.

Immune thrombocytopenia results from antiplatelet antibodies that identify platelets for early destruction. Treatment is indicated when patients have signs or symptoms of spontaneous bleeding or when the platelet count drops below 50,000/mL. The initial treatment approach with glucocorticoids is similar to that used for hemolytic anemia. For patients with chronic thrombocytopenia or for those who cannot achieve an acceptable long-term dose of prednisone, steroid-sparing agents, including azathioprine,[1] mycophenolate mofetil,[1] danazol,[1] rituximab,[1] and intravenous immunoglobulin[1] can be used in doses similar to those used for hemolytic anemia. Dapsone,[1] cyclosporine (Sandimmune, Neoral),[1] and cyclophosphamide (Cytoxan)[1] have also been used.

Thrombotic thrombocytopenia purpura may occur in SLE, and it must be differentiated from immune thrombocytopenia because treatment requires emergent plasmapheresis. Manifestations of thrombotic thrombocytopenia purpura include fever,

---

[1] Not FDA approved for this indication.
[2] Not available in the United States.

microangiopathic hemolysis, and central nervous system and renal abnormalities.

Antiphospholipid antibodies include the lupus anticoagulant, anticardiolipin antibodies, and β_2-glycoprotein. They are associated with coagulopathy, thrombocytopenia, late-trimester miscarriage, and heart valve abnormalities. Antiphospholipid antibodies that can be determined with blood testing but are not associated with thromboembolism do not require treatment. Low-dose aspirin[1] may be considered but has not been shown to prevent future thrombosis. Hydroxychloroquine[1] 200 mg twice daily has been shown to reduce the risk. Patients with antiphospholipid antibodies who develop thromboembolism need lifelong treatment with warfarin (Coumadin). A goal international normalized ratio (INR) remains controversial because different studies advocate for high-intensity warfarin (INR >3) or low-intensity therapy (INR >2). For women who have suffered a miscarriage determined to be related to antiphospholipid antibodies, low-dose aspirin and heparin 5000 units SQ twice daily may increase the likelihood of a successful pregnancy.

Treatment of Renal Manifestations
Many patients with SLE have mild to severe renal involvement. Diagnosis by renal biopsy is important to establish the type of kidney involvement. Lupus nephritis is considered one of the more severe manifestations of the disease, and treatment is aimed at preventing renal failure. Treatment should be coordinated with a rheumatologist or nephrologist.

Class I disease requires no specific therapy. The class IIb pattern with more than 1 g of proteinuria can be treated with moderate-dose prednisone (20 mg/day for 6 weeks to 3 months), followed by tapering. Class III and IV patterns of disease have the same prognosis and are treated similarly with high-dose prednisone (1 mg/kg/day) for at least 6 weeks before tapering, based on clinical response, by 10 mg a week to a maintenance of 10 to 15 mg/day. In addition to prednisone, cytotoxic therapy is initiated with cyclophosphamide[1] 0.5 to 1 g/m^2 of body surface area monthly for 6 months and tapered to every 3 months, based on clinical response, for a total of 2 to 3 years. Cyclophosphamide has serious toxicities, including hemorrhagic cystitis, bone marrow suppression, infertility, teratogenicity, and increased risk of malignancy. 2-Mercaptoethane sulfonate sodium (Mesna)[1] can be given with each infusion to minimize bladder toxicity. Class V disease can be treated with prednisone alone, similar to class IIb disease, unless there are coexisting features of class III or IV disease, for which treatments outlined previously should be implemented.

An acceptable alternative to cyclophosphamide for class III and IV disease is mycophenolate mofetil[1] 2 to 3 g/day in divided doses combined with corticosteroids (dosing outlined earlier). This appears to be an effective therapy with fewer side effects than traditional therapy.

Treatment of Nervous System Manifestations
Neuropsychiatric involvement is common in patients with lupus. Symptoms can range from mild to severe and include headache, aseptic meningitis, neuropathy, myelopathy, cognitive dysfunction, seizures, cerebritis, and stroke. A thorough evaluation is necessary to define the cause of nervous system dysfunction and differentiate it from a medication side effect. For seizures, antiepileptic therapy is used, preferably in coordination with a neurologist. Lupus cerebritis and transverse myelitis are two of the more serious manifestations that need to be treated emergently with aggressive immunosuppression in coordination with a rheumatologist or neurologist. Treatment includes high-dose corticosteroids and cyclophosphamide,[1] similar to treatment for lupus nephritis.

Dermatomyositis and Polymyositis
Clinical Features
Dermatomyositis may affect skin and muscle. Cutaneous dermatomyositis manifests with violaceous erythema of characteristic areas, including the periorbital skin (i.e., heliotrope rash), upper back (i.e., shawl sign), dorsal hands (i.e., Gottron's papules), scalp, lateral thighs (i.e., Holster sign), and periungual skin, where dilated capillary loops and erythema are observed. Patients may report muscle weakness. As in lupus, a punch biopsy of an actively inflamed cutaneous lesion shows characteristic features.

Evaluation of patients with cutaneous dermatomyositis is not complete without assessment for systemic involvement. Serum aldolase is the most specific marker for myositis, and it can be used as a measure of response to treatment. Creatinine kinase and alanine aminotransferase levels may be elevated but are not specific indicators. An electromyogram shows dampening of signals, and a muscle biopsy shows a characteristic pattern of myositis. Inflammatory lung disease, diagnosed by the characteristic pattern on chest computed tomography, bronchoalveolar lavage, or biopsy, may be life limiting and therefore should be treated aggressively, similar to lung disease in scleroderma. Adult patients should have age-appropriate cancer screening because dermatomyositis is a paraneoplastic phenomenon in 10% to 50% of patients.

Some patients present with characteristic cutaneous dermatomyositis but no systemic involvement (i.e., dermatomyositis sine myositis). The risk of concurrent or subsequent cancer development is thought to be increased. These patients require monitoring for systemic involvement that may develop over time.

Treatment
Patients with dermatomyositis need photoprotection similar to patients with lupus. Periodic evaluation by clinical examination and review of systems allows for early intervention for developing visceral or muscle involvement.

Cutaneous dermatomyositis is treated the same as lupus (see earlier). Dermatomyositis with systemic involvement is initially treated with immunosuppression using prednisone at doses of 1 mg/kg/day. Steroid-sparing agents are incorporated early in the disease and include antimalarials (methotrexate,[1] azathioprine,[1] and mycophenolate mofetil[1]) at doses that are used in treating lupus.

Scleroderma
Clinical Features
Scleroderma is a sclerosing condition of skin or viscera, or both. The cause is unknown, but transforming growth factor-β plays a role. Type I and III collagens are excessively produced, as are other substances, including glycosaminoglycans, tenascin, and fibronectin.

Cutaneous scleroderma without Raynaud's phenomenon or clinically relevant systemic involvement is also known as *morphea*. Morphea has different distribution patterns, including guttate, linear, segmental, or diffuse distribution, but it is always characterized by indurated plaques that are inflammatory initially, have an advancing inflammatory ("lilac") border as they progress, and then become hyperpigmented. The cutaneous lesions may restrict movement of joints and can cause restricted growth of underlying structures, particularly when they develop in childhood.

Systemic sclerosis may affect the respiratory, renal, cardiovascular, genitourinary, and gastrointestinal systems and vascular structures. Raynaud's phenomenon may be the first presenting symptom of systemic sclerosis, and it can be severe, leading to digital ulcerations and autoamputation. The American College of Rheumatology has defined criteria for the diagnosis.

Tests for antinuclear antibodies are positive in approximately 95% of patients, who typically present with a homogeneous or speckled pattern. A nucleolar pattern is more specific for systemic sclerosis. Anticentromere antibodies are present in 60% to 90% of patients with limited disease but are rare in diffuse disease. Topoisomerase I (Scl-70) antibodies are positive in 30% of

---

[1]Not FDA approved for this indication.

[1]Not FDA approved for this indication.

patients with diffuse disease and are associated with pulmonary fibrosis. Anti-PM-Scl antibodies are present in overlap syndromes and are associated with myositis and renal involvement.

Treatment
Treatment of Limited Scleroderma
For limited scleroderma, treatment with topical medium-potency corticosteroids such as triamcinolone 0.1% ointment (Kenalog) plus calcipotriene (Dovonex)[1] 0.005% cream or intralesional triamcinalone[1] 20 mg/mL may slow progression of active lesions or improve the pruritus and cutaneous stiffness that typify cutaneous scleroderma. For rapidly evolving disease, prednisone[1] 1 mg/kg/day and methotrexate[1] 15 to 20 mg/week may help slow progression of disease. UVA[1] given over 36 treatments at doses of 30 to 60 mJ/cm^2 or PUVA (oral methoxsalen [8-MOP] 10 mg taken 2 hours before treatment with UVA light) can soften the existing plaques of morphea.

Treatment of Systemic Sclerosis: Raynaud's Phenomenon
First-line treatment for Raynaud's phenomenon is preventive, with cold avoidance and the use of warming techniques. If pharmacotherapy is required, extended-release calcium channel blockers such as nifedipine (Procardia XL)[1] starting at 30 mg/day or amlodipine (Norvasc)[1] starting at 5 mg/day may be useful. If this is not helpful, the α-blocker prazosin (Minipress)[1] 1 mg three times daily or the angiotensin receptor blocker losartan (Cozaar)[1] 50 mg daily may be helpful. Antiplatelet therapy with low-dose aspirin[1] (81 mg/day) or dipyridamole (Persantine)[1] 50 to 100 mg three or four times daily may be useful. Topical vasodilators such as nitroglycerin ointment (Nitro-Bid)[1] applied to the base of the affected finger three times daily can be helpful in refractory disease. Digit-threatening ischemia may be treated with an intravenous prostaglandin such as alprostadil (Prostin VR)[1] or iloprost (Ilomedine),[5] which require peripheral or central access. Patients with severe recurrent digital ischemia may ultimately benefit from surgical sympathectomy.

Treatment of Gastrointestinal Manifestations
The most common gastrointestinal manifestation is esophageal reflux caused by esophageal dysmotility. Proton pump inhibitors such as omeprazole (Prilosec)[1] 20 mg twice daily should be used and may prevent the development of esophageal strictures. Prokinetic drugs such as metoclopramide (Reglan)[1] 10 mg four times daily can be helpful. Erythromycin[1] 500 mg three or four times daily can help esophageal and gastric hypomotility. Small bowel hypomotility can lead to bacterial overgrowth, resulting in malabsorption and diarrhea. Rotating antibiotics that include metronidazole (Flagyl),[1] ciprofloxacin (Cipro),[1] and amoxicillin/clavulanate (Augmentin)[1] can be used.

Treatment of Pulmonary Manifestations
Inflammatory lung disease occurs commonly in patients with scleroderma and can be life limiting. Cyclophosphamide[1] at doses of up to 2 mg/kg/day for up to 2 years may slow progression of pulmonary disease. Pulmonary hypertension occurs more commonly in limited systemic sclerosis than in diffuse disease. Symptomatic patients may receive treatment with prostacyclin analogues, which require continuous infusions. The endothelin receptor antagonist bosentan (Tracleer)[1] can be given orally starting at 62.5 mg twice daily. Liver tests should be monitored frequently. At this point, care is typically coordinated with a cardiologist to monitor disease progression and treatment response. Anticoagulation for pulmonary hypertension may improve survival because of the frequent occurrence of pulmonary arterial thrombosis.

[1] Not FDA approved for this indication.
[5] Investigational drug in the United States.

Treatment of Renal Manifestations
Angiotensin-converting enzyme (ACE) inhibitors (e.g., captopril [Capoten[1]] beginning at 6.25 mg three to six times daily and titrated for blood pressure control) have dramatically reduced the incidence of renal failure and death due to renal crisis. Avoidance of prednisone at doses greater than 15 mg/day is also important in reducing the risk of renal crisis.

[1] Not FDA approved for this indication.

References
Atzeni F, Bendtzen K, Bobbio-Pallavicini F, et al: Infections and treatment of patients with rheumatic diseases, Clin Exp Rheumatol 26(Suppl. 48):S67–73, 2008.
Dziadzio M, Denton CP, Smith R: Losartan therapy for Raynaud's phenomenon and scleroderma, Arthritis Rheum 42(12):2646–2655, 1999.
Ginzler EM, Dooley MA, Aranow C, et al: Mycophenolate mofetil or intravenous cyclophosphamide for lupus nephritis, N Engl J Med 353(21):2219–2228, 2005.
Iorizzo LJ, Jorizzo JL: The treatment and prognosis of dermatomyositis: An updated review, J Am Acad Dermatol 59:99–112, 2008.
Matucci-Cerinic M, Steen VD, Furst DE, et al: Clinical trials in systemic sclerosis: Lessons learned and outcomes, Arthritis Res Ther 9(Suppl. 2):S7, 2007.
Nihtyanova SI, Denton CP: Current approaches to the management of early active diffuse scleroderma skin disease, Rheum Dis Clin North Am 34:161–179, 2008.
Pisoni CN, Sanchez FJ, Karim Y, et al: Mycophenolate mofetil in systemic lupus erythematosus: Efficacy and tolerability in 86 patients, J Rheumatol 32:1047–1052, 2005.
Steen VD: The many faces of scleroderma, Rheum Dis Clin North Am 34:1–15, 2008.
Subcommittee for Scleroderma Criteria of the American Rheumatism Association Diagnostic and Therapeutic Criteria Committee: Preliminary criteria for the classification of systemic sclerosis (scleroderma), Arthritis Rheum 23:581–590, 1980.
Tan EM, Cohen AS, Fries JF, et al: The 1982 revised criteria for the classification of lupus erythematosus, Arthritis Rheum 25:1271–1272, 1982.
Wallace DD: Lupus Erythematosus, ed 7, Philadelphia, 2006, Lippincott Williams & Wilkins.

FIBROMYALGIA

Method of
Timothy Sowder, MD; Jeffrey Michael Foster, DO; and Andrea L. Nicol, MD, MSc

CURRENT DIAGNOSIS

- Fibromyalgia (FM) is a common condition, seen in 2% to 8% of the population, depending on the diagnostic criteria used.
- Hallmark symptoms of FM typically include widespread body pain, cognitive difficulties ("fibro fog"), poor sleep, and fatigue. Other associated symptoms may also include headaches, abdominal or pelvic pain, and symptoms of depression or anxiety.
- FM may occur independently of any other medical conditions, but is also known to associate with other painful conditions such as osteoarthritis and autoimmune disorders such as lupus and rheumatoid arthritis.
- No blood tests or imaging modalities are useful for diagnosing FM; however, tender point examination and questionnaires are available for aiding in diagnosis.

CURRENT THERAPY

- Treatment should be multidisciplinary and focus on symptom management, lifestyle modifications, and psychological interventions.
- A variety of on-label and off-label medications are available to mechanistically address the altered pain processing underlying FM.

- Physical therapy, exercise, and psychological treatments such as cognitive behavioral therapy are of the utmost importance in adequate management of FM symptoms.
- Seeing patients frequently to monitor medications, address side effects, and provide motivational interviewing and care is important to providing optimal patient pain relief and minimizing poor outcomes.

Epidemiology

The global prevalence of fibromyalgia (FM) has been estimated to be 2.7% (4.2% female, 1.4% male), but studies have produced varying results. Historically, studies have been conducted using the 1990 American College of Rheumatology (ACR) diagnostic criteria, which required pain to be present on palpation of at least 11/18 tender points to confirm a diagnosis of FM. Using these criteria, prevalence estimates range from 0.4% to 8.8% with 2.0% in the USA (3.4% of females and 0.5% of males, ratio ~7:1). The problems with these criteria include difficulty reproducing tender points, significantly higher rates in women (possibly due to increased number of tender points in women or a higher pressure pain threshold in males), and a strong correlation with various measures of distress and negative affect. In 2010 the ACR released updated criteria that do not require a tender point assessment. These new criteria have yielded prevalence estimates of 7.7% in women and 4.9% in men for a ratio of 1.6:1, which is similar to that seen in other chronic pain conditions. The prevalence is similar in different countries, cultures, and ethnic groups; there is no evidence that FM has a higher prevalence in industrialized countries and cultures. There are also concerns about underdiagnosis of FM with only 12% to 28% of subjects identified during population-based surveys as fulfilling the ACR 1990 criteria having ever been diagnosed with FM.

Risk Factors

There are both genetic and environmental risk factors associated with the development of FM. FM has been thought to affect mostly women with initial studies predicting that women were up to seven times more likely to develop FM. More recent studies using updated criteria have found less of a discrepancy but still indicate an increased risk with women being 1.5 to 2 times more likely to be affected than men. FM can affect people of all ages, including children. Many patients are diagnosed when they are young or middle aged, but studies show that prevalence rises with age, peaking in people greater than 60 years old. It is postulated that perhaps widespread chronic pain in older patients is more likely to be attributed to osteoarthritis or other degenerative conditions instead of FM, however, the two conditions are known to coexist. Patients diagnosed with certain conditions like rheumatoid arthritis and lupus have been noted to be more likely to develop FM than others. Obesity, poor sleep, low physical activity levels, and decreased job or life satisfaction are potentially modifiable risk factors. There are many other conditions associated with FM, though the degree of contribution to actual disease development has yet to be determined. Individuals with FM are more likely have psychiatric disorders, including depression, anxiety, obsessive-compulsive disorder, and posttraumatic stress disorder. A history of childhood, adolescent, or adulthood abuse or traumatic events have also been linked with the development of FM and other centralized pain syndromes. Maladaptive cognitive features are poor prognostic factors for FM and can include catastrophizing and fear-avoidance of movement and activity. Lower education and other indicators of lower social status have been thought to place patients at an increased risk for FM, though other studies did not find a significant difference in developed and wealthy areas versus rural and poor areas.

Pathophysiology

FM can be thought of as a centralized pain state, where "centralized" refers to amplification of pain emanating from the central nervous system. Evidence suggests that dysfunction in central nervous system pain processing mechanisms underlie this condition and include central amplification of pain and nonpainful stimuli (including auditory, visual, and olfactory). Typical manifestations of central amplification include allodynia (pain resulting from a non-noxious stimulus) and hyperalgesia (increased sensitivity to a painful stimulus), and temporal summation (progressive increase in the pain response to repetitive painful stimulus). This term "centralized pain" does not exclude that an individual's peripheral nervous system and its nociceptive input may be contributing to the patient's overall pain symptoms, but rather that they feel greater levels of pain than would be normally expected based on the degree of peripheral nociceptive input. However, it must be noted that many patients with FM do not have any identifiable structural or functional abnormalities in the periphery that would explain their widespread pain and associated symptoms. The concept of central amplification helps describe the heterogenous clinical features of FM as many of the same neurotransmitters that control sensory sensitivity and pain also control mood, memory, fatigue, and sleep. A variety of quantitative research methods have been employed to establish that central amplification is involved in the pathophysiology of FM, including quantitative sensory testing and functional, chemical, and structural brain neuroimaging. Functional magnetic resonance imaging (MRI) has corroborated that nonnoxious stimuli such as mild pressure activates brain regions involved in pain processing compared with healthy controls. It has also been found that endogenous pain inhibitory pathways do not effectively operate in patients with FM. This defective inhibition is postulated to exist due to altered homeostasis of inhibitory and excitatory neurotransmitters.

Clinical Manifestations

The patient with FM can experience a wide variety of symptoms, including pain, fatigue, sleep disturbance, cognitive dysfunction, and mood alterations. These patients typically present with chronic widespread pain for at least 3 months that is not fully explained by injury or inflammation. This pain is typically identified as being "all over," but drawings by patients show various localized areas of pain, which may migrate in intensity from time to time. Somatic pain is typically the dominant feature; however, visceral pain (including abdominal and pelvic pain) and headaches are also commonly seen. Most frequently, the affected areas include the shoulders, arms, lower back, buttocks, and thighs. Widespread pain in the joints is also common. The patients most generally experience pain that is throbbing, achy, and tender. This pain is often accompanied by generalized hypersensitivity, allodynia, and hyperalgesia, which is indicative of the underlying central amplification. Other symptoms can include numbness, tingling, burning, cramps, and sensitivity to light and sound. Exacerbating factors for these patients' pain include emotional distress, weather changes, sleeping problems, and strenuous activity. A total of 70% to 90% of patients with FM sleep fewer hours, have more frequent waking, and report nonrestorative sleep. They also suffer from significant fatigue, weakness, and stiffness that are worse in the morning and improve as the day progresses. A total of 76% of patients report mental confusion, forgetfulness, and concentration difficulties. This cognitive dysfunction is frequently described as being more bothersome than their widespread pain. These symptoms are so pervasive and disruptive that they are commonly referred to as "fibro fog." In addition, there is an affective component to the cognitive dysfunction that is usually described by patients as feeling fatigued and exhausted all the time, irrespective of how much sleep they get. Depression, anxiety, and posttraumatic stress disorder are comorbidities with high prevalence in this patient population, and their various symptoms can also be present in the patient with FM.

Diagnosis

FM is a condition with distinctive clinical characteristics that allow for it to be diagnosed in the primary care setting. Although many practitioners may have concern that the diagnosis of FM is controversial or that it may label patients in a negative manner, studies suggest that the opposite is true. Establishing the diagnosis of FM can actually provide substantial validity and relief for patients for their previously unexplained symptoms. Prompt diagnosis is a vital component of effective FM management and is linked with patients having greater satisfaction in health, which in turn leads to decreased health care utilization and its associated costs.

In the clinical setting, FM should be considered as a diagnosis in any patient presenting with chronic widespread or multifocal pain. It is commonly comorbid in patients with other chronic pain syndromes, those with thyroid dysfunction, and patients with rheumatic diseases. There exists other co-occurring pain syndromes that have been linked to the same pathophysiology as FM that may also spark a clinicians' suspicion for FM such as irritable bowel syndrome, interstitial cystitis, migraine headache, temporomandibular disorder, and chronic pelvic or genitourinary pain (e.g., interstitial cystitis, vulvodynia). It is very important to note that FM should *not* be considered a diagnosis of exclusion.

A thorough history including asking about pain during childhood and adolescence, other comorbid pain symptoms, a history of childhood or adulthood abuse, or other traumatic events will help elucidate whether FM should be considered in the differential diagnosis. An excellent physical exam including musculoskeletal, neurologic, assessment of tenderness or significant pain to palpation, and allodynia should always be performed. Laboratory tests are not necessary or useful to establish the diagnosis of FM, besides possibly helping sort through the differential diagnoses. Basic laboratory evaluation may include vitamin D levels, thyroid panels, erythrocyte sedimentation rate, C-reactive protein, and blood count or blood chemistries to guide an assessment of potentially treatable causes of diffuse musculoskeletal pain. Detailed serologic studies are not necessary unless the patient has other signs and symptoms of other potential comorbid diseases. No imaging studies are specific in diagnosing FM, and one must be careful in performing radiographs or other imaging studies, as these can have findings that are associated with the degenerative aging process, but may not be the actual cause of the patient's ongoing pain symptoms.

The 1990 ACR tender point exam has been historically used to "diagnose" FM; however, it was originally developed to be used for research and was never intended to be used in clinical practice. Revised versions of diagnostic criteria were published in 2010 and again in 2016. These revised criteria do not require a tender point exam to elucidate a diagnosis and may be ascertained with a self-report questionnaire (Table 1). These criteria rapidly assess widespread pain symptoms and associated symptoms of poor sleep, cognitive difficulties, fatigue, and mood problems. Once diagnosed, treatment for FM can be initiated immediately, even if further tests or referrals to specialists are pending.

Differential Diagnosis

While the diagnosis of FM can be difficult and time-consuming, providing the patient with an answer to their issues can decrease healthcare costs by decreasing biological testing and imaging, decreasing the number of visits, and decreasing the number and dosage of drugs prescribed. With such a wide variety of possible symptomatic expressions of FM, it is important to address the differential diagnoses in a systematic way. Arthralgias are commonly seen in osteoarthritis and spondyloarthritis, but are also seen in rheumatic diseases like rheumatoid arthritis, Sjögren syndrome, systemic lupus erythematous, and polymyalgia rheumatica. Inflammatory, metabolic, and drug-induced myopathies and myalgias should also be ruled out. Myofascial pain syndrome, tendonitis, and bursitis are common pathologies that cause pain in localized areas. Neurologic disorders such as multiple sclerosis and myasthenia gravis should be considered in addition to radiculopathies, and both peripheral and compressive neuropathies that could complicate the picture. Viral infections and Lyme disease should be considered as potential infectious causes.

TABLE 1	American College of Rheumatology 2016 Revised Fibromyalgia

Criteria

A patient satisfies modified 2016 fibromyalgia criteria if the following three conditions are met:

(1) Widespread pain index (WPI) ≥ 7 and symptom severity scale (SSS) score ≥ 5 OR WPI of 4–6 and SSS score ≥ 9.
(2) Generalized pain, defined as pain in at least 4 of 5 regions, must be present. Jaw, chest, and abdominal pain are not included in generalized pain definition.
(3) Symptoms have been generally present for at least 3 months.

Ascertainment

(1) WPI: note the number of areas in which the patient has had pain over the last week. In how many areas has the patient had pain? Score will be between 0 and 19.
Left upper region (Region 1)
  Jaw, left
  Shoulder girdle, left
  Upper arm, left
  Lower arm, left
Right upper region (Region 2)
  Jaw, right
  Shoulder girdle, right
  Upper arm, right
  Lower arm, right
Left lower region (Region 3)
  Hip (buttock, trochanter), left
  Upper leg, left
  Lower leg, left
Right lower region (Region 4)
  Hip (buttock, trochanter), right
  Upper leg, right
  Lower leg, right
Axial region (Region 5)
  Neck
  Upper back
  Lower back
  Chest
  Abdomen
(2) SSS score
  Fatigue
  Waking unrefreshed
  Cognitive symptoms
For the each of the 3 symptoms above, indicate the level of severity over the past week using the following scale:
  0 = No problem
  1 = Slight or mild problems, generally mild or intermittent
  2 = Moderate, considerable problems, often present and/or at a moderate level
  3 = Severe: pervasive, continuous, life-disturbing problems
  The SSS score: is the sum of the severity scores of the 3 symptoms (fatigue, waking unrefreshed, and cognitive symptoms) (0–9) plus the sum (0–3) of the number of the following symptoms the patient has been bothered by that occurred during the previous 6 months:
(1) Headaches (0–1)
(2) Pain or cramps in lower abdomen (0–1)
(3) And depression (0–1)

The final symptom severity score is between 0 and 12

The fibromyalgia severity (FS) scale is the sum of the WPI and SSS

A diagnosis of fibromyalgia is valid irrespective of other diagnoses. A diagnosis of fibromyalgia does not exclude the presence of other clinically important illnesses.

Endocrinopathies like hypothyroidism, Cushing syndrome, and hyperparathyroidism can cause weakness, but are unlikely to cause the significant widespread pain seen in FM. There are other disorders that frequently overlap or co-occur with FM that should be optimally treated in conjunction. These include depression, anxiety, obsessive-compulsive disorder, posttraumatic stress disorder, tension headaches, migraines, temporomandibular disorder, chronic fatigue syndrome, irritable bowel syndrome, interstitial cystitis (painful bladder syndrome), chronic prostatitis, and vulvodynia. It is important for any clinician to distinguish that the patient's symptoms are not explained by another pathology or systemic disorder because treatment of these entities can vary greatly. However, the 2016 Revised Fibromyalgia Criteria does not exclude the diagnosis of FM if other conditions are present. Each of these problems should be considered as variables and optimally treated when attempting to diagnose this complex syndrome.

Treatment

FM is best approached by using an integrated, multidisciplinary approach where pharmacologic and nonpharmacologic treatments are provided in parallel. Engaging and motivating the patient toward their treatment goals as an active participant in their care is vital for success. As stated before, FM can be diagnosed and treated in the primary care setting. Referral to specialists should only be necessary when pain is refractory to therapy (e.g., comprehensive pain management clinic), those in whom the diagnosis is uncertain (e.g., to a rheumatologist or neurologist depending on symptoms), or those with significant comorbid mood or psychiatric disturbances. Forming treatment teams can be very useful and should include clinicians with expertise in exercise/physical activity (e.g., physical therapists), patient education, and pain psychology.

Most comprehensive guidelines on treatment of FM generally recommend that all patients should receive education on their condition, the importance of being an active participant in their care, and that setting reasonable and attainable goals and expectations for treatment. Patients need to be informed that instead of searching for treatments to cure the condition, that management of the condition should focus on pain reduction (not complete pain relief), increased physical functioning, and improved quality of life. This management should rely heavily on stress reduction, exercise and physical activity, adequate sleep, and improving function through cognitive restructuring (e.g., reducing catastrophizing, increasing self-efficacy). Pharmacologic treatments can be effective in alleviating some of the symptoms of FM, but rarely will patients achieve significant improvements without embracing these essential self-management strategies.

In the United States, there are three drugs currently approved by the US Food and Drug Association (FDA) for the treatment of FM: (1) pregabalin (Lyrica), (2) milnacipran (Savella), and (3) duloxetine (Cymbalta). These drugs mechanistically treat FM through either increasing the activity of inhibitory neurotransmitters (milnacipran and duloxetine) or to decrease the activity of excitatory neurotransmitters (pregabalin). Table 2 highlights the FDA-approved medications in the pharmacologic treatment of FM. Careful initiation and titration are recommended to improve patient compliance and response, given the incidence of side effects or drug-drug interactions. There are a variety of commonly utilized drugs other than those listed previously, although none of them have an FDA approval for the FM indication. These other medications have been shown in a variety of research studies to provide pain and symptom relief in FM and include gabapentin (Neurontin)[1], tricyclic antidepressants (e.g., nortriptyline [Pamelor][1], amitriptyline [Elavil][1]), cyclobenzaprine (Flexeril)[1], and venlafaxine (Effexor)[1]. Basic analgesics such as acetaminophen and nonsteroidal antiinflammatories (NSAIDs) have little evidence supporting effectiveness for FM. Other emerging therapies such as low-dose naltrexone (ReVia, Vivitrol)[1] warrant further investigation and should only be used in refractory cases by those who are familiar with its use. There exists no evidence that mu-opioid agonists are helpful in the long-term treatment of FM and ultimately increase central amplification overtime, thereby increasing the potential for worsening pain and functioning whilst placing the patient at risk for dependence and addiction. Clinicians and patients

TABLE 2	Comparison of FDA-approved Pharmacologic Therapies for Fibromyalgia				
DRUG	DATE OF FDA APPROVAL	MECHANISM OF ACTION	AVAILABLE STRENGTHS	DOSING	COMMON SIDE EFFECTS
Duloxetine (Cymbalta)	June 16, 2008	Serotonin norepinephrine reuptake inhibition	20 mg; 30 mg; 60 mg	• 60 mg/day recommended total dose (doses higher than 60 mg rarely helpful for pain) • Start 30 mg/day for 1 week or longer and then may increase to 60 mg/day	Dry mouth, somnolence, nausea, constipation, decreased appetite, hyperhidrosis
Milnacipran (Savella)	January 14, 2009	Serotonin norepinephrine reuptake inhibition	12.5 mg; 25 mg; 50 mg; 100 mg; convenience starter pack	• Convenience starter pack dosing: Start 12.5 mg daily × 1 day, then 12.5 mg bid × 2 days, then 25 mg bid × 4 days, then 50 mg bid • Max dose 100 mg bid (200 mg/day)	Nausea, constipation, hot flush, hyperhidrosis, vomiting, palpitations, increased heart rate, dry mouth, hypertension
Pregabalin (Lyrica)	June 21, 2007	Non-selective alpha-2-delta calcium channel blocker	25 mg; 50 mg; 75 mg; 100 mg; 150 mg; 200 mg; 225 mg; 300 mg	• Start at 75 mg bid (can start much lower in sensitive or older patient population) • May increase to 150 mg bid within 1 week • Max dose 225 mg bid (450 mg/day)	Dizziness, somnolence, dry mouth, peripheral edema, blurred vision, weight gain, abnormal thinking/cognitive difficulties

should recognize that in many cases, treatment with pharmacologic agents may be ineffective. The choice of drug should always be discussed with the patient and should focus on targeting the most bothersome symptoms. Oftentimes multiple types of drugs/drug combinations are needed. If a drug is trialed and does not lead to clinically meaningful relief after four weeks at the full recommended dose, it should be tapered or stopped, and an alternative drug trialed.

Nonpharmacologic treatment for FM consists of psychological and educational interventions, in addition to physical modalities and should be an integral part of a comprehensive FM treatment plan. Education should be a foundational intervention applied immediately with diagnosis or early in the patient's treatment plan, and should consist of information on the underlying pain mechanisms causing clinical pain and associated symptoms (e.g., central nervous system pain and sensory amplification) and information on the nature of the condition (e.g., nonprogressive, chronic, and lifelong with episodic flares, risk of other comorbid conditions). This will provide a strong foundation to then add psychological therapies, which are typically behavioral based and focused on acceptance theories. Cognitive behavioral therapy has been shown to be effective for the treatment of FM and focuses on the link between pain, mood, thoughts, and behavior, and trying to unravel negative coping mechanisms such as catastrophizing and poor self-efficacy. Mind-body therapies, including stress reduction, biofeedback, and mindfulness, have also shown good benefit for FM.

Physical activity, including active and passive modalities, is perhaps the most important nonpharmacologic treatment for FM. Physical therapy, including warm-water aquatherapy, can be utilized initially to help patients improve their conditioning and obtain education on how to incorporate movement and activity into their daily lives. Among different exercise interventions, aerobic exercise has been shown to be the most beneficial. Patients should start with low-to-moderate intensity activities (such as walking, stationary cycling, or swimming). Over time, patients can increase their intensity and duration over time to a goal of at least 20 min/day at least two to three times weekly. It is important to counsel patients on pacing themselves and that initially they may have more soreness or pain as they gradually build their physical conditioning and strength. Continuation of the exercise regimen is of paramount value as ongoing exercise has been associated with maintenance of improvements in FM. Passive forms of physical activity such as balneotherapy (heated spa treatments), manipulation, massage, transcutaneous electrical stimulation, and ultrasound have only weak evidence to support their use. Complementary and alternative medicine options that may be considered include acupuncture, yoga, tai chi, and qi gong meditation, but there are few high-quality evidence studies to support their use as first-line therapy.

Monitoring

No laboratory or imaging monitoring is required in the treatment of FM. Regular/frequent outpatient engagement with patients is recommended—to discuss the comprehensive care plan and focus on patient goals for treatment, as increased outpatient engagement has been shown to reduce morbidity and mortality (including risk of suicide) in patients with FM.

References

Arnold LM, Gebke KB, Choi EHS: Fibromyalgia: management strategies for primary care providers, *Int J Clin Pract* 70(2):99–112, 2016.
Borchers AT, Gershwin ME: Fibromyalgia: A critical and comprehensive review, *Clinic Rev Allerg Immunol* 49:100–151, 2015.
Clauw DJ: Fibromyalgia: A clinical review, *JAMA* 311(15):1547–1555, 2014.
Perrot S: Fibromyalgia: A misconnection in a multi-connected world? *Eur J Pain,* 2019, Available at: https://doi.org/10.1002/ejp.1367, [Epub ahead of print].
Rahman A, Underwood M, Carnes D: Fibromyalgia: *BMJ* 348:g1224, 2014.
Talotta R, Bazzichi L, Di Franco M, et al: One year in review 2017: fibromyalgia, *Clin Exp Rheumatol* 35(Suppl. 105):S6–S12, 2017.
Wolfe F, Clauw DJ, Fitzcharles M, et al: 2016 Revisions to the 2010/2011 fibromyalgia diagnostic criteria, *Semin Arthritis Rheum* 46(3):319–329, 2016.

JUVENILE IDIOPATHIC ARTHRITIS

Method of
Ashley Cooper, MD

CURRENT DIAGNOSIS

- Juvenile idiopathic arthritis (JIA) is a clinical diagnosis. JIA is diagnosed when objective signs of arthritis persist in a child for at least 6 weeks in the absence of another identifiable cause.
- Children who present with musculoskeletal pain without accompanying objective signs of joint inflammation (swelling or painful, limited range of motion) are unlikely to have arthritis. In many children with JIA, swelling and joint limitation are more prominent than pain.
- Laboratory testing has limited value in diagnosing JIA. In some cases, no laboratory tests are needed to make the diagnosis. When clinically indicated, laboratory tests are used to exclude other causes of arthritis such as infection (including Lyme disease in endemic areas), malignancy, or underlying systemic autoimmune disease.
- The antinuclear antibody (ANA), rheumatoid factor (RF), and anticitric citrullinated peptide (anti-CCP) have prognostic but *not* diagnostic value in JIA. These tests should not be drawn to evaluate musculoskeletal pain in children in the absence of objective signs of arthritis.

CURRENT THERAPY

- Medical therapy is individualized for each child based on severity and number of affected joints and comorbidities. The goal of treatment is to completely control joint inflammation to minimize symptoms and prevent damage.
- Many rheumatologists use a step-up treatment approach, titrating medication until inactive disease is achieved. In children with severe arthritis, early combination therapy is sometimes used. With appropriate use of currently available medications, most children with JIA can achieve clinically inactive disease.
- Current treatment options include scheduled nonsteroidal antiinflammatory drugs (NSAIDs), intraarticular corticosteroid injections, disease-modifying antirheumatic drugs (DMARDs, most commonly methotrexate), and biologic response modifiers (such as antitumor necrosis factor alpha, anti-interleukin-1, or anti-interleukin-6 therapy).
- With the currently available medications, many children with JIA do not require systemic corticosteroids. Steroids should not be prescribed to a child presenting with joint pain or swelling of unclear etiology.
- Optimal timing and approach to medication discontinuation in patients who have achieved inactive disease are unclear. Relapse rates are high after medication discontinuation in most JIA subtypes.
- A partnership between the child's rheumatologist and primary care provider is key to safe use of immune-modulating medications. Optimal management includes:
  - Medication toxicity monitoring with periodic laboratory studies;
  - Prompt evaluation of infectious symptoms in immunosuppressed patients;
  - Administration of age-appropriate vaccines (with avoidance of live virus vaccines in patients on immunosuppression);

- Counseling of adolescents to avoid alcohol while on methotrexate and pregnancy while on teratogenic medications.
- Children with JIA should remain physically active and be allowed to continue participating in sports and leisure activities as tolerated. Physical and/or occupational therapy is indicated for patients with limited mobility, deconditioning, or compromised activities of daily living.
- Regular screening for uveitis is an essential part of JIA management to allow prompt treatment of this sight-threatening complication.

Juvenile idiopathic arthritis (JIA) is an umbrella term that encompasses multiple forms of chronic, immune-mediated arthritis that begin in childhood. The classification system currently used for JIA was established in 1995 by the International League of Associations for Rheumatology (ILAR). By replacing the term *juvenile rheumatoid arthritis* with *juvenile idiopathic arthritis* and defining additional subtypes, the ILAR criteria better reflect the clinical heterogeneity among children with arthritis. Absence of the term "rheumatoid" from the current nomenclature appropriately highlights that most cases of juvenile arthritis are not simply early onset rheumatoid arthritis (RA), as only 5% of all children with JIA have rheumatoid factor (RF) positive polyarticular disease.

The subtypes of JIA are summarized in Table 1 and include oligoarticular, polyarticular (RF negative and RF positive), enthesitis-related (a childhood-onset spondyloarthropathy closely related to ankylosing spondylitis), psoriatic, and systemic arthritis.

Although each of these conditions has a distinct phenotype, the presence of chronic inflammatory arthritis is the unifying feature and sine qua non of JIA. A careful history and physical exam are the most important tools in diagnosis. A complete exam of all joints should be performed in children with possible JIA as the pattern of affected joints impacts disease classification. Additional affected joints are often identified on exam that have not been apparent to patients and parents. Common pitfalls in diagnosis of arthritis in children include the following:

- *Diagnosing JIA in the absence of objective clinical signs of arthritis (joint inflammation).* Most children who present to the primary care office with joint pain (even chronic pain) do not have JIA. Isolated pain in the absence of objective findings of arthritis such as swelling predicts against JIA or other chronic rheumatic disease.
- *Attempting to rule in JIA with laboratory studies.* ANA tests can be positive in up to 30% of healthy children, and the most common cause of a positive RF in children is recent viral infection. Due to the high frequency of positive results in children without rheumatic disease, these tests should not be drawn to evaluate for arthritis in the setting of normal exam findings.
- *Attempting to rule out JIA with laboratory studies.* Arthritis is a clinical diagnosis. If a child presents with chronic joint swelling, limited range of motion or contractures, one should not be falsely reassured by normal labs. Many children with arthritis have completely normal inflammatory markers and a negative ANA, and 95% of children with JIA are RF negative.

Risk Factors/Prevention

All JIA subtypes are generally thought to result from an aberrant immune response to an environmental trigger in a genetically predisposed person. A monozygotic twin concordance of 25% to 40% and increased autoimmunity in family members of children with JIA suggest a significant genetic contribution to disease development. Recent genome-wide association studies have revealed susceptibility loci for JIA, though differences in genetic factors exist between clinical JIA subtypes. Strong genetic associations are rare for most JIA subtypes and many identified risk loci are associated with multiple autoimmune diseases. The exception is that 80% to 90% of children with enthesitis-related arthritis (ERA) are human leukocyte antigen (HLA) B27 positive. Testing

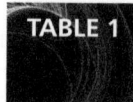

TABLE 1 International League of Associations for Rheumatology Classification Criteria for Juvenile Idiopathic Arthritis

JIA CLASSIFICATION CRITERIA

JIA Definition:
Inflammatory arthritis in at least one joint that begins before age 16, persists at least 6 weeks, and has no other identifiable cause.

JIA SUBTYPE	DESCRIPTION
Oligoarthritis	Arthritis affects 1–4 joints in the first 6 months
• Persistent	Never extends beyond 4 joints
• Extended	Extends to affect 5 or more joints after first 6 months
Polyarthritis	Arthritis affects 5 or more joints in the first 6 months
• RF negative	
Enthesitis-Related Arthritis	Arthritis and enthesitis, OR
	Arthritis or enthesitis with at least 2 of the following:
	• Signs of sacroiliitis,
	• Positive HLA-B27,
	• Onset in a boy age 6 or older,
	• Acute anterior uveitis,
	• HLA-B27-related disease in a first-degree relative.
Psoriatic Arthritis	Arthritis and psoriasis, OR
	Arthritis and at least 2 of the following:
	• Dactylitis,
	• Nail pitting or onycholysis,
	• Psoriasis in a first-degree relative.
Systemic JIA	Arthritis in at least 1 joint with at least 2 weeks of fever that is daily for at least 3 days, with at least one of the following:
	• Evanescent erythematous rash,
	• Generalized lymphadenopathy,
	• Hepatomegaly and/or splenomegaly,
	• Serositis.
Undifferentiated	Fulfills criteria for no category or 2 or more categories

JIA, Juvenile idiopathic arthritis.
Adapted from Petty RE, Southwood TR, Manners P, et al. International League of Associations for Rheumatology classification of juvenile idiopathic arthritis: second revision, Edmonton, 2001. *J Rheumatol.* 2004;31(2):390–392.

for specific HLA alleles currently has no diagnostic utility in JIA. For the interested reader, Hersh and Prahalad recently reviewed the genetics of JIA, and Yasin and Schulert published a detailed review of the genetics and pathophysiology of systemic JIA (SJIA).

There is no known prevention for JIA.

Pathophysiology

Synovitis in JIA is characterized by synovial hypertrophy, edema, and hypervascularity. A mixed inflammatory infiltrate of T and B lymphocytes, plasma cells, macrophages, and dendritic cells is found in the synovial lining of affected joints. Infiltrating mononuclear cells produce proinflammatory cytokines and chemokines that contribute to bone and cartilage erosion and perpetuate recruitment of inflammatory cells.

SJIA is uniquely characterized by significant innate immune activation, including increased production of the proinflammatory cytokines interleukin-1 (IL-1) and 6 (IL-6). Some experts suggest that SJIA may be better classified as an autoinflammatory disease.

Given their unique clinical phenotypes, the epidemiology, clinical manifestations, diagnosis, and management of the JIA subtypes will each be discussed separately. Some general principles of diagnosis and management reviewed in "Current Diagnosis and Therapy", previously discussed, and introduced in the oligoarticular JIA section are applicable to all JIA subtypes.

Oligoarticular Juvenile Idiopathic Arthritis

Epidemiology

Oligoarticular JIA is the most common JIA subtype, comprising 40% to 50% of all cases, with an incidence of approximately 1 in 10,000 children per year. Peak age of onset is 1 to 4 years, with a female predominance. It is most commonly seen in children of Northern European descent.

Clinical Manifestations

Children with oligoarticular JIA present with arthritis in one to four joints, without spread to more than four joints in the first 6 months of disease. Oligoarthritis typically affects large joints in an asymmetrical pattern. The most common presentation is arthritis of a single knee. Swelling is the predominant symptom, often with little or no apparent pain early in the disease course. Affected joints may have a limited range of motion or contractures. A relatively painless limp is common, and is sometimes the first symptom apparent to parents. Stiffness is worse in the morning or after inactivity, though may be difficult for children to describe. Children with oligoarthritis may experience a persistent oligoarticular course (limited to four or fewer affected joints throughout the child's life) or an extended articular course (spread to five or more joints after the first 6 months of disease).

Diagnosis

A careful history and exam are key to diagnosis. Persistent joint swelling for more than 6 weeks, joint contracture, and/or gait disturbance are the most common presenting symptoms of oligoarticular JIA. Physical exam reveals joint effusion or thickened synovium indicating joint inflammation. Some children may also have warmth, decreased range of motion, contracture, or pain with range of motion on exam. Atrophy of adjacent muscles can be seen in chronic arthritis. Children with oligoarticular JIA are otherwise well-appearing. Severe pain (especially with nighttime waking), extremely red or hot joints, *migratory* swelling, fevers, rash, pallor, or a generally ill-appearing child suggest an alternative diagnosis.

All forms of JIA are diagnosed on the basis of objective signs of arthritis, a history of at least 6 weeks of persistent symptoms, and exclusion of alternative diagnoses *as appropriate based on the patient's clinical picture*. As there is no single test that can confirm the diagnosis of JIA, the value of lab testing is limited to excluding other diagnoses and for prognostic purposes in confirmed cases of JIA (see "Complications"). Radiographs have limited diagnostic value with the exception of detecting other conditions such as malignancy. MRI or musculoskeletal ultrasound can be useful in cases of equivocal or challenging physical exam (such as in obese patients).

Differential Diagnosis

In some patients with a classic clinical picture, no specific workup for other diagnoses is needed. Prompt evaluation by a pediatric rheumatologist is key to confirming the presence of arthritis, determining an appropriate individualized workup, and rapidly initiating treatment if a diagnosis of JIA is established.

Features that suggest the need to evaluate for alternative diagnoses include the following:

- Atypical demographics (age, ethnicity)—may suggest a different JIA subtype such as ERA in older children (see "Enthesitis-Related Arthritis").
- Travel history—may suggest the need to evaluate for Lyme arthritis or tuberculosis in patients residing in or traveling to endemic areas.
- Atypical clinical features—severe pain, constitutional symptoms such as weight loss, fevers, fatigue, or an ill appearance should prompt consideration of infection, malignancy, inflammatory bowel disease, or systemic collagen vascular disease such as lupus in a child with arthritis. Acute, subacute, or migratory arthritis suggests an infectious or postinfectious cause

(including rheumatic fever). Episodic joint swelling, especially after trauma, may suggest a bleeding disorder or intra-articular vascular malformation.

Treatment

Treatment of JIA aims to completely control joint inflammation to control symptoms and mitigate the risk of joint damage. In oligoarticular JIA, either scheduled nonsteroidal antiinflammatory drugs (NSAIDs) or intraarticular corticosteroid injections are used as first line therapy. NSAIDs must be administered at antiinflammatory doses on a scheduled basis to control inflammation, and may take 6 to 8 weeks to be effective. Naproxen (Naprosyn) is often preferred due to twice daily dosing and available liquid formulation. Steroid joint injections can control inflammation rapidly and are often used for patients with contractures or severe arthritis to more rapidly restore physical function. Intraarticular steroid injections should not be repeated more frequently than every 3 months. In patients with arthritis refractory to NSAIDs or steroid injections, traditional or biologic disease modifying antirheumatic drugs (DMARDs), such as methotrexate (Trexall) and tumor necrosis factor (TNF) inhibitors, can be used (some are off-label) in a stepwise fashion until disease control is achieved. DMARDs should be prescribed and monitored by a rheumatologist.

Monitoring

JIA disease control is monitored by a rheumatologist on the basis of history and physical exam. The frequency of follow-up visits varies depending on the patient's disease course and medications. Assessments of functional status should be performed to identify patients who would benefit from physical and occupational therapy service or school accommodations. Eye screening for uveitis is a critical part of JIA monitoring (see "Complications"). Medication toxicity monitoring depends on the medication used:

- Daily NSAIDs: complete blood count (CBC), comprehensive metabolic panel (CMP), and urinalysis every 6 to 12 months.
- Methotrexate: CBC and CMP at baseline, 1 month after starting or dose escalation, and then every 3 months on stable doses. Urine pregnancy screening should be considered in girls of reproductive age.
- Biologic DMARDS: Similar lab screening to methotrexate, with some variation depending on medication. Testing for tuberculosis should be performed prior to starting biologic medications.

Patients on immunosuppressive medications should be evaluated promptly for symptoms of infection. They should avoid live virus vaccines, but receive all other age-appropriate vaccinations including an annual flu vaccine.

Complications

Articular complications include joint limitation, contractures, and muscle atrophy, leading to chronic disability and pain, though these complications are less common with currently available treatments. A complication of arthritis unique to the growing child is local growth disturbance, most commonly seen as leg length discrepancy as a result of knee arthritis. Inflammation near the open growth plate can cause overgrowth of the affected limb in young children or premature growth plate closure leading to a shorter limb in the adolescents.

Chronic anterior uveitis is a common complication of JIA, particularly oligoarticular and RF negative polyarticular JIA. Chronic uveitis is treatable but carries a high risk of morbidity including cataract, glaucoma, synechiae (adhesions leading to an irregular pupil), band keratopathy (corneal calcium deposits), and blindness. Chronic uveitis is often completely asymptomatic until damage has occurred. Because it can only be detected by slit lamp exam performed by an eye doctor, regular screening is critical to early detection, treatment, and prevention of permanent damage. Uveitis is more likely to occur early in the course of disease, in patients who are ANA positive, and who have an early age of arthritis onset. Well-established screening recommendations guide the frequency of eye exams, ranging from every 3 to 12 months, depending on risk factors. Risk stratification for uveitis is the only use of ANA testing in patients with JIA. Uveitis may occur independent of active arthritis, so eye screening is a critical part of health maintenance for people with JIA throughout their lives. All children diagnosed with uveitis should see an ophthalmologist with experience treating uveitis. Topical corticosteroids are first-line therapy for anterior uveitis, though long-term use is not advisable given the risk of cataracts and glaucoma. Methotrexate[1] and the TNF inhibitors adalimumab (Humira) and infliximab (Remicade)[1] are used widely in children with refractory uveitis. Some patients require more aggressive treatment for uveitis than for arthritis.

Polyarticular Juvenile Idiopathic Arthritis
Epidemiology
Polyarticular arthritis has two subtypes. RF negative polyarthritis has two peaks of onset (at 1 to 4 years and in adolescence) and comprises 20% of all JIA. It is more common in girls and occurs in all ethnicities. RF positive polyarthritis makes up only 5% of JIA, has a peak onset of 9 to 11 years, and is more common in girls and in nonwhites.

Clinical Manifestations
Children with polyarthritis present with evidence of arthritis (swelling, morning stiffness, pain, limited range of motion) in five of more joints. Young children may present with gait disturbance or loss of milestones, while older children may present with prolonged morning stiffness or difficulty with activities of daily living and fine motor tasks. Large and small joints in the extremities are affected (often symmetrically). Long-standing disease can produce bony overgrowth of the small joints in the hands or joint deformities including wrist subluxation and boutonniere deformities of the fingers. Arthritis of the cervical spine (presenting with limited extension) and temporomandibular joint (TMJ; presenting with decreased mouth opening, jaw deviation, or micrognathia) are common and cause significant morbidity. Mild to moderate systemic symptoms, including fatigue and weight loss, may be present; however, high grade fevers should not occur.

Diagnosis
Diagnosis hinges on the presence of arthritis in five or more joints on physical exam (typically with some degree of wrist and hand involvement), at least 6 weeks of symptoms, and exclusion of other causes. There are no confirmatory tests; however, in patients with polyarticular JIA diagnosed clinically, the RF and anticitric citrullinated peptide (anti-CCP) have prognostic value. RF and anti-CCP positivity are associated with a more severe, erosive course. Some children with polyarticular JIA have normal inflammatory markers, while others have a moderately elevated erythrocyte sedimentation rate (ESR) and anemia of chronic disease. These findings are more useful for assessing overall health and monitoring response to therapy than in establishing an initial diagnosis, as they are nonspecific.

Differential Diagnosis
Reactive arthritis may present with polyarticular joint swelling, but is typically acute in onset and characterized by more pain than is seen in JIA. The arthritis of acute rheumatic fever is typically exquisitely painful and has a unique migratory pattern. While patients with polyarticular JIA may experience an *additive* arthritis pattern early in the disease course, *migratory* arthritis (i.e., swelling resolving completely in one joint and moving to another) is not seen in JIA. In patients with extreme pain, bone pain, pallor, or severe fatigue, malignancy such as leukemia or neuroblastoma should be considered.

Polyarthritis can occur as a manifestation of other underlying autoimmune diseases, including systemic lupus erythematosus, mixed connective tissue disease, or inflammatory bowel disease. The best approach to evaluating for these conditions

is a thorough history and physical exam. Oral ulcers, Raynaud phenomenon, or malar or discoid rashes raise concern for lupus. Because ANA tests are nonspecific and have a high positive rate in both the healthy and JIA populations, an ANA test in isolation is not helpful in evaluating for lupus unless it is negative (which essentially excludes lupus). In cases in which the history or physical raises concern for lupus, using a combination of several laboratory studies is more helpful. A reasonable initial workup for lupus when clinical suspicion is high includes an ANA, specific lupus antibodies (Smith, double-stranded DNA), ESR, C3 and C4 levels, CBC to evaluate for cytopenias, a urinalysis, creatinine, and blood pressure measurement.

Inflammatory bowel disease can present with inflammatory arthritis. Inflammatory bowel disease (IBD) should be considered in patients with significant oral ulcers, chronic abdominal pain and/or diarrhea, weight loss, significantly elevated ESR, or anemia.

Treatment
The goals of treatment are the same as for oligoarticular disease, although children with polyarticular JIA often require more aggressive medical therapy to attain inactive disease. Scheduled NSAIDs are often started first line or in conjunction with other medications for pain relief, but rarely are effective as monotherapy. Intraarticular steroid injections may be used in combination with systemic therapy for severely affected or critical joints, but monotherapy with steroid injections is not a viable approach to treating this disease.

Most children with polyarticular JIA require treatment with DMARDs for disease control. There are two general approaches to initiation of medications: step-up therapy and early aggressive (combination) therapy. The choice of approach may be driven by provider and/or patient preference or severity of disease. In a step-up approach, methotrexate is most commonly used as the first DMARD. Methotrexate (10 to 15 mg/m^2 or 0.4 to 1 mg/kg) once weekly is administered orally or subcutaneously, with subcutaneous dosing preferred by many pediatric rheumatologists on the basis of possible improved absorption and mitigation of side effects.

Biologic medications shown to be effective in JIA refractory to methotrexate include TNF inhibitors (etanercept [Enbrel], adalimumab [Humira], infliximab [Remicade][1], and others not yet FDA approved in children), the IL-6 inhibitor tocilizumab (Actemra), and the T cell costimulation inhibitor abatacept (Orencia). Selection of an initial biologic medication can be driven by a variety of factors including patient/parent preference, logistics of administration, side effects, comorbid medical conditions, and (in our current health system) insurance restrictions. The anti-CD20 medication rituximab (Rituxan)[1] is sometimes used in patients with RF positive disease, usually after failure of other medications. Medications with other biologic targets, including Janus kinase inhibitors, are currently under investigation in juvenile arthritis.

In patients with severe polyarticular JIA, an early aggressive approach, such as first-line combination therapy with methotrexate and a TNF inhibitor with or without adjunctive NSAIDs, intraarticular steroid injections, or a short oral steroid bridge, is sometimes used. With earlier aggressive use of DMARDs, treatment with systemic corticosteroids can now be limited to short courses or avoided altogether in most children. While systemic steroids can produce rapid improvements in pain, symptoms return quickly after discontinuation and their side effect profile makes long-term use unacceptable. Systemic steroids should *never* be initiated in a child presenting with musculoskeletal pain of unknown etiology, given the danger of corticosteroids in undiagnosed infection or malignancy.

Monitoring
Monitoring of clinical disease and medications (NSAIDs, methotrexate, TNF inhibitors) is the same as described for oligoarthritis. Other biologic medications have similar monitoring requirements,

including testing for latent tuberculosis (TB) prior to initiation. Some biologics have additional recommended laboratory monitoring parameters. Given the expertise needed to safely prescribe and monitor DMARDs, these medications should only be prescribed to children with JIA by a rheumatologist. In patients with systemic inflammation or anemia at presentation, these labs should be followed as adjunctive markers of disease activity, but normalization should not falsely reassure that arthritis is well controlled if the joint exam indicates otherwise. Children with polyarticular JIA who develop fever while on immunosuppression should be assessed promptly for infection.

Complications

Articular complications in polyarticular JIA include joint contractures, deformities, growth disturbances, and progressive, erosive disease. Cervical spine, TMJ, hip, and wrist involvement are associated with higher morbidity. Fortunately, with earlier aggressive treatment, severe joint destruction and severe physical disability are now less common. Surgical interventions are sometimes required for patients with severe micrognathia (mandibular distraction or reconstruction techniques), joint destruction (joint replacements), or severe growth disturbances (limb inequality procedures).

Children with polyarticular JIA can also develop chronic uveitis. Similar to oligoarticular JIA, age of onset, duration of disease, and ANA status are risk factors for development of uveitis and direct frequency of eye screening. The exception is that uveitis is rare in RF positive polyarticular JIA; thus eye screening is needed only once yearly in this subtype.

Enthesitis-Related Arthritis
Epidemiology
ERA is the only JIA subtype more common in boys, makes up 9% to 19% of all JIA, and has a peak age of onset of 10 to 13 years.

Clinical Manifestations
ERA is a childhood form of spondyloarthropathy and closely related to ankylosing spondylitis. Spondyloarthropathies are characterized by axial arthritis, although in children peripheral arthritis precedes axial disease, sometimes by years. Peripheral arthritis in ERA preferentially affects the lower extremities, often asymmetrically. Arthritis of the hips and sacroiliac joints, tenosynovitis (inflammation of tendon sheaths), and *enthesitis* (inflammation at the bony insertions of tendons, ligaments, or fascia) are common findings. *Tarsitis,* diffuse swelling of the dorsum of the foot, is relatively unique to ERA. Pain is more prominent in ERA than other JIA subtypes. Axial arthritis develops in some patients in late adolescence or adulthood. Uveitis in ERA is acute and symptomatic (with a red, photophobic eye), distinct from uveitis in other forms of JIA.

Diagnosis
ERA usually presents as monoarthritis or oligoarthritis in the lower extremities (hips, knees, ankles). Diagnosis is made on the basis of arthritis on exam with a history supporting a chronic course. HLA-B27 positivity can support the diagnosis, though the HLA-B27 is not a diagnostic test (as some ERA patients are B27 negative and many B27 positive individuals are healthy). Though most children do not have sacroiliitis or spinal arthritis at presentation, findings of inflammatory spinal arthritis on radiographs or magnetic resonance imaging strongly suggest this diagnosis.

Differential Diagnosis
School-aged children with ERA often present with arthritis of a single knee or ankle. In addition to the diagnostic considerations outlined above for oligoarthritis, ERA must be distinguished from oligoarticular JIA itself. Clues to diagnosis in this clinical scenario are older age (recall that the peak age of onset of oligoarticular JIA is age 1 to 4), male gender, and supporting clinical features if present (tenosynovitis, enthesitis, acute uveitis).

In children presenting with hip symptoms, infectious and orthopedic conditions (including slipped capital femoral epiphysis or

Perthes) should be considered. Rarely, older adolescents present with sacroiliitis. Low back stiffness, worse in the morning, helps distinguish from infectious and orthopedic conditions, though imaging is usually required to make this distinction with confidence. The vast majority of children with chronic low back pain have mechanical rather than inflammatory pain.

Treatment
The general approach to treatment of ERA is similar to polyarticular JIA, though for patients with sacroiliitis or spinal arthritis, TNF inhibition should be considered early in the disease course.

Monitoring
Monitoring is very similar to polyarticular JIA with a few exceptions:
1. Children with ERA should be monitored closely for development of axial arthritis. This may include a combination of the following approaches: querying symptoms of inflammatory back pain, eliciting sacroiliac pain on exam, measuring spine mobility (with a modified Schober test), and/or imaging sacroiliac joints with x-ray or magnetic resonance imaging (MRI).
2. Eye exams are only required once yearly and as indicated based on symptoms as uveitis in ERA is usually symptomatic.

Complications
Acute uveitis occurs in some patients with ERA, and often responds to topical corticosteroids. Patients who develop a red or photophobic eye should be evaluated promptly by an eye doctor. Arthritis of the spine, sacroiliac joints, and hips can be difficult to control, sometimes leading to joint destruction, even in the setting of prompt and aggressive therapy. In adulthood, these patients are at risk for progressive, ascending ankylosis of the spine.

Juvenile Psoriatic Arthritis
Epidemiology
Juvenile psoriatic arthritis comprises approximately 10% of JIA, is more common in girls, and has two peaks of onset: preschool and late childhood.

Clinical Manifestations
Psoriatic arthritis usually presents with peripheral joint involvement and can occur in a monoarticular, oligoarticular, or polyarticular pattern. Both small and large joints can be affected, often in an asymmetrical pattern. *Dactylitis,* or a sausage digit, is a unique feature of psoriatic arthritis not seen in other forms of JIA. Dactylitic fingers and toes exhibit diffuse swelling that extends beyond individual joints. Arthritis of the distal interphalangeal (DIP) joints is also unique to psoriatic arthritis among children with JIA. There is some clinical overlap between psoriatic arthritis and ERA. Enthesitis and tenosynovitis are prevalent features and sacroiliitis can occur in up to 30% of adolescents. Nail changes, including pitting, horizontal ridges, and onycholysis, are common, and overt psoriasis occurs in about half of children. Both chronic uveitis (with risk factors similar to patients with oligo- and polyarticular JIA) and acute uveitis (in HLA-B27 positive patients) can occur.

Diagnosis
Unlike adults, children with psoriatic arthritis often present with arthritis prior to skin disease. In patients with chronic arthritis and psoriasis, the diagnosis is relatively straightforward. In those with chronic arthritis without psoriasis, clinical clues to diagnosis include dactylitis, psoriatic nail changes (pitting or onycholysis), or a first-degree relative with psoriasis.

Differential Diagnosis
Depending on the pattern of joint involvement, differential diagnosis includes other forms of JIA (oligoarticular, polyarticular, ERA) and other conditions listed previously in the differential of

these JIA subtypes. Small joint involvement or dactylitis help distinguish psoriatic from oligoarticular JIA in young children with less than five affected joints.

Treatment

The treatment approach is similar to polyarticular JIA, though for patients with sacroiliitis, enthesitis, or dactylitis, TNF inhibition has the most well-established efficacy.

Monitoring

Monitoring is similar to other forms of JIA including eye screening for chronic uveitis described for oligo- and polyarthritis and monitoring for axial arthritis described for ERA. In addition, patients who have not developed skin manifestations should be monitored for development of psoriasis.

Complications

Articular and ocular complications are similar to other JIA subtypes, though children with psoriatic arthritis often have poorer functional outcomes and lower rates of remission off medication than those with oligo- or polyarticular JIA.

Systemic Juvenile Idiopathic Arthritis
Epidemiology

SJIA occurs in children of all ages and into adulthood (Still disease in adults). It is the only form of JIA that affects boys and girls equally. SJIA makes up 10% to 20% of JIA. It occurs in all ethnicities, with increased prevalence in some Asian countries including Japan.

Clinical Manifestations

SJIA is characterized by fever, rash, and arthritis. Fevers in SJIA are high grade, typically spiking once (quotidian) or twice (double quotidian) daily with return to normal temperature between fevers. The rash seen in SJIA is salmon-colored or erythematous, macular or urticarial, sometimes with associated Koebner phenomenon. A unique feature of the SJIA rash is its *evanescent* nature: it appears with fever and resolves or fades during afebrile periods. The arthritis in SJIA can affect any number of joints, in any pattern, and is not always present at disease onset. In some patients, the latent period between onset of systemic features and arthritis is weeks or months. Many patients exhibit nonspecific symptoms, including fatigue, irritability, and myalgia during fevers.

Children with SJIA have significant systemic inflammation during periods of disease activity. Profoundly elevated white blood count, platelet count, ESR, CRP, and anemia are common.

SJIA is truly a systemic disease, with some patients exhibiting lymphadenopathy, hepatosplenomegaly, and serositis (pleural or pericardial effusions). The most feared complication of SJIA is macrophage activation syndrome (MAS; see "Complications").

Diagnosis

SJIA is diagnosed based on the presence of quotidian fevers, evanescent Stills rash, arthritis, and systemic inflammation, with exclusion of similar conditions. SJIA often leads to inpatient evaluation, given patients' high grade fevers and ill appearance. Children who lack arthritis at the time of presentation are challenging to diagnose. In practice, SJIA is often presumptively diagnosed before arthritis has been present for 6 weeks (and sometimes in the absence of arthritis), as the severity of this disease can necessitate urgent treatment.

Differential Diagnosis

SJIA has a broad differential diagnosis that includes infectious (viral, bacterial), oncologic (leukemia, neuroblastoma), and inflammatory conditions (Kawasaki, polyarteritis nodosa, inflammatory bowel disease, among others). Involvement of infectious disease and oncology consultants can help exclude these mimics, particularly if treatment with corticosteroids is being considered.

Additional workup, including infectious studies and bone marrow biopsy, is appropriate in cases of diagnostic uncertainty.

Treatment

The treatment paradigms have evolved more for SJIA than any other JIA subtype over the last decade. Traditionally, children with SJIA were treated with systemic corticosteroids, resulting in the full spectrum of anticipated morbidities (growth delay, infections, osteoporosis, etc.). Traditional DMARDs and TNF inhibitors are significantly less effective than for other JIA subtypes. Targeted therapy with inhibition of IL-1 (with anakinra [Kineret][1] or canakinumab [Ilaris]) or IL-6 (with tocilizumab [Actemra]) is the emerging standard of care, though optimal timing of these medications is unclear. Many pediatric rheumatologists are now using IL-1 or IL-6 blockade first line or after a failed NSAID trial to avoid or minimize corticosteroids. Systemic corticosteroids continue to have a role in severe disease or MAS. Other treatments for MAS include cyclosporine (Neoral)[1] and etoposide (Toposar)[1].

Monitoring

Monitoring is similar to polyarticular JIA, with a few exceptions. As uveitis is rare in SJIA, eye exams are needed only annually. Laboratory markers of systemic inflammation are useful in monitoring disease activity and evaluating for impending MAS, which can develop even when disease otherwise appears well controlled. Given the serious and life-threatening nature of this disease, all children with SJIA should be followed closely by a pediatric rheumatologist or an adult rheumatologist with experience managing SJIA.

Complications

Articular complications of SJIA are similar to polyarticular JIA, though the arthritis of SJIA is often aggressive and destructive. There is emerging evidence that earlier treatment with targeted biologics may prevent progression to chronic polyarthritis.

MAS is a serious complication of SJIA, characterized by unregulated production of proinflammatory cytokines, macrophage proliferation, and hemophagocytic activity in the bone marrow and other organs. MAS is a potentially fatal rheumatologic emergency. It is often suspected on the basis of rapidly worsening clinical status and the development of continuous fever. Laboratory findings include a profoundly elevated ferritin, elevated lactate dehydrogenase and transaminases, falling blood cell counts, and paradoxically low or falling ESR and fibrinogen in the setting of other signs of systemic inflammation. MAS is currently considered a secondary form of hemophagocytic lymphohistiocytosis (HLH).

---

[1]Not FDA approved for this indication.

References

Aeschlimann FA, Chong S, Lyons TW, et al: Risk of serious infections associated with biologic agents in juvenile idiopathic arthritis: a systematic review and meta-analyses, *J Pediatr* 204:162–171, 2019.

Clarke SLN, Sen ES, Ramanan AV: Juvenile Idiopathic arthritis-associated uveitis, *Pediatric Rheumatol Online J* 14:27, 2016.

Crayne CB, Beukelman T: Juvenile idiopathic arthritis: oligoarthritis and polyarthritis, *Pediatr Clin N Am* 65:657–674, 2018.

Hersh AO, Prahalad S: Genetics of juvenile idiopathic arthritis, *Rheum Dis Clin N Am* 43:435–448, 2017.

Lee JJL, Schneider R: Systemic juvenile idiopathic arthritis, *Pediatr Clin N Am* 65:691–709, 2018.

Petty RE, Southwood TR, Manners P, et al: International League of Associations for Rheumatology classification of juvenile idiopathic arthritis: second revision, Edmonton, 2001, *J Rheumatol* 31(2):390–392, 2004.

Shoop-Worrall SJW, Kearsley-Fleet L, Thomson W, Verstappen SMM, Hyrich KL: How common is remission in juvenile idiopathic arthritis: a systematic review, *Semin Arthritis Rheum* 47:331–337, 2017.

Wong KO, Bond K, Homik J, Ellsworth JE, Karkhaneh M, Ha C, Dryden DM: Antinuclear antibody, rheumatoid factor, and cyclic-citrullinated peptide tests for evaluating musculoskeletal complaints in children: Comparative Effectiveness Review No. 50, *Agency for Healthcare Research and Quality*, 2012, Available at https://effectivehealthcare.ahrq.gov/sites/default/files/pdf/musculoskeletal-complaints-tests-children_research.pdf. Accessed 1 January 2019.

Yasin S, Schulert GS: Systemic juvenile idiopathic arthritis and macrophage activation syndrome: update on pathogenesis and treatment, *Curr Opin Rheumatol* 30:514–520, 2018.

OSTEOARTHRITIS

Method of
Rachel Chamberlain, MD; Jacob Christensen, DO; and Christopher Bossart, MD

CURRENT DIAGNOSIS

- Risk factors for osteoarthritis (OA) include age, gender, genetics, and anatomic factors, which are nonmodifiable; modifiable risk factors include body mass index (BMI), tobacco use, trauma, physical activity, and muscle strength.
- OA is diagnosed using both clinical and radiologic information.
- Clinical signs and symptoms include joint pain, crepitus, mild swelling, and joint line tenderness to palpation. Symptoms wax and wane and may be related to activity but can be present at varying times of day.
- The Kellgren-Lawrence Classification system can help determine the grade of OA, but the ultimate determination of the severity is based on clinical factors.

CURRENT THERAPY

- First-line therapy for OA includes exercise, physical therapy, and weight loss (if the patient is overweight or obese).
- Nonsteroidal antiinflammatory drugs (NSAIDs) are the best studied pharmacologic treatment for OA pain. Their use must be balanced by their side effects and the patient's comorbid conditions.
- Injections of corticosteroids may be used for OA pain management, but their pain relief effects are not long term.
- Hyaluronic acid injections can be considered in patients with mild to moderate OA of the knee, but this is an expensive therapy and evidence of effectiveness is mixed.
- No current treatment either in systemic medications or injections alters the course of OA. Research in the long-term benefits of biologic agents is ongoing.
- Total joint replacement is an expensive but definitive treatment for many patients with OA. The referring clinician should consider the patient's overall health and help optimize the patient's health for a successful outcome when referring for a total joint replacement.

Osteoarthritis (OA), also known as degenerative joint disease, is the most common form of arthritis worldwide. OA is a significant cause of morbidity, disability, and decreased quality of life. It is one of the leading contributors to global years lived with disability (YLDs) by Global Disease Burden studies. It is the leading cause of lower extremity disability. OA affects about one in eight people in the United States, or 27 to 31 million, and about 250 million people worldwide, with the most commonly affected joints being the knees, hips, hands, feet, and spine. As the age of the population and the rates of obesity increase, the economic impact of OA also increases. It is estimated that OA costs 1% to 2.5% of GDP in developed countries, with the majority of cost for treatment (85%) coming from joint replacement surgeries.

OA has been previously characterized pathologically by varying levels of cartilage involvement. One may find fissures and microfibrillations in mild or early disease, and erosive destruction of the joint surfaces may be seen in more advanced disease. However, it is recognized that the effects of OA can be seen throughout the entire joint including the bone, synovium, menisci, and ligaments.

Pathogenesis
The pathogenesis of OA remains unclear. For decades, the traditional belief was that OA was a "wear and tear" condition associated with the cumulative stress of aging. This theory has not been shown to be true, or at least it is not an accurate depiction of "the whole story." Research investigating other possible mechanisms is gaining traction. More recent research areas of focus include what role inflammatory mediators, genetics, metabolic factors, proteases, and biomarkers may play in the development of OA.

Risk Factors
Despite the pathogenesis of OA being unclear, a number of factors have been identified to be associated with increased risk. These risk factors include age, gender, body mass index (BMI), genetics, tobacco smoking, trauma, chronic overuse, anatomic factors, and muscle strength.

Age—There is a clear correlation between aging and development of OA. It is also clear that the aging of joint tissues and the development of OA are separate and distinct processes. There are a number of aging changes within the joint that may contribute to development of OA including: thinning of articular cartilage, reduced hydration, accumulation of advanced glycation end-products (AGEs), and abnormal calcification ("chondrocalcinosis"). Based on population based radiographic surveys from the Framingham study, the prevalence of knee OA in patients aged 63 to 94 was 33%, and symptomatic knee OA was 9.5%.

Gender—OA is more common in women than men. Some have postulated that the correlation between age and OA explains the why OA is more common in the postmenopausal years; however, there is some evidence to suggest decreased estrogen exposure in women could also be a contributing factor.

BMI—Being overweight or obese has been well documented as a strong risk factor for development of OA. This is likely both related to increased mechanical forces and metabolic changes associated with obesity. Weight loss has also been shown to reduce the risk of developing knee OA.

Genetics—Twin studies have shown a genetic contribution of about 40% to 70% depending on the site of OA. There exists substantial heterogeneity depending on the site of involvement, and there is also racial variation, which makes studying this genetic component more difficult.

Trauma and chronic overuse—Trauma, which includes both major injuries and surgery, increases the risk of OA. For example, history of anterior cruciate ligament (ACL) tear in the knee is associated with increased risk of OA development regardless of whether surgical reconstruction is done. The mechanism for this is not completely understood. Chronic overuse as is seen in some occupations carries an increased risk of development of OA. For example, professional soccer players have an increased risk of developing knee OA, and professional baseball pitchers have a higher risk of developing elbow OA.

Biomechanical factors—Joint structural abnormalities may increase the risk of developing OA. The understanding of the role of muscle strength in OA is expanding. It is known that patients with knee and hip OA have reduced muscle strength in the surrounding muscles. However, it has been thought previously that this was a consequence of the symptoms of OA causing decreased activity, muscle atrophy, and subsequent weakness. There is more recent evidence to suggest that muscle weakness may actually predate the onset of knee OA.

Clinical Features
OA is characterized clinically by insidious onset, usage-related joint pain, which can be accompanied by mild stiffness. Pain can be present at varying times of day. Mild swelling may be present in OA; however, large effusion and history of trauma or injury should prompt further workup. Patients may complain of limitation in range of motion, as well as a sensation of giving way or buckling (particularly in knee OA). Tenderness to palpation along the joint lines is a common physical exam finding. Joint deformity is a sign of advanced disease. Symptoms are typically slowly progressive as is the disease course.

OA severity can be graded based on radiographic criteria or a combination of radiographic criteria and symptom severity. Perhaps the most commonly used radiographic criteria is the

Kellgren-Lawrence method, classifying OA severity into grades 0 to 4 based on presence of joint space narrowing, osteophyte formation, and sclerosis of subchondral bone (Table 1). This method is certainly useful, though it should be mentioned that there are limitations to this method—namely, that there is somewhat poor correlation between radiographic findings and symptoms. It is estimated that up to 50% of people with radiographic findings of OA do not have any symptoms.

Current Therapy

Treatment for OA is individualized based on patient symptoms, values, needs, goals, and response to therapies. There is no single treatment for OA, which reliably and consistently manages symptoms on its own. Therefore, a combination of therapeutic approaches is used in order to optimize function, minimize pain, and in some cases modify the process of damage to the joint. In general, safer treatments should be considered first before trying other treatments with higher risk profiles. Treatments can be placed into four categories: nonpharmacologic, pharmacologic, nonsurgical, and surgical interventions.

Nonpharmacologic Therapies

Nonpharmacologic therapies represent the mainstay of treatment for OA initially. These therapies include education, exercise, weight management, braces, assistive devices, psychologic therapies, manual medicine, and alternative therapies.

Education—It is important to inform patients about their diagnosis, the modifiable risk factors for their specific case, and their expected prognosis. Information should be provided regarding the various treatment options including their risks, benefits, costs, and alternatives. Doing this helps encourage active shared decision making and combat some of the common misconceptions about OA management. Patient involvement in setting goals and self-managing their condition improves adherence and can make a significant difference in patients' view of their disease.

Exercise—The goal of exercise therapy is reduction in pain and improvement in joint function. Various forms of exercise exist, and physical activity in general should be encouraged, providing it is done with patient symptoms as a guide. The forms of exercise with the best evidence for improvement, particularly in knee OA, are aerobic exercise and resistance strength training. Perhaps the most readily available form of aerobic exercise is walking, and formal walking programs have been shown to significantly improve OA symptoms, as well as quadriceps strength. Aquatic exercise has also been shown to be beneficial, and has the added benefit of decreased weight-bearing stress on joints.

Weight loss—In overweight and obese patients (BMI > 25), a reduction of 10% of baseline body weight has been shown to decrease OA-related joint pain. This is true of patients with knee and hip OA, but may also be beneficial in patients with OA of the

hands in light of evidence that increased BMI is a risk factor for development of hand OA. Again, this may be partially related to metabolic changes.

Braces and assistive devices—Walking aids, such as a walking stick or cane, as well as knee braces for patients with joint malalignment, may be helpful, and should be considered as an adjunct treatment in appropriate patients. OA of the thumb is particularly amenable to splinting to improve pain.

Psychologic therapies—Chronic pain from OA can have significant effects on a patient's ability to function. Often as patients feel less able to perform the activities they enjoy, their mood is adversely affected, which in turn negatively affects their pain symptoms. There is some evidence that psychological interventions, such as cognitive behavioral therapy, are helpful in this regard.

Manual medicine—Manual techniques, whether performed by a physical therapist, doctor of osteopathic medicine (DO), massage therapist, or chiropractor, typically focus on improvement/maintenance of range of motion as well as joint mobility. There is some limited evidence to suggest manual manipulation may improve pain scores, particularly when combined with exercise therapy. However, more research in this area is needed.

Alternative therapies—There is currently insufficient evidence to recommend the use of acupuncture, therapeutic ultrasound, and neuromuscular electrical stimulation for treatment of OA.

Pharmacotherapy

Despite the fact that nonpharmacologic agents are first line, many patients with OA require drug therapy. Although no available medications predictably reverse or halt the inexorable progression of the disease, some medications do reduce pain and inflammation, enhancing the patient's quality of life.

Analgesics—The most common nonnarcotic analgesic agent currently used for OA is acetaminophen (Tylenol). The recommended dose for OA is 1 g administered every 8 hours or three to four times daily (not to exceed 4 g/day). However, even at a high dose, studies are mixed if acetaminophen is effective for OA pain. Adverse effects are rare, but caution must be exercised in patients who have preexisting renal or liver conditions. Duloxetine (Cymbalta) 60 mg daily is approved by the US Food and Drug Administration (FDA) for mild to moderate pain resulting from OA. In a double-blind, randomized, placebo-controlled study of patients with chronic pain due to OA of the knees, there was significant improvement with duloxetine versus the placebo. In treating OA, the regular use of opioids is not recommended or supported. Tramadol (Ultram) is commonly used, particularly in patients who have contraindications to nonsteroidal antiinflammatory drugs (NSAIDs), but we suggest caution in prescribing even this medication given potential for tolerance. While for years it has been suggested that opioids improve quality of life and function in patients with chronic pain from OA, there is no evidence to support this in OA. Opioids may be needed occasionally for intense pain, but the benefits are limited compared to the risks of tolerance, opioid misuse, addiction, overdose, and death.

Nonsteroidal antiinflammatory drugs—Pain in OA patients is often not adequately controlled with pure analgesics, whereas NSAIDs in adequate dosage can provide significant clinical improvement. The 2013 AAOS Guidelines on nonsurgical management of knee OA recommend NSAIDs with a strong strength of recommendation. If simple analgesics fail to provide adequate relief, one of the many currently available NSAIDs may be tried. Clinical trials with naproxen (Anaprox), diclofenac (Voltaren), and sulindac (Clinoril) showed significantly greater improvement when compared with high-dose acetaminophen. The chief limiting factor in the use of NSAIDs is the possible induced gastric pathologic changes, disturbed renal function, and potential increased cardiac events. In addition, many patients with OA may be on other platelet inhibiting medications and interactions should be taken into consideration. For patients ages 75 and above, topical NSAIDs are advised over oral given less toxicity and adverse effects. Cost and compliance also must be given consideration.

TABLE 1	Kellgren Lawrence Radiographic Classification of Osteoarthritis of the Knee
Grade 1	Doubtful joint space narrowing, possible osteophytic lipping
Grade 2	Definite osteophytes, possible joint space narrowing
Grade 3	Moderate osteophytes, definite joint space narrowing, some sclerosis, possible bone-end deformity
Grade 4	Large osteophytes, marked joint space narrowing, severe sclerosis, definite bone ends deformity

Data from Kellgren JH, Lawrence JS. Radiological assessment of osteo-arthrosis. *Ann Rheum Dis.* 1957;16:494–502.

Many of the NSAIDs are now available in dosage forms that can be given once or twice daily, which helps overcome the issue of noncompliance.

Cyclooxygenase 2 inhibitors—COX-2 inhibitors block prostaglandin synthesis and inflammatory mediators without the COX-1 effect of inhibiting gastric mucosal protection. In the United States, the COX-2–specific inhibiting NSAID that is FDA approved is celecoxib (Celebrex). It is equivalent to the older nonselective NSAIDs with regard to therapeutic effectiveness, but the risk of gastrointestinal injury and adverse effects on platelet aggregation is lessened. The risk of renal side effects is probably comparable with that of the conventional NSAIDs. A trial assessing the effect of celecoxib on cardiovascular events found a slightly higher risk of cardiovascular events, but primarily only at higher doses (400 mg/day or greater). In addition, celecoxib can be used with low-dose aspirin (81 mg) daily and anticoagulants, including warfarin. It is important to take into consideration that the cost of Celebrex is several times that of traditional NSAIDs.

Glucosamine and chondroitin sulfate—Glucosamine and chondroitin sulfate are over-the-counter dietary supplements that have gained moderate press touting their possible symptom-modifying effects. However, there is no significant evidence demonstrating that either of these used alone or in combination prevents or reduces arthritis in the knee. A Cochrane review shows mild improvement in pain scores at short-term follow-up with glucosamine compared with placebo, however only with certain preparations of the product. At this point, multiple organizations including the American College of Rheumatology and American Academy of Orthopedic Surgeons cannot recommend their use in treating OA.

Turmeric—Turmeric[7] has been used for treatment of many inflammatory disease processes, including OA, with modest improvement in pain. Curcumin[7] is the primary constituent within turmeric, and there is thought that regular intake can protect joints in individuals with OA. The studies to date are small and limited in number, but they do show modest reduction in pain among those with OA. Larger studies would be needed in order for a definitive recommendation to be made but given its low side effect profile and risk of adverse effects it seems to be a reasonable addition to treatment. However, turmeric may interact with other antiplatelet therapies, and this should be considered individually for each patient.

Disease-modifying drugs—To date, there are no known medications that reliably slow or stop the disease process of OA, and disease modifying antirheumatic drugs (DMARDs) are not recommended in the treatment of OA.

Intra-articular Injections

Corticosteroid injections (CSI)—Early in symptomatic OA it is preferable to attempt to control symptoms by nonpharmacologic therapy and with oral therapy, rather than by local injection. CSI are commonly used for OA. Steroids are strong antiinflammatory medications, and there is reasonable evidence that CSI decreases pain in the short term. There remain concerns that CSI may damage cartilage and therefore hasten the advancement of OA. Clinical trials remain mixed. However, when noninvasive therapies are not controlling OA pain or a patient has an OA flair, CSI can provide relief. CSI is thought to be relatively safe to be given three to four times per year, although this is an expert opinion and not based in sound evidence. The remote risk of introducing infection from the procedure is minimized by adhering to a meticulous aseptic technique. CSI is thought to be less problematic than systemic steroids when it comes to side effects such as raising blood sugar, but caution should be used in patients with diabetes, particularly uncontrolled DM. While arthrocentesis of a painful arthritic joint is commonly done, there is little evidence that this is an effective therapy, particularly after the short term.

Hyaluronic acid—Intra-articular hyaluronic acid (HA) injections have been approved by the FDA since 1997 as a medical device for OA of the knee. The clinical use of intra-articular HA in painful OA of the knee was introduced in Europe in the 1990s. The mechanism of action of HA is not completely understood, but it is thought to restore normal viscoelastic properties to the pathologically altered synovial fluid. Other possible beneficial effects include protection of the chondrocytes, antiinflammatory effects, and possible improvement of the mechanics of joint motion. Unfortunately, in non-industry-funded studies, head-to-head comparisons often fail to show superiority over cortisone and placebo injections. In addition, HA does not change the course of OA. Numerous preparations of FDA-approved HA products are in wide use in the United States. Initially, all HA products were extracted from rooster combs; however, that is no longer the case. In approximately 2% to 8% of patients injected with avian derived product, a subsequent pseudoseptic reaction can occur, mimicking an infected joint. Newer HA products are not animal-derived preparations but rather are developed from biological fermentation of streptococcal bacteria. In the United States, these products are only approved for knee OA. Drawbacks of intra-articular HA products include mixed evidence, cost, and less efficacy in patients with morbid obesity or severe (Kellrgan Lawrence Grade 4) OA.

Platelet rich plasma (PRP)—PRP injections have become popular in recent years. However, as many of these procedures are not covered by insurance, their use has been limited secondary to the expense of these treatments. There are some studies suggesting increased efficacy in functional improvement when compared to HA products. However, the data are still lacking, and it is hard to make clear conclusions at this point.

Stem cells—Stem cell injections have become an intriguing area of research. The thought that intra-articular injections of stem cells can help improve/restart chondrogenesis, and regeneration of damaged cartilage is actively being researched. However, a recent systematic review of the literature shows only a low level of evidence for its use, all of which were studies deemed to be at high risk for bias. At this time, it is not considered a mainstay treatment for OA in the United States.

Surgical Management of Osteoarthritis

Surgical management of arthritis varies by which joint is affected, with knee arthritis being most common, followed by hip. Knee arthroscopy should not be used to manage knee OA and/or degenerative meniscus tears in the setting of OA, as there is little to no improvement compared with exercise. Hemiarthroplasty can be considered in patients with unicompartmental knee arthritis, and may carry less risks than total knee arthroplasty (TKA). In addition, a valgus-producing proximal tibial osteotomy may be beneficial in patients with symptomatic medial compartment knee OA. Total joint arthroplasty is an expensive surgery, though often well covered by insurance companies. The surgeries carry significant risks, including cardiovascular events, deep vein thrombosis, and prosthesis infection, which can lead to long hospitalizations for intravenous antibiotics and repeat surgeries. Not all patients have the pain relief and function improvement expected from total joint arthroplasty (TJA).

When referring a patient to orthopedic surgery for consideration of a total hip or knee arthroplasty, the clinician may be able to help prepare the patient to optimize their surgical outcome. This includes, but is not limited to, helping a patient with smoking cessation, weight loss, and diabetes control. Ideally, a patient would be tobacco/nicotine free for at least 8 weeks prior to surgery, would have a BMI less than 40, and would have a hemoglobin A1C ≤7.0. In addition, the referring clinician should take into consideration that patients with chronic pain and/or opioid use, depression and anxiety, liver cirrhosis/hepatitis C, and other chronic conditions may not have optimal outcomes from total joint replacement. It is acceptable to delay total knee arthroplasty up to 8 months to improve these modifiable risk factors without decreasing the patient's benefit from total joint arthroplasty. Arthroplasty procedures are also performed for arthritis of the shoulder, elbow, wrist, thumb, and ankle with varying degrees of

---

[7] Available as dietary supplement.

evidence for pain and quality of life improvement. Surgical techniques and prostheses are undergoing advancements and improving patient outcomes for the less commonly done arthroplasty surgeries, and clinicians can expect this technology to continue to advance in the future.

Conclusions

OA remains a very common source of pain and disability throughout the world and also carries a significant financial burden. The pathophysiology of OA is more complex than previously believed, and is not fully understood. OA has both modifiable and nonmodifiable risk factors. Nonmodifiable risk factors include age, gender, and genetic risk/family history. Modifiable risk factors include weight loss in patients who are overweight or obese, eliminating tobacco exposure, trauma and overuse, and control of metabolic syndrome.

Nonpharmacologic therapy for OA is first-line treatment and includes education and management of patient expectations, weight loss, exercise, and physical therapy. Braces and assistive devices, cognitive behavioral therapy, manual therapy, and alternative therapy may also be considered but have less definitive evidence.

Pharmacologic therapy is usually required for OA, with acetaminophen being first line. Clinicians should educate patients on high dose acetaminophen and safe amounts to take to achieve therapeutic effect without danger to liver. NSAIDs are often more effective at controlling pain from OA, but do carry a higher risk profile for gastrointestinal bleeding, renal dysfunction, and cardiovascular events. Herbal medications such as glucosamine chondroitin and turmeric may also be beneficial but studies are mixed. Opioids should be avoided in management of OA pain, as there is no evidence that they improve function and quality of life (as previously proposed) but do carry very serious side effects.

Nonsurgical interventions such as intra-articular injections can be beneficial in managing pain from OA. It is important to counsel patients that none of the current injection therapies have data that they change the course of the disease process; they only help control pain and improve function. Corticosteroid injections often give the patient good pain relief but are often not long lasting. HA injections may also be beneficial, but many studies show equivocal pain improvement compared with cortisone and the cost is much greater. Studies are still ongoing at biologic agent injections such as PRP and stem cell therapies, and data is mixed. It is unclear if these expensive, non-FDA-approved therapies are beneficial at this time.

Total joint arthroplasty is the definitive treatment for OA, with the best data in hip followed by knee arthroplasty. These surgeries carry significant risks, especially in the older population that OA most commonly affects. In addition, surgery is very expensive and associated with significant time loss from work. Patients' chronic medical conditions should be well controlled prior to a total joint arthroplasty, to minimize risks of poor outcomes or adverse effects.

References

American Academy of Orthopedic Surgeons: Management of Osteoarthritis of the Hip Evidence-Based Clinical Practice Guideline. Available at: https://www.aaos .org/uploadedFiles/PreProduction/Quality/Guidelines_and_Reviews/OA%20Hip %20CPG_3.13.17.pdf. Accessed 15 March 2019.

Bartels EM, Juhl CB, Christensen R, et al: Aquatic exercise for the treatment of knee and hip osteoarthritis, *Cochrane Database of Systematic Reviews* 2016, Available at: https://doi.org/10.1002/cca.1312.

Brown GA: AAOS Clinical Practice Guideline: Treatment of osteoarthritis of the knee: evidence-based guideline, 2nd Edition, *Journal of the American Academy of Orthopaedic Surgeons* 21(9):577–579, 2013, Available at: https://doi. org/10.5435/jaaos-21-09-577.

Conaghan, P. I56. DMARDs in Osteoarthritis: What is the evidence? *Rheumatology,* 53(suppl_1):i12–i13, 2014, Available at: https://doi.org/10.1093/rheumato logy/keu061.003

Dadabo J, Fram J, Jayabalan P: Noninterventional therapies for the management of knee osteoarthritis, *The Journal of Knee Surgery* 32(01):046–054, 2018, Available at: https://doi.org/10.1055/s-0038-1676107.

Dai WL, et al: Efficacy of platelet-rich plasma in the treatment of knee osteoarthritis: a meta-analysis of randomized controlled trials, *Arthroscopy* 33(3):659–670. e1, 2017 Mar, Available at: https://doi.org/10.1016/j.arthro.2016.09.024, Epub 2016 Dec 22. Review. PubMed PMID: 28012636.

Fransen M, Mcconnell S, Harmer AR, Esch MV, Simic M, Bennell KL: Exercise for osteoarthritis of the knee, *Cochrane Database of Systematic Reviews*, 2015, Available at: https://doi.org/10.1002/14651858.cd004376.pub3.

Henrotin Yves, et al: Curcumin: a new paradigm and therapeutic opportunity for the treatment of osteoarthritis: curcumin for osteoarthritis management, *SpringerPlus* 2(1), 2013, Available at: https://doi.org/10.1186/2193-1801-2-56.

Hochberg MC, Altman RD, April KT, et al: American College of Rheumatology 2012 recommendations for the use of nonpharmacologic and pharmacologic therapies in osteoarthritis of the hand, hip, and knee, *Arthritis Care & Research* 64(4):465–474, 2012, Available at: https://doi.org/10.1002/acr.21596.

Kohn MD, Sassoon AA, Fernando ND: Classifications in Brief: Kellgren-Lawrence Classification of Osteoarthritis, *Clin Orthop Relat Res* 474(8):1886–1893, 2016, Available at: https://doi.org/10.1007/s11999-016-4732-4.

Lin KY, et al: Intra-articular injection of platelet-rich plasma is superior to hyaluronic acid or saline solution in the treatment of mild to moderate knee osteoarthritis: a randomized, double-blind, triple-parallel, placebo-controlled clinical trial, *Arthroscopy* 35(1):106–117, 2019 Jan, Available at: https://doi.org/10.1016/j. arthro.2018.06.035. PubMed PMID: 30611335.

McGrory B, Weber K, Jevsevar D, Sevarino K: Surgical management of osteoarthritis of the knee, *Journal of the American Academy of Orthopaedic Surgeons* 24(8), 2016, Available at: https://doi.org/10.5435/JAAOS-D-16-00159.

Moyer RF, Birmingham TB, Bryant DM, et al: Valgus bracing for knee osteoarthritis: a meta-analysis of randomized trials, *Arthritis Care & Research* 67(4):493–501, 2015, Available at: https://doi.org/10.1002/acr.22472.

Nakagawa Yasuaki, et al: Short-term effects of highly-bioavailable curcumin for treating knee osteoarthritis: a randomized, double-blind, placebo-controlled prospective study, *Journal of Orthopaedic Science* 19(6):933–939, 2014, Available at: https://doi.org/10.1007/s00776-014-0633-0.

Oneill TW, Mccabe PS, Mcbeth J: Update on the epidemiology, risk factors and disease outcomes of osteoarthritis, *Best Practice & Research Clinical Rheumatology* 32(2):312–326, 2018, Available at: https://doi.org/10.1016/j.berh.2018.10.007.

Pas HI, Winters M, Haisma HJ, et al: Stem cell injections in knee osteoarthritis: a systematic review of the literature, *Br J Sports Med* 51(15):1125–1133, 2017 Aug, Available at: https://doi.org/10.1136/bjsports-2016-096793, Epub 2017 Mar 3. Review. PubMed PMID: 28258177.

Sanders TL, Pareek A, Kremers HM, et al: Long-term follow-up of isolated ACL tears treated without ligament reconstruction, *Knee Surgery, Sports Traumatology, Arthroscopy* 25(2):493–500, 2016, Available at: https://doi.org/10.1007/ s00167-016-4172-4.

Siemieniuk RAC, Harris IA, Agoritsas T, et al: Arthroscopic surgery for degenerative knee arthritis and meniscal tears: a clinical practice guideline, *BMJ* 357, 2017, Available at: https://doi.org/10.1136/bmj.j1982.

Smithers CJ, Young AA, Walch G: Reverse shoulder arthroplasty, *Curr Rev Musculoskelet Med* 4(4):183–190, 2011, Available at: https://doi.org/10.1007/s12178-011-9097-4.

Towheed TE, Maxwell L, Anastassiades TP, et al: Glucosamine therapy for treating osteoarthritis, *Cochrane Database Syst Rev* (2)CD002946, 2005 Apr 18, Review. PubMed PMID: 15846645.

Tsoukas D, Fotopoulos V, Basdekis G, Makridis KG: No difference in osteoarthritis after surgical and non-surgical treatment of ACL-injured knees after 10 years, *Knee Surgery, Sports Traumatology, Arthroscopy* 24(9):2953–2959, 2015, Available at: https://doi.org/10.1007/s00167-015-3593-9.

OSTEOPOROSIS

Method of

Alexei DeCastro, MD; Scott Bragg, PharmD; and Peter J. Carek, MD, MS

CURRENT DIAGNOSIS

- Evaluation of risk factors for osteoporosis and related fractures is always recommended.
- Screening for osteoporosis with bone mineral density (BMD) testing in women age 65 years and older is recommended.
- In women younger than 65 years old with equal or increased risk of osteoporosis compared with 65-year-old women, BMD testing is recommended.
- Current evidence is insufficient to recommend screening for osteoporosis in men.
- Determination of BMD is indicated for those with osteoporotic fractures to determine the severity of the disorder and to help guide future treatment decisions.
- Clinical and laboratory work-up of secondary causes of osteoporosis should be pursued in all patients with osteoporosis.
- Vertebral fracture assessment and trabecular bone scores could be considered in addition to BMD testing to augment fracture risk assessment.

CURRENT THERAPY

- A comprehensive nutritional assessment targeting normal body weight and adequate ingestion of calcium and vitamin D is recommended.
- New evidence does not show major benefit in taking calcium and vitamin D for primary prevention in adults over age 50. For secondary prevention, calcium intake should be at least 1200 mg/day, including supplements, when necessary. Vitamin D consumption should at least be 800–1000 IU daily to prevent insufficiency.
- Weight-bearing and muscle-strengthening exercises are important tools to reduce the risk of falls and fracture.
- Pharmacologic treatment of osteoporosis is indicated for postmenopausal women and men age 50 years and older with a clinical diagnosis of osteoporosis (i.e., hip or vertebral fractures without major trauma) or radiographic evidence of osteoporosis (i.e., bone mineral density [BMD] T-scores ≤–2.5 at the lumbar spine, femoral neck, or total hip) after proper evaluation.
- Pharmacologic treatment of osteoporosis is indicated for postmenopausal women and men age 50 years and older with low bone mass and high 10-year fracture risk. The 10-year fracture risk is considered high if the 10-year hip fracture probability is 3% or more or if the 10-year probability of a major osteoporosis-related fracture is 20% or more based on the fracture risk assessment tool (FRAX) from the US-adapted algorithm from the World Health Organization.
- Treatment of premenopausal women and men less than 50 years old with antiresorptive therapy is controversial. Z-scores of ≤–2.0 indicate osteoporosis. However, antiresorptive treatment is often reserved for glucocorticoid-induced osteoporosis in patients with moderate to high fracture risk or patients with multiple fragility fractures.
- The drugs currently approved by the Food and Drug Administration (FDA) for treating osteoporosis include bisphosphonates (i.e., alendronate [Fosamax], ibandronate [Boniva], risedronate [Actonel], zoledronic acid [Reclast]), calcitonin (Miacalcin), raloxifene (Evista), denosumab (Prolia), parathyroid hormones (i.e., teriparatide [Forteo], abaloparatide [Tymlos]), and romosozumab [Evenity]).
- It is unclear how frequently BMD testing should be repeated in patients undergoing screening or when monitoring therapeutic response to treatment. Assessing treatment response may vary based upon the severity of osteoporosis, the standard error seen with imaging measurements, and the osteoporosis treatment used to prevent fractures. Normally, BMD testing is repeated every 2 to 3 years after the initiation of pharmacotherapy, but shorter or longer intervals could be reasonable.

Osteoporosis is a skeletal disease characterized by low bone mass and structural deterioration of bone tissue, which is associated with decreased bone strength and increased susceptibility to fractures. Its clinical relevance is increasing because healthcare professionals are caring for more older adults and the morbidity and mortality associated with the disease. The signs and symptoms of osteoporosis, such as back pain, height loss, and thoracic kyphosis, not only are usually late manifestations of previously unrecognized vertebral fractures but also can be important risk indicators for future fractures. A challenge to primary care clinicians is to find the best screening method(s) to identify patients at highest risk for fracture who would benefit from a preventive or therapeutic intervention.

The World Health Organization (WHO) has defined osteoporosis as a condition in which bone mineral density (BMD) assessed by dual-energy x-ray absorptiometry (DEXA) at the lumbar spine or hip is decreased compared with a young-adult reference population. Osteoporosis is seen in postmenopausal women or men over age 50 with a BMD of 2.5 standard deviations (SDs) below normal (T-score ≤–2.5). Low bone mass, previously known as osteopenia, is a milder degree of bone loss seen in the same populations (T-score of –1.0 to –2.4). Although the risk of fracture increases significantly with decreasing BMD, large observational studies have demonstrated that osteoporotic fractures can occur across a wide spectrum of BMDs. These events may be related not only to bone quantity but also to bone quality, a component not measured by DEXA scans. Qualitative determinants of bone strength include trabecular bone scores, microcracks, mineralization defects, bone geometry, cell death, changes in bone size, and changes in bone turnover. Even though a low BMD defines osteoporosis, a fragility fracture (i.e., fracture without trauma or a low-trauma fall) also can be used to clinically diagnose osteoporosis.

Although there is no universally accepted screening tool for patients at risk for osteoporotic fracture, the WHO and US Preventive Services Task Force (USPSTF) recommend screening in women greater than 65 years old and in women younger than 65 who are at equal or increased risk of osteoporosis compared with an average 65-year-old woman (Level B). To identify patients at increased risk, they use a decision support tool to calculate the 10-year risk of a hip fracture and a major osteoporotic fracture. The fracture risk assessment tool (FRAX) considers several major independent risk factors, including BMD of the femoral neck, previous fracture history, family history of fracture, age, sex, ethnicity, glucocorticoid use, alcohol abuse, current smoking status, and possible secondary osteoporosis causes. Nevertheless, many women with osteoporosis go unrecognized and untreated. In one study, it was reported that less than 50% of women with a fragility fracture were diagnosed with osteoporosis within 1 year of the fracture and even fewer treated with pharmacologic therapy for osteoporosis based on information from claims databases. Another study showed overscreening of patients at low risk (46% for women 50 to 59 and 59% for women 60 to 64 without risk factors) and underscreening of patients at high risk (58% for women 65 to 74 and 43% for women ≥75).

Epidemiology

Osteoporosis is the most common metabolic disorder of the skeleton. The estimated prevalence of osteoporosis is highest in Hispanic Americans, followed by non-Hispanic whites, and lowest in non-Hispanic blacks. Worldwide, 200 million women suffer from osteoporosis, and those women have an estimated 65% lifetime risk of a fragility fracture. In men with osteoporosis, the lifetime risk of a fragility fracture is estimated at 42%. In the United States, approximately 8 million women and 2 million men have osteoporosis, and another 34 million people have low bone mass. After the fourth decade of life, fracture rates in women are twice those in men. In addition, hip fracture has a seasonal influence, with an increase during winter months in temperate countries. Hip fractures are reported to cause a mortality rate of 10% to 20% at 12 months, but they cause a higher rate of deaths in men than women. Up to 25% of those with hip fractures require long-term nursing care.

Screening

Risk factors for osteoporosis should be considered at well visits or during all visits in high-risk individuals. Nonmodifiable risk factors are genetic background, advancing age, female sex, low socioeconomic status, Hispanic Americans or non-Hispanic whites, personal history of fracture, and family history of fracture in a first-degree relative. Modifiable risk factors consist of low body weight, hormonal deficiencies, smoking, alcohol abuse, an inactive lifestyle, and a diet low in calcium and vitamin D. In addition, certain medications affect skeletal homeostasis and increase fracture risk. Patients taking high-risk medications such as glucocorticoids, immunosuppressive medications, anticonvulsants, sex hormone deprivation therapy, thyroid hormone, and proton pump inhibitors should routinely be assessed. Other comorbid illnesses (e.g., chronic kidney disease, hyperthyroidism, rheumatoid arthritis) increase the risk of secondary osteoporosis, but may be managed to an extent with better control of the underlying condition and more frequent screening.

Several decision support tools are available to help identify patients who are at high risk for osteoporosis and fracture. The most common risk assessments include the fracture risk assessment tool (FRAX), the simple calculated osteoporosis risk estimation, the osteoporosis self-assessment tool, and the osteoporosis risk assessment instrument. However, the USPSTF guideline recommends using FRAX because it incorporates the most risk factors and provides a 10-year absolute fracture risk. FRAX uses readily available information such as age, body mass index, parental fracture history, comorbid conditions that cause secondary osteoporosis, and tobacco and alcohol use. The FRAX tool also incorporates DEXA results but does not require this information to estimate fracture risk. The USPSTF recommends screening with a DEXA scan in all women 65 years and older and postmenopausal women less than 65 years old if their 10-year fracture risk with FRAX is 9.3% or higher. The other decision support tools to assess the need for a DEXA scan may be reasonable as well because they rely on fewer factors and have comparable sensitivity and negative predictive values.

The National Osteoporosis Foundation (NOF) and the International Society for Clinical Densitometry recommend screening all men 70 years and older, and men 50 to 69 years of age based on risk factors. However, the USPSTF guidelines state that insufficient evidence is available to support screening for osteoporosis in men. Other screening risk assessments, such as vertebral imaging and trabecular bone scores, may be considered in addition to DEXA scans to help identify asymptomatic vertebral fractures or to quantify bone microarchitecture. These techniques may help better characterize 10-year fracture risk or guide pharmacologic treatment decisions, although neither vertebral imaging nor trabecular bone scores are discussed in the USPSTF guidelines because of limited data with these screening modalities. It remains unclear how frequently patients should be rescreened after having an initial DEXA scan indicating normal, reduced, or severely reduced BMD.

Pathophysiology

Although osteoporosis is often thought of as synonymous with decreased BMD, this association is not always present. Several factors can lead to decreased bone strength, including small bone size, increased length of the femoral neck, cortical porosity, decreased viability of osteocytes, and others.

Peak bone mass is the maximum bone mass achieved in life and typically occurs in the patient's third decade of life. Differences in the peak bone mass may be secondary to genetic, hormonal, and environmental variables. Increases in body size and skeletal load also play a role in determining peak bone mass. Physical activity during childhood also enhances bone mass, whereas chronic diseases during childhood may decrease BMD. The contribution of genetic variants is unclear because osteoporosis is a polygenic disease and the individual genetic variants that have been identified seem to have small effect on fracture risk and BMD. Hispanic Americans and Asian Americans have lower BMDs than non-Hispanic whites or non-Hispanic blacks. However, lower hip fracture rates are reported in Asian Americans and non-Hispanic blacks. Some of these differences in fracture risk can be predicted by BMD, but other factors also influence fracture risk.

Age-related bone loss is a significant factor in the development of osteoporosis. Bone resorption begins to overtake bone formation with advancing age. Men, however, are less likely to develop bone loss because of greater bone gain during puberty and no

sudden loss of sex hormones. Hormonal deficiency causes bone loss by unbalancing the homeostasis normally present and the bone remodeling rate (i.e., osteoclast-induced bone resorption vs. osteoblast-supported bone formation). Estrogen loss initially affects trabecular bone after menopause. After a few years, bone loss continues to occur more slowly and primarily affects cortical sites. This slower phase is associated with a decreased number of osteoblasts and a slower bone formation rate. It is also theorized that androgen loss has detrimental effects on BMD, but it is uncertain how much. Still, both sex hormone deficiencies play a role in bone loss in both men and women. Also, there is evidence that aging itself seems to be an independent risk factor for bone loss. Other contributing factors include loss of muscle strength and coordination, which increase the risk for falls and fragility fractures. Triclosan, an endocrine-disrupting antibacterial agent, has been associated with lower BMD in the femur and lumbar spine and osteoporosis. The association is more pronounced in postmenopausal women. Although the US Food and Drug Administration (FDA) has prohibited the sale of triclosan in "consumer antiseptic washes" since 2017, it may still be found in many soaps, toothpastes, and mouthwashes.

Clinical Manifestations

There are typically no clinical manifestations of osteoporosis until a patient actually has a fracture. The signs and symptoms associated with osteoporosis correspond to direct or indirect manifestations of these fractures. Patients may have height loss, back pain, and thoracic kyphosis after experiencing a vertebral fracture. Moreover, manifestations from thoracic kyphosis could include dyspnea, from pulmonary restrictive lung disease, or constipation. Significant pain is often seen with both vertebral fractures and hip fractures although some patients may present with asymptomatic vertebral fractures that can be clinically inconspicuous. Functional disability is common after a fracture and many times requires rehabilitation to improve long-term functional status.

Diagnosis

Osteoporosis is diagnosed either clinically or radiographically. It can be established after the occurrence of a fragility fracture, such as a low-trauma fracture of appendicular or axial bones, excluding the skull. The initial evaluation includes a history to assess for clinical risk factors for fracture, evaluation for secondary conditions that contribute to bone loss, a physical examination, basic laboratory tests, and assessment of medications that increase fracture risk. Most cases of osteoporosis are diagnosed by a DEXA scan of the total hip, femoral neck, or lumbar spine, with a T-score of −2.5 or below. Bone mass measurements by DEXA must be interpreted in relation to the patient's age, ethnicity, fracture history, family background, previous medication use, timing of menopause, and other concomitant disorders.

Other techniques for measuring bone mass besides DEXA scans exist. These include ultrasound of the calcaneus, wrist, and finger and computed tomography of the spine or peripheral quantitative computed tomography of the wrist and tibia. However, these modalities may be limited by factors such as availability, radiation exposure, and cost. DEXA scans give an accurate and precise estimate of BMD and have been proven, cost-effective tools.

DEXA results are expressed as a T-score and a Z-score. The T-score was established by the WHO and is the number of SD difference between the patient's BMD and a sex- and ethnicity-matched young-adult reference population. The T-score should be used in the evaluation of men age 50 and older and postmenopausal women. The T-score provides an indication of the risk for developing fractures because of the association of fractures with decreasing BMD. A T-score that is −2.5 SD or more is diagnostic of osteoporosis; a T-score that is between −1.0 and −2.4 SD below the mean is defined as low bone mass, also known as *osteopenia*. A T-score of −2.5 SD or below plus a fragility fracture is termed *severe osteoporosis*. BMD measurements may be different across various bone sites in the same patient. These discrepancies may likely be related to differences in skeletal compartments (trabecular vs. cortical) at distinct sites. The lowest T-score of the lumbar spine, femoral neck, and total hip should be used to classify the degree of osteoporosis.

The Z-score is the number of SDs the patient's BMD differs from a reference population matched for age in addition to sex and ethnicity. A low Z-score of −2.0 SD or below may identify patients who need further evaluation for secondary causes of osteoporosis or even osteoporosis treatment. Z-scores should be used in the evaluation of adult men younger than age 50, premenopausal women, and children. Less evidence exists for characterizing the severity of disease or need for osteoporosis treatment in these populations making patient care decisions difficult. For example, there is no great way to compare the BMD of a child to an adult who has achieved peak bone mass or determine at what Z-score treatment is warranted. Further research is needed to identify appropriate groups to screen with Z-scores and if osteoporosis treatment changes patient-oriented outcomes.

Biochemical markers reflect the activity of the bone-remodeling unit. These markers, such as urinary pyridinoline and deoxypyridinoline, are called *bone turnover markers*. Their roles in the management of osteoporosis have not been well established. Future use of these biochemical markers may be helpful in determining risk and for monitoring patients treated with medications for osteoporosis.

Differential Diagnosis

Because osteoporosis is radiographically or clinically identified from a history, the differential focuses on a comprehensive workup of potential secondary causes of osteoporosis. If evaluation does not support a clear secondary cause, there is currently little evidence for additional testing in postmenopausal women. However, in premenopausal and perimenopausal women, additional testing could be considered if there is no clear cause found by history and physical examination. More than 50% of men with vertebral collapse fractures are reported to have secondary causes of osteoporosis. Common causes of osteoporosis in men are long-term use of glucocorticoids, hypogonadism, alcohol abuse, myeloma, and comorbidities (e.g., celiac disease, hyperthyroidism, hyperparathyroidism). It is important to note most recommendations for screening and diagnosis are based on expert opinion.

Prevention

Prevention of osteoporosis is important because bone loss with aging is difficult to correct. Treatment stabilizes the disease by increasing BMD, reducing fracture risk, and restoring bone strength. Lower peak bone mass established in early adulthood may determine bone strength and fracture risk decades later. Therefore prevention starts with good nutrition, maintenance of a healthy body weight, and weight-bearing exercise to optimize bone mass during bone-forming years. Other lifestyle factors that can be modified are discouraging cigarette smoking and excessive alcohol intake. Medications that may be harmful to bone health should be closely monitored and used for the minimum duration.

Calcium and vitamin D are both physiologically vital in bone formation. However, studies are conflicting on the benefits of primary prevention using calcium and vitamin D[1] in older adults. Some studies have shown increases in BMD and reduction of fracture risk in high risk adult patients given both calcium and vitamin D. As a result, the NOF recommends 1200 mg of elemental calcium and 800 to 1000 IU of vitamin D daily for postmenopausal women. However, several recent studies do not support dietary or supplemental calcium or vitamin D to reduce the risk of fractures or to increase BMD in older adults when used in primary prevention.

Treatment

Nonpharmacologic Therapy

Nondrug therapy includes addressing risk of falls, diet, exercise, and smoking. Vision deficits, gait abnormalities, cognitive impairment, dizziness, and balance problems need to be addressed to prevent falls. Performing a formal home safety evaluation and modifying the patient's living environment by improving lighting and removing loose rugs can enhance safety. Physical therapy evaluation and treatment can address both balance and gait issues. Medications need to be reviewed that pose a risk of falls due to their side-effect profile.

Ensuring adequate nutrition is an initial approach in treating osteoporosis, especially calcium and vitamin D. Studies showing the efficacy of calcium on fracture primary prevention are mixed, with some meta-analyses showing benefit and others showing no effect. Although primary prevention benefit is unclear, adequate calcium and vitamin D consumption should be encouraged when used with antiresorptives to reduce the risk of hypocalcemia with bisphosphonates and to ensure optimal efficacy of these agents. Because optimal doses are not established, a daily intake of at least 1200 mg of calcium and 800 to 1000 IU of vitamin D[1] is recommended for all women with osteoporosis by the NOF based on historic recommended dietary amounts. Calcium and vitamin D supplements are often used because of low dietary consumption of each and reduced sun exposure with aging. Both calcium carbonate and calcium citrate can be used, but caution should be used because of constipation and gastrointestinal upset. Concerns about renal adverse events, particularly nephrolithiasis, exist with excessive dietary and/or supplemental calcium. There is also theoretical concern that excessive calcium administration could increase the risk of myocardial infarction via coronary calcification although there are no strong data supporting this concern.

The appropriate vitamin D level remains unclear, with mixed evidence and different experts advocating for different goal values. Some studies suggest that a serum 25-hydroxyvitamin D level of at least 30 ng/mL is needed to reduce falls and to improve physical function in the elderly. However, some experts advocate for treating only severely low 25-hydroxyvitamin D values <20 ng/mL because of mixed evidence with slightly low vitamin D values. In patients with confirmed vitamin D insufficiency, administration of 50,000 IU of oral ergocalciferol (vitamin D_2 [Drisdol])[1] given once-weekly for 8 to 12 weeks is thought to be safe and effective. A repeat serum 25-hydroxyvitamin D value should be used after this treatment course to determine the need for further high dose supplementation versus starting a maintenance dose. However, a more recent study has shown that high-dose vitamin D may increase the risk of falls, so caution should be used.

Regular physical activity with aerobic, weight-bearing, and resistance exercises are effective in increasing spine BMD. Patients should exercise at least 30 minutes three times per week. However, there is no evidence that high-intensity exercise provides greater benefit. Smoking cessation and moderate alcohol consumption should be stressed to reduce the risk for fracture as well.

Pharmacologic Treatment

All drugs approved by the FDA for osteoporosis reduce vertebral fracture risk. Many of the antifracture effects of these medications are not due to an increase in BMD but rather to an improvement in qualitative measures of bone strength. The drugs approved by the FDA to treat or prevent osteoporosis are noted in Table 1.

The mechanisms of each class of osteoporosis agent are slightly different and primarily work through decreasing bone resorption by inhibiting osteoclasts or increasing bone formation by stimulating osteoblasts. The bisphosphonates (e.g., alendronate [Fosamax], risedronate [Actonel], ibandronate [Boniva], zoledronic acid [Reclast]) impair osteoclastic resorption through the inhibition of farnesyl diphosphate synthase, a key enzyme that supports osteoclast activity. Estrogen, raloxifene ([Evista], a selective estrogen receptor modulator or SERM), and bazedoxifene/conjugated equine estrogen [Duavee] inhibit osteoclastogenesis

---

[1]Not FDA approved for this indication.

			CLINICAL EVIDENCE OF EFFICACY		
MEDICATION	**ROUTE**	**DOSE**	**VERTEBRAL**	**HIP**	**NONVERTEBRAL**
Alendronate (Fosamax)	Oral	Oral 10 mg daily or 70 mg weekly	+	+	+
Risedronate (Actonel)	Oral	5 mg daily or 35 mg weekly	+	+	+
Zoledronic acid (Reclast)	IV	5 mg yearly	+	+	+
Ibandronate (Boniva)	Oral	150 mg monthly	+	–	–
	IV	3 mg every 3 months	+	–	–
Denosumab (Prolia)	SubQ	60 mg every 6 months	+	+	+
Abaloparatide (Tymlos)	SubQ	80 mcg daily	+		+
Teriparatide (Forteo)	SubQ	20 mcg daily	+		+
Romosozumab (Evenity)	SubQ	210 mg monthly	+		+
Raloxifene (Evista)	Oral	60 mg daily	+	–	–
Bazedoxifene/ conjugated equine estrogen (Duavee)[1]	Oral	20/0.45 mg daily	+		
Conjugated equine estrogen (Premarin)[1]	Oral	0.3–1.25 mg daily	+	+	+
Calcitonin (Miacalcin)	Nasal	200 IU daily	+	–	+
	IM or SubQ	100 IU daily	+	–	+

TABLE 1 Osteoporosis Treatment Dosing and Effectiveness on Fracture Risk Reduction

[1]Not FDA approved for treating established osteoporosis. Only FDA approved to prevent fractures in postmenopausal women.
IM, Intramuscular; *IU,* international units; *IV,* intravenous; *SubQ,* subcutaneous.

through blocking the receptor activator of nuclear factor κB ligand/osteoprotegerin (OPG) system expressed on osteoblasts that signal the production of osteoclasts. Denosumab (Prolia), a monoclonal antibody, works similarly to estrogen by inhibiting the receptor activator of nuclear factor κB ligand system for osteoclast formation. Calcitonin (Miacalcin) works through a different mechanism by inhibiting osteoclast activity through the calcitonin receptor. Parathyroid hormones (i.e., teriparatide [Forteo], abaloparatide [Tymlos]) stimulate osteoblast bone formation, increasing calcium absorption in the gastrointestinal track, and promoting renal tubular calcium reabsorption. Lastly, romosozumab (Evenity), a new class of monoclonal antibody, inhibits sclerostin which is a protein that regulates bone metabolism. By inhibiting sclerostin, romosozumab will increase osteoblast activity and reduce osteoclast activity.

There are different approved indications for bisphosphonates in patients with osteoporosis. Alendronate and risedronate are indicated for the prevention and treatment of postmenopausal osteoporosis, treatment of osteoporosis in men, and treatment of glucocorticoid-induced osteoporosis. Ibandronate is approved only for prevention and treatment of postmenopausal females with osteoporosis. Daily and intermittent doses of ibandronate have demonstrated benefit on reducing only vertebral fractures, which limits its use because other bisphosphonates have better evidence at reducing vertebral, nonvertebral, and hip fractures. Zoledronic acid 5 mg by intravenous (IV) administration is approved for once-yearly treatment of postmenopausal osteoporosis, and 5 mg IV administered once every other year is approved to prevent osteoporosis. Zoledronic acid is the only osteoporosis therapy shown to reduce all-cause mortality and may be a preferred option in those who cannot tolerate or are nonadherent with oral therapy in addition to its potential mortality benefits. In patients with an osteoporotic hip fracture, it is essential that they receive treatment with a bisphosphonate after surgery to modify the subsequent risk of fracture at any site. There have been concerns that bisphosphonates started soon after surgery could disrupt bone remodeling and fracture healing, but current evidence shows that early administration of bisphosphonates does not delay fracture healing. Therefore they should be given soon after surgery to reduce subsequent fractures.

Side effects of oral bisphosphonates include esophageal and gastric irritation, musculoskeletal pain, and hypocalcemia. They must be taken with a full glass of water, and a 30- to 60-minute wait is required before eating or reclining to lower the risk of upper gastrointestinal adverse effects. Intravenous bisphosphonates are associated with hyperthermia, episcleritis, uveitis, and hypocalcemia. The proper duration of bisphosphonate therapy is unknown. Low-risk patients may consider discontinuing therapy after 3 to 5 years once the risks and benefits are weighed. High-risk patients (e.g., patients with a *T*-score still below –2.5, having recent fragility fractures) could have continued benefit on reducing vertebral fractures with bisphosphonates out to 10 years, but other types of fracture do not seem to be reduced and the risk of long-term complications (e.g., atypical fractures, osteonecrosis of the jaw, atrial fibrillation, myocardial infarction, esophageal cancer) may increase.

The reports of atypical femur fractures with bisphosphonates, particularly alendronate, appear rare but are seen more frequently when used longer than 5 years. Young women are particularly prone to these fractures, which often require surgical intervention. Prodromal symptoms that have been linked to this syndrome include proximal femur pain and evidence of previous stress fracture or cortical thickness on x-ray. Osteonecrosis of the jaw is another one of the most feared complications seen with long-term bisphosphonate use, but again it is also very rare. The actual incidence of both atypical fractures and osteonecrosis of the jaw are difficult to predict because these are largely point estimates from cohort studies with so few events seen in randomized trials.

Denosumab, 60 mg subcutaneously twice a year, is a human monoclonal antibody approved for treatment of men and postmenopausal women with osteoporosis who are at high risk for fracture. In a large trial involving more than 7000 postmenopausal women, denosumab was administered for 3 years and showed significant efficacy in reducing the risk of vertebral, nonvertebral, and hip fractures compared to placebo. The safety profile of denosumab has been demonstrated in long-term trials, although there was a reported modest increase in skin infections with continued use. Long-term risks of atypical fractures and osteonecrosis of the jaw have been reported with denosumab similar to bisphosphonates, so it is recommended to reevaluate the need for continued treatment after 3 to 5 years.

Estrogen is an effective therapy at reducing all types of fracture and is often reserved for women unable to use other options because of potential serious consequences. These complications include thromboembolism, stroke, myocardial infarction, and some types of cancer. Raloxifene, on the other hand, improves BMD and reduces the risk of vertebral fractures, but not nonvertebral or hip fractures. Unfortunately, it can exacerbate the vasomotor symptoms of menopause and increases the risk of thromboembolic events. Raloxifene may be considered in postmenopausal women with osteoporosis who cannot tolerate bisphosphonates, have no vasomotor symptoms, have a low risk of venous thromboembolism, and have a high breast cancer risk. A new selective estrogen receptor modulator, bazedoxifene plus conjugated equine estrogens (Duavee), has been approved for prevention of postmenopausal osteoporosis and vasomotor symptoms with menopause. It might prove to be an alternative to raloxifene, but it is still associated with many of the serious precautions seen with estrogen therapy.

Parathyroid hormones (i.e., teriparatide, abaloparatide) have recognized antifracture effects on both vertebral and nonvertebral sites. Currently, therapy with either treatment should be limited to 2 years and reserved for patients at the highest fracture risk or refractory to other antiresorptives. There are slight differences in FDA indications with teriparatide being approved for postmenopausal women, men, or in patients with glucocorticoid-induced osteoporosis; abaloparatide has only been approved for postmenopausal women. The maximum 2-year duration is based on reports of increased risk of osteosarcoma, which has only been seen in laboratory animals exposed to high doses. Consequently, parathyroid hormones are contraindicated in patients with risk of osteosarcoma, such as those with Paget disease of the bone, previous skeletal radiation, or unexplained elevations of alkaline phosphatase. Adverse effects may include orthostatic hypotension, hypercalcemia, nausea, arthralgia, risk of renal stones, and leg cramps. In addition to its approved indications, some experts recommend using one of the anabolic options in patients who experience an atypical fracture or patients who have not improved on bisphosphonates. No evidence exists for combining anticatabolic and anabolic classes of drugs at the same time. However, it is recommended that after a period of 2 years of using parathyroid hormones, sequential therapy with an antiresorptive should be started to avoid posttreatment bone loss.

Romosozumab (Evenity) is a monoclonal antibody that works by binding and inhibiting sclerostin. Sclerostin is a glycoprotein that inhibits osteoblast bone formation and to a lesser degree, increases osteoclast bone resorption. There is robust evidence showing better effectiveness at reducing hip, vertebral, and nonvertebral fractures when compared head-to-head with alendronate over 24 months. It was originally rejected by the FDA because of concern about increasing the risk of myocardial infarction and stroke but it was officially approved in April 2019 for postmenopausal women at high fracture risk. The increased risk of cardiovascular events is still a concern, but ongoing studies are being performed to determine its long-term safety. Romosozumab will likely be reserved for patients at the highest risk for osteoporotic fracture because of its safety concerns and high costs. If used in patients, romosozumab is given as two consecutive subcutaneous injections every month for up to 1 year and then other antiresorptive medications are recommended as sequential therapy similar to using parathyroid hormones.

References

Bilezikian JP: Efficacy of bisphosphonates in reducing fracture risk in postmenopausal osteoporosis, *Am J Med* 122(Suppl. 2):S14–S21, 2009.

Bischoff-Ferrari HA, Dawson-Hughes B, Orav J, et al: Monthly high-dose vitamin D treatment for the prevention of functional decline: a randomized clinical trial, *JAMA Intern Med* 176(2):175–183, 2016.

Bischoff-Ferrari HA, Dawson-Hughes B, Staehelin HB, et al: Fall prevention with supplemental and active forms of vitamin D: a meta-analysis of randomised controlled trials, *BMJ* 339:b3692, 2009.

Bolland MJ, Leung W, Tai V, et al: Calcium intake and risk of fracture: systematic review, *BMJ* 351:h4580, 2015.

Chen SJ, Chen YJ, Cheng CH, et al: Comparisons of different screening tools for identifying fracture/osteoporosis risk among community-dwelling older people, *Medicine (Baltimore)* 95(20):e3415, 2016.

Committee to Review Dietary Reference Intakes for Vitamin D and Calcium: *Dietary reference intakes for calcium and vitamin D*, Washington, DC, 2010, Institute of Medicine.

Draft Recommendation Statement: *Osteoporosis to Prevent Fractures: Screening*, 2017. Available at: https://www.uspreventiveservicestaskforce.org/Page/Document/draft-recommendationstatement/osteoporosis-screening1. Accessed 9 March 2018.

Fink HA, MacDonald R, Forte ML, et al. Long-term drug therapy and drug holidays for osteoporosis fracture prevention: a systematic review. Comparative Effectiveness Review No. 218. (Prepared by the Minnesota Evidence-based Practice Center under Contract No. 290-2015-00008-I) AHRQ Publication No. 19-EHC016-EF. Rockville, MD, 2019, Agency for Healthcare Research and Quality.

Hippisley-Cox J, Coupland C: Predicting risk of osteoporotic fracture in men and women in England and Wales: prospective derivation and validation of QFracture scores, *BMJ* 339:b4229, 2009.

Karinkanta S, Piirtola M, Sievanen H, et al: Physical therapy approaches to reduce fall and fracture risk among older adults, *Nat Rev Endocrinol* 6(7):396–407, 2010.

Ketteler M, Block GA, Evenepoel P, et al: Diagnosis, evaluation, prevention, and treatment of chronic kidney disease–mineral and bone disorder: synopsis of the Kidney Disease: Improving Global Outcomes 2017 clinical practice guideline update, *Ann Intern Med* 168:422–430, 2018.

Khosla S, Melton LJ: Clinical practice: osteopenia, *N Engl J Med* 356:2293–2300, 2007.

Lyles KW, Colon-Emeric CS, Magaziner JS, et al: Zoledronic acid and clinical fractures and mortality after hip fracture, *N Engl J Med* 357:1799–1809, 2007.

Moyer V: To supplement or not to supplement: the U.S. Preventive Services Task Force recommendations on calcium and vitamin D, *Ann Intern Med* 158:691–696, 2013.

Nguyen ND, Ahlborg HG, Center JR, et al: Residual lifetime risk of fractures in women and men, *J Bone Miner Res* 22:781–788, 2007.

Ralston SH, Uitterlinden AG: Genetics of osteoporosis, *Endocrine Reviews* 31:629–662, 2010.

Rosen CJ: Clinical practice. Postmenopausal osteoporosis, *N Engl J Med* 353:595, 2005.

Rosen CJ: Bone remodeling, energy metabolism, and the molecular clock, *Cell Metab* 7:7–10, 2008.

Saag K, Petersen J, Brandi ML, et al: Romosozumab or alendronate for fracture prevention in women with osteoporosis, *N Engl J Med* 377:1417–1427, 2017.

Schousboe JT, Taylor BC, Fink HA, et al: Cost-effectiveness of bone densitometry followed by treatment of osteoporosis in older men, *JAMA* 298:629–637, 2007.

Sweet, et al: Diagnosis and management of osteoporosis, *Am Fam Physician* 92:261–268, 2015.

Uitterlinden AG, Ralston SH, Brandi ML, et al: The association between common vitamin D receptor gene variations and osteoporosis: a participant-level meta-analysis, *Ann Intern Med* 145:255–264, 2006.

U.S. Department of Health and Human Services: *Bone health and osteoporosis: a report of the surgeon general*, Rockville, MD, 2004, U.S. Department of Health and Human Services, Office of the Surgeon General.

Wells GA, Cranney A, Peterson J, et al: Alendronate for the primary and secondary prevention of osteoporotic fractures in postmenopausal women, *Cochrane Database Syst Rev* 1:CD001155.

Zhao J, Zeng X, Wang J, Liu L: Association between calcium or vitamin D supplementation and fracture incidence in community-dwelling older adults, *JAMA* 318:2466–2482, 2017.

PAGET'S DISEASE OF BONE

Method of
Ian R. Reid, MD

CURRENT DIAGNOSIS

- Suspect the presence of Paget's disease in those patients with bone pain, bone deformity, isolated elevation of alkaline phosphatase, or lytic/sclerotic lesions on radiographs.
- Paget's disease is diagnosed from plain radiographs.
- Bone scintigraphy identifies the affected bones and allows some assessment of disease activity.
- Biochemical markers of bone turnover allow more precise assessment of turnover and response to therapy.
- Serum total alkaline phosphatase activity is the most cost-effective marker, although bone-specific alkaline phosphatase and procollagen type I N-terminal propeptide (PINP) are marginally more sensitive.

CURRENT THERAPY

- Zoledronate (zoledronic acid, Reclast) 5 mg given as a single infusion over 15 minutes; retreatment is seldom required within 5 years.
- Alendronate (Fosamax) 40 mg/day for 6 months; retreatment may be required between 2 and 6 years.
- Risedronate (Actonel) 30 mg/day for 2 months; retreatment may be required between 1 and 5 years.

Paget's disease is a focal skeletal condition in which one or more bones has a clearly circumscribed area of increased turnover (Figure 1A). Either osteoblasts or osteoclasts may predominate at a given time, resulting in sclerosis or lysis, respectively. Areas that are initially lytic often become sclerotic later, and it is common to see both changes within the same bone (see Figure 1B). Unaffected areas of the skeleton are completely normal, in marked contrast to some rare congenital conditions which are sometimes (inappropriately) referred to as early-onset or juvenile Paget's disease. Such conditions (e.g., familial expansile osteolysis, idiopathic hyperphosphatasia) have different etiologies, clinical presentations, and responses to treatment when compared to Paget's disease.

Etiology

Within pagetic bone, there is a loss of the usual tight control of bone cell function, and the bone-resorbing cells (osteoclasts) and bone-forming cells (osteoblasts) both exhibit overactivity. In the case of osteoclasts, this leads to local areas of bone loss, which can result in deformity or fracture. Osteoblast overactivity leads to the random laying down of new bone, which is disorganized in its structure, mechanically inadequate, and prone to deformity. Osteoblast overactivity can also lead to bone expansion, resulting in bone pain, premature arthritis (if it affects articular surfaces), and nerve compression (e.g., in the spine or skull). Figure 1B shows the effects of osteoblast and osteoclast overactivity on the structure of an affected tibia. The disease progresses along a long bone at a rate of about 1 cm per year, so most patients have had active disease for 1 or more decades before presentation. Typically, the disease progresses until the entire bone is involved. However, Paget's disease does not spread from one bone to another, so the number of affected bones remains constant throughout the disease course.

Paget's disease sometimes runs in families, and about 10% of patients are reported to have an affected relative. This observation has led to much work seeking genetic associations of the condition. It is now apparent that mutations of the gene for sequestosome 1 are associated with Paget's disease in some families. Other research has focused on possible environmental causes, and a slow viral infection has been suggested. Evidence that the prevalence of Paget's disease has decreased in recent decades would be consistent with altered exposure to an environmental agent. However, both the genetic and environmental hypotheses fail to account for the focal nature of the condition, which in some ways resembles a benign neoplasm.

Altered gene expression in osteoblasts and bone marrow stromal cells from pagetic bone has been demonstrated recently, including increased levels of dickkopf-1, interleukin-1, and interleukin-6. These changes are likely to result in stimulation of osteoclast proliferation and inhibition of osteoblast growth, leading to development of the characteristic lytic bone lesions. This work suggests that the key abnormality may reside in the osteoblast, rather than the osteoclast, as was assumed in the past. Uncertainties remain regarding the primary abnormality giving rise to this condition.

Epidemiology

Paget's disease is classically a condition of older adults, most patients being older than 60 years of age at diagnosis. There is a

Figure 1 **A,** Bone scintigram in a patient with Paget's disease, demonstrating the multifocal nature of the condition and the presence of normal bone at other sites. **B,** Tibia affected by Paget's disease. The upper tibia is of increased density and width as a result of osteoblast overactivity, whereas the lower part of the affected bone shows a lytic region *(between arrows)* resulting from osteoclastic bone resorption. Below this, the bone is normal. (Copyright I. R. Reid, used with permission.)

male preponderance in some studies. It is overwhelmingly a condition of individuals with European forebears, particularly from the United Kingdom and Western Europe (excluding Scandinavia), where about 6% to 7% of the older population is affected. Among older white Americans, the prevalence is about 2%. There is evidence that prevalence and disease severity are both declining, possibly reflecting change in an environmental etiologic factor. It is extremely uncommon in individuals with predominantly Asian or Polynesian ancestry, although it is observed in some black populations.

Clinical Presentation

The most common symptoms attributable to Paget's disease are bone and joint pain. The bone pain is typically worse at rest and may trouble patients particularly at night. With skull involvement, pounding headaches can result. If Paget's disease leads to deformity of joint surfaces, premature arthritis occurs. This is particularly common at the hips. Deformity in long bones can occur, and involvement of the radius or weight-bearing bones of the lower limb often manifests in this way. Microfractures, which can be very painful, sometimes occur over the convexity of a deformed, weight-bearing bone. These can progress to complete fractures. Fractures can also occur through an area of active lytic disease in a weight-bearing bone.

Deafness is a common manifestation of Paget's disease and is caused by involvement of the bones of the middle ear or compromise of the eighth cranial nerve. More rarely, other neurologic syndromes can arise from nerve entrapment, including paraplegia as a result of spinal cord involvement.

Some pagetic patients are asymptomatic and are diagnosed because of an incidental finding of elevated circulating levels of alkaline phosphatase. The diagnosis may also result from an incidental radiographic finding, such as in studies of the urinary tract. Commonly, only one or two bones are involved, although disease may be more widespread. The pelvis, vertebral bodies, long bones, and skull are the most common sites, but almost any bone can be involved.

Diagnosis

Serum alkaline phosphatase, the most widely available marker of osteoblast activity, is usually elevated; however, if only one bone is involved, this test can be normal. In any patient with an elevation of alkaline phosphatase, it is important to determine whether this is coming from liver or bone. This question is usually addressed by other liver function tests, although assays of bone-specific alkaline phosphatase and of other osteoblast-specific markers (e.g., procollagen type I N-terminal propeptide [PINP]) are available. If the elevation of alkaline phosphatase is bony in origin, it is important to rule out other bone conditions such as metastatic cancers (e.g., breast, prostate). This is usually done by identifying the sites of skeletal abnormality on a bone scintigram and then obtaining plain radiographs of the abnormal areas.

Paget's disease has a characteristic appearance on plain radiographs, showing either bony rarefaction or sclerosis (depending on whether the osteoclastic or osteoblastic phase is predominating), disorganization of trabecular architecture, and the other abnormalities already discussed (e.g., deformity). Bone biopsy is not usually necessary to confirm the diagnosis.

Other biochemical markers of osteoblast or osteoclast activity, such as breakdown products of bone collagen, have been used in Paget's disease. Total alkaline phosphatase, bone alkaline phosphatase, PINP or N-terminal telopeptide of type I collagen (NTX) identified more than 95% of pagetic subjects in one cohort of pagetic subjects, although the poorer precision of NTX reduced its utility in monitoring the effects of treatment. Osteocalcin, C-telopeptide of type I collagen, and urinary free deoxypyridinoline are less useful for assessment of baseline activity and monitoring response to therapy. Total alkaline phosphatase remains the most widely used test because of its low cost and wide availability.

Treatment

Treatment of Paget's disease almost always relies on the potent bisphosphonates. These compounds have a very high affinity for the bone surface, where they remain for years. They are ingested by osteoclasts when bone is resorbed and inhibit a key enzyme in the mevalonate pathway, farnesyl pyrophosphate synthase. This results in disruption of the osteoclast cytoskeleton and cell death. Bisphosphonates are preferentially taken up at sites of high bone turnover, which accounts for their utility as bone scintigraphy agents, and therefore target active pagetic bone.

The injectable bisphosphonate pamidronate (Aredia, generic) has been used for many years in the treatment of Paget's disease. It is typically given as a series of infusions of 60 to 90 mg, each administered over a period of 1 to 2 hours. Pamidronate produces partial or complete remissions of disease activity that last for up to several years. The first administration of the drug may be accompanied by mild flu-like symptoms, which settle over 24 to 48 hours and usually do not recur. Their resolution can be hastened by the use of paracetamol (acetaminophen, Tylenol) or similar agents.

More recently, potent oral bisphosphonates such as alendronate (Fosamax, generic) and risedronate (Actonel, generic) have become widely used. These are administered daily over periods of 2 to 6 months and produce good disease control. The duration of treatment chosen in the pivotal clinical trials was arbitrary to some extent, and individual patients may require longer or shorter initial courses to achieve remission. Oral bisphosphonates have a very low bioavailability. Therefore, they must be taken in a fasting state, with a glass of water, and at least 30 minutes before consumption of food or other fluids. Positively charged ions (including calcium supplements, antacids, and mineral supplements) bind avidly to bisphosphonates and impair their absorption, so they must be taken at a different time of day. Potent bisphosphonates can cause irritation to the upper gastrointestinal tract and should not be prescribed to patients with inflammation or ulceration in that region. Patients should remain upright for 30 minutes after taking oral bisphosphonates to minimize the risk of reflux and associated esophagitis or ulceration.

The preferred treatment at present is the more potent intravenous bisphosphonate zoledronate (Reclast, generic), which is administered in a single dose of 5 mg over 15 minutes. It has been compared with the standard 2-month course of risedronate in two randomized, controlled trials. At 6 months, 96% of patients receiving zoledronate had a therapeutic response, compared with 74% of those randomized to risedronate ($P < 0.001$). Alkaline phosphatase levels normalized in 89% of patients in the zoledronate group and in 58% of those in the risedronate group ($P < 0.001$). Zoledronate showed a more rapid onset of action and superior effects on quality-of-life measures. Perhaps the most impressive data with zoledronate have been those from the open follow-up of responders in these studies. Six years after drug administration, relapse had occurred in 0.7% of those receiving zoledronate but in 20% of risedronate-treated patients. Therefore, zoledronate produces much more sustained responses to therapy than have hitherto been possible.

Potent bisphosphonates can cause mild hypocalcemia, which is usually asymptomatic and not a cause for concern. However, in patients with marked vitamin D deficiency, hypocalcemia can be more severe and sustained. Therefore, it is important to ensure that patients are vitamin D sufficient before receiving these drugs—a serum 25-hydroxyvitamin-D level greater than 40 nmol/L is more than adequate. Many physicians prescribe calcium to patients receiving bisphosphonate therapy (given in the evening if the oral bisphosphonate is given in the morning) as a further protection against hypocalcemia.

In the past, the weak bisphosphonate etidronate (Didronel) was used to treat Paget's disease. This is much less effective than the agents discussed previously. If used in high doses or for more than a few months, it carries the risk of producing osteomalacia, which can lead to bone pain and fractures. Therefore, it no longer has a place in the treatment of Paget's disease. Calcitonin (Miacalcin Injection) has also been relegated to an historical role only, because its efficacy is much less than that of the potent bisphosphonates and its effects are rapidly reversed after cessation of therapy. Denosumab (Prolia)[1] has some efficacy, but also appears to be inferior to zoledronate.

There are several philosophical approaches to Paget's disease management, none of which is strictly evidence based. There is general agreement that patients with symptoms attributable to Paget's disease should receive treatment. This is clear-cut in patients who have bone pain at the site of a pagetic lesion, but it is a common observation that antipagetic drugs can produce variable degrees of improvement in pain from joints adjacent to pagetic bone. Patients with neurologic complications from spinal cord or other nerve entrapments also improve with antipagetic therapy.

Treatment aimed at preventing complications of Paget's disease is variably endorsed, because there is no clinical trial evidence that treatment prevents the progression of deformity, the development of pagetic symptoms, or fracture. However, it is clear that treatment leads to a restoration of normal bone histology (Figure 2) and radiographic healing of lytic lesions and that, in the absence of such intervention, both bone lysis and deformity progress. It seems unreasonable to withhold safe therapies that are able to halt histologic and radiologic disease progression. Therefore, many experienced physicians endorse the provision of antipagetic therapy for individuals with lytic lesions in long bones; lesions at sites that are likely to lead to neurologic complications, arthritis, or deformity; or involvement of the skull that could compromise hearing. Expert opinion also supports the use of antipagetic therapy before elective surgery on pagetic bone, because this approach reduces the vascularity of pagetic bone and results in less perioperative blood loss. On the other hand, Paget's disease in asymptomatic patients whose future risk of complications is thought to be low (e.g.,

---

[1]Not FDA approved for this indication.

Figure 2 Section of a bone trabecula affected by Paget's disease, viewed under polarized light to show orientation of lamellae. In the center of the trabecula, the collagen fibers are chaotically laid down (woven bone), consistent with active Paget's disease. Over the outer surfaces, collagen is organized in parallel lamellae, indicating the restoration of normal bone microarchitecture after treatment with alendronate. (Reprinted with permission from: Reid IR, Nicholson GC, Weinstein RS, et al: Biochemical and radiologic improvement in Paget's disease of bone treated with alendronate: A randomized, placebo-controlled trial. Am J Med 1996;101:341–48.)

with involvement of the ilium) is commonly managed without specific pharmaceutical intervention, although the availability of a safe, single-dose treatment with zoledronate is increasing the inclination to treat.

When providing treatment targeted at these goals, it is important to consider how adequacy of therapy can be judged. In the case of patients with pain, maximal relief of pain is an important endpoint. Lytic lesions should be treated and monitored with sequential radiographs until healing is apparent. Activity at other sites can be assessed indirectly with biochemical markers of bone turnover, although these are much less sensitive in patients with monostotic disease. In this context, there can be considerable residual activity at a single affected site without the markers being abnormal. Bone scintigrams provide the most sensitive method of assessing local disease activity.

In the past, Paget's disease caused substantial morbidity in the elderly population. However, it is now possible to achieve adequate and sustained disease control with use of intravenous zoledronate. Prompt use of these agents, when indicated, can be expected to halt disease progression and to effectively prevent the development of significant complications from this condition.

References

Kanis JA: *Pathophysiology and Treatment of Paget's Disease of Bone*, London, 1991, Martin Dunitz.
Lyles KW, Siris ES, Singer FR, et al: A clinical approach to diagnosis and management of Paget's disease of bone, *J Bone Miner Res* 16:1379–1387, 2001.
Miller PD, Brown JP, Siris ES, et al: A randomized, double-blind comparison of risedronate and etidronate in the treatment of Paget's disease of bone, *Am J Med* 106:513–520, 1999.
Ralston SH, Langston AL, Reid IR: Pathogenesis and management of Paget's disease of bone, *Lancet* 372:155–163, 2008.
Reid IR, Davidson JS, Wattie D, et al: Comparative responses of bone turnover markers to bisphosphonate therapy in Paget's disease of bone, *Bone* 35:224–230, 2004.
Reid IR, Miller P, Lyles K, et al: Comparison of a single infusion of zoledronic acid with risedronate for Paget's disease, *N Engl J Med* 353:898–908, 2005.
Reid IR, Nicholson GC, Weinstein RS, et al: Biochemical and radiologic improvement in Paget's disease of bone treated with alendronate: A randomized, placebo-controlled trial, *Am J Med* 101:341–348, 1996.
Selby PL, Davie MWJ, Ralston SH, et al: Guidelines on the management of Paget's disease of bone, *Bone* 31:366–373, 2002.

POLYMYALGIA RHEUMATICA AND GIANT CELL ARTERITIS

Method of
Mark A. Matza, MD, MBA; and John H. Stone, MD, MPH

 CURRENT DIAGNOSIS

Polymyalgia Rheumatica
- Age is greater than 50 years.
- Symptoms include pain, aching, or stiffness in the bilateral shoulders, neck, hips, or thighs in the absence of weakness.
- Constitutional symptoms such as fever, fatigue, and weight loss can be present. Peripheral arthritis occasionally occurs.
- Giant cell arteritis (GCA) symptoms are present in approximately 20% of cases.
- Acute-phase reactants (erythrocyte sedimentation rate and C-reactive protein concentration) are typically elevated, but a wide range of values is observed, from normal values to dramatic elevations.
- Ultrasound can be used to assess for synovitis, tenosynovitis, or bursitis in the shoulder girdle.

Giant Cell Arteritis
- Age is greater than 50 years.
- Acute-phase reactants (erythrocyte sedimentation rate and C-reactive protein concentration) are typically elevated, but a wide range of values is observed, from normal values to dramatic elevations.
- Symptoms include new-onset headaches (often temporal), scalp tenderness, jaw or tongue claudication, and vision changes such as diplopia, amaurosis fugax, or blindness.
- Constitutional symptoms such as fever, fatigue, and weight loss are often present.
- Approximately 50% of patients with GCA also have polymyalgia rheumatic either concurrently or before diagnosis.
- Temporal arteries may be bulging, irregular, or tender on examination, but they may also be normal. Bruits can often be auscultated in the presence of large-vessel disease.
- Imaging with computed tomography, magnetic resonance, or positron emission tomography–computed tomography angiography can be used to evaluate for aortic arch involvement.
- Ultrasound scanning of the temporal arteries can be used to assess for the characteristic "halo sign."
- Temporal artery biopsy is the diagnostic test of choice for patients presenting with cranial symptoms, but false-negative results may occur.

 CURRENT THERAPY

Polymyalgia Rheumatica
- Prednisone at a dose of 15 to 20 mg/day (or equivalent) is used initially, with tapering to begin after one month of treatment. The starting dose should be continued for 1 full month to suppress the disease effectively and then tapered to 10 mg by the end of month 2 of treatment. Prednisone can then be tapered off at the rate of 1 mg/month for a total prednisone duration of approximately 1 year.
- Should symptoms recur with tapering, the last effective dose of prednisone can be resumed.
- Tocilizumab (Actemra)[1] can be considered should symptoms be refractory to glucocorticoid taper.

Giant Cell Arteritis

- Treatment should not be delayed while awaiting temporal artery biopsy.
- Prednisone[1] at a dose of 1 mg/kg or approximately 60 mg (or equivalent) should be started if the diagnosis is suspected.
- Pulse dose methylprednisolone[1] (1 gm daily for 3 days) should be initiated if vision changes occur.
- Tocilizumab (Actemra) should be started as soon as possible in the absence of contraindications such as diverticulitis. Most patients with GCA should be treated with the combination of tocilizumab and prednisone from the start of therapy; that is, prednisone treatment should begin immediately, and tocilizumab treatment initiated as soon as approval is obtained.
- All patients with GCA should be treated with aspirin[1] (81 mg/day) in addition to tocilizumab and prednisone.
- Glucocorticoids can be tapered to discontinuation over a period of 4 to 6 months if tocilizumab is used concomitantly with prednisone. Patients treated with glucocorticoid monotherapy require longer prednisone treatment courses. Prophylaxis for glucocorticoid-induced osteoporosis with bisphosphonates, calcium, and vitamin D should be considered. Among patients treated with one year of weekly subcutaneous tocilizumab who achieve remisson and discontinue glucocorticoids, more than 40% are able to maintain treatment-free remissions for at least two years after stopping tocilizumab.

[1]Not FDA approved for this indication.

Polymyalgia rheumatica (PMR) and giant cell arteritis (GCA) are related and often overlapping systemic inflammatory disorders that typically affect patients older than 50 years of age. Women are more commonly affected than men, and whites more so than blacks and Hispanics. Both conditions are characterized by elevated acute phase reactants. Symptoms range from proximal muscle aching to blindness. Most patients respond swiftly to glucocorticoid treatment, but many patients fail to maintain disease control during or after prednisone tapers. Interleukin-6 receptor blockade with tocilizumab (Actemra) has been confirmed to be effective for the treatment of GCA in a randomized clinical trial and is approved by regulatory agencies all over the world. Tocilizumab should be used in combination with glucocorticoids in most patients with GCA and in patients with PMR who are unable to maintain steroid-induced remissions.

Polymyalgia Rheumatica

Clinical Presentation

PMR is characterized by symmetric proximal joint pain that typically occurs in the context of elevated inflammatory markers and nearly always targets patients older than 50 years of age. Symptom onset can be swift, but patients sometimes delay seeking medical attention for days to weeks. Morning stiffness is generally prolonged greater than 45 minutes. Patients have a negative rheumatoid factor and negative assays for anti-CCP antibodies. Other joints can be affected, manifesting as hand, wrist, or knee arthritis. Constitutional symptoms can be seen with weight loss, fatigue, and low-grade fever. The frequency of PMR increases with age and the disorder is encountered most often in whites. Physical examination demonstrates tenderness and limited active range of motion of the shoulder and hip girdle. Patients typically have substantially better range of motion with passive limb movements.

Diagnosis

Diagnosis is made on the basis of the clinical presentation and physical examination. The response to prednisone is also often a telling indication of PMR: most patients experience dramatic clinical improvements within 24 to 48 hours. Most patients have elevated acute phase reactants, but these markers are not dramatically increased in all patients and are normal in some. Ultrasound can be used to detect synovitis, tenosynovitis, or bursitis. GCA occurs in approximately 20% of patients with PMR. Therefore these patients should be queried closely to detect any symptoms that suggest GCA, namely headaches, scalp tenderness, jaw claudication, and visual disturbances.

A minority of patients with presentations of PMR eventually declare their true underlying inflammatory arthritis to be rheumatoid arthritis (RA). Such patients can convert from seronegative to seropositive (i.e., positive rheumatoid factor or anti-CCP antibodies) at some point in follow-up. The presence of distal joint symptoms might help predict the evolution to RA, but the development of RA cannot be predicted if seronegative at baseline.

Treatment

Patients with PMR are treated with antiinflammatory medications. Prednisone at a dose of 15 to 20 mg (or prednisone equivalent) is often used initially. Symptoms should dramatically improve within 1 to 2 days, but some patients require a few days longer to achieve clear responses. Although patients with PMR respond essentially universally to appropriate doses of glucocorticoids, treatment failures over the course of glucocorticoid tapers or after discontinuation are common. A dose of 10 mg should be achieved relatively quickly by 2 months unless refractory. After 10 mg, the prednisone taper should be slowed, and the dose decreased by approximately 1 mg per month based on symptoms and inflammatory markers. Should symptoms recur, prednisone can be increased to the last effective dose and the taper again slowed by approximately 1 mg every 2 months.

Most patients can taper off prednisone completely; however, in some a low dose of prednisone may be required to prevent the recurrence of symptoms. For patients with PMR who require excessive prednisone to maintain disease control, interleukin-6 receptor blockade with tocilizumab[1] should be considered.

Giant Cell Arteritis

Clinical Presentation

GCA is a large vessel vasculitis with a predilection for the proximal aorta and its primary branches, particularly the vessels of the head and neck. Essentially every patient is older than 50 years of age at diagnosis, and the disease incidence increases with each decade. Symptoms, often referred to as "cranial symptoms" (to be distinguished from symptoms of large-vessel vasculitis), can include new-onset headaches, scalp tenderness, jaw or tongue claudication, diplopia, and vision changes.

Visual symptoms, the most worrisome effects of GCA because they may herald irreversible blindness in one or even both eyes, often consist of amaurosis fugax or the sudden onset of monocular blindness through the mechanism of anterior ischemic optic neuropathy or central retinal artery occlusion. Permanent vision loss occurs in at least one eye in approximately 15% of untreated patients. Unfortunately, vision loss frequently occurs as the symptom that finally brings the patient to medical attention, at a time when preventive treatment is too late.

Approximately 40% of patients with GCA also have PMR, characterized by pain and stiffness in the shoulder and hip girdles and occasionally by more distal joint involvement (e.g., the wrists). Conversely, 20% of those with PMR eventually develop GCA. Patients can have fevers and constitutional symptoms such as weight loss and fatigue. GCA is a common cause of fever of unknown origin in the elderly. Extracranial vasculitis can occur in the proximal aorta and its branches and can ultimately lead to aortic aneurysm formation. Among the primary branches of the aorta, the subclavian arteries are involved most commonly. Bruits auscultated above or below the clavicle are a key physical examination finding, as is a reduction in the upper extremity pulses. Intracranial vessels are seldom affected in GCA, but an important exception is occasional posterior vertebrobasilar circulation involvement, which can lead to strokes.

[1]Not FDA approved for this indication.

Diagnosis

GCA is diagnosed based on a combination of the clinical presentation, inflammatory markers (i.e., erythrocyte sedimentation rate [ESR] and CRP), imaging, and biopsy. The temporal arteries may be bulging, irregular, or tender on examination; however, they may also be normal on examination, even if temporal artery biopsy subsequently confirms the presence of GCA. Bruits can be auscultated should the proximal aorta be involved. The ESR is greater than 50 mm/hr in most cases, but population-based studies confirm that the ESR is <50 mm/hr in approximately 10% of patients. Aortic arch involvement can be detected with imaging modalities such as computed tomography, magnetic resonance, or positron emission tomography–computed tomography angiography. Imaging abnormalities on cross-sectional imaging typically include long segments of smooth arterial narrowing and concentric thickening of the arterial wall. Temporal artery duplex ultrasound scanning may reveal a characteristic "halo sign," caused by edema within and around the blood vessel wall. Temporal artery biopsy is the test of choice for diagnosis; however, false-negative results can occur for a variety of reasons in GCA, including the fact that the arterial involvement is often segmental (i.e., characterized by "skip lesions").

Treatment

Treatment with high-dose glucocorticoids should not be delayed to obtain a temporal artery biopsy. A dose of prednisone[1] 1 mg/kg or approximately 60 mg (or prednisone equivalent) should be initiated promptly when a diagnosis of GCA is considered. Lower doses (e.g., 40 mg/day) can be used for individuals who are frail and elderly. If visual involvement has occurred, pulse dose methylprednisolone[1] 1000 mg daily for 3 days can be initiated followed by high-dose oral glucocorticoids. The optimal duration of a prednisone taper in GCA is not certain. In one randomized clinical trial, the percentage of patients achieving sustained disease remission at 1 year was essentially the same regardless of whether patients received a 6-month or 12-month prednisone taper. Sustained remissions were achieved in only 14% and 18% of patients, respectively. Thus, although high-dose glucocorticoids are effective at controlling GCA and inducing remission in most patients, the great majority of patients experience disease flares whenever prednisone is tapered to a lower dose (e.g., less than 15 mg/day) or discontinued.

The interleukin-6 receptor blocker tocilizumab (Actemra) is now approved worldwide for the treatment of GCA in combination with glucocorticoids. The addition of tocilizumab leads to substantial improvement in the rate of glucocorticoid-free remissions at 1 year and a reduction in the cumulative prednisone dose by approximately 50%. Tocilizumab can be administered either intravenously (8 mg/kg each month) or subcutaneously (165 mg each week). The high rate of treatment failure with regimens involving prednisone alone suggests that all patients without contraindications to tocilizumab should be treated with the combination of tocilizumab and prednisone initially, followed by an aggressive prednisone taper designed to discontinue prednisone within 4 to 6 months. In a trial of the interleukin-6 receptor blocker tocilizumab, 42% of patients who completed one year of weekly tocilizumab were able to discontinue treatment and maintain treatment-free remissions for at least two years. Some patients, on the other hand, may require ongoing tocilizumab or even tocilizumab plus prednisone to maintain disease control. Patients who are not able to discontinue prednisone entirely can usually be controlled well with the combination of tocilizumab and low-dose prednisone.

Aspirin[1] (81 mg/day), which has been shown in retrospective studies and a meta-analysis to reduce the incidence of vision loss, should be used in all patients without contraindications. Prophylaxis for glucocorticoid-induced osteoporosis with bisphosphonates, calcium, and vitamin D should be considered, particularly since GCA tends to afflict elderly individuals, many of whom have significant comorbidities at baseline, including osteoporosis. Prophylaxis for *Pneumocystis jiroveci* pneumonia may also

be considered in appropriate clinical circumstances, particularly when prolonged or recurrent courses of high-dose glucocorticoids are required.

References

Banz Y, Stone JH: Why do temporal arteries go wrong? Principles and pearls from a clinician and a pathologist, *Rheumatology* 57:ii3–ii10, 2018.

Buttgereit F, Dejaco C, Matteson EL, Dasgupta B: Polymyalgia rheumatica and giant cell arteritis: a systematic review, *JAMA* 315(22):2442–2458, 2016.

Koster MJ, Matteson EL, Warrington KJ: Large-vessel giant cell arteritis: diagnosis, monitoring and management, *Rheumatology* 57:ii32–ii42, 2018.

Stone JH, Tuckwell K, Dimonaco S, et al: Trial of tocilizumab in giant-cell arteritis, *N Engl J Med* 377(4):317–328, 2017.

Vodopivec I, Rizzo JF: Ophthalmic manifestations of giant cell arteritis, *Rheumatology* 57:ii63–ii72, 2018.

PSORIATIC ARTHRITIS

William Tillett, MBChB, PhD; and Laura C. Coates, MBChB, PhD

CURRENT DIAGNOSIS (SUMMARY)

- Psoriatic arthritis (PsA) is a form of inflammatory arthritis genetically associated with the spondylarthritides (SpA) (e.g., ankylosing spondylitis, reactive arthritis [ReA], inflammatory bowel disease [IBD], arthritis).
- It is usually diagnosed in the presence of psoriasis (personal or family history), negative rheumatoid factor, and other typical features such as dactylitis and nail involvement.
- Presentation is highly heterogeneous with potential involvement in multiple domains (arthritis, enthesitis, dactylitis and axial disease, skin plaques and nail dystrophy), as well as SpA-related extra-articular manifestations (IBD and uveitis).

CURRENT THERAPY

- Therapy of PsA aims to control musculoskeletal inflammation (arthritis, enthesitis, dactylitis, and axial disease) and cutaneous manifestations (skin plaques and nail dystrophy).
- Treatment usually follows a step up approach with non-steroidal antiinflammatory drugs (NSAIDs), topical therapies (for skin plaques), conventional synthetic disease-modifying antirheumatic drugs (DMARDs; e.g., methotrexate [Trexall], leflunomide)[1] and biologics (inhibitors of TNF, IL12/23, IL17, IL23) and targeted synthetic DMARDs (apremilast and janus kinase [JAK] inhibitors).
- PsA is commonly associated with comorbidities such as depression and increased cardiovascular risk with elements of the metabolic syndrome which may impact on therapeutic choice.

[1]Not FDA approved for this indication.

Epidemiology

Psoriatic arthritis (PsA) is a destructive inflammatory arthritis occurring in up to 20% people with psoriasis. Psoriasis affects approximately 2% to 3% of the US population. The exact prevalence of PsA among the general population has been difficult to estimate due to the heterogeneous nature of the disease and variety of different classification criteria. The lowest prevalence estimates come from Japan (0.001%) and highest from Italy (0.42%). Data from recent studies have been more consistent with prevalence estimates of 0.16% in North America and 0.19% in the United Kingdom. PsA affects men and women equally and can develop at any age but typically occurs in the 10 to 15 years after the diagnosis of psoriasis, usually between the ages of 30 and 50 years. The incidence of developing PsA among people with psoriasis is approximately 2% per year. In a

---

[1]Not FDA approved for this indication.

recent prospective study of patients with psoriasis, 51 of 464 patients developed PsA over an 8-year follow-up period.

Risk Factors

A number of risk factors have been identified that appear to increase the risk of developing PsA. The presence of HLAB27 is an established genetic risk factor. Increased rates of PsA are seen among those with more severe psoriasis (relative risk [RR] 5.4 P = 0.006). The site of psoriasis may also be important, and some reports suggest that intergluteal and scalp psoriasis confer an increased risk of developing PsA. Nail psoriasis (pitting, onycholysis, subungual hyperkeratosis, and oil drop discoloration) is also associated with an increased likelihood of developing PsA. Nail dystrophy occurs in 80% of patients with PsA but only 20% patients with psoriasis alone. Obesity is a well-documented risk factor for developing both psoriasis and PsA. The higher the body mass index (BMI), the higher the risk of developing arthritis. Alcohol is a potentially modifiable risk factor with associated increased rates of both psoriasis and arthritis. Data relating to smoking as a risk factor are mixed, with reports suggesting both increased risk and a potentially protective effect.

Pathophysiology

Genetics

The exact etiology of PsA remains uncertain. Genetics are known to play a central role. However, the number of genes identified do not account for the strong heritability seen clinically. Approximately 40% of people with PsA will have a first-degree relative with the condition. PsA appears to have a stronger association with HLA-B and HLA-C alleles, whereas psoriasis is associated with HLA-C. HLA-Cw6, B57, DR7, and B17 are all associated with early onset psoriasis. HLA-B7, HLA-B27, DR4, 38, and DR7 are associated with PsA. HLA-B39, B27, and DR7 are associated with more progressive/destructive disease, whereas HLA-B22 appears to be protective.

Immunopathology

Tissue specific autoantibodies have not yet been identified. The inflammatory arthritis is characterized by hypervascularity, hypertrophy/tissue proliferation, and inflammatory cell infiltrate. Lymphocytes (particularly Th17 cells) and dendritic cells are known to play an important role. The cytokine profile for PsA shows a predominance of TNF-α, IL-1, and IL-10.

Infection and Trauma

The temporal link between infections and the development of PsA raises the possibility of a pathological role of bacteria or viruses. There are higher rates of both psoriasis and PsA in HIV endemic areas, and psoriasis is often more extensive among patients with HIV. The gut microbiome is an area of current interest where disturbance of the normal microbiota is being investigated as a possible immunological trigger. Finally, a small number of epidemiological studies have made the association with trauma and the subsequent development of PsA, but reports are inconclusive.

Prevention

There are no known strategies to prevent the development of PsA. Preventive strategies focus on early diagnosis and prevention of damage accumulation, loss of function, and disability. The treatment of comorbid conditions, pre-drug-treatment screening, and drug dose optimization to minimize drug exposure are important prevention strategies.

Early diagnosis and treatment strategies focus on the prevention of damage and subsequent disability. Untreated inflammation results in damage to the articular surface and surrounding tissues with subsequent loss of movement, pain, limitation of function, and reduced quality of life. Erosion of the surface of the bone, narrowing of the joint space, and new bone formation (osteoproliferation) cause pain, reduced movement, and physical dysfunction. Observational studies have suggested that delay of diagnosis by as little as 6 months results in more damage and worse physical function.

In the United Kingdom, annual screening of patients with psoriasis for arthritis is recommended using the Psoriasis Epidemiology Screening Tool (PEST) questionnaire. The questionnaire asks patients with psoriasis if they have ever had pain in their joints, if a doctor has ever told them they have arthritis, if they have had nail pitting, if they have had pain in their heel, and if they have ever had a completely sausage-like swelling of a finger or toe without reason. A score of 3 or more is positive.

Clinical Manifestations

PsA is classified with the seronegative spondyloarthropathies that include axial spondyloarthritis (AxSpA), Reactive Arthritis (ReA), and Inflammatory Bowel Disease (IBD) arthritis. The seronegative spondyloarthropathies share many of the clinical and genetic features, such as HLAB27 association, enthesopathy (inflammation at the tendon and ligament insertion to the bone), association with uveitis, spondyloarthritis, and asymmetric peripheral arthritis.

The classical patterns of PsA are listed in the following, although there is often overlap between these groups:

- Polyarthritis (five or more joints);
- Oligoarthritis (four or fewer joints);
- Monoarthritis (one joint);
- Spondyloarthritis (axial disease);
- PsA Mutilans (digital shortening/telescoping due to onycholysis).

Polyarthritis is the most common form occurring in approximately 60% cases, whereas mutilans only occurs in 5% cases.

The signs of PsA are heterogeneous and include the following:

Psoriasis—In its most common plaque form, the skin lesions of psoriasis are characterized by scaly plaques on the extensor surfaces. Psoriasis can be hidden in the scalp, ear, natal cleft, and umbilicus. Most patients develop their psoriasis before developing arthritis, but a small proportion, approximately 10%, will develop psoriasis after their arthritis. A proportion of patients present with musculoskeletal symptoms but are unaware they have skin psoriasis, which can be subtle in sites such as the hairline, intergluteal region, behind the ear, or umbilicus. Other patterns of psoriasis include guttate (small spots which can be widespread), palmar-plantar (palms and soles), and inverse (affecting the flexural creases).

Nail dystrophy—pitting (fine pits), onycholysis (lifting of the distal nail plate), hyperkeratosis (thickening of the nail plate), and oil drop discoloration (salmon-colored spots) are the most common nail manifestations of psoriasis. Other features include leukonychia, Beau lines, and longitudinal ridging. Nail pitting can be clinically subtle but a helpful sign to distinguish PsA from other types of arthritis. Nail dystrophy itself is associated with an increased risk of developing arthritis and can be the only manifestation of psoriasis.

Joint disease—Inflammatory arthritis is the hallmark of PsA. The joints appear swollen and hot and are stiff and painful. The recognized patterns of joint involvement are inflammatory polyarthritis (5 or more joints involved, which may be symmetric or asymmetric in distribution), oligoarticular (<5 joints), monoarticular (one joint), axial (spondyloarthritis), and mutilans (digital shortening due to onycholysis).

Enthesitis—Inflammation at the insertion of the tendon or ligament to the bone (rather than the mid portion of the tendon which is more likely to be an overuse tendinopathy) may be a sign. Many sites can be affected by enthesitis. However, the most readily assessable are the Achilles insertion to the calcaneus, the lateral epicondyle of the elbow, and the medial condyle of the femur. Enthesitis is not commonly seen in rheumatoid arthritis and can be a useful distinguishing sign. The assessment of enthesitis can be challenging, as many entheseal insertions correlate anatomically with myofascial tender points seen in fibromyalgia. Ultrasound can be helpful to examine for sonographic features of enthesitis, such as insertional hypervascularity, osteoproliferation, and erosion.

Dactylitis—Also known as "sausage finger," dactylitis is the swelling of an entire digit. Dactylitis occurs on 50% of patients with PsA at some point in their disease. The inflammation is at the joint, tendon and extracapsular tissues.

Spondyloarthritis—Spondyloarthritis affects up to 50% of patients with PsA, but cohort studies have suggested only half of these patients have symptoms of inflammatory back pain. Inflammatory back pain typically occurs before the age of 40 years, will wake people in the second half of the night, are characteristically stiff in the morning, and feel better with exercise and nonsteroidal antiinflammatory drugs. The radiographic features are of sacroiliitis (sclerosis, erosions, and fusion), which can be asymmetrical, and syndesmophytes (bone formation which can be fine or chunky), which can flow between vertebrae, causing fusion.

Other manifestations include uveitis (approximately 30% patients, RR 3.5 compared to the general population), metabolic syndrome (elevated BMI, hypertension, and dyslipidemia), IBD (Crohn disease, RR 2.9 compared to the general population), and depression.

Diagnosis

In the absence of specific antibodies, the diagnosis of PsA remains clinical. The Classification Criteria for Psoriatic Arthritis (CASPAR) criteria were developed for use in clinical trials to ensure a consistent trial population and have also been shown to apply in the clinical setting as diagnostic criteria (Box 1).

Differential Diagnosis

The other seronegative spondyloarthropathies are in the primary differential diagnosis.

The absence of an infectious trigger or concurrent IBD discount ReA and IBD arthritis. The presence or history of psoriasis (or a first-degree relative with psoriasis) is the most useful distinguishing feature in differentiating from axial spondyloarthritis.

Osteoarthritis is a common and clinically challenging differential, particularly in the hands. Young age of onset, the presence of nail psoriasis at the affected ray, and radiographic features of PsA are the most useful distinguishing features.

Gout is an important differential for two reasons. First, a history of a swollen toe is often mistaken as gout (or podagra). Second, uric acid is commonly mildly elevated in patients with PsA. A careful history and examination for other clinical features of PsA can be helpful, such as history of psoriasis, nail dystrophy at the affected toe, enthesitis, or axial symptoms. Ultrasound to examine for sonographic features of crystal deposition or aspiration to examine for crystals may be required. Concurrent gout and PsA are rare but recognized.

Investigations to support the diagnosis include:

- Rheumatoid factor (RhF) and anticyclic citrullinated peptide (ACPA or Anti-CCP) are usually negative.

| **BOX 1** | The Classification Criteria for Psoriatic Arthritis Criteria |

Confirmed inflammatory articular disease (joint, spine, or entheseal) with at least three points from the following features;
1. Current psoriasis (two points).
2. A past personal history or family history of a first-or second-degree relative with psoriasis (one point each).
3. Dactylitis (one point).
4. Juxtaarticular new bone formation (ill-defined ossification near joint margins—excluding osteophyte formation—on plain hand and feet radiographs; one point).
5. Rheumatoid factor negativity (one point).
6. Psoriatic nail dystrophy (onycholysis, pitting, and hyperkeratosis observed on current physical examination; one point).

- Inflammatory markers such as C-reactive protein (CRP), plasma viscosity (PV), and erythrocyte sedimentation rate (ESR) can often be normal, and do not exclude inflammatory joint disease.
- Plain radiographs can be helpful to distinguish PsA from rheumatoid arthritis (RA) or osteoarthritis (OA). The plain radiographic features of PsA are erosions, joint space narrowing, osteoproliferation (bone formation), ankyloses (fusion), and, in the mutilans form of the disease, osteolysis (bone resorption).
- Magnetic resonance imaging (MRI) and ultrasound are both frequently used to assess for spondyloarthritis and articular and entheseal inflammation, respectively.

Therapy (or Treatment)

The treatment of PsA aims to control inflammation related to the disease to improve symptoms, maximize function, and prevent long-term complications. Different therapies may be chosen dependent on the domains of disease (arthritis, skin, nails, enthesitis, dactylitis, axial disease) that are active in any one individual patient. In general, treatment of PsA follows a step-up approach with treatment escalated in case of non-response to the previous therapy. Ideally treatment should follow a treat-to-target approach where a treatment target, such as minimal disease activity (MDA), is reassessed at each visit, and therapy is assessed if the target is not met. This approach has been shown to improve disease control in the tight control of PsA (TICOPA) trial.

Nonsteroidal antiinflammatory drugs are used frequently to help manage pain and stiffness but do not seem to have a significant effect on the disease course. Particularly in the early stages of disease or in the case of disease flares, parenteral steroids (intra-articular or intramuscular) are used to control inflammation quickly, although there can be a risk of psoriasis flare on withdrawal of systemic steroids. The mainstay of therapy in PsA are disease-modifying antirheumatic drugs (DMARDs), which are grouped into three categories:
1. Conventional synthetic DMARDs (methotrexate, sulfasalazine,[1] leflunomide[1])
2. Biologic DMARDs (tumor necrosis factor [TNF] inhibitors, interleukin 12/23, 17, or 23 inhibitors)
3. Targeted synthetic DMARDs (phosphodiesterase 4 [PDE4] and janus kinase [JAK] inhibitors)

Conventional synthetic DMARDs (csDMARDs) are commonly used to treat skin psoriasis and peripheral arthritis. The use of these drugs is based on their efficacy in psoriasis and in rheumatoid arthritis, although the data supporting their efficacy in PsA are relatively lacking. The most commonly used csDMARD is methotrexate, although the placebo-controlled MIPA (Methotrexate In PsA) trial did not show a significant effect of methotrexate over placebo. Many rheumatologists discounted these data, due to flaws in the study design (low target dose used, poor completion rate). Interestingly in the supplementary data from the study, it seemed that patients with polyarticular disease responded much better to methotrexate than those with oligoarthritis. This may be due to a differential response in different forms of arthritis, but it most likely relates to the sensitivity of the outcome measures used. There is, however, proven efficacy for the use of methotrexate in psoriasis so this drug is useful to manage patients with both peripheral arthritis and active psoriasis. Sulfasalazine is also commonly used and does have a number of studies supporting its efficacy. However, a Cochrane review in 2000 summarized the results of these studies and concluded that while it was effective, the effect size was relatively small. Leflunomide is the conventional DMARD with the strongest trial data. The TOPAS study in 2004 confirmed efficacy of leflunomide versus placebo but came shortly before breakthrough trials with biological therapies with superior results.

Despite the mixed data on the csDMARDs and their effect on clinical measures of disease activity, none of them have any proven

---

[1]Not FDA approved for this indication.

effect on disease progression in the form of radiographic damage. Observational studies have suggested that early use of therapies and higher dosages used in more recent years may be associated with less radiographic damage, but this has not been formally tested. There is very limited data in treating other domains of PsA, such as enthesitis and dactylitis, where only small open label studies are available. In axial PsA, as in other axial spondylarthritides, there is no evidence of efficacy of conventional drugs, and treatment algorithms rely on biological therapies.

A number of biological DMARDs (bDMARDS) have proven efficacy in PsA and have been licensed for use in this condition. There are five different TNF inhibitors (adalimumab, certolizumab, etanercept, infliximab, golimumab), which have all shown efficacy across the key domains of PsA, including arthritis, enthesitis, dactylitis, skin, and nails. They have all shown long-term efficacy and retardation of radiographic damage, confirming their effect on structural progression. In most of the studies, around 50% of the patients were also receiving a concomitant csDMARD (usually methotrexate). However, in PsA, in contrast to rheumatoid arthritis, there has not been a significant difference in efficacy seen with combination treatment over monotherapy biologics. Recently a randomized trial addressed this point, comparing methotrexate monotherapy, etanercept monotherapy, and the combination in a placebo-controlled trial. This study confirmed superiority of both etanercept arms over methotrexate monotherapy but did not find a difference in effect with concomitant use of csDMARDs.

As a secondary outcome in the PsA studies, there has been a significant difference seen in enthesitis and dactylitis using clinical measures. In the PsA studies and in specific psoriasis studies, the efficacy of TNF inhibitors has been proven for both skin and nail disease. As yet, there are no specific studies in axial PsA, but data in axial spondyloarthritis and/or ankylosing spondylitis has confirmed the efficacy of TNF inhibitors for spinal symptoms.

A number of interleukin inhibitors have been licensed for the treatment of PsA. Ustekinumab (Stelara; a p40 antibody that blocks the action of IL-12 and IL-23) is particularly effective for psoriasis, with proven superiority over TNF inhibitors. It also has evidence of efficacy for peripheral arthritis, enthesitis, and dactylitis. Surprisingly, however, despite a small positive open label study, a randomized trial in axial spondyloarthritis was halted early, with no evidence of efficacy over placebo. Thus the phenotype of disease must be considered when choosing a therapy.

IL-17A inhibitors (secukinumab [Cosentyx] and ixekizumab [Taltz]) are now licensed for PsA and secukinumab for ankylosing spondylitis, providing an alternative biologic option for those with PsA. These drugs showed even higher responses in skin psoriasis, with head-to-head studies confirming superiority over ustekinumab and TNF inhibitors. Additional drugs targeting the Th17 pathway are in development. Bimekizumab[5] blocks both IL-17A and IL-17F and has positive phase II trial results. Further studies will show if dual blockade is superior to blocking IL-17A alone. Brodalumab (Siliq)[1], a human antibody against the IL-17 receptor, would also block different forms of IL-17 and has positive phase 2 data in PsA.

A number of specific IL-23 inhibitors are also in development following from data with ustekinumab. These bind to the p19 subunit, providing specific blockade of IL-23 only, and have been shown to have impressive efficacy in skin psoriasis. Phase 2 data are available in PsA, with evidence of efficacy in peripheral arthritis, but again studies in ankylosing spondylitis and axial spondyloarthritis have been halted due to lack of efficacy in the spinal domain.

In recent years, a third class of drugs, the targeted synthetic DMARDs (tsDMARDs), have also become available for the treatment of PsA. Apremilast (Otezla) is a phosphodiesterase 4 inhibitor with proven modest efficacy in the treatment of peripheral arthritis, psoriasis, enthesitis, and dactylitis. Although responses seem lower than the biologic drugs, apremilast has a very reassuring safety profile with no requirement for regular blood monitoring. The other group of tsDMARDs in development focus on targeting the JAK pathway. Tofacitinib (Xeljanz) is licensed for treatment of peripheral arthritis, with comparable improvements in arthritis outcomes to adalimumab, which was included in the study as an internal control. Tofacitinib also shows modest efficacy on skin psoriasis, although it is not specifically licensed for psoriasis. Other JAK inhibitors, with different selectivity for JAK pathways, are in phase II and III studies.

In all cases, the aim of treatment should be to minimize disease activity. The choice of therapy can be difficult, as there is a lack of head-to-head comparison studies and many of the newer biologic or tsDMARDs appear to have similar efficacy in arthritis. In cases with significant psoriasis, an argument could be made for IL12/23, IL17, or IL23 inhibitors, where superior efficacy has been shown. For those with axial disease, proven efficacy is limited to TNF and IL17 inhibitors. In other cases, the choice of medication often depends on comorbidities, where therapies may be contraindicated (IL17 inhibitors worsening active IBD) or helpful (TNF inhibitors).

Monitoring

Monitoring of PsA may include assessment of clinical disease activity measures, patient reported outcomes, laboratory tests, and imaging. The majority of day-to-day disease monitoring consists of clinical outcome measures, often combined with patient reported outcomes.

Ideally all domains of disease should be assessed to allow optimal choice of therapy. To assess arthritis, a full 68/66 joint count is required, rather than reduced joint counts used in rheumatoid arthritis. Dactylitis is usually evident when joints are examined. Enthesitis can be assessed clinically looking for tenderness and swelling at the site of key tendon attachments. In cases of doubt, ultrasound imaging can be helpful to look for inflammation and increased blood flow. Although rheumatologists are focused on musculoskeletal signs, when treating patients with PsA, they should also assess skin and nail manifestations. This can be a relatively brief assessment, such as a body surface area of skin psoriasis affected; it is important not to underestimate the impact of skin involvement on patient's quality of life.

Multiple patient reported outcomes are available to measure the patient perspective in PsA, including questionnaires assessing pain, function, work disability, and other impacts. The majority of these are research tools, and they are often combined with physician assessed clinical measures to form composite scores. In clinical practice, some questionnaire may be used to assess the patient perspective and encourage dialogue with patients.

As mentioned previously, treatment recommendations now state that a treat-to-target approach should be implemented in routine care of PsA. Recommendations state that the treatment target should ideally be remission with the alternative target of low disease activity if remission is not feasible. Additional recommendations on treat to target have highlighted that the target of therapy should include both musculoskeletal and skin manifestations of disease. Thus the MDA criteria have been recommended for the target of treatment, as these include measures of arthritis, psoriasis, enthesitis and patient reported pain, global activity, and functional ability.

Management of Complications

PsA is associated with a number of comorbidities. It is part of the spectrum of spondyloarthritis and has associated extra-articular manifestations (EAMs), including potential overlap with IBD and uveitis. The involvement of these other systems is important to recognize to aid diagnosis and then comanage patients to optimize outcome. Often therapies for PsA are also licensed for treatment of EAMs, allowing treatment of the disease as a whole.

Other comorbidities, not directly related to the disease complex, are also prominent in patients with psoriasis and PsA. Depression and anxiety are prevalent in up to half of the population and are

[1] Not FDA approved for this indication.
[5] Investigational drug in the United States.

important to address to maximize quality of life and also to aid adherence to therapy. Patients with psoriasis and PsA also have a much higher risk of metabolic syndrome and associated cardiovascular comorbidity. There are higher rates of obesity, diabetes, hypertension, hyperlipidemia, and associated complications such as nonalcoholic fatty liver disease and cardiovascular events. The cardiovascular risk seems to be higher in those with severe active disease and provides another argument for effective control of inflammation. Beyond controlling disease, patients need support and interventions to manage their other risk factors such as weight, smoking, blood pressure, and lipid control.

References

Charlton R, Green A, Shaddick G: On behalf of the PROMPT study group. Risk of uveitis and inflammatory bowel disease in people with psoriatic arthritis: a population-based cohort study, *Annals of the Rheumatic Diseases* 77:277–280, 2018.

Coates LC, Kavanaugh A, Mease PJ, et al: Group for research and assessment of psoriasis and psoriatic arthritis: Treatment recommendations for psoriatic arthritis 2015, *Arthritis Rheumatol* 68(5):1060–1071, 2016 May.

Coates LC, Moverley AR, McParland L, et al: Effect of tight control of inflammation in early psoriatic arthritis (TICOPA): a UK multicentre, open-label, randomised controlled trial, *Lancet* 386(10012):2489–2498, 2015.

Ogdie A, Weiss P: The epidemiology of psoriatic arthritis, *Rheum Dis Clin North Am* 41(4):545–568, 2015.

Taylor W, Gladman D, Helliwell P, et al: Classification criteria for psoriatic arthritis: Development of new criteria from a large international study, *Arthritis & Rheumatism* 54:2665–2673, 2006.

Tillett W, Charlton R, Nightingale A, et al: Interval between onset of psoriasis and psoriatic arthritis comparing the UK Clinical Practice Research Datalink with a hospital-based cohort, *Rheumatology* 56(12):2109–2113, 1 Dec 2017.

Van den Bosch F, Coates L: Clinical management of psoriatic arthritis, *Lancet* 391(10136):2285–2294, 2018 Jun 2.

Veale DJ, Fearon U: The pathogenesis of psoriatic arthritis, *Lancet* 391:2273–2284, 2018.

RHEUMATOID ARTHRITIS

Method of
Megan Krause, MD

CURRENT DIAGNOSIS

- Clinical diagnosis based on combination of history, examination, and supporting laboratory studies.
- Presentation is typically chronic symmetric polyarticular inflammatory arthritis.
- While not required for diagnosis, supporting laboratory studies include positive rheumatoid factor (RF), positive anticitrullinated protein antibodies (ACPA), elevated C-reactive protein (CRP), and elevated sedimentation rate (ESR).
- Radiographs can be normal at diagnosis. Findings of periarticular osteopenia and erosions are supportive of diagnosis of rheumatoid arthritis (RA).

CURRENT THERAPY

- Methotrexate (Otrexup, Rasuvo, Rheumatrex) initial dose typically 10 to 15 mg weekly with an increase based on disease activity up to 25 mg weekly orally or subcutaneously in conjunction with daily folic acid[1] 1 mg orally daily.
- Hydroxychloroquine (Plaquenil) 5 mg/kg orally per day with maximum of 400 mg daily.
- Sulfasalazine (Azulfidine-EN) initially dose typically 500 mg orally once daily or 500 mg twice daily, increasing up to goal dose of 1000 to 1500 mg twice daily.
- Leflunomide (Arava) 10 to 20 mg orally once daily.
- Azathioprine (Imuran) initial 1 mg/kg/day orally with increasing dose based on response to maximum of 2.5 mg/kg/day.
- Janus kinase inhibitors
  - Tofacitinib (Xeljanz) immediate release 5 mg orally twice daily or extended release 11 mg orally once daily.
  - Baricitinib (Olumiant) 2 mg orally once daily.
  - Upadacitinib (Rinvoq) 15 mg once daily.
- Tumor necrosis factor (TNF) inhibitors
  - Adalimumab (Humira) 40 mg subcutaneous every other week.
  - Certolizumab (Cimzia) 400 mg subcutaneous at week 0, 2, and 4, then 200 mg every other week or 400 mg every 4 weeks.
  - Etanercept (Enbrel) 50 mg subcutaneous every week.
  - Golimumab (Simponi, Simponi Aria)
    - Subcutaneous: 50 mg subcutaneous every 4 weeks
    - Intravenous: 2 mg/kg intravenous (IV) at week 0, 4, and then every 8 weeks
  - Infliximab (Remicade) 3 mg/kg intravenous at week 0, 2, and 6 and then every 8 weeks but, if persistent disease activity, dose can be adjusted between 3 and 10 mg/kg every 4 to 8 weeks.
- Interleukin 6 (IL6) receptor inhibitors
  - Tocilizumab (Actemra)
    - Subcutaneous: if less than 100 kg: 162 mg every other week, increase to weekly if persistent disease activity; if more than 100 kg: 162 mg every week.
    - Intravenous: 4 mg/kg every 4 weeks, can be increased to 8 mg/kg every 4 weeks if persistent disease activity.
  - Sarilumab (Kevzara) 200 mg subcutaneous every 2 weeks.
- T cell co-stimulation inhibitors
  - Abatacept (Orencia)
    - Subcutaneous: 125 mg once weekly (with or without IV loading dose).
    - Intravenous: if less than 60 kg: 500 mg; if 60 to 100 kg: 750 mg; if more than 100 kg: 1000 mg with initial dosing at week 0, 2, and 4, and then every 4 weeks.
- B cell inhibitor
  - Rituximab (Rituxan) 1000 mg IV day 1 and 15, subsequent doses can be repeated at 24 weeks.
- Interleukin 1 receptor inhibitor
  - Anakinra (Kineret) 100 mg subcutaneous every day.

[1]Not FDA approved for this indication.

Epidemiology

Individuals can develop rheumatoid arthritis (RA) at any age, but a peak incidence is between 50 and 75 years. Women are affected at a frequency of two to three times greater than men. It is estimated that the prevalence is approximately 1% in the United States. However, the risk varies based on the race/ethnicity distribution of the population studied. Some Native American populations such as Chippewa and Pima can reach up to 5%.

Risk Factors

The exact pathogenesis of RA is not completely understood. It is likely the consequence of the interplay of multiple factors, including genetic predisposition and epigenetic factors, along with environmental exposures that result in the systemic inflammatory process. The environmental factors are diverse and are likely not the same in all individuals. Cigarette smoking has been identified as a significant risk factor. Periodontal disease also is associated with development of RA. Silica is an example of an associated occupational exposure.

Multiple genetic risk factors have been identified. The shared epitope, referring to a specific sequence at the HLA-DRB1 locus, which is involved with antigen presentation, has been one of the most studied. Other genetic factors have been identified but individually contribute a small increase in risk.

Pathophysiology

The combination of genetics, epigenetic factors, and environmental exposures lead to downstream consequences of loss of tolerance to self. Both the innate and adaptive immune systems are activated in this process. Diverse immune cells including T cells, B cells, macrophages, and dendritic cells are involved in the pathogenesis. The production of cytokines contributes to the wide variety of downstream tissue targets that lead to the diverse clinical manifestations of RA. While RA frequently is diagnosed based on presentation of inflammatory arthritis, the production of cytokines and interplay of multiple cell types leads to the multiorgan dysfunction.

Prevention

It is not understood how to prevent the development of RA. Limiting known risk factors such as smoking and maintaining periodontal health would be reasonable recommendations.

Clinical Manifestations
Articular Manifestations

Classically, individuals will present with symmetric inflammatory polyarthritis (affecting five or more joints) frequently affecting the wrists, metacarpophalangeal joints (MCPs), proximal interphalangeal joints (PIPs), and metatarsophalangeal joints (MTPs). Both small and large joints can be affected. The distal interphalangeal joints (DIPs) and the lumbar spine are spared.

On examination, the joints can be warm, erythematous, swollen, and tender. Range of motion of joints is frequently limited. The synovitis on exam can be described as boggy in contrast to bony hypertrophic changes of osteoarthritis.

Extraarticular Manifestations

One of the consequences of the systemic nature of RA is that the symptoms are not limited to the joints. The extraarticular manifestations can have significant impact both in terms of morbidity and mortality. High clinical suspicion is required, and evaluation is necessary to differentiate toxicity of medications versus a manifestation of RA. More data are required to understand how the advances in therapy will impact the extraarticular manifestations.

Individuals with RA can develop subcutaneous nodules, which sometimes can be independent of disease activity. Rarely, individuals can develop a paradoxical increase in rheumatoid nodules with methotrexate.

Individuals can present with significant dryness of the mouth consistent with secondary Sjögren syndrome. Some of these individuals will have positive autoantibodies, such as SSA/Ro and SSB/La.

Pulmonary manifestations can be quite varied and have important implications for treatment. Pleural disease can be seen and can include pleural effusions and pleurisy. Pulmonary nodules can also be present. Interstitial lung disease can present in wide ranging patterns, including usual interstitial pneumonia (UIP), nonspecific interstitial pneumonia (NSIP), organizing pneumonia, and constrictive bronchiolitis.

Cardiac manifestations can include accelerated coronary artery disease. If the joint symptoms preclude significant exertion, patients may not present with classic angina. Pericardial disease can range from pericarditis, pericardial effusion, and constrictive pericarditis. Depending on the location, rheumatoid nodules affecting the heart can be associated with valve dysfunction and conduction abnormalities.

Episcleritis and scleritis can be associated with RA. A dreaded ocular complication of RA is peripheral ulcerative keratitis and corneal melt; this requires emergent ophthalmologic evaluation.

Frequently hematologic abnormalities can be associated with RA. Anemia of chronic disease, leukocytosis, and thrombocytosis can be frequently seen. A minority of individuals will develop Felty syndrome, which includes clinical manifestations of splenomegaly, leukopenia (frequently neutropenia), and frequent infections.

Entrapment syndromes such as carpal tunnel syndrome can be a presenting symptom of RA or develop over the course of the disease. In the case of carpal tunnel syndrome, it is the result of compression of the median nerve due to swelling of the flexor tendons.

RA can affect the cervical spine. The atlantoaxial joint can be prone to subluxation, which can result in myelopathy. A high clinical suspicion is required, as individuals may not present with neck pain and joint damage can obscure examination findings such as reflexes.

An increasingly rare manifestation is vasculitis secondary to RA. This can have multiple manifestations but can include cutaneous ulcers and mononeuritis multiplex.

Diagnosis

Rheumatoid arthritis is a clinical diagnosis based on the pattern of clinical and laboratory findings. Rarely at presentation, individuals can present with monoarticular (one joint) or oligoarticular (two to four joints), but typically when observed over time, individuals will have polyarticular involvement.

Tests to aid diagnosis include the RF, which refers to an immunoglobuin M (IgM) directed against immunoglobulin G (IgG). It is a nonspecific test and can be elevated related to age, as well other diseases that can mimic RA, such as hepatitis C. ACPA have the advantage of being more specific than RF with specificity as high as 95%. Individuals are considered to have seropositive RA when either RF or ACPA is positive; this occurs in approximately 70% to 80% of individuals. Acute phase reactants including CRP and ESR, when elevated, are supportive of the diagnosis but not required of the diagnosis. Anemia of chronic disease, thrombocytosis, and leukocytosis can also be supportive of the diagnosis but are nonspecific.

The American College of Rheumatology (ACR) and European League Against Rheumatism (EULAR) have developed classification criteria. Domains included the pattern of joint involvement, serology status (RF and ACPA), acute phase reactants (CRP and ESR), and duration of symptoms (cutoff of 6 weeks).

At presentation, x-rays can be normal. The earliest abnormality in RA on x-ray evaluation of the joints includes soft tissue swelling and periarticular osteopenia. Additional changes on x-rays include symmetric joint space narrowing and marginal erosions. If erosions are present at diagnosis, this is associated with a worse prognosis.

Differential Diagnosis

The differential diagnosis is broad for RA. Multiple infections can cause polyarticular joint pain. Viral etiologies can include hepatitis B, hepatitis C, and HIV. Parvovirus B19 can also be a mimic of RA; joint pain can be a prominent feature in adults in contrast to children who rarely have joint involvement. Typically the arthritis of parvovirus B19 will resolve spontaneously over a few weeks. Travel history is also an important element of the history; for example, Chikungunya and Dengue can present with arthritis symptoms. Rubella, both the illness and vaccine, can be associated. Bacterial infection such as endocarditis and Lyme disease can present with oligoarticular/polyarticular joint pain. Rheumatic fever is also in the differential and can present with migratory joint pain.

Inflammatory arthritis can be a manifestation of other systemic rheumatologic conditions including seronegative spondyloarthropathy (psoriatic arthritis, arthritis secondary to inflammatory bowel disease, reactive arthritis, and ankylosing spondylitis). The pattern of involvement can be helpful, as seronegative spondyloarthropathy frequently presents in an asymmetric, large joint predominant, and lower extremity predominant fashion. Inflammatory arthritis can develop secondary to connective tissue disease such as systemic lupus erythematosus and systemic sclerosis. ANCA-associated vasculitis can also present with arthritis. Paraneoplastic syndromes can present with joint pain including hypertrophic osteoarthropathy.

Treatment

The goals of treatment of RA are to address both the short term and long term complications of RA. The overarching principle is "treat to target." The goal of therapy should be to achieve clinical remission or low disease activity. The treatment approach must be individualized and consider the comorbidities of the patient. The significant cost of the medications must also be considered in therapy decisions.

Analgesics and Nonsteroidal Antiinflammatory Drugs

Analgesics and nonsteroidal antiinflammatory agents can be utilized to help address breakthrough pain. However, these agents should not be the foundation of treatment. Their role can be used to help control symptoms while a maintenance strategy with conventional disease-modifying antirheumatic drugs (DMARDs) and/or biologics is being established, as there is delay to the full clinical benefit of these medications. Since these medications do not alter the natural history of the disease, they should not be used in isolation.

In patients with extensive damage related to RA, these medications can have a role in helping address pain. DMARDs and biologics are unable to address pain related to damage.

Glucocorticoids

Glucocorticoids are frequently used due to their rapid onset of action, which distinguishes them from DMARDs and biologics. These are frequently utilized at initial diagnosis or with flares of established disease. However, the side effects of corticosteroids limit their use. Corticosteroids should not be utilized in isolation to treat RA. Corticosteroids can be given in multiple administration forms, including oral, intramuscular, and intraarticular. The choice of which to use is dependent on the individual patient's scenario.

Conventional Disease Modifying Antirheumatic Drugs

Conventional DMARDs are immunosuppressants with the goal of inducing and maintaining remission of patients with RA.

Methotrexate

Methotrexate (Otrexup, Rasuvo, Rheumatrex), in the absence of contraindications, is typically the first-line medication utilized for RA. The exact mechanism specifically for RA is incompletely understood. Methotrexate inhibits dihydrofolate reductase which results in reduction of DNA synthesis and, as a result, cell replication. However, this is not the role in isolation as daily folic acid[1] is prescribed to help counter the side effects and does not reverse the therapeutic benefit. Methotrexate also increases the release of adenosine which leads to reduction of inflammation.

Methotrexate can be given in both oral and subcutaneous administration forms. Typically, the starting dose is 10 to 15 mg weekly with titration depending on clinical response, up to 25 mg weekly. At higher doses, gastrointestinal absorption can be limited, and this can be a situation to prefer the subcutaneous form.

Common side effects can include oral ulcers, nausea, fatigue, increased infection risk, cytopenias, and hepatotoxicity. Methotrexate requires routine blood monitoring specifically for cytopenia and hepatotoxicity. The toxicity of methotrexate is increased in the setting of renal dysfunction, and in the setting of renal dysfunction there should be consideration of dose reduction versus choosing an alternative agent.

Methotrexate is a teratogen. The recommendation is to wait 3 months from stopping methotrexate before trying to conceive.

Hydroxychloroquine

Hydroxychloroquine (Plaquenil) has multiple mechanisms of action including inhibition of antigen presentation via interference of toll-like receptors and acidification of lysosomes.

It is an oral medication with the dose range of 200 to 400 mg daily. It is a weight-based regimen, and when using real body weight, the dose is 5 mg/kg with the maximum of 400 mg daily.

Side effects can include photosensitive rash, hypoglycemia, hearing loss, and retinal toxicity. Hydroxychloroquine can deposit in the retina which can ultimately lead to vision loss if not identified. Individuals are recommended to have routine eye examinations so changes related to hydroxychloroquine,

[1] Not FDA approved for this indication.

including bull's eye maculopathy, can be identified and hydroxychloroquine can then be discontinued if necessary. Eye comorbidities, such as macular degeneration, may complicate the ability to monitor for hydroxychloroquine toxicity and would need to be discussed with patient's eye provider.

Sulfasalazine

The exact mechanism of action of sulfasalazine (Azulfidine-EN) in RA is not currently well understood.

It is an oral medication that is utilized twice daily. The dose is typically started at 500 mg once or twice daily with titration of dose to 1000 to 1500 mg twice daily.

Side effects include rash, gastrointestinal side effects, cytopenias, and hepatoxicity. Laboratory monitoring is required to monitor for cytopenia and hepatotoxicity.

Leflunomide

Leflunomide (Arava) inhibits dihydroorotate dehydrogenase, which results in the reduction of pyrimidine synthesis and ultimately reduction of cellular replication.

It comes in an oral form. A loading dose is not required and frequently not used, as it can result in a side effect of diarrhea. Leflunomide has a very long half-life due to its entrance in the enterohepatocyte circulation.

Side effects include diarrhea, cytopenias, hepatoxicity, and increased infection risk. It requires routine laboratory monitoring for cytopenia and hepatotoxicity. It is contraindicated in pregnancy.

A cholestyramine (Questran)[1] washout procedure can be utilized to eliminate leflunomide when needed for a time sensitive scenario, such as a woman wanting to pursue pregnancy.

Azathioprine

Azathioprine (Imuran) is an inhibitor of purine synthesis and as a result of cellular replication.

It is an oral medication and the dosing is weight based. Azathioprine is typically started at 1 mg/kg/day and can be escalated up to a maximum of 2.5 mg/kg/day.

Side effects can include cytopenias, rash, nausea, diarrhea, and pancreatitis. Azathioprine requires routine monitoring for cytopenias and hepatotoxicity. A thiopurine methyltransferase (TPMT) level can be checked prior to initiation for assessment of the metabolism of azathioprine. If there are reduced levels of TPMT activity, then one would need to consider using a reduced dose or an alternative agent.

Azathioprine has been less commonly used as other agents have become available. Interstitial lung disease secondary to RA is one scenario in which it is still utilized.

Synthetic Disease Modifying Antirheumatic Drugs

Janus kinase (JAK) Inhibitors

Tofacitinib (Xeljanz), baricitinib (Olumiant), and upadacitinib (Rinvoq) are targeted small molecules that inhibit Janus kinases (JAKs). Inhibition blocks intracellular signaling of cytokine receptors and results in decreased gene activation.

Both are oral medications. Side effects can include cytopenia, hepatotoxicity, and cholesterol elevation. Routine lab monitoring is required to monitor for these complications. There are rare reports of bowel perforation, and currently there is a recommendation to avoid in the setting of diverticulitis.

Biologics

Biologics refer to the complex chemical structure of these medications. Biologics can be used in combination with conventional DMARDs.

TNF Inhibitors

TNF inhibitors inhibit the effect of TNF alpha, a proinflammatory cytokine. There are five different TNF inhibitors: etanercept (Enbrel), adalimumab (Humira), certolizumab (Cimzia), golimumab (Simponi), and infliximab (Remicade).

Etanercept has a component of the TNF receptor, allowing it to bind TNF alpha, and prevents it from binding to TNF receptors. The remaining are monoclonal antibodies targeting TNF alpha. Etanercept, adalimumab, certolizumab, and golimumab come in a subcutaneous form. Golimumab and infliximab are available as an infusion. Biosimilars, referencing their similar structure and as a result function but not identical their corresponding biologic, are now available for some of the TNF inhibitors (e.g., Inflectra [infliximab-dyyb] and Renflexis [infliximab-abda] are biosimilar to infliximab).

Side effects include injection site/infusion reactions. Patients must be counseled on infection risk to wide-ranging organisms, ranging from bacterial, viral, fungal, and mycobacterial. Individuals must undergo tuberculosis testing prior to initiation of therapies. There were initial concerns regarding lymphoma in the setting of TNF inhibitor use, but it is likely that the underlying RA drives the risk primarily. TNF inhibitors can be associated with exacerbations of congestive heart failure. Multiple sclerosis would be a contraindication to TNF inhibitors.

Interleukin 6 Receptor Inhibitor (Tocilizumab and Sarilumab)

Tocilizumab (Actemra) and sarilumab (Kevzara) are both interleukin 6 (IL6) receptor inhibitors, which prevents activation of the receptors of IL6. This prevents the downstream activation of targets of IL6, a proinflammatory cytokine.

Tocilizumab comes as both infusion and subcutaneous versions. Sarilumab comes as a subcutaneous version.

Side effects include cytopenia, particularly neutropenia and thrombocytopenia, hepatotoxicity, and elevated cholesterol. Routine monitoring is necessary. Injection site/infusion reactions are also a risk. The infection concerns are similar to TNF inhibitors, with the risk pertaining to diverse organisms. Due to rare reports of bowel perforations, it is recommended to be avoided in the setting of diverticulitis.

T Cell Coactivation Inhibition

Abatacept (Orencia) prevents T cell coactivation by binding the costimulating signal (CD80/86) on antigen presenting cells and preventing it from binding T cells. Administration forms include subcutaneous injection and intravenous infusions. Side effects include injection/infusion site reactions. Infection risk is also a concern with abatacept. Higher rates of chronic obstructive pulmonary disease (COPD) exacerbations have been described with patients on abatacept.

B Cell Inhibition

Rituximab (Rituxan) depletes B cells by targeting CD20, which is present on B cells.

It is an intravenous medication. The timing of subsequent doses is typically 6 months.

The risks of rituximab include infusion reactions. Infection risk is a concern with rituximab, particularly considering the long timeframe of effect. Careful attention must be given to prevent hepatitis B reactivation. Even in patients with evidence of natural immunity via cleared infection, they would be a candidate for hepatitis B reactivation prophylaxis. Progressive multifocal leukoencephalopathy (PML) related to JC virus has been reported in patients receiving rituximab for the indication of RA. The risk is very low, and in multiple reports, patients were also on additional immunosuppressants such as chemotherapy.

Interleukin 1 Inhibition

Anakinra (Kineret) is an inhibitor of the IL1 receptor preventing the downstream activation of IL1, a proinflammatory cytokine. Risks are similar to other biologics in terms of infection, injection site reaction, cytopenia, and nausea. It is a daily subcutaneous injection.

Combination Therapy

Combination therapy is frequently utilized for treatment of RA. An indication to proceed with combination therapy is when disease activity is persistent despite therapeutic dosing with a single agent. A frequently used combination therapy is termed "triple therapy." This refers to the combination of methotrexate, sulfasalazine, and hydroxychloroquine. A single biologic can be utilized in combination with conventional DMARDs, most frequently methotrexate. Two biologics are not recommended to be utilized together, due to concern with increased infection risk.

Choice of Therapy

Multiple factors must be weighed in terms of the choice of therapy for RA. If there are no contraindications, methotrexate is typically used as the first choice. If there is an insufficient response to a maximized dose of methotrexate, including use of subcutaneous methotrexate, then combination therapy is frequently utilized. If methotrexate is unable to be tolerated, then leflunomide could be considered in its place. The combination therapy to be utilized with methotrexate could include triple therapy versus methotrexate in combination with a biologic or synthetic DMARD (JAK inhibitors). Triple therapy has been compared with methotrexate plus biologic therapy in multiple studies and overall thought to be equivalent in terms of achieving clinical response. The choice between the two is dependent on discussion with the patient. Consideration for the forms of administration would need to be taken into account. Comorbidities of the patient can restrict choices. Another consideration is cost and insurance coverage for different medications. Currently, there is not available testing to inform choice of therapy in a personalized manner beyond consideration of comorbidities.

When patients have consistently achieved clinical remission, there can be consideration for reduction in treatment. There is increased risk of flare of disease when reducing medications. Patients would need to be counseled regarding this risk and monitored closely.

Special Scenarios
Pregnancy

As RA can affect women of childbearing age, understanding the goals in terms of pregnancy and breastfeeding must be understood for patients with RA. Methotrexate and leflunomide would be contraindicated in the setting of pregnancy. Methotrexate is associated with known congenital abnormalities. The recommendation would be to stop methotrexate 3 months prior to contraception. Leflunomide has a much longer half-life and the level could be checked and, if elevated, then could use cholestyramine washout. If there is a possibility of pregnancy, then hydroxychloroquine or sulfasalazine are frequently used options in this setting. TNF inhibitors have been utilized in pregnancy. The recommendations would be to stop TNF inhibitors over the course of pregnancy with the specific TNF inhibitors having different recommendations; certolizumab is not felt to cross the placenta due to its chemical structure, and in some individuals, this is continued throughout the pregnancy. Less information is available about the safety of other biologics in pregnancy and, if possible, would be avoided until further information is known.

Patients frequently have improvement in their clinical symptoms during pregnancy, which emphasizes the importance of an individualized approach during pregnancy. Patients should be counseled on the risk for flare in the postpartum setting.

Breastfeeding

Data is limited regarding the effects of medications for RA and breastfeeding. The potential benefits of breastfeeding would need to be weighed with potential risk. Methotrexate and leflunomide are avoided during breastfeeding. An individualized approach is necessary in conjunction with the patient and obstetrician.

Malignancy

Data is limited regarding the ideal choice of therapy in the setting of a history of malignancy. DMARDs are frequently preferred over biologics in the setting of prior malignancy. Specifically in the setting of lymphoproliferative disorders, if a biologic is indicated due to disease activity, rituximab is preferred over other biologic choices. Individualized decisions must be made in conjunction with the patient and their hematologist/oncologist.

Preoperative Management

Due to the risk of atlantoaxial instability in RA, particularly in long-standing disease, patients prior to surgery should be screened for this complication. Cervical spine x-rays with flexion and extension views would be recommended. The results should be reviewed with an anesthesiologist to assist with planning for positioning during surgery.

Management of immunosuppressant medications must be reviewed with the surgeon and take into account the nature of surgery as well as the pharmacokinetics of the immunosuppressants. Data are limited on the ideal management of immunosuppressants in this setting. Guidelines have been published in the setting of total hip and knee arthroplasty.

Monitoring

There are two components of monitoring for patients with RA. The first is to assess for disease activity both from the standpoint of the joints as well as extraarticular manifestations. From the joint perspective, there are multiple disease activity scores that can be utilized. Some rely solely on patient reported outcomes. Others are a combination of patient reported outcomes, exam findings, and provider global assessment. Swollen joint counts and tender joint counts are frequently utilized. Specifically for laboratory monitoring of disease activity, ESR and CRP can be utilized but do not trend with disease activity in all patients. ACPA and RF do not trend with disease activity and thus the values do not need to be repeated if positive.

Separately, drug toxicity must be assessed including clinical symptoms and laboratory monitoring. In addition, monitoring for development of infection is also necessary.

Management of Complications

If drug toxicity develops, depending on the nature of toxicity, the medication dose should either be reduced or discontinued. If the side effect likely reflects a class effect, consider an agent in a different drug class. If infection occurs while on immunosuppressant therapy, these medications should be held at least until the infection has resolved. Restarting would be dependent on the clinical scenario, including the nature of the infection and the specific treatment for RA.

References

Aletaha D, Neogi T, Silman AJ, et al: 2010 Rheumatoid Arthritis Classification Criteria: an American College of Rheumatology/European League Against Rheumatism Collaborative Initiative, *Arthritis Rheum* 62:2569–2581, 2010.

Aletaha D, Smolen JS: Diagnosis and management of rheumatoid arthritis: a review, *JAMA* 320:1360–1372, 2018.

Anderson J, Caplan L, Yazdany J, et al: Rheumatoid arthritis disease activity measures: American College of Rheumatology recommendations for use in clinical practice, *Arthritis Care Res (Hoboken)* 64:640–647, 2012.

Goodman SM, Springer B, Guyatt G, et al: 2017 American College of Rheumatology/American Association of Hip and Knee Surgeons guideline for the perioperative management of antirheumatic medication in patients with rheumatic diseases undergoing elective total hip or total knee arthroplasty, *Arthritis Care Res* 69:1111–1124, 2017.

Hochberg M: *Rheumatology*, Seventh edition, Philadelphia, PA, 2019, Elsevier.

Singh JA, Saag KG, Bridges Jr SL, et al: 2015 American College of Rheumatology guidelines for the treatment of rheumatoid arthritis, *Arthritis Care Res (Hoboken)* 68:1–25, 2016.

Smolen JS, Landewe R, Bijlsma J, et al: EULAR recommendations for the management of rheumatoid arthritis with synthetic and biologic disease-modifying antirheumatic drugs: 2016 update, *Ann Rheum Dis* 76:960–977, 2017.

13 Sexually Transmitted Diseases

CHLAMYDIA TRACHOMATIS

Method of
Tracy L. Williams, MD

CURRENT DIAGNOSIS

- Screen all sexually active woman 25 years of age or younger for *C. trachomatis* annually regardless of symptoms per the CDC recommendations.
- Symptomatic patients should be tested regardless of gender.
- Reinfection with *C. trachomatis* is common.
  - Retest all patients who have a history of *C. trachomatis* or *N. gonorrhea* at 3 to 6 months following treatment, regardless of whether their partner(s) were treated.
  - If the patient does not follow up at 3 to 6 months, then retest upon presentation for medical care within the first 12 months posttreatment.
- Patients who screen positive for *C. trachomatis* need to be screened for gonorrhea, syphilis, and HIV.
- Perform test of cure on pregnant patients at 3 to 4 weeks posttreatment and repeat in 3 to 6 months, preferably in the third trimester if the pregnant woman was diagnosed during the first trimester.
- Rescreen pregnant patients for other sexually transmitted infections (STIs) 3 months posttreatment including gonorrhea, syphilis, and HIV.

CURRENT THERAPY

- Azithromycin (Zithromycin) 1 g orally in a single dose or doxycycline (Vibramycin) 100 mg orally twice a day for 7 days are the recommended regimens for nonpregnant patients and for presumptive treatment for *C. trachomatis*.
- All of the patient's recent sexual partners need referral and treatment.
  - The patient's last sexual contact should be referred and treated if it has been more than 60 days since the patient had a sexual partner.
  - The partner needs to be treated for *C. trachomatis* even if his or her personal STI results are negative.
- Counsel patients and their partners to abstain from sexual contact until 7 days after one-dose therapy or after the final dose of the 7-day regimen.
- The CDC recommends that patients who test positive for gonorrhea should also receive presumptive treatment for *C. trachomatis* because coinfection is common.

Epidemiology
Chlamydia trachomatis is the most common notifiable sexually transmitted infection (STI) in the United States, with an incidence of over 1.5 million cases per year according to the Centers for Disease Control and Prevention (CDC) in 2015. Women age 15 to 19 years are the most commonly affected, followed by women age 20 to 24. The incidence of *C. trachomatis* has steadily climbed yearly since it became a federally mandated notifiable disease; part of this is an artifact of improved screening practices that are discovering disease in asymptomatic patients.

C. trachomatis costs an estimated $2.4 billon annually. Cost-benefit analyses have consistently shown prioritizing screening efforts in asymptomatic women to be cost-effective.

Risk Factors
The risk of contracting *C. trachomatis* increases with: multiple sexual partners; unprotected sex including vaginal, oral, and anal intercourse; anal-receptive intercourse; and men having sex with men. The risk increases in the presence of other coinfections including human immunodeficiency virus (HIV) or herpes simplex virus (HSV). African Americans have a fourfold higher incidence compared to their white counterparts (13% versus 2.4%, respectively).

Pathophysiology
Chlamydia trachomatis is an obligate intracellular parasite. It is found only in human cells, but can live on fomites for up to 30 hours. Previous infections do not yield protection against future infections with *C. trachomatis*. *C. trachomatis* does not infect the squamous epithelium of the vaginal vault, but can infect the urethra, the squamocolumnar junction of the cervix, the rectal mucosa, and the oropharynx.

Prevention
Prevention depends on screening of asymptomatic patients, who make up a large portion of the infected population. The United States Preventive Task Force (USPSTF) recommends annual screening of all sexually active women younger than 25 years of age and for older women at increased risk. The United States Preventive Services Task Force (USPSTF) has similar recommendations but uses age 24 years and younger.

The CDC and the USPSTF found insufficient evidence to recommend routine screening of men based on cost-effectiveness, efficacy, and practicality, but screening of symptomatic men or men in areas with high prevalence of *Chlamydia*, including men having sex with men, men in correctional facilities, and men visiting STI clinics, is recommended. Overall, screening of men is recommended so long as it does not detract resources from the screening of women. Symptomatic patients should be tested regardless of gender.

Men who have sex with other men are at high risk for bacterial and viral STI. The CDC STI screening recommendation in this group is an annual test for urethral infection with *C. trachomatis* and *N. gonorrhea*. The preferred methodology is testing the urine using nucleic acid amplification technique (NAAT). Men who have receptive anal intercourse are recommended to have annual anal screening for both *C. trachomatis* and *N. gonorrhea*. Men who have oral receptive sex are also advised to have pharyngeal screening for *N. gonorrhea* but not *C. trachomatis*. The NAAT is only Food and Drug Administration (FDA)–approved on urine in the above scenarios but is used off-label in laboratories that have met all regulatory requirements.

Patients who screen positive for *Chlamydia* need to be screened for other STIs, including gonorrhea, syphilis, and HIV.

953

Abstinence and monogamous relationships are ideal to help prevent the transmission of *C. trachomatis*. Safer sex practices to limit the spread of *C. trachomatis* include the consistent use of condoms. Epidemiologic studies show that people often base their decision to use condoms on their perception of their partner's risk. Given the high prevalence of asymptomatic *C. trachomatis* infections in certain American populations, selective condom use is not an effective strategy.

Clinical Manifestations

Most infections are asymptomatic. However, some women will report vaginal discharge, postcoital or intermenstrual bleeding, or lower abdominal pain. Men are more commonly symptomatic than women and may report dysuria or urethral discharge.

Untreated *C. trachomatis* in women has significant health sequelae. Approximately 40% of women with untreated *Chlamydia* go on to develop pelvic inflammatory disease (PID). Women with PID may become infertile (20%), develop debilitating chronic pelvic pain (18%), or suffer ectopic pregnancy (9%).

Men do not tend to suffer as severe sequelae from *C. trachomatis*. The most common illness is urethritis, but men may also suffer epididymitis, proctitis, and conjunctivitis. Reactive arthritis is also more common in men.

Diagnosis

Tests used for detection of *C. trachomatis* can be divided into molecular (NAAT, DNA probing, and hybrid capture), antigen detection (direct immunofluorescence and enzyme immunoassay), and cell culture.

The most reliable method of testing for *C. trachomatis* is NAAT. It is FDA-approved for use on vaginal/endocervical secretions, male intraurethral swabs, and first-catch urine. It is not FDA-approved for rectal or orophyngeal use but is used off label in laboratories as described above. The primary benefit of NAAT is the lack of a need for viable organisms to induce a positive test result; this increases its sensitivity to more than 95% because of the ability to detect *C. trachomatis* even if only one copy of the targeted RNA or DNA is present. Its specificity is also desirable at 99%.

C. trachomatis cell culture is used as the reference standard for all testing but has many limitations, including expense, long turnaround time (72 hours), and transport and specimen storage requirements. Its sensitivity is 80% to 85%. It is not readily available.

Limiting barriers to screening is important. If testing in the clinic is difficult to arrange, self-collected vaginal swab specimens perform at least as well as other approved specimens using NAAT. First-catch urine NAAT testing is also more acceptable to many patients, particularly asymptomatic men and women who do not otherwise need a pelvic examination.

Differential Diagnosis

Infection with *Chlamydia* is often asymptomatic but is included in the differential diagnosis of various organ system complaints. It should be ruled out in any sexually active patient presenting with urethritis, mucopurulent cervicitis, epididymitis, and proctitis. There is significant overlap in the symptoms caused by *C. trachomatis* with *N. gonorrhea*, so testing for both bacteria with NAAT is preferred. Other agents that are included in the differential diagnosis after *C. trachomatis* and *N. gonorrhea* have been ruled out include: *Trichomonas vaginalis*, HSV, adenovirus, *Mycoplasma* species, and *Ureaplasma*. More specifically, persistent urethritis after treatment with doxycycline (Vibramycin) can be caused by infection with *T. vaginalis* or doxycycline-resistant *Urea urealyticum* or *Mycoplasma genitalium*.

C. trachomatis should be ruled out in newborn infants with conjunctivitis in the first 30 days of life or pneumonia at 1 to 3 months of life, especially if they were born to mothers with untreated chlamydial infections.

Treatment

Recommendations for treatment regimens are summarized in Box 1. The benefit of using single-dose azithromycin (Zithromycin) is the ability to directly observe the patient taking the therapy. The 7-day

---

BOX 1   *Chlamydia trachomatis*: Recommended Treatment Regimens by Clinical Syndrome

Cervicitis or urethritis or for presumptive treatment in nonpregnant patient*
- Azithromycin (Zithromycin) 1 g orally in a single dose
or
- Doxycycline (Vibramycin) 100 mg orally twice a day for 7 days
Alternative regimens (one of the following)
- Erythromycin base (E-Mycin) 500 mg orally four times a day for 7 days
or
- Erythromycin ethylsuccinate (EES) 800 mg orally four times a day for 7 days
or
- Levofloxacin (Levaquin)[1] 500 mg orally once daily for 7 days
or
- Ofloxacin (Floxin) 300 mg orally twice a day for 7 days
Pregnant patient with cervicitis or urethritis*
- Azithromycin 1 g orally in a single dose
or
- Amoxicillin 500 mg orally three times a day for 7 days
Alternative regimens
- Erythromycin base 500 mg orally four times a day for 7 days
or
- Erythromycin base[†] 250 mg orally four times a day for 14 days
or

- Erythromycin ethylsuccinate 800 mg orally four times a day for 7 days
or
- Erythromycin ethylsuccinate[†] 400 mg orally four times a day for 14 days
Epididymitis
- Ceftriaxone (Rocephin) 250 mg IM in a single dose
plus
- Doxycycline 100 mg orally twice a day for 10 days
Ophthalmia neonatorum or C. trachomatis pneumonia
- Erythromycin base or ethylsuccinate 50 mg/kg/day orally divided into 4 doses daily for 14 days[‡]
Recommended regimen for children who weigh <45 kg
- Erythromycin base or ethylsuccinate 50 mg/kg/day orally divided into 4 doses daily for 14 days
Recommended regimen for children who weigh ≥45 kg but who are <8 years old
- Azithromycin 1 g orally in a single dose
Recommended regimens for children aged ≥8 years
- Azithromycin 1 gram orally in a single dose
or
- Doxycycline 100 mg orally twice a day for 7 days
Inpatient and outpatient PID
- Please refer to PID chapter for treatment regimens

Providers should consult the Centers for Disease Control and Prevention's website at http://cdc.gov/std/treatment for up-to-date treatment recommendations.
[1]Not FDA approved for this indication.
*Consider concurrent treatment for gonococcal infection if prevalence of gonorrhea is high in the patient population under assessment.
[†]The lower-dose and longer-treatment option with erythromycin can be considered if gastrointestinal tolerance is an issue.
[‡]Infants <6 weeks of age who are treated with erythromycin should be followed for signs and symptoms of infantile hypertrophic pyloric stenosis.

course of doxycycline (Vibramycin) has comparable cure rates to azithromycin, but decreased compliance.

Presumptive treatment for *C. trachomatis* should be considered for high-risk patients with cervicitis. High-risk patients include women up to 25 years old, those with new or multiple sexual partners, those who engage in unprotected sex, especially if follow-up cannot be ensured, and those for whom a relatively insensitive diagnostic test is used in place of NAAT.

The CDC also recommends presumptive treatment for patients being treated for *N. gonorrhea*. Coinfection is common, as illustrated in a study that found 20% of men with *N. gonorrhea* and 42% of women with *N. gonorrhea* were also infected with *C. trachomatis*. Cotreatment is also recommended in the hope that it will impede the development of antimicrobial-resistant *N. gonorrhea*.

Chlamydia trachomatis is a reportable infectious disease. The patient is instructed to refer all of his or her sexual partners for testing and treatment if they have had sexual contact during the previous 60 days. If the patient has not been sexually active for the last 60 days, then the patient is to refer his or her most recent sexual contact. The patient's recent sexual partners should be treated empirically even if their personal STI evaluation returns negative results. The patient and his or her sexual partners should be counseled to abstain from sexual activity for 7 days post treatment. Reinfection, rather than recurrence, is the more common etiology of repeat *C. trachomatis* infection.

Expedited partner therapy is an option in certain cases. This entails the patient delivering the antibiotic to his or her partner(s) without a physician first seeing the patient. Patients are to give their partners written materials on the importance of following up with a physician if any signs of complications occur (e.g., pelvic pain in women or testicular pain in men). It can be used effectively in certain situations but is not routinely recommended in men who have sex with men because of the high risk for coexisting infections, especially undiagnosed HIV infection, in their partners. Please refer to the CDC website (www.cdc.gov/std/ept) to check on legality in individual states. In general, utilizing the traditional patient-physician model is preferred.

Infants born to women with untreated *C. trachomatis* infection are at increased risk for vertical transmission. Prophylactic treatment with oral erythromycin (E-Mycin) for *C. trachomatis* is not recommended. The state-mandated standard erythromycin eye ointment (Ilotycin) that all newborns receive is still indicated. Overall, infants born to infected mothers need to be closely monitored for any signs and symptoms of infection and treated appropriately.

Intrauterine devices (IUDs) have regained popularity in the United States after they were implicated in causing PID in the 1970s. The IUD has evolved and now the risk of PID appears increased only in the first three weeks postinsertion. If *C. trachomatis* or PID is contracted with an IUD in place, practitioners must decide if the IUD should be removed. Research has found insufficient evidence to mandate removal, but close follow-up is mandatory.

Monitoring
Repeat testing is recommended for all patients treated for *C. trachomatis* at 3 to 6 months regardless of the treatment status of the patient's partner(s) because reinfection is so common. If the patient does not follow up at 3 to 6 months, he or she should be retested upon presentation for medical care within the first 12 months posttreatment.

Test of cure, which is testing at 3 to 4 weeks posttreatment, is recommended only for pregnant patients. Testing for cure earlier than 3 to 4 weeks increases the rate of false positive results. If the initial diagnosis was in the first trimester of pregnancy, testing should be repeated in 3 to 6 months, preferably in the third trimester. Rescreening for other STIs should be performed upon retesting for *Chlamydia*.

Complications
C. trachomatis is a major public health concern because it results in serious health complications and sequelae. In women it can cause PID, endometritis, ectopic pregnancy, infertility, salpingitis, and perihepatitis (Fitz-Hugh-Curtis syndrome). In men it is associated with postgonococcal or nongonococcal urethritis and epididymitis. Reactive arthritis can occur in both men and women.

C. trachomatis is especially problematic in pregnancy because it is associated with an increased risk of preterm labor and preterm premature rupture of membranes. Infants born to women infected with *Chlamydia* risk suffering pneumonia and conjunctivitis.

C. trachomatis pneumonia can present as an afebrile pneumonia often with a staccato cough without wheezing between 1 and 3 months of life. *C. trachomatis* conjunctivitis, also known as ophthalmia neonatorum, is uncommon in the United States, but worldwide it is the number one cause of blindness. It usually presents within the 5th and 12th day of life but can present at up to 1 month of age. State-mandated prophylactic eye ointment given to babies at birth mainly helps prevent gonococcal ophthalmia; it does not prevent perinatal transmission of *Chlamydia* from mother to infant. Therefore the screening of pregnant women and ultimate treatment of their *Chlamydia* during pregnancy is the best method of preventing complications in newborn infants.

References
Bebear C, de Barbeyrac B: Genital *Chlamydia trachomatis* infections, *Clin Microbiol Infect* 15:4–10, 2009.
Blas MM, Canchihuaman FA, Alva IE, et al: Pregnancy outcomes in women infected with *Chlamydia trachomatis*: a population-based cohort study in Washington State, *Sex Transm Infect* 83:314–318, 2007.
Centers for Disease Control and Prevention (CDC). Sexually Transmitted Disease Surveillance 2015. Available at: http://www.cdc.gov/std/stats15 [accessed February 7, 2017].
Centers for Disease Control and Prevention (CDC). Sexually transmitted diseases treatment guidelines 2015. MMWR Recomm Rep 2015;64(No. 3):[55–60].
Honey E, Augood C, Templeton A, et al: Cost effectiveness of screening for *Chlamydia trachomatis*: a review of published studies, *Sex Transm Infect* 78:406–412, 2002.
Johnson RE, Newhall WJ, Papp JR, et al: Screening tests to detect *Chlamydia trachomatis* and *Neisseria gonorrhoeae* infections—2002, *MMWR Recomm Rep* 51(RR-15):1–38, 2002.
Kramer A, Schewebke I, Kampf G: How long do nosocomial pathogens persist on inanimate surfaces? A systematic review, *BMC Infect Dis* 6:130, 2006.
LeFevre ML: U.S. Preventive Services Task Force. Screening for chlamydia and gonorrhea: U.S. Preventive Services Task Force recommendation statement, *Ann Intern Med.* 161(12):902–910, 2014.
Lyss SB, Kamb ML, Peterman TA, et al: *Chlamydia trachomatis* among patients infected with and treated for *Neisseria gonorrhoeae* in sexually transmitted clinics in the United States, *Ann Intern Med* 139:178–185, 2003.

CONDYLOMATA ACUMINATA

Method of
M. Chantel Long, MD

CURRENT DIAGNOSIS

- Condylomata acuminata are usually flesh-colored, brown, or gray and can be flat, plaquelike, or exophytic papules, giving them the classic "cauliflower" appearance.
- The lesions may be single or multiple and can range in size from minute to several centimeters in diameter.
- When the appearance of the lesion is typical, confirmatory tests are usually unnecessary.
- Suspicious lesions or uncertain diagnoses warrant biopsy to rule out malignancy.

CURRENT THERAPY

- In the absence of dysplasia, treatment of subclinical human papilloma virus infection is not recommended.

- The goal of therapy is to eliminate symptoms, namely clinically apparent warts, rather than address the underlying HPV infection.
- Common treatment options include podofilox (Condylox), imiquimod (Aldara, Zyclara), sinecatechins (Veregen), podophyllin resin (Podocon-25), trichloroacetic acid (Tri-Chlor), cryotherapy, and surgery.

Epidemiology

Condylomata acuminata, commonly known as genital warts, is a sexually transmitted disease caused by the human papilloma virus (HPV). It is estimated that 20 million people are infected with HPV in the United States, with the highest prevalence in adolescents and young adults. Lifetime incidence of HPV infection is greater than 50% and appears to be increasing, making it the most common sexually transmitted disease.

Risk Factors

Risk factors associated with HPV infection include sex with an infected partner, early age at first sexual intercourse, multiple sexual partners, history of sexually transmitted infections, cigarette smoking, and lack of condom use. The majority of patients whose sexual partner has condyloma will themselves develop condyloma within 3 months. An even larger percentage of people are believed to develop subclinical infection.

Pathophysiology

About 90% of warts are caused by HPV types 6 and 11; condyloma can be coinfected with types 16, 18, 31, 33, 35, and 45, which have oncogenic potential. Genital skin appears to be less susceptible to the oncogenic potential of HPV compared to the transformation zones of the cervix and anal canal.

The virus is easily transmitted via sexual contact. Vertical transmission and autoinoculation are possible. The average incubation period between infection and appearance of condyloma ranges from 3 months to several years. Condyloma can persist or recur after therapy, undergo malignant transformation, or spontaneously regress.

Prevention

Prevention options include HPV vaccination, abstinence, routine condom use, and limiting sexual partners. Once patients have condyloma, they should be encouraged to use condoms consistently. Educate patients that condoms can decrease transmission but might not completely prevent infection.

Two HPV vaccine series are currently available in the United States. Gardasil is a quadrivalent HPV vaccine indicated for male and female patients aged 9 to 25 years for prevention of cervical cancer and genital warts. Cervarix is the bivalent vaccine indicated for female patients aged 9 to 25 years for prevention of cervical cancer.

Clinical Manifestations

Most genital warts are asymptomatic on presentation, although patients can present with complaints of a "bump." Localized irritation, pruritus, pain, or bleeding can occur, and symptoms may vary based on the location and size of the lesions. Usually, the warts appear flesh-colored, brown, or gray and can be flat, plaquelike, or exophytic papules, giving them the classic "cauliflower" appearance. The lesions may be single or multiple and range in size from minute to several centimeters in diameter. Flat HPV lesions might not be grossly visible.

The majority of HPV infections are either subclinical or unrecognized. Clinically apparent disease might represent only a small portion of the actual infected area.

Diagnosis

When the clinical appearance of the lesion is typical, confirmatory tests are usually unnecessary. The entire anogenital tract should be examined because of the widespread nature of HPV. A magnifying glass and anoscopy may be helpful for thorough detection and examination. Application of dilute 3% to 5% acetic acid solution to the skin surface can help detect subtle HPV lesions by producing an acetowhitening of the condyloma; however, this is not a specific test and is not routinely recommended. Pap smears or tissue biopsy can provide histopathologic confirmation of the diagnosis. Biopsy is recommended to rule out malignancy in any suspicious lesions, such as large or rapidly growing condyloma; pigmented, atypical, friable, bleeding, or ulcerated lesions; sites of previous treatment failure; areas of recurrence; acetowhite lesions; or lesions in immunocompromised patients. Although costly and not recommended, HPV identification via DNA testing can be performed.

Differential Diagnosis

Table 1 outlines the differential diagnosis for condylomata acuminata.

Treatment

In the absence of dysplasia, the Centers for Disease Control and Prevention recommends no treatment of subclinical HPV infection. The goal of treatment is to eliminate symptoms, namely clinically apparent warts, rather than address the underlying HPV infection. Current treatments do not eradicate the virus.

Ideally, treatment of condyloma should continue until all warts are gone. A repeated course of therapy is often required to achieve a wart-free state. Recurrence may be due to latent HPV in the surrounding normal tissue, HPV reinfection, or improper selection or use of a therapy modality. Nearly all treatment regimens have similar efficacy and rates of intolerance and toxicity. All are known to cause local pain and irritation. Any given treatment has a 40% to 80% rate of wart clearance and up to a 50% recurrence rate. It is unknown whether eliminating warts will decrease infectivity of current or future sexual partners.

The factors to consider when deciding on treatment include location and size of the warts, the patient's tolerance and preference, cost, convenience, and the clinician's preference. Patient-applied options allow the patient greater control; however, this requires good compliance, and the warts must be accessible by the patient or caregiver. Provider-applied treatments are good choices for large treatment areas. Data regarding the efficacy of using more than one modality at a time are lacking. It is common practice for health care providers to combine treatment modalities. Table 2 outlines current

TABLE 1 Differential Diagnosis	
LESION	**APPEARANCE**
Verruca vulgaris	Occurs anywhere Tends to be thicker, drier, and hyperkeratotic
Molluscum contagiosum	Occurs anywhere Smooth, round papules with central umbilication
Seborrheic keratoses	Occurs anywhere Multiple waxy, rough, hyperpigmented papules
Condyloma latum	Moist, rounded, white papules of syphilis
Pearly penile papules	Smooth, uniform, small, 1–2 mm at corona, benign
Vestibular papillae	Both sides of vulva, female equivalent of pearly penile papules
Lichen planus	Purplish, pruritic rash or flat-topped polygonal papules
Nonpigmented nevi	Occurs anywhere Flat or raised, reddish or flesh colored

TABLE 2	Treatment Regimens				
DRUG	**USE ON**	**ADVANTAGES**	**DISADVANTAGES**	**INSTRUCTIONS**	
Patient Applied					
Podofilox 0.5% gel or solution (Condylox)	Moist warts	Relatively inexpensive	Avoid in pregnancy Avoid on mucous membranes Do not exceed 10 cm² area Do not exceed 0.5 mL daily; can have systemic side effects	Apply bid × 3 d, then 4 d off Repeat weekly May use for 4–6 cycles	
Imiquimod 5% cream (Aldara)	Dry or moist warts		Avoid with large warts >10 cm² Requires compliance Hypo- or hyperpigmentation of treated skin can occur	Apply nightly on dry warts Apply every other night on moist warts Use up to 16 wk Wash off after 6–10 h	
Sinecatechins 15% ointment (Veregen)	Dry warts		Avoid in pregnancy Avoid in immunocompromised patients	Apply tid Use up to 16 wk Do not wash off	
Provider Applied					
Podophyllin resin (Podocon-25, Podofilm)	Moist warts	Use on large warts May use on urethral meatus	Avoid in pregnancy Do not exceed 10 cm² area Do not exceed 0.5 mL daily; can have systemic side effects	Apply thin layer with cotton tip Allow to air dry Repeat weekly Leave on for 4 h Do not cover May leave on overnight if tolerated	
Trichloroacetic acid (TCA) (Tri-Chlor 80%)	Small, few Moist warts	May use on vagina, cervix May use on anal warts May use in pregnancy	Avoid with dry and large warts	Apply sparingly with cotton tip Air dry Repeat weekly to every other week Do not allow to "run" on normal skin Neutralize with soap or sodium bicarbonate	
Cryotherapy	Small, few, flat Dry or moist	May use in pregnancy May use liquid nitrogen in vagina, meatus, anus	Avoid with large warts Avoid cryoprobe use in vagina or anus	Freeze q1–2 wk Freeze 1–2 mm border May offer/need local anesthesia	
Surgery	Small or large Dry or moist	May use on anal warts Use on large warts and large treatment areas	Avoid in patients with bleeding disorder	Scissors, shave biopsy, punch excision, curettage, cautery, laser	
Interferon-α-2b injections (Intron A)	Refractory warts		Expensive Flulike side effects	Multiple intralesional injections Several times a week Often requires specialty referral	
Laser vaporization	Refractory warts	May use on intraurethral and large warts as well as large treatment areas	Expensive	Requires specialty referral	

therapy regimens. Topical fluorouracil (Efudex)[1] is no longer recommended. Failure to respond after four treatments or failure to clear within 3 months warrants a change in therapy modality and possible reevaluation of the diagnosis.

Advise patients to abstain from sexual activity while undergoing treatment for genital warts.

Monitoring

Counseling of patients regarding prevention and recognition of condyloma as well as screening and treatment of sexual partners should be part of the comprehensive management plan. One should consider testing for other sexually transmitted diseases because they often coexist with HPV. Encourage patients to discuss their HPV diagnosis with sexual partners. Asymptomatic partners likely harbor a subclinical infection, and examination for genital warts is appropriate if lesions are suspected. Discuss the need for smoking cessation and regular physician examinations, including Pap smears, as ways to prevent early HPV-related neoplasm.

Complications

Anogenital HPV infection with high-risk genotypes is associated with squamous cell carcinoma of the cervix, vagina, vulva, penis, and anus. Persistent HPV infection is the most important risk factor for development of cervical intraepithelial neoplasia and cancer.

[1] Not FDA approved for this indication.

References

American Academy of Pediatrics. Human papillomavirus. In: Pickering LK, Baker CJ, Kimberlin DW, Long SS, editors. Red Book: 2009 Report of the Committee on Infectious Diseases. 28th ed. Elk Grove Village, IL: American Academy of Pediatrics; 2009. p. 477–483.

Centers for Disease Control and Prevention: *Epidemiology and Prevention of Vaccine-Preventable Diseases. The Pink Book*, ed 12, Washington, DC, 2011, Public Health Foundation.

Centers for Disease Control and Prevention: 2010 Sexually transmitted diseases treatment guidelines, *MMWR* 59:1–5, 2010. 69–78.

Centers for Disease Control and Prevention. Human papillomavirus: HPV information for clinicians. Available at www.cdc.gov/std/hpv/Provider6-2005/ApF1-DesignA.pdf [accessed August 6, 2015].

Gilbert SM, Lambert SM, Weiner D: Extensive condylomata acuminata of the penis: Medical and surgical management, *Infect Urol* 16:65–76, 2003.

Kodner CM, Nasrat S: Management of genital warts, *Am Fam Physician* 70:2335–2342, 2004.

Figure 1 Chancroid. This photo shows an early chancroid ulcer on the penis along with accompanying regional inguinal adenopathy. (Courtesy of Dr. Pirozzi, Centers for Disease Control and Prevention.)

GENITAL ULCER DISEASE: CHANCROID, GRANULOMA INGUINALE, AND LYMPHOGRANULOMA

Method of,
Todd Stephens, MD

Chancroid, granuloma inguinale, and lymphogranuloma venereum (LGV) are important genital ulcer diseases that should be included in the differential diagnosis of patients presenting with anal or genital ulcers with or without inguinal adenopathy. Syphilis and herpes simplex virus testing should be considered on all such patients because of similarities in clinical presentation. Testing or treatment for other potential sexually transmitted infections (STIs), including HIV, should be considered given the high risk for concomitant infection.

Chancroid

History

Chancroid, also called soft sore, was first distinguished from the hard chancre of syphilis by Ricord in 1838. Ducrey, in Naples, demonstrated that inoculation of material from the chancroid ulcer into the skin of the forearm could reproduce the ulcer, and he went on to identify the causative organism, which bears his name.

Epidemiology

Chancroid is an important cause of genital ulceration in most countries of the developing world, accounting for about 10 million cases annually. Chancroid was diagnosed in 60% of patients who had genital ulcers and who presented to STI clinics in Africa before the HIV epidemic. Now, herpes simplex lesions represent a higher percentage. The prevalence of this disease is highest among commercial sex workers, and the presence of chancroid lesions significantly increases the risk of transmission of HIV. Although generally rare in industrialized countries, there have been several well-documented outbreaks in urban centers of North America, particularly among men who have sex with men.

Etiology

Chancroid is caused by *Haemophilus ducreyi*, a small anaerobic Gram-negative bacillus that forms streptobacillary chains on Gram stain and grows only on enriched media.

Clinical Features

After an incubation of 3 to 7 days, a papule appears that soon ulcerates, leaving a soft ulcer with an undermined edge and a purulent base. Vesicles are not seen. About half of patients develop unilateral inguinal adenopathy (Figure 1). Both the adenopathy and the lesions are very painful. Lesions can be single or multiple, and atypical presentations occur. Kissing lesions often occur on adjacent cutaneous surfaces. Not infrequently, a giant ulcer develops with several smaller satellite ulcers around the periphery, which can mimic the ulcerative phase of herpes simplex. More than half of the lesions occur on the prepuce, particularly in uncircumcised men. In women, the majority of lesions are on the fourchette, labia, and perianal area. Adenopathy can progress to bubo formation with tender, overlying erythema. These buboes can rupture and produce inguinal abscesses.

Diagnosis

Gram stain of smears obtained from the ulcer base has been advocated in the past for diagnosis, but this lacks both sensitivity and specificity. The preferred diagnostic modality is swabs for culture from the ulcer base or undermined edge. These are plated directly on enriched media (GC agar and Mueller-Hinton agar base) and incubated for 72 hours in an atmosphere of 5% carbon dioxide at 33°C. Polymerase chain reaction (PCR) and immunochromatography tests are also available.

Treatment

The Centers for Disease Control and Prevention (CDC) recommend a syndromal management approach in which a positive diagnosis is suggested if the patient has one or more painful ulcers and no evidence of syphilis or herpes simplex virus. Ulcers with painful adenopathy are pathognomonic (Table 1 lists antimicrobial treatment). The safety and efficacy of azithromycin (Zithromax) for pregnant and lactating women have not been established. Ciprofloxacin (Cipro)[1] is contraindicated during pregnancy and lactation. No adverse effects of chancroid on pregnancy outcome have been reported. Serologic testing for syphilis, HIV, and other appropriate STIs should be performed. Chancroidal ulcers should be kept clean with regular washing in soapy water and kept dry. Fluctuant buboes might require incision and drainage, which is preferable over needle aspiration. Treatment of all sexual partners within 60 days should be pursued, and treatment is similar to that for the source patient. Patients should not engage in sexual activity until the ulcers are healed.

Granuloma Inguinale (Donovanosis)

History

Granuloma inguinale was first recognized in India, where Donovan observed, in an oral lesion of the disease, the bodies that bear his name. There is considerable confusion about terminology between this disease and LGV, because various similar synonyms have been used inconsistently. Adding to the confusion, Donovan's name is associated with two tropical diseases that he discovered: leishmaniasis, with the discovery of intracellular protozoan inclusions that bear his name (Leishman-Donovan bodies), and granuloma inguinale (whose intracellular inclusions were believed to be caused by protozoa but are now known to be caused by bacteria).

---

[1] Not FDA approved for this indication.

TABLE 1 Clinical Features and Treatment Summary of Chancroid, Granuloma Inguinale, and Lymphogranuloma Venereum

FEATURES AND TREATMENT	CHANCROID	GRANULOMA INGUINALE	LYMPHOGRANULOMA VENEREUM
Clinical Features			
Incubation period	3–7 days	3–40 days	1–28 days
Primary lesion	Papule	Papule	Papule or vesicle
Ulcerative lesion painful	Yes	No	No
Lymphadenopathy	Yes (unilateral)	No	Yes (unilateral or bilateral)
Base	Purulent	Raised, easily bleeds	Nonvascular
Border	Round, raised, undermined edges	Irregular, expansion along skin folds	Irregular, ragged
Treatment			
Treatment of choice (any of the options listed)	Azithromycin (Zithromycin) 1 g Ciprofloxacin (Cipro)[1] 500 mg bid × 3 d Ceftriaxone (Rocephin)[1] 250 mg IM once	Azithromycin[1] 1 g PO on day 1 followed by 500 mg PO daily for 3 weeks Doxycycline (Vibramycin) 100 mg bid × 3 wks	Azithromycin[1] 1 g weekly × 3 wk Doxycycline 100 mg bid × 3 wk
Alternative treatment (any of the options listed)	Erythromycin (Ery-Tab)[1] 500 mg qid × 7 d	Azithromycin[1] 1 g PO qwk × 3 wk Erythromycin[1] 500 mg qid × 3 wk Ciprofloxacin[1] 750 mg bid × 3 wk Trimethoprim/Sulfamethoxazole[1]: One double-strength (160 mg/800 mg) tablet PO bid × 3 wk	Erythromycin[1] 500 mg qid × 3 wk

[1]Not FDA approved for this indication.

Epidemiology

Endemic areas are localized to a few specific areas of the tropics, particularly India, Papua New Guinea, Brazil, and the eastern part of South Africa, particularly Durban. Commercial sex workers and men are primarily involved.

Etiology

The disease is caused by an encapsulated Gram-negative coccobacillus *Klebsiella granulomatis* (previously known as *Calymmatobacterium* or *Donovania granulomatis*).

Clinical Features

A firm, painless papule or nodule is the presenting sign of granuloma inguinale. The incubation period is variable from 3 to 40 days from inoculation. This nodule quickly ulcerates, and the base is highly vascular, is beefy red, and bleeds easily. Lymphadenopathy is not part of the clinical presentation of this disease, distinguishing granuloma inguinale from chancroid and LGV. However, the ulcer can be easily confused with chancroid, condyloma lata, ulcerated verrucous warts, and squamous carcinoma. Untreated, the ulcers slowly expand, particularly along skin folds toward the inguinal region or anus (Figure 2). The ulcers are flat and raised and have slightly hypertrophic margins, but the bases are typically free of pus and necrotic debris. Less-common presentations include extragenital lesions involving the neck and mouth; cervical lesions that resemble carcinoma; and involvement of the uterus, tubes, and ovaries, producing hard masses, abscesses, or frozen pelvis.

Diagnosis

Diagnosis requires the demonstration of intracellular Donovan bodies from Giemsa or Wright staining of smears taken from a swab of the ulcer base or from biopsy material.

Treatment

See Table 1 for antimicrobial treatment. Treatment should be continued until lesions are resolved and, if possible, a little longer to reduce the risk of relapse.

Figure 2 Granuloma inguinale. (Source: NEHC http://www.nhec.med.navy.mil/hp/sharp/std_pictures.htm)

Lymphogranuloma Venereum

History

LGV was first differentiated from syphilis in 1906 by Wasserman, though the first full description of the disease was given by Durand, Nicolas, and Favre in 1913. In 1925, Frei developed an intradermal skin test that gave positive responses in most LGV patients. The term "tropical bubo" was associated with the disease later.

Epidemiology

LGV is largely confined to the tropics and is not a common STI. The global overall incidence is in a decline. It is seen more commonly in men, but since 2004, there has been a resurgence manifesting as proctitis in North America and Europe among HIV-positive men who have sex with men.

Figure 3 Lymphogranuloma venereum. **A,** Small ulcerative lesion near corona of penis *(arrow).* **B,** Bilateral inguinal adenopathy, with developing groove sign as adenopathy expands above and below the inguinal ligament. (**A** courtesy Ronald Ballard, Reproduced with permission from The Diagnosis and Management of Sexually Transmitted Infections in South Africa, 3rd ed., Johannesburg, South African Institute for Medical Research, 2000. **B** courtesy Connexions (http://cnx.org/content/m14883/latest/Case_10-pres1-1.jpg).

Etiology
LGV is a chlamydial infection caused by the invasive L1, L2, and L3 serovars of *Chlamydia trachomatis*, an intracellular gram-negative bacterium.

Clinical Features
LGV is essentially a systemic disease whose natural course is divided into three distinct phases. The initial phase of LGV is normally an inconspicuous genital lesion beginning as a typically small, painless papule or vesicle occurring 1 to 28 days after inoculation. This papule or vesicle quickly ulcerates and heals without a scar, and it often goes unrecognized by the patient (Figure 3). However, the second phase of LGV is the development of increasingly painful lymphadenopathy, often with fever and malaise. The lymphadenopathy progresses to bubo formation over 1 to 2 weeks. When a sexually active adult patient presents with an inguinal bubo not associated with genital ulcers, LGV is an important diagnosis to consider. The infected nodes are usually unilateral (bilateral in a third of cases) and often coalesce into a matted mass that can project outwards above or below the inguinal ligament, producing the pathognomonic groove sign present in 20% of patients with LGV. The buboes are likely to rupture, forming multiple sinuses. Untreated, LGV can cause extensive lymphatic damage, resulting in elephantiasis of the genitalia. Anal involvement, likewise, can lead to perirectal abscesses, fistulas, and rectal strictures. These complications represent the late phase of LGV.

Diagnosis
The diagnosis of LGV can only be confirmed using PCR methods of smears, scrapings, or aspirated material. Alternatively, the ability to perform micro-immunofluorescence serology testing using a fluorescein-conjugated monoclonal antibody and viewing the slide with a fluorescence microscope can demonstrate the inclusion bodies within the cytoplasm of macrophages. Gram staining by itself lacks appropriate sensitivity or specificity. Additional laboratory findings include leukocytosis, elevated erythrocyte sedimentation rate, and increases in immunoglobulin G and cryoglobulins.

Treatment
Antimicrobial treatment is summarized in Table 1. Needle aspiration or incision and drainage of fluctuant buboes may be required for symptomatic relief but are not routinely recommended for treatment because drainage can delay healing. Fistula openings should receive sterile dressings. One of the primary goals of treatment of LGV is to prevent long-term complications such as anogenital strictures or fistulas. Plastic surgical operations may be of benefit in cases with extensive rectal strictures or elephantiasis of the genitalia. However, these surgical interventions should only be performed after a prolonged course of antibiotics. Scars should be monitored to detect malignant change.

Management of Sex Partners
Any person having had sexual contact with a patient with LGV within 60 days before the onset of the patient's symptoms should be examined and presumptively treated with azithromycin[1] 1 gram orally as a single dose or doxycycline 100 mg orally twice a day for seven days. Symptomatic patients should be treated with longer treatment regimens.

References
Centers for Disease Control and Prevention, Workowski KA, Berman SM: Sexually transmitted diseases treatment guidelines, 2006 *MMWR Recomm Rep* 55(RR-11):1–94, Aug 4; 2006. Available at http://www.cdc.gov/std/treatment/default.htm (accessed August 6, 2015).
Habif T: In *Clinical Dermatology*, ed 4, Philadelphia, 2004, Mosby, pp 325–329.
Leppard B: In *An Atlas of African Dermatology*, Oxon, UK, 2002, Radcliffe Medical Press, p 69. 151, 237.
Ndinya-Achola JO, Kihara AN, Fisher LD, et al: Presumptive specific clinical diagnosis of genital ulcer disease (GUD) in a primary health care setting in Nairobi, *Int J STD AIDS* 7(3):201–205, 1996.
Richens J, Mabey DC: Sexually transmitted infections (excluding HIV). In Cook GC, Zumla AI, editors: *Manson's Tropical Diseases*, ed 22, London, 2009, Saunders, pp 403–434.
Ronald A: Chancroid. In Hunter GW, Strickland GT, Magill AJ, editors: *Hunter's Tropical Medicine and Emerging Infectious Diseases*, ed 8, Philadelphia, 2000, WB Saunders, pp 367–369.

GONORRHEA

Method of
John Brill, MD, MPH

CURRENT DIAGNOSIS

- Gonorrhea is caused by the gram-negative diplococcus *Neisseria gonorrhoeae.*
- Asymptomatic gonococcal infections are common in men and women, particularly in extragenital locations.
- Molecular tests are more sensitive than culture for diagnosis, particularly in extragenital locations.
- All patients diagnosed with gonorrhea should be tested for other sexually transmitted infections, including HIV.
- Annual screening for *N gonorrhoeae* infection is recommended for all sexually active women aged <25 years and for older women at increased risk for infection.

CURRENT THERAPY

- The combination of ceftriaxone (Rocephin) 250 mg intramuscularly *and* azithromycin (Zithromax) 1 g by mouth is the first-line treatment for gonorrhea. Ceftriaxone alone should not be used to treat gonorrhea, even when concomitant chlamydia testing is negative.

- Azithromycin is preferred as the second agent over doxycycline (Vibramycin) because of enhanced compliance and better antimicrobial activity.
- Only immunoglobulin E–mediated allergic reaction to PCN or cephalosporins (anaphylaxis, Stevens-Johnson syndrome, or toxic epidermal necrolysis) should contraindicate use of ceftriaxone.

Gonorrhea is a sexually transmitted infection caused by the gram-negative diplococcus *Neisseria gonorrhoeae*, or gonococcus (GC).

Epidemiology

Gonorrhea is the second-most common reportable human infection in the United States, with 468,514 cases of gonorrhea reported to the Centers for Disease Control and Prevention (CDC) in 2016, an 18.5% increase from 2015. The actual number of cases is estimated to be at least double those reported because of asymptomatic cases and underreporting. Regional rates vary widely from 20 (Vermont) to 480 (District of Columbia) per 100,000 population. The estimated annual US health care costs related to GC infections is $162 million.

Risk Factors

Risk factors for infection include unprotected intercourse, adolescent and young adult age, new/multiple sexual partners, and exchanging sex for money or drugs. Gonococcal infection is strongly associated with other sexually transmitted infections (STIs) (Figure 1). In fact, at a county population level, HIV infection rate carries the highest association with GC rates, superseding all other socioeconomic and demographic risk factors. Additional risk factors for gonorrhea include inconsistent condom use among persons who are not in mutually monogamous relationships, previous or coexisting sexually transmitted infections, and exchanging sex for money or drugs. Military recruits, incarcerated persons and persons receiving care at public STI clinics are also at high risk. A significant ethnic disparity in GC rates is seen, with rates in black men 8.9 times higher than in white men and black women and 8.4 times higher than in white women in 2016; however, these proportions have been decreasing since 2011 (Figure 2).

Pathophysiology

N gonorrhoeae infects non-cornified epithelial cells, such as the urethra, endocervix, rectum, oropharynx, and conjunctiva. The bacteria divide by binary fission every 20 to 30 minutes, thus the rapid emergence of symptoms. *N gonorrhoeae* attaches to different types of mucus-secreting epithelial cells via a number of alterable structures located on the surface of gonococci, and additionally uses several mechanisms to counter the immune system. *N gonorrhoeae* is primarily spread by infected secretions (oral, urethral) coming into contact with mucosal surfaces. Maternal-child transmission is well established; hence, the recommendation to treat all newborns prophylactically with erythromycin (Ilotycin) 0.5% ophthalmic ointment.

Screening and Prevention

The United States Preventive Service Task Force recommends annual screening for *N gonorrhoeae* infection in all sexually

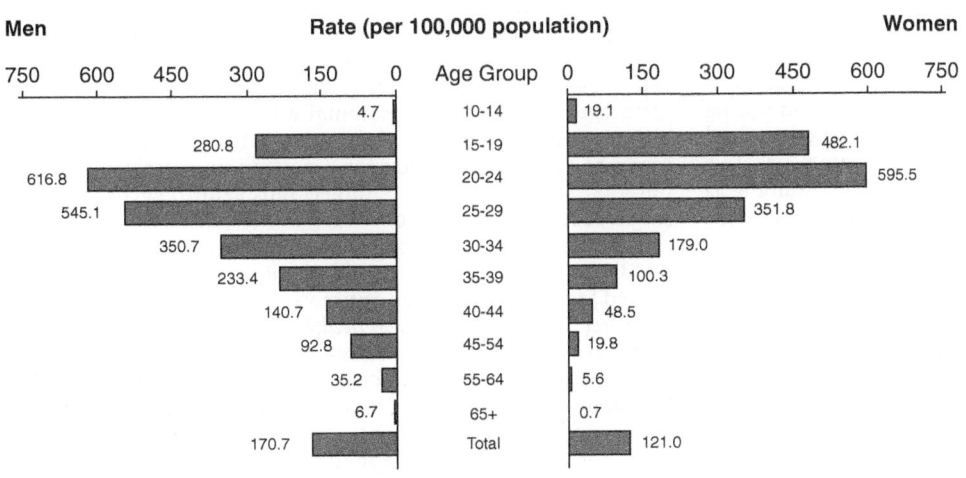

Gonorrhea – Rates of Reported Cases by Age Group and Sex, United States, 2016

Figure 1 Rates of reported cases by age group and sex, United States 2016.

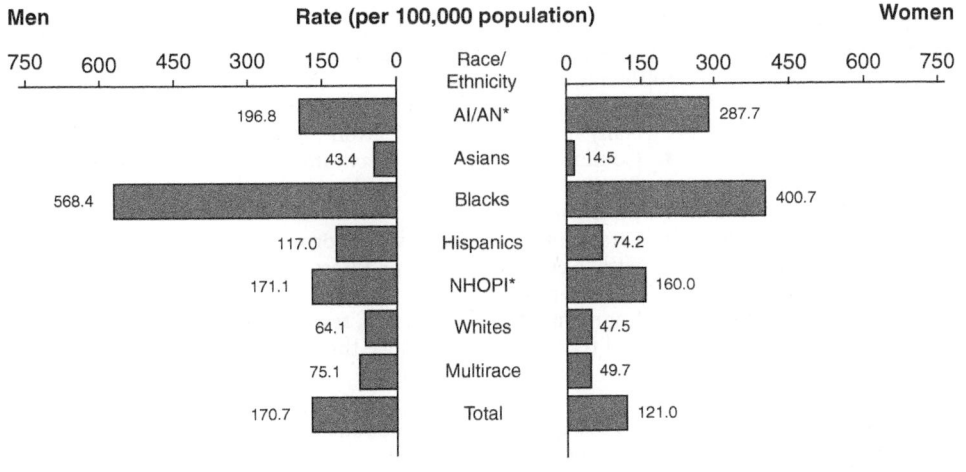

Figure 2 Ethnic disparity rates per population.

active women aged <25 years and for older women at increased risk for infection (e.g., those who have a new sex partner, more than one sex partner, a sex partner with concurrent partners, or a sex partner who has an STI); a "B" recommendation. The United States Preventive Service Task Force concludes that the current evidence is insufficient to assess the balance of benefits and harms of screening for gonorrhea in men; an "I" recommendation.

Men who have sex with men (MSM) without consistent condom use are at high risk for gonorrhea infection, and the CDC recommends screening of sexually active MSM at least annually at anatomic sites of exposure. Mucosa that is infected by GC is more susceptible to HIV, even in asymptomatic states, raising the impetus for screening and treatment. Because the bacterium is an obligate human pathogen with adult transmission only via sexual contact, avoidance of intimate contact with an infected person is the optimal mode of prevention. Male latex condoms, used correctly and consistently, are highly effective at preventing GC transmission; polyurethane male and female condoms are effective when intact but have higher breakage rates.

Clinical Manifestations

The most common symptom of genital GC infection is a mucopurulent urethritis or cervicitis. In men, genital GC typically manifests with urethral discharge and dysuria 2 to 5 days after exposure; however, approximately 30% of urethral infections are asymptomatic. About half of genitally infected women will show symptoms, most commonly vaginal discharge, dysuria, and itching, generally 5 to 10 days after exposure. The great majority of rectal and pharyngeal infections are asymptomatic. GC can also present as ocular and disseminated infection. Except for neonatal infections believed to arise from perinatal transmission, diagnosis of gonococcal infection in infants and children should trigger a sexual abuse investigation, including multisite testing.

Diagnosis

Laboratory diagnosis of GC can be made by gram staining of urethral secretions in symptomatic men, by culture of endocervical or urethral specimens, or by nucleic acid amplification testing (NAAT) of urine or the target location. Gram staining of urethral discharge showing leukocytes with intracellular gram-negative diplococci is extremely specific and sensitive. Gram staining is not sensitive enough to rule out infection in symptom-free men or in extra-urethral locations. NAAT has largely replaced culture and appears to be more than twice as sensitive as culture in extragenital locations. The increased sensitivity of NAATs is due to their ability to produce a positive test result from as little as a single copy of the target DNA. False-positive test results can occur with nucleic acid amplification testing, especially if NAAT is not cleared by the Food and Drug Administration for use with these specimens or if it is ordered too soon after treatment, because NAATs do not require viable organisms. Although this higher sensitivity has allowed the use of less invasively collected specimens, such as first-catch urine, specific site testing or pharyngeal or rectal specimens will detect up to 80% more infections than urine screening alone, highlighting the importance of a careful exposure history and consideration of multiple-site screening in high-risk populations. Recent literature has also demonstrated that approved self-collection vaginal swabs are accurate and highly acceptable to patients.

Differential diagnosis

Differential diagnosis of gonorrheal genital infections includes *Chlamydia trachomatis* (CT), *Mycoplasma genitalium*, *Trichomonas vaginalis*, and herpes simplex infection. In women, yeast vaginitis and bacterial vaginosis should be considered. Coinfection is common and cannot be ruled out on clinical grounds; therefore co-testing for CT and trichomonas should be done in all patients, and all patients should be offered testing for HIV, syphilis, and hepatitis.

Gonococcal conjunctivitis is typically purulent and unilateral but again cannot be distinguished clinically from other bacterial infections. Because gonococcal eye infections in adults generally result from autoinoculation, this diagnosis should prompt testing at other exposure sites.

Therapy

The 2015 CDC guidelines recommend ceftriaxone (Rocephin) *and* azithromycin (Zithromax) for the treatment of gonorrhea, even if the concomitant chlamydia testing result is negative. Ideally the dual treatment should be carried out under direct observation or at least in the same day. Unfortunately, primary care clinician awareness of recommendations for dual therapy is suboptimal, especially in clinicians who do not pursue continuing education in this area. Use of azithromycin as the second antimicrobial is preferred to doxycycline (Vibramycin) because of the convenience and compliance advantages of single-dose therapy and the substantially higher prevalence of gonococcal resistance to tetracycline than to azithromycin among surveillance study isolates. Tetracycline resistance is associated with cefixime (Suprax) resistance, underscoring the importance of using azithromycin as the second agent if oral therapy is used.

Data are limited regarding alternative regimens for treating gonorrhea among persons who have either a cephalosporin or immunoglobulin E–mediated penicillin allergy. Potential therapeutic options are dual treatment with gemifloxacin (Factive)[1] 320 mg by mouth plus oral azithromycin 2 g (single dose of each) or dual treatment with single doses of intramuscular gentamicin (Garamycin)[1] 240 mg plus oral azithromycin 2 g. The 2-g dose[3] of azithromycin has significantly higher efficacy than 1 g and can be used as solo therapy if no other options are available.

Expedited partner therapy (EPT) is a strategy of treating sex partners of patients with GC or chlamydia without examining the partner. EPT is advocated by the CDC to decrease reinfection rates, particularly where the likely alternative is no care. In 2018, all US states except Kentucky and South Carolina allowed EPT as an exception to scope of practice legislation requiring an established clinician-patient relationship. A challenge for EPT with gonorrhea is the need for parental administration of one of the components of the preferred therapy, ceftriaxone. If oral therapy seems to be the only option for a partner to be treated, cefixime (Suprax, 400 mg single-dose tablet) plus azithromycin (1- or 2-g single dose) should be used.

Treatment has been complicated by emerging resistance. In 2013 the CDC released Antibiotic Resistance Threats in the United States, which named antibiotic-resistant gonorrhea among the *three most urgent public health threats* in the country. Currently at least 30% of US isolates are resistant to at least 1 tested drug, most commonly tetracyclines, fluoroquinolones, or PCN. Resistant strains are much more frequent outside of the United States, underlining the importance of travel history, and are also more common in MSM. Cephalosporin resistance has stabilized following the recommendations for dual therapy, raising optimism that this strategy will maintain efficacy of these agents.

Monitoring

Test of cure after treatment is not recommended except for the following circumstances:

- Use of a non-preferred antibiotic regimen for treatment, especially for pharyngeal infection
- Continued intercourse <7 days after treatment of any/all partners
- Pregnant women (if treated early in pregnancy, also retest in third trimester)
- Persistent symptoms 3 weeks or more after treatment. Testing with NAAT in a shorter interval after treatment may result in false-positive test results because of the presence of DNA fragments. In this situation, testing should be repeated for CT and trichomonas to reduce the potential for false-negative ini-

---

[1] Not FDA approved for this indication.
[3] Exceeds dosage recommended by the manufacturer.

tial test results. For continued symptomatic genital infections despite appropriate therapy, culture with sensitivity testing is recommended.

- Suspected internationally acquired infection
- Culture sensitivity testing showed decreased susceptibility to cephalosporins

Because of a high rate of reinfection, persons treated for gonorrhea should be retested 3 months after treatment regardless of whether they believe their sex partners were treated. If the 3-month retesting does not occur, clinicians should retest whenever the individual next presents for care within 1 year of initial treatment.

Management of Complications

In men younger than 40, GC causes about 30% of cases of epididymitis, marked by unilateral testicular pain and swelling. Uncommon male complications of *N gonorrhoeae* include inguinal lymphadenitis, penile edema, periurethral abscess or fistula, accessory gland infection (Tyson's glands), balanitis, urethral stricture, and perhaps prostatitis. Female complications of gonorrhea are more frequent and burdensome and include pelvic inflammatory disease, potentially leading to infertility or ectopic pregnancy in women. Disseminated gonococcal infections may occur in up to 2% of untreated patients. Certain gonococcal strains are more likely to cause disseminated gonococcal infections. Although patients are bacteremic, many appear nontoxic. Symptoms and signs may include fevers, myalgias, arthralgias, asymmetrical polyarthritis, and a characteristic dermatitis consisting of a small number (<30) of skin lesions on the distal extremities that begin as papules and progress to pustules and ulcerations. Rarely, meningitis and endocarditis may occur. Hospitalization and consultation with an infectious-disease specialist are recommended.

References

Andreatos N, Grigoras C, Shehadeh F, et al: The impact of HIV infection and socioeconomic factors on the incidence of gonorrhea: a county-level, US-wide analysis, *PLoS ONE [Electronic Resource]* 12(9):e0183938, 2017.

Arias M, Jang D, Gilchrist J, et al: Ease, comfort, and performance of the HerSwab Vaginal Self-Sampling Device for the detection of *Chlamydia trachomatis* and *Neisseria gonorrhoeae*, *Sex Transm Dis* 43:125–129, 2016.

Bornstein M, Ahmed F, Barrow R, Risley JF, Simmons S, Workowski KA: Factors associated with primary care physician knowledge of the recommended regimen for treating gonorrhea, *Sex Transm Dis* 44:13–16, 2017.

CDC: Sexually Transmitted Diseases (STDs)> Gonorrhea. Available at https://www.cdc.gov/std/gonorrhea/default.htm. Accessed April 18, 2018.

Grov C, Cain D, Rendina HJ, Ventuneac A, Parsons JT: Characteristics associated with urethral and rectal gonorrhea and chlamydia diagnoses in a US national sample of gay and bisexual men: results from the One Thousand Strong Panel, *Sex Transm Dis* 43:165–171, 2016.

Kirkcaldy RD, Harvey A, Papp JR, et al: *Neisseria gonorrhoeae* Antimicrobial Susceptibility Surveillance—The Gonococcal Isolate Surveillance Project, 27 Sites, United States, 2014, *MMWR Morb Mortal Wkly Rep* 65(7):1–19, 2016.

United States Preventive Services Task Force: Final Recommendation Statement: *Chlamydia and Gonorrhea Screenings*. Available at https://www.uspreventiveservicestaskforce.org/Page/Document/RecommendationStatementFinal/chlamydia-and-gonorrhea-screening. Accessed April 18, 2018.

NONGONOCOCCAL URETHRITIS

Method of
Robert S. Freelove, MD

CURRENT DIAGNOSIS

- Urethritis is diagnosed by the presence of mucopurulent/purulent urethral discharge, >5 WBC/hpf on Gram stain of urethral secretions, a positive leukocyte esterase test or ≥10 WBC/hpf on microscopic examination of first-void urine.
- Testing first-void urine/urethral discharge using NAAT has replaced culture as the "gold standard" in diagnosis of chlamydial NGU.

- Test for cure is indicated in pregnant women and should wait at least 3 to 4 weeks after treatment.
- Patients with confirmed Chlamydia infection should be rescreened 3 to 6 months after treatment.

CURRENT THERAPY

- Treatment of choice is azithromycin (Zithromax) 1 g orally in a single dose.
- Other first-line treatment is doxycycline (Vibramycin) 100 mg orally twice a day for 7 days.
- If test results are not immediately available, patients should receive concurrent treatment for gonorrhea with ceftriaxone (Rocephin) 250 mg IM.
- Expedited partner therapy should be offered where allowed.
- Persistent symptoms in compliant patients who have not been reexposed can be treated with metronidazole (Flagyl) 2 g orally in a single dose.

Epidemiology

Chlamydia trachomatis is the most common pathogen identified in nongonococcal urethritis (NGU) in men. Other potential causes include *Mycoplasma genitalium, Trichomonas vaginalis*, herpes simplex virus, adenovirus, and urethral trauma. Chlamydia is the most commonly reported sexually transmitted infection (STI) in the United States. Determining the exact prevalence of *C. trachomatis* infection is difficult, because most infected individuals are asymptomatic. Additionally, although screening commonly occurs in women, empiric treatment without confirmatory testing is routinely extended to sexual partners of those who test positive. While 1,307,893 cases were reported to the CDC in 2010, the estimated prevalence is 2.8 million.

Risk Factors

C. trachomatis infection is associated with young age (less than 25 years), multiple sex partners, history of prior STI, low condom use, cervical ectopy, lower socioeconomic status, and low/intermediate education. Insertive oral sex among men who have sex with men is associated with urethritis caused by HSV or adenovirus. Posttraumatic urethritis is 10 times more likely in patients using latex catheters than silicone catheters for intermittent catheterization.

Pathophysiology

Urethritis is inflammation of the urethra caused by infection or traumatic injury. The term *nongonococcal urethritis* is typically reserved to describe an STI of the male urethra with a negative Gram stain of urethral discharge, most commonly due to *Chlamydia*. In women, urethral infection often accompanies chlamydial cervicitis.

C. trachomatis is an obligate intracellular parasite with a two-phase life cycle: an extracellular, nonreplicating, infectious elementary body; and an intracellular, replicating, noninfectious reticulate body. A cycle can take 3 to 5 days, requiring prolonged courses of treatment. Immunity to infection is relatively short-lived, contributing to reinfection or persistent infection.

Prevention

Primary prevention of NGU relies on education regarding chlamydial infection targeted at adolescents and young adults. Education should include promotion of behavioral changes aimed at reducing the risk of acquiring and transmitting STIs such as abstinence from sexual activity, delaying coitarche, reducing the number of sexual partners, and consistent and correct condom use.

Because most infections in males and females are asymptomatic, screening at-risk individuals is a cornerstone of secondary prevention. As most reproductive complications of *Chlamydia* infection occur in women, the CDC recommends annual screening of all sexually active, nonpregnant women 25 years old or younger and sexually active older women with a new partner or multiple partners. Because of the potential for maternal complications and transmission to the neonate, the CDC also recommends screening all pregnant women regardless of age. The CDC reserves screening of males for those at highest risk, including men attending STI clinics, under age 30 in the military, in correctional facilities, whose partners test positive, and who have sex with men. The United States Preventive Services Task Force recommends screening all sexually active and pregnant women age 24 or younger; recommends screening women age 25 or older only if they are at increased risk, whether or not they are pregnant; and concludes that there is insufficient evidence to assess benefits and harms of screening in men.

Clinical Manifestations

Many patients with NGU are asymptomatic, including up to 42% of men and 75% of women. The most common complaints are of urethral discharge and/or dysuria, usually appearing 1 to 3 weeks after exposure. The discharge can be watery, mucoid, or mucopurulent (Figure 1). The dysuria is commonly described as a burning sensation. Men may also have some itching and/or redness at the urethral meatus. Symptoms appear 1 to 3 weeks after exposure. Physical examination should include inspection for inguinal lymphadenopathy, ulcers, and/or urethral discharge.

Diagnosis

Urethritis is diagnosed clinically based on the presence of mucopurulent or purulent urethral discharge, greater than 5 WBC/hpf on Gram stain of urethral secretions, a positive leukocyte esterase test on first-void urine or 10 WBC/hpf or greater on microscopic examination of first-void urine sediment. All patients who have confirmed or suspected urethritis should be tested for both gonorrhea and chlamydia, and consideration should be given to check for other STIs. *C. trachomatis* cannot be cultured on artificial media and instead requires a tissue culture. However, nucleic acid amplification techniques (NAAT) are both sensitive and specific

and have replaced culture as the "gold standard" in diagnosis of chlamydial NGU. Testing can be performed on urethral specimens or on urine. Performing the testing on urine avoids invasive sampling of the urethra and may improve patient acceptance. Testing first-morning void improves detection rate.

Differential Diagnosis

The differential diagnoses include gonococcal urethritis, urinary tract infection (UTI), and urethritis caused by *M. genitalium*, HSV, and *T. vaginalis*. The incubation period for gonococcal urethritis is typically shorter and the discharge is more copious and purulent. UTIs usually cause more dysuria as well as other urinary symptoms, and bacteria can often be identified on Gram stain during urinalysis.

Therapy (or Treatment)

Treatment for chlamydial urethritis should be initiated immediately after diagnosis, ideally observed and in the health-care provider's office to ensure compliance. Recommended first-line agents are azithromycin (Zithromax) 1 g orally in a single dose or doxycycline (Vibramycin) 100 mg orally twice a day for 7 days. Alternative regimens include erythromycin base (Ery-Tab) 500 mg orally four times a day for 7 days; or erythromycin ethylsuccinate (E.E.S.) 800 mg orally four times a day for 7 days; or ofloxacin (Floxin) 300 mg orally twice a day for 7 days; or levofloxacin (Levaquin) 500 mg orally once daily for 7 days. Patients with confirmed urethritis in whom test results are not already known or immediately available should also be treated empirically for gonorrhea with ceftriaxone (Rocephin) 250 mg intramuscularly in a single dose. All sexual partners should be referred for evaluation and treatment. Alternatively, expedited partner therapy (EPT), providing prescriptions or medications to the patient to take to his/her partner, should be offered where allowed; EPT has been shown to increase partner treatment and reduce reinfection. Patients with symptoms of persistent or recurrent infection can be re-treated with the initial regimen if they were not compliant with treatment or have been reexposed to an untreated partner. If the patient was compliant and was not reexposed, he or she should be treated with metronidazole (Flagyl) 2 g orally in a single dose; or tinidazole (Tindamax) 2 g orally in a single dose plus azithromycin (Zithromax) 1 g orally in a single dose.

Monitoring

Testing for cure is not recommended except in pregnant women or those in whom therapeutic compliance is in question, and must wait for at least 3 to 4 weeks after treatment, because NAAT may be positive in the presence of dead organisms. All patients with *Chlamydia* infection should be screened again 3 to 6 months after treatment.

Complications

In men, untreated chlamydial NGU can lead to epididymitis and/or prostatitis. Reactive arthritis is an uncommon complication in men, as is Reiter syndrome (arthritis, conjunctivitis/uveitis, urethritis, mucocutaneous lesions). In women, concurrent cervicitis can lead to PID. Transmission to newborns can result in conjunctivitis or pneumonia.

References

Workowski KA, Berman S: Centers for Disease Control and Prevention. Sexually transmitted diseases treatment guidelines, 2010, *MMWR* 59(RR-12):1–110, 2010.

Centers for Disease Control and Prevention. STD trends in the United States: 2010 national data for gonorrhea, chlamydia, and syphilis. Table. http://www.cdc.gov/std/stats10/tables/trends-table.htm; [accessed 05.08.13].

Centers for Disease Control and Prevention: *Expedited partner therapy in the management of sexually transmitted diseases*, Atlanta, GA, 2006, US Department of Health and Human Services.

U.S. Preventive Services Task Force: Screening for chlamydial infection: U.S. Preventive Services Task Force Recommendation Statement, *Ann Intern Med* 147:128–133, 2007.

Figure 1 Mucopurulent urethral discharge in patient with NGU.

SYPHILIS

Method of
Jennifer Frank, MD

CURRENT DIAGNOSIS

- Serologic testing includes both nontreponemal-specific testing (VDRL and RPR) and treponemal-specific testing (FTA-Abs [fluorescent treponemal antibody absorption] and TP-PA [*Treponema pallidum* particle agglutination]).
- Cerebrospinal fluid testing (VDRL [Venereal Disease Research Laboratory], protein, cell count) is performed to diagnose neurosyphilis.

CURRENT THERAPY

- Penicillin is first-line therapy for all types and stages of syphilis.
- Penicillin is the only recommended treatment for pregnant women and for congenital syphilis. Penicillin-allergic patients should undergo desensitization.

Epidemiology

The rate of primary and secondary syphilis reached a low point (2.1 per 100,000) in 2000 and has increased since that time, reaching a rate of 9.5 per 100,000 in 2017; this represented an 11% increase from 2016 and is the highest rate since 1993. The recent increase in rates has occurred in both men and women, in all regions, in all age groups between 15 years and older, and in all ethnicities. Men who have sex with men (MSM) have the highest rates of primary and secondary syphilis. Seventy-two percent of states saw an increased rate from 2016 to 2017; the West continues to have the overall highest rate. Congenital syphilis is also increasing with a rate of 23.3 cases per 100,000 live births in 2017, a 43% increase from 2016; this represents a steady increase since 2012 and mirrors the increased rates among women.

Risk Factors

MSM and HIV-positive persons are at highest risk for primary and secondary syphilis. Other risk factors include living in the certain geographic areas in the United States or an urban area, and being born to a mother infected with syphilis.

Pathophysiology

Syphilis is caused by infection with the spirochete *Treponema pallidum* subspecies *pallidum* (Figure 1). The average incubation period is 21 days (range 3-90 days). Primary infection manifests with signs and symptoms at the site of infection; secondary and tertiary syphilis manifest with systemic signs and symptoms. Syphilis is primarily sexually transmitted but may be transmitted perinatally or through nonsexual cutaneous transmission Previous infection does not confer long-term immunity.

Prevention

Prevention includes both avoiding initial infection and preventing disease progression through early detection and treatment. Transmission of syphilis can be reduced (although not eliminated) by using condoms. Screening for syphilis in pregnancy combined with treatment of infected women reduces perinatal transmission. Screening high-risk populations may prevent spread of infection.

Screening

The US Preventive Services Task Force recommends screening people at increased risk for syphilis. Screening HIV-infected men or MSM every 3 months increases rates of detection. All pregnant women should be screened for syphilis at the first prenatal visit. Women at increased risk should be rescreened in the third trimester, at delivery, and after any potential exposure to an infected partner.

Clinical Manifestations

Primary syphilis manifests as a chancre at the site of inoculation. The chancre, a painless ulcer with sharp borders, is usually solitary and associated with regional lymphadenopathy. Atypical presentations include extragenital location (most commonly oral or anal) and the presence of pain or multiple lesions. Secondary syphilis characteristically manifests with a generalized rash with variable features four to eight weeks after onset of primary syphilis (Figure 2). The palms and soles are affected in the majority of patients. Typically, the rash is maculopapular or papulosquamous and nonpruritic. Other clinical manifestations include highly infectious flat lesions (condyloma lata), fever, malaise, sore throat, headache, myalgias, alopecia, and, rarely, renal, bone, eye, or liver involvement. Latent syphilis, by definition, has no clinical manifestations. Ocular syphilis can occur during any stage of syphilis and has been reported in 20 states in the last few years. Patients with syphilis should be screened for any visual symptoms or eye complaints.

Tertiary syphilis, which is rare, is a late manifestation in untreated people and includes neurosyphilis, cardiovascular, and gummatous disease. Gummas are nodular lesions that vary in size and location. They can ulcerate and cause local tissue destruction. Cardiovascular syphilis most commonly manifests as aortitis of the ascending aorta. The clinical manifestations of neurosyphilis are numerous and include meningitis with or without vascular involvement, dementia, tabes dorsalis (posterior column involvement with ataxia and bowel and bladder dysfunction), and ocular or otologic involvement.

Congenital syphilis has early (birth to 2 years) and late (2 to 20 years) clinical manifestations. Early signs include hepatosplenomegaly, rash, fever, neurosyphilis, pneumonitis, rhinitis, generalized lymphadenopathy, hepatitis, ascites, hematologic disease, renal disease, periostitis, and osteochondritis. Late manifestations (present in 40% of untreated patients) include skeletal deformities, neurologic disease (deafness), dental abnormalities, and ocular abnormalities.

Diagnosis

Diagnosis of primary syphilis may be optimally diagnosed by specific testing of the skin lesion or exudate as it can take several weeks for treponemal antibodies to develop. There are three methods for testing of exudate: direct fluorescent antibody testing, PCR testing, and darkfield microscopy; all have limited availability. Serologic testing is done using nontreponemal (VDRL or RPR) and treponemal testing (multiple types, including FTA-ABS and TPPA) because both tests have limitations; it may take several weeks for antibodies to develop. Nontreponemal testing may be falsely positive with other medical conditions, but antibody titers correlate with disease activity and therefore can indicate response to treatment. Nontreponemal tests usually become nonreactive after successful treatment. A serofast reaction can occur in which the nontreponemal test stays reactive. Treponemal tests are specific for syphilitic infection but usually stay reactive regardless of treatment or disease status. Treponemal test antibody titers do not match the level of disease activity and therefore cannot be used to monitor treatment response. Reverse sequence testing has been used in which a treponemal specific test is the initial screening test, followed by a non-treponemal test. Reverse sequence testing has a higher false-positive rate with the initial screening step of testing but identifies more cases of syphilis, particularly early infection, previously treated infection, or long-standing infection. If reverse sequence screening is used, a third treponemal specific test using different antigens should be used to confirm the results.

Neurosyphilis is diagnosed based on clinical signs and symptoms using laboratory testing to support a clinical diagnosis. No single test can be used to diagnose all patients with

Figure 1 *Treponema pallidum* on darkfield microscopy.

Figure 2 Syphilis skin lesion.

neurosyphilis, which means that neurosyphilis is usually diagnosed by a combination of serologic testing, testing of cerebrospinal fluid (CSF), and clinical evaluation. Laboratory testing includes reactive serologic testing; cerebrospinal fluid (CSF) VDRL (Venereal Disease Research Laboratory) testing, which is specific but not sensitive; and CSF positive for white blood cells or protein, or both. The CSF FTA-ABS (fluorescent treponemal antibody absorption) test is sensitive but less specific than CSF VDRL testing. Patients with latent, tertiary, or neurosyphilis should be tested for HIV infection.

Differential Diagnosis

Syphilis, which can affect every organ system, has historically been called the great mimicker. Syphilis is on the differential diagnosis of, most commonly, conditions causing genital ulcers or lesions, conditions causing systemic rashes affecting the palms and soles, conditions causing ocular and otologic manifestations (uveitis, sudden visual changes, hearing loss), and conditions causing dementia, meningitis, or ataxia.

Treatment

Penicillin G is the preferred treatment for all stages of syphilis; other forms of penicillin (oral penicillin, combinations of benzathine and procaine [Bicillin CR]) are not effective. The stage and extent of clinical disease determine which preparation is used, the dosage, and the length of treatment (Table 1). In penicillin-allergic patients, antibiotic alternatives exist for all types and stages of syphilis except for syphilis in pregnancy and congenital syphilis.

Neurosyphilis is ideally treated with penicillin. Alternative treatment of primary and secondary syphilis and early latent syphilis includes doxycycline (Vibramycin) 100 mg orally twice a day or tetracycline 500 mg orally four times daily for 14 days.

TABLE 1 CDC Recommendations for Treatment of Syphilis

STAGE	RECOMMENDED PENICILLIN TREATMENT	
	PENICILLIN	DOSAGE
Primary and secondary syphilis	Benzathine penicillin G (Bicillin LA)	2.4 million U IM once
Early latent syphilis (acquired within previous 12 mo)	Benzathine penicillin G	2.4 million U IM once
Late latent syphilis	Benzathine penicillin G	2.4 million U IM weekly × 3 doses
Tertiary syphilis	Benzathine penicillin G	2.4 million units IM weekly × 3 doses
Neurosyphilis	Aqueous crystalline penicillin G *or*	3–4 million U q4h
	Continuous infusion *or*	18–24 U daily IV × 10–14 d (preferred)
	Procaine penicillin (Wycillin) *plus*	2.4 million U IM
	Probenecid	500 mg PO qid
Congenital Syphilis		
Proven or highly probable disease	Aqueous crystalline penicillin G *or*	100,000–150,000 U/kg/d (divided 50,000 U/kg/dose) IV q12h × first 7 d of life, then q8h for total of 10 d of treatment
	Procaine penicillin G	50,000 U/kg/dose IM daily × 10 d
Normal examination but mother inadequately treated	Aqueous crystalline penicillin G *or*	100,000–150,000 U/kg/d (divided 50,000 U/kg/dose) IV q12h × first 7 d of life, then q8h for total of 10 days of treatment
	Procaine penicillin G *or*	50,000 U/kg/dose IM daily × 10 d
	Benzathine penicillin G	50,000 U/kg/dose IM once
Normal examination, serologic titers ≤4× the maternal titer, and mother adequately treated during pregnancy	Benzathine penicillin G	50,000 U/kg/dose IM once

Abbreviation: CDC = Centers for Disease Control and Prevention.

Ceftriaxone (Rocephin)[1] 1 g daily IM or IV for 10 to 14 days is also used, although data is limited regarding optimal dose and treatment duration. Azithromycin (Zithromax)[1] 2 g orally as a single dose may be used when treatment with both penicillin and doxycycline is contraindicated, although treatment failures have been reported and azithromycin is not appropriate treatment for MSM, HIV-infected patients, or in pregnancy. Penicillin-allergic patients with late latent syphilis can be treated with doxycycline 100 mg orally twice daily or tetracycline 500 mg orally four times daily for 28 days, recognizing that there is limited data to support this treatment. Treatment of penicillin-allergic patients with tertiary syphilis should be done is consultation with a specialist. Ceftriaxone[1] 2 g given IV or IM daily for 10 to 14 days has been described for the treatment of neurosyphilis in penicillin-allergic patients.

The Jarisch-Herxheimer reaction is an acute febrile reaction (with accompanying headache, myalgias, and other symptoms) occurring within 24 hours of treatment of syphilis. It is more common in early stages of syphilis and rare in newborns.

Monitoring

No definite criteria exist for either cure of syphilis or treatment failure. It is recommended that nontreponemal antibody titers be followed every 6 months, and patients should be periodically reexamined for clinical signs or symptoms of syphilitic infection. Treatment failure is probable in patients with either persistent or recurrent clinical signs or symptoms or a sustained fourfold increase in nontreponemal antibody titer (compared to maximum titer at time of treatment). Treatment failure is possible if nontreponemal antibody titers fail to decline fourfold within 6 months after treatment. Suspected treatment failure warrants retesting for neurosyphilis and HIV infection. Patients with HIV infection, with congenital syphilis, who are pregnant, or who have neurosyphilis warrant closer and more-specific laboratory and clinical follow-up. Full recommendations can be found in the Centers for Disease Control and Prevention (CDC) treatment guidelines (http://www.cdc.gov/std/tg2015/syphilis.htm).

---

[1] Not FDA approved for this indication.

Complications

Complications of syphilis are primarily related to neurologic involvement, tertiary syphilis, or late manifestations of congenital syphilis.

References

ACOG. Clinical Practice: Syphilis Resurgence Reminds Us of the Importance of STD Screening and Treatment during Prenatal Care, Available at https://www.acog.org/About-ACOG/ACOG-Departments/ACOG-Rounds/May-2017/Syphilis-Resurgence.

Cantor AG, Pappas M, Daeges M, Nelson HD: Screening for syphilis: updated evidence report and systematic review for the US Preventive Services Task Force, JAMA 315:2328–2337, 2016.

Centers for Disease Control and Prevention. 2015 Sexually Transmitted Diseases Treatment Guidelines. Available at: http://www.cdc.gov/std/tg2015/syphilis.htm.

Centers for Disease Control and Prevention: Discordant results from reverse sequence syphilis screening—five laboratories, United States, 2006–2010, MMWR Morbid Mortal Wkly Rep 60:133–137, 2011.

Centers for Disease Control and Prevention, Association of Public Health Laboratories: Laboratory diagnostic testing for Treponema pallidum, Expert Consultation Meeting Summary Report, January 13–15, 2009, Atlanta, GA. Available at: http://www.aphl.org/aphlprograms/infectious/std/Documents/ID_2009Jan_Laboratory-Guidelines-Treponema-pallidum-Meeting-Report.pdf. 2009.

Centers for Disease Control and Prevention: Clinical Advisory: Ocular Syphilis in the United States. Available at, https://www.cdc.gov/std/syphilis/clinicaladvisoryos2015.htm; 2015.

Centers for Disease Control and Prevention. 2017 Sexually Transmitted Disease Surveillance. Available at https://www.cdc.gov/std/syphilis/stats.htm.

Centers for Disease Control and Prevention: Discordant results from reverse sequence syphilis screening: five laboratories, United States, 2006–2010, MMWR Morb Mortal Wkly Rep. 60(5):133–137, 2011.

Kent ME, Romanelli F: Reexamining syphilis: an update on epidemiology, clinical manifestations, and management, Ann Pharmacother 42:226–236, 2008.

Koss CA, Dunne EF, Warner L: A systematic review of epidemiologic studies assessing condom use and risk of syphilis, Sex Trans Dis 36:401–405, 2009.

Lautenschlager S: Cutaneous manifestations of syphilis, Am J Clin Dermatol 7:291–304, 2006.

Marra CM: Update on neurosyphilis, Curr Infect Dis Rep 11:127–134, 2009.

New York City Department of Health and Mental Hygiene, and the New York City STD PreventionTraining Center: The diagnosis and management of syphilis: an update and review. March 2019. www.nycptc.org.

Woods CR: Congenital syphilis—persisting pestilence, Pediatr Infect Dis 28:536–537, 2009.

USPSTF: Syphilis Infection in Nonpregnant Adults and Adolescents: Screening; June 2016.

14 Diseases of the Skin

ACNE VULGARIS

Method of
Daniel J. Van Durme, MD, MPH; and Lisa M. Johnson, MD

CURRENT DIAGNOSIS

- Acne vulgaris is primarily found in teenagers and young adults and is characterized by microcomedones that develop into open and closed comedones (blackheads and whiteheads) as well as inflammatory papules and pustules, or nodules and cysts.
- Acne vulgaris lesions are primarily on the face, neck, upper arms, back, and chest.
- Acneiform lesions are typically found in various stages, with many patients having a predominant type.

CURRENT THERAPY

- Acne therapy targets abnormal hyperkeratinization, excess sebum production, colonization by *Propionibacterium acnes*, and inflammation. Therapy involves prevention of new lesions and control over a long period of time with response generally seen in 6 to 8 weeks.
- Numerous topical and oral medications have demonstrated efficacy for patients with acne; there is little evidence for which is best.
- Benzoyl peroxide is an excellent starting agent owing to extensive safety and efficacy studies, its demonstrated benefit in controlling *P. acnes*, and some benefits in controlling abnormal keratinization and inflammation.
- Topical retinoids should also be considered as starting agents owing to their demonstrated benefits in controlling abnormal keratinization leading to microcomedones, a primary lesion in acne.
- Topical antibiotics such as clindamycin (Cleocin-T) and erythromycin (Akne-Mycin) should be used in combination with topical retinoids for more efficacy or with benzoyl peroxide to decrease the likelihood of bacterial resistance.
- Oral antibiotics such as doxycycline (Vibramycin) should be used if acne is widespread or unresponsive to topical agents.
- Oral contraceptives have proven benefits for most types of acne.
- Oral isotretinoin (Accutane, Claravis) can be very effective and even cures many patients, but the teratogenic and other side effects are profound and mandate use with extreme caution.

Acne (or acne vulgaris) and rosacea (previously called acne rosacea and sometimes adult acne) are often thought of together. However, they actually represent different pathophysiologic processes and require different therapeutic approaches.

Epidemiology

Acne is a chronic inflammatory dermatosis that is most common in adolescents, affecting approximately 85% of teenagers with the average age of onset being 11 to 12 years of age, peaking at ages 15 to 17, and decreasing with age. It is typically worse in male patients. The severity varies widely. Although significant physical scarring is uncommon, the psychological burden may be severe and includes depression, anxiety, social withdrawal, and suicidal ideation. More severe forms of acne are found in those with a genetic predisposition and those with earlier onset.

Prevention

Cigarette smoking raises acne risk, and the severity increases in a dose-dependent fashion. There are many myths, anecdotes, and limited (flawed) studies regarding acne and its triggers, but there is no good evidence to date to support the roles of chocolate, greasy foods, or other dietary factors in causing acne. There is some evidence that dairy products (particularly milk) might contribute to acne, but others have questioned the strength of these studies.

Pathophysiology

The pathophysiology of acne involves androgens as a major contributing factor, and thus acne starts with puberty. Four intersecting pathophysiologic processes are involved in acne, and the sequence and degree of contribution of each factor is still under study. The lesions begin with abnormal keratinization of the pilosebaceous glands that are more concentrated on the face, neck, and trunk. The keratin that lines the opening of the glands becomes more cohesive; this blocks the gland from being able to adequately excrete the sebum, and the plugged opening dilates. This leads to a closed comedone (whitehead) or open comedone (blackhead). Additional factors include the proliferation of the gram-positive *Propionibacterium acnes* (*P. acnes*) and an increase in inflammatory mediators, such as cytokines, leukotrienes, lymphocytes, and macrophages, which lead to the papules and pustules of inflammatory acne. Finally, the abnormal and excess production of sebum, particularly triggered by androgens, can play a key role as well, notably in nodulocystic acne.

Diagnosis

Diagnosis is generally straightforward, especially in teenagers. Dermatologic lesions include open and closed comedones, pustules, inflammatory papules, nodules, and cysts. Lesions are primarily found on the face, neck, upper arms, back, and chest. They are typically found in various stages, and many patients have a predominant type.

Clinical Manifestations

Clinical manifestations include open and closed comedones (blackheads and whiteheads), inflammatory papules and pustules, and in severe cases, nodules and cysts. There are several proposed classification schemes to help identify the numbers and types of lesions. Perhaps the most useful combines an estimate of the numbers of lesions with a descriptor of the lesions and location. Thus, a patient can have mild (few lesions) papulopustular acne of the face and severe (many lesions) comedonal acne on the back and shoulders. This classification helps to identify optimal treatment and provide a better description to assess response to therapy.

Differential Diagnosis

Differential diagnosis should include drug-induced acne (especially from steroids), which can be identified by seeing all lesions at nearly the same stage of development. Rosacea should also be considered in the differential diagnosis of acne vulgaris, though the age of onset and symptomatology are usually distinguishing.

Treatment

Treatment of acne begins with careful patient education and often involves a negotiation of management with teenagers who are taking responsibility for their health for the first time. It is increasingly important to address myths and misperceptions that they might hear from others or find on the Internet (such as the use of toothpaste for acne as seen on YouTube). Additionally, it is key to set realistic expectations about how acne can be controlled with the regular use of a variety of agents and how it can take 6 to 8 weeks to see improvement. If these issues are not addressed, the likelihood of adherence and long-term improvement are low.

Medical treatment should begin with a benzoyl peroxide agent because these are available over the counter and have an extensive history of safety and efficacy. They are available in a wide range of vehicles (soaps, lotions, gels); strengths vary from 2.5% to 10%. Many patients go straight to the maximum strength and report significant irritation, so it is important to educate that higher strengths dry the skin but are otherwise no more effective against *P. acnes* than the lower strengths. Patients should be advised that this reflects the base of treatment upon which other agents are added. Benzoyl peroxide plays a key role as a combination with both topical and oral antibiotics in preventing the development of bacterial resistance. If necessary, the patient can use it every other day to develop a tolerance to any irritation and gradually work up to once- or twice-daily dosing.

Topical retinoids (tretinoin [Retin-A, Renova, Avita], adapalene [Differin], or tazarotene [Tazorac]) are all extremely effective for abnormal keratinization and comedone development and thus treat existing lesions and prevent the development of new lesions. These can be irritating and come in a variety of strengths. Patients might need to start at the lowest strength with every-other-day dosing and work up to the highest strength needed and tolerated. Some formulations of tretinoin (primarily generic products) are not photo stable and should be applied in the evening. All are contraindicated in pregnancy.

Salicylic acid preparations are comedolytic and can be used for patients who cannot tolerate either benzoyl peroxide or topical retinoids, although salicylic acid preparations have not been shown to be as effective.

For patients with moderate inflammatory and comedonal lesions, it can be appropriate to start both benzoyl peroxide and topical retinoids at the initial visit; however, the applications should be separated in time because the benzoyl peroxide will inactivate the retinoid. An effective regimen (if tolerated) is a benzoyl peroxide wash in the morning and topical retinoid at bedtime.

Antibiotics should be added if response to topical benzoyl peroxide and retinoids is inadequate at the 6- to 8-week follow-up visit. Topical clindamycin (Cleocin-T) and erythromycin (Akne-Mycin) have demonstrated efficacy and can be used twice a day at the same time as the benzoyl peroxide. There are also combination agents that conveniently add the two agents into a single preparation: clindamycin 1% plus benzoyl peroxide 5% gel (BenzaClin, Duac) and erythromycin 3% plus benzoyl peroxide 5% gel (Benzamycin). They are more expensive, however.

Oral antibiotics should be started if the acne is moderate to severe, if it is too widespread to reasonably cover with topical antibiotics, or if there is an inadequate response after 6 to 8 weeks of topical antibiotics. Effective oral agents include the tetracyclines, macrolides, and trimethoprim-sulfamethoxazole (TMP-SMX [Bactrim])[1]; however, side effects of each must be considered, and bacterial resistance is an increasing issue.

Doxycycline (Vibramycin) at 100 mg/day is generally considered the optimal antibiotic despite some issues with photosensitivity. Minocycline (Minocin) at 100 mg twice daily has side effects that include pigment deposition in skin, mucous membranes, and teeth (as well as rare autoimmune hepatitis and other problems). TMP-SMX (Bactrim, Septra DS)[1] taken twice daily also has side effects to consider but can be useful when other agents are not tolerated. Macrolides, particularly erythromycin (Ery-Tab),[1] have had the most problems with bacterial resistance. For this reason, they should be reserved for pregnant patients or when other agents cannot be used and should always be used with benzoyl peroxide to minimize that resistance. All oral agents should be used in combination with benzoyl peroxide and/or a topical retinoid but not in combination with topical antibiotics. If significant improvement is noted, oral agents should be decreased after 3 to 4 months and stopped in order to attempt maintenance control with topical agents.

Oral contraceptives can be very helpful in female patients with moderate acne owing to their antiandrogenic effects, which decrease sebum production. There are currently 4 combined oral contraceptives approved by the FDA for the treatment of acne. They are ethinyl estradiol/norgestimate (Orthotricyclen), ethinyl estradiol/norethindrone acetate/ferrous fumarate (Estrostep Fe, Tilia Fe, Tri-Legest Fe), ethinyl estradiol/drospirenone (Yasmin, Yaz), and ethinyl estradiol/drospirenone/levomefolate (Beyaz, Rajani).

Several other topical agents have shown benefit for acne, including azelaic acid (Azelex, Finacea) used twice a day. It seems less effective than other agents, but can be useful when multiple types of lesions are present. It can also cause gradual hypopigmentation, which may be helpful in those with inflammatory hyperpigmentation. Topical sulfacetamide 10% (Klaron)[1] applied twice daily has also shown benefit.

Oral isotretinoin (Accutane, Claravis) has demonstrated marked benefit for patients with severe recalcitrant acne, even inducing a full remission. It is a potent teratogen and has a host of other significant side effects, including cheilitis, epistaxis, photosensitivity, and many others. Prescribed at 0.5 to 2 mg/kg per day over 20 weeks, it is like chemotherapy for acne. It is extremely tightly regulated, and both prescribers and patients must register with the iPledge program in order to write for the medicine and to receive the prescriptions. See www.ipledgeprogram.com. When all the precautions are managed, it can be an extremely effective option for the patients with the worst cases of acne.

[1] Not FDA approved for this indication.

References

Gannon M, Underhill M, Wellik KE: Which oral antibiotics are best for acne? *J Fam Pract* 60:290–292, 2011.
Strauss JS, Krowchuk DP, Leyden JJ, et al: Guidelines of care for acne vulgaris management, *J Am Acad Dermatol* 56:651–663, 2007.
Titus S, Hodge J: Diagnosis and treatment of acne, *Am Fam Physician* 86:734–740, 2012.
Knutsen-Larson S, Dawson AL, Dunnick CA, et al: Acne vulgaris: Pathogenesis, treatment, and needs assessment, *Dermatol Clin* 30:99–106, 2012.

ATOPIC DERMATITIS

Method of
Peck Y. Ong, MD

CURRENT DIAGNOSIS

- Itch must be present for the diagnosis of atopic dermatitis. In addition, the diagnosis must include three or more of the following criteria (U.K. Working Party's Diagnostic Criteria for Atopic Dermatitis):
  - History of generalized dry skin
  - Visible flexural dermatitis
  - Onset of the skin condition before 2 years (not used for patients younger than 4 years)

[1] Not FDA approved for this indication.

- History of itchy skin involving the following areas: elbows, behind knees, front of ankles, or around the neck
- History of asthma or allergic rhinitis (or for children younger than 4 years, history of atopic disease in a first-degree relative)

 CURRENT THERAPY

- Bathe or shower for 10 to 20 minutes daily and pat dry gently.
- Follow immediately by applying an emollient on unaffected areas and an antiinflammatory medication on affected areas.
- Use topical corticosteroids as a first-line antiinflammatory medication; alternative medications are topical calcineurin inhibitors, topical phosphodiesterase 4 inhibitor or dupilumab (Dupixent).
- Avoid environmental triggers such as extreme heat, humidity, or dryness.
- Avoid food allergens that may cause anaphylaxis. Consult an allergist regarding the interpretation of serum-specific IgE tests or food challenge.
- Treat skin infection only when clinical signs are present (e.g., oozing, impetigo).
- Severe, generalized infection or vesicular lesions may indicate herpes simplex virus infection; persistent fever may indicate invasive *S. aureus* infection.

Atopic dermatitis (AD) is a chronic inflammatory skin disease that is characterized by itch and a predilection of eczema on extensor areas in young infants or flexural areas in older children and adults. In the United States, AD affects about 15% of children and 2% of adults. For more than 85% of patients, AD begins during the first 5 years, but 50% of the children with AD improve significantly or outgrow the disease by age 7. The persistence of AD depends on various factors: early onset, severity, family history of AD, personal history of asthma, and food or inhalant allergies.

The itch associated with AD causes significant discomfort in these patients and often leads to sleep loss and to poor school or work performance. The quality of life of children with generalized AD is worse than that for children with diabetes, epilepsy, asthma, cystic fibrosis, or renal disease. The maternal stress in taking care of children with moderate to severe AD is equivalent to that associated with care of children with diabetes, Rett syndrome, profound deafness, or the need for enteral feeding.

Pathophysiology

AD is caused by a combination of genetic and environmental factors. Patients with AD have a defective skin barrier. This leads to a loss of skin hydration and susceptibility to environmental triggers. There is evidence that the skin barrier defects of AD are caused by genetic mutations. Studies have shown that many AD patients carry a genetic mutation in filaggrin, a protein with important barrier function.

Potential external triggers of AD include microbial pathogens and environmental allergens. Almost 100% of AD skin lesions are colonized by *Staphylococcus aureus*, which may produce toxins that trigger immune response in the skin. As a result, AD patients produce an increased amount of pro-allergic cytokines, such as interleukin-4 (IL-4), IL-5, and IL-13, in their skin. These cytokines lead to an increased infiltration of inflammatory T cells and eosinophils. IL-4 and IL-13 also are important for the production of serum IgE, the level of which is elevated in AD patients.

Diagnosis and Clinical Assessment

Most AD patients can be diagnosed by clinical history and physical examination. Typical presentation includes itch, dryness, flexural

TABLE 1 Differential Diagnoses of Atopic Dermatitis

DISEASE CATEGORY	DIFFERENTIAL DIAGNOSES
Dermatologic diseases	Contact dermatitis, seborrheic dermatitis, psoriasis, dyshidrotic eczema, eosinophilic pustular folliculitis, ichthyosis vulgaris
Neoplastic diseases	Cutaneous T-cell lymphoma, Langerhans cell histiocytosis
Immunodeficiencies	Hyper-IgE syndrome, severe combined immunodeficiency, Omenn syndrome, IPEX (immune dysregulation, polyendocrinopathy, enteropathy X-linked) syndrome
Infectious diseases	Scabies, cutaneous candidiasis, tinea versicolor
Nutritional deficiencies	Acrodermatitis enteropathica (zinc deficiency), essential fatty acid deficiency, biotin deficiency
Multisystemic disorders	Netherton syndrome, dermatitis herpetiformis

dermatitis, early age of onset, and atopy such as multiple food allergies. Patients with generalized eczema or adult-onset eczema can present as a diagnostic challenge. The differential diagnosis includes immunodeficiency (e.g., hyper-IgE syndrome, Omenn syndrome), malignancy (e.g., cutaneous T-cell lymphoma), zinc deficiency (i.e., acrodermatitis enteropathica), and celiac-associated dermatitis (i.e., dermatitis herpetiformis) (Table 1). AD children seldom present with failure to thrive, unless they are under severe dietary restriction. Failure to thrive should therefore prompt further investigation. Punch skin biopsies may be needed when the diagnosis is still unclear.

The prevalence of mild, moderate, and severe AD is 80%, 18%, and 2%, respectively. Most patients with mild to moderate disease have flexural, extensor, or facial involvement, whereas patients with severe disease often present with total-body involvement with or without erythroderma (Figure 1). Validated scales for assessing the severity of AD include Scoring of Atopic Dermatitis (SCORAD) and Eczema Area and Severity Index (EASI). These scoring systems or a simplified diagram documenting the extent of dermatitis are useful for more objective follow-up of the patient's progress.

Management of Atopic Dermatitis and Associated Conditions

Daily Maintenance Care

Changes in humidity can adversely affect AD symptoms. Dry conditions lead to increased transepidermal water loss and dry AD skin. Extreme heat, humidity, and sweating may lead to irritation of AD skin. AD patients are at increased risk for contact or irritant dermatitis, which may occur with over-the-counter topical skin medications that contain multiple ingredients. Wool or synthetic acrylic fabrics may also be irritating to AD skin.

To improve barrier function, AD patients should bathe or shower for 10 to 20 minutes once or twice daily, followed immediately by gently drying the skin and applying an emollient on the unaffected areas and a topical antiinflammatory medication on the affected areas. A petrolatum-based emollient is recommended in infants and young children because of its occlusive property. In older children and adults, the ointment may not be tolerated well because of its greasy feel, and another emollient or moisturizer may be chosen based on the patient's preference or experience.

Itch may continue to be a problem even if the rash has improved. The mechanisms of itch in AD are not fully understood but do not appear to be mediated solely by histamine. The use of first-generation antihistamines (diphenhydramine [Benadryl][1] and hydroxyzine [Vistaril]) in AD largely depend on their sedative

[1] Not FDA approved for this indication.

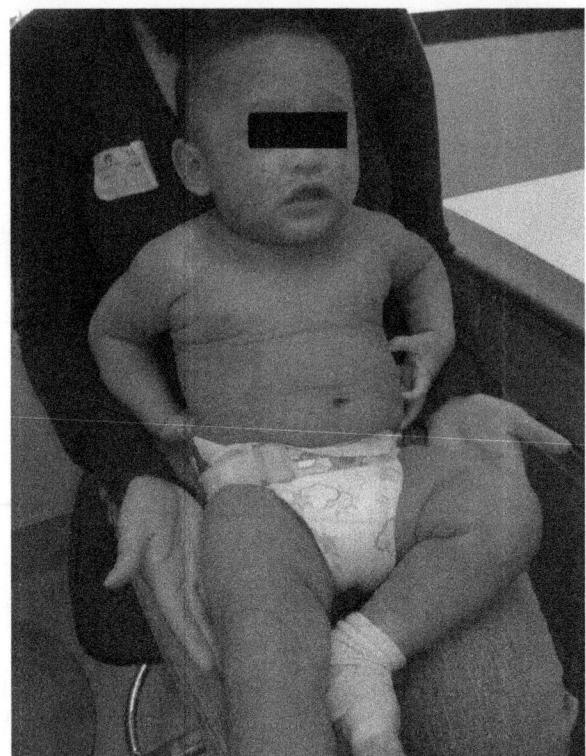

Figure 1 Generalized atopic dermatitis.

effects and are best used at bedtime. The second-generation, non-sedating antihistamines such as loratadine (Claritin)[1] and cetirizine (Zyrtec)[1] have not proved helpful in treating AD. Low-dose doxepin has been used anecdotally to treat itching in AD.

Topical and Systemic Medications

The first-line medication for AD is a topical corticosteroid (TCS). For mild AD, a TCS with group VI and VII potency (Table 2) may suffice. However, for moderate to severe AD, a TCS with at least group III to V potency is chosen to increase efficacy and to shorten the duration of need for these medications.

The use of TCS is confronted with various obstacles, including rare side effects such as skin atrophy, but mostly patients' or parents' misunderstanding of TCS. Studies have shown that twice-daily use of fluticasone propionate (Cutivate) 0.05% cream (group V) and desonide (DesOwen, Tridesilon) 0.05% ointment or aqueous gel (group V and VI, respectively) continuously up to 1 month in young children with AD results in no significant adverse effect. It is therefore important to clarify for patients or parents the safety and side effects based on the potency of the TCS.

Topical calcineurin inhibitors (TCI) (pimecrolimus [Elidel] 1% cream and Protopic/tacrolimus ointment) are alternative nonsteroidal antiinflammatory medications for AD. Elidel is indicated for mild to moderate AD in patients older than 2 years, whereas 0.03% and 0.1% Protopic are indicated for moderate to severe AD in patients 2 to 15 years old and in patients 16 years old or older, respectively. Both Elidel and Protopic have an FDA black box warning saying that their long-term use may be associated with cancer risk. However, a recent large longitudinal study has failed to confirm this risk. These medications continue to be useful alternatives for skin areas that are prone to atrophy, including the face, axillae, and groins.

A third class of topical medication, phosphodiesterase 4 inhibitor (crisaborole [Eucrisa] 2% ointment), has been approved by the FDA for patients 2 years and older with mild to moderate AD. A biologic dupilumab (Dupixent), which targets IL-4 and IL-13, has also been approved by the FDA for patients 12 years and older with moderate to severe AD.

---

[1] Not FDA approved for this indication.

TABLE 2 Classification of Topical Corticosteroids Based on Potency

GROUP	TOPICAL CORTICOSTEROIDS
I (most potent)	Clobetasol propionate 0.05% (Temovate) (cream, ointment, gel), betamethasone dipropionate, augmented 0.05% (Diprolene) (cream, ointment), diflorasone diacetate 0.05% (Psorcon) (ointment)
II	Amcinonide 0.1% (Cyclocort) (ointment), betamethasone dipropionate 0.05% (Diprosone) (ointment), mometasone furoate 0.1% (Elocon) (ointment), halcinonide 0.1% (Halog) (cream), fluocinonide 0.05% (Lidex) (gel, cream, ointment), desoximetasone (Topicort) (0.05% gel, 0.25% cream, 0.25% ointment)
III	Fluticasone propionate 0.005% (Cutivate) (ointment), amcinonide 0.1% (Cyclocort) (lotion, cream), diflorasone diacetate 0.05% (Florone) (cream), betamethasone valerate 0.1% (Valisone) (ointment)
IV	Flurandrenolide 0.05% (Cordran) (ointment), mometasone furoate 0.1% (Elocon) (cream), triamcinolone acetonide 0.1% (Kenalog) (cream), fluocinolone acetonide 0.025% (Synalar) (ointment), hydrocortisone valerate 0.2% (Westcort) (ointment)
V	Flurandrenolide 0.05% (Cordran) (cream), fluticasone propionate 0.05% (Cutivate) (cream), hydrocortisone butyrate 0.1% (Locoid) (cream), fluocinolone acetonide 0.025% (Synalar) (cream), desonide 0.05% (Tridesilon) (ointment), betamethasone valerate 0.1% (Valisone) (cream), hydrocortisone valerate 0.2% (Westcort) (cream), prednicarbate 0.1% (Dermatop) (cream)
VI	Alclometasone dipropionate 0.05% (Aclovate) (cream, ointment), fluocinolone acetonide 0.01% (Synalar) (solution, cream) (Derma-Smoothe/FS Oil), Desonide 0.05% (Tridesilon) (cream and aqueous gel)
VII (least potent)	Hydrocortisone 1%/2.5% (lotion, cream, ointment).

Data from Stoughton RB. Vasoconstrictor assay—specific applications. In Maibach HI, Surber C, editors. *Topical Corticosteroids.* Basel, Switzerland: Karger, 1992, pp 42–53.

Wet-wrap treatment, phototherapy, and systemic immunosuppressive therapies (e.g., cyclosporine [Sandimmune, Neoral],[1] azathioprine [Imuran],[1] methotrexate [Trexall],[1] and mycophenolate mofetil [CellCept])[1] are alternatives, but not approved by FDA, for severe AD patients. Because of the potential serious adverse effects associated with these treatments, referral to an allergist or dermatologist is recommended before their initiation.

Systemic corticosteroids usually are not recommended for AD because of their known adverse effects, including stunted growth in children, adrenal suppression, osteoporosis, and cataracts. A rebound of AD symptoms is common after the medication is stopped. If a systemic corticosteroid is used, it should be tapered over a short period (e.g., a week) while topical antiinflammatory treatment is intensified.

The efficacy and side effects of the following medications have not been established in AD: intravenous immunoglobulin (IVIG),[1] anti-IgE (omalizumab [Xolair]),[1] probiotics,[7] montelukast (Singulair),[1] Chinese medicinal herbs,[7] and fish oils.[1]

---

[1] Not FDA approved for this indication.
[7] Available as a dietary supplement.

TABLE 3	Predictability of ImmunoCAP-Specific IgE							
REACTION*	MILK	SOY	EGG	WHEAT	PEANUT	FISH	TREE NUTS
Reaction highly probable	>15 kU/L	>60 kU/L	>7 kU/L	>80 kU/L	>14 kU/L	>20 kU/L	>15 kU/L
Reaction highly probable (young children)	>5 kU/L (<1 y)		>2 kU/L (<2 y)				

*Because of their high positive predictive values, quantitative serum-specific IgE antibodies are used in the diagnosis of food allergies.

Food Allergies

At least 30% of children with moderate to severe AD have one or more food allergies, compared with 4% to 6% of the general population. Accurate diagnosis of food allergies in AD patients is crucial because it can prevent life-threatening anaphylaxis or unnecessary food restriction.

The diagnosis of food allergy involves one or more of the following: history taking, skin tests, serum-specific IgE tests, and food challenge. History taking is helpful in the diagnosis of food allergy in most patients. It is often useful to begin by asking the patients whether they have any problems or reactions with any of the seven food allergens: milk, egg, peanut, wheat, soybean, seafood, and tree nuts. These foods account for more than 90% of food allergies. Almost all food allergic reactions occur in the first hour. AD patients may complain of immediate worsening of itching after ingestion. Symptoms of anaphylactic reactions include throat-clearing, cough, shortness of breath, vomiting, dizziness, fainting, and headache, which may be attributed to hypotension. Most food allergic reactions also manifest with skin symptoms, including hives, swelling, or generalized itching.

Skin tests are useful in the context of negative test results because they have a negative predictive value of more than 95%. A positive test result has only a 50% positive predictive value.

Quantitative serum-specific IgE antibodies (ImmunoCAP, Phadia) have become useful in the diagnosis of food allergies because of their high positive predictive values (Table 3). These tests are also useful for deciding whether a food challenge is necessary to confirm the diagnosis.

Although history, skin tests, and serum-specific IgE values are useful in the diagnosis of food allergy, a double-blind, placebo-controlled food challenge remains the gold standard in diagnosing food allergy. Food challenge should be done in consultation with an allergist because of the risk of anaphylaxis.

Patients with confirmed food allergy should avoid any amount of the food allergen. Parents or patients should be instructed to read food allergen labels carefully. All packaged foods in the United States are required to label the contents of milk, eggs, peanuts, wheat, soybeans, fish, shellfish, or tree nuts. Organizations, such as the Food Allergy Research & Education, can provide patients and parents with useful information on potential hidden food allergens and alternative food sources.

AD children often have multiple food allergies, including cow's milk and soy, and the use of a hydrolyzed or amino acid–based formula can provide an alternative source of nutrition. For these patients, consultation with a dietitian can be helpful in managing food avoidance and nutrition needs.

Patients or parents of children with anaphylactic reactions should be prescribed and instructed on the use of an epinephrine autoinjector (EpiPen or Auvi-Q 0.15 mg for patients who weigh more than 15 kg but less than 30 kg; 0.3 mg for patients who weigh 30 kg or more, while Auvi-Q 0.1 mg for patients who weigh 7.5–15 kg).

Infants with severe AD who consume peanut products early have a 86% relative risk reduction in the development of peanut allergy. For any infants with AD under a year, clinicians should consider introducing peanut products early in their diet according to the guidelines of National Institute of Allergy and Infectious Disease, or consult an allergist.

Infections

Most AD patients are colonized by *S. aureus* on their skin lesions or in their nostrils. The frequency of colonization increases with AD severity. Exacerbation of AD is frequently associated with

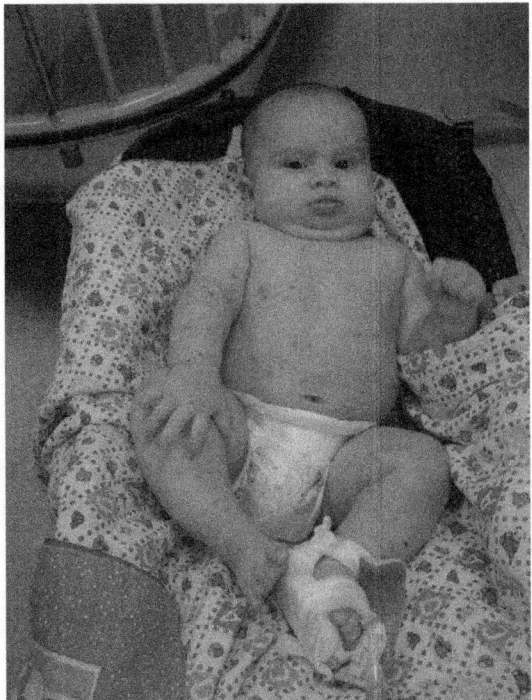

Figure 2 Eczema herpeticum.

secondary *S. aureus* skin infections. Other common skin pathogens in AD include group A β-hemolytic *Streptococcus* and herpes simplex virus (HSV), which causes eczema herpeticum (Figure 2). Many reports have documented invasive *S. aureus* infections such as bacteremia, septic arthritis, osteomyelitis, and endocarditis in AD patients. Persistent fever or focal limb pain should alert the physician to the possibility of these infections.

The reasons for the high rate of bacterial colonization and skin infections in AD are not completely understood. A defective skin barrier and decreased cutaneous innate immunity (i.e., deficiency in natural skin antibiotics) likely contribute to the frequency of skin infections in patients with AD.

Because of the concern about increasing bacterial resistance, antibiotics are not recommended for treating *S. aureus* colonization in patients with AD. Treating AD patients with methicillin-resistant *S. aureus* (MRSA) can be challenging, due to possibly recolonization from family contacts. Decolonization may be effective but controversial.

Inhalant Allergies and Asthma

Eighty-five percent of AD infants have concurrent respiratory allergies or are at risk for allergic rhinitis or asthma. However, whether inhalant allergens lead to a worsening of AD remains controversial. Randomized, double-blind, placebo-controlled studies have shown positive and negative effects of house dust mites (HDM) as a trigger for AD symptoms. Because there is no serious side effect associated with the use of HDM-proof bed and pillow encasings, unless cost is an issue, these encasings are recommended for AD patients with HDM sensitization. Further research is needed to confirm the role of inhalant allergens, including furry pets and pollens, as triggers for AD.

Investigational Treatments for Atopic Dermatitis

Because of the concern about potential side effects associated with existing therapies of AD, several agents are being investigated for the treatment of AD. They include anti-IL-13, anti-IL-22, anti-IL-31, and Janus kinase (JAK) inhibitors. Kappa opiod receptor agonists, systemic chymase inhibitors, and cannabinoid receptor agonists are potential anti-itch medications for AD. With improved understanding of the pathophysiology of AD, treatments for AD are likely going to be personalized in the future.

References

Beattie PE, Lewis-Jones MS: A comparative study of impairment of quality of life in children with skin disease and children with other chronic childhood diseases, *Br J Dermatol* 155:145–151, 2006.

Beck LA, Thaçi D, Hamilton JD, et al: Dupilumab treatment in adults with moderate-to-severe atopic dermatitis, *N Engl J Med* 371:130–139, 2014.

Du Toit G, Roberts G, Sayre PH, et al: Randomized trial of peanut consumption in infants at risk for peanut allergy, *N Engl J Med* 372:803–813, 2015.

Eichenfield LF, Basu S, Calvarese B, et al: Effect of desonide hydrogel 0.05% on the hypothalamic-pituitary-adrenal axis in pediatric subjects with moderate to severe atopic dermatitis, *Pediatr Dermatol* 24:289–295, 2007.

Elias PM: Barrier-repair therapy for atopic dermatitis: corrective lipid biochemical therapy, *Expert Rev Dermatol* 3:441–452, 2008.

Faught J, Bierl C, Barton B, Kemp A: Stress in mothers of young children with eczema, *Arch Dis Child* 92:683–686, 2007.

Friedlander SF, Hebert AA, Allen DB, for the Fluticasone Pediatrics Safety Study Group: Safety of fluticasone propionate cream 0.05% for the treatment of severe and extensive atopic dermatitis in children as young as 3 months, *J Am Acad Dermatol* 46:387–393, 2002.

Margolis DJ, Abuabara K, Hoffstad OJ, et al: Association between malignancy and topical use of pimecrolimus, *JAMA Dermatol* 151(6):594–599, 2015.

Ong PY: New insights in the pathogenesis of atopic dermatitis, *Pediatr Res* 75: 171–175, 2014.

Sampson HA: The evaluation and management of food allergy in atopic dermatitis, *Clin Dermatol* 21:183–192, 2003.

Sun D, Ong PY: Infectious complications in atopic dermatitis, *Immunol Allergy Clin North Am* 37:75–93, 2017.

Togias A, Cooper SF, Acebal ML, et al: Addendum guidelines for the prevention of peanut allergy in the United States: report of the National Institute of Allergy and Infectious Diseases-sponsored expert panel, *J Allergy Clin Immunol* 139:29–44, 2017.

BACTERIAL DISEASES OF THE SKIN

Method of
Dennis L. Stevens, MD, PhD

CURRENT DIAGNOSIS

- Most infections are superficial and local and not associated with systemic toxicity.
- Deeper infections may involve many layers of the soft tissues, including fascia and muscle.
- Systemic toxicity is always present in deeper infections.
- Rapid advancement of the local infection with areas of necrosis indicates more serious infections, including necrotizing and gangrenous processes.
- Streptococci and clostridial microorganisms are the cause of most gangrenous infections.
- Mixed aerobic and anaerobic microflora cause most necrotizing infections.

CURRENT THERAPY

- Local care and oral antibiotics chosen for the suspected or culture-proven pathogens are the usual treatments for most limited skin infections.
- Infections that show evidence of rapid advancement associated with bullae, blebs, crepitus, or necrosis require parenterally administered antibiotics and prompt surgical débridement.

- Morbidity and mortality rates associated with the deeper infections increase with delays in antibiotic therapy and surgical débridement.
- Antibiotic therapy should be guided by clinical presentation and changed if necessary when culture and sensitivity studies are available.

The spectrum of bacterial diseases of the skin ranges from superficial, localized, easily recognized, and treated skin eruptions to deep, aggressive, gangrenous, or necrotizing infections that may appear innocuous at first but quickly become life threatening. The prompt recognition and treatment of these infections are paramount in limiting morbidity and mortality. A healthy respect for the aggressiveness of gangrenous and necrotizing infections of the skin and soft tissues is developed by first harboring a high index of suspicion to provide early recognition and appropriate treatment before overwhelming clinical infection occurs.

Common Infections

Impetigo

Impetigo is the most common bacterial infection of the skin. It is highly contagious and can occur at any age from infancy to adulthood, but it is most common in preschool-age children. There are two classic forms of impetigo: nonbullous and bullous. Both forms have a predominantly staphylococcal cause, but they manifest with different morphologic characteristics.

Nonbullous (crusted) impetigo can be recognized by the development of a serous, yellow-brown exudate, which dries into a golden crust. Lesions rarely elicit pain but can be associated with erythema and pruritus. They are most common on exposed areas such as the hands, feet, face, and legs and are often associated with a minor traumatic event such as an insect bite, abrasion, or laceration. Crusted impetigo is usually caused by a heavy mixed flora of staphylococci and streptococci. Streptococcal impetigo has been associated with the postinfectious sequelae of poststreptococcal glomerulonephritis.

The bullous variety usually manifests as a rapidly spreading papule, which may progress to a thin-walled vesicle if the lesion is infected with *Staphylococcus aureus*, an organism that produces an exfoliative toxin. These lesions occur most often in warm, moist areas of the body. Predisposing factors include warm ambient temperatures, humidity, poor hygiene, and crowded living conditions.

Treatment of impetigo begins with eradication of the environmental factors thought to be influential in its development. Aggressive lesion débridement with mesh gauze sponges or brushes and antibacterial soap is encouraged. Special attention to hygiene and disinfection of towels and bedding are also necessary. Topical antibiotic treatment with mupirocin (Bactroban) or bacitracin[1] has been effective in mild to moderate cases. In more extensive cases, oral antibiotic therapy with a penicillinase-resistant synthetic penicillin (oxacillin) is the treatment of choice (Table 1). However, a high percentage of methicillin-resistant strains of *S. aureus* (MRSA) are isolated in institutional and community settings. Patients should be treated for at least 5 to 7 days. If no improvement is seen, lesions should be cultured and antibiotics adjusted appropriately.

Systemic complications from impetigo are very uncommon. Cellulitis has occurred but is usually susceptible to systemic antibiotic therapy. Septicemia and staphylococcal scaled skin syndrome are rare complications of impetigo. When they occur, systemic therapy is indicated.

Folliculitis

Folliculitis is a pyoderma that arises within a hair follicle. The process is known as a furuncle (boil) when the infection extends beyond the hair follicle. These lesions occur most frequently in the moist areas of the body and in areas subject to friction and perspiration.

---

[1]Not FDA approved for this indication.

TABLE 1	Suggested Antibiotic Therapy for Gram-Positive Bacterial Isolates	
ISOLATE	**ORAL**	**PARENTERAL**
GABHS	Penicillin G or V Erythromycin First-generation cephalosporin	Penicillin G Ampicillin/sulbactam (Unasyn) First-generation cephalosporin
Staphylococcus aureus (methicillin sensitive)	Penicillinase-resistant synthetic penicillin (Oxacillin)	First-generation cephalosporin Clindamycin (Cleocin) Oxacillin
Staphylococcus aureus (methicillin resistant)	Linezolid (Zyvox)	Vancomycin (Vancocin) Daptomycin (Cubicin) Linezolid (Zyvox) Ceftaroline (Teflaro)
Clostridial species	Penicillin G or V Clindamycin (Cleocin) Metronidazole (Flagyl)	Penicillin G Clindamycin Metronidazole

Abbreviation: GABHS = group A β-hemolytic *Streptococcus*.

Host factors known to predispose one to folliculitis include obesity, blood dyscrasias, defects in neutrophil function, immune deficiency states (e.g., diabetes, transplantation-related immunosuppression, acquired immunodeficiency syndrome [AIDS]), and treatment with corticosteroids or cytotoxic agents. The offending organism in most immunocompetent patients is *S. aureus*; however, when immunosuppression impairs host defenses, gram-negative organisms (*Klebsiella*, *Enterobacter*, and *Proteus* species) can be involved. *Pseudomonas* species such as *aeruginosa* or *cepacia* are associated with hot-tub folliculitis, which involves numerous hair follicles. It is usually self-limited, resolving in 7 to 10 days.

Successful treatment of folliculitis depends on correcting the predisposing factors that promote the development of this condition. For patients with localized disease, topical wound care including antibiotics such as mupirocin (Bactroban) is effective. Patients with furunculosis or multiple lesions with surrounding erythema of more than 2.5 cm should be treated with orally administered systemic antibiotics that are effective against *S. aureus*. Any fluctuant nodules or abscesses should be incised and drained. Patients with recurrent furunculosis should have their nares cultured for methicillin-susceptible *Staphylococcus aureus* (MSSA) or MRSA because nose rubbing and self-inoculation are the usual means of developing infection. This not only determines which type of *Staphylococcus* is causing the infection, but illustrates to the patient the importance of self-inoculation. Intranasal bacitracin or mupirocin (Bactroban) and daily baths with chlorhexidine (Hibiclens) or hexachlorophene (PHisoHex) (adults only) may break the cycle of nasal colonization and reinfection.

Cellulitis

Cellulitis is an acute infection of the skin and underlying soft tissues. It commonly begins as a hot, red, edematous, sharply defined eruption and may progress to lymphangitis, lymphadenitis, or in severe cases, necrotizing fasciitis and gangrene. Cellulitis usually occurs in local skin trauma caused by insect bites, abrasions, surgical wounds, contusions, or other cutaneous lacerations. Immunosuppressed patients are particularly susceptible to the progression of cellulitis to regional or systemic infections, and these patients should be treated aggressively with systemic antibiotics, drainage, and débridement when indicated. Cellulitis is 20-fold more common in patients with chronic venous stasis or lymphedema. Recurrent cellulitis may occur in patients at the exact site of saphenous donor site surgery.

Initial presentation is that of a rapidly expanding, tender, erythematous, indurated area of skin. An ascending lymphangitis may be present, especially in cellulitis involving an extremity often associated with regional lymphadenopathy. Systemic signs and symptoms can eventually evolve and when present, mandate hospitalization and treatment with systemic antibiotics. Offending organisms are most commonly group A β-hemolytic *Streptococcus* (GABHS), other group A species, and group C and group G streptococcal species. The IDSA guidelines suggest that *S. aureus* is associated with purulent infections (e.g., localized abscesses, furuncles, or carbuncles) and not really cellulitis which is, of course, non-purulent. The redness around an abscess is not cellulitis but merely local inflammation. This is an important consideration in selecting treatment options. In diabetic patients, cellulitis can be caused by group B *Streptococcus*.

Localized processes are treated with oral antibiotics (see Table 1). If fever, septicemia, or other signs of advancement to deeper tissues are present, the patient should be admitted to the hospital for blood and wound cultures, parenteral antibiotics (see Table 1), and observation. If a prompt response is not observed after parenteral antibiotic treatment, surgical exploration of the involved area may be indicated to establish an etiologic diagnosis and rule out the presence of necrotic or gangrenous tissue. Immunosuppressed patients or patients with recurrent cellulitis should be extensively examined to exclude chronic sources of infection, and these patients should be treated with parenteral antibiotics until the cellulitis resolves, followed by 5 to 7 days of oral antibiotics.

Abscess

Local skin signs and symptoms such as pain (dolor), redness (rubor), warmth (calor), and swelling (tumor) often denote an abscess and, like furunculosis, is usually caused by *S. aureus*. Loss of function associated with fluctuation may also indicate abscess formation. Localization of purulent fluid necessitates surgical drainage and local wound care. The administration of oral or parenteral antibiotic therapy should not be used routinely after incision and drainage of localized abscesses. They should be administered only when clinically indicated, and antibiotic therapy should be based on culture and sensitivity testing. Some recent studies suggest that oral treatment with trimethoprim/sulfamethoxazole (Bactrim)[1] improves resolution by about 24 hours and lessens but does not prevent the recurrence of infection.

Life-Threatening Infections
Group A β-Hemolytic Streptococcal Gangrene

Group A β-hemolytic streptococcal gangrene is an extremely rapidly progressing skin and soft tissue infection commonly caused by *Streptococcus pyogenes*. These organisms secrete hemolysins and streptolysins O and S, which are cardiotoxic, leukocytic, and responsible for the characteristic hemolysis. Gangrene results when the cutaneous blood vessels thrombose, a finding that is often associated with intense local pain. The involved skin is initially erythematous and indurated and quickly evolves to hemorrhagic blebs with focal necrotic zones. The potential for extensive tissue loss and mortality exists, especially if treatment is delayed. Prompt, aggressive tissue débridement and antibiotic therapy are necessary for a favorable outcome (see Table 1).

Synergistic Necrotizing Cellulitis

Synergistic necrotizing cellulitis (SNC) is an extremely aggressive, often lethal, polymicrobial infection of the skin and soft tissues that exhibits progressive invasion superficial to fascial planes. This condition may initially begin as a benign process with scant indication of its impending severity. The initial lesion is typically an erythematous, tender pustule or abscess with a small area of necrosis. The benign appearance of this lesion belies the widespread and aggressive tissue destruction that has occurred beneath it.

Direct inspection through skin incisions reveals extensive gangrene of the superficial tissues and fat that rarely involves the underlying fascia and muscles. These lesions characteristically exude a thin, brown, malodorous discharge, which manifests mixed flora with abundant polymorphonuclear leukocytes with a Gram stain.

---

[1] Not FDA approved for this indication.

Crepitus, which is caused by the accumulation of gas in the tissue produced by facultative or obligate anaerobes, can be palpated in 25% of patients, and it mandates immediate surgical attention.

The most common site of involvement is the perineum, which is involved in 50% of patients with SNC. Predisposing factors include perirectal abscess and ischiorectal abscess, both of which may track to the deeper structures of the pelvis, leading to abscess formation and subsequent septicemia. The thigh and leg are involved in approximately 40% of patients. This infection can occur after amputation and is usually associated with diabetes mellitus (75% of cases) or peripheral vascular disease (50% of cases). The relative immunosuppression and poor circulation that accompany these significant causes of morbidity are also responsible for upper extremity and neck SNC, which account for the remaining 10% of cases.

Synergistic necrotizing cellulitis is commonly caused by mixed flora originating in the gastrointestinal tract. Coliforms are the most prevalent aerobes (*Escherichia coli*, *Klebsiella*, *Proteus*), and anaerobic flora include *Bacteroides*, *Peptostreptococcus*, *Clostridium*, and *Fusobacterium*. The primary treatment modality is aggressive débridement of nonviable skin and subcutaneous tissues. This may involve several operations and dressing changes under general anesthesia, which should be performed until all necrotic tissue is removed. Rotation or free myocutaneous flaps and split-thickness skin grafting may cover areas of tissue loss when necessary. If the perineum is involved, fecal diversion by colostomy may be necessary to facilitate healing. Empiric parenteral antibiotics effective against polymicrobial gram-positive and gram-negative aerobic and anaerobic flora are also a mainstay of therapy. However, antibiotic coverage must be modified as soon as culture and susceptibility testing reveal specific offending organisms (Table 2) to reduce the emergence of resistant organisms.

Clostridial Myonecrosis

Clostridial myonecrosis (i.e., gas gangrene) is a destructive infectious process of muscle associated with infections of the skin and soft tissues. It is often associated with local crepitus and systemic signs of toxemia, which are caused by the anaerobic, gas-forming bacilli of the *Clostridium* species. This infection most often occurs after abdominal operations on the gastrointestinal tract; penetrating trauma, such as gunshot wounds, and frostbite can also expose muscle, fascia, and subcutaneous tissues to these organisms. Common to all these conditions is an environment containing tissue necrosis, low oxygen tension, and sufficient amounts of amino acids and calcium to allow germination of clostridial spores and production of the lethal α toxin.

Clostridia are gram-positive, spore-forming, obligate anaerobes that are widely found in soil contaminated with animal excreta.

They have also been isolated in the human gastrointestinal tract and skin, most importantly in the perineum and oropharynx. *Clostridium perfringens* is the most common isolate (in 80% of cases) and is among the fastest growing clostridial species, having a generation time under ideal conditions of approximately 16 minutes. This organism produces collagenases and proteases that cause widespread tissue destruction and produces α toxin, which is associated with the high mortality rate of clostridial myonecrosis. The α toxin, a phospholipase C, causes platelet-neutrophil complexes, vascular obstruction, and extensive compromised vascular perfusion, leading to necrosis of the muscle and overlying fascia, skin, and subcutaneous tissues.

Historically, clostridial myonecrosis was a disease associated with battle injuries, but 60% of current cases occur after trauma: 50% after automobile accidents and the remainder after crush injuries, industrial accidents, and gunshot wounds. Mortality can be the result of a failure to recognize that clostridial infection is underway, which leads to a delay in the débridement of devitalized tissues. Patients often complain of a sudden onset of pain at the site of trauma or surgical wound, which increases rapidly in severity and extends beyond the original borders of the wound. The skin initially exhibits tense edema, but its pale appearance progresses to a magenta hue. Hemorrhagic bullae and a thin, watery, foul-smelling discharge are common. A Gram stain examination of wound discharge reveals abundant gram-positive rods with a paucity of leukocytes.

The diagnosis of gas gangrene is based on the appearance of the muscle on direct visualization by surgical exposure, because many changes are not apparent when inspected through a small traumatic wound. Initially, the muscle is pale, edematous, and unresponsive to stimulation. As the disease process continues, the muscle becomes frankly gangrenous, black, and extremely friable. This occurs as a late event and is often accompanied by septicemia and shock. Despite profound hypotension and impending organ failure, these patients may be remarkably alert and extremely sensitive to their surroundings. They feel their impending doom and often panic just before slipping into toxic delirium and eventually into coma.

The clinical features should arouse suspicion early in the course, so the disease can be recognized and treated with aggressive surgical débridement. Gas in the wound is a relatively late finding, and by the time crepitation is observed, the patient may be near death. Approximately 15% of blood cultures are positive, but this is also a late finding. Serum creatinine kinase levels, although relatively nonspecific, are always elevated in cases with muscle involvement.

The mortality rate for gas gangrene is as high as 60%. It is highest in cases involving the abdominal wall and lowest in those affecting the extremities. Among the signs that prognosticate a poor outcome are leukopenia, thrombocytopenia, hemolysis, and severe renal failure. Myoglobinuria is common and can contribute significantly to worsening renal function. Frank hemorrhage may also be present and indicates disseminated intravascular coagulation.

Successful treatment of this life-threatening infection depends on early recognition and débridement of devitalized and infected tissues. Hyperbaric oxygen and systemic antibiotics are important adjuncts. Surgical intervention should include wide débridement of all necrotic tissue and amputation if extremities are involved. Hyperbaric oxygen (100% O_2 at 3 atm) has been reported to reduce associated tissue loss and mortality; however, core treatment is surgical débridement, and it should never be delayed to arrange for hyperbaric oxygen treatments. In animal studies of gas gangrene, hyperbaric oxygen was not efficacious, whereas clindamycin (Cleocin) treatment had dramatic effects in reducing mortality. A parenteral antibiotic is directed toward the offending organism (see Table 1). Clindamycin[1] is the treatment of choice because of its ability to suppress toxin production. Cardiovascular collapse mandates careful monitoring of intravenous fluid resuscitation, which may require large volumes. Failure to adequately resuscitate these patients compromises therapy by limiting oxygen delivery and antibiotic distribution to the affected tissues and may promote progression to multisystem organ failure.

TABLE 2	Suggested Parenteral Antibiotic Therapy for Mixed Infections
ORGANISMS	**PRIMARY CHOICE**
Aerobic (must include an agent effective against anaerobic organisms)	Amikacin (Amikin) Aztreonam (Azactam) Ceftriaxone (Rocephin) Ciprofloxacin (Cipro) Gentamicin (Garamycin) Levofloxacin (Levaquin) Tobramycin (Nebcin)
Anaerobic (must include an agent effective against aerobic organisms)	Clindamycin (Cleocin) Metronidazole (Flagyl)
Aerobic and anaerobic	Ampicillin/sulbactam (Unasyn) Imipenem/cilastatin (Primaxin) Meropenem (Merrem) Piperacillin/tazobactam (Zosyn) Tigecycline (Tygacil)

---

[1]Not FDA approved for this indication.

A less life-threatening form of this disease is known as clostridial cellulitis. In this process, the bacterial tissue invasion is primarily superficial, extending to the fascial layer without muscle involvement. Prompt recognition and treatment can reduce morbidity and mortality. Spontaneous gas gangrene caused by *Clostridium septicum* can occur in the absence of trauma in patients with gastrointestinal lesions such as carcinoma of the colon.

Necrotizing Fasciitis

Necrotizing fasciitis is an aggressive soft tissue infection involving the fascia with extensive undermining and tracking along anatomic planes. Necrotizing fasciitis is probably an incorrect designation, since tissue from the deep muscles to the epidermis is generally destroyed. A better designation would likely be necrotizing infection. This process usually occurs in patients with significant comorbidity, such as diabetes mellitus or peripheral vascular disease, but it is also seen in obese or malnourished patients and intravenous drug abusers. Cellulitis is a frequent occurrence, and progressive necrosis to subcutaneous tissue results from thrombosis of the perforating vessels. Necrotizing fasciitis can be caused by single organisms such as GABHS and staphylococci (MRSA), *Vibrio vulnificus* or *Aeromonas hydrophila*, or a combination of a variety of organisms, including aerobic streptococci, staphylococci, and coliforms, as well as anaerobic *Peptostreptococcus* and *Bacteroides*. Ninety percent of these infections have a polymicrobial cause, and it is common to culture up to five organisms from the fascial planes involved with this infection.

Polymicrobial necrotizing fasciitis most commonly evolves from a benign-appearing skin lesion (80% of cases). Minor abrasions, insect bites, injection sites, and perirectal abscesses have been implicated. Rare cases have been reported in women with Bartholin's gland abscess, from which the infection has spread to fascial planes of the perineum and thigh. The remaining 20% of patients have no visible skin lesion. Surgical procedures, especially bowel resections, and penetrating trauma can be complicated by superficial wound infections that evolve into necrotizing fasciitis. The infection commonly involves the buttocks and perineum, which results from untreated perirectal abscesses or decubitus ulcers; intravenous drug abusers commonly participate in "skin popping," which leads to infections of the upper extremities.

Fifty percent of group A streptococcal necrotizing fasciitis patients have a portal of entry such as an insect bite, slivers, surgical procedures, or burns, whereas the other 50% have no portal of entry, and the infection begins at the exact site of nonpenetrating trauma, such as a muscle strain or bruise. This idiopathic form, commonly known as spontaneous necrotizing fasciitis, is particularly dangerous because of the frequent delay in diagnosis.

For those with a portal of entry, the initial presentation is a slowly advancing cellulitis that progresses to a firm, tense, woody feel of the subcutaneous tissues. This entity may be distinguished from other aggressive anaerobic soft tissue infections (e.g., SNC) by the brawny, pale, erythematous appearance of the skin overlying subcutaneous tissues that are unyielding, making fascial planes and muscle groups indistinguishable during palpation. Often, a broad, erythematous tract along the route of the underlying fascial plane can be discerned through the skin. If an open wound exists, probing the edges with a blunt instrument permits ready dissection of the superficial fascia well beyond the wound margins, and this is the most important diagnostic feature of necrotizing fasciitis. On direct inspection, the fascia is swollen and dully gray in appearance, with stringy areas of fat necrosis. A thin, brown exudate can be expressed from the wound, but frank purulent drainage is rare. These wounds are remarkably insensate when found and mandate immediate débridement.

As with other gangrenous soft tissue infections, the most important component of the treatment plan is aggressive, total débridement of all devitalized and necrotic tissue. This often necessitates frequent operations and dressing changes. Wide débridement and parenteral antibiotics have a profound effect on survival, and limited or staged débridement has no place in the treatment of this very aggressive, life-threatening infection. Parenteral antibiotics (see Table 2) should be directed against the polymicrobial aerobic and anaerobic microorganisms isolated from these infections. Every effort should be made to quickly identify the offending organisms, and antibiotic therapy should be changed accordingly.

In patients with no defined portal of entry, severe pain at the site of previous nonpenetrating trauma is common. Early in the course, there may be no cutaneous evidence of infection. Severe pain and fever may be the only presenting symptoms. These patients usually have a slightly elevated white blood cell count with a left shift and an elevated pulse. Later, erythema, induration, and warmth occur and may rapidly progress to violaceous skin, ecchymosis, and blister formation. A markedly elevated creatine phosphokinase level in a patient with any erythematous rash may suggest a necrotizing process. By the time these late cutaneous findings are present, most patients have evidence of shock and organ failure. Misdiagnosis and delay in diagnosis are common and associated with significant morbidity and mortality. Surgical exploration with débridement of infected and necrotic tissue in addition to systemic antibiotic therapy directed toward the aerobic *Streptococcus* organism can result in decreased morbidity and mortality (see Table 1).

Special Circumstances

Fournier's Gangrene

Fournier's gangrene is a necrotizing fasciitis that originates as a necrotic black area on the scrotum of male patients or the labia of female patients, and it most often has a cryptogenic origin. In my experience, Fournier's gangrene occurs more commonly without a predisposing event or after routine, uncomplicated hemorrhoidectomy. Less commonly, this condition has occurred after urologic manipulation or as a late complication of deep anorectal suppuration.

Fournier's gangrene is characterized by necrosis of the skin and soft tissues of the scrotum or perineum and is associated with a fulminant, painful, and severely toxic infection. Definitive diagnosis is made by identification of a necrotic black area on the scrotum associated with local and systemic signs of infection. Left untreated, death ensues from uncontrolled, severe systemic sepsis and multiple-organ failure. Prompt recognition and treatment can minimize tissue loss, especially the skin and soft tissues of the scrotum or labia and perineum, and may prevent complete loss of genitalia.

The infection is often polymicrobial, as with necrotizing fasciitis, with several species of aerobic and anaerobic bacteria predominating. Successful treatment is based on early recognition and vigorous surgical débridement, occasionally including diversion of the fecal stream. Empiric treatment is appropriate until results of culture and susceptibility testing are available (see Table 2). The therapeutic benefit of hyperbaric oxygen treatments has not been proved, and it should be used only as an adjunct to surgical débridement.

Ecthyma Gangrenosum

Occasionally, hospitalized patients with overwhelming pseudomonal septicemia develop a patchy dermal and subcutaneous necrosis. Although sepsis caused by *Pseudomonas aeruginosa* is often indistinguishable from other types of gram-negative sepsis, a characteristic skin lesion may develop with erythematous macular eruptions that quickly become bullous with central ulceration and necrosis. This lesion may resemble a decubitus ulcer with the characteristic black eschar. There are usually multiple lesions occurring in different stages of development. They may concentrate on the extremities or the gluteal region. These lesions may be distinguished from the lesions of pyoderma gangrenosum (a noninfectious dermatosis) by their association with clinical signs of infection (i.e., fever and leukocytosis) in addition to the isolation of *P. aeruginosa* from culture of the lesion.

Treatment is primarily administration of antimicrobial therapy effective against the *Pseudomonas* organism and by débridement of the multiple lesions. This may lessen the bacterial burden, perhaps allowing greater antibiotic efficacy.

Sea Water and Fresh Water Infections

Infections caused by *V. vulnificus* and *A. hydrophilia* can be extremely aggressive, with necrosis often occurring within hours and necessitating rapid, wide débridement. Although infections caused by these organisms cannot be differentiated from those caused by mixed infections, a history of exposure to sea water (*V. vulnificus*) or fresh water (*A. hydrophila*) and the rapidity with which the infection spreads often suggest the cause of the infection. The antibiotics of choice for *V. vulnificus* infection are doxycycline (Vibramycin) or tetracycline and an aminoglycoside. In patients with impaired renal function, chloramphenicol (Chloromycetin) may be used. *A. hydrophila* is susceptible to cephalosporins such as ceftazidime (Fortaz), cefuroxime (Ceftin), and fluoroquinolones such as levofloxacin (Levaquin) and ciprofloxacin (Cipro).

Conclusion

The many types of soft tissue infections caused by bacteria may be distinguished by their presenting signs, symptoms, and body location and by the time course of the pathologic processes unique to each. Early recognition is of paramount importance to an effective treatment plan, which most often includes aggressive surgical débridement and specific antimicrobial therapy. This approach can often minimize tissue damage and promote recovery.

References

Adinolfi MF, Voros DC, Moustoukas NM, et al: Severe systemic sepsis resulting from neglected perineal infections, *South Med J* 76:746–749, 1983.

Craig ML, Hardin WD Jr, Fox LS, et al: Ecthyma gangrenosum: A deadly complication, *Hosp Physician* 23:65–71, 1987.

Moustoukas NM, Nichols RL, Voros D: Clostridial sepsis: Usual clinical presentations, *South Med J* 78:440–445, 1985.

Nichols RL, Florman S: Clinical presentations of soft-tissue infections and surgical site infections, *Clin Infect Dis* 33(Suppl 2):84–93, 2001.

Nichols RL: Postoperative infection in the age of drug-resistant gram-positive bacteria [review], *Am J Med* 104(Suppl 5A):11S–16S, 1998.

Singer AJ, Talan DA: Management of skin abscesses in the era of methicillin-resistant Staphylococcus aureus, *N Engl J Med* 370(11):1039–1047, 2014.

Stevens DL, Bisno DL, Chambers HF, et al: Practice guidelines for the diagnosis and management of skin and soft tissue infections: 2014 update by the Infectious Diseases Society of America, *Clin Infect Dis* 50(2):e10–e52, 2014.

Stevens DL, Bryant AE: Necrotizing soft-tissue infections, *N Engl J Med* 377:2253–2265, 2017.

BULLOUS DISEASES

Method of
Diya F. Mutasim, MD

CURRENT DIAGNOSIS

- Clinical
- Histology (always required)
- Direct immunofluorescence (always required)
- Indirect immunofluorescence (sometimes required)
- Antibody specificity for the antigen by enzyme-linked immunosorbent assay (ELISA) (rarely required)

CURRENT THERAPY

- Topical steroids
- Systemic glucocorticoids
- Steroid-sparing (adjuvant) immunosuppressive agents
  - Azathioprine (Imuran)[1]
  - Mycophenolate mofetil (Cellcept)[1]
  - Methotrexate (Trexall)[1]
  - Cyclosporine (Neoral)[1]
  - Cyclophosphamide (Cytoxan)[1]
  - Dapsone
  - Tetracycline (Sumycin)[1]
- Other
  - Niacinamide, nicotinamide[1]
  - High-dose intravenous immunoglobulin (IVIg) (Gammagard)[1]
  - Rituximab (Rituxan)[1]
  - Plasmapheresis, immunoapheresis

[1]Not FDA approved for this indication.

Epidemiology

The primary lesion in bullous diseases is a vesicle or a bulla. Autoimmune bullous diseases result from immune dysregulation that increases with age, hence the incidence of autoimmune bullous diseases is higher in the elderly. This group of disorders is heterogeneous, and generalizations about the epidemiology cannot be made.

Risk Factors

In general, predisposition to autoimmune bullous diseases is genetic and manifests as loss of tolerance toward self antigens followed by a T-cell and B-cell response resulting in antibody production. Age may be a risk factor in the development of bullous pemphigoid and mucous membrane pemphigoid. Pemphigus vulgaris has a higher incidence among persons of Jewish ancestry.

Pathophysiology

Autoimmune bullous diseases result from an immune response against proteins of desmosomes or the epidermal (or other epithelial) basement membrane. The pemphigus group of diseases is associated with antibodies to different desmosomal proteins. There is strong direct experimental evidence that these antibodies cause acantholysis and blister formation directly without significant participation of cellular components of the immune system. The subepidermal autoimmune bullous diseases, however, result from antibodies against one or more components of the basement membrane that activate the complement system. The latter results in chemoattraction of inflammatory cells, particularly eosinophils and neutrophils, to the basement membrane, as well as activation of local mast cells with degranulation of their cytoplasmic granules, resulting in the release of mediators that further attract inflammatory cells. Both complement and inflammatory cells are required for blister formation. Experimental animals that lack complement or leukocytes fail to develop lesions when injected with patients' serum antibodies.

Prevention

There are no methods for preventing autoimmune bullous diseases. These disorders result from genetically controlled immune dysregulation.

Clinical Manifestations

Clinical manifestations are described for each disease separately under the section on therapy.

Complications

Severe blistering can lead to extensive erosions that heal slowly, especially in the elderly and in those with nutritional deficiencies or systemic disease. Slow healing of extensive erosions predisposes patients to considerable loss of fluids and electrolytes as well as secondary bacterial infection and sepsis. Superficial erosions can become ulcers owing to increased local pressure in immobile and bedridden patients. Temperature regulation can also be compromised following loss of large areas of epidermis. Over the past several decades, mortality from bullous disease has decreased significantly. At present, the common causes of death are complications of the pharmacologic agents used in the treatment.

Diagnosis

The diagnosis of autoimmune bullous diseases requires clinical evaluation, histopathology, direct immunofluorescence, and indirect immunofluorescence. The ideal specimen for direct immunofluorescence should be from normal-appearing skin immediately adjacent to a lesion (perilesional skin). Immunofluorescence tests are usually performed in specialized immunopathology laboratories and are best interpreted by a dermatopathologist with special expertise in the area of immunofluorescence and autoimmune bullous diseases.

Differential Diagnosis

An accurate diagnosis is essential for predicting the course and prognosis of a disease as well as for choosing therapy. Autoimmune bullous diseases overlap clinically and histologically, hence the need for immunofluorescence studies. For example, epidermolysis bullosa acquisita can have clinical and histologic overlap with both bullous pemphigoid and linear IgA disease. The three diseases, however, have different courses and therapeutic responses and may be easily differentiated on the basis of immunofluorescence tests.

Treatment
Principles

Because autoimmune bullous disorders result from immune dysregulation, the principle of treatment is immune modulation. Immune modulation can be accomplished by several methods: blocking antibody production by B cells and plasma cells, eliminating antibodies from the circulation, suppressing inflammation, or inducing resistance of target epithelial cells to separation and blister formation. Antibody production by B cells and plasma cells may be blocked by destroying the B cell lineage or suppressing activation of T or B cells. The former is accomplished by the drug rituximab (Rituxan) and, to a lesser degree, cyclophosphamide (Cytoxan), and the latter may be accomplished by many immunosuppressive agents including corticosteroids, azathioprine (Imuran), cyclosporine (Neoral), cyclophosphamide, methotrexate (Trexall), and mycophenolate mofetil (Cellcept). Antibodies may be eliminated from circulation by plasmapheresis, high-dose intravenous immunoglobulin (IVIg, Gammagard), and immunoadsorption.

Inflammation that is required for blister formation, especially in subepidermal bullous diseases, may be suppressed by several agents. These include systemic and topical corticosteroids, dapsone, tetracyclines, erythromycin, nicotinamide, and etanercept (Enbrel). Although not yet available, agents that experimentally inhibit signal transduction and agents that inhibit apoptosis can induce resistance of the target epidermal or epithelial cell to separation (acantholysis) and blister formation.

The choice of agents in therapy of bullous diseases requires evaluation of both disease-specific parameters and patient-specific parameters. Disease-specific parameters include the pathophysiology of the disease and its severity; patient-specific parameters include age and concomitant illness such as diabetes, hypertension, active infection, or cancer. There are very few controlled studies that provide high-quality evidence for bullous disease therapy. This is primarily a result of the rarity of many of these disorders. Because of the relative frequency of bullous pemphigoid, some controlled studies have been performed on the disease in Europe. Most of the evidence for bullous disease therapy is available from case reports, case series, and personal experience.

Pharmacologic Treatment
Glucocorticoids

Glucocorticoids (prednisone, prednisolone) have both antiinflammatory and immunosuppressive effects. Long-term use of glucocorticoids is associated with well-known adverse effects.

Azathioprine

Azathioprine (Imuran)[1] interferes with de novo purine synthesis and hence DNA synthesis. This results in suppression of T-cell function and a decrease in B-cell antibody production. In low doses (1–2 mg/kg/day), azathioprine is usually well tolerated. In higher doses (2–4 mg/kg/day), bone marrow may be suppressed, resulting in leukopenia (most commonly) and, less commonly, thrombocytopenia and anemia. Severe bone marrow suppression can occur in patients who are homozygous deficient for the enzyme thiopurine methyltransferase. Other adverse effects include hepatotoxicity and gastrointestinal toxicity as well as pancreatitis and are all dose related. Allopurinol (Zyloprim) is contraindicated in patients receiving azathioprine because it results in an increase in the blood level of azathioprine.

Mycophenolate Mofetil

Mycophenolate mofetil[1] is a purine analogue antimetabolite that inhibits inosine monophosphate dehydrogenase, resulting in suppression of purine and DNA synthesis and hence suppression of both T and B cell function. Mycophenolate mofetil is usually well tolerated.

Methotrexate

Methotrexate[1] is an antimetabolite and a folic acid analogue. Its metabolites inhibit folate-dependent enzymes of de novo purine and thymidylate synthesis. This results in the suppression of DNA and RNA synthesis, which causes decreased lymphocyte function and hence immune modulation.

Cyclophosphamide

Cyclophosphamide[1] is an alkylating agent that binds DNA, resulting in cell cycle arrest, DNA repair, and cell death. The most susceptible cells reside in rapidly proliferating tissues. The toxicity of cyclophosphamide is significantly higher than that of azathioprine, mycophenolate mofetil, and methotrexate. Acute myelosuppression is common, with a nadir at 6 to 10 days and recovery in 2 to 3 weeks. Both cellular and humoral immunity are suppressed.

Cyclosporine

Cyclosporine[1] significantly suppresses cellular immunity and preferentially inhibits antigen-triggered signal transduction in T lymphocytes, which results in decreased expression of several lymphokines. Cyclosporine forms complexes with the receptor protein cyclophilin in the cytoplasm. The complex binds and inhibits calcineurin, resulting in failure of T cells to respond to antigenic stimulation.

Several drugs can interact with cyclosporine and influence its blood level. Agents that can increase cyclosporine blood level include calcium channel antagonists (diltiazem [Cardizem], nicardipine [Cardene], and verapamil [Calan]), systemic antifungal agents (fluconazole [Diflucan], itraconazole [Sporanox], and ketoconazole [Nizoral]), antibacterials (clarithromycin [Biaxin], erythromycin), methylprednisolone (Medrol), other drugs (allopurinol [Zyloprim], bromocriptine [Parlodel], danazol [Danocrine], metoclopramide [Reglan], colchicine [Colcrys], and amiodarone [Cordarone]), and grapefruit juice.

Dapsone

Dapsone is highly effective in neutrophil-mediated conditions. The mechanism of action of dapsone is not well understood. Its clinical benefit in inflammatory conditions probably results from inhibition of neutrophil chemotaxis. Dapsone is associated with multiple potential adverse effects that include dose-related hemolysis, methemoglobulinemia (which is common and may be severe in patients who are genetically predisposed), and agranulocytosis (not dose-related and usually occurs in the first 3 months of therapy).

Tetracycline

Tetracycline (Sumycin),[1] doxycycline (Vibramycin),[1] and minocycline (Minocin)[1] have been used interchangeably for the treatment of subepidermal, inflammation-mediated, bullous diseases. Their mechanism of action is not clear.

Niacinamide (Nicotinamide)

Niacinamide[1] is a vitamin whose mechanism of action in cutaneous disorders including autoimmune bullous diseases is not known.

High-Dose Intravenous Immunoglobulin

IVIg[1] is a purified human source of immunoglobulin that is given as a slow infusion over 6 to 8 hours. Treatment is repeated every 3 to 4 weeks. IVIg is highly expensive.

Rituximab

Rituximab[1] is a chimeric monoclonal antibody against CD20 on the surface of pre-B, mature B, and malignant B cells and is not expressed on stem, pro-B or plasma cells. B cells are depleted primarily by antibody-dependent cellular cytotoxicity and, to a lesser degree, by complement-dependent cytotoxicity or apoptosis. Rituximab is given in different regimens, including 375 mg/m²/week (approximately 500 mg for an average-size adult) for 4 consecutive weeks, or 1000 mg once or on two occasions 2 weeks apart.

Plasmapheresis and Immunoapheresis

Plasmapheresis and immunoapheresis are procedures that aim to physically remove pathogenic antibodies. Plasmapheresis consists of withdrawing the patient's blood, filtering cellular elements from the plasma, and returning the cellular components to the patient. Immunoapheresis consists of exposing the patient's plasma to an immunoglobulin-binding matrix that contains the disease-specific antigen. Plasmapheresis and immunoapheresis are usually used in patients who are resistant to other therapies. Plasmapheresis or immunoapheresis is accompanied by immunosuppressive drugs to prevent the rebound phenomenon of excessive antibody production.

Treatment of Individual Disorders

Pemphigoid

There are three forms of pemphigoid: bullous pemphigoid (primary skin involvement); mucous membrane pemphigoid (primary mucosal disease), previously referred to as cicatricial pemphigoid; and pemphigoid gestationis (bullous pemphigoid in pregnant women), previously called herpes gestationis. The pemphigoid group of diseases shares the histology of a subepithelial vesicle with usually eosinophil-rich infiltrate, skin-bound IgG and C3 along the basement membrane, and circulating IgG antibodies against two hemidesmosomal proteins of the basement membrane.

Bullous Pemphigoid. Bullous pemphigoid affects primarily persons older than 60 years and is rarely reported in children. Lesions have a predilection for the inner thighs, groin, axillae, neck, and abdomen. The course of bullous pemphigoid is variable. The disease is self-limited within 5 years, and the mortality from the disease is low.

Because blisters in bullous pemphigoid result from an abnormal immune response that is mediated by inflammatory cells, therapy for bullous pemphigoid should suppress inflammation or the immune response. Potent topical steroids may be considered for patients with localized disease. Although potent topical steroids lead to rapid resolution of a lesion at its earliest manifestation, they are impractical for patients with generalized disease because they do not prevent new lesions. Patients with generalized bullous pemphigoid require systemic therapy. Glucocorticoids are the most commonly used agents. Prednisone (or methylprednisolone) is sufficient as the only therapy in most cases. The dose varies between 0.2 and 0.5 mg/kg/day depending on the severity of the disease, the age of the patient, and the patient's general health status. A clinical response is usually obtained within 1 to 2 weeks and is manifested by healing of existing lesions and cessation of new blister formation. The dose is then gradually decreased by relatively large amounts initially (approximately 10 mg) and smaller amounts

(2.5–5 mg) subsequently. If the patient develops a flare of lesions during the tapering phase, the dose may be increased to the previous level or higher and maintained longer before further, slower tapering. In many patients, prednisone may be decreased to 5 mg every day or completely discontinued after 6 months.

For patients who require a high dose of steroid for either clearing or maintenance, adjuvant therapy with another agent should be considered in order to avoid the long-term adverse effects of corticosteroids. These drugs include azathioprine[1] (1–3 mg/kg/day in two equally divided doses), mycophenolate mofetil[1] (1000–3000 mg/day or 40 mg/kg/day in two divided doses), and methotrexate[1] (10–15 mg/week). The dose of the second drug may be decreased a few months after clinical remission, slowly tapered, and ultimately discontinued. Dapsone[1] and sulfapyridine[1] are used less commonly and may be effective. Dapsone may be commenced at 25 to 50 mg/day and increased as needed by 25 mg every week until a beneficial effect is obtained. The maximum dose of dapsone is 250 mg/day.

Plasmapheresis and high-dose IVIg[1] are reserved for more resistant cases. Antibiotics of the tetracycline family as well as erythromycin[1] have been used alone or in combination with niacinamide[1] and have been shown to have some benefit. The dose of tetracycline[1] is 500 mg four times daily and niacinamide 500 mg three times daily. Minocycline[1] or doxycycline[1] in a dose of 100 mg twice daily may be substituted for patients who do not tolerate tetracycline. In my view, a tetracycline with niacinamide is indicated in two situations. In mild cases, the combination alone can lead to a clinical remission. In patients with extensive disease, the addition of this combination to prednisone can have a corticosteroid-sparing effect.

Mucous Membrane Pemphigoid. Therapy for mucous membrane pemphigoid varies with the disease location, extent, and severity. In limited oral disease, local therapy with topical anesthetic agents and topical glucocorticoids in addition to oral hygiene can suffice. The steroid may be applied under occlusion with a prosthetic device or may be injected intralesionally. Patients with extensive oral involvement can require systemic therapy.

Dapsone[1] is effective in some patients with oral mucous membrane pemphigoid. The drug may be started at 50 mg daily and increased gradually. Tetracyclines,[1] with or without niacinamide,[1] may be effective. In patients with severe oral disease and in patients with ocular, pharyngeal, or laryngeal involvement, systemic glucocorticoids, in combination with cyclophosphamide[1] are indicated. In my experience, most patients have an excellent response, with a prolonged remission after treatment with the combination of prednisone (1 mg/kg/day for 6 months) and cyclophosphamide (1–2 mg/kg/day for 18–24 months).

Azathioprine[1] and mycophenolate mofetil[1] are generally less effective but may be used if there are contraindications to steroid or cyclophosphamide use. High-dose IVIg[1] may be used for patients who are refractory to other therapy.

Patients with severe ocular scarring might benefit from cryotherapy ablation of eyelashes. Ocular surgery is contraindicated when the disease is active. Surgical intervention may cause severe flares of the disease.

Epidermolysis Bullosa Acquisita

Unlike bullous pemphigoid and other subepidermal autoimmune bullous diseases, epidermolysis bullosa acquisita is generally resistant to therapy. The disease waxes and wanes, with periods of exacerbation and remission. Trauma contributes to blister formation, especially in the classic form of epidermolysis bullosa acquisita. The inflammatory form of epidermolysis bullosa acquisita responds more easily to therapy than the classic form.

Because of the neutrophil predominance in the inflammatory form, patients might respond to dapsone.[1] The drug may be started at a dose of 50 mg daily and increased by 50 mg every week until clinical remission (usually 100–250 mg). The dose is maintained

---

[1] Not FDA approved for this indication.

[1] Not FDA approved for this indication.

for several months. If the patient remains in remission, the dose may be decreased slowly and ultimately discontinued. Colchicine[1] 0.6 mg two or three times daily is variably effective. Patients who do not tolerate or do not respond to colchicine and dapsone may be treated with oral glucocorticoids such as prednisone in a dose of 0.5–1 mg/kg/day in divided doses. The response is variable. If there is no response to glucocorticoids or the patient develops adverse effects, cyclosporine[1] 4–6 mg/kg/day may be initiated and is usually associated with a rapid response. Once disease activity is controlled, the dose may be slowly decreased. Cyclosporine should be discontinued if there is no response in a few weeks.

The duration of treatment varies with the course of the disease. The same agents used for the inflammatory form may be used for the classic form. The latter is generally more resistant to treatment. Patients who fail to respond may be treated with immunosuppressive agents such as azathioprine,[1] cyclophosphamide,[1] mycophenolate,[1] or methotrexate[1] in a manner similar to pemphigus vulgaris, bullous pemphigoid, or mucous membrane pemphigoid. Patients who are resistant to these agents may be treated with extracorporeal photochemotherapy or with IVIg[1] alone or in conjunction with plasmapheresis.

Dermatitis Herpetiformis

Dermatitis herpetiformis results from an immune response to gluten and manifests as pruritic papulovesicles over the elbows, knees, buttocks, and scalp. A gluten-free diet is extremely helpful and is often associated with a marked decrease in the requirement for pharmacologic therapy. A strict gluten-free diet can result in complete remission of the disease without requiring dapsone. Reinstitution of gluten-containing diet results in rapid recurrence of the disease.

Many patients find a strict gluten-free diet too restrictive and instead choose pharmacologic therapy. The drug of choice is dapsone. Treatment is initiated with dapsone 50 mg daily and is increased by 25 to 50 mg every week as needed and as tolerated. The average daily maintenance dose is 100 mg. Some patients require slowly increasing doses several years later, likely secondary to increased deposition of IgA in the skin that results in increased disease activity.

In patients who are intolerant or allergic to dapsone, therapy with sulfapyridine may be considered. The initial dose is 500 mg three times daily and may be increased slowly to 2 g three times daily. The response to sulfapyridine is not as predictable as that to dapsone. Patients who are allergic to dapsone often tolerate sulfapyridine.

Patients who are intolerant or allergic to dapsone and sulfapyridine may be treated with colchicine,[1] cholestyramine (Questran),[1] heparin,[1] tetracycline,[1] or nicotinamide.[1] These agents are much less effective than dapsone and sulfapyridine. Topical steroids are only minimally effective.

Linear Immunoglobulin A Disease

Linear IgA disease is mediated by neutrophils and clinically mimics bullous pemphigoid and dermatitis herpetiformis. Dapsone[1] is the first-line agent. The drug may be started at 25 to 50 mg daily and increased by 25 to 50 mg every 1 to 2 weeks until an effective dose is reached. Patients with early disease tend to respond to lower doses of dapsone.

Sulfapyridine[1] is an alternative agent for patients who cannot tolerate dapsone. The starting dose is 500 mg twice daily and may be increased by 1000 mg every 1 to 2 weeks until the disease is adequately controlled. Colchicine[1] 0.6 mg 2–3 times daily may also be used if a patient is allergic to dapsone. Glucocorticoids may be added if patients do not respond completely to these agents.

Tetracyclines in combination with niacinamide[1] have been reported to be effective. The dose of tetracycline[1] is 500 mg 4 times daily. Alternatively, doxycycline[1] or minocycline[1] 100 mg twice daily may be used. The dose of niacinamide is 500 mg three times daily. Cyclosporine[1] or high-dose IVIg[1] may be used in resistant cases.

Pemphigus

Pemphigus Vulgaris. Pemphigus vulgaris often manifests with erosions in the oral cavity that may be followed by skin blisters. Successful therapy suppresses the production of pathogenic autoantibodies. Therefore immunosuppressive drugs are used. A positive clinical response is associated with a decrease in or absence of pathogenic circulating autoantibodies in the serum and then absence of bound autoantibodies in the skin. There has been a dramatic decrease in the mortality of pemphigus vulgaris owing to the increasing availability of immunosuppressive drugs and glucocorticoids, as well as earlier diagnosis and treatment.

Unless there is an absolute contraindication, the initial therapy of pemphigus vulgaris is systemic glucocorticoid. Prednisone is the most commonly used agent. The initial dose is 1 mg/kg/day divided into two or three doses. Most patients obtain remission within 4 to 12 weeks. The dosage is maintained for 6 to 10 weeks, then decreased by 10 to 20 mg every 2 to 4 weeks. If there is no recurrence, the patient is maintained on 5 mg daily or every other day for several years. Pulsed-steroid therapy with intravenous methylprednisolone, 1 g daily for 3 consecutive days, is reserved for severe cases. The goal of this approach is to quickly achieve the immunosuppressive effects of glucocorticoids while avoiding the long-term side effects.

If prednisone fails to induce a remission, or if the patient develops serious adverse effects, adjuvant immunosuppressive drugs should be instituted. My practice is to initiate adjuvant therapy concomitant with steroid therapy to decrease the total dose of glucocorticoid used. The glucocorticoid is tapered rapidly and the patient is maintained on the steroid-sparing agent for 24 to 36 months. The most commonly used steroid-sparing immunosuppressive drugs are azathioprine[1] and mycophenolate mofetil.[1] Cyclophosphamide[1] is used for resistant cases at a dose of 2 to 3 mg/kg/day, azathioprine at a dose of 3 to 5 mg/kg/day, and mycophenolate at a dose of 2 to 3 g daily (or 40 mg/kg/day in two divided doses). Methotrexate[1] may also be used, but it is generally less effective than other treatments.

The response of pemphigus vulgaris to cyclosporine[1] is controversial. High-dose IVIg[1] has a rapid onset of action and appears most effective when used as an adjuvant to conventional therapy, especially as a steroid-sparing agent. Plasmapheresis is used in refractory cases. To avoid the rebound phenomenon (increased production of autoantibodies), immune suppression (usually with cyclophosphamide) is used concomitantly with plasmapheresis. Rituximab[1] has been used successfully in several cases of pemphigus vulgaris and other autoimmune bullous diseases. For resistant cases, extracorporeal photochemotherapy may be considered.

Pemphigus Foliaceous. The principles and practice of managing pemphigus foliaceous are similar to those for pemphigus vulgaris.

Paraneoplastic Pemphigus. Paraneoplastic pemphigus is a unique intraepidermal blistering disease associated with antibodies against a unique set of skin and internal organ antigens. The most common associated neoplasms are lymphoproliferative. The management of paraneoplastic pemphigus consists of the treatment of the underlying neoplasm as well as immune suppression. Surgical excision of benign neoplasms such as thymoma and Castleman's disease can result in clinical and serologic improvement. In patients with malignant neoplasms, treatment of the associated neoplasm might not result in remission. Generally, skin lesions respond more rapidly than mucosal lesions.

Systemic glucocorticoids are often used as the first-line agent in a dose of 1 to 2 mg/kg/day. Patients usually have a partial response and rarely have complete resolution of lesions. Other immunosuppressive drugs have been used with variable success. These include mycophenolate mofetil,[1] azathioprine,[1] and cyclosporine.[1]

Rituximab[1] has been reported to be effective in a case of paraneoplastic pemphigus associated with CD20-positive follicular lymphoma and in a case of paraneoplastic pemphigus associated with follicular non-Hodgkin's lymphoma. Immunoapheresis has been used successfully occasionally.

Bullous Diseases

---

[1] Not FDA approved for this indication.

[1] Not FDA approved for this indication.

References

Bystryn JC, Jiao D, Natow S: Treatment of pemphigus with intravenous immuno-globulin, *J Am Acad Dermatol* 47:358–363, 2002.

Herron MD, Zone JJ: Treatment of dermatitis herpetiformis and linear IgA bullous dermatosis, *Dermatol Ther* 15:374–381, 2002.

Kirtschig G, Middleton P, Hollis S, et al: Interventions for bullous pemphigoid, *Cochrane Database Syst Rev*(3):CD002292, 2005.

Kirtschig G, Murrell D, Wojnarowska F, Khumalo N: Interventions for mucous membrane pemphigoid and epidermolysis bullosa acquisita, *Cochrane Database Syst Rev*(1):CD004056, 2003.

Mutasim DF: Treatment considerations while awaiting the ideal bullous pemphigoid trial, *Arch Dermatol* 138:404, 2002.

Mutasim DF: Management of autoimmune bullous diseases: Pharmacology and therapeutics, *J Am Acad Dermatol* 51:859–877, 2004.

Mutasim DF: Autoimmune bullous dermatoses in the elderly: An update on patho-physiology, diagnosis and management, *Drugs Aging* 7:1–19, 2010.

Nousari HC, Sragovich A, Kimyai-Asadi A, et al: Mycophenolate mofetil in auto-immune and inflammatory skin disorders, *J Am Acad Dermatol* 40:265–268, 1999.

Rogers RS 3rd, Seehafer JR, Perry HO: Treatment of cicatricial (benign mucous membrane) pemphigoid with dapsone, *J Am Acad Dermatol* 6:215–223, 1982.

Wojnarowska F, Kirtschig G, Highet AS, et al: Guidelines for the management of bullous pemphigoid, *Br J Dermatol* 147:214–221, 2002.

NONMELANOMA CANCER OF THE SKIN

Method of
Julia Dai, MD; and Diana Bolotin, MD, PhD

CURRENT DIAGNOSIS

- Skin cancers are polymorphous in appearance, ranging from small papules and plaques to nodules and tumors of different colors, sizes, and consistencies.
- The surface may be smooth, scaly, ulcerated, or crusted.
- A common feature is that all of these skin neoplasms grow continuously and relapse when superficially treated.
- The distinction between skin cancers and benign neoplasms or inflammatory dermatoses may be difficult for the nonder-matologist to make.

CURRENT THERAPY

- For the majority of nonmelanoma skin cancers, localized treatments are sufficient and include cryotherapy, immuno-therapy, topical chemotherapy, and photodynamic therapy.
- Surgical techniques include electrodesiccation and curettage, simple excision, and Mohs micrographic surgery, which offers intraoperative confirmation of complete tumor removal and maximal cure rates.
- The Mohs procedure is indicated for more-aggressive tumors, for tumors in certain anatomic locations, and in immunosup-pressed patients.
- Rarely, sentinel lymph node dissection and adjuvant thera-pies, such as radiation and chemotherapy, are warranted.

Nonmelanoma skin cancer (NMSC) is a heterogeneous group of skin malignancies that includes basal cell cancer (BCC) and squa-mous cell cancer (SCC). These are the most common skin cancers and NMSC in the stricter sense of the definition (Figure 1). The more-inclusive use of the term NMSC also includes malignant neo-plasms of adnexal, fibrohistiocytic, and vascular origin, as well as Merkel cell carcinoma and metastatic tumors. The vast majority of NMSCs are slowly growing and locally invasive neoplasms that are often diagnosed and treated by dermatologists. Management of the more aggressive tumors often requires a team approach to diagnosis, treatment, and clinical follow-up (Table 1).

Basal Cell Carcinoma

BCC accounts for the majority of NMSC seen in the United States and is increasingly diagnosed in younger patients. Light skin com-plexion and history of ultraviolet (UV) light exposure are the pre-dominant risk factors for BCC in the majority of the population. Intermittent intense UV light exposures early in life, but not cumu-lative UV light exposure, pose the highest risk factor for develop-ing BCC later in life. Other risk factors for BCC include exposure to ionizing radiation, psoralen photochemotherapy, arsenic, and smoking. A history of BCC also increases one's risk for develop-ing a subsequent BCC. Immunosuppression, especially in recipi-ents of solid-organ transplants, presents a significant risk factor for BCC. Inherited genodermatoses such as Gorlin, Bazex, and Rombo syndromes, xeroderma pigmentosum, and some forms of albinism are predisposing factors for BCC as well. Mutations in *PTCH1* that are found in Gorlin syndrome have been shown to be an early event underlying BCC pathogenesis.

Clinically, BCC is most commonly found on the head and neck region, though any part of the body can develop this tumor. The presentation varies depending on the histologic subtype of the tumor. Although many histologic variants of BCC exist, the most common subtypes are superficial, nodular and micronodu-lar, morpheaform, and metatypic. The histologic heterogeneity results in variable clinical findings. Superficial BCC typically forms an erythematous scaly patch or plaque. Nodular BCC is the more classic-appearing lesion, a pink pearly nodule with or without central crust or ulcer. Unlike these subtypes, morphea-form BCC clinically resembles an ill-defined scar; it is the most histologically aggressive variant with a tendency for deep local invasion. Metatypic BCC is also known as basosquamous carci-noma, because it has histologic features of both BCC and SCC, though it is distinguished from the latter by molecular markers. This subtype also has a tendency for more-aggressive growth.

Although it is potentially locally destructive, BCC rarely metas-tasizes. Successful treatment of this tumor involves its local eradi-cation. A number of treatment options exist and depend on the histologic subtype of the tumor. For small, superficial tumors, a nonsurgical approach can suffice, though nonsurgical treatment often carries a higher risk of recurrence than surgical treatment. Nonsurgical options include topical 5-fluorouracil (Efudex 5%), topical imiquimod (Aldara), liquid nitrogen cryotherapy, photo-dynamic therapy, and local radiation therapy.

Electrodesiccation and curettage (ED&C) is an option that has a high cure rate for small and superficial tumors (95% to 98%). Standard excision with adequate margins is an appropriate sur-gical treatment providing good cure rates, especially for tumors with nonaggressive histologic pattern. Mohs micrographic sur-gery (MMS) offers the advantage of precise margin examination during excision and therefore carries the lowest overall rate of recurrence. This tissue-sparing procedure is also advantageous in terms of reconstruction on cosmetically sensitive regions. MMS is indicated to treat recurrent tumors, those in immunosuppressed patients, aggressive histologic variants, and BCCs located on cer-tain areas of the face known to carry a higher risk of recurrence.

Although locally advanced and metastatic BCCs are uncom-mon, treatment with targeted molecules such as vismodegib (Eri-vedge) have demonstrated clinical efficacy.

Squamous Cell Carcinoma

Cutaneous SCC is the second most common skin malignancy. Its incidence is rising among both men and women in the United States. Development of SCC is intimately linked to the cumulative ultraviolet radiation exposure of the patient via a mechanism that combines DNA damage with immunosuppres-sion. History of ionizing radiation exposure is a risk factor as well. Similar to BCC, occupational exposures such as arsenic can also predispose one to SCC. Patients with xeroderma pig-mentosum or oculocutaneous albinism also are at higher risk for SCC.

Chronic inflammation or injury can predispose to epidermal malignant transformation. Examples of this phenomenon are

Figure 1 Clinical images of skin cancers. (A) Squamous cell carcinoma in sun-exposed skin of a 102-year-old African American woman. (B) Depressed scarlike appearance of a morpheaform basal cell carcinoma on the nose. (C) This firm tumor on the abdomen is a dermatofibrosarcoma protuberans. (D) Violaceous plaques on the instep in an elderly Greek man typical for endemic Kaposi sarcoma.

TABLE 1	Overview of Therapeutic Modalities for the Management of Skin Cancers	
THERAPEUTIC MODALITY	**NEOPLASM**	**COMMENT**
Cryotherapy	AK, SCC in situ Superficial BCC Kaposi sarcoma	Versatile, but operator dependent
Topical 5-fluorouracil (Efudex)	AK, SCC in situ Superficial BCC	Will treat preclinical AK
Topical imiquimod (Aldara)	AK Superficial BCC	Flulike adverse effects can occur
Photodynamic therapy	AK, SCC in situ Superficial BCC	SCC and BCC are off-label uses
Electrodesiccation and curettage	AK, SCC BCC	
Excision	All	
Mohs micrographic surgery	BCC, SCC MAC, sebaceous carcinoma DFSP, AFX Angiosarcoma EMPD, MCC	Preferred for certain types of invasive tumors (e.g., morpheaform BCC), on high-risk regions (e.g., nose, lip), and settings (e.g., recurrence, immunosuppressed patient)
Radiation therapy	BCC, SCC Kaposi sarcoma, angiosarcoma MCC Inoperable tumors	Careful risk-to-benefit evaluation

AFX, Atypical fibroxanthoma; *AK,* actinic keratosis; *BCC,* basal cell carcinoma; *DFSP,* dermatofibrosarcoma protuberans; *EMPD,* extramammary Paget disease; *MAC,* microcystic adnexal carcinoma; *MCC,* Merkel cell carcinoma; *SCC,* squamous cell carcinoma.

SCC developing within scars from burns, in chronic ulcers and skin overlying osteomyelitis, and in persistent lichen sclerosus or lichen planus. These tumors have a more-aggressive behavior and higher rates of metastasis.

Human papilloma virus (HPV) predisposes to SCC. Verrucous carcinoma, a well-differentiated subtype of SCC, has a well-documented association with HPV types 6 and 11.

Transplant patients are at high risk for SCC that correlates with the degree of immunosuppression. In fact, SCC development is up to 250 times greater in the immunosuppressed compared to the general population, whereas BCC increases to a lesser extent with immunocompromise. A more common association between HPV and SCC has been noted in the immunocompromised population

and might account for the disproportional increase of SCC over BCC in this population.

As with BCC, history of previous SCC has been found to be a risk factor for developing a subsequent SCC. This risk appears especially pronounced in smokers.

Unlike BCC, SCC often has a precursor lesion: actinic keratosis. Histologically, actinic keratosis demonstrates partial thickness atypia of the epidermis, and patients often describe it as waxing and waning. Full-thickness histologic atypia is seen in SCC in situ (Bowen disease), whereas invasive SCC penetrates the basement membrane to invade underlying dermis. Histologically, the degree of differentiation of SCC tends to correlate with its clinical behavior. Well-differentiated lesions tend toward local invasion, as opposed to poorly differentiated SCC, which more commonly is infiltrative.

The typical clinical presentation of SCC is that of a hyperkeratotic pink plaque. More-advanced lesions may be nodular and can ulcerate. In most cases, SCC shows only local invasion; however, perineural invasion and rarely metastasis are more likely with SCC than BCC. The central face, temples, and scalp present high-risk zones for recurrence and metastasis.

Treatment of SCC involves modalities similar to those used for BCC. Cryotherapy is the mainstay of treatment for actinic keratosis. Topical treatment with 5-fluorouracil (Carac 0.5%, Fluoroplex 1%, Fluorouracil 2 or 5%, Efudex 5%) alone or in combination with calcipotriol (Dovonex)[1]; imiquimod (Aldara or Zyclara); ingenol mebutate (Picato); or photodynamic therapy is often used as field therapy to depopulate large regions of the skin of actinic keratosis lesions. Continued sun protection has been shown to be of benefit to prevent progression from actinic keratosis to SCC, especially in the immunocompromised population. Systemic retinoids, such as acitretin (Soriatane)[1] and nicotinamide[7] have also been used for the prevention and reduction of NMSC, particularly in high-risk populations. SCC in situ may be treated with ED&C. Excision with a clear surgical margin is often used in treatment of SCC on the trunk or extremities, but MMS yields the highest cure rates, especially in high-risk areas such as the face and scalp. Adjuvant radiotherapy, surgical excision, and targeted approaches with anti-PD-1 monoclonal antibodies may be used alone or in combination for more-aggressive tumors. Overall, the prognosis for a patient with cutaneous SCC depends heavily on location, degree of histologic differentiation, invasion, and metastasis.

Neoplasms of Adnexal Origin
The adnexal structures of the skin include the pilosebaceous unit as well as apocrine and eccrine glands and ducts. A great number of benign and malignant tumors of adnexal origin occur in the skin. Most of the adnexal malignancies are rare. Sebaceous carcinoma and microcystic adnexal carcinoma (MAC) are two of the more common adnexal carcinomas that have an aggressive nature and may be subtle at presentation.

Sebaceous Carcinoma
Sebaceous carcinoma is an aggressive malignancy that is most commonly found on the head and neck region. More specifically, it is one of the more common tumors of the eyelid and periocular area. Due to its nonspecific clinical presentation it is often treated as chalazion before biopsy and diagnosis. Population-based risk factors associated with development of sebaceous carcinoma include older age and European ethnicity. History of irradiation and immunosuppression predisposes to sebaceous carcinoma development, similar to BCC and SCC. Sebaceous carcinoma is one of the cutaneous neoplasms characteristic of Muir-Torre syndrome, which results from mutations in DNA mismatch repair genes and is associated with multiple sebaceous neoplasms and internal malignancy.

Clinical diagnosis of sebaceous carcinoma is difficult, and therefore progressive or nonresolving eyelid lesions require biopsy. Treatment of sebaceous carcinoma is primarily surgical. Wide local excision with 5- to 6-mm margins or MMS is indicated. A lower rate of recurrence with MMS (11.1%) has been shown as compared to local excision (32%). Close follow-up is indicated to monitor for recurrence and metastasis.

Microcystic Adnexal Carcinoma
MAC is another adnexal malignancy with predilection for the head and neck. In the United States it is most prevalent in the white population and on the left side of the body, suggesting UV irradiation as a risk factor. Although it can be seen in a wide age range of patients, older patients have a higher risk of developing MAC. The low incidence of this tumor makes it difficult to

evaluate other risk factors, though cases have been reported in immunosuppressed patients and those with a history of radiation therapy.

Clinically, MAC occurs as a slowly growing, pink- to flesh-colored ill-defined plaque. Paresthesia and/or numbness are common complaints and have been attributed to the high degree of perineural invasion by this tumor. MAC is a locally aggressive tumor with an unpredictable pattern of infiltrative growth. Histologically, MAC exhibits both pilar and sweat duct differentiation, deep invasion with a desmoplastic stromal response, and perineural invasion.

Surgical excision is the standard of care treatment for MAC, and radiation as an adjunct therapy is reported in a few cases. Because this tumor can extend for centimeters subclinically, MMS is favored as the first-line surgical treatment because it allows complete examination of the surgical margins intraoperatively and has been reported to have a lower recurrence rate than standard excision.

Fibrohistiocytic Malignancies
Fibrohistiocytic tumors of the skin are derived from the mesenchymal tissue and range from those of intermediate malignant potential to aggressive pleomorphic sarcomas. Of these overall rare malignancies, dermatofibrosarcoma protuberans (DFSP) and atypical fibroxanthoma are more frequently encountered.

Dermatofibrosarcoma Protuberans
DFSP is the most common fibrohistiocytic malignancy of the skin. It occurs at various ages ranging from infancy to older adulthood. The pathogenesis of DFSP involves a translocation between chromosomes 17 and 22 that fuses the collagen type 1 α1 gene (COL1A1) with the platelet-derived growth factor B-chain gene (PDGFB). This fusion gene results in overexpression of PDGFB, which acts as a potent growth stimulant for mesenchymal cells. In general slowly growing, DFSPs are locally invasive and infiltrative rather than metastatic. Therefore, treatment of this tumor is primarily surgical.

A high recurrence rate has been noted in a number of studies and is attributed to the infiltrative growth of the tumor. MMS reduces recurrence rates, and is often recommended. DFSP is thought to be a radiosensitive tumor, and adjunctive radiation therapy has been successful used both pre- and postoperatively. The discovery of COL1A1-PDGFB fusion has led to trials of imatinib (Gleevec) therapy as an adjunct to surgery for DFSP. So far, a limited number of clinical reports have demonstrated regression of DFSPs during treatment with imatinib. Larger studies and long-term follow-up are needed to determine whether this warrants a change to the current treatment recommendations.

Atypical Fibroxanthoma
Atypical fibroxanthoma is a low-grade sarcoma of the skin. This locally invasive tumor favors sun-damaged skin of the head and neck region in older adults. Patients with xeroderma pigmentosum have a higher risk for developing atypical fibroxanthoma. It has a nonspecific clinical presentation, and a biopsy with histopathology is needed for diagnosis. Histologically, this tumor often exhibits marked pleomorphism and frequent mitoses. Often immunohistochemical staining is necessary for definitive diagnosis. Surgery is the treatment of choice for atypical fibroxanthoma. Either wide local excision or MMS may be used, though lower recurrence rates have been reported with MMS. Despite the pleomorphic microscopic appearance, this tumor rarely metastasizes, and the prognosis with appropriate treatment is favorable.

Vascular Malignancies
Vascular neoplasms of the skin are rare. Kaposi sarcoma (KS) and angiosarcoma, both increasingly encountered in healthy older adults as well as immunosuppressed patients, are discussed here.

---

[1]Not FDA approved for this indication.
[7]Available as dietary supplement

Kaposi Sarcoma

Controversy exists regarding the nature of cell proliferation seen in KS. Some regard it as a true malignancy, and others view it as a reactive proliferation. Four types of KS exist: KS of elderly men of Jewish and Mediterranean origin, African endemic KS, immunosuppression-associated KS, and AIDS-associated KS. Infection with human herpesvirus 8 (HHV 8) is involved in the pathogenesis of all types of KS. Clinical findings include non-blanching purpuric patches and plaques that can progress to nodules with ulceration. KS can be isolated to the skin or can become disseminated to the lymph nodes and viscera. Diagnosis is established with histopathology and immunostaining. Management of KS is complex owing to the varied clinical course of the four subtypes. In cases of localized lesions, surgery, cryotherapy, or laser treatment may be useful. Radiotherapy can also be used for localized disease. Patients with disseminated KS are generally treated with chemotherapy. In AIDS-associated KS, institution of HIV medications has been shown to effect resolution of KS.

Angiosarcoma

Angiosarcoma is a more rare but aggressive vascular cutaneous malignancy that tends to metastasize and carries a poor prognosis. Clinically, angiosarcoma favors the head and neck area of elderly men; it can also arise within sites of previous radiation therapy or chronic lymphedema. No association between angiosarcoma and HHV8 has been found. Patients present with an asymptomatic enlarging purpuric plaque that can eventually develop a nodular component. Angiosarcoma may have multifocal involvement that is often not appreciated clinically. The treatment for angiosarcoma involves wide local excision and postoperative radiation. The overall prognosis is poor, and distant metastasis-free 5-year survival rates range between 20% and 37%.

Other Nonmelanoma Skin Cancers
Merkel Cell Carcinoma

Merkel cell carcinoma (MCC) is a rare but often fatal NMSC that derives from cutaneous neuroendocrine cells. Fair skin and a history of exposure to UV light are risk factors for developing MCC. Like many other NMSCs, MCC favors the head and neck and is much more common in the elderly. Immunosuppression appears to be a risk factor for MCC development because its incidence is significantly increased in patients with AIDS and recipients of organ transplants. Polyomavirus has been implicated in the pathogenesis of MCC.

This malignancy is often metastatic upon presentation. Clinically, it occurs as a nonspecific, red asymptomatic papule or nodule. A biopsy with immunohistochemical analysis is diagnostic. The therapy for MCC involves surgery with wide local excision or MMS. Sentinel lymph node biopsy can be performed for staging purposes but should be considered on a case-by-case basis. MCC is sensitive to radiation therapy, which is a recommended adjuvant treatment for patients with lymph node involvement. Palliative chemotherapy often produces a response; however, recurrence is common. Preliminary data indicates a promising signal with checkpoint immunotherapy in patients with advanced disease, though prognosis remains poor for metastatic disease or lymph node involvement.

Paget Disease

Paget disease refers to intraepidermal spread of adenocarcinoma. Two types are seen in the skin: mammary Paget disease and extramammary Paget disease (EMPD). Mammary Paget disease is most commonly seen in women and has a strict association with adenocarcinoma of the breast. The lesions are usually unilateral scaly red plaques that favor the nipple. Often the underlying tumor is not clinically present but is detected through imaging. Other dermatoses of the nipple can resemble mammary Paget disease, and therefore definitive diagnosis requires biopsy and immunohistochemistry. Surgical excision along with appropriate treatment of the breast cancer is the recommended treatment. Prognosis depends on the extent of breast cancer at diagnosis, though it appears to be worse for breast cancer patients with mammary Paget disease than those without.

EMPD consists of two types of disease: type I disease, which is associated with distant adenocarcinoma, and type II, primary cutaneous EMPD. Both are very rare but, like mammary Paget disease, have a female predominance. Most commonly EMPD is found in the genital or perianal region; however, other areas of the skin can be affected less frequently. Clinically, EMPD manifests as a well-demarcated red plaque that can become erosive. Long-standing disease can spread from the groin to the trunk, mimicking an inflammatory dermatosis. Definitive diagnosis is based on biopsy findings, and further work-up includes extensive screening for associated internal malignancy. Treatment relies on surgical excision with wide margins. MMS can be used to examine margins intraoperatively. Prognosis for type I EMPD depends on the extent of underlying tumor, but that for type II is favorable.

Cutaneous Metastases

Metastasis to the skin often heralds the systemic spread of an internal malignancy. Primary malignancy underlying the skin metastasis tends to differ by sex and age. In men, lung cancer is the most common source of skin metastasis, whereas breast cancer is the more common primary tumor in women. The head and neck are favored as sites of skin metastasis in men but the trunk is favored in women.

The clinical presentation of skin metastasis is varied and often nonspecific. A new, asymptomatic cutaneous or subcutaneous nodule may be the reason for a biopsy that reveals metastasis of an unknown primary tumor. Diagnosis is made by histopathology and appropriate molecular staining. Specific clinical patterns of metastasis may be encountered. Inflammatory carcinoma can be seen with cutaneous breast cancer metastases. Occasionally, neoplastic infiltration leads to localized areas of alopecia. Zosteriform distribution of skin metastasis has been reported with breast, colon, or SCC.

Leukemia cutis refers to skin involvement with acute myelogenous leukemia, chronic myelogenous leukemia, myelodysplastic syndromes, chronic lymphocytic leukemia, or adult T-cell lymphoproliferative diseases. In rare cases, skin involvement precedes bone marrow disease and is termed *aleukemic leukemia cutis*. In chronic leukemias, skin involvement tends to predict disease progression into the acute phase. Children appear to have a higher incidence of leukemia cutis as compared to adults but have a better overall prognosis.

Metastatic skin tumors are distinguished from primary cutaneous malignancies histologically. Treatment is always geared toward the primary malignancy. Regardless of type of neoplasm or site of metastasis, spread of an internal malignancy to the skin carries a poor prognosis.

References

Alam M, Ratner D: Cutaneous squamous-cell carcinoma, *N Engl J Med* 344(13):975–983, 2001.

Billings SD, Folpe AL: Cutaneous and subcutaneous fibrohistiocytic tumors of intermediate malignancy: An update, *Am J Dermatopathol* 26(2):141–155, 2004.

Buitrago W, Joseph AK: Sebaceous carcinoma: The great masquerader: Emerging concepts in diagnosis and treatment, *Dermatol Ther* 21(6):459–466, 2008.

Chen L, Aria AB, Silapunt S, Migden MR: Emerging nonsurgical therapies for locally advanced and metastatic nonmelanoma skin cancer, *Dermatol Surg* 45(1):1–16, 2019.

Cho-Vega JH, Medeiros LJ, Prieto VG, Vega F: Leukemia cutis, *Am J Clin Pathol* 129(1):130–142, 2008.

Christenson LJ, Borrowman TA, Vachon CM, et al: Incidence of basal cell and squamous cell carcinomas in a population younger than 40 years, *JAMA* 294(6):681–690, 2005.

Cumberland L, Dana A, Liegeois N: Mohs micrographic surgery for the management of nonmelanoma skin cancers, *Facial Plast Surg Clin North Am* 17(3):325–335, 2009.

Dasgupta T, Wilson LD, Yu JB: A retrospective review of 1349 cases of sebaceous carcinoma, *Cancer* 115(1):158–165, 2009.

Dubina M, Goldenberg G: Viral-associated nonmelanoma skin cancers: A review, *Am J Dermatopathol* 31(6):561–573, 2009.

Eisen DB, Michael DJ: Sebaceous lesions and their associated syndromes: Part I, *J Am Acad Dermatol* 61(4):549–560, 2009.

Fan H, Oro AE, Scott MP, Khavari PA: Induction of basal cell carcinoma features in transgenic human skin expressing Sonic Hedgehog, *Nat Med* 3(7):788–792, 1997.

Feng H, Shuda M, Chang Y, Moore PS: Clonal integration of a polyomavirus in human Merkel cell carcinoma, *Science* 319(5866):1096–1100, 2008.

Hussein MR: Skin metastasis: A pathologist's perspective, *J Cutan Pathol* 37(9):e1–320, 2010.

Kamino H, Jacobson M: Dermatofibroma extending into the subcutaneous tissue. Differential diagnosis from dermatofibrosarcoma protuberans, *Am J Surg Pathol* 14(12):1156–1164, 1990.

Kanitakis J: Mammary and extramammary Paget's disease, *J Eur Acad Dermatol Venereol* 21(5):581–590, 2007.

Karagas MR, Stukel TA, Greenberg ER, et al: Risk of subsequent basal cell carcinoma and squamous cell carcinoma of the skin among patients with prior skin cancer. Skin Cancer Prevention Study Group, *JAMA* 267(24):3305–3310, 1992.

Lee DA, Miller SJ: Nonmelanoma skin cancer, *Facial Plast Surg Clin North Am* 17(3):309–324, 2009.

Lehmann P: Methyl aminolaevulinate-photodynamic therapy: a review of clinical trials in the treatment of actinic keratoses and nonmelanoma skin cancer, *Br J Dermatol* 156(5):793–801, 2007.

Lemm D, Mugge LO, Mentzel T, Hoffken K: Current treatment options in dermatofibrosarcoma protuberans, *J Cancer Res Clin Oncol* 135(5):653–665, 2009.

Maddox JS, Soltani K: Risk of nonmelanoma skin cancer with azathioprine use, *Inflamm Bowel Dis* 14(10):1425–1431, 2008.

Marcet S: Atypical fibroxanthoma/malignant fibrous histiocytoma, *Dermatol Ther* 21(6):424–427, 2008.

McGuire JF, Ge NN, Dyson S: Nonmelanoma skin cancer of the head and neck. I: Histopathology and clinical behavior, *Am J Otolaryngol* 30(2):121–133, 2009.

Mendenhall WM, Mendenhall CM, Werning JW, et al: Cutaneous angiosarcoma, *Am J Clin Oncol* 29(5):524–528, 2006.

Prieto VG, Shea CR: Selected cutaneous vascular neoplasms, A review, *Dermatol Clin* 17(3):507–520, 1999, viii.

Rockville Merkel Cell Carcinoma Group: Merkel cell carcinoma: Recent progress and current priorities on etiology, pathogenesis, and clinical management, *J Clin Oncol* 27(24):4021–4026, 2009.

Rubin AI, Chen EH, Ratner D: Basal-cell carcinoma, *N Engl J Med* 353(21):2262–2269, 2005.

Schwartz RA, Micali G, Nasca MR, Scuderi L: Kaposi sarcoma: a continuing conundrum, *J Am Acad Dermatol* 59(2):179–206, 2008.

Smeets NW, Krekels GA, Ostertag JU, et al: Surgical excision vs Mohs' micrographic surgery for basal-cell carcinoma of the face: Randomised controlled trial, *Lancet* 364(9447):1766–1772, 2004.

Spencer JM, Nossa R, Tse DT, Sequeira M: Sebaceous carcinoma of the eyelid treated with Mohs micrographic surgery, *J Am Acad Dermatol* 44(6):1004–1009, 2001.

Ulrich C, Jurgensen JS, Degen A, et al: Prevention of non-melanoma skin cancer in organ transplant patients by regular use of a sunscreen: A 24 months, prospective, case-control study, *Br J Dermatol* 161(Suppl. 3):78–84, 2009.

Wetter R, Goldstein GD: Microcystic adnexal carcinoma: a diagnostic and therapeutic challenge, *Dermatol Ther* 21(6):452–458, 2008.

Yu JB, Blitzblau RC, Patel SC, et al: Surveillance, Epidemiology, and End Results (SEER) database analysis of microcystic adnexal carcinoma (sclerosing sweat duct carcinoma) of the skin, *Am J Clin Oncol* 33(2):125–127, 2010.

CONTACT DERMATITIS

Method of
James A. Yiannias, MD; Genevieve L. Egnatios, MD; and Heidi E.K. Mullen, DO

CURRENT DIAGNOSIS

- Gather a detailed history on skin exposures, including the use of these items:
  - Irritants
  - Alkalis: soaps, detergents, cleansers
  - Acids
  - Hydrocarbons: petroleum, oils
  - Solvents
  - Allergens
  - Nickel sulfate
  - Balsam of Peru (Myroxilon pereira, fragrance)
  - Fragrance mix
  - Quaternium-15 (formaldehyde-releasing preservative)
  - Neomycin
  - Bacitracin
  - Formaldehyde
  - Cobalt chloride (metals, personal products)
- Examine the skin for the location and pattern of eruption:
  - Eyelid: nail polish
  - Postauricular scalp: perfume
  - Perioral area: chewing gum, toothpaste
  - Trunk: dyes, clothing finish
  - Wrist: nickel, chrome
  - Waistline: rubber
  - Feet: shoes
  - Wounds: topical antibiotic ointment
- Perform Patch Testing:
  - T.R.U.E. TEST with 35 allergens (note: one common allergen, benzalkonium chloride, is not included in this panel)
- Customized series with 70 or more allergens

CURRENT THERAPY

- Avoid irritants and allergens, using the prepared patient handout.
- Consult the SkinSAFE shopping list of skin-care products free of top 10 most common allergens (if patch testing is not performed).
- Consult a customized SkinSAFE shopping list of skin-care products free of the patient's contact allergens, based on patch test results.
- Topical corticosteroids can be applied.
- Hydrocortisone 2.5% (Hytone) can be applied twice daily on the face, neck, axillae, groin, and intertriginous areas.
- Triamcinolone 0.1% (Kenalog) can be applied twice daily on the body.
- For severe reactions, short-term, higher-potency steroids can be applied (e.g., clobetasol [Clobex] 0.05% twice daily).
- Sedating antihistamines can be taken: doxepin (Sinequan)[1] 10 to 20 mg nightly 2 hours before bed.
- Steroid-sparing topical agents can be applied: tacrolimus 0.1% (Protopic), pimecrolimus 1% (Elidel), crisaborole 2% (Eucrisa)
- For severe, acute episodes, systemic corticosteroids can be taken in a several-week, tapering course (e.g., prednisone 60 mg for 5 days, 40 mg for 5 days, and 20 mg for 5 days).
- Longer-term systemic therapy is possible for severe or recalcitrant disease.
- Phototherapy is suggested, with narrowband ultraviolet B.
- Azathioprine (Imuran) can be taken 1 to 3 mg/kg daily.
- Mycophenolate mofetil (CellCept) can be taken 2 to 3 g daily.
- Methotrexate can be taken 10 to 25 mg weekly.
- Cyclosporine (Neoral) can be taken 2.5 to 5 mg/kg daily.
- Dupilumab (Dupixent) can be taken by injection at 600 mg initially and then 300 mg every other week.

[1]Not FDA approved for this indication.

Dermatitis typically manifests as papules and vesicles with weeping and oozing that can become lichenified and scaly when chronic. When this clinical picture is secondary to an exogenous substance coming into contact with the skin, it is termed *contact dermatitis*. Further delineation leads to irritant versus allergic contact dermatitis, although in practice these often overlap.

Irritant contact dermatitis is not an allergic process. It represents damage to the skin from repeated and cumulative exposure to an agent. Irritants do not require prior sensitization. A decreased barrier function of the skin—for example, with frequent hand washing—can predispose or exacerbate the condition. Examples include alkalis (in soaps, detergents, and cleansers), acids (in germicides, dyes, and pigments), hydrocarbons (in petroleum and oils), and solvents.

Allergic contact dermatitis is an immunologic process classified as a type IV cell-mediated delayed hypersensitivity reaction.

Poison ivy is a classic example. It requires an initial exposure to the contactant in which sensitization occurs but without outward physical effect. Subsequent exposure can elicit a striking response that is independent of the amount of the contactant.

From 1994 to 2016 the most common contact allergens have changed little. Based on studies performed by the North American Contact Dermatitis Group (NACDG) and the Mayo Clinic Contact Dermatitis Group (MCCDG), the allergens most consistently in the top 10 were nickel sulfate, balsam of Peru, fragrance mix, quaternium-15, neomycin, bacitracin, formaldehyde, and cobalt chloride (Box 1). However, in the past few years, two additional preservatives have gained prominence: methylisothiazolinone (MI) and benzalkonium chloride. Common sources of exposure to nickel include costume jewelry, snaps, zippers, and other metal objects. Balsam of Peru and fragrance mix are markers for fragrance sensitivity. Sources of exposure to formaldehyde include skincare products, household products, and the resins in plastics and clothing. Quaternium-15 is a formaldehyde-releasing preservative and may be found in items such as skincare products, paper, inks, and photocopier toner. Neomycin and bacitracin are topical antibiotics available alone and in combination with polymyxin (Neosporin), antifungals, and corticosteroids. Cobalt is found with other metals, including zinc, and in items such as jewelry, crayons, hair dye, and antiperspirants. MI is a common preservative found in personal care products and may be used in combination with another preservative, methylchloroisothiazolinone (MCI/MI). Benzalkonium chloride is commonly used in the healthcare field as a cleanser, antiseptic, and preservative, but is also found in personal care products such as wipes and an increasing number of skin care products.

Others less consistently in the top 10 during that period were methyldibromo glutaronitrile, gold sodium thiosulfate, potassium dichromate, p-phenylenediamine, thiuram mix, methylisothiazolinone/methylchloroisothiazolinone (MCI/MI), and propolis. Methyldibromo glutaronitrile is a preservative and can be found in healthcare and personal products. Clinically relevant sources of gold may be found in jewelry and dental appliances. Potassium dichromate is used in cement, leather, and steel surfaces. Permanent hair dyes are the usual source of p-phenylenediamine. Thiuram mix is in rubber and some personal products. Propolis is another marker of fragrance sensitivity.

Each year since 2000, the American Contact Dermatitis Society has designated an allergen of the year, designed to spotlight allergens, common or not, that are rising in significance. For 2019, non-allergen parabens have been chosen and for 2020, isobornyl acrylate. Parabens are preservatives commonly found in cosmetics, foods, pharmaceuticals, dentifrices, and suppositories. The adhesive, isobornyl acrylate, is often used in medical devices, such as insulin pumps, and can also be found in acrylic nails. Other designated allergens of the year have been alkyl glucosides, cobalt chloride, benzophenones, MI, acrylates, dimethyl fumarate, neomycin, mixed dialkyl thioureas, nickel, fragrance, p-phenylenediamine, corticosteroids, cocamidopropyl betaine, bacitracin, thimerosal, gold, disperse blue, and propylene glycol. Alkyl glucosides are surfactants that are pervasive in consumer products including cosmetics. Benzophenones, such as oxybenzone, are chemical ultraviolet light filters that are found in sunscreens and personal care products. Artificial nails, dentures, and bone cement contain acrylates, but these substances are only allergenic when in the liquid, powder, or paste forms. Dimethyl fumarate is a biocide in furniture, shoes, and textiles. It is often placed in little paper packets with these items. Rubber products and shoe glue are common sources of mixed dialkyl thioureas. Shampoos often contain cocamidopropyl betaine as a lathering agent. Thimerosal is a preservative for medications and personal-care products, including contact lens solution. Disperse blue is a fabric dye. Patients with an allergy to disperse dyes may also react to p-phenylenediamine. Propylene glycol is a common ingredient in personal care products, topical corticosteroids and other medications, and foods.

BOX 1   Top 10 Most Common Allergens

North American Contact Dermatitis Group
1. Nickel sulfate
2. Methylisothiazolinone (MI)
3. Fragrance mix
4. Formaldehyde 2%
5. Methylchloroisothiazolinone/methylisothiazolinone (MCI/MI)
6. Balsam of Peru
7. Neomycin
8. Bacitracin
9. Formaldehyde 1%
10. p-Phenylenediamine

Mayo Clinic Contact Dermatitis Group
1. Nickel sulfate
2. Methylisothiazolinone (MI)
3. Balsam of Peru
4. Neomycin
5. Cobalt chloride
6. Benzalkonium chloride
7. Fragrance mix I
8. Potassium dichromate
9. Bacitracin
10. Methylchloroisothiazolinone/methylisothiazolinone (MCI/MI)

From DeKoven and colleagues, 2018, and Veverka and colleagues, 2018.

Diagnosis

The evaluation of a patient with suspected contact dermatitis begins with the history. Specific questions directed at the patient's occupation, hobbies, and home routine will be helpful. Examination should note the location and pattern of the eruption. Although eyelid dermatitis may be seen in the atopic patient, nail polish may be the source of the offending allergen. Dyshidrotic eczema occurs as vesicles along the lateral aspects of the fingers, whereas eczematous changes along the dorsal hands are more commonly due to an allergen. Other distributions as clues include postauricular scalp (perfume), perioral area (chewing gum, toothpaste), trunk (dyes or clothing finish), wrist (nickel or chrome), waistline (rubber), feet (shoes), and history or presence of wounds (topical antibiotic ointment).

Patch testing can confirm or reveal a contact allergy. It involves placement of allergens against the skin of the patient's back for 48 hours. An initial reading is then done, with follow-up readings typically at 96 hours. Prepared series include the thin-layer, rapid-use epicutaneous test (T.R.U.E. TEST), which consists of 35 allergens and 1 negative control (www.truetest.com); customized series, such as the NACDG Standard Series with 70 allergens and the Mayo Clinic's Standard Series with 73 allergens, must be manually assembled. The majority of dermatologists performing patch testing use T.R.U.E. TEST. Note that benzalkonium chloride MI and propolis are not included in that panel. Overall, the NACDG estimates that 25% to approximately 40% of allergic reactions would have been missed by the T.R.U.E. TEST based on their data for 2015–2016.

In addition to ascertaining degree of positivity, relevance must be determined. This involves collaborating with patients to assess the likelihood that they are currently exposed to the positive antigen.

Treatment

Ideally, the allergen(s) will be identified and avoided. Realistically, compliance is a challenge. To assist patients in avoiding antigens in skin-care products, SkinSAFE was created in 1999. It includes approximately 18,550 ingredients and 40,495 individual over-the-counter and prescription skin-care products. Once the patient's allergens have been identified with patch testing, they can

Introduction

Eczema, also known as dermatitis, is an inflammation of the skin due to dryness, irritation, or possible external allergy. Eczema/dermatitis is not contagious.

Some skin care products contain fragrance even though the package says "fragrance free" or "unscented." Therefore, please choose the skin care products as listed below by their *exact brand name*.

Suggestions

Soaps/Cleansing

- Vanicream cleansing bar
- Free and Clear liquid cleanser
- Aveeno moisturizing bar for dry skin fragrance
- Free or Aveeno advanced care body wash
- Oilatum unscented soap
- Neutrogena original formula fragrance-free (bar or liquid)

Any of the shampoos listed in this brochure may be used as your hand or body soap.

- Vanicream shave cream for sensitive skin

Moisturizers

- Vanicream, Vanicream Lite
- Aveeno daily moisturizing lotion fragrance Free
- Plain Vaseline, Vaniply
- DML unscented
- Use moisturizers twice daily.
- All of the above are OK to use on the face.
- After showering, blot excess water with hands and apply cream. Do not use a towel to dry.
- Robathol bath oil

Deodorants

- Almay unscented antiperspirants
- Plain cornstarch from the grocer can be used.

Shampoo

- Free and Clear shampoo and conditioner
- DHS clear shampoo and DHS conditioner
- If you have dandruff, use DHS sal shampoo or Neutrogena T-SAL shampoo (not T-Gel).
- Conditioners can be used as "leave on" hair gel.

Hairspray

- Fragrance-free hairspray such as Free and Clear hairspray
- Caution: Hairsprays labeled as "unscented" may not be fragrance free.

Laundry and Home Care

- Unscented laundry detergents (Tide free, Cheer free and gentle, All free clear, Arm & Hammer unscented, Wisk free, Purex unscented)
- Wash all new clothes and linens five times before using.
- Old clothes and fabrics are preferred.
- Use white vinegar in rinse cycle to help remove soap.

Hand, Nail, and General Skin Care Tips

- Wear cotton gloves under rubber/vinyl gloves for any activities where hand-wetting is expected.
- Trim nails short. Long nails are dangerous to skin, especially when sleeping.

Sunscreens

- Vanicream sunscreen #30 or #60

Make-ups/cosmetics

- If you would like a list of make-ups and cosmetics that are free of the most common allergy-causing ingredients, ask your provider about a "virtual patch testing" printout from our Mayo CARD program.

Avoid

Soaps/Cleansing

- No hot water (use lukewarm).
- Avoid hot tubs.
- No rubbing alcohol.

Moisturizers

- No creams, lotions, oils or powders other than those recommended in this brochure.
- No Neosporin, triple antibiotic, or bacitracin antibiotic ointments.

Fragrances

- No perfumes, colognes, after shave, or pre-shave on any part of body/clothing.

Laundry and Home Care

- No fabric softener in washer.
- Bounce unscented fabric softener sheets in dryer if desired.
- No washing machine water softener such as Calgon (in-house water softeners are acceptable).
- White vinegar may be used as a general household cleaner.

Hand, Nail, and General Skin Care Tips

- No wetting of hands more than five times a day.
- Avoid tight-fitting clothes unless your doctor has advised you to wear a pressure garment such as support hose.
- No scrubbing! No loofah! No pumice stone!
- Do not pull off dead skin. Snip with scissors instead.

Figure 1 Sample of prepared handout (used at Mayo Clinic Arizona) with recommendations for the patient on hypoallergenic skin-care products.

be entered into the database, and a list of products free of those substances is generated. The patient should be reminded that even small and infrequent exposures can perpetuate the eczema.

Topical corticosteroids applied twice daily are helpful in hastening resolution and may also be used for disease control when the allergen is unknown. Low-potency corticosteroids such as 2.5% hydrocortisone (Hytone) are recommended for the thinner skin of the face, neck, axillae, groin, and intertriginous areas. Mid-potency steroids such as triamcinolone 0.1% (Kenalog, Kenonel) are appropriate for the thicker skin of the body. Short-term use of higher-potency steroids may be necessary if the reaction is severe. If there is significant pruritus, sedating antihistamines such as doxepin (Sinequan) 10 to 20 mg taken nightly 2 hours before bedtime can provide relief. Steroid-sparing topical immunomodulators such as tacrolimus (Protopic), pimecrolimus (Elidel), and crisaborole (Eucrisa) may be helpful adjuncts. Treatment for severe acute episodes can entail a several-week tapering course of systemic corticosteroids, especially if the eruption is widespread. Other longer-term systemic therapies for severe or resistant disease include phototherapy or systemic immunosuppressants such as azathioprine (Imuran), mycophenolate mofetil (CellCept), methotrexate, cyclosporine (Neoral), or dupilumab (Dupixent).

It may take many weeks before the skin reverts to a normal appearance despite successful avoidance of antigens. A prepared handout with concrete recommendations for the patient on truly hypoallergenic skincare is beneficial. A sample of that used at Mayo Clinic Arizona is shown in Figure 1.

If patch testing is not performed, an initial approach may be to instruct the patient on avoiding the most common contact allergens via such a handout and prescribing symptomatic treatment including topical and oral therapies. SkinSAFE can generate a shopping list of products free of the top 10 allergens as identified by the NACDG and the MCCDG. Patients may access SkinSAFE independently (at www.skinsafeproducts.com, Apple App Store, or Google Play Store under "SkinSAFE") to generate this list or build customized lists free of fragrances, common preservatives, parabens, nickel, lanolin, coconut, and topical antibiotics. In 35% of patients, simply using products free of the top 10 allergens can prompt clearance. Some physicians follow these measures for several months, especially if the eruption is mild, before pursuing formal patch testing.

An excellent primer for the physician interested in learning more about contact allergy diagnosis and management is *Contact and Occupational Dermatology*.

References

Bruze M, Zimerson E: Dimethyl fumarate, *Dermatitis* 22:3–7, 2011.
Castanedo-Tardana MP, Zug KA: Methylisothiazolinone. *Dermatitis* 24:2–6, 2013. Available at: https://doi.org/10.1097/ DER.0b013e31827edc73.
DeKoven JG, Warschaw EM, Belsito DV, et al: North American Contact Dermatitis Group patch test results 2013-2014, *Dermatitis* 28:33–46, 2017, Available at: https://doi.org/10.1097/DER.0000000000000225.
DeKoven JG, Warschaw EM, Zug KA, et al: North American Contact Dermatitis Group patch test results: 2015-2016, *Dermatitis* 29:297–309, 2018, Available at: https://doi.org/10.1097/DER.0000000000000417.
Heurung AR, Raju SI, Warshaw EM: Benzophenones, *Dermatitis* 25:3–10, 2014. Available at: https://doi.org/10.1097/ DER.0000000000000025.
Jacob SE, Scheman A, McGowan MA: Allergen of the Year: Propylene Glycol, *Dermatitis*, 2017 Available at: https://doi.org/10.1097/DER.0000000000000315.
Macneil JS: Henna tattoo ingredient is allergen of the year, *Skin & Allergy News*, March 1, 2006, Available at: http://www.skinandallergynews.com/index.php?id=372&cHash=071010&tx_ttnews%5Btt_news%5D=559. Accessed 12 February 2014.
Marks JG, Elsner P, DeLeo VA: *Contact and Occupational Dermatology*, 3rd ed, St. Louis, 2002, Mosby.
Nelson SA, Yiannias JA: Relevance and avoidance of skin-care product allergens: Pearls and pitfalls, *Dermatol Clin* 27:329–336, 2009.
Sasseville D: Acrylates. *Dermatitis* 23:3–5, 2012. Available at: https://doi.org/10.1097/DER.0b013e31823d5cd8.
Splete H: Dermatologists name isobornyl acrylate contact allergen of the year, *Dermatology News*. March 5, 2019, Available at: https://www.mdedge.com/dermatology/article/195656/contact-dermatitis/dermatologists-name-isobornyl-acrylate-contact.
Thin-layer rapid-use epicutaneous test (T.R.U.E. TEST). Available at, https://www.smartpractice.com/shop/wa/category?cn=Products-T.R.U.E.-TEST&id=508222&m=SPA Accessed June 11, 2019.
Veverka KK, Hall MR, Yiannias JA, et al: Trends in patch testing with the mayo clinic standard series, 2011-2015, *Dermatitis* 29(6):310–315, 2018, Available at: https://doi.org/10.1097/DER.0000000000000411.
Warshaw EM, Belsito DV, Taylor JS, et al: North American Contact Dermatitis Group patch test results: 2009 to 2010, *Dermatitis* 24, 2013, 50–9.
Warshaw EM, Maibach HI, Taylor JS, et al: North American Contact Dermatitis Group patch test results: 2011-2012, *Dermatitis* 26(1):49–59, 2015, Available at: https://doi.org/10.1097/DER.0000000000000097.
Wentworth AB, Yiannias JA, Keeling JH, et al: Trends in patch test results and allergen changes in the standard series: A Mayo Clinic 5-year retrospective review. January 1, 2006, through December 31, 2010, *J Am Acad Dermatol* 70:269–275. e4, 2014. Available at: https://doi.org/10.1016/j.jaad.2013.09.047.
Yiannias J: Virtual patch testing: Data driven empiric contact allergen avoidance. In *American College of Allergy, Asthma and Immunology Annual Scientific Meeting, November 11, 2013*, Baltimore, MD, 2013.

CUTANEOUS T-CELL LYMPHOMAS, INCLUDING MYCOSIS FUNGOIDES AND SÉZARY SYNDROME

Method of
Gary S. Wood, MD

CURRENT DIAGNOSIS

For Cutaneous T-cell Lymphomas, obtain the following:
- History: duration and pace of lesion development
- Skin examination: extent of patches, plaques, tumors, and ulcers
- Extracutaneous examination: status of lymph nodes, liver, and spleen
- Laboratory: complete blood cell count, differential, and lesional biopsy results
- Imaging: CT or fused PET/CT scans of the chest, abdomen, and pelvis (not needed for early stage mycosis fungoides)

CURRENT THERAPY

Guidelines Are Primarily for Mycosis Fungoides and Sézary Syndrome:
- Stages IA–IIA: skin-directed therapy with potent topical corticosteroids, topical mechlorethamine (Mustargen),[1] or phototherapy; radiation therapy or topical bexarotene (Targretin) in selected cases
- Stages IIB–IVB: skin-directed therapy plus one or more systemic therapies, such as interferon alfa-2b (Intron A),[1] bexarotene (Targretin), vorinostat (Zolinza), denileukin diftitox (Ontak), or methotrexate; photopheresis for erythrodermic cases
- Combination therapies are often used in intermediate- and advanced-stage disease.
- Multiagent chemotherapy is usually not an effective long-term treatment strategy.

---

[1] Not FDA approved for this indication.

989

Cutaneous T-Cell Lymphomas

Classification

Virtually every subtype of T-cell lymphoma involves the skin primarily or secondarily. The principal types of primary cutaneous T-cell lymphomas (CTCLs) recognized in the World Health Organization and European Organization for Research and Treatment of Cancer classification include mycosis fungoides (MF) and its leukemic variant, the Sézary syndrome (SS); CD30+ large cell lymphoma and lymphomatoid papulosis (LyP); CD30− large cell lymphoma; and pleomorphic CD4+ small or medium cell variants (Table 1). All other primary CTCLs comprise only a few percent of the total. This discussion focuses on MF and SS because they account for up to 75% of primary cutaneous cases.

TABLE 1	Classification of Primary Cutaneous T-Cell Lymphomas	
CTCL TYPE	PROPORTION OF PRIMARY CTCL (%)	5-YEAR SURVIVAL RATE (%)
MF and variants	60	85
SS	3	35*
CD30+ large cell/LyP	25	<95
CD30− large cell	2	15
Pleomorphic small/ medium cell**	8	99
Miscellaneous	<1	Variable

Abbreviations: CTCL = cutaneous T-cell lymphoma; MF = mycosis fungoides; SS = Sézary syndrome.
*The 5-year survival rate depends on the criteria used to define SS, and it may be as low as 10%.
**Now regarded as a lymphoproliferative disorder, not lymphoma.

Standard Diagnosis and Staging Methods

The evaluation of CTCL patients begins with a thorough clinical history and physical examination. Key elements of the history include the pace and nature of disease development, the presence or absence of spontaneous regression of lesions, prior therapy, and ingestion of drugs (e.g., anticonvulsants, antihistamines, other agents with antihistaminic properties) that have been associated with pseudolymphomatous skin eruptions that can mimic CTCLs. The review of systems should establish the presence of lymphoma-associated constitutional symptoms (e.g., fever of unknown origin, night sweats, weight loss, fatigue). In addition to general aspects, the physical examination should document the type and distribution of skin lesions and whether there is lymphadenopathy, hepatosplenomegaly, or edema of extremities (i.e., potential sign of lymphatic obstruction).

Histopathologic analysis of representative lesional skin biopsy specimens is the primary means of confirming the clinical diagnosis. Biopsy specimens should be deep enough to include the deepest portions of the cutaneous lymphoid infiltrates because these areas often exhibit the most diagnostic features. Putative extracutaneous involvement should be confirmed by biopsy if it is relevant to clinical management.

Routine blood tests include a complete blood cell count, differential review, and general chemistry panel. A "Sézary prep" is used to assess peripheral blood involvement.

Internal nodal and visceral involvement by lymphoma usually is assessed with chest radiography, computed tomography (CT), or combined positron emission tomography and CT (PET/CT) scans of the chest, abdomen, and pelvis. These radiologic studies usually are not needed for patients with early forms of MF (i.e., nontumorous skin lesions without evidence of extracutaneous involvement assessed by physical examination); however, they are usually obtained during the workup of other types of CTCLs. The role of immunopathologic and molecular biologic assays in the diagnosis and staging of CTCLs is discussed later.

An algorithm for the diagnosis of early MF has been proposed by the International Society for Cutaneous Lymphomas (ISCL) (see Pimpinelli et al. in References). It relies on a combination of clinical, histopathologic, immunopathologic, and clonality criteria. This differs from former approaches that have been based primarily on histopathologic criteria.

Mycosis Fungoides, Sézary Syndrome, and Variants
Clinical Features

MF classically manifests as erythematous, scaly, variably pruritic, flat patches or indurated plaques, often favoring the most sun-protected areas. The patches or plaques may progress to cutaneous tumors and involvement of lymph nodes or viscera,

although this usually does not occur as long as the skin lesions are reasonably well controlled by therapy. SS manifests as total-body erythema and scaling (i.e., erythroderma), generalized lymphadenopathy, hepatosplenomegaly, and leukemia. Large-plaque parapsoriasis is essentially the prediagnostic patch phase of MF. Lesions may exhibit poikiloderma (i.e., atrophy, telangiectasia, and mottled hyperpigmentation and hypopigmentation) and have then been referred to as *poikiloderma atrophicans vasculare.*

Follicular mucinosis refers to a papulonodular eruption in which hair follicles are infiltrated by T cells and contain pools of mucin. In hairy areas, this may result in alopecia. Follicular mucinosis may exist as a lesional variant of MF (i.e., follicular MF) or as a clinically benign entity (i.e., alone or associated with other lymphomas).

Granulomatous slack skin is a variant of MF that manifests with pendulous skin folds in intertriginous areas. Lesional skin biopsy specimens contain atypical T cells in a granulomatous background.

Pagetoid reticulosis manifests as a solitary or localized, often hyperkeratotic plaque containing atypical T cells that are frequently confined to a hyperplastic epidermis. Some authorities regard it as a variant of unilesional MF, whereas others think it is a distinct entity.

Other variants of MF include hypopigmented, palmoplantar, bullous, and pigmented purpuric forms. The latter form shows clinicopathologic overlap with the pigmented purpuric dermatoses. *Tumor d'emblée* MF is an outmoded concept used in the past to refer to supposed cases of MF that manifested as cutaneous tumors in the absence of patches or plaques. Most experts now prefer to classify such cases as other forms of CTCL, depending on their histopathologic features.

Histopathologic and Cytologic Features

A well-developed plaque of MF contains a bandlike, cytologically atypical lymphoid infiltrate in the upper dermis that infiltrates the epidermis as single cells and cell clusters known as Pautrier's microabscesses. The atypical lymphoid cells exhibit dense, hyperchromatic nuclei with convoluted, cerebriform nuclear contours and scant cytoplasm. The term *cerebriform* comes from the brain-like ultrastructural appearance of these nuclei. In more advanced cutaneous tumors, the infiltrate extends diffusely throughout the upper and lower dermis and may lose its epidermotropism. In the earlier patch phase of the disease, the infiltrate is sparser, and lymphoid atypia may be less pronounced. In some cases, it may be difficult to distinguish early patch-type MF from various types of chronic dermatitis. The presence of lymphoid atypia and absence of significant epidermal intercellular edema (i.e., spongiosis) help to establish the diagnosis of early MF.

Involvement of lymph nodes by MF begins in the paracortical T-cell domain and may progress to complete effacement of nodal architecture by the same types of atypical lymphoid cells that infiltrate the skin. These cells can be seen in low numbers in the peripheral blood of many MF patients; however, those with SS develop gross leukemic involvement, usually defined as at least 1000 tumor cells/mm^3. These cells are known as Sézary cells, and they are traditionally detected by manual review of the peripheral blood smear (the so-called Sézary prep). They may also be defined by various immunophenotypic criteria.

Immunophenotyping

Cellular antigen expression is usually assessed by immunoperoxidase methods for tissue biopsy specimens and by flow cytometry for blood specimens. Almost all cases of MF or SS begin as phenotypically and functionally mature CD4+ T-cell neoplasms of skin-associated lymphoid tissue (SALT). MF and SS express homing markers consistent with "effector memory" and "central memory" T cells, respectively. They express the SALT-associated homing molecule cutaneous lymphocyte antigen (CLA) and most mature T-cell surface antigens, with the exceptions of CD7 and CD26, which are often absent. As disease progresses, the tumor cells often dedifferentiate and lose one or more mature T-cell markers, such as CD2, CD3, or CD5.

Cases typically express the α/β form of the T-cell receptor. At least in advanced cases, the cytokine profile is consistent with the T_H2 subset of CD4+ T cells (i.e., production of interleukin [IL]-4, IL-5, and IL-10 rather than T_H1 cytokines such as IL-2 and interferon-γ). Expression of the high-affinity IL-2 receptor (CD25, TAC) ranges widely, with most cases showing a variable minority of lesional CD25+ cells. Tumor cells can be induced to express a regulatory T-cell phenotype (Treg) in vitro. MF cases that express CD8+ or other aberrant phenotypes occur occasionally but behave like conventional cases. They should not be confused with rare aggressive CTCLs exhibiting cytotoxic T-cell differentiation.

In addition to tumor cells, MF and SS lesions contain a minor component of immune accessory cells (i.e., Langerhans cells and macrophages) and CD8+ T cells with a cytolytic phenotype. This presumed host response correlates positively with survival and tends to decrease as lesions progress. A favorable response to therapy such as photopheresis appears to correlate with normal levels of circulating CD8+ cells.

Molecular Biology

Well-developed MF or SS is a monoclonal T-cell lymphoproliferative disorder. Southern blotting or polymerase chain reaction (PCR) assays demonstrate monoclonal T-cell receptor gene rearrangements. The greater sensitivity of PCR assays allows the demonstration of dominant clonality in many early patch-type lesions of MF. These assays sometimes detect dominant clonality in lesional skin showing only chronic dermatitis histopathologically. These cases are called *clonal dermatitis* and may represent the earliest manifestation of MF because several have progressed to histologically recognizable MF within a few years. However, some cases of clinicopathologically defined early-phase MF lack a detectable monoclonal T-cell population until later in their clinical course. Next generation high throughput T-cell receptor sequencing is emerging as a more sensitive and quantitative alternative to other molecular assays of T-cell clonality.

In addition to aiding initial diagnosis, gene rearrangement analysis has facilitated staging and prognosis. Because some patients without MF or SS can have low levels of circulating Sézary-like cells and because not all cases of peripheral blood involvement in MF or SS exhibit morphologically recognizable tumor cells, the demonstration of dominant clonality that matches the clone in lesional skin has proved to be a useful diagnostic adjunct. The same holds true for assessing lymph node involvement. T-cell receptor gene rearrangement analysis of MF and SS lymph nodes is more sensitive than histopathology and possesses at least some prognostic relevance.

TNMB Staging

Although several proposed methods have used a weighted extent approach to more accurately determine the MF or SS tumor burden, the preferred approach is the tumor–node–metastasis–blood (TNMB) system, which is detailed in Tables 2 and 3. The original tumor (skin), lymph nodes, and metastasis (visceral organs) version of this system has been modified by the ISCL to incorporate the extent of blood involvement (B classification) into the staging process. Table 2 shows the TNMB classification relevant to MF and SS, and Table 3 shows how this information is used to determine the stage of disease. The prognostic relevance of this staging system has been supported by numerous studies, and use of the TNMB helps to guide the selection of therapies. For example, early-stage MF is the most amenable to control with topically directed treatments, whereas advanced MF or SS with extracutaneous involvement usually requires systemic therapies or topical plus systemic combinations.

Treatment

Treatment guidelines for CTCL published by the National Comprehensive Cancer Network can be found at www.nccn.org.

TABLE 2	TNMB Classification of Mycosis Fungoides and Sézary Syndrome
Skin (T)	
T1	Patches and/or plaques; <10% body surface area
T2	Patches and/or plaques; ≥10% body surface area
T3	Tumors with/without other skin lesions
T4	Generalized erythroderma
Lymph Nodes (N)	
N0	Not clinically enlarged; histopathology not required
N1	Clinically enlarged; histopathologically negative
N2	Clinically enlarged; histopathologically equivocal
N3	Clinically enlarged; histopathologically positive
Visceral Organs (M)	
M0	No involvement
M1	Involvement
Peripheral Blood (B)	
B0	Atypical cells ≤5% of lymphocyte
B1	Atypical cells >5% of lymphocytes
B2	Atypical cells ≥1000/mm³

T1 and T2 can be subclassified as patch only vs. plaque +/– patch. N and B categories can be subclassified as clone positive or negative.

TABLE 3	TNMB Staging System for Mycosis Fungoides and Sézary Syndrome			
STAGE	**SKIN**	**LYMPH NODES**	**VISCERA**	**BLOOD**
IA	T1	N0	M0	B0–1
IB	T2	N0	M0	B0–1
IIA	T1–2	N1–2	M0	B0–1
IIB	T3	N0–2	M0	B0–1
IIIA	T4	N0–2	M0	B0
IIIB	T4	N0–2	M0	B1
IVA-1	T1–4	N0–2	M0	B2
IVA-2	T1–4	N3	M0	B0–2
IVB	T1–4	N0–3	M1	B0–2

Modified from Olsen E, Vonderheid E, et al: Revisions to the staging and classification of mycosis fungoides and Sézary syndrome: A proposal of the International Society for Cutaneous Lymphomas (ISCL) and the cutaneous lymphoma task force of the European Organization of Research and Treatment of Cancer (EORTC). Blood 2007;110(6):1713–1722.

Rather than cure, which is attained in less than 10% of cases, the goal of MF and SS therapy is to reduce the impact of the skin disease on quality of life. For most patients, this is achieved by reducing pain, itch, and infection and improving clinical appearance. Appearance is affected by the disfigurement of the eruption and by the profound degree of scale shedding in some patients. Because the natural history of early-stage MF predicts a virtually normal life span, the goal of treatment must be directed at quality of life. For more advanced stages, prolongation of life expectancy may be a reasonable treatment goal.

Regardless of presentation, relief of symptoms should be addressed early. For dryness and scaling, the use of emollient ointments is indicated. These include petrolatum, Aquaphor, and commercially available shortening such as Crisco (an inexpensive alternative).[1] For modest dryness, creams (e.g., Nivea, Cetaphil, Eucerin) can be adequate and more acceptable to patients. Mild superfatted soaps such as Dove and Oil of Olay are recommended. Soap substitutes such as Cetaphil are also acceptable. Pruritus can be addressed with oral agents such as hydroxyzine (Atarax) or diphenhydramine (Benadryl)[1] 2 to 5 mg/kg/day and divided into four daily doses. Antipruritics work better when used on a regular basis rather than on an as-needed basis. Nonsedating antihistamines tend to be less effective. Measures to reduce dryness also help to reduce pruritus. Secondary infection needs to be treated with appropriate antibiotics. Their selection is guided by results of skin cultures but usually involves coverage of gram-positive organisms.

Phototherapy

Two main phototherapeutic regimens are used to treat CTCLs. Ultraviolet B radiation (290–320-nm broad band or 311-nm narrow band) can be used for patients with patches but not those with well-developed plaques or tumors. Seventy percent of patients achieve total clinical remission, usually within about 3 to 5 months. Another 15% achieve partial remission. Narrow-band UVB usually is more effective than broadband UVB and achieves maximal responses more rapidly.

Psoralen–ultraviolet A (PUVA) photochemotherapy uses oral 8-methoxypsoralen (8-MOP)[1] 0.6 mg/kg as a photosensitizer before UVA (320–400 nm) exposure. Sixty-five percent of patients with patch or plaque disease achieve complete remissions, and 30% have partial responses to this modality. For most patients, maximal responses are achieved within 3 months, and after 5 months, it is unlikely that further improvement will be gained. Limitations of these modalities include actinic damage, photocarcinogenesis, retinal damage (if eyes are not protected), and the inconvenience of getting to phototherapy centers. PUVA also has the risk of nausea and a theoretical risk of cataract induction without proper eye protection.

During the clearing phase of treatment, phototherapy treatments usually are administered three times per week. After resolution of skin lesions, treatment frequency is usually tapered gradually to once weekly for UVB and once every 4 to 6 weeks for PUVA. These maintenance regimens are often continued for months to years because abrupt cessation of phototherapy is commonly associated with rapid relapse, which is probably related to the persistence of microscopic disease after clinical clearing.

Topical Therapy

Like phototherapeutic regimens, topical therapies are appropriate for disease confined to the skin (stage I). Topical corticosteroids are frequently used for CTCLs, often before diagnosis. Low-potency formulations are useful on the face and skin folds. Medium-potency preparations are appropriate for the trunk and extremities. High-potency formulations are useful for recalcitrant lesions; however, prolonged use of such potent agents can cause local atrophy and adrenal suppression. Roughly half of patients achieve complete remissions, and most others have partial remissions. Response duration varies widely with the individual pace of disease and patient compliance. Topical corticosteroids are particularly useful as a means to relatively quickly ameliorate severe signs and symptoms and as an adjuvant therapy in combination with other primary treatments.

Mechlorethamine (nitrogen mustard, HN$_2$, Mustargen) is applied topically in an aqueous solution or in an ointment, such as Aquaphor. Although these forms are not FDA approved for this indication, a 0.016% gel formulation (Valchlor) is now commercially available and FDA approved. The aqueous form is prepared at home and involves a daily dose totaling 10 mg in 60 mL water. The ointment form is prepared by a pharmacist in 1-pound lots at a concentration of 10 mg mechlorethamine per 100 g ointment. Only the amount of ointment needed to apply a thin layer is used. Either formulation is usually applied at bedtime to lesional skin for limited disease or to the entire skin surface (excluding the head unless it is also involved) for more extensive disease. It is then showered off every morning using soap and water. Results are similar to those from PUVA. Advantages include therapy at home and availability in all regions of the country. Disadvantages are daily preparation (aqueous form only), daily application, and possible allergic contact dermatitis (more common with the aqueous preparation). Maximal efficacy is expected within 6 months. Mild flare-ups of disease may occur during the first few months of treatment and probably represent inflammation of subclinical skin lesions, analogous to the clinical accentuation of actinic damage during topical therapy with 5-fluorouracil (Efudex). As with phototherapy, topical mechlorethamine is tapered gradually after remission is achieved in an effort to delay clinical relapse.

Carmustine (BCNU, BiCNU)[1] is applied to the total skin surface as an alcohol/aqueous solution (10–20 mg in 60 mL).[6] Complete responses are seen in 85% of patients with stage IA disease (<10% involvement) and 50% of patients with stage IB disease (>10% involvement). Another 10% of patients obtain partial responses. Advantages include those described for nitrogen mustard and reports of success with application only to lesional skin. Disadvantages include skin irritation followed by telangiectasia formation and possible bone marrow suppression necessitating blood monitoring.

A topical gel formulation of the retinoid X receptor (RXR)–specific retinoid, bexarotene (Targretin), is useful for localized or limited skin lesions. The principal side effect is local irritation.

Radiotherapy

Conventional radiotherapy for mycosis fungoides therapy has been used for approximately 100 years. It is useful in the treatment of isolated, particularly problematic lesions such as recalcitrant tumors or ulcerated plaques. In addition to benefit from the photons delivered by radiotherapy, electron beam therapy (0.4 Gy per week for 8–9 weeks) is also useful for CTCL therapy. An approximately 85% complete response rate of skin disease with a median duration of 16 months is expected with electron beam therapy. An advantage is an excellent rate of complete response. Disadvantages include limited access to required equipment and expertise and cutaneous toxic effects, such as alopecia, sweat gland loss, radiation dermatitis, and skin cancers. As with other skin-directed therapy, the benefit for internal disease is limited. Cumulative toxicity also limits the number of courses a patient may receive. Localized electron beam therapy is also useful for treating cases of limited-extent MF and in treating selected problematic MF lesions in patients who are otherwise responding to therapy. After completion of total-skin electron beam therapy, patients require maintenance therapy such as topical mechlorethamine[6] or phototherapy to prolong remission. Low dose radiotherapy is emerging as an effective alternative to conventional regimens.

Apheresis-Based Therapy

Leukapheresis and particularly lymphocytapheresis (6000–7000 mL of blood treated three times per week initially, then according to response) have been used in the treatment of SS patients. Benefit has been reported in several case reports and small case series; however, response rates are not possible to determine. Photopheresis (i.e., extracorporeal photochemotherapy) describes an apheresis-based therapy in which circulating lymphocytes are first exposed to a psoralen (orally or extracorporeally) and then exposed to UVA extracorporeally. In contrast to leukapheresis, in which leukocytes are discarded, all cells are returned to the patient's circulation during photopheresis. Response rates in erythrodermic patients are 33% to 50%, and median survival for SS patients is prolonged from 30 months to

---

[1] Not FDA approved for this indication.

[1] Not FDA approved for this indication.
[6] May be compounded by pharmacists.

more than 60 months. In recent years, extracorporeal photoche-motherapy has been used increasingly in conjunction with one or more systemic therapies to enhance efficacy. The toxicity of the systemic agents is diminished because they are often used in combination at reduced doses.

Cytokine Therapy

Interferon alfa-2a (Roferon-A) or alfa-2b (Intron-A)[1] (1 to 100 × 10[6] units) is given subcutaneously or intralesionally every other day to once weekly. A standard starting dose is 3 × 10[6] units three times per week. Response rates are approximately 55%, with complete responses occurring in 17% of patients. Advantages include the relative ease of delivery. Disadvantages include anorexia, fever, malaise, leukopenia, and risk of cardiac dysrhythmia. Interferon alfa-2a or alfa-2b combined with narrow-band UVB or PUVA is effective for many patients with generalized skin lesions unresponsive to phototherapy alone.

Tumor-Associated Antigen-Directed Therapies

Various specific tumor-associated antigens have been targeted with antibody-based therapy. The response rate typically is low, and response durations are short. Less specific targets are CD4, CD5, and IL-2 receptors. Of this class of agent, the most promising is denileukin diftitox (Ontak, DAB389 IL-2) (9–18 µg per/kg/day IV on 5 consecutive days, every 3 weeks). This agent is a fusion protein combining IL-2 and diphtheria toxin. Cells bearing the IL-2 receptor (in the lesions of at least one half of MF patients) bind and internalize the drug. The drug also may destroy Treg cells that are CD25[+] and suppress immune responses. Inside the cell, the toxin portion of the molecule disrupts protein synthesis, leading to cell death. Approximately 10% of patients achieve complete responses, and total response rates of near 40% have been reported. Half of responders and 20% of nonresponders experienced decreased pruritus. Adverse events include capillary leak syndrome, flulike symptoms, and allergic reactions. Combination therapy with denileukin diftitox and multiagent chemotherapy is being explored for advanced disease. Alemtuzumab (Campath)[1] is an antibody directed against CD52. It has shown benefit in advanced-stage disease. This agent can be used alone or in conjunction with multiagent chemotherapy. Brentuximab vedotin (Adcetris)[1] is an anti-CD30 antibody linked to the microtubule toxin monomethyl auristatin E. It can be effective in those cases of MF that express sufficient CD30. Mogamulizumab (Poteligeo) is an antibody directed against CCR4. It is approved for relapsed or refractory MF or SS after at least one other systemic therapy. Pembrolizumab (Keytruda)[1] is an antibody directed against PD1. It can be of benefit for relapsed or refractory MF or SS. Mogamulizumab (Poteligeo) is an antibody directed against CCR4. It is approved for relapsed or refractory MF or SS after at least one other systemic therapy. Pembrolizumab (Keytruda)[1] is an antibody directed against PD1. It can be of benefit for relapsed or refractory MF or SS.

Systemic Chemotherapy

Various regimens of single-agent and multiagent chemotherapy have been used in the treatment of MF and SS. Oral methotrexate, chlorambucil (Leukeran)[1] with or without prednisone,[1] and etoposide (VePesid)[1] have shown therapeutic activity. The best response has been in erythrodermic patients treated with methotrexate (5 to 125 mg weekly),[3] who have shown a 58% response rate. The combination of low-dose methotrexate and interferon alfa has been reported to yield a high response rate in advanced-stage MF and SS.

The use of multiagent regimens is controversial because of the small number of patients treated with any given regimen. There is even some evidence that for some populations of CTCL patients, survival may be reduced. For individual patients with advanced disease, however, cyclophosphamide (Cytoxan),[1] doxorubicin (Adriamycin),[1] vincristine (Oncovin),[1] and prednisone[1] (CHOP regimen) can provide some short-term palliation. In some cases, CHOP has successfully eradicated large cell transformation of MF and returned patients to their more clinically indolent patch or plaque baseline disease. Idarubicin (Idamycin)[1] in association with etoposide, cyclophosphamide, vincristine, prednisone, and bleomycin (Blenoxane)[1] (VICOP-B regimen) has demonstrated response rates of 80% (36% complete response rate) for patients with stage II through IV disease and 84% for MF patients, with a median duration of response longer than 8 months. Other regimens have been used with more modest success.

Several purine nucleoside analogues have been used for CTCL treatment, including erythrodermic variants. These include 2-chlorodeoxyadenosine (cladribine [Leustatin],[1] with a response rate of 28%), 2-deoxycoformycin (pentostatin [Nipent],[1] with a response rate of 39%), and fludarabine (Fludara).[1] Toxicities include pulmonary edema, bone marrow and immune suppression, and neurotoxicity.

Retinoids

Retinoids have therapeutic activity against MF and SS alone and in combination with other therapies, such as interferon alfa or PUVA (the latter combination is called Re-PUVA). Arotinoid,[5] acitretin (Soriatane),[1] and 13-cis-retinoic acid (isotretinoin [Accutane])[1] have various degrees of efficacy, and they typically are used in conjunction with other modalities. A newer RXR-specific retinoid, bexarotene, has an overall response rate of about 40% and can be used alone or in combination with phototherapy and other systemic agents such as interferon alfa-2. Disadvantages of bexarotene therapy include signs of hypothyroidism and vitamin A toxicity, particularly hyperlipidemia.

Enzyme Inhibitors

Vorinostat (Zolinza) is the first histone deacetylase inhibitor to be FDA approved for MF and SS. The overall response rate approaches 40% using a standard oral dose of 400 mg/day. Side effects include gastrointestinal symptoms, thrombocytopenia, and cardiac conduction abnormalities. Rhomidepsin (Isotodax) is an intravenously administered histone deacetylase inhibitor recently approved by the FDA for MF and SS. Forodesine[5] is a purine nucleoside phosphorylase inhibitor that preferentially affects T cells because they contain relatively high concentrations of this enzyme. Forodesine is undergoing clinical trials for MF and SS in the United States and appears to have a response rate of about 40%.

Miscellaneous Therapies

Various other therapies have been tried for MF and SS with modest success. Nonmyeloablative allogeneic stem cell transplantation has led to favorable responses in some patients; however, the total number treated is small. Cyclosporine (Sandimmune)[1] has been used for MF and SS. Transient improvement is followed by worsened survival due to immunosuppression, and it is not a recommended therapy. Thymopentin[5] has given excellent results in SS patients (i.e., 40% complete response rate and 35% partial response rate, with a median duration of response of 22 months). The lack of follow-up reports in recent decades leaves the status of this therapy in question.

Selection of Therapy

Initial choices among conventional treatments for MF and SS depend on the types of lesions and the stage of disease. Disease subsets are followed by recommended initial treatments in parentheses: unilesional or localized MF (local radiation therapy), patch MF (broad- and narrow-band UVB, PUVA, mechlorethamine), patch/plaque MF (PUVA, mechlorethamine), thick plaque/tumor MF (electron beam radiation therapy, interferon alfa-2, bexarotene, histone deacetylase inhibitors), erythrodermic MF/SS (photopheresis), and nodal or visceral MF or SS (interferon alfa-2,

---

[1]Not FDA approved for this indication.
[3]Exceeds dosage recommended by the manufacturer.

[1]Not FDA approved for this indication.
[5]Investigational drug in the United States.

bexarotene, histone deacetylase inhibitors, denileukin diftitox, experimental systemic therapies, systemic chemotherapy).

Second-line therapeutic choices often involve interferons, retinoids, or histone deacetylase inhibitors, usually in combination with primary modalities. Multimodality combinations, often at reduced doses, are used commonly to treat patients with stage IIB or more advanced disease. Medium-potency topical corticosteroids, such as 0.1% triamcinolone cream or ointment (Kenalog),[1] are useful adjuncts to many different therapies. The optimal use of newer therapeutic agents in various subtypes and stages of MF and SS is still being established. Evidence-based guidelines for MF and SS therapy have been developed by the National Comprehensive Cancer Network (NCCN) (www.nccn.org).

Lymphoproliferative Disorders Associated with Mycosis Fungoides and Sézary Syndrome

Types and Clinical Features

Patients with MF or SS are at increased risk for large T-cell lymphomas, lymphomatoid papulosis, and Hodgkin's disease. Molecular biologic analysis has shown that these disorders and MF often share the same clonal T-cell receptor gene rearrangement when they arise in the same individual. As a consequence, they are considered to be subclones of the original MF tumor clone. The development of large T-cell lymphoma in a patient with MF or SS is referred to as *large cell transformation of MF*. This occurs in up to 20% of cases in some series and is associated with a median survival of only 1 to 2 years. One half of these large T-cell lymphomas are CD30[+]; however, the generally favorable prognosis of primary cutaneous CD30[+] anaplastic large cell lymphoma may not extend to these secondary forms of CD30[+] lymphoma. These patients may need to be treated with systemic chemotherapy such as CHOP or with experimental systemic therapies appropriate for advanced-stage CTCL.

Lymphomatoid papulosis manifests as recurrent, usually generalized crops of spontaneously regressing, erythematous papules that can exhibit crusting or vesiculation before resolution. It is the clinically benign end of a disease continuum that has primary cutaneous CD30[+] anaplastic large cell lymphoma at its other extreme. Intermediate forms of disease can occur. Histopathologically, lesions contain a mixed-cell infiltrate, including large, atypical T cells that resemble Reed-Sternberg cells and their mononuclear variants (so-called type A) or large MF-type cells (so-called type B). Type A cells are CD30[+]. A type C form is also recognized. It has sheets of type A cells histologically mimicking CD30[+] large T-cell lymphoma but is different from it clinically. A type D variant containing CD8[+] CD30[+] large atypical cells has also been described recently, as well as a few other rare subtypes. All types of lymphomatoid papulosis behave similarly. Patients with lymphomatoid papulosis sometimes respond to tetracycline[1] or erythromycin[1] (500 mg PO bid), presumably on the basis of antiinflammatory activity. Most cases improve within 1 month with low-dose methotrexate (10–20 mg PO every week). PUVA and narrow-band UVB given three times per week are other therapeutic options.

Treatment

In most cases, non-MF/SS CTCLs are treated with radiation therapy (with or without complete surgical excision) if they are localized or with various multiagent systemic chemotherapy regimens if they are generalized. The roles of other agents remain to be defined, except that studies have proved that methotrexate (10–40 mg PO every week) is effective therapy for most cases of primary cutaneous CD30[+] anaplastic large cell lymphoma. Therapies being investigated for this lymphoma include anti-CD30 antibodies, alone or conjugated to toxins. One of these antibody conjugates (brentuximab vedotin [Adcetris]) is FDA approved for systemic CD30[+] lymphomas and Hodgkin's disease. Denileukin diftitox[2] has been reported to be effective against some subcutaneous panniculitic T-cell lymphomas.

---

[1]Not FDA approved for this indication.
[2]Not available in the United States.

References

Olsen E, Vonderheid E, et al: Revisions to the staging and classification of mycosis fungoides and Sézary syndrome: A proposal of the International Society for Cutaneous Lymphomas (ISCL) and the cutaneous lymphoma task force of the European Organization of Research and Treatment of Cancer (EORTC), *Blood* 110(6):1713–1722, 2007.

Pimpinelli N, Olsen EA, Santucci M, et al: Defining early mycosis fungoides, *J Am Acad Dermatol* 53(6):1053–1063, 2005.

Richardson SK, Lin JH, Vittorio CC, et al: High clinical response rate with multimodality immunomodulatory therapy for Sézary syndrome, *Clin Lymphoma Myeloma* 7(3):226–232, 2006.

Vonderheid EC, Bernengo MG, Burg G, et al: Update on erythrodermic cutaneous T-cell lymphoma: Report of the International Society for Cutaneous Lymphomas, *J Am Acad Dermatol* 46(1):95–106, 2002.

Willemze R, Jaffe ES, Burg G, et al: WHO-EORTC classification for cutaneous lymphomas, *Blood* 105(10):3768–3785, 2005.

Wood GS, Greenberg HL: Diagnosis, staging, and monitoring of cutaneous T-cell lymphoma, *Dermatol Ther* 16(4):269–275, 2003.

CUTANEOUS VASCULITIS

Method of
Molly A. Hinshaw, MD; and Susan Lawrence-Hylland, MD

CURRENT DIAGNOSIS

- Cutaneous vasculitis can be limited to skin (leukocytoclastic vasculitis) or associated with systemic disease.
- Perform punch biopsy of intact, nonulcerated skin lesion.
- "Vasculitis" on skin biopsy describes vessel appearance and is not a clinical diagnosis.
- Thorough review of systems and physical examination are necessary to evaluate for systemic vasculitis.

CURRENT THERAPY

Leukocytoclastic Vasculitis
- First identify instigating factors: infection, medications.
- Care is symptomatic. Lesions typically remit without treatment.
- If needed, short course of prednisone may be given and tapered over 3 to 6 weeks.

All Forms of Vasculitis
- Treat underlying systemic vasculitis.

Vasculitis is an inflammatory-mediated destruction of blood vessels. The systemic vasculitides have historically been differentiated by their involvement of small, medium, or large blood vessels. Names used to describe isolated cutaneous vasculitis have included hypersensitivity vasculitis and leukocytoclastic vasculitis (LCV). In 1990, the American College of Rheumatology proposed five criteria for the classification of hypersensitivity vasculitis: age older than 16 years, possible drug trigger, palpable purpura, maculopapular rash, and skin biopsy showing neutrophils around vessel. At least three out of five criteria yield a sensitivity of 71% and specificity of 84%. In 1994, a new nomenclature proposed at the Chapel Hill International Consensus Conference in North Carolina further classified vasculitis (Box 1). The term "hypersensitivity vasculitis" was not used, because most vasculitides that would have previously been in this category fall into either microscopic polyangiitis or cutaneous LCV. LCV is vasculitis restricted to the skin without involvement of vessels in other organs. Cutaneous vasculitis may be a clue to systemic vasculitis and guides the clinician to a comprehensive evaluation (Table 1).

Vasculitis can affect almost any organ, and once affected, end organs can become dysfunctional. Such dysfunction may be as innocuous as cutaneous, tender, transient papules or as devastating as a stroke. A thorough evaluation of the patient with a complete review of systems, physical examination, laboratory evaluation, and clinical follow-up allows a distinction to be made between the different forms of vasculitis.

Leukocytoclastic Vasculitis

Epidemiology
LCV is common. The incidence and prevalence are unknown. Mean age of onset ranges from 34 to 49 years of age. The female-to-male ratio ranges from approximately 2:1 to 3:1.

BOX 1   Chapel Hill Consensus 1994 Classification of Vasculitis

Large-Vessel Vasculitis
Giant cell arteritis
Takayasu's arteritis

Medium-Vessel Vasculitis
Classic polyarteritis nodosa
Kawasaki's disease

Small-Vessel Vasculitis
Churg-Strauss syndrome
Cutaneous leukocytoclastic vasculitis
Essential cryoglobulinemia
Henoch-Schönlein purpura
Microscopic polyangiitis (polyarteritis)
Wegener's granulomatosis

Risk Factors
LCV is often secondary to a known trigger including infection, drug ingestion, or malignancy. LCV can also be a presenting feature of autoimmune disease.

Pathophysiology
LCV is best characterized as immune complex–mediated inflammatory destruction of the postcapillary venules of any organ. The exact mechanisms of vascular destruction is unknown.

Clinical Manifestations
LCV typically manifests as nonblanchable macules that evolve to papules or, less commonly, pustules and ulcers (Figure 1). Clues to the diagnosis include a monomorphous, ruddy-brown appearance owing to leakage of hemosiderin pigment from vessels. Lesions measure a few millimeters to a few centimeters in diameter. LCV is often localized to the lower extremities but may be diffuse. Pruritus, pain, or burning of the skin lesions are indicators that the patient might have a vasculitis extending beyond LCV.

Diagnosis
To confirm a clinical impression of LCV, perform a punch biopsy in the center of a nonulcerated cutaneous lesion that is less than 24 to 48 hours old and submit the sample in 10% formalin (standard medium). It is important to biopsy an intact, nonulcerated active lesion (Figure 2) because ulcers can show histologic features simulating vasculitis regardless of whether the patient has true vasculitis or not.

Pathology reveals a mononuclear or polymorphonuclear inflammation of the small blood vessels (called LCV), most prominent in the postcapillary venules. The appearance may be necrotizing or non-necrotizing.

TABLE 1   Diseases with Cutaneous Vasculitis as a Component of Their Presentation

DISEASE	SKIN LESIONS	CLUES AND CONFIRMATION
Urticarial vasculitis	Individual lesions look like urticaria but last >24 h; typical urticaria last a few hours, always <24 h Pruritus, burning of skin lesions	May be associated with connective tissue disease, medications, low complement, viral infections (e.g., hep B, hep C, EBV) Skin biopsy
Henoch-Schönlein purpura	Wheals progress to petechia, ecchymoses and palpable purpura Lesions are in gravity-dependent or pressure-dependent areas such as legs or the buttocks in toddlers	Arthralgia or arthritis, hematuria, abdominal pain, melena Skin biopsy and DIF for IgA
Essential mixed cryoglobulinemia	Palpable purpura	Peripheral neuropathy, GN Hep C positive Serum cryoglobulins
Wegener's granulomatosis	Palpable purpura, hemorrhagic lesions, petechiae, skin ulcers	c-ANCA >80% Pulmonary hemorrhage, GN Biopsy affected organ
Churg-Strauss syndrome	Maculopapular rash, palpable purpura, hemorrhagic lesions, subcutaneous nodules, livedo reticularis or Raynaud's disease	ANCA (50%) Asthma, allergic rhinitis Eosinophilia >1.5 × 10⁹/L Pulmonary infiltrates, pulmonary neuropathy Biopsy affected organ
Microscopic polyangiitis	Palpable purpura, hemorrhagic lesions, petechiae, skin ulcers, splinter hemorrhages	p-ANCA >60% Pulmonary hemorrhage, GN Biopsy affected organ
Polyarteritis nodosa	Livedo reticularis, tender nodules, skin ulcers, bullae or vesicles	Hypertension, elevated creatinine, abdominal pain, constitutional symptoms (fever) Abnormal angiogram Biopsy affected organ

Abbreviations: c-ANCA = classic antineutrophil cytoplasmic antibody; DIF = direct immunofluorescence; EBV = Epstein-Barr virus; GN = glomerulonephritis; hep = hepatitis; Ig = immunoglobulin; p-ANCA = protoplasmic-staining antineutrophil cytoplasmic antibody.

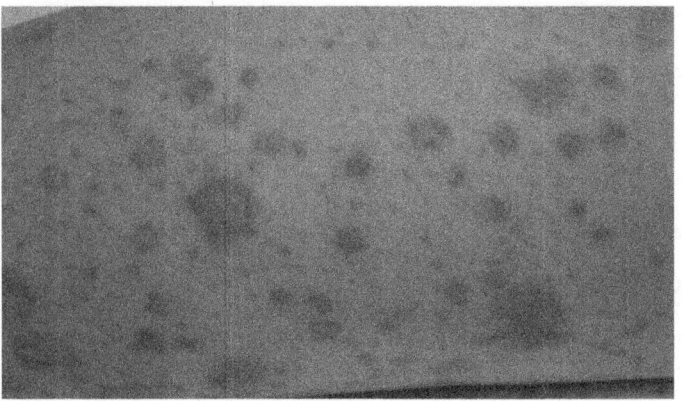

Figure 1 Leukocytoclastic vasculitis: palpable, purpuric, nonblanching, erythematous to ruddy-brown thin papules. Additional secondary changes include small pustules (pustular vasculitis) or shallow, small ulcerations.

Figure 2 Biopsy of intact clinical lesion of leukocytoclastic vasculitis. Histology shows destruction of postcapillary venules with fibrin deposition, degenerate inflammatory cells, and extravasated erythrocytes.

Differential Diagnosis

LCV manifests as erythematous papules or occasionally as papulopustules that can simulate a variety of entities (see Table 1). The review of systems and physical examination should be directed to evaluate for diseases that have cutaneous vasculitis as a component of their presentation (see Table 1). All patients with LCV should have a urinalysis to evaluate for hematuria as a sign of kidney involvement, with subsequent evaluation and management if identified.

Treatment

The primary goal in the management of LCV is to identify and treat instigating factors, including infection and medications. Supportive treatment includes resting, elevating legs, and wearing support hose. When review of systems, physical examination, and urinalysis do not reveal associated systemic diseases, treatment of LCV is generally not necessary. Lesions typically remit without treatment. In rare patients with symptomatic, extensively pustular, or progressive lesions, a short course of prednisone[1] dosed at 1 mg/kg/day initially and tapered over 3 to 6 weeks may be used, although no controlled trials have been performed using oral corticosteroids for isolated LCV. Rapid steroid taper can lead to rebound. Systematic evaluation of the use of other medications, such as colchicine[1] or dapsone,[1] to treat isolated LCV has not been performed.

---

[1]Not FDA approved for this indication.

Monitoring

Patients with LCV are at risk for recurrent or chronic vasculitis. In addition, apparent LCV can occur as a systemic disease that is not recognizable at the first episode. Patients with persistent or recurrent LCV require follow-up to ensure disease clearance, to monitor for medication side effects, and to evaluate for evolving disorders known to be associated with cutaneous vasculitis (see Table 1).

Complications

Isolated LCV generally resolves without sequelae. However, pustular or ulcerative LCV may be complicated by local sequelae such as cutaneous ulcerations and scars.

Cutaneous Vasculitis Associated with Systemic Vasculitis

Cutaneous vasculitis may be a component of the presentation of multiple diseases (see Table 1). When a clinician reads a pathology report from a biopsy of a skin lesion that states "vasculitis," it is important to realize that this term is a descriptor of the histopathology. It is the clinician's challenge to determine whether "vasculitis" is as potentially innocuous as LCV or part of a more severe systemic disease. Symptoms that are clues to a systemic process can include fever, arthralgias, myalgias, anorexia, abdominal pain, pulmonary abnormalities, or neurologic symptoms.

Skin biopsy may aid in the diagnosis of a systemic vasculitis (Henoch-Schönlein purpura), but biopsy of an affected end organ may be necessary to confirm a diagnosis. Pathology focuses on the confirmation of vasculitis in a small, medium, or large vessel.

Aside from Henoch-Schönlein purpura, treatment of systemic vasculitis is typically much more aggressive than treatment of LCV and should be pursued in conjunction with involvement of a rheumatologist, nephrologist, or pulmonologist. Systemic disease leads to severe complications including renal failure, pulmonary damage, permanent vascular disease, or neurologic insult depending on the viscera affected.

References

Gayraud M, Guillevin L, le Toumelin P, et al: Long-term followup of polyarteritis nodosa, microscopic polyangiitis, and Churg-Strauss syndrome: Analysis of four prospective trials including 278 patients, *Arthritis Rheum* 44:666–675, 2001.

Hannon CW, Swerlick RA: Vasculitis. In Bolognia J, Jorizzo J, Rapini R, editors: Dermatology, vol 1. St Louis, 2003, Mosby, pp 381–402.

Hoffman GS, Kerr GS, Leavitt RY, et al: Wegener granulomatosis: An analysis of 158 patients, *Ann Intern Med* 116:488–498, 1992.

Jennette JC, Thomas DB, Falk RJ: Microscopic polyangiitis (microscopic polyarteritis), *Semin Diagn Pathol* 18:3–13, 2001.

Jenette JC, Falk RF, Andrassy K, et al: Nomenclature of systemic vasculitides. Proposal of an international consensus conference, *Arthritis Rheum* 37(2):187–192, 1994.

DISEASES OF THE HAIR

Method of
Dirk M. Elston, MD

CURRENT DIAGNOSIS

- A sudden increase in shedding most commonly represents telogen effluvium.
- Hair thinning is more likely to represent pattern alopecia.
- Scarring alopecia generally requires a biopsy for diagnosis.
- Most medically significant hirsutism results from polycystic ovarian syndrome.
- New-onset virilization suggests the possibility of a tumor.

CURRENT THERAPY

- Pattern alopecia in men is treated with oral finasteride (Propecia), topical minoxidil (Rogaine for Men), or both.
- Pattern alopecia in women is treated with antiandrogens (such as spironolactone [Aldactone][1]), topical minoxidil (Women's Rogaine), or both. Platelet-rich plasma injections may be of benefit in both men and women.
- Alopecia areata can require intralesional corticosteroid injections, topical immunotherapy, or therapy with agents such as methotrexate (Trexall)[1] or Janus kinase (JAK) inhibitors.
- A scalp biopsy is critical to guide therapy in scarring alopecia.
- Hirsutism may be treated with laser epilation or systemic antiandrogens. Topical eflornithine (Vaniqa) can slow regrowth of facial hair.

[1] Not FDA approved for this indication.

Epidemiology

Hair disorders are common, with more than half of the population affected by pattern alopecia and the prevalence of hirsutism varying significantly by ethnicity.

Risk Factors

Most causes of alopecia and hirsutism are genetically determined.

Pathophysiology

Pattern alopecia relates to increased sensitivity to dihydrotestosterone. Telogen effluvium relates to an alteration in the normal hair cycle, with many hairs shedding synchronously. Alopecia areata represents an inflammatory insult directed against melanocytes in the hair bulb. There is strong evidence that the disease is mediated by T_H1 lymphocytes. Polycycstic ovarian syndrome is an insulin-resistance syndrome resulting in excess production of androgens.

Prevention

Little can be done to prevent hair disorders, so the focus is generally on diagnosis and treatment.

Clinical Manifestations

Pattern alopecia manifests with apical scalp thinning. In men, receding of the hairline at the temples is typical, whereas women demonstrate widening of the part but retain the anterior hairline. Telogen effluvium manifests with diffuse shedding of telogen hairs (hairs with a nonpigmented bulb). Alopecia areata typically occurs with patchy hair loss. Shed hairs demonstrate tapered fracture at the base. Syphilitic alopecia resembles alopecia areata but often affects smaller areas, with only partial hair loss, resulting in a moth-eaten appearance. Scarring alopecia shows permanent areas of smooth alopecia lacking follicular openings.

Polycystic ovarian syndrome manifests with evidence of anovulation and excess androgen production. Signs of virilization suggesting a possible tumor include new onset of hirsutism, deepening of the voice, change in body habitus, and clitoromegaly.

Diagnosis

Alopecia

The first step is to determine if a hair shaft abnormality exists (Box 1). This is particularly important in black patients, in whom trichorrhexis nodosa is a common cause of hair loss. Trichorrhexis nodosa results from overprocessing of the hair. Hair density is normal at the level of the scalp, but hairs break off, leaving patches of short hair.

The next step is to determine if telogen effluvium exists. Telogen effluvium manifests with increased shedding of hairs with a blunt nonpigmented bulb (Figure 1), and it commonly follows an illness, surgery, delivery, or crash diet by 3 to 5 months. Hairs

| BOX 1 | Diagnosis of Alopecia |

Trichodystrophy
Types
Trichorrhexis nodosa
Inherited trichodystrophies
Fractures

Causes
- Alopecia areata
- Chemotherapy
- Heavy metal

Determine Type
Anagen Effluvium
Tapered fractures can be caused by
- Alopecia areata
- Chemotherapy
- Heavy metal
Loose anagen can be caused by
- Loose anagen syndrome
- Easily extractable anagen in scarring alopecia

Telogen Effluvium
Increased shedding of club hairs can be caused by
- Diet, illness
- Pregnancy
- Medication
- Papulosquamous disorders
- Pattern alopecia

Diagnosis
Laboratory Studies
Iron
Thyroid stimulating hormone
Endocrine studies in virilized women

Biopsy
Nonscarring types
- Telogen effluvium
- Pattern alopecia
- Alopecia areata
Scarring types
- Lupus erythematosus
- Lichen planopilaris
- Folliculitis decalvans

Other Permanent Alopecia
Idiopathic pseudopelade
Morphea

can often be easily extracted with a gentle hair pull or 1 minute of combing. The presence of tapered fracture suggests alopecia areata, syphilis, or heavy metal poisoning. Alopecia areata can result in diffuse hair loss, but it more commonly manifests with well-defined round patches of hair loss. The skin is either normal or salmon pink. Syphilis more often shows a moth-eaten pattern of alopecia (Figure 2).

Most patients with hair loss need only limited laboratory testing or none at all. Thyroid disorders and iron deficiency are common, and testing for them is relatively inexpensive. I recommend them when telogen effluvium is present. Their presence can also accelerate the course of pattern alopecia, and it is reasonable to test for them in women with this disorder. Thyroid-stimulating hormone is the best screen for thyroid disorders. The role of iron deficiency in telogen hair loss is controversial, but iron deficiency is common, easily established, and inexpensive to correct. Iron status also serves as an indicator of overall nutritional status. Although a low ferritin level proves iron deficiency, ferritin behaves as an acute phase reactant and a normal level does not rule out iron deficiency. Therefore I recommend measurement of ferritin, serum iron, iron binding capacity, and saturation.

Figure 1 Telogen hair on *left*, anagen hair on *right* for comparison.

A scalp biopsy is required in any patient with scarring alopecia. It may also be necessary in other patients if history and physical examination do not establish a diagnosis and the alopecia is progressive. The scalp biopsy should be performed with a 4-mm biopsy punch oriented parallel to the direction of hair growth. Collagen hemostatic sponge (Gelfoam and others) can be placed into the resulting hole to stop bleeding and eliminate the need for sutures. The biopsy should be done in a well-established but still active area of inflammation if one can be identified. A combination of vertical and transverse sections increases the diagnostic yield and is usually recommended. In patients with scarring alopecia, half of the vertically bisected specimen should be sent for direct immunofluorescence. An additional biopsy of an end-stage scarred area can demonstrate characteristic patterns of scarring with an elastic tissue stain. This can help distinguish among causes of scarring alopecia such as lupus erythematosus (Figure 3), lichen planopilaris, pseudopelade, and folliculitis decalvans.

Hirsutism

Patients with *new-onset* virilization should be evaluated to rule out an ovarian or adrenal tumor. Ovarian and adrenal imaging studies and a total testosterone level are the best screens. A total testosterone more than 200 ng/dL or dehydroepiandrostenedione sulfate (DHEAS) more than 8000 ng/dL suggests tumor. In patients with physical signs of Cushing's disease, a 24-hour urine cortisol should be obtained. Most patients with *chronic* medically significant hirsutism have polycystic ovarian syndrome (PCOS). The diagnosis is established by means of history and physical examination, and the most important laboratory tests are serum lipids and fasting glucose to establish associated cardiac risk factors. A clinical diagnosis of PCOS requires the presence of hirsutism, acne or pattern alopecia, and evidence of anovulation (fewer than 9 periods per year or cycles longer than 40 days). Ratios of luteinizing hormone (LH) to follicle-stimulating hormone (FSH) have poor sensitivity and specificity for diagnosing PCOS. Imaging for ovarian cysts seldom affects management.

Differential Diagnosis

Syphilis can mimic alopecia areata, and serologic testing should be performed in any sexually active patient with a new diagnosis of alopecia areata. Correct diagnosis of scarring alopecia depends of a thorough examination for other cutaneous signs of lupus erythematosus or lichen planus as well as the results of a skin biopsy.

Tinea capitis can occur as inflammatory boggy areas with hair loss (kerion) or with subtle seborrheic-type scale and black-dot areas of hair loss. A potassium hydroxide (KOH) examination

Figure 2 Moth-eaten syphilitic alopecia.

Figure 3 Scarring alopecia secondary to chronic cutaneous lupus erythematosus.

can be performed by rubbing the affected area with moist gauze and examining broken hairs that cling to the gauze.

Hirsutism should be distinguished from hypertrichosis. Hirsutism is a male pattern of hair growth occurring in a woman and is hormonal in nature. Hypertrichosis is excess hair growth that occurs outside of an androgen-dependent distribution. It can be found in metabolic disorders such as porphyria or may be a sign of internal malignancy (Figure 4).

Non-classic 21-hydroxylase deficiency accounts for up to 10% of patients with medically significant hirsutism. Screening with a baseline morning 17-OH-progesterone is associated with many false positive results. A stimulated 17-OH-progesterone is more specific, but the results of testing seldom affect management because outcomes with dexamethasone (Decadron)[1] are no better than with spironolactone (Aldactone)[1].

Treatment

Alopecia

Telogen effluvium commonly resolves spontaneously once the cause has been eliminated. Poor diet and papulosquamous

---

[1]Not FDA approved for this indication.

Figure 4 Malignant hypertrichosis secondary to ovarian cancer.

Diseases of the Hair

diseases of the scalp such as seborrheic dermatitis and psoriasis can perpetuate a telogen effluvium and should be treated. The importance of a diet containing adequate protein and trace minerals should be emphasized. Seborrheic dermatitis responds to topical corticosteroids. Medicated shampoos containing selenium sulfide (Selsun Blue) or zinc pyrithione (T-gel Daily Control) can be helpful. Scalp psoriasis can require more potent topical steroids such as fluocinonide solution (Lidex) and calcipotriene (Dovonex) applied on weekends or daily. Systemic agents such as methotrexate (Trexall)[1] at doses of 7.5 to 20 mg once weekly may be required to control severe scalp psoriasis.

Pattern alopecia in men is mediated by dihydrotestosterone (DHT). Men with pattern alopecia may be treated with daily topical minoxidil 2% to 5% (Rogaine for Men) or oral finasteride (Propecia) at a dose of 1 mg daily. In women, the pathogenesis is complex, and adrenal androgens may play a larger role. Finasteride is of little benefit in the majority of women with pattern alopecia. Spironolactone[1] 100 mg twice daily can be helpful. In women of childbearing potential, spironolactone should always be used in conjunction with an oral contraceptive. Side effects are uncommon but can include urinary frequency, irregular periods, dyspareunia, and nausea. Most patients demonstrate a minor increase in serum potassium. Those with kidney failure are at risk for life-threatening potassium retention. Topical 2% minoxidil (Women's Rogaine) can also be of benefit, and some women derive added benefit from the 5% formulation. All patients with pattern alopecia should be evaluated for superimposed causes of telogen effluvium such as inadequate diet and seborrheic dermatitis.

Tinea capitis is often overlooked in adults and black children, in whom the manifestations of inflammation can be subtle. Black dot and seborrheic tinea are common in black children. Patchy hair loss is an important clue to the diagnosis. Treatment is summarized in Table 1.

Localized patches of alopecia areata respond to intralesional injections of triamcinolone hexacetonide (Aristospan) (2.5–5 mg/mL) given once per month. Approximately 0.1 mL/cm² is injected to a maximum of 3 mL during any one session. Minoxidil[1] solution produces slow regrowth in some patients who cannot tolerate other treatments. Anthralin (Dritho-Scalp 0.5%)[1] is sometimes used in children. It is applied 30 minutes before showering. It can stain skin and anything else it touches.

Topical immunotherapy with dinitrochlorobenzene (DNCB)[1], squaric acid dibutylester (SADBE)[1] or diphenylcyclopropenone (DPCP)[1] is more effective than either minoxidil or anthralin. DNCB is mutagenic in the Ames assay and none of the topical immunotherapies are currently approved for human use. A 2% solution of the sensitizer is applied to the arm in acetone to induce initial sensitization. Subsequently, diluted solutions, starting at about 0.001%, are applied weekly to the scalp with a

cotton-tipped applicator. Roughly 20% to 60% of patients have responded to this regimen in various studies.

Biologic agents have been disappointing, but methotrexate[1] in psoriatic doses (7.5–20 mg weekly for an adult) can be effective. Sulfasalazine (Azulfidine)[1] is sometimes effective in doses ranging from 500 to 1500 mg three times a day.[3] Tofacitinib (Xeljanz)[1] and other Janus kinase (JAK) inhibitors can be effective in patients with refractory alopecia areata. Patients should be encouraged to read about new therapies on the National Alopecia Areata Foundation website (www.naaf.org).

Early, aggressive therapy for discoid lupus erythematosus is recommended to prevent permanent scarring. Topical corticosteroids are rarely sufficient. Intralesional injections are performed in a manner similar to that described above. Initial control of severe disease can be achieved with a single 3-week tapered course of oral prednisone at a dose of 60 mg daily for the first week, 40 mg daily for the second week, and 20 mg daily for the third week. Intralesional steroid injections or a systemic steroid-sparing agent are required for maintenance therapy. Systemic agents that can be effective include antimalarials, dapsone[1], methotrexate[1], mycophenolate mofetil (CellCept)[1], and thalidomide (Thalomid)[1]. I generally begin treatment with hydroxychloroquine (Plaquenil)[1] at a dose of 400 mg daily for an adult. Dapsone is used at a dose of 100 mg daily for an adult. Thalidomide has been used effectively at doses of 50 to 100 mg daily, but peripheral neuropathy and teratogenicity limit its use. Mycophenolate mofetil is used at a dose of 1 gram twice daily, and methotrexate is used at doses of 7.5 to 20 mg weekly.

End-stage cicatricial alopecia is best treated by scalp reduction and hair transplantation. The disease can flare up in response to surgery, and it is best to plan a 3-week tapered course of prednisone[1] as described to help prevent the flare.

Lichen planopilaris is treated in a manner similar to lupus, except that hydroxychloroquine[1] is of less benefit and oral retinoids (Soriatane[1] at doses of 25 to 50 mg daily) are more likely to be successful. Topical calcineurin or JAK inhibitors can be effective in achieving and maintaining remission. A few months of pioglitazone (Actos)[1] may induce remission in a subset of patients, and the frontal fibrosing alopecia variant can respond to dutasteride (Avodart)[1]. Patients should be aware of the risks associated with each of these treatments, including bladder cancer and hypospadias in a male fetus. Mycophenolate mofetil[1] 1 g twice daily is often effective when other treatments fail and oral JAK inhibitors and low dose naltrexone (Revia)[1] are being investigated. Excimer laser and other forms of phototherapy can also be effective for lichen planopilaris, but are contraindicated in lupus erythematosus.

ANTIFUNGAL AGENT	DOSAGE	USUAL DURATION OF THERAPY
TABLE 1 Treatment of Tinea Capitis		
Griseofulvin (Fulvicin U/F)	Required dosages are often higher than reflected in the product label; 4–10 mg/kg/d is a good starting dosage	1 mo or more
Fluconazole (Diflucan)[1]	5–6 mg/kg/d	1 mo or more
Itraconazole (Sporanox)[1]	3–5 mg/kg/d	1 wk, repeated monthly until cured
Terbinafine (Lamisil)	Patient <20 kg: 62.5 mg/d Patient 20–40 kg: 125 mg/d Patient >40 kg: 250 mg/d	1 mo or more

[1]Not FDA approved for this indication.

[1]Not FDA approved for this indication.
[3]Exceeds dosage recommended by the manufacturer.

Folliculitis decalvans manifests with crops of pustules that result in permanent scarring. Patients respond to weekend applications of clobetasol (Clobex, Olux) together with prolonged use of antistaphylococcal antibiotics such as doxycycline (Doryx)[1] 100 mg twice daily.

Hirsutism

Treatment options include laser epilation, eflornithine (Vaniqa) cream to reduce the rate of hair growth, or spironolactone[1] at a starting dose of 100 mg twice daily as described for pattern alopecia. Cyproterone acetate is used in some countries but is not available in the United States. Other options that are less commonly used include insulin sensitizers, flutamide (Eulexin)[1], metformin (Glucophage)[1], and leuprolide (Lupron)[1] plus estrogen.

Monitoring

Patients treated with topical or intralesional corticosteroids should be monitored for cutaneous atrophy. Those on hydroxychloroquine should be monitored for ocular toxicity, including corneal deposits and retinal damage, although these are very rare at usual doses. They should also be monitored periodically for thrombocytopenia, agranulocytosis, and hepatitis. Patients beginning dapsone therapy should be screened for G6PD deficiency. Potential side effects include hemolysis, methemoglobinemia, and neuropathy. Monitoring includes periodic blood count assessment and measurement of strength and sensation. Mycophenolate mofetil can produce pancytopenia, and blood counts should be monitored. Methotrexate is cleared by the kidneys, and kidney function should be assessed at baseline. Periodic assessment of liver function tests and blood count is warranted, as is a yearly chest radiograph. I also monitor procollagen 3 terminal peptide levels quarterly to assess the risk of hepatic fibrosis. Patients on antiandrogen therapy should be monitored for dyspareunia resulting from vulvar atrophy.

Complications

Patients with pattern alopecia and polycystic ovarian syndrome have a greater risk of metabolic syndrome with cardiac complications. They should be evaluated for lipid abnormalities and glucose intolerance and treated appropriately.

---

[1]Not FDA approved for this indication.

References

Brown J, Farquhar C, Lee O, et al: Spironolactone versus placebo or in combination with steroids for hirsutism and/or acne, *Cochrane Database Syst Rev* (2): CD000194, 2009.

Buzney E, Sheu J, Buzney C, Reynolds RV. Polycystic ovary syndrome: a review for dermatologists: Part II. Treatment. *J Am Acad Dermatol* 2014 Nov;71(5):859. e1–859.e15.

Durdu M, Özcan D, Baba M, Seçkin D: Efficacy and safety of diphenylcyclopropenone alone or in combination with anthralin in the treatment of chronic extensive alopecia areata: A retrospective case series, *J Am Acad Dermatol* 72:640–650, 2015.

Elston DM, Ferringer T, Dalton S, et al: A comparison of vertical versus transverse sections in the evaluation of alopecia biopsy specimens, *J Am Acad Dermatol* 53(2):267–272, 2005.

Gentile P, Garcovich S, Scioli MG, et al: Mechanical and controlled PRP injections in patients affected by androgenetic alopecia, *J Vis Exp*, (131) Jan 27, 2018.

Giordano S, Romeo M, di Summa P, et al: A meta-analysis on evidence of platelet-rich plasma for androgenetic alopecia, *Int J Trichology* 10(1):1–10, 2018 Jan-Feb.

Pasquali R, Gambineri A. New perspectives on the definition and management of polycystic ovary syndrome. *J Endocrinol Invest*. 2018 Jan 23. doi: https://doi.org/10.1007/s40618-018-0832-1. [Epub ahead of print] Review. PubMed PMID: 29363047.

Sebastian MR, Wiemann CM, Bacha F, Alston-Taylor SJ. Diagnostic evaluation, comorbidity screening, and treatment of Polycystic Ovary Syndrome in adolescents in three specialty clinics. *J Pediatr Adolesc Gynecol*, 2018 Jan 31. doi: https://doi.org/10.1016/j.jpag.2018.01.007. pii:S1083-3188(18)30015-9. [Epub ahead of print] PubMed PMID: 29408736.

Somani N, Turvy D: Hirsutism: an evidence-based treatment update, *Am J Clin Dermatol* 15(3):247–266, 2014 Jul.

Tsuboi R, Arano O, Nishikawa T, et al: Randomized clinical trial comparing 5% and 1% topical minoxidil for the treatment of androgenetic alopecia in Japanese men, *J Dermatol* 36(8):437–446, 2009.

DISEASES OF THE MOUTH

Method of
Wendy S. Hupp, DMD

CURRENT DIAGNOSIS

High-Risk Conditions
- Obvious soft tissue enlargement that could lead to trismus or airway compromise: acute exacerbation of odontogenic infections; rapid onset, swelling, purulence, broken or decayed teeth.
- Suspicion of oral cancer: mucosal surface color change, slowly progressing enlargement, asymptomatic or with nonhealing ulcer, incidental finding, use of tobacco and alcohol.

Opportunistic Infections
- Necrotizing ulcerative gingivitis (trench mouth): compromised host resistance, generalized dental pain, usually acute onset, bleeding gums, fetid odor.
- Oral candidiasis: compromised host resistance, chronic or recurring course, bad taste, generalized burning sensation, superficial change in mucosal appearance (white or red).

Dry Mouth
- Salivary dysfunction (xerostomia): patient's perception of dry mouth, difficulty swallowing or speaking, tooth sensitivity as a result of new decay or receding gums; related to medication use or autoimmune gland dysfunction.

Acute-Onset Oral Ulcers
- Aphthous stomatitis: recurring episodes, formation of one or more superficial oral ulcers, located on nonbound mucosa, healing in approximately 7 to 10 days.
- Primary herpetic gingivostomatitis: acute onset of systemic viral infection features, including fever, and multiple oral vesicles, degenerating into ulcers; resolution in 7 to 10 days.
- Recurrent herpes: recurring episodes, acute formation of vesicles collapsing to ulcers, located on exposed lip, or bound mucosa; healing in 7 to 10 days.
- Erythema multiforme: acute onset of oral ulcers, triggering event, mild systemic features such as fever, characteristic skin lesions; resolution in 2 to 4 weeks.

Chronic Oral Ulcers
- Erosive lichen planus and lichenoid reaction: reticular appearance at periphery of ulcers, buccal mucosa affected, may cause desquamative gingivitis, skin lesions possible.
- Mucous membrane pemphigoid: typically desquamative gingivitis presentation, possible eye and genital ulcers, skin lesions unlikely.
- Pemphigus vulgaris: ulcers of irregular shape and jagged peripheral contour, possible skin lesions.

Osteonecrosis of the Jaw
- Radiation related: resulting from treatment of oral or head and neck cancer.
- Medication related: secondary to antiresorptives used to treat osteoporosis or bone metastases in cancer patients; bisphosphonates, antiangiogenics, receptor activator of nuclear factor kappa-B ligand (RANKL) inhibitors.
- More common in the mandible: exposed bone that persists for more than 8 weeks; may be asymptomatic with localized soft tissue irritation, rough edges of necrotic bone may be irritating; can progress to osteomyelitis and physiologic fractures.

Topical Management of Oral Ulcerations
- Ice chips as needed to help with pain.
- Diphenhydramine (Benadryl)[1] liquid 12.5 mg/5 mL (50/50 mix) with liquid antacid[1] (Maalox, Kaopectate, etc.), rinse with 1 to 2 teaspoons every 2 hours then spit; for pain.
- Triamcinolone acetonide 0.1% in oral paste (Oralone): dab a small amount on the lesion to provide a protective film, 2 to 4 times a day until ulcers are healed.
- Dexamethasone (Decadron)[1] elixir 0.5 mg/5 mL: rinse with 1 teaspoon for 2 minutes and spit out after meals and at bedtime until ulcers are healed.

Management of Resistant Ulcers With Topical Ultrapotent Corticosteroid Preparations
- Clobetasol propionate (Temovate)[1] 0.05%: apply a thin film to affected area after meals and at bedtime until healed.
- Halobetasol propionate (Ultravate)[1] 0.05%.

Management of Ulcers That Cannot Be Controlled With Topical Preparations
- Prednisone[1] 5- to 20-mg tablets; take 60 mg per day by mouth as needed to control ulcers; no taper indicated if less than 2 weeks of daily use; topical corticosteroid should be titrated to maintain control of ulcers.
- Methylprednisolone 4 mg tablets (Medrol Pak)[1] are used to control ulcers, taken with tapered doses, then topical corticosteroid should be titrated to maintain control of ulcers.

Management of Osteonecrosis of the Jaw
- Antibiotics if purulent exudate is present.
- Pain medication as needed.
- Conservative resection of hard tissue may be necessary (referred to oral surgeon).

Management of Dry Mouth
- Saliva substitute, sugarless mints or gum, ice chips as needed.
- Cholinergic agonist, e.g., pilocarpine (Salagen) 5 to 10 mg by mouth 30 minutes before meals, not to exceed 30 mg per day.

---

[1] Not FDA approved for this indication.

Patients often consult the physician with problems in the orofacial region, including those that are clearly dental in nature. For these problems, the intervention may simply be to treat the pain and/or infection until definitive treatment can be provided by a dentist. These problems may include a broken tooth or restoration with sharp edges that causes soft tissue injury; infected or traumatized nerves with spontaneous pain; or focal infections that cause swelling (likely to be less painful) or acute pain when the pressure of the purulent exudate is trapped within the bone at the apex of the root of the tooth.

Oral manifestations of systemic disease, such as pyostomatitis vegetans (Crohn disease), or mucosal petechiae (idiopathic thrombocytopenic purpura) are uncommon, and can pose difficult diagnostic challenges. Similarly, adverse oral reactions to therapeutic medications are inconsistent and may be unavoidable, for example, xerostomia, dysgeusia, and gingival overgrowth. These issues may best be handled in concert with the patient's dentist. Regional conditions, such as headache, cranial neuralgia, or sinusitis, may cause oral complaints, and vice versa. The diagnosis and treatment of these conditions is not discussed in this chapter.

Nevertheless, there are a few orofacial conditions that have serious implications and should be addressed by the physician rather than referred to the dentist. These conditions are addressed in the Current Diagnosis box. The Current Therapy box includes recommended treatment; if resolution does not occur in a reasonable amount of time, for example 2 weeks, the diagnosis must be questioned. For biopsy confirmation of potential oral neoplasms and autoimmune disorders, an oral pathologist is preferred.

Odontogenic Infection

With few exceptions, disseminated bacterial infections of odontogenic origin represent a dramatic, acute exacerbation of a chronic, asymptomatic infection. A variety of dental conditions are possible causes, such as a periodontal abscess, an abscess within the supportive bone resulting from the pulpal necrosis of a carious tooth, or an infection of the gingiva surrounding a partially erupted third molar. The patient often describes a history of one or more prior acute episodes of bacterial infection symptoms from the site, followed by resolution. The degree of swelling, lymphadenopathy, pain, and fever is proportional to the risk of potential complications such as septicemia. Of particular concern is evidence of the rapid progression of diffuse swelling into the floor of the mouth and neck because of the risk of respiratory distress (i.e., Ludwig angina), or superiorly from the anterior portion of the maxilla because of the possibility of cavernous sinus thrombosis.

Definitive dental treatment to eliminate the underlying infectious source is the treatment goal after the acute, disseminated infection has been controlled. Penicillin is still considered the empiric antibiotic choice for disseminated odontogenic bacterial infections in individuals with no history of adverse reaction, and clindamycin (Cleocin) is used for those hypersensitive to penicillin. Many patients mistakenly assume that empiric antibiotic treatment can eliminate the infection in the same sense that antibiotic treatment can cure bacterial sinusitis or pharyngitis. The patient should be informed that improvement of an acute odontogenic infection after antibiotic treatment is not curative and that dental care to eliminate the underlying cause is necessary. One or more courses of antibiotics without elimination of the source increase the probability of the emergence of more virulent, antibiotic-resistant pathogens. More aggressive treatment, including intravenous antibiotics and surgical drainage in a hospital setting, must be considered in cases of rapid progression or extensive swelling, particularly if the anterior maxilla or submandibular areas are involved and in instances of compromised host resistance.

Suspicion of Oral Cancer

About 90% of oral cancers are squamous cell carcinoma (SCC), but sarcoma, adenoma, and metastatic tumors of solid organs are also found. Although the 5-year survival rate of oral SCC has improved over the past decade, it still hovers about 50%. Many patients deny the presence of a lump or mass until it becomes painful, and even then first seek care from a physician instead of a dentist or oral surgeon. Routine oral examination is still the best weapon against morbidity and mortality, as there are no diagnostic tests that are satisfactory.

Oral cancer has been called the great imitator, for it can appear as many different oral conditions. It can be red, white or pigmented, exophytic, nodular, or ulcerative, smooth-surface or verrucous, and occur in any location of the oral cavity. The greatest suspicion is associated with an older patient, likely male, who uses tobacco and alcohol. The most common sites are the floor of the mouth and the lateral borders of the tongue, with the great majority being unilateral. Recently an increase in younger patients (less than 40 years old) has been tied to the presence of human papilloma virus, although no etiology has been confirmed.

Biopsy is indicated for lesions that show induration, are tied to underlying structures, are nontender, slow-growing, and especially if simple treatment of ulceration or infection has not eliminated the problem. The decision to obtain a biopsy of an oral lesion should be made with consideration of the substantial positive impact that early detection has on a disease with an otherwise unfavorable prognosis.

Necrotizing Ulcerative Gingivitis

Necrotizing ulcerative gingivitis (NUG) is a characteristic, potentially destructive infection of the dental supportive tissues caused by a predominance of fusiform bacteria and spirochetes. Some combination of psychologic stress, compromised immune function, malnutrition, or other condition of diminished host resistance dramatically increases the risk of NUG. This is suggested by the colloquial phrase *trench mouth* used to refer to this infection, because it was frequently observed among debilitated soldiers during World War I. It has also been called Vincent infection and acute NUG (ANUG).

Acute onset of poorly localized, severe dental pain, and a putrid taste are typically the patient's chief complaints. Onset usually corresponds with a significant alteration in the general health or emotional status, although a more chronic course of variably pronounced symptoms can be expected with protracted conditions, such as acquired immunodeficiency syndrome (AIDS). Visual features of NUG include necrotic deterioration of the gingiva with pronounced peripheral erythema and a superficial pseudomembrane. The tissue around the mandibular anterior teeth is most severely affected in most cases, and the gingiva often appears "punched out" from between the teeth. The gingival necrosis produces the characteristic fetid breath that is far more pungent than that caused by typical gingivitis. The putrid odor in combination with the acute onset and poor localization of pain is usually a more reliable basis for diagnosis than visual findings. Additional features, such as fever and cervical lymphadenopathy, are proportional to the severity of the oral findings.

Treatment of NUG consists of the combination of supportive care, antimicrobial measures, and improvement in the underlying compromising health conditions. Supportive care is nonspecific and includes rest, fluid intake, and a soft but nutritious diet. Warm saline, dilute hydrogen peroxide, and chlorhexidine gluconate (Peridex) are effective antimicrobial rinses. Penicillin and metronidazole (Flagyl) are the empiric systemic antibiotics of choice. Ultimately the most effective antimicrobial treatment is the combination of thorough dental cleaning of the teeth, with debridement of the necrotic soft tissue, and improved oral hygiene. Resolution of NUG, including complete healing of the gingival tissue, is strikingly rapid in most instances if this is accomplished, and underlying health status improves. Persistence or recurrence of NUG after debridement suggests the possibility of human immunodeficiency virus (HIV) infection or another undiagnosed compromising condition.

Oral Candidiasis

Oral candidiasis is a superficial fungal infection of the oral mucosa that is clinically similar to vaginal candidiasis in many respects. With isolated exceptions, the infection is caused by the fungus *Candida albicans*, which can be identified in the mouths of approximately 50% of healthy adults. The risk of oral candidiasis is increased by one or more factors of compromised host resistance: decreased local resistance, compromised immune function, or uncontrolled systemic disease. Frequently encountered examples of decreased local resistance include poor oral hygiene, xerostomia, wearing dentures that provide an organism reservoir or limit hygiene, and recent antibiotic therapy that has altered the normally competitive oral bacteria. The combination of one or more of these local factors with a systemic condition that causes compromised immune status or constitutional compromise dramatically increases the risk of clinical apparent infection. Common examples include AIDS, corticosteroid therapy, severe anemia, and poorly controlled diabetes mellitus.

Oral candidiasis lesions can have four distinct appearances. The most characteristic form is the pseudomembranous, curd-like plaques of thrush that wipe off with cotton gauze leaving a sore, erythematous mucosal surface. The erythematous or atrophic form of oral candidiasis produces a thin, "beefy" appearance often affecting the dorsum of the tongue or mucosa that supports a denture. The third type of lesion is the formation of fissures similar to those of tinea pedis that usually are at the corners of the mouth and are referred to as angular cheilitis. The fourth is a hyperplastic form that produces a patchy, white thickening of the surface epithelium that does not rub off and that appears similar to the hyperkeratosis of chronic frictional irritation. Oral candidiasis often produces more than one lesion form simultaneously in different areas of the mouth, which may be a confirmational finding. Patients often describe only a little discomfort or a mild burning sensation from affected sites, and also bad taste.

The clinical course of the infection may be acute, chronic, or cyclic in severity, depending on the nature of the underlying causes. The combination of clinical appearance, suspected compromised host status, and improvement after empiric treatment provides an adequate basis for the diagnosis. Exfoliative cytology provides definitive evidence of the infection in more equivocal situations.

Antifungal treatment eliminates oral candidiasis in most instances, but recurrences or a chronic, subclinical course can be expected if the predisposing condition remains unchanged. This implies that treatment of superficial oral candidiasis may not be justified in such instances, if the affected individual is asymptomatic, because the only realistic treatment goal is elimination of symptoms. That decision must be weighed against the possibility of spread to the esophagus.

Options for routine topical treatment of oral candidiasis include clotrimazole (Mycelex) troches, or nystatin (Mycostatin pastilles),[6] and use should continue for 1 week after resolution of symptoms. Several considerations can complicate effectiveness. Patients with xerostomia have difficulty dissolving the troches or pastilles and prefer a nystatin rinse. Concurrent management of the dry mouth (discussed later) increases the effectiveness of topical antifungal treatment for candidiasis. Limiting the *Candida* organism reservoir in the denture acrylic can be accomplished for those who wear dentures, by soaking them overnight in most commercial denture soaking solutions, mouthwashes such as Listerine, or chlorhexidine gluconate (Peridex). These products are adequately fungicidal, and keeping the denture out overnight disrupts adherence and colonization of candidal organisms. Some patients are more compliant about managing the denture problem by applying a thin layer of nystatin ointment[1] or clotrimazole cream (Lotrimin)[1] to the denture before wearing. Direct application of these preparations also promotes rapid resolution of angular cheilitis. Systemic administration of ketoconazole (Nizoral)[1] or fluconazole (Diflucan)[1] is an alternative for patients who cannot manage topical treatment, or for severely immunocompromised individuals in the interest of controlling oral symptoms and minimizing the risk of spread to the esophagus.

Xerostomia

Xerostomia is defined by the patient's subjective perception of "dry mouth" rather than by any objective parameter. The amount of saliva is decreased, and its character typically is altered to a more viscous, ropey consistency. The condition is common because salivary function is adversely affected by so many routinely encountered influences, including many frequently prescribed medications, smoking, methamphetamine abuse, several common systemic diseases, and radiation exposure for cancer treatment in the orofacial region. In addition to these influences, primary Sjögren syndrome is characterized by chronic dry eyes and dry mouth caused by autoimmune-mediated acinar degeneration. Secondary Sjögren syndrome is defined as oral and ocular dryness concurrent with an autoimmune connective tissue disorder such as rheumatoid arthritis.

The subjective response of different individuals to a mild or moderate degree of oral dryness varies considerably. Many patients who appear to produce adequate saliva complain of dryness, whereas others who seem unusually dry during oral examination have no complaints. Most patients with an advanced degree of dryness find the continual "cotton mouth" sensation and other consequences to be a significant quality-of-life issue. Decreased saliva production causes difficulty speaking, chewing, and swallowing, in addition to painful abrasion of the mucosa by coarse foods. Beyond the physical irritation, limited saliva alters the sense of taste and the enjoyment of food. Saliva contributes to

---

[1] Not FDA approved for this indication.
[6] May be compounded by pharmacists.

oral health by providing antimicrobial components such as lactoperoxidase and IgA antibodies, and it has a significant flushing and cleansing function. Xerostomia causes a rampant and rapidly progressive pattern of dental decay that is particularly destructive, even for previously caries-resistant individuals. This is compounded if the patient compensates for the dryness by drinking sucrose-rich soft drinks or sucking on hard candy. Similarly, periodontitis tends to progress rapidly, despite normally effective treatment, if saliva production is limited. Xerostomia is also associated with complaints of generalized soreness of the mouth caused by frequent and persistent episodes of oral candidiasis.

Management of xerostomia is challenging and often frustrating for the patient and the clinician. The treatment for severe, irreversible xerostomia, as in cases of head and neck radiotherapy, is essentially symptomatic. Different patients prefer different combinations of compensation methods. Sipping water throughout the day is the single most effective and simplest way to counter loss of saliva. Some patients report additional improvement with the use of commercially available saliva substitutes, although many do as well with water and ice chips. Most patients soon learn to avoid abrasive foods, irritating commercial mouth rinses that contain alcohol, and highly flavored toothpastes in favor of less irritating alternatives. Use of a humidifier at night is often beneficial. Comprehensive dental treatment should be recommended to limit the progression and severity of dental caries and periodontitis. Smoking and compensation by drinking sucrose-rich soft drinks, sports drinks, drinks that contain caffeine, and highly acidic citric juices should be discouraged.

Additional options beyond the previous recommendations are available for those who have some residual salivary function. Drinking ample water moistens the mucosa and maintains general hydration, which maximizes the residual saliva production. Sugar-free gum or hard candy significantly stimulates saliva flow. Alternative medications that are equally effective therapeutically but less likely to cause xerostomia may be substituted in some cases to treat conditions such as hypertension.

Several cholinergic agonists are available, including cevimeline (Evoxac), pilocarpine (Salagen), and bethanechol (Urecholine)[1]. Titration of dosage is usually necessary to optimize saliva flow while minimizing frequent adverse effects such as excessive sweating and gastritis. Many patients discontinue treatment because of these and less common side effects that become more troublesome than the xerostomia. Contraindications such as glaucoma and the risk of serious complications such as arrhythmia must also be considered.

Aphthous Stomatitis

Recurrent aphthous stomatitis, colloquially known as *canker sores*, is a common condition of complex immune-mediated pathogenesis. Patients describe recurring episodes of painful ulcers that often follow triggering events such as minor tissue abrasion, eating certain foods, or episodes of emotional stress. The phrase *minor aphthous stomatitis* differentiates the most common, mild form of the disease from the more severe major and herpetiform variations. Most authorities believe these categorizations are somewhat artificial distinctions within a continuum of a single process. Similar ulcers are a feature of Behçet syndrome, but are of minor diagnostic and treatment significance compared with the other manifestations of this rare, multisystem condition.

The clinical features of minor recurrent aphthous stomatitis are characteristic. One or more painful ulcers develop soon after a short prodromal period of burning or itching at the affected site. The round or oval superficial ulcers exhibit a uniform, yellowish white, pseudomembranous surface with an erythematous peripheral halo at the sharply delineated ulcer margin. Typical size is less than 10 mm in diameter, and lesions affect only unbound oral mucosal surfaces of the lips, cheeks, floor of the mouth, or soft palate. This distribution specifically excludes the bound surfaces of the gingiva, hard palate, and the dorsum of the tongue. This feature is valuable for differentiating aphthous stomatitis from

the intraoral recurrent herpetic lesions (discussed later) that affect only bound surfaces.

Aphthous lesions typically heal within 7 to 10 days, and most patients describe a long clinical course of symptom-free periods of various durations interrupted by episodes of ulcer formation. Lesion-free periods of weeks, months, or even years typically distinguish recurrent aphthous stomatitis from autoimmune conditions such as erosive lichen planus (discussed later) that produce a continuous course of oral ulcers.

The major form of recurrent aphthous stomatitis produces ulcers of similar appearance, but the lesions are larger, require a longer healing time, often heal with scarring, and form so frequently that at least one ulcer is usually present. The herpetiform variant is characterized by a cluster of numerous smaller (1 to 3 mm) ulcers that often coalesce into a single, large lesion, and the ulcers are described as exceptionally painful.[1] The clustering distribution explains the somewhat misleading herpetiform designation for this nonviral condition. This form of aphthous stomatitis may affect keratinized and nonkeratinized surfaces, which in addition to the clustering distribution may lead to confusion with recurrent herpes simplex lesions.

Minor recurrent aphthous stomatitis is more irritating than serious, and treatment beyond symptomatic management is usually not justified. Patients soon learn to avoid their particular trigger event as much as possible, and many find relief during outbreaks from over-the-counter preparations such as Orabase with benzocaine 20%, or by rinsing with soothing, coating products such as bismuth subsalicylate (Kaopectate).[1] Rinses containing a variety of ingredients, such as diphenhydramine[1], tetracycline[1], aloe,[7] and chlorhexidine gluconate (Peridex)[1], have been reported to promote ulcer healing in some cases. Treatment with corticosteroids (see Current Therapy box), however, is more consistently effective, and is justified for major and herpetiform variants, as well as for particularly severe or frequent outbreaks of minor aphthous lesions.

Orofacial Herpes Simplex Infection

Most herpes simplex infections of the oral mucosa are caused by herpes simplex virus type 1 (HSV-1). A much smaller proportion of oral cases results from the type 2 herpes simplex virus that typically causes genital lesions. Transmission occurs by direct contact or contaminated saliva, and serologic studies demonstrate that as much as 90% of the population has been infected by age 50.

The initial infection, referred to as acute herpetic gingivostomatitis or primary herpes, usually affects children and causes acute onset of cervical lymphadenopathy, chills, and fever similar to many acute viral infections. The distinguishing manifestation is the formation of multiple, painful oral vesicles that rapidly rupture. The resulting ulcers most prominently affect the gingiva, lips, and tongue but may occur on any oral surface. Primary herpes in adults is more likely to cause complaints of pharyngitis rather than oral ulcers, which makes distinguishing it from other systemic viral infections unlikely. The severity of primary herpes varies from virtually subclinical or indistinguishable from nonspecific viral infections, to debilitating. The distinguishing oral lesions are probably seen only in severe cases, because relatively few seropositive individuals recall the oral ulcers of the primary infection when questioned. Symptoms resolve within 5 days to 2 weeks, depending on the severity of the manifestations, and significant complications such as encephalitis or keratoconjunctivitis are rare.

The HSV-1 virus becomes latent within the sensory neurons that supply the primary infection site. Episodes of recurrent lesions may develop after the primary infection, a pattern similar to the recurring genital lesions caused by HSV-2. The frequency, severity, and course of these outbreaks vary widely among individuals, and at least one-half of HSV-1 seropositive individuals rarely or never suffer recurrent lesions. Those who do often associate occurrence with causative events, such as sun exposure of

---

[1] Not FDA approved for this indication.

[1] Not FDA approved for this indication.
[7] Available as a dietary supplement.

the exposed lip, abrasion of the surface, or an illness such as a nonspecific viral infection. This explains the colloquial terms *cold sore* and *fever blister* used to describe the most common presentation affecting the exposed lip, which is referred to as herpes labialis.

The typical episode begins with a prodromal sensation of burning or itching at the site near the vermillion border, followed by formation of one or more vesicles within 24 hours. The vesicles soon rupture, forming a coalesced crust that heals after 7 to 10 days. A few individuals suffer similar recurrent herpes lesions of the intraoral mucosa. Intraoral herpes lesions produce features of pain, onset, recurrent course, and healing time that are similar to those for aphthous stomatitis, which may present some differential diagnostic uncertainty. The diagnosis can be made in most cases based on the affected surface. Aphthous lesions are usually limited to the unbound mucosa of the lips, cheeks, soft palate, and floor of the mouth, whereas the intraoral ulcers of recurrent herpes simplex infection are limited to the bound mucosa of the gingiva and hard palate.

Treatment of primary herpes simplex infection for immuno-competent individuals is supportive and symptomatic, as for any acute systemic viral infection. In cases of significant oral discomfort, a rinse consisting of a 1:1 mixture of diphenhydramine (Benadryl)[1] elixir 12.5 mg/5 mL and a liquid antacid, or bismuth subsalicylate (Pepto-Bismol)[1] used as needed, provides some relief by coating the ulcers. The use of systemic antiviral medication such as acyclovir (Zovirax) and valacyclovir (Valtrex) is not recommended for primary infections, except for immunocompromised patients to reduce the risk of systemic dissemination.

Most individuals affected by secondary herpes lesions suffer relatively few episodes, and no treatment is warranted. Patients prone to frequent lip lesions after sun exposure soon learn the preventive value of sunscreen lip balms, but the advice may be helpful to those who have not made the association. For patients who experience numerous secondary herpetic episodes, the systemic administration of valacyclovir (Valtrex) can be used therapeutically during the prodromal stage or prophylactically. The one-day dosing is 2 g by mouth 12 hours apart. For immunocompromised patients, valacyclovir 1 g twice a day[1] or famciclovir (Famvir) 500 mg twice a day are recommended for 10 days.

Erythema Multiforme

Erythema multiforme, which is discussed in greater detail elsewhere in this textbook, is characterized by shallow oral ulcers and characteristic "target" skin lesions. Outbreaks of secondary herpetic lesions have been implicated as a frequent trigger for erythema multiforme. A prodrome of mild fever, malaise, sore throat, and headache may precede the appearance of the oral ulcers and skin lesions. The shallow oral ulcers usually affect the lips, tongue, or soft palate and are less likely to develop on the gingiva or hard palate. Ulcers gradually heal after 2 to 4 weeks, and approximately 20% of affected individuals experience multiple episodes. Certain medications, especially antibiotics, have also been implicated as triggers for erythema multiforme. Medication exposure is the typical stimulus for the onset of Stevens-Johnson syndrome and toxic epidermal necrolysis, which by similar allergic mechanisms produce much more extensive, generalized epithelial sloughing.

Treatment of the oral lesions of erythema multiforme is somewhat controversial. Topical and systemic corticosteroids have been recommended in the past based largely on the presumed pathogenesis of the lesions. However, little evidence exists to demonstrate the effectiveness of this approach. Supportive care usually is adequate and includes a less abrasive diet, maintaining hydration, use of analgesics, and use of a soothing, coating rinse (1:1 mixture of Benadryl[1] elixir and Kaopectate[1])[6]. Patients who experience recurring episodes may benefit from herpes simplex virus suppression with acyclovir or valacyclovir. More extensive epithelial sloughing or rapid progression suggesting

Stevens-Johnson syndrome or toxic epidermal necrolysis requires hospitalization and systemic corticosteroids.

Erosive Lichen Planus and Similar Autoimmune Ulcerative Conditions of the Oral Mucosa

Several diseases cause oral ulcers by autoimmune-mediated degeneration at or near the epithelial–connective tissue interface. In some patients, painful oral ulceration is the only presenting feature of the disease. For other patients, the oral pain is only an occasional or secondary complaint. However, with few exceptions, a chronic course of oral pain for months or years without complete remission is described by the patient. The location and severity may change over time with cyclic formation of new ulcers and concurrent healing of others, but the dominant trend is a chronic, protracted, or progressive course with little or no complete relief. This continuous course distinguishes the ulcers caused by autoimmune diseases from those of other conditions, such as aphthous stomatitis, which characteristically have an episodic pattern of occurrence. As with autoimmune diseases in general, the demographic pattern tends toward middle-aged women. Definitive diagnosis typically relies on biopsy results, but the differential diagnosis is often narrowed by the appreciation of additional findings, such as lesions of the skin or other mucous membranes, and by laboratory tests, such as obtaining an antinuclear antibody (ANA) titer. Lichenoid drug reactions can occur in any patient at anytime during the administration of a medication, although onset of ulcers associated with a new prescription is often indicative of a causative agent.

Distinguishing between chronic oral ulcers from four conditions—erosive lichen planus (ELP), lichenoid drug reaction, mucous membrane pemphigoid (MMP), or pemphigus vulgaris (PV)—can be assisted by reviewing the location and appearance of the ulcers, and the history of the condition.

ELP is relatively common, and oral lesions may occur before the characteristic skin lesions in many patients. In the mouth, the nonerosive lichen planus is characterized by a reticular white lacy expression on the buccal mucosa that may be visualized more easily by drying the tissue with a gauze. Erosions may be related to stressful experiences or exposure to certain foods or dental materials. The erosive lesions of ELP and the lichenoid drug reaction are indistinguishable, so history is helpful relating the chronologic onset of a medication. Many medications are implicated in the etiology of lichenoid drug reactions, including commonly prescribed thiazide diuretics, nonsteroidal antiinflammatory drugs, and penicillins.

Mucous membrane pemphigoid (MMP) has also been referred to as *cicatricial pemphigoid* and *benign MMP*. The typical presentation of MMP is a chronic course of primarily gingival vesicles and bullae that rapidly degenerate into ulcers, usually occurring on the gingival tissue, although any intraoral area may be affected. The patient may also have genital and conjunctival mucous membrane lesions. The incidence of the eye lesions approaches nearly 25% of affected individuals during the protracted disease course, and these lesions may cause blindness in severe cases.

Of the four characteristic forms of pemphigus, only PV causes oral lesions to any clinically significant degree. Approximately one-half of patients develop oral ulcers before the appearance of skin lesions. Most PV oral lesions are found on the marginal gingiva in the upper and lower premolar regions. They appear as bands of beefy red ulceration about 2 mm wide that bleed very easily and are painful when the patient attempts to brush or floss. Initial vesicle or bulla formation is unusual with oral PV, in contrast to MMP, and the peripheral striations described with ELP are absent. The oral ulcers caused by PV tend to show slow progression without healing over time, in contrast to the cyclic variation of concurrent healing and lesion formation characteristic of ELP and MMP.

The oral ulcers caused by all of the conditions in this group respond to corticosteroid medications in the recommended therapeutic approach as described in the Current Therapy box. Several pivotal issues about these conditions and treatment with corticosteroids are important for successful management:

---

[1] Not FDA approved for this indication.
[6] May be compounded by pharmacists.

- Ulcers from infectious diseases (fungal or viral) should not be treated with corticosteroids as this may worsen the condition.
- Most patients will not be cured, but the erosive nature of these ulcers will be controlled and therefore the pain will be reduced.
- Oral candidiasis is a frequent complication of corticosteroid treatment, and this risk is increased with any concurrent condition such as xerostomia. Candidiasis can be detected early with periodic recall evaluation and by exfoliative cytology in suspected situations. Understanding the typical oral candidiasis symptoms increases the patient's awareness of the need to return for treatment.
- Empiric topical corticosteroid treatment should be discontinued for 2 weeks if a biopsy becomes necessary for a definitive diagnosis.

Every effort should be made to identify and discontinue use of causative or irritating agents. Examples such as the link of acidic foods with aphthous ulcers are obvious to the patient, but many are more subtle. One example is cinnamon flavoring agents in many foods, mouthwashes, and toothpastes. Others are irritating to the mucosa but are mistakenly perceived as beneficial. Hydrogen peroxide, phenol preparations, and alcohol-based mouth rinses that "seem to be doing some good" because they are painful and consequently assumed to be killing bacteria are examples that should be avoided by patients with oral ulcers.

Corticosteroid Treatment of Immune-Mediated Oral Ulcers

Corticosteroid management of oral ulcers is similar to the approach for immune-mediated skin lesions. The therapeutic goal is lesion and symptom control, because disease cure or spontaneous remission is unlikely. This should be understood by the patient to avoid unreasonable expectations. Healing of ulcers should be achieved with as little corticosteroid medication as possible. Topical corticosteroids should be tried first, limiting systemic administration to "bursts" as needed to control outbreaks of refractory ulcers followed by maintenance with topical treatment. Long-term systemic corticosteroid administration should be considered only as a last resort. The severity of lesions in these conditions typically varies with time, which means that the need for treatment beyond topical control also varies. Understanding several issues unique to the oral cavity can increase treatment effectiveness:
- Application of the topical corticosteroid after eating and at bedtime and avoiding frequent snacks promote adherence, absorption, and effectiveness.
- Low- and intermediate-potency topical corticosteroid preparations such as triamcinolone (Kenalog) and dexamethasone (Decadron) tend to be less than optimally effective in the oral environment. Initial trial with a higher-potency preparation is justifiable because significant systemic absorption through the oral mucosa is minimal. The use of ultrapotent topical corticosteroids is reserved for persistent ulcers if some systemic absorption is acceptable.
- Titration of a topical steroid should be explained to the patient so that the least amount of steroid to keep the lesions from recurring can be found by experimenting with the interval of use.

Osteonecrosis of the Jaw

Due to the limited blood supply in the mandible, there is a greater risk of osteonecrosis of the jaw (ONJ) than in the maxilla. Many patients who have received radiation to treat head and neck or oral cancer may have an increased risk of ONJ due to the proximity of the mandible to the field of treatment. Secondary to the use of bisphosphonates and other antiresorptive drugs such as denosumab (Prolia), a small number of patients will develop an area of necrotic bone that persists for 8 weeks or more. Often the patient will first complain of an area that feels rough to the tongue on the medial side of the mandible. This is difficult to see because the tongue is in the way, but physicians who prescribe the medications for osteoporosis or metastatic tumors to the bone should be aware of the risk and use a tongue depressor to better visualize the area during examination. Some patients on these medications will have spontaneous development of the condition due to the forces put on the bone during each bite. Others will need dental surgery and the nonhealing area will appear after a tooth is extracted.

While some studies show that a drug holiday from these medications reduces the risk, there appears to be no way to evaluate this. The blood tests that show bone turnover by measuring c-telopeptide (CTX) activity are not specific, and although these tests correlate to improvement in osteoporosis, there has not been any evidence that predicts which patient will develop ONJ.

Treatment is to prescribe systemic antibiotics when there is purulent exudate, with the use of pain medication as needed. Antimicrobial mouthwash such as chlorhexidine gluconate (Peridex) is helpful to eliminate plaque when it is uncomfortable to brush. For extensive areas of necrotic bone, the oral surgeon should be consulted for conservative resection of the affected bone.

References

American Association of Oral and Maxillofacial Surgeons: Medication-Related Osteonecrosis of the Jaw—2014 Update. Available at https://www.aaoms.org/docs/govt_affairs/advocacy_white_papers/mronj_position_paper.pdf. [Accessed 18 July 2019].

Glick M: *Burket's Oral Medicine: Diagnosis and Treatment*, ed 12, Shelton Conn. 2015, People's Medical Publishing House-USA.

Hupp WS, Migliorati CA, Brennan MT, editors: *AAOM Clinician's Guide "The Dentist's Role in the Management of the Cancer Patient."*, Seattle, Wash, 2011, American Academy of Oral Medicine.

Neville BW, Damm DD, Allen CM, Chi AC: *Oral and Maxillofacial Pathology*, ed 4, St Louis, 2015, Elsevier Health Sciences.

Siegel MA, Sollecito TP, Stoopler ET: *Treatment of Common Oral Conditions*, 8th ed, Seattle, Wash, 2018, American Academy of Oral Medicine.

DISEASES OF THE NAILS

Method of
David de Berker, MRCP

Anatomy

The nail plate arises from the nail matrix and grows out attached to the nail bed (Figure 1). The plate is inert and physiologically comparable to the stratum corneum as a structure composed of modified corneocytes containing a high proportion of keratins specific to the hair and nail differentiation that provide the hard and flexible characteristics of the appendage. The matrix is clinically visible as the lunula or half moon in the radial digits, particularly in the thumb. It usually is concealed by the proximal nail fold in digits further round to the little finger and in the toes. The proximal nail fold is a flap of skin that provides a cover to the base of the nail and is adherent to it, with a seal at the distal edge of the nail fold in the form of the cuticle. The lateral nail folds provide a soft tissue boundary to the nail sides. Distally, the nail is firmly attached to the nail bed, with a specialized configuration of epidermis that serves the purpose of minimizing the risk of separation of the nail from the nail bed. Such lifting is called *onycholysis* and is seen in a range of inflammatory and traumatic diseases. Once established, onycholysis can result in pain and loss of function of the digit.

Physiology

Fingernails grow at approximately 3 mm a month, with a faster rate on the dominant hand, on larger digits, in men, in pregnant women, and possibly in warmer weather. The rate diminishes with age from about 45 years. It is slower in toenails, with a rate of approximately 1 mm a month, which can mean that it takes 12 months or more for a big toenail to grow out fully. This has significance for the assessment of the outcome of treatment interventions. It can take several months before a result can be assessed, and in the instance of treatment of onychomycosis it can mean that the treatment has been stopped before the benefits have been fully appreciated.

Function

Fine manipulation, picking up small objects, or scratching an itch or a sticky label are all common uses of a nail. All these functions can be lost in nail disease. Where many nail diseases are associated with soft tissue inflammation of the digit tip or nail fold, there can also be pain that limits function further.

Diseases

Onychomycosis

Onychomycosis is the infection of the nail plate and nail bed with fungus. Pathogenic fungi can damage the nail plate and its attachments. Fungus can also be present in an altered nail but not be the cause of the altered appearance in that it is biologically normal for fungus to occupy cracks in a damp space where there is organic material. Dermatophyte fungi (e.g., *Trichophyton* sp.) are more likely to be pathogenic than nondermatophytes, also referred to as molds (e.g., *Fusarium* sp.). *Candida* sp. also commonly colonizes rather than gives rise to an active onychomycosis with nail changes. However, when a nondermatophyte becomes established as a pathogen, it is often more difficult to eradicate than a dermatophyte and may well manifest with associated biological or occupational factors in the patient (e.g., working with soil, wet work).

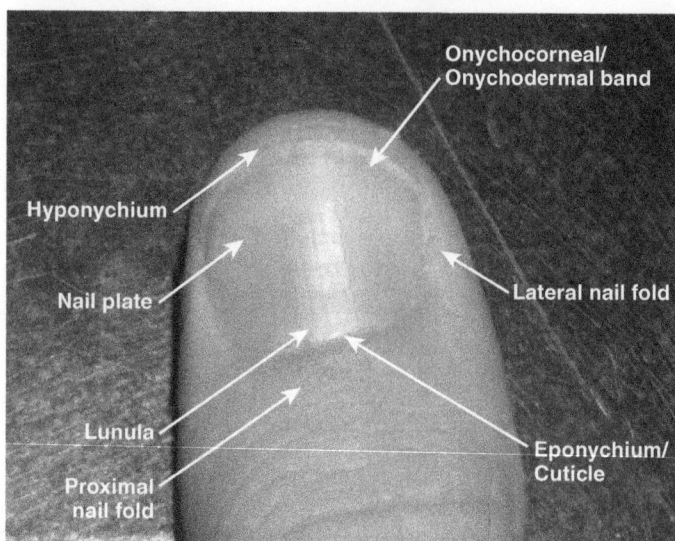

Figure 1 Surface anatomy of the nail.

CURRENT DIAGNOSIS: ONYCHOMYCOSIS

- Make an objective diagnosis with KOH, culture, or clipping for periodic acid–Schiff.
- Onychomycosis is much more common on the toenails than the fingernails.
- The most common organisms are *Trichophyton rubrum* and *Trichophyton mentagrophytes.*
- *Candida* only rarely causes onychomycosis. It is primarily a colonizer where the local environment is conducive.
- Nondermatophyte molds (e.g., *Aspergillus* and *Fusarium* spp.) are unusual causes of onychomycosis in the United States. Repeat tests showing the same organisms and ruling out other causes are required before initiating treatment.

Clinical Features and Diagnosis

Fungal invasion of nail alters the color and integrity of the nail. It may also alter attachment to the nail bed and the shape of the nail. The main color change is the development of shades of yellow or cream that are not transparent, in contrast with the normal color of the nail. Patterns of onychomycosis are described according to the dominant aspect of the infection.

Distal or distolateral onychomycosis is the most common, with the patient's history revealing the progress of a yellow discoloration that has extended gradually over many months or years from the free edge proximally up the nail bed or up one margin. This is usually associated with debris beneath the nail: subungual hyperkeratosis. Diagnosis relies on laboratory confirmation by obtaining a sample of nail and subungual debris for microscopy and mycological culture to provide the identity of the fungus, from which its role and likely sensitivities can be determined. Nail plate histology and polymerase chain reaction assay can be used as second-line tests.

Superficial white onychomycosis can manifest as small white powdery islands within the surface of the nail plate or as larger confluent areas. Scraping with a semisharp blade can demonstrate that it is limited to the dorsal aspect of the nail, and this sample can be sent to mycology for confirmation of the pathogen. It is a form of onychomycosis more common in children, who as a rule do not often suffer from onychomycosis.

Proximal white subungual onychomysis is a variant of onychomycosis seen relatively more often on the fingernails and in people with immunosuppression, either through medication or as part of disease such as HIV. The infection manifests as a white

appearance arising proximal to the rim of the proximal nail fold and beneath the nail plate. With time, as the nail grows out, there may be disturbance of the dorsal nail plate, and disease may progress to the distal free edge with nail destruction.

Dermoscopy can enhance clinical diagnosis with spikes, dots, or jagged borders of nail plate discoloration.

All forms of infection can combine or progress to result in a nail that is almost or entirely overtaken with fungal infection, creating a variant known as *total dystrophic onychomycosis.*

CURRENT THERAPY: ONYCHOMYCOSIS

- Oral treatment should be reserved for patients with mycological confirmation, with emphasis on those at risk for complications (diabetics, immunosuppressed patients, those at risk for secondary bacterial cellulitis).
- Topical treatment is disappointing when used in isolation, except in cases of superficial white onychomycosis. When used in combination with oral therapy, it can increase the cure rate by about 10%.
- Oral treatment is more successful than topical treatment. Terbinafine (Lamisil) 250 mg PO once a day for 6 weeks for a fingernail and 3 months for a toenail in adults is the first-line treatment. Itraconazole (Sporanox), dosed 200 mg daily or 200 mg twice daily pulsed 1 week per month, is the next most successful agent. Additional caution is needed for those on concurrent medication or who have liver disease.
- Newer antifungals are not established, and laser treatment is not fully evaluated.
- Nondermatophytes are not always pathogenic, but when they are, they can be difficult to effectively treat.
- Patients are at high risk for recurrence. Post-treatment prevention of tinea pedis is important to prevent reinfection.

Treatment

All national guidelines on the management of onychomycosis require that the clinical diagnosis be confirmed by microscopy of the nail for fungi and preferably also by mycological culture before commencing systemic treatment. It is common to see patients who have been treated for nonfungal disease with antifungal treatment, which wastes patients' time and money and puts them at needless risk of serious adverse effects if they take oral therapy. Polymerase chain reaction assays are available as an alternative to routine mycology but remain unable to determine the difference between a pathogenic and saprophytic role.

TABLE 1 Nail Psoriasis: Clinical Features and Diagnosis

CLINICAL FEATURE	FOCUS OF DISEASE	TREATMENT MODALITY	OPTIONS
Pitting	Proximal matrix	Potent topical steroid to nail fold	Clobetosone dipropionate[2]
		Tazarotene (Tazorac)[1] to nail fold	
		Steroid injection	Triamcinolone acetonide (10 mg/mL)
Onycholysis	Nail bed	Clip back and treat topically	Steroid and or vitamin D analogues
		Antiseptic finger soaks for secondary infection (e.g., *Candida* and *Pseudomonas*)	
		Systemic therapy	Cyclosporine (Sandimmune), methotrexate (Trexall), fumaric acid esters,[2] acitretin (Soriatane), biologicals
Salmon patch or oily patch		No topical therapy	
Transverse ridging and undulations	Proximal nail fold	Potent topical steroid, vitamin D analogues	See pitting
		Steroid injection	Triamcinolone acetonide (10 mg/mL)
Subungual hyperkeratosis	Nail bed	Steroid injection	Triamcinolone acetonide (10 mg/mL)
		Systemic therapy	Cyclosporine, methotrexate, fumaric acid esters, acitretin, biologicals
Nail shedding	Matrix and nail bed	Systemic therapy	Cyclosporine, methotrexate, fumaric acid esters, acitretin, biologicals

[1]Not FDA approved for this indication.
[2]Not available in the United States.

The main oral treatment for dermatophyte fungi is terbinafine (Lamisil). Itraconazole (Sporanox) is the main alternative. The concomitant treatment with a topical antifungal agent such as amorolfine 5% (Curanail, Loceryl)[2] or ciclopirox 8% (Penlac) can increase the rate of success, which in a trial environment is between 50% and 80% depending on accepted end points. Treatment of co-existent tinea pedis can almost double the efficacy of efinaconazole 10% solution (Jublia) when used topically on nail. There is a significant relapse or reinfection rate in the following 5 years. Ongoing intermittent management of tinea pedis is likely to help prevent this and some patients choose to use a topical therapy intermittently on the nail.

Topical therapy alone has a smaller chance of success in dermatophytes, but it can be effective, especially if combined with thorough debridement by the dermatologist or with the help of a podiatrist with a nail burr and curette. Topical therapy can also be undertaken in combination with surgical or chemical avulsion (50% urea paste in yellow soft paraffin), and this is of value in nondermatophytes, where the fungi are less susceptible to common oral treatments. Voriconazole (Vfend)[1] and other emerging systemic antifungals might have a place in complex nondermatophyte onychomycosis, and normally they would be used in collaboration with a clinical microbiologist. Laser therapy remains under evaluation.

Candidal onychomycosis responds to both of the main oral agents, but it is very prone to relapse if the circumstances that gave rise to the infection remain in place.

Psoriasis
Nail involvement in psoriasis is seen in 80% of psoriasis patients at some point in the course of their disease. In those with significant involvement, it results in pain and loss of function in more than 50%. Nail disease usually is in tandem with skin involvement and in particular with arthropathy of the distal interphalangeal joint, where the inflammation of the joint contributes to a zone of disease that alters matrix function.

Clinical Features and Diagnosis
A personal or family history of psoriasis assists in interpretation of the signs. Sometimes, nail psoriasis occurs in isolation, and clinical signs alone provide the diagnosis or may be supported by a nail unit biopsy. The presence of fungus does not rule out an underlying diagnosis of psoriasis, especially on a big toenail, where fungus has been noted in 27% of psoriatic nails. Nail psoriasis has features that reflect the focus of disease within the nail unit.

Treatment
Treatment requires close attention to hand care, which entails avoiding manicure or work practices that are likely to exacerbate the problem. Typical issues are the clearance of debris from beneath the nail with a sharp instrument that elicits the isomorphic reaction with further psoriasis. Manipulation of the cuticle does the same, and having long nails results in leverage on the nail plate with minor trauma to exacerbate onycholysis. So the rules are:
- No clearance of debris except with a gentle soft nail brush
- No trimming or manipulation of the cuticle
- All nails to be as short as possible.
- General hand care with protection from solvents and wet work and use of plenty of emollient

Where potent topical steroid is to be used (Table 1), it is best applied at night only and for 2 to 3 months. Nail steroid injections have the theoretical risk of rupture of the tendon of the distal interphalangeal joint if undertaken frequently and so are usually done up to several months apart; my practice is to provide a ceiling of four injections per digit. As a rule, all systemic agents work, including biologicals, but their use is rarely justified by nail disease alone. It can be argued that cyclosporine (Sandimmune) in 3-month pulses is good for younger people with no kidney problems, methotrexate (Trexall) might suit older people, and acitretin (Soriatane) may suit those with hypertrophic nail disease. But most choices will be determined by the additional characteristics of the patient and the psoriasis elsewhere.

Idiopathic Onycholysis
Onycholysis is the separation of the nail from the nail bed, with a cleavage that commences at the free edge and progresses proximally.

Diseases of the Nails

[1]Not FDA approved for this indication.
[2]Not available in the United States.

CURRENT DIAGNOSIS: ONYCHOLYSIS

- Primary onycholysis and chronic paronychia are diagnoses of exclusion.
- Onychomycosis, psoriasis, lichen planus, and drug reactions all must be ruled out before diagnosis.
- Primary onycholysis and chronic paronychia are more common on the fingernails than the toenails, in women, in adults, in those who use nail cosmetics, and in those who have recurrent exposure to moisture or chemicals.
- Both primary onycholysis and chronic paronychia represent breakdown in the normal barrier of the nail apparatus.
- Onycholysis results from breakdown of the onychocorneal band or nail bed–nail plate connection. Chronic paronychia is associated with loss of cuticle and inflammation of the nail folds.
- In both scenarios, moisture, contact irritants, contact allergens, colonizing yeast, and bacteria invade the exposed nail apparatus and contribute to a cycle of inflammation.

Clinical Features and Diagnosis

Most patients with onycholysis also have psoriasis. However, for some with problems of nail attachment, the cause is multifactorial and it might not be possible to provide a unifying diagnosis. A subtype of onycholysis occurs in people who undertake manicure vigorously and have long nails. Such people are troubled by the debris beneath a nail and significantly damage the area by scraping material out with a sharp object. This then creates more pathology, a bigger split, and the accumulation of more debris managed by physical manipulation. It is common for people with such cosmetic sensibilities to have long nails, which then exacerbates the onycholysis further through the mechanics of creating a large lever represented by the overhanging margin of the nail. The principle is shared with the wrench in your tool set: The longer the arm on the wrench, the easier it is to exert a torsion force on the point of contact. In this instance the contact is the margin of attachment with the nail bed.

Clipping for mycology is usually undertaken and sometimes reveals *Candida* sp. This is not causal, but is a colonizing microbe in the warm onycholytic space.

CURRENT THERAPY: ONYCHOLYSIS

- It is important not to misdiagnose the presence of yeast (especially *Candida*) as a primary infection or pathogen.
- It almost always represents a colonizer. Treatment of the yeast is therefore secondary.
- Avoidance is the mainstay of treatment. Avoid all wet work and exposure to acids, bases, and chemicals by wearing cotton gloves under heavy-duty vinyl gloves.
- Avoid nail manipulation except for regular plate trimming. No nail salon. Keep the plate trimmed to its proximal-most attachment point. Avoid obvious triggers and traumas to the nail apparatus.
- Where an allergic reaction to nail lacquer is ruled out, some people may find the concealing effect of a colored lacquer helpful.
- Use a potent topical steroid, sometimes under occlusion for paronychia in the first month.
- It can take up to 6 months for the nail apparatus to normalize.

Treatment

Treatment principles are shared with psoriasis (see earlier). The presence of *Candida* sp. on mycology might tempt the clinician to try itraconazole (Sporanox)[1] systemically. However, it rarely helps, although the removal of one factor in the pathology can help other treatments to improve the situation. Success mainly requires avoidance of all physical exacerbating factors and clipping back the separated nail to treat the exposed nail bed with moderate-potency topical steroid. Antiseptic soaks can help if clipping back is not an option or there is significant microbial colonization.

Lichen planus

Lichen planus of the nail has features in common with psoriasis in that it can involve all the different structures of the nail unit and give rise to a range of features accordingly. The area of greatest concern is when it manifests with features of scarring, which can cause permanent loss or splits in nails, with considerable cosmetic and physical handicap.

Clinical Features and Diagnosis

In common with its presentation on the skin, nail lichen planus can be hypertrophic, with thickened nails, or it can be atrophic, with patterns of pronounced pitting that coalesce and eventually fragment the nail. In some instances the disease is very focal and the matrix pathology results in complete loss of nail production, with scarring sequelae. If this occurs with normal matrix remaining on either side, a pterygium may be the outcome, with a scar and nail split being bordered by viable nail spurs like wings. This is normally irreversible, and any suggestion of this pattern of disease should prompt rapid and usually systemic treatment. The potential for side effects with systemic therapy, which may be prolonged, means that I favor a diagnostic biopsy when there is any doubt or when presentation is with nail disease alone. Sometimes, clinical corroboration with mucosal, skin, or scalp disease allows certainty without a biopsy. Biopsy is best taken of nail bed, matrix, and nail fold to ensure it is representative and does not miss the diagnosis.

Treatment

The general protective and topical steroid therapies used in psoriasis can apply in lichen planus. If systemic therapy is needed, oral or intramuscular steroid injection can be used and represent flexible and effective therapy. The duration of the treatment means that monitoring of blood pressure, glucose, and weight may be indicated and bone protection might be needed. Regimens[1] vary, but oral prednisolone[1] 0.25 to 0.5 mg/kg for 4 to 6 weeks, tapering in the 2 weeks following, normally reverses active disease. It also allows assessment of what may be the irreversible scarred element, although nail growth rate means that this judgment should wait until a further 4 to 6 weeks after the end of treatment. Acitretin (Soriatane)[1] and cyclosporine (Sandimmune)[1] also can be used in lichen planus and may be better where patient morbidity does not allow prolonged or repeated oral steroids. Locally injected steroids may be used to address areas of focal scaring but seldom result in full cure.

Eczema

Eczema of the nail folds or nail bed may be associated with eczema elsewhere on the hand or foot and can cause nail unit disturbance in a manner similar to psoriasis. Special patterns of eczema can be relevant for allergic contact sensitivity.

Clinical Features and Diagnosis

The most common pattern of nail changes in eczema is where the nail fold is inflamed as part of an irritant hand eczema or as part of atopic eczema. This acts as a focus of inflammation that in turn disturbs matrix function owing to their adjacency. The nail then suffers transverse ridges and alterations of color, which reflect the fluctuating inflammation. Where the eczema is more directed at the digit tip, the nail bed is more likely to be involved, which in turn results in onycholysis. Both patterns often manifest most in

---

[1] Not FDA approved for this indication.

the dominant hand because trauma, or simply use, increases the likelihood of pathology.

Occupational factors can be important both for analysis of the cause and for helping patients manage the global situation because they can suffer degrees of incapacitation. Where the occupation plays a part in the pathology, such as irritants in a health care or food-preparation worker, it may be necessary to review career choices. Hairdressers, beauticians, and engineers in certain fields come into contact with a wide range of contact sensitizers. The use of nail cosmetics alone can be relevant. Consider patch testing.

Treatment

Treatment is as for eczema elsewhere and shares many of the points made for managing psoriasis of the nail unit:
- Avoidance of irritants, trauma, nail manipulation, and frequent wetting
- Use of copious thick emollient
- Topical steroid tailored to severity
- Hand protection

Infective and chronic paronychia can be a complicating factor in nail unit eczema and requires additional systemic antibiotics in some instances.

Paronychia

Paronychia means inflammation of the proximal or lateral nail folds. There can be an infective component, and there is often a traumatic or eczematous background pathology.

Clinical Features and Diagnosis

An acute paronychia manifests as a focus of redness, pain, and sometimes a point of purulent collection and discharge in the nail fold. There may be a history of preceding trauma or, in children, of nail biting.

Chronic paronychia is seen with a raised, bolstered proximal nail fold, loss of cuticle, and transverse ridges in the nail extending up the nail plate, indicating many months of fluctuating inflammation. There is an account of episodic pain and sometimes discharge of pus. Antibiotics or antifungals alone do not settle the pathology.

Treatment

Acute paronychia is primarily infective and will subside after management of the bacterial infection and the associated wound or inflamed focus. Chronic paronychia has substantial crossover with an irritant hand eczema, and management is as for hand eczema. The low level of infection is secondary to the loss of cuticle and loss of barrier function in a digit that has substantial exposure to microbes. Where wet work is a factor, *Candida* sp. may be found, but short-term eradication with systemic therapy does not resolve the chronic problem. Management is with a potent steroid, sometimes under tape occlusion. Evening (10 minutes) antiseptic soaks can help diminish the risk of infective exacerbation, but once a cuticle has re-formed and the nail fold is flat, the risk greatly reduces.

If there is a failure to respond to this regimen, the diagnosis might need challenging. Periungual squamous cell carcinoma can manifest in this manner and requires nail or nail fold biopsy for assessment.

Ingrown Toenail

An ingrown nail represents a conflict between the shape of the nail and the soft tissues surrounding it. This conflict can be highlighted by an episode or period of trauma such as sport or new shoes, or may be a sustained anatomical state. It is compounded by cutting the nail short at the distolateral corner such that the nail fold overlaps the end of the nail. Symptoms arise through the soft tissue inflammation, which can sometimes be complicated by bleeding or infection. Treatment is directed at the acute inflammation and subsequently at the anatomy if needed.

CURRENT DIAGNOSIS: INGROWN TOENAIL

- Common risk factors include incorrect nail cutting, wide feet, narrow-toed shoes, lateral plate malalignment, and lateral nail fold hypertrophy.
- Neonates and infants demonstrate distal nail ingrowing, which is separate in pathogenesis and treatment from the disease in adolescents and adults.
- Ingrown nails can be graded on a scale from I to III, with I being erythema and swelling with drainage from the nail fold and III being associated with exuberant overgrowth of granulation tissue over and around the ingrown nail plate.

Clinical Features and Diagnosis

Ingrowing can occur at any nail margin, with the most common site being the lateral nail fold in the big toe of someone in the second or third decade of life. At this site, it is the angle of the distal and lateral nail that becomes embedded in the lateral nail fold to create a puncture wound. The inflammation that follows creates a more bulky lateral nail fold and a positive feedback loop such that resolution typically requires medical intervention.

In a newborn or in a nail regrowing after loss, ingrowing can occur at the free edge as it meets the distal digit pulp. Proximally, an incompletely shed nail may be displaced upwards to embed into the ventral aspect of the proximal nail fold, with a pattern of pain and inflammation that matches ingrowing at other sites. This is called *retronychia*. All variants can evolve to create a mass resembling a pyogenic granuloma coupled with ooze and potential for secondary infection and local cellulitis.

CURRENT THERAPY: INGROWN TOENAIL

- Infantile disease should be treated with warm soaks with antiseptic followed by massage of the nail and distal phalangeal tuft.
- Adolescent and adult disease should be addressed with correct nail plate cutting and shoes. For mild disease, twice daily antiseptic soaks, topical steroids, 20% to 40% topical urea cream (Keralac, Carmol), and cotton wisps or dental floss under the aggravating part of the lateral nail plate will decrease inflammation, improve symptoms, and normalize the nail plate without surgery.
- For more advanced cases, use twice-daily warm soaks and oral antibiotics (with signs of infection), followed by lateral plate avulsion and lateral matricectomy (either chemical or surgical).

Treatment

Mild acute ingrowing can be treated with antiseptic soaks, potent topical steroid, and oral antibiotic if infection is suspected. Causal footwear or activities should be avoided and shoes with a high toe box to accommodate the tips of the toes should be worn. It may be possible to insert a pledget of cotton, wool, or similar substance between the embedding edge of nail and the damaged soft tissue. Advice on square end nail cutting to avoid an overshort nail is important.

If this conservative approach does not work, surgery is indicated. This is normally ablation of the lateral 3 to 4 mm of nail matrix and can be done with 85% aqueous phenol to create a chemical burn or with excision. The latter requires considerable skill for a reliable outcome because the apex of the horn of the matrix is difficult to access, and a remnant, if left, results in a spicule of nail regrowth that will continue to cause problems. Phenol, however, tends to find the entire exposed matrix because it is a liquid flowing into a crevice and does not need precise placement.

Distal embedding normally settles with conservative measures, and proximal ingrowing with retronychia requires avulsion. Avulsion is not the treatment for lateral or distal ingrowing because it results in recurrence of the problem as the nail regrows in most instances.

Single Digit Dystrophy

Dystrophy of a single nail is relatively common.

CURRENT THERAPY: SINGLE DIGIT DYSTROPHY

- Once a biopsy has been obtained it is possible to pursue one of the three avenues of definitive treatment: antimicrobial, immunosuppressive, or surgical. Each option is directed at infection, inflammation, or neoplasm, respectively, and each is counterproductive for management of either of the other two diagnostic groupings.

Clinical Features and Diagnosis

Dystrophy in a single digit can have any appearance, but the important thing for the clinician is that single-digit dystrophies include the uncommon but significant category of skin cancer. The most common of these is in situ squamous cell carcinoma (SCC), but the main other diagnosis is melanoma, either with a longitudinal melanonychia or as amelanotic melanoma with a lesion resembling a pyogenic granuloma. Both SCC and melanoma are infamous for having a late diagnosis in the digit, and the reason for this is lack of awareness shared by patient and clinician.

Following exclusion of inflammatory dermatoses by history and body examination and of onychomycosis by multiple clippings, the area should be biopsied for histology of matrix and nail bed. The classic biopsy is the lateral longitudinal biopsy, although this should be tailored to the perceived focus of pathology. It is best undertaken by someone familiar with nail pathology and the procedure, because there is a further risk of false reassurance of a negative biopsy if the sample is too small or directed at the wrong area of the nail unit.

CURRENT DIAGNOSIS: SINGLE DIGIT DYSTROPHY

- Nail dystrophy on a single digit represents a risk factor for squamous cell carcinoma or melanoma of the nail unit.
- This is more common on a finger than a toe, where trauma is more often the explanation on a toe.
- When history, examination, and investigations do not provide a clear diagnosis, then a nail unit biopsy is indicated to exclude neoplasm and direct definitive treatment.

Treatment

Where malignancy is detected, treatment is normally surgery. Topical therapy for in situ SCC does not work well owing to obstruction of the involved surfaces beneath the nail. The crevices created by the nail folds make photodynamic therapy ineffective.

References

Dalle S, Depape L, Phan A, et al: Squamous cell carcinoma of the nail apparatus: Clinicopathological study of 35 cases, Br J Dermatol 156:871–874, 2007.
de Berker D: Clinical practice, Fungal nail disease, N Engl J Med 360:2108–2116, 2009.
de Berker DA, Lawrence CM: A simplified protocol of steroid injection for psoriatic nail dystrophy, Br J Dermatol 138:90–95, 1998.
Jiaravuthisan MM, Sasseville D, Vender RB, et al: Psoriasis of the nail: Anatomy, pathology, clinical presentation, and a review of the literature on therapy, J Am Acad Dermatol 57:1–27, 2007.
Piraccini BM, Saccani E, Starace M, et al: Nail lichen planus: response to treatment and long term follow-up, Eur J Dermatol 20:489–496, 2010.
Sánchez-Regaña M, Sola-Ortigosa J, Alsina-Gibert M, et al: Nail psoriasis: A retrospective study on the effectiveness of systemic treatments (classical and biological therapy), J Eur Acad Dermatol Venereol 25:579–586, 2011.

ERYTHEMA MULTIFORME

Method of
Chad Douglas, MD, PharmD

CURRENT DIAGNOSIS

- Acute cutaneous target-like papules, plaques, and bullae
- Oral mucosal lesions can be present
- Predominance in young adults
- Most often associated with acute or chronic herpes simplex virus (HSV-1) infection
- Less commonly associated with medications such as sulfonamide and penicillin antibiotics

CURRENT THERAPY

- Treat any underlying infection and discontinue any potential offending medications
- Mild disease: symptomatic care with oral antihistamines, topical corticosteroids
- Severe and persistent disease: prednisone, cyclosporine (Neoral and Sandimmune)[1] azathioprine (Imuran)[1]
- Recurrent episodes: prophylaxis with HSV antiviral agents

[1]Not FDA approved for this indication.

Epidemiology

Erythema multiforme (EM) is an acute, mucocutaneous, immune-mediated hypersensitivity disorder. This rare self-limiting disorder has an estimated incidence of 0.01% to 1% and predominately occurs in young adults between the ages of 20 and 40. Up to 20% of cases occur in children and adolescents.

Risk Factors

Erythema multiforme is most commonly associated with viral, fungal, and atypical bacterial infections. More than 60% of infection-associated cases of erythema multiforme occur with herpes simplex virus (HSV), most commonly HSV-1. Mycoplasma pneumonia is the second most common infectious organism associated with erythema multiforme and up to 5% of patients with this atypical pneumonia develop EM. Most cases of recurrent erythema multiforme are associated with acute HSV infections or reactivation of chronic HSV infections. The second most common cause of erythema multiforme are medications. Medication accounts for 10% to 20% of erythema multiforme cases and is referred to as drug-induced EM (DIEM). The most common medication classes in DIEM are sulfonamides, penicillins, nonsteroidal antiinflammatory agents, and aromatic amine anticonvulsants such as carbamazepine (Tegretol), phenytoin (Dilantin), and phenobarbital. Drug-induced erythema multiforme is considered a separate and distinct entity from hypersensitivity and cutaneous adverse drug reactions such as maculopapular erythema, Stevens-Johnson syndrome (SJS), and toxic epidermal necrolysis (TEN).

Pathophysiology

The pathophysiology of erythema multiforme has been extensively delineated in herpes-associated EM (HAEM). HSV DNA fragments are transported to distant skin sites by peripheral blood mononuclear cells. HSV genes within these fragments express various enzymes including DNA polymerase that leads to recruitment of CD4+ TH1 cells. These CD4+ TH1 cells release interferon-gamma (INF-gamma) that initiates an inflammatory cascade with the sequestration of circulating monocytes, natural killer (NK) cells, and lymphocytes as well as recruitment of autoreactive T-cells. This extensive immune response leads to keratinocyte destruction.

In contrast, the pathophysiology of drug-induced erythema multiforme involves tumor necrosis factor α (TNF-α) production that leads to epidermal destruction. Human leukocyte antigen polymorphisms have not been extensively characterized in DIEM, as they have been in more classic immune-mediated cutaneous drug hypersensitivity reactions such as SJS and TEN.

Prevention

There is no current prevention for erythema multiforme; however, the knowledge of infectious agents and medications that can cause EM can help one identify patients who could be at risk for development of this condition. Future studies in the advancement of pharmacogenetics may potentially identify human leukocyte antigen polymorphisms that could predispose patients to HAEM or DIEM.

Clinical Manifestations and Diagnosis

Erythema multiforme is a self-limited eruption that most often appears in a symmetric distribution on distal extremities with frequent involvement of dorsal surfaces of the hands and extensor surfaces of extremities. Prodromal syndrome such as fever, chills, malaise, and arthralgia can occur but are rare. Lesions often burn or itch and progress from distal areas of the body toward proximal regions. Initial lesions are usually sharply demarcated red or pink macules that can resemble hives or early stages of SJS. Unlike hives, these lesions become fixed and do not migrate. Mucosal involvement and skin sloughing is less common than with SJS. The macules become popular and may gradually enlarge into plaques that are several centimeters in diameter. Lesions often contain three concentric zones including a central darker red region, a pale pink edematous zone, and a peripheral red ring. These characteristic "target" or "iris" lesions may only contain a central dark red region with a lighter peripheral ring and may not appear until several days after onset of the eruptions. Lesions of multiple morphology are usually present, thus the name "multiforme." Mucosal lesions, when present, are red and edematous and often involve blister formation. These lesions are usually limited to the oral cavity and affect the lips, inside of cheeks, and the tongue. Typically, lips are swollen with hemorrhagic crusting. Erythema multiforme associated with mycoplasma pneumonia may present with mucosal lesions alone without cutaneous manifestations. Diagnosis is most often made clinically in patients with characteristic lesions and a preceding or concurrent infection that is known to be commonly associated with EM. A clinical diagnosis can also be made in patients with characteristic lesions who are taking a commonly associated medication. Rarely, a skin biopsy is needed to rule out other conditions, although there is no single diagnostic histologic feature specific to erythema multiforme. Erythema multiforme usually resolves spontaneously within 3 to 5 weeks.

Differential Diagnosis

Early erythema multiforme lesions can resemble urticaria, drug eruptions, viral exanthem, maculopapular erythema as well as early stages of Stevens-Johnson syndrome and toxic epidermal necrosis. Bullous lesions may resemble bullous pemphigoid and target lesions may resemble pityriasis rosea or vasculitis.

Treatment

Although erythema multiforme is self-limiting, early identification and treatment of the causative infectious agent or immediate discontinuation of an offending medication can reduce the severity and duration of the condition. Symptomatic treatment with oral first-generation antihistamines (diphenhydramine [Benadryl] 25 to 50 mg po q 6 hours prn or hydroxyzine [Atarax] 25 to 100 mg po q 6 hours prn) and mid-potency topical corticosteroids (triamcinolone [Kenalog] 0.1% cream) will usually suffice for mild disease. More severe disease including cases with mucosal involvement as well as recurrent EM can be treated with prednisone, cyclosporine (Neoral, Sandimmune),[1] or azathioprine (Imuran).[1] The use of dapsone[1] and antimalarial

agents in severe disease has demonstrated varying success. Recurrent erythema multiforme is most often associated with HSV-1, and herpes viral suppressive therapy with acyclovir (Zovirax)[1] or valacyclovir (Valtrex)[1] has been shown to be effective. Valacyclovir (Valtrex) is given once daily until the patient is recurrence free for 4 months. The valacyclovir (Valtrex) dose is then reduced with eventual discontinuation. Although reintroduction of an offending medication does not frequently cause recurrence of erythema multiforme, caution should still be advised when considering the future use of such medication or other medications within the same drug class.

Monitoring and Complications

Mucosal involvement may limit a patient's ability to eat or drink and close monitoring is advised in such cases. This can be of particular concern in pediatric patients. Skin lesions are usually not associated with scarring but postinflammatory hyperpigmentation can occur and often take several months to resolve.

---

[1]Not FDA approved for this indication.

References

Anquier-Durant A, Mockenhaupt M, et al: Correlations between clinical patterns and causes of erythema multiforme majus, Stevens-Johnson syndrome, and toxic epidermal necrolysis: results of an international prospective study, *Arch Dermatol* 138(8):1019–1024, 2002 Aug.

Aurelian L, Ono F, Burnett J: Herpes simplex virus (HSV)-associated erythema multiforme (HAEM): a viral disease with an autoimmune component, *Dermatol Online J* 9(I), 2003.

Kokuba H, Aurelian L, Burnett J: Herpes simplex virus associated erythema multiforme (HAEM) is mechanistically distinct from drug-induced erythema multiforme: interferon-gamma is expressed in HAEM lesions and tumor necrosis factor-alpha in drug-induced erythema multiforme lesions, *J Invest Dermatol* 113:808–815, 1999.

Lamoreux MR, Sternbach MR, Hsu WT: Erythema Multiforme, *Am Fam Physician* 74(11):1883–1888, 2006 Dec 1.

Ono F, Sharma BK, Smith CC, et al: CD34+ Cells in the peripheral blood transport herpes simplex virus DNA fragments to the skin of patients with erythema multiforme (HAEM), *J Invest Dermatol* 124:1215–1224, 2005.

Sokumbi O, Wetter DA: Clinical features, diagnosis, and treatment of erythema multiforme: a review for the practicing dermatologist, *Int J Dermatol* 51:889–902, 2012.

Svensson CK, Cowen EW, Gaspari AA: Cutaneous drug reactions, *Pharmacol Rev* 53(3):357–379, 2001 Sep.

FUNGAL INFECTIONS OF THE SKIN

Method of
Therese Holguin, MD; and Kriti Mishra, MD

CURRENT DIAGNOSIS

- Dermatophyte infections
  - Non-hair-bearing (glabrous) skin diagnostic techniques are scraping of leading edge of scale with glass slide onto glass slide, cover slip, and apply 10% potassium hydroxide (KOH) to edge of coverslip. Heat the bottom of slide slightly, clean off with tissue, and view under microscope without condenser. Counterstain with chlorazol black E or Parker blue-black ink may help visualize hyphae.
  - Hair-bearing skin may require a tissue biopsy with special fungal stains to confirm diagnosis.
  - Culture of scale, hair, and nail fragments sent to laboratory in a sterile urine cup and clearly marked "for dermatophyte culture" is an additional testing method. Nail fragments can be sent in formalin for periodic acid-Schiff (PAS) staining (a quick-turnaround test).
- Tinea versicolor
  - Stratum corneum removal with a glass slide against a glass slide and KOH examination as above is done for diagnosis. Cultures require a special media and lab needs notification this is the organism suspected.

- Candida cutaneous infections
  - Unroofing a pustule by scraping gently with a 15 blade and spreading contents onto a glass slide for KOH evaluation will review the characteristic yeast and pseudohyphae. Culture is usually not necessary.

CURRENT THERAPY

- Dermatophyte infections
  - Non-hair-bearing skin mild infections are treated with topical agents if severe and widespread; systemic and topical agents together will provide higher cure rate. Prevent reinfection of feet by wearing sandals when possible, especially in public places, alternating shoes, and keeping feet dry. For groin infections, dry well after showering and put socks on before underwear.
  - Hair-bearing skin and hair infections require systemic therapy for cure. Nail infections may be cured with newer topical agents.
- Tinea versicolor
  - Topical treatment with topical agents such as selenium sulfide lotion applied for 10 minutes for 2 weeks, neck to knees, is a cheap and effective treatment. Systemic agents may be needed for resistant cases. Prevention may require maintenance therapy with topical agents during warm and humid months.
- Candida cutaneous infections
  - Topical agents such as nystatin or ketoconazole cream are an effective choice. Prevention of intertrigo is somewhat successful if care to dry thoroughly after showering in body fold areas is done routinely. Zinc-talc shake lotion may be used once or twice daily.

Dermatophyte (tinea) infections are a group of filamentous fungal infections of the skin, hair, and nails and can be noninflammatory or inflammatory. The route of acquisition for dermatophytes is either person to person (anthropophilic), or from animals (zoophilic). Geophilic dermatophytes grow in soil and are a rare source of infection in humans. The causative organisms are of three genera: *Microsporum, Trichophyton, and Epidermophyton.*

Dermatophytoses are the most common fungal infections worldwide, affecting 20% to 25% of the world population. The predominant agents have changed over time by geography and population based on migration of populations, hygiene practices, and therapeutic breakthroughs (griseofulvin [Gris-PEG]). Clinical classification is based on site of infection. Tinea pedis refers to infection of the feet, tinea manuum the hands, tinea cruris the groin, and tinea corporis the skin excluding already mentioned sites plus scalp and nails. Tinea unguium (onychomycosis) refers to nail infection, tinea barbae to beard area, tinea faciei the face, and tinea capitis the scalp and hair. Virulence of the infection is dependent on underlying factors suppressing immunity (diabetes, cancer, HIV infection). Dissemination can be seen in the immunosuppressed.

Superficial infections of the skin and mucous membranes caused by yeasts are caused by *Candida* species. Also common are infections due to lipophilic yeast fungus *Malassezia.*

Superficial Mycoses Dermatophytes

Tinea Capitis

The populations most at risk are children, with boys more commonly than girls. The onset of puberty and change in the relative composition of unsaturated fatty acids in sebum is protective. African Americans and Hispanics have an increased incidence of *Trichophyton tonsurans.* Pet exposure is associated with

Figure 1 Black dot tinea.

infections of *Microsporum canis.* Infection with *Trichophyton schoenleinii (favus),* still seen in less well-developed countries, is of characteristic cup-shaped crusts, scutula.

The usual presentation of tinea capitis is of scale and itch on the scalp with broken-off hairs with a "black dot" appearance (Figure 1) or an inflamed boggy plaque, referred to as a *kerion.* Inflammatory presentations are most often seen in zoophilic infections. Patches of alopecia are common.

Tools for diagnosis include potassium hydroxide (KOH) preparation of scale or hair tweezed from affected patch to be examined microscopically. The Wood's light will show fluorescence with ectothrix infections (organism on outside of shaft) but not endothrix infections (spores on inside of shaft). Samples for culture are obtained by rubbing a wet cotton-tipped applicator over the affected area and applying this or pulled hairs onto the dermatophyte test medium or other medium if species identification is required in resistant cases. The differential diagnosis includes seborrheic dermatitis, psoriasis, folliculitis, pediculosis, secondary syphilis, discoid lupus erythematosus, lichen planus, lichen simplex chronicus, trichotillomania, alopecia areata, and other inflammatory follicular conditions.

Tinea Faciei and Barbae

Frequently misdiagnosed, infection of the face or beard is rare. Beard infections (tinea sycosis or barber's itch) can be deep and inflammatory and are seen in agricultural workers, especially those working with farm animals. Discoid lupus is a commonly mistaken diagnosis, and biopsies are sometimes required to differentiate.

Tinea Corporis

"Ringworm" is a layman's descriptive term of the characteristic clinical findings of dermatophyte infections. The term accurately portrays the appearance of an erythematous annular plaque with a scaly, raised, leading edge (Figure 2). Severe infections may herald new HIV infection or be secondary to topical immunosuppressant such as calcineurin inhibitors or, more commonly, steroids. KOH examination sampling should be taken from the leading edge. The differential diagnosis includes pityriasis rosea, impetigo, inflammatory dermatoses such as psoriasis and seborrheic dermatitis, and syphilis.

Tinea Cruris

More common in men and when humidity is high, "jock itch" or "crotch itch" involves the upper thigh, intertriginous area, and peripheral spread into the perineum and perianal areas. The scrotum is rarely involved. The usually well-defined border may display scale, papules, or pustules.

The differential diagnosis includes a bacterial infection, erythrasma, candidiasis, intertrigo, psoriasis, and dermatitis. Morphology of the rash and expected involvement of other cutaneous sites is useful to eliminate these possible diagnoses. The origin of

TABLE 1 Treatment

INFECTION	CHILDREN	ADULTS	TOPICAL	COMMENTS
Tinea capitis	Terbinafine (Lamisil granules)[2] first-line Age 4+ 4–6 weeks (granules can be added to nonacidic food) <25 kg 125 mg/d 25–35 kg 165.5mg/d >35 kg 250 mg/d Griseofulvin second line *Ultramicrosize* (Gris-PEG) Age 2+ 8 weeks (can sprinkle on apple sauce) 5–15 mg/kg/d, single or 2 divided doses, max 750 mg/d Fluconazole (Diflucan) [1] Age >14 days 3–6 mg/kg PO/IV q24h×6 weeks; Alt: 6 mg/kg PO/IV qweek×8-12 weeks Itraconazole (Sporanox)[1] 4–6 weeks 3–5 mg/kg/day (with full meal) or pulse regimen with capsules (5 mg/kg/d for 1wk times 3 pulses 3 wk apart), and with oral solution (3 mg/kg/d for 1 wk times 3 pulses, ie, 1 wk per mo)	Terbinafine (Lamisil tab)[1] 4–6 weeks 250 mg/d Fluconazole (Diflucan)[1] 50 mg/d (4–7 weeks) or 150 mg/week (4 weeks) Itraconazole (Sporanox)[1] 4 weeks 100–200 mg/d	Antifungal shampoos: selenium sulfide (antidandruff), ciclopirox (Loprox), and zinc pyrithione (Head & Shoulders) (twice-weekly with systemic treatment)	Systemic therapy: baseline CBC and Liver function tests. Repeat if >6 weeks. Griseofulvin contraindicated in pregnancy and restrictions for becoming or fathering after course. Avoid alcohol during treatment. Itraconazole has negative inotropic effect and can prolong Q-T interval. Ketoconazole has risks of fatal liver damage and adrenal insufficiency (not recommended)
Tinea corporis, Tinea cruris, Tinea pedis, Tinea mannum, Tinea faciei, Tinea barbae	Terbinafine[1] Age 2+ 2 weeks <20 kg 62.5 mg/d 20–40 kg 125 mg/d >40 kg 250 mg/d Itraconazole[1] 2 weeks 5 mg/kg/day divided qd-BID Griseofulvin ultramicrosize Age 2+ 2–8 weeks 5–15 mg/kg/day divided qd-BID; Max: 750 mg/day	Terbinafine[1] 2–4 weeks 250 mg/d Itraconazole[1] 1 week 200 mg/d Fluconazole[1] 2–4 weeks 150–300 mg/week Terbinafine 250 mg plus itraconazole 200 mg for 3 weeks (resistant cases)[1]	Terbinafine (Lamisil) Butenafine (Lotrimin-Ultra) Naftifine (Naftin) Clotrimazole (Lotrimin) Econazole (Spectazole) Ketoconazole (Nizoral) Sertaconazole (Ertaczo) Luliconazole (Luzu) Eberconazole (Ebernet) 2–6 weeks once or twice daily	Systemic treatment is reserved for widespread, resistant, or severe disease. Monitor for drug interactions and adverse effects.
Tinea unguium	Children may respond completely to antifungal topical lacquer or solutions without systemic therapy. Terbinafine Age 2+ 6 weeks fingernails 12 weeks toenails <20 kg 62.5 mg/d 20–40 kg 125 mg/d >40 kg 250 mg/d Itraconazole 1week of each month for 3–5 months, 2 pulses for fingernails and 3 for toenails 5 mg/kg/d Fluconazole[1] Age >14 d 6 mg/kg PO/IV/wk×12–16 weeks for fingernails and 18–26 for toenails Griseofulvin Not considered as useful as would have to have daily dosing for 6–12 months. Cure rate poor.	Terbinafine 250 mg/d (fingernails for 6 weeks 12 weeks for toenails) or 250 mg/d for 4 weeks off 4 weeks for 2 pulses for toenails Itraconazole 200 mg/d 12 weeks or 200mg BID for 1 week off 3 weeks (2× for fingernails and 3× for toenails) pulse therapy Fluconazole[1] 150–300 mg/week (6–9 months fingernails 9–18 months toenails)	Lacquers: Amorolfine (Curanail, Loceryl, Locetar, Odenil)[2] and Ciclopirox (Penlac) Hydrolacquer: Cicloprox Solution: Efinaconazole (Jublia) and Tavaborole (Kerydin) 48–60 weeks	Lacquers are debrided and reapplied daily. Hydrolacquers are removable with washing and reapplied daily. Conventional oral therapy followed by topical for maintenance may help prevent recurrence. Lasers and photodynamic therapy if available are considered third-line options. Surgical options include chemical (40%–50% urea compound), or surgical nail avulsion.

Abbreviations: BID = two times daily; CBC = complete blood count; IV = intravenous; PO = orally.
[1]Not FDA approved for this indication.
[2]Not available in the United States.

Figure 2 Tinea corporis.

the infection is believed to be autoinoculation from tinea pedis or onychomycosis.

Tinea Manuum and Pedis

A classic finding of "one hand and two feet" involvement is useful to lead one to consider tinea manuum (Figure 3). The organism involved in the infection determines the amount of inflammation resultant. Whereas *Trichophyton rubrum* produces a dry scale with erythema of hands and feet (moccasin-type), *Trichophyton interdigitale* (previously known as *Trichophyton mentagrophytes*) often leads to a painful, itchy, blistering eruption of the feet. Other signs of *T interdigitale* include interdigital maceration and superficial infection of the toenails with a distinct white appearance (white superficial onychomycosis). Toe-web infection with gram-negative bacteria may be consequential. Hyperhidrosis is often a precursor to this type of infection. An idiopathic reaction "dermatophytid" is a fairly common pruritic rash of small blisters involving the palms and sometimes the sides of the feet.

Onychomycosis

Fungal infections of the nail are caused by dermatophytes (tinea unguium), yeasts, and nondermaphytic molds. It is common in the general population, accounting for 50% of skin fungal infections. Risk factors include advanced age, diabetes, circulatory disorders, and family history. There are three major subtypes of onychomycosis: distal lateral subungual onychomycosis, white superficial onychomycosis, and proximal subungual onychomycosis. Distal lateral subungual onychomycosis is the most common subtype and is caused by the anthropophilic dermatophytic fungus, *T rubrum*. Symptoms include an initial discoloration of the distal corner of the nail that may be white, gray, or brown caused by accumulation of keratinous debris under the nail that eventually spreads to involve the entire nail. Other common features are onycholysis, or splitting of the nail from the bed, nail thickening, and impaired nail growth. The diagnosis typically involves KOH, mycologic laboratory confirmation (culture), and biopsy. Yeast onychomycosis is most commonly caused by *Candida albicans* and typically involves fingernails of hands frequently exposed to moisture. Nondermaphytic molds primarily involve toenails. Though not life threatening, onychomychosis can significantly impair an individual's quality of life with concerns such as issues cutting the nails and cosmetic disfigurement.

Pityriasis Versicolor

This superficial fungal infection of the skin is caused by a dimorphic lipophilic fungus, *Malassezia* species, which is part of the physiological skin flora. Certain environmental, genetic, and immunologic factors can predispose the fungus to convert to its pathogenic hyphal form and development of disease. It grows best in warm, humid climates; thus there has been a higher prevalence reported in tropical climates. Furthermore, potential hormonal

Figure 3 Tinea manuum.

changes during adolescence can increase sebum production and allow for *Malassezia* to thrive, and the prevalence is even further increased in active adolescents. The pathophysiology may also be related to an impaired immune system.

The diagnosis is usually made clinically, but the presentation may vary; it classically consists of a well-demarcated rash with fine scale and thin plaques. The rash may be hyperpigmented, hypopigmented, or erythematous. Typically, the rash appears on the torso but may become widespread. The lesions may be mildly pruritic or asymptomatic. If KOH is performed on skin scrapings, numerous spores and hyphae can be visualized ("spaghetti and meatball" appearance). Treatment options include topical antifungals, including azoles and terbinafine, selenium sulfide (antidandruff), and zinc pyrithione (Head & Shoulders). Oral azole antifungals can be used; systemic treatment is not first-line therapy because of side effects.

Candidiasis

A dimorphic commensal fungus inhabiting skin, mouth, and reproductive tract, candidiasis, is found in up to 70% of healthy individuals. *Candida* infection of the skin usually involves moist or occluded areas such as the groin, axillae, and diaper area in the young. Candidal intertrigo classically presents as erythematous and macerated plaques with peripheral scaling. Satellite lesions help differentiate candidal lesions from other conditions. Skin lesions are typically nontender but may develop central pallor or become hemorrhagic in patients with thrombocytopenia. Primary treatment is topical azole and polyene (nystatin) antifungals that are well tolerated. Adjunct therapy with low-dose topical corticosteroids may be used for associated pruritis and pain. Systemic antifungal therapy is rarely used but may be used for refractory disease.

References

Asz-Sigall D, Tosti A, Arenas R: Tinea unguium: diagnosis and treatment in practice, *Mycopathologia* 182:95–100, 2017.

Chen X, Jiang X, Yang M, et al: Systemic antifungal therapy for tinea capitis in children: an abridged cochrane review, *J Am Acad Dermatol* 76:368–374, 2017.

Gupta A, Foley K, Versteeg S: New antifungal agents and new formulations against dermatophytes, *Mycopathologia* 182:127–141, 2017.

Gupta AK, Kogan N, Batra R: Pityriasis versicolor: a review of pharmacological treatment options: expert opinion on pharmacotherapy, *Expert Opin Pharmacother* 6:165–178, 2005.

Hay R: Tinea capitis: current status, *Mycopathologia* 182:87–93, 2017.

Kyriakis KP, Terzoudi S, Palamaras I, et al: Pityriasis versicolor prevalence by age and gender, *Mycoses* 49:517–518, 2006.

Nenoff P, Krüger C: Ginter-Hanselmayer, et al: Mycology—an update. part 1: Dermatomycoses: Causative agents, epidemiology and pathogenesis, *J Dtsch Dermatol Ges* 12:188–209, 2014.

Perlroth J, Choi B, Spellberg B: Nosocomial fungal infections: epidemiology, diagnosis, and treatment, *Med Mycol* 45:321–346, 2007.

Priyanka S, Mala B, Gurvinder P, et al: Evaluation of efficacy and safety of oral terbinafine and itraconazole combination therapy in the management of dermatophytosis, *J Dermatol Treat*, 2019. https://doi.org/10.1080/09546634.2019.16 12835.

Solís-Arias MP, García-Romero MT: Onychomycosis in children: a review, *Int J Dermatol* 56:123–130, 2017.

KELOIDS

Method of
Leslie A. Greenberg, MD

CURRENT DIAGNOSIS

- Clinical characteristics: firm, raised, papular, plaque-like, nodular, and tumorous scar tissue that extends beyond the initial wound borders. May be painful or pruritic and disfiguring.
- Location: more commonly found on ears, upper back and chest, and upper arms.
- Cause: results from an abnormal healing process after skin trauma or inflammation.
- Histologic characteristics: abnormally functioning dermal fibroblasts and overproduction of extracellular matrix result in markedly thickened bundles of hyalinized collagen arranged in a haphazard fashion.

CURRENT THERAPY

Medical Therapies
- Intralesional corticosteroids (triamcinolone acetonide [Kenalog])
- Interferon alfa (IFN-alfa2b [Intron A])[1]
- Intralesional fluorouracil (5-FU, Adrucil)[1]

Surgical Therapies
- Cryotherapy
- Primary excision

Physical Modalities
- Pressure therapy
- Radiation therapy
- Laser therapy

Miscellaneous Therapies
- Silicone gel sheeting or gel

[1]Not FDA approved for this indication.

Keloids are common, benign fibroproliferative lesions resulting from altered wound healing caused by abnormalities of fibroblast function and extracellular matrix overproduction. Lesions may be painful and severely disfiguring—at times limiting range of motion. Histologically, keloids are foci of brightly eosinophilic-staining collagen bundles laid haphazardly.

Keloids may be papular, plaque-like, nodular, or tumorous. The term *keloid* is derived from the Greek word meaning "tumor-like." A keloid extends beyond the site of injury. Keloids tend to shrink over time, but rarely resolve.

Epidemiology
Keloids occur more commonly in people of African and Asian descent. There may be a familial or genetic contribution to keloid development as an autosomal dominant inheritance with incomplete penetrance. Keloids may be intentionally induced for cosmetic purposes. For example, the ancient Olmec of Mexico in pre-Columbian times are one ethnic group which has used keloid scarification as an intentional means of decoration.

Pathophysiology
Unlike scars, keloids are made up of markedly thickened bundles of collagen that are arranged in a haphazard fashion. Normal scar tissue formation, in contrast, consists of fibrillary bundles of collagen that are aligned parallel to the skin surface.

The pathogenesis of keloid formation is unknown. Fibroblast proliferation and increased collagen synthesis are due to over-expression of growth factors. Growth factor production fails to self-regulate and does not turn off once the wound is well healed. Alteration of programmed fibroblast apoptosis has been implicated. It has been suggested that keloid fibroblasts fail to undergo physiologically programmed cell death and thereby produce extra connective tissue. Genetic factors are likely involved, and studies have identified four susceptibility loci.

Keloids represent the end stage of an inflammatory process that starts after a traumatic disruption of skin integrity. Over a period of weeks, abnormally functioning fibroblasts replace the granulation tissue associated with the early stages of healing. At that point, a distinctive morphologic scar or keloid may be noticeable. After a keloid is fully formed, it may look the same for years or it may enlarge over time.

Risk Factors
Certain populations are at higher risk to develop keloids. Dark-skinned individuals such as those of Asian, African, and Hispanic descent have a 15-fold increased risk to develop keloids compared to light-skinned individuals. Skin insults such as lacerations, secondarily infected skin lesions, surgery, or ear piercings challenge the body's healing processes and may result in keloids, although keloids may also form without an inciting trauma. Keloids are more commonly found on the ears, upper back and chest, and upper arms. Ongoing tension or movement across the wound healing site may predispose to keloid formation. Genetics are a factor, as there are reports of familial cases with varied modes of inheritance, indicating multiple genetic disorders that may influence keloid formation. Patients with specific rare inherited conditions like Goeminne syndrome and Rubinstein-Taybi syndrome are at increased risk of keloid formation. Age affects propensity to make a keloid with the highest incidence in individuals age 10 to 20 years. Keloids are rarely found in newborns or the elderly.

Prevention
The best treatment is prevention of unnecessary trauma or surgery, including ear piercing and elective cosmetic surgery. Early treatment of acne helps decrease inflamed pustules and papule formation, which, when located at the posterior neck, may become acne keloidalis nuchae. Patients with acne keloidalis nuchae should avoid shaving the neck region and instead should use scissors to trim hair no shorter than one-eighth of an inch. Consider varicella vaccination (Varivax)[1] to decrease keloid risk of chickenpox lesions. Lack of ultraviolet (UV) B light may increase risk of keloid formation. In fact, using UV A1 phototherapy may be a promising treatment of keloids. Other environmental preventive measures are to keep the wound moist, as well as avoid sun exposure and tension on the wound.

Clinical Manifestations
Keloids are firm, rubbery, raised, papular, plaque-like, nodular, and tumorous scar tissue that extends beyond the initial wound borders. Frequently lesions are pruritic, are tender to palpation, and may be the source of sharp, shooting pains. Location is more often on the ears, jaw, neck, shoulders, upper back, and presternal chest. Keloids may be disfiguring and, in rare instances (e.g., location over a joint), may impair function.

[1]Not FDA approved for this indication.

Diagnosis

The clinical diagnosis of a keloid is usually apparent. Rarely is histologic confirmation necessary. Lesions may continue to grow for weeks to months. Keloids on the ears, neck, and abdomen tend to be pedunculated whereas those on the central chest and extremities are usually raised with a flat surface. Most keloids are round, oval, or oblong with regular margins; however, some have a claw-like configuration with irregular borders.

Differential Diagnosis

Hypertrophic scars appear different than keloids because the wound healing is linear, stays within the boundaries of the original wound site, and may be transiently indurated or tender to palpation. Hypertrophic scars are as prevalent in light- or dark-skinned individuals and as a rule tend to flatten significantly over time without treatment.

Giant cell fibroblastoma is a low-grade sarcoma considered a juvenile form of dermatofibrosarcoma protuberans. It is uncommon and locally aggressive. Histology shows multinucleated cells with hyperchromatic nuclei and infiltrating sheets of spindle-shaped fibroblasts.

Lobomycosis is a chronic fungal infection occurring in tropical areas of Latin America. It appears as localized slow-growing nodules in exposed skin.

Dermatofibrosarcoma protruberans is an uncommon, locally aggressive cutaneous soft tissue sarcoma that may present as a plaque-like area of cutaneous thickening that may be violet-red or blue at the margins. Rarely, this may arise within a preexisting scar or tattoo. Definitive diagnosis usually requires a core needle or incisional biopsy.

Treatment

Goals of therapy should be discussed with the patient. Often goals are cosmetic and functional improvement, reduction of scar volume and relief of pain and itching at the site.

Intralesional Corticosteroid. Injections of intralesional corticosteroids are considered first-line therapy for keloids. A systematic review showed that up to 70% of cases respond with flattening of lesions, though the recurrence rate is up to 50% at 5 years. For local anesthesia, apply liquid nitrogen for 10 to 15 seconds or lidocaine-prilocaine cream (EMLA) under occlusion for 1.5 hours before injection. Do not use liquid nitrogen for more than 30 seconds, or permanent hypopigmentation may result. Use triamcinolone acetonide (Kenalog) 10 mg/mL. Space injections approximately 0.5 to 1.0 cm apart. Use a ½-inch, 30-gauge Luer-Lok (twist-on) needle with bevel directed up toward the skin and a tuberculin syringe to allow injection under pressure. Wear a face shield to avoid contact with back-pressure spray. Inject within the bulk of the lesion with enough triamcinolone to make the keloid blanch, usually 0.1 to 0.5 mL. Multiple injections may be needed. Injections may be given monthly until the desired degree of involution and/or symptomatic relief is achieved. If no change occurs after one injection with triamcinolone acetonide 10 mg/mL, increase the strength to 40 mg/mL (Figure 1). If no change occurs after three or four injections, consider referral to a plastic surgeon or dermatologist for surgical excision.

Surgical Excision. Surgical excision of a keloid may help aesthetically and symptomatically, though lesions tend to recur and may result in more extensive scarring. After excision, immediately inject the base of the surgical site in multiple sites with triamcinolone acetonide 20 mg/mL. Use a 30-gauge needle and then occlude the excision site with a pressure dressing such as Elastoplast. Corticosteroid injections should then be repeated at 2-week intervals over a course of 3 to 4 months.

Silicon Gel Sheeting. The use of silicon sheeting may be effective for treatment of symptoms such as pain and itching for established keloids. It may also be used early in wound healing to prevent keloids at the site of new injuries. In some trials, silicone sheeting was effective in 70% to 80% of cases to avoid keloid formation. Sheeting is placed on top of the keloid, taped into place, and left on for 12 to 24 hours per day. The sheet is washed daily and replaced

Figure 1 A, A keloid on the back. B, The scar after four intralesional injections of corticosteroid 10 mg/mL at 4 weeks apart. Note side effects of skin atrophy and hypopigmentation. (Reprinted with permission from Manuskiatti W: Current management of hypertrophic scars and keloids. *Siriraj Hosp Gaz* 2003;55:249–258.)

every 10 to 14 days. Consider effectiveness after 2 to 6 months of therapy. Over-the-counter and prescription self-drying silicone gel formulations are an alternative for exposed or larger areas.

Cryosurgery. Cryotherapy can be used in conjunction with intralesional corticosteroids. This is widely available, is effective, and has an excellent safety profile. A 10- to 30-second freeze-thaw cycle can be repeated up to three times per treatment session and repeated every 4 to 6 weeks until response occurs. One major permanent side effect is hypopigmentation, which may be most apparent in darker-skinned patients.

Pressure Therapy. When pressure (to an area of possible keloid formation) is applied early in the healing process, it may decrease keloid formation. This is thought to occur due to decrease in oxygen tension of the wound by occluding small blood vessels and decreasing fibroblast proliferation. The optimal pressure should be 20–30 mm Hg for 12–24 hours per day for 6–12 months. Zimmer splints are inexpensive, molded earring-like pressure therapy that may be effective treatment for keloids following ear piercing.

Radiation Therapy. It is the biologically effective dose (BED) that influences the effectiveness in preventing recurrence. Differing amounts of BED are delivered depending on the radiation source used. Long-term risks of radiation such as malignancy are under investigation. Radiation therapy is effective in reducing keloid recurrence with improvement rates of 70% to 90% when used after surgical excision. Recurrence rates of keloids after radiation therapy are 13% to 33%.

Intralesional 5-Fluorouracil (5-FU). Intralesional 5-FU has been used for scars that do not respond to intralesional corticosteroids. Schedule intralesional injections of 5-FU (Adrucil)[1] 50 mg/mL with a volume of 0.5 to 2.0 mL per session for every four weeks up to 12 weeks. Intralesional 5-FU has been shown to improve keloids by 50% and is considered to work best on small keloids. Injections may be painful and may cause hyperpigmentation. 5-FU is can be mixed with triamcinolone acetonide for keloids

[1] Not FDA approved for this indication.

Figure 2 A, A scar developing after cesarean section. **B,** The scar after two pulsed dye laser treatments 8 weeks apart.

resistant to triamcinolone alone: 0.1 mL of triamcinolone acetonide 40 mg/mL can be mixed with 0.9 mL of 5-FU 50 mg/mL and injected weekly for 8 weeks. Pulsed dye laser has been used in combination with intralesional injection of a mixture of 5-FU and steroid with cumulative beneficial effect.

Pulsed Dye Laser. Pulsed dye laser therapy and neodymium-yttrium-aluminum-garnet (Nd: YAG) laser may minimize the erythema and telangiectasias of keloids. One study showed effectiveness of treatment with a combination of pulsed dye laser and intralesional steroid on recalcitrant keloid scars (Figure 2). These patients noted a 60% decrease in height of keloid, 40% improvement in erythema, and 75% decrease in pain and itching. Presternal scars may not benefit appreciably. It is speculated that the laser helped make the scar edematous and softer so that the intralesional steroid could work better.

Monitoring. Surveillance of scars during wound healing is important to alert the provider that keloids may be forming. Appropriate, focused, and timed treatment can then be performed. In a patient with keloid history, using prophylactic therapy may be instituted when a new wound is incurred. Close follow-up monitoring is vital during immediate and aggressive treatment.

Complications. Patients should be advised that keloids can be recalcitrant to all types of therapy. If a keloid recurs (especially if ablative methods such as electrosurgery are used), it may be more disfiguring than the original lesion. Trauma to the keloid may predispose the lesion to erosion and localized bacterial infection.

References

Asilian A, Darougheh A, Shariati F: New combination of triamcinolone, 5-fluorouracil, and pulsed-dye laser for treatment of keloids and hypertrophic scars, *Dermatol Surg* 32:907, 2006.

Derm101.com. Scars, keloids, and anetodermas. Available at www.derm101.com/clinical-atlas/scars-keloids-and-anetodermas; (accessed August 2, 2016).

Kelly AP: Update on the management of keloids, *Semin Cutan Med Surg* 28:71–76, 2009.

Kontochristopoulos G, Stefanaki C, Panagiotopoulos A, et al: Intralesional 5-fluorouracil in the treatment of keloids: an open clinical and histopathologic study, *J Am Acad Dermatol* 52(3 Pt 1):474, 2005.

Medscape.com. Keloid and hypertrophic scar differential diagnosis. Available at http://emedicine.medscape.com/article/1057599-differential; [accessed 06.10.17].

Nakashima M, Chung S, Takahashi A, et al: A genome-wide association study identifies four susceptibility loci for keloid in the Japanese population, *Nat Genet* 42:768, 2010.

Shaffer JJ, Taylor SC, Cook-Bolden F: Keloidal scars: a review with a critical look at therapeutic options, *J Am Acad Dermatol* 46:63, 2002.

Van Leeuwen MC, van der Wal MB, Bulstra AE, et al: Intralesional cryotherapy for treatment of keloid scars: a prospective study, *Plast Reconst Surg Glob Open* 3:e437, 2015.

MELANOMA

Method of
Vesna Petronic-Rosic, MD, MSc, MBA

CURRENT DIAGNOSIS

- ABCDEs:
  - Asymmetry of lesion.
  - Border irregularity, bleeding, or crusting.
  - Color change or variegation.
  - Diameter larger than 6 mm or growing lesion.
  - Evolving: Surface changes or symptomatic.
- The "ugly duckling" sign: A mole that looks or feels different compared to surrounding moles.
- Total-body photography and dermoscopy.
- Excisional biopsy with narrow margins.
- Interpretation by physician experienced in the microscopic diagnosis of pigmented lesions.
- Molecular analyses (rarely).
- Appropriate staging workup.
- Genetic testing when appropriate (rarely).

CURRENT THERAPY

- Early diagnosis and appropriate surgical therapy is the gold standard.
- Complete excision must be achieved with appropriate margins based on tumor thickness.
- Sentinel lymph node biopsy may be offered to patients with melanoma 1 to 4 mm thick, with clinically unaffected regional nodes, and without distant metastases.
- Dissection of the lymph node basin may be offered to patients with micronodal or macronodal metastases.
- Adjuvant therapy may be considered for stage III disease.
- Stage IV treatment depends on location and extent of metastatic disease and may include surgical resection, chemotherapy, biological therapy, or radiation therapy.

Melanoma is a malignancy of pigment-producing cells (melanocytes). Melanocytes are located predominantly in the skin but are also found in the eyes, ears, gastrointestinal tract, leptomeninges, and oral and genital mucous membranes.

Epidemiology

Even though melanoma accounts for less than 5% of skin cancer cases, it causes most skin cancer deaths. U.S. incidence figures estimate that there were about 108,230 new cases of melanoma in 2017: 48,290 in situ (noninvasive) and 59,940 invasive (33,910 in men and 26,030 in women). The American Cancer Society's most recent estimates for melanoma in the United States for 2019 are 96,480 new cases with 7,230 deaths. The prevalence of melanoma in the United States has doubled over the three decades from 1982 to 2011, from 11.2 per 100,000 population to 22.7 per 100,000. In 2011, the melanoma incidence rate was 19.7 per 100,000, and the death rate was 2.7 per 100,000. Overall, the lifetime risk for developing melanoma is about 1 in 50 for whites,

1 in 1000 for blacks, and 1 in 200 for Latin Americans. At current rates, 1 in 63 Americans will develop an invasive melanoma over a lifetime.

Risk Factors

A large number of nevi is the strongest risk factor for melanoma in persons of European ancestry. Atypical mole syndrome is another risk factor. Exposure to ultraviolet light is a major risk factor, especially in persons who have fair hair and skin, who have solar damage, who had sunburns and short sharp bursts of sun exposure in childhood, and who used tanning beds. Tanning beds appear more detrimental when used before the age of 20 years. The International Agency for Research on cancer has classified indoor tanning devices as "carcinogenic to humans" based on extensive review of scientific evidence. Familial risk factors include mutations in *CDKN2A*(p16INK4a), which are associated with increased risks for both melanoma and pancreatic cancer; they are transmitted in an autosomal dominant fashion and account for approximately 20% to 50% of familial melanoma cases. In recent years, mutations in BRCA1-associated protein 1 (BAP1), shelterin complex, microphthalmia-associated transcription factor (MITF), and phosphatase and tensin homolog (PTEN) have also been associated with melanoma and internal organ cancers. Organ transplant recipients have an increased risk for melanoma. Genodermatoses with a defect in DNA repair (such as xeroderma pigmentosum) increase risk for melanoma.

Pathophysiology

Transformation of normal melanocytes into melanoma cells likely involves a multistep process of progressive genetic mutations that alter cell proliferation, differentiation, and death and affect susceptibility to the carcinogenic effects of ultraviolet radiation. Primary cutaneous melanoma can develop in preexisting melanocytic nevi, but more than 60% of cases likely appear de novo.

Melanomas arising in skin that is chronically sun damaged show molecular features that distinguish them from melanomas arising in skin that is not sun damaged. These features might determine tumor behavior and potential response to new targeted drugs. About 70% of melanomas arising in skin that is not sun damaged carry *BRAF* mutations. Genetic studies have shown that 50% of familial melanomas and 25% of sporadic melanomas may be due to mutations in the tumor suppressor gene *p16*. Linkage studies have identified chromosome 9p21 as the site of the familial melanoma gene.

Prevention

Early detection of thin cutaneous melanoma is the best means of reducing mortality. Patients with a history of melanoma should be educated regarding sun-protective clothing and sunscreens, skin self-examinations for new primary melanoma, possible recurrence within the surgical scar, and screening of first-degree relatives, particularly if they have a history of atypical moles.

Clinical Manifestations

Early signs of melanoma include the ABCDEs:
- Asymmetry of lesion
- Border irregularity, bleeding, or crusting
- Color change or variegation
- Diameter larger than 6 mm or growing lesion
- Evolving: Surface changes or symptomatic

The "ugly duckling" sign is also useful to recognize lesions that look or feel different compared to surrounding moles.

Lentigo maligna (melanoma in situ) begins as an irregular tan-brown macule that slowly expands on sun-damaged skin of elderly persons. Long-term cumulative sun exposure confers the greatest risk. Progression to invasive lentigo maligna melanoma is estimated to be 30% to 50%.

Superficial spreading melanoma, the most common type in light skin, represents approximately 70% of all melanomas. Peak incidence is in the fourth and fifth decade. Superficial spreading melanoma can arise in a preexisting melanocytic nevus that slowly changes over several years; it most commonly affects intermittently

sun-exposed areas with the greatest nevus density (upper backs of men and women and lower legs of women). Pigment varies from black and blue-gray to pink or gray-white, and the borders are irregular. Absence of pigmentation often represents regression.

Nodular melanoma represents 15% of all melanomas. The median age at onset is 53 years. Clinically, a uniform blue-black, blue-red, or red nodule usually begins de novo and grows rapidly. About 5% are amelanotic. The most common sites are the trunk, head, and neck.

Acral lentiginous melanoma accounts for 10% of melanomas overall but is the most common type among Japanese, African Americans, Latin Americans, and Native Americans. The median age is 65 years, with equal gender distribution. It occurs on the palms or soles or under the nails and is on average 3 cm in diameter at diagnosis. Clinically, the lesion is a tan, brown-to-black, flat macule with color variegation and irregular borders. It does not appear to be linked to sun exposure.

Diagnosis

Excisional biopsy with narrow margins is recommended for diagnosis. Incisional biopsy is acceptable when suspicion for melanoma is low, the lesion is large, or it is impractical to perform a complete excision. It is believed not to be detrimental if subsequent therapeutic surgery is performed within 4 to 6 weeks. Dermoscopy and total body photography are adjunctive noninvasive diagnostic techniques. Routine laboratory tests and imaging studies are not required for asymptomatic patients with primary cutaneous melanoma 4 mm or less in thickness for initial staging or routine follow-up. Indications for such studies are directed by a thorough medical history and complete physical examination.

Histologic interpretation should be performed by a physician experienced in the microscopic diagnosis of pigmented lesions. Molecular analyses for evidence of gene mutations, DNA copy-number abnormalities, or changed protein expression are useful adjunctive tools in the assessment of histologically ambiguous primary melanocytic tumors. It is now known that melanomas from sun-damaged skin, non-sun-damaged skin, or mucosal or acral surfaces harbor distinct molecular phenotypes. Specifically, activating mutations in BRAF are present in approximately 40% to 60% of advanced melanomas, especially those arising from non-sun-damaged skin, and result in activation of the RAS/RAF/MEK/ERK pathway, providing a constitutive growth signal.

The new revised American Joint Committee on Cancer (AJCC) staging system was published in 2017 (Tables 1 and 2). Key changes in the eighth edition of the AJCC Cancer Staging Manual include: 1) tumor thickness measurements to be recorded to the nearest 0.1 mm, not 0.01 mm; 2) definitions of T1a and T1b are revised (T1a, <0.8 mm without ulceration; T1b, 0.8-1.0 mm with or without ulceration or <0.8 mm with ulceration), with mitotic rate no longer a T category criterion; 3) pathological (but not clinical) stage IA is revised to include T1b N0 M0 (formerly pathologic stage IB); 4) the N category descriptors "microscopic" and "macroscopic" for regional node metastasis are redefined as "clinically occult" and "clinically apparent"; 5) prognostic stage III groupings are based on N category criteria and T category criteria (i.e., primary tumor thickness and ulceration) and increased from three to four subgroups (stages IIIA-IIID); 6) definitions of N subcategories are revised, with the presence of microsatellites, satellites, or in-transit metastases now categorized as N1c, N2c, or N3c based on the number of tumor involved regional lymph nodes, if any; 7) descriptors are added to each M1 subcategory designation for lactate dehydrogenase (LDH) level (LDH elevation no longer upstages to M1c); and 8) a new M1d designation is added for central nervous system metastases. This evidence-based revision of the AJCC melanoma staging system will guide patient treatment, provide better prognostic estimates, and refine stratification of patients entering clinical trials.

Five-year and 10-year survival rates based on the TNM classification range from 99% and 98% for patients with T1a N0 M0 melanomas to 82% and 75%, respectively, for patients with T4b N0 M0 melanomas.

Tumor (T)

Classification	Thickness (mm)	Ulceration Status
TX: Primary tumor thickness cannot be assessed (e.g., diagnosis by curettage)	Not applicable	Not applicable
T0: No evidence of a primary tumor or the site of the primary tumor is unknown (e.g., in a patient who presents with an axillary metastasis with no known primary tumor)	Not applicable	Not applicable
Tis	Not applicable	Not applicable
T1	≤1.0 mm	Unknown or unspecified
T1a	<0.8 mm	Without ulceration
T1b	<0.8 mm	With ulceration
	0.8–1.0 mm	With or without ulceration
T2	>1.0–2.0 mm	Unknown or unspecified
T2a	>1.0–2.0 mm	Without ulceration
T2b	>1.0–2.0 mm	With ulceration
T3	>2.0–4.0 mm	Unknown or unspecified
T3a	>2.0–4.0 mm	Without ulceration
T3b	>2.0–4.0 mm	With ulceration
T4	>4.0 mm	Unknown or unspecified
T4a	>4.0 mm	Without ulceration
T4b	>4.0 mm	With ulceration

Nodes (N)

Classification	Number of Metastatic Nodes	Nodal Metastatic Burden
NX	Regional nodes not assessed (e.g., sentinel lymph node [SLN] biopsy not performed, regional nodes previously removed for another reason); Exception: pathological N category is not required for T1 melanomas, use clinical N information	
N0	0	NA
N1	1	a: Clinically occult b: Clinically apparent

Classification	Number of Metastatic Nodes	Nodal Metastatic Burden
N2	3	a: Clinically occult b: Clinically apparent
N3	4 + metastatic nodes or matted nodes or in transit metastases/ satellites with metastatic nodes	c: In transit metastases/ satellites without metastatic nodes

Metastases (M)

Classification	Site	Serum LDH
M0	No distant metastasis	NA
M1a	Distal skin, subcutaneous, or nodal metastasis	Normal
M1b	Lung metastasis	Normal
M1c	All other visceral metastasis	Normal
	Any distant metastasis	Elevated

Note: Micrometastases are diagnosed after sentinel lymph node biopsy. Macrometastases are defined as clinically detectable nodal metastases confirmed pathologically. *Abbreviations:* is, in situ; NA, not applicable.

Differential Diagnosis

The differential diagnosis includes melanocytic nevus, angioma, pigmented basal cell carcinoma, pyogenic granuloma, seborrheic keratosis, Kaposi's sarcoma, and hematoma (especially for acral lentiginous melanoma).

Treatment

Early diagnosis combined with appropriate surgical therapy is currently the only curative treatment. For melanoma in situ, wide excision with 0.5 to 1.0 cm margins is recommended; lentigo maligna histologic subtype may require >0.5 cm margins to achieve histologically negative margins because of characteristically broad subclinical extension. Surgical margins for invasive melanoma should be at least 1 cm and up to 2 cm clinically measured around the primary tumor; clinically measured surgical margins do not need to correlate with histologically negative margins. Margins may be modified to accommodate individual anatomic or functional considerations. The recommended margins are

Tumor thickness	Clinically measured surgical margin	Strength of recommendation	Level of evidence
In situ	0.5–1.0 cm	C	III
≤ 1.0 mm	1 cm	A	I
1.01–2.0 mm	1–2 cm	A	I
≥ 2.0 mm	2 cm	B	I,II,III

Strength of Recommendations: A,B,C Level of Evidence: I,II,II (https://www.aad.org/practicecenter/quality/clinical-guidelines/melanoma/surgical-management, accessed 04.08.2018)

The recommended deep margin is muscle fascia. Wider margins and Mohs' micrographic surgery can reduce the risk of contiguous subclinical spread for the desmoplastic variant of melanoma.

Sentinel lymph node biopsy (SLNB) provides accurate staging information for patients with clinically unaffected regional nodes and without distant metastases. The status of SLN is the most important prognostic indicator for disease-specific survival in patients with primary cutaneous melanoma; the impact of SLNB on overall survival remains unclear. Candidates for SLNB include patients with newly diagnosed primary cutaneous melanoma who

TABLE 2 Pathology Staging for Cutaneous Melanoma and Survival Rates

PATHOLOGY STAGING

STAGE	T	N	M	5-YEAR SUR-VIVAL	10-YEAR SUR-VIVAL
0	Tis	N0	M0		
IA	T1a	N0	M0	99%	98%
	T1b	N0	M0	99%	96%
IB	T2a	N0	M0		
IIA	T2b	N0	M0	82%	
	T3a	N0	M0	79%	
IIB	T3b	N0	M0	68%	
	T4a	N0	M0		
IIC	T4b	N0	M0	82%	75%
IIIA	T1a/b-T2a	N1b, N1c	M0	93%	
	T1a/b-T2a	N2a	M0		
IIIB	T0	N1a	M0	59%	
	T1a/b-T2a	N1b/c or N2b	M0		
	T2b/T3a	N1a-N2b	M0		
IIIC	T0	N2b, N2c, N3b, or N3c	M0		
	T1a-T3a	N2c or N3a/b/c	M0		
	T3b/T4a	Any N≥N1	M0		
	T4b	N1a-2c	M0		
IIID	T4b	N3a/b/c	M0	32%	
IV	Any T, Tis	AnyN	M1		

Pathology staging includes microstaging of the primary melanoma and pathologic information about the regional lymph nodes after partial (i.e., sentinel node biopsy) or complete lymphadenectomy. Pathologic stage 0 or stage IA patients are the exception; they do not require pathologic evaluation of their lymph nodes.
Adapted from Balch et al. (2009) and Gershenwals et al. (2017) http://onlinelibrary.wiley.com/doi/10.3322/caac.21409/full

are clinically node-negative and, based on primary tumor characteristics, are predicted to be at intermediate risk or high risk of harboring occult nodal disease. In cases of positive SLNB or clinically detected regional nodal metastases (palpable, positive cytology, or histopathology), radical removal of lymph nodes of the involved basin is indicated. There is clinical trial evidence suggesting that the survival outcome for patients who are sentinel node-positive is improved if an immediate regional lymphadenectomy is done.

For resectable local or in-transit recurrences, excision with a clear margin is recommended. For numerous or unresectable in-transit metastases of the extremities, isolated limb perfusion or infusion with melphalan may be considered.

Radiotherapy is indicated in select patients with lentigo maligna melanoma, as an adjuvant in select patients where re-resection is not feasible, with regional metastatic disease, and for palliation, especially in bone and brain metastases.

Numerous adjuvant therapies have been investigated for the treatment of localized cutaneous melanoma following complete surgical removal. Adjuvant interferon (IFN) alfa-2b (Intron A) is the only adjuvant therapy approved by the FDA for high-risk melanoma that affects outcome after surgery. No survival benefit has been demonstrated for adjuvant chemotherapy, nonspecific (passive) immunotherapy, radiation therapy, retinoid therapy, vitamin therapy, or biologic therapy.

Various experimental melanoma vaccines show promise in the adjuvant setting, although caution is needed because four phase III trials (E1694, MMAIT-III [Canvaxin], MMAIT-IV, and EORTC 18961) showed a deleterious effect of the experimental vaccine compared with control intervention. Considerable effort is now being focused on selecting patients on the basis of molecular profiling and on combining agents targeting melanoma-specific aberrations in signaling and apoptotic pathways to overcome the many resistance mechanisms in melanoma cells.

Metastatic melanoma is an aggressive, immunogenic, and molecularly heterogeneous disease. In the last two decades, treatment of melanoma took a dramatic turn with the discovery of targeted therapy aimed at the mutations in the mitogen-activated protein kinase (MAPK) pathway and immune checkpoint inhibitors. In 2011, US Food and Drug Administration (FDA) approved ipilimumab (Yervoy), an anti-cytotoxic T-lymphocyte antigen-4 (CTLA-4) antibody for metastatic melanoma therapy. Since then, novel drugs including antibodies to programmed cell death 1 (PD-1) such as pembrolizumab (Keytruda) and nivolumab (Opdivo), both approved in 2014; selective BRAF inhibitors such as vemurafenib (Zelboraf), approved in 2011; dabrafenib (Tafinlar), approved in 2013; and MEK inhibitor trametinib (Mekinist), approved in 2013; have greatly extended the potential of immunotherapy and molecular targeted therapy for advanced melanoma. Despite showing initial promise, resistance and poor duration of response have limited their effectiveness as monotherapies. Combining BRAF inhibitors with MEK inhibitors such as trametinib delays the development of resistance. The greatest survival improvement was observed with the combination of BRAF plus MEK inhibitors as well as with PD1 blockers with or without CTLA-4 blockers, respectively, with these two treatment strategies showing similar survival outcomes. For first-line therapy, averaged survival proportions of patients alive at 12 months were 74.5% with BRAF plus MEK inhibitor treatment versus 71.9% with PD-1 blockade. The use of combination immunotherapy may provide improved outcomes in patients over single-agent checkpoint blockade. On October 1, 2015, the FDA announced accelerated approval of a combination of immunotherapy drugs for the frontline treatment of advanced melanoma. The drugs, ipilimumab and nivolumab, are two immune checkpoint inhibitors that "release the brakes" on the immune system, allowing it to mount a stronger and more effective attack against cancer. The FDA based its approval on results from a clinical trial showing that patients who received the combination had better responses than those who received ipilimumab alone. In 2017, The FDA granted accelerated approval to pembrolizumab as a second-line treatment for all metastatic solid tumor types classified as MSI-hi (high microsatellite instability) or dMMR (deficient DNA mismatch repair). This was the first time the FDA has ever approved any treatment based on a biomarker rather than an organ-specific tumor type. Since then, the FDA has approved multiple new applications for existing medications, such as pembolizumab for adjuvant treatment of melanoma with involvement of lymph nodes following complete resection. For an up to date listing, see www.fda.gov.

Although melanoma has traditionally been regarded as a uniformly fatal malignancy, personalized treatment of this cancer relies on the recognition of its genetic heterogeneity and our ability to pharmacologically target these specific and recurrent changes. Recent advances in the treatment of melanoma have come from the understanding that melanoma is a large family of molecularly distinct diseases. Emerging evidence suggests that different melanoma subtypes may each be driven by diverse mechanisms of progression, associated with differing mechanisms of tumor escape and specific immunosuppression, innate immune cell activation, and altered T-cell trafficking into tumor sites that in turn modulate response to immunotherapies.

Monitoring

Most metastases occur in the first 1 to 3 years after treatment of the primary tumor, and an estimated 4% to 8% of patients with a history of melanoma develop another primary melanoma, usually within the first 3 to 5 years following diagnosis. The risk of new primary melanoma increases in the presence of multiple dysplastic nevi and family history of melanoma. Consider cancer genetics consultation in patients with three or more melanomas in aggregate in first-degree or second-degree relatives on the same side of the family, families with three or more cases of melanoma or pancreatic cancer on the same side of the family, and (in low-incidence countries) patients with three or more primary melanomas.

The frequency of monitoring is as follows: For patients with melanoma smaller than 1 mm: every 3 months for 1 year, then every 6 to 12 months for 4 years, then annual examinations thereafter. For patients with melanoma larger than 1 mm: every 3 months for 1 to 2 years, then every 6 months until the fifth year, then annual examinations thereafter.

Follow-up visits for all patients should include a thorough history, review of systems, complete skin examination, and examination of lymph nodes. In patients at high risk for metastatic disease or with an abnormal examination, appropriate imaging studies, laboratory studies, or biopsies may be indicated. Evidence to support the use of routine imaging and laboratory studies in asymptomatic patients with a normal physical examination remains controversial and is left to the discretion of the physician.

Complications

Metastasis may occur locally in the regional lymph node basins, or it can occur distally in the skin (away from the melanoma scar), the remote lymph node(s), the viscera, and skeletal and central nervous system sites.

References

Abbasi NR, Shaw HM, Rigel DS, et al: Early diagnosis of cutaneous melanoma: revisiting the ABCD criteria, *JAMA* 292:2771–2776, 2004.

American Cancer Society: *Overview: Skin cancer: Melanoma,* Available at http://www.cancer.org/%20cancer/skincancer-melanoma/index. (accessed 6-24-15).

Atkins M: Immunotherapy combinations with checkpoint inhibitors in metastatic melanoma: current approaches and future directions, *Semin Oncol* 42(Suppl. 3):S12–S19, 2015.

Balch CM, Gershenwald JE, Soong SJ, et al: Final version of 2009 AJCC melanoma staging and classification, *J Clin Oncol* 27:6199–6206, 2009.

Davar D, Tarhini AA, Kirkwood JM: Adjuvant immunotherapy of melanoma and development of new approaches using the neoadjuvant approach, *Clin Dermatol* 31:237–250, 2013. https://doi.org/10.1016/j.clindermatol.2012.08.012, Review. Erratum in: *Clin Dermatol* 2013;31:501.

Griewank KG, Ugurel S, Schadendorf D, et al: New developments in biomarkers for melanoma, *Curr Opin Oncol* 25:145–151, 2013.

Guy Jr GP, Thomas CC, Thompson T, Watson M, Massetti GM, Richardson LC: Centers for Disease Control and Prevention (CDC): Vital signs: melanoma incidence and mortality trends and projections—United States, 1982–2030, *MMWR Morb Mortal Wkly Rep* 64(21):591–596, 2015.

Pasquali S, Chiarion-Sileni V, Rossi CR, Mocellin S: Immune checkpoint inhibitors and targeted therapies for metastatic melanoma: a network meta-analysis, *Cancer Treat Rev* 54:34–42, 2017 Mar. https://doi.org/10.1016/j.ctrv.2017.01.006. Epub 2017 Feb 2. Review. PubMed PMID: 28189914.

Pasquali S, Hadjinicolaou AV, Chiarion Sileni V, Rossi CR, Mocellin S: Systemic treatments for metastatic cutaneous melanoma, *Cochrane Database Syst Rev* 2018 Feb 6;2:CD011123. https://doi.org/10.1002/14651858.CD011123.pub2. Review. PubMed PMID: 29405038.

Ross MI, Gershenwald JE: Sentinel lymph node biopsy for melanoma: a critical update for dermatologists after two decades of experience, *Clin Dermatol* 31:298–310, 2013. https://doi.org/10.1016/j.clindermatol.2012.08.004.

Sladden MJ, Balch C, Barzilai DA, et al: Surgical excision margins for primary cutaneous melanoma, *Cochrane Database Syst Rev* 2009, CD004835.

Soura E, Eliades PJ, Shannon K, Stratigos AJ, Tsao H: Hereditary melanoma: update on syndromes and management: genetics of familial atypical multiple mole melanoma syndrome, *J Am Acad Dermatol* 74(3):395–407, 2016. https://doi.org/10.1016/j.jaad.2015.08.038.

Ugurel S, Röhmel J, Ascierto PA, et al: Survival of patients with advanced metastatic melanoma: the impact of novel therapies, *Eur J Cancer* 53:125–134, 2016. https://www.cancer.org/content/dam/cancer-org/research/cancer-facts-and-statistics/annual-cancer-facts-and-figures/2017/cancer-facts-and-figures-2017.pdf (accessed 04.08.17).

NEVI

Method of

Jane M. Grant-Kels, MD; and Michael Murphy, MD

CURRENT DIAGNOSIS

Benign Melanocytic Lesions
- Symmetrical
- Sharply demarcated border
- Uniform color
- Diameter usually 6 mm or less and stable

Malignant Melanocytic Lesions
- Asymmetrical
- Poorly circumscribed border
- Variegated in color
- Diameter often >6 mm and increasing (changing or evolving)

CURRENT THERAPY

- Acquired melanocytic nevus: No treatment is required unless the lesion is asymmetrical or has an irregular border, change or variegation in color, or change in diameter. Symptomatic lesions should be biopsied.
- Recurrent melanocytic nevus: No treatment required if the original biopsy was benign.
- Halo melanocytic nevus: No treatment, but excision is recommended if atypical clinical features are identified.
- Congenital melanocytic nevus: Removal based on melanoma risk, cosmetics, and functional outcome. If not excised, routine follow-up with the use of photography, dermoscopy, and computer assistance is recommended.
- Blue nevus: No treatment, but excision is recommended if atypical clinical features are identified.
- Spitz nevus: If clinically unusual, a complete excisional biopsy is recommended.
- Dysplastic nevus: If only one lesion is present, excision may be considered. Patients with many dysplastic nevi require close surveillance, with removal of any lesion suspicious for melanoma.

Melanocytic nevi, or moles, are benign neoplasms composed of melanocytes. Melanocytic nevus cells are derived from melanocytes. Compared with melanocytes, nevus cells are not dendritic, are larger, and contain more abundant cytoplasm, often with coarse melanin granules. Nevus cells tend to aggregate into groups or nests. Melanocytic nevi are extremely common and can be found on almost everyone, anywhere on the cutaneous surface. This article discusses the most common types of melanocytic nevi: acquired melanocytic nevi, recurrent melanocytic nevi, halo melanocytic nevi, congenital melanocytic nevi (CMN), blue nevi, Spitz nevi, and dysplastic melanocytic nevi.

Melanocytic nevi demonstrate both heterogeneous clinical and molecular characteristics, but share common "driver" mutations with melanoma. Acquired melanocytic nevi and dysplastic nevi commonly harbor oncogenic mutations in BRAF, which is the predominant oncogene in melanoma. CMN and blue nevi frequently exhibit NRAS mutations and GNAQ/GNA11 mutations, respectively. Spitz nevi and atypical Spitz tumors often show HRAS and BAP1 alterations, in addition to rearrangements in other kinase genes. These early "driver" mutations are believed to initiate the development of benign melanocytic nevi.

Acquired Melanocytic Nevi

Acquired melanocytic nevi are subdivided into junctional, compound, and intradermal types based on the location of the nevus cells. By definition, these lesions are not present at birth but can begin to appear in early childhood, usually after 6 to 12 months of age. Peak ages of appearance of melanocytic nevi are 2 to 3 years of age in children and 11 to 18 years in adolescents. Although nevi can appear at any age, it is relatively unusual for new melanocytic nevi to develop in middle-aged or older adults. With time, nevi can spontaneously regress. Consequently, patients in their ninth decade of life usually demonstrate few melanocytic nevi. An average white adult has 10 to 40 melanocytic nevi, but African Americans have far fewer, averaging only 2 to 8.

The number and location of melanocytic nevi have been shown to be associated with sun exposure, immunologic factors, and genetics. Consequently, melanocytic nevi are most numerous on the sun-exposed skin of the head, neck, trunk, and extremities, but they are only rarely found on covered areas such as the buttocks, female breasts, and scalp. Evidence suggests that patients with an increased number of melanocytic nevi (>50) might have an increased risk of melanoma.

Melanocytic nevi appear in a sequential fashion. Junctional melanocytic nevi arise during childhood as flat, dark macules. Histologically, an increase in single or nested melanocytes is located at the dermoepidermal junction. With time, some of the junctional nests of melanocytes migrate into the dermis (compound melanocytic nevi). Clinically, compound melanocytic nevi are elevated and less heavily pigmented than junctional melanocytic nevi. Ultimately, all of the nevus cells migrate into the dermis (intradermal melanocytic nevi), resulting in the development of a tan or skin-colored dome-shaped papule. Melanocytic nevi can be flat or elevated and even polypoid, papillomatous, or verrucous, and can demonstrate a range of color from skin-tone to black, but they are characteristically uniform in color, symmetrical, well marginated, and usually smaller than 6 mm in diameter.

All melanocytic lesions of clinical concern should be examined with a dermatoscope—a handheld instrument with a magnified lens and a light source similar to an ophthalmoscope. This instrument allows evaluation of colors and microstructures not visible to the naked eye, helps determine whether pigmented lesions are melanocytic or nonmelanocytic, and aids in distinguishing whether melanocytic pigmented lesions are likely to be malignant. Used by an experienced physician with proper training, the dermatoscope improves diagnostic accuracy by 20% to 30%. Another useful technology is reflectance confocal microscopy (RCM), as it safely offers noninvasive imaging of skin lesions at cellular-level magnification and is reported to reduce unnecessary biopsies by 50% to 60%. RCM utilizes a low-energy laser light that focuses on a specific area of tissue; the magnitude of backscattering of light depends on the differences in refractive indices of various structures in the skin. The horizontal images of the skin afford review of a lesion up to 8 mm × 8 mm in diameter and extend 200 to 300 μm into the skin.

It is unnecessary to surgically remove all melanocytic nevi because they are benign neoplasms of melanocytes. However, indications for removal include ABCDE (asymmetry, irregular border, variegation or change in color, change in diameter, or evolving), symptoms (e.g., pruritus), evidence of inflammation or irritation, cosmetic issues, and patient anxiety. Melanocytic nevi on acral, genital, or scalp skin that appear benign do not require surgical removal. Shave biopsies are appropriate therapy for lesions considered clinically benign. However, if a lesion is being removed because of concern regarding the possibility of malignancy, an excisional biopsy (biopsy of choice) or incisional biopsy (including a deep scoop) that extends to the subcutaneous tissue is indicated. All melanocytic lesions should be submitted to a dermatopathologist for histologic review. A history of recent sun exposure or trauma should be conveyed to the dermatopathologist because such external trauma can induce reactive atypical histologic findings.

Recurrent Melanocytic Nevi

Recurrent melanocytic nevi are melanocytic nevi that have previously been incompletely removed (either iatrogenically or traumatically) and have recurred weeks to months later. Irregular brown pigmentation is clinically noted within the scar site. If the original biopsy demonstrated a benign melanocytic nevus, re-treatment is unnecessary unless the aforementioned indications are present. However, these nevi can demonstrate pseudomelanomatous histologic features. Therefore if the repigmented area is excised, the dermatopathologist should be notified of the clinical history and, if possible, the slides from the original biopsy should be obtained and reviewed to ensure that the lesion is not histologically misdiagnosed.

Halo (Melanocytic) Nevi

Halo (melanocytic) nevi are melanocytic nevi in which a white rim or halo has developed. This phenomenon most commonly occurs around compound or intradermal nevi and is histologically associated with a dense, bandlike inflammatory infiltrate. The white halo area is histologically characterized by diminished or absent melanocytes and melanin. Approximately 20% of patients with halo nevi also exhibit vitiligo.

Although a halo can develop around many lesions in the skin, the most important differential diagnosis is between a halo nevus and melanoma with a halo. The halo and the central melanocytic proliferation of halo nevi are symmetrical, round or oval, and sharply demarcated. Halo nevi most commonly occur in adolescence as an isolated event, but approximately 25% to 50% of affected persons have two or more.

The clinical course of halo nevi is variable. With time, the halo can repigment while the central nevus persists. Alternatively, the melanocytic nevus can regress completely and leave a depigmented macule that can persist or repigment over months or years.

Halo nevi do not require surgical excision unless atypical clinical features suggest the possibility of an atypical melanocytic lesion. It is advisable (particularly in adults, in whom halo nevi are less common) to perform a complete cutaneous examination with and without the aid of a Wood's lamp to rule out any associated atypical pigmented or regressed lesions. All patients should be advised to use sunscreens or protective clothing because of the increased risk of sunburn in the depigmented halo region.

Congenital Melanocytic Nevi

By definition, CMN are present at birth. Arbitrarily, they have been classified into small (<1.5 cm), medium (1.5 to 20 cm), and large (>20 cm) lesions. Terms such as *bathing trunk* or *garment-type* nevi refer to CMN that cover a significant portion of the cutaneous surface.

The approximate incidence of small congenital nevi is 1% of all live births. Large congenital nevi are rare and reported in only 1 in 20,000 births. Histologically, some congenital nevi have distinguishing histologic features (melanocytic nevus cells that extend into the deeper dermis as well as the subcutis and melanocytic nevus cells arranged periadnexally, angiocentrically, within nerves, and interposed between collagen bundles). However, these features have been identified in some acquired melanocytic nevi and are absent in some congenital nevi (especially small ones). In addition, the history obtained from the patient or their parents is often inaccurate. Consequently, it can be very difficult in some cases to distinguish a small congenital nevus from an acquired nevus.

Congenital nevi can give rise to dermal or subcutaneous nodular melanocytic proliferations. The vast majority of these lesions, particularly in the neonatal period, are biologically benign, despite a worrisome clinical presentation and atypical histologic features. Genetic analysis has shown that benign melanocytic proliferations within congenital nevi harbor aberrations qualitatively and quantitatively different from those seen in melanoma.

Patients with multiple CMN (two or more, of any site or size) are at risk for extracutaneous (i.e., endocrine, metabolic, neurological) manifestations, termed *CMN syndrome*. The primary significance of congenital nevi is related to the potential risk for progression to melanoma. Essentially, the larger the nevus, particularly if accompanied by multiple small CMN, the greater the risk of progression to melanoma. Historically, even small nevi were estimated to exhibit a lifetime melanoma risk of 5%. However, recent prospective studies suggest that small and medium congenital nevi are associated with a low risk that may approximate the risk of acquired nevi. Conversely, large congenital nevi have a lifetime risk of melanomatous progression of approximately 6.3%. Up to two-thirds of melanomas that arise within these giant congenital nevi have a nonepidermal origin (arising mainly in the deep dermis and subcutis with high Breslow thickness on presentation), thus making clinical observation for malignant change difficult. Approximately 50% of these melanomas occur in the first 5 years of life, 60% in the first decade, and 70% before 20 years of age. Patients with large congenital nevi, especially those that involve posterior axial locations (head, neck, back, or buttocks) and are associated with satellite congenital nevi, are at increased risk for neurocutaneous melanosis (melanosis of the leptomeninges) and primary central nervous system (CNS) melanoma. Recent data suggest that in up to one-third of these patients, the primary melanoma develops within the CNS rather than the skin. The risk of melanoma appears to be higher in those with congenital abnormalities of the CNS (12% vs. 1% to 2% without CNS changes).

For large congenital nevi that involve a posterior axial location, screening magnetic resonance imaging (MRI) is indicated to characterize congenital disease, if any, and act as a baseline should the child present with new neurological symptoms at a later stage. If clinical symptoms or MRI indicate neurocutaneous melanosis, excision of the large nevus should be postponed until 2 years of age (the median age of neurologic symptoms). Patients with neurocutaneous melanosis have a greater than 50% mortality rate within 3 years. The risk and morbidity of multiple, staged excisions of a large CMN is not appropriate in patients with symptomatic neurocutaneous melanosis. All other large CMN are candidates for excision as soon as general anesthesia is considered a relatively safe risk. Other issues that need to be considered before undertaking staged excisions include cosmetic issues, functional outcome, and psychosocial issues. The staged excisions are usually started after 6 months of age for nevi on the trunk and extremities and later for those on the scalp to allow closure of the fontanelle. If removal is not undertaken, follow-up with monthly self-examination, photography, dermoscopy, confocal laser microscopy, and computer assistance are recommended.

For small congenital nevi, routine excision is not always recommended because the risk of melanoma is lower, and if it occurs, it usually arises within the epidermis after puberty. If the lesions are not excised, follow-up by alternating visits to a dermatologist and primary care physician along with serial photography are indicated. Inasmuch as small congenital nevi typically enlarge with the growth of the child and can change in appearance with time, educating families on benign, predictable changes in contradistinction to potentially alarming changes is extremely important. If a lesion enlarges or changes suddenly or if parental anxiety or cosmetic issues arise, excision should then be contemplated for even small congenital nevi. Elective excision is best done when the patient is approximately 8 years old. With the use of topical anesthetic cream EMLA (eutectic mixture of local anesthetics: 2.5% lidocaine plus 2.5% prilocaine) or topical 4% lidocaine (ELA-Max), children of this age are usually cooperative and unscathed by the procedure.

Blue Nevi

Blue nevi occur primarily on the face and scalp, in addition to the dorsal surfaces of the hands and feet, as well-circumscribed, slightly raised or dome-shaped bluish papules that are usually less than 1 cm in diameter. Although these lesions are usually acquired in childhood and adolescence, rare congenital lesions have been reported. Histologically, blue nevi demonstrate a combination of intradermal spindle or dendritic melanin-pigmented melanocytes and melanophages with dermal fibrosis. The blue appearance of these lesions is a function of both the depth of the melanin in the dermis and the Tyndall phenomenon: longer wavelengths of light penetrate the deep dermis and are absorbed by the lesional melanin, and shorter wavelengths (e.g., blue) are reflected back. Blue nevi that are clinically stable and that do not demonstrate atypical features do not require removal.

Spitz Nevi

Nevi of large spindle and epithelioid cells (Spitz nevi) are relatively uncommon. In Australia, an annual incidence of 1.4 per 100,000 people has been recorded. Most Spitz nevi are noted in children and adolescents: One-third occur before the age of 10 years, one-third between the ages 10 to 20 years, and one-third past the age of 20 years. Rarely, lesions can occur in patients older than 40 years. Seven percent of Spitz nevi have been reported as congenital.

Four clinical types of Spitz nevi are recognized: light-colored soft Spitz nevi that can resemble a pyogenic granuloma; light-colored hard Spitz nevi that can resemble a dermatofibroma; dark Spitz nevi that must be distinguished from other melanocytic lesions, including melanoma; and disseminated or agminated Spitz nevi. Spitz nevi are typically smaller than 6 mm in diameter and dome shaped, with a smooth pink or tan surface and sharp borders. Although they can occur anywhere on the cutaneous surface except mucosal or palmoplantar areas, they are most commonly seen on the face (especially in children) and legs (especially in women). Spitz nevi in adults are usually more heavily melanized than those in children.

Dermatoscopy or epiluminescent microscopy (examination of lesions with enhanced light and a dermatoscope) helps magnify the images in vivo and can assist in establishing the clinical diagnosis of some Spitz nevi. Histologically, the lesion can demonstrate features similar to those of melanoma, which earned the lesion its original designation by Sophie Spitz as a melanoma of childhood. Because Spitz nevi can be histologically difficult to distinguish from melanoma, if a biopsy is performed on a lesion because of parental, cosmetic, or transitional concern, complete excision with clear margins is recommended. Spitz nevi show fundamental genomic differences compared with melanoma, consistent with the generally benign behavior of these lesions. Spitz nevi typically demonstrate no or only a very restricted set of chromosomal aberrations (i.e., 11p gain in a subset of Spitz nevi). A distinct subset of atypical Spitz tumors is characterized by BRAF mutation and loss of BAP1 expression.

Dysplastic Melanocytic Nevi

Dysplastic melanocytic nevi, or Clark's nevi, or nevi with architectural disorder and cytologic atypia, can occur sporadically as an isolated lesion or lesions or as part of a familial autosomal dominant syndrome. When such lesions occur sporadically, they are considered a marker for a patient who is at increased risk of melanoma (6% risk vs. an approximate 0.6% risk in the normal white population in the United States). In association with a family history or personal past medical history of melanoma, patients with dysplastic melanocytic nevi should be considered to have a significant risk of melanoma. One first-degree family member with melanoma is associated with a lifetime risk of melanoma of 15% for the patient with dysplastic melanocytic nevi. Two or more first-degree family members with melanoma place a patient with dysplastic melanocytic nevi at a lifetime risk of developing melanoma that approaches 100%. Less commonly, dysplastic melanocytic nevi can progress to melanoma. Such progression has been documented by serial photography. However, these data are confounded by the fact that clinically and histologically dysplastic melanocytic nevi may be difficult to distinguish from an early melanoma.

Dysplastic melanocytic nevi are clinically distinguished from common acquired melanocytic nevi by a diameter usually larger than 6 mm, an irregular border, asymmetry, and variable color with possible shades of brown, red, pink, and black; dysplastic melanocytic nevi can be flat, with or without a raised center (fried egg appearance). The lesions begin to appear in mid-childhood and early adolescence. New lesions can appear throughout the patient's life. In addition to the back and extremities, these lesions can occur on sun-protected areas, including the scalp, buttocks, and female breasts. Dysplastic melanocytic nevi can be few or numerous, with hundreds of lesions.

Histologically, dysplastic melanocytic nevi show both architectural disorder: extension of the junctional component beyond the dermal component (shouldering); bridging of nests between adjacent rete ridges; papillary dermal concentric and lamellar fibroplasia; and a variable lymphocytic infiltrate with vascular ectasias. They also show cytologic atypia of melanocytes: increased nuclear size, hyperchromasia, dispersion, or variation of nuclear chromatin patterns, and the presence of nucleoli. Although there is some discordance in the histologic grading of dysplastic melanocytic nevi among expert dermatopathologists, there is some evidence to support the use in clinical practice of a two-tier grading system: Grade A are dysplastic melanocytic nevi with mild or moderate cytologic atypia, and grade B are dysplastic melanocytic nevi with severe cytologic atypia. The probability of having a personal history of melanoma in any given patient with dysplastic melanocytic nevi correlates with the grade of cytologic atypia in melanocytic nevi cells. In addition, the presence of severe cytologic atypia in dysplastic melanocytic nevi correlates with a significantly greater risk of melanoma development (19.7%) compared with moderate (8.1%) or mild (5.7%) cytologic atypia.

Management of these patients is difficult. Dysplastic melanocytic nevi are not uncommon. Reportedly, as many as 4.6 million people in the United States have one or more sporadic dysplastic melanocytic nevi. Familial dysplastic melanocytic nevi are estimated to involve 50,000 patients in the United States. The risk of melanoma for these patients is probably on a continuum and correlated with their family history of melanoma or dysplastic melanocytic nevi, personal history of melanoma, number of acquired and dysplastic melanocytic lesions, and history of sun exposure. Removal of all dysplastic melanocytic nevi is inappropriate inasmuch as the chance of any single lesion becoming malignant is small and, in addition, the melanoma can arise de novo.

In cases of mild and moderate dysplastic nevi with microscopically positive margins and no concerning residual clinical lesion, observation, rather than reexcision, is a reasonable management option. All severely dysplastic nevi should be reexcised. Partial biopsy of any pigmented lesion that is suspicious for melanoma can lead to delayed melanoma diagnosis and is discouraged.

Management includes patient education and total body photography for comparison at future skin examinations. Patients should avoid the sun and use sunscreens and protective clothing. These patients should have regular biannual or quarterly examinations of the entire integument, including the oral, genital, and perianal mucosa, the scalp, and an ophthalmologic examination. Comparison with the previous total body photographs and use of the dermatoscope can be helpful. Any lesions that are suspicious for melanoma should be excised. Examination of first-degree family members (parents, siblings, and children) of patients with melanoma or dysplastic melanocytic nevi is recommended to identify other persons at high risk.

References

Argenziano G, Catricala C, Ardigo M, et al: Dermoscopy of patients with multiple nevi, *Arch Dermatol* 147:46–49, 2011.
Arumi-Uria M, McNutt NS, Finnerty B: Grading of atypia in nevi: correlation with melanoma risk, *Mod Pathol* 16:764–771, 2003.
Bauer J, Bastian BC: Distinguishing melanocytic nevi from melanomas by DNA copy number changes: comparative genomic hybridization as a research and diagnostic tool, *Dermatol Ther* 19:40–49, 2006.
de Snoo FA, Kroon MW, Bergman W, et al: From sporadic atypical nevi to familial melanoma: risk analysis for melanoma in sporadic atypical nevus patients, *J Am Acad Dermatol* 56:748–752, 2007.
Ferrara G, Soyer HP, Malvehy J, et al: The many faces of blue nevus: a clinicopathologic study, *J Cutan Pathol* 34:543–551, 2007.
Gelbard AN, Tripp JM, Marghoob AA, et al: Management of Spitz nevi: a survey of dermatologists in the United States, *J Am Acad Dermatol* 47:224–330, 2002.
Goodson AG, Florell SR, Boucher KM, et al: Low rates of clinical recurrence after biopsy of benign to moderately dysplastic melanocytic nevi, *J Am Acad Dermatol* 62:591–596, 2010.
King R, Hayzen BA, Page RN, et al: Recurrent nevus phenomenon: a clinicopathologic study of 357 cases and histologic comparison with melanoma with regression, *Mod Pathol* 22:611–619, 2009.
Kinsler VA, O'Hare P, Bulstrode N, et al: Melanoma in congenital melanocytic naevi, *Br J Dermatol* 176:1131–1143, 2017.
Naeyaert JM, Brochez L: Dysplastic nevi, *N Engl J Med* 349:2233–2240, 2003.
Price HN, Schaffer JV: Congenital melanocytic nevi: when to worry and how to treat: facts and controversies, *Clin Dermatol* 28:283–302, 2010.
Que K, Grant-Kels JM, Longo C, Pellacani G: Basics of confocal microscopy and the complexity of diagnosing skin tumors: new imaging tools in clinical practice, diagnostic workflows, cost-estimate and new trends, *Dermatol Clinics* 34:367–375, 2016.
Roh MR, Eliades P, Gupta S, Tsao H: Genetics of melanocytic nevi, *Pigment Cell Melanoma Res* 28:661–672, 2015.
Sommer LL, Barcia SM, Clarke LE, Helm KF: Persistent melanocytic nevi: a review and analysis of 205 cases, *J Cutan Pathol* 38:503–507, 2011.
Tetzlaff MT, Reuben A, Billings SD, et al: Toward a molecular-genetic classification of spitzoid neoplasms, *Clin Lab Med* 37:431–448, 2017.

PAPULOSQUAMOUS ERUPTIONS

Method of
Tam T. Nguyen, MD

CURRENT DIAGNOSIS

- Psoriasis can be clinically described as erythematous plaques with silvery white scales.
- Severity is rated as mild (< 5% body surface area [BSA]), moderate (5%–10% BSA), or severe (>10% BSA).
- Most cases are mild chronic plaques involving the extensor surfaces.
- Involvement of scalp and palmar and plantar surfaces is classified as severe.
- Psoriasis is commonly comorbid with several conditions, including cardiovascular disease, depression, and metabolic disorders.

CURRENT THERAPY

- Class I/II (super-potent) topical steroid is the mainstream treatment of mild to moderate psoriasis.
- For moderate to severe cases, systemic treatment with methotrexate is the gold standard.
- Narrowband ultraviolet B (UVB) remains a safe treatment option for all patients including children and pregnant women.
- Several immunomodulators or biologicals including etanercept (Enbrel) have been proved very effective therapy. Biologicals can be given as monotherapy or in combination with other modalities for very recalcitrant cases.
- Treatment of comorbid conditions is paramount.

Epidemiology

Psoriasis, a common chronic idiopathic inflammatory disorder, affects 2% to 3% of Americans. The number of persons affected by this condition has more than doubled from 1970 to 2000. It is a chronic disorder that can involve many organ systems including skin, mucosa, the gastrointestinal tract, and joints. Although the onset of psoriasis can occur at any age, there is a bimodal distribution peaking in young adults in their early 20s and again in persons in their 50s. There is an equal prevalence among male and female patients, but the incidence is higher in men among younger adult populations.

Risk Factors

There is a strong family history and association with HLA-Cw6, HLA-B13, and HLA-B27. Psoriatic genes appear to be located on four key genes called pSOR1-4, which show an autosomal dominant pattern. There are about 36 gene loci associated with psoriasis. The genome-wide association study (GWAS) showed that the genes STAT3 and STAT5 regulate the cytokines associated with psoriasis. In addition to the genetic etiology, environmental triggers, such as drugs, infection, and stress, also have a role in the pathogenesis of the psoriasis. Psychogenic stress from home and school is especially common in pediatric cases. Lithium and β-blockers are two well-known triggers of psoriasis. Certain conditions, such as Crohn's disease and multiple sclerosis, predispose patients to developing psoriasis.

Pathophysiology

Even though the exact mechanism is unknown, psoriasis is a disease of T cells that leads to abnormal epidermal differentiation and hyperproliferation. Normal skin has epidermal turnover of about 21 to 28 days, but psoriatic skin turns over every 3 to 4 days. Several cytokines, including IL-12 and IL-23, are part of the immune-mediated disease.

Diagnosis

Although most psoriatic lesions have characteristic scaly and silvery plaques, the lesions can be misleading. Refer to Box 1 for the differential diagnosis. Psoriasis has several subtypes including erythrodermic, pustular, and vulgaris. Psoriasis vulgaris has several subtypes including chronic plaque, guttate (Figure 1), and inverse psoriasis. More than 80% to 90% of psoriasis cases are the chronic plaque psoriasis. Therefore this chapter focuses on this subtype.

Severity of psoriasis is classified based on the body surface area (BSA) involved. There are several severity instruments, such as Koo-Menter Psoriasis, for assessing the severity. One of the best validated tools is the Psoriasis Area Severity Index (PASI). These instruments are used to classify the condition according to coverage of body surface area (BSA) as either mild (< 5% of BSA), moderate (5%–10% of BSA), or severe (>10% of BSA). BSA can be estimated using the rule of 9s. Each upper extremity and the head is 9%, and the chest, back, and each lower extremity are 18%. For children, similar rules apply, except that each lower extremity is 13.5%. When the lesions involve difficult regions such as hands, feet, face, scalp, and genitalia, they are treated as severe regardless of the amount of BSA they cover.

Fortunately, more than 70% to 75% of cases are classified as mild to moderate, and there is no need for blood work. However, when psoriasis is associated with comorbidities, such as depression and heart disease, or when systemic medications cause serious side effects, it may be reasonable to get basic laboratory tests such as a complete blood count with platelet (CBC), chemistry, liver function tests (LFTs), cholesterol panel, hepatitis B and C, uric acid, and erythrocyte sedimentation rate (ESR). For patients at high risk, consider HIV testing. Also, consider evaluating for tuberculosis with a PPD test. These laboratory tests are even more crucial when considering treating with immunosuppressants like methotrexate (Trexall) and biological agents. Liver biopsy should be done if methotrexate is used at a cumulative dose of 3.5 to 4 g. Equally important, patients' quality of life needs to be assessed, which can be done with an instrument called the Dermatology Life Quality Index (DLQI).

Differential Diagnosis

The differential diagnosis of psoriasis is lengthy and can be tricky. Box 1 lists the differential diagnosis of psoriasis.

Clinical Manifestations

Most presentations of psoriasis are asymptomatic. When symptomatic, the most common clinical manifestation is pruritus. Other possible symptoms include fever and malaise, especially for more extensive disease. When psoriasis involves the joints, patients can

---

| BOX 1 | Differential Diagnosis of Psoriasis |

Plaque-like
Eczema
Fungal infection
Squamous cell carcinoma
Subacute cutaneous lupus erythematous

Guttate
Secondary syphilis
Pityriasis rosea

Erythrodermic
Pityriasis rubra pilaris
Drug eruptions

Pustular
Candidiasis
Acute generalized exanthematic pustulosis

Inverse
Intertrigo
Cutaneous T-cell lymphoma

Figure 1 Guttate psoriasis with droplike, discrete papules and small plaques with scales.

Figure 2 Chronic plaque psoriasis on the extensor surfaces.

have pain and stiffness in the involved joints; many of these cases involve the distal interphalangeal joints. On physical examination, the lesions are well-circumscribed dark pink to red plaques with silvery to white scales (Figures 2 and 3). Scales can be absent in certain locations, such as the intertriginous area (gluteal folds) (Figures 4 and 5). The margins are sharp and distinct, especially

Figure 3 Chronic plaque psoriasis with classic silvery scales.

Figure 4 Chronic plaque psoriasis with limited scales.

Figure 5 Chronic plaque psoriasis without

over extensor surfaces such as the elbows and knees (see Figure 2). Lesions also can involve the sacral area, nails, scalp, and the genitalia. If psoriasis forms under a nail, onycholysis (lifting of the nail plate) can occur with pitting and subungual keratosis.

When the scales are removed, several distinctive minute blood droplets appear, called the Auspitz sign. Use caution when removing the scales because it can be painful. When new lesions form at a site of trauma, it is called the Koebner phenomenon. Diagnosis can be made clinically. However, when in doubt, biopsy the lesion, which will show a thickened epidermis with an absent granular cell layer. The stratum corneum is hyperkeratotic, with classic infiltration of neutrophils.

If this inflammatory process affects the joints, psoriatic arthritis ensues. Although this article does not discuss psoriatric arthritis, it is important to recognize when it occurs. Unlike rheumatoid arthritis, the distal interphalangeal (DIP) joints are regularly involved, but it can affect any joints. Psoriatric arthritis only occurs in 4% to 42% of patients with psoriasis. Diagnosis can be made with the CASPAR criteria, which evaluates five possible presentations, including having psoriasis, nail dystrophy, negative rheumatoid factor, dactylitis, and radiographic evidence.

Treatment

Corticosteroids remain the mainstay for psoriasis therapy; they reduce inflammation, decrease mitosis, and reduce erythema. Because most cases are mild to moderate, the first-line therapy to consider is topical corticosteroids. Even for severe cases that require systemic treatment, topical steroids should still be considered as a first-line adjuvant therapy. Because psoriatic lesions are thickened, it is critical to go directly to super-potent steroids (class I), such as clobetasol (Clobex) (refer to Box 2 for steroid potency). When the localized lesions are lichenified and do not respond to potent topical corticosteroids, using steroid-impregnated tapes (flurandrenolide tape [Cordran]), which function as an occlusive wrap, can help. However, for areas of thinner skin, such as mucosa and lesions on the face, use less-potent topical steroids. Use caution when using class 1 steroids owing to all the potential side effects, including skin atrophy, hypopigmentation, telangiectasis, striae, and potential systemic absorption. In addition to the possible side effects, tachyphylaxis (reduced efficacy with prolonged use) can occur. Therefore it is crucial to limit the use of potent topical steroids to less than 12 weeks.

One way to reduce the use of topical steroids is by using the vitamin D_3 analogue class, such as calcipotriene (Dovonex). This class of drugs inhibits epidermal proliferation and stimulates cellular differentiation. It is considered as effective as medium-potency corticosteroids, without the side effects. However, one drawback is that it takes about 8 weeks to be effective. Therefore it should not be used for acute psoriatic eruptions. More often it is used in combination with topical steroids, since topical calcipotriene in combination with high dose topical steroids like betamethasone (Enstilar) works better than either alone. It is generally well tolerated topically, but about 10% of patients experience burning and itching or hypercalcemia.

Other topical applications include tazarotene (Tazorac) and anthralin (Dritho-Crème HP 1%, Dritho-Scalp 0.5%). Tazarotene is an acetylenic retinoid and can be as effective as high-potency topical corticosteroids. However, its use is limited owing to the side effects of erythema, burning, pruritus, and peeling. Therefore it is best to combine it with corticosteroids to reduce the irritation. In addition, tazarotene can stain clothing, and it is less popular owing to the side effects (redness and irritation on skin as well as staining) and the feel and smell of the solutions. However, it is a good alternative to topical corticosteroids.

For a limited number of thickened lesions, consider intralesional steroid injections, such as a single intralesional injection of a mid-potency steroid (e.g., triamcinolone acetonide or Kenalog-10, 5–10 mg/mL). Most injected plaques clear completely and remain in remission for months. However, as with other steroid injections, side effects of skin atrophy and telangiectasis can occur. Therefore the face and intertriginous areas should not be injected because of the increased risk of side effects.

For severe and recalcitrant cases, systematic medications are needed. One of the gold standards in the United States and many other countries is methotrexate (Trexall) because it is available as a generic. Its exact mechanism is unknown; initially it was believed to inhibit proliferation, but more-recent studies describe an antiinflammatory property. The most common serious side effect of this drug is hepatotoxicity (as many as 33% of patients show some liver disease). Therefore it is crucial to screen for alcohol dependency, liver disease, and obesity. Standard practice is to check baseline CBC and liver function enzymes, and then repeat these laboratory tests after 1 month of therapy. Methotrexate is highly teratogenic; hence it is absolutely contraindicated in pregnancy. After stopping the medication, men should wait at least 3 months and women should wait one ovulatory cycle before attempting to conceive.

There are two methods for initiating methotrexate. Most patients start at an initial dose of 7.5 mg (3 tabs of 2.5 mg) weekly; in pediatric cases dosage[1] is 0.2 to 0.7 mg/kg weekly. Others start at a higher dosage of 0.4 to 0.5 mg/kg weekly. Unfortunately, there is no current study to compare the two methods. With either dosing regimen, do not exceed 30 mg per week. Methotrexate depletes the body's storage of folic acid, so it is important to supplement folic acid 1 mg daily except the day when methotrexate is taken. The methotrexate can be titrated upward every 2 to 4 weeks.

Unlike methotrexate, which can take several weeks before it becomes effective, cyclosporine (Neoral), a calcineruin inhibitor, is rapidly effective for severe cases. It is dosed at a low dose of 2 to 5 mg/kg/day divided into two doses and increased slowly every 2 to 4 weeks. Maintenance dosage is about 3 to 5 mg/kg/day. A main concern for this drug is nephrotoxicity. As long as the use of cyclosporine is limited to 1 year, it is generally safe. However, kidney function still needs to be monitored regularly. Cyclosporine has been associated with an increased risk of squamous cell carcinoma, especially when the patient has a history of psoralen plus ultraviolet A (PUVA) therapy.

Although not FDA-approved, azathioprine (Imuran) has been a successful systemic medication for psoriasis. Generally, it is initially dosed at 0.5 mg/kg. If there is cytopenia, then the dosage can be increased by 0.5 mg/kg/day every 4 to 6 weeks as needed. Another dosing method is based on thiopurine methyltransferase (TPMT) levels. If the TPMT is less than 5.0 U, do not use azathioprine. If the level is between 5 and 13.7 U, the maximum daily dose should be 0.5 mg/kg/daily. If the TMPT level is between 13.7 and 19.0 U, then the maximum daily dose may be increased to 1.5 mg/kg. There is only one FDA-approved phosphodiesterase type-4 inhibitor (PDE4), apremilast (Otezla). Taken orally twice a day, this drug inhibits PDE4 leading to increased intracellular cAMP levels.

Acitretin (Soriatane) and isotretinoin (Claravis)[1] are retinoids, which are vitamin A derivatives. Although acitretin is more commonly used, either may be used and requires a period of 3 to 6 months to achieve results. However, these retinoids are generally less effective than methotrexate and cyclosporine. Though they are less effective and a longer time is required for this class of agents to work, their main benefits include no malignancy potential and no immunosuppression. Therefore these drugs are safe in patients with HIV and other immunosuppressive conditions. Unfortunately, acitretin and isotretinoin are highly teratogenic. Both male and female patients need to be drug free for 1 year for isotretinoin and 3 years for acitretin before they conceive. For other possible treatment agents, refer to Box 3.

In recent years, immunomodulators or biologicals have revolutionized the treatment course of psoriasis. Generally, criteria for this class of therapy are PASI greater than 10 and failure of other therapies or a contraindication to other therapies such as methotrexate. Most agents are limited to 1 to 2 years of use because most studies have not been evaluated beyond 2 years. Tuberculosis should be evaluated (PPD and possibly chest x-ray) before starting these biologics. All the medications in this class should be avoided in pregnancy. Alefacept (Amevive)[2] and efalizumab (Raptiva) are T-cell inhibitors. Efalizumab (Raptiva) was withdrawn from the market in 2009 owing to reported cases of progressive multifocal leukoencephalopathy. Another class is tumor necrosis factor (TNF). Etanercept (Enbrel), one of the first TNF inhibitors,

---

[1] Not FDA approved for this indication
[2] Not available in the United States.

BOX 3 Other Treatment Modalities for Moderate to Severe Psoriasis

Fumaric acid esters[2]: First-line therapy in a couple of European countries

Hydroxyurea (Hydrea)[1]: A good option because there is no liver or kidney toxicity; however, be cautious of bone marrow suppression

Leflunomide (Arava)[1]

Mycophenolate mofetil (Cellcept)[1]: good choice for HIV patients and patients with immunobullous disorders

Retinoic acid metabolism–blocking agents: liarozole[2] and talarozole (Rombozale)[5]

Alitretinoin topical (Panretin)[1]

Sulfasalazine (Azulfidine)[1]

Tacrolimus (Prograf)[1]

6 thioguanine (Tabloid)[1]

---

[1] Not FDA approved for this indication.
[2] Not available in the United States.
[5] Investigational drug in the United States.

---

should not be used in patients with multiple sclerosis. Three monoclonal antibodies include infliximab (Remicade), adalimumab (Humira), and golimumab (Simponi), and all are TNF inhibitors. In recent years, a new class of biologics that inhibit interleukin (IL)-12 and IL-23 has shown promising results. Ustekinumab (Stelara) was first approved within this class, followed by guselkumab (Tremfya). Secukinumab (Cosentyx), a new biological for plaque psoriasis is a recombinant, high-affinity, fully humanized IgG monoclonal antibody that selectively binds and neutralizes interleukin-17A (IL-17A). Additional two IL-17A inhibitors, ixekizumab (Taltz) and brodalumab (Siliq), have been approved for use.

Etanercept (Enbrel) blocks TNF-α. It is generally dosed at 50 mg SC twice weekly for 12 weeks and then 50 mg weekly. Patients can self-administer the drug; laboratory monitoring is not required. There are limited data beyond 2 years. Etanercept is the preferred drug for children. Infliximab (Remicade) blocks both soluble and bound TNF-α. Its dosage is 3 to 5 mg/kg IV on weeks 0, 2, and 6, and then every 6 to 8 weeks. Medication generally is infused over 2 hours. It is approved for 1 year. In a comparative study, infliximab was found to be superior to methotrexate. TNF does not appear to increase the risk of herpes zoster but could be associated with an increase in melanoma.

Adalimumab (Humira) blocks both soluble and bound TNF-α. Initiate the dose at 40 mg SC every 2 weeks, although some patients require dosing every 7 to 10 days. Alternatively, the initial dose may be 80 mg followed by 40 mg. Patients may self-administer the injections. As with infliximab, before initiating treatment, obtain a PPD (and consider chest x-ray as well). Antibodies can develop within the first 28 weeks, which will decrease the efficacy of the drug. Both infliximab, which has been in use for many years, and adalimumab have limited long-term safety data beyond 1 year. Some data suggest an increase in cancer risk beyond 1 year. Adalimumab is FDA approved for psoriatic arthritis.

Alefacept (Amevive), a T-cell inhibitor, is dosed at 15 mg IM or IV once a week for 12 weeks. Its efficacy follows the rule of thirds: It works well in about one-third of cases, does not work at all in one-third of cases, and the rest fall in between. After a cycle of 12 weeks, the courses may be repeated as needed. However, it is crucial initially to monitor T-cell counts biweekly. A newer agent, ustekinumab (Stelara), has been shown to improve lesions in 66% to 76% of cases. It is initially dosed at 45 to 90 mg SC at weeks 0 and 4, depending on body weight. Maintenance is every 12 weeks. Besides ustekinumab, another Il-12/IL-23 inhibitor, guselkumab (Tremfya), was approved in 2017 and is dosed at 100 mg/mL SC in weeks 0 and 4, then every 8 weeks.

When these therapies are contraindicated, one alternative is phototherapy. This is the reason many patients report decreased symptom severity during the summer months due to the natural UV light. Phototherapy started with photochemotherapy with oral or topical psoralens combined with UVA light (PUVA). Although phototherapy is very effective for psoriasis, even in very thick lesions, recent studies have shown an increased risk of skin cancer. Therefore PUVA has become less popular since the advent of UVB radiation treatment, especially with narrow-band UVB (NB-UVB). NB-UVB is equally effective as PUVA and does not have the risk of skin cancer. The exact mechanism is unknown, but it is believed to affect DNA and to suppress IL-17 and IL-23, creating photoproducts that interfere with cell cycle progression. NB-UVB is first-line course of therapy for pregnant and pediatric patients. There are two methods for initiating NB-UVB phototherapy: the skin type protocol, which is easier to execute; and the minimum erythema dose (MED), which is more detailed but more accurate. Refer to Table 1 for treatment protocols. Both protocols generally require 30 to 35 treatments with the optimal frequency of three times a week.

Given all the treatment options (refer to Box 4), the choice of the treatment regimen depends on several factors. First, the severity of the psoriasis must be determined as well as the social and emotional impact of the condition. Another consideration is financial, including the insurance coverage, copayment, and deductibles. The lowest-cost treatment is methotrexate, and alefacept is the highest. The patient's conveniences and preferences should be discussed. If the severity is only mild to moderate without much emotional impact, topical steroid and vitamin D analogue should be considered the first options. Other topicals include tar (Balnetar, Psoriasin, Scytera), anthralin (Dritho-Crème HP, Dritho-Scalp), and tretinoin (Retin-A)[1]. If the degree is severe and/or the patient has emotional impact, systemic medications should be used. Most insurance plans will probably require that the patient try at least one oral medication before employing the biologicals. If systemic therapy is used, consider combining it with phototherapy (if possible). If there is no improvement within 2 to 4 months, the regimen should be changed to biologicals. Other combinations may be employed for better resolution.

For healthy patients, any of these therapies may be tried. Unfortunately, there are limitations with children, pregnant women, and patients trying to conceive. For pediatric patients, topical agents should be tried first, followed by UVB monotherapy. If the plaques are still recalcitrant, add either methotrexate (Trexall) or phototherapy. If phototherapy is not available and topical agents have failed, consider using methotrexate or cyclosporine (Neoral). Other options for pediatric patients include adalimumab (Humira) and etanercept (Enbrel). For pregnant women and patients trying to conceive, first try topical agents followed by UVB (ideally narrowband). This combination remains the safest option. If stronger options are needed, the only class B drugs are systemic steroids, adalimumab, alefacept (Amevive), infliximab (Remicade), and ustekinumab (Stelara). An absolute contraindication in this population is the retinoid class, such as isotretinoin (Claravis)[1] and acitretin (Soriatane).

Complications

Patients suffering from psoriasis cope with the physical appearance of their lesions as well as the associated mental anguish associated with many other chronic ailments. Furthermore, psoriasis is associated with other chronic diseases, such as abdominal obesity, metabolic syndrome, and atherogenic dyslipidemia. Weight loss can improve the appearance of psoriatic plaques. Patients with psoriasis are more likely to have coronary artery disease, elevated blood pressure, obesity, and insulin resistance. Treating psoriasis decreases the cardiovascular risks. There is an increased risk of malignancy, such as lymphoma. Substance abuse and smoking are common among these patients as well.

---

[1] Not FDA approved for this indication.

| TABLE 1 | Methods for Initiating Narrow-Band Ultraviolet B (NB-UVB) Therapy and Subsequent Dosing of Phototherapy |

| THERAPY | MED NB-UVB PROTOCOL | | | | | | MED NB-UVB PROTOCOL |
	TYPE 1	TYPE 2	TYPE 3	TYPE 4	TYPE 5	TYPE 6	
Initial dose	130 mJ/cm²	220 mJ/cm²	260 mJ/cm²	330 mJ/cm²	350 mJ/cm²	400 mJ/cm²	Start with 50%–70% MED The starting dose should be based on the provider's comfort and the patient's history of response to light; e.g., start closer to 70% if the patient has a history of tanning and start closer to 50% if the patient has a history of burning; most centers start at 70%

Subsequent Doses

Severe erythema	No treatment. When burn resolves, decrease by 50% of last dose and then increase dose by 10%						
Mild erythema	Same dose	Same dose	Same dose	Same dose	Same dose	Same dose	Decrease dose by 20%
Barely perceptible erythema	—	—	—	—	—	—	Same (erythmogenic) or slight decrease (suberythmogenic)
No erythema: increase dose by	15 mJ/cm²	25 mJ/cm²	40 mJ/cm²	45 mJ/cm²	60 mJ/cm²	65 mJ/cm²	20%

Dosing Schedule

Optimal schedule	3 ×/wk (M, W, F) is the optimal schedule because less is not as effective and more does not improve the resolution. Subsequent treatments should not be less than 24 hours from the last treatment. For the treatment of eczema, no clear guideline to the frequency. Some use 5 ×/wk.

Dose Adjustments for Missed Days

MISSED DAYS	DOSE ADJUSTMENT
1–7	Increase doses per skin type
8–11	Same dose
12–14	Decrease by 2 treatments' worth
15–20	Decrease by 25%
21–27	Decrease by 50%
28 +	Start over

| BOX 4 | Treatment Options for Psoriasis |

Topical
Steroid
Tar (e.g., Balnetar, Psoriasin, Scytera)
Anthralin (Dritho-Crème HP, Dritho-Scalp)
Calcipotriene (Dovonex)
Calcitriol (Vectical)
Adapalene (Differin)[1]
Tazarotene (Tazorac)
Tretinoin (Retin-A)[1]
Calcineurin inhibitors (pimecrolimus [Elidel][1], tacrolimus [Protopic][1])

Oral or Systemic
Methotrexate (Trexall)
Acitretin (Soriatane)/Isotretinoin (Claravis)[1]

Cyclosporine (Neoral)
Mycophenolate mofetil (Cellcept)[1]

Immunomodulators
Alefacept (Amevive)[2]
Etanercept (Enbrel)
Infliximab (Remicade)
Adalimumab (Humira)
Ustekinumab (Stelara)
Secukinumab (Cosentyx)
Ixekizumab (Taltz)
Brodalumab (Siliq)

Phototherapy
UVA
UVB

[1] Not FDA approved for this indication.
[2] Not available in the United States.

References

Ahlehoff O, et al: Cardiovascular disease event rates in patients with severe psoriasis treated with systemic anti-inflammatory drugs: a Danish real-world cohort study, *J Intern Med* 273:197–204, 2012.

American Academy of Dermatology Work Group: Menter A, Korman NJ, Elmets CA, et al: Guidelines of care for the management of psoriasis and psoriatic arthritis: section 6. Guidelines of care for the treatment of psoriasis and psoriatic arthritis: case-based presentations and evidence-based conclusions, *J Am Acad Dermatol* 65(1):137–174, 2011.

Callen JP, Krueger GG, Lebwohl M, et al: AAD: AAD consensus statement on psoriasis therapies, *J Am Acad Dermatol* 49(5):897–899, 2003.

Dubertret L: Retinoids, methotrexate and cyclosporine, *Curr Probl Dermatol* 38:79–94, 2009.

Foulkes AC, Grindlay DJ, Griffiths CE, Warren RB: What's new in psoriasis? An analysis of guidelines and systematic reviews published in 2009–2010, *Clin Exp Dermatol* 36(6):585–589, 2011 Aug quiz 588–9.

Gottlieb A, Korman NJ, Gordon KB, et al: Guidelines of care for the management of psoriasis and psoriatic arthritis: section 2, *Psoriatic arthritis: overview and guidelines of care for treatment with an emphasis on the biologics*, *J Am Acad Dermatol* 58(5):851–864, 2008.

Herrier RN: Advances in the treatment of moderate-to-severe plaque psoriasis, *Am J Health Syst Pharm* 68(9):795–806, 2011.

Jensen P, Zachariae C, Christensen R, et al: Effect of weight loss on the severity of psoriasis: a randomized clinical study, *JAMA Dermatol* 149:795–801, 2013.

Johnson-Huang LM, Suárez-Fariñas M, Sullivan-Whalen M, et al: Effective narrow-band UVB radiation therapy suppresses the IL-23/IL-17 axis in normalized psoriasis plaques, *J Invest Dermatol* 130(11):2654–2663, 2010.

Kalb RE, Strober B, Weinstein G, Lebwohl M: Methotrexate and psoriasis: 2009 National Psoriasis Foundation Consensus Conference, *J Am Acad Dermatol* 60:824–837, 2009.

Kimball AB, Gladman D, Gelfand JM, et al: National Psoriasis Foundation: National Psoriasis Foundation clinical consensus on psoriasis comorbidities and recommendations for screening, *J Am Acad Dermatol* 58:1031–1142, 2008.

Kuhn A, Patsinakidis N, Luger T: Alitretinoin for cutaneous lupus erythematosus, *J Am Acad Dermatol* 67(3):e123–6, 2012.

Menter A, Gottlieb A, Feldman SR, et al: Guidelines of care for the management of psoriasis and psoriatic arthritis: section 1. Overview of psoriasis and guidelines of care for the treatment of psoriasis with biologics, *J Am Acad Dermatol* 58:826–850, 2008.

Ormerod AD, Campalani E, Goodfield MJ: BAD Clinical Standards Unit: British Association of Dermatologists guidelines on the efficacy and use of acitretin in dermatology, *Br J Dermatol* 162:952–963, 2010.

Trueb RM: Therapies for childhood psoriasis, *Curr Probl Dermatol* 38:137–159, 2009.

Tsoi LC, et al: Identification of 15 new psoriasis susceptibility loci highlights the role of innate immunity, *Nat Genet* 44:1341–1348, 2012.

PARASITIC DISEASES OF THE SKIN

Method of
Andreas Katsambas, MD, PhD; and Clio Dessinioti, MD, MSc, PhD

CURRENT DIAGNOSIS

Cutaneous Amebiasis
- Purulent, foul-smelling nodules, ulcers, cysts, sinuses
- Microscopic identification of *Entamoeba histolytica* in stool or biopsy samples
- Molecular methods

Cutaneous Leishmaniasis
- Ulcerated nodule (i.e., volcano sign)
- Identification of *Leishmania* parasites by direct examination or culture from the lesion aspirate or biopsy
- Montenegro skin test
- In vitro lymphocyte proliferation assay
- Polymerase chain reaction

Trypanosomiasis
Chagas' Disease
- Chagoma: painful erythematous nodule
- Regional adenopathy
- Cardiomyopathy, megaesophagus, megacolon
- Microscopic examination of *Trypanosoma cruzi* in blood, lymph node biopsy, or skin biopsy or culture

African Sleeping Sickness
- Trypanosome chancre: painful, inflammatory nodule
- Regional adenopathy
- Fever, generalized pruritic eruption with erythematous annular plaques
- Central nervous system involvement
- Microscopic identification of *Trypanosoma brucei* in chancre fluid, lymph node aspirates, blood, bone marrow, cerebrospinal fluid

Cutaneous Toxoplasmosis
- Roseola, urticaria, prurigo-like nodules
- Isolation of *Toxoplasma gondii* in the skin

Ascariasis
- Urticaria
- Identification of adult worm or eggs in stool

Cutaneous Larva Migrans
- Creeping eruption
- Intense pruritus

Cysticercosis
- Subcutaneous nodules
- Isolation of *Taenia solium* in skin lesion
- Serologic tests

Dracunculiasis
- Ruptured blister with prolapsing worm

Filariasis
Lymphatic Filariasis
- Fever with lymphangitis and lymphadenitis
- Chronic pulmonary infection
- Progressive lymphedema leading to massive tissue thickening, especially of the legs and scrotum (i.e., elephantiasis)
- Microscopic identification of microfilariae in blood

Onchocerciasis (River Blindness)
- Subcutaneous nodules, dermatitis, "leopard skin," "lizard skin," lymphedema
- Identification of microfilariae in skin snips
- Blindness

Loiasis (Calabar Swellings)
- Pruritus, localized subcutaneous swellings
- Serpiginous lesion on the conjunctivae
- Microscopic identification of microfilariae in blood

Schistosomiasis (Snail Fever)
- Pruritic papules, edema
- Fever, lymphadenopathy, diarrhea
- Bilharziasis cutanea tarda: pruritic, grouped papules
- Identification of the eggs in stool, urine, biopsy of affected tissues
- Enzyme-linked immunosorbent assay (ELISA) tests

Cercarial Dermatitis (Swimmer's Itch)
- Extremely pruritic erythematous macules, papules, vesicles on body areas exposed to infested water

Human Scabies
- Pruritus worsening at night
- Papules, excoriations, nodules, burrows on genitals, interdigital spaces, axillae, wrists
- Microscopic identification of mites or eggs or feces from burrows or papules

Pediculosis
Pediculosis Capitis
- Intense pruritus of the scalp
- Nape dermatitis
- Identification of lice and nits on the hair

Pediculosis Corporis (Vagabond's Itch)
- Intense pruritus, erythema, urticarial lesions, papules, nodules, and excoriations
- Identification of lice and nits on clothing

Pediculosis Pubis
- Pruritus
- Blue macules
- Identification of lice and nits on pubic hair

CURRENT THERAPY

Cutaneous Amebiasis
- Metronidazole (Flagyl) 750 mg PO three times daily for 7 to 10 days, or
- Tinidazole (Tindamax) 2 g once PO daily for 5 days, followed by iodoquinol (Aloquin) 650 mg PO three times daily for 20 days or paromomycin (Humatin) 25 to 35 mg/kg/day PO in three doses for 7 days

Cutaneous Leishmaniasis
- Sodium stibogluconate (Pentostam)[10] 20 mg/kg/day IV or IM for 20 days, or
- Meglumine antimoniate (Glucantime)[1] 20 mg/kg/day IV or IM for 20 days, or
- Miltefosine (Impavido) 2.5 mg/kg/day PO (up to 150 mg/day) for 28 days, or
- Topical paromomycin, a formulation of 15% paromomycin and 12% methylbenzethonium chloride in soft white paraffin (Lesheutan)[1,6] applied twice daily for 10 days or
- Pentamidine (Pentam 300)[1] 2 to 3 mg/kg IV or IM daily or every second day for four to seven doses

Trypanosomiasis
Chagas' Disease (American Trypanosomiasis)
- Nifurtimox (Lampit)[10] 8 to 10 mg/kg/day PO in three or four doses for 90 to 120 days, or
- Benznidazole (Radanil, Rochagan)[10] 5 to 7 mg/kg/day PO in two doses for 60 to 120 days

East African Sleeping Sickness
- Suramin (Germanin)[10] 100 to 200 mg (test dose) IV, then 1 g IV on days 1, 3, 7, 14, 21
- For late disease with involvement of the central nervous system, melarsoprol (Mel-B)[10] 2 to 3.6 mg/kg/day IV for 3 days; after 7 days, 3.6 mg/kg/day for 3 days; repeat after 7 days

West African Sleeping Sickness
- Pentamidine (Pentam 300)[1] 4 mg/kg/day IM for 10 days, or
- Suramin (Germanin)[10] 100 to 200 mg (test dose) IV, then 1 g IV on days 1, 3, 7, 14, 21
- For late disease with involvement of the central nervous system, melarsoprol (Mel-B)[10] 2.2 mg/kg/day IV for 10 days, or
- For late disease with involvement of the central nervous system, eflornithine (Ornidyl)[10] 400 mg/kg/day IV in four doses for 14 days

Cutaneous Toxoplasmosis
- Self-limited disease; treatment not needed in healthy, non-pregnant persons
- For pregnant women or immunocompromised patients: pyrimethamine (Daraprim) 25 to 100 mg/day PO for 3 to 4 weeks (plus leucovorin 10–25 mg with each dose of pyrimethamine) and sulfadiazine[1] 1 to 1.5 g PO four times daily for 3 to 4 weeks

Ascariasis
- Albendazole (Albenza)[1] 400 mg PO once, or
- Mebendazole (Vermox) 100 mg PO twice daily for 3 days or 500 mg once, or
- Ivermectin (Stromectol)[1] 150 to 200 µg/kg PO once

Cutaneous Larva Migrans
- Ivermectin (Stromectol)[1] 200 µg/kg PO once; a second dose may be needed, or
- Albendazole (Albenza)[1] 400 mg daily PO for 3 days
- Topical thiabendazole[2] 10% to 15% applied three times daily for 5 to 7 days for a limited number of lesions

Dracunculiasis
- Slow extraction of the worm, which is facilitated by metronidazole (Flagyl)[1] 250 mg PO three times daily for 10 days

Filariasis
Lymphatic Filariasis
- Diethylcarbamazine (DEC, Hetrazan)[10] 6 mg/kg/day PO in three doses for 12 days, or
- Ivermectin (Stromectol)[1] 200 µg/kg PO once together with albendazole (Albenza)[1] 400 mg PO once; kills only the microfilaria, not the adult worms
- For patients with microfilaria in the blood, DEC as follows: day 1: 50 mg; day 2: 50 mg three times daily; day 3: 100 mg three times daily; days 4 through 14: 6 mg/kg in three doses

Onchocerciasis
- Ivermectin (Stromectol) 150 µg/kg PO once for 6 to 12 months, until asymptomatic
- DEC: contraindicated because it may lead to blindness

Loiasis
- DEC[10] 6 mg/kg/day PO in three doses for 12 days
- For patients with microfilaria in the blood, DEC as follows: day 1: 50 mg; day 2: 50 mg three times daily; day 3: 100 mg three times daily; days 4 through 14: 9 mg/kg in three doses

Schistosomiasis
- Praziquantel (Biltricide) 40 mg/kg/day[3] in two doses for 1 day (S. haematobium and S. mansoni) and 60 mg/kg/day[3] in three doses for 1 day (S. japonicum, S. mekongi)

Human Scabies
- Permethrin (Acticin, Elimite) 5% cream rinse, applied for 10 hours; a second application 7 to 10 days later, or
- Benzyl benzoate 25% solution[6] applied topically; second application 7 to 10 days later, or
- Crotamiton 10% (Eurax) applied twice daily for 2 days; second application 7 to 10 days later
- Sulfur 6% to 10% ointment in petrolatum[6]
- Ivermectin (Stromectol)[1] 200 µg/kg PO once: treatment of choice for crusted scabies

Pediculosis
Pediculosis Capitis
- Malathion (Ovide) 0.5% lotion, applied for 8 to 12 hours before being washed off; approved for children older than 6 years, or
- Permethrin (Nix) 1% lotion, applied to shampooed hair and washed off after 10 minutes; second application 7 to 10 days later; approved for children older than 2 years
- Pyrethrins with piperidyl butoxide (RID) applied for 10 minutes
- Benzyl benzoate 25% solution[6]
- Lindane shampoo: for recalcitrant disease, associated with serious reactions not to be used in children
- Ivermectin 0.5% lotion (Sklice), apply to dry hair and scalp then rinse off after 10 minutes

Pediculosis Corporis
- Disinfection of clothes

Pediculosis Pubis
- Same treatment as pediculosis capitis: three times daily

---

[1]Not available in the United States.
[2]Not available in the United States.
[3]Exceeds dosage recommended by the manufacturer.
[6]May be compounded by pharmacists
[10]Available in the United States from the Centers for Disease Control and Prevention.

Parasitic diseases are a common cause of morbidity and mortality, particularly in tropical and developing countries. They may be caused by protozoa, helminths, or arthropods. Because of the immigration of persons from tropical and subtropical countries worldwide and the travel of people from industrialized to tropical regions, parasitic diseases may be found in temperate climates. Skin lesions may provide important diagnostic clues for parasitic infections, and they are reviewed in the following sections, along with updated treatment guidelines.

Diseases Caused by Protozoa
Cutaneous Amebiasis
Intestinal amebiasis is caused by *Entamoeba histolytica*, which may rarely invade the skin and cause cutaneous amebiasis. The disease is transmitted by ingestion of food or water contaminated with cyst forms of the parasite and through fecal exposure during sexual contact.

Cutaneous amebiasis develops at the site of the invasion of the parasites into the skin from an underlying amebic abscess, usually at the perianal area or the abdominal wall. Cutaneous findings include purulent, foul-smelling nodules, cysts, and sinuses, which are associated with regional adenopathy and dysentery. Skin lesions grow rapidly and may lead to death if left untreated.

Diagnosis of cutaneous amebiasis is confirmed by microscopic identification of *E. histolytica* in the stool and in aspirates or biopsy samples obtained during colonoscopy, during surgery, or from the border of an ulcer. Treatment of choice for extraintestinal amebiasis is oral metronidazole (Flagyl) 750 mg PO three times daily for 7 to 10 days or tinidazole (Tindamax). Tinidazole was FDA approved in 2004 for the treatment of intestinal amebiasis in adults (2 g/day for 3 days) and children older than 3 years, and it appears to be as effective as, and better tolerated than, metronidazole. Either treatment should be followed by iodoquinol (Aloquin) 650 mg PO three times daily for 20 days or paromomycin 25 to 35 mg/kg/day PO divided in three doses for 7 days.

Leishmaniasis

Leishmaniasis results from the infection with intracellular protozoan parasites belonging to the genus *Leishmania*. Leishmania parasites are transmitted to humans and other mammalian hosts (e.g., dogs, rodents) during feeding by infected female phlebotomine sandflies that serve as vectors. The parasites exist as promastigotes in the midgut of sandflies and as amastigotes (i.e., Leishman-Donovan bodies) within macrophages of humans and other mammals. Based on the extent and the severity of involvement in the human host, leishmaniasis may be clinically classified as cutaneous leishmaniasis, diffuse cutaneous leishmaniasis, mucocutaneous leishmaniasis, and visceral leishmaniasis.

Cutaneous leishmaniasis (New World or Old World form) begins as a small erythematous papule at the site of the bite of the sandfly, which evolves into an ulcerated nodule with a raised and indurated border (i.e., volcano sign) (Figure 1). The lesions gradually heal with a depressed scar. Diffuse cutaneous leishmaniasis is characterized by widespread cutaneous involvement without visceralization. Mucocutaneous leishmaniasis (known as espundia in South America) affects the skin, the mucosa, and the cartilages of the upper respiratory tract (especially the nose and the larynx) and may result in severe disfigurement. Visceral leishmaniasis results from the involvement of the bone marrow, spleen, and the liver, and it may lead to death if left untreated. It manifests with fever, splenomegaly, pancytopenia, and wasting. Post–kala azar dermal leishmaniasis may appear within a year after visceral disease independent of treatment, and it is characterized by macules, papules, and nodules, which are usually hypopigmented.

Diagnosis of leishmaniasis is based on finding the parasites in the skin from the lesion aspirate or biopsy by direct examination or culture. The leishmanin (Montenegro) skin test shows past and current infections, and it detects the inflammatory response in the skin after injection of phenol-killed parasites into the dermis. A past or current infection is also documented by an in vitro lymphocyte proliferation assay that requires a drop of blood from a finger prick. Polymerase chain reaction (PCR) techniques may be used to identify different *Leishmania* species. Circulating antibody levels are not considered a useful diagnostic sign.

Cutaneous leishmaniasis is usually self-limited and may not require treatment. Treatment of cutaneous leishmaniasis is indicated in case of numerous lesions or when lesions affect the face to avoid scarring. Therapies include sodium stibogluconate (Pentostam)[10] 20 mg/kg/day IV or IM for 20 days. Meglumine antimoniate (Glucantime)[2] 20 mg/kg/day IV or IM for 20 days or miltefosine (Impavido) for 28 days may be used. In 2014, FDA approved oral miltefosine for the treatment of cutaneous leishmaniasis caused by *L. braziliensis*, *L. paramensis*, and *L. guyanensis* in adults and adolescents who are not pregnant or breastfeeding. The FDA-approved treatment regimen for persons who weigh from 30 to 44 kg is one 50-mg oral capsule of miltefosine twice a day (total

Figure 1 Cutaneous leishmaniasis is characterized by an ulcerated nodule with a raised and indurated border (i.e., volcano sign).

of 100 mg per day) for 28 consecutive days. The approved regimen for persons who weigh at least 45 kg (99 pounds) is one 50-mg capsule three times a day (total of 150 mg per day) for 28 consecutive days. Miltefosine is contraindicated in pregnant women during treatment and for 5 months thereafter. Alternatively, intralesional injections of antimonials 1 mg/kg once weekly, cryotherapy, local heat, oral ketoconazole (Nizoral)[1], topical amphotericin B[2], pentamidine (Pentam)[1] 2 to 3 mg/kg IV or IM daily or every second day for four to seven doses, or topical paromomycin[1,6] (applied twice daily for 10–20 days) may be used.

The production of antileishmanial antibodies does not correlate with resolution of the disease. Infection and recovery are associated with lifelong immunity to reinfection by the same species of *Leishmania*, although interspecies immunity may also exist.

Trypanosomiasis

There are three types of trypanosomiasis:
- American trypanosomiasis or Chagas' diseases, caused by *Trypanosoma cruzi*
- East African sleeping sickness, caused by *Trypanosoma brucei rhodesiense*
- West African sleeping sickness, caused by *Trypanosoma brucei gambiense*

American trypanosomiasis (i.e., Chagas' disease) is caused by the parasite *T. cruzi*, and it is endemic in Central and South America. The disease is transmitted by the bite of infected "cone-nosed" insects, by transfusion of infected blood, by organ transplantation, and across the placenta. During the acute stage, Chagas' disease manifests with a painful erythematous nodule, known as chagoma, which is associated with regional adenopathy. The chronic stage manifests with cardiomyopathy, megaesophagus, and megacolon. Diagnosis is confirmed by microscopic identification of the parasite in fresh anticoagulated blood, in blood smears, by lymph node biopsy or skin biopsy, or by culture. Treatment includes benznidazole (Radanil, Rochagan)[10] 5 to 7 mg/kg/day PO in two doses for 60 to 90 days or nifurtimox (Lampit)[10] 8 to 10 mg/kg/day PO in three or four doses for 90 to 120 days.

African trypanosomiasis (i.e., East and West African sleeping sickness) occurs in Africa and is transmitted by the bite of infected male and female tsetse flies. It manifests with a highly inflammatory, painful, red or violaceous, indurated nodule surrounded by an erythematous halo, called trypanosome chancre, at the site of the inoculation of the parasites. There is regional adenopathy. Later, the chancre resolves spontaneously, and the patient has fever, malaise, a generalized pruritic eruption with erythematous annular plaques or urticarial lesions, and central nervous system (CNS) involvement with personality changes, apathy, somnolence, coma, and death.

[2] Not available in the United States.
[10] Available in the United States from the Centers for Disease Control and Prevention.

[1] Not FDA approved for this indication.
[2] Not available in the United States.
[6] May be compounded by pharmacists.
[10] Available in the United States from the Centers for Disease Control and Prevention.

Diagnosis is based on the identification of trypanosomes by microscopic examination in chancre fluid, affected lymph node aspirates, blood, bone marrow, or in the late stages of infection, cerebrospinal fluid.

Treatment of East African sleeping sickness consists of suramin (naphthylamine sulfonic acid, Germanin)[10] 100 to 200 mg (test dose) IV and then 1 g IV on days 1, 3, 7, 14, and 21. For late disease with CNS involvement, melarsoprol B (a trivalent organic arsenical, Mel-B)[10] is used in the following dosage regimen: 2 to 3.6 mg/kg/day IV for 3 days; after 7 days, 3.6 mg/kg/day for 3 days; and the latter repeated after 7 days. For West African sleeping sickness, treatment of choice is pentamidine isethionate (Pentam 300)[1] 4 mg/kg/day IM for 10 days or suramin (Germanin)[10] as used for East African sleeping sickness. For late disease with involvement of the CNS, eflornithine (Ornidyl)[10] 400 mg/kg/day IV in four doses for 14 days is used.

Cutaneous Toxoplasmosis

Systemic toxoplasmosis (congenital or acquired) is caused by the parasite *Toxoplasma gondii*, and it usually is transmitted from contact with infected cats. The disease may also be acquired by eating raw or undercooked meats from infected animals. Cutaneous involvement is rare. It manifests with punctate macules or ecchymoses in the congenital form, and the acquired form manifests with roseola and erythema multiforme lesions, urticaria, prurigo-like nodules, and maculopapular lesions. Diagnosis of cutaneous toxoplasmosis is confirmed by isolation of the parasite in the skin. Treatment is not needed for healthy nonpregnant patients because symptoms resolve in a few weeks. Treatment for pregnant women or immunocompromised patients includes pyrimethamine (Daraprim) 25–100 mg/d PO for 3–6 wks together with sulfadiazine[1] 1–15 g PO qid for 3–6 wks. Leucovorin[1] should be taken with each dose of pyrimethamine.

Diseases Caused by Helminths
Ascariasis

Ascariasis is caused by *Ascaris* species, mainly *Ascaris lumbricoides*. It is transmitted by the ingestion of eggs in soil contaminated with human feces. Skin involvement of ascariasis manifests with urticaria. Diagnosis is based on finding the adult worm or eggs in the feces. Treatment includes albendazole (Albenza)[1] 400 mg PO once or mebendazole (Vermox) 100 mg PO twice daily for 3 days (or 500 mg once) or ivermectin (Stromectol)[1] 150 to 200 µg/kg PO once.

Cutaneous Larva Migrans

Cutaneous larva migrans is also known as creeping eruption, with the first term describing a syndrome and the second a clinical sign found in various conditions. The syndrome cutaneous larva migrans is caused when various nematode larvae (i.e., hookworms, such as *Ancylostoma braziliense*, *Ancylostoma caninum*, *Bunostomum phlebotomum*) of dogs, cats, and other mammals penetrate and migrate through the skin. Cutaneous larva migrans is transmitted by skin contact to soil contaminated with animal feces. In humans, larvae are unable to reach internal organs and eventually die. Cutaneous larva migrans manifests with intensely pruritic, papular lesions, which evolve as the larvae migrate to a characteristic linear, minimally elevated, serpiginous tract that moves forward in an irregular pattern. Diagnosis is easily made clinically and is supported by a travel history or by possible exposure in an endemic area.

Treatment of choice consists of ivermectin (Stromectol)[1] at a single dose of 200 µg/kg. In case of treatment failure, a second dose usually suffices. Ivermectin has an excellent safety profile, without any notable adverse events, and it has been used in millions of individuals in developing countries during onchocerciasis and filariasis control operations. It is contraindicated in children who weigh less than 15 kg (or are younger than 5 years) and in pregnant or breastfeeding women. Alternatively, repeated courses of oral albendazole (Albenza)[1] 400 mg daily for 3 days may be used. Treatment with oral thiabendazole (Mintezol)[2] 50 mg/kg daily for 2 to 4 days has been associated with adverse events such as dizziness, nausea,

vomiting, and intestinal cramps, and it is therefore not recommended. In the absence of multiple or widespread lesions, topical treatments may be considered, such as topical thiabendazole[2] 10% to 15%, applied three times daily for 5 to 7 days, which has similar efficacy with oral ivermectin and no adverse events.

Cysticercosis

Cysticercosis is caused by the larval stage (i.e., cysticerci) of the pork tapeworm *Taenia solium*, and it is the most common helminthic infection of the CNS. It is transmitted by ingesting eggs in food, in water, or on hands contaminated with human feces. Cutaneous manifestations are subcutaneous nodules that occur mainly on the extremities and trunk. There may be involvement of the CNS (i.e., seizures), eye, intestines, skeletal muscle, heart, kidneys, lung, and liver. Diagnosis is confirmed by isolation of the parasite in a nodule and by serologic tests.

Treatment options include surgery, albendazole (Albenza) 400 mg PO twice daily for 8 to 30 days, or praziquantel (Biltricide)[1] 100 mg/kg/day PO in three doses for 1 day and then 50 mg/kg/day in three doses for 29 days. Any cysticercocidal drug may cause irreparable damage when used in the presence of ocular or spinal cysts.

Dracunculiasis

Dracunculiasis is caused by the nematode *Dracunculus medinensis*. It is transmitted by drinking water with copepods (i.e., tiny aquatic arthropods) infected with the larvae of *D. medinensis*. In the human stomach, copepods release the larvae that mature and migrate to the skin, causing an erythematous papule or blister. The blister ruptures, and the female worm can often be seen prolapsing through the skin. Treatment includes extraction of the worm combined with wound care. Metronidazole (Flagyl)[1] 250 mg PO three times daily for 10 days may be efficacious and facilitates removal of the worm.

Filariasis

Filariasis is caused by nematodes (i.e., roundworms) that inhabit the lymphatics and subcutaneous tissues. The most common filarial infections include lymphatic filariasis, onchocerciasis, and loiasis.

Lymphatic Filariasis

Lymphatic filariasis is caused by *Wuchereria bancrofti*, *Brugia malayi*, and *Brugia timori*, and it is transmitted by mosquitoes. Adult worms result in a chronic inflammatory cell infiltrate around lymphatic vessels, causing their dilatation, hypertrophy, and obstruction. Many patients are asymptomatic, but some may develop fever with lymphangitis and lymphadenitis, chronic pulmonary infection, and progressive lymphedema leading to massive tissue thickening, especially of the legs and scrotum (i.e., elephantiasis). The overlying skin is thickened. Diagnosis is based on microscopic identification of the microfilariae in the blood and affected tissues.

Treatment consists of diethylcarbamazine (DEC, Hetrazan)[10] in the following regimen: 50 mg on day 1, 50 mg three times daily on day 2, 100 mg three times daily on day 3, and 6 mg/kg in three doses on days 4 through 14. Prophylaxis with DEC 500 mg/day for 2 days each month is effective against *W. bancrofti* infection for travelers in endemic areas.

Onchocerciasis

Onchocerciasis (i.e., blinding filariasis) is caused by the filarial nematode *Onchocerca volvulus*, which is transmitted by the blackflies *Simulium*. It may manifest with subcutaneous onchocercid nodules, acute or chronic dermatitis, depigmentation (i.e., leopard skin), and skin atrophy (i.e., lizard skin), and in later stages, it may manifest with lymphadenopathy and lymphedema. The microfilariae have a predilection for the eyes, and the infection can lead to blindness (i.e., river blindness). Diagnosis is based on identification of microfilariae in skin snips.

[1]Not FDA approved for this indication.
[2]Not available in the United States.

[1]Not FDA approved for this indication.
[10]Available in the United States from the Centers for Disease Control and Prevention.

Treatment consists of ivermectin (Stromectol) 150 μg/kg PO every 6 to 12 months until asymptomatic. DEC is contraindicated as it may lead to blindness.

Loiasis

Loiasis (i.e., Calabar swellings) is caused by the parasite *Loa loa*, which is transmitted by deerflies (*Chrysops*). Cutaneous manifestations include pruritus, urticaria, and Calabar swellings, which are erythematous, warm, subcutaneous swellings associated with the migration of the worm through the subcutaneous tissues. Occasionally, there is subconjunctival migration of the adult worm, producing a migrating serpiginous lesion on the conjunctivae. Diagnosis is confirmed by identification of microfilariae in the blood by microscopic examination.

DEC[10] is the treatment of choice in the following regimen: 50 mg on day 1, 50 mg three times daily on day 2, 100 mg three times daily on day 3, and 9 mg/kg/day in three doses on days 4 through 14. Ivermectin (Stromectol)[1] may cause encephalopathy in patients with a heavy *L. loa* infection. Prophylaxis with DEC is effective for *L. loa* in adults who travel in endemic areas.

Schistosomiasis

Schistosomiasis (i.e., snail fever) in humans is caused mainly by the trematodes *Schistosoma haematobium*, *Schistosoma japonicum*, and *Schistosoma mansoni*. All trematodes have a life cycle that involves the snail as an intermediate host. The infective cercariae leave the snail, swim, and penetrate the human skin, causing a pruritic papular dermatosis. The disease is transmitted by exposure to contaminated water with live cercariae or by drinking infested water. Skin findings of acute schistosomiasis include pruritic schistosomal dermatitis due to a hypersensitivity response to the cercariae and edema of the face, extremities, genitals, and trunk. Schistosomal fever (i.e., Katayama fever), lymphadenopathy, and diarrhea may also develop. Late skin findings (i.e., bilharziasis cutanea tarda) appear in patients with visceral disease and include firm, pruritic, grouped papules. Secondary infection, ulceration, and development of squamous cell carcinoma may follow. Diagnosis is confirmed by identification of the eggs in the urine or stool, by biopsy of affected tissues, or by enzyme-linked immunosorbent assay (ELISA).

Treatment includes praziquantel (Biltricide) 40 mg/kg/day[3] in two doses for 1 day (for *S. haematobium* and *S. mansoni*) or 60 mg/kg/day[3] in three doses for 1 day (for *S. japonicum*).

Cercarial Dermatitis

Cercarial dermatitis (i.e., swimmer's itch) is caused by cercariae (i.e., larvae) of nonhuman schistosomes that penetrate the skin and die without invading other tissues. It is transmitted by contact with fresh or salt water contaminated with cercariae. It manifests with extremely pruritic, erythematous macules of sudden onset, which evolve into papules, vesicles, and urticarial lesions located on parts of the body directly exposed to the water, while sparing clothed areas. Cercarial dermatitis is a self-limited disease, and treatment is symptomatic with topical steroids and oral antihistamines.

Diseases Caused by Arthropoda
Human Scabies

Scabies is a common skin infestation caused by the mite *Sarcoptes scabiei*, which is an obligate human parasite. Scabies is transmitted by direct contact with an infested individual or by contact with bedding and clothing. The incubation period for scabies is about 3 weeks, and reinfestation results in symptoms within 1 to 3 days. Scabies is characterized by pruritus that usually worsens at night. Papules, nodules, excoriations, and burrows may be found. Lesions are usually located on interdigital spaces, wrists, ankles, axillae, waist, and genitals. Scabies manifests as red-brown nodules that represent a hypersensitivity response. In adults, the head is usually spared, whereas the involvement of the scalp, palms, and soles is common in infants.

Crusted or Norwegian scabies manifests with hyperkeratotic papules or plaques of the hands and feet (often with nail involvement) and an erythematous scaly eruption on the face, neck, scalp, and trunk. Because pruritus is often absent, this disease can be misdiagnosed as psoriasis, eczema, or an adverse drug reaction. Lesions contain thousands of mites and are highly contagious. Crusted scabies mainly affects immunocompromised patients (e.g., patients with human immunodeficiency virus infection), mentally retarded persons, or debilitated patients.

Diagnosis is based on the microscopic identification of mites or their eggs or feces from burrows or papules. Treatment should be applied from the neck down in adults, and in infants, application should include the scalp and face (avoiding the eyes and mouth).

Treatment includes 5% permethrin (Elimite) applied for 10 hours and repeated after 1 week. A 25% benzyl benzoate solution[6] is also efficacious in adults, and because of low toxicity, it is recommended in a lower concentration (10%) for children older than 4 months and for women during pregnancy. Sulfur ointments in petrolatum[6] at concentrations of 6% to 10% may be used for scabies in children and pregnant women. Alternative treatments for scabies include crotamiton 10% (Eurax) applied once daily for 2 days, or ivermectin (Stromectol)[1] as a single- or two-dose regimen of 200 μg/kg/dose can be used. Aggressive treatment with ivermectin at a single dose of 200 μg/kg, repeated after 2 weeks with or without topical 5% permethrin cream (two applications, 1 week apart) and keratolytics (5% salicylic acid ointment[1] applied twice daily) is the treatment of choice for crusted scabies. All sexual and close personal and household contacts within the preceding 6 weeks should be treated simultaneously. Bedding and clothing should be decontaminated (i.e., machine washed and dried using the hot cycle or dry cleaned) or removed from body contact for at least 3 days, because the mite dies when separated from the human host.

Pediculosis

Pediculosis (i.e., lice) is a contagious dermatosis, caused by lice, which are blood-sucking, wingless insects and are obligate human parasites. Two species of lice infest humans causing three clinical forms of infestation: *Pediculus humanus capitis* (i.e., head louse), *Pediculus humanus corporis* (i.e., body louse), and *Phthirus pubis* (i.e., pubic louse). The body louse is the only louse that can carry human disease, including rickettsioses and epidemic typhus.

Pediculosis Capitis

Pediculosis capitis is caused by *P. humanus capitis*, and it is transmitted by close contact or by fomites with combs, brushes, towels, and hats. It manifests with pruritus (due to the saliva of the louse), excoriations, nape dermatitis, secondary bacterial infection, and cervical and suboccipital lymphadenopathy. Diagnosis is based on identification of lice and eggs or nits on the hair and on fluorescence of nits with Wood's light. Visible nits are deposited on the hair shaft, close to the scalp. After adequate treatment, nits found at 1.0 to 1.5 cm from the scalp are not alive.

Topical pediculicides should be applied according to the package instructions. Treatment includes malathion (Ovide) 0.5% lotion applied for 8 to 12 hours or permethrin (Nix) 1% cream rinse applied to shampooed hair for 10 minutes. A second application with permethrin is recommended 1 week later to kill hatching progeny. Alternatively, pyrethrins with piperidyl butoxide (RID) can be applied and washed off after 10 minutes. Benzyl benzoate 25% solution[6] is mainly a scabicide, but it may also be used as a

---

[1]Not FDA approved for this indication.
[3]Exceeds dosage recommended by the manufacturer.
[10]Available in the United States from the Centers for Disease Control and Prevention.

---

[1]Not FDA approved for this indication.
[6]May be compounded by pharmacists.

pediculicide. Ivermectin lotion 0.5% (Sklice) was approved by the FDA in 2012 for treatment of head lice in persons 6 months of age and older, using a fine-toothed comb. Bedding, clothing, and headgear should be decontaminated (as for scabies) or removed from body contact for 2 weeks. Information for managing head lice can be found at the National Pediculosis Association web site (http://www.headlice.org).

Pediculosis Corporis

Pediculosis corporis (i.e., vagabond's itch) is caused by *P. humanus corporis*, which lives and reproduces in the lining of clothes and leaves the clothing only for feeding from the skin. This disease is usually found among vagabonds. Transmission occurs mainly through contact with contaminated clothing or bedding. Clinical manifestations include pruritus, excoriations, and small, red macules that usually occur on the back. Clothes should be examined carefully for lice.

Treatment is the same as for pediculosis capitis. Dry heat or washing in hot water followed by ironing is effective in killing the lice and their ova in clothing. Items that cannot be washed should be removed from body contact for 2 weeks.

Pediculosis Pubis

Pediculosis pubis is caused by *P. pubis* and affects the pubic hair. However, if left untreated, it may also affect very hairy regions of the chest, abdomen, axillary region, and especially in children, the eyelashes, edge of the scalp, and eyebrows. Patients present with pruritus. Useful diagnostic signs include small, blue-gray macules on the trunk, thighs, and axillae (i.e., taches bleuâtres or maculae ceruleae) due to conversion of bilirubin to biliverdin by the saliva of the louse and a brown "dust" found on underclothing due to the excreta of the insects. *P. pubis* is transmitted mainly by sexual contact, but it also may be transmitted by clothing or from parents to children.

Patients with pubic lice should be evaluated for other sexually transmitted diseases. Treatment of pediculosis pubis is the same as for pediculosis capitis. Bedding and clothing should be decontaminated (as for scabies) or removed from body contact for 2 weeks. Attention should be paid to treating sexual partners within the previous month because they are a common cause of reinfestation. For infested eyelashes and eyebrows, ophthalmic-grade petrolatum ointment may be used two to four times daily for 10 days, and lice and nits should be carefully removed from the eyelashes with forceps.

References

Centers for Disease Control (CDC): Disease exposure while traveling, Available at: http://www.cdc.gov/travel/ (accessed August 15, 2014).
Centers for Disease Control (CDC): Leishmaniasis, Available at: http://www.cdc.gov/parasites/leishmaniasis/health_professionals/index.html#tx (accessed March 1, 2015).
Centers for Disease Control: Malathion, Available at: http://www.cdc.gov/parasites/lice/head/gen_info/faqs_malathion.html (accessed March 1, 2015).
Gorkiewicz-Petkow A: Scabicides and pediculicides. In Katsambas AD, Lotti TM, editors: *European Handbook of Dermatological Treatments*, 2nd ed., Berlin, 2003, Springer, pp 775–779.
Goyal NN, Wong GA: Psoriasis or crusted scabies, *Clin Exp Dermatol* 33:211–212, 2008.
Heukelbach J, Feldmeier H: Epidemiological and clinical characteristics of hookworm-related cutaneous larva migrans, *Lancet Infect Dis* 8:302–309, 2008.
Klaus SN, Frankenburg S, Dhar AD: Leishmaniasis and other protozoan infections. In Freedeberg IM, Eisen AZ, Wolff K, et al, editors: *Fitzpatrick's Dermatology in General Medicine*, 6th ed., New York, 2003, McGraw-Hill, pp 2215–2224.
Lucchina LC, Wilson ME: Cysticercosis and other helminthic infections. In Freedeberg IM, Eisen AZ, Wolff K, et al, editors: *Fitzpatrick's Dermatology in General Medicine*, 6th ed., New York, 2003, McGraw-Hill, pp 2225–2259.
Paller AS, Mancini AJ: Bites and infestations. In *Hurwitz Clinical Pediatric Dermatology*, 3rd ed., Philadelphia, 2006, Saunders, pp 479–501.
Stone SP: Scabies and pediculosis. In Freedeberg IM, Eisen AZ, Wolff K, et al, editors: *Fitzpatrick's Dermatology in General Medicine*, 6th ed., New York, 2003, McGraw-Hill, pp 2283–2289.
Tsoureli-Nikita E, Campanile G, Hautmann G, et al: Pediculosis. In Katsambas AD, Lotti TM, editors: *European Handbook of Dermatological Treatments*, 2nd ed., Berlin, 2003, Springer, pp 775–779.
Wadowski L, Balasuriya L, Harper HN, et al: Lice update: new solutions to an old problem, *Clin Dermatol* 33:347–354, 2015.

Method of

Rebat M. Halder, MD; and Ahmad Reza Hossani-Madani, MD, MS

CURRENT DIAGNOSIS

Hyperpigmentation

- Ephelides: Multiple, small (1–4 mm), light to dark brown macules with poorly defined margins that occur on sun-exposed areas of the body
- Solar lentigines: Light brown to dark brown macular hyperpigmented lesions that are induced by natural or artificial sources of radiation and that can coalesce; they are located on face, neck, forearms, and hands
- Melasma: Arcuate or polycyclic light to dark brown macules that coalesce into patches on face, neck, or forearms
- Postinflammatory hyperpigmentation: Dark patches or macules with indistinct margins at the location of an inciting inflammatory event

Hypopigmentation

- Pityriasis alba: two to three round, well-defined, pale macules with overlying powdery white scales, ranging in size from 0.5 to 5 cm in diameter, that transition to smooth, hypopigmented macules
- Vitiligo: Sharply demarcated, depigmented, milky white macules in a localized or generalized distribution
- Idiopathic guttate hypomelanosis: Multiple circular, smooth, small macules that are porcelain white, with occasional black dots, found on sun-exposed areas of upper and lower extremities
- Postinflammatory hypopigmentation: Off-white or tan macules, with ill-defined borders at the site of an inciting inflammatory event

CURRENT THERAPY

Hyperpigmentation

- Ephelides: Hydroquinone 4% (Epiquin Micro, Lustra) or glycolic plus kojic acid combination (Brown Spot Night Gel) plus maximum UVA-blocking sunscreen in the morning and tretinoin 0.025% cream (Retin-A)[1] in the evening
- Solar lentigines: Hydroquinone 4% (Epiquin Micro, Lustra) plus tretinoin 0.05% cream (Retin-A)[1] in the evening; cryotherapy; laser therapy
- Melasma: Monotherapy with hydroquinone 4% twice daily or tretinoin 0.05% in the evening; double therapy with hydroquinone 4% twice daily plus tretinoin 0.05% in the evening; triple therapy with fluocinolone acetonide 0.01% plus hydroquinone 4% plus tretinoin 0.05% (Tri-Luma Cream) in the evening
- Postinflammatory hyperpigmentation: Treat inciting event; hydroquinone 4% alone or in combination with topical steroid.

Hypopigmentation

- Pityriasis alba: Emollients, lubricants, sunscreen; tacrolimus 0.1% ointment (Protopic)[1] twice daily or mild nonhalogenated steroid for face and medium potency steroid for body; phototherapy (PUVA or UVB) for extensive disease
- Vitiligo: In patients with less than 20% body surface area (BSA) involvement, treat with cosmetics, topical (potent or very potent steroid or calcineurin inhibitor trial for less than 2 months), topical PUVA, or excimer laser. If local treatment fails, the surgical approach may be used if the patient has less than 20% BSA involvement. For patients with more than

Definition

The word *chromophore* is defined as elements that impart color to the skin. Hyperchromias describe abnormally darker skin, and hypochromias describe abnormally lighter skin. Pigmentation refers to melanotic causes of skin color change, differentiating it from skin color changes due to blood, carotene, bilirubin, or other causes. Hyperpigmentation refers to an increase in melanin production, melanocyte number, or both in the skin. Hypopigmentation refers to decrease of melanin, melanocytes, or both in the skin. Depigmentation refers to the absence of both melanin and melanocytes. Deposition of melanin in the epidermal layers visibly appears as a yellow to brownish hue. Dermal deposition appears as blue or blue-gray, with mixed epidermal and dermal melanin deposition appearing gray or blue-brown.

Evaluation

A thorough history and visual inspection of the pigmentary disorder can provide useful clues to the diagnosis, particularly recognition of pigmentary patterns (diffuse, circumscribed, linear, or reticulated). Further examination may be achieved by using the Wood's lamp to differentiate epidermal from dermal melanin.

General Recommendations for All Pigmentary Disorders

Broad-spectrum sunscreen with an SPF of 30 is recommended, in addition to wearing protective clothing. Avoiding prolonged sun exposure is also desired, if possible.

Hyperpigmentation

Ephelides

Description

Ephelides (freckles) are multiple, small (1–4 mm), light to dark brown macules with poorly defined margins that occur on sun-exposed areas of the body (face, upper back, arms). They are more commonly found in children (fading with age), fair-skinned persons, and those with red or blonde hair (especially those of Celtic ancestry). A relationship has been shown between painful sunburns in youth and development of ephelides, and the macules become darker with greater UV exposure. They are thought to be genetic in origin, following an autosomal dominant pattern, and are strongly associated with variants in the melanocortin-1-receptor (MC1R). Ephelides are significant because they are associated with an increased risk of melanoma and nonmelanoma skin cancer, perhaps serving as a marker for sun susceptibility.

Treatment

Although treatment is not necessary, modalities include either hydroquinone 4% (Epiquin Micro, Lustra) or glycolic plus kojic acid combination (Brown Spot Night Gel) plus maximum ultraviolet A (UVA)-blocking sunscreen in the morning and tretinoin 0.1% cream (Retin-A)[1] in the evening. Other therapies have included cryotherapy, lasers, and chemical peels.

[1]Not FDA approved for this indication.

Solar Lentigo (Lentigo Senilis Et Actinicus)

Description

Solar lentigines are pigmented spots that share morphologic similarities with ephelides, making differentiation difficult. They are defined as light brown to dark brown macular hyperpigmented lesions induced by natural or artificial sources of radiation, which can coalesce. The incidence increases with age, and more than 90% of white persons older than 50 years demonstrate lesions. They appear most often on the face, neck, forearms, and hands. They can occur in nonclassic locations in those receiving phototherapy (such as the penis). Histologically, they differ from ephelides by the presence of epidermal hyperplasia, increased melanocyte number, and elongation of the rete ridges.

Treatment

Although treatment is not necessary, two different modalities have been used: physical therapies and topical therapies. Physical therapies include cryotherapy and lasers, and topical treatments include retinoids or combinations of agents. Liquid nitrogen may be used with a cotton swab for 5 to 10 seconds to induce lightening. Recurrence rates may be as high as 55% at 6 months. Side effects include atrophy with longer cryoprobe application, postinflammatory hyper- or hypopigmentation, and pain. The Q-switched Nd:YAG (532 nm) laser, among others, has been used with success.

Melasma

Description

Melasma is a hypermelanosis of the face, neck, and forearms that occurs with a higher incidence in women of African American, Latin American, and Asian descent. It appears on sun-exposed areas as arcuate or polycyclic macules that coalesce into patches. Epidermal melanin deposition causes a brownish appearance, and dermal melanin appears bluish. Combined epidermal and dermal melanin deposition appears gray. It is distributed in a central facial (65%), malar (20%), or mandibular (15%) pattern. It is more commonly seen in women and those with darker skin, but it can also be found in men. Contributing factors include a genetic predisposition, pregnancy, oral contraceptive use, endocrine dysfunction, hormonal treatment, UV light exposure, cosmetics, and phototoxic drugs.

Treatment

First-line treatment for melasma consists of broad-spectrum sunscreen with greater than SPF 30 coverage in addition to monotherapy with hydroquinone 4% twice daily or tretinoin 0.1% once daily. Double therapy with hydroquinone 4% twice daily plus tretinoin 0.05% may prove efficacious after an unsuccessful trial of monotherapy. If that fails, triple therapy may be attempted, with fluocinolone acetonide 0.01%, hydroquinone 4%, and tretinoin 0.05% (Tri-Luma) once daily being effective. Side effects of triple therapy include erythema, desquamation, burning, dryness, and pruritus at the site of application; telangiectasia; perioral dermatitis; acne breakouts; and hyperpigmentation. Chemical peels, superficial and medium depth, and Q-switched 1064 nm Nd:YAG laser may also be used for patients whose topical treatments have failed.

Postinflammatory Hyperpigmentation

Description

Postinflammatory hyperpigmentation is a very common condition that occurs as a result of a previous or ongoing inflammatory process, most commonly acne vulgaris, atopic dermatitis, infections, and phototoxic reactions and as a result of treatment with topical medications, chemical peels, and lasers. Postinflammatory hyperpigmentation occurs more commonly in persons with darker skin pigmentation and appears as dark patches or macules with indistinct margins at the location of the inciting inflammatory event.

Treatment

Primary treatment is aimed at treating the inciting cause of the hyperpigmentation. Additional effective therapies include 4% hydroquinone alone or in combination with a topical steroid.

Combination treatment includes fluocinolone acetonide 0.01%, hydroquinone 4%, tretinoin 0.05% (Tri-Luma)[1] once daily. Treatment must be temporarily stopped if irritation occurs. Broad-spectrum sunscreen should also be employed.

Hypopigmentation or Depigmentation

Pityriasis Alba

Description

Pityriasis alba is a childhood or adolescent condition that affects all races. It begins as an erythematous macule with ill-defined borders. The erythema fades after a few weeks, leaving two or three round, well-defined, paler macules with overlying powdery white scale, ranging in size from 0.5 cm to 5 cm in diameter. These eventually transition to smooth, hypopigmented lesions, which are generally located on the face. The pathogenesis of this disorder is unknown.

Treatment

Pityriasis alba is thought to be a self-limited skin disease. However, general treatment guidelines include use of emollients and lubricant, use of sunscreen, and decreasing sun exposure. Lesions limited to the face may be treated with hydrocortisone 1%[1] or other mild, nonfluorinated steroid. More potent steroids may be used for lesions on the body, including hydrocortisone valerate 0.2% (Westcort)[1] or alclometasone dipropionate 0.05% (Aclovate)[1]. However, these can lead to atrophy if used over an extended period. Newer, safer, effective alternatives include tacrolimus 0.1% ointment (Protopic)[1] twice daily. Side effects include a burning sensation that fades over time. Extensive disease that is not amenable to topical therapy might benefit from photochemotherapy (psoralen plus UVA [PUVA] or UVB alone).

Vitiligo

Description

Persons with vitiligo acquire sharply demarcated, depigmented macules in a localized or generalized distribution. These macules appear milky white as compared with the surrounding normally pigmented skin. Lesions can increase in size. There is no predilection for race or sex, and three-quarters of patients generally present before the age of 30 years.

Treatment

General recommendations include the use of sunscreen, avoidance of the sun, and use of protective clothing. Treatments for localized vitiligo (<20% of body surface area) include cosmetics, a 2-month trial of topical treatment (potent or very potent corticosteroid or calcineurin inhibitor), excimer laser, or topical PUVA. Adults who have failed treatments for localized vitiligo may be considered for narrow-band UVB, oral PUVA, or surgical treatment, which includes split-skin grafting, transfer of suction blisters, or autologous epidermal suspensions added to dermabraded skin (followed by UVB). Surgical candidates should have localized, limited involvement and should not demonstrate lesion enlargement or Koebner phenomenon for 12 months prior to treatment. Patients with more than 20% body involvement may be considered for narrow-band UVB (311 nm) or oral PUVA. Those with greater than 50% body involvement or disfiguring facial involvement may be considered for complete depigmentation with monobenzyl ether of hydroquinone 20% (monobenzone 20% [Benoquin]). Children are generally not offered surgical treatment, and oral PUVA is relatively contraindicated in children younger than 10 years.

Idiopathic Guttate Hypomelanosis

Description

This is an acquired, asymptomatic leukoderma with multiple, circular, smooth, small macules that have a porcelain white color.

---

[1]Not FDA approved for this indication.

Black dots are occasionally observed within the macules. The macules increase in number with age, but they generally do not increase in size. They are most commonly located on sun-exposed areas of the upper and lower extremities.

Treatment

Treatments have included cryotherapy, dermabrasion, surgical minigrafting, and intralesional steroids; however, none of these have shown consistent acceptable results. Phototherapy has not been shown to be effective.

Postinflammatory Hypopigmentation

Description

Postinflammatory hypopigmentation is the result of an inciting inflammatory event leading to lesions that are off-white or tan, with ill-defined borders. This entity is noticed more commonly in those with darker skin.

Treatment

Hypopigmentation resolves with treatment of the underlying condition. Topical cosmetics may be useful. Topical corticosteroids tacrolimus 0.1% ointment (Protopic)[1] and topical PUVA therapy may also be used in patients who have lesions in cosmetically distressing areas.

---

[1]Not FDA approved for this indication.

References

Cestari T, Arellano I, Hexsel D, Ortonne JP: Melasma in Latin America: option for therapy and treatment algorithm, *J Eur Acad Dermatol Venereol* 23:760–772, 2009.

Gupta AK, Gover MD, Nouri K, Taylor S: The treatment of melasma: a review of clinical trials, *J Am Acad Dermatol* 55:1048–1065, 2006.

Halder RM, Richards GM: Management of dyschromias in ethnic skin, *Dermatol Ther* 17:151–157, 2004a.

Halder RM, Richards GM: Topical agents used in the management of hyperpigmentation, *Skin Therapy Lett* 9:1–3, 2004b.

Hexsel DM: Treatment of idiopathic guttate hypomelanosis by localized superficial dermabrasion, *Dermatol Surg* 25:917–918, 1999.

Lin RL, Janniger CK: Pityriasis alba, *Cutis* 76:21–24, 2005.

Nordlund JJ, Boissy RE, Hearing VJ, et al, editors: *The Pigmentary System: Physiology and Pathophysiology*, ed 2nd, Malden, MA, 2007, Blackwell Publishing.

Nordlund JJ, Cestari TF, Chan F, Westerhof W: Confusions about color: a classification of discolorations of the skin, *Br J Dermatol* 156(Suppl. 1):S3–S6, 2007.

Ortonne JP, Pandya AG, Lui H, Hexsel D: Treatment of solar lentigines, *J Am Acad Dermatol* 54:S262–S271, 2006.

Ploysangam T, Dee-Ananlap S, Suvanprakorn P: Treatment of idiopathic guttate hypolemanosis with iquid nitrogen: light and electron microscopic studies, *J Am Acad Dermatol* 23:681–684, 1990.

Rigopoulos D, Gregoriou S, Charissi C, et al: Tacrolimus ointment 0.1% in pityriasis alba: an open-label randomized, placebo-controlled study, *Br J Dermatol* 155:152–155, 2006.

Taylor SC, Burgess CM, Callender VD, et al: Postinflammatory hyperpigmentation: evolving combination treatment strategies, *Cutis* 78:S6–S19, 2006.

PREMALIGNANT SKIN LESIONS

Method of
Daniel Stulberg, MD; and Katarzyna Wilamowska, MD, PhD

 CURRENT DIAGNOSIS

Actinic Keratoses
- Scaly white or flesh-colored lesions often with palpably rough surface
- Individuals with light skin and hair color are at high risk
- Most common on face, hands, and sun-exposed skin

Actinic Cheilitis
- Scale, thickening or fissures on the lips
- Lower lip more commonly involved than upper lip

Porokeratoses
- Macular lesions with slight scale or rice-paper appearance and hyperkeratotic border
- Disseminated superficial actinic porokeratoses (DSAP) predominant type–autosomal dominant transmission

Human Papillomavirus Disease
- Verrucous or papular flesh-colored lesions
- Genital, perineal, perirectal, or oral locations are at risk of malignancy

Atypical Nevi
- Multiple irregularly pigmented nevi in the familial atypical mole and melanoma syndrome
- Numerous, often raised nevi, especially with shades of red, brown, and black

CURRENT THERAPY

Actinic Keratoses or Cheilitis
- Cryosurgery first line if limited number of lesions
- Topical medications for extensive actinic change with multiple lesions
- 5-fluorouracil (Carac, Efudex) typically 2–3 weeks, although multiple protocols/variations
- Diclofenac sodium (Solaraze) longer protocol, less effective
- Imiquimod (Aldara, Zyclara) longer protocol, less effective
- Ingenol mebutate (Picato) 3-day course limited by maximum of 25-cm² treatment area and expense of medication
- Less commonly, laser, curettage, retinoids, photosensitizing medications followed by light therapy

Porokeratoses
- See treatment options for actinic keratoses

Actinic keratoses are the most common precancerous skin lesions seen in usual practice. If untreated, it is estimated that from 0.1% to 10% of these lesions will progress to squamous cell carcinoma that requires significantly more aggressive treatment. Fortunately, effective treatment is available, although it can cause significant discomfort. Risk factors for developing actinic keratoses are similar to those of developing basal cell carcinoma (BCC), squamous cell carcinoma (SCC), and, to a certain extent, melanoma skin cancer. These risk factors include lighter skin colors, family history of actinic keratoses or nonmelanoma skin cancer, exposure to sunlight, ultraviolet radiation, use of tanning beds, and immunosuppression from disease, or immunosuppressant medications to prevent organ transplant rejection.

There are several other conditions or situations that can increase risk of precancerous and cancerous skin lesions. The first is arsenic. This is rare in developed countries and, other than avoiding arsenic exposures, is treated as outlined below for actinic keratoses. The human papilloma virus (HPV) can lead to papillomatous lesions and genital and oropharyngeal. Individuals with the familial atypical mole and melanoma syndrome (FAMMS), previously called atypical nevus syndrome, have multiple abnormal-appearing nevi and a family history of melanoma. Patients with atypical nevi and more than one first-degree relative with melanoma have a risk of melanoma approaching 100%.

Actinic keratoses should be treated to reduce the risk of progression to squamous cell carcinoma unless the patient has a limited life expectancy and the clinician determines that, based on the condition of the patient and their comorbidities, the discomfort of treatment would outweigh the benefits for the patient. Avoiding sun exposure and using broad-brimmed hats, sunscreen, and protective clothing while outdoors can reduce the risk of additional lesions. Unfortunately, because of the long lead time between sun exposure and onset of disease, most patients

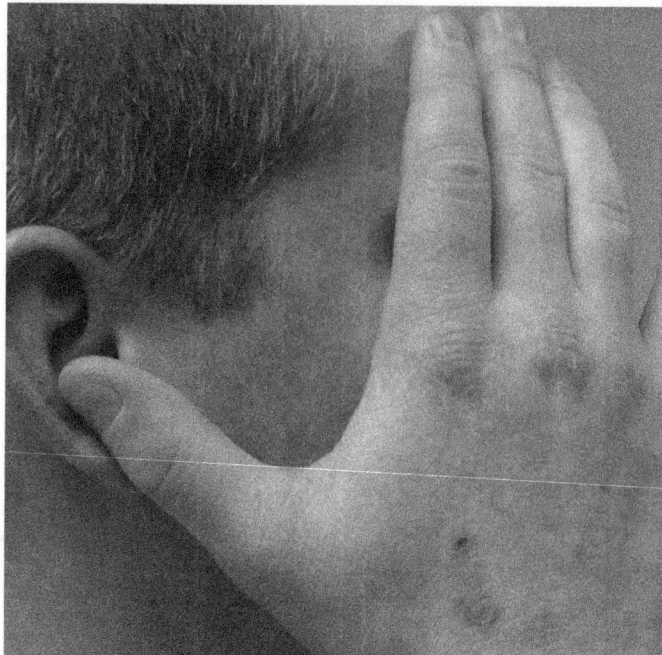

Figure 1 Early onset of actinic keratoses in young man with high-risk skin type.

will continue to develop more actinic keratoses due to the underlying skin damage. Patients should be counseled regarding the occurrence of additional precancerous and cancerous skin lesions and should be examined every 6 to 12 months, or even more frequently depending on the amount of disease burden, their individual risk factors, and clinical judgment.

There are several rare inherited genetic disorders that predispose patients to precancerous and cancerous cutaneous lesions, grouped under genodermatoses. Xeroderma pigmentosum (XP) is an autosomal recessive disorder where homozygotes have severe sun sensitivity due to inability to repair sun-damaged DNA, leading to development of BCCs, SCCs, and melanomas in early childhood. Basal cell nevus syndrome, another autosomal dominant disorder, is characterized by developmental anomalies and tumors, especially BCCs, starting in the fourth decade of life. Oculocutaneous albinism results from a group of autosomal recessive disorders of melanin biosynthesis. This deficiency leads to reduced or absent pigmentation of skin, hair, and eyes, leading to early photodamage.

Nevus sebaceous presents as a waxy yellow or brown congenital plaque or plaques. Around the time of puberty the plaque can thicken and develop into benign or, less commonly, malignant tumors. In addition to these specific disorders, patients with chronic ulceration, burn scars, radiation therapy fields, and inflammatory conditions including discoid lupus, lichen planus, lichen sclerosis, and lymphedema are at risk of developing skin cancers in affected areas.

Actinic Keratoses and Actinic Cheilitis
Clinical Manifestations
Actinic keratoses (AKs) are an abnormal proliferation of keratinocytes and a precursor of squamous cell carcinoma. Over time, 0.1% to 10% of the lesions will progress to squamous cell carcinoma. AKs present as rough or scaly white or flesh-colored lesions, often with a slightly erythematous base (Figure 1). A combination of visual inspection of the skin and tactile examination is useful to diagnose these lesions. Often they are easier to identify by gently palpating the patient's skin for their characteristic rough surface on sun-exposed areas. If there is significant underlying erythematous thickened tissue, the clinician should consider whether the lesion has already progressed to squamous cell carcinoma, and potentially proceed with biopsy (Figure 2). Patients frequently note that they have scratched off a lesion but

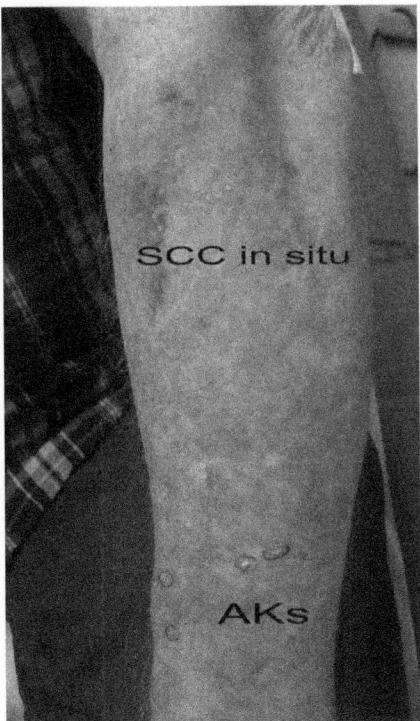

Figure 2 Sun-damaged skin with multiple actinic keratoses and squamous cell carcinoma in situ, a.k.a. Bowens disease.

Figure 3 Treating multiple actinic keratoses with cryosurgery.

Figure 4 BID 5- fluorouracil at 3 weeks.

it returns over time, and many patients who have had multiple AKs become very adept at pointing them out to their clinician.

Actinic cheilitis is the same precancerous process when it occurs on the lips. It is more common on the lower lip, which catches the sun's rays more directly. The lip becomes rough, or the patient notes that it is always chapped. Dyshidrotic chapped lips can be in the differential diagnosis. A trial of topical lip balm may be initiated, and if the rough surface does not resolve, actinic cheilitis is the likely diagnosis. If there is ulceration or significant thickening of the lip, biopsy should be performed because of the possibility of squamous cell carcinoma of the lip.

Treatment

For patients with a limited number of lesions, destruction with cryosurgery is a quick and effective treatment with success rates generally above 95%. Cryosurgery can be performed using a variety of tools. Liquid nitrogen spray devices provide the coldest temperatures and fastest treatment in clinical practice. Other useful options include nitrous oxide spray devices, evaporative refrigerant liquids, mechanically cooled metal probes via refrigerant technology or compressed nitrous oxide or carbon dioxide devices or using a swab dipped in liquid nitrogen. Treatment protocols vary based on the instrument. For liquid nitrogen spray, there are multiple sized apertures available and freezing protocols based on clinician preference and lesion size. One protocol is to hold the spray tip 1 to 2 cm from the AK, spray until the lesion is frozen and keep frozen for 6 seconds, allow the lesion to thaw, and repeat the cycle. For clinical efficiency it is useful to treat several lesions in succession to allow the earlier lesions to thaw before repeating the freeze (Figure 3). Counsel the patient that the cold spray does cause discomfort and even feels like a burning or stinging sensation. After treatment, the lesions typically become erythematous, have slight swelling, and sometimes will blister. If they blister, topical petrolatum and an adhesive bandage may be used to protect the healing wound. If lesions do not resolve after adequate cryosurgery, consider biopsy for possible squamous cell carcinoma, which will require more aggressive treatment. Patient discomfort of cryosurgery varies. Most individuals will tolerate up to 15 lesions, although some patients will only tolerate cryosurgery of a few lesions, and some will

tolerate treatment of dozens of lesions. Patients can return for additional cryosurgery on subsequent visits, or, if they have a very high density of lesions, topical agents may be more efficient to treat large areas with multiple lesions. The lips can be treated with cryosurgery or topical agents for actinic cheilitis. Because of the risk of swelling and discomfort, a lighter freeze protocol may be useful for the lips.

Topical chemotherapy with 5-fluorouracil (Carac, Efudex) has been used to treat AKs successfully for decades. It is particularly useful for field or blanket therapy in patients with multiple lesions and is very effective in clearing more than 90% of the lesions in treated areas. There are multiple variations in treatment protocols, and it is manufactured in 0.5% and 5% topical creams and 2% and 5% topical solutions. One option is to apply 5% 5-fluorouracil to the affected areas twice daily for 2 weeks until there is significant inflammation, often erosions and exudate (Figures 4 and 5). If there has been no reaction, the treatment can be extended out to 3 weeks. There is significant discomfort with this treatment protocol, which can be lessened by not treating the patient's entire affected areas all at once. Starting with treatment of one forearm and allowing that to heal before proceeding to

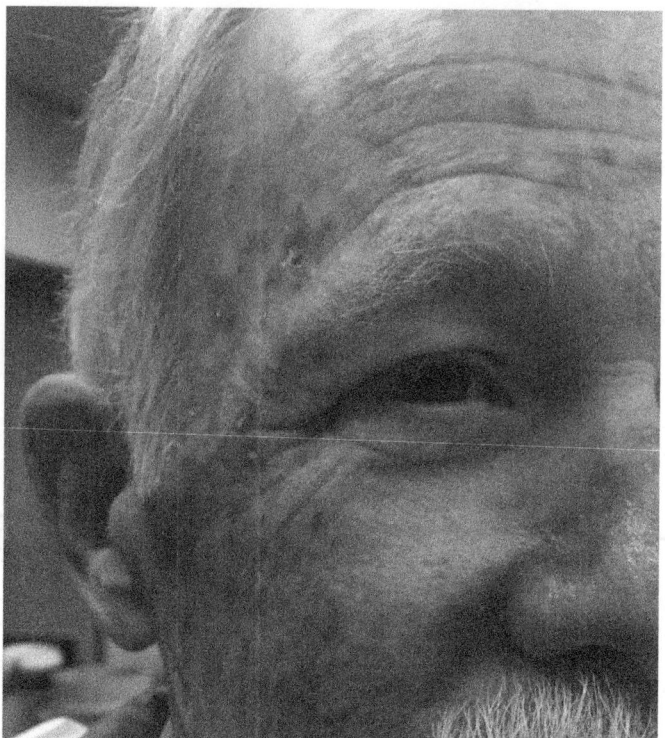

Figure 5 Daily 5-fluorouracil at 5 weeks.

Figure 6 Porokeratosis with rice-paper appearance and peripheral ridge a.k.a. cornoid lamella.

the next forearm can be a useful way of starting and allowing the patient to get some familiarity with its use before starting it on a portion of their face or scalp. Treating the entire face or scalp can be very uncomfortable, so treating only one portion at a time and waiting until that heals before treating another area may be helpful. Because of photo sensitivity and increased risk of sunburn, it is preferable to perform treatment during the winter months or use strict sun avoidance. The 0.5% 5-fluorouracil formulation may be better tolerated on the lips for actinic cheilitis. Patients should be counseled to expect significant inflammation. It may also be useful to advise them that as a topical chemotherapy, this medication targets the lesions and typically does not cause inflammation of unaffected skin.

Because of the amount of inflammation with 5-fluorouracil, other topical treatments have been developed. They cause less inflammation but unfortunately also have lower efficacy rates. These other treatments include topical imiquimod (Aldara, Zylara), diclofenac (Solaraze), and ingenol mebutate (Picato). Imiquimod is used at bedtime twice a week for 16 weeks. Diclofenac is used twice daily for 8 to 12 weeks and is typically better tolerated. Both of these are less effective than topical 5-fluorouracil. Ingenol mebutate is used once daily for only 3 days. Its use is limited currently by its high cost and only being approved to use for 25 cm², approximately a 2″ × 2″ area, which is extremely small compared with the large amount of skin usually affected by AKs and an efficacy of less than 50%.

Outside of typical primary care practices, several other options exist. Photodynamic therapy can be used after a sensitizing application of aminolevulinic acid (Levulan) or methyl aminolevulinate (Metvixia). Nonselective chemical peels, dermabrasion, and ablative lasers can be used for field therapy to an entire area, treating both lesions and unaffected skin in the treatment field. Individual lesions may be treated with laser, trichloroacetic acid (Tri-Chlor),[1] or curettage.

Nicotinamide[1,7] 500 mg orally BID has been shown to reduce the rate of developing additional lesions in patients already affected by actinic keratoses. The medication needs to be continued to maintain its effect.

[1] Not FDA approved for this indication.
[7] Available as a dietary supplement.

Porokeratoses

Clinical Manifestations

Although much less common than actinic keratoses, porokeratoses also have malignant potential. Disseminated superficial actinic porokeratoses, like AKs, present on sun-exposed areas. They usually present as atrophic or rice-paper–appearing lesions surrounded by a slightly raised border (Figure 6). The plaque form (i.e., Mibelli's porokeratosis) is large and progressive, and the linear type may be generalized or segmental. Both of these types often manifest very early in life. Malignant transformation occurs mostly commonly in the linear type, followed by the Mibelli type. It is rare in the disseminated type and has not been reported in the punctate type.

Treatment

Disseminated superficial porokeratosis can be treated with locally destructive methods as outlined above for actinic keratoses and surgical excision.

Management of Complications

Treatment with cryosurgery is expected to cause local inflammation including possible vesicles and erosions. Topical petrolatum under an adhesive dressing or applied multiple times per day if used without a dressing can facilitate moist wound healing. Cryosurgery can cause hypopigmentation, which can be cosmetically distressing for patients with darker skin types and can predispose to sunburn in any skin type. Inflammation from topical medications for actinic keratoses can be soothed by application of petrolatum. Secondary infections, impetigo, and cellulitis are uncommon but possible after cryosurgery or inflammation associated with topical products. Antibiotics to cover methicillin-resistant *Staphylococcus aureus* and *Streptococcus spp.*, should be prescribed if needed. Reactivation of herpes labialis can occur when treating the lips. Prophylactic antiviral therapy may reduce the risk of an outbreak in patients with history of herpes labialis.

References

Ameluz for actinic keratoses: *Med Lett Drugs Ther* 58(1509):155–156, 2016.

Bolognia JL, Jorizzo J, Schaffer JV, editors: *Dermatology*, New York, 2012, Elsevier.

Damian DL: Nicotinamide for skin cancer chemoprevention, *Australas J Dermatol* 58:174–180, 2017.

de Berker D, McGregor JM, Hughes BR: British Association of Dermatologists Therapy Guidelines and Audit Subcommittee. guidelines for the management of actinic keratoses, *Br J Dermatol* 156:222–230, 2007.

James WD, Berger TG, Elston DM, editors: *Andrews' Diseases of the Skin—Clinical Dermatology, 11th ed*, Philadelphia, 2011, Saunders.

Martin G: The impact of the current United States guidelines on the management of actinic keratosis: is it time for an update? *J Clin Aesthet Dermatol* 3(11):20–25, 2010.

Philipp-Dormston WG, Müller K, Novak B, et al: NMSC-QoL Study Group:Patient-reported health outcomes in patients with non-melanoma skin cancer and actinic keratosis: results from a large-scale observational study analyzing effects of diagnoses and disease progression, *J Eur Acad Dermatol Venereol*. 2017 Nov 17.

Poulin Y, Lynde CW, Barber K, et al: Canadian non-Melanoma Skin Cancer Guidelines Committee. Non-melanoma skin cancer in Canada Chapter 3: Management of Actinic Keratoses, *J Cutan Med Surg* 19:227–238, 2015.

Wood GS, Gunkel J, Stewart D, et al: Nonmelanoma skin cancers. In Abeloff MD, Armitage JO, Niederhuber JE, Kastan MB, editors: *Abeloff's Clinical Oncology*, 4th ed, Philadelphia, 2008, Churchill Livingstone.

PRESSURE INJURY

Method of
Rebecca M. Wester, MD

CURRENT DIAGNOSIS

- In April 2016, the National Pressure Ulcer Advisory Panel redefined the definition: pressure injury replaces the terms "pressure ulcer," "decubitus ulcer," and "bed sores."
- Pressure injury develops from pathologic changes in combination with localized skin and underlying soft tissue damage, typically over a bony prominence or associated with a medical device. Skin can be intact or have an open ulcer.

CURRENT THERAPY

- Treatment is based on the stage and characteristics of the pressure injury.
- Nutrition and pressure relief are important interventions.
- Host-specific factors have profound effects on the healing process and have a greater influence than what is put on the wound.

Epidemiology

Most pressure injuries develop during acute hospitalizations, in spite of the adoption of national pressure ulcer prevention guidelines. Prevalence rates for pressure injuries have changed little over the past two decades. Hospitalized patients in intensive care or undergoing cardiovascular or hip surgery have higher rates.

End-stage skin failure occurs when hypoperfusion occurs at the end of life. The prevalence of pressure injuries is 11% to 18% for palliative care patients, nearly double in comparison with hospital rates. Pressure injuries impose a significant burden, not only on the patient but also on the entire health care system. To put it into perspective, the cost of treating 10 pressure injuries is equivalent to 5 knee replacements, 6 hip replacements, 9 pacemakers, or 5 bypass operations.

Risk Factors

External factors that lead to the development of pressure injuries include pressure, shearing forces, friction, and moisture. Interaction of these external factors with host-specific factors such as immobility, sensory loss, incontinence, reduced perfusion, and compromised nutritional status culminates in tissue damage. Decreased skin perfusion resulting from hypotension, anemia, shock, or peripheral artery disease is increasingly recognized as an important cause of pressure ulcers. Other risk factors are cerebrovascular disease, cardiovascular disease, recent lower extremity fractures, medications, and diabetes.

Pressure ulcer risk assessment. The Braden and Norton scales are commonly used for pressure risk assessment. These scales assess risk factors such as physical and mental condition, mobility, moisture, continence, and nutrition. However, they are weak predictors of risk of ulcers and may be no better at reducing risk than clinical judgment.

Pathophysiology

Pressure alone is not sufficient to cause an ulcer; it's the addition of the confounding host-specific factors that ultimately leads to tissue damage. Superficial lesions are primarily the result of moisture and friction. Exposure to moisture in the form of perspiration, urine, or feces can lead to skin maceration. Friction occurs when patients are dragged across an external surface. This results in an abrasion with damage to the most superficial layer of skin. Friction contributes mostly to stage 2 pressure injuries, with limited contributions to stage 3 to 4 pressure injuries because it does not cause the necrotic changes associated with deep tissue injury. Pressure injuries are greatest over bony prominences where weight-bearing points come in contact with external surfaces and immobilization devices. Pressure over a bony prominence tends to result in a cone-shaped distribution, with the most affected tissues located deep, adjacent to the bone–muscle interface. Thus the extent of injury to deep tissues is often much greater than perceived from the visible ulcer on the skin surface. Typically, stage 3 to 4 pressure injuries start as a deep tissue injury that may then progress to the surface. There is little evidence to suggest that a stage 4 pressure injury develops as a gradual progression from stage 1 to stage 4.

Differential Diagnosis

Besides pressure injuries, other chronic skin ulcers are arterial ulcers, venous stasis ulcers, and diabetic ulcers: arterial ulcers occur in distal digits or over bony prominences, venous stasis ulcers occur on the lateral aspect of the lower leg in the setting of chronic edema, and diabetic ulcers occur in regions of callous formations. Traumatic injuries such as abrasions, skin tears, or burns are not pressure injuries; nor are surgical incision sites. Only pressure injuries are staged; never stage a wound that arises from a different etiology.

Diagnosis

Staging is done according to the National Pressure Ulcer Advisory Panel Pressure Injury Staging System:

Stage 1: Nonblanchable erythema of intact skin. May appear differently in darkly pigmented skin. Color changes do not include purple or maroon discoloration; this indicates deep tissue injury.

Stage 2: Partial-thickness skin loss with exposed dermis. The wound bed is viable, pink or red, and moist, and may also present as an intact or ruptured serum-filled blister. Adipose (fat) is not visible and deeper tissues are not visible. Granulation tissue, slough, and eschar are not present. This stage should not be used to describe moisture-associated skin damage (MASD) including incontinence-associated dermatitis (IAD), intertriginous dermatitis (ITD), medical adhesive–related skin injury (MARSI), or traumatic wounds (skin tears, burns, abrasions).

Stage 3: Full-thickness skin loss. Adipose (fat) is visible in the ulcer and granulation tissue and rolled skin edges are often present. Slough or eschar may be visible. The depth of tissue damage varies by anatomic location; areas of significant adiposity can develop deep wounds. Undermining and tunneling may occur. Fascia, muscle, tendon, ligament, cartilage, and bone are not exposed. If slough or eschar obscures the extent of tissue loss, then it is an unstageable pressure injury.

Stage 4: Full-thickness skin and tissue loss. Exposed or directly palpable fascia, muscle, tendon, ligament, cartilage, or bone is in the ulcer. Slough or eschar may be visible. Rolled edges, undermining, and tunneling often occur. Depth varies by anatomic location. If slough or eschar obscures the extent of tissue loss, then it is an unstageable pressure injury.

Unstageable: Obscured full-thickness skin and tissue loss. The extent of tissue damage within the ulcer cannot be determined because it is obscured by slough or eschar. If slough or eschar is removed, a stage 3 or 4 pressure injury will be revealed. Stable eschar (dry, adherent, intact, without erythema or fluctuance) on the heel or ischemic limb should not be softened or removed.

Deep tissue injury: Persistent, nonblanchable, deep red, maroon, or purple discoloration. May appear as a dark wound bed or blood-filled blister. Pain and temperature skin changes often precede skin color changes. Discoloration may appear differently in darkly pigmented skin. The wound may evolve rapidly from intense or prolonged pressure and shear forces at the bone–muscle interface. The wound may evolve rapidly to reveal the actual extent of injury or may resolve without tissue loss. If necrotic tissue, subcutaneous tissue, granulation tissue, fascia, muscle, or other underlying structure is visible, then it is a full-thickness pressure injury (unstageable or stage 3 or 4). Do not use deep tissue injury to describe vascular, traumatic, neuropathic, diabetic, or dermatologic conditions.

Medical device–related pressure injury: Results from the use of devices designed and applied for diagnostic or therapeutic purposes. The resultant pressure injury generally conforms to the pattern or shape of the device. The injury should be staged using the staging system.

Mucosal membrane pressure injury: Found on mucous membranes in patients with a history of a medical device in use at the location of the injury. Owing to the anatomy of the tissue, these ulcers cannot be staged.

Therapy

Pressure relief. Position the patient frequently at fixed intervals to relieve pressure over compromised areas. There is no evidence to suggest an optimal interval at which to reposition patients, although every 2 hours is recommended based on expert opinion. Advanced static support surfaces (mattress overlays and foam, gel, or air mattresses) rather than standardized hospital mattresses should be used to prevent pressure injuries in high-risk patients. Check the pressure-relieving devices for "bottoming out" by inserting your hand (palm up) between the device and the bed under the patient's sacral area. The device is considered ineffective if you are unable to slide your hand freely. For immobile individuals, offload the heels by "floating the heels" with pillows under the patient's legs.

Pain. Dressing changes hurt. Use individualized pain management.

Assessment of nutrition/hydration. Pressure injuries occur in sicker individuals in whom overall intake may be reduced by coexisting illness. If adequate dietary intake is compromised, supplemental vitamins/minerals at the recommended daily allowance (RDA) should be considered. Protein supplementation may improve outcomes in the treatment of pressure ulcers, as per current guidelines. However, a 2014 Cochrane review concluded that there is no clear evidence that nutritional interventions (i.e., dietary supplementation) reduce the number of people who develop pressure injuries or help the healing of existing pressure injuries. There is no evidence to support the use of vitamin C or zinc to treat pressure injuries in patients who are not deficient in these nutrients. There is no difference in healing rates associated with supratherapeutic doses of vitamin C or zinc. The decision to use tube feeding must consider the patient's wishes, overall goal of care, and complications of tube feeding. Recent studies surprisingly observed that the use of tube feedings increased the incidence of pressure injuries and was associated with poorer healing. Tube feeding is associated with agitation, increased use of physical and chemical restraints and worsening of ulcers in individuals with severe dementia.

Removal (débridement) of necrotic tissue. Débridement by any of several methods (Table 1) may improve the time to a clean wound bed, but the effect of débridement on the time to healing remains to be determined.

XIV Diseases of the Skin

1042

TABLE 1	Débridement Methods

Mechanical: Wet-to-dry dressings; removes both devitalized and viable tissues; causes pain
Surgical (sharp): Scalpel, scissors, or forceps to remove devitalized tissue; quick and effective by skilled clinician; should be used when infection is suspected; causes pain
Enzymatic: Topical débriding agent to dissolve the necrotic tissue; appropriate when there are no signs or symptoms of local infection
Autolytic: Synthetic dressing to allow the devitalized tissue to self-digest from the enzymes found in the ulcer fluids; recommended for those who cannot tolerate débridement; may take a long time to be effective; commonly used with palliative wounds
Biosurgery: Larvae to digest devitalized tissue; quick and effective; good option for those who cannot tolerate surgical débridement; limited by access to larvae

TABLE 2	Pressure Injury Dressing Types	
DRESSING	**RECOMMENDATIONS**	
Hydrocolloid	Light to moderate exudate ulcers	
	Clean stage 2 or shallow (noninfected) stage 3 ulcers	
	Consider using filler dressing beneath in deep ulcers to fill dead space	
Transparent film	Partial thickness with minimal exudate ulcers or closed wounds	
	Consider for autolytic débridement	
	Consider as secondary dressing with alginate or other wound filler that will likely remain in the ulcer for an extended time (3–5 days)	
	Do not use on moderately to heavily exudative ulcers	
	Do not use as cover dressing over enzymatic débriding agents	
Hydrogel	Full thickness with minimal or no exudate (stage 3 or 4) ulcers	
	Consider use on shallow, minimally exudate ulcer	
	Consider amorphous hydrogel for granulating noninfected ulcers	
	Consider for dry ulcer beds	
Alginate	Full thickness with moderate to heavy exudate ulcers with cavities (stage 3 or 4)	
	Consider in clinically infected ulcer with concurrent treatment for the infection	
Foams	Exudate stage 2 and shallow stage 3 ulcers	
	Avoid using single small piece pf foam in exudate ulcer with cavities	
	Consider gelling foam in heavily exuding ulcers	
Silver impregnated	Clinically infected or heavily colonized Avoid prolonged use; discontinue when wound infection is controlled	

Promotion of healing (reepithelialization). Pressure injuries should be cleansed with saline or tap water, and slough and necrotic tissue débrided (see Table 1). The choice of a particular dressing depends on the wound characteristics, such as amount of exudate, dead space, or wound infection. A hydrocolloid, foam, or other nonadherent dressing that promotes a moist wound environment should be used (Table 2). Follow manufacturer recommendations regarding frequency of dressing changes.

Monitoring

Measurement. After staging the pressure injury, measure the length, width, and depth of ulcers. Document the presence of exudate, necrotic tissue, eschar, slough, undermining, and tunneling. Presence of healing tissue (pink granulation or epithelialization) should be recorded as well. Measurement frequency depends on the patient's care location, whether it's the hospital, a long-term care facility, or home care.

Infection. All pressure ulcers are colonized with bacteria. Never swab a chronic ulcer. The presence of bacteria alone does not indicate active infection, only colonization. Edema, odor, and purulent discharge are nonspecific. Worsening pain, erythema at wound edges, and warmth are signs of advancing cellulitis. Fever or delirium may be the only signs of infection. Systemic rather than topical antibiotics should be used to treat an infected pressure ulcer. Consider osteomyelitis when bone is exposed.

References

The cost of pressure injuries. Available at http://www.cobro.co.nz/cms/the cost of pressure injuries [accessed February 14, 2017].

Don't recommend percutaneous feeding tubes in patients with advanced dementia; instead offer oral assisted feeding. Available at http://www.choosingwisely.org [accessed February 14, 2017].

Langer G, Fink A: Nutritional interventions for preventing and treating pressure ulcers, *Cochrane Database Syst Rev* 6, 2014:CD003216.

Lyder CH: *Pressure ulcers and wound care. Geriatric Review Syllabus: A Core Curriculum in Geriatrics Medicine*, ed 8th, New York, 2013, American Geriatrics Society.

National Pressure Ulcer Advisory Panel. Available at http://www.npuap.org [accessed January 3, 2017].

Raetz JG, Wick KH: Common questions about pressure ulcers, *Am Fam Physician* 92(10):888–894, 2015.

Thomas DR: Clinical management of pressure ulcers, *Clin Geriatr Med* 29:397–413, 2013.

Thomas DR: Does pressure cause pressure ulcers? An inquiry into etiology of pressure ulcers, *J Am Med Dir Assoc* 11:397–405, 2010.

PRURITUS ANI AND VULVAE

Method of
Muhammad Ahmad Ghazi, MD

CURRENT DIAGNOSIS

- Anogenital pruritis is primarily idiopathic; most secondary etiologies can be divided into dermatologic, anogenital conditions, and systemic causes.
- Good history and physical examination are important for accurate diagnosis.
- Laboratory tests and procedures to diagnose the cause of pruritis ani and vulvae should be tailored to individual patients based on their presentation.

CURRENT THERAPY

- Initial treatment is usually conservative, and clinicians should focus on reassurance, education about hygienic practices, regular bowel movements, avoidance of moisture and irritants, and a trial of topical corticosteroids.
- Anogenital conditions such as hemorrhoids, fissures, skin tags, and fistulas—if present—must be treated first.
- Pruritus vulvae secondary to lichen planus, lichen sclerosus, and lichen simplex chronicus usually require superpotent topical steroid treatment.
- Refractory cases of pruritus ani may benefit from injectable treatments of methylene blue.[1]
- Suspicious lesions of vulva and perineum that are resistant to initial treatment must be biopsied to rule out malignancy.

[1]Not FDA approved for this indication.

BOX 1	Common Causes of Pruritus Ani

Acute

Idiopathic up to 25% of cases
Fecal contamination:
Poor hygiene
Fecal incontinence
Anal sphincter dysfunction
Anorectal pathology: 10% to 50% of cases
Hemorrhoids, perianal fissures, pilonidal sinus, perianal abscess, rectal prolapse, polyps, and papilloma
Mechanical factors:
Excessive washing, rubbing, synthetic undergarments
Infectious:
Erythrasma (corynebacterium infection), Candida, dermatophytosis, herpes simplex, human papilloma virus, HIV, syphilis
Parasitic:
Scabies, pinworm
Dermatoses:
Allergic or contact dermatitis, psoriasis, drug eruptions
Dietary factors:
Tomatoes, chilis, coffee, beer, soda, dairy, chocolate, tea, citrus fruits

Chronic

Dermatoses:
Allergic or contact dermatitis, psoriasis, lichen planus, lichen simplex chronicus, lichen sclerosis, Hailey-Hailey disease
Inflammatory:
Inflammatory bowel disease (ulcerative colitis and Crohn's disease)
Malignant:
Anal squamous cell cancer
Extramammary Paget's disease
Lymphoma/leukemia
Metabolic:
Diabetes mellitus, chronic liver disease and chronic kidney disease, celiac disease, iron deficiency anemia, hypovitaminosis A, B, D, E
Miscellaneous:
Hyperhidrosis
Neuropathic pruritus
Psychogenic (anxiety related)

Pruritus ani and vulvae is not a disease per se; rather, it is a symptom or manifestation of an underlying disease or the result of poor personal hygienic practices. Pruritus is derived from the Latin *prurire*, which means "to itch." Pruritis ani is literally an unpleasant sensation leading to scratching the skin around the anal opening. Anogenital pruritus is a commonly ignored skin condition. Symptoms range from mild to severe and can be complicated by sleep disturbances, anxiety, depression, and social embarrassment. Pruritus ani and vulvae can be primary, in which case there is no identifiable cause, or be secondary to an underlying condition. Most of the secondary causes are anorectal, including hemorrhoids, fistulas, and fissures. Psoriasis, lichen sclerosus, and lichen simplex chronicus are common secondary dermatological causes of pruritus in the vulvar region.

Epidemiology

Pruritus ani is a common condition with an estimated prevalence of 1% to 5% of the population. It affects all ages and both genders. Male to female prevalence of pruritus ani is about 4:1. Symptoms are worse at night and in warm, moist climates. Pruritus vulvae is seen in women of all ages. Young females usually present with an infectious etiology while the primary disease is more common in postmenopausal women. Genital pruritus in men is rare and usually presents with balanitis.

Risk Factors

Poor personal hygiene, chronic diarrhea, obesity, high-risk sexual behaviors, and immunodeficiency states predispose a person to pruritus in the anogenital area. Heat, sweating, and tight undergarments may exacerbate the condition. A proposed list of causative factors is included in Boxes 1 and 2.

Pathophysiology

The itching sensations of pruritus ani and vulvae are mediated by unmyelinated C fibers, which are distributed densely in the perineal region at the dermal-epidermical junction of the skin. Irritants

BOX 2 | Common Causes of Pruritus Vulvae in Women

PREPUBERTAL AGE

Poor hygiene
Sensitization of vulvar skin: soaps,
    deodorants
Contact dermatitis
Parasitic infestations: Pinworms
    (*Enterobius vermicularis*),
    pediculosis, scabies
Bacterial infections (Group A
    beta hemolytic infections and
    Escherichia coli)
Vaginal candidiasis (rare in this age
    group)
Lichen sclerosis
Suspected child sexual abuse (based
    on evidence of genital trauma)

REPRODUCTIVE AGE

Vaginitis
Trichomonas
Bacterial vaginosis
Candidiasis
Rarely tinea cruris
Herpes simplex type II
HIV, syphilis
Dermatitis
Atopic dermatitis
Contact dermatitis
Psoriasis
Lichen planus
Lichen simplex chronicus
Lichen sclerosis
Seborrheic dermatitis
Pregnancy
Vulvar itching is worsened because of vulvar
    engorgement; pregnancy also predisposes women
    to vaginal discharge and candidiasis
Systemic diseases:
Diabetes, renal and liver diseases
Miscellaneous
Vulvar intraepithelial neoplasia (HPV)
Mechanical trauma
Idiopathic

POSTMENOPAUSAL AGE

Urinary or fecal incontinence
Menopause: Lack of estrogen
    leads to loss of skin elasticity
    and makes it prone to itching
Atrophic vaginitis
Lichen sclerosis
Paget's disease of vulvae
Vaginal malignancy (squamous
    cell cancer)

---

in stool (exotoxins, intestinal lysosymes, endopeptidase, trypsins) and increased alkalinity of certain foods such as tomatoes, chocolate, and caffeine contribute to the perianal itching that precedes scratching. The itch-scratch cycle is mediated by several mechanical and inflammatory mediators, including histamine, kallikrein, bradykinin, trypsin, serotonin, and neuropeptides. The resulting nerve impulse is carried via spinothalamic tract to the thalamus, where the itching sensation is perceived. Intestinal transit time and altered anal sphincter pressure are influenced by certain foods that predispose people to perianal seepage and pruritus.

Pruritus vulvae is the result of increased permeability of the dermis resulting from a structurally thin strateum corneum as compared to the rest of the vulvar skin. Factors aggravating the pruritus include constant friction, rubbing, anatomic location, occlusion, moistness, fear of uncleanliness in women, and excessive washing. The most common cause of pruritus vulvae is vulvar dermatitis or eczema, which affects one-third to half of all women presenting with this complaint. Dermatitis or eczema can be endogenous and the result of familial disposition, and it manifests as atopic dermatitis. Exogenous dermatitis such as contact dermatitis can be allergic, given that a trigger (allergen) might induce an immune response or contact irritant dermatitis. Common irritants include soaps, shampoos, vaginal creams, alcohol, tea tree oil,[7] douches, vaginal hygiene products, vaginal contraceptives, sanitary pads, nylon underwear, and toilet paper. Chemical allergens contributing to contact dermatitis in the genital area include benzocaine, neomycin, ethylenediamide, propylene glycol, latex dyes, nickels, semen, lanolin, perfumes, and tampons.

Clinical Manifestations

Perianal and vulvar itching, erythema, excoriations, fissures, hemorrhoids, pinworms, and fecal incontinence may be noticed on inspection of the perineal area. In the acute phase, skin redness of varying degrees is visible. Excoriations from the skin from itching may be present. Fissures in the labial folds may be present. Superinfection with yeast or bacteria may complicate the presentation.

Chronic anogenital dermatitis usually presents as erythema of varying degrees, and papillae appear in the labial folds. Hypo- or hyperpigmentation of the skin or thickening of the labial skin might develop over time, causing "lichenification," which leads to lichen simplex chronicus.

Diagnosis of Pruritus Ani and Vulvae

A detailed history of bowel habits and personal hygiene (including products used, such as perfumes); dietary habits (e.g., caffeine consumption); and previous medical, psychiatric, and surgical history help elucidate the cause of pruritus ani. The patient should be asked about personal or family history of hives, asthma, conjunctivitis, or atopy when allergic dermatitis is suspected. Other relevant questions of history include recent use of antibiotics, clothing preferences, family history of cancers, other family members with similar symptoms (pinworms and scabies), rectal bleeding, change in bowel habits, or sexual preference (anal receptive intercourse). For pruritus vulvae, the patient should be asked about any history of itching, burning sensation, vaginal discharge, postcoital bleeding, or dysperunia.

Physical Examination

Inspection with a bright light and a chaperone is recommended. Palpation includes a digital rectal exam and a female pelvic examination in case of pruritus vulvae. Wet preparation of vaginal secretions for Candida, bacterial vaginosis, potassium hydroxide testing, and cultures for *Neisseria gonorrhoeae* and chlamydia are recommended. Microscopic examination of scrapings will help to differentiate the parasitic and fungal infections.

Laboratory Tests

Laboratory tests should not be done routinely in all cases and should be tailored to the patient's history and physical examination. Below is a list of laboratory tests that should be considered when diagnosing possible causes of anogenital pruritus:
1. CBC (complete blood count) helps to differentiate between parasitic and infectious cases and diagnoses anemia (a possible cause of chronic pruritus ani)

---

[7]Available as dietary supplement.

2. Chemistry profile (to identify systemic causes such as hepatic and kidney diseases)
3. Urinalysis to screen for infection and systemic diseases such as diabetes
4. DNA polymerase chain reaction probe for gonorrhea and chlamydia
5. Cellophane tape test to look for pinworms
6. Stool for ova and parasites
7. Test for diabetes mellitus and HIV if suspected
8. Anal Pap smear for HPV is indicated if there is a history of anal receptive intercourse

Procedures

Anoscopy and proctoscopy are indicated to diagnose hemorrhoids and perianal fistulae. Colposcopic examination of the perineum may provide a detailed view of local pathology.

Colonoscopy is indicated for patients over 40 with a family history of colon cancers. Patch testing should be performed to diagnose allergic contact dermatitis. A skin biopsy is indicated in case of ulcerated skin lesions, refractory cases, and suspicious lesions to rule out malignancy. A 3 to 6 mm punch biopsy is recommended.

Differential Diagnosis

A broad range of clinical problems can be enumerated in the differential diagnosis, including (but not limited to) allergic skin reactions, infections, parasitic infestations, chronic liver disease, diabetes, and neoplasms; chronic conditions such as psoriasis or dermatitis; infections such as condylomata accuminata; and skin cancers such as Bowen's disease, squamous cell cancer, Paget's disease, or melanoma.

Prevention and Treatment

General Principles of Treatment

The goal of treatment should be the resolution of symptoms, restoration of skin anatomy, and prevention of recurrence. The most important step in the management of pruritus ani and vulvae is reassurance and patient education (Figure 1). An informed and educated patient tends to deal with symptom-related anxiety better. To identify and treat the cause, it should be understood that pruritus ani and vulvae are commonly idiopathic, and conservative measures are usually sufficient to treat the condition. However, secondary causes need to be identified and treated.

Anorectal conditions such as hemorrhoids, fistulas, and fissures may require surgical treatment and consultation. Antidiarrheals should be used in cases of loose stool. A high-fiber diet should be started.

Women presenting with vulvar pruritus should be screened and treated for vaginal infection (e.g., one dose of oral fluconazole [Diflucan] 150 mg for vulvovaginal candidiasis; metronidazole [Flagyl] 500 mg oral twice daily for 7 days for bacterial vaginosis). Dermatological conditions such as psoriasis and dermatitis are treated with topical steroids. Hormone replacement therapy can be used in cases of menopause. Topical estrogen creams are better alternatives for symptomatic relief.

Patients should be instructed to gently cleanse the perianal area twice daily and after each bowel movement. Sitz baths with plain warm water are recommended for perianal pruritus. The perianal area should be patted dry after washing. Patients with vulvar pruritus should avoid tight undergarments, jeans, and panty hose. The use of laundry detergents, bubble baths, feminine douches, or sprays containing protease should be discouraged. Women with a predisposition to vulvar dermatitis should wear loose pants. Panty liners should be avoided and replaced with tampons or cotton cloth. Vulvae should be washed gently; women should avoid vigorous rubbing or cleaning. Patients with vulvar pruritus should use a bland moisturizer as a soap substitute to avoid irritation resulting from chemicals. The vulva should be dried before wearing underwear, and excessive perspiration should be controlled with talcum powder. Patients should be encouraged to manage incontinence and maintain an ideal body weight. Cornstarch should be avoided, as it can lead to bacterial colonization and exacerbation of symptoms.

Dietary modifications (for anal pruritus) are imperative, including limitations on the consumption of chocolate, tea, coffee, citrus fruits, and alcoholic beverages. Eating yogurt is recommended, especially while on antibiotics, to prevent diarrhea and worsening of perianal seepage.

Emollients such as aqueous creams or petrolatum or emulsifying ointments treat itching and dry skin, which can prevent erosion and ulcer formation. These agents can be used irrespective of the etiology of pruritus. Zinc oxide (Desitin) cream is used topically to prevent excoriations in cases of perianal and vulvar pruritus. Combination products such as zinc oxide/bacitracin (rash relief antibacterial), zinc oxide/menthol (Calmoseptine), and zinc oxide/miconazole (Vusion) are available and can be used for symptomatic relief. Topical anesthetics (lidocaine 5% [L-M-X5 Anorectal, Topicaine 5]) may be used twice a day to help with acute symptoms. Topical benzocaine (Vagisil Anti-Itch Creme) should be avoided, as it is a strong irritant and allergen. Cool compresses and gel packs can help. Ice should not be used, as it can cause frostbite.

Antihistamines should be used to improve sleep, and patients should wear cotton gloves at night to prevent itching while asleep. Nails should be cut short, and nail varnish should be avoided. Sedating antihistamines might help (e.g., hydroxyzine [Vistaril] 50 mg PO at bedtime; doxepin [Sinequan][1] 10 to 100 mg at bedtime; citalopram [Celexa][1] 20 to 40 mg during the daytime). Citalopram can also help with underlying anxiety symptoms, but caution is advised in the elderly and patients at risk of arrhythmias, because citalopram can cause QT interval prolongation. Any suspicious lesions of the vulvae and perineum should be biopsied to rule out underlying malignancy.

Pharmacologic Treatments

For mild pruritus ani, 1% to 2.5% hydrocortisone (Hydrocort) topical ointment is effective. Pramoxine (Prax, Senna Sensitive) can also be used alone or in combination with topical hydrocortisone cream (Analpram-HC, Pramosone). 1% Hydrocortisone/1% iodoquinol (Vytone) can be used as an antiinflammatory treatment for external use in the anal and vulvar area. Topical capsaicin cream 0.006%[3] has been used in cases of refractory itching and can be combined with topical hydrocortisone cream[3] to avoid hypersensitivity. This strength of capsaicin cream is not commercially available. Mild topical corticosteroid ointments are sufficient to treat the perianal pruritus, and superpotent steroids should be avoided, as the skin is thin and there is a risk of ulcer formation. Methylene blue[1] injections are reserved for long-standing, intractable pruritus ani. Methylene blue 0.5% to 1% 5 to 30 mL mixed with normal saline and local anesthetics is injected intradermally, subcutaneously, and intracutaneously in the perianal skin to produce hypoesthesia. This treatment may be repeated, and studies report a success rate of 80% to 90%. Possible complications associated with methylene blue injections include cellulitis, transient urinary incontinence, urinary retention, skin abscess and skin necrosis. Long term effectiveness of these injections need further prospective studies.

For moderate vulvar disease, 0.1% triamcinolone (Kenalog) ointment is recommended. For severe cases and thickened skin, the superpotent steroid topical clobetasol (Temovate) or halobetasol (Ultravate) 0.05% ointments can be used. The use of these superpotent steroid creams should be limited and reserved for the resistant cases of pruritus vulvae, lichens simplex chronicus, lichen sclerosus, or resistant lichen planus. Vulvar lichen and lichen planus should be treated over the long term with superpotent steroids for adequate response and treatment. A very thin layer of steroid cream should be used, and patients should be educated about the side effects of the

---

[1] Not FDA approved for this indication.
[3] Exceeds dosage recommended by the manufacturer.

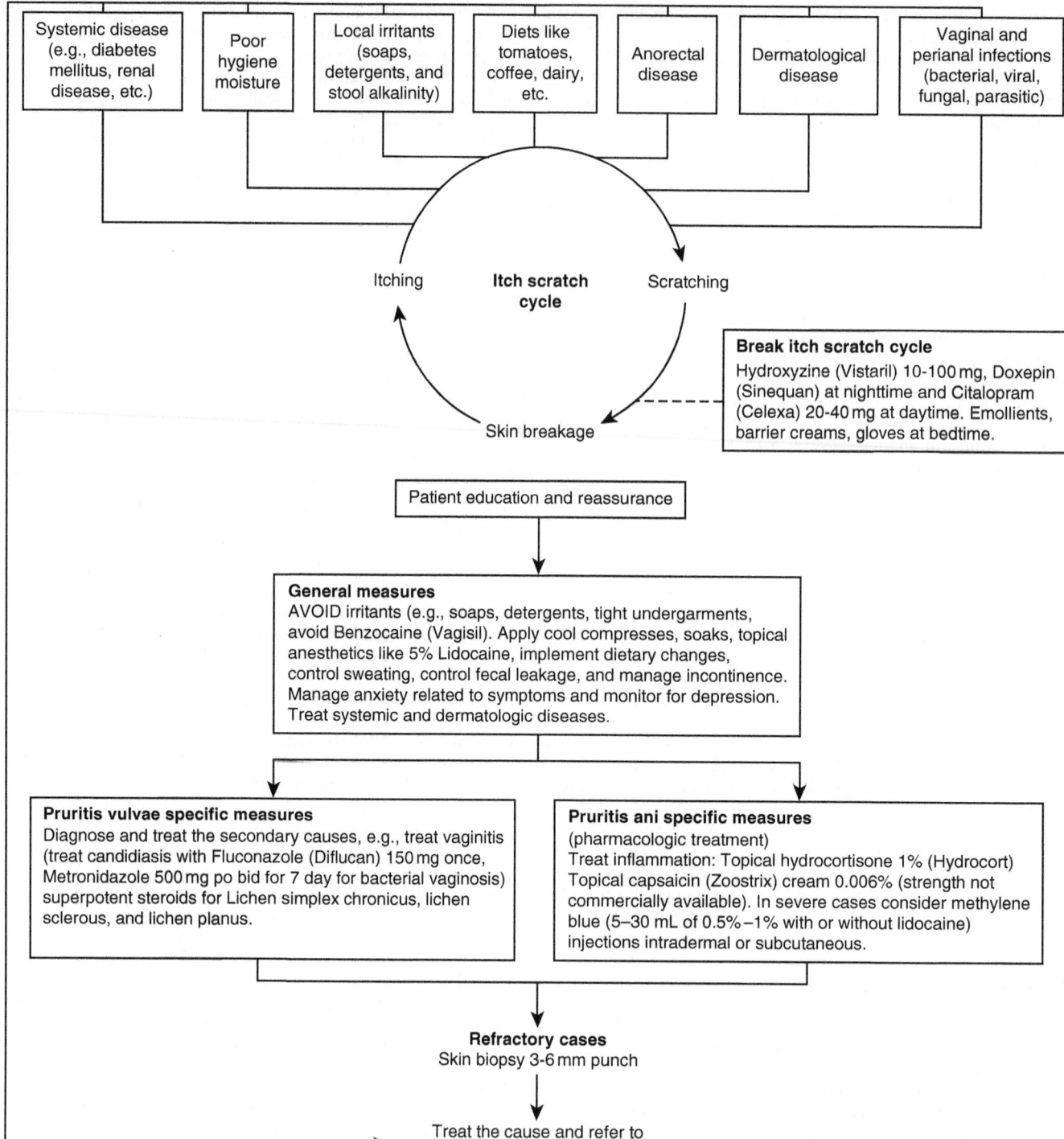

Figure 1 Pathogenesis and management of pruritus ani and vulvae.

medication before starting the treatment. For vulvar lichen planus and lichen sclerosus, superpotent steroids are used topically once or twice daily for 2 to 3 months; three times a week for 1 month; then once or twice per week for the long term. For lichen simplex chronicus, treatment is twice daily for 2 weeks and then once daily for 2 weeks. It then moves to three times per week.

Topical calcineurin inhibitors 1% pimecrolimus cream (Elidel)[1] or 0.03% to 1% tacrolimus ointment (Protopic)[1] may be used for refractory cases as steroid-sparing agents. A common side effect of these agents is a burning sensation, so their use is controversial in cases of lichen sclerosis and lichen planus. Lichen sclerosis has 2-5% increased risk of developing squamous cell cancer,

therefore clinical monitoring is recommended every 6–12 months and suspicious lesions must be biopsied.

In cases of neuropathic pruritus ani and vulvae, amitriptyline (Elavil)[1] 10 to 150 mg at bedtime is suggested. Other options are gabapentin (Neurontin)[1] 300 to 3600 mg up to three times a day (maximum daily dose is 3600 mg); pregabalin (Lyrica)[1] 75 to 400 mg/day; and mirtazapine (Remeron)[1] 7.5 to 15 mg at bedtime. In resistant and rare cases in which none of the above mentioned treatments is effective, radiation treatment may be indicated to destroy nerve endings. Naltrexone[1], an opioid antagonist has shown effectiveness in reducing itching episodes after one week of treatment in a case study. Several experimental treatments, such as

---

[1] Not FDA approved for this indication.

[1] Not FDA approved for this indication.

laser phototherapy, alcohol injection therapy, radiation, and surgery, have not been studied and are not recommended routinely.

Complications

Pruritus ani and vulvae can lead to myriad complications, including lichenification, skin excoriations, ulcers, secondary bacterial infections, and abscess formation.

Referral

For undiagnosed and resistant skin conditions, patients should be referred to a dermatologist. Persistent anal itching, a change in bowel habits, and rectal bleeding should prompt a referral to a gastroenterologist and colorectal specialist. Pruritus vulvae with vaginal bleeding and weight loss are indications for referral to a gynecologist.

Monitoring and Prognosis

Most cases of pruritus ani and vulvae are treated with general measures that lead to a full recovery. Long-term use of corticosteroids should be discouraged, and periodic monitoring for side effects, including skin erosions and bleeding, is advisable based on reported symptoms. The idiopathic disease usually persists and depicts a relapsing remitting course.

References

Al-Ghnaniem R, Short A, Pullen A: 1% Hydrocortisone ointment is an effective treatment of pruritus ani: A pilot randomized controlled crossover trial, *Int J Colorectal Dis* 22:1463–1467, 2007.
Family Practice Notebook: *Pruritus vulvae.* Available at http://www.fpnotebook.com/gyn/vulva/vlvrprts.htm, 2013 (accessed December 14, 2013).
Jones DJ: ABC of colorectal disease. Pruritus ani, *BMJ* 1305:575–577, 1992.
Margesson LJ: Overview of treatment of vulvovaginal disease, *Skin Therapy Lett* 16:5–7, 2011.
Margesson L, Danby WF: Pruritus ani and vulvae. In *Conn's Current Therapy 2013*: Philadelphia, 2012, Elsevier. pp 276–278.
Markell KW, Billingham RP: Pruritus ani: Etiology and management, *Surg Clin North Am* 90:125–135, 2010.
Mentes BB: Intradermal methylene blue injection for the treatment of intractable idiopathic pruritus ani: Results of 30 cases, *Tech Coloproctol* 8:11–14, 2004.
Reidy T, Rafferty JF: Management of pruritus ani. In *Current Surgical Therapy*, Philadelphia, 2011, Elsevier Mosby, pp 243–246.
Siddiqi S, Vijay V, Ward M, et al: Pruritus ani, *Ann R Coll Surg Engl* 90:457–463, 2008.
Stermer E, Sukhotnic I, Shoul R: Pruritus ani: An approach to an itching condition, *J Pediatr Gastroenterol Nutr* 48:513–516, 2009.
Weichert GE: An approach to the treatment of anogenital pruritus, *Dermatol Ther* 17:129–133, 2004.

PSYCHOCUTANEOUS MEDICINE

Method of
Ladan Mostaghimi, MD

Psychocutaneous medicine explores the interactions between mind and skin. The spectrum of patients ranges from those who are delusional and refuse to see a psychiatrist to those who are depressed because of chronic disfiguring skin problems. The relationship between chronic skin diseases and psychological factors has been known for many years. In the first reference to psychocutaneous medicine from 1200 BC, the physician to the Prince of Persia speculated that his patient's skin disease (possibly psoriasis based on the description) was related to his anxiety about succeeding his father. Research in psychoneuroimmunology has better defined the relationship between skin and mind. This chapter discusses common psychodermatologic disorders and their treatment.

Classification

The five general categories encountered in psychocutaneous medicine are as follows:
- Psychophysiologic disorders: Emotional factors can exacerbate a skin disorder, such as psoriasis.
- Primary psychiatric disorders: Patients have no primary skin disorder, and the cutaneous signs are self-induced, such as delusions of parasitosis. This category includes primary psy-

Figure 1 Onychotillomania of toenails.

Figure 2 Onychotillomania of fingernails.

chiatric disorders such as delusions of dysmorphosis, a variant of body dysmorphic disorder, and pathologic skin grooming behaviors (i.e., trichotillomania, onychotillomania [Figures 1 and 2], pathologic skin picking [Figure 3], and nail biting).
- Secondary psychiatric disorders: A chronic, disfiguring skin disorder causes psychological problems.
- Cutaneous sensory disorders: Patients have purely sensory complaints, such as pruritus, burning, stinging, and biting, without visible primary skin disease or an underlying medical condition.
- Use of psychotropic medications for dermatologic conditions such as urticaria or postherpetic neuralgia.

Another, more practical classification of psychocutaneous conditions is based on the underlying psychopathology such as depression, anxiety, obsessive-compulsive disorder (OCD), delusional disorders, trichotillomania, excoriation disorder (skin picking), and body dysmorphic disorder. Standardized self-rating questionnaires are available for different conditions. These questionnaires can be administered and rated by office staff before the visit with the physician. This classification system can also help with treatment choices and follow-up plans.

An important area of psychocutaneous medicine's contribution to dermatology is assessing quality of life of patients with and without treatments. Research in this area guides clinicians on their treatment choices and risks/cost benefits of medications. With new accountable care measures, psychocutaneous medicine experts potentially could play an important role in designing quality-of-care measures in dermatology clinics.

Finally, for psychocutaneous research to be successful, the use of needs assessment surveys is important. The first sample of these surveys was published in the *International Journal of Dermatology* in 2009.

Figure 3 Skin picking at rough spots of skin.

Delusions of Parasitosis

CURRENT DIAGNOSIS

- The patient has false fixed beliefs about being infested.
- Look for the matchbox sign: samples of excoriated pieces of skin, scabs, clothing lint, or other debris are kept in bags, in plastic wrap, on adhesive tape, or in matchboxes by the patient and brought to the physician for examination to detect suspected parasites.
- Determine the type of delusional disorder: primary or secondary such as mood disorder with delusional features.
- For secondary delusions, determine the possible causes and contributing factors, such as substance abuse, organic brain pathology, pernicious anemia, hypothyroidism or hyperthyroidism, and systemic lupus erythematosus (SLE).
- Determine the extent of damage to the skin and history of skin infections.

CURRENT THERAPY

- In secondary delusional disorders, treatment of the main disorder will help to clear the delusions.
- Psychosocial intervention. Work with families. Provide a good support system.
- Evaluate and monitor safety for the patient, family members, and health care providers.
- Some patients may try to get rid of parasites by burning their belongings or their body, or by using toxic substances, damaging their skin and causing serious toxicity.
- Treatment may include psychoeducation and cognitive-behavioral therapy (CBT).
- Neuroleptics/antipsychotic medications:
  - Pimozide (Orap)[1] is a first-generation antipsychotic frequently used by dermatologists.
  - There are case reports of second-generation antipsychotics working well in these situations.
- The treatment needs to be customized based on each patient's profile and medication side effects.

[1]Not US Food and Drug Administration (FDA) approved for this indication.

Delusions of parasitosis falls under the *Diagnostic and Statistical Manual of Mental Disorders*, Fifth Edition (DSM-5) category of delusional disorder somatic type.

These patients have false fixed beliefs that they are infested by parasites. To meet the diagnostic criteria, the problem should last at least a month and should not be part of schizophrenia manifestations. Apart from the impact of the delusions, the patient's functioning is not markedly impaired and behavior is not always odd or bizarre.

Besides delusions about infestation, patients may have delusions of having foreign material in their skin (e.g., strings coming out of skin, materials getting crystalized under skin). Tactile and olfactory hallucinations, if present, are related to the main delusional theme.

Other delusional disorders for which a patient would seek dermatology advice are delusion of bromhidrosis (i.e., patients are convinced they have a foul odor that no one else can perceive) and the delusion of dysmorphosis (i.e., patients are convinced that they have a defect in their appearance that no one else can appreciate). The delusion of dysmorphosis is part of body dysmorphic disorder–delusional variant and it is differentiated in DSM-5 from other somatic delusions because it responds to the same treatments as the nondelusional variant of body dysmorphic disorder.

Another group of patients with delusions of parasitosis consists of patients with psychotic mood disorders such as depression or bipolar disorder and false fixed somatic beliefs. If the patient has mood symptoms in addition to delusional symptoms, treatment of the mood problem may correct the delusional beliefs. For about 12% of patients, the delusion of parasitosis is shared by a family member or significant other. This condition is called folie à deux (i.e., two-person shared madness) or folie partagé (i.e., shared delusions).

The DSM-5, published in May 2013, recommends eliminating the requirement that the delusion must be nonbizarre. The American Psychological Association (APA) also decided to change the "shared delusions." Instead, if the criteria are met for delusional disorder, that diagnosis is used. If shared beliefs are present but the criteria are not met, then the term "other specified schizophrenia spectrum and other psychotic disorder" is used.

The patient with delusions of parasitosis usually has multiple superficial excoriations or deep wounds owing to manipulating the skin to try to remove the parasites. Physicians should be alert to the matchbox sign. In the matchbox sign, many samples of excoriated pieces of skin, scabs, clothing lint, or other debris are kept in bags, in plastic wrap, on adhesive tape, or in matchboxes by the patient and brought to physician's office for examination to detect suspected parasites. The patient can become very agitated when the physician denies the presence of any infestation after physical examination or assessment of the samples collected and brought in.

The physician should rule out substance abuse disorders. Some substances, especially amphetamines, cocaine, and phencyclidine (PCP), can cause formication and organic delusional syndrome in some patients. Organic reasons such as temporal lobe epilepsy or other brain pathology, neurosyphilis, pernicious anemia, hypothyroidism or hyperthyroidism, and SLE should be investigated, especially in older patients and if any neurologic symptoms are identified during the physical examination.

Treatment consists of antipsychotic or neuroleptic medications. For patients with psychotic mood disorder, treatment of the mood disorder usually improves the delusional symptoms. Depending on the amount of distress that the delusions are causing, treatment may start with a combination of a neuroleptic medication and an antidepressant, with subsequent tapering off of the neuroleptic and continuation of the antidepressant alone. Second-generation neuroleptics cause problems with weight gain and metabolic syndrome and require regular monitoring during treatment (Table 1). To facilitate acceptance of the treatment, it is important for the physician to have a good rapport with patients and address their concerns; at the same time, the physician must not accept or feed into patients' delusions by giving the impression that the delusion is believed to be real. Statements such as the following may encourage patients to accept treatment: "I'll be very honest with you; what you are telling me is very unusual. In most cases of infectious diseases, the doctors are able to easily identify the culprit. In your case, we have not found anything.

	BASELINE	4 WEEKS	8 WEEKS	12 WEEKS	QUARTERLY	ANNUALLY	EVERY 5 YEARS
TABLE 1 Recommended Monitoring for Patients on Atypical Antipsychotics According to the American Diabetic Association Consensus Statement on Diabetes Care 2004							
Personal/family history	+					+	
Weight (body mass index [BMI])	+	+	+	+	+		
Waist circumference	+					+	
Blood pressure	+			+		+	
Fasting plasma glucose	+			+		+	
Fasting lipid profile	+			+			+

Modified with permission from the American Diabetes Association. *Diabetic Care* 27:596–601, 2004. Copyright 2004 American Diabetes Association.

Although we will keep looking to find the culprit, if any, I know it is difficult to live with this condition and we have medications that can help alleviate the symptoms you are experiencing."

If the patient refuses psychotropic medications, he or she should be monitored for safety. If at any point the safety of the patient, family, or physician is threatened owing to dangerous behaviors related to delusional beliefs, local mental health providers should be consulted regarding institution of a court order for involuntary commitment for treatment.

Pimozide (Orap)[1] is a first-generation antipsychotic that dermatologists have traditionally used for delusions of parasitosis. However, most antipsychotic medications can help this condition. Physicians should be familiar with the first- and second-generation antipsychotics (Tables 2 and 3) and their side effect profiles and select the treatment that is best tailored to each patient. Notice the US Food and Drug Administration (FDA) warning on increased risk of stroke with the use of neuroleptics in elderly patients with Alzheimer disease.

A detailed, step-by-step approach to treating patients with delusions of parasitosis is discussed in *Cutis* (see references).

In recent years the Internet has been helpful in contributing to medical education and multiple other aspects of the physician's life. At the same time, the Internet has served as a medium to attract patients who feel their concerns are not validated by the medical community. Doctors are confronted with patients visiting their office with a self-diagnosis of diseases that do not exist in the medical literature.

One example of these "Internet-borne diseases" is "Morgellons disease" or, as the Centers for Disease Control and Prevention (CDC) named it, "unexplained dermopathy." In 2001, a former medical research laboratory technician believed that a nonhealing wound on her 2-year-old son's lip was due to an unknown parasite, called the disease "Morgellons," and started a foundation and website under that name. Very soon multiple patients self-identified with the symptoms, which included different-color fibers coming out of one's skin. The campaign spread rapidly. Both the Internet and mainstream media were involved in publicity for the new disease. The advocacy led Congress to request that the CDC investigate the cause of the disease. The CDC started the investigation but avoided calling the disease by its Internet name and named it "unexplained dermopathy." In January 2012, the CDC published the results of its investigation in the Public Library of Science online journal *PLoS ONE*, stating that "no common underlying medical condition or infectious source was identified, similar to more commonly recognized conditions such as delusional infestation." The prevalence reported in the CDC report was 3.65 per 100,000 enrollees.

Even after the CDC report, many patients continued to advocate for an infectious cause and argue against a noninfectious cause. Even though the Morgellons Research Foundation site has closed, other online sites are still active. These sites advise patients about how to talk to their physicians so they are not labeled as delusional and how to request more testing. Online advice includes instructions on avoiding the matchbox sign at the first visit. One such site is that of the Charles Holman Foundation. This foundation is invested in finding an organic cause for Morgellons disease. Physicians funded by this foundation have recently published articles referenced in PubMed. Their most recent theory is that Morgellons disease is a form of Lyme disease. The problem with this is that some patients become even more fixated in their delusions. Patients with negative Lyme tests may claim that Lyme testing is not diagnostic. This further delays appropriate treatment.

Our clinical approach is to do a complete physical examination and necessary laboratory testing. If we do not find a culprit and we believe the patient has somatic delusions, we give the patient the correct diagnosis and work closely with the patient and his or her family to treat the delusions. In the long run this will decrease individual and family suffering. It will also reduce unnecessary health care costs and doctor shopping.

Dermatitis Artefacta (Factitious Dermatitis), Neurotic Excoriation, and Acne Excoriée

CURRENT DIAGNOSIS

- Determine the type of problem: patient's need to assume sick role, secondary gain, or impulsive skin picking (neurotic excoriation and acne excoriée).
- Assess the severity and degree of scarring, which may require intensive treatment.

CURRENT THERAPY

- For dermatitis artefacta, the patient should be confronted in a nonjudgmental, empathetic way. Provide supportive dermatologic care for the skin and refer the patient for appropriate psychological interventions.
- For acne excoriée and neurotic excoriation, rule out underlying psychopathology and use a combination of therapy (CBT or behavioral therapy) and medications that help impulsive behavior such as selective serotonin reuptake inhibitors (SSRIs), serotonin-norepinephrine reuptake inhibitors (SNRIs), buspirone (BuSpar), anticonvulsants, naltrexone (ReVia), N-acetylcysteine (NAC), and neuroleptics, depending on the extent of the problem and scarring.
- There are no FDA-approved medications for this type of impulse control/compulsive behavior, and use of suggested medications should be based on the risk/benefit assessment for each patient.

[1] Not FDA approved for this indication.

TABLE 2	Medications Used in Psychocutaneous Disorders		
CLASS	**NAME**	**DOSAGE RANGE**	**SIDE EFFECTS TO MONITOR**
First-generation neuroleptics	Pimozide (Orap)*	1 mg daily in divided doses, gradually increase up to 0.2 mg/kg per day or maximum dose of 10 mg/d Perform CYP2D6 genotyping when the daily dose in adults is > 4 mg	Multiple drug–drug interactions due to metabolism through CYP4501A2 and CYP3A4; prolonged QT interval; torsades de pointes; GI, hematologic, hepatic, neurologic (tardive dyskinesia, neuroleptic malignant syndrome, extrapyramidal symptoms, acathisia); drug-induced SLE and priapism
	Haloperidol*	0.5–3 mg two to three times daily	Neurologic side effects, QT prolongation, drug–drug interactions
Second-generation neuroleptics	Olanzapine (Zyprexa)*	2.5–max 20 mg/d	Common side effects of second-generation neuroleptics include QT prolongation; neurologic side effects (extrapyramidal symptoms, tardive dyskinesia, neuroleptic malignant syndrome); risk of neurologic side effects is less with second-generation neuroleptics (least for quetiapine) but still exists; metabolic syndrome (needs regular monitoring; see Table 1); drug–drug interactions; blood dyscrasias (periodically assess and consider D/C if ANC <1000 or if unexplained decrease of WBC count)
	Risperidone (Risperdal)*	1–4 mg/d max 8 mg/d Age >65 keep max daily dose at 4 mg/d Doses above max recommended are rarely more effective and have more side effects	
	Aripiprazole (Abilify)*	2–max 30 mg/d	
	Quetiapine (Seroquel)*	25–max 800 mg/d in divided doses	
	Ziprasidone (Geodon)*	20–80 mg bid	
Antidepressants/ antianxiety SSRIs	Sertraline (Zoloft)*	50–200 mg/d	Each SSRI has its own side effect profile (e.g., fluoxetine may prolong QT interval; citalopram has dose depending QT interval prolongation with FDA warning on recommended dosage; fluvoxamine may cause Stevens-Johnson syndrome) Overall watch for sweating, GI symptoms, sexual side effects, myalgia, sleep problems, tremor, dizziness, bleeding tendencies, hyponatremia (rare), seizure (rare), manic episode, suicidal ideation, and suicide (rare); watch for drug–drug interactions
	Citalopram (Celexa)*	20–40 mg/d Do not exceed 20 mg for adults over age 60 or poor CYP2C19 metabolizers	
	Escitalopram (Lexapro)*	10–20 mg/d 10 mg/d in geriatric patients	
	Fluoxetine (Prozac)*	20–60 mg/d	
	Paroxetine (Paxil)*	20–50 mg/d, max 40 mg/d if age >60	
	Fluvoxamine,* works best in OCD	50–300 mg/d in divided doses (bid)	
Antidepressants/ antianxiety SNRIs	Venlafaxine,* extended-release form available (Effexor XR) Helpful in peripheral neuropathies	37.5–225 mg/d	Hypertension, sweating, GI symptoms, blurred vision, sexual side effects, hyponatremia, bleeding tendencies, neuroleptic malignant syndrome, serotonin syndrome, hepatitis (rare), drug–drug interactions
	Duloxetine (Cymbalta)* Also for treatment of fibromyalgia	30–60 mg/d, may increase to 120 mg/d but rarely more effective	Sweating, GI symptoms, sleep problems, bleeding tendencies, hepatotoxicity, fatigue, drug–drug interactions
Antidepressants/ antianxiety other	Trazodone,* helps insomnia and sometimes itching	50–400 mg/d	Sweating, weight change, GI symptoms, neurologic symptoms, blurred vision, hypertension, hypotension (rare), cardiac dysrhythmia (rare), priapism, seizure, drug–drug interactions

| TABLE 2 | Medications Used in Psychocutaneous Disorders—cont'd | | |

CLASS	NAME	DOSAGE RANGE	SIDE EFFECTS TO MONITOR
	Mirtazapine (Remeron),* helps insomnia and itching with higher affinity for histamine receptors than doxepin	15–45 mg/d	Increased appetite, hyperlipidemia, somnolence, neurologic disorders, agranulocytosis and neutropenia (rare), seizure, drug–drug interactions
	Bupropion (Wellbutrin),* sustained-release and extended-release forms available	100–450 mg/d in divided doses	Hypertension, tachycardia, arrhythmia, pruritus, urticaria, GI symptoms, arthralgia, myalgia, neurologic symptoms, agitation, anger outbursts, menstrual problems, Stevens-Johnson syndrome, anaphylaxis, drug–drug interactions
	Buspirone (BuSpar)* works for anxiety problems	5–60 mg/d in divided doses	Nausea, blurred vision, nervousness, angry behavior, neurologic symptoms, congestive heart failure (rare), MI (rare), CVA (rare), drug–drug interactions
Tricyclic antidepressants for pruritus and hives	Doxepin* Topical 5% doxepin cream (Zonalon) has FDA approval for pruritus (for atopic dermatitis and lichen simplex chronicus)	25–300 mg/d in single and divided doses for depression, 10–25 mg/d for pruritus Topical: every 3–4 h max for 8 days; do not use under occlusion	Weight gain, GI symptoms, neurologic symptoms, blurred vision, urinary retention, arrhythmia (rare), blood pressure changes, bleeding tendencies, hematologic changes, drug–drug interactions
Tricyclic antidepressant for trichotillomania	Clomipramine (Anafranil)*	25–250 mg/d	Weight gain or loss, GI symptoms, blurred vision, neurologic symptoms, urinary retention, MI, orthostatic hypotension, hematologic side effects, hepatotoxicity
Neuropathic pain treatments Tricyclic antidepressant	Amitriptyline*	10–150 mg/d	Weight gain, GI symptoms, neurologic symptoms, blurred vision, cardiac dysrhythmia, hematologic symptoms, hepatic symptoms, CVA, drug–drug interactions
Antiepileptic medications	Gabapentin (Neurontin) FDA approved for postherpetic neuralgia	100 mg at night, gradually increase to up to 1800 mg daily in divided doses if needed	Myalgia, peripheral edema, neurologic symptoms, angry behavior, mood swings, problems with thinking, Stevens-Johnson syndrome, seizure, drug–drug interactions
	Pregabalin (Lyrica) FDA approved for neuropathic pain and postherpetic neuralgia. Also treatment of fibromyalgia	50 mg tid with gradual increase up to 600 mg/d in divided doses	Peripheral edema, weight gain, GI symptoms, ataxia, somnolence, blurred vision, euphoria, problems with thinking, angioedema
	Carbamazepine (Tegretol)*	50–1200 mg/d in divided doses for blood levels of 4–12 mcg/mL	Hyponatremia, severe blood dyscrasias (rare but needs regular CBC monitoring), toxicity over therapeutic ranges, atrioventricular block, cardiac dysrhythmia, congestive heart failure, syncope, hypertension or hypotension, GI symptoms, hepatitis, SLE, skin rash, Stevens-Johnson syndrome, TEN, psoriasis, acne, angioedema, nephrotoxicity, drug–drug interactions
	Lamotrigine (Lamictal)* helps impulsive behavior and neuropathic pain	25–200 mg/d in divided doses; do not increase to >50 mg/every 2 weeks	Headaches, sleep problems, diplopia, ataxia, GI symptoms, rhinitis, photosensitivity, rash, Stevens-Johnson syndrome, TEN, angioedema, hypersensitivity reactions, neutropenia, DIC, hematologic problems, hepatic failure, pancreatitis, rhabdomyolysis, teratogenicity, drug–drug interactions
Miscellaneous treatments for intractable pruritus	Thalidomide (Thalomid)* (also used in Behçet syndrome)	50–200 mg/d	Severe birth defects in pregnancy, edema, skin rash, GI symptoms, leukopenia, thrombotic disorder, peripheral neuropathy, Stevens-Johnson syndrome, TEN, seizure, pulmonary embolism, hypocalcemia, tremor, somnolence, drug–drug interactions
	Naltrexone (ReVia)* Vivitrol (IM Naltrexone)* Usually used for alcohol dependence and not in dermatology	50 mg/d 380 mg/mo IM	GI symptoms, headaches, anxiety, hepatic damage, opioid withdrawal (rare), drug–drug interactions

Continued

| TABLE 2 | Medications Used in Psychocutaneous Disorders—cont'd | | |

CLASS	NAME	DOSAGE RANGE	SIDE EFFECTS TO MONITOR
	Cyclosporine (Sandimmune)* Monitor drug level	4–5 mg/kg per day	Hirsutism, pruritus in some patients, GI symptoms, neurologic symptoms (headaches, tremor, seizures, progressive multifocal encephalopathy [rare], coma [rare]), hepatotoxicity, nephrotoxicity, infections, hyperkalemia, hypomagnesemia, hypertension, anaphylaxis, lymphoproliferative disorder, drug–drug interactions
Benzodiazepines (sometimes used for burning mouth syndrome)	Clonazepam (Klonopin)*	0.25 mg at night with gradual increase. Usual dosage for neuralgia is 2–4 mg/d	Sialorrhea, ataxia, dizziness, somnolence, impaired cognition, aggravation of seizure, depression, behavioral problems, respiratory depression

*Not FDA approved for psychocutaneous disorders.
Abbreviations: ANC = absolute neutrophil count; bid = twice a day; CBC = complete blood count; CVA = cerebrovascular accident; D/C = discontinuation; DIC = disseminated intravascular coagulopathy; FDA = US Food and Drug Administration; GI = gastrointestinal; IM = intramuscular; MI = myocardial infarction; SLE = systemic lupus erythematosus; SNRI = serotonin-norepinephrine reuptake inhibitor; SSRI = selective serotonin reuptake inhibitor; TEN = toxic epidermal necrolysis; WBC = white blood cell.

| TABLE 3 | New Medications With Potential Use in Psychocutaneous Medicine but No FDA Approval for Any of the Psychocutaneous Ailments | | |

CLASS	NAME	DOSAGE RANGE	SIDE EFFECTS TO MONITOR
Antidepressants/ antianxiety Other	Vilazodone hydrochloride (Viibryd)* SRI plus 5-HT1A partial agonist, like buspirone	10 mg/d × 7 d Then 20 mg/d × 7 d Then 40 mg/d Not tested in children	GI side effects: most frequent, diarrhea and nausea, occasionally vomiting; dry mouth; dizziness; insomnia; rare but serious: palpitation, ventricular premature beats, suicidal thoughts, and serotonin syndrome.
	Desvenlafaxine (Pristiq)*; SNRI	50 mg/d Not to exceed 100 mg/d Needs to be tapered gradually at discontinuation by increasing the dosage interval Dose adjustment needed for renal impairment	Increased sweating in 10%–20% of patients May cause increase in triglycerides and cholesterol. Also watch for GI side effects, fatigue, blurred vision, proteinuria, anxiety. Rare but serious side effects including hypertension in 1%–2% and other cardiac effects to monitor, hyponatremia, GI hemorrhage, hypersensitivity reactions, seizure, mania, suicidal thoughts, withdrawal symptoms.
	Milnacipran (Savella)*; SNRI, pain reliever FDA application is only for fibromyalgia.	Start 12.5 mg daily Maximum dose 100 mg bid daily Dose adjustment needed for renal impairment, avoid using in hepatic disease	Increased blood pressure (2%–19.5%), tachycardia, palpitations, increased sweating (9%), sweats (12%), GI side effects, headache. Rare but serious: abnormal bleeding, serotonin syndrome, worsening of depression and suicidality, withdrawal symptoms.
	Selegiline transdermal (Emsam)*; MAOI FDA label for major depressive disorder and Parkinson disease.	6, 9, 12 mg patch/24 h May increase 3 mg/24 h every 2 weeks not to exceed 12 mg/24 h	Need to have low-tyramine diet. Decreased systolic pressure, orthostatic hypotension, application site reaction (24%), weight loss, diarrhea, indigestion, headache, insomnia, dry mouth. Rare but serious: atrial fibrillation, hypertensive crisis (with tyramine-containing food), suicidal thoughts.
New second-generation neuroleptics	Paliperidone (Invega)* A major active metabolite of risperidone IM form: Invega Sustenna FDA approved for schizophrenia and schizoaffective disorder	Start with extended-release tablets 6 mg/d and gradually increase to maximum of 12 mg/d Adjust dose for renal impairment For injectable Sustenna form dosage range is 39–234 mg IM once a month after initial titration	Tachycardia (up to 16%), hyperprolactinemia (45%–49%), weight gain (2%–19%), GI side effects, akathisia, dyskinesia, dystonia, EPS and parkinsonism, somnolence, tremor, anxiety, nasopharyngitis (up to 5%). Rare but serious: prolonged QT interval (7%), agranulocytosis, leukopenia, priapism, dysphagia, and TD.
	Asenapine (Saphris)* FDA indications: bipolar I, acute mixed or manic episodes, and schizophrenia	Sublingual medication No titration is needed 5–10 mg bid	Weight gain (3%–5%), oral hypoesthesia (5%), akathisia, dizziness, EPS, somnolence. Rare but serious: QT prolongation, hypersensitivity reactions, angioedema, neuroleptic malignant syndrome. TD is not listed but is always a possibility.

TABLE 3	New Medications With Potential Use in Psychocutaneous Medicine but No FDA Approval for Any of the Psychocutaneous Ailments—cont'd		
CLASS	**NAME**	**DOSAGE RANGE**	**SIDE EFFECTS TO MONITOR**
	Lurasidone (Latuda)*	Initial dose titration not required 40 to maximum of 160 mg/d taken with food (350 calories), needs dose adjustment in renal and hepatic impairment	Nausea, akathisia, EPS, parkinsonism, somnolence. Rare but serious: orthostatic hypotension, syncope, agranulocytosis, CVA, seizure, TD, transient ischemic attack, suicidal thoughts, neuroleptic malignant syndrome.
	Iloperidone (Fanapt)* FDA approval: schizophrenia	1 mg bid on day 1 and titrate to maximum of 12 mg bid Do not use in patients with hepatic impairment	Weight gain (1%–18%), orthostatic hypotension (3%–5%), tachycardia, dizziness, somnolence, GI problems, nasal congestion, fatigue, hyperprolactinemia (26%). Rare but serious: prolonged QT interval, syncope (0.4%), hyperglycemia, CVA, transient ischemic attack, suicidal intent. TD is a risk in all neuroleptics. Risk differs per medication.
Miscellaneous For pathologic grooming behaviors (trichotillomania, skin picking, nail biting)	N-acetylcysteine (NAC) (Acetadote)*	1200–2400 mg/d	GI (nausea, indigestion), abdominal pain, headache, worsening of asthma. In long-term treatment needs to be taken with a multivitamin plus vitamin C.

*Not FDA approved for this indication.

Each year there are new medications added to this list, for example, cariprazine (Vraylar), brexpiprazole (Rexulti), pimavanserin (Nuplazid), aripiprazole lauroxil (Aristada, long-acting injection form of aripiprazole). These new medications are not FDA approved for psychocutaneous disorders and they should be used with extreme caution, recognizing that their mechanism of action and side effect profile for treatment of psychocutaneous disorders are unclear.

Abbreviations: CVA = cerebrovascular accident; EPS = extrapyramidal symptoms; FDA = US Food and Drug Administration; GI = gastrointestinal; IM = intramuscular; MAOI = monoamine oxidase inhibitor; SNRI = serotonin-norepinephrine reuptake inhibitor; SRI = serotonin reuptake inhibitor; TD = tardive dyskinesia. Please note that the information on tables is summarized and not comprehensive; refer to drug databases such as the *Physician's Desk Reference* for a complete list of side effects and black-box warnings.

Dermatitis Artefacta or Factitious Dermatitis

Dermatitis artefacta (i.e., factitious dermatitis) refers to intentional production of skin lesions to satisfy a psychological need. This could be achieved by different methods, such as excoriation, burning, or injection of toxic substances. Patients usually deny the self-induced nature of the problem. Clinically the lesions are located in reachable areas of the skin and can mimic any skin disease.

The DSM-5 has two subtypes of factitious disorder: factitious disorder imposed on self and factitious disorder imposed on another (previously, factious disorder by proxy). The DSM-5 proposes the grouping of the factitious disorders with the somatic symptom disorders to facilitate research on the broad spectrum of symptom reporting by patients, from feigning symptoms to experiencing symptoms with no clinical findings.

Factitious dermatitis usually occurs in patients with underlying psychopathology. After a diagnosis is made, the physician needs to discuss it with the patient in a nonjudgmental, empathetic way. Supportive dermatologic care should be provided for wounds, and the patient should be referred for psychological evaluation. Antidepressant and antianxiety medications can help to treat underlying depression and anxiety. Supplementary therapies include biofeedback, relaxation, acupuncture, hypnosis, CBT, behavioral therapy, and family therapy if the family members are involved in care.

Neurotic Excoriation and Acne Excoriée

Patients with acne excoriée create excoriations by repetitive scratching or skin picking. Women are affected more than men. Patients scratch and pick at their acne, an insect bite, dermatitis, or other bumps or rough spots of the skin (Figure 4). Any part of the skin that is not smooth or is pruritic (Figures 4 and 5) can be a target. However, patients may inflict excoriations without the trigger of any skin pathology because the condition is a psychological process with dermatologic manifestations. Patients usually have ritualistic picking habits and report building of tension before picking and release of tension after picking.

Figure 4 Bruising of skin due to severe scratching in atopic dermatitis.

Figure 5 Scarring alopecia from chronic picking and new onset of lichenplanopilaris around the scar on the scalp.

Often patients with neurotic excoriations complain of pruritus. In this case a pruritus workup to rule out causes such as iron deficiency and gluten sensitivity is important.

The DSM-5 has recognized that pathologic skin picking is a prevalent and disabling condition (see Figures 3 and 4). The DSM-5 (as opposed to the DSM-IV, where skin picking was classified under impulse control disorders not otherwise specified) has skin picking classified under obsessive-compulsive and related disorders.

For any self-injurious behavior, patients must be screened for underlying psychopathologies such as personality disorders. However, in many patients, the behavior results from an impulse control problem or is a compulsive act in response to stressors or simply part of excessive grooming.

In addition to treatment of the underlying psychopathology, a combination of behavioral therapy and medications that help with impulsive behavior is used. The success of treatment depends on the patient's motivation to avoid scarring and to replace the self-injurious behavior with better behavior, including gentle skin care. Motivational interviewing could help patients explore and resolve their ambivalence and participate fully in treatment. Patients need to replace picking with other relaxing behaviors that are not harmful to skin, such as breathing relaxation or use of stress balls, Chinese exercise balls, Greek worry beads, stuffed animals, or Silly Putty. In finding appropriate replacement behavior, the physician should remember that tactile stimulation is important in these patients' anxiety relief.

Another therapy model for skin pickers is to consider chronic picking as an addiction and apply addiction therapy models to picking. Self-help groups and websites such as Pickers Anonymous (http://www.stoppickingonme.com) could help with treatment.

There is no FDA-approved medication for this condition. The use of different classes of medications is mostly based on case reports. The first step is to use an SSRI, such as fluoxetine (Prozac), sertraline (Zoloft), paroxetine (Paxil), or citalopram (Celexa), or an SNRI, such as venlafaxine (Effexor XR) or duloxetine (Cymbalta). Dosage and side effect profiles are provided in Table 2. If this is insufficient, the physician can add antianxiety medications, such as buspirone (BuSpar), and some of the newer anticonvulsant medications, such as lamotrigine (Lamictal). In the case of severe picking, such as in patients with Prader-Willi syndrome, multiple infections and scarring can occur. Naltrexone (ReVia), as well as the occasional use of neuroleptics such as aripiprazole (Abilify) and quetiapine (Seroquel), can help to break the cycle of scratching and give time for behavioral treatments to take effect. Once the patient has improved, medications can be tapered and discontinued, but he or she may need to stay on a maintenance dose of medications.

Prurigo Nodularis and Lichen Simplex Chronicus

CURRENT DIAGNOSIS

- Prurigo nodularis (Figure 6): hard nodules that are 1 to 5 cm in diameter with hyperpigmentation and warty or excoriated surface
- Lichen simplex chronicus: lichenification (thickening) of the skin
- Different histopathology for prurigo nodularis and lichen simplex chronicus
- Drug history to rule out pruritus induced by medications or drugs of abuse
- Complete blood cell count to rule out lymphoma and polycythemia rubra vera
- Iron studies
- Renal function tests (blood urea nitrogen [BUN], creatinine, and electrolytes) to rule out renal failure
- Liver function tests to rule out chronic obstructive biliary disease

- Serology for hepatitis
- Test for diabetes mellitus
- Thyroid and parathyroid hormone levels
- Total serum immunoglobulin E (IgE) levels for atopy
- Patch test if allergies are suspected
- HIV test and purified protein derivative (PPD) (if indicated)
- Rapid plasma reagin (RPR) test
- Skin biopsy and direct and indirect immunofluorescence assays to rule out immunobullous and autoimmune diseases
- Stool check for parasites
- Gastrointestinal and serum testing to rule out malabsorption and gluten sensitivity
- Psychological evaluation
- Chest x-ray and computed tomography (CT) scan if lymphoma is suspected

CURRENT THERAPY

- Topical antipruritic creams such as topical doxepin (Zonalon), Sarna Anti-Itch, Eucerin Calming Cream; topical steroids or intralesional steroid injection.
- Topical capsaicin (Zostrix)[1]
- Topical vitamin D₃ derivative (calcipotriene [Calcitrene])[1]
- Cryosurgical treatment for a small number of prurigo nodularis lesions
- For lichen simplex chronicus, some reports of efficacy of tacrolimus (Protopic)[1]
- Narrowband or broadband ultraviolet B (UVB) light more effective than UVA
- Psychosocial and therapy interventions to break the itch/scratch cycle
- Psychotropic medications to help with itching and sleep: mirtazapine (Remeron),[1] doxepin,[1] or trazodone[1]
- In resistant cases, other treatments such as naltrexone (ReVia),[1] cyclosporine (Sandimmune),[1] thalidomide (Thalomid),[1] and lenalidomide (Revlimid)[1]

[1]Not FDA approved for this indication.

Clinically, prurigo nodularis (i.e., chronic circumscribed nodular lichenification, picker's nodules) is a chronic, severe itch accompanied by 1- to 5-cm hard nodules with smooth or warty surfaces and a hyperpigmented periphery (Figure 6). The new lesions are usually red and inflamed, whereas the old lesions are pigmented. The lesions may also be excoriated. Lesions are mostly located on the extensor surface of limbs, but they can also be located on the face, scalp, and trunk. Histopathology evaluation shows lichenification, a dense infiltrate in dermis and neural hyperplasia, and proliferation of Schwann cells.

A good history and physical examination should include a medication history because pruritus is a side effect of many classes of medications (e.g., diuretics, angiotensin-converting enzyme [ACE] inhibitors, beta-blockers, antidepressants).

Laboratory testing (see Current Diagnosis box) is required before treatment. CT scans and chest radiographs are obtained if lymphoma is suspected. In chronic cases laboratory testing needs to be repeated at regular intervals since in some diseases itch may be the first sign and other symptoms may take some time to appear.

Topical treatments with antipruritic creams are not very helpful. Potent topical steroids such as betamethasone dipropionate (Diprosone) ointment under occlusion or intralesional injection of steroids such as triamcinolone acetonide (Kenalog-10) may be successful, but they have the risk of skin atrophy. Topical capsaicin (0.025%–0.1% Zostrix),[1] a component of red pepper, can help in early stages. In some cases topical vitamin D₃ derivative (calcipotriene [Calcitrene][1]) may help.

Figure 6 Prurigo nodularis.

For diffuse and resistant forms of prurigo nodularis, broadband and narrowband UVB and UVA can be effective. Narrowband UVB is more effective and has fewer side effects than UVA.

Also, for resistant forms, cyclosporine (Sandimmune)[1] 4 mg/kg per day can help. It should be continued for at least 6 months (see Table 2).

Thalidomide (Thalomid)[1] 200 to 400 mg in different studies has been an effective treatment for prurigo nodularis. Thalidomide is difficult to obtain because of its teratogenicity, and it does have serious side effects such as irreversible peripheral neuropathies. A similar compound, lenalidomide (Revlimid)[1] 5 mg/day, with less potential for peripheral neuropathy, was effective in one case of a patient resistant to all the other treatments.

Naltrexone (ReVia),[1] an opioid antagonist, 50 mg/day is effective in some cases. It has an FDA black-box warning on hepatotoxicity.

More recently low-dose Naltrexone (ReVia)[1] (1.5 mg qhs × 7 days then 3 mg qhs × 7 days then 4.5 mg qhs) has been reported to be effective in some autoimmune/inflammatory disorders and some pruritic conditions.

Another treatment that has had some success is the synthetic retinoid etretinate (Tigason),[2] but it was removed from the US market because of the high risk of birth defects. Other synthetic retinoids such as acitretin (Soriatane)[1] may be considered in severe resistant cases. They all have serious teratogenicity risk.

Psychological intervention is important in breaking the itch/scratch cycle. Help can be obtained with techniques such as biofeedback, in which subjects learn how to consciously control their automatic responses; hypnosis; CBT; and supportive counseling.

Some psychotropic medications can help with excessive itching and compulsive scratching, including doxepin[1] (10 mg at bedtime, can be increased up to 25 mg; the recommended dose for pruritus is lower than the dose for the treatment of depression, anxiety, or alcoholism, where it can be increased up to a maximum of 300 mg daily in divided doses), mirtazapine (Remeron)[1] (15–45 mg at night), and trazodone[1] (50–400 mg in divided doses). Doxepin is a tricyclic medication, and because it has the potential to cause cardiac arrhythmias, it should not be used in patients with a recent myocardial infarction (MI). Patients need to have periodic cardiovascular evaluations if they use tricyclic medications long term. Antidepressants should not be used in patients with bipolar disorder without a mood stabilizer, owing to the risk of triggering a manic episode. All antidepressants have an FDA black-box warning for increased risk of suicidality in children,

---

[1]Not FDA approved for this indication.
[2]Not available in the United States.

adolescents, and young adults under age 24. Patients need to be closely monitored.

Lichen Simplex Chronicus

Lichen simplex chronicus (i.e., circumscribed neurodermatitis) is characterized by lichenification of skin due to chronic excessive scratching or rubbing. Clinically, it appears as plaques of thickened skin with hyperpigmentation and accentuated skin lines. The most commonly affected areas are the occipital scalp, sides of the neck, ankles, genital areas, and extensor forearms. Itch is the main symptom. The histopathologic pattern in lichen simplex chronicus is different from that of prurigo nodularis and does not show the neural hyperplasia.

The physician must rule out the underlying diseases that may cause pruritus. The treatment for lichen simplex chronicus is similar to that for prurigo nodularis. In addition to other treatments, topical tacrolimus (Protopic) has shown efficacy in some cases of lichen simplex chronicus. Short-term topical 5% doxepin cream (Zonalon) can be used for lichen simplex chronicus (see Table 2).

Trichotillomania

CURRENT DIAGNOSIS

- Hair loss is caused by repeated hair pulling, producing oddly shaped patches of alopecia with broken hair and no signs of inflammation.
- Other areas besides the scalp may be affected.
- The age of onset and underlying psychopathology should be determined.
- If patient denies hair pulling, rule out other causes of alopecia.

CURRENT THERAPY

- In children, trichotillomania is usually self-limited and parents should be reassured. Psychotherapeutic interventions are helpful.
- In adolescents and adults, first-line treatment is psychotherapy: CBT or behavioral therapy and habit reversal. Improving coping mechanisms with stress is helpful.
- Case reports and small double-blind studies have shown the efficacy of clomipramine (Anafranil)[1] and SSRIs.
- Depending on the extent of the problem, augmentation with neuroleptics can be considered, but because of the important side effect profiles of these medications, their risks and benefits should be carefully considered.
- Before using antidepressants, patients should be screened for a family history of bipolar disorder or personal history of previous manic episodes.

Trichotillomania is partial hair loss caused by repeated hair pulling. Clinically, the patient has patches of alopecia with broken hair. The broken hairs are of different lengths and there is no inflammation of the scalp. The affected area has an unusual shape. A hair-pull test is negative. The hair-pull test consists of grasping between 40 and 60 hairs between the thumb and index finger and pulling them with moderate traction while moving the fingers toward the distal shaft. If less than 10% of the hair is pulled off, the test is negative. Trichotillomania can involve areas other than the scalp, and patients may pull hair in many sites. Trichotillomania can occur in any age group. In children, it is usually benign and self-limited, but in adults it usually accompanies other psychopathologies and requires psychological intervention. The lifetime prevalence rate is about 0.5% to 3.5%, and the prevalence in some reports is as high as 4.4%.

Trichotillomania was classified with impulse control disorders in the DSM-IV TR. In contrast, in the DSM-5, trichotillomania is classified with obsessive-compulsive and related disorders. If a patient denies hair pulling, other causes of alopecia, especially alopecia areata, need to be ruled out.

In children, trichotillomania may occur during periods of increased stress, such as arrival of a new sibling, parents' divorce/separation, or stressful events at school. It is usually self-limited, and parents should be reassured. In preadolescents and young adults, the diagnosis needs to be established first, followed by psychotherapeutic interventions; behavioral modification usually works well. Psychopharmacologic treatments should be reserved for last. Because of the FDA blackbox warning about the increased risk of suicide and suicidal behavior with use of antidepressants in children, adolescents, and young adults, these patients should be referred to a psychiatrist if needed.

In adults, trichotillomania often accompanies other psychopathology and the treatment of the underlying illness helps to resolve the condition. Habit reversal therapy usually works better than negative feedback. Habit reversal therapy teaches the patient to monitor the behavior and the triggering factors and to replace the harmful habit with another habit. Working on increasing coping skills for stress is also helpful. Relaxation and other stress relief techniques are helpful, especially in patients with underlying anxiety. The Trichotillomania Learning Center (http://www.trich.org) is a good source of information for patients.

Psychotropic medications can be used if psychotherapy alone is not enough. Most reports of effective medications are based on open-label studies. In a small, double-blind comparison, clomipramine (Anafranil) 180 mg to 250 mg/day showed greater efficacy than desipramine (Norpramin).[1] There have been some open-label studies showing the efficacy of fluoxetine (Prozac),[1] but these results were not reproduced in double-blind placebo-controlled trials. Other SSRIs, such as sertraline (Zoloft),[1] fluvoxamine (Luvox), and paroxetine (Paxil),[1] have shown efficacy in case reports and open-label studies. In some augmentation trials adding haloperidol (Haldol),[1] pimozide (Orap),[1] or olanzapine (Zyprexa)[1] was beneficial for patients taking fluoxetine or clomipramine. Small studies using haloperidol or lithium[1] have shown some efficacy. Because of important side effects such as tardive dyskinesia with haloperidol and the narrow therapeutic window with lithium, it is best to use these medications judiciously. Olanzapine (Zyrexa)[1] has been tested as monotherapy in a double-blind study and was effective. Note that before antidepressants are prescribed for these patients, it is important to screen them for bipolar disorder.

In 2009, Grant et al. evaluated N-acetylcysteine (NAC) (Acetadote),[1] a glutamatergic agent that restores extracellular glutamate concentration in the nucleus accumbens and blocks compulsive behavior, 1200 to 2400 mg/day in a double-blind placebo-controlled trial for trichotillomania for a 12-week period. Fifty-six percent of patients were much or very much improved, compared with 16% for placebo. Side effects were mild and short term, mostly affecting the gastrointestinal system (e.g., nausea, indigestion, abdominal pain) and causing headache. NAC may worsen asthma and should not be used in patients with asthma. If taken for an extended period of time, the authors recommend taking supplemental zinc, copper, and other trace minerals, as well as two to three times the typical amount of vitamin C. It is recommended to take NAC with a multivitamin plus vitamin C. In a small case series, NAC has shown efficacy in pathologic skin picking and nail biting as well.

Trichotillomania, skin picking, and nail biting can be considered as pathologic grooming behaviors. A review of available literature shows probable sufficient evidence from randomized controlled trials for the use of naltrexone (ReVia),[1] NAC, and

olanzapine[1] for trichotillomania; the SSRIs fluoxetine (Prozac)[1] and citalopram (Celexa)[1] for pathologic skin picking; and clomipramine for nail biting.

Cutaneous Sensory Disorders

CURRENT DIAGNOSIS

- Patients have a sensation of burning and itching in different areas of skin and mucous membranes, with no signs and symptoms of inflammation.

CURRENT THERAPY

- Rule out possible causes of abnormal sensations: infection, allergic reactions (e.g., dental fillings), vitamin and mineral deficiencies, iron deficiency or overload, diabetes, Sjögren syndrome, nerve injuries, medications, and neoplasia.
- Treat the primary cause of the abnormal sensation if found.
- In cases of idiopathic abnormal sensations, some medications may help: tricyclic antidepressants, gabapentin (Neurontin),[1] pregabalin (Lyrica),[1] SNRIs, and SSRIs.

Cutaneous sensory disorders are part of chronic pain syndromes, with pain occurring in different parts of the skin or mucous membranes. Disorders include burning mouth syndrome and vulvodynia (i.e., burning and itching of the vagina).

Burning mouth syndrome is a burning sensation that happens more frequently in middle-aged women. It affects the tongue more frequently, but other parts of the mouth may be affected. It can be associated with dry mouth and a metallic taste in the mouth.

The physician should rule out local problems (e.g., dental disorders, allergic reactions, infection) and systemic problems, such as vitamin B, folate, iron, and zinc deficiencies; diabetes; autoimmune problems such as Sjögren syndrome; nerve injury; side effects of medications, including antivirals, antiretrovirals, antiepileptics, hormones, and ACE inhibitors; and medications causing dysgeusia, such as asenapine (Saphris) and eszopiclone (Lunesta).

The workup needs a thorough physical examination, medication history, and laboratory workup, as well as screening for depression and anxiety. Mood problems may result from chronic pain issues.

The primary cause needs to be treated. In idiopathic cases, therapy to help relaxation, coping-skills training, and biofeedback may help. There is no FDA-approved medication for this condition, but medications used to treat neuropathies may help. These include gabapentin (Neurontin), which can be started at 100 mg at night for 3 days and gradually increased to 100 mg three times a day. The dosage can be adjusted to 300 to 600 mg three times a day as tolerated up to a maximum of 1800 mg. Tricyclics such as amitriptyline (10–25 mg orally at bedtime, may be increased every week to a maximum dosage of 150 mg/day) can be given. SNRIs such as venlafaxine extended-release form (Effexor XR) can be given as 37.5 mg in the morning with a gradual weekly increase to the maximum of 225 mg daily, and duloxetine (Cymbalta) can be given as 30 mg daily and increased to 60 mg in 1 week; dosages over 60 mg per day are rarely more effective. Clonazepam (Klonopin) 2 to 4 mg at night may help in some cases but it is habit forming and could cause memory problems as well as increase risk of fall in elderly patients. Up to two-thirds of patients report spontaneous partial recovery within 6 to 7 years of onset.

---

[1]Not FDA approved for this indication.

Vulvodynia is burning and pain in the vulvar area. Infectious, neoplastic, and inflammatory causes need to be ruled out. Depression and the impact on quality of life should be evaluated. Biofeedback and gabapentin or amitriptyline have been helpful in some cases.

Depression and anxiety lower the pain threshold, and their treatment can help patients with chronic pain syndromes to better cope with their pain and have a higher pain threshold.

Medications for Pain and Itching

Some of the psychotropic medications can be used for various dermatologic conditions, such as urticaria or postherpetic neuralgia. The older tricyclic medications have specific effects on pain or itching.

When itching is the main symptom, doxepin[1] has a much higher affinity for histamine receptors than do conventional antihistamines. It has a long half-life, and taking it once at night can control the daytime itching. The effective antipruritic dosage is usually 10 to 25 mg at night, but it could be increased at weekly intervals as needed. Amitriptyline[1] works best for disorders with pain as their main symptoms, such as burning mouth syndrome or postherpetic neuralgia. The usual dosage is 10 to 25 mg orally at bedtime, but it may be increased every week to a maximum dosage of 150 mg/day. Because tricyclic medications can affect cardiac conduction, patients need to have stable cardiovascular status. Periodic testing is required during long-term treatment. These drugs should not be used with other medications that prolong the QT interval, such as cisapride (Propulsid). They should not be prescribed during the immediate recovery period after an MI, and they should not be used at the same time as monoamine oxidase inhibitors. Patients need to be instructed to avoid driving owing to the drowsiness side effect of tricyclics.

Other medications that could help with pain symptoms include the following:

- Gabapentin (Neurontin)[1] is started at 100 mg at night, increased every 3 days to 300 mg at night, and then increased weekly to 900 to 1800 mg daily in three to four divided doses as tolerated.
- Pregabalin (Lyrica) is started with 50 mg taken orally three times daily and increased to 100 mg three times daily within 1 week based on efficacy and tolerability. If patients with postherpetic neuralgia do not experience sufficient pain relief in 2 to 4 weeks and are tolerating the medication well, the dosage can be increased to 300 mg twice daily or 200 mg three times daily (600 mg/day).
- SNRIs such as duloxetine (Cymbalta) 60 mg daily have FDA approval for diabetic neuropathy and fibromyalgia. Venlafaxine extended-release capsule (Effexor XR), which has a mechanism of action similar to that of duloxetine, can be started at 37.5 mg in the morning, with a gradual weekly increase to a maximum of 225 mg daily, for pain symptoms, though it is not FDA approved for pain treatment.
- There are some reports that SSRIs can help pain symptoms.
- Recent research has focused attention on the interaction between the pain and itch neurobiologic pathways. The potential to block different variants of opioid receptors may lead to new therapies such as novel uses of butorphanol (Stadol), a kappa-agonist that comes in the form of nasal spray.
- The substance P/neurokinin 1 (NK1) antagonist aprepitant (Emend)[1] can potentially be used for the treatment of pain.
- Another potential treatment for pruritus, nalfurafine (Remitch),[2] is under testing. This is a novel derivative of the opioid receptor antagonist naltrexone. It is a selective kappa-opioid receptor agonist and has a potent antipruritic effect in different types of pruritus.
- In our experience of resistant cases of postherpetic neuralgia, applications of small amounts of the following compound cream a couple times a day on the painful area is helpful: amitriptyline 2% and ketamine 0.5% in a Vanicream base.[1]

[1]Not FDA approved for this indication.
[2]Not available in the United States.

Body Dysmorphic Disorder in Dermatology

CURRENT DIAGNOSIS

- Patients have excessive preoccupation with an imagined defect or a slight flaw in their appearance. The problem is not perceived by, or appears slight to, others.
- Patients have rituals and repetitive behaviors in response to the appearance concern.
- Preoccupation causes clinically significant impairment in functioning and is not better accounted for by another mental illness.

CURRENT THERAPY

- Rule out other mental illnesses or causes (e.g., severe depression with bodily focus, delusional disorder, substance abuse).
- CBT and high-dose SSRIs have been shown to be effective.
- Clomipramine (Anafranil)[1] is more effective than desipramine (Norpramin).[1]
- In severe cases, augmentation with an antipsychotic such as ziprasidone (Geodon)[1] has been effective in case series.

[1]Not FDA approved for this indication.

Body dysmorphic disorder (BDD) is an excessive preoccupation with an imagined defect or a slight flaw in appearance. It is a severe, underrecognized problem. Patients are unwilling to discuss the symptoms owing to a sense of shame. Concerns about physical appearance vary across cultures and affect the presentation of BDD. Patients most commonly focus on the hair, skin, and nose, but they may focus on other areas of the body as well. These patients usually seek dermatology or plastic surgery help. There is a high rate of depression and suicidal ideation. More than 50% of patients experience suicidal ideation.

BDD usually starts early in the teenage years and rarely starts after age 55. Potentially patients could be between the ages of 6 and 80, but they are mostly in their 30s. Prevalence in dermatology is about 9% to 12%. Correct diagnosis and treatment are important because dermatology or surgical interventions usually are not effective. Patients are often unhappy with the results, and this may lead to litigation and suicidal ideation. Retrospective studies have shown that even when patients are satisfied with the intervention results, they focus their attention on other parts of their body.

Feusner et al. performed interesting neuroimaging studies with functional magnetic resonance imaging (fMRI) in patients with BDD compared with normal controls. Researchers studied subjects' processing of images using fMRI and showed that patients with BDD had an abnormal focus on details and tiny abnormalities and failed to process the images holistically. Studies also showed that compared with controls, patients with BDD had an activation of the amygdala, a structure that is involved in the processing of many emotions, including fear, while viewing faces. Patients usually demonstrate ritualistic grooming behavior, excessive mirror checking, and reassurance seeking. They try to camouflage the perceived defect. Some may have skin picking in an effort to get rid of a perceived imperfection. They may also compulsively tan to cover acne or pale skin.

Patients with acne and BDD usually have mild acne and often doctor shop in hopes of receiving aggressive treatments such as isotretinoin (Accutane). They also seek laser and other cosmetic treatments to treat the perceived acne scars.

Once the diagnosis is suspected, screening questionnaires should be used; also, a visual analog scale should be used by both the patient and the physician to rate the perceived defect. This could help clarify the diagnosis by showing the discrepancy between the two ratings. Treatment consists of a combination of pharmacotherapy and CBT.

Therapy should be tailored to BDD and is different from OCD or social anxiety. It is important to show sympathy for the patient's suffering, but do not try to reassure the patient that the perceived defect does not exist. This approach will only reinforce patients' reassurance-seeking behavior and will not change their perception.

SSRIs are effective in treatment, but usually high doses for at least 12 to 14 weeks are necessary to have results. Clinical follow-up of ritualistic behaviors helps to assess the response to treatment. For resistant cases, augmentation with antipsychotics may be helpful, but these medications do not have FDA approval for this indication.

References

Bjornsson AS, Didie ER, Phillips KA: Body dysmorphic disorder, *Dialogues Clin Neurosci* 12:221–232, 2010.

Epcrates Database. Available at http://www.epocrates.com (accessed August 2, 2016).

Feusner JD, Townsend J, Bystritsky A, Bookheimer S: Visual information processing of faces in body dysmorphic disorder, *Arch Gen Psychiatry* 64:1417, 2007.

Grant JE, Odlauq BL, Kim SW: Lamotrigine treatment of pathologic skin picking: An open-label study, *J Clin Psychiatry* 68:1384, 2007.

Grant JE, Stein DJ, Woods DW, et al: *Trichotillomania, Skin Picking, and Other Body-Focused Repetitive Behaviors*, Washington, DC, 2011, American Psychiatric Publishing.

Harth W, Gieler U, Kusnir D, Tausk FA: *Clinical Management in Psychodermatology*, Berlin, 2010, Springer.

Kanavy H, Bahner J, Korman NJ: Treatment of refractory prurigo nodularis with lenalidomide, *Arch Dermatol* 148:794–796, 2012.

Koo JY: Psychotropic agents in dermatology, *Dermatol Clin* 11:215, 1993.

Koo JY, Lee CS: *Psychocutaneous Medicine*, New York, 2003, Marcel Dekker.

Koo JY, Lee CS: Psychocutaneous diseases. In Bolognia JL, Jorizzo JL, Rapini RP, editors: *Dermatology*, Philadelphia, 2008, Elsevier.

Kowahara T, Henry L, Mostaghimi L: Needs assessment survey of psychocutaneous medicine, *Int J Dermatol* 48:1066–1070, 2009.

Lotti T, Buggiani G, Prignano F: Prurigo nodularis and lichen simplex chronicus, *Dermatol Ther* 21:42, 2008.

Madhavi S: Burning mouth syndrome. In *Ferri's Clinical Advisor*, editor: Philadelphia, 2009, Elsevier.

Micromedex Database. Available at http://www.micromedex.com (accessed August 2, 2016).

Mostaghimi L: Treating patients with delusions of parasitosis: A blueprint for clinicians, *Cutis* 86:65–68, 2010.

Odlaug BL, Grant JE: N-acetyl cysteine in the treatment of grooming disorders, *J Clin Psychopharmacol* 27:227–229, 2007.

Pearson ML, Selby JV, Katz KA, et al: Clinical, epidemiologic, histopathologic and molecular features of an unexplained dermopathy, *PLoS One* 7:29908, 2012.

ROSACEA

Method of
Daniel J. Van Durme, MD, MPH; and Lisa M. Johnson, MD

CURRENT DIAGNOSIS

- Rosacea is most common in adults aged 30 to 50 years and can have any of four overlapping presentation types: facial flushing and erythema with telangiectasias, inflammatory papules and pustules, ocular dryness and irritation, and nasal sebaceous gland hypertrophy leading to fibrotic changes and rhinophyma.
- Common exacerbating factors include alcohol, heat, spicy foods, and sunlight.

CURRENT THERAPY

- Therapy is best chosen on the basis of severity and predominant manifestation(s).
- Avoidance of known triggers is key for all four types, especially the erythematotelangiectatic type.

- Topical antibiotics (metronidazole [Metrogel], azelaic acid [Finacea], sodium sulfacetamide, and sulfur [Sulfacet-R]) are appropriate for milder forms of papulopustular rosacea. Oral antibiotics (doxycycline [Oracea], minocycline [Minocin],[1] erythromycin [Ery-Tab],[1] azithromycin [Zithromax],[1] or metronidazole [Flagyl][1]) are used for more severe cases. Isotretinoin (Accutane, Claravis)[1] can be effective in treating very severe and refractory rosacea.
- Ocular rosacea can be treated with increased eyelid hygiene, adding topical or oral antibiotics if needed.
- Rhinophyma (sebaceous gland hypertrophy and fibrosis) needs surgical management.

[1]Not FDA approved for this indication.

Rosacea is a common facial dermatosis found primarily in adults aged 30 to 50 years, particularly those of northern European or Celtic descent.

Diagnosis

Rosacea can have any of four primary manifestations, and although these overlap, most patients tend toward one predominant type. Facial erythema and flushing that also has telangiectasia is called erythematotelangiectatic type. The papulopustular type has inflammatory papules, small pustules, and occasionally small nodules. The presentation of papulopustular rosacea differs from acne vulgaris because the onset is in the 30- to 50-year-old age group instead of adolescence, and comedones are not present in papulopustular rosacea. When the sebaceous glands get markedly hypertrophic and fibrotic, this is called *phymatous type* and can lead to profound disfigurement of the nose, called rhinophyma. The ocular type involves dryness of the eyes with decreased tear production, blepharitis, and conjunctivitis.

Treatment

One key aspect of management is to have the patient maintain a careful diary for the purpose of determining and then avoiding his or her own triggers. Common triggers include alcohol, heat, certain foods, sunlight, stress, and menstruation, among others. Broad-spectrum sunblock (UVA and UVB) should be used daily. Cosmetics with a red-neutralizing green pigment can help appearance.

Topical 1% ivermectin cream (Soolantra) which is applied to the face once daily, has received approval for use in rosacea; in part, it was developed on the understanding that there is a potential etiologic role of the *Demodex* mite in the induction of rosacea. Brimonidine tartrate 0.33% gel (Mirvaso) is a selective alpha^2-adrenergic receptor agonist with vasoconstrictive activity, has been approved for the treatment of nonpersistent facial erythema in adults 18 years and older with rosacea.

The erythematotelangiectatic type of rosacea is the most difficult to treat, although benefit can be found with topical antibiotics such as metronidazole 0.75% to 1% cream, lotion, or gel (Metrogel, Noritate) or azelaic acid cream (Azelex)[1] or gel (Finacea) applied once or twice daily. Sodium sulfacetamide with sulfur is made by several manufacturers, and some brands (Sulfacet-R) include a pigmenting agent to help hide the erythema. The sulfur component can also help in cases of coexisting seborrheic dermatitis. Persistent telangiectasias can be effectively treated with laser ablation.

Papulopustular rosacea can respond to topical antibiotics, but when it is moderate to severe, oral antibiotics are indicated. Doxycycline (Adoxa)[1] 50 to 100 mg taken once or twice a day for 2 to 3 months can markedly decrease symptoms, and then the patient can switch to topical agents for long-term maintenance as needed. Minocycline (Minocin)[1] 50 to 100 mg, erythromycin[1] 250 to 500 mg, and lower-dose metronidazole (Flagyl)[1]

[1]Not FDA approved for this indication.

250 mg can each be taken once or twice a day as alternatives. Resistant cases can be treated with azithromycin (Zithromax)[1] 500 mg three times weekly in the first month; 250 mg three times weekly in the second month; and 250 mg twice weekly in the third month. Side effects can limit longer-term use of these agents, especially metronidazole.

Patients resistant to conventional treatment can be treated with oral isotretinoin (Claravis)[1] (at low dose 0.1–0.3 or "classic" dose of 0.5–1.0 mg/kg/day) for 16 weeks. Isotretinoin has many severe side effects and is tightly regulated. Both prescribers and patients must register with the iPledge program in order to prescribe and to receive the prescriptions. See www.ipledgeprogram.com.

Ocular rosacea can often be controlled with increased eyelid hygiene, washing with warm water and baby (no-tears) shampoo twice a day along with artificial tears. Long-term consumption of omega-3 fatty acids[7] may improve meibomian-gland dysfunction. Topical ophthalmic cyclosporine drops (Restasis)[1], applied as one drop to the eye twice daily (twelve hours apart) demonstrate statistically significant improvement in common signs and symptoms compared with artificial tears. If severe, it can be treated with topical erythromycin[1] or metronidazole ointment[1] or oral antibiotics such as tetracycline[1] or azithromycin[1]. If severe, it can be treated with topical erythromycin ointment (Ilotycin)[1] or oral antibiotics. If it still persists, ophthalmology referral is necessary.

The disfigurement of rhinophyma is often of concern to patients with rosacea. They can be reassured that this is uncommon; women can be further reassured that it is much more common in men. Oral isotretinoin[1] (at the dose of O.3 to 1 mg per kg per day for 12 to 28 weeks), may be effective in reducing nasal volume in early disease. Recurrence is likely after discontinuation, and mucinous and fibrotic changes are unresponsive to this type of therapy. Surgical techniques including laser- or light-based therapies (pulsed dye laser, intense pulsed light, carbon dioxide laser), electrosurgery, dermabrasion, tangential excision, electroscalpel, loop cautery, and scissor sculpting are effective in correcting or minimizing phymatous changes.

---

[1] Not FDA approved for this indication.
[7] Available as a dietary supplement.

References

Goldgar C, Keahey DJ, Houchins J: Treatment options for acne rosacea, *Am Fam Physician* 80:461–468, 2009.
Powell FC: Clinical practice: Rosacea, *N Engl J Med* 352:793–803, 2005.
Wollina U: Rosacea and rhinophyma in the elderly, *Clin Dermatol* 29:61–68, 2011.

STEVENS-JOHNSON SYNDROME AND TOXIC EPIDERMAL NECROLYSIS

Method of
Scott Worswick, MD

CURRENT DIAGNOSIS

- A diagnosis of toxic epidermal necrolysis (TEN) can be rendered when the body surface area (BSA) involved contains more than 30% denuded skin.
- A diagnosis of Stevens-Johnson Syndrome (SJS) can be rendered when less than 10% of the BSA involves denuded skin.
- SJS-TEN overlap is diagnosed when the involved BSA is between 10% and 30% BSA.
- Patients with SJS, SJS-TEN overlap, and TEN should have involvement of not only the cutaneous surface but also at least one mucosal region (most commonly the oral mucosa). Cases do exist with no mucosal involvement but this is rare and should prompt consideration of an alternate diagnosis.
- A thorough drug history and skin biopsy (ideally using the fresh-frozen technique) are essential when considering a diagnosis of SJS or TEN.

CURRENT THERAPY

- Conservative therapy is a cornerstone of therapy for all patients. This includes appropriate wound care, monitoring for fluid loss and electrolyte imbalance, thorough daily skin exams, and monitoring of vital signs to rule out concurrent infection.
- A dermatologist should be involved in the care of all hospitalized patients with Stevens-Johnson Syndrome and toxic epidermal necrolysis. In the appropriate clinical context, ophthalmology and OBGYN should also be involved. Depending on hospital resources, ICU and/or plastic surgery and the burn unit should be involved early in the care of these patients.
- Classically, systemic corticosteroids and intravenous immunoglobulin (IVIG)[1] were utilized in the management of these patients. New data suggest either cyclosporine (Neoral, Sandimmune)[1] or etanercept (Embrel)[1] may improve overall outcomes.

[1] Not FDA approved for this indication.

Epidemiology

Toxic epidermal necrolysis (TEN) is a rare diagnosis, only afflicting approximately one patient per million per year (most studies cite this incidence rate, though one study from the United States did cite an incidence rate as high as 12.7 per year). Stevens-Johnson Syndrome (SJS) and SJS-TEN overlap affect approximately five per million patients per year. The overall mortality varies greatly among different studies but is currently estimated to be ~25% for TEN. It can affect patients of any age, and most data regarding therapy are stratified by age into pediatric and adult cohorts. There are some experts who feel there may be a viral trigger or cofactor for the disease because prevalence increases in the spring.

Risk Factors

Common implicated agents include sulfonamide antibiotics as well as more recently described penicillin and cephalosporin antibiotics, aromatic anticonvulsants, allopurinol (Zyloprim), and nonsteroidal antiinflammatory drugs (NSAIDs). Numerous other medications have been reported to trigger the disease and some other common offending agents include the anti-programmed death-1 and anti-cytotoxic T-lymphocyte-associated protein 4 chemotherapeutic agents, dapsone and nevirapine (Viramune). The most important intervention is to determine and remove the offending agent as some studies cite an increase in mortality of 34% per day if the offending agent is not removed from the patient's regimen.

Certain tests can be performed after hospitalization in selected cases to determine the most likely offending agent if unknown. For example, patch testing can be done, and in the case of carbamazepine-induced SJS-TEN, has a sensitivity greater than 70%. Likewise, if multiple drugs are suspected as potential inciting agents, it may be worth checking the patient's human leukocyte antigen (HLA) types and correlating this with his/her ethnicity to make an educated guess about likely agent (if a patient has three potential inciting agents including allopurinol, the patient is of Asian descent, and HLA-typing reveals positive HLA-B5801, it could be concluded with a higher level of certainty that allopurinol is the most likely agent).

Less common triggers include vaccines such as MMR and less commonly the meningococcal, varicella and influenza vaccines, herpes, and ultraviolet light. These are more likely to be implicated in patients with target lesions or low body surface area (BSA) involvement and are exceedingly rare in patients diagnosed with full-blown TEN. An important trigger to consider in the work-up is mycoplasma, which can be responsible for causing mycoplasma-induced rash and mucositis (MIRM). MIRM is a clinical mimicker common in pediatric patients, which is characterized by lower BSA but worse mucosal involvement (typically involving two sites and usually including the ocular mucosa in dramatic fashion).

In addition to the causes of SJS and TEN described previously, there are risk factors that seem to predispose patients to the disease. These include: HIV (some studies cite a thousand-times increased chance of developing TEN among HIV-positive patients, even when controlled for the number and type of medications these patients were exposed to), lupus, female gender, Asian or African ethnicity, patients undergoing brain cancer treatment with corticosteroids and radiation, and certain HLA types. For example, one recent meta-analysis found that certain HLA-B subtypes predispose Asian patients to the development of carbamazepine-induced TEN, including HLA-B1502, HLA-B4001, HLA-B4601, and HLA-B5801. Other studies have identified HLA-B1502 as a risk factor for aromatic anticonvulsant-induced TEN among various Asian populations, HLA-B5801 as a risk factor for allopurinol-induced TEN among Asians, HLA-C0401 for nevirapine-induced TEN among patients in Malawi, and HLA type B3802, A29, B12, and DR7 as a risk factor among Europeans for sulfonamide-induced TEN.

Pathophysiology

As described previously, an immunologic basis for the development SJS and TEN is hypothesized given the fact that certain HLA types among certain groups predispose them to development of the disease. There currently exist four theories to explain how small drugs might interact with HLA and T-cell receptors (TCRs) to initiate a chain of events leading to SJS/TEN.

In the hapten theory (which has been validated in the case of penicillin-induced drug reactions), it is presumed that the drug molecule combines with an endogenous peptide and this is presented to the HLA molecule and recognized by the TCR. In the p-i model (pharmacologic interaction with the immune receptors), which has been validated in carbamazepine-HLA-B1502 interactions, the drug itself binds directly, reversibly, and noncovalently to HLA and/or TCR. In the altered peptide repertoire model, it is proposed that the drug binds to the peptide-binding groove of the HLA molecule thereby altering the overall binding ability of the HLA molecule. Lastly, in the altered TCR repertoire model, it is suggested that some drugs (such as sulfamethoxazole) can bind directly to the TCR (but not with the HLA molecule) and thereby alter the conformation of the TCR giving them the ability to bind to self-HLA.

Regardless of the type of interaction that allows a drug to alter the way HLA and TCR react to self, patients with TEN exhibit increased activity of natural killer (NK) cells and specific T lymphocytes (NK T-cells and CD* + cytotoxic T-cells). These cells mediate keratinocyte cell death via a cascade of events including Fas–FasL binding and procaspase-8 activation, increased tumor necrosis factor-α and interferon-γ levels, and activation of the perforin-granzyme-granulysin apoptosis pathway.

Differential Diagnosis

Patients with SJS and TEN typically complain of skin pain before the eruption begins. A prodrome consisting of low-grade fever, malaise, and/or flu-like symptoms is not uncommon. Within days some degree of mucosal involvement (which can take the form of dusky erythema, bullae/vesicles, denuded mucosal surface(s), dysuria, ocular erythema, pain with defecation, or pain with swallowing) is almost universal, while the extent of cutaneous involvement can vary dramatically but should include either a dusky erythema with eventual vesicles, bullae, or denuded skin, or less commonly targetoid lesions. The majority of patients with SJS and TEN present with painful red-purple (dusky) patches or macules that progress over the span of a few days. Areas that began with dusky erythema develop superimposed bullae, vesicles, or denuded skin.

Most patients with SJS and TEN do not present with typical targets on cutaneous exam. Such lesions are characterized by a small red central papule surrounded by a white ring and finally most peripherally by another ring of erythema. These lesions characterize erythema multiforme, which is much more commonly the result of herpes rather than drug allergy. However, there are rare reported cases of SJS and TEN that do include or are even dominated by cutaneous typical or atypical targets.

The main differential diagnosis for patients with classic dusky erythema, mucosal involvement, and skin pain includes acute graft-versus-host disease (GVHD), bullous lupus, generalized fixed drug eruption (FDE), cutaneous burns, paraneoplastic pemphigus (PNP), in pediatric patients MIRM, and in infants infection with the Chikungunya virus. The majority of these entities can be ruled out by clinical history alone, as patients with acute GVHD should have had a recent transplant and patients with PNP a concurrent malignancy. Dramatic mucosal involvement, in any age group, should prompt work-up for mycoplasma; when MIRM is suspected it should be treated with empiric antibiotics and in severe cases IVIG[1]. Patients with a known malignancy (particularly chronic lymphocytic leukemia [CLL], lymphoma, Castleman disease, sarcoma, or thymoma) and/or of older age and with significant mucosal disease should have, in addition to a biopsy, a direct immunofluorescence (DIF) performed and serum drawn for indirect immunofluorescence and ELISA performed to rule out PNP. It is important to check a DIF as well in any patients with joint pain or other symptoms suggestive of systemic lupus erythematosus (SLE), as well as antinuclear antibody (ANA), anti-Sjogren's syndrome–related antigen (SSA), and anti-Sjogren's Syndrome Type B (SSB), anti-dsDNA and anti-Smith. Likewise, if you are evaluating an infant who has no medication exposure and is from an endemic area, it is important to check serum titers for the Chikungunya virus.

Diagnosis

Determining the inciting agent is as important as making a quick diagnosis of TEN. A thorough drug history is essential including prn medication usage (frequently patients do not report their NSAID use or a recent antibiotic exposure). If SJS or TEN is suspected and the inciting agent is known, it is important to immediately inform the patient and his/her family of the suspected allergy and add it to the patient's medication allergy list. Dermatology should be consulted and when possible/necessary will ideally perform a skin biopsy to be processed emergently using the fresh-frozen technique (results can be ready within 30 minutes). Hematoxylin and eosin staining will also be done on permanent sections (and these results are available 1 to 3 days later depending on the site/lab).

After making a diagnosis of SJS or TEN, a practitioner can employ a scoring system called SCORTEN to estimate the patient's mortality. In this system a patient receives one point if he/she is aged above 40 years, BSA greater than 10%, history of concurrent malignancy within 2 years, serum blood urea nitrogen greater than 28 mg/dL, glucose greater than 252 mg/dL, bicarbonate level less than 20 mEq/L, and heart rate more than 120 beats per minute during the first 24 hours. With each increasing point, mortality increases such that a score of 2 confers an expected mortality of 12%; a score of 3 equates to a 35% mortality; a score of 4 with a 58% mortality; and a score of 5 or higher with an expected 90% chance of mortality.

Therapy
Medical Therapy

Classic therapy for SJS and TEN was with systemic corticosteroids but this has fallen out of favor in the United States due to recent meta-analyses suggesting no improvement in outcomes. Likewise, IVIG[1] was a mainstay of therapy in the early 21st century, but a large review from Europe found a worsened mortality in patients given IVIG compared with those given steroids or supportive care alone. Other data are conflicting with some studies suggesting that a 4-day dose of daily 1 g/kg IV[1] provides a mortality benefit, with other studies finding no improvement.

More recent success seems to have come from the utilization of etanercept (Enbrel)[1] or cyclosporine (Neoral, Sandimmune)[1] in the treatment of this disease. In 2014 a group from Italy treated 10 patients with one 50 mg subcutaneous dose and found not only a 0% mortality despite an expected mortality of 47%, but also decreased time to re-epithelialization. Likewise, in 2018 a Taiwanese group found an improved mortality benefit of etanercept over corticosteroids among 96 patients.

---

[1]Not FDA approved for this indication.

Similarly, data emerging in the last decade have suggested that cyclosporine also confers a mortality benefit. In 2010 a British case series found a 0% mortality in patients receiving 3 mg/kg per day orally despite a predicated ~30% mortality based on SCORTEN. Another study cites a significantly decreased time to re-epithelialization (3.67 days) among patients who survived after receiving cyclosporine at a dose of 3 to 4 mg/kg per day.

Adjuvant Mucosal Therapies

Patients with SJS/TEN can suffer from long-term skin/hair/nail complications including post-inflammatory hyperpigmentation, photosensitivity (70% of patients according to one study), chronic pruritus, eruptive nevi, nail changes, hypertrophic scars, and telogen effluvium. They also have a significant morbidity when their mucosal surfaces are severely involved with disease. Ocular complications can include ectropion, trichiasis, ankyloblepharon, corneal scarring, and even blindness. To some extent these complications are minimized by a choice of systemic therapy to mediate disease (i.e., either etanercept or cyclosporine). However, other measures can also be employed including amniotic membrane grafting by ophthalmology (which has been shown in a randomized controlled trial to improve multiple ocular outcome measures), topical steroid application, oxygen therapy, and bronchodilators. Likewise, urogenital sequelae occur in about one in four patients and can include adhesions leading to dyspareunia or even total vaginal fusion. Therefore involvement of gynecology or urology in the care of any patient with genital SJS/TEN is essential.

Monitoring

It is important to remember that the cutaneous examination of a patient with TEN differs greatly depending on the time of exam relative to the onset of eruption. With onset it is possible the patient will only complain of pain and have no skin lesions whatsoever. Within days a typical exam would include florid oral mucosal involvement with areas of skin showing dusky erythematous macules or patches. Over the next few days, most of the cutaneous lesions will evolve and become vesicles, bullae, or entire surfaces will denude. Monitoring for efficacy of chosen therapy means being aware of what is expected in terms of progression (that some or all areas that were dusky will denude), and ensuring that no new dusky areas develop.

The most common cause of death in patients with TEN is infection, so checking daily white blood cell counts and following vitals every 2 to 4 hours if not more frequently is essential. Fevers can occur simply as the result of the disease process itself, but any fever should prompt blood, urine, and sputum cultures. Prophylactic antibiotics have not been shown to improve outcomes but when an infection is suspected it must be treated immediately.

References

Canavan TN, Mathes EF, Friedan I, et al: Mycoplasma pneumonia-induced rash and mucositis as a syndrome distinct from Stevens-Johnson syndrome and erythema multiforme: A systematic review, *JAAD* 72(2):239–245, 2015.
Chahal D, Aleshin M, Turegano M, et al: Vaccine-induced TEN: A case and systematic review, *Dermatology Online Journal* 24(1), 2018.
Chen CB, Abe R, Pan RY, et al: An updated review of the molecular mechanisms in drug hypersensitivity, *Journal of Immunology Research*, 2018.
Conner C, McKenzie E, Owen C: The use of cyclosporine for SJS-TEN spectrum at the University of Louisville: A case series and literature review, *Dermatology Online Journal* 24(1), 2018.
Lee HY, Walsh SA, Creamer D: Long-term complications of SJS/TEN: The spectrum of chronic problems in patients who survive an episode of SJS/TEN necessitates multidisciplinary follow-up, *British Journal of Dermatology* 177:924–935, 2017.
Paradisi A, et al: Etanercept therapy for TEN, *JAAD* 71(2):278–283, 2014.
Schneck J, et al: Effects of treatment on the mortality of SJS and TEN: A retrospective study on patients included in the prospective EuroSCAR Study, *JAAD* 58(1):33–40, 2008.
Valeyrie-Allanore L, Wolkenstein P, Brochard L, et al: Open trial of ciclosporin treatment for SJS and TEN, *British Journal of Dermatology* 163(4):847–853, 2010.
Wang CW, Yang LY, Chen CB, et al: Randomized, controlled trial of TNF-alpha antagonist in CTL-mediated severe cutaneous adverse reactions, *J Clin Invest* 128(3):985–996, 2018.
Wang Q, Sun S, Xie M, et al: Association between the HLA-B alleles and carbamazepine-induced SJS/TEN: A meta-analysis, *Epilepsy Research* 135:19–28, 2017.

SUNBURN

Method of
Warwick L. Morison, MD

CURRENT DIAGNOSIS

- Sunburn appears 3 to 4 hours after exposure to sunlight or an artificial source of UV radiation such as a sunlamp.
- The redness of skin is diffuse and continuous, unlike rashes, which are often discontinuous.
- Sunburns are graded as pink, red, and blistering.

CURRENT THERAPY

- Prevention is the best approach to management and consists of a package of measures: avoiding over-exposure, using sunscreens, and wearing protective clothing.
- Treatment of a sunburn consists of cool baths and use of moisturizing creams.
- Topical and systemic corticosteroids do not alter the course of a sunburn.

Sunburn is a common problem, particularly in fair-skinned white persons, caused by excessive exposure to ultraviolet (UV) radiation from sunlight or artificial sources such as sunlamps. When induced by sunlight, it is mainly due to UVB (280–320 nm) radiation plus a smaller contribution from UVA (320–400 nm) radiation. Sunburn is also described as erythema, and it appears 3 to 4 hours after exposure, reaches a maximum at 12 to 18 hours, and usually settles after 72 to 96 hours. In severe reactions with blistering, complete resolution can take a week or more.

Sunburns are graded as pink, red, and blistering. In contrast, thermal burns are graded by degree (first, second, and third), but this classification should not be applied to sunburns because thermal burns have quite different sequelae, such as scarring and death, which are extremely rare consequences of a sunburn. Keratoconjunctivitis, or ocular sunburn, can also be caused by UV radiation and it follows a similar time course.

There are two facets to management of sunburn: prevention and treatment. Because there is no effective treatment for an established sunburn, most emphasis should be placed on prevention.

Prevention

Skin color and the capacity of a person to tan will determine how important it is for an individual person to take preventive measures. However, even dark-skinned people can sunburn provided the exposure dose is sufficiently high. Skin color, past history of sunburn, and likely exposure should therefore be used as a guide in advising people about protection. Protection from sunlight is often equated with use of sunscreens, but this approach is too narrow, and protection should consist of a package of measures: avoiding overexposure to sunlight, using sunscreens, and wearing protective clothing.

Avoidance of Exposure

Simple avoidance of excessive exposure to a threshold dose of UV radiation is often the best advice for fair-skinned people. Scheduling outdoor activities for before 10 am and after 4 pm will avoid the peak UV irradiance period and still permit enjoyment of the outdoors. This advice should be accompanied by several warnings. Sitting in the shade or under a beach umbrella only reduces exposure by about 70%. A cloudy day is often the setting for the worst sunburns because even complete white cloud cover reduces UV exposure by only about 50%.

Clothing is not always an effective protector. If it is possible to see through a fabric, UV radiation can also penetrate to a significant extent. The geographic location of exposure must also be considered because UV radiation may be twice as intense at the equator as compared with much of continental North America.

Sunscreens

There are now a great number of sunscreens on the market, and they contain numerous active ingredients. If this is not enough to cause confusion, some are not even labeled as sunscreens: sunblocks and tanning lotions are other terms. However, the informed physician need only know four properties of a sunscreen: the sun protection factor (SPF), the spectrum of protection, the base, and whether or not it is water resistant.

The SPF is an index of the amount of protection provided by the sunscreen. For example, a fair-skinned person who normally begins to sunburn after a 10-minute exposure to sunlight should be able to tolerate up to 150 minutes of exposure after application of an SPF 15 sunscreen.

There are several provisos for this statement. To provide the stated protection, a sunscreen must be applied 10 minutes before exposure to allow binding to skin proteins to occur, and it must be applied in an adequate amount. Several studies have shown that under ideal circumstances in which sunscreen is supplied freely and the subject is observed while making the application, most people only use one half the required amount. Ordinary use probably provides much less protection. As a rough guide, one ounce of sunscreen is necessary to cover a 70-kg adult in a bathing suit; in other words, a four ounce bottle of sunscreen only provides four applications.

Sunscreens vary in the amount of the solar spectrum for which they provide protection. All sunscreens provide protection against UVB radiation and the shorter end of UVA radiation. Some sunscreens claim to provide broad-spectrum protection against UVB and UVA radiation and contain avobenzone or titanium dioxide to protect against the longer wavelengths in the UVA spectrum. Ecamsule (Mexoryl SX), a recently approved sunscreen active, provides good absorption in the middle of the UVA spectrum; a sunscreen containing this, avobenzone, and octocrylene—an absorber of UVB radiation—provides very good broad-spectrum protection.

The base of a sunscreen is also important because it often determines whether or not a sunscreen will be used. Men usually prefer alcohol-based lotions because they dry quickly and leave a dry and nongreasy film. Women usually prefer lotions or creams because they give a moisturizing feel to the skin.

Finally, a sunscreen may be labeled water resistant or very water resistant. Because almost all outdoor pastimes involve perspiring or contact with water, a very water-resistant sunscreen should be selected.

A fair-skinned person should always use a sunscreen with an SPF 15 or higher. People who tan well and never burn are probably adequately protected with an SPF of 8 to 10. People with black or brown skin probably do not need sunscreens except for extreme occupational or social exposure.

A few myths should be dismissed. There is no effective oral sunscreen. Many have been tested and all have failed. Self-tanning preparations are not sunscreens. They do provide the appearance of a tan and are safe to use but they provide no significant protection against UV radiation.

Protective Clothing

There has been significant progress in recent years in the development, testing, and classification of UV-protective clothing. Akin to the SPF for sunscreens, such clothing is labeled with an ultraviolet protective factor (UPF), and a fabric with a UPF of 50 blocks transmission of 98% of UV radiation. A hat with a 3-inch brim all around completes the package of protection.

Protective Tanning

The proliferation of suntan parlors has generated a lot of interest in protective tanning, with much misinformation provided by the commercial interests involved. Little scientific information is available to provide a guide as to whether protective tanning is of any value in preventing the long-term hazards of excessive exposure to sunlight, namely skin cancer and premature aging of the skin. Certainly, preventive tanning using multiple suberythemal doses of UV radiation can prevent sunburn, but the cost in terms of chronic damage is unknown.

Most tanning salons claim to use only UVA radiation in their tanning beds, but this claim is false. All so-called UVA tanning beds emit some UVB radiation, the most damaging wavelengths, and in addition, UVA radiation, especially in large doses, can produce the same damaging effect as UVB radiation. Furthermore, a UVA-induced tan is not very protective and at most has an SPF of 6 to 8.

A person who tans well and never burns might gain some protection from sunlight by preventive tanning without incurring too much damage. However, the risk-to-benefit ratio for people who do sunburn is probably very unfavorable.

Treatment

When a person has a sunburn, general supportive measures are the only approach to treatment. Cold compresses and cool baths with bath oil provide some relief. Frequent application of moisturizing creams help alleviate dryness. Blistering of the skin can lead to secondary infection and require use of an antibiotic cream. Rarely, an extremely severe sunburn necessitates hospitalization and management as a thermal burn.

Topical corticosteroids reduce erythema by causing vasoconstriction, but this effect is temporary and does not reduce epidermal damage. Systemic corticosteroids, even in very large doses, do not alter the course of a sunburn. Nonsteroidal antiinflammatory drugs, if given at the time of exposure or beforehand, reduce the degree of erythema over the first 24 hours but do not change epidermal damage. Of course, few people lying on the beach anticipate an excessive exposure, so they are unlikely to embark on such preventive measures.

URTICARIA AND ANGIOEDEMA

Method of
Joyce M.C. Teng, MD, PhD

CURRENT DIAGNOSIS

- Acute and chronic urticaria have the same features, including erythematous, edematous papules or wheals with central pallor that last less than 24 to 48 hours.
- Laboratory assessments are not recommended for acute urticaria in the absence of evidence suggesting underlying systemic illness.
- Limited laboratory studies are indicated for chronic urticaria only if there are signs of systemic disease.
- Serum measurements of C4 and C1-esterase inhibitor are the recommended initial tests if hereditary or acquired angioedema are suspected.
- Skin biopsy should be considered to rule out urticarial vasculitis if an individual lesion is painful and persists for more than 2 to 3 days with accompanying ecchymosis or petechiae.

CURRENT THERAPY

- Primary treatment of urticaria and angioedema is removal of triggering factors and initiation of therapy for symptomatic relief.
- Oral antihistamines are the cornerstones of therapy. The application of first-generation H_1-antihistamines may be limited by central nervous system and anticholinergic side effects.

- Nonsedating second generation antihistamine are often used as first line therapy.
- Systemic corticosteroids and immunosuppressive therapy, especially cyclosporine (Neoral),[1] have been used successfully in cases that are refractory to the maximum dose of antihistamines.
- Fresh-frozen plasma infusions along with standard airway precautions have been recommended for angioedema patients with laryngeal edema.
- A subcutaneous C1 esterase inhibitor injection (Haegarda) has been used successfully to prevent attack in hereditary angioedema.

[1]Not FDA approved for this indication.

TABLE 1	Mechanisms in Urticaria and Angioedema	
DISORDER	**CAUSES**
Immunoglobulin-mediated urticaria	Ig-E mediated: food, medication, insect bites, contact allergen, aeroallergens, other causes Urticaria associated with autoimmunity: antinuclear antibodies (ANAs), thyroid autoantibodies, other causes
Direct activation of mast cell degranulation	Physical stimuli: exercise, heat, cold, pressure, aquagenic, solar radiation, etc. Other agents: opiates, antibiotics (e.g., vancomycin [Vancocin]), radiocontrast, ACTH (Cortrosyn), muscle relaxants
Complement-mediated	Viral infections, parasites, blood transfusion
C1-esterase inhibitor deficiency	Genetic and acquired angioedema, paraproteinemia
Reduced kinin metabolism	Angiotensin-converting enzyme (ACE) inhibitors
Reduced arachidonic acid metabolism	Aspirin

Urticaria, or hives, is a common cutaneous eruption that occurs in up to 25% of the general population sometime during their lives.[1] It is characterized by transient, circumscribed, pruritic, erythematous papules or plaques, often with central pallor. Individual lesions often coalesce into large wheals on the trunk and extremities that may resolve over a few hours without leaving any residual skin changes. The process is mediated by mast cells in the superficial dermis.

Angioedema is a similar process occurring in deep dermis or subcutaneous tissue. Angioedema may occur independently, accompanied by urticaria, or as a component of anaphylaxis. It is characterized by localized swelling that develops over minutes to hours and resolves within 24 to 48 hours. Common locations of angioedema include the mucosa and areas with loose connective tissue, such as the face, eyes, lips, tongue, and genitalia. Patients usually do not have pruritus, but they may have pain and a sensation of warmth. Angioedema is usually a benign process that resolves without sequelae unless it involves the larynx. African Americans are disproportionately affected, representing up to 40% of the hospital admissions for angioedema.

Classification
Urticaria can be classified as acute or chronic, depending on the duration. Acute urticaria usually lasts for less than 6 weeks and is commonly triggered by infection, medication, insect bite, and food (Table 1). The chronic form, lasting more than 6 weeks, accounts for approximately 30% of cases of urticaria, and no clear causes can be identified in more than 80% of these cases. Stress however has been identified as a trigger in some of the cases. A significant number of patients with chronic urticaria may have persistent symptoms for more than 10 years. Approximately 40% of patients with chronic urticaria have associated angioedema, although the incidence of laryngeal edema is low.

Diagnosis
Urticaria is diagnosed clinically in most cases. A detailed history, physical examination, and complete review of systems are essential for diagnosing patients with urticaria and angioedema. The history should include the distribution and characteristics of lesions (e.g., pain, pruritus), duration of skin eruption, accompanying angioedema, airway involvement and other associated systemic symptoms (e.g., fever, arthralgia, swelling joints, refusal to walk by children). Patients should also be questioned about changes in dietary habits, stress, recent exposures, infection, and newly administered medications, including antibiotics, over-the-counter analgesia, and hormones.

Laboratory assessment is usually not helpful in diagnosing patients with acute urticaria who lack any history or clinical findings to suggest an underlying disease process. A limited number of diagnostic tests are indicated in the evaluation of patients with chronic urticaria when there is sign of systemic disease associated, such as a complete blood cell count with differential white blood

cell count, an erythrocyte sedimentation rate (ESR) or C-reactive protein (CRP) determination, a thyroid-stimulating hormone (TSH) level, antithyroglobulin and antimicrosomal antibodies, antinuclear antibodies (ANA), folate, B12, ferritin, liver function test, and hepatitis B and C serologies. A detailed review of systems may help to narrow the focus of the screening test.

A skin biopsy of an early lesion should be performed to rule out urticarial vasculitis if the affected individual has skin lesions that are painful and last for more than 2 to 3 days with residual ecchymosis or petechiae. In patients with angioedema, prominent edema of the interstitial tissue may be demonstrated by biopsy. It is associated with antibodies against C1q, which leads to persistent complement activation and low serum C3, C4. Serum measurements of C4 and C1-esterase inhibitor are recommended initial tests if hereditary or acquired angioedema is suspected. Hereditary angioedema is caused by deficiency (type I) or dysfunction (type II) of C1-esterase inhibitor protein. A C1q level should be obtained to screen for the acquired form of angioedema if the affected individual is middle-aged.

Treatment
More than two thirds of cases of urticaria are self-limited. Spontaneous remission of chronic urticaria and angioedema is also common. The primary objective of management is to identify and discontinue the offending trigger. A patient presenting with angioedema must first be assessed for signs of airway compromise. Medical therapy is indicated for those who are symptomatic.

Antihistamines remain the first-line therapy for most patients with urticaria, because the primary complaint of pruritus is predominantly mediated by histamine released from mast cells. First-generation antihistamines such as hydroxyzine (Atarax or Vistaril 25–50 mg every 6 hours), diphenhydramine (Benadryl 25–50 mg every 6 hours), cyproheptadine (Periactin 4 mg three times daily), and chlorpheniramine[1] (Chlor-Trimeton 4 mg every 6 hours) are potent and have the quickest onset of action. However, the treatments are often limited by their sedating and anticholinergic side effects. Many first-generation antihistamines are available over the counter, providing accessible first-line therapy for patients. Patients with urticaria that lasts for several days should be considered for treatment using second-generation antihistamines such as loratadine (Claritin[1] 10 mg twice daily[3]), desloratadine[1] (Clarinex 5 mg twice daily[3]), cetirizine[1] (Zyrtec 10 mg twice daily[3]), levocetirizine[1] (Xyzal 5 mg daily), and fexofenadine[1] (Allegra 180 mg twice daily[3]). Doxepin (Sinequan),[1] an H_1- and H_2-receptor antagonist, is seven times more potent than hydroxyzine in suppression of wheal and flare responses. Because of its central nervous system side effects, combined use of doxepin with a first-generation antihistamine should be restricted. Topical 5% doxepin cream (Zonalon)[1] may help to suppress pruritus in patients with localized urticaria.

Systemic prednisone at 30 to 40 mg in a single morning dose is sufficient to suppress acute urticaria in adults. Tapering should be gradual over a 3- to 4-week period by decreasing the dosage 5 mg every 3 to 5 days to minimize rebound. Alternate-morning dosing when reaching 20 mg daily may help to minimize the steroid side effects. Methylprednisolone (Solu-Medrol 40 mg) should be given intravenously as initial therapy to patients with angioedema. This may be followed by a tapering oral course. Chronic therapy is to be avoided. Three months of treatment with cyclosporine (Neoral)[1] at 3 to 5 mg/kg can be given safely to patients who are refractory to corticosteroid therapy or have difficulty tapering their therapy. Close monitoring for hypertension and renal insufficiency is necessary during the treatment.

Leukotriene inhibitors such as zileuton (Zyflo[1] 600 mg four times daily), zafirlukast (Accolate[1] 20 mg twice daily), and montelukast (Singulair[1] 10 mg once daily) may be effective for patients with autoimmune urticaria. Successful treatment of chronic urticaria with anti-IgE (omalizumab [Xolair][1]) has been reported but the medication is approved by the FDA for moderate to severe allergic asthma only for patients above 12 years of age.

Proper management of underlying autoimmune thyroid disease or autoimmune collagen vascular diseases has been beneficial for patients with associated urticaria. Life-threatening angioedema triggered by angiotensin-converting enzyme (ACE) inhibitors has been successfully treated with infusion of fresh-frozen plasma. Hereditary angioedema can be prevented with tranexamic acid[1] or modified androgens. Intravenous C1-esterase inhibitor (Cinryze) or icatibant (Firazyr), a bradykinin B2 antagonist, can be administered to prevent acute attacks. Subcutaneous injection of C1-esterase inhibitor (Haegarda) has been approved by FDA in 2017 to prevent hereditary angioedema attacks. Treatments with methotrexate[1], warfarin (Coumadin),[1] plasmapheresis, and intravenous immunoglobulin (Baygam)[1] have been reported for severe, refractory[1] urticaria. These treatments are administered only by specialists on an individual basis. Non-pharmacotherapeutic means such as frequent use of skin emollients, avoidance of hot shower, scrubbing, and excessive sun exposure should also be recommended as part of management plans.

---

[1] Not FDA approved for this indication.
[3] Exceeds dosage recommended by the manufacturer.

Bailey E, Shaker M: An update on childhood urticaria and angioedema, *Curr Opin Pediatr* 20(4):425–430, 2008.
Champion RH, Roberts SO, Carpenter RG, Roger JH: Urticaria and angio-oedema. A review of 554 patients, *Br J Dermatol* 81(8):588–597, 1969.
Joint Task Force on Practice Parameters: The diagnosis and management of urticaria: A practice parameter. Part II. Chronic urticaria/angioedema, *Ann Allergy Asthma Immunol* 85(2):521–544, 2000.
Kaplan AP, Joseph K, Maykut RJ, et al: Treatment of chronic autoimmune urticaria with omalizumab, *J Allergy Clin Immunol* 122(3):569–573, 2008.
Lin RY, Cannon AG, Teitel AD: Pattern of hospitalizations for angioedema in New York between 1990 and 2003, *Ann Allergy Asthma Immunol* 95(2):159–166, 2005.
Longhurst H, Cicardi M, Craig T, et al: Prevention of hereditary angioedema attacks with a subcutaneous C1 inhibitor, *N Engl J Med* 376(12):1131–1140, 2017 Mar 23.
Maurer M, Rosen K, Shieh HJ: Omalizumab for chronic urticaria, *N Engl J Med* 386:2530, 2013. https://doi.org/10.1056/JEJMc1305687.
Nizami RM, Baboo MT: Office management of patients with urticaria: An analysis of 215 patients, *Ann Allergy* 33(2):78–85, 1974.
Powell RJ, Du Toit GL, Siddique N, et al: BSACI guidelines for the management of chronic urticaria and angio-oedema, *Clin Exp Allergy* 37(5):631–650, 2007.

VENOUS ULCERS

Method of
Jose A. Jaller, MD; and Robert S. Kirsner, MD, PhD

CURRENT DIAGNOSIS

- Venous ulcers are the most common cause of lower-extremity ulceration.
- Valvular incompetence, vein distention, muscular weakness, and/or a decrease in the range of motion of the ankle may lead to venous insufficiency.
- The mechanism of cutaneous ulceration resulting from venous insufficiency remains unclear.
- The typical location for a venous ulcer is on the medial malleolus.
- Complications of chronic venous ulcers are cellulitis and less often squamous cell carcinoma.
- Compression is the gold standard of treatment of venous disease.

CURRENT THERAPY

- Compression therapy is used to deliver a graded compression of 30–40 mm Hg at the ankle. Arterial disease should be excluded prior to full compression.
- Systemic medications as adjuvant therapy to compression bandages include aspirin[1,] pentoxifylline (Trental), or micronized purified flavonoid fraction (Daflon 500 mg)[2.]
- Other treatments, along with compression, include engineered skin, placental and skin grafts, electrical stimulation, locally derived growth factors, and venous surgery.
- The lifelong use of elastic compression stockings (30–40 mm Hg) is the mainstay of prevention.

[1]Not FDA approved for this indication.
[2]Not available in the United States.

Ulcers resulting from venous insufficiency are the most common cause of leg ulceration. Many definitions exist for a chronic wound, which ultimately reflect the demographics, incidence, and prevalence data available. The Wound Healing Society classifies wounds as *acute* if they sustain restoration of anatomic and functional integrity in an orderly and timely process and *chronic* if they do not. Venous leg ulcers (VLUs) are more frequently seen in the elderly population; however, about 1 in 5 primary VLUs occur in patients under 40 years of age. Personal or family history of venous disease, obesity, smoking, advanced age, female sex, hypertension, and leg injuries are strong risk factors to the development of VLUs.

Epidemiology

Venous insufficiency affects approximately 5% of the world's population and about 2% of the American population. VLUs affect 1% to 2% of adults in the United States, accounting for over 2 million lost workdays annually. The associated pain, inability to perform daily activities, and social stigma due to the appearance and odor of the wounds drastically diminish patients' quality of life. Moreover, the high cost of treatment, time off work, and hospital admissions forge a massive economic burden in the healthcare system. Seventy percent of all leg ulcers result solely from venous disease, and an additional 20% of patients have mixed arterial and venous disease. A recent report that used claims data from 2013 private and governmental insurance companies revealed that wounds and ulcers had the highest direct

US healthcare cost of all skin diseases ($12 billion) and caused approximately 21% of all deaths related to skin condition, second only to cutaneous cancers.

Pathophysiology

In the lower extremities, the venous system comprises the deep and superficial veins. Blood flows from the superficial to the deep veins through the communicating or perforating veins to ultimately reach the heart. Veins contain unidirectional valves that prevent blood return or reflux. During calf muscle relaxation, the pressure difference (high pressure in the superficial veins) allows blood flow from the superficial to deep veins. When a healthy individual contracts the calf muscles, a high pressure develops in the deep vein system, allowing blood to flow from the deep veins to the heart. If the calf muscle contraction is restricted or the one-way valves are deficient, the system fails to adequately return venous blood to the heart, leading to venous hypertension (also known as sustained ambulatory high pressure).

The pathway to developing an ulcer due to venous insufficiency is unclear, albeit several hypotheses have been considered since the beginning of the 20th century. In the early 1980s, Browse and Burnard suggested that venous hypertension could lead to endothelial distention, causing extravasation of fibrinogen into the interstitial fluid, which results in "pericapillary fibrin cuff" formation around the capillary vessels. Fibrin cuffs act as a barrier to diffusion of oxygen and nutrients, causing ischemia and ulcer formation. A few years later, Coleridge-Smith and colleagues suggested that venous hypertension could lead to decreased capillary perfusion, resulting in leukocyte trapping. The trapped leukocytes release proteolytic enzymes, which result in free radical formation and capillary damage. The increased capillary permeability causes extravasation of fibrinogen and other metabolites, which leads to the formation of a fibrin cuff around the capillaries and ultimately ischemia.

Further studies supported the presence of increased levels of monocyte aggregation. Claudy and colleagues showed that leukocyte activation caused release of tumor necrosis factor alpha ($TNF-\alpha$), ultimately leading to pericapillary fibrin cuff formation. In 1993, Falanga and Eaglstein observed that fibrin cuffs were discontinuous around capillaries and therefore did not form a barrier to oxygen and nutrients causing ischemia. They also postulated the "trap" hypothesis, which suggests that venous hypertension causes endothelial cell distention leading to extravasation of macromolecules (i.e., α_2-macroglobulin and fibrinogen) into the dermis. Moreover, α_2-macroglobulin can bind to growth factors, such as $TNF-\alpha$ and transforming growth factor beta (TGF-β), making them unavailable for wound repair. Patients with venous disease may have other factors that contribute to venous ulcer formation, such as systemic alteration in fibrinolysis and arteriovenous shunting. Despite all previously conducted studies and hypotheses, further research is needed to explain the mechanism of cutaneous ulceration resulting from venous insufficiency.

Evaluation and Diagnosis

VLUs are diagnosed clinically; however, blood flow imaging, pathology, and microbiologic cultures can aid to rule out other conditions. Clinical signs, such as wound location, associated venous disease, and past personal history of venous ulcers, are paramount for the diagnosis. VLUs are typically located on the lower leg, particularly in the medial lower leg or medial malleolus. The ulcer usually begins as a blister or erosion on the skin that hinders healing and develops into a full-thickness lesion, or ulcer. Ulcer borders are irregular and usually smooth. The base of the ulcer may be covered with granulation tissue, yellow slough, or both. Venous ulcers are associated with the presence of pigmentation, erythema, dermatitis, edema, and induration (i.e., lipodermatosclerosis) of the surrounding skin and with varicose veins in the lower leg. Hemosiderin deposition resulting from red blood cell extravasation and iron-related stimulation of melanocytes cause the surrounding hyperpigmentation.

Lipodermatosclerosis is caused by sclerosis of the dermis and subcutaneous tissue. The presence of lipodermatosclerosis has been associated with a greater impairment of fibrinolysis in patients with venous ulcers and may be a poor prognostic factor for restriction of leg movement. Other known prognostic factors are duration and size of the ulcer and history of venous surgery. Ulcers present for longer than 6 months and larger than 5 cm in diameter tend to be more refractory to therapy.

A diagnosis of venous ulcers may be based on clinical presentation. The findings of a lower leg ulcer associated with lipodermatosclerosis or varicose veins, or both, suggest a venous ulcer. Other common findings include atrophie blanche (i.e., porcelain white scars with telangiectasia and dyspigmentation) and dermatitis. Venous dermatitis is associated with erythema, eczema, pruritus, and scaling of the skin. Contact dermatitis surrounding the ulcer may result from the use of topical agents.

Even though venous insufficiency should be confirmed with a variety of techniques, including duplex ultrasound or plethysmography, the presence or absence of arterial disease is a more important factor dictating treatment and prognosis. Treatment with compression bandages is the mainstay of therapy and should be used cautiously in patients with arterial disease. A simple, noninvasive measurement to assess peripheral arterial disease is the ankle brachial index (ABI). This value is calculated by dividing the systolic pressure in the ankle by the systolic pressure in the arm. An ABI of less than 0.9 indicates peripheral vascular disease and represents an independent risk factor for vascular disease in other vascular beds, such as the coronary arteries. Care must be taken with diabetic or elderly patients who may have a falsely negative ABI value. All patients with an abnormal ABI value should be further evaluated. Consider a vascular consultation, magnetic resonance angiography (MRA), angioplasty, and stent bypass.

To aid in the exclusion of any underlying disease (e.g., hematologic disease, diabetes), initial laboratory tests should include complete blood cell (CBC) count with a differential count, chemistry panel, hemoglobin A1C, prealbumin and albumin determinations, liver function tests, and levels of homocysteine, proteins C and S, antithrombin III, and factor V Leiden.

Several vascular studies help in the diagnosis and severity of venous disease. Color duplex ultrasound is usually the initial study done to assess venous reflux in the lower extremities. Continuous-wave Doppler studies may yield false-negative results because it may be difficult to differentiate between the superficial and deep venous system. Air plethysmography and photoplethysmography are helpful in evaluating venous reflux and calf muscle dysfunction. Invasive venography is the gold standard to assess venous reflux, but it is used only as a last resort because of its invasive properties.

The CEAP classification was developed in 1994 by the American Venous Forum (AVF) to standardize the diagnosis and treatment of venous disease. It was based on clinical manifestations (C), etiologic factors (E), anatomic distribution of disease (A), and underlying pathophysiologic findings (P).

Complications

Main complications of long-term or chronic venous ulcers are cellulitis, osteomyelitis, and squamous cell carcinoma. A finding of exposed tendon or bone, in addition to suggesting an underlying osteomyelitis, suggests an ulcer with a nonvenous cause.

Radiographs and biopsy for histology and culture are appropriate first steps in evaluation. Consult an orthopedic surgeon for further analysis and treatment, which may include a bone biopsy and bone débridement.

Treatment

Compression is the gold standard of treatment of venous disease. After arterial disease has been excluded, reversal of the effects of venous hypertension through compression bandages and leg elevation is the cornerstone of therapy.

The goal of compression therapy is to deliver sustained graded compression with 30 to 40 mm Hg at the ankle. These bandages are applied circumferentially from the toes to the knees (involving the heel) with the foot dorsiflexed. The optimal method to deliver this pressure is through multilayered elastic compression dressings. Elastic compression dressings deliver compression during ambulation (i.e., walking) and at rest, accommodate to reduction in edema, and are superior to single-layered dressings. Inelastic compression (short-stretch compression) may deliver similar results but appear to require greater sophistication by those applying them to accomplish this. Inelastic bandages, which do not deliver compression at rest, may be advantageous[1] in patients with arterial disease or patients who do not tolerate full compression (e.g., elderly). Highly pressured compression stockings are as effective as compression wrappings; however, patients' compliance is a significant limitation.

Systemic medication as adjuvant therapy to compression bandages, such as pentoxifylline[1] (Trental 400 to 800 mg three times daily[3]), aspirin[1], or micronized purified flavonoid fraction (MPFF, Daflon 500 mg[2] [diosmin[7] 90% and hesperidin[7] 10%]) have shown to be superior to compression bandages alone with regard to the rate of healing. The use of pentoxifylline as adjuvant therapy to compression in venous ulcers has been shown to be very beneficial.

Wound bed preparation was proposed as a way to help the healing process. It is a multistep process that improves the wound bed by removing necrotic and fibrinous wound tissue, increasing the amount of granulation tissue, and decreasing edema, chronic wound fluid (i.e., exudate), and bacterial burden.

The decision of which wound dressing to use will depend on the amount of wound drainage. Occlusive dressings should be used for dry to mildly exudative wounds, providing a moist environment for healing. A variety of types of occlusions may be used, and the choice depends on several factors, including the location of the wound and the amount of fibrinous slough and exudate present. Foam, gel, and calcium alginate dressings are highly absorbent dressings and should be used for moderate-to-severe exudating wounds. Sharp wound debridement should be performed to remove any devitalized tissue. Fear of excessive infection with the use of occlusive dressings is unfounded. Topical antiseptics and cleansing agents should be used with caution because they may increase the time required for healing. Topical agents such as cadexomer iodine (Iodosorb), silver-impregnated dressings, and topical anesthetics are alternatives that do not prolong healing. These topical agents should be considered when the wound appears contaminated, but not infected. Wound infections should be treated like cellulitis, with systemic antibiotics.

Up to 50% of venous ulcers may be refractory to compression therapy alone. This refractory subset may be predicted by baseline characteristics (size and duration) and by a decrease in size with 2 to 4 weeks of treatment (Figure 1). Other available treatments include tissue-engineered skin, autologous skin, electrical stimulation, treatment with locally delivered growth factors, and venous surgery. Three categories exist for skin grafts: autologous, allogeneic (cultured), and artificial (tissue-engineered skin). Three different techniques have been used for autologous skin grafts: epidermal skin graft (only epidermis and no dermis), split-thickness skin graft (all the epidermis and a portion of the dermis), and full-thickness skin graft (complete dermis and epidermis). The use of artificial, or bioengineered grafts, has risen in the past decades.

Apligraf is a bilayered engineered living skin composed of keratinocytes and fibroblasts from neonatal foreskin that is approved by the US Food and Drug Administration for treatment of venous

Figure 1 Simplified algorithm for the diagnosis and treatment of patients with venous ulcers. *ABI*, Ankle-brachial index; *MPFF*, micronized purified flavonoid fraction; *SCC*, squamous cell carcinoma.

leg and diabetic neuropathic foot ulcers. Likewise, other synthetic skin grafts have used animal tissue to generate this sophisticated dressing. Surgical treatment of incompetent superficial and perforator veins along with standard of care (i.e., compression) reduce the risk of recurrence.

After healing occurs, patients with venous insufficiency are at risk for recurrence. The lifelong use of elastic compression stockings (30 to 40 mm Hg) is the mainstay of therapy, but early intervention after recurrence is critical. Health professionals need to understand the importance of further research to ultimately minimize the psychological, physical, and socioeconomic impact that ulcers caused by venous insufficiency have on patients and society.

References

Abbade LP, Lastória S: Venous ulcer: Epidemiology, physiopathology, diagnosis and treatment, *Int J Dermatol* 44:449–456, 2005.

Browse NL, Burnand KG: The cause of venous ulceration, *Lancet* 2:243–245, 1982.

Claudy AL, Mirshahi M, Soria C, et al: Detection of undegraded fibrin and tumor necrosis factor alpha in venous leg ulcers, *J Am Acad Dermatol* 25:623–627, 1991.

Coleridge-Smith PD, Thomas P, Scurr JH, et al: Causes of venous ulceration: A new hypothesis? *Br Med J* 296:1726–1727, 1988.

Falanga V, Eaglstein WH: The trap hypothesis of venous ulceration, *Lancet* 341:1006–1008, 1993.

Jull A, Arroll B, Parag V, Waters J: Pentoxyphilline for treating venous leg ulcers, *Cochrane Database Syst Rev* (3):CD001733, 2007.

Kirsner R: Wound bed preparation, *Ostomy Wound Manage* (Feb. Suppl.):2–3, 2003.

Kirsner RS, Falanga V: Techniques of split-thickness skin grafting for lower extremity ulcerations, *J Dermatol Surg Oncol* 19:779–783, 1993.

Kirsner RS, Pardes JB, Eaglstein WH, Falanga V: The clinical spectrum of lipodermatosclerosis, *J Am Acad Dermatol* 28:623–627, 1993.

Lazarus GS, Cooper DM, Knighton DR, et al: Definitions and guidelines for assessment of wounds and evaluation of healing, *Arch Dermatol* 130:489–493, 1994.

Lim HW, Collins SAB, Resneck JS Jr., et al: The burden of skin disease in the United States, *J Am Acad Dermatol* 76 (5):958–972.e952, 2017.

Olin JW, Beusterien KM, Childs MB, et al: Medical costs of treating venous stasis ulcers: Evidence from a retrospective cohort study, *Vasc Med* 4:1–7, 1999.

Phillips TJ, Machado F, Trout R, et al: Prognostic indicators in venous ulcers, *J Am Acad Dermatol* 43:627–630, 2000.

Singer AJ, Tassiopoulos A, Kirsner RS: Evaluation and management of lower-extremity ulcers, *N Engl J Med* 377(16):1559–1567, 2017.

Trent JT, Falabella A, Eaglstein WH, Kirsner RS: Venous ulcers: Pathophysiology and treatment options, *Ostomy Wound Manage* 51:38–54, 2005.

---

[1] Not FDA approved for this indication.
[2] Not available in the United States.
[3] Exceeds dosage recommended by the manufacturer.
[7] Available as dietary supplement.

VIRAL DISEASES OF THE SKIN

Method of
Sylvia L. Brice, MD

CURRENT DIAGNOSIS

Herpes Simplex Viruses 1 and 2
- Clinical: Grouped vesicles or erosions, especially in perioral or anogenital location
- Laboratory: Tzanck smear, viral culture, antigen detection, PCR, gG-based type-specific serology

Varicella-Zoster Virus
- Clinical: Papules, pustules, vesicles in diffuse (varicella) or dermatomal (herpes zoster) distribution
- Laboratory: Tzanck smear, antigen detection, viral culture, PCR

Hand-Foot-and-Mouth Disease
- Clinical: Papulovesicles on oral mucosa, hands, feet following fever, constitutional symptoms
- Laboratory: PCR

Parvovirus B19
- Clinical: "Slapped cheeks" reticular erythema on trunk or extremities following fever, constitutional symptoms; arthralgias, arthritis, purpuric eruptions; transient aplastic crisis, fetal hydrops
- Laboratory: B19 specific IgM serology, PCR

Molluscum Contagiosum
- Clinical: Few to multiple 1- to 4-mm umbilicated flesh-colored papules
- Laboratory: Histopathology if clinical appearance atypical

Orf
- Clinical: One to several solid to vesicular nodules on hands, forearms; history of exposure to sheep, goats, cattle
- Laboratory: Histopathology if clinical appearance atypical; PCR

Abbreviation: NSAID = nonsteroidal antiinflammatory drug.

CURRENT THERAPY

Herpes Simplex Viruses 1 and 2
- Acyclovir (Zovirax), valacyclovir (Valtrex), famciclovir (Famvir)
- For acyclovir resistance: foscarnet (Foscavir),[1] cidofovir (Vistide)[1]

Varicella-Zoster Virus
- Acyclovir, valacyclovir, famciclovir
- For acyclovir resistance: foscarnet,[1] cidofovir[1]

Hand-Foot-and-Mouth Disease
- Supportive care

Parvovirus B19
- Supportive care, IVIg (Gammagard)[1]

Molluscum Contagiosum
- Surgical or chemical methods of destruction
- Immunomodulators (imiquimod [Aldara],[1] cimetidine [Tagamet][1])

Orf
- Self-limited

[1]Not FDA approved for this indication.
Abbreviation: HSV = herpes simplex virus; IVIg = intravenous immunoglobulin.

Herpes Simplex Viruses 1 and 2

Herpes simplex virus types 1 and 2 (HSV-1 and HSV-2) are the most closely related members of the human herpesvirus family, and the skin lesions they produce are clinically indistinguishable. Clusters of tense blisters on an erythematous base often quickly evolve into erosions or ulcerations with associated crusting. Lesions can develop at any mucocutaneous site but are typically found in the perioral or anogenital regions. Both HSV-1 and HSV-2 are transmitted by direct mucocutaneous contact with an infected host. Following viral replication in the skin or mucosa, intact viral nucleocapsids travel via sensory neurons to the corresponding dorsal root ganglia to establish latency. Later, a variety of stimuli can trigger reactivation. The virus travels back along the sensory neurons to the mucocutaneous surface to replicate and induce active or subclinical infection. In the case of subclinical infection, no active skin lesions are evident, but infectious particles are present, a state known as asymptomatic shedding. Although the viral titer is much lower than during clinically active disease, asymptomatic shedding of the virus in oral and genital secretions is thought to be responsible for the majority of cases of HSV transmission.

Primary, initial nonprimary (also known as first episode), and recurrent are terms used to further define the nature of the HSV infection. A *primary* infection refers to a patient's first infection with either type of HSV at any site. These patients are seronegative initially but subsequently develop HSV type-specific antibodies. A patient who is already infected with one HSV type and then develops an infection with the alternate type experiences an *initial nonprimary* or first-episode infection (e.g., the first episode of genital herpes in a patient with a prior history of orofacial herpes). These patients are seropositive for one type-specific HSV antibody (e.g., HSV-1) and later develop antibodies specific for the alternate HSV type (e.g., HSV-2). A *recurrent* infection is one that occurs at a site of prior infection. These patients are seropositive for HSV-1 or HSV-2, or both. Because most primary infections, whether oral or genital, are asymptomatic, the first evidence of disease often represents a recurrent or initial nonprimary infection.

Orofacial Herpes Simplex Virus Infection

Orofacial HSV, also known as herpes labialis, fever blisters, or cold sores, is commonly acquired during childhood or adolescence. Symptomatic primary disease usually takes the form of gingivostomatitis with or without additional lesions on the cutaneous perioral surfaces. Fever, malaise, and tender lymphadenopathy may also be present. In recurrent episodes, clusters of blisters erupt along the vermillion border of the lips, and subsequent erosions and crusting persist for several days up to 2 weeks. Lesions can develop anywhere in the perioral area, especially on the cheeks. In men, a viral folliculitis of the beard area (herpetic sycosis) may be mistaken for a bacterial process because it is often pustular. The presence of a prodrome and recurrence in the same site are clues to the correct diagnosis. Although recurrent intraoral lesions of HSV can occur, they are uncommon in immunocompetent persons. Exposure to ultraviolet light is a common trigger factor for herpes labialis, as is fever or intercurrent infection.

Genital Herpes Simplex Virus Infection

When symptomatic, primary genital herpes often involves bilaterally distributed lesions in the anogenital area with associated fever, inguinal adenopathy, and dysuria or urinary retention. Aseptic meningitis can also occur. The lesions often persist for 2 to 3 weeks or longer. Nonprimary infections are usually less severe and have fewer constitutional symptoms. Recurrent episodes tend to be milder and shorter in duration. Often, there is a prodrome of tingling or burning followed by the development of localized vesicles that can quickly rupture, leaving nonspecific erosions or ulcerations. The lesions may be anywhere within the anogenital region but tend to recur close to the same area in subsequent episodes. The time between exposure and development of primary disease is estimated to be from 3 to 14 days. However, more often the first clinical indication of disease is a recurrence, which can occur weeks to years after the initial infection. Prior infection with HSV-1 provides some protection against acquisition of HSV-2.

Based on seroepidemiologic evidence, it is estimated that approximately 17% of the United States population aged 14 to 49 years are infected with HSV-2. In most of these persons, this disease has not been officially diagnosed and they are unaware that they are infected. Nevertheless, they experience asymptomatic shedding and unknowingly transmit the disease to sexual partners. Interrupting this cycle of transmission has become a major focus among health care providers who work with these patients. A combination of patient education and appropriate use of systemic antiviral agents may be gradually having some impact on this epidemic. Recommendations for patients with genital herpes include avoiding sex with uninfected partners when active lesions or prodromal symptoms are present and routinely using latex condoms to minimize transmission during periods of asymptomatic shedding. Chronic suppressive doses of oral antiviral agents (Table 1), including acyclovir (Zovirax), valacyclovir (Valtrex), and famciclovir (Famvir), significantly reduce the frequency of clinical recurrences as well as the rate of asymptomatic shedding and may be recommended together with these other practices to reduce the risk of transmission.

Although HSV-2 is the etiologic agent in a majority of cases of genital herpes infections, an increasing number of genital herpes infections are caused by HSV-1. Symptomatic recurrences and asymptomatic shedding are less frequent with genital HSV-1 infection than with genital HSV-2 infection, and this distinction becomes important for patient counseling and prognosis.

Other Mucocutaneous Herpes Simplex Virus Infections

Eczema herpeticum, also known as Kaposi's varicelliform eruption, represents a cutaneous dissemination of HSV usually seen in patients with atopic dermatitis or other underlying skin disease. Herpetic vesicles develop over an extensive mucocutaneous surface, most often the face, neck, and upper trunk, presumably spreading from a recurrent oral HSV infection or asymptomatic shedding from the oral mucosa. Eczema herpeticum can also develop in the presence of genital HSV. As with other HSV infections, eczema herpeticum may be recurrent. In addition, patients can develop localized, recurrent HSV in previously involved areas. Because of the extensive and inflammatory nature of the process and the possible secondary bacterial infection, the underlying viral etiology may be obscured. A history of eczema and recurrent HSV in the patient and careful observation for the grouped vesicles or erosions can be key to the correct diagnosis.

Herpetic whitlow refers to HSV infection of the hand, usually one or more distal digits. Previously thought to be limited to health care professionals with exposure to oral secretions of their patients, it is now recognized that autoinoculation from orolabial or genital HSV contributes to a significant number of cases.

Herpes gladiatorum is a problem seen most commonly in athletes who participate in close contact sports such as wrestling. Typically transmitted from active herpes labialis or asymptomatic shedding in oral secretions of an infected opponent, herpes gladiatorum often affects the head, neck, or shoulders and may be recurrent. In the wrestler with frequent outbreaks, chronic suppressive therapy may be recommended.

Diagnosis

Viral culture remains a common and acceptable method for diagnosing HSV infection. This method is sensitive when specimens are obtained from lesions that have not yet become too dry or crusted, usually during the first 2 to 3 days after onset. An adequate sample, obtained by unroofing the blister and swabbing the base, increases the likelihood of an accurate result. Antigen detection tests can remain positive even after lesions have dried, as long as the specimen includes epithelial cells and not just debris. For this method, a scraping from the lesion is usually smeared on a glass slide to be sent to the laboratory. Not all antigen detection methods are designed to distinguish HSV-1 from HSV-2.

Polymerase chain reaction (PCR) is highly sensitive and has become routinely available for diagnosis of mucocutaneous HSV infections. PCR may also be useful for detection of asymptomatic shedding.

The Tzanck smear (cytologic detection) is both insensitive and nonspecific but may be of use in some clinical settings. It does not differentiate HSV types or HSV from varicella-zoster virus (VZV).

Serologic testing for HSV was previously of limited use because it could not reliably differentiate HSV-1 from HSV-2. Because they share significant genetic homology, HSV-1 and HSV-2 code for a number of common proteins that are not antigenically distinct. However, they also code for type-specific proteins that can be used to differentiate them. Current tests based on detecting type-specific viral glycoprotein G (gG-based, type-specific assays) are accurate and should be requested for this purpose. A positive HSV-2 serology may be useful in confirming the diagnosis of genital herpes in a patient with a negative viral culture or with unrecognized or asymptomatic disease. Alternatively, a negative serology can help exclude the diagnosis of HSV in a patient with chronic, nonspecific oral or genital symptoms.

Varicella Zoster Virus

VZV, another member of the human herpesvirus family, produces two specific patterns of disease in the skin. The primary infection results in varicella, also known as chickenpox, a widespread vesicular eruption usually seen in the pediatric population. Following the primary infection, VZV establishes latency in the dorsal root ganglia until some later point, when reactivation can occur. The ensuing unilateral dermatomal distribution of blisters, often preceded by neuralgic pain, is known as herpes zoster or shingles. Herpes zoster is especially common in patients older than 50 years, but it may be seen at any age. It is also seen more commonly in immunocompromised patients, such as organ transplant recipients or patients infected with HIV. Herpes zoster is no longer considered a marker for underlying cancer, and evaluation for occult malignancy in an otherwise asymptomatic patient is not indicated. A single recurrence of herpes zoster, usually in the same dermatome, may occur, but this is uncommon in immunocompetent individuals. Additional recurrences, however, suggest a dermatomal form of HSV, and laboratory assessment for this possibility may be indicated.

The most common dermatomes involved with herpes zoster are in the thoracolumbar (T3-L2) and trigeminal (V1) regions. Skin lesions typically evolve from papules to vesicles and pustules, and then to crusted erosions, before healing approximately 2 to 4 weeks after onset. The associated neuropathic pain commonly persists after the lesions have healed. Pain that continues for more than 3 months after the skin lesions resolve is referred to as postherpetic neuralgia, one of the most common and debilitating complications of this infection.

Several clinical presentations of herpes zoster deserve additional attention. Ophthalmic zoster, with lesions along the tip, side, or base of the nose indicating involvement of the nasociliary branch of the trigeminal nerve (Hutchinson's sign), may be associated with increased risk for ocular complications. Prompt initiation of a systemic antiviral agent (Table 2) and evaluation by an ophthalmologist are recommended. Disseminated zoster, with more than a few lesions outside the primary and immediately adjacent dermatomes, can indicate visceral involvement and its associated complications. The term *zoster sine herpete* describes patients with neuropathic pain resembling zoster but without any skin lesions. The diagnosis can be supported by demonstration of increased IgG antibody titers between the acute and convalescent phases. Chronic zoster is seen predominantly in HIV-infected persons. Single or multiple warty growths can persist for weeks or months in areas of skin previously involved by typical lesions of varicella or herpes zoster.

Chronic zoster is often resistant to acyclovir. Tissue biopsy and viral cultures, with further testing for antiviral resistance, may aid in assessment.

Herpes Zoster
Diagnosis
Diagnosis of herpes zoster is often made on clinical grounds alone. A Tzanck smear can provide additional support of the viral etiology. With atypical presentations, however, the diagnosis is best confirmed by real time PCR. An antigen detection method can be used if active blisters are present. Both are rapid and differentiate VZV from HSV. Viral cultures is insensitive but may be required if there is a need to assess possible antiviral resistance. Basic VZV serology is rarely useful for diagnosis.

Treatment
There are three systemic antiviral agents routinely used for the treatment of HSV and VZV infections: acyclovir, valacyclovir, and famciclovir. All three are highly effective and generally well tolerated. Because they inhibit only actively replicating viral DNA, they have no impact on latent infection. Recommendations for antiviral treatment of mucocutaneous HSV infections and herpes zoster, localized topical measures, and available formulations are outlined in Tables 1 to 5. Optimal antiviral dosage schedules for less-common HSV infections, such as herpetic whitlow, have not been determined. The doses outlined in Table 1 for either episodic or chronic suppressive therapy can be used as a guideline in these cases.

Acyclovir became available more than 25 years ago and continues to be widely used. Inside an infected host cell, acyclovir must be phosphorylated—first by a virally encoded enzyme (thymidine kinase) and then by host-cell enzymes—to the active form of the drug, acyclovir triphosphate. As a nucleotide analogue, acyclovir triphosphate is incorporated into replicating viral DNA, abruptly terminating further synthesis of that viral DNA chain. Acyclovir triphosphate also interferes with viral DNA replication by directly inhibiting viral DNA polymerase. Valacyclovir is an oral prodrug of acyclovir and has a much higher bioavailability. After ingestion, valacyclovir is rapidly metabolized to acyclovir, and the subsequent mechanism of action is as just described. Famciclovir is an oral prodrug of penciclovir (Denavir), designed for greater bioavailability. Similar to acyclovir, penciclovir must first be phosphorylated by viral thymidine kinase and then by cellular enzymes to penciclovir triphosphate. In this active form, penciclovir triphosphate interferes with viral DNA synthesis and replication by inhibiting viral DNA polymerase. Famciclovir has greater bioavailability and a longer intracellular half-life than acyclovir. For all three agents, the required activation by viral thymidine kinase and the preferential inhibition of viral DNA synthesis contribute to the highly specific antiviral activity.

If taken as recommended, acyclovir, valacyclovir, and famciclovir are generally comparable in their safety and effectiveness. Valacyclovir and famciclovir offer the convenience of less-frequent dosing. Dosing for all three should be adjusted in the presence of renal insufficiency (see Table 5).

Although antiviral therapy does not decrease the incidence of postherpetic neuralgia, all three agents decrease the time for lesion healing and shorten the overall duration of pain if initiated within 48 to 72 hours after the onset of herpes zoster. Valacyclovir and famciclovir appear to be more effective than acyclovir for this purpose, presumably because of easier dosing. An otherwise healthy person younger than 50 years who has discrete involvement on the trunk and mild to moderate pain might benefit minimally or not at all from this intervention, especially if it is initiated after 72 hours of lesion onset. However, patients who are older than 50 years, are immunosuppressed, have involvement in the ophthalmic distribution, or have more-extensive lesions or severe pain should receive systemic antiviral therapy, even if the 72-hour deadline has expired. Adequate pain control, often requiring opiates, is also important.

TABLE 1	Recommendations for Systemic Antiviral Treatment of Mucocutaneous Herpes Simplex Virus Infection	
EPISODE	**DRUG**	**DOSAGE**
Genital Herpes Simplex Virus		
Primary or first episode	Acyclovir	Mild to moderate: 400 mg PO tid[3] or 200 mg PO 5 ×/d × 7–10 d Severe: 5 mg/kg IV q8h × 5 d
	Valacyclovir	1 g PO bid × 7–10 d
	Famciclovir[1]	250 mg PO tid × 10 d
Recurrent episode (start at prodrome)	Acyclovir	400 mg PO tid × 5 d[3] or 800 mg PO bid × 5 d[3] or 800 mg PO tid × 2 d[3]
	Valacyclovir	500 mg PO bid × 3 d *or* 1 g daily × 5 d
	Famciclovir	1 g PO bid × 1 d *or* 125 mg PO bid × 5 d
Chronic suppression	Acyclovir	>6 outbreaks per year: 400 mg PO bid *or* 200 mg PO tid Adjust up or down according to response
	Valacyclovir	6–10 outbreaks per year: 500 mg PO qd ≥10 outbreaks/year: 1 g PO qd
	Famciclovir	≥6 outbreaks/year: 250 mg PO bid
Orofacial Herpes Simplex Virus		
Primary or first episode	Acyclovir[1]	15 mg/kg 5 ×/d × 7 d
	Valacyclovir[1]	1 g bid × 7 d
	Famciclovir[1]	500 mg bid × 7 d
Recurrent episode (start at prodrome)	Acyclovir[1]	400 mg PO 5 ×/d × 5 d
	Valacyclovir	2 g PO bid × 1 d
	Famciclovir	1500 mg in 1 dose
Chronic suppression	Acyclovir[1]	400 mg PO bid-tid
	Valacyclovir[1]	500 mg–1 g PO qd
Orolabial or Genital Herpes Simplex Virus in Immunosuppressed Patients		
Recurrent or suppressive	Acyclovir[1]	400 mg PO tid *or* 5–10 mg/kg IV q8h
	Valacyclovir	500 mg–1 g PO bid
	Famciclovir	500 mg PO bid

[1]Not FDA approved for this indication.
[3]Exceeds dosage recommended by the manufacturer.

The addition of systemic corticosteroids to the antiviral regimen is not recommended for uncomplicated herpes zoster. Corticosteroids may be of benefit in herpes zoster complicated by facial paralysis, cranial polyneuropathy, or acute retinal necrosis. Corticosteroids should not be used without concomitant systemic antiviral therapy.

Vaccination with a herpes zoster vaccine substantially reduces the incidence of both herpes zoster and postherpetic neuralgia. There are two herpes zoster vaccines available. The live attenuated vaccine (ZVL/Zostavax) has been in use since 2006 and

TABLE 2	Recommendations for Systemic Antiviral Treatment of Herpes Zoster	
	DOSAGE	
DRUG	IMMUNO-COMPETENT PATIENTS	IMMUNO-SUPPRESSED PATIENTS
Acyclovir	800 mg PO 5 × per d × 7–10 d	800 mg PO 5 × per d × 10 d* 10 mg/kg/dose IV q8h × 7–10 d*
Valacyclovir	1 g PO tid × 7 d	1 g PO tid × 10 d*
Famciclovir	500 mg PO tid × 7 d	500 mg PO tid × 10 d*

*Continue until there are no new lesions for 48 h.

is given as a single intramuscular injection. The Zoster Vaccine Recombinant, Adjuvanted (RZV/Shingrix) received FDA approval in October 2017, for immunocompetent adults 50 years and older. RZV is a non-live recombinant glycoprotein E vaccine and requires 2 doses given intramuscularly 2–6 months apart. The U.S. Advisory Committee on Immunization Practices (ACIP) currently recommends the use of RZV for immunocompetent adults aged 50 years or older for the prevention of herpes zoster and related complications. The ACIP also recommends RZV for adults aged 50 years or older who previously received the live-attenuated herpes zoster vaccine (ZVL/Zostavax) and either RZV or ZVL for adults aged 60 years or older (RZV is preferred).

Despite widespread use of these antiviral agents, antiviral resistance is rarely a problem in the immunocompetent population. However, it does arise in the setting of immunosuppression. The basis for the resistance is most commonly a mutation in the gene coding for thymidine kinase. Less often there is a mutation in the viral DNA polymerase. In either case, all three standard drugs become ineffective. Alternative antiviral agents available for treatment of acyclovir-resistant HSV and VZV infections include foscarnet (Foscavir)[1] and cidofovir (Vistide).[1]

Hand-Foot-and-Mouth Disease

Hand-foot-and-mouth disease is typically a disease of childhood. The most common etiologic agent is a nonpolio enterovirus, Coxsackie A16, and transmission is via the oral–oral or fecal–oral route. It is highly contagious. Several days after exposure, a prodrome of low-grade fever, malaise, abdominal pain, or respiratory symptoms can develop, followed by the appearance of papulovesicles on the palate, tongue, or buccal mucosa. Similar lesions can subsequently develop on the feet and hands. The eruption persists for 7 to 10 days and then resolves. Treatment is symptomatic. Nail dystrophies including onychomadesis (separation of the proximal portion of the nail plate from the nail bed) and Beau's lines (horizontal grooves in the nail plate) may be seen 2–4 weeks later.

Since 1997, outbreaks of hand-foot-and-mouth disease caused by enterovirus 71 have been reported in Asia and Australia. Although hand-foot-and-mouth disease associated with Coxsackie A16 infection is typically a mild illness, hand-foot-and-mouth disease caused by enterovirus 71 has shown a higher incidence of neurologic involvement, including fatal cases of encephalitis.

An atypical hand-foot-and-mouth disease with more widespread cutaneous involvement has been reported as associated with Coxsackievirus A6. There is a predilection for areas commonly involved in atopic dermatitis, such as the antecubital and popliteal fossae and this presentation may be confused with eczema herpeticum or VZV infection. Diagnosis of these more atypical cases may require laboratory assessment. This could

include antigen detection or PCR to exclude HSV and VZV. Reverse Transcription PCR (RT-PCR) of vesicle fluid, oropharyngeal swab or stool specimen may be used to confirm the enterovirus infection.

Parvovirus B19

Cutaneous manifestations of parvovirus B19 infection include the childhood exanthem known as erythema infectiosum (fifth disease) and, less commonly, petechial or purpuric eruptions. The virus is transmitted primarily via respiratory secretions and, to a much lesser extent, through blood or blood products. The host cells for viral replication are erythroid progenitor cells, which subsequently undergo cell lysis.

A child with erythema infectiosum typically develops a low-grade fever and nonspecific upper respiratory symptoms approximately 2 days before the onset of rash. The rash has been described as having a slapped-cheeks appearance, with prominent redness over the malar eminences. This is followed by a pink-to-red lacy or reticular eruption over the trunk and extensor surfaces of the arms and legs. The rash usually lasts a week to 10 days but can transiently recur over months in response to precipitating factors such as sunlight, exercise, and bathing. Diagnosis of erythema infectiosum is usually made on clinical grounds, and treatment is symptomatic. By the time the rash appears and the diagnosis has been made, the child is no longer infectious. Much less commonly parvovirus B19 infection may manifest as a papular-purpuric eruption with edema, erythema, and patecchiae in a "gloves and socks" distribution on the hands and feet.

Infection with parvovirus B19 in older adolescents and adults often manifests with arthralgias or arthritis rather than a rash. In certain patient populations, parvovirus B19 infections may be associated with complications including transient aplastic crisis, chronic anemia, and hydrops fetalis. In these less-typical presentations, serology (anti-B19 IgM or documented seroconversion) may be needed for diagnosis. Intravenous immunoglobulin (IVIg [Gamimune N][1]) is used successfully for treatment of chronic or persistent infection in immunosuppressed patients.

Molluscum Contagiosum

Molluscum contagiosum are benign umbilicated papules caused by infection with the *Molluscipoxvirus*, a member of the poxvirus family. Lesions are limited to the mucocutaneous surface and typically appear in clusters on the face, trunk, and skin fold areas in children and on thighs, lower abdomen, and suprapubic areas in sexually active adults. Large numbers of lesions in an extensive distribution may be seen in the immunosuppressed population.

Transmission routinely occurs by skin-to-skin contact with an infected host, but transmission from contaminated fomites has been reported. Autoinoculation commonly occurs. Diagnosis is usually based on clinical examination, but histopathology of atypical lesions may be used for confirmation.

Because molluscum contagiosum tends to be self-limited, treatment is not always recommended, but it can reduce the risk of autoinoculation and transmission to others. Treatment modalities are primarily aimed at destroying the lesions, similar to those used for verruca vulgaris (Table 6). In the case of sexual transmission, evaluation for other sexually transmitted diseases may be indicated.

Orf and Milker's Nodules

Orf (also known as ecthyma contagiosum) and milker's nodules are caused by the closely related *Parapoxvirus*, a member of the poxvirus family. The virus responsible for orf is widespread in sheep and goats, whereas the virus causing milker's nodules is found in cattle. Transmission to humans is by direct

---

[1]Not FDA approved for this indication.

[1]Not FDA approved for this indication.

TABLE 3 Topical Treatment Options for Mucocutaneous Herpes Simplex Virus and Varicella Zoster Virus Infections

TREATMENT	COMMENT
Cool, moist compresses using tap water or aluminum acetate 1:20 to 1:40 (Burow's solution, Domeboro, Bluboro)	Good for moist, oozing lesions to accelerate drying Apply wet dressing to involved skin and cover with a dry cloth to allow evaporation
Calamine lotion or similar shake lotion containing alcohol, menthol, and/or phenol; Aveeno colloidal oatmeal	Useful as drying and antipruritic agent May be applied after wet dressing
Bacitracin,[1] Polysporin, mupirocin[1] (Bactroban)	Use if there is concern for localized secondary bacterial infection
2% Viscous lidocaine, compounded suspensions[1,6] (e.g., Kaopectate[1] or Maalox,[1] diphenhydramine,[1] lidocaine)	Useful for temporary pain relief of oral or genital mucosal involvement
Acyclovir ointment	Used together with systemic antiviral agents, may be of benefit to immunocompromised individuals for localized HSV
Penciclovir (Denavir) cream	Can decrease the duration of lesions in herpes labialis by half a day if applied every 2h while awake for 4 days beginning at the first sign of disease
Acyclovir buccal tablet (Sitavig) 50 mg	Can decrease the duration of herpes labialis by 0.8 days if single tablet is applied within 1 hour of prodromal symptom

[1]Not FDA approved for this indication.
[6]May be compounded by pharmacists.
Abbreviation: HSV = herpes simplex virus.

TABLE 4 Formulations of Acyclovir, Valacyclovir, and Famciclovir

DRUG	ORAL	TOPICAL	INTRAVENOUS
Acyclovir	200, 400, 800 mg 50 mg buccal tablet	5% Ointment (5g, 15g, 30g) 5% cream (5 g)	Yes
Valacyclovir	500 mg, 1 g	No	No
Famciclovir	125, 250, 500 mg	No	No
Penciclovir (Denavir)	No	1% cream (1.5 g, 5 g)	No

Viral Diseases of the Skin

TABLE 5 Recommended Antiviral Dose Modification in Patients with Impaired Renal Function

| CREATININE CLEARANCE (ML/MIN) | GENITAL HERPES SIMPLEX VIRUS | | | HERPES ZOSTER | HERPES LABIALIS |
	INITIAL	RECURRENT	SUPPRESSION		
Acyclovir (Zovirax)					
>25	200 mg 5 ×/d	200 mg 5 ×/d	400 mg q12h	800 mg 5×/d	
10–24	200 mg 5 ×/d	200 mg 5 ×/d	400 mg q12h	800 mg q8h	
<10	200 mg q12h	200 mg q12h	200 mg q12h	800 mg q12h	
Valacyclovir (Valtrex)					
>50	1 g q12h	500 mg q12h	500 mg-1 g q24h	1 g q8h	2 g PO bid for 1 d
30–49	1 g q12h	500 mg q12h	500 mg-1 g q24h	1 g q12h	1 g PO bid for 1 d
10–29	1 g q24h	500 mg q24h	500 mg q24-48h	1 g q24h	500 mg bid for 1 d
<10	500 mg q24h	500 mg q24h	500 mg q24-48h	500 mg q24h	500 mg single dose
Famciclovir (Famvir)					
>60		125 mg q12h	250 mg q12h	500 mg q8h	
40–59		125 mg q12h	250 mg q12h	500 mg q12h	
20–39		125 mg q24h	125 mg q12h	500 mg q24h	
<20		125 mg q24h	125 mg q24h	250 mg q24h	
>60	1 g bid × 1 d				1500 mg single dose
40–59	500 mg bid × 1 d				750 mg single dose
20–39	500 mg single dose				500 mg single dose
<20	250 mg single dose				250 mg single dose

TABLE 6	Treatment Options for Molluscum Contagiosum
TREATMENT	**COMMENT**
Cryotherapy (liquid nitrogen)	Freeze individual lesions for 5–10 sec Repeat PRN in 2–3 wk
Curettage	Entire lesion may be removed using a curette; this results in bleeding Removal of central core with toothpick or other pointed instrument is also effective
Cantharidin (Cantharone)[1]	Blister-inducing agent: Apply to lesion with toothpick, air dry Cover with tape or adhesive bandage Patient to wash area after 24 h (or sooner if significant pain)
Podophyllin (25% in tincture of benzoin)[1]	Cytotoxic agent: Apply to lesion with toothpick Patient to wash off after 4–6 h Contraindicated in pregnancy
Podofilox (Condylox 0.5% gel or solution)[1]	Done by patient: Apply bid for 3 consecutive d/wk × 2–4 wk Contraindicated in pregnancy
Salicylic acid/lactic acid (Occlusal, Duofilm)[1]	Done by patient: Apply daily
Imiquimod (Aldara) 5% cream[1,2]	Done by patient: Apply daily 5 consecutive d/wk Leave on overnight Continue for 8–12 wk
Cimetidine (Tagamet)[1]	30 mg/kg/d PO × 6–12 wk Can boost cell-mediated immunity
Candida antigen (Candin)[1]	Intralesional injection 0.3 mL[3]

[1]Not FDA approved for this indication.
[2]Not available in the United States.
[3]Exceeds dosage recommended by the manufacturer.

contact with infected animals or recently vaccinated animals and is usually seen several days and up to 2 weeks after exposure. Preexisting skin trauma or other disruption of the normal cutaneous barrier enhances the risk of transmission. Barrier precautions and proper hand hygiene are important preventive measures.

Orf and milker's nodules most commonly appear as one to several nodules on the dorsal aspect of the hands or forearms. Lesions evolve through several clinical stages over a period of 3 to 5 weeks, ranging from solid red nodules to vesicular, exudative, or wartlike tumors. As with other poxvirus infections, lesions of orf often demonstrate central umbilication. Regional lymphadenopathy and lymphangitis are commonly seen.

Diagnosis is based on a history of exposure and clinical examination. Tissue biopsy for histopathology or electron microscopy may also be used. Orf virus infection can resemble skin lesions associated with potentially life-threatening zoonotic infections such as tularemia, cutaneous anthrax, and erysipeloid. Should this be a concern, definitive diagnostic testing using PCR is available through the Centers for Disease Control and Prevention (CDC).

In general, the lesions of orf are self-limited, resolving within 4 to 6 weeks, and treatment is not routinely required. However, immunocompromised persons can develop more progressive and destructive lesions requiring therapeutic intervention such as topical cidofovir[1,6] or imiquimod (Aldara).[1]

[1]Not FDA approved for this indication.
[6]May be compounded by pharmacists.

Reference

Advisory Committee on Immunization Practices Recommended Immunization Schedule for Adults Aged 19 Years or Older—United States, 2018, *MMWR* 67(5):158–160, 2018.
Bergqvist C, Kurban M, Abbas O: Orf virus infection, *Rev Med Virol* 27(4), 2017.
Centers for Disease Control and Prevention: Sexually Transmitted Diseases Treatment Guidelines, 2010. *MMWR* 59(RR-12), 2010. Available at http://www.cdc.gov/STD/treatment/2010.
Cernik C, Gallina K, Brodell RT: The treatment of herpes simplex infections: an evidence-based review, *Arch Intern Med* 168(11):1137–1144, 2008.
Dayan RR, Peleg R: Herpes zoster - typical and atypical presentations, *Postgrad Med* 129(6):567–571, 2017.
Gnann JW, Whitley RJ: Genital herpes, *N Engl J Med* 375:666–674, 2016.
Nassef C, Ziemer C, Morrell DS: Hand-foot-and-mouth disease: a new look at a classic viral rash, *Curr Opin Pediatr* 27(4):486–491, 2015.
Qiu J, Soderlund-Venermo M, Young NS: Human parvoviruses, *Clin Microbiol Rev* 30(1):43–113, 2017.
Sacks HS: Review: Adjuvant recombinant subunit vaccine prevents herpes zoster more than live attenuated vaccine in adults ≥ 50 years, *Ann Intern Med* 170(4):JC14, 2019.
van der Wouden JC, van der Sande R, Kruithof EJ, et al: Interventions for cutaneous molluscum contagiosum, *Cochrane Database Syst Rev* 17;5:CD004767, 2017.

WARTS (VERRUCAE)

Method of
M. Chantel Long, MD

CURRENT DIAGNOSIS

- Common warts: rough, hyperkeratotic, firm papules usually found on the extremities.
- Flat warts: small, flat, pink or flesh-colored papules on the face, arms, or legs.
- Plantar and palmar warts: callus-like lesions that disrupt skin lines on the soles or palms.
- Mosaic warts: large clusters of warts.
- Filiform warts: small, finger-like lesions on the face.
- Genital warts: flesh to brown colored, flat or exophytic, found in the anogenital region.
- Differential diagnoses: seborrheic keratoses, molluscum contagiosum, keratoacanthoma, squamous cell carcinoma, acrochordon, amelanocytic melanoma, calluses, and corns.

CURRENT THERAPY

- Approximately 20% of warts spontaneously resolve within 3 months and 60% within 2 years in a healthy person.
- Salicylic acid and dimethyl ether.
- Cryotherapy.
- Cantharidin (Cantharone).[1,6]
- Surgical removal.
- Pulsed-dye laser.
- Immunotherapy: topical imiquimod (Aldara),[1] intralesional *Candida* antigen (Candin).[1]
- Photodynamic therapy.

[1]Not FDA approved for this indication.
[6]May be compounded by pharmacists.
Note: Cantharidin and Candin are not FDA approved. Aldara is approved for genital and perianal warts only.

Verrucae, commonly known as cutaneous warts, are benign skin growths caused by the human papillomavirus (HPV). Cutaneous warts are divided into common warts, plantar warts, flat warts, and genital warts. Common warts account for 70% of all cutaneous warts. Two-thirds of untreated common warts spontaneously regress within 2 years, but previously infected individuals have a higher rate of developing new warts than those who were never infected.

Epidemiology
It is estimated that 10% of the general population has cutaneous warts, and warts are one of the most common reasons for dermatologic visits. Transmission occurs through direct contact with an infected person or indirectly through fomites. As a result, warts are seen with greater frequency among groups of people in close contact, such as schoolchildren. Thus, warts are more common in adolescents with a frequency estimated as high as 20%. Since the extent of infection is determined by the immune response, warts are also more common in immunocompromised patients. Autoinoculation is possible by scratching the lesions, often leading to a linear pattern.

Pathophysiology
Warts are caused by HPV. More than 100 genotypes of HPV have been identified, and the virus is prevalent. HPV causes both clinical and subclinical infections and plays a role in certain cutaneous malignancies, including squamous cell carcinoma. It is found in the basal layer of the epidermis but replicates in the superficial, well-differentiated layer of the skin. The cellular proliferation gives rise to thick, hyperkeratotic lesions generally known as warts. The warts can occur anywhere on the skin or mucous membranes.

Clinical Manifestations
Most warts are asymptomatic, though patients often present with complaints of a "bump." Usually, the warts appear flesh-colored, brown, or gray and can be flat to exophytic, giving them the classic "cauliflower" appearance. The lesions may be single or multiple and may range in size from miniscule to several centimeters in diameter. Localized irritation, pruritus, pain, or bleeding may occur. Symptoms vary based on the location and size of the lesions.

Several types of warts occur with variations in appearance, site of infection, and the specific type of HPV involved. Common warts (verrucae vulgaris) are white to flesh-colored, rough, hyperkeratotic, raised, and firm, usually found on the extremities. They disrupt normal skin lines on the fingers and toes and are most associated with HPV types 1, 2, and 4. Flat warts (verrucae plana) are caused by HPV types 3, 10, or 28 and are tan to flesh colored. They are small, 1 to 3 mm in diameter, flat, sharply demarcated growths that appear in large numbers on the face, arms, or legs. They usually occur in a linear arrangement related to local trauma, such as shaving. Butcher warts are associated with HPV type 7 and have a thick, raised, exophytic appearance. They are most common in workers who regularly handle raw meat or fish. Plantar and palmar warts (verrucae plantaris and verrucae palmaris) are hard, thickened, callus-like lesions that disrupt skin lines on the soles or palms. They are associated with HPV types 1, 2, 4, 27, and 57. They are usually flesh colored, covered with callus, and can be painful, especially when located on pressure points. If warts coalesce into a plaque, this is termed a *mosaic* wart. Filiform warts are slender, finger-like growths most commonly seen on the face, especially around the eyelids, nose, and mouth. Periungual warts are common warts impinging on and growing under toenails or fingernails. Genital warts (condyloma acuminatum) are flesh colored to brown, flat or exophytic lesions, occurring in anogenital regions. Mucosal papillomas are warts that occur on mucous membranes, usually in the mouth or vagina, and tend to be white in color.

Epidermodysplasia verruciformis is a rare, autosomal recessive disorder that leads to widespread reddish brown, flat papules on the trunk, hands, face, and extremities. These warts have malignant potential, especially on sun-exposed areas. It is estimated that one-third may become malignant. These patients present in childhood. Chronically infected with multiple types of HPV, including types 3, 5, 8, 9, 12, 14, 15, 17, 19 to 25, 36 to 38, 47, 49, and 50, the warts have lifelong persistence. Another related

disease is verrucous carcinoma. This is a slow-growing variant of squamous cell carcinoma that occurs in the oral mucosa, anogenital region, or plantar surface. These warts are associated with HPV types 6 and 11.

Risk Factors
Risk factors most associated with verrucae include immunosuppression and close contact. Due to their decreased immune response, immunocompromised hosts are at increased risk not only for infection, but also for malignant transformation of the warts. Pregnancy, previous wart infection, and handling raw meat or fish are also known risk factors.

Differential Diagnosis
The differential diagnosis of warts includes seborrheic keratoses, molluscum contagiosum, keratoacanthoma, squamous cell carcinoma, acrochordon, amelanocytic melanoma, porokeratosis, calluses, and corns.

Diagnosis is based on clinical findings. When the clinical appearance of the lesion is typical, no other confirmatory tests are usually necessary. Paring down the stratum corneum, or outer layer of skin, may reveal black dots, which are thrombosed or bleeding capillaries, and helps confirm the diagnosis. If needed, tissue biopsy can provide histopathologic confirmation. In immunocompromised patients, biopsy is recommended to rule out squamous cell carcinoma in any suspicious lesions, which includes large or rapidly growing, pigmented, atypical, friable, bleeding, or ulcerated lesions.

Treatment
Approximately 20% of warts spontaneously resolve within 3 months and 60% within 2 years in a healthy person. Therefore, treatment is not always necessary. Current treatments do not eradicate the virus and do not guarantee resolution. Most patients seek treatment because of the physical appearance, discomfort, or interference with daily and social functioning, especially if located on the palms, digits, or soles. The American Academy of Dermatology established reasoning for wart treatment, including the desire of the patient; for symptoms of pain, bleeding, itching, or burning; for disabling or disfiguring lesions; for large numbers or large size of lesions; for a desire to prevent spread to unblemished skin; and because of a concomitant immunocompromised condition. Immunosuppressed patients are at higher risk for developing numerous warts and require treatment to prevent progression to squamous cell carcinoma. It is often more difficult to eradicate warts in an immunosuppressed host.

Many therapeutic modalities are available for the treatment of warts. No single therapy is universally effective. Warts can resolve, recur, shrink, or grow despite therapy. It is likely that all wart therapies work by triggering an immune response to the presence of papillomavirus in the skin. Treatment of warts must be individualized and often more than one modality is needed to achieve resolution. Conservative, less painful, and less expensive treatments are preferred.

Treatment methods are divided into the categories of home remedies, over-the-counter treatments, and office-based therapies. Office-based treatments include destructive methods, surgical or laser procedures, immunologic intervention, and combination therapy.

Home Remedies
Home remedies include applications of tea tree oil,[7] garlic extract,[7] duct tape,[1] and hyperthermic therapy. One study comparing cryotherapy with duct tape occlusion of common warts showed resolution in 85% of the children treated by occlusion, compared with 60% in the liquid nitrogen group. Proper protocol involves covering the wart with duct tape, which is left in place for 6 days. Then the site should be soaked, pared down with an

---

[1] Not FDA approved for this indication.
[7] Available as dietary supplement.

emery board, and left uncovered overnight. This is repeated for a total of eight cycles. Another common home remedy is hyperthermic therapy. This involves immersing the affected area in a 45°C water bath for 30 minutes three times per week. It is a safe and inexpensive option.

Over-the-Counter Treatment

The most common over-the-counter option used by patients is one of the salicylic acid products, such as Compound W, Duofilm, Occlusal-HP, and Mediplast. These keratolytic products are offered as a solution, gel, cream, or pad in concentrations from 10% to 60%. They can be quite successful when used consistently and as directed in motivated patients. Repeated application, with pumice stone or callus file use, results in cure rates of 60% to 80%, but takes several weeks to work.

More recently, several over-the-counter wart-freezing therapies have become available. One such option is dimethyl ether, marketed as Compound W Freeze Off or Dr. Scholl's Freeze Away. These are available in aerosol form for wart treatment, which can be repeated every 2 weeks. Dimethyl ether achieves a temperature of –57°C, which is markedly higher than the –196°C temperature obtained with liquid nitrogen. This results in a more shallow depth of destruction. Because salicylic acid and dimethyl ether treatments destroy the infected epidermis and cause an immune reaction, they can be irritating and tedious, prompting many patients to seek medical care.

Office-based Treatment

Office-based treatments are largely destructive, immunomodulating, or both. Destructive treatments include cryosurgery, surgical excision, laser therapy, or repeated application of topical chemotherapy agents, such as salicylic acid, cantharidin (Cantharone),[1,6] podophyllin (Podocon),[1] or 5-fluorouracil (Efudex).[1] The most commonly used physician office-based treatment is cryotherapy with liquid nitrogen. It can be applied by a cotton-tipped applicator or cryogun. The wart and a 1 to 2 mm margin are frozen for 10 to 30 seconds. The freeze should be repeated once after a thaw of 20 seconds. If the warts are thick, they can initially be pared down. The patient is told that a blister will result and should be left intact if possible. Treatment should be repeated every 3 to 4 weeks until normal skin markings return. Cryotherapy has demonstrated a 60% to 80% cure rate. If warts persist beyond 3 months of therapy, another method of treatment should be selected.

Another option is cantharidin (Cantharone) in a 0.7% colloidal solution. It is a chemical derived from blister beetles that is painless on application and well tolerated by children. It causes epidermal necrosis with blistering after application and occlusion for 8 hours. It is applied in the office and repeated every 4 weeks. Although not Food and Drug Administration (FDA) approved, it is a commonly used technique and can be compounded by a pharmacist. It is useful for treatment of common, periungual, and plantar warts in children, and the cure rate approaches 80%. Unfortunately, an occasional "donut wart," a ring of new warts surrounding the cleared original site, occurs.

Surgery is used for large, solitary warts, and is more direct. Large common warts of the hands or extremities are more easily treated if they are debulked surgically. This method is not recommended for plantar warts because of scarring. Surgical removal followed by electrodesiccation and curettage is effective but requires local anesthesia and can result in scarring.

Other destructive methods of wart removal usually are reserved for resistant, multiple lesions, or recalcitrant warts in immunosuppressed patients. This often requires specialty referral. Acids, including bichloroacetic and trichloroacetic acid (Tri-Chlor),[1] should be applied by a skilled practitioner because they are known to cause pain on application, ulceration, and even scarring. Laser therapy, most often with a pulsed-dye laser (PDL) or carbon dioxide (CO_2) laser, provides selective photothermolysis of blood vessels within the wart, which compromises blood supply and results in necrosis. The PDL method is less aggressive and less painful than CO_2 vaporization. These treatments cause minimal damage to normal skin. Overall, both therapies are generally well tolerated, but local anesthesia may be necessary. Although more expensive, these methods have cure rates ranging from 45% to 90%. Photodynamic therapy (PDT) is useful for patients with multiple recalcitrant warts, especially patients who are immunosuppressed. PDT involves a topical photosensitizer applied by a trained provider. It is activated by visible light, resulting in tissue destruction. Studies of this method have been promising.

Immune modulation alone or in combination with destructive methods is helpful in treating resistant warts. The self-applied immunomodulator imiquimod (Aldara) was initially approved for treatment of genital warts. It is also used anecdotally to treat flat and common warts by inducing cytokines, including interferon production, at the site of application. A thin coat is applied at bedtime and then washed off after 6 to 10 hours. It is usually applied three times weekly and combined with cryotherapy or salicylic acid.

Intralesional immunotherapy, which includes *Candida* antigen (Candin),[1] interferon alfa-2b (Intron A),[1] bleomycin,[1] and MMR vaccine,[1] is an effective option for treatment in some patients. *Candida* antigen injection (Candin) is considered a first-line therapy in children with large or multiple warts and a second-line therapy for patients with resistant warts. It is well tolerated. *Candida* antigen is commercially available as a 1:1000 dilution. Using a 30-gauge needle and tuberculin syringe, one can inject 0.2 to 0.3 mL directly into the wart. Pretesting is unnecessary, side effects are minimal, and more than 75% of patients treated with a series of three injections have clearing of the injected and distant warts. Intralesional interferon alfa-2b (Intron A) has been used successfully to treat genital warts and warts that have not responded to conventional therapies. The clearance rate varies from 36% to 62%, but it requires multiple injections in a physician's office, is expensive, and can cause systemic adverse effects such as flu-like symptoms. Intralesional bleomycin is effective but expensive and causes severe pain. The MMR vaccine is used off-label for intralesional injection and often combined with lidocaine for comfort.

Other topical immunomodulators, such as squaric acid dibutylester (SADBE)[1,6] or diphencyprone,[1,6] are contact sensitizers that induce an allergic dermatitis through type IV hypersensitivity reactions. Although time consuming, treatment with SADBE is well tolerated and a good choice for recalcitrant warts in children. Other topical products available for off-label treatment include retinoids, formaldehyde compounds, and 5-fluorouracil (Efudex).[1] These agents interfere with epidermal proliferation, effect a nonspecific antiviral action, or inhibit mitosis, leading to keratinocyte and viral death. All of these choices usually require specialty referral.

Oral immunomodulation with high-dose cimetidine (Tagamet)[1] has been proposed. It is postulated to enhance cell-mediated immune response. Evidence has been anecdotal. Daily doses of 30 to 40 mg/kg have been used divided twice a day to four times a day for 8 to 12 weeks.

To ensure resolution and no recurrence of warts, the patient and practitioner must often make compromises in regard to convenience, discomfort, and scarring. The factors to consider when deciding on treatment include wart location and size, patient tolerance and preference, cost, convenience, and clinician preference. Patient-applied options allow the patient greater control; however, this requires good compliance and the warts must be accessible by the patient or caregiver. Provider-applied treatments are good choices for large treatment areas. Data regarding the efficacy of using more than one modality at a time are lacking. It is common practice for health care providers to combine treatment modalities. Table 1 outlines current therapy regimens.

---

[1] Not FDA approved for this indication.
[6] May be compounded by pharmacists.

[1] Not FDA approved for this indication.
[6] May be compounded by pharmacists.

TABLE 1 | Treatment Regimens

DRUG	AVAILABLE AS	MECHANISM OF ACTION	DISADVANTAGES	INSTRUCTIONS
Patient Applied				
Salicylic acid (Compound W, Duofilm, Occlusol-HP, or Mediplast)	Solution, gel, lotion, cream, plaster, pad 10%–60% concentration	Keratolytic that destroys the infected epidermis while irritation stimulates an immune response	Local irritation Requires multiple applications Requires compliance Wart may need to be pared down to increase penetration	Apply nightly until clear, usually for weeks to months
Dimethyl ether (Compound W, Freeze Off, Dr. Scholl's Freeze Away)	OTC in spray canister	As above	Local irritation Requires compliance Blistering may occur	May treat every 2 weeks Total of four treatments per wart advised
Retinoids (Accutane, Retin-A, Soriatane)[1]	Soriatane (10 and 25 mg tabs), Accutane (10, 20, and 40 mg tabs), Retin-A cream/gel	Antimitotic that interferes with epidermal proliferation	Systemic with mucocutaneous dryness, elevated triglycerides, abnormal liver enzymes Avoid use in pregnancy Local irritation and dryness	Take PO daily If topical form, apply nightly
Imiquimod (Aldara)[1]	Cream 5%	Immunomodulator that mediates cytokines	Irritation, erythema, pruritus, scarring, hyperpigmentation	Apply 3 times/wk on mucosal skin Apply daily on keratinized skin
Cimetidine (Tagamet)[1]	Tablets (200, 300, 400 mg) Liquid (300 mg/5 mL)	Immunomodulator that may enhance immune response	Unclear efficacy Diarrhea Many drug-drug interactions	30–40 mg/kg daily, divided bid–qid for 8–12 weeks
Provider Applied				
Cryotherapy	Cryogun or cotton-tip application	Destroys infected dermis, induces inflammation, and leads to stimulated immune response	Pain, erythema, blistering, hypopigmentation, scarring Onychodystrophy if not careful with periungual warts	Freeze for 10–30 seconds with a 1–2 mm border, allow to thaw, then repeat May offer/need local anesthesia May repeat every 3–4 weeks
Candida antigen injections (Candin)[1]	1:1000 dilution	Immunomodulator	Discomfort	Intralesional injection of 0.2–0.3 mL
Trichloroacetic acid (TCA)[1]	Solution, up to 50%	Destroys infected epidermis; best for mucosal surfaces	Pain	Apply sparingly with cotton tip, air dry Repeat weekly to every other week Do not allow to "run" on normal skin Neutralize with soap or sodium bicarbonate
Cantharidin (Cantharone)[1]	Colloidal solution 0.7%, compounded	Destroys epidermis, leads to blister formation Is painless, good for kids	Avoid on face Blistering will occur	Apply with fine applicator to wart only and have patient wash off after 6–8 hr
Surgery		Surgical removal	Avoid if bleeding disorder Often requires anesthesia Scarring	Surgical excision followed by curettage and cauterization
Interferon alpha-2b (Intron A)[1] injections		Immunomodulator	Expensive Flu-like side effects	Multiple intralesional injections several times a week Often requires specialty referral
Laser vaporization		Destroys epidermis	Expensive Requires local anesthesia	Requires specialty referral

[1]Not FDA approved for this indication.
Abbreviations: bid=twice a day; OTC=over-the-counter; PO=orally; qid=four times a day.

Patient Education

Counseling of patients regarding the goal and length of treatment is necessary. Patients should be educated that current treatments do not eradicate HPV, and therefore the objective of therapy is elimination of symptoms. They also need to understand that a repeated course of therapy is often required and it may take weeks to months to achieve desired results. Each treatment should be reviewed in detail, including risks and benefits. Subsequently, the management should be tailored depending on the wart, patient, and practitioner.

References

Cockayne S, Hewitt C, Hicks K, et al: Cryotherapy versus salicylic acid for the treatment of plantar warts: a randomized controlled trial, *BMJ* 342:d3271, 2011.

Kwok CS, Holland R, Gibbs S: Efficacy of topical treatments for cutaneous warts: a meta-analysis and pooled analysis of randomized controlled trials, *Br J Dermatol* 65:233–246, 2011.

Leung L: Recalcitrant nongenital warts, *Aust Fam Physician* 40–42, 2011.

Simonart T, De Maertelaer V: Systemic treatments for cutaneous warts: a systematic review, *J Dermatolog Treat* 23:72–77, 2012.

Yelverton CB: Warts. In *Manual of dermatologic therapeutics*, ed 7th, Philadelphia, 2007, Lippincott Williams & Wilkins. pp 233–240.

Urogenital Tract

ACUTE KIDNEY INJURY

Method of
Sarah Burns, DO, MS

CURRENT DIAGNOSIS

- Acute kidney injury (AKI) is a common diagnosis seen in the outpatient setting, in the emergency department, and in hospitalized patients.
- AKI is defined by increase in serum creatinine by ≥0.3 mg/dL within 48 hours, increase ≥1.5 times the baseline creatinine within 7 days, or oliguria.
- Identify the underlying cause of AKI, denoted by pathophysiologic etiology (prerenal, intrinsic, and postrenal) to determine therapy.

CURRENT THERAPY

- Treat any reversible causes identified.
- Ensure hemodynamic stability.
- Correct any imbalances in electrolytes or in acid-base standing.
- Avoid nephrotoxins and renally dose all medications if glomerular filtration rate (GFR) is decreased.
- Prompt consultation to specialists to determine if renal replacement treatment is appropriate.

Background/Definitions

Acute kidney injury (AKI) is a diverse syndrome defined by a sudden decrease in kidney function shown by a rise in serum creatinine and/or decrease in urine output. This sudden decrease in renal function affects fluid balance, electrolyte balance, acid-base balance, and waste elimination. The older term "acute renal failure" has been supplanted by AKI. The term "AKI" reflects a lack of strict separation between normal renal function and complete failure of the kidneys.

Previously there was no standard definition for diagnosing AKI and there were more than 30 different definitions in the literature. In 2004, Risk, Injury, Failure, Loss, and End-stage kidney disease (RIFLE) criteria were proposed, evolving into the AKI Network (AKIN) criteria in 2007. In 2012, these validated criteria were adapted into international clinical practice guidelines released by Kidney Disease: Improving Global Outcomes (KDIGO). While KDIGO criteria are widely used in research, there are parts of the definition that have not been validated. However, most experts endorse the use of KDIGO criteria for the diagnosis and management of AKI.

KDIGO criteria denote AKI when there is an increase in serum creatinine greater than or equal to 0.3 mg/dL within 48 hours, or an increase greater than or equal to 1.5 times the baseline

creatinine within 7 days, or a decrease in urine volume to less than 0.5 mL/kg/h over 6 hours. To further describe the severity of AKI, there are stages (Table 1) describing the amount of change in serum creatinine from baseline. Multiple studies have demonstrated that increasing severity of AKI is associated with increased mortality and worse kidney function in the future.

Epidemiology

AKI is commonly found in hospitalized patients and the incidence appears to be increasing over time in the United States. A 2013 meta-analysis for all hospitalized patients worldwide showed an overall incidence of AKI in 21.6% of patients. With the KDIGO definition, this study showed that 1 in 5 adults and 1 in 3 children worldwide experience AKI during a hospital stay. A 2015 multinational cross-sectional study of AKI in intensive care unit (ICU) patients showed AKI occurred in 57.3% of ICU patients. Additionally, it has been observed that rises in serum creatinine are associated with adverse patient outcomes, increased mortality, longer length of hospital stay, and higher healthcare costs. AKI also has been shown to be an independent risk factor for mortality.

There are multiple factors, based on several observational studies, that may affect the chance of developing AKI. These factors vary between individuals, and it is not clear why one factor would cause an individual to develop an AKI and another not to. As delineated by KDIGO clinical practice guidelines, the following increase the risk of AKI: critical illness, sepsis, shock, burns, trauma, major surgery including cardiac surgery, nephrotoxic drugs, iodinated radiocontrast agents, and poisonous animals and plants. KDIGO clinical practice guidelines indicate that certain patient populations are susceptible to AKI and they include the following: volume depletion, older age, female sex, black race, chronic kidney disease (CKD), other chronic diseases (including heart, lung, and liver), diabetes mellitus, cancer, and anemia.

Etiology

The causes of AKI can be broadly divided by the pathophysiologic etiology, specifically prerenal, intrinsic, and postrenal causes (Box 1). Prerenal AKI from renal hypoperfusion is the most common cause of AKI in the community setting. Acute tubular necrosis (ATN; an intrinsic etiology) is the most common cause of hospital-acquired AKI. While the cause of AKI is traditionally classified by the portion of the kidney affected, it should be noted that diseases may cross these pathophysiologic boundaries. Therefore AKI may be multifactorial.

Prerenal

Prerenal AKI is caused by renal hypoperfusion due to a decrease in the arterial volume. Recall that autoregulation will help maintain the kidney's glomerular filtration rate (GFR) by blunting changes in blood flow by various mechanisms. Ultimately, autoregulation can only compensate for a degree in decreased renal perfusion. For example, in those with CKD, these autoregulatory mechanisms are diminished which increases the susceptibility of developing an AKI on CKD. Decreased arterial volume occurs in renal vasoconstriction which is caused by sepsis (early in course), hepatorenal syndrome, iodinated contrast, medications such as norepinephrine or vasopressin, nonsteroidal antiinflammatory drugs, and angiotensin-converting enzyme inhibitors. Intravascular volume depletion reduces the arterial volume to the kidneys and is caused by gastrointestinal losses, hemorrhage, diuretic use, cirrhosis, nephrotic syndrome, and burns. Renal hypoperfusion is also due to reduction in cardiac output which is seen in shock, pericardial disease, heart failure, pulmonary embolism, pulmonary hypertension, and sepsis. Systemic vasodilation is another cause of renal hypoperfusion and is due to sepsis, cirrhosis, anaphylaxis, and drugs. Increased abdominal pressure as seen in abdominal compartment syndrome can be another cause of prerenal AKI.

The clinical presentation of prerenal AKI is variable and dependent on the cause. The cause should be investigated first with an excellent history and physical exam. Prerenal causes may be suspected in patients with dehydration, gastrointestinal losses such as vomiting or diarrhea, sweating, other insensible losses, increased ostomy output, bleeding, dizziness, or syncope. Prerenal causes should be suspected in patients with chronic medical conditions, such as heart failure or cirrhosis. All medications (current, recently used, prescribed, over the counter) should be investigated in every patient suspected to have an AKI from any cause. Further work-up is discussed below. Prerenal AKI may improve rapidly if the underlying cause is treated, if the volume status is improved, and/or if the offending medication is removed.

Intrinsic

Intrinsic AKI can be divided into the component of the kidney that is affected, which includes diseases of the vasculature, the glomeruli, the tubules, and the interstitium. Vascular causes are uncommon and include those that affect the small vessels and those that affect the large vessels. Small vessels are affected by vasculitides, scleroderma, and malignant hypertension. Large vessels are affected by aneurysms, infarct from aortic dissection, venothrombosis, and atheroembolism especially in the setting of recent vascular surgery or arterial catheterization.

Glomerular diseases originate from inflammation of the vessels and the glomeruli, and may be a manifestation of an infection, of a vasculitis, or of a rheumatologic disorder. Glomerular diseases are divided into nephritic and nephrotic diseases, determined by less than 3 g of proteinuria per day or more than 3 g of proteinuria per day, respectively. Rapid progressive glomerulonephritis (RPGN) is an acute cause of AKI that may be seen in the hospital and always presents with a nephritic pattern. Nephrotic patterns of AKI are rarely encountered in hospitalized patients.

Tubular and interstitial diseases commonly cause AKI specifically from damage due to ischemia, endogenous or exogenous nephrotoxins, medications, or infections. Tubulointerstitial diseases include ATN, acute interstitial necrosis, cast nephropathy, acute urate nephropathy, crystalline nephropathy, and acute phosphate nephropathy. The most common AKI in hospitalized

TABLE 1	Staging of Acute Kidney Injury (based on Kidney Disease: Improving Global Outcomes).	
STAGE	**SERUM CREATININE**	**URINE OUTPUT**
1	≥0.3 mg/dL increase OR 1.5–1.9 times baseline	<0.5 mL/kg/h for 6–12 h
2	2–2.9 times baseline	<0.5 mL/kg/h for ≥12 h
3	3 times baseline OR Increase in creatinine to ≥4 mg/dL OR Starting renal replacement therapy	<0.3 mL/kg/h for ≥24 h OR Anuria for ≥12 h

BOX 1 Etiology of Acute Kidney Injury by Pathophysiology.

Prerenal Causes
- Hypovolemia due to true or effective intravascular volume depletion
  - Hemorrhage of any cause, gastrointestinal (GI) losses (diarrhea, vomiting), diuretics, burns, cirrhosis, nephrotic syndrome
- Diminished cardiac output or pump failure
  - Shock, pericardial disease, heart failure, pulmonary embolism, pulmonary hypertension, and sepsis
- Systemic vasodilation
  - Sepsis, cirrhosis, anaphylaxis, and drugs
- Vasoconstriction of renal vessels
  - Sepsis (initially), hepatorenal syndrome, iodinated contrast, medications such as norepinephrine (Levophed) and vasopressin, nonsteroidal antiinflammatory drugs, and angiotensin-converting enzyme inhibitors
- Increased abdominal pressure
  - Abdominal compartment syndrome

Intrinsic Causes
- Intrinsic renal vascular disease
  - Small: vasculitides, thrombotic thrombocytopenic purpura, scleroderma, atheroembolic disease, and malignant hypertension
  - Large: infarct from aortic dissection, systemic thromboembolism, renal artery aneurysm, and renal vein thrombosis
- Intrinsic renal glomerular disease
  - Nephritic: proliferative glomerulonephritis (e.g., rapidly progressive glomerulonephritis)
  - Nephrotic: nonproliferative glomerulonephritis

- Intrinsic tubular and interstitial disease
  - Acute tubular necrosis
    - Angiotensin-converting enzyme inhibitors/angiotensin II receptor blockers plus nonsteroidal antiinflammatory drugs, radiocontrast or other nephrotoxins, after cardiac surgery, sepsis/shock or prerenal state, and rhabdomyolysis
  - Acute interstitial nephritis
    - Nonsteroidal antiinflammatory drugs, aspirin, omeprazole (Prilosec), thiazide diuretics, furosemide, allopurinol (Zyloprim), penicillin, vancomycin, and cephalosporins
  - Cast nephropathy
    - Multiple myeloma
  - Acute urate nephropathy
    - Tumor lysis syndrome
  - Crystalline nephropathy
    - IV acyclovir (Zovirax)
  - Acute phosphate nephropathy after phosphate bowel prep

Postrenal Causes
- Extrinsic
  - Benign prostatic hyperplasia
  - Metastatic cancer
  - Retroperitoneal fibrosis
  - Neurogenic bladder
- Intrinsic
  - Calculi
  - Crystals
  - Blood clots

- Vancomycin
- Aminogylcosides
- Penicillin
- Piperacillin and tazobactam (Zosyn)
- Cephalosporins
- Heme pigments
- Cisplatin
- Radiocontrast
- Pentamidine (Pentam)
- Foscarnet (Foscavir)
- Cidofovir (Vistide)
- Tenofovir (Viread)
- IV immunoglobulin
- Mannitol
- Synthetic cannabinoids
- Nonsteroidal antiinflammatory drugs
- Angiotensin-converting enzyme inhibitors
- Aspirin
- Omeprazole (Prilosec)
- Thiazide diuretics
- Furosemide (Lasix)
- Allopurinol (Zyloprim)

patients is due to ATN. ATN occurs from prolonged renal hypoperfusion and tissue ischemia or from endogenous or exogenous nephrotoxic exposure. Common endogenous nephrotoxins include hemolysis, rhabdomyolysis, tumor lysis syndrome, and multiple myeloma. Common exogenous nephrotoxins include radiocontrast, aminoglycosides, ethylene glycol, cisplatin, and methotrexate. Common nephrotoxins associated with AKI are listed in Box 2. Cast nephropathy is attributable to excess immunoglobulin light chains in multiple myeloma. Excess cellular contents released into circulation after chemotherapy can cause acute urate nephropathy in tumor lysis syndrome, less common nowadays with the prophylactic use of allopurinol (Zyloprim) or rasburicase (Elitek) prior to chemotherapy administration. Intravenous acyclovir (Zovirax) causes crystalline nephropathy. Oral sodium phosphate solution (Fleet) given for a bowel preparation for colonoscopy can cause acute phosphate nephropathy through an unclear mechanism.

The clinical presentation of intrinsic AKI is variable and dependent on the cause. The cause should be investigated first with an excellent history and physical exam. Vascular causes of intrinsic AKI should be suspected in recent vascular surgery, recent arterial catheterization, anticoagulation, atheroembolic disease, flank pain, or trauma. Glomerular causes of intrinsic AKI should be suspected in patients with systemic lupus erythematosus, systemic sclerosis, rash, arthritis, HIV infection, hepatitis C viral infection, cough, sinusitis, hematuria, hemoptysis, or weight loss. ATN should be suspected in patients with exposure to nephrotoxins, hypotension, trauma, or exposure to radiocontrast agents. AIN should be suspected in medication use or if there is a rash, fever, infection, or arthralgias. Further work-up is described in the following. Management and prognosis are variable and depend on the underlying cause.

Postrenal

Postrenal AKI is due to obstruction of any cause in the urinary tract, within the kidney itself or from the ureter, bladder, bladder neck, or urethra. The most common cause is due to obstruction of the bladder neck, either structural or functional, such as seen in benign prostatic hyperplasia. Other causes include extrinsic compression from metastatic cancer, neurogenic bladder, or retroperitoneal fibrosis, or intrinsic obstruction from calculi, crystals, or blood clots.

The clinical presentation of postrenal causes of AKI with variable urine output from anuria to polyuria, hematuria (if clots are present or malignancy is suspected), dysuria, urgency, increased frequency, weak stream, nocturia, spinal cord injuries, or long-standing poorly controlled diabetes. An excellent history and physical exam will start the investigation of the cause. It is important to diagnosis and treat postrenal causes promptly to avoid long-term damage and improve the chance for recovery.

Approach to Diagnosis

The cause of AKI should always be approached in a patient-centered manner. The diagnostic work-up will depend on clinical context, severity, and duration of AKI in addition to comorbid conditions. For patients in the outpatient setting with new onset or rapidly worsening GFR, close follow-up is warranted and these patients should likely be hospitalized for daily monitoring of laboratory studies and clinical status especially if urgent or emergent treatment is warranted.

Careful review of the medical record can aid in determining trends in serum creatinine, assisting in the determination of an acute, acute on chronic, or chronic process. Once an acute process is identified, then the evaluation of AKI should be categorized into prerenal, intrinsic, or postrenal cause to determine further work-up and ultimately treatment. At minimum, the clinician should obtain urinalysis, urine microscopy, laboratory studies including complete blood count, and metabolic panel with creatinine and electrolytes. Prerenal causes are more suggestive when blood urea nitrogen (BUN):creatinine ratio is greater than 20, when urine specific gravity is elevated, or when urine sodium is low. A renal ultrasound may be useful to obtain to assess for postrenal causes including obstruction, and can specifically give information on cortical thickness, differences in densities in cortex and medulla, integrity of the collecting system, and kidney size. Postvoid residual may be considered and placement of urinary catheter if obstruction is suspected. While a patient's urine output is an important clinical indicator, it is not necessarily kidney specific. Urine output may increase, decrease, or maintain irrespective of the insult affecting the kidneys. Trends in urine output can be useful when determining possible causes of AKI.

Measurements of fractional excretion of sodium (FeNa) or urea (FeUr) have not consistently been shown to have clear clinical correlations. FeNa is defined by the following formula:

$$FeNa = 100 \times \frac{(urinary\ sodium \times serum\ creatinine)}{(serum\ sodium \times urinary\ creatinine)}$$

FeNa less than 1% suggests prerenal and FeNa greater than 2% suggests ATN. Despite the claims that a FeNa calculation can determine prerenal AKI versus ATN, there is no absolute FeNa value that is always diagnostic of prerenal disease. There are many limitations in using FeNa, including that there are other causes of AKI that have a calculated FeNa of less than 1% (including some occasions of ATN). Additionally, single measurements of creatinine may be misleading, given that serum creatinine can vary even in a given day. Patients with CKD have impaired sodium handling and in the setting of prerenal disease, will have a FeNa that is greater than 1%. However, this FeNa value should not preclude the clinician from addressing the underlying issue (for example, hypovolemia causing prerenal AKI in a patient with known CKD) solely based on a FeNa percentage. FeNa is not sensitive or specific enough in the inpatient population and therefore is not generalizable to the average hospitalized patient. The entirety of a patient's presentation should allow the clinician to determine the cause of AKI.

Approach to Treatment

The cause of AKI will determine the treatment. If history and exam are pointing toward prerenal volume depletion as the mechanism of AKI, then intravenous fluids should be administered. This does not apply to prerenal AKI from heart failure or cirrhosis. Hypovolemia and hypotension should be addressed with balanced crystalloid solutions (for example, lactated Ringer's) which will reduce the risk of severe hyperchloremic metabolic acidosis that can occur with saline solutions. The optimal rate of infusion of fluids depends on the clinical status of the patient and comorbidities with expert recommendation to consider one to three liters of fluid to start and to avoid volume overload. Concern for sepsis or infection should be treated appropriately including cultures as indicated, intravenous fluid resuscitation, and antibiotics. Urinary obstruction should be treated and depending on the site of obstruction, a patient may need placement of a urinary catheter or percutaneous nephrostomy tube. Depending on the patient's GFR, any medication given should be renally dosed. All nephrotoxic insults should be avoided. Diuretics should be used in the setting of volume overload, such as in acute decompensated heart failure causing AKI, and it should be noted that diuretics do not specifically affect AKI recovery or have a survival benefit. If there are life-threatening abnormalities or imbalances due to AKI including volume overload, hyperkalemia, acidemia, or uremia, then prompt consultation is warranted to a nephrologist and likely to a critical care specialist. In these cases, renal replacement therapy or another hemodialysis modality will likely be considered. The ideal timing to starting dialysis in patients with AKI is unknown and the mortality benefit to early initiation of dialysis also is unclear. As already mentioned, in patients with acute decompensated heart failure, diuretics are utilized and inotropes may also be necessary to achieve improvement in renal perfusion in the setting of decreased cardiac output. In patients with liver disease and concomitant AKI, hepatorenal syndrome may be considered as the underlying cause of AKI; however, it is a diagnosis of exclusion and is treated in the ICU with norepinephrine (Levophed)[1] or on the general medical floor with midodrine (Proamatine)[1], octreotide (Sandostatin)[1], and albumin[1]. Acute interstitial nephritis should be treated with the withdrawal of the inciting medication or agent, and if there is no improvement in some days, patients may benefit from glucocorticoids. ATN has no one specific treatment, as it is dependent on the underlying cause (ischemia or nephrotoxins).

Prognosis and Outcomes

AKI is associated with adverse patient outcomes, increased mortality, longer length of hospital stay, and higher healthcare costs. The duration of AKI tends to vary between 7 and 21 days. Some patients with AKI recover kidney function within days and some require dialysis for months. After an episode of AKI, patients are at increased risk for CKD and end-stage renal disease (ESRD). Patients with CKD who experience AKI are more likely to advance to ESRD. Some patients may never return to their baseline kidney function. Irreparable decline in kidney function is more likely in patients of advanced age, those with CKD, and those with heart failure. Mortality rates range from 16% to 50% according to stage of AKI and also depend on cause of AKI, concurrent comorbid conditions such as sepsis, lung or liver failure, and cerebrovascular events. Patients who are discharged after a hospitalization during which AKI occurred warrant close follow-up. The KDIGO clinical practice guideline, in their expert opinion, recommended that clinicians evaluate patients 3 months after AKI for resolution of AKI or new onset CKD or worsening of pre-existing CKD.

Developing Issues—Biomarkers

New biomarkers, not yet in widespread clinical use, have been studied for the aim of earlier identification and therefore earlier treatment of AKI. There has been an ongoing search for a sensitive and specific marker of renal injury early on in the AKI syndrome course. Several biomarkers have been evaluated including neutrophil gelatinase–associated lipocalin (NGAL), kidney injury molecule 1 (KIM-1), cystatin C, IL-18, liver-type fatty acid–binding protein (L-FABP), tissue inhibitor of metalloproteinase-2 (TIMP-2), and IGF-binding protein 7 (IGFBP7). TIMP-2 and IGFBP7 have recently been studied and validated in the prediction of onset of severe AKI as defined by KDIGO stage with better

accuracy than other biomarkers. Nearly all identified biomarkers are affected by one or many factors. Cystatin C, validated as an alternative biomarker for GFR, is affected by malignancy, thyroid problems, and cigarette smoking. TIMP-2 and IGFBP7 do not appear to be affected by any factors. Additional study is needed to better understand how to incorporate these biomarkers in identifying and intervening on AKI. A renal "troponin" may indeed be identified in the future.

References

Alge JL, Arthur JM: Biomarkers of AKI: A review of mechanistic relevance and potential therapeutic implications, *Clin J Am Soc Nephrol* 10(1):147–155, 2015, Available at: https://doi.org/10.2215/CJN.12191213.

Balogun R: Fractional excretion of sodium, urea, and other molecules in acute kidney injury - UpToDate. Available at: https://www-uptodate-com.libproxy.unm.edu/contents/fractional-excretion-of-sodium-urea-and-other-molecules-in-acute-kidney-injury?search=fena&source=search_result&selectedTitle=1~40&usage_type=default&display_rank=1#H791015361. Accessed 25 February 2019.

Cooper CM, Fenves AZ, Cooper CM: Before you call renal: Acute kidney injury for hospitalists, *Journal of Hospital Medicine* 10(6), 2015, Available at: https://doi.org/10.1002/jhm.2325.

Hoste EAJ, Bagshaw SM, Bellomo R, et al: Epidemiology of acute kidney injury in critically ill patients: the multinational AKI-EPI study, *Intensive Care Med* 41(8):1411–1423, 2015, Available at: https://doi.org/10.1007/s00134-015-3934-7.

Levey AS, James MT: Acute kidney injury, *Annals of Internal Medicine* 167(9):ITC66, 2017, Available at: https://doi.org/10.7326/AITC201711070.

Ostermann M, Joannidis M: Acute kidney injury 2016: diagnosis and diagnostic workup, *Crit Care* 20(1):299, 2016, Available at: https://doi.org/10.1186/s13054-016-1478-z.

Pahwa AK, Sperati CJ: Urinary fractional excretion indices in the evaluation of acute kidney injury: Urinary excretion indices in AKI, *Journal of Hospital Medicine* 11(1):77–80, 2016, Available at: https://doi.org/10.1002/jhm.2501.

Rahman M, Shad F, Smith MC: Acute kidney injury: a guide to diagnosis and management, *Acute Kidney Injury* 86(7):9, 2012.

Sharfuddin AA, Weisbord SD, Palevsky PM, Molitoris BA: Acute kidney injury. In *Brenner and Rector's The Kidney*, 10th ed., Philadelphia, PA, 2016, Elsevier, pp 958–1011.e19. Available at: http://www.clinicalkey.com/#!/content/book/3-s2.0-B9781455748365000031X. Accessed 22 February 2019.

Susantitaphong P, Cruz DN, Cerda J, et al: World incidence of AKI: A meta-analysis, *CJASN* 8(9):1482–1493, 2013, Available at: https://doi.org/10.2215/CJN.00710113.

Wald R: Changing incidence and outcomes following dialysis-requiring acute kidney injury among critically ill adults: a population-based cohort study-clinical key, *American Journal of Kidney Diseases* 65(6):870–877, 2015.

Wasung ME, Chawla LS, Madero M: Biomarkers of renal function, which and when? *Clinica Chimica Acta* 438:350–357, 2015, Available at: https://doi.org/10.1016/j.cca.2014.08.039.

Yu MK, Kamal F, Chertow GM: Updates in management and timing of dialysis in acute kidney injury, *Journal of Hospital Medicine* 7, February 2019, Available at: https://doi.org/10.12788/jhm.3105.

Section 2: AKI Definition, *Kidney International Supplements* 2(1):19–36, 2012, Available at: https://doi.org/10.1038/kisup.2011.32.

CHRONIC KIDNEY DISEASE

Method of
Kashif Abad, MD; and Mark Unruh, MD, MS

CURRENT DIAGNOSIS

- The estimated glomerular filtration rate (eGFR) is the generally accepted, best index of kidney function. Normal eGFR varies according to age, sex, and body size; in young adults, it is approximately 125 mL/min per 1.73 m² and declines with age.
- Chronic kidney disease (CKD) is defined as GFR < 60 mL/min/1.73 m² as well as elevated markers of kidney damage. The most common marker of kidney damage is urine albumin.
- The most common method to access GFR is serum creatinine combined with CKD-EPI equation. If possible, determine the underlying cause of CKD and consider referral to a nephrologist for management if GFR < 30 mL/min/1.73 m²

---

[1]Not FDA approved for this indication.

- Initiate treatment to delay or prevent disease progression, including an angiotensin-converting enzyme inhibitor (ACEI) or an angiotensin receptor blocker (ARB) to reduce blood pressure to < 130/80 mm Hg and urine total protein excretion to as low as possible but at least < 1 g/day.
- Prevent or treat biochemical or clinical abnormalities including serum potassium, calcium, bicarbonate, calcium, phosphorous, parathyroid hormone, and hemoglobin.
- Evaluate for presence of comorbid conditions such as hypertension, diabetes, and cardiovascular disease.

TABLE 1 Risk Factors for the Development or Progression of Kidney Disease

Albuminuria
Hypertension
Episodes of acute kidney injury
Underlying cause of kidney disease (e.g., diabetic nephropathy)
Obesity
Hyperlipidemia
Smoking
High-protein diet
Metabolic acidosis
Hyperphosphatemia
Hyperuricemia
Hyperglycemia

Chronic kidney disease is the term used to describe patients with decrease in glomerular filtration rate (GFR) or kidney damage such as albuminuria; there are different levels of CKD. CKD has been classified by cause, kidney function, and severity of albuminuria. *Kidney damage* is defined as structural or functional abnormalities of the kidney, initially without decreased GFR, which over time can lead to decreased kidney function. Markers of kidney damage include abnormalities in the composition of the blood or urine or abnormalities in imaging tests. *End-stage renal disease (ESRD)* or *kidney failure* is the term used to describe patients who have advanced renal failure requiring renal replacement therapy (i.e., either hemodialysis/peritoneal dialysis or transplantation). CKD has been associated with higher costs of care and risk of death.

Most chronic kidney disease demonstrates an inexorable progression. The rate of decline could be estimated as much as 7-10 mL/min/year in those with an untreated diabetic nephropathy. Electrolyte homeostasis, causes of progressive decline in function, and manifestations of kidney failure are similar enough across the different pathologies that we can think of common underlying routes to progression, symptoms, and hopefully amelioration of CKD. These interventions often do not reverse kidney disease; rather, they slow the progression of kidney disease. Therefore earlier diagnosis and treatment may delay kidney death so that a patient can avoid undergoing dialysis, transplantation, and the complication of kidney failure.

Prevalence of Chronic Kidney Disease
Estimates are that there are 30 times as many subjects with chronic kidney disease as compared to ESRD. Approximately 14.7% of the US adult population is thought to have some form of chronic kidney disease. Of note, the majority of those with stage 1 and 2 kidney disease may not even be aware of their kidney disease. Furthermore, more than 75 million are thought to have an increased risk of developing CKD. Only a fraction of patients understand that they have CKD, so it is crucial that to convey this to them so that they can take steps to slow the progression of CKD.

Risk Factors for CKD
The non-modifiable risk factors are important for risk stratification by screening and for understanding the pathophysiology of CKD progression (Table 1). These risk factors include ethnicity, which is a risk factor for many kidney diseases. For example, African-American patients with diabetes have a two-to-three-fold higher risk of developing kidney failure compared to white patients. Modifiable risk factors are important for both understanding disease progression and as a possible option for prevention or therapy. For example, the heavy consumption of analgesics has been associated with the development of kidney failure. The number of patients that develop kidney disease and at risk for developing kidney disease will increase with the increasing prevalence of diabetes and aging of the population.

Approach to the Diagnosis of Chronic Kidney Disease
In clinical practice, the serum creatinine and blood urea nitrogen (BUN) concentrations are commonly used as indicators of GFR.

The laboratory measurement of creatinine and urea is accurate and reliable, although normal values may vary slightly from lab to lab. Creatinine production varies with muscle mass, and therefore changes in lean body weight influence the serum creatinine level. For example, a body builder may have an elevated Cr but normal renal function and vice versa for a cachectic elderly woman with muscle atrophy. When using the plasma creatinine to assess GFR, it is also important to keep in mind the semi-logarithmic relationship between the serum creatinine concentration and GFR. Kidney Disease International Global Outcomes (KDIGO) Guideline on Chronic Kidney Disease currently recommends using the Chronic Kidney Disease Epidemiology (CKD-EPI) 2009 creatinine equation: The CKD-EPI equation is currently the most accurate way to estimate GFR from serum creatinine.

CKD-EPI CREATININE EQUATION:

$$GFR = 141 \times \min (S_{cr}/\kappa, 1)^\alpha \times \max(S_{cr}/\kappa, 1)^{-1.209} \times 0.993^{Age} \times 1.018 \text{ [if female]} \times 1.159 \text{ [if black]}$$

where: S_{cr} is serum creatinine in mg/dL,
κ is 0.7 for females and 0.9 for males,
α is −0.329 for females and −0.411 for males,
min indicates the minimum of S_{cr}/κ or 1, and
max indicates the maximum of S_{cr}/κ or 1.

Formulas derived from studies of large groups of patients—such as those by Cockroft and Gault and the Modification of Diet in Renal Disease (MDRD) in which GFR was correlated with other factors (e.g., body weight, age, and serum albumin)—are sufficiently accurate to use for clinical purposes.

The recent classification of CKD includes a measure of albuminuria. A spot albumin/creatinine ratio serves as a very important biomarker. Higher levels of albuminuria are linked to progression of CKD, higher frequency of acute kidney injury, higher rates of dialysis, and higher risk of death.

There are novel estimating equations that use a range of new biomarkers to estimate kidney function. The most widely used is Cystatin C, which can be used to estimate GFR in patients with extremes of age or body habitus. Cystain C is a low-molecular-weight cysteine protease inhibitor produced in all nucleated cells and has a constant level of production but rises with poor renal function. Hence, Cystatin C may serve to improve the estimates of GFR in a number of settings. However, Cystatin C levels have been associated with thyroid levels and inflammation, so providers should interpret this biomarker with caution in these settings.

Management of Chronic Kidney Disease
Staging of CKD
The purpose of CKD staging is to guide management, including stratification of risk for progression and complications of CKD. Staging of CKD should be done according to Figure 1 and Table 2 and based on:
- Cause of disease
- Six categories of eGFR (G stages)
- Three levels of albuminuria (A stages)

The GFR is the generally accepted best index of kidney function. Chronic kidney disease (CKD) is defined as GFR less than

Prognosis of CKD by GFR and Albuminuria Categories: KDIGO 2012

			Persistent albuminuria categories Description and range		
			A1	A2	A3
			Normal to mildly increased	Moderately increased	Severely increased
			<30 mg/g <3 mg/mmol	30-300 mg/g 3-30 mg/mmol	>300 mg/g >30 mg/mmol
GFR categories (ml/min/ 1.73 m²) Description and range	G1	Normal or high	≥90		
	G2	Mildly decreased	60-89		
	G3a	Mildly to moderately decreased	45-59		
	G3b	Moderately to severely decreased	30-44		
	G4	Severely decreased	15-29		
	G5	Kidney failure	<15		

Very dark gray (G1/G2 and A1): low risk (if no other markers of kidney disease, no CKD); Light gray (G3a and A1; G1/G2 and A2): moderately increased risk; Medium gray (G3b and A1; G3a and A2; G1/G2 and A3): high risk; Medium dark gray (G4/G5 and A1; G3b/G4/G5 and A2; G3a/G3b/G4/G5 and A3): very high risk.

Figure 1 Prognosis of CKD by GFR and albuminuria.

60 mL/min per 1.73 m² as well as markers of kidney damage. In the United States the most common marker of kidney damage is urine albumin. Other markers are kidney cysts or pathologic changes in the kidney, for example. The severity of CKD is also determined by the level of GFR.

CKD Stage 3 (moderately decreased GFR)

Stage 3 CKD (a GFR of 30 to 59 mL/min per 1.73 m²) has been subdivided into GFR stages 3a (G3a – GFR 45 to 59 mL/min per 1.73 m²) and 3b (G3b – GFR 30 to 44 mL/min per 1.73 m²) to more accurately reflect the continuous association between lower GFR and risk for mortality and adverse kidney outcomes.

CKD Stage 4 (Severely decreased GFR)

GFR 15–29 mL/min per 1.73 m²

CKD Stage 5 (Kidney failure)

G5 – GFR <15 mL/min per 1.73 m² or treatment by dialysis

Referral to a nephrologist is recommended when eGFR <30 mL/min per 1.73 m² and/or urine albumin creatinine ratio is >300 mg/g, with earlier referral recommended in specific cases. Early referral to a nephrologist is associated with improved outcomes once patients initiate dialysis.

General Approach to Treatment of Chronic Kidney Disease

Treatment of CKD is divided according to modalities that are specific to the underlying disorder and those that are used to treat all patients with CKD.

The physician treating the patient with CKD has two goals: preventing or delaying progression of CKD and alleviating the electrolyte and hormonal abnormalities that can lead to symptoms or complications. The provider can use the CKD classification system shown in Figure 1 to educate patients and highlight the need for adhering to strategies to slow the rate of CKD progression.

Strategies to Slow Progression of CKD

Since we have a better understanding of the progression of kidney disease, we can effectively slow progression. Rather than losing 10 ml/min/year of kidney function as an untreated Type 1 diabetic, those with adequate disease control can forestall the need for dialysis by slowing the rate of progression anywhere from 2 to 6 mL/min/year. This makes a dramatic difference to the individual and to society in terms of quality of life and costs to the health care system. Treat the underlying cause by identifying reversible factors such as volume depletion, uncontrolled hypertension, obstructive uropathy and nephrotoxins.

Blood Pressure Management

In addition to the use of an ACE-I or ARB, management of hypertension in CKD first entails salt-depleting therapy with a salt-restricted diet and diuretic therapy (Table 3). Patients frequently require additional therapy to combat the enhanced vasoconstriction and to attempt to slow the rate of CKD progression. The KDIGO Blood Pressure guidelines have recommended a target blood pressure of <130/80 for those with advance kidney disease. Among patients with diabetes and CKD, these guidelines recommended a blood pressure target <140/90 based largely on results from the ACCORD study. Lastly, there is a real opportunity to improve care due to gaps in awareness, treatment, and control of BP among patients with CKD. Although BP treatment has been shown to slow progression of CKD, there is a substantial number of CKD patients with poor BP control. Around 30% of CKD patients are not aware of their BP. Of those that are aware, substantial portions are untreated. Few of those that are treated, are controlled. Only one-fifth of the patients with CKD stages 3–4 have awareness, treatment, and control of BP.

TABLE 2 — Chronic Kidney Disease Classification Based on Glomerular Filtration Rate and Albuminuria

GFR STAGES	EGFR (ML/MIN/1.73M2)	TERMS
G1	>90	Normal or high
G2	60–89	Mildly decreased
G3a	45–59	Mildly to moderately decreased
G3b	30–44	Moderately to severely decreased
G4	15–29	Severely decreased
G5	<15	Kidney failure (add D if treated by dialysis)

ALBUMINURIA STAGES	ALBUMIN/CREATININE RATIO (MG/G)	TERMS
A1	<30	Normal to mildly increased
A2	30–300	Moderately increased
A3	>300	Severely increased

*Chronic kidney disease is defined as either GFR ≤60 mL/min/1.73 m2 for ≥ 3 months or structural or functional abnormalities manifested by presence of markers of kidney damage in blood, urine, or imaging studies.† Uremic symptoms include nausea, vomiting, anorexia, metallic taste, pericarditis, peripheral neuropathy, central nervous system changes including difficulty with concentration, and seizures.

Angiotensin-Converting Enzyme Inhibitors and Angiotensin Receptor Blockers

Angiotensin-converting enzyme inhibitors (ACE-Is) and angiotensin receptor blockers (ARBs) are preferred anti-hypertensive agents for the treatment of blood pressure among patients with CKD, particularly patients with albuminuria. Ang II plays a key role in the progression of glomerulosclerosis, and there is a large amount of experimental data in both animals and people that blocking AngII mitigates progressions. This is thought to be due to a reduction in the glomerular capillary hypertension, reduction in proteinuria, and a diminution of the Ang II fibrosing effects. ACE-I and ARB both are likely to delay progression of kidney disease and have cardiovascular benefits. Some studies have examined the possibility of using both together in treatment of chronic kidney disease, with results suggesting more harm than benefit owing to higher rates of hyperkalemia and acute kidney injury among patients receiving dual therapy. The ACE/ARBs substantially delay progression of kidney failure. There does not appear to be a point where you should discontinue ACE/ARB medications unless after starting these medicines there is a significant rise in creatinine. When an ACE-I or ARB causes a rise in creatinine >30%, the agent should be held to investigate potential renal artery stenosis or volume depletion.

Dietary Protein Restriction

The role of dietary protein restriction in renoprotective strategies for CKD patients remains controversial. Kidney Disease Improving Global Outcomes (KDIGO) suggests daily restriction in protein intake to 0.8 g/kg for CKD patients, although a very-low-protein diet has been associated with increased mortality over the long term. One study had shown a benefit with nuts and other healthy protein foods in reducing the progression and mortality from CKD.

In spite of the fact that inconclusive results of the largest controlled clinical trial done to investigate protein restriction in CKD, the Modified Diet in Renal Disease (MDRD) study, a benefit of moderate protein restriction was suggested by a long-term follow-up analysis. Several prior and subsequent studies and meta-analyses appear to support the role of low protein in retarding progression of CKD and delaying initiation of maintenance dialysis therapy.

Overall, most experts believe that, despite the absence of observed benefit in the MDRD trial, systematic reviews suggest that protein restriction may be beneficial, and the balance of evidence suggests a benefit of moderate dietary protein restriction.

TABLE 3 — Recommendations for the Treatment of Patients With CKD

BLOOD PRESSURE CONTROL IN CKD	MAINTAIN BLOOD PRESSURE < 130/80 MM HG < 140/90 FOR DIABETIC CKD
Reduce proteinuria by administering angiotensin-converting enzyme inhibitors (ACEIs) or angiotensin receptor blockers (ARBs)	Decrease urine protein excretion as low as possible, at least < 1 g/day
Control phosphate concentration with phosphate binders, using non–calcium-containing binders when possible	Maintain serum phosphate toward the normal range in CKD
Maintain vitamin D level by administration of vitamin D analogs	Maintain 25-OH vitamin D levels at 30 ng/mL by administration of cholecalciferol (D_3) or ergocalciferol (D_2)
Prevent hyperparathyroidism with vitamin D analogs or calcimimetics	Maintain parathyroid levels between 150–600 (2–9 × normal)
Correct anemia with erythropoiesis-stimulating agents and iron replacement as needed	Maintain hemoglobin between 10 and 11 mg/dL. Keep iron saturation (iron/TIBC) > 20%
Administer diuretics to control hypertension and volume overload	Maintain euvolemia when possible
Control serum potassium with dietary restriction, diuretics, and/or potassium exchange resin as necessary	Maintain serum potassium < 5.0 mEq/L
Prevent malnutrition with adequate calories and protein intake	Maintain protein intake between 0.6 and 1 g/kg in CKD and between 1 and 1.3 g/kg on dialysis
Control metabolic acidosis with administration of sodium bicarbonate or sodium citrate	Maintain serum bicarbonate > 22 mEq/L but < 26 mEq/L

Limiting protein intake is also associated with favorable laboratory and metabolic effects, including reduction of blood urea nitrogen levels, uremic toxins, and acid load, in addition to reduced phosphorus load with better control of metabolic bone disorders. Protein restriction may be particularly effective in diseases characterized by hyperfiltration, such as diabetes and certain glomerulopathies.

In patients with CKD, a balanced and individualized dietary approach based on low-protein diet should be carefully monitored, with periodic follow-up for adequate caloric intake and surveillance to optimize protein malnutrition with body weight as well as serum albumin.

Avoid Nephrotoxic Medications

Avoid nephrotoxins and note that both prescription and over-the-counter medications can have delterious kidney effects. The most concerning nephrotoxins over the counter are NSAIDS, antacids, proton pump inhibitors, and a number of herbal medications (licorice, Cat's Claw). Several prescription medications can be deleterious to the kidney. Noteworthy are the calcineurin inhibitors such as cyclosporine (Sandimmune) and tacrolimus (Prograf), which cause progressive renal insufficiency. We know this because solid-organ transplants have a high rate of kidney failure. Other medications such as aminoglycosides and amphotericin (Fungizone) or the use of IV contrast have detrimental effects on the hospitalized patient.

Clinical Manifestations of Kidney Failure

P. A. Piorry coined the word *urémie* in 1847 to indicate problems caused by "contaminating the blood with urine." The basic abnormality is the presence of waste products that are not being eliminated by the kidney. In current use, the term *uremia* reflects a clinical syndrome associated with loss of kidney function. Uremic symptoms in advanced CKD result both from kidney excretory failure (retention of urea, certain hormones, polyamines, trace elements, serum proteases, so-called "middle molecules," pyridine derivatives, B_2 microglobulin, etc.) and from the loss of metabolic and endocrine functions normally performed by the kidney. Uremia is thought to be in part due to protein intake, since a low-protein diet mitigates some of the symptoms. While we know that some of the uremic toxins are partially dialyzable, the exact etiology of uremia remains unknown.

Uremia also relates a loss of metabolic and endocrine functions normally performed by the intact kidney. Hence, kidney failure is a multisystem disorder (see Table 4). The measurement of kidney function can be variable, and that degree of variability makes it difficult to use as the only factor in clinical decision making. Therefore, as CKD progresses, clinicians tend to regularly assess the subjective symptoms associated with uremia. In particular, uremia has been described in the following systems: neurologic (sleep, memory), GI (appetite, nausea, dysguesia), and dermatologic (itching). If the severity of these symptoms cannot be managed by symptomatic therapy, then that would be an indication for starting dialysis. Furthermore, if a dialysis patient has these symptoms, it may reflect an inadequate treatment, and the dialysis dose will have to be increased. Of note, the usual physical signs of kidney failure can be rapidly assessed during an exam: blood pressure, pericardial rub, edema, and crackles on lung exam.

Measures Designed to Treat Comorbidity in Kidney Disease
Anemia (Table 5)

Anemia may be managed in patients with CKD by first ruling out other causes of anemia such as GI bleeding and iron deficiencies. Iron deficiency is common in patients with CKD and may be evaluated with a total iron saturation (TSAT) and ferritin. Low ferritin (<100ng/mL) and TSAT (<20) in patients with moderate to advanced CKD indicate an absolute iron deficiency. Iron deficiency may be treated using the oral or intravenous route. After iron stores are restored, if the anemia persists and other causes are ruled out, then a erythropoiesis-stimulating agent (ESA) such as erythropoietin (Procrit, Epogen) may be used. For CKD

patients, the uses of ESAs are shown to reduce the need for blood transfusions and modestly improve quality of life. The risks of ESA use include an increase in cardiovascular events, hypertension, and cancer progression. For CKD patients the recommendations are to initiate therapy if the Hgb are below 10g/dL with an individualized decision for a target based on risks and benefits. In many cases, providers target a hemoglobin between 10 mg/dL and 11 mg/dL and avoid exceeding levels >12 mg/dL.

Metabolic Acidosis

Metabolic acidosis develops in CKD when the eGFR drops below 30 mL/min. Recent studies have linked metabolic acidosis in CKD to protein wasting, loss of bone, and sympathetic activation.

TABLE 4   Signs and Symptoms of Kidney Failure

CARDIOVASCULAR COMPLICATIONS	ENDOCRINE DISORDERS
Hypertension	Secondary hyperparathyroidism
Ischemic cardiac disease	Glucose intolerance (uremic diabetes)
Pericardial disease	Hyperlipidemia
Congestive heart failure	Sexual dysfunction/infertility
Hematologic Abnormalities	**Immunologic Defects**
Anemia	Lymphocytopenia, leukopenia
Bleeding tendency	Decreased antibody responses
	Decreased cell-mediated response
	Increased susceptibility to infection
Neuropsychiatric Abnormalities	**Dermatologic Abnormalities**
Peripheral neuropathy	Pruritus, uremic pigmentation,
CNS disturbances	uremic frost, calciphylaxis, nail changes
Seizures	
Sleep disorders	
Musculoskeletal Abnormalities	Gastrointestinal Abnormalities
Bone disease	Anorexia, nausea, vomiting
Myopathies	Upper tract disease: gastritis, duodenitis,
Carpal Tunnel Syndrome	

TABLE 5   Factors to Consider in the Management of Patients With CKD

Contributors to the loss of kidney function
Hypertension
Diabetes mellitus
Dietary salt intake
Proteinuria
Metabolic acidosis
Complications of chronic kidney disease
Anemia
Platelet dysfunction
Abnormal bone and mineral metabolism (e.g., secondary hyperparathyroidism)
Lipid abnormalities (elevated cholesterol and triglycerides)
Metabolic acidosis
Volume overload
Electrolyte disturbances (e.g., hyperkalemia)
Cardiovascular disease

Observational studies have also linked metabolic acidosis to a higher rate of CKD progression and increased risk of death. There are a large number of ongoing studies testing whether oral sodium bicarbonate supplementation in CKD preserves renal function, and bicarbonate supplementation has been widely adopted for metabolic acidosis in CKD. A standard dose used in clinical trials for CKD patients has been sodium bicarbonate 0.5 mEq/kg/day. The supplemental bicarbonate may be titrated up or down depending on serum bicarbonate and symptoms. If bicarbonate is not tolerated by patients, then clinicians could try Shohl's solution (citric acid/sodium citrate), as citrate is converted to bicarbonate by the liver. Currently, a reasonable target serum bicarbonate for patients with moderate to advanced CKD would be >22mEq/L and <26mEq/L.

Divalent Ion Metabolism

CKD is associated with abnormalities of divalent ions (Ca^{++}, P) and of the hormones that regulate the concentration of these minerals in body fluids. It is of note that the dysregulation of these divalent ions has also attracted attention as a possible source of cardiovascular disease, since those with CKD are found to have calcium deposition and a calcification of heart valves. Lastly, failed management of divalent ions may lead to calcific uremic arteriolopathy, or calciphylaxis. Calciphylaxis is a rare syndrome characterized by the development of painful nodules in the soft tissue that indurate and ulcerate. This disorder has no uniformly effective treatment and has a high mortality rate. Serum phosphorus is controlled by administration of phosphate binders usually starting with calcium citrate (Citracal) or acetate (PhosLo). If these are not successful or if patients have elevated serum calcium levels, then sevelamer (Renagel) or lanthanum (Fosrenol) can be used alone or in combination with calcium binders. Physicians should aim to maintain serum phosphorus levels between 2.7 and 4.6 mg/dL in CKD stage 3 and 4 and between 3.5 and 5.5 mg/dL in CKD stage 5. Defining the target PTH level in the setting of CKD remains a challenge because of end-organ resistance to PTH. Parathyroid hormone levels should be maintained between 150 and 600 pg/mL (2–9 × normal) in end-stage renal disease and patients on dialysis. Suppression of parathyroid hormone secretion can be achieved by administration of various vitamin D analogs in combination with calcimimetic agents such as cinacalcet (Sensipar). Serum calcium levels should be monitored closely. Low 25-OH vitamin D levels have been documented in a large number of individuals both with and without renal failure. In patients with renal impairment this can contribute to the abnormal 1,25-OH vitamin D levels. Measurement of 25-OH vitamin D levels should be obtained in all patients with CKD and estimated GFR less than 60 mL/min/1.73 m². If levels are below 30 ng/mL, ergocalciferol (D_2) or cholecalciferol (D_3) should be given at sufficient doses to maintain it above this level.

Hyperkalemia

The clinical consequence of hyperkalemia includes cardiac toxicity, muscle weakness, and death. The target potassium concentration for patients with CKD should remain in the normal range, and patients should be monitored during treatment with ACEIs or ARBs. Management of a high serum potassium in patients with CKD should include a low-potassium diet. If there is a sudden increase, it may be due to use of salt substitutes, large amounts of juice, or eating high-potassium foods. It may be helpful to get a nutrition consult to help the patient maintain a low-potassium diet and have a nutritionist be aware of differences in diverse foods, since both noni and coconut juice are high in potassium. In addition, review medications for those associated with hyperkalemia and consider decreasing the dose of ACEI or ARB. Diuretics also may be used to decrease serum potassium levels in CKD, with loop diuretics the most widely used for patients with an eGFR<30mL/min. Lastly, potassium binding agents may be used to control serum potassium levels in patients with advanced CKD. The potassium exchange resin, sodium polystyrene sulfonate (Kayexalate), or one of the newer exchange resins patriromer (Veltassa) decreases serum potassium levels.

Volume Overload

Sodium retention contributes to hypertension and edema among patients with CKD. In order to adequately address volume overload, both the intake and sodium excretion may need to be addressed in patients with CKD. Patients should adhere to a low-sodium diet, which is often complicated by other dietary restrictions (low-potassium, low-phosphate, ADA diet). Given the complexity of diet in CKD, use of a nutritionist with expertise in kidney-related diets can help both volume overload and the other complications of CKD. In addition to sodium restriction, patients may need to use a diuretic for blood pressure and volume management. In the setting of an eGFR<30mL/min, loop diuretics are often used to address volume overload. The loop diuretics such as furosemide (Lasix) should be dosed frequently enough to maintain a negative sodium balance. If the loop diuretic at higher doses is not adequately addressing volume overload, then an additional distal tubule diuretic such as metolazone (Zaroxolyn) may be used to increase urinary sodium excretion. It should be noted that increasing sodium excretion may cause acute kidney injury of CKD patients, particularly in the setting of ACEI/ARB and other diuretics. In this case, the patients will often respond to reducing the diuretic dose with close monitoring.

Chronic Kidney Disease–Mineral Bone Disorder (CKD-MBD)

Chronic kidney disease–mineral bone disorder (CKD-MBD) is a systemic disorder of mineral and bone metabolism associated with CKD due to hyperphosphatemia from diminished kidney phosphorus excretion and hypocalcemia due to impaired kidney production of active 1, 25-(OH)2 D leading to secondary hyperparathyroidism. Elevations in serum fibroblast growth factor 23 (FGF23), metabolic bone disease, soft tissue calcifications, and other metabolic derangements are associated with morbidity and mortality in CKD. The management of CKD-MBD is complex due to homeostatic system and multiple treatment options without definitive randomized trials. The ideal strategy should be normalizing serum calcium, phosphate, PTH, and metabolic acidosis while minimizing the risks associated with the therapies. The various treatment options for hyperphosphatemia and secondary hyperparathyroidism include dietary phosphorus restriction, phosphate binders, calcitriol (Rocaltrol) or other active vitamin D analogues, calcimimetics, adequate hemodialysis, and parathyroidectomy. The optimal PTH level in the setting of CKD remains a challenge and has not been prospectively determined. KIDIGO guidelines recommend that PTH be kept between two to nine times the upper limit of normal for the assay.

Cardiovascular Disease

While >10 million American adults are estimated to have a GFR<60 mL/min (i.e., CKD 3 or worse), far fewer are on dialysis or have received a transplant. Why is there a disparity between the number receiving renal replacement therapies and the number with CKD? Most patients with CKD die from cardiovascular disease (CVD) prior to requiring dialysis or transplantation. On dialysis, the risk of death from CVD remains 10–100 times higher than the general population. A 25-year-old man on hemodialysis has approximately the same risk of dying from heart disease as an 80-year-old without CKD. Traditional risk factors account for only a portion of the CVD risk associated with CK. Traditional risk factors include age, diabetes, lipids, hypertension, and smoking, among others. Many nontraditional risk factors are believed to play a role in increasing CVD risk in CKD. Some of these risk factors are anemia, volume overload, hyperparathyroidism, calcium/phosphate disturbances, uremia, and malnutrition/inflammation often associated with CKD. The exact role these nontraditional risk factors play is an actively researched area. In general, consider patients with CKD high-risk patients for CVD, and CKD is considered by some to be a coronary equivalent. Data indicate that patients with lower GFRs (<45 mL/min) and microalbuminuria/proteinuria carry a very high CVD risk (~ equivalent to a prior history of coronary disease). This is important when seeing a patient in the emergency room for chest pain or when evaluating a patient pre-operatively for surgery, etc. Treatment focuses on optimizing management of known CVD risk factors and being alert for harbingers of active CVD. Those caring for CKD patients must address CVD risk management. Primary prevention focuses on blood pressure, exercise, +/- aspirin, +/- statins. The data available for cardiovascular risk management is limited in part owing to the exclusion of patients with significant CKD in many large studies. Hence, the utility of ASA and statins (if any) in this setting is not well established. CKD patient's often present with atypical symptoms of CVD, a high index of suspicion is important.

References

Fox CS, Matsushita K, Woodward M, Bilo HJ, Chalmers J, Heerspink HJ, Lee BJ, Perkins RM, Rossing P, Sairenchi T, Tonelli M, Vassalotti JA, Yamagishi K, Coresh J, de Jong PE, Wen CP, Nelson RG: Associations of kidney disease measures with mortality and end-stage renal disease in individuals with and without diabetes: a meta-analysis, Chronic Kidney Disease Prognosis Consortium, *Lancet* 380(9854):1662–1673, 2012 Nov 10, https://doi.org/10.1016/S0140-6736(12)61350-6, Epub 2012 Sep 24. Review. Erratum in: *Lancet* 2013 Feb 2;381(9864):374, 2013 Feb 2. PMID: 23013602.

Kalantar-Zadeh K, Fouque D: *Nutritional Management of Chronic Kidney Disease*, N Engl J Med. 377(18):1765–1776, 2017 Nov 2, https://doi.org/10.1056/NEJMra1700312, Review. PMID:29091561.

KDIGO 2017: Clinical Practice Guideline Update for the Diagnosis, Evaluation, Prevention, and Treatment of Chronic KidneyDisease–Mineral and Bone Disorder (CKD-MBD), 2017.

KDOQI: Clinical practice guidelines and clinical practice recommendations for diabetes and chronic kidney disease, *Am J Kidney Dis* 49:S1–S54, 2007.

Klahr S, et al: The effects of dietary protein restriction and blood-pressure control on the progression of chronic renal disease. Modification of Diet in Renal Disease Study Group, *N Engl J Med* 330:877, 1994.

Kovesdy CP, Appel LJ, Grams ME, Gutekunst L, McCullough PA, Palmer BF, Pitt B, Sica DA, Townsend RR: Potassium Homeostasis in Health and Disease: A Scientific Workshop Cosponsored by the National Kidney Foundation and the American Society of Hypertension, *Am J Kidney Dis* 70(6):844–858, 2017 Dec. https://doi.org/10.1053/j.ajkd.2017.09.003, Epub 2017 Oct 10. PMID: 29029808.

Kraut JA, Madias NE. Metabolic Acidosis of CKD: Am J Kidney Dis 67(2):307–317, 2016 Feb. https://doi.org/10.1053/j.ajkd.2015.08.028. Epub 2015 Oct 23. An Update.

Levey AS, Stevens LA, Schmid CH, Zhang YL, Castro 3rd AF, Feldman HI, Kusek JW, Eggers P, Van Lente F, Greene T, Coresh J: CKD-EPI (Chronic Kidney Disease Epidemiology Collaboration): A new equation to estimate glomerular filtration rate, *Ann Intern Med* 150:604–612, 2009.

Navaneethan SD, Schold JD, Arrigain S, Jolly SE, Wehbe E, Raina R, Simon JF, Srinivas TR, Jain A, Schreiber Jr MJ, Nally Jr JV: Serum bicarbonate and mortality in stage 3 and stage 4 chronic kidney disease, *Clin J Am Soc Nephrol* 6(10):2395–2402, 2011 Oct. https://doi.org/10.2215/CJN.03730411, Epub 2011 Sep 1. PMID: 21885787.

Pfeffer MA, Burdmann EA, Chen CY, Cooper ME, de Zeeuw D, Eckardt KU, Feyzi JM, Ivanovich P, Kewalramani R, Levey AS, Lewis EF, McGill JB, McMurray JJ, Parfrey P, Parving HH, Remuzzi G, Singh AK, Solomon SD, Toto R, TREAT Investigators: A trial of darbepoetin alfa in type 2 diabetes and chronic kidney disease, *N Engl J Med* 361(21):2019–2032, 2009 Nov 19, https://doi.org/10.1056/NEJMoa0907845. Epub. 2009 Oct 30. PMID: 19880844.

Webster AC, Nagler EV, Morton RL, Masson P: Chronic Kidney Disease, *Lancet* 389(10075):1238–1252, 2017 Mar 25, https://doi.org/10.1016/S0140-6736(16)32064-5. Epub 2016 Nov 23.

Wright Jr JT, Williamson JD, Whelton PK, Snyder JK, Sink KM, Rocco MV, Reboussin DM, Rahman M, Oparil S, Lewis CE, Kimmel PL, Johnson KC, Goff Jr DC, Fine LJ, Cutler JA, Cushman WC, Cheung AK, Ambrosius WT: A Randomized Trial of Intensive versus Standard Blood-Pressure Control, *SPRINT Research Group*, N Engl J Med. 373(22):2103–2116, 2015 Nov 26. https://doi.org/10.1056/NEJMoa1511939, Epub 2015 Nov 9. Erratum in: *N Engl J Med* 377(25):2506, 2017 Dec 21.

MALIGNANT TUMORS OF THE UROGENITAL TRACT

Method of
Peter E. Clark, MD

CURRENT DIAGNOSIS

Carcinoma of the Prostate
- Average-risk patients can be offered screening with prostate-specific antigen (PSA) testing and digital rectal examination (DRE) at 55 years of age, high-risk patients with a strong family history, and African American patients at age 40 years.
- Patients with an elevated PSA or abnormal DRE are referred for discussion regarding risks, benefits, and alternatives to biopsy of the prostate.
- Diagnosis is made with transrectal ultrasound-guided biopsy of the prostate.
- Staging with bone scanning is done for patients with high-grade tumors (Gleason grade 4 or 5), PSA levels greater than 20 μg/mL, elevated alkaline phosphatase levels, or bone pain.

Renal Cell Carcinoma
- Hematuria is the single most common sign, occurring in up to 60% of cases. Flank pain and a palpable mass can also occur, but the classic triad of hematuria, flank pain, and a palpable abdominal mass is present in only 10% of cases. Other common signs and symptoms are fever, anemia, thrombocytosis, hypercalcemia, and an elevated sedimentation rate.
- Most tumors are asymptomatic and are detected incidentally on radiographic imaging (renal ultrasonography, computed tomography [CT] scanning, or magnetic resonance imaging).

Benign Renal Tumors
- Angiomyolipomas have a characteristic appearance of fat within the lesion on CT scans.
- Angiomyolipomas may occur sporadically or as part of the tuberous sclerosis complex.
- Tuberous sclerosis is characterized by benign tumors within the cerebellum, mental retardation, epilepsy, and adenoma sebaceum. Angiomyolipomas occur in half of these patients and are typically bilateral and multifocal, making management more challenging.
- Oncocytomas are benign renal tumors that account for 5% to 10% of solid renal lesions.
- Oncocytomas can be more round and of uniform density, or they may have a central scar or spoke-wheel appearance on CT scan. However, no feature can reliably distinguish these tumors from a malignant renal tumor.
- Oncocytomas should be diagnosed only histologically; they are characterized by eosinophilic granular, mitochondria-laden cells.
- In general, a non–fat-containing, solid renal mass should be considered malignant until proven otherwise.

Tumors of the Renal Pelvis and Ureter
- Tumors arising in the renal pelvis account for 10% of all renal tumors and approximately 5% of all urothelial carcinomas.
- Ureteral tumors account for 25% of upper tract urothelial carcinomas.
- These tumors are more common in men than in women.
- Cigarette smoking is strongly associated with an increased risk, as are analgesic abuse and cyclophosphamide (Cytoxan).
- The most common presenting symptom is hematuria.
- Diagnostic work-up usually includes CT urography, urinary cytology, and cystoscopy.
- Cytologic examination of the urine has a high specificity but poor sensitivity, particularly for low-grade lesions.
- Between 3% and 5% of patients with bladder cancer have associated upper tract urothelial carcinoma. This risk is increased in patients with carcinoma in situ (CIS) or high-grade disease, in whom the risk can be as high as 20%.
- Patients with upper tract urothelial carcinoma have a 30% to 70% risk of developing bladder cancer.

Urothelial Carcinoma of the Bladder
- Painless, gross hematuria is the most common presenting symptom.
- Twenty percent of patients present with only microscopic hematuria.
- Irritative voiding symptoms such as frequency, urgency, or dysuria may also suggest a malignancy, particularly CIS.
- Patients with suspected bladder cancer should undergo an evaluation of their upper tracts (typically by CT), cystoscopy, and cytologic examination of the urine (or another urine-based tumor marker study).

- Transurethral biopsy or resection confirms the diagnosis.
- Ninety percent of bladder cancers are urothelial carcinoma, and 75% are non–muscle-invasive (superficial) at presentation.

Urethral Carcinoma
- Urethral carcinoma is the only urologic malignancy that is more common in females than in males.
- Fifty percent of cases are associated with urethral stricture.
- Urethral carcinoma may manifest as hematuria, obstructive voiding, or a palpable mass.
- Transurethral biopsy is usually required for diagnosis.

Penile Cancer
- Squamous cell carcinoma of the penis occurs most commonly in the sixth decade of life.
- Symptoms are related to ulceration, necrosis, suppuration, and hemorrhage of the penile lesion.
- The diagnosis is established by biopsy.
- Clinical evaluation of patients with penile cancer includes physical examination with palpation of the inguinal region, chest radiography, CT of the abdomen and pelvis.

Testicular Cancer
- Testicular cancer is relatively rare overall, but it is the most common malignancy in men between the ages of 15 and 35 years, with 8090 new cases occurring annually.
- Testicular cancer often manifests as a painless, enlarging testicular mass.
- Malignant tumors of the testis can be divided into those originating from the germinal cells (seminomatous and nonseminomatous germ cell tumors), rare tumors from the supporting cells (Leydig cells and Sertoli cells), and rare metastases from another primary site.
- Ninety-five percent of tumors originating in the testis are germ cell tumors. Fewer than 10% of all germ cell tumors arise from extragonadal primary sites such as the mediastinum or retroperitoneum.
- Human β-chorionic gonadotropin and α-fetoprotein are accurate and relatively specific tumor markers for testicular cancer.

 ## CURRENT THERAPY

Carcinoma of the Prostate
- Potentially curative treatment is generally offered to men with at least a 10-year life expectancy.
- Treatment options for clinically localized T1c and T2 tumors include active surveillance/watchful waiting, radiation therapy (external irradiation and brachytherapy), cryotherapy, High Intensity Focused Ultrasound (HIFU) and surgery (open and laparoscopic).
- Treatments for locally advanced tumors (T3/T4) or high-risk cancer patients include surgery and external irradiation in combination with androgen-deprivation therapy (ADT).
- Treatment for patients with metastatic disease (N1–2 or M1) includes initial ADT and later potentially chemotherapy, alternate forms of ADT, or immunotherapy.
- Follow-up includes history, physical examination, and monitoring of prostate-specific antigen at least every 6 months for 2 years and then annually. Any abnormalities may be more fully evaluated with appropriate imaging.

Renal Cell Carcinoma
- Treatment for localized masses is almost always surgical excision via radical or partial nephrectomy. Both operations may be performed with an open or a laparoscopic approach.
- Partial nephrectomy should be attempted in patients who have a solitary kidney, bilateral disease, or renal insufficiency.

- Partial nephrectomy is the preferred operation for patients who have lesions 4 cm or smaller and a normal contralateral kidney, with local recurrence rates of less than 5%.
- Minimally invasive approaches including percutaneous radiofrequency ablation and cryotherapy are acceptable alternatives to carefully selected patients.
- Up to 25% of patients have metastatic disease at diagnosis. Sites of metastasis, in decreasing frequency, include lungs, lymph nodes, liver, bone, and adrenal gland.
- Chemotherapy and radiation therapy provide little to no survival benefit, with radiation only palliating painful metastases.
- The mainstay of treatment in the past was immunotherapy, with 5-year survival rates of 10% to 20%. Immunotherapy now relies on high dose IL-2 (interleukin-2, Proleckin). In select cases and more recently the checkpoint inhibitor nivolumab (Opdivo) for second line therapy.
- Modern therapies for advanced or metastatic RCC include targeted therapies such as the oral tyrosine kinase inhibitors such as sunitinib (Sutent), pazopanib (Votrient), axitinib (Inlyta), and sorafenib (Nexavar), and the mammalian target of rapamycin (mTOR) inhibitors, temsirolimus (Torisel) and everolimus (Afinitor).
- Evidence suggests improved survival for those undergoing nephrectomy before systemic immunotherapy for metastatic disease.

Benign Renal Tumors
- For angiomyolipomas, management should be individualized. With asymptomatic lesions smaller than 4 cm, observation with annual imaging is reasonable.
- For patients with a symptomatic angiomyolipoma or one larger than 4 cm, surgical excision should be considered, although angioembolization is another option. Angioembolization can be used to stabilize a patient with acute hemorrhage secondary to an angiomyolipoma.

Tumors of the Renal Pelvis and Ureter
- Distal ureteral tumors can be managed with distal ureterectomy and ureteroneocystostomy.
- High-grade, multifocal, or high-stage tumors are optimally treated by nephroureterectomy with removal of a cuff of bladder at the ureteral orifice.
- Laparoscopic nephroureterectomy is the preferred surgical approach, allowing for complete tumor removal and often quicker convalescence.
- Carefully selected patients, especially those who have bilateral disease or a functionally solitary kidney, can be managed with endoscopic tumor ablation.

Urothelial Carcinoma of the Bladder
- Treatment depends on tumor stage.
- Superficial (Ta) low-grade cancers are managed with transurethral resection, with or without a single, immediate postresection instillation of a chemotherapeutic agent, typically mitomycin-C (Mutamycin).
- Carcinoma in situ or high-grade stage Ta tumors that involve the lamina propria (stage T1) and recurrent tumors are managed with transurethral resection and intravesical agents such as thiotepa (Thioplex), doxorubicin (Adriamycin), and mitomycin-C[1] or intravesical bacillus Calmette-Guérin (Tice BCG).
- Bladder surveillance is mandatory, because the recurrence rate in the bladder can be as high as 50% at 5 years.
- Surveillance protocols vary but typically include cystoscopy and urinary tumor studies (usually cytology) every 3 months for the first 2 years, semiannually in years 3 to 5, and annually thereafter.
- Periodic evaluation of the upper tracts should be performed, usually by computed tomographic (CT) urography.
- Superficial disease that progresses or is refractory to conservative management, as well as tumors that invade the bladder muscle (stages T2–T4), is best managed by radical cystectomy and urinary diversion.

- Urinary diversion may be either incontinent (conduit) or continent (orthotopic or continent cutaneous).
- Five-year recurrence-free survival rates are 60% to 85% after cystectomy for organ-confined disease (stages T2a–T2b). For extravesical disease (stages T3a to T4), the 5-year survival rate decreases to 40% to 60%; for node-positive disease it is less than 30%.
- Patients with T2–T4 disease should be strongly considered for combination therapy with surgery plus chemotherapy, either in the neoadjuvant or the adjuvant setting. Recent randomized trials have suggested an approximately 5% survival advantage for neoadjuvant chemotherapy plus surgery, compared with surgery alone.
- Patients with M1 disease are usually treated with chemotherapy.
- The standard regimen over the past decade has been MVAC: methotrexate (Trexall),[1] vinblastine (Velban),[1] doxorubicin (Adriamycin), and cisplatin (Platinol); however, durable complete response rates are less than 15%.
- Newer agents such as gemcitabine (Gemzar)[1] along with cisplatin appear to offer similar response rates and reduced toxicity.
- The checkpoint inhibitor atezolizumab (Tecentriq) is now approved as immunotherapy for patients who have failed first line chemotherapy.

Urethral Carcinoma

- Treatment of the primary tumor is surgical excision and varies based on the location and stage of the tumor.
- In men, urethrectomy can be performed via a perineal incision.
- Proximal tumors of the bulbar urethra are often managed with cystoprostatectomy and en bloc urethrectomy.
- Among women, for tumors of the proximal urethra and tumors with extension into adjacent structures, cystectomy with en bloc urethrectomy and anterior vaginectomy along with pelvic lymphadenectomy is usually required.
- Radiation therapy is also reported to provide local control in selective cases.

Penile Cancer

- Small penile cancers limited to the prepuce can be treated by circumcision alone.
- Partial penectomy is used to treat smaller (2–5 cm) distal penile tumors. The remaining penis should be long enough to permit voiding in the standing position. The 5-year cure rate for patients treated with partial penectomy is 70% to 80%.
- Larger distal penile lesions and proximal tumors require total penectomy and perineal urethrostomy. If the scrotum, pubis, or abdominal wall is involved, radical en bloc excision may be necessary.
- Many patients have inguinal lymphadenopathy at presentation. However, inguinal lymph node enlargement before excision of the primary tumor may be the result of infection and not metastatic disease. Therefore clinical assessment of the inguinal region should be delayed 4 to 6 weeks.
- If inguinal lymphadenopathy persists or with high-risk features, there is a high likelihood of metastatic disease, and ilioinguinal lymphadenectomy should be performed. The procedure is performed on the contralateral side if the initial side contains tumor and could be simultaneously performed or staged on inpatients with high risk disease.
- Irradiation of the primary tumor and regional lymph nodes is an alternative to surgery in patients with small (≤2 cm), low-stage tumors.
- Mohs' surgery is another alternative for small lesions (≤2 cm).

Testicular Cancer

- All patients with suspected testicular tumors should undergo a radical orchiectomy through an inguinal approach and early, high ligation of the spermatic cord.
- Serum tumor markers should be measured before surgery and are used for disease staging and to monitor for recurrence.

- Radiographic staging should include, at a minimum, a CT scan of the abdomen and pelvis and chest radiography.
- Seminoma is the most common histologic form of germ cell tumor and generally carries a better prognosis than other variants. Standard therapy for low-stage (T1, 2a, or 2b) disease is orchiectomy with active surveillance, short course chemotherapy, or adjuvant radiation therapy to the retroperitoneum. Relapse is relatively rare, occurring in 4% of patients with stage 1 and 10% of patients with stage 2 disease. Relapses after radiation therapy can be salvaged in more than 90% of cases through systemic chemotherapy. The long-term cure rate for low-stage seminoma is approximately 99%.
- Nonseminomatous germ cell tumors (NSGCTs) include embryonal cell carcinomas, choriocarcinomas, yolk sac carcinomas, teratomas, and mixed germ cell tumors. As with pure seminoma, the cure rate for low-stage NSGCTs is high (>95%) in patients with stage 1 disease.
- Surveillance, retroperitoneal lymph node dissection (RPLND), and adjuvant chemotherapy are standard treatment options for stage 1 NSGCT.
- RPLND is a major abdominal operation in which lymph nodes from the retroperitoneum are removed, from the renal hilum down to the level of the common iliac artery, with lateral margins being confined by the ureters.
- Adjuvant chemotherapy after RPLND should be considered if any lymph node is larger than 2 cm in diameter, if at least six nodes are involved, or if there is extranodal invasion.
- Patients with persistently increased concentrations of α-fetoprotein, human β-chorionic gonadotropin, or both but without other clinical evidence of disease after orchiectomy usually have systemic disease and are treated with chemotherapy.
- Approximately one third of patients require up-front chemotherapy. Those with clinical stage 2c disease (or higher), primary retroperitoneal germ cell tumors, or mediastinal seminomas treated with radiation therapy should undergo systemic, cisplatin-based, multiagent chemotherapy.
- Postchemotherapy RPLND for seminoma is typically reserved for patients with residual masses larger than 3 cm. For NSGCT, some groups reserve postchemotherapy RPLND for patients who do not have substantial tumor shrinkage (>90% shrinkage of retroperitoneal nodes and no residual nodes >1.5 cm) and those with teratomatous elements in the primary tumor. Others advocate surgery for all patients with initial bulky retroperitoneal disease. All agree that a clear, residual mass after chemotherapy in the setting of NSGCT warrants postchemotherapy RPLND.
- Multimodal therapy has allowed 90% to 95% of testicular cancer patients to be cured, even in the face of metastatic disease.

[1]Not FDA approved for this indication.

Carcinoma of the Prostate

Prostate cancer is the most common noncutaneous solid malignancy among men in the United States, and it is second only to lung cancer with respect to cancer-related death. In 2008, there were an estimated 186,320 new cases of prostate cancer and 28,660 deaths due to this disease. Because prostate cancer is predominantly a disease of the elderly, its incidence may be expected to rise over time as the US population ages.

There is a familial predisposition to prostate cancer, which is more common among those with a first-degree relative who also has the disease, and it appears to be more common among African American men than among Caucasian men. Environmental factors that have been associated with an increased risk of prostate cancer include a high-fat Western-style diet, as compared with a high-soy Asian diet, and low levels of vitamin D.

Hereditary prostate cancer is relatively rare but may account for up to 40% of tumors among young men with the disease. One of several genes found in families with hereditary prostate cancer is hereditary prostate cancer 1 (*HPC1*), which is located on the long arm of chromosome 1. Translocations leading to fusion of two genes (TMPRSS2:ERG gene fusion) has also been implicated in a large number of sporadic prostate cancers.

Diagnosis

The vast majority of prostate cancers are adenocarcinomas. There is a large discrepancy between the risk of finding incidental prostate cancer at autopsy (estimated to be as high as 75% by age 80 or older) and the risk of having the disease clinically diagnosed (lifetime risk, approximately 1 in 6). Most men with early-stage prostate cancer diagnosed in the modern era have no specific disease-related symptoms. Benign prostatic hypertrophy is often found in association with prostate cancer and is also more common in men as they age, but there is no known causal relationship between the two. Prostate cancer can rarely manifest with pelvic pain, bladder outlet obstruction, or ureteral obstruction from locally advanced disease or with bone pain from distant metastatic disease.

The advent and widespread use of the serum prostate-specific antigen (PSA) test as a screening tool for prostate cancer has resulted in a stage migration, with most men now diagnosed with early-stage disease. This has been associated with better recurrence-free survival rates after definitive local therapy. Certain groups, such as the American Urologic Association and the American Cancer Society, have advocated that physicians offer screening with a serum PSA determination and digital rectal examination for men older than 55 years of age and for African American men and those with a family history of prostatic cancer starting at age 40 years. However, these recommendations are not uniformly accepted; the US Preventive Services Task Force recently gave a grade D recommendation for routine screening with PSA for prostate cancer. It is generally accepted that the decision to screen for prostate cancer should be made in individuals with at least 10 years of life expectancy.

Serum PSA is specific for the prostate but is not specific for cancer. It is secreted by both benign and malignant prostatic epithelial cells. The PSA may be elevated in men with a variety of prostate-related conditions, such as prostatitis, benign prostatic hypertrophy, urinary tract infection, or prostatic cancer. Until recently, a PSA level lower than 4.0 ng/mL was considered normal, and in younger men a value of greater than 2.5 ng/mL could perhaps be considered abnormal. More recently, it has become clear that there is no true cutoff value for PSA. Instead, the association between PSA and prostate cancer risk is a continuum. Even at a PSA of essentially zero, there is still a 6% chance of having prostate cancer on biopsy.

The majority of the serum PSA is bound to protease inhibitors such as α_1-antichymotrypsin, whereas a fraction is unconjugated or free. The relative proportion of free serum PSA can be used to improve the specificity of PSA for diagnosis of prostate cancer by biopsy. Benign prostatic hypertrophy is associated with a higher proportion of free PSA, and patients with greater 25% free serum PSA are less likely to harbor prostate cancer. The precise cutoff point associated with prostate cancer is controversial and ranges from 10% to 20% or higher. Development of new tests to improve PSA specificity, such as measurement of complexed PSA or early pro-forms of PSA, is an area of ongoing investigation.

The most common method used to diagnose prostate cancer is a transrectal ultrasonography (TRUS)-guided prostate biopsy. TRUS allows for accurate localization of the zonal anatomy of the prostate and can accurately measure its size. It therefore acts as a guide for the biopsy, because prostatic cancers typically reside in the peripheral zone, and biopsies are concentrated within that zone. Although prostate cancer can manifest as hypoechoic lesions on TRUS, the tumors usually are not visible. TRUS lacks both sensitivity and specificity and should not be used as a screening test.

The most common grading system used to estimate the degree of tumor differentiation is the Gleason grading system. The two most common Gleason grade patterns (on a scale of 1 to 5) are summed to give a score between 2 and 10. Tumors with Gleason scores between 2 and 6 are well differentiated and have a better prognosis, whereas those with Gleason scores between 8 and 10 are poorly differentiated and have a worse prognosis. Gleason score 7 is associated with intermediate differentiation and prognosis. The majority of cancers found in the modern era are well to intermediately differentiated (Gleason score 5 to 7).

Staging of prostatic cancer defines the local, regional, and distant extent of disease. The tumor-node-metastasis (TNM) staging system is the most commonly used method. The most common clinical stage in the modern era is that of nonpalpable tumors detected because of a concerning PSA result (stage T1c). The primary staging modality for local disease is the digital rectal examination. This may be supplemented by pelvic magnetic resonance imaging in selected cases where there is significant concern for locally advanced disease based on the digital rectal examination. Although PSA only roughly correlates with the overall disease burden, bone metastasis is quite uncommon among patients whose PSA value is less than 20 ng/mL. Therefore a radionucleotide bone scan in the absence of symptoms is not required routinely if the PSA value is less than 10 ng/mL and the Gleason sum is 7 or less. Computed tomography (CT) scanning is not routinely used, because grossly positive nodes are detected rarely with a clinically localized tumor.

Lymph node staging is important in selecting patients for therapy. CT scanning may show enlarged lymph nodes in patients with high-volume or high-grade primary tumor but has poor sensitivity and specificity. Laparoscopic pelvic lymphadenectomy can provide adequate sampling of the pelvic lymph nodes in those patients not selecting surgery. More commonly, lymph node dissection is performed concomitantly at the time of radical prostatectomy.

Treatment

There is no one optimal treatment for clinically localized prostatic cancer, so therapy must be individualized. Among men with a life expectancy of less than 10 years, observation alone may be appropriate. Carefully selected men with low-risk prostate cancer may choose active surveillance rather than curative treatment but must be rigorously monitored for evidence of worsening disease.

Surgery and radiation therapy are the most commonly used curative modalities. For low-risk, organ-confined tumors, the 15-year disease-free survival rates are greater than 90% among patients treated with surgery. Moreover, the survival outcome is similar after radiation therapy and after surgery. However, properly done prospective, randomized comparisons among similarly staged patients have not been done. Radiation therapy can be delivered as external-beam radiotherapy or as brachytherapy using radioactive seeds (iodine 125 or palladium 103) implanted directly into the prostate. Cryotherapy (i.e., freezing of the prostate) is another approved treatment for men with prostatic carcinoma that is becoming more widely accepted as an alternative treatment option. More recently, High Intensity Focused Ultrasound (HIFU) has been approved for use in the United States, although experience with this modality in the US is limited compared to Europe.

Radical prostatectomy, or surgical removal of the prostate, may be performed via an open incision or by a laparoscopic technique. Traditionally, an open surgery is performed through an anterior, retropubic approach or, less commonly, through a perineal incision. Laparoscopic and, in particular, robot-assisted radical prostatectomy is being performed with increasing frequency. The benefits of a robot-assisted approach may include reduced blood loss, sooner return to normal function, and possibly better functional outcomes and better surgical margin rates (although the latter two have not been definitively demonstrated to this point). In patients who were sexually active before therapy, preservation of the neurovascular bundles is often undertaken in an attempt to maintain postoperative sexual function. For patients with organ-confined disease, the prognosis is excellent, with a life expectancy similar to that of men without prostatic cancer. For those patients with positive surgical margins or positive lymph nodes on final pathology, consideration can be given to delivering, respectively, adjuvant irradiation or androgen-deprivation therapy (ADT).

Serum PSA should rapidly become undetectable after radical prostatectomy, because, in theory, all PSA-producing tissue has been removed. After radiation therapy or cryotherapy, the PSA is expected to reach low levels over time and then remain stable. An increasing serum PSA is evidence of tumor recurrence. There is controversy about when to initiate ADT in men with a rising PSA level after treatment.

Prostatic cancer, at least initially, is an androgen-sensitive disease. Therefore the primary first-line treatment for metastatic prostate cancer is ADT. Suppression of serum testosterone can be achieved by orchiectomy (i.e., surgical castration). Alternatively, medical castration may be considered. Luteinizing hormone–releasing hormone analogues effectively suppress testosterone to the castrate range within 1 month after administration by suppressing central nervous system secretion of luteinizing hormone. There is increasing awareness that ADT can be associated with significant long-term morbidity, including vasomotor reflex changes (hot flushes), loss of libido, erectile dysfunction, osteoporosis, anemia, muscle wasting, gynecomastia, and possibly cognitive changes and increased risk of cardiovascular disease. The choice to use ADT must, therefore, be carefully balanced based on the individual patient's overall risk of prostate cancer–related morbidity and mortality versus ADT-related morbidity.

Most patients with metastatic disease initially respond to ADT, but almost inexorably the disease progresses despite ongoing ADT, to become castration resistant prostate cancer (CRPC). At that point, the median survival time is less than 2 years. The standard chemotherapy for CRPC is docetaxel (Taxotere) plus prednisone, and prospective randomized trials have demonstrated a modest survival benefit among patients so treated. An alternative for asymptomatic or minimally symptomatic men with metastatic CRPC include sipuleucel-T (Provenge), a novel cellular immunotherapy-based intervention, abiraterone acetate (Zytiga) and enzaluamide (Xtandi). Several options now exist for men with metastatic CRPC who have failed prior docetaxel therapy including cabazitaxel (Jevtana), abiraterone acetate (Zytiga), enzalutamide (Xtandi), and Radium-223 dichloride (Xofigo). Another approved drug is mitoxantrone (Novantrone) for palliative relief of symptomatic bone pain from CRPC. Radiation therapy can be used effectively to palliate focal sites of bone metastases. The mechanisms by which prostatic carcinoma escapes hormonal control and becomes castrate resistant represent an area of ongoing intensive research.

Tumors of the Renal Parenchyma

Malignant tumors of the renal parenchyma are of either primary or metastatic origin. Primary renal tumors may be benign or malignant. The most common tumor of primary renal cell carcinoma (RCC) is conventional (clear cell) RCC; other tumor types, such as papillary, chromophobe, collecting duct, and medullary carcinomas and sarcomas, occur infrequently. The most common benign renal tumors are angiomyolipomas and oncocytomas. The latter, in particular, are generally indistinguishable from malignant lesions on radiographic imaging. Metastatic lesions (e.g., from lung, breast, melanoma, or ovary) may occur, and primary lymphoma may be present in the kidney.

Renal Cell Carcinoma

RCC is the most common primary neoplasm of the kidney, accounting for more than 85% of all primary renal tumors. There were an estimated 54,390 newly diagnosed cases of RCC in the United States in 2008, and an estimated 13,010 people died of this disease. RCC represents approximately 3% of all adult malignancies and usually manifests between 40 and 60 years of age, although it can be found in younger age groups. It has a 2:1 male-to-female preponderance and in both sporadic and familial forms is associated with aberrations of the von Hippel–Lindau (VHL) gene and protein.

RCC is thought to arise from cells of the proximal convoluted tubule. The most consistent genetic aberration found in most cases of sporadic, conventional RCC are aberrations in the *VHL* gene. No specific agent has been implicated as the cause of RCC, although tobacco products are associated with an approximately twofold increased risk of being diagnosed with the disease. Patients, and particularly younger patients, with end-stage renal disease who develop acquired cystic disease of the kidney also have an increased risk of RCC. Between 1% and 2% of these patients develop RCC, so annual renal ultrasonography is reasonable as a screening tool in this population, with confirmatory studies such as CT for complex or suspicious lesions.

Diagnosis

The most common sign associated with RCC in 29% to 60% of cases is hematuria. The classic triad of flank pain, hematuria, and a palpable abdominal mass is relatively rare, occurring in fewer than 10% of cases. Other common symptoms and signs include fever, anemia, hypercalcemia, thrombocytosis, and elevated erythrocyte sedimentation rate, lactate dehydrogenase, or alkaline phosphatase. Currently, there are no reliable, commercially available tumor markers for RCC. Most often, these tumors are incidentally diagnosed on radiographic imaging performed for unrelated or nonspecific purposes.

The most commonly used staging system for RCC is the TNM staging system. It allows for a distinction between venous involvement and nodal invasion and stratifies the extent of each stage. RCC can involve the renal vein and vena cava and may even extend into the right atrium. Locally, it can directly invade surrounding structures such as the adrenal gland and colon. Five-year survival rates range from 80% to 90% for stages T1 N0 M0 (<7cm) and T2 N0 M0 (>7cm), 40% to 60% for stage T3 N0 M0, and 10% to 20% for N1–3 and M1 disease.

Treatment

Surgical excision of the tumor is the primary treatment for RCC. The classic procedure was a radical nephrectomy, in which the kidney was removed en bloc within Gerota's fascia and the ipsilateral adrenal gland and lymph nodes. This was routinely performed as an open procedure (flank, transabdominal, or thoracoabdominal incision). Adrenalectomy is now generally reserved for upper-pole tumors, very large tumors, or lesions that directly extend into the adrenal gland. Although these operations are increasingly performed through a laparoscopic approach, an open approach is usually preferred if there is extensive involvement of the inferior vena cava. In rare cases with supradiaphragmatic tumor extension within the cava, cardiopulmonary bypass may be required for tumor extraction.

A partial nephrectomy has become a standard approach for surgical excision of renal parenchymal tumors, particularly for individuals with solitary kidneys, those with bilateral masses, and those with compromised renal function. It has become the preferred operation for patients who have lesions of 4 cm or smaller and a normal contralateral kidney, because local recurrence rates are less than 5%, and partial (rather than radical) nephrectomy is associated with a lower long-term risk of chronic renal failure. As with radical nephrectomy, there is a growing experience with laparoscopic approaches to partial nephrectomy. There are also several, minimally invasive approaches that are being utilized with increasing frequency including radiographically guided, percutaneous thermal tumor ablation using radiofrequency ablation or cryotherapy. These modalities are typically reserved for older patients or poor surgical candidates.

Up to 25% of patients initially present with metastatic disease. Sites of metastasis of RCC, in decreasing frequency of occurrence, include lung, lymph nodes, liver, bone, and adrenal gland. Chemotherapy and irradiation have little to no survival benefit, with radiation therapy only palliating painful metastases. The mainstay of treatment in the past was immunotherapy, with 5-year survival rates of 10% to 20%. Modern therapies for advanced or metastatic RCC now include the so-called targeted therapies, such as the oral tyrosine kinase inhibitors, sunitinib (Sutent), pazopanib (Votrient), axitinib (Inlyta), and sorafenib (Nexavar), and the mammalian target of rapamycin (mTOR) inhibitors, temsirolimus (Torisel) and everolimus (Afinitor). More recently the checkpoint inhibitor nivolumab (Opdivo) has been approved for use in metastatic RCC. Evidence suggests improved survival among those patients who undergo nephrectomy before systemic immunotherapy.

Benign Renal Tumors

Although they are not as frequent as malignant tumors, benign solid masses are also seen in the kidney. Angiomyolipomas can often be diagnosed radiographically based on the appearance of fat by CT scan. They can occur sporadically or as part of an inherited familial syndrome, tuberous sclerosis. The latter entity is characterized by mental retardation, benign tumors of the cerebellum, epilepsy, adenoma sebaceum, and angiomyolipomas. Approximately 50% of patients with tuberous sclerosis develop angiomyolipomas, most of which are bilateral and multifocal. The management of angiomyolipoma is controversial and should be individualized. Asymptomatic tumors smaller than 4 cm can generally be observed with annual radiographic imaging. Symptomatic lesions (bleeding, pain, rapid growth) and lesions larger than 4 cm should be considered for surgical excision, although angioembolization is another option. Acute hemorrhage from an angiomyolipoma can often be managed or at least stabilized by angioembolization.

Oncocytomas are the most common solid, benign renal tumors and account for 5% to 10% of solid renal lesions. Although these lesions tend to have a more uniform density than RCC and can have a characteristic central scar or spoke-wheel appearance on CT, there is no radiographic feature that reliably distinguishes an oncocytoma from a malignant renal lesion. Oncocytoma is therefore a diagnosis that should be made only on histologic analysis. The tumors characteristically exhibit eosinophilic, granular cells packed with mitochondria. Oncocytomas are thought to arise from the distal portion of the renal tubule.

Metastatic Renal Lesions

The most common primary malignancy to metastasize to the kidney is lung cancer, although cancers of the ovary, breast, or bowel, melanoma, and lymphoma can do so as well. Lymphoma of the kidney is almost always a manifestation of systemic disease. The management is therefore grounded in systemic chemotherapy, with surgery reserved for palliative symptom relief. However, approximately 15% of renal lymphomas manifest with a solitary renal mass as the sole radiographic manifestation. These lesions can be challenging to manage and difficult to distinguish from RCC preoperatively.

Tumors of the Renal Pelvis and Ureter

Approximately 10% of all renal tumors originate in the renal pelvis rather than the renal parenchyma. These account for 5% of all urothelial carcinomas (the majority of which arise in the bladder). Of the upper tract urothelial carcinomas, approximately one fourth arise in the ureter and the remainder in the renal pelvis. Urothelial carcinoma of the upper urinary tract is more common in men than in women and more common in whites than in blacks. Environmental exposures associated with a higher risk of developing upper tract urothelial carcinoma include analgesic abuse, cyclophosphamide (Cytoxan), and a strong association with tobacco abuse.

Among patients with bladder cancer, approximately 3% to 5% develop upper tract urothelial carcinoma. This can increase to as high as 20% among those with carcinoma in situ (CIS) or high-grade disease. Conversely, approximately 30% to 70% of patients with a history of upper tract urothelial carcinoma go on to develop bladder cancer. As a consequence, these patients require ongoing periodic cystoscopic surveillance. The incidence

of bilateral upper tract tumors is 2% to 5%. Other histologic tumor types that can manifest in the upper urinary tract include squamous cell carcinoma (SCC) and adenocarcinoma. Although they are rare, the risk is increased among patients with a history of recurrent, refractory urinary tract infections or staghorn calculi.

Diagnosis

The most common presenting symptom for upper tract urothelial tumors is hematuria. For patients with adequate renal function, the evaluation for hematuria includes CT urography, urinary cytology (or another urinary-based tumor marker), and cystoscopy. Urinary cytology has a high specificity but a generally poor sensitivity, particularly for low-grade disease. Other urinary tumor markers, such as NMP-22, and fluorescent in situ hybridization approaches typically have better sensitivity but are not as specific. A retrograde ureteropyelogram may be helpful in patients with poor renal function who cannot receive intravenous contrast agents. In general, if a suspicious mass is seen on CT or other imaging, a ureteroscopy is typically performed with biopsy or brushings to establish the diagnosis. The TNM system is the standard for staging.

Treatment

Disease isolated to the distal ureter is most often managed with distal ureterectomy and ureteroneocystostomy. High-grade or high-stage disease and multifocal disease isolated to one side are optimally managed in most cases by excision of that upper tract system via a radical nephroureterectomy, including excision of the distal portion of the ureter and complete excision of the ureteral orifice together with a cuff of bladder. Traditionally, these procedures were done via open incisions (one or two separate incisions, depending on the surgeon), but laparoscopy is increasingly being used to decrease patient morbidity and improve surgical recovery. In selected patients who have low-grade, low-stage disease with a small overall disease burden, an endoscopic approach using laser or electrocautery to destroy the tumors may be considered. This is also a strong consideration for those patients with bilateral disease or involvement of a functionally solitary renal unit. Most often, retrograde endoscopic approaches via ureteroscopy are employed, although in highly selected cases antegrade percutaneous approaches can be used.

Carcinoma of the Bladder

Urothelial Carcinoma of the Bladder

Bladder carcinoma is the fifth most common malignancy in the United States, with more than 68,810 new cases diagnosed annually. It is almost three times more common in men than in women, in whom it is the fourth most common cancer. Because of its propensity to recur, particularly in patients with superficial disease, it is the second-most prevalent cancer. High-grade bladder cancer is a deadly disease and is the fifth most common cause of cancer deaths among men. There is a well-established relationship between the development of bladder cancer and a variety of carcinogens. Perhaps the most widespread factor is tobacco abuse. Cigarette smoking is thought to account for up to half of all bladder cancers in men. Bladder cancer is also associated with other, less frequent occupational exposures, such as in the rubber and oil refinery industries. It is also associated with exposure to the chemotherapeutic agent, cyclophosphamide (Cytoxan); exposed patients have up to a ninefold increased risk of developing bladder cancer, most likely related to a urinary metabolite of cyclophosphamide, acrolein.

Approximately 90% of bladder malignancies are urothelial carcinomas. Of these, the majority (70%) are papillary, 10% are sessile, and 20% demonstrate mixed morphology. Although roughly three quarters of bladder cancer patients present with non-muscle invasive, or superficial, disease, approximately 20% to 25% progress to muscle invasion over time. Nevertheless, 80% to 90% of patients with muscle-invasive disease had it at initial presentation. A strong correlation exists between tumor grade and stage; most well-differentiated tumors are superficial, and most poorly differentiated tumors are invasive. CIS is a poorly differentiated urothelial carcinoma that grows as a sheet confined to the urothelium. CIS may be found as a solitary or multifocal process and is associated with invasive carcinoma in 25% of cases, where it portends a poor prognosis. Between 10% and 20% of patients treated with cystectomy for diffuse or refractory CIS are found to have microscopic muscle-invasive disease.

Diagnosis

Gross painless hematuria is the most common presenting sign of bladder cancer. However, approximately 1 in 5 patients have only microscopic hematuria. Other symptoms that can be indicative of urothelial carcinoma (in particular, CIS) include irritative voiding symptoms such as frequency, urgency, and dysuria. Patients who present with symptoms and signs concerning for urothelial carcinoma should undergo an evaluation that includes cystoscopy, urinary tumor marker study (typically, urinary cytology), and evaluation of the upper tracts (typically by CT urography). The diagnosis is usually confirmed at the time of transurethral resection or biopsy.

Treatment

The management options for urothelial carcinoma are heavily dependent on the stage and grade of disease. The TNM system is recommended for staging. For most non-muscle invasive, low-grade tumors, transurethral resection, with or without a single, immediate instillation of a chemotherapeutic agent such as mitomycin-C (Mutamycin),[1] is all that is required. This must then be followed by careful, ongoing surveillance by cystoscopy, urinary tumor studies (typically cytology), and periodic upper tract imaging. For patients with high-grade disease (including CIS) and tumors that superficially invade the lamina propria (stage T1) or are rapidly recurrent tumors, adjuvant treatment with intravesical agents such as thiotepa (Thioplex), doxorubicin (Adriamycin), and mitomycin-C (Mutamycin)[1] or intravesical bacillus Calmette-Guérin (Tice BCG) may be indicated. In the United States, the most frequently used agent for this purpose, particularly for CIS, is intravesical BCG.

Patients with superficial disease must undergo regular surveillance, because the recurrence rate is as high as 50% at 5 years. Surveillance protocols vary but typically include cystoscopy and urinary tumor studies (usually urinary cytology) every 3 months for 2 years, then every 6 months for 3 years, and annually thereafter. Periodic evaluation of the upper tracts, typically by CT urography, is warranted, because there is a 3% to 5% incidence of development of upper tract urothelial carcinoma among patients with bladder urothelial carcinoma.

The risk of disease progression in patients with low-grade, low-stage (Ta) urothelial carcinoma is less than 5% to 10%. This risk increases as the stage and grade of the tumor increase. Patients who have muscle-invasive disease (stage T2 or higher), either at presentation or with progression after therapy for superficial disease, are best treated by radical cystectomy and urinary diversion. A thorough pelvic lymphadenectomy should be performed at the time of surgery. The precise limits of dissection for the lymphadenectomy remain somewhat controversial, although the latest data suggest that patients who have more lymph nodes removed fare better.

High-grade bladder cancer is a potentially lethal disease. There are an estimated 14,100 deaths due to bladder cancer annually. Among patients with organ-confined (pT2a-pT2b), muscle-invasive disease who undergo cystectomy, the 5-year recurrence-free survival rates are between 60% and 85%. For patients undergoing radical cystectomy who have extravesical extension of their disease (pT3-pT4 disease), the 5-year recurrence-free survival rates are lower, 40% to 60%. Patients with lymph node–positive disease fare the worst, with 5-year recurrence-free survival rates of 20% to 30%.

Patients with muscle-invasive bladder cancer should be considered for multimodal therapy (i.e., chemotherapy in addition to surgery). The standard regimen over the past decade has been MVAC: methotrexate (Trexall),[1] vinblastine (Velban),[1] doxorubicin (Adriamycin), and cisplatin (Platinol). This can be delivered either before surgery (neoadjuvant) or in the postsurgery setting (adjuvant). There is level 1 evidence to support MVAC chemotherapy combined with cystectomy for muscle-invasive bladder cancer, although the survival benefit across studies is only on the order of 5% to 10%. Newer agents, such as gemcitabine (Gemzar)[1] along with cisplatin, appear to offer similar response rates and reduced toxicity and are often used currently in lieu of MVAC. Cytotoxic chemotherapy produces response rates of 50% to 70% in patients with advanced or metastatic disease; however, the durable, long-term, complete response rates at 5 years are no more than 15% across series. The checkpoint inhibitor, atezolizumab (Tecentriq) had recently been approved in the second line for the systemic treatment of mestastatic bladder cancer.

Urinary diversion may be accomplished after cystectomy in several ways, but the fundamental categories are incontinent and continent forms. Incontinent forms of diversion include ileal and colon conduits, both of which require that the patient wear an external collection appliance. Continent forms of diversion include the continent cutaneous diversion, which requires creation of a low-pressure reservoir (often of colon) and a catheterizable efferent limb with an associated valve mechanism to prevent urine leakage. More recently, emphasis has shifted to continent diversions in which the low-pressure reservoir is anastomosed to the native urethra. These orthotopic neobladders may be crafted from colon or ileum and offer the opportunity to avoid any external collection devices and, usually, any need for catheterization. Such devices may improve patients' quality of life after surgery, although this has not been formally demonstrated in a randomized trial.

Adenocarcinoma of the Bladder

Adenocarcinomas account for fewer than 2% of bladder cancers. They can be found in three settings: as primary lesions in the bladder, as metastases or local extensions from another site, or as primary urachal carcinomas. They are typically invasive and poorly differentiated and carry a poor prognosis. Adenocarcinomas may be found in association with bladder augmentation cystoplasties and are the most common form of bladder cancer in patients born with bladder exstrophy. The treatment of choice is typically radical cystectomy, pelvic lymphadenectomy, and urinary diversion.

Squamous Cell Carcinoma of the Bladder

SCC accounts for approximately 6% of bladder cancers in the United States but more than 75% of bladder cancers in Egypt. SCC is associated with chronic bladder inflammation from a variety of sources. These include chronic indwelling Foley catheters, recurrent or refractory bladder infections, and bladder diverticula or stones. In Egypt, approximately 80% of SCCs are associated with *Schistosoma haematobium* infestation. These bilharzia-associated SCCs of the bladder tend to occur in patients 10 to 20 years earlier than in the United States.

SCC of the bladder often carries a poor prognosis and is usually best treated by radical cystectomy. After surgery, this form of bladder cancer has a higher propensity for local recurrence, compared with urothelial carcinomas. SCC of the bladder is typically resistant to cytotoxic chemotherapy, particularly the regimens frequently used for urothelial carcinoma. The benefit of neoadjuvant radiation therapy before cystectomy remains to be proven, at least for the non-bilharzial SCC typically found in the United States.

---

[1] Not FDA approved for this indication.

[1] Not FDA approved for this indication.

Urethral Carcinoma

Diagnosis

Urethral carcinoma is unusual in that it is more common in women than in men. It is a disease of the elderly, typically occurring after 60 years of age. The etiology remains to be determined, but approximately half of the cases are associated with urethral stricture disease. In women, there is an association with urethral malakoplakia and urethral caruncles. The usual presenting symptom in this circumstance is a papillary or fungating urethral mass and hematuria. A number of scenarios warrant a more thorough evaluation for possible urethral carcinoma, including a palpable urethral mass, an obstruction that does not respond to conventional management, development of a urethral abscess or fistula, presence of microscopic or gross hematuria, and the development of inguinal adenopathy.

Treatment

The primary treatment of urethral carcinoma is most often surgical excision, with the approach and the extent of surgery driven by both gender and the location of the mass relative to the sphincteric complex (likelihood of postoperative continence). For example, cystectomy with en bloc urethrectomy and anterior vaginectomy along with pelvic lymphadenectomy is usually required for tumors located in the proximal urethra or tumors with extension into adjacent structures. In selected cases, radiation therapy can provide local control. In locally advanced disease, multimodality treatment with chemotherapy and either surgical excision or radiation therapy provides the optimal chance for long-term cure, although there is no standard regimen to date.

Penile Cancer

Diagnosis

Penile cancer is relatively rare in the United States. Penile carcinoma has been associated with retained phimotic foreskin and poor personal hygiene. It is rare among men who are circumcised before puberty and occurs most commonly in the sixth decade of life. The symptoms relate directly to the mass itself and can include ulceration, pain, necrosis, foul odor, hemorrhage, and suppuration of the lesion. The clinical evaluation of patients with penile cancer involves a thorough physical examination including of the phallus and careful attention to palpation of the inguinal lymph nodes. Additional studies may include radiographic testing with chest radiography, CT scan of the abdomen and pelvis, and bone scan.

Treatment

Treatment is usually dictated by the tumor stage (TNM system), size, and location. Small tumors that are confined to the prepuce can often be managed by circumcision alone. Smaller tumors on the distal shaft can be treated by partial penectomy, provided that a normal tissue margin can be achieved and there is enough penile length remaining to permit voiding in the standing position. Among patients treated by partial penectomy, the 5-year recurrence-free survival rate is 70% to 80%. Large lesions and tumors on the proximal shaft may require total penectomy and perineal urethrostomy to achieve adequate local tumor control. If there is involvement of local structures such as the scrotum or pubis, radical en bloc resection may be required. Achieving negative margins is critical, because local recurrence of the disease can rarely be salvaged by radiation or chemotherapy.

Although many patients have inguinal lymphadenopathy at presentation, inguinal lymph node enlargement before excision of the primary tumor may be the result of infection and not metastatic disease. Clinical assessment of the inguinal region is therefore typically delayed for 4 to 6 weeks. Lymphadenopathy that persists or develops de novo raises the strong possibility of lymph node metastases, and an ilioinguinal lymphadenectomy should be performed. If inguinal lymphadenopathy resolves, lymph node dissection may not be necessary. It is often necessary to perform bilateral inguinal lymphadenectomy, particularly in patients with

high-risk disease, for whom this should be considered regardless of the presence or absence of palpable nodes. Radiation of the primary tumor and regional lymph nodes is an alternative to surgery in carefully selected patients with small (≤2 cm), low-stage tumors. Similarly, Mohs' surgery is an option for small tumors, particularly ones at the base that otherwise might require a total penectomy.

Testicular Cancer

Malignant tumors of the male gonads can be divided into neoplasms originating from the germinal cells, rare tumors from the supporting cells (Leydig cells and Sertoli cells), and rare metastases from another primary site. The germinal neoplasms include seminomatous and nonseminomatous germ cell tumors (NSGCTs). Ninety-five percent of tumors originating in the testis are germ cell tumors. Fewer than 10% of all germ cell tumors arise from extragonadal primary sites such as the mediastinum and retroperitoneum. Testicular cancer is relatively rare overall, but it is the most common malignancy in men between the ages of 15 and 35 years, with 8090 new cases occurring annually.

Testicular cancer represents one of the great success stories in modern medicine. The mortality rates for testis cancer have decreased from more than 50% before the 1970s to less than 10% in the modern age. This is the result of a variety of advances, including more effective multiagent chemotherapy, improved surgical techniques, and better methods to diagnose and monitor the disease (e.g., CT scans, tumor markers). Testicular cancer currently serves as a paradigm for the multimodal treatment of malignancies.

Germ cell tumors are substantially more prevalent in Caucasians than in African Americans, by a margin of at least 5:1. Indeed, a report from the US military indicated a relative incidence of 40:1. The exact etiology of germ cell tumors is not fully understood. Familial clustering has been demonstrated, particularly among siblings. Two conditions associated with a higher risk for germ cell tumors are cryptorchidism and Klinefelter's syndrome, the latter associated with disease arising from the mediastinum. Orchidopexy for cryptorchidism does not appear to reduce the risk of neoplasia, but it does improve the ability to monitor the testis.

Diagnosis

A painless testicular mass in a patient of the appropriate age group should be considered a primary testicular tumor until proven otherwise. A substantial number of testicular tumors manifest with less specific symptoms, including diffuse testicular pain, swelling, hardness, or some combination of these findings. A tumor can be difficult to distinguish from an infectious epididymo-orchitis. However, because the latter is more common than a testicular tumor, a short trial of antibiotics is often undertaken. If symptoms do not abate or the findings do not revert to normal within 2 to 4 weeks, testicular sonography is indicated to identify any underlying testicular mass. A radical inguinal orchiectomy with early, high ligation of the spermatic cord at the internal ring is required for all patients with a suspected testicular tumor.

Testicular cancers typically first spread to regional, retroperitoneal lymph nodes below the level of the renal vessels. The primary nodal landing zone for right-sided tumors lies between the aorta and the inferior vena cava (interaortocaval nodes), whereas for left-sided tumors it is lateral to the aorta (para-aortic). Other frequent sites of metastases include the left supraclavicular lymph nodes and the lungs. Standard initial metastatic evaluation should include a CT scan of the abdomen and pelvis and chest radiography. Enlarged lymph nodes (>1–2 cm) in the primary lymphatic drainage areas (landing zones) of the affected side are involved by metastatic disease in approximately 70% of cases. CT imaging of the chest is required if mediastinal, hilar, or lung parenchymal disease is suspected. Serum tumor markers should be measured before orchiectomy and should include human β-chorionic gonadotropin (β-hCG), α-fetoprotein (AFP), and the less-specific marker, lactate dehydrogenase.

Treatment

All suspected testicular tumors should be treated with a radical orchiectomy through an inguinal approach and early, high ligation of the spermatic cord. β-hCG and AFP are relatively specific tumor markers for testicular cancer. They have substantially improved the ability to monitor the disease and to intervene early in the event of recurrence. They, along with lactate dehydrogenase, should be measured before orchiectomy. AFP production is restricted to NSGCTs, specifically tumors that contain at least a component of embryonal carcinoma or yolk sac tumor. Patients with an increased AFP and pure seminoma on pathologic examination of the orchiectomy specimen are still considered to have an NSGCT. Increased serum β-hCG can occur with seminomatous and nonseminomatous tumors. Increased concentrations of β-hCG are seen in 40% to 60% of patients with metastatic NSGCT and in 15% to 20% of patients with metastatic seminomas. Lactate dehydrogenase is less specific but has independent prognostic value in patients with advanced germ cell tumors. Serum lactate dehydrogenase is increased in approximately 60% of patients with NSGCT and in 80% of those with seminomatous germ cell tumors.

Persistently elevated concentrations of AFP and β-hCG, even in the absence of radiographic or clinical findings, implies active disease and is sufficient cause to initiate systemic therapy, provided that false-positive elevations have been ruled out. The serum half-life of β-hCG is 5 to 7 days, and that for AFP is 30 hours. A slow decrease in serum levels after orchiectomy also implies metastatic disease.

Seminoma is the most common histologic form of germ cell tumor and generally carries a better prognosis than other variants. Standard therapy for low-stage (T1, 2a, or 2b) disease is orchiectomy followed by active surveillance, chemotherapy, or radiation therapy to the retroperitoneal and possibly the ipsilateral pelvic lymph nodes, depending on clinical stage and patient preference. Relapse is relatively rare, occurring in 4% of patients with stage 1 and 10% of patients with stage 2 disease. Relapses can be salvaged in more than 90% of cases by systemic chemotherapy. The long-term cure rate for low-stage seminoma is approximately 99%.

NSGCTs include embryonal cell carcinomas, choriocarcinomas, yolk sac carcinomas, teratomas, and mixed germ cell tumors. As with pure seminoma, the cure rate is high (>95%) in patients with stage 1 disease. Retroperitoneal lymphatic metastases may be found in 20% of patients who have no lymphatic or vascular invasion or invasion into the tunica albuginea, spermatic cord, or scrotum at the time of orchiectomy, even if CT scans are negative for lymphadenopathy. There are three options for low-stage NSGCT after orchiectomy in the absence of radiographic evidence of lymphadenopathy and with normalized serum tumor markers: surveillance, two cycles of chemotherapy, and nerve-sparing retroperitoneal lymph node dissection (RPLND). Patients with clinical stage 1 disease but embryonal histology or the presence of lymphovascular invasion or extension beyond the tunica albuginea have a higher risk of relapse (>30%) with surveillance and should be considered for primary RPLND.

Although RPLND is a major abdominal operation, it offers the best way to control disease within the retroperitoneum. Lymph nodes are removed from the level of the renal hilum caudad to the level of the aortic bifurcation. The lateral margins are the ureters. Historically, this operation was associated with loss of ejaculatory function due to ligation of the sympathetic nerve fibers in the region. With modern, nerve-sparing techniques, ejaculatory function can be preserved in more than 95% of patients. Patients with persistently elevated AFP or β-hCG after orchiectomy most likely have metastatic disease, even in the absence of radiographically detectable lesions. These patients usually should go on to systemic chemotherapy first, rather than RPLND or two cycles of chemotherapy.

Clinical stage 2 NSGCTs can be managed by either RPLND or primary chemotherapy, depending on several factors. Those patients who are without marker elevation, are asymptomatic, and have small-volume retroperitoneal-only disease can be offered primary RPLND. Those with persistently elevated tumor markers, symptomatic disease, or more bulky retroperitoneal disease usually undergo systemic chemotherapy. Local recurrence in the retroperitoneum after a properly performed RPLND is rare (<10%).

Adjuvant chemotherapy after RPLND should be considered if any lymph node is more than 2 cm in diameter, if six or more nodes are involved, or if there is extranodal invasion. Cure rates are not different in those who do or do not receive adjuvant chemotherapy, but the former group require fewer cycles of chemotherapy and fewer additional surgeries.

Approximately one third of patients require up-front chemotherapy. Those patients with clinical stage 2c disease (or higher), primary retroperitoneal germ cell tumor, or mediastinal seminomas treated with radiation therapy should all undergo systemic, cisplatin-based, multiagent chemotherapy.

Postchemotherapy RPLND for seminoma is typically reserved for patients with residual masses more than 3 cm in size or a positive PET scan. For NSGCT, this issue is more controversial. Some groups reserve this treatment for patients who do not have substantial tumor shrinkage (>90% shrinkage of retroperitoneal nodes and no residual nodes >1.5 cm) and for those with teratomatous elements in the primary tumor. Others advocate surgery for all patients with initial bulky retroperitoneal disease, regardless of the response to chemotherapy. All agree that a clear residual mass after chemotherapy in the setting of NSGCT warrants a postchemotherapy RPLND.

The first successful combination chemotherapy regimens for testicular cancer included cisplatin, vinblastine, and bleomycin (Blenoxane) and resulted in complete remission in 70% to 80% of patients with metastatic disease. Studies have shown that prolonged maintenance chemotherapy is unnecessary, and etoposide (VePesid) has largely replaced vinblastine (because it is less toxic and probably more efficacious). Serious adverse effects of chemotherapy include neuromuscular toxic affects, myelosuppression, bleomycin-induced pulmonary fibrosis, Raynaud's phenomenon, and secondary malignancy.

Leydig cell tumors are generally benign tumors that make up between 1% and 3% of all testicular tumors. The majority of cases occurs in men aged 20 to 60 years old, although roughly one fourth are diagnosed before puberty. After radical orchiectomy, the prognosis is usually good, with recurrences rarely reported.

Gonadoblastoma is a rare tumor that occurs almost exclusively in patients with a history of gonadal dysgenesis. They account for fewer than 1% of all testicular neoplasms and can occur at any age from infancy to beyond 70 years, although most patients are diagnosed before age 30. Initial management is with radical orchiectomy. Because of a 50% incidence of bilateral disease, a contralateral gonadectomy is generally warranted. The prognosis after orchiectomy is usually excellent.

Lymphoma is the most common secondary neoplasm of the testicle and the most common testicular neoplasm in men older than 50 years of age, with a median age at presentation of 60 years. Although survival is often poor for patients with bilateral disease and those presenting with lymphoma at other sites who later experience a testicular relapse, the prognosis is substantially better for patients presenting with primary testicular lymphoma confined to the testicle.

Disclaimer

The views expressed in this article are those of the author and do not reflect the official policy or position of the United States Army, the Department of Defense, or the US government.

References

Barocas DA, Clark PE: Bladder cancer, *Curr Opin Oncol* 20:307–314, 2008.

Damber JE, Aus G: Prostate cancer, *Lancet* 371:1710–1721, 2008.

Flechon A, Rivoire M, Droz JP: Management of advanced germ-cell tumors of the testis, *Nat Clin Pract Urol* 5:262–276, 2008.

Jemal A, Siegel R, Ward E, et al: Cancer statistics, 2008, *CA Cancer J Clin* 58:71–96, 2008.

Rini BI, Rathmell WK, Godley P: Renal cell carcinoma, *Curr Opin Oncol* 20:300–306, 2008.

PRIMARY GLOMERULAR DISEASE

Method of
Saeed Kamran Shaffi, MD, MS

CURRENT DIAGNOSIS

- Hematuria, proteinuria, hypoalbuminemia, hyperlipidemia, and elevated blood urea nitrogen and creatinine levels are the main laboratory abnormalities seen in patients with primary glomerular diseases.
- Our ability to diagnose some of the glomerular diseases and to monitor their disease-activity has improved with the recent discovery of disease-specific serum and kidney biopsy markers.

CURRENT THERAPY

- The goals of management of a primary glomerular disease patient are:
  - To diagnose the glomerular abnormality
  - To slow the progression of chronic kidney disease and subsequent development of end-stage kidney disease
  - To manage and ameliorate the symptoms of the glomerular disease
  - To prevent complications of primary glomerular diseases and the therapies used for their management, such as infection, thrombosis, coronary vascular disease, osteoporosis, and trace metal deficiencies

Clinical Presentation

The clinical presentation of the primary glomerular diseases can be grouped into syndromes, which are listed in Box 1.

Nephrotic syndrome: The disease-defining symptoms of the nephrotic syndrome are >3.5 g/day of proteinuria in adults, serum albumin of <3 g/L, and edema. Hyperlipidemia and thrombophilia are often present.

Sub-nephrotic proteinuria: These patients have proteinuria of <3.5 g/day without hypoalbuminemia, edema, and hyperlipidemia.

Acute nephritic syndrome: Nephritic syndrome presents as microscopic hematuria, which is defined as >3 red blood cells (RBC) per high-power field (HPF). Patients with the nephritic syndrome also have a varying amount of proteinuria and may have an elevated creatinine level indicating a decline in the glomerular filtration rate (GFR).

Asymptomatic microhematuria: Hematuria is seen on urine analyses; however, these patients do not develop progressive kidney dysfunction.

Rapidly progressive glomerulonephritis (RPGN): Rapidly progressive glomerulonephritis is a syndrome associated with a rapid decline in renal function over the course of a few days, weeks, or months. On the kidney biopsy, RPGN presents as glomerular crescents which are seen due to the disruption of the glomerular basement membrane with fluid spillage in the Bowmans space

BOX 1 — Clinical Presentation of Glomerular Diseases

Nephrotic syndrome
Sub-nephrotic proteinuria
Acute nephritic syndrome
Asymptomatic microhematuria
Rapidly progressive glomerulonephritis
Slowly progressive chronic nephritis

TABLE 1 — Causes and Clinical Presentation of the Primary Glomerular Diseases

CAUSES OF PRIMARY GLOMERULAR DISEASE	PRESENTATION
Minimal change disease	Nephrotic syndrome
Primary focal segmental glomerulosclerosis	Usually nephrotic syndrome, rarely nephritic syndrome
Primary membranous glomerulonephritis	Nephrotic syndrome
IgA nephropathy	Usually nephritic syndrome, sometimes microscopic hematuria or gross hematuria
Postinfectious glomerulonephritis	Nephritic syndrome
Membranoproliferative glomerulonephritis due to alternate complement pathway abnormalities (dense deposit disease and C3 glomerulonephritis)	Nephritic syndrome
Fibrillary glomerulonephritis	Nephritic or nephrotic syndrome
Thin basement membrane disease	Asymptomatic microscopic hematuria

resulting in extracapillary cellular proliferation and crescent formation.

Slowly progressive nephritic syndrome: Some of the glomerular diseases have a smoldering course with persistent hematuria and proteinuria that may eventually lead to CKD and end-stage kidney disease.

Causes of primary glomerular diseases: Table 1 lists the causes of primary glomerular diseases.

Diagnosis of the Primary Glomerular Diseases

Glomerular disease is suspected when a clinician notices hematuria, proteinuria, or an abnormal blood urea nitrogen or creatinine level. It is paramount to rule out other conditions which can present with similar abnormalities.

Hematuria: It is imperative to differentiate between the glomerular and nonglomerular hematuria (Box 2 and Figure 1).

Proteinuria: Proteinuria is often seen in primary glomerular diseases. Urinary protein and albumin excretion in an adult should not exceed 150 mg/day, and 30 mg/g, respectively. Reduction in proteinuria—especially when sustained longitudinally—is associated with better clinical outcomes. In clinical practice, a spot urine protein to creatinine (P/C) ratio or albumin to creatinine ratio is

BOX 2 — Signs of Glomerular Hematuria.

>22% dysmorphic* RBCs on optical and >40% on phase contrast microscopy

In the setting of hematuria and dysmorphic RBCs, an immunoreactive albumin excretion of >0.59 mg/mg total protein excretion is strongly suggestive of glomerular hematuria.

The newer generation of the automated urine analysis machines (sediMAX) may automate the phase-contrast microscopy detection of dysmorphic RBCs without loss of precision.

*Red blood cells in the glomerular hematuria develop membrane abnormalities when they pass through the inflamed glomerular membranes and are called dysmorphic. A certain type of dysmorphic RBC, with characteristic membrane blebs called acanthocytes, are strongly correlated with glomerular hematuria.

Figure 1 Dysmorphic red blood cells (Phase contrast microscopy 40× magnification). *Yellow arrow* shows a normal RBC with smooth membranes. *Black arrows* show dysmorphic RBCs with protruding cell membranes.

often used for the assessment of the proteinuria; however, the concordance between the spot and the 24-hour urine collection is poor. On the other hand, 24-hour urine collection is cumbersome, is not feasible in children, and is associated with significant under- and overcollection even in highly motivated patients. Therefore, a spot urine (P/C) ratio is adequate for proteinuria surveillance; however, a 24-hour urine collection for proteinuria assessment should be considered when the use of therapeutic agents that can cause significant morbidity is being contemplated for proteinuria reduction.

GFR assessment: The best method to estimate GFR in patients with glomerular diseases is not known. Assessment of the longitudinal trends in the estimated GFR (eGFR) in this population rather than small variations in eGFR value may provide the clinicians with a better guide of renal status compared to a single value in isolation.

Kidney biopsy: Apart from a few situations such as serum anti-phospholipase A 2 receptor positivity in a high biopsy risk patient and steroid responsive nephrotic syndrome in children, which is almost always due to minimal change nephropathy, a kidney biopsy is essential for the diagnosis of primary glomerular diseases. Kidney biopsy not only provides a definitive diagnosis of the primary glomerular abnormality in most of the patients but also informs the clinician of the prognosis by quantifying the degree of the irreversible changes such as glomerulosclerosis, interstitial fibrosis, and tubular atrophy.

General Management of Primary Glomerular Diseases

Primary glomerular diseases may manifest as symptoms (Box 3) which are debilitating.

Treatment of Primary Glomerulonephritis

Edema: Dietary sodium restriction (1.5 to 2 g or 60 to 80 mmol/day) is the first step for edema management due to nephrotic syndromes. Oral loop diuretics (Table 2) should be used if the sodium

BOX 3	Symptoms in the Primary Glomerular Diseases

Edema
Hypertension
Hyperlipidemia
Hypercoagulable state
Chronic kidney disease
Trace metal and vitamin deficiencies
Endocrine hormonal abnormalities
Infection risk

restriction does not ameliorate the symptoms. Use of diuretics with better oral bioavailability and longer half-life may be more effective in edema management (see Table 2). Gut wall edema in patients with severe nephrotic syndrome may preclude effective diuresis with orally administered diuretics in which case intravenous loop diuretics alone or combined with a thiazide diuretic (e.g., metolazone [Zaroxolyn]) may be tried. Use of loop diuretics with intravenous albumin (Albuminar)[1] to maximize diuresis is controversial with some reports showing beneficial while others showing equivocal results; this strategy can be considered in patients with severe diuretic resistance.

Hypertension: Optimal control of hypertension in patients with a glomerular disease may decrease cardiovascular morbidity and mortality, and slow the progression of CKD. There is limited evidence for sodium restriction and angiotensin-converting enzyme inhibitors (ACEi) or angiotensin receptor blockers (ARBs) use to achieve a goal BP target of <125/75 mm Hg in patients with >1g/day of proteinuria.

Hyperlipidemia: Patients with primary glomerular diseases are at a higher risk of developing hyperlipidemia and cardiovascular events. Hyperlipidemia should be treated aggressively to the same targets as the general population.

Hypercoagulable states: Patients with glomerular diseases are at significant risk of thromboembolism due to the alterations in the pro-coagulant and anticoagulant factors. The incidence of thromboembolism has been reported as high as 8% to 44%, and 5% to 62% in nephrotic syndrome and membranous glomerulonephritis, respectively. Anticoagulation should be considered in patients with a low serum albumin (below 2 to 2.5 g/dL) along with one of the following: >10 g/d of proteinuria; BMI of >35 kg/m^2; family history and genetic disposition of thromboembolism; New York Heart Association Class III or IV congestive heart failure; recent abdominal or orthopedic surgery; prolonged immobilization. The Chapel Hill group has devised an online calculator to aid the clinicians in deciding about the use of anticoagulation in patients with membranous glomerulonephritis.

Case-reports have described aspirin[1], warfarin (Coumadin)[1], or direct-acting oral anticoagulant (DOAC) use for thromboembolism prevention in patients with nephrotic syndrome; however, care should be taken regarding appropriate dosing for renal function, use of medications with the least renal clearance (apixaban [Eliquis])[1], and cognizance of interaction of the anticoagulants with other medications that may inhibit their metabolism.

Chronic kidney disease: Studies have shown that complete remission of proteinuria is associated with preservation of renal function and end-stage kidney disease. Disease-modifying therapies, which will be described later, should be used to prevent the development of renal fibrosis which is irreversible.

Trace metal deficiency: Patients with primary glomerular diseases who have nephrotic syndrome may have deficiencies of iron, copper, zinc, and selenium. Twenty-five hydroxyvitamin D [25-(OH)D] deficiency is extremely common in patients with nephrotic syndrome, is due to urinary loss of 25(OH)D, and is often difficult to treat unless the patient achieves complete remission. Treatment of 25(OH)D deficiency is outlined in Box 4 and is similar to that in the general population.

Endocrine abnormalities: Loss of hormone-binding proteins and albumin in patients with proteinuric glomerular diseases leads to various endocrine abnormalities. Low T4 levels are seen in approximately 50% of nephrotic syndrome patients with preserved renal function due to urinary loss of thyroid-binding globulin; however, these patients are usually euthyroid due to no impairment in the conversion of T4 to T3. On the other hand, glomerular disease patients with low GFRs have a diminished T3 level due to decreased conversion of T4 to T3; however, unlike

---

[1]Not FDA approved for this indication.

TABLE 2   Pharmacokinetics of Loop Diuretics

NAME	RELATIVE POTENCY	ORAL BIOAVAIL-ABILITY	HALF-LIFE (HOURS)	ELIMINATION ROUTE	COMMENTS
Furosemide (Lasix)	1	~60%	~1.5	~65% renal, 25% metabolism	Renal disease prolongs half-life
Bumetanide (Bumex)	40	~80	~0.8	~62% renal, 38% metabolism	Liver disease prolongs half-life
Torsemide (Demadex)	3	~80%	~3.5	~20% renal, 80% metabolism	Liver disease can prolong half-life

other chronic illnesses, the conversion of T4 to metabolically inactive reverse T3 (rT3) is not enhanced.

Risk of infections: Chronic kidney disease, nephrotic syndrome, and use of the immunosuppressive medications are some of the risk factors that increase the propensity to develop infections in patients with primary glomerular diseases. Patients should be up to date on their vaccinations to mitigate infection risk (Box 5).

Pneumocystis jirovecii prophylaxis should be administered to patients who are on >20 mg of prednisone and/or on immunosuppressive medications that affect the T cells such as corticosteroids and cyclophosphamide (Cytoxan).

Therapy of Specific Glomerular Diseases
Minimal-Change Disease
Minimal-change disease is the most common cause of nephrotic syndrome in children (90%) and is a rare cause in adults (10%). No abnormality is detected on plain light microscopic evaluation of the kidney; however, the electron microscopy shows diffuse foot process effacement. A child presenting with nephrotic syndrome is assumed to have a minimal-change disease and does not require a kidney biopsy. In adults, minimal-change disease is a rare occurrence and is usually diagnosed with a kidney biopsy. Most cases of minimal-change disease are idiopathic, although secondary causes such as drugs (nonsteroidal antiinflammatory drugs [NSAIDs]), hematological malignancies, and thymoma are associated with this condition. Therapy of minimal-change disease is shown in Box 6.

Primary Focal Segmental Glomerulosclerosis
Primary focal segmental glomerulosclerosis is a pathological term denoting patchy glomerulosclerosis and is thought to be due to an unknown permeability factor which causes proteinuria, hypertension, and kidney dysfunction. This condition should be differentiated from the secondary glomerulosclerosis (focal or global) which is a sequela of previous kidney injury. Reduction in proteinuria is associated with better

renal survival and is the goal of therapy. Box 7 shows the therapies used for the management of primary focal segmental glomerulosclerosis.

Primary Membranous Glomerulonephritis
Idiopathic membranous glomerulonephritis is the second most common cause of nephrotic syndrome in the US adults. This condition is characterized by diffuse subepithelial deposits seen on kidney biopsy. Our understanding of the pathophysiology of the idiopathic membranous glomerulonephritis was revolutionized in 2009 with the discovery of elevated M-type phospholipase-A(2) receptor [PLA2R], an antigen expressed in the human podocytes, antibody in the serum and the immune deposits in the glomeruli of the vast majority of patients. Antibodies against thrombospondin type 1 domain-containing 7A (THSD7A) have been found in PLA2R negative idiopathic membranous patients (2% to 4%). Serum anti-PLA2R antibody levels are measured by commercial laboratories and are used to monitor idiopathic membranous glomerulonephritis disease activity—a rise in titer is associated with relapse while a fall is associated with remission. Box 8 details the treatment strategies used for the management of primary membranous glomerulonephritis.

IgA Nephropathy
IgA nephropathy is the leading cause of glomerulonephritis worldwide. Mistracking of the poorly O-glycosylated IgA1 produced by the intestinal mucosal cells into the circulation and production of IgA and IgG antibodies play a cardinal role in the pathogenesis of IgA nephropathy. The antigen-antibody complexes deposit in the kidneys and cause a mesangial (M) and endocapillary (E) proliferative glomerulonephritis which can lead to glomerulosclerosis (S) and tubular atrophy (T). At times, IgA nephropathy can also present as crescentic glomerulonephritis (C). The MEST-C classification of the kidney biopsy provides useful information regarding disease prognostication. The secondary cause of IgA nephropathy such as HIV and cirrhosis should be ruled out. IgA nephropathy often has a smoldering

---

BOX 4   Treatment of Vitamin D Deficiency in Primary Glomerular Diseases

25(OH)D level less than 12 ng/mL: treat with 50,000 international units (IU) of vitamin D2 (ergocalciferol)[1] or vitamin D3 (cholecalciferol)[1] orally once a week for 6 to 8 weeks followed by 800–1000 IU/day of vitamin D3 for maintenance therapy. Higher doses of daily vitamin D3 may be necessary if the levels remain low (<30 ng/mL) 3 months after therapy initiation.

25(OH)D levels between 12 and 20 ng/mL: treat with 800–1000 IU/day of vitamin D3. Repeat levels in 3 months. Higher vitamin D3 doses may be necessary if the levels are below the normal range (30–50 ng/mL).

25(OH)D level between 20 and 30 ng/mL: replace with 600–800 IU of vitamin D3 daily.

[1]Not FDA approved for this indication.

BOX 5   Recommended Immunization in Patients With Glomerular Diseases

Hepatitis A vaccine (Havrix, VAQTA)
Hepatitis B vaccine (Engerix-B, Recombivax HB)
Haemophilus influenzae type B conjugate vaccine (Hib [ActHIB, Hiberix])
Annual trivalent inactivated influenza vaccine
1 dose thirteen-valent pneumococcal conjugate vaccine (PCV13 [Prevnar 13]) followed in 8 weeks by a 23-valent pneumococcal polysaccharide vaccine (PPSV23 [Pneumovax 23]), then repeat PPSV23 in 5 years since the last dose; at age 65 years or older, administer 1 dose PPSV23 at least 5 years after the most recent PPSV23
Meningococcal Vaccine against sero-group (A, C, W and Y; Menactra, Menveo)[1]

[1]Not FDA approved for this indication.

BOX 6 Minimal-Change Disease Therapy

Prednisone 1 mg/kg (maximum 80 mg) or alternate-day single dose of 2 mg/kg (maximum 120 mg) for 4–16 weeks. Taper slowly in 6 months if complete remission (proteinuria <300 mg/g) is achieved in 4 weeks.

Most patients respond to corticosteroids but 25% of treated patients have frequent relapses and 30% become steroid dependent (two relapses during or within 2 weeks of completing steroid therapy). No response to steroids in 8–16 weeks should be considered steroid resistance.

Second-line agents are calcineurin inhibitors, oral cyclophosphamide (Cytoxan), or rituximab (Rituxan)[1]

[1]Not FDA approved for this indication.

BOX 7 Primary Focal Segmental Glomerulosclerosis Therapy

First line: Prednisone 1 mg/kg q day or 2 mg/kg every alternate day. Continue high-dose steroids for 4–16 weeks until complete remission is achieved, followed by a taper in 6 months.

Second line: Calcineurin inhibitors for patients who cannot tolerate prednisone.

Third line: Mycophenolate mofetil (MMF [CellCept]).[1]

Adrenocorticotropic hormone (ACTH) gel (Corticotropin [HP Acthar]).[1]

[1]Not FDA approved for this indication.

---

course presenting as a nephritic syndrome with progressive loss of kidney function that may lead to end-stage kidney disease. Recently, it has been shown that decreasing proteinuria to <1 g/day results in better renal survival and has become one of the goals of care. Box 9 shows the therapeutic options for IgA nephropathy.

Many new therapeutic options are being developed for the management of IgA nephropathy. A phase 3 clinical trial to study the effects of a molecule that inhibits the lectin-binding pathway of the complement system is currently being conducted. Another trial studied the effects of oral budesonide (Entocort EC)[1] in patients with IgA nephropathy and showed that this agent reduced proteinuria significantly compared to placebo and a phase 3 study is currently being planned.

Postinfectious Glomerulonephritis

Acute postinfectious glomerulonephritis presents as nephritic syndrome, acute kidney injury, and low serum complement levels and is more common in children and young adults. This condition was classically described in the convalescence of scarlet fever, but other bacteria, viruses, and protozoa can also cause this condition. Kidney biopsy shows diffuse proliferative glomerulonephritis with prominent mesangial and subepithelial deposits that on immunofluorescence microscopy show positivity for C3 and IgG. It can also present as crescentic glomerulonephritis which portends a poor prognosis. The treatment of renal failure due to postinfectious glomerulonephritis is symptomatic. The primary infection that caused postinfectious glomerulonephritis should be treated appropriately if present at the time of diagnosis. Children have an excellent prognosis with the recovery of kidney function in the vast majority of the patients. However, adults with this condition have a poor renal prognosis with 30% of the patients developing CKD. The outcomes are particularly worse for patients with severe proteinuria with two out of three patients developing progressive kidney dysfunction.

[1]Not FDA approved for this indication.

BOX 8 Primary Membranous Glomerulonephritis Therapy

Maximal ACEi or ARB
Watchful waiting for 6 months with maximization of ACEi or ARB. Factors associated with low likelihood of achieving spontaneous remission are persistence of >4 g/day of proteinuria with no response to antihypertensive/antiproteinuric therapy in 6 month; presence of life threatening nephrotic syndrome; more than 30% increase in serum creatinine; and a high PLA2R titer.

Oral cyclophosphamide[1] and prednisone with or without intravenous methylprednisolone (Solumedrol) pulses in alternate months for 6 months. Some centers use cyclophosphamide and prednisone together for 3 months, while others eliminate prednisone altogether.

Calcineurin inhibitors are as effective as cyclophosphamide in inducing remission; however, the risk of relapse after medication discontinuation is high.

Rituximab[1] has similar rates of complete remission as cyclophosphamide, however, the complete remission rate is lower. Furthermore, rituximab-treated patients are less likely to develop adverse events than cyclophosphamide-treated groups.

[1]Not FDA approved for this indication.
ACEi, Angiotensin-converting enzyme inhibitors; *ARB*, angiotensin receptor blockers.

BOX 9 IgA Nephropathy Therapy

Maximum ACEi/ARB therapy to bring the proteinuria to <1 g/day.

Patients who continue to have >1 g/day of proteinuria, despite maximum ACEi/ARB inhibition for >6 months with a BP of <125/75 mm Hg, should receive a 6-month course of corticosteroids if their eGFR is >50 mL/min/1.73 m². Recent data show that patients with eGFR <50 mL/min/1.73 m² may benefit from corticosteroid therapy; however, they may experience higher serious adverse events.

Patients with IgA nephropathy in whom >50% glomeruli show crescents should be treated with corticosteroids and cyclophosphamide.[1]

[1]Not FDA approved for this indication.
ACEi, Angiotensin-converting enzyme inhibitors; *ARB*, angiotensin receptor blockers; *eGFR*, estimated GFR.

Membranoproliferative Glomerulonephritis due to Alternate Complement Pathway Abnormalities

Membranoproliferative glomerulonephritis (MPGN) is a pathological phenotype seen on kidney biopsy characterized by endocapillary proliferative glomerulonephritis, increased mesangial matrix, and thickening of the glomerular basement membranes. Various infectious, autoimmune, vascular, and neoplastic processes can lead to this type of glomerular injury. MPGN is now classified on the basis of disease mechanism rather than the histological findings with an emphasis of staining intensity of C3 and IgG on immunofluorescence microscopy. Presence of both C3 and IgG point toward an immune-complex-mediated process. Predominant C3 staining on immunofluorescence with minimal IgG staining indicates abnormalities in the alternate complement pathway that cause dense deposit disease (DDD) and C3 glomerulonephritis (C3GN). These are rare conditions affecting children and young adults and present as nephritic syndrome, renal function abnormalities, and hypertension. Laboratory data abnormalities include low C3 levels with normal C4 levels (alternate complement pathway abnormality), presence of antibodies (C3 nephritic factor, anti-factors H, B, or I), gene mutations of the alternate complement pathway proteins (complement factor H and I-related protein gene mutations), diminished serum factors that regulate the alternate complement pathway (serum factor H, B, I, and serum membrane cofactor protein [MCP]), and elevated terminal complement pathway constituents (C5b-9). Treatment options for DDD and C3GN are listed in Box 10.

Fibrillary Glomerulonephritis

Fibrillary glomerulonephritis is an uncommon condition primarily affecting adults. Kidney biopsy shows amyloid-like deposits; however, they are Congo-Red negative and thus are not truly amyloid. Electron-microscopy shows characteristic findings of randomly organized fibrils sized 10 to 30 nm. One-third of the patients with fibrillary glomerulonephritis have another disorder such as autoimmune disease, malignancy, and monoclonal gammopathy. Recently, our understanding of the pathophysiology of idiopathic fibrillary glomerulonephritis improved significantly with the identification of DnaJ homolog subfamily B member 9 (DNAJB9)—a member of the molecular chaperone gene family—in fibrillary deposits. Almost all the patients with fibrillary glomerulonephritis showed positive immunohistochemistry to DNAJB9 while all the patients with amyloidosis were negative. The disease usually presents as nephritic syndrome. The prognosis is generally poor with most of the patients developing end-stage kidney disease. Antiproteinuric therapy with ACEi/ARB and immunosuppression have been tried with variable results with the patients with milder disease (non-nephrotic range proteinuria and preserved eGFR) more likely to achieve complete remission.

References

Agrawal S, Zaritsky JJ, Fornoni A, Smoyer WE: Dyslipidaemia in nephrotic syndrome: mechanisms and treatment, *Nat Rev Nephrol* 14(1):57–70, 2018 Jan.

Cattran DC, Kim ED, Reich H, et al: Membranous nephropathy: quantifying remission duration on outcome, *J Am Soc Nephrol JASN* 28(3):995–1003, 2017 Mar.

Floege J, Barbour SJ, Cattran DC, et al: Management and treatment of glomerular diseases (part 1): conclusions from a Kidney Disease: Improving Global Outcomes (KDIGO) Controversies Conference, *Kidney Int* 95(2):268–280, 2019 Feb.

Harris RC, Ismail N: Extrarenal complications of the nephrotic syndrome, *Am J Kidney Dis Off J Natl Kidney Found* 23(4):477–497, 1994 Apr.

Improving Global Outcomes (KDIGO) Glomerulonephritis Work Group: Kidney Disease: KDIGO Clinical Practice Guideline for Glomerulonephritis, *Kidney Inter Suppl* 2:139–274, 2012.

Lee T, Biddle AK, Lionaki S, et al: Personalized prophylactic anticoagulation decision analysis in patients with membranous nephropathy, *Kidney Int* 85(6):1412–1420, 2014 Jun.

Nasr SH, Vrana JA, Dasari S, et al: DNAJB9 is a specific immunohistochemical marker for fibrillary glomerulonephritis, *Kidney Int Rep* 3(1):56–64, 2017 Aug 8.

Ponticelli C, Glassock R: *Treatment of primary glomerulonephritis*, North America, 2009, ESCCO eBook Subscription Academic Collection.

Radice A, Trezzi B, Maggiore U, et al: Clinical usefulness of autoantibodies to M-type phospholipase A2 receptor (PLA2R) for monitoring disease activity in idiopathic membranous nephropathy (IMN), *Autoimmun Rev* 15(2):146–154, 2016 Feb.

Reich HN, Troyanov S, Scholey JW, Cattran DC: Remission of proteinuria improves prognosis in IgA nephropathy, *J Am Soc Nephrol* 18(12):3177–3183, 2007 Dec 1.

Rovin BH, Caster DJ, Cattran DC, et al: Management and treatment of glomerular diseases (part 2): conclusions from a Kidney Disease: Improving Global Outcomes (KDIGO) Controversies Conference, *Kidney Int* 95(2):281–295, 2019 Feb.

PYELONEPHRITIS

Method of
Patricia D. Brown, MD

CURRENT DIAGNOSIS

- Abrupt onset of fever, flank pain, and costovertebral angle tenderness with or without symptoms of cystitis are classic presenting features.
- Patients with lower UTI symptoms or laboratory evidence of UTI accompanied by flank pain, fever, or signs of systemic toxicity such as GI complaints should be managed as having APN.
- Urinalysis with microscopic examination should be performed in all patients with suspected APN. Absence of pyuria is strong evidence against the diagnosis.
- A urine culture should be obtained in all patients with APN. Blood cultures should be obtained in those who are hospitalized.
- Patients should be categorized into those with uncomplicated and those with complicated infections.

Abbreviation: APN = acute pyelonephritis; GI = gastrointestinal; UTI = urinary tract infection.

CURRENT THERAPY

- Hospitalization is recommended for patients unable to tolerate oral intake, those with severe pain, and those with signs of severe sepsis. Hospitalization is generally recommended for patients with complicated infections and for all pregnant women.
- Parenteral regimens for hospitalized patients include an aminoglycoside, third-generation cephalosporin, or fluoroquinolone, with oral switch therapy selected on the basis of culture and susceptibility data.
- Initial empiric therapy for outpatients is a fluoroquinolone.
- Imaging is not recommended for patients with uncomplicated infections. Pre- and postcontrast computed tomographic scans should be obtained in those who fail to respond within 72 hours to appropriate antibiotic therapy.

Acute pyelonephritis (APN) is a urinary tract infection (UTI) that involves the renal parenchyma, also referred to as *upper tract UTI*. Most episodes of APN occur as a result of ascending infection from the bladder; patients with APN might or might not have symptoms of concomitant cystitis. Rarely, pyelonephritis occurs secondary to hematogenous seeding of the kidney as a result of infection elsewhere, most commonly endocarditis due to *Staphylococcus aureus* or disseminated fungal infection.

Epidemiology

Surprisingly little is known about the epidemiology of APN. Similar to cystitis, APN (and hospitalization for APN) is more common in women than men; men have been reported to have higher in-hospital mortality. In contrast to cystitis, risk factors for pyelonephritis are not well defined. A study of nonpregnant women 18 to 49 years of age found risk factors for APN included factors known to be risk factors for acute cystitis, including frequency of sexual intercourse, recent UTI, diabetes, and maternal UTI history. The incidence of bacteremia in patients with APN is reported to be 11% to 53% in various studies; risk factors for bacteremia are not well established. In one study, age greater than 65 years, vomiting, pulse greater than 110 beats per minute, segmented neutrophils greater than 90%, and pyuria with greater than 50 leukocytes per high-powered field were independent risk factors for bacteremia in women with uncomplicated APN.

Similar to lower UTI, APN can be further classified into complicated or uncomplicated infection. The factors that make an episode of APN a complicated UTI are outlined in Box 1.

Clinical Presentation

The classic presenting features of APN include abrupt onset of fever, flank pain, and costovertebral angle tenderness with or without symptoms of lower UTI including dysuria, urgency, and frequency. Unfortunately, there is no single constellation of signs or symptoms that is pathognomonic for APN. When localization studies have been performed on patients with symptoms of acute cystitis, 30% to 50% have been shown to have APN. Women who present with symptoms that have been present more than 7 days and those with a recent history of UTI are more likely to have APN. Flank pain is reported in approximately one-half of patients with APN but also occurs in almost 20% of patients with cystitis. Fever is present in one half of patients with APN, but less than 5% of patients with cystitis. Nausea, vomiting, and diarrhea occur commonly in patients with APN, and gastrointestinal (GI) symptoms can dominate the presenting complaints.

In general, patients who present with lower urinary tract symptoms or laboratory evidence of urinary tract infection accompanied by fever, flank pain or tenderness, or signs of systemic toxicity, such as GI symptoms, should be treated for APN.

The diagnosis can be particularly challenging in the frail elderly patient, because symptoms such as frequency, urgency, and incontinence are often chronic in this patient population and unrelated to active UTI. Change in mental status may be the only presenting complaint. Because the prevalence of bacteriuria in this patient population is high, particularly among those with chronic indwelling catheters, UTI must be a diagnosis of exclusion.

Acute pelvic inflammatory disease can have a presentation similar to APN. Pelvic examination should be performed on all sexually active women to exclude this diagnosis.

The differential diagnosis of APN is outlined in Box 2.

Diagnosis

Urinalysis, ideally with microscopic examination, using a clean-catch, midstream specimen, should be performed in all patients with suspected APN. Pyuria is a key finding in the diagnosis of UTI, and the absence of pyuria is strong evidence against a diagnosis of APN. Direct microscopic examination under high power of the urinary sediment from a centrifuged specimen should reveal more than 10 leukocytes per high-powered field. The presence of white blood cell (WBC) casts is highly specific for localization of the infection to the kidney, but it is inadequately

sensitive to exclude the diagnosis of APN. The dipstick test for leukocyte esterase is used as a rapid screening test to detect significant pyuria; the sensitivity is reported to be 75% to 96%, with a specificity of 94% to 98%. Because of the lower range of the reported sensitivity of the dipstick test, microscopic examination to exclude significant pyuria should be obtained in patients with suspected APN.

The presence of nitrite in the urine, detected by a dipstick test, has a reported sensitivity of 35% to 85% and a specificity of 92% to 100% for UTI. Microscopic examination of a gram-stained, centrifuged urine specimen revealing at least one bacterium per oil-immersion field correlates with more than 10^5 colony-forming units (cfu)/mL of bacteria, with a sensitivity of 95%. Although this is the standard definition of significant bacteriuria, it has been shown that women with UTI can have levels of bacteriuria as low as 10^2 cfu/mL.

Although the microbiology of APN has remained predictable, significant changes in antimicrobial susceptibility patterns have occurred. Therefore, in contrast to recommendations for acute uncomplicated cystitis, a urine culture should be obtained in all patients with suspected APN. The need to obtain blood cultures has been debated, because blood cultures rarely yield a pathogen different from what was isolated from the urine. Bacteremia has been reported in 11% to 53% of patients hospitalized with APN. Bacteremic patients have a longer length of stay, and one report suggests that this is due to a longer time to resolution of fever. Many experts continue to recommend that blood cultures be obtained as part of the diagnostic evaluation of patients who are ill enough to require hospitalization; blood cultures are not necessary for those who will be managed as outpatients.

The role of diagnostic imaging in the management of APN is discussed later. In some cases with an atypical presentation, imaging may be helpful to confirm the diagnosis of APN. In this setting, pre- and postcontrast computed tomography (CT) is the imaging procedure of choice in adults.

Microbial Etiology

Most cases of APN are caused by *Escherichia coli*. Other enterobacteriaceae, including *Klebsiella* species and *Proteus* species, are also occasionally implicated. Other gram-negative pathogens such as *Pseudomonas*, *Serratia*, *Enterobacter*, and *Acinetobacter* should be considered in health care–associated infections. *Enterococcus* is an uncommon pathogen in community-acquired infections, but it must be considered in health care–associated infections, including vancomycin-resistant enterococci. Other gram-positive pathogens include *Streptoccocus agalactiae* and *Staphylococcus* species. Although a common cause of acute cystitis in young women, *Staphylococcus saprophyticus* is a rare cause of pyelonephritis; the finding of *Staphylococcus aureus* in a urine culture should always prompt a search for an extrarenal source of infection that might have served as a source of hematogenous seeding. A Gram stain of the urine is a simple and rapid test to exclude a gram-positive pathogen as the etiology of APN and guide the initial selection of empiric therapy.

The emergence of resistance to trimethoprim-sulfamethoxazole (TMP-SMX [Bactrim]) among *E. coli* has had a major impact on the approach to initial empiric antimicrobial therapy for APN. It is clear that the prevalence of resistance varies depending on geographic region, and clinicians often do not have access to meaningful local resistance data. Recent reports of increasing fluoroquinolone resistance among uropathogens are of great concern, although overall resistance rates in North America remain low. Also concerning is the increasing prevalence of extended-spectrum β-lactamase (ESBL) *E.coli* and *Klebsiella* species, although these are mainly a concern in health care-associated infections in the U.S. Risk factors for infection with ESBL producing organisms are poorly defined however recent infection or colonization with an ESBL producing organism should be considered a risk factor for this pathogen. Other potential risk factors include older age, frequent antibiotic use in the preceding year and recent APN in patients with underlying diabetes. Carbapenemase-producing Enterbacteriaceae are also now reported in health care-associated complicated infections.

Treatment

The first decision in the management of patients with APN is whether or not the patient requires hospitalization. Although prospective randomized trials are lacking, several retrospective studies as well as several prospective nonrandomized trials suggest that outpatient management is safe for many patients. Hospitalization should be considered for patients who cannot tolerate oral intake or who have severe pain or signs of severe sepsis. A strategy of initial management in the emergency department or an observation unit with an initial dose of parenteral antibiotic therapy, intravenous fluids, and symptomatic treatment of nausea and pain may be used in select patients to avoid hospital admission. Patients who will be treated as outpatients should have a stable social situation and the ability to contact the physician and return promptly if their symptoms worsen. Hospitalization is generally recommended for patients with complicated infections. Most experts believe that pregnant women with APN should always be hospitalized.

There are surprisingly few prospective randomized trials of the treatment of pyelonephritis. For patients who require hospitalization, parenteral therapy with an aminoglycoside, a third-generation cephalosporin, or a fluoroquinolone is recommended. At my institution we discourage fluoroquinolones for this indication because there are other effective alternatives and we wish to minimize the use of these very broad-spectrum agents in the hospital setting. Although resistance to TMP-SMX among uropathogenic *E. coli* appears to have leveled off and might actually be decreasing, this agent should not be used for empiric therapy of APN. If a ESBL-producing organism is suspected, empiric therapy should include a carbapenem. Because risk factors for ESBL-producing organisms are not well defined, consideration for coverage of these pathogens should be given in all patients with APN who have severe sepsis or septic shock. Multi-drug resistant pathogens may require treatment with newer B-lactam/B-lactamase inhibitor drugs such as ceftazidime-avibactam (Avycaz), ceftolozane-tazobactam (Zerbaxa), or meropenem-vaborbactam (Vabomere).

If a gram-positive pathogen is suspected or suggested by the results of urine Gram stain, ampicillin or ampicillin-sulbactam (Unasyn) with or without an aminoglycoside can be used. Patients should receive intravenous therapy until they are clinically improving and able to reliably tolerate oral intake; oral therapy can be chosen based on the results of urine culture and susceptibility data. TMP-SMX, a fluoroquinolone, and ampicillin are all potential candidates for oral switch therapy. The narrowest spectrum, least expensive agent to which the isolated pathogen is susceptible should be chosen. Despite in vitro susceptibility data, first- and second-generation cephalosporins have a poor track record in the treatment of APN and are

generally not recommended, with the exception of pyelonephritis in pregnancy.

Bacteremic patients might take longer to respond but do not require more prolonged parenteral therapy. The total duration of therapy for pyelonephritis is generally 14 days. Seven days of therapy with ciprofloxacin for uncomplicated APN has been shown to be effective as has 5 days of therapy with high-dose (750 mg daily) levofloxacin, and these regimens are endorsed by the current guidelines. Longer courses of therapy may be required for select patients with complicated pyelonephritis. For outpatients, initial empiric therapy with a fluoroquinolone is recommended, with adjustment of therapy, if needed, based on the results of urine culture. All of the currently available fluoroquinolones can be used, with the exception of moxifloxacin (Avelox), which does not achieve adequate levels in the urine. Although it is useful in the treatment of cystitis, norfloxacin (Noroxin) is not recommended for the treatment of APN because it does not achieve sustained tissue or serum levels. Suggested antimicrobial dosing regimens for APN are outlined in Box 3.

Imaging

Imaging is generally not needed in patients with uncomplicated APN. For patients with complicated infections (e.g., history of stones, prior renal surgery), renal ultrasound with abdominal plain films is considered an acceptable alternative to excretory urography. For patients with diabetes or other immunocompromise and for patients who fail to respond after 72 hours of appropriate antibiotic therapy, pre- and postcontrast CT is the imaging procedure of choice.

Follow-up

Most patients will respond to appropriate antibiotic therapy. Follow-up urine cultures to document microbiological response are not recommended in patients who have responded clinically.

References

Foxman B, Klemstine KL, Brown PD: Acute pyelonephritis in US hospitals in 1997: hospitalization and in-hospital mortality, *Ann Epidemiol* 13:144–150, 2003.

Gupta K, Hooton TN, Naber K, et al: International clinical practice guidelines for the treatment of acute uncomplicated cystitis and pyelonephritis in women: a 2010 update by The Infectious Diseases Society of America and the European Society for Microbiology and Infectious Diseases, *Clin Infect Dis* 52:e103–e120, 2010.

Kim KS, Kim K, Jo YH, et al: A simple model to predict bacteremia in women with acute pyelonephritis, *J Infect* 63:124–130, 2011.

Nikolaidis P, Dogra VS, Goldfarb S, et al: ACR appropriateness criteria–acute pyelonephritis, *J Am Coll Radiol* 15(11S):S232–S239, 2018.

Pappas PG: Laboratory in the diagnosis and management of urinary tract infections, *Med Clin North Am* 75:313–325, 1991.

Sandberg T, Skoog G, Hermansson AB, et al: Ciprofloxacin for 7 days versus 14 days in women with acute pyelonephritis: a randomised, open-label and double-blind, placebo-controlled, non-inferiority trial, *Lancet* 380:484–490, 2012.

Scholes D, Hooton TM, Roberts PL, et al: Risk factors associated with acute pyelonephritis in healthy women, *Ann Intern Med* 142:20–27, 2005.

NEPHROLITHIASIS

Method of
William J. Somers, MD

CURRENT DIAGNOSIS

- Renal calculi can present acutely or more often are discovered as an incidental finding on an unrelated radiologic study.
- Ureteral calculi present with either acute onset of excruciating flank pain or a gradual onset preceded by generalized abdominal discomfort.
- Renal colic pain can radiate from ipsilateral flank to lower abdomen, often mimicking pain from cholecystitis, appendicitis, or ovarian conditions such as torsion or ruptured ovarian cysts.
- Physical exam will reveal an anxious patient experiencing sharp, excruciating costovertebral pain. Pain commonly occurs in waves. Percussion of the flank reveals exquisite tenderness. The patient cannot find a comfortable resting position.
- Computed tomography (CT) scan without intravenous contrast (CT stone protocol) is the definitive diagnostic study. Abdominal plain film and renal ultrasonography are not as accurate as CT.
- Urinalysis may demonstrate either microscopic or gross hematuria. Pyuria in the absence of bacteriuria is common and does not always indicate infection.
- Nausea, vomiting, and low-grade fever are common. Temperature over 101°F suggests infection and is an acute urologic emergency.

CURRENT THERAPY

- Asymptomatic renal stones can be managed electively with observation or surgical intervention.
- Once the acute episode is controlled with intravenous analgesics, and the patient is discharged from the emergency room, ureteral obstruction can be managed with oral analgesics, liberal oral fluid intake, and expectant observation if the patient is afebrile and the stone is 5 mm or less in size.
- A follow-up renal ultrasound should be obtained 2 weeks after the first presentation of symptoms. If hydronephrosis persists or if the stone has not passed, refer the patient to a urologist.
- Fever and/or leukocytosis, regardless of a clean urine, indicates possible pyonephrosis, a surgical emergency, and the patient should be hospitalized for definitive treatment.
- Patients who are calcium stone formers should be encouraged to maintain a low sodium, low protein, normal calcium diet, and increase oral intake of fluids to 2 L daily.
- Patients who are recurrent calcium stone formers should be offered thiazide diuretics in addition to maintaining the dietary measures to limit stone formation.
- Patients who form uric acid stones should be encouraged to maintain a liberal oral intake of fluids and try to maintain an alkaline urine with potassium citrate (Urocit-K).

Pathophysiology

Urine exists in four states: **undersaturated,** in which no crystals will form; **metastable,** a state where concentration of salts is high but urine inhibitors prevent supersaturation; **saturated,** where addition of salts will not dissolve; and **supersaturated,** which is an unstable solution and crystals can form spontaneously. Urine is generally in a supersaturated state.

The generally accepted theory describing stone formation begins with spontaneous crystallization in a supersaturated urine.

This tiny crystal nucleus then attaches to a cell membrane in the collecting tubule. This nidus then attracts other crystals and cell debris forming a tiny calcification, which gradually grows larger as these particles continue to adhere to the mass. Some of these calcifications break off and proceed to the collecting system or remain in the renal tubules indefinitely.

Another theory suggests that spontaneous crystallization occurs at damaged sites along the nephron. Crystals attach to the damaged cell wall, remain fixed in place, and attract further crystal accumulation. Initial cell damage is believed to occur from high calcium oxalate levels based on studies that implicate oxalate as the sole cause for renal tubule cell damage. Pak 1976 showed that the calcium oxalate concentration is four times higher in urine than its solubility in water. This higher concentration may have an adverse effect on the cells, an interesting but as yet unproved theory.

Historically Randall plaques were believed to provide a base for crystal nucleation in the collecting system. These plaques are located in the loop of Henle just below the urothelium in the renal papillae. As they grow, they erode through the urothelium forming a nidus for crystal attachment and growth.

Since a supersaturated salt solution will spontaneously generate crystal formation, there must be some inherent factors that inhibit crystal formation. Citrate, magnesium, and pyrophosphates are the major stone inhibitors naturally found in urine. Citrate is the major inhibitor. Citrate complexes with calcium, reducing its availability and thus preventing spontaneous precipitation of calcium oxalate as well as inhibiting the calcium crystal nucleation. Magnesium binds to oxalate, also reducing its availability to bind with calcium.

Other inhibitors such as Tamm-Horsfall proteins have been identified, but their role is not fully understood.

Calcium Stones

Calcium stones are the most common type of stone in the United States. Hypercalciuria is the first step in stone formation. Thirty percent to 40% of calcium is absorbed in the small intestine, and about 10% from the colon. The kidney filters 270 mmol of calcium daily and absorbs all except for approximately 4 mmol. The active form of vitamin D is the most potent stimulator of intestinal calcium absorption. Calcium transport is regulated at three sites: intestine, bone, and kidney. Low calcium intake stimulates increased calcium absorption, which stimulates parathyroid hormone (PTH). PTH regulates the conversion of 25-hydroxyvitamin D to 1,25-dihydroxyvitamin D or calcitriol. PTH also stimulates the mobilization of calcium from bone through the action of osteoclasts and increases the absorption of calcium from renal tubules.

The classic model for hypercalciuria describes three types:

1. Absorptive hypercalciuria, the most common form, occurs in 55% of stone formers and is caused by increase in intestinal absorption of calcium. Absorptive hypercalciuria can be categorized as Type 1, in which urinary calcium remains high despite a low calcium diet, and Type 2, in which urinary calcium is normalized on a low calcium diet.
2. Resorptive hypercalciuria, identified in approximately 5% of stone formers, is usually seen in patients with hyperparathyroidism. Excessive PTH secretion causes increased production of calcitriol (1,25-dihydroxyvitamin D) which causes increased intestinal absorption of calcium. These patients present with hypercalciuria, hypercalcemia, and reduced phosphatemia. Patients with serum calcium levels above 10 should be evaluated for hyperparathyroidism.
3. Renal hypercalciuria, commonly referred to as renal leak hypercalciuria, is caused by a defect in calcium reabsorption in the proximal tubule. It is characterized by high fasting urine calcium levels, normal serum calcium levels, and elevated PTH.

Other causes for hypercalcemia include sarcoidosis, granulomatous diseases, malignancy, and glucocorticoid use. Malignancy is the most common cause for hypercalcemia in hospitalized patients. Of the malignancies, lung and breast are most common. It is believed the tumors produce cytokines and other factors which cause bone destruction through the action of osteoclasts, resulting in bone destruction and subsequent hypercalcemia. Glucocorticoids stimulate the release of PTH. Nephrolithiasis is common in patients with Cushing syndrome.

Calcium Stones and Calcium and Vitamin D Supplementation

If a patient develops de novo kidney stones while taking calcium and vitamin D supplements, order a 24-hour urine collection for calcium, phosphorus, uric acid, and citrate. If this demonstrates hypercalciuria, refer to a nutritionist for dietary guidance. Suggest that dietary calcium is a more natural way of increasing calcium levels, whereas calcium supplements could increase the risk. I would also question the need for taking both supplements.

Oxalate

Oxalates cause increased urinary saturation of calcium oxalate, which in turn can cause calcium oxalate stone formation. Primary hyperoxaluria is an autosomal recessive disorder responsible for end-stage renal failure before the age of 15 in 50% of young patients.

Enteric hyperoxaluria is the most common cause of acquired hyperoxaluria. It is associated with chronic diarrheal conditions, loss of large segments of small bowel, and intrinsic bowel disease. Loss of fat absorption in these patients results in increased oxalate absorption. Oxalate readily binds to calcium, which can ultimately initiate stone formation.

Renal Tubular Acidosis

Renal tubular acidosis (RTA) describes a defect in urinary acidification resulting in a metabolic acidosis. Hypokalemia, elevated urine pH, hypocitraturia, and hypercalciuria can lead to stone formation. There are three common types of RTA. Type 1, or distal, RTA patients are at high risk for stone formation. Calcium phosphate stones are associated with Type 1 patients which should prompt the physician to further diagnostic testing. Treatment can decrease the rate of stone formation. Type 2, or proximal, RTA is not associated with nephrolithiasis. Type 4 RTA is not commonly associated with stones, but they can occur.

Uric Acid Stones

Uric acid stones are unique in that they can be dissolved medically. Uric acid is the end product of purine metabolism. Humans lack the enzyme uricase which is the final step in the metabolism of uric acid to allantoin. Uric acid is not readily soluble in normally acidic urine. Hyperuricosuria is found in patients with gout, type 2 diabetes, and Lesch-Nyan syndrome. Alkalinizing urine is the primary treatment for asymptomatic uric acid renal stones.

Prevention

The time-honored key to prevention for all stones is increased water intake. Multiple studies have shown increasing oral intake of fluids to produce a 2 to 2.5 L daily urine output is the most efficient and least expensive way to prevent most stones. Additional measures include a low salt diet, limiting protein, and avoiding foods with high oxalate content.

When available, the stone should be analyzed to provide a diagnosis and a specific plan tailored to the type of stone and underlying pathologic cause if present. A complete medical history should be obtained which can identify an underlying cause such as hyperparathyroidism, Cushing syndrome, type 2 diabetes, antiviral medication, and so on. The American Urological Association has published guidelines for prevention and management of nephrolithiasis, which are summarized in the following.

Common misconceptions about the type of fluid patients should be drinking include avoiding alcohol, coffee, colas, wine, and beer. Only one study reported a decrease in the recurrence

rate when patients avoided colas but the rate was so low it was not clinically significant. In general, there is no definite consensus on avoidance of certain fluids or the selection of certain fluids to help prevent recurrent calcium oxalate stones.

Contrary to popular belief, a low-calcium diet is associated with an increase in calcium oxalate stones. It is believed that low calcium intake results in increased oxalate absorption from the gut and higher levels of urinary oxalate. Recommendations suggest daily calcium intake of 1 to 2 g. A low-sodium diet has been shown to decrease urinary calcium excretion but in general, compliance with a low-sodium diet is difficult. A high-oxalate diet has been shown to increase stone recurrence. Patients should be counseled to limit foods high in oxalate. Oxalate content of various foods is readily available through online searches. Here again, a 1- to 2-g daily intake of calcium seems to offset the risk of stone recurrence in these patients with high urinary oxalate levels. Calcium supplements in older women may lead to a higher risk of stone disease, but there are conflicting reports. If a patient is taking supplements, baseline 24-hour urine collections should be obtained to monitor urinary calcium levels and make dietary adjustments as needed. Since urinary citrate is a stone inhibitor, patients should be encouraged to add fruits and vegetables to their diet. There is no hard evidence that drinking lemonade or adding lemon to tap water prevents recurrent stone formation. Animal protein intake contributes to an acidic urine, which promotes stone formation. Patients should limit their weekly intake of meats, cheese, eggs, and fish.

There are no definitive studies demonstrating a beneficial effect of reducing a high purine diet with lower uric acid stones formation. But in general, patients with recurrent calcium or uric acid stones and a diet high in purines may benefit from reducing their intake of high purine foods. These include various seafoods, shellfish, water fowl, organ meats, game meats, pork, and poultry. Simply restricting red meats without limiting other high purine foods is not beneficial.

For those patients who have failed dietary measures or those that continue to form stones after altering their diets, medical therapy is indicated.

Thiazide diuretics are the gold standard for treatment of recurrent calcium oxalate stones. Chlorthalidone[1] 25 mg daily, hydrochlorothiazide[1] 50 mg daily, and indapamide[1] 2.5 mg daily are all well tolerated. (Patients should be monitored for hypokalemia.) Potassium citrate (Urocit-K) 10 to 20 mEq daily can be prescribed for patients with recurrent calcium oxalate stones, uric acid stones, and cystine stones. Sodium citrate is an alternate choice but risks creating a higher urinary calcium load. A baseline 24-hour urinary citrate level and follow-up study 6 months later will determine if therapy is effectively raising urinary citrate levels. Uric acid stones can be dissolved with aggressive urinary alkalinization using potassium citrate. Patients with hyperuricosuria and recurrent calcium oxalate or uric acid stones should be offered allopurinol (Zyloprim) 300 mg daily. Patients with cystine stones should be managed with high fluid intake, urinary alkalinization with potassium citrate, and reduction in sodium and protein intake. Thiol drugs should be prescribed if dietary measures fail. Alpha-mercaptopropionyl glycine (tiopronin, Thiola) 800 mg daily in 3 divided doses is the standard treatment. An alternative preparation D-penicillamine (Cuprimine) is associated with more severe side effects and should be a second-line choice.

Struvite stones occur in the presence of chronic urinary infection. Treatment of the stone with sterilization of the urinary tract is the best option. If surgery is not an option, suppressive antibiotic therapy may help.

According to one recent study only one in three patients will follow recommendations to prevent recurrent stones.

Diagnosis

A CT scan without intravenous contrast is the most accurate way of diagnosing renal and ureteral stones. It is the first choice for

---

[1] Not FDA approved for this indication.

suspected renal or ureteral stones. An abdominal plain film is an unreliable and inaccurate diagnostic tool. It should never be ordered in an acute situation. Small 1- to 2-mm stones are difficult to see on plain films. Uric acid stones, cystine stones, and triamterene stones are radiolucent and seldom visible on plain films. Renal ultrasound is a good tool to identify and follow hydronephrosis but it does not accurately identify renal stones and cannot be used to follow ureteral stones. It too does not play a role in the acute situation. A CT stone protocol is readily available in medical centers and outpatient facilities. It can be performed in less than 15 minutes and no preparation is required. Diagnosis is instantaneous and accurate. MRI has been used to diagnose ureteral stones in pregnant females but interpretation is dependent on the experience of the radiologist and his or her familiarity with the technique. It is not frequently used for this purpose.

Differential Diagnosis

Asymptomatic nephrolithiasis is usually discovered as an incidental finding on an unrelated radiological study. Intense renal shadowing on abdominal ultrasound is suggestive for renal stone. A calcification overlying the renal shadow on an abdominal plain film can suggest renal stone, but the differential includes arterial calcifications, stomach or intestinal contents, calcified lymph nodes, renal cell tumors, cholelithiasis, etc. Pelvic calcifications seen on plain films can be ascribed to phleboliths, ovarian calcifications, prostate calcifications, appendoliths, vascular calcifications, bladder stones, and so on. Needless to say, plain films should not be expected to provide an accurate diagnosis. Unless the renal stone is obstructing the renal pelvis, it does not cause pain. Patients who present with back pain and nonobstructing renal stones should not be treated for renal colic. Further diagnostic evaluation is indicated.

In contrast to asymptomatic renal stones, ureteral stones almost always present with dramatic onset of excruciating pain. The diagnosis is almost instantaneous. Renal colic is localized to either costovertebral area. Nausea and vomiting are common. Pain is not relieved by changing position. As the stone progresses distally the pain can mimic multiple acute abdominal conditions. The differential diagnosis of right lower quadrant abdominal pain includes:

- Acute appendicitis
- Ovarian conditions (e.g., rupture, ectopic pregnancy)
- Incarcerated inguinal hernia
- Cholecystitis
- Testicular torsion
- Diverticulitis, but very rarely

The differential for left lower quadrant pain is the same as for right lower quadrant pain, with the exception of appendicitis and cholecystitis, for obvious reasons. Diverticulitis is more commonly seen in the descending colon than in the ascending colon.

Treatment

Renal Stones

Asymptomatic renal stones pose a dilemma whether to treat or not. One of the largest retrospective studies evaluated the natural history of these stones based on location, and size of the stone. In more than 3 years of active observation, they found 60% of stones remained asymptomatic, 7% passed spontaneously, and 20% were operated on for pain. Less than 30% of the stones caused renal colic. Most studies determined lower pole stones did not pass spontaneously but grew faster in size than stones in the upper collecting system. These upper pole stones also passed more spontaneously. Patients should be offered treatment of renal stones if larger than 5 mm and in the upper pole of the kidney. Lower pole stones can be followed if the patient is not anxious to have treatment or if the stone has been present for years without change in size or location. Stones 10 mm or larger should be treated regardless of position. These stones could pass spontaneously and will require emergency surgery. All staghorn calculi should be treated unless comorbidities prevent surgical intervention. Autonephrectomy is the ultimate outcome for untreated staghorn calculi.

Once a decision is made to treat a renal stone, the next step is to decide which method is best for the patient. Factors to consider are size of the stone, stone composition, location, number of stones, and body habitus.

Rigid and flexible ureteroscopy with holmium laser disintegration of stones is rapidly replacing electrocorporeal shockwave lithotripsy (ESWL) for both ureteral and renal calculi. The success rate for stone destruction and removal is higher than ESWL. ESWL is indicated for renal and ureteral stones less than 20 mm. However the clearance rate after ESWL is only 60%.

Percutaneous nephrostolithotomy (PNL) is the best choice for these larger stones. All staghorn and partial staghorn calculi should be treated by PNL.

Medical dissolution treatment should be offered to patients with uric acid or cystine stones. Unfortunately, compliance to a medical and dietary regimen is dismal and most will need surgical intervention.

Ureteral Stones

It is generally accepted that stones less than 5 mm will pass spontaneously over 3 months. Most stones pass sooner than that.

The following is a general guide for treatment of the acute episode:

- CT stone protocol to identify the number, size, and location of the stone(s)
- Intravenous narcotic and antiemetic if necessary
- Urinalysis to evaluate for bacteria. Pyuria and hematuria are common and not signs of infection. If bacteria are present obtain culture and begin empiric antibiotics.
- Abdominal plain film. If the stone is visible this will provide a way to follow the stone.
- CBC, electrolytes
- Hydronephrosis will be present but does not dictate treatment.

Once pain is controlled, the patient is able to tolerate fluids by mouth, laboratory tests are acceptable, and the patient can be discharged with oral narcotics and possibly an alpha blocker. Oxycodone 5 mg PO q4-6 hours is a good choice for pain control. Tamsulosin (Flomax)[1] 0.4 mg PO daily has been shown in many studies to assist in spontaneous stone passage, but recent research has called this into question.

A randomized double-blind, placebo-controlled clinical trial study published in 2018 found no benefit for prescribing tamsulosin for stones less than 9 mm.

A Cochrane review meta-analysis published just before the previously mentioned study came to the conclusion that alpha blockers likely increase stone clearance rates but also slightly increase the risk of major adverse advents—retrograde ejaculation, lightheadedness, and hypotension. They also found alpha-blockers to be less effective in stones less than 5 mm.

Urologic dogma holds that stones less than 5 mm have spontaneous passage rates of higher than 90%. Stones in the distal ureter have a 98% passage rates. I believe most urologists doubt 9-mm stones will pass with or without the concomitant use of tamsulosin unless the patient has passed these large stones previously. Surgical intervention, either ureteroscopy or ESWL, is usually the preferred treatment option.

Since there is no clear choice, I believe a 6-week course of tamsulosin is reasonable. The patient should be followed every 2 weeks. If the stone has not passed by then, surgical intervention should be discussed with the patient.

Patients with any of the following signs and/or symptoms should be admitted and urologic consultation obtained as soon as possible:

- Fever and leukocytosis, or signs of sepsis
- Solitary kidney
- Uncontrolled pain or vomiting
- Bilateral ureteral stones
- Stones larger than 5 to 7 mm
- Uretero-pelvic junction stones larger than 5 mm

---

[1] Not FDA approved for this indication.

The choice to insert a ureteral stent depends on the urologist and his or her assessment of the situation. There are no strict rules, but insertion of stent is left to the discretion of the urologist.

Once the patient is discharged, he/she should be encouraged to drink as much fluids as possible and strain the urine for the stone. If the stone is visible on plain film, the patient should return to the office in 2 weeks for a renal ultrasound and abdominal plain film. If the stone is progressing and the patient is not experiencing significant pain, observation can continue. If the renal sonogram demonstrates increasing hydronephrosis, urologic consultation is indicated.

If the stone has not passed within 30 days, urologic consultation should be obtained. It is not uncommon for a patient to pass the stone and not see it in the urinary stream. Renal sonogram is very useful to identify resolution of the hydro nephrosis in these cases.

Once the patient collects the stone, it should be sent for analysis. A follow-up renal sonogram should be obtained 6 to 8 weeks after passage to identify any residual silent hydronephrosis. If hydronephrosis is present, urologic consultation should be obtained.

Complications

The most serious complication of nephrolithiasis is pyonephrosis, infected urine behind an obstructing stone. This is a urologic emergency requiring immediate drainage of the obstructed kidney. A percutaneous nephrostomy is the quickest way to achieve drainage.

Stones can become lodged in the ureter and remain asymptomatic. They eventually become impacted. The urothelium surrounds and covers the stone, trapping it in place over time. Silent hydronephrosis continues until the kidney eventually becomes atrophic and nonfunctioning. This is the reason why either a CT or renal sonogram must be obtained 6 to 8 weeks after patient passes a stone or is no longer symptomatic.

Failure to identify treatable conditions such as hyperparathyroidism, hyperuricemia, and cystinuria contribute to recurrent stone formation and morbidity associated with stone passage.

Surgical complications from ureteroscopy include pain, hemorrhage, infection, ureteral perforation, and ureteral avulsion. Ureteral avulsion should never occur and is the most feared complication by every urologist. Ureteral stents can usually manage any other ureteral complication.

Complications from ESWL include hemorrhage, perirenal hemorrhage, failure to disintegrate the stone, and retained stone fragments. Some studies have shown an association between uncomplicated ESWL and delayed onset of diabetes and hypertension.

Monitoring

Stone patients should have yearly radiologic studies for at least the first 5 years after they present with a stone. There is a 50% chance they will develop another stone during that time. CT is the most accurate but abdominal plain films are useful if the stone(s) are visible. There is no place for renal sonogram for monitoring patients. If the stone burden increases over time urologic consultation should be obtained.

If a 24-hour urine collection is obtained and dietary or medical treatment is recommended the metabolic evaluation should be repeated 6 months later to determine if the plan is effective. Not surprisingly, most patients will not comply with the recommendations. Periodic 24-hour metabolic evaluations every few years is a good way to remind patients to self-monitor their fluid intake and modify their diets if necessary.

References

Assimos D, et al: Surgical management of Stones. American Urological Association/Endourological Society Guideline, Part 1, *J Urol* 196:1153-1160, 2016

Campschroer T, et al: Alpha-blockers as medical expulsive therapy for ureteric stones: a Cochrane systematic review, *BJU Int* 122(6):932–945, 2018.

Kidney Stones, American Urological Association July 2016

Meltzer AC, Burrows PK, Wolfson AB, et al: Effect of tamsulosin on passage of symptomatic ureteral stones: a randomized clinical trial, *JAMA Intern Med* 178(8):1051–1057, 2018, Available at: https://doi.org/10.1001/jamainternmed.2018.2259.

Medical Management of Kidney Stones: AUA Guideline March 2014, Pearle, M et. al.

TRAUMA TO THE GENITOURINARY TRACT

Method of
Bahaa S. Malaeb, MD; and Yooni Yi, MD

The genitourinary tract is involved in 3% to 10% of trauma cases. The kidney, followed by the bladder and urethra, are the most commonly involved genitourinary organs. In most cases, injury to the genitourinary tract is not isolated, and the initial evaluation of the urologic injuries should emphasize the context of the patient's associated injuries that might be more pressing or life-threatening. Still, early involvement of the urologist is prudent to help plan further interventions. The spectrum of genitourinary injuries is widespread, and management can range from immediate repair to temporization with delayed reconstruction. The goal of a urologist in the trauma setting is to establish urinary drainage in order to optimize kidney function, minimize hemorrhage, and control urinary extravasation to reduce associated complications such as infection or ileus.

Renal Trauma

Renal injury occurs in 1% to 5% of all trauma cases. Blunt impact accounts for the majority of renal injuries (90%–95%) and causes damage secondary to direct organ injury or disruption of the kidney from its attachments (e.g., renal hilum and ureteropelvic junction). Penetrating trauma most commonly is caused by stabbing or gunshot wounds. The damage from penetrating injury can be limited to the tract of the stab wound, or it can be more extensive secondary to necrosis from energy transfer and the blast effect of high-velocity bullets. The history is crucial in the diagnosis of renal injury and should include the mechanism of trauma as well as any preexisting kidney disease or condition that might contribute to worsening renal function. Hematuria has a very poor correlation with degree of injury, because disruption of the ureteropelvic junction, arterial disruption or thrombosis, and other severe injuries can exist in a setting with no hematuria.

The American Association for the Surgery of Trauma (AAST) classifies renal injuries into five grades (Figures 1 and 2):
- Grade 1: Nonexpanding subcapsular hematoma/contusion with absence of parenchymal injury
- Grade 2: Less than 1 cm laceration into the renal cortex, not extending into the collecting system, with a nonexpanding hematoma confined to the perirenal fascia
- Grade 3: Greater than 1 cm laceration, extending through the renal cortex and medulla but not the collecting system
- Grade 4: Laceration extending to the collecting system with urinary extravasation or a segmental vascular injury with contained hematoma; renal artery thrombosis
- Grade 5: Shattered kidney or renal pedicle avulsion

Renal injury should be suspected in any trauma patient who has a penetrating injury with gross or microscopic hematuria

Figure 1 Computed tomography scan demonstrating large right perirenal hematoma and thrombosed posterior segmental artery. This was classified as a grade IV renal injury.

Figure 2 American Association for the Surgery of Trauma grading system for traumatic renal injuries: grade I, renal contusion and subcapsular hematoma; grade II, cortical laceration and perirenal hematoma; grade III, laceration into medulla or segmental renal artery thrombosis without a parenchymal injury; grade IV, laceration involving the collecting system, with or without a devascularized segment and contained vascular injury; grade V, renal artery thrombosis, avulsion of the renal pedicle, and shattered kidney. From McAninch JW [ed]: Traumatic and Reconstructive Urology. Philadelphia, WB Saunders, 1996.

(≤3 red blood cells per high-power field), a blunt injury with gross hematuria, or a blunt injury with microscopic hematuria and shock (systolic blood pressure <90 mm Hg). In addition, imaging of the urinary tract should be obtained in children who have more than 50 red blood cells per high-power field even in the absence of hypotension.

In a stable patient, radiographic evaluation should consist of computed tomographic (CT) scanning with intravenous contrast and delayed images showing opacification of the collecting system and ureters. In the absence of a CT scan in a patient who is transported directly to the operating room for exploration, an intraoperative single-film intravenous pyelogram can be performed to confirm that two functioning kidneys are present; however, the poor quality of the images makes them unreliable for staging purposes.

Kidney exploration is indicated for the unstable patient in whom renal injury is thought to be the reason for a life-threatening and persistent hemorrhage. Another absolute indication for renal exploration and revascularization is renal artery hilar avulsion or renal artery thrombosis, if bilateral or in a solitary kidney. In patients undergoing exploratory laparotomy for associated injuries, renal exploration should be performed only in the presence of an expanding or pulsatile hematoma. Exploration of a nonexpanding, nonpulsatile hematoma is associated with a higher rate of nephrectomy and should be avoided. Almost all other injuries can be managed conservatively or with minimally invasive methods.

Nonoperative management consists of supportive care with intravenous hydration, antibiotics, bedrest, and serial measurements of hemoglobin and hematocrit. Patients can ambulate after they are clinically stable, gross hematuria has resolved, and the hemoglobin and hematocrit have been relatively constant over 24 hours.

Routine early follow-up imaging for grades 1 to 3 blunt renal injury is unnecessary. Any imaging should be motivated by a change in the patient's clinical situation or laboratory values. Grade 4 renovascular injuries can be followed up clinically. Follow-up imaging is indicated for patients with grade 4 or 5 injuries with urinary extravasation to assess for worsening urinoma or hematoma that might require further intervention. Additionally, there should be periodic monitoring of blood pressure following renal trauma.

Figure 3 Intravenous pyelogram demonstrating extravasation of urine from right mid-ureter.

Ureteral Trauma

Trauma to the ureter is rare, most likely because of its retroperitoneal and bony pelvis location, its relatively small caliber, and its mobility. The etiology of ureteric trauma is mostly iatrogenic (75% of all ureteric injuries); 73% of iatrogenic injuries occur secondary to gynecologic procedures, and the remainder are divided between general surgery and urologic procedures. Ureteral injury should be suspected in all cases of penetrating trauma to the abdomen, especially with high-velocity projectiles, because of the blast effect.

The AAST has classified ureteric injuries into five grades of severity:

- Grade 1: Hematoma only
- Grade 2: Injury involving less than 50% of the circumference of the ureter
- Grade 3: Injury involving greater than or equal to 50% of the circumference of the ureter
- Grade 4: Complete transection with less than 2 cm of devascularization
- Grade 5: Complete transection with more than 2 cm of devascularization

The diagnosis usually is made intraoperatively if a high suspicion of ureteric injury is present or postoperatively by imaging obtained for investigation of fistula formation or clinical signs of upper tract obstruction. Hematuria is not a sensitive marker for ureteral injury, therefore lack of hematuria does not portend a lack of ureteral injury. For noniatrogenic injuries, imaging should be obtained in patients who had rapid deceleration or penetrating injuries to the flank. Imaging modalities used are usually intravenous pyelography, CT scanning with intravenous contrast and delayed images, and retrograde pyelography. Findings indicative of ureteral injury include contrast extravasation, ureteral narrowing, and delayed peristalsis (Figure 3). Alternatively, the ureters may be interrogated intraoperatively by using direct inspection, by injecting intravenous methylene blue[1] and watching for leakage of dye, or by passing a ureteral catheter (if it passes easily, an injury is unlikely).

---

[1]Not FDA approved for this indication.

Grade 1 and 2 injuries can be managed initially by placement of a ureteral stent. If grade 2 or 3 injuries are identified immediately during exploration for a suspected ureteric injury, they can be managed by primary closure of the ureteric injury over an internal stent and placement of a nonsuction abdominal drain, as long as there is no associated thermal injury or necrosis. Grade 3 to 5 injuries usually require débridement of nonviable ends with reanastomosis over an internal ureteral stent or more complicated surgical procedures involving mobilization of the bladder and reimplantation of the ureter into the bladder. In an unstable patient, ureteral repair may be managed with temporary urinary drainage and a definitive repair in a delayed fashion. The type of ureteral repair depends on the amount of devitalized tissues and the location of the injury (proximal, middle, or distal ureter). Ureteroureterostomy, transureteroureterostomy, ureterocalicostomy, renal autotransplantation, ureteroneocystostomy with or without Boari flap or psoas hitch, and bowel interposition are all treatment options for various degrees of ureteral injuries.

Bladder Trauma

Blunt trauma accounts for 67% to 86% of bladder injuries resulting from external trauma, and up to 97% of those patients have associated pelvic fractures. The most common cause of blunt trauma is motor vehicle crashes. Penetrating trauma accounts for 14% to 33% of traumatic bladder injuries. The incidence of iatrogenic injury varies by procedure but is highest for hysterectomy and other obstetric and gynecologic procedures (up to 61 per 1000 cases). In cases of blunt trauma, injury should be suspected in patients who have pelvic fractures, suprapubic pain and inability to void, ileus, absent bowel sounds, or abdominal distention. For iatrogenic injuries, any urine in the field, visible laceration in bladder, or gas distention of the urinary drainage bag in laparoscopic surgery warrants further investigation. It is important to delineate whether a bladder injury involves intraperitoneal or extraperitoneal rupture. Intraperitoneal rupture occurs at the level of the bladder dome, where the muscular support is weakest (Figures 4 and 5).

Figure 4 Intraperitoneal bladder rupture. Note contrast extravasating from the dome of the bladder and outlining the small intestine as well as the left colon.

The diagnostic test of choice is a CT cystogram, in which the bladder is filled with contrast to capacity (350–400 mL instilled by gravity). In children, the volume instilled is 60 mL plus 30 mL per year of age up to a maximum of 300 mL. Passive filling of the bladder by clamping of the catheter is associated with unacceptably high rates of false-negative tests. Plain film cystography is an alternative, but a single anteroposterior film is insufficient; postdrainage films and, preferably, oblique views should be obtained as well. In both settings, retrograde urethrography should be performed, if there is a suspicion of urethral injury, before placement of a Foley catheter.

Most extraperitoneal bladder ruptures can be managed with Foley catheter drainage for 7 to 10 days. Bladder neck involvement, concomitant vaginal or rectal injuries, presence of bone fragments in the bladder, or bladder wall entrapment necessitates surgical intervention. Intraperitoneal ruptures should be managed with surgical exploration because of the associated ileus and peritonitis caused by urine leak. In contrast, all penetrating bladder injuries should be explored and repaired because of the risk of necrosis and nonhealing. Bladder repair is performed with a multiple-layer closure and catheter drainage for 7 to 10 days.

Urethral Trauma

Traumatic injury to the urethra occurs in 10% of patients who sustain a pelvic fracture. Female urethral injuries are very rare. The male urethra is anatomically divided into a posterior part (prostatic and membranous urethra) and an anterior part (bulbous urethra, penile/pendulous urethra, and fossa navicularis). Injury to the anterior urethra occurs mostly from blunt trauma, penetrating injuries, or instrumentation. Posterior urethral injuries are usually associated with pelvic fractures but can occur secondary to blunt, penetrating, or iatrogenic injury.

Classic signs of urethral injury include blood at the meatus, a high-riding prostate on rectal examination, and perineal or scrotal ecchymosis. Imaging is indicated with any of these signs. The imaging study of choice is a retrograde urethrogram, and it should be performed before placement of a urethral catheter is attempted. In the absence of any signs, the diagnosis is most frequently made when retrograde urethrography is performed to investigate difficulty with urethral catheter placement (Figure 6).

The AAST grading system does not distinguish between anterior or posterior injury but classifies urethral injuries as follows:

- Grade 1: Contusion and blood at the meatus with normal urethrogram
- Grade 2: Stretch injury with no extravasation of contrast
- Grade 3: Partial disruption with contrast extravasating at the injury site but still reaching the bladder
- Grade 4: Complete disruption with contrast not reaching the bladder; urethral defect of less than 2 cm
- Grade 5: Complete disruption with urethral defect greater than 2 cm or complex injury involving the bladder neck, prostate, rectum, or vagina

Grade 1 and 2 injuries can be managed conservatively by placement of a urethral catheter. Management of grade 3 urethral injury should initially emphasize stabilization of the patient, because extensive bleeding could be present in cases of severe injury to the pelvis. Placement of a catheter may be attempted even if there is a suspicion of partial urethral injury. If this is met with difficulty, a suprapubic tube may be placed.

In cases of complete disruption, prompt urinary drainage should be established either by placement of a suprapubic catheter or with primary realignment. Primary realignment involves endoscopic passage of a guidewire across the defect and placement of a catheter over the guidewire. Immediate open repair is rarely indicated unless complex injury extends into the bladder, rectum, or vagina and the patient is undergoing surgery for associated injuries. Immediate exploration is recommended for anterior urethral injuries associated with penetrating trauma or penile fractures. Physicians should continue to follow patients for possible complications such as incontinence or stricture formation.

Figure 5 Extraperitoneal bladder rupture seen on computed tomographic cystogram.

Figure 6 Retrograde urethrogram diagnostic of partial bulbar urethral transaction resulting from straddle injury.

Trauma to the External Genitalia

Injury to the scrotum is most frequently secondary to blunt trauma and can cause subcutaneous hematoma, hematocele, or testicular injury. Scrotal swelling and patient discomfort can make separation of testicular injury from extratesticular scrotal trauma difficult on physical examination. Therefore, one should have a low threshold for further investigation with ultrasound. A heterogeneous echo pattern in the testicular parenchyma on ultrasonography suggests testicular injury (Figure 7). Visualization of a tear in the tunica albuginea is less accurate. Ultrasound studies additionally provide information about any compromise in testicular blood flow.

Scrotal exploration should be performed whenever testicular injury is suspected. If the tunica is ruptured and there is extrusion of seminiferous tubules, the extruded tubules should be débrided, hemorrhage controlled, and the tunica closed. Testicular salvage rates are high (90%) when the scrotum is explored acutely but drop by half if exploration is delayed. Another indication for scrotal exploration is a large hematocele; evacuation of the hematoma can decrease the morbidity associated with protracted recovery and resolution of the hematoma and can occasionally identify a manageable source of bleeding. Scrotal exploration should also be performed in cases of inconclusive ultrasound findings or whenever the clinical suspicion for testicular injury is high.

Trauma to the penis can range in severity from a contusion to complete amputation. In cases of penile amputation, stabilization of the patient is important, and the need for transfusion should be addressed. Immediate microreimplantation is the management technique of choice if available. The severed penile fragment should be immediately placed in normal saline and bag over ice to help preserve the fragment for reimplantation. Penile fracture occurs after blunt injury to the erect penis, usually incurred during sexual intercourse. Patients often report a "crack" or a

Figure 7 Testis ultrasound image demonstrating heterogeneous architecture characteristic of testicular rupture.

"pop" followed by severe pain and detumescence. Penile fractures involve rupture of the tunica albuginea. The hematoma is usually limited to the penis, unless the injury also involves Buck's fascia, causing ecchymosis and bruising that involves the scrotum as well. It is important to rule out associated urethral injury, which occurs in 10% of the cases. Surgical exploration, closure of the fascial defect, and repair of any associated urethral injury should be done acutely.

In females, blunt trauma to the vulva is rare. Injuries to genitalia can be associated with sexual assault and must be evaluated in that context. Consequently, vaginal smears should be taken, and the vagina should be thoroughly inspected with a speculum and with the patient under anesthesia.

Trauma resulting in skin loss, such as burns, large abrasions, and avulsions, should be explored and débrided in an effort to stage the injury and decrease the risk of complications such as Fournier's gangrene and urinoma. Delayed reconstruction can be performed after stabilization and proper delineation of viable versus nonviable tissues. The reconstructive options include mobilization of local flaps or skin grafts.

An understanding of the mechanism of injury is important to establish clinical suspicion of urologic trauma. Radiologic imaging is essential in making the correct diagnosis and managing it appropriately. Early diagnosis minimizes patient morbidity.

Studies of prospective design are clearly lacking for urologic trauma. Consolidation of the experience of major trauma institutions nationwide in a consortium for multi-institutional protocols could be the answer to this lack of prospective data.

References

Brandes S, Coburn M, Armenakas N, McAninch J: Diagnosis and management of ureteric injury: An evidence-based analysis, *BJU Int* 94(3):277–289, 2004.

Chapple C, Barbagli G, Jordan G, et al: Consensus statement on urethral trauma, *BJU Int* 93(9):1195–1202, 2004.

Gomez RG, Ceballos L, Coburn M, et al: Consensus statement on bladder injuries, *BJU Int* 94(1):27–32, 2004.

Lynch TH, Martínez-Piñeiro L, Plas E, et al: European Association of Urology: EAU guidelines on urological trauma, *Eur Urol* 47(1):1–15, 2005.

Malcolm JB, Derweesh IH, Mehrazin R, et al: Nonoperative management of blunt renal trauma: Is routine early follow-up imaging necessary? *BMC Urol* 8:11, 2008.

Morey AF, Metro MJ, Carney KJ, et al: Consensus on genitourinary trauma: External genitalia, *BJU Int* 94(4):507–515, 2004.

Phonsombat S, Master VA, McAninch JW: Penetrating external genital trauma: A 30-year single institution experience, *J Urol* 180(1):192–195, 2008. discussion 195–196.

Santucci RA, Fisher MB: The literature increasingly supports expectant (conservative) management of renal trauma: A systematic review, *J Trauma* 59(2):493–503, 2005.

Santucci RA, Wessells H, Bartsch G, et al: Evaluation and management of renal injuries: Consensus statement of the renal trauma subcommittee, *BJU Int* 93(7):937–954, 2004.

URETHRAL STRICTURE DISEASE

Method of
Hadley Wyre, MD and Sable Shew, MD

CURRENT DIAGNOSIS

- Perform a thorough history and physical examination, delineating past trauma, instrumentation, and sexual history, as well as a complete genitourinary examination.
- Patients with urethral stricture will commonly present with obstructive symptoms of weak urinary stream, straining to urinate, and even frank urinary retention.
- In-office testing consists of urinalysis and urine culture for evaluation of infection, as well as uroflowmetry and postvoid residual bladder ultrasound to evaluate urine flow rate and emptying ability.
- Retrograde urethrogram remains the gold standard for diagnosis of urethral stricture disease.

CURRENT THERAPY

- In the acute setting of urinary retention, the ideal management would be placement of a suprapubic tube to avoid manipulation of the stricture; however, dilation and catheter placement may be appropriate or necessary in some patients.
- Depending on the patient, goals of care should be delineated regarding treatment of stricture disease; that is, definitive therapy versus chronic management of stricture symptoms.
- Endoscopic treatments are available and include urethral dilation and direct visualization internal urethrotomy; however, repeat attempts at these approaches have a low long-term success rate.
- Surgical management includes both anastomotic and augmentation urethroplasty—both of which are more invasive than endoscopic approaches but are known to have improved long-term patency rates.

Urethral stricture disease affects 0.6% of the male population and can be classified in multiple ways: anterior versus posterior, benign versus malignant, extrinsic versus intrinsic, and congenital versus acquired. The urethra is a conduit for urine from the bladder to outside of the body. In males, the anterior urethra (region encircled by corpus spongiosum) begins at the meatus and includes the fossa navicularis, penile urethra, and bulbar urethra—strictures here are the result of scarring of the urethral epithelium and surrounding spongy tissue, termed spongiofibrosis. As this scarring narrows the urethral lumen, symptoms become noticeable. Typically, the urethral lumen must narrow to less than 14 French for this scarring to be the cause of any voiding symptoms. Anterior urethral stricture can be secondary to iatrogenic injury, infections, penile/perineal trauma, pelvic fractures, and self-instrumentation. In the posterior urethra, including the membranous urethra, prostatic urethra, and bladder neck, narrowing is termed contracture or stenosis and is the result of a distraction injury sustained during pelvic trauma or prior surgical procedures of the prostate (Figure 1).

Diagnosis

Often patients with strictures will present with obstructive voiding symptoms including weak or intermittent stream, postvoid dribbling, straining to urinate, or overt urinary retention. Nonobstructive symptoms include postvoid fullness, urinary tract infections, and pelvic pain. A thorough history, including a detailed social/sexual history, and physical examination should be done,

and any prior trauma to or instrumentation of the genitourinary tract noted. The physical examination should be comprehensive, with the genital examination examining for palpable strictures in the anterior urethra.

Laboratory workup should include urinalysis and urine culture for evaluation of infection, as well as a basic metabolic panel to evaluate for any renal function compromise. It is possible to perform an assessment of voiding symptoms in a clinic setting with the use of postvoid ultrasound and uroflowmetry. Once the patient has voided to completion, an ultrasound measurement of postvoid residual urine volume can objectively estimate the patient's ability to evacuate and alert the provider to overt retention. Uroflowmetry is the measurement of flow rate of urine—findings that suggest significant stricture include an elongated voiding time and a low maximal flow rate, essentially flattening the flow curve to a plateau appearance.

The gold standard in urethral stricture diagnosis remains the retrograde urethrogram. Radiocontrast is administered via catheter in a retrograde fashion, filling the urethra and opacifying it—this study is especially helpful for evaluating the length, location, and severity of strictures in the anterior urethra. Additionally, an antegrade study, or voiding cystourethrogram, can be performed to allow for visualization of the bladder neck, prostatic urethra, and membranous urethra. In addition to cystoscopic evaluation for direct visualization of the stricture, ultrasound of the penis/perineum can be used to further delineate characteristics of the stricture. Biopsy is occasionally performed to rule out malignancy as a cause of the stricture (Figure 2).

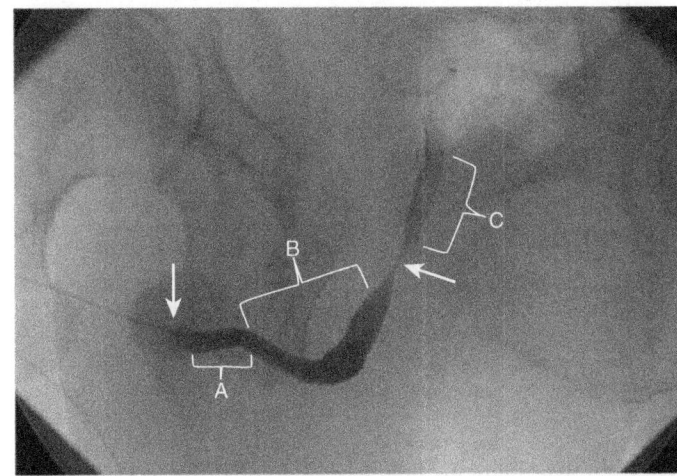

Figure 1 Anatomy of male urethra. (A) Penile urethra. (B) Bulbar urethra. (C) Prostatic urethra. White arrow by A=fossa navicularis; white arrow between B and C=membranous urethra.

Figure 2 Bulbar urethral stricture visualized on retrograde urethrogram.

Acute Treatment

Acutely, the main complication from a urethral stricture is frank urinary retention, which may be associated with a decline in renal function. Typically a urethral catheter cannot be placed because of obstruction from the stricture. In the setting of overt urinary retention, a suprapubic tube is often placed at the bedside or in the operating room to allow for rapid decompression of the urinary system without manipulating the stricture. There are times where suprapubic tube placement may not be possible, and it is therefore reasonable to dilate the stricture and place a urethral catheter to drain the urine. However, manipulation of the stricture can lead to an increase in the length of the stricture and complexity of the eventual repair.

Long-Term Treatment

Multiple modalities exist for the treatment of urethral stricture disease, with varying success rates and complication rates. A thorough discussion between the patient and provider, considering the patient's goals for either cure or symptom management, life expectancy, and stricture qualities, is vital to ensuring that an appropriate care plan is developed. Prior to proceeding with any treatment, it is essential to evaluate the urethra proximal to and distal to the stricture with the modalities mentioned earlier; this is to ensure removal of all affected tissue and prevent recurrence.

Conservative management with urethral dilation is appropriate as a first attempt at treatment of a short stricture with minimal spongiofibrosis, with the ultimate goal of stretching rather than tearing tissue to open the lumen without increasing the scarring present. Direct visualization internal urethrotomy (DVIU) is opening of a stricture—by laser, cold knife, or hot knife—to release the scar and allow the urethra to heal at a larger diameter over a catheter. Long-term success rates for DVIU have been reported at 20% to 30% for short strictures with minimal spongiofibrosis. It is important to note that the success rate of repeat DVIU is close to 0%, and after failure, the patient should be referred for definitive surgical repair.

Surgical management includes operations to excise the scar and perform urethral anastomosis, and tissue transfer reconstruction with harvesting of distant tissue—typically oral mucosa—for urethral augmentation. Anastomotic urethroplasty is best for short strictures, 1 to 2 cm in length, while augmentation urethroplasty can be utilized for much longer defects. For any type of urethral reconstruction, restricture is the most common complication, as well as sexual dysfunction and ejaculatory dysfunction. Other treatment options include long-term suprapubic tube drainage, perineal urethrostomy, and urinary diversion, depending on each patient's individual case and discussion with the patient's surgeon. Regardless of modality, clinicians should monitor patients for symptomatic recurrence of strictures.

References

Albers P, Fichtner J, Bruhl P, et al: Long-term results of internal urethrotomy, *J Urol* 156:1611–1614, 1996.
Andrich DE, Mundy AR: The nature of urethral injury in cases of pelvic fracture urethral trauma, *J Urol* 165:1492–1495, 2001.
Bhargava S, Chapple CR, Bullock AJ, et al: Tissue-engineered buccal mucosa for substitution urethroplasty, *BJU Int* 93:807–811, 2004.
Fichtner J, Filipas D, Fisch M, et al: Long-term outcome of ventral buccal mucosa onlay graft urethroplasty for urethral stricture repair, *Urology* 64:648–650, 2004.
Hudak SJ, Atkinson TH, Morey AF: Repeat transurethral manipulation of bulbar urethral strictures is associated with increased stricture complexity and prolonged disease duration, *J Urol* 187(5):1691–1695, 2012.
Kellner DS, Fracchia JA, Armenakas NA: Ventral onlay buccal mucosal grafts for anterior urethral stricture: Long-term followup, *J Urol* 171:726–729, 2004.
McCallum RW, Colapinto V: The role of urethrography in urethral disease. Part I. Accurate radiological localization of the membranous urethra and distal sphincters in normal male subjects, *J Urol* 122:607–611, 1979.
McCammon KA, Zuckerman JM, Gerald HJ: Surgery of the penis and urethra. In Wein A, et al, editors: *Campbell-Walsh Urology*, 11th edition, Philadelphia, 2016, Elsevier, pp 907–945.
Rosen MA, Nash PA, Bruce JE, et al: The actuarial success rate of surgical treatment of urethral strictures, *J Urol* 151:370, 1994.

URINARY INCONTINENCE

Method of
Simon Patton, MD; and Renee M. Bassaly, DO

CURRENT DIAGNOSIS

- Urinary incontinence is broadly categorized as stress urinary incontinence or urgency urinary incontinence.
- The diagnosis can often be determined by a careful history and physical examination but can be aided with noninvasive methods such as a bladder diary.
- It is important to rule out any other potential causes of incontinence including urinary tract infection, urinary retention, or medication side effect.

CURRENT THERAPY

- Modest weight loss has been shown to help both forms of incontinence and is an important first-line therapy.
- Urgency urinary incontinence can initially be managed with lifestyle modifications including timed voiding and avoidance of bladder irritants, as well as physical therapy. Further options include medications (anticholinergics or B_3 agonists).
- Third-line therapy for urgency urinary incontinence includes sacral neuromodulation, botulinum toxin injections, and tibial nerve stimulation.
- Stress urinary incontinence can be managed conservatively with home Kegel exercises or formal pelvic floor training with physical therapy. Mechanical urethral support using a disposable tampon-like device or incontinence pessary is another non-invasive option.
- Surgical management of stress urinary incontinence is midurethral slings, principally using synthetic mesh. I would include Burch and autologous sling.

Epidemiology

Urinary incontinence is a very common problem particularly in the female population, with incidence roughly twice that of male patients (30% vs. 17%). The exact incidence may be difficult to know, however, because this is a sensitive subject that patients may not volunteer unless solicited. The annual cost of treating incontinence is estimated to be $24 billion, and annually 260,000 women undergo surgery for stress incontinence.

Risk Factors

Risk factors vary between genders. Women are at greater risk due to anatomic differences, principally a shorter urethral length. Other risk factors include increased age, parity, obesity, diabetes, smoking, and pelvic radiation. In male patients a history of prostate surgery or an enlarged prostate are potential risk factors. Urinary tract symptoms including incontinence may represent manifestations of neurologic disorders including history of stroke, multiple sclerosis, or spinal cord injury.

Pathophysiology

The bladder consists of a smooth muscular reservoir (the detrusor muscle), two inlets (the ureters), and an outlet (the urethra). Urine from the kidneys enters the bladder via the ureters and exits via the urethra, which is itself a muscular tube consisting of smooth and striated muscle. Bladder function has two phases: storage and emptying. During the storage phase, the bladder collects urine; this phase involves relaxation of the detrusor muscle and contraction of the urethral muscle, all of which is under sympathetic and voluntary control. The emptying phase involves relaxation of the urethral muscles and contraction of the detrusor, which is mediated by the parasympathetic system. Under normal circumstances, emptying is voluntarily initiated in the adult.

In women, the bladder and urethra are supported by the anterior vaginal wall, which, in turn, is suspended by connective tissue attachments from the pelvic floor muscles. Continence is maintained when the urethral closure pressure exceeds the detrusor pressure. Adequate support from the anterior vaginal wall is required to maintain this relationship during periods of increased intraabdominal pressure. Consequently, urinary continence depends on the relative relaxation of the detrusor, the contraction of urethral muscles, and the support of the anterior vaginal wall. Incontinence can ensue when these relationships are disrupted.

Prevention

The pelvic floor musculature plays an important role in the maintenance of continence, and as such, pelvic floor physical therapy directed at these muscles has been shown to improve continence in both postmenopausal women and younger postpartum women, at least in the short term. Physical therapy in the male population has not been studied as a prevention strategy. One modifiable risk factor for incontinence is obesity, and even a modest weight loss of 10% has been shown to help improve continence status.

Clinical Manifestation

Urinary incontinence can be a sign, symptom, as well as a diagnosis. Urinary incontinence falls into two broad categories: stress incontinence and urge incontinence. Stress urinary incontinence occurs when urethral closure pressure cannot increase sufficiently to compensate for a sudden increase in intraabdominal pressure, as from laugh, cough, or Valsalva maneuver. Urgency urinary incontinence occurs when an unintended bladder contraction creates an insuppressible urge to void, leading to urinary leakage. When patients have signs or symptoms of both stress and urge incontinence, it is referred to as *mixed urinary incontinence.*

Diagnosis

Diagnosis rests principally on a careful history and physical examination. A thorough history is important to solicit what causes a patient to leak. Leakage with laughing, coughing, sneezing, exercise, or similar exertion would likely be stress urinary incontinence. Leakage associated with an urge that is difficult to defer is likely urgency urinary incontinence. If patients have both symptoms, then they likely have mixed urinary incontinence. If a patient complains of symptoms of mixed incontinence, a careful history to determine which is most bothersome is important. If the patient has difficulty knowing what has caused their leakage, a 3-day bladder diary recording liquid consumed, times and amounts voided, and leakage events with associated symptoms can help with diagnosis and treatment.

Other pertinent components to a thorough history include surgery to the spinal cord, bladder neck, or pelvic floor, which may lead to obstruction; neurologic disease (e.g., multiple sclerosis or a spinal cord lesion); or psychiatric disease (e.g., dementia, which may limit the ability to recognize a need to void). Musculoskeletal function, with emphasis on mobility, should be reviewed. A detailed medication history will identify any medications that may affect urine output or bladder function. It is important to also elicit any other symptoms that may coexist with incontinence and signal pelvic floor dysfunction, including nocturia, fecal incontinence, or constipation.

After a thorough history, a detailed physical examination is necessary. A focused genitourinary examination includes inspection of the external genitalia. Eliciting reflexes from the S2-S4 nerve roots will help determine whether there is any neurologic component. In female patients, perform a pelvic examination and look for any prolapse or pelvic masses and note whether any atrophy is present. Palpation of the urethra allows for evaluation of any urethral masses or possible diverticula. Lastly, assessment of pelvic floor musculature is important, evaluating for any pain or discomfort in the levator ani muscles and assessing the patient's ability to perform a proper Kegel exercise. In males, performance

of a digital rectal examination is recommended to evaluate for any prostatic masses or hypertrophy.

The physical examination provides an opportunity for diagnosis as well; asking the patient to cough or perform a Valsalva maneuver allows for the direct visualization of stress incontinence if present. Additionally, this provides an opportunity in female patients to evaluate for prolapse and assess urethral mobility. Historically, this was done by placing a cotton swab in the urethra to observe for hypermobility seen with >30 degrees of mobility on strain from baseline. However, because of patient discomfort, this test is not routinely performed. After completing the physical examination, one must perform a urinalysis to rule out any infectious etiology and at times perform a post-void residual (either with a bladder scan or with catheterization) to evaluate for any possible voiding dysfunction. If the patient has a more complex history because of prior urologic surgery, neurologic disease, or is difficult to diagnose on history and physical alone, then complex urodynamic testing may be indicated.

Differential Diagnosis

The differential diagnosis for urinary incontinence includes stress urinary incontinence, urgency urinary incontinence, and a mixture of the two as mentioned above. Other causes of undesired leakage of urine include overflow (due to urinary retention), functional (due to impaired mobility or mental capacity), as well as a fistula or diverticulum. A patient with a fistula most commonly presents with the complaint of constant persistent urinary leakage. In the industrialized world these generally form after genitourinary surgery, whereas in developing countries trauma from childbirth is the primary cause. A diverticulum may present with a painful anterior vaginal wall mass as well as irritative voiding symptoms such as urinary frequency, urgency, dysuria, and postvoid dribbling. Other causes of lower urinary tract symptoms such as urgency, frequency, and dysuria include urinary tract infection, uncontrolled diabetes, or urinary tract malignancy.

Therapy
Stress Urinary Incontinence

Nonsurgical options for treatment of stress urinary incontinence include strengthening of the pelvic musculature through Kegel exercises and mechanical support of the urethra. Kegel exercises may be performed by the patient at home, although some patients may have difficulty identifying the muscles to perform them properly. Formal training with a pelvic floor physical therapist can help the patients learn to identify the muscles (sometimes using biofeedback devices) and contract them appropriately. Proper contraction of the levator ani muscles provides improved support for the bladder and urethra and helps decrease leakage.

Mechanical support of the urethra and bladder neck can be accomplished using an incontinence pessary or a disposable incontinence tampon. Pessaries are ring-shaped silicone devices with a knob that is meant to sit under the urethra. Patients are fitted for the correct size in the office. Patients must be followed up for at 3 to 6 month intervals to ensure the pessary has not caused any erosions or excoriations. This can be avoided by teaching patients how to insert and remove the pessary themselves or prescribing a vaginal estrogen cream in postmenopausal patients. A disposable option is available over the counter as well. It comes in three sizes, and the patients can fit themselves at home with the starter pack. Once they find the correct size, it can be placed when the patient desires and may be kept in place for up to 8 hours. Some patients choose this option if they only have stress incontinence during certain times (i.e., exercise).

If conservative therapies do not adequately address their complaints, surgical options are available. The general principle of restoring support to the urethra is the same as in conservative therapies. This can be accomplished by placing a sling under the urethra. The sling material can be lightweight polypropylene mesh or fascia (either autologous or cadaveric). The most commonly used type is the synthetic mesh and it is placed either retropubically or through the obturator membrane. Both methods have been shown to have a high rate of satisfaction with a low complication rate.

Stress incontinence in men is much less common but can also be treated with slings placed at the bulbar urethra. Artificial urinary sphincters can also be implanted that compress the urethra and can be controlled by the patient.

Urgency Urinary Incontinence

Lifestyle modifications are a good first-line therapy for patients with urgency urinary incontinence. Drinking an appropriate amount of fluids and avoiding foods and beverages that are known to irritate the bladder can provide significant relief. Additionally, performing timed voiding can help retrain the bladder. Formal training with a pelvic floor physical therapist has also been shown to significantly decrease incontinence episodes. It is important to note, however, that just performing Kegel exercises is often not adequate in these patients and can in fact worsen their symptoms if they already have tightly held, nonrelaxing pelvic floor musculature.

Pharmacologic therapy consists of anticholinergic medications or beta 3 agonists. Anticholinergic medications target the muscarinic receptors on the bladder; however, they are not specific and can cause significant dry mouth, dry eyes, and constipation, side effects that lead to a high discontinuation rate. Patients are unable to take this class of medication if they have closed-angle glaucoma. Additionally, there have recently been some concerns raised about long-term use leading to cognitive decline. The beta 3 agonists also work to slow down detrusor contractions but do so by targeting a different receptor. They have been shown to raise blood pressure and so are precluded in patients with uncontrolled severe hypertension; all patients should routinely check their blood pressure after starting one of these medications.

Third-line therapies for urgency urinary incontinence include sacral neuromodulation, tibial nerve stimulation, and intradetrusor injection of botulinum toxin A. Sacral neuromodulation has been approved by the Food and Drug Administration for this indication, as well as fecal incontinence and voiding dysfunction. It consists of a lead placed in the S3 foramen and connected to a pacemaker-like device that is implanted in the adipose of the buttocks. Patients are then able to control some of the settings (including program and amplitude) from an external device. The sacral nerve roots can also be stimulated via the tibial nerve. Treatments involve a small, acupuncture-sized needle placed in the tibial nerve followed by 30 minutes of stimulation. These are carried out at weekly treatments for 12 weeks followed by monthly maintenance therapy. Botulinum toxin A, a neurotoxin that works by decreasing the presynaptic release of acetylcholine, can be injected directly into the detrusor muscle. A risk of this treatment is urinary retention, which requires that patients be able to perform self-catheterization.

Mixed Urinary Incontinence

If a patient presents with components of both stress and urgency, eliciting first which symptom is the most bothersome allows for appropriate tailoring of treatment. It is important to remind patients that even a modest weight loss of 10% can help reduce bothersome urinary symptoms by up to 60%. As noted above, physical therapy can help address both type of incontinence as a valuable first-line therapy.

Overflow Incontinence

If a patient is diagnosed with overflow incontinence, then management is directed at maintaining an empty bladder through self-catheterization. In male patients, if the retention is due to prostatic hypertrophy, then pharmacologic therapy with α-agonists or 5α reductase inhibitors may be warranted. If medication fails to improve their symptoms, then surgical treatment with ablation (microwave or radiofrequency) or resection is indicated.

Complications

Urinary incontinence can cause significant morbidity in terms of financial as well as psychological burdens on patients. In addition to causing rashes and skin breakdown, incontinence also leads to depression, isolation, anxiety, depression, and increased risk of falls. Incontinence is one of the leading causes of institutionalization in the elderly. As the population ages, the incidence of incontinence will continue to increase, making its diagnosis and treatment increasingly important.

References

Abrams P, Cardozo L, Fall M, et al: The standardisation of terminology of lower urinary tract function: report from the Standardisation Sub-committee of the International Continence Society, *Neurourol Urodyn* 21:167–178, 2002.

AUGS: Consensus Statement: Association of Anticholinergic Medication Use and Cognition in Women With Overactive Bladder, *Female Pelvic Med Reconstr Surg* 23:177–178, 2017.

Hay-Smith EJ, Herderschee R, Dumoulin C, Herbison GP: Comparisons of approaches to pelvic floor muscle training for urinary incontinence in women, *Cochrane Database Syst Rev* 2011;(12:CD009508.

Hersh L, Salzman B: Clinical management of urinary incontinence in women, *Am Fam Physician* 87:634–640, 2013, Review. Erratum in: Am Fam Physician 2013;88:427.

Hu TW, Wagner TH, Bentkover JD, et al: Costs of urinary incontinence and overactive bladder in the United States: a comparative study, *Urology* 63:461–465, 2004.

16 Men's Health

URINARY TRACT INFECTIONS IN THE MALE

Method of
Donald A. Neff, MD

CURRENT DIAGNOSIS

- Urinary tract infection (UTI) can involve any portion of the urinary tract.
- Infection at any site in the urinary tract places the entire system at risk of infection.
- Urinary tract infections can be broadly categorized as uncomplicated or complicated.
- Although uncommon, men can have uncomplicated UTI.
- Urologic evaluation is recommended for UTI in young boys.
- Detailed workup of uncomplicated UTI in the adult male is usually not needed.
- Urinalysis is useful to establish presumptive diagnosis.
- Urine culture with sensitivities is helpful to document infection and guide therapy.
- Screening urine cultures in asymptomatic individuals should be avoided.

CURRENT THERAPY

- The goal of treatment is elimination of infection from the urinary tract.
- Prompt initiation of treatment can prevent the spread of infection to other portions of the urinary tract.
- Management of complicated UTI should include imaging of the upper urinary tract.
- Efforts should be made to control underlying risk factors in patients with complicated UTI.
- For complicated UTI, repeat culture after treatment may be helpful to document clearance of infection.
- Repeat urine culture after treatment of uncomplicated UTI is unnecessary.

Definitions

Standardized terminology for the diagnosis and treatment of urinary tract infection (UTI) is helpful for communication between healthcare providers. Box 1 outlines standardized wording for the common terminology used to discuss UTIs.

Introduction

UTIs are one of the most common bacterial infections in humans, defined as an inflammatory response of the urothelium to bacterial invasion. Infections of the urinary tract encompass a wide variety of diagnoses depending on the specific anatomic site of infection, the common denominator being bacterial invasion of genitourinary organs and tissues. Any site within the urinary tract may be involved including the kidney (pyelonephritis), ureters (ureteritis), bladder (cystitis), prostate (prostatitis), epididymis (epididymitis), and urethra (urethritis). Once any part of the urinary tract is infected, the rest of the urinary tract is placed at risk for infection through ascending or descending bacterial spread. Due in part to the relative rarity of UTI in adult males, evaluation and management of UTI in this population is hampered by the lack of high quality empirical data on which to guide treatment decisions.

Incidence and Epidemiology

UTI in males is not a reportable disease, and therefore the incidence is difficult to assess in the United States. For both sexes, UTI accounts for 7 million office visits and 400,000 hospitalizations annually. In men, UTI accounts for 0.6% of all office visits. During infancy, the incidence of symptomatic UTIs is higher in boys than in girls and is related to circumcision status. Bacteria adhere to the inner prepuce, allowing easier access to the meatus followed by ascending infection. Neonatal circumcision reduces the rate of UTI in boys by over 90%. After the neonatal period, symptomatic UTI is uncommon in men until middle age. The incidence then increases to approach 10% by age 61, 14% in ages 61 to 70, 26% in ages 71 to 80, and 42% over age 81.

Pathophysiology

In the modern era most infections of the urinary tract occur via the ascending route. This begins with colonization of the perineum, usually with fecal bacteria. These bacteria then move from the perineal area to the urethra, to the bladder, ureter, and eventually can ascend to the kidney. Fecal flora is a common source of infection, and *Escherichia coli* is the most common cause of UTIs accounting for 85% of community-acquired and 50% of hospital-acquired infections. Hematogenous seeding does occur, however this is uncommon in anatomically and physiologically normal individuals. The kidney may be secondarily infected by *Staphylococcus aureus* or *Candida* fungemia. In certain geographic areas, tuberculosis of the urinary tract is still seen and reaches the urinary tract organs hematogenously. Infection is facilitated by prior renal damage or obstruction of the urinary tract.

Adherence of bacteria to the uroepithelium is an essential step in the pathogenesis of UTI. Bacterial virulence factors such as adhesins, Type-1 pili, and P pili facilitate adherence to receptors on uroepithelial cells. Some individuals are genetically predisposed to infection, with increased uroepithelial receptivity to adherence of bacteria resulting in increased susceptibility to infection. Once within the bladder, uropathogenic bacteria are internalized into the intracellular space of superficial urothelial cells. In this space, the bacteria are more protected from the immune response and form intracellular bacterial communities, eventually forming protective biofilms. Bacteria then escape from the intracellular space into the urinary lumen, where they readhere and reinvade the uroepithelium. Once the inoculum is sufficient, a host immune response occurs. This response involves multiple cell types including neutrophils, macrophages, and other immunocytes along with associated cytokines. This inflammatory response results in the symptoms of UTI. Indeed, the levels of certain inflammatory factors have been correlated with the severity of symptoms.

BOX 1   Urinary Track Infection Standardized Terminology

Bacteriuria: Presence of bacteria in the urine. This may be symptomatic or asymptomatic. Asymptomatic bacteriuria may not require treatment.

Pyuria: Presence of white blood cells (WBCs) in the urine. Suggests infection or inflammatory response of the urothelium. Sterile pyuria is lack of bacterial growth in presence of WBCs in the urine, and should warrant further investigation to determine the underlying cause.

Urinary tract infection (UTI): Inflammatory response of urothelium to bacterial invasion.

Uncomplicated UTI: Infection in a healthy patient with anatomically and functionally normal urinary tract. These infections respond promptly to appropriate treatment.

Complicated UTI: Infection associated with an anatomically or functionally abnormal urinary tract. The host may be immunocompromised. Risk factors for complicated UTI include male gender, advanced age, diabetes, immunosuppression, recent antibiotic use, the presence of an indwelling urinary catheter, recent instrumentation, and recent hospitalization.

Colonization: Presence of bacteriuria in the urine and absence of inflammatory response. Often seen in patients with indwelling urinary catheters. Generally, colonization does not require treatment. Overtreatment of the colonized urinary tract will select for bacterial resistance.

Isolated UTI: Infection in patient with no or remote prior history.

Recurrent UTI: Infection that occurs after successful treatment of a prior infection. May be bacterial persistence or reinfection. Persistence is suggested by growth of the same organism. Reinfection usually shows growth of different types of organisms.

Unresolved UTI: Generally due to bacterial persistence. Repeated infection with same organism with similar resistance profile.

The urinary tract has natural defenses in place to resist adherence and ascension of bacteria. Normal urogenital flora forms a barrier to colonization by uropathogenic bacteria. Inhibitory urinary factors include osmolality, urea, organic acid concentration, and pH. Uromodulin is a protein present in the urine that binds to type-1 pili, preventing binding of bacteria to the urothelium. Regular and complete emptying of the bladder helps expel bacteria and keep bacterial inoculum low.

Clinical Manifestations

The specific clinical symptoms of UTI depend on the anatomic site of infection. Urethritis presents with dysuria, urinary urgency and frequency, and penile discharge. The penis may be tender or swollen. Associated inguinal lymphadenopathy may be present. Epididymitis usually presents as unilateral testicular pain that is gradual in onset. The scrotum is swollen, warm, and erythematous. Scrotal cellulitis may be present. Acute prostatitis includes fevers, chills, dysuria, and pelvic pain. Urinary hesitancy and weak stream are often seen due to swelling of the prostate gland. Cystitis is associated with dysuria, urinary urgency, and urinary frequency. There may be associated suprapubic pain or gross hematuria. Pyelonephritis is associated with the classical triad of fevers, chills, and flank pain. In the elderly, symptoms may not be as clear. Generalized abdominal pain, increased confusion, and altered mental status may be the presenting signs of UTI in these individuals.

Differential Diagnosis

The differential diagnosis of UTI should be focused on the anatomic location of symptoms. Urethritis can be caused by multiple organisms, and sexually transmitted diseases should be considered. Lower urinary tract symptoms (urgency, frequency) associated with cystitis can also be seen with bladder stones or bladder tumors. Sterile pyuria should prompt investigation for stone, tuberculosis, and malignancy. Flank pain may be due to urinary tract obstruction due to stone, trauma, or musculoskeletal sources.

Clinical Evaluation

The foundation for evaluation of a patient with UTI remains a thorough history and physical examination. A detailed surgical history is helpful to determine risk factors for complicated UTI. A urinalysis is essential in the evaluation of urinary symptoms, and can provide information for a preliminary diagnosis. Normal urine should be free of bacteria and inflammation. False negatives can occur early in the clinical course or when a patient has taken antimicrobial therapy prior to obtaining the urine specimen. False positives may be caused by contamination or over-the-counter remedies such as phenazopyridine (AZO Urinary Pain Relief, Uricalm Max), which can cause a positive nitrites reaction on urinary dipstick evaluation. The decision to obtain urine culture should be based on the clinical picture. For an uncomplicated UTI, a urine culture is seldom necessary. If symptoms fail to improve, or if the patient has risk factors for complicated UTI, a culture is strongly recommended to determine the underlying organism and antimicrobial sensitivities. Proper collection and storage of the urine specimen can minimize the potential for false results.

Localization of the anatomic source of an infection within the lower urinary tract of males can be challenging. The Meares-Stamey four glass urinary tract localization test has been well described. First, the patient is asked to void 5 to 10 cc into a sterile container (VB1). A second mid-stream specimen is then obtained (VB2). A prostatic massage is then performed by digital rectal exam (DRE), and the expressed prostatic secretions (EPS) are collected. Finally, the post–prostate massage urine is collected. The four specimens are then sent separately for culture and sensitivity. VB1 represents urethral flora, VB2 represents bladder urine flora, and EPS and VB3 represent prostatic flora. The four-glass test can be expensive, cumbersome, and is often of low diagnostic yield. An alternate approach is a modified Meares-Stamey 2 glass test, which is easier and less costly to perform. This is performed by collecting a urine specimen pre–prostate massage and then a second specimen post–prostate massage. The premassage specimen represents bladder flora, and the postmassage specimen represents the prostatic flora.

Due to the rarity of urinary infection in boys outside of the neonatal period, urologic investigation is essential for the evaluation of UTI in the pediatric population to rule out structural abnormalities. These include vesicoureteral reflux, posterior urethral valves, congenital ureteropelvic junction obstruction, ureterocele, and megaureter. Early diagnosis and therapy will help to prevent scarring and preserve renal function. A history of constipation should be elucidated, as bowel-bladder dysfunction places boys at risk of UTI. The optimal imaging approach to the pediatric patient is controversial. Traditionally, the combination of renal-bladder ultrasound and voiding cystourethrogram (VCUG) has been used to assess both the upper and lower urinary tracts. In the modern era, provided the renal bladder ultrasound is normal, VCUG may be safely deferred. A nuclear medicine scan can be useful to determine differential renal function and identify the presence of obstruction of the upper urinary tract.

For adults, the use of radiographic investigations is again based on the unique clinical picture of a given patient. For uncomplicated UTI, particularly in otherwise healthy men whose infections resolve easily, detailed investigations, including imaging, are often not necessary. Complicated infections require further investigation to search for an infectious nidus or anatomic abnormality. These include patients with a recurrent or unresolved infection or patients with aforementioned risk factors. CT urography is a complete study of the upper urinary tract and includes a noncontract phase, a nephrographic phase, and delayed images to evaluate the upper urinary drainage system. This study allows for assessment of renal stones, masses, impaired, or altered drainage and is the imaging study of choice in patients with normal renal function. For patients with poor renal function, renal-bladder ultrasound is a reasonable alternative. Measurement of postvoid residual is helpful to determine if retention of urine in the bladder is causing urinary stasis.

Treatment

Elimination of the infecting organism from the urinary tract is the goal of therapy for UTI. There is limited data to guide duration of treatment of UTI in males, with many treatment strategies extrapolated from studies performed in females. Although traditionally men have been considered to always have complicated UTIs, an afebrile man with a first UTI and no complicating factors can be considered to have an uncomplicated UTI.

In general, empirical selection of antimicrobial therapy should be selected to target the pathogen being treated, with local resistance patterns taken into consideration. Uncomplicated infections should be anticipated to resolve promptly with appropriate therapy. Duration of therapy for these types of infections in men is not well established, but 5 to 7 days of treatment is reasonable depending on the antibacterial agent chosen. Prompt initiation of broad spectrum therapy in complicated UTIs will help to prevent further dissemination of the infection and the development of sepsis. Treatment can later be tailored to the results of culture and sensitivities. Complicated infections require longer duration of therapy, 10 to 14 days. In the setting of multidrug-resistant isolates, parenteral therapy may be required for the duration of treatment. For patients with bacterial persistence after treatment, a thorough urologic evaluation should be performed, followed by an attempt to eliminate the source of bacteria if possible.

Monitoring and Prevention

In most patients with UTI, routine repeat culture of urine after therapy is not indicated. However, if patients thought to have uncomplicated UTI do not improve as expected, a urine culture should be obtained to guide therapy. Similarly, rapid recurrence of symptoms after initial improvement should prompt repeat urine culture. Antibiotic prophylaxis in males is generally not warranted, and prevention should be directed at elimination or treatment of the underlying cause if possible. For example, initiation of medications to treat incomplete bladder emptying due to benign prostatic hypertrophy, or surgical treatment of an infected urinary stone, would be of higher yield than suppressive antibiotics.

Management of Complications

Complications in patients with UTI should be managed according to the clinical setting. The decision to admit a patient to the hospital is dictated by multiple factors. Nontoxic patients who can take medications by mouth may be safely managed as outpatients. Immunosuppressed or diabetic patients may warrant admission for observation. These patients, and those with other risk factors for complicated UTI, may progress rapidly to sepsis and admission to the ICU may be necessary. Patients who develop perinephric or prostatic abscess will require either percutaneous or surgical drainage.

Special Considerations

Patients with chronic indwelling catheters will nearly always be colonized with bacteria. Screening cultures are not indicated and should be avoided. In general, bacterial colonization of the urinary tract should not be treated unless symptoms develop. It is often counterproductive to attempt clearance of bacteria in this population as overtreatment will select for bacterial resistance. Further, elimination of benign colonizing bacteria from the urinary tract in these individuals often allows more virulent bacteria to establish residence. Antimicrobial prophylaxis is not indicated. Treatment strategies in these individuals should be focused on the underlying factors leading to the need for catheter drainage. These include institution of clean intermittent catheterization

when possible, or more frequent changing of the indwelling catheter if necessary.

Another special consideration is the presence of a bacterial UTI in an obstructed urinary system. This most commonly occurs when a kidney stone causes ureteral obstruction in the setting of pyelonephritis. These patients can rapidly progress to sepsis. Prompt drainage of the affected renal unit either by ureteral stent or percutaneous nephrostomy tube, along with institution of appropriate antimicrobial therapy, is essential in the management of these patients.

References

Simmering JE, et al: The increase in hospitalizations for urinary tract infections and the associated costs in the United States, 1998–2011, *Open Forum Infectious Diseases* 4(1), 2017, Available at: https://www.ncbi.nlm.nih.gov/pmc/articles/PMC5414046/. Accessed 23 January 2019.

Detweiler K, et al: Bacteria and urinary infections in the elderly, *Urol Clin North Am* 42(4):561–568, 2015 Nov.

Subcommittee on Urinary Tract Infection Reaffirmation of AAP Clinical Practice Guideline: The diagnosis and management of the initial urinary tract infection in febrile infants and young children 2–24 months of age, *Pediatrics December* 138(6), 2016.

Foxman B: Epidemiology of urinary tract infections: incidence, morbidity, and economic costs, *The American Journal of Medicine* 113(Suppl 1A):5S–13S, 2002 Jul 8.

Nicolle L: Uncomplicated urinary tract infection in adults including uncomplicated pyelonephritis urol, *Clin N Am* 35:1–12, 2008.

Schaeffer AJ, et al: Infections of the Urinary Tract. In Wein AJ, editor: *Campbell-Walsh Urology* Philadelphia, 2015, Elsevier, pp 237–303.

Schappert SM: Ambulatory care visits of physician offices, hospital outpatient departments, and emergency departments: United States, 1995, *Vital Health Stat* 13:1–38, 1997.

BENIGN PROSTATIC HYPERPLASIA

Method of
Judd W. Moul, MD; and Brian M. Whitley, MD

Epidemiology

Benign prostatic hyperplasia (BPH) was generally a topic only of interest to urologists up to about 20 years ago, when several classes of medical therapy became available. Once widespread direct-to-consumer medical advertising hit the airwaves, the public's lexicon included "BPH" and men and their families were being educated about it. When combined with the aging population, the obesity epidemic, and subsequent health consequences, BPH becomes a very important disease process. As other countries have improved their standards of living, BPH has become one of the most common health conditions of the aging man worldwide.

From a practical standpoint, BPH and its symptoms are very uncommon before the age of 40 years. By ages 60 years and 85 years, the histologic prevalence of BPH at autopsy is 50% and 90%, respectively. The symptoms of BPH are now referred to as lower urinary tract symptoms (LUTS). At age 70 years, about 40% of men report LUTS and by age 75 years, the incidence of LUTS increases to 50%.

The diagnosis and treatment of BPH has always been in the realm of the specialty of urology, and this remains the case. However, as more medical and surgical therapies have been introduced and prostate-specific antigen (PSA) testing for prostate cancer has become commonplace, urologists are working more closely with internists, family physicians, generalists, and physician extenders to jointly manage these patients.

Pathophysiology

Even though BPH is common, we know very little about the true pathophysiology. However, we do know that men who were castrated before puberty do not develop BPH, and we also know that it is a progressive disease of aging. Before the 1980s, BPH was generally thought of as a static condition of a gradually growing prostate gland that caused progressive bladder outlet obstruction. In fact, it was common to use the "donut hole" analogy with patients, explaining to them that the prostate is like a donut surrounding the bladder neck and outlet. With aging and prostate growth, the donut hole gets smaller, causing progressive obstruction. In the era when transurethral resection of the prostate (TURP) was the only effective treatment, this simple static explanation was sufficient.

From the 1980s onward, our understanding has advanced to recognize that BPH has both a static obstructive and a dynamic component under neural control. The donut hole now has to have electrical wires attached to it with the ability to adjust the current. In addition, the contribution of the bladder to LUTS has been well recognized as a key contributor to the dynamic component of BPH and LUTS.

The static growth and proliferation of the periurethral tissue into BPH is under androgenic stimulation. Specifically, the main male hormone testosterone is converted to the more active metabolite dihydrotestosterone (DHT) by the enzyme 5α-reductase in the prostatic stromal and epithelial cells. 5α-Reductase occurs in two forms, type 1 and type 2. Only type 2 is present in the prostate and genitalia. This is critical for the understanding of one of the two main classes of medical therapy for BPH, the 5α-reductase inhibitors (5-ARIs), medications that block the conversion of testosterone to DHT.

The dynamic component of BPH and LUTS is based on autonomic input to the smooth muscles in the lower urinary tract, including the bladder, prostate, and urethra. These areas have a large concentration of α1-adrenergic receptors that, when stimulated, cause increased smooth muscle tone. This increased tone leads to increased urethral resistance and contributes to the bladder outlet obstructive symptoms of BPH. This physiology leads to the basis for the other main class of drugs to treat BPH, the α1-adrenergic blockers.

Symptoms

LUTS include urinary frequency, decreased force and caliber of the urinary stream, hesitancy, straining to void, urgency, and nocturia. The degree of impact may range from minimal bother to frank urinary retention with renal failure. Most urologists now use a standardized self-administered questionnaire, such as the International Prostate Symptom Score (IPSS) (Figure 1), to elicit symptoms and bother in a typical male population with suboptimal health-seeking behavior.

It is now very common for men to be referred to urology for a collection of age-related issues including elevated PSA, LUTS, BPH, or erectile dysfunction (ED). Commonly, the PSA or ED brings the patient to the attention of the healthcare system for the first time in years and may be the first opportunity to influence men on healthy living and health maintenance as they enter middle or older vulnerable ages. Recognizing this, all healthcare providers should keep this in mind and try to perform a broader men's health assessment while the patient is captive.

Diagnosis

The diagnosis of BPH is generally made based on symptoms or the IPSS standardized patient-self-administered questionnaire combined with a digital rectal examination, PSA blood test, urinalysis, and, in some cases, a cystoscopy. The differential diagnosis can include urinary tract infection (UTI), prostatitis, urinary stones in the lower urinary tract, urethral stricture disease, neurogenic or overactive bladder, prostate or bladder cancer, and even congestive heart failure. Some common medications, such as over-the-counter cold medicines containing α-adrenergic agents, can exacerbate LUTS and can even put a man into acute urinary retention if he has underlying BPH.

A properly performed digital rectal examination is critical to master in the diagnosis of BPH. Because the posterior prostate gland is located adjacent to the rectum and about 3 to 5 cm internal to the anus, the experienced clinician can gain valuable information. The authors prefer the patient to bend over the examining table with toes pointed slightly inward, the knees bent slightly forward, and the forehead and arms resting on the table. The examiner uses a liberally lubricated gloved index finger to palpate the posterior side of the prostate for size estimate and for any induration or nodularity that might indicate the presence of prostate cancer. In this case, referral to an urologist is mandatory.

The size of the prostate is measured either by estimating the weight in grams or the volume in cubic centimeters. Models have been developed to teach clinicians how to gauge size and consistency. In general, a normal size prostate is 20 to 25 g (or cm^3) in middle-aged men. A size of 25 to 30, 30 to 50, and greater than 50 g (or cm^3) is a general guide to mild, moderate, and severe BPH. However, size does not necessarily correlate to symptoms, and both symptom score and size estimate should be reported. The size gauges the histologic condition and the symptoms indicate the LUTS and the bother index, which are both important for individualized treatment.

The laboratory assessment should include a urinalysis to rule out hematuria. Like an abnormal digital rectal examination, a urinalysis that shows persistent red blood cells should prompt referral to a urologist for cystoscopic and upper urinary tract assessment. A urinalysis suggesting UTI should be followed up with a urine culture. If the patient presents in acute or chronic urinary retention and especially if there is a high postvoid or post-catheter residual bladder volume, a serum creatinine and blood urea nitrogen should be obtained. Severe BPH sometimes causes hydronephrosis and renal insufficiency, and rarely it causes renal failure. In-office bladder ultrasound scanners are very useful to quickly assess residual urine.

Contemporary diagnosis of BPH involves obtaining a PSA result. The latest guidelines from the American Urological Association (http://www.auanet.org) regarding the use of PSA testing are very helpful. Although the traditional upper limit of normal for PSA testing has been 4.0 ng/mL, recent guidelines base more on changes in PSA levels over time, considering that most men with BPH will have prior PSA results. In the specific setting of using PSA to help manage BPH, the best data come from the PLESS trial (Proscar Long-Term Efficacy and Safety Study), where a PSA of 0 to 1.3 ng/mL, 1.4 to 3.2 ng/mL, and greater than 3.2 ng/mL was associated with small, medium, and large prostate glands (assuming prostate cancer has been ruled out) and predicted therapeutic response to finasteride (Proscar) (see later section).

Treatment

Treatment of BPH is always individualized to the patient and involves evaluation of symptoms and bother along with objective findings from examination and laboratory results. Current treatments range from periodic monitoring without treatment to treatment of extreme cases with open enucleative surgery.

Active Surveillance and Watchful Waiting

For many men, especially those with lower symptom scores and little bother, annual monitoring with digital rectal examination, PSA, urinalysis, and symptom assessment are all that is required. Many men are happy to be reassured that they do not have clinically significant prostate cancer and are glad to hear that no immediate treatment is necessary.

Complementary and Alternative Medicine

The use of complementary and alternative medicine supplements is very common and physicians should ask patients about their use just as they ask about prescription medications. There are now many "prostate" and "men's health" supplements containing a variety of chemicals that include zinc[1], saw palmetto[7], vitamin E[1], vitamin D[1], and selenium[7], among others. Aside from a few European clinical trials of saw palmetto, the use of supplements to help BPH is speculative. One challenge is quality assurance of dose and ingredients of these agents that are not FDA-regulated. Although not for BPH, the NIH-funded SELECT trial (Selenium and Vitamin E Cancer Prevention Trial) to determine whether vitamin E or selenium, or both, would prevent prostate cancer is

---

[1] Not FDA approved for this indication.
[7] Available as dietary supplement.

International Prostate Symptom Score (I-PSS)

Patient Name: _____ Date of birth: _____ Date completed _____

In the past month:	Not at all	Less than 1 in 5 times	Less than half the time	About half the time	More than half the time	Almost always	Your score
1. Incomplete emptying How often have you had the sensation of not emptying your bladder?	0	1	2	3	4	5	
2. Frequency How often have you had to urinate less than every two hours?	0	1	2	3	4	5	
3. Intermittency How often have you found you stopped and started again several times when you urinated?	0	1	2	3	4	5	
4. Urgency How often have you found it difficult to postpone urination?	0	1	2	3	4	5	
5. Weak stream How often have you had a weak urinary stream?	0	1	2	3	4	5	
6. Straining How often have you had to strain to start urination?	0	1	2	3	4	5	
	None	1 Time	2 Times	3 Times	4 Times	5 Times	
7. Nocturia How many times did you typically get up at night to urinate?	0	1	2	3	4	5	
Total I-PSS score							

Score   1–7: *Mild*   8–19: *Moderate*   20–35: *Severe*

Quality of life due to urinary symptoms	Delighted	Pleased	Mostly satisfied	Mixed	Mostly dissatisfied	Unhappy	Terrible
If you were to spend the rest of your life with your urinary condition just the way it is now, how would you feel about that?	0	1	2	3	4	5	6

Figure 1 International Prostate Symptom Score (IPSS) questionnaire. (Available from the Urological Sciences Research Foundation at http://www.usrf.org/questionnaires/AUA_SymptomScore.html [accessed August 10, 2017].)

illustrative. Neither supplement had any effect on prostate cancer (or BPH to our knowledge). With the lack of robust trial data for the plethora of supplements, the evidence-based medicine answer to patients is clear.

Medical Therapy

α-Blocker Medications

The use of α-adrenergic blocking oral agents to treat BPH has been commonplace since the 1980s. These agents are directed at the dynamic component of BPH and LUTS by relaxing the smooth muscle tissue in the bladder neck and prostate. In simple terms, they relax the bladder outlet, resulting in better urinary flow.

Initial agents, such as prazosin (Minipress)[1], were not selective blockers and were also used to treat hypertension. Furthermore, these early agents were not long-acting and had to be taken multiple times per day, which severely limited their practical clinical utility. The next generation in the class were doxazosin (Cardura) and terazosin (Hytrin), which were longer-acting agents only dosed once a day. However, they were not selective and also lowered blood pressure, so titration was necessary. The third and current generation agents are selective blockers that treat BPH but do not lower blood pressure when used at recommended doses. The three in this class are tamsulosin (Flomax), alfuzosin (Uroxatral), and silodosin (Rapaflo).

In general, clinicians use α-blockers in men with smaller prostate glands (≤30 to 35 g or cm³), in younger men, and in patients where rapid effect is needed. Side effects of this class can include headache, dizziness, asthenia, drowsiness, and retrograde ejaculation, with alfuzosin reported to have the lowest rate of retrograde ejaculation among these drugs. The α-blockers are also now frequently used to relieve the dysfunctional voiding which is believed to contribute significantly to some cases of prostatitis.

[1] Not FDA approved for this indication.

5α-Reductase Inhibitors

The 5α-reductase inhibitors have been available since the early 1990s. Finasteride (Proscar) was the first agent in this class (5 mg/daily) and is a type 2 inhibitor. Dutasteride (Avodart; 0.5 mg/daily) is a type 1 and type 2 inhibitor and was approved in 2002. Both drugs prevent the conversion of testosterone to the more active metabolite DHT in the prostate. This inhibition results in involution of BPH tissue and prostate shrinkage. On average, most men achieve 20% to 40% reduction in prostate size after at least 6 months of use. In general, these agents are most effective in men with prostate glands more than 30 g (or cm³). Both drugs are expected to result in lower PSA levels by about 50% after 6 months of use. This is critical to take into account when screening for prostate cancer. If the PSA level does not fall by about one-half and the patient has been compliant with medication, the patient should be referred for urological evaluation. In follow-up of men on finasteride or dutasteride, PSA is generally doubled in assessing risk for prostate cancer. However, the use of PSA velocity or doubling-time and other prostate cancer screening tools are still valid as long as the effect on PSA is appreciated.

There are two key clinical trials that are important. The MTOPS trial (Medical Therapy of Prostate Symptoms) showed that the combination of an α-blocker (doxazosin) and a 5α-reductase inhibitor (finasteride) was more effective than either alone or placebo in treatment of BPH and LUTS. The PCPT (Prostate Cancer Prevention Trial) showed that finasteride lowered the rate of prostate cancer by 25% over placebo in a large 7-year study. The REDUCE trial (Reduction by Dutasteride of Prostate Cancer Events) confirmed the prostate chemoprevention benefit of this class of drugs, showing that dutasteride also lowered the rate of prostate cancer by 23% over placebo. In 2010 the FDA ruled that dutasteride would not be approved for prostate cancer prevention, citing safety concerns in this prevention setting. In 2013, the long-term follow up of the PCPT showed that there was no excess mortality associated with long-term finasteride use compared to placebo, proving the long term safety of this therapy.

Urologists frequently use 5α-reductase inhibitors to treat chronic hematuria due to an enlarged prostate after exclusion of more worrisome etiologies such as renal or bladder cancer and may also prescribe these agents before prostate surgeries or procedures for BPH to lessen surgical bleeding.

Minimally Invasive Procedures

In the past 35 years, a series of minimally invasive procedures have appeared in practice with the goals of reducing prostatic obstruction while preserving sexual function with normal erections and ejaculation. Balloon dilation, transurethral microwave therapy (TUMT), and transurethral needle ablation (TUNA) have all fallen from favor due to lack of durable effect in improving LUTS. Two newer minimally invasive procedures have, however, shown durability in multiyear randomized clinical trials. The prostatic urethral lift procedure (UroLift) utilizes small, permanently implanted anchors placed cystoscopically that physically retract and compress the obstructing lobes of the prostate and can provide near immediate improvement in flow rates and symptom scores. Alternatively, the Rezum thermal ablation procedure utilizes radiofrequency-generated water vapor (103°C) injected cystoscopically into the prostate tissue resulting in gradual resorption of treated prostate tissue and significant improvements in flow rates and symptom scores over the course of weeks following the procedure. Both procedures carry the benefits of very low rates of ED and retrograde ejaculation, however it remains unknown whether either procedure will provide long-lasting relief of LUTS similar to more invasive surgical procedures. High-intensity focused ultrasound was granted FDA approval in 2015 for ablation of prostate tissue, but has not gained wide use for BPH management and is more frequently utilized in the treatment of prostate cancer.

Surgical Therapy

Transurethral resection of prostate (TURP) remains the gold-standard treatment for men who have failed to improve on medical therapy, who dislike or are intolerant of medication side effects, or who have developed urinary retention, renal failure secondary to BPH, or large bladder calculi. TURP is associated with relatively low rates of incontinence and ED, however retrograde ejaculation is an expected permanent outcome for most men undergoing this surgery. Evolutions of the traditional TURP procedure now utilize saline irrigation thereby reducing the risk of hyponatremia during the procedure. Several laser technologies (Greenlight, Holmium, or Thulium) utilized for enucleation or vaporization of prostate tissue have resulted in reduction in hospital stay, transfusion rates, and catheter duration compared to TURP and are recommended treatment options for medically complex men requiring anticoagulant therapy. Finally, for men with severe BPH and very large glands (>150 g), simple prostatectomy performed robotically or via small suprapubic incision remains a valuable and highly effective surgical treatment. As with radical prostatectomy used for prostate cancer, open or robotic prostatectomy for BPH should be performed by urologic surgeons who are highly experienced in this area.

Summary

With the widespread acceptance of medical therapies for BPH in the 1980s and 1990s, treatment paradigms rapidly shifted away from surgical treatment of bothersome voiding symptoms. A growing number of studies have suggested an association between medical therapies for LUTS and development of dementia. These studies are controversial and preliminary, however it is common in my practice to encounter elderly men using two or three medications for management of symptoms. With the increasing awareness of the risks of polypharmacy and with the advent of new minimally based procedures for BPH, many of which can be performed in-office, the pendulum seems to be swinging back toward earlier consideration for surgical treatment of BPH.

References

Barkin J: Benign prostatic hyperplasia and lower urinary tract symptoms: evidence and approaches for best case management, *Can J Urol* (18 Suppl)14–19, 2011.

Biester K, Skipka G, Jahn R, et al: Systematic review of surgical treatments for benign prostatic hyperplasia and presentation of an approach to investigate therapeutic equivalence (non-inferiority), *BJU Int* 109:722–730, 2012.

Dahm P, Brasure M, MacDonald R, et al: Comparative effectiveness of newer medications for lower urinary tract symptoms attributed to benign prostatic hyperplasia: a systemic review and meta-analysis, *Eur Urol* 71:570–581, 2017.

Djavan B, Kazzazi A, Bostanci Y: Revival of thermotherapy for benign prostatic hyperplasia, *Curr Opin Urol* 22:16–21, 2012.

Gravas S, Bachmann A, Reich O, et al: Critical review of lasers in benign prostatic hyperplasia (BPH), *BJU Int* 107:1030–1043, 2011.

Lepor H, Kazzazi A, Djavan B: α-Blockers for benign prostatic hyperplasia: the new era, *Curr Opin Urol* 22:7–15, 2012.

Nicholson TM, Ricke WA: Androgens and estrogens in benign prostatic hyperplasia: past, present and future, *Differentiation* 82:184–199, 2011.

Roehrborn C, Barkin J, Gange S, et al: Five year results of the prospective randomized controlled prostatic urethral L.I.F.T. study, *Can J Urol* 24(3):8802–8813, 2017.

Roehrborn C, Gange S, Gittelman M, et al: Convective thermal therapy: durable 2-year results of randomized controlled and prospective crossover studies for treatment of lower urinary tract symptoms due to benign prostatic hyperplasia, *J Urol* 197(6):1507–1516, 2017.

Slater S, Dumas C, Bubley G: Dutasteride for the treatment of prostate-related conditions, *Expert Opin Drug Saf* 11:325–330, 2012.

EPIDIDYMITIS AND ORCHITIS

Method of
Robin A. Walker, MD

CURRENT DIAGNOSIS

- Subacute or gradual onset of scrotal pain and swelling that occasionally radiates to lower abdomen. Typically unilateral; however, inflammation can spread to opposite testicle.

- Fever and urinary tract symptoms (e.g., dysuria, frequency, urgency, hematuria) may be present.
- Testicle should be in normal position with cremasteric reflex intact (rule out torsion).
- Pain is relieved by elevation of testicle (Prehn sign).
- Ultrasound with Doppler is readily available and has high sensitivity and specificity for ruling out testicular torsion; however, referral to urology should not be delayed if torsion is suspected.
- Urinalysis should be obtained, preferably on first-void urine.
- Send urine for culture, especially when sexually transmitted disease (STD) is not suspected.
- Nucleic acid amplification assays for *Gonorrhea* and *Chlamydia* can be run on urine or urethral specimens.

 ## CURRENT THERAPY

- Sexually active men 14 to 35 years old: ceftriaxone (Rocephin)[1] 250 mg IM once and doxycycline (Vibramycin)[1] 100 mg twice daily for 10 days. Azithromycin (Zithromax)[1] 1 g PO for one dose may be substituted for doxycycline if compliance is questionable.
- Oral cephalosporins and fluoroquinolones are no longer recommended for gonococcal infections.
- For older men or when enteric organisms are thought to be the most likely cause: levofloxacin (Levaquin)[1] 500 mg orally twice daily for 10 days, or ofloxacin (Floxin)[1] 300 mg orally twice daily for 10 days.
- Cultures, if obtained, should be followed and treatment adjusted accordingly.
- Patients should follow up in 2 to 3 days. Pain should improve in 1 to 3 days with treatment. Failure to improve should elicit reevaluation of the diagnosis and therapy, and consideration should be given to other causes such as a testicular tumor/cancer, abscess, infarction, and tuberculosis (TB) or fungal pathogens.
- Sexual partners should be referred for evaluation and treatment if there was intercourse in the preceding 60 days from onset of symptoms.
- Education should occur regarding prevention of STDs.

[1]Not US Food and Drug Administration (FDA) approved for this indication.

Epidemiology

Epididymitis is most common in males 18 to 35 years of age, but can occur in all ages. There are approximately 600,000 cases per year in the United States, and these accounted for 1 in 144 outpatient visits in men (2002 data).

In men 35 years of age or younger who are sexually active, the most common pathogens are *Chlamydia trachomatis* and *Neisseria gonorrhoeae*. In those older than 35, the cause is most likely urinary tract pathogens such as *Escherichia coli*. In men who perform insertive anal intercourse, coliform bacteria are common causative agents. Other less common pathogens include TB, fungal infections, and viruses. Cytomegalovirus has been identified as a cause in patients with HIV.

In boys ages 2 to 13 the incidence is approximately 1.2 per 1000 and is most commonly a postinfectious inflammatory reaction to pathogens such as enteroviruses, adenoviruses, and mycoplasma pneumonia. If a bacterial pathogen is isolated, a urologic workup for any anatomic abnormalities is warranted.

Other uncommon noninfectious causes of epididymitis include vasculitides and medications such as amiodarone (Pacerone).

Orchitis is less common than epididymitis and is most often associated with concurrent epididymitis, occurring in approximately 60% of men with epididymitis. In prepubertal boys, orchitis is usually a sequela of mumps infection. Between 20% and 30% of men with mumps develop orchitis.

Risk Factors

The predominant risk factor for epididymitis is unprotected sexual intercourse. Additionally, trauma from strenuous physical activity, bicycle or motorcycle riding, and prolonged sitting can predispose to epididymitis. Risk factors in prepubertal boys and men over age 35 are related to anatomic abnormalities (e.g., prostatic obstruction, posterior urethral valves, meatal stenosis), recent instrumentation, or urogenital tract surgery (e.g., vasectomy). In prepubertal boys, recent infections can predispose to a postinfectious inflammatory reaction in the epididymis.

Pathophysiology

Infective epididymitis is usually caused by retrograde ascent of pathogens, most commonly bacterial. Noninfectious epididymitis can be autoimmune or can be associated with known syndromes (e.g., Behçet disease) or a side effect of medications, most notably amiodarone (Pacerone). If symptoms last longer than 3 months, the patient meets the diagnostic criteria for chronic epididymitis.

Clinical Manifestations

The typical presentation is subacute onset of unilateral scrotal pain. Any acute onset of pain requires careful consideration of possible testicular torsion. The pain in epididymitis can radiate to the lower abdomen. Fever and urinary tract symptoms such as increased frequency, dysuria, and hematuria are frequently present. The cremasteric reflex is preserved and the testicle should be in its normal anatomic position. The epididymis is tender, swollen, and often indurated. Pain is relieved on testicular elevation (Prehn sign). Over time, scrotal wall erythema and a reactive hydrocele may appear and infection can spread from the epididymis to the testicle (orchitis), as well as to the opposite testicle.

Epididymitis secondary to noninfectious causes tends to have a more gradual onset of symptoms.

Viral orchitis from mumps is characterized by abrupt onset of unilateral testicular pain with swelling that typically occurs between 4 and 7 days after the development of parotitis. About 75% of patients with orchitis will also have fever and one third will complain of dysuria.

Diagnosis

Diagnosis can be made by a careful history and physical examination; however, laboratory testing can help confirm epididymitis. Urine should be obtained for analysis and culture, preferably from a first-void sample. The presence of leukocyte esterase and 10 or more white blood cells (WBCs) per high-power field is suggestive for urethritis, helping to differentiate from testicular torsion.

Nucleic acid amplification tests for *N. gonorrhoeae* and *C. trachomatis* should be run on all sexually active men 35 years of age or younger and those over 35 who are at increased risk. These can be run on urine or urethral samples. A Gram stain of urethral discharge should demonstrate 5 or more WBCs per high-power field. Gonococcal infection is established by the presence of WBCs containing intracellular gram-negative diplococci. Depending on risks, consideration should be given to testing for the presence of other STDs.

Color Doppler ultrasound is a readily available study with a sensitivity and specificity for testicular torsion ranging between 89% and 100%. However, imaging should not delay immediate referral to a specialist if torsion is clinically suspected.

Differential Diagnosis

- Testicular torsion: duration less than 6 hours, absence of cremasteric reflex, diffuse testicular tenderness. Elevation of the testis usually exacerbates discomfort.
- Orchitis: testicular tenderness and swelling, normal cremasteric reflex.

Therapy/Treatment

In sexually active men ages 14 to 35, empiric treatment should be started for suspected epididymitis before laboratory results are available. The current recommended regimen is ceftriaxone (Rocephin)[1] 250 mg IM once plus doxycycline (Vibramycin)[1] 100 mg orally twice daily for 10 days. If compliance is questionable or the patient is allergic to doxycycline, azithromycin (Zithromax)[1] 1 g orally once can be substituted. The Centers for Disease Control and Prevention (CDC) no longer recommends fluoroquinolones or oral cephalosporins for the treatment of gonococcal infections.

For men 35 years of age or older, and when a coliform pathogen is suspected, treatment consists of levofloxacin (Levaquin)[1] 500 mg orally for 10 days or ofloxacin (Floxin)[1] 300 mg orally twice daily for 10 days.

Most patients can be treated in the outpatient setting. Inpatient treatment is recommended for suspicion of abscess, intractable pain, signs of sepsis, or failure of outpatient care. Symptomatic care consists of pain control with supportive garments, analgesics, rest, and cold packs.

Orchitis, when not associated with epididymitis infection, is typically treated in a supportive manner with hot or cold packs, rest, nonsteroidal antiinflammatory drugs, and scrotal elevation. Symptoms from viral-associated orchitis typically resolve in 3 to 10 days.

Complications

Complications include sepsis, abscess formation, extension of infection, and infertility.

---

[1] Not FDA approved for this indication.

References

Centers for Disease Control and Prevention: *Sexually transmitted diseases treatment guidelines*, 2010. Available at http://www.cdc.gov/std/treatment/2010/epididymitis.htm. [accessed 08.09.14].

Centers for Disease Control and Prevention: Update to CDC's sexually transmitted diseases treatment guidelines, 2006; fluoroquinolones no longer recommended for treatment of gonococcal infections, *MMWR Morb Mortal Wkly Rep* 56:332–336, 2007.

Centers for Disease Control and Prevention: Update to CDC's sexually transmitted diseases treatment guidelines, 2010; oral cephalosporins no longer recommended treatment for gonococcal infections, *MMWR Morb Mortal Wkly Rep* 61:590–594, 2012.

Kaver I, Matzkin H, Braf ZF: Epididymo-orchitis: A retrospective study of 121 patients, *J Fam Pract* 30:548–552, 1990.

Remer EM, Casalino DD, Arellano RS, et al: ACR appropriateness criteria; acute onset of scrotal pain—without trauma, without antecedent mass, *Ultrasound Q* 28:47–51, 2012.

Trojian TH, Lishnak TS, Meiman D: Epididymitis and orchitis: An overview, *Am Fam Physician* 79:583–587, 2009.

ERECTILE DYSFUNCTION

Method of
Aleksandr Belakovskiy, MD; Joel J. Heidelbaugh, MD; and Karl T. Rew, MD

CURRENT DIAGNOSIS

- Questionnaire
  - Sexual Health Inventory for Men (SHIM) [also called International Index of Erectile Function (IIEF-5)] https://www.baus.org.uk/_userfiles/pages/files/Patients/Leaflets/SHIM.pdf
- Assessment of risk factors
  - Tobacco use
  - Diabetes
  - Hypertension
  - Hyperlipidemia
- Obesity
- Iatrogenic causes
- Psychogenic causes
- Physical exam including vitals, body mass index (BMI), genital exam, and assessment for secondary sex characteristics
- Relationship between erectile dysfunction, endothelial dysfunction, and coronary heart disease

CURRENT THERAPY

- Lifestyle modifications including tobacco cessation, weight loss, increased exercise
- Sexual health counseling
- Medication modification if taking medications known to contribute to erectile dysfunction
- Pharmacotherapy (Table 1)
  - Oral phosphodiesterase type 5 (PDE-5) inhibitors: avanafil (Stendra), sildenafil (Viagra), tadalafil (Cialis), and vardenafil (Levitra, Staxyn)
  - Prostaglandin: alprostadil; either by intracavernosal injection (Caverject, Edex) or as an intraurethral suppository (Muse)
    - Requires a test dose in the office and instruction on technique for proper administration
- Vacuum erectile devices
- Referral for surgical management
  - Penile implants

Erectile dysfunction is the inability to attain or maintain a penile erection sufficient for sexual satisfaction.

Epidemiology

Numerous studies have investigated the prevalence of erectile dysfunction in men of various ages. Based on the most recent studies, worldwide prevalence increases with age. For men under age 40 the prevalence is 1% to 10%; for ages 40 to 49 it is 2% to 15%; for men ages 50 to 59 it is mixed, ranging from 15% to 40%; for ages 60 to 69 it is 20% to 40%; and for men 70 and older it is 50% to 100%. Among men in the United States the prevalence is 22% overall. This is higher than the 16% prevalence for seven other countries found in a study comparing the United States to Brazil, Mexico, United Kingdom, Germany, France, Italy, and Spain. Accurate diagnosis of erectile dysfunction has varied over time, with current literature favoring the use of validated questionnaires such as the Sexual Health Inventory for Men (SHIM; https://www.baus.org.uk/_userfiles/pages/files/Patients/Leaflets/SHIM.pdf).

Risk Factors

A number of medical conditions can predispose to erectile dysfunction. Numerous studies have demonstrated the correlation between cardiovascular disease and the incidence of erectile dysfunction. Risk factors that predispose to cardiovascular disease also play similar roles in erectile dysfunction, including increasing age, diabetes, hypertension, hyperlipidemia, tobacco use, and obesity.

Certain classes of medications can contribute to the development of erectile dysfunction. One of the most common is the antidepressants, specifically selective serotonin reuptake inhibitors (SSRIs) and serotonin norepinephrine reuptake inhibitors (SNRIs). Common antihypertensive medications can also contribute to or exacerbate erectile dysfunction, including beta blockers, alpha blockers, calcium channel blockers, and thiazides. Other medication classes that should be considered in patients with erectile dysfunction include opiates, first-generation antihistamines, and benzodiazepines.

Risk factors for psychogenic erectile dysfunction should also be evaluated. Psychogenic erectile dysfunction can occur at any age, but it is frequently seen in men under age 40, and it often occurs in men with anxiety, stress, depression, or a history of sexual abuse. Assess for healthy sexual partnerships by asking about performance anxiety and sexual desire discrepancy, both of which are common contributors to erectile dysfunction. Clues that erectile dysfunction may have a psychogenic component include the ability to have normal erections with masturbation, and the continued presence of nocturnal erections. If needed for evaluation, nocturnal tumescence testing can be performed.

Tobacco, alcohol, opioids, and substances such as marijuana and cocaine can cause erectile dysfunction. All substance use should be assessed. Many other health issues can contribute to erectile dysfunction, including a history of prostate or pelvic surgery, radiation therapy, or trauma; gonadal, thyroid, or other diseases that affect hormone levels; testicular pain; and chronic diseases that affect general health and well-being.

Pathophysiology
The pathophysiology of erectile dysfunction depends on the etiology of the condition. Many men have multiple potential causes. Psychogenic erectile dysfunction is due to nonorganic causes, while individuals with risk factors for cardiovascular disease primarily have etiologies stemming from vascular disease. Iatrogenic erectile dysfunction due to medication use or prior surgery may be caused by inhibition of the parasympathetic nervous system or other mechanisms of action.

Erectile dysfunction can be a warning sign of silent cardiovascular disease. The relationship between erectile dysfunction and the risk factors for coronary heart disease was noted in the Massachusetts Male Aging Study. The endothelial dysfunction that can precede the clinical stage of atherosclerotic disease is recognized as an additional risk factor for erectile dysfunction in men without symptoms of cardiovascular disease. Endothelial function is mediated by nitric oxide, which is also the mechanism responsible for the vascular dilatation required to obtain and maintain an erection. A man with erectile dysfunction should be considered at risk for cardiovascular disease until proven otherwise.

Prevention
Erectile dysfunction prevention is centered around treating modifiable risk factors. Treatment of overweight and obesity with dietary changes and increased aerobic exercise can aid in the prevention of erectile dysfunction. For tobacco users, cessation should be strongly encouraged. Bupropion (Zyban) and varenicline (Chantix) can be used for smoking cessation with limited risk of exacerbating erectile dysfunction. Nicotine replacement therapy can be used as a bridge to help with tobacco cessation. Appropriate treatment of comorbid diseases, including diabetes, hypertension, and hyperlipidemia can also aid in prevention. Sexual health counseling that focuses on good partner communication and healthy relationship dynamics can help prevent psychogenic erectile dysfunction.

Clinical Manifestations
Many men are uncomfortable mentioning problems of sexual function. Some men will report erectile dysfunction without providing information on the specifics of their concern. It is important for physicians to proactively ask about sexual function, and to clarify if a patient's concern is with achieving or maintaining an erection, or if it may be related to ejaculation or low libido. Low libido can be secondary to stress, mood disorders, hypogonadism, or other causes. The evaluation and potential treatments will differ based on the specific concern. Questionnaires such as the SHIM (https://www.baus.org.uk/_userfiles/pages/files/Patients/Leaflets/SHIM.pdf) can provide additional information to help distinguish the specific clinical manifestation.

Diagnosis
The history provides the majority of information needed for the diagnostic evaluation, including a review of known medical and surgical history, use of medications and substances, an assessment of current relationship satisfaction, and a questionnaire such as the SHIM. The history should include risk factor evaluation, assessment for any history of cardiovascular disease, diabetes, hypertension, hyperlipidemia, or mood disorders, as well as a review of medications that might contribute to erectile dysfunction. A physical exam should also be performed, including evaluation of blood pressure, body mass index, secondary sex characteristics, and a genital exam.

The role of laboratory studies is limited. In individuals who lack secondary sex characteristics, as well as those with refractory symptoms despite PDE-5 inhibitor use, check a morning total testosterone to assess for hypogonadism. Limited evidence supports obtaining a morning total testosterone in all men with erectile dysfunction. If the initial morning total testosterone is low, it should be repeated at least once in several months to confirm the diagnosis. If morning testosterone levels are normal in a patient with high likelihood of hypogonadism, a free testosterone or bioavailable testosterone can be checked to help account for the effects of sex hormone–binding globulin. If evidence of hypogonadism is found, additional testing to distinguish primary versus secondary hypogonadism should be done. Hemoglobin A1c and a lipid panel may be helpful if there is a suspicion for underlying diabetes, hyperlipidemia, or cardiovascular disease contributing to erectile dysfunction. If a review of symptoms elicits a suspicion for hypothyroidism, checking a thyroid stimulating hormone level may be indicated. Consultation with a urologist, endocrinologist, or men's health specialist may be helpful when the etiology is unclear.

Differential Diagnosis
In men presenting with concern for erectile dysfunction, the differential diagnosis is geared toward deciphering the underlying cause. As previously mentioned, there are numerous potential contributing factors to erectile dysfunction. It is important to assess for both organic and psychogenic causes. The history should include asking about nocturnal tumescence, as well as the ability to achieve and maintain an erection with and without a partner. If erectile dysfunction occurs regardless of situation, this is more likely to indicate an organic etiology. If it occurs primarily with a partner, further evaluation of the relationship is indicated. As mentioned above, numerous factors can predispose to erectile dysfunction, and related diagnoses may include cardiovascular disease, tobacco use, diabetes, hypertension, hyperlipidemia, obesity, and metabolic syndrome. Medications should also be reviewed, because they can cause iatrogenic erectile dysfunction in some patients.

Therapy (or Treatment)
Lifestyle modifications play an important role in both the prevention and treatment of erectile dysfunction. Weight reduction for overweight or obese men (BMI >25 kg/m^2) and increased exercise for all men can improve SHIM scores. Underlying illnesses such as hyperlipidemia, hypertension, and diabetes should be adequately controlled in order to decrease their potential impact on erectile dysfunction. Another important consideration is tobacco cessation; current or former smoking increases the risk of erectile dysfunction. Sexual health counseling is often helpful for individuals and couples dealing with erectile dysfunction, no matter what the etiology is. Referral to a mental health professional or sexuality expert may be beneficial.

Pharmacologic treatment begins with oral PDE-5 inhibitors. They prevent the breakdown of cyclic guanosine monophosphate (cGMP) and allow increased nitric oxide levels, causing smooth muscle relaxation of the corpora cavernosa, and helping to sustain an erection. This requires a functional libido as well as intact vasculature in order to achieve an erection. There are four PDE-5 inhibitors currently approved in the United States for treatment of erectile dysfunction: avanafil (Stendra), sildenafil (Viagra), tadalafil (Cialis), and vardenafil (Levitra, Staxyn) (see Table 1). There are no significant differences in safety or benefit among these medications. Tadalafil has a longer duration of action than the others.

TABLE 1 Pharmacotherapy for Erectile Dysfunction

GENERIC NAMES	BRAND NAMES	SIZES	TYPICAL DOSING	COMMENTS
Oral Phosphodiesterase Type 5 (PDE-5) Inhibitors				
avanafil	Stendra	50-, 100-, 200-mg tablet	50–200 mg by mouth once daily as needed, 1 h before sexual activity	Use lowest effective dose. Contraindicated with nitrates.
sildenafil	Viagra	25-, 50-, 100-mg tablet	25–100 mg by mouth once daily as needed, 1 h before sexual activity	Use lowest effective dose. Contraindicated with nitrates.
tadalafil	Cialis	2.5-, 5-, 10-, 20-mg tablet	5–20 mg by mouth once daily as needed, 1 h before sexual activity OR 2.5–5 mg by mouth once daily without regard to sexual activity	Use lowest effective dose. Contraindicated with nitrates. Has a longer duration of action than other PDE-5 inhibitors.
vardenafil	Levitra Staxyn	5-, 10-, 20-mg tablet 10-mg oral dissolving tablet	5–20 mg by mouth once daily as needed, 1 h before sexual activity	Use lowest effective dose. Contraindicated with nitrates. Available as a 10 mg oral dissolving tablet (Staxyn)
Prostaglandin				
alprostadil injectable	Caverject 20 mcg/mL, 40 mcg/mL vials	Caverject Impulse 10 mcg/0.5 mL, 20 mcg/0.5 mL prefilled syringes Edex 10 mcg/mL, 20 mcg/mL, 40 mcg/mL cartridges	Initiate dose at 1.25 or 2.5 mcg intracavernosally and titrate does with no more than 2 doses per 24 hours (maximum dose: 40 mcg [Edex], 60 mcg [Caverject]). Self administration: maximum 3 times/week with 24 hours between doses	Provide an in-office test dose and instruction in proper technique for administration. Use lowest effective dose.
alprostadil intraurethral	Muse	125-, 250-, 500-, 1000-mcg urethral suppositories	Initiate dose at 125 or 250 mcg intraurethrally and titrate dose on separate occasions in physician's office. Maximum 2 suppositories per 24 hours for self-administration	Provide an in-office test dose and instruction in proper technique for administration. Use lowest effective dose.

PDE-5 inhibitors are usually taken on an as-needed basis, with onset of effects typically within about 1 hour of ingestion. The lowest effective dose should be used to reduce the risk of adverse reactions. Higher doses do not lead to a linear increase in beneficial effect, but can increase the risk of adverse reactions. Tadalafil, because of its longer duration of action, can be taken daily at a lower dose with similar efficacy to as-needed dosing. The duration of adverse effects may be longer with daily use.

The most common adverse reactions to PDE-5 inhibitors include headache, flushing, dyspepsia, dizziness, nasal congestion, visual disturbance, and myalgias. Overall, these adverse reactions tend to be mild to moderate in nature and are similar across all four medications. Special consideration should be given to individuals who take nitrate-containing medications; the combination of a PDE-5 inhibitor with nitrates can cause severe hypotension that may be life threatening.

Testosterone is not an effective monotherapy for erectile dysfunction. However, for men with confirmed hypogonadism, the combination of a PDE-5 inhibitor with testosterone replacement may be effective.

If patients do not have adequate symptom relief with lifestyle modification, sexual health counseling, and oral PDE-5 inhibitor use, the prostaglandin alprostadil (Caverject, Edex, Muse) can be considered. Alprostadil works by relaxing arterial smooth muscle and is available in intraurethral and injectable preparations (see Table 1). The intraurethral formulation (Muse) is a dissolvable suppository placed in the urethra with an applicator. The injectable form (Caverject, Edex) is injected directly into one side of the corpora cavernosa. Alprostadil can be used as a single agent or in combination with a PDE-5 inhibitor. If the patient is amenable to a trial of alprostadil, an in-office test dose should be administered to find the lowest effective dose and to teach proper administration technique. Some patients may not be suitable candidates if they are not comfortable with injections or intraurethral insertion. Alprostadil should be avoided in patients who have sickle cell anemia or other risk factors for priapism.

If pharmacological therapies are ineffective or contraindicated, patients may elect to use a vacuum erectile device. These prescription devices are placed over the penis and a vacuum pump removes air from inside the device, creating an influx of blood into the penis and leading to an erection. A ring is then slid from the base of the vacuum tube onto the penis to constrict the outflow of blood and maintain the erection. To avoid ischemic injury, the ring should only be used for up to 30 minutes. Adverse effects of vacuum erectile devices may include the erect penis feeling cool or cold to the touch due to the restricted blood flow, and bending at the base of the penis due to the application of the constricting ring. Overall, these devices have a fairly high satisfaction rate. Caution should be used when considering a vacuum erectile device for patients who are taking anticoagulants or have bleeding disorders.

For patients with erectile dysfunction refractory to the above treatments, surgical implantation of a penile prosthesis can be offered. Penile prostheses come in several forms, including inflatable devices and persistently semirigid implants. Patients and their partners should be counseled regarding risks and benefits to ensure realistic postsurgical expectations. Risks include scarring, penile shortening, recurrent infections, and mechanical failure requiring removal.

Monitoring
A validated questionnaire such as the SHIM (https://www.baus.org.uk/_userfiles/pages/files/Patients/Leaflets/SHIM.pdf) is a simple and reliable tool for monitoring ongoing symptoms. A periodic clinical evaluation, including a review of all supplements and medications, can be helpful to identify potential causes of symptoms and any adverse reactions.

Management of Complications
The majority of adverse reactions with PDE-5 inhibitors are mild to moderate in nature and can be limited by using the lowest effective dose. PDE-5 inhibitors are contraindicated in

patients taking nitrates because of the significant risk of life-threatening hypotension. If accidentally ingested, the patient should be monitored by healthcare professionals. The risk also depends on which specific agent was ingested, as the duration of action differs between medications. While the risk of prolonged erection (priapism) is low with PDE-5 inhibitors, men with erections lasting greater than 4 hours should seek emergency attention.

The major potential complication of alprostadil is a prolonged erection lasting greater than 4 hours, which will require emergent urological treatment. Penile fibrosis is also a risk that has been reported in 4.9% of patients using alprostadil at 4 years.

Treatment with exogenous testosterone impairs spermatogenesis and should be avoided in men who are trying to conceive or are interested in future fertility.

The major complication of vacuum erectile devices is ischemic injury, generally when the constricting ring is left in place for greater than 30 minutes at a time. Any suspicion for ischemic injury should also prompt emergent urologic intervention.

Patients with penile implants are prone to recurrent infections or mechanical failure, potentially requiring removal of the device.

References

Burnett AL, Nehra A, Breau RH, et al: Erectile dysfunction: AUA Guideline, J Urol 200(3):633–641, 2018 Sep, Available at: https://doi.org/10.1016/j.juro.2018.05.004, Epub 2018 May 7.

Buvat J, Büttner H, Hatzimouratidis K, et al: Adherence to initial PDE-5 inhibitor treatment: randomized open-label study comparing tadalafil once a day, tadalafil on demand, and sildenafil on demand in patients with erectile dysfunction, J Sex Med 10(6):1592–1602, 2013.

Costa P, Grandmottet G, Mai HD, Droupy S: Impact of a first treatment with phosphodiesterase inhibitors on men and partners' quality of sexual life: results of a prospective study in primary care, J Sex Med 10(7):1850–1860, 2013.

Ghanem HM, Salonia A, Martin-Morales A: SOP: physical examination and laboratory testing for men with erectile dysfunction, J Sex Med 10(1):108–110, 2013.

Khayyamfar F, Forootan SK, Ghasemi H, Miri SR, Farhadi E: Evaluating the efficacy of vacuum constrictive device and causes of its failure in impotent patients, Urol J 10(4):1072–1078, 2014.

Martin-Morales A, Haro JM, Beardsworth A, Bertsch J, Kontodimas S: Therapeutic effectiveness and patient satisfaction after 6 months of treatment with tadalafil, sildenafil, and vardenafil: results from the erectile dysfunction observational study (EDOS), Eur Urol 51(2):541–550, 2007.

Mccabe MP, Sharlip ID, Lewis R, et al: Incidence and prevalence of sexual dysfunction in women and men: a consensus statement from the Fourth International Consultation on Sexual Medicine 2015, J Sex Med 13(2):144–152, 2016.

Mulhall JP, Trost LW, Brannigan RE, et al: Evaluation and management of testosterone deficiency: AUA Guideline, J Urol 200(2):423–432, 2018 Aug, Available at: https://doi.org/10.1016/j.juro.2018.03.115, Epub 2018 Mar 28.

Rosen RC, Fisher WA, Eardley I, et al: The multinational Men's Attitudes to Life Events and Sexuality (MALES) study: I. Prevalence of erectile dysfunction and related health concerns in the general population, Curr Med Res Opin 20(5):607–617, 2004.

Selvin E, Burnett AL, Platz EA: Prevalence and risk factors for erectile dysfunction in the US, Am J Med 120(2):151–157, 2007.

PROSTATE CANCER

Method of
William G. Nelson, MD, PhD

CURRENT DIAGNOSIS

- Serum prostate-specific antigen (PSA) testing, with or without digital rectal examination (DRE), can be used for prostate cancer screening for men beginning at age 50 years until age 70 years.
- Prostate cancer screening carries significant risks of over-diagnosis and over-treatment of clinically insignificant prostate cancers.
- The diagnosis of prostate cancer is usually made via ultrasound-guided transrectal core needle biopsies that sample the prostate; magnetic resonance imaging (MRI) is increasingly used to direct core biopsies to regions of the prostate suspicious for harboring aggressive prostate cancers.

- Histologic grade (Gleason score) and anatomic stage carry prognostic information needed for treatment decision making.
- Metastatic prostate cancer can be evaluated using 99mTc-methylene diphosphonate (MDP) of 18F-sodium fluoride (NaF) bone scans, abdominopelvic computed tomography (CT) scan or magnetic resonance imaging (MRI), and 11C-choline or 18F-fluciclovine positron emission tomography (PET) studies

CURRENT THERAPY

- Options for management of localized prostate cancer include active surveillance, radical prostatectomy, external beam radiation therapy, brachytherapy, and proton radiotherapy.
- Androgen deprivation therapy (ADT) using gonadotrophic hormone-releasing hormone analogs is a mainstay of systemic prostate cancer treatment.
- CYP17 inhibitors and androgen receptor antagonists can be used to further ablate androgen signaling in castration-resistant prostate cancer (CRPC).
- Taxane chemotherapy, given along with ADT for hormone-sensitive metastatic prostate cancer or at the time of progression to CRPC, improves survival.
- The α–particle-emitting calcium mimetic 223Ra can palliate painful bony metastases.
- Poly(ADP-ribose) polymerase (PARP) inhibitors may be effective in up to 20% of men with CRPC who carry germline and/or somatic mutations in homologous recombination repair genes (BRCA1, BRCA2, ATM, and others).

Prostate cancer comprises the most commonly diagnosed cancer among men in the United States, with an estimated 174,650 new cases and 31,620 deaths expected for 2019. Some 1 in 8 men can expect to be diagnosed with prostate cancer at some point during life, though the risk of dying from the disease is only about 1 in 37. African-American men suffer disproportionately with the disease, exhibiting more than twice the age-adjusted mortality as Caucasians.

The prostate itself is a male sex accessory gland located adjacent to the rectum in the pelvis and surrounding the urethra to supply secretions to the ejaculate. Why it should spawn so many cancers has proven enigmatic. The prostate can be divided into three zones, a *peripheral zone* where most prostate cancers arise, a *transition zone* near the urethra prone to benign enlargement (benign prostatic hyperplasia/hypertrophy [BPH]), and a *central zone*. Under the influence of the male androgenic hormones testosterone (T) and dihydrotestosterone (DHT), normal epithelial cells produce the serine protease prostate-specific antigen (PSA; encoded by the gene *KLK3*). The appearance of PSA in the bloodstream tends to indicate epithelial barrier dysfunction within the prostate, attributable to three highly prevalent conditions in aging men in the US: inflammation (prostatitis), BPH, or prostate cancer. Blood testing for PSA has emerged as a common screening tactic for prostate cancer, necessarily confounded by the near ubiquitous coexistence of prostatitis and BPH.

Most men present with prostate cancer apparently confined to the prostate gland, often detected by PSA screening. Though usually indolent, when aggressive, prostate cancer tends to spread to bony sites, causing pain by undermining bone architecture through stimulating osteoblastic activity, a phenomenon readily evident via 99mTc-methylene diphosphonate (MDP) of 18F-sodium fluoride (NaF) bone scanning. Men dying of prostate cancer also manifest metastasis to lymph nodes, liver, the dura, and elsewhere.

Men diagnosed with prostate cancer today confront a large and often confusing array of treatment options. The typical man diagnosed with the disease is at least 65 years of age or older; the risks and benefits associated with different treatment choices in this age range are relevant not only for prostate cancer specialty care, but for general medical care as well. The 5-year survival for a man with localized prostate cancer is >95%, underscoring the need for balancing prostate cancer treatment selection with other health priorities.

Epidemiology

Heredity plays as significant a role in prostate cancer development as for any other common cancer. Analyses of concordance for prostate cancer between monozygotic (identical) versus dizygotic (fraternal) twins have consistently found excess prostate cancers among the identical twins despite similar environmental exposures, leading to the estimate that as many as 42% of prostate cancer cases may be attributable to inheritance. Two sets of inherited susceptibility genes merit special attention for prostate cancer treatment. Germline defects in DNA double-strand break repair genes, such as *BRCA1*, *BRCA2*, *ATM*, and others, or in DNA mismatch repair genes, such as *MSH2*, *MLH1*, MSH6, and *PMS2*, may increase the risk of developing prostate cancer or of exhibiting metastatic prostate cancer progression. Defective DNA repair in prostate cells has important treatment implications. When germline DNA repair gene defects are accompanied by somatic alterations at the remaining allele, crippling of DNA double-strand break repair can serve as an indication for treatment with poly(ADP-ribose) polymerase (PARP) inhibitors, while loss of DNA mismatch repair constitutes an indication for treatment with immune checkpoint inhibitors. With a growing role in prostate cancer treatment decision making, germline testing for DNA repair gene defects has become increasingly common for men with the disease. Of course, the detection of defective DNA repair genes in a man with prostate cancer should also alert his physician to consider cascade genetic testing of relatives as abnormal repair gene carriers could be at risk for breast, ovarian, colorectal, or other cancers.

Evidence for a critical contribution of the environment to prostate cancer is as strong as is the case for an impact of heredity. Prostate cancer incidence and mortality vary widely throughout the world, and migrants from low-risk regions to high-risk regions tend to adopt higher prostate cancer predilection within a single generation. Whether the high rates of prostate cancer in the US reflect ingestion of food carcinogens, such as the heterocyclic amines and polycyclic aromatic hydrocarbons in over-cooked meats (known to cause prostate cancer in rodents), or reflect inadequate intake of tomatoes and cruciferous vegetables, replete with antioxidant micronutrients (known to protect against prostate cancer in model studies), has not been established. Whatever the etiology of the disease, prostates removed at autopsy from high-risk parts of the world display an astonishing abundance both of chronic inflammation and of undiagnosed prostate cancers. And, in rodent models, exposures that cause prostate cancer also trigger chronic prostatic inflammation, connecting the two disease processes. In the US, asymptomatic prostatitis arises in nearly all men as they age, leading to the appearance of proliferative inflammatory atrophy (PIA) lesions, the earliest histologic precursors to prostate cancer. In turn, small prostate cancers ultimately appear in as many as 64% of men age 60 to 70 years. Fortunately, the majority of these cancers pose little threat to health or to life. Nonetheless, this reservoir of indolent asymptomatic disease in the midst of chronically inflamed prostates complicates prostate cancer screening, early detection, and treatment, leading to significant over-diagnosis and over-treatment of the disease.

Risk Factors

Key risk factors for prostate cancer include age, family history, African ancestry, a diet rich in saturated fats and red meats, and a sedentary lifestyle, all features that may motivate the use of prostate cancer screening as a part of routine primary care. The most widely used screening strategies feature blood testing for PSA with or without digital rectal examination (DRE), usually

beginning at age 50 to 55 years or earlier for African-American men, for men with a strong family history, or for men known to be carriers of prostate cancer risk genes. Unfortunately, even though the benefits of screening for reducing prostate cancer progression to metastasis and prostate cancer mortality have been demonstrated in a large randomized trial, prostate cancer screening remains highly controversial. The United States Preventive Services Task Force (USPSTF) formally recommends against prostate cancer screening (assigning a grade D), reasoning that detection of asymptomatic prostate cancer leads to unnecessary treatment of the majority of cases that will never progress to threaten health or life. The USPSTF concern is that the harms of unnecessary treatment outweigh the benefits.

Pathophysiology

Nearly all of the exposures that can cause prostate cancers in laboratory mice and rats, ranging from charred meat carcinogens to estrogens to various "hit-and-run" infectious agents, trigger chronic inflammatory changes in prostate tissues that lead to PIA. Some fraction of PIA lesions, likely those exhibiting morphologic atypia and containing somatic genome alterations, in turn progress to prostatic intraepithelial neoplasia (PIN) and to prostate cancer.

The normal prostate contains an epithelium able to contribute secretions to the ejaculate. The epithelium features *(i)* basally located cells, expressing cytokeratins K5 and K14, and p63; *(ii)* columnar secretory cells, expressing the androgen receptor (AR), PSA, cytokeratins K8 and K18, and prostate-specific membrane antigen (PSMA); and *(iii)* neuroendocrine cells, producing chromogranin A, neuron-specific enolase, and synaptophysin. PIA lesions arising in response to epithelial damage give rise to "intermediate cells" that express markers characteristic of both basal and luminal cells. The cellular target of transformation is likely such an "intermediate cell"; the resultant PIN or prostate cancer cells exhibit many of the phenotypic characteristics of columnar secretory cells, including the expression of AR, PSA, and PSMA, and acquire expression of new gene products, such as α-methylacyl-CoA racemase (AMACR). For this reason, many prostate pathologists use immunohistochemical staining for basal cells (antibodies against cytokeratins K5/K14 and p63) and for neoplastic prostate cells (antibodies against AMACR) to aid in prostate cancer diagnosis; prostate cancer cells tend to be cytokeratin K5/K14-negative, p63-negative, and AMACR-positive.

Prostate cancer cells acquire a number of somatic genome and epigenome alterations. Fusion translocations of an androgen-regulated gene, *TMPRSS2*, to genes encoding various members of the E26 transformation-specific (ETS) family of transcription factors are the most common somatic genetic changes in prostate cancers. Somehow, these gene fusions allow prostate cancer cells to coopt androgen signaling to drive neoplastic transformation and malignant progression. As a result, interference with androgen signaling forms the foundation for most advanced prostate cancer treatments. When such translocations are not present, other somatic alterations, such as mutations in *SPOP*, are more frequent. Hypermethylation of *GSTP1*, encoding detoxification enzyme for carcinogens and oxidants, can be detected in >90% of cases. DNA methylation changes at other loci are also very common. The somatic defects in genes and gene function somehow allow prostate cancer cells to proliferate, escape terminal differentiation, and survive to grow in ectopic sites, such as in bones, lymph nodes, and other organs. Two notable somatic gene defects, mutations or deletions in *TP53* and in *PTEN*, have been consistently associated with malignant prostate cancer progression.

Prevention

There are no established drugs that prevent prostate cancer, although there have been three very large randomized clinical trials of agents for prostate cancer prevention. One such trial aimed to test predictions from epidemiologic studies and earlier small clinical trials that inadequate intake of the micronutrients selenium and vitamin E might lead to increased prostate cancer risk. The trial, called Selenium and Vitamin E Cancer Prevention Trial (SELECT), enrolled men 55 years or older (50 years or older for African Americans) with an unremarkable DRE and a serum PSA of 4.0 ng/mL or less to treatment with the micronutrients for 7 to 12 years (randomized to 200 μg selenomethionine daily, 400 IU α-tocopherol daily, the combination, or neither). Unfortunately, the study failed to show any reduction in prostate cancer, instead revealing a slight increase in prostate cancer incidence among men taking vitamin E. As a result, high-level intake of selenium, vitamin E, and other nutritional supplements for the purpose of prostate cancer prevention should be discouraged.

The two other large randomized trials tested the propensity for the 5α-reductase inhibitors finasteride (Proscar)[11] and dutasteride (Avodart)[1] to prevent prostate cancer development. In one of the studies, called the Prostate Cancer Prevention Trial (PCPT), finasteride (5 mg daily or a placebo) was given to healthy men age 55 years and older, with a normal DRE and a serum PSA of 3.0 ng/mL or less, for 7 years. During the trial, men with increasing PSA values or an abnormal DRE were subjected to prostate biopsy. At the end of the trial, biopsies were planned for all of the men. The results were a decrease in prostate cancer detection from 24.4% of men receiving a placebo to only 18.4% of men treated with finasteride, but an increase in more aggressive high-grade prostate cancers in men receiving finasteride versus placebo from 6.4% to 5.1%.

Similar results were encountered with dutasteride in the other trial, called Reduction by Dutasteride of Prostate Cancer Events (REDUCE), where men with an elevated serum PSA between 2.5 to 10.0 ng/mL and a recent negative prostate biopsy were given dutasteride (0.5 mg daily) or a placebo for 4 years, with prostate biopsies obtained after 2 and 4 years on study. Overall, prostate cancer was reduced from 25.1% to 19.9% for men taking dutasteride, but high-grade prostate cancer was increased in these men from <0.1% to 0.5%. Data from PCPT and REDUCE clearly indicated that 5α-reductase inhibitors are better at preventing low-grade cancers than high-grade cancers. Whether the development of high-grade cancers was actually increased in either trial, or whether these cancers were just more easily detected, has been controversial, and the Food and Drug Administration (FDA) has not approved either finasteride or dutasteride for prostate cancer prevention. In 2019, long-term follow-up of participants in the PCPT revealed no increases in prostate cancer mortality accompanying finasteride treatment, likely affirming the general safety of 5α-reductase inhibitor treatment for BPH and male pattern baldness, and reanimating discussions about how 5α-reductase inhibitors might be used to lower the overall burden of prostate cancer in some way.

Clinical Manifestations

Most men present for prostate cancer care after a diagnosis triggered by prostate cancer screening and are thus initially asymptomatic. Local progression of the disease can result in lower urinary tract symptoms of voiding obstruction or irritation, in urinary tract infections and urosepsis, in erectile dysfunction, in hematospermia, and in diminished ejaculate volume. Metastatic prostate cancer dissemination most often involves the skeleton, resulting in bone pain and low blood counts, and involves pelvic lymph nodes and nearby lymphatics, resulting in lower extremity edema or retroperitoneal fibrosis, respectively.

Diagnosis

Prostate cancer diagnosis is typically made using transrectal ultrasound (TRUS)-guided prostate biopsy. The technique involves the repeated firing of an 18-gauge needle from a spring-loaded gun through a port on the TRUS probe. To sample prostate tissue, the biopsy needle passes through the rectum into the prostate, and fluoroquinolone antibiotics are typically administered before the biopsy procedure. Hematuria and/or hematospermia occur commonly after prostate biopsy. Hospital admissions, usually the

result of an infection, are rare but can be needed in up to 7% of men with significant comorbidities. Importantly, TRUS does not delineate the locations of prostate cancers within the prostate. For this reason, the numbers and sites of biopsies placed during a prostate biopsy procedure, typically 10 to 12 directed laterally into the peripheral zone of the gland, are designed to minimize the chance of missing life-threatening high-grade cancers.

Increasingly, magnetic resonance imaging (MRI) has been employed to better direct prostate biopsies, hoping to reduce detection of low-grade cancers that pose little threat to life and to more accurately sample high-grade disease. Multiparametric MRI (mpMRI) incorporates T2-weighted anatomic imaging, diffusion-weighted imaging, and contrast enhancement to highlight suspicious areas in the prostate for biopsy. The technique generates a standardized "suspicion" score for individual lesions, using the Prostate Imaging–Reporting and Data System (PI-RADS). The MR image itself can then be used to direct TRUS biopsies via coregistration (or "fusion") of the acquired mpMRI data with real-time TRUS. Biopsies obtained by MRI/TRUS fusion are becoming more widespread, especially for men who need a repeat biopsy because of a persistently elevated or rising serum PSA.

The histologic grade and anatomic stage of newly diagnosed prostate cancer carry important prognostic information useful for treatment planning. Recently, prostate cancer grade "groups" (1, best prognosis and 5, worst prognosis) have been introduced into clinical practice as risk tools for localized prostate cancer. These "groups" are derived from Gleason scoring as conducted by an expert genitourinary pathologist. The Gleason score represents the sum of the two most common histologic patterns of growth exhibited by the cancer within the prostate; the pattern designations range from pattern 3 to pattern 5 (there are no patterns 1 or 2), providing Gleason scores from 6 to 10. The disease stage focuses on the extent of tumor in the prostate itself (T1, not palpable by DRE; T2, palpable by DRE; T3, extending outside the prostate itself; and T4, invading adjacent pelvic structures), in regional lymph nodes (N0, no lymph node metastases; N1, lymph node metastases), and in distant sites (M0, no distant metastases; M1, metastases). Staging tools include a number of imaging modalities, including abdominopelvic CT or MR images and nuclear medicine scans for soft tissue and for bone, using ^{11}C-choline, ^{18}F-fluciclovine, or ^{18}F-sodium fluoride. A new generation of nuclear medicine scans targeting PSMA are working their way toward FDA approval.

Differential Diagnosis

The critical issue surrounding the diagnosis and staging of many men with prostate cancer is whether the disease is at risk to progress to threaten life or whether it is so indolent as to not need treatment. Most men with indolent disease indicated by a Gleason score of 6 do not need immediate treatment, and many may never need treatment. Instead, these men can be monitored using *active surveillance*, with serum PSA tests twice yearly, DREs each year, and MR images and/or prostate biopsies as necessary or after 2 to 4 years. This surveillance strategy aims to detect higher Gleason score prostate cancer if it appears. Gleason score greater than 7 tends to be an indication for curative local disease treatment with surgery or radiation therapy. Deferring aggressive local therapy as part of active surveillance appears safe, and as a result, active surveillance has become a common approach to prostate cancer care. By avoiding aggressive intervention until and unless necessary, active surveillance is distinct from observation or watchful waiting approaches, which are typically reserved for men with significant comorbidities and limited life expectancy.

Therapy

For localized prostate cancer with Gleason score greater than 7, curative treatments include radical prostatectomy, interstitial brachytherapy, and external beam radiation therapy. Most radical prostatectomies these days are performed using a robot-assisted laparoscopic approach. Urinary incontinence and erectile function after the procedure vary greatly between surgeons, with

---

[1] Not FDA approved for this indication.

as many as 20% of men describing some level of urine leakage 2 years after radical prostatectomy, and at least 26% of men reporting significant sexual dysfunction a year after surgery. Ideally, following surgery, the serum PSA should fall to an undetectable level and remain so in perpetuity if the procedure resulted in prostate cancer cure. Two thirds of men subjected to radical prostatectomy remain free of PSA recurrence 15 years after surgery. A rising serum PSA after surgery is a sign that prostate cancer has recurred or persisted somewhere. Nonetheless, such a PSA rise may not herald imminent overt metastasis or death. In one analysis, only 30% of men with a rising serum PSA postsurgery had suffered with metastatic prostate cancer by 8 years after the initial PSA increase. The rate of serum PSA rise can be informative; a rapid doubling of serum PSA values is usually associated with a greater threat of symptomatic disease progression.

Prostate brachytherapy provides for direct irradiation of localized prostate cancer, via implantation of radioactive sources into the prostate using image guidance. The procedure itself is fairly convenient, able to be completed as an outpatient within a couple of hours using spinal anesthesia. The most common radioactive sources used are ^{125}I (iodine) and ^{103}Pd (palladium) and as many as a hundred seeds might be implanted. In general, though the ^{125}I seeds decay more slowly than the ^{103}Pd seeds, prostate brachytherapy implants are essentially inert by 10 months after insertion into the prostate. Complications of brachytherapy for prostate cancer differ from those of radical prostatectomy and of external beam radiotherapy, with irritative voiding symptoms reported by at least half of men in the first few months after implant placement. These symptoms tend to abate after a year or so, persisting in some 15% to 20% of men. Long-term side effects can include urethral stricture, incontinence, erectile dysfunction, and rectal irritation. Relative contraindications to prostate brachytherapy include large prostate size (requires a lot of seeds or use of androgen deprivation to shrink the prostate), preimplant obstructive urinary symptoms (greatly worsen after implantation), and history of transurethral surgery for symptomatic BPH (tends to lead to incontinence).

A series of technical innovations have improved both the efficacy and safety of external beam radiation therapy, including CT-based treatment planning, the use of multileaf collimators in modern linear accelerators, and improvements in treatment planning software. Three-dimensional conformal radiation therapy (3D-CRT) allows creation of more accurate target volumes using reconstructions of pelvic CT images, better sparing vulnerable structures such as the bladder and the rectum. Intensity-modulated radiation therapy (IMRT) even further optimizes dose distribution for prostate cancer treatment, by controlling the intensity of radiation dose, in addition to the shape of the volume designated for treatment. Despite more accurate deposition of radiation doses to the prostate, side effects of external beam radiation therapy remain mostly rectal toxicity (early irritation and late rectal bleeding), late urethral strictures, and erectile dysfunction. External beam radiation can also be used as adjuvant therapy for prostate cancer with positive surgical margins after radical prostatectomy or as salvage therapy for local prostate cancer recurrence after surgery.

Proton beam radiotherapy has become available at a limited number of treatment centers. The physical properties of protons allow them to deposit energy very precisely, with little radiation dose to skin and little radiation scatter to nearby tissues. This behavior is ideal for cancers located in close proximity to sensitive structures in the body, such as at the base of the skull, near the eye, and elsewhere. For prostate cancer, proton radiotherapy has emerged as an effective treatment for localized disease, but whether this approach offers an improvement over conventional external beam radiation using 3D-CRT with IMRT awaits the results of an ongoing randomized clinical trial.

Systemic approaches to prostate cancer include agents targeted at androgen signaling, taxane chemotherapy, radiopharmaceuticals, and PARP inhibitors. Disruption of androgen signaling has been a mainstay of advanced prostate cancer care for seven

decades. Originally accomplished by surgical removal of the testes, and later by the administration of estrogens, androgen deprivation therapy (ADT), involving a reduction in circulating testosterone levels to <50 ng/mL, is now more commonly achieved by inhibition of pituitary gonadotropin production using luteinizing hormone–releasing hormone (LHRH) analogs that cause suppression of testosterone production. The LHRH analogs are all available in long-acting injectable depot formulations (goserelin [Zoladex] 10.8 mg depot every 3 months, leuprolide [Lupron Depot] 22.5 mg depot every 3 months, and triptorelin [Trelstar] 3.75 mg depot monthly) and antagonists (degarelix [Firmagon] 240 mg depot initially followed by 80 mg depot monthly). The benefits of ADT are evident in most men by a decline in the serum PSA, a shrinkage of metastatic cancer deposits, and improvements in symptoms, such as bone pain, that accompany metastatic prostate cancer progression. Side effects often include hot flashes, bone loss, reduced libido, decreased muscle mass, increased fat, and fatigue. An increased risk for cardiovascular disease is also suspected.

Ultimately, most men on ADT for advanced prostate cancer progress to castration-resistant prostate cancer (CRPC). Nonetheless, the prostate cancers in many men with CRPC remain addicted to androgen signaling and continue to produce PSA, which requires an activated AR. In this setting, two strategies have emerged to ablate androgen signaling more completely. One involves the use of the AR antagonists enzalutamide ([Xtandi] 160 mg daily) and apalutamide ([Erleada] 240 mg daily). Each is approved by the FDA for CRPC; enzalutamide is approved for CRPC with or without overt metastases and apalutamide for CRPC without overt metastases. A second approach involves inhibition of adrenal steroid biogenesis to further reduce circulating levels of androgenic hormones. Abiraterone ([Zytiga] 1000 mg daily with 5 mg prednisone twice daily), a CYP17 inhibitor, suppresses extragonadal androgen production and provides an effective treatment for CRPC. A second CYP17 inhibitor, orteronel[5] (400 mg twice daily with 5 mg prednisone twice daily), is in the midst of clinical trials seeking registration by the FDA. Both of the CYP17 inhibitors must be administered along with replacement corticosteroids (5 mg prednisone twice daily).

ADT can be used as adjuvant therapy along with prostate radiotherapy, as initial treatment for prostate cancer recurrence manifest as a rapidly rising serum PSA in the absence of overt metastases following surgery or radiotherapy, and as treatment for established metastatic prostate cancer, with or without taxane chemotherapy. Of these three indications, the use of ADT for men with disease recurrence after primary therapy remains somewhat controversial. The concern is that the benefits may not be much better than waiting to initiate ADT until overt metastases can be detected, while the hazards, including bone loss, possible risk for cardiovascular complications, and poor quality-of-life are significant. Careful monitoring of PSA rises and periodic use of imaging studies may allow for introduction of ADT before symptoms of metastatic prostate cancer appear. Nuclear medicine scans with agents targeting PSMA may find a use in this setting. Another tactic for ADT with a rapidly rising serum PSA after primary therapy has been intermittent administration. Intermittent ADT appears to control prostate cancer progression as well as continuous ADT, and to provide some minor improvement in quality-of-life. Finally, a novel strategy now in clinical trials for men with advanced prostate cancer exposed to ADT for at least 6 months is the administration of androgenic hormones. This approach can lower serum PSA levels in more than half of men treated and improve quality-of-life.

Of all the cytotoxic chemotherapy drugs used for advanced prostate cancer, agents targeting intracellular microtubules have exhibited disproportionate activity. Prostate cancer cells tend to have low growth rates, rendering most antineoplastic drugs that interfere with cell replication less effective than for other cancers.

---

[5] Investigational drug in the United States.

Taxane drugs, including docetaxel (Taxotere) and cabazitaxel (Jevtana), disrupt microtubule function in both replicating and nonreplicating cells. In nonreplicating prostate cancer cells, the taxane drugs may hinder the trafficking of AR and other critical gene regulatory proteins into the cell nucleus, triggering apoptosis. Both docetaxel (75 mg/m² every 3 weeks given along with prednisone 10 mg daily) and cabazitaxel (25 mg/m² every 3 weeks given along with prednisone 10 mg daily) are effective treatments for CRPC, able to lower serum PSA, reduce measurable volumes of cancer seen on imaging studies, and prolong disease survival. Docetaxel toxicity includes significant neutropenia, ankle edema, peripheral neuropathy, hair loss, and nail changes. Cabazitaxel, which was more effective than docetaxel for multidrug-resistant tumor cells in preclinical studies and better able to penetrate the blood–brain barrier, was initially used to treat docetaxel-resistant CRPC. In that setting, cabazitaxel caused more substantial neutropenia than docetaxel and was associated with more diarrhea and asthenia. A randomized trial comparing docetaxel to cabazitaxel as first-line treatment for metastatic CRPC revealed similar overall survival for either treatment and docetaxel remains the preferred first-line chemotherapy option. Six doses of docetaxel given every 3 weeks is now frequently used along with ADT for men with metastatic hormone-sensitive prostate cancer, significantly prolonging overall survival when compared to ADT alone in two large randomized clinical trials. In addition to the taxanes docetaxel and cabazitaxel, the topoisomerase poison mitoxantrone (Novantrone) is approved by the FDA as an agent capable of improving quality-of-life for men with CRPC.

Palliation of symptomatic bone metastases in men with CRPC can be achieved using the α–particle-emitting calcium mimetic ²²³Ra. The agent has a brief half-life ($t_{1/2}$ = 11.4 days) and a marked proclivity for skeletal uptake; an estimated 40% to 60% of administered ²²³Ra ends up in bones. ²²³Ra (50 kBq/kg) is typically given in six injections at 4-week intervals. Side effects include nausea, vomiting, diarrhea, leg swelling, and low blood counts. More recently, ¹⁷⁷Lu- and ²²⁵Ac-labeled PSMA ligands have been introduced into the care of men with CRPC. Early trials hint at marked beneficial treatment responses. Nonetheless, significant xerostomia resulting from salivary gland toxicity (a site of PSMA expression) bedevils the use of these agents so far. Attempts to optimize radiolabeled PSMA ligand dosing to limit salivary gland damage, to prevent radioisotope uptake by the salivary gland, and to improve treatment for salivary gland dysfunction, postradioactive PSMA ligand administration are ongoing.

The up to 20% of men with CRPC who carry germline and/or somatic mutations in homologous recombination repair genes (*BRCA1*, *BRCA2*, *ATM*, and others) derive significant benefit from treatment with PARP inhibitors. PARPs are enzymes that contribute to several steps in DNA repair. Inhibition of PARP in cells with homologous recombination deficiency results in "synthetic lethality" and apoptosis. This phenomenon has been exploited successfully for the treatment of ovarian and breast cancers carrying defective homologous recombination repair genes. The PARP inhibitors olaparib ([Lynparza][1] 300 mg twice daily), rucaparib ([Rubraca][1] 600 mg twice daily), and niraparib ([Zejula][1] 300 mg daily) have all shown early evidence of activity in the treatment of CRPC with deficient homologous recombination repair; clinical trials for FDA registration are ongoing. Common side effects of PARP inhibitors include gastrointestinal symptoms and fatigue.

Two additional systemic treatment approaches merit attention. First, for CRPC arising in the setting of DNA mismatch repair deficiency, like other cancers with DNA mismatch repair defects, the immune checkpoint inhibitor pembrolizumab ([Keytruda][1] 200 mg every 3 weeks) can be effective at achieving significant and durable treatment responses. Major side effects include "autoimmune breakthrough events" such as colitis, pneumonitis, and hypophysitis. Immune checkpoint inhibitor therapy otherwise shows very little activity against prostate cancers. Second, for men with CRPC manifest as small cell neuroendocrine cancer, treatment with chemotherapy doublet regimens like cisplatin or carboplatin and etoposide may be helpful.

Monitoring

Men treated for clinically localized prostate cancer by surgery or radiation therapy are monitored for cancer recurrence principally by serum PSA testing every 6 to 12 months and by DRE yearly. A newly detectable or rising serum PSA can trigger a more complete evaluation using bone scans, abdominopelvic CT or MR imaging, and ¹¹C-choline or ¹⁸F-fluciclovine PET studies. ¹⁸F-deoxyglucose PET imaging is not helpful. If necessary, a prostate biopsy may be undertaken in the setting of disease recurrence after radiation therapy.

Metastatic prostate cancer treatment can be monitored using serial serum PSA determinations and repeated imaging at known and/or symptomatic sites of disease. In addition, whether used for nonmetastatic or metastatic prostate cancer, ADT carries a substantial risk of osteoporosis. As such, men should be subjected to dual energy X-ray absorptiometry (DEXA) scanning. For men with a low fracture risk, calcium (1000 mg) and vitamin D (400 IU) supplements may suffice, but for men facing a higher probability of bone fracture, treatment with agents such as denosumab ([Prolia] 60 mg every 6 months), zoledronic acid ([Reclast][1] 4 mg no more often than monthly), or alendronate ([Fosamax][1] 70 mg once weekly) should be considered along with calcium and vitamin D. Men receiving ADT should also be screened for diabetes and for cardiovascular disease, conditions that are common among men in the age range for prostate cancer.

Management of Complications

Men who are survivors of prostate cancer face a number of health challenges that comprise long-term side effects of the treatment(s) they received. Surgery tends to disrupt urinary and sexual functions. Stress incontinence may be the most common urinary problem, though more severe incontinence can occur. Urinary symptoms, such as urgency, frequency, and nocturia can arise; sometimes these symptoms herald the appearance of a urethral stricture at the site of the anastomosis of the bladder neck to the urethra during surgery. Urethral strictures related to scarring can be distinguished from cancer recurrence and treated via dilation by a urologist. Sexual problems include difficulties achieving erections sufficient for intercourse and a change in sexual experience attributable to lack of ejaculation and to differences in orgasms. Frank discussions about sexual function after primary prostate cancer treatment can aid in sexual recovery. Some urologists have attempted to use phosphodiesterase type 5 inhibitors (sildenafil [Viagra][1] 50 mg, vardenafil [Levitra][1] 10 mg, and tadalafil [Cialis][1] 5 mg) early after surgery to augment restoration of erectile function. These drugs have also been used successfully by some men to improve erections months and years after surgery. Radiation therapy late effects can also include urinary and sexual difficulties, and can involve the rectum in inflammation, pain, bleeding, and incontinence. Minor rectal symptoms can be alleviated using stool softeners, but more severe complications require the attention of a gastroenterologist or colorectal surgeon. Hyperbaric oxygen may help some men with radiation proctitis as a late effect of prostate cancer treatment.

ADT causes a diverse collection of long-term side effects, including loss of libido, erection problems, hot flashes, weight gain and obesity, mood changes/depression, anxiety/distress, gynecomastia, anemia, osteoporosis (see previously), diabetes/metabolic syndrome, and decreased lean muscle mass. Increased physical activity and dietary changes appropriate for obesity can be helpful. Careful attention and screening for psychological stress and depression should be a routine aspect of prostate cancer survivorship care. Even men likely cured of prostate cancer by surgery or radiation therapy frequently suffer with significant

---

[1] Not FDA approved for this indication.

[1] Not FDA approved for this indication.

"PSA anxiety" around the time of follow-up vigilance to detect disease recurrence. Hot flashes, which occur in as many as 40% of men on ADT, can be treated using selective serotonin reuptake inhibitors such as paroxetine ([Paxil][1] 10 to 20 mg daily), serotonin and norepinephrine uptake inhibitors such as venlafaxine ([Effexor XR][1] 75 mg daily), or the anticonvulsant gabapentin ([Neurontin][1] 600 mg or more daily).

---

[1] Not FDA approved for this indication.

References

Antonarakis ES, Feng Z, Trock BJ, et al: The natural history of metastatic progression in men with prostate-specific antigen recurrence after radical prostatectomy: long-term follow-up, *BJU Int* 109:32–39, 2012.

De Marzo AM, Platz EA, Sutcliffe S, et al: Inflammation in prostate carcinogenesis, *Nat Rev Cancer* 7:256–269, 2007.

Mateo J, Carreira S, Sandhu S, et al: DNA repair defects and olaparib in metastatic prostate cancer, *N Engl J Med* 373:1697–1708, 2015.

Nelson WG, Antonarakis ES, Carter HB, De Marzo AM, DeWeese TL: Prostate cancer. In Niederhuber JE, Armitage JO, Doroshow JH, Kastan MB, Tepper JE, editors: *Abeloff's Clinical Oncology*, 6th edition, Philadelphia, 2018, Churchill Livingstone.

Nelson WG, De Marzo AM, Isaacs WB: Prostate cancer, *N Engl J Med* 349:366–381, 2003.

Nuhn P, De Bono JS, Fizazi K, et al: Update on systemic prostate cancer therapies: management of castration-resistant prostate cancer in the era of precision oncology, *Eur Urol* 75:88–99, 2019.

Sanda MG, Dunn RL, Michalski J, et al: Quality of life and satisfaction with outcome among prostate-cancer survivors, *N Engl J Med* 358:1250–1261, 2008.

Siegel RL, Miller KD, Jemal A: Cancer statistics, 2019, *CA Cancer J Clin* 69:7–34, 2019.

Viswanathan SR, Ha G, Hoff AM, et al: Structural alterations driving castration-resistant prostate cancer revealed by linked read genome sequencing, *Cell* 174:433–447, 2018.

PROSTATITIS

Method of
C.R. Powell, MD

CURRENT DIAGNOSIS

- The work up for prostatitis begins with a thorough history and physical as well as a urinalysis and urine culture. Diagnosis is based on symptoms (Figure 1) and tenderness on digital rectal exam. There is a controversial role for prostate massage and culture of expressed prostatic secretions.
- Urinalysis and mid-stream urine culture are important to distinguish bacterial from non-bacterial causes, but is not necessary for the diagnosis of prostatitis.
- Prostatitis is categorized as acute or chronic. It has been further characterized by the United States National Institutes of Health (NIH) National Institute of Diabetes, Digestive, and Kidney disorders (NIDDK) into four categories: acute bacterial, chronic bacterial, chronic pelvic pain syndrome (also called chronic nonbacterial prostatitis), and asymptomatic (Table 1).
- Chronic prostatitis is defined as duration longer than 3 months and typically manifests with pelvic pain and lower urinary tract symptoms.

CURRENT THERAPY

- The majority of prostatitis falls under the category of chronic prostatitis/chronic pelvic pain syndrome and monotherapy has not proven effective.
- Fluoroquinolone antibiotics are first-line therapy for acute and chronic *bacterial* prostatitis, which are thought to comprise <10% of all cases. Ciprofloxacin (Cipro) and levofloxacin

(Levaquin) have demonstrated cure rates of 73% to 75% in one RCT with culture-proven prostatitis.
- Trimethoprim/sulfamethoxazole (Bactrim)[1] can be considered first-line therapy but local antibiotic resistance patterns should be considered prior to empiric treatment.
- First-generation cephalosporins, doxycycline (Vibramycin)[1], tetracycline (not available in most areas), azithromycin (Zithromax)[1], clarithromycin (Biaxin)[1] are all second-line agents.
- Acute prostatitis may require inpatient admission and IV antibiotics depending on severity and presence of sepsis. Urinary retention may require suprapubic tube urinary drainage as a Foley catheter may worsen prostate inflammation.
- The role of antibiotics in the treatment of *chronic pelvic pain syndrome* is less clear. Treatment directed at *specific phenotypes* has improved outcomes. The U.P.O.I.N.T. treatment philosophy has garnered much interest in the urologic community and is used to phenotype subjects and to direct multimodal therapy.

---

[1] Not FDA approved for this indication.

Epidemiology

The prevalence of prostatitis is approximately 8.2% (range: 2.2% to 9.7%). It accounts for 8% of visits to urologists, and up to 1% of visits to primary care physicians. It has been estimated to cost the patient more than $6300 annually in direct costs, with the estimated national cost in the United States to diagnose and treat prostatitis being $84 million, not including pharmaceutical spending.

Risk Factors

The risk factors for prostatitis include urinary tract infection, elevated post-void residual (urinary retention), recent history of prostate biopsy, urinary catheterization, unprotected anal intercourse, recent urethral instrumentation such as cystoscopy, and condom catheter use.

Pathophysiology

Prostatitis is commonly associated with infection, but can also describe noninfectious chronic pelvic pain as well as asymptomatic histologic evidence of sterile inflammation. The causes for acute and chronic *bacterial* prostatitis (CBP) include prior genitourinary infections such as epididymitis/orchitis, infection resulting from prostate needle biopsy, and recent urinary tract infection. Other predisposing factors include obstruction of urine from urethral stricture, BPH, or neurogenic causes. A causative organism can be found in <10% of prostatitis cases. The causative organisms include: *Escherichia coli* (most common at 65% to 80% of infections), *Pseudomonas aeruginosa*, *Serratia* species, *Klebsiella* species, and *Enterobacter aerogenes*. Gram positive organisms include enterococci. Organisms isolated from patients with recent history of lower urinary tract instrumentation or manipulation exhibit more resistance to ciprofloxacin and cephalosporins. For these patients ciprofloxacin is often inadequate. A combination of cephalosporins and aminoglycosides is appropriate. Patients with a history of HIV infection should prompt investigation for atypical pathogens. The cause of chronic pelvic pain syndrome (CPPS)/chronic non-bacterial prostatitis (NIH category 3) is less well understood, as is asymptomatic prostatitis (NIH category 4).

Prevention

Prophylactic antibiotic dose is appropriate prior to urologic procedures, particularly prostate needle biopsy according to the American Urological Association Best Practice Statement for Urologic Surgery (http://www.auanet.org). Pre-procedure rectal swabs to assess resistance patterns are now considered in select cases where resistance is more likely.

Clinical Manifestations

Figure 1 details some symptoms of prostatitis, separated by domain.

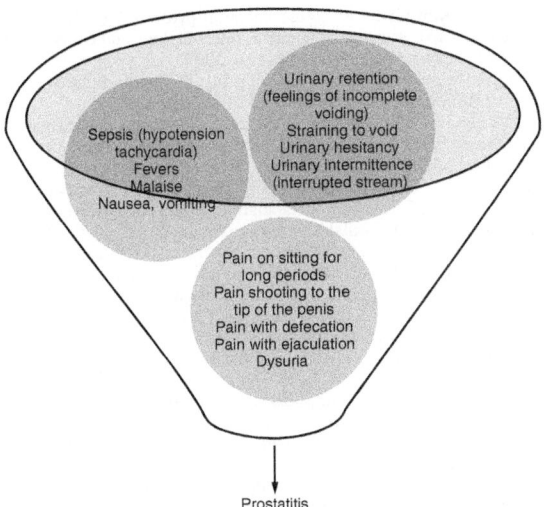

Figure 1 Symptoms associated with prostatitis.

Diagnosis

Diagnosis of acute and CBP is primarily based on history, physical examination, urine culture, and urine specimen testing pre- and post-prostatic massage. If acute bacterial prostatitis is suspected prostatic massage should not be performed as this might be harmful. Sexually active men younger than 35 years and older men who engage in high-risk sexual behaviors should be tested for *Neisseria gonococcus* and *Chlamydia trachomatis* as well. The presence of leukocytes in the semen, first voided urine, midstream urine, expressed prostatic secretions, or post-prostatic massage urine did not correlate with symptoms when studied in a prospective manner. Bacterial localization studies, such as the Meares-Stamey 4-glass test, are useful in sub-categorizing type 3 CPPS but have unclear significance in the acute clinical setting.

Differential Diagnosis

The differential diagnosis of prostatitis includes acute cystitis, benign prostatic hyperplasia (BPH), prostate cancer, urinary tract stones, bladder cancer, prostatic abscess, enterovesical fistula, foreign body within the urinary tract, voiding dysfunction, and inflammatory conditions of the bladder such as interstitial cystitis/painful bladder syndrome.

Therapy (or Treatment)

Treatment depends on the NIH-NIDDK Prostatitis Classification Category. For those with **acute prostatitis**, oral ciprofloxacin (Cipro)[1] 500 mg orally, twice daily for 4 to 6 weeks or levofloxacin (Levaquin)[1] 500 mg orally, once daily for 4 to 6 weeks is appropriate for non-septic appearing patients. Trimethoprim/sulfamethoxazole (Bactrim, Septra)[1], 160 mg/800 mg orally twice daily for 4 to 6 weeks is also appropriate, depending on local antibiotic resistance patterns. Patients appearing septic (hypotension, tachycardia, high fevers) should be admitted to the hospital and started on broad-spectrum antibiotics such as ampicillin 2 g intravenous every 6 hours and an aminoglycoside such as gentamicin 1 mg/kg intravenous every 8 hours. Aminoglycosides should be monitored and adjusted based on serum peak and trough levels. Aminoglycosides should be used cautiously in patients with azotemia. Prostatic abscess should be considered if patients do not improve within 24 to 48 hours. Prostatic abscesses are urologic emergencies and can be drained with transurethral resection of the prostate, ultrasound-guided transrectal needle drainage, or CT-guided needle drainage. Urinary retention should be treated with suprapubic catheter drainage in cases of acute prostatitis. **Chronic bacterial prostatitis** is treated with the same oral agents as acute bacterial prostatitis. For the treatment of **chronic pelvic pain syndrome**

antibiotics play a less clear role, but fluoroquinolone antibiotics used empirically for 4 to 6 weeks have been effective in previously untreated patients. There is little value to repeated courses of antibiotics if the first course is not effective. There is conflicting evidence for α-blockers such as tamsulosin (Flomax 0.4 mg orally once per night)[1]. The interested reader is referred to a review article by Nickel 2010, wherein a multidisciplinary approach is advocated taking into account a more detailed 6 domain phenotype with therapy directed at the relevant phenotype(s). This is known as UPOINT. These phenotype domains include Urinary (broken down into voiding and storage symptoms), Psychosocial (subdivided into depression and catastrophizing), Organ specific (divided into bladder and prostate), Infection (noted in the urine or expressed prostatic secretions), Neurologic (divided into focal and systemic), and Tenderness (muscle). Categorizing patients according to these domains may allow clinicians to personalize treatment using a multimodal approach involving physical therapy, psychiatry, and medication.

Other therapies have been described with low-quality evidence for efficacy. These are included below as an alternative treatment option for patients who do not respond to the interventions and strategies outlined above. 5-α-reductase inhibitors (Finasteride [Proscar])[1] have demonstrated slight improvement over placebo in 2 underpowered RCTs, but carry a 10% to 15% risk of adverse event including "partial impotence." Chronic opioid therapy (COT) is appealing to some, but as the United States Centers for Disease Control (CDC) has noted, the harms outweigh the benefits for most causes of chronic pain. Its use should be discouraged. Celecoxib (Celebrex)[1] has demonstrated no benefit over placebo in one RCT utilizing the NIH-CPSI instrument as the validated endpoint. Allopurinol (Zyloprim)[1] has demonstrated a slight benefit versus placebo in an underpowered RCT that utilized a non-validated questionnaire as the clinical endpoint. Pentosan polysulfate (Elmiron)[1] has demonstrated a slight benefit in the NIH-CPSI quality-of-life domain compared to placebo, but not in other endpoints. Twenty-two of 100 men (22%) withdrew from the study due to adverse events such as diarrhea, headache, and nausea. One very small RCT (*n* = 20) comparing sham treatment versus transurethral microwave therapy (TUMT) of the prostate, a treatment for BPH, reported 7 of 10 patients having at least 50% improvement, measured by non-validated "global assessment" endpoint. Transurethral resection of the prostate (TURP) has also been discussed but no RCT exists having the intent to treat men with chronic prostatitis. It is an untested option for men in whom all other treatment modalities have failed, but has a long history of ameliorating obstructive and irritative lower urinary tract symptoms (LUTS) which often accompany CP/CPPS.

Monitoring

Monitoring is based on symptoms. In cases of acute prostatitis treated with appropriate antibiotics, persistent fevers should prompt a work up for prostatic abscess. The NIH-Chronic Prostatitis Symptom Index (CPSI) patient-reported questionnaire can be used to quantify symptoms over time. It is available online at http://www.prostatitis.org/symptomindex. html. prostate specific antigen (PSA) testing plays no role in the treatment or monitoring of prostatitis, but should be considered if risk factors for prostate cancer are present such as a prostate nodule or family history. PSA testing is affected by acute inflammation and should be postponed until a few months after the symptoms of prostatitis have resolved.

Complications

Acute prostatitis can progress to urosepsis and hypotension. CBP might have the ability to progress to CPPS and become a source of pain for years.

[1] Not FDA approved for this indication.

[1] Not FDA approved for this indication.

TABLE 1	National Institutes of Health Consensus Classification of Prostatitis
CATEGORY	**DESCRIPTION**
I. Acute bacterial prostatitis	Acute infection of the prostate gland with positive urine or semen cultures. Symptoms present for less than 3 months
II. Chronic bacterial prostatitis	Chronic infection of the prostate gland with positive urine or semen cultures. Symptoms present for greater than 3 months
III. Chronic pelvic pain syndrome	Chronic pelvic pain in the absence of bacterial infection localized to the prostate. Symptoms present for greater than 3 months.
A. Inflammatory	Significant WBC count in the prostatic secretions, urine, or semen
B. Noninflammatory	Insignificant WBC count in the prostatic secretions, urine, or semen
IV. Asymptomatic prostatitis	WBC count elevated and/ or bacteria in the prostatic secretions, urine, semen, or histologic specimens of prostate tissue

WBC, White blood cells.

References

Bowen DK, Dilubanza E, Schaefer A: Chronic bacterial prostatitis and chronic pelvic pain syndrome, *Clinical Evidence* 8:1802, 2015.

Bundrick W, Heron SP, Ray P, et al: Levofloxacin versus ciprofloxacin in the treatment of chronic bacterial prostatitis: a randomized double-blind multicenter study, *Urology* 62:537–541, 2003.

Clemens JQ, Markossian T, Calhoun EA: Comparison of economic impact of chronic prostatitis/chronic pelvic pain syndrome and interstitial cystitis/painful bladder syndrome, *Urology* 73(4):743–746, 2009, Available at: https://doi.org/10.1016/j.urology.2008.11.007.

Collins MM, Stafford RS, O'Leary MP, Barry MJ: How common is prostatitis? A national survey of physician visits, *J Urol* 159(4):1224–1228, 1998.

Ha US, Kim ME, Kim CS, et al: Acute bacterial prostatitis in Korea: clinical outcome, including symptoms, management, microbiology and course of disease, *Int J Antimicrob Agents* 31(Suppl 1):S96–101, 2008.

Krieger JN, Lee SW, Jeon J, Cheah PY, Liong ML, Riley DE: Epidemiology of prostatitis, *Int J Antimicrob Agents* 31(Suppl 1):S85–90, 2008.

Leskinen M, Lukkarinen O, Marttila T: Effects of finasteride in patients with inflammatory chronic pelvic pain syndrome: a double-blind, placebo-controlled, pilot study, *Urology* 53:502–505, 1999.

Li S, Huang X, Chen Z, et al: Neutrophil CD64 expression as a biomarker in the early diagnosis of bacterial infection: a meta-analysis. [Meta-Analysis Review], *Int J Infect Dis* 17(1):e12–23, 2013, Available at: https://doi.org/10.1016/j.ijid.2012.07.017.

Litwin MS, McNaughton-Collins M, Fowler FL Jr., et al (2002). "Prostatatitis: The National Institutes of Health Chronic Prostatitis Symptoms Index (NIH-CPSI)." Retrieved 12/26/2012, 2012, Available at: http://www.prostatitis.org/nih-cpsi.html.

Litwin MS, McNaughton-Collins M, Fowler Jr FJ, et al: The National Institutes of Health chronic prostatitis symptom index: development and validation of a new outcome measure. Chronic Prostatitis Collaborative Research Network, *J Urol* 162(2):369–375, 1999.

Nickel JC, Downey J, Pontari MA, Shoskes DA, Zeitlin SI: A randomized placebo-controlled multicentre study to evaluate the safety and efficacy of finasteride for male chronic pelvic pain syndrome (category IIIA chronic nonbacterial prostatitis), *BJU Int* 93:991–995, 2004.

Nickel JC, Forrest JB, Tomera K, et al: Pentosan polysulfate sodium therapy for men with chronic pelvic pain syndrome: a multicenter, randomized, placebo controlled study, *J Urol* 173:1252–1255, 2005.

Nickel JC, Shoskes DA: Phenotypic approach to the management of the chronic prostatitis/chronic pelvic pain syndrome, *BJU Int* 106(9):1252–1263, 2010.

Nickel J, Sorensen R: Transurethral microwave thermotherapy for nonbacterial prostatitis: a randomized double-blind sham controlled study using new prostatitis specific assessment questionnaires, *J Urol* 155:1950–1955, 1996.

Persson B, Ronquist G, Ekblom M: Ameliorative effect of allopurinol on nonbacterial prostatitis: a parallel double-blind controlled study, *J Urol* 155:961–964, 1996.

Pontari MA, Joyce GF, Wise M, McNaughton-Collins M: Prostatitis, *J Urol* 177(6):2050–2057, 2007.

Qian L, Li SB, Zhou Y, Teng SJ, Guo JJ: Determination of CD64 for the diagnosis of bacterial chronic prostatitis, *Am J Reprod Immunol*, 2015https://doi.org/10.1111/aji.12391.

Roberts RO, Lieber MM, Rhodes T, Girman CJ, Bostwick DG, Jacobsen SJ: Prevalence of a physician-assigned diagnosis of prostatitis: the Olmsted County study of urinary symptoms and health status among men, *Urology* 51:578–584, 1998.

Schaeffer AJ, Knauss JS, Landis JR, et al: Leukocyte and bacterial counts do not correlate with severity of symptoms in men with chronic prostatitis: the National Institutes of Health Chronic Prostatitis Cohort Study, *J Urol* 168(3):1048–1053, 2002.

Sharp VJ, Takacs EB, Powell CR: Prostatitis: diagnosis and treatment, *Am Fam Physician* 82(4):397–406, 2010.

Wolf SJ Jr, Bennett CJ, Dmochowski RR, et al: (2008, 1/1/2012). "Urologic Surgery Antimicrobial Prophylaxis." Transrectal prostate biopsy. Retrieved 12/26/2012, 2012, from http://www.auanet.org/content/media/antimicroprop08.pdf.

Zhao WP, Zhang ZG, Li XD, et al: Celecoxib reduces symptoms in men with difficult chronic pelvic pain syndrome (Category IIIA), *Braz J Med Biol Res* 42:963–967, 2009.

17 Women's Health

ABNORMAL UTERINE BLEEDING

Method of
Sarina Schrager, MD, MS

CURRENT DIAGNOSIS

- Anovulation and pelvic structural abnormalities are the most common causes of abnormal vaginal bleeding in reproductive-age women.
- All women with abnormal bleeding should have a pregnancy test.
- A pelvic ultrasound will detect many structural causes of abnormal bleeding.
- Either a pelvic ultrasound or endometrial biopsy is appropriate for evaluation of postmenopausal bleeding.

CURRENT THERAPY

- Unstable women with acute heavy vaginal bleeding should be admitted to hospital for intravenous (IV) estrogen therapy (Premarin) or surgical intervention.
- Treatment of anovulatory bleeding includes ovulation induction if a woman desires pregnancy and hormonal cycle control if she does not.
- Anovulatory women are at risk for endometrial hyperplasia or carcinoma due to unopposed estrogen and should have regular progesterone-induced withdrawal bleeds.
- Treatment of menorrhagia can include nonsteroidal antiinflammatory drugs (NSAIDs), tranexamic acid (Lysteda), or insertion of a levonorgestrel intrauterine device (IUD) (Mirena).

Epidemiology

Abnormal vaginal bleeding is a common complaint in primary care. The prevalence of some type of abnormal bleeding is between 10% and 30% among women of reproductive age. Anovulatory bleeding is more common in women who are perimenopausal and who are overweight. The estimated direct and indirect costs of abnormal bleeding are $1 billion and $12 billion annually, respectively. Abnormal bleeding is also a common reason for women to be referred to gynecologists and is an indication for up to 25% of all gynecologic surgery.

Pathophysiology

Normal menstrual bleeding is defined as regular vaginal bleeding that occurs at intervals from every 21 to 35 days. A normal menstrual cycle is ovulatory, with two distinct phases: the follicular phase and the luteal phase. The follicular phase is the first half of the cycle. The luteal phase occurs after ovulation, when the corpus luteum develops in anticipation of a possible pregnancy. Table 1 defines vocabulary to describe different patterns of abnormal bleeding.

The pathologic abnormality in anovulatory cycles is a lack of ovulation, which produces an unopposed estrogen state. The luteal phase of the menstrual cycle is dominated by progesterone, which is only produced after ovulation. This lack of progesterone contributes to irregular endometrial growth and nonuniform bleeding. In a normal cycle, the entire endometrium sloughs off during menstruation. In an anovulatory cycle, different sections of endometrium outgrow their blood supply at different times and bleed erratically. Anovulatory bleeding (also referred to as dysfunctional uterine bleeding) is unpredictable in timing and amount of bleeding.

The most common structural abnormalities that cause abnormal bleeding are endometrial polyps, leiomyomas, adenomyosis, and hyperplasia or malignancy.

Abnormal bleeding is also common in women who use hormonal contraception, usually due to endometrial abnormalities from exogenous hormones. Women who take combination estrogen/progestin contraception often have intermenstrual bleeding for the first 3 months of treatment. Missed pills are a very frequent cause of abnormal bleeding. In women using progestin-only methods, the abnormal bleeding usually is caused by progestin-induced endometrial atrophy.

Diagnosis

All women with abnormal bleeding should have a thorough history and physical examination and a pregnancy test. If the pregnancy test is negative, the next step is to determine whether her cycles are ovulatory or anovulatory. Table 2 describes characteristics of ovulatory cycles. Laboratory evaluation includes looking for causes of anovulation (Table 3), assessing for anemia with a hemoglobin and hematocrit level, and consideration of getting a pelvic ultrasound to look for structural abnormalities.

In menorrhagia, evaluation for a coagulation disorder (most commonly von Willebrand disease), liver failure, or chronic renal failure is also indicated. Evaluation in an acute bleeding episode (usually due to anovulatory bleeding) should include a hemoglobin and hematocrit if the bleeding is heavy assessment of volume status, and an endometrial biopsy. Postmenopausal bleeding is related to an increased risk of endometrial hyperplasia and cancer and should be evaluated with a transvaginal ultrasound to look at the endometrial thickness (under 4 mm is reassuring) or an office endometrial biopsy. Table 4 describes the steps in evaluation of a woman with abnormal bleeding.

Treatment

If a woman presents with heavy bleeding and exhibits any signs or symptoms of hypovolemia, she should be admitted to the hospital and either treated with IV conjugated estrogen (Premarin) to stop the bleeding or have a surgical procedure (such as dilation and curettage). If the bleeding is heavy but the woman is stable and her hemoglobin and hematocrit are close to normal, outpatient treatment with high-dose oral contraceptive pills (OCPs), estrogen, cyclic progesterone, NSAIDs, or tranexamic acid (Lysteda) is indicated. Women with structural abnormalities causing menorrhagia should be referred for possible surgical treatment.

TABLE 1	Causes of Abnormal Uterine Bleeding (ACOG)
PALM (structural causes)	**COEIN (non-structural causes)**
Polyp	Coagulopathy
Adenomyosis	Ovulatory dysfunction
Leiomyoma	Endometrial
Malignancy and hyperplasia	Iatrogenic
	Not yet classified

TABLE 2	Signs and Symptoms of Ovulatory Cycles	
Regular cycle length	Presence of premenstrual stress (PMS) symptoms
Dysmenorrhea	Mittelschmerz (pain at ovulation)
Changes in cervical mucus	Biphasic temperature curve
Premenstrual breast tenderness	Positive test result from luteinizing hormone (LH) predictor kit

TABLE 3 — Causes of Anovulatory Cycles

Hypothalamic
- Weight loss
- Eating disorders
- Female athlete triad
- Chronic illness
- Stress
- Excessive exercise

Polycystic ovary syndrome

Thyroid disorders

Hyperprolactinemia

Idiopathic chronic anovulation

Medication-induced (i.e., after discontinuation of hormonal contraceptives)

TABLE 4 — Clinical Evaluation of a Woman With Abnormal Bleeding

OVULATORY BLEEDING	ANOVULATORY BLEEDING
History, physical examination, pregnancy test	History, physical examination, pregnancy test

In menorrhagia:
• Consideration of liver function tests, BUN/Cr, CBC, coagulation profile
  • Pelvic ultrasound to exclude uterine fibroids
  • Sonohysterogram to exclude polyps or adenomyosis
  • Endometrial biopsy (especially if age >45) to exclude endometrial hyperplasia
	Laboratory studies:
	• TSH
	• Prolactin
	• CBC (if acute bleeding episode or frequent heavy bleeding)
	• Consideration of endometrial biopsy (especially if age >45) to exclude hyperplasia or malignancy
	• Evaluation for other symptoms of PCOS

In intermenstrual bleeding: • Pap smear, cervical cultures	Screen for eating disorder, stress, female athlete triad

Abbreviations: BUN/Cr=blood urea nitrogen/creatinine; CBC=complete blood count; Pap=Papanicolaou smear; PCOS=polycystic ovary syndrome; TSH=thyroid-stimulating hormone.

TABLE 5 — Treatment Options for Abnormal Vaginal Bleeding

Anovulation: cycle control with estrogen/progestin contraception, DMPA, levonorgestrel IUD (Mirena), or scheduled progestin-induced withdrawal bleeds, ovulation induction with clomiphene citrate (Clomid), and referral to gynecologist if pregnancy desired

Acute bleeding episode—outpatient: administration of high-dose OCPs (up to 4 per day) for 5–7 days with subsequent continuous cycling with OCPs for at least 1 month, administration of oral estrogen to acutely stop bleeding, or administration of oral progesterone to acutely stop bleeding

Acute bleeding episode—inpatient: IVF, supportive care, IV estrogen therapy, consultation for surgical intervention

Menorrhagia—treatment with NSAIDs, tranexamic acid (Lysteda), insertion of levonorgestrel IUD, referral for endometrial ablation or surgical treatment of structural abnormality

On combination estrogen/progestin contraception: supportive care for first 3 months, assessment of adherence to pill regimen, add supplemental estrogen, change to a method with a higher dose of estrogen or a different class of progestin

On progestin-only contraception: add supplemental estrogen or combination oral contraceptive pill and NSAID to decrease bleeding

Abbreviations: DMPA=depot medroxyprogesterone acetate (Depo-Provera); IUD=intrauterine device; IV=intravenous; IVF=in vitro fertilization; NSAID=nonsteroidal antiinflammatory drug; OCP=oral contraceptive pill.

Treatment of women with ovulatory bleeding is indicated if the woman is anemic or is bothered by her bleeding pattern. However, treatment of anovulation with some type of progesterone is necessary to reduce the risk of endometrial hyperplasia or carcinoma. All women with chronic anovulation should have regular progesterone-induced withdrawal bleed. OCPs, monthly cycling of progesterone, and continuous administration of progestin contraception (e.g., depot medroxyprogesterone acetate [Depo-Provera] or levonorgestrel IUD [Mirena]) are all effective treatments (Table 5).

Treatment of women with abnormal bleeding on OCPs involves education and support to try to get them through the first 3 months on the pills. After that, consideration of supplemental estrogen, changing to a higher dose of an estrogen pill, changing to a pill with a different class of progestin, use of a supplemental NSAID to decrease the amount of bleeding, decreasing the hormone free interval, or changing to a nonhormonal type of contraception are all potential treatments.

References

Abdel-Aleem H, d'Arcangues C, Vogelsong KM, et al: Treatment of vaginal bleeding irregularities induced by progestin only contraceptives, *Cochrane Database Syst Rev*(4), 2007. CD003449.

ACOG: Practice bulletin no 128: Diagnosis of abnormal uterine bleeding in reproductive-aged women, *Obstet Gynecol* 120:197–206, 2012.

ACOG: Practice bulletin no. 136. Management of abnormal uterine bleeding associated with ovulatory dysfunction. *Obstet Gynecol* 122(1):176–185, 2013.

Ely JW, Kennedy CM, Clark EC, et al: Abnormal uterine bleeding: a management algorithm, *J Am Board Fam Med* 19:590–602, 2006.

Liu Z, Doan QV, Blumenthal P, et al: A systematic review evaluating health-related quality of life, work impairment, and health-care costs and utilization in abnormal uterine bleeding, *Value Health* 10:183–194, 2007.

Naoulou B, Tsai MC: Efficacy of tranexamic acid in the treatment of idiopathic and non-functional heavy menstrual bleeding: a systematic review, *Acta Obstet Gynecol* 91:529–537, 2012.

Schrager S: Abnormal bleeding associated with hormonal contraception, *Am Fam Physician* 65:2073–2080, 2002. 2083.

Sweet MG, Schmidt-Dalton TA, Weiss PM, et al: Evaluation and management of abnormal uterine bleeding in premenopausal women, *Am Fam Physician* 85:35–43, 2012.

AMENORRHEA

Method of
Colleen Loo-Gross, MD, MPH

CURRENT DIAGNOSIS

- In the absence of physiologic causes (e.g., pregnancy, lactation, and menopause), four conditions account for the majority of amenorrhea cases: polycystic ovary syndrome, hypothalamic amenorrhea, hyperprolactinemia, and primary ovarian insufficiency.
- Most causes of amenorrhea can be identified through a detailed history, physical examination, and laboratory evaluation.
- Müllerian agenesis is the most common cause of anatomic malformations associated with amenorrhea.
- In the evaluation of amenorrhea, it is important to exclude physiologic causes such as pregnancy and lactation, as well as potential iatrogenic causes (e.g., hormonal contraception, chemotherapy and radiation therapy, and medications that may cause hyperprolactinemia).
- Initial laboratory evaluation should include follicle-stimulating hormone (FSH), thyroid-stimulating hormone (TSH), and prolactin levels.
- In amenorrheic women less than 40 years of age, an elevated FSH level in the menopausal range indicates primary ovarian insufficiency.
- A low or normal FSH value in amenorrhea without evidence of anatomic cause suggests chronic anovulation, most commonly attributed to hypothalamic amenorrhea or polycystic ovary syndrome.
- In cases of elevated prolactin level (with no evidence of thyroid disease), MRI is warranted to assess for a possible pituitary tumor.

CURRENT THERAPY

- The underlying cause of amenorrhea should be treated accordingly.
- For those with an estrogen deficient state, cyclic hormone therapy may be indicated, and adequate calcium and vitamin D intake are essential to reduce the risk of osteoporosis.
- Fertility considerations should be addressed in all causes of amenorrhea.
- Psychosocial support, such as counseling services and peer support groups, is an important aspect of management.

Amenorrhea is defined as the absence of menses. Its prevalence, when not related to pregnancy or lactation, is approximately 3% to 4% among premenopausal women. Amenorrhea is further categorized into primary amenorrhea (prior to menarche) and secondary amenorrhea (following menarche). Evaluation for primary amenorrhea should be initiated when menarche has not occurred by 15 years of age, or sooner for females without onset of menses within 5 years of thelarche. Evaluation should also be considered when thelarche has not occurred by 13 years of age. Secondary amenorrhea is the lack of menses for 3 months in females with preceding regular cycles or 6 months in those with irregular menstrual cycles.

Etiology
There are a number of potential etiologies of amenorrhea. In the absence of physiologic causes (e.g., pregnancy, lactation, and menopause), four conditions account for the majority of amenorrhea cases: polycystic ovary syndrome (PCOS), hypothalamic amenorrhea, hyperprolactinemia, and primary ovarian insufficiency. The approximate frequency of common causes of primary and secondary amenorrhea are shown in Tables 1 and 2. Other considerations may also include adrenal disease, adrenal hyperplasia, chronic disease, Cushing syndrome, androgen-secreting tumors, central nervous system infections, and a history of trauma (such as traumatic brain injury).

With primary amenorrhea, anatomic defects and chromosomal abnormalities (with associated primary ovarian insufficiency) are often causative factors. Anatomic abnormalities may cause amenorrhea due to obstruction along the genital outflow tract. With Müllerian agenesis, incomplete development of the Müllerian duct embryologically results in a range of defects due to agenesis or atresia of the uterus and/or vagina, though ovarian function is usually unaffected. Müllerian agenesis is a common cause of primary amenorrhea among females who present with normal signs of adrenarche and breast development. In primary ovarian insufficiency, amenorrhea occurs as the result of ovarian follicle depletion or dysfunction. It comprises 2% to 10% of cases of amenorrhea.

Excluding pregnancy, the most common causes of secondary amenorrhea are hypothalamic amenorrhea and PCOS. Functional hypothalamic amenorrhea occurs in the presence of hypothalamic-pituitary-ovarian axis suppression, without evidence of organic cause. In these cases, the regulatory pulsatile secretion of gonadotropin-releasing hormone (GnRH) is affected, leading to abnormally low levels of estrogen.

Evaluation
Most causes of amenorrhea can be identified through a detailed history, physical examination, and laboratory evaluation. It is important to exclude physiologic causes of amenorrhea such as pregnancy and lactation, as well as potential iatrogenic causes (for example, hormonal contraception, chemotherapy and radiation therapy, and medications that may cause hyperprolactinemia such as antipsychotics, antidepressants, opiates, and metoclopramide [Reglan]). The incidence of amenorrhea is approximately 12% in women taking antipsychotic medications, due to the resultant increase in prolactin levels.

History
Obtaining a detailed history is an important component in the evaluation of amenorrhea. The presence of vasomotor symptoms, such as hot flashes, may be indicators of primary ovarian insufficiency, whereas reports of headache or vision changes may prompt further evaluation for possible central nervous system tumor or empty sella syndrome. Women with anatomic causes of amenorrhea, such as transverse vaginal septum, imperforate hymen, and isolated absence of the vagina or cervix, may report cyclic pelvic pain, which occurs due to blood accumulation behind the outflow tract obstruction and in some cases, associated endometriosis. Anosmia may be an indication of the rare Kallmann syndrome, which presents with amenorrhea due to GnRH deficiency and is associated with abnormal development of the olfactory bulb.

Additional history details should include assessment of mood and stress, weight changes, nutrition and eating patterns, and exercise routines, with evaluation for a possible eating disorder or other cause of an overall energy deficit. Abnormal historical findings such as these may be suggestive of functional hypothalamic amenorrhea. It is also important to assess for signs or symptoms of thyroid disease and of other potential chronic medical conditions.

Family history may also provide useful information. A positive family history for delayed menarche may suggest constitutional delay of puberty as the cause of amenorrhea, though this is considered a diagnosis of exclusion. A family history of primary ovarian insufficiency is also worth noting, given the related genetic predisposition. Moreover, early menopause in family members is a risk factor associated with primary ovarian insufficiency.

Physical Examination
About 15% of those with primary amenorrhea have an abnormality noted on genital examination. Both internal and external

TABLE 1 Common Causes of Primary Amenorrhea

CATEGORY	APPROXIMATE FREQUENCY (%)
Breast development present	30
Müllerian agenesis	10
Androgen insensitivity	9
Transverse vaginal septum	2
Imperforate hymen	1
Constitutional delay of puberty	8
No breast development: high FSH	40
46,XX	15
46,XY	5
Abnormal karyotype	20
No breast development: low FSH	30
Constitutional delay of puberty	10
Prolactinoma	5
Kallmann syndrome	2
Other CNS etiology	3
Stress, weight loss, eating disorders	3
Polycystic ovary syndrome	3
Congenital adrenal hyperplasia	3
Other	1

CNS, Central nervous system; FSH, follicle-stimulating hormone.
Adapted from Practice Committee of American Society for Reproductive Medicine. Current evaluation of amenorrhea. *Fertil Steril.* 2008;90:S219–S225.

TABLE 2 Common Causes of Secondary Amenorrhea

CATEGORY	APPROXIMATE FREQUENCY (%)
Low or normal FSH	66
Stress, weight loss, eating disorders	
Non-specific hypothalamic causes	
Chronic anovulation, including PCOS	
Hypothyroidism	
Cushing syndrome	
Pituitary tumor, empty sella, Sheehan syndrome	
Gonadal failure: high FSH	12
46,XX	
Abnormal karyotype	
Hyperprolactinemia	13
Anatomic	7
Asherman syndrome (intrauterine synechiae)	
Other hyperandrogenic states	2
Ovarian tumor	
Non-classic congenital adrenal hyperplasia	
Undiagnosed	

FSH, Follicle-stimulating hormone; PCOS, polycystic ovary syndrome.
Adapted from Practice Committee of American Society for Reproductive Medicine. Current evaluation of amenorrhea. *Fertil Steril.* 2008;90:S219–S225.

genitalia should be examined. A shortened vagina is associated with conditions such as Müllerian agenesis (which may present with a range of defects resulting from incomplete embryologic development of the Müllerian duct), imperforate hymen, transverse vaginal septum, cervical atresia, or other uterine anomalies. In some cases, the vagina may appear as no more than a small dimple.

Additional physical findings may also help guide the evaluation of amenorrhea. Dysmorphic features should be noted, such as a webbed neck or short stature, which may be suggestive of Turner syndrome. Galactorrhea may warrant evaluation for a pituitary tumor. Clinical evidence of self-induced vomiting may be suggestive of a hypothalamic etiology of amenorrhea.

The physical examination should further assess for secondary sexual characteristics, such as the presence of pubic hair and also breast development, which is an indicator of endogenous estrogen effect. Conversely, the presence of thin vaginal mucosa is a sign of low endogenous estrogen level. Signs of hirsutism, acne, and male pattern alopecia are indicators of androgen excess, which may suggest hyperandrogenic etiologies of amenorrhea such as PCOS. Body mass index (BMI) also helps to differentiate PCOS from other causes of amenorrhea (such as functional disorders of the hypothalamus) given its typical presentation with obesity.

Laboratory Studies

When the etiology of amenorrhea is not evident after completing a thorough history and physical examination, additional assessment is warranted. Initial laboratory evaluation should include levels of follicle-stimulating hormone (FSH), thyroid-stimulating hormone (TSH), and prolactin. Abnormal thyroid levels should be managed accordingly. An elevated prolactin level without apparent cause necessitates further investigation with diagnostic imaging of the pituitary gland.

In amenorrheic women less than 40 years of age, an elevated FSH level in the menopausal range indicates primary ovarian insufficiency. The FSH level should be repeated at least 1 month following the initial result for confirmation. For women less than 30 years of age with identified primary ovarian insufficiency, a karyotype should be obtained to assess for possible chromosomal abnormality. Karyotype analysis may be considered for those over 30 years of age as well. In cases when the cause is not identified, particularly in women who also have a family history of primary ovarian insufficiency, premutation carrier testing for the fragile X gene (*FMR1*) should be considered.

A low or normal FSH value in amenorrheic women without evidence of anatomic cause suggests chronic anovulation, most commonly attributed to hypothalamic amenorrhea or PCOS. In principle, hypothalamic amenorrhea would be associated with low estradiol levels, and PCOS would more often be associated with normal estradiol levels. However, estradiol levels fluctuate and testing is not recommended to help distinguish between these diagnoses. Similarly, the progesterone challenge test for withdrawal bleeding is not considered a reliable indicator of estrogen levels, given both high false positive and false negative rates.

Imaging Studies

In certain situations, further evaluation with imaging may be indicated, such as the use of ultrasound, magnetic resonance imaging (MRI), or hysteroscopy to assess for a potential anatomic abnormality. Examples include the absence of the uterus in primary amenorrhea, as may be seen with Müllerian agenesis and 46,XY conditions like androgen insensitivity syndrome, or the presence of intrauterine synechiae (Asherman syndrome) in those with prior procedural instrumentation of the uterus. In cases of an elevated prolactin level (with no evidence of thyroid disease), MRI is warranted to assess for a possible pituitary tumor, which is present in 50% to 60% of women with hyperprolactinemia.

Diagnoses and Management
Anatomic Causes

Müllerian agenesis is the most common cause of anatomic malformations associated with amenorrhea, comprising approximately

10% of primary amenorrhea cases. In addition to malformations along the genital tract, over half of Müllerian agenesis cases may also present with other congenital abnormalities, such as urinary tract or skeletal defects (e.g., scoliosis, vertebral arch anomalies, and wrist hypoplasia). Thus, it is important to assess for the presence of coexisting congenital anomalies in those with Müllerian agenesis. Renal ultrasound and spinal X-ray imaging should be considered in these women.

A less common cause of anatomical defects in the uterus or vagina is complete androgen insensitivity, which accounts for 5% of primary amenorrhea. Other anatomic defects leading to primary amenorrhea include transverse vaginal septum (2% of cases), imperforate hymen (1% of cases), and isolated absence of the vagina or cervix. In women with prior history of procedural interventions involving the uterus or cervix, intrauterine synechiae (Asherman syndrome) and cervical stenosis should also be considered as potential etiologies of amenorrhea. In cases of Asherman syndrome, treatment often involves hysteroscopy for lysis of the intrauterine adhesions.

Women with Müllerian agenesis typically present with normal secondary female sexual characteristics, in the setting of anatomic defects in all or some aspects of the uterus and vagina. Women with complete androgen insensitivity may also present with vaginal defects, though in addition they have a family history suggestive of androgen insensitivity, lack of pubarche, and may present with inguinal hernias or masses containing testes. Complete androgen insensitivity is an X-linked recessive condition and is confirmed by an elevated serum testosterone level in the male range and karyotype analysis (46,XY). Of note, complete androgen insensitivity confers an increased risk of gonadal malignancy, and treatment includes gonadal removal, typically after completion of growth and breast development. Hormonal replacement therapy is indicated following prophylactic gonadal removal for the maintenance of bone health.

The first-line treatment for Müllerian agenesis includes vaginal dilation to achieve elongation, a nonsurgical, patient-controlled therapy that has a success rate above 90%. Surgery to create a vagina is much less commonly required and reserved for rare cases. Psychosocial support is another important aspect of treatment for these individuals. Fertility considerations should also be addressed. In those with Müllerian agenesis who desire children, options may include assisted reproductive technology with gestational surrogacy or adoption. With regard to ongoing care, routine cervical cancer screening is not typically indicated given the absence of a cervix in these women.

Primary Ovarian Insufficiency

Persistently elevated FSH levels in the menopausal range indicate impaired ovarian function, consistent with primary ovarian insufficiency. Other terms to describe this condition have been previously used, including premature ovarian failure, premature menopause, and primary ovarian failure. This condition may affect 1% to 5% of women, though the etiology is not always known.

Congenital causes are a factor in some cases of primary ovarian insufficiency, with certain chromosomal abnormalities leading to gonadal dysgenesis, an example being Turner syndrome (45,X). Chromosomal abnormalities are identified in 50% of adolescents without comorbidities who present with primary amenorrhea and in 13% of women 30 years of age or younger who present with secondary amenorrhea. With regard to management, it is important to remember that the incidence of gonadal malignancy is up to 25% for women with a Y chromosome. Accordingly, in 46,XY women with lack of gonadal function as evidenced by elevated FSH levels and absence of hormone secretion, gonadal removal is indicated at the time of diagnosis.

Primary ovarian insufficiency has shown associated genetic predisposition, and premutation carrier testing for fragile X syndrome should be considered in these women when another cause has not been identified. Among those with a normal karyotype, 6% of women with primary ovarian insufficiency are found to

have premutation of the *FMR1* (fragile X) gene. Additionally, primary ovarian insufficiency may also be seen with various endocrinopathies, such as hypoparathyroidism and hypoadrenalism, or autoimmune disease. Specifically, approximately 4% of cases have adrenal or ovarian antibodies, and autoimmune disorders may be found in up to 40% of women with primary ovarian insufficiency, most commonly thyroid disease.

For women with primary ovarian insufficiency, infertility should be addressed, though up to 10% may have temporary remission with spontaneous conception. It is unclear whether oral contraceptives are as effective in this population, so alternative methods such as barrier contraception or intrauterine device options are more appropriate for pregnancy prevention. Genetic predisposition for this condition should also be addressed. Consultations with reproductive endocrinology and fertility specialists are indicated when pregnancy is desired, as options are limited beyond donor *in vitro* fertilization. Psychosocial counseling and support should be offered as well.

Annual visits are recommended in those with primary ovarian insufficiency. Given the increased cardiovascular risk associated with the early estrogen deficient state, steps should be taken to ensure optimized cardiovascular health, including routine screening for hypertension and a lipid panel at least every 5 years. Furthermore, hormonal treatment until the typical age of menopause is appropriate both to support bone health as well as to develop and maintain secondary sexual characteristics. The estrogen deficient state in this condition poses risk to the attainment of peak bone mass. Thus, weight-bearing exercise as well as adequate calcium (1300 mg per day) and vitamin D (400 to 1000 IU per day) intake are also important aspects of management to reduce the risk of osteoporosis. With regard to hormone therapy in these cases, additional potential benefits include decreased risk of ischemic heart disease, less cardiovascular mortality, and vasomotor symptom control. Of note, combined oral contraceptives provide higher levels of hormones than are necessary for this purpose and are not recommended in this setting. A more appropriate regimen would include daily estradiol (e.g., 100 µg dose in transdermal [Alora, Dotti, Minivelle, Vivelle] or oral form [Estrace], though the latter confers a relatively higher thromboembolism risk), with 12 days of cyclic progesterone monthly (e.g., medroxyprogesterone acetate [Provera] 10 mg). For those still undergoing pubertal growth and maturity, specialized care is recommended, as hormone therapy should begin with estrogen before the introduction of progesterone, with the purpose of mimicking hormonal levels associated with development.

Hyperprolactinemia and Pituitary Causes

Another potential etiology of amenorrhea or oligomenorrhea is an elevated prolactin level, which inhibits the release and thus the effect of gonadotropins. Specifically, the presence of hyperprolactinemia suppresses GnRH secretion. When hyperprolactinemia is identified, in the absence of other potential causes such as medications or thyroid disease, an MRI of the head is warranted for further evaluation. Among women who present with amenorrhea and elevated prolactin, 50% to 60% are associated with a pituitary tumor. Additionally, pituitary disorders including Sheehan syndrome, pituitary gland necrosis, and empty sella syndrome may also be causes of anovulation and amenorrhea, as well as other pituitary or central nervous system tumors and organic diseases.

Regarding treatment for hyperprolactinemia, dopamine agonists may be used to aid in decreasing prolactin levels, regardless of the presence of pituitary tumor. This has an effect on the subsequent restoration of menses. In cases of pituitary adenoma, surgical resection may be warranted.

Hypothalamic Amenorrhea

The most common cause of chronic anovulation is functional hypothalamic amenorrhea, often associated with stress, weight loss, poor nutrition, and strenuous exercise. In these cases, suppression of the normal hypothalamic-pituitary-ovarian axis occurs as a result of an overall energy deficit, though the exact pathophysiology remains unclear. A much less common cause of hypothalamic amenorrhea is isolated gonadotropin deficiency, such as that seen in Kallmann syndrome (primary GnRH deficiency).

Multidisciplinary care should be considered in the approach to treatment of functional hypothalamic amenorrhea. Appropriate nutrition rehabilitation and reduction of strenuous exercise are important aspects of management for these women, and restoration of menses usually occurs following correction of the energy deficit. Furthermore, treatment should address stress reduction and psychosocial health, which may also play a role in the resumption of menses. As for pharmacologic management, evidence suggests that the use of leptin may help restore GnRH pulsatility and thus ovulation and menses, given its regulatory role in hypothalamic dysfunction. For those with hypothalamic amenorrhea desiring pregnancy, treatment options for ovulation induction may be pursued, typically with GnRH or gonadotropin therapy.

Similar to primary ovarian insufficiency, hypothalamic amenorrhea is associated with an estrogen deficient state, so affected women are at increased risk for osteoporosis. Bone density screening may be considered. In addition to nutrition rehabilitation and a decrease of strenuous activity, it is important to ensure adequate calcium and vitamin D intake with supplementation. Cyclic hormone therapy at physiologic doses may be considered for optimizing bone health, such as in cases where correction of the underlying cause of hypothalamic amenorrhea is not easily achieved. However, the potential beneficial effects on bone density in these cases are limited in the absence of appropriate nutrition rehabilitation. Furthermore, the use of bisphosphonates in the premenopausal population is not recommended given the limited data available and concern for potential teratogenic risks. Thus, treatment should primarily focus on addressing the underlying cause of hypothalamic amenorrhea.

Polycystic Ovary Syndrome

Chronic anovulation and amenorrhea may also occur with PCOS, though these women are more likely to present with oligomenorrhea. The presence of obesity and concomitant signs of androgen excess help distinguish PCOS from hypothalamic amenorrhea. Typically, a higher BMI is associated with PCOS, while normal or low BMI is more often associated with functional hypothalamic amenorrhea. According to the Rotterdam Consensus Criteria from 2003, the diagnosis of PCOS requires at least two of the following: (1) signs of androgen excess, (2) the presence of polycystic ovaries, and (3) ovulatory dysfunction. However, the 2006 Androgen Excess Society criteria for PCOS differ slightly from these guidelines, specifically requiring hyperandrogenism as one of the diagnostic conditions, along with ovarian dysfunction (oligo-anovulation and/or polycystic ovaries) and exclusion of other androgen excess or related disorders. The evidence of hyperandrogenism may be established by clinical findings (e.g., hirsutism, acne, male pattern alopecia) or laboratory measurement. Generally, serum androgen levels in those with PCOS do not exceed twice the upper limit of normal range, so further investigation for other etiologies of hyperandrogenism would be warranted in these cases.

The management of women with PCOS includes monitoring for insulin resistance and glucose intolerance, dyslipidemia, and cardiovascular risk, with subsequent interventions as indicated for any identified comorbidities. Treatment also involves healthy lifestyle modifications directed at dietary changes, exercise, and weight loss, given the association of PCOS with obesity. Furthermore, low-dose combined oral contraceptives are recommended to reduce the risk for endometrial cancer in the setting of chronic anovulation. Pharmacotherapy with metformin (Glucophage)[1] is another important treatment consideration, which may provide beneficial effects on ovulation, menstrual abnormalities, and androgen levels, in addition to its known effects on improving glucose tolerance.

---

[1]Not FDA approved for this indication.

References

American College of Obstetricians and Gynecologists: Committee Opinion No. 728. Müllerian agenesis: diagnosis, management, and treatment, *Obstet Gynecol* 131:e35–42, 2018.

American College of Obstetricians and Gynecologists: Committee Opinion No. 605. Primary ovarian insufficiency in adolescents and young women, *Obstet Gynecol* 123:193–197, 2014.

Gordon CM: Clinical practice: Functional hypothalamic amenorrhea, *N Engl J Med* 363(4):365–371, 2010.

Klein DA, Poth MA: Amenorrhea: An approach to diagnosis and management, *Am Fam Physician* 87(11):781–788, 2013.

Practice Committee of American Society for Reproductive Medicine: Current evaluation of amenorrhea, *Fertil Steril* 90:S219–S225, 2008.

BACTERIAL INFECTIONS OF THE URINARY TRACT IN WOMEN

Method of
Kinder Fayssoux, MD

CURRENT DIAGNOSIS

- Acute cystitis is the most common urologic disorder in women.
- *Escherichia coli* and *Staphylococcus saprophyticus* are the causative agents for 80% of community acquired urinary tract infections (UTIs).
- *E. coli* is also the most common uropathogen in the nosocomial setting.
- Anatomic risk factors include short urethra, the proximity of the urethra to the anus, and the colonization of the periurethral mucosa with bowel flora.
- Other risk factors include previous UTI, sexual intercourse, and, separately, the use of spermicide, pregnancy, diabetes, incontinence, cystocoele, and incomplete emptying of the bladder and dysfunctional voiding (defined as abnormal bladder emptying in the absence of neurologic disease).
- Postmenopausal women are also at increased risk if they are estrogen deficient.
- Acute cystitis typically presents with abrupt onset of dysuria, increased frequency, and/or urgency. Less frequently a patient will present with hematuria, suprapubic discomfort, or back/costovertebral angle pain. If a fever is present, it is usually less than 38.9°C (102°F).
- Acute pyelonephritis can evolve from either asymptomatic bacteriuria or from an ascending bladder infection.
- Symptoms usually include fever usually greater than 38.9°C (102°F) with chills, nausea/vomiting, dysuria, increased frequency, urgency, and costovertebral angle (CVA) tenderness (usually unilateral).
- *E. coli* is the major pathogen in acute pyelonephritis and treatment depends on severity and pregnancy status.

CURRENT THERAPY

- Empiric therapy for uncomplicated UTIs should be dependent on the most recent antibiotic guidelines and the uropathogen resistance patterns in a community.
- In a community with >20% incidence of resistant *E. coli*, nitrofurantoin (Macrobid) 100 mg bid for 7 days is the treatment of choice with quinolones as second-line therapy.

- In a community with <20% *E. coli* resistance, trimethoprim/sulfamethoxazole 160/800 (Bactrim DS) PO twice daily for 3 days is also acceptable as first-line therapy with quinolones still considered as second-line therapy.
- Phenazopyridine (Pyridium), a smooth muscle relaxant, can be prescribed for spasm relief.
- Fungal UTIs or candiduria should be treated with fluconazole (Diflucan) 200 mg daily for 2 weeks.
- Outpatient treatment guidelines for acute pyelonephritis are the same as for uncomplicated UTI except the duration of antimicrobial therapy is longer (10–14 days).
- Inpatient treatment for acute pyelonephritis is typically IV levofloxacin (Levaquin) (750 mg daily) or ampicillin (1 g every 6 h).
- Acute pyelonephritis should resolve in 48 to 72 hours, if patients are not getting better, imaging should be undertaken with ultrasound or CT scan to assess for renal abscess or urethral obstruction.

Acute Cystitis (Urinary Tract Infection)

Acute cystitis is the most common urologic disorder among women. It represents 4% of all outpatient visits. Of these visits, 52% present to a primary care clinic and 23% to the emergency department. The annual health care costs associated with urinary tract infections (UTIs) are roughly 1.6 billion and climbing. Antimicrobial prescriptions for UTIs account for 15% of all outpatient prescriptions. One-third of all women will have at least one symptomatic UTI by age 24, with more than half of all women having at least one during their lifetime.

Acute cystitis can be defined as uncomplicated or complicated. Uncomplicated cystitis is defined as a UTI in patients with normal urinary tract anatomy without a contributing medical condition such as diabetes mellitus, neurogenic bladder, pregnancy, renal insufficiency, immune deficiency, recent antibiotic use, recent genitourinary instrumentation, spinal cord injury, ureteral obstruction, or nephrolithiasis. Complicated cystitis is defined as a UTI in patients with abnormal urinary tract anatomy or with one of the aforementioned medical conditions. These patients generally require urine culture as part of the initial work-up to guide antimicrobial therapy and often additional condition specific evaluation and treatment.

Acute cystitis is caused by ascending bacteria of perineal/urethral/fecal origin through the urethra into the bladder and renal systems. *Escherichia coli* and *Staphylococcus saprophyticus* are the causative agents for 80% of community acquired UTIs (complicated and uncomplicated). *E. coli* is also the most common uropathogen in the nosocomial setting. Other known uropathogens include *Pseudomonas spp*, *Klebsiella spp*, *Proteus*, *Corynebacterium urealyticum*, and *Providencia*. Fungal UTIs caused by *Candida spp*, *Aspergillus spp*, and *Cryptococcus neoformans* are also increasingly encountered. These are usually caused by indwelling urinary devices and seen more frequently in diabetics. Other populations prone to fungal UTIs include patients who are immunocompromised, hospitalized, or elderly.

There are numerous risk factors for acute cystitis, several specific to women. Risk factors unique to women include several related to their anatomy. These anatomic differences are the primary reason for the increased incidence of UTI in women when compared to men and include the female's relatively short urethra (when compared to the male counterpart), the proximity of the urethra to the anus, and the colonization of the periurethral mucosa with bowel flora.

Other risk factors include previous UTI, sexual intercourse, and, separately, the use of spermicide, pregnancy, diabetes, incontinence, cystocoele, and incomplete emptying of the bladder and dysfunctional voiding (defined as abnormal bladder emptying in the absence of neurologic disease). Postmenopausal women are also at increased risk if they are estrogen deficient.

Dysfunctional voiding has an unknown etiology and results in increased external sphincter activity during voluntary voiding which results in reflux, increasing chances of UTI.

Commonly advised behavioral modifications thought to decrease the risk of UTI (e.g., postcoital voiding, increased fluid intake, avoidance of urinary holding, douching, front-to-back wiping, proper tampon/sanitary napkin use, and loose/cotton underwear) have been supported by the literature.

Acute cystitis typically appears as an abrupt onset of dysuria, increased frequency, and/or urgency. Less frequently a patient will present with hematuria, suprapubic discomfort, or back/costovertebral angle pain. If a fever is present, it is usually less than 38.9°C (102°F).

Obtaining a good history that assesses for risk factors and symptoms is important in diagnosing acute cystitis. In a woman who presents with one or more symptoms of UTI (dysuria, frequency, urgency, hematuria), the probability of infection is already 50%. A urine dipstick is a useful diagnostic test, with a positive (+) nitrite or leukocyte esterase result increasing the chances of infection. The combination of positive nitrite *and* leukocyte esterase results has the highest diagnostic correlation with UTI. Physical examination findings may include suprapubic tenderness or costovertebral angle tenderness, although these are unlikely in an uncomplicated UTI scenario.

The gold standard for diagnosis of acute cystitis is a culture that has 10^2 to 10^3 colony-forming units of a single uropathogen from a clean catch or catheterized urine specimen. However, research has shown that, for uncomplicated cystitis, ordering cultures and sensitivities makes little difference in treatment while increasing cost of care. Thus, it is reasonable to start empiric treatment without a culture and sensitivities in a patient presenting with uncomplicated UTI.

The differential diagnosis for an uncomplicated UTI includes:
- Vaginitis/vaginal infections: can cause dysuria
  - *Gardnerella*, *Candida albicans*, and *Trichomonas*
- Urethritis: can cause dysuria/frequency
  - STDs (*Chlamydia trachomatis*, gonorrhea, herpes simplex)
  - Pelvic floor spasm (leads to urethral spasm/irritability)
- Interstitial cystitis
- Malignancy
- Renal tuberculosis

Differentiating between sexually transmitted infections (STI), vaginal infections, and UTIs can be difficult because symptoms and signs commonly overlap. History elements that should prompt a pelvic examination and laboratory evaluation for pathogens are complaints of a vaginal discharge or vaginal irritation/pruritus. Persistent hematuria should raise the concern for underlying malignancy or renal tuberculosis, and further evaluation should be done.

Empiric therapy for uncomplicated UTIs should be dependent on the most recent antibiotic guidelines and the uropathogen resistance patterns in a community. In a community with >20% incidence of resistant *E. coli*, nitrofurantoin (Macrobid) 100 mg bid for 7 days is the treatment of choice with quinolones as second-line therapy. In a community with <20% *E. coli* resistance, trimethoprim/sulfamethoxazole 160/800 (Bactrim DS) PO twice daily for 3 days is also acceptable as first-line therapy with quinolones still considered as second-line therapy. Phenazopyridine (Pyridium), a smooth muscle relaxant, can be prescribed for spasm relief and is usually only necessary for the first 24 hours after treatment is initiated. Fungal UTIs or *candiduria* should be treated with fluconazole (Diflucan) 200 mg daily for 2 weeks.

For a complicated UTI, a culture must always be obtained and the patient should be evaluated in the context of his or her specific comorbid condition before treatment.

Acute Pyelonephritis

Acute pyelonephritis can evolve from either asymptomatic bacteruria or from an ascending bladder infection. Although it can progress from an uncomplicated cystitis, it more commonly presents from a complicated cystitis in the setting of other medical conditions such cholelithiasis, urinary obstruction, malformations, or pregnancy.

Symptoms usually include fever usually greater than 38.9°C (102°F) with chills, nausea/vomiting, dysuria, increased frequency, urgency, and CVA tenderness (usually unilateral). These symptoms can present on a spectrum from mild to severe. *E. coli* is the major pathogen, and treatment depends on severity and pregnancy status. Pregnant patients or patients with moderate to severe nausea/vomiting that would interfere with oral antibiotic treatment should be hospitalized and have blood cultures done in addition to urine culture. Patients with mild symptoms and the ability to tolerate oral antibiotics can be treated as on an outpatient basis with a urine culture obtained before initializing treatment. Outpatient treatment guidelines are the same as for uncomplicated UTI, except the duration of antimicrobial therapy is longer (10–14 days). Inpatient treatment is typically IV levofloxacin (Levaquin 750 mg daily) or ampicillin (1 g every 6 h). Once the inpatient is able to tolerate oral antibiotics and the infection is felt to be controlled, he or she can be switched to oral antibiotics and discharged to complete a 14-day course of treatment as an outpatient.

Symptoms should resolve in 48 to 72 hours; if patients are not getting better, imaging should be undertaken with ultrasound or CT scan to assess for renal abscess or urethral obstruction.

Urethritis

Urethritis usually has a gradual onset and is accompanied with milder symptoms of dysuria, frequency, urgency, or hematuria. It can also occur with a vaginal discharge and complaints of dyspareunia and vaginal pruritus depending on cause. Chalmydial, gonorrheal, candidal and trichomonal urethritis is usually accompanied by a vaginal discharge. Candidal urethritis can also be associated with pruritus and dyspareunia. If urethritis is suspected, a pelvic examination and further laboratory work-up is necessary.

Asymptomatic Bacteruria

Asymptomatic bacteruria is defined as the presence of 100,000 microorganisms/milliliter of urine without any symptoms of cystitis.

No screening should be performed in healthy nonpregnant women, elderly living in the community, diabetic women, institutionalized elderly, or persons with spinal cord injury. Pregnant women are the exception. They should be screened; positive cultures need to be treated, as there is an increased likelihood of asymptomatic bacteruria turning into UTI or pyelonephritis because of vesicoureteral reflux and urinary stasis resulting from increased progesterone levels.

Recurrent Cystitis

Recurrent cystitis is defined as at least three episodes of uncomplicated UTI with one or more documented positive (+) cultures in 12 months. It can be due to relapse or reinfection. Relapse is defined as infection occurring with the same organism as a previous UTI. Reinfection is when symptoms return after treatment and a completely symptom-free interval along with a negative urine culture or when the second infection is caused by a different organism. Most recurrent cystitis tends to be caused by reinfection.

In patients presenting with recurrent cystitis, an age-based evaluation is a good place to start. Adolescents who are not sexually active should be evaluated for congenital abnormalities. Premenopausal females should be questioned about the temporal relationship of the onset of UTI to increased frequency/recent sexual intercourse, spermicide use (with or without condom or diaphragm), or renal stones. Postmenopausal females should be evaluated for decreased estrogen/vaginal atrophy, incontinence, incomplete bladder emptying, cystocoeles, and prolapse.

If a complete and thorough evaluation is done, complicating factors are ruled out, modifiable factors are treated, and recurrent cystitis still remains a problem, then treatment should be considered. Treatment options include continuous antibiotics, postcoital therapy, or self-initiated treatment at the first sign or symptom of an infection.

Gross hematuria or persistent microscopic hematuria should increase suspicion for an underlying malignancy. Also, recurrent cystitis symptoms in a setting of negative cultures may suggest mycobacterial infection or interstitial cystitis.

Catheter Associated Urinary Tract Infection

Catheter-associated UTI is defined as a UTI in a patient who had an indwelling urethral catheter within 48 hours of onset of infection. Indwelling urinary catheters and clean intermittent catheterization are associated with the highest rates of bacteriuria; after 1 month of either there is almost 100% risk of bacteriuria. Formation of a bacterial biofilm on the catheter is thought to be the mechanism of infection in this setting.

No treatment is recommended for asymptomatic patients, and neither prophylactic antibiotics nor routine UA and culture are recommended for this population. For symptomatic patients, the first step is to determine whether the catheter can be removed. If it cannot, then it should be replaced. In addition, a blood and urine culture (taken from a new catheter) should be obtained. Initial treatment is the same as for an uncomplicated UTI as discussed earlier. Confirmation of susceptibility should be confirmed with culture results.

References

Litza JA, Brill JR: Urinary tract infection, *Primary Care Clinical Office Practice* 37:491–507, 2010.
Minardi D, d'Anzeo G, Cantoro D, et al: Urinary tract infections in women: Etiology and treatment options, *Int J Gen Med* 4:333–343, 2011.
Finer G, Landau D: Pathogenesis of urinary tract infections with normal female anatomy, *Lancet* 4:631–634, 2004.
Foster RT: Office gynecology uncomplicated urinary tract infections in women. Obstet Gynecol Clin 35:235–48.
Berek JS: *Berek and Novak's Gynecology*, Philadelphia, 2012, Lippincott. p. 570–71.
Essentials evidence plus: Urinary tract infection (adults), Available at http://essentialevidenceplus.com, accessed August 16, 2016.
Essentials evidence plus: Urethritis (female), http://essentialevidenceplus.com, Accessed August 16, 2016.
Bent SN, Nallamothu BK, Simel DL, et al: Does this woman have an acute uncomplicated urinary tract infection? *JAMA* 287:2701–2710, 2002.
Wagenlehner F, Weidner W, Naber K: An updated on uncomplicated urinary tract infections in women, *Curr Opin Urol* 19:368–374, 2009.
Dielubaza EJ, Schaeffer AJ: Urologic issues for the internist- urinary tract infections in women. Med Clin North Am 95:27–41.
Giesen LG, Cousins G, Dimitrov BD, et al: Predicting acute uncomplicated urinary tract infections in women: A systematic review of the diagnostic accuracy of symptoms and signs, *BMC Fam Pract* 11:78, 2010. Available at http://www.biomedcentral.com/1471-2296/11/78. accessed August 16, 2016.

BENIGN BREAST DISEASE

Method of
Lauren Nye, MD

CURRENT DIAGNOSIS

- Mammography is used for breast cancer screening, and it is recommended to begin screening in women at average risk for breast cancer between ages 40 and 50.
- Benign breast disease may present with an abnormality on screening breast imaging or with a breast symptom such as breast mass or nipple discharge.
- Nonproliferative breast lesions are not associated with an increased risk of breast cancer.
- Proliferative breast lesions without atypia are associated with a slightly increased risk for breast cancer, while proliferative lesions with atypia are associated with a significantly increased risk for breast cancer.
- Factors contributing to a woman's breast cancer risk include family history, personal health history, and modifiable lifestyle factors.

- Some benign breast lesions do not need any further intervention after diagnosis, while others may require surgical excision to rule out malignancy.
- Women at high risk for breast cancer may warrant additional breast screening or begin screening at an earlier age.
- Women at high risk for breast cancer should be counseled on risk reduction strategies including lifestyle modification.
- Chemoprevention agents include tamoxifen, raloxifene (Evista), and aromatase inhibitors.

Breast health is an important aspect of women's health care and includes breast cancer screening and evaluation of breast concerns. Benign breast disease can be identified on a biopsy done for an abnormal screening test, a palpable breast mass, nipple discharge, or other breast concerns. Benign breast disease may be associated with an increased risk for breast cancer. Women at high risk for breast cancer should be considered for additional breast cancer screening recommendations and risk reduction strategies.

Presentation and Workup

Patients can present with benign breast disease after an abnormality detected on screening imaging or after workup for breast symptoms such as a palpable mass, breast pain, or spontaneous nipple discharge. In women who are considered at average risk for breast cancer based on medical and family history, screening includes history and physical examination by their health care provider, clinical breast examination, and breast imaging. Breast awareness should be encouraged, but formal breast self-examinations in average-risk women have not been shown to have a breast cancer mortality benefit, although in women who performed self-breast examinations, a greater number of benign breast lesions were detected.

Breast Cancer Screening

Women at average risk for breast cancer should begin screening mammography between age 40 and 50. The 2016 updated recommendations of the U.S. Preventive Services Task Force (USPSTF) recommend biennial screening mammography for women ages 50 to 74; the decision to start screening mammography prior to age 50 should be individualized. The 2015 American Cancer Society (ACS) breast cancer screening guidelines for women at average risk include a strong recommendation to begin screening mammography at age 45 and a qualified recommendation to begin at age 40, and continuing as long as the woman is in good overall health and life expectancy is 10 years or greater. The most updated recommendation from the National Comprehensive Cancer Network (NCCN) and the American College of Radiology (ACR) is for annual screening mammography beginning at age 40. The standard for breast cancer screening is the digital mammogram; however, in recent years digital breast tomosynthesis has become more prevalent and available to women at breast imaging centers. Digital breast tomosynthesis has both a higher breast cancer detection rate and a lower recall rate compared to the digital mammogram for breast cancer screening. In women with heterogeneously dense breast or dense breast tissue on screening mammogram, the risks and benefits of supplemental screening should be discussed as high breast density limits mammogram sensitivity.

Normal and abnormal findings on breast imaging are reported using the universal classification system by the ACR's classification: the Breast Imaging Reporting and Data System (BI-RADS). Table 1 includes the BI-RADS categories, the risk of malignancy, and the recommended follow-up. BI-RADS 0 indicates an incomplete assessment and that further workup is needed, typically with additional imaging recommendations. BI-RADS 3 lesions are considered probably benign based on appearance and a mammogram and/or

TABLE 1	Breast Imaging Reporting and Data System (BI-RADS) Mammography Classification		
BI-RADS CATEGORY	DEFINITION	RISK FOR MALIGNANCY	RECOMMENDED FOLLOW-UP
0	Incomplete assessment	N/A	Further imaging
1	Negative study	N/A	Routine mammogram screening
2	Benign	N/A	Routine mammogram screening
3	Probably benign	≤ 2%	Repeat imaging in 6 months
4	Suspicious	> 2%–95% depending on degree of suspicion	Biopsy recommended
5	Highly suggestive of malignancy	≥ 95%	Biopsy recommended
6	Known biopsy-proven malignancy	N/A	Appropriate action should be taken

ultrasound in 6 months is recommended for follow-up. BI-RADS 4 and BI-RADS 5 lesions are suspicious or highly suggestive of malignancy, respectively, and a biopsy of the lesion is recommended.

Palpable Breast Mass

In patients who present with a palpable breast mass, workup is determined by patient age, menopausal status, and degree of suspicion of breast mass. Figure 1 outlines the algorithm for evaluation of a woman with a breast mass. In women younger than age 30 with a mass of low clinical suspicion, it would be appropriate to consider observation over one to two menstrual cycles prior to moving on to ultrasound imaging if the mass persists. If no mass is detected on ultrasound, short-term clinical follow-up is recommended. Diagnostic mammography with ultrasound may be considered in women younger than age 30 who have a mass of high clinical suspicion or increased breast cancer risk. In postmenopausal women and women ages 30 and older, a clinically palpable breast mass should be evaluated with a diagnostic mammogram and ultrasound. A patient identified to have a simple cyst on imaging can return to age-appropriate breast screening. A solitary complicated cyst should be aspirated or be followed in short-term follow-up for stability. Multiple complicated cysts are considered a benign finding and do not require aspiration or short-term follow-up. Routine cytology of aspirated fluid is not recommended. If the mass persists after aspiration of a complicated cyst or if initial imaging shows a mass of high clinical suspicion or a complex cystic and solid mass, ultrasound-guided biopsy of the mass is recommended.

The sonographic description of a simple cyst is a round or oval circumscribed mass with acoustic enhancement and lacking any solid components or Doppler signals. A nonsimple cyst may be complicated or a complex cystic and solid mass. A complicated cyst is round or oval and circumscribed but may show low-level internal echoes without demonstrating vascular flow, while a complex cystic and solid mass may have thick septations, thick and irregular walls, and an internal solid component and display internal echoes, internal blood flow, and lack of posterior wall enhancement.

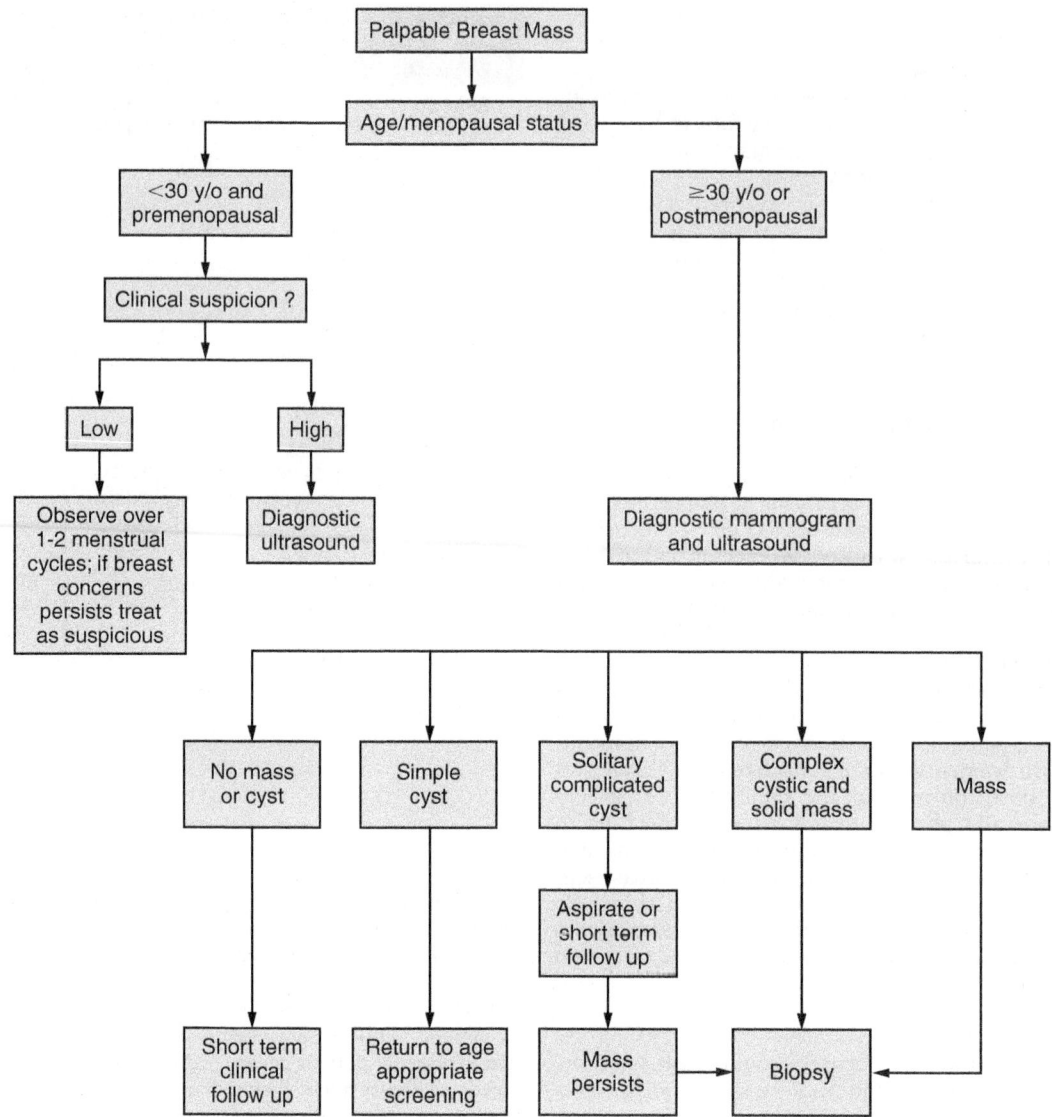

Figure 1 Algorithm for evaluation of a woman with a breast mass.

Nipple Discharge

Some women may present with nipple discharge without a palpable mass. Concerning features for pathologic nipple discharge include spontaneous, unilateral, single-duct discharge that is reproducible on examination and discharge that is clear, serous, sanguineous, or serosanguinous. Nonspontaneous nipple discharge or multiduct discharge in women is likely physiologic and the most common cause is duct ectasia. Women should be educated on avoiding further breast compression to illicit the discharge, ensure they are up to date on age-appropriate breast cancer screening, and review potential medications that could cause nipple discharge. In women with spontaneous pathologic single-duct nipple discharge, the most common etiology is an intraductal papilloma. The most common malignant explanation would be ductal carcinoma in situ (DCIS). The workup should include diagnostic mammography and ultrasound for women ages 30 or older and at least a diagnostic ultrasound women younger than 30 years old. Suspicious or highly suspicious imaging findings warrant biopsy. If initial imaging does not explain the nipple discharge, consider ductogram or magnetic resonance imaging (MRI) for further evaluation. In some cases duct excision may be recommended; otherwise, the patient should have short-term follow-up with clinical breast examination and imaging.

Benign Lesions

Benign breast diseases can be categorized as nonproliferative, proliferative without atypia, proliferative with atypia, and miscellaneous other conditions such as fat necrosis, various types of mastitis, pseudoangiomatous stromal hyperplasia, fibrous mastopathy, amyloid deposits, and dermatologic conditions. Table 2 outlines the benign breast lesions. A study by Dupont and Page in the 1980s and a review by Hartmann et al. in 2005 found that nonproliferative breast disease was not associated with an increased risk for breast cancer. Proliferative breast disease without atypia is associated with a slightly increased risk for breast cancer but less than two times the average population risk. Proliferative breast disease with atypia is associated with a significantly increased breast cancer risk that can be four to five times higher than the average population risk.

Nonproliferative Lesions

Nonproliferative breast lesions are also known as fibrocystic disease or change and include duct ectasia, fibrosis, and apocrine metaplasia. In women without a significant family history of breast cancer, nonproliferative breast lesions are not associated with an increased breast cancer risk. In the study by Dupont and Page including 3303 patients with benign breast disease, only 2.2% of the patients with nonproliferative lesions had breast cancer at a mean follow-up of 17 years. The Hartmann study of 9087 women followed for a median of 15 years found that the strength of family history was an independent risk factor, and in women with nonproliferative lesions the relative risk of breast cancer was 1.27. No increased risk was found in women with no family history.

TABLE 2	Benign Breast Lesions	
NONPROLIFERATIVE LESIONS	PROLIFERATIVE LESIONS WITHOUT ATYPIA	PROLIFERATIVE LESIONS WITH ATYPIA
Apocrine metaplasia	Fibroadenomas	Atypical ductal hyperplasia
Breast cysts	Microglandular adenosis	Atypical lobular hyperplasia
Columnar cell change	Moderate or florid usual ductal hyperplasia	
Duct ectasia	Papilloma	
Fibrosis	Radial scar	
	Sclerosing adenosis	

Ductal ectasia and breast cysts are common findings. Occasionally the ectatic ducts are surrounded with periductal inflammation, which can occur in nonlactating women when the duct becomes congested with debris. This can lead to periductal mastitis that requires treatment with antibiotics. Breast cysts are most common in perimenopausal women but can occur in premenopausal women and postmenopausal women on hormone replacement therapy. Breast cysts may present in women with fibrocystic breast disease, which women may report as nodular breast tissue and is caused by microcystic formation and stromal proliferation of the breast. Apocrine metaplasia, in which acini and cysts are lined with large columnar cells that resemble the apocrine sweat glands, is not an uncommon finding. The individual cells are large with abundant granular eosinophilic cytoplasm. The apical aspects of these cells have a rounded protrusion into the cyst spaces. Columnar cell change is characterized by enlargement of the terminal duct lobular units and dilated acini without atypia.

Proliferative Lesions Without Atypia

Proliferative breast lesions without atypia include fibroepithelial lesions such as fibroadenomas, moderate or florid usual ductal hyperplasia, microglandular and sclerosing adenosis, papillomas, and radial scars. Proliferative breast lesions without atypia are associated with a slightly increased risk of breast cancer compared to the average risk of the population, with a relative risk estimated between 1.8 and 1.9. These lesions are not currently considered to put a woman at high risk for breast cancer unless other risk factors are present such as family history.

Fibroadenomas are benign processes containing glandular and fibrous tissue. Fibroadenomas were originally classified as nonproliferative lesions (including in the Hartmann study) but are now typically considered proliferative breast lesions. Simple fibroadenomas without associated proliferative disease are not associated with an increased risk for breast cancer, while complex fibroadenomas and those with coinciding proliferative disease are associated with a slight increase in breast cancer risk. Fibroadenomas are most common in young premenopausal women and can fluctuate in size with changes in hormones. They do not routinely need to be excised unless they are enlarging or have associated symptoms such as tenderness.

The normal number of the epithelial linings within the breast is two. Epithelial hyperplasia has a spectrum of changes from mild to severe presenting with an escalating scale of complexity. Usual ductal hyperplasia (UDH) is an increased number of cells within the duct that will vary in size and shape but will appear benign and without atypia. Microglandular adenosis and sclerosing adenosis are lesions with an increased number of glandular elements within fibrous stroma. Microglandular and sclerosing adenosis may be associated with microcalcifications and/or a mass on mammography.

Classic papillomas are masslike lesions that occur within large ducts close to the subareolar area. Histologically, they are composed of arborizing fronds of fibrovascular stroma lined by epithelial cells with a stalk attaching the mass to the wall of the cyst within which they arise. They can appear as a mass on mammography or present with unilateral nipple discharge. Papillomas can be associated with hyperplasia with and without atypia or DCIS, and in those cases, surgical excision is recommended to rule out malignancy.

Radial scars or complex sclerosing lesions are a pathologic diagnosis but can cause abnormalities on breast imaging including mass, nonmass enhancement, or architectural distortion. Histologically, they have a central fibroelastic core with radiating and branching ducts and lobules at the periphery. The etiology of these lesions is unknown. Depending on the size and presentation, surgical excision may be recommended to rule out underlying malignancy.

Proliferative Lesions With Atypia

Proliferative lesions with atypia include atypical ductal hyperplasia (ADH) and atypical lobular hyperplasia (ALH). These atypical hyperplasia lesions are characterized by an abundance of monotonous-appearing epithelial cells partially filling a duct and/or lobule. The presence of atypical hyperplasia is a risk factor for future breast cancer and is associated with a relative risk of breast cancer between four and five times the general population risk. The risk of breast cancer over the 25 years following the biopsy demonstrating atypical hyperplasia is estimated at 30%. The number of foci of atypia present in the specimen can stratify the risk, with one focus being a lower risk compared to three or more foci of atypia. These patients should be managed in a multidisciplinary fashion to include assessment of concordance between radiology and pathology. The standard management for atypical hyperplasia including ADH and ALH is surgical excision to rule out underlying malignancy; however, select patients who have concordance with imaging may be appropriate for screening in lieu of surgical excision.

Miscellaneous Benign Breast Conditions

Pseudoangiomatous stromal hyperplasia (PASH) is a lesion of a stromal proliferation with anastomosing spaces, with the dense hyalinized stroma intermixed with glandular components. These spaces could appear as vascular structures to the untrained pathologist. PASH may appear similar to an angiosarcoma but can be differentiated by the lack of atypia and mitosis. PASH can present with a palpable mass, with a mammogram abnormality, or as an incidental finding. Historically this lesion commonly underwent excision; however, depending on the size of the lesion, concordance with imaging, and other risk factors, PASH may be appropriately monitored with follow-up imaging.

Fat necrosis is secondary to trauma or injury to the breast. Fat necrosis typically presents with a painless breast mass and appears as an ill-defined dense mass on breast imaging. A biopsy is recommended to rule out malignancy; however, no further treatment is necessary.

High-Risk Evaluation and Management

The lifetime risk of breast cancer for women in the United States is approximately one in eight. There are elements of a woman's personal or family history that may increase her risk for breast cancer and potentially warrant additional screening and management. Risk factors that contribute to a women's lifetime risk of breast cancer include family history of breast and/or ovarian cancer, genetic mutations associated with hereditary breast cancer, reproductive history, personal history of multiple breast biopsies or a breast biopsy showing atypical hyperplasia or lobular carcinoma in situ (LCIS), and dense breast tissue on mammography. Women who received thoracic radiation prior to age 30 are also at an increased risk for breast cancer. Modifiable risk factors for breast cancer include increased body mass index, sedentary lifestyle, alcohol intake, and hormone replacement therapy with estrogen and progesterone. Breast cancer risk assessment tools are available to estimate a woman's risk and include the modified

Gail Model and family history–based models such as Claus, BRCAPRO, BOADICEA, and Tyrer-Cuzick. In women with a strong family history of breast or ovarian cancer, genetic counseling should be offered.

Women considered at high risk for breast cancer include those with a Gail Model 5-year breast cancer risk of greater than or equal to 1.7%, a lifetime risk of breast cancer of greater than 20% based on a family history–based model, or a history of thoracic radiation prior to age 30, as well as women harboring a deleterious genetic mutation associated with breast cancer or a personal history of atypical hyperplasia or lobular carcinoma in situ. Women at high risk for breast cancer may be eligible for additional screening including earlier age at initiation of screening imaging and consideration of annual breast MRI.

Women at high risk for breast cancer should be counseled on screening recommendations and risk reduction strategies. Lifestyle modifications associated with decreased breast cancer risk include breastfeeding, achieving a healthy body mass index, limiting alcohol consumption, and exercising regularly. Some women may be considered for risk-reducing surgery. Chemoprevention may also be an option for women at high risk for breast cancer.

Chemoprevention

Risk-reducing agents, also known as chemoprevention, are appropriate to consider in women with atypical hyperplasia, LCIS, or a 5-year breast cancer risk of greater than or equal to 1.7%. Risk-reducing agents include tamoxifen, raloxifene (Evista), and aromatase inhibitors (exemestane [Aromasin][1] and anastrozole [Arimidex][1]). Chemoprevention is taken daily for 5 years and associated with a potential risk reduction of 40% to 65%. No survival benefit has been demonstrated in women who take chemoprevention, and the risks and benefits of each therapy should be discussed. Tamoxifen is a selective estrogen receptor modulator (SERM) and is the only agent available for premenopausal women. Tamoxifen should not be recommended to women who are currently pregnant or considering future pregnancy owing to potential teratogenic effects. The National Surgical Adjuvant Breast and Bowel Project (NSABP) Breast Cancer Prevention Trial (NSABP P-1) of tamoxifen 20 mg daily for 5 years verses placebo included both pre- and postmenopausal women at high risk for breast cancer and demonstrated a reduced risk of invasive breast cancer of 49%. In this study tamoxifen was associated with an increased rate of endometrial cancer, deep vein thrombosis, pulmonary embolism, and stroke, and these events were more frequent in women over the age of 50. Raloxifene is a second-generation SERM. The STAR trial (NSABP P-2) randomized postmenopausal women at high risk for breast cancer to 5 years of tamoxifen 20 mg daily versus raloxifene 60 mg daily. Raloxifene was demonstrated to be as effective as tamoxifen at reducing the risk of invasive breast cancer but not noninvasive breast cancer. Raloxifene was associated with a lower rate of venous thromboembolic events and endometrial cancer. Aromatase inhibitors were studied in postmenopausal women for breast cancer prevention in the MAP.3 (exemestane) and IBIS-II (anastrozole) trials. Exemestane 25 mg daily for 5 years was associated with a 65% relative reduction in annual incidence of breast cancer compared to placebo. Anastrozole 1 mg daily for 5 years reduced the incidence of estrogen receptor–positive breast cancers by over 50% compared to placebo with a hazard ratio (HR) of 0.47. In both trials, musculoskeletal complaints and vasomotor symptoms were more common in the aromatase inhibitor groups. Vaginal dryness and decreased libido are also common side effects of aromatase inhibitors. There is potential for a decrease in bone mineral density while taking an aromatase inhibitor; however, no increased fracture rate was seen in either trial. In postmenopausal women, age and comorbidities along with bone health should be considered when selecting a risk-reducing agent.

---

[1]Not U.S. Food and Drug Administration (FDA) approved for this indication.

References

Ciatto S, Houssami N, Bernardi D, et al: Integration of 3D digital mammography with tomosynthesis for population breast-cancer screening (STORM): a prospective comparison study, *Lancet Oncol* 14(7):583–589. 2013. https://doi.org/10.1016/S1470-2045(13)70134-7. PubMed PMID:23623721.

Cuzick J, Sestak I, Forbes JF, et al: Investigators I-I. Anastrozole for prevention of breast cancer in high-risk postmenopausal women (IBIS-II): an international, double-blind, randomised placebo-controlled trial, *Lancet* 383(9922): 1041–1048, 2014. https://doi.org/10.1016/S0140-6736(13)62292-8. PubMed PMID: 24333009.

Dupont WD, Page DL: Risk factors for breast cancer in women with proliferative breast disease, *N Engl J Med* 312(3):146–151, 1985. https://doi.org/10.1056/NEJM198501173120303 PubMed PMID: 3965932.

Fisher B, Costantino JP, Wickerham DL, et al: Tamoxifen for prevention of breast cancer: Report of the National Surgical Adjuvant Breast and Bowel Project P-1 Study, *J Natl Cancer Inst* 90(18):1371–1388, 1998. PubMed PMID: 9747868.

Goss PE, Ingle JN, Ales-Martinez JE, et al: Investigators NCMS. Exemestane for breast-cancer prevention in postmenopausal women, *N Engl J Med* 364(25):2381–2391, 2011. https://doi.org/10.1056/NEJMoa1103507. PubMed PMID: 21639806.

Hartmann LC, Sellers TA, Frost MH, et al: Benign breast disease and the risk of breast cancer, *N Engl J Med* 353(3):229–237, 2005. https://doi.org/10.1056/NEJMoa044383. PubMed PMID: 16034008.

Oeffinger KC, Fontham ET, Etzioni R, et al: American Cancer Society. Breast cancer screening for women at average risk: 2015 guideline update from the American Cancer Society, *JAMA* 314(15):1599–1614, 2015. https://doi.org/10.1001/jama.2015.12783. PubMed PMID: 26501536; PMCID: PMC4831582.

Siu AL: Force USPST. Screening for breast cancer: U.S. Preventive Services Task Force Recommendation Statement, *Ann Intern Med* 164(4):279–296, 2016. https://doi.org/10.7326/M15-2886. PubMed PMID: 26757170.

Thomas DB, Gao DL, Ray RM, et al: Randomized trial of breast self-examination in Shanghai: final results, *J Natl Cancer Inst* 94(19):1445–1457, 2002. PubMed PMID: 12359854.

Vogel VG, Costantino JP, Wickerham DL, et al: National Surgical Adjuvant Breast and Bowel Project. Effects of tamoxifen vs raloxifene on the risk of developing invasive breast cancer and other disease outcomes: the NSABP Study of Tamoxifen and Raloxifene (STAR) P-2 trial, *JAMA* 295(23):2727–2741, 2006. https://doi.org/10.1001/jama.295.23.joc60074. PubMed PMID: 16754727.

▰ BREAST CANCER

Method of
Lauren Nye, MD; and Takae Brewer, MD

CURRENT DIAGNOSIS

- Mammography is used for breast cancer screening, and it is recommended to begin screening in women at average risk for breast cancer between ages 40 and 50.
- Women with an elevated risk for breast cancer may be considered for additional high-risk screening that can include breast magnetic resonance imaging (MRI) or other supplemental screening in addition to annual mammography.
- Individuals with a palpable breast mass or breast symptom concerning for malignancy and those with an abnormal screening mammogram need diagnostic breast imaging.
- Diagnostic breast imaging that is suspicious or highly suggestive of malignancy should undergo core needle biopsy.

CURRENT THERAPY

- Breast cancer is a heterogeneous disease and requires a multidisciplinary approach and multimodality therapy.
- The treatment of early-stage breast cancer may include local therapy such as surgery and radiation, as well as systemic therapy including chemotherapy, endocrine therapy, and biologic therapy.
- Metastatic breast cancer is treated with systemic therapy, and the goal of treatment is disease control and preserving quality of life.
- Breast cancer survivors may have multiple long-term complications of therapy that need to be addressed, including vasomotor symptoms, osteoporosis, lymphedema, and increased cardiac risk factors.

Overview

Breast cancer is the most common cancer and the third leading cause of death among women in the United States. Breast cancer is a heterogeneous disease for which a personalized approach is important in the evaluation and treatment of each individual. Furthermore, the multidisciplinary team is vital in the management of breast cancer and can include a medical oncologist, surgical oncologist, plastic surgeon, radiation oncologist, pathologist, supportive services, and the patient's personal physician. At the conclusion of treatment and active surveillance, the patient typically returns to their primary care physician for continued survivorship care.

Epidemiology

It is estimated that there were 252,710 new cases of breast cancer in 2017, comprising 15% of all new cancer cases. The estimated deaths from breast cancer in the same year were 40,610, accounting for 6.8% of all cancer deaths. Female breast cancer is most commonly diagnosed among women from 55 to 64 years of age with the median age at diagnosis of 62. Although rare, male breast cancer comprises of 1% of all breast cancer cases in the United States. The incidence of breast cancer has risen slowly by 0.3% annually, whereas the mortality rate has been falling by 1.8% each year. The 5-year relative survival improved rate by 16% over 30 years, from 74% in 1980 to 90.9% in 2010.

Risk Factors

Well-recognized risk factors for breast cancer include older age, female sex, white race, obesity, high exposure to hormones (either exogenous or endogenous), personal and family history of breast cancer, inherited genetic mutations, certain benign breast disease (e.g., atypical hyperplasia and LCIS), previous history of radiation therapy to the chest, as well as lifestyle factors such as alcohol consumption and obesity.

Individuals who carry a BRCA1 or BRCA2 mutation are at a significantly higher risk for developing breast cancer. In a case-control study by Couch et al. in 2017 of more than 65,000 women with breast cancer, genetic mutations associated with an increased risk of breast cancer were identified in 10.2% of cases. The most common gene mutations identified included BRCA1, BRCA2, ATM, CHEK2, PALB2, BARD1, and RAD51D. Individuals with a strong family history of cancer should be considered for genetic counseling and testing for appropriate risk stratification.

Prevention

For women at an average risk for breast cancer, lifestyle modifications including regular aerobic exercise, maintaining a healthy weight, and limiting alcohol are most important for breast cancer prevention. In addition, complying with breast cancer screening recommendations provides opportunity for early detection and decreased mortality. Women at average risk for breast cancer should begin screening mammography between age 40 and 50. The United States Preventive Task Force (USPSTF) updated recommendations in 2016 recommend biennial screening mammography for women aged 50 to 74 years, and the decision to start screening mammography prior to age 50 should be individualized. The 2015 American Cancer Society (ACS) breast cancer screening guidelines for women at average risk include a strong recommendation to begin screening mammography at age 45 and a qualified recommendation to begin at age 40, and continuing as long as in good overall health and life expectancy is 10 years or greater. The most updated recommendations from the National Comprehensive Cancer Network (NCCN) and the American College of Radiology (ACR) are for annual screening mammography beginning at age 40. The standard for screening breast imaging is the digital mammogram; however, in recent years digital breast tomosynthesis has become more prevalent and available to women at breast imaging centers. Digital breast tomosynthesis has both a higher breast cancer detection rate and lower recall rate compared with the digital mammography for breast cancer screening.

Women who are at an increased risk for breast cancer may be considered for additional screening and prevention measures. Risk factors that increase a women's risk include having a known genetic mutation associated with hereditary breast cancer, having a family history of breast cancer in a first- or second-degree relative, especially premenopausal breast cancer or male breast cancer, having a personal history of a breast biopsy with atypical hyperplasia or lobular carcinoma in situ, having a personal history of chest radiation before age 30, or having a high breast density. Several breast cancer assessment tools are available for evaluation for women who are at a higher risk of developing breast cancer than the average population (e.g., Gail, Tyrer-Cuzick, Claus, BRCAPRO, BOADICEA models). Women with a lifetime risk of breast cancer greater than 20% on a family history–based model or women with a genetic mutation or prior chest radiations may be eligible for additional annual screening with breast MRI. Certain high-risk populations may benefit from risk-reducing therapies such as chemoprevention and prophylactic mastectomy, especially for high-penetrance mutation carriers.

Clinical Manifestations

Women with DCIS and early-stage breast cancer may be asymptomatic. The most common symptoms of breast cancer include the following:
- New palpable mass in the breast or axilla
- Skin changes such as dimpling, erythema, irritation, edema, thickening, Peau d'orange (Figure 1)
- Nipple retraction
- Abnormal nipple discharge
- New asymmetric appearance of breast

Differential Diagnosis

Differential diagnoses include benign conditions such as fibroadenoma, papilloma, breast cyst, mastitis, as well as malignant conditions such as breast lymphoma, sarcoma, neuroendocrine tumors, leukemia, and skin metastasis from breast or other primary tumors.

Diagnosis

Once breast malignancy is suspected clinically, either by palpation or breast imaging (Figure 2), further evaluation is warranted. Women with an abnormal mammogram should undergo further diagnostic imaging, which may include diagnostic mammography, ultrasonography, or breast MRI. Normal and abnormal findings on breast imaging are reported using the universal classification system by the American College of Radiology—Breast Imaging Reporting and Data System (BI-RADS). BI-RADS 0 indicates an incomplete assessment and further workup is needed, typically with additional imaging recommendations. BI-RADS 1 and BI-RADS 2 lesions are negative or benign, respectively.

Figure 1 Peau d'orange of the breast.

Figure 2 Breast cancer on mammogram.

BI-RADS 3 lesions are considered probably benign based on appearance and a mammogram or ultrasound scan in 6 months is recommended for follow-up. BI-RADS 4 and BI-RADS 5 lesions are suspicious or highly suggestive of malignancy, respectively, and a biopsy of the lesion is recommended. Core need biopsy is the recommended approach for tissue sampling. The pathology report from a biopsy of a primary breast cancer will typically include the histology and tumor prognostic markers. These histologic subtypes of breast cancer include ductal, lobular, mixed, metaplastic, as well as the more favorable histologic subtypes of tubular, mucinous, and papillary.

Once a breast cancer is diagnosed, appropriate clinical staging is done, directed by a medical oncologist or surgical oncologist. This may include further breast imaging to characterize the extent of the tumor, axillary staging with ultrasound to assess for abnormal-appearing lymph nodes, and clinical examination with consideration of whole-body staging with computed tomography (CT) scan of the chest, abdomen, and pelvis depending on the size and lymph node involvement of the primary breast cancer. Bone scanning or positron emission tomography (PET/CT) may also be considered in some circumstances. Staging of the breast cancer is done in accordance with the American Joint Committee on Cancer (AJCC) staging system. The most updated version, the AJCC Cancer Staging Manual, Eight Edition, was published in December 2017 and includes anatomic stage groups, clinical prognostic stage groups, and pathologic prognostic stage groups. All patients should have a clinical prognostic stage documented as part of their treatment plan, and those with surgery as initial treatment may also have a pathologic prognostic stage. The updated staging guidelines also include biomarker testing results within the staging system.

Pathophysiology

Breast cancer is a heterogeneous disease. Malignant cells arise from neoplastic proliferation of epithelial cells in the ducts or lobules of the breast. If neoplastic cells are confined inside of the duct or lobule, the lesion is termed ductal or lobular in situ, respectively. Ductal carcinoma in situ (DCIS) is a precursor lesion that can potentially develop into invasive carcinoma (Figure 3). Invasive carcinoma is classified into four distinct molecular subtypes: luminal A, luminal B, basal-like, and HER2 enriched. More frequently we use the tumor receptor markers of the breast cancer to guide therapy, namely estrogen receptor (ER), progesterone receptor (PR), and HER-2 overexpression. Hormone receptor–positive breast cancer, meaning progesterone or estrogen receptor–positive, is the most common type of breast cancer, comprising more than 65% of all breast cancers and in general has less aggressive

disease course with a long survival, even in the metastatic setting. In contrast, hormone receptor negative and HER-2 negative breast cancer, also known as triple negative breast cancer (TNBC), tends to be more aggressive and has a much poorer outcome, especially in the advanced setting. Although the natural course of HER-2 overexpressed disease tends to be aggressive, HER-2 positive breast cancer now has a longer survival time since the advent of effective HER-2 directed therapies.

Treatment

Breast cancer is a complex disease and requires multidisciplinary management, as well as a tailored therapy plan depending on the stage, histologic subtype, and prognostic tumor marker status. Current modalities for treating breast cancer include local therapy such as surgery and radiation therapy, as well as systemic therapy including chemotherapy, endocrine, and biologic therapy.

Early-stage breast cancer is treated with surgery (lumpectomy or mastectomy) with or without radiation therapy. Women who undergo lumpectomy and radiotherapy have equivalent outcomes to those receiving mastectomy. Axillary lymph nodes are typically evaluated by sentinel lymph node biopsy and/or axillary lymph node dissection depending on initial clinical findings and lymph node involvement with metastases on pathologic review. For selected cases, preoperative (neoadjuvant) treatment with chemotherapy or endocrine therapy are used. Neoadjuvant chemotherapy is indicated for inoperable or locally advanced breast cancer such as inflammatory breast cancer, extensive primary tumor extending to the chest wall or skin, bulky or matted axillary lymph nodes, and extraaxillary lymph node involvement. In the setting of operable breast cancer, neoadjuvant systemic treatment may be recommended to optimize surgical outcomes in the setting of a large tumor or to allow for breast-conserving surgery.

After the definitive surgical management, adjuvant systemic therapy may be offered to reduce the risk of local and distant recurrence. Chemotherapy is considered for those at high risk for recurrence, characterized by large tumor size, positive lymph nodes, high-grade histology, or a triple negative (hormone receptor negative, HER2 negative) breast cancer. For hormone receptor–positive, HER2-negative, axillary node-negative breast cancer, the 21-gene recurrence score is widely used to evaluate for the potential benefit of adjuvant chemotherapy. HER2-positive breast cancer is treated with HER2-directed biologic agents along with chemotherapy followed by maintenance therapy with anti-HER2 agents such as trastuzumab (Herceptin), pertuzumab (Perjeta), and adotrastuzumab emtansine (Kadcyla). When an anthracycline chemotherapy or HER2 antibody therapy is indicated, baseline cardiac function evaluation by either echocardiogram or multigated acquisition (MUGA) scan must be obtained before treatment and will be regularly monitored during the treatment with trastuzumab. Radiation therapy, if indicated, is typically offered after chemotherapy.

After local treatment of hormone receptor–positive breast cancer with or without chemotherapy, adjuvant endocrine therapy is recommended for a minimum of 5 years with either a selective estrogen-receptor modulator (SERM) such as tamoxifen (Nolvadex), an aromatase inhibitor such as anastrozole (Arimidex), letrozole (Femara) or exemestane (Aromasin), or a selective estrogen receptor degrader (SERD) such as fulvestrant (Faslodex). In general, the choice of endocrine therapy agents is based on the menopausal state and side effects profiles. Adjuvant endocrine therapy is associated with an approximate 50% reduction in breast cancer recurrence.

Locally recurrent disease without distant metastasis can be managed with a curative intent. Combination of local therapies and systemic treatment may be used depending on the clinical scenario. Metastatic (stage IV) breast cancer with distant metastasis is not curable and is managed with the intent of disease control while maintaining quality of life and requires systemic therapy. Local therapies such as surgery and radiation therapy are indicated for palliative purposes when appropriate.

(a)

N

(b)

IS

Figure 3 Breast adenocarcinoma histopathology of ductal carcinoma in situ and invasive breast cancer.

Hormone-positive metastatic breast cancer with bone-only involvement or small tumor burden can be treated with endocrine therapy. Recently the advent of combination therapy with cyclin-dependent kinases (CDK4/6) inhibitors has emerged as a promising agent for hormone receptor–positive, metastatic disease. In combination with endocrine therapy, CDK inhibitors demonstrated longer progression-free survival, and in some cohorts an overall survival benefit. The mTOR inhibitor can be also used in this setting in combination with endocrine therapy. The mTOR inhibitor is known to overcome endocrine resistance, although toxicity (e.g., mucositis and gastrointestinal side effects) may limit its use.

Metastatic HER2-positive breast cancer is treated with HER2-directed agents and chemotherapy. Additional strategies include drug antibody conjugates or dual HER2 blockade such as trastuzumab (Herceptin) and pertuzumab (Perjeta) or lapatinib (Tykerb) with chemotherapy, which demonstrate superior progression-free survival compared with a single HER2 agent added to chemotherapy. For HER2-positive and hormone receptor–positive disease, dual HER-2 targeted therapy combined with an aromatase inhibitor may be beneficial.

Although single chemotherapy is preferred for metastatic disease, combined chemotherapy may be indicated for diseases with high tumor burden or in visceral crisis. Management of metastatic breast cancer may also include germline genetic testing for a BRCA1 or BRCA2 mutation and/or genomic testing of the tumor to identify potential molecular targets unique to the individual or tumor. In 2018, the FDA approved olaparib (Lynparza) and talazoparib (Talzenna), which are a poly-ADH ribose polymerase (PARP) inhibitor, for the treatment of metastatic HER2-negative, BRCA-associated breast cancer. Further targeted therapies may be explored in the setting of a clinical trial.

For patients with bone metastasis, bone-targeted therapy such as denosumab (Xgeva) or intravenous bisphosphonates are given to reduce skeletal-related events, such as pathologic fractures. Patients with poor dentition or oral hygiene who need future dental procedures during treatment are at increased risk for osteonecrosis of the jaw; thus dental evaluation is important before initiating bone-directed therapy.

Monitoring and Survivorship

The majority of breast cancer patients are treated with curative intent and enjoy long-term survival. The risk of recurrence, however, is a realistic concern for many years after definitive therapy, especially for women with locally advanced or node-positive disease. Once the patient has completed definitive treatment, careful history taking and physical examination are the most important aspects of surveillance. Patients are advised to have an office visit up to 4 times yearly for the first 5 years, then annually. The monitoring for recurrence by laboratory and radiologic tests should be kept minimal in the non-metastatic setting unless clinically indicated.

Women should continue to undergo annual screening mammography for their remaining breast tissue. If they were receiving high-risk screening with a breast MRI based on a genetic mutation, this may also be continued after breast cancer treatment. Annual gynecologic assessment is recommended for women on tamoxifen because of the associated increased risk of uterine cancer, which typically presents with abnormal bleeding in postmenopausal women. Patients on aromatase inhibitor should have a bone mineral density completed at baseline and then annually while receiving treatment with an aromatase inhibitor. Bone-modifying agents such as intravenous bisphosphonates or RANK ligand inhibitors may be used for management or prevention of osteoporosis while on aromatase inhibitor therapy.

In addition, women receiving adjuvant endocrine therapy may experience menopause-related symptoms such as vasomotor symptoms, vaginal dryness, and sexual dysfunction. Patients are encouraged to discuss these symptoms with their physician because they can frequently be managed with non-hormone–based approaches. Venlafaxine (Effexor)[1], oxybutynin (Ditropan)[1], and gabapentin (Neurontin)[1] have demonstrated efficacy in management of hot flashes, as well as cognitive behavioral therapy and avoiding triggers. Vaginal moisturizers and lubricants can be applied to help alleviate symptoms of vaginal dryness. Laser therapy may also be considered in some circumstances.

Long-term complications after definitive treatment may include lymphedema and self-image issues after surgery, skin changes after radiation therapy and persistent neuropathy, prolonged hair loss, fatigue, cognitive impairment, and a small risk of developing leukemia and myelodysplastic syndrome (MDS) after chemotherapy.

Heart disease remains the leading cause of death in US women. Those women who have undergone treatment for breast cancer may be at a higher risk for myocardial events depending on their baseline risk factors and the treatment they received. Accumulating evidence suggests that lifestyle modifications including regular exercise, achieving a healthy body mass index, limiting alcohol intake, and abstaining from tobacco products lead to optimal outcomes for breast cancer survivors.

---

[1] Not FDA approved for this indication.

References

Baselga J, Cortes J, Kim SB, et al: Pertuzumab plus trastuzumab plus docetaxel for metastatic breast cancer, *N Engl J Med* 366:109–119, 2012.

Couch FJ, Shimelis H, Hu C: Associations between cancer predisposition testing panel genes and breast cancer, *JAMA Oncol* 3(9):1190–1196, 2017.

Davies C, Pan H, Godwin J, et al: Long-term effects of continuing adjuvant tamoxifen to 10 years versus stopping at 5 years after diagnosis of oestrogen receptor-positive breast cancer: ATLAS, a randomized trial, *Lancet* 381(9869):805–816, 2013.

Finn RS, Crown JP, Lang I, et al: The cyclin-dependent kinase 4/6 inhibitor palbociclib in combination with letrozole versus letrozole alone as first-line treatment of oestrogen receptor-positive, HER2-negative, advanced breast cancer (PALOMA-1/TRIO-18): a randomized phase II study, *Lancet Oncol* 16(1):25–35, 2015.

Fisher B, Anderson S, Bryant J, et al: Twenty-year follow-up of a randomized trial comparing total mastectomy, lumpectomy, and lumpectomy plus irradiation for the treatment of invasive breast cancer, *N Engl J Med* 347:1233–1241, 2002.

Noone AM, Howlander N, Krapcho M, et al: SEER Cancer Statistics Review, 1975-2015, National Cancer Institute. Bethesda, MD, https://seer.cancer.gov/csr/1975_2015/, based on November 2017 SEER data submission, posted to SEER website, April 2018.

Slamon DJ, Leyland-Jones B, Shak S, et al: Use of chemotherapy plus a monoclonal antibody against HER2 for metastatic breast cancer that overexpresses HER2, *N Engl J Med* 344:783–792, 2001.

Sparano JA, Gray RJ, Makower DF, et al: Prospective validation of a 21-gene expression assay in breast cancer, *N Engl J Med* 373:2005–2015, 2015.

Verma S, Miles D, Gianni L, et al: Trastuzumab emtansine for HER2-positive advanced breast cancer, *N Engl J Med* 367:1783–1791, 2012.

CANCER OF THE ENDOMETRIUM

Method of
Locke Uppendahl, MD; and Boris Winterhoff, MD

CURRENT DIAGNOSIS

- The high incidence of uterine cancer in developed countries reflects increased obesity rates.
- The progression from atypical hyperplasia to adenocarcinoma is a consequence of prolonged, unopposed estrogen exposure.
- Approximately 90% of women with uterine cancer report abnormal uterine bleeding, with postmenopausal bleeding the most common.
- Over 95% of uterine cancers are diagnosed in women 40 years or older.
- In most uterine cancer cases, the tumor is confined to the uterine corpus at the time of diagnosis and portend a good prognosis.
- Uterine carcinomas are classified into two broad histologic categories: the estrogen related endometrioid (Type I) and nonestrogen related (Type II) tumors.

CURRENT THERAPY

- Comprehensive surgical staging with total hysterectomy, bilateral salpingo-oophorectomy, and bilateral pelvic and para-aortic lymphadenectomy is a critical component for the diagnosis and management of all endometrial cancers.
- The utility and extent of lymph node dissection in endometrial cancer is controversial.
- The decision for adjuvant therapy is based on the risk of relapse and persistent disease.
- Surgery alone is usually curative for women with early-stage, low-risk disease.
- Adjuvant vaginal brachytherapy is recommended for early-stage endometrial cancers that demonstrate pathologic features known to increase risk of vaginal cuff recurrence, such as high-grade, deep myometrial invasion, cervical involvement, or presence of lymphovascular space invasion.
- Women with advanced-stage (stage III or IV) or recurrent endometrial cancer are frequently treated with systemic, platinum-based chemotherapy

Epidemiology

In the United States, uterine cancer is the most common gynecologic malignancy of the female genital tract, with an estimated 63,230 new cases and 11,350 deaths expected for 2018. Approximately 1 in 35 women will develop invasive cancer over their lifetime, with an average age of diagnosis of 62 years. The high incidence observed in developed countries is attributable to increased obesity rates and other risk factors.

Uterine cancer is one of the few malignancies where survival has not improved since the mid-1970s. In fact, death rates for uterine cancer rose in 2011 through 2015 by 2% per year. The 5-year survival rate for all stages is 22% lower for black women compared to white women. This large disparity likely reflects a delay in diagnosis in this population.

Classification

Uterine cancers arising from the lining of the uterus are called endometrial carcinoma and are classified into two broad histologic categories: the estrogen related endometrioid (Type I) and nonestrogen related (Type II) tumors.

Type I tumors

Type I tumors are the predominant form of endometrial cancer, comprising approximately 80% of new diagnoses. They include tumors of endometrioid histology and often arise in the background of atypical endometrial hyperplasia. Type I tumors are more indolent, diagnosed at earlier stages, occur in younger women, and overall portend a favorable prognosis. Patients with high-grade (grade 3) endometrioid adenocarcinoma have a less favorable prognosis. The average age at diagnosis is approximately 63 years old, with nearly 70% of the tumors confined to the uterus at time of diagnosis.

Recent, comprehensive genomic characterization has identified a number of genetic alterations associated with type I tumors. The loss of function in the DNA mismatch repair (MMR) enzymes MLH1, MSH2, MSH6, and PMS2 results in the inability to properly detect and repair abnormal DNA sequences. This leads to mutations in genes that have microsatellite repeats. Microsatellite instability (MSI) is found in approximately one-third of type I tumors and can be as a result of germline or sporadic mutations. Other commonly mutated genes include *PTEN*, *CTNNB1*, *PIK3CA*, *ARID1A*, and *KRAS*.

Type II tumors

In contrast to type I tumors, other endometrial cancers are unrelated to unopposed estrogen exposure. Type II cancers include clear cell and serous histology tumors. They are diagnosed more frequently among older, non-obese, non-white women and portend an unfavorable prognosis due to the later stage in diagnosis and the aggressive nature of the tumor.

Serous carcinoma of the endometrium represents ~10% of endometrial carcinomas but accounts for 40% of all endometrial cancer-related deaths. They often invade deep into the myometrium and demonstrate the ability for early peritoneal spread. Uterine serous carcinomas are molecularly distinct and are characterized by high genomic instability (high copy number alterations), low mutational burden, and *TP53* mutations. Newer evidence demonstrates dysregulation of the *Her2/neu* oncogene in 27% of cases. Clear cell carcinomas, another rare but aggressive subtype, represent ~5% of endometrial carcinomas. The 5-year overall survival rates for serous and clear cell carcinomas are 41% and 65%, respectively. Recently, genomic characterization identified approximately 25% of grade 3 endometrioid tumors cluster with serous carcinomas, with very high somatic copy-number alterations. Nearly 90% of these tumors have *TP53* mutations. Novel mutations in *TAF1* have been implicated in a subset of clear cell carcinomas.

Risk Factors

Type I tumors are strongly linked to long-term, unopposed exposure to estrogen. Therefore risk factors include any excessive exogenous (hormonal therapy, tamoxifen [Nolvadex]) or endogenous (obesity, chronic anovulation, estrogen-secreting tumors) estrogen exposure to the uterine lining. In the United States, the high prevalence of obesity has increased the incidence of uterine cancer over the past two decades. A BMI 25 to < 30 kg/m^2 confers a relative risk of 1.5 to develop endometrial cancer, compared to 7.1 for BMI > 40 kg/m^2. Other risk factors for type I tumors include nulliparity, diabetes mellitus, and hypertension.

Tamoxifen (Nolvadex) is a selective-estrogen receptor modulator (SERM) used in the treatment and prevention of breast cancer. The drug functions as an antagonist in the breast but has agonist effects on the endometrium. The risks of endometrial cancer associated with tamoxifen, although very low, are well documented in the literature.

Lynch / Hereditary Non-Polyposis Colorectal Cancer (HNPCC) syndrome is caused by mutations in DNA mismatch-repair genes *MLH1*, *MSH2*, *MSH6*, and *PMS2*. The lifetime risk of developing colorectal and endometrial cancer is 25–50% and 15–71% (depends on mutated gene), respectively.

Pathophysiology

The World Health Organization (WHO) has recently clarified the classification of endometrial hyperplasia, differentiating between only two categories: (1) hyperplasia without atypia and (2) atypical hyperplasia / endometrioid intraepithelial neoplasia. Multiple studies have demonstrated the progression of atypical hyperplasia to adenocarcinoma is a consequence of prolonged, unopposed estrogen exposure.

Prevention

Over 95% of uterine cancers are diagnosed in women 40 years or older. Therefore abnormal uterine bleeding in these women should prompt evaluation with endometrial biopsy or dilatation and curettage (D&C). Depending on age and reproductive desire, women with endometrial hyperplasia may be treated with removal of estrogen stimulus, the periodic use of progestins, or by hysterectomy to prevent the onset of uterine cancer. For women with atypical hyperplasia, hysterectomy is the treatment of choice, because coexistent adenocarcinoma may be present in 40% of cases. In addition, this group of women carries a 30% risk of developing invasive carcinoma later in life. Finally, women with a uterus should never receive estrogen-only hormone replacement therapy (HRT). The addition of a progestin to HRT can prevent endometrial hyperplasia and subsequent endometrial cancer.

Despite no current scientific evidence, women diagnosed with Lynch syndrome should consider annual screening with endometrial sampling and transvaginal ultrasound, beginning between ages of 30 and 35 years. Hysterectomy with or without oophorectomy is an option after childbearing to deter the risk of endometrial cancer.

Clinical Manifestations

Abnormal uterine bleeding is often the only presenting symptom in women diagnosed with endometrial cancer. Upwards of 90% of women diagnosed with endometrial cancer report abnormal uterine bleeding, with postmenopausal bleeding the most common. However, postmenopausal bleeding has many etiologies, and only ~15% of these women will have endometrial cancer.

For pre- and perimenopausal women, the diagnosis is more challenging and often delayed. For this group of women, intermenstrual bleeding, prolonged, heavy bleeding, or the absence of menses for several months interrupted with episodes of bleeding warrants investigation.

Finally, Papanicolaou smears demonstrate malignant cells in only ~50% of women with underlying endometrial cancer. This highlights the ineffectual screening method of indirectly sampling the endometrium. To date, no screening method for the general population is recommended.

Diagnosis

Diagnosis of endometrial cancer is confirmed with a histological specimen. All women suspected of having uterine cancer due to abnormal uterine bleeding should have their endometrium sampled via biopsy. Most often, this can be done in the clinic with a rigid or flexible catheter. With this technique, reported detection rates for postmenopausal and premenopausal are 99.6% and 91%, respectively. However, there is approximately a 10% false-negative rate with endometrial biopsy. Therefore a negative biopsy result in women highly suspicious for endometrial cancer should undergo exam under anesthesia and curettage. Finally,

transvaginal ultrasound demonstrating an endometrial thickness of 5 mm or more in a postmenopausal woman requires endometrial sampling.

Women taking tamoxifen should be counseled about the increased risk of endometrial cancer and to report any abnormal vaginal bleeding so they can be thoroughly evaluated. However, no evidence supports the screening of asymptomatic women with ultrasound or serial endometrial sampling.

Staging

Due to the high incidence of lymph node metastases, the Cancer Committee of the International Federation of Gynecology and Obstetrics (FIGO) replaced a clinical staging system with a surgical staging system in 1988. The current, updated in 2009 FIGO staging system is detailed in Table 1.

Treatment

Comprehensive surgical staging with exploration of the abdominal cavity, total hysterectomy with bilateral salpingo-oophorectomy, and bilateral pelvic and para-aortic lymphadenectomy are critical components for the diagnosis and management of all endometrial cancers. For type II tumors, meticulous surgical staging with the addition of collection of peritoneal washings for cytology, omentectomy ± peritoneal biopsies is required, since metastatic disease is often only identified microscopically. In cases with gross metastatic disease, cytoreductive surgery may be required. Surgical staging can be performed by laparotomy, laparoscopy, or robotically assisted procedure.

The utility and extent of lymph node dissection in endometrial cancer is controversial. Different strategies, including universal, selective, and sentinel lymph node mapping, are currently used. The universal method performs uniform comprehensive surgical staging for nearly all patients with endometrial cancer. This method allows for the most complete information postoperatively to make adjuvant decisions, but a significant percentage of women will develop lymphedema secondary to the nodal dissection. A common selective approach involves avoiding lymph node dissection in patients who have grade 1 or 2 endometrioid histology with < 50% myometrial invasion and tumor size < 2 cm, since these patients have < 1% risk of nodal metastases. Finally, an alternative approach utilizing sentinel lymph node mapping with indocyanine green dye is becoming more popular. Early studies have demonstrated promising results in decreasing morbidity while optimizing the pathological assessment of nodes in these women. Regardless the strategy, the presence of pelvic or para-aortic lymph node

TABLE 1	Carcinoma of the Endometrium
Stage I: Tumor confined to uterine corpus	
IA	Tumor limited to endometrium or < 50% myometrial invasion
IB	≥50% myometrial invasion
Stage II: Extension to cervical stroma	
II	Cervical stromal invasion
Stage III: Local and/or regional spread	
IIIA	Tumor invades serosa and/or adnexa
IIIB	Vaginal and/or parametrial extension
IIIC1	Pelvic lymph node involvement
IIIC2	Para-aortic lymph node involvement
Stage IV: Distant spread	
IVA	Tumor invades bladder and/or rectal mucosa
IVB	Distant metastases, including abdominal spread and/or inguinal lymph nodes

Tumor grade, cell type, and presence/absence of malignant cytology in pelvic washings should be reported along with stage.

metastases remains one of the most important prognostic factors for endometrial cancer.

Following surgery, women are stratified by age and pathologic features to determine their risk for recurrence and the need for adjuvant therapy.

Adjuvant Therapy

The decision for adjuvant therapy is difficult and is based on the risk of relapse and persistent disease. In general, women with stage IA, grade 1 or 2 endometrioid adenocarcinoma have a favorable prognosis, and no adjuvant radiation is necessary following surgery. Early-stage endometrial carcinomas with risk factors for recurrence, stage II-IV cancers, and all serous and clear cell carcinomas often require adjuvant therapy in the form of radiation, chemotherapy, or a combination of both.

Early-Stage Disease

Surgery alone is usually curative for women with early-stage, low-risk disease. Women with early-stage, high-risk or high-intermediate risk factors are often recommended adjuvant radiation. The treatment can be in the form of external beam radiation therapy or vaginal brachytherapy. All serous and clear cell carcinomas of the uterus are recommended to receive adjuvant platinum-based combination chemotherapy regardless of stage. Adjuvant systemic therapy in patients with high-risk, early-stage endometrioid carcinoma remains controversial.

Metastatic Disease

Approximately 10–15% of patients will present with metastatic disease at presentation. Surgical cytoreduction is the preferred treatment approach if complete resection is achievable because it is associated with improved progression-free and overall survival. This would be followed by adjuvant platinum-based combination chemotherapy. The most common regimens are carboplatin (Paraplatin)[1] plus paclitaxel (Taxol)[1] or the triple drug combination of cisplatin (Platinol)[1], doxorubicin (Adriamycin)[1], and paclitaxel.

Patients who are not candidates for surgical cytoreduction either due to grossly metastatic disease or too poor a surgical candidate have a poor prognosis, with 5-year relative survival of < 20%. These patients should be offered systemic chemotherapy generally with palliative intent. Radiation therapy to achieve local control in the pelvis to palliate bleeding, discharge, and pain is often performed.

Recurrent Disease

Local recurrences, distance metastases, and simultaneous local and distant metastases are found in 50%, 29%, and 21%, respectively. Isolated vaginal recurrences are often salvaged with either surgery or radiation.

Distant recurrent endometrial cancer portends a poor prognosis. Systemic chemotherapy is given with a palliative intent, with the most active agents including platinums, taxanes, and anthracyclines.

Combination Chemotherapy and Radiation Therapy. Several studies have evaluated combining chemotherapy and radiation therapy in advanced-stage endometrial cancer. Most recently, a randomized phase III trial compared cisplatin and tumor volume directed irradiation followed by four cycles of chemotherapy (experimental arm) against six cycles of chemotherapy (control arm). While the overall survival is immature, the study reported no increase in recurrence-free survival in optimally debulked, stage III or IV endometrial cancer.

Our experience involves using a "sandwich" method of irradiation between rounds of chemotherapy for advanced or recurrent endometrial cancer. The phase II trial demonstrated an overall 5-year survival of 79% with acceptable toxicity. The optimal sequencing of chemotherapy and radiation warrants further development.

Hormone Therapy

Prior to endometrial cancer, the risk of endometrial hyperplasia and the development into carcinoma can be significantly reduced with administration of a progestin. After the development of carcinoma, patients whose tumors test positive for estrogen receptor (ER) and progesterone receptor (PR) are associated with longer survival, with PR being a stronger predictor than ER. However, the role of adjuvant progestins in stage I or II endometrial cancer has not been demonstrated to be of value and may worsen cardiovascular disease. Progestins are commonly used in advanced or recurrent well-differentiated endometrial cancers. Oral megestrol acetate (Megace) and medroxyprogesterone acetate (Provera)[1] are two of the most commonly used progestins.

The SERM tamoxifen[1] has been used to treat patients with recurrent endometrial cancer, with response rates seen in ~22% of patients. The aromatase inhibitors anastrozole (Arimidex)[1] and letrozole (Femara)[1] were investigated in recurrent and metastatic endometrial cancer and demonstrated minimal activity.

Targeted Therapy

Multiple novel agents are being evaluated in clinical trials for use in treatment against endometrial cancer. Bevacizumab (Avastin)[1] is a monoclonal antibody directed against vascular endothelial growth factor (VEFG) that is active in endometrial cancer. Recent randomized trials demonstrated a benefit with the addition of bevacizumab to carboplatin and paclitaxel in first-line and second-line treatment of advanced, metastatic, and recurrent endometrial cancer. Results from phase 3 trials are needed prior to adopting as standard of care.

Pembrolizumab (Keytruda)[1] is an immune checkpoint inhibitor that has FDA approval for the use in advanced solid tumors demonstrating MMR deficiency or MSI. In patients with endometrial cancer, it is often used following progression on platinum-based chemotherapy in women with MMR or MSI tumors.

Trastuzumab (Herceptin)[1] and lapatinib (Tykerb)[1] are anti–human epidermal growth factor 2 (HER2) are investigational agents being tested as single agents and in combination with chemotherapy in some endometrial cancers, although the results thus far are not encouraging. The mechanistic Target of Ramamycin (mTOR) inhibitors everolimus (Zortress)[1] and ridaforolimus (MK-8669)[5] have been used to treat advanced-stage and recurrent endometrial cancers, with mixed response.

Monitoring

Surveillance recommendations for endometrial cancer are stratified by risk of recurrence, and most women diagnosed and treated for endometrial cancer will fall into the low-risk category. High risk for recurrence is defined as advanced stage or grade 3 endometrioid, serous, or clear cell histology. Follow-up recommendations for low-risk women involve a history and physical examination, including a speculum and pelvic examination, scheduled every 6 months for the first 2 years, then yearly. Women with high risk of recurrence should have the same follow-up recommendations at intervals of 3 months for the first 2 years, every 6 months in years 2–5, then yearly. Pap test/cytology, CA 125, and routine radiographic imaging are not recommended. Women suspected of recurrence should have imaging performed.

---

[1] Not FDA approved for this indication.
[5] Investigational drug in the United States.

References

The American College of Obstetricians and Gynecologists Committee Opinion no. 631: Endometrial intraepithelial neoplasia, *Obstet Gynecol* 125(5):1272–1278, 2015.

de Boer SM, et al: Adjuvant chemoradiotherapy versus radiotherapy alone for women with high-risk endometrial cancer (PORTEC-3): final results of an international, open-label, multicentre, randomised, phase 3 trial, *Lancet Oncol* 19(3):295–309, 2018.

---

[1] Not FDA approved for this indication.

Geller MA, et al: A phase II trial of carboplatin and docetaxel followed by radiotherapy given in a "Sandwich" method for stage III, IV, and recurrent endometrial cancer, *Gynecol Oncol* 121(1):112–117, 2011.

Kandoth C, et al: Integrated genomic characterization of endometrial carcinoma, *Nature* 497(7447):67–73, 2013.

Pecorelli S: Revised FIGO staging for carcinoma of the vulva, cervix, and endometrium, *Int J Gynaecol Obstet* 105(2):103–104, 2009.

Salani R, et al: An update on post-treatment surveillance and diagnosis of recurrence in women with gynecologic malignancies: Society of Gynecologic Oncology (SGO) recommendations, *Gynecol Oncol* 146(1):3–10, 2017.

CANCER OF THE UTERINE CERVIX

Method of
Lucybeth Nieves-Arriba, MD; and Peter G. Rose, MD

CURRENT DIAGNOSIS

- New recommendations for cytology screening recommend starting screening at 21 years of age.
- Initial workup must include a biopsy.
- Imaging techniques including magnetic resonance imaging and positron emission tomography–computed tomography can assist in treatment planning.

CURRENT THERAPY

- Despite recent availability of human papillomavirus (HPV) vaccination (Gardasil[2], Gardasil 9, Cervarix[2]) and advances in screening, cervical cancer remains a significant global health problem, especially in underserved populations.
- Improved understanding of the disease has allowed more conservative treatment of selected patients with early-stage disease.
- For advanced and high-risk cervical cancer, chemoradiation has had a significant impact on survival.

[2]Not available in the United States.

Epidemiology

Worldwide, cervical cancer is the fourth most common cancer in women. It is the greatest cancer killer of young women and the most common cause of death from cancer in women in the developing world. Worldwide in 2018, among the 570,000 new cases of cervical cancer, the highest incidence rates were in Africa, Central and South America, and Asia. In the United States, it is estimated that approximately 13,240 new cases were diagnosed and 4170 patients died from cervical cancer in 2018. Significant disparities in incidence and stage at time of diagnosis have been identified among different ethnic groups—African Americans, Asian Americans, European Americans, and Latin Americans—in the United States. Factors that increase the risk of cervical cancer include early age at first coitus, multiple sexual partners, history of sexually transmitted diseases, low socioeconomic status, cigarette smoking, immunosuppression, and Fanconi syndrome.

Pathophysiology

Cervical cancer occurs secondary to viral transformation of the surface (epithelial) cells by high-risk types of the human papillomavirus (HPV), and it is the only gynecologic cancer that can be prevented by regular screening. Persistent infection with high-risk HPV has been identified as the essential factor in the pathogenesis of the majority of cervical cancers. The virus's ability to transform human epithelium has been associated with the expression of two viral gene products, E6 and E7, which interact with p53 (a tumor-suppressor protein) and retinoblastoma protein (pRB), respectively, and affect control mechanisms of the cell cycle.

The prevalence of genital HPV infection in the world is estimated to be 400 million. Data from the National Health and Nutrition Examination Survey (NHANES) estimate the prevalence of HPV infection among girls and women in the United States aged 14 to 59 years is 26.8%. In about 90% of cases, the high-risk HPV infection is cleared by the immune system within 16 months. HPV infections in girls and younger women are more likely transient and therefore less likely to be associated with significant cervical lesions.

Prevention and Screening

Advances in molecular biology have allowed the development of viral-like particles using the L1 protein (major immunogenic capsid protein) of the HPV virus. Currently approved HPV vaccines include: Gardasil (2006)[2], Cervarix (2009)[2], and Gardasil 9 (2014). These vaccines are approved to use in girls/boys and women/men between the ages of 9 and 26 years. The FDA expanded its approval in 2018 to include men and women between 27 and 45 years old. Awareness of the importance of HPV vaccination has increased but vaccination rates for US adolescents are still not at goal with only 48.6% vaccinated as of 2017.

The current standard screening algorithm in the United States for preventing cervical cancer is presented in Table 1. Women with abnormal cytology are referred for a colposcopic examination. The colposcopic examination is used to guide biopsies of the exocervix, and in most cases an endocervical biopsy is also performed. The biopsy results then determine the type of follow-up and or therapy required.

Staging

The International Federation of Gynecology and Obstetrics (FIGO) defined the most commonly accepted staging of cervical cancer. This staging is based on a careful clinical examination and the results of specific radiologic studies and procedures. FIGO's latest update (2009) is summarized in Table 2.

In cervical cancer, primary lesions initially progress to lymphatics in the parametrium and pelvic nodes and then extend laterally to the pelvic side wall, bladder, and rectum. The two major spread patterns identified in cervical cancer include direct extension and lymphatic spread.

Diagnosis

The initial workup for cervical cancer depends on whether a cervical lesion is visible. Patients without a visible cervical lesion require a cone biopsy to diagnose stage IA1 or IA2 tumor. Patients with a cervical lesion are assessed by history and physical examination and possibly by examination under anesthesia for biopsy, cystoscopy, sigmoidoscopy, and conventional imaging (chest x-ray, intravenous pyelogram). Other imaging modalities including computed tomography (CT), magnetic resonance imaging (MRI), and fluorodeoxyglucose positron emission tomography (FDG-PET) are useful in evaluating nodal or other metastatic sites but are not incorporated in the FIGO staging system owing to their limited availability worldwide. MRI performed significantly better than CT in detecting parametrial invasion, presence of bladder or rectal invasion, and identification of women suitable for fertility-preserving surgery. PET-CT is the most sensitive modality in

[2]Not available in the United States.

TABLE 1 Cervical Cytologic Screening Guidelines from the American College of Obstetricians and Gynecologists

AGE (YEAR)	RECOMMENDATION FOR CYTOLOGIC SCREENING	COMMENTS
Younger than 21	Avoid screening	
21 to 29	Screen every 3 years	
30 to 65 or 70	May screen every 3 years	This recommendation applies only to women with 3 consecutive cytologic tests; exceptions include women with HIV infection, compromised immunity, a history of cervical intraepithelial neoplasia grade 2 or 3, or exposure to DES in utero.
	Screen every 5 years	Pap + HPV co-testing use
Between 65 and 70	May discontinue screening	This recommendation applies only to women with ≥3 consecutive negative cytologic tests and no abnormal tests in the preceding 10 years; exceptions include women with multiple sexual partners.

DES, Diethylstilbestrol.

Adapted from American College of Obstetricians and Gynecologists (ACOG). Cervical cancer screening and prevention. American College of Obstetricians and Gynecologists (ACOG); (ACOG practice bulletin; no. 168); 2016.

TABLE 2 Revised FIGO Staging for Carcinoma of the Cervix

STAGE	CRITERIA
Stage I	
I	The carcinoma is strictly confined to the cervix
IA	Invasive carcinoma, which can be diagnosed only by microscopy, with deepest invasion ≤5 mm and largest extension ≥7 mm
IA1	Measured stromal invasion of ≤3 mm in depth and extension of ≤7 mm
IA2	Measured stromal invasion of >3 mm in depth and extension of >7 mm
IB	Clinically visible lesions limited to the cervix or preclinical cancers greater than stage IA
IB1	Lesion >5 mm depth of stromal invasion and <2 cm greatest dimension
IB2	Lesion 2 cm to <4 cm in greatest dimension
1B3	Lesion >4 cm in dimension
Stage II	
II	Cervical carcinoma invades beyond the uterus, but not to the pelvic wall or to the lower third of the vagina
IIA	Without parametrial invasion
IIA1	Clinically visible lesion ≤4 cm in greatest dimension
IIA2	Clinically visible lesion >4 cm in greatest dimension
IIB	With obvious parametrial invasion
Stage III	
III	The tumor extends to the pelvic wall and/or involves lower third of the vagina and/or causes hydronephrosis or nonfunctioning kidney
IIIA	Tumor involves lower third of the vagina, with no extension to the pelvic wall
IIIB	Extension to the pelvic wall and/or hydronephrosis or nonfunctioning kidney
IIIC1	Pelvic lymph node metastasis only
IIIC2	Para-aortic lymph node metastasis
Stage IV	
IV	The carcinoma has extended beyond the true pelvis or has involved (biopsy proven) the mucosa of the bladder or rectum; a bullous edema, as such, does not permit a case to be allotted as stage IV
IVA	Spread of the growth to adjacent organs
IVB	Spread to distant organs

Adapted from Bhatla N, Berek JS, Cuello Fredes M, et al. Revised FIGO Staging for carcinoma of cervix uteri. Int J Gynaecol Obstet. 2019;145:129–135.

identifying nodal metastasis or metastatic disease assisting with radiotherapy planning and evaluation of metabolic response to therapy. A 3-month posttherapy PET scan is highly predictive of long-term survival outcome.

Treatment

Multiple factors including tumor stage, size, histologic features (lymphovascular space invasion [LVSI], nonsquamous components, and depth of cervical stromal invasion), and evidence of lymph node metastasis influence the choice of treatment for cervical cancer. Patients with stage IA1 cervical cancer have undergone a cone biopsy and pathology demonstrates 3 mm of invasion or less, less than 7 mm width, no LVSI, and negative margins. Patients with this extent of disease can safely be treated with a less-radical hysterectomy, an extrafascial hysterectomy. Pelvic lymphadenectomy is not recommended owing to the low risk of pelvic node metastasis (<1%). In patients who desire to retain fertility, a cone biopsy may be considered. Wright and colleagues reported on 1409 women from the SEER database who were younger than 40 years and had stage IA1 cancer. The 5-year survival was 98% among 568 who underwent cone biopsy alone versus 99% among 841 who underwent hysterectomy.

Patients with stage IA2 to IB1 are generally treated with radical hysterectomy; in patients who are not candidates for surgery owing to comorbidities, radiation therapy is used. In patients with high-risk criteria after surgery—positive surgical margin, parametrial involvement, and positive pelvic nodes—cisplatin-based[1] chemoradiation, based on a positive randomized trial, is recommended. Those with intermediate risk factors including tumor size, cervical stromal invasion, and lymphovascular invasion had an improved progression-free survival with adjuvant radiation.

Radical trachelectomy—laparoscopic, vaginal, or open—in conjunction with lymphadenectomy is a reasonable alternative treatment for select young patients with stage IA2 and IB1 who desire to maintain their childbearing capacity. The criteria used for patient selection include early-stage cervical cancer with a lesion less than 2 cm, no lymphovascular invasion, and no lymph node metastasis. Reports comparing radical trachelectomies with matched controls identified increased complications (25% vs. 3%) and overall less-radical dissection.

Treatment of stage IB2 cancer of the cervix varies depending on the bulkiness and shape of the lesion. Surgery and chemoradiation therapy have advantages and disadvantages. Finan and colleagues reported that up to 72% of patients with stage IB2 disease who were

[1] Not FDA approved for this indication.

TABLE 3 | Randomized Trials of Cisplatin-Based Chemoradiation

| TREATMENT | STAGE | SURVIVAL | | | SIGNIFICANCE |
		TYPE	PERCENTAGE (%)		
Gynecology Oncology Group 85					
RT/5-FU* infusion/bolus cisplatin*	IIB-IVA	3 y PFS	67		P = .033
RT/oral HU*			57		
Gynecology Oncology Group 109					
Rad hyst/RT	IA2-IIA	Est. 4-y	63		P = .003
Rad hyst/RT/cisplatin*/5-FU*			80		
Radiation Therapy Oncology Group 9001					
RT	IIB-IVA	DFS	40		P < .001
RT/5-FU*/cisplatin*			67		
Gynecology Oncology Group 120					
RT + cisplatin*	IIB-IVA	3-y PFS	67		P < .001
RT + cisplatin*/5-FU*/HU*			64		
RT + HU*			47		
Gynecology Oncology Group 123					
RT + TAH	IB2	3 y PFS	74		P < .001
RT + cisplatin* + TAH			83		
Di Silvestro et al.					
RT + cisplatin	IB2-IVA	3 y PFS	64		P = .7869
RT + cisplatin + TPZ			63		
Pearcey et al.					
RT + cisplatin*	IB-IVA >5 cm	5-y DFS	62		P = .42
RT			58		

DFS, Disease-free survival; *5-FU*, fluorouracil (Adrucil); *HU*, hydroxyurea; *PFS*, progression free survival; *rad hyst*, radical hysterectomy; *RT*, radiotherapy; *TAH*, total abdominal hysterectomy.

*Not FDA approved for this indication.

treated with surgery received adjuvant radiation owing to high-risk factors identified in pathologic evaluation of specimens. In a randomized Gynecologic Oncology Group trial, 94% of patients with IB2 cervical cancer who underwent radical hysterectomy had high or intermediate risk factors warranting adjuvant radiation.

In 1999 the National Cancer Institute (NCI) initiated a clinical alert recommending that concurrent cisplatin-based chemotherapy be given with radiotherapy to women with cervical cancer based on five randomized studies, and this established a new standard of care (Table 3).

It is estimated that approximately 35% of patients with invasive cervical cancer will have recurrent or persistent disease, with most recurrences occurring in the first 2 years following primary therapy. Recurrence can be expected in 10% to 20% of patients treated with radical hysterectomy in contrast to 30% to 50% treated for more-advanced disease primarily with radiation plus concurrent chemotherapy. The site of the recurrence can direct further treatment. Patients with central pelvic recurrences after surgery are candidates for curative radiation; after primary treatment with radiation therapy patients may be candidates for curative radical surgery (exenteration). Prognosis is more favorable for patients undergoing exenteration when there is a small (<3 cm) central recurrence, no sidewall involvement, and longer than 2 years of disease-free interval. Those with small recurrences limited to the cervix or upper vagina can occasionally be treated with radical hysterectomy and upper vaginectomy.

However, most recurrences are distant, involving the lung, bone, abdominal cavity, and supraclavicular lymph nodes. Recurrences within irradiated areas have a poor response to therapy (0% to 5%). Recurrences in the nonirradiated areas respond better to chemotherapy, with response rates of 25% to 70%. The use of chemotherapy in the treatment of recurrent cervical cancer is challenging because agents are only moderately active and patients can present with renal impairment secondary to obstructive uropathy, resulting in altered excretion with increased toxicity from chemotherapeutic agents. Table 4 compares results of randomized chemotherapy trials for the treatment of recurrent cervical cancer.

New treatment strategies for recurrent disease include immunotherapy with multiple ongoing trials at this time.

Conclusion

Adherence to current screening guidelines should allow early cervical cancer or precancerous detection. However, most patients with cervical cancer have not participated in regular screening and present with a variety of disease extents.

	STUDY	STAGE	RESPONSE RATE (%)	PROGRESSION-FREE SURVIVAL (MO)	OVERALL SURVIVAL (MO)
TABLE 4	Phase III Trials Comparing Cisplatin Doublets and Cisplatin Alone to Treat Metastatic or Recurrent Cervical Carcinoma				
Gynecology Oncology Group 110					
Cisplatin[1]		IVB or recurrent	18	3.2	8
Cisplatin/mitolactol[8]			21	3.3	7.3
Cisplatin/ifosfamide (Ifex)[1]			31	8.3	4.6
Significance			$P = .004$	$P = .003$	$P = .835$
Gynecology Oncology Group 149					
Cisplatin/bleomycin[1]/ifosfamide		IVB or recurrent	31	5.1	8.4
Cisplatin/ifosfamide			32	4.6	8.5
Significance			$P = .42$	$P = .495$	$P = .79$
Gynecology Oncology Group 169					
Cisplatin		IVB or recurrent	19	2.8	8.8
Cisplatin/paclitaxel (Taxol)[1]			36	4.8	9.7
Significance			$P = NS$	$P = NS$	$P = NS$
Gynecology Oncology Group 179					
Cisplatin		IVB or recurrent	13	2.9	6.5
Cisplatin/topotecan (Hycamtin)[1]			27	4.6	9.4
Cisplatin/methotrexate[1]/vinblastine (Velban)[1]/doxorubicin (Adriamycin)[1]					
Significance			$P = .004$	$P = .014$	$P = .017$
Gynecology Oncology Group 204					
Cisplatin/paclitaxel versus cisplatin/vinorelbine (Navelbine)[1]				HR[†] = 1.35	NR
Cisplatin/gemcitabine (Gemzar)[1]				HR[†] = 1.43	NR
Cisplatin/topotecan		IVB or recurrent		HR[†] = 1.28	NR
Gynecology Oncology Group 240					
Cisplatin/paclitaxel		IVB or recurrent	45%	5.9	13.3
Paclitaxel/topotecan			27%		
Cisplatin/paclitaxel/Bevacizumab			50%	8.2	17.0
Paclitaxel/topotecan/Bevacizumab			47%	HR = 0.67	HR = 0.71

NR, Not reported; NS, not significant.
[1]Not FDA approved for this indication.
[8]Orphan drug in the United States.
[†]Hazard ratio for PFS for experimental arms to cisplatin/paclitaxel.

References

American Cancer Society: *Cancer facts and figures*, Available at http://www.cancer.org/Research/CancerFactsFigures/CancerFactsFigures/index. Accessed 28 May 2019.

American College of Obstetricians and Gynecologists (ACOG): Cervical Cancer Screening and Prevention. Practice Bulletin #168. ACOG, *Obstet Gynecol* 128, 2016, e111-30.

Bhatla N, et al: Revised FIGO staging for carcinoma of the cervix uteri, *Int J Gynaecol Obstet* 145:129–135, 2019.

Bloss JD, Blessing JA, Behrens BC, et al: Randomized trial of cisplatin and ifosfamide with or without bleomycin in squamous carcinoma of the cervix: A Gynecologic Oncology Group study, *J Clin Oncol* 20:1832–1837, 2002.

Covens A, Shaw P, Murphy J, et al: Is radical trachelectomy a safe alternative to radical hysterectomy for patients with stage IA-B carcinoma of the cervix? *Cancer* 86:2273–2279, 1999.

DiSilvestro PA, Ali S, Craighed PS, et al: Phase III randomized trial of weekly cisplatin and irradiation versus cisplatin and tirapazamine and irradiation in stages IB2, IIA, IIB, IIIB and IVA cervical carcinoma limited to the pelvis: a Gynecologic Oncology Group study, *J Clin Oncol* 32(5):458–464, 2014.

Dunne EF, Unger ER, Sternberg M, et al: Prevalence of HPV infection among females in the United States, *JAMA* 297(8):813–819, 2007.

Finan MA, Decesare S, Fiorica JV, et al: Radical hysterectomy for stage IB1 vs IB2 carcinoma of the cervix: does the new staging system predict morbidity and survival? *Gynecol Oncol* 62(2):139–147, 1996.

Keys HM, Bundy BN, Stehman FB, et al: Cisplatin, radiation, and adjuvant hysterectomy compared with radiation and adjuvant hysterectomy for bulky stage IB cervical carcinoma, *N Engl J Med* 340(15):1154–1161, 1999, Erratum in N Engl J Med 1999;341(9):708.

Long 3rd HJ, Bundy BN, Grendys EC, et al: Randomized phase III trial of cisplatin with or without topotecan in carcinoma of the uterine cervix: A Gynecologic Oncology Group study, *J Clin Oncol* 23(21):4626–4633, 2005.

Monk BJ, Sill MW, McMeekin DS, et al: Phase III trial of four cisplatin-containing doublet combinations in stage IVB, recurrent, or persistent cervical carcinoma: A Gynecologic Oncology Group study, *J Clin Oncol* 27(28):4649–4655, 2009.

Moore DH, Blessing JA, McQuellon RP, et al: Phase III study of cisplatin with or without paclitaxel in stage IVB, recurrent, or persistent squamous cell carcinoma of the cervix: A Gynecologic Oncology Group study, *J Clin Oncol* 22(15):3113–3119, 2004.

Morris M, Eifel PJ, Lu J, et al: Pelvic radiation with concurrent chemotherapy compared with pelvic and para-aortic radiation for high-risk cervical cancer, *N Engl J Med* 340(15):1137–1143, 1999.

National Cancer Institute: *Cervical cancer*, Available at: http://www.cancer.gov/cancertopics/types/cervical. Accessed 27 May 2019.

Omura GA, Blessing JA, Vaccarello L, et al: Randomized trial of cisplatin versus cisplatin plus mitolactol versus cisplatin plus ifosfamide in advanced squamous carcinoma of the cervix: A Gynecologic Oncology Group study, *J Clin Oncol* 15(1):165–171, 1997.

Pearcey R, Brundage M, Drouin P, et al: Phase III trial comparing radical radiotherapy with and without cisplatin chemotherapy in patients with advanced squamous cell cancer of the cervix, *J Clin Oncol* 20(4):966–972, 2002.

Peters 3rd WA, Liu PY, Barrett 3rd RJ, et al: Concurrent chemotherapy and pelvic radiation therapy compared with pelvic radiation therapy alone as adjuvant therapy after radical surgery in high-risk early-stage cancer of the cervix, *J Clin Oncol* 18(8):1606–1613, 2000.

Rose PG, Bundy BN, Watkins EB, et al: Concurrent cisplatin-based radiotherapy and chemotherapy for locally advanced cervical cancer, *N Engl J Med* 340(15):1144–1153, 1999.

Tewari KS, Sill MW, Long HR, et al: Improved survival with bevacizumab in advance cervical cancer, *N Engl J Med* 370(8):734–743, 2014.

Whitney CW, Sause W, Bundy BN, et al: Randomized comparison of fluorouracil plus cisplatin versus hydroxyurea as an adjunct to radiation therapy in stage IIB-IVA carcinoma of the cervix with negative para-aortic lymph nodes: A Gynecologic Oncology Group and Southwest Oncology Group study, *J Clin Oncol* 17(5):1339–1348, 1999.

Wright JD, Nathavithrana R, Lewin SN, et al: Fertility-conserving surgery for young women with stage IA1 cervical cancer: Safety and access, *Obstet Gynecol* 115(3):585–590, 2010.

CONTRACEPTION

Method of
Rachel A. Bonnema, MD, MS; and Abby L. Spencer, MD, MS

CURRENT THERAPY

- Combined estrogen and progesterone methods (e.g., pills, patch, ring) are effective and commonly used. They provide excellent cycle control and decreased rates of ectopic pregnancy, pelvic inflammatory disease, and endometrial and ovarian cancer, and they can be used in extended-cycle methods for patients who desire fewer than 12 periods per year.
- The use of estrogen has been associated, albeit rarely, with the development of deep vein thrombosis, myocardial infarction, and stroke; estrogen should not be used in smokers older than 35 years, in patients with diabetes with end-organ damage, coronary artery disease, migraines with aura, or a known hypercoagulable condition.
- For women with a contraindication to estrogen, progestin-only methods are safe to use.
- Long-acting reversible contraception (LARC) such as an implant or intrauterine device (IUD) is safe and extremely effective and should be considered in all women, including nulliparous women.

Nearly half of all pregnancies in the United States are unplanned, a rate higher than the rate in other developed countries. Primary care physicians need up-to-date knowledge on contraceptive counseling for women to provide the best match between patient and contraceptive method, in part because providers frequently need to supply contraceptives to women who have particular medical comorbidities. Newer contraceptive preparations are now available, including long-acting implants and altered oral formulations, which differ from traditional oral contraceptives in their hormonal dosages, cycle length, and hormone-free intervals.

Nonhormonal Methods

Nonhormonal methods of contraception include barrier methods and the copper intrauterine device (IUD). These methods are safe, easily available, inexpensive, and reversible. Common barrier methods include male and female condoms, spermicides, vaginal sponges, diaphragms, and cervical caps (Table 1). Only condom use has been consistently found to protect against sexually transmitted diseases including HIV, and condom use may reduce risks of cervical cancer as well. Barrier methods have the lowest efficacy rates of all contraceptive methods, and users should also be counseled about emergency contraception (EC). The copper IUD is an extremely effective form of long-acting reversible contraception (LARC) and is a particularly attractive option for a woman with contraindications to hormone use desiring effective contraception.

Combined Hormonal Contraception

Combined hormonal contraception (CHC) contains estrogen (ethinyl estradiol) and a progestin and works primarily by preventing the surge of luteinizing hormone and thereby preventing ovulation. CHC can be delivered as an oral contraceptive pill (OCP), as a vaginal ring (NuvaRing), or as a transdermal patch (Xulane). Risks, benefits, side effects, and contraindications of CHC are thought to be largely similar across delivery methods.

There are many noncontraceptive benefits to CHC, including first-line treatment for dysfunctional uterine bleeding, dysmenorrhea, and menorrhagia. Benefits in addition to menstrual control include reduction in the risks for, and symptoms of, endometriosis, ovulatory pain, ovarian cysts, benign breast disease, premenstrual syndrome, and premenstrual dysphoric disorder. CHC also reduces risk of ovarian and endometrial cancers; these risk reductions extend for years after stopping CHC. The most common side effects of CHC are outlined in Table 2. The risk of venous thromboembolism (VTE) may be higher in obese women, smokers, and those who use certain progestins such as desogestrel or drospirenone. This risk is lower, however, than the risk of VTE associated with pregnancy, and the absolute risk of VTE among CHC users remains small.

CHCs can be used safely by women who have a range of medical conditions, including well-controlled hypertension, uncomplicated diabetes, migraines *without* aura in women less than age 35, and a family history of breast cancer, to name a few. CHC use is contraindicated in women who have a history of migraine headache with aura at any age, or in women over age 35 with any migraine, owing to elevated risk for stroke. Owing to the increased risk of a cardiovascular event, CHC is also contraindicated in women with moderate hypertension, diabetes with end-organ damage, or known cardiovascular disease and in women who smoke after age 35 years. Other contraindications include a personal history of breast cancer, an estrogen-dependent tumor, unexplained vaginal bleeding, stroke, known thromboembolic disorder, or known VTE. Elevated risk of VTE and negative effect on lactation restrict the use of CHC in the first 6 weeks after delivery.

Combined Oral Contraceptive Pills

There are dozens of formulations of OCPs, which differ by their estrogen dosage, progestin type and dosage, and hormone delivery schedule. OCPs can be monophasic, where each pill contains the same amount of hormones, or multiphasic, where pills contain different amounts of hormones throughout the monthly cycle. The different formulations offer patients options in cycle length, hormone levels, duration of withdrawal bleeding, and side-effect profile. Women should be educated to take their pill at the same time each day; this becomes even more critical in OCPs containing lower dosages of estrogen (20 μg). If a pill is missed, it should be taken as soon as the woman remembers. If 2 days of pills are missed, she should take two pills daily for 2 days in a row and use a backup method. If 3 days of pills are missed, she should discard the pill pack and use a backup method. At that point, it should be discussed whether to start a new pack or to change contraceptive methods.

Traditional OCP regimens include 21 days of hormones, followed by 7 days of placebo pills during which women get their menses. Other women desire fewer days of menses or fewer than 12 menses per year. For these women, extended-cycle OCP regimens can be offered that shorten the placebo period to 4 days, offer a placebo week every 4 months, or eliminate the placebo week altogether. Extended-cycle regimens have other benefits, including decreased hormone withdrawal symptoms such as headaches, tiredness, bloating, excessive bleeding, or menstrual pain.

In addition to estrogen dose and scheduling, it is also important to consider the progestin component, which theoretically may affect libido, weight gain, acne, and hirsutism. These choices, however, must be balanced with the potential increased risk for VTE; levonorgestrel-containing OCPs have a long track record and are associated with a lower risk of VTE than other progestins such as desogestrel, gestodene, and drospirenone.

Contraceptive Patch

Norelgestromin/ethinyl estradiol (Xulane) is a thin transdermal patch delivering a daily dose of 35 μg/d ethinyl estradiol and 150 μg/d norelgestromin. Patches should be changed weekly for 3

TABLE 1 Nonhormonal Contraception

	BARRIER METHODS			INTRAUTERINE DEVICE
	CONDOM (MALE/FEMALE)	DIAPHRAGM OR CERVICAL CAP	SPONGE	COPPER IUD
Duration	Female condom can be inserted up to 8 h before intercourse; male condoms must be changed with each act of intercourse	Can be placed up to 6 h before intercourse and should be removed within 6 h after	Can be left in for 30 h and through multiple acts of intercourse	Approved for up to 10 years
Typical-use failure rate*	15%	15%	15%	Less than 0.1%
Side effects and considerations	High failure rates: condom can break, slip; Acceptability by partner may be limited	Requires expert fitting; Needs to be refitted after childbirth; Requires dexterity and self-placement by patient; Use with spermicide increases efficacy but can lead to risk of UTIs, increased risk of toxic shock syndrome, and potential increased risk of HIV transmission	May increase risk of UTIs; Use with spermicide increases efficacy but can lead to risk of UTIs, increased risk of toxic shock syndrome, and potential increased risk of HIV transmission	Bleeding and cramping with menses initially; Low risk of ectopic pregnancy, premature delivery, perforation, or expulsion; Avoid with active infection, undiagnosed genital bleeding, cervical cancer, or Wilson disease
Consider in:	Patients at risk for STIs; Patients without access to medical care and who are looking for nonhormonal, reversible, and convenient methods of contraception	Women who are looking for nonhormonal, reversible, and convenient methods of contraception	Women who are looking for nonhormonal, reversible, and convenient methods of contraception; Patients without access to medical care	Women with contraindication to hormones or who desire hormone-free, long-acting, reversible contraception; Women in need of EC followed by long-term effective contraception

*Trussel J. Contraceptive failure in the United States. *Conception.* 2011;83:397–404.

EC, Emergency contraception; *HIV,* human immunodeficiency virus; *IUD,* intrauterine device; *UTI,* urinary tract infection.

TABLE 2 Hormonal Contraception

	COMBINATION ESTROGEN-PROGESTIN		PROGESTIN-ONLY		
	TRADITIONAL OCPS	EXTENDED CYCLE OCPS	PILL	INJECTION	IMPLANT/IUD
Duration / Reversibility	Daily pill / Immediate	Daily pill / Immediate	Daily pill with no hormone-free interval / Immediate	3 months / Variable	3–5 years / Immediate
Typical-use failure rate*	9%	9%	9%	6%	0.05%–0.8%
Side effects†	Spotting, nausea, headache, breast tenderness, breakthrough bleeding, VTE, stroke, MI	Spotting, increased unscheduled bleeding, nausea, VTE, stroke, MI	Spotting, unscheduled bleeding, or absence of bleeding; headaches, nausea, mood changes, breast tenderness, depression, enlarged ovarian follicles	Spotting, unscheduled bleeding, or absence of bleeding; weight gain, depression, reversible decrease in BMD	Spotting, unscheduled bleeding, or absence of bleeding
Consider in:	Women with dysmenorrhea, menorrhagia, irregular menstrual periods, acne, hirsutism, or polycystic ovary syndrome	Women who do not desire monthly periods. Fewer withdrawal bleeds per year and shorter placebo may offer particular benefit for women with estrogen withdrawal symptoms, dysmenorrhea, or endometriosis	Women with contraindication to estrogen, hypercoagulable states, dysmenorrhea, migraine with aura, or breast-feeding	Women with contraindication to estrogen, seizure disorder, hypercoagulable states, dysmenorrhea, migraine with aura, or breast-feeding	Women with contraindication to estrogen, seizure disorder, hypercoagulable states, dysmenorrhea, migraine with aura, or breast-feeding

*Trussell J. Contraceptive failure in the United States. *Contraception.* 2011;83:397–404.

†Note: For all combination methods, must have no contraindication to estrogen.

BMD, Bone mineral density; *IUD,* intrauterine device; *MI,* myocardial infarction; *OCP,* oral contraceptive pill; *VTE,* venous thromboembolism.

weeks on "patch change day" followed by a patch-free week during which menses occur. Only one patch should be worn at a time, and no more than 7 days should pass during the patch-free week. The patch has decreased efficacy in women who weigh more than 90 kg. Most of the noncontraceptive benefits, side effects, cardiovascular risks, and contraindications are similar to those of other forms of CHC, but there may be an increased risk of VTE in patch users compared to users of OCPs. Studies are controversial as to the actual increase in risk associated with patch use, but did prompt the updating of the drug label to indicate a higher risk of VTE. Of note, the VTE risk associated with patch use is lower than that associated with pregnancy.

Vaginal Ring

Etonogestrel/ethinyl estradiol (NuvaRing) is a soft plastic ring that is inserted vaginally by the patient, usually for 3 weeks, and then removed for 1 week at which time menses occur. A new ring is inserted 7 days after the last was removed even if bleeding is not complete. The ring releases 15 μg of ethinyl estradiol and 0.12 mg of etonogestrel daily for 3 to 5 weeks, so it can be kept in longer than 3 weeks for women who desire the benefits of extended-cycling use discussed previously. Each ring releases approximately half the level of hormones as the average OCP without affecting efficacy. If the ring falls out (as occurs in 2.5% of women per year), it can be rinsed and reinserted without a change in efficacy. Unlike the patch, the ring is not affected by excess weight. Most women find the ring easy to insert and remove and comfortable to retain during intercourse. The vaginal ring has been associated with an increase in leukorrhea. Otherwise, its noncontraceptive benefits, side effects, cardiovascular risks, and contraindications are similar to those of other forms of CHC.

Progestin-Only Contraceptives

Progestin-only contraceptives are of particular benefit for women who have a contraindication to estrogen, because progestin-only methods have decreased medical risks associated with their use including no increased risk of stroke, myocardial infarction, or VTE. All progestin-only methods have a similar method of action: ovulation is variably inhibited, cervical mucus is thickened, and the endometrial lining undergoes histologic alterations making implantation less likely. Owing to the fact that many of the progestin-only methods are long acting, they tend to have lower failure rates as opposed to CHCs (see Table 2). All progestin-only methods are appropriate for breast-feeding women.

Pill

Progestin-only pills (POPs) are taken without a hormone-free interval and fertility returns immediately on discontinuation. In fact, most experts believe fertility can return in as little as 3 hours after a missed dose; thus a woman should be counseled to use a backup method if she is 3 or more hours late in taking her dose. Given this small window for error, this method should be prescribed only to patients who can adhere closely to a daily pill schedule. Additionally, women should be counseled that while taking the POP, normal menstrual patterns may include anything from amenorrhea to menometrorrhagia. This unpatterned bleeding is likely one of the greatest obstacles to wider use of progestin-only oral contraception. Owing to the fact that POPs have demonstrated no significant negative effects on breastfeeding, POPs are most commonly used in the postpartum period and can be prescribed immediately postpartum. POPs may have similar effects as other progestin-only methods in decreasing the frequency of sickle cell crises; however, unlike depot medroxyprogesterone acetate (DMPA, Depo-Provera) injections, certain anticonvulsants may lower effectiveness of the POP so other methods may be more beneficial in women with seizure disorders.

Injectable

The intramuscular DMPA injection (Depo-Provera) is given every 12 weeks and has a typical-use failure rate of 6%. A lower dose of DMPA (104 mg in Depo-SubQ Provera) has been approved for subcutaneous injection. Women with seizure disorders are particularly good candidates for DMPA injections because, unlike other forms of contraception, the efficacy of DMPA is not affected by enzyme-inducing antiepileptic drugs. Depo-Provera may also decrease seizure frequency, providing additional benefit for patients who have a seizure disorder. DMPA reduces serum estradiol levels, which can adversely affect bone health. In 2004, the United States Food and Drug Administration (FDA) issued a black box warning that women who use Depo-Provera may lose significant bone mineral density (BMD) and recommended that use be limited to less than 2 years unless other methods are inadequate. Since that time, data have shown that although there is a clear association between DMPA use and decreased BMD, the BMD loss was reversible with discontinuation of use and there is no increased risk of fracture with use of DMPA. The World Health Organization has recommended that there be no restriction on the use of Depo-Provera in women ages 18 to 45. According to recent consensus guidelines, clinicians should advise patients about the risk for BMD loss but can reassure them about reversibility with discontinuation.

Intrauterine System

The levonorgestrel intrauterine system (LNG-IUS) is a highly effective contraceptive method long considered to be reversible sterilization owing to its excellent efficacy in preventing pregnancy and quick return to fertility after its removal. There are now multiple formulations of LNG IUS that prevent pregnancy up to 3 years (Skyla) and 5 years (Kyleena, Liletta, Mirena). Mirena is an IUS that releases approximately 20 μg/d of LNG and is effective for 5 years. Skyla is a lower dose LNG-IUS that releases approximately 14 mcg/d of LNG and is effective for 3 years. The LNG-IUS is ideal for women who require highly effective contraception and is particularly beneficial for women requiring a progestin-only contraception. Its relatively low cost over time is another factor for patients to consider. Numerous studies have confirmed the effectiveness of the LNG-IUS for reduction of menstrual blood loss in menorrhagia, leiomyomas, and pain caused by endometriosis. In fact, the LNG-IUS (Mirena) recently received FDA approval for the indication of menorrhagia and has also been shown to decrease menorrhagia even in women on anticoagulation. Insertion of the LNG-IUS requires a trained provider. At the time of placement, women may have cramping and pain; a rare complication of placement is uterine wall rupture. Although women will likely develop amenorrhea, they should be counseled about initial irregular bleeding and spotting.

Implant

There is one single-rod subdermal implant available in the United States called Nexplanon that is a highly effective long-term contraceptive containing the progestin etonogestrel (ENG). The rod is implanted in the upper arm and remains active for 3 years. ENG does not cause a hypoestrogenic state and thus this method is not considered to have any significant effect on BMD. ENG implantation can be done as a simple procedure by a trained provider under local anesthetic with a preloaded, disposable applicator. Women experience a quick return to normal cycles after implant removal, and there have been no reports of infertility after removal. Similar to other progestin-only forms of contraception, irregular bleeding is the major side effect of the ENG implant. The most common bleeding pattern associated with the implant is infrequent, irregular bleeding. Unfortunately, there is no method to predict bleeding response for an individual patient after ENG implantation, so this is an important counseling point, particularly since the highest rate of discontinuation is during the first 8 to 9 months of use, primarily owing to frequent bleeding.

Permanent

Permanent birth control methods include vasectomy and female sterilization by various procedures. These methods are highly effective (typical failure rate 0.15% to 0.5%); however, they are permanent, and can be associated with regret. Each sterilization procedure has advantages and disadvantages that should be considered by the patient before choosing which one to use.

Emergency Contraception

Familiarity with EC is critical both for women who are having unprotected sex and for those who are using methods with higher failure rates. EC use has not been shown to reduce compliance with other first-line methods. EC primarily acts by inhibiting or delaying ovulation, and works before implantation; if a fertilized egg has already implanted, EC will not work. EC includes pills (comprised of estrogen + progestin, progestin only, and antiprogestins) and copper IUD placement (inserted up to 5 days after unprotected intercourse); EC pills are most effective when taken in the first 12 hours, but have gradually decreasing effectiveness for up to 120 hours after intercourse. The most commonly used and most accessible form of EC in the United States contains levonorgestrel only (Plan B One Step) and is over the counter without age restrictions.

Counseling

When counseling patients about their contraceptive choices, it is important that providers are aware of their role in giving information and allowing patients to make informed decisions. The only effective contraceptive is one that a patient is willing to use consistently and correctly, and the choice of contraception is ultimately the patient's decision. Providers must educate patients regarding the advantages and disadvantages of each method that is medically appropriate for them. Discussing a patient's preferences for menstrual frequency and tolerance for scheduled and unscheduled bleeding will be important in deciding which contraceptive will best fit her needs. Providers should counsel patients on expected side effects as well as expectant management strategies. Every effort should be made to remove barriers to initiation, including having no requirement for a pelvic examination or Pap smear before initiation. Using the conversation about contraceptives to also discuss safe sex is ideal.

References

ACOG Committee on Practice Bulletins—Gynecology: ACOG practice bulletin. No. 73: use of hormonal contraception in women with coexisting medical conditions, *Obstet Gynecol* 107:1453–1472, 2006.

Curtis KM, Tepper NK, Jatlaoui TC, et al: U.S. Medical Eligibility Criteria for Contraceptive Use, 2016, *MMWR Recomm Rep* 65(No. RR-3):1–104, 2016. https://doi.org/10.15585/mmwr.rr6503a1.

Finer LB, Zolna MR: Unintended pregnancy in the United States: incidence and disparities, 2006, *Contraception* 84:478–485, 2011.

Lanza LL, McQuay LJ, Rothman KJ, et al: Use of depot medroxyprogesterone acetate contraception and incidence of bone fracture, *Obstet Gynecol* 121:593–600, 2013.

Parkin L, Sharples K, Hernandez RK, et al: Risk of venous thromboembolism in users of oral contraceptives containing drospirenone or levonorgestrel: nested case control study based on UK General Practice Research Database, *BMJ* 340:d2139, 2011.

Petitti DB: Combination estrogen-progestin oral contraceptives, *N Engl J Med* 349:1443–1450, 2003.

Spencer AL, Bonnema RA, McNamara MC: Helping women choose appropriate hormonal contraception: update on risks, benefits, and indications, *Am J Med* 122:497–506, 2009.

Trussel J: Contraceptive failure in the United States, *Conception* 83:397–404, 2011.

World Health Organization: Cardiovascular disease and use of oral and injectable progestogen-only contraceptives and combined injectable contraceptives. Results of an international, multicenter, case-control study. World Health Organization Collaborative Study of Cardiovascular Disease and Steroid Hormone Contraception, *Contraception* 57:315–324, 1998.

DYSMENORRHEA

Method of
Linda Speer, MD

CURRENT DIAGNOSIS

- Primary dysmenorrhea (painful menses without underlying pathology) is common among adolescents and young women. It usually begins shortly after menarche.
- Diagnosis of primary dysmenorrhea can be made based on typical history of crampy pelvic pain during the first 1 to 3 days of the menstrual cycle. Pelvic examination is not required.

- Secondary dysmenorrhea (with underlying pathology) should be considered in cases that do not match the typical history, begin later in life, and/or are refractory to treatment.
- The most common cause of secondary dysmenorrhea is endometriosis. The clinical standard for diagnosis of endometriosis is laparoscopic confirmation. Ultrasound imaging is useful in some cases.

CURRENT THERAPY

- Nonsteroidal antiinflammatory drugs (NSAIDs) are well-established first-line therapy for treatment of primary dysmenorrhea. None has been confirmed as superior to others.
- Cyclooxygenase-2 (COX-2) inhibitors are effective and have fewer gastrointestinal side effects but may be less effective than NSAIDs.
- Oral contraceptives and the levonorgestrel intrauterine system (Mirena)[1] reduce dysmenorrhea.
- Other effective therapies include topical heat, high-frequency transcutaneous electrical nerve stimulation (TENS), and several herbal preparations.
- Treatments for endometriosis as a secondary cause of pelvic pain and dysmenorrhea include hormonal suppression of the endometrial tissue, conservative laparoscopic surgical debulking, and hysterectomy in selected cases.

[1]Not FDA approved for this indication.

Dysmenorrhea is defined as painful menses. Primary dysmenorrhea occurs without underlying pathology, typically beginning soon after menarche. It is common in adolescent girls, with prevalence ranging from 20% to 90% depending on measurement methods; about 15% of adolescents describe their dysmenorrhea as severe. The median duration of each episode is 2 days beginning with the onset of menses. During adolescence, dysmenorrhea leads to high rates of school absence and activity nonparticipation. According to representative national survey data in the United States, 14% of adolescent girls aged 12 to 17 years frequently miss school because of menstrual cramps.

A prospective cohort study showed that the prevalence and severity of dysmenorrhea was lower at 24 years of age than at 19 years of age. At 24 years of age, 67% of the women still experienced dysmenorrhea, and 10% reported pain severity that limited daily activity. The prevalence and severity of dysmenorrhea were reduced in women who were parous at 24 years and nulliparous at 19 years, but they were unchanged in women who were still nulliparous or women who had had a miscarriage or abortion.

There is a significant correlation between the severity of dysmenorrhea and the amount of menstrual flow. Survey data demonstrate that depression and anxiety are associated with menstrual pain and suggest that loss of social support is a significant contributor to menstrual symptoms. The severity of dysmenorrhea is not associated with height, weight, or regularity of the menstrual cycle. A relationship to smoking has been found inconsistently. Physical activity has been studied and found not to be associated with any pain parameter.

Secondary dysmenorrhea typically starts later in life after the onset of an underlying causative condition, most often endometriosis. The association between dysmenorrhea and endometriosis is uncertain for women with minimal disease. However, based on a study of more than 1000 women with laparoscopically confirmed endometriosis, chronic pelvic pain, dyspareunia, and dysmenorrhea are in fact related to the extent of endometriosis.

Diagnosis

For adolescents who present with complaints typical for primary dysmenorrhea, treatment may be started empirically without a pelvic examination or diagnostic studies. Sexually active adolescents and young women should be screened for chlamydia and gonorrhea, which can be done with either urine or a genital sampling.

For adolescents and women who do not have a history consistent with primary dysmenorrhea or who are refractory to treatment, endometriosis may be suspected. The gold standard for diagnosis is laparoscopy and biopsy. Ultrasound may also be useful, especially to identify endometriomas.

Treatment

Nonsteroidal Antiinflammatory Drugs

A Cochrane review of randomized, controlled trials (RCTs) concluded that among women with primary dysmenorrhea, NSAIDs were significantly more effective for pain relief than placebo or acetaminophen (Tylenol). No specific NSAID was shown to be superior to others for either pain relief or safety. However, the available evidence had little power to detect such differences, because most individual comparisons were based on few small trials. In one study in which diclofenac (Voltaren) 100 mg was compared with placebo for treatment of primary dysmenorrhea, the authors found that leg strength and aerobic capacity were maintained at the level found during luteal phase when women took diclofenac for dysmenorrhea, but they were reduced during menses in the placebo group.

COX-2 Inhibitors

Several COX-2 inhibitors have been evaluated for treatment of dysmenorrhea in RCTs. Celecoxib (Celebrex) 200 mg was compared with naproxen sodium (Naprosyn) 550 mg and placebo for treatment of dysmenorrhea and found to be superior to placebo but not as effective as naproxen. Etoricoxib (Arcoxia)[5] 120 mg daily was found to be better than placebo and equivalent to mefenamic acid (Ponstel) for treatment of primary dysmenorrhea with less nausea and epigastric pain than mefenamic acid. Lumiracoxib (Prexige)[5] 200 mg daily was compared with naproxen 500 mg twice daily and placebo for treatment of primary dysmenorrhea and found to reduce pain more than placebo and similar to naproxen.

Oral Contraceptives

In a systematic review of NSAIDs and oral contraceptives (OCs) for treatment of dysmenorrhea that included 10 placebo-controlled RCTs of NSAIDs, two RCTs of OCs and six prospective observational studies of OCs, the authors concluded that both are effective. In a study of women with laparoscopically proven endometriosis, low-dose ethinyl estradiol and norethisterone (norethindrone) decreased dysmenorrhea associated with endometriosis as compared with placebo (with pain assessment on a verbal rating scale from 0 to 3). There was also a significant reduction in volume of endometriomas with OCs but not placebo.

Levonorgestrel Intrauterine System

The levonorgestrel intrauterine system (LNG-IUS), Mirena, reduces menstrual bleeding and dysmenorrhea, which can be a desirable side effect for women desiring long-term contraception. In an uncontrolled case series of women treated with LNG-IUS for adenomyosis, dysmenorrhea diminished continuously during the 3-year study from a mean 78 mm to a mean 12 mm on a 100-mm visual analog scale. Overall satisfaction with treatment was 73%. Depot medroxyprogesterone acetate[1] (Depo-Provera) is similarly effective, but it is less likely to be well tolerated owing to unpredictable bleeding, weight gain, and mood changes.

Nifedipine

In one uncontrolled study, nifedipine[1] (Procardia) 20 to 40 mg given orally reduced myometrial activity and relieved dysmenorrhea.

This drug could be considered as an adjunct in severe cases of primary dysmenorrhea after ruling out endometriosis.

Transcutaneous Electrical Nerve Stimulation

In a study comparing transcutaneous electrical nerve stimulation (TENS) with interferential current for treatment of dysmenorrhea, each group received application of the modality for 20 minutes while experiencing dysmenorrhea. Both groups improved significantly from baseline without significant difference between them. High-frequency TENS has been found to be effective for the treatment of dysmenorrhea in a number of small trials. Low-frequency TENS does not appear to be effective.

Topical Heat and Infrared Light

Two meta-analyses have concluded that topical heat is likely an effective therapy based on several small low-to-moderate-quality studies. In a trial comparing far-infrared emitting belt versus placebo belt for treatment of primary dysmenorrhea, both with concurrent application of topical heat, both groups improved, and the duration of the analgesic effect was significantly longer in the group treated with the infrared belt.

Complementary and Alternative Medicine Approaches
Herbal

Several herbal remedies have been studied in RCTs for treatment of dysmenorrhea and found to be effective as compared with placebo or NSAIDs. They include *Psidii guajava* extract[7] 6 mg/day, French maritime pine bark extract (pycnogenol),[7] ginger root powder[7] 250 mg 4 times daily, salix extract (willow bark) 400 mg daily, and cinnamon one 1000 mg capsule daily. A pilot study of oral lactobacillus capsules (probiotic)[7] suggests that it may also be helpful.

Acupressure and Acupuncture

The evidence for the effectiveness of acupuncture is not conclusive. In unblinded studies women experience clinically relevant reduction in pain scores, a mean of more than 10 points on a 100-point scale, which could be due to placebo effect. In fact, in a well-designed RCT of electro-acupuncture at the Sanyinjiao point (the point expected to be related to uterine pain) compared to an unrelated nonacupoint or no acupuncture, the only significant differences were with the no-acupuncture group as measured with a visual analogue rating scale.

Adequate blinding is also an issue among studies of acupressure. For example, in an RCT comparing auricular seed acupressure versus adhesive tape only for treatment of primary dysmenorrhea the acupressure group (but not the tape only group) had instructions to massage the seed 15 times, three times daily for 20 days. Menstrual pain decreased significantly in the acupressure group. Several other studies suggest that acupressure at the Sanyinjiao point or Taichong point is more effective than no intervention or inadequately blinded control groups. Because acupressure is a low-cost and harmless intervention, it may be worth considering even if the pain reduction is a placebo response. It appears to be less effective than analgesics.

Yoga and Other Physical Activity

Yoga is another alternative approach with low cost and little risk that may be worth considering despite weak evidence for effectiveness. In one unblinded RCT, three yoga poses (cat, cobra, and fish) were studied for treatment of primary dysmenorrhea. Participants randomized to the intervention group were told to do the yoga poses during luteal phase and complete a questionnaire regarding menstrual characteristics. The control group was asked to complete the questionnaire only. There was significant reduction in intensity and duration of pain in the yoga group compared with baseline and with the control group.

---

[1] Not FDA approved for this indication.
[5] Investigational drug in the United States.

---

[7] Available as dietary supplement.

Two meta-analyses have concluded limited quality evidence suggests that physical activity interventions reduce the duration and intensity of primary dysmenorrhea, perhaps more than oral analgesics.

Spinal Manipulation

Overall there is no evidence to suggest that spinal manipulation is effective in the treatment of primary and secondary dysmenorrhea.

Surgical Treatment

Surgical treatment may be considered in severe and refractory cases of pelvic pain including dysmenorrhea. Laparoscopic uterosacral nerve ablation (LUNA, $n=35$) alone has been compared with LUNA plus presacral neurectomy ($n=32$). There were no differences between groups for relief of dysmenorrhea at 3-, 6-, and 12-month follow-up, but more surgical complications were experienced with neurectomy.

Treatment of Endometriosis

Treatment of endometriosis may start with use of NSAIDs, hormonal contraceptives, and/or LNG-IUS.[1] However, often endometriosis is diagnosed after those first-line therapies have failed. Debulking of the ectopic endometrial tissue during laparoscopy can relieve pain.

Other treatments involve hormonal suppression of endometrial tissue. Danazol is a 19-nortestosterone derivative with a long history of use for treatment of endometriosis pain at a dosage of 400 to 800 mg daily for 6 months, but it is often poorly tolerated owing to androgenic side effects. Oral progestin regimens (medroxyprogesterone acetate[1] [DepoProvera] up to 100 mg daily[3] or norethindrone [Aygestin] up to 15 mg daily) may be used to suppress menses for a 6-month course. Other accepted therapies include gonadotropin-releasing hormone (GnRH) agonist analogues such as leuprolide (Lupron). Aromatase inhibitors have been shown to be effective in a systematic review of several small RCTs. Etonogestrel subdermal implant[1] (Nexplanon) has been evaluated in an uncontrolled case series and found to be associated with pain relief.

In severe refractory cases, hysterectomy may be considered.

---

[1] Not FDA approved for this indication.
[3] Exceeds dosage recommended by the manufacturer.

References

Akin MD, Weingand KW, Hengehold DA, et al: Continuous low-level topical heat in the treatment of dysmenorrhea, *Obstet Gynecol* 97:343–349, 2001.

Alonso C, Coe CL: Disruptions of social relationships accentuate the association between emotional distress and menstrual pain in young women, *Health Psychol* 20:411–416, 2001.

Andersch B, Milsom I: An epidemiologic study of young women with dysmenorrhea, *Am J Obstet Gynecol* 144:655–660, 1982.

Andersson KE, Ulmsten U: Effects of nifedipine on myometrial activity and lower abdominal pain in women with primary dysmenorrhoea, *Br J Obstet Gynaecol* 85:142–148, 1978.

Armour M, Smith CA, Steel KA, Macmillan F: The effectiveness of self-care and lifestyle interventions in primary dysmenorrhea: a systematic review and meta-analysis, *BMC Complement Altern Med* 19:22, 2019.

Bazarganipour F, Lamyian M, Heshmat R, et al: A randomized clinical trial of the efficacy of applying a simple acupressure protocol to the Taichong point in relieving dysmenorrhea, *Int J Gynaecol Obstet* 111:105–109, 2010.

Brown J, Pan A, Hart RJ: Gonadotrophin-releasing hormone analogues for pain associated with endometriosis, *Cochrane Database Syst Rev*(12), 2010. CD008475.

Chantler I, Mitchell D, Fuller A: Diclofenac potassium attenuates dysmenorrhea and restores exercise performance in women with primary dysmenorrhea, *J Pain* 10:191–200, 2009.

Daniels S, Robbins J, West CR, Nemeth MA: Celecoxib in the treatment of primary dysmenorrhea: Results from two randomized, double-blind, active- and placebo-controlled, crossover studies, *Clin Ther* 31:1192–1208, 2009.

Daniels S, Gitton X, Zhou W, et al: Efficacy and tolerability of lumiracoxib 200 mg once daily for treatment of primary dysmenorrhea: Results from two randomized controlled trials, *J Womens Health (Larchmt)* 17:423–437, 2008.

Davis AR, Westhoff CL: Primary dysmenorrhea in adolescent girls and treatment with oral contraceptives, *J Pediatr Adolesc Gynecol* 14:3–8, 2001.

Doubova SV, Morales HR, Hernández SF, et al: Effect of a *Psidii guajavae folium* extract in the treatment of primary dysmenorrhea: A randomized clinical trial, *J Ethnopharmacol* 110:305–310, 2007.

Harada T, Momoeda M, Taketani Y, et al: Low-dose oral contraceptive pill for dysmenorrhea associated with endometriosis: A placebo-controlled, double-blind, randomized trial, *Fertil Steril* 90:1583–1588, 2008.

Harlow SD, Park M: A longitudinal study of risk factors for the occurrence, duration and severity of menstrual cramps in a cohort of college women, *Br J Obstet Gynaecol* 103:1134–1142, 1996.

Jahangirifar M, Taebi M, Dolatian M: The effect of cinnamon on primary dysmenorrhea: A randomized, double-blind clinical trial, *Complement Ther Clin Pract* 33:56–60, 2018.

Jensen JT: Noncontraceptive applications of the levonorgestrel intrauterine system, *Curr Womens Health Rep* 2:417–422, 2002.

Juang CM, Chou P, Yen MS, et al: Laparoscopic uterosacral nerve ablation with and without presacral neurectomy in the treatment of primary dysmenorrhea: A prospective efficacy analysis, *J Reprod Med* 52:591–596, 2007.

Jo J, Lee SH: Heat therapy for primary dysmenorrhea: A systematic review and meta-analysis of its effects on pain relief and quality of life, *Sci Rep* 8:16252, 2018.

Kashefi F, Ziyadlou S, Khajehei M, et al: Effect of acupressure at the Sanyinjiao point on primary dysmenorrhea: A randomized controlled trial, *Complement Ther Clin Pract* 16:198–202, 2010.

Khodaverdi S, Mohammedbeigi R, Khaled M, et al: Beneficial effects of oral lactobacillus on pain severity in women suffering from endometriosis: A pilot placebo-controlled randomized clinical trial, *Int J Fertil Steril* 13:178–183, 2019.

Klein JR, Litt IF: Epidemiology of adolescent dysmenorrhea, *Pediatrics* 68:661–664, 1981.

Lee CH, Roh JW, Lim CY, et al: A multicenter, randomized, double-blind, placebo-controlled trial evaluating the efficacy and safety of a far infrared-emitting sericite belt in patients with primary dysmenorrhea, *Complement Ther Med* 19:187–193, 2011.

Liu CZ, Xie JP, Wang LP, et al: Immediate analgesia effect of single point acupuncture in primary dysmenorrhea: A randomized controlled trial, *Pain Med* 12:300–307, 2011.

Matthewman G, Lee A, Kaur JG, Daley AJ: Physical activity for dysmenorrhea: a systematic review and meta-analysis of randomized controlled trials, *Am J Obstet Gynecol* 219:255e.1-e.20, 2018.

Marjoribanks J, Proctor M, Farquhar C, Derks RS: Nonsteroidal anti-inflammatory drugs for dysmenorrhoea, *Cochrane Database Syst Rev*(1), 2010. CD001751.

Mirbagher-Ajorpaz N, Adib-Hajbaghery M, Mosaebi F. The effects of acupressure on primary dysmenorrhea: A randomized controlled trial. Complement Ther Clin Pract 2011;17:33–26.

Moen MH, Stokstad T: A long-term follow-up study of women with asymptomatic endometriosis diagnosed incidentally at sterilization, *Fertil Steril* 78:773–776, 2002.

Momoeda M, Taketani Y, Terakawa N, et al: Is endometriosis really associated with pain? *Gynecol Obstet Invest* 54(Suppl. 1):18–21, 2002.

Nawathe A, Patwardhan S, Yates D, et al: Systematic review of the effects of aromatase inhibitors on pain associated with endometriosis, *BJOG* 115:818–822, 2008.

Ozgoli G, Goli M, Moattar F: Comparison of effects of ginger, mefenamic acid, and ibuprofen on pain in women with primary dysmenorrhea, *J Altern Complement Med* 15:129–132, 2009.

Proctor ML, Smith CA, Farquhar CM, Stones RW: Transcutaneous electrical nerve stimulation and acupuncture for primary dysmenorrhoea, *Cochrane Database Syst Rev* 2(1), 2002. CD002123.

Proctor ML, Hing W, Johnson TC, Murphy PA: Spinal manipulation for primary and secondary dysmenorrhoea, *Cochrane Database Syst Rev*(3), 2006. CD002119.

Raisi Dehkordi Z, Rafaieian-Kopaei M, Hosseina-Baharanchi FS: A double-blind controlled crossover study to investigate the efficacy of salix extract on primary dysmenorrhea, *Complement Ther Med* 44:102–109, 2019.

Rakhshaee Z. Effect of three yoga poses (cobra, cat and fish poses) in women with primary dysmenorrhea: A randomized clinical trial. J Pediatr Adolesc Gynecol 2011;24:192–6.

Ranong CN, Sukcharoen N: Analgesic effect of etoricoxib in secondary dysmenorrhea: A randomized, double-blind, crossover, controlled trial, *J Reprod Med* 52:1023–1029, 2007.

Selak V, Farquhar C, Prentice A, Singla A: Danazol for pelvic pain associated with endometriosis, *Cochrane Database Syst Rev*(4), 2007. CD000068.

Sheng J, Zhang WY, Zhang JP, Lu D: The LNG-IUS study on adenomyosis: A 3-year follow-up study on the efficacy and side effects of the use of levonorgestrel intrauterine system for the treatment of dysmenorrhea associated with adenomyosis, *Contraception* 79:189–193, 2009.

Strinić T, Buković D, Pavelić L, et al: Anthropological and clinical characteristics in adolescent women with dysmenorrhea, *Coll Antropol* 27:707–711, 2003.

Sundell G, Milsom I, Andersch B: Factors influencing the prevalence and severity of dysmenorrhoea in young women, *Br J Obstet Gynaecol* 97:588–594, 1990.

Suzuki N, Uebaba K, Kohama T, et al: French maritime pine bark extract significantly lowers the requirement for analgesic medication in dysmenorrhea: A multicenter, randomized, double-blind, placebo-controlled study, *J Reprod Med* 53:338–346, 2008.

Telimaa S, Puolakka J, Rönnberg L, Kauppila A: Placebo-controlled comparison of danazol and high-dose medroxyprogesterone acetate in the treatment of endometriosis, *Gynecol Endocrinol* 1:13–23, 1987.

Tugay N, Akbayrak T, Demirtürk F, et al: Effectiveness of transcutaneous electrical nerve stimulation and interferential current in primary dysmenorrhea, *Pain Med* 8:295–300, 2007.

Wang MC, Hsu MC, Chien LW, et al: Effects of auricular acupressure on menstrual symptoms and nitric oxide for women with primary dysmenorrhea, *J Altern Complement Med* 15:235–242, 2009.

Witt CM, Reinhold T, Brinkhaus B, et al: Acupuncture in patients with dysmenorrhea: A randomized study on clinical effectiveness and cost-effectiveness in usual care, *Am J Obstet Gynecol* 198:166, 2008, e1–8.

Wong CL, Lai KY, Tse HM. Effects of SP6 acupressure on pain and menstrual distress in young women with dysmenorrhea. Complement Ther Clin Pract 2009;16:64–9.

Yisa SB, Okenwa AA, Husemeyer RP: Treatment of pelvic endometriosis with etonogestrel subdermal implant (Implanon), *J Fam Plann Reprod Health Care* 31:67–70, 2005.

Zahradnik HP, Hanjalic-Beck A, Groth K. Nonsteroidal anti-inflammatory drugs and hormonal contraceptives for pain relief from dysmenorrhea: A review. Contraception 2010;81:185–96.

ENDOMETRIOSIS

Method of
Zachary Kuhlmann, DO

CURRENT DIAGNOSIS

- Clinical symptoms associated with endometriosis include chronic pelvic pain, dysmenorrhea, dyspareunia, and infertility.
- A pelvic sonogram may be helpful to aid in diagnosis of endometriosis. Care should be taken to exclude other gynecologic and non-gynecologic etiologies of pain.
- Diagnostic laparoscopy may reveal powder burn–like lesions, adhesions, endometriomas, or other signs of endometriosis on inspection.
- The gold standard to make a pathologic diagnosis of endometriosis requires a tissue biopsy of a suspected lesion.

CURRENT MANAGEMENT

- Initial therapy for endometriosis includes NSAIDs, progesterones, combined OCPs, danazol (Danocrine), GnRH agonists, and GnRH antagonists.
- Diagnostic laparoscopy with excision or ablative techniques are often used to treat endometriosis.
- It is reasonable to consider empiric medical therapy with a GnRH agonist before surgery in some situations.
- Hysterectomy with bilateral salpingo-oophorectomy is definitive surgical treatment for endometriosis.

Endometriosis is a common and benign gynecologic condition diagnosed when endometrial tissue is found outside the uterus. Common places for endometrial tissue to implant include the peritoneum and ovaries, although endometriosis can occur outside the pelvis as well. Other locations for endometriosis to be found include the rectovaginal septum, bowel, bladder, pleura, abdominal wall, and even the brain in rare cases. Endometriosis is an estrogen-dependent, inflammatory disorder.

Epidemiology
Endometriosis affects between 5% to 10% of women of reproductive age. Women who experience infertility may have a prevalence of endometriosis of up to 50%, and women with chronic pelvic pain may experience a prevalence of endometriosis well over 80%.

Risk Factors
There appears to be an inheritable component for endometriosis. Women who have a first-degree relative affected by endometriosis may have a 6 to 7 times higher incidence than women without an affected relative. Other risk factors for endometriosis include menarche before age 11 and extremes of cycle length (either short or long cycles). Women who breastfeed for long durations, women who have more children, and women who exercise regularly may see a reduction in their risk of endometriosis.

Pathophysiology
There are many theories regarding the origin of endometriosis. Perhaps the most popular hypothesis proposes that retrograde menstruation allows for endometrial tissue to be passed back through the fallopian tubes and implant into the pelvis. Another theory suggests that coelemic metaplasia occurs. In this theory, it is thought that the differentiation of mesothelial cells into endometrial cells results in endometriosis lesions. It is also thought that hematogenous or lymphatic spread is a plausible explaination for endometriosis. Endometrial cells may be deposited from the vascular or lymphatic vessels onto tissues outside the uterus. One final theory for the etiology of endometriosis involves bone marrow. Cells originating from the bone marrow may differentiate into endometrial tissue outside the uterus.

No matter how endometriosis originates, the immune system plays a pivotal role in the disease process. Endometriosis is associated with an overproduction of estrogen, prostaglandins, and cytokines. Estrogen is overproduced by an increase in aromatase activity. Cyclooxygenase-2 (COX-2) activity is also increased, which stimulates prostaglandin production. Endometriosis is also associated with progesterone resistance, and that magnifies the effect of estrogen in an already estrogen-rich environment. This inflammatory cascade leads to an increase in cytokines and macrophages. The cytokines increase the presence of macrophages and lymphocytes in the peritoneum.

The chronic inflammation identified in endometriosis may cause pain by stimulating the nerve endings or affect the neural innervations of the uterus. Fallopian tube function and sperm function may be adversely affected by the inflammatory cytokines. Also, the fallopian tubes may be completely blocked in some cases of endometriosis.

Clinical Manifestations
Many clinical symptoms have been associated with endometriosis. Cyclical pain is often described with endometriosis. Some of the more commonly recognized symptoms include dysmenorrhea, chronic pelvic pain, dyspareunia, and infertility. Dysmenorrhea can be described as primary or secondary. The dysmenorrhea with endometriosis is classically described as secondary dysmenorrhea because it is associated with a pathologic diagnosis. Primary dysmenorrhea is when there is painful menstruation in the absence of pelvic pathology. Examples of chronic pelvic pain with endometriosis may include other visceral symptoms such as dyschezia or dysuria. Hematuria, diarrhea, constipation, and chronic back pain may all be symptoms associated with endometriosis.

Interestingly, the extent of disease may not necessarily correlate with the severity of symptoms. Some women with a small foci of endometriosis may have excruciating symptoms, whereas others with extensive endometriosis may only experience mild symptoms.

Exam findings consistent with a diagnosis of endometriosis may include uterosacral ligament nodulartiy/tenderness and presence of an adnexal mass. Tenderness in the cul-de-sac with a fixed and immobile uterus may also indicate presence of endometriosis. Cyclical hemoptysis has been reported with endometriosis. Endometriotic implants have also been located in scars, so the presence of cyclical pain in an abdominal incision may lead to suspicion of endometriosis.

Diagnosis/Differential Diagnosis
The diagnosis of endometriosis is made surgically. The gold standard to make a diagnosis of endometriosis is to have a pathologic specimen from a tissue biopsy of a suspected lesion. Histology will reveal endometrial glands and stroma and inflammation. If a biopsy is not performed, surgical findings consistent with an endometriosis diagnosis include lesions that look like black powder burns and nonclassical red or white lesions. Endometriomas have also been described as a classic surgical finding of endometriosis. Endometriomas are an ovarian structure filled with endometriosis and are colloquially described as chocolate cysts because when they rupture, it appears as though chocolate syrup flows out of the cyst. Endometriomas appear on sonographic imaging as cysts with homogenous internal echoes. Although rare, endometriosis can sometimes be found in the bladder. If bladder involvement is suspected, such as the case of cyclical hematuria, a cystoscopy may be of benefit for diagnosis. Although surgery remains the mainstay of diagnosis for endometriosis, some studies suggest there is a low correlation between the severity of symptoms, the amount of endometriosis visualized on surgical inspection, and diagnostic histologic findings.

TABLE 1 — Differential Diagnosis for Chronic Pelvic Pain Based on Organ Systems

GYNECOLOGIC	GASTROINTESTINAL	URINARY	MUSCULOSKELETAL
Endometriosis	Irritable bowel syndrome	Urinary tract infection	Fibromyalgia
Adenomyosis	Diverticuli	Interstitial Cystitis	Ankylosing spondylitis
Cervicitis	Crohn's	Malignancy	Arthritis
Leiomyoma	Ulcerative Colitis	Renal lithiasis	Muscle strains
Ovarian cysts	Gastroenteritis		
Pelvic adhesive disease	Hemorrhoids		
Hydrosalpinx/tubal disease			
Pelvic congestion syndrome			

Pelvic imaging may be helpful in the evaluation of endometriosis, especially in the presence of an adnexal mass. In patients with pelvic pain or disorders of menstruation, a sonogram is usually the preferred imaging modality for the pelvis. Computed tomography (CT) may help delineate the size and characteristic of an adnexal mass and is likely most useful to rule out other pathology or surrounding organ involvement. The usefulness of magnetic resonance imaging (MRI) is limited in the evaluation of endometriosis and should be reserved for extreme cases where specific organ involvement such as the bladder or bowel is suspected. MRI may also be useful in evaluating specific musculoskeletal conditions.

There is no good serum marker to make the diagnosis of endometriosis. CA-125 levels may be elevated in endometriosis, but there are many other inflammatory conditions that cause an elevation in CA-125 levels.

When initially evaluating for endometriosis, one should consider a thorough differential diagnosis for causes of chronic pelvic pain. Table 1 lists the differential diagnosis for chronic pelvic pain. A basic approach to the patient with chronic pelvic pain should include a detailed history and physical, urinalysis, gonorrhea/chlamydia cultures, consideration of pelvic sonogram, and serum or urine beta human chorionic gonadotropin (Bhcg). If after careful evaluation, endometriosis is at the top of the differential diagnosis for the patient's pelvic pain, then discussion with the patient regarding empiric treatment or diagnostic workup should occur.

Medical Therapy

The goal of medical intervention for endometriosis is the treatment of pain. A reasonable approach to treating the patient with suspected endometriosis is to give a trial of empiric medical therapy. Although endometriosis is a surgical diagnosis, some patients with suspected endometriosis may wish to avoid surgery. Medical therapy is usually preferred for those patients who would like to preserve fertility and who are interested in delaying childbearing while managing their symptoms.

The combined oral contraceptive pill (OCP) is a usual first-line therapy for the treatment of suspected or diagnosed endometriosis. A 3- to 6-month trial with empiric treatment with OCPs is a reasonable time frame to assess effectiveness of medical treatment. OCPs should be avoided in patients that have contraindications to OCPs including pregnancy, history of thrombosis, liver disease, migraine with aura, uncontrolled hypertension, and those patients that smoke and are over the age of 35 years.

Other medications used to treat endometriosis include danazol (Danocrine), nonsteroidal anti-inflammatory drugs (NSAIDs), progestins, and gonadotropin releasing hormone (GnRH) agonists and antagonists. NSAIDs may improve the pain and dysmenorrhea associated with endometriosis. Danazol is an effective treatment for endometriosis. The side effect profile for danazol limits its use. Danazol has been associated with masculinizing symptoms, which can include acne and hair growth. Danazol should be avoided in pregnancy because the masculinizing effects could be detrimental to a female infant.

Physicians commonly prescribe progestins in three different ways to treat endometriosis: injectable, oral, or intrauterine. Injectable medroxyprogesterone (Depo-SubQ Provera 104) is approved by the Food and Drug Administration (FDA) for the treatment of endometriosis. Depo-Provera's side effects may include weight gain, bleeding, amenorrhea, and slow return to fertility. Patients using Depo-Provera may initially experience irregular bleeding but often develop amenorrhea after the second dose is administered. Return to fertility after Depo-Provera is discontinued can also pose a problem. Oral agents such as norethindrone acetate (Aygestin) have also been approved by the FDA for the treatment of endometriosis. The levonorgestrel-containing intrauterine device (IUD) (Mirena)[1] is approved only for contraception and the treatment of menorrhagia, but it may still be an effective treatment for endometriosis.

The GnRH agonists are among the most effective medications available to treat endometriosis. The side effects of GnRH agonists include menopausal-like symptoms such as vaginal dryness, hot flashes, and osteopenia. The addition of add-back therapy may help ameliorate some of the GnRH agonist symptoms. Typically, add-back therapy involves the use of progestins concurrently with a GnRH agonist. Practice patterns vary; some providers may start add-back therapy immediately when a patient is started on a GnRH agonist. It is recommended that add-back therapy be initiated after 6 months of GnRH agonist use if it was not started previously. In addition to progestins, the combination of progestins and estrogen have been used for add-back therapy. The maximum duration of GnRH agonist treatment is typically 12 months. Another class of medication to treat endometriosis is the GnRH antagonist, currently available as elagolix (Orilissa). Advantages to this medication are that it is in an oral form and available in multiple doses. Studies showed estradiol suppression in a dose dependent manner. Common side effects include hot flashes, headaches, and nausea. Although add-back therapy is widely used in GnRH agonists, it has not been studied with the GnRH antagonists. When using this medication, consideration of a nonhormonal contraception would be recommended.

Surgical Therapy

The goal of surgery for endometriosis is to relieve pain and/or infertility. One of the first questions the provider must answer is when to perform surgery. Surgery may be indicated if medical treatment has failed. Other times, the severity of symptoms or presence of large endometriomas may direct a provider to consider surgery sooner.

Laparoscopy is a common surgical approach for patients with confirmed or suspected endometriosis. At the time of laparoscopy,

[1]Not FDA approved for this indication.

the surgeon can assess the uterus, ovaries, and surrounding viscera for pathology. When endometriosis is encountered on laparoscopy, common approaches are to excise or ablate the lesions. Excision of endometriosis allows for a pathologic diagnosis. If the provider elects to ablate the lesions, this can be performed through electrocautery or laser. In addition to diagnosing and treating endometriosis, further evaluation of patients with infertility can be done at the time of laparoscopy. Tubal function can be assessed through a chromotubation where dye is passed through the fallopian tubes to prove the tubes are patent. Although laparotomy allows for thorough evaluation of the pelvis, it is usually reserved for cases of confirmed endometriosis where the extent of adhesions and distorted anatomy makes laparoscopy unsafe.

Endometriomas present an array of challenges when noted at the time of surgery. The decision to drain the cyst versus perform a cystectomy during surgery must be made by the surgeon. A general approach is to use a "3-centimeters (cm) rule" to help guide management decisions. Patients with an endometrioma greater than 3 cm may benefit from cystectomy, whereas endometriomas less than 3 cm may be managed by drainage and ablation. Although removing the endometrioma through cystectomy may confer a decreased risk or recurrence, the risk of damaging healthy ovarian tissue is ever present. Other confounders to consider are future fertility plans of the patient, severity of symptoms, and previous treatments for endometriosis.

In a patient who has completed childbearing or has no desire for future fertility, hysterectomy with a bilateral salpingo-oophorectomy (BSO) may be considered for treatment of endometriosis. Studies suggest that hysterectomy alone is less effective at curing pain than hysterectomy with a BSO. Although hysterectomy with BSO offers definitive treatment for endometriosis, surgery does not guarantee resolution of pain. Many routes may be considered for surgery, including laparoscopic, robotic-assisted laparoscopic, or laparotomy with a total abdominal hysterectomy/BSO. Although vaginal hysterectomy is a common and preferred route of surgery, the distorted anatomy and presence of adhesions often associated with endometriosis tends to discourage many surgeons from performing vaginal hysterectomies for endometriosis.

Monitoring

Patients diagnosed with endometriosis may require frequent monitoring of symptoms. Routine visits with a physician may help determine the effectiveness of current treatment regimens. Physicians should consider what the patient's goals of treatment are: Does the patient want resolution of pain or infertility or both? Individualized plans may help each patient achieve their goals of treatment. As with any diseases involving chronic pain, care should be taken to regularly assess patients with endometriosis for depression.

References

ACOG Practice Bulletin Number 114. Management of Endometriosis. 2010.
Bulun SE: Endometriosis, *N Engl J Med* 360:268–279, 2009.
Cramer DW, Missmer SA: The epidemiology of endometriosis, *Ann N Y Acad Sci* 955:11–22, 2002.
Davis L, Kennedy SS, Moore J, Prentice A: Oral contraceptives for pain associated with endometriosis, *Cochrane Database Syst Rev* 2007;(3):Cd001019.
Dlugi AM, Miller JD, Knittle J: Lupron depot (leuprolide acetate for depot suspension) in the treatemnt of endometriosis: a randomized, placebo-controlled, double-blind study, *Fert Steril* 54:419–427, 1990.
Guidance LC, Kao LC: Endometriosis, *Lancet* 364:1789–1799, 2004.
Olive DL, Pritts EA: The treatment of endometriosis: a review of the evidence, *Ann N Y Acad Sci* 955:360–372, 2002.
Pittaway DE, Fayez JA: The use of CA-125 in the diagnosis and management of endometriosis, *Fertil Steril* 46:790–795, 1986.
Rawson JM: Prevalence of endometriosis in asymptomatic women, *J Reprod Med* 36:513–515, 1991.
Ripps BA, Martin DC: Endometriosis and chronic pelvic pain, *Gynecol Clin North Am* 20:709–717, 1993.
Surrey E, Taylor HS, et al: Long-term outcomes of elagolix in women with endometriosis, *Obstetrics and Gynecology* 132:147–160, 2018.
Sutton CJ, Ewen SP, Whitelaw N, Haines P: Prospective, randomized, double blind, controlled trial of laser laparoscopy in the treatment of pelvic pain associated with minimal, mild, and moderate endometriosis, 62:696–700, 1994.
Walter AJ, Hentz JG, Magtibay PM, Cornella JL, Magrina JF: Endometriosis: correlation between histologic and visual findings at laparoscopy, *Am J Obstet Gynecol* 184:1407–1411, 2001.

INFERTILITY

Method of
Jessica Kanter, MD; and Michael P. Diamond, MD

CURRENT DIAGNOSIS

- Infertility is defined as the inability to conceive with regular intercourse after 12 months in couples in which the female partner is younger than 35 or after 6 months in couples in which the female partner is over 35.
- The incidence of infertility is increasing.

CURRENT THERAPY

- Assisted reproductive technologies are being used with increasing frequency and with increasing success rates.

Epidemiology

Infertility is defined as the failure to conceive after 12 months of regular, unprotected intercourse. In couples where the female partner's age exceeds 35 years, evaluation may begin after just 6 months of infertility owing to the time sensitive nature of the problem. In some circumstances, diagnostic evaluation and therapeutic intervention is warranted at an earlier time. Infertility affects approximately 15% of couples. Many of these patients present to their primary care physician. Timely evaluation and potential referral to an infertility subspecialist is prudent.

Risk Factors

There are numerous risk factors that contribute to infertility. The most common is age. However, it is necessary to evaluate other potential contributing factors to infertility as these may lead to narrowing of the differential diagnosis and a more targeted subsequent treatment plan. For example, a history of sexually transmitted infections (STIs), especially chlamydia, and episodes of pelvic inflammatory disease have been associated with tubal factor infertility in women. Metabolic disorders such as obesity and polycystic ovarian syndrome, which may lead to anovulation are an increasingly prevalent concern and a major risk factor for infertility. Finally, certain genetic diseases such as Fragile X, Turner syndrome, cystic fibrosis, and Klinefelter disease may also lead to inability or difficulty in conceiving.

Pathophysiology

The pathophysiology of infertility should be grouped first by male and female factors and then by component of their respective reproductive tracts. One must not discount the fact that multiple factors may coexist. Unexplained infertility has been reported to be accountable for 8% to 28% of infertility in couples; however, in intensively evaluated couples the rate is likely to be 25%.

Prevention

Some etiologies of infertility may be preventable. Many cases of tubal factor infertility may be prevented by protecting against transmission of STIs. Barrier contraception is essential to prevent STIs, particularly in high-risk individuals with an early age of coitarche and/or those with multiple sexual partners. Even with highly efficacious forms of contraception such as intrauterine devices, long-acting injectable progestins, and progestin-containing subdermal implants, providers must counsel their patients that barrier contraception is still of the utmost importance in preventing STI transmission.

There are also various medical therapies, particularly those related to cancer treatment, that may be detrimental to fertility. In these cases, oncofertility consultation prior to treatment will optimize fertility preservation. For men, sperm cryopreservation is a relatively easy, noninvasive method. For women, oocyte or embryo preservation, experimental approaches to medically induced ovarian suppression, and ovarian transposition are all tools to have in the arsenal for women undergoing gonadotoxic chemotherapy or radiation therapy.

Finally, fertility should also be considered when managing tubal ectopic pregnancy in women. Medical therapy, when not contraindicated, is an excellent option in the compliant patient with an ectopic pregnancy. When surgery is necessary, salpingostomy may be considered when possible in lieu of salpingectomy in an attempt to preserve tubal function.

Clinical Manifestations

Infertile patients generally present with failure to conceive after a variable time of home intercourse. The definition of infertility is subdivided into primary and secondary infertility. Primary infertility means the patient has not borne children in the past. Secondary infertility means the patient has successfully procreated in the past.

Diagnosis

The diagnosis of infertility begins with a thorough history and physical examination. It is important to remember that a history must be obtained from both partners during this evaluation. The male partner assessment begins with a semen analysis. Textbooks often suggest two semen analyses, preferably separated in time by at least 1 month.

Female partner assessment can include determination of ovarian reserve by hormonal evaluation of antimüllerian hormone (AMH) or cycle day 3 follicle-stimulating hormone (FSH). Frequently, prolactin and thyroid-stimulating hormone (TSH) are also obtained, as is a measure of ovulation such as a mid-luteal progesterone level. Other labs may be ordered if clinically indicated, such as androgens in women with hirsutism. Tubal patency is assessed by sonohysterograms or hysterosalpingogram. These imaging tests also allow assessment of the uterine cavity for uterine contour and any abnormalities including fibroids or polyps. Sonography may also be useful in identifying müllerian anomalies or anomalies of the basic structure of the uterus; the gold standard for use of imaging modalities for identifying these anomalies is magnetic resonance imaging. In cases where other pelvic pathology such as endometriosis and adhesions are suspected, diagnostic laparoscopy may be considered. Chromotubation during laparoscopy may be performed. Finally, for both partners, karyotype analysis may be considered.

Differential Diagnosis

When determining a differential diagnosis, both male and female factors must be considered.

Male Factors

The most common etiologies of male-factor infertility are oligospermia and azoospermia. The etiologies leading to these diagnoses are broad and varied, and include genetic conditions such as cystic fibrosis (leading to congenital absence of the vas deferens).

Female Factors

Female factors for infertility are numerous and most easily subdivided by system.

Ovulatory Dysfunction

Inability to produce a viable oocyte each month can be related to several factors. First, anovulation may occur, meaning oocytes are present in the ovaries but none are released on a regular basis. This can be related to hormonal ovarian suppression (e.g., hyperprolactinemia) and metabolic disturbances (e.g., polycystic ovarian syndrome). Alternatively, an oocyte may not be produced

secondary to paucity of oocytes owing to age, genetic factors, or prior insults to the ovaries such as radiation therapy. In addition to the aforementioned AMH and day 3 FSH and serum estradiol to assess ovarian function, ultrasound may be employed to evaluate antral follicle count, another marker of ovarian reserve.

Tubal Factor

The fallopian tubes are responsible for transporting the oocyte from the ovaries to the uterine cavity. For this to occur, at least one fallopian tube must be patent. Perhaps the most common etiology of tubal factor infertility is a history of pelvic inflammatory disease, with one of the most common inciting agents being *Chlamydia trachomatous. C. trachomatis* is particularly problematic in women as the initial infection may be asymptomatic. Other tubal infertility may arise from prior tubal ligation, other tubal surgery, history of ectopic pregnancy with salpingectomy or salpingostomy, or scarring of the tubal lumen.

Uterine Factor

Any irregularities within the uterine cavity may also lead to infertility, generally secondary to poor implantation of the fertilized embryo. Some such etiologies may be present from birth, namely müllerian anomalies and uterine septae. The abnormally shaped uterine cavity in these anomalies reduces the opportunity for normal implantation and embryo growth.

During the course of a woman's life, she may develop benign intrauterine growths including polyps and leiomyomas that can reduce the opportunity for normal embryo implantation. Finally, prior uterine surgery may damage the endometrium and myometrium, as in Asherman syndrome, or cause uterine cavity scarring, called synechiae.

Combined

One must not forget that multiple etiologies in a wide variety of combinations may be at play in female-factor infertility.

Unexplained

Perhaps the most frustrating of all diagnoses is unexplained infertility. In couples who have had a negative fertility workup, a specific etiology of infertility is never revealed. There is new, burgeoning research in the area of sperm microRNA that may identify male-factor infertility in men with otherwise normal semen analyses. Although not currently in wide use, such studies may be of great utility in the future.

Prior Diagnosis

As the field of infertility is becoming understood to an increasingly greater degree, there are prior diagnoses that have fallen out of favor. One such diagnosis is cervical factor insufficiency. It was previously evaluated by the postcoital test, in which a sample of cervical mucous would be taken after intercourse and was evaluated for presence of motile sperm. This test has fallen out of favor owing to subjectivity, lack of reproducibility, and poor correlation with future fertility.

Also out of favor is the prior diagnosis of luteal phase deficiency (LPD), previously defined as inadequate endogenous progesterone production during the luteal phase of the menstrual cycle. No clinical tests have proven reliable for LPD, nor have any treatments demonstrated any significant improvement in fertility.

Treatment

The mainstay of therapy is first treating underlying disorders such as obesity, thyroid disease, hyperprolactinemia, and so forth. Lifestyle modifications should be recommended to all women, including folate supplementation[1] (at least 400 μg daily), caffeine reduction, and weight loss for those who are overweight or obese. Other known causes of infertility that require surgical management may include intrauterine pathology (e.g., polyps, fibroid

---

[1]Not FDA approach for this indication.

tumors) or repair of a hydrosalpinx distally blocked fallopian tube filled with serous fluid.

With a normal male partner semen analysis, the first step in intervention is generally an oral agent to induce ovulation combined with intrauterine insemination. Options for induction include clomiphene citrate (Clomid) and off-label use of letrozole (Femara), an aromatase inhibitor. If this fails, therapy can proceed to treatment with injectable gonadotropins (i.e., FSH and luteinizing hormone) to stimulate development of ovarian follicles and ovulation with intrauterine insemination or in vitro fertilization. Various additional procedures may include assisted hatching of the embryo with the hope to increase implantation rates, intracytoplasmic sperm injection to increase fertilization rates of the oocytes, particularly in the setting of male factor infertility, and preimplantation genetic screening to evaluate for embryo genetic anomalies, particularly in women of advanced maternal age.

Monitoring
To reduce risks associated with ovulation induction and ovarian stimulation, monitoring of serum estradiol and follicular development is performed. Monitoring provides the ability to minimize the occurrence of multiple gestation and complications associated with ovarian hyperstimulation syndrome.

References
Gelbaya TA, Potdar N, Jeve YB, Nardo LG: Definition and epidemiology of unexplained infertility, *Obstet Gynecol Surv* 69(2):109–115, 2014.

Jodar M, Sendler E, Moskovtsev SI, et al: Absence of sperm RNA elements correlates with idiopathic male infertility, *Sci Transl Med* 7(295):295–296, 2015. Available at: https://doi.org/10.1126/scitranslmed.aab1287.

Practice Committee of American Society for Reproductive Medicine: Current clinical irrelevance of luteal phase deficiency: A committee opinion, *Fertil Steril* 103(4):e27–e32, 2015.

Practice Committee of American Society for Reproductive Medicine: Diagnostic evaluation of the infertile female: A committee opinion, *Fertil Steril* 98(2):302–307, 2012.

Sharlip ID, Jarow JP, Belker AM, et al: Best practice policies for male infertility, *Fertil Steril* 77(5):873–882, 2002.

MENOPAUSE

Method of
Andrew M. Kaunitz, MD; and JoAnn E. Manson, MD, DrPH

CURRENT DIAGNOSIS

- In women who meet clinical criteria for menopause who present for management of vasomotor symptoms (VMS), checking follicle-stimulating hormone (FSH) and estradiol levels is not necessary. However, if no recent level is available, checking a thyroid-stimulating hormone (TSH) level to rule out thyroid disease is appropriate.
- Occasionally, nonmenopausal conditions can masquerade as menopausal VMS.
- Although genitourinary syndrome of menopause (GSM) can be presumptively diagnosed based on a characteristic history, a pelvic examination can help exclude other vulvovaginal conditions that can present with similar symptoms.
- Although laboratory assessment is not necessary to establish that GSM is present, vaginal pH is typically higher than 5.0.

CURRENT THERAPY

- Estrogen represents the most effective therapy for VMS and related symptoms.
- Oral and transdermal estrogen have similar efficacy in treating menopausal VMS.

- Estrogen plus progestin therapy (EPT) is appropriate when treating menopausal symptoms in women with an intact uterus.
- For healthy symptomatic women younger than age 60 or within 10 years of menopause onset, the benefits of systemic hormone therapy (HT) outweigh risks.
- Conjugated estrogen (CE) 0.45 mg combined with the selective estrogen receptor modulator bazedoxifene 20 mg (Duavee) (without concomitant use of a progestational agent) is approved to treat VMS and prevent osteoporosis in women with an intact uterus.
- Low-dose paroxetine mesylate (Brisdelle) 7.5 mg is the only nonhormonal formulation approved to treat VMS. Off-label use of venlafaxine (Effexor) is also effective in treating VMS. These agents are less effective, however, than standard-dose hormone therapy.
- Arbitrary discontinuation of systemic HT when women turn 65 is not evidence based. Although controversial, extended use of systemic HT may be appropriate in well-counseled women for treatment of persistent VMS, prevention of bone loss, and prevention/treatment of atrophic genital changes. Women considering extended use of systemic HT should be aware that with a longer duration of EPT, the risk of breast cancer increases. If genitourinary syndrome of menopause (GSM)/atrophic changes represent the only indication for HT, local low-dose vaginal estrogen is appropriate, and highly effective.

Epidemiology
Menopause, the permanent cessation of menstruation caused by loss of ovarian function, occurs at a mean age of 51 to 52 years. With increases in life expectancy, it is projected that by 2020, more than 50 million US women will be older than 51 years.

Risk Factors
Spontaneous menopause represents a natural event. Spontaneous menopause occurs at a younger age in women who smoke or undergo hysterectomy with ovarian conservation. Chemotherapy, radiation therapy, or bilateral oophorectomy can induce menopause.

Clinical Manifestations and Pathophysiology
Often described by women as hot flashes or night sweats, VMS represent the most bothersome symptoms of menopause and the most common reason women present for care at the time of the menopausal transition. VMS often include a sudden sensation of heat in the face, neck, and chest, and persist for several minutes or less. VMS may cause flushing, chills, anxiety, and sleep disruption. VMS are caused by estrogen withdrawal and are associated with pulsatile luteinizing hormone secretion and decreased endorphin concentration in the hypothalamus, as well as increased release of norepinephrine and serotonin. VMS occur in almost three quarters of women during the late perimenopausal transition, and are more prevalent among the groups listed in Box 1. The median duration of moderate to severe VMS is approximately 10 years.

GSM, also known as vulvovaginal or genital atrophy, signifies the progressive changes in the vulva, vagina, and urethra resulting from estrogen deficiency. GSM, which characteristically causes vaginal dryness and pain with sex, represents a common condition that adversely impacts health, sexuality, and quality of life in menopausal women.

Diagnosis
Although FSH levels increase and estradiol levels decline in menopausal women, such testing is not necessary when late perimenopausal or postmenopausal women report characteristic VMS as described previously. Because thyroid disease is common in women and can cause symptoms that mimic VMS, checking a TSH level is appropriate in women seeking treatment for VMS.

Although GSM can be presumptively diagnosed based on a characteristic history, a pelvic examination can help exclude other vulvovaginal conditions that can present with similar symptoms (see next section). Physical examination findings characteristic of GSM are listed in Box 2. Although laboratory assessment is not necessary to establish that GSM is present, vaginal pH is typically higher than 5.0.

Differential Diagnosis

Nonmenopausal conditions that can masquerade as menopausal VMS include anxiety disorders, thyroid disease, autoimmune conditions, carcinoid syndromes, diabetic autonomic dysfunction/hypoglycemia, insulinoma/pancreatic tumors, epilepsy, infections, including tuberculosis, mast cell disorders, and new-onset hypertension, as well as use of certain selective serotonergic reuptake inhibitors or serotonin-norepinephrine reuptake inhibitors.

Lichen sclerosus, chronic candidiasis, contact dermatitis, and lichen planus represent vulvar conditions that might be confused with GSM.

Therapy

Estrogen represents the most effective therapy for VMS and related symptoms. Higher doses are more effective; oral and transdermal formulations have comparable efficacy. Many estrogen formulations/doses are also approved for prevention of osteoporosis. Because estrogen-only therapy (ET) in women with an intact uterus increases the risk of endometrial neoplasia, estrogen plus progestin therapy (EPT) is appropriate when treating VMS in women with a uterus. In the United States, the most commonly used oral estrogens for systemic treatment of VMS are estradiol (E2, Estrace) and conjugated equine estrogens (CEE, Premarin). Standard doses of these estrogens are 1.0 mg and 0.625 mg, respectively; lower and higher doses are available. Weekly and twice-weekly skin patches and other transdermal E2 formulations are available; estradiol patches releasing 0.05 mg and 0.0375 mg daily are considered standard dose; and lower- and higher-dose patches are available. A 3-month vaginal systemic E2 ring (Femring) for treatment of VMS is also available; the ring releasing 0.05 mg E2 daily is considered the standard dose.

In the United States, the progestational agents most commonly prescribed to accompany systemic ET in women with an intact uterus are medroxyprogesterone acetate (MPA [Provera], available in 2.5-mg, 5-mg, and 10-mg doses) and micronized progesterone (Prometrium) 100-mg and 200-mg capsules. Micronized progesterone is formulated with peanut oil. With standard-dose estrogen, an appropriate daily dose of MPA or micronized progesterone used continuously is 2.5 mg and 100 mg, respectively.

Because micronized progesterone has a hypnotic effect, it should be taken at night. A variety of oral estrogen–progestin formulations, all of which have demonstrated endometrial safety, are available in different doses and combine CEE with MPA (Prempro); E2 or ethinyl E2 with norethindrone acetate (Activella, Femhrt); or E2 with drospirenone (Angeliq) or norgestimate (Prefest). Transdermal estrogen–progestin combination formulations combine E2 with norethindrone acetate (CombiPatch) or levonorgestrel (Climara Pro). The North American Menopause Society regularly updates and posts tables listing all formulations approved in the United States or Canada for treating menopausal symptoms (see references) (http://www.menopaus e.org/docs/default-source/professional/nams-ht-tables.pdf?sfvrs n=18.pdf). Although off-label use of testosterone can increase sexual desire in menopausal women, efficacy is achieved only with supraphysiologic doses, which may cause hyperandrogenic adverse effects.

CE 0.45 mg combined with the selective estrogen receptor modulator bazedoxifene 20 mg (Duavee) (without the concomitant use of a progestational agent) is approved to treat VMS and prevent osteoporosis in women with an intact uterus and does not increase the incidence of uterine bleeding or endometrial hyperplasia. This novel combination formulation may be useful for women with an intact uterus who choose not to use progestin, including those intolerant of progestin side effects.

Among US women using HT, approximately one-third are using compounded HT; most users are not aware these formulations are not evaluated or approved by the FDA. FDA-approved HT is preferable to compounded HT unless a specific FDA-approved formulation is not available.

Nonhormonal therapy with paroxetine (Paxil)[1], escitalopram (Lexapro)[1], citalopram (Celexa)[1], venlafaxine (Effexor)[1], desvenlafaxine (Pristiq)[1], gabapentin (Neurontin)[1], and pregabalin (Lyrica)[1] are more effective than placebo but less effective than HT in treating VMS. Low-dose paroxetine mesylate (Brisdelle) 7.5 mg is the only nonhormonal formulation approved to treat VMS. Lowering the ambient temperature, use of fans, wearing layered clothing, and avoiding tobacco, alcohol, and caffeine represent common sense measures for women bothered by VMS. In a clinical trial, clinical hypnosis was found more effective than placebo in addressing VMS. Although over-the-counter herbal formulations including soy and black cohosh have been widely used to treat VMS, these have not been found to be more effective than placebo.

When clinicians identify GSM, they should advise women that (unlike VMS) without proactive management, GSM progresses. If severe symptoms are not present, recommending use of over-the-counter lubricants (or substances such as coconut or olive oil) for sexual activity, as well as regular use of vaginal moisturizers, is helpful. Such women should also be advised that regular sexual activity may help improve symptoms and prevent progression. If other indications for systemic HT such as treatment of VMS or prevention of osteoporosis are present, systemic HT is effective in treating GSM. However, if GSM represents the only indication for HT, local low-dose vaginal estrogen is appropriate and highly effective treatment. Vaginal estrogen also reduces the risk of recurrent urinary tract infections and overactive bladder symptoms in menopausal women. In the United States, two low-dose creams, estradiol (Estrace) and CEE (Premarin), are available. Although package labeling provides instructions for patients regarding dose and schedule, in practice, most women use a fraction of an applicator vaginally (and often also benefit from digital application to vestibular tissues) one to three times weekly. Some women find use of vaginal estrogen creams to be messy. Vaginal tablets (Vagifem) equivalent to 10 mcg E2 are inserted vaginally with an applicator nightly for 2 weeks, then twice weekly for maintenance. Vaginal 4 mcg or 10 mcg E2 inserts (Imvexxy) are placed digitally nightly for 2 weeks, then twice weekly for maintenance. The

---

[1] Not FDA approved for this indication.

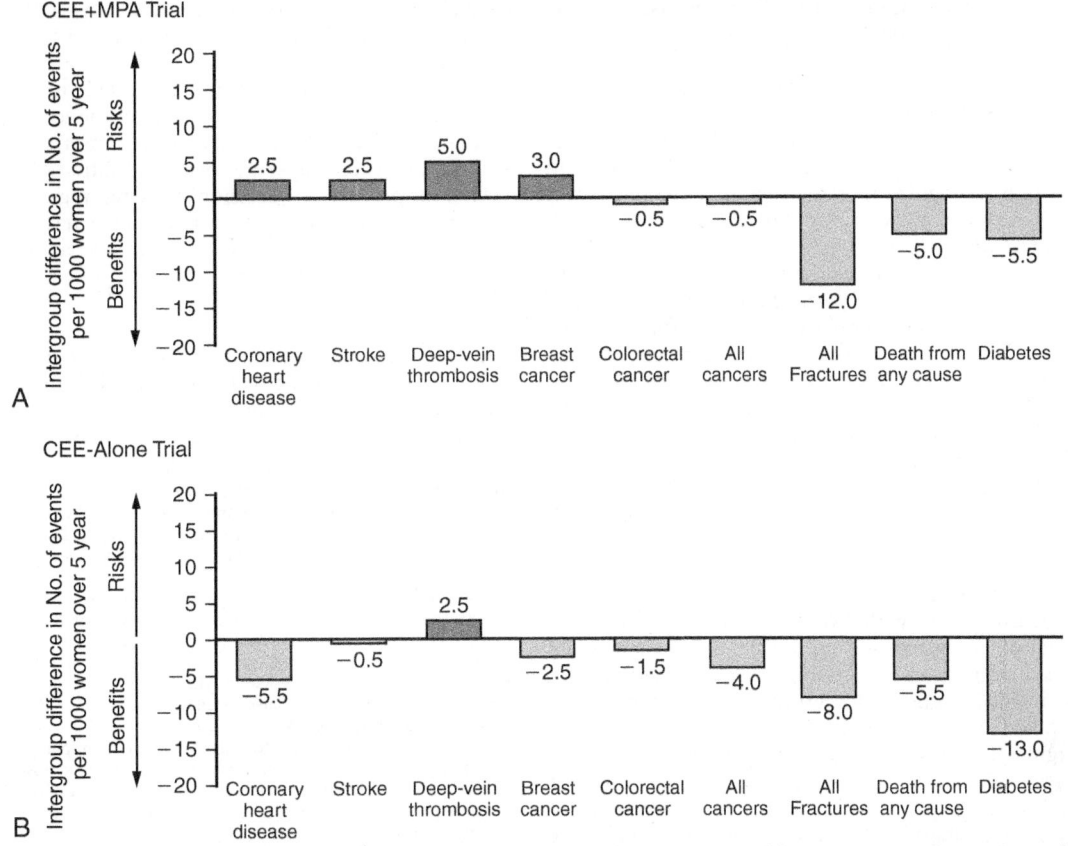

Figure 1 Benefits and risks of the two hormone therapy formulations evaluated in the Women's Health Initiative. Results are shown for the two formulations, conjugated equine estrogens (CEEs) alone (B) or in combination with medroxyprogesterone acetate (A; MPA), for women 50 to 59 years of age. Risks and benefits are expressed as the difference in number of events (number in the hormone therapy group minus the number in the placebo group) per 1000 women over 5 years. (Data are from Manson JE, Chlebowski RT, Stefanick ML, et al. Menopausal hormone therapy and health outcomes during the intervention and extended poststopping phases of the Women's Health Initiative randomized trials. *JAMA* 2013;310:1353.)

3-month low-dose E2 vaginal ring (Estring) releases 7.5 mcg E2 daily. A systemic selective estrogen receptor modulator, ospemifene (Osphena), improves symptoms of GSM; some users report VMS. In late 2016, the FDA approved vaginal dehydroepiandrosterone (DHEA, prasterone) (Intrarosa) for treatment of GSM.

Monitoring

For most women using systemic HT, monitoring serum estrogen levels is not indicated. However, when women continue to report bothersome symptoms despite escalating HT doses, monitoring can be useful. In contrast to fluctuating serum estrogen levels in women using oral estrogen, transdermal ET results in relatively steady-state levels; serum E2 levels of 40 to 100 pg/mL represent a reasonable target range.

Side Effects of Systemic Hormone Therapy

Breast tenderness, bloating, and uterine bleeding represent common side effects of ET. Although lowering the ET dose may reduce side effects, this may cause VMS to increase. Progestins cause dysphoria in some women. Prescribing a different progestin, prescribing progestins sequentially, off-label use of a progestin intrauterine device (Skyla, Kyleena, Mirena, Liletta), or use of the CEE/bazedoxifene combination formulation (Duavee) or antidepressant therapy may be useful in this setting.

Safety of Hormone Therapy

Findings from the Women's Health Initiative (WHI) study of oral CEE and MPA, CEE alone, and other recent randomized clinical trials have helped to clarify the benefits and risks of combination estrogen–progestin and estrogen-alone therapy. A 2013 WHI report detailed findings from the two HT trials with a median 13 years of cumulative follow-up. Since initial findings of the WHI were first published in 2002, use of systemic HT has dramatically

decreased, owing to misinterpretation of WHI findings, which has generated anxiety and confusion among clinicians and women. Importantly, absolute risks of adverse events related to hormone therapy were much lower for younger women (ages 50 to 59) than for older women (Figure 1). Overall, for healthy women with bothersome VMS younger than age 60 and/or within 10 years of menopause onset, the benefits of HT for women outweigh risks.

With respect to coronary heart disease (CHD), HT's impact varies by age of users. Among women who initiate HT before age 60 and/or within 10 years of menopause, HT does not increase (and may reduce) risk. In contrast, among women older than age 60 and/or more than 10 years following menopause onset, HT appears to increase CHD risk.

With respect to stroke, the WHI found that CEE alone or with MPA increased risk; however, for women younger than age 60, the absolute increase in risk was small (see Figure 1).

With respect to venous thromboembolism (VTE), including pulmonary embolism, oral estrogen with or without progestin increases risk, particularly within 2 years of HT initiation. Absolute risks of VTE are higher for women initiating HT more than 10 years following menopause onset. Observational studies have consistently found that in contrast to oral HT, HT with transdermal (e.g., skin patch) estrogen elevates VTE risk less (if at all) compared with oral HT. Because oral estrogen and body mass index represent independent risk factors for VTE, transdermal estrogen may be preferable for women at elevated baseline VTE risk, including obese women. Personal and familial risk of cardiovascular disease, stroke, and VTE should be considered when initiating HT. Low-dose vaginal estrogen has not been found to elevate the risk of CHD, stroke, VTE, breast or endometrial cancer. With respect to breast cancer risk, WHI results diverged, with increased risk in the CEE-plus-MPA group and borderline reduced risk in the CEE-alone group. With 13 years of follow-up, a modest elevation of risk (hazard ratio 1.28) persisted in the CEE-plus-MPA group in all participant age strata. To put the elevated risk of breast cancer observed among women randomized to CEE plus MPA into perspective, the attributable risk with combination hormone therapy is less than one additional case of breast cancer diagnosed per 1000 users of combination hormone therapy annually. Another way to put this elevated hazard ratio into perspective is to recognize that the hazard ratio of 1.28 is slightly higher than that seen with one daily glass of wine, and less than that noted with two daily glasses. With long-term follow-up of WHI participants randomized to CEE alone, a significantly reduced risk of breast cancer (hazard ratio = 0.79) emerged over this time period. During cumulative 18-year follow-up of participants in the WHI hormone therapy trials, all-cause mortality rates did not differ appreciably between the intervention and control groups in the overall cohort. The hazard ratio (HR) for all-cause mortality among women assigned hormone therapy compared to those assigned placebo was 0.99 (95% CI, 0.94 to 1.03) in the overall pooled cohort; HRs were 1.02 (95% CI, 0.96 to 1.08) with CEE + MPA and 0.94 (95% CI, 0.88 to 1.01) with CEE alone.

Although trials up to 2 years' duration found that CEE plus bazedoxifene did not increase risk of breast cancer, long-term trials are needed. In women with *BRCA1* or 2 mutations, limited observational data suggest that use of HT does not increase breast cancer risk, suggesting that mutation carriers should not defer risk-reducing salpingo-oophorectomy owing to concerns that HT to treat VMS would be unsafe.

Low-dose vaginal ET may be used as long as needed, including indefinitely; routine use of concomitant progestin therapy for endometrial protection is not recommended. In the absence of reported spotting or bleeding, routine endometrial surveillance during use of vaginal ET is not recommended. However, clinicians should recognize that endometrial safety data for currently marketed formulations are based on 1-year trials, with no trials assessing the safety of longer-term administration available.

Current package labeling for low-dose vaginal estrogen, as for all systemic HT formulations, includes a boxed warning that refers to endometrial cancer, myocardial infarction, stroke, invasive breast cancer, pulmonary emboli, and dementia. This warning reflects safety concerns associated with findings from clinical trials of systemic HT, and does not reflect current evidence regarding local low-dose vaginal estrogen. At the time this chapter was being prepared, the FDA was considering a proposal to modify package labeling so that it better reflects the safety profile of vaginal estrogen.

A personal history of breast cancer is listed as a contraindication to use of all systemic and local low-dose vaginal HT (other contraindications to use of HT are listed on package labeling). However, one study found that use of the low-dose estrogen vaginal ring does not cause persistently elevated serum estradiol levels in breast cancer survivors using aromatase inhibitors; some oncologists prescribe this ring off-label to treat symptomatic atrophy in breast cancer survivors (including those using aromatase inhibitors), periodically checking serum estradiol levels. Nonetheless, many oncologists caution against use of vaginal HT in breast cancer survivors. In package labeling for vaginal DHEA (Intrarosa), a personal history of breast cancer is not listed as a contraindication.

Extended Use/Discontinuation of Systemic Hormone Therapy

Although controversial, extended use of systemic HT may be appropriate for treatment of persistent VMS, prevention of bone loss, and prevention/treatment of GSM in well-counseled women. Extended use of systemic HT should not be confused with initiation of systemic HT by women older than age 60 or more than 10 years following menopause onset, a practice that is known to be associated with elevated risk of CHD (see previous section on safety). Women considering extended use of systemic HT should be aware that with longer duration of EPT, the risk of breast cancer increases. Since older age is an independent risk factor for venous thromboembolism, use of transdermal estrogen

formulations should be considered in this setting. Arbitrary discontinuation of systemic HT when women turn 65 is not evidence based.

When women discontinue systemic HT, loss of bone mass and progression of GSM/atrophic genital changes occur. The likelihood of recurrent VMS in this setting appears similar with abrupt and gradual (dose-tapering) discontinuation of HT.

One approach to decision making regarding treatment of menopausal symptoms is available in a free mobile app called MenoPro (dual mode for clinicians and patients, downloadable on iPhone, iPad, and Android devices).

Financial Disclosure

Dr. Kaunitz serves on advisory boards for AMAG, Mithra, and Pfizer. His department receives research funding from Allergan, Bayer, Endoceutics, Medicines360, and Mithra. Dr. Manson does not report any potential conflicts of interest.

References

Bhupathiraju SN, Grodstein F, Stampfer MJ, et al: Vaginal estrogen and chronic disease in the Nurses' Health Study, *Menopause* 26:2019.
Kaunitz AM, Manson JE: Clinical expert series: management of menopausal symptoms, *Obstet Gynecol* 126:859, 2015.
Manson JE, Ames JM, Shapiro M, et al: Algorithm and mobile app for menopausal symptom management and hormonal/ non-hormonal therapy decision making: a clinical decision-support tool from the North American Menopause Society, *Menopause* 2(3):247, 2014.
Manson JE, Aragaki AK, Rossouw JE, et al: Menopausal hormone therapy and long-term all-cause and cause-specific mortality: the Women's Health Initiative randomized trials, *JAMA* 310:927, 2017.
Manson JE, Chlebowski RT, Stefanick ML, et al: Menopausal hormone therapy and health outcomes during the intervention and extended poststopping phases of the Women's Health Initiative randomized trials, *JAMA* 310:1353, 2013.
Manson JE, Kaunitz AM: Menopause management: getting clinical care back on track, *N Engl J Med* 374:803, 2016.
Melisko ME, Goldman ME, Hwang J, et al: Vaginal testosterone cream vs estradiol vaginal ring for vaginal dryness or decreased libido in women receiving aromatase inhibitors for early-stage breast cancer: a randomized clinical trial, *JAMA Oncol* 3:313–319, 2017.
North American Menopause Society: Approved Prescription Products for Menopausal Symptoms in the United States and Canada. Available at: http://www.menopause.org/docs/default-source/professional/nams-ht-tables.pdf?sfvrsn=18.pdf. Accessed 25 November 2016.
North American Menopause Society: The 2017 hormone therapy position statement of the North American Menopause Society, *Menopause* 24:728–753, 2017.
Trabuco EC, Moorman PG, Algeciras-Schimnich A, et al: Association of ovary-sparing hysterectomy with ovarian reserve, *Obstet Gynecol* 127:819, 2016.
Vinogradova Y, Coupland C, Hippisley-Cox J: Use of hormone replacement therapy and risk of venous thromboembolism: nested case-control studies using the QResearch and CPRD databases, *BMJ* 364, 2019.

OVARIAN CANCER

Method of
Michelle A. Roett, MD, MPH

CURRENT DIAGNOSIS

- The U.S. Preventive Services Task Force (USPSTF), American Academy of Family Physicians and American College of Obstetricians and Gynecologists recommend against routine screening for ovarian cancer in asymptomatic women. Screening for ovarian cancer may lead to significant harms, including invasive surgical interventions for women without cancer.
- The USPSTF recommends that women with family history associated with increased risk for deleterious mutations in *BRCA1* and *BRCA2* should be referred for genetic counseling and evaluation for *BRCA* testing.
- The Society of Gynecologic Oncology (AAGL) recommends against screening low-risk women with cancer antigen (CA) 125 or ultrasound for ovarian cancer. The American College of Physicians recommends against routine screening pelvic examinations in asymptomatic women.

Epidemiology

Ovarian cancer accounts for only 3% of cancers in women in the United States but results in more deaths than any other gynecologic cancer. Ovarian cancer has an age-adjusted incidence of 11 per 100,000 women, slightly decreased in recent years. In 2015, an estimated 224,940 women were living with ovarian cancer. According to the National Cancer Institute, 22,530 new cases of ovarian cancer and 13,980 deaths were expected in the United States in 2019.

Caucasian women have the highest incidence rate of ovarian cancer followed by Hispanic, Asian/Pacific Islander, African American, and American Indian/Alaska Native women. Caucasian women are more likely to die of ovarian cancer than any other group. AI/AN and African American women have the second and third highest rates of death from ovarian cancer, followed by Hispanic and Asian/Pacific Islander women. African American women with advanced epithelial ovarian cancer are more likely to die than their Caucasian counterparts (Hazard Ratio 1.27). Hispanic women have intermediate incidence and death rates compared to non-Hispanic women. Similar to other cancers affecting women, incidence of ovarian cancer and associated mortality increase with age, with women over 50 years of age experiencing the highest incidence. However, varying types of ovarian cancer may be diagnosed at any age, from infancy onward.

Risk Factors

Women at highest risk of ovarian cancer have a family history, associated genetic syndrome, or specific genetic mutation. For women of Ashkenazi Jewish descent, increased-risk family history refers to having one first-degree relative with breast or ovarian cancer or two second-degree relatives on the same side of the family. For other women increased-risk family history refers to having two or more first- or second-degree relatives with a history of ovarian cancer, a combination of breast and ovarian cancer among first- or second-degrees relatives, breast cancer in a male relative, one first-degree relative with bilateral breast cancer, or three or more first- or second-degree relatives with breast cancer.

Women with hereditary breast and ovarian cancer syndrome have an autosomal dominant mutation in the *BRCA1* or *BRCA2* gene. This occurs in one in every 500 women. Hereditary breast and ovarian cancer syndrome increases the risk of breast, ovarian, pancreatic, and prostate cancers, and is associated with up to 54% lifetime risk of ovarian cancer. Hereditary nonpolyposis colorectal cancer syndrome (Lynch II) is also autosomal dominant, increases risk of breast, colorectal, endometrial and ovarian cancers, and is associated with up to 12% lifetime risk of ovarian cancer.

Early age of menarche and later age at menopause are both associated with increased risk of ovarian cancer. Current smoking status increases risk of mucinous epithelian ovarian cancer (RR 2.22), along with former smoking (RR 2.02). Other risk factors including 7-fold increased risk from taking 12 or more monthly cycles of clomiphene, or taking fertility drugs used in in-vitro fertilization (RR 1.59).

Pathophysiology

While earlier evidence suggested that ovarian cancer frequently developed from ovarian surface epithelium or cortical inclusion cysts, recent studies suggest that serous carcinoma originates from distal fallopian tube epithelium. The age distribution of patients with ovarian cancer corresponds with the type of ovarian tumor. Germ cell tumors commonly occur in adolescents or patients under 1 year of age. Stromal cell tumors may occur at any age but include types more common in adolescence, such as androblastomas. Epithelial cell tumors commonly affect patients 50 years of age and older.

Ovarian cancer primarily spreads based on proximity to the uterus and opposite ovary, followed by intraperitoneal metastasis. Death usually arises from complications associated with local spread. Distant metastases may spread to the lungs, liver, adrenal glands, or spleen. In 2014, the International Federation of Gynecology and Obstetrics redefined stages of ovarian cancer to include ovarian, peritoneal and fallopian tube cancers because of similarities in their origins and treatment. FIGO staging guides treatment and prognosis to complement tumor-node-metastasis (TNM) staging defined by the American Joint Committee on Cancer. Stage II includes pelvic extension of an ovarian tumor, with a 60% to 80% 5-year survival rate. The 5-year survival rate is greatly diminished for stages III and IV. Some 85% of ovarian cancer cases are diagnosed in Stage III, which is associated with 20% survival. Stage III includes metastasis to the peritoneum outside the pelvis, primary peritoneal cancer, and/or metastasis to retroperitoneal lymph nodes. Stage IV is associated with less than 10% survival and includes distant metastases.

Prevention

The U.S. Preventive Services Task Force recommends again routine screening for ovarian cancer in asymptomatic women. The USPSTF also recommends that primary care clinicians screen women who have any family members with breast, ovarian, tubal or peritoneal with a validated screening tool to identify a significant family history with increased risk for BRCA-1 or BRCA-2 mutations. If the screening is positive, the patient should be referred for genetic counseling, and if indicated by counseling, BRCA testing. Screening with serum cancer antigen 125 (CA-125) level or transvaginal ultrasound does not reduce deaths from ovarian cancer and may lead to significant harms, including possibly unnecessary major surgical interventions in women without cancer. The most protective factors decreasing risk of ovarian cancer include older age at menarche, hormonal contraceptive use, multiparity, and younger age at menopause, primarily by decreasing the frequency of ovulation. Oral contraceptives (OR 0.75) and tubal ligation (OR 0.63) both decrease risk with longer duration. IUD use for up to 4 years is also protective (OR 0.53), but risk increases with IUD in place for more than 10 years (OR 1.4). Statin use for more than 5 years also reduces risk (RR 0.48). Multiple dietary interventions may be associated with lower risk of ovarian cancer. Drinking two or more cups of tea per day is associated with lower risk of ovarian cancer compared to one cup or less per day. A low-fat, high-fiber diet and a diet with increased vegetable consumption are both associated with decreased risk of ovarian cancer. Ovarian cancer is effectively reduced in women with *BRCA* mutations (NNT = 36) and hereditary nonpolyposis colorectal cancer syndrome (NNT = 28) by prophylactic bilateral salpingo-oophorectomy (BSO). Given the risk of ovarian cancer and 60% lifetime risk of endometrial cancer, total abdominal hysterectomy with BSO may be considered for patients with hereditary nonpolyposis colorectal cancer syndrome.

Clinical Manifestations

Although presenting symptoms for ovarian cancer may be nonspecific, the most common symptom is abdominal pain. Children and teenagers may also present with irregular menses, precocious puberty, or hirsutism. Any one of six symptoms for more than 12 days per month for less than 1 year has a 56.7% sensitivity for early ovarian cancer and 79.5% sensitivity for advanced stage ovarian cancer. These symptoms include abdominal pain, pelvic pain, increased abdomen size, bloating, difficulty eating, and early satiety. For patients with a pelvic mass, an irregular or enlarged ovary more than 10 cm, a nodular or fixed pelvic mass, or bilateral lesions more significantly increase suspicion of ovarian cancer. For women more than 3 years postmenopausal, ovaries are normally significantly diminished in size and often nonpalpable.

Diagnosis

Ovarian cancer patients with primarily gastrointestinal symptoms such as nausea, vomiting, diarrhea, and constipation tend to be diagnosed at a later stage than patients presenting with primarily gynecologic symptoms such as abnormal vaginal bleeding or pain. Diagnostic evaluation involves consideration of nonspecific signs and symptoms (Table 1). Women over 40 with persistent or unexplained symptoms should undergo laboratory evaluation including complete blood count, comprehensive metabolic panel, and CA-125. Pelvic inflammatory disease, endometriosis, functional ovarian cysts, menstruation, pregnancy, ascites, and other malignancies may cause elevated CA-125 levels.

Unfortunately, early detection is limited because CA-125 is elevated in only 50% of stage I tumors, but 90% of advanced stage ovarian cancer. Highest estimates of sensitivities, specificities, and positive predictive values are most applicable to postmenopausal women with known adnexal mass. An elevated CA-125 level (more than 200 U/mL in a premenopausal women, more than 35 U/mL in postmenopausal women) with an adnexal mass warrants evaluation by a gynecologic oncologist. OVA-1 is an FDA-approved panel measuring five biomarkers: CA-125, transferrin, prealbumin, apolipoprotein A1, and beta-2 microglobulin. Scored results identify ovarian cancer with 93% sensitivity and 43% specificity. Doppler transvaginal ultrasound for patients with adnexal masses has up 86% sensitivity and up to 91% specificity for ovarian cancer. Suspicious findings include a complex mass with both solid and cystic areas, extramural fluid, echogenicity, wall thickening, septa, or papillary projections, or an increased number and tortuosity of vessels on Doppler evaluation. Gadolinium-enhanced magnetic resonance imaging is useful for further delineation of indeterminate masses seen on ultrasonography.

Differential Diagnosis

The differential diagnosis for the signs and symptoms is broad, based on the nonspecific nature of presenting complaints. The differential for an adnexal mass may include a benign ovarian tumor, metastatic lesion, ovarian cyst or torsion, tubo-ovarian abscess, endometrioma or endometriosis, and rarely a pelvic kidney or pedunculated uterine fibroid.

Therapy or Treatment

Treatment for ovarian cancer is surgical debulking followed by chemotherapy. Chemotherapy before debulking surgery is associated with similar outcomes. Radiation may be used for palliative therapy or postchemotherapy localized disease. Surgical staging involves total abdominal hysterectomy, BSO, and the removal of pelvic and para-aortic lymph nodes and omentum.

Monitoring

Ovarian cancer of low malignant potential presents at stage I in 82% of cases typically between 30 and 50 years old, allowing for consideration of fertility-sparing measures, such as unilateral salpingo-oophorectomy. Adjuvant chemotherapy is reserved for patients with postoperative residual disease. Surgical treatment completion with total abdominal hysterectomy and unilateral salpingo-oophorectomy should be considered after the reproductive years. Positron emission tomography scans are useful for evaluation of increased CA-125 in known ovarian cancer in combination with computed tomography.

TABLE 1	Diagnostic Findings Associated With Ovarian Cancer

History	Physical Examination
• Abdominal fullness	• Abdominal mass
• Back pain	• Inguinal lymphadenopathy
• Bowel obstruction	• Pelvic or adnexal mass
• Constipation	• Sister Mary Joseph nodule
• Diarrhea	• Seborrheic keratoses (Leser-Trélat sign) sudden onset
• Early satiety	• Laboratory tests for patient with known adnexal mass:
• Fatigue	• CA-125 levels > 200 U/mL (200 arb U/L) in premenopausal women
• Nausea	• CA 125 > 35 U/mL (35 arb U/L) in postmenopausal women
• Pelvic pain	• Increased β–human chorionic gonadotropin*
• Shortness of breath	• Increased serum alpha-fetoprotein*
• Subacute cerebellar degeneration	• Increased neuron-specific enolase*
• Trousseau syndrome (unexplained spontaneous, recurrent, or migratory venous thrombotic events)	• Increased lactate dehydrogenase*
• Ureteral obstruction	
• Urinary symptoms	

Family History
- Bilateral breast cancer
- Early-onset breast cancer (younger than 50 years)
- Male breast cancer
- Personal or family history of colon or endometrial cancer
- Two or more first- or second-degree relatives with ovarian cancer

*Primarily used to evaluate adnexal masses during adolescence.

References

ABIM Foundation. Choosing Wisely. Available at http://www.choosingwisely.org/wp-content/uploads/2015/01/Choosing-Wisely-Recommendations.pdf. Accessed July 4, 2018.

American Cancer Society: *Cancer facts and figures 2015*, Atlanta, 2015, American Cancer Society.

American College of Obstetricians and Gynecologists: ACOG committee opinion: number 280, December 2002. The role of the generalist obstetrician-gynecologist in the early detection of ovarian cancer, *Obstet Gynecol* 100:1413–1416, 2002.

American College of Obstetricians and Gynecologists: ACOG practice bulletin. Management of adnexal masses, *Obstet Gynecol* 110:201–214, 2007.

Barney SP, Muller CY, Bradshaw KD: Pelvic masses, *Med Clin North Am* 92:1143–1161, 2008.

Doubeni CA, Doubeni ARB, Myers AE: Diagnosis and management of ovarian cancer, *Am Fam Physician.* 93(11):937–944, 2016.

Ducie J, Dao F, Considine M, Olvera N, Shaw PA, Kurman RJ, Shih IM, Soslow RA, Cope L, Levine DA: Molecular analysis of high-grade serous ovarian carcinoma with and without associated serous tubal intra-epithelial carcinoma, *Nat Commun* 8:990, 2017.

Ellenson LH, Pirog EC: The female genital tract. In Kumar V, Abbas AK, Aster AC, et al: *Robbins and Cotran pathologic basis of disease*, 9th ed., Philadelphia, 2005, Elsevier.

Finch A, Beiner M, Lubinski J, et al: for the Hereditary Ovarian Cancer Clinical Study Group: Salpingo-oophorectomy and the risk of ovarian, fallopian tube, and peritoneal cancers in women with a *BRCA1* or *BRCA2* mutation, *JAMA* 296:185–192, 2006.

Funt SA, Hann LE: Detection and characterization of adnexal masses, *Radiol Clin North Am* 40:591–608, 2002.

Goff BA, Mandel LS, Drescher CW, et al: Development of an ovarian cancer symptom index: possibilities for earlier detection, *Cancer* 109:221–227, 2007.

Han LY, Coleman RL: Ovarian cancer staging, *Oper Tech Gen Surg* 9:53–60, 2007.

Howell EA, Egorova N, Hayes MP, Wisnivesky J, Franco R, Bickell N: Racial disparities in the treatment of advanced epithelial ovarian cancer, *Obstet Gynecol* 122(5):1025–1032, 2013.

Larsson SC, Holmberg L, Wolk A: Fruit and vegetable consumption in relation to ovarian cancer incidence: the Swedish mammography cohort, *Br J Cancer* 90:2167, 2004.

Larsson SC, Wolk A: Tea consumption and ovarian cancer risk in a population-based cohort, *Arch Intern Med* 165:2683, 2005.

Li LL, Zhou J, Qian XJ, Chen YD: Meta-analysis on the possible association between in vitro fertilization and cancer risk, *Int J Gynecol Cancer* 23(1):16–24, 2013.

Liu Y, Qin A, Li T, Qin X, Li S: Effect of statin on risk of gynecologic cancers: a meta-analysis of observational studies and randomized controlled trials, *Gynecol Oncol* 133(3):647–655, 2014.

Morrison J, Swanton A, Collins S, et al: Chemotherapy versus surgery for initial treatment in advanced ovarian epithelial cancer, *Cochrane Database Syst Rev* 4: 2007. CD005343.

Moyer VA: Risk assessment, genetic counseling, and genetic testing for BRCA-related cancer in women: U.S. preventive services task force recommendation statement, *Ann Intern Med* 160(4):271–282, 2014.

Moyer VA: Screening for ovarian cancer: U.S. Preventive Services Task Force reaffirmation recommendation statement, *Ann Intern Med* 157:900–904, 2012.

National Comprehensive Cancer Network: Genetic/familial high-risk assessment: breast and ovary, http://www.nccn.org/professionals/physician_gls/pdf/genetics_screening.pdf; 2014. Accessed July, 4 2018.

Ness RB, Dodge RC, Edwards RP, et al: Contraception methods, beyond oral contraceptives and tubal ligation, and risk of ovarian cancer, *Ann Epidemiol* 21(3):188–196, 2011.

Noone AM, Howlader N, Krapcho M, Miller D, Brest A, Yu M, Ruhl J, Tatalovich Z, Mariotto A, Lewis DR, Chen HS, Feuer EJ, Cronin KA, editors. *SEER Cancer Statistics Review*. Bethesda, MD: National Cancer Institute; 1975-2015.

Prentice RL, Thomson CA, Caan B, et al: Low-fat dietary pattern and cancer incidence in the Women's health initiative dietary modification randomized controlled trial, *J Natl Cancer Inst* 99:1534, 2007.

Qaseem A, Humphrey LL, Harris R, Starkey M, Denberg TD: Clinical Guidelines Committee of the American College of Physicians. Screening pelvic examination in adult women: a clinical practice guideline from the American College of Physicians, *Ann Intern Med* 161(1):67–72, 2014.

Ryerson AB, Eheman C, Burton J, et al: Symptoms, diagnoses, and time to key diagnostic procedures among older U.S. women with ovarian cancer, *Obstet Gynecol* 109:1053–1061, 2007.

Sanner K, et al: Ovarian epithelial neoplasia after hormonal infertility treatment: long-term follow-up of a historical cohort in Sweden, *Fertil Steril* 91(4):1152–1158, 2009 Apr.

SEER Cancer Stat Facts: *Ovarian Cancer*. Bethesda, MD: National Cancer Institute. Available at https://seer.cancer.gov/statfacts/html/ovary.html. Accessed July 4, 2018.

Smith LH, Morris CR, Yasmeen S, et al: Ovarian cancer: can we make the clinical diagnosis earlier? *Cancer* 104:1398–1407, 2005.

Tworoger SS, Gertig DM, Gates MA, et al: Caffeine, alcohol, smoking, and the risk of incident epithelial ovarian cancer, *Cancer* 112:1169, 2008.

Ueland FR, Desimone CP, Seamon LG, Miller RA, Goodrich S, Podzielinski I, et al: Effectiveness of a multivariate index assay in the preoperative assessment of ovarian tumors, *Obstet Gynecol* 117(6):1289–1297, 2011.

U.S. Cancer Statistics Working Group. *United States Cancer Statistics: 1999–2014 Incidence and Mortality Web-based Report*. Atlanta, GA: Department of Health and Human Services, Centers for Disease Control and Prevention, and National Cancer Institute; 2017. Available at https://gis.cdc.gov/Cancer/USCS/DataViz.html. Accessed July 4, 2018.

Yang HP, Anderson WF, Rosenberg PS, et al: Ovarian cancer incidence trends in relation to changing patterns of menopausal hormone therapy use in the United States, *J Clin Oncol* 31:2146–2151, 2013.

Young RH, Clement PB, Scully RE: The ovary. In Sternberg SS, Antonioli DA, Mills SE, et al, editors: *Diagnostic surgical pathology*, 2nd ed., New York, 1994, Raven Press.

CURRENT THERAPY

Empiric treatment for pelvic inflammatory disease (PID) should be initiated in any woman at risk for sexually transmitted infections if:
- Pelvic or lower abdominal pain is present;
- Cervical motion tenderness *OR* uterine tenderness *OR* adnexal tenderness is found on pelvic examination;
- No other cause for the pain can be identified.

Inpatient therapy for PID:
- Regimen A: either cefotetan (Cefotan) 2 g IV every 12 hours *OR* cefoxitin (Mefoxin) 2 g IV every 6 hours *PLUS* doxycycline (Vibramycin) 100 mg PO/IV every 12 hours.
- Regimen B: clindamycin (Cleocin) 900 mg IV every 8 hours *PLUS* gentamicin (Garamycin) 2 mg/kg of body weight loading dose followed by 1.5 mg/kg of body weight IV/IM every 8 hours. A single daily dose of 3 to 5 mg/kg of body weight IV/IM can also be used.
- Alternate regimen: ampicillin/sulbactam (Unasyn) 3 g IV every 6 hours *PLUS* doxycycline (Vibramycin) 100 mg PO/IV every 12 hours.

Outpatient therapy for PID:
- Ceftriaxone (Rocephin) 250 mg IM single dose *PLUS* doxycycline (Vibramycin) 100 mg PO every 12 hours for 14 days *WITH/WITHOUT* metronidazole (Flagyl) 500 mg PO every 12 hours for 14 days.
- *OR*
- Cefoxitin (Mefoxin) 2 g IM and probenecid (Benemid) 1 g PO both given concurrently as a single dose *PLUS* doxycycline (Vibramycin) 100 mg PO every 12 hours for 14 days *WITH/WITHOUT* metronidazole (Flagyl) 500 mg PO every 12 hours for 14 days.
- *OR*
- Other parenteral third-generation cephalosporins: either ceftizoxime (Cefizox) 1 g IM single dose *OR* cefotaxime (Claforan) 1 g IM single dose *PLUS* doxycycline (Vibramycin) 100 mg PO every 12 hours for 14 days *WITH/WITHOUT* metronidazole (Flagyl) 500 mg PO every 12 hours for 14 days.
- Alternative treatment options are available for those who have penicillin or cephalosporin allergy.

PELVIC INFLAMMATORY DISEASE

Method of
Amy E. Curry, MD

CURRENT DIAGNOSIS

- Pelvic inflammatory disease is a clinical diagnosis based on suspicious clinical findings in a woman who is at risk.
- Patients may be asymptomatic. Symptoms may range from nonspecific complaints including lower abdominal pain, vaginal discharge, dyspareunia, and irregular uterine bleeding to high fever, vomiting, and lower abdominal tenderness with rebound.
- Physical examination findings may include vaginal and endocervical discharge, as well as cervical motion, uterine and adnexal tenderness, and adnexal fullness.
- Cultures should be performed for *Chlamydia trachomatis* and *Neisseria gonorrhoeae*, the two most commonly implicated organisms, though a variety of infectious agents may be causative.

Pelvic inflammatory disease (PID) is a polymicrobial infection of any or all of the upper genital tract organs in women. It is initiated by a community-acquired sexually transmitted agent and can involve the uterus, fallopian tubes, and ovaries, as well as adjacent pelvic structures.

Epidemiology
In the United States, the diagnosis of PID accounted for 90,000 initial visits to physician offices between 2007–2016 and 4.4% of women (2.5 million) 18 to 44 years of age reported a history of PID based on 2013-2014 survey data.

Risk Factors
The single greatest risk factor for PID is a history of multiple sex partners. Other risk factors include 15 to 25 years of age, a male partner with symptoms of a sexually transmitted infection (STI) such as dysuria or urethral discharge, history of previous PID, inconsistent use of condoms, African American ethnicity, and use of vaginal douching. Any phenomenon that disrupts the mucus barrier of the endocervical canal can also potentially facilitate PID, such as menses, bacterial vaginosis, or intrauterine instrumentation. Accordingly, the risk of an intrauterine device causing PID usually occurs during the first 3 weeks following insertion and rarely thereafter.

Pathophysiology

PID occurs when bacteria from the vagina ascend into the normally sterile environment of the upper genital tract. This typically occurs in the setting of a *Neisseria gonorrhoeae* or *Chlamydia trachomatis* infection. Ascending bacteria can include anaerobes, especially those implicated in bacterial vaginosis, group A and B *Streptococcus*, *Escherichia coli*, *Klebsiella*, *Proteus mirabilis*, *Haemophilus influenzae*, *Peptococcus*, genital *Mycoplasma*, *Actinomycosis*, and cytomegalovirus. Methicillin-resistant *Staphylococcus aureus* has been reported to cause PID, but rarely. Once present, this polymicrobial infection can remain asymptomatic or cause endometritis, salpingitis, oophoritis, peritonitis, perihepatitis, or tubo-ovarian abscesses.

Clinical Presentation

PID may be asymptomatic. It may have an indolent presentation of low-grade fever, weight loss, and nonspecific abdominal pain. A more symptomatic presentation of PID includes bilateral lower quadrant abdominal pain, recent onset of dyspareunia, abnormal vaginal bleeding, and vaginal discharge. On physical examination, the patient may have fever, decreased bowel sounds, diffuse lower abdominal tenderness with rebound tenderness, and/or right upper quadrant tenderness. During the pelvic examination, purulent vaginal or endocervical discharge, vaginal mucosa redness, and cervical irritation or friability may be noted. Cervical motion pain or tenderness of the adnexa or uterus during the bimanual examination is strongly suggestive of PID.

There are several diagnostic findings that support the diagnosis of PID: the presence of abundant white blood cells or clue cells in vaginal or cervical mucus; the presence of an STI, especially gonorrhea or chlamydia; an elevated erythrocyte sedimentation rate or C-reactive protein; an elevated serum white blood cell count; evidence of endometritis on endometrial biopsy; findings of thickened, fluid-filled fallopian tubes, free fluid in the pelvis, or a tubo-ovarian abscess on transvaginal sonography or magnetic resonance imaging; or evidence of pelvic organ inflammation on laparoscopic exploration.

Diagnosis

Unfortunately, no single element of the history, finding on physical examination, laboratory test result, or diagnostic procedure has both the sensitivity and the specificity to help the clinician accurately diagnose PID. Consequently, PID remains a diagnosis based primarily on clinical suspicion in at-risk women.

Differential Diagnosis

The differential diagnosis of PID includes ectopic pregnancy, inflammatory bowel disorders, ovarian cysts and cyst rupture, ovarian torsion, appendicitis, endometriosis, proctitis, urinary tract infections, diverticulitis, constipation, or functional pain related to current or past abuse.

Treatment

The 2015 Centers for Disease Control and Prevention (CDC) treatment guidelines for STIs are outlined in the Current Diagnosis and Current Therapy boxes. These guidelines recommend empiric treatment for PID in all at-risk women who meet the criteria listed and encourage health care providers to "maintain a low threshold for the diagnosis" and treatment of PID due to "the potential for significant damage to the reproductive health of women."

Treatment guidelines are based on the patient's need for inpatient versus outpatient care. The Pelvic Inflammatory Disease Evaluation and Clinical Health (PEACH) trial demonstrated no difference in the reproductive outcomes of women with mild-to-moderate PID who were randomized to inpatient treatment versus those randomized to outpatient treatment.

Indications for inpatient treatment of PID include the following: pregnancy; failed trial or intolerance to oral medications; signs of severe PID such as high fever, nausea, vomiting, or intractable abdominal pain; complicated PID (e.g., peritonitis, perihepatitis); and pelvic abscesses. The need for surgical intervention or diagnostic exploration to rule out other abdominal pathology would also mandate inpatient treatment. In those patients requiring inpatient treatment, any one of the parenteral antibiotic regimens as outlined above may be administered, depending on the patient's history of allergies and the cost and availability of treatment options. When possible, the use of oral doxycycline (Vibramycin) is preferred over intravenous (IV) infusion due to the pain of IV infusion and the similar bioavailability of the oral form as compared to IV administration. Treatment should also include appropriate analgesia, antiemetics, antipyretics, IV fluids, and rest. Patients may be transitioned from parenteral to oral therapy after 24 hours of sustained clinical improvement including lack of fever. Further completion of a total of 14 days of treatment with oral medications is recommended. Those patients treated with either regimen A or the alternative regimen should be transitioned to oral doxycycline (Vibramycin) 100 mg every 12 hours. Those treated with regimen B should be transitioned to oral doxycycline (Vibramycin) 100 mg every 12 hours or oral clindamycin (Cleocin) 450 mg every 6 hours. If a tubo-ovarian abscess is present, the patient should be transitioned preferably to oral clindamycin (Cleocin) 450 mg every 6 hours for a total of 14 days of treatment. Alternatively, oral doxycycline (Vibramycin) 100 mg every 12 hours with oral metronidazole (Flagyl) 500 mg every 8 hours for a total of 14 days of treatment may also be used.

In patients not meeting criteria for inpatient treatment, any of the outpatient treatment regimens as outlined above may be used, the choice being again dependent on the cost and availability of treatment options. The addition of metronidazole (Flagyl) is recommended due to cephalosporin limitations in anaerobic coverage and in the case of *Trichomonas* or bacterial vaginosis infections. The addition of metronidazole (Flagyl) is also recommended if there is a history of recent uterine instrumentation.

In patients who are at a high risk for gonorrheal infection and who have a history of anaphylaxis to penicillin (urticaria, angioedema, stridor, hypotension, or desquamation), recommended treatment options include the following: hospitalization for regimen B parenteral antibiotic treatment; azithromycin (Zithromax) 2 g PO administered as a single dose along with either levofloxacin (Levaquin) 500 mg PO every 24 hours for 14 days or moxifloxacin (Avelox) 400 mg PO every 24 hours for 14 days. If these patients are at a low risk of gonorrhea, either levofloxacin (Levaquin) 500 mg PO every 24 hours or ofloxacin (Floxin) 400 mg PO every 24 hours with or without metronidazole (Flagyl) 500 mg PO every 12 hours for 14 days may be used.

In patients with a history of mild, non-anaphylactic reaction to penicillin, ceftriaxone (Rocephin) or cefoxitin (Mefoxin) can be safely administered as there is negligible cross-reactivity between penicillin and these cephalosporins. The patient should be observed for another 1 hour after the second dose.

Regardless of the treatment regimen used, patients should be advised to abstain from intercourse until treatment is completed and they are free of symptoms. In patients with an intrauterine device (IUD), there are inconclusive data to recommend its removal, unless clinical improvement does not occur, but close clinical follow-up is warranted. There is no difference in the treatment regimens for PID in women with a history of HIV.

Patient Monitoring and Counseling

Patients treated with an outpatient regimen should be evaluated for clinical improvement within 48 to 72 hours. If no improvement is noted, the patient should be hospitalized for parenteral antibiotics and further diagnostic evaluation. All patients should be counseled on the need to complete the full course of antibiotic treatment to decrease the potential complications of PID. Patients should be informed of the cause of their infection, if known, and the need for any sexual partners to be tested and treated. Testing for HIV, syphilis, and hepatitis B and C should also be offered. If the patient is an appropriate candidate, immunization against hepatitis B (Engerix-B, Recombivax HB) and human papillomavirus (Gardasil 9) should also be offered. In order to decrease future PID episodes, patients should be advised on the need for safe sex practices and the recommendation for future routine screening for chlamydia and gonorrhea.

Complications

Complications of PID include recurrence of the infection, infertility secondary to fallopian tube scarring, chronic pelvic pain, and ectopic pregnancy. Extension of the infection can also occur, potentially causing pelvic abscesses, peritonitis, and perihepatitis (Fitz-Hugh-Curtis syndrome).

References

Campagna JD, Bond MC, Schabelman E, Hayes BD. The use of cephalosporins in penicillin-allergic patients: a literature review, *J Emerg Med* 42(5):612–620, 2012.

Centers for Disease Control and Prevention. STD surveillance 2017-STDs in women and infants. Available at: https://www.cdc.gov/std/stats17/womenandinf.htm#pid (Accessed May 29, 2019)

Gradison M. Pelvic inflammatory disease. *Am Fam Physician* 85(8):791–796, 2012.

Kreisel K, Torrone E, Bernstein K, Hong J, Gorwitz R: Prevalence of pelvic inflammatory disease in sexually experienced women of reproductive age United States, 2013–2014, *MMWR Morb Mortal Wkly Rep* 66(3):80–83, 2017.

Ness RB, Soper DE, Holley RL, et al: Effectiveness of inpatient and outpatient treatment strategies for women with pelvic inflammatory disease: results from the pelvic inflammatory disease evaluation and clinical health (PEACH) randomized trial, *Am J Obstet Gynecol* 186:929–937, 2002.

Tepper NK, Steenland MW, Gaffield ME, Marchbanks PA, Curtis KM. Retention of intrauterine devices in women who acquire pelvic inflammatory disease: a systematic review, *Contraception* 87(5):655–660, 2013.

PREMENSTRUAL SYNDROME

Method of
Ellen W. Freeman, PhD

CURRENT DIAGNOSIS

- Confirm that symptoms occur premenstrually and abate following menses.
- Confirm that symptoms are clinically significant and impair daily activities and/or cause problems for the woman.
- Obtain a medical history and conduct a physical examination to determine that other disorders are not causing the symptoms.
- Assess depression, stress, substance abuse, and other diagnoses that could cause the symptoms.
- Ask the woman to maintain a daily symptom report for two or more menstrual cycles to confirm the reported symptoms and their relation to the menstrual cycle.
- Perform laboratory tests only as needed to confirm general good health or rule out other suspected conditions.

CURRENT THERAPY

SSRI	Range Studied (mg)	Mean Dose (mg/d)
Citalopram (Celexa[1])	10–30	20
Escitalopram (Lexapro[1])	10–20	15
Fluoxetine (Prozac,[1] Sarafem*)	10–60	20
Paroxetine (Paxil[1])	10–30	20
Paroxetine-CR* (Paxil-CR)	12.5, 25	NA[†]
Sertraline (Zoloft*)	50–150	75
SNRI		
Venlafaxine (Effexor[1])	37.5–200	112.5

[1]Not FDA approved for this indication.
*FDA approved for the indication of premenstrual dysphoric disorder (PMDD).
[†]Not applicable because of fixed-dose study.

The premenstrual syndromes (PMS) are characterized by mood, behavioral, and physical symptoms that occur from several days to 2 weeks before menses and remit with the menstrual flow. The term *PMS* as used by clinicians and the general public is generic, imprecise, and commonly applied to numerous symptoms. Included symptoms range from the mild and normal physiologic changes of the menstrual cycle to clinically significant symptoms that limit or impair normal functioning. In recent years, randomized controlled trials and other well-designed studies have defined diagnostic criteria for PMS and identified effective treatments for this disorder.

Based on scientific evidence at this time, serotonergic antidepressants are considered the primary treatment for clinically significant PMS, and particularly its severe form termed *premenstrual dysphoric disorder* (PMDD). This review focuses on PMS and its treatment with serotonergic antidepressants. It is not a comprehensive review of all treatments or associated literature. Other recent reviews may guide the reader to further information and other treatments for PMS and PMDD.

Symptoms

Numerous symptoms were traditionally attributed to PMS. This plethora is related in part to the absence of a clear diagnosis that distinguishes PMS from other comorbid conditions. Many disorders, both physical and psychiatric, are exacerbated premenstrually or occur as a comorbid disorder with PMS. When a careful diagnosis is made to distinguish PMS from other conditions, a much smaller group of symptoms appear to be typical of the disorder (Box 1).

Mood symptoms are usually the main complaint (irritability, anxiety, tension, mood swings, feeling out of control, depression), but behavioral symptoms (e.g., decreased interest, fatigue, poor concentration, poor sleep) and physical symptoms, most commonly breast tenderness and abdominal swelling, are also present. Multiple studies suggest that irritability is the cardinal symptom of PMS. Although depressive symptoms such as low mood, fatigue, sleep difficulties, and poor concentration are frequent complaints of women with PMS, the growing evidence indicates that PMS is not a simple variant of depression but has distinct mechanisms that differ from those of depressive disorders.

Prevalence

Surveys indicate that PMS is among the most common health problems reported by reproductive-age women. Current estimates from epidemiologic data indicate that up to 30% of women experience severe and clinically significant premenstrual symptoms, although only 6% to 8% of menstruating women meet the stringent and predominantly dysphoric criteria for PMDD.

BOX 1	Symptoms of Premenstrual Syndrome

Affective
- Irritability
- Anxiety
- Angry outbursts
- Confusion
- Social withdrawal
- Depression

Somatic
- Abdominal bloating
- Breast tenderness or swelling
- Swelling of extremities
- Headache
- Joint or muscle pain

From the American College of Obstetricians and Gynecologists (ACOG), FAQ057, May 2015.

Morbidity

The morbidity of PMS is related to its severity, chronicity, and resulting distress that affect work, personal relationships, or daily activities. The level of impairment is significantly above community norms and similar to that of other health problems such as major depressive disorder. Studies consistently demonstrate that the greatest impairment or distress resulting from PMS is in relationships with the partner or children and in the effectiveness of work.

Etiology

The etiology of PMS remains undefined, although the monthly cycling of the reproductive hormones appears to have an essential role in the disorder. While circulating levels of the hormones are in normal range, the dominant theory is that some women have an underlying vulnerability to the normal fluctuations of one or more of these hormones. It is further believed that PMS involves central nervous system–mediated interactions of the reproductive steroids with neurotransmitters. A current review of the genetic etiology found only limited evidence for the genetic basis of PMDD, with both familial and candidate gene studies having negative or conflicting results. The principal research evidence at this time supports the involvement of reproductive hormones, serotonergic dysregulation, and possibly dysregulation of GABAergic receptor functioning. Recent evidence suggested a pathophysiological role of beta-adrenergic mechanisms in the clinical pain of PMS.

Diagnosis

A diagnosis of PMS is determined primarily by the *timing* and the *severity* of the symptoms. These factors, together with an assessment of whether other physical or psychiatric disorders may account for the symptoms, are more important for the diagnosis than the particular symptoms, which are typically nonspecific and must be assessed for their relationship to the menstrual cycle.

Box 2 lists the diagnostic criteria for PMS presented by the American College of Obstetricians and Gynecologists. These criteria indicate that PMS symptoms must be experienced during the 5 days before menses and abate during the menstrual flow. The symptoms should cause identifiable impairment or distress, be confirmed by prospective reports recorded daily by the woman for at least two to three consecutive menstrual cycles, and not be accounted for by other disorders.

To diagnose PMS, a medical history should be obtained and a complete physical with gynecologic examination performed. PMS is understood to occur in ovulatory menstrual cycles; cycles that are irregular or outside the normal range are an indication for further gynecologic investigation. Comorbid conditions such as dysmenorrhea, endometriosis, uterine fibroids, pelvic inflammatory disease, thyroid disorders, migraine, diabetes, mood disorders, substance abuse, and numerous other possibilities should be identified. It may be difficult to determine whether the symptoms under investigation are an exacerbation of a comorbid condition or superimposed on another condition. In either case, the usual recommendation is to treat the ongoing condition first, then reassess and possibly add treatment for the symptoms that arise premenstrually.

The diagnostic criteria for PMDD are listed in the *Diagnostic and Statistical Manual of Mental Disorders,* Fifth Edition *(DSM-V)* and are intended to diagnose a severe, dysphoric form of PMS. Importantly, the Food and Drug Administration (FDA) has approved medications only for the indication of PMDD and not for the indication of PMS at the present time. Briefly, the PMDD criteria require 5 of 11 *listed* symptoms including at least one mood symptom. Physical symptoms, regardless of the number, are considered a single symptom in meeting the diagnostic criteria. The 11 PMDD symptoms are depressed mood, anxiety or tension, mood swings, anger or irritability, decreased interest, concentration difficulties, fatigue, appetite change or food cravings, sleep disturbance, feeling overwhelmed, and physical symptoms. At least five of these symptoms must *each* be severe premenstrually and abate with the menstrual flow. The symptoms must markedly interfere with functioning, be confirmed by daily symptom reports for at least two menstrual cycles, and not be an exacerbation of another physical or mental disorder.

No laboratory test identifies PMS or PMDD and none should be routinely performed for diagnosis. Laboratory tests that indicate or confirm other possible disorders are useful if suggested by the individual woman's symptom presentation or medical findings.

The key diagnostic tool for evaluating premenstrual symptoms is the daily symptom report. The diagnostic criteria for both PMS and PMDD include a daily symptom report that is maintained by the woman for at least two menstrual cycles to confirm that the woman's reported symptoms are linked to the menstrual cycle in the requisite pattern. Numerous symptom reports appropriate for this diagnosis are identified in the medical literature. It is important that the ratings indicate the severity of each symptom (and not simply check the presence or absence of symptoms).

It is informative to use two visits for the diagnostic evaluation. Although counterintuitive, seeing the patient following menses when PMS symptoms have abated is instructive. If symptoms are absent, it provides strong evidence for the diagnosis. If symptoms are present in the follicular phase, the type and severity of the symptoms are important diagnostic information for identifying other physical or mental disorders that may be the primary focus of treatment.

Treatment

Selective Serotonin Reuptake Inhibitors

Serotonergic antidepressants are the primary treatment for severe PMS and PMDD at this time. Modulating serotonergic function is consistent with a leading theoretical view that the normal gonadal steroid fluctuations of the menstrual cycle are associated with an abnormal serotonergic response in vulnerable women. A meta-analysis of randomized controlled trials of selective serotonin reuptake inhibitors (SSRIs) in treatment of PMS and PMDD determined that these drugs were an effective first-line therapy, with both a statistically significant and clinically meaningful difference from placebo. The FDA has approved fluoxetine (Sarafem), sertraline (Zoloft), and controlled-release paroxetine (Paxil CR) for the indication of PMDD. Other randomized, placebo-controlled, double-blind trials show efficacy of citalopram (Celexa[1]), escitalopram (Lexapro[1]), venlafaxine (Effexor[1]) (a selective serotonin-norepinephrine reuptake inhibitor [SNRI]), and clomipramine (Anafranil[1]) (a tricyclic antidepressant) for treatment of PMS and PMDD, but they are not FDA approved for this indication.

Effective doses of SSRIs are consistently at the low end of the dose range for depressive disorders in all reports of PMS and PMDD treatments. Significant response is often seen in the first menstrual cycle of treatment, with smaller increments with or without dose adjustments in the second and third treatment cycles. If there is not sufficient response in the first treated

---

BOX 2	Diagnosis of Premenstrual Syndrome

Presenting symptoms:
- Consistent with premenstrual syndrome
- Restricted to the luteal phase
- Cause impairment or distress
- Not an exacerbation of another disorder
- Confirmed by 2-3 consecutive cycles of daily symptom rating

From the American College of Obstetricians and Gynecologists (ACOG), FAQ057, May 2015.

[1]Not FDA approved for this indication.

menstrual cycle, the dose should be increased in the next cycle unless precluded by side effects.

Side effects are common with the initiation of an SSRI but are usually transient and abate within 1 to 2 weeks of continued treatment. The most common side effects include headache, nausea, insomnia, fatigue or lethargy, diarrhea, decreased concentration, dizziness, and decreased libido or delayed orgasm. The sexual side effects of SSRIs have received considerable attention, although it is often difficult to determine the extent to which sexual effects are related to the medication or to preexisting conditions. The incidence of decreased sexual interest or delayed orgasm in the few published reports of PMS patients is approximately 9% to 16%, which is notably lower than the rates reported with the use of SSRIs by depressed patients. Another important issue is the lack of any well-controlled clinical trials of SSRI treatment for PMS and PMDD in adolescents. Whether SSRIs are safe and effective for this indication in women younger than 18 years is not demonstrated.

Luteal Phase Dosing

The use of medication only in the symptomatic luteal phase of the menstrual cycle is particularly important in PMS because of the cyclic pattern of the symptoms, which occur only in the premenstrual phase and abate following menses. Efficacy of luteal phase administration of the SSRIs is demonstrated in multiple trials: three large multicenter, randomized, placebo-controlled trials that examined fluoxetine (Sarafem), paroxetine (Paxil), and sertraline (Zoloft); a trial that directly compared continuous and luteal phase administration of sertraline; and multiple preliminary studies.

Luteal phase administration of an SSRI is typically initiated 14 days prior to the expected onset of menstrual bleeding and concluded within several days of bleeding, using a taper for increased doses. As with continuous dosing, the SSRI doses are usually at the low end of the dose range.

A preliminary study compared symptom-onset dosing (mean of 6 days before menses) to luteal-phase dosing and found no difference between the two dosing regimens in improvement overall, although there was suggestion that women with more severe symptoms may respond better to full luteal-phase dosing. A recent RCT of sertraline in symptom-onset dosing suggested greater improvement with sertraline compared to placebo, but results were inconsistent and varied with the symptom scale. Importantly, however, this study showed that cessation of symptom-onset treatment was not associated with discontinuation symptoms.

Side effects may be less frequent with an intermittent dosing regimen because they may not occur when not taking the medication. However, some women experience recurring side effects when dosing is resumed.

Insufficient Response to Selective Serotonin Reuptake Inhibitors

Approximately 60% of PMS and PMDD patients in controlled studies respond well to an SSRI. There are no clear predictors of response. An adequate trial of an SSRI for PMS and PMDD is at least two menstrual cycles at a dose level of demonstrated efficacy, with a third cycle when there is partial response. If a woman has an insufficient response or unacceptable side effects, it is reasonable to try another SSRI. Although the SSRIs are similar in their structure and have similar response rates and side-effect profiles, an individual patient may respond better to one SSRI versus another.

Other approaches to a poor treatment response include augmenting the SSRI with another medication to address the nonresponding symptoms, but there is no systematic information on this in PMS or PMDD treatment. Switching to another class of medication, such as anxiolytics, is suggested, but no data indicate whether nonresponders to SSRIs will respond to another class of medication. Nonresponse may also be related to other comorbid disorders. A thorough review of the diagnosis and adjustments of the premenstrual doses of medication for both the primary disorder and PMS should be considered before pursuing other treatments.

Other Treatments

Hormonal

In spite of the evidence for hormonal involvement in PMS and PMDD, traditional oral contraceptives (OCs) do not show efficacy for the disorder. However, some data indicate that shortening or omitting the placebo week in the traditional OC pill pack may effectively treat PMS and PMDD. The FDA has approved the oral contraceptive YAZ (ethinyl estradiol 20 mcg/drospirenone 3 mg), a 24/4-day combination pill, to treat PMDD. The continuous daily use of an OC (without a hormone-free interval) suppresses ovulation-related hormone cyclicity. Continuous daily levonorgestrel 90 mcg/ethinyl estradiol 20 mcg (Amethyst[1]) has been evaluated for continuous use up to one year and may be useful for managing the symptoms of PMDD. A Cochrane review of estrogen preparations for management of PMS found only five randomized controlled trials out of more than 500 reports. The evidence was considered low-quality, inconclusive with regard to effectiveness, and too limited to provide answers regarding the safety of these preparations for the indication of PMS.

Gonadotropin-releasing hormone (GnRH) agonists such as depot leuprolide (Lupron)[1] and buserelin[2] (Suprefact) are effective for PMS and PMDD but are of limited usefulness because of the risks associated with low estrogen levels that result from these treatments. Although add-back therapy using low-lose estrogen and progesterone together with the GnRH agonist did not appear to reduce efficacy in a meta-analysis, there are no definitive data on the safety and efficacy of this approach in long-term treatment. The historic use of progesterone has failed to show efficacy for the mood and behavioral symptoms of PMS in numerous controlled trials.

Anxiolytics

Alprazolam (Xanax)[1] and buspirone (Buspar)[1] showed modest efficacy for PMS in some studies but not others. Although these medications offer an alternative to antidepressants, the response rates appear much lower, and it is not known whether a PMS patient who does not respond to antidepressants will respond to an anxiolytic. The risk of dependency with alprazolam should be considered. Dosing should be strictly limited to the luteal phase, and the patient should have no history of substance abuse.

Nonpharmacologic

Calcium supplementation[1] (500 mg daily; 600 mg twice daily) reduced PMS symptoms significantly more than placebo in several clinical trials. Improved symptoms included anxiety, depression, water retention, and somatic changes. Calcium offers a dietary supplement approach that may be beneficial for some women with PMS, although there are no predictors of which women will respond well to this therapy. Vitex agnus castus (chasteberry[7]) appears to be a safe and effective treatment for PMS or PMDD in randomized controlled trials. Other complementary and alternative therapies may be helpful for some women, but there is no consistent evidence of their efficacy for PMS.

Behavioral treatments that facilitate coping or reduce stress may reduce PMS symptoms. Cognitive-behavioral therapy is effective for PMS, and in one study it was as effective as the SSRI fluoxetine after 6 months of treatment.

Treatment Duration

The published studies of treatment efficacy for PMS and PMDD are based on acute treatment of 2 to 3 months' duration. Several investigations suggest that PMS symptoms are likely to return within several months after medication is stopped. It also appears that PMS symptoms do not resolve spontaneously but continue for many years. These observations of PMS as a chronic condition and the swift return of symptoms following the cessation of medication suggest that treatment can be expected to be long term. In a controlled study that compared

---

[1]Not FDA approved for this indication.
[2]Not available in the United States.
[7]Available as dietary supplement.

4 months to 1 year of SSRI treatment, approximately half of the patients who improved with SSRI treatment relapsed within 6 to 8 months after discontinuing medication. Longer treatment was marginally better at preventing relapse. Patients with more severe symptoms before treatment were the most likely to relapse, while patients who experienced symptom remission with treatment were least likely to relapse.

Conclusions

The SSRIs are currently the first-line treatment for severe PMS and PMDD. Continuous dosing and luteal phase dosing regimens are similarly effective for these disorders when the symptoms are clearly limited to the luteal phase of the menstrual cycle. Hormonal treatments have lacked consistent scientific evidence of their efficacy or safety or both for PMS treatment. Several new oral contraceptives that decrease or omit the placebo interval, calcium supplementation, and cognitive behavioral therapy may provide an effective alternative to antidepressant medications. Evidence indicates that long-term maintenance of the medication may be required for PMS and PMDD.

References

American College of Obstetricians and Gynecologists: *Guidelines for women's health care: a resource manual*, 4th ed., Washington, DC: American College of Obstetricians and Gynecologists, 2014.

American College of Obstetricians and Gynecologists: *Patient Education FAQ057*, Washington, DC, American College of Obstetricians and Gynecologists, May 2015.

American Psychiatric Association: *Diagnostic and statistical manual of mental disorders. 5th ed.* (DSM-5), Arlington, VA:P American Psychiatric Association , 2013.

Cerqueira RO, Frey BN, Leclerc E, et al: Vitex agnus casus for premenstrual syndrome/premenstrual disphoric disorder: a systematic review, *Arch Women's Ment Health* 20(6):713–719, 2017.

Freeman EW: Luteal phase administration of agents for the treatment of premenstrual dysphoric disorder, *CNS Drugs* 18(7):453–468, 2004.

Freeman EW, Rickels K, Sammel MD, et al: Time to relapse after short-term or long-term treatment of severe premenstrual syndrome with sertraline, *Arch Gen Psychiatry* 66(5):537–544, 2009.

Hall E, Steiner M: Psychiatric symptoms and disorders associated with reproductive cyclicity in women: advances in screening tools, *Women's Health* 11(3):397–415, 2015.

Jang SH, Kim DI, Choi M-S: Effects and treatment methods of acupuncture and herbal medicine for premenstrual syndrome/premenstrual dysphoric disorder: systematic review, *BMC Compl Alternative Med* 14(11), 2014. Available at http://www.biomedcentral.com/1472-6882/14/11.

Lopez LM, Kaptein AA, Helmerhorse FM: Oral contraceptives containing drospirenone for premenstrual syndrome, *Cochrane Database Syst Rev* (2): CD006586, 2012 Feb 15.

Maharaj S, Trevino K: A comprehensive review of treatment options for premenstrual syndrome and premenstrual dysphoric disorder, *J Psychiatr Prac* 21(5):334–350, 2015.

Marjoribanks J, Brown J, O'Brien PMS, et al: Selective serotonin reuptake inhibitors for premenstrual syndrome (Review), *Cochrane Libr* 6:21–32, 2013.

McEvoy K, Osborne LM, Nanavati J, et al: Reproductive affective disorders: a review of the genetic evidence for premenstrual dysphoric disorder and postpartum depression, *Curr Psychiatry Rep* 94(19):94–106, 2017.

Naheed B, Kuiper JH, Uthman OA, et al: Non-contraceptive oestrogen-containing preparations for controlling symptoms of premenstrual syndrome, *Cochrane Database Syst Rev*, 2017 Mar 3. CD010503.

Whelan AM, Jurgens TM, Naylor H: Herbs, vitamins and minerals in the treatment of premenstrual syndrome: a systematic review, *Can J Clin Pharmacol* 16:c407–c429, 2009.

FEMALE SEXUAL DYSFUNCTION

Method of
Melissa Hague, MD

CURRENT DIAGNOSIS

- Sexual pain is a common cause of distress for women and their partners, with up to 50% of women experiencing distress at some point in their lifetime.
- Women may present with a complaint of decreased libido, but on further questioning may have significant pain with sex that is causing or contributing to decreased desire.
- Always ask about relationship stress, pain, and ability to achieve climax when discussing sexual distress with female patients.
- Many medications interfere with libido, as does a patient's lifestyle and overall health status.
- Like many medical concerns, female sexual dysfunction is a complex, multifactorial problem that should be addressed with a holistic multidisciplinary approach.

CURRENT THERAPY

- You cannot treat decreased libido in a patient who is having sexual pain without addressing the source of the pain.
- Determine the cause of sexual pain and once this has been adequately addressed you may consider a treatment plan for decreased libido.
- Consider the approach to sexual pain from the outside working in. Start with skin or vulvar causes such as lichen sclerosis, atrophy, or herpes. Work in toward the pelvic floor and consider muscle or nerve pain as a cause. Once you have considered these as a source of pain and not found a problem, you can consider a bimanual exam and see if pain occurs with cervical or uterine motion, or if there is evidence of pelvic mass.
- Realize that patients that have suffered sexual trauma such as abuse or rape will need a multidisciplinary approach that may include a physician, physical therapist, and counselor or sex therapist to help them with pain and libido concerns.
- Physical therapists trained in the treatment of pelvic floor dysfunction are an essential part of the team approach to treatment of patients with neuromuscular pelvic floor pain or dyspareunia.
- Mindfulness is a tool utilized by therapists to help patients struggling with anorgasmia to improve the sexual experience.
- Engaging the partner in developing a treatment plan for sexual pain or decreased libido is important to obtain endorsement from the patient. This is especially the case if you are recommending abstaining from sex for a period of time to allow for healing.

Epidemiology

The prevalence of female sexual function concerns in the primary care clinic is difficult to quantify. Depending on which article you read, the prevalence is between 30% and 100% throughout the lifespan of a woman. The emotional toll that low libido, sexual pain, and anorgasmia take on women and their partners is significant. Patients experiencing sexual pain may be hesitant to discuss their concerns, or may have had a negative experience with a health care provider in the past when they tried to discuss concerns. On average, patients see more than six health care providers before the source of their sexual pain or libido concerns are adequately addressed. The occurrence of sexual concerns is higher in patients with depression, chronic pain, cancer diagnosis, bowel or bladder problems, and arthritis as well as in the postmenopausal years.

The general topic of female sexual function can be difficult to address in the primary care setting. When a patient presents for an annual exam, for example, and she says she is having pain with intercourse, it can cause anxiety on the part of the practitioner. This is often not a visit that can be accomplished in a 10-minute slot, so do not hesitate to tell the patient that you want to make sure you have adequate time to address her concern. If this was not the reason for her visit, consider asking her to schedule a visit when you have more time available so that you can best help her. Having a basic knowledge about a systematic approach to female sexual pain can help the practitioner have confidence in discussing this area of distress with women and their partners. We will approach this from two different areas of concern: decreased libido and sexual pain.

Pathophysiology, Diagnosis, Treatment: Decreased Libido

If a patient comes in complaining of decreased sex drive, you must consider many issues and life concerns that can impact intimacy. At the heart of hypoactive sexual desire disorder (HSDD) is an imbalance between excitatory (dopamine and norepinephrine) and inhibitory (serotonin) neurotransmitters in key regions of the brain. The difficulty in women is that libido is impacted by psychosocial factors such as relationship concerns, physical concerns such as obesity or arthritis, medical conditions, and medications. In research that includes women complaining of decreased libido, 30% may improve with placebo alone. This tells us how important addressing the psychosocial problems can be. The first question to consider is very simple and very powerful, "Do you like your partner?" This question alone can open up lines of communication and help sort out the cause of decreased desire (Table 1). If the patient indicates that her relationship is not currently rewarding or that she does not get along well with her partner, there is no pill that will solve desire concerns. Help the patient see that intervention in the form of counseling from a qualified provider may provide the best treatment for sexual concerns, or at least offer a good starting point. Make sure to follow your first question with the next question, "Does sex hurt?" If a woman has sexual pain, she may avoid sexual encounters. Helping the patient understand that sexual pain is not normal and is treatable may help her open up to you about the other important considerations for diagnosis including onset, duration, circumstances in which the pain occurs, and associated factors. You may also need to assess her willingness and desire to address the problem of pain. Some women are resistant to discussing their pain due to a history of poor medical encounters with physicians, previous trauma, or a foundational religious or cultural belief system surrounding sex. As stated previously, treatment for this condition is best guided by a careful history and discussion with the patient. If libido has been a concern for a significant period of time, encourage the patient to see a qualified counselor. Creating a list of resources available in your area is helpful to have on hand. If the patient previously had what she considers a good sex drive and this is a new problem, consider new medications, trauma, or recent events that may have triggered the onset of pain. See the list of medications impacting libido (Table 2). Although this is not exhaustive, if the patient is on more than one medication that affects sex drive you may need to work with her to adjust medications. If she is premenopausal and not on any medications, treatment for HSDD includes psychosocial intervention, lifestyle adjustment, and medications. Lifestyle adjustments may include changing her schedule so there is time for intimacy, as many patients are too busy to allow for

adequate time for arousal and a positive sexual experience. Also keep in mind the positive effect exercise has on sex drive, both directly by increasing norepinephrine and indirectly by improving stamina and self-image. Dietary considerations are also important, as women who are overweight or obese may suffer from low libido due to self-image, fatigue from hyperinsulinemia or diabetes, and gastrointestinal or other issues. Currently, there are two FDA approved treatments for HSDD: flibanserin (Addyi), which is a daily medication, and bremelanotide (Vyleesi), which is an episodic injectable medication. Both need to be prescribed by physicians experienced with the medication, indications, and potential side effects. Many other medications have been used to improve libido (see Table 2). Another consideration in women being treated for depression is to switch them from an inhibitory medication to one that may have a positive effect on libido. Encouraging patients to have open communication with their partners about what leads to pleasure and what does not is essential when addressing desire and arousal.

Pathophysiology, Diagnosis, Treatment: Sexual Pain

Dyspareunia can have many origins. The layered approach described by Dr. Coady is a systematic way to consider evaluation and also helps us understand the pathophysiology of this often complex problem (Table 3). Consider that the pain can be due to skin concerns or changes, neurologic problems, muscle pain, bowel conditions, bladder pain, medications (such as chemotherapy), and medical problems such as endometriosis or enlarged uterus. A careful history and exam are the most important diagnostic tools when helping discern the cause for sexual pain.

There are many different ways to evaluate a patient for pain with sex, and specifically, pain with intercourse. When you take a history in a patient complaining of sexual pain it is important to glean from her the duration, inciting factors, alleviating factors, previous treatment, and what she thinks is causing the pain. Understanding if she has primary (never had a sexual encounter without pain) or secondary (new onset, previous pain-free encounters) dyspareunia is also important. Primary sexual pain can be caused by a history of sexual trauma, tight hymenal ring, skin-level concerns such as atrophy, herpes, or lichen sclerosis, pelvic floor muscle pain, or internal pain such as endometriosis, ovarian cysts, or other pelvic organ pathology. Secondary sexual pain can include the same causes, but may be easier to treat depending on the sequence of events that led to the patient's onset of pain. When taking a history of the patient's pain, it is important to ask her if the pain is only on penetration or occurs through the entire encounter. Pain that only occurs with deeper penetration may be more likely pelvic floor muscle pain or endometriosis,

TABLE 1	Decreased Libido Diagnosis

Psychological: Do you like your partner?
- If they do not have a good relationship, you have an opportunity to point them to resources in your community to help them. Consider referral to a local marriage and family therapist or sex therapist to intervene.

Physical: Does sex hurt?
- If a woman is experiencing sexual pain she will also suffer from low libido as her brain is trying to protect her body from further trauma. Once you discover there is pain, work toward diagnosis or referral to a specialist.

Neurologic: Are you able to achieve climax?
- If a woman is unable to orgasm, she may have lower desire. Acknowledging her lack of climax and the distress it is causing is the first step in helping her decide if she wishes to explore this area further with a specialist.

TABLE 2	Treatment of Decreased Libido	
MAY INHIBIT DESIRE OR AROUSAL	**MAY IMPROVE DESIRE OR AROUSAL**	
SSRIs	Flibanserin (Addyi)	
Antipsychotics	Bremelanotide (Vyleesi)	
Benzodiazepines	Buspirone (BuSpar)	
TCAs	Bupropion (Wellbutrin)	
Lithium	Naltrexone/bupropion	
Phenytoin (Dilantin)	(Contrave)	
Trazodone (Desyrel)	SNRIs	
OCP	Transdermal testosterone	
Narcotics	Topical (vulvar/vaginal) estrogen	
Beta blockers	Topical (vulvar) testosterone	
Digoxin	Hormonal therapy in	
Spironolactone (Aldactone)	postmenopausal women	
Antihistamines		
Anticholinergics		

Abbreviations: OCP = oral contraceptive pill; SNRIs = serotonin–norepinephrine reuptake inhibitors; SSRIs = selective serotonin reuptake inhibitors; TCAs = tricyclic antidepressants.

TABLE 3	Sexual Pain Pathophysiology
CAUSES OF SEXUAL PAIN: THE LAYERED APPROACH	
Surface layer: lichen sclerosis, herpes, atrophy	
Nerve layer: localized provoked vestibulodynia, pudendal neuralgia	
Myofascial layer: chronic pain or acute secondary to injury	
Organ layer: ovarian cyst, endometriosis	
Body-wide systems: gastrointestinal, psychological (history of trauma or abuse)	

whereas pain that occurs with any touch points you toward vulvar causes such as lichen sclerosis or atrophic changes.

Once you have gathered a careful history, it is important to perform a careful exam. Start with a very careful inspection of the vulva. Note the presence of labia minora—if absent or blunted, this may be consistent with atrophy. Note the clitoral hood—if it is retracted or adhesions are noted the patient may have lichenification. A bright light and magnification (such as a colposcope) are often helpful in careful visualization. If no abnormalities are noted on careful inspection, look at the introitus. Patients with localized provoked vestibulodynia (LPV) may have an area of erythema at the 6 o'clock position of the introitus, just external to the hymenal ring. Show the patient a cotton swab and tell her you are going to touch areas on the vulva and you want her to tell you if anything hurts. With light pressure (depressing about 1 mm), touch the patient's thigh, slowly working inward to the labia. Touch the clitoris, the area around the urethra, and the area just external to the hymenal ring. Lastly, touch the area around the anus, as the rectal branch of the pudendal nerve could be the cause of pain. If she has significant pain on palpation with the swab along Hart's line, note the location of the pain and consider referral to a specialist who can address LPV. If the exam is normal and her pain does not appear to be external, do a careful exam of the pelvic floor. One way to do this is to insert one finger and gently palpate the muscles of the pelvic floor one at a time. A careful review of the anatomy of this area is helpful. If you are not comfortable evaluating for pelvic floor pain, referral to a sexual pain specialist or pelvic floor physical therapist is appropriate. If the patient does not seem to have pain on palpation of the pelvic floor muscles, performing a bimanual exam can be helpful; however, great care must be taken to avoid further trauma. I do not often do a bimanual exam on patients with a complaint of sexual pain as their pain is often elicited by the previously described exam. A speculum is rarely useful for these patients and should be avoided if they are complaining of pain with intercourse as you may cause her more pain and further discourage the patient from seeking medical help.

Your treatment plan for sexual pain must be guided by the differential diagnosis you develop following a careful history and exam. For skin concerns, clobetasol topical is the treatment for lichenification that includes lichen sclerosis and lichen simplex chronicus. If nerve or pelvic floor muscle pain is noted, sending the patient to a qualified physical therapist is a good first step. If this fails, or if the patient desires medication to help with the discomfort while working with a therapist, vaginal diazepam (Valium) can be utilized. The patient uses 10 mg at HS and is encouraged to use this as needed to help with more severe discomfort as many of the patients that have dyspareunia also have generalized pelvic floor pain that may interfere with sleep or activities of daily living. If physical therapy does not provide relief, a sexual medicine specialist may perform dry needling or trigger point injections to help with the pain. If the cause does not seem to be related to either skin or pelvic floor pain an ultrasound may help to identify ovarian masses or uterine enlargement and the patient may need referral to a gynecologist for surgical intervention. In cases of gastrointestinal dysfunction such as constipation or diarrhea, consider treatment of this dysfunction as it could lead to improvement in dyspareunia.

A Note About Atrophy

When considering atrophic or hypoestrogenic changes many clinicians think of a postmenopausal woman. When it comes to sexual pain, however, do not forget that atrophy can be seen in premenopausal women in the setting of cancer treatment, post-oophorectomy patients, and patients who have been on combined oral contraceptive pills for a period of time. Each of these patients may require a unique approach to treatment. For instance, if a woman is experiencing atrophy due to treatment of a nonhormonal cancer such as leukemia, treating her with systemic or local hormonal therapy is likely the most appropriate approach. If she is currently being treated for certain breast cancers, however, you should first consider nonhormonal treatments such as moisturizers and lubricants. When considering hormonal treatment options for these patients there is good evidence that vaginal and topical estrogen is quite safe when used appropriately. The lowest possible dose for the shortest duration is recommended in these patients and often providers will feel more comfortable considering hormonal therapies in consultation with the patient's oncologist. Be aware that many patients that are breastfeeding or are taking combination oral contraceptives may also experience atrophic changes that cause pain during sexual encounters. For these patients, topical vulvar hormones are often quite effective in relieving symptoms.

References

Coady D: Chronic sexual pain: a layered guide to evaluation, *Contemporary OB/GYN* 60:18–28, 2015.

Goldstein A, editor: *Female Sexual Pain Disorders Evaluation and Management*, Hoboken, 2009, Wiley-Blackwell.

Goldstein AT, Belkin ZR, Krapf JM, et al: Polymorphisms of the androgen receptor gene and hormonal contraceptive induced provoked vestibulodynia, *J Sex Med* 11:2764–2771, 2014.

Shifren JL, Monz BU, Russo PA, et al: Sexual problems and distress in United States women: Prevalence and correlates, *Obstet Gynecol* 112:970–978, 2008.

Stein A: *Heal Pelvic Pain: A Proven Stretching, Strengthening, and Nutrition Program for Relieving Pain, Incontinence, IBS, and Other Symptoms Without Surgery*, New York, 2009, McGraw Hill, 785–802.

UTERINE LEIOMYOMA

Method of
James W. Haynes, MD; and Theodore T. Tsaltas, MD

CURRENT DIAGNOSIS

- Uterine leiomyomas are the most common pelvic tumors in women.
- Risk factors include African American ethnicity, family history, obesity, decreased physical activity, nulliparity, and early menarche.
- Exact pathophysiologic mechanism is unknown but tumors consist of swirls of smooth muscle cells and fibroblasts.
- The primary clinical manifestations of uterine fibroids include heavy menstrual bleeding and pelvic pain.
- Ultrasonography is the primary diagnostic test of choice when fibroids are suspected.
- Differential diagnoses include adenomyosis, ectopic pregnancy, endometrial polyp, endometriosis, pregnancy, endometrial carcinoma, uterine sarcoma, and metastatic disease.

CURRENT THERAPY

- Therapy for uterine leiomyomas is based on symptoms, uterine size, and future fertility desires.
- Nonsurgical treatment options include nonsteroidal anti-inflammatory, progestational, and gonadotropin-releasing hormonal pharmaceutical agents.

- Indications for surgical treatment include uterine size >12 weeks, anemia from menometrorrhagia, soiling of clothing or bedding from menometrorrhagia, intractable dysmenorrhea or dyspareunia, and urinary or bowel obstruction.
- The definitive treatment option is hysterectomy with laparoscopic/robotic vaginal route being preferred.
- Other viable surgical interventions include myomectomy, uterine artery embolization, radio frequency focused ablation, and endometrial ablation.

Epidemiology

Uterine leiomyomas (fibroids) are the most common pelvic tumors in women. Thirty to fifty percent of premenopausal women have ultrasound evidence of fibroids without symptoms. Leiomyomas rarely occur prior to puberty, incidence increases with age, peaks at age 50, and decreases after menopause. African American women have a two- to threefold incidence compared to Caucasians, Asian, and Hispanic women who have similar frequencies of fibroids. African American women have an earlier onset of disease with an average age of onset 5 years earlier when compared to Caucasian women. Additionally, African American women have larger and more numerous fibroids compared to Caucasian women.

Risk Factors

Table 1 includes risk factors for uterine fibroid development. Consumption of vegetables and fruits, physical activity, dark-meat fish, vitamin D, and vitamin A is associated with a decreased risk of fibroids. Data are conflicting with respect to oral contraceptives and smoking, whereas breastfeeding, vitamin C, vitamin E, and folates have no association with the development of fibroids.

Pathophysiology

Uterine leiomyomas histologically consist of smooth muscle cells and fibroblasts, which ultimately form round, hard tumors. The exact pathologic mechanism of disease is unknown but a smooth muscle cell mutation has been hypothesized.

Prevention

There are currently no proven therapies that prevent uterine fibroid formation. Identification of the genes responsible for fibroid growth in patients genetically predisposed to fibroids could possibly lead to genomic-mediated prevention of fibroids.

Clinical Manifestations

Fifty to eighty percent of uterine fibroids are asymptomatic. Heavy menstrual bleeding and pelvic pain are the most common symptoms associated with uterine fibroids. Additional symptoms include secondary dysmenorrhea, abdominal distention, pelvic pressure, urinary symptoms (urgency, frequency, incontinence, and hydronephrosis), and bowel dysfunction, including constipation, back pain, dyspareunia, and infertility.

Diagnosis

Physical examination of the abdomen and pelvis may elucidate an enlarged uterus secondary to uterine fibroids. Transvaginal ultrasonography is 90% to 99% sensitive in the detection of uterine fibroids but may miss small or subserosal fibroids. Hysteroscopy or sonohysterography increase diagnostic sensitivity for subserosal myomas.

Differential Diagnosis

Diagnostic possibilities in patients presenting with symptoms of uterine fibroids include adenomyosis, ectopic pregnancy, endometrial polyp, endometriosis, pregnancy, endometrial carcinoma, uterine carcinosarcoma, uterine sarcoma, and metastatic disease.

Treatment of Myomas

Myomas are benign lesions; hence, there is no *a priori* requirement for treatment. Management is based on symptoms and

TABLE 1	Uterine Fibroid Risk Factors

African American descent
First-degree relative with uterine fibroid
Early menarche
Less than three obstetric deliveries
Five years since last birth
Obesity
Metabolic syndrome
Decreased physical activity
Childhood trauma
Beef, red meat, and ham
Vitamin D deficiency
Alcoholic beverages (especially beer)
Caffeine intake (younger women)
Hormone replacement therapy

TABLE 2	Treatment Options for Management of Uterine Leiomyomas

Definitive surgery
  Hysterectomy (various methods)
Palliative/uterine conserving surgery
  Myomectomy (open or laparoscopic)
  Hysteroscopic myomectomy
  Uterine artery embolization
  Radio frequency focused ablation
Symptomatic treatment
  Nonsteroidal antiinflammatory drugs (NSAIDs)
  Progestational agents
  Gonadotropin-releasing hormone (GnRH) agonists
  Endometrial ablation

patient's wishes. Three parameters control recommendations—uterine size, severity of symptoms, and the patient's interest in childbearing.

Table 2 outlines the limited number of options for management.

The indications for surgical intervention are tailored to the patient's individual problems and preferences. Common indicators for surgical intervention include uterine size >12 weeks (>14 weeks for some insurers to cover), anemia from menometrorrhagia, soiling of clothing or bedding from menometrorrhagia, intractable dysmenorrhea, dyspareunia or abdominal discomfort, and urinary or bowel obstruction.

The choice of procedure is strongly constrained by a patient's desire for future childbearing. This precludes hysterectomy and procedures that destroy the endometrial cavity to stop bleeding, such as endometrial ablations. Uterine conservation may prove impossible, or have marked complications, if the number of myomas is large.

Hysterectomy

Although multiple newer treatments have been introduced, hysterectomy remains the single most common management strategy. It is definitive, ending mass impingement symptoms, bleeding, pain, urinary frequency, and constipation with a single intervention. Recurrence of myomas is extremely rare after hysterectomy.

The route of hysterectomy remains under debate. When possible, a vaginal hysterectomy is the preferred route, as it has the lowest morbidity of all types. More than two-thirds of hysterectomies for myomas are still done by the open abdominal route, despite laparoscopy and robotic surgery having been repeatedly demonstrated as equivalent or superior for blood loss and complications.

Surgical complications of hysterectomy are common, but significant complications are rare. The most common problems are urinary tract infection (~25%) and superficial wound disruptions. More serious complications include deep venous thrombosis and pulmonary embolism, anaerobic pelvic cellulitis, and pneumonia. Organ injury to bowel, bladder, blood vessel, or ureter occurs in approximately 1 in 500 cases, 1 in 1000 for vaginal procedures. Bleeding sufficient to require transfusion occurs in about 1% of hysterectomies.

Myomectomy

Myomectomy is the procedure of choice for symptomatic myomas in women desiring fertility preservation. Myomas may be removed abdominally, vaginally, laparoscopically, or via hysteroscopy, depending on their size and location. Myomectomy does not necessarily lead to future cesarean delivery, but if uterine cavity integrity is violated or there is an extensive dissection, it then becomes mandatory.

Laparoscopic procedures are much less invasive, but require significant skill. Closure of myomectomy defects is also difficult and time consuming. Hysteroscopic resection is an elegant technique applicable only to intracavitary myomas.

Between 40% and 75% of patients undergoing myomectomy will have a future hysterectomy. Complication rates from open myomectomy are significantly higher than for hysterectomy, accounted for by fever and blood loss.

Uterine Artery Embolization

Uterine artery embolization (UAE) now accounts for approximately 3% of myomectomies. The method uses injectable microspheres placed under fluoroscopic guidance. It is effective for isolated myomas of moderate size (up to 5 cm), although lesions up to 9 cm have been treated by UAE. It is an outpatient procedure done in interventional radiology suites without entering the abdominal cavity.

There are several significant problems with UAE that have limited its broad application. Inflammatory mediators released by myoma necrosis can cause substantial cramping and bowel symptoms. Lesion defects cannot be closed, leading to uterine wall defects with secondary placental implantation abnormalities and uterine rupture in pregnancy. Vascular anatomy is quite variable, and microspheres can be injected into any of the branches of the internal iliac. This can lead to necrosis of bladder, buttock, or vulva. Limitations in available facilities as well as trained and experienced operators, combined with the significant complications, have limited usage of UAE.

Radio Frequency Ablation

This technique uses focused, high-frequency radio wave or ultrasound to cause mechanical destruction of myomas. It is an uncommon technique because of limited facilities and experienced practitioners. It does not have the potentially disfiguring complications of UAE but does have all its other problems, as well as risk of destruction of normal uterine tissue.

Observation

Since myomas are benign they may be observed if indications for hysterectomy noted above are not met. In this setting, the goal is symptom control. Cramping may be managed with nonsteroidal antiinflammatory drugs (NSAIDs). Acetaminophen (Tylenol) has less than 30% of the peripheral antiinflammatory activity of ibuprofen (Advil, Motrin), so that ibuprofen, aspirin, and other NSAIDs are much preferred. The individual drug choice relies with the patient and physician.

Bleeding can be improved with oral contraceptives, medroxyprogesterone (Provera), or tranexamic acid (Lysteda). In pooled results, tranexamic acid was more effective than medroxyprogesterone injection (Depo-Provera)[1] used over an equivalent time, reducing menstrual blood loss by 30%. Depo-Provera also provides contraception and uterine mass shrinkage at the expense of breakthrough bleeding.

Gonadotropin-releasing hormone (GnRH) agonists are extremely effective in affecting uterine mass shrinkage. Volume reduction up to 70% is possible with a 3-month course. Myoma re-expansion is, however, prompt and returns to original size. GnRH agonists are thus not suitable for treatment of myomas. Rather, they are best used to shrink myomas prior to surgery, making their removal easier and faster. As Depo-Provera achieves almost as much shrinkage, few insurers cover GnRH agonists for this purpose.

Managing Complications

Complications other than pain and bleeding are uncommon. Uterine mass and distortion can become so great as to obstruct venous return from the legs and pelvis, leading to deep venous thrombosis. Obstipation can occur, requiring manual disimpaction. More frequently, but still uncommon, urinary obstruction with retention or inability to void is possible.

The most frequent problem during observation of myomas is degeneration. Myomas are monoclonal tumors and thus have only a single, primary blood supply. If their growth outstrips available perfusion, the myocytes undergo necrosis. This can be quite painful. Management consists of NSAIDs, heavy hydration, rest, and occasional use of opioids. If initial interventions fail, inpatient management may be necessary for pain control. Intramuscular ketorolac (Toradol) materially reduces pain and can be used in an outpatient setting.

Leiomyomatosis peritonealis disseminata is a very rare condition where myomatous change occurs along the smooth muscle of the internal iliac arterioles. It can produce pelvic congestion, altered perfusion, and deep venous thrombosis. Management is by hysterectomy followed by GnRH agonists for 3 to 6 months. Complete resolution is the norm.

Myomas do not undergo malignant degeneration, but the frequency of uterine sarcoma is generally expressed as a proportion of all myoma cases. Uterine sarcomas are rare, with incidental discovery in a myomatous uterus in about 1 in 1000 myomatous uteri. Early epidemiologic studies on power morcellators indicated a rate of sarcoma in myomatous uteri of up to 1%. Larger studies have clearly shown this is a massive overstatement. Many hospitals are accordingly again allowing the use of power morcellation for myomectomy and laparoscopic removal of large hysterectomy specimens.

Some situations with myomas require prompt attention. Sudden, rapid uterine growth in a woman over 40 years of age should prompt consideration for sarcoma. Similarly, such tumors should not be morcellated but removed intact, either by open surgery or a laparoscopy with mini-lap.

Myomas can be confused with thecoma-fibromas, a benign ovarian tumor. The thecoma-fibroma is usually stone hard and heavily calcified on ultrasound, but can be so large and firm that it cannot be distinguished from a myoma. Laparoscopy can distinguish the lesions.

References

Al-Hendy A, Myers ER, Stewart E: Uterine fibroids: burden and unmet medical need, *Semin Reprod Med* 35:473–480, 2017.

Alternatives to Hysterectomy in the Management of Leiomyomas, *Am Coll Obstet Gyn Practice Bulletin* 96, August 2008.

De La Cruz MD, Buchanan EM: Uterine fibroids: diagnosis and treatment, *Am Fam Phys* 95(2):100–107, 2017.

Emanuel MH, Wamsteker K, Hart AA, et al: Long-term results of hysteroscopic myomectomy for abnormal uterine bleeding, *Obstet Gynecol* 93(5):743–748, 1999 May.

Lumsden MA, Hamoodi I, Gupta J, Hickey M: Fibroids: diagnosis and management, *BMJ* 35:h4887, 2015.

Palomba S, Zupi E, Falbo A, et al: A multicenter randomized, controlled study comparing laparoscopic versus minilaparotomic myomectomy: reproductive outcomes, *Fertil Steril* 88(4):933–941, 2007.

Pavone D, Clemenza S, Sorbi F, Fambrini M, Petraglia F: Epidemiology and risk factors of uterine fibroids, *Best Prac and Research Clin Obs Gynaecology* 46:3–11, 2018.

Spies JB, Bruno J, Czeyda-Pommersheim F, et al: Long-term outcome of uterine artery embolization of leiomyomata, *Obstet Gynecol* 106(5):933–939, 2005.

Tanos V, Berry KE: Benign and malignant pathology of the uterus, *Best Prac and Research Clin Obs Gynaecology* 46:12–30, 2018.

Wallach EE, Vlahos NF: Uterine myomas: an overview of development, clinical features, and management, *Obstet Gynecol* 104(2):393–406, 2004.

---

[1]Not FDA approved for this indication.

VULVAR NEOPLASIA

Method of
Christine Conageski, MD

CURRENT DIAGNOSIS

- Most cystic lesions are benign. Excision is reserved for symptomatic cysts and suspicious Bartholin's gland cysts, especially in women older than 40 years of age.
- All solid lesions should be biopsied for diagnostic purposes.
- Multifocal disease requires multiple biopsies to rule out invasive disease.
- Most premalignant and malignant lesions cause pruritus, discomfort, or a noticeable lesion.
- The vagina and cervix in women with dysplastic or malignant vulvar lesions should be evaluated.

CURRENT THERAPY

- Benign solid lesions should be excised.
- After ablative treatment of vulvar intraepithelial neoplasia (VIN), excise any residual lesions to rule out occult invasive disease.
- Avoid podophyllin and 5-fluorouracil in women of reproductive potential.
- Rule out synchronous neoplasms in women with Paget's disease.
- Invasion more than 1 mm requires radical excision and lymph node evaluation.

The female external genitalia includes the mons pubis, labia majora, labia minora, clitoris, perineal body, and the structures of the vaginal introitus or vestibule. Whether benign or malignant, vulvar neoplasms are uncommon, occur at all ages, and have varying characteristics. Therefore liberal use of biopsies is usually required for diagnosis and treatment decisions.

Benign Cystic Neoplasms

Benign cystic lesions of the vulva include Bartholin's duct cyst, sebaceous and epidermal inclusion cysts, mucinous cysts, Skene duct cysts, and cysts of the canal of Nuck. Bartholin's duct cyst, located in the posterior labia near the vaginal introitus, is most common. Treatment is usually not required in asymptomatic young women (<40 years). If the cyst is symptomatic or infected, however, drainage, marsupialization or use of a Word catheter, is indicated. Bartholin's gland carcinomas are rare, especially in women younger than 40 years of age. But if the mass feels firm or nodular, it should be biopsied.

Sebaceous and epidermal inclusion cysts are also common. They are prone to infection but rarely malignant. If an infection develops, they should be incised and drained. Mucinous cysts are rare and possibly arise from the minor vestibular glands. They are located anteriorly on the vulva, typically on the inner labia minora. Skene duct cysts are located next to the urethra. Excision of these cysts is necessary only if symptomatic.

Cysts of the canal of Nuck are located in the anterior portion of the labia majora at the termination of the insertion of the round ligament. These cysts represent herniation of the peritoneum through the inguinal canal and contain peritoneal fluid. If symptomatic, excision must be accompanied by closure of the fascial defect to prevent recurrence.

Benign Solid Neoplasms

The benign solid tumors of the vulva include fibromas, myomas, lipomas, hidradenomas, syringomas, myoblastomas, vestibular adenomas, and angiomas, among others. Benign pigmented lesions, such as nevi and seborrheic keratoses, may occasionally be found. Malignancy is rare, but most should be excised for diagnostic and therapeutic purposes.

Condyloma Acuminatum

Vulvar condyloma acuminatum is a sexually transmitted verrucous lesion of the vulva caused by human papilloma virus (HPV), most frequently types 6 and 11. These lesions are warty growths that frequently cover large areas of the vulva. Smoking and immunosuppression are risk factors. Representative biopsies should be obtained to document disease and rule out malignancy. Wide local excision can be used for small lesions, although these growths are usually best treated by ablation to avoid morbdity associated with excision.

Chemical ablative techniques include self or provider-administered medications. Self-administered medications include topical podofilox (0.5%, Condylox) or imiquimod (5%, Aldara). Podofilox is applied twice daily for 3 days, repeated weekly for 4 weeks and imiquimod is applied three times per week for up to 16 weeks. It is primarily an immune modulator. Providers may instead choose in-office application of trichloroacetic acid (Tri-Chlor), 5-fluorouracil[1] (1%, Fluoroplex or 5%, Efudex),[1] or podophyllin. Podophyllin and 5-fluorouracil should not be used in women who could become pregnant. Surgical ablative therapies include CO_2 laser vaporization and use of the Cavitron ultrasonic aspirator (CUSA), especially for extensive disease.

Intraepithelial Neoplasms of the Vulva

Vulvar Intraepithelial Neoplasia

Vulvar intraepithelial neoplasia (VIN) is a dysplastic condition of the squamous epithelium whose incidence is increasing, especially in younger women. There are two pathologically distinct types of VIN, usual and differentiated types.

The usual type has a strong association with HPV infections and thus shares similar risk factors with cervical intraepithelial neoplasias (CIN). These risk factors include early first intercourse, multiple sexual partners, smoking, and immunosuppression. Up to 22% of women have concurrent CIN lesions and up to 71% have had a previous, concomitant or subsequent history of vaginal intraepithelial neoplasia. Differentiated VIN is not associated with HPV and is found in relation to vulvar dermatoses such as lichen sclerosus. Differentiated VIN typically occurs in older women with a mean age of 67 years compared to 47.8 years in usual type VIN. Symptoms of both types include pruritus (most common), pain, a noticeable lesion, and discoloration. Most patients with HPV-related disease have multifocal lesions. Typical findings are raised white, gray, red, or mottled lesions; application of 4% acetic acid for several minutes can help identify faint lesions and outline abnormal vascular patterns. Diagnosis of VIN is made by punch biopsies through full thickness of the epithelium to rule out invasion. Usual and differentiated VIN have very different cancer progression risks, 5.7% for HPV-mediated VIN and 32.8% for differentiated VIN. Differentiated VIN, also, has a shorter time to progression, 22.8 months compared to 41.4 months.

Treatment of VIN can be categorized into excisional and ablative therapies. Management should be individualized to each patient taking into account risk of progression, distribution of disease and histologic features on biopsy. Often a combination of medical and surgical management is appropriate. Patients at risk for microinvasion (unifocal disease, raised lesions, older age, and prior radiation) should have the lesion excised completely if possible. Skinning vulvectomy is rarely used because of psychological and sexual consequences related to scarring and disfigurement.

The ablative therapies can be divided into mechanical and chemical. The mechanical method most commonly used is the CO_2 laser, although use of the CUSA is also described. Both can

---

[1] Not FDA approved for this indication.

TABLE 1	Recurrence of Vulvar Intraepithelial Neoplasia III
TREATMENT METHOD	**% RECURRENCE**
Chemical ablation	20–40
Mechanical ablation	20–40
Wide local excision	
Negative margin	15–25
Positive margin	30–45

TABLE 2	Incidence of Regional Node Metastases by Tumor Diameter
TUMOR DIAMETER (CM)	**% POSITIVE INGUINAL NODES**
<1	1–15
5–20	
25–35	
35–50	
≥50	≥50

TABLE 3	Incidence of Regional Node Metastases by Depth of Tumor Invasion
DEPTH OF INVASION (MM)	**% POSITIVE INGUINAL NODES**
<1	1–5
1–3	10–15
3–5	15–30
5–10	30–45

ablate large or multifocal lesions successfully with an excellent cosmetic and functional outcome. The chemical method most commonly used is topical 5-fluorouracil (5%, Efudex).[1] Because of its teratogenic potential, it should not be used in women who could become pregnant. It can be applied on two consecutive nights weekly for 10 weeks. An alternative ablative therapy is use of imiquimod[1] (Aldara), as described earlier. Because of the irritation caused by these topical therapies, many patients have problems with treatment compliance. Residual disease should be excised to rule out invasion.

Patients with VIN frequently have recurrent disease, regardless of the treatment method used (Table 1). Continued smoking increases this risk, so patients should be counseled in smoking cessation. In those patients whose cancers recur and are retreated, subsequent 5-fluorouracil prophylaxis, with a single application biweekly, is used successfully to minimize further recurrences.

Paget's Disease

Paget's disease of the vulva is an uncommon condition characterized by a patchy, eczematoid lesion that frequently covers much of the vulva. Most patients are postmenopausal and present with complaints of pruritus. Although Paget's disease is an in situ disease process, 15% to 25% of patients have an underlying malignancy, usually an adenocarcinoma of the apocrine glands but occasionally an invasive Paget's. In addition, up to 30% of patients have a synchronous adenocarcinoma of the breast, colon, rectum, or upper genital tract. Screening for these cancers is therefore recommended. To assess for invasion, the lesion should be excised via wide local excision or simple vulvectomy with at least 5 mm of the adjacent subcutaneous tissue. Achieving negative margin status is frequently difficult. However, the risk of recurrence is approximately 30% whether margins are negative or positive. Thus expectant management, reserving treatment for symptomatic recurrences, is usually recommended.

Invasive Vulvar Lesions

Less than 5% of gynecologic cancers arise on the vulva. Over 90% are squamous cell carcinomas. The etiology of this type appears mixed. The differentiated type is more common, occurs in older women (age 60–69, mean age 65) and is associated with vulvar dystrophies. The classic or usual type is predominantly associated with HPV-16. These women are slightly younger (age 45–52 years) and present with earlier stage disease. Other histologic types are melanomas (5%–10%), basal cell carcinomas (2%–3%), adenocarcinomas

(1%), and sarcomas (1%–2%). Most patients present with a combination of symptoms, including pruritus, discomfort, and complaints of a mass. Examination frequently reveals a suspicious lesion, which should be biopsied for diagnosis. Vulvar cancers typically spread by local extension and lymphatic dissemination. Factors that influence dissemination include tumor size (Table 2), depth of invasion (Table 3), lymphovascular space invasion, and tumor grade. Staging is surgical and classified using the tumor, nodes, and metastasis (TNM) system as well as the International Federation of Gynecology and Obstetrics (FIGO) system (Table 4).

Squamous Cell Carcinomas and Adenocarcinomas

Surgical management of squamous cell carcinomas and adenocarcinomas depends on the size, depth of invasion, and location of the lesion. The vulvar lesion is managed with a radical excision. Management of the groins is based on depth of invasion. Lesions with invasion of less than 1 mm (Stage IA) have minimal risk of lymphatic spread (<1%) and do not require lymphadenectomy. All others require surgical assessment of the lymph nodes. Lesions less than 2 cm in size of the primary tumor, greater than 2 cm from the vulvar midline and are of squamous histology require only unilateral lymphadenectomy. Those without these characteristics or have palpable lymph nodes of the contralateral side require bilateral assessment. This surgical approach is associated with significant morbidity including disfigurement, wound breakdown, and problems with lymphocysts and chronic lymphedema. For patients with very large lesions or lesions in sensitive areas such as the clitoris, preoperative radiation, followed by less radical excision of residual disease, may minimize problems with the vulvar wound. Current investigations are ongoing in the use of sentinel lymph node dissections as a method of minimizing the groin morbidity without sacrificing survival. Positive vulvar margins or metastases to lymph nodes are managed with postoperative radiation. Survival depends on stage at diagnosis (Table 5).

Verrucous Carcinoma

Verrucous carcinoma is a large exophytic tumor that resembles giant condyloma acuminatum. It is a variant of squamous carcinomas but has an excellent prognosis because of the lack of metastases. Verrucous carcinomas have a high tendency to recur and should be managed with radical local excision.

Malignant Melanoma

Malignant melanoma is the second most common vulvar malignancy. Most patients have disease on the mucosal surfaces of the vulvar introitus, clitoris, and labia minora. The vulvar lesion is treated by radical excision, but management of the groins is controversial. The risk of spread is significant with a tumor thickness greater than 0.75 mm, but survival at 5 years is only approximately 10% with groin node metastases. Some argue against node dissection for this reason. However, given some long-term survivors with modern melanoma therapy, either lymphadenectomy or sentinel lymph node dissection, as is done for other cutaneous melanomas, appears indicated.

Basal Cell Carcinoma

Basal cell carcinomas typically occur in elderly white women, are commonly located on the labia majora, and have characteristics

TABLE 4 Staging Vulvar Carcinoma

TNM CATEGORIES	FIGO STAGES	
T Primary tumor		
T0		No evidence of primary tumor
Tis		Carcinoma in situ
T1	I	Confined to vulva
T1a	IA	Lesions ≤2 cm in size, confined to the vulva or perineum and with stromal invasion ≤1 mm
T1b	IB	Lesions >2 cm in size OR any size with stromal invasion >1.0 mm, confined to the vulva or perineum
T2	II	Tumor of any size with extension to adjacent perineal structures (lower/distal 1/3 urethra, lower/distal 1/3 vagina, anal involvement)
T2	III	Tumor of any size with or without extension to adjacent perineal structures (lower/distal 1/3 urethra, lower/distal 1/3 vagina, anal involvement) with positive inguinofemoral lymph nodes
T3	IVA	Tumor of any size with extension to any of the following: upper/proximal 2/3 of urethra, upper/proximal 2/3 vagina, bladder mucosa, rectal mucosa, or fixed to pelvic bone
T3	IVB	Any distant metases including pelvic lymph nodes

TNM CATEGORIES	FIGO STAGES	
N Regional lymph nodes		
N0		No lymph node metastases
N1		One or two regional lymph nodes with the following features:
N1b	IIIAi	One lymph node metastasis, ≥ 5 mm
N1a	IIIAii	One to two lymph node metastases, < 5 mm
N2	IIIB	Regional lymph node metastasis with the following features:
N2b	IIIBi	Two or more lymph node metastases, ≥ 5 mm
N2a	IIIBii	Three or more lymph node metastases, <5 mm
N2c	IIIC	Lymph node metastasis with extracapsular spread
N3	IVA	Fixed or ulcerated regional lymph node metastasis

TNM CATEGORIES	FIGO STAGES	
M Distant metastases		
M0		No distant metastases
M1	IVB	Distant metastasis (including pelvic lymph node metastasis)

Abbreviations: TNM = tumor, node, metastasis; FIGO = International Federation of Gynecology and Obstetrics.

TABLE 5 Survival Rate by FIGO Stage for Patients With Invasive Squamous Cell Vulvar Cancer

FIGO STAGE	OVERALL SURVIVAL (PERCENT)		
	One year	Two years	Five years
I	96.4	90.4	78.5
II	87.6	73.2	58.8
III	74.7	53.8	43.2
IV	35.3	16.9	13.0

Abbreviation: FIGO = International Federation of Gynecology and Obstetrics.

similar to basal cell carcinomas at other sites. Treatment is wide local excision only because metastases are rare. Basal cell carcinomas are prone to local recurrence, however. A malignant squamous component must be ruled out because it should be managed as a squamous cell carcinoma.

Sarcomas

Leiomyosarcoma is the most common vulvar sarcoma and usually arises in the labia majora. Malignant fibrous histiocytoma is the second most common. Management of these lesions is radical vulvar excision.

References

Beller U, Quinn MA, Benedet JL, et al: Carcinoma of the vulva, *Int J Gynaecol Obstet* 95:S7, 2006.
Garland SM: Imiquimod, *Curr Opin Infect Dis* 16:85–89, 2003.
Homesley HD, Bundy BN, Sedlis A, et al: Prognostic factors for groin node metastasis in squamous cell carcinoma of the vulva (a Gynecologic Oncology Group study), *Gynecol Oncol* 49:279–283, 1993.
Hording U, Junge J, Lundvall F: Vulvar intraepithelial neoplasia III: a viral disease of undetermined progressive potential, *Gynecol Oncol* 56(2):276, 1995.
Krebs HB: The use of topical 5-fluorouracil in the treatment of genital condylomas, *Obstet Gynecol Clin North Am* 14(2):559–568, 1987.
Modesitt SC, Waters AB, Walton L, et al: Vulvar intraepithelial neoplasia III: Occult cancer and the impact of margin status on recurrence, *Obstet Gynecol* 92(6):962–966, 1998.
Phillips GL, Bundy BN, Okagaki T, et al: Malignant melanoma of the vulva treated by radical hemivulvectomy, a prospective study of the Gynecologic Oncology Group, *Cancer* 73:2626–2632, 1994.
Tebes S, Cardosi R, Hoffman M: Paget's disease of the vulva, *Am J Obstet Gynecol* 187:281–284, 2002.
Trimble CL, Trimble EL, Woodruff JD: Diseases of the vulva. In Hernandez E, Atkinson BE, editors: *Clinical Gynecologic Pathology*, Philadelphia, 1995, WB Saunders, pp 1–90.
Van de Nieuwehnof, et al. Vulvar squamous cell carcinoma development after diagnosis of VIN increases with age. *Eur J Canc* 45:851, 2009.
Wright VC, Chapman WB: Colposcopy of intraepithelial neoplasia of the vulva and adjacent sites, *Obstet Gynecol Clin North Am* 20(1):231–255, 1993.

VULVOVAGINITIS

Method of
Michael A. Malone, MD; and Vasudha Jain, MD

 CURRENT DIAGNOSIS

- Bacterial vaginosis: pH > 4.5; 20% clue cells, malodorous "fishy" discharge.
- Vulvovaginal candidiasis: pH 4–4.5; pseudohyphae, blastospores, thick curd-like discharge, vulvar inflammation.
- Trichomonas vaginitis: pH 5–6; motile, flagellated trichomonads, many white blood cells (WBCs), purulent discharge, vulvovaginal inflammation.

CURRENT THERAPY

TABLE 1 Characteristics for Different Causes of Vaginitis

	TYPICAL PH	DISCHARGE CHARACTERISTICS
Bacterial vaginosis	> 4.5	Thin, homogeneous, "fishy smelling" gray discharge.
Trichomonas	5–6	Greenish-yellow purulent malodorous discharge
Vulvovaginal candidiasis	4–4.5	Thick, white, adherent, "cottage cheese-like" discharge

TABLE 2 Common Findings With Each Cause of Vaginitis

FINDING	DISCHARGE WITH AN ODOR	INFLAMMATION	VULVAR INVOLVEMENT
Bacterial vaginosis	Yes	No	No
Candidiasis	No	Yes	Yes
Trichomonas	Yes	Yes	Yes

Vulvovaginitis is the general term for disorders of the vulva and vagina caused by infection, inflammation, or changes in the normal vaginal flora. Common symptoms include vulvovaginal erythema, discomfort, odor, and vaginal discharge. From a medical perspective, vaginitis is considered a relatively benign problem. However, it can cause physical discomfort, potential pregnancy risks, and, with chronic vaginitis, body image problems and sexual dysfunction. Despite a large percentage of patients who self-treat with over-the-counter treatments, vaginal symptoms are one of the most common reasons for gynecological consultation. A health care provider is consulted in the majority of women with symptoms of vaginitis, accounting for 10 million office visits a year in the United States.

This article addresses the most common causes of vaginitis, which account for over 90% of cases.

Differential Diagnosis

The common causes of vaginitis include bacterial vaginosis (40%–50% of cases), candidiasis (20%–25%), and trichomoniasis (15%–20%). Less common causes of these symptoms include vaginal atrophy, cervicitis, foreign body, irritants and allergens, and desquamative inflammatory vaginitis.

Clinical Manifestations

Common symptoms of vulvovaginitis include vulvovaginal erythema, discomfort, odor, and vaginal discharge. History can help differentiate the cause of the vaginitis. For example, a patient's lack of itching makes candidiasis less likely, while lack of perceived odor makes bacterial vaginosis unlikely and candidiasis more likely. However, none of the findings from the history alone allows a definitive diagnosis, as there is considerable overlap in symptoms among the different etiologies. Inspecting the vulva on examination can be helpful in determining the diagnosis. The vulva is often inflamed by candidiasis and trichomoniasis, but not by bacterial vaginosis. The characteristics of the vaginal discharge, if present, may help distinguish the type of infection (Table 1). However, the appearance of the discharge is unreliable and should not be the sole basis for diagnosis.

Diagnosis

Identifying the etiology of vaginitis is primarily based on patient history, pelvic examination, vaginal pH measurement (Table 2), whiff test, speculum examination, and microscopic evaluation of any discharge. Microscopic examination is used to look for hyphae, motile trichomonads, epithelial cells studded with adherent coccobacilli (clue cells), and increased numbers of polymorphonuclear leukocytes (PMNs). Initial office evaluation correctly results in a diagnosis of 60% of *Candida* vulvovaginitis, 70% of trichomoniasis, and 90% of bacterial vaginosis. If microscopy is negative, culture for *Candida* species or polymerase chain reaction (PCR) testing for *Trichomonas vaginalis* (the choice is dictated by the clinical findings) is important because microscopy is not sufficiently sensitive to exclude these diagnoses in symptomatic patients. Bacterial cultures are not indicated in women with vaginal discharge. In fact, they are frequently misleading, since a large variety of bacterial species colonize the vagina.

Trichomoniasis

Trichomoniasis is caused by the protozoan *T. vaginalis*, and most men and women who are infected do not have any symptoms. Symptomatic disease is characterized by purulent, malodorous, greenish-yellow discharge, which may be accompanied by burning, pruritus, dysuria, and/or dyspareunia, and postcoital bleeding. Although all of the common causes of vulvovaginitis have been associated with other sexually transmitted infections, trichomoniasis is the only one that is actually sexually transmitted. *T. vaginalis* can be identified in 70% of the male sexual partners of infected women, although carriage in men is often self-limited. *T. vaginalis* infection causes genital inflammation that increases the risk of HIV acquisition. Trichomonas infection increases the risk of complications in pregnancy. In a 2014 systematic review and meta-analysis of the association between *T. vaginalis* and perinatal outcomes, the risk of preterm birth was increased by 42% among infected women. The risks of premature rupture of membranes and delivery of a small for gestational age infant also increased. Although it should be treated when identified, whether the successful treatment of trichomonas in pregnancy affects or decreases these risks is unclear.

The diagnosis of trichomonas is based on laboratory testing including motile trichomonads on wet mount, positive culture, positive nucleic acid amplification test, and positive rapid antigen test (Box 1). As with other types of vaginitis, none of the clinical features of trichomoniasis is sufficiently sensitive or specific to allow a diagnosis based upon signs and symptoms alone. The presence of motile trichomonads on wet mount is diagnostic of infection, but they are identified in only 50% to70% of culture-confirmed cases. There should not be significant delay in viewing the wet prep slide for trichomonas as they only remain motile for 10 to 20 minutes after collection. Other findings suggestive, but not diagnostic, of trichomonas include an elevated vaginal pH (> 4.5) and an increase in PMNs on saline microscopy. Fixation and staining is not useful as trichomonads may lose morphologic characteristics during this process.

Culture (sensitivity over 80%) can be useful with a high clinical suspicion, but an absence of motile trichomonads on wet mount.

However, PCR detection has become the new gold standard for diagnosis of trichomoniasis and can be used with a urine or vaginal specimen. Rapid and point-of-care tests are available for the diagnosis of Trichomonas vaginalis in women and men with sensitivities of 83%–86% compared with nucleic acid amplification tests (NAATs) and can be performed in approximately 15 min. (Gaydos 2017) Papanicolaou (Pap) smear should not be used as a diagnostic test or screen for trichomoniasis. However, asymptomatic women with trichomonads identified on a Pap smear can be treated empirically or further evaluated by wet mount, PCR detection, or culture.

Treatment of trichomoiasis

The nitroimidazoles, metronidazole (Flagyl) and tinidazole (Tindamax), are the only medications approved by the FDA for the treatment of trichomoniasis. In randomized clinical trials, the recommended metronidazole regimens have resulted in cure rates of approximately 90% to 95%, and the recommended tinidazole regimen has resulted in cure rates of approximately 86% to 100%. Topically applied antimicrobials such as metronidazole gel (MetroGel Vaginal)[1] are unlikely to achieve therapeutic levels in the urethra or perivaginal glands and are not recommended. Sex partners of patients with *T. vaginalis* should be treated. Treatment of patients and sex partners results in relief of symptoms, microbiologic cure, and reduction of transmission.

Bacterial Vaginosis (BV)

Bacterial vaginosis is caused by a shift in the normal bacterial vaginal flora with a decrease of lactobacilli and overgrowth of *Gardnerella vaginalis*, *Mycoplasma hominus*, and anaerobes. The normal acidic (pH 4–4.5) vaginal environment helps maintain the normal vaginal flora and inhibits growth of pathogenic organisms. Disruption of the normal ecosystem can lead to conditions favorable for development of bacterial vaginosis. Factors that are associated with bacterial vaginosis include multiple sex partners, a new sex partner, sexual activity, phase of the menstrual cycle, contraceptive choice, pregnancy, foreign bodies, estrogen level, sexually transmitted diseases, antibiotics, and douching.

In contrast to trichomonas and candidiasis, bacterial vaginosis is associated with only minimal inflammation and minimal irritative symptoms. Clinical indicators of bacterial vaginosis include Amsel's criteria (Box 2). If two or three of the criteria are present, the clinical diagnosis of bacterial vaginosis can be made with a 90% sensitivity and 77% specificity. The presence of more than 20% clue cells on microscopy is the most reliable single finding predictor of BV. The use of culture for the diagnosis of bacterial vaginosis is not useful or recommended because the organisms that tend to overgrow are normal vaginal flora.

Use of a Gram-stained smear of vaginal discharge is the diagnostic gold standard for diagnosis of BV, but is typically performed only in research studies. In clinical practice, the diagnosis of BV is usually based on Amsel criteria, which is easy to use at the point-of-care. Using Gram's stain as the standard for diagnosing BV, the sensitivity of Amsel criteria is over 90% and has a specificity of 77%. It may have false positives with trichomonas,

as the first three Amsel criteria findings are sometimes present in patients with trichomoniasis. Commercial tests for diagnosis of BV are not commonly used, given the reliability and ease of Amsel criteria, but can be useful when microscopy is not available.

Changes suggesting bacterial vaginosis reported on a Pap smear do have good specificity but do not require treatment unless the patient is symptomatic (sensitivity 49%, specificity 93%). BV has been diagnosed using a swab of vaginal discharge obtained by the patient or clinician without speculum examination. However, omission of the speculum examination results in under-diagnosis and therefore is not ideal.

In pregnant patients, bacterial vaginosis has been associated with premature rupture of membranes (PROM), prematurity, chorioamnionitis, and low birth weight. In symptomatic patients, the treatment of bacterial vaginosis decreases those risks. In asymptomatic pregnant women, however, the effectiveness of treatments in reducing pregnancy-related risk is uncertain. There conflicting data on treatment of bacterial vaginosis in high-risk women and no evidence of risk reduction in low-risk women. Therefore the current data does not support universal screening and treatment of asymptomatic patients during pregnancy.

Treatment of Bacterial Vaginosis

Treatment is recommended for women with symptoms (Box 3). Besides relief of symptoms, potential benefits to treatment include reduction in the risk of acquiring sexually transmitted diseases (STDs). Because of positive results for much of the Amsel criteria with both BV and trichomonas (and lack of microscopy sensitivity for trichomonas), using a metronidazole regimen that covers both of these diagnoses (500 mg twice a day × 7 days)[1] may be reasonable when a patient meets the Amsel criteria. Treatment of male sex partners has not been beneficial in preventing the recurrence of BV. No data support the use of douching for treatment or symptomatic relief and it may increase the risk for relapse. Metronidazole appears to be safe in pregnancy, as multiple studies and meta-analyses have shown no association between its use during pregnancy and teratogenic or mutagenic effects in newborns. Several studies have evaluated the clinical and microbiologic efficacy of using intravaginal lactobacillus formulations to treat BV and restore normal flora, but further research is needed to determine possible utility.

Vulvovaginitis Candidiasis (VVC)

Candida is considered part of the normal vaginal flora, but overgrowth of the organism and penetration of superficial epithelial cells can result in vulvovaginitis. Vulvovaginal candidiasis often presents with marked inflammation, scant discharge, itching, dysuria, and dyspareunia (Box 4). Vulvar pruritus is typically the dominant symptom and erythema, excoriations, and fissures of the vulva and vagina may be present. There is often little or no discharge; when present, it is classically white, thick, adherent, and clumpy (cottage cheese-like) with no or minimal odor. The diagnosis of vulvovaginal candidiasis is based on history, examination findings, and the presence of *Candida* on wet mount or culture.

[1] Not FDA approved for this indication.

BOX 3 — Treatment of Bacterial Vaginosis

Recommended Treatment Regimens
Metronidazole 500 mg orally twice a day for 7 days[1]
Metronidazole gel (MetroGel-Vaginal) 0.75%, one full
 applicator (5 g) intravaginally, once a day for 5 days
Clindamycin (Cleocin) cream 2%, one full applicator (5 g)
 intravaginally at bedtime for 7 days

Alternative Regimens
Tinidazole (Tindamax) 2 g orally once daily for 2 days
Tinidazole 1 g orally once daily for 5 days
Clindamycin 300 mg orally twice daily for 7 days[1]
Clindamycin ovules 100 mg intravaginally once at bedtime for
 3 days

Recommended Regimens for Pregnant Women
Metronidazole 500 mg orally twice a day for 7 days
Metronidazole 250 mg orally three times a day for 7 days
Clindamycin 300 mg orally twice a day for 7 days

[1] Not FDA approved for this indication.

BOX 5 — Recommended Regimens for Uncomplicated VVC

Over-the-Counter Intravaginal Agents:
Butoconazole (Femstat, Mycelex), clotrimazole (Gyne-Lotrimin),
miconazole (Monistat), tioconazole (Vagistat)

Prescription Intravaginal Agents:
Butoconazole (Gynazole-1) 2% cream 5 g intravaginally for 1
 day
Nystatin 100,000-unit vaginal tablet, one tablet for 14 days
Terconazole (Terazol-7, Zazole): 0.4% cream 5 g intravaginally
 for 7 days
Terconazole (Terazol-3, Zazole): 0.8% cream 5 g intravaginally
 for 3 days
Terconazole (Terazol-3, Zazole) 80 mg vaginal suppository, one
 suppository for 3 days

Oral Agent:
Fluconazole (Diflucan) 150 mg oral tablet, one tablet in single
dose

BOX 4 — Classification of Vulvovaginal Candidiasis (VVC)

Uncomplicated VVC
Sporadic or infrequent vulvovaginal candidiasis
Mild-to-moderate vulvovaginal candidiasis
Likely to be *C. albicans*
Non-immunocompromised women

Complicated VVC (if any of below apply)
Recurrent vulvovaginal candidiasis (> 4 episode in 1yr)
Severe vulvovaginal candidiasis (extensive vulvar erythema,
 edema, excoriation, and fissure formation)
Non-albicans candidiasis
Women with uncontrolled diabetes, debilitation, or
 immunosuppression

BOX 6 — Treatment Regimens of Complicated Vulvovaginal Candidiasis (VVC)

Recurrent VVC Initial Regimen:
Any topical agent 7 to 14 days
OR
Fluconazole: 100, 150, or 200 mg orally once daily every third
 day for three doses[3]

Maintenance Regimens
Fluconazole 100- or 200-mg tab: 1 tab PO every week for 6
 months[3]

Alternative Maintenance Regimens:
Clotrimazole 200-mg suppository (Gyne-Lotrimin 3): 1
 suppository intravaginally qhs 2 x/week[3]
Butoconazole 2% cream (Femstat-3, Mycelex-3): 1 applicator
 (5 g) intravaginally qhs for 3 days

Severe VVC:
Any topical azole intravaginally once daily for 7 to 14 days
OR
Fluconazole 150 mg in two sequential doses (second dose 72
 hours after initial dose)[3]

[3] Exceeds dosage recommended by the manufacturer.

Candida albicans accounts for 80% to 92% of episodes of vulvovaginal candidiasis; *Candida glabrata* is the next most common species. For the diagnosis of a specific *Candida* species, a culture must be obtained, but culture is not necessary for diagnosis if microscopy shows yeast. A culture should be obtained in women with clinical features of vulvovaginal candidiasis, normal vaginal pH, and negative microscopy and in women with persistent or recurrent symptoms. Many of the women with recurrent symptoms have non-albicans infection resistant to azoles. If the wet mount is negative and *Candida* cultures cannot be done, empiric treatment can be considered for symptomatic women with any sign of VVC on examination.

Treatment of Vaginal Candidiasis
Asymptomatic women and sexual partners do not require treatment. The treatment regimen is based on whether the woman has an uncomplicated infection (90% of patients) or complicated infection (Box 5). Treatment with oral or topical azoles results in symptom relief in 80% to 90% of patients who complete therapy, and are more effective than nystatin. Intravaginal antifungals are available over the counter, although unnecessary or inappropriate use of these preparations is common and can lead to a delay in appropriate treatment. In pregnant women, topical azole therapies, applied for 7 days, are recommended. Oral azole therapy should be avoided in pregnancy, as case reports have described a pattern of birth defects after first trimester exposure to high dose oral azole therapy.

Candida glabrata should be considered in those who do not respond to recommended therapy or have multiple recurrences.

Candida glabrata does not form pseudohyphae or hyphae and is not easily recognized on microscopy, making diagnosis difficult without culture. The optimal treatment of non-albicans vulvovaginal candidiasis, such as *C. glabrata*, remains unknown but recommended regimens include an azole drug for a longer duration of therapy (7–14 days) (Box 6). If recurrence occurs, 600 mg of boric acid in a gelatin capsule[1,6] administered vaginally once daily for 2 weeks is recommended.

Severe vulvovaginitis is characterized by extensive vulvar erythema, edema, excoriation, and fissure formation. It is associated with lower clinical response rates in patients treated with short courses of topical or oral therapy. Recurrent vulvovaginal candidiasis (RVVC) is usually defined as four or more symptomatic episodes in 1 year. Routine treatment of sex partners in women with RVVC is controversial and does not appear effective. Vaginal cultures should be obtained from patients with RVVC to confirm the clinical diagnosis and to identify unusual

[1] Not FDA approved for this indication.
[6] May be compounded by pharmacists.

species (including non-albicans species), particularly *Candida glabrata*. Each episode of RVVC caused by *Candida albicans* tends to respond well to short-duration oral or topical azole therapy. However, for recurrent infections, some specialists recommend a longer duration of therapy before initiating a maintenance antifungal regimen. Suppressive maintenance antifungal therapies are effective in preventing episodes, but 30% to 50% of women will have recurrent disease when maintenance therapy is stopped.

Immunocompromised populations including pregnant women, diabetics with poorly controlled diabetes, women with HIV or other immunocompromised disease, and patients receiving immunosuppressive therapy need special considerations. This population does not respond well to short duration treatment and requires longer courses of 7–14 days. Vulvovaginitis due to *Candidia albicans* is common in pregnancy and only topical azoles for 7 days are recommended.

References

Anderson MR, Klink K, Cohrssen A: Evaluation of vaginal complaints, *JAMA* 291:1368–1379, 2004.

Centers for Disease Control and Prevention: Sexually transmitted diseases treatment I guidelines, 2010, *MMWR* 59(RR12):1–110, 2010. Available at: http://www.cdc.gov/std/treatment/2010 (accessed August 10, 2015).

Edwards T, Burke P, Smalley H, Hobbs G: *Trichomonas vaginalis*: clinical relevance, pathogenicity and diagnosis, *Crit Rev Microbiol* 10:1–12, 2014.

Gaydos CA, Klausner JD, Pai NP, Kelly H, Coltart C, Peeling RW: Rapid and point-of-care tests for the diagnosis of Trichomonas vaginalis in women and men, *Sex Transm Infect.* 93(S4):S31–S35, 2017.

Hainer BL, Gibson MV: Vaginitis, *Am Fam Physician* 83:807–815, 2011.

Huppert JS, Hesse EA, Bernard MC: Accuracy and trust of self-testing for bacterial vaginosis, *J Adolesc Health* 51:400–405, 2012.

Landers DV, Wiesenfeld HC, Heine RP: Predictive value of the clinical diagnosis of lower genital tract infection in women, *Am J Obstet Gynecol* 190:1004–1010, 2004.

Nyirjesy P: Management of persistent vaginitis, *Obstet Gynecol* 124(6):1135–1146, 2014.

Seæa AC, Miller WC, Hobbs MM, et al: *Trichomonas vaginalis* infection in male sexual partners: implications for diagnosis, treatment, and prevention, *Clin Infect Dis* 44:13–22, 2007.

Senok AC, Verstraelen H, Temmerman M, Botta GA: Probiotics for the treatment of bacterial vaginosis, *Cochrane Database Syst Rev* 2009, CD006289.

Silver BJ, Guy RJ, Kaldor JM, et al: *Trichomonas vaginalis* as a cause of perinatal morbidity: a systematic review and meta-analysis, *Sex Transm Dis* 41:369–376, 2014.

Singh RH, Zenilman JM, Brown KM, et al: The role of physical examination in diagnosing common causes of vaginitis: a prospective study, *Sex Transm Infect* 89:185–190, 2013.

Vulvovaginitis

18 | Pregnancy and Antepartum Care

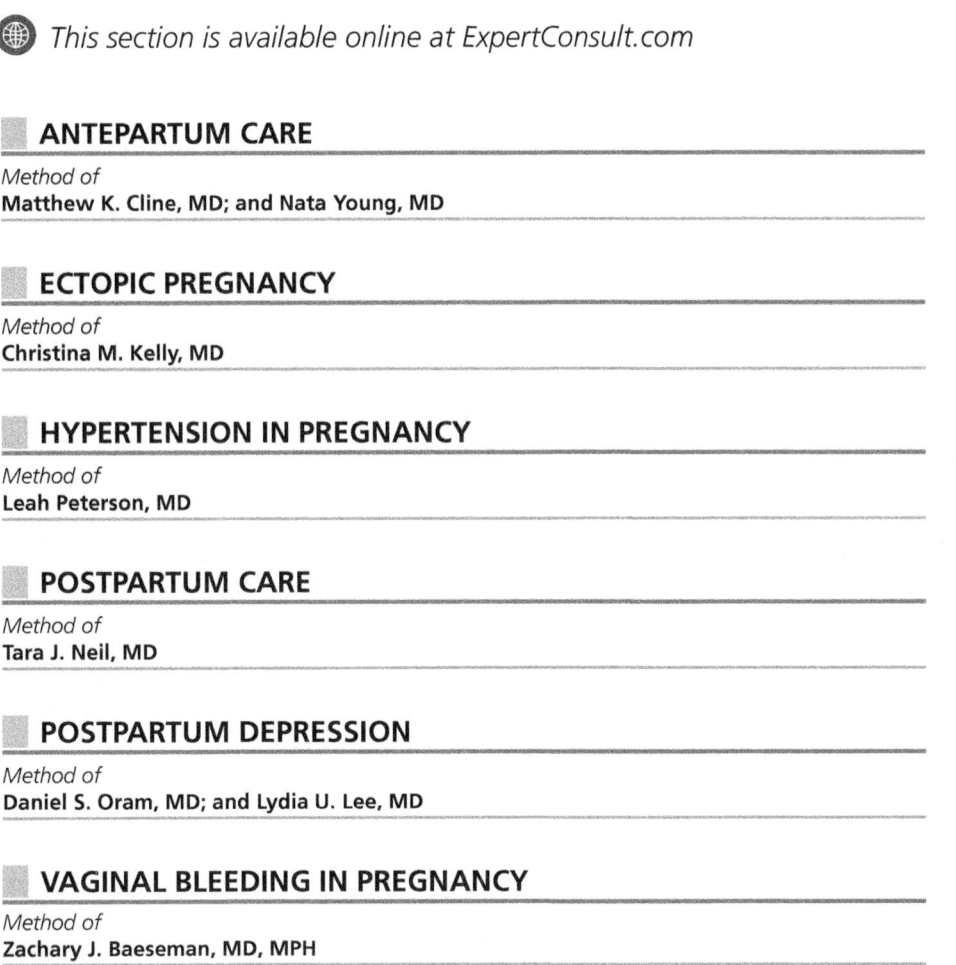

This section is available online at ExpertConsult.com

19 Children's Health

ACUTE LEUKEMIA IN CHILDREN

Method of
Patrick Brown, MD; and Stephen P. Hunger, MD

The word "leukemia" is derived from the Greek roots *leukos* (white) and *haima* (blood). Leukemia, cancer of the blood-forming cells, is characterized by a marked proliferation of abnormal leukocytes in the bone marrow and blood that may be associated with widespread infiltration in extramedullary sites including the central nervous system (CNS), testes, thymus, liver, spleen, and lymph nodes.

Classification

The first level of classification of leukemia is *acute* versus *chronic*. Acute leukemia is characterized by the predominance of very immature white blood cell precursors, or blasts, and is an aggressive, rapidly fatal disease if left untreated. Chronic leukemia is characterized by proliferation of relatively mature white blood cells and is typically an indolent disease.

The second level of classification is *lymphoid* versus *myeloid*, depending on whether the leukemic cells display characteristics of lymphocyte precursors or myelocyte (granulocyte, erythrocyte, monocyte, or megakaryocyte) precursors. Acute lymphoblastic leukemia (ALL) and acute myeloid leukemia (AML) account for the overwhelming majority of pediatric leukemias. Chronic leukemias are uncommon in pediatrics.

ALL and AML are further subclassified by morphology and expression of cell surface antigens using flow cytometry. For ALL, classification is largely based on cell surface and cytoplasmic marker expression (Table 1). AML cases are classified by characteristic chromosomal abnormalities (if present) or by light microscopic morphology in cases where these specific chromosomal changes are absent (Box 1).

Epidemiology

The incidence of childhood cancer is 14 cases per 100,000 children younger than 16 years of age per year, which translates into approximately 11,000 new cases per year in the United States. Leukemia accounts for approximately 30% of childhood cancers, making it the most common form of childhood cancer. The distribution of the major forms of leukemia is vastly different in children than in adults (Figure 1). In general, children are far more likely to have acute leukemia, and ALL is much more common than AML. In adults, most cases of leukemia are chronic, and AML is much more common than ALL.

The incidence of the various forms of leukemia varies by age in both children and adults (Figure 2). This is especially true for childhood ALL, for which there is a marked incidence peak in the 2- to 4-year-old age group. This ALL age peak is primarily found in children living in industrialized nations, leading to speculation that a common environmental exposure, coupled with age-related immunologic susceptibility, is at least partially responsible for many cases of ALL. Except for a small peak in infants, the incidence of AML is fairly constant in childhood but rises quickly in later adulthood.

Prognosis

One of the most dramatic success stories in modern medicine is the improvement in survival of children with ALL over the past four decades. Leukemia was once a uniformly fatal diagnosis, with less than a 5% to 10% cure rate until the mid to late 1960s. Today, approximately 85% of children with ALL are cured. The improved prognosis has been built on pioneering observations on the efficacy of multiagent systemic therapy and the importance of presymptomatic CNS treatment in the late 1960s and early 1970s. Further successive, incremental improvements in outcome have been achieved due to clinical trials conducted by large single centers and national and international cooperative groups that have successfully enrolled a high percentage of eligible children.

Similar approaches have unfortunately not been quite so successful in improving the prognosis of children with AML. Although approximately one half of children with AML are cured today, this has been accomplished by intensifying therapy to the point that the toxic death rate in the early phases of therapy is about 10%. Current research in AML is therefore focusing on developing novel molecularly targeted agents that hold the promise of improving efficacy and limiting toxicity.

Etiology

The question "What is the cause of leukemia?" can be considered on a few different levels. First, what is wrong with *this child* that caused the child to develop leukemia? Second, what is wrong with *the leukemia cell* that causes it to behave so badly? Third, what is wrong with *the leukemia cell's genes* that cause the cell to behave that way?

Predispositions

The answer to the first question is unknown in the vast majority of cases. Attempts to correlate various genetic features or environmental or infectious exposures with risk of childhood leukemia have been largely uninformative. It is presumed that children are particularly susceptible to ALL because of the marked expansion and genetic rearrangement of lymphocytes that occurs during early childhood as the result of exposure to a multitude of immunogenic antigens for the first time. The proliferation required to meet the constant demand for granulocytes, erythrocytes, and platelets is likely a setup for the development of AML in children.

Although a number of constitutional and single-gene disorders are known to confer an increased risk of childhood leukemia (Table 2), in total, these are involved in only a very small minority of cases. The most common of these is Down syndrome. Children with Down syndrome have a 10- to 20-fold increased risk of leukemia, with an approximately equal incidence of ALL and AML. The peak age at onset of leukemia for children with Down syndrome is earlier than for other children. Approximately 30% of Down syndrome children with AML have the megakaryoblastic form (M7AML), a subtype that is extremely rare in children without Down syndrome. In the newborn period, Down syndrome patients can present with transient myeloproliferative disease, a disorder distinguishable from congenital AML primarily by its spontaneous resolution within 3 months. Children with Down syndrome tend to present with biologically favorable subtypes of leukemia, but they also suffer increased toxicity from therapy. On balance, the prognosis of leukemia in Down syndrome patients is similar to that in other children.

The only environmental exposures that are known to predispose to leukemia are ionizing radiation (such as was seen with

TABLE 1 Classification of Childhood Acute Lymphoblastic Leukemia

ALL SUBTYPE	PHENOTYPIC MARKER				%	COMMENT
	CD19	CD10	CLG	SLG		
Pre-pre B	+	–	–	–	5	Mostly infants, poor prognosis, frequent *KMT2A* 11q23 rearrangements
Early pre-B	+	+	–	–	63	Common ALL, young children, good prognosis
Pre-B	+	+	+	–	16	Older children, good prognosis with intense therapy
B-cell	+	+	+	+	4	Burkitt leukemia, *MYC/Ig* fusion genes, good prognosis with lymphoma-type therapy
T-cell	–	–	–	–	12	Adolescents, anterior mediastinal mass, CNS involvement, good prognosis with intense therapy

Abbreviations: ALL = acute myeloid leukemia; clg = cytoplasmic immunoglobulin; slg = surface immunoglobulin; CNS = central nervous system.

BOX 1 Classification of Childhood Acute Myeloid Leukemia (World Health Organization Criteria)

Acute Myeloid Leukemia with Recurrent Genetic Abnormalities
Acute myeloid leukemia with t(8;21)(q22;q22), *(RUNX1/RUNX1T1)*
Acute myeloid leukemia with abnormal bone marrow eosinophils and inv(16)(p13q22) or t(16;16)(p13;q22), *(CBFβ/MYH11)*
Acute promyelocytic leukemia with t(15;17)(q22;q12), *(PML/RARA)*, and variants
Acute myeloid leukemia with 11q23 *(KMT2A)* abnormalities

Acute Myeloid Leukemia, Not Otherwise Categorized
Acute myeloid leukemia, minimally differentiated (FAB M0)
Acute myeloid leukemia without maturation (FAB M1)
Acute myeloid leukemia with maturation (FAB M2)
Acute myelomonocytic leukemia (FAB M4)
Acute monoblastic/acute monocytic leukemia (FAB M5)
Acute erythroid leukemia (FAB M6)
Acute megakaryoblastic leukemia (FAB M7)

Abbreviation: FAB = French–American–British classification.

Cellular Pathogenesis

Three major characteristics of leukemia cells distinguish them from normal hematopoietic cells. They proliferate rapidly, they do not differentiate, and they have defects in apoptosis. This results in a growth advantage for leukemia cells, leading to progressive replacement of the normal bone marrow with a massive clonal population of poorly differentiated leukemic blasts. Another characteristic of leukemia cells is their tendency to spread throughout the body and infiltrate organs other than the bone marrow. This is discussed in more detail in the section on clinical presentation.

Molecular Pathogenesis

As is true of most human cancers, development of leukemia is a multihit process. The initiating or permissive mutation (first hit) in childhood ALL often occurs in utero or early infancy, which is the peak of lymphocyte expansion and recombinase activity.

The initiating events are typically chromosomal rearrangements that activate expression of cellular proto-oncogenes by fusing them to transcriptionally active immunoglobulin or T-cell receptor genes or by joining two genes from different chromosomes to create a new fusion gene that encodes a chimeric protein with unique functional properties. The most common of these sentinel chromosomal rearrangements are translocations (exchanges of genetic material between chromosomes), which can serve as a unique marker of the malignant clone. Retrospective studies of blood obtained at birth and preserved on filter paper used for diagnosis of genetic disorders (Guthrie cards) of children who developed leukemia in early childhood have shown that leukemia-associated fusion genes were present at birth in a large percentage of children, including some who did not develop leukemia for one or more years.

In ALL, the promotional mutation (second hit) likely occurs during the proliferative stress generated by immune responses to exogenous antigens. Because these are maximal in the 2- to

atomic bomb survivors) and prior exposure to certain chemotherapy drugs (cyclophosphamide [Cytoxan], etoposide [Vepesid]). There is good evidence that in utero exposure to maternal diagnostic radiation also increases the risk of childhood cancer (including leukemia), particularly if the exposure is in the first trimester. Other environmental or infectious exposures remain unproved as risk factors for childhood leukemia, including electromagnetic fields from power lines.

Figure 1 Relative incidence of four major leukemia subtypes in children and adults. *Abbreviations:* ALL = acute lymphoblastic leukemia; AML = acute myeloid leukemia; CLL = chronic lymphoblastic leukemia; CML = chronic myeloid leukemia.

Figure 2 Age-specific incidence of acute lymphoblastic leukemia *(ALL)* and acute myeloid leukemia *(AML)* in children and in adults *(inset)*.

TABLE 2	Summary of Known Constitutional and Heritable Childhood Leukemia Predispositions		
DISORDER	**INHERITANCE**	**MALIGNANCY TYPE**	**COMMENTS**
Ataxia-telangiectasia	AR	ALL, NHL	*ATM* gene mutations lead to defective DNA repair
Bloom's syndrome	AR	AML, ALL	Chromosomal instability, sister chromatid exchanges
Down syndrome	Sporadic	AML, ALL	See text
Li-Fraumeni syndrome	AD	AML, ALL, many others	*p53* mutations; leukemias less common than solid tumors
Fanconi's anemia	AR	AML	Chromosomal instability, increased sensitivity to DNA damage
Kostmann's syndrome	AR	AML	G-CSF receptor mutations lead to agranulocytosis
Neurofibromatosis type 1	AD	AML, JMML, MPNST	*NF1* gene mutations lead to enhanced *RAS* signaling

AD, Autosomal dominant; *ALL*, acute lymphoblastic leukemia; *AML*, acute myeloid leukemia; *AR*, autosomal recessive; *G-CSF*, granulocyte colony-stimulating factor; *JMML*, juvenile myelomonocytic leukemia; *MPNST*, malignant peripheral nerve sheath tumor; *NHL*, non-Hodgkin lymphoma.

4-year-old age group, this is thought to explain the age peak of childhood ALL during these years. The lack of such a peak in AML suggests that the promotional mutations can occur at any time or are not triggered by immune stimulation. Examples of specific genetic hits known to be associated with the development of childhood leukemia are summarized in Table 3.

Clinical Presentation

Most symptoms and signs of childhood leukemia are the result of the propensity of leukemia cells to replace the bone marrow and infiltrate multiple other organs throughout the body. It is estimated that approximately 10^9 (1 trillion) leukemia cells are present in the child's body at diagnosis.

The replacement of normal bone marrow is responsible for the characteristic abnormal blood counts, which in most cases include the triad of neutropenia, anemia, and thrombocytopenia. Depending on the number of circulating leukemic blasts in the peripheral blood, the total white blood cell count may be low, normal, or high. The neutropenia is often profound (absolute neutrophil count <500/μL), and is associated with an increased risk of serious infection. Blood cultures and broad-spectrum intravenous antibiotic coverage are indicated in any patient with newly diagnosed leukemia and fever. Anemia is often manifested by fatigue, lethargy, headache, pallor, and, in extreme cases, congestive heart failure that may be precipitated by vigorous transfusion or intravenous hydration. Thrombocytopenia often leads to bruising and petechiae; however, clinically significant hemorrhage is uncommon in industrialized countries. Platelet transfusion is indicated for bleeding or for very low platelet counts (<10,000–20,000/μL).

Infiltration of organs other than the bone marrow with leukemia cells is responsible for additional presenting clinical features. Box 2 summarizes the organ systems most often involved in leukemia and the typical clinical manifestations.

Medical Emergencies in Childhood Leukemia

Newly diagnosed leukemia in a child is a medical emergency. There are several potentially life-threatening complications that may be present at diagnosis or can develop within a short time after diagnosis. The need to diagnose and treat potential infection in patients who are febrile and neutropenic was discussed earlier.

Tumor lysis syndrome (TLS) is a complication resulting from the rapid lysis of large numbers of tumor cells, releasing intracellular contents. Although TLS is seen most often after initial treatment with chemotherapy, it can also be present before therapy is initiated due to spontaneous lysis. Risk factors include high white blood cell (WBC) count, lymphadenopathy, hepatosplenomegaly, high mitotic index, and a diagnosis of ALL (especially Burkitt's leukemia or lymphoma and T-cell ALL). TLS is

TABLE 3	Summary of Common Leukemogenic Genetic Events	
ACUTE LYMPHOBLASTIC LEUKEMIA		**ACUTE MYELOID LEUKEMIA**

Chimeric Transcription Factors

t(12;21): *ETV6-RUNX1* fusion	t(8;21): *RUNX1-RUNX1T1* fusion
t(1;19): *TCF3-PBX1* fusion	t(15;17): *PML-RARA* fusion
t(4;11), et al: *KMT2A* fusions	t(9;11), et al: *KMT2A* fusions
t(8;14), t(8;22), t(2;8): Ig-MYC fusions	inv(16): MYH11-CBFB
T-cell receptor fusions	

Mutationally Activated Oncogenes

t(9;22): *BCR-ABL1* fusion	*FLT3* mutation
JAK2 mutation	*RAS* mutation
CRLF2 fusion	*KIT* mutation

Altered Tumor-Suppressor Genes

CDKN2A deletion	*NPM1* mutation
IKZF1 mutation	*WT1* mutation
TP53 mutation	*CEBPA* mutation

BOX 2	Summary of Clinical Manifestations of Childhood Leukemia*

Bone Marrow
Pancytopenia, bone pain

Reticuloendothelial System
Lymphadenopathy
  Hepatosplenomegaly

Thymus
Anterior mediastinal mass (T-cell leukemia)

Bones
Bone pain is common
  Fractures and chloromas are rare

Gums
Gingival hypertrophy (M4 and M5 AML)

Skin
Leukemia cutis and chloromas (M2, M4, and M5 AML, infant ALL)

Central Nervous System
Meningitis
  Cranial nerve palsies
  Rarely intracranial epidural or orbital chloromas (M4 and M5 AML, T-cell ALL)

Kidneys
Often infiltrated or enlarged
  Rarely acute renal failure (except in tumor lysis syndrome)

Genitourinary
Testicular enlargement (T-cell ALL)

---

*See Box 1 for descriptions of classifications.
Abbreviation: ALL = acute lymphoblastic leukemia; AML = acute myeloid leukemia; TBSA = total body surface area.

---

characterized by the triad of hyperuricemia (from breakdown of purines by xanthine oxidase), hyperkalemia, and hyperphosphatemia (with secondary hypocalcemia). Renal insufficiency can develop due to the nephrotoxic effects of precipitated urate crystals in the renal tubules; in severe cases, dialysis may be necessary.

Management consists of aggressive hydration to reduce tubular uric acid concentration. The xanthine oxidase inhibitor allopurinol (Zyloprim) is routinely used during the first 3 to 7 days of leukemia treatment to decrease uric acid production. Rasburicase (Elitek) (recombinant urate oxidase) is a new agent used in severe cases of TLS to almost instantaneously convert uric acid to the more soluble allantoin. Frequent electrolyte monitoring with standard management of abnormal levels is essential.

Hyperleukocytosis becomes a potential clinical problem when the WBC count rises above 100,000/μL. Markedly elevated WBCs lead to increased blood viscosity that can produce sludging of blood in the brain, lungs, kidneys, and other organs, causing clinical features such as depressed level of consciousness, stroke, intracranial hemorrhage, respiratory distress, hypoxia, diffuse pulmonary infiltrates, and renal insufficiency. The risk of hyperviscosity is higher with AML than ALL, because myelolasts are generally larger and stickier than lymphoblasts (likely due to increased expression of integrins and other mediators of cell–cell adherence on the surface of myeloblasts). Management consists of treating the leukemia as soon as possible and performing exchange transfusion or leukopheresis in cases where symptoms are prominent.

Life-threatening bleeding is another potential complication of leukemia. Although all patients with thrombocytopenia are at risk, patients with concomitant coagulopathy due to disseminated intravascular coagulation (DIC) are at particularly high risk. The leukemia subtype most commonly complicated by DIC and serious bleeding is acute promyelocytic leukemia (APL). This association results from the release of thromboplastin from the cytoplasmic granules in promyelocytic blasts. Aggressive blood product support and early treatment with the differentiation-inducing agent all-*trans* retinoic acid (ATRA) has been shown to decrease the risk of bleeding in APL. Despite these measures, up to 10% of patients die of bleeding complications during the initial weeks of therapy, and additional patients suffer lasting morbidity from retinal hemorrhages and nonfatal central nervous system hemorrhages.

Tracheal compression and superior vena cava syndrome can result from large anterior mediastinal masses, which are commonly present in T-cell ALL but are rare in other forms of leukemia. Patients can present with respiratory distress, cough, orthopnea, headaches, syncope, dizziness, facial swelling, or plethora. A chest x-ray should be performed to assess the mediastinum in any patient suspected to have ALL. If the mediastinum is enlarged, a CT is indicated to assess airway patency. This evaluation must precede any attempts at sedation for diagnostic procedures, because even light sedation can precipitate acute airway collapse. Diagnostic material should be obtained by the least invasive method possible before treatment. If necessary, emergent airway compromise can be treated with radiation or steroids, or both.

Differential Diagnosis

Although leukemia should be considered in cases of isolated neutropenia, anemia, or thrombocytopenia, the vast majority of leukemia patients present with depressions in more than one cell line. In suspected cases of immune thrombocytopenic purpura (ITP), for example, a careful review of the peripheral blood smear should be performed to rule out the presence of circulating leukemic blasts. Routine bone marrow aspiration is not necessary for children with ITP, but it should be performed in patients with atypical features, such as concomitant anemia or neutropenia, hepatosplenomegaly, bone pain, or significant weight loss. Treatment of ITP with corticosteroids should only be instituted after evaluation by an experienced hematologist.

Pancytopenia can be caused by diseases other than leukemia. Some viral infections have a propensity to suppress bone marrow function and cause low peripheral blood cell counts, including Epstein-Barr virus (EBV), herpes simplex virus (HSV), influenza, hepatitis viruses, and HIV. Infectious mononucleosis from EBV infection can be particularly difficult to differentiate from leukemia, because patients often have hepatosplenomegaly and circulating atypical lymphocytes (which can appear very similar to leukemic blasts). Pancytopenia on the basis of bone marrow failure (from acquired aplastic anemia or rare inherited bone marrow failure syndromes) can be distinguished from leukemia by bone marrow biopsy for assessment of overall marrow cellularity. Certain solid tumors have a tendency to metastasize to the bone marrow and cause cytopenias, including neuroblastoma, rhabdomyosarcoma, and retinoblastoma, but it is rare for pancytopenia to be the primary presenting feature in these cases.

Joint pain, fever, hepatosplenomegaly, and pallor are common presenting features in both systemic-onset juvenile idiopathic arthritis (JIA) and leukemia. A bone marrow aspirate should be performed to rule out leukemia before treatment with steroids in suspected cases of systemic-onset JRA.

Risk Stratification

In the last several years, treatment decisions for children with newly diagnosed acute leukemia have been based on the concept of risk stratification. Using factors identified during clinical trials to predict a high or low risk of relapse, patients are separated into risk groups before the start of treatment or at the end of the first month of induction therapy. The treatment plan is then tailored to the degree of risk. The desired result is that patients with relatively low-risk disease can be treated with less toxic therapy without compromising cure rates, and patients with high-risk disease receive more-intensive, potentially toxic therapy. The risk groups are currently defined based on several criteria and differ for ALL and AML. Different centers and cooperative groups typically employ different risk-stratification strategies.

In ALL, the initial risk assessment is based on two simple clinical parameters that are available immediately at the time of diagnosis (the National Cancer Institute [NCI] or Rome criteria): WBC count (>50,000/µL is high risk), and age (<1 year or >9 years is high risk). Further refinement of risk assignment is often based on a combination of leukemia phenotype (B- vs T-lineage), the presence of certain sentinel cytogenetic lesions, and how quickly the patient's leukemia responds to the first few weeks of therapy (rapid clearance of leukemia cells from the blood or marrow is associated with a lower risk of relapse).

Low-risk cytogenetic features include hyperdiploidy (≥50 chromosomes in the leukemia cells) or trisomies of specific chromosomes and the presence of a t(12;21) that results in TEL/AML1 fusion. High-risk cytogenetic features include hypodiploidy (<44 chromosomes in the leukemia cells) and the presence of either an 11q23 (MLL gene) rearrangement or a t(9;22), or Philadelphia chromosome, that creates a BCR/ABL fusion gene.

Early response has historically been measured by the response to a prednisone prophase that includes a single dose of intrathecal methotrexate and 7 days of prednisone, or by the percentage of blast cells remaining in the bone marrow after 7 to 14 days of multiagent therapy. Over the past 10 to 15 years, measures of tumor burden remaining in the marrow at the end of induction therapy (minimal residual disease) have been shown to be highly predictive of outcome and have been integrated into risk-stratification schemata of all of the major leukemia cooperative groups.

In AML, risk stratification is based largely on cytogenetics. Low-risk features include a t(8;21), which results in the AML1/ETO fusion, and either inv(16) or a t(16;16), both of which create the CBFβ/MYH11 fusion. High-risk features include monosomy 7 and abnormalities in the long arm of chromosome 5. In addition to these cytogenetic abnormalities, failure to achieve remission with induction chemotherapy is another high-risk feature in AML. All other cytogenetic abnormalities, as well as normal cytogenetics (which are seen in approximately 60% of cases), are considered intermediate risk. More recently, a specific type of genetic mutation in the tyrosine kinase gene FLT3 has been identified as another high-risk feature. This type of FLT3 mutation (called an internal tandem duplication [ITD]) occurs in 10% to 15% of childhood AML.

Treatment

There are significant differences in the specific treatments for ALL and AML, so they will be discussed separately. Table 4 summarizes the most salient features of the treatment for each.

Acute Lymphoblastic Leukemia

Treatment for ALL generally occurs in four phases: remission induction, CNS preventive therapy, consolidation, and

TABLE 4	Summary of Treatment for Childhood Leukemia	
CHARACTERISTICS	**ACUTE LYMPHOBLASTIC LEUKEMIA**	**ACUTE MYELOID LEUKEMIA**
Remission Induction		
Chemotherapy	4 wk with prednisone or dexamethasone, vincristine, PEG asparaginase, daunorubicin (not all cases)	Two courses (6–8 wk) with cytarabine (Ara-C), doxorubicin[1], others (e.g., etoposide[1], thioguanine)
Toxic death rate	Low (<3%)	High (>10%)
Remission rate	>98%	75%–85%
CNS Preventive Therapy		
Intrathecal chemotherapy	Methotrexate	Cytarabine
Cranial irradiation	For high risk (blasts in CSF at diagnosis and/or high WBC count)	None
Consolidation		
Chemotherapy	Combinations of various drugs (not cross-resistant) Intensity/duration based on risk stratification	Based on cytogenic/molecular risk group and minimal residual disease (MRD) Low risk: 2–3 additional courses Intermediate risk: If MRD-negative, treat as low risk; if MRD positive, treat as high risk High risk: BMT for patients with best available donor
Maintenance		
Chemotherapy	Low-dose oral (6-mercaptopurine and methotrexate) Total duration of therapy 2–3 y	No maintenance therapy (does not improve survival)

Abbreviations: BMT = bone marrow transplant; CNS = central nervous system; CSF = cerebrospinal fluid; HLA = human leukocyte antigen; WBC = white blood cell.
[1]Not FDA approved for this indication.

maintenance. Remission induction in ALL typically lasts 4 to 6 weeks and includes three to five systemic agents. Common to almost all regimens are a corticosteroid (either prednisone [Deltasone] or dexamethasone [Decadron]), vincristine (Vincasar), and PEG asparaginase (Oncaspar), which compose the three-drug induction. An anthracycline, typically daunorubicin (Cerubidine), is also included in many regimens (four-drug induction), with other agents such as cyclophosphamide (Cytoxan) or etoposide (VePesid)[1] used in a small minority of centers. More than 98% of children enter remission by the end of 4 weeks of induction therapy, and the mortality rate from toxicity during induction therapy is generally less than 2% to 3% in industrialized countries.

The concept that the CNS could be a sanctuary site for leukemia emerged in the mid 1960s when the introduction of multiagent systemic chemotherapy led to high remission rates, but a majority of patients relapsed within 6 to 12 months, with many of these recurrences being limited to the CNS. Routine introduction of presymptomatic CNS radiation in the late 1960s and early 1970s led to substantial increases in cure rates to approximately 50%. Modern CNS preventive therapy includes periodic administration of intrathecal chemotherapy (usually methotrexate) starting at the time of the first diagnostic lumbar puncture. Systemic agents with improved CNS penetration (dexamethasone rather than prednisone, higher doses of intravenous methotrexate) might also play an important role in CNS control. Cranial irradiation is currently reserved for patients at the highest risk for CNS relapse (e.g., those with high diagnostic WBC count or leukemic blasts in CSF at diagnosis). Over time, CNS radiation has been given to fewer and fewer ALL patients; some groups believe that it can be eliminated for all patients. With these modern strategies, the risk of isolated CNS relapse is less than 5%.

Following the induction of remission, patients receive additional chemotherapy designed to consolidate the remission. The intensity and duration of the consolidation phase are risk based, and alternating cycles of non–cross-resistant chemotherapy drugs are typically used. These consolidation or intensification phases typically last about 6 months and often include a reinduction phase similar to the first month of treatment.

It has been clearly demonstrated that the risk of relapse in ALL can be reduced with an extended phase of continuous low-dose chemotherapy (maintenance) that lasts until 2 to 3 years from the time of diagnosis. Oral 6-mercaptopurine (Purinethol) and methotrexate are used universally, with variable administration of intrathecal chemotherapy. Some centers or groups also employ periodic doses of vincristine and 5- to 7-day pulses of prednisone or dexamethasone. The optimal frequency of intrathecal chemotherapy treatments and vincristine and steroid pulses is uncertain and might depend on the intensity of therapy delivered during the induction and consolidation phases.

Acute Myeloid Leukemia

Remission induction in AML typically consists of two courses of very intensive chemotherapy with cytarabine (Tarabine) and doxorubicin (Adriamycin)[1], often combined with thioguanine (Tabloid) or etoposide. Remission rates are 75% to 85%, with about one half of the failures due to resistant leukemia and the others to mortality from toxicity (usually infection).

Similar to ALL, CNS preventive therapy in AML begins at diagnosis with intrathecal chemotherapy (usually cytarabine) and continues with additional periodic intrathecal treatments during consolidation. High-dose cytarabine, which is a key component of most AML treatment regimens, also contributes to CNS treatment. Cranial radiation is not typically administered by most groups to children with AML, except for treatment of chloromas (solid masses of leukemia cells) that do not resolve with chemotherapy.

Consolidation in AML is risk dependent. High-risk patients can be identified who have less than a 20% to 25% chance of cure with intensive chemotherapy. Most groups consider these patients to be candidates for BMT. If a matched sibling is unavailable, then alternative donor sources (e.g., matched unrelated bone marrow or umbilical cord blood) are usually offered. For low-risk patients, for whom the cure rate with chemotherapy alone approaches 70%, BMT is usually not offered in first remission, even for patients with a matched sibling donor. In addition, relapses in low-risk patients, unlike relapses in intermediate-risk or high-risk patients, can often be successfully treated with BMT in second remission, justifying reservation of BMT for use as a salvage therapy for low-risk patients. Consolidation in these cases consists of two to three additional chemotherapy courses that are slightly less intense and usually consist of cytarabine combined with drugs not used in induction, such as mitoxantrone (Novantrone) and L-asparaginase. For intermediate-risk patients, minimal residual disease (MRD) testing at the end of induction is increasingly being used to determine whether to consolidate with chemotherapy or BMT. Unlike ALL, most groups have found no benefit to extended maintenance therapy in children with AML.

Relapse

The most common site of relapsed leukemia is the bone marrow (with or without concomitant CNS involvement). Less common are isolated extramedullary relapses (CNS or testicular relapse in ALL, chloromas in AML). For both ALL and AML, a critical determinant of outcome following relapse is the time from diagnosis to relapse.

ALL patients who relapse within 18 months of initial diagnosis have a dismal outcome, with only about one half able to attain a second remission and less than 10% overall cure rate; the outcome is marginally better for those who relapse between 18 and 36 months after diagnosis. ALL patients with such early relapses are typically treated with 3 to 4 months of intensive therapy in an attempt to achieve a second remission and attain further cytoreduction, followed by BMT using a matched sibling or unrelated donor. In contrast, children with ALL who relapse more than 3 years after initial diagnosis have an approximately 95% chance of entering a second remission, and 40% to 45% can be cured with intensive chemotherapy; these patients are generally considered to be candidates for matched sibling, but not unrelated donor, BMT in second remission.

Overall, relapsed AML has a dismal outcome (long-term survival approximately 20%), and the approach is to attempt to reinduce remission and then proceed to BMT or investigational treatments. Even in this setting, there is clearly an improved outcome for patients who relapse after a prolonged initial remission (>12 months from the end of remission-induction therapy) compared with patients who have refractory disease or who relapse after a shorter period of remission.

New treatment strategies are urgently needed for patients with relapsed ALL and AML, because the current regimens produce poor results and are associated with a great deal of toxicity. The major clinical trial groups are testing novel and targeted therapies in these patient populations.

Late Effects

Approximately 70% of children with leukemia are cured of their disease. As the numbers of long-term survivors of childhood leukemia has grown, there has been increasing interest in assessing the late effects of leukemic therapy. In childhood ALL, with cure rates of 85%, a major effort is being made in ongoing clinical trials to reduce the intensity of therapy for lower-risk patients, with the hope of reducing late effects of therapy without compromising high cure rates. The most common late effects of leukemia therapy, with the known treatment-related risk factors and recommended diagnostic approach for each, are summarized in Table 5. Many pediatric oncology centers have developed late-effects

---

[1]Not FDA approved for this indication.

TABLE 5 Summary of Late Effects of Leukemia Treatment

LATE EFFECT	TREATMENT-RELATED RISK FACTORS	DIAGNOSTIC APPROACH
Bone	Avascular necrosis, osteonecrosis	X-ray and/or MRI of major joints for persistent pain
Cardiac dysfunction	Anthracyclines: cardiomyopathy (risk related to cumulative dose, higher risk in AML)	ECG or echocardiogram every 3 y (cardiomyopathy can occur decades after treatment)
Cataracts	CNS RT	Yearly eye examination
CNS and psychosocial	CNS RT, IT chemotherapy: learning problems, neurocognitive dysfunction	Yearly educational assessment, neurocognitive testing
Dental abnormalities	CNS RT	Dental examination at age 5
Endocrine and reproductive	CNS RT: pituitary dysfunction Alkylators: primary gonadal failure	Yearly growth curves, TSH, LH, FSH LH, FSH, estradiol or testosterone, semen analysis
Hepatic dysfunction	Methotrexate, 6-mercaptopurine, 6-thioguanine: late hepatic fibrosis	Yearly LFTs
Secondary neoplasms	CNS RT: brain tumors Alkylators or epipodophyllotoxins: secondary AML	MRI for symptoms Yearly CBC

Abbreviations: ALL = acute lymphoblastic leukemia; AML = acute myeloid leukemia; CNS = central nervous system; ECG = electrocardiogram; FSH = follicle stimulating hormone; IT = intrathecal; LFT = liver function test; LH = luteinizing hormone; MRI = magnetic resonance imaging; RT = radiation therapy; TSH = thyroid-stimulating hormone.

programs to conduct surveillance for the development of these problems and provide follow-up care to patients who develop late complications of therapy.

References

Brown P, Small D: FLT3 inhibitors: A paradigm for the development of targeted therapeutics for paediatric cancer, *Eur J Cance* 40:707–721, 2004.

Gaynon PS, Qu RP, Chappell RJ, et al: Survival after relapse in childhood acute lymphoblastic leukemia: Impact of site and time to first relapse—the Children's Cancer Group Experience, *Cancer* 82:1387–1395, 1998.

Gibson BE, Wheatley K, Hann IM, et al: Treatment strategy and long-term results in paediatric patients treated in consecutive UK AML trials, *Leukemia* 19:2130–2138, 2005.

Greaves MF, Wiemels J: Origins of chromosome translocations in childhood leukaemia, *Nat Rev Cancer* 3:639–649, 2003.

Hitzler JK, Zipursky A: Origins of leukaemia in children with Down syndrome, *Nat Rev Cancer* 5:11–20, 2005.

Meshinchi S, Alonzo TA, Stirewalt DL, et al: Clinical implications of FLT3 mutations in pediatric AML, *Blood* 108:3654–3661, 2006.

Moghrabi A, Levy DE, Asselin B, et al: Results of the Dana—Farber Cancer Institute ALL Consortium Protocol 95–01 for children with acute lymphoblastic leukemia, *Blood* 109:896–904, 2007.

Mrozek K, Heinonen K, Bloomfield CD: Clinical importance of cytogenetics in acute myeloid leukaemia, *Best Pract Res Clin Haematol* 14:19–47, 2001.

Pinkel D, Simone J, Hustu HO, Aur RJ: Nine years' experience with "total therapy" of childhood acute lymphocytic leukemia, *Pediatrics* 50:246–251, 1972.

Pui CH, Cheng C, Leung W, et al: Extended follow-up of long-term survivors of childhood acute lymphoblastic leukemia, *N Engl J Med* 349:640–649, 2003.

Pui CH, Evans WE: Treatment of acute lymphoblastic leukemia, *N Engl J Med* 354:166–178, 2006.

Pui CH, Mahmoud HH, Rivera GK, et al: Early intensification of intrathecal chemotherapy virtually eliminates central nervous system relapse in children with acute lymphoblastic leukemia, *Blood* 92:411–415, 1998.

Pui CH, Sandlund JT, Pei D, et al: Improved outcome for children with acute lymphoblastic leukemia: Results of Total Therapy Study XIIIB at St Jude Children's Research Hospital, *Blood* 104:2690–2696, 2004.

Ries LAG, Melbert D, Krapcho M, et al: *SEER Cancer Statistics Review, 1975–2004*, Bethesda, Md, 2007, National Cancer Institute.

Schrappe M, Reiter A, Zimmermann M, et al: Long-term results of four consecutive trials in childhood ALL performed by the ALL-BFM study group from 1981 to 1995. Berlin–Frankfurt–Munster, *Leukemia* 14:2205–2222, 2000.

Stahnke K, Boos J, Bender-Gotze C, et al: Duration of first remission predicts remission rates and long-term survival in children with relapsed acute myelogenous leukemia, *Leukemia* 12:1534–1538, 1998.

Wakeford R, Little MP: Risk coefficients for childhood cancer after intrauterine irradiation: A review, *Int J Radiat Biol* 79:293–309, 2003.

Woods WG, Kobrinsky N, Buckley JD, et al: Timed-sequential induction therapy improves postremission outcome in acute myeloid leukemia: A report from the Children's Cancer Group, *Blood* 87:4979–4989, 1996.

Woods WG, Neudorf S, Gold S, et al: A comparison of allogeneic bone marrow transplantation, autologous bone marrow transplantation, and aggressive chemotherapy in children with acute myeloid leukemia in remission, *Blood* 97:56–62, 2001.

ADOLESCENT HEALTH

Method of
Kari R. Harris, MD

CURRENT DIAGNOSIS

- In addition to general medical care, it is important to identify psychosocial health concerns at all adolescent visits.
- The key components of a psychosocial history are addressed in the HEADS private and confidential interview.
- Conducting a Home/Education/Employment/Activities/Accident Prevention/Diet/Disordered Eating/Drugs/Depression/Suicide/Self-harm/Sex/Sleep/Social Media (HEADS) interview is standard practice for adolescent care: it should be part of all adolescent well-checks and used, as time permits, in acute visits for teens who have high-risk behaviors or have no regular health care.
- High-acuity areas identified from the HEADS interview include substance use, disordered eating, sexual activity, and mental health.
- Depression screening should be part of well visits for all patients between 12 and 21 years of age.
- Substance use screening should be included in all adolescent well visits.
- HIV universal screening should be completed initially between 15 and 18 years of age and the need for re-screening reassessed annually.
- Immunization status should be assessed at every visit, with routine and catch up vaccines provided.

CURRENT THERAPY

- Long-acting reversible contraception (LARC) provides safe and effective contraception for teenagers.
- Emergency contraception should be offered within 5 days of unprotected sexual activity.
- Treatment for teens is often multidisciplinary involving subspecialists, mental health providers, medical or psychiatric inpatient units, and county welfare or health departments.

Setting the Stage for the Adolescent Visit

Comprehensive care for adolescents includes screening for high-risk behaviors in addition to routine medical care. To facilitate open communication, providers should be clear about consent and confidentiality policies in their practices. This can be achieved by discussing policies with patients and parents/caretakers during young adolescent visits (11–14 years) and by providing materials documenting the policies and practices such as a standard letter to parents. Policies can also be displayed in the office, provided in practice newsletters and materials, and made available through patient access portals.

Adolescent visits differ from early childhood visits in several important respects. At the beginning of the visit, time should be spent with both the teen and his/her parent or caregiver clarifying medical history and current concerns. The adolescent should then be offered time without the parent or caregiver present to discuss sensitive issues, including reproductive and mental health. At the end of the visit, the parent/caregiver should be provided with a summary of the visit, limited to the non-confidential portion, and including recommendations and arrangements for follow-up appointments.

Consent and Confidentiality Laws—Consent Does Not Equal Confidential

Consent and confidentiality laws vary by state. Most states allow minors to consent for reproductive health care, including testing and treatment for sexually transmitted infections. Most states also allow providers to prescribe contraceptives to minors. Many states have a "mature minor" statute that allows physicians to provide care if they deem the adolescent patient mature and capable of understanding the medical care. These laws give teens autonomy to consent to their own health care and they also enable care to be provided when a parent is unable to attend the appointment.

While consent and confidentiality laws are related, they are separate entities. Many states allow minors to consent for specific health services but do not prohibit a provider from informing the teen's parent/caretaker about that service. Even if allowed by law, expert consensus holds that such disclosures should only be made when in the best interest of the minor patient. The disclosure should not compromise future health care. Many teens will not seek reproductive health care if they have to involve a parent, making confidentiality necessary for comprehensive adolescent health care.

Confidentiality is limited when a minor patient is in direct harm such as intimate partner violence, sexual coercion or rape, certain pregnancy, suicidality, or self-harm. In such instances, a parent/caretaker should become involved, unless he/she is the perpetrator or some other extraordinary circumstances exist. Local authorities or social welfare agencies may also need to be contacted. These necessary breeches in confidentiality to protect safety must be explained beforehand to the patient and be included in written policies. Any breach of confidentiality must be carried out in a professional manner, explained sensitively to the patient and others, and well documented. Every attempt must be made not to compromise future care.

Information on consent and confidentiality laws for each state is available at the Guttmacher Institute website (guttmacher.org).

The HEADS Interview

The HEADS acronym provides a structured psychosocial history-taking tool that also screens for high-risk behaviors (Table 1). Although several variations of HEADS have been described, they all cover the most common risk categories for adolescents. Progressing from the least invasive topics to the most sensitive issues, HEADS covers all essential categories (see Table 1).

When using the HEADS interview tool, it is important to build rapport with the patient. The teen deserves explanation of why they are being asked personal questions and every attempt should be made to increase patient comfort and trust. The interview begins with questions regarding hobbies, school, and home life. Once rapport is established, questions proceed to more sensitive issues. Questioning should be open-ended, nonassuming and nonjudgmental. This allows for honest answers and does not discriminate among patients.

Home/Education/Employment/Activities/Accident Prevention

These topics begin the confidential interview with the least risky activities for adolescents. Although grouped together in this text, each category deserves its own time and questions (see Table 1). All adolescents should have a trusted adult with whom they can discuss concerns. Safety at home and school safety, including any bullying or coercion regardless of site or circumstances, should be discussed and addressed. Current school performance, concerns, grades and post-graduation goals should be discussed. After-school employment has benefits but can also negatively impact academic performance, mood, or family dynamics. These should be screened for and addressed if present. Healthy after-school activities should be encouraged. Predictably, adolescent illegal activity, drug use, and sexual activity peak during after-school hours. Participation in organized, supervised, extracurricular activities has been shown to decrease these risky behaviors and confer positive health and emotional benefits. Accidents remain the leading cause of death for this age group and prevention should be emphasized. Safety should be assessed at this time as well as throughout the course of the interview as it applies to each topic.

Diet/Disordered Eating

Nutritional health problems are of concern with adolescents. Many lifestyle habits, especially regarding nutrition, are formed during this period. Asking the teen to describe his/her typical diet provides insight on potential areas for improvement. Limiting portion sizes, avoiding excessive or late night snacking, and replacing sugary drinks with water is common advice for teens. This portion of the interview provides opportunity to screen for body image distortion or disordered eating. The growth chart should be reviewed and any significant weight changes discussed.

Drugs (Substance Use)

When asking about riskier behaviors, it is important to have rapport and trust. The subject of substance use can be broached by asking if peers use substances. Because alcohol, marijuana, electronic vaping, and tobacco use is so prevalent among high school students (reported by 60%, 35%, 42%, and 29%, respectively), this initial question can make a teen more comfortable moving on to talk about personal use. The CRAFFT acronym is a brief and effective screening tool designed specifically for use with adolescents and helps the provider determine if further conversation or evaluation regarding substance use is warranted. The questions are broken into part A and B. If a patient answers "yes" to any questions in A, then part B questions are asked. If the patient answers "yes" to two or more questions of part B, the screen is positive and further evaluation is recommended (Table 2). If necessary, referral should be made to a qualified mental health provider for treatment. Substance use is a leading cause of morbidity and mortality for teens in the United States, and teens who use substances at an early age are more likely to become addicted. Substance use should not be ignored or minimalized by providers. Counseling on prevention should contain a clear message of nonuse.

Depression/Suicide/Self-Harm

Depression screening is recommended at all well visits beginning at age 12. Several screening tools are available. Questions covering loss of interest in normal activities and feeling depressed, down, or hopeless open the door to more specific questions regarding signs and symptoms of depression. In addition to depressive feelings, teens should be explicitly screened for suicidal intention, past attempts, plans, self-harm, and safety. If a teen discloses an unsafe environment, law enforcement should be included in an immediate plan of care. If a teen is actively suicidal, then immediate inpatient treatment is warranted. Outpatient treatment for mental health disorders in teens includes cognitive-behavioral therapy with or without medication. For most teens, parental involvement is necessary when treating mental health disorders. If the provider feels the teen is unsafe due to their own actions or those of others, then the confidential interview is no longer appropriate and the caretaker must be included in the next stage of management.

TABLE 1 — HEADS Acronym With Sample Questions

H	Home	Who lives with you at home? Tell me about your relationships at home. Are you safe at home? Do you have a trusted adult to confide in at home? Do you have your own space at home? Have there been any changes at home?
E	Education	What grade are you in and what school? Is your school safe? Tell me about your friends. Does anyone bother you at school? How are your grades? Do you have any problems with school? Have you ever gotten in trouble for missing school? Do you plan to graduate? What do you want to do after graduation?
	Employment	Are you working? Do you like your job? Do you help your family with finances? Do you feel stressed because of work? is your family stressed by your work? How many hours a week do you work?
A	Activities	What do you do for fun? Who do you hang out with? Tell me what you do after school. Are you in any organized after-school or summer activities? Tell me about your hobbies. Do you have a religious preference?
	Accident prevention	Tell me about your activities. Do you wear a seatbelt? Do you wear a helmet while biking or using an all-terrain vehicle? Have you ever ridden with someone while they were under the influence of drugs or alcohol, or have you ever driven under the influence?
D	Diet/Disordered eating	Tell me about your diet. Do you eat breakfast daily? How many fruits and vegetables do you eat? How do you feel about your weight? Do you like the way you look? Have you ever not eaten to try to lose weight? Do you ever feel guilty about what you have eaten? Have you ever skipped meals or thrown up on purpose after you have eaten?
	Drugs	Have you seen drugs at your school? Do any of your friends smoke, drink alcohol, or use other drugs? Have you ever tried drugs? Have you ever been in trouble because of drug use?
	Depression	Do you ever feel sad, down, or depressed? Have you ever felt like you had nothing to look forward to? Do you still like to do the things you used to do?
S	Suicide/self-harm	Have you ever been so upset you have wanted to hurt yourself? Have you ever cut yourself? Have you ever thought about killing yourself or someone else?
	Sex	Are you in a relationship? When is the last time you had sex? Did you use a condom? Are you using anything to prevent pregnancy? Have you ever been tested for STIs? How many partners have you had? Tell me about your partner (age, gender, etc). Do you feel safe with your partner? Have you ever been forced to have sex or do something you were not comfortable with?
	Sleep	What time do you go to bed? Where is your cell-phone when you go to sleep? When do you wake up in the morning?
	Social Media	What social media sites do you have profiles on? Are you friends with people you do not know in real life? How much time do you spend on social media? Does this affect your grades? Tell me about your privacy settings. Do you have any trusted adults that can access your social media sites?

Adapted from: Klein, DA, Goldenring, JM. HEEADSSS 3.0: The psychosocial interview for adolescents updated for a new century fueled by media. Contemporary Pediatrics. 2014. Available at http://contemporarypediatrics.modernmedicine.com/contemporary-pediatrics/news/probing-scars-how-ask-essential-questions?page=full [accessed Oct 13, 2014].

TABLE 2 — CRAFFT Substance Use Disorder Screening Tool for Adolescents

PART A

During the past 12 months did you:
1. Drink any alcohol (more than a few sips)?
2. Smoked any marijuana or hashish?
3. Use anything else to get "high"?

If all answers in part A are negative then ask only question 1 of Part B.
If any answer to part A is positive then ask all 6 questions of Part B.

PART B

C	Have you ever ridden in a **CAR** driven by someone (including yourself) who was "high" or had been using alcohol or other drugs?
R	
A	
F	Do you ever use alcohol or other drugs to **RELAX**, feel better about yourself, or fit in?
F	Do you ever use alcohol or other drugs while you are **ALONE**?
T	Do you ever **FORGET** things you did while using alcohol or other drugs?
	Do your **FAMILY** or **FRIENDS** ever tell you that you should cut down on your drinking or drug use?
	Have you ever gotten into **TROUBLE** while you were using alcohol or other drugs?

The CRAFFT Screening Tool, The Center for Adolescent Substance Abuse Research (CeASAR), Children's Hospital Boston, 2009. Available at http://www.ceasar.org/CRAFFT/index.php [accessed August 17, 2017].

Sex

Nearly half of high school students have had sex. Of those, only about a quarter used reliable contraception at their last intercourse. Adolescents and young adults account for the majority of gonorrhea and chlamydia cases each year. Risk factors for morbidity related to sexual activity include early sexual initiation, increasing number of partners, substance use prior to sex, and unprotected sexual acts. Teenagers and men who have sex with men are the highest population groups at risk for sexually transmitted infections (STIs). STI screening should be discussed for those at risk. Recommendations are outlined in Table 3.

When discussing the sensitive issue of sex with teens, it is important to use neutral terms and remain nonjudgmental. It is also important to include gender identity in the history. Sexual history should include age of first sexual encounter, age of partner(s), gender of partner, number of partners, type of sexual activities, date of last sexual activity, and contraceptive and barrier use. Quality of relationships should also be assessed, as 7% of high school students report that they have experienced sexual dating violence including sexual coercion and rape. As with substance use, providers should relay a clear message of abstinence as the safest method to prevent morbidity.

Teens should be counseled on contraceptive options, emphasizing that LARC (intrauterine contraception and implants) is safe and the most reliable contraception available for teens. Quick-start contraception (prescribing or providing contraception at the current appointment) should be strongly considered to improve adherence in sexually active teens. The possibility of pregnancy

TABLE 3 Laboratory Screening and Procedure Recommendations

SCREENING	AGE	TEST/PROCEDURE	COMMENTS
Dyslipidemia	9–11 17–21	Nonfasting lipid profile	Once between 9 and 11 years and again between 17 and 21 years with annual risk assessment (NHLBI, AAP) Insufficient evidence for screening (USPSTF)
Hemoglobin/hematocrit	11–21	Verbally screen for risk	No routine testing recommended
Human immunodeficiency virus (HIV)	15–18	HIV 1–2 immunoassay	At least once if ≥ 15 years with more frequent screening if high-risk. (CDC, USPSTF, AAP) Screen MSM at least annually (CDC)
Chlamydia	Females < 25	NAAT at site of potential infection	Screen all sexually active women < 25 years at risk (USPSTF) or annually and MSM at least annually. (CDC)
Gonorrhea	Females < 25	NAAT at site of potential infection	Screen all sexually active women < 25 years at risk (USPSTF) and MSM at least annually (CDC)
Syphilis*	Adolescents at increased risk	Serology with confirmatory testing if positive	Screen persons at increased risk (USPSTF). Screen MSM at least annually (CDC)
Cervical dysplasia screening	21 years	Pap smear	Other indications for pelvic exam still apply but routine Pap testing < 21 years is not recommended (USPSTF, AAP)
Immunizations	All ages	Routine vaccinations per CDC guidelines	Immunization status should be assessed and routine and catch up vaccines provided at all adolescent visits

Abbreviations: AAP = American Academy of Pediatrics; CDC = Center for Disease Control and Prevention; MSM = Men who have sex with men; NAAT = nucleic acid amplification testing; NIHLB = National Heart, Lung, and Blood Institute; Pap smear = Papanicolaou smear; USPSTF = U.S. Preventive Services Task Force.
also consider screening high risk adolescents for Hepatitis B infection with HbsAg (USPSTF).

should be reasonably ruled out prior to providing contraception by taking a careful sexual history including last menstrual period, date of last sex, and method of contraception; lab work may also be considered (see the U.S. Selected Practice Recommendations for Contraceptive Use for guidance on how to reasonably rule out pregnancy https://www.cdc.gov/reproductivehealth/contraception/contraception_guidance.htm). If a patient has been recently sexually active, most non-intrauterine contraceptives have not been shown to harm an existing pregnancy. Nevertheless, counseling regarding this risk is important prior to initiating contraception, and pregnancy testing should be performed 2-4 weeks following contraception initiation. For patients who have had unprotected sex in the past 5 days, emergency contraception should be discussed and offered at the time of quick start contraception. Concurrent barrier contraception should be stressed. Aside from abstinence, male condoms are the most effective way of preventing STIs.

Sleep/Social Media

The conclusion of this format of the HEADS interview concerns less sensitive topics and allows for a comfortable close to the interview. Sleep is problematic for many teens and can usually be improved with better sleep hygiene. Encourage all teens to have a consistent sleep and wake time and 8 to 10 hours of sleep daily. Caffeinated beverages should be limited. Daily exercise should be recommended. The teen's bedroom should be free from distractions including screened electronic devices.

Social media and cell phones are now integral to popular culture. While these offer benefits to teens, use should be limited. Both social media and cell phones contribute to unintentional injuries, especially with distracted driving. In addition, personal information being shared on the internet through electronic media opens the teen up to vulnerability. Lastly, both can act as significant distractions from academic work, family time, and sleep. Discuss safe and appropriate use of electronic devices with patients and summarize to parents.

Summary

In addition to providing routine health care to teens, providers should focus on the psychosocial history. The HEADS acronym provides a tool for providers to approach these sensitive topics systematically. This interview should take place privately, respecting the teen's ability to consent for certain care, and when able, keeping care confidential. Providers should be familiar with the laws regarding consent and confidentiality of minors in their state. Although teens should be allowed access to confidential health care, providers must be aware that often the best care includes a trusted adult. Parents should be involved in their teen's care when appropriate. Once teens have been assessed for high-risk behaviors, problematic behaviors should be addressed and low-risk behaviors should be commended and encouraged.

References

American Academy of Pediatrics Committee on Practice and Ambulatory Medicine, Bright Futures: Recommendations for Preventive Pediatric Health Care, Committee on practice and ambulatory medicine, bright futures periodicity schedule workgroup, *Pediatrics* 2017: (No. RR-3). Available at https://www.aap.org/en-us/documents/periodicity_schedule.pdf [accessed Feb 10, 2018].

Centers for Disease Control and Prevention: Sexually Transmitted Diseases Treatment Guidelines, 2015, *MMWR Recomm Rep* 64:1–137, 2015. Available at https://www.cdc.gov/std/tg2015/ [accessed 02.10.18].

Cohen DA, Farley TA, Taylor SN, et al: When and where do youths have sex? The potential role of adult supervision, *Pediatrics* 110: Available at http://pediatrics.aappublications.org/content/110/6/e66.long [accessed 02.10.18].

Curtis KM, Jatlaoui TC, Tepper NK, et al: U.S. Selected Practice Recommendations for Contraceptive Use, 2016, *MMWR Recomm Rep* 65(No. RR-4):1–66, 2016. https://doi.org/10.15585/mmwr.rr6504a1 [accessed 14 March 2017].

Daniels SR, Benuck I, Christakis DA, et al: Expert panel on integrated guidelines for cardiovascular health and risk reduction in children and adolescents: summary report. National Heart, Lung, and Blood Institute. Available at http://www.nhlbi.nih.gov/health-pro/guidelines/current/cardiovascular-health-pediatric-guidelines/summary.htm [accessed 03.10.14].

Guttmacher Institute: *State policies in brief: an overview of minors' consent law*, Oct 1, 2014. Available at https://www.guttmacher.org/statecenter/spibs/spib_OMCL.pdf [accessed 10.13.14].

Kann L, McManus T, Harris WA, et al: Youth risk behavior surveillance—United States, 2017. *MMWR Surveill Summ* 67(No. SS-8):1–114, 2018.

Klein DA, Goldenring JM: HEEADSSS 3.0: the psychosocial interview for adolescents updated for a new century fueled by media, *Contemp Pediatr*, 2014. Available at http://contemporarypediatrics.modernmedicine.com/contemporary-pediatrics/news/probing-scars-how-ask-essential-questions?page=full [accessed 10.13.14].

Performing preventive services: a bright futures handbook, 2010, American Academy of Pediatrics Available at http://brightfutures.aap.org/pdfs/preventive%20services%20pdfs/physical%20examination.pdf [accessed 10.13.14].

The CRAFFT Screening Tool: The Center for Adolescent Substance Abuse Research (CeASAR), Children's Hospital Boston, 2009. Available at http://www.ceasar.org/CRAFFT/index.php [accessed 10.28.14].

U.S. Preventive Services Task Force. Recommendations for Primary Care Practice. Available at https://www.uspreventiveservicestaskforce.org/Page/Name/recommendations [accessed 02.10.18].

ASTHMA IN CHILDREN

Method of
Susan M. Pollart MD, MS; Katharine C. DeGeorge MD, MS; and Amanda Kolb, MD

CURRENT DIAGNOSIS

- Recurrent wheeze, cough, and shortness of breath are typical asthma symptoms.
- A personal or family history of atopy is associated with an increased risk of developing asthma.
- Atopy, allergic rhinitis, eczema, or nasal polyps are common comorbidities in patients with asthma.
- Specifically ask about symptom triggers such as allergens, irritants, exercise, stress, cold, or infection.
- At initial diagnosis, outline symptom frequency, intensity, and timing to classify severity.
- Physical examination of asthmatic children is often normal, but mucosal edema of nasal turbinates, eczematous skin rashes, tachypnea, tachycardia, expiratory wheezes, and lung hyperexpansion may be observed.
- In children older than 5 years, spirometry revealing an obstructive pattern at least partially reversible with bronchodilators confirms the diagnosis. In children younger than 5 years, diagnosis is based on history, physical examination, and a trial of antiasthma medications.
- Chest x-ray, complete blood count (CBC), and IgE levels are not routinely recommended but may be useful in certain situations.

CURRENT THERAPY

- The goal of asthma management is to reduce impairment of activities and decrease risk of exacerbations.
- Initial assessment of asthmatics should focus on symptom frequency, timing, and effect on activities.
- The four central components of management are frequent assessment and monitoring, patient education, controlling environmental triggers, and appropriate use of medication.
- Short-acting inhaled β₂-adrenergic receptor agonists such as albuterol (Proventil HFA) are the mainstay of acute therapy in an episode of bronchoconstriction. Additionally, anticholinergics such as ipratropium bromide (Atrovent HFA)[1] and systemic steroids are important components of managing an acute exacerbation. Magnesium sulfate[1], epinephrine (Adrenalin)[1], and terbutaline (Brethine)[1] are reserved for refractory cases, and terbutaline is only approved for children 12 years and older.
- Inhaled corticosteroids are the most effective daily controller medications for children. Long-acting β₂-agonists, leukotriene-receptor antagonists, and mast cell stabilizers are commonly used adjunctive therapies.
- Visits should be scheduled frequently in the outpatient setting to reassess symptom severity, adjust medications accordingly, and emphasize patient education.
- Consider increasing medication therapy only after assessing the patient's adherence and technique with medications. Consider a step-down in therapy only after 3 months of adequate control of symptoms.
- Involve both children and their caregivers in designing a written asthma action plan to empower patients in recognizing and managing escalating symptoms.
- Refer to a pulmonologist or allergist if there is any question regarding diagnosis or if symptoms are not adequately controlled with standard treatment. Consultation by a pulmonologist is recommended for children aged 5 years or older at ≥step 4 of therapy (or ≥step 3 in children younger than 5 years).

[1]Not FDA approved for this indication.

Epidemiology

Asthma prevalence in the United States has been on the rise since the 1990s. It is currently estimated that 9.6% of children younger than 18 years (7.1 million children) carry the diagnosis of asthma. Male sex, African American or Puerto Rican ethnicity, and lower socioeconomic status are associated with an increased risk of developing asthma. Prevalence estimates for these groups are as high as 11% to 16%.

Asthma has a significant impact on both school attendance and healthcare expenditures. According to the National Health Statistics Report in 2007, children made 640,000 emergency department visits and were hospitalized 157,000 times due to asthma. In 2008, it was estimated that there were 10.5 million missed school days, and about 5% of children reported long-term limitations on their usual activities due to asthma symptoms.

Although no significant difference in asthma prevalence between urban areas and suburban or rural areas has been found, there do seem to be broader geographic trends with higher prevalence in the Northeast and Midwest. Mortality rates remain low, but preventable deaths attributable to asthma exacerbations persist.

Risk Factors

No clear precipitating factors have been associated with the onset of asthma in children, but multiple risk factors for the development of this disease have been identified. Perhaps the strongest link is that between a family history of atopy, atopic dermatitis in infancy, or elevated serum immunoglobulin (Ig)E levels and subsequent sensitization to aeroallergens at 5 years of age. Recent observational data support an association with both prenatal exposure to acid-suppressive drugs and the use of antibiotics or acid-suppressive drugs in the first 6 months of life. Other identified associations include sensitization to dust mites, preterm birth, exposure to tobacco smoke, and certain respiratory infections such as respiratory syncytial virus (RSV).

Pathophysiology

Asthma is a chronic disease with recurrent episodes of reversible airway obstruction. It is thought to consist of three major pathophysiologic components: bronchoconstriction, airway inflammation, and bronchial hyperresponsiveness. Bronchoconstriction results from bronchial smooth muscle contraction in response to exposure to allergens, irritants, stress, infection, exercise, or certain medications such as aspirin and nonsteroidal antiinflammatory drugs (NSAIDs). Inflammation occurs via the T helper 2-(T_H2) and IgE-mediated pathways. Examination of the airways of asthmatics reveals inflammatory infiltrates consisting of neutrophils, eosinophils, lymphocytes, and activated mast cells. These mast cells release histamine along with other inflammatory mediators, causing airway edema, mucous hypersecretion, and airway hyperresponsiveness to environmental stimuli. Over time, remodeling can occur with airway thickening and smooth muscle hyperplasia, with a resulting decline in lung function and reduced response to therapeutic interventions.

Long-term observational studies have suggested that declining lung function is most commonly seen in children with symptom onset before 3 years of age. It still remains unclear whether older children or adults experience the same reductions in lung function.

Prevention

Primary prevention of asthma is a much-studied topic, yet few studies have successfully identified effective strategies for preventing asthma. The effect of breast-feeding on asthma prevalence has been a focus of extensive research. Much of the literature regarding breast-feeding as primary prevention for asthma suggests a protective effect of breast-feeding, but this has not been borne out consistently. A Cochrane review of 5 trials (952 pregnant or lactating mothers) found no evidence that avoidance of antigens (milk, eggs, nuts) by breast-feeding mothers during pregnancy or lactation decreased asthma or eczema in children through the study period of 18 months.

There is conflicting evidence regarding allergen avoidance to prevent the onset of asthma, although reducing exposure to inhalant allergens such as mites and pet dander can improve symptoms in patients with diagnosed asthma.

Based on the best available evidence, breast-feeding should be encouraged for its many known health benefits and potential protective effect on developing asthma. Avoidance of household dust mite aeroallergen or specific single food allergen exposure during pregnancy, breast-feeding, or first years of life is not routinely recommended for primary prevention of asthma. The topic of primary prevention of asthma warrants further study to clearly establish feasible preventive measures.

Clinical Manifestations

Asthma is characterized by recurrent episodes of wheezing, chest tightness, and shortness of breath. Asthma can also manifest as a chronic dry cough, especially if occurring at night. Young children commonly present with chronic cough alone, a form of asthma called cough-variant asthma. Wheezing that recurs in the setting of specific, predictable triggers is also a manifestation of asthma.

Diagnosis

A focused history revealing recurrent episodes of wheezing, shortness of breath, or cough suggests asthma and merits further investigation. In infants, the symptoms of asthma can involve difficulty feeding. Parents might also report intermittent grunting or loud breathing.

When taking the history, it is important to ask about symptom triggers, time course, and frequency of symptoms to assess severity. It is also important to discuss any family history of atopy, asthma, eczema, or nasal polyps. Triggers such as exposure to inhalant allergens (mold, dust, pollen, pet dander), irritants (chemicals, cigarette smoke), weather changes, intense emotion, physical activity, and viral illnesses should be elicited specifically (Box 1).

Begin the physical examination with measurements of height and weight and inspection of the growth chart. Most children do not have a significant growth or height reduction as a result of asthma. If a child's growth chart demonstrates a marked decrease in growth velocity, it is prudent to seriously consider alternative diagnoses.

1200

| BOX 1 | Asthma Triggers. |

Allergens
- Animal dander
- Pollen
- Dust mites
- Mold

Chemical irritants
- Tobacco smoke
- Wood stove smoke
- Air pollution
- Cleaning chemicals
- Gases

Medications
- Aspirin
- Nonsteroidal antiinflammatory drugs
- β-Blockers

Other
- Gastroesophageal reflux
- Exercise
- Respiratory infection
- Extremes of emotion
- Stress
- Changes in weather
- Cold air

Owing to the intermittent nature of asthma symptoms, children with asthma often have an entirely normal examination. Upper airway findings can include nasal polyps or mucosal edema of nasal turbinates. The skin examination might reveal signs of atopic dermatoses such as eczema or urticaria. Lung examination may be remarkable for wheezing, hyperexpanded barrel chest, increased respiratory rate, or tachycardia, depending on severity of symptoms. The American Academy of Allergy, Asthma, and Immunology recommends spirometry as a useful means of obtaining objective data on lung function and presence of obstructive disease for the diagnosis of asthma prior to trial of medications in patients over the age of 5 years, a recommendation that is part of the Choosing Wisely campaign.

Spirometry before and after short-acting β-agonist inhalation should show reversibility of obstruction in a patient with asthma. A rise in forced expiratory volume in 1 second (FEV_1) of 200 mL and 12% above baseline after bronchodilator is consistent with reversible obstruction. In children younger than 5 years, such studies might not be feasible. In these cases, diagnosis is based on history and physical. A trial of bronchodilator is helpful in establishing the diagnosis as well as ruling out other possible etiologies of symptoms.

A common presenting symptom of asthma in children is chronic cough. In cough-variant asthma, spirometry may be entirely normal. A trial of antiasthma medication that results in resolution of cough confirms the diagnosis.

Peak flow meters are useful in monitoring symptom severity but should not be used to make a diagnosis owing to wide variations in individual results and normal values.

Chest x-ray should be considered when ruling out alternative diagnoses but is not recommended in routine diagnostic testing for asthma. Allergy skin testing can identify potentially avoidable inhalant indoor allergens and, when appropriate, guide immunotherapy. Finally, checking a complete blood count with differential and serum IgE levels is not clearly indicated in making a diagnosis but may be useful in guiding treatment. Eosinophilia (greater than 4%) can indicate the need for controller medications, and patients with high levels of IgE have been shown to have a particularly good response to inhaled corticosteroids.

Finally, fractional exhalation of nitrous oxide (FeNO) may have an emerging role in diagnosing asthma and monitoring response to treatment. A 2016 Cochrane review of nine randomized controlled trials suggested that using FeNO levels to tailor treatment may decrease exacerbations overall, including severe exacerbations requiring oral corticosteroids.

Differential Diagnosis

The differential diagnosis of recurrent respiratory symptoms is broad and must be considered when initiating diagnostic workup. When creating a list of other diagnoses, it can be useful to consider the airway from the top down, as is shown in Box 2. Also keep in mind that the age of the patient and the chronicity of symptoms can point to certain diagnoses in your differential.

Treatment

To treat asthma in children appropriately, the severity of symptoms must first be assessed. This initial evaluation should be followed by an ongoing assessment that monitors response to therapy. The general tenets of asthma treatment are to reduce the functional limitations caused by asthma symptoms and decrease the risk of exacerbations, decline in lung function, and side effects of medications. The Expert Panel Report 3 of the National Asthma Education and Prevention Program describes a patient-oriented and clinically relevant approach to asthma management. Emphasis is placed on organized primary care visits and patient education. It is important to plan routine visits with a child's pediatrician or family doctor until symptoms are adequately controlled.

Once the diagnosis of asthma is made in a child, symptom severity should be assessed. To determine severity, the frequency of daytime symptoms, nighttime symptoms, frequency of using

Upper Airway
Allergic rhinitis
Sinusitis

Large Airway Obstruction
Vocal cord dysfunction
Laryngotracheomalacia (infants)
Tracheal stenosis (infants)
Vascular rings
Tracheal webs
Inhaled foreign body
Tumor or enlarged lymph nodes compressing airway

Small Airway Obstruction
Viral bronchiolitis
Pneumonia
Obliterative bronchiolitis
Cystic fibrosis
Bronchopulmonary dysplasia
Heart failure

Other
Gastroesophageal reflux disease
Swallowing mechanism dysfunction leading to aspiration

From National Heart, Lung, and Blood Institute, National Asthma Education and Prevention Program. Expert Panel Report 3: Guidelines for the diagnosis and management of asthma. Summary report 2007. http://www.nhlbi.nih.gov/guidelines/asthma/asthgdln.htm. Accessed March 13, 2018.

short-acting β_2-agonists, impairment of activities, frequency of exacerbations requiring oral steroids, and lung function must be considered (Table 1). Once severity has been classified, treatment can be started based on the stepwise approach outlined in Table 2. This stepwise approach is intended to be a guideline only. Clinical judgment is necessary when applying these guidelines to the individual patient. Children 12 years and older may be assessed and treated according to the guidelines described for adults.

Assessing adequacy of symptom control is essential to the management of asthma. At each follow-up visit, discussion should focus on how often the patient is having asthma symptoms and how much those symptoms are interfering with normal activities. Tools such as the Asthma Control Test (ACT) or the Childhood Asthma Control Test are helpful in measuring symptom control in a standardized fashion. Symptom assessment determines adequacy of control and guides changes in treatment, as shown in Tables 2 and 3. Frequency of primary care visits depends on severity of symptoms and can initially occur every 2 to 6 weeks. As control improves, visits may be decreased to every 1 to 6 months. At each visit, medications can be reviewed, doses adjusted, and education reiterated on recognizing symptoms and using medication and spacers.

Only after at least 3 months of adequate control should a decrease in therapy be considered. When stepping down, do so gradually, with frequent reassessment for reemerging symptoms. In the same way, therapy should be increased only after ensuring that the patient has been adherent with medications and is using the inhaler properly and that comorbid conditions have been addressed.

Referral to a pulmonologist or allergist is recommended if there is any question about the accuracy of diagnosis or if symptoms are difficult to control. The National Heart, Lung, and Blood Institute (NHLBI) recommends consultation if a child older than 5 years requires step 4 or higher level of therapy (step 3 or higher therapy in children younger than 5 years).

Allergen avoidance is currently recommended in the management of all asthmatics, but there is limited evidence that these interventions are effective. Various studies have analyzed the effects of controlling dust mite exposure with specially designed mattress and pillow covers and the use of air filtration units to reduce the burden of airborne pet dander. None of these studies have demonstrated clear benefits in decreasing symptoms. One nonblinded, randomized controlled trial, however, did suggest that removal of mold and improved ventilation in homes affected by mold can reduce symptoms of wheezing, rhinitis, and need for asthma medications.

Yearly inactivated influenza vaccination is recommended for all children with asthma to reduce the risk of complications due to influenza, although any clinically significant benefit for asthma symptoms is questionable. The live attenuated influenza vaccine (LAIV, FluMist) is typically not offered to children with asthma due to limited safety data in this population, although one trial of 2229 children and adolescents with asthma demonstrated better prevention of influenza with LAIV than injectable vaccine and no differences in asthma symptoms or exacerbations. Pneumococcal vaccination is recommended for all children and, based on limited data, appears to reduce asthma exacerbations in those with asthma. Finally, management of comorbid conditions has been implicated in improving asthma control. Sinusitis, allergic rhinitis, gastroesophageal reflux disease (GERD), and obesity are thought to contribute to asthma symptoms. Research has shown, however, that treatment of GERD with lansoprazole (Prevacid) in children with poorly controlled asthma not only had no effect on asthma symptoms but also led to a significant increase in respiratory infections.

Medications

Asthma management requires both fast-acting rescue medications and long-term controller medications. The goal of therapy is to find a daily controller medicine that reduces symptoms to such a degree that rescue medications are needed only rarely. Patients and their caretakers must be educated regarding the different roles of these two classes of medication to ensure the best possible outcome and the patient's safety.

Rescue Medications

Fast-acting bronchodilators are important in both the mildest and the most-severe forms of asthma. Short-acting β_2-adrenergic receptor agonists lead to smooth muscle relaxation and airway dilation. Racemic albuterol (Proventil) is a commonly used member of this group, but levalbuterol (Xopenex) is an alternative. Initially levalbuterol was thought to have fewer side effects, but studies have shown similar tolerability between racemic albuterol and levalbuterol. There is no significant difference in efficacy between these medications. Short-acting β_2-adrenergic receptor agonists should be reserved for relief of acute symptoms. Frequent use is discouraged and can indicate inadequate control of symptoms. See Table 4 for usual dosing of rescue medications.

Controller Medications

Inhaled corticosteroids are the most effective long-term controller medications. Some commonly used inhaled corticosteroids are fluticasone (Flovent), budesonide (Pulmicort), beclomethasone (Qvar), mometasone (Asmanex), and flunisolide (Aerospan). No single formulation of inhaled corticosteroid is superior to another. These medications reduce frequency of exacerbations and hospitalizations and are superior to leukotriene receptor antagonists and mast cell stabilizers. They are available as both metered-dose inhalers and dry-powder inhalers. A significant concern related to their use in children, however, is their effect on bone density and growth. High- and medium-dose inhaled corticosteroids have been linked to reduced growth velocity, but several studies have shown that at low doses they do not consistently or significantly affect growth. A systematic review and meta-analysis of effects of asthma and ICS on final adult height concluded that ICS does not significantly affect final adult height. To minimize potential side effects, continuous monitoring, reevaluation, and consideration of step-down treatment is imperative.

Long-acting β-agonists include salmeterol (Serevent) and formoterol (Foradil). They are an adjunctive therapy to

TABLE 1 Classification of Asthma Severity.

COMPONENTS OF SEVERITY	AGE (YEAR)	INTERMITTENT	PERSISTENT		
			MILD	MODERATE	SEVERE
Impairment					
Symptoms	All	≤2 days/week	>2 day/week but not daily	Daily	Throughout the day
Nighttime awakenings	0–4	0	1–2 times/month	3–4 times /month	>1 times /week
	≥5	≤2 times /month	3–4 times /month	>1 times /week but not nightly	Often 7 times /week
SABA for symptom control	All	≤2 days/week	>2 days/week but not daily	Daily	Several times /day
Interference with normal activity	All	None	Minor limitation	Some limitation	Extremely limited
Lung Function		Normal FEV$_1$ between exacerbations			
FEV$_1$ (predicted) or PEF (personal best)	≥5	>80%	>80%	60%–80%	<60%
FEV$_1$/FVC	5–11	>85%	>80%	75%–80%	<60%
	≥12	Normal	Normal	Reduced 5%	Reduced >5%
Risk					
Exacerbations requiring oral corticosteroids	0–4	≤1/year	≥2 times in 6 months or ≥4 wheezing episodes/year lasting >1 day *and* risk factors for persistent asthma		
	5–11	≤1/year	≥2 times/yearfnlowast*		
	≥12	≤1/year			
Starting Treatment					
Recommended step	0–4	Step 1	Step 2	Step 3	Step 3
	5–11	Step 1	Step 2	Step 3	Step 3 or 4
	≥12	Step 1	Step 2	Step 3	Step 4 or 5
	All				Consider short course of oral corticosteroids
	All	In 2–6 weeks, evaluate level of asthma control and adjust therapy accordingly. For children 0–4 years, if no clear benefit is observed in 4–6 weeks, stop treatment and consider alternative diagnosis or adjusting therapy			

*Consider severity and interval since last exacerbation. Frequency and severity can fluctuate over time for patients in any severity category. Relative annual risk of exacerbations may be related to FEV1.

FEV$_1$, Forced expiratory volume in 1 second; *FVC*, forced vital capacity; *PEF*, peak expiratory flow; *SABA*, short-acting β$_2$-adrenergic receptor agonist.
From National Heart, Lung, and Blood Institute. National Asthma Education and Prevention Program Expert Panel Report 3: Guidelines for the Diagnosis and Management of Asthma. NIH Publication Number 08-5846. Washington, DC: National Heart, Lung, and Blood Institute; 2007.

inhaled corticosteroids and should be considered in step 3 of management of symptoms in children aged 5 to 11 years and in step 4 in children 0 to 4 years old. Long-acting β-agonists carry a risk of increased asthma-related deaths, intubations, and hospitalizations when used alone. This risk was most prominent in children 4 to 11 years of age. Long-acting β-agonists should never be used as monotherapy and are not recommended for use during exacerbations. In combination with inhaled corticosteroids, however, long-acting β-agonists have been shown to increase asthma control days and improve lung function, but safety data are unclear based on a systematic review in 2012. For children younger than 5 years, data are lacking.

Leukotriene-receptor antagonists, including montelukast (Singulair) and zafirlukast (Accolate), are another adjunctive therapy to inhaled corticosteroids. They reduce symptoms by blocking the inflammatory cascade initiated by mast cells. In the mildest forms of asthma, they may be used as an alternative to inhaled corticosteroids if the steroids are not well tolerated or there is difficulty with administration. They are also effective in decreasing symptoms of exercise-induced asthma.

Mast cell stabilizers such as cromolyn sodium (Intal) or nedocromil (Tilade)[2] have a role similar to that of the leukotriene-receptor antagonists. They reduce inflammation by preventing mast cells from initiating the inflammatory cascade. They are safe and well tolerated in children, but the efficacy of inhaled sodium cromoglycate (Intal) has been brought into question after a systematic review found insufficient evidence to demonstrate sodium cromoglycate's superiority over placebo. The nedocromil inhaler has been discontinued owing to difficulties with manufacturing inhaler propellant.

Immunotherapy consists of subcutaneous injections of extracts from allergens intended to desensitize a patient to specific allergic triggers. This should occur in consultation with an allergist and may be considered at steps 2 through 6 of asthma treatment in children ages 5 to 11 years if asthma symptoms are predominantly allergic.

Immunomodulators are reserved for the most refractory cases of asthma. Omalizumab (Xolair, an anti-IgE agent) functions by blocking the binding of IgE to mast cells and basophils. It is

[2] Not available in the United States.

TABLE 2 Levels of Asthma Control.

COMPONENTS OF CONTROL	AGE (YEAR)	WELL CONTROLLED	NOT WELL CONTROLLED	VERY POORLY CONTROLLED
Impairment				
Symptoms	0–4	≤2 day/week but ≤1 times/day	>2 day/week or multiple times on ≤2 day/week	Throughout the day
	5–11			
	≥12	≤2 day/week	>2 day/week	
Nighttime awakenings	0–4	≤1 times/month	>1 times/month	>1 times/week
	5–11	≤1 times/month	≥2 times/month	≥2 times/week
	≥12	≤2 times/month	1–3 times/week	≥4 times/week
Interference with normal activity	All	None	Some limitation	Extremely limited
SABA for symptoms	All	≤2 day/week	>2 day/week	Several times/day
Lung Function				
FEV$_1$ (predicted) or PEF (personal best)	≥5	>80%	60%–80%	<60%
FEV$_1$/FVC	5–11	<80%	75%–80%	<75%
Validated Questionnaires				
ATAQ	≥12	0	1–2	3–4
ACQ	≥12	≤0.75	≥1.5	N/A
ACT	≥12	≥20	16–19	≤15
Risk				
Exacerbations requiring oral corticosteroids	0–4	≤1 times/year	2–3 times/year	>3 times/year
	5–11	≤1 times/year	≤2 times/year	
	≥12	≤1 times/year	Consider severity and interval since last exacerbation	
Reduction in lung growth	5–11	Evaluation requires long-term follow-up care		
Loss of lung function	≥12	Evaluation requires long-term follow-up care		
Treatment-related adverse effects	All	Medication side effects can vary in intensity from none to very troublesome and worrisome		
Recommended Treatment				
Recommended treatment actions	All	Maintain current step Regular follow-up q1–6 months Consider stepping down if well controlled for ≥3 months	Step up 1 step	Step up 1–2 steps and consider short course of oral corticosteroids
			Before stepping up, review adherence to medication, inhaler technique, environmental control, comorbid conditions If an alternative treatment option was used in a step, discontinue and use the preferred treatment for that step Reevaluate the level of asthma control in 2–6 weeks and adjust therapy accordingly For side effects, consider alternative treatment options	

ACQ, Asthma control questionnaire; ACT, asthma control test; ATAQ, asthma therapy assessment questionnaire; FEV$_1$, forced expiratory volume in 1 second; FVC, forced vital capacity; ICS, inhaled corticosteroid; PEF, peak expiratory flow; SABA, short-acting β$_2$-adrenergic receptor agonist.

From National Heart, Lung, and Blood Institute: National Asthma Education and Prevention Program Expert Panel Report 3: Guidelines for the Diagnosis and Management of Asthma. NIH Publication Number 08-5846. Washington, DC: National Heart, Lung, and Blood Institute; 2007.

effective in children with allergic triggers for their asthma but carries a risk of anaphylaxis, and the FDA, as of 2014, has associated its use with an increase in cardiovascular and cerebrovascular events. In 2013, the National Institute for Health and Care Excellence (NICE) issued a recommendation that omalizumab be reserved for children age 6 and older who have frequent need for oral steroids (more than three courses in prior 12 months) and who have failed optimized therapy. Optimized therapy is defined as a full trial of inhaled high-dose corticosteroid, long-acting β$_2$ agonist, leukotriene receptor antagonist, theophyllines, and oral steroids.

Early data from a randomized controlled trial suggests improved FEV$_1$ in children with severe symptomatic asthma with the addition of the anticholinergic drug tiotropium (Spiriva Respimat Inhaler) to an established regimen of medium- or high-dose inhaled steroids plus 1 or 2 other asthma control medications. More studies are needed to determine clinical benefit, however.

Theophylline (Theochron) was previously a mainstay of asthma management but is no longer a first-line medication. With the development of alternative treatments and because of theophylline's risk for toxicity, theophylline now has a lesser role

TABLE 3 Stepwise Treatment of Asthma in Children Younger than 12 Years.

STEP	0–4 YEARS OLD	5–11 YEARS OLD
Step 1: Intermittent	SABA as needed	SABA as needed
Step 2: Mild persistent	Add low-dose daily ICS *or* cromolyn *or* montelukast (Singulair)	Add low-dose daily ICS *or* cromolyn, LTRA, nedocromil (Tilade)* *or* theophylline
Step 3: Moderate persistent	Increase ICS to medium dose	Increase ICS to medium dose *or* continue low-dose ICS *plus* either LTRA, LABA, or theophylline
Step 4: Severe persistent	Medium-dose ICS *plus* either LABA or montelukast	Medium-dose ICS *plus* LABA, *or* medium-dose ICS *plus* either LTRA or theophylline
Step 5: Severe persistent	High-dose ICS *plus* either LABA or montelukast	High-dose ICS *plus* LABA, *or* high-dose ICS *plus* LTRA *or* theophylline
Step 6: Severe persistent	Step 5 *plus* oral glucocorticoids	Step 5 *plus* oral glucocorticoids
Step-Down Therapy	Step-Up Therapy	
If control is adequate for 3 months, may consider gradual decrease in treatment Reassess every 1–3 months	SABA use >2 times /week can indicate inadequate control Check for triggers, medication adherence, medication technique, comorbid disease before increasing therapy	

Children ≥12 years: May be treated according to adult guidelines.
Children 5–11 years: Consider subcutaneous allergen immunotherapy if the child has allergic asthma in steps 2 to 6.
All children: Treat comorbid conditions to improve asthma control.
For exacerbations that occur at all levels:
SABA 2–4 puffs every 4–6 h for 24 h with physician consultation.
Consider 3- to 10-day course of oral glucocorticoids for moderate to severe exacerbation.

*Not available in the United States.
ICS, Inhaled corticosteroid; *LABA*, long-acting β-agonist; *LTRA*, leukotriene receptor antagonist; *SABA*, short-acting β2-adrenergic receptor agonist.
From National Heart, Lung, and Blood Institute: National Asthma Education and Prevention Program Expert Panel. Report 3: Guidelines for the Diagnosis and Management of Asthma. NIH Publication Number 08-5846. Washington, DC: National Heart, Lung, and Blood Institute; 2007.

TABLE 4 Usual Dosing of Rescue Medications.

DRUG	BRONCHOSPASM*	ACUTE EXACERBATION†
Albuterol (Proventil HFA, AccuNeb)	>4 years old: 2 inhalations q4–6 h prn >2 years old (min 15 kg): 0.083% nebulized soln (AccuNeb) inhaled over 5–15 min 3–4 times daily prn	4–8 inhalations q20 min × 3 doses, then q1–4 h prn; add mask in children <4 years 0.15 mg/kg (min 2.5 mg) q20min × 3 doses, then 0.15–0.3 mg/kg up to 10 mg q1–4 h prn
Levalbuterol (Xopenex)	Age 0–4 years: 0.31–1.25 mg nebulized soln q4–6 h prn Age 5–11 years: 0.31–0.63 mg q8h prn	0.075 mg/kg (min 1.25 mg) q20min × 3 doses, then 0.075–0.15 mg/kg up to 5 mg q1–4 h prn

*Symptoms of obstruction, cough, wheeze, breathlessness.
†Symptoms of obstruction not responsive to initial SABA use.
SABA, Short-acting β2-adrenergic receptor agonist; *soln*, solution.
Information from Micromedex Healthcare Series. http://www.micromedex.com.

in asthma management. Currently it is used as an alternative treatment in the chronic management of patients with symptoms refractory to or intolerant of standard therapies. Use of this medication requires frequent monitoring of drug serum levels. It can cause nausea, vomiting, or tachyarrhythmias if dosing is too high. See Table 5 for usual dosing of controller medications.

Acute Asthma Exacerbations

Exacerbations consist of worsening wheezing, cough, or shortness of breath. They can vary in severity from mild to life threatening. When deciding how to treat a patient in an exacerbation, use the history and physical examination to determine severity. As in all emergency situations, first assess airway, breathing, and circulation. In a life-threatening exacerbation, the patient can appear confused or obtunded, may be bradycardic, and can have minimal respiratory effort, indicating imminent respiratory arrest. A child in a severe exacerbation can appear short of breath even at rest, may be agitated, and might only be speaking one word at a time. The child is likely tachycardic and tachypneic, with obvious use of accessory muscles. In certain cases, lung examination might not reveal wheezing owing to severe impairment of aeration; only after treatment does the wheezing become audible as air movement improves. In mild to moderate exacerbations, the patient

might only be short of breath with walking, might speak in short phrases or full sentences, and can appear anxious but not necessarily agitated. Lung examination can reveal wheezing.

The cornerstone of treatment of asthma exacerbations is rapid recognition of symptoms, correction of hypoxemia, and early initiation of short-acting β2-adrenergic receptor agonists and corticosteroids. Oxygen administration should be employed to maintain oxygen saturation at greater than 94%. Short-acting β-agonists are essential to relieve bronchoconstriction and may be combined with ipratropium (Atrovent)[1], especially if the patient is not responsive to initial therapy with a short-acting β2-adrenergic receptor agonist alone. Ipratropium should not be used as single agent, as it is less efficacious than β2 agonists alone as well as combined β2 agonist–ipratropium. Combined anticholinergics and short-acting β-agonists were shown to decrease the rate of hospitalization in children when used during initial treatment for an exacerbation with a NNT of 16; however, benefit did not persist with continuing use during hospitalization. In 2006, a systematic review showed that metered-dose inhalers with a spacer are as effective in administering β-agonists as nebulizers are in children older than 2 years. It was noted in the same study that

[1] Not FDA approved for this indication.

TABLE 5	Usual Dosing of Controller Medications		
DRUG	**FORMAT**	**DOSING**
Fluticasone	HFA: 44, 110, 220 μg per puff DPI: 50, 100, 250 μg per inhalation	Low: 88–176 μg BID Medium: 176–440 μg BID High: > 440 μg BID
Fluticasone-salmeterol	DPI 100 μg/50 μg MDI 45 μg/25 μg	> 5 y: DPI 100 μg/50 μg BID MDI 90 μg/50 μg BID
Budesonide	DPI90 or 180 μg/inhalation	Low: 90–180 μg BID Medium: 180–360 μg BID High: 540–720 μg TID–QID
Budesonide-formoterol	HFA MDI 80 μg/4.5 μg per inhalation	80 μg/4.5 μg–160 μg/ 9 μg BID
Beclomethasone HFA	40 or 80 μg per puff	Low: 80–160 μg BID Medium: 160–320 μg BID High: > 320 μg BID
Mometasone aerosol DPI	110, 220 μg per puff	110 μg daily is max per guidelines for 4–11 yR
Flunisolide HFA	80 μg per puff	5–11 y: 80–160 μg BID >12 y: 160–320 μg BID
Montelukast	4 mg or 5 mg chewable tablet 4 mg granule packets	< 5 y: 4 mg hs 6–14 y: 5 mg hs
Zafirlukast	10 mg tablet	Ages 5–11 y: 10 mg BID
Cromolyn sodium	Nebulized soln (20 mg/2 mL), MDI[2] 800 μg	> 2 y: nebulized soln: inhale 20 mg qid Age > 2: MDI: 2 puffs QID
Theophylline	Liquids, sustained-release tablets and capsules	Starting dose: 10 mg/kg/d < 1 y: max dose 0.2 × (age in weeks) + 5 = mg/kg/d ≥ 1 y: max dose 16 mg/kg/day

cap, Capsule; *DPI*, dry powder inhaler; *HFA*, hydrofluoroalkane; *MDI*, metered-dose inhaler; *soln*, solution.
[2]Not available in the United States.
Information from Lexicomp. http://online.lexi.com

length of stay in the emergency department was reduced in those using the spacers.

Corticosteroids given systemically are also considered rescue medications, although the onset of action is 1 to 2 hours and duration of action is 18 to 36 hours. They work primarily as antiinflammatories and are an important treatment in exacerbations. Early use of systemic steroids, either oral or intravenous, reduced rates of relapse and decreased admissions to the hospital. The greatest benefit of systemic steroids was seen in patients having a severe attack and those who were not already on a course of steroids. Studies have shown that oral steroids are as effective as intravenous or intramuscular preparations. Even a short course of oral steroids can reduce relapse and decrease the need for rescue inhalers. Systemic corticosteroids should be continued for 3 to 10 days after an exacerbation. A taper is not necessary if the course is less than 1 week or less than 10 days in a patient who is also using an inhaled corticosteroid (ICS). Prolonged use of systemic corticosteroids carries significant risk for side effects such as adrenal suppression, osteoporosis, reduced growth, and cataracts, and thus their use should be minimized. Despite some evidence that use of ICS in acute exacerbations can reduce hospital admission rates, mounting data do not support treatment with increased doses of ICS (2 to 5 times maintenance dose) in children with acute asthma exacerbations, as rates of oral corticosteroid use do not appear to be reduced, yet the magnitude of increased cumulative ICS dose with this practice raises concern for potential height restriction.

Use of intravenous magnesium sulfate[1] (a smooth muscle relaxer) should be reserved for severe exacerbations only. Its use has not been shown to reduce admission rates in milder exacerbations but can improve lung function in those with only a partial response to short-acting β-agonists. Similarly, subcutaneous

epinephrine[b] and subcutaneous terbutaline (Brethine)[1] should be reserved for emergency department settings when patients are not responding to short-acting β₂-adrenergic receptor agonists, anticholinergics, or corticosteroids, or when air entry is so diminished that inhaled medications are not effective.

Finally, not enough evidence exists to make a recommendation regarding routine use of antibiotics during an acute asthma exacerbation. In some circumstances, when there are findings consistent with bacterial infections (such as consolidation on chest x-ray), their use may be warranted. See Table 6 for usual dosing of medications used in acute exacerbations.

Monitoring

Asthma is a dynamic disease whose symptoms fluctuate based on a number of variables. Routine scheduled appointments with a pediatrician or family physician are essential to monitor symptoms and adjust therapy. Initial management can require visits every 2 to 6 weeks; as control of symptoms improves, the interval may be increased to every 3 to 6 months.

Patient education is essential to successfully controlling this disease. Education should be focused on the theory behind controller and rescue medications, the importance of medication compliance, and how to administer these medications properly. Newer trial data support improved inhaler adherence with the use of electronic reminders such as mobile phone alarms. The National Asthma Education and Prevention Program Expert Panel 3 emphasizes the importance of asthma action plans to empower patients in recognizing and treating escalating symptoms of asthma. Action plans also provide recommendations on reducing exposure to irritants, allergens, and triggers. Some plans are based on peak flow levels, but studies show that symptom-based written action plans are better at decreasing acute care visits. Examples of asthma action plans can be found on the National Heart, Lung, and Blood Institute website.

[1]Not FDA approved for this indication.

[1]Not FDA approved for this indication.

TABLE 6 Usual Dosing of Medications Used in Exacerbations

DRUG	DOSING
Chronic Management	
Corticosteroids (methylprednisolone, prednisolone, prednisone)	0.25–2 mg/kg daily or every other day
Acute Exacerbation	
Ipratropium bromide (DuoNeb)[1]	Age 0–5 years: 250 µg nebulized × 2, then q4h prn Age 5–11: 500 µg nebulized × 2, then q4h prn
Corticosteroids (methylprednisolone, prednisolone, prednisone)	1–2 mg/kg/day (max 60 mg/day) in 2 divided doses × 3–10 days
Severe Acute Exacerbation	
Not Responding to SABAs	
Magnesium sulfate[1]	25–50 mg/kg IV up to 2 g over 10–20 min
Terbutaline[1]	0.01 mg/kg SC q20min for 3 doses, then every 2–6 hr prn
Epinephrine[1]	0.01 mg/kg up to 0.3–0.5 mg SC q20min for 3 doses
Related to Allergic Reaction	
Epinephrine	1:1000: 0.01 mL/kg SC (max 0.3 mL)

[1]Not FDA approved for this indication.

SABA = Short-acting β_2-adrenergic receptor agonist.

Complications

The most worrisome complications of asthma include reduced lung function, pneumonia, pneumothorax, and death. More common complications include chronic cough, fatigue due to poor sleep, missed school days and worse academic performance, and limited ability to participate in sports.

References

Brightling CE, Bradding P, Symon FA, et al: Mast-cell infiltration of airway smooth muscle in asthma, N Engl J Med 346:1699–1705, 2002.

British Thoracic Society/Scottish Intercollegiate Guidelines Network (BTS/SIGN): Guideline on the management of asthma Guideline, 2016, Available at http://www.brit-thoracic.org.uk/document-library/clinical-information/asthma/btssign-asthma-guideline-2016. Accessed 11 March 2018.

Burr ML, Matthew IP, Arthur RA, et al: Effects on patients with asthma of eradicating visible indoor mould: a randomised controlled trial, Thorax 62:767–772, 2007.

Cates CJ, Jefferson T, Rowe BH: Vaccines for preventing influenza in people with asthma, Cochrane Database Syst Rev (2), 2008.

Centers for Disease Control and Prevention (CDC): Vital signs: Asthma prevalence, disease characteristics, and self-management education: United States, 2001–2009, MMWR Morb Mortal Wkly Rep 60(17):547–552, 2011. Available at: http://www.ncbi.nlm.nih.gov/pubmed/21544044. Accessed 12 March 2018.

Chen LH, Chen SS, Liang L, Li CC: Effects of asthma and inhaled corticosteroids in children on the final adult height: a systemic review and meta-analysis, Zhongguo Dang Dai Er Ke Za Zhi 17(11):1242–1247, 2015.

Courtney U, McCarter D, Pollart S: Childhood asthma: Treatment update, Am Fam Physician 71:1959–1968, 2005.

Dicpinigaitis PV: Chronic cough due to asthma: ACCP evidence-based clinical practice guidelines, Chest 129:75S–79S, 2006.

Elward K, Pollart S: Medical therapy for asthma: Updates from the NAEPP guidelines, Am Fam Physician 82(10):1242–1251, 2010.

Fleming DM, Crovari P, Wahn U, et al: Comparison of the efficacy and safety of live attenuated cold-adapted influenza vaccine, trivalent, with trivalent inactivated influenza virus vaccine in children and adolescents with asthma, Pediatr Infect Dis J 25(10):860–869, 2006.

Global Initiative for Asthma (GINA): GINA Report, Global Strategy for Asthma Management and Prevention, Available at: http://ginasthma.org/gina-reports, 2017. Accessed 11 March 2018.

Holbrook JT, Wise RA, Gold BD: Lansoprazole for children with poorly controlled asthma: a randomized controlled trial, JAMA 307(4):373–381, 2012.

Irazuzta JE, Chiriboga N: Magnesium sulfate infusion for acute asthma in the emergency department, J Pediatr (Rio J) 93, 2017.

Jackson DJ, Bacharier LB, Mauger DT, et al: Quintupling inhaled glucocorticoids to prevent childhood asthma exacerbations, N Engl J Med 378:891–901, 2018.

Kramer MS, Kakuma R: Maternal dietary antigen avoidance during pregnancy or lactation, or both, for preventing or treating atopic disease in the child, Cochrane Database Syst Rev (3), CD000133.

Lai T, Wu M, Liu J, et al: Acid-suppressing drug use during pregnancy and the risk of childhood asthma: a meta-analysis, Pediatrics 141(2), e 20170889, 2018.

Lemanske RF, Mauger DT, Sorkness CA, Jackson DJ: Step up therapy for children with uncontrolled asthma receiving inhaled corticosteroids, N Engl J Med 362(11):975–985, 2010.

Maas T, Kaper J, Sheikh A, et al: Mono and multifaceted inhalant and/or food allergen reduction interventions for preventing asthma in children at high risk of developing asthma, Cochrane Database Syst Rev (3), CD006480.

McCowan C, Neville R, Thomas G, et al: Effect of asthma and its treatment on growth: four year follow up of cohort of children from general practices in Tayside, Scotland, BMJ 316(7132):668–672, 1998.

McIvor RA, Kaplan A, Koch C: Montelukast as an alternative to low dose inhaled corticosteroids in the management of mild asthma(the SIMPLE trial): an open label effectiveness trial, Can Respir J 16:11A–21A, 2009.

Mitre E, Susi A, Kroop LE, et al: Association between use of acid-suppressive medications and antibiotics during infancy and allergic diseases in early childhood, JAMA Pediatr 172(6):e180315, 2018.

Morton RW, Elphick HE, Rigby AS, et al: STAAR: a randomised controlled trial of electronic adherence monitoring with reminder alarms and feedback to improve clinical outcomes for children with asthma, Thorax 72(4):347–354, 2017.

National Asthma Education and Prevention Program, National Heart, Lung, and Blood Institute (NHLBI). Expert panel report 3: guidelines for the diagnosis and management of asthma. NHLBI website. Available at: https://www.nhlbi.nih.gov/files/docs/guidelines/asthgdln.pdf. [Accessed March 11, 2018].

National Heart Lung, Blood Institute: Asthma action plan, Available at http://www.nhlbi.nih.gov/health/public/lung/asthma/asthma_actplan.pdf. Accessed 13 March 2018.

Petsky HL, Kew KM, Chang AB: Exhaled nitric oxide levels to guide treatment for children with asthma, Cochrane database Syst Rev 11:CD011439, 2016.

Pollart S, Compton R, Elward K: Management of acute asthma exacerbations, Am Fam Physician 84:40–47, 2011.

Pollart S, Elward K: Overview of changes to asthma guidelines: Diagnosis and screening, Am Fam Physician 79:761–767, 2009.

Prevention strategies for asthma—primary prevention, CMAJ 173(Suppl. 6):S20–S24, 2005.

Sheik A, Alves B, Dhami S: Pneumococcal vaccine for asthma (Cochrane Review). The Cochrane Library Issue 2. Ed. Chichester, UK, 2009, John Wiley and Sons, Ltd.

Sokol KC, Sharma G, Lin Y-L, Goldblum RM: Choosing wisely: adherence by physicians to recommended use of spirometry in the diagnosis and management of adult asthma, Am J Med 128(5):502–508, 2015.

Toelle B, Ng K: Eight year outcomes of the Childhood Asthma Prevention Study, J Allergy Clin Immunol 126:388–389, 2010.

ATTENTION-DEFICIT/HYPERACTIVITY DISORDER

Method of
Scott E. Moser, MD

CURRENT DIAGNOSIS

- Diagnosis is clinical and based on DSM-5 criteria for inattentive symptoms, hyperactive/impulsive symptoms, or combined symptoms with onset by age 12 years.
- For the inattentive presentation, symptoms must include 6 of the following 9 (5 of 9 if age >17 years): fails to give attention to details, difficulty sustaining attention, does not seem to listen, does not follow through, difficulty organizing, avoids mental effort, loses things, easily distracted, and forgetful in daily activities.
- For hyperactive/impulsive presentation, 6 of the following must be documented (5 of 9 for age >17years): fidgets, leaves seat, runs about or climbs excessively, difficulty playing quietly, "on the go/driven by a motor," talks excessively, blurts answers before the end of questions, difficulty awaiting turn/waiting in line, interrupts/intrudes on others.
- Clinical diagnosis relies on use of standardized questionnaires and must account for potential comorbid psychological or learning problems.

CURRENT THERAPY

- For all patients older than age 6 years, stimulants are the primary treatment unless contraindicated.
- Important second line or adjunctive medications include atomoxetine (Strattera), guanfacine (Intuniv), clonidine (Kapvay), venlafaxine [1](Effexor), and bupropion (Wellbutrin).[1]
- Behavioral therapies are important adjuncts to medication for best outcomes.

[1]Not FDA approved for this indication.

Epidemiology/Pathophysiology

Attention-deficit/hyperactivity disorder (ADHD) is one of the most commonly diagnosed conditions in childhood, affecting at least 5% of school-age children. It is more commonly diagnosed in boys than girls at a 2:1 ratio, a difference that may be exaggerated by bias inherent in the standardized questionnaires used to detect ADHD.

Risk Factors

DSM-5 categorizes ADHD among the neurodevelopmental disorders based on its heritability of about 75%, chromosomal pattern evidence, and brain metabolism studies in the control centers for attention (prefrontal cortex) and motor activity (temporal lobe). In addition to genetic factors, several environmental factors have been associated: maternal smoking or alcohol use, pregnancy/delivery complications, psychosocial adversity, and exposure to environmental toxins including PCBs and pesticides. Food additives and television viewing have been studied without consistent evidence that they contribute.

Clinical Manifestations and Diagnosis

ADHD is a clinical diagnosis based on the criteria described in Diagnostic and Statistical Manual of Mental Disorders, 5th Edition: DSM-5 (DSM-5). In spite of growing evidence for characteristic findings in chromosomal and brain metabolism studies, there are no genetic, biochemical, or imaging tests validated for clinical use in making the diagnosis. Thus a clinician considering the diagnosis should review the explicit DSM-5 criteria.

DSM-5 recognizes three presentations: predominantly inattentive, predominantly hyperactive/impulsive, and a combined presentation. The use of the word "presentation" in DSM-5 is a change from the use of the word "type" in DSM-4, recognizing that the predominant symptoms can change modestly over time. ADHD begins in childhood, so to make the diagnosis after age 12, evidence must be found for significant symptoms before that age. At any age, the symptoms must be present in at least two different settings (home, school, work, etc.) and clearly interfere with social, academic, or occupational functioning. The symptoms cannot be better explained by another mental disorder (e.g., mood disorder, anxiety disorder, substance abuse).

To meet criteria for the inattentive presentation, the patient must exhibit age-inappropriate levels of at least six of the following nine symptoms: (1) fails to give attention to details or makes careless mistakes, (2) difficulty sustaining attention, (3) does not seem to listen when addressed, (4) does not follow through on instructions/fails to finish schoolwork or chores, (5) difficulty organizing tasks/activities, (6) avoids/refuses to engage in tasks that require sustained mental effort, (7) loses items necessary for tasks or activities, (8) easily distracted by extraneous stimuli, (9) forgetful in daily activities/routines.

To meet criteria for the hyperactive/impulsive presentation, the patient must exhibit age-inappropriate levels of at least six of the following nine symptoms: (1) often fidgets or squirms in seat, (2) leaves seat inappropriately, (3) runs or climbs excessively, (4) unable to play quietly, (5) "on the go" or "driven by a motor," (6) talks excessively, (7) blurts out answers before a question is completed, (8) difficulty waiting their turn, (9) interrupts or intrudes on others.

The combined presentation requires meeting criteria for both the inattentive and hyperactive/impulsive presentations.

Patients age 17 years and older need to meet only five of the nine criteria in a presentation category. DSM-5 includes examples of adult equivalents of the criteria. For example, inattention criterion (6) reads, "Often avoids, dislikes, or is reluctant to engage in tasks that require sustained mental effort (e.g., schoolwork or homework; for older adolescents and adults, preparing reports, completing forms, reviewing lengthy papers)." Several of the symptoms must have been present before 12 years of age. For most patients, the hyperactivity improves by adolescence, but patients continue to have challenges with inattention and impulsivity as adults unless adequately treated.

The mainstay of diagnosis is the use of standardized questionnaires completed by parents, teachers, or other observers. The diagnosis of ADHD requires that the patient manifest symptoms in multiple environments, so it is important to obtain questionnaires from as many observers as is realistic. Each of the commercially available questionnaires has advantages and disadvantages such that clinicians should cooperate with local school and mental health partners regarding which forms to use. Commonly used scales include the Conners, Vanderbilt, Achenbach, and others. In addition to making the diagnosis of ADHD, these scales can give clues to comorbid conditions and alternative diagnoses.

When gathering the history, it is important to obtain specific examples of behaviors rather than general labels. For example, "doesn't pay attention" could mean "spends the day staring out the window" or "slumps in his chair and doesn't respond to questions for several minutes." Because there are no specific diagnostic tests for ADHD, ordering laboratory studies and imaging is individualized based on the clinician's suspicion of comorbid or alternative diagnoses as described below.

Making the diagnosis of ADHD is more complicated in adults than in children for several reasons, including the challenges of recall bias by patients, difficulty obtaining information from other observers, less well-validated symptom questionnaires, and potential drug seeking for stimulants. Therefore clinicians should be wary and consider consultation with an experienced mental health colleague in these cases.

Careful evaluation that includes documentation of meeting DSM-5 criteria for ADHD prior to initiating treatment is important for both patients and clinicians. Studies have demonstrated that a lack of adequate documentation by physicians is common. Because the main treatment for ADHD includes use of Drug Enforcement Agency (DEA) Schedule II agents, the stimulants, the clinician is wise to perform a careful evaluation and document their findings well.

Differential Diagnosis

Comorbid learning disorders occur in as many as one-third of patients with ADHD, and comorbid oppositional defiant disorder and conduct disorder are also exceedingly common. Thus comorbidity is the rule rather than the exception, implying that when considering the differential diagnosis, clinicians must answer not only, "Could this be ADHD *or* something else?" They must also consider, "Could this be ADHD *and* something else?"

In addition to the potential comorbidities noted above, other common and important psychological conditions that share manifestations with ADHD or may be comorbid with ADHD include bipolar disorder, depression, anxiety, intellectual disability, and autism spectrum disorder. In adolescents and adults, substance use disorders are also common.

A large number of medical and neurologic conditions share some manifestations with ADHD, including absence seizure disorder, tics, hearing problems, sleep disorders, lead intoxication, allergies, and side effects of medications, particularly those used to treat asthma or allergies. A history of physical or sexual abuse is common. Children who live in a chaotic home environment or attend an unstructured school can exhibit ADHD-like symptoms or have their symptoms of ADHD exacerbated. Parental psychopathology or chemical dependency may complicate

TABLE 1	Patient and Parental Resources for the Management of ADHD

www.chadd.org/Resources from the national support group for children and adults with ADHD.

www.add.org/Resources from the ADD Association, a national ADHD adult support group.

www.nimh.nih.gov/health/topics/attention-deficit-hyperactivity-disorder-adhd/index.shtml Information on ADHD from the National Institutes of Mental Health, including a link to current ADHD clinical trials.

Taking Charge of ADHD, Third Edition: The Complete, Authoritative Guide for Parents by Russell A. Barkley (2013). Book recommending environmental changes to structure the schedule and behavior of children with ADHD.

Smart but Scattered: The Revolutionary Executive Skills Approach to Helping Kids Reach Their Potential, by Peg Dawson and Richard Guare (2009). Book recommending routines and study skills to maximize functioning in children with ADHD.

symptomatology Therefore a careful social, developmental, and medical history and physical examination are important to making the diagnosis with individualized testing on the basis of the clinical suspicion of alternative or comorbid conditions. In cases where the clinician suspects complex or comorbid conditions, referral for neuropsychological assessment should be considered.

Treatment

The best treatment outcomes have been demonstrated with a combination of stimulant medication and behavioral interventions. This evidence comes primarily from studies of school-age children. Because of concerns about accurate diagnosis in children younger than 6 years old and less evidence of stimulant efficacy in younger children, guidelines encourage great caution in starting medications before age 6, relying primarily on behavioral therapy in younger children. As soon as ADHD is diagnosed, the clinician should point patients and families to reliable sources of education about the disorder, especially because so much misinformation is circulating among the public (Table 1). Regardless of the treatment plan, it is important to establish communication links between physician, family, school, and mental health partners to address the myriad of complications and consequences that often develop. Regular follow-up that includes assessment of the effectiveness of treatment is important in the management of this chronic condition. Treatment in adolescents and adults is similar to that in children with exceptions noted in the text below and in Table 2. Table 2 includes all the medications with current FDA approval for treatment of ADHD. In general, clinicians should not exceed FDA maximum doses because this practice increases the risk of side effects with little evidence of improved efficacy.

Finally, because ADHD has a high rate of inheritance, parents of affected children often also have the disorder. The clinician should remain vigilant for ways this can complicate management, including treatment nonadherence, parental denial, or inconsistency with behavioral interventions.

Stimulants

The psychostimulants are first-line treatment for all presentations of ADHD at all ages, age 6 years and older. Their mechanism of action is thought to be primarily due to inhibition of reuptake of dopamine and norepinephrine in the prefrontal cortex, a key to regulating attention, behavior, and emotion. Children with ADHD who take stimulants have longer attention spans, are less impulsive and distractible, perform better in school, and have better relationships with family and peers than those who do not.

All the stimulants are DEA Schedule II agents because of their abuse potential, which makes prescribing more challenging than nonstimulant alternatives. In spite of this, the stimulants remain the medications of first choice due to their strong record of efficacy and safety. The stimulants are grouped into two major categories: methylphenidate and the amphetamines. Both categories

of stimulants are available in a variety of dosing options including short-acting, long-acting, and very long-acting preparations (Table 2). Standard methylphenidate and dextro-amphetamine maintain therapeutic levels for only 3 to 4 hours, necessitating multiple doses throughout the day. Therefore the longer-acting preparations have become much more popular. Many of the longer-acting drug choices achieve their prolonged effect because of technological modifications of their surface coating, resulting in slow intestinal release of the active medication. As a result, it is important that patients avoid breaking or chewing these pills. Exceptions are preparations utilizing micronized beads in capsules (methylphenidate ER [Metadate CD], dexmethylphenidate XR [Focalin XR], mixed amphetamine salts [Adderall XR], lisdexamfetamine [Vyvanse]), suspensions (methylphenidate ER suspension [Quilivant XR], dextroamphetamine solution [Pro-Centra]), or tablets designed to be chewed (methylphenidate ER Chewable Tablets [Quilichew ER]). The preparations of encapsulated beads can be emptied into apple sauce or other soft food for children unable to swallow pills.

The effectiveness of stimulants is great enough that if the initial trial of a stimulant is not effective or is poorly tolerated, evidence-based guidelines generally encourage the trial of a stimulant from the other category before resorting to a nonstimulant. When converting from one class of stimulant to another, 1 mg of amphetamine is roughly equivalent to 2 mg of methylphenidate.

Common side effects of stimulants include loss of appetite, abdominal pain, headache, irritability, and weight loss. These side effects are often transient and can be minimized by using a low starting dose and increasing the dosage gradually. Stimulants can exacerbate tics or seizure disorders. A rare but serious side effect is sudden cardiac death. The risk is so rare and unpredictable that current guidelines do not recommend routine electrocardiographic or other screening tests before initiating therapy. However, it is prudent to carefully assess cardiac risk factors prior to initiating treatment.

Apart from the kinetics of short-acting versus longer-acting options and the various routes of administration (e.g., pills, suspensions, dermal patches), two stimulants have specific niches. Dexmethylphenidate is the active isomer of methylphenidate. Theoretically, this may improve the side effect profile, although clinical evidence for this is lacking. Because it is the active isomer, the therapeutic conversion is 1 mg of dexmethylphenidate approximates 2 mg of methylphenidate. Lisdexamfetamine is a prodrug of dextroamphetamine. It was developed to reduce the risk of abuse, but the DEA has maintained its Schedule II designation.

Parents are often concerned about whether the use of a DEA-controlled substance might increase the risk of their child developing a substance use disorder as they mature. Current evidence is reassuring in this regard in that appropriate treatment with stimulants likely decreases that risk.

Stimulants are also first-line treatment for ADHD in adults, though the evidence from controlled studies is not as strong as with children. As indicated in Table 2, for women who clearly benefit from treatment with stimulants and who are pregnant or could become pregnant, methylphenidate is considered the safest choice.

Nonstimulants

All of the nonstimulants are second-line agents or adjuncts to stimulant treatment. The most important agent in this class is atomoxetine (Strattera). It should be titrated up over days to weeks and may require 4 weeks to see the full benefit. Usually, once-daily dosing is effective, but genetically fast metabolizers may require multiple daily doses. Common side effects include loss of appetite, headache, and drowsiness. One benefit of atomoxetine is that it is not a DEA-scheduled agent so it is more convenient to prescribe than a stimulant. Also, it does not exacerbate tics. A downside to atomoxetine is it carries a black box warning of increased risk of suicidality, especially during the first months of treatment. A rare but serious potential side effect is

TABLE 2 Common ADHD Medications

CATEGORY	GENERIC NAME	SELECTED BRAND NAME EXAMPLES	ONSET	THERAPEUTIC EFFECT	PREGNANCY RISK	COMMENTS
Stimulants						
	Methylphenidate				No known teratogenicity based on animal data	Variety of dosing options as noted
	Short-acting	Ritalin	20 min	3–4 hrs		Requires multiple doses to last through school day
	Long-acting	Metadate CD	30 min	8 hrs		Single dose to last through school day but may require afternoon boost for homework; capsule contents may be sprinkled on food
		Quillivant XR	20 min	8–10 hrs		Liquid suspension
		QuilliChew ER	30 min	8 hrs		Chewable tablet
	Very long-acting	Concerta	1–2 hrs	12–14 hrs		Single dose to last entire day but more likely to interfere with sleep
		Daytrana patch	2–4 hrs	>20 hrs		Must be removed before bedtime
	Dexmethylphenidate	Focalin	20 min	3–4 hrs	Caution in pregnancy due to inadequate data to assess risk	Bioactive isomer may reduce side effects
		Focalin XR	20 min	8 hrs		Capsule contents may be sprinkled on food
	Amphetamine/ dextroamphetamine				Avoid in pregnancy due to risk of teratogenicity and neonatal complications including premature delivery	
		Adderall	20 min	6–8 hrs		
		Adderall XR	30–60 min	12–14 hrs		Capsule contents may be sprinkled on food
	Dextroamphetamine				Avoid in pregnancy due to risk of teratogenicity and neonatal complications including premature delivery	
		Dexedrine	20 min	3–4 hrs		Requires multiple doses to last through school day
		ProCentra	20 min	4–6 hrs		Oral suspension
	Lisdexamfetamine	Vyvanse	30 min	10–12 hrs	No human data but avoid in pregnancy based on limited human data with amphetamines	Prodrug with theoretically less abuse potential; capsule contents may be sprinkled on food
Nonstimulants						
	Atomoxetine	Strattera	1 hr	Variable	Caution in pregnancy; inadequate human data to assess risk; no known harm	Usually once daily dosing; fast metabolizers may need twice daily dosing

Continued

TABLE 2 Common ADHD Medications—cont'd

CATEGORY	GENERIC NAME	SELECTED BRAND NAME EXAMPLES	ONSET	THERAPEUTIC EFFECT	PREGNANCY RISK	COMMENTS
	Clonidine, extended-release	Kapvay	30–60 min	8–16 hrs	Caution in pregnancy; risk of low birth weight; risk of fetal death from animal data	Dose at bedtime
	Guanfacine, extended-release	Intuniv	30–60 min	16–24 hrs	Caution in pregnancy; no known risk of fetal harm	Dose at bedtime
	Venlafaxine[1]	Effexor			Caution in pregnancy especially in third trimester due to potential withdrawal or serotonin syndrome	
	Bupropion[1]	Wellbutrin (immediate release, 12 hr extended release, 24 hr extended release)			Caution in pregnancy; risk of congenital heart defects inconclusive	Extended release forms not approved for children <12 years old

[1]Not FDA approved for this indication.

hepatotoxicity. Atomoxetine should be considered first-line therapy in patients with a comorbid tic disorder, significant anxiety disorder, or recent substance abuse.

Clonidine (Kapvay) and guanfacine (Intuniv) are alpha-adrenergic agonists that are helpful adjuncts to treating hyperactivity or aggression that does not adequately respond to a stimulant alone. Because a side effect is drowsiness, nighttime dosing can actually improve sleep. Use of extended-release formulations allows for single daily dosing. Patients should be monitored for development of hypotension or bradycardia. Because of the risk of rebound hypertension, these agents should be tapered slowly rather than stopped abruptly.

In controlled trials, the serotonin-norepinephrine reuptake inhibitors (SNRIs) have demonstrated effectiveness for ADHD, and one agent in this category is venlafaxine (Effexor).[1] SNRIs are particularly useful adjuncts in patients with significant mood instability, common in adolescents. Prescribers should use caution due to the black box warning regarding potential increased suicide risk.

Bupropion (Wellbutrin)[1] has been shown to be somewhat effective in treating ADHD, and its value is similar to that of the SNRIs as adjuncts in special situations. Like the SNRIs, it has a black box warning regarding increased suicidality risk.

Several tricyclic antidepressants have demonstrated efficacy for ADHD in controlled trials, but their use is limited due to side effects and lack of FDA approval. Selective serotonin reuptake inhibitors (SSRIs) have not demonstrated effectiveness for ADHD and should only be considered for comorbid mood disorders. Other mood stabilizers and atypical antipsychotics should generally be reserved for use by specialists.

Behavior Therapy and Educational Interventions
For younger children the emphasis is on behavior training for parents and teachers. All parents should receive instruction in common behavioral mistakes such as overreliance on negative reinforcement instead of positive and too long a delay in dispensing rewards. Most parents benefit from specific training in parenting techniques or support groups. As children enter adolescence and beyond, cognitive behavior therapies, group therapy with peers, and individual coaching approaches show the most promise. Educational placement and classroom interventions

are also important. The diagnosis of ADHD, at the very least, deserves consideration for special classroom accommodations under federal law for this chronic handicapping condition. If the child is still failing in spite of these accommodations, consideration should be given for special education placement. Patients of all ages may benefit from counseling regarding adequate physical activity and good sleep hygiene.

Monitoring
Once satisfactory response to treatment is established, children on stimulants should continue to be seen at least every 6 months for height and weight checks to be sure they are continuing to grow normally and for blood pressure and pulse checks, watching for onset of hypertension or tachycardia. Guidelines typically recommend annual consideration of a medication holiday to evaluate the need for continued treatment. Children typically require gradually increasing doses during the school years, then some tapering of the dose in late adolescence.

Management of Complications
Children with suspected comorbid psychiatric conditions and those who do not respond to initial treatment should be referred to a specialist.

References
AACAP. Practice parameter for the assessment and treatment of children and adolescents with attention-deficit/hyperactivity disorder, *J Am Acad Child Adolesc Psychiatry* 46(7):894–921, 2007.

ADHD: Clinical Practice Guideline for the Diagnosis, Evaluation, and Treatment of Attention-Deficit/Hyperactivity Disorder in Children and Adolescents. Subcommittee on Attention-Deficit/Hyperactivity Disorder, Steering Committee on Quality Improvement and Management, *Pediatrics* 128(5):1007–1022, 2011.

American Psychiatric Association: Diagnostic and Statistical Manual of Mental Disorders, Fifth Edition. Arlington, VA, American Psychiatric Association, 2013.

Biederman J, Wilens T, Mick E, Spencer T, Faraone S: Pharmacotherapy of attention-deficit/hyperactivity disorder reduces risk for substance use disorder, *Pediatrics* 104(2):1–5, 1999.

Fabiano GA, Pelham Jr. WE, Coles EK, et al: A meta-analysis of behavioral treatments for attention-deficit/hyperactivity disorder. *Clin Psychol Rev* 29:129–140, 2009.

Gould MS, Walsh BT, Munfakh JL, et al: Sudden death and use of stimulant medications in youth, *Am J Psychiatry* 166:992–1001, 2009.

MTA Cooperative Group: A 14-month randomized clinical trial of treatment strategies for attention-deficit/hyperactivity disorder. Multimodal Treatment Study of Children with ADHD, *Arch Gen Psychiatry* 56:1073–1086, 1999.

[1]Not FDA approved for this indication.

BRONCHIOLITIS

Method of
Danae D. Goerl, MD

CURRENT DIAGNOSIS

- Clinical diagnosis made in children less than 2 years old with symptoms of congestion and rhinorrhea associated with lower respiratory tract findings that may include wheezing, crackles, tachypnea, or increased work of breathing.
- Viral polymerase chain reaction (PCR) assays are available, but are not routinely needed to establish diagnosis.
- Chest x-ray not indicated for evaluation of bronchiolitis. Consider in children with severe respiratory distress or lung findings concerning for alternate diagnosis.

CURRENT THERAPY

- Treatment remains supportive care: supplemental oxygen for oxygen saturation less than 90%, fluids to maintain hydration, and suction of the nasal passages.
- No indication for corticosteroids, racemic epinephrine, or albuterol therapy.

Bronchiolitis, or viral pneumonia in children less than 2 years old, is one of the most common diseases encountered in pediatric medicine. Respiratory syncytial virus (RSV) causes most cases of bronchiolitis; however, other viruses cause similar symptoms. Approximately 90% of children will be infected with RSV by the time they are 2 years old. Despite the high number of infants affected, there are no curative therapies and no medication has been shown to shorten the course of bronchiolitis.

Epidemiology and Virology

Most epidemiologic data has been reported about RSV. RSV is the most common virus that causes bronchiolitis; however, other viruses including human rhinovirus, influenza, human metapneumovirus, parainfluenza, and adenovirus may cause bronchiolitis. Outbreaks caused by RSV vary by season. In the United States, the incidence of RSV is typically highest between November and April, and regional variability does occur. Approximately 800,000 children in the United States require outpatient medical attention during the first year of life due to RSV, and between 2% and 3% of all children younger than 12 months of age are hospitalized with a diagnosis of bronchiolitis.

Risk Factors

Certain conditions put infants at risk for severe presentation of the illness. These are listed in Box 1.

Pathophysiology

Bronchiolitis is a viral infection that affects the lower respiratory tract. These viruses may only affect epithelial cells of the nasal passages and cause strictly upper respiratory symptoms. However in approximately 30%–40% of patients, the lower respiratory tract will become affected. When the bronchioles are involved, shedding of respiratory epithelium, impaired ciliary function, and edema occur. As the viral-infected epithelium is sloughed into the lumen of the airway, obstruction of the airway occurs and leads to alveolar collapse or atelectasis distal to the obstruction.

Clinical Manifestations

The virus initially causes upper respiratory symptoms such as rhinorrhea, congestion, and cough that are present for 2 to 3 days.

Fever may also occur. As the lower airways become involved, mucous plugging and atelectasis may cause tachypnea, and increased work of breathing demonstrated by nasal flaring, costal retractions, or grunting. On physical examination, clinicians may auscultate crackles and wheezes that are typically symmetric and bilateral. If ventilation and perfusion mismatch occur, the child will become hypoxemic. There is a spectrum of clinical presentations ranging from nonlabored breathing with mild crackles heard on exam to apnea and rarely respiratory failure. Infants may also appear clinically dehydrated if the increase in respiratory effort causes poor feeding.

Diagnosis

The diagnosis of bronchiolitis is made clinically by history and physical examination. Commercial viral polymerase chain reaction (PCR) assays that are obtained via nasopharyngeal swab are available; however, these are not routinely indicated. There are some clinical situations when viral testing may be useful. When the clinician suspects that the child has influenza, viral PCR may be used to determine need for oseltamivir (Tamiflu). Additionally, if a patient is receiving monthly palivizumab (Synagis) prophylaxis and is hospitalized with bronchiolitis, the clinician should obtain viral testing. If the patient has RSV, this would be an indication to discontinue monthly prophylaxis due to the low likelihood of a second RSV infection in the same year.

Chest x-ray is not indicated in routine evaluation of bronchiolitis. Obtaining a chest x-ray is unlikely to change management of the patient, and may lead to inappropriate use of antibiotics. If the child is ill enough to be admitted to the intensive care unit or if there is a clinical concern for an alternate diagnosis such as bacterial pneumonia, radiographs may be warranted.

Differential Diagnosis

Other respiratory conditions must be considered when a child presents with clinical features of bronchiolitis. One clinical challenge when evaluating a patient with bronchiolitis is to distinguish it from asthma or recurrent viral-induced wheezing. Severe bronchiolitis early in life is associated with an increased risk of asthma. It is unclear whether bronchiolitis early in life results in injury that alters normal lung development and predisposes the child to subsequent wheezing, or whether certain infants have a preexisting abnormality of the immune response or of airway function that causes them to have both severe bronchiolitis and recurrent wheezing. Infants who have risk factors for asthma including eczema, and personal or family history of asthma associated with recurrent wheezing, may be difficult to clearly diagnose with viral bronchiolitis.

The differential diagnosis also includes other infections such as bacterial pneumonia caused by community acquired or atypical organisms, aspiration pneumonia, or pertussis. Undiagnosed congenital cardiac defects with heart failure may also present similarly to bronchiolitis, with tachypnea, increased work of breathing, and crackles heard on lung auscultation. Other diagnoses to consider include foreign body aspiration, congenital pulmonary abnormalities, or vascular rings.

Treatment

The treatment for bronchiolitis remains supportive therapy.
Supportive measures include:

BOX 1	Infants at Risk for Severe Presentation of Bronchiolitis

- Age younger than 3 months
- History of prematurity
- History of congenital cardiac abnormalities or chronic lung disease
- Infants whose immune systems are compromised

TABLE 1 Summary of Evidence for Treatment of Bronchiolitis

MEDICATION	RECOMMENDATION	EVIDENCE QUALITY
Systemic corticosteroids	Not recommended	Cochrane systematic review shows that corticosteroids do not significantly reduce outpatient admissions when compared with placebo and do not reduce length of stay for inpatient admissions
Epinephrine	Not recommended	Cochrane meta-analysis systematically evaluated the evidence and found no evidence for utility in the inpatient setting
Albuterol	Not recommended	Meta-analyses and systematic reviews have shown that bronchodilators improve clinical symptom scores, but they do not affect disease resolution, need for hospitalization, or length of stay
Hypertonic saline	May consider	May decrease inpatient length of stay (LOS) in settings where LOS is greater than 3 days (typical US length of stay is 2.4 days)
Oxygen therapy	Provide supplemental oxygen if oxyhemoglobin saturation is <90%	
Nutrition and hydration	Administer IV or NG fluid for infants unable to maintain hydration orally	

Adapted from AAP Clinical Practice Guideline: The Diagnosis, Management and Prevention of Bronchiolitis. 2014.

- Supplemental oxygen to keep oxygen saturations greater than 90%.
- Hydration via intravenous fluids or nasogastric tube for children unable to maintain oral hydration.
- Nasal suctioning, though often provided for patients with bronchiolitis, has not been well studied. One study published in JAMA Pediatrics in 2013 concluded that in patients admitted with bronchiolitis, the use of deep suctioning in the first 24 hours after admission and lapses greater than 4 hours between suctioning events were associated with longer length of stay.

Outpatient Management

Outpatient management includes parental education about the expected clinical course of the illness, providing return precautions, and close follow up for infants at risk for severe disease. Information can be given to parents regarding supportive measures they can provide at home, including clearing the nasal passages prior to feeding, appropriate antipyretic therapy if fever is causing the infant discomfort, and discouraging over-the-counter decongestants for children less than 2 years old.

Inpatient Management

Admission to the hospital should be considered for infants who appear ill, hypoxemic with oxygen saturation <90% on room air, those with respiratory distress characterized by tachypnea with respiratory rate >70 breaths per minute, retractions, grunting, or apnea. Hospitalization is also indicated for infants who are dehydrated.

Medications including albuterol, corticosteroids, and racemic epinephrine have been studied, but have not been shown to cure the disease, prevent hospitalization, or shorten the course in patients hospitalized with bronchiolitis. Multiple studies have been conducted recently examining the role of nebulized hypertonic saline (3%) to determine if it decreases hospitalization when given in the emergency department or if it shortens hospital stays. Evidence is not considered strong enough at this point to advocate for routine use of hypertonic saline in the United States. In 2014, the American Academy of Pediatrics published clinical practice guidelines that summarize the most recent evidence regarding diagnosis and treatment (Table 1). Chest physiotherapy is not recommended when managing hospitalized patients with bronchiolitis. A Cochrane Review evaluated nine randomized controlled trials in hospitalized patients and found no benefit to chest percussion or chest vibration. Antibiotic therapy is only indicated in the case of secondary bacterial infection.

The data reviewed does not extend to patients admitted to the intensive care unit with bronchiolitis.

Prevention

Immunoprophylaxis

Palivizumab (Synagis) is an immunoglobulin G monoclonal antibody directed against a surface protein of RSV. It was approved by the FDA in 1998 after a randomized controlled trial demonstrated a reduction in the rate of hospitalization related to RSV in premature infants. In July 2014, the American Academy updated the recommendations for patients that may benefit from palivizumab. This replaced the Red Book Guidelines published in 2012. The current recommendation is that palivizumab prophylaxis be limited to:

- Infants born before 29 weeks' gestation.
- Infants with hemodynamically significant congenital cardiac disease.
- Infants diagnosed with chronic lung disease of prematurity. This is defined by an oxygen requirement of more than 21% FiO_2 for the first 28 days of life with continued requirement of supplemental oxygen, diuretic therapy, or chronic corticosteroid therapy.

If criteria for palivizumab therapy are met, the infant will receive one shot per month, 15 mg/kg per dose, for 5 months. The shots are administered during RSV season, which is typically from November until March, but may vary based on the region. Palivizumab prophylaxis is not indicated past 12 months of age except for infants with chronic lung disease of prematurity, who may benefit from therapy through a second RSV season.

Breastfeeding

Breastfeeding has many proven benefits in the neonatal period. This extends to respiratory infections. Studies have demonstrated decreased risk of hospitalization with respiratory infections, as well as shorter hospital stays for bronchiolitis in infants who are breastfed.

Complications

Complications from bronchiolitis include secondary bacterial infections such as acute otitis media or bacterial pneumonia. Respiratory failure requiring mechanical ventilation and intensive care unit admission may also occur. Though bronchiolitis is a disease associated with high morbidity, the mortality is low. Death from respiratory failure in bronchiolitis is rare, accounting for 5.3 deaths per 100,000 children below 12 months in the United States.

References

American Academy of Pediatrics Committee on Infectious Diseases, American Academy of Pediatrics Bronchiolitis Guidelines Committee: Updated guidance for palivizumab prophylaxis among infants and young children at increased risk of hospitalization for respiratory syncytial virus infection, *Pediatrics* 134:415–420, 2014.

Hall CB, Weinberg GA, Iwane MK, et al: The burden of respiratory syncytial virus infection in young children, *N Engl J Med* 360:588–598, 2009.

Hasegawa K, Tsugawa Y, Brown D, et al: Trends in bronchiolitis hospitalizations in the United States, 2000–2009, *Pediatrics* 132:28–36, 2013.

Meissner HC: Viral bronchiolitis in children, *N Engl J Med* 374:62–72, 2016.

Ralston SL, Lieberthal AS, Meissner HC, et al: Clinical practice guideline: the diagnosis, management, and prevention of bronchiolitis, *Pediatrics* 134:1474–1502, 2014.

Thompson WW, Shay DK, Weintraub E, et al: Mortality associated with influenza and respiratory syncytial virus in the United States, *JAMA* 289:179–186, 2003.

DIABETES MELLITUS IN CHILDREN

Method of
Gregory Goodwin, MD

CURRENT DIAGNOSIS

- Random glucose >200 mg/dL and symptoms (polyuria, polydipsia)
- Fasting glucose >126 mg/dL
- 2-hour glucose >200 mg/dL after glucose tolerance test
- Hemoglobin A1c >6.5%
- Diabetic ketoacidosis: pH <7.3, serum bicarbonate <15 mmol/L

CURRENT TREATMENT

Type 1 Diabetes
- Basal/bolus regimen**: rapid-acting insulin* before meals and long-acting insulin† at bedtime
- Insulin pump therapy**: continuous infusion of short-acting insulin
- NPH insulin at breakfast and bedtime, rapid-acting insulin before meals
- Premixed insulins (75/25‡, 50/50§) at breakfast and dinner
- Total daily insulin dose (TDD): 0.25–1.0 units/kg/d
- Basal/bolus: 50% long-acting, 50% rapid-acting
- NPH/rapid acting: ⅔ TDD in A.M., ⅓ TDD P.M.
- A.M. & P.M. dose: ⅔ NPH, ⅓ rapid-acting
- Premixed insulins: ⅔ A.M., ⅓ before dinner

Diabetic Ketoacidosis
- Fluids: 10 to 20 mL/kg normal saline × 1, repeat if shock/poor perfusion. Ongoing fluids: ½ normal saline with 20 mEq/L KCL and 20 mEq/L KPhos at 1.5 to 2.0 × maintenance fluids.
- Regular insulin infusion: 0.05 to 0.1 units/kg/h
- Add dextrose (5% to 10%) when glucose <300 mg/dL.
- Urgent consultation with center experienced in treatment of pediatric ketoacidosis (if not available on-site)

Type 2 Diabetes
1) Aggressive dietary modification
2) Metformin (Glucophage): 500 to 1000 mg bid, titrate up to avoid gastrointestinal side effects
3) 1) & 2) plus insulin therapy: either as single long-acting insulin at bed or full basal bolus regimen until stable glucose control

---

*Rapid-acting insulin: lispro, aspart, glulisine.
†Long-acting insulin: glargine, detemir, degludec.
‡75% intermediate-acting insulin, 25% rapid-acting insulin.
§50% intermediate-acting insulin, 50% rapid-acting insulin.
**Preferred treatment.

Type 1 Diabetes: Introduction

Type 1 diabetes mellitus (T1DM) results from progressive autoimmune destruction of insulin-producing (β-cell) cells of the pancreatic islets that ultimately leads to insulin deficiency resulting in hyperglycemia and in some cases ketoacidosis.

The precise cause of T1DM remains elusive, but an association with human lymphocytic antigens (HLA) has been known for decades. Whole genome-wide linkage studies have identified up to 60 genes associated with T1DM, and many are related to the immune response. The strongest linked genes to T1DM are HLA and insulin.

However, identical twin studies show a concordance rate of 30% to 60%, suggesting that unidentified environmental factors make up the remaining risk. Environmental factors implicated in T1DM risk include viral infections, toxins (nitrosamines), and dietary factors such as early exposure to cow's milk and cereals in infancy. However, recent prospective studies showed no advantage of using elemental formulas or delaying introduction of gluten until 1 year of life in infants at increased risk for development of T1DM. A large meta-analysis of 24 studies of over 4000 participants showed an almost 10-fold risk of RT-PCR determined enteroviral infections in T1D patients versus controls, while the TEDDY study showed an almost 50% conversion of high-risk infants and children to expressing islet cell antibodies when more than five respiratory infections were reported in the preceding 9 months.

Epidemiology

The prevalence of type 1 diabetes is about {1/300} (0.3%) in the United States, with significant global and racial variations. The presence of a first-degree relative with T1DM, such as a sibling or parent, increases the chances of developing T1DM to 3% to 6%.

The highest incidence rates of T1DM in children are seen in early adolescence (10 to 14 years), followed by early childhood ages 5 to 9 years. The youngest age of onset of T1DM can be seen in infants <1 year of age but usually not before 6 months.

The incidence of T1DM has been increasing steadily by 2% to 5% per year over the past several decades in the United States, Europe, and Australia, further implicating environmental causes for this disorder. Interestingly, in some but not all studies, the youngest age group (0 to 4 years) demonstrates the highest rates of rising incidence of T1DM.

Presentation

The classic symptoms of diabetes are polyuria, polydipsia, and nocturia, which is the result of an osmotic diuresis induced by hyperglycemia. Symptoms can be present from days to months, but the majority of patients present after 1 to 2 weeks of symptoms. Weight loss is a common finding on presentation, because insulin plays an important role in protein and fat synthesis, and therefore insulin deficiency results in loss of muscle and fat stores. Weight loss also occurs because calorie loss from high concentrations of glucose in the urine can be substantial.

Abdominal pain, nausea, and vomiting are classic signs of ketoacidosis that can often be misdiagnosed as gastroenteritis. Approximately 70% of patients with new-onset diabetes have hyperglycemia without ketoacidosis at presentation, whereas ~25% to 30% of cases present in diabetic ketoacidosis (DKA), although there can be significant variations from various centers internationally.

Diagnosis

A random glucose >200 mg/dL in the presence of classic symptoms of diabetes is diagnostic of diabetes. A fasting glucose >126 mg/dL is also diagnostic of diabetes; however, rarely is a fasting glucose or a glucose tolerance test necessary in the diagnosis of T1DM.

A venous pH <7.3 or a serum bicarbonate <15 mmol/L is diagnostic of DKA in the presence of hyperglycemia. Distinguishing type 1 from type 2 diabetes can sometimes be difficult at presentation, particularly in an overweight adolescent. In this circumstance islet cell autoantibodies are useful in distinguishing the two forms of diabetes. Islet cell autoantibodies include anti-glutamic

Treatment Options for Type 1 Diabetes

Regimen	12 am 6am noon 6 pm		comments
Basal-bolus		Rapid-acting insulin* Long-acting insulin#	Fixed basal dose Rapid-acting insulin with meals Ideal for insulin pens
Insulin pump		rapid acting Basal rate	Adjustable basal rate Ease of bolusing insulin Risk for infusion site failure
NPH and short-acting insulin		NPH rapid acting	Fewer insulin injections No lunch injection Usually suboptimal control
Fixed mixed insulins (e.g. 75/25)		75/25 insulin injection	Two injections per day—fixed doses Usually inadequate coverage Use only in most challenging cases

Figure 1 Treatment options for patients with type 1 diabetes. # Long-acting insulin: glargine (Lantus, Basaglar), degludec (Tresiba), detemir (Levemir). *Rapid-acting insulin: lispro (Humalog), aspart (Novolog), glulisine (Apidra). Note: {75/25}premixed insulin consists of 75% intermediate insulin (NPH) and 25% rapid-acting insulin, lispro (Humalog). Third-row arrows: NPH injections; fourth-row arrows 75/25 injections.

acid decarboxylase (GAD), anti-insulin, anti-insulinoma autoantigen 2 (IA-2), and anti-zinc transporter 8 (ZnT8). These antibodies are available in most commercial laboratories, but results are usually not available until weeks after initial presentation. The safest course of action in most pediatric patients with new-onset diabetes is to treat with insulin until islet antibodies and other parameters such as endogenous insulin production as assessed by c-peptide levels are available.

Treatment of Type 1 Diabetes Mellitus
Type 1 Diabetes Mellitus (Without Ketoacidosis or After Ketoacidosis has Resolved)
Insulin is the mainstay of treatment for T1DM. Intensive insulin therapy has become the standard of care for patients with T1DM. Typically a long-acting basal insulin such as glargine (Lantus, Basaglar), detemir (Levemir), or degludec (Tresiba), along with premeal boluses of rapid-acting insulin such as lispro (Humalog), aspart (NovoLog, Fiasp), or glulisine (Apidra), are instituted (Figure 1).

Required total daily insulin dosing (TDD) is dependent on age at presentation, pubertal stage, and the presence of acidosis at diagnosis. Total daily insulin requirements range from ~0.25 to 1.0 units/kg per day (Table 1). Long-acting or basal insulin is typically 50% of TDD, and the remaining 50% is bolus insulin. Bolus rapid-acting insulin dosing is calculated by the following formulas (Figure 2):

To cover meal carbohydrates, a *carbohydrate ratio* is derived from the following formula: 500/total daily insulin dose.

To correct hyperglycemia, a *correction factor* is derived from the following formula: 1500/total daily insulin dose. Correction doses should not be given more frequently than every 3 hours.

For new-onset patients, a *target glucose* of 150 mg/dL is assigned, whereas more established patients typically use 120 mg/dL. Correction at bedtime or during the night should be less aggressive, and a higher target may be assigned—for example, 150 to 200 mg/dL.

TABLE 1	Suggested Total Daily Insulin Dosage in New-Onset Type I Diabetes
PATIENT CATEGORY	INSULIN DOSE (UNITS/KG/DAY)
Prepubertal without DKA	0.25–0.5
Prepubertal with DKA	0.5–0.75
Pubertal without DKA	0.5–0.75
Pubertal with DKA	0.75–1.0

DKA, Diabetic ketoacidosis.

Patient Example 1

- 6 y.o. girl presents with 2 week history of polydipsia and polyuria.
- She is otherwise well with a normal exam.
- Serum glucose in the ER is 425 mg/dl and serum bicarbonate is 20.
- Weight in the ER: 20 kg

- Total daily insulin =
  - 20 kg X 0.3 u/kg/d = 6 units.
- ~50% basal = 3.0 units (glargine, degludec)
- Target = 150
- Carbohydrate ratio: 500/6 = 83~80
- Correction factor: 1500/6 = 250

Figure 2 New-onset type 1 diabetes in a 6-year-old girl who is not in diabetic ketoacidosis (DKA). Total daily insulin dosage is determined by multiplying body weight by recommended dosage requirements for a prepubertal girl who is not in DKA. One-half of total daily insulin dose is given as long-acting insulin, which is 3.0 units in this example. Carbohydrate ratio and correction factors are calculated using formulas provided in text. Calculated ratios can be adjusted up to 10% to simplify calculations.

Carbohydrate ratios, correction factors, and targets are adjusted on the basis of fasting and postprandial glucose levels. High postprandial glucose levels would require a lower carbohydrate ratio. High blood glucose levels that do not correct after a correction dose has been given would require a lowering of

Patient Example 2

- 8 y.o. boy—2 week history of polydipsia, polyuria and vomiting for for the past 24 hours.
- In doctors office: glucose 380 mg/dl and urine ketones are large.
- In emergency room serum HCO3 9, anion gap 25.
- Admitted to ICU for insulin drip, IV fluids, and frequent monitoring.
- At 7 am the following morning: glucose 120, HCO3 20.
- Weight: 25
- Family would like to avoid insulin at lunch as school nurse not available.

- Total daily dose 0.6 X 25 kg = 15 units
- 2/3 am = 10 units
  - 2/3 NPH ~ 6.5 units
  - 1/3 rapid acting 3.5 units
- 1/3 pm = 5 units
  - 1/3 rapid acting ~ 1.5 units before dinner
  - 2/3 NPH 3.5 units at bedtime
- Supplement with sliding scale: 0.5 unit rapid-acting insulin per 50 mg/dl above 200 mg/dl.

Figure 3 An 8-year-old boy who presents in diabetic ketoacidosis. Treated with insulin drip overnight and acidosis resolved by the morning. Parents desire regimen that does not require insulin at lunch time. Total daily insulin dose—see Table 1.

Patient Example 3

- 14 y.o. boy with cognitive delays presents with 3-week history of polydipsia and polyuria and 10 lb weight loss.
- Glucose 625 mg/dl in ER
- Bicarbonate 19 meq/l.
- Tanner 4 on exam
- Weight 44 kg
- Parents also have cognitive impairments

- Total daily dose: 44 kg X 0.6 u/kg/d = 26.4 units per day.
- Medical team decides fixed mixed 75/25 insulin regimen may be best.
- 2/3 TDD given before breakfast = 17 units
- 1/3 before dinner = 9 units
- Sliding scale rapid acting: 1 unit per 50 mg/dl over 200 mg/dl.

Figure 4 A 14-year-old boy with intellectual impairments presents with new-onset type 1 diabetes without diabetic ketoacidosis. Because of cognitive delays in patient and parents, a simplified two-injection regimen is derived using above calculations. Regimen may be supplemented with sliding scale of rapid-acting insulin.

the correction factor. High morning fasting glucose levels would require an increase in the long-acting insulin dose.

Implicit in recommending the above treatment regimen is (1) the patient or family's ability to count carbohydrates correctly and (2) the family's ability to calculate insulin dosing correctly using carbohydrate ratio, correction factor, and target. If the patient or family is unable or unwilling to perform these calculations, then a simplified insulin regimen should be devised using fixed doses of intermediate-acting insulin and a sliding scale of rapid-acting insulin (see Figure 1).

Less complex insulin regimens include NPH and rapid-acting insulin given at breakfast, dinner, and bedtime (Figure 3). NPH and rapid-acting insulin are given at breakfast (no insulin at lunch if glucose <200 mg/dL), rapid-acting insulin at dinner, and NPH at bedtime. This regimen can be used to avoid giving insulin at lunchtime. Typically, ⅔ of the daily dose is given in the morning, with ⅔ NPH, ⅓ rapid-acting, and ⅓ of daily dose given in evening. The evening dose is divided, with ⅓ rapid-acting before dinner and ⅔ NPH at bedtime. The patient should, however, consume a relatively fixed amount of carbohydrate at each meal. Consistency in meal content and portion sizes is very important in overall glycemic control. A simplified sliding scale of rapid-acting insulin may be added to the NPH and rapid-acting insulin regimen.

In certain challenging cases in which there are significant compliance or cognitive deficits, fixed doses of premixed intermediate- and rapid- or short-acting insulin such as Humalog mix {75/25} can be used before breakfast and before dinner (Figure 4). Pre-mixed {75/25} insulin preparations come in vials or pens and consist of 75% intermediate-acting (NPH) and 25% rapid-acting (lispro) insulins. Insulin pens are a very convenient way to give insulin, but in some cases, because of patient preference or insurer restrictions, dosing by syringe is preferred or required.

Treatment of Diabetic Ketoacidosis

There are critical differences in the treatment of DKA between children and adults. A major complication of the treatment of

TABLE 2	Formulas for Calculation of Maintenance Fluids for Infants and Children.
For infants 3.5–10 kg, daily fluid requirement = 100 mL/kg
For children 11–20 kg, daily fluid requirement = 1000 mL + 50 mL/kg for every kg over 10
For children >20 kg, daily fluid requirement = 1500 mL + 20 mL/kg for every kg over 20, up to a maximum of 2400 mL daily

DKA in children is cerebral edema, a complication rarely seen in adults. Although a relatively infrequent complication (<1% of DKA episodes), cerebral edema can be associated with serious morbidity and mortality.

Risk factors for the development of cerebral edema include new-onset diabetes, younger age at diagnosis, longer duration of symptoms before diagnosis, and severity of acidosis—manifested as DKA with hypocapnia, high blood urea nitrogen, bicarbonate boluses, and a failure for the corrected serum sodium to rise as treatment for DKA progresses. For these reasons, aggressive fluid resuscitation and boluses of bicarbonate are avoided in the treatment of pediatric DKA.

Judicious fluid replacement with a bolus of normal saline—initially 10 mL/kg and, if necessary, a second 10-mL/kg bolus of saline solution—may be given in the first hour of treatment. Thereafter ½ normal saline with 20 to 40 (usually 40) mEq/L of potassium chloride or potassium phosphate at a fluid rate of no more than 1.5 to 2.0 × maintenance is administered (Table 2). Dextrose (5% to 10%) should be added to the intravenous fluids when the serum glucose is between 250 to 300 mg/dL to prevent hypoglycemia and interruption of the insulin drip. Although fluid deficit estimates in DKA are between 5% and 10% of body weight, intravascular volume is often preserved in the hyperosmolar state, and hence hypovolemic shock is uncommon in DKA. The goal is to replace the fluid deficit slowly over 24 to 48 hours. Frequent neurologic checks are highly recommended in the first 24 hours of treatment. Altered mental status or development of a severe headache during treatment for DKA are potentially serious signs of cerebral edema.

Insulin plays a critical role in the treatment of DKA, not only in lowering serum glucose levels but also in the paramount role of shutting down ketogenesis in the liver. The standard insulin drip for pediatric DKA is 0.1 units/kg per hour; however, treatment with 0.05 units/kg per hour has been used effectively as well. Please note that human regular insulin remains the standard insulin in the intravenous treatment of DKA.

Once the acidosis has resolved as reflected by a normal anion gap and serum bicarbonate >15 mmol/L and pH >7.35, discontinuation of the insulin drip can be considered. Please note that hyperchloremic non-anion gap acidosis (HCO_3 <15 but normal anion gap <12) can occur during the recovery phase of DKA. Hyperchloremic metabolic acidosis is likely due to large amount of chloride administered in intravenous fluids as both NaCl and KCL supplementation. For this reason, many centers typically give 50% of the potassium replacement as potassium phosphate. Subcutaneous insulin can be started per the "Treatment of T1DM" section of this chapter once the acidosis is resolved and the patient can tolerate oral intake. The most convenient time to do so is just before a meal.

Importantly, treatment of pediatric DKA should ideally occur in centers with experienced pediatric intensivists, endocrinologists, and nursing staff. If referral to a pediatric center is not practical, then early contact with a pediatric endocrinologist for treatment guidance is highly recommended.

Finally, the most common causes of pediatric DKA are (1) new-onset diabetes presenting in DKA and (2) known T1DM usually due to infusion site failure in either a patient on an insulin pump or missed long-acting insulin injections in a patient on insulin injections. Infections including gastroenteritis and febrile illnesses are infrequently the exclusive cause of DKA in pediatrics.

Diabetes Self-Management Education

Children and adolescents with type 1 diabetes should receive outpatient care through multidisciplinary teams, which include an endocrinologist, certified diabetes educator, nurse, registered dietician, and licensed clinical social worker. Provision of comprehensive education at the time of diagnosis is essential, because this is a time when the patient and family are most receptive and impressionable. Patients who do not receive proper early education often fall into suboptimal diabetes care habits that can be hard to undo once established.

Important educational topics that must be rapidly learned by the family and patient in addition to glucose monitoring and insulin administration include diet and carbohydrate counting, prevention and treatment of hypoglycemia, emergency glucagon, exercise and hypoglycemia, prevention of ketoacidosis, and sick day management. Learning to count carbohydrates accurately is a particularly challenging skill to master.

Mental Health Considerations in Type 1 Diabetes Mellitus

Diabetes "burnout" issues are common in the treatment of youth with diabetes, particularly during the adolescent years. Conflicts between parents and teens can often arise during this time, and it is important for the parents to maintain a healthy supporting role with their child or teenager in an age and developmentally appropriate manner. Recognition of relatively common mental health comorbidities, such as depression, anxiety, and eating disorders, is essential to the overall well-being of the pediatric patient with T1DM.

Goals of Therapy for Patients With Type 1 Diabetes Mellitus

The number-one goal of the diabetes healthcare team is to prevent readmission to the hospital for severe hypoglycemia or ketoacidosis. Resumption of the full range of daily activities, including returning to school and work, as well as engaging in essentially all meaningful activities that preceded the diagnosis of diabetes, is to be expected.

Although the goal hemoglobin A1c in the pediatric age group is <7.5%, less than 25% of pediatric patients in the United States are able to achieve that goal. The average hemoglobin A1c in the pediatric population is approximately 8.2%, whereas in 19-year-olds the average hemoglobin A1c is 9.2%.

The Diabetes Control and Complications Trial (DCCT) in 1993 showed convincingly that lowering the hemoglobin A1c from 9% to 7.1% resulted in significantly less diabetes-related retinopathy, nephropathy, and neuropathy. Most patients in the DCCT trial who were randomized to the intensive-treated group used insulin pumps to achieve tighter control, but tight control was achieved with injectable insulin regimens as well.

Sick Day Management

Patients with T1DM who have development of intercurrent infectious illnesses are prone to hyperglycemia with ketosis and also hypoglycemia, depending on the nature of the individual illness. Blood glucose levels should be monitored every 1 to 3 hours during illnesses. Rapid-acting insulin may need to be administered every 2 to 4 hours for hyperglycemia, especially in the presence of serum or urine ketones. Rapid-acting insulin can be dosed at 0.1 to 0.2 units/kg/dose in this setting. Improvement in hyperglycemia and particularly in ketosis using the above treatment regimen can be invaluable in preventing ketoacidosis or hospitalization. Patients with persistent vomiting who are unable to keep fluids down need to be referred to the emergency department for intravenous hydration and assessment for DKA.

For patients on an insulin pump, ketosis with nausea and vomiting is often a sign that the insulin infusion set is not properly functioning. Insulin therefore should be given by syringe or pen device until the ketones have cleared and a new infusion set has been placed.

Poor oral intake during a gastrointestinal illness may result in hypoglycemia. Frequent small volumes of sugar-containing fluids such as juice or sports drinks may be necessary to keep the blood glucose >70 mg/dL, and basal insulin requirements may need to be decreased by 10% to 50%. Low-dose glucagon may be used in the setting of recurrent hypoglycemia and poor oral intake. Glucagon can be dosed at 1 unit on an insulin syringe for every year of age, using a standard 1-mg/mL glucagon preparation. The dose may be repeated every 15 minutes as needed. In some cases, persistent low glucose levels (<70 mg/dL) in the setting of recurrent vomiting may be best managed in an emergency department or hospital setting where intravenous dextrose-containing fluids are readily available.

Risk for Additional Autoimmune Disorders

Patients with one autoimmune disorder are at increased risk for development of one or more additional autoimmune conditions. Children and adolescents with T1DM are particularly at risk for thyroid and celiac disorders. Screening for thyroid disorders with serum TSH and free T_4 should occur in the first 6 months after T1DM diagnosis and every 1 to 2 years thereafter. Celiac disorder should also be screened in the first year after diabetes diagnosis. Most cases of celiac disorder are detected within the first 5 years after diagnosis of T1DM, and the majority of cases are asymptomatic. Recent American Diabetes Association recommendations include screening for celiac disorder at diagnosis and again at 2 and 5 years after diagnosis. Elevated serum tissue transglutaminase levels should be referred to a pediatric gastroenterologist. Because the diagnosis of celiac disorder is a lifelong condition, obtaining a small bowel biopsy is advised. Autoimmune adrenal (Addison) disease rarely occurs with T1DM but has the unique presentation of recurrent hypoglycemia, necessitating significant reductions in daily insulin requirements. Sending simultaneous ACTH and cortisol levels on a morning blood specimen usually will render the diagnosis of Addison disease.

Screening for Complications of Type 1 Diabetes Mellitus

Microvascular complications of T1DM are infrequent in the pediatric age group, although background retinopathy and microalbuminuria become more prevalent in the late-adolescent and young-adult age ranges. Proactive early screening regimens are advocated to detect diabetes complications early so that medical interventions can prevent more serious diabetes-related complications such as proliferative retinopathy and end-stage renal disease.

Annual screening for microalbuminuria with a random urine specimen should be performed at puberty or at age >10 years once the child has had diabetes for 5 years. Elevated urine albumin/urine creatinine (>30 mg/gm creatinine) ratios should be repeated 2 to 3 times over a 6-month period to confirm the diagnosis, because transient microalbuminuria is a common finding. Variables such as exercise or recent illness can lead to microalbuminuria, and therefore repeating the study after recovery and on a first morning specimen will often be normal. In addition, individuals with the benign condition of orthostatic albuminuria can be identified by finding completely normal albumin excretion on a first morning-voided specimen, whereas a random specimen will often be frankly proteinuric. When urinary albumin/creatinine ratios are found to be consistently elevated, then treatment with an angiotensin converting enzyme inhibitor is recommended. Referral to a pediatric nephrologist should be obtained in complex cases.

Annual dilated eye examinations are recommended after age 10 or at pubertal onset (whichever comes first) once the patient has had diabetes for 3 to 5 years. Referral to an eye care professional with expertise in diabetic retinopathy is recommended.

Cardiovascular risk factors including blood pressure and lipid profiles should be monitored in patients with T1DM. Blood pressure should be obtained at each visit.

High blood pressure is defined as systolic or diastolic blood pressure >90th percentile, and hypertension is defined as >95th percentile for age, sex, and height. Blood pressure measurements should be obtained using an appropriate cuff size, particularly in the overweight patient. White-coat hypertension can be problematic in the adolescent population. Such patients will often demonstrate elevated heart rate as a clue to stress-induced hypertension. Monitoring blood pressure in a nonthreatening environment, such as at home, using an accurate home blood pressure monitor may be helpful. Twenty-four–hour home blood pressure monitoring can be very useful when white-coat hypertension is suspected.

Initial management of high blood pressure includes salt restriction and weight control measures. For persistent hypertension, treatment with an antihypertensive medication (lisinopril) may be necessary.

Obtain non-fasting total and high-density lipoprotein cholesterol shortly after diagnosis once glucose control has been established. If total cholesterol is high, then obtain a fasting morning lipid panel. If low-density lipoprotein (LDL) cholesterol is <100, then repeating in 5 years is reasonable. For elevated LDL cholesterol >100, dietary measures are taken, along with efforts to improve metabolic control. For patients >10 years of age with an LDL cholesterol >130 to 160 and in whom lifestyle changes resulted in inadequate lowering of LDL cholesterol, statin therapy may be considered. Referral to a pediatric preventive cardiology program would also be appropriate.

Technological Changes in Type 1 Diabetes Mellitus Care

Technological changes have revolutionized the care of patients with T1DM. Unheralded changes such as the emergence of ultrafine lancet technology coupled with glucose test strips requiring less than 10 μL of blood resulted in rapid essentially painless fingerstick glucose monitoring. Ultrafine insulin syringes and pen needles helped usher in widespread adoption of intensive insulin regimens with rapid-acting insulin taken before all meals and snacks.

The insulin pump further advanced diabetes care in making insulin dosing before meals and snacks even less challenging, especially for children. The development of a tubeless insulin pump (Omnipod) led to an even wider array of insulin pump choices.

Continuous glucose monitoring (CGM) has evolved into a very powerful and widely used technology in T1DM. Subcutaneous fluid glucose levels are determined every 5 minutes and provide the user with meaningful feedback to influence diabetes self-management decisions in a real-time fashion. Particularly useful are alarm functions for impending low glucose levels that can be invaluable in the prevention of hypoglycemia. Alarms for hyperglycemia are also used regularly with this technology. The accuracy of glucose determinations by CGM technology is now approaching subcutaneous blood glucose technology, and the improved accuracy has led the US Food and Drug Administration (FDA) to approve insulin-dosing decisions based on CGM data (Dexcom G5 and G6). It is important to remember, however, that subcutaneous glucose levels lag behind whole blood glucose levels by about 15 minutes. This fact is particularly important when glucose levels are changing rapidly, so the user is advised to pay attention to the glucose trend. Alarms for predictive hypoglycemia are also available in some CGM technology platforms.

A drawback to CGM technology has been the need to calibrate the device accurately with periodic fingerstick glucose checks. Calibration must be done correctly, or inaccurate CGM glucose data will result. Ideally calibrations should be done when glucose levels are not changing, which for some individuals with high glucose variability may not be practical. However, the Dexcom G6 that was released to market in 2018 and the Abbot Libre are factory calibrated and no longer require consumer calibration. Remarkably, patients using calibration-free CGM may no longer be required to check fingerstick glucose levels! A CGM sensor placed on the arm or abdomen will last 7 to 14 days before needing to be changed.

The most remarkable technological changes emerging in the care of patients with T1DM is the coupling of CGM and insulin pump technologies to provide hybrid closed-loop insulin pump therapy (Medtronic 670G insulin pump) or suspending insulin delivery when hypoglycemia has occurred or is likely to occur (Tandem Basal IQ). *Hybrid closed-loop* refers to the fact that some aspects of management such as carbohydrate counting and manual bolusing for meals are still required.

The first hybrid closed-loop insulin pump was FDA approved in 2016 (Medtronic 670G). This technology involves coupling the Medtronic Guardian sensor with the 670G insulin pump using algorithms that will deliver microboluses of insulin, depending on sensor glucose levels. Conversely, insulin delivery can be halted when the rate of falling glucose predicts hypoglycemia or the patient is in the hypoglycemic range. However, carbohydrate counting and entry of carbohydrate content of meals must be manually entered by the user before meals. Prevention of postprandial hyperglycemia can be achieved by pre-bolusing rapid-acting insulin 10 to 30 minutes before eating. Pre-bolusing of rapid-acting insulin is particularly difficult in view of modern lifestyles. Hybrid closed-loop technology can be particularly useful for overnight glycemic control, when many patients and families are most fearful of hypoglycemia. The Medtronic 670G, however, has proven to be very challenging in the "real world" setting due to technical problems with the Guardian sensor but also due to frequent calibration requirements and forced exits from hybrid closed loop insulin delivery. In our center, more than 40% of patients discontinued use of the Medtronic hybrid closed loop insulin delivery system for these reasons. Medtronic plans to upgrade their HCL system with fewer calibration requirements and fewer forced exits from automatic insulin delivery in their next generation hybrid closed loop system. A number of additional hybrid closed-loop systems are currently in clinical trials or awaiting FDA approval (Omnipod Horizon, Tandem Control IQ, Beta Bionic iLet), and the diabetes community can look forward to further remarkable technological advancements in the near future.

Type 2 Diabetes in Children

Since the 1990s, type 2 diabetes mellitus (T2DM) in the <18-year-old age group has risen dramatically. The increased incidence of type 2 diabetes has coincided with the obesity epidemic. Children from minority populations (non-Hispanic black, Hispanic, Native Americans) and those patients with a positive family history of T2DM are at the greatest risk. The majority of pediatric T2DM is found in adolescents and children >10 years of age.

Diagnosis of T2DM can be made with a fasting glucose >126 mg/dL, random glucose >200 mg/dL, and oral glucose tolerance test 2-hour glucose >200 mg/dL. A hemoglobin A1c >6.5% is indicative of diabetes as well and is particularly convenient in the outpatient setting. An elevated fasting or random glucose and an elevated hemoglobin A1c are diagnostic of T2DM in high-risk patients.

Pediatric patients with T2DM are often symptom free at diagnosis but can present acutely with classic diabetes symptoms and even ketosis or mild ketoacidosis. Distinguishing the latter group from T1DM can be difficult initially, but the absence of beta cell antibodies and very stable glycemic control after diagnosis are often telltale signs of T2DM.

In individuals who present with marked hyperglycemia (hemoglobin A1c >8.5%), ketosis, or both, stabilization with insulin initially may be required. Basal bolus regimens using a combination of long- and short-acting insulins can be instituted. Insulin resistance may be quite significant at the time of diagnosis, and relatively high doses of insulin can be required to achieve target glucose levels.

Metformin (Glucophage) is the mainstay of treatment for T2DM treatment for T2DM in the <18-year-old age group. Maximal dosing is 1000 mg bid or 2000 mg/day of the extended-release preparation. Gastrointestinal side effects are relatively common, and metformin should be taken with meals. Initial dosing can be 500 mg bid or 1000 mg extended-release daily, and the dose can be titrated upward as needed and tolerated. Bear in mind that dietary modifications such as weight control and exercise are of fundamental importance in the treatment of T2DM. Liraglutide (Victoza) a glucagon-like peptide (GLP-1) agonist was FDA approved for the treatment of T2DM for patients > 10 years of age in 2019. GLP-1 agonist are associated with early satiety, weight loss, and improved glycemic control in adult T2DM; however, side effects such as nausea are common, and an increased risk of pancreatitis is well recognized. Given the limited pediatric experience with GLP-1 agonists, health care practitioners should use cautiously and perhaps limit use to pediatric T2DM patients who have suboptimal outcomes with metformin and insulin.

Adherence to a healthy diet in combination with metformin alone, insulin therapy, or both often results in very stable glycemic control in T2DM in pediatrics. In many cases, bolus short-acting insulin and even long-acting insulin therapy can be withdrawn safely 6 to 12 months after diagnosis. However, resumption of lax dietary and self-care habits can result in significant decline in glycemic control and the need to restart insulin. Therefore patients with T2DM need to be as vigilant as patients with T1DM with regular monitoring of glucose levels and follow-up visits every 3 to 6 months with their healthcare team.

Monogenic or Maturity Onset Diabetes of Youth (MODY)

Single-gene mutations leading to diabetes are referred to as *MODY diabetes* or *monogenic diabetes*. Up to 14 individual forms of MODY diabetes have been described, although ~80% of cases are due to glucokinase and *HNF1A* and *HNF1B* gene mutations. Patients can be diagnosed at any age but usually are diagnosed before age 35 years. Routine laboratory testing or laboratory testing during an illness may lead to detection of MODY diabetes incidentally. Patients with MODY are often lean, and the family history may reveal two to three affected generations. Testing for islet cell antibodies is universally negative.

Glucokinase diabetes is a very mild form of MODY diabetes that is nonprogressive and does not require treatment, whereas HNF alpha and beta forms of MODY diabetes are progressive, and these patients can develop long-term complications of diabetes. HNF diabetes is uniquely sensitive to sulfonylureas, and hence the diagnosis can be life changing in an individual who has been treated with insulin prior to definitive diagnosis.

Genetic panels for MODY diabetes are available commercially, and genetic testing is increasingly covered by insurance companies in the United States. It is important to test for both mutations and deletions of the most common forms of MODY. A full list of laboratories that offer MODY testing is available at the NCBI Genetic Testing Registry (http://www.ncbi.nlm.nih.gov/gtr/).

Neonatal diabetes can also be due to monogenic forms of diabetes, and these infants are usually diagnosed before 6 to 9 months of age. Testing for monogenetic forms of diabetes should be considered in infants <9 to 12 months of age whose islet cell auto-antibodies are negative. Single gene mutations in the K-ATP channel of the beta cell leading to neonatal diabetes can be remarkably responsive to oral sulfonylureas.

References

American Diabetes Association: Children and adolescents: Standards of medical care in diabetes—2018, *Diabetes Care* 41(Suppl 1):S126–S136, 2018.

Copeland KC, Zeiter P, Geffner M, et al: Characteristics of adolescents and youth with recent-onset type 2 diabetes: the TODAY cohort at baseline, *J Clin Endocrinol Metab* 96:159–167, 2011.

Delli AJ, Lernmark A: Type 1 (insulin-dependent) diabetes mellitus: Etiology, pathogenesis, prediction, and prevention. In *Endocrinology: Adult and Pediatric*, 7th ed., Saunders, 2016.

International Consensus on Use of Continuous Glucose Monitoring, *Diabetes Care* 40:1631–1640, 2017.

Levitsky L, Misra M: Epidemiology, presentation and diagnosis of type 1 diabetes in children and adolescents. Up To Date. Available at Up To Date. Accessed October 4, 2019.

Miller KM, Foster NC, Beck RW, et al: Current state of type 1 diabetes treatment in the US: updated data from the T1D Exchange Clinic Registry, *Diabetes Care* 38:971–978, 2015.

Sperling MA, Tamborlane WR, Sperling MA, et al: In *Pediatric Endocrinology*, 4th ed., Philadelphia, 2014, Elsevier, pp 847–900.

The Environmental Determinants of Diabetes Study: Available at: https://teddy.epi.usf.edu/. Accessed October 4, 19.

The National Center for Monogenic Diabetes at the University of Chicago Monogenic Diabetes Registry. Available at Monogenic https://monogenicdiabetes.uchicago.edu/. Accessed October 4, 19.

White NH: Long-term outcomes in youth with diabetes mellitus, *Pediatr Clin North Am* 62:889–909, 2015.

Wolfsdorf JI: The International Society of Pediatric and Adolescent Diabetes guidelines for management of ketoacidosis: do the guidelines need to be modified? *Pediatric Diabetes* 15:277–286, 2014.

Wolfsdorf JI, Garvey K: Diabetes mellitus in children. In Jameson L, DeGroot L, editors: *Endocrinology Adult and Pediatric*, 7th ed., Philadelphia, 2016, Saunders, pp 854–882.

Writing Group for the TRIGR Study Group: Effect of hydrolyzed infant formula vs conventional formula on the risk of type 1 diabetes, *JAMA* 319:38, 2018.

Yeung W, Rawlinson W, Craig M: Enterovirus infection and type 1 diabetes mellitus: Systematic review and meta-analysis of observational molecular studies, *BMJ: British Medical Journal* 342(7794):421, 2011.

ENCOPRESIS

Method of
Sarah Houssayni, MD

CURRENT DIAGNOSIS

- Voluntary or involuntary passage of stools into inappropriate places at least once a month for 3 consecutive months once a chronologic or developmental age of 4 years has been reached.
- Encopresis can be primary when it persists from infancy onward or secondary when it appears after toilet training.
- The behavior is not due to the direct effects of a substance such as a laxative or a general medical condition except those associated with constipation.
- Distinguishing subtypes is essential because treatment differs:
  - Retentive encopresis: occurs as a result of involuntary leakage of liquid stools due to severe constipation and impaction.
  - Nonretentive encopresis: children pass bowel movements into their underwear due to their refusal to use the toilet.
  - Children occasionally fail to wipe after bowel movements and the secondary soiling should be distinguished from encopresis.

CURRENT THERAPY

Retentive Encopresis
Initial Disimpaction
- Hyperphosphate enemas (Pedia-Lax Enema) (one daily for 2 or 3 days):
  - Less than 1 year old: 60 mL.[3]
  - Greater than 1 year old: 6 mL/kg, up to 135 mL twice.[3]
- Glycerin suppositories (Glycerin Pediatric Suppositories) for infants and toddlers.

Older Children—Slow Disimpaction
- Polyethylene glycol with electrolytes (Golytely, Colyte)[1] ingested over 2–3 days: 25 mL/kg/hr up to 1 L/hr until stooling clear bowel movements. (This is not approved for bowel cleansing for children.)
- Over 5–7 days:
  - Mineral oil[1] 3 mL/kg twice a day for 1 week. (Mineral oil is not approved for use in children younger than 6 years of age.)
  - Lactulose[1] 2 mL/kg twice a day for 1 week.
  - Magnesium hydroxide (Milk of Magnesia) 2 mL/kg twice a day for 1 week.
  - Polyethylene glycol without electrolyte (MiraLax)[1] 1.5 g/kg/day for 3 days.

Maintenance Therapy

- Polyethylene glycol 3350 (MiraLax)[1] age greater than 1 month: 0.7 g/kg divided into 1–2 doses daily.
- Lactulose or sorbitol 70% solution age greater than 1 month: 1–3 mL/kg/day divided into 1–2 doses daily for 1–3 months.
- Sennosides (Senna, Senna-GRX, Senexon) are habit forming, doses vary greatly in the different available formulations, and they can only be used for short-term treatment. Give at bedtime for a morning bowel movement. Dose is 5 mL (1 tablet) for 1-[1] to 5-year-olds and 2 tablets for 5- to 15-year-olds for a maximum of three tablets daily. (Sennosides are not approved for use in children younger than 2 years of age.)
- Glycerin enemas and bisacodyl suppositories (Dulcolax) can be used for short-term constipation treatment.
- Glycerin/saline enema in patients greater than 10 years of age: 20–30 mL/day (solution of 1/2 glycerin and 1/2 normal saline).
- Bisacodyl suppositories in patients greater than 10 years of age: 10 mg daily.

Nonretentive Encopresis

- **NO** medical treatment.
- Clean up soiling immediately, involve the child.
- Ensure adequate water and dietary fiber intake.
- Avoid use of stool softeners and laxatives.
- **STOP** all reminders, make child responsible for own toilet habits.
- Use rewards when child defecates in toilet.
- Refer to health care professional when refractory (refuses to sit on toilet and older than 5 years of age, refuses to take medication, is older than 8 years of age with nonretentive encopresis).

[1]Not FDA approved for this indication.
[3]Exceeds dosage recommended by the manufacturer; manufacturer-recommended doses are: 5–11 y, 1 bottle (60 mL); 2–4 y, half bottle (30 mL); <2 y, do not use.

Encopresis is the voluntary or involuntary passage of stools at least once a month for 3 consecutive months once a chronologic or developmental age of 4 years has been reached. Encopresis is classified as primary when it persists from infancy onward or secondary when it appears after toilet training. Retentive encopresis occurs as a result of involuntary leakage of liquid stools due to severe constipation and fecal impaction. Nonretentive encopresis occurs in children who pass stool into their underwear due to their refusal to use the toilet. It is important to distinguish between the types of encopresis, because treatment differs.

Epidemiology

The prevalence of encopresis is reported to be 4% in 5- to 6-year-olds and 1.5% in 11- to 12-year-olds. Affected boys outnumber girls by a factor of anywhere from 3:1 to 5:1 depending on the source. Encopresis tends to decrease with age. A large number of children with encopresis go unreported due to the shame associated with the condition and underdiagnosis of the condition.

Diagnosis

The diagnosis of encopresis includes the following four criteria: (1) Repeated passage of feces into inappropriate places such as in clothing or on the floor, whether intentional or involuntary. (2) At least one event a month for at least 3 months. (3) A chronologic age of at least 4 years or an equivalent developmental level. (4) The behavior is not due exclusively to the direct physiologic effects of a substance such as a laxative or a general medical condition other than constipation.

Differential Diagnosis

Retentive encopresis is organic in less than 5% of the affected patients. Organic causes include hypothyroidism, hypercalcemia, cerebral palsy, abnormal anatomy of the anus, Hirschsprung's disease, cystic fibrosis, and neuropathy with secondary impaired voiding sensation. Spinal cord conditions such as tethered cord, spina bifida occulta, and spinal cord dysplasia affect stooling through diminished bowel sensation and secondary fecal retention.

Pathophysiology

Patients who are severely constipated hold stools back because of the pain associated with defecation. This becomes a vicious cycle of constipation, rectal dilation, and secondary encopresis. Frequently, emotional problems emerge due to the fear and shame associated with the problem. Control issues with parents trying to take the stooling issues at hand may worsen the constipation problem.

From 10% to 20% of encopretic patients are not constipated. They are frequently preschoolers or school-age children who are postponing their bowel movements too long because they are distracted or because they associate the bathroom with an unpleasant experience (i.e., fear or disgust).

Clinical Manifestations

History

The history should assess for size and consistency of stools, as well as stooling intervals. Families often confuse soiling with stooling, leading to inaccurate reporting of the frequency of bowel movements. Characteristic symptoms of retentive and nonretentive encopresis differ (Table 1).

In retentive encopresis the physician may elicit a history of difficult or painful defecation, crying with bowel movements, and posturing that suggests the child is deliberately holding back stools due to the pain associated with passage.

Children may suddenly become still or hide during play, cross their legs, grimace, or shift their position in an attempt to retain stools. The physician should assess for a history of enuresis and urinary tract infections, anorexia, sensations of bloating, fullness, and abdominal pain leading to the patient's avoidance of food and weight loss. Obtain a dietary history including fiber, fluid, and dairy intake. The historian needs to inquire about streaks of blood on toilet paper and underwear. With retentive encopresis, when the child does pass stool, it may be of large caliber and hard, indicative of constipation.

With nonretentive encopresis, the history often reveals bowel movements of normal size and consistency passed into the underwear once or twice a day. Symptoms of constipation are usually absent. A history of behavioral problems, child-parent struggles, and history of abuse may be elicited. Toilet avoidance is common.

TABLE 1	Characteristic Symptoms of Retentive and Nonretentive Encopresis

Retentive Encopresis

- Constipation
- Stained underwear
- Fewer than three bowel movements per week
- Large-caliber or hard stools
- Abdominal pain, reports of bloated sensation
- Odor of feces from leakage onto underwear
- Difficult or painful defecation
- Enuresis
- Overflow incontinence
- Anorexia

Nonretentive Encopresis

- Passage of stools in inappropriate places without presence of constipation
- Refusal to sit on toilet even though old enough to (older than 5 years, even older than 8 years at times)
- Refusal to take medications
- Child may be depressed

Patients with encopresis eventually develop secondary emotional problems, which can be elicited from the history taking.

Physical Examination

Retentive Encopresis

In retentive soiling the physical examination should assess for abdominal distention and tenderness on palpation. A mass can be occasionally felt in the midline in the suprapubic area. This mass of hardened fecal matter most commonly involves the rectosigmoid area and can sometimes extend throughout the entire colon. If the patient is anxious or in pain and tightens the rectus abdominis, this mass can be missed. Rectal examination is a must; it can be done with minimal discomfort. Rectal examination assesses the dilation of the rectum, which may be 6 to 10 cm wide. It is usually packed with stools with clay-like consistency. Visually inspect the anal opening for tone, fissure, and hemorrhoids.

Nonretentive Encopresis

The child with nonretentive encopresis typically has a normal abdominal examination, is likely to have a rectal vault that is not dilated, and the stool will be of normal caliber and consistency. The rectal vault may be empty if the child has just passed a bowel movement. The anal opening may reveal protruding fecal material in children who are deliberate stool holders.

Treatment

Encopresis is treated through a multistep approach. First, clearing the colon of fecal material will allow the dilated rectal vault and rectosigmoid colon to return to normal. The rectal cleanout can be achieved in different ways (see Current Therapy). Enemas and stool softeners are often used in combination.

Maintenance is achieved by keeping stools soft and ensuring daily bowel movements with mineral oil and hyperosmolar agents (e.g., Miralax[1]) that are very safe and can be used from a very young age and are not habit forming. The goal is painless stools once or twice a day with no associated withholding behavior.

Education is key for families so that they understand the physiology and process of stool elimination. Frustration is associated with failure, guilt, and depression and should be replaced with a positive attitude if success is to be achieved.

- Patients should sit daily on the toilet for 5 minutes after meals twice a day.
- Families need to keep a record of the events, as well as a record for success.
- Soiled underwear should be changed as soon as noticed and the child should be cleaned and changed in a timely, emotionally neutral fashion.
- As soon as compliance wanes, the problem is expected to return and is sometimes worse than the previous episode.
- The care provider's continued involvement in titrating medication with the patient's symptoms is necessary.
- Pain-related impaction can be cured in the majority of cases with medical management of the initial presentation. The success rate is reported to be about 70% with psychogenic impaction.
- With nonretentive encopresis, behavioral modification is essential. Stress reduction, effective coping techniques, relaxation training, and a combination of individual and family therapy is sometimes indicated.

---

[1] Not FDA approved for this indication.

References

Baker SS, et al: Clinical practice guideline. Evaluation and treatment of constipation in infants and children: recommendations of the North American Society for Pediatric Gastroenterology, Hepatology and Nutrition, *J Pediatr Gastroenterol Nutr* 43:e1–e13, 2006.
Becker A, Ruby M, El Khatib D, et al: Central nervous system processing of emotions with faecal incontinence, *Acta Paediatr* 100:e267–e747, 2011.
Boris NM, Dalton R, et al: *Encopresis, Nelson Textbook of Pediatrics*, ed 19, Philadelphia, 2011, Saunders.
Brazzelli M, Griffiths P: Behavioral and cognitive interventions with or without other treatments for the management of faecal incontinence in children, Art. No. CD002240, *Cochrane Database Syst Rev*(2), 2006. https://doi.org/10.1002/14651858.CD002240.pub3.
Coelho DP: Encopresis. A medical and family approach, *Pediatr Nurs* 37:107–112, 2011.
Har AF, Groffie JM: Encopresis, *Pediatr Rev* 31:368–374, 2010.
Raghumath N, Glassman MS, Halata MS, et al: Anorectal motility abnormalities in children with encopresis and chronic constipation, *J Pediatr* 158:293–296, 2011.

EPILEPSY IN INFANTS AND CHILDREN

Method of
Adam L. Hartman, MD

CURRENT DIAGNOSIS

- At initial diagnosis, determine whether the event was a seizure or not.
- If appropriate, diagnose an epilepsy *syndrome*.
- Age of onset aids in the development of a differential diagnosis.

CURRENT THERAPY

- Selection of an antiseizure medicine should be made based on the type of seizure.
- General principles include the use of a single agent at the lowest effective dose with the goal of no side effects.
- Epilepsy can be associated with comorbidities, including depression and anxiety. Successful management includes referrals and/or management of these and associated psychosocial issues.

A seizure can be defined as clinical signs or symptoms resulting from abnormal neuronal firing. Epilepsy is defined as either (1) at least two unprovoked seizures occurring >24 hours apart; (2) one unprovoked seizure and a probability of further seizures similar to the general recurrence risk (at least 60%) after two unprovoked seizures, occurring over the next 10 years; or (3) diagnosis of an epilepsy syndrome. There may be associated psychological, social, and cognitive consequences. Approximately 3% to 5% of the US population have had a seizure (mostly febrile seizures). Nearly 1% of the US population are being treated actively for seizures at any given time. Infants and children represent one of the two major peaks in seizure incidence, making this a very common diagnosis in pediatric practice.

Risk Factors

The primary risk factors for epilepsy in any age group include a history of meningitis, encephalitis, brain trauma, complicated perinatal course, and febrile seizures. Other risk factors for seizures include cortical or developmental malformations, certain inborn errors of metabolism or genetic syndromes, congenital infections, stroke, intracranial hemorrhage, acute metabolic abnormalities, and drug withdrawal.

Pathophysiology

Because the primary abnormality is abnormal neuron firing, many different types of pathology can lead to seizures. Abnormalities in neuronal networks (e.g., cortical malformations), structure (e.g., abnormal dendrite structure in trisomy 21), or ion channels (e.g., *KCNQ2*) can lead to seizures. In many cases, an underlying cause of seizures cannot be identified. Some forms of epilepsy have been linked to various genetic mutations, although the exact relationship between specific genotypes and phenotypes is unclear for most.

Clinical Manifestations

Broadly speaking, the clinical manifestations of seizures vary depending on which brain structures are involved. Although most people think of seizures only as generalized tonic–clonic seizures (GTCS), a wide variety of signs and symptoms can be caused by seizures. Furthermore, a GTCS may be the initial manifestation of a seizure (i.e., as seen in primary generalized epilepsy) or it may be the end result of a seizure that started in one brain location and then spread to the rest of the brain (e.g., a focal-onset seizure with spread to other broad cortical regions of the brain). These two broad categories (generalized versus focal onset) are approached somewhat differently from a diagnostic and therapeutic perspective.

Signs of a generalized seizure (i.e., those involving abnormal neuronal firing in both sides of the brain) include loss of interaction or staring (absence seizures), myoclonus, tonic posturing, and/or tonic–clonic seizures. Signs of focal-onset seizures can involve specific regions controlling motor, sensory, or autonomic function, a loss of interaction and/or awareness, or automatisms (chewing, lip smacking, repetitive hand motions), to name a few. Patients with focal seizures might have an aura (a warning sign just prior to the seizure). The aura is an altered sensory function that can include salty or metallic taste, tingling sensations, rising sensation in the abdomen, déjà vu, jamais vu, sense of fear, or a nonspecific feeling that something is about to happen. After a seizure, patients also can have a period of postictal lethargy, confusion, or irritability.

The initial symptoms or signs of a seizure are the most important in determining whether a seizure is generalized or focal in origin because they often localize the anatomic site of pathology. Thus, it is the beginning of a seizure, rather than its end, that is most useful in making a specific diagnosis.

Diagnosis and Management

History and Physical Examination

A detailed history is usually more valuable than any expensive test in diagnosing a seizure or epilepsy. In addition to a description of the actual event, it is useful to inquire about subtle signs that might not be recognized by observers as a seizure, including staring spells, myoclonic jerks, loss of time, and unexplained nocturnal tongue biting, enuresis, or emesis. The presence of postictal weakness can help localize the hemisphere of onset after a focal seizure, even if secondarily generalized. Making the diagnosis of a specific epilepsy syndrome allows the clinician to develop a plan for further diagnosis and treatment and to counsel about prognosis. On physical examination, any signs of focal neurologic deficits can indicate an underlying lesion. A skin examination might identify a neurophakomatosis, such as tuberous sclerosis complex or Sturge Weber syndrome.

Diagnostic Studies

In selected cases, typical clinical findings in the right clinical context strongly support the diagnosis of epilepsy, but an electroencephalogram (EEG) may be required to confirm the diagnosis. Even if the patient does not have a seizure during the EEG recording, interictal findings (when the patient is not having a seizure) can provide enough evidence to make the diagnosis of epilepsy. Under ideal circumstances, a single EEG can detect epileptiform activity in a patient with untreated generalized epilepsy about 75% of the time, making it a very sensitive test. In contrast, an EEG can detect epileptiform activity in a patient with focal-onset seizures only 50% of the time (although this number increases to about 90% after three EEGs have been done). Conversely, a normal interictal EEG (particularly one that includes sleep and provocative maneuvers such as intermittent photic stimulation and hyperventilation) in an untreated patient suggests, but is not necessarily diagnostic of, a focal rather than generalized onset.

Other ancillary studies can show underlying structural lesions that lead to epilepsy or provide physiologic information. Magnetic resonance imaging (MRI) can be useful in detecting lesions such as tumors, cortical dysgenesis, and strokes (both ischemic and hemorrhagic). Recent advances in image analysis have substantially improved the ability to find subtle regions of cortical dysgenesis that may be the source of seizures. Positron-emission tomography (PET) scans may show regions of abnormal metabolism that might not be evident on MRI. Another nuclear medicine study, single photon emission tomography (SPECT), can be used to identify the region of onset of a seizure. Functional MRI (fMRI) studies show regions involved in a specific task (e.g., motor or language).

Magnetoencephalography, when combined with MRI, can be useful in detecting areas of abnormal electrical activity that might not be evident on a scalp EEG recording. Neuropsychology evaluations can aid in localization of regions of dysfunction and also aid in determining risk for loss of function if surgery is performed. The intracarotid amobarbital (Amytal)[1] test (Wada test) or intracarotid methohexital (Brevital)[1] test is used to lateralize language function and memory; fMRI is being investigated as a replacement for aspects of this invasive test. Some institutions use intracranial electrodes to localize the onset of a seizure prior to a surgical resection and to identify regions of eloquent neurologic function (regions where critical function would be lost if they were resected).

Specific Epilepsy Syndromes

Some of the more common syndromes are described here, listed by typical age at presentation.

Neonatal Seizures

Seizures in neonates can be caused by any type of neurologic pathology, including infections (prenatal or postnatal), strokes, hemorrhages, electrolyte abnormalities, cortical dysgenesis, inborn errors of metabolism (including vitamin B_6 dependency), genetic syndromes, drug (illicit and licit) withdrawal, and medications. Some neonatal seizure syndromes (benign idiopathic neonatal seizures and benign familial neonatal seizures) are benign in terms of resolution of seizures; early infantile epileptic encephalopathy (Ohtahara syndrome) and early myoclonic encephalopathy frequently are refractory to medical treatment and have a poor prognosis for development. Neonatal seizures should be managed in conjunction with specialists.

Febrile Seizures

Febrile seizures are the most common type of seizure, occurring in 3% to 5% of people in the United States. Febrile seizures, even though they can recur, are not diagnostic of epilepsy because they are provoked (i.e., by fever). With an onset between 1 month and 5 years of age (and almost always outgrown by 6 to 7 years of age), these seizures can be generalized or focal in onset. Meningitis and encephalitis also can manifest with seizures and fever and thus are exclusion criteria for febrile seizures because the prognosis and treatment are completely different. Febrile seizures that last longer than 15 minutes, have a focal onset, or occur more than once in a febrile illness are complex febrile seizures (only one of the three criteria are needed to make the diagnosis). Patients with complex febrile seizures are at a higher risk for developing epilepsy, although the overall risk is still low (4%). In patients who lack all three of these factors (i.e., simple febrile seizures), routine imaging, blood work, lumbar puncture, and EEG are not necessary for diagnosing the cause of the seizure. Rather, the workup should be guided by other concerns, such as dehydration, concern for occult bacteremia, or, in the appropriate clinical context, meningitis.

Approximately one-third of patients have a recurrence of a febrile seizure. Factors that increase the recurrence risk include

---

[1]Not FDA approved for this indication.

very young age at onset, family history of febrile seizures, low-grade fever at onset of the seizure, frequent febrile illnesses, or the occurrence of the seizure in the first hour of the fever. Febrile seizures always are outgrown, so typically long-term seizure prophylaxis is not used. Oral diazepam (Valium) prophylaxis, started at the onset of fever, prevents febrile seizures but can lead to excessive sedation. Patients who have prolonged febrile seizures can benefit from rectal diazepam gel (Diastat) or other benzodiazepines given soon after the onset of a febrile seizure to prevent additional prolonged seizures or febrile status epilepticus. A similarly good prognosis is seen in infants and children who have febrile seizures in the setting of acute gastroenteritis (whether febrile or not). The risk of epilepsy is increased after a febrile seizure in the setting of a complex febrile seizure, abnormal development, frequent febrile seizures, or a family history of epilepsy.

Infantile Spasms

With an onset typically around 4 to 8 months of age, infantile spasms consist of a triad of typical seizures (head drops and brief flexor and/or extensor spasms occurring in clusters around sleep transitions), a highly disorganized multifocal EEG pattern called hypsarrhythmia, and developmental delays. Between 70% and 90% of patients have identifiable underlying neurologic pathology associated with this syndrome. This is one of the most medically intractable epilepsy syndromes, and the prognosis for seizure control and development is very poor, except in a small subset of patients with no identifiable underlying pathology. Treatment typically is with corticosteroids (prednisolone [Orapred][1] or ACTH [Acthar HP]), or vigabatrin (Sabril), which is commonly the first-line treatment in infants with tuberous sclerosis complex (Box 1).

Dravet Syndrome

The typical presentation for Dravet syndrome is a prolonged febrile seizure involving one side of the body (hemiclonic) or recurrent GTCS in a previously normal infant. After a relatively quiescent period, seizures (including myoclonic, focal, and absence) may appear in the second year of life. Additional features include developmental abnormalities, ataxia, and extrapyramidal signs. Seizures induced by heat (either with fevers or exogenous) may be noted.

Genetic testing for mutations in the *SCN1A* gene is recommended because this eliminates the need for other extensive testing for an underlying diagnosis and allows the clinician to prognosticate. The EEG may be normal initially but later shows generalized spike-and-wave complexes and may show focal abnormalities. Treatment typically is with antiseizure medications; drugs that block sodium channels are typically avoided because they may exacerbate seizures. The ketogenic diet may be useful. Heated environments might need to be avoided and accommodations (e.g., air-conditioned buses and classrooms) may be recommended in some cases.

Lennox–Gastaut Syndrome

Typically occurring between the ages of 1 and 8 years, Lennox–Gastaut syndrome is characterized by mixed seizure types, a markedly abnormal EEG, and abnormal development. Virtually any type of brain pathology can be seen as an antecedent of Lennox–Gastaut syndrome. The syndrome of infantile spasms is a common antecedent. Patients with Lennox–Gastaut syndrome typically have combinations of tonic, atonic, and absence seizures, although focal-onset seizures and GTCS also occur. The EEG shows slow (less than 2.5 Hz) spike-and-wave complexes and occasionally a paroxysmal fast pattern, although background slowing also is very common. The vast majority of patients have developmental delays. Diagnosis is made in the setting of typical findings. Seizures are very difficult to control, but treatment commonly includes medicines and/or nonpharmacologic options (see Box 1). The prognosis for seizure control and development is poor. The differential diagnosis of Lennox–Gastaut syndrome

also includes Doose syndrome, which is characterized by myoclonic and astatic seizures (although other seizure types can occur). In Doose syndrome, patients often have normal development and a good prognosis once seizures are controlled.

Childhood and Juvenile Absence Epilepsy

Most clinicians are familiar with childhood and juvenile absence epilepsy. The typical age of onset is 4 to 14 years, and there is a slight female predominance. The most common type of seizure is an absence seizure, characterized by staring and loss of interaction lasting 5 to 20 seconds, occurring tens to hundreds of times per day. Patients also can have GTCS (particularly if they present later in childhood) and/or myoclonic seizures. There is no aura and there are no postictal behavior changes. Absence seizures can be induced with 3 to 4 minutes of hyperventilation at the bedside. The interictal EEG shows a 3 Hz generalized spike-and-wave pattern. Treatment includes ethosuximide (Zarontin) if the patient has not had a GTCS (see Box 1). Valproate (Depakene) is the first choice if the patient has had a GTCS. Nearly two-thirds of patients grow out of their seizures by young adulthood.

"Benign" Epilepsy With Centrotemporal Spikes and "Benign" Occipital Epilepsy

One of the more common epilepsies in childhood, "benign" epilepsy with centrotemporal spikes (also known commonly as Rolandic epilepsy), first occurs between the ages of 3 and 13 years. The typical seizure involves the face and/or hand, but GTCS also are common. The most common time for a seizure is within the first few hours of sleep, but a minority of patients only have daytime seizures. The diagnosis is made based on a typical seizure history and EEG (which shows spikes over bilateral central and temporal regions). Learning disabilities, which may be very subtle, are fairly common in patients with this syndrome, so extra vigilance is warranted (and this is the reason for quotation marks around the word "benign").

"Benign" occipital epilepsy (also known as Panayiotopoulos syndrome) can occur between the ages of 1 and 14 years (with a peak at 4 to 5 years) with autonomic symptoms such as emesis, pallor, flushing, or tachycardia, as well as focal-onset or generalized seizures. Patients also can have visual symptoms. The EEG can show sharp waves in the occipital regions, but abnormal activity has been reported in other brain regions as well.

Because most patients have fewer than six seizures in both syndromes, medicine usually is not prescribed. Seizures typically are outgrown by adolescence. Patients with frequent seizures are treated with medicine. Gastaut occipital epilepsy (not to be confused with Lennox–Gastaut syndrome) occurs in older children and can require medication treatment because of seizure recurrence.

Juvenile Myoclonic Epilepsy

The most common form of generalized seizures in adolescents, juvenile myoclonic epilepsy first occurs between the ages of 12 and 20 years. Most patients have brief myoclonic seizures that tend to cluster in the early morning hours (but may occur at any time of day). Patients often are unaware that these are seizures but on careful questioning report loss of control of a toothbrush or spoon. Many patients also have absence seizures. The interictal EEG typically shows a 4 to 5 Hz generalized spike-and-wave pattern. The prognosis for lifelong remission of seizures is poor, although most patients' seizures are controlled easily with medicines (see Box 1). There is a subgroup of patients (many of whom previously had childhood absence epilepsy) whose seizures are very challenging to control.

Other Epilepsy Syndromes With a Poor Prognosis

Landau–Kleffner syndrome and epileptic encephalopathy with continuous spike-and-wave during sleep are syndromes characterized by mild seizures, nearly continuous epileptiform activity during sleep, and neuropsychological deterioration. Progressive myoclonus epilepsy represents a family of disorders characterized by medically intractable epilepsy (commonly including myoclonic

---

[1]Not FDA approved for this indication.

always bad. Rasmussen syndrome is characterized by medically intractable epilepsy, progressive unilateral neurologic deficits, and cortical atrophy on MRI. Because they are so rare, any suspicion of these diagnoses should prompt referral to a pediatric epilepsy center with expertise in diagnosing and managing these conditions.

Tumors

Brain tumors can manifest with seizures and are covered in a separate chapter. Certain developmental tumors are seen with an increased frequency in pediatric epilepsy clinics, including dysembryoplastic neuroepithelial tumors (DNET) and gangliogliomas. These tumors typically manifest with seizures and can be associated with malformations of cortical development. EEG can show abnormalities over the involved region but can be falsely localizing as well. MRI shows the location of the tumor but can underestimate the extent of surrounding abnormal tissue. If seizures are not controlled with medicine, or if there is progression in tumor size, resection surgery is recommended.

Cortical Dysgenesis

Abnormal brain development can lead to inappropriately wired brain circuitry, which can be the underlying substrate for seizures. Two forms of abnormal cortical development include lissencephaly (abnormally smooth, or simplified, gyral pattern) and polymicrogyria. Another form of cortical dysgenesis, the malformations of cortical development, is graded based on both dyslamination of the normal six-layer neocortex and the occurrence of abnormal cell types (including balloon cells). EEG shows epileptiform abnormalities over the involved region. MRI shows the anatomic location of the involved tissue in more severe cases but may be normal if the abnormality is mild. In patients with focal abnormalities, if seizures are not controlled with medicine, resection surgery is an option. Patients with more extensive abnormalities can try nonpharmacologic options if medicines do not work.

Mesial Temporal Lobe Epilepsy With Hippocampal Sclerosis

The mesial temporal structures (particularly the hippocampus) can become scarred, and the remaining neurons develop abnormal connections. This can lead to medically intractable seizures. EEG shows interictal epileptiform activity over the temporal head regions. Imaging studies show atrophic mesial temporal structures with increased signal on T2-weighted FLAIR (fluid-attenuated inversion recovery) images. A temporal lobectomy should be considered as an option for patients who do not respond to two appropriately chosen and tolerated medications for seizure control.

Comorbidities

The definition of epilepsy includes comorbidities, which in turn can have a significant impact on quality of life. Clinicians must actively probe for these underlying conditions in order to optimize outcomes. People with epilepsy have increased rates of depression and anxiety compared to the general population. Developmental disorders and learning disabilities are more common in children with epilepsy, as are attention-deficit/hyperactivity disorder and migraines. Once identified, these conditions should be managed by clinicians experienced with their treatment.

Differential Diagnosis

The differential diagnosis of seizures depends largely on age. In infants, opisthotonic posturing can be seen in gastroesophageal reflux disease (Sandifer syndrome). Some infants have benign myoclonus or shuddering attacks. The EEG in all these disorders is normal, but the diagnosis can be made based on the history. Apparent life-threatening events can appear to be seizures, although apnea rarely is the only manifestation of a seizure. Hyperekplexia is an exaggerated startle response that can be due to abnormal glycine receptor subunits in the spinal cord. Because of potential involvement of the diaphragm, this disorder can be lethal. In children, stereotypies can be paroxysmal and persistent, but the behaviors during these episodes are typical enough that the diagnosis usually is made based on the history.

seizures) and significant neurologic deterioration. Underlying diagnoses include myoclonus epilepsy with ragged red fibers (MERRF), Unverricht–Lundborg disease, and Lafora's disease, among others. Gelastic (laughing) seizures can be caused either by hypothalamic hamartomas or temporal lobe seizures. The prognosis depends on response to medication and/or surgery but is not

Breath-holding spells may be associated with an older infant or toddler who is upset, followed by unresponsiveness and either facial pallor or mild cyanosis, lasting less than 1 to 3 minutes. These episodes are typical enough that the history is all that is usually needed to make the diagnosis. Children with pallid breath-holding spells are at higher risk for vasovagal syncope in the adolescent and young adult ages.

Night terrors, one of the parasomnias, occur in toddlers and young children. Persistent screaming (lasting minutes to 1 hour) and lack of memory of the event are seen commonly; the latter raises a question of whether the child had a seizure. Most commonly, these are outgrown by the late preschool years.

Patients with syncope may have a few mild clonic twitches, but this typically does not represent epilepsy. Screening orthostatic blood pressures should be done to rule out one of the orthostatic syndromes. Consideration also should be given to an electrocardiogram or a cardiology consultation in the appropriate clinical context.

Older children and adolescents can have psychogenic nonepileptic events, also known as psychogenic nonepileptic seizures. Considered to be a form of a conversion disorder (DSM-5), the diagnosis is made by noting a normal EEG during a typical clinical episode (and thus should be referred to a neurologist for diagnosis). Cognitive behavioral therapy is helpful in some patients. This is a very important diagnosis to make so that patients receive appropriate treatment and are not exposed to medicines where the risks outweigh the benefits.

In all age groups, focal lesions such as infarctions, hemorrhages, and infections should be considered in the differential diagnosis, although the diagnostic workup should be guided by the history and physical examination.

Treatment

The goals for treatment are to maximize efficacy and minimize side effects. Medication is the first line of therapy for most patients. Nearly 70% to 80% of children are treated successfully by one of the first two medications tried. Practically speaking, neurologists try to use a single agent at the lowest tolerated dosage. Suggested medicines for the epilepsy syndromes discussed previously are listed in Box 1. Details about specific medicines are listed in Table 1. If one of the first two medicines tried does not work, there are three major options.

TABLE 1	Summary of New Commonly Used Antiseizure Drugs				
DRUG	MAINTENANCE DOSAGE*	STARTING DOSAGE*	HALF-LIFE (H)	COMMON SIDE EFFECTS	SERIOUS IDIOSYNCRATIC SIDE EFFECTS
Brivaracetam (Briviact)	> 16 y, 25–100 mg bid	50 mg bid	9	Agitation, behavioral disinhibition, dizziness	Suicidality
Cannabidiol (Epidiolex)	5 mg/kg bid (can go up to 10 mg/kg bid)	2.5 mg/kg bid	56–61	Somnolence, decreased appetite, diarrhea, transaminase elevations (check before initiating therapy), fatigue, rash, sleep disorders, infections	Severe encephalopathy leading to respiratory depression and oversedation, hepatic injury, suicidality
Clobazam (Onfi)	> 2 y, < 30 kg: 10 mg bid > 2 y, > 30 kg: 20 mg bid	> 2 y, < 30 kg: 5 mg/d > 2 y, > 30 kg: 5 mg bid	Parent drug: 36–42 Active metabolite: 71–82	Sedation irritability Needs to be tapered off slowly	Respiratory depression, benzodiazepine withdrawal, Stevens–Johnson syndrome
Eslicarbazepine (Aptiom)	4-17 y (11-21 kg), 400-600 mg once/day 4-17 y (22-31 kg), 500-800 mg once/day 4-17 y (32-38 kg), 600-900 mg once/day 4-17 y (>38 kg), 800-1200 mg once/day >17 y, 800–1600 mg once/day	4-17 y (11-21 kg), 200 mg once/day 4-17 y (22-31 kg), 300 mg once/day 4-17 y (32-38 kg), 300 mg once/day >4 y (>38 kg), 400 mg once/day	13–20	Somnolence, dizziness, hyponatremia, thyroid dysfunction	Stevens-Johnson, toxic epidermal necrolysis, withdrawal seizures if stopped abruptly
Lacosamide (Vimpat)	4-16 y (11-<30 kg), 3-6 mg/kg bid 4-16 y (30-50 kg), 2-4 mg/kg bid >4 y (>50 kg), 100–200 mg bid	4-16 y (<50 kg), 1 mg/kg bid >4 y (≥50 kg), 50 mg bid	13	Somnolence, fatigue, headache	Cardiac conduction abnormalities, Stevens-Johnson syndrome, cytopenias
Levetiracetam (Keppra)	20–60 mg/kg/d	10 mg/kg/d, incr in 10-mg/kg increments	6–8	Agitation, behavioral disinhibition, rashes	Suicidal ideation
Oxcarbazepine (Trileptal)	30–60 mg/kg/d	8–10 mg/kg/d, incr by 10–15 mg/kg increments	Parent drug: 2 Metabolite: 9	Hyponatremia, somnolence, lethargy, dizziness, blurred vision	Rash
Perampanel (Fycompa)	> 12 y, 8–12 mg at bedtime	> 12 y, 2–4 mg at bedtime	105 h	Somnolence, headaches	Serious psychiatric and behavior reactions
Rufinamide (Banzel)	45 mg/kg/d	10 mg/kg/d	6–10	Nausea, vomiting, somnolence	Seizures, QT shortening

DRUG	MAINTENANCE DOSAGE*	STARTING DOSAGE*	HALF-LIFE (H)	COMMON SIDE EFFECTS	SERIOUS IDIOSYNCRATIC SIDE EFFECTS
Vigabatrin (Sabril)	50–150 mg/kg/d	50 mg/kg/d	7.5 (5.7 in infants)	Headache, dizziness, fatigue, tremor, swallowing problems, T2-weighted or DWI hyperintensities	Vision loss
Zonisamide (Zonegran)	> 16 y: 100–600 mg/d	> 16 y: 100 mg once/day	63	Somnolence, irritability, cognitive slowing, weight loss, renal stones, oligohidrosis	Rash

*Dosages should not exceed maximum adult dosages.
Abbreviations: DWI = diffusion-weighted imaging; incr = increase.

1. Trials of Additional Medication

Although the first two medicines might not work, new medicines often are introduced into the market. Clinical trials often show that a modest number of patients respond well to newer medicines, although the positive response to newer medicines is no greater overall than response to older medicines, despite lower rates of adverse effects and drug–drug interactions.

2. Surgery

Any patient who fails to respond to two medications should be assessed for surgery. In patients with a potentially resectable lesion, surgery offers the greatest chance of seizure freedom. Ideal surgical candidates have identifiable lesions on imaging studies and a seizure onset zone that is distinct from eloquent cortex. Patients without identifiable lesions or those with multifocal or generalized seizures are poor candidates for resection surgery. Options for these patients include the vagus nerve stimulator, which has outstanding compliance and adherence because it is surgically implanted. Although this device significantly decreases seizure frequency in some patients, it only rarely leads to seizure freedom. Neurostimulation devices, some of which also include seizure detectors, are being introduced into clinical practice for adults and will be used in children in the future.

3. Diet Therapy

The concept of fasting to improve seizure control dates back to Hippocrates, but in modern times, dietary management of epilepsy is implemented using a high-fat, low-carbohydrate (adequate protein) ketogenic diet. A modified Atkins diet and a low glycemic index treatment have been used successfully as well. These diets require varying degrees of clinical supervision at centers experienced in their implementation.

Monitoring

Seizure calendars (which can take the form of notebooks or Internet-based tools) are very useful for tracking frequency of events, especially if they are completed on a daily basis. There has been a recent explosion in wearable devices and other types of biotechnology for monitoring seizures and vital signs during seizures (for home use). Monitoring for medication-related adverse effects and comorbidities should continue during treatment. In addition, some comorbidities can occur even if seizures have stopped; there is good evidence for this in patients with childhood absence epilepsy, which typically is considered a "benign" syndrome because seizures typically resolve by adulthood. Patients taking certain medicines are screened periodically for evidence of renal and/or hepatic abnormalities and abnormal blood cell counts. Scenarios for testing drug levels include the following:

- Assessing adherence to a prescribed drug regimen
- Testing whether symptoms result from drug toxicity

- Determining whether a patient can benefit from higher amounts of medicine when the administered doses are already high (i.e., fast metabolizers)

Reminders about seizure-related safety should be reinforced periodically. GTCS counseling typically includes instructions about safety for the patient, including protecting the head and airway (putting the patient on his or her side to prevent aspiration) and not putting anything in the patient's mouth. Other safety topics include water safety and wearing helmets, as well as discouraging participation in certain sports (e.g., scuba diving). Periodic assessments of bone health should be considered for patients taking enzyme-inducing or enzyme-inhibiting medicines. Patients of an appropriate age should be counseled about local driving laws. Adolescent girls should be counseled about the effect of antiseizure medicines on hormonal forms of contraception (and vice versa). Consideration should be given to prescribing folate in this group, as well.

Complications

Single GTCS can lead to trauma (e.g., from a fall), tongue biting, pneumothorax, fractures of the vertebrae or limbs, and joint dislocations. A brief physical examination can rule out the more serious complications of a single GTCS. Adverse effects of medications are listed in Table 1. Surgical resections can lead to a variety of neurologic deficits, depending on which tissue is involved. Vagus nerve stimulator surgery can lead to hoarseness and coughing. Unsupervised diet therapy also can have adverse effects; such therapy should be undertaken only by centers with experience. Rarely, patients with epilepsy can die unexpectedly from no apparent cause, known as sudden unexplained death in epilepsy (SUDEP). The cause is unknown, but most (not all) patients have epilepsy that is resistant to medications. Counseling about this condition should be provided by an epilepsy expert.

References

Baldin E, Hauser WA, Buchhalter JR, et al: Yield of epileptiform electroencephalogram abnormalities in incident unprovoked seizures: a population-based study, *Epilepsia* 55:1389–1398, 2014.

Dang LT, Silverstein FS: Drug treatment of seizures and epilepsy in newborns and children, *Pediatr Clin North Am* 64:1291–1308, 2017.

El Achkar CM, Olson HE, Poduri A, et al: The genetics of the epilepsies, *Curr Neurol Neurosci Rep* 15:39, 2015.

Fisher RS, Acevedo C, Arzimanoglou A, et al: ILAE official report: a practical clinical definition of epilepsy, *Epilepsia* 55:475–482, 2014.

Go CY, Mackay MT, Weiss SK, et al: Child Neurology Society, American Academy of Neurology: Evidence-based guideline update: medical treatment of infantile spasms. Report of the Guideline Development Subcommittee of the American Academy of Neurology and the Practice Committee of the Child Neurology Society, *Neurology* 78:1974–1980, 2012.

Muthugovindan D, Hartman AL: Pediatric epilepsy syndromes, *Neurologist* 16:223–237, 2010.

Scheffer IE, Berkovic S, Capovilla G, et al: ILAE classification of the epilepsies: position paper of the ILAE Commission for Classification and Terminology, *Epilepsia* 58:512–521, 2017.

Subcommittee on Febrile Seizures, American Academy of Pediatrics: Neurodiagnostic evaluation of the child with a simple febrile seizure, *Pediatrics* 127:389–394, 2011.

PEDIATRIC FAILURE TO THRIVE

Method of
Gretchen Homan, MD

CURRENT DIAGNOSIS

- Pediatric failure to thrive (PFTT), also known as weight faltering, refers to failure to gain weight at an appropriate rate over time.
- History taking, physical examination, and growth chart data are used to identify PFTT.
- Weight below the fifth percentile with a negative growth trend over time indicates potential PFTT.
- Weight measurements declining across two major percentiles may indicate PFTT.
- Failure to gain or maintain weight is the earliest indication of PFTT, but length and head circumference may be impacted and should always be monitored.

CURRENT THERAPY

- Successful treatment includes addressing all causes, including underlying medical problems.
- Hospitalization is generally not indicated, and serial clinic visits can be used to monitor weight gain and maintenance.
- Growth chart parameters can help set a goal weight. Daily weight gain goals can be identified to monitor treatment over weeks to months.
- The majority of patients respond to generalized techniques for increased calories combined with frequent outpatient monitoring of progress.
- Consulting with a dietitian or using detailed nutrition calculations can provide specific guidance for protein and calorie goals in complicated cases.

In pediatric failure to thrive (PFTT), also known as weight faltering, the child fails to gain weight at an appropriate rate; this failure is documented over time. The concept has been recognized for over a century, but there is still no consensus on terminology or a definition. Historically, the terms *organic* and *nonorganic* were used to identify PFTT, and they were attributed to medical conditions and psychosocial causes, respectively. Insufficient usable nutrition is now regarded as the underlying cause of PFTT. It can be due to problems with calorie intake or absorption or both. Approximately 80% of children with PFTT are diagnosed by age 18 months. For older children, the preferred term is *poor weight gain*.

Epidemiology

In the United States, PFTT occurs in approximately 5% to 10% of children seen in primary care and in up to 5% of children admitted to the hospital. An estimated 20% to 30% of cases are undiagnosed. PFTT is a condition rather than a specific diagnosis, and imprecise diagnostic criteria complicate estimating its incidence and prevalence. Some children show a decrease in their weight curves followed by weight maintenance on the new curve; although this occurs in approximately 25% of children, it is not considered weight faltering.

Risk Factors

Risk factors for PFTT can be medical and/or psychosocial. In up to 80% of cases, no obvious medical etiology is identified. Any disease process has the potential to cause PFTT. Prenatal predisposing factors include exposure to toxins, intrauterine growth retardation, and poor maternal nutrition. Infants born prematurely are at high risk for PFTT. Premature infants need to catch up in growth over months to years and should not be expected to reach normal peer percentiles too quickly, as this could have negative implications for healthy weight in adult life. Any medical problem that interferes with or inhibits calorie intake and absorption of nutrients can cause PFTT, as can any condition that creates increased caloric demand. Leading medical causes include development delay, congenital anomalies such as cleft lip and/or palate, genetic conditions such as cystic fibrosis or celiac disease, and childhood cancers and related treatments.

Poverty is the most powerful psychosocial risk factor for PFTT, as it limits access to appropriate nutrition. Healthcare providers should be aware of "food deserts" in their communities as well as families within their practice that are food insecure. Children of families with increased life stresses, social isolation, poor parenting skills, or substance abuse are at increased risk for PFTT. Personal nutritional beliefs and practices can also limit nutrition, leading to PFTT. Examples include prolonged exclusive breast feeding or avoidance of multiple food categories for cultural or religious reasons.

Pathophysiology

Inadequate caloric intake, malabsorption, or increased metabolic demand, either as isolated entities or concurrently, can lead to PFTT. Caloric intake may be impaired by use of diluted formula, poor feeding habits, neglect, or mechanical feeding difficulties. Inadequate nutrient absorption can be caused by a range of diseases or conditions that affect the gastrointestinal tract, including celiac disease, cystic fibrosis and other pancreatic diseases, milk protein allergy, inborn errors of metabolism, and chronic infections. Increased energy needs and potential caloric deficit leading to PFTT can occur in children with chronic infections, congenital heart or lung disease, hyperthyroidism, malignancy, renal failure, inflammatory conditions, and HIV.

Prevention

Prevention of PFTT begins with prenatal care and maternal health, especially limiting potential exposure to toxins, optimizing maternal nutrition, and conducting routine pregnancy screenings. Being aware of potential genetic conditions facilitates planning appropriate support for the family. State-mandated newborn screening tests provide opportunities for early intervention in patients at risk for PFTT. Routine well-child visits in the first 2 years of life provide surveillance for growth and anticipatory guidance regarding nutrition to support development. Connecting families with appropriate community resources can help provide high-risk children and families with access to nutritional resources. Supporting overall good health with patient education and general preventive services, including oral health and immunization, is essential to reducing the risk of FTT.

Clinical Manifestations

PFTT is defined by problems with weight as a documented trend over time. The Centers for Disease Control and Prevention (CDC) recommend that the World Health Organization growth charts be used to document growth for children under age 2 years and that the CDC growth charts be used for children ages 2 years and older. The majority of PFTT patients show at least one of three characteristics: weight below the 5th percentiles for age and sex, weight drop of two major percentiles, or weight less than the 80th percentile of ideal body weight. Some infants may benefit from a PFTT evaluation when their daily weight gain is less than expected for age and sex but does not yet meet these criteria. If weight faltering persists, length and then head circumference are impacted, and these indicate severe PFTT.

Patients with PFTT can generally be diagnosed as outpatients. Laboratory evaluation or imaging is not generally required. Detailed history taking and physical examination, along with the growth chart information, are sufficient to identify PFTT. A delay in development coupled with weight faltering noted on the growth chart comprise the clinical presentation of severe or

TABLE 1	Techniques to Increase Calories	
AGE	**CALORIE SOURCE ADJUSTMENT**	**FEEDING TECHNIQUE**
Infant – breast fed	• Increase feeds up to 12 in 24 hours • Pump after feeds and use expressed breast milk (EBM) to supplement nursing; add formula powder to expressed breast milk	• Evaluate and ensure proper latch/position • Feed both breasts with each feeding • Work to keep baby awake for complete feeding • Do not allow feeds to persist beyond 30 minutes total
Infant – formula fed	• Increase calorie concentration by mixing formula powder with less water, from 19/20 to 24/26 kcal; monitor for tolerance • Evaluate feeding volume and frequency to avoid over- or underfeeding; rule of thumb feeds average 1 oz/h (e.g., 3 oz/3 h)	• Evaluate for intolerance and change formula if needed; consider predigested proteins • Use proper bottle nipple speed • Avoid bottle propping
Toddler	• Add butter, dips such as ranch or mayonnaise, and cheese to foods • Use high-calorie foods and offer proteins such as cheese, peanut butter, avocados, and high-fat yogurts • Encourage a variety of healthy foods such as fruits, vegetables, proteins, and grains • Consider supplement drinks or shake powders to mix 1–2 times/day	• Structured mealtimes in a high chair with adult supervision and without distractions (e.g., television, other children) • Evaluate toddler's ability to self-feed effectively; intervene and teach if needed • Aim for 3 meals with 3 snacks daily • Minimize fruit juices • Offer water with meals and offer foods before milk or supplement drinks

prolonged PFTT. The aim of the physical examination is to identify any underlying or contributing medical condition that could impair nutrition and/or increase metabolic demands. The clinician should observe for any dysmorphic features and look for signs of abuse or neglect. Signs of malnutrition may become evident when PFTT is allowed to persist. The most severely affected children show edema, wasting, hepatomegaly, rash, or skin and hair changes.

Differential Diagnosis

Prematurely born infants and those with intrauterine growth retardation may be mistaken for patients with PFTT. These infants and children may meet the diagnostic criteria for delay on standard growth charts (values less than the 5th percentile) for age and sex. Ongoing monitoring for underlying medical conditions, regular developmental assessments, and evaluation of the social support network for each patient can provide reassurance that the child does not have PFTT and is expected to "catch up" in growth parameters within 18 to 36 months.

Genetic short stature and constitutional growth delay should be ruled out by reviewing the midparental height and growth patterns for delays. Radiologic testing for bone age may be helpful when confirming constitutional growth delay.

Therapy

PFTT can have one or multiple causes or complicating factors. Each issue should be addressed in the context of the overall health of the child and family. Any underlying medical condition must be diagnosed and treated. Children with a history of choking or oral motor dysfunction may benefit from a speech therapist evaluation and treatment program. Hospitalization is rarely indicated but may be helpful if there are complicating medical or social problems or if outpatient treatment has failed. Outpatient therapy is centered on increasing calorie intake with appropriate food options (Table 1). Equations can be used to calculate estimated calorie and protein needs by age and sex for both normal and catch-up growth. To simplify this process, a generalized list of targets is provided in Table 2. When available, a dietitian can define the required protein and calorie goals for catch-up growth initially and over the remaining treatment period. Alternatively, the primary care physician can use the growth chart to determine the desired weight goal for age and plan for a daily weight gain goal over weeks or months. The techniques described in Table 1 can be used to initiate treatment. Frequent visits are necessary. At each visit, the child's measurements should be done on the same well-calibrated scale to provide reliable data for clinical decision making about appropriate weight gain and maintenance. Patients

TABLE 2	Estimated Calorie Needs by Age
AGE	**KCAL/KG/DAY**
Preterm infant	115–130; up to 150 for very low birth weight infants
Full-term infant • 0–2 months • 3 months • 4–35 months	• 104–107 • 95 • 82
Toddler	70–80

Add 5–20 kcal/kg/day for catch-up growth, depending on tolerance and desired rate of recovery.

who are unable to grow with these interventions may benefit from either short-term nasogastric tube feedings or more long-term gastric tube feedings.

Monitoring

Children with PFTT may require more frequent monitoring than the scheduled routine well-child visits. Young infants can be seen weekly or monthly and older patients every 2 to 4 months. At these visits, patients should be weighed and measured, preferably without clothing, by trained staff using routinely calibrated devices and standardized techniques to ensure the most accurate measurements. The clinician should review the patient's growth charts, diet and activity history, any changes in the social and medical history, and perform a physical examination. Recent acute illness may slow or reverse growth progress and should be addressed. It may take months for malnourished patients to show and maintain growth recovery. Patients who were born prematurely or with intrauterine growth retardation may require years to catch up. Depending on the underlying cause of PFTT, relapse is possible.

Complications

Weight loss or deceleration is the earliest clinical indicator for PFTT; if allowed to persist, height and length can be affected. Eventually, head size and brain growth can be impaired. At this level of severity, PFTT puts cognitive development and achievement of milestones in jeopardy. Immune system function may be impaired during a malnourished state, thus putting affected patients at risk for infections. Social and emotional health may also be impacted. Research is ongoing to understand the long-term effects of PFTT.

References

Black MM, Dubowitz H, Krishnakumar A, Starr Jr RH: Early intervention and recovery among children with failure to thrive: follow-up at age 8, *Pediatrics* 120:59–69, 2007.

Cole SZ, Lanham JS: Failure to thrive: an update, *Am Fam Physician* 83:829–834, 2011.

Emond AM, Blair PS, Emmett PM, Drewett RF: Weight faltering in infancy and IQ levels at 8 years in the Avon Longitudinal Study of Parents and Children, *Pediatrics* 120:e1051–8, 2007.

Engorn B, Flerlage J, editors: *The Harriet Lane Handbook: A Manual for Pediatric House Officers*, 20th ed., Philadelphia, 2014, Elsevier Saunders.

Kleinman RE, Greer FR, editors: Failure to thrive. In *Pediatric Nutrition*, 7th ed., Elk Grove Village, IL, 2014, American Academy of Pediatrics, pp 663–700.

Olsen EM, Petersen J, Skovgaard AM, et al: Failure to thrive: the prevalence and concurrence of anthropometric criteria in a general infant population, *Arch Dis Child* 92:109–114, 2007.

Rybak A: Organic and nonorganic feeding disorders, *Ann Nutr Metab* 66(suppl 5):16–22, 2015.

Shields B, Wacogne I, Wright CM: Weight faltering and failure to thrive in infancy and early childhood, *BMJ* 345:e5931, 2012.

Wright CM, Parkinson KN, Drewett RF: How does maternal and child feeding behavior relate to weight gain and failure to thrive? Data from a prospective birth cohort, *Pediatrics* 117:1262–1269, 2006.

Yoo SD, Hwang EH, Lee YJ, Park JH: Clinical characteristics of failure to thrive in infant and toddler: organic vs. nonorganic, *Pediatr Gastroenterol Hepatol Nutr* 16:261–268, 2013.

NOCTURNAL ENURESIS

Method of
Alexander K.C. Leung, MBBS

Note: This chapter has been published in part in *Common Problems in Ambulatory Pediatrics: Specific Clinical Problems,* volume 1, with permission from Nova Science Publishers, Inc.

CURRENT DIAGNOSIS

- Nocturnal enuresis is defined as involuntary nighttime bedwetting in a child at least 5 years of age.
- Primary nocturnal enuresis is present when the child has never achieved a period of nighttime dryness greater than 6 consecutive months. Secondary nocturnal enuresis is present when the child has experienced a period of nighttime dryness of at least 6 consecutive months.
- The most common causes of primary nocturnal enuresis are a deep sleep pattern, nocturnal polyuria, and a small-capacity bladder or nocturnal detrusor overactivity.
- A urinalysis is warranted to rule out urinary tract infection, glycosuria, and a defect in the ability to concentrate urine.
- Ultrasound examination of the bladder (prevoid and postvoid) can be used to evaluate bladder dysfunction and functional bladder capacity.

CURRENT THERAPY

- Desmopressin (DDAVP, 1-deamino-8-arginine vasopressin) is indicated as a first-line therapy for children with monosymptomatic nocturnal enuresis associated with nocturnal polyuria and normal bladder function.
- Enuretic alarm is indicated as a first-line therapy for children with monosymptomatic nocturnal enuresis associated with a small bladder capacity or in children with severe enuretic symptoms refractory to desmopressin therapy.
- Behavioral therapy such as encouraging the child to urinate frequently during the daytime, emptying the bladder before bedtime, and restricting fluid in the evening may increase the success rate of pharmacologic therapy or enuretic alarm therapy.

Nocturnal enuresis is defined as involuntary nighttime bedwetting in a child at least 5 years of age. Primary nocturnal enuresis is present when the child has never achieved a period of nighttime dryness greater than 6 consecutive months. Secondary nocturnal enuresis is present when the child has experienced a period of nighttime dryness of at least 6 consecutive months. For the majority of children with secondary nocturnal enuresis, the pathogenesis is no different from that of primary nocturnal enuresis.

Nocturnal enuresis is a common problem that is frustrating for children, parents, and physicians alike. The condition may affect the child's self-esteem and may lead to reduced social interaction and behavioral problems.

Epidemiology

It has been estimated that 15% to 25% of 5-year-old children and 5% to 10% of 7-year-old children have nocturnal enuresis. Without specific treatment, approximately 15% of affected children become dry each year. The male-to-female ratio is approximately 3:1.

Risk Factors

Encopresis, daytime wetting (diurnal enuresis), and male gender are significant risk factors. Constipation, emotional stress, developmental delay, bladder dysfunction, sleep deprivation, adenotonsillar hypertrophy, and attention-deficit/hyperactivity disorder also play a role.

Pathogenesis

The most common causes of primary nocturnal enuresis are a high arousal threshold, nocturnal polyuria, and a small-capacity bladder or nocturnal detrusor overactivity. Although these causes may overlap, it is important to conceptualize them separately, because this differentiation will help the physician to understand the problem, to educate both the parents and child, and to plan an appropriate treatment program.

It has been shown that enuretic children have a high arousal threshold and a reduced prepulse inhibition of startle. In most children, arousability from sleep improves with maturation of the central nervous system.

In most circumstances, the rate of secretion of antidiuretic hormone from the posterior pituitary gland is increased at night. This circadian variation is usually established when the child is 3 to 4 years old. Some children with primary nocturnal enuresis have a lack of this circadian variation with an abnormally low nocturnal secretion of antidiuretic hormone with resultant nocturnal polyuria. Other causes of nocturnal polyuria include fluid and solute overload in the evening.

Children with a small-capacity bladder or nocturnal detrusor overactivity often have primary nocturnal enuresis. Conditions that may reduce the functional bladder capacity include cystitis and constipation.

There is a strong genetic component to nocturnal enuresis. The child of parents who were both enuretic has a 77% chance of developing enuresis. If one parent was enuretic, there is up to a 44% occurrence rate. If neither parent was enuretic, the occurrence rate is only 15%. Twin studies also support a genetic basis for nocturnal enuresis: the concordance rate is much higher in monozygotic twins (68%) when compared with dizygotic twins (36%). Linkage studies have suggested possible genetic markers for primary nocturnal enuresis located on chromosomes 12, 13, and 22.

A neurogenic bladder is one of the few anatomic abnormalities that can cause primary nocturnal enuresis. Congenital urethral obstruction is another infrequent anatomic cause of primary nocturnal enuresis. The enuresis in these children is due to an overflow phenomenon from a poorly compliant bladder. The most common cause of urethral obstruction in the male is posterior urethral valves. Girls and boys with significant congenital urethral stenosis may also present with this problem. An ectopic ureter or vesicovaginal fistula is an infrequent anatomic cause of primary nocturnal enuresis in girls.

A defect in the ability of the kidney to concentrate urine can cause primary nocturnal enuresis. The causes of concentrating defects include any cause of chronic renal failure and diabetes insipidus.

Diagnosis
History
Onset and Frequency
The timing of the onset and the frequency of nocturnal enuresis are important historical clues to the etiology. Secondary nocturnal enuresis and intermittent nocturnal enuresis are not usually associated with structural abnormalities in the urinary tract. Nocturnal enuresis due to a structural abnormality of the urinary tract is usually present from birth and is not associated with periods of remission.

Timing, Frequency, and Volume per Episode
A history of soaking absorbent underpants in the morning suggests nocturnal polyuria. Parents of children with nocturnal polyuria often remark that the volume of urine associated with the enuretic episode or the first morning void is very large. Frequent episodes of nocturnal enuresis with a small volume of urine suggest bladder dysfunction such as may occur with a urethral obstruction or a neurogenic bladder. Several episodes of nocturnal enuresis with a large volume suggest diabetes mellitus or diabetes insipidus. Constant wetting suggests an ectopic ureter or vesicovaginal fistula.

Associated Symptoms
Nocturnal enuresis associated with daytime urinary frequency, urgency, incontinence, and difficulties in initiating the urinary stream suggests urethral obstruction. Daytime urinary frequency, urgency, incontinence, squatting behavior, constipation, encopresis, gait disturbance, and a history of spina bifida or spinal trauma suggest a neurogenic bladder. Constant dampness in the underwear by day and night in a female suggests an ectopic ureter or vesicovaginal fistula. Secondary nocturnal enuresis associated with dysuria, urinary frequency, urgency, fever, suprapubic/loin pain, or cloudy, foul-smelling urine suggests a urinary tract infection. Polyuria, polydipsia, polyphagia, and weight loss suggest diabetes mellitus. Polyuria, polydipsia, and episodes of dehydration in a child with a history of central nervous system disease suggest diabetes insipidus. A history of constipation is important because the condition is associated with a reduced functional bladder capacity.

Volume of First Morning Void
Most children with nocturnal enuresis void only a small or average amount of urine in the morning after an enuretic episode. A large volume of urine voided following a significant episode of nocturnal enuresis may be a clue to the presence of low nocturnal secretion of antidiuretic hormone.

Soundness of Sleep
Children with nocturnal enuresis often sleep more deeply than other family members. Some children only wet when they are overtired. Conversely, children who are usually enuretic may be continent during periods of wakeful sleep such as during intercurrent illnesses.

Past Health
A child with a history of a structural abnormality of the urinary tract or neurogenic bladder may have nocturnal enuresis due to these causes. A history of spinal trauma may indicate a neurogenic bladder as a cause of enuresis. A history of central nervous system disorder may indicate neurogenic diabetes insipidus. Certain medications such as methylxanthines and caffeine may be associated with nocturnal enuresis.

Family History
A family history of nocturnal enuresis should be sought because nocturnal enuresis tends to run in the family. A family history of diabetes mellitus, diabetes insipidus, or kidney disease suggests the corresponding disorder. Any stressful events in the family such as birth of a sibling and parental disharmony should be explored, especially in children with secondary nocturnal enuresis.

Physical Examination
Height and weight should be measured and plotted onto standard growth charts. All children should have their blood pressure checked, which, if elevated, might indicate renal disease. A thorough physical examination should include examination of the abdomen and genitalia and a complete neurologic examination. In chronic constipation, fecal masses are often palpable in the left lower quadrant of the abdomen and in the suprapubic area.

In the majority of children with primary nocturnal enuresis, the physical examination is unremarkable. An abnormal physical examination is only present when primary nocturnal enuresis is due to a structural cause. A myelomeningocele is usually obvious at birth; however, subtle spinal defects may also be associated with primary nocturnal enuresis. A midline tuft of hair, an exaggerated dimple, or a birthmark in the area of the lumbosacral spine; a gait abnormality; absence of anal wink; or abnormal motor power, tone, reflexes, or sensation in the lower extremities suggests a neurogenic bladder. A palpably enlarged bladder or kidney and a weak or dribbling urinary stream suggests urinary obstruction, such as may result from posterior urethral valves.

Laboratory and Imaging Studies
A urinalysis is warranted to rule out urinary tract infection, diabetes mellitus, and a defect in the ability to concentrate urine. Ultrasound examination of the bladder (prevoid and postvoid) can be used to evaluate bladder dysfunction and functional bladder capacity.

Treatment
One essential part of the treatment plan of every child with primary nocturnal enuresis should be compassion and support from both the family and physician. It is important to clarify to parents that the child is not at fault and to specify that punishment for bedwetting is inappropriate. The child and family can be reassured that in the absence of structural defect, primary nocturnal enuresis tends to resolve with time.

Simple behavioral strategies such as encouraging the child to urinate frequently during the daytime, emptying the bladder before bedtime, and limiting fluid and solute intake in the evening are often recommended. Caffeinated beverages should be avoided, particularly in the evening. Some authors recommend waking the child 1.5 to 2 hours after bedtime to go to the bathroom. Star charts and reward systems need to reinforce positive behavior. Behavioral therapy may increase the success rate of pharmacologic therapy or enuretic alarm therapy.

Desmopressin (DDAVP, 1-deamino-8-arginine vasopressin) is an analogue of vasopressin that has a profound antidiuretic activity without pressor activity. The medication acts on the V2 receptors of the renal tubules and increases the reabsorption of fluid from the renal tubules, thereby decreasing the amount of urine produced. The medication is indicated as a first-line therapy for children with monosymptomatic nocturnal enuresis associated with nocturnal polyuria and normal bladder function. Desmopressin is available in a sublingual lyophilisate (melt) preparation,[2] as well as a tablet. The bioavailability of the lyophilisate (melt) preparation is approximately 60% greater than that of the tablet formulation. The recommended dose of desmopressin is 120 to 240 μg melt and 200 to 400 μg tablet. The former is usually given 30 minutes to 1 hour before bedtime, and the latter is usually given 1 hour before bedtime. Side effects are rare and include symptomatic hyponatremia with water intoxication. When desmopressin is prescribed, patients should be instructed to avoid high fluid intake in the evening.

---

[2]Not available in the United States.

Imipramine (Tofranil), a tricyclic agent with antimuscarinic property, may be helpful in children who have not responded to desmopressin alone. Presumably, the medication decreases the amount of time spent in rapid eye movement sleep, stimulates antidiuretic hormone secretion, and relaxes the detrusor muscle. The recommended starting dose is 25 mg for children 6 to 12 years of age and 50 mg for those older than 12 years, given 1 to 2 hours before bedtime. If necessary, the dose may be increased gradually to a maximum of 50 mg in children 6 to 12 years of age and 75 mg for those older than 12 years. However, potential side effects (anxiety, depression, dizziness, headache, drowsiness, lethargy, sleep disturbance, dry mouth, anorexia, vomiting, skin rashes) and serious adverse effects (hepatotoxicity, cardiotoxicity) with overdose limit their use.

Monotherapy with oxybutynin (Ditropan),[1] an anticholinergic and antispasmodic agent that decreases uninhibited bladder contraction, is not effective in treating monosymptomatic nocturnal enuresis. The medication can be added, however, as a second-line drug in the treatment of children with both diurnal and nocturnal enuresis. The dose is 5 mg administered 1 hour before bedtime.

Enuretic alarm is indicated as a first-line therapy for children with monosymptomatic nocturnal enuresis associated with a small bladder capacity or nocturnal detrusor overactivity. Randomized controlled trials have demonstrated that the enuretic alarm has greater efficacy than other forms of treatment. The enuretic alarm is triggered when a sensor in the sheets or night clothes gets wet; a bell or buzzer is thereby activated. Presumably, alarm therapy startles the child and improves arousal from sleep either by classical conditioning or avoidance conditioning. A disadvantage of alarm therapy is that it takes a couple of weeks to take effect. As such, alarms should be used for at least 6 weeks in children who do not respond before discontinuing their use. Because success depends on a cooperative, motivated child, conditioning therapy with an alarm device is generally used in children over 6 years of age.

It has been shown that combination of alarm and desmopressin works better than either treatment alone. Such treatment may be considered for children with refractory nocturnal enuresis.

When an anatomic abnormality or defect in urinary concentration ability is present, the underlying problem may require specific dietary, pharmacologic, or surgical treatment. Any underlying constipation should also be treated.

---

[1]Not FDA approved for this indication.

References

Brown ML, Pope AW, Brown EJ: Treatment of primary nocturnal enuresis in children: a review, *Child Care Health Dev* 37:153–160, 2011.

Glazener CM, Evans JH: Desmopressin for nocturnal enuresis in children, *Cochrane Database Syst Rev* 3, 2002. CD002112.

Glazener CM, Evans JH, Pero RE: Alarm interventions for nocturnal enuresis in children, *Cochrane Database Syst Rev* 2, 2005. CD002911.

Kamperis K, Hagstroem S, Rittig S, et al: Combination of the enuresis alarm and desmopressin: Second line treatment for nocturnal enuresis, *J Urol* 179:1128–1131, 2008.

Leung AK: Nocturnal enuresis. In Leung AK, editor: *Common Problems in Ambulatory Pediatrics: Specific Clinical Problems*, vol 1. New York, 2011, Nova Science Publishers, pp 161–171.

Lottmann H, Froeling F, Alloussi S, et al: A randomized comparison of oral desmopressin lyophilisate (MELT) and tablet formulations in children and adolescents with primary nocturnal enuresis, *Int J Clin Pract* 61:1454–1460, 2007.

Nevéus T: Nocturnal enuresis—theoretic background and practical guidelines, *Pediatr. Nephrol* 26:1207–1214, 2011.

Robson WL: Evaluation and management of enuresis, *N Engl J Med* 360:1429–1436, 2009.

Robson WL, Leung AK, van Howe R: Primary and secondary nocturnal enuresis: similarities in presentation, *Pediatrics* 115:956–959, 2005.

Robson WL, Leung AK, Norgaard JP: The comparative safety of oral versus intranasal desmopressin in the treatment of children with nocturnal enuresis, *J Urol* 178:24–30, 2007.

Van de Walle J, Rittig S, Bauer S, et al: Practical consensus guidelines for the management of enuresis, *Eur J Pediatr* 171:971–983, 2012.

NORMAL INFANT FEEDING

Method of
Amy Seery, MD

CURRENT THERAPY

- Breast milk is considered the best nutritional source for all infants including preterm infants.
- Breast-feeding is strongly encouraged, but many mothers require support from a multidisciplinary medical team to achieve success.
- There are few absolute contraindications to breast-feeding but these include maternal HIV, infant galactosemia, herpetic lesions on the breast, maternal use of illicit drugs, and mothers undergoing some types of chemotherapy.
- Maternal medications should be individually reviewed for safety during breast-feeding.
- Newborns should be fed at least every 3 hours during the day and every 4 hours during the night.
- Breast-fed infants can go up to 10 days between stools. This is a normal stooling pattern so long as the infant shows no signs of distress or illness.

The newborn period is defined as birth through the 28th day of life. During this time, newborns primarily feed, grow, and sleep. Therefore adequate nutrition carries special significance during this phase of life. This chapter focuses on available options for newborn nutrition (e.g., breast milk and commercial formulas), information medical caregivers can use when counseling families, definitions of adequate quality and quantity of nutritional sources, and assessing for appropriate intake in terms of growth.

Breast-feeding and Breast Milk

Breast-feeding is the nutritional source of choice as recommended by the American Academy of Pediatrics (AAP), the Canadian Pediatric Society, and the American Academy of Family Physicians. Caregivers should always respect the choice of the mother and support her during her bonding period with her newborn infant. However, because many misconceptions exist regarding breast-feeding, it is practical for caregivers to inquire about a mother's reasons if she chooses to use formula to feed her infant. She may have several concerns about breast-feeding including returning to work, the logistics of pumping, or her modesty, or she may consider breast-feeding to be "antiquated." Breast-feeding may be contrary to cultural and ethnic beliefs of the mother. For example, some Hispanic women are concerned that when breast-feeding they might inadvertently pass on negative emotions to their newborn. Because Somalian mothers attribute special powers to Western medicine and infant formulas, they often breast-feed but supplement with formula to ensure their infant gets everything that modern medicine can offer. With proper education and support, many mothers find breast-feeding to be a more reasonable option than they first thought.

Thanks to the efforts of several organizations promoting the health benefits of breast-feeding, even mothers who choose to formula feed recognize breast milk as the best nutritional option for their infant. But even after making the decision to breast-feed, some mothers continue to struggle with the actual undertaking of breast-feeding. There remains in our culture the inaccurate belief that something so "natural" must be easy to do. Many first-time mothers are easily frustrated and discouraged during the first few attempts at breast-feeding because they have unreasonable expectations based on the media and popular culture. With more and more women willing to try breast-feeding after delivery, adequate support and teaching should be provided by the entire medical team.

Thanks to multiple initiatives and ongoing education efforts, breast-feeding rates have been increasing in the US and are currently at their highest rates since World War II. Healthy People 2020 has a goal for a national breast-feeding initiation rate of 81.9%, and the actual rate of breast-feeding initiation in 2012 was 80.0%. Targets for exclusive breast-feeding at 3 months and 6 months are 46% and 25% respectively. The actual rate reported at 3 months is 43.3% and at 6 months is 21.9%. The rate for any breast-feeding at 12 months old is 29.2% though the goal is 34.1%. While significant progress has been made, especially in the last decade, there is still substantial room for further improvement. The biggest disparities in breast-feeding rates are among racial and ethnic minorities. Special attention should be made by medical teams to provide sufficient support and education to these women.

Breast milk is considered the ideal source of nutrition for all newborns, including premature infants, in a large part owing to its contents. There is a greater ratio of whey to casein in breast milk than in formula. Whey is associated with better absorption and digestion, as well as faster gastrointestinal transit times. There are also several specific proteins found only in breast milk, such as lactoferrin, lysozyme, and secretory immunoglobulin A, that aid in immune defense in the gut. Breast milk also contains long-chain polyunsaturated fatty acids (PUFAs) that aid in neural and visual development. Infants given formulas that contain long-chain PUFAs have serum concentrations that never match those of breast milk–fed infants, but there is also no known minimum amount needed to achieve benefit.

There is also a difference in the intestinal microflora seen in infants fed breast milk versus those fed formula. Larger percentages of *Lactobacillus* and *Bifidobacterium* species are found in infants fed breast milk, whereas *Bacteroides* spp and enterobacteria are in more abundance in formula-fed counterparts. Newer evidence suggests this difference in the diversity of gut microflora accounts for the stronger immune systems seen in breast-fed infants.

Breast milk has the benefit of containing several nonnutritive substances that are advantageous for young infants including maternal antibodies, growth regulators, digestive enzymes, and hormones. Breast milk has been associated with a reduced risk for many chronic illnesses including asthma, food and environmental allergies, diabetes mellitus, eczema, cardiovascular disease, and obesity. There is a reduction in the number of short-term illnesses of childhood including acute respiratory and gastrointestinal illnesses, as well as otitis media.

Newer research shows an association between being fed breast milk and having higher IQ scores later in childhood.

The act of breast-feeding offers several benefits to the infant. There is a sense of security and closeness that comes from skin-to-skin contact and the resultant interaction between infant and mother. Nursing can also reduce the opportunities and risk for bottle-propping and overfeeding. Breast-feeding allows nutrition to be more immediately available with minimal preparation work compared to the mixing and warming of formula. Breast milk is a much cheaper alternative to supplemental formulas. Breast-feeding can also lead to health benefits for the mother such as decreased risk of ovarian and breast cancers, as well as diabetes mellitus type II.

There are very few contraindications to breast-feeding. Contraindications include maternal HIV, active herpetic lesions on the breast (herpetic lesions elsewhere are not a contraindication), maternal use of illicit drugs, women undergoing chemotherapy with antimetabolite agents, and mothers with active tuberculosis. Nearly all over-the-counter medications are safe to take during breast-feeding. Some prescription medications are contraindicated, although safe substitutes are usually available. Providers can use the online National Library of Medicine's Drugs and Lactation Database (LactMed) to check safety and provide up-to-date counseling. Infants with galactosemia should not be breast-fed or bottle fed with milk products.

Infant Formulas

Commercially available infant formulas became widely used during World War II when there was a large influx of women into the national workforce. Since that time, infant formulas have been continuously improved upon and contain all the necessary energy and nutrient requirements for full-term infants up to the age of 6 months. According to the AAP there are three indications for the use of formulas:

- An alternative primary nutritional source for infants whose mothers choose not to or are unable to breast-feed
- A supplementary nutritional source for mothers with an inadequate supply of breast milk
- A nutritional source in infants with a medical condition in which breast-feeding is contraindicated (e.g., galactosemia)

Commercial formulas usually come in three distinct preparations, including ready-to-feed, concentrated liquid, and powder. All three preparations yield 20 kcal per fluid ounce when prepared correctly, the same amount of energy per volume found in breast milk. Powder preparations are generally the least expensive. An advantage to formulas over breast-feeding is the ability to increase caloric density for an infant with increased metabolic needs (e.g., infants with congenital heart defects). Breast-feeding mothers have the option to breast pump and add a fortifier if needed to achieve similar increases in caloric density.

Formulas carry the risk of improper preparation, whether intentional or accidental. Caregivers might choose to dilute the formula secondary to financial pressures or to concentrate formula preparations in a desire to have a larger infant, because some cultures equate larger infant size and weight with better health. Either change can be dangerous to the infant. Diluting leads to an excess of free water with an insufficient solute load (e.g., hyponatremia) and concentrating can conversely lead to hypernatremia. Nevertheless, formulas remain an appropriate alternative when desired by the infant's mother or when medically indicated (Table 1).

Micronutrients

Both breast milk and formula contain most of the micronutrients needed by infants. Calcium and phosphorus are found in lower concentrations in breast milk but are more bioavailable than the minerals present in formulas. Therefore there is no difference in bone mineral concentrations in both sets of infants. Iron, zinc, and copper serum levels are sufficient during the first 6 months of life in breast-fed infants, although tissue stores are gradually depleted. After 6 months breast-feeding should be supplemented with complementary foods to prevent outcomes such as iron deficiency anemia.

Vitamin K, necessary to prevent hemorrhagic disease, is produced by the digestive actions of intestinal flora. For this reason, most infants at the time of birth are given a single intramuscular dose to provide adequate amounts until intestinal flora concentrations are more mature and dietary supplementation with solid food begins at 6 months.

Vitamin D needs historically have been achieved with adequate sunlight exposure. However, with appropriate use of sunscreens and sunlight avoidance, most infants are at risk for vitamin D deficiency. Vitamin D is not passed in sufficient quantities in breast milk, and the content in formulas is so low that the daily recommended amount of 400 IU is only achieved when infants are consuming a volume typical of a 6-month old. Therefore supplementation should be recommended for all infants regardless of skin color and nutritional source to help prevent rickets. The recommendation is 400 IU of vitamin D for all pediatric age groups beginning after the first 2 weeks of life.

Neither formula-fed nor breast-fed infants usually require supplementation with water. In fact, providing infants with excess free water can lead to hyponatremia, seizures, and death. If there is concern that the infant is constipated or overheated, caregivers can provide up to a tablespoon of water daily to infants younger than 4 months old.

TABLE 1 Infant Formulas and their Indications

CLASS	BRAND NAMES	CALORIES (KCAL PER OZ)	CARBOHYDRATE SOURCE	PROTEIN SOURCE	INDICATIONS
Breast milk	—	20	Lactose	Human milk	Preferred for all infants
Term formula	Gerber Good Start Gentle	20	Lactose	Cow's milk	Appropriate for most infants
Term formula with DHA and ARA	Enfamil Premium Infant; Good Start Protect; Similac Advanced	20	Lactose	Cow's milk	Marketed to promote eye and brain development
Preterm formula	Enfamil Premature; Similac Special Care 24 with Iron	24	Lactose	Cow's milk	<34 wk gestational age Weight <1800 g
Enriched formula	Enfacare; Similac Neosure	22	Lactose	Cow's milk	34–36 wk gestational age Weight ≥1800 g
Soy formula	Enfamil Prosobee; Good Start Soy; Similac Isomil	20	Corn-based	Soy	Congenital lactase deficiency, galactosemia
Lactose-free formula	Similac Sensitive	20	Corn-based	Cow's milk	Congenital lactase deficiency, primary lactase deficiency, galactosemia
Hypoallergenic formula	Similac Alimentum; Enfamil Nutramigen; Enfamil Pregestimil	20	Corn or Sucrose	Hydrolyzed proteins	Milk protein allergy
Nonallergenic formula	Elecare; Neocate Infant; Nutramigen AA	20	Corn or Sucrose	Amino acids	Milk protein allergy
Antireflex formula	Enfamil AR; Similac Senstive for Spit-Up	20	Lactose (thickened with rice starch)	Cow's milk	Gastroesophageal reflux

Abbreviations: ARA=arachidonic acid; DHA=docosahexaenoic acid.
Adapted from O'Connor NR. Infant formula. Am Fam Physician 2009;79:565–70.

Defining Adequate Intake

To determine whether a newborn is receiving adequate nutrition, physicians should ask the caregiver how often feedings are occurring, for how long (for breast-fed infants), and how much is eaten (for formula-fed infants) and should assess the number of wet diapers and stools daily. Initially infants should consume 10 to 15 mL per feeding for the first 24 to 36 hours, gradually increasing to 30 to 45 mL by the fourth day of life. Breast-fed infants should feed 15 to 20 minutes each side. At the time of discharge to home, all newborns should be feeding 8 to 12 times a day, or every 2 to 3 hours. This interval can be increased to every 4 hours at night, and parents should be encouraged to wake any infants who sleep for longer than this duration. If an infant has lost more than 10% of his or her birth weight, the care team should consider delaying discharge to review the infant's nutritional status and feeding habits. Caregivers should be attentive to infant cues of hunger and satiety to provide an ideal feeding pattern for each infant.

Voiding and stooling patterns change with age and can also be influenced by the infant's diet. All newborns should have at least one wet diaper and one stool within the first 24 hours of life. If this does not occur, close observation and further workup are indicated to rule out structural or metabolic abnormalities. During the first week of life, infants usually void and stool with every feeding or even more often. Beyond the first week, infants should have at least 4 to 6 voids daily regardless of diet. Formula-fed infants might have one stool every other day up to 2 to 3 stools daily. Because of the higher percentage of protein that is absorbed in breast milk, breast-fed infants can go up to 10 days between stools. Physicians should review with families the signs

and symptoms (emesis, refusal to feed, lethargy, inconsolability, and abdominal distention) that indicate an infant with infrequent stooling should be medically evaluated. Breast-fed infants also have stools that are described as loose, yellow, and seedy. Caregivers should be educated that this is a normal stool color and consistency and is not considered diarrhea.

Medical providers can also calculate an infant's nutritional needs and compare to the actual intake. Nutritional needs are represented as kcal/kg per day (KKD). The following formula can be used:

$$KKD = \frac{Volume\ in\ mL\ consumed\ in\ 24h}{Weight\ in\ kg} \times \frac{20\ kcal/oz}{30}$$

During the first 3 months of life, infants should consume an intake that equals 90 to 135 kcal/kg per day. This intake goal should lead to a weight gain of approximately 25 to 30 g daily. From 3 to 6 months of age, infants gain at a slightly slower rate of approximately 15 to 20 g per day (Table 2). For example, a

TABLE 2 Expected Growth Velocities during Infancy

AGE	WEIGHT GAIN (g/d)	LENGTH (cm/mo)	HEAD CIRCUMFERENCE (cm/wk)
0–3 mo	25–30	2.5	0.5
3–6 mo	15–20	2.5	0.5
6–12 mo	10	1.25	0.25

2-month-old who weighs 6 kg should consume between 810 mL to 1215 mL daily.

At subsequent visits an infant can be assessed for adequate growth using standardized, gender-specific growth curves. Attention should be paid to growth parameters including weight, length, head circumference, and weight-for-length. Weight-for-length charts are used during the first 2 years of life as a gross equivalent to body-mass-index charts used for children older than 2 years. For years, practices defined adequate weight gain using growth charts as designed by the National Center for Health Statistics (NCHS), a branch of the Centers for Disease Control and Prevention (CDC). These charts were last updated in 2000 and unfortunately still reflect means for a population with a predominance of formula-fed infants. The World Health Organization (WHO) has since completed the Multi-Centre Growth Reference Study to better establish growth norms for infants and children who are breast-fed throughout the first year of life. A provider who is uncertain whether an exclusively breast-fed infant is meeting minimum growth requirements should refer to these charts before automatically encouraging caregivers to begin formula supplementation. Growth failure is usually considered a weight less than the third percentile or a drop of two or more percentiles in a short time (Figures 1 to 8, available on Expert Consult).

Overfeeding of newborns is unfortunately common, although bottle-fed infants are at a greater risk compared with breast-fed infants. Several factors can contribute to overfeeding, including lack of caregiver experience and support, as well as cultural biases such as the desire to have a chubbier infant. Many caregivers are unable to recognize infant cues for hunger and satiety and misinterpret cries or other vocalizations as a request for food. Medical providers should teach families about the rooting and sucking reflex and explain that some forms of sucking provide the infant with a means for self-soothing and are not signals that the infant is hungry (nonnutritive vs nutritive sucking).

Introduction of Complementary Foods

It remains controversial when solid foods should be added to the diet of an infant. The WHO recommends waiting until 6 months old. The AAP encourages waiting until an infant is 4 months old before adding solids and encourages continued breast-feeding until at least 1 year of age. However, some families want to start solids sooner than 4 months of age for a variety of reasons. A common explanation is "helping the baby sleep better at night." Only by 4 months will infants have attained sufficient muscle strength and coordination to keep their head upright when seated and to protect their own airway during feedings that contain solid foods. Families should be encouraged to wait at least until 4 months old before introducing solids, usually starting with rice cereal. Introduction of solids should not be delayed for much longer than 6 months, especially for breast-fed infants, because this is typically when micronutrient stores have been depleted and dietary supplementation with solid foods is needed. Only one new solid should be introduced every 3 to 5 days so infants can be monitored for adverse food reactions.

Either formula or breast milk should continue to be offered until 12 months old, at which time infants can be transitioned to whole-fat cow's milk. Low-fat milk does not provide toddlers with sufficient lipid concentrations for adequate brain development or the required caloric density for general growth. Large quantities of fruit juices should be avoided throughout infancy and childhood because they provide little nutritional value.

Summary

The majority of term infants are born ready and able to begin feeding, but it is up to providers to know available nutritional options, normal feeding patterns, and means for measuring adequate intake and growth. Providers and other members of the care team also need to be able to counsel caregivers about best practices when feeding infants. When infants are suspected to be overfed or underfed, it may take a multidisciplinary approach by physicians, nurses, dieticians, speech therapists, lactation counselors, and social workers to help patients and their families.

Head circumference-for-age BOYS
Birth to 2 years (percentiles)

World Health Organization

WHO Child Growth Standards

Figure 1 Head circumference for age: boys.

Length-for-age BOYS
Birth to 2 years (percentiles)

WHO Child Growth Standards

Figure 2 Length for age: boys.

Weight-for-age GIRLS
Birth to 2 years (percentiles)

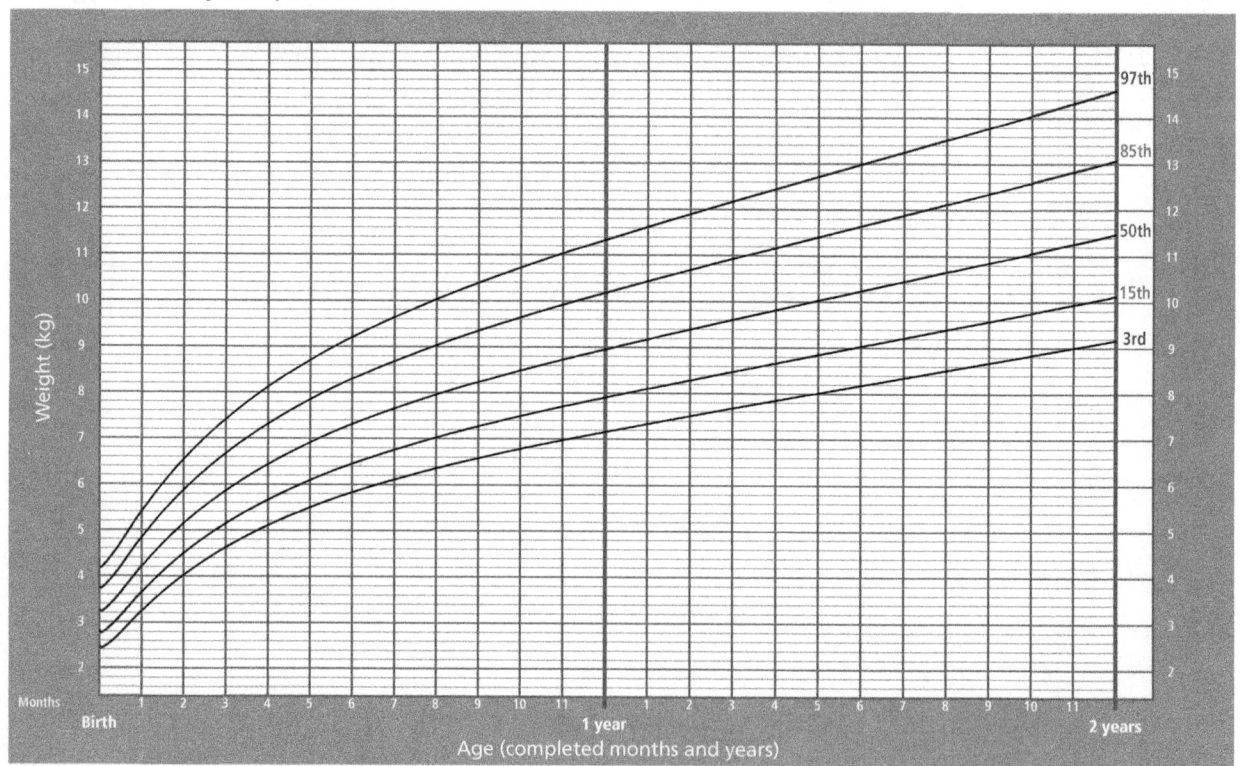

WHO Child Growth Standards

Figure 3 Weight for age: girls.

Weight-for-length GIRLS
Birth to 2 years (percentiles)

World Health Organization

WHO Child Growth Standards

Figure 4 Weight for length: girls.

Head circumference-for-age GIRLS
Birth to 2 years (percentiles)

World Health Organization

WHO Child Growth Standards

Figure 5 Head circumference for age: girls.

Weight-for-length BOYS
Birth to 2 years (percentiles)

Figure 6 Weight for length: boys.

Weight-for-age BOYS
Birth to 2 years (percentiles)

Figure 7 Weight for age: boys.

Length-for-age GIRLS
Birth to 2 years (percentiles)

WHO Child Growth Standards

Figure 8 Length for age: girls.

References

American Academy of Family Physicians. Breastfeeding, Family Physicians Supporting (Position Paper). Available at http://www.aafp.org/online/en/home/policy/policies/b/breastfeedingpositionpaper.htm; [accessed August 17, 2017].

American Academy of Pediatrics, HealthyChildren.Org. Feeding and Nutrition, 0 to 12 Months. Available at http://www.healthychildren.org/English/ages-stages/baby/feeding-nutrition/Pages/default.aspx; [accessed August 17, 2017].

Duncan P: *Bright Futures: Guidelines for Health Supervision of Infants, Children, and Adolescents*, 3rd ed., Elk Grove Village, IL, 2007, American Academy of Pediatrics.

Kleinmann RE: *Pediatric Nutrition Handbook*, ed 6, Elk Grove Village, IL, 2008, American Academy of Pediatrics.

McInerny TK: *AAP Textbook of Pediatric Care*, ed 1, Elk Grove Village, IL, 2009, American Academy of Pediatrics.

National Library of Medicine. Drugs and Lactation Database. Available at http://toxnet.nlm.nih.gov/cgi-bin/sis/htmlgen?LACT; [accessed August 17, 2017].

O'Connor NR: Infant formula, *Am Fam Physician* 79:565–570, 2009.

USPSTF. Primary care interventions to support breastfeeding- USPSTF recommendation statement, *JAMA* 316(16):1688–1693, 2016.

World Health Organization. The WHO Multicentre Growth Reference Study. Available at http://www.who.int/childgrowth/mgrs/en/; [accessed August 17, 2017].

PARENTERAL FLUID THERAPY FOR INFANTS AND CHILDREN

Method of
Aaron Friedman, MD

CURRENT DIAGNOSIS

- Maintenance fluid therapy is designed to replace the next 24 hours' anticipated losses from sensible and insensible losses in an otherwise healthy, euvolemic patient with normal kidney function.

- In a patient with extracellular volume loss, the percentage of body weight lost should be used as a guide to the volume needed for restoration.

- Serum sodium in patients with dehydration should be measured at the time of presentation and also after restoration fluid has been provided. The further correction of serum sodium will be much easier in a patient with a normalized extracellular volume.

CURRENT THERAPY

- Maintenance fluid therapy should not be used as a restoration or replacement fluid.

- Restoration fluid therapy can be given over short periods with a plan for complete restoration, in the majority of patients, within 24 hours.

- When treating hyponatremia or hypernatremia, the goal should be to change the serum sodium by *no more than* 10 mmol/L in a 24-hour period.

- When calculating how much water (in the case of hypernatremia) or how much sodium (in the case of hyponatremia) to provide a patient in order to restore sodium into the normal range, remember the calculation is based on the *total body water*, which is 60% of body weight, and the aim is to get to the closest serum sodium considered normal; for example, sodium 135 mmol/L for hyponatremia and sodium 145 mmol/L for hypernatremia.

- Replacement fluid therapy for patients with abnormal losses—gastrointestinal or urinary losses—should be based on measurement of the lost fluid volume and fluid electrolyte content.

TABLE 1 — Approach to Determine Parenteral Fluids and Electrolytes for a 24-Hour Period

WEIGHT (KG)	WATER (ML)	NA (MEQ/L)	K (MEQ/L)
0–10	100/kg	3/100 mL	2/100 mL
11–20	1000 + 50/kg 11–20 kg	3/100 mL	2/100 mL
>20	1500 + 20/kg >20 kg	3/100 mL	2/100 mL
Examples			
15-kg child	1250	37 mEq/1250 mL	25 mEq/1250 mL
30-kg child	1700	51	34

Note: For sodium, potassium, and chloride, milliequivalents (mEq) and milliosmoles (mOsm) are the same.

TABLE 2 — Hourly Administration of Fluids

CHILD'S WEIGHT (kg)	VOLUME OF WATER PER HOUR
≤10	4 ml/kg
11–20	40 mL + 2 mL/kg for every kilogram 11–20
>20	60 mL + 1 mL/kg for every kilogram >20

Children receive three types of parenteral fluid therapy: maintenance therapy, restoration therapy, and replacement therapy. Maintenance fluid therapy provides the typical anticipated fluid and electrolyte losses seen in otherwise normal, euvolemic children. Restoration fluid therapy restores fluid volume previously lost. Replacement fluid therapy keeps up with ongoing abnormal fluid losses, such as ongoing losses from the gastrointestinal tract or abnormal urinary losses.

Maintenance Fluid Therapy

In 1957, Holliday and Segar proposed an approach to providing parenteral fluids and electrolytes to hospitalized children who are not permitted to eat or drink. The formulation was based on calories expended, presumed the patient did not have previous fluid losses (was euvolemic), and had normal kidney function. The surrogate for calories is weight because calories expended correlates to weight in grams. Therefore, the anticipated fluid losses for the upcoming 24 hours would come from urine excreted, water lost during breathing, and fluids lost from sweating. The prescription includes two components: water and electrolytes. Table 1 describes the approach recommended by Holliday and Segar to determine parenteral fluids and electrolytes for a 24-hour period. It includes determining the amount of water to be provided based on weight as a surrogate for calories expended and it includes electrolytes to be provided. The electrolytes are sodium and potassium. Sodium is given at 2 to 3 mmol per 100 mL water provided, and potassium is given at 2 mmol per 100 mL water provided, with each provided as the chloride salt. Once the amount is calculated, the hourly rate can be determined by dividing the final calculation by 24.

The prepared solution that most closely resembles this maintenance prescription is 0.2 NS (0.2 normal saline, or 154 mmol sodium and chloride per liter) with 20 mEq KCl/L of fluid. Often glucose is added at 50 g/L (D_5W) or 5 g/100 mL. This provides some readily available calories to reduce catabolism. Note also that D_5W has an osmolality of nearly 300 mOsm/kg H_2O, essentially the same as plasma. This allows safe administration of the solution, because a markedly hypotonic solution administered into a vein could result in lysis of cells (especially red cells) in the vicinity of the infused hypotonic solution.

Another approach for calculating the water with the appropriate electrolytes to be provided is 1500 mL/m²/24 hours. This approach requires measuring the child's height and weight to determine square meters and is less convenient. The volume provided by the approach in Table 1 and the 1500 mL/m² calculation are equivalent.

Another approach is to determine the hourly need of water bearing the electrolytes to be provided, the same as Holliday and Segar. The hourly approach to determining volume is shown in Table 2. Using this approach, maintenance fluid therapy for a 15-kg child would be infused at a rate of 50 mL/hour:

$$(4 \text{ mL/kg/h} \times 10 \text{ kg}) + (2 \text{ mL/kg/h} \times 5 \text{ kg})$$

Maintenance fluid therapy was designed to provide water and electrolytes to cover *future* (anticipated) loss, particularly from urine, expired air, and sweat. Unfortunately, since the publication of maintenance fluid therapy guidelines by Holliday and Segar, the formulation has often been misused. Maintenance fluid therapy should *not* be used as a fluid prescription for *restoring* extracellular fluid volume previously lost, for example, as a result of vomiting, diarrhea, or burns. It is almost always *not* an appropriate solution for *replacing* abnormal losses from the gastrointestinal tract, urinary tract, and so on. The volume calculation and the electrolyte concentrations are *not* appropriate to calculate a restoration solution or replacement solution.

The primary reason that a hypotonic solution such as maintenance fluids, as described by Holliday and Segar, is problematic for use as a restoration solution is the nonosmotic release of antidiuretic hormone (ADH, also called AVP [arginine vasopressin]). Since the mid 1950s it has been known that ADH is released from the hypothalamus under two different physiologic stimuli. One is an increase in serum and extracellular osmolality, usually greater than 290 mOsm/kg H_2O, termed *osmotic stimulus.* The other is a nonosmotic stimulus, usually the result of a fall in extracellular fluid volume or the perception of such a fall by volume receptors mainly in the thorax.

Since the 1950s we have come to learn that a large number of other stimuli can act as a nonosmotic stimulus to ADH release. These include, but are not limited to, a wide range of medications (antihypertensives, some antineoplastics, barbiturates), stress, central nervous system (CNS) injury or surgery, positive pressure ventilation, malignancy, and intrathoracic infection or malignancy. Under these conditions, ADH levels will be high and the administration of a hypotonic solution even at calculated maintenance doses could result in a fall in serum sodium and serum osmolality, on occasion to levels that might cause serious CNS injury, seizures, and even CNS herniation and death. Even in the early 1960s, when the precise reasons for the nonosmotic release of ADH were not well known, the risk of developing hyponatremia when providing the full volume prescribed in maintenance fluid therapy in the face of a concentrated urine and low urine volumes (signaling ADH release) was well known. The recommendation was to reduce the volume of fluid provided to approximately 50% of the standard calculated amount.

More recently, some have recommended, to prevent the development of hyponatremia, that all maintenance fluid therapy should be delivered as isotonic (normal) saline. The volume portion of the Holliday–Segar formulation is not altered, but the solution recommended in this approach is isotonic saline. The full impact of this approach on all types of hospitalized children is still unknown. It

TABLE 3 Signs of Volume Depletion

SIGN	MILD (1%–4%)	MODERATE (5%–7%)	SEVERE (>7%)
	DEGREE OF DEPLETION		
Skin	Normal	Cool	Cool, mottled
Capillary refill	Normal	Decreased	Markedly decreased
Skin turgor	Normal	Loose	Tenting
Buccal mucosa	Slightly dry	Dry	Parched
Eyes	Normal	Sunken	Markedly sunken
Fontanel*	Normal	Sunken	Markedly sunken
Pulse	Normal (full)	Rapid	Rapid, thready
Urine output	Normal	Decreased	Oliguria (<1 mL/kg/h)
Systolic blood pressure	Normal	Normal, low	Low, shock

*Infants <9 mo of age.

seems clear that patients in the perioperative period should receive normal saline in anticipation of the potential need for extracellular volume restoration. This approach does not guarantee that hyponatremia or hypernatremia will be totally prevented.

Restoration Fluid Therapy

Many children require parenteral fluids because of an inability to take fluids by mouth or due to abnormal fluid losses, such as from vomiting and diarrhea, excessive urinary losses, burns (excessive fluid losses from skin), or third spacing (the extravasation of fluid from the extracellular spaces such as the abdominal or thoracic cavity). In these situations, patients are at risk for serious extracellular volume depletion and even plasma volume depletion, which, left untreated, can result in hypotension or shock.

The parenteral fluid therapy for volume depletion should aim to first replace extracellular volume depletion. How much fluid to provide can be estimated by a long-standing approach using clinical signs to estimate the percentage of reduction in body weight associated with fluid losses (Table 3). In general, these losses can be replaced with a solution that restores extracellular fluid (isotonic saline or lactated Ringer's solution). In situations of prolonged fluid losses (more than 7 days), partial replacement with isotonic saline followed by a slower replacement with a more hypotonic solution with added potassium may be warranted. Table 3 outlines the clinical approach to assessing a patient's degree of volume depletion as a percentage of body weight.

Once the percentage of volume depletion is determined and the decision is made to use parenteral fluids based on moderate to severe volume depletion and ongoing vomiting, thus decreasing the effectiveness of oral rehydration, then rapid parenteral volume repletion is usually safe and effective. Replacing 50% of the determined volume depletion in 1 to 4 hours is appropriate, with the remaining replacement in the subsequent 4 to 16 hours. This should result in restored volume and improvement in the signs and symptoms demonstrated or reported by the patient. Often, partial restoration of extracellular volume depletion improves gastrointestinal symptoms and allows a switch to the oral route for completing volume restoration.

Example: A 15-kg patient presents with a 3-day history of vomiting and diarrhea. Physical examination suggests 5% volume depletion. The patient has ongoing vomiting, and parenteral fluids will be started. Volume depletion of 5% is 750 mL of fluid:

$$0.5 \times 15 \text{ kg (body weight)}$$

A commonly used volume expansion technique is to provide isotonic saline, 20 mL/kg, in a bolus (over 30 minutes to 1 hour). This amount of 300 mL (15 kg × 20 mL/kg) is approximately 2% of body weight and in this example is less than 50% of the determined volume depletion. The plan, therefore, is 375 mL (50%) over 1 to 2 hours of isotonic saline (or lactated Ringer's solution) parenterally, then 375 mL of the same solution over the next 4 to 6 hours.

Replacement Fluids

As a general rule of thumb, unusual losses—gastrointestinal or renal, for example—should be replaced with a solution of comparable electrolyte concentration and of comparable volume. The most precise way to determine the needed solution is to measure the concentration of solutes such as sodium, potassium, chloride, or bicarbonate lost in emesis, diarrhea, or urine. Emesis contains sodium at 10 to 40 mmol/L and even less potassium (5–20 mmol/L) but large amounts of chloride (90–150 mmol/L). Diarrheal fluid typically contains sodium at 40 to 90 mmol/L, potassium at 10 to 50 mmol/L, and up to 40 or 50 mmol/L of bicarbonate. Cholera patients can excrete sodium up to 140 mmol/L. When possible, the volume of loss should be measured so a replacement fluid solution volume can be planned.

The safe approach to the patient with ongoing losses is first to restore extracellular volume to normal using normal saline or lactated Ringer's solution as noted earlier. During extracellular volume restoration, measure the output and electrolyte content of abnormal losses, preferably over a 12- to 24-hour period. Once this is known, then replacement of ongoing losses should be provided as a separate solution, the volume and electrolyte concentration determined by the measurements of each. Provide the replacement solution over the next 12 to 24 hours. For example, a patient with diarrhea is found to be producing 300 mL of diarrheal fluid over 12 hours. The measured sodium concentration is 80 mmol/L, potassium is 20 mmol/L, and bicarbonate is 40 mmol/L. The solution that will nearly approximate the losses is 0.2 NS (34 mmol/L of sodium and of chloride) with 20 mmol/L of potassium and 40 mmol/L of sodium bicarbonate. The solution will contain 74 mmol/L of Na, 20 mmol/L of K and 40 mmol/L of bicarbonate. The solution would be infused at a rate of 25 mL/hour. The advantage of providing this separately from maintenance or restoration fluids is that the rate of infusion or even the electrolyte content can be changed to address just the replacement needs without having to change all the intravenous solutions.

Hyponatremia and Hypernatremia

Hyponatremia (serum sodium <135 mmol/L) and hypernatremia (serum sodium >145 mmol/L) are often associated with volume depletion. Hypernatremia is nearly exclusively associated with volume depletion, and hyponatremia can be seen in situations of volume expansion such as vasopressin excess (syndrome of inappropriate antidiuretic hormone [SIADH]) or congestive heart failure, kidney failure, or liver failure. At times, the need to normalize the serum sodium concentration requires parenteral intervention.

Approach to Hyponatremia

Symptomatic hyponatremia can occur if the serum sodium falls rapidly, but usually not until the serum sodium falls below 125 mmol/L. The symptoms associated with hyponatremia include anorexia, anxiety, agitation, ataxia, weakness, lethargy, disorientation, depressed deep tendon reflexes, seizures, coma, and death (usually the result of CNS herniation).

In situations where hyponatremia is associated with volume depletion, restoration of volume with isotonic saline often raises the serum sodium. When extracellular fluid volume is normal or expanded (such as situations when SIADH is at play), a four-fold approach to hyponatremia should be considered:
1. Treat the underlying condition.
2. Reduce water intake. In particular, if parenteral fluids are being provided, reduce or eliminate the use of hypotonic fluids.

3. Increase water excretion. This is usually done with loop diuretics such as furosemide (Lasix 0.5–1 mg/kg IV) to achieve a more rapid response.
4. Hypertonic saline IV is a step reserved for symptomatic patients. The most readily available hypertonic saline solution is 3% normal saline (sodium concentration of 513 mmol/L or approximately 0.5 mmol/mL). The desired outcome is to raise the serum sodium sufficiently to improve symptoms, but never more than 10 mmol/L in a 24-hour period. There is no need to raise the serum sodium beyond the lower limit of normal or 135 mmol/L. The desired increase in the serum sodium concentration should not exceed a maximum of 10 mmol/L.

The addition of sodium into the extracellular space will result in a shift of water from the intracellular to the extracellular space. Thus, the entire water space will be affected. The following example demonstrates how to calculate the amount of hypertonic saline to infuse in the face of severe hyponatremia:

A patient weighing 15 kg has a serum sodium of 125 mmol/L and experiences a seizure. The patient is felt to be euvolemic. Thus, hypertonic saline infusion is being considered. How should this be prescribed? Raise the serum sodium to 135 mmol/L from 125 mmol/L:

Change in serum sodium (mmol/L) × body weight (kg)
× 0.6 (total body water space) = $10 \times 15 \times 0.6 = 90$ mmol

Because hypertonic saline is approximately 0.5 mmol/mL, if 90 mmol is the amount of sodium calculated to raise the serum sodium and osmolality, then 180 ml of 3% saline is needed.

An alternative way to calculate the maximum 3% saline to use is: The maximum change in serum sodium is 10, the body weight is 15 kg, the water space is 1.2 ($0.6 \times 2 = 1.2$; i.e., 2 ml/mmol sodium in 3% saline), so:

$$10 \times 15 \times 1.2 = 180 \text{ mL of } 3\% \text{ saline}$$

Once the amount is calculated, the rate of administration should be no more than 2 to 4 mL/kg/hour, with measurements of the serum sodium at 2-hour intervals. Usually symptoms improve before there is a full 10-mmol rise in serum sodium. This rate should not result in a change of greater than 1 to 2 mmol/hour. If a change faster than this is seen, slow or stop the infusion immediately.

Approach to Hypernatremia

Hypernatremia (serum sodium >145 mmol/L) is seen with volume depletion. The extremely rare situation of pure salt overload is seen in babies receiving improperly mixed formula or intensive care patients receiving concentrated blood products and IV solutions. In these situations the patients do not show evidence of volume depletion, and urinary sodium excretion (and fractional excretion of sodium) is very high. In the overwhelming majority of patients who are volume depleted, hypernatremia signals volume losses of *at least* 10% of body weight. The classic teaching is that hypernatremic patients appear less-severely volume depleted than they actually are. This is attributed to the increased osmolality protecting the extracellular space at the cost of intracellular space. Intracellular volume contains two thirds of total body water, and the decreased volume in the intracellular space means nearly all cells in the body (importantly, including in the brain) are smaller than normal.

The approach to hypernatremia is first to restore volume using isotonic saline. Providing 40 to 50 mL/kg of isotonic saline over 4 hours will improve extracellular volume and is unlikely to markedly reduce the serum sodium. Restoring extracellular volume will improve organ perfusion, especially perfusion of the gut and the kidney. This will improve the likelihood of being able to use the gut for fluid replacement and improve glomerular filtration rate and overall kidney function so as to be able to restore volume and safely return serum sodium and osmolality to normal. The major consequence of a too-rapid fall in serum sodium or osmolality is cerebral edema, the result of smaller-than-normal cell volume too rapidly expanded by IV (especially hypotonic) fluids.

Following the first infusion, as noted earlier, consider providing 30 to 40 mL/kg of isotonic fluid over the next 20 hours (to complete a 24-hour treatment plan) to continue replenishing extracellular volume. Check the serum sodium and serum osmolality frequently, at 2- to 4-hour intervals in the first 24 to 48 hours if the serum sodium is greater than 155 mmol/L at presentation. As with hyponatremia, it is important not to change (in this case, drop) the serum sodium by more than 10 mmol/L in 24 hours or to change the serum osmolality by more than 20 mOsm/kg H2O in 24 hours. To determine how much water is necessary to lower the serum sodium, the following formula is often used:

Actual serum sodium – desired serum sodium
(not to exceed 10) × body weight in kg × 4 mL

For a 15-kg child with a serum sodium of 155:

$$10 \times 15 \times 4 = 600 \text{ mL of water}$$

The safe approach to reducing the water deficit is to provide no more than half of the water deficit in the first 24 hours as a solution of 5% dextrose (D_5W) with potassium of 20 to 30 mmol/L. The intracellular fluid compartment is rich in potassium, and patients with hypernatremic dehydration have had considerable intracellular volume loss and have lost potassium, usually through urinary losses. The same approach may be considered in day 2 and following. Certain caveats are important here. First, as noted earlier, frequent measurements of serum sodium and serum osmolality are necessary to prevent too rapid a decline. Because the maintenance prescription is very hypotonic in the first 24 hours, at least, replacing volume loss should be the first priority. Once the patient approaches a normal volume status and serum sodium, providing maintenance *may* be appropriate. Patients with hypertonicity (hypernatremic dehydration) are very thirsty. Any fluid they consume by mouth must be measured and monitored lest their oral consumption along with parenteral fluids exceed the safe amount recommended.

Intravenous Electrolyte Replacements

At times, IV replacement of other electrolytes may be necessary. The IV replacement of potassium, in situations where the serum potassium concentration falls below 2.5 mmol/L or where oral replacement cannot be used, can be given as potassium chloride or potassium phosphate at a dose of no more than 0.5 mmol/kg/hour. The concentration of potassium in the solution infused should not exceed 40 mmol/L in a peripheral vein because potassium infusions are painful and sclerosing. Higher concentrations under the appropriate circumstances could be given through a central vein.

On occasion, IV administration of calcium or phosphate (or both) is clinically indicated. IV calcium is considered in patients with tetany, usually a serum calcium <6.5 mg/dL with a normal serum albumin. For IV calcium administration to correct symptomatic hypocalcemia, in older children the recommendation is 10 to 20 mL of a 10% calcium gluconate solution over 15 minutes to reduce or stop symptoms such as tetany or seizures. In neonates and young children, 10 to 20 mg/kg or 1 to 2 mL/kg of a 10% calcium gluconate solution administered at a rate of 1 mL/min with cardiac monitoring is recommended. For more chronic administration, 50 to 75 mg/kg/24 hours of calcium gluconate is recommended. Rapid calcium administration temporarily lowers the serum phosphate and can lead to arrhythmia, hence the cardiac monitoring.

Hypophosphatemia might require parenteral administration of phosphate. This approach is usually reserved for patients with a serum phosphate less than 1 mg/dL. The recommended dosage of elemental phosphorus is 2.5 to 5 mg/kg (0.08 to 0.16 mmol/kg) over 6 to 8 hours. This administration can lower serum calcium, so frequent testing of both the serum phosphorus and calcium is appropriate.

Finally, bicarbonate may be given intravenously. Usually the IV solution of bicarbonate should not exceed a concentration of 45 mmol/L. For example, in certain clinical conditions alkalinization of the urine is desired to prevent crystal or stone formation. The usual prescription is 1 to 2 mmol/kg body weight in 24 hours.

Higher infused concentrations of bicarbonate (seen in patients with proximal tubule disease or injury as noted with certain chemotherapeutic agents) should be given into a central vein under careful monitoring. Calcium and bicarbonate should not be given in the same solution.

References

Feld LG, Friedman AL, Massengil SF: Disorders of water metabolism in fluid and electrolytes. In Feld LG, Kaskel FJ, editors: *Pediatrics*, Totowa, NJ, 2010, Humana Press, pp 3–47.

Friedman AL, Ray PE: Maintenance fluid therapy. What it is and what it is not, *Pediatr Nephrol* 23:677–680, 2008.

Gauer OH, Henry JP: Circulatory basis of fluid volume control, *Physiol Rev* 43:423–481, 1963.

Holliday MA, Segar WE: The maintenance need for water in parenteral fluid therapy, *Pediatrics* 19:823–832, 1957.

Moritz ML, Ayus JC: Prevention of hospital acquired hyponatremia, a case for using isotonic saline, *Pediatrics* 111:227–230, 2003.

Nelville KA, Sondeman DJ, Rubenstein A, et al: Prevention of hyponatremia during maintenance intravenous fluid administration: A prospective, randomized study of fluid type versus fluid rate, *J Pediatr* 156:313–319, 2010.

Robertson GL: Antidiuretic hormone. Normal and disordered function, *Endocrinol Metab Clin North Am* 30:671–684, 2001.

PEDIATRIC SLEEP DISORDERS

Method of
Julie M. Baughn, MD

CURRENT DIAGNOSIS

- Sleep disorders are common in children.
- Evaluation of pediatric sleep disorders in children begins with a thorough sleep history.
- Overnight polysomnography is most commonly used to evaluate for sleep-disordered breathing
- Other diagnostic tools include the multiple sleep latency test (MSLT), oximetry, sleep logs, and actigraphy.
- Common sleep disorders in children include obstructive sleep apnea, insomnia, restless legs syndrome, and delayed sleep phase syndrome.

CURRENT THERAPY

- For most children tonsillectomy and adenoidectomy are an effective treatment for obstructive sleep apnea.
- Behavioral therapy is essential to treating insomnia.
- Only in select circumstances are medications used to treat children with sleep disorders.

Introduction

Pediatric sleep medicine has grown as the importance of sleep in the developing child has been recognized along with the impact that insufficient or disrupted sleep can have on cognitive development and behavior. The American Academy of Sleep Medicine (AASM) and the American Academy of Pediatrics (AAP) have recently published guidelines and practice parameters addressing several aspects of pediatric sleep medicine. Pediatric sleep disorders have unique societal impact; both the child's and the family's sleep can be affected when a disorder is present. The aim of this chapter is to offer a practical approach to the diagnosis and treatment of the most common pediatric sleep disorders, discuss diagnostic tools available, and discuss recommended treatment.

Developmental Aspects of Sleep

Pediatric sleep disorders also have the unique challenge of dealing with sleep issues that are subject to change based on the child's developmental age. The amount of sleep required by age has been described in a recent AASM consensus statement (Table 1). The sleep architecture of the child characteristically changes as he or she develops. The portion of rapid eye movement (REM) sleep declines from 50% at birth to 25% to 30% in adolescence. The proportion of slow-wave sleep is highest in early childhood and continues to decline throughout life. The pattern of sleep and sleep requirement also change. Neonates may not develop a regular sleep-wake pattern until about 3 months of age. Most infants are capable of sleeping through the night by about 6 months of age, but many may continue to waken. Naps are typically given up somewhere between 3 and 5 years of age. Most adolescents, due to many societal and social constraints, do not get a requisite 8 to 10 hours of sleep at night.

Clinical Approach
Taking a Sleep History

There are several key elements to obtaining a sleep history in children. The mnemonic BEARS (*B*edtime problems, *E*xcessive daytime sleepiness, *A*wakenings during the night, *R*egularity and duration of sleep, and *S*leep-disordered breathing) has been offered as a practical starting point for obtaining a history, tailoring questions to both parent and child where appropriate (Table 2).

The primary sleep complaint should be obtained in the child's or parent's own words. Once the primary complaint is detailed, the presence/absence of snoring, the presence of restlessness at sleep initiation and during sleep, and the child's sleep-wake patterns during school should be gathered. The presence or absence of a bedtime routine and the details of that routine should be noted. A child's sleep environment should be carefully queried. A child who shares his or her bedroom, sleeps in his or her parents' bed, or ends up sleeping on a couch in front of the television may lead to specific sleep complaints. A history of whether there is more than one household involved (i.e., shared custody) is particularly important.

Sleepiness in children can be a particularly challenging symptom to evaluate. It is normal physiologically for children to nap until age 5. Other clues to daytime sleepiness that can be obtained in children include behavior issues, hyperactivity, excessive napping, or napping after age 5 years (intentionally or unintentionally). School-age children often display symptoms of behavioral problems or inattentiveness rather than sleepiness. Sleep-wake patterns on school days, weekends, and vacations need to be detailed. Often the child's most natural sleep pattern will emerge over the summer months.

Determining the child's sleep hygiene or good sleep practices is important in diagnosing and treating sleep disorders. Principles of good sleep hygiene are listed in Table 3.

Past Medical History/Family History

A history of prematurity, trisomy 21, velopharyngeal cleft palate repair, or hypotonia is each associated with an increased risk of sleep-disordered breathing. A past history of adenotonsillectomy for snoring is important information to obtain. Chronic nasal obstruction can cause maxillary hypoplasia. Arnold-Chiari malformation, myelomeningocele, or a brainstem lesion can predispose to central sleep apnea due to impaired central respiratory drive. Chronic health issues can also be associated with sleep disruption and consequently with behavioral problems associated with sleep.

A family history of obstructive sleep apnea (OSA), insomnia, or restless legs syndrome (RLS) is important; a family history of RLS can be used to support a diagnosis of RLS in the child. In particular, questioning the mother if she had symptoms of RLS during any of her pregnancies can be helpful because this is a common time for RLS to present or worsen. Morning or evening preferences (i.e., "night-owl" or "lark" tendencies) can also have a familial element. In addition, sleepwalking can be found to occur in families.

Focused Physical Examination

The physical examination in a child presenting with a sleep complaint should include a general assessment. Presence/absence of sleepiness, fatigue, and irritability/hyperactivity are all important. Height, weight, and body mass index (BMI) should be recorded. Children with OSA can have poor growth and even failure to thrive. Obesity is a risk factor for OSA. Special attention to a child's craniofacial features is important because these may make a child more at risk for sleep-disordered breathing. Assessment of tonsil size, oropharyngeal crowding (using the Mallampati or Friedman classification systems can be useful), and presence of maxillary/mandibular hypoplasia can all offer clues to an airway that may predispose to OSA. The practitioner should evaluate for evidence of nasal obstruction by noting mouth breathing and signs of allergy (i.e., allergic shiners, nasal crease).

Diagnostic Tools

Polysomnography

The AASM has published practice parameters on both the respiratory and nonrespiratory indications for polysomnography (PSG) in pediatric patients. In this chapter, a sleep study or PSG will refer only to an in-laboratory attended study, because home monitoring currently has not been sufficiently evaluated in the pediatric population. PSG in children entails spending the night at a sleep center. A parent or caregiver must also spend the night. During the night, the child's sleep characteristics, respiratory function, and movement are analyzed. This is done by the following measures: electroencephalography (EEG), electromyography (EMG) of chin and limbs, airflow by thermistor and nasal pressure, end-tidal or transcutaneous carbon dioxide measurements, and induction plethysmography to measure respiratory effort. Scoring of a PSG performed on a child is done using pediatric scoring rules set forth by the AASM.

The most common indication for a sleep study in children is OSA. PSG can be used to both diagnose OSA and treat sleep apnea with continuous positive airway pressure (CPAP). PSG can also be used to evaluate for elevated periodic limb movements of sleep, and in rare cases to characterize abnormal nocturnal behavior such as evaluation of parasomnias or nocturnal seizures.

Overnight Oximetry

The gold standard for diagnosis of pediatric OSA is PSG. Overnight oximetry has been suggested as an alternative screening tool for pediatric sleep-disordered OSA. Although an abnormal oximetry will suggest OSA, a normal oximetry does not rule out OSA. Children can have sleep apnea that is severe and still maintain normal oxygenation. In a study by Brouillette and colleagues (2000), when a positive oximetry graph was present (defined by three or more desaturation clusters and at least three desaturations < 90%) in a referred population, the positive predictive value for OSA on PSG was 97%. A negative or inconclusive oximetry by this definition did not rule out OSA and there was still a 47% chance OSA was present on PSG.

Sleep Logs/Actigraphy

Sleep logs can be effective in demonstrating a child's sleep-wake patterns. Actigraphy is often done in conjunction with a sleep log. Actigraphy is a portable wristband that measures movement. The absence of movement over a certain time period is used as a surrogate marker of sleep, and the presence of movement over a certain time period is used as a surrogate for wakefulness. Some devices also measure ambient light exposure. Used in conjunction with actigraphy sleep logs can be extremely helpful in demonstrating discrepancies between perceived and actual sleep, and are

TABLE 1	Sleep Requirements in Children by Age
AGE	**AVERAGE SLEEP DURATION IN 24 HOURS (OVERNIGHT AND NAPS)**
Infants (4 to 12 months)	12 to 16 hours
Children (1-2 years)	11-14 hours
Children (3-5 years)	10–13 hours Most give up naps between 3 and 5 years
Children (6-12 years)	9–12 hours
Teenagers (> 12 years13-18 years)	9 hours8-10 hours

Paruthi S, Brooks LJ, D'Ambrosio C, et al. Consensus Statement of the American Academy of Sleep Medicine on the Recommended Amount of Sleep for Healthy Children: Methodology and Discussion, *J Clin Sleep Med* 2016; 12(11):1549-1561.

TABLE 2	BEARS Mnemonic: A Screening Tool for Sleep Disorders in Children		
	PRESCHOOL (2–5 YEARS)	**SCHOOL-AGE (6–12 YEARS)**	**ADOLESCENT (13–18 YEARS)**
Bedtime problems	Does your child have any problems going to bed? Falling asleep?	Does your child have any problems at bedtime? (P) Do you have any problems going to bed? (C)	Do you have any problems falling asleep at bedtime? (C)
Excessive daytime sleepiness	Does your child seem overly tired or sleepy during the day? Does your child still take naps?	Does your child have difficulty waking in the morning, seem sleepy during the day, or take naps? (P) Do you feel tired a lot? (C)	Do you feel sleepy a lot during the day? In school? While driving? (C)
Awakenings during the night	Does your child wake up a lot at night?	Does your child seem to wake up a lot at night? Any sleepwalking or nightmares? (P) Do you wake up a lot at night? Have trouble getting back to sleep? (C)	Do you wake up a lot at night? Have trouble getting back to sleep? (C)
Regularity and duration of sleep	Does your child have a regular bedtime and wake time? What are they?	What time does your child go to bed and get up on school days? Weekends? Do you think your child is getting enough sleep? (P)	What time do you usually go to bed on school nights? Weekends? How much sleep do you usually get? (C)
Sleep-disordered breathing	Does your child snore a lot or have difficulty breathing at night?	Does your child have loud or nightly snoring or any breathing difficulties at night? (P)	Does your teenager snore loudly or nightly? (P)

Abbreviations: C = child; P = parent.
From Owens JA, Dalzell V: Use of the "BEARS" sleep screening tool in a pediatric residents' continuity clinic: A pilot study. Sleep Med 2005;6:63–69.

helpful in demonstrating insufficient sleep and circadian rhythm disorders. Those that measure light as well can aid in uncovering sleep hygiene issues.

Multiple Sleep Latency Test
The multiple sleep latency test (MSLT) is a daytime study used to objectively measure sleepiness. It is often used to aid in the diagnosis of narcolepsy or hypersomnia. It is a set of four to five scheduled naps that typically occur the day after an overnight sleep study. Often 2 weeks of actigraphy are done before the MSLT to determine sleep-wake patterns.

Common Pediatric Sleep Diagnoses and Treatment
Obstructive Sleep Apnea
Epidemiology
Up to one-fifth of children can have intermittent snoring. Prevalence rates of OSA range from 1.2% to 5.7%. OSA is most common in children 2 to 8 years of age corresponding to the peak age of adenotonsillar hypertrophy. Due to the rise in childhood obesity there is now a corresponding rise in older children diagnosed with OSA.

Pathophysiology
The pharynx has many roles, including swallowing, speaking, and maintaining airway patency. Pharyngeal size is determined by the bones and soft tissue. The soft tissue is affected by the size of the tonsils and adenoids, as well as adipose tissue. Airway patency is maintained during wakefulness; a small airway can become vulnerable during sleep resulting in partial or total closure of the airway, hypoxemia, hypercapnia, and an arousal that results in opening of the airway and termination of the obstructive event. This leads to sleep disruption and daytime consequences. OSA in children likely results from a combination of narrowing of the upper airway, abnormal upper airway tone, and genetic factors.

Clinical Manifestation
OSA in adults is typically associated with daytime sleepiness. Associations have been made with hypertension, stroke, and metabolic syndrome. In children, OSA may not present with daytime

---

TABLE 3	Principles of Sleep Hygiene in Children

The child's bedroom should be dark and quiet.
Bedtime routines should be strictly enforced. Routines should be relaxing and only 20 to 30 minutes in length.
The time of morning awakening should be firmly and consistently structured.
Bedroom temperatures should be kept comfortably cool (< 75 °F).
Environmental noise should be minimized as much as possible. Background music and/or white noise may inhibit extraneous noise.
Children should not go to bed hungry and may have a snack before bedtime.
Excessive fluids before bedtime may result in bladder distention and arousal and disrupt sleep.
Children should learn to fall asleep alone (i.e., without their parents' presence in the room).
Vigorous activity should be avoided before bedtime.
A bath is often a stimulating activity for children. If bedtime struggles are present after a child's bath, it may be moved to the morning or separated from the child's bedtime by at least 2 hours.
Methylxanthine-containing beverages and food (e.g., caffeinated beverages/colas, tea, chocolate) should be avoided several hours before bedtime.
Parents should read labels on all over-the-counter and prescription medications. Some may contain alcohol or caffeine and may disrupt sleep.
Naps should be developmentally appropriate. Brief naps may be refreshing, but prolonged naps or napping too frequently may result in significant accumulation of sleep during the day and make it more difficult to fall asleep at night.

Modified from Sheldon SH, Ferber R, Kryger M (eds): Principles and Practice of Pediatric Sleep Medicine. Philadelphia: Elsevier Saunders, 2005.

---

sleepiness. Children may present with daytime inattention and/or neurocognitive and behavioral issues. Symptoms include snoring with or without apneic pauses or gasps. Restless sleep or secondary enuresis may also be noted. Parents may comment on increased work of breathing while sleeping. Other associations include poor growth, obesity, hypertension, and systemic inflammation.

Diagnosis
The gold standard for diagnosis of pediatric OSA is an in-laboratory attended PSG by an accredited sleep laboratory. History and physical examination lack sensitivity and specificity in predicting which children with snoring have OSA. However, a history of loud snoring, tonsillar hypertrophy, and abnormal oximetry is strongly suggestive of the diagnosis of OSA (see above). History alone cannot distinguish children with OSA from those with primary snoring. Criteria for the diagnosis of OSA in children are met when there is one or more apnea or hypopnea events per hour identified using scoring criteria by the AASM.

Differential Diagnosis
Other forms of sleep-disordered breathing are not as common as OSA. Sleep-related hypoventilation can occur in patients with neuromuscular weakness. Central hypoventilation syndromes are rare, but should be considered in children with persistent gas exchange abnormalities without additional explanation. Sleep-related hypoxemia can be present in pediatric patients with chronic lung disease. Central sleep apnea should be thought of in patients with brainstem abnormalities or Arnold-Chiari malformation. Sleep-related seizures may be difficult to differentiate from OSA in infants and an extended EEG montage may be necessary during their sleep study. Normal breathing patterns of infants and children should also be identified; brief (less than 10 seconds), central respiratory pauses that are self-resolving (and without significant desaturation) are common in normal children in either REM sleep or post-arousal/post-sigh.

Treatment
Treatment of OSA in most children is adenotonsillectomy. Recent guidelines from the AAP recommend an overnight sleep study in children where the practitioner had a clinical suspicion of OSA before adenotonsillectomy. Children with mild OSA preoperative can be monitored clinically postoperatively. Children with moderate to severe OSA, as well as children with craniofacial abnormalities, neurologic disorders, and obesity, should have a follow-up PSG to demonstrate resolution of OSA after surgery. Children who are not candidates for adenotonsillectomy may be treated with CPAP and use may have an impact on neurobehavioral outcomes. Treatment with CPAP therapy in children requires close follow-up because pressure needs may change with growth.

Difficulty with Sleep Initiation and Night Wakings
Epidemiology
Bedtime problems and night wakings occur in up to 30% of children.

Clinical Manifestations
The diagnosis of insomnia includes difficulty going to sleep and/or staying asleep, the complaint that sleep is not of good quality, and the report of poor daytime functioning. The sleep complaints of infants and young children are often in the words of their parent or caregiver.

In preschool-age children both bedtime problems and night wakings are common and characterized by two types of behavioral insomnia of childhood: sleep-onset association type and limit-setting type. The definition of the *sleep-onset association type*, as defined in the ICSD-3, includes the following: sleep initiation is an extended process, associations are demanding, if the associations are not present sleep onset is delayed, and awakenings require caregiver intervention. The *limit-setting type* involves difficulty initiating or maintaining sleep, there is bedtime stalling or refusal, and the caregiver does not set sufficient and appropriate limits around this behavior. Children with frequent and prolonged night wakings have the sleep-onset association type. They often require an intervention by the caretaker to reinitiate sleep. Both problems can be present at once. Children who have difficulty going to sleep and provide resistance to bedtime have the limit-setting type. Parents of these children may complain of daytime behavioral issues due to the parent's inability to set limits during the day as well.

Diagnosis
Diagnosis is made from the history in the majority of cases. An overnight sleep study may be indicated in cases where another sleep disorder is suspected.

Differential Diagnosis
The differential diagnosis of insomnia or behavioral insomnia of childhood includes sleep disorders such as OSA, RLS, or nocturnal seizures. These disorders can prompt nocturnal awakenings or make sleep initiation difficult. If there is clinical suspicion of one of these disorders, an overnight sleep study may be indicated.

Treatment
Behavioral interventions have been shown to be effective in treating all forms of insomnia. In older children, primary and secondary insomnia can be effectively treated with cognitive-behavioral therapy. This often includes stimulus control and sleep restriction. Stimulus control includes maintaining a regular sleep-wake pattern and using the bed and bedroom only for sleeping. It involves getting out of bed if sleep is not initiated within about 20 minutes. Sleep restriction includes minimizing the time in bed to be only sleeping. It often includes delaying bedtime to the child's actual sleep onset, and then over time gradually advancing the bedtime. Sleep hygiene should be effectively addressed, including development of a relaxing bedtime routine, maintaining a regular sleep-wake pattern, and eliminating electronic use before bedtime.

There are several treatments of behavioral insomnia of childhood sleep-onset association type. No one treatment has been found to be superior. The goal of all of these methods is for the child to fall asleep in his or her crib or bed on the child's own. These include extinction (i.e., "cry it out"), which is often not palatable to caregivers. There is the graduated extinction method, which has parents ignoring crying or protests for specified periods of increasingly longer intervals. Some prefer an even more gradual approach of sitting next to the child's bed in a chair and over several days to weeks moving that chair across the room and out of the room. A consistent bedtime routine should also be implemented. Use of a transitional object can be helpful. Treatment of the limit-setting type includes firm limit setting. Positive reinforcement and limiting negative reinforcement should be used. The use of a reward system can be helpful. Effectively addressing behavioral treatment of sleep issues can be challenging for the primary care provider because of time constraints.

Restless Legs Syndrome/Willis Ekbom Disease
Epidemiology
Prevalence rates for pediatric RLS/WED have ranged from 1% to 6%.

Risk Factors
Risk factors include a family history and a history of anemia or iron deficiency. Attention-deficit/hyperactivity disorder (ADHD) is associated with RLS.

Pathophysiology
Decreased dopamine has been suggested in the pathophysiology of RLS/WED. Iron is a cofactor in the synthesis of dopamine

and treatment of iron deficiency or low ferritin, if present, may improve symptoms.

Diagnosis
Diagnosis of pediatric RLS/WED is a clinical diagnosis. It is made using the adult criteria set forth in the ICSD-3 but with some modification for children due to developmental issues. It consists of the child reporting an urge to move the legs, usually accompanied by an uncomfortable sensation; this urge or sensation worsens during rest or inactivity; the sensations are improved or resolved by movement; the sensations are present or worsen in the evening or night. If a child cannot express a description in his or her own words, diagnosis can be made using two out of the following three criteria: a sleep disturbance for age, a family history of RLS, and a periodic limb movement index on PSG of > 5 per hour. Because of this last criterion, a sleep study can be helpful in children to make this diagnosis. There can be an association with sleep initiation and maintenance difficulties.

Differential Diagnosis
Differential diagnosis of RLS should include insomnia, sleep-disordered breathing, or neurologic or musculoskeletal etiologies for the discomfort.

Treatment
Nonpharmacologic treatment of RLS includes good sleep hygiene, moderate exercise a few hours before bedtime, and avoidance of substances that are associated with worsening of RLS symptoms, including caffeine, alcohol, antihistamines, and antiemetics. A serum ferritin should be drawn in all children with RLS and if < 50 ng/mL, treatment with 6 mg/kg/day of oral elemental iron should be considered. Oral iron absorption is enhanced by vitamin C and impaired by calcium. Gastrointestinal upset and constipation can be common side effects. Compliance can be difficult. A serum ferritin should be rechecked at 3 months to evaluate therapy. Referral to a sleep medicine specialist should be made if lifestyle and oral iron therapy have been unsuccessful. There are no FDA-approved medications for the treatment of RLS in children. Dopamine agonists, gabapentin (Neurontin),[1] clonazepam (Klonopin)[1], and clonidine (Catapres)[1] have been used to treat pediatric RLS.

Delayed Sleep Phase Syndrome
Epidemiology
Delayed sleep phase syndrome (DSPS) occurs most commonly in adolescents and young adults.

Clinical Manifestations
Symptoms usually present in adolescents but can occur in younger children. Adolescents with DSPS consistently have sleep onset at a later time, typically after midnight. They have difficulty initiating sleep earlier. They do not have difficulty maintaining sleep. They have difficulty waking in the morning unless able to sleep until their preferred time, which is typically after 10 AM. They may have sleepiness during the daytime if forced to rise early (i.e., for school); however, during long vacations or summer breaks when allowed to sleep to preferred wake time they feel refreshed. Children who already have a preferred evening preference may find this exacerbated in adolescence. Poor school performance can be present.

Diagnosis
Diagnosis is made from history; actigraphy and sleep logs are also useful. An overnight sleep study may be indicated if another sleep disorder is suspected (e.g., OSA).

Differential Diagnosis
The differential diagnosis includes insomnia, poor sleep hygiene, insufficient sleep, mood disorder, OSA, and RLS.

---

[1] Not FDA approved for this indication.

Treatment

Treatment is typically behavioral and includes good sleep hygiene. Typically either the patient's sleep-wake schedule is advanced (if there is less than 3 hours between actual and desired bedtime) by 15 minutes every 2 to 3 days until the goal bedtime is achieved. Rise time is advanced as well and if set at the desired wake time initially it should facilitate the advancement of the bedtime by increasing sleep drive. If the desired bedtime of the adolescent is greater than 3 hours from the current bedtime, phase delay can be considered. Bedtime is delayed by 2 to 3 hours each day until the target bedtime is reached. Timing of this therapy should be considered, because it will interfere with school or other daytime activities. Parental or caregiver support is necessary, as well as commitment by the adolescent.

Once the new pattern is established weekends must not differ from weekdays by more than 1 to 2 hours. This is particularly important for the rise time. Relapse is common if strict sleep-wake patterns are not adhered to, a problem common on vacations.

Both bright light exposure and melatonin have been used to help reset the circadian rhythm. Exposure to bright light in the morning is encouraged and can be as simple as increasing sun exposure in the morning. Light boxes using 2500 to 10,000 lux can be used in the morning for 20 to 30 minutes. Exposure to light in the evening should be limited. A small dose of melatonin[7] (0.5 mg) can be used in the early evening (about 5 hours before desired bedtime) to attempt to physiologically advance sleep onset. If the timing is not optimal for both light and melatonin, the phase delay can be worsened; consultation with a sleep physician should be considered.

Parasomnias

Parasomnias can occur out of both non-REM (NREM) and REM sleep. Those occurring out of NREM sleep include sleepwalking, sleep terrors, and confusional arousals. They typically occur in the first one-third of the night, when NREM-3 sleep is most prevalent, and are not recalled the next day. They can be part of normal development, but depending on their nature, they can be distressing to caregiver and child. Parasomnias occurring out of REM sleep include nightmares and REM-sleep behavior disorder (RBD). Nightmares are commonly recalled and have been associated with anxiety in children. Nightmares typically peak in the school-age child. RBD is rare in children but has been reported; it involves the loss of atonia that occurs in REM sleep and consequently dreams are "acted out."

Risk Factors

Poor sleep hygiene, insufficient sleep, irregular sleep-wake patterns, and a positive family history are all risk factors. Sleep disruption from sleep-disordered breathing or periodic limb movements of sleep can exacerbate parasomnias.

Differential Diagnosis

The differential diagnosis should include nocturnal seizures. In addition, if another sleep disorder is present, parasomnias can be exacerbated.

Treatment

Safety is most important in children with parasomnias, and it is important that the child's sleep environment is kept clear of things that could cause injury. Door alarms can be effective. The child should not be awakened during the episode. The event should not be referred to the next morning because this can cause distress for the child. Maintaining good sleep hygiene and regular sleep-wake patterns is important. If the events occur at a predictable time each night, the caregiver can do planned awakenings 30 minutes before the event typically occurs for several weeks. This may abolish the episodes. It can also have the effect of pushing the episode to later in the night. Pharmacologic treatment with a small dose of a benzodiazepine (e.g., 0.5 mg of clonazepam [Klonopin][1] at bedtime) may be indicated in severe cases with the drug tapered slowly after episodes are suppressed.

Hypersomnias

A full discussion of primary hypersomnias (including narcolepsy) in children is beyond the scope of this chapter. Consideration for a primary hypersomnia should be made in a child who is sleepy after common causes of sleepiness such as insufficient sleep and obstructive sleep apnea have been ruled out. Symptoms of narcolepsy include disrupted nocturnal sleep, hallucinations on going to sleep or waking up, and sleep paralysis. Daytime sleepiness is present with "sleep attacks" both during quiet activities and while active. Cataplexy may also be present and is defined by loss of muscle tone without loss of consciousness. It should be noted that onset of narcolepsy is often in adolescence or as a young adult. Diagnosis is often delayed because the symptoms are attributed to other conditions. Treatment of pediatric hypersomnia is done under the supervision of a sleep specialist and often involves use of stimulants.

---

[1]Not FDA approved for this indication.

References

Aurora RN, Lamm CI, Zak RS, et al: Practice parameters for the non-respiratory indications for polysomnography and multiple sleep latency testing for children, *Sleep* 35:1467–1473, 2012.

Aurora RN, Zak RS, Karippot A, et al: Practice parameters for the respiratory indications for polysomnography in children, *Sleep* 34:379–388, 2011.

Berry RB, Brooks R, Gamaldo C, et al: *The AASM Manual for the Scoring of Sleep and Associated Events*, Westchester, Illinois, 2012, American Academy of Sleep Medicine.

Brouillette RT, Morielli A, Leimanis A, et al: Nocturnal pulse oximetry as an abbreviated testing modality for pediatric obstructive sleep apnea, *Pediatrics* 105:405–412, 2000.

Kaditis A, Kheirandish-Gozal L, Gozal D: Algorithm for the diagnosis and treatment of pediatric OSA: a proposal of two pediatric sleep centers, *Sleep Med* 13:217–227, 2012.

Kirk V, Baughn J, D'Andrea L, et al: American Academy of Sleep Medicine Position Paper for the Use of a Home Sleep Apnea Test for the Diagnosis of OSA in Children, *J Clin Sleep Med* 13(10):1099–1203.

Kotagal S, Nichols CD, Grigg-Damberger MM, et al: Non-respiratory indications for polysomnography and related procedures in children: an evidence-based review, *Sleep* 35:1451–1466, 2012.

Lloyd R, Tippmann-Peikert M, Slocumb N, et al: Characteristics of REM sleep behavior disorder in childhood, *J Clin Sleep Med* 8:127–131, 2012.

Marcus CL, Brooks LJ, Draper KA, et al: Diagnosis and management of childhood obstructive sleep apnea syndrome, *Pediatrics* 130:576–584, 2012a.

Marcus CL, Brooks LJ, Draper KA, et al: Diagnosis and management of childhood obstructive sleep apnea syndrome, *Pediatrics* 130:e714–e755, 2012b.

Marcus CL, Radcliffe J, Konstantinopoulou S, et al: Effects of positive airway pressure therapy on neurobehavioral outcomes in children with obstructive sleep apnea, *Am J Respir Crit Care Med* 185:998–1003, 2012.

Mindell JA, Barrett KM: Nightmares and anxiety in elementary-aged children: is there a relationship? *Child Care Health Dev* 28:317–322, 2002.

Mindell JA, Owens J: *A clinical guide to pediatric sleep: diagnosis and management of sleep problems*, Philadelphia, 2003, Lippincott Williams & Wilkins.

Mindell JA, Owens J: *A clinical guide to pediatric sleep: diagnosis and management of sleep problems*, ed 2, Philadelphia, 2010, Lippincott Williams & Wilkins.

Morgenthaler T, Alessi C, Friedman L, et al: Practice parameters for the use of actigraphy in the assessment of sleep and sleep disorders: an update for 2007, *Sleep* 30:519–529, 2007.

Morgenthaler T, Kramer M, Alessi C, et al: Practice parameters for the psychological and behavioral treatment of insomnia: an update. An American Academy of Sleep Medicine report, *Sleep* 29:1415–1419, 2006.

Owens JA, Dalzell V: Use of the "BEARS" sleep screening tool in a pediatric residents' continuity clinic: a pilot study, *Sleep Med* 6:63–69, 2005.

Paruthi S, Brooks LJ, D'Ambrosio C, et al: Consensus Statement of the American Academy of Sleep Medicine on the Recommended Amount of Sleep for Healthy Children: Methodology and Discussion, *J Clin Sleep Med* 12(11):1549–1561, 2016.

Picchietti D, Allen RP, Walters AS, et al: Restless legs syndrome: prevalence and impact in children and adolescents—the Peds REST study, *Pediatrics* 120:253–266, 2007.

Sateia MJ, editor: *The International Classification of Sleep Disorders*, 3rd ed, Westchester, Illinois, 2014, American Academy of Sleep Medicine.

Sheldon SH, Ferber R, Kryger M, editors: *Principles and Practice of Pediatric Sleep Medicine*, Philadelphia, 2005, Elsevier Saunders.

St Louis EK, Morgenthaler TI: Sleep disorders. In Bope E, Kellerman R, editors: *Conn's Current Therapy 2013*, Philadelphia, 2013, Saunders Elsevier.

---

[7]Available as dietary supplement.

RESUSCITATION OF THE NEWBORN

Method of
Stacey A. Hinderliter, MD; and David S. Gregory, MD

CURRENT DIAGNOSIS

- The transition from intrauterine to extrauterine life at birth requires effective breathing by the infant to expand the lungs and oxygenate the blood. All newborn infants are at risk for delays in this process, prompting a need for resuscitation.
- The fetal and newborn response to hypoxia is to develop apnea. If primary apnea is diagnosed, it can be corrected by gentle stimulation and oxygen delivery. If hypoxia persists, secondary apnea will occur. It is not readily apparent whether a newborn has primary or secondary apnea, and the approach to resuscitation therefore requires that any apneic event be treated using the same sequence of interventions.
- The initial steps of newborn resuscitation include drying the infant, providing warmth, suctioning the airway, and providing gentle stimulation. Infants who do not respond to these interventions need more assistance. Establishment of effective ventilation spontaneously by the newborn or with assistance by positive-pressure ventilation is the most important step in newborn resuscitation.
- Reassessment of the infant's heart rate, respiratory effort, pulse oximeter reading or color, and tone every 30 seconds during resuscitation is crucial to determine the next appropriate intervention. Apgar scoring should *not* be used to guide newborn resuscitation. Pulse oximetry in the delivery room should be used to guide oxygen therapy. Temperature of the infant should be monitored.
- If application of positive-pressure ventilation does not improve the infant's heart rate, chest compressions or drug therapy, or both, may be required. A team approach is needed to coordinate these interventions, and ongoing reassessment is necessary to determine cardiorespiratory and hemodynamic status. Subsequent assessment and treatment should be performed in an intensive care setting.

CURRENT THERAPY

- Term gestation infants who are breathing and crying with good muscle tone do not need newborn resuscitation.
- Initial resuscitation includes drying the infant, providing warmth, suctioning the mouth and nose, and giving gentle stimulation.
- If the infant is breathing vigorously but has central cyanosis, oxygen should be administered. Pulse oximetry should be used to guide oxygen therapy.
- If the infant is apneic, breathing slowly, or gasping, positive-pressure ventilation (PPV) with a mask and bag should be administered.
- If the infant's heart rate drops below 60 beats/min, chest compressions should be initiated using the two-thumb technique.
- If the heart rate remains less than 60 beats/min despite PPV and chest compressions, IV epinephrine (Adrenalin) should be given using an umbilical venous catheter.
- Reassessment of the newborn every 30 seconds during resuscitation is required to adjust therapy as indicated. The best indicator of successful resuscitation is an increase in heart rate.

The changes that occur in the transition from fetus to newborn are unmatched in any other time of life. Most newborns manage to make this transition on their own, but about 10% require some assistance. Approximately 1% of newborns require extensive resuscitative measures to survive. The approach to resuscitation in infants is similar to that in adults, consisting of evaluation and intervention when needed for the infant's airway, breathing, and circulation. Every birth should be attended by personnel trained in neonatal resuscitation. Specific training and certification are offered by the American Academy of Pedatrics/American Heart Association's Neonatal Resuscitation Provider (NRP) course. This chapter has been updated based on the NRP 7th edition.

Transition from Fetal to Extrauterine Life

The environment of the fetus differs greatly from that of the infant after birth. The fetus depends on receiving oxygen and nutrients from the mother through the placental circulation. The fetus experiences relative hypoxia and almost constant body temperature in the amniotic fluid. The fetal lungs are filled with fluid and do not participate in the exchange of oxygen and carbon dioxide. Several adaptations in the fetus permit survival in this environment.

Oxygenated blood from the mother enters the fetus by means of the placenta through the umbilical vein. Most of this oxygenated blood bypasses the liver through the ductus venosus and enters the inferior vena cava. On entering the right atrium, this oxygenated blood is directed toward the patent foramen ovale into the left atrium, bypassing the fetal lungs. Fetal blood also passes through the right atrium into the right ventricle and then into the pulmonary artery. The vascular resistance and blood pressure of the pulmonary vessels in the fetal lung are higher than in the aorta and systemic circulation; most of the blood is therefore shunted away from the lungs through the ductus arteriosus into the ascending aorta. Only a small amount of fetal blood passes through the lungs to the left atrium and then to the left ventricle. The umbilical arteries branch off from the internal iliac arteries and return fetal blood to the placenta. The functional organ for gas exchange of oxygen and carbon dioxide in the fetus is the placenta.

At birth, the newborn is no longer connected to the placenta, and the lungs become the only source of oxygen. The first breaths of the infant cause the fluid in the lung alveoli to be replaced with air. The umbilical arteries and veins constrict at birth and are eventually clamped. This increases the vascular resistance and blood pressure of the systemic circulation. As the oxygen level in the alveoli increases, the blood vessels in the lung start to relax, decreasing pulmonary vascular resistance. Blood in the pulmonary artery travels toward the lung and away from the ductus arteriosus because the blood pressure in the systemic circulation is higher than that in the pulmonary circulation. Increased blood flow to the lungs allows the oxygen from the alveoli to enter the infant's blood, increasing the P_{O_2}. Oxygenated blood enters the left heart through the pulmonary vein and is delivered to the rest of the infant's tissues through the aorta.

Although the initial steps in this transition occur within a few minutes of birth, the entire process may not be completed for several hours to days. The ductus venosus, foramen ovale, and ductus arteriosus remain potentially patent and do not completely involute for days or weeks. Changes in the infant's systemic and pulmonary pressures can result in blood flow through these channels in the infant.

Transition can be prevented or delayed in several circumstances. The infant may not breathe adequately, in which case the lung fluid is not forced out of the alveoli. Material such as meconium may block air from entering the alveoli. If the lungs do not fill with air, hypoxia will quickly develop. Systemic hypotension due to excessive blood loss, poor cardiac function, or bradycardia prevents the change in the direction of blood flow that is necessary to promote blood flow into the lungs. Failure of the lungs to expand or hypoxia can prevent relaxation of the pulmonary blood vessels, resulting in a high pulmonary vascular resistance. This leads to decreased blood flow to the lungs and worsening of hypoxia.

Risk Factors for Newborn Resuscitation

A number of prenatal and intrapartum factors are associated with a higher chance that the infant will have a delay in transition and require resuscitation (Table 1). However, some infants *with no risk factors* need resuscitation; therefore, preparations for neonatal resuscitation should be made during all deliveries.

Reaction to Hypoxia and Asphyxia

Normally at birth, the newborn makes vigorous efforts to breathe. The process of leaving the warm, dark, and liquid environment in utero is replaced by cold air, dryness, and bright lights. Drying the infant with towels and wiping the mouth and nose are all the assistance that most newborns require. The end result of any mechanism that delays transition is a period of hypoxia for the fetus or newborn infant. Laboratory studies have shown that the first sign of oxygen deprivation in the newborn is a change in the breathing pattern. After an initial period of rapid breathing attempts, cessation of breathing occurs. This is called *primary apnea*. Stimulation by drying the infant or slapping the feet can cause breathing to resume. If hypoxia continues after primary apnea has occurred, the infant will make attempts at gasping and then stop breathing. This is called *secondary apnea*. Stimulation does not affect secondary apnea. Assisted ventilation is necessary to provide breaths to the newborn to reverse the hypoxia. The infant's heart rate starts to decrease when primary apnea occurs. The heart rate increases with stimulation if the infant has primary apnea, and blood pressure is maintained. With continued hypoxia, the heart rate continues to drop, and hypotension develops. If assisted ventilation is not adequate to increase the infant's heart rate, chest compressions will be required.

When a newborn becomes apneic, it is not readily apparent whether the infant has primary or secondary apnea. The approach to resuscitation therefore requires that any apneic event in a newborn be treated using the same sequence of interventions. If the apneic infant responds to simple stimulation, the diagnosis is primary apnea, and no further intervention is required. If the infant does not improve with stimulation, secondary apnea has occurred, and more intensive intervention is needed.

Sequence of Newborn Resuscitation
Initial Steps and Basic Resuscitation

Resuscitation of the newborn starts the rapid assessment of three characteristics: Is the infant at term gestation, does the infant have good tone, and is the infant crying and breathing? The answers to these questions will affect the approach to care. Resuscitation when fluid is meconium stained is discussed later in this chapter. The information presented here refers to term infants with clear amniotic fluid. More information regarding the care of premature infants is discussed in a later section.

The infant at term who is crying and breathing with good muscle tone does not need resuscitation and should not be separated from the mother. Current evidence suggests cord clamping should be delayed for at least 30–60 seconds for most vigorous term and preterm infants unless there is evidence of placental abruption or bleeding. The baby should be dried, placed skin-to-skin with the mother, and covered with dry linen to maintain temperature. Ongoing observation for breathing, activity, and color should continue while the infant is with the mother. If the infant is not term, is not crying and breathing, or does not have good muscle tone, newborn resuscitation should begin with the initial steps: providing warmth, positioning and clearing (if needed) the airway, drying and stimulating the infant.

The newborn should be placed under a radiant warmer to prevent heat loss and to allow easy observation. Although warm blankets or towels can be used to dry the infant, they should not be left in place to cover the infant. The newborn should be placed on the back with the neck slightly extended in the "sniffing" position (Figure 1). This facilitates air entry into the lungs by lining up the posterior pharynx, larynx, and trachea. Hyperextension or hyperflexion of the neck can obstruct air entry into the lungs.

If the newborn is crying vigorously, secretions can be removed by wiping the nose and the mouth with a towel. Routine suctioning should be avoided. Gentle suctioning of the mouth and nose with a bulb syringe or suction catheter is *only* indicated when there is obvious obstruction to spontaneous breathing or when there is a need for positive-pressure ventilation. Deep or vigorous suctioning can be detrimental to the infant because of stimulation of the vagus nerve, causing bradycardia or apnea. The mouth should be suctioned before the nose to prevent aspiration if the infant gasps during suctioning.

TABLE 1	Risk Factors for Newborn Resuscitation
PRENATAL FACTORS	**INTRAPARTUM FACTORS**
Maternal	Placental
Diabetes, preexisting	Placenta previa
Chronic hypertension	Abruption of the placenta
Infection	Premature or prolonged rupture of
Cardiac, renal, pulmonary,	membranes
thyroid, or neurologic	Chorioamnionitis
disease	Fetal
Drug therapy	Macrosomia
Substance use	Low birth weight
Lack of prenatal care	Breech or other abnormal
Age <16 or >35 years	presentation
Previous fetal or neonatal	Persistent fetal bradycardia
death	Non-reassuring fetal heart rate
Pregnancy	patterns
Bleeding in second or third	Labor
trimester	Premature labor
Pregnancy-induced	Precipitous labor
hypertension	Prolonged labor (>24 h)
Toxemia	Prolonged second stage of labor
Gestational diabetes	(>2 h)
Fetal anemia or	Prolapsed cord
isoimmunization	Emergency cesarean section
Polyhydramnios	Forceps or vacuum-assisted
Oligohydramnios	delivery
Fetal hydrops	Other
Postterm gestation	Meconium-stained amniotic fluid
Multiple gestation	General anesthesia
Size-date discrepancy	Narcotics given within 4 h of
Diminished fetal activity	delivery
Fetal malformation or	Uterine hyperstimulation
abnormality	Severe intrapartum bleeding

Figure 1 The sniffing position. Positioning the infant on the back with the neck slightly extended brings the posterior pharynx, larynx, and trachea in line (*white line*) to facilitate air entry into the lungs.

Drying the infant, slapping the feet, and rubbing the back are appropriate forms of stimulation. More forceful methods of stimulation can harm the infant. Primary apnea, if present, will respond to stimulation in less than 30 seconds. Prolonged apnea will require positive-pressure ventilation (PPV).

Evaluating the infant's response to resuscitation is essential. The Apgar score is a traditional method for evaluating newborn status at 1 and 5 minutes after delivery. However, effective resuscitation demands that evaluation of the newborn's status not be delayed until 1 minute of age, and Apgar scores therefore should *not* be used to guide resuscitative efforts. Within 30 seconds of delivery, the infant's need for PPV must be assessed. Establishment of effective ventilation spontaneously by the newborn or with assistance by PPV is the most important step in newborn resuscitation. The respiratory status, heart rate, and color or oximetry reading should be determined. The chest wall should move with each breath, and the newborn should be breathing spontaneously. Although heart rate can be assessed by feeling for a pulse at the base of the umbilical cord, this method can be unreliable. Auscultation with a stethoscope is the preferred method during initial resuscitation. The heart rate should be greater than 100 beats/min. Peripheral cyanosis (i.e., blueness of the hands and feet) is acceptable in the initial period after delivery. Central cyanosis in which the lips and trunk are blue indicates hypoxemia and the need for more resuscitation efforts. A pulse oximeter can provide continuous assessment of the oxygen saturation and is the optimal method for monitoring the infant's state of oxygenation. Pulse oximetry often displays lower heart rate readings during the first 2 minutes of life. Placement of 3-lead ECG as soon as possible to monitor the infant's heart rate during resuscitation may be beneficial. The initial steps of stabilization, reassessment, and establishing ventilation should be completed within the first minute of life (the "Golden Minute"). The oximeter probe should be placed on the newborn's right wrist or hand to detect preductal saturation. A pulse oximeter should be used to confirm the perception of central cyanosis. Temperature should be monitored during newborn resuscitation. The normal range is an axillary temperature of 36.5–37.5°C.

Respiratory Support and Positive-Pressure Ventilation

If the infant is breathing with a heart rate higher than 100 beats/min but has central cyanosis, free-flowing oxygen delivery is indicated. This can be administered with a facemask or by holding oxygen tubing or a flow-inflating bag and mask close to the infant's face. *A self-inflating bag and mask cannot be used to give free-flowing oxygen.* If the newborn is apneic, not breathing effectively, or has a heart rate less than 100 beats/min, PPV using a self-inflating bag, flow-inflating (or anesthesia) bag, or a T-piece resuscitator is required. Use of a flow-inflating bag requires a compressed gas source and considerable practice to be used effectively. A T-piece resuscitator needs special equipment and a compressed gas source. Most delivery rooms are equipped with self-inflating bags (Figure 2) because they are easy to use and can be fitted with a pressure-release valve to decrease overinflation. A reservoir must be used with a self-inflating bag to provide 100% oxygen.

Positive pressure ventilation (PPV) should begin using room air for term newborns. The facemask should cover the infant's nose, mouth, and tip of chin, but not the eyes (Figure 3). Multiple sizes should be available. A tight seal between the infant's skin and the facemask is needed, but excessive pressure can bruise the face. The mask can be held in place using the thumb and index finger in a C-shaped position on top of the mask, with the remaining fingers in an E-shaped position below the infant's chin (Figure 4). Inspiratory pressures of 20 to 25 cm H_2O are usually needed when squeezing the bag to make the infant's chest rise. A pressure gauge can be connected to the self-inflating bag for monitoring inspiratory pressure. The heart rate and color of the infant should rapidly improve if enough pressure is being given. An assistant can also use a stethoscope to listen to breath sounds for air movement. Breaths should be given at a rate of 40 to 60 breaths/min.

Traditionally, 100% oxygen has been used in newborn resuscitation. However, several randomized, controlled studies enrolling term and near-term infants have shown that room air can be used initially with oxygen as a backup if room air fails. A meta-analysis of these trials showed a benefit for the use of room air. Providing oxygen at concentrations between room air and 100% requires the use of compressed air, oxygen, and blenders by experienced personnel. A pulse oximeter with a probe designed for use in newborns can be used to guide oxygen administration during newborn resuscitation. It will take 1 to 2 minutes to apply the pulse oximeter probe to the infant's right palm or wrist (preductal site) and get a consistent reading. The pulse oximeter may not

Figure 2 Self-inflating bag with infant mask and reservoir. This type of device is available in most delivery rooms.

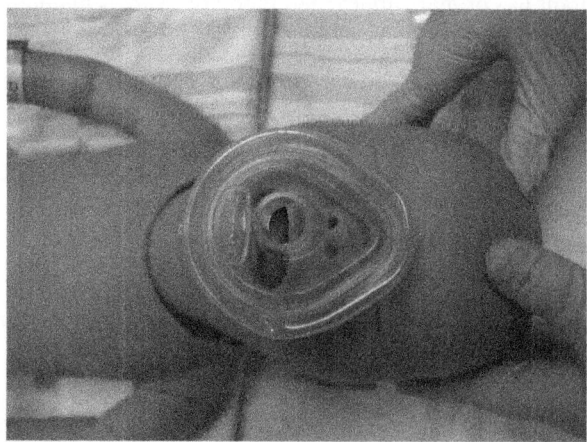

Figure 3 Facemask. Choose a size that covers the infant's mouth and nose.

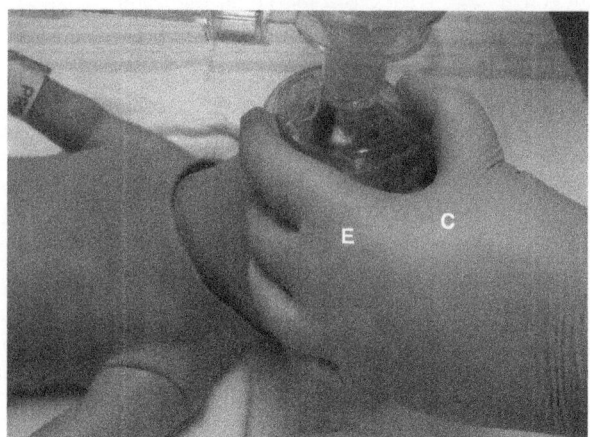

Figure 4 Facemask placement. The thumb and index finger are held in a C-shaped position on top of the mask, and the remaining fingers are held in an E-type position under the chin.

TABLE 2	Titrated Oxygen Saturations After Birth
1 minute	60-65%
2 minutes	65-70%
3 minutes	70-75%
4 minutes	75-80%
5 minutes	80-85%
10 minutes	85-95%

function during states of very poor cardiac output or perfusion. In these situations, observation for central cyanosis will be necessary. The infant's oxygen saturation may remain in the 70% to 80% range for several minutes after birth. Oxygen may be titrated to the interquartile range of preductal saturations measured in healthy babies following vaginal birth at sea level (see Table 2). If blended oxygen is not available, room air should be used for resuscitation. If the infant's heart rate does not respond to positive pressure ventilation with room air after 90 seconds, 100% oxygen should then be used.

After 30 seconds of PPV, the infant should be reevaluated. Once PPV is started, an electronic cardiac monitor is the preferred method to measure heart rate. Ventilation with a bag and mask can be stopped when the newborn has a heart rate higher than 100 beats/min, spontaneous breathing, improved color, and good muscle tone. Supplemental oxygen should still be given to the infant. If the newborn is not improving, use the acronym "MR SOPA" to correct the technique of PPV: M=mask adjustment to check seal, R=reposition head in sniffing position, S=suction mouth and nose, O=open mouth with infant's jaw lifted forward, P=increase pressure up to 30-40 cm H_2O, A=consider using an alternative airway such as endotracheal (ET) intubation.

ET intubation is a technical skill that must be learned and practiced to maintain competency. Effective ventilation can be given with a bag and mask approach to most newborns. This skill is easily mastered and maintained. If an infant is responding well to bag and mask ventilation, it can be continued for longer periods; however, some air may escape into the esophagus and into the stomach. This may cause gastric distention, which can prevent full expansion of the lungs and cause vomiting and aspiration. An orogastric tube can be placed in the stomach and left open to air to vent any air introduced into the infant's stomach during bag and mask ventilation.

Chest Compressions

Before beginning chest compressions, intubation is strongly recommended to provide effective ventilation. After 30 seconds of effective PPV, the heart rate should be assessed. If the heart rate dips below 60 beats/min, chest compressions are needed to support the circulation. The two-thumb technique (Figure 5) is recommended. The two-thumb technique generates higher blood pressure and coronary perfusion with less rescuer fatigue. It can also be continued with the rescuer at the head of the bed if access to the abdomen is needed. If chest compressions are required, 100% oxygen should be given by PPV. Two people are required to give PPV and chest compressions effectively. To coordinate the breaths and chest compressions, three compressions are given followed by one breath, and this sequence is repeated to give the infant 90 compressions and 30 breaths/min. The thumbs are placed on the lower third of the infant's sternum but above the xyphoid process. The sternum is depressed to a depth of one third of the infant's anteroposterior chest diameter. The purpose of chest compressions is to squeeze the heart between the sternum and the spine, forcing blood in and out of the heart and to the body. The direction of the compressions should be perpendicular to the chest surface, and the thumbs should not be lifted off of the chest after the correct placement is obtained. Incorrect methods during chest compressions can cause rib fracture and liver laceration.

Figure 5 Two-thumb technique. The hands encircle the torso, and the thumbs are placed on top of the lower sternum above the xyphoid process and below a line drawn between the nipples *(white line)*.

After 60 seconds of chest compressions, the infant's heart rate, breathing, pulse oximeter reading or color, and tone are reassessed. If the heart rate is higher than 60 beats/min, chest compressions can be stopped, although PPV may still be needed. If the heart rate is not improving, the following problems must be considered: ventilation is not adequate, 100% oxygen concentration is not being given, or the compressions may not be deep enough or well coordinated with the breaths. If the arrest is suspected to be of primary cardiac etiology, a compression ratio of 15 compressions to 2 breaths may be more effective.

Medications for Newborn Resuscitation

If the newborn heart rate remains below 60 beats/min despite 30 seconds of effective PPV and 60 seconds of chest compressions, epinephrine (Adrenalin) can be used to stimulate the newborn heart. Fewer than 2 of 1000 infants will require this step in resuscitation. *IV administration of epinephrine is preferred.*

A catheter can be quickly inserted into the umbilical vein for intravenous access. A 3.5 or 5 F catheter prefilled with saline and connected to a 3-way stopcock is inserted about 2 to 4 cm into the umbilical vein using sterile technique. After blood is aspirated, insertion of the catheter is stopped, and the epinephrine is given rapidly, followed by a saline flush. The concentration of epinephrine used in neonatal resuscitation is 1:10,000. The intravenous dose is 0.01 to 0.03 mg/kg (0.1 to 0.3 mL/kg) (Table 3). A dose of epinephrine may be considered through the ET tube during the umbilical vein catheterization process but there is no evidence of benefit. The ET dose of epinephrine is 0.05 to 0.1 mg/kg (0.5 to 1 mL/kg).[1] *These higher doses are for ET use only.* Because lung absorption of epinephrine varies, the intravenous route using the umbilical vein is preferred. The intraosseous route can also be used.

During umbilical vein cannulation, PPV and chest compressions are continued. More personnel will be needed to place the catheter and draw up the medications and saline flushes. After an intravenous dose of epinephrine, the infant's heart rate, respirations, color or oximeter reading, and tone are reevaluated. The heart rate should increase to more than 60 beats/min. If the heart rate does not respond, the dose of epinephrine can be repeated every 3 to 5 minutes. The effectiveness of ventilation and compressions should be reassessed. If the infant appears pale, has delayed capillary refill, or decreased pulses, shock may be present. Infant blood loss might have occurred during delivery from placental problems or other sources. Administration of an isotonic crystalloid solution such as normal saline or Type O negative blood at 10 mL/kg over 5 to 10 minutes can improve circulation. Ringer's lactate is no longer recommended for newborns. Volume expansion should be used cautiously because there is evidence from animal studies for poorer outcomes when it is used in the absence of hypovolemia. Rapid infusion of large volumes has been associated with intraventricular hemorrhage in premature infants.

TABLE 3 Drugs for Newborn Resuscitation

DRUG	CONCENTRATION	DOSE	INDICATIONS	COMMENTS
Epinephrine	1:10,000	0.01–0.03 mg/kg IV = 0.1–0.3 mL/kg IV route preferred 0.05–0.1 mg/kg ETT[1]	Asystole Bradycardia that does not improve with PPV and chest compressions Shock	May repeat every 3–5 min. No evidence for giving epinephrine via ETT.
Volume expanders	Normal saline O negative blood	10 mL/kg IV	Hypovolemia	Crossmatch blood to mother if possible Repeat if needed
Glucose	10% Dextrose	2–5 mL/kg IV	Hypoglycemia	Monitor glucometer or venous glucose levels

Abbreviations: ETT = endotracheal tube; IV = intravenous.
[1]Not FDA approved for this indication.

Newborns, especially premature infants, are at risk for hypoglycemia. Blood from the infant's heel or the umbilical vein can be tested at the bedside and intravenous 10% dextrose (2 to 5 mL/kg) given for low blood glucose. No specific glucose level has been associated with a poorer outcome. There is no evidence that use of sodium bicarbonate benefits the neonate, and its use during resuscitation in the delivery room is not recommended.

After resuscitation, newborns should be monitored in an intensive care setting. These infants are at risk for several complications, such as infection, metabolic abnormalities, and seizures. Infants of 36 weeks' gestation or older with moderate to severe hypoxic-ischemic encephalopathy may benefit from induced hypothermia under clearly defined protocols.

Special Considerations

Some newborns do not respond to resuscitation because of specific problems. Infants with upper airway obstruction from micrognathia can be helped by a nasopharyngeal airway and placement of the infant in the prone position. Choanal atresia can be treated by placing an oral airway. Absence of breath sounds on one side of the chest can indicate a pneumothorax, requiring needle aspiration of the chest. An infant with a scaphoid abdomen and decreased breath sounds may have a diaphragmatic hernia. These infants should be intubated, and PPV by mask and bag should not be used. If the mother has received narcotics shortly before the delivery, the narcotic may be the cause of respiratory depression in the infant. These infants need *PPV and respiratory support.* Naloxone is no longer recommended as part of initial resuscitative efforts in the delivery room. Heart rate and oxygenation should be supported by PPV.

Endotracheal Intubation

During neonatal resuscitation, endotracheal intubation may be indicated in the following circumstances: cases in which bag and mask ventilation is ineffective or prolonged, if chest compressions are performed, and in special situations such as congenital diaphragmatic hernia or extremely low birth weight infants. Intubation of the newborn requires preparation that can be performed while the infant is being ventilated by bag and mask. The ET tube should not be placed unless the glottis is visualized by direct laryngoscopy. To ensure that the tube is in the trachea, a carbon dioxide (CO_2) detector should be used. Listening for equal breath sounds and looking for vapor condensation in the ET tube during exhalation can help, but an increase in the infant's heart rate or a positive detection of CO_2 is most reliable. It should be noted that poor or absent pulmonary blood flow may result in the absence of CO_2 detection despite tube placement in the trachea. The best indicator for effective ventilation is an increase in the newborn's heart rate.

Intubation should be performed as quickly as possible, with a goal of 30 seconds from insertion of the laryngoscope to the connection of the ET tube to the resuscitation bag. Complications of intubation include worsening of hypoxia and bradycardia,

pneumothorax, contusions, perforation of the trachea or esophagus, and infection. After the infant has been intubated, deterioration in the infant's status should prompt an organized sequence to assess the adequacy of ventilation using the mnemonic DOPE: *Dislodged* (D): Is the tube in the right bronchus or out of the trachea?

Obstructed (O): Is the tube obstructed by secretions or blood?
Pneumothorax (P) and *esophagus* (E): Is the tube in the esophagus?

An alternative to intubation for infants ≥34 weeks gestation and ≥2000 grams is placement of a laryngeal mask airway. This type of airway does not require laryngoscopy. A soft inflatable mask that is attached to a flexible airway tube is placed in the hypopharynx such that the air in the tube is directed into the larynx and away from the esophagus. However, this type of airway cannot be used to suction the trachea nor to give endotracheal drugs. Its use has not been evaluated during chest compressions.

Premature Infants

Infants born before 37 weeks' gestation are at increased risk for complications and the need for resuscitation. Premature lungs may lack surfactant, making ventilation difficult. Very low birth weight (less than 1500 g) infants will need additional warming techniques such as prewarming the delivery room, covering the baby in plastic wrapping, and placing the baby under a radiant warmer and/or an exothermic mattress; however, iatrogenic hyperthermia (axillary temperature >38°C) should be avoided. Immature brain development may decrease the drive to breathe. Weak muscles make respiratory efforts less effective. Thin skin and decreased subcutaneous fat make temperature regulation a challenge. Premature infants often have infections such as pneumonia or sepsis. The blood vessels in their brains are fragile and can easily bleed during periods of blood pressure variation. The lower birth weights of premature newborns also require smaller sizes of equipment for resuscitation such as facemasks, suction catheters, endotracheal tubes, and umbilical catheters. Initial oxygen concentrations between room air and 30% should be used to protect the premature infant from oxygen toxicity. The use of continuous positive airway pressure (CPAP) in premature infants who are breathing spontaneously but with difficulty following birth may reduce the need for intubation, mechanical ventilation, and surfactant use. If PPV is needed, it is preferable to use a device that can deliver positive end expiratory pressure (PEEP). Many personnel trained in newborn resuscitation should be present at the delivery of a high-risk premature infant.

Meconium Staining of the Amniotic Fluid

Meconium is formed in the newborn gastrointestinal system during gestation. Intrauterine stress can cause release of meconium into the amniotic fluid. Aspiration of meconium-stained amniotic fluid into the lungs can result in severe pneumonitis and lung injury. The approach to resuscitation for an infant born in

TABLE 4	Equipment for Newborn Resuscitation

TYPE OF USE	EQUIPMENT
General	Sterile towels Radiant warmer or heat lamps Pulse oximeter Cardiorespiratory monitor Sterile gowns, gloves
Airway	Bulb syringe Suction catheters (5, 8, 10, 12, 14F) Suction source with manometer Oral and nasopharyngeal airways (newborn sizes) Laryngoscope and straight blades sizes 0 and 1 Endotracheal tubes (sizes 2.5, 3.0, 3.5)
Ventilation	Face masks (premature, newborn, and infant sizes) Self-inflating bag (450–750 mL) with oxygen reservoir and manometer Oxygen source Orogastric tubes (8, 10F) Carbon dioxide (CO_2) indicator Chest tubes (8 and 10F)
Circulation	Umbilical catheters (3.5 and 5F) Umbilical catheter tray (sterile scissors, scalpel, forceps, umbilical tape) Three-way stopcock Syringes (1, 3, 5, 10 mL) No 88.5679 Normal saline Epinephrine 1:10,000 10% Dextrose

TABLE 5	Important Changes in Newborn Resuscitation based on Neonatal Resuscitation Program 7th edition.

1. Delayed cord clamping of 30-60 seconds is recommended for vigorous term and preterm infants.
2. Routine intubation and tracheal suctioning is no longer recommended for nonvigorous infants born in MSAF.
3. Positive pressure ventilation of term newborns begins in room air. For preterm newborns, oxygen should be started between room air and 30%.
4. Oxygen therapy should be titrated using pulse oximeter readings of the preductal oxygen saturation on the right hand.
5. The most important indicator of effective PPV is a rising heart rate.
6. Once PPV is started, an electronic monitor should be used to assess heart rate.
7. Intubation to provide effective PPV is strongly recommended prior to starting chest compressions.
8. The preferred technique for chest compressions is the two thumb method.
9. Epinephrine should not be given until after the infant has received 30 seconds of PPV that inflates the lungs and 60 seconds of chest compressions, and the heart rate is still <60 beats/minute.
10. Ringer's lactate is no longer recommended to treat hypovolemia during newborn resuscitation.
11. Temperature should be monitored during resuscitation with a goal of axillary temperature between 36.5° and 37.5°C.

meconium stained amniotic fluid (MSAF) has been revised. There is no evidence that the consistency of meconium-stained fluid (i.e., thick or thin) has an effect on the outcome of the newborn.

Crying and Vigorous Infant

If the newborn born in MSAF has normal respiratory effort and muscle tone with a heart rate higher than 100 beats/min, *gentle* mouth and nose suctioning can be performed using a bulb syringe or suction catheter. Deep and prolonged suctioning should be avoided. ET intubation is not required for vigorous infants with meconium-stained amniotic fluid.

Nonvigorous Infant

Routine endotracheal intubation and tracheal suctioning is no longer recommended for nonvigorous newborns born in MSAF, however, the resuscitation team should include someone skilled in endotracheal intubation. If the newborn is gasping or apneic and has poor muscle tone, the initial steps of routine resuscitation should be started—provide warmth, dry the infant, position the airway, and provide gentle mouth and nose suctioning. If there is no response, PPV should be started using a bag and mask. If bag and mask ventilation is not effective, intubation should be performed. There is no evidence that suctioning the trachea of nonvigorous newborns born in MSAF prevents morbidity or mortality. It is possible that the main cause of meconium aspiration into the lungs is due to intrauterine fetal gasping.

Newborn Resuscitation Outside of the Delivery Room

Resuscitation of infants born at home, in an emergency room, in an ambulance, or otherwise outside of a delivery room setting should proceed according to the same principles as in the delivery room. Providing warmth, wiping the airway, and providing stimulation are usually adequate measures. Establishing effective ventilation using a bag and mask is the most important step if the infant fails to breathe on its own. Emergency providers should be familiar with resuscitation of the newborn, and basic equipment (Table 4) should be available.

Withholding and Withdrawing Newborn Resuscitation

Newborns should be offered resuscitation at delivery except in extreme circumstances. Newborn resuscitation should not be used if the infant has a condition that is incompatible with survival, such as a confirmed gestational age of less than 22 completed weeks, birth weight less than 400 g, or congenital anomalies associated with certain death or extreme morbidity.

In most situations, initial resuscitation can provide time to observe the infant's response to interventions and to discuss the infant's condition with the parents. Techniques for obstetric dating of pregnancies are accurate only to ±1 to 2 weeks, and estimates of fetal weight are accurate only to ±100 to 200 g. Care must be taken before deciding to withhold resuscitation from a newborn. Ongoing conversation between parents and medical caregivers allows mutual decision making. Withdrawal of care is indicated if continued support is futile. After 10 minutes of asystole (heart rate of 0), newborns are very unlikely to survive.

References

American Academy of Pediatrics Committee on Fetus and Newborn: EF Bel. Non-initiation or withdrawal of intensive care for high-risk newborns, *Pediatrics* 119:401, 2007.

American Academy of Pediatrics/American Heart Association. 2015 Guidelines for Cardiopulmonary Resuscitation and Emergent Cardiovascular Care of the Neonate. Available at http://eccguidelines.heart.org [Accessed April 2, 2016]. (Table 5).

Aschner JL, Poland RL: Sodium bicarbonate: Basically useless therapy, *Pediatrics* 122:831, 2008.

Bassam H, Mercer BM, Livingston JC, et al: Outcome after successful resuscitation of babies born with Apgar scores of 0 at both 1 and 5 minutes, *Am J Obstet Gynecol* 182:1210, 2000.

Chettri S, Adhisivam B, Bhat V: Endotracheal suction for nonvigorous neonate born through meconium stained amniotic fluid: A randomized controlled trial, *J Pediatr* 166:1208–1213, 2015.

Field DJ, Dorling JS, Manktelow BN, et al: Survival of extremely premature babies in a geographically defined population: Prospective cohort study of 1994–99 compared with 2000–05, *BMJ* 336:1221, 2008.

Halliday HL: Endotracheal intubation at birth for preventing morbidity and mortality in vigorous, meconium-stained infants born at term, *Cochrane Database Syst Rev*(1), 2001. CD000500.

Kattwinkel J, Perlman J: The neonatal resuscitation program: the evidence evaluation process and anticipating edition 6, *Neoreviews* 11, 2010. e673.

Weiner GM, Zaichkin J, Kattwinkel J, editors: *Textbook of Neonatal Resuscitation*, 7th ed., Elk Grove Village, IL, 2016, American Academy of Pediatrics and American Heart Association.

Wiswell TE, Gannon CM, Jacob J, et al: Delivery room management of the apparently vigorous meconium-stained neonate: Results of the multicenter, international collaborative trial, *Pediatrics* 105:1, 2000.

URINARY TRACT INFECTIONS IN INFANTS AND CHILDREN

Method of
Ellen R. Wald, MD

The urinary tract is the most common site for serious bacterial infections in infants and young children. Urinary tract infections (UTIs) are more common than bacterial meningitis, bacterial pneumonia, and bacteremia.

Infection of the urinary tract may involve only the bladder, or only the kidney, or both. In general, infections of the bladder (cystitis), while causing substantial morbidity, are not regarded as serious bacterial infections. In contrast, infections that involve the kidney (pyelonephritis) can cause acute morbidity and lead to scarring with rare consequences of hypertension, preeclampsia, and chronic renal disease.

Diagnosis

The diagnosis of UTI may be suggested by certain signs and symptoms, but culture of the urine is the gold standard. Because culture results are not available for at least 24 hours, there has been considerable interest in evaluating tests that may predict the results of urine culture, so that appropriate therapy can be initiated at the first encounter with the symptomatic patient. The tests that have received the most attention are urine microscopy for white blood cells and bacteria and biochemical analysis of leukocyte esterase and nitrite, which can be assessed rapidly by dipstick.

Several studies have concluded that both the presence of any bacteria on Gram staining of an uncentrifuged urine sample and dipstick analysis for leukocyte esterase perform similarly in children from birth through 12 years of age and are helpful in identifying individuals with UTI. Other recent studies done involving young infants (<2 months of age) and older infants (<12 months and 1–24 months) concluded that a hemocytometer white blood cell count of 10 or more cells/μL provides the most valuable cutoff point for identifying infants for whom urine culture is warranted.

The definition of a positive urine culture depends on the method used to collect the specimen. This variable definition reflects the fact that urine that has passed through the urethra may be contaminated by bacteria present in the distal urethra. If the urine is obtained by the clean-catch method, a positive culture is defined as equal to or greater than 10^5 colony-forming units (CFU)/mL. If the specimen is obtained by catheterization of the urethra, a positive culture is defined as equal to or greater than 5×10^4 CFU/mL. Finally, if a urine culture is obtained by suprapubic aspiration, a method that bypasses the potential source of contamination, a positive culture is defined as recovery of any bacteria from the urine.

Imaging

Imaging studies have been the standard of care for young children with a first UTI for the past decade. Commonly, a renal ultrasound study is performed to evaluate the gross anatomy of the urinary tract (size and shape of the kidneys, duplication or dilatation of the ureters). A voiding cystourethrogram (VCUG) is done to determine whether vesicoureteral reflux is present. This practice has rested on the assumption that continuous prophylactic antimicrobial therapy is effective in reducing the incidence of reinfection of the kidney and renal scarring that may occur in children with vesicoureteral reflux. The 2011 guidelines on diagnosis and management of urinary tract infection in infants and children 2–24 months of age issued by the American Academy of Pediatrics recommend postponing performance of the VCUG until the second infection (unless there is a major abnormality of the renal ultrasound).

Treatment

In general, there are many choices for the antibiotic treatment of UTIs in children. If a child is toxic in appearance or vomiting (thereby precluding oral antimicrobials), admission to the hospital for parenteral therapy is appropriate. Many would recommend a third-generation cephalosporin, such as ceftriaxone (Rocephin) 50 mg/kg/d given once daily or cefotaxime (Claforan) 25 mg/kg/dose every 6 hours, until the emesis has resolved and the patient can be treated orally. Otherwise, children, even those with presumed pyelonephritis, do well on oral therapy.

For the child who is to receive oral therapy, the choices are amoxicillin potassium clavulanate (Augmentin) 30 mg/kg/dose given every 12 hours[3]; a second- or third-generation cephalosporin such as cefuroxime (Ceftin)[1] 50 mg/kg/dose twice daily,[3] cefpodoxime (Vantin)[1] 5 mg/kg/dose given twice daily, cefdinir (Omnicef)[1] 7 mg/kg/dose given twice daily, or cefixime (Suprax) 10 mg/kg/dose once daily[3]; or sulfamethoxazole-trimethoprim (Bactrim) 6 mg/kg/day of trimethoprim given once daily. There has been a tendency during the past several years for the prevalence of antimicrobial resistance to increase. The overall resistance to antibiotics varies geographically, and it is essential for the practitioner to be familiar with local antibiotic resistance patterns. In patients with suspected acute pyelonephritis, amoxicillin (Amoxil), cephalexin (Keflex), and sulfamethoxazole-trimethoprim should be avoided as presumptive therapy because of the potentially high rate of antibiotic resistance.

The optimal duration of therapy for children with UTI has been somewhat controversial. If the diagnosis of pyelonephritis is known or suspected, 10 days of treatment is conventional. Shorter courses of therapy have been successful in adult women with infection of the lower urinary tract. A recent meta-analysis conducted by the Cochrane Database of Systematic Reviews evaluated 10 trials (652 children) with lower-tract UTI. There was no significant difference in frequency of positive urine cultures between short-term (2–4 days) and standard (7–14 days) duration of oral antibiotic therapy for cystitis in children, either early after treatment or at 1 to 15 months after treatment. Furthermore, there was no difference between groups in the development of resistant organisms at the end of treatment or in the incidence of recurrent UTIs. Accordingly, in cases in which the diagnosis of cystitis is assured, 4 days of antimicrobial therapy is sufficient.

Voiding Dysfunction

Voiding dysfunction is a broad term indicating a voiding pattern that is abnormal for the child's age. This is a condition that should be considered in all children who are diagnosed as having a UTI after toilet training has been accomplished. Constipation plays a significant role in some children with voiding dysfunction, and attention to this comorbidity sometimes results in resolution of recurrent UTIs.

Prophylaxis

For children who are thought to be at very high risk for recurrent UTIs and potential scarring, prophylactic treatment with sulfamethoxazole-trimethoprim or nitrofurantoin (Macrodantin) should be considered. These groups include children with high degrees of vesicoureteral reflux (grades 4 and 5), those with frequent and closely spaced UTIs without reflux, and, occasionally, those who have urologic abnormalities.

The RIVUR study, Randomized Intervention for Children with Vesicoureteral Reflux (VUR), was undertaken in 2007 to determine whether antimicrobial prophylaxis with SMX-TMP is effective in preventing recurrent UTI in infants and children with reflux of any grade. The study showed a modest benefit of prophylaxis with regard to febrile episodes of UTI but no difference in scarring. There is no question of the biologic plausibility of prophylactic antimicrobial therapy in preventing recurrent UTI; however, adverse effects, emergence of antimicrobial resistance, and difficulties with long-term adherence to prophylactic strategies present barriers to effectiveness.

---

[1]Not FDA approved for this indication.
[3]Exceeds dosage recommended by the manufacturer.

References

Gorelick MH, Shaw KN: Screening tests for urinary tract infection: A meta-analysis, *Pediatrics* 104:e54, 1999.

Hellerstein S, Linebarger JS: Voiding dysfunction in pediatric patients, *Clin Pediatr* 42:43–49, 2003.

Hoberman A, Charron M, Hickey RW, et al: Imaging studies after a first febrile urinary tract infection in young children, *N Engl J Med* 348:195–202, 2003.

Hoberman A, Wald ER, Hickey RW, et al: Oral versus initial intravenous therapy for urinary tract infections in young febrile children, *Pediatrics* 104:79–86, 1999.

Hoberman A, Wald ER, Reynolds EA, et al: Pyuria and bacteriuria in urine specimens obtained by catheter from young children with fever, *J Pediatr* 124:513–519, 1994.

Huicho L, Campos-Sanchez M, Alamo C: Metaanalysis of urine screening tests for determining the risk of urinary tract infection in children, *Pediatr Infect Dis J* 21:1–11, 2002.

Michael M, Hodson EM, Craig JC, et al: Short versus standard duration oral antibiotic therapy for acute urinary tract infection in children, *Cochrane Database Syst Rev*(1), 2009. CD003966 [First published in 2003].

RIVUR Trial Investigators, Hoberman A, Greenfield SP, Mattoo TK, et al: Antimicrobial prophylaxis for children with vesicoureteral reflux, *N Engl J Med* 370:2367–2376, 2014.

Subcommittee on Urinary Tract Infection: Steering Committee on Quality Improvement and Management, Roberts KB. Urinary tract infection: clinical practice guideline for the diagnosis and management of the initial UTI in febrile infants and children 2 to 24 months, *Pediatrics* 128:595–610, 2011.

Subcommittee on Urinary Tract Infection: Reaffirmation of AAP clinical practice guideline: The diagnosis and management of the initial urinary tract infection in febrile infants and young children 2-24 months of age, *Pediatrics* 138(6):e20163026, 2016.

Williams G, Craig JC: Long-term antibiotics for preventing recurrent urinary tract infection in children, *Cochrane Database Rev*, 2019.

20 Physical and Chemical Injuries

BURNS

Method of
Bradley E. Barth, MD

CURRENT DIAGNOSIS

- Calculate percentage of burns – use a diagram for accuracy
- Chemical burns – be aware of treatment differences based on the substance involved
- Ocular injury – check for injury and consult ophthalmology
- Cyanide exposure – check for and treat cyanide toxicity in victims of structure fires

CURRENT THERAPY

- The first, immediate treatment is to stop the burning
- Cool water irrigation (NOT ice or ice water)
- Standard airway, breathing, and circulation resuscitation applies
- Resuscitation fluids should be calculated on the basis of surface area of deep partial and deeper burns (does not include superficial burns)
- Topical treatment is the mainstay for most wounds
- Update tetanus vaccination if needed
- Consult poison control center for chemical injuries or toxic gas exposure
- Hydroxocobalamin (CYANOKIT) is the treatment of choice for cyanide exposure
- Develop transfer relationship with burn center

Epidemiology

Annually in the United States, there are nearly 500,000 burns that are significant enough to require emergency treatment or admission to the hospital, and about 4000 deaths attributable to fire or fire-related inhalation injuries. The vast majority of the annual 40,000 injuries that require admission to the hospital are treated in a specialized burn center. Worldwide there are over 265,000 deaths annually due to fire-related injuries, with over 90% of these occurring in low- and middle-income countries.

Risk Factors

Burns are distributed across the spectrum of age, although their types and mechanisms vary with age. Burns tend to be more common in males. Males tend to get burned by flames, while females are more likely to sustain scald or heat contact wounds. Old and very young persons are more likely to sustain injury due to inability to get away from either a flame or heat contact. Alcohol use and other substance use are associated with an increased risk of burn injury. Burns tend to cluster in lower socioeconomic groups and are much more common in countries with lower incomes.

Pathophysiology

The injuries that result from burns are thought to be due to a combination of immediate tissue injury, the resulting inflammatory cascade, immediate and delayed cellular and humoral effects, and the delayed effects of changes in gene expression induced by the earlier injuries. The immediate injury is divided into three zones. The most severely injured is the central zone of necrosis; this area is surrounded by the zone of stasis, which is surrounded by the zone of hyperemia (Figure 1). The zone of necrosis is composed of coagulated tissue that will progress to rapid cell death and eschar formation. The outer zone of hyperemia has increased blood flow and minimal tissue damage and will almost certainly heal. The middle zone of stasis is the region where blood flow has ceased within the capillary bed. Depending on subsequent actions over the next 24 to 48 hours, this area either will worsen to necrotic tissue or may re-epithelialize to healing. The immediate postinjury efforts are focused on salvaging this area.

Burning Tissue

As heat transfers to tissue, damage begins to occur as cellular temperature rises above 44 °C. Once the internal cellular temperature reaches 60 °C, the cell will die. Generally, once the heat source is removed from the skin, the tissue temperature rapidly returns to normal, but the tissue injury does not stop at that point. Within seconds of the injury, arterioles begin to spasm, and red blood cells aggregate within the vessels. Histologic changes are visible within 15 minutes, and tissue edema begins. Tissue edema typically peaks 6 to 12 hours postinjury.

It is much easier for a burn injury to penetrate through the dermal layers in thin skin than in thick skin, leading to more severe injury in the former with a similar degree of heat transfer. These injuries pose a particular risk in infants and children as well as the elderly.

Shortly after the burning stops, processes of both inflammation and healing begin. There is a complex interplay of inflammatory mediators, immune cell action, and changes in gene expression that will continue over the following weeks to months and will play a role in how the wound heals.

Prevention

Public safety initiatives have done a great deal to decrease the risk of burn injury in the developed world. Often patient visits provide opportunities for educational interventions, especially if for a minor burn. Campaigns to decrease hot water heater temperatures in homes have helped reduce scald injuries. Safety plugs for electrical outlets decrease the risk of electrical injury in children. Smoke detectors and planned and practiced escape routes increase the likelihood of escaping from structure fires. Reminders to check smoke detectors and to change the batteries with the seasonal clock change ensure that devices are functional. Child-resistant lighters and safety matches, especially when stored out of reach of children, increase fire safety. Keeping screens or safety devices around fireplaces and fire pits may decrease injuries as well. Avoiding activities with fuel and flames, especially while intoxicated, will also decrease fire injuries.

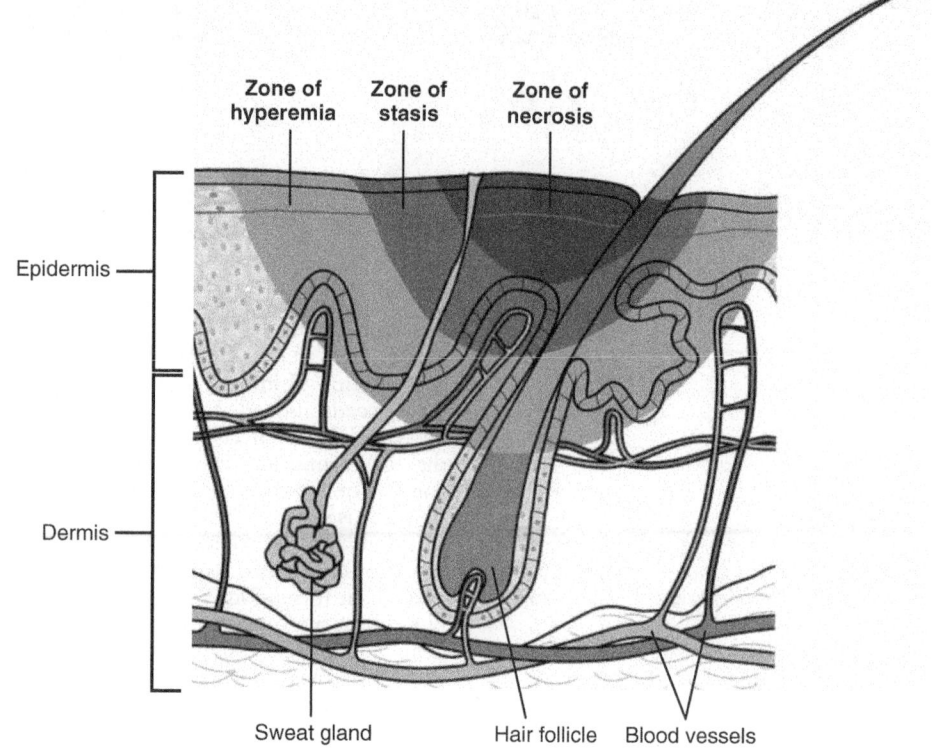

Figure 1 Burn injury.

TABLE 1	Types of Burns					
DEPTH	**ANATOMY**	**APPEARANCE**	**SENSATION**	**TIME**	**TREATMENT**	
Superficial	Epidermis only	Pink or red and dry, blanches	Painful	Days	Topical	
Superficial partial thickness	Epidermis and upper papillary dermis	Pink, clear blisters, moist surface, blanches	Painful	14–21 days	Debride and topical medication	
Deep partial thickness	Epidermis, papillary dermis, and lower reticular dermis	Pink or red, moist surface, blisters, may be hemorrhagic, does not blanch	Painful, may have decreased sensation	Weeks or may progress to full thickness	Debride, topical medication, possible surgery	
Full thickness	Epidermis, dermis, and into underlying tissue	White or brown, dry, leathery, does not blanch	Insensate	Weeks, and heals by contraction and scarring	Surgical	

Clinical Manifestations

Descriptions of burns are based on the depth of the injury and the extent of coverage (Table 1). Superficial burns involve the epidermis alone. These injuries are typically painful and erythematous, and they will heal without scarring. These injuries are not included in calculations of the percentage total body surface area (TBSA) burned. Superficial partial thickness burns involve the entire epidermis and extend down to the papillary region of the upper dermis. These injuries are painful, erythematous, and moist, and they form blisters. Deep partial thickness burns involve the entire epidermis and extend deeper into the lower reticular dermis. These wounds are typically painful and whitish, and they have less weeping and blanching than superficial partial thickness wounds. Full-thickness burns extend through the entire dermis and destroy nerves and other deep structures. These wounds are insensate, stiff, and white or tan, and they do not blanch. Wounds of this depth cannot heal spontaneously and will have significant scarring and contracture if not surgically managed.

Areas of burn that have extensive or circumferential deep partial thickness or full-thickness burns are at risk for development of restrictive eschars. Thickened areas of eschar can restrict circulation, leading to compartment syndrome; in areas of the neck and chest, they can restrict respiration, leading to hypoventilation. Ideally, burn patients can reach burn centers before an escharotomy is required, but an escharotomy will be required emergently in some cases.

Inhalation injury is a source of significant morbidity in burn patients. The initial injury may not seem particularly severe, but edema can develop rapidly in the airway, which makes delayed airway management perilous. Early intubation may be necessary.

Special Situations

Ocular Injuries

Patients with any signs of burns to the face, complaints of eye pain, or inability to communicate should undergo eye examinations with fluorescein staining. If corneal burns are identified, appropriate antibiotic ointment should be started, and consultation with an eye specialist should be obtained.

Nonaccidental Trauma

Up to 6% of burns in children are secondary to physical abuse. Burns caused by abuse are more likely to occur in males and

TABLE 2	Chemical Burns*	
CHEMICAL	**TREATMENT**	**SPECIAL NOTES**
Dry chemical	Brush or remove as much chemical as possible, then copious irrigation	Obtain material safety data sheet information on exposure
Liquid chemical	Copious irrigation	
Ocular injury	Copious irrigation with Lactated Ringer's solution, measure pH early and repeat frequently	
Elemental metals (e.g., sodium, magnesium)	Cover with mineral oil if available, physically remove as soon as possible, irrigate with water if no other options	Water causes an intense exothermic reaction, but tissue damage occurs with continued contact
Strong alkalis (pH 10–12; e.g., lye, bleach, cement [calcium oxide], ammonia)	Copious irrigation, continue until pH normalizes, but at least 1 hour; may require 12 or more hours	Current recommendations are not to try to neutralize, but research is continuing
Petroleum	Irrigation, mild soap solution	May be seen in vehicle trauma patients
Hydrofluoric acid	Irrigation, topical calcium gluconate (Calgonate) mixed with water-based lubricant (e.g., K-Y jelly), intradermal or intravenous calcium gluconate	Associated with pain out of proportion to appearance, fluoride ion can cause hypocalcemia and death
Phenol	Polyethylene glycol (PEG) (Miralax)[1] stops phenol burn more quickly than water; if PEG is not available, use high-flow, low-pressure, copious irrigation	

*Consider contacting a burn center or poison control center for assistance with chemical injury treatment.
[1]Not FDA approved for this indication.

children with developmental delays and may result in a delay in seeking care. Other concerning findings are burns that have clear lines of demarcation (e.g., cigarette burns, dunking, radiator, grill, curling iron), that are symmetric on both extremities, or spare the flexor creases with deep surrounding burns. If nonaccidental trauma is suspected, it must be reported, and the child must be kept in a safe place until authorities have cleared the child to go home.

Chemical Burns
The risk and degree of injury caused by chemical burns vary greatly, depending on the substance involved as well as on the concentration of the material and the duration of exposure. The Centers for Disease Control and Prevention has a website that provides information on treatment for chemical injuries: http://www.atsdr.cdc.gov/mmg/index.asp. General precautions for chemical burns are to decontaminate as quickly as possible while avoiding rescuer contamination or injury. For dry or powdered chemicals, remove as much chemical physically while it is still in the dry form by brushing or other mechanical removal. After mechanical removal, or for liquid contamination, dilute the chemical and continue the removal process by using water. Water should be used via copious, high-flow, low-pressure irrigation for at least 20 minutes. If feasible, check the pH of the contaminated area and continue irrigation until it returns to normal. In most cases, removal and irrigation are more important to neutralizing the chemical because using neutralizing agents can make the injury worse in some cases. Evaluate the patient for possible inhalation or ocular injury as well. There are important exceptions to typical management, some of which are listed in Table 2.

Electrical Injuries
Injuries with electrical sources vary based on the type of circuit (alternating vs direct current), amperage, voltage, tissue resistance, duration of exposure, and path of current through the body. High voltage (≥1000 V) tends to cause more thermal tissue injury and often causes concomitant traumatic injuries. Depending on the path of electricity, there may be significant internal injuries beneath normal-appearing skin, especially in high-voltage cases. Significant injuries should be treated more like crush injuries, as the extent of the internal injuries is difficult to assess. Cutaneous burns due to electrical injury can be treated similarly to thermal burns. During the initial evaluation of electrical injury,

patients should undergo electrocardiography and cardiac monitoring, and obtaining serum levels of myoglobin, creatine kinase, and troponin, as well as coagulation studies, should be considered, in addition to liver and pancreas enzyme levels in patients with intra-abdominal injuries. In cases of multiple victims of a lightning strike, a reverse triage process occurs whereby care is provided first to the patients who appear to be in cardiac arrest, as cardiopulmonary resuscitation and defibrillation may save their lives if applied early enough.

Therapy (or Treatment)
First Aid and Office Management
The initial management for burn injuries consists of stopping further injury by removing the heat source and providing cooling. Remove the patient from the burning area in the event of flame injury. If the patient's clothing is on fire, it is important to stop the burning and remove hot clothing as quickly as possible. Hot liquid or scald injuries especially require prompt removal of overlying clothing, as the clothing will trap the heat, which will continue the burning damage. After the heat source is removed, copious cool water should be used to irrigate the injured area, and any constricting jewelry should be removed immediately. The ideal temperature for cool water irrigation is not clear, but it is likely between 15 °C and 25 °C (59 °F–77 °F); colder temperatures can be damaging. The cooling irrigation can be continued for up to 20 minutes. Early wound cooling decreases the temperature of the injured area quickly to halt the burning process, but irrigation has been shown to be beneficial even after the wound has returned to a normal temperature. Cooling the wound is thought to be effective up to 3 hours after the injury. It is unclear why cool water irrigation improves burn outcomes; heat removal and edema prevention appear to play a role, but they also appear to lead to alterations in gene expression that decrease injury and improve healing. After cooling the injured area, the initial treatment is to cover the wounds with a clean, thin cloth or sterile sheets while the patient awaits further care. Ensure that the patient's tetanus vaccination is up to date.

Superficial burns or superficial partial thickness burns can generally be treated on an outpatient basis, with important exceptions (>10% TBSA; very young or old patient, circumferential injury; hand, face, or genital area burns). Debride any ruptured blister tissue, clean the wounds with mild soap and water or dilute antiseptic solution, and dress the wound. Wound dressings may include topical antibiotic cream or ointment, silver impregnated nylon or bismuth tribromophenate, and petrolatum impregnated gauze (Xeroform). Topical bacitracin or triple-antibiotic ointment is often used. Silver sulfadiazine cream 1% (Silvadene) is also commonly used, but avoid use on the face as it can lead to pigmented scarring. The management of intact blisters is controversial; however, if a blister appears fragile or likely to rupture, unroof and debride the wound before dressing the wound. If the blister is in thicker skin or appears stable, most recommendations are to aspirate the blister fluid and dress the wound. Occlusive dressings over mild burns have also been shown to improve healing. Dressings should be changed as dictated by the dressing choice. Some silver products and occlusive bandages may be left in place for several days; most traditional dressings need to be changed daily, or more frequently if needed.

Burns are painful injuries and often require early, aggressive pain control, such as with nonsteroidal anti-inflammatory medications, opioid medications, and acetaminophen. It is important to remember to provide additional analgesia as needed for dressing changes and wound care. Pruritus and neuropathic pain may occur as the wound heals, these are often treated with adjunct pain medications such as gabapentin (Neurontin),[1] and diphenhydramine (Benadryl).[1]

Wounds that are of deep partial thickness or deeper usually require some form of surgical management and should be referred for specialized care. Early surgical management has been demonstrated to be beneficial. Prophylactic antibiotics should not be used for burn management, as they have been shown to be harmful.

Hospital Management

For patients with more severe injuries, follow the traditional algorithm of assessing and stabilizing the respiratory and circulatory system first, then proceeding with a complete history and physical examination, including comorbid conditions, allergies, medications, and other past medical history. If possible, identify the mechanisms and circumstances surrounding the injury, including agents involved, duration of exposure, and situation, including possibility of inhalation injury or enclosed space involvement. Assess whether there are chemical or electrical burns and any associated trauma. The social history may play an important role in disposition and management decisions.

Patients who were in an enclosed space or structure fire or who were otherwise exposed to high levels of smoke or toxins should be assessed for carbon monoxide and cyanide injuries. Lactate, troponin, and carboxyhemoglobin levels should be checked in patients at risk for carbon monoxide or cyanide exposure. A patient at risk for cyanide exposure who has a decreased level of consciousness, hypotension, or a lactate level greater than 9 should receive 5 g (or 70 mg/kg to a maximum of 5 g) of hydroxocobalamin (Cyanokit) intravenously. If the patient is in cardiac arrest or does not improve with the initial dose, a total of 10 g should be given.

A patient with carbon monoxide exposure should have a carboxyhemoglobin level obtained and be placed on 100% oxygen as soon as possible, typically delivered via a non-rebreather face mask. Carbon monoxide binds tightly to hemoglobin, and by increasing the oxygen concentration in the lungs and blood, the half-life of carboxyhemoglobin is greatly reduced. With oxygen levels typically delivered by non-rebreather face mask, the half-life of carboxyhemoglobin is 74 minutes. This leads to the recommendation that after 6 hours on 100% oxygen, if the patient is asymptomatic, treatment can be stopped. It is unnecessary to use arterial blood or to repeat carboxyhemoglobin levels. Patients with carbon monoxide poisoning may experience delayed neurologic sequelae. Hyperbaric oxygen therapy may reduce the risk of delayed neurologic sequelae in appropriately selected patients. Although controversial, this therapy is thought to be most helpful if it occurs within 12 hours after the end of the patient's exposure, but patients may benefit up to 24 hours after exposure. If possible, consult with a physician capable of

TABLE 3	Symptoms of Carbon Monoxide Exposure*
Headache
Dizziness
Nausea
Vomiting
Confusion
Fatigue
Chest pain
Shortness of breath
Loss of consciousness

*It is important to note that carboxyhemoglobin levels do not correlate well with symptoms or with severity of exposure. Arterial blood gas samples are not superior to venous blood samples.

providing hyperbaric oxygen therapy or with a poison control center for patients with carboxyhemoglobin levels greater than 10, symptoms consistent with carbon monoxide exposure, or pregnant patients (Table 3).

Patients with inhalation injuries can develop rapidly progressing airway swelling. The initial evaluation of burn patients should include assessment for perioral injury, singed facial or nasal hair, and soot or swelling in the oral or hypopharyngeal cavities. These findings, other indications of airway swelling, or difficulty breathing should prompt early placement of a definitive airway. Delay may make placement of an endotracheal tube difficult or impossible.

Burn Management

After evaluation and stabilization of the respiratory and circulatory status of the patient, and after stabilizing acute traumatic injuries, the next step is to evaluate the extent of the burn injuries. Removing the heat source and cooling the injured areas remain a priority. Burned areas can be cooled with cool water irrigation or saline-soaked gauze. Because patients with extensive wounds can be at risk of developing hypothermia during this phase, it is important to raise the ambient temperature in the resuscitation room or use warm blankets to maintain normothermia. The extent of the burns should be determined. The "rule of nines" diagram is an accepted mechanism for approximating the percentage of TBSA burned in adults, but it tends to overestimate. Because children have a proportionally larger head and torso, diagrams have been adapted for use in pediatric populations. The Lund-Browder chart has been adapted for use with patients of all ages (Figure 2). It can also be useful to diagram the areas of burn by estimated depth. For determination of burn severity, calculation of transfer criteria, and fluid resuscitation, only the areas of deep partial thickness and deeper burns are added together to determine TBSA. Use of a diagram is recommended because TBSA is frequently overestimated when providers estimate the extent of burned areas. Overestimating TBSA burned leads to excessive fluid administration and the complications that accompany fluid overload.

Burn Center Referral Criteria

It is important to identify the regional burn referral center and to establish a line of communication with it before a burn patient is encountered, in order to know of the center's suggested criteria for transfer (Table 4). In general, the following criteria are recommended for transfer to a burn center: burns greater than 10% of TBSA; inhalation injury; burns with significant associated mechanical injury; burns of the face, hands, feet, perineum, or genitalia or across major joints; full-thickness burns of any size; and circumferential burns. Burns that warrant a discussion with a burn center for possible transfer or outpatient follow-up

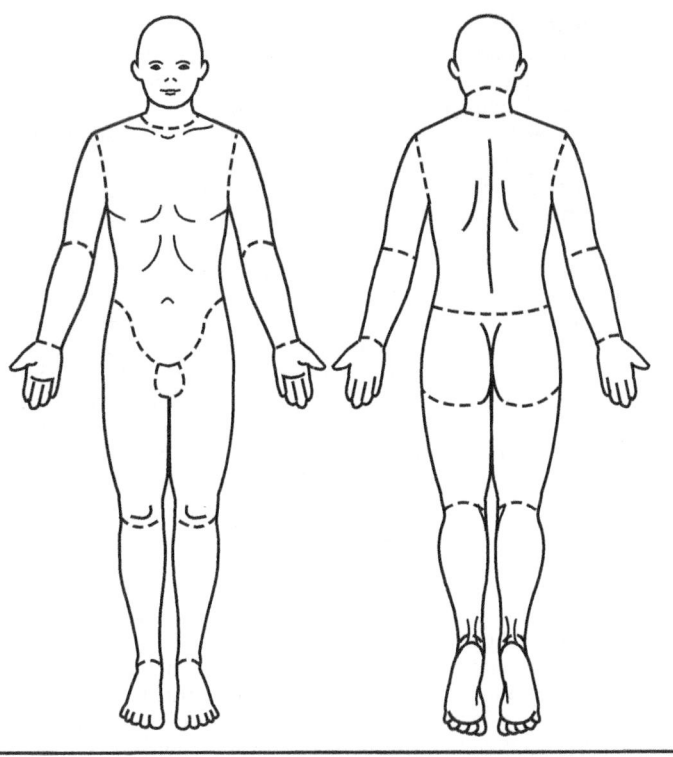

	Birth 1 yr.	1–4 yrs.	5–9 yrs.	10–14 yrs.	15 yrs.	Adult	Burn size estimate
Head	19	17	13	11	9	7	
Neck	2	2	2	2	2	2	
Anterior trunk	13	13	13	13	13	13	
Posterior trunk	13	13	13	13	13	13	
Right buttock	2.5	2.5	2.5	2.5	2.5	2.5	
Left buttock	2.5	2.5	2.5	2.5	2.5	2.5	
Genitalia	1	1	1	1	1	1	
Right upper arm	4	4	4	4	4	4	
Left upper arm	4	4	4	4	4	4	
Right lower arm	3	3	3	3	3	3	
Left lower arm	3	3	3	3	3	3	
Right hand	2.5	2.5	2.5	2.5	2.5	2.5	
Left hand	2.5	2.5	2.5	2.5	2.5	2.5	
Right thigh	5.5	6.5	8	8.5	9	9.5	
Left thigh	5.5	6.5	8	8.5	9	9.5	
Right leg	5	5	5.5	6	6.5	7	
Left leg	5	5	5.5	6	6.5	7	
Right foot	3.5	3.5	3.5	3.5	3.5	3.5	
Left foot	3.5	3.5	3.5	3.5	3.5	3.5	

Total BSAB _____

Figure 2 Lund-Browder classification of burn size.

include burns in children; patients with comorbid conditions that will impact healing; and patients with special social, emotional, psychological, or rehabilitative needs.

Monitoring

Critically ill burn patients should be monitored in an intensive care setting while awaiting transfer to a burn center. In addition to monitoring of respiratory and circulatory status, a Foley catheter should be placed to monitor urinary output and for intermittent assessment of bladder pressure to evaluate for the development of intra-abdominal compartment syndrome.

Because burned tissue increases insensible fluid losses, burn victims have increased fluid requirements. Various formulas are available for calculating approximate fluid requirements, but all require careful monitoring of the results and progress of fluid resuscitation. Patients who receive more than 250 mL/kg in the first 24 hours are at increased risk of developing fluid-related complications. The American Burn Association Consensus Statement formula is used to guide initial fluid management. The starting fluid requirements are 2 to 4 mL/kg of Lactated Ringer solution per TBSA percent value, with half given in the first 8 hours and the rest over the next 16 hours (e.g., for an 80-kg patient with a 35% TBSA deep and deep partial burn, the calculation would be $3 \, \text{mL/kg} \times 80 \, \text{kg} \times 35 = 8400 \, \text{mL}$, for a rate of 525 mL/h in first 8 hours, followed by 265 mL/h for the next 16 hours). Urine output should be monitored hourly and maintained between 0.5 and 1 mL/kg/h. If a patient's urine output is greater than 1 mL/kg/h, the rate of fluid administration should be decreased by 20% and

TABLE 4 Burn Center Referral Criteria

Partial thickness burns greater than 10% TBSA

Full-thickness burns

Burns to high-risk areas, such as the face, hands, feet, genitals, perineum, or major joints

Circumferential burns

Electrical burns, including lightning strikes

Chemical burns

Inhalation injury

Preexisting conditions known to impair healing and increase risk of mortality

Burns in combination with traumatic injury (e.g., fracture, traumatic brain injury) whereby the burn is the leading risk for patient mortality

Burn injury in patients who will require special social, emotional, or long-term rehabilitative intervention

Burns in a setting unequipped (personnel, equipment, or unit) to care for critically ill children

Available from: http://www.ameriburn.org/BurnUnitReferral.pdf. Accessed June 19, 2016.

Abbreviation: TBSA=total body surface area.

TABLE 5 Fluid Administration and Calculation

80-kg male patient with a burn of 35% TBSA full-thickness and partial thickness burns:

$80\,kg \times 35 \times 3\,mL/kg = 8400\,mL$ in first 24 hours

$8400\,mL/24\,hours \div 2 = 4200\,mL$ in first 8 hours, 4200 mL in next 16 hours

Initial rate of 525 mL/h over first 8 hours, then switching to a rate of 265 mL/h over next 16 hours

Expected urine output is 0.5–1 mL/kg/h

$80\,kg \times 0.5\,mL/kg/h = 40\,mL/h$

$80\,kg \times 1\,mL/kg/h = 80\,mL/h$

So, for our 80-kg patient, we would expect 40–80 mL of urine every hour. In hours 1 and 2 of resuscitation, the patient has 65 mL of urine per hour. In hour 3 of resuscitation, the patient has 90 mL of urine per hour. We would then decrease the fluid administration rate by 20%, or

$525\,mL/h - (0.20 \times 525) = 420\,mL/h$

Thus, the rate of administration of lactated Ringer solution would change from 525 mL/h to 420 mL/h and continue to be monitored and recorded hourly, with continued adjustments based on hourly urine output.

Abbreviation: TBSA=total body surface area.

continued to be monitored hourly. If the urine output is less than 0.5 mL/kg/h, the rate of fluid administration should be increased by 20% and continued to be monitored (Table 5).

Unfortunately, ensuring adequate urine output does not necessarily guarantee adequate fluid resuscitation. In addition to using urine output as an indicator of resuscitation adequacy, other modes of monitoring can be used to help guide fluid resuscitation (hemodynamic monitoring, echocardiography, gastric tonometry, or other devices). Whether they lead to any increased improvement or survivability is not clear, however.

Transfer

Burn centers typically manage more than 200 burn patients annually and have specially trained physicians, nurses, and ancillary personnel who are focused on treating burn patients. Severely burned patients who are treated at specialized centers have better outcomes. It is recommended that hospitals and clinics have agreements with burn centers for the management of complicated patients and patients who meet criteria for burn center transfer.

Complications

Pain management for burns may require multiple modalities because the type of pain varies, depending on where the patient is in the cycle of treatment and healing. There are three types of pain that need to be treated during the care of a burn patient: background pain, breakthrough pain, and long-term pain. Background pain is present from the onset of the injury, and the pain is typically intensified during procedures. There will also be episodes of breakthrough pain. Depending on the severity of the injury, initial pain and background pain may be treated with acetaminophen, nonsteroidal anti-inflammatory drugs (e.g., ibuprofen, naproxen sodium), or opioids. Procedural pain may require bolus dosing of opioids or other adjunctive medications such as ketamine[1] (0.1–0.2 mg/kg IV). Long-term pain may respond to medications such as gabapentin, clonidine, or others.

Psychosocial recovery from burns is impacted by the preexisting conditions and the resilience of the patient. Preexisting mental health, substance abuse, and other medical and psychosocial issues complicate the patient's recovery from burns. Risk factors for burn injury include poverty, a history of abuse or neglect, substance abuse, serious mental illness, and risk for suicide or assault. Psychiatric recovery is negatively affected by posttraumatic stress disorder, depression, learning disorders, substance abuse, stigma, and disability. Individual resilience, social support, and education or occupation also impact patient outcomes.

The patient's age and stage of life at the time of injury impact recovery as well. Younger victims have a longer remaining lifespan to live with the scarring and disfigurement. Pediatric patients often have fewer comorbid medical conditions, which can speed their recovery and limit disability, and they tend to heal more quickly, but their injuries may have a significant impact on their body image development, self-confidence, and interpersonal relationship building. The family may be of assistance in recovery from the injury, but family members, too, may experience stress and psychological concerns related to the injury to a child. Adults and older patients have to deal with the impact of the injury on their identity and their ability to return to their preinjury roles.

Some patients and caregivers may develop posttraumatic stress disorder related to the injury or to postinjury treatment. It is thought that early multidisciplinary interventions may decrease this risk, but the research is unclear. Some patients will require long-term, continued outpatient treatment.

Hypertrophic scarring is the most common complication related to healing of burn wounds, but scar contracture and pruritus are common complications as well. It is thought that hypertrophic scarring may be decreased with early, appropriate surgical repair, but it still can occur. The development of hypertrophic scarring is multifactorial; it is likely a result of a complex interplay of humoral and cellular immunity causing an inappropriate response to healing tissue. Multiple host and injury factors contribute, but protracted healing of a partial thickness injury is a common theme. There are some experimental therapies for manipulating different components of the host response, but none has clearly proven to be beneficial.

Scar contracture results from tissue loss at the time of injury and tissue-healing properties. Burn injuries are more complicated than other traumatic wounds because the destroyed tissue is surrounded by profoundly damaged tissue. As a result of this tissue injury, there is increased collagen deposition resulting from

---

[1] Not FDA approved for this indication.

changes in inflammation, proliferation, and remodeling at the cellular and extracellular matrix levels. Hypertrophic scars tend to form within the first month after injury and may improve over the first 6 months, but then tend not to show significant changes after that time. Burn treatment and scar prevention consist of tissue replacement, tissue rehabilitation, and tension release. Early and existing scars are often treated with compression garments and silicone sheets. It is thought that these may alter and improve remodeling of the extracellular matrix and thereby improve scarring. In some cases, surgical release of tension may be necessary.

References

American Burn Association: *Burn incidence and treatment in the United States*, 2015. Available at http://www.ameriburn.org/resources_factsheet.php (accessed 06.03.16).

Cancio LC: Initial assessment and fluid resuscitation of burn patients, *Surg Clin North Am* 94:741–754, 2014.

de Castro RJ, Leal PC, Sakata RK: Pain management in burn patients, *Braz J Anesthesiol* 63:149–153, 2013.

Forjuoh SN: Burns in low- and middle-income countries: A review of available literature on descriptive epidemiology, risk factors, treatment, and prevention, *Burns* 32:529–537, 2006.

Haines E, Fairbrother H: Optimizing emergency management to reduce morbidity and mortality in pediatric burn patients, *Pediatr Emerg Med Pract* 12:1–23, 2015. quiz 24–5.

Lavrentieva A: Critical care of burn patients: New approaches to old problems, *Burns* 42:13–19, 2016.

MacLennan L, Moiemen N: Management of cyanide toxicity in patients with burns, *Burns* 41:18–24, 2015.

Marx JA, Hockberger RS, Walls RM: *Rosen's emergency medicine: Concepts and clinical practice*, ed 8, Philadelphia, 2014, Elsevier Saunders.

Monseau AJ, Reed ZM, Langley KJ, Onks C: Sunburn, thermal, and chemical injuries to the skin, *Prim Care* 42:591–605, 2015.

Retrouvey H, Shahrokhi S: Pain and the thermally injured patient—a review of current therapies, *J Burn Care Res* 36:315–323, 2015.

Robinson EP, Chhabra AB: Hand chemical burns, *J Hand Surg Am* 40:605–612, 2015. quiz 613.

Sheridan RL, Greenhalgh D: Special problems in burns, *Surg Clin North Am* 94:781–791, 2014.

Stoddard Jr FJ, Ryan CM, Schneider JC: Physical and psychiatric recovery from burns, *Surg Clin North Am* 94:863–878, 2014.

Tredget EE, Levi B, Donelan MB: Biology and principles of scar management and burn reconstruction, *Surg Clin North Am* 94:793–815, 2014.

Wright EH, Harris AL, Furniss D: Cooling of burns: Mechanisms and models, *Burns* 41:882–889, 2015.

DISTURBANCES DUE TO COLD[a]

Method of
Jerrold B. Leikin, MD; Scott M. Leikin, DO; Frederick K. Korley, MD; and Ernest Wang, MD

CURRENT DIAGNOSIS

- Accidental hypothermia may be classified as mild, moderate, or severe.
- The measured temperature should be the core body temperature.
- The method of rewarming depends on the severity of the temperature drop.
- The complications of rewarming include arrhythmias, rewarming-related hypotension, core temperature after drop, and rhabdomyolysis.
- Patients can be declared dead only after they are warm.

---

[a] Portions of this chapter have been previously printed in *Conn's Current Therapy* 2009–2012. The content of this chapter has also appeared in *Disease-a-Month* 2012;58(1):6–32.

CURRENT THERAPY

Mild Hypothermia: 32.2°C (90°F) to 35°C (95°F)
- Start passive external rewarming; remove wet clothing.
- Ambient temperature should exceed 21.0°C (70.0°F).
- Cover patient with insulating material.

Moderate Hypothermia: 28°C (82.4°F) to 32.2°C (90°F)
- Start active external rewarming; use radiant heat.
- Use thermal mattresses and electric heating blankets.
- Use forced-air heating blankets.
- Perform active core rewarming; use warmed humidified oxygen.
- Give warmed intravenous saline.
- Give bladder, colonic, and gastric irrigation.
- Start pleural cavity lavage.
- Avoid alcohol, caffeine, and nicotine (tobacco).

Severe Hypothermia: Less than 28°C (82.4°F)
- Begin aggressive active core rewarming; use warmed, humidified oxygen.
- Give warmed intravenous saline.
- Give bladder, colonic, and gastric irrigation.
- Start pleural cavity lavage.
- Perform peritoneal lavage or dialysis.
- Perform extracorporeal warming or heated cardiopulmonary bypass.

Frostnip
- Gentle rewarming, generally in a water bath of 104°F to 108°F (40°C to 42°C).
- It is usually self-resolving.

Frostbite
- Immerse in warm (not hot) water.
- Débride broken vesicles.
- Do not débride hemorrhagic or intact blisters.
- Apply topical aloe vera[7] or antibiotic ointment.
- Use nonsteroidal antiinflammatory drugs (NSAIDs) for pain.
- Update tetanus status.
- Do not rub or massage the affected area.
- Do not use a heating pad or heat lamp; affected areas can be easily burned.
- Avoid alcohol and tobacco products.

Chilblain
- Rewarm gently.
- Nifedipine (Procardia)[1] may be useful.

Trench foot
- Dry the foot.
- Rewarm gently.
- Use NSAIDs for pain.

---

[1] Not FDA Approved for this indication.
[7] Available as dietary supplement.

Accidental Systemic Hypothermia

Hypothermia is classically defined as a reduction in the body's core temperature below 95.0°F (35.0°C). Most reported cases of hypothermia are due to environmental exposure to low ambient temperatures (accidental hypothermia). Other causes of hypothermia include sepsis, severe hypothyroidism (myxedema coma), acute spinal cord injury, diabetic ketoacidosis, multisystem trauma, and prolonged cardiac arrest.

Epidemiology

Risk factors for developing hypothermia include extremes of age (elderly people might not be able to remove themselves from cold environments, and young children lose heat more rapidly because of their increased total body surface area), major trauma, homelessness, psychiatric illness, and drug and alcohol abuse (Box 1).

BOX 1 — Factors Predisposing to Hypothermia or Frostbite

Physiologic

Decreased heat production
Age extremes (infants, elderly)
Dehydration or malnutrition
Diaphoresis or hyperhidrosis
Endocrinologic insufficiency
Hypoxia
Insufficient fuel
Overexertion
Physical conditioning
Prior cold injury
Trauma (multisystem or extremity)

Increased heat loss
Burns
Dermatologic malfunction
Cold infusions
Emergency resuscitation
Poor acclimatization or conditioning
Shock
Vascular diseases

Impaired thermoregulation
Central nervous system trauma or disease
Metabolic disorders
Pharmacologic or toxicologic agents
Sepsis
Spinal cord injury

Psychological
Fatigue
Fear or panic
Hunger
Intense concentration on tasks
Intoxicants
Mental status or attitude
Peer pressure

Environmental
Altitude with or without associated conditions
Ambient temperature or humidity
Duration of exposure
Heat loss (conductive, evaporative, radiative, convective)
Quantity of exposed surface area
Wind chill factor

Mechanical
Constricting or wet clothing or boots
Inadequate insulation
Immobility or cramped positioning

Cold-related deaths also are reported in military combatants and outdoor winter sports participants. Several drugs and chemicals can predispose to hypothermia (Box 2). Alcohol is the most common intoxicant associated with hypothermia because of its ability to cause cutaneous vasodilation, impairment of shivering, and impairment of adaptive behavior.

Between 1979 and 2002, 16,555 deaths in the United States, an average of 689 per year, were attributed to exposure to low environmental temperatures. In 2002, of the 646 hypothermia-related deaths reported, 66% occurred in male patients, 52% of all decedents were aged 65 years or younger, 45% of the deaths occurred among white male patients, and 14% occurred among black male patients. The states of Alaska, New Mexico, North Dakota, and Montana had the largest overall death rates from hypothermia in 2002. The lowest recorded core temperature in a pediatric survivor of accidental hypothermia is 57.9°F (14.4°C) and the lowest in an adult survivor is 56.7°F (13.7°C).

Pathophysiology

The normal range of human core temperature is 97.5°F (36.4°C) to 99.5°F (37.5°C). Humans are thus warm-blooded and are normally able to maintain their body temperature by heat-generating mechanisms and heat-conserving behavior. These compensatory responses, however, can be overwhelmed under extreme environmental conditions, leading to hypothermia.

The anterior hypothalamus coordinates the nonshivering heat conservation and dissipation mechanisms, and the posterior hypothalamus coordinates shivering thermogenesis. Heat loss usually occurs by four mechanisms: About 55% to 65% of heat is lost by radiation, 25% to 30% by evaporation from the skin and respiratory tract, and 10% to 15% by conduction and convection. The amount of heat lost via conduction is markedly increased in cold-water immersion (by about 32-fold). Each organ system is affected uniquely by hypothermia.

Skin

Cutaneous blood flow is regulated by the individual's thermoregulatory needs, modulated by neural control through the arteriovenous anastomoses located in the extremities. Sympathetic tone is increased, which leads to arteriovenous constriction, which is maximum at 59°F (15°C). Cold-induced dermal vasodilatation can occur at 50°F (10°C).

Cardiovascular System

One of the initial heat-conserving mechanisms is peripheral vasoconstriction to decrease blood flow to the skin. There are also initial increases in heart rate and blood pressure owing to a catecholamine surge. At core temperatures below 82.4°F (28.0°C), bradycardia can result from a decrease in spontaneous depolarization of the pacemaker cell firing. The myocardium also becomes irritable, predisposing it to bradyarrhythmias and hypotension. Cardiac output decreases to approximately 45% at 77°F (25°C).

Atrial arrhythmias can occur with a slow ventricular response, and they can precede ventricular arrhythmias and asystole at core temperatures below 77.0°F (25.0°C). The characteristic Osborn or J waves (a hump seen at the QRS-ST junction) may be seen on the electrocardiogram (ECG) at core temperatures below 89.6°F (32.0°C). The development of the Osborn wave appears to be related to lower blood pH, low serum bicarbonate, and higher serum creatinine levels. Orthostasis also commonly occurs. Risk factors for development of cardiac arrest include core temperature under 82.4°F (28°C), ventricular arrhythmia development, and systolic blood pressure under 90 mm Hg.

Renal System

Renal blood flow is affected by peripheral vasoconstriction, causing the glomerular filtration rate to fall and contributing to metabolic acidosis. Antidiuretic hormone activity is usually inhibited. This can result in intravascular volume depletion, subsequent vasodilation, increased renal blood flow, and, ultimately, acute renal failure. Urinary output can increase threefold, and this may be accentuated with concomitant ethanol use.

Respiratory System

At core temperatures below 82.4°F (28°C), minute ventilation, tidal volume, respiratory rate, and thoracic elasticity all are reduced; bronchorrhea can occur, with a loss of cough and gag reflexes leading to an increased risk for aspiration. Carbon dioxide production drops by one-half for every 14°F (8°C) drop in temperature, and oxygen consumption is reduced by 75% at 72°F (22°C). Apnea can then result.

Central Nervous System

Cerebral metabolism is depressed 6% to 7% per 1°C decrease in core temperature. Cerebrovascular autoregulation remains intact until below 77.0°F (25.0°C), which helps maintain cortical blood flow. Electroencephalographic activity is clearly not prognostic, but it is abnormal below 92°F (33°C); burst suppression can occur at 71.6°F (22°C) and it silences around 66.2°F to 68.0°F

BOX 2   Drugs and Chemicals That Can Cause Hypothermia

Medicinals

Acetaminophen (Tylenol)
N-Acetylcysteine (Mucomyst)
β-Adrenergic blocking agents
Alprostadil (Caverject, Muse)
Amphotericin B (Fungizone)
Atropine
Azithromycin (Zithromax)
Baclofen (Lioresal)
Barbiturates
Benzodiazepines
Bethanechol (Urecholine)
Biperiden (Akineton)
Bromocriptine (Parlodel)
Carbamazepine (Tegretol)
Chloral hydrate (Noctec)
Chlorpromazine (Thorazine)
Clobazam (Onfi)
Clonidine (Catapres)
Colchicine (Colcrys)
Delorazepam (Dadumir)[2]
Diazepam (Valium)
Diltiazem (Cardizem)
Enflurane
Erythromycin
Ethchlorvynol (Placidyl)[2]
Ethyl alcohol
Fenoprofen (Nalfon)
Fluphenazine (Prolixin)
Fosphenytoin (Cerebyx)
Gallium nitrate (Ganite)
Glutethimide (Doriden)[2]
Guanabenz (Wytensin)
Guanfacine (Tenex)
Haloperidol (Haldol)
Halothane (Fluothane)
Heroin
γ-Hydroxybutyrate (as sodium salt [Xyrem])
Ibuprofen (Advil, Motrin)
Immune globulin
Insulin preparations
Interferon β-1b (Betaseron)
Iobitridol (Xenetix)[2]
Iopanoic acid (Telepaque)
Ipsapirone
Isoflurane (Forane)
Lincomycin (Lincocin)
Lithium (Eskalith, Lithobid)
Lormetazepam
Loxapine (Loxitane)
Magnesium sulfate
Maprotiline (Ludiomil)
Mefenamic acid (Ponstel)
Melatonin
Methyldopa (Aldomet)
Methyprylon (Noludar)[2]
Moricizine (Ethmozine)

Morphine sulfate
Naphazoline (Naphcon)
Nitrofurantoin (Macrodantin)
Nitrous oxide
Olanzapine (Zyprexa)
Omeprazole (Prilosec)
Oseltamivir (Tamiflu)
Oxcarbazepine (Trileptal)
Oxymetazoline (Afrin)
Penicillin V
Phencyclidine (PCP)
Phenol
Phenytoin (Dilantin)
Pilocarpine (Salagen)
Pipamperone
Prazosin (Minipress)
Propoxyphene (Darvon)[2]
Procarbazine (Matulane)
Propylthiouracil (PTU)
Quinine (Quinamm)
Rauwolfia serpentine
Reserpine
Risperidone (Risperdal)
Salicylate
Spectinomycin (Trobicin)[2]
Terazosin (Hytrin)
Tetracycline (Sumycin)
Tetrahydrozoline (Visine, Opti-Clear)
Thioridazine (Mellaril)
Topiramate (Topamax)
Tretinoin (topical) (Retin-A)
Triazolam (Halcion)
Tricyclic antidepressants
Valproic acid and derivatives (Depakene)
Zinc sulfate

Nonmedicinals

Acrylamide
Aldicarb
Amitraz
Ashwagandha
Barium
Bis(chloromethyl) ether
Boron hydrides
Bromophos
Cadmium oxide
Carbon disulfide
Carbon monoxide
Castor pornace
Chloralose
Chlorfenvinphos
Chlorpyrifos
Copper fumes
Coumaphos
Cyanide
Diazinon Dichlorvos
Dicrotophos

Dioxathion
Disulfoton
Ethanol
Ether
Ethion
Fensulfothion
Fenthion
Hexachlorobenzene
Hyaluronidase (Hylenex)
Hydrochloric acid
Hydrogen sulfide
Isopropyl alcohol
Lewisite
Lobelia
Mace
Malathion
Mephedrone
Metal fume fever
Methidathion
Methiocarb
Methomyl
Methyl bromide
Methylene chloride
Methylparathion
Nickel carbonyl
Parathion
Profenofos
Pyrimidifen
Sarin
Sodium azide
Terbufos
Tetraethyl pyrophosphate
Tetrafluoroethylene
Thiocyanates
Vacor
Zinc fumes (zinc oxide)

Biologicals

Ackee fruit poisoning
Brown recluse spider
Ciguatera food poisoning
Clostridium perfringens
Clupeotox
Copperhead envenomation
Cotton mouth envenomation
Delphinium
Grayanotoxin ("Mad Honey")
Lobelia
Marijuana (Cannabis)
Monkshood
Nutmeg
Salmonella food poisoning
Selenious acid fume
Star of Bethlehem (Hippobroman longiflora)
Streptococcus food poisoning
Tetrodotoxin food poisoning
White chameleon

[2]Not available in the United States.

(19.0°C to 20.0°C). Most patients are unconscious at a core temperature of 82.4°F to 86°F (28°C to 30°C).

Coagulation
Because of depression of enzymatic activity of the activated clotting factors, clotting time (particularly partial thromboplastin time [PTT]) is prolonged. At 84°F (29°C), a 50% increase of PTT can be expected. Thrombocytopenia also commonly occurs due to bone marrow suppression along with splenic and hepatic platelet sequestration, which can be exacerbated by cryoglobinemia.

Clinical Presentation
Accidental hypothermia is classified as mild at body temperatures of 90°F (32.2°C) to 95°F (35°C), moderate at body temperatures of 82.4°F (28.0°C) to 90°F (32.2°C), or severe at body temperatures less than 82.4°F (28°C).

In general, a patient's symptoms depend on the severity of the temperature drop. Patients with mild hypothermia can develop vigorous shivering and cold diuresis. Those with moderate hypothermia can have a paradoxical decrease in shivering, slurred speech, hyporeflexia, and confusion. They are also at risk for intravascular thrombosis. Splanchnic vasoconstriction, gastric erosions, hepatic necrosis, and pancreatitis can occur. Prominent laboratory abnormalities include leukopenia (from splenic sequestration), thrombocytopenia (during rewarming), hypoglycemia, respiratory or metabolic acidosis, and hyperkalemia. In pregnant patients, fetal bradycardia can occur in response to maternal hypothermia, but long-term sequelae are unknown.

During severe hypothermia, shivering gives way to rigor, minute ventilation decreases, and heart rate and cardiac output decrease. Cardiac instability can be seen at this stage and can manifest in the form of arrhythmias, heart blocks, and eventually asystole. Neurologically, the patient's mental status declines. The patient might attempt to undress (paradoxical undressing) and might respond only to painful stimuli, have decreased gag reflexes, and eventually become apneic. Generally, at about 68.0°F (20.0°C), patients become totally neurologically unresponsive, lose corneal and ocular reflexes, and can have a flat electroencephalogram (EEG).

Emergency Department Evaluation
Typically, the source of hypothermia is revealed from the patient's history; however, it is very important to rule out secondary causes of hypothermia, such as sepsis, hypothyroidism, central nervous system lesions, and hypoglycemia, among others. All patients arriving in the emergency department with hypothermia need a complete evaluation to rule out traumatic injuries and drug or toxin ingestion or overdose.

As in all resuscitation, attention should be paid to the ABCs (airway, breathing, and circulation). Successful neurologic recovery has been documented following 5 hours of cardiopulmonary resuscitation (CPR) in the setting of profound accidental hypothermia (62.4°F or 16.9°C). Ideally, in patients in cardiac arrest, CPR should be maintained throughout the pre-hospital period. In a patient with a core temperature of under 28°C, evidence supports alternating 5 minutes of CPR with less than or equal to 5 minutes without CPR, if feasible. With a core temperature under 20°C, data supports alternating 5 minutes of CPR with less than or equal to 10 minutes without CPR. Respiratory failure should be treated with endotracheal intubation and mechanical ventilation. Hypotension can be treated initially with warmed fluids. Placing the patient in a warm environment, removing all cold and wet clothes, and remembering to cover up the patient after he or she has been exposed should help prevent further heat loss.

The temperature should be confirmed by checking a core temperature (e.g., rectal, bladder, or esophageal), using a thermometer capable of recording very low temperatures. Patients should be placed on a cardiac monitor and an ECG should be obtained. Laboratory testing is especially useful in the postresuscitative period, when complications begin. Laboratory tests should include a complete blood count (CBC), a chemistry panel with liver function tests, creatine phosphokinase (CPK) to evaluate for rhabdomyolysis, a coagulation profile, blood type and screen, an arterial blood gas, and a drug screen. A Foley catheter should be placed to assess urinary output.

Rewarming Strategies
There are several methods of rewarming. The method of choice usually depends on the severity of hypothermia. During rewarming, the patient should be placed on a cardiac monitor with frequent measurements of blood pressure and temperature (via a rectal probe) for easy detection of complications of rewarming, such as rewarming-related hypotension, arrhythmias, and core temperature after-drop. It should be noted that the human body is capable of raising the body temperature through heat generation by approximately 1°C/h.

Passive External Warming
Passive external warming is ideal for patients with mild hypothermia (greater than 93°F or 34°C) who are otherwise healthy. It uses the patient's endogenous heat production for rewarming and it involves simple, logical passive maneuvers that minimize heat dissipation. When using this method, all wet clothing should be removed and the patient should be covered with insulating materials. Patients warmed easily using this method can be safely discharged.

Active External Rewarming
Active external rewarming should be considered for patients with core temperatures between 86°F and 92°F (30°C to 34°C). It involves exposing the patient's skin to exogenous heat sources. Radiant heat, thermal mattresses, electric heating blankets, and forced-air heating blankets are some of the available techniques. The rate of temperature rise is approximately 2.7°F to 7.2°F (1.5°C to 4°C) per hour.

This method has several disadvantages. First, burn injuries can occur to the vasoconstricted skin. Second, any sort of immersion can hinder monitoring and other resuscitative activities. Finally and most important, active external rewarming produces a phenomenon called *core-temperature after-drop*. This refers to a drop in core temperature resulting from sudden peripheral vasodilation. This causes cold, acidic blood to return to the core. Hypotension and potentially fatal dysrhythmias can result. Focusing on rewarming the trunk only (rather than the trunk and extremities) can prevent these temperature gradients. In general, active external rewarming is used in conjunction with active core rewarming.

Active Core Rewarming
Active core rewarming involves techniques to deliver direct heat internally. It should be used in patients with moderate to severe hypothermia (under 86°F or 30°C). The simplest method entails the administration of heated, humidified oxygen at 107.6°F to 114.8°F (42.0°C to 46.0°C) and intravenous saline solution warmed to 109.4°F (43.0°C). Saline should be administered via a central line at 150 to 200 mL/h. Gastric, bladder, and colonic irrigations have been used, but their relatively small surface areas usually limit their effect. Urinary bladder or gastric lavage (which is rarely used due to aspiration potential and electrolyte shifts) can rewarm at an hourly rate of 0.9°F to 1.8°F (0.5°C to 1°C).

Another method of active core rewarming is pleural irrigation using two large-bore (36°F or greater) thoracostomy tubes. One tube is placed at the midclavicular line and is connected to saline at 107.6°F (42.0°C). The other tube is placed at the posterior axillary line and connected to a chest tube drainage kit.

A more-aggressive method of active core rewarming is via peritoneal lavage and dialysis. This can be accomplished using a standard diagnostic peritoneal lavage kit and introducing an 8-F catheter into the peritoneum using the Seldinger technique. The crystalloid dialysate should be warmed at 104.0°F to 113.0°F (40.0°C to 45.0°C). This method affords the added advantage of allowing the serum potassium level to be adjusted.

The most efficient and physiologic active core rewarming method is via extracorporeal warming or heated cardiopulmonary bypass. This is the method of choice for the most-severe cases, patients with severe rhabdomyolysis, and patients who require CPR. Survival rates with no chronic neurological sequelae as high as 75% have been documented. Excellent recovery has been documented from a nasopharyngeal temperature of 13.8°C (and a serum potassium of 11.3 mmol/L) due to drowning with a submersion time of at least 83 minutes in icy sea water with slow rewarming with extracorporeal membrane oxygenation. Extracorporeal life support can be an effective rewarming tool in patients with prolonged cardiac arrest from accidental hypothermia, particularly in the absence of asphyxia, trauma, or severe hyperkalemia. Veno-arterial extracorporeal membrane oxygenation (VA-ECMO) is increasingly utilized for its ability to gradually increase core body temperature while providing respiratory and hemodynamic support. It should be considered, especially in pediatric patients or in individuals requiring prolonged support. Survival rates as high as 40% (with good neurologic outcome) have been documented.

Most arrhythmias are corrected by rewarming. Atrial dysrhythmias often occur during rewarming and generally resolve without treatment. Atropine is typically ineffective for cold-associated bradydysrhythmias. Ventricular tachycardia and fibrillation require electrocardioversion and the use of bretylium (not available in the United States) if it is available. Dopamine, epinephrine[1], and vasopressin (Pitressin)[1] may be effective vasopressors. External pacing may be ineffective. Empiric antibiotics may be given. However, the empiric use of levothyroxine (Synthroid)[1] and corticosteroids may be hazardous. Phenytoin (Dilantin)[1] might have cardiac-depressant qualities in the moderately hypothermic patient. Box 3 demonstrates drugs with possible decreased metabolism or clearance with resultant increase in toxicity in hypothermia.

For hypothermia due to myxedema coma, levothyroxine (Synthroid) should be administered intravenously (at a dose of 250 to 500 μg over 30 to 60 seconds). Daily intravenous injections of 100 μg may be required for up to 7 days. Hydrocortisone (Solu-Cortef)[1] (200 to 400 mg IV daily) administration should also be considered. Other active core rewarming techniques are usually not required.

Indicators of grave prognosis include development of profound hyperkalemia (serum potassium greater than 10 mEq/L), elevated serum creatinine, serum sodium, serum lactate concentration, or lower prothrombin time, underlying medical conditions, intravascular thrombosis (fibrinogen less than 59 mg/dL), pH less than 6.5, and a core temperature less than 82.4°F (28.0°C). Submersion in cold water for over 10 minutes is associated with a poor prognosis; if the water is less than 43°F (6°C), survival is unlikely to occur if submerged for over 90 minutes.

Peripheral Cold Injuries
Peripheral cold injuries span a spectrum ranging from minimal to severe tissue damage. Freezing and nonfreezing syndromes can

cause these injuries. About 500 patients with frostbite are hospitalized yearly in the United States, with about an 80% male demographic and lower extremity predominance. The average length of stay in critical care units and total hospital stay is approximately 7 and 10 days, respectively. Frostnip and frostbite are caused by exposure to freezing temperatures. *Frostnip* refers to the numbness and blue-white discoloration of the face and extremities that occur during exposure to freezing temperatures. It is a precursor to frostbite. It is characterized by reversible skin changes, including blanching and numbness with no permanent tissue damage, unlike frostbite. Nonfreezing injuries depend on whether the ambient environment during exposure was wet (trench or immersion foot) or dry (pernio or chilblain).

Pathophysiology
During exposure to cold temperatures, the core body temperature is preserved to the detriment of the extremities. Frostbite occurs in four stages: prefreeze, freeze–thaw, vascular stasis, and late ischemic stages. The prefreeze phase occurs when the temperature of the extremities falls below 50.0°F (10.0°C) and cutaneous sensation is lost. Vasoconstriction also occurs along with leakage of intracellular fluid into the interstitium.

The freeze–thaw phase begins at the freezing point of water (32.0°F or 0°C) with the formation of ice crystals extracellularly. This further enhances the exit of water from the intracellular space under osmotic forces, resulting in cell shrinkage and, ultimately, damage. During the vascular stasis phase, plasma leakage and formation of ice crystals continue. Arachidonic acid breakdown products are then released from underlying damaged tissue. Both prostaglandin $F_{2\alpha}$ and thromboxane A_2 produce platelet aggregation, leukocyte immobilization, and vasoconstriction.

Endothelial cells are sensitive to cold injury, and the microvasculature becomes distorted and clogged, leading to tissue ischemia. The late ischemic phase is characterized by ischemia, thrombosis, continued shunting, gangrene, autonomic dysfunction, and denaturation of tissue proteins. The tissue can eventually mummify and demarcate more than 60 to 90 days later.

Clinical Presentation of Local Extremity Issues
Frostnip and Frostbite
The face and ears are the most common sites prone to cold injury, followed by the hands and feet. Patients with frostnip usually have blanching and numbness of their fingertips. The skin has a firm or waxy texture. Often the patient is unaware of these changes. Frostnip is usually reversible. Frostbite has been classified as superficial, affecting the skin and subcutaneous tissue, or deep, affecting the bones, joints, and tendons. When a superficial frostbite is rewarmed, the skin can form a clear blister; however, when a deep frostbite is rewarmed, it can form a hemorrhagic blister. This classification, however, has no therapeutic or prognostic value given that frostbites can initially appear benign. Many weeks can pass before the demarcation between viable and nonviable tissues becomes apparent. Facial frostbite, with skin blistering, can also occur following halogenated (especially fluorinated) hydrocarbon inhalation abuse. This can appear initially as angioneurotic edema if it involves the oral mucosa membranes. Acute compartment syndrome of the foot and ankle, associated with gangrenous toe changes, have been described.

Although no prognostic factors can be entirely predictive, favorable factors include retained sensation, normal skin color, and clear rather than cloudy fluid in the blisters, if present. Poor prognostic features include nonblanching cyanosis, firm skin, and dark, fluid-filled blisters. Patients can present with pain, numbness, and a clumsy "chunk of wood" sensation in the affected extremity. The pain is initially described as a dull ache and evolves to become a throbbing sensation in about 48 to 72 hours.

Chilblain
Chilblain, also referred to as perniosis, results from repetitive exposure to cold, dry air. It manifests as painful erythematous

---

[1] Not FDA approved for this indication.

nodules or cyanotic lesions often referred to as cold sores. These lesions usually develop on exposed surfaces after a delay of 12 to 14 hours and are characterized by pruritus and burning paresthesias. Young women, especially those with Raynaud phenomenon and/or a low body mass index, are at risk.

Chilblains are located on acral skin associated with cold exposure. They are usually located on the dorsum of the fingers, toes, and thighs, where blisters or ulcerations can develop in very severe cases. Perivascular lymphocytic infiltration with vacuolation of the basal layer is often seen on histologic analysis, especially when it is associated with an autoimmune disease (particularly lupus erythematosus).

Susceptibility to chilblains increases when the ambient temperature is less than 10°C and relative humidity is 60%.

Trench Foot and Immersion Foot

Trench foot occurs as a result of prolonged exposure (about 10 to 15 hours) to a damp, cold, nonfreezing environment (with temperature as high as 15°C or 59°F). It has been classically described among soldiers in World War I, many of whom were confined to cold and damp trenches for prolonged periods. Symptoms include numbness and painful paresthesias that can progress to a throbbing and burning sensation. Initial evaluation reveals a cold, pale extremity, with or without vesicles or bullae. Inflammatory serum markers, such as erythrocyte sedimentation rate (ESR) or C-reactive protein (CRP), may be elevated.

Immersion foot may be considered the sailor's counterpart to trench foot. It occurs after prolonged immersion in cold water at temperatures above freezing.

Treatment

Treatment of frostbite should begin with removing all wet or frozen clothing. For patients with moderate or severe hypothermia, initial resuscitative efforts should be geared toward raising their core temperature. The patient should be moved to a warm environment and all wet clothing should be removed. The frozen extremity should be rewarmed by immersion in circulation water at 98.6°F to 102.2°F (37.0°C to 39.0°C) for about 15 to 30 minutes. Given the risks of thermal injury, the frozen parts should not be exposed to direct or dry heat (such as hair dryers, heating pads, or heat lamps). Do not rub or massage the affected area. The process should be continued until the extremity appears warm and well perfused. Following rewarming, the extremity should be air dried and elevated. Because of the pain associated with reperfusion, there may be the temptation to abruptly abort the rewarming process. This can, however, promote further tissue damage.

Because the pain is usually prominent at night, amitriptyline (Elavil)[1] at an initial dosage of 10 to 25 mg and a maximum of 100 mg may be helpful. Gabapentin (Neurontin)[1] also may be an alternative therapy. Parenteral analgesic medications—nonsteroidal antiinflammatory drugs (NSAIDs) and opioids—may be administered as needed to make this process more tolerable. Ibuprofen at a dose of 12 mg/kg twice daily (400 mg in adults twice daily, which can be increased to a maximum of 600 mg daily) may be helpful for its analgesic and antiinflammatory effects.

Almost all authors agree that hemorrhagic blisters should not be débrided because of the risk of secondary desiccation of deep dermal layers, extending the injury. Débriding broken vesicles or bullae is also widely accepted; however, clear, intact vesicles may be broken and débrided or left intact. Topical aloe vera ointment (Dermaide Aloe)[7] or topical antibiotic ointments may be applied. Cold extremity wounds are not considered tetanus prone.

The injured tissue should be loosely covered with sterile, dry, nonadherent dressing. Hands and feet may be splinted and elevated to reduce edema. Because the damaged tissue is tetanus prone, patients whose tetanus status has not been updated may require a tetanus booster (Td).

Adjunctive agents that have been used for their antithrombotic and vasodilative properties with varying success include heparin[1], steroids[1], NSAIDs[1], dimethylsulfoxide (DMSO, Rimso-50)[1], nonionic detergents[1], dipyridamole (Persantine)[1], calcium channel blockers[1], thrombolytics, pentoxifylline (Trental)[1], and phenoxybenzamine (Dibenzyline)[1]. Hyperbaric oxygen with thrombolytic therapy has been used to treat severe frostbite of the hand. Negative pressure wound therapy, following blister excision, has been demonstrated to be beneficial in treating infant frostbite hand injures. Following rewarming, intravenous tissue plasminogen activator (TPA, Activase)[1] with an initial bolus followed by a 6- to 12-hour infusion has been utilized effectively with systemic anticoagulation and/or anti-platelet therapy to follow. Intra-arterial TPA (Activase)[1] has also been utilized. Surgical consultation is appropriate for guiding long-term management, because some patients might need débridement of infections or skin grafts for nonhealing wounds. A sympathetic nerve block (sympathectomy) can relieve painful and refractory vasospasms.

A familial association of chilblain (associated with contractual arachnodactyly) has been described in Italy. Chilblain (pernio) may be treated with nifedipine[1] at an oral dose of 20 mg three times daily. Oral prednisolone (Millipred)[1], 0.5 mg/kg in two divided doses over 2 weeks, and topical glucocorticoids have been used to treat perniosis; pentoxyfylline[1] (1200 mg/day in three divided doses for 2 weeks) has also been demonstrated to be effective. Acupuncture treatment (once weekly for 12 weeks) has been used to decrease cold sensitivity due to second-degree frostbite in the fingertips.

Sequelae

Late sequelae of frostbite include cold hypersensitivity, arthritis, numbness, chronic pain, ulceration, decreased sensation, and functional loss of the extremity. This is a result of early neuronal damage and abnormal sympathetic tone. Patients with chronic symptoms should be advised to avoid nicotine and cold exposure while using NSAIDs. Tissue demarcation can occur 60 to 90 days after initial injury. Amputation decisions should be deferred unless there is supervening sepsis or gangrene. The ultimate tissue salvage after a spontaneous slough usually far exceeds the most optimistic initial estimates. A medical simulation flow diagram is presented in Figure 1.

---

[1]Not FDA approved for this indication.

[1]Not FDA approved for this indication.
[7]Available as dietary supplement.

Figure 1 Hypothermia simulation flow diagram.

References

Albright JT, Lebovitz BL, Lipson R, et al: Upper aerodigestive tract frostbite complicating volatile substance abuse, *Int J Pediatr Otorhinolaryngol* 1:63–67, 1999.

Boada A, Bielsa I, Frenandez-Figueras MT, et al: Perniosis: clinical and histopathological analysis, *Am J Dermatopathol* 32(1):19–23, 2010.

Bottie Y, Lavolaine J, Bouzat P, et al: Neurologic recovery from profound accidental hypothermia after 5 hours of cardiopulmonary resuscitation, *Crit Care Med* 42:e167–e170, 2014.

Brandao RA, St John JM, Langan TM, et al: Acute compartment syndrome of the foot due to frostbite: literature review and case report, *Journal of Foot and Ankle Surgery* 57(2):382–387, 2018.

Bright F, Gilbert JD, Winskog C, Byard RW: Additional risk factors for lethal hypothermia, *J Forensic Leg Med* 20(6):595–597, 2013.

Bush JS, Watson S: Trench foot (updated 2018 Jan 12). In Stat Pearls (Internet), Treasure Island, FL, 2018 Jan, Stat Pearls Publishing, Available from http://www./ncbi.nim.nih.gov/books/NBK482364/.

Centers for Disease Control and Prevention (CDC): Hypothermia-related deaths—United States, 2003–2004, *MMWR Morb Mortal Wkly Rep* 54:173–175, 2005.

Danzl D: Hypothermia, *Semin Respir Crit Care Med* 23:57–68, 2002.

Danzl DF: Accidental hypothermia. In Auerbach PS, editor: *Wilderness Medicine*, 5th ed, St. Louis, 2007, Mosby, pp 125–160.

Eroglu O, Serbest S, Kufeciler T, Kalkan A: Osborn wave in hypothermia and relation to mortality, *Am J Emerg Med* 37(6):1065–1068, 2019.

Fudge J: Exercise in the cold. Preventing and managing hypothermia and frostbite injury, *Sports Health* 8(2):133–139, 2016.

Gilbert M, Busund R, Skagseth A, et al: Resuscitation from accidental hypothermia of 13.7°C with circulatory arrest, *Lancet* 355:375–376, 2000.

Gomez CR: Disorders of body temperature, *Handbook of Clinical Neurology* 120:947–957, 2014.

Handford C, Thomas O, Imray CHE: Frostbite, *Emerg Clin N Am* 35:281–299, 2017.

Herzog E, Shapiro J, Aziz EF, et al: Pathway for the management of survivors of out-of-hospital cardiac arrest, *Crit Pathw Cardiol* 9:49–54, 2010.

Higginson R: Causes of hypothermia and the use of patient-rewarming techniques, *Br J Nursing* 27(21):1222–1224, 2018.

Imray CH, Richards P, Greeves J, et al: Nonfreezing cold-induced injuries, *J R Army Med Corps* 157:79–84, 2011.

Jones LM, Coffey RA, Natwa MP, Bailey JK: The use of intravenous TPA for the treatment of severe frostbite, *Burns* 43(5):1088–1096, 2017.

Kurbat RS, Pollack Jr CV: Facial injury and airway threat from inhalant abuse: a case report, *J Emerg Med* 16(2):167–169, 1998.

Linford A, Valtonen J, Hult M, et al: The evolution of the Helsinki frostbite management protocol, *Burns* 43:1455–1463, 2017.

Lloyd EL: Accidental hypothermia, *Resuscitation* 32:111–124, 1996.

Lorentzen AK, Davis C, Penninga L: Interventions for frostbite injuries, *Cochrane Database Syst Rev* (3):CD012980, 2018. Available from: https://doi.org/10.1002/14651858.CD012980,2018.

Mazur P, Kosinski S, Podsiadlo P, et al: Extracorporeal membrane oxygenation of accidental deep hypothermia - current challenges and future perspectives, *Ann Cardiothoracic Surg* 8(1):137–142, 2019.

McCauley RD, Killyon GW, Smith Jr DJ, et al: Frostbite and other cold-induced injuries. In Auerbach PS, editor: *Wilderness Medicine*, 5th ed, St. Louis, 2007, Mosby, pp 195–210.

Mommse P, Andruszkow H, Fromke C, et al: Effects of accidental hypothermia on posttraumatic complications and outcome in multiple trauma patients, *Injury* 44:86–90, 2013.

Monti M, Mommi V, Forte MB, et al: Olazapine-associated hypothermia: a case report of a rare event, *Italian Journal of Medicine* 12:67–69, 2018.

Noaimi AA, Fadheel BM: Treatment of perniosis with oral pentoxyfylline in comparison with oral prednisolone plus topical clobetasol ointment in Iraqi patients, *Saudi Med J* 29:1762–1764, 2008.

Norheim AJ, Alraek T: Acupuncture for frostbite sequel—a case report, *European Journal of Integrative Medicine* 17:102–106, 2018.

Nygaard RM, Endorf FW. Frostbite in the United States: an examination of the national burn repository and national trauma data back. *Journal of Burn Case and Research*.irx048, Available from: https://doi.org/10.1093/jbcr/irx048

Paal P, Gordon L, Strapazzon G, et al: Accidental hypothermia-an update, *Scandinavian Journal of Trauma, Resuscitation and Emergency Medicine* 24(1):111, 2016, 10-1186/S13049-016-0303-7.

Parna SL, Wisco OJ: What is your diagnosis? Perniosis (chilblain), *Cutis* 84:27–29, 2009.

Piga M, Vacca A, Cauli A, et al: Familial chilbain and late contractual arachnodactyly: a novel association? *Joint Bone Spine* 7:205–208, 2009.

Plumb J, Thomas RG, Corneli HM: Facial frostbite associated with intentional inhalation of a commercial dusting product, *Clin Toxicol* 49:529, 2011.

Pratsinis A, Devuyst O, Leroux JC: Peritoneal dialysis beyond kidney failure? *Journal of Controlled Release,* Available from: https://doi.org/10.1016/j.jconrel.2018.01.017.

Raza N, Sajid MD, Suhail M, et al: Onset of chilblains in relation to weather conditions, *J Ayub Med Coll Abbottabad* 20:17–20, 2008.

Saczkowski RS, Brown DJA, Abu-Laban RB, et al: Prediction of survival in accidental hypothermia requiring extracorporeal life support: an individual patient meta analysis, *Resuscitation,* Available from: https://doi.org/10.1016/1.resuscitation.2018.03.028.

Ulrich AS, Rathlev NK: Hypothermia and localized cold injuries, *Emerg Med Clin North Am* 22:281–298, 2004.

Urbanic RC, Mazzaferri EL: Thyrotoxic crisis and myxedema coma, *Heart Lung* 7:435–447, 1978.

Wexler A, Zavala S: The use of thrombolytic therapy in the treatment of frostbite injury, *Journal of Burn Care and Research* 38(5):e877–e881, 2017.

Wiersinga WM: Myxedema and coma (Severe Hypothyroidism) [Updated 2018 Apr 25]. In Feingold KR, Anawalt B, Boyce A, et al: Endotext [Internet]. South Dartmouth (MA), MDText.com, Inc., 2000, Available from: https://www.ncbi.nlm.nih.gov/books/NBK279007/.

HEAT-RELATED ILLNESS

Method of
Paul Cleland, MD

CURRENT DIAGNOSIS

- Heat illness is a spectrum of illness which is usually seen among athletes in hot and humid environments.
- Children, elderly and poorly acclimatized individuals are at increased risk for developing exertional heat illness (EHI).
- Exercise-associated cramps are intense, prolonged, painful muscle spasms that occur during physical activity.
- Heat exhaustion is an elevation in core temperature (<104°F) without central nervous system (CNS) dysfunction resulting in a collapse or difficulty continuing activity.
- Heat stroke is a life-threatening illness characterized by elevation in core temperature (≥104°F) with CNS dysfunction (altered consciousness, seizure, coma) and usually end-organ damage.

CURRENT THERAPY

- Acclimatization is key for prevention of EHI.
- Heat illness is most effectively managed by immediate recognition of the signs and symptoms and proper diagnosis.
- Core temperature measurement MUST be done with a rectal thermometer.
- Exercise-Associated Collapse
  - Continue walking after race to prevent development.
  - Position the patient in a Trendelenburg position and start fluid administration.
- Heat exhaustion
  - Rapid cooling with ice bags to areas adjacent to large vasculature (groin, neck, axilla).
  - Oral or intravenous (IV) fluid administration to correct for hydration deficit.
- Heat stroke
  - Ensure the ability to maintain adequate circulation, airway, and breathing.

- Rapid cooling with ice-water immersion is the most effective way to cool.
- Goal of cooling is to reduce and maintain temperature below 101°F.
- May require transport to hospital if patient does not reduce temperature effectively or return to normal mental status after 30 minutes of medical treatment.

Heat illness is a continuum of disease that can affect a wide array of individuals including athletes, firefighters, construction workers, military, and others. Exertional heat illness (EHI) is a leading cause of death among young athletes and may be on the rise with possible climate change and increasing popularity of mass events such as marathons. Knowledge of the risk factors presented by the patient and the environment can provide clinicians with a better understanding toward prevention of heat illness. Early recognition and treatment of EHI can lead to significant reduction in the morbidity and mortality associated with this disease.

In the United States, most cases of EHI occur in summer months. Elevations in the ambient temperature and humidity as well as athletic deconditioning are predominant contributing factors. There is a rising incidence of heat illness associated with decreased heat acclimation and an increase in the wet-bulb globe temperature (WBGT). High school and collegiate athletic programs that have protocols in place to stop practice or reduce duration or frequency in certain heat situations have shown a decreased incidence of heat illness compared to those that do not.

It is important to understand the pathophysiology of the regulation of heat within the body to gain an accurate picture of heat illness. The human body has a great capacity to withstand drastic reductions in temperature to tolerate cold. However, only mild increases in core temperature can results in severe consequences. Heat is generated by normal metabolic processes that occur continuously in our bodies and is also absorbed from the environment. Exercise generates additional heat from the skeletal muscles. As a core temperature rise is detected in the hypothalamus, signals are sent out to induce sweating and cutaneous vasodilation. Blood is then shunted to the skin and exercising skeletal muscle. Under normal conditions, the body can dissipate heat through evaporation, radiation, convection, and conduction. Evaporation is the primary means of heat dissipation and occurs as water is converted from its liquid to its vapor form but becomes ineffective above a relative humidity of 75%. Radiation, convection, and conduction are also methods to dissipate heat but are decreasingly effective as the ambient temperature approaches the skin's temperature. When the physiologic cooling mechanisms fail, heat is continually produced, and the core temperature increases. As the temperature rises, cell damage occurs and a systemic inflammatory response ensues, releasing cytokines throughout the body. Blood is shunted to the peripheral circulation leading to organ hypoperfusion and ischemia. Organ failure and disseminated intravascular coagulation (DIC) will develop and eventually result in death.

The injury that occurs as a result of heat illness can be mitigated by acclimatization of the patient and is the most important factor to thrive in hot and humid conditions. Acclimatization occurs as the body is repeatedly exposed to certain levels of stress and then makes compensatory changes to allow for better performance the next time the body is under duress. This process occurs over 1 to 2 weeks of exposure to new conditions and appears to be lost with re-exposure to the previous climate for about the same time period. There are several key changes that occur as the body is exposed to heat, including: production of heat shock proteins which give cells the ability to resist heat-stress, decreased sweat temperature threshold, increased sweat production, decreased salt concentration in sweat, and increased skin blood flow. These factors all serve to aid the athlete under high-risk heat conditions to improve performance and alleviate potential heat illness. It is recommended that the athlete spend at least 2 weeks acclimatizing

TABLE 1   Substances That May Increase Risk of Heat Illness

- Amphetamines
- Anticholinergic agents
- Antiepileptic agents
- Antihistamines
- Benzodiazepines
- Beta blockers
- Calcium channel blockers
- Cocaine
- Decongestants
- Diuretics
- Ergogenic stimulants
- Ethanol
- Laxatives
- Lithium
- Phenothiazines
- Tricyclic antidepressants

Data from Bouchama, Wexler

to the environment mimicking both temperature and humidity for maximal outcome. If an athlete returns to a more temperate environment after training, such as an air-conditioned room, they would not see the same benefit as they would with exposure to the conditions for 24 hours a day. If possible, air-conditioning should be restricted to nighttime only when the athlete is resting.

Risk Factors

Although each person has unique genetic traits that determine how their body reacts to specific conditions, there are known congenital and acquired risk factors that may preclude an individual toward development of EHI. Exposure to a hot and humid environment may be the most obvious risk factor as ambient heat is transferred to the body and elevated humidity impairs the body's ability to dissipate heat. Poor conditioning, lack of acclimatization, obesity, and dehydration are all contributors that have been shown to increase the incidence of EHI. The use of prescription medications, supplements, and recreational drugs (Table 1) may cause disturbances in the capacity to dissipate heat or cause a production of heat. Creatine supplementation does not appear to impair heat dissipation or cause a negative impact on hydration.

Children are at increased risk of developing heat illness for several physiologic reasons. A larger surface area to mass ratio allows for more heat absorption from the environment. Children also produce more heat compared to their adult counterparts due to higher basal metabolic rates. Fluid is conserved more efficiently than adults and consequently children have lower sweat rates, as they depend more on non-evaporative forms of heat transfer for cooling. Children can make the same physiologic changes of acclimatization that adults can, though it appears to occur at a slower rate.

Environmental characteristics such as heat and humidity may play the largest role in development of heat illness. The wet bulb globe temperature index (WBGT) is a tool that assesses the overall environmental conditions and can accurately predict the development of EHI in a particular setting and allows for modification of work or athletic events. The WBGT is a measurement of temperature, relative humidity, and radiant heat from the sun and ground and is recommended over the use of the heat index. A dangerous clinical situation is likely to develop when activities are performed with an elevated WBGT. It is recommended that endurance events be adjusted when the WBGT exceeds 82°F (28°C) and that only events where adequate rest and recovery is observed may continue.

Heat Edema

Heat edema is caused by vasodilation of blood vessels resulting in swelling that is typically observed in the hands and feet. The core temperature of the body is not elevated. Treatment begins with removal from the hot environment, elevation of the extremities, and may involve use of compression with stockings or wrapping. Diuretics are not recommended.

Heat Cramps

Also known as exercise-associated cramps, heat cramps present as intense pain, spasm, and prolonged muscle contraction as athletes undergo high intensity activity. Although they are termed "heat cramps," they are known to occur in cool settings as well, such as swimming and winter sports. The pathophysiology has not been entirely agreed upon but seems to stem from a neurogenic response to muscle fatigue in conjunction with fluid and electrolyte losses. To make the diagnosis, no signs of other illness may be present such as rhabdomyolysis, sickle cell disease or trait, or heat stroke, and it is important to remember to take a thorough medical history to avoid pitfalls in the diagnosis.

Management consists of stretching and massaging the affected muscle and oral replacement of fluid and electrolytes. IV fluids and benzodiazepines may be used for refractory cases. One study has shown that ingestion of pickle juice at 1 mL/kg may cause a faster recovery from electrically induced muscle cramps when compared to deionized water. This would owe to the theory of a neurogenic-mediated process, as the recovery occurred before the contents of the pickle juice had time to reach the sites of action in the cramping skeletal muscle with discontinuation of cramping seen at an average of 85 seconds compared to deionized water at 134 seconds.

Exercise-Associated Collapse

Also termed Exercise-Associated Postural Hypotension, exercise-associated collapse (EAC) is an inability of the athlete to maintain a standing posture due to hypotension that develops commonly *after* an endurance event. Blood in circulation pools in the lower extremities as the athlete finishes the event and discontinues exercising. The skeletal muscles in the lower extremities normally exert a pressure on the corresponding vasculature, but as exercise ceases, the blood pools cause an unexpected drop in cranial blood pressure, triggering collapse. Heat may play an indirect role in the development of EAC, but the terms "heat syncope" and "heat collapse" are incorrect because there is no elevation in the athlete's core temperature. Athletes may develop dizziness, nausea, and vomiting as a result of the rapid drop in blood pressure.

Athletes should be encouraged to continue activity such as walking or light activity at the end of events (rather than abrupt cessation or standing in place) to continue normal blood flow to avoid a sudden collapse, risking injury. If an athlete does collapse, treatment should begin with laying the patient supine in a Trendelenburg position, keeping the legs and pelvis elevated. Administration of oral fluids containing glucose and electrolytes is helpful. Intravenous fluid administration should be reserved for those with elevated pulse (>100 bpm) or hypotension (<110 SBP) and not responding to oral fluid intake. Generally, these athletes will respond favorably within 10 to 30 minutes and should be allowed to leave under their own power.

Heat Exhaustion

Heat exhaustion occurs when the cardiovascular system is unable to provide adequate output to the body to continue to perform activity as a result of fatigue produced by exercise and environmental heat stress. This is clinically manifested most often by collapse or difficulty continuing activity that occurs *before* the event has finished. Core body temperature (rectal) is commonly elevated between 98.6°F and 104°F. It may be accompanied by nausea, vomiting, diarrhea, headache, muscle cramping, tachycardia, hypotension, weakness, dehydration, and electrolyte depletion. Dehydration can be difficult to judge clinically as the only reliable assessment of dehydration is measurement of water loss that occurs through pre-weight and post-weight measurements. A clear distinction between heat exhaustion and heat stroke is the development of CNS dysfunction such as an altered level of consciousness, delirium, or seizure. Confusion may be present but should be mild and resolve quickly with treatment measures.

Athletes with heat exhaustion should be removed from the heat and placed in a cool, shaded, or air-conditioned environment.

Vital signs including a rectal temperature should be measured to ensure the proper diagnosis is made and to be able to monitor cooling status. Any excess clothing should be removed, and the athlete should be placed in a Trendelenburg position or supine with feet elevated. Cooling may be performed initially with placement of ice bags over the groin, axilla, and neck, and water or ice-soaked towels over the head, trunk, and extremities. Immersion in an ice bath, tub of cold water, or simply running cold water from a hose over the athlete may be necessary, but these measures tend to be more for comfort as heat exhaustion is not life threatening. Oral administration of an electrolyte-containing solution is helpful to restore adequate hydration and assists in returning the cardiac output to normal. Intravenous fluid would be beneficial to individuals who do not respond or are not able to take oral fluids. Athletes who do not respond to these measures should be transported to a hospital to monitor for other developing conditions.

Heat Stroke and Heat Injury

Heat stroke is defined as a core body temperature elevated above 104°F associated with central nervous system dysfunction and end-organ damage. The CNS dysfunction can be observed in several ways, including: confusion, delirium, aggression or irritability, seizures, altered consciousness, and coma. Heat stroke can occur as classic heat stroke (non-exertional) or exertional heat stroke. Classic heat stroke usually afflicts the elderly population in the summer season and can be related to a lack of access to adequate air-conditioning. Heat is continually absorbed from the environment and may be poorly dissipated secondary to other medical conditions and medications that preclude cooling. Exertional heat stroke is seen in a younger and more athletic population and does not necessarily occur in hot and humid environments. Other signs and symptoms are similar to those seen in heat exhaustion, but vital sign abnormalities are more likely to be present. The presence or absence of sweating does not make a diagnosis of heat stroke. Examining a collapsed individual can be difficult and the differential diagnosis can extend beyond heat exhaustion and heat stroke to include cardiac arrhythmia and exercise-associated hyponatremia. It is important to maintain a degree of suspicion for those athletes who present with collapse but do not have an elevated core temperature.

The term heat injury is not currently recognized by the World Health Organization as a diagnosis but was created by the US military physicians to further categorize patients suffering from heat illness. Heat injury is diagnosed as an elevation in core temperature above 104°F with associated end-organ damage but lacks the CNS dysfunction seen in heat stroke. Organs most commonly affected with heat stroke or injury include the liver, kidneys, and skeletal muscle (rhabdomyolysis).

Individuals who present with heat stroke should be assessed beginning with basic life support measures. Secure the airway and make sure adequate circulation and breathing are maintained. An initial set of vital signs including a rectal temperature should be performed and repeated throughout the course of treatment. If a rectal thermometer is not available, do not use other methods to determine temperature, as these are inaccurate to measure core temperature in athletes who have been exercising. If available, rapid assessment of serum electrolytes including sodium and glucose should be done, especially with longer endurance events such as marathons. Rapid cooling should commence as soon as possible after the diagnosis is made, as the prognosis worsens the longer the core temperature is elevated. The most effective cooling measure is ice-water immersion and expected cooling rates are about 1°F per 3 minutes or 1°C per 5 minutes of immersion. Measurement with a rectal thermistor allows for continuous monitoring but if this is not available, measurement by a rectal thermometer should be done approximately once every 10 minutes. Cooling should continue until the core temperature reaches

101°F. If no rectal thermometer is available, cool until the athlete begins to shiver or about 15 to 20 minutes. If other interventions need to be performed (intubation, administration of IV medications or fluid) and ice-water immersion is not practical, other cooling tactics such as ice bags to the groin, axilla, and neck, and placement of ice or water-soaked towels to the rest of the body should be performed. Fluid resuscitation should be performed but careful attention should be paid to fluid overload as pulmonary edema can develop with rapid administration of IV fluids. Despite rapid reduction in core temperature, these individuals are still at risk for organ damage and transport to the hospital is usually necessary, where appropriate monitoring and lab evaluation can be performed. Transport to the hospital is always required in patients who do not regain consciousness within 30 minutes of appropriate cooling and medical intervention, or if appropriate response to cooling is not achieved.

Return to Play

The prognosis for returning to physical activity after an episode of EHI is dependent upon the individual and the severity of the illness incurred. Athletes who develop heat cramps or EAC should be allowed to return to activity as soon as they feel capable. Decisions about returning those who develop heat exhaustion or heat stroke are more complicated. These athletes should avoid physical activity for at least 7 days. All lab abnormalities should be corrected, and the athlete should feel physically and psychologically capable of returning. Once these conditions are met, a gradual progression of activity can begin in a cool or temperate environment. Acclimatization occurs over a period of approximately 2 weeks as activity is increased in duration and intensity and the individual is gradually reexposed to heat. Once the athlete can perform full-intensity workouts for 2 to 4 weeks in the heat, they may be returned to competition. For individuals who fail to acclimatize at 4 weeks or who have had multiple episodes of EHI, an exercise-heat tolerance test should be performed.

References

American College of Sports Medicine, Armstrong LE, Casa DJ, et al: American College of Sports Medicine Position Stand. Exertional heat illness during training and competition, *Medicine & Science in Sports & Exercise* 39:556–572, 2007.

Asplund CA, O'Connor FG: Challenging return to play decisions: heat stroke, exertional rhabdomyolysis, and exertional collapse associated with sickle cell trait, *Sports Health* 8(2):117–125, 2016 Mar-Apr.

Boeckmann M, Rohn I: Is planned adaptation to heat reducing heat-related mortality and illness? A systematic review, *BMC Public Health* 14:1112, 2014 Oct 28.

Bouchama A, Knochel JP: Heat Stroke, *New England Journal of Medicine* 346(25):1978–1988, 2002. June 20.

Brukner P, Karim K, Noakes T: Exercise in the Heat. *In Brukner & Khan's Clinical Sports Medicine*, 4th ed., Sydney, 2012, McGraw-Hill, pp 1132–1143.

Cooper ER, Ferrara MS, Casa DJ, et al: Exertional heat illness in american football players: when is the risk greatest? *Journal of Athletic Training* 51(8):593–600, 2016.

Gaudio FG, Grissom CK: Cooling methods in heat stroke, *Journal of Emergency Medicine* 50(4):607–616, 2016 Apr.

Ishimine, P. Heat Stroke in Children. *UpToDate*. N.p., 26 Oct. 2016. Web. 1 Jan. 2017.

Lopez RM, Casa DJ, McDermott BP, et al: Does creatine supplementation hinder exercise heat tolerance or hydration status? A systematic review with meta-analyses, *J Athl Train*. 44(2):215–223, 2009 Mar.

Maron BJ, Doerer JJ, Haas TS, et al: Sudden deaths in young competitive athletes: analysis of 1866 deaths in the United States, 1980-2006, *Circulation* 119(8):1085–1092, 2009.

Miller KC, Mack GW, Knight KL, et al: Reflex inhibition of electrically induced muscle cramps in hypohydrated humans, *Medicine & Science in Sports & Exercise* 42(5):953–961, 2010. May.

O'Connor FG, Casa DJ. Exertional heat illness in adolescents and adults: epidemiology, thermoregulation, risk factors, and diagnosis. *UpToDate*. N.p., 12 Nov 2018. Web. 22 July 2019.

Wexler RK: Evaluation and treatment of heat-related illnesses, *American Family Physician* 65:2307–2314, 2002.

Yeargin SW, Kerr ZY, Casa DJ, et al: Epidemiology of exertional heat illnesses in youth, high school, and college football, *Medicine & Science in Sports & Exercise* 48(8):1523–1529, 2016 Aug.

Zurawlew MJ, Walsh NP, et al: Post-exercise hot water immersion induces heat acclimation and improves endurance exercise performance in the heat, *Scandinavian Journal of Medicine & Science in Sports* 26(7):745–754, 2016 Jul.

HIGH ALTITUDE ILLNESS

Method of
Adrienne N. Kovalsky, DO, MPH; and Ryan M. Commins, MD

CURRENT DIAGNOSIS

Acclimatization
- Symptoms include exertional dyspnea, increased respiratory rate, polyuria, peripheral edema, and insomnia.

High Altitude Headache (HAH)
- New-onset headache that fulfills at least two of the following:
  - Develops in temporal relation to altitude gain above 2500 m (8000 ft)
  - Worsens in conjunction with continued ascent and/or resolves within 24 hours of descent below 2500 m (8000 ft)
  - Includes at least two of the following characteristics: bilateral; mild or moderate intensity; aggravated by exertion, movement, straining, coughing, and/or bending

Acute Mountain Sickness (AMS)
- New-onset headache occurs within 12 hours of altitude gain above 2500 m (8000 ft), and
- Anorexia, nausea, vomiting, fatigue, weakness, dizziness, or lightheadedness (see Box 3).

High Altitude Cerebral Edema (HACE)
- Mental status changes or ataxia with preexisting AMS, or
- Mental status changes and ataxia without a prodrome of AMS

High Altitude Pulmonary Edema (HAPE)
- Relative hypoxemia in the setting of at least two signs or symptoms from each of the following lists:
  - Resting dyspnea, cough, weakness, decreased exercise performance, and chest tightness or congestion
  - Wheezing, rales, tachypnea, tachycardia, or central cyanosis

CURRENT THERAPY

Insomnia or Sleep Disturbance
- Acetazolamide (Diamox)[1] 125 mg PO at bedtime is recommended.
- Consider diphenhydramine (Benadryl) 50 mg at bedtime, zolpidem (Ambien) 5–10 mg at bedtime, or temazepam (Restoril) 15 mg at bedtime for patients with no history of altitude illness.

High Altitude Headache
- Medications for headache include ibuprofen (Advil) 600–800 mg PO every 8 hours, acetaminophen (Tylenol) 650–1000 mg PO every 6 hours, enteric-coated aspirin (Ecotrin) 325–650 mg PO every 4 hours, oxygen by nasal cannula at 1–2 L/min, or acetazolamide[1] 125 mg PO twice daily.

Acute Mountain Sickness, Mild
- Avoid respiratory depressants, strenuous activity, or further ascent until the patient is asymptomatic.
- Acetazolamide 125–250 mg PO twice daily may be tried.
- Symptomatic treatment as for headache and nausea.

Acute Mountain Sickness, Moderate to Severe
- Stop ascent and rest until asymptomatic AND:
  - Administer acetazolamide 250 mg PO twice daily.
  - Oxygen (1–2 L) or hyperbaric chamber 2–4 psi may be used if available.
  - Consider dexamethasone (Decadron)[1] 4 mg PO or IM every 6 hours as an adjunct or if acetazolamide is contraindicated.

- Monitor for mental status changes, confusion, or ataxia and descend immediately at onset.
- If symptoms are severe, or if there is no response to 24 hours of therapy, immediate descent of at least 500 m or to last asymptomatic altitude is the definitive treatment.

High Altitude Cerebral Edema
- Prepare for evacuation or emergent descent of at least 1000 m (3,280 ft).
- Administer dexamethasone[1] 8 mg PO, IM, or IV once followed by 4 mg every 6 hours.
- Consider adding acetazolamide[1] 250 mg PO twice daily as an adjunct.
- Early recognition and treatment are essential.

High Altitude Pulmonary Edema
- Bed rest with oxygen 4–6 L by nasal cannula.
- If the patient is not improving or if HAPE is severe, descend at least 500 m, avoiding exertion.
- Use a hyperbaric chamber at 2–4 psi if oxygen is unavailable or the patient is unable to descend.
- If oxygen is unavailable or the patient is unable to descend, or if the patient is not responding to either:
  - Give nifedipine (Procardia)[1] 10 mg PO once and 30 mg extended-release PO every 12 to 24 hours[3] (contraindicated in HACE).
  - Consider adding tadalafil (Cialis)[1] 10 mg PO twice daily[3], sildenafil (Viagra)[1] 50 mg PO thrice daily[3], or salmeterol (Serevent)[1] 125 µg inhaled twice daily[3].
  - It is not advisable to use both nifedipine and a phosphodiesterase inhibitor; if this becomes necessary, carefully monitor blood pressure and stagger doses to prevent potential cerebral hypoperfusion.

Concurrent High Altitude Pulmonary and Cerebral Edema
- As always, immediate descent and supplemental oxygen therapy are critical.
- Treatment as for HAPE with the addition of dexamethasone.[1]

---

[1]Not FDA approved for this indication.
[3]Exceeds dosage recommended by the manufacturer.

The appeal of travel to high altitude is vast. For many it is tourism, skiing, or mountaineering, but for others it is far more fundamental, as many travel to high altitudes for work. The number of people residing at elevations higher than 1500 m has risen significantly in the last two decades, and is approximately 440 million worldwide. While elevation greater than 1500 m (5000 ft) is generally considered high altitude (Denver, for example, is 1609 m or 5,278 ft), most high altitude illness occurs above 2500 m or 8000 ft. It is at these altitudes that the effects of hypoxia and decreasing barometric pressure start to be seen. Elevation greater than 5500 m (18,000 ft) is considered extreme altitude. Many persons become symptomatic during the adaptive process known as acclimatization, and some develop acute high altitude syndromes, including acute mountain sickness (AMS), high altitude cerebral edema (HACE), and high altitude pulmonary edema (HAPE). These syndromes are often preventable, but they have the potential to cause significant morbidity and mortality for the patient and for those involved in risky rescue efforts by land or air.

Epidemiology and Risk Factors
The incidence of altitude illnesses is highly variable and commonly idiosyncratic. At 3000 m (~10,000 ft) the incidence of AMS ranges from 4% to 58%, whereas the incidence of HAPE and HACE generally is less than 1%. The occurrence of altitude illness depends on the rate of ascent, altitude of residence, exertion, prior history of altitude illness, and individual susceptibility. For each 1000 m (3,280 ft) above 2500 m (8,000 ft) the rate of AMS increases 13%. The most predictive risk factor for AMS is previous AMS, and the risk of recurrence in similar elevations

is as high as 60%. Physical fitness does not alter susceptibility, whereas obesity is a risk factor. Tobacco smoking, asthma, and diabetes do not confer any additional risk. Certain medical conditions including chronic obstructive pulmonary disease, pulmonary hypertension, congestive heart failure, coronary artery disease, sickle cell disease, and sleep apnea increase risk of developing altitude illness. Stable and well-controlled conditions such as hypertension and diabetes do not appear to increase the risk for altitude illness. A more detailed discussion of some of these diseases is included later in the text.

Physiologic Adaptation and Pathophysiology

Hypoxia inducible factors (HIFs) are a family of transcription regulators that respond to level of oxygenation and ultimately control the physiologic response to hypoxia. In hypoxic conditions, they are able to increase transcription of hypoxia-responsive genes. The HIFs have a wide range of effects including increasing glycolysis and angiogenesis, stimulating erythropoiesis, regulating endothelial nitric oxide synthase, and controlling ventilation.

The physiologic response to altitude rests along one end of a spectrum of compensatory mechanisms that can evolve into to high altitude syndromes. The pathophysiology of AMS and HACE is incompletely understood, but hypoxemia and changes in the brain itself have been implicated. Hypoxemia is thought to increase cerebral blood flow though it is unclear whether there is a true difference in cerebral blood flow in patients with and without AMS. Hypoxemia may also increase vascular permeability through various mechanisms. Changes that occur in the brain include edema, increased ICP, vascular distention due to increased intravascular pressure, and release of nociceptive chemicals or substances. The development of HAPE is usually preceded by an excessive rise in the pulmonary artery pressure in response to hypoxic vasoconstriction. However, other factors including alveolar inflammation, impaired sodium and water reabsorption by the alveolar epithelium and uneven hypoxic vasoconstriction may also play a role.

In the first few hours at high altitude, peripheral chemoreceptors are activated by hypoxia, leading to an increased respiratory rate. The increased minute ventilation reduces the dilutional effects of CO_2 in the alveolar air and causes a respiratory alkalosis. This subsequent alkalosis also improves oxygen binding in the lung but ultimately slows respiration. After 24 to 48 hours the kidneys excrete excess bicarbonate, normalizing the elevated pH that would otherwise prevent an adequate increase in respiration. This is the basis for acclimatization.

Periodic breathing is also more likely to occur at higher elevations owing to hypoxia and the resulting respiratory alkalosis. Altitude-dependent diuresis causes transient hemoconcentration in the first 1 to 2 days, with true erythropoiesis starting at 4 to 5 days. Long-term residence at altitude can cause polycythemia, increasing the risk for tissue infarction. With permanent residence at high altitude there is evidence that cognitive development may be slowed in children and that neuropsychological function is impaired in adults. Permanent residents will see improved maximal oxygen consumption at lower elevations. The most complex effects of hypobaric hypoxia are seen in the lung and the brain and are not completely understood.

Prevention

High altitude illness is a morbid and potentially fatal disease, and preventive measures should be employed. The most reliable way to prevent altitude illness is through graded ascent, thereby allowing sufficient time for acclimatization. A conservative guideline for activities above 2500 m (8,000 ft) is increasing sleep altitude by no more than 300 m (1000 ft) in a 24-hour period and with an additional rest day every 1000 m (3,280 ft). If symptoms of AMS are noted, no further ascent should be attempted until they resolve in order to prevent more severe illness or evolution of HACE or HAPE. Additional preventive measures should be taken and are of particular importance for persons planning rapid ascent, whether on foot or flying directly into altitudes of

---

| BOX 1 | Prevention of High Altitude Sickness |

Ascent above 2500 m (8,000 ft) should be at a gradual rate of 300 m per 24 hours, with an additional rest day for every 1000 m (3,280 ft) gain

With rapid ascent above 2500 m (8,000 ft), light activity may be helpful with acclimatization, but strenuous activity should be avoided for at least 48 hours.

Avoid respiratory depressants such as alcohol until acclimatized.

Five days of comparable altitude exposure should be undertaken within 2 months of ascent.

For AMS or HACE, begin prophylaxis 1 or 2 days before starting ascent:

- Acetazolamide 125 mg PO bid
- Dexamethasone[1] 2 mg q6 or 4 mg q12 h for patients with sulfa allergy
- Prophylaxis is strongly recommended for patients with a history of AMS or HACE or for rapid ascent.

For persons with a history of HAPE, begin prophylaxis 1 day before starting ascent:

- Nifedipine[1] 30 mg BID[3]
- Salmeterol[1] (adjuct) 125 µg inhaled bid[3]
- Dexamethasone[1] 8 mg PO bid
- Tadalafil (Cialis)[1] 10 mg PO bid[3]
- Sildenafil (Viagra)[1] 50 mg PO tid[3]

Stop ascent with onset of even mild AMS to prevent evolution to HACE.

Abbreviations: AMS = acute mountain sickness; HACE = high altitude cerebral edema; HAPE = high altitude pulmonary edema.
[1]Not FDA approved for this indication.
[3]Exceeds dosage recommended by the manufacturer.

2500 m (8,000 ft) or greater. Light activity can accelerate acclimatization, but strenuous exertion should be avoided in the first 2 days. Pre-exposure of 5 days of comparable altitude within 2 months of ascent is protective. CNS depressants such as alcohol are thought to worsen effects of altitude, particularly overnight when respiration is already more depressed, and they should be avoided. Abrupt cessation of caffeine intake in chronic users may provoke withdrawal symptoms that can mimic AMS. If available, residing and working in an oxygen-enriched environment may also help reduce the incidence of AMS. Refer to Box 1 for a summary.

Medical prophylaxis should be considered when graded ascent is not possible, whether on foot or flying directly into altitudes of 2500 m (8,000 ft) or greater, and for persons with any history of prior altitude illness returning to the same elevation. Prophylaxis is also advised for ascent profiles that are considered moderate to high risk in patients with unknown susceptibility, including planned ascent to more than 3000 m (10,000 ft) in one day, rapid ascent greater than 500 m (1,640 ft) per day above 3000 m (10,000 ft), or very rapid ascent to a final altitude greater than 4000 m (13,000 ft). This should be started the day prior to beginning ascent and continue until at a stable altitude for at least 2 to 4 days. If further ascent is undertaken, or if symptoms recur, prophylaxis can be restarted at any point.

The most effective medication for prophylaxis of AMS and HACE is acetazolamide (Diamox) 125 mg PO twice daily starting 1–2 days before ascent. This is a central-acting respiratory stimulant that causes a metabolic acidosis and ultimately facilitates acclimatization. Patients should be warned about side effects and possible allergy (Box 2). Dexamethasone (Decadron)[1] 2 mg every 6 hours or 4 mg every 12 hours also is effective, though its mechanism is not completely understood. Unlike with acetazolamide,

---

[1] Not FDA approved for this indication.

BOX 2   Medications for AMS, HACE, and HAPE

Acetazolamide

Acetazolamide (Diamox) is a central-acting respiratory stimulant that causes a metabolic acidosis and ultimately facilitates acclimatization. It is effective in preventing and treating AMS and HACE.[1] Patients should be warned about side effects, including paresthesias, flat taste of carbonated beverages, and polyuria, particularly at night. Persons with a history of asthma, sulfonamide allergy, anaphylaxis, or penicillin allergy should try this medication under the supervision of a medical professional prior to departure. It should not be used in type 1 diabetics due to the risk for ketoacidosis. It also should not be used in chronic lung disease if FEV_1 is less than 25% predicted, in patients on potassium-wasting diuretics, or on long-term high doses of aspirin.

Dexamethasone

Dexamethasone (Decadron)[1] is also effective in the prevention and treatment of AMS and HACE, though its mechanism is not completely understood. Unlike with acetazolamide, symptoms can recur after stopping treatment, and it does not facilitate acclimatization. It is not recommended for prophylaxis of AMS unless acetazolamide is contraindicated, though it is the drug of choice for treatment of HACE. Use is cautioned in diabetics due to hyperglycemia and in patients at risk for amebiasis or strongyloides.

Nifedipine

Nifedipine (Procardia)[1] is a calcium channel blocker that inhibits pulmonary vasoconstriction secondary to hypoxia at high altitude and is used in treatment and prevention of HAPE. Caution should be used with other antihypertensives due to risk for hypotension. Medications that inhibit the cytochrome P450 3A4 pathway, including macrolides, doxycycline, and azoles, may increase plasma concentrations and also precipitate hypotension. Ginkgo biloba[7] may also increase levels of nifedipine and cause hypotension and should be avoided.

Tadalafil (Cialis) and sildenafil (Viagra)

These are phosphodiesterase inhibitors[1] that cause pulmonary vasodilation and are used in preventing HAPE. They should not be used in conjunction with nitrates due to risk for significant hypotension, nor with alpha-blockers due to orthostatic hypotension. Medications that inhibit the cytochrome P450 3A4 pathway, including macrolides, doxycycline, and azoles, may increase plasma concentrations and also precipitate hypotension.

Abbreviations: AMS = acute mountain sickness; HACE = high altitude cerebral edema; HAPE = high altitude pulmonary edema
[1]Not FDA approved for this indication.
[7]Available as a dietary supplement.

---

symptoms can recur after stopping dexamethasone, and it does not facilitate acclimatization. It is not recommended for prophylaxis unless acetazolamide is contraindicated, and it is best saved for treatment of severe AMS or HACE. Ginkgo biloba[7] is no better than placebo at preventing AMS. Ibuprofen (Advil)[1] has not been shown to prevent AMS but does prevent high altitude headache.

Prophylaxis of HAPE has been studied in preventing recurrence in persons with a history of HAPE, though it also would be prudent to consider prophylaxis for anyone undertaking very rapid ascent. Numerous agents have been evaluated in patients with history of HAPE and are listed in Box 1. Nifedipine (Procardia)[1]

is the preferred medication for prevention, with salmeterol (Serevent)[1] as a potential adjunct if there is significant history of HAPE and anticipated rapid ascent profile.

Symptomatic Acclimatization and Disrupted Sleep

Many people experience symptoms of normal adaptation that do not always herald illness, but they should nonetheless always be completely evaluated. Expected symptoms include exertional dyspnea, polyuria, peripheral and facial edema, and nocturnal awakenings and insomnia. The most common side effects of normal acclimatization are disrupted sleep and mild peripheral edema. Acetazolamide[1] 125 mg at bedtime has been shown to decrease nocturnal oxygen saturation and lessen awakenings (see Box 2). Diphenhydramine (Benadryl)[1] 25 to 50 mg may also be used, but it does not have the same benefits. Studies have shown that zolpidem (Ambien)[1] 10 mg and temazepam (Restoril)[1] 15 mg are probably safe, but because studies have been small and targeted, these medications probably should be avoided whenever possible, particularly in persons with a history of altitude illness.

High Altitude Headache

Headache is a common occurrence and does not always evolve into AMS. The headache is generally bilateral, and throbbing is exacerbated with coughing, bending, straining, and exertion, and is often worst early in the morning. There should be no other associated symptoms. Onset can occur within 1 hour but usually begins within 6 to 10 hours. Numerous medications are effective for treatment, including analgesics and medications used in prophylaxis of AMS. See the Current Therapy box for a complete listing.

High Altitude Syndromes

Acute Mountain Sickness

In the setting of a recent gain in altitude, AMS is defined as headache with at least one of the following: anorexia, nausea, or vomiting; fatigue or weakness; or dizziness or lightheadedness. Clinically, a lack of headache with otherwise suggestive symptoms should not rule out AMS. As with high altitude headache, onset can occur within 1 hour but usually begins within 6 to 10 hours. Other symptoms can include decreased urine output, lassitude, and ataxia. All symptoms typically resolve within 2 to 3 days, though on occasion at higher altitudes symptoms can persist for days or weeks without progression or resolution. Examination is normal and no diagnostic studies are indicated. The differential includes dehydration, exhaustion, hangover, viral illness, carbon monoxide poisoning, caffeine withdrawal, migraine, and meningitis. Early recognition of AMS is essential in order to begin appropriate measures that might help prevent evolution to the potentially fatal HACE, which exists along the same spectrum.

If mild, AMS can be monitored at a stable altitude with no further ascent undertaken. Analgesics and antiemetics are effective for managing symptoms. Acetazolamide may be considered for mild AMS and is recommended for moderate to severe symptoms. Dexamethasone[1] may be added, or used in substitution if intolerant of or allergic to acetazolamide, for a short course (less than 5 days) while acclimatizing. Low-flow supplemental oxygen and hyperbaric chambers can be used as an adjunct for moderate to severe symptoms. Descent is advised for symptoms that progress after 24 hours of rest or treatment or for symptoms that are severe or stable but prolonged in order to prevent evolution to HACE, but graded ascent can be resumed once symptoms resolve. Immediate descent should be undertaken for ataxia, altered mental status, or any signs or symptoms of pulmonary edema. Refer to the Current Therapy box for dosing and summary.

High Altitude Cerebral Edema

In the setting of a recent gain in altitude, HACE is defined as a change in mental status and/or ataxia in a person with AMS, or

---

[1]Not FDA approved for this indication.
[7]Available as a dietary supplement.

[1]Not FDA approved for this indication.

both mental status changes and ataxia in a person without AMS. There may be changes in mood or hallucinations. It generally progresses over 1 to 3 days, but it can also cause loss of consciousness within 12 hours. Examination has nonfocal neurologic findings with confusion. Papilledema may be seen, and rales are often present from concurrent HAPE. If computed tomography (CT) or magnetic resonance imaging (MRI) is available acutely, findings would be consistent with vasogenic edema. If a lumbar puncture is performed, increased opening pressure is usually present.

Differential diagnosis is similar to that for AMS but should be expanded to include diabetic ketoacidosis, hypoglycemia, electrolyte imbalances, brain tumor, stroke, acute psychosis, and seizure. After a long term at altitude or any length of time at very high altitudes blood can become hyperviscous and increasingly thrombogenic, so in these circumstances stroke should rise on the differential.

Early recognition is crucial in management of HACE to prevent evolution to irreversible disease. The most important element of treatment is descent of at least 1000 m (3,280 ft). Supplemental oxygen and hyperbaric bags may be used during descent and are imperative if descent is not possible. Dexamethasone[1] should be initiated, and should be continued after descent if symptoms persist. Acetazolamide[1] may be added. Dosages are listed in the Current Therapy box.

High Altitude Pulmonary Edema

In the setting of a recent gain in altitude, HAPE is diagnosed with at least two of resting dyspnea, cough, weakness or decreased exercise performance, and chest tightness or congestion and two of wheezing or rales, tachypnea, tachycardia, or central cyanosis. There may also be an associated low-grade temperature elevation. Cough is initially dry but in late stages is productive of pink or bloody sputum. Onset often occurs during sleep, usually the second night at altitude, and often after the use of sleep aids that cause respiratory depression. It rarely occurs after 4 or 5 days at a stable altitude and should resolve within 48 hours of descent.

Examination is significant for rales that can begin in the right axilla and progress diffusely and for low-grade temperature elevation. Hypoxia, often very pronounced, is noted on pulse oximetry; oxygen levels will be disproportionately low for a given elevation. If available, chest radiography typically demonstrates bilaterally diffuse patchy opacities without pulmonary vascular changes, though initially they may be seen in the right middle lobe. Computed tomography of the chest typically shows a patchy peripheral and nodular distribution of edema. Ultrasound may be more readily available than radiography in remote locations and through the use of the comet-tail technique may be helpful in identifying HAPE and differentiating from pneumonia or other conditions.

HAPE can occur in conjunction with severe AMS or HACE. Differential includes heart failure, acute myocardial ischemia, pulmonary embolus, asthma, bronchitis, and pneumonia. Among the altitude illnesses, HAPE is associated with the highest rate of mortality but, unlike HACE, it is unlikely to cause long-term sequelae if treated appropriately. As with all altitude illness, removing the hypoxic stimulus is the central principle in management, and with HAPE it is also the most effective. This can be done with descent, supplemental oxygen, or a hyperbaric chamber. If available, supplemental oxygen and bed rest may be sufficient. If the pulmonary edema is severe, descent is the definitive treatment and should be undertaken without delay. Exertion and cold stress should be avoided during descent. Nifedipine (Adalat, Procardia)[1] and salmeterol (Serevent)[1] may be of benefit in treatment of HAPE, but they are not as effective as oxygen or descent and should be used as an adjunct or if no other alternatives exist. Dual vasodilating agent use (nifedipine[1] and a phosphodiesterase inhibitor[1]) is not recommended, but if attempted when no alternatives exist, doses should be staggered and blood pressure

carefully monitored to prevent potentially disastrous hypotension and cerebral hypoperfusion. Refer to the Current Therapy box for dosing. Reascent may be considered 2 to 3 days after resolution, but risk of recurrence is significantly higher.

Other High Altitude Disorders
Upper Respiratory Disorders

Rhinorrhea, chronic cough, and noninfectious pharyngitis and bronchitis are commonly seen at high altitude and very prevalent at extreme altitude. Sputum is often purulent. Onset of high altitude bronchitis and chronic cough is generally after strenuous activity, and use of a balaclava to increase humidification of inhaled air may help prevent this. Symptoms may become severe enough to cause rib fracture. Comprehensive studies on the most effective treatment are lacking, but symptomatic therapies may be helpful, including decongestant nasal sprays, inhaled corticosteriods and beta agonists, and codeine-based cough medications; the latter should never be used in the pediatric population or in combination with other opiate medications or benzodiazepines. Infectious upper respiratory syndromes should remain in the differential; however, viral etiologies are most common with judicious consideration of antibiotic therapy.

High Altitude Retinopathy (HAR)

Hypoxia is known to cause hyperemia and engorgement of the retinal vessels at any elevation, and will be seen above 2500 meters (8,000 ft) in the setting of hypobaric hypoxia. Evolution to retinal hemorrhage indicates the presence of high altitude retinopathy (HAR) and may occur above 4000 meters (13,000 ft). Macular or vitreous hemorrhage, disc edema, and cotton wool spots can be seen in more severe HAR. There may be a delay between ascent and onset of hemorrhage. The retinopathy is generally asymptomatic; however, scotomas and visual field deficits may occur, particularly with macular hemorrhage.

Lower oxygen saturation, higher ascent, strenuous exertion, and longer duration at high altitude are associated with HAR. Higher baseline intraocular pressure, hypercoagulable disorders, and aspirin and NSAID use also appear to be risk factors. Slower ascent and improved acclimatization are protective. Acetazolamide does not appear to affect incidence. Recent research has not shown a definitive correlation between HAR and AMS or HACE.

Most HAR will resolve within days to weeks of descent. Rarely visual deficits have persisted longer. Descent is recommended for any premacular hemorrhage due to higher risk to central vision and unclear long-term prognosis, as well as any new visual deficits. Given the potential risk of worsening retinopathy, diabetics and other patients with risk for or preexisting retinopathy should avoid travel to elevations greater than 4000 meters (13,000 ft), and consult with their ophthalmologist if such travel is unavoidable or if any travel is intended above 2500 meters (8,000 ft).

Chronic High Altitude Diseases

Residence above 2500 meters (8,000 ft) in the United States is rising, and numbers in the hundreds of millions worldwide. Prevalence is dependent on many factors, most notably residence altitude and ethnicity. Ethnic groups with longer history of high altitude residence, such as Tibetans, have improved adaptation and lower prevalence compared to other ethnic groups at the same elevation. Prevalence increases with increasing altitude, even among more adapted ethnic groups.

Chronic Mountain Sickness (CMS). Symptoms include headache, dizziness, dyspnea, palpitations, insomnia, fatigue, arthralgias, myalgias, distal peripheral paresthesias, anorexia, and cognitive dysfunction. Diagnosis is made by excessive erythrocytosis (hemoglobin greater than 19 g/dL in women or 21 g/dL in men) in the setting of severe hypoxemia (there is not yet consensus on threshold value, but less than <85% is highly suggestive), normal pulmonary function tests, and chronic residence above 2500 meters (8,000 ft). Pulmonary hypertension and heart failure may also be present. Patients with a history of

---

[1] Not FDA approved for this indication.

antecedent chronic pulmonary disease such as COPD or other medical condition that may account for hypoxia are excluded from this diagnosis, as the presentation cannot be fully attributed to altitude, though consideration for a diagnosis of secondary CMS may be made. Phlebotomy, optimally with isovolemic hemodilution, provides temporary benefit and may result in more significant recurrence and is not recommended as a long-term solution. Consideration may be made for severe symptoms or as a short-term bridge to permanent resettlement at lower elevation. Supplemental oxygen, slow breathing technique, a supervised mild to moderate exercise regimen, and intermittent pulses of acetazolamide[1] 250 mg per day for three weeks have all been found to help. Other medications are still being studied. Strenuous activity should be avoided. Definitive therapy is migration to lower elevations, upon which CMS will slowly resolve, but will reappear upon return to high altitude. Periodic travel to lower altitude is recommended if permanent migration is not possible.

High Altitude Pulmonary Hypertension (HAPH). Symptoms include cough, dyspnea, cyanosis, and insomnia, and may include physical findings of right heart failure. Diagnosis is made by a mean pulmonary artery pressure greater than 30 mmHg or systolic pulmonary artery pressure greater than 50 mmHg measured at altitude of residence with moderate hypoxemia, absence of excessive erythrocytosis, and chronic residence above 2500 meters (8,000 ft) after the exclusion of chronic lung disease and other causes of pulmonary hypertension. Screening diagnosis should be made by echocardiography and confirmed via invasive measurement. As with CMS, definitive therapy is migration to low altitude. If this is not feasible, calcium channel blockers and phosphodiesterase inhibitors may be of benefit. Early referral to a pulmonary hypertension specialist is recommended.

Additional Considerations

Traveling to high altitude with children, during pregnancy or in the setting of chronic medical conditions includes additional considerations, some of which are summarized below. Patients should include consultation with the patient's pediatrician, obstetrician, or specialist prior to travel. Complete medication list, including as-needed prescriptions for travel, such as antibiotics, should be carefully reviewed for interactions, contraindications, and dose adjustments prior to prescribing medications for prevention or treatment of altitude illness. Refer to Box 2 for a limited summary.

Children

Susceptibility of the pediatric population to altitude illness is comparable to that of the adult population. Travel to high altitude should not be undertaken in first 4 to 6 weeks or in prematurity. It should also be avoided in any children with history of cardiopulmonary conditions, Down syndrome, at increased risk for pulmonary hypertension, or a recent upper respiratory illness. Presentation will generally mimic that in adults; however, assessment of nonverbal children is more complicated with criteria including fussiness, decreased playfulness, decreased appetite, and sleep disturbance. Physical findings are similar to the adult population and may also include agitation, productive cough, cyanosis, and tachycardia. Management and prevention are comparable with the following dosage adjustments: acetazolamide* 2.5 mg/kg every 12 hours can be used for prevention and treatment of both AMS and HACE[1]. Dexamethasone[1] 0.15 mg/kg every 6 hours should be used for treatment of severe AMS and HACE, in conjunction with descent. Medications to prevent and treat HAPE have not been adequately studied in the pediatric population.

Pregnant Women

Women who travel to high altitude during pregnancy are at higher risk for preterm labor, but the rate of complications does not appear to be significantly changed in the setting of uncomplicated low-risk pregnancy, and travel to 2500 meters (8,000 ft) is likely safe. While exercise during pregnancy is associated with better outcome, it should be minimized the first few days at high altitude while acclimatizing, and strenuous exertion should be avoided. Most medications used for the treatment of high altitude illness are rated category C for pregnancy, and priority should be made for descent rather than medical management of altitude illness. Travel to high altitude should be avoided in any pregnancy that is complicated or not low risk. Residence at high altitude during pregnancy is associated with a decrease in birth rate in proportion to the increase in altitude, as well as increased complications, although highland ancestry is protective.

Hypertension

Blood pressure response to high altitude is variable. Adequately controlled hypertension should not confer any additional risk for altitude illness. Any patient requiring more than one medication or maximum dose of one medication should travel with a blood pressure cuff and monitor their blood pressure. These patients should also develop an algorithm with their physician for how to manage elevated blood pressure and when to decrease or hold doses.

Coronary Artery Disease (CAD)

All patients with known history or antecedent symptoms should undergo risk stratification, cardiac stress testing, and consult with their cardiologist. Patients with stable CAD who are able to exercise will likely tolerate travel to high altitude. It is advisable to avoid exertion until acclimatized, or for at least 4 to 5 days. Subsequent exertion should be below tolerated exertion at their elevation of residence, and strenuous exercise should be avoided. Other patients, including those with abnormal stress tests, angina, or acute coronary syndrome within six months without revascularization, should not travel to altitude.

Heart Failure

High altitude may increase risk for decompensation of chronic heart failure, and patients with poorly compensated heart failure should avoid travel. If heart failure is stable and controlled, patients may tolerate travel to altitude less than 3000 meters, but physical activity should remain below what is tolerated at their altitude of residence. These patients should monitor their body weight and develop an algorithm with their physician for how to adjust diuretics for increasing edema or weight gain.

Respiratory Conditions

Asthma. Allergic asthma will likely improve at high altitude, but asthma that is exercise- or cold-induced may be made worse. An optimized pre-travel medical regimen should be continued, and these patients should travel with additional rescue medications, including bronchodilators and corticosteroids. Patients should travel with an up-to-date asthma action plan and know where to seek medical attention for an exacerbation that cannot be managed independently. Travel should be avoided in moderate persistent or severe asthma, history of hospitalization, or recent exacerbation.

Chronic Obstructive Pulmonary Disease (COPD). Studies evaluating patients with COPD at high altitude are limited, and data from commercial flights assess exposure of insufficient duration to evaluate risk for high altitude illness. Those who are chronically hypoxemic may have some tolerance to hypobaric hypoxia due to their adaptations to chronic hypoxia. Data is more limited on patients with chronic carbon dioxide retention, and these patients should avoid travel to high altitude. Those with an $FEV_1 < 1$ liter should travel with supplemental oxygen. If FEV_1 is 1–1.5 liters, patients should be assessed by their pulmonologist for possible initiation of supplemental oxygen after arrival

---

[1] Not FDA approved for this indication.
* Acetazolamide is approved for use in children aged 12 years and older only.

at altitude. If supplemental oxygen is already being utilized, the anticipated increase in flow rate may be estimated by the ratio of higher to lower barometric pressure. Patients who have dyspnea at rest or with minimal exertion should not travel to altitudes higher than residence. High-altitude travel also should be avoided if there is a history of frequent recurrent exacerbations or hospitalizations. The home medical regimen should be optimized, and patients should travel with additional rescue medications and inhalers. All patients should travel with a pulse oximeter and seek medical attention for new persistent respiratory symptoms, hypoxia, or fatigue. Acetazolamide should not be used in patients with severe COPD or history of CO_2 retention.

Pulmonary Hypertension. Patients with pulmonary hypertension are at increased risk for developing HAPE and should be educated about the clinical presentation and treatment of HAPE. If mean pulmonary arterial pressure is 35 mm Hg or greater, or if systolic pulmonary arterial pressure is 50 mm Hg or greater, patients should travel with supplemental oxygen. If not on vasodilator therapy, these patients should also be started on nifedipine[1] 30 mg SR BID. Those with milder pulmonary hypertension should monitor oxygen saturation and consider prophylaxis with nifedipine[1] 30 mg SR BID. Pre-travel evaluation by a pulmonary hypertension specialist is recommended.

Sleep Apnea. Patients with obstructive sleep apnea tend to do better at high altitudes than those with central sleep apnea, but both of these populations should continue CPAP while at altitude. Older machines may lack pressure-compensating features and thus need intended CPAP pressure adjusted at high altitude. In patients not using CPAP, acetazolamide prophylaxis is recommended.

Other Considerations. Travel to high altitude should be avoided in patients with obesity hypoventilation or bilateral carotid body resection. If such travel is unavoidable, supplemental oxygen should be used and any home use of CPAP should be continued while at altitude.

Diabetes Mellitus

Patients with controlled type 1 diabetes do not appear to be at higher risk for AMS. Those with type II diabetes may be at higher risk for AMS, possibly related to other underlying risk factors and the metabolic syndrome. The elevated risk for cerebrovascular accident in diabetics may be further increased at high altitude. The prevalence of diabetes is lower at higher altitudes.

Metabolism and glucose control will change at altitude. Basal metabolic rate will increase, appetite may be suppressed, and absorption may be slowed, but hypoxia also causes hyperglycemia. Close glucose monitoring is imperative. Glucose-monitoring devices may lose accuracy, though glucose dehydrogenase-based glucometers may have more reliable performance. Malfunction risk is decreased if devices are kept warm. Acetaminophen may cause hyperglycemia, and care should be taken in use for HAH. Hydration is also particularly important for diabetic patients, particularly type 1, which can be self monitored by urine output and color.

Despite the above changes at altitude that suggest later administration of prandial insulin, there may also be a delay in the effects of rapid-acting insulin with increasing elevation, which may require earlier administration. This will also be affected by rate of ascent, acclimatization, exertion, and of course diet. Given this variability and individual response, patients should track their specific responses upon ascent and factor this in during descent, particularly if rapid, as is often the case. Glucose should be checked at a greater frequency to assess response, and any insulin administration should be adjusted accordingly. Continuous glucose monitoring may help track trends but, given the lag time compared to capillary testing and lack of studies at high altitude, probably only be used in conjunction with capillary testing.

In Type 1 diabetes, travel to altitude induces hyperglycemia initially and with any acute hypoxia or further ascent. After acclimatization there is a decrease in fasting glucose, and a further drop with exertion. The initial hypoxia-induced hyperglycemia may contribute to ketonuria as well as ketoacidosis, particularly with rapid ascent. This is particularly notable at very high to extreme elevations, and increased exertion and decreased appetite at these elevations may not be adequate to compensate for this hyperglycemia. Risk for DKA is increased due to these metabolic effects of altitude as well as the increased risk infectious diarrhea in some high-altitude regions, changes in diet, and certain medications. As symptoms of AMS, HACE, and diarrheal illness may mimic DKA, onset of symptoms of AMS or HACE, diarrhea in the setting of hyperglycemia, or suspected DKA warrants immediate descent.

Use of an insulin pump at altitude in controlled type 1 diabetics appears safe without significant pump dysfunction, though with rapid pressure changes such as cabin pressurization during air travel there have been reports of bubble formation affecting insulin delivery. It is advisable to also carry injectable insulin in case of pump failure. Use of acetazolamide is not advisable for type 1 diabetics due to increased risk for acidosis and diuresis increasing risk for dehydration. Dexamethasone should also be avoided due to the risk for hyperglycemia. This should be reserved for treatment of severe AMS, HACE, or if descent is not possible but emergent descent is a priority.

Type 2 diabetics do not appear to have the same extent of glycemic changes, though they may also experience hyperglycemia with initial ascent and hypoxia. Once acclimatized, they may need to decrease doses of sulfonylurea medications and insulin due to increased basal metabolic rate. It may be safe to use acetazolamide with caution in type 2 diabetes if not on insulin. Dexamethasone will cause hyperglycemia.

All travel companions should be educated on the signs and symptoms of hyper- and hypoglycemia, diabetic ketoacidosis (DKA) if applicable, overlap between these and AMS, HACE, and gastrointestinal illness, and how these conditions should be managed. Patients with poorly controlled or brittle diabetes should not travel to high altitude. Sedentary patients are advised to discuss cardiac stress testing with their physician.

References

Antony KM, Ehrenthal D, Evensen A, et al: Travel during pregnancy: considerations for the obstetric provider, *Obstet Gynecol Surv* 72(2):97–115, 2017.

Barthelmes D, Bosch MM, Merz TM, et al: Delayed appearance of high altitude retinal hemorrhages, *PLoS ONE* 6(2):1–7, 2011.

Bartsch P, Maggiorini M, Ritter M, et al: Prevention of high-altitude pulmonary edema by nifedipine, *N Engl J Med* 325:1284–1289, 1991.

Butler FK, Harris DJ, Reynolds RD: Altitude retinopathy on Mount Everest, *Ophthalmology* 99(5):739–746, 1992.

Campbell AD, McIntosh SE, Nyberg A, et al: Risk stratification for athletes and adventurers in high-altitude environments: recommendations for preparticipation evaluation, *Wilderness Environ Med* 26:S30–S39, 2015.

Ghofrani HA, Reichenberger F, Kohstall M, et al: Sildenafil increased exercise capacity during hypoxia at low altitudes and at Mount Everest base camp: a randomized, double-blind, placebo-controlled crossover trial, *Ann Intern Med* 141:169–177, 2004.

Hackett PH, Roach RC: High-altitude medicine and physiology. In Auerbach PS, editor: *Wilderness Medicine*, 6th ed., Philadelphia, 2012, Mosby, pp 2–33.

Ho TY, Kao WF, Lee SM, et al: High-altitude retinopathy after climbing Mount Aconcagua in a group of experienced climbers, *Retina* 31(8):1650–1655, 2011.

Joy E, Van Baak K, Dec KL, et al: Wilderness preparticipation evaluation and considerations for special populations, *Wild Env Med* 26:576–591, 2015.

Leon-Velarde F, Maggiorini M, Reeves JT, et al: Consensus statement on chronic and subacute high altitude diseases, *High Alt Med Biol* 6(2):147–157, 2005.

Luks AM: Should travelers with hypertension adjust their medications when traveling to high altitude, *High Alt Med Biol* 10:11–15, 2009.

Luks AM, Hackett PH: High altitude and common medical problems. In Swenson ES, Bartsch P, editors: *High Altitude: Human Adaptation to Hypoxia*, New York, 2014, Springer, 2014, pp. 449–477.

Luks AM, Swenson ER: Medication and dosage considerations in the prophylaxis and treatment of high-altitude illness, *Chest* 133:744–755, 2008.

Luks AM, Swenson ER, Bärtsch P: Acute high-altitude sickness, *Eur Respir Rev.* 26(143):214–220, 2017.

Maggiorini M, Brunner-La Rocca HP, Peth S, et al: Both tadalafil and dexamethasone may reduce the incidence of high-altitude pulmonary edema, *Ann Intern Med* 145:497–506, 2006.

---

[1] Not FDA approved for this indication.

Matejko B, Gawrecki A, Wrobel M, et al: Type 1 diabetes at high altitude: performance of personal insulin pumps and patient metabolic control, *Diabetes Technol Ther* 19(10):600–602, 2017.

McFadden DM, Houston CS, Sutton JR, et al: High-altitude retinopathy, *JAMA*
245(6):581–586, 1981.

del Mol P, de Vries ST, de Koning EJ, et al: Physical activity at altitude: challenges
for people with diabetes: a review, *Diabetes Care* 37(8):2404–2413, 2014.

Oelz O, Maggiorini M, Ritter M, et al: Nifedipine for high altitude pulmonary oede-
ma, *Lancet* 2:1241–1244, 1989.

Richards P, Hillebrandt D: Clinicians corner. The practical aspects of insulin at high
altitude, *High Alt Med Biol* 14:197–204, 2013.

Roach RC, Hackett PH, Oelz O, et al: The 2018 Lake Louise Acute Mountain Sickness Score, *High Alt Med Biol.* 19:1–4, 2018.

Schneider M, Bernasch D, Weymann J, et al: Acute mountain sickness: influence
of susceptibility, pre-exposure and ascent rate, *Med Sci Sports Exerc* 34:1886–
1891, 2002.

West JB: Physiological effects of chronic hypoxia, *N Engl J Med* 376(20):1965–
1971, 2017.

Woolcott OO, Adler M, Bergman RN: Glucose homeostasis during short tern and
prolonged exposure to high altitudes, *Endocr Rev* 36(2):149–173, 2015. (for elevation ref)

Zafren K, Reeves JT, Schoene R: Treatment of high-altitude pulmonary edema by
bed rest and supplemental oxygen, *Wilderness Environ Med* 7(2):127–132, 1996.

MARINE POISONINGS, ENVENOMATIONS, AND TRAUMA

Method of
Allen Perkins, MD, MPH

CURRENT DIAGNOSIS

- History of exposure is necessary for diagnosis.
- Ingested toxins can cause unusual symptoms, predominately gastrointestinal.
- Jellyfish envenomation is very painful but almost always self-limited.
- Trauma management follows principles of dirty wounds.
- Specific marine pathogens should be covered if contamination is suspected.

CURRENT THERAPY

Ingestions
- Avoidance is the best strategy.
- Early decontamination with activated charcoal (Actidose-Aqua) can reduce duration of symptoms.
- Symptomatic care is generally sufficient.

Jellyfish
- Remove visible stingers.
- Control pain with topical analgesia.

Trauma
- Avoiding water at feeding time can help avoid injury.
- If envenomation is suspected, consider hot water immersion.
- Tetanus status should be checked.
- Antibiotic coverage should take marine pathogens into account.

The United States has more than 80,000 miles of coastline, and more people are enjoying water-dependent recreation activities such as scuba diving, snorkeling, and surfing. As a consequence, people are more likely to suffer trauma, envenomation, or poisoning related to an encounter with a marine creature, which will come to the attention of a physician. The science of marine medicine is limited; hence, treatment of these conditions is largely based on case reports and expert opinion; very few randomized, controlled studies are available. Misdiagnosis is common, especially when the patient has returned from vacationing or when the patient has been poisoned by improperly handled seafood. This article describes common ailments and injuries occurring as a consequence of direct contact with sea creatures and discusses management and prevention.

Ingestions
Ciguatera
Epidemiology
Ciguatera poisoning is the most commonly reported marine toxin disease in the world. It is caused by human ingestion of reef fish that have bioaccumulated sufficient amounts of the dinoflagellate *Gambierdiscus toxicus*, either through direct ingestion or through ingestion of smaller reef fish. Although limited to tropical regions, it is heat and cold tolerant, is lipid soluble, and can survive transport to other areas. The toxin becomes more concentrated as it passes up the food chain; fish such as amberjack, grouper, and snapper pose less of a risk than predatory fish such as barracuda and moray eel. Ciguatera poisoning affects at least 50,000 people worldwide annually, and there are several thousand cases of poisoning in Puerto Rico, the U.S. Virgin Islands, Hawaii, and Florida each year.

Clinical Features
Patients can exhibit a primarily gastrointestinal (diarrhea, abdominal cramps, and vomiting), neurologic (parasthesias, diffuse pain, blurred vision), cardiac (bradycardia), or mixed pattern of symptoms. Additionally, a cold sensation reversal, in which a patient perceives the cold temperatures as a hot sensation and vice versa, occurs in 80% of patients and is considered pathognomonic for ciguatera poison (Box 1).

The attack rate is high. As many as 80% to 100% of people who ingest affected fish develop symptoms depending on the size of the fish and the toxin load. Ingestion of internal organs where the toxin accumulates (e.g., liver, roe) is associated with more severe symptoms, but avoiding these organs is not protective. The symptoms are also related to the number of exposures over time, and patients typically have more severe symptoms with subsequent exposures. There is no age-related susceptibility, and no immunity is acquired through exposure.

Symptoms typically begin 1 to 6 hours after ingestion, although a delay of 12 to 24 hours can occur. Duration is 7 to 14 days, and neurologic symptoms occasionally persist for months to years. Chronic ciguatera syndrome can also occur as a constellation of symptoms such as general malaise, depression, headaches, muscle aches, and dysesthesias in the extremities. Patients with chronic disease report recurrences with ingestion of fish, ethanol, caffeine, and nuts up to 6 months after the acute illness resolves.

Diagnosis
The diagnosis should be entertained in any patient who has neurologic, gastrointestinal, or cardiac symptoms and a history of ingesting predatory fish within the past 24 hours. The symptom constellation can be similar to other ingestions, such as certain shellfish toxins, and differentiation requires knowledge of the patient's diet for the previous day. Additionally, scombroid and type E botulinum poisoning should be considered, but these are unlikely if the patient did not ingest ill-appearing game. Other poisonings, such as organophosphates, can produce a similar symptom complex. There are no currently available clinical assays to assist in making the diagnosis, which is based on clinical suspicion and knowledge of the patient's diet history.

Treatment
If ciguatera poisoning is suspected soon after ingestion, I would consider gut decontamination with activated charcoal (Actidose-Aqua) because it can reduce the toxin load and subsequent symptoms. Initial symptomatic treatment typically consists of fluid replacement to replace gastrointestinal losses.

BOX 1 Symptom Patterns Associated With Ciguatera Poisoning

Gastrointestinal Pattern
Onset 15 minutes to 24 hours, typically worsens, lasts 1–2 days and resolves
- Nausea and/or vomiting
- Profuse, watery diarrhea
- Abdominal pain

Neurologic Pattern
Onset up to 24 hours after ingestion, commonly nonphysiologic pattern, can last several months
- Numbness and paresthesias
- Vertigo
- Ataxia
- Severe weakness or lethargy
- Severe myalgia
- Decreased vibration and pain sensations
- Diffuse pain pattern
- Cold sensation reversal
- Coma

Cardiovascular Pattern
Onset up to 24 hours after ingestion is uncommon but occurs rapidly
- Bradycardia
- Hypotension
- Cardiovascular collapse

Atropine (AtroPen) is used in patients who have bradycardia. Temporary electrical pacing may be used for refractory symptoms, and pressors may be needed in cases of severe hypotension. Neurologic symptoms are problematic because of their extended course as well as their severity. Mannitol (Osmitrol)[1] is often cited as effective in reducing the duration of neurologic symptoms, but I would use it with caution because the only double-blind trial failed to show any benefit. There are many local remedies used throughout the world that are said to be successful, which likely attests to the self-limited course of the ingestion in most cases. Table 1 offers more details regarding treatments currently used for ciguatera poisoning.

Prevention
Prevention is difficult except by avoiding ingestion of affected reef fish. The toxin is not deactivated by cooking, freezing, smoking, or salting. There are no outward signs of ciguatera: The fish look, taste, and smell normal. Although several commercial assays are available, they are neither sensitive nor specific enough to be relied on to prevent ciguatera poisoning.

To decrease the risk of ciguatera poisoning, I recommend the following steps: Avoid warm-water reef fish, especially those caught where ciguatera poisoning is known to occur; avoid moray eel injection; avoid ingesting large game fish; avoid consuming the internal organs; and limit the amount of initial ingestion if you are in an area where ciguatera is known to occur. Additionally, patients travelling to distant locales should be made aware that, although the vast majority of cases result from direct ingestion, there have been cases of ciguatera passed through sexual contact and through breast milk, so they should be wary of body fluid contact if ciguatoxin is endemic to the area, if for no other reasons.

Scombroid
Epidemiology
Scombroid poisoning (also known as histamine fish poisoning) results from improper handling of certain fish between the time the fish is caught and the time it is cooked. In the United States it is most common in Hawaii and California. Improper preservation and refrigeration lead to histamine and histamine-like substances being produced in the dark meat of certain fish through a conversion of histadine to histamine by bacterial decarboxylases. Members of the family Scombridae, such as tuna and mackerel, contain the highest amounts of this substance, but both scombroid and nonscombroid fish have been associated with the disease. The production of toxins requires the introduction of bacteria during the handling process, primarily during storage at high temperatures. It is the total amount of histamine, the presence of other biogenic amines, and individual susceptibility that determine the severity of the symptoms.

Clinical Features
The patient develops a histamine reaction 20 to 30 minutes after ingestion. Symptoms can be cutaneous, gastrointestinal, neurologic, or hemodynamic, or any combination of these. Cutaneous symptoms include flushing, urticaria and conjunctival injection, and localized edema; gastrointestinal symptoms include dry mouth, nausea, vomiting, diarrhea, and abdominal cramping; neurologic symptoms include severe headache and dizziness; and hemodynamic symptoms include palpitations and hypotension. In severe cases there can be bronchospasm and respiratory distress. These symptoms typically come on rapidly (within several minutes) and last less than 6 to 8 hours. Flushing is the most consistent clinical sign, occurring on exposed areas so it typically resembles sunburn. Diarrhea is also very common, occurring in 75% of symptomatic patients.

Diagnosis
As with ciguatera, the diagnosis is one of history. If the time between ingestion and illness is short and the patient has ingested a type of fish previously implicated in scombroid, then a tentative diagnosis can be made. The diagnosis is often confused with an allergic reaction. It can be distinguished from allergy by the lack of a previous allergic reaction as well as by testing the remaining fish for histamine, although testing is rarely warranted.

Treatment
Treatment is the same as for any histamine reaction, the cornerstone of which is antihistamine. Diphenhydramine (Benadryl) 50 mg for adults and 0.5–1 mg/kg/dose for children, repeated every 4 hours until symptoms abate, is delivered either intravenously or intramuscularly in severe cases and orally for milder cases. For severe cases, cimetidine (Tagamet)[1] 300 mg for adults, 20 mg/kg for children, either orally or intravenously, might be added for more complete histamine-receptor blockade. In cases where ingestion was recent, consider induced emesis using syrup of ipecac: 15 mL for children younger than 12 years or 30 mL otherwise. Most patients require only reassurance, and pharmacologic treatment will be unnecessary. It should be stressed to the patient that this is not an *allergic* reaction to fish, because the histamine is exogenous. Prevention is possible in regions where food storage and preparation are monitored through identification and removal of suspect fish.

Other Ingested Toxins
In addition to the toxins just discussed, ingestion of certain other marine creatures can lead to problems.

Ingestion of bivalves harvested from contaminated waters has been associated with hepatitis A, Norwalk virus, *Vibrio parahaemolyticus* and *Vibrio vulnificans* infections, the latter two particularly problematic and occasionally fatal in immunocompromised patients. I counsel patients likely to be immunocompromised, including diabetics and those with known liver disease, to avoid uncooked bivalves.

Shellfish are occasionally known to contain one or more of several toxins acquired through bioaccumulation of certain algae. These dinoflagellates tend to bloom in summer months.

[1]Not FDA approved for this indication.

[1]Not FDA approved for this indication.

TABLE 1	Treatment for Ciguatera Poisoning	
DRUG	**DOSE**	**INDICATION**
Activated charcoal (Actidose-Aqua)	Children <1 y: 1 g/kg	Gut emptying and decontamination
	Children 1–12 y: 25–50 g	
	Adults: 25–100 g	More effective in first hour
Antiemetics (no preference)	Administer per dosing recommendations	Intractable nausea and/or vomiting
Intravenous fluid bolus and infusion (normal saline or lactated Ringer's as initial)	Per volume replacement protocols	Hypovolemia
Atropine (AtroPen)	0.5–1.0 mg IV every 3–5 min to a maximum dose of 0.04 mg/kg per episode	Bradycardia
	Maximum total dose: 3 mg for adults, 2 mg for adolescents, 1 mg for young children	
Pressors: Dopamine (Intropin), dobutamine (Dobutrex), epinephrine	Varies with clinical response	Hypotension, shock
Antihistamines (no preference)	Administer per dosing recommendations	Pruritus
Mannitol (Osmitrol)[1]	1 g/kg of a 20% solution given IV over several h	Neurologic symptoms, double-blind study did not show benefit
	Adult dose: 25–100 g, titrate to urinary output of 100 mL/h	
Amitriptyline (Elavil)[1]	25–75 mg PO bid for patients >25 kg	Pruritus, dysesthesias

[1]Not FDA approved for this indication.

The symptoms occur immediately after ingestion and last several hours and are typically neurologic or gastrointestinal, or both. The shellfish poisoning syndromes are known as paralytic, neurologic, diarrheal, or amnestic depending on the predominant symptom. The care is typically supportive. Public health officials typically monitor local mollusk populations fairly carefully and alert the public to possible hazards.

Ingestion of the flesh of certain puffer fish has been associated with tetrodotoxin poisoning. The flesh of the fish (fugu) is considered a delicacy. The toxin builds up in internal organs such as the liver and the roe. If the toxin is ingested, it is likely to be fatal, but there are certified chefs who are trained in avoiding the toxin when preparing the dish. Despite this precaution, as many as 50 deaths occur in Japan annually from exposure to this toxin. Avoiding this puffer fish and avoiding the ingestion of certain other exotic animals (such as the blue-ringed octopus) eliminate the risk of acquiring this toxin.

Envenomations

Many marine creatures are venomous, and beachgoers experience clinically significant envenomations with some regularity. Jellyfish and related creatures (Cnidarians), sea urchins (Echinodermata), and stingrays (Chondrichthyes) are some of the more commonly identified marine animals involved with envenomations.

Jellyfish

These invertebrates have stinging cells called *nematocytes*, which carry nematocysts that continue to function when separated from the larger organism. For example, jellyfish nematocysts can sting if the tentacle is separated and after the jellyfish is dead. The venom is antigenic and causes a reaction of a dermatonecrotic, hemolytic, cardiopathic, or neurotoxic nature. The severity of the reaction depends on several variables, including the number of nematocysts that discharge, the toxicity of the coelenterate involved, and each patient's unique antigenic response.

Clinical Features

Although occasionally fatal as a consequence of an anaphylactic response in the United States and Caribbean, the primary concern in these areas with contact is pain, which is almost always self-limiting. Other, less common symptoms include parasthesias, nausea, headaches, and chills. The symptoms may last up to 2 to 3 days. Certain Pacific jellyfish primarily found in the waters around Australia have a more potent toxin and are much more likely to cause death (which is still very uncommon). Additionally, the Irukandji syndrome, which occurs in the Pacific, is a suite of symptoms including muscle spasms, vomiting, hypertension, incessant coughing, and occasionally heart failure and brain hemorrhage. Almost all exposed people, regardless of the geographic location, do not have a severe reaction, and the principles of first aid are primarily the same throughout the world.

Treatment

In my experience, treatment is mostly concerned with limiting pain and neurologic symptoms, because anaphylaxis and other severe reactions are rare, and the following general guidelines can be applied. In the field, either the victim or a companion should remove any visible tentacles. To do so requires using care, with gloves or forceps being optimal to prevent further stings. If a towel is used, any nematocysts remaining on the towel can still discharge. Salt water can be used to wash off the nematocysts. Urine, household vinegar, fresh water, and rubbing with sand should be avoided.

Should the victim present to the physician's office or emergency department, topical lidocaine (4%)[1] should be liberally applied for 30 minutes or until the pain subsides, followed by removal of the nematocysts, usually through use of the gloved hand or with forceps. Another method for removing the nematocysts is to apply shaving cream or baking soda slurry to the area and scrape off the nematocysts with a razor. Applications of cold, in the form of an ice pack, and immersion in hot water have variously been shown to improve pain, but because of the self-limited nature of the discomfort, it is hard to gauge an optimum therapy. Either is probably acceptable until the patient is comfortable. Meat tenderizer has been found to be ineffective. Local anesthetics, antihistamines, and steroids are all used to control prolonged symptoms, based on anecdotal experience. Antibiotics are not

[1]Not FDA approved for this indication.

generally necessary. In the rare cases of cardiovascular collapse, supportive care and principles of treatment of anaphylaxis should be followed. A delayed hypersensitivity reaction can occur 1 to 3 days out, which will almost certainly be self-limited and can be treated with oral antihistamines and topical steroids if symptoms are severe.

Sea bather's itch is a form of jellyfish sting caused by the larvae of the thimble jellyfish. It is characterized by a painful, itchy rash under the edges of the bathing suit or wet suit. It can occasionally progress to a papular rash. Topical steroids can be used to relieve symptoms.

Prevention

Prevention is mostly a matter of common sense. Staying away from the organism (the tentacles can extend several meters from the body of the organism) and staying out of the water when jellyfish are known to be present are the most effective. There is a commercially available product, Safe Sea, which has been shown to reduce the number of nematocyst discharges and thus the severity of the sting should a swimmer need to be in the water when jellyfish are present. Wetsuits and other protective gear are ineffective.

Echinoderms

The Echinoderm family includes sea urchins. Urchins have toxin-coated spines that break off, leaving calcareous material in the wound, which can potentially cause infection. Symptoms include local pain, burning, and local discoloration. The discoloration is thought to be a temporary tattooing of the skin resulting from dye in the spines; absence of a spine is indicated if the discoloration spontaneously resolves within 48 hours. Theoretically, hot water disables the toxin, although there is no evidence in humans that it is effective. If a spine is present and easily accessible, it should be removed with fingers or forceps. If it is close to a joint or neurovascular structure, it should be surgically removed. If the spines do not cause symptoms, retained pieces will likely reabsorb into the skin.

Stingrays

Although many fish are venomous, stingrays are the most clinically important, accounting for an estimated 1500 mostly minor injuries in the United States annually. These creatures partially bury themselves in the shallow, sandy bottom of the ocean, leading water enthusiasts to accidentally step on them or grab at what they think is a seashell.

Clinical Features

Stingrays have a spine at the base of their tail, which contains a venom gland. The spine, including the venom gland, is broken off and may be left in the resulting wound. The venom has vasoconstrictive properties that can lead to cyanosis and necrosis with poor wound healing and infection. Symptoms can include immediate and intense pain, salivation, nausea, vomiting, diarrhea, muscle cramps, dyspnea, seizures, headaches, and cardiac arrhythmias. Fatalities are rare and mostly a consequence of exsanguination at the scene or penetration of a vital organ.

Treatment

Home care should include rinsing the area thoroughly with fresh water if available (salt water if not) and removing any foreign body. If the damage is minimal, the victim may soak the wound in warm water at home. The victim should watch for signs of infection and seek care for excessive bleeding, retained foreign body, or infection.

For severe wounds that lead the victim to seek medical attention, treatment should include achieving hemostasis followed by submersion of the affected region in hot but not scalding water (42–45 °C, 108–113 °F) for 30 to 90 minutes or until the pain resolves. Spines and stingers are typically radiopaque, so radiographs or an ultrasound should be obtained if a retained spine is suspected. The wound should be thoroughly cleansed, and delayed closure should be allowed. Tetanus immunization status should be reviewed and updated as appropriate. Surgical exploration may be necessary to remove residual foreign bodies. Prophylactic antibiotics are typically not necessary unless there is a residual foreign body or if the patient is immunosuppressed. If the wound becomes infected, *Staphylococcus* and *Streptococcus* species are the most common pathologic organisms. Unique to the marine environment are *Vibrio vulnificus* and *Mycobacterium marinum*, and antibiotic coverage should include coverage for all of these (Table 2).

Other Venomous Sea Creatures

Seasnakes are venomous creatures found most commonly in the Indo-Pacific area. Bites are uncommon (and envenomation is even less common), but should they occur, the toxin is very potent. The care is supportive. There is antivenom, which may be available in areas where the snakes are endemic.

Certain other fish and octopi have been associated with envenomation and occasional death. Most are tropical such as the

TABLE 2	Antibiotic Choices in Marine Injuries		
		DOSAGE	
DRUG	**PEDIATRIC**		**ADULT**
Outpatient Management			
Ciprofloxacin (Cipro)[1]	20–30 mg/kg/day PO × 14 d[1]		500 mg PO bid × 14 d
Levofloxin (Levaquin)[1]			750 mg PO qd × 14 d
Doxycycline (Vibramycin, Doryx)	>8 y: 2.2 mg/kg PO qd × 14 d		100 mg bid × 14 d
Inpatient Management			
	Preferred		
Ceftazidime (Fortaz, Tazicef) *plus*	150 mg/kg/d q8h		1 g IV q8h
PO or IV quinolone or doxycycline	150 mg/kg/d q8h		1 g IV q8h
Alternative			
Gentamicin *plus*	Typically based on institutional protocol and adjusted based on serum levels		Typically based on institutional protocol and adjusted based on serum levels
TMP-SMX (Bactrim, Cotrim, Septra)	8–10 mg/kg/d TMP		8–10 mg/kg (lean body mass)/d TMP

[1]Not FDA approved for this indication.
Abbreviation: TMP-SMX = trimethoprim-sulfamethoxazole.

stonefish, scorpionfish, and rabbitfish and the blue-ringed octopus. Certain varieties of catfish have venom as well. Envenomations are rare, and if they occur, treatment is based on good first-aid principles and antivenom where available (mostly in tropical areas).

Certain cone shells contain a toxin that can be fatal. This toxin is injected by the mollusk into the victim from a proboscis, which it extends from the small end of the cone. Treatment is primarily supportive.

Trauma

Abrasions, bites, and lacerations are usually the result of a marine animal's instinct to protect itself against a perceived danger. The most commonly involved marine animals are octopi, sharks, moray eels, and barracuda. The trauma alone creates problems for patients, but the trauma can be further complicated by envenomation. It is often difficult to identify the marine animal involved in the attack. Treatment is for the most part symptomatic, with local cleansing and topical dressing usually sufficing. If the wound becomes infected, antibiotics should cover common organisms (see Table 2).

Environmental Hazards

Abrasions from the ambient environment are also common. These wounds should be thoroughly cleansed with soap and water and a topical antibiotic applied, because the wounds can contain toxins and are commonly contaminated with bacteria. Coral contains nematocysts and also has very sharp edges. Scuba divers in particular suffer from coral cuts in the course of their recreational diving. If these wounds become infected, coverage for *Vibrio* species should be included as well.

Sharks

Although shark attacks receive a lot of publicity, there are only around 50 such attacks worldwide annually and they result in fewer than 10 deaths. The majority of the deaths are in South Africa. Typically these attacks involve the tiger, great white, gray reef, and bull sharks. Attacks occur in shallow water within 100 feet of shore during the evening hours when sharks tend to feed. Common sense dictates avoiding areas where aggressive shark feeding has been noted.

Sequelae of a shark attack range from abrasions to death from hemorrhage. Abrasions and lacerations can occur when sharks brush or aggressively investigate humans. Soft tissue damage, fractures, and neurovascular damage result from such attacks. The majority of attacks result in minor injuries that require simple suturing. Morbidity increases in wounds that are greater than 20 cm or where more than one myofascial compartment is lost. General principles of first aid in marine animal injuries are found in Box 2. Although it would seem self-evident, practices such as urinating on the injury, applying oil or gasoline to injuries, and application of any strong oxidizing agents, such as strong bases or acids, should be counseled against when doing patient education regarding self-care.

References

Birsa L, Verity P, Lee R: Evaluation of the effects of various chemicals on discharge of and pain caused by jellyfish nematocysts, *Comp Biochem and Physiol Part C: Toxicology & Pharmacology* 151:426–430, 2010.

Centers for Disease Control and Prevention. *Vibrio vulnificus* after a disaster. Available at http://emergency.cdc.gov/disasters/vibriovulnificus.asp (accessed August 19, 2015).

Edmonds C: Marine animal injuries. In Bove AA, editor: *Bove and Davis' Diving Medicine*, 4th ed., Philadelphia, 2004, Saunders, pp 287–318.

Fleming LE: Ciguatera fish poisoning. In *National Institute of Environmental Health Sciences, Marine and Freshwater Biomedical Sciences Center*, 2006.

Isbister GK: Venomous fish stings in tropical northern Australia, *Am J Emerg Med* 19:561–565, 2001.

Lahey T: Invasive *Mycobacterium marinum* infections, *Emerg Infect Dis [serial online]* 2003. November; Available at http://wwwnc.cdc.gov/eid/article/9/11/03-0192_article.htm (accessed August 19, 2015).

Lehane L, Olley J: *Histamine (scombroid) fish poisoning: A review in a risk-assessment framework*, Canberra, Australia, 1999, National Office of Animal and Plant Health.

Lynch PR, Bove AA: Marine poisonings and intoxications. In Bove AA, editor: *Bove and Davis' Diving Medicine*, 4th ed., Philadelphia, 2004, Saunders, pp 287–318.

Perkins A, Morgan S: Poisonings, envenomations, and trauma from marine creatures, *Am Fam Physician* 69:885–890, 2004.

Thomas C, Scott SA: *All Stings Considered: First Aid and Medical Treatment of Hawaii's Marine Injuries*, Honolulu, 1997, University of Hawaii Press.

Thomas CS, Scott SA, Galanis DJ, Goto RS: Box jellyfish *Carybdea alata* in Waikiki. The analgesic effect of Sting-Aid, Adolph's meat tenderizer and fresh water on their stings: a double-blinded, randomized, placebo-controlled clinical trial, *Hawaii Med J* 60:205–210, 2001.

Thomas CS, Scott SA, Galanis DJ, Goto RS: Box jellyfish *Carybdea alata* in Waikiki. Their influx cycle plus the analgesic effect of hot and cold packs on their stings to swimmers at the beach: a randomized, placebo-controlled, clinical trial, *Hawaii Med J* 60:100–107, 2001.

MEDICAL TOXICOLOGY

Method of
Howard C. Mofenson, MD; Thomas R. Caraccio, PharmD; Michael McGuigan, MD; and Joseph Greensher, MD

Introduction and Epidemiology

According to the national Toxic Exposure Surveillance System (TESS), over 2.4 million potentially toxic exposures were reported last year to Poison Control Centers throughout the United States. Poisonings were responsible for 1183 deaths and more than 500,000 hospitalizations. Poisoning accounts for 2% to 5% of pediatric hospital admissions, 10% of adult admissions, 5% of hospital admissions in the elderly (>65 years of age), and 5% of ambulance calls. In one urban hospital, drug-related emergencies accounted for 38% of the emergency department visits. An evaluation of a medical intensive care unit and step-down unit over a 3-month period indicated that poisonings accounted for 19.7% of admissions.

The largest number of fatalities resulting from poisoning reported to the TESS are caused by analgesics. The other principal toxicologic causes of fatalities are antidepressants, sedative hypnotics/antipsychotics, stimulants/street drugs, cardiovascular agents, and alcohols. Less than 1% of overdose cases reaching the hospitals result in fatality. However, patients presenting in deep coma to medical care facilities have a fatality rate of 13% to 35%. The largest single cause of coma of inapparent etiology is drug poisoning.

Pharmaceutical preparations are involved in 50% of poisonings. The number one pharmaceutical agent involved in exposures is acetaminophen. The severity of the manifestations of acute poisoning exposures varies greatly depending on whether the poisoning was intentional or unintentional. Unintentional exposures make up 85% to 90% of all poisoning exposures. The majority of cases are acute, occurring in children younger than 5 years of age, in the home, and resulting in no or minor toxicity. Many are actually ingestions of relatively nontoxic substances that require minimal medical care. Intentional poisonings, such as suicides,

---

BOX 2

Management of Marine Trauma
Remove the victim from the water.
Ensure airway control.
Control bleeding.
Do not remove the wet suit if the victim is wearing one.
Attempt to identify the animal involved in the injury.
If the injury is severe, transport the victim to a hospital.
If envenomation is suspected, consider hot water immersion.
Irrigate the wound with normal saline.
Perform surgical débridement of the wound as appropriate.
If sutures must be placed, place them loosely and allow drainage. Primary suturing should be avoided in puncture wounds, crush injuries, and wounds in the distal extremities.
Start appropriate antibiotics if indicated.

constitute 10% to 15% of exposures and may require the highest standards of medical and nursing care and the use of sophisticated equipment for recovery. Intentional ingestions are often of multiple substances and frequently include ethanol, acetaminophen, and aspirin. Suicides make up 54% of the reported fatalities. About 25% of suicides are attempted with drugs. Sixty percent of patients who take a drug overdose use their own medication and 15% use drugs prescribed for close relatives. The majority of the drug-related suicide attempts involve a central nervous system (CNS) depressant, and coma management is vital to the treatment.

Assessment and Maintenance of the Vital Functions

The initial assessment of all patients in medical emergencies follows the principles of basic and advanced cardiac life support. The adequacy of the patient's airway, degree of ventilation, and circulatory status should be determined. The vital functions should be established and maintained. Vital signs should be measured frequently and should include body core temperature. The assessment of vital functions should include the rate numbers (e.g., respiratory rate) and indications of effectiveness (e.g., depth of respirations and degree of gas exchange). Table 1 gives important measurements and vital signs.

Level of consciousness should be assessed by immediate AVPU (Alert, responds to Verbal stimuli, responds to Painful stimuli, and Unconscious). If the patient is unconscious, one must assess the severity of the unconsciousness by the Glasgow Coma Scale (Table 2).

If the patient is comatose, management requires administering 100% oxygen, establishing vascular access, and obtaining blood for pertinent laboratory studies. The administration of glucose, thiamine, and naloxone, as well as intubation to protect the airway, should be considered. Pertinent laboratory studies include arterial blood gases (ABG), electrocardiography (ECG), determination of blood glucose level, electrolytes, renal and liver tests, and acetaminophen plasma concentration in all cases of intentional ingestions. Radiography of the chest and abdomen may be useful. The severity of a stimulant's effects can also be assessed and should be documented to follow the trend.

The examiner should completely expose the patient by removing clothes and other items that interfere with a full evaluation. One should look for clues to etiology in the clothes and include the hat and shoes.

Prevention of Absorption and Reduction of Local Damage

Exposure

Poisoning exposure routes include ingestion (76.8%), dermal (8%), ophthalmologic (5%), inhalation (6%), insect bites and stings (4%), and parenteral injections (0.5%). The effect of the toxin may be local, systemic, or both.

Local effects (skin, eyes, mucosa of respiratory or gastrointestinal tract) occur where contact is made with the poisonous substance. Local effects are nonspecific chemical reactions that depend on the chemical properties (e.g., pH), concentration, contact time, and type of exposed surface.

Systemic effects occur when the poison is absorbed into the body and depend on the dose, the distribution, and the functional reserve of the organ systems. Shock and hypoxia are part of systemic toxicity.

Delayed Toxic Action

Therapeutic doses of most pharmaceuticals are absorbed within 90 minutes. However, the patient with exposure to a potential toxin may be asymptomatic at this time because a sufficient amount has not yet been absorbed or metabolized to produce toxicity at the time the patient presents for care.

Absorption can be significantly delayed under the following circumstances:

1. Drugs with anticholinergic properties (e.g., antihistamines, belladonna alkaloids, diphenoxylate with atropine [Lomotil], phenothiazines, and tricyclic antidepressants).
2. Modified release preparations such as sustained-release, enteric-coated, and controlled-release formulations have delayed and prolonged absorption.
3. Concretions may form (e.g., salicylates, iron, glutethimide, and meprobamate [Equanil]) that can delay absorption and prolong the toxic effects. Large quantities of drugs tend to be absorbed more slowly than small quantities.

Some substances must be metabolized into a toxic metabolite (acetaminophen, acetonitrile, ethylene glycol, methanol, methylene chloride, parathion, and paraquat). In some cases, time is required to produce a toxic effect on organ systems (*Amanita phalloides* mushrooms, carbon tetrachloride, colchicine, digoxin [Lanoxin], heavy metals, monoamine oxidase inhibitors, and oral hypoglycemic agents).

| | | | | | | BLOOD PRESSURE | | | |
| | | | | | | | HYPERTENSION | | |
AGE	BODY SURFACE AREA (M²)	WEIGHT (KG)	HEIGHT (CM)	PULSE (BPM) RESTING	HYPOTENSION	SIGNIFICANT	SEVERE	RESPIRATORY RATE (RPM)
Newborn	0.19	3.5	50	70–190	<60/40	>96	>106	30–60
1mo–6mo	0.30	4–7	50–65	80–160	<70/45	>104	>110	30–50
6mo–1y	0.38	7–10	65–75	80–160	<70/45	>104	>110	20–40
1–2y	0.50–0.55	10–12	75–85	80–140	<74/47	>112/74	>118/82	20–40
3–5y	0.54–0.68	15–20	90–108	80–120	<80/52	>116/76	>124/84	20–40
6–9y	0.68–0.85	20–28	122–133	75–115	<90/60	>122/82	>130/86	16–25
10–12y	1.00–1.07	30–40	138–147	70–110	<90/60	>126/82	>134/90	16–25
13–15y	1.07–1.22	42–50	152–160	60–100	<90/60	>136/86	>144/92	16–20
16–18y	1.30–1.60	53–60	160–170	60–100	<90/60	>142/92	>150/98	12–16
Adult	1.40–1.70	60–70	160–170	60–100	<90/60	>140/90	>210/120	10–16

TABLE 1 Important Measurements and Vital Signs

Data from Nadas A: Pediatric Cardiology, 3rd ed. Philadelphia, WB Saunders, 1976; Blumer JL (ed): A Practice Guide to Pediatric Intensive Care. St Louis, Mosby, 1990; AAP and ACEP: Respiratory Distress in APLS Pediatric Emergency Medicine Course, 1993; Second Task Force: Blood pressure control in children–1987, Pediatr 79:1, 1987; Linakis JG: Hypertension. In Fliesher GR, Ludwig S (eds); Textbook of Pediatric Emergency Medicine, 3rd ed. Baltimore, Williams & Wilkins, 1993.

TABLE 2	Glasgow Coma Scale		
SCALE	ADULT RESPONSE	SCORE	PEDIATRIC, 0–1 YEARS
Eye opening	Spontaneous	4	Spontaneous
	To verbal command	3	To shout
	To pain	2	To pain
	None	1	No response
Motor response			
To verbal command	Obeys	6	
To painful stimuli	Localized pain	5	Localized pain
	Flexion withdrawal	4	Flexion withdrawal
	Decorticate flexion	3	Decorticate flexion
	Decerebrate extension	2	Decerebrate flexion
	None	1	None
Verbal response: adult	Oriented and converses	5	Cries, smiles, coos
	Disoriented but converses	4	Cries or screams
	Inappropriate words	3	Inappropriate sounds
	Incomprehensible sounds	2	Grunts
	None	1	Gives no response
Verbal response: child	Oriented	5	
	Words or babbles	4	
	Vocal sounds	3	
	Cries or moans to stimuli	2	
	None	1	

Data from Teasdale G, Jennett B: Assessment of coma impaired consciousness. Lancet 2:83, 1974; Simpson D, Reilly P: Pediatric coma scale. Lancet 2:450, 1982; Seidel J: Preparing for pediatric emergencies. Pediatr Rev 16:470, 1995.

Initial Management

1. Stabilization of airway, breathing, and circulation and protection of same.
2. Identification of specific toxin or toxic syndrome.
3. Initial treatment: D50W; consider thiamine, naloxone (Narcan), oxygen, and antidotes if needed.
4. Physical assessment.
5. Decontamination: Gastrointestinal tract, skin, eyes.

Decontamination

In the asymptomatic patient who has been exposed to a toxic substance, decontamination procedures should be considered if the patient has been exposed to potentially toxic substances in toxic amounts.

Ocular exposure should be immediately treated with water irrigation for 15 to 20 minutes with the eyelids fully retracted. One should not use neutralizing chemicals. All caustic and corrosive injuries should be evaluated with fluorescein dye and by an ophthalmologist.

Dermal exposure is treated immediately with copious water irrigation for 30 minutes, not a forceful flushing. Shampooing the hair, cleansing the fingernails, navel, and perineum, and irrigating the eyes are necessary in the case of an extensive exposure. The clothes should be specially bagged and may have to be discarded. Leather goods can become irreversibly contaminated and must be abandoned. Caustic (alkali) exposures can require hours of irrigation. Dermal absorption can occur with pesticides, hydrocarbons, and cyanide.

Injection exposures (e.g., snake envenomation) can be treated with venom extractors. Venom extractors can be used within minutes of envenomation, and proximal lymphatic constricting bands or elastic wraps can be used to delay lymphatic flow and immobilize the extremity. Cold packs and tourniquets should not be used and incision is generally not recommended. Substances of abuse may be injected intravenously or subcutaneously. In these cases, little decontamination can be done.

Inhalation exposure to toxic substances is managed by immediate removal of the victim from the contaminated environment by protected rescuers.

Gastrointestinal exposure is the most common route of poisoning. Gastrointestinal decontamination historically has been done by gastric emptying: induction of emesis, gastric lavage, administration of activated charcoal, and the use of cathartics or whole bowel irrigation. No procedure is routine; it should be individualized for each case. If no attempt is made to decontaminate the patient, the reason should be clearly documented on the medical record (e.g., time elapsed, past peak of action, ineffectiveness, or risk of procedure).

Gastric Emptying Procedures

The gastric emptying procedure used is influenced by the age of the patient, the effectiveness of the procedure, the time of ingestion (gastric emptying is usually ineffective after 1 hour postingestion), the patient's clinical status (time of peak effect has passed or the patient's condition is too unstable), formulation of the substance ingested (regular release versus modified release), the amount ingested, and the rapidity of onset of CNS depression or stimulation (convulsions). Most studies show that only 30% (range, 19% to 62%) of the ingested toxin is removed by gastric emptying under optimal conditions. It has not been demonstrated that the choice of procedure improved the outcome.

A mnemonic for gathering information is STATS:

S—substance
T—type of formulation
A—amount and age
T—time of ingestion
S—signs and symptoms

The examiner should attempt to obtain AMPLE information about the patient:

A—age and allergies
M—available medications
P—past medical history including pregnancy, psychiatric illnesses, substance abuse, or intentional ingestions
L—time of last meal, which may influence absorption and the onset and peak action
E—events leading to present condition

The intent of the patient should also be determined.

The Regional Poison Center should be consulted for the exact ingredients of the ingested substance and the latest management. The treatment information on the labels of products are notoriously inaccurate.

Ipecac Syrup

Syrup of ipecac–induced emesis has virtually no use in the emergency department. Although at one time it was considered most useful in young children with a recent witnessed ingestion, it is no longer advised in most cases. Current guidelines from the American Association of Poison Control Centers have significantly limited the indications for inducing emesis because the risk most often exceeds the benefit derived from this procedure. The Poison Control Center should be called if inducting emesis is being considered.

Contraindications or situations in which induction of emesis is inappropriate include the following:
- Ingestion of caustic substance
- Loss of airway protective reflexes because of ingestion of substances that can produce rapid onset of CNS depression (e.g., short-acting benzodiazepines, barbiturates, nonbarbiturate sedative-hypnotics, opioids, tricyclic antidepressants) or convulsions (e.g., camphor [Ponstel], chloroquine [Aralen], codeine, isoniazid [Nydrazid], mefenamic acid, nicotine, propoxyphene [Darvon], organophosphate insecticides, strychnine, and tricyclic antidepressants)
- Ingestion of low-viscosity petroleum distillates (e.g., gasoline, lighter fluid, kerosene)
- Significant vomiting prior to presentation or hematemesis
- Age under 6 months (no established dose, safety, or efficacy data)
- Ingestion of foreign bodies (emesis is ineffective and may lead to aspiration)
- Clinical conditions including neurologic impairment, hemodynamic instability, increased intracranial pressure, and hypertension
- Delay in presentation (more than 1 hour postingestion)

The dose of syrup of ipecac in the 6- to 9-month-old infant is 5 mL; in the 9- to 12-month-old, 10 mL; and in the 1- to 12-year-old, 15 mL. In children older than 12 years and in adults, the dose is 30 mL. The dose can be repeated once if the child does not vomit in 15 to 20 minutes. The vomitus should be inspected for remnants of pills or toxic substances, and the appearance and odor should be documented. When ipecac is not available, 30 mL of mild dishwashing soap (not dishwasher detergent) can be used, although it is less effective.

Complications are very rare but include aspiration, protracted vomiting, rarely cardiac toxicity with long-term abuse, pneumothorax, gastric rupture, diaphragmatic hernia, intracranial hemorrhage, and Mallory-Weiss tears.

Gastric Lavage

Gastric lavage should be considered only when life-threatening amounts of substances were involved, when the benefits outweigh the risks, when it can be performed within 1 hour of the ingestion, and when no contraindications exist.

The contraindications are similar to those for ipecac-induced emesis. However, gastric lavage can be accomplished after the insertion of an endotracheal tube in cases of CNS depression or controlled convulsions. The patient should be placed with the head lower than the hips in a left-lateral decubitus position. The location of the tube should be confirmed by radiography, if necessary, and suctioning equipment should be available.

Contraindications to gastric lavage include the following:
- Ingestion of caustic substances (risk of esophageal perforation)
- Uncontrolled convulsions, because of the danger of aspiration and injury during the procedure
- Ingestion of low-viscosity petroleum distillate products
- CNS depression or absent protective airway reflexes, without endotracheal protection
- Significant cardiac dysrhythmias
- Significant emesis or hematemesis prior to presentation
- Delay in presentation (more than 1 hour postingestion)

Size of Tube. The best results with gastric lavage are obtained with the largest possible orogastric tube that can be reasonably passed (nasogastric tubes are not large enough to remove solid material). In adults, a large-bore orogastric Lavacuator hose or a No. 42 French Ewald tube should be used; in young children, orogastric tubes are generally too small to remove solid material and gastric lavage is not recommended.

The amount of fluid used varies with the patient's age and size. In general, aliquots of 50 to 100 mL per lavage are used in adults. Larger amounts of fluid may force the toxin past the pylorus. Lavage fluid is 0.9% saline.

Complications are rare and may include respiratory depression, aspiration pneumonitis, cardiac dysrhythmias as a result of increased vagal tone, esophageal-gastric tears and perforation, laryngospasm, and mediastinitis.

Activated Charcoal

Oral activated charcoal adsorbs the toxin onto its surface before absorption. According to recent guidelines set forth by the American Academy of Clinical Toxicology, activated charcoal should not be used routinely. Its use is indicated only if a toxic amount of substance has been ingested and is optimally effective within 1 hour of the ingestion. Because of the slow absorption of large quantities of toxin, activated charcoal may be beneficial after 1 hour postingestion.

Activated charcoal does not effectively adsorb small molecules or molecules lacking carbon (Table 3). Activated charcoal adsorption may be diminished by milk, cocoa powder, and ice cream.

There are a few relative contraindications to the use of activated charcoal:
1. Ingestion of caustics and corrosives, which may produce vomiting or cling to the mucosa and falsely appear as a burn on endoscopy.
2. Comatose patient, in whom the airway must be secured prior to activated charcoal administration.
3. Patient without presence of bowel sounds.

Note: Activated charcoal was shown not to interfere with effectiveness of N-acetylcysteine in cases of acetaminophen overdose, so it is no longer contraindicated as was thought in the past.

The usual initial adult dose is 60 to 100 g and the dose for children is 15 to 30 g. It is administered orally as a slurry mixed with water or by nasogastric or orogastric tube. *Caution:* Be sure the tube is in the stomach. Cathartics are not necessary.

Although repeated dosing with activated charcoal may decrease the half-life and increase the clearance of phenobarbital,

TABLE 3	Substances Poorly Adsorbed by Activated Charcoal
C	Caustics and corrosives
H	Heavy metals (arsenic, iron, lead, mercury)
A	Alcohols (ethanol, methanol, isopropanol) and glycols (ethylene glycols)
R	Rapid onset of absorption (cyanide and strychnine)
C	Chlorine and iodine
O	Others insoluble in water (substances in tablet form)
A	Aliphatic hydrocarbons (petroleum distillates)
L	Laxatives (sodium, magnesium, potassium, and lithium)

dapsone, quinidine, theophylline, and carbamazepine (Tegretol), recent guidelines indicate there is insufficient evidence to support the use of multiple-dose activated charcoal unless a life-threatening amount of one of the substances mentioned is involved. At present there are no controlled studies that demonstrate that multiple-dose activated charcoal or cathartics alter the clinical course of an intoxication. The dose varies from 0.25 to 0.50 g/kg every 1 to 4 hours, and continuous nasogastric tube infusion of 0.25 to 0.5 g/kg/h has been used to decrease vomiting.

Gastrointestinal dialysis is the diffusion of the toxin from the higher concentration in the serum of the mesenteric vessels to the lower levels in the gastrointestinal tract mucosal cell and subsequently into the gastrointestinal lumen, where the concentration has been lowered by intraluminal adsorption of activated charcoal.

Complications of treatment with activated charcoal include vomiting in 50% of cases, desorption (especially with weak acids in intestine), and aspiration (at least a dozen cases of aspiration have been reported). There are many cases of unreported pulmonary aspirations and "charcoal lungs," intestinal obstruction or pseudoobstruction (three case reports with multiple dosing, none with a single dose), empyema following esophageal perforation, and hypermagnesemia and hypernatremia, which have been associated with repeated concurrent doses of activated charcoal and saline cathartics. Catharsis was used to hasten the elimination of any remaining toxin in the gastrointestinal tract. There are no studies to demonstrate the effectiveness of cathartics, and they are no longer recommended as a form of gastrointestinal decontamination.

Whole-Bowel Irrigation

With whole-bowel irrigation, solutions of polyethylene glycol (PEG) with balanced electrolytes are used to cleanse the bowel without causing shifts in fluids and electrolytes. The procedure is not approved by the US Food and Drug Administration (FDA) for this purpose.

Indications. The procedure has been studied and used successfully in cases of iron overdose when abdominal radiographs reveal incomplete emptying of excess iron. There are additional indications for other types of ingestions, such as with body-packing of illicit drugs (e.g., cocaine, heroin).

The procedure is to administer the solution (GoLYTELY or Colyte), orally or by nasogastric tube, in a dose of 0.5 L per hour in children younger than 5 years of age and 2 L per hour in adolescents and adults for 5 hours. The end point is reached when the rectal effluent is clear or radiopaque materials can no longer be seen in the gastrointestinal tract on abdominal radiographs.

Contraindications. These measures should not be used if there is extensive hematemesis, ileus, or signs of bowel obstruction, perforation, or peritonitis. Animal experiments in which PEG was added to activated charcoal indicated that activated charcoal-salicylates and activated charcoal-theophylline combinations resulted in decreased adsorption and desorption of salicylate and theophylline and no therapeutic benefit over activated charcoal alone. Polyethylene solutions are bound by activated charcoal in vitro, decreasing the efficacy of activated charcoal.

Dilutional treatment is indicated for the immediate management of caustic and corrosive poisonings but is otherwise not useful. The administration of diluting fluid above 30 mL in children and 250 mL in adults may produce vomiting, reexposing the vital tissues to the effects of local damage and possible aspiration.

Neutralization has not been proven to be either safe or effective.

Endoscopy and surgery have been required in the case of body-packer obstruction, intestinal ischemia produced by cocaine ingestion, and iron local caustic action.

Differential Diagnosis of Poisons on the Basis of Central Nervous System Manifestations

Neurologic parameters help to classify and assess the need for supportive treatment as well as provide diagnostic clues to the etiology. Table 4 lists the effects of CNS depressants, CNS stimulants, hallucinogens, and autonomic nervous system anticholinergics and cholinergics.

CNS depressants are cholinergics, opioids, sedative-hypnotics, and sympatholytic agents. The hallmarks are lethargy, sedation, stupor, and coma. In exception to the manifestations listed in Table 4, (a) barbiturates may produce an initial tachycardia; (b) convulsions are produced by codeine, propoxyphene (Darvon), meperidine (Demerol), glutethimide, phenothiazines, methaqualone, and tricyclic and cyclic antidepressants; (c) benzodiazepines rarely produce coma that will interfere with cardiorespiratory functions; and (d) pulmonary edema is common with opioids and sedative-hypnotics.

The CNS stimulants are anticholinergic, hallucinogenic, sympathomimetic, and withdrawal agents. The hallmarks of CNS stimulants are convulsions and hyperactivity.

There is considerable overlapping of effects among the various hallucinogens, but the major hallmark manifestation is hallucinations.

Guidelines for In-Hospital Disposition

Classification of patients as high risk depends on clinical judgment. Any patient who needs cardiorespiratory support or has a persistently altered mental status for 3 hours or more should be considered for intensive care.

Guidelines for admitting patients older than 14 years of age to an intensive care unit, after 2 to 3 hours in the emergency department, include the following:

1. Need for intubation
2. Seizures
3. Unresponsiveness to verbal stimuli
4. Arterial carbon dioxide pressure greater than 45 mm Hg
5. Cardiac conduction or rhythm disturbances (any rhythm except sinus arrhythmia)
6. Close monitoring of vital signs during antidotal therapy or elimination procedures
7. The need for continuous monitoring
8. QRS interval greater than 0.10 second, in cases of tricyclic antidepressant poisoning
9. Systolic blood pressure less than 80 mm Hg
10. Hypoxia, hypercarbia, acid-base imbalance, or metabolic abnormalities
11. Extremes of temperature
12. Progressive deterioration or significant underlying medical disorders

Use of Antidotes

Antidotes are available for only a relatively small number of poisons. An antidote is not a substitute for good supportive care. Table 5 summarizes the commonly used antidotes, their indications, and their methods of administration. The Regional Poison Control Center can give further information on these antidotes.

Enhancement of Elimination

The acceptable methods for elimination of absorbed toxic substances are dialysis, hemoperfusion, exchange transfusion, plasmapheresis, enzyme induction, and inhibition. Methods of increasing urinary excretion of toxic chemicals and drugs have been studied extensively, but the other modalities have not been well evaluated.

In general, these methods are needed in only a minority of cases and should be reserved for life-threatening circumstances when a definite benefit is anticipated.

Dialysis

Dialysis is the extrarenal means of removing certain substances from the body, and it can substitute for the kidney when renal failure occurs. Dialysis is not the first measure instituted; however, it may be lifesaving later in the course of a severe intoxication. It is needed in only a minority of intoxicated patients.

TABLE 4   Agents with Central Nervous System (CNS) Effects

AGENTS	GENERAL MANIFESTATIONS	AGENTS	GENERAL MANIFESTATIONS
CNS Depressants		**Hallucinogens**	
Alcohols and glycols (S-H)	Bradycardia	Amphetamines‡	Tachycardia and dysrhythmias
Anticonvulsants (S-H)	Bradypnea	Anticholinergics	Tachypnea
Antidysrhythmics (S-H)	Shallow respirations	Cardiac glycosides	Hypertension
Antihypertensives (S-H)	Hypotension	Cocaine	Hallucinations, usually visual
Barbiturates (S-H)	Hypothermia	Ethanol withdrawal	Disorientation
Benzodiazepines (S-H)	Flaccid coma	Hydrocarbon inhalation (abuse)	Panic reaction
Butyrophenones (Syly)	Miosis	Mescaline (peyote)	Toxic psychosis
β-Adrenergic blockers (Syly)	Hypoactive bowel sounds	Mushrooms (psilocybin)	Moist skin
Calcium channel blockers (Syly)		Phencyclidine	Mydriasis (reactive)
Digitalis (Syly)			Hyperthermia
Opioids			Flashbacks
Lithium (mixed)			
Muscle relaxants		**Anticholinergics**	
Phenothiazines (Syly)		Antihistamines	Tachycardia, dysrhythmias (rare)
Nonbarbiturate/benzodiazepine glutethimide, methaqualone, methyprylon, sedative–hypnotics (chloral hydrate, ethchlorvynol, bromide)		Antispasmodic gastrointestinal preparations	Tachypnea
		Antiparkinsonian preparations	Hypertension (mild)
Tricyclic antidepressants (late Syly)		Atropine	Hyperthermia
		Cyclobenzaprine (Flexeril)	Hallucinations ("mad as a hatter")
CNS Stimulants		Mydriatic ophthalmologic agents	Mydriasis (unreactive) ("blind as a bat")
Amphetamines (Sy)	Tachycardia	Over-the-counter sleep agents	Flushed skin ("red as a beet")
Anticholinergics*	Tachypnea and dysrhythmias	Plants (*Datura* spp.)/mushrooms	Dry skin and mouth ("dry as a bone")
Cocaine (Sy)	Hypertension	Phenothiazines (early)	Hypoactive bowel sounds
Camphor (mixed)	Convulsions	Scopolamine	Urinary retention
Ergot alkaloids (Sy)	Toxic psychosis	Tricyclic/cyclic antidepressants (early)	Lilliputian hallucinations ("little people")
Isoniazid (mixed)	Mydriasis (reactive)		
Lithium (mixed)	Agitation and restlessness	**Cholinergics**	
Lysergic acid diethylamide (H)	Moist skin	Bethanechol (Urecholine)	Bradycardia (muscarinic)
Hallucinogens (H)	Tremors	Carbamate insecticides (Carbaryl)	Tachycardia (nicotinic effect)
Mescaline and synthetic analogues		Edrophonium	Miosis (muscarinic)
Metals (arsenic, lead, mercury)		Organophosphate insecticides (Malathion, parathion)	Diarrhea (muscarinic)
Methylphenidate (Ritalin) (Sy)		Parasympathetic agents (physostigmine, pyridostigmine)	Hypertension (variable)
Monoamine oxidase inhibitors (Sy)		Toxic mushrooms (*Clitocybe* spp.)	Hyperactive bowel sounds
Pemoline (Cylert) (Sy)			Excess urination (muscarinic)
Phencyclidine (H)†			Excess salivation (muscarinic)
Salicylates (mixed)			Lacrimation (muscarinic)
Strychnine (mixed)			Bronchospasm (muscarinic)
Sympathomimetics (Sy) (phenylpropanolamine, theophylline, caffeine, thyroid)			Muscle fasciculations (nicotinic)
Withdrawal from ethanol, β-adrenergic blockers, clonidine, opioids, sedative–hypnotics (W)			Paralysis (nicotinic)

Abbreviations: H = hallucinogen; S-H = sedative–hypnotic; Sy = sympathomimetic; Syly = sympatholytic; W = withdrawal.

*Anticholinergics produce dry skin and mucosa and decreased bowel sounds.

†Phencyclidine may produce miosis.

‡The amphetamine hybrids are methylene dioxymethamphetamine (MDMA, ecstasy, "Adam") and methylene dioxyamphetamine (MDA, "Eve"), which are associated with deaths.

TABLE 5 Initial Doses of Antidotes for Common Poisonings

ANTIDOTE	USE	DOSE	ROUTE	ADVERSE REACTIONS/COMMENTS
N-Acetyl Cysteine (NAC, Mucomyst): Stock level to treat 70kg adult for 24h: 25 vials, 20%, 30mL	Acetaminophen, carbon tetrachloride (experimental)	140mg/kg loading, followed by 70mg/kg q4h for 17 doses 150mg/kg in 200mL of D_5W over 1h, then 50mg/kg in 1 liter D_5W over 16h	PO IV	Nausea, vomiting. Dilute to 5% with sweet juice or flat cola. Useful for those who cannot tolerate oral route.
Atropine: Stock level to treat 70kg adult for 24h: 1g (1 mg/mL) in 1, 10mL)	Organophosphate and carbamate pesticides: bradydysrhythmics, β-adrenergics, calcium channel blockers/nerve agents	*Child:* 0.02–0.05 mg/kg repeated q5–10min to max of 2mg as necessary until cessation of secretions *Adult:* 1–2 mg q5–10 min as necessary. Dilute in 1–2mL of 0.9% saline for ET instillation. *IV infusion dose:* Place 8mg of atropine in 100mL D_5W or saline. Conc. = 0.08 mg/mL; dose range = 0.02–0.08mg/kg/h or 0.25–1mL/kg/h. Severe poisoning may require supplemental doses of IV atropine intermittently in doses of 1–5 mg until drying of secretions occurs.	IV/ET	Tachycardia, dry mouth, blurred vision, and urinary retention. Ensure adequate ventilation before administration.
Calcium Chloride (10%): Stock level to treat 70kg adult for 24h: 10 vials 1g (1.35 mEq/mL)	Hypocalcemia, fluoride, calcium channel blockers, β-blockers, oxalates, ethylene glycol, hypermagnesemia	0.1–0.2 mL/kg (10–20mg/kg) slow push q10min up to max 10 mL (1g). Since calcium response lasts 15 min, some may require continuous infusion 0.2mL/kg/h up to maximum of 10mL/h while monitoring for dysrhythmias and hypotension.	IV	Administer slowly with BP and ECG monitoring and have magnesium available to reverse calcium effects. Tissue irritation, hypotension, dysrhythmias from rapid injection. Contraindications: digitalis glycoside intoxication.
Calcium Gluconate (10%): Stock level to treat 70kg adult for 24h: 20 vials 1g (0.45 mEq/mL)	Hypocalcemia, fluoride, calcium channel blockers, hydrofluoric acid; black widow envenomation	0.3–0.4 mL/kg (30–40mg/kg) slow push; repeat as needed up to max dose 10–20mL (1–2g).	IV	Same comments as calcium chloride.
Infiltration of Calcium Gluconate	Hydrofluoric acid skin exposure	Dose: Infiltrate each square cm of affected dermis/subcutaneous tissue with about 0.5mL of 10% calcium gluconate using a 30-gauge needle. Repeat as needed to control pain.	Infiltrate	
Intra-arterial Calcium Gluconate	Hydrofluoric acid skin exposure	Infuse 20mL of 10% calcium gluconate (not chloride) diluted in 250 mL D_5W via the radial or brachial artery proximal to the injury over 3–4h.		Alternatively, dilute 10mL of 10% calcium gluconate with 40–50mL of D_5W.
Calcium Gluconate Gel: Stock level: 3.5g	Hydrofluoric acid skin exposure	2.5g USP powder added to 100mL water-soluble lubricating jelly, e.g., K-Y jelly or Lubifax (or 3.5 mg into 150mL). Some use 6g of calcium carbonate in 100g of lubricant. Place injured hand in surgical glove filled with gel. Apply q4h. If pain persists, calcium gluconate injection may be needed (above).	Dermal	Powder is available from Spectrum Pharmaceutical Co. in California: 800-772-8786. Commercial preparation of Ca gluconate gel is available from Pharmascience in Montreal, Quebec: 514-340-1114.
Cyanide Antidote Kit: Stock level to treat 70kg adult for 24h: 2 Lilly Cyanide Antidote kits	Cyanide Hydrogen sulfide (nitrites are given only)	Amyl nitrite: 1 crushable ampule for 30sec of every min. Use new amp q3min.	Inhalation	If methemoglobinemia occurs, do not use methylene blue to correct this because it releases cyanide.
	Do not use sodium thiosulfate for hydrogen sulfide	May omit step if venous access is established.		
	Individual portions of the kit can be used in certain circumstances (consult PCC)			

Continued

TABLE 5   Initial Doses of Antidotes for Common Poisonings—cont'd

ANTIDOTE	USE	DOSE	ROUTE	ADVERSE REACTIONS/COMMENTS
	Cyanide Hydrogen sulfide (nitrites are given only) Do not use sodium thiosulfate for hydrogen sulfide Individual portions of the kit can be used in certain circumstances (consult PCC)	Sodium nitrite: *Child:* 0.33 mL/kg of 3% solution if hemoglobin level is not known, otherwise based on tables with product. *Adult:* up to 300 mg (10 mL). Dilute nitrite in 100 mL 0.9% saline, administer slowly at 5 mL/min. Slow infusion if fall in BP.	IV	If methemoglobinemia occurs, do not use methylene blue to correct this because it releases cyanide.
	Do not use sodium thiosulfate for hydrogen sulfide Individual portions of the kit can be used in certain circumstances (consult PCC)	Sodium thiosulfate: *Child:* 1.6 mL/kg of 25% solution, may be repeated q30–60 min to a maximum of 12.5 g or 50 mL in adult. Administer over 20 min.	IV	Nausea, dizziness, headache. Tachycardia, muscle rigidity, and bronchospasm (rapid administration).
Dantrolene Sodium (Dantrium): Stock level to treat 70 kg adult for 24 h: 700 mg, 35 vials (20 mg/vial)	Malignant hyperthermia	2–3 mg/kg IV rapidly. Repeat loading dose every 10 min. If necessary up to a maximum total dose of 10 mg/kg. When temperature and heart rate decrease, slow the infusion 1–2 mg/kg q6h for 24–28h until all evidence of malignant hyperthermia syndrome has subsided. Follow with oral doses 1–2 mg/kg four times a day for 24 h as necessary.	IV/PO	Hepatotoxicity occurs with cumulative dose of 10 mg/kg. Thrombophlebitis (best given in central line). Available as 20 mg lyophilized dantrolene powder for reconstruction, which contains 3 g mannitol and sodium hydroxide in 70-mL vial. Mix with 60 mL sterile distilled water without a bacteriostatic agent and protect from light. Use within 6 hours after reconstituting.
Deferoxamine (Desferal): Stock level to treat 70 kg adult for 24 h: 17 vials (500 mg/amp)	Iron	IV infusion of 15 mg/kg/h (3 mL/kg/h: 500 mg in 100 mL D₅W) max 6 g/d Rates of >45 µg/kg/h if conc >1000 µg/dL.	Preferred IV: avoid therapy >24h	Hypotension (minimized by avoiding rapid infusion rates) DFO challenge test 50 mg/kg is unreliable if negative.
Diazepam (Valium): Stock level to treat 70 kg adult for 24 h: 200 mg, 5 mg/mL; 2, 10 mL	Any intoxication that provokes seizures when specific therapy is not available (e.g., amphetamines, PCP, barbiturate and alcohol withdrawal) Chloroquine poisoning	*Adult,* 5–10 mg IV (max 20 mg) at a rate of 5 mg/min until seizure is controlled. May be repeated 2 or 3 times. *Child,* 0.1–0.3 mg/kg up to 10 mg IV slowly over 2 min.	IV	Confusion, somnolence, coma, hypotension. Intramuscular absorption is erratic. Establish airway and administer 100% oxygen and glucose.
Digoxin-Specific Fab Antibodies (Digibind): Stock level to treat 70 kg adult for 24 h: 20 vials	Digoxin, digitoxin, oleander tea with the following: (1) Imminent cardiac arrest or shock (2) Hyperkalemia >5.0 mEq/L (3) Serum digoxin >5 ng/mL (child) at 8–12 h post ingestion in adults (4) Digitalis delirium (5) Ingestion over 10 mg in adults or 4 mg in child (6) Bradycardia or second- or third-degree heart block unresponsive to atropine (7) Life-threatening digitoxin or oleander poisoning	(1) If amount ingested is known total dose × bioavailability (0.8) = body burden. The body burden + 0.6 (0.5 mg of digoxin is bound by 1 vial of 38 mg of Fab) = # vials needed. (2) If amount is unknown but the steady state serum concentration is known in ng/mL: Digoxin: ng/mL: (5.6 L/kg Vd) × (wt kg) = µg body burden. Body burden + 100 = mg body burden/0.5 = # vials needed. Digitoxin body burden = ng/mL × (0.56 L/kg Vd) × (wt kg) Body burden + 1000 = mg body burden/0.5 = # vials needed. (3) If the amount is not known, it is administered in life-threatening situations as 10 vials (400 mg) IV in saline over 30 min in adults. If cardiac arrest is imminent, administer 20 vials (adult) as a bolus.	IV	Allergic reactions (rare), return of condition being treated with digitalis glycoside. Administer by infusion over 30 min through a 0.22-µ filter. If cardiac arrest imminent, may administer by bolus. Consult PCC for more details.

Agent (Stock)	Indication	Dose	Route	Precautions/Adverse Effects
Dimercaprol (BAL in Peanut Oil): Stock level to treat 70 kg adult for 24 h: 1200 mg (4 amps—100 mg/mL 10% in oil in 3 mL amp)	Chelating agent for arsenic, mercury, and lead	3–5 mg/kg q4h usually for 5–10d	Deep IM	Local infection site pain and sterile abscess, nausea, vomiting, fever, salivation, hypertension, and nephrotoxicity (alkalinize urine).
2,3 Dimercaptosuccinic Acid (DMSA Succimer): 100 mg/capsule:20 capsules	Used as a chelating agent for lead, especially blood lead levels >45 µg/dL. May also be used for symptomatic mercury exposure	10 mg/kg 3 × daily for 5 days followed by 10 mg/kg 2 × daily for 14 days	PO	Precautions: monitor AST/ALT; use with caution in G6PD-deficient patients. Avoid concurrent iron therapy. Relatively safe antidote, rarely severe, uncommon minor skin rashes may occur.
Diphenhydramine (Benadryl): Antiparkinsonian action. Stock level to treat a 70 kg adult for 24 h: 5 vials (10 mg/mL, 10 mL each)	Used to treat extrapyramidal symptoms and dystonia induced by phenothiazines, phencyclidine, and related drugs	*Children:* 1–2 mg/kg IV slowly over 5 min up to maximum 50 mg followed by 5 mg/kg/24h orally divided every 6h up to 300 mg/24h. *Adults:* 50 mg IV followed by 50 mg orally four times daily for 5–7d. *Note:* Symptoms abate within 2–5 min after IV.	IV	Fatal dose: 20–40 mg/kg. Dry mouth, drowsiness.
Ethanol (Ethyl Alcohol): Stock level to treat 70 kg adult for 24 h: 3 bottles 10% (1 L each)	Methanol, ethylene glycol	10 mL/kg loading dose concurrently with 1.4 mL/kg (average) infusion of 10% ethanol (consult PCC for more details)	IV	Nausea, vomiting, sedation. Use 0.22-µ filter if preparing from bulk 100% ethanol.
Flumazenil (Romazicon): Stock level to treat 70 kg adult for 24 h: 4 vials (0.1 mg/mL, 10 mL)	Benzodiazepines (may also be beneficial in the treatment of hepatic encephalopathy)	Administer 0.2 mg (2 mL) IV over 30 sec (pediatric dose not established, 0.01 mg/kg), then if desired consciousness is not achieved, administer 0.3 mg (3 mL) over 30 sec, then wait 3 min for response, then if desired consciousness is not achieved, administer 0.5 mg (5 mL) over 30 sec at 60-sec intervals up to a maximum cumulative dose of 3 mg (30 mL) (1 mg in children). Because effects last only 1–5 h, if patient responds, monitor carefully over next 6h for resedation. If multiple repeated doses, consider a continuous infusion of 0.2–1 mg/h.	IV	Nausea, vomiting, facial flushing, agitation, headache, dizziness, seizures, and death. It is not recommended to improve ventilation. Its role in CNS depression needs to be clarified. It should not be used routinely in comatose patients. It is **contraindicated** in cyclic antidepressant intoxications, stimulant overdose, long-term benzodiazepine use (may precipitate life-threatening withdrawal), if benzodiazepines are used to control seizures, in head trauma.
Folic Acid (Folvite): Stock level to treat 70 kg adult for 24 h: 4 100-mg vials	Methanol/ethylene glycol (investigational)	1 mg/kg up to 50 mg q4h for 6 doses	IV	Uncommon
Fomepizole (4-MP, Antizol): Stock level to treat 70 kg adult: 4 1.5-mL vials (1 g/mL)	Ethylene glycol Methanol	Loading dose: 15 mg/kg (0.015 mL/kg) IV followed by maintenance dose of 10 mg/kg (0.01 mL/kg) q12h for 4 doses, then 15 mg/kg q12h until ethylene glycol levels are <20 mg/dL. Fomepizole can be given to patients undergoing hemodialysis (dose q4h).	IV	Suggested: co-administer folate 50 mg IV (child 1 mg/kg), thiamine 100 mg/d (child 50 mg), and pyridoxine 50 mg IV/IM q6h until intoxication is resolved. Monitor for urinary oxalate crystals. Adverse reactions include headache, nausea, and dizziness. Antizole should be diluted in 100 mL 0.9% saline or D5W and mixed well. Antizole should not be given undiluted.

Continued

TABLE 5 Initial Doses of Antidotes for Common Poisonings—cont'd

ANTIDOTE	USE	DOSE	ROUTE	ADVERSE REACTIONS/COMMENTS
Glucagon: Stock level to treat 70 kg adult for 24 h: 10 vials, 10 units	β-Blocker, calcium channel blocker	3–10 mg in adult, then infuse 2–5 mg/h (0.05–0.1 mg/kg in child, then infuse 0.07 mg/kg/h) Large doses up to 100 mg/24 h used	IV	Use D₅W, not 0.9% saline, to reconstitute the glucagon (rather than diluent of Eli Lilly, which contains phenol). Vomiting precautions.
Magnesium Sulfate: Stock level to treat 70 kg adult for 24 h: approx 25 g (50 mL of 50% or 200 mL of 12.5%)	Torsades de pointes	*Adult:* 2 g (20 mL or 20%) over 20 min. If no response in 10 min, repeat and follow by continuous infusion 1 g/h. *Children:* 25–50 mg/kg initially and maintenance is 30–60 mg/kg/24 h (0.25–0.5 mEq/kg/24 h) up to 1000 mg/24 h. (Dose not studied in controlled fashion.)	IV	Use with caution if renal impairment is present.
Methylene Blue: Stock level to treat 70 kg adult for 24 h: 5 amps (10 mg/10 mL)	Methemoglobinemia	0.1–0.2 mL/kg of 1% solution, slow infusion, may be repeated q30–60 min	IV	Nausea, vomiting, headache, dizziness.
Naloxone (Narcan): Stock level to treat 70 kg adult for 24 h: 3 vials (1 mg/mL, 10 mL)	Comatose patient; decreased respirations <12; opioids	In postoperative opioid depression reversal, IV 0.1–0.5 μg/kg q2 min as needed and may repeat up to a total dose of 1 μg/kg In suspected overdose, administer IV 0.1 mg/kg in a child younger than 5 years of age up to 2 mg; in older children and adults administer 2 mg every 2 min up to a total of 10–20 mg. Can also be administered into the endotracheal tube. If no response by 10 mg, a pure opioid intoxication is unlikely. If opioid abuse is suspected, **restraints** should be in place before administration; initial dose 0.1 mg to avoid withdrawal and violent behavior. The initial dose is then doubled every minute progressively to a total of 10 mg. A continuous infusion has been advocated because many opioids outlast the short half-life of naloxone (30–60 min). The naloxone infusion hourly rate to produce a response is equal to the effective dose required (improvement in ventilation and arousal). An additional dose may be required in 15–30 min as a bolus.	IV, ET	**Larger doses** of naloxone may be required for more poorly antagonized synthetic opioid drugs: buprenorphine (Buprenex), codeine, dextromethorphan, fentanyl, pentazocine (Talwin), propoxyphene (Darvon), diphenoxylate, nalbuphine (Nubain), new potent "designer" drugs, or long-acting opioids such as methadone (Dolophine). **Complications.** Although naloxone is safe and effective, there are rare reports of complications (<1%) of pulmonary edema, seizures, hypertension, cardiac arrest, and sudden death. The infusions are titrated to avoid respiratory depression and opioid withdrawal manifestations. Tapering of infusions can be attempted after 12 h and when the patient is stable.
Physostigmine (Antilirium): Stock level to treat 70 kg adult for 24 h: 2–4 mg (2 mL each)	Anticholinergic agents (not routinely used, only indicated if life-threatening complications)	*Child:* 0.02 mg/kg slow push to max 2 mg q30–60 min *Adult:* 1–2 mg q5 min to max 6 mg.	IV	Bradycardia, asystole, seizures, bronchospasm, vomiting, headaches. Do not use for cyclic antidepressants.
Pralidoxime (2PAM, Protopan): Stock level to treat 70 kg adult for 24 h: 12 vials (1 g per 20 mL)	Organophosphates/nerve agents	Child ≤12 y, 25–50 mg/kg max (4 mg/min); >12 y, 1–2 g/dose in 250 mL of 0.9% saline over 5–10 min. Max 200 mg/min. Repeat q6–12 h for 24–48 h. Max adult 6 g/d. Alternative: Maintenance infusion 1 g in 100 mL, of 0.9% saline at 5–20 mg/kg/h (0.5–12 mL/kg/h) up to max 500 mg/h or 50 mL/h. Titrate to desired response. End point is absence of fasciculations and return of muscle strength.	IV	Nausea, dizziness, headache; tachycardia, muscle rigidity, bronchospasm (rapid administration).

Antidote	Indications	Route	Dose	Comments
Pyridoxine (Vitamin B₆): Stock level to treat 70 kg adult for 24 h: 100 mg/mL 10% solution. For a 70 kg patient, 10 g = 10 vials	Seizures from isoniazid or *Gyromitra* mushrooms, ethylene glycol	IV	*Isoniazid: Unknown amount ingested:* 5 g (70 mg/kg) in 50 mL D₅W over 5 min + diazepam 0.3 mg/kg IV at rate of 1 mg/min in child or 10 mg dose at rate up to 5 mg/min in adults. Use different site (synergism). May repeat q5–20 min until seizure controlled. Up to 375 mg/kg have been given (52 g). *Known amount:* 1 g for each gram isoniazid ingested over 5 min with diazepam (dose above). *Gyromitra mushroom:* Child 25 mg/kg or 2–5 g, adults IV over 15–30 min to max 20 g	After seizure is controlled, administer remainder of pyridoxine 1 g/1 g isoniazid total 5 g as infusion over 60 min. Adverse reactions uncommon; do not administer in same bottle as sodium bicarbonate. For *Gyromitra* mushrooms, some use PO 25 mg/kg/d early when mushroom ingestion is suspected.
Sodium Bicarbonate (NaHCO₃): Stock level to treat 70 kg adult for 24 h: 10 ampules or syringes (500 mEq)	Tricyclic antidepressant cardiotoxicity (QRS >0.12 sec; ventricular tachycardia, severe conduction disturbances); metabolic acidosis: phenothiazine toxicity *Salicylate:* to keep blood pH 7.5–7.55 (not >7.55) and urine pH 7.5–8.0. Alkalinization recommended if salicylate conc. >40 mg/dL in acute poisoning and at lower levels if symptomatic in chronic intoxication, 2 mEq/kg will raise blood pH 0.1 unit	IV	*Ethylene glycol:* 100 mg IV daily. 1–2 mEq/kg undiluted as a bolus. If no effect on cardiotoxicity, repeat twice a few minutes apart *Adult* with clear physical signs and laboratory findings of acute moderate or severe salicylism: Bolus 1–2 mEq/kg followed by infusion of 100–150 mEq NaHCO₃ added to 1 L of 5% dextrose at rate of 200–300 mL/h *Child:* Bolus same as adult followed by 1–2 mEq/kg in infusion of 20 mL/kg/h 5% dextrose in 0.45% saline Add potassium when patient voids Rate and amount of the initial infusion, if patient is volume depleted: 1 h to achieve urine output of 2 mL/kg/h and urine pH 7–8 In mild cases without acidosis and urine pH >6, administer 5% dextrose in 0.9% saline with 50 mEq/L or 1 mEq/kg NaHCO₃, as maintenance to replace ongoing renal losses. If acidemia is present and pH <7.2, add 2 mEq/kg as loading dose followed by 2 mEq/kg q3–4 h to keep pH at 7.5–7.55. If acidemia is present, recommend isotonic NaHCO₃, 3 ampules to 1 L of D₅W at 10–15 mL/kg/h or sufficient to produce normal urine flow and a urine pH of 7.5 or higher	Monitor sodium, potassium, and blood pH because fatal alkalemia and hyponatremia have been reported. Monitor both urine and blood pH. Do not use the urine pH alone to assess the need for alkalinization because of the paradoxical aciduria that may occur. Adjust the urine pH to 7.5–8 by NaHCO₃ infusion. After urine output established, add potassium 40 mEq/L.
	Long-acting barbiturates: Phenobarbital and primidone (Mysoline). *Note:* Alkalinization is ineffective for the short- or intermediate-acting barbiturates	IV	NaHCO₃; 2 mEq/kg during the first hour or 100 mEq in 1 L of D₅W with 40 mEq/L potassium at a rate of 100 mL/h in adults Adequate potassium is necessary to accomplish alkalinization	Additional sodium bicarbonate and potassium chloride may be needed. Adjust the urine pH to 7.5–8 by NaHCO₃ infusion.
Thiamine: 100 mg/mL, 2 vials	Thiamine deficiency, ethylene glycol poisoning, alcoholism	IV/IM	100 mg IV followed with 100 mg V/IM for 5–7 days in an alcoholic and followed by 100 mg/d orally	
Vitamin K₁ (Aqua Mephyton): 10 mg/1–5 mL; 5-mg tablets	Warfarin anticoagulant or rodenticide toxicity	PO/SC, IV	Oral 0.4 mg/kg/dose child, 10–25 mg adults. If evidence of bleeding, administer vitamin K, SC, IV 0.6 mg/kg/dose child and up to 25–50 mg adults for 6 hours depending on severity	Give vitamin K daily until PT/INR are normal. Examine stools and urine for evidence of bleeding.

Abbreviations: ALT = alanine aminotransferase; amp = ampule; AST = aspartate aminotransferase; BAL = British anti-Lewisite; BP = blood pressure; conc. = concentration; ECG = electrocardiogram; ET = endotracheal; G6PD = glucose-6-phosphate dehydrogenase; IM = intramuscular; IV = intravenous; PCC = poison control center; PO = oral; PT = prothrombin time; SC = subcutaneous.

TABLE 6	Plasma Concentrations Above Which Removal by Extracorporeal Measures Should Be Considered			
DRUG	**PLASMA CONCENTRATION**	**PROTEIN BINDING (%)**	**VOLUME DISTRIBUTION (L/KG)**	**METHOD OF CHOICE**
Amanitin	NA	25	1.0	HP
Ethanol	500–700 mg/dL	0	0.3	HD
Ethchlorvynol	150 µg/mL	35–50	3–4	HP
Ethylene glycol	25–50 µg/mL	0	0.6	HD
Glutethimide	100 µg/mL	50	2.7	HP
Isopropyl alcohol	400 mg/dL	0	0.7	HD
Lithium	4 mEq/L	0	0.7	HD
Meprobamate (Equanil)	100 µg/mL	0	NA	HP
Methanol	50 mg/dL	0	0.7	HD
Methaqualone	40 µg/dL	20–60	6.0	HP
Other barbiturates	50 µg/dL	50	0–1	HP
Paraquat	0.1 mg/dL	poor	2.8	HP > HD
Phenobarbital	100 µg/dL	50	0.9	HP > HD
Salicylates	80–100 mg/dL	90	0.2	HD > HP
Theophylline		0	0.5	
Chronic	40–60 µg/mL			HP
Acute	80–100 µg/mL			HP
Trichlorethanol	250 µg/mL	70	0.6	HP

Abbreviations: HD = hemodialysis; HP = hemoperfusion; HP > HD = hemoperfusion preferred over hemodialysis.
Data from Winchester JF: Active methods for detoxification. In Haddad LM, Winchester JF (eds). Clinical Management of Poisoning and Drug Overdose, 2nd ed. Philadelphia, WB Saunders, 1990; Balsam L, Cortitsidis GN, Fienfeld DA: Role of hemodialysis and hemoperfusion in the treatment of intoxications. Contemp Manage Crit Care 1:61, 1991.
Note: Cartridges for charcoal hemoperfusion are not readily available anymore in most locations. So hemodialysis may be substituted in these situations. In mixed or chronic drug overdoses, extracorporeal measures may be considered at lower drug concentrations.

Peritoneal dialysis uses the peritoneum as the membrane for dialysis. It is only 1/20 as effective as hemodialysis. It is easier to use and less hazardous to the patient but also less effective in removing the toxin; thus it is rarely used except in small infants.

Hemodialysis is the most effective dialysis method but requires experience with sophisticated equipment. Blood is circulated past a semipermeable extracorporeal membrane. Substances are removed by diffusion down a concentration gradient. Anticoagulation with heparin is necessary. Flow rates of 300 to 500 mL/min can be achieved, and clearance rates may reach 200 or 300 mL/min.

Dialyzable substances easily diffuse across the dialysis membrane and have the following characteristics: (a) a molecular weight less than 500 daltons and preferably less than 350; (b) a volume of distribution less than 1 L/kg; (c) protein binding less than 50%; (d) high water solubility (low lipid solubility); and (e) high plasma concentration and a toxicity that correlates reasonably with the plasma concentration. Considerations for hemodialysis and hemoperfusion are cases of serious ingestions (the nephrologist should be notified immediately), and cases involving a compound that is ingested in a potentially lethal dose and the rapid removal of which may improve the prognosis. Examples of the latter are ethylene glycol 1.4 mL/kg 100% solution or equivalent and methanol 6 mL/kg 100% solution or equivalent. Common dialyzable substances include alcohol, bromides, lithium, and salicylates.

The patient-related criteria for dialysis are (a) anticipated prolonged coma and the likelihood of complications; (b) renal compromise (toxin excreted or metabolized by kidneys and dialyzable chelating agents in heavy metal poisoning); (c) laboratory confirmation of lethal blood concentration; (d) lethal dose poisoning with an agent with delayed toxicity or known to be metabolized into a more toxic metabolite (e.g., ethylene glycol, methanol); and (e) hepatic impairment when the agent is metabolized by the liver, and clinical deterioration despite optimal supportive medical management. Table 6 gives plasma concentrations above which removal by extracorporeal measures should be considered.

The contraindications to hemodialysis include the following: (a) substances are not dialyzable; (b) effective antidotes are available; (c) patient is hemodynamically unstable (e.g., shock); and (d) presence of coagulopathy because heparinization is required.

Hemodialysis also has a role in correcting disturbances that are not amenable to appropriate medical management. These are easily remembered by the "vowel" mnemonic:
A—refractory acid-base disturbances
E—refractory electrolyte disturbances
I—intoxication with dialyzable substances (e.g., ethanol, ethylene glycol, isopropyl alcohol, methanol, lithium, and salicylates)
O—overhydration
U—uremia

Complications of dialysis include hemorrhage, thrombosis, air embolism, hypotension, infections, electrolyte imbalance, thrombocytopenia, and removal of therapeutic medications.

Hemoperfusion

Hemoperfusion is the parenteral form of oral activated charcoal. Heparinization is necessary. The patient's blood is routed extracorporeally through an outflow arterial catheter with a filter-adsorbing cartridge (charcoal or resin) and returned through a venous catheter. Cartridges must be changed every 4 hours. The blood glucose, electrolytes, calcium, and albumin levels; complete blood cell count; platelets; and serum and urine osmolarity must be carefully monitored. This procedure has extended extracorporeal removal to a large range of substances that were formerly either poorly dialyzable or nondialyzable. It is not limited by molecular weight, water solubility, or protein binding, but it is limited by a volume distribution greater than 400 L, plasma concentration, and rate of flow through the filter. Activated charcoal cartridges are the primary type of hemoperfusion currently available in the United States.

The patient-related criteria for hemoperfusion are (a) anticipated prolonged coma and the likelihood of complications; (b) laboratory confirmation of lethal blood concentrations; (c) hepatic impairment when an agent is metabolized by the liver; and (d) clinical deterioration despite optimally supportive medical management.

The contraindications are similar to those for hemodialysis.

Limited data are available as to which toxins are best treated with hemoperfusion. Hemoperfusion has proved useful in treating glutethimide intoxication, phenobarbital overdose, and carbamazepine, phenytoin, and theophylline intoxication.

Complications include hemorrhage, thrombocytopenia, hypotension, infection, leukopenia, depressed phagocytic activity of granulocytes, decreased immunoglobulin levels, hypoglycemia, hypothermia, hypocalcemia, pulmonary edema, and air and charcoal embolism.

Hemofiltration

Continuous arteriovenous or venovenous hemodiafiltration (CAVHD or CVVHD, respectively) has been suggested as an alternative to conventional hemodialysis when the need for rapid removal of the drug is less urgent. These procedures, like peritoneal dialysis, are minimally invasive, have no significant impact on hemodynamics, and can be carried out continuously for many hours. Their role in the management of acute poisoning remains uncertain, however.

Plasmapheresis

Plasmapheresis consists of removal of a volume of blood. All the extracted components are returned to the blood except the plasma, which is replaced with a colloid protein solution. There are limited clinical data on guidelines and efficacy in toxicology. Centrifugal and membrane separators of cellular elements are used. It can be as effective as hemodialysis or hemoperfusion for removing toxins that have high protein binding, and it may be useful for toxins not filtered by hemodialysis and hemoperfusion.

Plasmapheresis has been anecdotally used in treating intoxications with the following agents: paraquat (removed 10%), propranolol (removed 30%), quinine (removed 10%), L-thyroxine (removed 30%), and salicylate (removed 10%). It has been shown to remove less than 10% of digoxin, phenobarbital, prednisolone, and tobramycin. Complications include infection; allergic reactions including anaphylaxis; hemorrhagic disorders; thrombocytopenia; embolus and thrombus; hypervolemia and hypovolemia; dysrhythmias; syncope; tetany; paresthesia; pneumothorax; acute respiratory distress syndrome; and seizures.

Supportive Care, Observation, and Therapy for Complications

Altered Mental Status

If airway protective reflexes are absent, endotracheal intubation is indicated for a comatose patient or a patient with altered mental status. If respirations are ineffective, ventilation should be instituted, and if hypoxemia persists, supplemental oxygen is indicated. If a cyanotic patient fails to respond to oxygen, the practitioner should consider methemoglobinemia.

Hypoglycemia

Hypoglycemia accompanies many poisonings, including with ethanol (especially in children), clonidine (Catapres), insulin, organophosphates, salicylates, sulfonylureas, and the unripe fruit or seed of a Jamaican plant called ackee. If hypoglycemia is present or suspected, glucose should be administered immediately as an intravenous bolus. Doses are as follows: in a neonate, 10% glucose (5 mL/kg); in a child, 25% glucose 0.25 g/kg (2 mL/kg); and in an adult, 50% glucose 0.5 g/kg (1 mL/kg).

A bedside capillary test for blood glucose is performed to detect hypoglycemia, and the sample is sent to the laboratory for confirmation. If the glucose reagent strip visually reads less than 150 mg/dL, one administers glucose. Venous blood should be used rather than capillary blood for the bedside test if the patient is in shock or is hypotensive. Large amounts of glucose given rapidly to nondiabetic patients may cause a transient reactive hypoglycemia and hyperkalemia and may accentuate damage in ischemic cerebrovascular and cardiac tissue. If focal neurologic signs are present, it may be prudent to withhold glucose, because hypoglycemia causes focal signs in less than 10% of cases.

Thiamine Deficiency Encephalopathy

Thiamine is administered to avoid precipitating thiamine deficiency encephalopathy (Wernicke-Korsakoff syndrome) in alcohol abusers and in malnourished patients. The overall incidence of thiamine deficiency in ethanol abusers is 12%. Thiamine 100 mg intravenously should be administered around the time of the glucose administration but not necessarily before the glucose. The clinician should be prepared to manage the anaphylaxis that sometimes is caused by thiamine, although it is extremely rare.

Opioid Reactions

Naloxone (Narcan) reverses CNS and respiratory depression, miosis, bradycardia, and decreased gastrointestinal peristalsis caused by opioids acting through μ, κ, and δ receptors. It also affects endogenous opioid peptides (endorphins and enkephalins), which accounts for the variable responses reported in patients with intoxications from ethanol, benzodiazepines, clonidine (Catapres), captopril (Capoten), and valproic acid (Depakote) and in patients with spinal cord injuries. There is a high sensitivity for predicting a response if pinpoint pupils and circumstantial evidence of opioid abuse (e.g., track marks) are present.

In cases of suspected overdose, naloxone 0.1 mg/kg is administered intravenously initially in a child younger than 5 years of age. The dose can be repeated in 2 minutes, if necessary up to a total dose of 2 mg. In older children and adults, the dose is 2 mg every 2 minutes for five doses up to a total of 10 mg. Naloxone can also be administered into an endotracheal tube if intravenous access is unavailable. If there is no response after 10 mg, a pure opioid intoxication is unlikely. If opioid abuse is suspected, restraints should be in place before the administration of naloxone, and it is recommended that the initial dose be 0.1 to 0.2 mg to avoid withdrawal and violent behavior. The initial dose is then doubled every minute progressively up to a total of 10 mg. Naloxone may unmask concomitant sympatho-mimetic intoxication as well as withdrawal.

Larger doses of naloxone may be required for more poorly antagonized synthetic opioid drugs: buprenorphine (Buprenex), codeine, dextromethorphan, fentanyl and its derivatives, pentazocine (Talwin), propoxyphene (Darvon), diphenoxylate, nalbuphine (Nubain), and long-acting opioids such as methadone (Dolophine).

Indications for a continuous infusion include a second dose for recurrent respiratory depression, exposure to poorly antagonized opioids, a large overdose, and decreased opioid metabolism, as with impaired liver function. A continuous infusion has been advocated because many opioids outlast the short half-life of naloxone (30 to 60 minutes). The hourly rate of naloxone infusion is equal to the effective dose required to produce a response (improvement in ventilation and arousal). An additional dose may be required in 15 to 30 minutes as a bolus. The infusions are titrated to avoid respiratory depression and opioid withdrawal manifestations. Tapering of infusions can be attempted after 12 hours and when the patient's condition has been stabilized.

Although naloxone is safe and effective, there are rare reports of complications (less than 1%) of pulmonary edema, seizures, hypertension, cardiac arrest, and sudden death.

Agents Whose Roles Are Not Clarified

Nalmefene (Revex), a long-acting parenteral opioid antagonist that the FDA has approved, is undergoing investigation, but its role in the treatment of comatose patients and patients with opioid overdose is not clear. It is 16 times more potent than naloxone, and its duration of action is up to 8 hours (half-life 10.8 hours, versus naloxone 1 hour).

Flumazenil (Romazicon) is a pure competitive benzodiazepine antagonist. It has been demonstrated to be safe and effective for reversing benzodiazepine-induced sedation. It is not recommended to improve ventilation. Its role in cases of CNS depression needs to be clarified. It should not be used routinely in comatose patients and is not an essential ingredient of the coma therapeutic regimen. It is contraindicated in cases of co-ingestion of cyclic antidepressant intoxication, stimulant overdose, and long-term benzodiazepine use (may precipitate life-threatening withdrawal) if benzodiazepines are used to control seizures. There is a concern about the potential for seizures and cardiac dysrhythmias that may occur in these settings.

Laboratory and Radiographic Studies

An electrocardiogram (ECG) should be obtained to identify dysrhythmias or conduction delays from cardiotoxic medications. If aspiration pneumonia (history of loss of consciousness, unarousable state, vomiting) or noncardiac pulmonary edema is suspected, a chest radiograph is needed. Electrolyte and glucose concentrations in the blood, the anion gap, acid-base balance, the arterial blood gas (ABG) profile (if patient has respiratory distress or altered mental status), and serum osmolality should be measured if a toxic alcohol ingestion is suspected. Table 7 lists appropriate testing on the basis of clinical toxicologic presentation. All laboratory specimens should be carefully labeled, including time and date. For potential legal cases, a "chain of custody" must be established. Assessment of the laboratory studies may provide a clue to the etiologic agent.

Electrolyte, Acid-Base, and Osmolality Disturbances

Electrolyte and acid-base disturbances should be evaluated and corrected. Metabolic acidosis (usually low or normal pH with a low or normal/high $Paco_2$ and low HCO_3) with an increased anion gap (AG) is seen with many agents in cases of overdose.

The AG is an estimate of those anions other than chloride and HCO_3 necessary to counterbalance the positive charge of sodium. It serves as a clue to causes, compensations, and complications. The AG is calculated from the standard serum electrolytes by subtracting the total CO_2 (which reflects the actual measured bicarbonate) and chloride from the sodium: $(Na - [Cl + HCO_3]) = AG$. The potassium is usually not used in the calculation because it may be hemolyzed and is an intracellular cation. The lack of anion gap does not exclude a toxic etiology.

The normal gap is usually 7 to 11 mEq/L by flame photometer. However, there has been a "lowering" of the normal AG to 7 ± 4 mEq/L by the newer techniques (e.g., ion selective electrodes or colorimetric titration). Some studies have found AGs to be relatively insensitive for determining the presence of toxins.

It is important to recognize anion gap toxins, such as salicylates, methanol, and ethylene glycol, because they have specific antidotes, and hemodialysis is effective in management of cases of overdose with these agents.

Table 8 lists the reasons for increased AG, decreased anion gap, or no gap. The most common cause of a decreased AG is laboratory error. Lactic acidosis produces the largest AG and can result from any poisoning that results in hypoxia, hypoglycemia, or convulsions.

Table 9 lists other blood chemistry derangements that suggest certain intoxications.

Serum osmolality is a measure of the number of molecules of solute per kilogram of solvent, or mOsm/kg water. The osmolarity is molecules of solute per liter of solution, or mOsm/L water at a specified temperature. Osmolarity is usually the calculated value and osmolality is usually a measured value. They are considered interchangeable where 1 L equals 1 kg. The normal serum osmolality is 280 to 290 mOsm/kg. The freezing point serum osmolarity measurement specimen and the serum electrolyte specimens for calculation should be drawn simultaneously.

The serum osmolal gap is defined as the difference between the measured osmolality determined by the freezing point method and the calculated osmolarity. It is determined by the following formula (BUN is blood urea nitrogen):

$$(Sodium \times 2) + (BUN/3) + (Glucose/20)$$

TABLE 7	Patient Condition/Systemic Toxin and Appropriate Tests
CONDITION	**TESTS**
Comatose	Toxicologic tests (acetaminophen, sedative-hypnotic, ethanol, opioids, benzodiazepine), glucose.
Respiratory toxicity	Spirometry, FEV_1, arterial blood gases, chest radiograph, monitor O_2 saturation
Cardiac toxicity	ECG 12-lead and monitoring, echocardiogram, serial cardiac enzymes (if evidence or suspicion of a myocardial infarction), hemodynamic monitoring
Hepatic toxicity	Enzymes (AST, ALT, GGT), ammonia, albumin, bilirubin, glucose, PT, PTT, amylase
Nephrotoxicity	BUN, creatinine, electrolytes (Na, F, Mg, Ca, PO_4), serum and urine osmolarity, 24-hour urine for heavy metals if suspected, creatine kinase, serum and urine myoglobin, urinalysis and urinary sodium
Bleeding	Platelets, PT, PTT, bleeding time, fibrin split products, fibrinogen, type and match

Abbreviations: ALT = alanine transaminase; AST = aspartate transaminase; BUN = blood urea nitrogen; ECG = electrocardiogram; FEV_1 = forced expiratory volume in 1 second; GGT = γ-glutamyltransferase; PT = prothrombin time; PTT = partial thromboplastin time.

TABLE 8	Etiologies of Metabolic Acidosis	
NORMAL ANION GAP HYPERCHLOREMIC	**INCREASED ANION GAP NORMOCHLOREMIC**	**DECREASED ANION GAP**
Acidifying agents	Methanol	Laboratory error[†]
Adrenal insufficiency	Uremia*	Intoxication—bromine, lithium
Anhydrase inhibitors	Diabetic ketoacidosis*	Protein abnormal
Fistula	Paraldehyde,* phenformin	Sodium low
Osteotomies	Isoniazid	
Obstructive uropathies	Iron	
Renal tubular acidosis	Lactic acidosis[†]	
Diarrhea, uncomplicated*	Ethanol,* ethylene glycol*	
Dilutional	Salicylates, starvation solvents	
Sulfamylon		

*Indicates hyperosmolar situation. Studies have found that the anion gap may be relatively insensitive for determining the presence of toxins.
[†]Lactic acidosis can be produced by intoxications of the following: carbon monoxide, cyanide, hydrogen sulfide, hypoxia, ibuprofen, iron, isoniazid, phenformin, salicylates, seizures, theophylline.

TABLE 9	Blood Chemistry Derangements in Toxicology
DERANGEMENT	**TOXIN**
Acetonemia without acidosis	Acetone or isopropyl alcohol
Hypomagnesemia	Ethanol, digitalis
Hypocalcemia	Ethylene glycol, oxalate, fluoride
Hyperkalemia	β-Blockers, acute digitalis, renal failure
Hypokalemia	Diuretics, salicylism, sympathomimetics, theophylline, corticosteroids, chronic digitalis
Hyperglycemia	Diazoxide, glucagon, iron, isoniazid, organophosphate insecticides, phenylurea insecticides, phenytoin (Dilantin), salicylates, sympathomimetic agents, thyroid vasopressors
Hypoglycemia	β-Blockers, ethanol, insulin, isoniazid, oral hypoglycemic agents, salicylates
Rhabdomyolysis	Amphetamines, ethanol, cocaine, or phencyclidine, elevated creatine phosphokinase

TABLE 10	Conversion Factors for Alcohols and Glycols		
ALCOHOLS/ GLYCOLS	**1 MG/DL IN BLOOD RAISES OSMOLALITY MOSM/L**	**MOLECULAR WEIGHT**	**CONVERSION FACTOR**
Ethanol	0.228	40	4.6
Methanol	0.327	32	3.2
Ethylene glycol	0.190	62	6.2
Isopropanol	0.176	60	6.0
Acetone	0.182	58	5.8
Propylene glycol	NA	72	7.2

Example: Methanol osmolality. Subtract the calculated osmolality from the measured serum osmolarity (freezing point method) = osmolar gap × 3.2 (one-tenth molecular weight) = estimated serum methanol concentration.
Note: This equation is often not considered very reliable in predicting the actual measured blood concentration of these alcohols or glycols.

This gap estimate is normally within 10 mOsm of the simultaneously measured serum osmolality. Ethanol, if present, may be included in the equation to eliminate its influence on the osmolal gap (the ethanol concentration divided by 4.6; Table 10).

The osmolal gap is not valid in cases of shock and postmortem state. Metabolic disorders such as hyperglycemia, uremia, and dehydration increase the osmolarity but usually do not cause gaps greater than 10 mOsm/kg. A gap greater than 10 mOsm/mL suggests that unidentified osmolal-acting substances are present: acetone, ethanol, ethylene glycol, glycerin, isopropyl alcohol, isoniazid, ethanol, mannitol, methanol, and trichloroethane. Alcohols and glycols should be sought when the degree of obtundation exceeds that expected from the blood ethanol concentration or when other clinical conditions exist: visual loss (methanol), metabolic acidosis (methanol and ethylene glycol), or renal failure (ethylene glycol).

A falsely elevated osmolar gap can be produced by other low molecular weight un-ionized substances (dextran, diuretics, sorbitol, ketones), hyperlipidemia, and unmeasured electrolytes (e.g., magnesium).

Note: A normal osmolal gap may be reported in the presence of toxic alcohol or glycol poisoning, if the parent compound is already metabolized. This situation can occur when the osmolar gap is measured after a significant time has elapsed since the ingestion. In cases of alcohol and glycol intoxication, an early osmolar gap is a result of the relatively nontoxic parent drug and delayed metabolic acidosis, and an anion gap is a result of the more toxic metabolites. The serum concentration is calculated as

$$mg/dL = mOsm \text{ gap} \times MW \text{ of substance divided by } 10.$$

Radiographic Studies

Chest and neck radiographs are useful for suspected pathologic conditions such as aspiration pneumonia, pulmonary edema, and foreign bodies and to determine the location of the endotracheal tube. Abdominal radiographs can be used to detect radiopaque substances.

The mnemonic for radiopaque substances seen on abdominal radiographs is CHIPES:
C—chlorides and chloral hydrate
H—heavy metals (arsenic, barium, iron, lead, mercury, zinc)
I—iodides
P—PlayDoh, Pepto-Bismol, phenothiazine (inconsistent)
E—enteric-coated tablets
S—sodium, potassium, and other elements in tablet form (bismuth, calcium, potassium) and solvents containing chlorides (e.g., carbon tetrachloride)

Toxicologic Studies

Routine blood and urine screening is of little practical value in the initial care of the poisoned patient. Specific toxicologic analyses and quantitative levels of certain drugs may be extremely helpful. One should always ask oneself the following questions: (a) How will the result of the test alter the management? and (b) Can the result of the test be returned in time to have a positive effect on therapy?

Owing to long turnaround time, lack of availability, factors contributing to unreliability, and the risk of serious morbidity without supportive clinical management, toxicology screening is estimated to affect management in less than 15% of cases of drug overdoses or poisonings. Toxicology screening may look specifically for only 40 to 50 drugs out of more than 10,000 possible drugs or toxins and more than several million chemicals. To detect many different drugs, toxic screens usually include methods with broad specificity, and sensitivity may be poor for some drugs, resulting in false-negative or false-positive findings. On the other hand, some drugs present in therapeutic amounts may be detected on the screen, even though they are causing no clinical symptoms. Because many agents are not sought or detected during a toxicologic screening, a negative result does not always rule out poisonings. The specificity of toxicologic tests is dependent on the method and the laboratory. The presence of other drugs, drug metabolites, disease states, or incorrect sampling may cause erroneous results.

For the average toxicologic laboratory, false-negative results occur at a rate of 10% to 30% and false-positives at a rate of 0% to 10%. The positive screen predictive value is approximately 90%. A negative toxicology screen does not exclude a poisoning. The negative predictive value of toxicologic screening is approximately 70%. For example, the following benzodiazepines may not be detected by some routine immunoassay benzodiazepine screening tests: alprazolam (Xanax), clonazepam (Klonopin), temazepam (Restoril), and triazolam (Halcion).

The "toxic urine screen" is generally a qualitative urine test for several common drugs, usually substances of abuse (cocaine and metabolites, opioids, amphetamines, benzodiazepines, barbiturates, and phencyclidine). Results of these tests are usually available within 2 to 6 hours. Because these tests may vary with each hospital and community, the physician should determine exactly which substances are included in the toxic urine screen of his or her laboratory. Tests for ethylene glycol, red blood cell cholinesterase, and serum cyanide are not readily available.

For cases of ingestion of certain substances, quantitative blood levels should be obtained at specific times after the ingestion to avoid

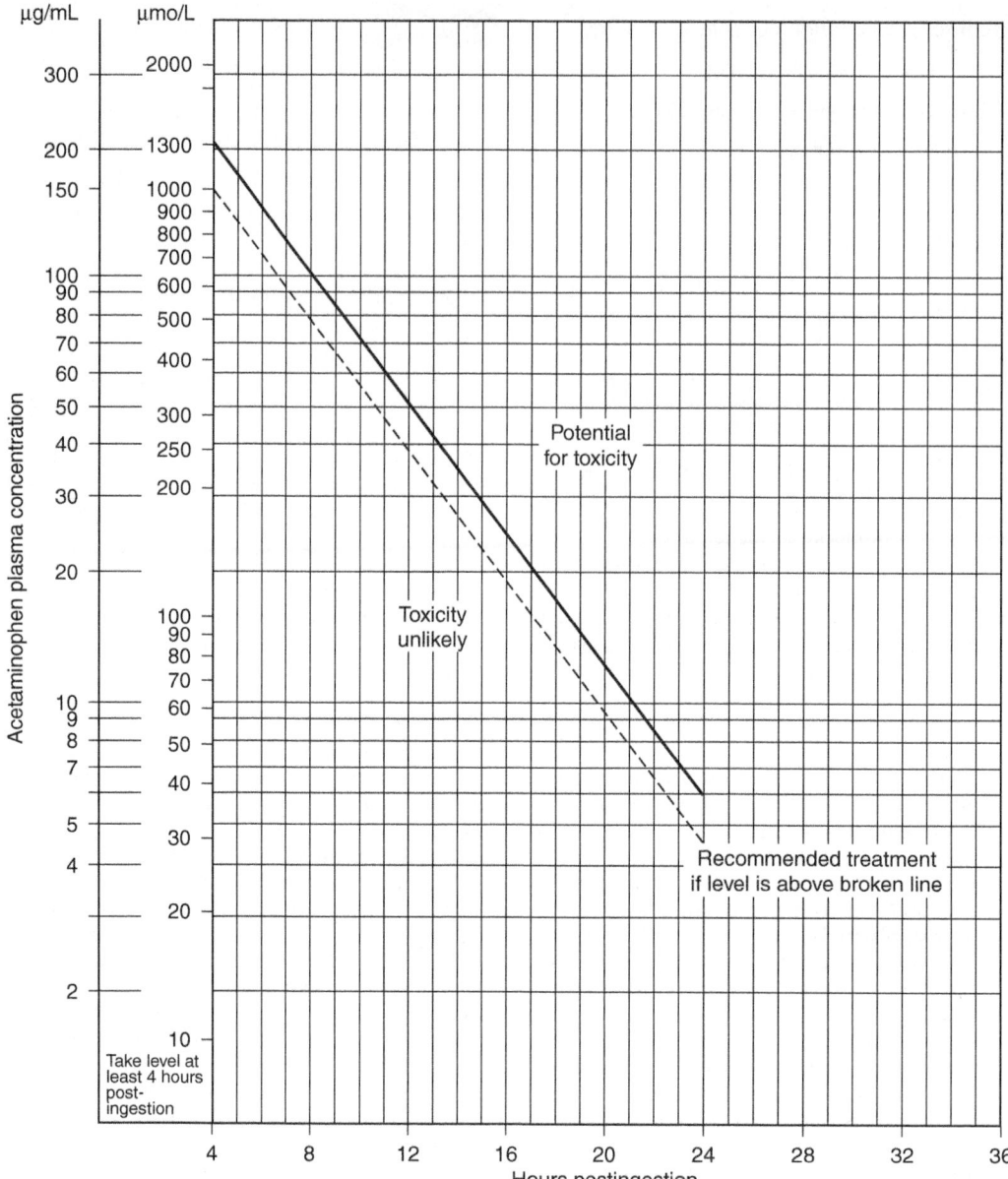

Figure 1 Nomogram for acetaminophen intoxication. *N*-acetylcysteine therapy is started if levels and time coordinates are above the lower line on the nomogram. Continue and complete therapy even if subsequent values fall below the toxic zone. The nomogram is useful only in cases of acute single ingestion. Levels in serum drawn before 4 hours may not represent peak levels. From Rumack BH, Matthew H: Acetaminophen poisoning and toxicity. *Pediatrics* 55:871, 1975.

spurious low values in the distribution phase, which result from incomplete absorption. The detection time for drugs is influenced by many variables, such as type of substance, formulation, amount, time since ingestion, duration of exposure, and half-life. For many drugs, the detection time is measured in days after the exposure.

Common Poisons
Acetaminophen (Paracetamol, *N*-Acetyl-Paraaminophenol)
Toxic Mechanism
At therapeutic doses of acetaminophen, less than 5% is metabolized by P450-2E1 to a toxic reactive oxidizing metabolite, *N*-acetyl-p-benzoquinoneimine (NAPQI). In a case of overdose, there is insufficient glutathione available to reduce the excess NAPQI into nontoxic conjugate, so it forms covalent bonds with hepatic intracellular proteins to produce centrilobular necrosis. Renal damage is caused by a similar mechanism.

Toxic Dose
The therapeutic dose of acetaminophen is 10 to 15 mg/kg, with a maximum of five doses in 24 hours for a maximum total

daily dose of 4 g. An acute single toxic dose is greater than 140 mg/kg, possibly greater than 200 mg/kg in a child younger than age 5 years. Factors affecting the P450 enzymes include enzyme inducers such as barbiturates and phenytoin (Dilantin), ingestion of isoniazid, and alcoholism. Factors that decrease glutathione stores (alcoholism, malnutrition, and HIV infection) contribute to the toxicity of acetaminophen. Alcoholics ingesting 3 to 4 g/d of acetaminophen for a few days can have depleted glutathione stores and require *N*-acetylcysteine therapy at 50% below hepatotoxic blood acetaminophen levels on the nomogram.

Kinetics
Peak plasma concentration is usually reached 2 to 4 hours after an overdose. Volume distribution is 0.9 L/kg, and protein binding is less than 50% (albumin).

Route of elimination is by hepatic metabolism to an inactive nontoxic glucuronide conjugate and inactive nontoxic sulfate metabolite by two saturable pathways; less than 5% is metabolized into reactive metabolite NAPQI. In patients younger than 6

TABLE 11	Protocol for *N*-Acetylcysteine Administration			
ROUTE	LOADING DOSE	MAINTENANCE DOSE	COURSE	FDA APPROVAL
Oral	140 mg/kg	70 mg/kg every 4 h	72 h	Yes
Intravenous	150 mg/kg over 15 min	50 mg/kg over 4 h followed by 100 mg/kg over 16 h	20 h	Yes

years of age, metabolic elimination occurs to a greater degree by conjugation via the sulfate pathway.

The half-life of acetaminophen is 1 to 3 hours.

Manifestations

The four phases of the intoxication's clinical course may overlap, and the absence of a phase does not exclude toxicity.

- Phase I occurs within 0.5 to 24 hours after ingestion and may consist of a few hours of malaise, diaphoresis, nausea, and vomiting or produce no symptoms. CNS depression or coma is not a feature.
- Phase II occurs 24 to 48 hours after ingestion and is a period of diminished symptoms. The liver enzymes, serum aspartate aminotransferase (AST) (earliest), and serum alanine aminotransferase (ALT) may increase as early as 4 hours or as late as 36 hours after ingestion.
- Phase III occurs at 48 to 96 hours, with peak liver function abnormalities at 72 to 96 hours. The degree of elevation of the hepatic enzymes generally correlates with outcome, but not always. Recovery starts at about 4 days unless hepatic failure develops. Less than 1% of patients with a history of overdose develop fulminant hepatotoxicity.
- Phase IV occurs at 4 to 14 days, with hepatic enzyme abnormalities resolving. If extensive liver damage has occurred, sepsis and disseminated intravascular coagulation may ensue.

Transient renal failure may develop at 5 to 7 days with or without evidence of hepatic damage. Rare cases of myocarditis and pancreatitis have been reported. Death can occur at 7 to 14 days.

Laboratory Investigations

The therapeutic reference range is 10 to 20 µg/mL. For toxic levels, see the nomogram presented in Figure 1.

Appropriate and reliable methods for analysis are radioimmunoassay, high-pressure liquid chromatography, and gas chromatography. Spectroscopic assays often give falsely elevated values: bilirubin, salicylate, salicylamide, diflunisal (Dolobid), phenols, and methyldopa (Aldomet) increase the acetaminophen level. Each 1 mg/dL increase in creatinine increases the acetaminophen plasma level 30 µg/mL.

If a toxic acetaminophen level is reached, liver profile (including AST, ALT, bilirubin, and prothrombin time), serum amylase, and blood glucose must be monitored. A complete blood cell count (CBC); platelet count; phosphate, electrolytes, and bicarbonate level measurements; ECG; and urinalysis are indicated.

Management

Gastrointestinal Decontamination. Although ipecac-induced emesis may be useful within 30 minutes of ingestion of the toxic substance, we do not advise it because it could result in vomiting of the activated charcoal. Gastric lavage is not necessary. Studies have indicated that activated charcoal is useful within 1 hour after ingestion. Activated charcoal does adsorb N-acetylcysteine (NAC) if given together, but this is not clinically important. However, if activated charcoal needs to be given along with NAC, separate the administration of activated charcoal from the administration of NAC by 1 to 2 hours to avoid vomiting.

N-Acetylcysteine (Mucomyst). NAC (Table 11), a derivative of the amino acid cysteine, acts as a sulfhydryl donor for glutathione synthesis, as surrogate glutathione, and may increase the nontoxic sulfation pathway resulting in conjugation of NAPQI. Oral NAC should be administered within the first 8 hours after a toxic amount of acetaminophen has been ingested. NAC can be started while one awaits the results of the blood test for acetaminophen plasma concentration, but there is no advantage to giving it before 8 hours. If the acetaminophen concentration result after 4 hours following ingestion is above the upper line on the modified Rumack-Matthew nomogram (see Figure 1), one should continue with a maintenance course. Repeat blood specimens should be obtained 4 hours after the initial level is measured if it is greater than 20 mg/mL, which is below the therapy line, because of unexpected delays in the peak by food and co-ingestants. Intravenous NAC (see Table 11) is approved in the United States.

There have been a few cases of anaphylactoid reaction and death by the intravenous route.

Variations in Therapy

In patients with chronic alcoholism, it is recommended that NAC treatment be administered at 50% below the upper toxic line on the nomogram.

If emesis occurs within 1 hour after NAC administration, the dose should be repeated. To avoid emesis, the proper dilution from 20% to 5% NAC must be used, and it should be served in a palatable vehicle, in a covered container through a straw. If this administration is unsuccessful, a slow drip over 30 to 60 minutes through a nasogastric tube or a fluoroscopically placed nasoduodenal tube can be used. Antiemetics can be used if necessary: metoclopramide (Reglan) 10 mg per dose intravenously 30 minutes before administration of NAC (in children, 0.1 mg/kg; maximum, 0.5 mg/kg/d) or ondansetron (Zofran) 32 mg (0.15 mg/kg) by infusion over 15 minutes and repeated for three doses if necessary. The side effects of these antiemetics include anaphylaxis and increases in liver enzymes.

Some investigators recommend variable durations of NAC therapy, stopping the therapy if serial acetaminophen blood concentrations become nondetectable and the liver enzyme levels (ALT and AST) remain normal after 24 to 36 hours.

There is a loss of efficacy if NAC is initiated 8 or 10 hours postingestion, but the loss is not complete, and NAC may be initiated 36 hours or more after ingestion. Late treatment (after 24 hours) decreases the rates of morbidity and mortality in patients with fulminant liver failure caused by acetaminophen and other agents.

Extended relief formulations (*ER* embossed on caplet) contain 325 mg of acetaminophen for immediate release and 325 mg for delayed release. A single 4-hour postingestion serum acetaminophen concentration can underestimate the level because ER formulations can have secondary delayed peaks. In cases of overdose of the ER formulation, it is recommended that additional acetaminophen levels be obtained at 4-hour intervals after the initial level is measured. If any level is in the toxic zone, therapy should be initiated.

It is recommended that pregnant patients with toxic plasma concentrations of acetaminophen be treated with NAC to prevent hepatotoxicity in both fetus and mother. The available data suggest no teratogenicity to NAC or acetaminophen.

Indications for NAC therapy in cases of chronic intoxication are a history of ingestion of 3 to 4 g for several days with elevated liver enzyme levels (AST and ALT). The acetaminophen blood concentration is often low in these cases because of the extended time lapse since ingestion and should not be plotted on the Rumack-Matthew nomogram. Patients with a history of chronic alcoholism or those on chronic enzyme inducers may also present with elevated liver enzyme levels and should be considered for NAC therapy if they have a history of taking acetaminophen on a chronic basis, because they are considered to be at a greater risk for hepatotoxicity despite a low acetaminophen blood concentration.

Specific support care may be needed to treat liver failure, pancreatitis, transient renal failure, and myocarditis.

Liver transplantation has a definite but limited role in patients with acute acetaminophen overdose. A retrospective analysis determined that a continuing rise in the prothrombin time (4-day peak, 180 seconds), a pH of less than 7.3 2 days after the overdose, a serum creatinine level of greater than 3.3 mg/dL, severe hepatic encephalopathy, and disturbed coagulation factor VII/V ratio greater than 30 suggest a poor prognosis and may be indicators for hepatology consultation for consideration of liver transplantation.

Extracorporeal measures are not expected to be of benefit.

Disposition
Adults who have ingested more than 140 mg/kg and children younger than 6 years of age who have ingested more than 200 mg/kg should receive therapy within 8 hours postingestion or until the results of the 4-hour postingestion acetaminophen plasma concentration are known.

Amphetamines
The amphetamines include illicit methamphetamine ("Ice"), diet pills, and formulations under various trade names. Analogues include MDMA (3,4 methylenedioxymethamphetamine, known as "ecstasy," "XTC," or "Adam") and MDA (3,4-methylenedioxyamphetamine, known as "Eve"). MDA is a common hallucinogen and euphoriant "club drug" used at "raves," which are all-night dances. Use of methamphetamine and designer analogues is on the rise, especially among young people between the ages of 12 and 25 years. Other similar stimulants are phenylpropanolamine and cocaine.

Toxic Mechanism
Amphetamines have a direct CNS stimulant effect and a sympathetic nervous system effect by releasing catecholamines from α- and β-adrenergic nerve terminals but inhibiting their reuptake.

Hallucinogenic MDMA has an additional hazard of serotonin effect (refer to serotonin syndrome in the SSRI section). MDMA also affects the dopamine system in the brain. Because of its effects on 5-hydroxytryptamine, dopamine, and norepinephrine, MDMA can lead to serotonin syndrome associated with malignant hyperthermia and rhabdomyolysis, which contributes to the potentially life-threatening hyperthermia observed in several patients who have used MDMA.

Phenylpropanolamine stimulates only the β-adrenergic receptors.

Toxic Dose
In children, the toxic dose of dextroamphetamine is 1 mg/kg; in adults, the toxic dose is 5 mg/kg. The potentially fatal dose of dextroamphetamine is 12 mg/kg.

Kinetics
Amphetamine is a weak base with pKa of 8 to 10. Onset of action is 30 to 60 minutes, and peak effects are 2 to 4 hours. The volume distribution is 2 to 3 L/kg.

Through hepatic metabolism, 60% of the substance is metabolized into a hydroxylated metabolite that may be responsible for psychotic effects.

The half-life of amphetamines is pH dependent—8 to 10 hours in acid urine (pH <6.0) and 16 to 31 hours in alkaline urine (pH >7.5). Excretion is by the kidney—30% to 40% at alkaline urine pH and 50% to 70% at acid urine pH.

Manifestations
Effects are seen within 30 to 60 minutes following ingestion.

Neurologic manifestations include restlessness, irritation and agitation, tremors and hyperreflexia, and auditory and visual hallucinations. Hyperpyrexia may precede seizures, convulsions, paranoia, violence, intracranial hemorrhage, psychosis, and self-destructive behavior. Paranoid psychosis and cerebral vasculitis occur with chronic abuse.

MDMA is often adulterated with cocaine, heroin, or ketamine, or a combination of these, to create a variety of mood alterations. This possibility must be taken into consideration when one manages patients with MDMA ingestions, as the symptom complex may reflect both CNS stimulation and CNS depression.

Other manifestations include dilated but reactive pupils, cardiac dysrhythmias (supraventricular and ventricular), tachycardia, hypertension, rhabdomyolysis, and myoglobinuria.

Laboratory Investigations
The clinician should monitor ECG and cardiac readings, ABG and oxygen saturation, electrolytes, blood glucose, BUN, creatinine, creatine kinase, cardiac fraction if there is chest pain, and liver profile. Also, one should evaluate for rhabdomyolysis and check urine for myoglobin, cocaine and metabolites, and other substances of abuse. The peak plasma concentration of amphetamines is 10 to 50 ng/mL 1 to 2 hours after ingestion of 10 to 25 mg. The toxic plasma concentration is 200 ng/mL. When the rapid immunoassays are used, cross-reactions can occur with amphetamine derivatives (e.g., MDA, "ecstasy"), brompheniramine (Dimetane), chlorpromazine (Thorazine), ephedrine, phenylpropanolamine, phentermine (Adipex-P), phenmetrazine, ranitidine (Zantac), and Vicks Inhaler (L-desoxyephedrine). False-positive results may occur.

Management
Management is similar to management for cocaine intoxication. Supportive care includes blood pressure and temperature control, cardiac monitoring, and seizure precautions. Diazepam (Valium) can be administered. Gastrointestinal decontamination can be undertaken with activated charcoal administered up to 1 hour after ingestion.

Anxiety, agitation, and convulsions are treated with diazepam. If diazepam fails to control seizures, neuromuscular blockers can be used and the electroencephalogram (EEG) monitored for nonmotor seizures. One should avoid neuroleptic phenothiazines and butyrophenone, which can lower the seizure threshold.

Hypertension and tachycardia are usually transient and can be managed by titration of diazepam. Nitroprusside can be used for hypertensive crisis at a maximum infusion rate of 10 µg/kg/min for 10 minutes followed with a lower infusion rate of 0.3 to 2 mg/kg/min. Myocardial ischemia is managed by oxygen, vascular access, benzodiazepines, and nitroglycerin. Aspirin and thrombolytics are not routinely recommended because of the danger of intracranial hemorrhage. It is important to distinguish between angina and true ischemia. Delayed hypotension can be treated with fluids and vasopressors if needed. Life-threatening tachydysrhythmias may respond to an α-blocker such as phentolamine (Regitine) 5 mg IV for adults or 0.1 mg/kg IV for children and a short-acting β-blocker such as esmolol (Brevibloc) 500 µg/kg IV over 1 minute for adults, or 300 to 500 µg/kg over 1 minute for children. Ventricular dysrhythmias may respond to lidocaine or, in a severely hemodynamically compromised patient, immediate synchronized electrical cardioversion.

Rhabdomyolysis and myoglobinuria are treated with fluids, alkaline diuresis, and diuretics. Hyperthermia is treated with external cooling and cool 100% humidified oxygen. More extensive therapy may be needed in severe cases. If focal neurologic symptoms are present, the possibility of a cerebrovascular accident should be considered and a CT scan of the head should be obtained.

Paranoid ideation and threatening behavior should be treated with rapid tranquilization using a benzodiazepine. One should observe for suicidal depression that may follow intoxication and may require suicide precautions.

Extracorporeal measures are of no benefit.

Disposition
Symptomatic patients should be observed on a monitored unit until the symptoms resolve and then observed for a short time after resolution for relapse.

Anticholinergic Agents
Drugs with anticholinergic properties include antihistamines (H_1 blockers), neuroleptics (phenothiazines), tricyclic antidepressants, antiparkinsonism drugs (trihexyphenidyl [Artane], benztropine [Cogentin]), ophthalmic products (atropine), and a number of common plants.

The antihistamines are divided into the sedating anticholinergic types and the nonsedating single daily dose types. The sedating types include ethanolamines (e.g., diphenhydramine [Benadryl], dimenhydrinate [Dramamine], and clemastine [Tavist]), ethylenediamines (e.g., tripelennamine [Pyribenzamine]), alkyl amines (e.g., chlorpheniramine [Chlor-Trimeton], brompheniramine [Dimetane]), piperazines (e.g., cyclizine [Marezine], hydroxyzine [Atarax], and meclizine [Antivert]), and phenothiazine (e.g., Phenergan). The nonsedating types include astemizole (Hismanal), terfenadine (Seldane), loratadine (Claritin), fexofenadine (Allegra), and cetirizine (Zyrtec).

The anticholinergic plants include jimsonweed (*Datura stramonium*), deadly nightshade (*Atropa belladonna*), henbane (*Hyoscyamus niger*), and antispasmodic agents for the bowel (atropine derivatives).

Toxic Mechanism
By competitive inhibition, anticholinergics block the action of acetylcholine on postsynaptic cholinergic receptor sites. The toxic mechanism primarily involves the peripheral and CNS muscarinic receptors. H_1 sedating-type agents also depress or stimulate the CNS, and in large overdoses some have cardiac membrane–depressant effects (e.g., diphenhydramine [Benadryl]) and α-adrenergic receptor blockade effects (e.g., promethazine [Phenergan]). Nonsedating agents produce peripheral H_1 blockade but do not possess anticholinergic or sedating actions. The original agents terfenadine (Seldane) and astemizole (Hismanal) were recently removed from the market because of the severe cardiac dysrhythmias associated with their use, especially when used in combination with macrolide antibiotics and certain antifungal agents such as ketoconazole (Nizoral), which inhibit hepatic metabolism or excretion. The newer nonsedating agents, including loratadine (Claritin), fexofenadine (Allegra), and cetirizine (Zyrtec), have not been reported to cause the severe drug interactions associated with terfenadine and astemizole.

Toxic Dose
The estimated toxic oral dose of atropine is 0.05 mg/kg in children and more than 2 mg in adults. The minimal estimated lethal dose of atropine is more than 10 mg in adults and more than 2 mg in children. Other synthetic anticholinergic agents are less toxic, and the fatal dose varies from 10 to 100 mg.

The estimated toxic oral dose of diphenhydramine (Benadryl) in a child is 15 mg/kg, and the potential lethal amount is 25 mg/kg. In an adult, the potential lethal amount is 2.8 g. Ingestion of five times the single dose of an antihistamine is toxic.

For the nonsedating agents, an overdose of 3360 mg of terfenadine was reported in an adult who developed ventricular tachycardia and fibrillation that responded to lidocaine and defibrillation. A 1500-mg overdose produced hypotension. Cases of delayed serious dysrhythmias (torsades de pointes) have been reported with doses of more than 200 mg of astemizole. The toxic doses of fexofenadine (Allegra), cetirizine, and loratadine (Claritin) need to be established.

Kinetics
The onset of absorption of intravenous atropine is in 2 to 4 minutes. Peak effects on salivation after intravenous or intramuscular administration are at 30 to 60 minutes.

Onset of absorption after oral ingestion is 30 to 60 minutes, peak action is 1 to 3 hours, and duration of action is 4 to 6 hours, but symptoms are prolonged in cases of overdose or with sustained-release preparations.

The onset of absorption of diphenhydramine is in 15 minutes to 1 hour, with a peak of action in 1 to 4 hours. Volume distribution is 3.3 to 6.8 L/kg, and protein binding is 75% to 80%. Ninety-eight percent of diphenhydramine is metabolized via the liver by N-demethylation. Interactions with erythromycin, ketoconazole (Nizoral), and derivatives produce excessive blood levels of the antihistamine and ventricular dysrhythmias.

The half-life of diphenhydramine is 3 to 10 hours.

The chemical structure of nonsedating agents prevents their entry into the CNS. Absorption begins in 1 hour, with peak effects in 4 to 6 hours. The duration of action is greater than 24 hours.

These agents are metabolized in the gastrointestinal tract and liver. Protein binding is greater than 90%. The plasma half-life is 3.5 hours. Only 1% is excreted unchanged; 60% of that is excreted in the feces and 40% in the urine.

Manifestations
Anticholinergic signs are hyperpyrexia ("hot as a hare"), mydriasis ("blind as a bat"), flushing of skin ("red as a beet"), dry mucosa and skin ("dry as a bone"), "Lilliputian type" hallucinations and delirium ("mad as a hatter"), coma, dysphagia, tachycardia, moderate hypertension, and rarely convulsions and urinary retention. Other effects include jaundice (cyproheptadine [Periactin]), dystonia (diphenhydramine [Benadryl]), rhabdomyolysis (doxylamine), and, in large doses, cardiotoxic effects (diphenhydramine).

Overdose with nonsedating agents produces headache and confusion, nausea, and dysrhythmias (e.g., torsades de pointes).

Laboratory Investigations
Monitoring of ABG (in cases of respiratory depression), electrolytes, glucose, and the ECG should be undertaken. Anticholinergic drugs and plants are not routinely included on screens for substances of abuse.

Management
For patients in respiratory failure, intubation and assisted ventilation should be instituted. Gastrointestinal decontamination can be instituted. Caution must be taken with emesis in cases of diphenhydramine (Benadryl) overdose because of the drug's rapid onset of action and risk of seizures. If bowel sounds are present for up to 1 hour after ingestion, activated charcoal can be given. Seizures can be controlled with benzodiazepines (diazepam [Valium] or lorazepam [Ativan]).

The administration of physostigmine (Antilirium) is not routine and is reserved for life-threatening anticholinergic effects that are refractory to conventional treatments. It should be administered with adequate monitoring and resuscitative equipment available. The use of physostigmine should be avoided if a tricyclic antidepressant is present because of increased toxicity. Urinary retention should be relieved by catheterization to avoid reabsorption of the drug and additional toxicity.

Supraventricular tachycardia should be treated only if the patient is hemodynamically unstable. Ventricular dysrhythmias can be controlled with lidocaine or cardioversion. Sodium bicarbonate 1 to 2 mEq/kg IV may be useful for myocardial depression and QRS prolongation. Torsades de pointes, especially when associated with terfenadine and astemizole ingestion, has been treated with magnesium sulfate 4 g or 40 mL 10% solution intravenously over 10 to 20 minutes and countershock if the patient fails to respond.

Hyperpyrexia is controlled by external cooling. Hemodialysis and hemoperfusion are not effective.

Disposition
Antihistamine H_1 Antagonists. Symptomatic patients should be observed on a monitored unit until the symptoms resolve, then observed for a short time (3 to 4 hours) after resolution for relapse.

Nonsedating Agents. All asymptomatic children who acutely ingest more than the maximum adult dose and all symptomatic children should be referred to a health care facility for a minimum of 6 hours' observation as well as cardiac monitoring. Asymptomatic adults who acutely ingest more than twice the maximum adult daily dose should be monitored for a minimum of 6 hours. All symptomatic patients should be monitored for as long as there are symptoms present.

Barbiturates

Barbiturates have been used as sedatives, anesthetic agents, and anticonvulsants, but their use is declining as safer, more effective drugs become available.

Toxic Mechanism

Barbiturates are γ-aminobutyric acid (GABA) agonists (increasing the chloride flow and inhibiting depolarization). They enhance the CNS depressant effect of GABA and depress the cardiovascular system.

Toxic Dose

The shorter-acting barbiturates (including the intermediate-acting agents) and their hypnotic doses are as follows: amobarbital (Amytal), 100 to 200 mg; aprobarbital (Alurate), 50 to 100 mg; butabarbital (Butisol), 50 to 100 mg; butalbital, 100 to 200 mg; pentobarbital (Nembutal), 100 to 200 mg; secobarbital (Seconal), 100 to 200 mg. They cause toxicity at lower doses than long-acting barbiturates and have a minimum toxic dose of 6 mg/kg; the fatal adult dose is 3 to 6 g.

The long-acting barbiturates and their doses include mephobarbital (Mebaral), 50 to 100 mg, and phenobarbital, 100 to 200 mg. Their minimum toxic dose is greater than 10 mg/kg, and the fatal adult dose is 6 to 10 g. A general rule is that an amount five times the hypnotic dose is toxic and an amount 10 times the hypnotic dose is potentially fatal. Methohexital and thiopental are ultrashort-acting parenteral preparations and are not discussed.

Kinetics

The barbiturates are enzyme inducers. Short-acting barbiturates are highly lipid-soluble, penetrate the brain readily, and have shorter elimination times. Onset of action is in 10 to 30 minutes, with a peak at 1 to 2 hours. Duration of action is 3 to 8 hours. The volume distribution of short-acting barbiturate is 0.8 to 1.5 L/kg; pKa is about 8. Mean half-life varies from 8 to 48 hours.

Long-acting agents have longer elimination times and can be used as anticonvulsants. Onset of action is in 20 to 60 minutes, with a peak at 1 to 6 hours. In cases of overdose, the peak can be at 10 hours. Usual duration of action is 8 to 12 hours. Volume distribution is 0.8 L/kg, and half-life is 11 to 120 hours. The pKa of phenobarbital is 7.2. Alkalinization of urine promotes its excretion.

Manifestations

Mild intoxication resembles alcohol intoxication and includes ataxia, slurred speech, and depressed cognition. Severe intoxication causes slow respirations, coma, and loss of reflexes (except pupillary light reflex).

Other manifestations include hypotension (vasodilation), hypothermia, hypoglycemia, and death by respiratory arrest.

Laboratory Investigations

Most barbiturates are detected on routine drug screens and can be measured in most hospital laboratories. Investigation should include barbiturate level; ABG; toxicology screen, including acetaminophen; glucose, electrolyte, BUN, creatinine, and creatine kinase levels; and urine pH. The minimum toxic plasma levels are greater than 10 µg/mL for short-acting barbiturates and greater than 40 µg/dL for long-acting agents. Fatal levels are 30 µg/mL for short-acting barbiturates and 80 to 150 µg/mL for long-acting agents. Both short-acting and long-acting agents can be detected in urine 24 to 72 hours after ingestion, and long-acting agents can be detected up to 7 days.

Management

Vital functions must be established and maintained. Intensive supportive care including intubation and assisted ventilation should dominate the management. All stuporous and comatose patients should have glucose (for hypoglycemia), thiamine (if chronically alcoholic), and naloxone (Narcan) (in case of an opioid ingestion) intravenously and should be admitted to the intensive care unit. Emesis should be avoided especially in cases of ingestion of the shorter-acting barbiturates. Activated charcoal followed by MDAC (0.5 g/kg) every 2 to 4 hours has been shown to reduce the serum half-life of phenobarbital by 50%, but its effect on clinical course is undetermined.

Fluids should be administered to correct dehydration and hypotension. Vasopressors may be necessary to correct severe hypotension, and hemodynamic monitoring may be needed. The patient must be observed carefully for fluid overload. Alkalinization (ion trapping) is used only for phenobarbital (pKa 7.2) but not for short-acting barbiturates. Sodium bicarbonate, 1 to 2 mEq/kg IV in 500 mL of 5% dextrose in adults or 10 to 15 mL/kg in children during the first hour, followed by sufficient bicarbonate to keep the urinary pH at 7.5 to 8.0, enhances excretion of phenobarbital and shortens the half-life by 50%. Diuresis is not advocated because of the danger of cerebral or pulmonary edema.

Hemodialysis shortens the half-life to 8 to 14 hours, and charcoal hemoperfusion shortens the half-life to 6 to 8 hours for long-acting barbiturates such as phenobarbital. Both procedures may be effective in patients with both long-acting and short-acting barbiturate ingestion. If the patient does not respond to supportive measures or if the phenobarbital plasma concentration is greater than 150 µg/mL, both procedures may be tried to shorten the half-life.

Bullae are treated as a local second-degree skin burn. Hypothermia should be treated.

Disposition

All comatose patients should be admitted to the intensive care unit. Awake and oriented patients with an overdose of short-acting agents should be observed for at least 6 asymptomatic hours; overdose of long-acting agents warrants observation for at least 12 asymptomatic hours because of the potential for delayed absorption. In the case of an intentional overdose, psychiatric clearance is needed before the patient can be discharged. Chronic use can lead to tolerance, physical dependency, and withdrawal and necessitates follow-up.

Benzodiazepines

Benzodiazepines are used as anxiolytics, sedatives, and relaxants.

Toxic Mechanism

The GABA agonists produce CNS depression and increase chloride flow, inhibiting depolarization.

Flunitrazepam (Rohypnol; street name "roofies") is a long-acting benzodiazepine agonist sold by prescription in more than 60 countries worldwide, but it is not legally available in the United States.

Toxic Dose

The long-acting benzodiazepines (half-life >24 hours) and their maximum therapeutic doses are as follows: chlordiazepoxide (Librium), 50 mg; clorazepate (Tranxene), 30 mg; clonazepam (Klonopin), 20 mg; diazepam (Valium), 10 mg in adults or 0.2 mg/kg in children; flurazepam (Dalmane), 30 mg; and prazepam, 20 mg.

The short-acting benzodiazepines (half-life 10 to 24 hours) and their doses include the following: alprazolam (Xanax), 0.5 mg, and lorazepam (Ativan), 4 mg in adults or 0.05 mg/kg in children, which act similar to the long-acting benzodiazepines.

The ultrashort-acting benzodiazepines (half-life <10 hours) are more toxic and include temazepam (Restoril), 30 mg; triazolam (Halcion), 0.5 mg; midazolam (Versed), 0.2 mg/kg; and oxazepam (Serax), 30 mg.

In cases of overdose of short- and long-acting agents, 10 to 20 times the therapeutic dose (>1500 mg diazepam or 2000 mg chlordiazepoxide) have been ingested with resulting mild coma but without respiratory depression. Fatalities are rare, and most patients recover within 24 to 36 hours after overdose. Asymptomatic unintentional overdoses of less than five times the therapeutic dose can be seen. Ultrashort-acting agents have produced respiratory arrest and coma within 1 hour after ingestion of 5 mg of triazolam (Halcion) and death with ingestion of as little as 10 mg. Midazolam (Versed) and diazepam (Valium) by rapid intravenous injection have produced respiratory arrest.

Kinetics
Onset of CNS depression is usually in 30 to 120 minutes; peak action usually occurs within 1 to 3 hours when ingestion is by the oral route. The volume distribution varies from 0.26 to 6 L/kg (LA, 1.1 L/kg); protein binding is 70% to 99%. For flunitrazepam, the onset of action is in 0.5 to 2 hours, oral peak is in 2 hours, and duration 8 hours or more. The half-life of flunitrazepam is 20 to 30 hours, volume distribution is 3.3 to 5.5 L/kg, and 80% is protein bound. Flunitrazepam can be identified in urine 4 to 30 days after ingestion.

Manifestations
Neurologic manifestations include ataxia, slurred speech, and CNS depression. Deep coma leading to respiratory depression suggests the presence of short-acting benzodiazepines or other CNS depressants. In elderly persons, the therapeutic doses can produce toxicity and can have an additive effect with other CNS depressants. Chronic use can lead to tolerance, physical dependency, and withdrawal.

Laboratory Investigations
Most benzodiazepines can be detected in urine drug screens. Quantitative blood levels are not useful. Some of the immunoassay urinary screens cannot detect all of the new benzodiazepines currently available. A consultation with the laboratory analyst is warranted if a specific case occurs in which the test result is negative but benzodiazepine use is suspected by the patient's history. Situations in which benzodiazepines may not be detected include ingestion of a low dose (e.g., <10 mg), rapid elimination, and a different or no metabolite. Some immunoassay methods can produce a false-positive finding for the benzodiazepines when nonsteroidal antiinflammatory drugs (tolmetin [Tolectin], naproxen [Aleve], etodolac [Lodine], and fenoprofen [Nalfon]) are used. If this is a concern, the laboratory analyst should be consulted.

In cases in which "date rape" drugs such as flunitrazepam are suspected, a police crime or reference laboratory should be consulted for testing.

Management
Emesis and gastric lavage should be avoided. Activated charcoal can be useful only if given early before the peak time of absorption occurs. Supportive treatment should be instituted but rarely requires intubation or assisted ventilation.

Flumazenil (Romazicon) is a specific benzodiazepine receptor antagonist that blocks the chloride flow and inhibitor of GABA neurotransmitters. It reverses the sedative effects of benzodiazepines, zolpidem (Ambien), and endogenous benzodiazepines associated with hepatic encephalopathy. It is not recommended to reverse benzodiazepine-induced hypoventilation. The manufacturer advises that flumazenil be used with caution in cases of overdose with possible benzodiazepine dependency (because it can precipitate life-threatening withdrawal), if cyclic antidepressant use is suspected, or if a patient has a known seizure disorder.

Disposition
If the patient is comatose, he or she must be admitted to the intensive care unit. If the overdose was intentional, psychiatric clearance is needed before the patient can be discharged.

β-Adrenergic Blockers (β-Blockers)
β-Blockers are used in the treatment of hypertension and of a number of systemic and ophthalmologic disorders. Properties of β-blockers include the factors listed in Table 12.

Lipid-soluble drugs have CNS effects, active metabolites, longer duration of action, and interactions (e.g., propranolol). Cardioselectivity is lost in overdose. Intrinsic partial agonist agents (e.g., pindolol) may initially produce tachycardia and hypertension. Cardiac membrane depressive effect (quinidine-like) occurs in cases of overdose but not at therapeutic doses (e.g., with metoprolol or sotalol). α-Blocking effect is weak (e.g., with labetalol or acebutolol).

Toxic Mechanism
β-Blockers compete with the catecholamines for receptor sites and block receptor action in the bronchi, the vascular smooth muscle, and the myocardium.

Toxic Dose
Ingestions of greater than twice the maximum recommended daily therapeutic dose are considered toxic (see Table 12). Ingestion of 1 mg/kg propranolol in a child may produce hypoglycemia. Fatalities have been reported in adults with 7.5 g of metoprolol. The most toxic agent is sotalol, and the least toxic is atenolol.

Kinetics
Regular-release formulations usually cause symptoms within 2 hours. Propranolol's onset of action is 20 to 30 minutes and peak is at 1 to 4 hours, but it may be delayed by co-ingestants. The onset of action with sustained-release preparations may be delayed to 6 hours and the peak to 12 to 16 hours. Volume distribution is 1 to 5.6 L/kg. Protein binding is variable, from 5% to 93%.

Metabolism
Atenolol (Tenormin), nadolol (Corgard), and sotalol (Betapace) have enterohepatic recirculation. The duration of action for regular-acting agents is 4 to 6 hours, but in cases of overdose it may be 24 to 48 hours. The duration of action for sustained-release agents is 24 to 48 hours.

The regular preparation with the longest half-life is nadolol, at 12 to 24 hours, and the one with the shortest half-life is esmolol, at 5 to 10 minutes.

Manifestations
See "Toxic Properties" and Table 12.

Highly lipid soluble agents produce coma and seizures. Bradycardia and hypotension are the major cardiac symptoms and may lead to cardiogenic shock. Intrinsic partial agonists initially may cause tachycardia and hypertension. ECG changes include atrioventricular conduction delay or asystole. Membrane-depressant effects produce prolonged QRS and QT interval, which may result in torsades de pointes. Sotalol produces a very prolonged QT interval. Bronchospasm may occur in patients with reactive airway disease with any β-blocker because the selectivity is lost in overdose. Other manifestations include hypoglycemia (because β-blockers block catecholamine counter-regulatory mechanisms) and hyperkalemia.

Laboratory Investigations
Measurements of blood levels are not readily available or useful. ECG and cardiac monitoring should be maintained, and blood glucose and electrolytes, BUN, and creatinine levels should be monitored, as well as ABG if there are respiratory symptoms.

Management
Vital functions must be established and maintained. Vascular access, baseline ECG, and continuous cardiac and blood pressure monitoring should be established. A pacemaker must be available. Gastrointestinal decontamination can be undertaken initially with activated charcoal up to 1 hour after ingestion. MDAC is no longer recommended, based on the latest guidelines. Whole-bowel irrigation can be considered in cases of large overdoses with sustained-release preparations, but there are no studies evaluating the efficacy of intervention.

| TABLE 12 | Pharmacologic and Toxic Properties of β-Blockers | | | | | | | |

B-BLOCKER	MAXIMUM SOLUBILITY	THERAPEUTIC PLASMA LEVEL	LIPID SOLUBIL-ITY	INTRINSIC SYM-PATHOMIMETIC ACTIVITY (PARTIAL AGONIST)	MEMBRANE STABILIZING EFFECT B-SELECTIVE B₁	MEMBRANE STABILIZING EFFECT B-SELECTIVE B₂	CARDIAC SELECTIVITY A-SELECTIVE
Acebutolol (Sectral)	800 mg	200–2000 ng/mL	Moderate	+	+	+	+
Alprenolol[2]	800 mg	50–200 ng/mL	Moderate	2+	+	−	−
Atenolol (Tenormin)	100 mg	200–500 ng/mL	Low	−	−	2+	−
Betaxolol (Kerlone)	20 mg	NA	Low	+	−	+	−
Carteolol (Cartrol)	10 mg	NA	No	+	−	−	−
Esmolol (Brevibloc) (Class II antidysrhythmic, IV only)			Low	−	−	+	−
Labetalol (Trandate)	800 mg	50–500 ng/mL	Low	+	+/−	−	+
Levobunolol (AKBeta eyedrop) (Eye drops 0.25% and 0.5%)	20 mg	NA	No	−	−	−	−
Metoprolol (Lopressor)			Moderate	−	−	2+	−
Nadolol (Corgard)	320 mg	20–40 ng/mL	Low	−	−	−	−
Oxyprenolol[2]	480 mg	80–100 ng/mL	Moderate	2+	+	−	−
Pindolol (Visken)	60 mg	50–150 ng/mL	Moderate	3+	+/−	−	−
Propranolol (Inderal) (Class II antidysrhythmic)	360 mg	50–100 ng/mL	High	−	2+	−	−
Sotalol (Betapace) (Class II antidysrhythmic)	480 mg	500–4000 ng/mL	Low	−	−	−	−
Timolol (Blocadren)	60 mg	5–10 ng/mL	Low	−	+/−	−	−

[2]Not available in the United States.

If there are cardiovascular disturbances, a cardiac consultation should be obtained. Class IA antidysrhythmic agents (procainamide, quinidine) and III (bretylium) are not recommended. Hypotension is treated with fluids initially, although it usually does not respond. Frequently, glucagon and cardiac pacing are needed. Bradycardia in asymptomatic, hemodynamically stable patients requires no therapy. It is not predictive of the future course of the disease. If the patient is unstable (has hypotension or a high-degree atrioventricular block), atropine 0.02 mg/kg (up to 2 mg) in adults, glucagon, and a pacemaker can be used. In case of ventricular tachycardia, overdrive pacing can be used. A wide QRS interval may respond to sodium bicarbonate. Torsades de pointes (associated with sotalol) may respond to magnesium sulfate and overdrive pacing. Prophylactic magnesium for prolonged QT interval has been suggested, but there are no data. Epinephrine must not be used because an unopposed α effect may occur.

Hypotension and myocardial depression are managed by correction of dysrhythmias, Trendelenburg position, fluids, glucagon, or amrinone (Inocor), or a combination of these. Hemodynamic monitoring with a Swan-Ganz catheter or arterial line may be necessary to manage fluid therapy.

Glucagon is the initial drug of choice. It works through adenyl cyclase and bypasses catecholamine receptors; therefore, it is not affected by β-blockers. Glucagon increases cardiac contractility and heart rate. It is given as an intravenous bolus of 5 to 10 mg[3] over 1 minute and followed by a continuous infusion of 1 to 5 mg/h

(in children, 0.15 mg/kg followed by 0.05 to 0.1 mg/kg/h). In large doses and in infusion therapy D₅W, sterile water, or saline should be used as a dilutant to reconstitute glucagon in place of the 0.2% phenol diluent provided with some drugs. Effects are seen within minutes. It can be used with other agents such as amrinone.

Amrinone (Inocor) inhibits phosphodiesterase enzyme, which metabolizes cyclic AMP. It is administered as a bolus of 0.15 to 2 mg/kg (0.15 to 0.4 mL/kg) intravenously, followed by infusion of 5 to 10 µg/kg/min.

Hypoglycemia should be treated with intravenous glucose. Life-threatening hyperkalemia is treated with calcium (avoid if digoxin is present), bicarbonate, and glucose or insulin. Convulsions can be controlled with diazepam or phenobarbital. If bronchospasm is present, β₂ nebulized bronchodilators are given.

Extraordinary measures such as intra-aortic balloon pump support can be instituted. Extracorporeal measures can be undertaken. Hemodialysis for cases of atenolol, acebutolol, nadolol, and sotalol (low volume distribution, low protein binding) ingestion may be helpful, particularly when there is evidence of renal failure. Hemodialysis is not effective for propranolol, metoprolol, and timolol.

Prenalterol[2] has successfully reversed both bradycardia and hypotension but is not currently available in the United States.

Disposition

Asymptomatic patients with history of overdose require baseline ECG and continuous cardiac monitoring for at least 6 hours with

---

[3]Exceeds dosage recommended by the manufacturer.

[2]Not available in the United States.

regular-release preparations and for 24 hours with sustained-release preparations. Symptomatic patients should be observed with cardiac monitoring for 24 hours. If seizures or abnormal rhythm or vital signs are present, the patient should be admitted to the intensive care unit.

Calcium Channel Blockers

Calcium channel blockers are used in the treatment of effort angina, supraventricular tachycardia, and hypertension.

Toxic Mechanism

Calcium channel blockers reduce influx of calcium through the slow channels in membranes of the myocardium, the atrioventricular nodes, and the vascular smooth muscles and result in peripheral, systemic, and coronary vasodilation, impaired cardiac conduction, and depression of cardiac contractility. All calcium channel blockers have vasodilatory action, but only bepridil, diltiazem, and verapamil depress myocardial contractility and cause atrioventricular block.

Toxic Dose

Any ingested amount greater than the maximum daily dose has the potential of severe toxicity. The maximum oral daily doses in adults and toxic doses in children of each are as follows: amlodipine (Norvasc), 10 mg for adults and more than 0.25 mg/kg for children; bepridil (Vascor), 400 mg for adults and more than 5.7 mg/kg for children; diltiazem (Cardizem), 360 mg for adults (toxic dose >2 g) and more than 6 mg/kg for children; felodipine (Plendil), 40 mg for adults and more than 0.56 mg/kg for children; isradipine (DynaCirc), 40 mg for adults and more than 0.4 mg/kg for children; nicardipine (Cardene), 120 mg for adults and more than 0.85 mg/kg for children; nifedipine (Procardia), 120 mg for adults and more than 2 mg/kg for children; nimodipine (Nimotop), 360 mg for adults and more than 0.85 mg/kg for children; nitrendipine (Baypress),[1] 80 mg for adults and more than 1.14 mg/kg for children; and verapamil (Calan), 480 mg for adults and 15 mg/kg for children.

Kinetics

Onset of action of regular-release preparations varies: for verapamil it is 60 to 120 minutes, for nifedipine 20 minutes, and for diltiazem 15 minutes after ingestion. Peak effect for verapamil is 2 to 4 hours, for nifedipine 60 to 90 minutes, and for diltiazem 30 to 60 minutes, but the peak action may be delayed for 6 to 8 hours. Duration of action is up to 36 hours. The onset of action for sustained-release preparations is usually 4 hours but may be delayed, and peak effect is at 12 to 24 hours. In cases of massive overdose, concretions and prolonged toxicity can develop.

Volume distribution varies from 3 to 7 L/kg. Hepatic elimination half-life varies from 3 to 7 hours. Patients receiving digitalis and calcium channel blockers run the risk of digitalis toxicity, because calcium channel blockers increase digitalis levels.

Manifestations

Cardiac manifestations include hypotension, bradycardia, and conduction disturbances occurring 30 minutes to 5 hours after ingestion. A prolonged PR interval is an early finding and may occur at therapeutic doses. Torsades de pointes has been reported. All degrees of blocks may occur and may be delayed up to 16 hours. Lactic acidosis may be present. Calcium channel blockers do not affect intraventricular conduction, so the QRS interval is usually not affected.

Hypocalcemia is rarely present. Hyperglycemia may be present because of interference in calcium-dependent insulin release. Mental status changes, headaches, seizures, hemiparesis, and CNS depression may occur.

Laboratory Investigations

Specific drug levels are not readily available and are not useful. Monitor blood sugar, electrolytes, calcium, ABG, pulse oximetry,

---

[1] Not FDA approved for this indication.

creatinine, and BUN, and also use hemodynamic monitoring, ECG, and cardiac monitoring.

Management

Vital functions must be established and maintained. Baseline ECG readings should be obtained and continuous cardiac and blood pressure monitoring maintained. A pacemaker should be available. Cardiology consultation should be sought.

Gastrointestinal decontamination with activated charcoal is recommended. If a large dose of a sustained-release preparation was ingested, whole-bowel irrigation can be considered, but its effectiveness has not been investigated.

If the patient is symptomatic, immediate cardiology consult must be obtained, because a pacemaker and hemodynamic monitoring may be needed. In the case of heart block, atropine is rarely effective and isoproterenol (Isuprel) may produce vasodilation. The use of a pacemaker should be considered early.

Hypotension and bradycardia can be treated with positioning, fluids, and calcium gluconate or chloride, glucagon, amrinone (Inocor), and ventricular pacing. Calcium salts must be avoided if digoxin is present. Calcium usually reverses depressed myocardial contractility but may not reverse nodal depression or peripheral vasodilation. Calcium chloride can be given in a 10% solution, 0.1 to 0.2 mL/kg up to 10 mL in an adult, or calcium gluconate in a 10% solution 0.3 to 0.4 mL/kg up to 20 mL in an adult. Administration is intravenous, over 5 to 10 minutes. One should monitor for dysrhythmias, hypotension, and the serum ionized calcium. The aim is to increase calcium 4 mg/dL to a maximum of 13 mg/dL. The calcium response lasts 15 minutes and may require repeated doses or a continuous calcium gluconate infusion 0.2 mL/kg/h up to maximum of 10 mL/h.

If calcium fails, glucagon can be tried for its positive inotropic and chronotropic effect, or both. Amrinone (Inocor), an inotropic agent, may reverse the effects of calcium channel blockers. An effective dose is 0.15 mg to 2 mg/kg (0.15–0.4 mL/kg) by intravenous bolus followed by infusion of 5 to 10 μg/kg/min.

In case of hypotension, fluids, norepinephrine (Levophed), and epinephrine may be required. Amrinone and glucagon have been tried alone and in combination. Dobutamine and dopamine are often ineffective.

Extracorporeal measures (e.g., hemodialysis and charcoal hemoperfusion) are not useful, but extraordinary measures such as intra-aortic balloon pump and cardiopulmonary bypass have been used successfully.

For cases of calcium channel blocker toxicity that fail to respond to aggressive management, recent studies demonstrate that insulin and glucose have therapeutic value. The suggested dose range for insulin is to infuse regular insulin at 0.5 IU/kg/h with a simultaneous infusion of glucose 1 g/kg/h, with glucose monitoring every 30 minutes for at least the first 4 hours of administration and subsequent glucose adjustment to maintain euglycemia (70 to 100 mg/dL). Potassium levels should be monitored regularly, as they may shift in response to the insulin.

Disposition

Patients who have ingested regular-release preparations should be monitored for at least 6 hours and those who have ingested sustained-release preparations should be monitored for 24 hours after the ingestion. Intentional overdose necessitates psychiatric clearance. Symptomatic patients should be admitted to the intensive care unit.

Carbon Monoxide

Carbon monoxide is an odorless, colorless gas produced from incomplete combustion; it is also an in vivo metabolic breakdown product of methylene chloride used in paint removers.

Toxic Mechanism

Carbon monoxide's affinity for hemoglobin is 240 times greater than that of oxygen. It shifts the oxygen dissociation curve to the left, which impairs hemoglobin release of oxygen to tissues and inhibits the cytochrome oxidase enzymes.

TABLE 13	Carbon Monoxide Exposure and Possible Manifestations

COHB SATURATION (%)	MANIFESTATIONS
3.5	None
5	Slight headache, decreased exercise tolerance
10	Slight headache, dyspnea on vigorous exertion, may impair driving skills
10–20	Moderate dyspnea on exertion, throbbing, temporal headache
20–30	Severe headache, syncope, dizziness, visual changes, weakness, nausea, vomiting, altered judgment
30–40	Vertigo, ataxia, blurred vision, confusion, loss of consciousness
40–50	Confusion, tachycardia, tachypnea, coma, convulsions
50–60	Cheyne-Stokes, coma, convulsions, shock, apnea
60–70	Coma, convulsions, respiratory and heart failure, death

Toxic Dose and Manifestations

Table 13 describes the manifestations of carbon monoxide toxicity. Exposure to 0.5% for a few minutes is lethal. Sequelae correlate with the patient's level of consciousness at presentation. ECG abnormalities may be noted. Creatine kinase is often elevated, and rhabdomyolysis and myoglobinuria may occur.

The carboxyhemoglobin (CoHB) expresses in percentage the extent to which carbon monoxide has bound with the total hemoglobin. This may be misleadingly low in the anemic patient with less hemoglobin than normal. The patient's presentation is a more reliable indicator of severity than the CoHB level. The manifestations listed in Table 13 for each level are in addition to those listed at the level above. The CoHB may not correlate reliably with the severity of the intoxication, and linking symptoms to specific levels of CoHB frequently leads to inaccurate conclusions. A level of carbon monoxide greater than 40% is usually associated with obvious intoxication.

Kinetics

The natural metabolism of the body produces small amounts of CoHB, less than 2% for nonsmokers and 5% to 9% for smokers.

Carbon monoxide is rapidly absorbed through the lungs. The rate of absorption is directly related to alveolar ventilation. Elimination also occurs through the lungs. The half-life of CoHB in room air (21% oxygen) is 5 to 6 hours; in 100% oxygen, it is 90 minutes; in hyperbaric pressure at 3 atmospheres oxygen, it is 20 to 30 minutes.

Laboratory Investigations

An ABG reading may show metabolic acidosis and normal oxygen tension. In cases of significant poisoning, the ABG, electrolytes, blood glucose, serum creatine kinase and cardiac enzymes, renal function tests, and liver function tests should be monitored. A urinalysis and test for myoglobinuria should be obtained. Chest radiograph can be useful in cases of smoke inhalation or if the patient is being considered for hyperbaric chamber. ECG monitoring should be maintained, especially if the patient is older than 40 years, has a history of cardiac disease, or has moderate to severe symptoms. Which toxicology studies are used is based on symptoms and circumstances. CoHB should be monitored during and at the end of therapy. The pulse oximeter has two wavelengths and overestimates oxyhemoglobin saturation in carbon monoxide poisoning. The true oxygen saturation is determined by blood gas analysis, which measures the oxygen bound to hemoglobin. The co-oximeter measures four wavelengths and separates out CoHB and the other hemoglobin binding agents from oxyhemoglobin. Fetal hemoglobin has a greater affinity for carbon monoxide than adult hemoglobin and may falsely elevate the CoHB as much as 4% in young infants.

Management

The first step is to adequately protect the rescuer. The patient must be removed from the contaminated area, and his or her vital functions must be established.

The mainstay of treatment is 100% oxygen via a non-rebreathing mask with an oxygen reservoir or endotracheal tube. All patients receive 100% oxygen until the CoHB level is 5% or less. Assisted ventilation may be necessary. ABG and CoHB should be monitored and the present CoHB level determined. *Note:* A near-normal CoHB level does not exclude significant carbon monoxide poisoning, especially if the measurement is taken several hours after termination of exposure or if oxygen has been administered prior to obtaining the sample.

The exposed pregnant woman should be kept on 100% oxygen for several hours after the CoHB level is almost 0, because carbon monoxide concentrates in the fetus and oxygen is needed longer to ensure elimination of the carbon monoxide from fetal circulation. The fetus must be monitored, because carbon monoxide and hypoxia are potentially teratogenic.

Metabolic acidosis should be treated with sodium bicarbonate only if the pH is below 7.2 after correction of hypoxia and adequate ventilation. Acidosis shifts the oxygen dissociation curve to the right and facilitates oxygen delivery to the tissues.

The decision to use the hyperbaric oxygen chamber must be made on the basis of the ability to handle other acute emergencies that may coexist in the patient and of the severity of the poisoning. The standard of care for persons exposed to carbon monoxide has yet to be determined, but most authorities recommend using the hyperbaric oxygen chamber under any of the following conditions:

- If the patient is in a coma or has a history of loss of consciousness or seizures
- If there is cardiovascular dysfunction (clinical ischemic chest pain or ECG evidence of ischemia)
- If the patient has metabolic acidosis
- If symptoms persist despite 100% oxygen therapy
- In a child, if the initial CoHB is greater than 15%
- In symptomatic patients with preexisting ischemia
- If there are signs of maternal or fetal distress regardless of CoHB level (infants and fetus are a special problem because fetal hemoglobin has greater affinity for carbon monoxide)

Although controversial, a neurologic-cognitive examination has been used to help determine which patients with low carbon monoxide levels should receive more aggressive therapy. Testing should include the following: general orientation memory testing involving address, phone number, date of birth, and present date; and cognitive testing, involving counting by 7s, digit span, and forward and backward spelling of three-letter and four-letter words. Patients with delayed neurologic sequelae or recurrent symptoms up to 3 weeks may benefit from hyperbaric oxygen chamber treatment.

Seizures and cerebral edema must be treated.

Disposition

Patients with no or mild symptoms who become asymptomatic after a few hours of oxygen therapy, have a carbon monoxide level less than 10%, and have normal physical and neurologic-cognitive examination findings can be discharged, but they should be instructed to return if any signs of neurologic dysfunction appear. Patients with carbon monoxide poisoning requiring treatment need follow-up neuropsychiatric examinations.

Caustics and Corrosives

The terms *caustic* and *corrosive* are used interchangeably and can be divided into acids and alkalis. The U.S. Consumer Product

Safety Commission Labeling Recommendations on containers for acids and alkalis indicate the potential for producing serious damage, as follows:

- Caution—weak irritant
- Warning—strong irritant
- Danger—corrosive

Some common acids with corrosive potential include acetic acid, formic acid, glycolic acid, hydrochloric acid, mercuric chloride, nitric acid, oxalic acid, phosphoric acid, sulfuric acid (battery acid), zinc chloride, and zinc sulfate. Some common alkalis with corrosive potential include ammonia, calcium carbide, calcium hydroxide (dry), calcium oxide, potassium hydroxide (lye), and sodium hydroxide (lye).

Toxic Mechanism

Acids produce mucosal coagulation necrosis and may be absorbed systemically; they do not penetrate deeply. Injury to the gastric mucosa is more likely, although specific sites of injury for acids and alkalis are not clearly defined.

Alkalis produce liquefaction necrosis and saponification and penetrate deeply. The esophageal mucosa is likely to be damaged. Oropharyngeal and esophageal damage is more frequently caused by solids than by liquids. Liquids produce superficial circumferential burns and gastric damage.

Toxic Dose

The toxicity is determined by concentration, contact time, and pH. Significant injury is more likely with a substance that has a pH of less than 2 or greater than 12, with a prolonged contact time, and with large volumes.

Manifestations

The absence of oral burns does not exclude the possibility of esophageal or gastric damage. General clinical findings are stridor; dysphagia; drooling; oropharyngeal, retrosternal, and epigastric pain; and ocular and oral burns. Alkali burns are yellow, soapy, frothy lesions. Acid burns are gray-white and later form an eschar. Abdominal tenderness and guarding may be present if perforation has happened.

Laboratory Investigations

If acid ingestion has taken place, the patient's acid-base balance and electrolyte status should be determined. If pulmonary symptoms are present, a chest radiograph, ABG measurement, and pulse oximetry are called for.

Management

It is recommended that the container be brought to the examination, as the substance must be identified and the pH of the substance, vomitus, tears, or saliva tested.

If the acid or alkali has been ingested, all gastrointestinal decontamination procedures are contraindicated except for immediate rinse, removal of substance from the mouth, and dilution with small amounts (sips) of milk or water. The examiner should check for ocular and dermal involvement. Contraindications to oral dilution are dysphagias, respiratory distress, obtundation, or shock. If there is ocular involvement one should immediately irrigate the eye with tepid water for at least 30 minutes, perform fluorescein stain of eye, and consult an ophthalmologist. If there is dermal involvement, one should immediately remove contaminated clothes and irrigate the skin with tepid water for at least 15 minutes. Consultation with a burn specialist is called for.

In cases of acid ingestion, some authorities advocate a small flexible nasogastric tube and aspiration within 30 minutes after ingestion.

Patients should receive only intravenous fluids following dilution until endoscopic consultation is obtained. Endoscopy is valuable to predict damage and risk of stricture. The indications are controversial, with some authorities recommending it in all cases of caustic ingestions regardless of symptoms, and others selectively using clinical features such as vomiting, stridor, drooling,

and oral or facial lesions as criteria. We recommend endoscopy for all symptomatic patients or patients with intentional ingestions. Endoscopy may be performed immediately if the patient is symptomatic, but it is usually done 12 to 48 hours postingestion.

The use of corticosteroids is considered controversial. Some feel they may be useful for patients with second-degree circumferential burns. They recommend starting with hydrocortisone sodium succinate (Solu-Cortef) intravenously 10 to 20 mg/kg/d within 48 hours and changing to oral prednisolone 2 mg/kg/d for 3 weeks before tapering the dose. We do not usually recommend using corticosteroids because they have not been shown to be effective.

Tetanus prophylaxis should be provided if the patient requires it for wound care. Antibiotics are not useful prophylactically. Contrast studies are not useful in the first few days and may interfere with endoscopic evaluation; later, they can be used to assess the severity of damage.

Emergency medical therapy includes agents to inhibit collagen formation and intraluminal stents. Esophageal and gastric outlet dilation may be needed if there is evidence of stricture. Bougienage of the esophagus, however, has been associated with brain abscess. Interposition of the colon may be necessary if dilation fails to provide an adequate-sized passage.

Management of inhalation cases requires immediate removal from the environment, administration of humid supplemental oxygen, and observation for airway obstruction and noncardiac pulmonary edema. Radiographic and ABG evaluation should be obtained when appropriate. Intubation and respiratory support may be required.

Certain caustics produce systemic disturbances. Formaldehyde causes metabolic acidosis, hydrofluoric acid causes hypocalcemia and renal damage, oxalic acid causes hypocalcemia, phenol causes hepatic and renal damage, and picric acid causes renal injury.

Disposition

Infants and small children should be medically evaluated and observed. All symptomatic patients should be admitted. If they have severe symptoms or danger of airway compromise, they should be admitted to the intensive care unit. After endoscopy, if no damage is detected, the patient may be discharged when he or she can tolerate oral feedings. Intentional exposures require psychiatric evaluation before the patient can be discharged.

Cocaine (Benzoylmethylecgonine)

Cocaine is derived from the leaves of *Erythroxylum coca* and *Truxillo coca*. "Body packing" refers to the placement of many small packages of contraband cocaine for concealment in the gastrointestinal tract or other areas for illicit transport. "Body stuffing" refers to spontaneous ingestion of substances for the purpose of hiding evidence.

Toxic Mechanism

Cocaine directly stimulates the CNS presynaptic sympathetic neurons to release catecholamines and acetylcholine, while it blocks the presynaptic reuptake of the catecholamines; it blocks the sodium channels along neuronal membranes; and it increases platelet aggregation. Long-term use depletes the CNS of dopamine.

Toxic Dose

The maximum mucosal local anesthetic therapeutic dose of cocaine is 200 mg or 2 mL of a 10% solution. Although CNS effects can occur at relatively low local anesthetic doses (50 to 95 mg), they are more common with doses greater than 1 mg/kg; cardiac effects can occur with doses greater than 1 mg/kg. The potential fatal dose is 1200 mg intranasally, but death has occurred with 20 mg parenterally.

Kinetics

Cocaine is well absorbed by all routes, including nasal insufflation, and oral, dermal, and inhalation routes (Table 14). Protein binding is 8.7%, and volume distribution is 1.5 L/kg.

Cocaine is metabolized by plasma and liver cholinesterase to the inactive metabolites ecgonine methyl ester and benzoylecgonine.

TABLE 14	Routes and Kinetics of Cocaine					
TYPE	ROUTE	ONSET	PEAK (MIN)	HALF-LIFE (MIN)	DURATION (MIN)
Cocaine leaf	Oral, chewing	20–30 min	45–90	—	240–360
Hydrochloride	Insufflation	1–3 min	5–10	78	60–90
	Ingestion	20–30 min	50–90	54	Sustained
	Intravenous	30–120 sec	5–11	36	60–90
Freebase/crack	Smoking	5–10 sec	5–11	—	Up to 20
Coca paste	Smoking	Unknown	—	—	—

Plasma pseudocholinesterase is congenitally deficient in 3% of the population and decreased in fetuses, young infants, the elderly, pregnant people, and people with liver disease. These enzyme-deficient individuals are at increased risk for life-threatening cocaine toxicity.

Ten percent of cocaine is excreted unchanged. Cocaine and ethanol undergo liver synthesis to form cocaethylene, a metabolite with a half-life three times longer than that of cocaine. It may account for some of cocaine's cardiotoxicity and appears to be more lethal than cocaine or ethanol alone.

Manifestations

The CNS manifestations of cocaine ingestion are euphoria, hyperactivity, agitation, convulsions, and intracranial hemorrhage. Mydriasis and septal perforation can occur, as well as cardiac dysrhythmias, hypertension, and hypotension (with severe overdose). Chest pain is frequent, but only 5.8% of patients have true myocardial ischemia and infarction. Other manifestations include vasoconstriction, hyperthermia (because of increased metabolic rate), ischemic bowel perforation if the substance is ingested, rhabdomyolysis, myoglobinuria, and renal failure. In pregnant users, premature labor and abruptio placentae can occur.

Body cavity packing should be suspected in cases of prolonged toxicity.

Mortality can result from cerebrovascular accidents, coronary artery spasm, myocardial injury, or lethal dysrhythmias.

Laboratory Investigations

Monitoring of the ECG and cardiac rhythms, ABG, oxygen saturation, electrolytes, blood glucose, BUN, creatinine, and creatine kinase levels should be maintained. One should monitor cardiac fraction if the patient has chest pain, as well as the liver profile, and the urine for myoglobin. Intravenous drug users should have HIV and hepatitis virus testing.

Urine should be tested for cocaine and metabolites and other substances of abuse, and abdominal radiographs or ultrasonogram should be ordered for body packers. If the urine sample was collected more than 12 hours after cocaine intake, it will contain little or no cocaine. If cocaine is present, cocaine has been used within the past 12 hours. Cocaine's metabolite benzoylecgonine may be detected within 4 hours after a single nasal insufflation and for up to 114 hours. Cross-reactions with some herbal teas, lidocaine, and droperidol (Inapsine) may give false-positive results by some immunoassay methods.

Management

Supportive care includes blood pressure, cardiac, and thermal monitoring and seizure precautions. Diazepam (Valium) is the drug of choice for treatment of cocaine toxicity agitation, seizures, and dysrhythmias; doses are 10 to 30 mg intravenously at 2.5 mg per minute for adults and 0.2 to 0.5 mg/kg at 1 mg per minute up to 10 mg for a child.

Gastrointestinal decontamination should be instituted, if the cocaine was ingested, by administration of activated charcoal. MDAC may adsorb cocaine leakage in body stuffers or body packers. Whole-bowel irrigation with polyethylene glycol solution (PEG) has been used in body packers and stuffers if the contraband is in a firm container. If the packages are not visible on plain radiographs of the abdomen, a contrast study or CT scan can help to confirm successful passage. Cocaine in the nasal passage can be removed with an applicator dipped in a non–water-soluble product (lubricating jelly) if this is done within a few minutes after application.

In body packers and stuffers, venous access must be secured, and drugs must be readily available for treating life-threatening manifestations until the contraband is passed in the stool. Surgical removal may be indicated if the packet does not pass the pylorus, in an asymptomatic body packer, or in the case of intestinal obstruction.

Hypertension and tachycardia are usually transient and can be managed by careful titration of diazepam. Nitroprusside may be used for severe hypertension. Myocardial ischemia is managed by oxygen, vascular access, benzodiazepines, and nitroglycerin. Aspirin and thrombolysis are not routinely recommended because of the danger of intracranial hemorrhage.

Dysrhythmias are usually supraventricular (SVT) and do not require specific management. Adenosine is ineffective. Life-threatening tachydysrhythmias may respond to phentolamine (Regitine) 5 mg IV bolus in adults or 0.1 mg/kg in children at 5- to 10-minute intervals. Phentolamine also relieves coronary artery spasm and myocardial ischemia. Electrical synchronized cardioversion should be considered for patients with hemodynamically unstable dysrhythmias. Lidocaine is not recommended initially but may be used after 3 hours for ventricular tachycardia. Wide complex QRS ventricular tachycardia may be treated with sodium bicarbonate 2 mEq/kg as a bolus. β-Adrenergic blockers are not recommended.

Anxiety, agitation, and convulsions can be treated with diazepam. If diazepam fails to control seizures, neuromuscular blockers can be used. The EEG should be monitored for nonmotor seizure activity. For hyperthermia, external cooling and cool humidified 100% oxygen should be administered. Neuromuscular paralysis to control seizures will reduce temperature. Dantrolene and antipyretics are not recommended. Rhabdomyolysis and myoglobinuria are treated with fluids, alkaline diuresis, and diuretics.

If the patient is pregnant, the fetus must be monitored and the patient observed for spontaneous abortion.

Paranoid ideation and threatening behavior should be treated with rapid tranquilization. The patient should be observed for suicidal depression that may follow intoxication and may require suicide precautions. If focal neurologic manifestations are present, one should consider the possibility of a cerebrovascular accident and obtain a CT scan.

Extracorporeal clearance techniques are of no benefit.

Disposition

Patients with mild intoxication or a brief seizure that does not require treatment who become asymptomatic may be discharged after 6 hours with appropriate psychosocial follow-up. If cardiac or cerebral ischemic manifestations are present, the patient should be monitored in the intensive care unit. Body packers and stuffers require care in the intensive care unit until passage of the contraband.

Cyanide

Hydrogen cyanide is a byproduct of burning plastic and wools in residential fires. Hydrocyanic acid is the liquefied form of hydrogen cyanide. Cyanide salts can be found in ore extraction. Nitriles, such as acetonitrile (artificial nail removers), are metabolized in the body to produce cyanide. Cyanogenic glycosides are present in some fruit seeds (such as amygdalin in apricots, peaches, and apples). Sodium nitroprusside, the antihypertensive vasodilator, contains five cyanide groups.

Toxic Mechanism
Cyanide blocks the cellular electron transport mechanism and cellular respiration by inhibiting the mitochondrial ferricytochrome oxidase system and other enzymes. This results in cellular hypoxia and lactic acidosis. *Note:* Citrus fruit seeds form cyanide in the presence of intestinal β-glucosidase (the seeds are harmful only if the capsule is broken).

Toxic Dose
The ingestion of 1 mg/kg or 50 mg of hydrogen cyanide can produce death within 15 minutes. The lethal dose of potassium cyanide is 200 mg. Five to 10 mL of 84% acetonitrile is lethal. Infusions of sodium nitroprusside in rates above 2 μg/kg per minute may cause cyanide to accumulate to toxic concentrations in critically ill patients.

Kinetics
Cyanide is rapidly absorbed by all routes. In the stomach, it forms hydrocyanic acid. Volume distribution is 1.5 L/kg. Protein binding is 60%. Cyanide is detoxified by metabolism in the liver via the mitochondrial thiosulfate-rhodanase pathway, which catalyzes the transfer of sulfur donor to cyanide, forming the less toxic irreversible thiocyanate that is excreted in the urine. Cyanide is also detoxified by reacting with hydroxocobalamin (vitamin B_{12a}) to form cyanocobalamin (vitamin B_{12}).

The cyanide elimination half-life from the blood is 1.2 hours. The elimination route is through the lungs.

Manifestations
Hydrogen cyanide has the distinctive odor of bitter almonds or silver polish. Manifestations of cyanide intoxication include hypertension, cardiac dysrhythmias, various ECG abnormalities, headache, hyperpnea, seizures, stupor, pulmonary edema, and flushing. Cyanosis is absent or appears late.

Laboratory Investigations
The examiner should obtain and monitor ABGs, oxygen saturation, blood lactate, hemoglobin, blood glucose, and electrolytes. Lactic acidemia, a decrease in the arterial-venous oxygen difference, and bright red venous blood occurs. If smoke inhalation is the possible source of cyanide exposure, CoHB and methemoglobin (MetHb) concentrations should be measured.

Cyanide levels in whole blood, red blood cells, or serum are not useful in the acute management because the determinations are not readily available. Specific cyanide blood levels are as follows: smokers have less than 0.5 μg/mL; a patient with flushing and tachycardia has 0.5 to 1.0 μg/mL, one with obtundation has 1.0 to 2.5 μg/mL, and one in coma or who has died has more than 2.5 μg/mL.

Management
If the cyanide was inhaled, the patient must be removed from the contaminated atmosphere. Attendants should not administer mouth-to-mouth resuscitation. Rescuers and attendants must be protected. Immediate administration of 100% oxygen is called for and oxygen should be continued during and after the administration of the antidote. The clinician must decide whether to use any or all components of the cyanide antidote kit.

The mechanism of action of the antidote kit is twofold: to produce methemoglobinemia and to provide a sulfur substrate for the detoxification of cyanide. The nitrites make methemoglobin, which has a greater affinity for cyanide than does the cytochrome oxidase enzymes. The combination of methemoglobin and cyanide forms cyanomethemoglobin. Sodium thiosulfate provides a sulfur substrate for the rhodanese enzyme, which converts

cyanide into the relatively nontoxic sodium thiocyanate, which is excreted by the kidney.

The procedure for using the antidote kit is as follows:
Step 1: Amyl nitrite inhalant perles is only a temporizing measure (forms only 2% to 5% methemoglobin) and it can be omitted if venous access is established. Alternate 100% oxygen and the inhalant for 30 seconds each minute. Use a new perle every 3 minutes.
Step 2: Sodium nitrite ampule is indicated for cyanide exposures, except for cases of residential fires, smoke inhalation, and nitroprusside or acetonitrile poisonings. It is administered intravenously to produce methemoglobin of 20% to 30% at 35 to 70 minutes after administration. A dose of 10 mL of 3% solution of sodium nitrite for adults and 0.33 mL/kg of 3% solution for children is diluted to 100 mL 0.9% saline and administered slowly intravenously at 5 mL/min. If hypotension develops, the infusion should be slowed.
Step 3: Sodium thiosulfate is useful alone in cases of smoke inhalation, nitroprusside toxicity, and acetonitrile toxicity and should not be used at all in cases of hydrogen sulfide poisoning. The administration dose is 12.5 g of sodium thiosulfate or 50 mL of 25% solution for adults and 1.65 mL/kg of 25% solution for children intravenously over 10 to 20 minutes.

If cyanide symptoms recur, further treatment with nitrites or the perles is controversial. Some authorities suggest repeating the antidotes in 30 minutes at half of the initial dose, but others do not advise this for lack of efficacy. The child dosage regimen on the package insert must be carefully followed.

One hour after antidotes are administered, the methemoglobin level should be obtained and should not exceed 20%. Methylene blue should not be used to reverse excessive methemoglobin.

Gastrointestinal decontamination of oral ingestion by activated charcoal is recommended but is not very effective because of the rapidity of absorption. Seizures are treated with intravenous diazepam. Acidosis should be treated with sodium bicarbonate if it does not rapidly resolve with therapy. There is no role for hyperbaric oxygen or hemodialysis or hemoperfusion.

Other antidotes include hydroxocobalamin (vitamin B_{12a}) (Cyanokit), which has proven effective when given immediately after exposure in large doses of 4 g (50 mg/kg) or 50 times the amount of cyanide exposure with 8 g of sodium thiosulfate. Hydroxocobalamin has FDA orphan drug approval.

Disposition
Asymptomatic patients should be observed for a minimum of 3 hours. Patients who ingest nitrile compounds must be observed for 24 hours. Patients requiring antidote administration should be admitted to the intensive care unit.

Digitalis
Cardiac glycosides are found in cardiac medications, common plants, and the skin of the Bufo toad.

Toxic Mechanism
Cardiac glycosides inhibit the enzyme sodium/potassium-adenosine triphosphatase ($Na^+, K^+, ATPase$), leading to intracellular potassium loss and increased intracellular sodium, and producing phase 4 depolarization, increased automaticity, and ectopy. There is increased intracellular calcium and potentiation of contractility. Pacemaker cells are inhibited, and the refractory period is prolonged, leading to atrioventricular blocks. There is increased vagal tone.

Toxic Dose
Digoxin total digitalizing dose, the dose required to achieve therapeutic blood levels of 0.6 to 2.0 ng/mL, is 0.75 to 1.25 mg or 10 to 15 μg/kg for patients older than 10 years of age; 40 to 50 μg/kg for patients younger than 2 years of age; and 30 to 40 μg/kg for patients 2 to 10 years of age.

The acute single toxic dose is greater than 0.07 mg/kg or greater than 2 or 3 mg in an adult, but 2 mg in a child or 4 mg in an adult usually produces only mild toxicity. One to 3 mg or more may be found in a few leaves of oleander or foxglove. Serious and fatal overdoses are more than 4 mg in a child and more than 10 mg in an adult.

Acute digitoxin ingestion of 10 to 35 mg has produced severe toxicity and death. Digitoxin therapeutic steady state is 15 to 25 ng/mL. In cases of chronic or acute-on-chronic ingestions in patients with cardiac disease, more than 2 mg may produce toxicity; however, toxicity can develop within therapeutic range on chronic therapy.

Patients at greatest risk of overdose include those with cardiac disease, those with electrolyte abnormalities (low potassium, low magnesium, low T_4, high calcium), those with renal impairment, and those on amiodarone (Cordarone), quinidine, erythromycin, tetracycline, calcium channel blockers, and β-blockers.

Kinetics

Digoxin is a metabolite of digitoxin. In cases of oral overdose, the typical onset is 30 minutes, with peak effects in 3 to 12 hours. Duration is 3 to 4 days. Intravenous onset is in 5 to 30 minutes; peak level is immediate, and peak effect is at 1.5 to 3 hours.

Volume distribution is 5 to 6 L/kg. The cardiac-to-plasma ratio is 30:1. After an acute ingestion overdose, the serum concentration is not reflective of tissue concentration for at least 6 hours or more, and steady state is 12 to 16 hours after last dose.

Sixty percent to 80% of the parent compound is excreted unchanged in the urine. The elimination half-life is 30 to 50 hours.

Manifestations

Onset of manifestations is usually within 2 hours but may be delayed up to 12 hours.

Gastrointestinal effects of nausea and vomiting are frequently present in cases of acute ingestion but may also occur in cases of chronic ingestion. The "digitalis effect" on ECG is scooped ST segments and PR prolongation; in cases of overdose, any dysrhythmia or block is possible but none are characteristic. Bradycardia occurs in patients with acute overdose with healthy hearts; supraventricular tachycardia occurs in patients with existing heart disease or chronic overdose. Ventricular tachycardia is seen only in cases of severe poisoning.

The CNS effects include headaches, visual disturbances, and colored halo vision. Hyperkalemia occurs following acute overdose and correlates with digoxin level and outcome. Among patients with serum potassium levels of less than 5.0 mEq/L, all survive. If the level is 5 to 5.5, 50% survive, and if the level is greater than 5.5, all die. Hypokalemia is commonly seen with chronic intoxication. Patients with normal digitalis levels may have toxicity in the presence of hypokalemia.

Chronic intoxications are more likely to produce scotoma, color perception disturbances, yellow vision, halos, delirium, hallucinations or psychosis, tachycardia, and hypokalemia.

Laboratory Investigations

Continuous monitoring of ECG, pulse, and blood pressure is called for. Blood glucose, electrolytes, calcium, magnesium, BUN, and creatinine levels should also be monitored. An initial digoxin level should be measured on patient presentation and repeated thereafter. Levels should be measured more than 6 hours postingestion because earlier values do not reflect tissue distribution. Digoxin clinical toxicity is usually associated with serum digoxin levels of greater than 3.5 ng/mL in adults.

An endogenous digoxin-like substance cross-reacts in most common immunoassays (not with high-pressure liquid chromatography) and values as high as 4.1 ng/mL have been reported in newborns, patients with chronic renal failure, patients with abnormal immunoglobulins, and women in the third trimester of pregnancy.

Management

A cardiology consult should be obtained and a pacemaker should be readily available.

In undertaking gastrointestinal decontamination, excessive vagal stimulation should be avoided (e.g., emesis and gastric lavage). Activated charcoal should be administered, and if a nasogastric tube is required for the activated charcoal, pretreatment

with atropine (0.02 mg/kg in children and 0.5 mg in adults) should be considered.

Digoxin-specific antibody fragments (Fab, Digibind) 38 mg binds 0.5 mg digoxin and then is excreted through the kidneys. The onset of action is within 30 minutes. Problems associated with Fab therapy are mainly from withdrawal of digoxin and worsening heart failure, hypokalemia, decrease in glucose (if the patient has low glycogen stores), and allergic reactions (very rare). Digitalis administered after Fab therapy is bound and may be inactivated for 5 to 7 days.

Absolute indications for Fab therapy include the following:
- Life-threatening malignant (hemodynamically unstable) dysrhythmias
- Ventricular dysrhythmias, unstable severe bradycardia, or second- or third-degree blocks unresponsive to atropine or rapid deterioration in clinical status
- Life-threatening digitoxin and oleander poisonings

Relative indications for Fab therapy include the following:
- Ingestions greater than 4 mg in a child and 10 mg in an adult
- Serum potassium level greater than 5.0 mEq/L
- Serum digoxin level greater than 10 ng/mL in adults or greater than 5 ng/mL in children 6 hours after an acute ingestion
- Digitalis delirium and thrombocytopenia response

Digoxin-specific Fab fragments therapy can be administered as a bolus through a 22-μm filter if the case is a critical emergency. If the case is less urgent, then it can be administered over 30 minutes. An empiric dose is 10 vials in adults and 5 vials in a child for an unknown amount ingested in a symptomatic patient with history of a digoxin overdose.

To calculate the dose in the case of a known ingestion, the following equation is used:

$$\text{Amount (total mg)} \times (0.8) \text{ body burden}$$

If liquid capsules were taken or the substance was given intravenously the 80% bioavailability figure is not used. Instead, the body burden divided by 0.5 (0.5 mg digoxin is bound by 1 vial of 38 mg of Fab) equals the number of vials needed.

If the amount is unknown but the steady state serum concentration is known, the following equations are used:

For digoxin:

$$\text{Digitoxin ng/mL} \times (5.6 \text{ L/kg Vd}) \times (\text{wt kg}) = \text{mg body burden}$$
$$\text{Body burden} \div 1000 = \text{mg body burden}$$
$$\text{Body burden}/0.5 = \text{number of vials needed}$$

For digitoxin:

$$\text{Digitoxin ng/mL} \times (0.56 \text{ L/kg Vd}) \times (\text{wt kg}) = \text{mg body burden}$$
$$\text{Body burden} \div 1000 = \text{mg body burden}$$
$$\text{Body burden}/0.5 = \text{number of vials needed}$$

Antidysrhythmic agents or a pacemaker should be used only if Fab therapy fails. For ventricular tachydysrhythmias, electrolyte disturbances should be corrected by the administration of lidocaine or phenytoin. For torsades de pointes, magnesium sulfate 20 mL 20% IV can be given slowly over 20 minutes (or 25 to 50 mg/kg in a child), titrated to control the dysrhythmia. Magnesium should be discontinued if hypotension, heart block, or decreased deep tendon reflexes are present. Magnesium is used with caution if the patient has renal impairment.

Unstable bradycardia and second-degree and third-degree atrio-ventricular block should be treated by Fab first. A pacemaker should be available if necessary. Isoproterenol should be avoided because it causes dysrhythmias. Cardioversion is used with caution, starting at a setting of 5 to 10 joules. The patient should be pretreated with lidocaine, if possible, because cardioversion may precipitate ventricular fibrillation or asystole.

Potassium disturbances are caused by a shift, not a change, in total body potassium. Hyperkalemia (>5.0 mEq/L) is treated with Fab only. Calcium must never be used, and insulin/glucose and sodium bicarbonate should not be used concomitantly with Fab because they may produce severe life-threatening hypokalemia.

TABLE 15 Summary of Alcohol and Glycol Features

	METHANOL	ISOPROPANOL	ETHANOL	ETHYLENE GLYCOL
Principal uses	Gas line antifreeze, Sterno, windshield de-icer	Solvent jewelry cleaner, rubbing alcohol	Beverage, solvent	Radiator antifreeze, windshield de-icer
Specific gravity	0.719	0.785	0.789	1.12
Fatal dose	1 mL/kg 100%	3 mL/kg 100%	5 mL/kg 100%	1.4 mL/kg
Inebriation	±	2+	2+	1+
Metabolic change		Hyperglycemia	Hypoglycemia	Hypocalcemia
Metabolic acidosis	4+	0	1+	2+
Anion gap	4+	±	2+	4+
Ketosis	Ketobutyric	Acetone	Hydroxybutyric	None
Gastrointestinal tract	Pancreatitis	Hemorrhagic gastritis	Gastritis	
Osmolality*	0.337	0.176	0.228	0.190

*1 mL/dL of substances raises freezing point osmolarity of serum. The validity of the correlation of osmolality with blood concentrations has been questioned.

Sodium polystyrene sulfonate (Kayexalate) should not be used. Hypokalemia must be treated with caution because it may be cardioprotective. Treatment can be administered if the patient has ventricular dysrhythmias or a serum potassium level less than 3.0 mEq/L and atrioventricular block.

Extracorporeal procedures are ineffective. Hemodialysis is used for severe or refractory hyperkalemia.

One must never use antidysrhythmic types Ia (procainamide, quinidine, disopyramide [Norpace], amiodarone [Cordarone]), Ic (propafenone [Rythmol], flecainide [Tambocor]), II (β-blockers), or IV (calcium channel blockers). Class Ib drugs (lidocaine, phenytoin [Dilantin], mexiletine [Mexitil], and tocainide [Tonocard]) can be used.

Disposition

Consultation with a poison control center and a cardiologist experienced with digoxin-specific Fab fragments is warranted. All patients with significant dysrhythmias, symptoms, elevated serum digoxin concentration, or elevated serum potassium level should be admitted to the intensive care unit.

Ethanol

Table 15 lists the features of alcohols and glycols.

Toxic Mechanism

Ethanol has CNS depressant and anesthetic effects. Ethanol stimulates the γ-aminobutyric acid (GABA) system. It promotes cutaneous vasodilation (contributes to hypothermia), stimulates secretion of gastric juice (gastritis), inhibits the secretion of the antidiuretic hormone, inhibits gluconeogenesis (hypoglycemia), and influences fat metabolism (lipidemia).

Toxic Dose

A dose of 1 mL/kg of absolute ethanol (100% ethanol, or 200 proof) gives a blood ethanol concentration of 100 mg/dL. A potentially fatal dose is 3 g/kg for children or 6 g/kg for adults. Children are more prone to developing hypoglycemia than adults.

Kinetics

Onset of action is 30 to 60 minutes after ingestion; peak action is 90 minutes on empty stomach. Volume distribution is 0.6 L/kg. The major route of elimination (>90%) is by hepatic oxidative metabolism. The first step is by the enzyme alcohol dehydrogenase, which converts ethanol to acetaldehyde. Alcohol dehydrogenase metabolizes ethanol at a constant rate of 12 to 20 mg/dL/h (12 to 15 mg/dL/h in nondrinkers, 15 to 30 mg/dL/h in social drinkers, 30 to 50 mg/dL/h in heavy drinkers, and 25 to 30 mg/dL/h in children). At very low blood ethanol concentration (>30 mg/dL), the metabolism is by first-order kinetics. In the

TABLE 16 Clinical Signs in the Nontolerant Ethanol Drinker

ETHANOL BLOOD CONCENTRATION (MG/DL)*	MANIFESTATIONS
>25	Euphoria
>47	**Mild incoordination,** sensory and motor impairment
>50	Increased risk of motor vehicle accidents
>100	Ataxia (legal toxic level in many localities)
>150	**Moderate incoordination,** slow reaction time
>200	Drowsiness and confusion
>300	Severe incoordination, stupor, blurred vision
>500	**Flaccid coma,** respiratory failure, hypotension; may be fatal

*Ethanol concentrations sometimes reported in %.
Note: mg% is not equivalent to mg/dL because ethanol weighs less than water (specific gravity 0.79). A 1% ethanol concentration is 790 mg/dL and 0.1% is 79 mg/dL. There is great variation in individual behavior at different blood ethanol levels. Behavior is dependent on tolerance and other factors.

second step, acetaldehyde is metabolized by acetaldehyde dehydrogenase to acetic acid, which is metabolized by the Krebs cycle to carbon dioxide and water. The enzyme steps are nicotinamide adenine dinucleotide-dependent, which interferes with gluconeogenesis. Less than 10% of ethanol is excreted unchanged by the kidneys. The relationship between blood ethanol concentration (BEC) and dose (amount ingested) can be calculated as follows:

$$\text{BEC (mg/dL)} = \text{amount ingested (mL)} \times$$
$$\% \text{ ethanol product} \times \text{SG (0.79)/Vd (0.6 L/kg)} \times \text{body wt (kg)}$$
$$\text{Dose (amount ingested)} = \text{BEC (mg/dL)} \times$$
$$\text{Vd (0.6)} \times \text{body wt (kg)/\% ethanol} \times$$
$$\text{specific gravity (0.79)}$$

Manifestations

Table 16 lists the clinical signs of acute ethanol intoxication.

Chronic alcoholic patients tolerate higher blood ethanol concentration, and correlation with manifestations is not valid. Rapid interview for alcoholism is the CAGE questions:
- C—Have you felt the need to Cut down?
- A—Have others Annoyed you by criticism of your drinking?

- G—Have you felt Guilty about your drinking?
- E—Have you ever had a morning Eye-opening drink to steady your nerves or get rid of a hangover?

Two affirmative answers indicate probable alcoholism.

Laboratory Investigations

The blood ethanol concentration should be specifically requested and followed. Gas chromatography or a breathalyzer test gives rapid reliable results if no belching or vomiting is present. Enzymatic methods do not differentiate between the alcohols. ABG, electrolytes, and glucose should be measured, the anion and osmolar gaps determined (measure by freezing point depression, not vapor pressure), and a check for ketosis made.

Management

The examiner should inquire about trauma and disulfiram use. The patient must be protected from aspiration and hypoxia. Vital functions must be established and maintained. The patient may require intubation and assisted ventilation.

Gastrointestinal decontamination plays no role in the management of ethanol intoxication.

If the patient is comatose, glucose should be administered intravenously, 1 mL/kg 50% glucose in adults and 2 mL/kg 25% glucose in children. Thiamine, 100 mg intravenously, is administered if the patient has a history of chronic alcoholism, malnutrition, or suspected eating disorders to prevent Wernicke-Korsakoff syndrome. Naloxone (Narcan) has produced a partial inconsistent response but is not recommended for known alcoholics.

General supportive care includes administration of fluids to correct hydration and hypotension and correction of electrolyte abnormalities and acid-base imbalance. Vasopressors and plasma expanders may be necessary to correct severe hypotension. Hypomagnesemia is frequent in chronic alcoholics. In case of hypomagnesemia, a loading dose of 2 g magnesium sulfate 10% is administered by intravenous solution over 5 minutes in the intensive care unit with blood pressure and cardiac monitoring and calcium chloride 10% on hand in case of overdose. This is followed with constant infusion of 6 g of 10% solution over 3 to 4 hours. Caution must be taken with the use of magnesium if renal failure is present.

Hypothermic patients should be warmed. See the section on disturbances caused by cold.

Hemodialysis can be used in severe cases when conventional therapy is ineffective (rarely needed).

Repeated or prolonged seizures should be treated with diazepam (Valium). The brief "rum fits" do not need long-term anticonvulsant therapy. Repeated seizures or focal neurologic findings may warrant skull radiographs, lumbar puncture, and CT scan of the head, depending on the clinical findings. Withdrawal is treated with hydration and large doses of chlordiazepoxide (Librium) 50 to 100 mg or diazepam (Valium) 2 to 10 mg intravenously; these doses may be repeated in 2 to 4 hours. Very large doses of benzodiazepines may be required for delirium tremens. Withdrawal can occur in presence of elevated blood ethanol concentration and can be fatal if left untreated.

Chest radiograph is warranted to determine whether aspiration pneumonia is present. Renal and liver function tests and bilirubin level measurement should be made.

Disposition

Clinical severity (e.g., intubation, assisted ventilation, aspiration pneumonia) should determine the level of hospital care needed. Young children with significant unintentional exposure to ethanol (calculated to reach a blood ethanol concentration of 50 mg/dL) should have blood ethanol concentration obtained and blood glucose levels monitored for hypoglycemia frequently for 4 hours after ingestion. Patients with acute ethanol intoxication seldom require admission unless a complication is present. However, intoxicated patients should not be discharged until they are fully functional (can walk, talk, and think independently), have suicide potential evaluated, have proper disposition environment, and have a sober escort.

Ethylene Glycol

Ethylene glycol is found in solvents, de-icers, radiator antifreeze (95%), and air-conditioning units. Ethylene glycol is a sweet-tasting, colorless, water-soluble liquid with a sweet aromatic fragrance.

Toxic Mechanism

Ethylene glycol is oxidized by alcohol dehydrogenase to glycolaldehyde, which is metabolized to glycolic acid and glyoxylic acid. Glyoxylic acid is metabolized to oxalic acid via a pyridoxine-dependent pathway to glycine and by thiamine and magnesium-dependent pathways to α-hydroxy-ketoadipic acid. The metabolites of ethylene glycol produce a profound metabolic acidosis, increased anion gap, hypocalcemia, and oxalate crystals, which deposit in tissues (particularly the kidney).

Toxic Dose

The ingestion of 0.1 mL/kg 100% ethylene glycol can result in a toxic serum ethylene glycol concentration of 20 mg/dL. Ingestion of 3.0 mL (less than 1 teaspoonful or swallow) of a 100% solution in a 10-kg child or 30 mL of 100% ethylene glycol in an adult produces a serum ethylene glycol concentration of 50 mg/dL, a concentration that requires hemodialysis. The fatal amount is 1.4 mL/kg of 100% solution.

Kinetics

Absorption is via dermal, inhalation, and ingestion routes. Ethylene glycol is rapidly absorbed from the gastrointestinal tract. Onset is usually in 30 minutes but may be delayed by co-ingestion of food and ethanol. The usual peak level is at 2 hours. Volume distribution is 0.65 to 0.8 L/kg.

For metabolism, see *Toxic Mechanism*.

The half-life of ethylene glycol without ethanol is 3 to 8 hours; with ethanol, it is 17 hours, and with hemodialysis it is 2.5 hours. Renal clearance is 3.2 mL/kg/min. About 20% to 50% is excreted unchanged in the urine. The relationship between serum ethylene glycol concentration (SEGC) and dose (amount ingested) can be calculated as follows:

$$0.12 \text{ mL/kg of } 100\% = \text{SEGC } 10 \text{ mg/dL}$$

Manifestations

Phase I. The onset of manifestations is 30 minutes to several hours longer after ingestion with concomitant ethanol ingestion. The patient may be inebriated. Hypocalcemia, tetany, and calcium oxalate and hippuric acid crystals in urine can be seen within 4 to 8 hours but are not always present. Early, before metabolism of ethylene glycol, an osmolal gap may be present (see *Laboratory Investigations*). Later, the metabolites of ethylene glycol produce changes starting 4 to 12 hours following ingestion, including an anion gap, metabolic acidosis, coma, convulsions, cardiac disturbances, and pulmonary and cerebral edema. Because fluorescein is added to some antifreeze, the presence of fluorescence may be a clue to ethylene glycol exposure. However, it has been shown that fluorescent urine is not a reliable indicator of ethylene glycol ingestion and should not be used as a screen.

Phase II. After 12 to 36 hours, cardiopulmonary deterioration occurs, with pulmonary edema and congestive heart failure.

Phase III. Phase III occurs 36 to 72 hours after ingestion, with pulmonary edema and oliguric renal failure from oxalate crystal deposition and tubular necrosis predominating.

Phase IV. Neurologic sequelae may occur rarely, especially in patients who fail to receive early antidotal therapy. The onset ranges from 6 to 10 days after ingestion. Findings include facial diplegia, hearing loss, bilateral visual disturbances, elevated cerebrospinal fluid pressure with or without elevated protein levels and pleocytosis, vomiting, hyperreflexia, dysphagia, and ataxia.

Laboratory Investigations

Blood glucose and electrolytes should be monitored. Urinalysis should look for oxalate ("envelope") and monohydrate ("hemp seed") crystals. Urine fluorescence is not reliable as a screen. ABG, ethylene glycol, and ethanol levels, plasma osmolarity (using freezing point depression method), calcium, BUN, and creatinine should be measured. A serum ethylene glycol concentration of 20 mg/dL is toxic (ethylene glycol levels are very difficult to obtain). If possible, a glycolate level should be obtained. Cross-reactions with propylene glycol, a vehicle in many liquids and intravenous medications (phenytoin [Dilantin], diazepam [Valium]), other glycols, and triglycerides, may produce spurious ethylene glycol levels. False-positive ethylene glycol values may occur with colorimetric or gas chromatography using an OV-17 column in the presence of propylene glycol.

The following equations can be used to calculate the osmolality, osmolal gap, and ethylene glycol level:

$$2(Na + mEq/L) + (Blood\ glucose\ mg/dL)/20 + (BUN\ mg/dL)/3 = Total\ calculated\ osmolality (mOsm/L)$$
$$Osmolar\ Gap = measured\ osmolality\ (by\ freezing\ point\ depression\ method) - calculate\ osmolality$$

A gap greater than 10 is abnormal. *Note:* if ethanol is involved, add ethanol level/4.6 to the calculated equation.

An increased osmolal gap is produced by the following common substances: acetone, dextran, dimethyl sulfoxide, diuretics, ethanol, ethyl ether, ethylene glycol, isopropanol, paraldehyde, mannitol, methanol, sorbitol, and trichloroethane. Table 10 gives the conversion factors for these substances.

Although a specific blood level of ethylene glycol in milligrams per deciliter can be estimated using the equation below, this is not considered to be a reliable method and should not take the place of obtaining a measured ethylene glycol blood concentration.

$$Osmolar\ gap \times conversion\ factor = serum\ concentration$$

Caution: The accuracy of the ethylene glycol estimated decreases as the ethylene glycol levels decrease. The toxic metabolites are not osmotically active, and patients presenting late may show signs of severe toxicity without an elevated osmolar gap.

The anion gap can be calculated using the following equation:

$$Na - (Cl + HCO_3) = anion\ gap$$

The normal gap is 8 to 12. Potassium is not used because it is a small amount and may be hemolyzed. Table 8 lists factors that may account for an increased or a decreased anion gap.

Management

Vital functions should be established and maintained. The airway must be protected, and assisted ventilation can be used, if necessary. Gastrointestinal decontamination has a limited role. Only gastric aspiration can be used within 60 minutes after ingestion. Activated charcoal is not effective.

Baseline measurements of serum electrolytes and calcium, glucose, ABGs, ethanol, serum ethylene glycol concentration (may be difficult to obtain readily in some institutions), and methanol concentrations should be obtained. In the first few hours, the measured serum osmolality should be determined and compared to calculated osmolality (see osmolality equation, earlier). If seizures occur, one should measure serum calcium (preferably ionized calcium) and treat with intravenous diazepam. If the patient has hypocalcemic seizures, he or she should also be treated with 10 to 20 mL 10% calcium gluconate (0.2 to 0.3 mL/kg in children) slowly intravenously, with the dose repeated as needed. Metabolic acidosis should be corrected with intravenous sodium bicarbonate.

Ethanol therapy should be initiated immediately if fomepizole (Antizol) is unavailable (see next paragraph). Alcohol dehydrogenase has a greater affinity for ethanol than ethylene glycol. Therefore, ethanol blocks the metabolism of ethylene glycol. Ethanol therapy is called for if there is a history of ingestion of 0.1 mL/kg of 100% ethylene glycol, serum ethylene glycol concentration is greater than 20 mg/dL, there is an osmolar gap not accounted for by other alcohols or factors (e.g., hyperlipidemia), metabolic acidosis is present with an increased anion gap, or there are oxalate crystals in the urine. Ethanol should be administered intravenously (the oral route is less reliable) to produce a blood ethanol concentration of 100 to 150 mg/dL. The loading dose is 10 mL/kg of 10% ethanol intravenously, administered concomitantly with a maintenance dose of 10% ethanol of 1.0 mL/kg/h. This dose may need to be increased to 2 mL/kg/h in patients who are heavy drinkers. The blood ethanol concentration should be measured hourly and the infusion rate should be adjusted to maintain a blood ethanol concentration of 100 to 150 mg/dL.

Fomepizole (Antizol, 4-methylpyrazole) inhibits alcohol dehydrogenase more reliably than ethanol and it does not require constant monitoring of ethanol levels and adjustment of infusion rates. Fomepizole is available in 1 g/mL vials of 1.5 mL. The loading dose is 15 mg/kg (0.015 mL/kg) IV; maintenance dose is 10 mg/kg (0.01 mL/kg) every 12 hours for four doses, then 15 mg/kg every 12 hours until the ethylene glycol levels are less than 20 mg/dL. The solution is prepared by being mixed with 100 mL of 0.9% saline or D5W (5% dextrose in water). Fomepizole can be given to patients requiring hemodialysis but should be dosed as follows:
Dose at the beginning of hemodialysis:
- If <6 hours since last Antizol dose, do not administer dose
- If >6 hours since last dose, administer next scheduled dose
Dosing during hemodialysis:
- Dose every 4 hours
Dosing at the time hemodialysis is completed:
- If <1 hour between last dose and end of dialysis, do not administer dose at end of dialysis
- If 1 to 3 hours between last dose and end of dialysis, administer one half of next scheduled dose
- If >3 hours between last dose and end of dialysis, administer next scheduled dose
Maintenance dosing off hemodialysis:
- Give the next scheduled dose 12 hours from the last dose administered

Hemodialysis is indicated if the ingestion was potentially fatal; if the serum ethylene glycol concentration is greater than 50 mg/dL (some recommend at levels of >25 mg/dL); if severe acidosis or electrolyte abnormalities occur despite conventional therapy; or if congestive heart failure or renal failure is present. Hemodialysis reduces the ethylene glycol half-life from 17 hours on ethanol therapy to 3 hours. Therapy (fomepizole and hemodialysis) should be continued until the serum ethylene glycol concentration is less than 10 mg/dL, the glycolate level is nondetectable (not readily available), the acidosis has cleared, there are no mental disturbances, the creatinine level is normal, and the urinary output is adequate. This may require 2 to 5 days.

Adjunct therapy involving thiamine, 100 mg/d (in children, 50 mg), slowly over 5 minutes intravenously or intramuscularly and repeated every 6 hours and pyridoxine, 50 mg IV or IM every 6 hours, has been recommended until intoxication is resolved, but these agents have not been extensively studied. Folate, 50 mg IV (child 1 mg/kg), can be given every 4 hours for 6 doses.

Disposition

All patients who have ingested significant amounts of ethylene glycol (calculated level above 20 mg/dL), have a history of a toxic dose, or are symptomatic should be referred to the emergency department and admitted. If the serum ethylene glycol concentration cannot be obtained, the patient should be followed for 12 hours, with monitoring of the osmolal gap, acid-base parameters, and electrolytes to exclude development of metabolic acidosis with an anion gap. Transfer should be considered for fomepizole therapy or hemodialysis.

Hydrocarbons

The lower the viscosity and surface tension of hydrocarbons or the greater the volatility, the greater the risk of aspiration. Volatile substance abuse has produced the "Sudden Sniffing's Death Syndrome," most likely caused by dysrhythmias.

Toxicologic Classification and Toxic Mechanism

All systemically absorbed hydrocarbons can lower the threshold of the myocardium to dysrhythmias produced by endogenous and exogenous catecholamines.

Aliphatic hydrocarbons are branched straight chain hydrocarbons. A few aspirated drops are poorly absorbed from the gastrointestinal tract and produce no systemic toxicity by this route. However, aspiration of very small amounts can produce chemical pneumonitis. Examples of aliphatic hydrocarbons are gasoline, kerosene, charcoal lighter fluid, mineral spirits (Stoddard's solvent), and petroleum naphtha. Mineral seal oil (signal oil), found in furniture polishes, is a low-viscosity and low-volatility oil with minimum absorption that never warrants gastric decontamination. It can produce severe pneumonia if aspirated.

Aromatic hydrocarbons are six carbon ring structures that are absorbed through the gastrointestinal tract. Systemic toxicity includes CNS depression and, in cases of chronic abuse, multiple organ effects such as leukemia (benzene) and renal toxicity (toluene). Examples are benzene, toluene, styrene, and xylene. The seriously toxic ingested dose is 20 to 50 mL in adults.

Halogenated hydrocarbons are aliphatic or aromatic hydrocarbons with one or more halogen substitutions (Cl, Br, Fl, or I). They are highly volatile and are abused as inhalants. They are well absorbed from the gastrointestinal tract, produce CNS depression, and have metabolites that can damage the liver and kidneys. Examples include methylene chloride (may be converted into carbon monoxide in the body), dichloroethylene (also causes a disulfiram [Antabuse] reaction known as "degreaser's flush" when associated with consumption of ethanol), and 1,1,1-trichloroethane (Glamorene Spot Remover, Scotchgard, typewriter correction fluid). An acute lethal oral dose is 0.5 to 5 mL/kg.

Dangerous additives to the hydrocarbons can be summed up with the mnemonic CHAMP: C, camphor (demothing agent); H, halogenated hydrocarbons; A, aromatic hydrocarbons; M, metals (heavy); and P, pesticides. Ingestion of these substances may warrant gastric emptying with a small-bore nasogastric tube.

Heavy hydrocarbons have high viscosity, low volatility, and minimal gastrointestinal absorption, so gastric decontamination is not necessary. Examples are asphalt (tar), machine oil, motor oil (lubricating oil, engine oil), home heating oil, and petroleum jelly (mineral oil).

Laboratory Investigations

The ECG, ABG, pulmonary function, serum electrolytes, and serial chest radiographs should be continuously monitored. Liver and renal function should be monitored in cases of inhalation of aromatic hydrocarbons.

Management

Asymptomatic patients who ingested small amounts of aliphatic petroleum distillates can be followed at home by telephone for development of signs of aspiration (cough, wheezing, tachypnea, and dyspnea) for 4 to 6 hours. Inhalation of any hydrocarbon vapors in a closed space can produce intoxication. The victim must be removed from the environment, have oxygen administered, and receive respiratory support.

Gastrointestinal decontamination is not advised in cases of hydrocarbon ingestion that usually do not cause systemic toxicity (aliphatic petroleum distillates, heavy hydrocarbons). In cases of ingestion of hydrocarbons that cause systemic toxicity in small amounts (aromatic hydrocarbons, halogenated hydrocarbons), the clinician should pass a small-bore nasogastric tube and aspirate if the ingestion was within 2 hours and if spontaneous vomiting has not occurred. Some toxicologists advocate ipecac-induced emesis under medical supervision instead of small-bore nasogastric gastric lavage; we do not.

Patients with altered mental status should have their airway protected because of concern about aspiration. The use of activated charcoal has been suggested, but there are no scientific data as to effectiveness and it may produce vomiting. Activated charcoal may, however, be useful in adsorbing toxic additives such as pesticides or co-ingestants.

The symptomatic patient who is coughing, gagging, choking, or wheezing on arrival has probably aspirated. The clinician should provide supportive respiratory care and supplemental oxygen, while monitoring pulse oximetry, ABG, chest radiograph, and ECG. The patient should be admitted to the intensive care unit. A chest radiograph for aspiration may be positive as early as 30 minutes after ingestion, and almost all are positive within 6 hours. Negative chest radiographs within 4 hours do not rule out aspiration.

Bronchospasm is treated with a nebulized β-adrenergic agonist and intravenous aminophylline if necessary. Epinephrine should be avoided because of susceptibility to dysrhythmias. Cyanosis in the presence of a normal arterial PaO_2 may be a result of methemoglobinemia that requires therapy with methylene blue. Corticosteroids and prophylactic antimicrobial agents have not been shown to be beneficial. (Fever or leukocytosis may be produced by the chemical pneumonitis itself.)

Most infiltrations resolve spontaneously in 1 week; lipoid pneumonia may last up to 6 weeks. It is not necessary to surgically treat pneumatoceles that develop because they usually resolve. Dysrhythmias may require α- and β-adrenergic antagonists or cardioversion.

There is no role for enhanced elimination procedures.

Methylene chloride is metabolized over several hours to carbon monoxide. See treatment of carbon monoxide poisoning. Halogenated hydrocarbons are hepatorenal toxins; therefore, hepatorenal function should be monitored. N-acetylcysteine therapy may be useful if there is evidence of hepatic damage.

Extracorporeal membrane oxygenation (ECMO) has been used successfully for a few patients with life-threatening respiratory failure. Surfactant used for hydrocarbon aspiration was found to be detrimental.

Disposition

Asymptomatic patients with small ingestions of petroleum distillates can be managed at home. Symptomatic patients with abnormal chest radiographic, oxygen saturation, or ABG findings should be admitted. Patients who become asymptomatic and have normal oxygenation and a normal repeat radiograph can be discharged.

Iron

There are more than 100 iron over-the-counter preparations for supplementation and treatment of iron deficiency anemia.

Toxic Mechanism

Toxicity depends on the amount of elemental iron available in various salts (gluconate 12%, sulfate 20%, fumarate 33%, lactate 19%, chloride 21% of elemental iron), not the amount of the salt. Locally, iron is corrosive and may cause fluid loss, hypovolemic shock, and perforation. Excessive free unbound iron in the blood is directly toxic to the vasculature and leads to the release of vasoactive substances, which produces vasodilation. In cases of overdose, iron deposits injure mitochondria in the liver, the kidneys, and the myocardium. The exact mechanism of cellular damage is not clear but is thought to be related to free radical formation.

Toxic Dose

The therapeutic dose is 6 mg/kg/d of elemental iron. An elemental iron dose of 20 to 40 mg/kg may produce mild self-limited gastrointestinal symptoms, 40 to 60 mg/kg produces moderate toxicity, more than 60 mg/kg produces severe toxicity and is potentially lethal, and more than 180 mg/kg is usually fatal without treatment. Children's chewable vitamins with iron have between 12 and 18 mg of elemental iron per tablet or 0.6 mL of liquid drops. These preparations rarely produce toxicity unless very large quantities are ingested and have never caused death.

Kinetics

Absorption occurs chiefly in the upper small intestine. Ferrous (+2) iron is absorbed into the mucosal cells, where it is oxidized to the ferric (+3) state and bound to ferritin. Iron is slowly released from ferritin into the plasma, where it binds to transferrin and is transported to specific tissues for production of hemoglobin (70%), myoglobin (5%), and cytochrome. About 25% of iron is stored in the liver and spleen. In cases of overdose, larger amounts of iron are absorbed because of direct mucosal corrosion. There is no mechanism for the elimination of iron (elimination is 1 to 2 mg/d) except through bile, sweat, and blood loss.

Manifestations

Serious toxicity is unlikely if the patient remains asymptomatic for 6 hours and has a negative abdominal radiograph. Iron intoxication can produce five phases of toxicity. The phases may not be distinct from one another.

Phase I. Gastrointestinal mucosal injury occurs 30 minutes to 12 hours postingestion. Vomiting starts within 30 minutes to 1 hour of ingestion and is persistent; hematemesis and bloody diarrhea may occur; abdominal cramps, fever, hyperglycemia, and leukocytosis may occur. Enteric-coated tablets may pass through the stomach without causing symptoms. Acidosis and shock can occur within 6 to 12 hours.

Phase II. A latent period of apparent improvement occurs over 8 to 12 hours postingestion.

Phase III. Systemic toxicity phase occurs 12 to 48 hours postingestion with cardiovascular collapse and severe metabolic acidosis.

Phase IV. Two to 4 days postingestion, hepatic injury associated with jaundice, elevated liver enzymes, and prolonged prothrombin time occur. Kidney injury with proteinuria and hematuria occur. Pulmonary edema, disseminated intravascular coagulation, and *Yersinia enterocolitica* sepsis can occur.

Phase V. Four to 8 weeks postingestion, pyloric outlet or intestinal stricture may cause obstruction or anemia secondary to blood loss.

Laboratory Investigations

Iron poisoning produces anion gap metabolic acidosis. Monitoring should include complete blood cell counts, blood glucose level, serum iron, stools and vomitus for occult blood, electrolytes, acid-base balance, urinalysis and urinary output, liver function tests, and BUN and creatinine levels. Blood type and match should be obtained.

Serum iron measurements taken at the proper time correlate with the clinical findings. The lavender top Vacutainer tube contains EDTA, which falsely lowers serum iron. One must obtain the serum iron measurement before administering deferoxamine. Serum iron levels of less than 350 μg/dL at 2 to 6 hours predict an asymptomatic course; levels of 350 to 500 μg/dL are usually associated with mild gastrointestinal symptoms; those greater than 500 μg/dL have a 20% risk of shock and serious iron toxicity. A follow-up serum iron measurement after 6 hours may not be elevated even in cases of severe poisoning, but a serum iron measurement taken at 8 to 12 hours is useful to exclude delayed absorption from a bezoar or sustained-release preparation. The total iron-binding capacity is not necessary.

Adult iron tablet preparations are radiopaque before they dissolve by 4 hours postingestion. A "negative" abdominal radiograph more than 4 hours postingestion does not exclude iron poisoning.

Patients who develop high fevers and signs of sepsis following iron overdose should have blood and stool cultures checked for *Yersinia enterocolitica*.

Management

Gastrointestinal decontamination should involve immediate induction of emesis in cases of ingestions of elemental iron of greater than 40 mg/kg if vomiting has not already occurred. Activated charcoal is ineffective. An abdominal radiograph should be obtained after emesis to determine the success of gastric emptying. Children's chewable vitamins and liquid iron preparations are not radiopaque. If radiopaque iron is still present, wholebowel irrigation with polyethylene glycol solution should be considered. In extreme cases, removal by endoscopy or surgery may be necessary because coalesced iron tablets produce hemorrhagic infarction in the bowel and perforation peritonitis.

Deferoxamine (Desferal) in a dose of about 100 mg binds 8.5 to 9.35 mg of free iron in the serum. The deferoxamine infusion should not exceed 15 mg/kg/h or 6 g daily, but faster rates (up to 45 mg/kg) and larger daily amounts have been administered and tolerated in extreme cases of iron poisoning (>1000 mg/dL). The deferoxamine-iron complex is hemodialyzable if renal failure develops.

Indications for chelation therapy are any of the following:
- Very large, symptomatic ingestions
- Serious clinical intoxication (severe vomiting and diarrhea [often bloody], severe abdominal pain, metabolic acidosis, hypotension, or shock)
- Symptoms that persist or progress to more serious toxicity
- Serum iron level greater than 500 mg/dL

Chelation should be performed as early as possible within 12 to 18 hours to be effective. One should start the infusion slowly and gradually increase to avoid hypotension.

Adult respiratory distress syndrome has developed in patients with high doses of deferoxamine for several days; infusions longer than 24 hours should be avoided.

The end point of treatment is when the patient is asymptomatic and the urine clears if it was originally a positive "vin rosö" color.

For supportive therapy, intravenous bicarbonate may be needed to correct the metabolic acidosis. Hypotension and shock treatment may require volume expansion, vasopressors, and blood transfusions. The physician should attempt to keep the urinary output at greater than 2 mL/kg/h. Coagulation abnormalities and overt bleeding require blood products or vitamin K. Pregnant patients are treated in a fashion similar to any other patient with iron poisoning.

Hemodialysis and hemoperfusion are ineffective. Exchange transfusion has been used in single cases of massive poisonings in children.

Disposition

The asymptomatic or minimally symptomatic patient should be observed for persistence and progression of symptoms or development of toxicity signs (gastrointestinal bleeding, acidosis, shock, altered mental state). Patients with mild self-limited gastrointestinal symptoms who become asymptomatic or have no signs of toxicity for 6 hours are unlikely to have a serious intoxication and can be discharged after psychiatric clearance, if needed. Patients with moderate or severe toxicity should be admitted to the intensive care unit.

Isoniazid

Isoniazid is a hydrazide derivative of vitamin B_3 (nicotinamide) and is used as an antituberculosis drug.

Toxic Mechanism

Isoniazid produces pyridoxine deficiency by increasing the excretion of pyridoxine (vitamin B_6) and by inhibiting pyridoxal 5-phosphate (the active form of pyridoxine) from acting with L-glutamic acid decarboxylase to form γ-aminobutyric acid (GABA), the major CNS neurotransmitter inhibitor, resulting in seizures. Isoniazid also blocks the conversion of lactate to pyruvate, resulting in profound and prolonged lactic acidosis.

Toxic Dose

The therapeutic dose is 5 to 10 mg/kg (maximum 300 mg) daily. A single acute dose of 15 mg/kg lowers the seizure threshold; 35 to 40 mg/kg produces spontaneous convulsions; more than 80 mg/kg produces severe toxicity. A fatal dose in adults is 4.5 to 15 g. The malnourished patients, those with a previous seizure disorder, alcoholic patients, and slow acetylators are more susceptible to isoniazid toxicity. In cases of chronic intoxication, 10 mg/kg/d produces hepatitis in 10% to 20% of patients but less than 2% at doses of 3 to 5 mg/kg/d.

Kinetics

Absorption from intestine occurs in 30 to 60 minutes, and onset is in 30 to 120 minutes, with peak levels of 5 to 8 μg/mL within 1 to 2 hours. Volume distribution is 0.6 L/kg, with minimal protein binding.

Elimination is by liver acetylation to a hepatotoxic metabolite, acetyl-isoniazid, which is then hydrolyzed to isonicotinic acid. In slow acetylators, isoniazid has a half-life of 140 to 460 minutes (mean 5 hours), and 10% to 15% is eliminated unchanged in the urine. Most (45% to 75%) whites and 50% of African blacks are slow acetylators, and, with chronic use (without pyridoxine supplements), they may develop peripheral neuropathy. In fast acetylators, isoniazid has a half-life of 35 to 110 minutes (mean 80 minutes), and 25% to 30% is excreted unchanged in the urine. About 90% of Asians and patients with diabetes mellitus are fast acetylators and may develop hepatitis on chronic use.

In patients with overdose and hepatic disease, the serum half-life may increase. Isoniazid inhibits the metabolism of phenytoin (Dilantin), diazepam, phenobarbital, carbamazepine (Tegretol), and prednisone. These drugs also interfere with the metabolism of isoniazid. Ethanol may decrease the half-life of isoniazid but increase its toxicity.

Manifestations

Within 30 to 60 minutes, nausea, vomiting, slurred speech, dizziness, visual disturbances, and ataxia are present. Within 30 to 120 minutes, the major clinical triad of severe overdose includes refractory convulsions (90% of overdose patients have one or more seizures), coma, and resistant severe lactic acidosis (secondary to convulsions), often with a plasma pH of 6.8.

Laboratory Investigations

Isoniazid produces anion gap metabolic acidosis. Therapeutic levels are 5 to 8 μg/mL and acute toxic levels are greater than 20 μg/mL. These levels are not readily available to assist in making decisions in acute overdose situations. One should monitor the blood glucose (often hyperglycemia), electrolytes (often hyperkalemia), bicarbonate, ABGs, liver function tests (elevations occur with chronic exposure), BUN, and creatinine.

Management

Seizures must be controlled. Pyridoxine and diazepam should be administered concomitantly through different IV sites. Pyridoxine (vitamin B_6) is given in a dose of 1 g for each gram of isoniazid ingested. If the dose ingested is unknown, at least 5 g of pyridoxine should be given intravenously. Pyridoxine is administered in 50 mL D_5W or 0.9% saline over 5 minutes intravenously. It must not be administered in the same bottle as sodium bicarbonate. Intravenous pyridoxine is repeated every 5 to 20 minutes until the seizures are controlled. Total doses of pyridoxine up to 52 g have been safely administered; however, patients given 132 and 183 g of pyridoxine have developed a persistent crippling sensory neuropathy.

Diazepam is administered concomitantly with pyridoxine but at a different site. They work synergistically. Diazepam should be administered intravenously slowly, 0.3 mg/kg at a rate of 1 mg/min in children or 10 mg at a rate of 5 mg/min in adults. After the seizures are controlled, the remainder of the pyridoxine is administered (1 g/1 g isoniazid) or a total dose of 5 g.

Phenobarbital or phenytoin is ineffective and should not be used.

In asymptomatic patients or patients without seizures, pyridoxine has been advised by some toxicologists prophylactically in gram-for-gram doses in cases of large overdoses (<80 mg/kg per dose) of isoniazid, although there are no studies to support this recommendation. In comatose patients, pyridoxine administration may result in the patient's rapid regaining of consciousness. Correction of acidosis may occur spontaneously with pyridoxine administration and correction of the seizures. Sodium bicarbonate should be administered if acidosis persists.

Hemodialysis is rarely needed because of antidotal therapy and the short half-life of isoniazid, but it may be used as an adjunct for cases of uncontrollable acidosis and seizures. Hemoperfusion has not been adequately evaluated. Diuresis is ineffective.

Disposition

Asymptomatic or mildly symptomatic patients who become asymptomatic can be observed in the emergency department for 4 to 6 hours. Larger amounts of isoniazid may warrant pyridoxine administration and longer periods of observation. Intentional ingestions necessitate psychiatric evaluation before the patient is discharged. Patients with convulsions or coma should be admitted to the intensive care unit.

Isopropanol (Isopropyl Alcohol)

Isopropanol can be found in rubbing alcohol, solvents, and lacquer thinner. Coma has occurred in children sponged for fever with isopropanol. See Table 10 for ethanol features of alcohols and glycols.

Toxic Mechanism

Isopropanol is a gastric irritant. It is metabolized to acetone, a CNS and myocardial depressant. It inhibits gluconeogenesis. Normal propyl alcohol is related to isopropyl alcohol but is more toxic.

Toxic Dose

A toxic dose of 0.5 to 1 mg/kg of 70% isopropanol (1 mL/kg of 70%) produces a blood isopropanol plasma concentration of 70 mg/dL. The CNS depressant potency is twice that of ethanol.

Kinetics

Onset of action is within 30 to 60 minutes, and peak is 1 hour postingestion. Volume distribution is 0.6 kg/L. Isopropyl alcohol metabolizes to acetone. Its excretion is renal.

Note: The serum isopropyl concentration and amount ingested can be estimated using the same equation as is used in ethanol kinetics and substituting the specific gravity of 0.785 for isopropyl alcohol.

Manifestations

Ethanol-like inebriation occurs, with an acetone odor to the breath, gastritis, occasionally with hematemesis, acetonuria, and acetonemia without systemic acidosis.

Depression of the CNS occurs: lethargy at blood isopropyl alcohol levels of 50 to 100 mg/dL, coma at levels of 150 to 200 mg/dL, potentially death in adults at levels greater than 240 mg/dL.

Hypoglycemia and seizures may occur.

Laboratory Investigation

Monitoring of blood isopropyl alcohol levels (not readily available in all institutions), acetone, glucose, and ABG should be maintained. The osmolal gap increases 1 mOsm per 5.9 mg/dL of isopropyl alcohol and 1 mOsm per 5.5 mg/dL of acetone. The absence of excess acetone in the blood (normal is 0.3 to 2 mg/dL) within 30 to 60 minutes or excess acetone in the urine within 3 hours excludes the possibility of significant isopropanol exposure.

Management

The airway must be protected with intubation, and assisted ventilation administered if necessary. If the patient is hypoglycemic, glucose should be administered. Supportive treatment is similar to that for ethanol ingestions.

Gastrointestinal decontamination has no role in the treatment of isopropanol ingestion. Hemodialysis is warranted in cases of life-threatening overdose but is rarely needed. A nephrologist should be consulted if the blood isopropanol plasma concentration is greater than 250 mg/dL.

Disposition

Symptomatic patients with concentrations greater than 100 mg/dL require at least 24 hours of close observation for resolution and should be admitted. If the patient is hypoglycemic, hypotensive, or comatose, he or she should be admitted to the intensive care unit.

Lead

Acute lead intoxication is rare and usually occurs by inhalation of lead, resulting in severe intoxication and often death. Lead fumes can be produced by burning of lead batteries or use of a heat gun to remove lead paint. Acute lead intoxication also occurs from exposure to high concentrations of organic lead (e.g., tetraethyl lead).

TABLE 17 Occupations Associated With Lead Exposure

Lead production or smelting
Production of illicit whiskey
Brass, copper, and lead foundries
Radiator repair
Scrap handling
Sanding of old paint
Lead soldering
Cable stripping
Worker or janitor at a firing range

Demolition of ships and bridges
Battery manufacturing
Machining/grinding lead alloys
Welding of old painted metals
Thermal paint stripping of old buildings
Ceramic glaze/pottery mixing

Modified from Rempel D: The lead-exposed worker. *JAMA* 262:533, 1989.

TABLE 18 CDC Questionnaire: Priority Groups for Lead Screening

1. Children age 6–72 months (was 12–36 months) who live in or are frequent visitors to older, deteriorated housing built before 1960.

2. Children age 6–72 months who live in housing built prior to 1960 with recent, ongoing, or planned renovation or remodeling.

3. Children age 6–72 months who are siblings, housemates, or playmates of children with known lead poisoning.

4. Children age 6–72 months whose parents or other household members participate in a lead-related industry or hobby.

5. Children age 6–72 months who live near active lead smelters, battery recycling plants, or other industries likely to result in atmospheric lead release.

TABLE 19 Sources of Lead

PRODUCT	LEAD CONTENT (%) BY DRY WEIGHT
Paint	0.06
Solder	0.6
Plastic additives	2.0
Priming inks	2.0
Plumbing fixtures	2.0
Pesticides	0.1
Stained glass panes	0.1
Wine bottle foils	0.1
Construction material	0.1
Fertilizers	0.1
Glazes, enamels	0.06
Toys/recreational games	0.1
Curtain weights	0.1
Fishing weights	0.1

Chronic lead poisoning occurs most often in children 6 months to 6 years of age who are exposed in their environment and in adults in certain occupations (Table 17). In the United States, the prevalence in children aged 1 to 5 years with a venous blood lead greater than 10 µg/dL decreased from 88.2% in a 1976–1980 survey to 8.9% in a 1988–1991 survey as a consequence of measures to reduce lead in the environment, particularly leaded gasoline. However, an estimated 1.7 million children between 1 and 5 years of age and more than 1 million workers in over 100 different occupations still have blood lead levels greater than 10 µg/dL.

Toxic Dose
In cases of chronic lead poisoning, a daily intake of more than 5 µg/kg/d in children or more than 150 µg/d in adults can give a positive lead balance. In 1991, the Centers for Disease Control and Prevention (CDC) recommended routine screening for all children younger than 6 years of age. In children a venous blood level greater than 10 µg/dL was determined to be a threshold of concern. The average venous blood level in the United States is 4 µg/dL. In cases of occupational exposure (see Table 17), a venous blood level greater than 40 µg/dL is indicative of increased lead absorption in adults.

Toxic Mechanism
Lead affects the sulfhydryl enzyme systems, the immature CNS, the enzymes of heme synthesis, vitamin D conversion, the kidneys, the bones, and growth. Lead alters the tertiary structure of cell proteins by denaturing them and causing cell death. Risk factors are mouthing behavior of infants and children and excessive oral behavior (pica), living in the inner city, a poorly maintained home, and poor nutrition (e.g., low calcium and iron). The CDC questionnaire given in Table 18 is recommended at every pediatric visit. If any answers to the CDC questionnaire are "positive," a blood screening test for lead should be administered. To be more accurate, however, identifying lead exposure studies have suggested that the questionnaire will have to be modified for each individual community because it has had poor sensitivity (40%) and specificity (60%) as it stands.

Table 19 lists sources of lead. The number one source is deteriorating lead-based paint, which forms leaded dust. Lead concentrations in indoor paint were not reduced to safer (0.06%) levels until 1978. Lead can also be produced by improper interior or exterior home renovation (scraping or demolition). It is found in pre-1960 built homes. The use of leaded gasoline (limited in 1973) resulted in residue from leaded motor vehicle emissions. Lead persists in the soil near major highways and in deteriorating homes and buildings. Vegetables grown in contaminated soil may contain lead.

Oil refineries and lead-processing smelters produce lead residue. Food cans produced in Mexico contain lead solder (95% do not in the United States). Lead water pipes (until 1950) and lead solder (until 1986) deliver lead-containing drinking water (calcium deposits, however, may offer some protection). Water at a consumer's tap should contain less than 15 parts per billion (ppb) of lead (Table 20).

For occupational exposure, see Table 17. The Occupational Safety and Health Administration (OSHA) standards require employers to provide showering and clothes changing facilities for personnel working with lead; however, businesses with fewer than 25 employees are exempt from the regulation. The OSHA lead standard of 1978 set a limit of 60 µg/dL for occupational exposure to lead. At a blood lead level of 60 µg/dL, a worker should be removed from lead exposure and not allowed back until his or her lead level is below 40 µg/dL. Many authorities believe that this level should be lower. The lead residue on the clothes of the workers may represent a hazard to the family. Other occupations that are potential sources of lead exposure include plumbers, pipe fitters, lead miners, auto repairers, shipbuilders, printers, steel welders and cutters, construction workers, and rubber product manufacturers.

Leaded pots to make molds for "kusmusha" tea represent lead exposure. Imported pottery lined with ceramic glaze can leach large amounts of lead into acids (e.g., citrus fruit juices).

Hobbies associated with lead exposure are listed in Box 1. Some "traditional" folk remedies or cosmetics that contain lead include the following:

- "Azarcon por empacho" ("Maria Louisa" 90% to 95% lead trioxide): a bright orange powder used in Hispanic culture, especially Mexican, for digestive problems and diarrhea.
- "Greta" (4% to 90% lead): a yellow powder "por empacho" ("empacho" refers to a variety of gastrointestinal symptoms), used in Hispanic cultures, especially Mexican.
- "Pay-loo-ah": an orange-red powder used for rash and fever in Southeast Asian cultures, especially among Northern Laos Hmong immigrants.

TABLE 20	Agency Regulations and Recommendations Concerning Lead Content		
AGENCY	**SPECIMEN**	**LEVEL**	**COMMENTS**
CDC	Blood (child)	$10\,\mu g/dL$	Investigate community
OSHA	Blood (adult)	$60\,\mu g/dL$	Medical removal from work
OSHA	Air	$50\,\mu g/m^3$	PEL*
	Air	$0.75\,\mu g/m^3$	Tetraethyl or tetramethyl
ACGIH	Air	$150\,\mu g/m^3$	TWA†
EPA	Air	$1.5\,\mu g/m^3$	Three-month average
EPA	Water	$15\,\mu g/L$ (ppb)	5 ppb circulating
EPA	Food	$100\,\mu g/d$	Advisory
FDA	Wine	300 ppm	Plan to reduce to 200 ppm
EPA	Soil/dust	50 ppm	
CPSC	Paint	600 ppm (0.06%) by dry weight	

*PEL = permissible exposure limit (highest level over an 8-hour workday).
†TWA = time-weighted average (air concentration for 8-hour workday and 40-hour workweek).
Abbreviations: ACGIH = American Conference of Governmental Industrial Hygienists; CDC = Centers for Disease Control and Prevention; CPSC = Consumer Product Safety Commission; EPA = Environmental Protection Agency; FDA = Food and Drug Administration; OSHA = Occupational Safety and Health Administration.

BOX 1	Hobbies Associated With Lead Exposure

Casting of ammunition
Collecting antique pewter
Collecting/painting lead toys (e.g., soldiers and figures)
Ceramics or glazed pottery
Refinishing furniture
Making fishing weights
Home renovation
Jewelry making, lead solder
Glass blowing, lead glass
Bronze casting
Print making and other fine arts (when lead white, flake white, chrome yellow pigments are involved)
Liquor distillation
Hunting and target shooting
Painting
Car and boat repair
Burning/engraving lead-painted wood
Making stained leaded glass
Copper enameling

- "Alkohl" (Al-kohl, kohl, suma 5% to 92% lead): a black powder used in Middle Eastern, African, and Asian cultures as a cosmetic and an umbilical stump astringent.
- "Farouk": an orange granular powder with lead used in Saudi Arabian culture.
- "Bint Al Zahab": used to treat colic in Saudi Arabian culture.
- "Surma" (23% to 26% lead): a black powder used in India as a cosmetic and to improve eyesight.
- "Bali goli": a round black bean that is dissolved in "grippe water," used by Asian and Indian cultures to aid digestion.

Cases of substance abuse involving lead poisoning have been reported, in which the patient sniffs leaded gasoline or uses improperly synthesized amphetamines.

Kinetics

Absorption of lead is 10% to 15% of the ingested dose in adults; in children, up to 40% is absorbed, especially in cases of iron deficiency anemia. With inhalation of fumes, absorption is rapid and complete. Volume distribution in blood (0.9% of total body burden) is 95% in red blood cells. Lead passes through the placenta to the fetus and is present in breast milk.

Organic lead is metabolized in the liver to inorganic lead. Its half-life is 35 to 40 days in blood; in soft tissue, the half-life is 45 days and in bone (99% of the lead), the half-life is 28 years. The major elimination route is the stool, 80% to 90%, and then renal 10% (80 g/d) and hair, nails, sweat, and saliva. Nine percent of organic lead is excreted in the urine per day.

Manifestations

Adverse health effects are given in Table 21 and include the following.

Hematologic. Lead inhibits γ-aminolevulinic acid dehydratase (early in the synthesis of heme) and ferrochelatase (transfers iron to ferritin for incorporation of iron into protoporphyrin to produce heme). Anemia is a late finding. Decreased heme synthesis starts at $>40\,\mu g/dL$. Basophilic stippling occurs in 20% of severe lead poisoning.

Neurologic. Segmental demyelination and peripheral neuropathy, usually of the motor type (wrist and ankle drop), occurs in workers. A venous blood level of lead greater than $70\,\mu g/dL$ (usually $>100\,\mu g/dL$), produces encephalopathy in children (symptom mnemonic "PAINT": P, persistent forceful vomiting and papilledema; A, ataxia; I, intermittent stupor and lucidity; N, neurologic coma and refractory convulsions; T, tired and lethargic). Decreased cognitive abilities have been reported with a venous blood level of lead greater than $10\,\mu g/dL$, including behavioral problems, decreased attention span, and learning disabilities. IQ scores may begin to decrease at $15\,\mu g/dL$. Encephalopathy is rare in adults.

Renal. Nephropathy as a result of damaged capillaries and glomerulus can occur at a venous blood level of lead greater than $80\,\mu g/dL$, but recent studies show renal damage and hypertension with low venous blood levels. A direct correlation between hypertension and venous blood level over $30\,\mu g/dL$ has been reported. Lead reduces excretion of uric acid, and high-level exposure may be associated with hyperuricemia and "saturnine gout," Fanconi's syndrome (aminoaciduria and renal tubular acidosis), and tubular fibrosis.

Reproductive. Spontaneous abortion, transient delay in the child's development (catch up at age 5 to 6 years), decreased sperm count, and abnormal sperm morphology can occur with lead exposure. Lead crosses the placenta and fetal blood levels reach 75% to 100% of maternal blood levels. Lead is teratogenic.

Metabolic. Decreased cytochrome P450 activity alters the metabolism of medication and endogenously produced substances. Decreased activation of cortisol and decreased growth are caused by interference in vitamin conversion (25-hydroxyvitamin D to 1,25-hydroxyvitamin D) at venous blood levels of 20 to $30\,\mu g/dL$.

Other Manifestations. Abnormalities of thyroid, cardiac, and hepatic function occur in adults. Abdominal colic is seen in children at doses greater than $50\,\mu g/dL$. "Lead gum lines" at the dental border of the gingiva can occur in cases of chronic lead poisoning.

Laboratory Investigations

Serial venous blood lead measurements are taken on days 3 and 5 during treatment and 7 days after chelation therapy, then every 1 to 2 weeks for 8 weeks, and then every month for 6 months. Intravenous infusion should be stopped at least 1 hour before blood lead levels are measured. Table 22 gives a classification of blood lead concentrations in children.

One should evaluate CBC, serum ferritin, erythrocyte protoporphyrin ($>35\,\mu g/dL$ indicates lead poisoning as well as iron deficiency and other causes), electrolytes, serum calcium and

TABLE 21	Summary of Lead-Induced Health Effects in Adults and Children	
BLOOD LEAD LEVEL (MG/DL)	AGE GROUP	HEALTH EFFECT
>100	Adult	Encephalopathic signs and symptoms
>80	Adult	Anemia
	Child	Encephalopathy Chronic nephropathy (e.g., aminoaciduria)
>70	Adult	Clinically evident peripheral neuropathy
	Child	Colic and other gastrointestinal symptoms
>60	Adult	Female reproductive effects CNS disturbance symptoms (i.e., sleep disturbances, mood changes, memory and concentration problems, headaches)
>50	Adult	Decreased hemoglobin production Decreased performance on neurobehavioral tests
	Adult	Altered testicular function Gastrointestinal symptoms (i.e., abdominal pain, constipation, diarrhea, nausea, anorexia)
	Child	Peripheral neuropathy*
>40	Adult	Decreased peripheral nerve conduction Hypertension, age 40–59 years Chronic neuropathy*
>25	Adult	Elevated erythrocyte protoporphyrin in males
15–25	Adult	Elevated erythrocyte protoporphyrin in females
>10	Child	Decreased intelligence and growth Impaired learning Reduced birth weight* Impaired mental ability
	Fetus	Preterm delivery

*Controversial.
From Anonymous: Implementation of the Lead Contamination Control Act of 1988. *MMWR Morb Mortal Wkly Rep* 41:288, 1992.

TABLE 22	Classification of Blood Lead Concentrations in Children
BLOOD LEAD (MG/DL)	RECOMMENDED INTERVENTIONS
<9	None
10–14	Community intervention Repeat blood lead in 3 months
15–19	Individual case management Environmental counseling Nutritional counseling Repeat blood lead in 3 months
20–44	Medical referral Environmental inspection/abatement Nutritional counseling Repeat blood lead in 3 months
45–69	Environmental inspection/abatement Nutritional counseling Pharmacologic therapy DMSA succimer oral or CaNa₂EDTA parenteral Repeat every 2 weeks for 6–8 weeks, then monthly for 4–6 months
>70	Hospitalization in intensive care unit Environmental inspection/abatement Pharmacologic therapy Dimercaprol (BAL in oil) IM initial alone Dimercaprol IM and CaNa₂EDTA together Repeat every week

Abbreviations: BAL = British anti-Lewisite; CaNa$_2$EDTA = edetate calcium disodium; DMSA = dimercaptosuccinic acid; IM = intramuscular.

phosphorus, urinalysis, BUN, and creatinine. Abdominal and long bone radiographs may be useful in certain circumstances to identify radiopaque material in bowel and "lead lines" in proximal tibia (which occur after prolonged exposure in association with venous blood lead levels greater than 50 μg/dL).

Neuropsychological tests are difficult to perform in young children but should be considered at the end of treatment, especially to determine auditory dysfunction.

Management

The basis of treatment is removal of the source of lead. Cases of poisoning in children should be reported to local health department and cases of occupational poisoning should be reported to OSHA. The source must be identified and abated and dust controlled by wet mopping. Cold water should be let to run for 2 minutes before being used for drinking. Planting shrubbery (not vegetables) in contaminated soil will keep children away.

Supportive care should be instituted, including measures to deal with refractory seizures (continued antidotal therapy, diazepam, and possibly neuromuscular blockers), and the hepatic and renal failure, and intravascular hemolysis in severe cases. Seizures are treated with diazepam followed by neuromuscular blockers if needed.

Lead does not bind to activated charcoal. One must not delay chelation therapy for complete gastrointestinal decontamination in severe cases. Whole-bowel irrigation has been used prior to treatment. Some authorities recommend abdominal radiographs followed by gastrointestinal decontamination if necessary before switching to oral therapy. Chelation therapy can be used for patients in whom venous blood level of lead is greater than 45 μg/dL in children and greater than 80 μg/dL in adults or in adults with lower levels who are symptomatic or who have a "positive" lead mobilization test result (not routinely performed at most centers) (Table 23).

Succimer (dimercaptosuccinic acid, DMSA, Chemet), a derivative of British anti-Lewisite (BAL), is an oral agent for chelation in children with a venous blood level of greater than 45 μg/dL. The recommended dose is 10 mg/kg every 8 hours for 5 days, then every 12 hours for 14 days. DMSA is under investigation to determine its role in children with a venous blood level less than 45 μg/dL. Although not approved for adults, it has been used in the same dosage. Monitoring should be maintained by CBC, liver transaminases, and urinalysis for adverse effects.

D-Penicillamine (Cuprimine) is another oral chelator that is given in doses of 20 to 40 mg/kg/d not to exceed 1 g/d. However, it is not FDA approved and has a 10% adverse reaction rate. Nevertheless, D-penicillamine has been used infrequently in adults and children with elevated venous blood lead levels.

Edetate calcium disodium (ethylene diaminetetra-acetic acid or CaNa₂EDTA Versenate) is a water-soluble chelator given intramuscularly (with 0.5% procaine) or intravenously. The

TABLE 23 Pharmacologic Chelation Therapy of Lead Poisoning

DRUG	ROUTE	DOSE	DURATION	PRECAUTIONS	MONITOR
Dimercaprol (BAL in oil)	IM	3–5 mg/kg q4–6h	3–5 days	G6PD deficiency Concurrent iron therapy	AST/ALT enzymes
CaNa$_2$EDTA (calcium disodium versenate)	IM/IV	50 mg/kg per day	5 days	Inadequate fluid intake Renal impairment Penicillin allergy	Urinalysis, BUN Creatinine Urinalysis, BUN
D-Penicillamine (Cuprimine)	PO	10 mg/kg per day increase 30 mg/kg over 2 weeks	6–20 weeks	Concurrent iron therapy; lead exposure Renal impairment	Creatinine, CBC
2,3-Dimercaptosuccinic acid (DMSA; succimer)	PO	10 mg/kg per dose 3 times daily 10 mg/kg per dose twice daily for 14 days	19 days	AST/ALT Concurrent iron therapy G6PD deficiency lead exposure	AST/ALT

Abbreviations: ALT = alanine aminotransferase; AST = aspartate transaminase; BAL = British anti-Lewisite; bid = twice daily; BUN = blood urea nitrogen; CBC = complete blood count; G6PD = glucose-6-phosphate dehydrogenase; IM = intramuscular; IV = intravenous; PO = oral; tid = three times daily.

calcium in the compound is displaced by divalent and trivalent heavy metals, forming a soluble complex, which is stable at physiologic pH (but not at acid pH) and enhances lead clearance in the urine. EDTA usually is administered intravenously, especially in severe cases. It must not be administered until adequate urine flow is established. It may redistribute lead to the brain; therefore, BAL may be given first at a venous blood lead level of greater than 55 µg/dL in children and greater than 100 µg/dL in adults. Phlebitis occurs at a concentration greater than 0.5 mg/mL. Alkalinization of the urine may be helpful. CaNa$_2$EDTA should not be confused with sodium EDTA (disodium edetate), which is used to treat hypercalcemia; inadvertent use may produce severe hypocalcemia.

Dimercaprol (BAL) is a peanut oil–based dithiol (two sulfhydryl molecules) that combines with one atom of lead to form a heterocyclic stable ring complex. It is usually reserved for patients in whom venous blood lead is greater than 70 µg/dL, and it chelates red blood cell lead, enhancing its elimination through the urine and bile. It crosses the blood-brain barrier. Approximately 50% of patients have adverse reactions, including bad metallic taste in the mouth, pain at the injection site, sterile abscesses, and fever.

A venous blood lead level greater than 70 µg/dL or the presence of clinical symptoms suggesting encephalopathy in children is a potentially life-threatening emergency. Management should be accomplished in a medical center with a pediatric intensive care unit by a multidisciplinary team including a critical care specialist, a toxicologist, a neurologist, and a neurosurgeon. Careful monitoring of neurologic status, fluid status, and intracranial pressure should be undertaken if necessary. These patients need close monitoring for hemodynamic instability. Hydration should be maintained to ensure renal excretion of lead. Fluids, renal and hepatic function, and electrolyte levels should be monitored.

While waiting for adequate urine flow, therapy should be initiated with intramuscular dimercaprol (BAL) only (25 mg/kg/d divided into 6 doses). Four hours later, the second dose of BAL should be given intramuscularly, concurrently with CaNa$_2$EDTA 50 mg/kg/d as a single dose infused over several hours or as a continuous infusion. The double therapy is continued until the venous blood level is less than 40 µg/dL.

As long as the venous blood level is greater than 40 µg/dL, therapy is continued for 72 hours and followed by two alternatives: either parenteral therapy with two drugs (CaNa$_2$EDTA and BAL) for 5 days or continuation of therapy with CaNa$_2$EDTA alone if a good response is achieved and the venous blood level of lead is less than 40 µg/dL. If one cannot get the venous blood lead report back, one should continue therapy with both BAL and EDTA for 5 days. In patients with lead encephalopathy, parenteral chelation should be continued with both drugs until the patient is clinically stable before changing therapy. Mannitol and dexamethasone can reduce the cerebral edema, but their role in lead encephalopathy is not clear. Surgical decompression is not recommended to reduce cerebral edema in these cases.

If BAL and CaNa$_2$EDTA are used together, a minimum of 2 days with no treatment should elapse before another 5-day course of therapy is considered. The 5-day course is repeated with CaNa$_2$EDTA alone if the blood lead level rebounds to greater than 40 µg/dL or in combination with BAL if the venous blood level is greater than 70 µg/dL. If a third course is required, unless there are compelling reasons, one should wait at least 5 to 7 days before administering the course.

Following chelation therapy, a period of equilibration of 10 to 14 days should be allowed and a repeat venous blood lead concentration should be obtained. If the patient is stable enough for oral intake, oral succimer 30 mg/kg/d in three divided doses for 5 days followed by 20 mg/kg/d in two divided doses for 14 days has been suggested, but there are limited data to support this recommendation. Therapy should be continued until venous blood lead level is less than 20 µg/dL in children or less than 40 µg/dL in adults.

Chelators combined with lead are hemodialyzable in the event of renal failure.

Disposition

All patients with a venous blood lead level of greater than 70 µg/dL or who are symptomatic should be admitted. If a child is hospitalized, all lead hazards must be removed from the home environment before allowing the child to return. The source must be eliminated by environmental and occupational investigations. The local health department should be involved in dealing with children who are lead poisoned, and OSHA should be involved with cases of occupational lead poisoning. Consultation with a poison control center or experienced toxicologist is necessary when chelating patients. Follow-up venous blood lead concentrations should be obtained within 1 to 2 weeks and followed every 2 weeks for 6 to 8 weeks, then monthly for 4 to 6 months if the patient required chelation therapy. All patients with venous blood level greater than 10 µg/dL should be followed at least every 3 months until two venous blood lead concentrations are 10 µg/dL or three are less than 15 µg/dL.

Lithium (Eskalith, Lithane)

Lithium is an alkali metal used primarily in the treatment of bipolar psychiatric disorders. Most intoxications are cases of chronic overdose. One gram of lithium carbonate contains 189 mg (5.1 mEq) of lithium; a regular tablet contains 300 mg (8.12 mEq) and a sustained-release preparation contains 450 mg or 12.18 mEq.

Toxic Mechanism

The brain is the primary target organ of toxicity, but the mechanism is unclear. Lithium may interfere with physiologic functions by acting as a substitute for cellular cations (sodium and potassium), depressing neural excitation and synaptic transmission.

Toxic Dose

A dose of 1 mEq/kg (40 mg/kg) of lithium will give a peak serum lithium concentration about 1.2 mEq/L. The therapeutic serum lithium concentration in cases of acute mania is 0.6 to 1.2 mEq/L, and for maintenance it is 0.5 to 0.8 mEq/L. Serum lithium concentration levels are usually obtained 12 hours after the last dose. The toxic dose is determined by clinical manifestations and serum levels after the distribution phase.

Acute ingestion of twenty 300-mg tablets (300 mg increases the serum lithium concentration by 0.2 to 0.4 mEq/L) in adults may produce serious intoxication. Chronic intoxication can be produced by conditions listed below that can decrease the elimination of lithium or increase lithium reabsorption in the kidney.

The risk factors that predispose to chronic lithium toxicity are febrile illness, impaired renal function, hyponatremia, advanced age, lithium-induced diabetes insipidus, dehydration, vomiting and diarrhea, and concomitant use of other drugs, such as thiazide and spironolactone diuretics, nonsteroidal antiinflammatory drugs, salicylates, angiotensin-converting enzyme inhibitors (e.g., captopril), serotonin reuptake inhibitors (e.g., fluoxetine [Prozac]), and phenothiazines.

Kinetics

Gastrointestinal absorption of regular-release preparations is rapid; serum lithium concentration peaks in 2 to 4 hours and is complete by 6 to 8 hours. The onset of toxicity may occur at 1 to 4 hours after acute overdose but usually is delayed because lithium enters the brain slowly. Absorption of sustained-release preparations and the development of toxicity may be delayed 6 to 12 hours.

Volume distribution is 0.5 to 0.9 L/kg. Lithium is not protein bound. The half-life after a single dose is 9 to 13 hours; at steady state, it may be 30 to 58 hours. The renal handling of lithium is similar to that of sodium: glomerular filtration and reabsorption (80%) by the proximal renal tubule. Adequate sodium must be present to prevent lithium reabsorption. More than 90% of lithium is excreted by the kidney, 30% to 60% within 6 to 12 hours.

Manifestations

The examiner must distinguish between side effects, acute intoxication, acute or chronic toxicity, and chronic intoxications. Chronic is the most common and dangerous type of intoxication.

Side effects include fine tremor, gastrointestinal upset, hypothyroidism, polyuria and frank diabetes insipidus, dermatologic manifestations, and cardiac conduction deficits. Lithium is teratogenic.

Patients with acute poisoning may be asymptomatic, with an early high serum lithium concentration of 9 mEq/L, and deteriorate as the serum lithium concentration falls by 50% and the lithium distributes to the brain and the other tissues. Nausea and vomiting may occur within 1 to 4 hours, but the systemic manifestations are usually delayed several more hours. It may take as long as 3 to 5 days for serious symptoms to develop. Acute toxicity and acute on chronic toxicity are manifested by neurologic findings, including weakness, fasciculations, altered mental state, myoclonus, hyperreflexia, rigidity, coma, and convulsions with limbs in hypertension. Cardiovascular effects are nonspecific and occur at therapeutic doses, flat T or inverted T waves, atrioventricular block, and prolonged QT interval. Lithium is not a primary cardiotoxin. Cardiogenic shock occurs secondary to CNS toxicity. Chronic intoxication is associated with manifestations at lower serum lithium concentrations. There is some correlation with manifestations, especially at higher serum lithium concentrations. Although the levels do not always correlate with the manifestations, they are more predictive in cases of severe intoxication. A serum lithium concentration greater than 3.0 mEq/L with chronic intoxication and altered mental state indicates severe toxicity. Permanent neurologic sequelae can result from lithium intoxication.

Laboratory Investigations

Monitoring should include CBC (lithium causes significant leukocytosis), renal function, thyroid function (chronic intoxication), ECG, and electrolytes. Serum lithium concentrations should be determined every 2 to 4 hours until levels are close to therapeutic range. Cross-reactions with green-top Vacutainer specimen tubes containing heparin will spuriously elevate serum lithium concentration 6 to 8 mEq/L.

Management

Vital function must be established and maintained. Seizure precautions should be instituted and seizures, hypotension, and dysrhythmias treated. Evaluation should include examination for rigidity and hyperreflexia signs, hydration, renal function (BUN, creatinine), and electrolytes, especially sodium. The examiner should inquire about diuretic and other drug use that increase serum lithium concentration, and the patient must discontinue the drugs. If the patient is on chronic therapy, the lithium should be discontinued. Serial serum lithium concentrations should be obtained every 4 hours until serum lithium concentration peaks and there is a downward trend toward almost therapeutic range, especially in sustained-release preparations. Vital signs should be monitored, including temperature, and ECG and serial neurologic examinations should be undertaken, including mental status and urinary output. Nephrology consultation is warranted in case of a chronic and elevated serum lithium concentration (>2.5 mEq/L), a large ingestion, or altered mental state.

An intravenous line should be established and hydration and electrolyte balance restored. Serum sodium level should be determined before 0.9% saline fluid is administered in patients with chronic overdose because hypernatremia may be present from diabetes insipidus. Although current evidence supports an initial 0.9% saline infusion (200 mL/h) to enhance excretion of lithium, once hydration, urine output, and normonatremia are established, one should administer 0.45% saline and slow the infusion (100 mL/h) for all patients.

Gastric lavage is often not recommended in cases of acute ingestion because of the large size of the tablets, and it is not necessary after chronic intoxication. Activated charcoal is ineffective. For sustained-release preparations, whole-bowel irrigation may be useful but is not proven. Sodium polystyrene sulfonate (Kayexalate), an ion exchange resin, is difficult to administer and has been used only in uncontrolled studies. Its use is not recommended.

Hemodialysis is the most efficient method for removing lithium from the vascular compartment. It is the treatment of choice for patients with severe intoxication with an altered mental state, those with seizures, and anuric patients. Long runs are used until the serum lithium concentration is less than 1 mEq/L because of extensive re-equilibration. Serum lithium concentration should be monitored every 4 hours after dialysis for rebound. Repeated and prolonged hemodialysis may be necessary. A lag in neurologic recovery can be expected.

Disposition

An acute asymptomatic lithium overdose cannot be medically cleared on the basis of single lithium level. Patients should be admitted if they have any neurologic manifestations (altered mental status, hyperreflexia, stiffness, or tremor). Patients should be admitted to the intensive care unit if they are dehydrated, have renal impairment, or have a high or rising lithium level.

Methanol (Wood Alcohol, Methyl Alcohol)

The concentration of methanol in Sterno fuel is 4% and it contains ethanol, in windshield washer fluid it is 30% to 60%, and in gas-line antifreeze it is 100%.

Toxic Mechanism

Methanol is metabolized by alcohol dehydrogenase to formaldehyde, which is metabolized to formate. Formate inhibits cytochrome oxidase, producing tissue hypoxia, lactic acidosis, and optic nerve edema. Formate is converted by folate-dependent enzymes to carbon dioxide.

Toxic Dose

The minimal toxic amount is approximately 100 mg/kg. Serious toxicity in a young child can be produced by the ingestion of 2.5 to 5.0 mL of 100% methanol. Ingestion of 5-mL 100% methanol by a 10-kg child produces estimated peak blood methanol of 80 mg/dL. Ingestion of 15 mL 40% methanol was lethal for a 2-year-old child in one report. A fatal adult oral dose is 30 to 240 mL 100% (20 to 150 g). Ingestion of 6 to 10 mL 100% causes blindness in adults. The toxic blood concentration is greater than 20 mg/dL; very serious toxicity and potential fatality occur at levels greater than 50 mg/dL.

Kinetics

Onset of action can start within 1 hour but may be delayed up to 12 to 18 hours by metabolism to toxic metabolites. It may be delayed longer if ethanol is ingested concomitantly or in infants. Peak blood methanol concentration is 1 hour. Volume distribution is 0.6 L/kg (total body water).

For metabolism, see *Toxic Mechanism*.

Elimination is through metabolism. The half-life of methanol is 8 hours; with ethanol blocking it is 30 to 35 hours; and with hemodialysis 2.5 hours.

Manifestations

Metabolism creates a delay in onset for 12 to 18 hours or longer if ethanol is ingested concomitantly. Initial findings are as follows:
- 0 to 6 hours: Confusion, ataxia, inebriation, formaldehyde odor on breath, and abdominal pain can be present, but the patient may be asymptomatic. *Note:* Methanol produces an osmolal gap (early), and its metabolite formate produces the anion gap metabolic acidosis (see later). Absence of osmolar or anion gap does not always exclude methanol intoxication.
- 6 to 12 hours: Malaise, headache, abdominal pain, vomiting, visual symptoms, including hyperemia of optic disc, "snow vision," and blindness can be seen.
- More than 12 hours: Worsening acidosis, hyperglycemia, shock, and multiorgan failure develop, with death from complications of intractable acidosis and cerebral edema.

Laboratory Investigation

Methanol can be detected on some chromatography drug screens if specified. Methanol and ethanol levels, electrolytes, glucose, BUN, creatinine, amylase, and ABG should be monitored every 4 hours. Formate levels correlate more closely than blood methanol concentration with severity of intoxication and should be obtained if possible.

Management

One should protect the airway by intubation to prevent aspiration and administer assisted ventilation as needed. If needed, 100% oxygen can be administered. A nephrologist should be consulted early regarding the need for hemodialysis.

Gastrointestinal decontamination procedures have no role.

Metabolic acidosis should be treated vigorously with sodium bicarbonate 2 to 3 mEq/kg intravenously. Large amounts may be needed.

Antidote therapy is initiated to inhibit metabolism if the patient has a history of ingesting more than 0.4 mL/kg of 100% with the following conditions:
- Blood methanol level is greater than 20 mg/dL
- The patient has osmolar gap not accounted for by other factors
- The patient is symptomatic or acidotic with increased anion gap and/or hyperemia of the optic disc.

The ethanol or fomepizole therapy outlined below can be used.

Ethanol Therapy. Ethanol should be initiated immediately if fomepizole is unavailable (see *Fomepizole Therapy*). Alcohol dehydrogenase has a greater affinity for ethanol than ethylene glycol. Therefore, ethanol blocks the metabolism of ethylene glycol.

Ethanol should be administered intravenously (oral administration is less reliable) to produce a blood ethanol concentration of 100 to 150 mg/dL. The loading dose is 10 mL/kg of 10% ethanol administered intravenously concomitantly with a maintenance dose of 10% ethanol at 1.0 mL/kg/h. This dose may need to be increased to 2 mL/kg/h in patients who are heavy drinkers. The blood ethanol concentration should be measured hourly and the infusion rate should be adjusted to maintain a concentration of 100 to 150 mg/dL.

Fomepizole Therapy. Fomepizole (Antizol, 4-methylpyrazole) inhibits alcohol dehydrogenase more reliably than ethanol and it does not require constant monitoring of ethanol levels and adjustment of infusion rates. Fomepizole is available in 1 g/mL vials of 1.5 mL. The loading dose is 15 mg/kg (0.015 mL/kg) IV, maintenance dose is 10 mg/kg (0.01 mL/kg) every 12 hours for 4 doses, then 15 mg/kg every 12 hours until the ethylene glycol levels are less than 20 mg/dL. The solution is prepared by being mixed with 100 mL of 0.9% saline or D_5W. Fomepizole can be given to patients requiring hemodialysis but should be dosed as follows:

Dose at the beginning of hemodialysis:
- If less than 6 hours since last Antizol dose, do not administer dose
- If more than 6 hours since last dose, administer next scheduled dose

Dosing during hemodialysis:
- Dose every 4 hours

Dosing at the time hemodialysis is completed:
- If less than 1 hour between last dose and end dialysis, do not administer dose at end of dialysis
- If 1 to 3 hours between last dose and end dialysis, administer one half of next scheduled dose
- If more than 3 hours between last dose and end dialysis, administer next scheduled dose

Maintenance dosing off hemodialysis:
- Give the next scheduled dose 12 hours from the last dose administered

Hemodialysis increases the clearance of both methanol and formate 10-fold over renal clearance. A blood methanol concentration greater than 50 mg/dL has been used as an indication for hemodialysis, but recently some toxicologists from the New York City Poison Center recommended early hemodialysis in patients with blood methanol concentration greater than 25 mg/dL because it may be able to shorten the course of intoxication if started early. One should continue to monitor methanol levels and/or formate levels every 4 hours after the procedure for rebound. Other indications for early hemodialysis are significant metabolic acidosis and electrolyte abnormalities despite conventional therapy and if visual or neurologic signs or symptoms are present.

A serum formate level greater than 20 mg/dL has also been used as a criterion for hemodialysis, although this is often not readily available through many laboratories. If hemodialysis is used, the infusion rate of 10% ethanol should be increased 2.0 to 3.5 mL/kg/h. The blood ethanol concentration and glucose level should be obtained every 2 hours.

Therapy is continued with both ethanol and hemodialysis until the blood methanol level is undetectable, there is no acidosis, and the patient has no neurologic or visual disturbances. This may require several days.

Hypoglycemia is treated with intravenous glucose. Doses of folinic acid (Leucovorin) and folic acid have been used successfully in animal investigations to enhance formate metabolism to carbon dioxide and water. Leucovorin 1 mg/kg up to 50 mg IV is administered every 4 hours for several days.

An initial ophthalmologic consultation and follow-up are warranted.

Disposition
All patients who have ingested significant amounts of methanol should be referred to the emergency department for evaluation and blood methanol concentration measurement. Ophthalmologic follow-up of all patients with methanol intoxications should be arranged.

Monoamine Oxidase Inhibitors
Nonselective monoamine oxidase inhibitors (MAOIs) include the hydrazines phenelzine (Nardil) and isocarboxazid (Marplan), and the nonhydrazine tranylcypromine (Parnate). Furazolidone (Furoxone) and pargyline (Eutonyl)[2] are also considered nonselective MAOIs. Moclobemide,[2] which is available in many countries but not the United States, is a selective MAO-A inhibitor. MAO-B inhibitors include selegiline (Eldepryl), an antiparkonsism agent, which does not have similar toxicity to MAO-A and is not discussed. Selectivity is lost in an overdose. MAOIs are used to treat severe depression.

Toxic Mechanism
Monoamine oxidase enzymes are responsible for the oxidative deamination of both endogenous and exogenous catecholamines such as norepinephrine. MAO-A in the intestinal wall also metabolizes tyramine in food. MAOIs permanently inhibit MAO enzymes until a new enzyme is synthesized after 14 days or longer. The toxicity results from the accumulation, potentiation, and prolongation of the cate-cholamine action followed by profound hypotension and cardiovascular collapse.

Toxic Dose
Toxicity begins at 2 to 3 mg/kg and fatalities occur at 4 to 6 mg/kg. Death has occurred after a single dose of 170 mg of tranylcypromine in an adult.

Kinetics
Structurally, MAOIs are related to amphetamines and catecholamines. The hydrazine peak levels are at 1 to 2 hours; metabolism is hepatic acetylation; and inactive metabolites are excreted in the urine. For the nonhydrazines, peak levels occur at 1 to 4 hours, and metabolism is via the liver to active amphetamine-like metabolites.

The onset of symptoms in a case of overdose is delayed 6 to 24 hours after ingestion, peak activity is 8 to 12 hours, and duration is 72 hours or longer. The peak of MAO inhibition is in 5 to 10 days and lasts as long as 5 weeks.

Manifestations
Manifestations of an acute ingestion overdose of MAO-A inhibitors are as follows:

Phase I. An adrenergic crisis occurs, with delayed onset for 6 to 24 hours, and may not reach peak until 24 hours. The crisis starts as hyperthermia, tachycardia, tachypnea, dysarthria, transient hypertension, hyperreflexia, and CNS stimulation.

Phase II. Neuromuscular excitation and sympathetic hyperactivity occur with increased temperature greater than 40°C (104°F), agitation, hyperactivity, confusion, fasciculations, twitching, tremor, masseter spasm, muscle rigidity, acidosis, and electrolyte abnormalities. Seizures and dystonic reactions may occur. The pupils are mydriatic, sometimes nonreactive with "ping-pong gaze."

Phase III. CNS depression and cardiovascular collapse occur in cases of severe overdose as the catecholamines are depleted. Symptoms usually resolve within 5 days but may last 2 weeks.

Phase IV. Secondary complications occur, including rhabdomyolysis, cardiac dysrhythmias, multiorgan failure, and coagulopathies.

[2]Not available in the United States.

Biogenic interactions usually occur while the patient is on therapeutic doses of MAOI or shortly after they are discontinued (30 to 60 minutes), before the new MAO enzyme is synthesized. The following substances have been implicated: indirect acting sympathomimetics such as amphetamines, serotonergic drugs, opioids (e.g., meperidine, dextromethorphan), tricyclic antidepressants, specific serotonin reuptake inhibitors (SSRIs; e.g., fluoxetine [Prozac], sertraline [Zoloft], paroxetine [Paxil]), tyramine-containing foods (e.g., wine, beer, avocados, cheese, caviar, chocolate, chicken liver), and L-tryptophan. SSRIs should not be started for at least 5 weeks after MAOIs have been discontinued.

In mild cases, usually caused by foods, headache and hypertension develop and last for several hours. In severe cases, malignant hypertension and severe hyperthermia syndromes consisting of hypertension or hyperthermia, altered mental state, skeletal muscle rigidity, shivering (often beginning in the masseter muscle), and seizures may occur.

The serotonin syndrome, which may be a result of inhibition of serotonin metabolism, has similar clinical findings to those of malignant hyperthermia and may occur with or without hyperthermia or hypertension.

Chronic toxicity clinical findings include tremors, hyperhidrosis, agitation, hallucinations, confusion, and seizures and may be confused with withdrawal syndromes.

Laboratory Investigations
Monitoring of the ECG, cardiac monitoring, CPK, ABG, pulse oximeter, electrolytes, blood glucose, and acid-base balance should be maintained.

Management
In the case of MAOI overdose, ipecac-induced emesis should not be used. Only activated charcoal alone should be used.

If the patient is admitted to the hospital and is well enough to eat, a nontyramine diet should be ordered.

Extreme agitation and seizures can be controlled with benzodiazepines and barbiturates. Phenytoin is ineffective. Nondepolarizing neuromuscular blockers (not depolarizing succinylcholine) may be needed in severe cases of hyperthermia and rigidity. If the patient has severe hypertension (catecholamine mediated), phentolamine (Regitine), a parenteral β-blocking agent, 3 to 5 mg intravenously, or labetalol (Normodyne), a combination of an α-blocking agent and a β-blocker, 20-mg intravenous bolus, should be given. If malignant hypertension with rigidity is present, a short-acting nitroprusside and benzodiazepine can be used. Hypertension is often followed by severe hypotension, which should be managed by fluid and vasopressors. *Caution:* Vasopressor therapy should be administered at lower doses than usual because of exaggerated pharmacologic response. Norepinephrine is preferred to dopamine, which requires release of intracellular amines.

Cardiac dysrhythmias are treated with standard therapy but are often refractory, and cardioversion and pacemakers may be needed.

For malignant hyperthermia, dantrolene (Dantrium), a nonspecific peripheral skeletal relaxing agent, is administered, which inhibits the release of calcium from the sarcoplasm. Dantrolene is reconstituted with 60 mL sterile water without bacteriostatic agents. Glass equipment must not be used, and the drug must be protected from light and used within 6 hours. Loading dose is 2 to 3 mg/kg intravenously as a bolus, and the loading dose is repeated until the signs of malignant hyperthermia (tachycardia, rigidity, increased end-tidal CO_2, and temperature) are controlled. Maximum total dose is 10 mg/kg to avoid hepatotoxicity.

When malignant hyperthermia has subsided, 1 mg/kg IV is given every 6 hours for 24 to 48 hours, then orally 1 mg/kg every 6 hours for 24 hours to prevent recurrence. There is a danger of thrombophlebitis following peripheral dantrolene, and it should be administered through a central line if possible. In addition one should administer external cooling and correct metabolic acidosis and electrolyte disturbances. Benzodiazepine can be used for sedation. Dantrolene does not reverse central dopamine blockade; therefore, bromocriptine mesylate (Parlodel) 2.5 to 10 mg should be given orally or through a nasogastric tube three times a day.

Rhabdomyolysis and myoglobinuria are treated with fluids. Urine alkalinization should also be treated.

Hemodialysis and hemoperfusion are of no proven value.

Biogenic amine interactions are managed symptomatically, similar to cases of overdose. For the serotonin syndrome cyproheptadine (Periactin), a serotonin blocker, 4 mg orally every hour for three doses, or methysergide (Sansert), 2 mg orally every 6 hours for three doses, should be considered. The effectiveness of these drugs has not been proven.

Disposition

All patients who have ingested more than 2 mg/kg of an MAOI should be admitted to the hospital for 24 hours of observation and monitoring in the intensive care unit because the life-threatening manifestations may be delayed. Patients with drug or dietary interactions that are mild may not require admission if symptoms subside within 4 to 6 hours and the patients remain asymptomatic. Patients with symptoms that persist or require active intervention should be admitted to the intensive care unit.

Opioids (Narcotic Opiates)

Opioids are used for analgesia, as antitussives, and as antidiarrheal agents and are illicit agents (heroin, opium) used in substance abuse. Tolerance, physical dependency, and withdrawal may develop.

Toxic Mechanism

At least four main opioid receptors have been identified. The μ receptor is considered the most important for central analgesia and CNS depression. The κ and δ receptors predominate in spinal analgesia. The σ receptors may mediate dysphoria. Death is a consequence of dose-dependent CNS respiratory depression or secondary to pulmonary aspiration or noncardiac pulmonary edema. The mechanism of noncardiac pulmonary edema is unknown.

Dextromethorphan can interact with MAOIs, causing severe hyperthermia, and may cause the serotonin syndrome (see *Selective Serotonin Reuptake Inhibitors*). Dextromethorphan inhibits the metabolism of norepinephrine and serotonin and blocks the reuptake of serotonin. It is found as a component of a large number of non-prescription cough and cold remedies.

Toxic Dose

The toxic dose depends on the specific drug, route of administration, and degree of tolerance. For therapeutic and toxic doses, see Table 24. In children, respiratory depression has been produced by 10 mg of morphine or methadone, 75 mg of meperidine, and 12.5 mg of diphenoxylate. Infants younger than 3 months of age are more susceptible to respiratory depression. The dose should be reduced by 50%.

Kinetics

Oral onset of analgesic effect of morphine is 10 to 15 minutes; the action peaks in 1 hour and lasts 4 to 6 hours. With sustained-release preparations, the duration is 8 to 12 hours. Opioids are 90% metabolized in the liver by hepatic conjugation and 90% excreted in the urine as inactive compounds. Volume

TABLE 24	Doses and Onset and Duration of Action of Common Opioids					
DRUG	**ADULT ORAL DOSE**	**CHILD ORAL DOSE**	**ONSET OF ACTION**	**DURATION OF ACTION**	**ADULT FATAL DOSE**
Camphored tincture of opium	25 mL	0.25–0.50 mL/kg (0.4 mg/mL)	15–30 min	4–5 h	NA
Codeine	30–180 mg	0.5–1 mg/kg	15–30 min	4–6 h	800 mg
	>1 mg/kg is toxic in a child, above 200 mg in adult >5 mg/kg fatal in a child				
Dextromethorphan	15 mg 10 mg/kg is toxic	0.25 mg/kg	15–30 min	3–6 h	NA
Diacetylmorphine; street heroin is less than 10% pure	60 mg	NA	15–30 min	3–4 h	100 mg
Diphenoxylate atropine (Lomotil)	5–10 mg	NA	120–240 min	14 h	300 mg
	7.5 mg is toxic in a child, 300 mg is toxic in adult				
Fentanyl (Duragesic)	0.1–0.2 mg	0.001–0.002 mg/kg	7–8 min	Intramuscular: ½–2 h	1.0 mg
Hydrocodone with APAP (Lortab)	5–30 mg	0.15 mg/kg	30 min	3–4 h	100 mg
Hydromorphone (Dilaudid)	4 mg	0.1 mg/kg	15–30 min	3–4 h	100 mg
Meperidine (Demerol)	100 mg	1–1.5 mg/kg	10–45 min	3–4 h	350 mg
Methadone (Dolophine)	10 mg	0.1 mg/kg	30–60 min	4–12 h	120 mg
Morphine	10–60 mg	0.1–0.2 mg/kg	<20 min	4–6 h	200 mg
	Oral dose is 6 times parenteral dose, MS Contin sustained-release prep				
Oxycodone APAP (Percocet)	5 mg	NA	15–30 min	4–5 h	NA
Pentazocine (Talwin)	50–100 mg	NA	15–30 min	3–4 h	NA
Propoxyphene (Darvon)	65–100 mg	NA	30–60 min	2–4 h	700 mg

distribution is 1 to 4 L/kg. Protein binding is 35% to 75%. The typical plasma half-life of opiates is 2 to 5 hours, but that of methadone is 24 to 36 hours. Morphine metabolites include morphine-3-glucuronide (inactive) and morphine-6-glucuronide (active) and normorphine (active). Meperidine (Demerol) is rapidly hydrolyzed by tissue esterases into the active metabolite normeperidine, which has twice the convulsant activity of meperidine. Heroin (diacetylmorphine) is deacetylated within minutes to 6-monacetylmorphine and morphine. Propoxyphene (Darvon) has a rapid onset of action, and death has occurred within 15 to 30 minutes after a massive overdose. Propoxyphene is metabolized to norpropoxyphene, an active metabolite with convulsive, cardiac dysrhythmic, and heart block properties. Symptoms of diphenoxylate overdose appear within 1 to 4 hours. It is metabolized into the active metabolite difenoxin, which is five times more active as a regular respiratory depressant agent. Death has been reported in children after ingestion of a single tablet.

Manifestations
Initially, mild intoxication produces miosis, dull face, drowsiness, partial ptosis, and "nodding" (head drops to chest then bobs up). Larger amounts produce the classic triad of miotic pupils (exceptions below), respiratory depression, and depressed level of consciousness (flaccid coma). The blood pressure, pulse, and bowel activity are decreased.

Dilated pupils do not exclude opioid intoxication. Some exceptions to the miosis effect include dextromethorphan (paralyzes iris), fentanyl, meperidine, and diphenoxylate (rarely). Physiologic disturbances including acidosis, hypoglycemia, hypoxia, and postictal state, or a co-ingestant may also produce mydriasis.

Usually, the muscles are flaccid, but increased muscle tone can be produced by meperidine and fentanyl (chest rigidity). Seizures are rare but can occur with ingestion of codeine, meperidine, propoxyphene, and dextromethorphan. Hallucinations and agitation have been reported.

Pruritus and urticaria are caused by histamine release by some opioids or by sulfite additives.

Noncardiac pulmonary edema may occur after an overdose, especially with intravenous heroin abuse. Cardiac effects include vasodilation and hypotension. A heart murmur in an intravenous addict suggests endocarditis. Propoxyphene can produce delayed cardiac dysrhythmias.

Fentanyl is 100 times more potent than morphine and can cause chest wall muscle rigidity. Some of its derivatives are 2000 times more potent than morphine.

Laboratory Investigations
For patients with overdose, one should obtain and monitor ABG, blood glucose, and electrolyte levels; chest radiographs; and ECG. For drug abusers, one should consider testing for hepatitis B, syphilis, and HIV antibody (HIV testing usually requires consent). Blood opioid concentrations are not useful. They confirm diagnosis (morphine therapeutic dose, 65 to 80 ng/mL; toxic, <200 ng/mL), but are not useful for making a therapeutic decision. Cross-reactions can occur with Vick's Formula 44, poppy seeds, and other opioids (codeine and heroin are metabolized to morphine). Naloxone 4 mg IV was not associated with a positive enzyme multiplied immunoassay technique urine screen at 60 minutes, 6 hours, or 48 hours.

Management
Supportive care should be instituted, particularly an endotracheal tube and assisted ventilation. Temporary ventilation can be provided by a bag-valve mask with 100% oxygen. The patient should be placed on a cardiac monitor, have intravenous access established, and have specimens for ABG, glucose, electrolytes, BUN, and creatinine levels, CBC, coagulation profile, liver function, toxicology screen, and urinalysis taken.

For gastrointestinal decontamination, emesis should not be induced, but activated charcoal can be administered if bowel sounds are present.

If it is suspected that the patient is an addict, he or she should be restrained first and then 0.1 mg of naloxone (Narcan) should be administered. The dose should be doubled every 2 minutes until the patient responds or 10 to 20 mg has been given. If the patient is not suspected to be an addict, then 2 mg every 2 to 3 minutes to total of 10 to 20 mg is administered.

It is essential to determine whether there is a complete response to naloxone (mydriasis, improvement in ventilation), because it is a diagnostic therapeutic test. A continuous naloxone infusion may be appropriate, using the "response dose" every hour. Repeat doses of naloxone may be necessary because the effects of many opioids can last much longer than naloxone does (30 to 60 minutes). Methadone ingestions may require a naloxone infusion for 24 to 48 hours. Half of the response dose may need to be repeated in 15 to 20 minutes, after the infusion has been started.

Acute iatrogenic withdrawal precipitated by the administration of naloxone to a dependent patient should not be treated with morphine or other opioids. Naloxone's effects are limited to 30 to 60 minutes (shorter than most opioids) and withdrawal will subside in a short time.

Nalmefene (Revex), an FDA-approved long-acting (4 to 8 hours) pure opioid antagonist, is being investigated, but its role in cases of acute intoxication is unclear and it could produce prolonged withdrawal. It may have a role in place of naloxone infusion.

Noncardiac pulmonary edema does not respond to naloxone, and the patient needs intubation, assisted ventilation, positive end-expiratory pressure, and hemodynamic monitoring. Fluids should be given cautiously in patients with opioid overdose because opioids stimulate the antidiuretic hormone.

If the patient is comatose, 50% glucose (3% to 4% of comatose opioid overdose patients have hypoglycemia) and thiamine should be given prior to naloxone. If the patient has seizures that are unresponsive to naloxone, one administers diazepam and examines for metabolic (hypoglycemia, electrolyte disturbances) causes and structural disturbances.

Hypotension is rare and should direct a search for another etiology. If the patient is agitated, hypoxia and hypoglycemia must be excluded before opioid withdrawal is considered as a cause. Complications to consider include urinary retention, constipation, rhabdomyolysis, myoglobinuria, hypoglycemia, and withdrawal.

Disposition
If a patient responds to intravenous naloxone, careful observation for relapse and the development of pulmonary edema is required, with cardiac and respiratory monitoring for 6 to 12 hours. Patients requiring repeated doses of naloxone or an infusion, or those who develop pulmonary edema, require intensive care unit admission and cannot be discharged from the intensive care unit until they are symptom free for 12 hours. Intravenous overdose complications are expected to be present within 20 minutes after injection, and discharge after 4 symptom-free hours has been recommended. Adults with oral overdose have delayed onset of toxicity and require 6 hours of observation. Children with oral opioid overdose should be admitted to the hospital for observation because of delayed toxicity. Some toxicologists advise restraining a patient who attempts to sign out against medical advice after treatment with naloxone, at least until the patient receives psychiatric evaluation.

Organophosphates and Carbamates
Cholinergic intoxication sources are insecticides (organophosphates or carbamates), some medications, and some mushrooms. Examples of organophosphate insecticides are malathion (low toxicity, median lethal dose [LD$_{50}$] 2800 mg/kg), chlorpyrifos, which has been removed from market (moderate toxicity), and

parathion (high toxicity, LD_{50} 2 mg/kg). Carbamate insecticides include carbaryl (low toxicity, LD_{50} 500 mg/kg), propoxur (moderate toxicity, LD_{50} 95 mg/kg), and aldicarb (high toxicity, LD_{50} 0.9 mg/kg). Pharmaceuticals with carbamate properties include neostigmine (Prostigmin) and physostigmine (Antilirium). Cholinergic compounds also include the "G" nerve war weapons tabun (GA), sarin (GB), soman (GB), and venom X (VX).

Toxic Mechanism

Organophosphates phosphorylate the active site on red cell acetylcholinesterase and pseudocholinesterase in the serum, neuromuscular and parasympathetic neuroeffector junctions, and in the major synapses of the autonomic ganglia, causing irreversible inhibition. There are two types of organophosphate intoxication: (a) direct action by the parent compound (e.g., tetraethylpyrophosphate), or (b) indirect action by the toxic metabolite (e.g., parathoxon or malathoxon).

Carbamates (esters of carbonic acid) cause reversible carbamylation of the active site of the enzymes. When a critical amount, greater than 50%, of cholinesterase is inhibited, acetylcholine accumulates and causes transient stimulation at cholinergic synapses and sympathetic terminals (muscarinic effect), the somatic nerves, the autonomic ganglia (nicotinic effect), and CNS synapses. Stimulation of conduction is followed by inhibition of conduction.

The major differences between the carbamates and the organophosphates are as follows: (a) carbamate toxicity is less and the duration is shorter; (b) carbamates rarely produce overt CNS effects (poor CNS penetration); (c) carbamate inhibition of the acetylcholinesterase enzyme is reversible and activity returns to normal rapidly; (d) pralidoxime, the enzyme regenerator, may not be necessary in the management of mild carbamate intoxication (e.g., carbaryl).

Toxic Dose

Parathion's minimum lethal dose is 2 mg in children and 10 to 20 mg in adults. The lethal dose of malathion is greater than 1375 mg/kg and that of chlorpyrifos is 25 g; the latter compound is unlikely to cause death.

Kinetics

Absorption is by all routes. The onset of acute ingestion toxicity occurs as early as 3 hours, usually before 12 hours and always before 24 hours. Lipid-soluble agents absorbed by the dermal route (e.g., fenthion) may have a delayed onset of more than 24 hours. Inhalation toxicity occurs immediately after exposure. Massive ingestion can produce intoxication within minutes.

Metabolism is via the liver. With some pesticides (e.g., parathion, malathion), the effects are delayed because they undergo hepatic microsomal oxidative metabolism to their toxic metabolites, the -oxons (e.g., paroxon, malaoxon).

The half-life of malathion is 2.89 hours and that of parathion is 2.1 days. The metabolites are eliminated in the urine and the presence of *p*-nitrophenol in the urine is a clue up to 48 hours after exposure.

Manifestations

Many organophosphates produce a garlic odor on the breath, in the gastric contents, or in the container. Diaphoresis, excessive salivation, miosis, and muscle twitching are helpful clues to diagnosis.

Early, a cholinergic (muscarinic) crisis develops that consists of parasympathetic nervous system activity. DUMBELS is the mnemonic for defecation, cramps, and increased bowel motility; urinary incontinence; miosis (mydriasis may occur in 20%); bronchospasm and bronchorrhea; excess secretion; lacrimation; and seizures. Bradycardia, pulmonary edema, and hypotension may be present.

Later, sympathetic and nicotinic effects occur, consisting of MATCH: muscle weakness and fasciculation (eyelid twitching is often present), adrenal stimulation and hyperglycemia, tachycardia, cramps in muscles, and hypertension. Finally, paralysis of the skeletal muscles ensues.

The CNS effects are headache, blurred vision, anxiety, ataxia, delirium and toxic psychosis, convulsions, coma, and respiratory depression. Cranial nerve palsies have been noted. Delayed hallucinations may occur.

Delayed respiratory paralysis and neurologic and neurobehavioral disorders have been described following certain organophosphate ingestions or dermal exposure. The "intermediate syndrome" is paralysis of proximal and respiratory muscles developing 24 to 96 hours after the successful treatment of organophosphate poisoning. A delayed distal polyneuropathy has been described with ingestion of certain organophosphates, such as triorthocresyl phosphate, bromoleptophos, and methomidophos.

Complications include aspiration, pulmonary edema, and acute respiratory distress syndrome.

Laboratory Investigations

Monitoring should include chest radiograph, blood glucose (nonketotic hyperglycemia is frequent), ABG, pulse oximetry, ECG, blood coagulation status, liver function, hyperamylasemia (pancreatitis reported), and urinalysis for the metabolite alkyl phosphate paranitrophenol. Blood should be drawn for red blood cell cholinesterase determination before pralidoxime is given. The red blood cell cholinesterase activity roughly correlates with clinical severity. Mild poisoning is 20% to 50% of normal, moderate poisoning is 10% to 20% of normal, and severe poisoning is 10% of normal (>90% depressed). A postexposure rise of 10% to 15% in the cholinesterase level determined at least 10 to 14 days after the exposure confirms the diagnosis.

Management

Protection of health care personnel with clothing (masks, gloves, gowns, goggles) and respiratory equipment or hazardous material suits, as necessary, is called for. General decontamination consists of isolation, bagging, and disposal of contaminated clothing and other articles. Vital functions should be established and maintained. Cardiac and oxygen saturation monitoring are needed. Intubation and assisted ventilation may be needed. Secretions should be suctioned until atropinization drying is achieved.

Dermal decontamination involves prompt removal of clothing and cleansing of all affected areas of skin, hair, and eyes. Ocular decontamination involves irrigation with copious amounts of tepid water or 0.9% saline for at least 15 minutes. Gastrointestinal decontamination, if the ingestion was recent, involves the administration of activated charcoal.

Atropine sulfate can be given as an antidote. It is both a diagnostic and a therapeutic agent. Atropine counteracts the muscarinic effects but is only partially effective for the CNS effects (seizures and coma). Preservative-free atropine (no benzyl alcohol) should be used. If the patient is symptomatic (bradycardia or bronchorrhea), a test dose should be administered, 0.02 mg/kg in children or 1 mg in adults, intravenously. If no signs of atropinization are present (tachycardia, drying of secretions, and mydriasis), atropine should be administered immediately, 0.05 mg/kg in children or 2 mg in adults, every 5 to 10 minutes as needed to dry the secretions and clear the lungs. Beneficial effects are seen within 1 to 4 minutes and maximum effect in 8 minutes. The average dose in the first 24 hours is 40 mg, but 1000 mg or more has been required in severe cases. Glycopyrrolate (Robinul) can be used if atropine is not available. The maximum dose should be maintained for 12 to 24 hours, then tapered and the patient observed for relapse. Poisoning, especially with lipophilic agents (e.g., fenthion, chlorfenthion), may require weeks of atropine therapy. An alternative is a continuous infusion of atropine 8 mg in 100 mL 0.9% saline at rate of 0.02 to 0.08 mg/kg/h (0.25 to 1.0 mL/kg/h) with additional 1 to 5 mg boluses as needed to dry the secretions.

Pralidoxime chloride (Protopam) has both antinicotinic and antimuscarinic effects and possibly also CNS effects. Successful treatment with pralidoxime chloride may allow a reduction in the dose of atropine. Pralidoxime acts to reactivate the phosphorylated cholinesterases by binding the phosphate moiety on the esteritic site and displacing it. It should be given early before "aging" of phosphate bond produces tighter binding. However, recent reports indicate that pralidoxime chloride is beneficial even several days after the poisoning. Improvement is seen within 10 to 40 minutes. The initial dose of pralidoxime chloride is 1 to 2 g in 250 mL 0.89% saline over 5 to 10 minutes, maximum 200 mg/min, in adults or 25 to 50 mg/kg, maximum 4 mg/kg/min, in children younger than 12 years of age. The dose can be repeated every 6 to 12 hours for several days. An alternative is a continuous infusion of 1 g in 100 mL 0.89% saline at 5 to 20 mg/kg/h (0.5 to 12 mL/g/h) up to 500 mg/h and titrated to desired response. Maximum adult daily dose is 12 g. Cardiac and blood pressure monitoring is advised during and for several hours after the infusion. The end point is absence of fasciculations and return of muscle strength.

Contraindicated drugs include morphine, aminophylline, barbiturates, opioids, phenothiazine, reserpine-like drugs, parasympathomimetics, and succinylcholine.

Noncardiac pulmonary edema may require respiratory support. Seizures may respond to atropine and pralidoxime chloride but often require anticonvulsants. Cardiac dysrhythmias may require electrical cardioversion or antidysrhythmic therapy if the patient is hemodynamically unstable. Extracorporeal procedures are of no proven value.

Disposition
Asymptomatic patients with normal examination findings after 6 to 8 hours of observation may be discharged. In cases of intentional poisoning, the patients require psychiatric clearance for discharge. Symptomatic patients should be admitted to the intensive care unit. Observation of milder cases of carbamate poisoning, even those requiring atropine, for 6 to 8 hours symptom-free may be sufficient to exclude significant toxicity. In cases of workplace exposure, OSHA should be notified.

Phencyclidine (Angel Dust)
Phencyclidine is an arylcyclohexylamine related to ketamine and chemically related to the phenothiazines. Originally a "dissociative" anesthetic banned in United States since 1979, it is now an illicit substance, with at least 38 analogues. It is inexpensively manufactured by "kitchen chemists" and is mislabeled as other hallucinogens. Improper phencyclidine synthesis may release cyanide when heated or smoked and can cause explosions.

Toxic Mechanism
The mechanism of phencyclidine is complex and not completely understood. It inhibits some neurotransmitters and causes a loss of pain sensation without depressing the CNS respiratory status. It stimulates α-adrenergic receptors and may act as a "false neurotransmitter." The effects are sympathomimetic, cholinergic, and cerebellar.

Toxic Dose
The usual dose of phencyclidine mixed with marijuana joints is 100 to 400 mg of phencyclidine. Joints or leaf mixtures contain 0.24% to 7.9% of PCP, 1 mg of PCP/150 leaves. Tablets contain 5 mg (the usual street dose). CNS effects at doses of 1 to 6 mg include hallucinations and euphoria, 6 to 10 mg produces toxic psychosis and sympathetic stimulation, 10 to 25 mg produces severe toxicity, and more than 100 mg has resulted in fatalities.

Kinetics
Phencyclidine is a lipophilic weak base, with a pKa of 8.5 to 9.5. It is rapidly absorbed when smoked and snorted, poorly absorbed from the acid stomach, and rapidly absorbed from the alkaline middle small intestine. It has an enterogastric

secretion and is reabsorbed in the small intestine. The onset of action when smoked is 2 to 5 minutes, with a peak in 15 to 30 minutes. With oral ingestion, the onset is in 30 to 60 minutes and when taken intravenously it is immediate. Most adverse reactions in cases of overdose begin within 1 to 2 hours. Its duration of action at low doses is 4 to 6 hours and normality returns in 24 hours; in large overdoses, fluctuating coma may last 6 to 10 days.

Volume distribution is 6.2 L/kg. Phencyclidine concentrates in brain and adipose tissue. Protein binding is 70%. The route of elimination is by gastric secretion, liver metabolism, and 10% urinary excretion of conjugates and free phencyclidine. Renal excretion may be increased 50% with urinary acidification. The half-life is 1 hour (in cases of overdose, it is 11 to 89 hours).

Manifestations
The classic picture is bursts of horizontal, vertical, and rotary nystagmus, which is a clue to diagnosis (occurs in 50% of cases), miosis, hypertension, and fluctuating altered mental state. There is a wide spectrum of clinical presentations.

Mild intoxication with 1 to 6 mg produces drunken and bizarre behavior, agitation, rotary nystagmus, and blank stare. Violent behavior and sensory anesthesia make these patients insensitive to pain, self-destructive, and dangerous. Most are communicative within 1 to 2 hours, are alert and oriented in 6 to 8 hours, and recover completely in 24 to 48 hours.

Moderate intoxication with 6 to 10 mg produces excess salivation, hypertension, hyperthermia, muscle rigidity, myoclonus, and catatonia. Recovery of consciousness occurs in 24 to 48 hours and complete recovery in 1 week.

Severe intoxication with 10 to 25 mg results in opisthotonus, decerebrate rigidity, convulsions, prolonged fluctuating coma, and respiratory failure. Patients in this category have a high rate of medical complications. Recovery of consciousness occurs in 24 to 48 hours, with complete normality in a month. Medical complications include apnea, aspiration pneumonia, cardiac arrest, hypertensive encephalopathy, hyperthermia, intracerebral hemorrhage, psychosis, rhabdomyolysis and myoglobinuria, and seizures. Loss of memory and "flashbacks" last for months. Phencyclidine-induced depression and suicide have been reported.

Fatalities occur with ingestions of greater than 100 mg and with serum levels greater than 100 to 250 ng/mL.

Laboratory Investigations
Marked elevation of creatine kinase level may occur. Values greater than 20,000 units have been reported. Urinalysis should be monitored and urine tested for myoglobin. One should monitor the blood for creatine kinase, uric acid (an early clue to rhabdomyolysis), BUN, creatinine, electrolytes (hyperkalemia), blood glucose (20% of patients have hypoglycemia), urinary output, liver function tests, ECG, and ABG if the patient has any respiratory manifestations. Measurement of phencyclidine in the gastric juice is called for because concentrations are 10 to 50 times higher than in blood or urine. Phencyclidine blood concentrations are not helpful. Phencyclidine may be detected in the urine of the average user for 10 days to 3 weeks after the last dose. In chronic users, it can be detected for over 1 month. The analogues of phencyclidine may not produce positive test results for phencyclidine in the urine. Cross-reactions with bleach and dextromethorphan may cause false-positive urine test results on immunoassay, and cross-reaction with doxylamine may produce a false-positive finding on gas chromatography.

Management
The patient should be observed for violent, self-destructive, bizarre behavior, and paranoid schizophrenia. Patients should be placed in a low sensory environment and dangerous objects should be removed from the area.

Gastrointestinal decontamination is not effective because phencyclidine is rapidly absorbed from intestines. Overtreating the mild intoxication should be avoided. There is insufficient evidence to support the use of MDAC. In cases of severe toxicity (stupor or coma), continuous gastric suction can be tried (with protection of the airway) because the drug is secreted into the gastric juice. The value of this procedure is controversial because of limited data.

The patient must be protected from harming himself or herself or others. Physical restraints may be necessary, but they should be used sparingly and for the shortest time possible because they increase risk of rhabdomyolysis. Metal restraints such as handcuffs should be avoided. For behavioral disorders and toxic psychosis, diazepam is the agent of choice. Pharmacologic intervention includes diazepam (Valium) 10 to 30 mg orally or 2 to 5 mg intravenously initially and titrated upward to 10 mg; however, up to 30 mg may be required. "Talk down" technique is usually ineffective and dangerous. Phenothiazines and butyrophenones should be avoided in the acute phase because they lower the convulsive threshold; however, they may be needed later for psychosis. Haloperidol (Haldol) administration has been reported to produce catatonia.

Seizures and muscle spasm are managed with diazepam, from 2.5 mg up to 10 mg. Hyperthermia (>38.5°C [101.3°F]) is treated with external cooling measures. Hypertension is usually transient and does not require treatment. In the case of emergent hypertensive crisis (blood pressure >200/115 mm Hg) nitroprusside can be used in a dose of 0.3 to 2 μg/kg/min. Maximum infusion rate is 10 μg/kg/min for only 10 minutes.

Acid ion trapping diuresis is not recommended because of the danger of myoglobin precipitation in the renal tubules. Rhabdomyolysis and myoglobinuria are treated by correcting volume depletion and ensuring a urinary output of greater than 2 mL/kg/h. Alkalinization is controversial because of reabsorption of phencyclidine.

Hemodialysis is beneficial if renal failure occurs; otherwise, the extracorporeal procedures are not beneficial.

Disposition
All patients with coma, delirium, catatonia, violent behavior, aspiration pneumonia, sustained hypertension greater than 200/115 mm Hg, and significant rhabdomyolysis should be admitted to the intensive care unit until asymptomatic for at least 24 hours. If patients with mild intoxication are mentally and neurologically stable and become asymptomatic (except for nystagmus) for 4 hours, they may be discharged in the company of a responsible adult. All patients must be assessed for suicide risk before discharge. Drug counseling and psychiatric follow-up should be arranged. Patients should be warned that episodes of disorientation and depression may continue intermittently for 4 weeks or more.

Phenothiazines and Nonphenothiazines (Neuroleptics)
Toxic Mechanism
Neuroleptics have complex mechanisms of toxicity, including (a) block of the postsynaptic dopamine receptors; (b) block of peripheral and central α-adrenergic receptors; (c) block of cholinergic muscarinic receptors; (d) quinidine-like antidysrhythmic and myocardial depressant effect in cases of large overdose; (e) lowering of the convulsive threshold; (f) effect on hypothalamic temperature regulation (Table 25).

Toxic Dose
Extrapyramidal reactions, anticholinergic effects, and orthostatic hypotension may occur at therapeutic doses. The toxic amount is not established, but the maximum daily therapeutic dose may result in significant side effects, and twice this amount may be potentially fatal. Chlorpromazine (Thorazine), the prototype, may produce serious hypotension and CNS depression at doses greater than 200 mg (17 mg/kg) in children and 3 to 5 g in an adult. Fatalities have been reported after 2.5 g of loxapine (Loxitane) and mesoridazine (Serentil) and 1.5 g of thioridazine (Mellaril).

Kinetics
These agents are lipophilic and have unpredictable gastrointestinal absorption. Peak levels occur 2 to 6 hours postingestion and have enterohepatic recirculation.

The mean serum half-life in phase 1 is 1 to 2 hours and the biphasic half-life is 20 to 40 hours. Volume distribution is 10 to 40 L/kg; protein binding is 92% to 98%. Chlorpromazine taken orally has an onset of action in 30 to 60 minutes, peak in 2 to 4 hours, and duration of 4 to 6 hours. With sustained-release preparations, the onset is in 30 to 60 minutes and duration is 6 to 12 hours.

Elimination is by hepatic metabolism, which results in multiple metabolites (some are active). Metabolites can be detected in urine months after chronic therapy. Only 1% to 3% is excreted unchanged in the urine.

Manifestations
In cases of phenothiazine overdose, anticholinergic symptoms may be present early but are not life-threatening. Miosis is usually present (80%) if the phenothiazine has strong α-adrenergic blocking effect (e.g., chlorpromazine), but anticholinergic activity mydriasis may occur. Agitation and delirium rapidly progress into coma. Major problems are cardiac toxicity and hypotension. The cardiotoxic effects are seen more commonly with thioridazine and its metabolite mesoridazine. These agents have produced the largest number of fatalities in patients with phenothiazine overdose. Cardiac conduction disturbances include prolonged PR, QRS, and QTc intervals, U- and T-wave abnormalities, and ventricular dysrhythmias, including torsades de pointes. Seizures occur mainly in patients with convulsive disorders or with administration of loxapine. Sudden death in children and adults has been reported.

Idiosyncratic dystonic reactions are most common with the piperidine group. Reactions are not dose-dependent and consist of opisthotonos, torticollis, orolingual dyskinesia, or oculogyric crisis (painful upward gaze). These reactions are more frequent in children and women. Neuroleptic malignant syndrome occurs in patients on chronic therapy and is characterized by hyperthermia, muscle rigidity, autonomic dysfunction, and altered mental state. There is one case reported with acute overdose. The loxapine syndrome consists of seizures, rhabdomyolysis, and renal failure.

Laboratory Investigations
Monitoring should include arterial blood gases, renal and hepatic function, electrolytes, blood glucose, and creatine kinase and myoglobinemia in neuroleptic malignant syndrome. Most of these agents are detected on routine screening. Quantitative serum levels are not useful in management. Cross-reactions with enzyme multiplied immunoassay technique tests occur with cyclic antidepressants. Phenothiazines give false-negative results on pregnancy urine tests using human chorionic gonadotropin as an indicator, and give false-positive results for urine porphyrins, indirect Coombs test, urobilinogen, and amylase.

Management
Vital functions must be established and maintained. All overdose patients require venous access, 12-lead ECG (to measure intervals), cardiac and respiratory monitoring, and seizure precautions. One should monitor core temperature to detect poikilothermic effect. If the patient is comatose, intubation and assisted ventilation may be required, as well as 100% oxygen, intravenous glucose, naloxone (Narcan), and thiamine.

Emesis is not recommended. Activated charcoal can be administered if ingestion was within 1 hour. MDAC has not been proven beneficial. A radiograph of the abdomen may be useful, if the phenothiazine is radiopaque. Haloperidol (Haldol) and trifluoperazine (Stelazine) are most likely to be radiopaque. Whole-bowel irrigation may be useful when a large number of pills are visualized on radiograph or if sustained-release preparations were taken, but whole-bowel irrigation has not been evaluated in patients with phenothiazine overdose.

TABLE 25 Neuroleptics and Properties

COMPOUND	ANTIPSYCHOTIC	ANTICHOLINERGIC	EXTRAPYRAMIDAL	HYPOTENSIVE AND CARDIOTOXIC	SEDATIVE
Phenothiazine					
Aliphatic 　Chlorpromazine (Thorazine) 　Promethazine (Phenergan)	1+	3+	2+	2+	3+
Piperazine 　Fluphenazine (Prolixin) 　Perphenazine (Trilafon) 　Prochlorperazine (Compazine) 　Trifluoperazine (Stelazine)	3+	1+	3+	1+	1+
Piperidine 　Mesoridazine (Serentil) 　Thioridazine (Mellaril)	1+	2+	1+	3+	3+
Nonphenothiazine					
Butyrophenone 　Haloperidol (Haldol)	3+	1+	3+	1+	1+
Dibenzoxazepine 　Loxapine (Loxitane)	3+	1+	3+	1+	2+
Dihydroindolone 　Molindone (Moban)	3+	1+	3+	1+	1+
Thioxanthenes 　Thiothixene (Navane) 　Chlorprothixene (Taractan)	3+	1+	3+	3+	1+

1+ = very low activity; 2+ = moderate activity; 3+ = very high activity.

Convulsions are treated with diazepam or lorazepam (Ativan). Loxapine (Loxitane) overdose may result in status epilepticus. If nondepolarizing neuromuscular blockade is required, pancuronium (Pavulon) or vecuronium (Norcuron) should be used (not succinyl-choline [Anectine], which may cause malignant hyperthermia), and EEG should be monitored during paralysis.

Patients with dysrhythmias should be monitored with serial ECGs. Unstable rhythms can be treated with electrical cardioversion. Class 1a antidysrhythmics (procainamide, quinidine, and disopyramide [Norpace]) must be avoided.

Hypokalemia predisposes to dysrhythmias and should be corrected aggressively. Supraventricular tachycardia with hemodynamic instability is treated with electrical cardioversion. The role of adenosine has not been defined. Calcium channel and β-blockers should be avoided.

Prolongation of the QRS interval is treated with sodium bicarbonate 1 to 2 mEq/kg by intravenous bolus over a few minutes. Torsades de pointes is treated with magnesium sulfate IV 20% solution 2 g over 2 to 3 minutes. If there is no response in 10 minutes, the dose is repeated and followed by a continuous infusion of 5 to 10 mg/min or given as an infusion of 50 mg/min for 2 hours followed by 30 mg/min for 90 minutes twice a day for several days, as needed. The dose in children is 25 to 50 mg/kg initially and maintenance dose is 30 to 60 mg/kg per 24 hours (0.25 to 0.50 mEq/kg per 24 hours) up to 1000 mg per 24 hours. Serum magnesium levels should be monitored.

To treat ventricular tachydysrhythmias in a stable patient, lidocaine is used. If the patient is unstable, electrical cardioversion is used. Patients with heart block with hemodynamic instability should be managed with temporary cardiac pacing.

Hypotension is treated with the Trendelenburg position and 0.9% saline. If the condition is refractory to treatment or there is a danger of fluid overload, vasopressors are administered. The vasopressor of choice is α-adrenergic agonist norepinephrine (Levophed), titrated to response. Epinephrine and dopamine should not be used because β-receptor stimulation in the presence of α-receptor blockade may provoke dysrhythmias and phenothiazines are antidopaminergic.

Hypothermia and hyperthermia are treated with external warming and cooling measures, respectively. Antipyretic drugs must not be used.

Management of the neuroleptic malignant syndrome includes the following actions:

- Immediately discontinuing the offending agent
- Hyperventilating the patient, using 100% humidified, cooled oxygen at high gas flows (at least 10 L/min) because of rapid breathing
- Administering a benzodiazepine to control convulsions and facilitate cooling measures
- Initiating appropriate mechanical cooling measures, which may include intravenous cold saline (not lactated Ringer's), ice baths, cold lavage of the stomach, bladder, and rectum, and a hypothermic blanket
- Correcting acid-base and electrolyte disturbances and treating significant hyperkalemia with hyperventilation, calcium, sodium bicarbonate, intravenous glucose, and insulin; hemodialysis may be necessary

In addition, dysrhythmias usually respond to correction of the underlying acid-base disturbances and hyperkalemia. If antidysrhythmic agents are required, calcium channel blockers must be avoided because they may precipitate hyperkalemia and cardiovascular collapse. Dantrolene sodium (Dantrium), which is a phenytoin derivative, inhibits calcium release from the sarcoplasmic reticulum and results in decreased muscle contraction. Dantrolene acts peripherally and does not reverse the rigidity or psychomotor disturbances resulting from the central dopamine blockade;

it therefore is often used in combination with bromocriptine. Bromocriptine mesylate (Parlodel) acts centrally as a dopamine agonist, as does amantadine hydrochloride (Symmetrel). Bromocriptine and dantrolene have been reported to be successful in combination with cooling and good supportive measures in malignant hyperthermia.

Dosing for these agents is as follows: dantrolene sodium at 2 to 3 mg/kg IV as a bolus, then 1 mg/kg/min to a maximum of 10 mg/kg or until the tachycardia, rigidity, increased end-tidal CO_2, and temperature elevation are controlled. *Note:* Hepatotoxicity occurs with doses greater than 10 mg/kg. To prevent symptom recurrence, 1 mg/kg should be administered every 6 hours for 24 to 48 hours after the episode. After that time, oral dantrolene can be used at a dose of 1 mg/kg every 6 hours for 24 hours as necessary. The patient should be observed for thrombophlebitis following intravenous dantrolene. It is best administered via a central line. Bromocriptine mesylate at 2.5 to 10 mg orally or via a nasogastric tube, three times a day, should be used in combination with dantrolene.

Idiosyncratic dystonic reaction can be treated with diphenhydramine (Benadryl) 1 to 2 mg/kg/dose intravenously over 5 minutes up to maximum of 50 mg intravenously; a response is noted within 2 to 5 minutes. This can be followed with oral doses for 4 to 6 days to prevent recurrence.

Extracorporeal measures (hemodialysis, hemoperfusion) are not effective in removing these agents.

Disposition

Asymptomatic patients should be observed for at least 6 hours after gastric decontamination. Symptomatic patients with cardiotoxicity, hypotension, and convulsions should be admitted to the intensive care unit and monitored for 48 hours.

Salicylates (Acetylsalicylic Acid, Salicylic Acid)
Toxic Mechanism

The primary toxic mechanisms include (a) direct stimulation of the medullary chemoreceptor trigger zone and respiratory center; (b) uncoupling oxidative phosphorylation; (c) inhibition of the Krebs cycle enzymes; (d) inhibition of vitamin K dependent and independent clotting factors; (e) alteration of platelet function; and (f) inhibition of prostaglandin synthesis.

Toxic Dose

Acute mild intoxication occurs at a dose of 150 to 200 mg/kg, moderate intoxication at 200 to 300 mg/kg, and severe intoxication at 300 to 500 mg/kg. Acute salicylate plasma concentration greater than 30 mg/dL (usually >40 mg/dL) may be associated with clinical toxicity. Chronic intoxication occurs at ingestions greater than 100 mg/kg/d for more than 2 days because of accumulation kinetics. Methyl salicylate (oil of wintergreen) is the most toxic form of salicylate. A dose of 1 mL of 98% contains 1.4 g of salicylate. Fatalities have occurred with ingestion of 1 teaspoonful in children and 1 ounce in adults. It is found in topical ointments and liniments (18% to 30%).

Kinetics

Acetylsalicylic acid and salicylic acid are weak acids with a pKa of 3.5 and 3.0, respectively. Acetylsalicylic acid is absorbed from the stomach, from the small bowel, and dermally. Onset of action is within 30 minutes. Methyl salicylate and effervescent tablets are absorbed more rapidly. Salicylate plasma concentration is detectable within 15 minutes after ingestion and peaks in 30 to 120 minutes. The peak may be delayed 6 to 12 hours in cases of large overdose, overdose with enteric-coated or sustained-release preparations, and development of concretions. The therapeutic duration of action is 3 to 4 hours but is markedly prolonged in cases of overdose.

Volume distribution is 0.13 L/kg for salicylic acid but increases as the salicylate plasma concentration increases. Protein binding is greater than 90% for salicylic acid at pH 7.4 and a salicylate plasma concentration of 20 to 30 mg/dL, 75% at a salicylate plasma concentration greater than 40 mg/dL, 50% at a salicylate plasma concentration of 70 mg/dL, and 30% at a salicylate plasma concentration of 120 mg/dL.

The half-life for salicylic acid is 3 hours after a 300 mg dose, 6 hours after a 1 g overdose, and greater than 10 hours after a 10 g overdose. Elimination includes Michaelis-Menten hepatic metabolism by three saturable pathways: (a) glycine conjugation to salicyluric acid (75%); (b) glucuronyl transferase to salicyl phenol glucuronide (10%); and (c) salicyl aryl glucuronide (4%). Nonsaturable pathways are hydrolysis to gentisic acid (<1%). Ten percent is excreted unchanged.

Acidosis increases the severity of the intoxication by increasing the non-ionized salicylate that can cross membranes and enter the brain cells. In kidneys, the unionized salicylic acid undergoes glomerular filtration, and the ionized portion undergoes tubular secretion in proximal tubules and passive reabsorption in the distal tubules. Renal excretion of salicylate is enhanced by alkaline urine.

Manifestations

The ingestion of concentrated topical salicylic acid preparations (e.g., wart remover) can cause mucosal caustic injury to the gastrointestinal tract. Occult salicylate overdose should be considered in any patient with unexplained acid-base disturbance.

The manifestations of acute overdose of salicylates are as follows:

Minimal Symptoms. Tinnitus, dizziness, and deafness may occur at high therapeutic salicylate plasma concentrations of 20 to 30 mg/dL. Nausea and vomiting may occur immediately because of local gastric irritation.

Phase I. Mild manifestations occur at 1 to 12 hours after ingestion with a 6-hour salicylate plasma concentration of 45 to 70 mg/dL. Nausea and vomiting followed by hyperventilation are usually present within 3 to 8 hours after acute overdose. Hyperventilation, an increase in both rate (tachypnea) and depth (hyperpnea), is present but it may be subtle. It results in a mild respiratory alkalosis with a serum pH greater than 7.4 and urine pH greater than 6.0. Some patients may have lethargy, vertigo, headache, and confusion. Diaphoresis may be noted.

Phase II. Moderate manifestations occur at 12 to 24 hours after ingestion with a 6-hour salicylate plasma concentration of 70 to 90 mg/dL. Serious metabolic disturbances, including a marked respiratory alkalosis with anion gap metabolic acidosis, dehydration, and urine pH less than 6.0, may occur. Other metabolic disturbances include hypoglycemia or hyperglycemia, hypokalemia, decreased ionized calcium, and increased BUN, creatinine, and lactate. Mental disturbances (confusion, disorientation, hallucinations) may occur. Hypotension and convulsions have been reported.

Phase III. Severe intoxication occurs more than 24 hours after ingestion with a 6-hour salicylate plasma concentration of 90 to 130 mg/dL. In addition to the above clinical findings, coma and seizures develop and indicate severe intoxication. Pulmonary edema may occur. Metabolic disturbances include metabolic acidemia (pH <7.4) and aciduria (pH <6.0). In adults, alkalosis may persist until terminal respiratory failure.

In children younger than 4 years of age, a mixed metabolic acidosis and respiratory alkalosis develop earlier (within 4 to 6 hours) than in adults because children have less respiratory reserve and accumulate lactate and other organic acids. Hypoglycemia is more common in children.

Fatalities occur at 6-hour salicylate plasma concentrations greater than 130 to 150 mg/dL and result from CNS depression, cardiovascular collapse, electrolyte imbalance, and cerebral edema.

Chronic salicylism is more serious than acute intoxication and the 6-hour salicylate plasma concentration does not correlate

TABLE 26   Fluid and Electrolyte Treatment of Salicylate Poisoning

TYPE OF SALICYLISM	METABOLIC DISTURBANCE	BLOOD PH	URINE PH	HYDRATING SOLUTION	AMOUNT OF NAHCO₃ (MEQ/L)	AMOUNT OF POTASSIUM (MEQ/L)
Mild	Respiratory alkalosis	>7.4	>6.0	5% Dextrose, 0.45% saline	50 (adult) 1 mEq/kg (child)	20
Moderate Chronic Child <4 years	Respiratory alkalosis Metabolic acidosis	>7.4	<6.0	5% Dextrose in water	100 (adult) 1–2 mEq/kg (child)	40
Severe Chronic Child <4 years	Metabolic acidosis Respiratory alkalosis	<7.4	<6.0	5% Dextrose in water	150 (adult) 2 mEq/kg (child)	60
CNS Depressant Co-ingestant	Respiratory acidosis	<7.4	<6.0	5% Dextrose in water	100–150*	60

*Correct hypoventilation.

Modified from Linden CH, Rumack BH: The legitimate analgesics, aspirin and acetaminophen. In Hansen Jr W (ed): *Toxic Emergencies*. New York, Churchill Livingstone, 1984.

well with the manifestations in both acute and chronic cases of intoxication. Chronic intoxication usually occurs with therapeutic errors in young children or the elderly with underlying illness, and the diagnosis is delayed because it is not recognized. Noncardiac pulmonary edema is a frequent complication in the elderly. The mortality rate is about 25%. Chronic salicylate poisoning in children may mimic Reye syndrome. It is associated with exaggerated CNS findings (hallucinations, delirium, dementia, memory loss, papilledema, bizarre behavior, agitation, encephalopathy, seizures, and coma). Hemorrhagic manifestations, renal failure, and pulmonary and cerebral edema may occur. The metabolic picture is hypoglycemia and mixed acid-base derangements. A chronic salicylate plasma concentration greater than 60 mg/dL with metabolic acidosis and an altered mental state is very serious.

Laboratory Investigations

All patients with intentional salicylate overdoses should have acetaminophen plasma level measured after 4 hours.

One should continuously monitor ECG, urine output, urine pH, and specific gravity. Every 2 to 4 hours in cases of severe intoxication, salicylate plasma concentration, glucose (in a case of salicylism, CNS hypoglycemia may be present despite normal serum glucose), electrolytes, ionized calcium, magnesium and phosphorus, anion gap, ABGs, and pulse oximeter should be monitored. Daily monitoring of BUN, creatinine, liver function tests, and prothrombin time should take place.

The therapeutic salicylate plasma concentration is less than 10 mg/dL for analgesia and 15 to 30 mg/dL for antiinflammatory effect. Cross-reaction with diflunisal (Dolobid) will give a falsely high salicylate plasma concentration. The Done nomogram is not considered accurate in evaluating acute or chronic salicylate intoxications.

Management

Treatment is based on clinical and metabolic findings, not on salicylate levels. Continuous monitoring of the urine pH is essential for successful alkalinization treatment. One should always obtain an acetaminophen plasma level.

Vital functions must be established and maintained. If the patient is in an altered mental state, glucose, naloxone, and thiamine are administered in standard doses. Depending on the severity, the initial studies include an immediate and a 6-hour postingestion salicylate plasma concentration, ECG and cardiac

monitoring, pulse oximeter, urine (analysis, pH, and specific gravity), chest radiograph, ABGs, blood glucose, electrolytes and anion gap calculation, calcium (ionized), magnesium, renal and liver profiles, and prothrombin time. Gastric contents and stool should be tested for occult blood. Bismuth and magnesium salicylate preparations may be radiopaque on radiographs. Consultation with a nephrologist is warranted in cases of moderate, severe, or chronic intoxication.

For gastrointestinal decontamination, activated charcoal is useful (each gram of activated charcoal binds 550 mg of salicylic acid) if a toxic dose was ingested up to 4 hours postingestion. MDAC is not recommended for salicylate intoxication.

Concretions may occur with massive (usually >300 mg/kg) ingestions. If blood levels fail to decline, prompt contrast radiography of the stomach may reveal concretions that have to be removed by repeated lavage, whole-bowel irrigation, endoscopy, or gastrostomy.

Fluids and electrolyte treatment of salicylate poisonings is given in Table 26. For shock, perfusion and vascular volume should be established with 5% dextrose in 0.9% saline, then the treatment can proceed with correction of dehydration and alkalinization.

For cases of acute moderate or severe salicylism (see Table 26), adults should receive a bolus of 1 to 2 mEq/kg of sodium bicarbonate (NaHCO₃) followed by an infusion of 100 to 150 mEq NaHCO₃ added to 500 to 1000 mL of 5% dextrose and administered over 60 minutes. Children should receive a bolus of 1 to 2 mEq/kg of NaHCO₃ followed by an infusion of 1 to 2 mEq/kg added to 20 mL/kg of 5% dextrose administered over 60 minutes. Potassium is added after the patient voids. The goal is to achieve a urine output of greater than 2 mL/kg/h and a urine pH of greater than 8. The initial infusion is followed by subsequent infusions (two to three times normal maintenance) of 200 to 300 mL/h in adults or 10 mL/kg/h in children. If the patient is acidotic and has a serum pH of less than 7.15, an additional 1 to 2 mEq/kg of NaHCO₃ is given over 1 to 2 hours; persistent acidosis may require 1 to 2 mEq/kg of bicarbonate every 2 hours. The infusion rate, the amount of bicarbonate, and the electrolytes should be adjusted to correct serum abnormalities and to maintain the targeted urine output and urinary pH. Diuresis is not as important as the alkalinization. Careful monitoring for fluid overload should take place for patients at risk of pulmonary and cerebral edema (e.g., the elderly) and because of inappropriate secretion of the antidiuretic hormone.

In patients with mild intoxication who are not acidotic and have a urine pH greater than 6, 5% dextrose in 0.45% saline should be administered as maintenance to replace ongoing fluid loss. Some toxicologists may consider adding sodium bicarbonate 50 mEq/L or 1 mEq/kg in some cases.

To achieve alkalinization, sodium bicarbonate is administered to produce a serum pH 7.4 to 7.5 and a urine pH greater than 8. Carbonic anhydrase inhibitors (acetazolamide [Diamox]) should not be used. If the patient is acidotic, additional bicarbonate may be required. About 2 mEq/kg raises the blood pH 0.1. In children, alkalinization may be a difficult problem because of the organic acid production and hypokalemia. Hypokalemic and fluid-depleted patients cannot be adequately alkalinized. Alkalinization is usually discontinued in asymptomatic patients with a salicylate plasma concentration less than 30 to 40 mg/dL but is continued in symptomatic patients regardless of the salicylate plasma concentration. A decreased serum bicarbonate but normal or high blood pH indicates respiratory alkalosis predominating over metabolic acidosis, and the bicarbonate should be administered cautiously. An alkalemic pH of 7.40 to 7.50 is not a contraindication to bicarbonate therapy because these patients have a significant base deficit in spite of elevated blood pH.

Potassium is added, 20 to 40 mEq/L, to the infusion after the patient voids. In cases of severe, late, and chronic salicylism, 60 mEq/L of potassium may be needed. When the serum potassium is below 4.0 mEq/L, 10 mEq/L should be added over the first hour. If the patient has hypokalemia less than 3 mEq/L and flat T waves and U waves, 0.25 to 0.5 mEq/kg up to 10 mEq/h is administered. Potassium should be administered under ECG monitoring. Serum potassium is rechecked after each rapidly administered dose. A paradoxical urine acidosis (alkaline serum pH and acid urine pH) indicates that potassium is probably needed.

Convulsions are treated with diazepam or lorazepam, but hypoglycemia, low ionized calcium, cerebral edema, and hemorrhage should first be excluded with a CT scan. If tetany develops, the NaHCO$_3$ therapy is discontinued and calcium gluconate 0.1 to 0.2 mL/kg 10% administered.

Pulmonary edema management consists of fluid restriction, high FiO$_2$, mechanical ventilation, and positive end-expiratory pressure.

Cerebral edema management consists of fluid restriction, elevation of the head, hyperventilation, osmotic diuresis, and administration of dexamethasone. Vitamin K$_1$ is administered parenterally to correct an increased prothrombin time (>20 seconds) and coagulation abnormalities. If the patient has active bleeding, fresh plasma and platelets are administered as needed. Hyperpyrexia is managed by external cooling measures, not antipyretics.

Hemodialysis is the choice for removal of salicylates because it corrects the acid-base, electrolyte, and fluid disturbances as well. The indications for hemodialysis include the following:

- Acute poisoning with salicylate plasma concentration greater than 100 mg/dL without improvement after 6 hours of appropriate therapy
- Chronic poisoning with cardiopulmonary disease and a salicylate plasma concentration as low as 40 mg/dL with refractory acidosis, severe CNS manifestations (coma and seizures), and progressive deterioration, especially in elderly patients
- Impairment of vital organs of elimination
- Clinical deterioration in spite of good supportive care and alkalinization
- Severe refractory acid-base or electrolyte disturbances despite appropriate corrective measures

Disposition

There are limitations of salicylate plasma levels and patients are treated on the basis of clinical and laboratory findings. Patients who are asymptomatic should be monitored for a minimum of 6 hours, and longer if enteric-coated tablets or massive overdose was taken or if there is suspicion of concretions. Those who remain asymptomatic with a salicylate plasma concentration less

than 35 mg/dL may be discharged following psychiatric evaluation, if indicated. Chronic salicylate-intoxicated patients with acidosis and an altered mental state should be admitted to the intensive care unit. Patients with acute ingestion and a salicylate plasma concentration less than 60 mg/dL and mild symptoms may be able to be treated in the emergency department. Patients with moderate and severe intoxications should be admitted to the intensive care unit.

Selective Serotonin Reuptake Inhibitors

Selective serotonin reuptake inhibitors (SSRIs) are primarily prescribed as antidepressants. SSRIs include fluoxetine (Prozac), paroxetine (Paxil), and sertraline (Zoloft).

Toxic Mechanism

The SSRIs interfere with the neuron reuptake of serotonin (5-hydroxytryptamine) at the presynaptic ganglia sites in the brain, increasing the activity of serotonin. SSRIs should not be used within 5 weeks of when a MAOI is given, nor should MAOI therapy be initiated or discontinued within 5 weeks of SSRI therapy.

Toxic Dose

The therapeutic oral dose of fluoxetine is 20 to 80 mg/d. No toxicity is seen in children with up to 3.5 mg/kg/dose orally. A fatal dose for adults is 6 g. The therapeutic dose for paroxetine is 20 to 50 mg/d. In 35 adult patients, none developed serious side effects after the ingestion of 10 to 1000 mg, and a study involving 35 children failed to demonstrate serious adverse effects at doses less than 180 mg. The therapeutic dose for sertraline is 50 mg to 200 mg/d. Patients have ingested up to 2.6 g without serious side effects. Overdose involving children who ingested less than 100 mg failed to cause adverse events.

Kinetics

Fluoxetine is well absorbed from the gastrointestinal tract and has a peak plasma concentration at 6 to 8 hours. Volume distribution is 20 to 42 L/kg; 95% is protein bound. The half-life is 4 days (for the demethylated active metabolite norfluoxetine, the half-life is 7 to 15 days). Elimination is 80% renal. Fluoxetine and other serotonin inhibitors are inhibitors of the cytochrome P450, CYP2D6 enzyme. Therefore interactions may occur with many other medications, such as antidysrhythmic class IC drugs (quinidine), phenytoin (Dilantin), haloperidol, lithium, tricyclic antidepressants (TCAs), β-blockers, codeine, and carbamazepine (Tegretol).

Paroxetine is almost completely absorbed from the gastrointestinal tract, with a peak in 2 to 8 hours. Protein binding is greater than 90%; volume distribution is 13 L/kg. Paroxetine undergoes extensive first-pass liver metabolism by oxidation and methylation to inactive metabolites. It inhibits the P450 system (see fluoxetine metabolism). The average half-life is 21 hours.

Sertraline peaks in 8 to 12 hours. Its volume distribution is 20 L/kg and protein binding is 98%. The average half-life of sertraline is 26 hours. It is metabolized to form a less-active metabolite, N-desmethylsertraline (half-life of 62 to 104 hours).

Manifestations

All SSRIs may cause serotonin syndrome, a potentially life-threatening reaction, if they are administered concurrently with an MAOI. Serotonin syndrome is caused by cerebral serotonergic stimulation and can cause severe hyperthermia, myoclonus, rhabdomyolysis, confusion, tremors, and a variety of psychological disturbances. In addition, cardiovascular complications and extrapyramidal side effects, including akathisia, dyskinesia, and Parkinson-like syndromes may occur. Also, increased suicidal ideation, seizures, sexual disorders, and hematologic disorders (platelet serotonin activity blockade leading to prolonged bleeding times) may develop. Inappropriate secretion of antidiuretic hormone resulting in hyponatremia may occur when SSRIs are administered to the elderly. This effect is usually seen within the first week of therapy.

Overdose effects are similar to the serotonin syndrome.

Laboratory Investigations

One should obtain a complete blood count (CBC), electrolytes, glucose levels, a coagulation profile, liver function tests, creatine kinase level, and an ECG.

Management

There is no specific antidote to SSRI intoxication.

Initial management consists of stabilizing vital functions, including thermoregulation. Supportive therapy and anticipation of potential life-threatening manifestations (hypotension, hyperthermia, seizures, coma, disseminated intravascular coagulation, ventricular tachycardia, and metabolic acidosis) are essential. Vital signs, EEG, creatine kinase, and blood chemistry should be monitored.

Benzodiazepines are administered to prevent and control muscle hyperactivity (diazepam [Valium] for seizures, clonazepam [Klonopin] for myoclonus). If benzodiazepine therapy fails to control muscle activity or seizures, anesthesia or nondepolarizing neuromuscular blockade may be necessary.

Electrolyte abnormalities and acid-base balance should be corrected. Fluids are used to maintain a urine output of greater than 2 mL/kg/h if there is a risk of myoglobinuria.

There are no data to support the use of gastrointestinal decontamination, although activated charcoal may be used if an ingestion has occurred within 1 hour. Hemodialysis and charcoal hemoperfusion are unlikely to be beneficial. Haloperidol (Haldol), phenothiazines, and other highly protein-bound drugs are to be avoided.

Benzodiazepine and cooling therapy can be used for hyperthermia. Serotonin antagonists, such as cyproheptadine (Periactin), may be useful in treating serotonin syndrome, although there are no controlled data. Dantrolene (Dantrium) and bromocriptine (Parlodel) are not recommended and may actually precipitate serotonin syndrome.

Disposition

Cases of ingestions in children up to 5 years of age of less than 180 mg of paroxetine (Paxil), less than 3.5 mg/kg of fluoxetine (Prozac), or less than 100 mg of sertraline (Zoloft) can be observed at home. Symptomatic patients should be admitted to the intensive care unit until asymptomatic for 24 hours. Asymptomatic patients should be observed for 6 hours. All patients should be assessed for risk of suicide before discharge. When taken chronically, SSRIs may increase cholesterol and triglycerides and decrease uric acid, so these test results should be followed.

Theophylline

Theophylline (Slo-Phyllin) is a methylxanthine alkaloid similar to caffeine and theobromine. Aminophylline is 80% theophylline. Theophylline is used in the acute treatment of asthma, pulmonary edema, chronic obstructive pulmonary disease, and neonatal apnea.

Toxic Mechanism

The proposed mechanisms of action include phosphodiesterase inhibition, adenosine receptor antagonism, inhibition of prostaglandins, and increase in serum catecholamines. Theophylline stimulates the central nervous, respiratory, and emetic centers and reduces the seizure threshold. It has positive cardiac inotropic and chronotropic effects, acts as a diuretic, relaxes smooth muscle, and causes peripheral vasodilation but cerebral vasoconstriction. Gastric secretions, gastrointestinal motility, lipolysis, glycogenolysis, and gluconeogenesis are all increased.

Toxic Dose

A single dose of 1 mg/kg produces a theophylline plasma concentration of approximately 2 μg/mL. The therapeutic range usually is 10 to 20 μg/mL. An acute, single dose greater than 10 mg/kg causes mild toxicity, a dose greater than 20 mg/kg causes moderate toxicity, and a dose greater than 50 mg/kg causes serious, possibly fatal toxicity. Fatalities occur at lower doses in patients with chronic toxicity, especially those with risk factors (see *Kinetics*).

Kinetics

The pKa is 9.5. Absorption from the stomach and upper small intestine is complete and rapid, with onset in 30 to 60 minutes. Peak theophylline plasma concentration occurs within 1 to 2 hours after ingestion of liquid preparations, 2 to 4 hours after ingestion of regular tablets, and 7 to 24 hours after ingestion of slow-release formulations. Volume distribution is 0.3 to 0.7 L/kg. Protein binding is 40% to 60% in adults, mainly to albumin (low albumin increases free active theophylline).

Elimination is 90% by hepatic metabolism to an active metabolite, 2-methyl xanthine. The half-life is 3.5 hours in a child and 4 to 6 hours in an adult. The half-life is shorter in smokers and patients taking enzyme-inducing drugs. Only 8% to 10% of the drug is excreted unchanged in the urine.

Risk factors that produce a longer half-life include age younger than 6 months or older than 60 years, use of enzyme-inhibitor drugs (calcium channel blockers, oral contraceptives, cimetidine [Tagamet], ciprofloxacin [Cipro], erythromycin, macrolide antibiotics, isoniazid), illness (persistent fever >38.9°C [>102°F]), viral illness, liver impairment, heart failure, chronic obstructive pulmonary disease, and influenza vaccination.

Manifestations

Acute toxicity generally correlates with blood levels; chronic toxicity does not (Table 27).

In the case of an acute, single, regular-release overdose, vomiting and occasionally hematemesis occur at low theophylline plasma concentrations. CNS stimulation includes restlessness, muscle tremors, and protracted tonic–clonic seizures, but coma is rare. Convulsions are a sign of severe toxicity and usually are preceded by gastrointestinal symptoms (except with sustained-release and chronic intoxications). Cardiovascular disturbances

TABLE 27 Theophylline Blood Concentrations and Acute Toxicity

PLASMA CONCENTRATION (MG/ML)	TOXICITY DEGREE	MANIFESTATIONS
8–10	None	Bronchodilation
10–20	Mild	Therapeutic range: nausea, vomiting, nervousness, respiratory alkalosis, tachycardia
15–25		35% have mild manifestations of toxicity
20–40	Moderate	Gastrointestinal complaints and central nervous system stimulation Transient hypertension, tachypnea, tachycardia; 80% will have some manifestations of toxicity
60–100	Severe	Convulsions, dysrhythmias Hypokalemia, hyperglycemia Ventricular dysrhythmias, protracted convulsions, hypotension, acid-base abnormalities

Reprinted and modified from Linden CH, Rumack BH: In Hansen Jr W (ed): *Toxic Emergencies.* New York, Churchill Livingstone, 1984. With permission from Elsevier.

include cardiac dysrhythmias (supraventricular tachycardia) and transient hypertension with mild overdoses, but hypotension and ventricular dysrhythmias with severe intoxications. Rhabdomyolysis and renal failure are occasionally seen. Children tolerate higher serum levels, and cardiac dysrhythmias and seizures occur at theophylline plasma concentrations greater than 100 μg/mL. Possible metabolic disturbances include hyperglycemia, pronounced hypokalemia, hypocalcemia, hypomagnesemia, hypophosphatemia, increased serum amylase, and elevation of uric acid.

Chronic intoxication, defined as multiple doses of theophylline over 24 hours, or cases in which interacting drugs or illness interfere with theophylline metabolism are more serious and difficult to treat. Cardiac dysrhythmias and convulsions may occur at theophylline plasma concentrations of 40 to 60 μg/mL and there is no correlation with TPC. The seizures occur without warning and are protracted and repetitive and may produce status epilepticus. Vomiting and typical metabolic disturbances do not occur.

Differences with slow-release preparations are that few or no gastrointestinal symptoms occur, peak concentrations and convulsions may be delayed 12 to 24 hours postingestion, and convulsions occur without warning.

Laboratory Investigations

Monitoring includes vital signs, pulse oximeter, ABG, hemoglobin, hematocrit (for gastrointestinal hemorrhage), ECG and cardiac monitor, renal and hepatic function, electrolytes, blood glucose, acid-base balance, and serum albumin. Gastric contents and stools should be tested for occult blood. Samples for theophylline plasma concentration measurement should be drawn within 1 to 2 hours after ingestion of liquid preparations, 2 to 4 hours after ingestion of regular-release formulations, and 4 hours after ingestion of slow-release formulations. One should check the serum albumin level because a decrease in albumin levels may cause manifestations of toxicity despite normal theophylline plasma concentration. A single theophylline plasma concentration reading may be misleading; therefore, theophylline plasma concentration measurement should be repeated every 2 to 4 hours to determine the trend until a declining trend is reached and then monitored every 4 to 6 hours until it is below 20 μg/mL.

Management

Vital functions must be established and maintained. If the patient is in a coma or has convulsions or vomiting, he or she should be intubated immediately. The theophylline plasma concentration is obtained and repeated every 2 to 4 hours to determine peak absorption, and a theophylline bezoar should be considered if the theophylline plasma concentration fails to decline. Consultation with a nephrologist about charcoal hemoperfusion is recommended.

Gastrointestinal decontamination is warranted in the case of an acute overdose, but emesis must not be induced. Activated charcoal is the choice decontamination procedure in a dose of 1 g/kg to all patients, followed with MDAC 0.5 g/kg every 2 to 4 hours until the theophylline plasma concentration is less than 20 μg/mL. MDAC is effective in treating acute, chronic, and intravenous overdoses. Activated charcoal shortens the half-life of theophylline by about 50% and may be indicated up to 24 hours following ingestion.

Whole-bowel irrigation with polyethylene-electrolyte solution has been recommended for cases of massive overdose, possible concretions, and ingestion of sustained-release preparations. If intractable vomiting occurs, the antiemetic metoclopramide (Reglan) (0.1 mg/kg adult dose), droperidol (Inapsine) (2.5 to 10 mg IV), or ondansetron (Zofran) (8 to 32 mg IV) is administered. Ondansetron, however, inhibits metabolism of theophylline after a few doses.

Convulsions are controlled with lorazepam (Ativan) or diazepam (Valium) and phenobarbital. Phenytoin (Dilantin) is ineffective. The convulsions in patients with chronic intoxication are often refractory and may require, in addition to anticonvulsants, neuromuscular paralyzing agents, sedation, assisted ventilation, and EEG monitoring.

Hypotension is treated with fluids and vasopressors, if necessary. Norepinephrine (Levophed) 0.05 μg/kg/min is preferred as the vasopressor over dopamine.

Supraventricular tachycardia with hemodynamic instability requires cardioversion. Low-dose β-blockers may be used but should not be used in patients with reactive airway disease or hypotension. Adenosine (Adenocard) is ineffective. For ventricular dysrhythmias, electrolyte disturbances should be corrected. Lidocaine is the treatment of choice but has the potential to cause seizures at toxic concentrations. Cardioversion may be needed.

Hematemesis is managed with sucralfate (Carafate) 1 g four times daily and/or Maalox TC 30 mL every 2 hours and blood replacement, if necessary. H_2 antihistamine blockers that are enzyme inhibitors are not used.

Fluid and metabolic disturbances should be corrected. Hyperglycemia does not require insulin therapy. Hypokalemia should be corrected cautiously, as it may be largely an intracellular shift and not total body loss. Usually adding 40 mEq potassium to a liter of fluid will suffice. The serum potassium level must be monitored closely.

Charcoal hemoperfusion is the management of choice for patients with serious intoxications. Hemoperfusion can increase the clearance twofold to threefold over hemodialysis, but hemodialysis can be used if hemoperfusion is not available. Criteria for charcoal hemoperfusion are as follows:

- Life-threatening events such as convulsions or dysrhythmias
- Intractable vomiting refractory to antiemetics
- Acute intoxications with a theophylline plasma concentration greater than 80 μg/mL or greater than 70 μg/mL 4 hours after overdose with a sustained-release formulation and greater than 40 μg/mL in the case of chronic intoxication
- Acute or chronic overdoses with a theophylline plasma concentration greater than 40 μg/mL, especially if the patient has risk factors that lengthen the half-life of the drug (see Kinetics)

Disposition

Patients with mild symptoms and a theophylline plasma concentration less than 20 μg/mL can be treated in emergency department and discharged when asymptomatic for a few hours. Any patient with acute ingestion and a theophylline plasma concentration greater than 35 μg/mL should be admitted to a monitored bed with seizure precautions and suicide precautions, if needed. If neurologic or cardiotoxic effects or a theophylline plasma concentration greater than 50 μg/mL is present, the patient should be admitted to the intensive care unit. A patient with an overdose of a sustained-release preparation, regardless of symptoms or initial theophylline plasma concentration, requires admission, monitoring, activated charcoal, and MDAC. In patients on chronic therapy, toxicity may occur at a lower theophylline plasma concentration, and these patients should not be discharged until they are asymptomatic for several hours.

Tricyclic and Cyclic Antidepressants

Historically, tricyclic antidepressants are an important cause of pharmaceutical overdose fatalities. The mortality rate was reduced from 15% in the 1970s to less than 1% in the 1990s because of a better understanding of the pathophysiology of these agents and improvements in management (Table 28).

Toxic Mechanism

The major mechanisms of toxicity of the tricyclic antidepressants are (a) central and peripheral anticholinergic effects; (b) peripheral α-adrenergic blockade; (c) quinidine-like cardiac membrane stabilizing action blockade of the fast inward sodium channels; and (d) inhibition of synaptic neurotransmitter reuptake in the

GENERIC NAME (TRADE NAME)	ADULT DAILY DOSE (MG)	THERAPEUTIC RANGE (NG/ML)	HALF-LIFE (HOURS)	TOXICITY		
				ANTICHOL	CNS	CARDIAC
Tertiary Amines						
Amitriptyline (Elavil)	75–300	120–250	31–46	3+	3+	3+
Imipramine (Tofranil)	75–300	125–250	9–24	3+	3+	2+
Doxepin (Sinequan)	75–300	30–150	8–24	3+	3+	2+
Trimipramine (Surmantil)	75–200	10–240	16–18	3+	3+	2+
Secondary Amines						
Nortriptyline (Pamelor)	75–150	50–150	18–93	2+	3+	3+
Desipramine (Norpramin)	75–200	75–160	14–62	1+	3+	3+
Protriptyline (Vivactil)	20–60	70–250	54–198	2+	3+	3+
Newer Cyclic Antidepressants						
Teracyclic			30–60	1+	2+	3+
Maprotiline (Ludiomil)	75–300	—	30–60	1+	2+	3+
Trizolopyridine, a noncyclic, produces less serious cardiac and CNS toxicity						
Trazodone (Desyrel)	50–600	700	4–7	1+	1+	1+
Monocyclic Aminoketones						
Bupropion (Wellbutrin)	200–400	—	8–24	1+	3+	1+
Dibenzazepine						
Clomipramine (Anafranil)	100–250	200–500	21–32	2+	2+	2+
Dibenoxazepine						
Amoxapine (Ascendin)	150–300	200–500	6–10	1+	3+	2+

Abbreviations: Antichol = anticholinergic effect; CNS = central nervous system effect primarily seizures; cardiac = cardiac effect.
Other drugs with similar structures are cyclobenzaprine, a muscle relaxant (similar to amitriptyline), and carbamazepine, an anticonvulsant (similar to imipramine); however, they cause less cardiac toxicity.

CNS presynaptic neurons. The tetracyclics, monocyclic aminoketones, and dibenzoxazepines possess convulsive activity and less cardiac toxicity in overdose than the older tricyclic antidepressants. Triazolopyridine has less serious cardiac and CNS toxicity.

Toxic Dose
The therapeutic dose of imipramine (Tofranil) is 1.5 to 5 mg/kg; a dose greater than 5 mg/kg may be mildly toxic; 10 to 20 mg/kg may be life threatening, although less than 20 mg/kg has produced few fatalities; greater than 30 mg/kg carries a 30% mortality rate; and at a dose greater than 70 mg/kg, patients rarely survive. In children 375 mg and in adults as little as 500 mg have been fatal. In adults, five times the maximum daily dose is toxic and 10 times is potentially fatal. Although major overdose symptoms are associated with plasma concentrations greater than 1 μg/mL (>1000 ng/mL), plasma tricyclic levels do not correlate well with toxicity; clinical signs and symptoms should guide therapy.

The relative dosage or potency equivalents are as follows: amitriptyline (Elavil) 100 mg = amoxapine (Asendin) 125 mg = desipramine (Norpramin) 75 mg = doxepin (Sinequan) 100 mg = imipramine (Tofranil) 75 mg = maprotiline (Ludiomil) 75 mg = nortriptyline (Pamelor) 50 mg = trazodone (Desyrel) 200 mg. This allows one to determine an equivalent dosage of an agent compared with another (see Table 28).

Kinetics
The tricyclic and cyclic antidepressants are lipophilic. They are rapidly absorbed from the alkaline small intestine, but absorption may be prolonged and delayed in cases of massive overdose owing to anticholinergic action. Onset varies from less than 1 hour (30 to 40 minutes) to, rarely, 12 hours. The peak serum levels are reached in 2 to 8 hours and the peak effect is in 6 hours but may be delayed 12 hours because of erratic absorption. The clinical effects correlate poorly with plasma levels.

Cyclic antidepressants are highly protein-bound to plasma glycoproteins, 98% at a pH 7.5 and 90% at 7.0. Volume distribution is 10 to 50 L/kg. The elimination route is by hepatic metabolism. The tertiary amines are metabolized into active demethylated secondary amine metabolites. The active secondary amine metabolites undergo a 15% enterohepatic recirculation and are metabolized over a period of days into nonactive metabolites. The intestinal bacterial flora may reconstitute the metabolites, which are active.

The half-life varies from 10 hours for imipramine to 81 hours for amitriptyline and 100 hours for nortriptyline. The active metabolites have longer half-lives.

Only 3% of the ingested dose is excreted in the urine unchanged.

Manifestations
There are reports of asymptomatic patients who, upon arrival to an emergency department, suddenly have a seizure, develop hemodynamically unstable dysrhythmias, and die shortly thereafter from ingestion of a tricyclic antidepressant. Most patients with severe toxicity develop symptoms within 1 to 2 hours, but symptoms may be delayed 6 hours after overdose.

Small overdoses produce early anticholinergic effects, agitation, and transient hypertension, which are not life-threatening. Large overdoses produce depression of the CNS and myocardium, convulsions, and hypotension. Death can occur within the first 2 to 6 hours following ingestion.

Some ECG screening tools for predicting cardiac or neurologic toxicity from ingestion of a tricyclic antidepressant have been developed: (a) a QRS greater than 0.10 second may produce seizures, and if greater than 0.16 second, 50% of patients may develop ventricular dysrhythmias (20% of these may be life-threatening) and seizures; (b) a terminal 40 msec of the QRS axis greater than 120 degrees in the right frontal plane may be associated with toxicity; or (c) a large R wave greater than 3 mm in

ECG lead aVR may predispose the patient to toxicity. The quinidine cardiac membrane stabilizing effect produces depression of myocardium, conduction, and ECG changes. The peripheral α-adrenergic blockade produces hypotension.

The secondary amines are metabolized to inactive metabolites. The tetracyclics produce a high incidence of cardiovascular disturbances and seizures. Monocyclic aminoketones produce seizures in doses greater than 600 mg. Dibenzoxazepines produce a syndrome of convulsions, rhabdomyolysis, and renal failure.

Laboratory Investigations

If the patient has altered mental status or ECG abnormalities, ABG, ECG, chest radiograph, blood glucose, serum electrolytes, calcium, magnesium, blood urea nitrogen, and creatinine levels, liver profile, creatine kinase level, urine output, and, in severe cases, hemodynamic monitoring are indicated. Levels of the tricyclic and cyclic antidepressants less than 300 ng/mL are therapeutic; levels greater than 500 ng/mL indicate toxicity, and levels greater than 1000 ng/mL indicate serious poisoning and are associated with QRS widening.

Management

Vital functions must be established and maintained. Even if the patient is asymptomatic, intravenous access should be established, vital signs and neurologic status monitored, and baseline 12-lead ECG and continuous cardiac monitoring obtained for at least 6 hours from admission or 8 to 12 hours postingestion. QRS interval should be measured on a limb lead ECG every 15 minutes for 6 hours postingestion.

For gastrointestinal decontamination, emesis should not be induced and gastric lavage should not be used. Activated charcoal is preferable. If the patient is in an altered mental state, the airway must be protected. Activated charcoal 1 g/kg is recommended up to 1 hour postingestion. Benefit from MDAC has not been demonstrated.

Alkalinization does not control seizures; diazepam or lorazepam should be used. Status epilepticus may require high-dose barbiturates or neuromuscular blockers with intravenous diazepam. If not successful, the patient can be paralyzed with short-term nondepolarizing neuromuscular blockers such as vecuronium (Norcuron), intubation, and assisted ventilation. A bolus of sodium bicarbonate is recommended as an adjunct to correct the acidosis produced by the seizures.

Sodium bicarbonate is administered in a dose of 1 to 2 mEq/kg undiluted as a bolus and repeated twice a few minutes apart, if needed, for "sodium loading" and alkalinization, which may increase protein binding from 90% to 98%. The sodium loading overcomes the sodium channel blockage and is more important than the alkalinization. Indications include (a) a QRS complex greater than 0.12 second, (b) ventricular tachycardia, (c) severe conduction disturbances, (d) metabolic acidosis, (e) coma, and (f) seizures. A continuous infusion of sodium bicarbonate is of limited usefulness for controlling dysrhythmias. Bolus therapy should be used as needed.

Hyperventilation alone has been recommended, but the pH elevation is not as instantaneous and there is compensatory renal excretion of bicarbonate; therefore, we do not recommend it. The combination of hyperventilation and sodium bicarbonate has produced fatal alkalemia and is not recommended. One should monitor serum potassium level (the sudden increase in blood pH can aggravate or precipitate hypokalemia), serum sodium, and ionized calcium levels (hypocalcemia may occur with alkalinization) and blood pH.

Specific cardiovascular complications should be treated as follows: Hypotension is treated with norepinephrine, a predominantly α-adrenergic drug, which is preferred over dopamine. Hypertension that occurs early rarely requires treatment. Sinus tachycardia usually does not require treatment. Supraventricular tachycardia in a patient who is hemodynamically unstable requires synchronized electrical cardioversion, starting at 0.25 to 1.0 watt-second per kilogram, after sedation. Ventricular tachycardia that persists after alkalinization requires intravenous

lidocaine or countershock if the patient is hemodynamically unstable. Ventricular fibrillation should be treated with defibrillation. Torsades de pointes is treated with magnesium sulfate IV 20% solution, 2 g over 2 to 3 minutes, followed by a continuous infusion of 1.5 mL 10% solution or 5 to 10 mg per minute. For the treatment of bradydysrhythmias, atropine is contraindicated because of the anticholinergic activity. Isoproterenol 0.1 µg/kg/min, used with caution, may produce hypotension. If the patient is hemodynamically unstable, a pacemaker is used.

Extraordinary measures, such as aortic balloon pump and cardiopulmonary bypass, have been successful.

Investigational treatments include FAB fragments specific for tricyclic antidepressant, which have been successful in animals. Prophylactic NaHCO3 to prevent dysrhythmias is also being investigated.

Physostigmine has produced asystole, and flumazenil has produced seizures. Both are contraindicated.

Disposition

A patient with an antidepressant overdose who meets any of the following criteria should be admitted to the intensive care unit for 12 to 24 hours: (a) ECG abnormalities except sinus tachycardia, (b) altered mental state, (c) seizures, (d) respiratory depression, and (e) hypotension. Low-risk patients include those in whom the above symptoms are absent at 6 hours postingestion, those who present with minor transient manifestations such as sinus tachycardia who subsequently become and remain asymptomatic for a 6-hour period, and asymptomatic patients who remain asymptomatic for 6 hours. These patients may be discharged if the ECG remains normal, they have normal bowel sounds, and they undergo psychiatric disposition.

Even if the patient is asymptomatic upon presentation to the health care facility, intravenous access should be established, vital signs and neurologic status monitored, a baseline 12-lead ECG obtained, and cardiac monitoring continued for at least 6 hours. *Caution:* In 25% of fatal cases, the patients were initially alert and awake at presentation. However, in most cases of fatality initially deemed as sudden cardiac death, the patient, upon reexamination, actually had symptoms that were missed.

Children younger than 6 years of age with non-intentional (accidental) exposures to amitriptyline (Elavil), desipramine (Norpramin), doxepin (Sinequan), imipramine (Tofranil), or nortriptyline (Aventyl) in a dose less than 5 mg/kg, who are asymptomatic and have what are deemed reliable caregivers, can be observed at home, with close poison control follow-up for 6 hours. Parents or caregivers should be given instructions regarding signs and symptoms to be alert for. Children who are symptomatic, or who ingested greater than 5 mg/kg, should be referred to the emergency department for monitoring, observation, and activated charcoal treatment.

SPIDER BITES AND SCORPION STINGS

Method of
Anne-Michelle Ruha, MD

CURRENT DIAGNOSIS

Black Widow Bite
- Target lesion, not always present
- Generalized pain and muscle cramps
- Hypertension, regional diaphoresis

Brown Recluse Bite
- Unlikely to occur outside of endemic areas
- Cyanotic or blistering wound within area of pallor surrounded by erythema
- Systemic loxoscelism associated with rash, fever, hemolysis, renal failure

Bark Scorpion Sting
- Absence of lesion or local inflammatory reaction
- Painful paresthesias
- Disconjugate, roving eye movements are characteristic
- Restlessness, agitation, and involuntary jerking of muscles

CURRENT THERAPY

Black Widow Bite
- Opioid analgesics to control pain
- Benzodiazepines to control muscle cramping and anxiety
- Anti-*Latrodectus* antivenom (Antivenin) for persistent severe symptoms

Brown Recluse Bite
- General wound care
- If surgical excision is required, perform after 6 to 8 weeks
- Antibiotics only if infected

Bark Scorpion Sting
- Close attention to airway
- Opioid analgesics to control pain
- Benzodiazepines to control agitation
- *Centruroides* (scorpion) Immune F(ab')$_2$

Spider Bites

The majority of spiders native to the United States are incapable of envenomating humans. Important exceptions are *Latrodectus* and *Loxosceles* spiders, which produce clinical envenomations that, on rare occasion, are life-threatening.

Brown Recluse Spider

The most famous and abundant *Loxosceles* spider in the United States is *Loxosceles reclusa*, known as the brown recluse or fiddleback spider, due to the violin-shaped marking on its cephalothorax. The brown recluse inhabits the midwestern United States, with a range extending from east Texas to west Georgia and reaching north to southern Iowa. Bites from this nonaggressive spider are defensive, and they generally occur when spiders become trapped in clothes or bedsheets. The risk of a bite, even in heavily infested homes, appears to be very small. Most diagnoses of brown recluse bites, including many published in the medical literature, are likely erroneous, occurring in nonendemic areas without identification of the spider. Other *Loxosceles* species found in the United States are even less likely to bite because they avoid human dwellings. Evidence supporting an association between other native spider species and necrotic wounds is weak.

Although the majority of brown recluse bites do not produce significant injury, some result in loxoscelism, which ranges from minor dermonecrosis to, very rarely, life-threatening illness. The venom component thought responsible for loxoscelism is sphingomyelinase D, which affects platelets and cell membranes and activates inflammatory mediators. The first signs of dermonecrosis are often erythema, pruritus, and pain at the bite site. Over hours the site becomes pale and edematous. Erythema can progress and spread gravitationally. A vesicle can develop, form an eschar, and slough over days to weeks. In the first days after the bite, a sunken bluish wound surrounded by a ring of pallor and then erythema is characteristic. Some patients develop a generalized maculopapular rash. Although most necrotic lesions are not serious, some can enlarge to 40 cm and leave a significant scar. Obese persons are at risk for more-severe lesions.

Very rarely, systemic loxoscelism develops within 48 hours of the bite, characterized by fever, myalgias, and hemolysis. Vomiting and diarrhea can occur, and some patients develop a diffuse erythroderma. Renal failure, disseminated intravascular coagulation, and death can result. Death from massive hemolysis is rare and is more likely to occur in children.

Diagnosis of loxoscelism depends on recognition of signs and symptoms in combination with positive identification of the spider when possible. Alternative etiologies for necrotic wounds are much more common than necrotic arachnidism, especially in nonendemic areas. The differential diagnosis of brown recluse bite is large and includes infectious causes, neoplastic disease, and vascular disease.

Treatment is supportive. Most wounds heal without intervention, although a scar might remain. Early surgical excision, dapsone,[1] hyperbaric oxygen, or prophylactic antibiotics cannot be recommended owing to lack of convincing evidence. Patients should receive tetanus prophylaxis (Td) and general wound care. In severe cases, healing can take months and require surgical intervention, which should occur 6 to 8 weeks following the bite after the wound is fully demarcated.

Black Widow Spiders

Latrodectus, or widow, spiders are, medically, the most important group of spiders in the world. Native black widow spiders are shiny black with a red hourglass pattern on their ventral surface. They can reside in or near human structures, leading to contact with humans and subsequent bites.

α-Latrotoxin in venom causes neurotransmitters to be released from synaptic vesicles. This results in a combination of neuromuscular and autonomic effects unique to *Latrodectus* bites, termed *latrodectism*. Bites are inconsistently felt, and they might or might not leave visible puncture marks and a target-like lesion. Pain can progress locally or become generalized within several hours. Severe muscle pain, particularly involving the abdomen and back, is common. Other findings include hypertension, tachycardia, tremor, localized or diffuse diaphoresis, periorbital edema, and urinary retention. Less commonly, vomiting, fever, priapism, paresthesias, and fasciculations occur. Rhabdomyolysis can result from increased muscle activity. Rarely, acute cardiomyopathy, cardiac ischemia, and pulmonary edema occur. Deaths are uncommon but reported.

Diagnosis of latrodectism is based on history of a spider bite and consistent clinical findings. In the absence of a witnessed bite, diagnosis can be difficult. Sudden onset and rapid progression of symptoms should raise suspicion. Infectious and surgical etiologies must be considered in a febrile or vomiting patient. Similar neuromuscular and autonomic findings might also be seen with intoxication by stimulant drugs and scorpion envenomations, and these should be considered in the differential.

Latrodectism typically resolves within 2 to 7 days. Opioid analgesics are often required to treat pain. Severe symptoms require intravenous opioids for adequate pain control and benzodiazepines for muscle spasms and anxiety. If symptoms are life-threatening or not controlled with these therapies, antivenom (Antivenin [*Latrodectus mactans*, equine origin], Merck, Boston, Mass.) should be considered. One vial reverses symptoms of envenomation. This whole-immunoglobulin product can produce acute hypersensitivity and should be administered in a monitored setting. Risks and benefits must be weighed before using this product. If antivenom is not an option or the patient is critically ill, care is supportive, including oxygen and airway support as needed, antihypertensives, antiemetics, and other symptomatic treatment.

Tarantulas

Tarantulas are common pets and are generally harmless. Bites may be painful, but envenomation by native species has not been reported. Most injury to humans resulting from interaction with tarantulas is secondary to trauma and inflammation caused by barbed abdominal hairs that the spiders eject defensively when

---

[1]Not FDA approved for this indication.

threatened. If the hairs embed in the skin, a rash and pruritus can result. They can also embed in the cornea or be transferred there by rubbing the eyes after handling a tarantula. Ophthalmia nodosa, iritis, and keratouveitis have all been reported following exposure to tarantula hairs.

Treatment of embedded corneal hairs entails referral to an ophthalmologist and removal of the hairs if possible. Topical steroids are generally recommended, and some authors also recommend topical antibiotics.

Scorpion Stings

The bark scorpion, *Centruroides sculpturatus*, is the only native scorpion capable of producing a life-threatening envenomation. This small (<3 inches), yellowish-brown scorpion is found throughout Arizona and in bordering areas of surrounding states.

The scorpion seeks cool, dark environments and commonly enters homes. It injects venom by thrusting its stinger, located at the tip of its tail, toward the victim. The neurotoxic venom increases release of neurotransmitters that act at the neuromuscular junction and autonomic nerve endings.

Most stings are minor, producing local pain and paresthesias. Less than 5% of stings result in neurotoxicity, and the majority of these occur in children. Stings typically do not produce a visible skin lesion, although on rare occasion a small red mark is noted. Pain is immediate, and in a grade 1 envenomation remains local and resolves quickly. Grade 2 envenomations involve pain and paresthesias distal from the sting site, which can persist for days to weeks.

Most severe envenomations affect children younger than 5 years. Symptoms develop within 5 to 45 minutes and can progress for 4 hours. Infants and toddlers can exhibit sudden agitation and crying and transient vomiting, and they might rub their face and ears in response to paresthesias. If the child is verbal, complaints of burning pain and sensation of tongue swelling are common. Sinus tachycardia, hypertension, low-grade fever, and hypersalivation are common, and some children develop stridor. Restlessness, agitation, and twisting of the trunk with thrashing of the extremities is typical, as are tongue fasciculations and dysconjugate eye movements, or opsoclonus. Patients are conscious but often keep their eyes closed owing to diplopia. Presence of cranial nerve findings or neuromuscular agitation constitute a grade 3 envenomation; both are present in grade 4 envenomation. Severe envenomation may be associated with pulmonary edema, rhabdomyolysis, and aspiration pneumonia. Respiratory failure can occur due to several factors, including loss of tongue and respiratory muscle control, hypersalivation, and use of respiratory depressant medications.

Diagnosis often relies on recognition of symptoms, because children might not report a sting. Characteristic findings in regions inhabited by this scorpion usually make diagnosis straightforward. Differential diagnosis includes seizures or amphetamine toxicity. If a suspected envenomation does not follow the expected clinical course, a urine drug screen should be obtained.

Patients with grade 4 envenomation must be monitored for respiratory compromise in an emergency department or intensive care unit. If available, treatment with the antivenom Centruroides (Scorpion) Immune F(ab')2 (Equine) Injection (Anascorp) should be considered. Anascorp reverses neurotoxicity within hours and often allows discharge home from the emergency department. In clinical trials Anascorp had an excellent safety profile; however, acute hypersensitivity reactions are possible, so antihistamines and epinephrine (Adrenalin) must be accessible. Serum sickness can also develop up to 3 weeks after receiving antivenom.

If antivenom is not an option, longer-acting medications (morphine and lorazepam [Ativan][1]) may be used to control pain and agitation. Intubation and mechanical ventilation is sometimes necessary owing to venom effects and respiratory depression from the medications used to control symptoms. While the

---

[1]Not FDA approved for this indication.

patient is intubated, continuous infusion of sedative, analgesic, and muscle relaxing agents may be necessary until signs and symptoms of envenomation resolve. This typically occurs within 24 hours, although residual medication effects can require prolonged observation.

References

Anascorp package insert: http://www.fda.gov/downloads/BiologicsBloodVaccines/BloodBloodProducts/ApprovedProducs/LicensedProductsBLAs/FractionatedPlasmaProducts/UCM266725.pdf.

Bernardino CR, Rapuano C: Ophthalmia nodosa caused by casual handling of a tarantula, *CLAO* 26(2):111–112, 2000.

Boyer LV, Theodorou AA, Berg RA, et al: Antivenom for critically ill children with neurotoxicity from scorpion stings, *N Engl J Med* 360(20):2090–2098, 2009.

Clark RF, Wethern-Kestner S, Vance MV, Gerkin R: Clinical presentation and treatment of black widow spider envenomation: A review of 163 cases, *Ann Emerg Med* 21(7):782–787, 1992.

Curry SC, Vance MV, Ryan PJ, et al: Envenomation by the scorpion *Centruroides sculpturatus*, *J Toxicol Clin Toxicol* 21(4–5):417–449, 1983-1984.

Furbee RB, Kao LW, Ibrahim D: Brown recluse spider envenomation, *Clin Lab Med* 26:211–226, 2006.

Vetter RS: Spiders of the genus *Loxosceles (Araneae, Sicariidae)*: A review of biological, medical and psychological aspects regarding envenomations, *J Arachnol* 36:150–163, 2008.

Vetter RS, Isbister GK: Medical aspects of spider bites, *Annu Rev Entomol* 53:409–429, 2008.

Vetter RS, Isbister GK: Do hobo spider bites cause dermonecrotic injuries? *Ann Emerg Med* 44(6):605–607, 2004.

Watts P, Mcpherson R, Hawksworth NR: Tarantula keratouveitis, *Cornea* 19(3):393–394, 2000.

VENOMOUS SNAKEBITE

Method of
Steven A. Seifert, MD

CURRENT DIAGNOSIS

Crotalinae (rattlesnake, copperhead, cottonmouth) bite

One or two fang puncture marks

Dry bites (nonenvenomation) may occur in up to 20%. If no local effects, no envenomation but patients should be observed for at least 8 to 10 hours

Envenomation produces pain and progressive swelling, often with an active, proximal leading edge, usually finished progressing by 24 hours

Edema and functional deficits may take many weeks to completely resolve

May include clear or hemorrhagic blisters

May include ecchymosis

Tissue necrosis and infection are rare and usually late (>2 days) complications

Abnormalities in hematologic clotting elements (platelets, fibrinogen, PT/INR) are variable, may result in significant bleeding, and may persist for more than two weeks

Typical findings in an endemic area may be sufficient as an indication for antivenom treatment

Coral snake bite

One or two fang puncture marks

Dry bites (nonenvenomation) may occur in up to 50%. Patients should be observed for 24 hours

Local effects, even with significant systemic envenomation, may be minimal to nil

Neurologic effects (progressive, descending paralysis) predominate and may require airway support

Motor effects may be poorly reversible once established and may persist for many weeks

CURRENT TREATMENT

Crotalinae bite
Opioid-level pain relief may be required
If signs of envenomation, either Anavip or CroFab may be considered first-line treatment for rattlesnake bites. CroFab currently has the only FDA-approved labeling for copperhead and cottonmouth bites
Allergic reactions are rare; no pre-testing or pre-treatments are needed
Maintenance doses are recommended for CroFab
Although the incidence of recurrent hematologic effects is lower with Anavip, post-discharge hematologic monitoring is needed for all patients
Wound care follow up may be required for tissue necrosis
Serum sickness incidence is low (<5%) and most symptoms are mild
Coral snake bite
Antivenom is in short and uncertain supply
Antivenom should be given at the earliest sign of neurologic toxicity to prevent progression

Two families of significantly venomous snakes are native to the United States. The Viperidae family (viperids) is composed of three genera and more than 30 species of rattlesnakes, copperheads, and cottonmouths. The Elapidae family (elapids) is composed of two genera and several species of coral snakes.

Each year, there are more than 5500 venomous snakebites by native species reported to United States' poison centers, with fewer than 10 deaths. Ninety-eight percent of these bites are from viperids. Currently, there are two antivenoms that are effective against viperid species. Crotalidae polyvalent immune Fab (ovine) antivenom (CroFab, Protherics, Brentwood, TN) is effective and indicated for all native species in this family. A second F(ab')2 antivenom, Crotalidae Immune F(ab')2 (Equine) (Anavip; Rare Disease Therapeutics, Inc., Franklin, TN) is specifically indicated for all North American rattlesnake envenomations. There is also a single antivenom (Antivenin [*Micrurus fulvius*], equine origin, Wyeth Laboratories, Marietta, PA) against coral snakes, which are usually easily recognized by their distinctive markings.

There are approximately 50 additional bites per year by a wide variety of nonnative venomous species of snakes housed in zoos, academic institutions, serpentariums, and private collections. Identification of the biting species in these cases is usually not an issue.

Diagnostic and Management Overview

Taking Action

Only a few actions can be undertaken in the field to reduce morbidity or mortality from a venomous snakebite. Most "treatments" that have been advocated—cutting, sucking, or applying tourniquets, heat, cold, or electricity—have no proven efficacy and are much more likely to result in additional tissue injury and delay of definitive therapy. Appropriate local injury management—primarily removal of jewelry, splinting of the extremity, and measures to retard venom entry into central circulation until definitive therapy, can be undertaken *in carefully selected cases*—and expeditious transport to a healthcare facility can produce optimal outcomes.

Definitive management for native venomous snakes in the United States is achieved with appropriate local wound care and antivenom, which is composed of antibodies raised in a host animal (horses or sheep) against snake venom components. Because native viperids inhabit every state except Maine, every hospital should stock or have ready access to one or both antivenoms.

No US Food and Drug Administration (FDA)–approved elapid antivenom is currently being manufactured in the United States. Older stocks of a previously produced antivenom (Antivenin) are still available at many hospitals in endemic areas (e.g., Florida, Georgia, Alabama, Louisiana, Texas), but they are rapidly being depleted, and existing stocks will eventually be consumed or pass their expiration dates. An experimental antivenom has completed a Phase 3 clinical trial but is not currently available. Foreign-produced antivenoms against related coral snake species may also have efficacy against United States snakes but should be used only in the unavailability of an FDA-approved drug and, ideally, with prior FDA approval.

An even more difficult situation results from exotic envenomations, for which the appropriate antivenom (if one exists) is certain to be a non-FDA-approved product and may be located at a zoo or other nonhealthcare source quite distant from the location of the envenomation.

Antivenom, local wound care, and symptomatic and supportive care are the mainstays of envenomation management. A regional poison center should be contacted for information and assistance in managing any venomous snake exposure, including locating an appropriate antivenom. Poison centers have personnel who are experienced at assessing and managing envenomations and have access to a database, the Antivenom Index, which lists sources of antivenoms for nonnative species. Poison centers can be contacted from anywhere in the United States by calling 1-800-222-1222.

Snake Identification

Beyond determining whether the victim has been bitten by a coral snake or a viperid, it may be useful to distinguish a rattlesnake bite from a copperhead or cottonmouth bite for the selection of the antivenom. A photo taken with a cell phone may be of some value to the treating physician, but it should be obtained only if it can be done safely and without causing a delay in transporting the patient. Viperid snakes are easily differentiated from coral snakes by virtue of the latter's distinctive color pattern of red, yellow, and black bands. It can be difficult to differentiate a coral snake from nonvenomous snakes that have similar markings. The ditty "red touches yellow, kills a fellow; red touches black, venom lack," which describes the red band being surrounded on either side by yellow or black, is accurate only for North American coral snakes. South American coral snakes may have the opposite pattern.

As all viperid envenomations are currently treated with a single product and the physical findings or laboratory evaluation is all that is required to determine that the snake is venomous, attempting to kill or capture the snake is unlikely to add additional information to treatment decisions but is likely to result in the individual being bitten a second time or other individuals becoming bite victims. Differences in the appearance of the bite wound (e.g., fang punctures, swelling, ecchymosis) and the observation of signs and symptoms are usually sufficient to determine whether the biting snake was venomous and to guide therapy.

Since approximately half of envenomations are associated with intentional interactions with snakes, remember this advice: "Red touches yellow, leave it alone. Red touches black, leave it alone. Slithers on the ground, LEAVE IT ALONE."

Factors Affecting Toxicity and the Severity of Envenomation

Many factors govern whether an envenomation occurs after a bite, the signs and symptoms that develop, and the overall severity of effects. Up to 25% of viperid bites and up to 50% of elapid bites do not result in an envenomation. Barriers to fang penetration and other factors may result in no venom being injected. Patients must be watched for a sufficient length of time (i.e., 8 hours in a viperid bite and 24 hours in a coral snakebite) to ensure that this has been the case.

If an envenomation has occurred, the family and species of snake generally determines the spectrum of symptoms and signs. The amount of venom, specific venom components, and the underlying health status of the victim determine severity.

Viperid Envenomations

Epidemiology and Recognition

Viperid snakes are distributed throughout North America, with the apparent exception of Maine. Bites are more common in southern states and during summer months, but they occur year-round and may occur at any time and in any location with captive collections. The various genera and species of viperids in the United States have relatively stable geographic ranges, with much overlap. Many different species of venomous snakes may inhabit any given area. Nonvenomous or mildly venomous colubrid snakes are also native to the United States. Viperids, also called pit vipers (i.e., rattlesnakes, copperheads, and cottonmouths), may be recognized by a, generally, triangular-shaped head, with the so-called pit (an infrared heat-detection organ) located approximately midway between the nostril and the eye, and pupils shaped like those of a cat (not round).

Pit vipers have large, movable fangs through which venom is injected into the victim. Because fangs are curved, venom is usually injected subcutaneously, rather than into deeper muscle compartments. Because of anatomic and other physical factors, bite wounds may appear as scratches or as one or more punctures. Envenomation may occur with any break in the skin.

Viperid venom is complex, consisting of dozens of proteolytic enzymes, small peptides, phospholipases, and other elements responsible for the spectrum of clinical effects seen. There is a great variability in this complex poison between species, within species, and even within a single specimen over the course of a season and lifespan.

Clinical Effects

The spectrum of clinical effects is based on the specific genus or species of viperid and is unpredictable, ranging in any given event from a nonenvenomation (a "dry bite"; up to 25% of bites) to life-threatening reactions. Viperid snake envenomation invariably results in tissue injury, manifested by pain and progressive swelling, and it may include ecchymosis, elevated tissue and compartment pressures, tissue necrosis, and tissue loss. The complete absence of local effects can be used as a reliable marker of nonenvenomation in a viperid bite as long as a sufficient period (8 to 10 hours) of observation has occurred.

Systemic effects may occur, including hematologic, neurologic, cardiovascular, and nonspecific findings. Rattlesnake envenomations are more likely to result in hematologic effects, such as thrombocytopenia, hypofibrinogenemia, or prolongation of the prothrombin time (PT) or activated partial thromboplastin time (aPTT), and are more likely to produce neurologic effects, such as muscle fasciculation or weakness, compared with copperhead or cottonmouth envenomations; however, these effects can be seen with any viperid snake. Hypotension from direct myocardial depression or from type 1 hypersensitivity (i.e., anaphylactic or anaphylactoid) reactions may occur with any viperid exposure. Nausea, vomiting, diaphoresis, anxiety, and other nonspecific effects may be seen.

Duration of Clinical Effects

Local effects may develop rapidly or may not be apparent for many hours. Progression may occur for 24 to 36 hours, with resolution of tissue injury occurring over 3 to 6 weeks. Complications of tissue necrosis or infection have their own timeframe of resolution. Hematologic effects usually begin within 1 to 2 hours of envenomation. If antivenom is given within this time frame, the detection of those effects may be masked and become apparent only after unbound antivenom has been eliminated from the body, usually 2 to 4 days after treatment. Hematologic effects may persist for 1 to 3 weeks after an envenomation. Neurologic and other systemic effects tend to occur within a few hours of envenomation and resolve over 24 to 36 hours.

Severity of Envenomation

Untreated, local injury worsens over time, with proximal progression of tissue injury. Hematologic effects can be profound, resulting in spontaneous hemorrhage. Hypotension may be profound and can result in death. Neurologic and other systemic effects are rarely life-threatening events. Owing to changes in basic medical care and healthcare systems, it is not directly applicable to compare case-fatality rates before the introduction of antivenom (1950) with what can be expected today. Currently, there are three to five deaths from snakebite per year in the United States.

Management
Determining Whether Envenomation Has Occurred and Its Severity

Owing to the unpredictability of envenomation and the variability of possible clinical effects, each viperid bite must be assessed and responded to individually (Box 1). It is important to determine whether an envenomation has occurred. If there are no signs or symptoms of envenomation, there is no indication for antivenom or other specific treatment. The severity of the envenomation helps to determine the amount of antivenom required to counter and neutralize venom effects, but this may not be immediately apparent because envenomations tend to progress over time, and what may at first appear to be mild venom effects may progress to a severe envenomation.

Initial Hospital Management

On arrival at the hospital, jewelry should be removed and the bitten extremity loosely splinted. The wound should be cleaned, and a radiograph should be obtained to rule out a foreign body (Box 2). Tetanus status should be updated if required. In the absence of other factors, the extremity should be maintained slightly below heart level until antivenom is started and then should be elevated. If there are immediate life-threatening effects (e.g., anaphylaxis, hypotension), the extremity should be placed in an inferior position and consideration given to impeding venom entry into central circulation by means of a lymphatic constriction band or pressure immobilization bandage, weighing the potential benefit against the possible risk of increased local tissue injury from increasing venom concentration and duration in the tissues. Patients often require opioid-level pain relief.

At least one large intravenous line should be initiated and crystalloid infused as required. Initial hospital therapy, including a first dose of antivenom, should be provided in an area capable of close monitoring of vital signs and capable of managing life-threatening reactions; this usually is an emergency department. Whether an intensive care unit (ICU) or similar patient care area is used for subsequent management depends on the clinical situation.

Indications for Antivenom

Owing to the safety of the current FDA-approved antivenoms and their ability to stop proximal progression of local tissue injury, all patients with signs of progressive local envenomation effects as well as those with significant systemic effects are candidates for treatment with antivenom. In areas where the ranges of rattlesnakes, copperheads, and/or cottonmouths overlap, Crotalidae Polyvalent Immune Fab (Ovine) antivenom (CroFab) is the only antivenom specifically indicated for the latter two snakes. Aside from the benefit in managing systemic venom effects, a recent study of Fab antivenom in the treatment of copperhead envenomation demonstrated that antivenom improved limb function at 14 days post envenomation.

Depending on the original indication for treatment (local effects, systemic effects, or both), initial control of envenomation effects is the goal of the loading dose of antivenom. Currently, there are two FDA-approved viperid antivenoms for North American pit viper envenomation: Crotalidae Polyvalent Immune Fab (Ovine) Antivenin (CroFab), and Crotalidae Immune F(ab')$_2$ (Equine), (Anavip). The incidence of type 1 reactions with CroFab and Anavip are low and generally mild and were found to be similar between products in the comparative trial. Pretreatment sensitivity testing is not required or recommended. There are rare reports of IgE-mediated type 1 hypersensitivity reactions on repeat exposure in individuals who were previously treated with CroFab, but most people who have been previously treated do not develop an adverse reaction to subsequent administrations. The incidence of type 3 hypersensitivity reactions ("serum sickness") with both antivenoms was approximately 2.5% in the comparative trial.

- Remove jewelry.
- Splint the extremity and maintain just below heart level.
- Expeditiously transport to a healthcare facility.
- Consider use of lymphatic constriction band (blood pressure cuff at 15–25 mm Hg) *for life-threatening effects only.*
- Obtain intravenous access if possible.
- Do not use cutting, sucking, heat, cold, or other local "therapies."

| BOX 2 | Hospital Diagnosis and Initial Management for Viperid Envenomation. |

- Remove jewelry.
- If an arterial or venous tourniquet has been placed, convert to a lymphatic constriction band.
- Obtain intravenous access, and use crystalloid as indicated.
- Obtain CBC with platelet count, PT or INR, aPTT, and fibrinogen level q6–12h for 1 day and then daily if values are abnormal. An initial D-dimer value (or fibrin degradation products) should be obtained to detect fibrinogenolytic activity that may not yet have produced hypofibrinogenemia. Multiple D-dimer determinations are not required beyond 2 h of envenomation and an elevated D-dimer is not an independent indication for antivenom. It is an indication of fibrinogenolytic activity and indicates the potential for late hypofibrinogenemia.
- Determine whether an envenomation has occurred.
- Determine severity based on the family or species of snake, age and health status of the victim, and development and rate of progression of signs and symptoms (e.g., local injury, hematologic abnormalities, hypotension and other systemic effects).
- Determine the tetanus vaccination status and update if necessary.
- Seek consultation from a poison center: 1-800-222-1222.
- If a pressure immobilization or lymphatic constriction band was placed before arriving at the hospital, determine whether antivenom is indicated, and remove the band after the antivenom infusion has started.
- If there are minimal or no signs of envenomation or if the bands are placed inappropriately, remove them under close observation.
- Determine whether antivenom is indicated and administered per protocol.
- Provide basic wound care (i.e., cleaning and radiograph), and determine whether local injury requires specific management.
- Determine whether hematologic or other systemic effects require specific management.

aPTT, Activated partial thromboplastin time; *CBC*, complete blood cell count; *INR*, international normalized ratio; *PT*, prothrombin time.

The half-life of CroFab is approximately 18 to 24 hours, which is considerably shorter than IgG or $F(ab')_2$ antivenoms, and it is responsible for the recurrence of hematologic effects in approximately 70% of patients with an initial coagulopathy. The half-life of Anavip, an equine-based $F(ab')_2$ antivenom, has a longer half-life of approximately 133 hours, and a lower risk of subacute coagulopathy.

For confirmed and progressive envenomations, antivenom is administered as an intravenous solution, with 4- to 6 vials of CroFab, or 10 vials of Anavip diluted into 250 mL of normal saline. The infusion should be started at 25 to 50 mL/h over the first 5 to 10 minutes and then the rate increased to finish by one hour if there is no reaction. If a type 1 reaction occurs, the infusion should be slowed or stopped, depending on the severity, and appropriate symptomatic treatment should be started with H_1- and H_2-blockers, epinephrine, corticosteroids, and other supportive measures, as required. It should be determined whether antivenom is still required, and if so, it should be restarted at a slower rate or higher dilution, or both.

Treatment of Local Tissue Injury

Monitoring of the proximal extent of the active leading edge of edema, usually seen as a raised, tender, and perhaps erythematous margin, is usually sufficient to document progressive local injury and an indication for antivenom. There is little to no value in circumferential measurements of extremities, although comparisons between right and left in large fleshy areas (e.g., the thigh) may be helpful in detecting a deeper envenomation. If the antivenom is given exclusively for local findings, the syndromic response to envenomation is deemed to be controlled if there is cessation of proximal progression of edema at the end of the infusion. There is often some redistribution of existing tissue edema, but uncontrolled proximal progression is usually seen as an active leading edge of edema. If antivenom is being given for hematologic effects, cessation of worsening or reversal should be seen. Often, thrombocytopenia rebounds dramatically. Hypofibrinogenemia may not rebound as quickly or merely stabilize because the liver must manufacture new fibrinogen. Although an elevated D-dimer value indicates fibrinogenolytic activity, it is not an independent indicator for antivenom treatment.

Other systemic effects may serve as indicators for antivenom use, and they should show control by the end of the initial infusion. If initial control is not deemed to have occurred, additional doses of antivenom should be administered until initial control is determined to have occurred. Most patients achieve initial control with 4 to 12 vials of Fab antivenom and 10 to 20 vials of $F(ab')_2AV$.

Maintenance Doses

Because of the rapid decline of antivenom levels resulting from the larger volume of distribution of Fab antivenoms, after initial control is achieved, maintenance dosing of 2 vials every 6 hours for three doses is commenced. This usually maintains adequate antivenom serum levels to prevent recurrence of local tissue injury progression. If progression of local effects does recur, an additional two vials of antivenom are usually sufficient to control local worsening. Routine maintenance dosing with Anavip is not recommended. In the comparative clinical trial of Anavip versus CroFab, additional antivenom was not required in any of the 38 patients who received placebo maintenance doses following initial control with Anavip. If required, however, 4 vials should be used. Tissue pressures may be increased, and elevated muscle compartment pressures may be identified when measured directly. My colleagues and I do not routinely measure tissue or compartment pressures. When pressures are measured and demonstrated to be elevated, it should be remembered that the mechanisms of these phenomena are different from other muscle compartment syndromes. For example, extensive edema in the subcutaneous space circumferentially in an extremity may elevate compartment pressures by extrinsic compression. Case reports and series suggest that additional antivenom and extremity elevation result in reduced tissue and compartment pressures. Intracompartmental injection of venom can result in a true compartment syndrome; however, there is no evidence that fasciotomy is beneficial in this setting, and there are animal data to suggest that it may result in worse clinical outcomes.

Bleb formation at the site of a bite is not an important sign in and of itself, although it may suggest significantly elevated tissue pressures resulting in dermal-epidermal separation or the presence of tissue necrosis. Bleb fluid may contain unneutralized venom. It is reasonable to unroof blebs at or near the bite site and to débride obviously necrotic tissue, which usually becomes apparent several days after the bite.

Antibiotics

The incidence of culture-proven infection in the United States viperid bites is low, probably less than 5%. There are no data to support the use of prophylactic antibiotics, and it is best to limit the opportunities for adverse drug effects. It is often difficult to distinguish inflammatory venom effects from infection starting on the second day after an envenomation. If antibiotics are prescribed, a first-generation, broad-spectrum agent should be used.

Long-Term Local Tissue Effects

The edema and tissue injury produced by most North American viperid envenomations usually resolves within 1 to 2 months, and a return to normal function can be anticipated; however, tissue necrosis or deep tissue injury may result in longer-term or even permanent structural and functional disability. Loss of tissue may occur, including digits and other parts of extremities, although this is rare and may be associated with pre-hospital application of tourniquets or other imprudent surgical interventions, delayed care, or complications such as infections. Some victims engage in behaviors that result in multiple envenomations, and this may increase the risks of long-term tissue injury.

Hematologic Abnormalities and Bleeding

One or more hematologic abnormalities may occur with native viperid envenomation (Box 3). Significant decreases in platelet count or fibrinogen concentrations are independent indications for antivenom treatment. Isolated, mild prolongations of PT or aPTT may not require antivenom treatment; however, these effects may be progressive or indicate an impending hypofibrinogenemia, and early antivenom treatment may prevent severe abnormalities. Even if platelets, fibrinogen, and intrinsic and extrinsic clotting systems are involved, the end result is not a true disseminated intravascular coagulopathy because there is no true intravascular coagulation. Sufficient platelets, fibrinogen, and thrombin are usually available for hemostasis, and clinically significant bleeding is rarely seen; however, severe depletion of individual clotting elements or a combination of hematologic abnormalities can result in bleeding.

The management of initial or persistent laboratory abnormalities is achieved with additional antivenom. Administration of blood products (e.g., fresh-frozen plasma [FFP], platelet concentrates, other blood products) should be reserved for clinically significant bleeding and be given in conjunction with additional antivenom because transfused elements are similarly likely to be consumed by venom activity. Ecchymosis in damaged tissues, expansion of the vascular volume from crystalloid administration, and red blood cell hemolysis from hemolytic venom factors may produce an anemia that may rarely require a red blood cell transfusion.

Recurrence of Hematologic Effects

Approximately 70% of patients who develop an initial hematologic effect will have a recurrence of those effects, usually beginning several days after initial treatment but which may not manifest for up to one week. The incidence of recurrence of hematologic abnormalities was 5% to 10% with Anavip, and 30% with CroFab in the comparative trial. One likely mechanism is recurrent unneutralized venomemia after elimination of unbound antivenom. Because Anavip has a longer half-life, it remains in circulation longer and thus provides longer protection against recurrence. Postdischarge hematologic abnormalities may be severe, or even appear to be occurring *de novo* if the patient was treated soon after envenomation, blunting the acute effects of the venom and masking the true severity of the envenomation.

Patients who present with severe early hematologic effects, an elevated D-dimer, an increase in the platelet count of more than 20% within 4 hours of the initial antivenom dose, or who are treated with antivenom within 1 to 2 hours of envenomation are at risk for severe recurrent effects and should be followed closely after discharge. Although the incidence of significant bleeding is low, even with profound laboratory abnormalities, it seems prudent to administer additional antivenom if the platelet count

BOX 3 Management of Hematologic Effects and Recurrence in Viperid Envenomation.

- CroFab
  - Administer 4–6 vials of antivenom (Crotalidae Polyvalent Immune Fab [Ovine, CorFab]) in rattlesnake, copperhead or cottonmouth envenomations, for significant abnormalities of platelet count, PT or INR, aPTT, or fibrinogen.
- Anavip
  - Administer 10 vials of antivenom (Crotalidae Immune $F(ab')_2$ (Equine), (Anavip) in rattlesnake envenomations for significant abnormalities of platelet count, PT or INR, aPTT, or fibrinogen.
- An elevated D-dimer value indicates accelerated fibrinogen breakdown and should prompt close monitoring of the fibrinogen concentrations, but it is not an independent indication to treat with antivenom. A single D-dimer should be obtained at > 4 h post envenomation.
- Administer additional antivenom in 4–6-vial (CroFab) or 10-vial (Anavip) increments until there is reversal of hematologic abnormalities. Replacement of platelets, clotting factors, or fibrinogen may be gradual, and a positive trend indicates neutralization of venom or replacement in excess of venom effect.
- Patients with initial hematologic effects or who were treated within 1–2 h of envenomation are at risk for recurrent effects 2–4 days after treatment and should be followed closely: every other day until no recurrence at 7 days or daily for declining parameters.
- Consider treating recurrent hematologic abnormalities with additional antivenom. Indications include platelets <25,000/mm³; fibrinogen <50 mg/dL; INR >5; aPTT >150 seconds; and lesser abnormalities involving more than one parameter.
- Consider readmission for severe abnormalities, other risk factors (e.g., uncontrolled hypertension, advanced age, other bleeding diatheses), or clinically significant bleeding.
- Administer blood products *plus* additional antivenom for significant bleeding.

---

aPTT, Activated partial thromboplastin time; *INR*, international normalized ratio; *PT*, prothrombin time.

is less than 25,000, the fibrinogen level is less than 50 mg/dL, the PT or aPTT values indicate nonclotting, there is a combination of significant defects in coagulation, or there are underlying medical conditions that make hemorrhage more likely, such as advanced age, hypertension, or a bleeding diathesis. Additional antivenom may be given for severe hematologic effects or abnormalities associated with significant bleeding. In patients who have been discharged and who are not actively bleeding, additional CroFab antivenom has been given in an outpatient setting and the patients followed daily. Such additional doses may be needed for more than 2 weeks. For patients who remain hospitalized or are readmitted, CroFab antivenom has been given by continuous IV infusion in a number of individual cases and small case series. An infusion initiated at 3 vials over 24 hours and titrated to clinical effect (up to 4 vials per 24 hours) was successful in reversing recurrent hematologic effects in all five cases reported in one series. Sterility and stability data for this product during prolonged administration is not currently available, however. If used in this way, sterile reconstitution and infusing 1 vial continuously over no more than 8 hours (3 vials per 24 hours) would be prudent. All patients treated in this way were able to have antivenom discontinued by 14 days and most were able to have it discontinued by 7 to 10 days.

There is insufficient data regarding the severity, duration, or management of postdischarge hematologic abnormalities with Anavip.

Disposition

Patients whose local effects are regressing and do not have complications, such as infection or necrosis, and whose hematologic and other systemic effects are controlled, may be discharged. Typically, this occurs between 36 and 48 hours after envenomation but may be delayed for up to a week. Patients with any venom-related hematologic abnormality during hospitalization (thrombocytopenia, hypofibrinogenemia, elevated D-dimer, or prolonged PT/international normalized ratio (PT/INR) or aPTT) should have at least one repeat set of labs within 7 days of treatment because there is a risk of recurrent effects or late, new onset of hematologic abnormalities. In my practice, I obtain one set of labs at 3 to 4 days in high-risk patients and a second at 5 to 7 days. Ongoing pain relief may be required, with an effort to transition to nonopioid agents during the first week, and the patient should be warned to watch for signs of serum sickness. Occupational or physical therapy should be arranged to maximize return of function, and follow-up for local and systemic effects should be arranged.

Elapid Envenomations

Epidemiology and Recognition

The US coral snakes can be recognized by their distinctive band pattern, with a red band seeming to be placed on top of a larger yellow band. This color pattern applies only to North American coral snakes. Each year, there are approximately 75 to 100 bites by coral snakes in the United States. Two genera and several species inhabit the United States, with the *Micrurus* genus responsible for most bites in Florida, Texas, Georgia, Louisiana, Alabama, and some neighboring states. A smaller genus, *Micruroides*, is found in Arizona and New Mexico, but it is responsible for very few bites, and there have been no reports of serious envenomations in recent years. Bites are more common during the warmer months.

Elapids have relatively short, fixed fangs, which may decrease the rate of envenomation. More than one puncture, deep punctures, and a history of the snake hanging on increases the risk of envenomation.

Clinical Effects

Envenomation by the coral snake primarily produces neurologic toxicity from presynaptic toxins, initially producing bulbar muscle weakness, ptosis, diplopia, and dysphagia. These effects can begin within 15 to 30 minutes or may be delayed up to 24 hours after an envenomation. Muscle weakness and paralysis progress to include respiratory muscles, and they can result in respiratory arrest and death. Typical of presynaptic toxins, effect progression can be arrested with the use of antivenom, but the effects are not rapidly reversed. Typically, there is no or little local tissue injury, and the absence of local injury cannot be used to exclude envenomation. Likewise, there is usually no effect on hematologic function, and other systemic effects are rare. Patients cannot be assumed to have eluded envenomation by a coral snake because they lack these symptoms, and patients should be observed for at least 24 hours before concluding that an envenomation has not occurred.

Because of changes in basic medical care and healthcare systems, it is not directly applicable to compare case-fatality rates before the introduction of antivenom (1967) with what can be expected today; however, at that time, the case-fatality rate was approximately 10%.

Management

Because of the potential for rapid progression of motor paralysis and respiratory compromise, the difficulty of reversing paralysis after it is established, and the lack of local effects, it is reasonable to attempt to retard venom progression into the circulation until a decision regarding antivenom can be made. A pressure immobilization band (i.e., elastic bandage wrapped from an extremity's tip to trunk with the degree of tension used for sprains) is used for this purpose for elapid envenomations elsewhere in the world (Boxes 4 and 5). In Australian studies, a pressure immobilization bandage has been shown to slow venom absorption and in

Venomous Snakebite

1341

those studies, bandage pressures have been between 40 and 70 mm Hg in the upper extremity and 55 to 70 mm Hg in the lower extremity; however, the proper technique requires training, and the infrequency of these bites makes teaching and retention of such skills problematic. A blood pressure cuff inflated to similar pressures may also retard venom entry into circulation, and it can be a more reliable and easily taught technique, although it has not been validated in clinical studies.

Standard wound care should be performed, including cleansing the wound, obtaining a radiograph, and updating the tetanus status, if required. Wound infection is uncommon, and prophylactic antibiotics are not recommended.

As the first signs of envenomation can be rapidly progressive neurotoxicity and because of the difficulty of reversing paralysis, some authorities have proposed administering antivenom in cases in which an envenomation is possible, before the appearance of any clinical symptoms. Others have pointed to the infrequency of respiratory muscle paralysis, resulting in the need for intubation and respiratory support, and to possible geographic differences in snake toxicity, and they have counseled observation and antivenom treatment only after envenomation has been confirmed by progressive symptoms. Recent analysis of the national database has not demonstrated a significant difference in clinical severity between Florida and Texas coral snake envenomations, which supports early treatment; however, shortages of the FDA-approved coral snake antivenom and delays in obtaining the experimental product or a non-United States antivenom is likely to result in delays of many hours before antivenom can be administered, if it is available at all. The expiration date for one lot of Wyeth North American Coral Snake Antivenin (Micrurus fulvius) (Equine Origin, Lot L67530) has been extended through January 31, 2020 (https://www.fda.gov/vaccines-blood-biologics/safety-availability-biologics/expiration-date-extension-north-american-coral-snake-antivenin-micrurus-fulvius-equine-origin-lot-1). Updated information can be obtained from the FDA website on Vaccines, Blood and Biologics (http://www.fda.gov/BiologicsBloodVaccines/). The designated poison center (1-800-222-1222) will have information on antivenom availability in the region. Aggressive and meticulous respiratory support, including intubation and ventilation that may be needed for days to weeks, should ultimately result in survival of even severe neurotoxic envenomations. If an FDA-approved coral snake antivenom is not available, there may be a clinical trial of an investigational coral snake antivenom in progress. Clinical trials can be located at: www.clinicaltrials.gov.

Exotic Snakebite

Epidemiology and Clinical Effects

In the United States, most exotic snake envenomations occur in private collections. These are not usually known to authorities or healthcare providers until an envenomation occurs, and they may involve the collection owner or family members, including children. They may occur in any locale, and victims may present to any healthcare facility.

Viperid and elapid snakes, which account for the bulk of venomous bites worldwide, have patterns of venom activity similar to those of their North American counterparts, with some variation and with generally greater toxicity for some non-United States species. Some nonnative elapids, such as cobras, mambas, black snakes, or taipans, produce much higher rates of respiratory paralysis and may produce much greater local tissue injury than US coral snakes. Similarly, envenomation from some nonnative viperids, such as *Bothrops, Echis,* or *Bitis* species, or from an African colubrid, such as the boomslang, results in a greater risk of bleeding. Some of these species may directly activate prothrombin (e.g., *Echis* species, *Bothrops* species) and factor X (e.g., *Vipera* species, *Dispholidus* species), leading to a true disseminated intravascular coagulopathy with intravascular thrombosis, marked organ dysfunction, and, potentially, death.

Management

The specific management of exotic envenomations is beyond the scope of this chapter. Not all venomous exotic snakes have antivenoms, and even for snakes with antivenoms, none may be available in the United States, but zoos stock antivenoms for snakes in their collections. An updateable online database, the Antivenom Index, lists these antivenoms and is accessible by regional poison centers. For information on exotic antivenoms and assistance in managing an exotic snake envenomation, the regional poison center should be contacted (1-800-222-1222).

References

Boyer LV, Seifert SA, Cain JS: Recurrence phenomena after immunoglobulin therapy for snake envenomations. Part 2. Guidelines for clinical management with Crotaline Fab antivenom, *Ann Emerg Med* 37:196–201, 2001.

Boyer LV, Seifert SA, Clark RF, et al: Recurrent and persistent coagulopathy following pit viper envenomation, *Arch Intern Med* 159(7):706–710, 1999.

Bush SP, Ruha AM, Seifert SA, et al: Comparison of F(ab')2 versus Fab antivenom for pit viper envenomation: a prospective, blinded, multicenter, randomized clinical trial, *Clin Toxicol (Phila)* 53(1):37–45, 2015 Jan, Available at: https://doi.org/10.3109/15563650.2014.974263, Epub 2014 Oct 31.

Bush SP, Seifert SA, Oakes J, et al: Continuous IV crotalidae polyvalent immune fab (ovine) (FabAV) for selected North American rattlesnake bite patients, *Toxicon* 69:29–37, 2013, Epub 2013 Mar 6 Available at: https://doi.org/10.1016/j.toxicon.2013.02.008.

Extension of Expiration Date of Coral Snake Antivenin: https://www.fda.gov/vaccines-blood-biologics/safety-availability-biologics/expiration-date-extension-north--american-coral-snake-antivenin-micrurus-fulvius-equine-origin-lot-1

Gerardo CJ, Quackenbush E, Lewis B, et al: The efficacy of crotalidae polyvalent immune fab (ovine) antivenom versus placebo plus optional rescue therapy on recovery from copperhead snake envenomation: a randomized, double-blind, placebo-controlled, clinical trial, *Ann Emerg Med* 70(2):233–244, 2017 Aug.

Gold BS, Barish RA, Dart RC: North American snake envenomation: Diagnosis, treatment, and management, *Emerg Med Clin North Am* 22(2):423–443, 2004, ix.

Kitchens CS, Van Mierop LH: Envenomation by the Eastern coral snake (*Micrurus fulvius fulvius*). A study of 39 victims, *JAMA* 258(12):1615–1618, 1987.

Seifert SA, Boyer LV: Recurrence phenomena after immunoglobulin therapy for snake envenomations. Part 1. Pharmacokinetics and pharmacodynamics of immunoglobulin antivenoms and related antibodies, *Ann Emerg Med* 37(2):189–195, 2001.

Seifert SA, Boyer LV, Dart RC, et al: Relationship of venom effects to venom antigen and antivenom serum concentrations in a patient with *Crotalus atrox* envenomation treated with a Fab antivenom, *Ann Emerg Med* 30(1):49–53, 1997.

Seifert SA, Kirschner RI, Martin N: Recurrent, persistent, or late, new-onset hematologic abnormalities in crotaline snakebite, *Clin Toxicol (Phila)* 49:324–329, 2011. Available at: https://doi.org/10.3109/15563650.2011.566883.

Seifert SA, Oakes JA, Boyer LV: Toxic Exposure Surveillance System (TESS)-based characterization of U.S. non-native venomous snake exposures, 1995–2004, *Clin Toxicol (Phila)* 45(5):571–578, 2007.

21 Preventive Health

IMMUNIZATION PRACTICES

Method of
Beth A. Damitz, MD

CURRENT DIAGNOSIS

- Single-agent and poly-agent variety vaccines are available in the United States.
- Vaccine-preventable diseases are occurring in the United States despite efforts.
- Vaccine registries and office-based strategies can increase vaccination rates.

CURRENT THERAPY

- Vaccination schedules are available through various sources such as the CDC, including catch-up dosing.
- Vaccines can prevent diseases that are still occurring in the United States.
- Vaccination registry participation can increase vaccination rates.
- Each office visit should be used as an opportunity to review and offer vaccines.
- Providers need to be aware of special populations such as breast-feeding and pregnant women, immunosuppressed persons, and health care workers who could need different vaccines.

Definitions and Background

Vaccination is one of the most successful and cost-effective ways to prevent infectious diseases. Immunization is the process of inducing immunity artificially by either active immunization or passive immunization. It also occurs naturally through transplacental transmission of antibodies to a fetus, which provides protection against many infectious diseases for the first few months of life.

Physiology of Vaccines

Vaccines prevent disease in the people who receive them and protect those who come into contact with unvaccinated individuals such as children too young to receive vaccines, those who cannot be immunized for medical reasons, and those who cannot make an adequate response to vaccination. Vaccines are preparations of proteins, polysaccharides, or nucleic acids of pathogens that are delivered to the immune system as single entities, as part of complex particles, or by live, attenuated agents to induce specific responses that inactivate, destroy, or suppress the pathogen.

Immunization Recommendations

The Advisory Committee on Immunization Practices (ACIP) sponsored by the Centers for Disease Control (CDC; https://www

.cdc.gov/vaccines/schedules/hcp/index.html), the American Academy of Pediatrics (AAP), and the American Academy of Family Practice (AAFP) work together to issue a national schedule for routinely recommended vaccinations. They recommend routine vaccination to prevent 17 vaccine-preventable diseases that occur in infants, children, adolescents, or adults. These recommendations are reviewed and revised periodically. These immunization schedules give ranges of target ages for vaccines to be given (Figures 1 to 3). They include single and combination vaccine products. Catch-up dosing and special-population schedules are also available (updated immunization schedules are available https://www.cdc.gov/vaccines/schedules/index.html).

Disease Prevention

Since the development of vaccines, we have seen a dramatic decrease in both cases and deaths from vaccine-preventable diseases. For example, in 1950, there were 319,124 cases and 468 deaths from measles. This dramatically decreased to 43 cases and zero deaths in 2007. Obviously, decrease in disease and death is paramount, but in addition is the decrease in cost burden to our health care system. For every $1 spent on measles, mumps, and rubella (MMR) vaccine, $21 is saved in direct medical costs of treating a case of measles.

Immunization Responsibility

Appropriate vaccination is the responsibility of the health care team and patient (and parents). Education is critical. This can be done through various dissemination techniques such as one-on-one counseling, posters in the office, health fairs, and handouts at school and work. An office-based strategy consists of nursing and physician education of updates and changes in vaccines, the ability to track patient immunization records through registries, sending reminder letters to patients that there are vaccines they are recommended to have, and adopting standing orders to take advantage of appropriate office visits to maximize vaccination opportunities.

There are many sources for keeping current on immunizations and vaccines including the CDC's *Morbidity and Mortality Weekly Report* (MMWR). For parents and patients, the vaccine information statement (VIS), which is made available by the CDC to inform patients about the risks and benefits of immunizations, is very helpful and by law must be distributed before administering any vaccine. After the patient reads the VIS, the physician can then give any further information or answer questions before administering the vaccine. This discussion should be documented in the patient's medical record, including the refusal to receive certain vaccines (i.e., informed refusal).

General Principles for Vaccine Scheduling

Optimal response to a vaccine depends on several factors, including the type of vaccine, age of the recipient, and immune status of the recipient. Simultaneous administration of vaccines increases the probability that a patient will be vaccinated fully by the appropriate age. Simultaneous administration of all age-appropriate doses of vaccines is recommended by the MMWR for children for whom no specific contraindications exist at the time of the visit. The use of combination vaccine preparations greatly reduces the overall number of injections a child or patient will

(FOR THOSE WHO FALL BEHIND OR START LATE, SEE THE CATCH-UP SCHEDULE [FIGURE 2]).

These recommendations must be read with the footnotes that follow. For those who fall behind or start late, provide catch-up vaccination at the earliest opportunity as indicated by the green bars in Figure 1. To determine minimum intervals between doses, see the catch-up schedule (Figure 2). School entry and adolescent vaccine age groups are shaded in gray.

Vaccine	Birth	1 mo	2 mos	4 mos	6 mos	9 mos	12 mos	15 mos	18 mos	19-23 mos	2-3 yrs	4-6 yrs	7-10 yrs	11-12 yrs	13-15 yrs	16 yrs	17-18 yrs
Hepatitis B[1] (HepB)	1st dose	←2nd dose→			←———— 3rd dose ————→												
Rotavirus[2] (RV) RV1 (2-dose series); RV5 (3-dose series)			1st dose	2nd dose	See footnote 2												
Diphtheria, tetanus, & acellular pertussis[3] (DTaP: <7 yrs)			1st dose	2nd dose	3rd dose		←———— 4th dose ————→					5th dose					
Haemophilus influenzae type b[4] (Hib)			1st dose	2nd dose	See footnote 4		←3rd or 4th dose, See footnote 4→										
Pneumococcal conjugate[5] (PCV13)			1st dose	2nd dose	3rd dose		←———— 4th dose ————→										
Inactivated poliovirus[6] (IPV: <18 yrs)			1st dose	2nd dose	←———— 3rd dose ————→							4th dose					
Influenza[7] (IIV)								Annual vaccination (IIV) 1 or 2 doses					Annual vaccination (IIV) 1 dose only				
Measles, mumps, rubella[8] (MMR)					See footnote 8		←———— 1st dose ————→					2nd dose					
Varicella[9] (VAR)							←———— 1st dose ————→					2nd dose					
Hepatitis A[10] (HepA)							←———— 2-dose series, See footnote 10 ————→										
Meningococcal[11] (MenACWY-D ≥9 mos; MenACWY-CRM ≥2 mos)						See footnote 11								1st dose		2nd dose	
Tetanus, diphtheria, & acellular pertussis[13] (Tdap: ≥7 yrs)														Tdap			
Human papillomavirus[14] (HPV)														See footnote 14			
Meningococcal B[12]														See footnote 12			
Pneumococcal polysaccharide[5] (PPSV23)												See footnote 5					

Legend:
- Range of recommended ages for all children
- Range of recommended ages for catch-up immunization
- Range of recommended ages for certain high-risk groups
- Range of recommended ages for high-risk groups
- Range of recommended ages for non-high-risk groups that may receive vaccine, subject to individual clinical decision making
- No recommendation

NOTE: The above recommendations must be read along with the footnotes of this schedule.

Figure 1 Recommended Immunization Schedule for Children and Adolescents Aged 18 Years or Younger—United States, 2019.

This figure should be reviewed with the accompanying footnotes. This figure and the footnotes describe indications for which vaccines, if not previously administered, should be administered unless noted otherwise.

Vaccine	19–21 years	22–26 years	27–49 years	50–64 years	≥65 years
Influenza[1]	1 dose annually				
Tdap[2] or Td[2]	1 dose Tdap, then Td booster every 10 yrs				
MMR[3]	1 or 2 doses depending on indication (if born in 1957 or later)				
VAR[4]	2 doses				
RZV[5] (preferred)				2 doses RZV (preferred)	
ZVL[5]				1 dose ZVL	
HPV–Female[6]	2 or 3 doses depending on age at series initiation		1 or 2 doses depending on indication		
HPV–Male[6]	2 or 3 doses depending on age at series initiation		1 or 2 doses depending on indication		
PCV13[7]	1 or 2 doses depending on indication				1 dose
PPSV23[7]	1 or 2 doses depending on indication				1 dose
HepA[8]	2 or 3 doses depending on vaccine				
HepB[9]	3 doses				
MenACWY[10]	1 or 2 doses depending on indication, then booster every 5 yrs if risk remains				
MenB[10]	2 or 3 doses depending on vaccine				
Hib[11]	1 or 3 doses depending on indication				

Recommended for adults who meet the age requirement, lack documentation of vaccination, or lack evidence of past infection

Recommended for adults with other indications

No recommendation

Figure 2 Recommended immunization schedule for adults aged 19 years or older by age group, United States, 2019.

This figure should be reviewed with the accompanying footnotes. This figure and the footnotes describe indications for which vaccines, if not previously administered, should be administered unless noted otherwise.

Vaccine	Pregnancy[1-6]	Immuno-compromised (excluding HIV infection)[3-7,11]	HIV infection CD4+ count (cells/µL)[3-7,9-10] <200	HIV infection CD4+ count (cells/µL)[3-7,9-10] ≥200	Asplenia, complement deficiencies[7,10,11]	End-stage renal disease, on hemodialysis[7,9]	Heart or lung disease, alcoholism[7]	Chronic liver disease[7-9]	Diabetes[7,9]	Health care personnel[3,4,9]	Men who have sex with men[6,8,9]
Influenza[1]	1 dose annually										
Tdap[2] or Td[2]	1 dose Tdap each pregnancy	1 dose Tdap, then Td booster every 10 yrs									
MMR[3]	contraindicated	contraindicated	contraindicated		1 or 2 doses depending on indication						
VAR[4]	contraindicated	contraindicated	contraindicated		2 doses						
RZV[5] (preferred)					2 doses RZV at age ≥50 yrs (preferred)						
— or —											
ZVL[5]	contraindicated	contraindicated	contraindicated		1 dose ZVL at age ≥60 yrs						
HPV-Female[6]	3 doses through age 26 yrs	3 doses through age 26 yrs			2 or 3 doses through age 26 yrs						
HPV-Male[6]	3 doses through age 26 yrs	3 doses through age 26 yrs			2 or 3 doses through age 21 yrs						2 or 3 doses through age 26 yrs
PCV13[7]					1 dose						
PPSV23[7]					1, 2, or 3 doses depending on indication						
HepA[8]					2 or 3 doses depending on vaccine						
HepB[9]					3 doses						
MenACWY[10]					1 or 2 doses depending on indication , then booster every 5 yrs if risk remains						
MenB[10]					2 or 3 doses depending on vaccine						
Hib[11]		3 doses HSCT recipients only			1 dose						

Recommended for adults who meet the age requirement, lack documentation of vaccination, or lack evidence of past infection

Recommended for adults with other indications

Contraindicated

No recommendation

Figure 3 Recommended immunization schedule for adults aged 19 years or older by medical condition and other indications, United States, 2019.

receive. However, care must be taken to ensure that the individual vaccine entities are not administered too early and are not administered too many at once. This can be a challenge when patients switch clinics or in times of vaccine shortages.

More often, dosing intervals longer than recommended are encountered in the office. With the exception of oral live typhoid vaccine (Vivotif Berna), an interruption in the vaccination schedule does not require restarting the entire series of a vaccine or toxoid or addition of extra doses. When an unknown or uncertain vaccination status is encountered, every effort should be made to access records. If this cannot be done in a reasonable amount of time, these persons should be considered susceptible and started on the age-appropriate vaccination schedule. Serologic testing for immunity is an alternative to vaccination; however, commercial serologic testing might not always be sufficiently sensitive or standardized for detection of vaccine-induced immunity, and research laboratory testing might not be readily available.

Route of Administration
There are two orally administered vaccines in the United States: rotavirus (Rotarix, RotaTeq) and typhoid vaccines. Rotavirus is licensed for infants and does not need to be repeated if the vaccine is spit up or vomited. Typhoid vaccine capsules should be taken as directed by the manufacturer. Live, attenuated influenza vaccine (LAIV, FluMist) is the only intranasal vaccine available. It does not need to be repeated if the person coughs or sneezes immediately after administration. With the exception of bacille Calmette-Guérin (BCG) vaccine and smallpox vaccine,[1] injectable vaccines are administered by the intramuscular or subcutaneous route.

Storage
In general, vaccines need to be stored in a refrigerator or freezer. When vaccines are inappropriately stored, they can lose potency. Refrigerator and freezer storage units must be properly monitored and maintained to assure vaccine integrity. Temperature logs should be maintained for 3 years unless state or local authorities require a longer time. Vaccines that have been stored at inappropriate temperatures should not be administered. An office protocol should be established for handling inappropriately stored vaccines, procedures for follow-up when these vaccines are inadvertently given, emergency vaccine retrieval and storage, handling vaccine shipments, maintaining a vaccine inventory log, and rotating vaccine stock to avoid expiration. Care should be taken to store similar vaccine products (sound-alike or lookalike) away from each other (on different shelves) or by color-coding labels. Diphtheria toxoid-, tetanus toxoid-, and acellular pertussis-containing vaccines are easily confused.

Vaccine Safety
Vaccines in the United States undergo extensive safety and efficacy evaluations through the FDA licensing process. Despite this rigorous process, adverse reactions can and do occur. Adverse reactions are reportable to the Vaccine Adverse Event Reporting System (VAERS). VAERS is a national reporting system created in 1990 to unify the collection of all reports of adverse events after vaccination. Its primary purpose is detecting new or rare vaccine adverse events, increases in rates of known side effects, and risk factors for particular types of adverse events.

In 1986, the National Childhood Vaccine Injury Act established the Vaccine Injury Compensation Program (VICP). It is a no-fault program that covers all routinely recommended childhood vaccines. Those claims may be based on a vaccine injury table, which lists the adverse events associated with vaccines and provides a rebuttable presumption of causation, or by proving by preponderance evidence that the vaccine caused an injury not on the table. The table was created to provide swift compensation to those possibly injured by vaccines.

The provider's role to help ensure safety of vaccination includes proper vaccine storage and administration, timing and spacing of vaccine doses, observation of contraindications and precautions, and reporting adverse events to the VAERS.

Contraindications and Adverse Events
A contraindication is a condition in a recipient that increases the chance of a *serious* adverse reaction. A precaution is a condition in a recipient that *might* increase the chance or severity of an adverse reaction or compromise the ability of the vaccine to produce immunity. Situations do arise when the benefits outweigh the risks of a side effect. The only contraindication applicable to all vaccines is a history of a severe allergic reaction (anaphylaxis) after a previous dose of vaccine or to a vaccine component unless the recipient has been desensitized. Children who experienced encephalopathy within 7 days after administration of a previous dose of DTP,[2] DTaP (Daptacel, Infanrix), or Tdap (Adacel, Boostrix) not attributable to another identifiable cause should not receive additional doses of a vaccine that contains pertussis. The following are *not* contraindications to vaccination:

- Minor illness
- Diarrhea
- Mild or moderate local reaction or fever following a prior dose
- Antimicrobial therapy
- Disease exposure or convalescence
- Pregnant or immunosuppressed person in the household
- Premature birth
- Breast-feeding

Vaccination should be deferred for persons with a moderate or severe acute illness. This precaution avoids causing diagnostic confusion between manifestations of the underlying illness and possible adverse effects of vaccination or superimposing adverse effects of the vaccine on the underlying illness.

Vaccine adverse reactions are classified as local, systemic, or allergic. Allergic reactions might be caused by the vaccine antigen, residual animal protein, antimicrobial agents, preservatives, stabilizers, or other vaccine components. Anaphylaxis is rare and usually begins within minutes of vaccine administration. Children who have had an apparent severe allergic reaction to a vaccine should be evaluated by an allergist to determine the responsible allergen and to make recommendations regarding future vaccination.

Barriers
Barriers to appropriate and timely vaccination include patients' misconceptions, false contraindications, complexity of the immunization schedules, religious or philosophical beliefs, and cost. The Vaccines for Children Program (VCP) is a federally funded program that provides free ACIP-recommended vaccines to adolescents and children younger than 19 years old. This program has reduced the barrier of cost.

Recording Vaccinations
Health care providers who administer vaccines covered by the National Childhood Vaccine Injury Act are required to ensure that the permanent medical record of the recipient indicates the date the vaccine was administered, the vaccine manufacturer, the vaccine lot number, and the name, address, and title of the person administering the vaccine. In addition, the provider is required to record the edition date of the VIS distributed and the date those materials were provided. Patients should also keep a record of the immunizations they receive, when they were received, and at what facility they received them. A permanent vaccination record card should be established for each newborn infant and maintained by the parent or guardian.

Immunization information systems (IIS), formerly referred to as immunization registries, are confidential population-based computerized information systems that collect and consolidate

---

[1]Available in the United States from the Centers for Disease Control and Prevention.

[2]Not available in the United States.

vaccination data from multiple health care providers within a geographic area. The CDC oversees a network of 64 IIS programs distributed throughout all 50 states, the District of Columbia, and eight U.S. territories. A fully operational IIS can prevent duplicate vaccinations, provide a complete record of immunizations if the patient has received vaccines from multiple sites, and offer catch-up and needed vaccine information. Although participation of a provider is voluntary, it is highly encouraged.

Special Populations
Children
Although infants are born with some level of immunoglobulin (Ig)G that is contributed from the mother via passive immunity, these levels generally decrease by 9 months of age, leaving them vulnerable to many infectious diseases. Infants begin developing IgG shortly after birth and continue to increase these levels throughout the first year of life, but they remain generally susceptible to infection until they achieve adult levels of IgG at 10 years of age. Therefore this age group is especially important to vaccinate.

Breast-feeding
Neither inactivated nor live virus vaccines administered to a lactating woman affect the safety of breast-feeding for women or their infants. Breast-feeding is a contraindication for small-pox vaccination of the mother because of the theoretical risk for contact transmission from mother to infant. Yellow fever vaccine (YF-VAX) should be avoided. Breast-fed infants should be vaccinated according to the recommended schedule.

Pregnancy
No evidence exists of risk to the fetus from vaccinating pregnant women with inactivated virus or bacterial vaccines or toxoids. Live vaccines, such as smallpox, MMR, and varicella (Varivax), pose a theoretical risk to the fetus and therefore are generally contraindicated during pregnancy. New recommendations from ACIP advise to give all pregnant women a Tdap in every pregnancy. New data indicate that maternal antipertussis antibodies are short-lived; therefore Tdap vaccination in one pregnancy will not provide high levels of antibodies to protect newborns during subsequent pregnancies. Alternatively, if Tdap is not administered during pregnancy, the woman should receive a dose of Tdap as soon as possible after delivery to ensure pertussis immunity and reduce the risk for transmission to the newborn regardless of when she last received a tetanus booster. Routine influenza vaccination is recommended for all women who are or will be pregnant (in any trimester) during influenza season, which usually occurs early October through late March.

Altered Immunocompetence
Persons with altered immunocompetence include those with primary and secondary causes of immunodeficiency as well as those with asplenia, chronic kidney disease, treatments with therapeutic monoclonal antibodies, and prolonged administration of high-dose corticosteroids. In general they should receive trivalent inactivated influenza virus (TIV, Fluzone) and age-appropriate polysaccharide-based vaccines (pneumococcal conjugate vaccine [PCV, Prevnar], pneumococcal polyvalent [PPSV, Pneumovax 23], meningococcal conjugate [MCV4, Menactra], meningococcal polysaccharide [MPSV4, Menomune] and haemophilus B conjugate [Hib, ActHib, PedvaxHib]). Persons with most forms of altered immunocompetence should not receive live vaccines (MMR, varicella, MMRV [ProQuad], LAIV, zoster [Zostavax], yellow fever, oral typhoid, BCG, and rotavirus).

Health Care Personnel
Health care personnel are considered to be at substantial risk for acquiring or transmitting hepatitis B, influenza, measles, mumps, rubella, pertussis, and varicella and should be counseled on appropriate vaccinations.

TRAVEL MEDICINE
Method of
Jane Zuckerman, MD; and Yael Paran, MD

International travel is increasing, with the global air passenger market forecast to grow by 3.9% per annum. In 2018, international tourist arrivals in all countries exceeded 1.4 billion persons; it is estimated that the number of flights worldwide will more than double in the next 20 years. Such statistics exemplify the ever-increasing need for the specialty of travel medicine to protect the health of all groups of travelers.

Eight percent of travelers seek health care assistance either while abroad or upon returning home, with 22% to 64% of travelers reporting some type of illness. Most of the latter are mild and self-limiting, with diarrhea, respiratory infections, and skin disorders being the most common; however, some illnesses can be severe in returning travelers. Approximately 4% of travelers who seek medical help have an acute potentially life-threatening infectious disease, the most common being *falciparum* malaria. The most common causes of death in travelers are noninfectious, with the leading causes of death being cardiovascular events among older travelers and motor vehicle accidents among younger travelers.

The goal of a travel medicine visit is to maximize health and to prevent illness while traveling through the use of appropriate drugs and immunizations. Knowledge of disease risk, current outbreaks, and local health conditions relevant to each destination is constantly changing; thus, the use of current, updated resources is essential. Table 1 lists several recommended information resources.

The preferred timing of a pretravel health consultation is usually 6 to 8 weeks before travel for most travelers but may be longer when travelers are going overseas for long-term employment or several months of travel. The pretravel health consultation should be structured and comprehensive. Table 2 lists items that might require consideration and discussion during consultation. Patients should be asked to arrive with documentation of previous vaccinations. The consultation should begin with details including information regarding the proposed travel itinerary, type of travel, purpose of travel, and planned activities and information regarding the patient's medical history, including age, underlying diseases, allergies, current medications, pregnancy status, and previous vaccination status. A useful "travel history form" is available on the Shoreland Travax website.

Vaccinations
When deciding which vaccination to recommend, several factors must be considered, including any specific potential risks associated with the travel itinerary, length of stay, and activities. For each vaccine-preventable disease (VPD), one should consider the prevalence and impact of the disease in question.

Routine Vaccinations
The travel health practitioner should confirm that the traveler is up to date with routine vaccinations. Most travelers from developed countries will have received routine childhood vaccinations or experienced the illnesses themselves and are therefore naturally immune. Nevertheless, some destinations require a booster immunization. In contrast, some travelers born in less developed countries might not have been fully immunized as children. The pretravel health consultation is a good "checkpoint" to verify routine vaccination status, which is important beyond the immediate requirement for travel. For example, measles, one of the most contagious diseases, is more common in developing countries because vaccine coverage is poor, leaving many susceptible to infection.

Measles-Mumps-Rubella Vaccine
Measles remains a serious cause of morbidity and mortality in the non-Western world. Importation of measles from regions that

TABLE 1	List of Information Resources for Risk Assessment of Travel.	
Centers for Disease Control and Prevention	Comprehensive travel reports and travel vaccination and preparation information including the Yellow Book with information on country-specific risks and travel advice	www.cdc.gov/travel/
Travax (Shoreland)	Commercial software-generated reports combining itinerary-specific recommendations on recommended travel vaccines and risks. Requires a fee.	www.shoreland.com
U.S. Department of State	Travel warnings	https://travel.state.gov/content/passports/en/alertswarnings.html
World Health Organization	General travel health information and access to its international travel guide and alerts	www.who.int/ith/en/

TABLE 2	Checklist of Items to Address in the Pretravel Consultation*
CATEGORY	**ISSUES THAT SHOULD BE ADDRESSED**
Patient risk assessment	Obtain history: itinerary, type of travel, personal medical history, age, underlying diseases, allergies, current medication, pregnancy status, previous vaccination status
Immunizations	Update routine immunization Provide routine travel immunization Provide destination-specific immunization
Malaria prophylaxis	If indicated: Provide malaria education and advice; discuss bite avoidance measures Prescribe antimalaria prophylaxis
Travelers' diarrhea	Prescribe self-treatment medication
Prevention against mosquito bites	Give advice regarding mosquito-borne disease Discuss personal protection measures
Rabies prevention	Give advice regarding behavior near animals Discuss measures to be taken if bitten or scratched by an animal—seek urgent medical advice Administer vaccine where indicated
Altitude sickness	Provide education Prescribe acetazolamide (Diamox) 125 mg orally twice a day, for 1 day before ascent, continuing for 2–3 days on arrival at maximum altitude.
Prevention of sexually transmitted diseases	Provide education regarding safe sex
Zika	Discuss potential risk of congenital Zika syndrome for pregnant women or women/men planning to conceive following return from an endemic area
Others	Deep venous thrombosis prevention Accident prevention Motion sickness

*Some of the recommendations are indicated only for specific destinations or specific at-risk groups.

report endemic disease such as Europe, Africa, and parts of Asia remains one of the main reasons for outbreaks in areas where there is interrupted transmission (like the Americas). Indeed, several cases have even been associated with transmission during air travel itself.

The measles-mumps-rubella (MMR) vaccine is routinely recommended for the following:

- All children from the age of 12 months. Younger children traveling to endemic areas might require a first dose of MMR vaccine at age 6 months but will still need the standard two-dose schedule after the age of 12 months to ensure immunity.
- Nonimmune children and adolescents who did not complete a childhood series.
- Adults born after 1956 in the United States (1970 or later in Canada and the United Kingdom; 1966 or later in Australia) without evidence of immunity, regardless of level of risk.
- If there is no record of prior immunization, you can either check for immunity (IgG) or give a booster vaccine. There is no harm in providing a dose of MMR vaccine for any patient who requests it provided there are no contraindications to the vaccine.

These groups should receive two doses of the vaccine after the age of 12 months, with at least 4 weeks having elapsed between the doses. The effectiveness of the individual measles, mumps, and rubella components of the MMR vaccine after one dose is 95% to 98%, 94%, and 95%, respectively. After two doses, more than 99% will be protected against measles and rubella (90% to 95% against mumps) for more than 20 years.

Poliovirus Vaccine

Owing to successful efforts to eradicate poliomyelitis, most of the world is now polio-free. As of 2016, Afghanistan and Pakistan are the only countries that still have endemic wild-type poliovirus infections, but outbreaks from importation of polio from endemic countries can occur. In 2012 and 2013, outbreaks of imported polio occurred in seven countries in Africa and the Middle East. In addition, a small number of developing countries continue to report cases of circulating vaccine-derived poliovirus (cVDPV). A single adult booster of poliovirus vaccine is recommended for travelers to endemic areas who have received the primary childhood series. A country is considered "endemic" when local disease is due to wild-type infection *or* to cVDPV. An inactivated, injectable poliovirus vaccine (IPV) (Ipol) is available for adults and children.

Since 2014, in view of the risk of international spread, the World Health Organization (WHO) has issued temporary polio vaccine exit recommendations under the authority of the International Health Regulations (IHR) for long-term travelers (staying > 4 weeks) and residents departing from countries with either wild poliovirus (WPV) transmission or cVDPV transmission. As of 2017, countries covered by the WHO vaccine exit recommendation are Afghanistan, Nigeria, Pakistan, Guinea, Laos, and Madagascar. These recommendations are likely to change from time to time. A small number of individual countries also require proof of polio vaccination prior to entering the country.

Tetanus-Diphtheria-Pertussis Vaccine

Unvaccinated or inadequately vaccinated travelers are at risk of contracting diphtheria in developing countries, as well as tetanus and pertussis anywhere in the world. The potential risk of exposure to pertussis is worldwide, with the highest rates of disease being found in developing countries where vaccine coverage is low. In recent decades there has also been a resurgence of pertussis in several developed countries despite adequate vaccine programs, including the United States. One explanation for this phenomenon involves waning of immunity in adulthood following receipt of the currently used acellular pertussis vaccine series given in childhood. Adolescents and adults who completed the childhood series of DTaP (Daptacel, Infanrix) and did not previously receive Tdap (Adacel, Boostrix) should receive a one-time Tdap vaccine before travel, instead of a Td booster, to booster their immunity against pertussis.

If more than 5 years have elapsed since the last booster dose, a tetanus-containing booster should be considered for persons going to remote areas where tetanus boosters may not be readily available, to eliminate the need for in-country vaccination after contaminated trauma. A Tdap booster is recommended every 10 years and can be given regardless of the interval from the last Td booster.

Varicella Vaccine

Varicella remains prevalent worldwide. The morbidity and mortality associated with varicella increases with age, with pregnant women and their unborn or newborn children being especially prone to severe sequelae. Travelers without either a history of the disease or documented immunity should consider receiving a course of the vaccine, especially if they will be living close to the local community. In several developed countries including the United States, varicella vaccine (VARIVAX) is now part of the routine childhood vaccine program, while most adults are immune to the disease because of past infection.

Influenza Vaccine

Influenza is the most common VPD among travelers. Travelers aged 6 months and older should receive the most up-to-date influenza vaccine available in their countries if traveling to an area where influenza is circulating at the time of their travel (year-round in tropical and subtropical areas, and winter months in temperate areas).

Pneumococcal Vaccine

The prevalence of pneumococcal disease is highest in developing countries. Since 2014, the Advisory Committee of Immunization Practices (ACIP) of the Centers for Disease Control and Prevention (CDC) recommends administration of pneumococcal conjugate vaccine (PCV13; Prevnar13) to all individuals 65 years or older who did not receive a pneumococcal vaccine in the past, followed by a dose of pneumococcal polysaccharide vaccine (PPSV23; Pneumovax) given 1 or more years later for immune-competent individuals and 8 or more weeks later for immune-compromised patients. This recommendation is not implemented in several developed countries, which continue to administer polysaccharide vaccine (PPSV23; Pneumovax) to otherwise healthy individuals 65 years or older.

Routine Travel Vaccination

Hepatitis A Vaccine

Hepatitis A is the second most common VPD in travelers after influenza. A vaccine for hepatitis A is recommended to people traveling to any developing country and even some industrialized countries where sanitary conditions are variable. The vaccine is recommended for travel of any duration and for any purpose.

Two hepatitis A vaccine preparations are available (Havrix, Vaqta), which are approved for administration in those aged 12 months or older. A combination of hepatitis A and B vaccines (Twinrix) is also available and is approved for people aged 18 years or older, with accelerated schedules available to provide protection for those traveling at short notice. A single dose of hepatitis A vaccine given any time before travel will provide complete protection for healthy persons. A booster dose is generally recommended at 6 to 12 months after the second dose to ensure long-term protection, but recent studies have shown that protection after only one dose can last for years. A 2012 position paper of the WHO stated that use of a single-dose schedule for hepatitis A can be considered; however, this does not apply to

immune-compromised individuals or at-risk groups, for whom a two-dose schedule is still recommended.

Typhoid Vaccine

Although hepatitis A and typhoid are both transmitted by contaminated food and water, hepatitis A is 100 times more common than typhoid in travelers. The Indian subcontinent seems to be a key focus of typhoid in travelers, accounting for more than 80% of travel-related cases in the United States. The efficacy of typhoid vaccines ranges from 50% to 80% in various published studies.

Typhoid vaccine is protective against *Salmonella enterica* serotype *typhi*, but not against paratyphoid fever, which is caused by strains of *Salmonella enterica* paratyphi A, B, and C. Typhoid vaccine is recommended to long-term travelers to developing countries and short-term travelers to South Asia, as well as for other destinations for high-risk groups such as travelers visiting friends and relatives and food adventurers.

Two vaccines are available: the oral live, attenuated typhoid vaccine (Ty21A, Vivotif Berna) and the injectable typhoid V1 polysaccharide vaccine (Typhim Vi). The oral vaccine, which consists of four capsules (one taken every other day), should be completed at least 1 week before travel, and the injectable vaccine should be given at least 1 week before travel.

Hepatitis B

Hepatitis B is endemic worldwide. In Asia, the Middle East, Eastern and Southern Europe, sub-Saharan Africa (excluding West Africa), and Russia, disease prevalence is intermediate (2% to 7%), while in West Africa, the prevalence is high (≥8%). The vaccine (Engerix-B, Recombivax HB) is recommended for long-stay travelers to intermediate- and high-prevalence areas, and for short stays for high-risk groups such as travelers who are likely to have new sexual partners during travel and those with underlying medical conditions that may cause them to seek medical care while abroad. Health care workers should be vaccinated for any destination, regardless of the period of travel. The availability of accelerated schedules of administration of monovalent and combination hepatitis B vaccines enables rapid protection to be given when necessary.

Geographically Targeted Vaccines

Yellow Fever Vaccine

Yellow fever is a mosquito-borne disease endemic in parts of sub-Saharan Africa and tropical South America. It is reported rarely in travelers, with only 10 cases documented during 1970–2013, and two more reported from 2016 to 2017. The risk of a traveler acquiring yellow fever varies with season, location, activities, and duration of travel. For a 2-week stay, the estimated risk for illness attributed to yellow fever for an unvaccinated traveler to West Africa is 50 cases per 100,000 population; for South America, the risk for illness is 5 cases per 100,000 population. The vaccine is recommended for personal protection of travelers to endemic areas. In addition, under WHO rules, any given country may routinely require vaccination for entry into its territory. Valid yellow fever vaccinations must be administered at an authorized site, recorded on a WHO standardized yellow card, and completed at least 10 days before entry. The aim of the regulation is to protect countries that have the mosquito vector, which can potentially introduce the virus by virtue of a viremic traveler.

Yellow fever vaccine (YF-VAX) is a live attenuated preparation that has been rarely associated with severe and even fatal adverse reactions—generally following a first dose to the individual. The overall rate of serious adverse reaction is 1 event per 250,000 doses. The likelihood of serious adverse events increases with age, with patients older than age 60 years having a much higher risk for severe adverse reaction than younger people, and in particular those with a history of thymus dysfunction or myasthenia gravis, which is associated significantly with a disease affecting the thymus gland (thymic hyperplasia or thymoma). The incidence of yellow fever-associated neurotropic disease (YEL-AND) is 17 per million doses in those older than 60 years of age and 4 per million in those younger than 60 years of age. The incidence of yellow fever-associated viscerotropic disease is 20.5 per million in those older than 60 years of age and 3 per million in those younger than 60 years of age. The decision on the need for administering yellow fever vaccine should consider the benefit from the vaccine versus the potential risk.

A change in the IHR since July 2016 now considers a valid yellow fever vaccination as effective for life, with no need for boosters at 10-year intervals. This also applies retrospectively to yellow fever vaccines given any time before 2016. The new policy also extends to the validity of the vaccine for personal protection, with no need for booster doses among healthy, immunecompetent individuals. A booster vaccine after 10 years is still recommended for specific high-risk individuals: long-term travelers, travelers to West Africa, and travelers to an area where there is a current outbreak.

Japanese Encephalitis

Japanese encephalitis (JE) is a mosquito-borne arbovirus disease found primarily in China, Korea, the Indian subcontinent, Southeast Asia, and the Western Pacific. JE has a mortality rate of up to 30% and is rarely reported in travelers. The risk varies according to destination, duration, season, and activities being undertaken. The risk is highest for travelers to rural areas, travel in the active transmission period, and travelers who plan nighttime outdoor activities. The overall incidence of JE among persons from nonendemic countries traveling to Asia is estimated to be less than 1 case per 1 million. Only 55 cases of travel-associated JE were reported between 1973 and 2008, with most cases reported from Thailand and Bali.

A killed-cell vaccine, IXIARO, is licensed in the United States for use in persons aged 2 months or older. Children 2 months to 2 years old are given half the dose used for adults. The vaccine is given as a two-dose series, at 0 and 28 days. Recent studies on accelerated vaccine schedules for travelers who are unable to receive the vaccine 28 days before departure have shown that a two-dose schedule of the vaccine given at an interval of 1 week provides good immunogenicity for up to 2 months postvaccination. Results for longer duration of protection using this accelerated schedule are currently unknown.

Rabies

Rabies exists worldwide, with only small pockets of the world being rabies-free. Disease rates are highest in Asia, Africa, and South and Central America. Dogs remain the primary vector, but bats are increasingly important sources. From 1990 to 2013, 66 cases of rabies were documented in travelers—40% from Asia, and 85% following canine exposure. Bites from animals during travel are common. Approximately 2700 travelers received care for animal-related exposures and required rabies postexposure prophylaxis at GeoSentinel clinics during a 15-year period (1997–2012). Of note, the median duration of stay for these travelers was less than 1 month. In another study, 1.6% of Israeli travelers traveling for more than a month had experienced an injury from a potentially rabid animal.

A three-dose preexposure course of rabies vaccine (Imovax Rabies, RabAvert) can be administered before travel. In the event of an exposure, persons vaccinated before exposure do not require human rabies immune globulin (HRIG [HyperRAB, Imogam Rabies]), which may be expensive, unavailable, or unreliable in the traveler's locale. Following an exposure and despite having received the three-dose preexposure course of vaccine, a traveler will still require two additional doses following an animal bite, administered as soon as possible. Children may be at higher risk for exposure to rabies because of more frequent contact with dogs and their failure to inform parents of incidental bites or scratches. Rabies vaccine is recommended for travelers based on age, destination, duration of stay, likelihood of activities that may lead to potential exposure to rabid animals, visiting remote areas, and the likely need for rabies vaccine and rabies immune globulin

for postexposure care. In light of the devastating consequences of rabies, the fact that animal bites, scratches, or licks over mucous membranes are common among travelers even during short trips; the difficulties in receiving rabies immune globulin in the developing world; and the fact that a one-time preexposure course of vaccine is "for life" suggest that the threshold for recommending rabies vaccine to travelers to the developing world should be low.

Meningococcal Vaccine

Meningococcal disease is endemic worldwide. The "meningitis belt" in sub-Saharan Africa is a hyperendemic area for meningococcal disease, with seasonal epidemics occurring during the dry season (December-June). The serogroups prevalent in the meningitis belt are A, C, W, and, to a smaller extent, X.

Meningococcal disease is rare in travelers (1:100,000 to <1:1,000,000 per month of travel). The vaccines recommended for travelers include quadrivalent conjugated preparations (Menactra, Menveo, and Nimenrix), which are recommended for travelers to the meningitis belt, travelers to areas with current outbreaks of meningococcal disease, and those who anticipate close contact with crowds or the local population in developing countries (e.g., aid workers in refugee camps).

Meningococcal vaccine is required for entry for pilgrims going to Saudi Arabia (Hajj or Umrah). The risk of meningococcal serogroup B may be underestimated as a potential public health hazard during the Hajj and Umrah, and with the availability of an effective vaccine against MenB, vaccination of pilgrims against MenB in addition to vaccination with meningococcal ACWY should be considered. Since serogroup B is common in industrialized countries but not in developing countries, the newly approved meningococcal vaccine for serogroup B (Bexsero, Trumenba) is not recommended for travelers in general, unless they fall into a high-risk group (e.g., asplenia). Attendance at a travel clinic, however, can present an opportunity to vaccinate against MenB.

Tick-Borne Encephalitis

Tick-borne encephalitis (TBE), an arboviral zoonosis transmitted primarily through the bite of *Ixodes* species ticks, is endemic in many popular tourist destinations in Europe, Eastern Europe, and parts of Asia including China, Japan, Russia, and Siberia. In Europe, the highest rates occur in Austria, Estonia, Lithuania, and Slovenia. TBE is an emerging infection, and since 1973 there has been an increase in TBE of nearly 400% in all endemic regions of Europe. Most cases of TBE occur between June and October, with a peak in July. The risk for travelers is difficult to quantitate, but recently published data suggests there is a higher risk than previously thought. A TBE vaccine is available and considered immunogenic and safe. In some countries in Europe, the vaccine is included in the routine immunization program, and it is highly effective in reducing TBE in disease-endemic areas. Vaccination is recommended even for short stays for travelers to disease-endemic areas in the transmission period and for those planning high-risk activities such as hiking and camping.

Cholera

Cholera is endemic in several countries in Asia, sub-Saharan Africa, and the Caribbean. Vaxchora, an oral live attenuated cholera vaccine, was approved for use by the FDA in 2016. The vaccine is recommended for aid and refugee workers and health care workers who are traveling to affected countries to support displaced populations.

Malaria

Malaria continues to kill millions of people worldwide. Malaria is transmitted by the *Anopheles* mosquito and involves five species of the parasite *Plasmodium*, with *Plasmodium falciparum* and *Plasmodium vivax* being the most common species. The mosquitoes that spread malaria are most active from dusk to dawn. Transmission of malaria occurs both in urban and in rural areas in the African continent and the Indian subcontinent. In South America, Central America, and the Caribbean, transmission of malaria occurs in rural areas. There is no transmission of malaria in areas above altitudes of 2500 m.

Malaria is the most common cause of fever in the returning traveler. Malaria is also by far the most common acute potentially life-threatening disease in travelers, constituting 76% of this group of diseases in an analysis of the GeoSentinel registry. In the United States, the overall trend of malaria cases has been increasing since 1973, with approximately 1700 cases each year. In a 2013 malaria surveillance report of the CDC, 82% of the cases were from the African continent (mostly from West Africa); 11% from Asia (mostly India); 6% from Central America, South America, and the Caribbean; and 1% from Oceania. Travelers visiting friends and relatives (e.g., people who emigrated from a malaria-endemic area and return to visit their homeland) are a major source of imported malaria because they often do not use prophylaxis when returning to the endemic country.

There is no vaccine available against malaria for travelers. Protection against malaria includes:
1. Using chemoprophylaxis where needed
2. Using personal protection/bite avoidance measures
3. Advising travelers to seek medical care if they have a febrile illness during or after travel

Malaria Chemoprophylaxis

Among patients diagnosed with malaria in the United States, only about a third report having taken chemoprophylaxis. Among those who do take chemoprophylaxis, adherence is poor. Distribution of malaria in a country is focal and can change greatly from one area to another. Malaria maps by country are available on the CDC website, and they are updated regularly and should be consulted before deciding whether chemoprophylaxis is recommended. In almost all areas with malaria, atovaquone-proguanil (Malarone), doxycycline, and mefloquine (Lariam) are equally effective against chloroquine-resistant *P. falciparum*. Although resistance to mefloquine limits its use in Southeast Asia, *P. falciparum* is resistant to chloroquine in most areas where this species occurs. Areas where the parasite is still chloroquine sensitive are Central America west of the Panama Canal, Haiti, the Dominican Republic, and most of the Middle East. As such, chloroquine is the drug of choice in these areas.

The traveler should be briefed on the side effects of any of the types of chemoprophylaxis, as well as when to start the medication before travel and how long to continue it once outside the endemic malarial zone. Travelers should be instructed if the drug is to be taken once daily (e.g., doxycycline [Vibramycin], atovaquone-proguanil [Malarone]) or once a week (e.g., mefloquine [Lariam], chloroquine), because serious instances of toxicity and drug failures have occurred when these drugs are taken improperly.

In 2013, the FDA added a "black box" warning to the mefloquine drug label because of the potential risk of serious psychiatric and neurologic side effects that can persist for long periods, or even for life, after the discontinuation of mefloquine.

Owing to its good safety profile, atovaquone-proguanil [Malarone] may be the drug of choice for malaria prophylaxis in most situations. Malarone (one 250 mg/100 mg tablet) is taken 1 day before entering and daily until 1 week after leaving the endemic area. Some experts believe that taking atovaquone-proguanil (Malarone) only until 1 day after leaving the endemic area is safe and can improve traveler compliance. This recommendation is based on several small studies and the fact that both atovaquone and proguanil kill early stages of *P. falciparum* in the liver and have a half-life elimination period of nearly 6 days.

It is important to remember that the aforementioned medications are not protective against dormant hepatic forms of two species of the malaria parasite (*P. vivax* or *P. ovale*), which can cause relapses of malaria months and even years after returning from travel.

Personal Protection/Bite Avoidance Measures

Travelers should be informed about the principles of malaria transmission and prevention, including avoiding outdoor exposure from dusk to dawn, wearing long-sleeved clothing to provide maximum cover of exposed areas of the body, using repellents, and sleeping in an air-conditioned room. If the traveler is unable to sleep in a sealed, air-conditioned room, permethrin-coated mosquito bed nets have been demonstrated to significantly reduce malaria incidence. Travelers can protect themselves by sleeping under well-made, treated bed nets and by employing a knock-down aerosol repellent to treat the room. Repellents containing DEET (30% to 35%) or picaridin (20% or above) are recommended. The concentration of DEET determines the length of protection; 35% DEET is effective from 6 to 8 hours, and concentrations of DEET of up to 30% are safe for children and infants older than 2 months when the eyes, hands, and mouth and mucous membranes are avoided.

Seeking Medical Care

Travelers should be advised to seek medical attention if they experience any symptoms that could be compatible with malaria (mainly fever and rigors) and about the need to tell their health care practitioner about where they have traveled. They should be aware of the fatal potential of this disease, the detrimental effect of delay in diagnosis and treatment, and the possibility of the disease appearing again, even months or years after leaving their destination (*P. vivax*, *P. malariae*, or *P. ovale*).

Travelers' Diarrhea

Travelers' diarrhea (TD) is the most common health problem encountered by travelers. TD is defined as passing three or more unformed stools in 24 hours, in addition to at least one additional symptom such as abdominal cramps, tenesmus, nausea, vomiting, fever, or fecal urgency. The condition usually has an abrupt onset. Most cases of TD are self-limited, lasting a median duration of 3 to 4 days. The risk of acquiring diarrhea ranges from 20% to 83% in travelers to the developing world and varies by location, individual, and length of stay. Of these factors, destination is most important, with South Asia and West/Central Africa being the destinations with the highest risk.

Most cases of TD are caused by bacterial pathogens, with *Escherichia coli* (mostly enterotoxigenic) being most common, followed by *Shigella*, *Campylobacter*, and *Salmonella*. Causative viral pathogens include noroviruses and rotavirus. Protozoa are uncommon causes of TD and are generally associated with a more gradual onset of diarrhea. Postinfectious irritable bowel syndrome (PI-IBS) following TD may occur in 3% to 17% of patients.

Prevention

TD is associated with the consumption of contaminated food and beverages and coming into contact with contaminated hands. Foods more often linked to diarrhea include reheated foods (such as quiche, rice, or casseroles), raw vegetables, raw meats (especially shellfish), unpasteurized milk products (also a source of brucellosis), buffet services, and raw berries. The key to food safety is keeping hot foods hot and following standard recommendations for food preparation; evidence that food restrictions reduce the likelihood of acquiring TD is weak. The importance of frequent handwashing should be stressed in addition to drinking clean, bottled water. Ice prepared from contaminated water can contaminate any drink. Water may be made safer at any altitude by bringing it to a boil and allowing it to cool while covered (boiling for 1 minute, or 3 minutes at altitudes above 2000 m). Halogenation with iodine or chlorine is also an acceptable means to treat water.

Treatment

TD is a self-limited disease. Mild to moderate cases can be treated with rehydration, antimotility agents such as loperamide (Imodium), or antisecretory agents such as bismuth subsalicylate (Pepto-Bismol). Since adult travelers with TD rarely lose significant quantities of electrolytes, specific replacement is rarely indicated. Children may experience more severe fluid and electrolyte losses, and oral rehydration remains paramount to any pediatric drug therapy, as does seeking immediate medical advice. Packets of oral rehydration salts (ORSs) are available in most pharmacies in the developing world. ORSs are rapidly absorbed from the intestine and can be useful even in the presence of vomiting.

Antibiotic therapy should be reserved only for severe cases. A recent study showed that the use of antibiotic therapy for TD

TABLE 3 Drugs for Treatment of Travelers' Diarrhea.

DRUG	ADULT DOSAGE	COMMENTS
Symptomatic Medication		
Bismuth subsalicylate (Pepto-Bismol)	Two tablets or 2 tablespoonfuls (1 dose cup, 30 mL), repeated half hourly, as needed. Do not exceed a total dose of 16 tablets, or 8 oz. of the liquid, in any 24-h period.	The maximum recommended dose is 240 mL/d (16 tabs)
Loperamide (Imodium)	2 caplets (2 mg each) for first dose, then 1 after each loose stool. Do not exceed 8 caplets (16 mg) in 24 h	Antiperistaltic drug Do not use if dysentery is diagnosed Sold "over the counter"
Antibiotics (Recommend only for Severe Cases)		
Ciprofloxacin (Cipro)	500 mg tab q12h × 3 days or 750 mg tab once at start of diarrhea symptoms	Do not use in pregnant women Do not use in children < 18 years
Azithromycin[1] (Zithromax)	1 g as a single oral dose or 500 mg once daily × 3 days	Drug of choice for quinolone-resistant *Campylobacter* strains Use for travelers' diarrhea in persons unable to use fluoroquinolones
Rifaximin (Xifaxan)	200 mg tab tid × 3 days	Nonabsorbable antibiotic Do not use for diarrhea complicated by fever or blood For patients 12 years of age or older Safety for adults ≥65 years has not been studied

[1]Not FDA approved for this indication.

increases the likelihood of gut colonization with extended-spectrum beta-lactamase-producing Enterobacteriaceae (ESBL-PE) among returning travelers. Rates of colonization with ESBL-PE for travelers treated with antibiotics for TD have reached 80% among those returning from Southeast Asia. Concomitant use of loperamide and antibiotics for TD has also been shown to increase the rate of colonization of ESBL-PE. Patients should be advised to restrict the use of antibiotics for self-treatment of TD only to severe cases, or for episodes associated with high fever or bloody stools.

Antibiotics can shorten the duration of illness. A quinolone is recommended as first-line treatment for most destinations. Azithromycin (Zithromax)[1] is preferred for Southeast Asia in view of an increased incidence of quinolone-resistant *Campylobacter* strains. Azithromycin is also the drug of choice for children and pregnant women. Most patients will improve after 24 hours of treatment with antibiotics, and if diarrhea persists beyond 24 hours, a 3-day course is recommended (Table 3).

Altitude Sickness

Altitude sickness can be fatal and, importantly, is preventable. For example, Nepal registers 2 to 3 deaths in travelers due to altitude sickness per week, with an estimated mortality rate of 7.7 per 100,000 trekkers. Travelers should be aware of the illness and must be educated to recognize and acknowledge the presence of symptoms when they first appear. Air travel to an elevated environment allows for sudden exposure, with little time for acclimatization. Rapid ascent (<24 hours) to altitudes over 2400 m is associated with altitude sickness. Common destinations at high altitudes include Cusco, Peru (3400 m); La-Paz, Bolivia (2650 m); Lhasa, Tibet (3700 m); and Quito, Ecuador (2800 m).

Ideally, ascent rates below 300 m per day to altitudes over 2400 m may reduce the risk of altitude sickness. Acute mountain sickness is characterized by headache, dyspnea, nausea, vomiting, insomnia, and changes in mental status. The condition may be reduced or prevented in adults by taking acetazolamide (Diamox), 125 mg orally twice a day, for 1 day before ascent, continuing for 2 to 3 days on arrival at maximum altitude. The risks for infants and children at high altitude remains controversial because acute mountain sickness can be more difficult to diagnose, with only nonspecific symptoms being present such as irritability, poor feeding, and sleeplessness. Increasing hydration, resting, and limiting exertion in

the first few days following arrival help acclimatization. The definitive treatment of all forms of altitude sickness is descent to a lower altitude. All travelers experiencing difficulty at altitude should be prepared to abandon their trip if symptoms persist or worsen.

Conclusion

With the ease of travel and the ever-increasing numbers of travelers exploring the world, the need for meeting the health needs of this diverse group of travelers continues to grow. Travel medicine specialist practitioners are ideally placed to identify and treat travel-related health problems, both before and after travel.

Acknowledgment

The authors and editors gratefully acknowledge the contributions of the previous author, Edward Dick, MD, MPH.

References

Air Passenger Forecasts. Global Report. Available at: https://www.iata.org/publications/Documents/global-report-sample1.pdf. Accessed 1 September 2017.

Cullen KA, Mace KE, Arguin PM: Malaria surveillance - United States, 2013, *MMWR Surveill Summ* 65:1–22, 2016.

Freedman DO: Protection of travelers. In Bennett JE, Raphael D, Blaser MJ, editors: *Mandell, Douglas, and Bennett's Principles and Practice of Infectious Diseases*, 8th Edition, Philadelphia, 2015, Saunders Elsevier, pp 3559–3567.

Freedman DO, Chen LH, Kozarsky PE: Medical considerations before international travel, *N Engl J Med* 375:247–260, 2016.

Freedman DO, Weld LH, Kozarsky PE: Spectrum of disease and relation to place of exposure among ill returned travelers, *N Engl J Med* 354:119–130, 2006.

Gautret P, Harvey K, Pandey P: Animal-associated exposure to rabies virus among travelers, 1997-2012, *Emerg Infect Dis* 21:569–577, 2015.

Gautret P, Parola P: Rabies in travelers, *Curr Infect Dis Rep* 16:394, 2014.

Grobusch MP: Malaria chemoprophylaxis with atovaquone-proguanil: Is a shorter regimen fully protective? *J Travel Med* 21(2):79–81, 2014.

Jelinek T, Burchard GD, Dieckmann S, et al: Short-term immunogenicity and safety of an accelerated pre-exposure prophylaxis regimen with Japanese encephalitis vaccine in combination with a rabies vaccine: A phase III, multicenter, observer-blind study, *J Travel Med* 22:225–231, 2015.

Jensenius M, Han PV, Schlagenhauf P, et al: Acute and potentially life-threatening tropical diseases in western travelers–A GeoSentinel multicenter study, 1996-2011, *Am J Trop Med Hyg* 88:397–404, 2013.

Kantele A, Lääveri T, Mero S: Antimicrobials increase travelers' risk of colonization by extended-spectrum betalactamase-producing Enterobacteriaceae, *Clin Infect Dis* 60:837–846, 2015.

Kantele A, Mero S, Kirveskari J: Increased risk for ESBL-producing bacteria from co-administration of loperamide and antimicrobial drugs for travelers' diarrhea, *Emerg Infect Dis* 22(1):117–120, 2016.

Leshem E, Meltzer E, Stienlauf S: Effectiveness of short prophylactic course of atovaquone-proguanil in travelers to sub-Saharan Africa, *J Travel Med* 21(2):82–85, 2014.

[1]Not FDA approved for this indication.

Leshem E, Pandey P: Clinical features of patients with severe altitude illness in Nepal, *J Travel Med* 15:315–322, 2008.

Meltzer E, Paran Y, Lustig Y: Travel-related tick-borne encephalitis, Israel, 2006-2014, *Emerg Infect Dis* 23:119–121, 2017.

Menachem M, Grupper M, Paz A: Assessment of rabies exposure risk among Israeli travelers, *Travel Med Infect Dis* 6:12–16, 2008.

Steffen R: Epidemiology of tick-borne encephalitis (TBE) in international travellers to Western/Central Europe and conclusions on vaccination recommendations, *J Travel Med* 23(4).

Steffen R, Hill DR, DuPont HL: Traveler's diarrhea: A clinical review, *JAMA* 313:71–80, 2015.

Yezli S, Alotaibi B: Meningococcal disease during the Hajj and Umrah mass gatherings: A, C, W, Y may be covered but don't forget the B and X factors, *Travel Med Infect Dis* 15:5–7, 2017.

22 Appendices

BIOLOGIC AGENTS REFERENCE CHART

Method of
James J. James, MD, DrPH; and James M. Lyznicki, MS, MPH

Biological weapons are devices used intentionally to cause disease or death through dissemination of microorganisms or toxins in food and water, by insect vectors, or by aerosols. Potential targets include human beings, food crops, livestock, and other resources essential for national security, economy, and defense. Unlike nuclear, chemical, and conventional weapons, the onset of a biological attack will probably be insidious. For some infectious agents, secondary and tertiary transmission could continue for weeks or months after the initial attack.

Initial detection of an unannounced biological attack will likely occur when an astute health professional notices an unusual case or disease cluster and reports his or her concerns to local public health authorities. Physicians and other health professionals should be alert to the following:
- Unusual temporal or geographic clustering of illnesses
- Sudden increase of illness in previously healthy persons
- Sudden increase in nonspecific illnesses such as pneumonia; flu-like illness; bleeding disorders; unexplained rashes, particularly in adults; neuromuscular illnesses; and diarrhea

To enhance detection and treatment capabilities, physicians and other health professionals in acute care settings should be familiar with the clinical manifestations, diagnostic techniques, isolation precautions, treatment, and prophylaxis for likely causative agents (e.g., smallpox, pneumonic plague, anthrax, viral hemorrhagic fevers). Table 1 provides a quick summary of diagnostic and treatment considerations for various infectious and toxic biological agents. For some of these agents, delay in medical response could result in a potentially devastating number of casualties. To mitigate such consequences, early identification and intervention are imperative. Frontline physicians must have an increased level of suspicion regarding the possible intentional use of biological agents as well as an increased sensitivity to reporting those suspicious to public health authorities, who, in turn, must be willing to evaluate a predictable increase in false-positive reports.

Medical response efforts require coordination and planning with emergency management agencies, law enforcement, health care facilities, and social services agencies. Health care agencies should ensure that physicians know whom to call with reports of suspicious cases and clusters of infectious diseases, and they should work to build a good relationship with the local medical community. Resource integration is absolutely necessary to
- Establish adequate capacity to initiate rapid investigation of an outbreak
- Educate the public
- Begin mass distribution of antibiotics and vaccines
- Ensure mass medical care
- Control public anger and fear

In an epidemic, overwhelming numbers of critically ill patients will require acute and follow-up medical care. Both infected persons and the worried well will seek medical attention, with a corresponding need for medical supplies, diagnostic tests, and hospital beds. The impact—or even the threat—of an attack can elicit widespread panic and civil disorder, overwhelm hospital resources, and disrupt social services.

Any suspicious or confirmed exposure to a biological weapons agent should be reported immediately to the local health department, local Federal Bureau of Investigation office, and the Centers of Disease Control and Prevention (770–488–7100).

TABLE 1   Quick Reference Chart on Biological Weapon Agents

DISEASE AND AGENT	DIAGNOSTIC CONSIDERATIONS				TREATMENT CONSIDERATIONS*		
	SIGNS AND SYMPTOMS	INCUBATION PERIOD	DIAGNOSIS	LETHALITY	TREATMENT	PROPHYLAXIS	COMMENTS
Bacteria							
Anthrax *Bacillus anthracis* (all forms)		1–5 d (perhaps ≤60 d)†	Gram stain and culture of blood, pleural fluid, cerebrospinal fluid, ascitic fluid, vesicular fluid, or lesion exudate Confirmatory serologic and PCR tests are available through public health laboratory network		Steroids may be considered for severe edema and for meningitis Penicillin¹ should be considered if strain is susceptible and does not possess inducible β-lactamases	Ciprofloxacin or doxycycline with or without vaccination If strain is susceptible, penicillin¹ or amoxicillin¹ (Amoxil) should be considered Anthrax Vaccine Adsorbed (BioThrax) Primary: 3 IM injections given at day 0, 1 month, and 6 months; booster: 6 and 12 months after completion of primary series and annually for persons who remain at risk	If meningitis is suspected, doxycycline may be less optimal because of poor CNS penetration
Cutaneous	Evolving skin lesion (face, neck, arms), progresses to vesicle, depressed ulcer, and black necrotic lesions			20% if untreated, otherwise rarely fatal			
Gastrointestinal	Nausea, vomiting, abdominal pain, bloody diarrhea, sepsis Widened mediastinum on chest radiograph is occasionally seen†			Approaches 100% if untreated, but data are limited Rapid, aggressive treatment can reduce mortality			
Inhalational	Abrupt onset of flulike symptoms, fever with or without chills, sweats, fatigue or malaise, non- or minimally productive cough, nausea, vomiting, dyspnea, headache, chest pain, followed in 2–5 d by severe respiratory distress, mediastinitis, hemorrhagic meningitis, sepsis, shock§ Widened mediastinum on chest radiograph is characteristic‡		Sputum is rarely positive	Once respiratory distress develops, mortality rates approach 90% Begin treatment when inhalational anthrax is suspected; do not wait for confirmatory testing‖	Combination therapy of ciprofloxacin or doxycycline plus one or two other antimicrobials should be considered¶		

Agent	Clinical features	Incubation	Diagnosis	Lethality	Treatment	Prophylaxis / Vaccine	Comments
Brucellosis *Brucella abortus, B. canis, B. melitensis, B. suis*	Nonspecific flulike symptoms, fever, headache, profound weakness and fatigue; GI symptoms such as anorexia, nausea, vomiting, diarrhea, or constipation	5–60 d, usually 1–2 mo	Blood and bone marrow culture (can require 6 wk to grow *Brucella*) Confirmatory culture and serologic testing available through public health laboratory network	Less than 5% even if untreated Tends to incapacitate rather than kill	Doxycycline plus streptomycin or rifampin[1] *Alternative therapies:* Ofloxacin[1] plus rifampin[1] Doxycycline plus gentamicin (Garamycin) TMP-SMX[1] plus gentamicin	Doxycycline plus streptomycin or rifampin No approved human vaccine	Osteoarticular complications are common
Inhalational (pneumonic) tularemia *Francisella tularensis*	Sudden onset of acute febrile illness, weakness, chills, headache, generalized body aches, elevated WBCs Pulmonary symptoms such as dry cough, chest pain or tightness with or without objective signs of pneumonia Progressive weakness, malaise, anorexia, and weight loss, potentially leading to sepsis and organ failure	3–5 d Range, 1–21 d	Largely clinical Culture of blood, sputum, biopsies, pleural fluid, bronchial washings (culture is difficult and potentially dangerous); confirmatory testing available through public health laboratory network	~30%–60% Fatal if untreated	Streptomycin or gentamicin (Garamycin) *Alternative therapies:* Ciprofloxacin[1] Doxycycline Chloramphenicol[1] (Chloromycetin)	Tetracycline Doxycycline Ciprofloxacin[1] Live, attenuated vaccine (USAMRIID, IND) given by scarification; currently under FDA review, limited availability	
Pneumonic plague *Yersinia pestis*	Acute onset of flulike prodrome: fever, myalgia, weakness, headache; within 24 h of prodrome, chest discomfort, cough with bloody sputum, and dyspnea By day 2 to 4 of illness, symptoms progressing to cyanosis, respiratory distress, and hemodynamic instability	1–10 d, typically 2–3 d	Gram stain and culture of blood, CSF, sputum, lymph node aspirates, bronchial washings Confirmatory serologic and bacteriologic tests available through public health laboratory network	Almost 100% if untreated 20%–60% if appropriately treated within 18–24 h of symptoms	Streptomycin, gentamicin (Garamycin) *Alternative therapies:* Doxycycline Tetracycline Ciprofloxacin[1] Chloramphenicol[1] (Chloromycetin) is first choice for meningitis except for pregnant women	Tetracycline Doxycycline Ciprofloxacin[1] Inactivated whole-cell vaccine licensed but not readily available; injection with boosters Vaccine not effective against aerosol exposure	Begin treatment when diagnosis of plague is suspected; do not wait for confirmatory testing
Rickettsia Q-fever *Coxiella burnetii*	Nonspecific febrile disease, chills, cough, weakness and fatigue, pleuritic chest pain Pneumonia is possible	2–14 d May be ≤40 d	Isolation of organism may be difficult; confirmatory testing via serology or PCR available through public health laboratory network	1%–3% Fatalities are uncommon even if untreated Relapsing symptoms can occur	Tetracycline Doxycycline	Tetracycline Doxycycline Inactivated whole-cell[2] vaccine (IND)	Skin test to determine prior exposure to *C. burnetii* is recommended before vaccination

Continued

TABLE 1 Quick Reference Chart on Biological Weapon Agents—cont'd

| DISEASE AND AGENT | DIAGNOSTIC CONSIDERATIONS | | | | TREATMENT CONSIDERATIONS* | | |
	SIGNS AND SYMPTOMS	INCUBATION PERIOD	DIAGNOSIS	LETHALITY	TREATMENT	PROPHYLAXIS	COMMENTS
Viruses							
Smallpox Variola major virus	Prodrome of high fever, malaise, prostration, headache, vomiting, delirium followed in 2–3 d by maculopapular rash uniformly progressing to pustules and scabs, mostly on extremities and face	7–17 d	Pharyngeal swab, vesicular fluid, biopsies, scab material for electron microscopy and PCR testing through public health laboratory network	30% in unvaccinated persons	Supportive care Cidofovir (Vistide) shown to be effective in vitro and in experimental animals infected with surrogate orthopox virus	Live, attenuated vaccinia vaccine derived from calf lymph; given by scarification (licensed, restricted supply) New vaccine being developed from tissue culture Vaccination given within 3–4 d following exposure can prevent or decrease the severity of disease	Requires astute clinical evaluation; may be confused with chickenpox, erythema multiforme with bullae, or allergic contact dermatitis Notify CDC Poxvirus Section at 404–639–2184
Viral Encephalitis							
All forms	Systemic febrile illness, with encephalitis developing in some populations Generalized malaise, spiking fevers, headache, myalgia		Clinical and epidemiologic diagnosis WBC count can show striking leukopenia and lymphopenia Confirmatory test and viral isolation available through public health laboratory network		Supportive care Analgesics, anticonvulsants as needed	Several IND vaccines, poorly immunogenic, highly reactogenic	Incidence of seizures and/ or focal neurologic deficits may be higher after biological attack
Eastern equine encephalitis		7–14 d		50%–75%			
Western equine encephalitis		7–14 d		10%			
Venezuelan equine encephalitis		2–6 d		<10%			

Viral Hemorrhagic Fevers

DISEASE AND AGENT	SIGNS AND SYMPTOMS	SYMPTOM ONSET	DIAGNOSIS	LETHALITY	TREATMENT	PROPHYLAXIS	COMMENTS
Arenaviruses (Lassa, Junin, and related viruses) Bunyaviruses (Hanta, Congo–Crimean, Rift Valley) Filoviruses (Ebola, Marburg) Flaviviruses (yellow fever, dengue, various tick-borne disease viruses)	Fever with mucous membrane bleeding, petechiae, thrombocytopenia, and hypotension in patients without underlying malignancies Malaise, myalgias, headache, vomiting, diarrhea possible	4–21 d	Confirmatory testing and viral isolation available through public health laboratory network	Variable depending on viral strain; 15%–25% with Lassa fever to ≤90% with Ebola	Supportive therapy Ribavirin (Virazole) A may be effective for Lassa fever, Rift Valley fever, Argentine hemorrhagic fever, and Congo–Crimean hemorrhagic fever	Ribavarin (Virazole)[1] is suggested for Congo–Crimean hemorrhagic fever and Lassa fever Yellow fever vaccine (YF-VAX) is the only licensed vaccine available Vaccines for some of the other VHFs exist but are for investigational use only	Call CDC Special Pathogens Office at 404-639-1115

Biological Toxins

DISEASE AND AGENT	SIGNS AND SYMPTOMS	SYMPTOM ONSET	DIAGNOSIS	LETHALITY	TREATMENT	PROPHYLAXIS	COMMENTS
Botulism *Clostridium botulinum* toxin	Blurred vision, diploplia, dry mouth, ptosis, fatigue As disease progresses, acute bilateral descending flaccid paralysis, respiratory paralysis resulting in death	1–5 d, typically 12–36h	Clinical Serum and stool should be assayed for toxin by mouse neutralization bioassay, which can take several days	60% without ventilatory support	Intensive and prolonged supportive care; ventilation may be necessary Trivalent equine antitoxin (serotypes A, B, E, – licensed, available from the CDC) should be administered immediately after clinical diagnosis	Pentavalent toxoid (A-E), yearly booster (IND, CDC) Not available to the public Antitoxin may be sufficient to prevent illness following exposure but is not recommended until patient is showing symptoms	Anaphylaxis and serum sickness are potential complications of antitoxin Aminoglycosides and clindamycin (Cleocin) A must not be used
Enterotoxin B *Staphylococcus aureus*	Acute onset of fever, chills headache, nonproductive cough	3–12h	Clinical Normal chest radiograph Serology on acute and convalescent serum can confirm diagnosis	Probably low (few data available for respiratory exposure)	Supportive care	No vaccine available	
Ricin toxin *Ricinus communis*	Weakness, nausea, chest tightness, fever, cough, pulmonary edema, respiratory failure, circulatory collapse, hypoxemia resulting in death (usually within 36–72h)	≤6–24h	Clinical and epidemiologic Confirmatory serological testing available through public health laboratory network	Mortality data are not available, but likely to be high with extensive exposure	Supportive care Treatment for pulmonary edema Gastric decontamination if toxin is ingested	No vaccine available	

Continued

TABLE 1 Quick Reference Chart on Biological Weapon Agents—cont'd

DISEASE AND AGENT	SIGNS AND SYMPTOMS	SYMPTOM ONSET	DIAGNOSIS	LETHALITY	TREATMENT	PROPHYLAXIS	COMMENTS
T-2 Mycotoxins *Fusarium Myrothecium Trichoderma Stachybotrys*	Abrupt onset of mucocutaneous and airway irritation and pain Can include skin, eyes, and GI tract; systemic toxicity can follow	Minutes to hours			Clinical support	No vaccine available	Soap and water washing within 4–6 h reduces dermal toxicity; washing within 1 h can eliminate toxicity entirely
Other filamentous fungi			Confirmation requires testing blood, tissue, and environmental samples	Severe exposure can cause death in hours to days			Consult with local health department regarding specimen collection and diagnostic testing procedures

Adapted from Lyznicki JL: AMA quick reference guide: Biological emergencies. In American Medical Association: Management of Public Health Emergencies. A Resource Guide for Physicians and Other Community Responders. Chicago, American Medical Association, 2005.

[1]Not FDA approved for this indication.

[2]Not available in the United States.

*Different situations can require different dosage and treatment regimens. Please consult other references and an infectious disease specialist for definitive dosage information, especially dosages for pregnant women and children.

†Data from 22 patients infected with anthrax in October and November 2001 indicate a median incubation period of 4 days (range, 4–7 days) for inhalational anthrax and a mean incubation of 5 days (range, 1–10 days) for cutaneous anthrax.

‡Chest radiograph abnormalities include paratracheal and hilar fullness and may be subtle. Consider chest computed tomography if diagnosis is uncertain.

§Limited data from the October and November 2001 anthrax infections indicate hemorrhagic pleural effusions to be strongly associated with inhalational anthrax; rhinorrhea was present in only 1/10 patients.

‖Limited data from the 2001 terrorist-related anthrax infections indicate that early treatment significantly decreased the mortality rate.

¶Other agents with in vitro activity suggested for use in conjunction with ciprofloxacin or doxycycline for treatment of inhalational anthrax include rifampin, vancomycin (Vancocin), imipenem (Primaxin), chloramphenicol (Chloromycetin), penicillin and ampicillin, clindamycin (Cleocin), and clarithromycin (Biaxin).

Abbreviations: CDC=Centers for Disease Control and Prevention; CNS=central nervous system; CSF=cerebrospinal fluid; GI=gastrointestinal; IND=investigational new drug; PCR=polymerase chain reaction; TMP-SMX=trimethoprim-sulfamethoxazole; USAMRIID=U.S. Army Medical Research Institute of Infectious Diseases; VHF=viral hemorrhagic fever; WBC=white blood cell. *Abbreviations:* CDC=Centers for Disease Control and Prevention; CNS=central nervous system; CSF=cerebrospinal fluid; GI=gastrointestinal; IND=investigational new drug; PCR=polymerase chain reaction; TMP-SMX=trimethoprim-sulfamethoxazole; USAMRIID=U.S. Army Medical Research Institute of Infectious Diseases; VHF=viral hemorrhagic fever; WBC=white blood cell.

POPULAR HERBS AND NUTRITIONAL SUPPLEMENTS

Method of
Miriam Chan, PharmD

Popular Herbs and Nutritional Supplements

HERB OR NUTRITIONAL SUPPLEMENT	COMMON USES	REASONABLE ADULT ORAL DOSAGE*	PRECAUTIONS AND DRUG INTERACTIONS
Aloe vera	Commonly found in skin products as a moisturizer Used topically to treat burns, wounds, skin infections, and inflammation Approved in Germany to use orally as a laxative Used orally for a variety of conditions, including diabetes, asthma, epilepsy, and osteoarthritis	For external use, apply aloe gel on the skin tid to qid For constipation, 40–170 mg of dried aloe juice or latex (corresponds to 10–30 mg hydroxyanthracene derivatives) taken in the evening For other conditions, no established dosage documented	Aloe gel is generally well tolerated and safe when used topically Aloe gel taken orally can cause hypoglycemia in patients who are concomitantly taking antidiabetic drugs Aloe juice or latex contains anthraquinone, a cathartic laxative and should not be taken by people with intestinal obstruction, acute intestinal inflammation, and ulcers Pregnant women should not take aloe latex because it may cause uterine contractions Oral use of aloe latex can cause abdominal cramps and diarrhea. Long-term use or abuse can cause electrolyte imbalances, albuminuria, hematuria, and pseudomelanosis coli. Prolonged use of high doses (≥1 g/d) can cause nephritis, acute renal failure, and death In 2002, the FDA banned the sale of aloe-containing laxative products in the United States because of the lack of safety data Aloe can decrease platelet aggregation and should be avoided at least 2 weeks before surgery
Astragalus	Used in combination with other herbs to support and enhance the immune system Used to prevent and treat common colds and upper respiratory infections Used for heart disease Widely used in China for chronic hepatitis and as an adjunctive therapy in cancer	Extract: 250–500 mg tid to qid standardized to 0.4% 4-hydroxy-3-methoxyisoflavone 7-sug Powdered root: 500–1000 mg tid Tincture (1:5) in 30% ethanol: 3–5 mL tid Decoction: 3–6 g of dried root per 12 oz water tid	Avoid using astragalus in organ transplant patients and those with autoimmune disorders Side effects include mild stomach upset and allergic reactions Astragalus can decrease the effects of cyclophosphamide and other immunosuppressants
Bilberry fruit	Often used orally to improve visual acuity and to treat degenerative retinal conditions Used orally to treat chronic venous insufficiency, varicose veins, and hemorrhoids Approved in Germany to use orally for acute diarrhea and topically for mild inflammation of the mucous membranes of mouth and throat	For eye conditions and circulation, 80–160 mg tid of the extract standardized to at least 25% anthocyanosides For diarrhea, 20–60 g/d of the dried, ripe berries or as a tea preparation (5–10 g of crushed dried berries in 150 mL water, brought to a boil for 10 min, then strained) For external use, 10% decoction	No known side effects reported with bilberry fruit and extract However, bilberry leaf taken in large quantities or used long term has been shown to cause wasting, anemia, jaundice, acute excitation, disturbances of tonus, and death in animals The anthocyanidin extracts from bilberry can increase the risk of bleeding in those taking warfarin or other blood thinners
Black cohosh root	Commonly used to relieve hot flashes and other menopausal symptoms Used to treat premenstrual discomfort and dysmenorrhea	20 mg bid of the rhizome extract standardized to triterpene glycosides Remifemin is the proprietary brand used in a number of clinical trials The German guidelines do not recommend its use for > 6 months	Black cohosh may have an estrogen-like effect and should be avoided in women with breast cancer Large doses may induce miscarriage and it is contraindicated during pregnancy It may cause GI disturbances, headache, and hypotension International case reports of liver dysfunction suspected to be associated with its use

Continued

HERB OR NUTRITIONAL SUPPLEMENT	COMMON USES	REASONABLE ADULT ORAL DOSAGE*	PRECAUTIONS AND DRUG INTERACTIONS
Black haw	To relieve uterine cramps and painful periods To prevent miscarriage and ease pain that follows childbirth	For menstrual pain, 5 mL of tincture in water, taken 3–5 times daily For prevention of miscarriage, 1–2 cups of tea per day (1 tsp of dried herb in 1 cup of boiling water, steeped for 10 min)	Black haw should not be used in pregnancy because of its uterine relaxant effects The salicylate constituent in black haw could trigger allergic reactions in individuals with aspirin allergies or asthma Black haw may aggravate tinnitus Large doses of black haw can prolong bleeding time The oxalic acid component of black haw can increase kidney stone formation in susceptible individuals Black haw can interact with warfarin and increase risk of bleeding
Cat's claw	Used primarily to reduce pain in osteoarthritis and rheumatoid arthritis Used for a variety of health conditions, including viral infections (e.g., herpes, HIV), Alzheimer disease, and cancer Used to support the immune system and promote kidney health Used to prevent and abort pregnancy	For osteoarthritis, 100 mg/d of the dry encapsulated extract For rheumatoid arthritis, 20 mg tid of the dry extract standardized to 1.3% pentacyclic oxindole alkaloids free of tetracyclic oxindole alkaloids For general uses, 1–3 cups of tea per day (1 g root bark boiled for 15 min in 250 mL of water) or 1 mL of tincture 2–3 times/d	Avoid using cat's claw during pregnancy or breastfeeding People with autoimmune diseases and transplant recipients should avoid cat's claw because of its immune stimulating effects Side effects include headaches, dizziness, and vomiting Cat's claw can lower blood pressure and cause hypotension when used with antihypertensive drugs Cat's claw can inhibit CYP3A4 enzyme and increase levels of drugs metabolized by this enzyme
Cannabidiol (CBD) (A cannabinoid extracted from the hemp plant and often made into an oil for use)	For relieving anxiety, insomnia, chronic pain, and many common ailments Epidiolex, a purified CBD solution, is the only prescription CBD approved by the FDA to treat Lennox-Gastaut syndrome or Dravet syndrome A variety of CBD products (oral, sublingual, inhaling, topical) are marketed and sold as dietary supplements and CBD-infused foods While the 2018 Farm Bill legalized CBD oil derived from the hemp plant containing ≤ 0.3% tetrahydrocannabinol (THC) at the federal level, all 50 states have laws legalizing CBD with varying degrees of restriction. CBD products are readily obtainable in most parts of the United States and have become the hot new products in states that have legalized medical marijuana Currently, the FDA does not allow CBD to be added in foods	No established dosage documented for CBD supplement There are concerns about the quality and purity of CBD products. Many have shown to be mislabeled and contain THC (>3%) and other contaminants (e.g., toxic chemicals including heavy metals and pesticides)	Marijuana contains THC and CBD. Unlike THC, pure CBD does not cause a "high" CBD may cause nausea, diarrhea, fatigue, and irritability High CBD doses are linked to elevated liver function tests Effects of cumulative CBD exposure are unknown Avoid CBD in pregnant or breastfeeding women Many potential drug interactions: Worsening sedation when combining with CNS depressants CBD inhibits CYP2C8, 2C9, and 2C19 enzymes and can increase levels of drugs such as carbamazepine, warfarin, amitriptyline, citalopram, phenytoin, and valproic acid CBD levels can be increased by CYP3A4 inhibitors, such as clarithromycin, ritonavir, and verapamil
Chamomile flower	Used orally to calm nerves and treat GI spasms and inflammatory diseases of the GI tract Used topically to treat wounds, skin infections, and skin or mucous membrane inflammation	1 cup of freshly made tea 3–4 times daily (1 tbsp or 3 g of dried flower in 150 mL boiling water for 5–10 min)	Chamomile can cause an allergic reaction, especially in people with severe allergies to ragweed or other members of the daisy family (e.g., echinacea, feverfew, and milk thistle) It should not be taken concurrently with other sedatives, such as alcohol or benzodiazepines

HERB OR NUTRITIONAL SUPPLEMENT	COMMON USES	REASONABLE ADULT ORAL DOSAGE*	PRECAUTIONS AND DRUG INTERACTIONS
Chaste tree berry (Chasteberry, Vitex)	For normalizing irregular menstrual periods and relieving premenstrual complaints For relieving menopausal symptoms For restoring fertility in women For treating acne associated with menstrual cycles For increasing breast milk production in lactating women	For menstrual irregularities and premenstrual complaints, 30–40 mg/d of the dried berries or an equivalent amount of aqueous-alcoholic extracts (50%–70% v/v) Dried fruit extract, standardized to 0.6% agnusides, is used in doses of 175–225 mg/d For other conditions, no established dosage documented	Chaste tree berry can have uterine stimulant properties and should be avoided in pregnancy Women with hormone-dependent conditions (e.g., breast, uterine, and ovarian cancers, and endometriosis and uterine fibroids) and men with prostate cancer should avoid chaste tree berry because it contains progestins Side effects include intramenstrual bleeding, dry mouth, headache, nausea, rash, alopecia, and tachycardia High doses (≥480 mg/d extract) can paradoxically decrease lactation Chaste tree berry is thought to have dopaminergic effects and can interact with dopamine antagonists, such as antipsychotics and metoclopramide Chaste tree berry can decrease the effects of oral contraceptives and hormone therapy
Chondroitin	Orally, used frequently in combination with glucosamine for osteoarthritis Topically, in combination with sodium hyaluronate, as a viscoelastic agent in cataract surgery	Oral: 200–400 mg tid	Occasional mild side effects include nausea, indigestion, and allergic reactions Chondroitin derived from bovine cartilage carries a potential risk of contamination with diseased animals
Chromium	For diabetes For hypercholesterolemia Commonly found in weight-loss products Also promoted for body building	For diabetes, 100 µg bid for ≤4 months or 500 µg bid for 2 months For hypercholesterolemia, 200 µg tid or 500 µg bid for 2–4 months For body building, 200–400 µg/d Chromium picolinate has been used in most studies, even though the chloride form is also available	Adverse effects are rare, but they include headaches, insomnia, sleep disturbances, irritability, and mood changes; some patients may also experience cognitive, perceptual, and motor dysfunction Long-term use of high doses (600–2400 µg/d) can cause anemia, thrombocytopenia, hemolysis, hepatic dysfunction, and renal failure Interstitial nephritis has been reported A few studies suggest that chromium can cause DNA damage Chromium competes with iron for binding to transferrin and can cause iron deficiency Antacids, H_2 blockers, and proton pump inhibitors can decrease the absorption of chromium
Coenzyme Q10	As adjunctive treatment for congestive heart failure, angina, hypertension, and diabetes Used for reducing cardiotoxicity associated with doxorubicin Used to treat statin-induced myopathy	For heart failure, 100 mg/d in 2 or 3 divided doses For angina, 50 mg tid For hypertension, 60 mg bid For diabetes, 100–200 mg/d	Mild adverse events include gastric distress, nausea, vomiting, and hypotension Doses >300 mg/d can cause elevated liver enzyme levels Coenzyme Q10 can reduce the anticoagulation effects of warfarin Oral hypoglycemic agents and HMG-CoA reductase inhibitors can reduce serum coenzyme Q10 levels
Cranberry	To prevent and treat UTIs or *Helicobacter pylori* infections that can lead to stomach ulcers To prevent dental plaque As an antioxidant to prevent cardiovascular disease and cancer	For UTIs, 150–600 mL of cranberry juice daily or 300–400 mg of standardized extract bid For other conditions, no dosage determined	Drinking excessive amounts of juice could cause GI upset or diarrhea Prolonged use of cranberry juice in large doses increases the risk of kidney stone formation because of its high oxalate content Cranberry can interact with warfarin and cause an increase in INR The effectiveness of proton pump inhibitors can be reduced by cranberry because of its acidity

HERB OR NUTRITIONAL SUPPLEMENT	COMMON USES	REASONABLE ADULT ORAL DOSAGE*	PRECAUTIONS AND DRUG INTERACTIONS
Creatine	To enhance muscle performance, especially during short-duration, high-intensity exercise	Loading dose of 20 g/d for 5–7 d followed by a maintenance dose of ≥2 g/d An alternative dosing of 3 g/d for 28 d has been suggested	Creatine can cause gastroenteritis, diarrhea, heat intolerance, muscle cramps, and elevated serum creatinine levels Creatine is contraindicated in patients taking diuretics Concurrent use with cimetidine, probenecid, or nonsteroidal antiinflammatory drugs increases the risk of adverse renal effects Caffeine can decrease creatine's ergogenic effects
Dehydroepiandrosterone (DHEA)	Replace low serum DHEA levels in adrenal insufficiency Treat SLE Reverse aging Used in many other conditions, including Alzheimer disease, depression, diabetes, menopause, osteoporosis, impotence, and AIDS Used to promote weight loss Used by bodybuilders to increase muscle mass	For replacement therapy, 25–50 mg/d For SLE, 200 mg/d For antiaging and osteoporosis, 50 mg/d For other conditions, no established dosage documented	Most common side effects are androgenic in nature and include acne, hair loss, hirsutism, and deepening of the voice Cases of hepatitis have been reported When used in high doses, DHEA can cause insomnia, manic symptoms, and palpitations DHEA at physiologic doses increases circulating androgens in women, but not in men; it also increases circulating estrogens in both men and women Avoid use of DHEA in individuals with a history of sex hormone–dependent malignancy Safety of DHEA in individuals aged < 30 years is unknown DHEA inhibits CYP3A4 enzyme and could increase serum concentrations of drugs metabolized by this enzyme (e.g., lovastatin, ketoconazole, itraconazole, and triazolam)
Dong quai root	Commonly used for the relief of premenstrual and menopausal symptoms Used as a "blood tonic" and a strengthening treatment for the heart, spleen, liver, and kidneys	For premenstrual and menopausal symptoms, 3–4 g/d in 3 divided doses For other conditions, no established dosage documented	Dong quai should not be used in pregnant women because of its uterine stimulant and relaxant effects Women with hormone sensitive conditions (e.g., breast, uterine, and ovarian cancers, and endometriosis and uterine fibroids) should avoid dong quai because of its estrogenic effects Drinking the essential oil of dong quai is not recommended because it contains a small amount of carcinogenic constituents Dong quai contains psoralens that can cause photosensitivity and photodermatitis Dong quai contains natural coumarin derivatives that can increase the risk of bleeding in those who are taking anticoagulant or antiplatelet drugs
Echinacea	As an immune stimulant, particularly for the prevention and treatment of the common cold and influenza Supportive therapy for lower urinary tract infections Used topically to treat skin disorders and promote wound healing	300 mg tid of *Echinacea pallida* root or 2–3 mL tid of expressed juice of *Echinacea purpurea* herb Do not use for >8 weeks because echinacea may suppress immunity if used long term	Echinacea should not be used in transplant patients and those with autoimmune disease or liver dysfunction Allergic reactions have been reported Adverse events are rare and include mild GI effects It should be discontinued as far in advance of surgery as possible Echinacea can decrease effectiveness of the immunosuppressants

HERB OR NUTRITIONAL SUPPLEMENT	COMMON USES	REASONABLE ADULT ORAL DOSAGE*	PRECAUTIONS AND DRUG INTERACTIONS
Ephedra (ma huang)	For diseases of the respiratory tract with mild bronchospasm Promoted for weight loss and performance enhancement	1 tsp or 2 g of dried herb (15–30 mg of ephedrine) in 240 mL boiling water for 10 min In Canada, the maximum allowable dosage of ephedrine is 8 mg per dose or 32 mg/d	Ephedra contains ephedrine, which has sympathomimetic activities; consequently, it should not be used in patients who have cardiovascular disease, diabetes, glaucoma, hypertension, hyperthyroidism, prostate enlargement, psychiatric disorders, or seizures Serious adverse effects, including seizures, arrhythmias, heart attack, stroke, and death, have been associated with the use of ephedra; as a result, the FDA banned the sale of ephedra-containing products in the United States. The ban does not apply to traditional Chinese herbal remedies Because of the cardiovascular effects of ephedrine, patients taking ephedra should discontinue use at least 24 h before surgery Concurrent use of ephedra and digitalis, guanethidine, monoamine oxidase inhibitors, or other stimulants, including caffeine, is not recommended
Evening primrose oil	For PMS, especially if mastalgia is present For treatment of atopic eczema Used for other medical conditions, including rheumatoid arthritis, menopausal symptoms, Raynaud phenomenon, Sjögren syndrome, and diabetic neuropathy	For PMS, 2–4 g/d For atopic eczema, 6–8 g/d For rheumatoid arthritis, 2.8 g/d These doses are based on products standardized to 9% γ-linolenic acid Daily dose can be given in divided doses	Evening primrose oil can increase the risk of pregnancy complications Side effects include indigestion, nausea, soft stools, and headache Seizures have been reported in patients with schizophrenia who were taking phenothiazines and evening primrose oil concomitantly Evening primrose oil can interact with anesthesia and cause seizures Concomitant use of evening primrose oil with anticoagulant and antiplatelet drugs can increase the risk of bleeding
Fenugreek seed	For diabetes and hypercholesterolemia For constipation, dyspepsia, gastritis, and kidney ailments Approved in Germany for use orally for loss of appetite and topically as a poultice for local inflammation	For loss of appetite, 1–2 g of the seed tid or 1 cup of tea (500 mg seed in 150 mL cold water for 3 h) several times a day Maximum 6 g/d For other conditions, no established dosage documented For topical use, 50 g powdered seed in 0.25 L of hot water to form a paste	Fenugreek can cause uterine contractions and should be avoided in pregnancy Individuals who have allergies to peanuts or soybeans might also be allergic to fenugreek Fenugreek can cause diarrhea and flatulence; it can also make urine smell like maple syrup Hypoglycemia can occur if fenugreek is taken in large amounts Repeated external applications can result in undesirable skin reactions Fenugreek contains small amounts of coumarins and can interact with anticoagulants and antiplatelet drugs High mucilage content of fenugreek can affect the absorption of oral drugs; therefore, fenugreek should not be taken within 2 h of other drugs
Feverfew	For migraine headache prophylaxis For treatment of fever, menstrual problems, and arthritis	Migraine prevention: 25–75 mg bid of the encapsulated dried leaf extract standardized to 0.2% parthenolide, for up to 4 months 2.08–18.75 mg tid for MIG-99 preparation (a carbon dioxide extract enriched with parthenolide) for 3–4 months For other conditions, no established dosage documented	Feverfew can induce menstrual bleeding and is contraindicated in pregnancy Fresh leaves can cause oral ulcers and GI irritation Sudden discontinuation of feverfew can precipitate rebound headache Feverfew can interact with anticoagulants and potentiate the antiplatelet effect of aspirin

HERB OR NUTRITIONAL SUPPLEMENT	COMMON USES	REASONABLE ADULT ORAL DOSAGE*	PRECAUTIONS AND DRUG INTERACTIONS
Fish oils (omega-3 fatty acids)	Commonly used in the treatment of hypertriglyceridemia Used to prevent CHD and stroke Used in many noncardiac conditions, including depression, diabetes, dysmenorrhea, rheumatoid arthritis, and IgA nephropathy Used to reduce the risk of developing age-related maculopathy, Alzheimer disease, and cancer Promotes visual and mental development in children	For hypertriglyceridemia, 3–5 g/d For cardioprotection, 1 g/d for patients with CHD; oily fish at least twice a week, or about 0.5 g/d for people with no known heart disease For other conditions, no established dosage documented Fish oils are composed of EPA and DHA; fish oil capsules vary widely in amounts and ratios of EPA and DHA; the most common fish oil capsules in the United States provide 180 mg of EPA and 120 mg DHA per capsule, and three capsules will provide about 1 g/d of omega-3 fatty acids	Common side effects include fishy aftertaste, GI disturbances, belching, halitosis, and heartburn High doses can cause nausea and loose stools Doses > 3 g/d can inhibit platelet aggregation, suppress immune function, worsen glycemic control, and raise LDL cholesterol levels Long-term use may be associated with weight gain Less well-controlled preparations can contain appreciable amount of organochloride contaminants Fish oil can increase the risk of bleeding in patients taking warfarin, an antiplatelet agent, or herbs that have antiplatelet constituents (e.g., garlic, ginkgo, and red clover) Fish oils can lower blood pressure and can have additive effects with antihypertensive agents Oral contraceptives can interfere with the triglyceride lowering effects of fish oils
Flaxseed	Orally, approved in Germany for chronic constipation, irritable bowel, and other colon disorders Often used orally for hypercholesterolemia and atherosclerosis Topically, approved in Germany for painful skin inflammation	For constipation, 1 tbsp (5 g) of whole or "bruised" seeds (not ground) in 150 mL of liquid 2–3 times daily For bowel inflammation, 2–3 tbsp of milled flaxseed soaked in 200–300 mL water and strain after 30 min For hypercholesterolemia, 1–2 tbsp flaxseed oil daily Topical: 30–50 g flaxseed flour as poultice or compress for a moist-heat direct application directly to the skin	Flaxseed should be taken with plenty of water to prevent possible intestinal blockage Patients with ileus should not take flaxseed High mucilage content of flaxseed can delay absorption of other drugs taken at the same time
Garlic	To lower blood pressure and serum cholesterol To prevent atherosclerosis	Fresh clove: one 4 g clove per day Tablet: 300 mg bid to tid standardized to 0.6%–1.3% allicin	Intake of large quantities can lead to stomach complaints Garlic has antiplatelet effects, so patients should discontinue use of garlic at least 7 d before surgery Concomitant use of garlic and anticoagulants can increase the risk of bleeding
Ginger root	As an antiemetic For prevention of motion sickness	Fresh rhizome: 2–4 g/d Powdered ginger: 250 mg 3–4 times daily Tea: 1 cup of tea tid (0.5–1 g dried root in 150 mL boiling water for 5–10 min)	Ginger should not be used by patients with gallstones because of its cholagogic effect It can inhibit platelet aggregation; cases of postoperative bleeding have been reported Large doses of ginger can increase bleeding time in patients taking antiplatelet agents
Ginkgo biloba leaf	To slow cognitive deterioration in dementia To increase peripheral blood flow in claudication To treat sexual dysfunction associated with the use of SSRIs	60–120 mg bid of extract Egb761 standardized to 24% flavonoids and 6% terpenoids	Adverse effects are rare and can include mild stomach or intestinal upset, headache, or allergic skin reaction Ginkgo can inhibit platelet aggregation; reports of spontaneous bleeding have been published Patients should discontinue ginkgo at least 36 h before surgery Concurrent use of ginkgo and anticoagulants, antiplatelet agents, vitamin E, or garlic can increase the risk of bleeding

HERB OR NUTRITIONAL SUPPLEMENT	COMMON USES	REASONABLE ADULT ORAL DOSAGE*	PRECAUTIONS AND DRUG INTERACTIONS
Ginseng root	As a tonic during times of stress, fatigue, disability, and convalescence To improve physical performance and stamina	Root: 1–2 g/d Tablet: 100 mg bid of extract standardized to 4%–7% ginsenosides A 2- to 3-week period of using ginseng followed by a 1- to 2-week "rest" period is generally recommended Ginseng is commonly adulterated, especially Siberian ginseng (eleuthero) products	Ginseng has a mild stimulant effect and should be avoided in patients with cardiovascular disease Tachycardia and hypertension can occur Overdosages can lead to ginseng abuse syndrome, characterized by insomnia, hypotonia, and edema Ginseng has estrogenic effects and can cause vaginal bleeding and breast tenderness Ginseng has been shown to inhibit platelets, so patients should discontinue ginseng use at least 7 d before surgery Ginseng should not be used with other stimulants Patients taking antidiabetic agents and ginseng should be monitored to avoid the hypoglycemic effects of ginseng Ginseng can interact with warfarin and cause a decreased INR Siberian ginseng can increase digoxin levels Ginseng can interact with phenelzine (a MAOI) resulting in insomnia, headache, tremulousness, and manic-like symptoms
Glucosamine	For osteoarthritis	500 mg tid with meals Glucosamine is available in the form of sulfate, hydrochloride, or N-acetyl salt; glucosamine sulfate is the form that has been used in most clinical studies	Side effects are generally limited to mild GI symptoms, including stomach upset, heartburn, diarrhea, nausea, and indigestion Glucosamine derived from marine exoskeletons may cause reactions in people allergic to shellfish Glucosamine may raise blood glucose level in patients with diabetes
Goldenseal	Often combined with echinacea to treat colds and other upper respiratory infections Used for diarrhea, dyspepsia, and gastritis Used topically as an eyewash, mouthwash, feminine cleansing product, and skin remedy	Oral: 0.5–1 g of the dried rhizome/root or 2–4 mL tincture (1:10, 60% ethanol) or 0.3–1 mL fluid extract (1:1, 60% ethanol) tid Eyewash: For trachoma infections, 2 drops of a 0.2% aqueous berberine solution tid × 3 week	Avoid using goldenseal during pregnancy and breast feeding; berberine, the principle constituent in goldenseal, can cause uterine contractions and neonatal jaundice Avoid using goldenseal in kidney failure because of inadequate urinary excretion of its alkaloids High dosages or long-term usage can lead to nausea, vomiting, headache, hypotension, bradycardia, leucopenia, and mucosal irritation Berberine can increase the risk of bleeding in patients taking warfarin or an antiplatelet agent Be aware that other herbs containing berberine, including Chinese goldthread and Oregon grape, are sometimes substituted for goldenseal
Grape seed	For conditions related to the heart and blood vessels, such as atherosclerosis, high blood pressure, high cholesterol, and poor circulation For vision problems, diabetic neuropathy or retinopathy, and swelling after an injury or surgery For cancer prevention and wound healing	For general health purposes, 100–300 mg daily of a standardized extract (95% oligomeric proanthocyanidin complexes)	Side effects include headache, dizziness, nausea, and dry, itchy scalp Concomitant use with warfarin or antiplatelet agents can increase risk of bleeding because of the tocopherol content of grape seed oil

Popular Herbs and Nutritional Supplements

1367

HERB OR NUTRITIONAL SUPPLEMENT	COMMON USES	REASONABLE ADULT ORAL DOSAGE*	PRECAUTIONS AND DRUG INTERACTIONS
Hawthorn leaf with flower	Commonly used in Germany to increase cardiac output in patients with New York Heart Association stage I and II heart failure	160–900 mg water-ethanol extract (30–169 mg procyanidins or 3.5–19.8 mg flavonoids) divided into 2–3 doses	Side effects include GI upset, palpitations, hypotension, headache, dizziness, and insomnia Concomitant use with CNS depressants can have additive CNS effects Hawthorn can potentiate effects of digoxin and vasodilators
Hops	For mood disturbances such as restlessness and anxiety For sleep disturbances Commonly found in combination products with other herbal sedatives	0.5 g of cut or powdered strobile in a single dose; can be taken as tea (0.5 g in 150 mL water), fluid extract 1:1 (0.5 mL), tincture 1:5 (2.5 mL), or dry extract 6–8:1 (60–80 mg) The preparation contains at least 0.35% (v/w) essential oil	Side effects are rare but include drowsiness and allergic reactions Hops is not recommended for use during pregnancy and lactation It can potentiate the sedative effect of CNS depressants (e.g., benzodiazepines, alcohol) and other herbal tranquilizers
Horse chestnut seed	To relieve symptoms of chronic venous insufficiency	250 mg bid of extract standardized to 50 mg aescin in delayed-release form Unsafe to ingest the raw seed, which contains significant amounts of the most toxic constituent, esculin	Mild GI symptoms, headache, dizziness, and pruritis have been reported Ingestion of high doses can cause renal, hepatic, and hematologic toxicity Concomitant use with anticoagulants can increase the risk of bleeding Horse chestnut can potentiate the effects of hypoglycemic drugs
Kava kava	As an anxiolytic for nervous anxiety, stress, and restlessness As a sedative to induce sleep	Herb and preparations equivalent to 60–120 mg/d of kava pyrones Most clinical trials have used 100 mg tid of extract standardized to 70% kava pyrones for anxiety disorders	Kava should not be used by patients with depression Kava should be avoided in pregnant or nursing women Kava can affect motor reflexes and judgment, so it should not be taken while driving and/or operating heavy machinery Accommodative disturbances have been reported; kava can exacerbate Parkinson disease Extended use can cause a temporary yellow discoloration of skin, hair, and nails Reports have linked kava use to at least 25 cases of severe liver toxicity; sale of products containing kava has been banned in Canada and several European countries Kava has been shown to have additive CNS depressant effects with benzodiazepines, alcohol, and herbal tranquilizers Kava can potentiate the sedative effects of anesthetics, so kava should be discontinued at least 24 h before surgery
Lutein	Commonly used to prevent AMD and cataracts Used to prevent skin cancer, breast cancer, and colon cancer Used to protect against cardiovascular disease	For AMD and cataracts, 6–20 mg/d of lutein from diet For other uses, no established dosage documented Foods containing high concentrations of lutein include kale, spinach, broccoli, and romaine lettuce Not known if supplemental lutein is as effective as natural lutein Supplemental lutein in the form of esters might require a higher fat intake for effective absorption than purified lutein	No major adverse effects and drug interactions have been reported

HERB OR NUTRITIONAL SUPPLEMENT	COMMON USES	REASONABLE ADULT ORAL DOSAGE*	PRECAUTIONS AND DRUG INTERACTIONS
Lycopene	Commonly used to prevent and treat prostate cancer Used for cancer prevention, arthrosclerosis prevention, and reduction of asthma symptoms	For decreasing the growth of prostate cancer, 15 mg supplement bid For prostate cancer prevention, at least 6 mg/d from tomato products (or ≥10 servings/wk) For other uses, no established dosage documented Heat processing converts lycopene in fresh tomatoes from the *trans-* to the *cis*-configuration. The *cis* isomer has better bioavailability Lycopene supplements usually do not specify the type and amount of isomers in their product labeling	Lycopene, when consumed in amounts found in foods, is generally considered to be safe Concomitant ingestion of beta-carotene can increase lycopene absorption Lycopene may reduce cholesterol levels and potentiate the effects of statins
Melatonin	For jet lag, insomnia, shift-work disorder, and circadian rhythm disorders For other medical conditions, including depression, multiple sclerosis, tinnitus, headache, and cancer	For jet lag, 5 mg at bedtime for 2–5 d beginning the day of return For sleep disorders, 0.3–5 mg taken 2 h before bedtime Avoid melatonin from animal pineal gland because of the possibility of contamination.	Avoid use in pregnancy because melatonin decreases serum luteinizing hormone concentrations and increases serum prolactin levels The common adverse reactions include headache, transient depressive symptoms, daytime fatigue and drowsiness, dizziness, abdominal cramps, irritability, and reduced alertness Concomitant use of melatonin with alcohol, benzodiazepines, or other CNS depressants can cause additive sedation Melatonin can affect immune function and may interfere with immunosuppressive therapy Concomitant use with other herbs that have sedative properties (e.g., chamomile, goldenseal, hop, kava, valerian) can produce additive CNS-impairing effects
Milk thistle fruit	As a hepatoprotectant and antioxidant, particularly for treatment of hepatitis, cirrhosis, and toxic liver damage Used in Europe for the treatment of hepatotoxic mushroom poisoning from *Amanita phalloides*	Average daily dose is 12–15 g of crude drug or formulations equivalent to 200–400 mg of silymarin	Adverse effects are rare but include diarrhea and allergic reactions Milk thistle can potentiate the hypoglycemic effect of antidiabetic agents
Peppermint	Commonly used for indigestion and irritable bowel syndrome (IBS) Used externally for myalgia and neuralgia	Indigestion: 1 tsp dried leaves in 1 cup of boiling water, steeped for 10 min; drink 4–5 times/d between meals IBS: 1–2 enteric coated cap (0.2 mL of peppermint oil/cap) 2–3 times/d. Take peppermint ≥2 h before or after an acid-reducing drug to ensure adequate absorption	Peppermint, in amounts normally found in food, is likely to be safe Larger supplemental amounts can cause side effects including heartburn, flushing, headache, and mouth sores Hypersensitivity reactions, contact dermatitis, and exacerbations of asthma may occur Peppermint can exacerbate symptoms in patients with gastroesophageal reflux disease (GERD) because it can relax the lower esophageal sphincter Peppermint tea has been shown to reduce free testosterone levels in men Peppermint can decrease the blood levels of cyclosporine and drugs that metabolized by the CYP3A4 isoenzyme
Probiotics	Prevent and treat antibiotic-associated diarrhea and acute infectious diarrhea Relieve symptoms of IBS Treat atopic dermatitis for at-risk infants	Dosage varies based on preparations *Lactobacillus* sp., *Bifidobacterium* sp., *Saccharomyces boulardii* are the most widely used organisms For *Lactobacillus* sp., 10 billion CFUs/d For *Lactobacillus* sp./*Bifidobacterium* sp., 100 million to 35 billion CFUs/d For *Saccharomyces boulardii*, 250–500 mg/d Quality of products varies among brands Refrigeration is required to maintain potency	Avoid use in short-gut syndrome and severe immunocompromised condition Common adverse effects include flatulence, mild abdominal discomfort, and, rarely, septicemia

HERB OR NUTRITIONAL SUPPLEMENT	COMMON USES	REASONABLE ADULT ORAL DOSAGE*	PRECAUTIONS AND DRUG INTERACTIONS
Red clover flower	Commonly used for conditions associated with menopause, such as hot flashes, cardiovascular health, and osteoporosis Used for PMS, benign prostate hyperplasia, and cancer prevention Used topically to treat psoriasis, eczema, and other rashes	For hot flashes, 40 mg/d of the isoflavones extract (Promensil) For other conditions, no established dosage documented	Red clover has estrogenic activity and should be avoided during pregnancy and lactation Women with hormone-dependent conditions (e.g., breast, uterine, and ovarian cancer, and endometriosis and uterine fibroids) and men with prostate cancer should also avoid taking red clover Side effects include headache, myalgia, nausea, and rash Red clover contains coumarin derivatives and can increase the risk of bleeding in those who are taking anticoagulants or antiplatelet drugs Preliminary report suggests that red clover might antagonize the effects of tamoxifen Some evidence suggests that red clover can increase the levels of drugs that metabolized by the cytochrome P450 3A4 isoenzyme (e.g., lovastatin, ketoconazole, itraconazole, fexofenadine, and triazolam)
SAMe (S-adenosyl-L-methionine)	For treatment of osteoarthritis, depression, fibromyalgia, and liver disease	For osteoarthritis, 200 mg tid For depression and fibromyalgia, 800 mg bid For liver disease, 600–800 mg bid	Common side effects include flatulence, nausea, vomiting, and diarrhea SAMe can cause anxiety in people with depression and hypomania in people with bipolar disorder Concurrent use of SAMe and other antidepressants can cause serotonin syndrome
Saw palmetto berry	To treat symptomatic benign prostatic hyperplasia and irritable bladder	160 mg bid of extract standardized to 85%–95% fatty acids and sterols	Adverse effects are rare but include headache, nausea, and upset stomach High doses can cause diarrhea
Soy	Commonly used for cholesterol reduction in combination with a low-fat diet Used for menopausal symptoms and for prevention of osteoporosis and cardiovascular disease in postmenopausal women	For lowering cholesterol, 25–50 g/d of soy protein For hot flashes, 20–60 g/d of soy protein For osteoporosis, 40 g/d of soy protein containing 90 mg isoflavones	Soy, when consumed as whole foods (e.g., tofu or soy milk), has minimal adverse effects Consumption of large amounts of soy can cause gastric complaints such as constipation, bloating, and nausea Long-term use of soy tablets containing isoflavones (150 mg/d for 5 years) has been shown to cause endometrial hyperplasia
St. John's wort	Used for treatment of mild to moderate depression May have antiinflammatory and antiinfective activities	300 mg tid of hypericum extract standardized to 0.3% hypericin	St. John's wort should not be used in pregnancy Side effects include dry mouth, GI upset, dizziness, fatigue, and constipation St. John's wort can induce photosensitivity, especially in fair-skinned individuals It can cause serotonin syndrome if used with other antidepressants, including SSRIs, or other serotonergic drugs It has been shown to induce CYP3A4 and decrease blood levels of many drugs such as indinavir, nevirapine, cyclosporine, digoxin, theophylline, simvastatin, oral contraceptive pills, and warfarin St. John's wort should be discontinued at least 5 d before surgery to avoid any potential drug interactions
Stinging nettle root	Approved in Germany for difficulty in urination in BPH stage 1 and 2	4–6 g/d of cut root; can be taken as tea (1.5 g in 150 mL boiling water for 10–20 min, tid), fluid extract 1:1 (1.5 mL tid), tincture 1:5 (5–7.5 mL tid), or dry extract 5.4–6.6:1 (0.22–0.33 g tid)	Occasionally, mild GI upsets may occur No known interactions with drugs

HERB OR NUTRITIONAL SUPPLEMENT	COMMON USES	REASONABLE ADULT ORAL DOSAGE*	PRECAUTIONS AND DRUG INTERACTIONS
Turmeric root	Approved by the German Commission E for dyspeptic conditions Used extensively in Ayurveda medicine for its antiinflammatory and antiarthritic effects Other uses include allergic rhinitis, depression, nonalcoholic fatty liver disease, osteoarthritis and cancer	For dyspeptic conditions: 1.5–3 g/d of cut root as tea infusion or equivalent preparations (e.g., powder, extract, tincture) The Commission E monograph requires turmeric to contain not less than 3% curcuminoids, calculated as curcumin and not less than 3% volatile oil	Side effects are uncommon and are generally limited to mild stomach distress Topical curcumin can cause allergic contact dermatitis Individuals with bile duct obstruction or gallstones should avoid curcumin due to its stimulating effects on the gallbladder
Valerian root	Used as a mild sedative for insomnia and anxiety	2–3 g of dried root or 1–3 mL of tincture, qd to several times per day Two clinical trials found 400–450 mg of the root extract effective for insomnia	Valerian has a bad odor and can cause morning drowsiness Long-term administration can lead to paradoxical stimulation, including restlessness and palpitations Because of the risk of benzodiazepine-like withdrawal, valerian should be tapered over a period of several weeks before surgery It can potentiate the sedative effect of CNS depressants (e.g., benzodiazepines, alcohol) and other herbal tranquilizers

*Doses presented in the table are adapted from the German Commission E Monographs and/or data from clinical trials. Products from different manufacturers vary considerably. A reliable product should have a label clearly stating the botanical name of the herb and milligram amount contained in the product. Standardized extracts should be used whenever possible and are often disclosed on the label of quality products.

AMD, Age-related macular degeneration; *BPH*, benign prostatic hyperplasia; *CFU*, colony-forming unit; *CHD*, coronary heart disease; *CNS*, central nervous system; *CYP3A4*, cytochrome P450 3A4; *DHA*, docosahexaenoic acid; *EPA*, eicosapentaenoic acid; *FDA*, Food and Drug Administration; *GI*, gastrointestinal; *HMG-CoA*, 3-hydroxy-3-methylglutaryl coenzyme A; *INR*, international normalized ratio; *LDL*, low-density lipoprotein; *MAOI*, monoamine oxidase inhibitor; *PMS*, premenstrual syndrome; *SLE*, systemic lupus erythematosus; *SSRIs*, selective serotonin reuptake inhibitors; *UTIs*, urinary tract infections.

References

Ang-Lee MK, Moss J, Yuan C: Herbal medicines and perioperative care, *JAMA* 286:208–216, 2001.

Bent S: Herbal medicine in the United States: Review and efficacy, safety, and regulation, *J Gen Intern Med* 23:854–859, 2008.

Blumenthal M, editor: *Herbal Medicines: Expanded Commission E monographs*, Austin, TX, 2000, American Botanical Council.

Blumenthal M, editor: *The ABC Clinical Guide to Herbs*, Austin, TX, 2003, American Botanical Council.

Ernst E: The risk-benefit profile of commonly used herbal therapies: Ginkgo, St John's wort, ginseng, Echinacea, saw palmetto, and kava, *Ann Intern Med* 136:42–53, 2002.

Gregory PJ, Worthington M, Shkayeva M, et al, editors: Natural Medicines (database online), Stockton, CA: 2018 Therapeutic Research Center. Available at https://naturalmedicines.therapeuticresearch.com/. (Assessed July 7, 2019).

Holland S, Silberstein SD, Freitag F, et al: Evidence-based guideline update: NSAIDs and other complementary treatments for episodic migraine prevention in adults: report of the Quality Standards Subcommittee of the American Academy of Neurology and the American Headache Society, *Neurology* 78(17):1346–1353, 2012.

Kligler B, Cohrssen A: Probiotics, *Am Fam Physician* 78:1073–1078, 2008.

Kronenberg F, Fugh-Berman A: Complementary and alternative medicine for menopausal symptoms: A review of randomized controlled trials, *Ann Intern Med* 137:805–813, 2002.

National Center for Complementary and Integrative Health: Herbs at a Glance. Available at https://nccih.nih.gov/health/herbsataglance.htm. Accessed 19 March 2018.

Smet P: Herbal remedies, *N Engl J Med* 347:2046–2056, 2002.

TOXIC CHEMICAL AGENTS REFERENCE CHART: SYMPTOMS AND TREATMENT

Method of
James J. James, MD, DrPH; and James M. Lyznicki, MS, MPH

Toxic chemical agents are poisonous vapors, aerosols, gases, liquids, or solids that have toxic effects on people, animals, or plants. Most of these agents are liquid at room temperature and are disseminated as vapors and aerosols. They may be released as bombs, sprayed from aircraft and boats, or disseminated by other means to intentionally create a hazard to people and the environment. Some of these agents are highly toxic and persistent, features that can render a site uninhabitable and require costly and potentially hazardous decontamination and remediation. Health effects range from irritation and burning of skin and mucous membranes to rapid cardiopulmonary collapse and death.

Efficient deployment of hazardous materials (HazMat) teams is critical to control a chemical agent attack. Although all major cities and emergency medical systems have plans and equipment in place to address this situation, physicians and other health professionals must be aware of principles involved in managing a patient or multiple patients exposed to these agents. Chemical-weapon agents have a high potential for secondary contamination from victims to responders. This requires that medical treatment facilities have clearly defined procedures for handling contaminated casualties, many of whom will transport themselves to the facility. Precautions must be used until thorough decontamination has been performed or the specific chemical agent is identified. Health care professionals must first protect themselves (e.g., by using protective suits, respiratory protection, and chemical-resistant gloves) because secondary contamination with even small amounts of these substances (particularly nerve agents such as VX) may be lethal.

Primary detection of exposure to chemical agents is based on the signs and symptoms of the potential victim (Table 1). Confirmation of a chemical agent, using detection equipment or laboratory analyses, takes considerable time and will not likely contribute to the early management of mass casualty victims. Several patients presenting with the same symptoms should alert physicians and hospital staff to the possibility of a chemical attack. If a chemical attack occurs, most victims will likely arrive within a short time. This situation differentiates a chemical attack from a biological attack involving infectious microorganisms. Additional diagnostic clues include the following:

- Unusual temporal or geographic clustering of illness
- Any sudden increase in illness in previously healthy persons
- Sudden increase in nonspecific syndromes (e.g., sudden unexplained weakness in previously healthy persons; dimmed or blurred vision; hypersecretion, inhalation, or burnlike syndrome)

A coordinated communication network is critical for transmitting reliable information from the incident scene to treatment facilities. Any suspicious or confirmed exposure to a chemical weapons agent should be reported to the local health department, local Federal Bureau of Investigation office, and the Centers for Disease Control and Prevention (770–488–7100).

TABLE 1 Quick Reference Chart on Chemical Weapon Agents

| CHEMICAL AGENT | DIAGNOSTIC CONSIDERATIONS | | | | | TREATMENT CONSIDERATIONS* | | | COMMENTS |
	SIGNS AND SYMPTOMS	SYMPTOM ONSET	ODOR	ACTION	TESTING	TREATMENT	ANTIDOTE	
Cyanides								
Cyanogen chloride (CK) Hydrogen cyanide (AC)	Nonspecific hypoxic and hypoxemic symptoms Resp: SOB, chest tightness, hyperventilation, resp arrest GI: nausea, vomiting CV: ventricular arrhythmias, hypotension, cardiac arrest, shock CNS: anxiety, headache, drowsiness, weakness, apnea, convulsions, seizure, coma Metabolic acidosis and increased concentration of venous oxygen (possibly also cyanosis)	Rapid, seconds to minutes	Bitter almond, musty, or chlorine-like	Binds cellular cytochrome oxidase, causing chemical asphyxia	Cyanide, thiocyanate, serum lactate levels Venous and arterial partial oxygen pressure	Immediate treatment of symptomatic patients is critical Hydroxycobalamin (vitamin B_{12a}) administered with thiosulfate[§,†] Activated charcoal[‡] for oral exposure Mechanical ventilation as needed Circulatory support with crystalloids and vasopressors Metabolic acidosis corrected with IV sodium bicarbonate Seizures controlled with benzodiazepines	Sodium nitrite and sodium thiosulfate; repeat one-half initial doses of both agents in 30 min if inadequate clinical response; amyl nitrate capsules are available for first aid until intravenous access is achieved Hydroxycobalamin (vitamin B_{12a}, Cyanokit)	Cyanide antidote kits are commercially available CNS effects may be confused with carbon monoxide and hydrogen sulfide poisoning
Incapacitating Agents								
Agent 15 3-quinuclidinyl benzilate (BZ)	Mydriasis, blurred vision, dry mouth, dry skin, possible atropine-like flush, initial rise in heart rate, decreased level of consciousness, confusion, disorientation, visual hallucinations, impaired memory	Hours 0–4 h: parasympathetic blockade and mild CNS effects 4–20 h: stupor with ataxia and hyperthermia 20–96 h: full-blown delirium Resolution phase: paranoia, deep sleep, reawakening, crawling, climbing automatisms, eventual reorientation	Odorless	Competitive inhibitor of acetylcholine muscarinic receptor		Support, intravenous fluids	Physostigmine salicylate (Antilirium)[‡]	
Nerve Agents								
Cyclohexyl sarin (GF) Sarin (GB) Soman (GD) Tabun (GA) VX	Most toxic of known chemical agents May be confused with organophosphate and carbamate pesticide poisoning	Vapor: seconds Liquid: minutes or hours Symptom onset may be delayed up to 18 h,	GB, VX: none GA: fruity GD: camphor-like	Irreversible acetylcholinesterase inhibitors	Erythrocyte or serum cholinesterase activity to confirm exposure	Rapid establishment of patent airway Early administration of 2-PAM is critical to minimize permanent agent inactivation of	Atropine[‡] and 2-PAM[‡] Additional doses until bronchial secretions are cleared and ventilation improved	Atropine,[‡] 2-PAM,[‡] and diazepam[‡] are available in autoinjector kits through

Agent	Signs/Symptoms	Onset	Examples/Notes	Treatment	Laboratory/Antidote	Comments
	Eyes: excessive lacrimation, miosis may be present; Resp: rhinorrhea, bronchospasm, resp failure; GI: hypersalivation, nausea, vomiting, diarrhea; Skin: localized sweating; Cardiac: sinus bradycardia; Skeletal muscles: fasciculations followed by weakness, flaccid paralysis; CNS: loss of consciousness, convulsions, apnea, seizures	particularly for localized exposures		Benzodiazepines to control nerve agent–induced seizures; Airway and ventilatory support as needed	acetylcholinesterase (i.e., "aging")	the U.S. military

Pulmonary or Choking Agents

Agent	Signs/Symptoms	Onset	Examples/Notes	Treatment	Antidote	Comments
Acrolein, Ammonia (NH$_3$), Chlorine (Cl), Choloropicrin (PS), Diphosgene (DP), Nitrogen oxides (NO$_x$), Perfluoroisobutylene (PFIB), Phosgene (CG), Sulfur dioxide (SO$_2$)	Degree of water solubility of the agent influences onset and severity of respiratory injury. Eye and airway irritation, dyspnea, chest tightness, rhinorrhea, hypersalivation, cough, wheezing. High-dose inhalation can cause laryngospasm, pneumonitis, and acute lung injury with delayed onset (≤48h) of acute resp distress syndrome. Chest radiograph: hyperinflation, noncardiogenic pulmonary edema	Rapid or delayed 1–24 h; rarely up to 72 h	CG: freshly mown hay or grass	Supportive measures; Specific treatment depends on the agent; IV fluids for hypotension; no diuretics; Ventilation with or without positive airway pressure; Bronchodilators for bronchospasm; Methylprednisolone[1] may be effective in preventing noncardiogenic pulmonary edema	No specific antidote	Easily absorbed via mucous membranes of eyes, nose, oropharynx. May be confused with inhalation exposure to industrial chemicals (e.g., HCl, Cl$_2$, NH$_3$)

Riot Control Agents

Agent	Signs/Symptoms	Onset	Examples/Notes	Treatment	Laboratory	Mechanism
Mace (CN), Tear gas (CS)	Metallic taste; Burning and pain on mucosal membranes and skin; Eyes: irritation, pain, tearing, blepharospasm; Airways: burning in nose and mouth, respiratory discomfort, bronchospasm (may be delayed 36h); Skin: tingling, erythema	Immediate	CN: apple blossom; CS: pepper	Supportive care; Irrigation as necessary; Persons with asthma, emphysema might need oxygen, inhaled bronchodilators, steroids, assisted ventilation; Lotions, such as calamine[1] for persistent erythema	No specific laboratory tests	SN2 alkylating agents

Continued

TABLE 1 Quick Reference Chart on Chemical Weapon Agents—cont'd

CHEMICAL AGENT	DIAGNOSTIC CONSIDERATIONS				TREATMENT CONSIDERATIONS*		COMMENTS
	SIGNS AND SYMPTOMS	SYMPTOM ONSET	ODOR	ACTION	TREATMENT	TESTING	ANTIDOTE	COMMENTS

CHEMICAL AGENT	SIGNS AND SYMPTOMS	SYMPTOM ONSET	ODOR	ACTION	TESTING	TREATMENT	ANTIDOTE	COMMENTS
	Nausea and vomiting are common CN can cause corneal opacification							
Vesicant or Blister Agents								
General	Clinical effects depend on extent and route of exposure	Effects may be delayed, appearing hours after exposure		Intracellular enzyme and DNA alkylating agents		Immediate decontamination Supportive care Thermal burn–type treatment Symptomatic management of lesions		Primary liquid hazard May be confused with skin exposure to caustic irritants (e.g., NaOH, NH₃)
Sulfur mustard (H) Distilled mustard (HD)	Skin: erythema and blisters (may be delayed ≤8h), pruritus Eye: irritation, conjunctivitis, corneal damage, lacrimation, pain, blepharospasm Resp: mild to marked acute airway damage, pneumonitis within 1–3 d, respiratory failure GI effects (nausea, vomiting diarrhea) may be present Bone marrow stem cell suppression leading to pancytopenia and increased susceptibility to infection Fever, sputum production	Delayed 2–48h	Garlic, horseradish, or mustard			Skin: silver sulfadiazine[1] Eye: homatropine[1] ophthalmic ointment Pulmonary: antibiotics, bronchodilators, steroids Colony-stimulating factor may be helpful for leukopenia Systemic analgesic and antipruritics Early use of PEEP or CPAP Maintain fluid and electrolyte balance (do not excessively fluid resuscitate as in thermal burns)		No specific antidote	Combination with lewisite (called mustard-Lewisite or HL) results in rapid effects of lewisite and delayed effects of mustard agents
Lewisite (L)	Skin: gray area of dead skin within 5min, erythema within 30min, blistering 2–3h, immediate irritation or burning pain on contact, severe tissue necrosis Eye: pain, blepharospasm, conjunctival and lid edema Airway: pseudomembrane formation, nasal irritation Intravascular fluid loss, hypovolemia, shock, organ congestion, leukocytosis	Immediate	Fruity or geranium					British anti-lewisite (BAL or dimercaprol)	More volatile than mustard Damages eyes, skin, and airways by direct contact

Agent	Signs and Symptoms	Onset	Odor	Classification	Laboratory Findings	Antidote	Treatment	Comments
Phosgene oxime (CX)	Burning, irritation, wheal-like skin lesions, eye and airway damage, conjunctivitis, lacrimation, lid edema, blepharospasm	Immediate	Freshly mown hay	Urticant, nonvesicant agent	No distinctive laboratory findings	No antidote	Parenteral methylprednisolone[1] may be effective in preventing noncardiogenic pulmonary edema. Experimental: aerosolized dexamethasone[1] and theophylline[1] for pulmonary involvement	Vapor extremely irritating; vapor and liquid cause tissue damage upon contact

Vomiting (Arsine-Based) Agents

Agent	Signs and Symptoms	Onset	Odor	Classification	Laboratory Findings	Antidote	Treatment	Comments
Adamsite (DM) Diphenylchlorarsine (DA) Diphenylcyanoarsine (DC)	Eyes: conjunctival irritation, tearing, and blepharospasm. Airways: sneezing, mucosal lung irritation, edema, progressive cough, wheezing. Cardiac: tachypnea, tachycardia. GI: intestinal cramps, emesis, diarrhea. Skin: erythema, edema at the site of dermal contact. CNS: depression, syncope	All rapidly acting within minutes	DA: none DC: garlic DM: burning fireworks	Arsine gas depletes erythrocyte glutathione and causes hemolysis	Chest radiograph to rule out chemical pneumonitis		Supportive care. Monitor for hemolysis. Wheezing or dyspnea: may need albuterol inhalation. Eye irrigation (water, normal saline, lactated Ringer's) in patients with ocular exposure. Treat repetitive emesis with IV hydration and antiemetics. Blood transfusion may be required. Exchange transfusion may be required. Hemodialysis may be useful in decreasing arsenic level and treating renal failure	Primary route of absorption is through respiratory system

Abbreviations: CNS=central nervous system; CPAP=continuous positive airway pressure; CV=cardiovascular; GI=gastrointestinal; 2-PAM=pralidoxime (2-pyridine aldoxime methyl chloride); PEEP=positive end-expiratory pressure; resp=respiratory; SOB=shortness of breath.

[1]Not FDA approved for this indication.
§Investigational drug in the United States.
*Different situations can require different treatment and dosage regimens. Please consult other references as well as a regional poison control center (800–222–1222), medical toxicologist, clinical pharmacologist, or other drug information specialist for definitive dosage information, especially dosages for pregnant women and children.
†Available in Europe.
Adapted from Lyznicki JL: AMA quick reference guide: Exposure to toxic chemical agents. In American Medical Association: Management of Public Health Emergencies. A Resource Guide for Physicians and Other Community Responders. Chicago, American Medical Association, 2005.

Index

Note: Page numbers followed by *f* indicate figures, *t* indicate tables, and *b* indicate boxes.

Index

1394

Index

HEIGHT IN FEET

HEIGHT IN CENTIMETERS

SURFACE AREA IN SQUARE METERS

WEIGHT IN POUNDS

WEIGHT IN KILOGRAMS